SELDIN AND GIEBISCH'S THE KIDNEY
PHYSIOLOGY AND PATHOPHYSIOLOGY

FIFTH EDITION

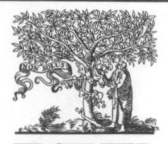

ELSEVIER
science & technology books

ELSEVIER

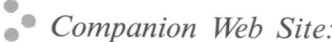

:• *Companion Web Site:*

http://booksite.elsevier.com/9780123814623

Seldin and Giebisch's The Kidney: Physiology and Pathophysiology, fifth edition
Robert J. Alpern, Orson W. Moe and Michael Caplan, Editors

Resources for Professors:

- All figures from the book available as both Power Point slides and .jpeg files

TOOLS FOR **ALL** YOUR **TEACHING NEEDS**
textbooks.elsevier.com

ELSEVIER

ACADEMIC PRESS

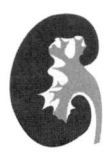

SELDIN AND GIEBISCH'S THE KIDNEY

PHYSIOLOGY AND PATHOPHYSIOLOGY

FIFTH EDITION

VOLUME 1

ROBERT J. ALPERN
Yale University School of Medicine
New Haven, CT, USA

ORSON W. MOE
The University of Texas Southwestern Medical Center at Dallas
Dallas, TX, USA

MICHAEL CAPLAN
Yale University School of Medicine, New Haven, CT, USA

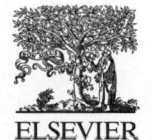

ELSEVIER

AMSTERDAM • BOSTON • HEIDELBERG • LONDON
NEW YORK • OXFORD • PARIS • SAN DIEGO
SAN FRANCISCO • SINGAPORE • SYDNEY • TOKYO

Academic Press is an imprint of Elsevier

Academic Press is an imprint of Elsevier

32 Jamestown Road, London NW1 7BY, UK
225 Wyman Street, Waltham, MA 02451, USA
525 B Street, Suite 1800, San Diego, CA 92101-4495, USA

Fifth edition 2013

Notice
No responsibility is assumed by the publisher for any injury and/or damage to persons or property
as a matter of products liability, negligence or otherwise, or from any use or operation of any methods,
products, instructions or ideas contained in the material herein. Because of rapid advances in the medical sciences, in particular, independent verification of diagnoses and drug dosages should be made

Medicine is an ever-changing field. Standard safety precautions must be followed, but as new research and clinical
experience broaden our knowledge, changes in treatment and drug therapy may become necessary or appropriate.
Readers are advised to check the most current product information provided by the manufacturer of each drug to be
administered to verify the recommended dose, the method and duration of administrations, and contraindications. It is
the responsibility of the treating physician, relying on experience and knowledge of the patient, to determine dosages
and the best treatment for each individual patient. Neither the publisher nor the authors assume any liability for any
injury and/or damage to persons or property arising from this publication

British Library Cataloguing-in-Publication Data
A catalogue record for this book is available from the British Library

Library of Congress Cataloging-in-Publication Data
A catalog record for this book is available from the Library of Congress

ISBN : 978-0-12-381462-3 (set)
ISBN : 978-0-12-397207-1 (volume 1)
ISBN : 978-0-12-397208-8 (volume 2)

For information on all Academic Press publications
visit our website at elsevierdirect.com

Typeset by MPS Ltd.
www.adi-mps.com

Printed and bound in United States of America

12 13 14 15 16 10 9 8 7 6 5 4 3 2 1

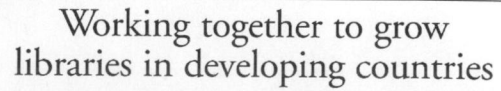

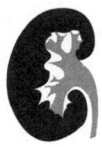

Dedication

This book is dedicated to Steven C. Hebert. Steve was at his heart a kidney physiologist, applying cutting edge technologies to address the most fundamental concepts of kidney function and disease. He was an extraordinary scientist, clinician, mentor, leader and friend.

CONTENTS

VOLUME 2

IV

PATHOPHYSIOLOGY OF RENAL DISEASE

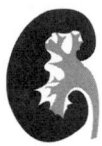

Foreword

The focus of these volumes ever since the publication of the first edition in 1985 has been on renal physiology, conceived broadly as the analysis of those processes by which the kidney maintains the volume and composition of the body in the face of varied intake, physiologic alterations and pathologic disturbances. The text began with a detailed exploration of the basic mechanisms and their regulation that underlie the exchanges of water and electrolytes across cell membranes of the body. The mechanisms used by the kidney to make appropriate renal homeostatic adjustments were next presented.

In the early texts the renal response was attributed to the whole organ rather than to discrete molecular processes. It was the application of the methods and theories of the generalizing sciences, physics and chemistry, to biologic systems that, in subsequent additions, facilitated a reduction of the explanatory system to the more basic level of molecular biology, thereby providing a more comprehensive understanding of the basic processes that permit the physiologic adjustments.

In this 5th edition, such new and powerful disciplines as genetics and cell biology have been deployed to deepen and widen further the explanatory framework. Not only have previous chapters been extensively updated, but new chapters have been added to incorporate additional disciplines. Individual chapters, for example, now provide detailed treatment of the significance of cilia; the role of stem cells is now given special consideration. Finally, there has been a significant expansion of the section of pathophysiology, incorporating the newer findings of cell biology and genetics.

In a sense, this new edition represents a significant advancement in the march of reduction to a more fundamental level of understanding of the normal and deranged function of the kidney.

Donald W. Seldin
Gerhard H Giebisch

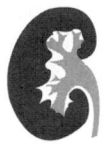

Preface

As described in its preface, the first edition of *The Kidney: Physiology and Pathophysiology*, published in 1985, focused on renal physiology, "conceived broadly as the study of those processes by which the kidney maintains the volume and composition of the body in the face of physiologic demands and pathologic disturbances." As noted in the fourth edition, science has since then become more reductionist, an evolution that has been reflected in the content of subsequent editions. Dissection of physiologic phenomena at the level of organs and cells has been enriched by descriptions of the roles of individual molecules. While this trend in science has continued, it has been complemented by a renewed focus on integrating these molecular functions to define their roles in cellular and organ physiology, as well as their role in body homeostasis and disease. A complete understanding of physiologic and pathophysiologic processes must include knowledge of individual molecules, as well as their integration into homeostatic systems that function to maintain body composition. A thorough understanding of physiologic mechanisms endows us with a greater understanding of pathophysiology and disease. Reciprocally, an understanding of disease states furnishes us with valuable information about normal physiology. The present edition continues to focus on describing the present state of knowledge of the molecules and the systems that contribute to normal physiologic function of the kidney, and the homeostatic mechanisms subserved by the kidney.

The present edition also concentrates on how these mechanisms malfunction, resulting in the diseased state. Again we will address the pathophysiology of disease states from the molecular to the system level. One of the appealing features of nephrology is the ability to utilize our understanding of normal physiology to elucidate principles of pathophysiology, and secondarily develop rational approaches to the diagnosis, treatment, and prevention of disease. Thus, the clinician addressing a patient with a fluid and electrolyte disorder need not memorize a list of possible causes or algorithms, but can logically deduce a solution through a thorough understanding of kidney function. As science continues to evolve, our understanding of the pathophysiologic basis of disease can now be applied to a much broader set of ailments. We continue, therefore, to broaden the scope of this book so as to place greater emphasis on mechanisms of disease.

The first section of the textbook begins with general principles of epithelial and non-epithelial transport and regulation. This extensive section of the book continues a tradition established in the first edition, but extends it to include a more extensive discussion of transport regulation.

The second section of the book describes the organization of the kidney with an increased emphasis on the glomerulus, as this field continues to evolve. There follows an in-depth review of renal growth and development, including a discussion of the role of stem cells in the kidney.

This is then followed by Section Three, describing mechanisms of fluid and electrolyte regulation and dysregulation. In no other book can one find this subject addressed with the depth and thoroughness found in this textbook. The Fifth Edition includes a more in-depth discussion of recently described families of transporters, integrating this information to describe their role in physiologic and pathophysiologic processes.

Section Four, the pathophysiology of renal disease, has been extended as our knowledge of renal dysfunctions and their contribution to renal ailments has expanded. Many chapters deal with common everyday clinical issues, but are presented in the context of pathophysiologic mechanisms. A series of chapters focus on mechanisms of progression of renal disease, as the importance of interrupting or forestalling this progression has assumed great importance in clinical nephrology. A thorough understanding of the roles of glomerular pressure, proteinuria, inflammation, and oxidants will help researchers and clinicians prevent renal failure, decreasing the need for dialysis and transplant.

The evolution of our understanding of kidney function and dysfunction derives from sequential discoveries made by a series of investigators, each benefiting from the accomplishments of their predecessors. The same can be said for this textbook. Originally conceived by two of the greatest renal physiologists of the twentieth century, Donald Seldin and Gerhard

Giebisch, it was passed on to Steve Hebert and one of the present editors. As the present editors, it is our hope to continue the book's commitment to science, and its role in our understanding and practice of nephrology, and in so doing to honor the previous editors for all that they have contributed to the book, to nephrology, to epithelial physiology, and to science in general.

List of Contributors

Dale R. Abrahamson, PhD Department of Anatomy and Cell Biology, University of Kansas Medical Center, Kansas City, KS, USA

Qais Al-Awqati, MB, ChB Departments of Medicine and Physiology, Columbia University, New York, NY, USA

Robert J. Alpern, MD Office of the Dean Yale, University School of Medicine, New Haven, CT, USA

Guillermo A. Altenberg, MD, PhD Department of Cell Physiology and Molecular Biophysics, and Center for Membrane Protein Research, Texas Tech University Health Sciences Center, Lubbock, Texas, TX, USA

Matthew A. Bailey, PhD British Heart Foundation Centre for Cardiovascular Science, University of Edinburgh, UK

Michel Baum, MD Departments of Pediatrics and Internal Medicine, University of Texas Southwestern Medical Center, Dallas, TX, USA

Daniel G. Bichet, MD, MSc Hôpital du Sacré-Coeur de Montréal, Departments of Medicine and Physiology, University of Montreal, Montréal, Québec, Canada

Roland C. Blantz, MD University of California and VA San Diego Healthcare System, San Diego, CA, USA

Matthew D. Breyer, PhD Biotechnology Discovery Research Eli Lilly and Company Indianapolis, IN and Division of Nephrology, Department of Medicine, Vanderbilt University, Nashville, TN

Richard M. Breyer Division of Nephrology, Department of Medicine, Vanderbilt University, Nashville, TN, USA

Paul T. Brinkkoetter University Hospital Cologne, Cologne, Germany

Kevin T. Bush, PhD Department of Pediatrics University of California San Diego, La Jolla, CA, USA

Lloyd Cantley, MD Section of Nephrology, Department of Internal Medicine, Yale University School of Medicine, New Haven, CT, USA

Chunhua Cao, MD, PhD Division of Nephrology, Department of Medicine, University of Maryland at Baltimore, Baltimore, MD, USA

Giovambattista Capasso, MD Chair of Nephrology, Department of Internal Medicine, Faculty of Medicine, Second University of Naples, Italy

Hayo Castrop, PhD Institute of Physiology, University of Regensburg, Germany

Laurence Chan, MD, PhD, FRCP University of Colorado Denver, Aurora, Colorado, USA

Davide Cina Samuel Lunenfeld Research Institute, Mount Sinai Hospital and Institute of Medical Science, Toronto, Ontario, Canada

Thomas M. Coffman, MD Division of Nephrology, Department of Medicine, Duke University and Durham VA Medical Centers, Durham, North Carolina, USA, Cardiovascular and Metabolic Disorders Research Program, Duke-NUS, Singapore

Steven D. Crowley, MD Division of Nephrology, Department of Medicine, Duke University and Durham VA Medical Centers, Durham, North Carolina, USA

Henrik Dimke, MSc Department of Biomedicine, University of Aarhus, Aarhus, Denmark; The Samuel Lunenfeld Research Institute, Mt. Sinai Hospital, Toronto, Ontario, Canada

Gilbert M. Eisner, Mb Georgetown University Medical Center, USA

Dominique Eladari, MD, PhD INSERM U872, Centre de Recherche des Cordeliers, Paris, France

David H. Ellison, MD Oregon Health & Science University & VA Medical Center, Portland, OR, USA

Hitoshi Endou, MD, PhD Department of Pharmacology and Toxicology, Kyorin University School of Medicine, Tokyo, Japan

Robin A. Felder, PhD University of Virginia Health Sciences Center, USA

Eric Féraille, MD, PhD Department of Cell Physiology and Metabolism and Service of Nephrology, University Medical Center, Geneva, Switzerland

Jørgen Frøkiær, MD, DMSc Water and Salt Research Center, Department of Clinical Physiology, Aarhus University Hospital-Skejby, Aarhus N, Denmark

Gerardo Gamba, MD, PhD Molecular Physiology Unit, Department of Nephrology and Mineral Metabolism, Instituto Nacional de Ciencias Médicas y Nutrición Salvador Zubirán, and Instituto de Investigaciones Biomédicas, Universidad Nacional Autónoma de México, Mexico City, Mexico

Jyothsna Gattineni, MD Department of Pediatrics, University of Texas Southwestern Medical Center, Dallas, TX, USA

Gerhard Giebisch, MD Dept. of Cellular & Molecular Physiology, Yale University School of Medicine, New Haven, CT, USA

Aleksandra Gmurczyk, MD The Feinberg School of Medicine, Northwestern University, Chicago, IL, USA

Joey P. Granger, PhD Department of Physiology and Biophysics and Department of Medicine, University of Mississippi Medical Center, MS, USA

Sian V. Griffin, MD University Hospital Wales, Health Park, Cardiff, Wales

William B. Guggino, PhD Department of Physiology, The Johns Hopkins University School of Medicine, Baltimore, MD, USA

Susan B. Gurley, MD, PhD Division of Nephrology, Department of Medicine, Duke University and Durham VA Medical Centers, Durham, North Carolina, USA

John E. Hall, PhD Department of Physiology and Biophysics and Department of Medicine, University of Mississippi Medical Center, MS, USA

Michael E. Hall, MD Department of Physiology and Biophysics and Department of Medicine, University of Mississippi Medical Center, MS, USA

Kenneth R. Hallows, MD, PhD Renal-Electrolyte Division, Department of Medicine and Department of Cell Biology and Physiology, University of Pittsburgh, Pittsburgh, PA, USA

Fiona Hanner Department of Physiology and Biophysics and Zilkha Neurogenetic Institute, University of Southern California Keck School of Medicine, Los Angeles, CA, USA

Raymond C. Harris, MD Division of Nephrology, Department of Medicine, Vanderbilt University, Nashville, TN, USA

Udo Hasler Department of Cell Physiology and Metabolism and Service of Nephrology, University Medical Center, Geneva, Switzerland

J. Kevin Hix, MD University of Rochester School of Medicine and Dentistry, Rochester, New York, USA

Chou-Long Huang, MD, PhD University of Texas, Southwestern Medical Center, Dallas, TX, USA

Edward J. Johns, BSc, PhD, DSc Department of Physiology, University College Cork, Cork, Republic of Ireland

Pedro A. Jose, MD, PhD Division of Nephrology, Department of Medicine, University of Maryland School of Medicine, USA

Brigitte Kaissling Institute for Anatomy, University of Zürich, Switzerland

Thomas R. Kleyman, MD Renal-Electrolyte Division, Department of Medicine and Department of Cell Biology and Physiology, University of Pittsburgh, Pittsburgh, PA, USA

Ulla C. Kopp, PhD Departments of Internal Medicine & Pharmacology, University of Iowa Carver College of Medicine, Iowa City, IA, USA

Wilhelm Kriz Department of Anatomy and Developmental Biology, Medical Faculty Mannheim, University of Heidelberg, Mannheim, Germany

Tae-Hwan Kwon Department of Biochemistry and Cell Biology, School of Medicine, Kyungpook National University, Taegu, Korea

Florian Lang Department of Physiology, University of Tübingen, Tübingen, Germany

Harold E. Layton Department of Mathematics, Duke University, Durham, NC, USA

Thu H. Le, MD Division of Nephrology, Department of Medicine, University of Virginia, Charlottesville, VA, USA

Richard P. Lifton Departments of Genetics and Internal Medicine, Howard Hughes Medical Institute, Yale University School of Medicine, New Haven, CT, USA

Johannes Loffing Institute of Anatomy, University of Zurich, Zurich, Switzerland

Yoshiro Maezawa Samuel Lunenfeld Research Institute, Mount Sinai Hospital, Toronto, Ontario, Canada

Gerhard Malnic Universidade de Sao Paulo, Instituto de Ciencias Biomedicas, Departamento de Fisiologie e Biofisica, Sao Paulo, Brazil

Karl S. Matlin, PhD Laboratory of Epithelial Pathobiology, Department of Surgery, University of Chicago, IL, USA

C. Charles Michel Department of Bioengineering, Imperial College, London, UK

Jeffrey H. Miner, PhD Department of Medicine, Renal Division, Washington University School of Medicine, St. Louis, MO, USA

Shigeaki Muto, MD, PhD Universidade de Sao Paulo, Instituto de Ciencias Biomedicas, Departamento de Fisiologie e Biofisica, Sao Paulo, Brazil

Søren Nielsen, MD, PhD Water and Salt Research Center, Department of Biomedicine, University of Aarhus, Aarhus, Denmark

Sanjay K. Nigam, MD Departments of Pediatrics, Cellular and Molecular Medicine, Medicine (Division of Nephrology and Hypertension), and Bioengineering, University of California San Diego, La Jolla, CA, USA

Man S. Oh, MD State University of New York, Downstate Medical Center, Brooklyn, NY, USA

Juan A. Oliver Department of Medicine, Columbia University, New York, NY, USA

Thomas L. Pallone, MD Division of Nephrology, Department of Medicine, University of Maryland at Baltimore, Baltimore, MD, USA

Biff F. Palmer, MD Professor of Internal Medicine, Department of Internal Medicine, Division of Nephrology, University of Texas Southwestern Medical Center, Dallas, TX, USA

Lawrence G. Palmer, PhD Department of Physiology & Biophysics, Weill Medical College of Cornell University, New York City NY, USA

János Peti-Peterdi, MD, PhD Department of Physiology and Biophysics and Zilkha Neurogenetic Institute, University of Southern California Keck School of Medicine, Los Angeles, CA, USA

Jay N. Pieczynski Department of Cell Biology, University of Alabama at Birmingham, Birmingham, AL, USA

Susan E. Quaggin Samuel Lunenfeld Research Institute, Mount Sinai Hospital; Institute of Medical Science; Division of Nephrology, St. Michael's Hospital University of Toronto, Toronto, Ontario, Canada

Luis Reuss, MD Department of Cell Physiology and Molecular Biophysics, and Center for Membrane Protein Research, Texas Tech University Health Sciences Center, Lubbock, Texas, TX, USA

Christopher J. Rivard, PhD University of Colorado Denver, Aurora, Colorado, USA

Gary L. Robertson, MD The Feinberg Medical School of Medicine, Northwestern University, Chicago, IL, USA

Robert M. Rosa, MD The Feinberg School of Medicine, Northwestern University, Chicago, IL, USA

Henry Sackin, PhD Department of Physiology & Biophysics, Rosalind Franklin University/The Chicago Medical School, North Chicago, IL, USA

Vaibhav Sahni, MD The Feinberg School of Medicine, Northwestern University, Chicago, IL, USA

Hiroyuki Sakurai, MD Department of Pharmacology and Toxicology, Kyorin University School of Medicine, Mitaka, Tokyo, Japan

Jeff M. Sands, MD Renal Division, Department of Medicine, Emory University School of Medicine, Atlanta, GA, USA

Lisa M. Satlin, MD Departments of Pediatrics and Medicine, Mount Sinai School of Medicine, New York, NY, USA

Laurent Schild Département de Pharmacologie et de Toxicologie, Université de Lausanne, Lausanne, Switzerland

Jürgen B. Schnermann, MD National Institute of Diabetes, and Digestive and Kidney Diseases, National Institutes of Health, Bethesda, MD, USA

Ute I. Scholl, MD Departments of Genetics and Internal Medicine, Howard Hughes Medical Institute, Yale University School of Medicine, New Haven, CT, USA

Takashi Sekine, MD Department of Pediatrics, Toho University School of Medicine, Ohashi Hospital, Tokyo, Japan

Donald W. Seldin, MD Department of Internal Medicine, University of Texas Southwestern Medical Center, Dallas, TX, USA

Stuart J. Shankland, MD University of Washington, Seattle, Washington, USA

Shaohu Sheng, MD Renal-Electrolyte Division, Department of Medicine, University of Pittsburgh, Pittsburgh, PA, USA

David G. Shirley, PhD UCL Centre for Nephrology, University College London Medical School, UK

Stephen M. Silver, MD Clinical Professor of Medicine, University of Rochester School of Medicine and Dentistry, Rochester, New York, USA

Martin Skott Department of Biomedicine, University of Aarhus, Aarhus, Denmark

Olivier Staub Department of Pharmacology & Toxicology, University of Lausanne, Lausanne, Switzerland

Richard H. Sterns, MD Rochester General Hospital and University of Rochester School of Medicine and Dentistry, Rochester, New York, USA

James D. Stockand, PhD Department of Physiology, University of Texas Health Science Center, San Antonio, TX, USA

Frederick W.K. Tam, PhD, FRCP Kidney and Transplant Institute, Imperial College School of Medicine, UK

Scott C. Thomson, MD University of California and VA San Diego Healthcare System, San Diego, CA, USA

Francesco Trepiccione Chair of Nephrology, Department of Internal Medicine, Faculty of Medicine, Second University of Naples, Italy

Robert J. Unwin, PhD, FRCP UCL Centre for Nephrology, University College London Medical School, UK

David L. Vesely, MD, PhD University of South Florida Cardiac Hormone Center, and James A. Haley Veterans Medical Center, Tampa, FL, USA

Wei Wang, MD University of Colorado Denver, Aurora, Colorado, USA

Wenhui Wang, MD Department of Pharmacology, New York Medical College, Valhalla, NY, USA

Alan M. Weinstein, MD Department of Physiology and Biophysics, Weill Medical College of Cornell University, New York, NY, USA

Paul A. Welling, MD Department of Physiology, University of Maryland School of Medicine, Baltimore, MD, USA

Scott S.P. Wildman, PhD Medway School of Pharmacy, The Universities of Kent and Greenwich at Medway, UK

Owen M. Woodward Department of Physiology, The Johns Hopkins University School of Medicine, Baltimore, MD, USA

Bradley K. Yoder, PhD Department of Cell Biology, University of Alabama at Birmingham, Birmingham, AL, USA

Alan S.L. Yu, MB, BChir Division of Nephrology and Hypertension, and The Kidney Institute, University of Kansas Medical Center, Kansas City, KS, USA

Miriam Zacchia Chair of Nephrology, Department of Internal Medicine, Faculty of Medicine, Second University of Naples, Italy

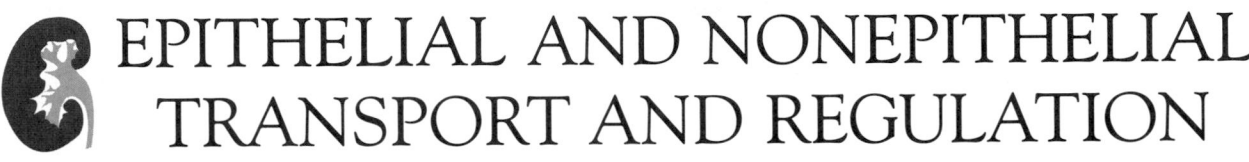

EPITHELIAL AND NONEPITHELIAL TRANSPORT AND REGULATION

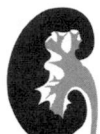

Epithelial Cell Structure and Polarity

Karl S. Matlin[1] and Michael J. Caplan[2]

[1]Laboratory of Epithelial Pathobiology, Department of Surgery, University of Chicago, IL, USA

[2]Department of Cellular and Molecular Physiology, Yale University School of Medicine, New Haven, CT, USA

INTRODUCTION

Many of the chapters in this volume are devoted to the mechanisms through which the nephron is able to convert the glomerular filtrate into concentrated urine that is responsive to the metabolic status of the organism as a whole. The multifactorial nature of this problem means it needs to be treated at several levels of resolution. A meaningful description of renal tubular functions requires an understanding of the nephron's properties as an integrated tissue, as well as those of its constituent parts, including the cells and molecules that contribute to its transport functions.

As detailed elsewhere in this volume, the nephron is a remarkably heterogeneous structure. Throughout its length, the renal tubule is notable for the marked variations in the morphologic and physiologic properties of its epithelial cells, reflecting the numerous and diverse responsibilities that neighboring segments are called on to fulfill. At the tissue level, the function of the kidney is critically dependent on the geometry and topography of the nephron. The precise juxtaposition of various epithelial cell types, which manifest distinct fluid and electrolyte transport capabilities, in large measure specifies the course of modifications to which the glomerular filtrate is exposed. This dependence on geometry also extends to renal function at the cellular level.

The Nature and Physiologic Implications of Epithelial Polarity

Despite their variations in form and function, all of the epithelial cells that line the nephron share at least one fundamental characteristic. Like their relatives in other tissues, all epithelial cells are polarized. The plasma membranes of polarized epithelial cells are divided into two morphologically and biochemically distinct domains.[1-6] In the case of the nephron, the apical surfaces of the epithelial cells face the tubular lumen. The basolateral surface rests on the epithelial basement membrane, and is in contact with the interstitial fluid compartment. The lipid and protein components of these two contiguous plasmalemmal domains are almost entirely dissimilar.[1-6] It is precisely these differences that account for the epithelial cell's capacity to mediate the vectorial transport of solutes and fluid against steep concentration gradients. Thus, the subcellular geometry of renal epithelial cells is critical to renal function.

The principal cell of the collecting tubule provides a useful illustration of the importance of biochemical polarity for renal function. As described in other contributions to this volume, the principal cell is required to resorb sodium against a very steep concentration gradient. It accomplishes this task through the carefully controlled placement of ion pumps and channels.[7-9] The basolateral plasma membrane of the principal cell, like that of most polarized epithelial cells, possesses a large complement of Na^+/K^+-ATPase. This basolateral sodium pump catalyzes the energetically unfavorable transport of three sodium ions out of the cell in exchange for two potassium ions, through the consumption of the energy embodied in one molecule of ATP.[10] The apical surface of the principal cell lacks sodium pump, but is equipped with a sodium channel, which allows sodium ions to move passively down their concentration gradient.[11] Through the action of the sodium pump the intracellular sodium concentration is kept low and the driving forces across the apical membrane favor the influx of sodium from the tubular fluid through the apical sodium channels. Thus, the combination of a basolateral Na^+/K^+-ATPase and an apical sodium channel lead to the vectorial movement of sodium from the tubule lumen to the interstitial space against its electrochemical gradient. This elegant mechanism is critically dependent upon the principal cell's biochemical polarity. If the sodium pump and the sodium channel occupied the same plasmalemmal domain, then the gradients generated by the former could not be profitably exploited by the latter. Thus, the vectorial resorption or secretion of solutes or fluid is predicated upon the asymmetric distribution of transport proteins in polarized epithelial cells.

The fact that epithelial cells manifest biochemical polarity implies that they are endowed with the capacity to generate and maintain differentiated subdomains of their cell surface membranes.[1-6] Newly synthesized membrane proteins must be targeted to the appropriate cell surface domain, and retained there following their delivery. During tissue development, cell division, and wound healing, plasmalemmal domains must be delimited and their biochemical character established. Clearly, specialized machinery and pathways must exist through which this energetically unfavorable compositional asymmetry can be supported. The nature of these specializations has been the subject of intense study for decades. While firm answers are not yet available, a number of fascinating model systems have been developed, and valuable insights have emerged. This chapter will focus on what is known of the processes through which tubular epithelial cells create their polarized geometry.

EPITHELIAL CELL STRUCTURE: MORPHOLOGY AND PHYSIOLOGY

The renal tubular epithelium is composed of a remarkably varied collection of cell types, ranging from the highly specialized glomerular epithelial cells with foot processes that faciliate filtration of the blood through the basement membrane, to the simple squamous epithelium of the loop of Henle. A detailed delineation of its morphologic diversity is beyond the scope of this chapter. However, certain essential features are shared among all cell types in the tubular epithelium and, indeed, most other epithelial cell types found in the body. Among these are a differentiated, microvillar apical surface facing the tubular lumen, a lateral surface specialized for cell–cell interactions and regulation of transepithelial permeability, and a basal surface that adheres to the basement membrane. Furthermore, as described previously, the basolateral plasma membrane is particularly important in ion transport, because it is the location of the Na^+/K^+-ATPase and the cell is able to modulate its surface area in response to the transport activity of individual cell types. The cell–cell adhesive relationships are responsible for the integrity of the epithelium, and also dictate the permeability of the epithelium to small molecules that, in part, give each segment of the epithelium its physiological identity. Furthermore, adhesion of epithelial cells to each other and to the basement membrane sends spatial signals to the cells essential for the establishment and maintenance of epithelial cell polarity. In the following sections the morphology and functional composition of the apical and basolateral domains of the plasma membrane will be described, after detailing the nature of the junctional complex that mediates cell–cell adhesion.

The Junctional Complex

All epithelial cells, including those of the kidney tubule, are joined together along the lateral surfaces by a series of intercellular junctions first noted by their characteristic ultrastructural appearance and relative locations on the lateral plasma membrane.[12,13] These include the tight junction or *zonula occludens*, the adherens junction (*zonula adherens* or intermediate junction), desmosomes, and gap junctions. In most mammalian epithelia the tight junction is located at the apical-most edge of the lateral membrane closely followed by the adherens junction. Desmosomes and gap junctions have less specific locations on the lateral membrane. Desomosomes and gap junctions will be described briefly, followed by a more comprehensive description of tight junctions and adherens junctions, because of their essential functions in the organization, physiology, and morphogenesis of epithelia.

Desmosomes are large, multiprotein complexes primarily responsible for the mechanical strength of cell–cell interactions.[14] They are formed after the assembly of adherens and tight junctions. By transmission electron microscopy they appear as discrete, focal concentrations of dense material in the cytoplasm of adjacent cells, as well as in the intercellular space.[13] In contrast to adherens and tight junctions, desmosomes do not form an adhesive belt around the entire epithelial cell, but are a kind of "spot weld" at various points on adjacent lateral membranes. They are composed of both integral membrane proteins of the cadherin family called desmogleins and desmocollins, and peripheral membrane proteins known as desmoplakins, as well as a variety of other protein constituents.[14] Adjacent cells adhere to each other through cadherin-mediated interactions. The peripheral components then provide mechanical stability to this interaction, via keratin intermediate filaments in the cytoplasm of each cell.[15] Ultrastructurally, these appear as a mass of hair-like protrusions interacting in parallel with each plaque and then splaying out into the cytoplasm.[13,14]

In this manner, desmosomes link all cells in the epithelium. While there is evidence that desmosomal components may play an active role in regulating some aspects of cell—cell adhesion and even gene expression,[16] in general their function is considered to be relatively passive.

Gap junctions are so named because of the characteristic 3 nm gap between adjacent cells that is evident using transmission electron microscopy.[17,18] Examination of freeze-fracture specimens, which permits visualization of the internal topography of membranes, reveals the gap junction as a discrete array of intramembranous particles or connexons.[17,18] Each connexon is composed of five identical connexins, a family of transmembrane proteins. Connexons on adjacent cells interact through their extracytoplasmic domains to form a series of low-resistance channels. These permit the passage of small molecules of less than 1 kDa, linking neighboring cells in the epithelium both electrically and metabolically. In the kidney, it is likely that gap junctions play important roles during morphogenesis and repair, although their precise functions have not been investigated in detail.[17,18]

Among the numerous functions subserved by epithelia, perhaps the most important is that of a barrier between the intra- and extracorporeal spaces. In the case of the kidney, the extracorporeal space is defined by the lumen of the renal tubule. That the chemical composition of urine differs substantially from that of the interstitial extracellular fluid bathing the epithelial basement membranes is evidence that the barrier provided by the tubular epithelium is tight to both small and large molecules. There are two components to this barrier, arranged in parallel.[19–21] The first is comprised of the apical and basolateral membranes of the epithelial cells, which together serve as a pair of series resistances to the flow of solutes across the epithelia. The second barrier is provided by the tight junction or *zonula occludens* that controls movement of molecules between the cells along the so-called paracellular pathway.[20–29]

The tight junction defines a border between the apical and basolateral plasma membranes. In columnar and cuboidal cells of the renal epithelium, it is found at the apical extremity of the lateral membrane and in the plane of the apical surface. Analysis by transmission electron microscopy originally suggested that the tight junction is a zone of partial fusion between the plasma membranes of adjacent cells.[13] Although this is no longer believed to be the case (see below), the ultrastructure of the junctions is consistent with this interpretation. When cells that have been treated with osmium are examined at high magnification, their membranes are distinguished by a characteristic pattern. The two leaflets of the lipid bilayer appear as a "unit membrane," defined by a pair of darkly stained parallel lines separated from one another by 5—10 nm.[30] In areas corresponding to the tight junction, the four parallel lines representing the two unit membrane of adjacent cells are replaced by three lines, which led to the suggestion that the two outer leaflets contributed by the neighboring cells have in some way merged to form a new trilaminar membrane structure.[12]

The putative outer leaflet fusion suggested by morphologic studies received some support from examination of lipid mobility in polarized epithelial cells. The mobility of outer leaflet lipids is restricted by the tight junction.[31,32] Labeled lipid probes inserted into the outer leaflets of epithelial apical or basolateral plasma membranes have unimpeded mobility within their respective domains, but cannot cross the tight junction.[31,32] Furthermore, outer leaflet lipids are unable to diffuse between neighboring epithelial cells through the tight junction. In contrast, inner leaflet lipids can apparently move freely between the two plasma membrane domains, suggesting that the tight junction presents no barrier to their diffusion. These observations are consistent with a model of the tight junction, in which the outer leaflets of the lipid bilayer participate in the formation of some junctional structure, while the inner leaflet remains unperturbed. These results also suggest that the lipid composition of the apical inner leaflet is necessarily identical to that of the basolateral one, because any differences would quickly be randomized by diffusion. Thus, the differences in lipid compositions of the apical and basolateral surfaces alluded to in the introduction to this chapter must be entirely contributed by the constituents of the outer leaflet.[32,33]

Electron microscopy has provided further insights into the structure of the tight junction. Examination of freeze-fracture replicas of epithelial cells reveals the tight junction to be composed of continuous branching and interwoven strands that surround the entire perimeter of the cell.[34] These strands appear as elevations in the P or cytoplasmic fracture face, and are matched by grooves in the E or external face. In some cell types the strands have a fibrillar appearance, and no discrete subunit structure can be resolved. In other cell types, and in samples not fixed with glutaraldehyde, the strands can appear more as a series of particles.[34] Although some early models postulated that the strands were composed of unusually structured lipids, it is now certain that they are primarily composed of integral membrane proteins (see below). Observations of a number of cell types with different amounts of transepithelial electrical resistance revealed a rough correlation between the number and complexity of the anastomosing strands and the degree of transepithelial electrical resistance. While this correlation certainly exists in at least some epithelia,[35] the amount of resistance is now known to be a function of the specific complement of proteins making up tight junctions in different cells.

The first tight junction protein identified was, appropriately, ZO-1 (zonula occludens-1).[36] ZO-1, however, turned out to be a cytoplasmic peripheral membrane protein, suggesting that other, integral transmembrane proteins capable of mediating cell–cell contact and the intermembrane permeability barrier must exist. Shortly thereafter, occludin, a multispanning membrane protein, was identified, followed by many other proteins.[21] It is now clear that the tight junction is an extremely complex structure composed of at least three different families of transmembrane proteins including: multiple claudins; occludin and other members of the MARVEL family; and the junctional adhesion molecules or JAMS.[21] Additional peripheral membrane proteins are also part of the tight junction, including ZO-1, -2, and -3, and cingulins. It is also evident that the functions of these protein complexes extend beyond regulating solute permeability to participation in epithelial cell polarization.[37]

Claudins are the most important tight junctional proteins controlling paracellular permeability of small molecules.[38–43] They are the major protein constituent of the tight junctional strands seen in freeze-fracture; expression of claudins in fibroblasts produces characteristic strands and promotes cell–cell adhesion.[21,38,41,43–45] The claudin family consists of at least 24 members in mammals. All are tetraspanning transmembrane proteins of $20-27$ kD, with two extracellular loops. With one exception, the cytoplasmic C-terminal sequence of claudins interacts with ZO-1, -2, and -3. Interacting claudins on neighboring epithelial cells create charge selective channels, with the overall permeability of the tight junction to ions dependent on the particular mix of claudins expressed in the cell.[21,44] This was illustrated dramatically in the renal epithelial cell line MDCK (Madin–Darby canine kidney) when expression of claudin 8, in addition to other endogenous claudins, reduced the paracellular movement of mono- and divalent cations without affecting the permeability of anions or uncharged solute molecules.[46] In the kidney tubular epithelium, cells of the proximal tubule, which has a transepithelial electrical resistance of $6-10$ Ωcm^2, express claudins 2, 6, 9, 10, and 11, while cells of the collecting duct, with a much higher resistance of 1000 Ωcm^2, express claudins 3, 4, 6, 7, 8, 10, and 14[29,47] (Figure 1.1). Other cell types along the nephron express other combinations, yielding a range of increasing resistances in the proximal-to-distal direction[29,47] (Figure 1.1).

The selective barrier created primarily by claudins is sometimes referred to as the "pore pathway," because it permits movement only of small ions and other uncharged small solute molecules. However, in at least some epithelia, there is also a kind of "leak pathway" that allows passage of larger molecules, including macromolecules.[21] The nature of the leak pathway and its regulation is poorly understood. Occludin, which is also a tetraspanning membrane protein unrelated to claudins, may play a role in the leak pathway, together with ZO-1 and the actin cytoskeleton. Even though it is counterintuitive, an electrically tight pore pathway can co-exist with an active leak pathway, although the molecular and structural basis of this has not been fully clarified.[21]

The tight junction is a structure whose function is highly dependent on interactions between integral and peripheral components and the actin cytoskeleton. ZO-1 and its family members are perhaps the most important class of proteins linking the various tight junctional proteins together.[36,48,49] ZO-1 contains multiple PDZ (PSD95-Dlg-ZO-1) protein interaction domains. These bind to both claudins and JAMs, while other regions of the molecule bind to occludin and actin. ZO-1 is also capable of binding to components usually identified with adherens junctions, and to a wide variety of signaling molecules.[21] While it is still valid to view the regulation of paracellular permeability as the primary function of the tight junction, it is more appropriate to think of the overall structure as a component of a larger apical junctional complex responsible for a multiplicity of adhesive, signaling, and membrane trafficking functions.

Originally, the tight junction was looked at as a stable, static structure in intact epithelia. Recent results using, among other approaches, expression of fluorescent tight junction proteins in cultured and intact epithelia, indicate that, in fact, the tight junction is highly dynamic.[50] In the intestine, the epithelial leak pathway will open to permit uptake of glucose beyond the capacity of the Na^+-glucose transporter in the apical membrane. This process is controlled by the actomyosin cytoskeleton, since drug-induced actin depolymerization, as well as activation of myosin light chain kinase (MLCK), compromises the epithelial barrier.[50–52] Breakdown in the barrier is accompanied by simultaneous endocytosis of occludin, both implicating occludin in the regulation of the leak pathway and further demonstrating the cell's capacity to reshape the junction. Tumor necrosis factor (TNF), which is involved in the pathogenesis of Crohn's disease, will cause barrier breakdown through a mechanism also dependent on MLCK.[50] Although these studies of tight junction plasticity have concentrated on the intestine, it would be surprising if similar mechanisms were not operable in the renal tubular epithelium, especially in the proximal tubule which morphologically resembles intestinal absorptive cells, and where uptake of a variety of filtered materials occurs.

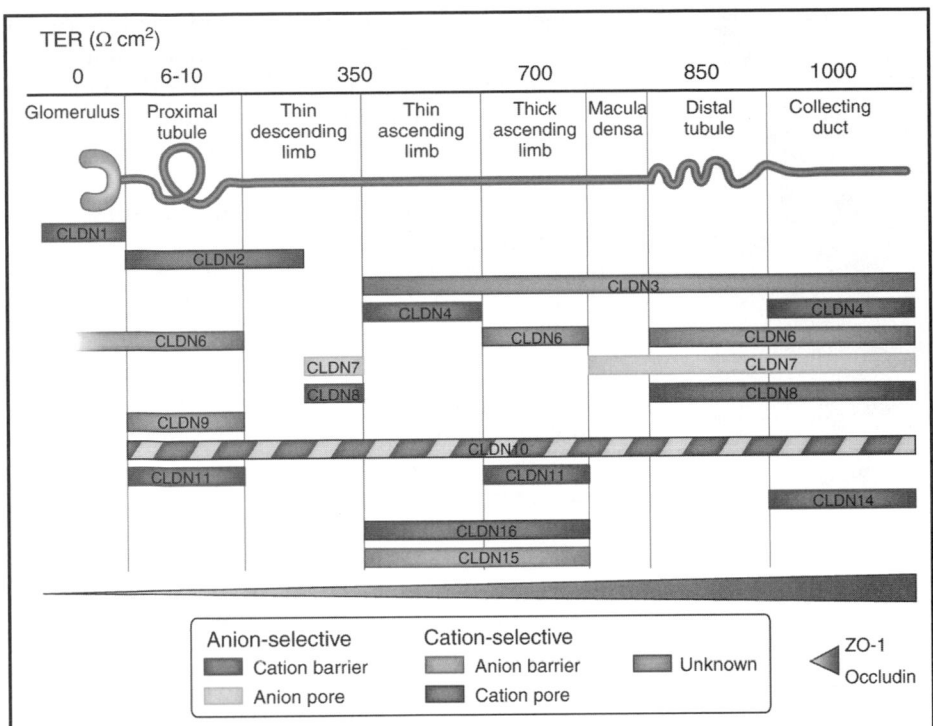

FIGURE 1.1 The relationship between transepithelial resistance and claudin subtype expression along the nephron. (*Reprinted from ref. [29].*)

The adherens junction, or *zonula adherens*, forms a belt just below the tight junction in most epithelial cells, connecting them via extracellular interactions and cytoplasmic linkages to the actin cytoskeleton (Figure 1.2). In the electron microscope, adherens junctions appear as a dense, somewhat amorphous concentration of submembranous staining, with a mass of impinging actin filaments.[13] The major adhesive component of the adherens junction is E-cadherin.[25,53,54] E-cadherin is a single-pass transmembrane protein that consists of a series of calcium-binding extracellular or EC repeat domains, and a cytoplasmic tail that interacts with members of the catenin family. In adherent cells E-cadherin is concentrated in the adherens junction, but can also be more diffusely distributed over the lateral plasma membrane. Adhesion between cells occurs through *trans* interactions between the EC1 domains contributed by different cells in the presence of calcium, which maintains the proper conformation of the extracellular part of E-cadherin. Interactions occur initially through individual molecules, but are then consolidated and strengthened through lateral interactions of individual units.

The stability of E-cadherin-mediated adhesion is dependent on the binding of catenins to the cytoplasmic tail of E-cadherin.[25,54] P120-catenin binds to a specific octapeptide located in the cytoplasmic juxtamembranous part of the cytoplasmic tail, and appears to be responsible for maintaining the stability of E-cadherin in the membrane, preventing its endocytosis and degradation. It is also involved in signaling related to cell motility,

and is a substrate for the Src-receptor tyrosine kinase. The second catenin that associates with E-cadherin is β-catenin, which binds to the carboxy terminus of the cytoplasmic tail in a phosphorylation-dependent manner.[25,54] Certain serine phosphorylations of E-cadherin increase the affinity of the β-catenin—E-cadherin interaction, while phosphorylation of serines on β-catenin disrupt the interaction with E-cadherin, and with α-catenin. In addition to its role in cell—cell adhesion, β-catenin is itself an important signaling molecule that is capable of entering the nucleus and regulating transcription of genes related to cell proliferation and differentiation.[16,55,56] Its function in transcription is carefully regulated by the Wnt signaling pathway by keeping the cytoplasmic concentration of β-catenin low, either through its interaction with E-cadherin or through its degradation by a mechanism dependent on a cytoplasmic "destruction complex" and ubiquitination.

In the adherens junction, β-catenin serves as a bridge between E-cadherin and α-catenin that, in turn, interacts with the actin cytoskeleton. In this manner, cell—cell adhesion through the adherens junction is given both a degree of mechanical stability and mobility through actomyosin contraction.[54] Originally the β-catenin—α-catenin—actin interaction was believed to be somewhat static, but recent evidence indicates that it is very dynamic. Alpha-catenin can exist as either a monomer or dimer, with the monomer able to bind β-catenin, but not actin, and the dimer able to bind actin, but not β-catenin. Three pools then exist in the cell: a monomer

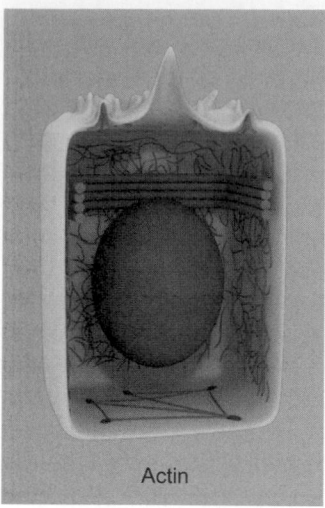

Actin   Microtubules

FIGURE 1.2   **The distribution of actin filaments and microtubules in polarized renal epithelial cells, based on the Madin−Darby canine kidney (MDCK) cell line.** *(Images courtesy of Jonathan Bowen and Elias T. Spoliotis, Drexel University, Philadelphia, Pennsylvania.)*

pool bound to β-catenin; a free cytoplasmic monomer pool; and a dimer pool bound to actin. As the adherens junction forms and consolidates, a high concentration of monomers is transported to a localized site on the membrane through β-catenin interactions. This then drives dimer formation and a dynamic linkage to the actin cytoskeleton. Localized concentration of α-catenin dimers can also inhibit Arp2/3, a mediator of actin branching essential for cell migration, and thus facilitate the transformation from a migrating cell to an adherent polarized cell during processes such as injury repair.[54] The recognition that the adherens junction is dynamic and plays a role in cell motility has helped to transform our view of epithelia from that of a static sheet of cells to one of interlocking cells capable of constant motion and remodeling, all the while maintaining a precise permeability barrier between the inside and outside compartments of the body.

The Apical Microvillar Surface

The apical brush border membrane is perhaps best epitomized by the one that graces the epithelial cells of the proximal tubule. Named for its appearance, the proximal tubular brush border is comprised of densely packed parallel microvilli which rise like the bristles of a brush from the level of the tight junctions to a height of 1 to 1.3 μm. The proximal tubular brush border is by far the most luxuriant to be found in the nephron; although the apical membranes of other renal epithelial cell types are endowed with small collections of microvillus-like structures, much less is known about the structural specializations characteristic of the apical membranes of more distal renal epithelial cells.[57]

The functions subserved by apical microvilli are not entirely clear. Certainly their most dramatic and obvious effect upon the properties of the apical membrane is manifest as a tremendous amplification of the apical membrane surface area. For the proximal tubule this amplification is in the order of 20-fold.[58,59] As is the case for the epithelia of the small intestine, it is through this redundancy that the proximal tubular epithelial cells markedly increase the efficiency of both their absorptive and degradative functions.

Physiologically, the proximal tubule is responsible for the resorption of ~60% of the filtered load of fluid and solutes.[60] Furthermore, it mediates the digestion of essentially all of the polysaccharides and peptides present in the glomerular filtrate, and transports the resultant sugars and amino acids from the lumen to the interstitial fluid space.[58] It is apparent, therefore, that the epithelial cells of the proximal tubule must be specially equipped, in order to cope efficiently with the comparatively enormous quantities of fluid and substrates that rapidly transit this nephron segment. The presence of an extravagant brush border greatly increases the fraction of the tubular fluid that comes into close contact with the enzymatic and transport systems arrayed on the microvillar surfaces prior to its passage from this tubule segment into the descending loop of Henle. Concomitantly, it proportionally multiplies the number of enzymatic and transport systems available to modify the substrates dissolved in the tubular fluid. Thus, the brush border membrane provides the scaffolding for the relatively massive arsenal of enzymatic and transport machinery required to accomplish the proximal tubule's function as a high-capacity and high-throughput absorptive system.

Ultrastructurally, a microvillus is composed of a bundle of ~19 parallel thin filaments that are linked to one another and to the overlying surface membrane by protein cross bridges.[61,62] The thin filaments extend well beyond the base of the microvillus, and are anchored in a dense matrix of fibers oriented parallel to the plane of the membrane. This meshwork, referred to as the terminal web, underlies the entire apical surface and anastomses with the filaments that radiate from the lateral desmosomes and zonulae adherens (Figure 1.2). The functional implications of these structural arrangements have become clearer as their components have been biochemically identified.[63,64]

The thin filaments that form the microvillar core are composed of actin[61,65] (Figure 1.2). Ultrastructural studies employing heavy meromyosin reveal that all of the filaments in the bundle share a single polarity, and are oriented with their nucleating end towards the microvillar tip. At their termination in the microvillar tip the filaments are received by an electron-dense cap whose molecular identity has yet to be established.[61]

As they emerge from the base of the microvillus, the actin filaments are caught up in the fibers of the terminal web (Figure 1.2). Fodrin, or non-erythroid spectrin, comprises one of the major components of this network.[61,64,66] It appears to function beneath the brush border as an actin fiber cross-linker. Another of the chief constituents of this fibrillar matrix is a non-muscle form of myosin II that belongs to the same myosin subfamily as its skeletal muscle counterpart. Bipolar myosin thick filaments appear to interact with the actin filaments as they sweep out of the microvillar sheath to join the terminal web.[61,65,67] Paired anti-parallel myosin filaments cross-link the actin filaments of neighboring microvilli to one another, forming a connection which bears close comparison to the actin—myosin arrangement characteristic of the striated muscle sarcomere. The analogy is strengthened by the presence in the microvillar rootlet of tropomyosin, a protein that functions in skeletal muscle to regulate the interaction between actin and myosin.[67,68]

This marked molecular similarity between the terminal web and the skeletal muscle contractile unit prompted speculation that this arrangement might also be functionally homologous. A number of investigators have postulated that activation of myosin-based contraction at the microvillar base might lead to microvillar shortening.[69] Repetitive activation of such a mechanism would lead to a piston-like extension and retraction of these membranous processes, which in turn might stir the surrounding tubular fluid. Such a mixing motion is certainly teleologically appealing, in that it would help to ensure that the tubular fluid is uniformly exposed to the enzymatic and transport systems of the proximal tubular apical membrane surface. No evidence for any such concerted and dynamic properties of microvilli has yet been gathered.

Biochemical studies have shed light on the identities and functional properties of some of the proteins which contribute to the interfibrillar cross bridges observed in transmission electron micrographic profiles of microvilli. Howe and Mooseker identified a protein of molecular weight 110 kDa that participates in cross-linking the filaments of intestinal microvilli to the plasma membrane.[70] This protein exhibits a high affinity for the calcium-binding protein calmodulin, which participates in the transduction of a number of calcium-regulated phenomena.[70] Of further interest was the fact that the 110 kDa protein manifests a myosin-like Mg-ATPase activity.[71] Addition of ATP to intact microvilli results in solubilization of the 110 kDa protein, and disruption of the cross-links between the actin filaments and the microvillar membrane.[72,73] Thus, attachment of the plasma membrane to the thin filaments may be regulated by ATP and calcium. The degree to which this putative capacity for structural modulation plays a role in microvillar function has yet to

be clarified. Subsequent molecular analysis revealed that the brush border 110 kDa protein belongs to the myosin I family of unconventional myosin molecules.[74,75] Unlike skeletal muscle myosin (which is assigned to the myosin II classification), brush border myosin I molecules possess a single globular head group, and do not form bipolar filaments.[71,72,76,77] Members of the myosin I family, including brush border myosin (myosin Ia), have been found to associate with the membranes of intracellular vesicles, prompting the hypothesis that these motor proteins serve to propel vesicles through the cytoplasm along actin filament tracks.[78,79] Co-localization studies have demonstrated that brush border myosin I and the microtubule-dependent motor protein dynein can be found together on the membranes of post-Golgi vesicles.[80] This observation has inspired the hypothesis that apically-directed vesicles depart the Golgi along microtubule tracks powered by the action of dynein. Upon their arrival at the actin-rich terminal web, they switch engines and are carried the rest of the way to the brush border by myosin I.[81] While brush border myosin I is abundantly expressed in intestinal epithelial cells, it may be present at lower levels in the renal proximal tubule.[82] Since the myosin I family is large and diverse, however, it is extremely likely that an as-yet-unidentified member of this class subserves similar structural and mechanical functions in the epithelial cells of the kidney.[83,84]

Another protein that apparently participates in the organization of the microvillus has a molecular weight of 95 kDa, and has been dubbed villin.[85] Villin belongs to a large family of actin-binding proteins.[86] Prominent in its structure is a pair of sequence domains that appear to be involved in associations with f-actin. The presence of this tandem repeat justifies the contention that villin mediates the bundling of actin fibers. It is interesting to note that villin is a calcium-binding protein, and that interaction with calcium alters its behavior in the presence of actin filaments.[87] In experiments carried out with purified villin in solution, it has been found that this protein bundles actin filaments when the free calcium concentration is less than 1 μM. When the calcium concentration rises to 10 μM, villin severs actin filaments into short protofilaments. At intermediate calcium concentrations, villin binds to actin filaments at their growing ends, forming a cap that prevents further elongation. Due to the dynamic nature of the microfilament polymer, this capping results in the formation of shortened filaments. It is not known whether these calcium-dependent activities of villin are manifest *in vivo*. If villin does indeed sever or shorten actin filaments within the living cell, it would seem likely that perturbations which produce elevations of intracellular calcium concentrations may lead to structurally significant alterations in the organization of the microvillar scaffolding. During embryonic development, villin is expressed throughout the cytoplasm of epithelial cells prior to the elevation of a brush border.[88] At later stages, villin becomes localized to the cytosolic surface of the apical membrane, and is subsequently incorporated into forming microvilli. This behavior has led to the suggestion that the localization of villin to the apical surface is a watershed event in the biogenesis of microvilli. Thus, the formation of inter-filamentous bridges, presumably mediated by villin, may be a critical first step in the organization of the microvillar infrastructure. Supporting this model are the results of experiments in which Caco-2 intestinal epithelial cells were stably transfected with a vector encoding antisense villin mRNA.[89] The consequent reduction in villin expression resulted in a loss of the brush border and mis-sorting of a subset of apical microvillar proteins. It must be noted, however, that results from gene knockout experiments argue against an obligate role for villin in microvillus formation.[90] Mice whose villin genes have been disrupted, and which produce no villin protein, are able nonetheless to generate morphologically and apparently physiologically normal brush borders. Presumably, other components of the microvillar infrastructure can shoulder the cross-linking and organizational duties normally performed by villin. Such functional redundancy is typical of biological systems endowed with architecture as esthetically elegant and complex as that which graces the microvillus.

While villin is limited in its distribution to those cell types endowed with brush borders, another actin-bundling component of the microvillus is present in numerous structures. Plastin-1, which is also known as fimbrin, is a 68 kDa polypeptide associated with the interfilamentous cross bridges that can also be detected in hair cell stereocilia and in ruffled borders.[91] Plastin-1 is clearly a multivalent actin-binding protein, and participates in the cross-linking of the microvillar actin filament array. Structural studies suggest that the cross-linking activity of plastin-1 constitutes the principal means through which the parallel actin filaments are interconnected in microvilli,[92] and the length and organization of brush borders are abnormal in plastin-1 knockout mice.[93] A third bundling protein, known as espin, also participates in the organization of the microvillar actin filaments.[94] While microvilli appear to form normally in the absence of espin,[95] espin overexpression leads to microvillar lengthening[96] by exerting subtle effects on the relative rates of actin filament polymerization and depolymerization. Simultaneous knockout of plastin-1, villin, and espin produces animals whose brush borders are short, and characterized by reduced numbers of disorganized actin filaments and mislocalized myosin. Interestingly, localization of enzymes that are normally concentrated in microvilli is markedly compromised in epithelial cells from these animals, suggesting that the organization of the

overlying plasma membrane is dependent upon the structural integrity of the microvillar actin bundle.[97]

Several other polypeptides, associated with the microvillus core and the terminal web, have also been identified. Among the most interesting and important of these is ezrin, a member of the ezrin–radixin–moesin family of proteins.[98] The C-terminal tails of these polypeptides bind to actin filaments, while their N-termini interact with proteins in the membrane. A number of proteins involved in the generation or regulation of intracellular second messengers associate in macromolecular complexes with ezrin–radixin–moesin family members, suggesting that in addition to functioning as linkers these proteins may also act as scaffolding for the assembly of components involved in signal transduction. Knockout of ezrin expression results in shortened and poorly formed brush border microvilli, and perturbations in the organization of the terminal web.[99] In addition, ezrin participates in forming complex molecular scaffolds that regulate and stabilize the expression of solute transport proteins in the apical membranes of renal epithelial cells.[100]

The terminal web mentioned above consists of three morphologically distinguishable domains. In addition to the cytoskeletal fibers that receive the rootlets of the microvilli, fibers that arise from desmosomes and the zonula adherens contribute to this meshwork. The desmosomal fibers consist primarily of 10 nm intermediate filaments composed of keratins.[15] At the level of the zonula adherens, the cell is ringed by a complex of randomly polarized actin filaments which also contains myosin and tropomyosin[67] (Figure 1.2). In vitro experiments have demonstrated that this ring has the capacity to contract circumferentially.[101] This capacity has led to the idea that contraction of the zonula adherens ring might contribute to the alterations in tight junctional permeability which have been observed in several epithelial systems in response to certain second messengers and osmotic stress, as described earlier.[20] Thus, activation of sodium-coupled glucose uptake in cultured intestinal epithelial cells has been shown to induce a decrease in transepithelial resistance. This effect is dependent upon the activity of myosin light chain kinase.[51,52] It is thought that by shortening in a "purse-string" fashion, these filaments might actually draw neighboring cells away from one another, and thus modify the structure and permeability of the occluding junctions. The relevance of this model to the functioning of renal epithelia has yet to be established.

The anisotropy and structural complexity that characterize the filamentous core of the microvillus apparently also extend to its overlying plasma membrane. The proteins embedded in, and associated with, the plasmalemma of the proximal tubule brush border are not uniformly distributed over its surface, but rather are restricted to specific subdomains. This lateral segregation is epitomized by the behavior of two trans-membrane polypeptides, maltase and gp330. The 300 kDa enzyme maltase is distributed over the entire surface of the microvilli themselves, but is absent from the intermicrovillar membrane regions.[102,103] In contrast, the heavily glycosylated gp330 (also known as megalin) is restricted in its distribution to these inter-microvillar regions. The restriction of megalin to the intermicrovillar regions appears to be mediated by its interactions with protein components of the endocytic machinery. Ultrastructural examination of the intermi-crovillar regions reveals the presence of coated pits. The cytosolic surface of the plasma membrane in these domains is coated with an electron dense material that biochemical and immunoelectron microscopic studies have demonstrated to be clathrin.[103] The presence in these intermicrovillar pits of morphologic and compo-sitional features associated with the process of endocy-tosis has led investigators to believe that this domain mediates the retrieval of large peptides and proteins from the proximal tubular fluid. The proximal tubular epithelial cells are responsible for capturing and degrading any proteins that pass through the glomeru-lar filtration barrier.[58] This function is apparently served by the profusion of coated pits and vesicles that decorate the surfaces of membranes at the microvillar base. Megalin is a member of the LDL receptor family and, together with cubulin, serves as a receptor that binds to and mediates the uptake of filtered proteins and peptides. Megalin knockout mice exhibit low molecular weight proteinuria, establishing the critical role for megalin as the proximal tubule's pre-eminent scavenger.

Finally, it is worth noting that most or all of the epi-thelial cells of the nephron are endowed with a single primary cilium (Figure 1.2). This non-motile cilium pos-sesses a ring of nine microtubules, but lacks the central pair of microtubules found in motile cilia. This primary cilium appears to serve sensory functions. Bending the primary cilium, in response to flow or mechanical sti-muli, induces calcium signaling in renal epithelial cells. Furthermore, the functional integrity of the primary cilium appears to be a prerequisite for the maintenance of normal renal tubular architecture. A number of cystic diseases of the kidney are attributable to mutations in genes encoding proteins found in cilia.[104−108] Similarly, mice in which expression of ciliary proteins has been disrupted develop cysts. The mechanisms through which loss of the cilium's mechanosensory functions leads to cystic transformation remain to be established.

The Basolateral Plasma Membrane

The rigid subservience of structure to function so elegantly exemplified by the apical microvillar membrane also extends to the basolateral surface of the epithelial plasma membrane. As was mentioned above, the basolateral membrane possesses the ion pumps that power the transepithelial resorption of solutes and water. The resorptive capacity of a given cell type is thus largely dependent on the quantity of ion pumps embedded within its basolateral mem-brane. This parameter appears, in turn, to be roughly proportional to the surface area encompassed by this membrane domain.[8] Consequently, renal epithelial cells that participate in resorption of large quantities of ions and fluid (such as those of the proximal tubule), as well as cells that carry out resorption of ions against steep concentration gradients (such as those of the thick ascending limb of the loop of Henle), are endowed with basolateral plasma membranes whose surface areas are amplified through massively redun-dant infoldings.

As was detailed in the discussion of the apical mem-brane, the lateral distribution of proteins within the plane of the basolateral membrane is not uniform. This fact is most dramatically illustrated by epithelial cell types that lack the deeply invaginated basolateral infold-ings discussed above. Studies have demonstrated that the Na$^+$/K$^+$-ATPase is concentrated in subdomains of the basolateral membranes of small intestinal epithelial cells.[109] The sodium pump is essentially restricted to the lateral membranes of these cells, and is absent from the basal surfaces that rest on the basement membrane. Dislodging these cells from the underlying basement membrane produces a redistribution of the sodium pump throughout the entire basolateral surface. These results suggest that the sodium pump is either actively or passively prevented from entering the basal domain of the plasma membrane, in some manner that is depen-dent on an intact interaction with the basement mem-brane. The meshwork of cytoskeletal elements associated with those sites at which the epithelial cell is anchored to the basement membrane may be too dense to allow membrane proteins such as the sodium pump to pene-trate. Conversely, cytoskeletal restraints whose integrity requires cell attachment to the basement membrane might retain the sodium pump within the lateral subdo-mains. In each of these scenarios, the cytoskeleton plays an important role in determining the subcellular distri-bution of a transmembrane protein. Research over the years has made it quite clear that the cytoskeleton plays a critical role in defining polarized domains, and in determining aspects of their protein compositions.[110−125]

The Basement Membrane

The basement membrane, while not strictly part of the epithelium, is such an essential contributor to epithelial function that it cannot be excluded from any comprehen-sive description of the renal epithelium. The basement membrane is a thin layer of secreted and assembled extracellular matrix that underlies all epithelia and endothelia in the body, and also surrounds skeletal muscle fibers and peripheral nerves.[126] In the past, the terms basement membrane and basal lamina were used inconsistently to describe morphological features of this layer, but there is no longer sufficient reason to distinguish these terms from each other, and they may be used interchangeably.[12] In the kidney, the tubular basement membrane is comparable to that found under other epithelia in the body, while that of the glomerulus is more complex and unusual.[127–129] In the glomerulus, the basement membrane is synthesized from proteins secreted by both podocytes and the closely apposed endothelium, resulting in a double-thick layer of matrix proteins that is an essential part of the glomerular blood filter. Diseases affecting the glomerular basement membrane often lead to compromise of the filter and proteinuria. Detailed discussion of this barrier and its specialized and distinctive composition is beyond the scope of our overall discussion of the biology of the renal epithelium, and will not be pursued in this chapter.

Basement membranes are visible by transmission electron microscopy of glutaraldehyde-fixed and heavy metal stained thin sections of epithelia, and classically appear as an electron dense layer (*lamina densa*) separated from an electron lucid (*lamina lucida*) layer adjacent to the basal epithelial surface.[12] While these morphological features were originally believed to have a structural basis, there is now evidence that they may be fixation artifacts. All basement membranes are composed of a common set of protein components which include laminins, type IV collagen, heparan sulfate proteoglycans, and nidogen, although the specific types of these can vary depending on both developmental stage and tissue, as well as accompanying pathology.[126] The most important component is probably laminin, because of its role in both assembly of the basement membrane and signaling.[130] Laminins consist of large ($\sim 400-800$ kDa) heterotrimeric secreted glycoproteins. In mammals, five α-, three β-, and three γ-subunits have been identified in at least 15 different heterotrimeric complexes. Prototypical laminins are cross-shaped molecules in which the short arms of the cross are contributed by the amino-termini of each subunit, and the stem by a coiled-coil made up of the carboxy-terminal halves of each subunit.[130] Typically, the amino-termini of each subunit consist of a globular LN or polymer domain that is involved in basement membrane assembly. The carboxy-terminus of the α-subunit is folded into a series of five globular domains (G1–5) that are essential for binding to the cell surface. Laminins are named according to their subunit composition, such that LM-511, the most common laminin in the kidney, is composed of the α5-, β1-, and γ1-subunits.[131] Like all collagens, collagen IV is a trimeric molecule composed of

combinations of various type IV α-subunits that fold into an elongated triple helix.[126] In contrast with fibrillar collagens such as collagen I, type IV collagen does not form bundles, because of the persistence of carboxy-terminal noncollagenous domains (NC1) and interruptions in the collagen repeats within the triple-helix forming regions that render the molecule more flexible. The most common types of proteoglycans found in the basement membrane are perlecan and agrin.[126] Each is a complex molecule that contains a variety of structural motifs resembling those found in laminins, in addition to substantial negatively-charged heparan sulfate polysaccharides. Nidogen (also called entactin) is a relatively small basement membrane protein that acts primarily to link laminin and collagen IV in the assembled structure. In addition to the core components of laminin, collagen IV, and proteoglycans, a variety of other minor components may also be present under particular, poorly-defined conditions, including extracellular matrix proteins normally considered to be primarily components of the interstitial matrix, such as fibronectin.

Basement membranes initially form during embryogenesis, and are then remodeled during development.[132,133] In addition, *de novo* basement membrane assembly may occur in adults following injuries that interrupt basement membrane continuity. Assembly is believed to occur through a mass-action process driven primarily by laminin polymerization.[126,130,134] Laminin molecules secreted by epithelial cells bind to receptors on the basal cell surface until the density of bound molecules permits formation of heterotrimeric complexes of α, β, and γ amino-terminal LN domains contributed by three different laminin molecules. The resulting structure is a polymerized network of molecules closely associated with the basal surface. Subsequently, collagen IV intercalates into this primary network to form a secondary network created by head-to-tail interactions between collagen IV molecules. The two networks are then linked through nidogen interactions between laminin and collagen, and other molecules, including notably proteoglycans, fill the spaces within the interlocked laminin and collagen networks.[126,130,134]

During pathological processes such as renal cyst formation and recovery from ischemic injury to the tubular epithelium, there is evidence that the atypical laminin isoform LM-332 is expressed.[135–138] This laminin consists of the α3-, β3-, and γ2-subunits, with both the α3- and γ2-subunits lacking amino-terminal LN domains, precluding the molecule from participating in typical network formation. The specific function of LM-332 in these pathological situations is unknown, but one hypothesis is that it interacts with prototypical laminins, such as LM-511, to terminate or even disrupt normal basement membrane assembly, facilitating remodeling of the basement membrane, and possibly signaling the epithelium to differentiate into a more plastic state suitable for injury repair.[139]

The basement membrane interacts with epithelial cells primarily by binding to the integrin family of extracellular matrix receptors. Integrins are a superfamily of cell adhesion receptors found in nearly all cells.[140] Each integrin consists of a heterodimer of α- and β-subunits, both of which are transmembrane glycoproteins. A total of 18 α- and 8 β-subunits are known in mammals, resulting in at least 24 heterodimers.[140] Although integrins are known primarily as receptors for extracellular matrix proteins, they may also participate in cell—cell adhesion.[141] Epithelial cells of the kidney and other organs typically express an array of integrins, including multiple forms with the β1-subunit, such as α2β1 and α3β1, as well as integrins with the β3-, β5-, and β6-subunits in combination with αV[142] (A. Manninen, personal communication). Many, if not all, epithelial cells also express integrin α6β4.[140,142] The β4-subunit is uniquely found in epithelial cells and, unlike most other epithelial integrins, interacts on the cytoplasmic side with cytokeratins, rather than the actin cytoskeleton. Integrin α2β1 is a collagen receptor, while α3β1 and α6β4 are receptors for multiple isoforms of laminin.[140] The various αV-containing integrins are receptors for ligands containing the binding sequence arginine—glycine—aspartate (RGD), such as fibronectin and vitronectin.[140] They may also play a role in activation of transforming growth factor β (TGFβ), which is important in epithelial repair and other processes.[143] The MDCK cell line, for example, expresses α2β1, α3β1, α6β4, and several αV-containing integrins, with α3β1 and α6β4 mediating adhesion to different laminins, and with αVβ3 (and possibly other αV integrins) activating TGFβ to turn on specific laminin expression during wound-healing.[143,144] In the kidney tubule, the complement of integrins expressed varies along the nephron, as does the expression of their extracellular matrix ligands, underlining their involvement not only in cell adhesion, but also in differentiation.[142]

In adherent cells, most integrins facilitate adhesion through dynamic interactions with the actin cytoskeleton.[145–148] Linkage to actin is mediated by adapter protein complexes that bind to integrin cytoplasmic tails and then to actin. Proteins found in these complexes include talin, which binds directly to integrins and activates their adhesive properties, paxillin, α-actinin, and vinculin.[145–148] Studies of migrating cells suggest that initial adhesive interactions occur through small "focal complexes" that form on leading lamellipodia and are linked to branched actin through the action of the Rac1, a small GTPase of the rho family. As the cell moves over these contacts, they mature into larger "focal adhesions" that associate with robust actin stress fibers (at least in culture) controlled by another GTPase RhoA and its effectors.[145–149] While the general

elements of this model have been somewhat validated in epithelial cells during wound healing, the status of focal complexes and focal adhesions in mature polarized epithelia of the kidney and elsewhere remain, for the most part, unexplored. As mentioned previously, α6β4 is a novel integrin, in that it is epithelial-specific and is capable of assembling adhesion complexes that interact with the cytokeratin cytoskeleton.[140] In normal skin, α6β4 is an essential part of hemidesmosomes.[150] These are large protein complexes containing a second transmembrane protein BP180 in addition to α6β4, as well as the cytoplasmic proteins BP230 and plectin that interact with cytokeratin filaments. The type of hemidesmosome found in the skin (type I) is visible as a dense plaque on the cytoplasmic surface of the basal plasma membrane under the electron microscope.[151] In the kidney such structures have not been reported. However, it is possible that a less developed type of hemidesmosome that is not apparent ultrastructurally (type II) is present in the kidney, although this has not been examined.[151]

In addition to their role in mechanical adhesion, focal complexes and focal adhesions are also platforms for signaling.[145–149] A variety of kinases including, notably, focal adhesion kinase (FAK) and members of the src family of tyrosine kinases, associate with integrin adhesion complexes and are activated by binding to the extracellular matrix. Subsequent signals then activate downstream serine/threonine kinases, such as integrin-linked kinase (ILK), and MAP kinases, such as ERK, to regulate a diverse range of processes including proliferation, migration, and apoptosis. Indeed, at least 180 different cytoskeletal, adapter, and signaling proteins are known to be associated with integrin adhesion complexes, depending on the cell type and circumstances.[149]

In addition to integrins, other membrane proteins are involved in epithelial cell adhesion to the extracellular matrix, including dystroglycan, a laminin receptor, and possibly a membrane-bound form of the Lutheran antigen.[129,130] There is evidence that glycolipids may also serve as transient laminin receptors.[152,153] While it is not proven that any of these receptors play a direct role in epithelial polarization, they may act indirectly by affecting assembly of the basal lamina.[152,153]

BIOGENESIS OF EPITHELIAL POLARITY

In the kidney, polarization of epithelial cells occur under two different circumstances: early development of the tubular epithelium; and repair of an existing epithelium following injury. In mammals, formation of the renal tubular epithelium is initiated by induction of the metanephric mesenchyme by the invading ureteric bud.[154] Following induction, cells of the mesenchyme form aggregates known as condensates, and these subsequently differentiate into polarized epithelial cells facing a central lumen. Extension of this lumen and further, more specialized, differentiation of epithelial cells eventually forms the nephron. In the case of injury by, for example, nephrotoxic substances or ischemia, the existing polarized tubular epithelium is disrupted in spots.[155,156] Cells at the periphery of these damaged areas then convert from relatively sessile cells polarized along an apical-to-basal axis to flatter, more migratory cells that now have front—rear rather than apical—basal polarity and the capacity to proliferate, enabling them to fill gaps in the epithelium. Once continuity has been achieved, apical—basal polarity is restored.[155,156] While front—rear and apical—basal polarization would seem to be quite distinctive, there is evidence that many of the important molecules and signals are shared. Indeed, as we are now beginning to understand, even front—rear polarization during injury repair is a close mechanistic cousin of apical—basal polarization.[157]

In the following sections, our current understanding of the mechanism of epithelial polarization will be described, after a brief introduction to the predominant experimental system used to study these processes.

In Vitro Systems

The kidney's complicated architecture and cellular heterogeneity renders it a poor substrate for studies designed to examine dynamic cell biological processes. Over the past four decades, the vast majority of research into the mechanisms through which epithelia generate and maintain their polarized phenotype has made use of several continuous lines of cultured epithelial cells. These cell lines retain many of the differentiated properties of their respective parent tissues in vitro. Thus, LLC-PK1 cells resemble the proximal tubule (although their precise origin is uncertain).[158] Similarly, Caco-2, HT-29, and T84 cells behave like their progenitors, the colonocytes of the large intestine.[158] Most importantly for this discussion, they manifest in culture the biochemical and morphologic features of the polarized state. Perhaps the best characterized and most heavily used of these culture models is the Madin—Darby canine kidney (MDCK) cell line (Figure 1.3). MDCK cells were originally derived from normal dog kidney in 1959, and grown in culture as a partially transformed line; that is, MDCK cells grow immortally as a monolayer and will not form tumors in nude mice.[159,160] Although their precise point of origin along the nephron is not entirely clear, their physiological and morphological properties suggest that they derive from cells of the thick ascending limb, distal tubule or collecting tubule.[161]

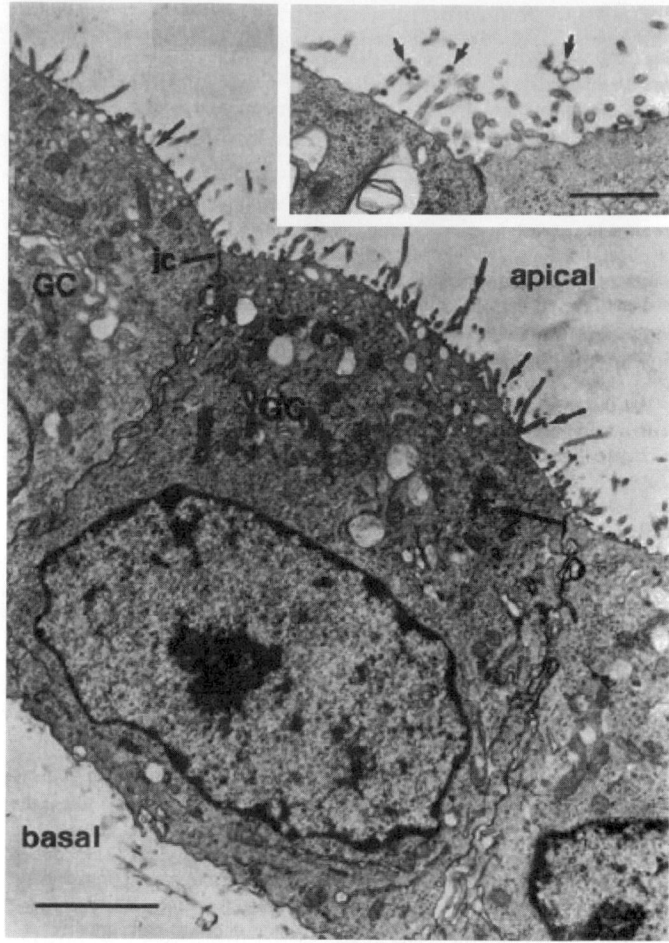

FIGURE 1.3 **Influenza virus buds from the apical surface of polarized MDCK cells.** MDCK cells were grown on a hydrated collagen gel, infected with influenza virus for 6 hours, and prepared for electron microscopy. The arrows denote mature virions which assemble at, and bud from, the apical surface. No virus particles are detected at the basal or lateral surfaces. Bar represents 3.0 μm (inset bar represents 1.0 μm) (GC: Golgi complex; jc: junctional complex). *(Reprinted with permission ref. [1].)*

The first clues to the polarized nature of the MDCK cell line came from the direct observation of these cells' capacity for vectorial transport. When grown on impermeable substrata, MDCK cells form domes (also called blisters or hemicysts).[162] Physiological studies have demonstrated that domes develop as a result of the transepithelial transport of solutes from the apical media to the basolateral surface.[163] Water that passively follows these solutes results in the generation of the fluid-filled blisters. It is fair to say that domes arise in regions where the cells have literally pumped themselves up off the dish. In keeping with this dramatic propensity for unidirectional solute movement, each MDCK cell manifests a polarized distribution of ion transport proteins, including several routes for sodium entry into its apical membrane, and approximately one million molecules of the

Na$^+$/K$^+$-ATPase in its basolateral plasmalemma.[164] The popularity of MDCK cells for polarity research developed out of the seminal observations of Rodriguez-Boulan and Sabatini in 1978.[165] In studies of enveloped virus budding from infected MDCK cells, these investigators found that influenza virus assembles at, and buds from, the apical cell surface (Figure 1.3). Of even greater significance was the demonstration that the spike glycoproteins which populate the membranes of these viruses accumulate preferentially at the cell surface from which budding is to occur.[166] Thus, the influenza hemagglutinin (HA) protein is predominantly on the apical surface early in infection. Similarly, the G protein of vesicular stomatitis virus (VSV) is almost exclusively basolateral in infected cells. The viral proteins provided investigators with the first experimentally manipulatable system for the study of membrane protein sorting. A large number of studies have subsequently elucidated the sorting of many endogenous MDCK cell proteins, as well as exogenous proteins expressed from vectors. This system remains the most thoroughly investigated paradigm and, as will be detailed below, has yielded important insights into the nature of pathways and signals that participate in membrane protein targeting and the overall biogenesis of epithelial polarity.

More recently, investigators have endeavored to develop new cell lines to study particular aspects of renal cell biology.[167–170] For example, immortalization genes from human papillomavirus or a hybrid between adenovirus and SV40 have been used to create permanent cell lines from human proximal tubule cells. These lines are of particular interest because of the proclivity of the proximal tubule to suffer injury following ischemic insult. The cell lines retain some differentiated characteristics of the proximal tubule, including expression of brush border markers and sodium dependent/phlorizin-sensitive sugar transport.[169,170] Cultures of cell lines derived in this fashion are not, however, always able to stably maintain the uniform morphology of a simple epithelium, limiting their usefulness for studies of epithelial polarity. More promising results have been obtained using cell lines derived from mice constitutively expressing immortalization factors as transgenes. Among these is the BUMPT-306 line derived from the mouse proximal tubule.[167,168] While certainly not perfect, this line does grow as a simple epithelium, and has the added advantage of providing an *in vitro* correlate to *in vivo* mouse experiments.

The study of epithelial polarization using cell lines has been facilitated by culturing cells in configurations that more closely resemble *in vivo* conditions (Figure 1.4 and 1.5). For example, many varieties of epithelial cells can be grown on permeable filter supports.[171,172] Originally, these were designed to mimic the Ussing chamber used

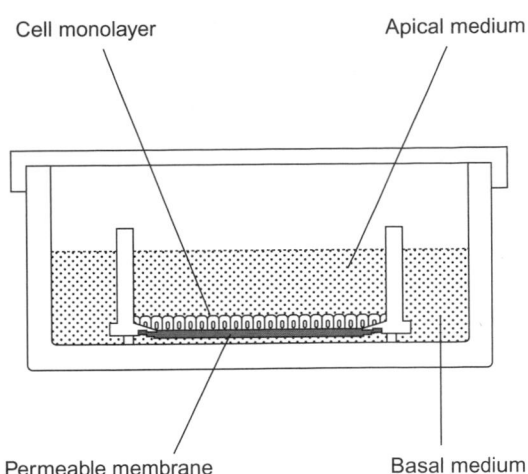

FIGURE 1.4 **Epithelial monolayers can be grown on permeable filter supports.** As depicted in the diagram, a porous filter, composed of cellulose acetate or polycarbonate, forms the bottom of a cylindrical cup. Epithelial cells are plated on top of the filter, and the cup is placed in a well filled with media. When the cells become confluent, the resultant monolayer forms a barrier between the media bathing the apical surface and the media in communication with the basolateral surface. This system thus provides investigators with simultaneous and independent access to both plasmalemmal domains.

for physiological studies, but later turned out to also be very useful for biochemical and morphological experiments. In their most common commercially-available configuration, these supports are composed of polycarbonate filters with pore sizes typically in the range of 0.4 μm that form the bottom cup. The cup is then suspended in a plastic well containing culture medium, and medium is also added to the inner compartment of the cup (Figure 1.4). Cells are plated on the upper surface of the filter. When a confluent monolayer is formed, it effectively creates a barrier between media compartments. The medium in the interior of the cup bathes the epithelial apical surface, whereas the basolateral surface communicates with the exterior media compartment through the pores of the filter (Figure 1.4). As epithelial cells in the kidney and other organs would normally receive most of their nutrition from the basolateral (serosal) surface, permeable supports are, in a sense, a more natural growth environment than impermeable tissue culture plastic or glass. Indeed, there is some evidence that epithelial cells are more polarized in filter cultures than on solid substrata.[173] Furthermore, the use of filters for the culture of epithelial cells permits investigators simultaneous and independent access to the apical and basolateral plasmalemma surfaces.[174–176] This useful capacity has been extensively exploited in the experiments described in the protein sorting section of this chapter.

In addition to permeable supports, a number of investigators also culture renal and other epithelial cell lines embedded in a gel of collagen type I or other

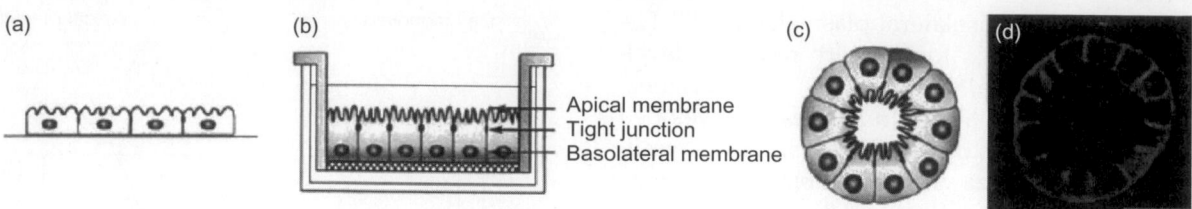

FIGURE 1.5   Two- and three-dimensional cultures of polarized epithelial cells. Epithelial cell lines may be grown on conventional impermeable substrata such as plastic or glass (a), or on permeable supports (b). In both cases, the provision of a flat, two-dimensional surface may provide spatial signals that normally would be generated by the cells themselves *in vivo*. In this regard, three-dimensional culture of cells in collagen gels, where a polarized cyst develops over 7 to 10 days (c), may more accurately represent the *in vivo* environment. In (d), an MDCK cell cyst is fluorescently labeled with antibodies to β-catenin to highlight the basolateral surface. *Reprinted with permission from ref. [178].*)

extracellular matrix molecules (Figure 1.5). These are called three-dimensional (3D) cultures, to distinguish them from more common two-dimensional (2D) cultures on either solid or permeable surfaces.[177,178] As with permeable supports, the idea behind 3D cultures is that placing the epithelial cell in an environment in which it is surrounded by extracellular matrix similar to that of the interstitium more closely resembles the *in vivo* environment. While that conclusion is subject to debate, there is no doubt that certain epithelial phenotypes are more readily expressed in 3D than in 2D cultures.[177,178] Nevertheless, these phenotypes are often slow to develop, frequently taking 7–10 days, and may occur asynchronously; this, and the inaccessibility of the cultures, somewhat limits their usefulness for biochemical studies. With the advent of high resolution confocal fluorescence microscopy and the wide array of fluorescent proteins and probes, the impact of this limitation is lessened. In the case of MDCK cells, individual suspended cells develop into polarized cysts or, when stimulated with certain growth factors, tubules. As will be described below, use of 3D cultures has led to important fundamental observations about epithelial cell polarization.[177,178] As a final note on the experimental use of 2D and 3D culture modalities, it is important to point out that formation of polarized cysts in 3D may be most closely analogous to the formation of the primordial kidney epithelium from condensed metanephric mesenchyme during development. In contrast, *in vitro* polarization of kidney epithelial cells in 2D cultures is more akin to the repair of existing kidney tubular epithelia following injury, a scenario that requires the spreading, migration, and proliferation of cells on a pre-existing surface to re-establish a contiguous epithelium.

Polarization Mechanisms: Spatial Cues from Cell Adhesion

It is now understood that not only epithelial cells but, indeed, all cell types are capable of polarizing in response to signals from the environment.[3,4,154,157,179,180]

Migrating cells of all types, for example, are polarized in the direction of migration in response to chemotactic or haptotactic gradients and even dividing cells can polarize through unequal division of their cytoplasm upon cytokinesis.[157,181] Epithelial cells are unique, in that their polar organization is stable over time and the apical—basal axis of polarity exhibited by each cell in the epithelium is parallel to the axes of its neighbors. These features permit epithelial cells to form an asymmetrically organized, semipermeable surface that defines the borders of tissues in complex organisms, and separates the inside of the body from the outside environment, while helping to create and maintain distinctly different milieus on each side.[182] The mechanism of epithelial cell polarization depends on specific spatial cues that cause the assembly and asymmetric reorganization of the intrinsic polarization machinery. The spatial cues are adhesive interactions between neighboring cells and the extracellular matrix, while the intrinsic machinery consists of primarily three polarity complexes called Par, Scribble, and Crumbs.[157,182] If the pattern of cell adhesion is asymmetric, then the response of the cell is asymmetric, and a polar phenotype results (Figure 1.6). This section will describe the specific nature of the cell—cell and cell—extracellular matrix adhesive interactions. The mechanisms by which adhesion is translated by the intrinsic polarization machinery into a polarized epithelial cell with distinct apical and basolateral plasma membrane domains will be presented in subsequent sections.

As mentioned previously, polarization of kidney epithelial cells occurs during initial differentiation of the primordial tubular epithelium from condensed mesenchyme, and after disruption of an existing mature epithelium following injury. These two situations are somewhat mimicked *in vitro* by, respectively, 3D culture and 2D culture of renal epithelial cell lines. It is important to recognize that the pattern of spatial cues provided by adhesive interactions is different in these two situations. In the developing kidney epithelium, cell—cell interactions in the condensed

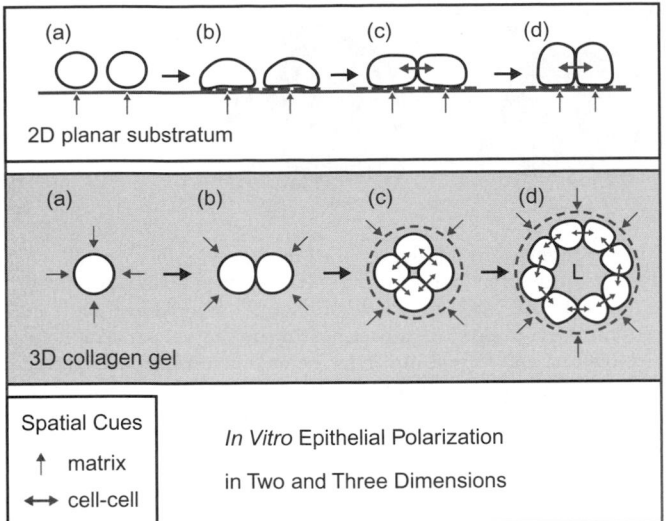

FIGURE 1.6 Geometry of spatial cues in two-dimensional and three-dimensional culture of epithelial cells. In two-dimensional culture (top) an asymmetric spatial cue is given by substratum adhesion as soon as contact occurs between the cell and the culture surface. A second spatial cue orthogonal to the first occurs when cell—cell contacts are initiated. In three-dimensional culture (bottom), the initial spatial cue impinging on single cells suspended in the collagen gel is isotropic. As soon as cell division takes place, an asymmetry is set up in which both the spatial cue from the collagen (and other secreted extracellular matrix proteins) and from cell—cell adhesion are asymmetric. The combination of asymmetric cues is required for full apical—basal polarization of epithelial cells.

mesenchyme are believed to precede meaningful cell matrix interactions[154] (Figure 1.7). These condensates are spatially differentiated: cells at the peripheries of the condensates have both a "free" plasma membrane domain facing the outside of the condensates and the undifferentiated mesenchyme, and an "attached" plasma membrane domain in contact with other cells of the condensate. Following this rudimentary polarization, the adherent mesenchymal cells in the condensate become more polarized, eventually forming a lumen and reorganizing into a simple epithelium attached to a basement membrane.[154,183] Similarly, in 3D collagen gel cultures of MDCK cells, individual cells are initially suspended in the gel. Spatial cues from collagen adhesion at this point are isotrophic rather than asymmetric, in that any signals impinging on the cell are unbiased with regard to direction (Figure 1.6). As soon as that cell divides, an asymmetric spatial cue is elicited from the resulting cell—cell adhesion, because the cells remain attached. This situation persists through subsequent divisions until at some point a basement membrane is formed, and the individual cells create a lumen.[178] In contrast, in a wounded epithelium and in 2D culture of epithelial cell lines, the persistent spatial cue from the extracellular matrix substratum is asymmetric, and then an

additional although qualitatively different asymmetric spatial cue develops as cell—cell adhesion is restored[139,157] (Figure 1.6). The take-home message from this discussion is that epithelial cells utilize both cell—cell and cell—extracellular matrix interactions as asymmetric spatial cues to polarize. The order in which these cues are provided to the cell may yield qualitatively different results but, in the end, both are required for full apical—basal polarization.

The hierachical relationship between cell—cell and cell—substratum interactions in epithelial cell polarization is illustrated best by a description of early experiments utilizing the MDCK cell line. MDCK cells cultured in suspension as individual cells lack polarized plasma membrane domains.[118,184] Upon attachment to a substratum in 2D culture, apical proteins are restricted to the free or apical surface, while basolateral proteins are distributed over the entire plasma membrane. This situation persists as the cell density increases and initial cell—cell contacts form until, as the cells reach confluency to form a true epithelium, basolateral proteins also become completely polarized.[118,185]

The relative roles of cell—cell and cell—substratum interactions can also be dissected by culturing MDCK cells in medium containing reduced amounts of calcium.[120,186,187] If cells are cultured on collagen-coated surfaces in medium with less than 5 μM calcium, they attach to the substratum but formation of cell—cell contacts mediated by the calcium-dependent adhesion protein E-cadherin is inhibited.[120,186,187] Cells assume a rounded morphology with no appreciable lateral membrane. In this situation, an immature apical surface forms. Microvilli are decreased in number, and expression of apical proteins on the cell surface, although reduced in quantity, remains polarized to the free surface.[186] Basolateral proteins, in contrast, are not polarized in cells cultured in medium containing low calcium concentrations. However, when the calcium concentration is raised to normal values (1.8 mM), then cell—cell contacts rapidly form and basolateral proteins polarize.[186]

The culturing of MDCK cells as multicellular aggregates in suspension also permits the relative effects of cell—cell and cell—substratum interactions to be independently evaluated. Under these conditions, which are different from the 3D culture described previously because the cells are surrounded only by culture medium, aggregated cells gradually form cysts with small central lumina.[184] In the absence of recognizable cell—substratum contact, both apical and basolateral polarization occurs, with the apical surface facing the outside of the cell aggregate. At this time, the tight junctional protein ZO-1 is found distributed over the entire lateral membrane, where cell—cell contacts occur. As the lumen forms, the cells secrete and deposit type IV collagen and laminin into the lumen.[184] Interaction with

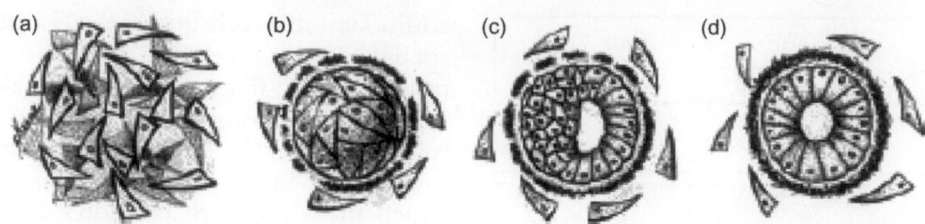

FIGURE 1.7 **Development of the kidney epithelium from induced mesenchyme.** The kidney epithelium develops *in vivo* following induction of the metanephric mesenchyme by the ureteric bud. The initial stages of differentiation from mesenchymal to epithelial cells may also be followed *in vitro* by organ culture. In this schematic view, induced mesenchymal cells are initially randomly oriented and show little cell—cell adhesion (a); Some mesenchymal cells adhere closely to each other and begin to produce a basement membrane at the periphery of the condensate (b); The cells of the condensate begin to reorganize into an epithelium and form a lumen as the basement membrane becomes more extensive (c); Finally, formation of the pretubular renal vesicle consisting of a polarized epithelium is complete, (d). *Redrawn with permission from ref. [154].*

this interior extracellular matrix then triggers redistribution of ZO-1 to the point of intersection between the apical and lateral membrane.[184] Thus, as in the reduced calcium experiments, cell—cell and cell—substratum interactions have somewhat independent but complementary effects on cell polarization.

The adherens junction provides the spatial cue from cell—cell interactions leading to polarization of epithelial cells. One of the most important components of the adherens junction is E-cadherin, the calcium-dependent homophilic cell adhesion molecule discussed previously. Suppression of E-cadherin expression by small-interfering RNAs prevents polarization, clearly implicating it in the polarization process.[188] However, other cell—cell adhesion proteins such as nectins and JAMs may be important as well. Nectins are transmembrane adhesion molecules containing immunoglobulin-like extracellular domains.[189] When epithelial cells transition from a migratory phenotype, as they exhibit during wound healing, nectins may be one of the earliest molecules in nascent cell—cell adhesions. Homophylic interaction of nectins between neighboring cells activates a variety of signaling pathways, among which are those involving the small GTPases Cdc42 and Rac1.[189,190] This, in turn, leads to reorganization of the cortical actin cytoskeleton and, consequently, facilitates the formation and stabilization of E-cadherin-mediated contacts, creating the mature adherens junction.[189] During this process, both nectins and JAMs may initiate the asymmetric activation of the intrinsic polarization machinery. Nectins and JAMs bind Par3, an element of the Par polarization complex (see below).[189,191,192] As the adherens junction matures, other polarization complexes bind and specification of the apical and basolateral plasma membrane domains occurs, with the dividing line located just at the adherens and tight junctions, collectively referred to as the apical junctional complex. At the same time, a complex of proteins known as the exocyst is also assembled at this location.[157,191,192] The exocyst is a kind of tethering

complex designed to capture transport vesicles carrying newly synthesized membrane proteins. Delivery of these proteins to this region of the plasma membrane then facilitates the development of the apical and basolateral surfaces.[193,194]

It is likely that the spatial cue emanating from cell—substratum adhesive interactions originates from integrin-mediated cell interactions with the basement membrane protein laminin. In the developing kidney, conversion of condensed mesenchyme into a polarized epithelium is dependent on laminin.[154,195,196] The laminin α1-subunit and integrin α6β1, a laminin receptor, are first detected in the induced mesenchyme following condensation.[129,154,195,196] Laminin localizes to the periphery of the condensate, suggesting that the crude polarization caused by condensation leads to polarized laminin secretion to the periphery. In organ culture antibodies against laminin α1 or the integrin α6-subunit block formation of a polarized epithelium from condensed mesenchyme, suggesting that their involvement in epithelial differentiation is critical.[154,196,197]

Results from a variety of other experimental systems generally support the conclusion that laminins and their integrin receptors play a role in epithelial polarization. Mutations in either integrin or laminin subunits lead to disruption of epithelial differentiation and polarization in the nematode *Caenorhabditis elegans*, and the fruit fly *Drosophila melanogaster*.[132] Expression of laminin in the early mouse embyro generally coincides with development of epithelial tissues. In embryoid bodies derived from cultures of aggregated embryonic stem (ES) cells, an LM-111 containing basement membrane forms between the endoderm and the polarizing inner cell mass cells. When ES cells deleted of both laminin γ1 alleles are aggregated into embryoid bodies, the inner cell mass forms, but does not polarize.[132] Laminin has also been implicated in the polarization of MDCK cells. When MDCK cells are cultured in 3D collagen gels for 7—10 days, they form polarized cysts with the apical surface facing the lumen, and the basal surface facing the extracellular matrix. Under these conditions, the cells secrete LM-511 and form a discrete layer closely associated with the basal surface, resembling an assembled basement membrane.[198,199] When MDCK cells are treated either with a function-blocking anti-β1 integrin antibody or express dominant-negative Rac1 during cyst formation, the laminin layer does not form properly, although laminin is secreted, and the cells display an inverted and somewhat disorganized polarity with apical antigens expressed on surfaces facing the extracellular matrix.[198,199] Addition of excess exogenous LM-111 to the collagen gel partially rescues both basement membrane assembly and correct polarization in cells expressing dominant-negative Rac1, possibly by driving laminin assembly adjacent to the basal plasma membrane.[198,199] Inverted polarization of the cyst caused by anti-β1 integrin can also be rescued by expression of constitutively-active Rac1.[198,199] These experiments suggest that a "serpentine" signaling pathway exists, leading from ligation of a β1 integrin outside the cell, to Rac1 activation inside the cell, to laminin assembly outside the cell, and finally to polarization. It is important to emphasize that the perturbations that lead to inverted polarity do not seem to affect the segregation of apical and basolateral proteins in individual cells, but instead affect the orientation of apical–basal axes in the cyst. It is unclear how intracellular signaling events can cause laminin assembly. Recent findings have implicated the polarization signaling molecule Par1b and dystroglycan, a non-integrin laminin receptor, in effecting laminin assembly, but the mechanisms are not apparent.[200,201]

Polarization Mechanisms: The Intrinsic Polarization Machinery

In epithelial cells, the intrinsic polarization machinery has traditionally been separated into three so-called polarity protein complexes that function collectively to control the formation of apical and basolateral domains of the plasma membrane.[191,192] Many of the components of the polarity complexes were initially identified in mutant screens in *Caenorhabditis elegans* and *Drosophila melanogaster*, but homologs that function in an essentially identical manner have also been identified in mammals. The first, and perhaps most important, polarity complex generally associated with apical surface determination is the Par complex composed of Par3, Par6, atypical protein kinase C (aPKC), and the small-GTPase Cdc42 (Figure 1.8). A second apical complex is the Crumbs complex, containing in mammals the transmembrane protein Crumbs (Crb3 in the kidney) associated with Lin-7 (PALS1), and PALS1-associated tight junction protein (PATJ). The final complex, which is located on the lateral surface in polarized

epithelia, is the Scribble complex composed of Scribble (SCRIB), discs large (Dlg), and lethal giant larvae (Lgl).[191,192] In the case of the Par and Crumbs complex, physical interactions between the components have been demonstrated, while interactions of Scribble complex components have been implied by genetic experiments. In addition to these polarity complexes, other proteins are involved in regulating apical–basal polarization in mammals or lower organisms including, in particular, Par1b and LKB1 (Par4). In the core polarity protein complexes, only aPKC and Cdc42 have enzymatic activities: the former a serine/threonine kinase; and the latter a GTPase-mediated molecular switch, while the others are largely scaffolds with a myriad of binding domains, including on many PDZ domains, that facilitate association with the apical junctional complex of the polarized cell.[191,192]

The mechanisms by which these complexes function to help establish and maintain apical–basal polarity is often described as a process of mutual antagonism or inhibition that creates and maintains a particular balance between the amounts of distinct apical and basolateral plasma membranes, with the "front line" of this battle being the apical junctional complex[191,192] (Figure 1.8). While the concept of mutual antagonism is not inaccurate, how this translates into intuitively comprehensible mechanisms has, until recently, not been obvious. Studies in *Drosophila* have highlighted the critical role of Par3 (Bazooka or Baz in *Drosophila*) and have, to some extent, called into question the idea of distinct, somewhat independently functioning polarization protein complexes.[191] A compelling model proposes that initiation of polarization commences when Par3 (Baz) associates with the region of cell–cell adhesion that will become the adherens junction, prior to the concentration of DE-cadherin (the *Drosophila* version of E-cadherin) in that location. Association is facilitated by phosphoinositides. Once the adherens junction forms, then Par3 binds Par6 and aPKC, and Cdc42 is activated. Activation of aPKC then leads to phosphorylation of Par3, as well as Crb and Lgl, following the delivery of Crb to the plasma membrane through vesicles. The phosphorylation of Par3 on serine 980 by aPKC weakens the interaction between Par3 and aPKC, as well as the interaction between Par3 and the Crb complex protein PALS1 (Lin-7, Stardust or Sdt in *Drosophila*). These changes permit formation of the apical complex Crb–PALS1–PATJ, while interactions between Crb and Par6 prevent association of Par3 with the forming apical surface. At the same time, Par1-mediated phosphorylation of Par3 creates binding sites for the scaffold 14-3-3, and the subsequent Par3-14-3-3 interaction further inhibits the association of Par3 with Par6/aPKC. Since Par1 is localized to the lateral surface, this prevents Par3 from assembling on the lateral surface.

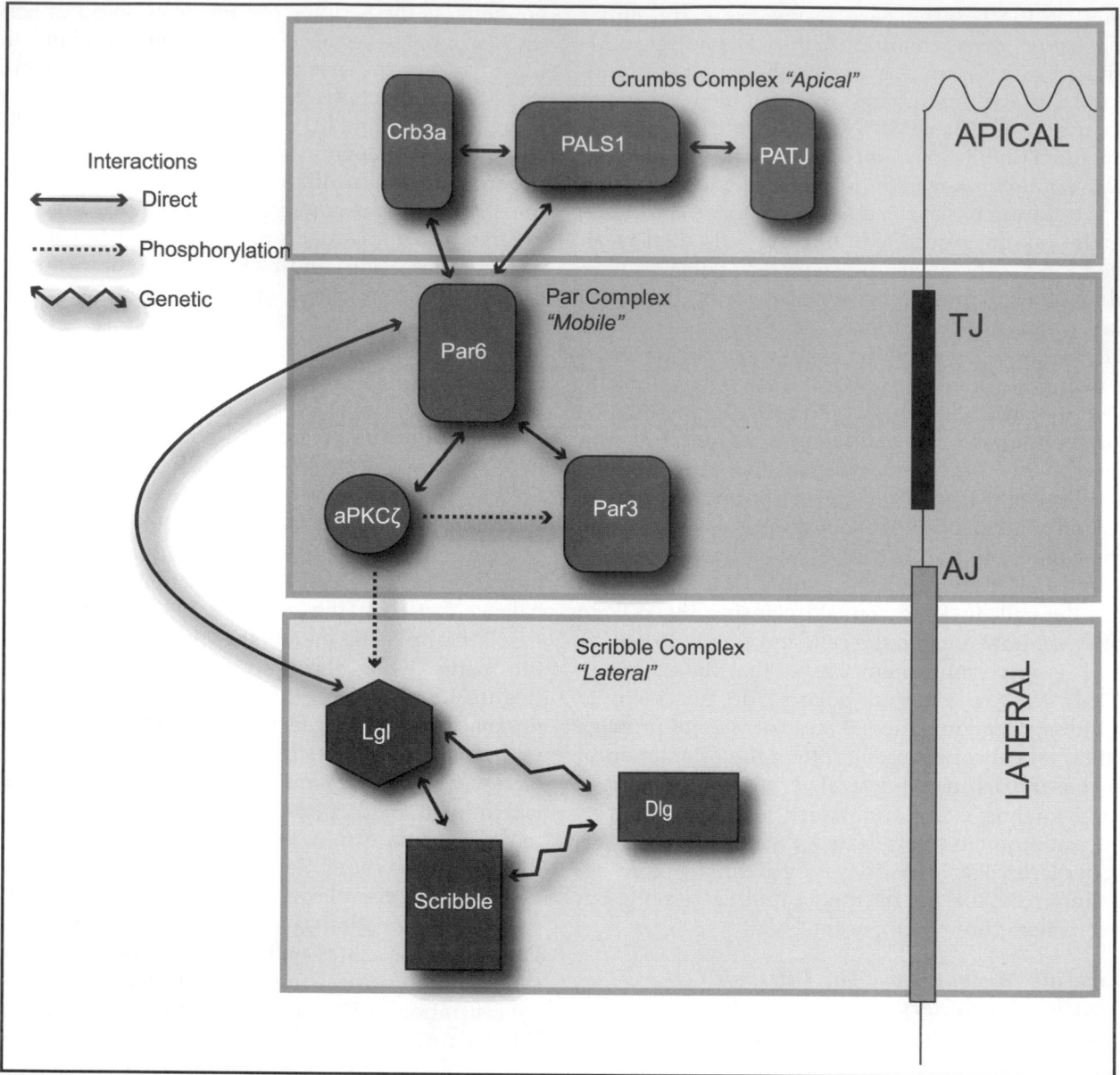

FIGURE 1.8 **Distribution of polarity complexes in polarized epithelial cells.** Solid lines indicate demonstrated physical interactions between components, while jagged lines indicate genetic interactions established from studies of invertebrate epithelial cells. *(Reprinted with permission from Laprise, J. and Margolis, B. (2011). AJP Renal Physiology 300, F589—F601.)*

Lgl is also phosphorylated by aPKC, which prevents its apical localization.[191] With Dlg and Scrib, it then contributes to maintaining the identity of the lateral membrane in a manner that is poorly understood.

In all likelihood this scenario, derived primarily from experiments on *Drosophila*, is also valid in renal epithelial cells. Studies in MDCK cells, in particular, have illuminated a number of steps and, in some instances, provided additional critical details. As mentioned previously, nascent cell—cell contacts may be initiated by nectins and JAMs prior to the coalescence, stabilization, and assembly of the adherens junction nucleated by E-cadherin and its associated proteins.[189,191,192] Nectins and JAM, which bind Par3, may serve to localize Par3 to the forming junction. In addition to its roles in facilitating the assembly of the other polarization complexes as described earlier, Par3 binds phosphoinositides in the membrane, as well as the phosphoinositide phosphatase PTEN (phosphatase and tensin homolog).[191,192] This phosphatase converts phosphatidylinositol $(3,4,5)P_3$ (PIP3) on the inner leaflet of the membrane to phosphatidylinositol $(4,5)P_2$ (PIP2). The latter lipid then facilitates the development of the apical surface by binding annexin2, which then recruits Cdc42, leading to the cascade of events involving aPKC described earlier.[202] The importance of the conversion of PIP3 to PIP2 in the formation of the apical surface was highlighted dramatically when exogenous PIP2 was added to the basolateral pole of mature MDCK cell cysts in 3D culture.[202] Incorporation of PIP2 into the basolateral plasma membrane led to gradual extension of the apical surface to the basal pole with collapse of the lumen.

The description of the polarization process so far has focused only on events initiated by cell—cell adhesion. However, as was described in the previous section, adhesion of epithelial cells to the basement membrane is also a key part of polarization, functioning particularly to orient the apical—basal axis in a coordinated fashion in neighboring cells. How basement membrane adhesion and, particularly, adhesion to laminin does this is not clear, but it likely involves the microtubule cytoskeleton (Figure 1.2). In individual MDCK cells adherent to a substratum in 2D culture, the organization of microtubules resembles that in other nonepithelial adherent cells, in that microtubule growth is initiated from a juxtanuclear centrosome or microtubular organizing center, and extends radially towards the cell surface.[203–205] Once cell—cell adhesion is initiated, the microtubule organizing activity begins to disperse to the cell periphery and, as the cell polarizes, it relocalizes diffusely to the apical surface.[203–205] In response to this, microtubules reassemble along the apical—basal axis with the plus (growing) ends pointing basally. Networks of microtubules also form roughly parallel to the basal and apical surfaces[203–205] (Figure 1.2). Reorganization of the microtubules depends on a family of GTPases known as septins, which provide directionality to the process,[206,207] while stabilization and anchoring depend on the plekstrin homology-like domain family A protein LL5, microtubule plus-end tracking proteins, and the APC (adenomatous polyposis coli) tumor suppressor.[208–211] LL5 anchors microtubule plus ends to the basal plasma membrane by associating with integrin-mediated cell adhesions to laminin.[208] Furthermore, the polarity protein Par1b, which has been implicated in assembly of the laminin network in the basement membrane, is also important in the formation of the apical surface in 3D cysts, reportedly through a mechanism that depends on signaling from the extracellular matrix.[212] Thus, there appears to be a signaling network linking laminin assembly and microtubule reorganization to formation of the apical surface in the correct location. How these microtubules mechanistically contribute to polarization is not clear, but it is known that they provide tracks for vesicle transport that are necessary for formation of the apical lumen through its population with specific proteins, a process facilitated by septins.[121,122,125]

Ultimately, cooperation of extrinsic spatial cues and the intrinsic polarization machinery creates a polarized cellular infrastructure composed of adhesive interactions, a spatially-differentiated cytoskeleton, and asymmetrically disposed signaling complexes. Completion of polarization, and its maintenance during cell and tissue function, then depends on the targeting of specific membrane proteins to the apical and basolateral plasma membrane domains. How this is accomplished is the subject of the following section.

Sorting Pathways

One of the first, and perhaps most easily addressed, questions presented by the phenomenon of epithelial polarity relates to where, within the cell, sorting occurs. The membrane proteins that populate the apical and basolateral plasmalemmal domains are all synthesized in association with the membranous elements of the rough endoplasmic reticulum (RER).[213] It has further been shown that after their co-translational insertion into the membranes of the RER, apically- and basolaterally-directed proteins share the same cisternae of the Golgi complex as they transit the secretory pathway en route to their respective sites of ultimate functional residence.[214,215] Immunoelectron microscopic studies performed on MDCK cells doubly infected with the VSV and influenza viruses revealed, through double labeling, that the influenza HA protein and the VSV G protein could be co-localized throughout the cisternae of the Golgi complex.[215]

This observation was confirmed and extended through a series of elegant biochemical studies. It had previously been shown that when cells are incubated at 20°C newly synthesized membrane proteins accumulate in the trans-most cisterna of the Golgi complex.[216,217] Elevating the temperature to 37°C relieves this block, and allows the proteins to proceed to the cell surface.[218] By examining the nature of the complex N-linked glycosylation associated with the VSV G protein, it was demonstrated that sialic acid residues are added in the 20°C compartment.[214] These investigators took advantage of the fact that in addition to the HA protein the membrane of the influenza virus contains a neuraminidase in their efforts to determine whether segregation of the apically directed influenza proteins from the basolaterally targeted VSV G protein occurs before or after the 20°C block compartment. They found that in singly infected cells incubated at 20°C, the VSV G protein became heavily sialylated. In contrast to this, when cells which had been doubly infected with both the VSV and influenza viruses were incubated at 20°C, little if any sialic acid could be detected on the newly synthesized VSV G protein.

These results demonstrate that as late as the 20°C block compartment, which corresponds to the trans-most cisterna of the Golgi complex, the newly synthesized apical neuraminidase and basolateral VSV G protein are still intermingled and capable of physical interaction. The segregation of these two classes of proteins from one another must, therefore, occur at or after this subcellular locus. It is interesting to note that immunoelectron microscopic studies of endocrine cells reveal that proteins destined for packaging in secretory granules are separated from those bound for constitutive delivery to the cell surface in the trans-most cisterna of the Golgi complex.[219–221] Observations such as these have prompted investigators to speculate that this compartment, which is referred to as the Trans Golgi Network (TGN), might be the site of several intracellular sorting events.[222] More recently, it has been shown that sorting may occur as well at the level of the recycling endosome. Loading endosomes with HRP-conjugated transferrin, and subsequently disrupting endosome function through the deposition of peroxidase reaction product, prevents the surface delivery of a subset of newly synthesized basolateral membrane proteins.[223] While the delivery of the VSV G protein to basolateral plasma membrane is prevented by this ablation of the recycling endosome, the delivery of the newly synthesized Na^+/K^+-ATPase to the basolateral surface is unaffected by this maneuver.[224] Thus, it would appear that proteins can pursue more than one route from the TGN to the basolateral membrane domain.

Three epithelial sorting pathways can be imagined (Figure 1.9).[1,2,158] In the direct model, sorting would take place prior to cell surface delivery. Segregation of basolateral from apical proteins would be completed intracellularly, and proteins would never appear, even transiently, in the inappropriate membrane domain. The random sorting scheme dictates that no separation of apical from basolateral proteins occurs prior to arrival at the cell surface. Following their insertion into the plasmalemma, proteins that find themselves in the wrong surface domain would be removed by endocytosis, and either transcytosed to the proper surface[225] or degraded. Finally, the indirect paradigm predicts that all newly synthesized plasmalemmal proteins initially appear together, either at the apical or basolateral membrane. The proteins for which this delivery is correct would be retained in that membrane domain, while those which had been mis-delivered would be internalized and transcytosed to their sites of ultimate functional residence.

These three models, although perhaps somewhat simplistic, are valuable for the relative ease with which they can be experimentally distinguished. Over the past two decades a great deal of effort has been invested in identifying which of these routes is, in fact,

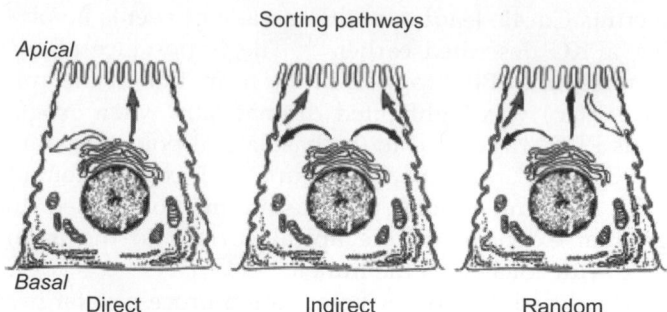

FIGURE 1.9 Three potential pathways for the sorting of membrane proteins in polarized epithelial cells. In the vectorial sorting scheme, apical and basolateral membrane proteins are separated from one another intracellularly and prior to plasmalemmal delivery (left). The indirect, or obligate, misdelivery model predicts that all newly synthesized plasma membrane proteins are carried together to a common cell surface domain. Proteins destined for the opposite surface are then internalized and transported to their appropriate destinations (middle). Finally, random sorting is defined by a complete lack of intracellular segregation. Apical and basolateral proteins are delivered without preference to both surfaces, and are subsequently redistributed by endocytosis and transcellular transport (right). Clear arrows represent vesicles carrying only basolateral proteins; hatched arrows denote vesicles carrying only apical proteins; and black arrows indicate vesicles carrying intermixed apical and basolateral membrane proteins. *Reprinted with permission from ref. [1].*

operational. The rather surprising answer appears to indicate that the sorting pathway pursued varies among different cell types, and even among different proteins within the same cell type.

Technical Approaches

Much of the early research into the nature of epithelial sorting pathways was carried out on MDCK cells that had been infected with the VSV or influenza viruses. The infected cells produced massive quantities of viral proteins, and retained their polarized distribution throughout at least the initial stages of the infection. These properties greatly facilitated the detection of cohorts of newly synthesized membrane proteins in the pulse chase protocols generally employed to monitor the polarity of cell surface delivery. Pulse labeling experiments demonstrated that the VSV G protein was not accessible to apically added antibodies at any point during its post-synthetic processing.[226] In the case of the influenza HA protein, the converse was true. Proteases[174] or antibody probes[227] added to the media compartment bathing the basolateral surfaces of MDCK cells grown on filters could not cleave or interact with this polypeptide during its journey to the apical cell surface. From these results, it was concluded that the direct model of sorting applied for at least these two proteins in MDCK cells.

Other labeling tools have also been brought to bear on the study of sorting pathways. The N-hydroxysuccinimidyl (NHS) derivative of biotin is a membrane impermeant molecule that will covalently combine with the ε-amino groups of exposed lysine residues.[228] Proteins thus modified are substrates for precipitation or detection with avidin-conjugated secondary reagents. These tools can be used to follow the fate of large numbers of membrane proteins that have been exposed at one or other cell surface to the NHS biotin compound. Using such a protocol, it has been demonstrated that several MDCK cell apical and basolateral membrane proteins are directly targeted to their appropriate membrane domains.[229,230]

Advances in the development of genetically encodable probes have also permitted sorting pathways to be visualized directly. By creating chimeras that incorporate photoactivatable versions of the green fluorescent protein (GFP), the trafficking of newly synthesized proteins of interest can be observed in intact cells in real-time.[231] Alternatively, the SNAP tag similarly permits newly synthesized cohorts of proteins to be observed in pulse chase protocols. The 20 kDa SNAP-Tag is a modified version of the DNA repair protein 0^6-alkylguanine-DNA alkyltransferase, which cleaves para-substituted benzyl guanines (BGs) by covalently transferring the substituted benzyl group to its active thiol.[232] The resulting thioether bond irreversibly prevents the reacted SNAP-Tag from participating in any further labeling reactions. Fluorescent BG derivatives allow for the labeling and detection of SNAP-Tagged fusion proteins in either live or fixed cells.[232,233] Through the combination of a "prepulse" blocking step with non-fluorescent BG, followed by selective labeling of newly synthesized protein with fluorescent BG, it is possible to follow a cohort of protein as it is synthesized and trafficked.[224]

Sodium Pump Targeting

Further support for the direct pathway paradigm in MDCK cells came from studies on the sorting of the endogenous Na^+/K^+-ATPase.[175] Filter grown MDCK cells which had been pulse-labeled with [35S]-methionine were exposed to the N-azidobenzoyl (NAB) derivative of ouabain at either their apical or basolateral surfaces during the course of a 90 minute chase. NAB-ouabain will bind to catalytically active sodium pumps with high affinity and, following UV photolysis, will become covalently incorporated into the protein backbone of the Na^+/K^+-ATPase α-subunit.[234–236] By analyzing immunoprecipitates prepared from these cells using an anti-ouabain antibody, it was possible to demonstrate that no sodium pump in a state competent to bind ouabain ever appears at the apical surface. Subsequent studies using a SNAP-tagged version of the Na^+/K^+-ATPase expressed in the same MDCK cell line recapitulated the finding that the newly synthesized pump traffics directly to the basolateral surface in these cells.[224]

Another investigation of sodium pump sorting in a different clonal line of MDCK cells made use of the NHS biotin surface-labeling technique, and arrived at a conclusion diametrically opposed to the one described above. The results of this study indicated that the Na^+/K^+-ATPase is randomly delivered to the apical and basolateral plasmalemmal surfaces.[237] The authors further suggested that stabilizing interactions with cytoskeletal elements which underly the basolateral, but not the apical, cell surface[112,114,119] result in a much longer residence time for pump inserted into the basolateral domain. These studies are thus consistent with a model in which sodium pump is not sorted intracellularly, but instead achieves its basolateral distribution through a mechanism based on random delivery followed by differential stabilization.

The apparent discrepancy among these studies appears to be attributable to differences in the pathways and processes through which these closely related cell lines achieve the polarized distribution of the Na^+/K^+-ATPase. While one line targets the pump directly to its basolateral destination, the other delivers it randomly and depends upon cytoskeletal interactions to stabilize only the basolateral pool.[238,239] Clearly, therefore, while cytoskeletal interactions may be sufficient to localize the Na^+/K^+-ATPase to the basolateral surface, they are not the sole mechanism involved in producing the sodium pump's anisotropic distribution. Instead, they may act as a failsafe mechanism to back up and reinforce the initial biosynthetic sorting of the Na^+/K^+-ATPase, to ensure that its polarized distribution is attained and maintained.

The preceding discussion suggests that the direct scheme cannot be applied to all epithelia or even to all MDCK cell clones. An alternative system has been shown to apply to the liver, for example. Cell fractionation studies performed on liver by Bartles et al. reveal that several apical membrane proteins appear in the fraction corresponding to the hepatocyte basolateral plasma membrane prior to being delivered to the apical surface.[240] This route has been especially well-documented for the polymeric immunoglobulin receptor (pIgR) expressed by hepatocytes. This 120 kDa polypeptide serves to carry dimeric IgA from the blood to the lumena of the bile cannaliculi. During its biosynthesis, the pIgR is transported directly from the TGN to the basolateral cell surface where it is available to bind dimeric IgA.[241,242] Independent of any interaction with IgA the receptor becomes phosphorylated in the basolateral plasmalemma, and the phosphorylated form is internalized and carried by a transcytotic vesicle to the apical, or canalicular, surface.[243] Following its insertion into the apical plasma membrane the ectodomain of the pIgR is cleaved and released into the bile as an 80 kDa protein referred to as secretory component.[241,242] Association with secretory component helps to protect the bound IgA from intestinal proteases. Coupled with other results,[240] the behavior of pIgR in hepatocytes supports the contention that apical membrane proteins arrive at their site of ultimate functional residence via obligate mis-delivery to the basolateral domain. This paradigm may not apply to all apical proteins in hepatocytes. Studies of the trafficking of apical members of the multidrug resistance (MDR) family of transport proteins indicate that these polytopic membrane proteins do not make an appearance at the basolateral surface en route to the apical membrane.[244,245] Thus, within a single polarized cell type multiple trafficking routes can be employed to target different proteins to the same place.

A combination of the direct and indirect paradigms seems to be involved in membrane protein delivery in cultured intestinal cells. The Caco-2 line of human colon carcinoma cells can be grown on filters and subjected to the NHS-biotin labeling protocol described above. Such experiments reveal that the basolateral protein followed is vectorially targeted.[246] Analysis of the apical polypeptides produced a somewhat more complicated picture. A fraction of these proteins appeared to transit through the basolateral plasmalemma prior to their apical delivery. The remainder of the apical proteins studied in this sampling were sorted intracellularly and inserted directly at the apical domain. Related and somewhat more complicated results have been gathered from studies on the biogenesis of brush border hydrolases by colonocytes *in situ*.[110,247,248]

To complete this already confusing picture it is necessary to return to a discussion of targeting studies in MDCK cells. A cDNA encoding the pIgR has been expressed by transfection in this cell line. Remarkably, the sorting pathway pursued by this protein in the cultured renal epithelium is apparently identical to the rather baroque scheme that characterizes its route in hepatocytes.[249] From the TGN, the pIgR travels to the basolateral surface from which it is internalized and subsequently transcytosed to the apical pole or recycled to the basolateral side. These observations demonstrate that an obligate mis-delivery pathway is either created or simply revealed in MDCK cells expressing the pIgR. Results from studies employing real-time imaging to follow the surface delivery of a class of newly synthesized apical proteins support the possibility that this indirect pathway does, in fact, exist constitutively in MDCK cells. As discussed in greater detail in the section on sorting signals, proteins whose attachments to the membrane are mediated by covalent linkage to glycosylphosphotidyl inositol (GPI)

lipids tend to accumulate in the apical domains of most varieties of polarized epithelial cells. A study that employed live cell imaging to track the sorting of GPI-linked proteins found that these proteins were delivered to the basolateral surface, after which they were endocytosed and carried to the apical plasmalemma.[250] It is worth noting, however, that subsequent studies found that several GPI-linked proteins were delivered directly to the apical membrane in MDCK cells, without making any detectable transient appearance at the basolateral surface.[251]

This apparent diversity of sorting pathways is perhaps not as surprising as it first appears. The relative flow of membranous vesicles from the Golgi complex to the two plasmalemmal surfaces in different epithelial cell types is likely to reflect a cell's biologic mission, as well as the nature of the environment in which it functions. It appears, for example, that although hepatocytes produce copious quantities of secretory proteins, none are released directly into the bile.[252] It has been proposed that newly synthesized membrane proteins depart the Golgi in the same transport vesicles that carry proteins destined for constitutive secretion.[158,252] Were this the case, then cells which do not produce a secretory content targeted for one or another membrane domain may also lack a direct traffic of membrane vesicles directed from the Golgi to that domain. The full complement of plasmalemmal proteins might thus be forced by default to share the same carrier out of the Golgi, and to be sorted by transcytosis subsequent to cell surface delivery. Some hepatic apical membrane proteins may transit through the basolateral surface, because there is very little non-stop cargo traveling from the TGN to the apical domain in this particular cell type. The apparent multiplicity of sorting pathways available to different proteins within the same cell type may reflect specializations relevant to these proteins' functions. Diversity may also arise from the nature of the signals and mechanisms that mediate these proteins' polarized distribution. The potential contribution of this latter influence will be referred to again in sections to follow. The lack of a single answer or unifying solution to the problem of sorting pathways is a theme that carries through the entire study of epithelial polarity. A number of equally effective mechanisms appear to have evolved for segregating membrane proteins into distinct domains. It remains to be determined how these differing approaches benefit their respective tissues and contribute to the maintenance of their unique functions.

Regulation of Renal Transport Protein Function by Endocytosis and Recycling

The delivery of a protein to its site of functional residence in a domain of the plasma membrane does not end that protein's involvement with the cellular sorting machinery. Cell surface proteins are subject to endocytic internalization, after which their fate is determined through processes that are mechanistically closely related to those that mediate biosynthetic sorting. Following their delivery to endosomes, endocytically internalized proteins can be recycled, meaning that they are returned to the same domain of the plasma membrane. Alternatively, they can be carried by transcytosis to the opposite plasma membrane domain. Finally, they can be targeted for degradation in the lysosome. The cellular machinery and molecular signals that govern these post-endocytic sorting processes appear to closely resemble those that mediate biosynthetic sorting.

From the perspective of the renal tubular epithelial cell, perhaps the most important implication of post-endocytic sorting relates to its role in the regulation of ion transport protein activity. The activities of a number of critically important transport proteins are controlled by regulated membrane insertion and endocytotic events.[253] Included on this list are the aquaporin 2 water channel (AQP2),[254] the ROMK potassium channel,[255] and the ENaC sodium channel of collecting duct principal cells[256]; the V-type proton ATPase of collecting duct intercalated cells[257]; the Na,Cl co-transporter (NCC) of the distal convoluted tubule[258]; the Na phosphate co-transporter (NaPi),[100] the Na proton exchanger (NHE3),[259] and the Na^+/K^+-ATPase of the proximal convoluted tubule.[260] These regulated trafficking events are precipitated by a variety of hormonal and physical stimuli, and involve the participation of a diverse collection of signaling cascades and trafficking proteins. While their details will be explored in far greater individual detail in the chapters that relate to each of the specific tubule segments and relevant transport systems, it is worth noting that these regulated trafficking processes exploit many of the biosynthetic sorting signals and components of the cellular trafficking machinery that are discussed in the following sections.

Sorting Signals

Rodriguez-Boulan and Sabatini's 1978 observation that viral spike glycoproteins are targeted to opposite domains of polarized epithelial cells[165,166] gave rise to the hypothesis that sorting signals — that is, the information required to direct a protein or proteins to a given subcellular location — might be wholly contained within the structure of the sorted proteins themselves. Evidence in favor of this contention has come from studies examining the distribution of viral membrane proteins expressed by transfection (rather than infection) in polarized cultured cells. A number of investigators have shown that the influenza HA protein, the VSV G protein, and related viral spike glycoproteins are sorted correctly in the absence of any other proteins encoded by viral genomes.[261–264] It is apparent, therefore, that all of the addressing information necessary to produce the polarized distributions of these polypeptides must be embodied within the proteins themselves. It has further been shown that this information is almost certainly associated with the protein backbone, rather than with any post-translational modification. Cells whose capacity to add asparagine-linked sugar residues has been impaired, either through mutation or via treatment with tunicamycin,[265,266] are nonetheless able to correctly target the viral spike proteins. Observations such as these have sparked an intensive search for the actual molecular information that specifies localization, and for the machinery that acts upon this information. It must be stated at the outset, however, that despite the rather confident and declarative tone of this section's heading the identification and characterization of epithelial sorting signals and mechanisms is far from complete.

Several distinct classes of signals have been found to specify basolateral sorting.[267] Perhaps the best characterized of these are short motifs that contain tyrosine residues and resemble or overlap with sequences involved in endocytosis. Work from a number of groups has suggested that sequences in the cytosolic tail of membrane proteins determine the rates at which these proteins are internalized. The presence of a tyrosine residue appears to be a critical determinant of the efficacy of an endocytosis signal.[268] The rapid endocytosis of both the LDL receptor and the transferrin receptor, for example, is dependent upon the presence of short, tyrosine-containing sequences in these proteins' cytoplasmic tails. Mutation of this tyrosine residue to any other amino acid vastly reduces the rates at which both of these proteins are internalized. The apically sorted influenza HA protein is normally endocytosed extremely slowly. Addition of a tyrosine residue to the cytosolic tail of the influenza HA protein causes it to behave like the LDL receptor or transferin receptor with respect to endocytosis — that is, it is rapidly internalized and recycled.[269] When this altered form of the HA protein is expressed in MDCK cells it is detected predominantly at the basolateral plasma membrane.[270] It would appear, therefore, that a signal that is permissive for endocytosis is also competent to mediate basolateral accumulation.

Studies of the VSV G protein reveal that its basolateral sorting is also driven by a tyrosine-containing motif.[271,272] Uptake measurements suggest, however, that the VSV G protein is internalized relatively slowly, suggesting that its tyrosine-based motif confers basolateral targeting, but not rapid endocytosis. Mutagenesis studies of the tyrosine-modified influenza HA protein, as well as several other basolateral membrane proteins, indicate that while internalization signals and basolateral sorting signals can share the same critical tyrosine residues, they are not identical.[273] Altering residues near the tyrosine can produce apically sorted influenza HA protein that is rapidly endocytosed, and basolateral HA protein that is internalized only slowly. Thus, basolateral and endocytosis signals can overlap, sharing one or more residues, but are clearly distinguishable from one another. Presumably, therefore, they must be interpreted by non-identical cellular machinery.

Data pointing to a similar conclusion have been gathered for Fc receptors.[274] One of the Fc receptor isoforms includes a di-leucine sequence in its cytoplasmic tail. This sequence has been shown to function as an endocytosis signal, and it also appears to confer basolateral targeting when the protein is expressed in polarized cells. Once again, alteration of residues flanking the di-leucine motif demonstrates that the sequence requirements for basolateral sorting are distinct from those that specify internalization.[275,276]

Tyrosine-containing basolateral sorting signals that are entirely distinct from recognizable endocytosis motifs have also been detected. The LDL receptor depends upon a basolateral sorting signal that bears no sequence resemblance to any known internalization motif.[276,277] Although this motif includes a tyrosine residue, mutation of that tyrosine to phenylalanine still permits basolateral localization. A distinct tyrosine-containing motif appears to mediate the internalization of the LDL receptor.[278] In the absence of the primary basolateral signal, this endocytosis motif can mediate a basolateral sorting function. Once again, however, with the exception of the tyrosine residue, the amino acids that contribute to the basolateral and endocytic aspects of this signal are distinct from one another.

Several basolateral sorting signals unrelated to tyrosine residues have also been reported. The well-characterized tyrosine-based endocytosis motif of the transferrin receptor is completely distinct from this protein's basolateral targeting signal, which resides in a different portion of the cytoplasmic tail. The peptide processing enzyme furin cycles between the trans-Golgi network and the basolateral plasmalemma. Its trafficking to the basolateral surface appears to be driven by residues that are associated with a casein kinase II phosphorylation site.[279,280] The invariant chain of the major histocompatibility class II complex is sorted to the basolateral membrane by virtue of the dihydrophobic sequence Met–Leu.[281] Once again, endocytic internalization of this molecule is conferred by a similar dihydrophobic sequence, Leu–Ile, which is present at another position on the cytoplasmic tail. All of the basolateral sorting motifs discussed thus far function in the context of membrane proteins that span

the bilayer once. As will be discussed below, a distinct cadre of molecular sequences appears to mediate the targeting of many ion transporters and other multi-spanning membrane proteins.

The list of identified basolateral sorting signals is considerably more extensive than the inventory of characterized apical membrane protein sorting signals. Perhaps the best studied member of this latter roster is not, in fact, a protein-based signal at all, but is instead constituted entirely of phospholipid. Glycophospholipid (or GPI)-linked proteins are synthesized as transmembrane polypeptides that are co-translationally inserted into the membrane of the RER.[282] While still associated with the ER, the GPI-linked protein's ectodomain is proteolytically removed and transferred to a preassembled structure composed of a complex glycan tethered to the membrane through its attachment to a molecule of phospholipid (frequently phosphotidylinositol). Previous work has shown that in polarized epithelial cells, most of the GPI-linked proteins reside in the apical plasmalemma.[230,283] Interestingly, the apical surface also plays host to most of the cell's complement of glycolipid.[284] Investigators prepared a construct in which the VSV G ectodomain was wedded to the transmembrane tail of Thy-1, which carries a signal for glycophospholipidation.[285] The resultant GPI-linked G protein is sorted to the apical membrane. The results of these and related experiments have generally been interpreted to indicate that a strong apical sorting signal is embodied in some component of the GPI linkage itself. The transmembrane domains of several single-spanning apical membrane proteins appear to carry information important for apical targeting. The transmembrane domains of the influenza virus neuraminidase and HA proteins, for example, are sufficient to mediate sorting to the apical surface when they are included in constructs expressed by transfection in MDCK cells.[286] As will be discussed below, the same mechanisms that are thought to be involved in recognizing the GPI tail as an apical sorting motif may also interpret signals embedded in transmembrane domains. Furthermore, transmembrane domain sorting signals may be important not only in the localization of single spanning membrane proteins, but may also determine the distributions of polytopic ion pumps such as the Na^+/K^+- and H^+/K^+-ATPases (see below). It should also be noted that the extracytoplasmic or ecto domains of several apical proteins appear to incorporate directional signals. Roth et al. have shown that the ectodomain of the influenza HA protein is sufficient to specify apical targeting.[287] When a cDNA construct encoding an anchor-minus form of the HA protein, which lacks both the cytosolic and transmembrane segments, is expressed in polarized cells it is secreted exclusively into the apical medium compartment. This is also true well for the polymeric immunoglobulin receptor.[288] These results suggest that a signal involved in apical sorting resides in the lumenal portion of the HA molecule, and that this signal remains interpretable when it is presented as a soluble protein or in association with portions of a basolateral membrane polypeptide. Finally, N-linked sugar groups, which are also present on the extracytoplasmic domains of membrane proteins, can in some circumstances contribute apical sorting information.[289] It is logical to conclude from this discussion that machinery necessary to read and interpret this putative ectodomain apical sorting information must be exposed at the lumenal surface of the organellar compartments involved in the segregation and targeting of newly synthesized membrane proteins.

As discussed above in the section on sorting pathways, not all of the plasma membrane proteins expressed by polarized epithelial cells pursue a direct course to their sites of ultimate functional residence. The polymeric immunoglobulin receptor (pIgR) for example, when examined in its native liver[241,242,290] or in transfected MDCK cells,[249] travels first to the basolateral surface and subsequently to the apical pole. A number of studies have examined the contributions that various portions of the pIgR molecule may make to this complicated sorting behavior. Anchor-minus ectodomain constructs of the pIgR are secreted apically from transfected MDCK cells.[288] Furthermore, deletion of the pIgR cytosolic tail results in a membrane protein that travels directly to the apical surface without ever appearing at the basolateral side.[291] These observations have led to the suggestion that the ectodomain of the pIgR receptor contains an apical sorting signal, and that this protein's cytosolic tail embodies information that is required for its initial appearance at the basolateral plasma membrane. Extensive mutational analysis reveals that a trio of amino acids in the sequence His, Arg, Val is primarily responsible for the vectorial targeting of the newly synthesized pIgR protein to the basolateral plasmalemma. This motif constitutes yet another addition to the growing collection of distinct amino acid sequences that can encode basolateral sorting.[292,293]

During its tenure at the basolateral membrane, the pIgR's cytosolic tail becomes phosphorylated on a serine residue. The phosphorylation event occurs both in liver[243] and in transfected MDCK cells.[294] Intriguing experiments demonstrated that the addition of this phosphate group acts as a switch that allows the apical sorting signal to predominate, and results in the protein's transcytosis to the apical side. Site directed mutagenesis has been performed on the cDNA encoding the pIgR in order to convert the serine of interest into either an alanine or an aspartate residue.[294] When expressed in MDCK cells, the wild-type, as well as the two mutant forms, are all initially targeted to the basolateral surface, and all three undergo endocytosis and

recycling at similar rates. Interestingly, however, while the wild-type receptor undergoes fairly rapid transcytosis, the alanine form remains largely associated with the basolateral plasma membrane. In contrast, the aspartate form is transcytosed at a rate that exceeds that characteristic of the non-mutant form. These observations suggest that the negative charge associated with the phosphate and aspartate residues permits or activates the incorporation of the pIgR into transcytotic vesicles, and thus initiates the protein's delivery to the apical surface. The mechanism through which this signal is detected and interpreted remains unclear.

The recognition and segregation of pIgR destined for transcytosis probably occurs in an endosome following internalization from the basolateral surface. The second sorting event involved in the targeting of the pIgR is thus almost certainly completed at a subcellular location distinct from the TGN. This behavior suggests that, once again, the sorting of apical from basolateral proteins need not occur exclusively on the exocytic pathway. The endosome or an endosome-related compartment appears competent to sense and act upon the sorting signals that are necessary for the pIgR's apical localization. It remains to be determined whether signals detected in the endosome correspond to the same ectodomain-associated information that mediates the apical secretion of an anchor-minus form of the pIgR. The segregation of this secretory form to the apical pathway almost certainly occurs during its passage through the Golgi, and is not likely to involve elements of the endocytic apparatus.

Most ion transport proteins and receptors span the membrane several times, and many are composed of multiple subunits. Their intricate structures complicate the search for sorting signals and increase the likelihood that multiple independent or hierarchical signals might be present. This is clearly the case for the gastric H,K-ATPase. Acid secretion in the stomach is mediated by the gastric H^+/K^+-ATPase. This dimeric ion pump is stored within an intracellular population of membranous vesicles, known as tubulovesicular elements (TVEs), in gastric parietal cells. Stimulation of acid secretion by secretagogues induces the TVEs to fuse with the parietal cell apical plasma membrane, resulting in the formation of deeply invaginated secretory canaliculi rich in H^+/K^+-ATPase. The cessation of acid secretion involves the retrieval of the H^+/K^+-ATPase from the cell surface, and the regeneration of the TVE storage compartment.[295] Both the α- and β-subunits of the H^+/K^+-ATPase belong to the large P-type ATPase gene family.[296] Their closest cousins in this collection are the corresponding α- and β-subunits of the Na^+/K^+-ATPase. Interestingly, while the H^+/K^+-ATPase functions at the apical surface of gastric parietal epithelial cells, the Na^+/K^+-ATPase is restricted in its distribution to the basolateral plasmalemma, in this and most other epithelial cell types.[297] The homology relating these ATPases has permitted the creation of chimeric ion pumps, whose subunits are composed of complementary portions of the H^+/K^+- and Na^+/K^+-ATPase α- and β-polypeptides. By expressing these constructs in cultured polarized epithelial cells it has been possible to determine the molecular domains of the ion pump subunit proteins that are responsible for their sorting. Through this analysis it has become clear that both the α- and β-subunit polypeptides of the H^+/K^+-ATPase contain molecular signals which can contribute to the targeting of the holo-enzyme.[298–300] Expression of a large number of progressively more refined α-subunit chimeras reveals that an eight amino acid sequence within the α-subunit of the H^+/K^+-ATPase is sufficient to specify apical sorting.[300] This domain is predicted to reside within a transmembrane helix, thus suggesting that protein–lipid or protein–protein interactions within the plane of the membrane are responsible for pump sorting.

The β-subunit of the H^+/K^+-ATPase contains a tyrosine-based sorting signal that functions to internalize the pump complex from the surface of the gastric parietal cell, and return it to an intracellular regulated storage compartment.[301] This internalization is responsible for the cessation of gastric acid secretion following the removal of secretagogue stimulation. This was demonstrated by generating a transgenic mouse which expresses an H^+/K^+-ATPase β-subunit lacking this endocytosis signal.[301] These animals are unable to re-internalize H^+/K^+-ATPase from the apical surfaces of their gastric parietal cells. Consequently, they produce elevated gastric acid secretion during the interdigestive period. Mice carrying the mutant β-subunit develop gastritis and gastric ulcerations, with histologic features that are essentially identical to those found in human disease. Examination of renal potassium clearance in these animals reveals that the same β-subunit sorting signal regulates active potassium resorption in the collecting tubule.[302]

Several studies have begun to define other signals employed in the polarized sorting of polytopic membrane proteins. Recently, for example, a novel motif has been identified in the cytoplasmic tail of the seven-membrane-span receptor rhodopsin that mediates this protein's apical sorting when it is expressed in MDCK cells.[303] Another member of the seven transmembrane G protein-coupled receptor family, the P2Y2 receptor, manifests an apical sorting signal in one of its extracellular loops.[304] Furthermore, studies of neurotransmitter re-uptake systems have demonstrated that the four members of the highly homologous GABA transporter gene family are differentially sorted in epithelial cells

and in neurons.[305,306] The GAT-1 and GAT-3 isoforms, which are restricted to axons when expressed endogenously or by transfection in neurons, are sorted to the apical membranes of epithelial cells. The GAT-2 and betaine transporters, which are 50–67% identical to GAT-1 and GAT-3, behave as basolateral proteins in epithelia, and are restricted to dendrites when expressed in neurons. Production of chimeric and deletion constructs have permitted the identification of very short amino acid sequences at the extreme C-terminal tails of these transporters which manifest targeting information. The nature of these sequences suggests that they may interact with polypeptides containing PDZ-type protein–protein interaction domains, raising the possibility that this association may play a direct role in the sorting of ion transport proteins.[307] A similar PDZ-dependent mechanism also appears to mediate the apical trafficking of CFTR.[308–311] The basolateral isoform of the Na,K,2Cl co-transporter, NKCC1, has recently been shown to be targeted to the basolateral surface by virtue of a di-leucine motif in its cytoplasmic C-terminal tail. The renal isoform of this protein, NKCC2, depends for its apical localization on a two non-contiguous stretch of amino acids that appear to collaborate to form a conformation-dependent signal in the context of the fully folded transporter's C-terminal domain. The mechanism through which this non-contiguous conformational determinant is recognized by the cellular sorting machinery has yet to be determined.[312]

Cell Type-Specific Sorting: Patterns

The message encoded within a membrane protein's sorting signal is dependent not only upon its own specific biochemical composition, but also upon the cellular context in which it is expressed. Several examples of membrane proteins that are differentially targeted in distinct epithelial cell types have been documented. The vacuolar H^+-ATPase, for example, accumulates at the apical surfaces of α-type intercalated cells, but at the basolateral plasmalemmas of β-type intercalated cells in the renal collecting duct.[313] Similarly, the Na^+/K^+-ATPase is basolateral in most epithelia, but behaves as an apical protein in cells derived from the neural crest, such as choroid plexus and retinal pigment epithelium.[314,315] Targeting of particular proteins or classes of proteins can also vary as a function of the differentiation states of epithelial cells. For example, the sorting of well-characterized polarity markers expressed in *Drosophila* via germ line transformation was followed in the developing *Drosophila* embryo. Human placental alkaline phosphatase (PLAP) is a glycosylphosphatidyl inositol (GPI)-linked protein that accumulates at the apical membranes of mammalian epithelial cells. A chimeric construct composed of the transmembrane and cytosolic portions of the vesicular stomatitis virus (VSV) G protein coupled to the ectodomain of PLAP has been found to behave as a basolateral protein when expressed in the MDCK cell system.[285] The subcellular distributions of these proteins were examined in the epithelial tissues of transgenic *Drosophila* embryos which expressed these proteins under the control of a heat shock promoter.[316] In the surface ectoderm both PLAP and PLAPG were restricted to the basolateral membranes throughout development. Internal epithelia derived from the surface ectoderm accumulated PLAP at their apical surfaces, while PLAPG retained its basolateral distribution. The redistribution of PLAP from the basolateral to the apical plasma membrane was found to be coincident with the invagination of the surface epithelium to form internal structures, suggesting that the sorting pathways which function in the epithelium of the *Drosophila* embryo are developmentally regulated.

In light of both the multiplicity of sorting signals presented in the preceding section, and the apparent potential for heterogeneity in their interpretation discussed above, it is natural to wonder whether any logic or consistency governs nature's solution to the deceptively simple problem of apportioning proteins among two separate membrane domains. Upon further reflection, however, the complexity and degeneracy of the "sorting code" can be seen as a tremendous virtue. Two different epithelial cell types may need to target a given membrane protein to opposite surfaces of their respective plasma membranes in order to fulfill their unique physiologic functions. These same functions may also require, however, that other membrane proteins occupy the same surface distributions in both cellular contexts. Thus, while the sodium pump occupies the apical membranes of the cells of the choroid plexus and the basolateral membranes of renal epithelial cells, receptors for basement membrane components are present at the basolateral surfaces of both cell types. If only a single class of basolateral sorting signal and a single class of apical sorting signal existed, then it would not be possible for a cell to selectively alter the distribution of one set of plasmalemmal proteins, without simultaneously altering the distributions of the entire population of the plasma membrane. In order to target the sodium pump to the apical surface, choroid plexus epithelial cells would be forced to target basement membrane receptors there as well. This would obviously constitute a wasteful compromise. In order to endow each epithelial cell type with the capacity to select individualized complements of proteins for its apical and basolateral domains, a dizzying multitude of sorting signals has evolved. Cells can thus customize the distributions of proteins among their plasmalemmal domains, without the constraints that would

be imposed by a limited number of sorting signals. According to this interpretation, sorting signals do not specify a specific destination such as apical or basolateral. Instead, they specify classes of proteins whose members are always sorted together. The membrane domain to which any one of these classes is sorted will depend upon the cellular context in which it is expressed, and will be determined by the idiosyncratic array of sorting machinery and pathways present in each individual epithelial cell type.

Sorting: Mechanisms

Extensive progress has been made in illuminating the mechanisms through which the sorting signals discussed above exert their effects and ensure the polarized delivery of newly synthesized plasma membrane proteins. The strong evidence for the existence of sorting signals leads quite naturally to the postulate that sorting receptors must exist that are capable both of recognizing these signals, and of transducing their messages to the relevant cellular machinery. Such receptors have, in fact, been demonstrated in the case of lysosomal enzyme sorting. Targeting of a newly synthesized hydrolase to the lysosome is mediated by the interaction between the enzyme's mannose-6-phosphate (man-6-p) recognition marker, and one of two receptors which bind man-6-p bearing ligands in the Golgi and mediate their segregation to pre-lysosomal endosomes.[317] Binding of newly synthesized lysosomal enzymes to the man-6-p receptors is pH-dependent. At the relatively neutral pH of the Golgi ligands are tightly bound, whereas in the acid environment of the pre-lysosomal endosome they are rapidly released. No such well-characterized receptor systems have yet emerged to explain the sorting behavior of secretory and membrane proteins in polarized cells. While sorting receptors for secretory proteins remain to be identified definitively, some progress has been made in understanding how such receptors might function. Lysosomotropic amines, such as NH_4Cl and chloroquine, elevate the lumenal pH of acidic organelles.[318] The resulting neutralization of acidic compartments can have profound effects on sorting. In the case of lysosomal enzyme targeting, addition of NH_4Cl raises the pH of the pre-lysosomal endosome, and thus prevents the acid-dependent unbinding of newly synthesized hydrolases from the man-6-p receptor.[317] In the continued presence of the drug, the Golgi becomes depleted of receptors available to complex with free ligand. Newly synthesized enzymes bearing the man-6-p recognition marker are thus secreted constitutively and by default. Experiments on cultured polarized epithelial cells suggest that a similar pH-dependent mechanism may function in the sorting of basolateral secretory proteins.[176]

Laminin and heparan sulfate proteoglycan are constituents of epithelial basement membranes.[130,319] Studies of MDCK cells grown on permeable filter supports revealed that both of these proteins are normally secreted predominantly into the basolateral medium compartment.[176] When secretion from cells treated with NH_4Cl was monitored, it was found that both proteins were released into both media compartments in roughly equal proportions. Removal of the drug reversed this effect and restored normal basolateral secretion. As mentioned above, studies have demonstrated that the secretory default pathway for MDCK cells — that is the route pursued by soluble proteins which lack any means of interacting with the cellular sorting machinery — is apical and basolateral.[176,261,320] It appears, therefore, that targeting of these two basolateral secretory proteins requires the participation of an intracellular acidic compartment. Elevation of the lumenal pH of this compartment reversibly blocks laminin and HSPG sorting, and results in their apical and basolateral default secretion.

Although the nature of the dependence of this sorting event on acidic compartments remains unknown, it is interesting to speculate that a mechanism similar to that which functions in lysosomal enzyme sorting may also be involved in routing basolateral secretory proteins. In such a model, binding or unbinding of laminin and HSPG from a sorting receptor would require the participation of an acidic organellar pH. Confirmation of this hypothesis will await the identification of such a pH-dependent binding protein with affinity for these and other basolaterally targeted proteins.[321] Finally, it is worth noting that the basolateral sorting of the Na^+/K^+-ATPase, and the apical sorting of the influenza HA protein and a complex of secretory polypeptides, occurs normally in the presence and absence of NH_4Cl.[175,176,322] It would appear, therefore, that different mechanisms are brought to bear in ushering different classes of proteins to their sites of ultimate functional residence.

Tyrosine-Based Motifs and Adaptors

Recent studies suggest that several different classes of soluble proteins may regulate the subcellular distributions of proteins bearing tyrosine-based signals. Perhaps the best understood of these are the adaptins.[323] The adaptins comprise a group of peripheral membrane proteins that mediate the interaction between transmembrane proteins and the clathrin skeletons of coated pits and vesicles. Adaptins recognize and bind to tyrosine-containing coated pit localization sequences and link the proteins bearing these motifs to the clathrin coat.[323–327] Adaptins can thus be considered to be among the most proximal elements of the endocytic sorting machinery — they recognize polypeptides endowed with endocytosis signals and ensure that they are incorporated into the specified internalization pathway. Distinct classes of adaptins function in the segregation of proteins into the coated structures associated with the trans-Golgi network, and into cell surface coated pits.[230] While AP2 adaptors mediate internalization of proteins from the cell surface, AP1 adaptor complexes participate in trafficking proteins out of the TGN. The μ-subunits of adaptor complexes appear to be responsible for interacting with tyrosine-based motifs.[325] Two isoforms of μ-subunits are found in AP1 complexes. The μ1a protein is ubiquitously expressed, and is found in both polarized and nonpolar cell types. The μ1b protein is instead found in only a subset of polarized cell types.[328] Proteins bearing tyrosine-based motifs are basolaterally sorted in MDCK cells, but accumulate apically in LLC-PK cells.[329] It was noted that MDCK cells express μ1b, whereas this protein is absent from LLC-PK cells. Remarkably, expression of μ1b in LLC-PK cells at least partially "normalizes" their sorting properties, so that many (but not all) membrane proteins containing tyrosine-based signals are directed to the basolateral surface.[330] Thus, μ1b constitutes perhaps the best characterized component of the sorting machinery. It is clearly capable of recognizing a class of sorting signals and acting upon the instructions that they convey. Consistent with the idea that clathrin adaptors play an important role in the sorting of at least some basolateral proteins, it has been demonstrated that knockdown of clathrin expression in cultured renal epithelial cells perturbs basolateral, but not apical, protein delivery.[331]

It is interesting to note that recent studies demonstrate that different proteins bind to and interpret the messages encoded by tyrosine-based and di-leucine endocytosis motifs. Overexpression of tyrosine-motif containing proteins can inhibit the endocytosis of other proteins carrying a similar endocytosis signal, presumably by competing for limited quantities of the adaptor proteins that cluster proteins bearing these signals into clathrin-coated pits. This intervention does not affect, however, the internalization of proteins endowed with di-leucine motifs, indicating that they must be recognized and interpreted by a different class of polypeptides.[332] It appears that the β-subunits of adaptor complexes interact with di-leucine motifs.[333] Finally, a very different type of protein has been shown to interact with a tyrosine-based proline-rich sequence in the C-terminal tails of epithelial sodium channel (ENaC) subunits. The Nedd-4 protein possesses a ubiquitin ligase domain, and through its interaction with the ENaC tails may lead to these channels' downregulation through degradation.[334]

The association of basolateral membrane proteins, such as the Na^+/K^+-ATPase with elements of the subcortical cytoskeleton,[112,119] has led to the speculation that this interaction may play a role in targeting. Evidence in support of this proposition was found in the studies, described above, which suggested that, at least in one MDCK cell clone, the Na^+/K^+-ATPase may be delivered in equal proportions to the apical and basolateral surface.[237] Apically delivered material may be rapidly degraded, whereas basolateral sodium pump would be stabilized through interaction with the cytoskeleton and consequently would turn over very slowly. The pump's polarized distribution would thus be the product of differential susceptibility to degradation, rather than sorting at the level of the Golgi. The degree to which stabilization through interaction with the cytoskeleton contributes to the polarized distribution of the sodium pump or any other proteins remains to be established.

Glycosphingolipid-Rich Membrane Domains

The observation that all of the glycolipids and GPI-linked proteins associated with epithelial cells tend to be found in the apical plasmalemmal domain led to the proposal that lipids may play a role in membrane protein sorting.[335] Since glycolipids and GPI-linked proteins are only associated with the outer leaflet of the plasma membrane, these molecules will be exposed at the lumenal face of the organelles of the biosynthetic pathway. Any sorting machinery that interacts with glycolipids, therefore, must do so either at the lumenal surface or within the plane of the membrane itself. These constraints have suggested to some investigators the possibility that lipid—lipid interactions are sufficient to segregate apically directed glycolipids and GPI-linked proteins into distinct patches during their residence in the Golgi. These self-assembled patches could then serve as the nuclei from which apically directed vesicles would bud. The biophysical properties of these patches might be involved in ensnaring other apically directed proteins, as well as the components necessary to appropriately target the resultant transit vesicle.[336] While evidence of lipid patches exists in both *in vitro* and *in vivo* systems,[284,337] their precise role in the sorting process remains to be elucidated. Independent of its applicability, however, this model is extremely interesting. It is a useful reminder that forces other than simple receptor—ligand interactions are likely to be involved in generating and maintaining the anisotropic protein distributions that define the polarized state.

As noted above, several proteins are targeted to the apical membrane by virtue of signals embedded within their transmembrane domains. The fact that the amino acid residues of a transmembrane domain may be in direct contact with lipid molecules suggests the possibility that they may mediate apical sorting through interactions with glycosphingolipid-rich membrane domains. According to this hypothesis, the composition of its transmembrane domain may permit a protein to partition into glycosphingolipid rich patches, and thus to become concentrated in a region of the membrane that will give rise to an apically directed transport vesicle. GPI-linked proteins which have become associated with glycosphingolipid-rich membrane domains are insoluble in 1% TritonX-100 at 4°C. When a cell lysate prepared in this fashion is fractionated on a sucrose gradient, insoluble proteins are found near the top of the gradient, whereas soluble proteins remain in the heavier fractions.[337] Interestingly, the transmembrane domain of the apical protein influenza neuraminidase carries apical sorting information, and also enables the protein to incorporate into insoluble material.

PDZ Domain-containing Proteins

As discussed above, the C-terminus of GABA transporter GAT-3 appears to be important for its apical localization in MDCK cells.[307] The final residues of this C-terminal tail, threonine, histidine, and phenylalanine (THF), are reminiscent of the sequences present at the extreme C-terminal tails of proteins known to associate with members of the membrane-associated guanylate kinase (MAGUK) family. The MAGUK proteins incorporate one or more copies of the PDZ domain, which is named for three of the proteins in which the sequence homology defining this protein—protein interaction motif were first identified; PSD-95/SAP90, Dlg, and ZO-1. Interactions between the PDZ domain of a MAGUK protein and the extreme cytoplasmic tail of an integral membrane polypeptide appear to be important in organizing the surface distributions of intrinsic membrane proteins.[338,339]

Observations obtained from a number of experimental systems provide further evidence for the involvement of PDZ domain-containing polypeptides in epithelial membrane protein sorting.[340] The LET-23 receptor tyrosine kinase is localized to the basolateral cell surfaces of vulvar epithelial cells in *C. elegans*. Genetic studies reveal that at least three proteins contribute to the generation or maintenance of this distribution. Mutation of the lin2, lin7 or lin10 genes leads to loss of LET-23 basolateral polarity. Each of the proteins encoded by these genes includes one or more PDZ domains. A mutation in the *Drosophila* discs lost protein, which contains multiple PDZ domains, also leads to the mis-localization of several apical and basolateral proteins in the epithelial structures of affected embryos.[341] It would appear, therefore, that PDZ domain-containing proteins may play a direct role in the polarized sorting of at least some membrane proteins or may be required for the generation or definition of polarized domains. These observations may be especially relevant to physiologic function of polarized renal epithelial cells, since a number of important ion transport proteins, including CFTR and NHE3, appear to interact with cytoplasmic proteins containing PDZ domains.[342–344] It seems likely that these interactions may play a role in establishing these proteins distributions, and hence in determining their capacity to participate in vectorial ion transport.

Finally, it is important to note that once proteins have been sorted into the vesicles that will carry them to the appropriate cell surface domain, these vesicles themselves need to be targeted appropriately. Presumably, the vesicular membranes include proteins that ensure that the vesicles will interact and fuse with only the proper domain of the epithelial plasmalemma. This recognition machinery is likely to include components of the membrane fusion machinery, such as vesicular SNARE (soluble NSF attachment receptor) proteins.[345] SNARE proteins present in both vesicular and target membranes form complexes that appear to be necessary for most normal cellular fusion processes. The extent to which different members of the SNARE family impart specificity to intracellular vesicular fusion events remains to be established.[346–348] Interestingly, however, a component of the machinery involved in vesicular targeting in yeast was identified in mammalian cells.[349] This Sec 6/8 "exocyst" complex appears to play a role specifically in the fusion of basolaterally-directed, but not apically-directed, post-Golgi carrier vesicles in epithelial cells.[350] It is likely that the number of "destination-specific" vesicular and plasma membrane proteins important for directing vesicular traffic in polarized cells will continue to grow.

Epithelial Cell Polarity and Renal Disease

Because kidney function is dependent on the polarity of tubular epithelial cells, any condition that compromises this polarity will lead to renal failure.[351,352] In general, this may occur through neoplastic processes, cell injury due to ischemia or nephrotoxicity, or through inherited genetic effects.[179,351] Each of these may affect the tubular epithelial cells, their surrounding environment including the basal lamina and interstitial compartment, or both.

Carcinogenesis

During neoplastic growth it can be appreciated on the basis of morphology alone that the changes in cell and tissue organization wrought by tumorigenesis are likely to affect cell polarity.[179] Model studies confirm this suspicion. When MDCK cells, which are not normally tumorigenic, are oncogenically transformed by introduction of the v-Ki-*ras* oncogene, they are converted from a simple epithelium to a multilayer, with great heterogeneity in overall cell morphology.[179]

Ultrastructural examination of these cells suggests that apical–basal polarity is severely compromised. Microvilli are diminished from the cells at the top layer, and organization of the cytoplasm is scrambled. Golgi complexes and centrosomes, which normally reside in an apical supranuclear location, are now randomly positioned.[179] Despite this apparent high degree of disorganization, immunocytochemical localization of specific antigens and physiological measurements suggests that polarity is not totally disrupted. Basolateral proteins, including Na^+/K^+-ATPase and the cell-adhesion molecule E-cadherin, are restricted to regions of cell–cell contact, as in normal polarized MDCK cells. Apical proteins, on the other hand, are randomly localized to the free surface of the multilayered epithelia, as well as to areas of cell–cell contact in cells throughout the multilayer. The tight junctional antigen ZO-1 is found typically at the point where the free and adherent surfaces of the uppermost cell layer meet, as well as at a number of sites within the multilayer.[179] The latter may be intercellular lumina or canaliculi connected to the upper surface. This localization probably reflects the presence of functional tight junctions, because the multilayer is both electrically tight and impermeant to inulin.

It is interesting to note that recent studies demonstrate that proteins encoded by tumor suppressor genes may function as key regulators of polarity. Mutations in the von Hippel–Lindau tumor suppressor gene can lead to renal cell carcinoma. While the primary function of the von Hippel–Lindau gene product (VHL) relates to the negative regulation of the activity of the hypoxia inducible factor (HIF) transcription factor, the VHL protein also appears to participate in the formation or stabilization of intercellular adhesive junctions.[353] Mutations in the gene encoding the LKB1 protein kinase are responsible for Peutz–Jaeger syndrome, an inherited form of tumor susceptibility associated with the development of numerous hamartomas. Epithelial cells expressing LKB1 that is constitutively activated are able to form polarized domains in the absence of cell–cell and cell–substratum contact.[354] Thus, proteins that participate in epithelial polarization may function as tumor suppressors by virtue of their capacity to control the growth and morphogenesis of the cells in which they are expressed.

Ischemic Injury

Other alterations in cell polarity may come about through the effect of renal ischemia on the tubular epithelium.[355–358] Ischemic episodes of less than 1 hour often do not lead to tubular necrosis but may, nevertheless, cause diminished sodium and water uptake by the proximal tubule.[359] Such brief ischemia compromises the polarity of tubular cells, resulting in the redistribution of a fraction of the Na^+/K^+-ATPase from the basolateral domain to the apical domain, preventing net sodium uptake by the tubule.[359,360] At the same time, leucine aminopeptidase moves from the apical to the basolateral domain, and also becomes intracellular, presumably through endocytosis. At later times, Na^+/K^+-ATPase and leucine aminopeptidase are randomly distributed on the plasma membrane of tubular epithelial cells, remaining attached to the basement membrane or exfoliated into the lumenal space. The mechanism leading to this loss of polarity is not known. It is possible that ischemia, which is known to affect mitochondria and other organelles and to possibly alter the permeability of the plasma membrane, may result in increased cytoplasmic calcium concentrations.[355,358] This, in turn, could disrupt elements of the cytoskeleton, perhaps affecting the maintenance of polarity. These may represent disruption or perturbation of the cortical actin cytoskeleton. In fact, *in vitro* studies with renal epithelial cell lines demonstrate that ATP depletion causes disassembly of the cytoskeleton and redistribution of actin from its normal locations in the cell cortex, terminal web, and microvilli to perinuclear cytoplasmic aggregates.[361,362] In addition, energy depletion can lead to the endocytic internalization and proteolytic cleavage of cell adhesion molecules such as E-cadherin.[363,364] Such alterations might affect transduction of spatial signals from the extracellular matrix to the polarization machinery along the lines previously discussed.

During reperfusion following renal ischemia, tubular epithelial cells detach from the basement membrane and accumulate in the lumen. It has been postulated that ischemia-induced depolarization of integrins from basal to apical domains of the plasma membrane contributes not only to cell detachment, but also to cell aggregation and tubular obstruction. According to this hypothesis, at early times post-ischemia, redistribution of integrins would loosen attachment of cells from the basal lamina, allowing some of them to detach.[365–367] Released cells would then aggregate and adhere to remaining tubular epithelial cells via their integrins. These would either bind directly to each other by homotypic interactions or associate through bridging matrix molecules. Collections of such aggregates would obstruct the tubules, causing oliguria and destruction of renal tissue.[365–367] In support of this hypothesis, integrins were observed to redistribute apically in oxidatively injured epithelial cell lines.[365] Even more compelling was the observation that infusion of RGD peptides, which block some integrin–matrix interactions, appeared to ameliorate the effects of ischemia-induced by clamping of the renal artery.[367,368] More recent *in vivo* findings utilizing a rat model of renal ischemia do not, however, support this hypothesis, at least with regard to β1 integrins.[156] Soon after reperfusion, β1 integrins redistributed from a strictly basal to basolateral location in cells of the S3 segment of the proximal tubule, but did not appear on the apical plasma membrane at this time.[156] Surprisingly, β1 integrins could not be detected by immunofluorescence in cells released from the basal lamina into the tubular lumen, precluding the possibility that they were mediating either cell aggregation or attachment of exfoliated cells to the residual tubular epithelium. Apical β1 integrins only appeared at later times post-ischemia, as cells lost polarity in the process of regeneration.[156]

Genetic Diseases of Proximal Tubule Apical Endocytosis: Dent's Disease and the Oculo Cerebral Renal Syndrome of Lowe

It is interesting to note that at least two genetic diseases with overlapping constellations of symptoms lead to perturbations of the proximal tubule's megalin-mediated scavenging activity that normally prevents the urinary loss of low molecular weight filtered proteins. Dent's disease is caused by inactivating mutations in the gene encoding the ClC5 protein, which functions as a chloride:proton exchanger in the membranes of proximal tubule epithelial cell endosomes.[369,370] ClC5 activity leads to the accumulation of chloride ions in these endosomes, which appears to be required for steps in the internalization or recycling of the proximal tubule endocytic machinery. The Oculo Cerebral Renal Syndrome of Lowe is caused by mutations in an inositol lipid phosphatase that participates in controlling the inventory of inositol phospholipids in subcellular membranes.[371] These inositol phospholipids help to establish the compartmental identity of subcellular membranes, and to facilitate the assembly of trafficking machinery on their cytosolic surfaces. While the precise mechanisms through which intra-endosomal chloride concentrations and intramembranous inositol phospholipid levels participate in the process of megalin endocytosis remain to be elucidated, it is clear that both of these parameters collaborate in generating or maintaining the proximal tubule epithelial cell's unusual active apical endocytic machinery.

Polycystic Kidney Disease

The progressive formation of renal cysts, which characterizes autosomal dominant polycystic kidney disease (ADPKD), has also been suggested to occur as a result of polarity defects. ADPKD is the most common potentially lethal dominant genetic human disease. Approximately 85% of all cases are linked to mutations in the PKD1 gene, with another 10% linked to PKD2.[108,372] While the specific functions of the proteins encoded by these genes are the focus of intense study, the behavior of cyst epithelial cells *in situ* and in culture is consistent with a role for the PKD proteins in directing epithelial differentiation. Whereas renal tubular epithelial cells normally mediate fluid and electrolyte absorption, cyst epithelial cells carry out net secretion.[373,374] It has been suggested that the proximal cause of renal cyst formation in polycystic kidney disease may be the mis-targeting of Na^+/K^+-ATPase to the apical plasmalemma.

According to this model, the presence of sodium pump at the apical surface leads to active apical ion secretion and the accumulation of lumenal cyst fluid.[375,376] Other studies suggest that mis-localization of Na^+/K^+-ATPase cannot be the primary driving force for cyst fluid accumulation. When examined in cyst cells in culture or *in situ*, the Na^+/K^+-ATPase was found to be exclusively basolateral.[377] Instead, the secretion appears to be driven by intracellular chloride accumulation via a basolateral $Na^+/K^+/^+2Cl^-$ co-transporter and apical chloride exit through the CFTR protein.[377] A similar mechanism is responsible for fluid secretion by the poorly differentiated epithelial cells lining the crypts of the small intestine. As these crypt cells migrate up the intestinal villus they mature functionally, metamorphosing from secretory into resorptive epithelial cells.[378] It has been suggested that the secretory phenotype is characteristic of immature epithelial cells, while more highly developed epithelial cells acquire the capacity to absorb fluid and electrolytes.[379] The physiologic similarities relating cyst and crypt epithelial cells has prompted the hypothesis that loss of appropriate PKD function results in the dedifferentiation of mature resorptive renal tubular epithelial cells into more primitive secretory cells. The precise mechanisms through the PKD1 and PKD2 mutations produce the dramatic pathology associated with ADPKD, and the potential role of epithelial differentiation and sorting pathways, remain to be determined.

Acknowledgments

K. S. Matlin and M. J. Caplan acknowledge support for the research in their laboratories through grants from the National Institutes of Health. They would also like to thank Aki Manninen for permitting the use of unpublished material, Jonathan Bowen and Elias T. Spoliotis for the images in Figure 1.2, and Ms. Ruth Crawford for assistance with the references.

References

[1] Caplan MJ, Matlin KS. Sorting of membrane and secretory proteins in polarized epithelial cells. In: Matlin KS, Valentich JD, editors. Functional epithelial cells in culture. New York: Alan R. Liss; 1989. p. 71–127.

[2] Matlin KS. The sorting of proteins to the plasma membrane in epithelial cells. J Cell Biol 1986;103:2565–8.

[3] Nelson WJ. Adaptation of core mechanisms to generate cell polarity. Nature 2003;422:766–74.

[4] Rodriguez-Boulan E, Nelson WJ. Morphogenesis of the polarized epithelial cell phenotype. Science 1989;245:718–25.

[5] Duffield A, Caplan MJ, Muth TR. Protein trafficking in polarized cells. Int Rev Cell Mol Biol 2008;270:145–79.

[6] Muth TR, Caplan MJ. Transport protein trafficking in polarized cells. Annu Rev Cell Dev Biol 2003;19:333–66.

[7] Koeppen BM, Giebisch G. Mineralcorticoid regulation of sodium and potassium transport by the cortical collecting duct. In: Graves JS, editor. Regulation and development of membrane transport processes. New York: John Wiley and Sons; 1985. p. 89–104.

[8] O'Neil RG. Adrenal steroid regulation of potassium transport. In: Giebisch GH, editor. Current topics in membranes and transport: potassium transport: physiology and pathophysiology. New York: Academic Press; 1987. p. 185–206.

[9] Schultz SG. Cellular models of epithelial ion transport. In: Andreoli TE, Hoffman JF, Fanestil DD, Schultz SG, editors. Physiology of membrane disorders. New York: Plenum Press; 1986. p. 519–34.

[10] Sweadner KJ, Goldin SM. Active transport of sodium and potassium ions: mechanism, function, and regulation. N Engl J Med 1980;302:777–83.

[11] Palmer LG, Frindt G. Amiloride-sensitive Na channels from the apical membrane of the rat cortical collecting tubule. Proc Natl Acad Sci USA 1986;83:2767–70.

[12] Fawcett DW. Bloom and Fawcett: a textbook of histology. Philadelphia: W.B. Saunders; 1986.

[13] Farquhar MG, Palade GE. Junctional complexes in various epithelia. J Cell Biol 1963;17:375–412.

[14] Schwarz MA, Owaribe K, Kartenbeck J, Franke WW. Desmosomes and hemidesmosomes: constitutive molecular components. Annu Rev Cell Biol 1990;6:461–91.

[15] Franke WW, Winter S, Grund C, Schmid E, Schiller DL, et al. Isolation and characterization of desmosome-associated tonofilaments from rat intestinal brush border. J Cell Biol 1981;90:116–27.

[16] Ben-Ze'ev A, Geiger B. Differential molecular interactions of beta-catenin and plakoglobin in adhesion, signaling and cancer. Curr Opin Cell Biol 1998;10:629–39.

[17] Simon AM. Gap junctions: more roles and new structural data. Trends Cell Biol 1999;9:169–70.

[18] Simon AM, Goodenough DA. Diverse functions of vertebrate gap junctions. Trends Cell Biol 1998;8:477–83.

[19] Fromter E, Diamond J. Route of passive ion permeation in epithelia. Nat New Biol 1972;235:9–13.

[20] Madara JL, Hecht G. Tight (occluding) junctions in cultured (and native) epithelial cells. In: Matlin KS, Valentich JD, editors. Functional epithelial cells in culture. New York: Alan R. Liss; 1989. p. 131–64.

[21] Shen L, Weber CR, Raleigh DR, Yu D, Turner JR. Tight junction pore and leak pathways: a dynamic duo. Annu Rev Physiol 2011;73:283–309.

[22] Anderson JM, Van Itallie CM. Physiology and function of the tight junction. Cold Spring Harb Perspect Biol 2009;1:a002584.

[23] Cereijido M, Ponce A, Gonzalez-Mariscal L. Tight junctions and apical/basolateral polarity. J Membr Biol 1989;110:1–9.

[24] Gonzalez-Mariscal L, Chavez de Ramirez B, Cereijido M. Tight junction formation in cultured epithelial cells (MDCK). J Membr Biol 1985;86:113–25.

[25] Hartsock A, Nelson WJ. Adherens and tight junctions: Structure, function and connections to the actin cytoskeleton. Biochim Biophys Acta 2008;1778:660–9.

[26] Schneeberger EE, Lynch RD. The tight junction: a multifunctional complex. Am J Physiol Cell Physiol 2004;286:C1213–28.

[27] Stevenson BR, Anderson JM, Bullivant S. The epithelial tight junction: Structure, function and preliminary biochemical characterization. Mol Cell Biochem 1988;83:129–45.

[28] Stevenson BR, Keon BH. The tight junction: morphology to molecules. Annu Rev Cell Dev Biol 1998;14:89—109.

[29] Denker BM, Sabath E. The biology of epithelial cell tight junctions in the kidney. J Am Soc Nephrol 2011;22:622—5.

[30] Hendler RW. Biological membrane ultrastructure. Physiol Rev 1971;51:66—97.

[31] Dragsten PR, Blumenthal R, Handler JS. Membrane asymmetry in epithelia: is the tight junction a barrier to diffusion in the plasma membrane? Nature 1981;294:718—22.

[32] van Meer G, Simons K. The function of tight junctions in maintaining differences in lipid composition between the apical and the basolateral cell surface domains of MDCK cells. EMBO J 1986;5:1455—64.

[33] van Meer G, Gumbiner B, Simons K. The tight junction does not allow lipid molecules to diffuse from one epithelial cell to the next. Nature 1986;322:639—41.

[34] Staehelin LA. Further observations on the fine structure of freeze-cleaved tight junctions. J Cell Sci 1973;13:763—86.

[35] Claude P, Goodenough DA. Fracture faces of zonulae occludentes from "tight" and "leaky" epithelia. J Cell Biol 1973;58:390—400.

[36] Stevenson BR, Siliciano JD, Mooseker MS, Goodenough DA. Identification of ZO-1: a high molecular weight polypeptide associated with the tight junction (zonula occludens) in a variety of epithelia. J Cell Biol 1986;103:755—66.

[37] Fanning AS, Van Itallie C, Anderson JM. Zonula occludens (ZO)-1 and -2 regulate apical cell structure and the zonula adherens cytoskeleton in polarized epithelia. Mol Biol Cell 2011;23(4):577—90.

[38] Angelow S, Ahlstrom R, Yu ASL. Biology of claudins. AJP: Renal Physiol 2008;295:F867—76.

[39] Balkovetz DF. Claudins at the gate: Determinants of renal epithelial tight junction paracellular permeability. Am J Physiol Renal Physiol 2006;290:F572—9.

[40] Colegio OR, Van Itallie CM, McCrea HJ, Rahner C, Anderson JM. Claudins create charge-selective channels in the paracellular pathway between epithelial cells. Am J Physiol Cell Physiol 2002;283:C142—7.

[41] Furuse M, Tsukita S. Claudins in occluding junctions of humans and flies. Trends Cell Biol 2006;16:181—8.

[42] Morita K, Furuse M, Fujimoto K, Tsukita S. Claudin multigene family encoding four-transmembrane domain protein components of tight junction strands. Proc Natl Acad Sci USA 1999;96:511—6.

[43] Van Itallie CM, Anderson JM. Claudins and epithelial paracellular transport. Annu Rev Physiol 2006;68:403—29.

[44] Furuse M. Molecular basis of the core structure of tight junctions. Cold Spring Harb Perspect Biol 2010;2:a002907-a.

[45] Furuse M, Sasaki H, Fujimoto K, Tsukita S. A single gene product, claudin-1 or -2, reconstitutes tight junction strands and recruits occludin in fibroblasts. J Cell Biol 1998;143:391—401.

[46] Furuse M, Furuse K, Sasaki H, Tsukita S. Conversion of zonulae occludentes from tight to leaky strand type by introducing claudin-2 into Madin—Darby canine kidney I cells. J Cell Biol 2001;153:263—72.

[47] Kiuchi-Saishin Y, Gotoh S, Furuse M, Takasuga A, Tano Y, et al. Differential expression patterns of claudins, tight junction membrane proteins, in mouse nephron segments. J Am Soc Nephrol JASN 2002;13:875—86.

[48] Haskins J, Gu L, Wittchen ES, Hibbard J, Stevenson BR. ZO-3, a novel member of the MAGUK protein family found at the tight junction, interacts with ZO-1 and occludin. J Cell Biol 1998;141:199—208.

[49] Jesaitis LA, Goodenough DA. Molecular characterization and tissue distribution of ZO-2, a tight junction protein homologous to ZO-1 and the *Drosophila* discs-large tumor suppressor protein. J Cell Biol 1994;124:949—61.

[50] Marchiando AM, Graham WV, Turner JR. Epithelial barriers in homeostasis and disease. Annu Rev Pathol 2010;5:119—44 Mechanisms of Disease

[51] Hecht G, Pestic L, Nikcevic G, Koutsouris A, et al. Expression of the catalytic domain of myosin light chain kinase increases paracellular permeability. Am J Physiol 1996;271:C1678—84.

[52] Turner JR, Rill BK, Carlson SL, Carnes D, Kerner R, Mrsny RJ, et al. Physiological regulation of epithelial tight junctions is associated with myosin light-chain phosphorylation. Am J Physiol 1997;273:C1378—85.

[53] Yap AS, Brieher WM, Gumbiner BM. Molecular and functional analysis of cadherin-based adherens junctions. Annu Rev Cell Dev Biol 1997;13:119—46.

[54] Nelson WJ. Regulation of cell—cell adhesion by the cadherin—catenin complex. Biochem Soc Trans 2008;36:149—55.

[55] Barth AI, Nathke IS, Nelson WJ. Cadherins, catenins and APC protein: interplay between cytoskeletal complexes and signaling pathways. Curr Opin Cell Biol 1997;9:683—90.

[56] Gumbiner B, Lowenkopf T, Apatira D. Identification of a 160-kDa polypeptide that binds to the tight junction protein ZO-1. Proc Natl Acad Sci USA 1991;88:3460—4.

[57] Griffith LD, Bulger RE, Trump BF. Fine structure and staining of mucosubstances on "intercalated cells" from the rat distal convoluted tubule and collecting duct. Anat Rec 1968;160:643—62.

[58] Maunsbach AB. Cellular mechanisms of tubular protein transport. Int Rev Physiol 1976;11:145—67.

[59] Welling LW, Welling DJ. Surface areas of brush border and lateral cell walls in the rabbit proximal nephron. Kidney Int 1975;8:343—8.

[60] Mandel LJ, Balaban RS. Stoichiometry and coupling of active transport to oxidative metabolism in epithelial tissues. Am J Physiol 1981;240:F357—71.

[61] Mooseker MS. Organization, chemistry, and assembly of the cytoskeletal apparatus of the intestinal brush border. Annu Rev Cell Biol 1985;1:209—41.

[62] Brown JW, McKnight CJ. Molecular model of the microvillar cytoskeleton and organization of the brush border. PLoS One 2010;5:e9406.

[63] McConnell RE, Benesh AE, Mao S, Tabb DL, Tyska MJ. Proteomic analysis of the enterocyte brush border. Am J Physiol Gastrointest Liver Physiol 2011;300:G914—26.

[64] Rodman JS, Mooseker M, Farquhar MG. Cytoskeletal proteins of the rat kidney proximal tubule brush border. Eur J Cell Biol 1986;42:319—27.

[65] Bretscher A, Weber K. Localization of actin and microfilament-associated proteins in the microvilli and terminal web of the intestinal brush border by immunofluorescence microscopy. J Cell Biol 1978;79:839—45.

[66] Glenney Jr. JR, Glenney P. Fodrin is the general spectrin-like protein found in most cells whereas spectrin and the TW protein have a restricted distribution. Cell 1983;34:503—12.

[67] Drenckhahn D, Groschel-Stewart U. Localization of myosin, actin, and tropomyosin in rat intestinal epithelium: immunohistochemical studies at the light and electron microscope levels. J Cell Biol 1980;86:475—82.

[68] Hirokawa N, Keller III TC, Chasan R, Mooseker MS. Mechanism of brush border contractility studied by the quick-freeze, deep-etch method. J Cell Biol 1983;96:1325—36.

[69] Mooseker MS. Brush border motility. Microvillar contraction in triton-treated brush borders isolated from intestinal epithelium. J Cell Biol 1976;71:417—33.

[70] Hayden SM, Wolenski JS, Mooseker MS. Binding of brush border myosin I to phospholipid vesicles. J Cell Biol 1990;111:443—51.

[71] Mooseker MS, Coleman TR. The 110-kD protein-calmodulin complex of the intestinal microvillus (brush border myosin I) is a mechanoenzyme. J Cell Biol 1989;108:2395−400.

[72] Coluccio LM, Bretscher A. Reassociation of microvillar core proteins: making a microvillar core *in vitro*. J Cell Biol 1989;108:495−502.

[73] Matsudaira PT, Burgess DR. Identification and organization of the components in the isolated microvillus cytoskeleton. J Cell Biol 1979;83:667−73.

[74] Garcia A, Coudrier E, Carboni J, Anderson J, Vanderkerkhove J, Mooseker M, et al. Partial deduced sequence of the 110-kD-calmodulin complex of the avian intestinal microvillus shows that this mechanoenzyme is a member of the myosin I family. J Cell Biol 1989;109:2895−903.

[75] Hoshimaru M, Nakanishi S. Identification of a new type of mammalian myosin heavy chain by molecular cloning. Overlap of its mRNA with preprotachykinin B mRNA. J Biol Chem 1987;262:14625−32.

[76] Cheney RE, Mooseker MS. Unconventional myosins. Curr Opin Cell Biol 1992;4:27−35.

[77] Mooseker MS, Cheney RE. Unconventional myosins. Annu Rev Cell Dev Biol 1995;11:633−75.

[78] Drenckhahn D, Dermietzel R. Organization of the actin filament cytoskeleton in the intestinal brush border: a quantitative and qualitative immunoelectron microscope study. J Cell Biol 1988;107:1037−48.

[79] McConnell RE, Tyska MJ. Leveraging the membrane − cytoskeleton interface with myosin-1. Trends Cell Biol 2010;20:418−26.

[80] Fath KR, Burgess DR. Golgi-derived vesicles from developing epithelial cells bind actin filaments and possess myosin-I as a cytoplasmically oriented peripheral membrane protein. J Cell Biol 1993;120:117−27.

[81] Fath KR, Trimbur GM, Burgess DR. Molecular motors are differentially distributed on Golgi membranes from polarized epithelial cells. J Cell Biol 1994;126:661−75.

[82] Barylko B, Wagner MC, Reizes O, Albanesi JP. Purification and characterization of a mammalian myosin I. Proc Natl Acad Sci USA 1992;89:490−4.

[83] Coudrier E, Kerjaschki D, Louvard D. Cytoskeleton organization and submembranous interactions in intestinal and renal brush borders. Kidney Int 1988;34:309−20.

[84] Coluccio LM. Identification of the microvillar 110-kDa calmodulin complex (myosin-1) in kidney. Eur J Cell Biol 1991;56:286−94.

[85] Bretscher A, Weber K. Villin: the major microfilament-associated protein of the intestinal microvillus. Proc Natl Acad Sci USA 1979;76:2321−5.

[86] Arpin M, Pringault E, Finidori J, Garcia A, Jeltsch JM, Vanderkerckhove J, et al. Sequence of human villin: a large duplicated domain homologous with other actin-severing proteins and a unique small carboxy-terminal domain related to villin specificity. J Cell Biol 1988;107:1759−66.

[87] Matsudaira PT, Burgess DR. Partial reconstruction of the microvillus core bundle: characterization of villin as a Ca^{++}-dependent, actin-bundling/depolymerizing protein. J Cell Biol 1982;92:648−56.

[88] Robine S, Huet C, Moll R, Sahuquillo-Merino C, Coudrieri E, Zweibaum A, et al. Can villin be used to identify malignant and undifferentiated normal digestive epithelial cells? Proc Natl Acad Sci USA 1985;82:8488−92.

[89] Costa de Beauregard MA, Pringault E, Robine S, Louvard D. Suppression of villin expression by antisense RNA impairs brush border assembly in polarized epithelial intestinal cells. EMBO J 1995;14:409−21.

[90] Pinson KI, Dunbar L, Samuelson L, Gumucio DL. Targeted disruption of the mouse villin gene does not impair the morphogenesis of microvilli. Dev Dyn 1998;211:109−21.

[91] Bretscher A, Weber K. Fimbrin, a new microfilament-associated protein present in microvilli and other cell surface structures. J Cell Biol 1980;86:335−40.

[92] Volkmann N, DeRosier D, Matsudaira P, Hanein D. An atomic model of actin filaments cross-linked by fimbrin and its implications for bundle assembly and function. J Cell Biol 2001;153:947−56.

[93] Grimm-Gunter EM, Revenu C, Ramos S, Hurbain I, Smyth N, Ferrary E, et al. Plastin 1 binds to keratin and is required for terminal web assembly in the intestinal epithelium. Mol Biol Cell 2009;20:2549−62.

[94] Bartles JR, Zheng L, Li A, Wierda A, Chen B. Small espin: a third actin-bundling protein and potential forked protein ortholog in brush border microvilli. J Cell Biol 1998;143:107−19.

[95] Zheng L, Sekerkova G, Vranich K, Tilney LG, Mugnaini E, et al. The deaf jerker mouse has a mutation in the gene encoding the espin actin-bundling proteins of hair cell stereocilia and lacks espins. Cell 2000;102:377−85.

[96] Loomis PA, Zheng L, Sekerkova G, Changyaleket B, Mugnaini E, et al. Espin cross-links cause the elongation of microvillus-type parallel actin bundles *in vivo*. J Cell Biol 2003;163:1045−55.

[97] Revenu C, Ubelmann F, Hurbain I, El-Marjou F, Dingli F, Loew D, et al. A new role for the architecture of microvillus actin bundles in apical retention of membrane proteins. Miol Biol Cell 2011;23(2):324−36.

[98] Bretscher A, Reczek D, Berryman M. Ezrin: a protein requiring conformational activation to link microfilaments to the plasma membrane in the assembly of cell surface structures. J Cell Sci 1997;110(Pt 24):3011−8.

[99] Saotome I, Curto M, McClatchey AI. Ezrin is essential for epithelial organization and villus morphogenesis in the developing intestine. Dev Cell 2004;6:855−64.

[100] Bacic D, Wagner CA, Hernando N, Kaissling B, Biber J, et al. Novel aspects in regulated expression of the renal type IIa Na/Pi-cotransporter. Kidney Int Suppl 2004;:S5−12.

[101] Burgess DR. Reactivation of intestinal epithelial cell brush border motility: ATP-dependent contraction via a terminal web contractile ring. J Cell Biol 1982;95:853−63.

[102] Kerjaschki D, Noronha-Blob L, Sacktor B, Farquhar MG. Microdomains of distinctive glycoprotein composition in the kidney proximal tubule brush border. J Cell Biol 1984;98:1505−13.

[103] Rodman JS, Seidman L, Farquhar MG. The membrane composition of coated pits, microvilli, endosomes, and lysosomes is distinctive in the rat kidney proximal tubule cell. J Cell Biol 1986;102:77−87.

[104] Lina F, Satlinb LM. Polycystic kidney disease: the cilium as a common pathway in cystogenesis. Curr Opin Pediatr 2004;16:171−6.

[105] Yoder BK, Mulroy S, Eustace H, Boucher C, Sandford R. Molecular pathogenesis of autosomal dominant polycystic kidney disease. Expert Rev Mol Med 2006;8:1−22.

[106] Mollet G, Silbermann F, Delous M, Salomon R, Antignac C, et al. Characterization of the nephrocystin/nephrocystin-4 complex and subcellular localization of nephrocystin-4 to primary cilia and centrosomes. Hum Mol Genet 2005;14:645−56.

[107] Lin F, Hiesberger T, Cordes K, Sinclair AM, Goldstein LS, Somlo S, et al. Kidney-specific inactivation of the KIF3A subunit of kinesin-II inhibits renal ciliogenesis and produces polycystic kidney disease. Proc Natl Acad Sci USA 2003;100:5286−91.

[108] Takiar V, Caplan MJ. Polycystic kidney disease: pathogenesis and potential therapies. Biochim Biophys Acta 2011;1812:1337−43.

[109] Amerongen HM, Mack JA, Wilson JM, Neutra MR. Membrane domains of intestinal epithelial cells: Distribution of Na$^+$/K$^+$-ATPase and the membrane skeleton in adult rat intestine during fetal development and after epithelial isolation. J Cell Biol 1989;109:2129–38.

[110] Achler C, Filmer D, Merte C, Drenckhahn D. Role of microtubules in polarized delivery of apical membrane proteins to the brush border of the intestinal epithelium. J Cell Biol 1989;109:179–89.

[111] McNeill H, Ozawa M, Kemler R, Nelson WJ. Novel function of the cell adhesion molecule uvomorulin as an inducer of cell surface polarity. Cell 1990;62:309–16.

[112] Morrow JS, Cianci CD, Ardito T, Mann AS, Kashgarian M. Ankyrin links fodrin to the alpha subunit of Na,K-ATPase in Madin–Darby canine kidney cells and in intact renal tubule cells. J Cell Biol 1989;108:455–65.

[113] Nelson WJ. Development and maintenance of epithelial polarity: a role for the submembranous cytoskeleton. In: Matlin KS, Valentich JD, editors. Functional epithelial cells in culture. New York: Alan R. Liss; 1989. p. 3–42.

[114] Nelson WJ, Hammerton RW. A membrane-cytoskeletal complex containing Na$^+$K$^+$-ATPase, ankyrin, and fodrin in Madin–Darby canine kidney (MDCK) cells: implications for the biogenesis of epithelial cell polarity. J Cell Biol 1989;108.893–902.

[115] Nelson WJ, Hammerton RW, McNeill H. Role of the membrane-cytoskeleton in the spatial organization of the Na,K-ATPase in polarized epithelial cells. Soc Gen Physiol Ser 1991;46:77–87.

[116] Nelson WJ, Hammerton RW, Wang AZ, Shore EM. Involvement of the membrane-cytoskeleton in development of epithelial cell polarity. Semin Cell Biol 1990;1:359–71.

[117] Nelson WJ, Shore EM, Wang AZ, Hammerton RW. Identification of a membrane-cytoskeletal complex containing the cell adhesion molecule uvomorulin (E-cadherin), ankyrin, and fodrin in Madin–Darby canine kidney epithelial cells. J Cell Biol 1990;110:349–57.

[118] Nelson WJ, Veshnock PJ. Dynamics of membrane-skeleton (fodrin) organization during development of polarity in Madin–Darby canine kidney epithelial cells. J Cell Biol 1986;103:1751–65.

[119] Nelson WJ, Veshnock PJ. Ankyrin binding to (Na^{++} K$^+$) ATPase and implications for the organization of membrane domains in polarized cells. Nature 1987;328:533–6.

[120] Nelson WJ, Veshnock PJ. Modulation of fodrin (membrane skeleton) stability by cell–cell contact in Madin–Darby canine kidney epithelial cells. J Cell Biol 1987;104:1527–37.

[121] Parczyk K, Haase W, Kondor-Koch C. Microtubules are involved in the secretion of proteins at the apical cell surface of the polarized epithelial cell, Madin–Darby canine kidney. J Biol Chem 1989;264:16837–46.

[122] Rindler MJ, Ivanov IE, Sabatini DD. Microtubule-acting drugs lead to the nonpolarized delivery of the influenza hemagglutinin to the cell surface of polarized Madin–Darby canine kidney cells. J Cell Biol 1987;104:231–41.

[123] Salas PJ, Vega-Salas DE, Hochman J, Rodriguez-Boulan E, Edidin M. Selective anchoring in the specific plasma membrane domain: a role in epithelial cell polarity. J Cell Biol 1988;107:2363–76.

[124] Grindstaff KK, Bacallao RL, Nelson WJ. Apiconuclear organization of microtubules does not specify protein delivery from the trans-Golgi network to different membrane domains in polarized epithelial cells. Mol Biol Cell 1998;9:685–99.

[125] Spiliotis ET, Hunt SJ, Hu Q, Kinoshita M, Nelson WJ. Epithelial polarity requires septin coupling of vesicle transport to polyglutamylated microtubules. J Cell Biol 2008;180:295–303.

[126] Yurchenco PD. Basement membranes: cell scaffoldings and signaling platforms. Cold Spring Harb Perspect Biol 2011;3: a004911-a.

[127] Miner JH. Organogenesis of the kidney glomerulus: focus on the glomerular basement membrane. Organogenesis 2011;7:75–82.

[128] Aumailley M. Structure and supramolecular organization of basement membranes. Kidney Int Suppl 1995;49:S4–7.

[129] Miner JH. Renal basement membrane components. Kidney Int 1999;56:2016–24.

[130] Miner JH, Yurchenco PD. Laminin functions in tissue morphogenesis. Annu Rev Cell Dev Biol 2004;20:255–84.

[131] Aumailley M, Bruckner-Tuderman L, Carter W, et al. A simplified laminin nomenclature. Matrix Biol 2005;24:326–32.

[132] Li S, Edgar D, Fassler R, Wadsworth W, Yurchenco PD. The role of laminin in embryonic cell polarization and tissue organization. Dev Cell 2003;4:613–24.

[133] Yurchenco PD, Patton BL. Developmental and pathogenic mechanisms of basement membrane assembly. Curr Pharm Des 2009;15:1277–94.

[134] Yurchenco P, Cheng Y. Laminin self-assembly: a three-arm interaction hypothesis for the formation of a network in basement membranes. Contrib Nephrol 1994;107:47–56.

[135] Joly D, Berissi S, Bertrand A, Strehl L, Patey N, et al. Laminin 5 regulates polycystic kidney cell proliferation and cyst formation. J Biol Chem 2006;281:29181–9.

[136] Joly D, Morel V, Hummel A, Ruello A, Nusbaum P, Patey N, et al. β4 integrin and laminin 5 are aberrantly expressed in polycystic kidney disease. Am J Pathol 2003;163:1791–800.

[137] Shannon MB, Patton BL, Harvey SJ, Miner JH. A hypomorphic mutation in the mouse laminin alpha5 gene causes polycystic kidney disease. J Am Soc Nephrol 2006;17:1913–22.

[138] Zuk A, Matlin KS. Induction of a laminin isoform and alpha (3)beta(1)-integrin in renal ischemic injury and repair *in vivo*. Am J Physiol Renal Physiol 2002;283:F971–84.

[139] Greciano PG, Moyano JV, Buschmann MM, Tang J, Lu Y, Rudnicki J, et al. Laminin 511 partners with laminin 332 to mediate directional migration of Madin–Darby canine kidney (MDCK) epithelial cells. Mol Biol Cell 2012;24:121–36.

[140] Hynes RO. Integrins: bidirectional, allosteric signaling machines. Cell 2002;110:673–87.

[141] Hemler ME. VLA proteins in the integrin family: structures, functions, and their role on leukocytes. Annu Rev Immunol 1990;8:365–400.

[142] Kreidberg JA, Symons JM. Integrins in kidney development, function, and disease. Am J Physiol Renal Physiol 2000;279: F233–42.

[143] Moyano JV, Greciano PG, Buschmann MM, Koch M, Matlin KS. Autocrine transforming growth factor-{beta}1 activation mediated by integrin {alpha}V{beta}3 regulates transcriptional expression of laminin-332 in Madin–Darby canine kidney epithelial cells. Mol Biol Cell 2010;21:3654–68.

[144] Schoenenberger CA, Zuk A, Zinkl GM, Kendall D, Matlin KS. Integrin expression and localization in normal MDCK cells and transformed MDCK cells lacking apical polarity. J Cell Sci 1994;107(Pt 2):527–41.

[145] Geiger B, Bershadsky A. Assembly and mechanosensory function of focal contacts. Curr Opin Cell Biol 2001;13:584–92.

[146] Zamir E, Geiger B. Components of cell–matrix adhesions. J Cell Sci 2001;114:3577–9.

[147] Zamir E, Geiger B. Molecular complexity and dynamics of cell–matrix adhesions. J Cell Sci 2001;114:3583–90.

[148] Zamir E, Katz BZ, Aota S, Yamada KM, Geiger B, et al. Molecular diversity of cell-matrix adhesions. J Cell Sci 1999;112(Pt 11):1655–69.

[149] Geiger B, Yamada KM. Molecular architecture and function of matrix adhesions. Cold Spring Harb Perspect Biol 2011;3: pii: a005033.

[150] Tsurata D, Hashimoto T, Hamill K, Jones JCR. Hemidesmosomes and focal contact proteins: functions and cross-talk in keratinocytes, bullous diseases and wound healing. J Derm Sci 2011;62:1–7.

[151] Zhang H, Labouesse M. The making of hemidesmosome structures *in vivo*. Dev Dyn 2010;239:1465–76.

[152] Li S, Liquari P, McKee KK, Harrison D, Patel R, Lee S, et al. Laminin-sulfatide binding initiates basement membrane assembly and enables receptor signaling in Schwann cells and fibroblasts. J Cell Biol 2005;169:179–89.

[153] Zinkl GM, Zuk A, van der Bijl P, van Meer G, Matlin KS. An antiglycolipid antibody inhibits Madin–Darby canine kidney cell adhesion to laminin and interferes with basolateral polarization and tight junction formation. J Cell Biol 1996;133:695–708.

[154] Ekblom P. Developmentally regulated conversion of mesenchyme to epithelium. FASEB J 1989;3:2141–50.

[155] Molitoris B, Wilson P, Schrier R, Simon FR. Ischemia induces partial loss of surface membrane polarity and accumulation of putative calcium ionophores. J Clin Invest 1985;76(6):2097–105.

[156] Zuk A, Bonventre JV, Brown D, Matlin KS. Polarity, integrin, and extracellular matrix dynamics in the postischemic rat kidney. Am J Physiol 1998;275:C711–31.

[157] Nelson WJ. Remodeling epithelial cell organization: transitions between front–rear and apical–basal polarity. Cold Spring Harb Perspect Biol 2009;1:a000513.

[158] Simons K, Fuller SD. Cell surface polarity in epithelia. Annu Rev Cell Biol 1985;1:243–88.

[159] Gausch CR, Hard WL, Smith TF. Characterization of an established line of canine kidney cells (MDCK). Proc Soc Exp Biol Med 1966;122:931–5.

[160] Madin SH, Darby NB. In: American type culture collection catalogue of strains II. Rockville, Maryland: American Type Culture Collection; 1975.

[161] Herzlinger DA, Easton TG, Ojakian GK. The MDCK epithelial cell line expresses a cell surface antigen of the kidney distal tubule. J Cell Biol 1982;93:269–77.

[162] Leighton J, Brada Z, Estes LW, Justh G. Secretory activity and oncogenicity of a cell line (MDCK) derived from canine kidney. Science 1969;163:472–3.

[163] Abaza NA, Leighton J, Schultz SG. Effects of ouabain on the function and structure of a cell line (MDCK) derived from canine kidney. I. Light microscopic observations of monolayer growth. In Vitro 1974;10:72–183.

[164] Cereijido M, Ehrenfeld J, Fernandez-Castelo S, Meza I. Fluxes, junctions, and blisters in cultured monolayers of epithelioid cells (MDCK). Ann NY Acad Sci 1981;372:422–41.

[165] Rodriguez Boulan E, Sabatini DD. Asymmetric budding of viruses in epithelial monlayers: a model system for study of epithelial polarity. Proc Natl Acad Sci USA 1978;75:5071–5.

[166] Rodriguez Boulan E, Pendergast M. Polarized distribution of viral envelope proteins in the plasma membrane of infected epithelial cells. Cell 1980;20:45–54.

[167] Jat PS, Noble MD, Ataliotis P, Tanaka Y, Yannoutsos N, Larsen L, et al. Direct derivation of conditionally immortal cell lines from an H-2Kb-tsA58 transgenic mouse. Proc Natl Acad Sci USA 1991;88:5096–100.

[168] Geng H, Lan R, Wang G, Siddiqi AR, Naski MC, Brooks AI, et al. Inhibition of autoregulated TGFbeta signaling simultaneously enhances proliferation and differentiation of kidney epithelium and promotes repair following renal ischemia. Am J Pathol 2009;174:1291–308.

[169] Racusen LC, Monteil C, Sgrignoli A, Lucskay M, Marouillat S, Rhim JG, Morin JP. Cell lines with extended *in vitro* growth potential from human renal proximal tubule: characterization, response to inducers, and comparison with established cell lines. J Lab Clin Med 1997;129:318–29.

[170] Ryan MJ, Johnson G, Kirk J, Fuerstenberg SM, Zager RA, et al. HK-2: an immortalized proximal tubule epithelial cell line from normal adult human kidney. Kidney Int 1994;45:48–57.

[171] Handler JS, Preston AS, Steele RE. Factors affecting the differentiation of epithelial transport and responsiveness to hormones. Fed Proc 1984;43:2221–4.

[172] Misfeldt DS, Hamamoto ST, Pitelka DR. Transepithelial transport in cell culture. Proc Natl Acad Sci USA 1976;73:1212–6.

[173] Fuller SD, Simons K. Transferrin receptor polarity and recycling accuracy in "tight" and "leaky" strains of Madin–Darby canine kidney cells. J Cell Biol 1986;103:1767–79.

[174] Matlin KS, Simons K. Sorting of an apical plasma membrane glycoprotein occurs before it reaches the cell surface in cultured epithelial cells. J Cell Biol 1984;99:2131–9.

[175] Caplan MJ, Anderson HC, Palade GE, Jamieson JD. Intracellular sorting and polarized cell surface delivery of (Na^+K^+)ATPase, an endogenous component of MDCK cell basolateral plasma membranes. Cell 1986;46:623–31.

[176] Caplan MJ, Stow JL, Newman AP, Madri J, Anderson HC, Farquhar MG, et al. Dependence on pH of polarized sorting of secreted proteins. Nature 1987;329:632–5.

[177] O'Brien LE, Zegers MM, Mostov KE. Opinion: building epithelial architecture: Insights from three-dimensional culture models. Nat Rev Mol Cell Biol 2002;3:531–7.

[178] Zegers MM, O'Brien LE, Yu W, Datta A, Mostov KE. Epithelial polarity and tubulogenesis *in vitro*. Trends Cell Biol 2003;13:169–76.

[179] Schoenenberger CA, Matlin KS. Cell polarity and epithelial oncogenesis. Trends Cell Biol 1991;1:87–92.

[180] Yeaman C, Grindstaff KK, Nelson WJ. New perspectives on mechanisms involved in generating epithelial cell polarity. Physiol Rev 1999;79:73–98.

[181] Macara IG, Mili S. Polarity and differential inheritance: Universal attributes of life? Cell 2008;135:801–12.

[182] Bryant DM, Mostov KE. From cells to organs: building polarized tissue. Nat Rev Mol Cell Biol 2008;9:887–901.

[183] Lelongt B, Ronco P. Role of extracellular matrix in kidney development and repair. Pediatr Nephrol 2003;18:731–42.

[184] Wang AZ, Ojakian GK, Nelson WJ. Steps in the morphogenesis of a polarized epithelium. II. Disassembly and assembly of plasma membrane domains during reversal of epithelial cell polarity in multicellular epithelial (MDCK) cysts. J Cell Sci 1990;95(Pt 1):153–65.

[185] Balcarova-Stander J, Pfeiffer SE, Fuller SD, Simons K. Development of cell surface polarity in the epithelial Madin–Darby canine kidney (MDCK) cell line. EMBO J 1984;3:2687–94.

[186] Vega-Salas DE, Salas PJ, Gundersen D, Rodriguez-Boulan E. Formation of the apical pole of epithelial (Madin–Darby canine kidney) cells: polarity of an apical protein is independent of tight junctions while segregation of a basolateral marker requires cell–cell interactions. J Cell Biol 1987;104:905–16.

[187] Vega-Salas DE, Salas PJ, Rodriguez-Boulan E. Modulation of the expression of an apical plasma membrane protein of Madin-Darby canine kidney epithelial cells: cell–cell interactions control the appearance of a novel intracellular storage compartment. J Cell Biol 1987;104:1249–59.

[188] Capaldo CT, Macara IG. Depletion of E-cadherin disrupts establishment but not maintenance of cell junctions in

Madin—Darby canine kidney epithelial cells. Mol Biol Cell 2007;18:189—200.

[189] Takai Y, Miyoshi J, Ikeda W, Ogita H. Nectins and nectin-like molecules: roles in contact inhibition of cell movement and proliferation. Nat Rev Mol Cell Biol 2008;9:603—15.

[190] Ehrlich J, Hansen M, Nelson W. Spatio-temporal regulation of rac1 localization and lamellipodia dynamics during epithelial cell—cell adhesion. Dev Cell 2002;3:259—70.

[191] Laprise P, Tepass U. Novel insights into epithelial polarity proteins in *Drosophila*. Trends Cell Biol 2011;21:401—8.

[192] Pieczynski J, Margolis B. Protein complexes that control renal epithelial polarity. AJP: Renal Physiology 2011;300:F589—601.

[193] Bryant D, Datta A, Rodriguez-Fraticelli A, Peranen J, Martin-Belmonte F, et al. A molecular network for de novo generation of the apical surface and lumen. Nat Cell Biol 2010;12 (11):1035—45 advance online publication:

[194] Macara IG, Spang A. Closing the GAP between polarity and vesicle transport. Cell 2006;125:419—21.

[195] Ekblom P. Formation of basement membranes in the embryonic kidney: an immunohistological study. J Cell Biol 1981;91(1):1—10.

[196] Klein G, Langegger M, Timpl R, Ekblom P. Role of laminin a chain in the development of epithelial cell polarity. Cell 1988;55:331—41.

[197] Sorokin L, Sonnenberg A, Aumailley M, Timpl R, Ekblom P. Recognition of the laminin E8 cell-binding site by an integrin possessing the alpha 6 subunit is essential for epithelial polarization in developing kidney tubules. J Cell Biol 1990;111:1265—73.

[198] O'Brien LE, Jou TS, Pollack AL, Zhang Q, Hansen SH, Yurchenco P, et al. Rac1 orientates epithelial apical polarity through effects on basolateral laminin assembly. Nat Cell Biol 2001;3:831—8.

[199] Yu W, Datta A, Leroy P, O'Brien LE, Mak G, Jou TS, et al. Beta1-integrin orients epithelial polarity via Rac1 and laminin. Mol Biol Cell 2005;16:433—45.

[200] Cohen D, Fernandez D, Lázaro-Diéguez F, Müsch A. The serine/threonine kinase Par1b regulates epithelial lumen polarity via IRSp53-mediated cell—ECM signaling. J Cell Biol 2011;192:525—40.

[201] Masuda-Hirata M, Suzuki A, Amano Y, Yamashita K, Ide M, Yamanaka T, et al. Intracellular polarity protein PAR-1 regulates extracellular laminin assembly by regulating the dystroglycan complex. Genes Cells 2009;14:835—50.

[202] Martin-Belmonte F, Gassama A, Datta A, Yu W, Rescher U, Gerke V, et al. PTEN-mediated apical segregation of phosphoinositides controls epithelial morphogenesis through Cdc42. Cell 2007;128:383—97.

[203] Bacallao R, Antony C, Dotti C, Karsenti E, Stelzer EH, et al. The subcellular organization of Madin—Darby canine kidney cells during the formation of a polarized epithelium. J Cell Biol 1989;109:2817—32.

[204] Bre MH, Kreis TE, Karsenti E. Control of microtubule nucleation and stability in Madin—Darby canine kidney cells: the occurrence of noncentrosomal, stable detyrosinated microtubules. J Cell Biol 1987;105:1283—96.

[205] Bre MH, Pepperkok R, Hill AM, Levilliers N, Ansorge W, Stelzer EH, et al. Regulation of microtubule dynamics and nucleation during polarization in MDCK II cells. J Cell Biol 1990;111:3013—21.

[206] Bowen JR, Hwang D, Bai X, Roy D, Spiliotis ET. Septin GTPases spatially guide microtubule organization and plus end dynamics in polarizing epithelia. J Cell Biol 2011;194:187—97.

[207] Spiliotis ET, Gladfelter AS. Spatial Guidance of cell asymmetry: septin GTPases show the way. Traffic (Copenhagen, Denmark) 2012;13(2):195—203.

[208] Hotta A, Kawakatsu T, Nakatani T, Sato T, Matsui C, et al. Laminin-based cell adhesion anchors microtubule plus ends to the epithelial cell basal cortex through LL5α/β. J Cell Biol 2010;189:901—17.

[209] Mogensen MM, Tucker JB, Mackie JB, Prescott AR, Nathke IS. The adenomatous polyposis coli protein unambiguously localizes to microtubule plus ends and is involved in establishing parallel arrays of microtubule bundles in highly polarized epithelial cells. J Cell Biol 2002;157:1041—8.

[210] Reilein A, Nelson WJ. APC is a component of an organizing template for cortical microtubule networks. Nat Cell Biol 2005;7:463—73.

[211] Reilein A, Yamada S, Nelson WJ. Self-organization of an acentrosomal microtubule network at the basal cortex of polarized epithelial cells. J Cell Biol 2005;171:845—55.

[212] Cohen D, Brennwald PJ, Rodriguez-Boulan E, Müsch A. Mammalian PAR-1 determines epithelial lumen polarity by organizing the microtubule cytoskeleton. J Cell Biol 2004;164:717—27.

[213] Walter P, Lingappa VR. Mechanism of protein translocation across the endoplasmic reticulum membrane. Annu Rev Cell Biol 1986;2:499—516.

[214] Fuller SD, Bravo R, Simons K. An enzymatic assay reveals that proteins destined for the apical or basolateral domains of an epithelial cell line share the same late Golgi compartments. EMBO J 1985;4:297—307.

[215] Rindler MJ, Ivanov IE, Plesken H, Rodriguez-Boulan E, Sabatini DD. Viral glycoproteins destined for apical or basolateral plasma membrane domains traverse the same Golgi apparatus during their intracellular transport in doubly infected Madin—Darby canine kidney cells. J Cell Biol 1984;98:1304—19.

[216] Matlin KS, Simons K. Reduced temperature prevents transfer of a membrane glycoprotein to the cell surface but does not prevent terminal glycosylation. Cell 1983;34:233—43.

[217] Saraste J, Kuismanen E. Pre- and post-Golgi vacuoles operate in the transport of Semliki Forest virus membrane glycoproteins to the cell surface. Cell 1984;38:535—49.

[218] Griffiths G, Pfeiffer S, Simons K, Matlin K. Exit of newly synthesized membrane proteins from the trans cisterna of the Golgi complex to the plasma membrane. J Cell Biol 1985;101:949—64.

[219] Orci L, Ravazzola M, Amherdt M, Perrelet A, Powell SK, Quinn DL, et al. The trans-most cisternae of the Golgi complex: a compartment for sorting of secretory and plasma membrane proteins. Cell 1987;51:1039—51.

[220] Tooze J, Tooze SA, Fuller SD. Sorting of progeny coronavirus from condensed secretory proteins at the exit from the transGolgi network of AtT20 cells. J Cell Biol 1987;105:1215—26.

[221] Tooze SA, Huttner WB. Cell-free protein sorting to the regulated and constitutive secretory pathways. Cell 1990;60:837—47.

[222] Griffiths G, Simons K. The trans Golgi network: sorting at the exit site of the Golgi complex. Science 1986;234:438—43.

[223] Ang AL, Taguchi T, Francis S, Folsch H, Murrells LJ, Pypaert M, et al. Recycling endosomes can serve as intermediates during transport from the Golgi to the plasma membrane of MDCK cells. J Cell Biol 2004;167:531—43.

[224] Farr GA, Hull M, Mellman I, Caplan MJ. Membrane proteins follow multiple pathways to the basolateral cell surface in polarized epithelial cells. J Cell Biol 2009;186:269—82.

[225] Matlin K, Bainton DF, Pesonen M, Louvard D, Genty N, et al. Transepithelial transport of a viral membrane glycoprotein implanted into the apical plasma membrane of Madin—Darby canine kidney cells. I. Morphological evidence. J Cell Biol 1983;97:627—37.

[226] Pfeiffer S, Fuller SD, Simons K. Intracellular sorting and basolateral appearance of the G protein of vesicular stomatitis

virus in Madin—Darby canine kidney cells. J Cell Biol 1985;101:470—6.

[227] Misek DE, Bard E, Rodriguez-Boulan E. Biogenesis of epithelial cell polarity: intracellular sorting and vectorial exocytosis of an apical plasma membrane glycoprotein. Cell 1984;39:537—46.

[228] Sargiacomo M, Lisanti M, Graeve L, Le Bivic A, Rodriguez-Boulan E. Integral and peripheral protein composition of the apical and basolateral membrane domains in MDCK cells. J Membr Biol 1989;107:277—86.

[229] Le Bivic A, Sambuy Y, Mostov K, Rodriguez-Boulan E. Vectorial targeting of an endogenous apical membrane sialo-glycoprotein and uvomorulin in MDCK cells. J Cell Biol 1990;110:1533—9.

[230] Lisanti MP, Le Bivic A, Saltiel AR, Rodriguez-Boulan E. Preferred apical distribution of glycosyl-phosphatidylinositol (GPI) anchored proteins: a highly conserved feature of the polarized epithelial cell phenotype. J Membr Biol 1990;113:155—67.

[231] Patterson GH, Lippincott-Schwartz J. A photoactivatable GFP for selective photolabeling of proteins and cells. Science 2002;297:1873—7.

[232] Keppler A, Kindermann M, Gendreizig S, Pick H, Vogel H, et al. Labeling of fusion proteins of O6-alkylguanine-DNA alkyltransferase with small molecules *in vivo* and *in vitro*. Methods 2004;32:437—44.

[233] Keppler A, Arrivoli C, Sironi L, Ellenberg J. Fluorophores for live cell imaging of AGT fusion proteins across the visible spectrum. Biotechniques 2006;41:167—70 72, 74-75

[234] Caplan MJ, Forbush III B, Palade GE, Jamieson JD. Biosynthesis of the Na,K-ATPase in Madin—Darby canine kidney cells. Activation and cell surface delivery. J Biol Chem 1990;265:3528—34.

[235] Forbush III B, Hoffman JF. Evidence that ouabain binds to the same large polypeptide chain of dimeric Na,K-ATPase that is phosphorylated from Pi. Biochemistry 1979;18:2308—15.

[236] Forbush III B, Kaplan JH, Hoffman JF. Characterization of a new photoaffinity derivative of ouabain: labeling of the large polypeptide and of a proteolipid component of the Na, K-ATPase. Biochemistry 1978;17:3667—76.

[237] Hammerton RW, Krzeminski KA, Mays RW, Ryan TA, Wollner DA, et al. Mechanism for regulating cell surface distribution of Na$^+$,K($^+$)-ATPase in polarized epithelial cells. Science 1991;254:847—50.

[238] Mays RW, Siemers KA, Fritz BA, Lowe AW, van Meer G, et al. Hierarchy of mechanisms involved in generating Na/K-ATPase polarity in MDCK epithelial cells. J Cell Biol 1995;130:1105—15.

[239] Gottardi CJ, Caplan MJ. Delivery of Na$^+$,K$^+$)-ATPase in polarized epithelial cells. Science 1993;260:552—4. Author reply 4-6.

[240] Bartles JR, Feracci HM, Stieger B, Hubbard AL. Biogenesis of the rat hepatocyte plasma membrane *in vivo*: comparison of the pathways taken by apical and basolateral proteins using subcellular fractionation. J Cell Biol 1987;105:1241—51.

[241] Hoppe CA, Connolly TP, Hubbard AL. Transcellular transport of polymeric IgA in the rat hepatocyte: biochemical and morphological characterization of the transport pathway. J Cell Biol 1985;101:2113—23.

[242] Sztul ES, Howell KE, Palade GE. Biogenesis of the polymeric IgA receptor in rat hepatocytes. II. Localization of its intracellular forms by cell fractionation studies. J Cell Biol 1985;100:1255—61.

[243] Larkin JM, Sztul ES, Palade GE. Phosphorylation of the rat hepatic polymeric IgA receptor. Proc Natl Acad Sci USA 1986;83:4759—63.

[244] Kipp H, Arias IM. Trafficking of canalicular ABC transporters in hepatocytes. Annu Rev Physiol 2002;64:595—608.

[245] Wakabayashi Y, Lippincott-Schwartz J, Arias IM. Intracellular trafficking of bile salt export pump (ABCB11) in polarized hepatic cells: constitutive cycling between the canalicular membrane and rab11-positive endosomes. Mol Biol Cell 2004;15:3485—96.

[246] Matter K, Brauchbar M, Bucher K, Hauri HP. Sorting of endogenous plasma membrane proteins occurs from two sites in cultured human intestinal epithelial cells (Caco-2). Cell 1990;60:429—37.

[247] Hauri HP, Quaroni A, Isselbacher KJ. Biogenesis of intestinal plasma membrane: posttranslational route and cleavage of sucrase-isomaltase. Proc Natl Acad Sci USA 1979;76:5183—6.

[248] Massey D, Feracci H, Gorvel JP, Rigal A, Soulie JM, et al. Evidence for the transit of aminopeptidase N through the basolateral membrane before it reaches the brush border of enterocytes. J Membr Biol 1987;96:19—25.

[249] Mostov KE, Deitcher DL. Polymeric immunoglobulin receptor expressed in MDCK cells transcytoses IgA. Cell 1986;46:613—21.

[250] Polishchuk R, Di Pentima A, Lippincott-Schwartz J. Delivery of raft-associated, GPI-anchored proteins to the apical surface of polarized MDCK cells by a transcytotic pathway. Nat Cell Biol 2004;6:297—307.

[251] Paladino S, Pocard T, Catino MA, Zurzolo C. GPI-anchored proteins are directly targeted to the apical surface in fully polarized MDCK cells. J Cell Biol 2006;172:1023—34.

[252] Hubbard AL, Stieger B, Bartles JR. Biogenesis of endogenous plasma membrane proteins in epithelial cells. Annu Rev Physiol 1989;51:755—70.

[253] Welling PA, Weisz OA. Sorting it out in endosomes: an emerging concept in renal epithelial cell transport regulation. Physiology (Bethesda) 2010;25:280—92.

[254] Lencer WI, Verkman AS, Arnaout MA, Ausiello DA, Brown D. Endocytic vesicles from renal papilla which retrieve the vasopressin-sensitive water channel do not contain a functional H$^+$ ATPase. J Cell Biol 1990;111:379—89.

[255] Fang L, Garuti R, Kim BY, Wade JB, Welling PA. The ARH adaptor protein regulates endocytosis of the ROMK potassium secretory channel in mouse kidney. J Clin Invest 2009;119:3278—89.

[256] Butterworth MB, Edinger RS, Frizzell RA, Johnson JP. Regulation of the epithelial sodium channel by membrane trafficking. Am J Physiol Renal Physiol 2009;296:F10—24.

[257] Schwartz GJ, Al-Awqati Q. Regulation of transepithelial H$^+$ transport by exocytosis and endocytosis. Annu Rev Physiol 1986;48:153—61.

[258] Mount DB. Regulated endocytosis of NCC. Am J Physiol Renal Physiol 2010;299:F297—9.

[259] Hu MC, Fan L, Crowder LA, Karim-Jimenez Z, Murer H, et al. Dopamine acutely stimulates Na$^+$/H$^+$ exchanger (NHE3) endocytosis via clathrin-coated vesicles: dependence on protein kinase A-mediated NHE3 phosphorylation. J Biol Chem 2001;276:26906—15.

[260] Pedemonte CH, Efendiev R, Bertorello AM. Inhibition of Na, K-ATPase by dopamine in proximal tubule epithelial cells. Semin Nephrol 2005;25:322—7.

[261] Gottlieb TA, Beaudry G, Rizzolo L, Colman A, Rindler M, Adesnik M, et al. Secretion of endogenous and exogenous proteins from polarized MDCK cell monolayers. Proc Natl Acad Sci USA 1986;83:2100—4.

[262] Jones LV, Compans RW, Davis AR, Bos TJ, Nayak DP. Surface expression of influenza virus neuraminidase, an amino-terminally anchored viral membrane glycoprotein, in polarized epithelial cells. Mol Cell Biol 1985;5:2181—9.

[263] Roth MG, Compans RW, Giusti L, Davis AR, Nayak DP, Gething MJ, et al. Influenza virus hemagglutinin expression is

polarized in cells infected with recombinant SV40 viruses carrying cloned hemagglutinin DNA. Cell 1983;33:435−43.

[264] Stephens EB, Compans RW, Earl P, Moss B. Surface expression of viral glycoproteins is polarized in epithelial cells infected with recombinant vaccinia viral vectors. EMBO J 1986;5:237−45.

[265] Green RF, Meiss HK, Rodriguez-Boulan E. Glycosylation does not determine segregation of viral envelope proteins in the plasma membrane of epithelial cells. J Cell Biol 1981;89:230−9.

[266] Roth MG, Fitzpatrick JP, Compans RW. Polarity of influenza and vesicular stomatitis virus maturation in MDCK cells: lack of a requirement for glycosylation of viral glycoproteins. Proc Natl Acad Sci USA 1979;76:6430−4.

[267] Carmosino M, Valenti G, Caplan M, Svelto M. Polarized traffic towards the cell surface: how to find the route. Biol Cell 2010;102:75−91.

[268] Davis CG, Lehrman MA, Russell DW, Anderson RG, Brown MS, et al. The J.D. mutation in familial hypercholesterolemia: amino acid substitution in cytoplasmic domain impedes internalization of LDL receptors. Cell 1986;45:15−24.

[269] Lazarovits J, Roth M. A single amino acid change in the cytoplasmic domain allows the influenza virus hemagglutinin to be endocytosed through coated pits. Cell 1988;53:743−52.

[270] Brewer CB, Roth MG. A single amino acid change in the cytoplasmic domain alters the polarized delivery of influenza virus hemagglutinin. J Cell Biol 1991;114:413−21.

[271] Thomas DC, Brewer CB, Roth MG. Vesicular stomatitis virus glycoprotein contains a dominant cytoplasmic basolateral sorting signal critically dependent upon a tyrosine. J Biol Chem 1993;268:3313−20.

[272] Thomas DC, Roth MG. The basolateral targeting signal in the cytoplasmic domain of glycoprotein G from vesicular stomatitis virus resembles a variety of intracellular targeting motifs related by primary sequence but having diverse targeting activities. J Biol Chem 1994;269:15732−9.

[273] Lin S, Naim HY, Roth MG. Tyrosine-dependent basolateral sorting signals are distinct from tyrosine-dependent internalization signals. J Biol Chem 1997;272:26300−5.

[274] Hunziker W, Mellman I. Expression of macrophage-lymphocyte Fc receptors in Madin−Darby canine kidney cells: polarity and transcytosis differ for isoforms with or without coated pit localization domains. J Cell Biol 1989;109:3291−302.

[275] Hunziker W, Fumey C. A di-leucine motif mediates endocytosis and basolateral sorting of macrophage IgG Fc receptors in MDCK cells. EMBO J 1994;13:2963−9.

[276] Matter K, Yamamoto EM, Mellman I. Structural requirements and sequence motifs for polarized sorting and endocytosis of LDL and Fc receptors in MDCK cells. J Cell Biol 1994;126:991−1004.

[277] Hunziker W, Harter C, Matter K, Mellman I. Basolateral sorting in MDCK cells requires a distinct cytoplasmic domain determinant. Cell 1991;66:907−20.

[278] Matter K, Hunziker W, Mellman I. Basolateral sorting of LDL receptor in MDCK cells: the cytoplasmic domain contains two tyrosine-dependent targeting determinants. Cell 1992;71:741−53.

[279] Jones BG, Thomas L, Molloy SS, Thulin CD, Fry MD, Walsh KA, et al. Intracellular trafficking of furin is modulated by the phosphorylation state of a casein kinase II site in its cytoplasmic tail. EMBO J 1995;14:5869−83.

[280] Simmen T, Nobile M, Bonifacino JS, Hunziker W. Basolateral sorting of furin in MDCK cells requires a phenylalanine-isoleucine motif together with an acidic amino acid cluster. Mol Cell Biol 1999;19:3136−44.

[281] Odorizzi G, Trowbridge IS. Structural requirements for major histocompatibility complex class II invariant chain trafficking in polarized Madin−Darby canine kidney cells. J Biol Chem 1997;272:11757−62.

[282] Cross GA. Eukaryotic protein modification and membrane attachment via phosphatidylinositol. Cell 1987;48:179−81.

[283] Lisanti MP, Caras IW, Davitz MA, Rodriguez-Boulan E. A glycophospholipid membrane anchor acts as an apical targeting signal in polarized epithelial cells. J Cell Biol 1989;109:2145−56.

[284] van Meer G. Polarity and polarized transport of membrane lipids in cultured epithelium. In: Matlin KS, Valentich JD, editors. Functional epithelial cells in culture. New York: Alan R. Liss; 1989. p. 43−69.

[285] Brown DA, Crise B, Rose JK. Mechanism of membrane anchoring affects polarized expression of two proteins in MDCK cells. Science 1989;245(4925):1499−501.

[286] Kundu A, Avalos RT, Sanderson CM, Nayak DP. Transmembrane domain of influenza virus neuraminidase, a type II protein, possesses an apical sorting signal in polarized MDCK cells. J Virol 1996;70:6508−15.

[287] Roth MG, Gundersen D, Patil N, Rodriguez-Boulan E. The large external domain is sufficient for the correct sorting of secreted or chimeric influenza virus hemagglutinins in polarized monkey kidney cells. J Cell Biol 1987;104:769−82.

[288] Mostov KE, Breitfeld P, Harris JM. An anchor-minus form of the polymeric immunoglobulin receptor is secreted predominantly apically in Madin−Darby canine kidney cells. J Cell Biol 1987;105:2031−6.

[289] Scheiffele P, Peranen J, Simons K. N-glycans as apical sorting signals in epithelial cells. Nature 1995;378:96−8.

[290] Mostov KE, Simister NE. Transcytosis. Cell 1985;43:389−90.

[291] Mostov KE, de Bruyn Kops A, Deitcher DL. Deletion of the cytoplasmic domain of the polymeric immunoglobulin receptor prevents basolateral localization and endocytosis. Cell 1986;47:359−64.

[292] Aroeti B, Kosen PA, Kuntz ID, Cohen FE, Mostov KE. Mutational and secondary structural analysis of the basolateral sorting signal of the polymeric immunoglobulin receptor. J Cell Biol 1993;123:1149−60.

[293] Reich V, Mostov K, Aroeti B. The basolateral sorting signal of the polymeric immunoglobulin receptor contains two functional domains. J Cell Sci 1996;109(Pt 8):2133−9.

[294] Casanova JE, Breitfeld PP, Ross SA, Mostov KE. Phosphorylation of the polymeric immunoglobulin receptor required for its efficient transcytosis. Science 1990;248:742−5.

[295] Wolosin JM, Forte JG. Stimulation of oxyntic cell triggers K^+ and Cl^- conductances in apical H^+K^+-ATPase membrane. Am J Physiol 1984;246:C537−45.

[296] Hersey SJ, Sachs G. Gastric acid secretion. Physiol Rev 1995;75:155−89.

[297] Dunbar LA, Caplan MJ. Ion pumps in polarized cells: Sorting and regulation of the Na^+, K^+- and H^+, K^+-ATPases. J Biol Chem 2001;276:29617−20.

[298] Gottardi CJ, Caplan MJ. An ion-transporting ATPase encodes multiple apical localization signals. J Cell Biol 1993;121:283−93.

[299] Muth TR, Gottardi CJ, Roush DL, Caplan MJ. A basolateral sorting signal is encoded in the alpha-subunit of Na-K-ATPase. Am J Physiol 1998;274:C688−96.

[300] Dunbar LA, Aronson P, Caplan MJ. A transmembrane segment determines the steady-state localization of an ion-transporting adenosine triphosphatase. J Cell Biol 2000;148:769−78.

[301] Courtois-Coutry N, Roush D, Rajendran V, McCarthy JB, Geibel J, Kashgarian M, et al. A tyrosine-based signal targets

H/K-ATPase to a regulated compartment and is required for the cessation of gastric acid secretion. Cell 1997;90:501—10.

[302] Wang T, Courtois-Coutry N, Giebisch G, Caplan MJ. A tyrosine-based signal regulates H-K-ATPase-mediated potassium reabsorption in the kidney. Am J Physiol 1998;275:F818—26.

[303] Chuang JZ, Sung CH. The cytoplasmic tail of rhodopsin acts as a novel apical sorting signal in polarized MDCK cells. J Cell Biol 1998;142:1245—56.

[304] Qi AD, Wolff SC, Nicholas RA. The apical targeting signal of the P2Y2 receptor is located in its first extracellular loop. J Biol Chem 2005;280:29169—75.

[305] Ahn J, Mundigl O, Muth TR, Rudnick G, Caplan MJ. Polarized expression of GABA transporters in Madin—Darby canine kidney cells and cultured hippocampal neurons. J Biol Chem 1996;271:6917—24.

[306] Pietrini G, Suh YJ, Edelmann L, Rudnick G, Caplan MJ. The axonal gamma-aminobutyric acid transporter GAT-1 is sorted to the apical membranes of polarized epithelial cells. J Biol Chem 1994;269:4668—74.

[307] Muth TR, Ahn J, Caplan MJ. Identification of sorting determinants in the C-terminal cytoplasmic tails of the gamma-aminobutyric acid transporters GAT-2 and GAT-3. J Biol Chem 1998;273:25616—27.

[308] Cheng J, Moyer BD, Milewski M, Loffing J, Ikeda M, et al. A Golgi-associated PDZ domain protein modulates cystic fibrosis transmembrane regulator plasma membrane expression. J Biol Chem 2002;277:3520—9.

[309] Milewski MI, Mickle JE, Forrest JK, Stafford DM, Moyer BD, Cheng J, et al. PDZ-binding motif is essential but not sufficient to localize the C terminus of CFTR to the apical membrane. J Cell Sci 2001;114:719—26.

[310] Moyer BD, Denton J, Karlson KH, Reynolds D, Wang S, Mickle JE, et al. PDZ-interacting domain in CFTR is an apical membrane polarization signal. J Clin Invest 1999;104:1353—61.

[311] Moyer BD, Duhaime M, Shaw C, Denton J, Reynolds D, et al. The PDZ-interacting domain of cystic fibrosis transmembrane conductance regulator is required for functional expression in the apical plasma membrane. J Biol Chem 2000;275:27069—74.

[312] Carmosino M, Gimenez I, Caplan M, Forbush B. Exon loss accounts for differential sorting of Na-K-Cl cotransporters in polarized epithelial cells. Mol Biol Cell 2008;19:4341—51.

[313] Al-Awqati Q. Plasticity in epithelial polarity of renal intercalated cells: Targeting of the H($^+$)-ATPase and band 3. Am J Physiol 1996;270:C1571—80.

[314] Alper SL, Stuart-Tilley A, Simmons CF, Brown D, Drenckhahn D. The fodrin-ankyrin cytoskeleton of choroid plexus preferentially colocalizes with apical Na$^+$K$^+$)-ATPase rather than with basolateral anion exchanger AE2. J Clin Invest 1994;93:1430—8.

[315] Gundersen D, Orlowski J, Rodriguez-Boulan E. Apical polarity of Na,K-ATPase in retinal pigment epithelium is linked to a reversal of the ankyrin-fodrin submembrane cytoskeleton. J Cell Biol 1991;112:863—72.

[316] Shiel MJ, Caplan MJ. Developmental regulation of membrane protein sorting in Drosophila embryos. Am J Physiol 1995;269: C207—16.

[317] Kornfeld S. Trafficking of lysosomal enzymes. FASEB J 1987;1:462—8.

[318] Maxfield FR. Weak bases and ionophores rapidly and reversibly raise the pH of endocytic vesicles in cultured mouse fibroblasts. J Cell Biol 1982;95:676—81.

[319] Martin GR, Timpl R. Laminin and other basement membrane components. Annu Rev Cell Biol 1987;3:57—85.

[320] Kondor-Koch C, Bravo R, Fuller SD, Cutler D, Garoff H. Exocytotic pathways exist to both the apical and the basolateral cell surface of the polarized epithelial cell MDCK. Cell 1985;43:297—306.

[321] Chung KN, Walter P, Aponte GW, Moore HP. Molecular sorting in the secretory pathway. Science 1989;243:192—7.

[322] Matlin KS. Ammonium chloride slows transport of the influenza virus hemagglutinin but does not cause mis-sorting in a polarized epithelial cell line. J Biol Chem 1986;261:15172—8.

[323] Pearse BM, Robinson MS. Clathrin, adaptors, and sorting. Annu Rev Cell Biol 1990;6:151—71.

[324] Beltzer JP, Spiess M. In vitro binding of the asialoglycoprotein receptor to the beta adaptin of plasma membrane coated vesicles. EMBO J 1991;10:3735—42.

[325] Ohno H, Stewart J, Fournier MC, Bosshart H, Rhee I, Miyatake S, et al. Interaction of tyrosine-based sorting signals with clathrin-associated proteins. Science 1995;269:1872—5.

[326] Pearse BM. Receptors compete for adaptors found in plasma membrane coated pits. EMBO J 1988;7:3331—6.

[327] Pearse BM. Assembly of the mannose-6-phosphate receptor into reconstituted clathrin coats. EMBO J 1985;4:2457—60.

[328] Ohno H, Tomemori T, Nakatsu F, Okazaki Y, Aguilar RC, Foelsch H, et al. MulB a novel adaptor medium chain expressed in polarized epithelial cells. FEBS Lett 1999;449: 215—20.

[329] Roush DL, Gottardi CJ, Naim HY, Roth MG, Caplan MJ. Tyrosine-based membrane protein sorting signals are differentially interpreted by polarized Madin—Darby canine kidney and LLC-PK1 epithelial cells. J Biol Chem 1998;273:26862—9.

[330] Folsch H, Ohno H, Bonifacino JS, Mellman I. A novel clathrin adaptor complex mediates basolateral targeting in polarized epithelial cells. Cell 1999;99:189—98.

[331] Deborde S, Perret E, Gravotta D, Deora A, Salvarezza S, Schreiner R, et al. Clathrin is a key regulator of basolateral polarity. Nature 2008;452:719—23.

[332] Marks MS, Woodruff L, Ohno H, Bonifacino JS. Protein targeting by tyrosine- and di-leucine-based signals: evidence for distinct saturable components. J Cell Biol 1996;135: 341—54.

[333] Rapoport I, Chen YC, Cupers P, Shoelson SE, Kirchhausen T. Dileucine-based sorting signals bind to the beta chain of AP-1 at a site distinct and regulated differently from the tyrosine-based motif-binding site. EMBO J 1998;17:2148—55.

[334] Staub O, Dho S, Henry P, Correa J, Ishikawa T, McGlade J, et al. domains of Nedd4 bind to the proline-rich PY motifs in the epithelial Na$^+$ channel deleted in Liddle's syndrome. EMBO J 1996;15:2371—80.

[335] Simons K, Wandinger-Ness A. Polarized sorting in epithelia. Cell 1990;62:207—10.

[336] Skibbens JE, Roth MG, Matlin KS. Differential extractability of influenza virus hemagglutinin during intracellular transport in polarized epithelial cells and nonpolar fibroblasts. J Cell Biol 1989;108:821—32.

[337] Arreaza G, Melkonian KA, LaFevre-Bernt M, Brown DA. Triton X-100-resistant membrane complexes from cultured kidney epithelial cells contain the Src family protein tyrosine kinase p62yes. J Biol Chem 1994;269:19123—7.

[338] Fanning AS, Anderson JM. PDZ domains and the formation of protein networks at the plasma membrane. Curr Top Microbiol Immunol 1998;228:209—33.

[339] Songyang Z, Fanning AS, Fu C, Xu J, Marfartia SM, Chishti AH, et al. Recognition of unique carboxyl-terminal motifs by distinct PDZ domains. Science 1997;275:73—7.

[340] Kim SK. Polarized signaling: basolateral receptor localization in epithelial cells by PDZ-containing proteins. Curr Opin Cell Biol 1997;9:853—9.

[341] Bhat MA, Izaddoost S, Lu Y, Cho KO, Choi KW, et al. Discs Lost, a novel multi-PDZ domain protein, establishes and maintains epithelial polarity. Cell 1999;96:833−45.

[342] Hall RA, Ostedgaard LS, Premont RT, Blitzer JT, Rahman N, Welsh MJ, et al. C-terminal motif found in the beta2-adrenergic receptor, P2Y1 receptor and cystic fibrosis transmembrane conductance regulator determines binding to the Na^+/H^+ exchanger regulatory factor family of PDZ proteins. Proc Natl Acad Sci USA 1998;95:8496−501.

[343] Short DB, Trotter KW, Reczek D, Kreda SM, Bretscher A, Boucher RC, et al. An apical PDZ protein anchors the cystic fibrosis transmembrane conductance regulator to the cytoskeleton. J Biol Chem 1998;273:19797−801.

[344] Wang S, Raab RW, Schatz PJ, Guggino WB, Li M. Peptide binding consensus of the NHE-RF-PDZ1 domain matches the C-terminal sequence of cystic fibrosis transmembrane conductance regulator (CFTR). FEBS Lett 1998;427:103−8.

[345] Ferro-Novick S, Jahn R. Vesicle fusion from yeast to man. Nature 1994;370:191−3.

[346] Ikonen E, Tagaya M, Ullrich O, Montecucco C, Simons K. Different requirements for NSF, SNAP, and Rab proteins in apical and basolateral transport in MDCK cells. Cell 1995;81:571−80.

[347] Inoue T, Nielsen S, Mandon B, Terris J, Kishore BK, et al. SNAP-23 in rat kidney: colocalization with aquaporin-2 in collecting duct vesicles. Am J Physiol 1998;275:F752−60.

[348] Low SH, Chapin SJ, Wimmer C, Whiteheart SW, Komuves LJ, Mostov KE, et al. The SNARE machinery is involved in apical plasma membrane trafficking in MDCK cells. J Cell Biol 1998;141:1503−13.

[349] Guo W, Roth D, Walch-Solimena C, Novick P. The exocyst is an effector for Sec4p, targeting secretory vesicles to sites of exocytosis. EMBO J 1999;18:1071−80.

[350] Grindstaff KK, Yeaman C, Anandasabapathy N, Hsu SC, Rodriguez-Boulan E, Scheller RH, et al. Sec6/8 complex is recruited to cell−cell contacts and specifies transport vesicle delivery to the basal-lateral membrane in epithelial cells. Cell 1998;93:731−40.

[351] Fish EM, Molitoris BA. Alterations in epithelial polarity and the pathogenesis of disease states. N Engl J Med 1994;330:1580−8.

[352] Stein M, Wandinger-Ness A, Roitbak T. Altered trafficking and epithelial cell polarity in disease. Trends Cell Biol 2002;12:374−81.

[353] Calzada MJ, Esteban MA, Feijoo-Cuaresma M, Castellanos MC, Naranjo-Suarez S, Temes E, et al. von Hippel-Lindau tumor suppressor protein regulates the assembly of intercellular junctions in renal cancer cells through hypoxia-inducible factor-independent mechanisms. Cancer Res 2006;66:1553−60.

[354] Baas AF, Kuipers J, van der Wel NN, Batlle E, Koerten HK, Peters PJ, et al. Complete polarization of single intestinal epithelial cells upon activation of LKB1 by STRAD. Cell 2004;116:457−66.

[355] Edelstein CL, Ling H, Schrier RW. The nature of renal cell injury. Kidney Int 1997;51:1341−51.

[356] Oliver J. Correlations of structure and function and mechanisms of recovery in acute tubular necrosis. Am J Med 1953;15:535−57.

[357] Oliver J, Mac DM, Tracy A. The pathogenesis of acute renal failure associated with traumatic and toxic injury; renal ischemia, nephrotoxic damage and the ischemic episode. J Clin Invest 1951;30:1307−439.

[358] Thadhani R, Pascual M, Bonventre JV. Acute renal failure. N Engl J Med 1996;334:1448−60.

[359] Molitoris BA, Chan LK, Shapiro JI, Conger JD, Falk SA. Loss of epithelial polarity: a novel hypothesis for reduced proximal tubule Na^+ transport following ischemic injury. J Membr Biol 1989;107:119−27.

[360] Spiegel DM, Wilson PD, Molitoris BA. Epithelial polarity following ischemia: a requirement for normal cell function. Am J Physiol 1989;256:F430−6.

[361] Bacallao R, Garfinkel A, Monke S, Zampighi G, Mandel LJ. ATP depletion: a novel method to study junctional properties in epithelial tissues. I. Rearrangement of the actin cytoskeleton. J Cell Sci 1994;107(Pt 12):3301−13.

[362] Golenhofen N, Doctor RB, Bacallao R, Mandel LJ. Actin and villin compartmentation during ATP depletion and recovery in renal cultured cells. Kidney Int 1995;48:1837−45.

[363] Mandel LJ, Doctor RB, Bacallao R. ATP depletion: a novel method to study junctional properties in epithelial tissues. II. Internalization of $Na^+,K(^+)$-ATPase and E-cadherin. J Cell Sci 1994;107(Pt 12):3315−24.

[364] Bush KT, Tsukamoto T, Nigam SK. Selective degradation of E-cadherin and dissolution of E-cadherin-catenin complexes in epithelial ischemia. Am J Physiol Renal Physiol 2000;278:F847−52.

[365] Gailit J, Colflesh D, Rabiner I, Simone J, Goligorsky MS. Redistribution and dysfunction of integrins in cultured renal epithelial cells exposed to oxidative stress. Am J Physiol 1993;264:F149−57.

[366] Goligorsky MS, Lieberthal W, Racusen L, Simon EE. Integrin receptors in renal tubular epithelium: new insights into pathophysiology of acute renal failure. Am J Physiol 1993;264:F1−8.

[367] Noiri E, Romanov V, Czerwinski G, Gailit J, DiBona GF, Som P, et al. Adhesion molecules and tubular obstruction in acute renal failure. Ren Fail 1996;18:513−5.

[368] Noiri E, Gailit J, Sheth D, Magazine H, Gurrath M, Muller G, et al. Cyclic RGD peptides ameliorate ischemic acute renal failure in rats. Kidney Int 1994;46:1050−8.

[369] Piwon N, Gunther W, Schwake M, Bosl MR, Jentsch TJ. ClC-5 Cl-channel disruption impairs endocytosis in a mouse model for Dent's disease. Nature 2000;408:369−73.

[370] Novarino G, Weinert S, Rickheit G, Jentsch TJ. Endosomal chloride-proton exchange rather than chloride conductance is crucial for renal endocytosis. Science 2010;328:1398−401.

[371] McCrea HJ, De Camilli P. Mutations in phosphoinositide metabolizing enzymes and human disease. Physiology (Bethesda) 2009;24:8−16.

[372] Chapin HC, Caplan MJ. The cell biology of polycystic kidney disease. J Cell Biol 2010;191:701−10.

[373] Grantham JJ. 1992 Homer Smith Award. Fluid secretion, cellular proliferation, and the pathogenesis of renal epithelial cysts. J Am Soc Nephrol 1993;3:1841−57.

[374] Sullivan LP, Wallace DP, Grantham JJ. Epithelial transport in polycystic kidney disease. Physiol Rev 1998;78:1165−91.

[375] Avner ED, Sweeney Jr. WE, Nelson WJ. Abnormal sodium pump distribution during renal tubulogenesis in congenital murine polycystic kidney disease. Proc Natl Acad Sci USA 1992;89:7447−51.

[376] Wilson PD, Sherwood AC, Palla K, Du J, Watson R, et al. Reversed polarity of $Na(^+)-K(^+)$-ATPase: mislocation to apical plasma membranes in polycystic kidney disease epithelia. Am J Physiol 1991;260:F420−30.

[377] Brill SR, Ross KE, Davidow CJ, Ye M, Grantham JJ, et al. Immunolocalization of ion transport proteins in human autosomal dominant polycystic kidney epithelial cells. Proc Natl Acad Sci USA 1996;93:10206−11.

[378] Freeman TC. Parallel patterns of cell-specific gene expression during enterocyte differentiation and maturation in the small intestine of the rabbit. Differentiation 1995;59:179−92.

[379] Sullivan LP, Grantham JJ. Mechanisms of fluid secretion by polycystic epithelia. Kidney Int 1996;49:1586−91.

2

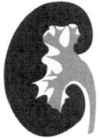

Mechanisms of Ion Transport across Cell Membranes

Luis Reuss and Guillermo A. Altenberg

Department of Cell Physiology and Molecular Biophysics, and Center for Membrane Protein Research,
Texas Tech University Health Sciences Center, Lubbock, Texas, TX, USA

INTRODUCTION

Ion transport by cell membranes serves two important purposes in pluricellular organisms, the maintenance of the volume and composition of the intracellular fluid, and the preservation and regulation of the volume and composition of the extracellular fluid. The first process involves fluxes between the cell interior and its surrounding medium ("homocellular" transport[91]), whereas the second one occurs because of transport across epithelial and endothelial cell layers (transcellular or "heterocellular" transport[91]). In addition, ion transport across intracellular membranes, which surround the nucleus and cytoplasmic organelles, is essential to generate and maintain ion concentration gradients between those organelles and the cytosol.

Needless to say, the narrowly regulated volume and ionic composition — inorganic cations (Na^+, K^+, H^+, Ca^{2+}, Mg^{2+}) and anions (Cl^-, phosphate, bicarbonate) — of the intracellular fluid is essential for cell survival, and for the cell's normal functions. A similar argument can be made for the extracellular fluid compartments, that is, whole body balances of water and the ions listed above are essential for the survival, growth, and development of the organism.

Our main focus in this chapter will be on the molecular mechanisms of ion transport by the plasma membranes of cells. The cell membrane is a phospholipid bilayer doped with abundant proteins. This structure is both a barrier between the cytoplasm and the extracellular fluid, and the pathway for ion and water transport between the two compartments. For most ions, the lipid bilayer is the barrier and membrane transport proteins are the pathway for these fluxes.

The Cell Interior and Extracellular Fluid Have Different Ionic Compositions

A crucial property of living cells is their capacity to maintain an internal (intracellular or cytosolic) composition different from that of the surrounding (extracellular) medium. As with all other ionic solutions, the cytosol and the extracellular fluid obey the principle of macroscopic (or bulk) electroneutrality, that is, the sum of cationic and anionic charges are the same in each compartment. As discussed below, there is a microscopic deviation from this principle at the membrane surfaces when there is a difference in electrical potential across the membrane, but the actual differences between anion and cation concentrations are extremely small.

The maintenance of ionic asymmetry between intracellular and extracellular compartments is based on the existence of the cell membrane (or plasma membrane), which separates the cell interior from its surroundings. As shown schematically in Figure 2.1, the membrane is a phospholipid bilayer, with high protein content. Membrane proteins can span the phospholipid bilayer (integral proteins, some of which span the membrane and are known as transmembrane proteins) or can be associated with the membrane surface (peripheral proteins). Transmembrane proteins perform many functions, including translocation of ions, nonelectrolytes, and water across the membrane (transport function, the main theme of this chapter); sensing and early transduction of extracellular events (signaling function); attachment to components of the cytoskeleton, the extracellular matrix or adjacent cells (adhesion function).

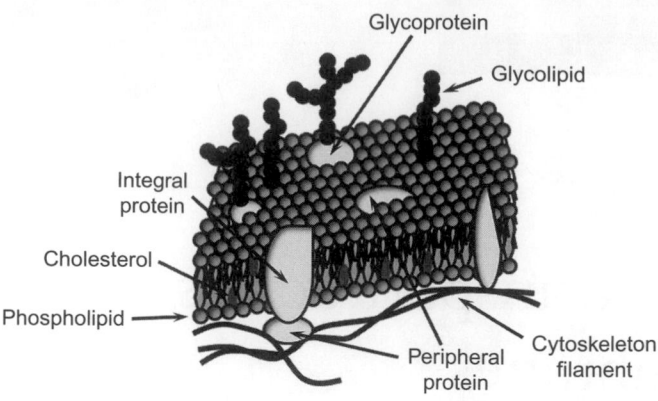

FIGURE 2.1 Structure of the plasma membrane. This two-dimensional representation of the plasma membrane is based on the fluid-mosaic model[95,96] modified according to recent observations.[30,59,71,94,112] The membrane is a lipid bilayer that contains integral and peripheral membrane proteins. The bilayer is largely made of phospholipids that have polar heads and hydrophobic tails. The hydrophobic tails face each other, while the polar head groups face the adjacent aqueous solutions (extracellular fluid and cytosol). In addition, the membrane contains glycolipids and cholesterol. The phospholipid compositions of the two leaflets differ; e.g., phosphatidyl inositol is more abundant in the inner leaflet. Additionally, certain areas of the membrane form *lipid rafts* (see text). A small fraction of the membrane surface area is occupied by either strongly-bound proteins (integral membrane proteins), some crossing the membrane one or more times (transmembrane proteins) or loosely attached (peripheral) membrane proteins. Membrane proteins can be glycosylated or have other post-translational modifications (not shown). Some membrane proteins are attached to components of the cytoskeleton or the exoskeleton, directly or via other proteins. Integral membrane proteins can associate forming oligomers, as well as macromolecular complexes.

Two properties of the cell membrane are needed to generate and maintain the intracellular ion composition essential for life: the barrier function and the transport function. This distinction is didactically convenient, although both functions are clearly linked. By the barrier function, the cell membrane prevents the flux of certain molecules; by the transport function, it translocates certain molecules. These two functions bring about a steady-state in which cell volume and composition are kept constant and appropriate for cell survival. Relative to the extracellular fluid, some substances are maintained at high concentrations (e.g., K^+ and ATP), whereas others are maintained at low concentrations (e.g., Ca^{2+} and Cl^-) inside the cell.

The cell interior is not homogeneous, but is rather a complex medium including a highly structured cytoplasm (cytosol and cytoskeleton) and numerous organelles. The latter are separated from the cytosol by their membranes. Exchanges between each organelle and the cytosol occur by mechanisms similar to those present in the plasma membrane. In this chapter, we will not address organelle membrane function.

The Plasma Membrane: Structure Related to Function

The plasma membrane, which is 3–8 nm thick, is largely formed by phospholipids, organized in a bilayer, and proteins. The main phospholipids are phosphatidylcholine and phosphatidylethanolamine, with lower levels of phosphatidylinositol, phosphatidylserine, and phosphatidylglycerol, and sterols (cholesterol, ergosterol, zymosterol).[6,63] The precise proportions vary among cells. Hydrophobic or amphipathic proteins are essential components of biological membranes. In most membranes, the w/w protein: lipid ratio is *ca.* 1, and therefore a membrane protein of *ca.* 40 kDa is surrounded by 50–55 lipid molecules.

Experimental work during the last two or three decades has ruled out the "fluid-mosaic" (Singer and Nicolson) model of membrane structure.[95,96] In this model, biological membranes are considered two-dimensional viscous phospholipid bilayers in which integral membrane proteins are randomly distributed and free to rotate and diffuse laterally. A main objection is the demonstration of asymmetry in the lipid composition of the membrane.[71] The current view is that the plasma membrane is a highly-organized and asymmetric structure composed of lipids and proteins.[30] There are lateral differences in lipid composition within a monolayer; sphingolipids, sterols, and phosphatidylcholine predominate on the extracellular leaflet, whereas the cytoplasmic leaflet is enriched in phosphatidylinositol, phosphatidylethanolamine, phosphatidylserine, and phosphatidic acid, which results in a negative charge that facilitates binding of peripheral and transmembrane proteins.[71] In addition, many membrane proteins cluster with others in microdomains, in which the lipid composition may differ from that of the bulk bilayer. These clusters are maintained by intramembrane lipid–lipid, protein–protein, and protein–lipid interactions, as well as interactions with intracellular molecules (cytoskeletal proteins) and extracellular components (extracellular matrix proteins and membrane proteins of adjacent cells). It is clear that the two monolayers also differ in composition. Lipid rafts are microdomains in the submicron range in which cholesterol and sphingolipids are enriched in the external leaflet, and cholesterol and phospholipids with saturated fatty acids in the internal leaflet of the plasma membrane. The surrounding bilayer is abundant in unsaturated fatty acids and contains more fluid than that in the raft.[59] Lipid rafts exclude certain proteins and organize others in specific oligomeric structures.[94] Rapid changes in composition and location in the membrane are essential for the role that lipid rafts play in signaling processes (e.g., receptor tyrosine kinases).

Phospholipids in the plasma membrane are not just a barrier and a "solvent" for membrane proteins, but play important roles in signaling processes. Inositol-1,4,5-triphosphate, diacylglycerol, and phosphatidylinositol-3,4,5-triphosphate (derived from phosphatidylinositol) are good examples.[9,72,73] Phosphatidylinositol 4,5-bisphosphate (PIP_2) exerts regulatory effects on a number of ion channels and other transport proteins. Its effects can be stimulatory or inhibitory and appear to require PIP_2 binding.[49,102] Other signaling molecules originating from plasma membrane phospholipids are arachidonic and docosahexaenoic acids, which are generated from phosphatidylethanolamine, phosphatidylcholine, and phosphatidylinositol by the action of phospholipase A_2. Certainly, being a dielectric is not the only function of the phospholipid moiety of the cell membrane.

This new notion of the structure of the plasma membrane[112] is based on results of biophysical studies, including fluorescence recovery after photo-bleaching, single-particle tracking techniques, optical trapping by laser tweezers, and fluorescence correlation spectroscopy. These methods, applied to cell membranes, have yielded quantitative dynamic information on the distribution, mobility, and compartmentalization of membrane proteins.[112] Biochemical, molecular, and physiological studies indicate that membrane transport proteins are not randomly distributed, but that they undergo homo- and hetero-associations,[59] and that these associations may have functional significance. A case in point is the proposed proximity between plasma membrane Ca^{2+} channels and Ca^{2+}-sensitive proteins, including Ca^{2+}-activated channels: Ca^{2+} entry results in a large, but highly localized, increase in intracellular $[Ca^{2+}]$, because of effective cytosolic buffering, and thus its signaling effects may be quite local.[70]

In summary, the current view of the structure of the plasma membrane is that of a compartmentalized two-dimensional structure, mosaic-like, with less fluidity than proposed by the Singer—Nicolson model. The phospholipids have signaling functions in addition to previously recognized ones. The mobility of membrane proteins may be restricted by the structure of the lipid domain, interactions with cytoskeletal proteins or other cytoplasmic components, and/or homo- and hetero-associations with other integral membrane proteins. Future studies of membrane transport proteins along these lines are likely to reveal important aspects of their function and regulation in health and disease (see Chapter 14).

The Plasma Membrane is Selectively Permeable

The barrier and transport functions of the plasma membrane are determined by its composition, mostly regarding lipids and integral transmembrane proteins

(for membrane structure, see references [59,95,96] and [112]; for a review of membrane proteins, see [103]). When the membrane is *permeable* to a specific molecule, then that molecule can cross the membrane. *Permeability* (cm s^{-1}) is a property of a specific membrane for a specific molecule. The amount of substance that crosses the membrane per unit of time and membrane area is the *flux*. Using radioactive techniques, unidirectional fluxes can be measured (e.g., in case of a cell, influx and efflux); the *net flux* is the difference between the two unidirectional fluxes. A finite net flux denotes the presence of either a net driving force across the membrane or an active process.

Permeation of a specific molecule can take place through the lipid phase (i.e., *solubility diffusion*) and/or through membrane proteins (i.e., *mediated transport*). Solubility diffusion always results in equilibrating transport, dissipating differences in concentration or electrochemical potential (see the section "Diffusion and Electrodiffusion," below). In contrast, mediated transport can either dissipate or generate differences in chemical or electrochemical potentials across the membrane. An example of mediated transport is the operation of the sodium pump, the Na^+,K^+-ATPase.

The lipid phase of the plasma membrane is hydrophobic, and therefore has high permeability for lipophilic molecules and low permeability for hydrophilic molecules. Thus, a protein-free phospholipid membrane has a high permeability for nonpolar small molecules such as O_2 and CO_2, a much lower permeability for uncharged small polar substances such as water, urea, and glycerol, and an extremely low permeability for ions and larger uncharged polar molecules, such as glucose. Most molecules are measurably permeable across plasma membranes. However, the diffusive permeability coefficients range over several orders of magnitude. It is thought that hydrophilic molecules permeate the membrane bilayer to some extent, because the thermal motion of the phospholipid molecules causes transient kinks in the bilayer structure.

Transport proteins can be classified in four groups, namely pores, channels, carriers (also referred to as transporters), and pumps (see next section). The expression of some transport proteins can be specific to tissue, cell, and sometimes membrane domain. Others are expressed in most, if not all, cell membranes. The functional significance of transport proteins is apparent in two realms. Some are primarily related to the establishment and maintenance of cellular composition (intracellular "homeostasis"), such as the Na^+,K^+-ATPase and K^+ channels in most animal cells. Others are primarily related to specific cell functions, such as excitability (e.g., the tetrodotoxin-sensitive, voltage-activated Na^+ channel in nerve and muscle), and transepithelial Na^+ transport (e.g., the amiloride-sensitive, voltage-insensitive Na$^+$ channel in the apical membrane of certain epithelial cells).

A *pore* is an aqueous communication between both sides of the membrane, accessible to both sides at all times — that is, it is always "open" (permeable). A *channel* is also an aqueous communication between the two sides of the membrane, but it opens and closes stochastically by changes in conformation called *gating*; when open, a channel is accessible from both sides of the membrane, when closed, it is impermeable. A *carrier* is a membrane transport protein whose permeation pathway is not simultaneously accessible to both sides of the membrane, but to one side at a time; changes in conformation change the orientation of the carrier, moving the transported ion to the other side; an appropriate simplified description is that a carrier has two gates and they are never open at the same time. Finally, a *pump* has the properties of a carrier, but in addition it is coupled to a metabolic energy source, in most cases hydrolysis of ATP.

MECHANISMS OF ION TRANSPORT

Ion Transport can be Active or Passive

The definitions of active and passive transport are thermodynamic. Passive transport occurs in the direction expected for the existing driving force, which in the case of ions involves the chemical gradient (given by the difference in concentration between the two sides of the membrane) and the electrical gradient (given by the transmembrane electrical potential difference or membrane voltage). In other words, passive transport is energetically downhill. In contrast, active transport takes place in the absence of or against the prevailing electrochemical gradient. In other words, active transport is energetically uphill, and therefore requires an energy input. Depending on the origin of this energy, one can distinguish two types of active transport.

Primary active transport is characterized by the direct use of metabolic energy, supplied by light, redox potential or ATP hydrolysis. In most cases of plasma membrane primary active transport in eukaryotic organisms, the energy is provided by the hydrolysis of ATP, a process catalyzed by the same molecule that performs the transport. Hence, in this case the transporter is also an ATP hydrolase (ATPase). Transporters responsible for primary active transport are referred to as pumps. In plasma membranes of most animal cells there can be expression of one or more of four ion-transporting ATPases. These are the Na$^+$,K$^+$-ATPase, H$^+$-ATPase, H$^+$,K$^+$-ATPase, and Ca^{2+}-ATPase.

Secondary active transport is characterized by the indirect use of metabolic energy. The energy stored in the electrochemical gradient of one substrate is utilized to transport actively another species (ion or molecule). In animal cells, including those from epithelia, secondary active transport is most frequently linked to Na$^+$ transport. The Na$^+$,K$^+$-ATPase establishes an electrochemical potential gradient for Na$^+$ across the plasma membrane, which includes chemical (high extracellular and low intracellular [Na$^+$]) and electrical components (cell electrically negative to the extracellular compartment), both contributing to a net driving force favoring Na$^+$ entry into the cell. This gradient is then utilized by carriers to actively transport other substrates, by coupling their translocation to that of Na$^+$ at the molecular level.

Depending on the directions of the fluxes, there are two kinds of secondary active transport: One is *co-transport* (or *symport*) in which the substrates move in the same direction, such as downhill for Na$^+$ and uphill for the co-transported substrate (e.g., Na$^+$-glucose co-transport). The other one is *countertransport* (also *antiport* or *exchange*), in which the fluxes are in opposite directions (e.g., Na$^+$–H$^+$ exchange). In most instances, secondary active transport involves only two species (Na$^+$ and another substrate), but in some cases there are three: an example is the Na$^+$-K$^+$-2Cl$^-$ co-transporter, an electroneutral symporter that is expressed principally in epithelial cells. This transporter accounts for uphill Cl$^-$ uptake, a step necessary for Cl$^-$ absorption (e.g., in the apical membrane of cells of the thick ascending limb of the loop of Henle) or Cl$^-$ secretion (e.g., in the basolateral membrane of crypt cells in the intestine and epithelial cells in the airway). For quantitative analyses of membrane transport processes, see Läuger,[64] Macey and Moura,[67] and Stein.[99]

Active and Passive Transport Processes can be Evaluated by Considering Direction of Electrochemical Potential Difference (Driving Force)

As stated above, passive transport is energetically downhill, driven by the pre-existing driving force; this force depends on the chemical or electrochemical gradient, for uncharged and charged solutes, respectively. Under isothermal conditions the driving force encompasses differences in concentration, electrical potential, and/or pressure across the membrane. Under these conditions, the electrochemical potential difference ($\Delta\overline{\mu}_j$) for the jth ion is given by Eq. (2.1):

$$\Delta\overline{\mu}_j = z_j V_m F + RT \ln\left(\frac{C_j^i}{C_j^o}\right) + \Delta P \overline{V}_j \qquad (2.1)$$

where z is the valence, V_m is the membrane voltage, F is the Faraday constant, R is the gas constant, T is the absolute temperature, C is the concentration, i and o refer to the two sides of the membrane (inside and outside, respectively), ΔP is the transmembrane hydrostatic pressure difference, and $\overline{V}_j$ is the ion's partial molar volume. The electrochemical potential has the three components defined above, given by the three terms on the right side of the equation. Across animal cell membranes, steady-state hydrostatic or osmotic pressure differences are small or nil (see Chapter 4), and therefore the third term of Eq. (2.1) is eliminated, yielding:

$$\Delta\overline{\mu}_j = z_j V_m F + RTln\left(\frac{C_j^i}{C_j^o}\right) \qquad (2.2)$$

This equation is used to evaluate the driving force for ion transport under isobaric conditions. In the case of nonelectrolytes, $z = 0$ and the first term of Eq. (2.2) can also be eliminated, yielding:

$$\Delta\mu_j = RTln\left(\frac{C_j^i}{C_j^o}\right) \qquad (2.3)$$

where $\Delta\mu_j$ denotes the chemical potential difference. This equation describes the driving force for nonelectrolyte transport.

From Eq. (2.2) (under isobaric and isothermal conditions), Ussing[111] derived the flux-ratio equation, a fundamental expression which provides a thermodynamic test for active or passive transport:

$$J_{in}/J_{out} = (C_i/C_o)exp(zV_mF/RT) \qquad (2.4)$$

where J is flux (the subscripts denote influx and efflux, respectively). The test proceeds as follows: the ratio of unidirectional fluxes (J_{in}/J_{out}) is determined experimentally, and the driving forces are measured; if the ratio deviates from the prediction given by Eq. (2.4), which evaluates the passive driving forces, then active transport is suspected. Deviations from the flux-ratio equation can also result from the presence of exchange diffusion and single-file diffusion, as discussed by Schultz.[90]

Pathways and Mechanisms of Passive Transport

Passive transport can be *via* the lipid bilayer (solubility diffusion) or *via* transmembrane proteins (mediated). Solubility diffusion is a permeation process that involves the movement of a molecule dissolved in the aqueous solution bathing one side of the membrane into the lipid phase of the membrane, then across the membrane, and then from the membrane lipid into the solution bathing the opposite side. Clearly, two processes are involved. The first one ("solubility") governs the fluxes at the solution–membrane interface, and depends on the relative solubility of the molecule in lipid and water, which can be quantified by the oil–water partition coefficient, β, a coefficient equal to the ratio of the molecule's steady-state concentrations in lipid and water. The second process ("diffusion") governs the solute translocation within the membrane lipid, which depends largely on the mass and shape of solute molecules. The lipid solubility of the molecule is the main factor determining its permeability via the lipid moiety of the membrane.

Mediated transport is the mode of transmembrane transport of substances with very low solubility in phospholipids, that is, charged and polar substances. The transport proteins provide a hydrophilic path across the membrane, through which the solute permeates or a narrow pore in which amino acid charges replace the water molecules surrounding the ion or polar molecule in free solution.

Diffusion and Electrodiffusion

Diffusion and electrodiffusion are the main processes of passive solute transport across homogeneous phases (e.g., lipid membranes or aqueous pores) by independent motion of the solute molecules. Diffusion applies to uncharged particles and electrodiffusion to ions. Although diffusion does not strictly apply to ion transport, its analysis is simpler and helps in understanding electrodiffusion.

Diffusion of a solute in aqueous solution is the result of the random thermal motion of solute molecules. In the absence of convection, if there are differences in concentration between different sectors of the solution, then random solute motion will tend to make its distribution homogeneous (equilibrating transport). All solute particles move randomly at uniform average velocities, dependent on the solution temperature. Hence, more particles will tend to move from regions of high concentration to sectors of low concentration than in the opposite direction, simply because there are more particles per unit volume in the high concentration regions. In other words, differences in concentration cause unequal unidirectional fluxes in a regime of diffusion because of differences in the number of particles flowing in each direction per unit of time, not because of different velocities of individual particles flowing in one direction or the other. In diffusion, the molecules move independently of each other and of other particles present in the solution, that is, there is no flux coupling. This is the *independence principle*.

Diffusion of a nonelectrolyte in solution is described by Fick's first law[34]:

$$J_s = -D_s\frac{dC_s}{dx} \qquad (2.5)$$

where J_s is the solute flux (moles $cm^2 sec^{-1}$), D_s is the solute diffusion coefficient ($cm^2 sec^{-1}$) and dC_s/d_x is the concentration gradient. The negative sign denotes the direction of the flux.

Fick's second law of diffusion[34] considers the time course of the process:

$$\frac{dC}{dt} = D_s \frac{d^2 C_s}{dx^2} \qquad (2.6)$$

where dC/dt is the rate of change in solute concentration, and x denotes distance.

The average time required by diffusing particles to cover a given distance is inversely proportional to the diffusion coefficient, and directly proportional to the square of the traveled distance. Einstein approximated the second law of diffusion with $\lambda = (D_s t)^{1/2}$, where λ is the traveled distance in the x-axis. The dependence of t on the square of the distance makes diffusion a very slow transport process for long distances. For a typical $D_s = 10^{-5}$ cm^2 sec^{-1}, it takes 1 millisecond for the solute to diffuse 1 μm, but it takes 1000 seconds (*ca.* 16.7 minutes) to diffuse 1 mm. Convective flow (see Chapter 9) is a much more effective mass transport mechanism for long distances.

Now we consider a thin lipid membrane of thickness δ_m separating two aqueous compartments (Figure 2.2). The solutions on both sides are well stirred, so that the solute concentrations are homogeneous in both. Inserting the solute partition coefficient (β_s) in Eq. (2.5) (β_s denotes lipid solubility relative to water solubility), we obtain the following expression for the solute flux:

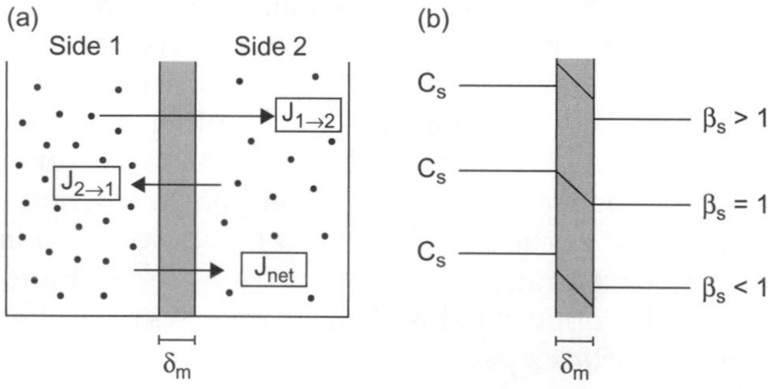

$$J_s = -\frac{D_s \beta_s}{\delta_m} \Delta C_s \qquad (2.7)$$

where ΔC_s is the solute concentration difference between the two solutions. Defining the solute permeability (P_s) as $P_s = D_s \beta_s / \Delta_m$, Eq. (2.7) reduces to:

$$J_s = -P_s \Delta C_s \qquad (2.8)$$

The diffusive permeability coefficient of the membrane relates the flux to the driving force and denotes the ease with which the membrane permits mass transfer of a particular species. Its units are cm s^{-1}, those of velocity. In the simple case of a nonelectrolyte, under isothermal and isobaric conditions, the permeability (P) of solute s is given by a rearrangement of Eq. (2.8): $P_s = J_s / \Delta C_s$. This is the phenomenological, experimentally determined permeability, calculated by dividing the steady-state solute flux by the difference between the solute concentrations of well-stirred bathing solutions. The other definition of diffusive permeability is mechanistic, and considers the factors involved in solubility diffusion, D_s, β_s, and δ_m, as described above.

The preceding discussion considers the specific case of solubility diffusion, but the phenomenological definition of permeability can be applied in principle to any transport mechanism. Of course, its interpretation varies. An important case is that of the permeation of certain hydrophilic nonelectrolytes through aqueous pores in the membrane. If the lipid bilayer is impermeable to the solute, then diffusive transport is entirely via the pores. The permeable area of this membrane (S_p) is only a fraction of the total membrane area, given (for 1 cm^2 of membrane) by $S_p = n\pi r^2$, where n is the density of homogeneous pores of radius r. The partition coefficient is unity (the solute is dissolved in water both inside and outside of the pore), and is hence eliminated from the equation:

$$P_s = n\pi r^2 D_s / L \qquad (2.9)$$

where L is the pore length (nearly equivalent to membrane thickness).

FIGURE 2.2 **Diffusion across a membrane.** (a) A membrane separates two aqueous solutions (1 and 2). The dots represent molecules of a solute to which the membrane is permeable; the solute concentration (C_s) is greater in solution 1. Solute molecules move randomly in each solution and collide with the membrane with a probability proportional to the concentration. Solutes collide, dissolve in, and diffuse across the membrane. The unidirectional fluxes ($J_{1 \to 2}$ and $J_{2 \to 1}$) are proportional to the solute concentrations in sides 1 and 2, respectively; the net flux (J_{net}) is proportional to the concentration difference. The concentration difference does not accelerate the molecules, and hence it is not a force, although it is usually referred to as the *chemical driving force*. Diffusion is a passive, equilibrating transport, i.e., net transport ceases when the concentrations on both sides of the membrane are equal. (b) Lines denote solute concentration profiles in the solutions and the membrane depending on the partition coefficient (β_s). When $\beta_s = 1$, solute concentration in the membrane boundaries are identical to those in the adjacent solutions; concentrations in the membrane are greater or smaller than those in the adjacent solution if β_s is greater or smaller than unity, respectively. The membrane thickness is denoted by δ_m.

Electrodiffusion

Electrodiffusion is the main mechanism of passive transport of ions in homogeneous media, that is, bulk aqueous solution or relatively large water-filled pores. Electrodiffusive transmembrane ion transport is a mediated transport process, but it is better discussed with diffusion for continuity. In large-diameter pores, electrodiffusion theory explains ion permeation very well. In ion channels, which have smaller diameter and are highly selective, there are significant interactions between the ions and the permeation pathway. For this reason, simple electrodiffusion theory is not entirely applicable to ion channels, but is nevertheless a useful approximation. For ion transport across a membrane, two factors determine the flux: the chemical potential difference (difference in concentration across the membrane) and the electrical potential difference (membrane voltage). The net ion flux (J_i) is given by the Nernst–Planck equation (see [50]). If a constant electrical field is assumed in the membrane and other assumptions are made, the Nernst–Planck equation can be solved, yielding the Goldman–Hodgkin–Katz (GHK) equation[41,51]:

$$J_i = -P_i \frac{z_i V_m F}{RT} \left[\frac{C_i^o - C_i^i \exp(V_m F/RT)}{1 - \exp(V_m F/RT)} \right] \quad (2.10)$$

where R, T, z, and F have their usual meanings, P is permeability, V_m is membrane voltage, C is concentration, the subscript i denotes the ith ion, and the superscripts i and o denote the two sides of the membrane.

Under zero current conditions, the GHK flux equation yields the membrane voltage as a function of the permeabilities and concentrations of all permeant ions. For the case of three monovalent permeant ions (Na$^+$, K$^+$, and Cl$^-$), the equation (GHK voltage equation) is:

$$V_m = -\frac{RT}{F} \ln \frac{P_{Na}[Na^+]_i + P_K[K^+]_i + P_{Cl}[Cl^-]_o}{P_{Na}[Na^+]_o + P_K[K^+]_o + P_{Cl}[Cl^-]_i} \quad (2.11)$$

where the brackets denote concentrations. Note that if the fraction including permeability coefficients and ion concentrations is inverted, then the sign of the right side of the equation is also inverted. We prefer the notation given here, because it gives the intracellular potential minus the extracellular potential, the convention used in electrophysiology. This also applies to the Nernst equation below.

Note that if only one ion is permeable, e.g., if P_{Na} and P_{Cl} are 0 in Eq. (2.11), then the membrane voltage becomes equal to the equilibrium potential for that ion, in this example K$^+$. The equilibrium potential is given by the Nernst equation[81]:

$$V_m = -\frac{RT}{F} \ln \frac{[K^+]_i}{[K^+]_o} \quad (2.12)$$

Under these conditions, the two compartments separated by the membrane are at a *steady-state* (the amounts of K$^+$ on each side remain constant with time), but also at *equilibrium*, which means that the net driving force for K$^+$ is zero, and hence the unidirectional fluxes are equal (Figure 2.3). In the case of cells, one frequently observes a steady-state K$^+$ distribution without equilibrium; the net efflux through channels is exactly balanced by influx via the Na$^+$,K$^+$-ATPase.

Another interesting point is that the Nernst equation indicates that if only one ion is permeable, then the

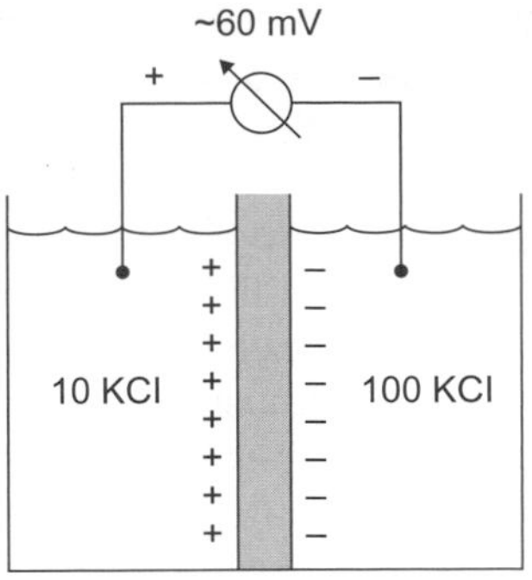

FIGURE 2.3 **Electrochemical equilibrium.** A membrane permeable to K$^+$ and impermeable to Cl$^-$ separates two KCl solutions of 10 mM and 100 mM concentrations, respectively. Because of the difference in concentrations, there is a chemical driving force for K$^+$ and Cl$^-$ fluxes from right to left. While the impermeant Cl$^-$ cannot move, the permeant K$^+$ moves across the membrane, and in doing so creates a difference in electrical potential across the membrane. The membrane becomes electrically charged by a tiny excess of K$^+$ on the left, and a tiny excess of Cl$^-$ on the right. This difference in electrical potential (the *transmembrane voltage*) opposes further K$^+$ flux, and a state is reached at which the chemical driving force and the electrical driving force for K$^+$ movement are equal and opposite. This condition, described by the Nernst equation (Eq. (2.12)), denotes electrochemical equilibrium.

membrane voltage is determined by the concentration ratio for that ion, not its absolute concentrations. In addition, the membrane voltage is independent of the absolute value of the ion permeability. As shown by the GHK voltage equation, in the case of a membrane permeable to more than one ion, the membrane voltage depends on the absolute concentrations and permeability coefficients of all permeant ions. The Nernst equation can be derived more directly from the definitions of electrochemical potential (Eq. (2.1)) and equilibrium ($\Delta \overline{\mu}_i = 0$).

The essential points concerning electrodiffusion are that ion fluxes across membranes are determined by both permeability and driving force, and that the driving force has chemical and electrical components. Hence, these three elements must be known to predict the direction and magnitude of the flux. For example, knowledge of the K$^+$ concentrations inside and outside a cell is insufficient to decide whether the ion is at equilibrium across the membrane or whether there is a passive driving force inwardly or outwardly directed. To establish this simple point, it is necessary to know the membrane voltage. However, knowledge of the electrochemical gradient is insufficient to predict the magnitude of the K$^+$ flux expected for this gradient; the K$^+$ permeability of the membrane must also be known.

Mediated Transport

This expression means that translocation across the membrane is not via the lipid bilayer, but via membrane transport proteins: pores, channels, carriers or pumps. Mediated transport is the process by which ions and polar nonelectrolytes undergo passive transport across the cell membrane. Hence, this mechanism is complementary to that provided by solubility diffusion, in that it is specialized for hydrophilic solutes, whereas solubility diffusion is more effective for lipophilic solutes. For certain solutes, both mechanisms may operate. Even for solutes with very low permeability across the phospholipid moiety of the membrane, a significant contribution of the diffusive flux may exist because of the large fractional area covered by phospholipids, in particular if there is also a low level of expression of the relevant transporters.

In mediated transport, specialized proteins spanning the membrane provide an aqueous environment that allows for the transmembrane flux of particles that are virtually insoluble in phospholipids. Recent advances have permitted the molecular identification of many of these proteins, as well as the genes that encode them. In addition to providing an aqueous environment for solute translocation, these molecules may undergo conformational changes during or related to the substrate translocation. The transport proteins underlying mediated transport can be classified in four groups: pores; channels; carriers; and pumps.

Thermodynamics of Mediated Passive Transport

Pores, channels, and carriers are membrane transport proteins that can only perform *overall* passive transport, meaning that the total energy employed in the transport is equal to or less than the energy available in the electrochemical gradients (see "Secondary Active Transport" section below). Carriers and channels do not use a metabolic energy supply for solute translocation. Some channels are activated by ATP binding and hydrolysis, but once they become permeable, ion translocation is passive and does not use metabolic energy. Some carriers are able to transport more than one solute in the same cycle. In this case, the energy stored in the electrochemical gradient for one of these solutes (accessory) can be employed for uphill transport of another (principal) solute, a process known as secondary active transport. Nevertheless, the total energy change is dissipative, that is, the energy stored in the accessory solute's electrochemical gradient is always greater than that used to actively transport the principal solute.

Kinetics of Mediated Passive Transport

The dependence of the transport rates on solute concentration are different in solubility diffusion and carrier-mediated transport. As shown in Figure 2.4, in diffusion the flux increases linearly with the

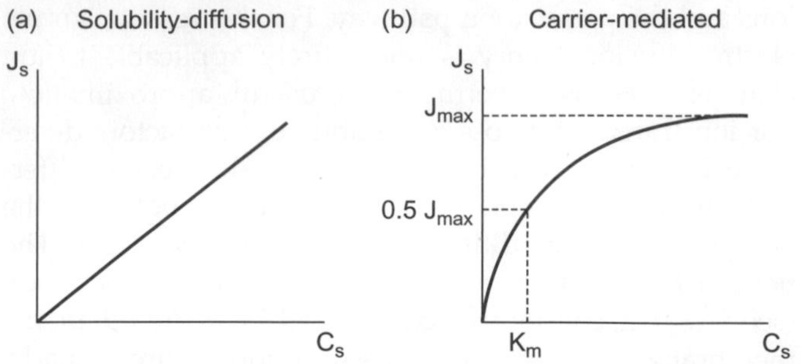

FIGURE 2.4 **Kinetics of diffusion and carrier-mediated transport.** Both graphs depict solute flux (J_s) as a function of solute concentration (C_s). In (a), the mechanism of translocation across the membrane is diffusion, which does not involve chemical reactions between solute and membrane. In (b), the mechanism of translocation is mediated (i.e., it involves a transport protein in the membrane). In (a), the flux is linear with the concentration, whereas in (b) it saturates, because of occupation of a finite number of sites by a solute that moves at a finite velocity. In the simplest case, the relationship in (b) is described by the Michaelis–Menten equation (Eq. (2.13)).

concentration, whereas in carrier-mediated transport it saturates. This is explained because transport occurs via a finite number of carrier molecules that can also operate at a finite rate. The simplest case of carrier-mediated transport can be described by the Michaelis–Menten equation; the two kinetic parameters are the maximum flux (J_{max}) and K_m, the concentration at which the flux is half-maximal (see Figure 2.4):

$$J_s = -\frac{C_s J_{max}}{C_s + K_m} \tag{2.13}$$

where J_s is the solute flux, and C_s is its concentration. For a detailed description of this, and more complex kinetic processes, see Segel.[92]

Modes of Coupled Transport

Coupled transport denotes the linked translocation of two or more species (ions and/or molecules) through a barrier. One can distinguish two coupling modes. *Molecular* coupling denotes carrier- or pump-mediated transport of more than one species by the same molecule. Examples shown in Figure 2.5a are the Na^+ and glucose fluxes via the Na^+-glucose co-transporter, and the Na^+ and K^+ fluxes via the Na^+K^+-ATPase. In addition, there is *thermodynamic* coupling. In this case, the fluxes of two or more species occur through different molecules, but are related to each other by electrochemical driving forces. For example, transepithelial Na^+ transport via cell membranes (apical membrane Na^+ channel in series with basolateral membrane Na^+ pump) can produce a transepithelial electrical potential difference responsible for a passive Cl^- flux via the intercellular (junctional) pathway. In this instance, the

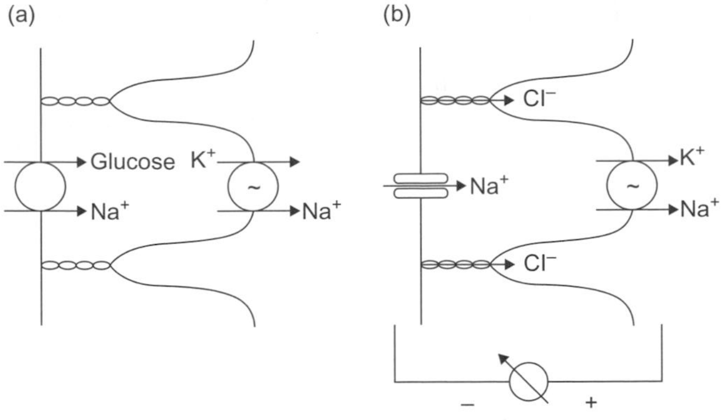

FIGURE 2.5 Modes of coupled transport. (a) Molecular coupling: glucose-absorbing epithelial cell (e.g., renal proximal tubule). Two cases of molecular coupling are depicted: the Na^+-glucose symporter (SGLT) at the apical membrane, and the Na^+,K^+-ATPase at the basolateral membrane. In both instances, the transport of two substrates occurs obligatorily in the same transport molecule. (b) Thermodynamic coupling: the epithelial cell depicted absorbs Na^+ by an electrogenic process that generates a lumen-negative transepithelial voltage. This voltage drives a paracellular, electrodiffusive Cl^- flux. The Na^+ and Cl^- fluxes occur via different pathways, and are linked by the driving force, not by binding to the same molecule.

coupling is not obligatory (if the potential difference is abolished, Cl^- transport ceases while Na^+ transport continues), and does not involve the Na^+ transport molecules. Instead, it corresponds to the parallel operation of two transporters linked by a driving force (Figure 2.5b). This apparently simple point has been a source of confusion in the transport literature (in particular of epithelial cells), where on occasion it has been incorrectly implied that all coupling is molecular.

Pathways and Mechanisms of Active Transport

Primary Active Transport

Primary active transport occurs in the absence of or against the existing electrochemical gradient, and is powered by metabolic energy, such as that originated by the exergonic hydrolysis of ATP (Figure 2.6). Ion pumps are the only molecules capable of performing primary active transport. Most ion pumps of interest to us are transport ATPases, bifunctional molecules that hydrolyze ATP and perform the translocation of the substrate against the prevailing electrochemical gradient. The Na^+,K^+-ATPase[85], Na^+-K^+ pump or Na^+ pump, was the first enzyme demonstrated to be an active ion transporter (reviewed in[97,98]). It is likely that the energy-consuming steps are the conformational changes of the pump protein required for the substrate translocation, that is, for making the substrate first inaccessible to the *cis* side, and then accessible to the *trans* side of the membrane.

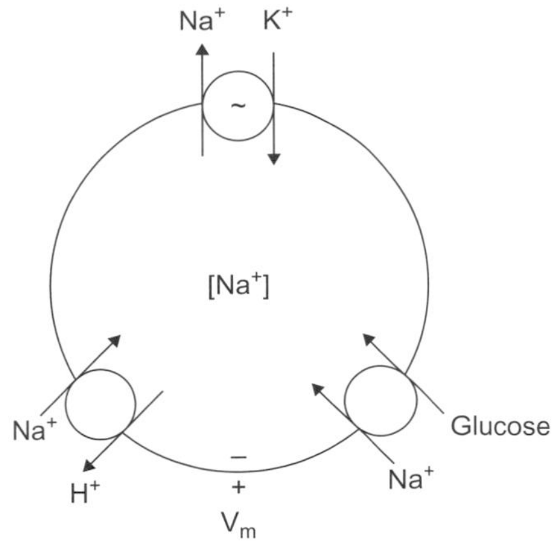

FIGURE 2.6 Active transport. The diagram represents a cell expressing three membrane transporters. Top: Primary-active transport of Na^+ and K^+ via the Na^+,K^+-ATPase. The energy for active transport is provided by the hydrolysis of ATP. The flux coupling is $3Na^+:2K^+$ per ATP molecule hydrolyzed. Bottom: Two mechanisms of secondary active transport. In both cases, the Na^+ electrochemical gradient (oriented inwards) is the driving force for the uphill movement of the other solute (glucose or H^+). On the right, Na^+-glucose co-transport via SGLT, the stoichiometry (Na^+:glucose) is 1:1 (SGLT2) or 2:1 (SGLT1). On the left, Na^+–H^+ exchange via NHE; the stoichiometry is 1:1. Note that the Na^+ driving forces operative in the two cases are different. Since Na^+–H^+ exchange is electroneutral, the driving force depends only on the difference in Na^+ concentrations. Since Na^+-glucose co-transport is electrogenic the driving force involves both the Na^+ chemical gradient and the membrane voltage. For a quantitative analysis, see text.

Secondary Active Transport

Secondary active transport is characterized by the indirect use of metabolic energy. The electrochemical gradient drives a downhill substrate flux, and part of this energy is utilized for the uphill flux of another substrate (Figure 2.6). The coupling between the two fluxes occurs in the same transport protein, and therefore there is molecular coupling.

In animal cells, secondary active transport is most frequently linked to Na^+ transport. The Na^+,K^+-ATPase establishes an electrochemical potential gradient for Na^+ across the plasma membrane, which includes a chemical (higher extracellular $[Na^+]$) and an electrical component (cell electrically negative to the extracellular compartment), both contributing to a net driving force (electrochemical gradient) favoring Na^+ entry into the cell. This energy is utilized to transport other substrates by coupling translocation to that of Na^+ at the molecular level.

Depending on the directions of the fluxes, there are two kinds of secondary active transport: *co-transport* (or *symport*), in which the substrates move in the same direction, such as downhill for Na^+ and uphill for the co-transported substrate (e.g., glucose); and *countertransport* (also *antiport* or *exchange*) in which the fluxes are in opposite directions. Secondary active transport may involve two substrates (Na^+ and another substrate) or more (e.g., the Na^+-K^+-$2Cl^-$ co-transporter). Sodium-glucose co-transport was the first secondary active transport mechanism studied experimentally, giving rise to the *Na$^+$ gradient hypothesis*.[16]

Transport by Na^+-glucose co-transporters and Na^+-Ca^{2+} exchangers is electrogenic, that is, there is net translocation of charge across the membrane in each cycle. The concentration ratios (intracellular/extracellular) for glucose and Ca^{2+}, respectively, depend on both the Na^+ concentration ratio and the membrane voltage (V_m). The equation describing the maximum substrate concentration ratio that can be obtained by co-transport is:

$$\frac{S_i}{S_o} = \left[\frac{A_o}{A_i}\right]^n \exp\left(\frac{-nzFV_m}{RT}\right) \qquad (2.14)$$

where S is the main substrate (glucose), A is the accessory substrate (Na^+), the subscripts i and o denote intra- and extracellular concentrations, respectively, n is the transport stoichiometry (number of A molecules/number of S molecules), z is the valence of the translocated species per cycle ($z = zA + zS$), V_m is the membrane voltage, and R, T, and F have their usual meanings. Changing to decimal power notation and inserting appropriate values for the constants, the exponent becomes $\sim nzV_m/60$. Hence, in the case of glucose transport via SGLT1 ($n = 2$), for $V_m = -60$ mV and Na^+ concentration ratio is 10, the maximum glucose concentration ratio (cell/lumen) is 10^4.

A similar equation describes the minimum concentration ratio of main substrate that can be achieved by an antiport:

$$\frac{S_i}{S_o} = \left[\frac{A_o}{A_i}\right]^n \exp\left(\frac{-nzFV_m}{RT}\right) \qquad (2.15)$$

where the symbols are the same as for Eq. (2.14). The difference is that the concentration ratios for A are inverted in these equations, denoting that in one case S and A are transported in the same direction, and in the other case they are transported in opposite directions. For the example of Na^+–Ca^{2+} exchange with $V_m = -60$ mV and Na^+ concentration ratio is 10, the minimum Ca^{2+} concentration ratio (cell/extracellular) is 10^{-6} for $n = 4$, the most likely stoichiometry.

ION TRANSPORT PROTEINS

Ion transport proteins are best classified in four groups: pores; channels; carriers (also called *transporters*); and pumps. Ion pores and channels are integral membrane proteins that when "open" communicate the aqueous solutions adjacent to the membrane, and permit ion flux in a direction determined by the electrochemical gradient. The permeant ion interacts little with the pore or channel, and thus the number of ions translocated per unit time (turnover number) is very high, typically 10^6–10^8 s^{-1}. Whereas pores are always open (ion conductive), ion channels undergo "gating," transitions between open (conductive) and closed (nonconductive) states. The part of the protein thought to move or change conformation during the gating is called the *gate*. Gating can be elicited by physical factors (changes in membrane voltage or mechanical stretch) or chemical factors (such as neurotransmitters or second messengers).

Carriers are also integral membrane proteins. In contrast with channels, the function of carrier proteins involves a chemical interaction with the transported ion, namely ion binding, which elicits conformational changes in the carrier, eventually resulting in the translocation of the ion across the membrane. Because of these interactions between the carrier and the transported ion, the transport rate is much slower than that of channels, typically 10^2–10^4 s^{-1}. The net ion flux through carriers is also determined by the electrochemical gradient, as in channels, but in a more complex fashion, because certain carriers can transport several ions in the same cycle.

Pumps are similar to carriers in that there are ion binding and conformational changes that cause ion translocation, but differ in that their function is coupled to a metabolic energy source, such as ATP hydrolysis. Pumps have low turnover numbers, similar to those of carriers.

Many ion transport proteins associate with so-called adapter proteins that appear to have two roles: to determine the subcellular location of the transport protein; and to facilitate its interaction with signal transduction components, including receptors, second messenger producing enzymes, and protein kinases. These adapter proteins often contain a specific protein–protein interaction domain called the *PDZ domain*.[82] Adapter proteins therefore contribute to the formation of macromolecular complexes of which ion transport proteins are important components.

During the last decade, atomic-resolution structures have been obtained by X-ray crystallography for a number of prototypical transport proteins, including bacterial pores,[21,89] prokaryotic ion channels,[26,28] the lac-permease of *Escherichia coli* carrier,[1,2] the mammalian sarcoplasmic-reticulum Ca^{2+} pump,[107,108] and several ATP-binding cassette (ABC) proteins.[4,19,53,113] These studies have provided detailed insight into the mechanism of the function of these specific transport proteins, as well as a framework in which to analyze other proteins. An example is the modeling of the cystic fibrosis transmembrane conductance regulator (CFTR) channel, based on the structure of other ABC proteins.[78]

As summarized in an excellent recent review,[74] the first atomic-resolution structure of an integral membrane protein, the reaction center from photosynthetic bacteria, was reported in 1985.[20] At that time there were 268 entries in the Protein Data Bank (PDB). In 2010, the PDB contained almost 60,000 entries, with about 700 of these being membrane proteins, and 80% of these belonging to the all-alpha type (i.e., the transmembrane regions are α helices, instead of the β sheets found in prokaryotic membrane proteins). Only *ca.* 250 of these structures are considered unique.[114]

An essential property of membrane proteins involved in ion transport is their selectivity, i.e., their capacity to "distinguish" between similar ions. This requires the ion pathway to have specific binding sites. In ion selective channels, the ion is at least partially dehydrated, with the binding sites providing favorable interactions, i.e., "replacing" the water molecules surrounding the ion in free solution. Selectivity results from a more favorable interaction of the site with one type of ion than another.[42] Ion-binding sites in transport proteins are formed by amino acid residues that provide charges of the opposite sign, with a size that specifically accommodates the ion. These sites have been identified in several crystal structures of transport proteins.[42] Small molecules selective for monovalent cations have been synthesized by changing the size of the cavity.[23,42]

Pores

Pores are wide conduits across biological membranes that are permanently open; they do not gate (Figure 2.7a). The best studied examples are those formed by bacterial porins, but they are also present in mitochondria (porins) and lymphocytes (perforin, a secretory product). It is also possible that most aquaporins are pores (see Chapters 4 and 41).

Bacterial pores formed by the transmembrane proteins called *porins* are radically different from animal membrane proteins, in that the transmembrane domains, instead of being α helices, are β sheets. For discussions of porin structures, see Delcour[21] and Schulz.[89]

Channels

Like pores, channels have the property of being accessible to both sides of the membrane at the same time, but this occurs only part of the time. Channels open and close stochastically. Gating may be determined by physical or chemical processes (see below), both requiring a sensing mechanism. In the open channel there is ion permeation with a characteristic selectivity for one or more ion species. Channels also have typical conductance (related to ion permeability),

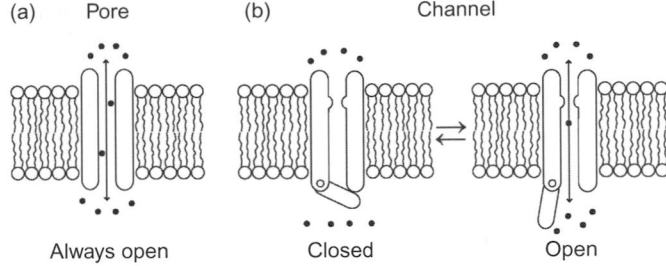

FIGURE 2.7 Pores and channels. (a) A pore is a transmembrane protein that forms an aqueous conduit across the membrane that is always accessible from both sides and never closed. Pores are generally of large diameter, and thus permit passive transport of small ions as well as larger hydrophilic solutes, driven by the electrochemical gradient across the membrane. (b) A channel is also a transmembrane protein that forms an aqueous conduit across the membrane. However, in contrast with a pore, it can have at least two conformations, closed and open. The change in conformation is depicted in the figure by a swiveling portion of the molecule, the gate. Gating is the process by which the channels open and close. When the channel is open, it is permeable (conductive), and its interior is accessible to both sides. When the channel is closed, it is impermeable. Channels are generally of smaller radius than pores, and exhibit varying degrees of ion selectivity. As in the case of pores, ion fluxes through channels are driven by the electrochemical gradient across the membrane.

physiological regulation, and inhibitor pattern. Hence, the functional "fingerprint" of a channel includes gating, sensing mechanism, conductance, selectivity, regulation, and pharmacological inhibition.

In channels, the main transport-related conformational change is the gating between open and closed states (Figure 2.7b). The gate is the portion of the channel protein that "moves" to cause channel opening and closure. When the channel is closed, it is impermeable, that is, nonconductive. When it is open, it is permeable or conductive, and allows ion fluxes, with a net flux that can also be expressed as the current carried by the ions. The flux, and hence the current, are determined by the permeability of the channel and the driving force, that is, the electrochemical gradient for the permeant ion. The channel persists in the open state for a given time and allows ion permeation without additional conformational changes during the opening. Hence, one conformational change (gating) allows for transport of a large number of ions, with no additional chemical modification of the protein. The open channel constitutes a water-filled conduit that spans the lipid bilayer communicating the two solutions separated by the membrane. The interior of the open channel is accessible from both solutions at the same time. The large number of ions that cross a channel per unit of time causes a measurable electrical current, allowing investigators to measure single channel events, net ion movements across individual molecules, either *in situ*, using the patch-clamp technique[88] or reconstituting purified channels and incorporating them in artificial planar bilayers.[75] The two channel conformations, open and closed, underlie the discrete levels observed in current records.

The total current (which denotes ion flux) via a population of channels of one kind in a membrane is given by:

$$I = N \cdot P_o \cdot g \cdot (V_m - E_i) \tag{2.16}$$

where I is the current, N is the number of functional channels in the membrane, P_o is the channel open probability (time open/total time), g is the single channel conductance (the reciprocal of resistance), V_m is the membrane voltage, and E_i is the permeant ion's equilibrium potential. Note that the term $g (V_m - E_i)$ denotes i, the single channel current. Equation (2.16) encompasses all mechanisms of channel function regulation: number of copies in the membrane; open probability (gating); conductance; and electrochemical driving force. The ion flux and the ion current through are related by the Faraday constant and the ion valence.

Whereas carriers can be uniporters, symporters or antiporters, channels can only be uniporters. There can be ion–ion interactions in channels, such as single file diffusion,[36,50] but molecular flux coupling, such as observed in carriers, does not occur. As is the case of carriers, channels exhibit substrate selectivity, typical pharmacological inhibition, and transport saturation, although the latter is more evident in carriers.

Plasma membrane ion channels are classified based on their selectivity. The most studied can be selective for K^+, Na^+, Ca^{2+}, H^+, Cl^-, cation or anions, or may be nonselective. Certain channels are highly selective for specific ions, whereas others discriminate less among different ions. The bases of selectivity are ion size and charge. It has been well-established that the Na^+, K^+, and Ca^{2+} channels of excitable membranes, as well as the epithelial Na^+ channel, K^+ channels, and Cl^- channels, are highly selective, where permeability ratios between two ions of the same charge and similar size can be 100 or more. As explained in more detail below, the structural basis of high selectivity channels is a very narrow region in the pore, called the *selectivity filter*, in which the dehydrated permeant ion is coordinated by dipoles in the protein.[69] Other ion channels are less selective. For example, gap junction channels, which communicate between adjacent cells, have cation–anion permeability ratios ranging from about 1 to 10, values similar to those of tight junctions of leaky (high permeability) epithelia. These channels are wider, the ions permeate in the hydrated state, and the cation–anion selectivity is probably governed by fixed charges facing the pore.

K^+-Selective Channels

All known K^+ channels belong to a single protein family, characterized by the highly conserved K^+ channel signature sequence,[48] which forms the selectivity filter. K^+ channels display high selectivity and high conduction rates. X-ray crystallographic studies performed in recent years have revealed the atomic structures of several K^+ channels. Roderick MacKinnon was awarded the 2003 Nobel Prize for Chemistry for this work. In this section, we summarize the current understanding of K^+ channel selectivity and conduction derived from structural studies. For a discussion of the gating process, see MacKinnon.[69]

The K^+ channel is formed by four subunits arranged around a central pore.[24,120] Each subunit consists of two transmembrane α helices (inner and outer, relative to the pore), and the pore helix, which is tilted and penetrates only half of the membrane thickness. Near the center of the membrane the pore forms a water-filled cavity that contains a hydrated K^+.[120] As shown in Figure 2.8, the selectivity filter, formed by the signature-sequence amino acids, is located between the central cavity and the extracellular solution. The filter consists of four layers of carbonyl oxygen atoms and a layer of threonine hydroxyl oxygen atoms, creating four K^+-binding sites (numbered one to four starting from the extracellular side). Thus, each dehydrated K^+ is surrounded by eight oxygen atoms, four "above" and four "below." The selectivity filter thus mimics the arrangement of the K^+ hydration shell, in which a single K^+ is surrounded on average by eight water molecules. The K^+ ions are "transferred" by diffusion from water to the selectivity filter, the hydration energy being compensated for by the binding energy in the filter. Sodium ions do not enter the selectivity filter,[119,120] because the selectivity filter binding energy cannot compensate for the Na^+ higher hydration energy. The small distances between the four K^+-binding sites cause electrostatic repulsion, so only two sites (one and three or two and four) are thought to be occupied at a time.[77] The electrostatic repulsion tends to balance the binding forces, thus ensuring a high turnover number.[69]

K^+ channels are present in the plasma membranes of virtually all cells. Their principal functions are generation of the resting membrane potential of the cell (inside negative), and performance of transepithelial K^+ transport, principally in renal and intestine epithelia. In addition, K^+ channels are involved in cell volume regulation, in the regulation of insulin secretion by pancreatic β-cells, and probably in cell growth and differentiation, although the latter functions remain controversial.

Na^+-Selective Channels

There are two broad classes of Na^+ channels: depolarization-activated Na^+ channels expressed in neurons and other excitable cells and the ENaC/degenerin ion family, which includes the epithelial Na^+ channel

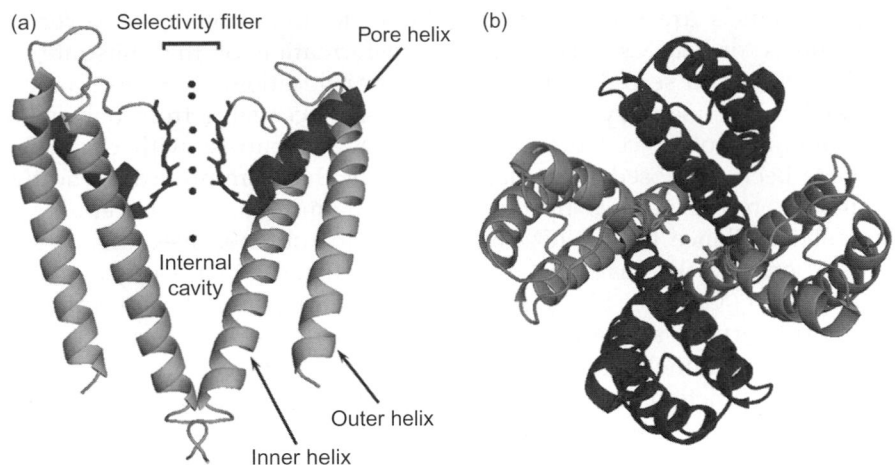

FIGURE 2.8 **Structure of a potassium channel.** (a) Side view of the KcsA channel showing only two subunits for simplicity. Two TM2 helices (pore helices) are shown in darker gray. The oxygens from backbone carbonyl groups at the selectivity filter coordinate K^+ (black circles) at four sites. There are two additional binding sites on the extracellular side (ions in transition), and one ion trapped in the internal cavity, presumably stabilized by the electrical dipole of the pore helices. (b) Tetrameric structure of the channel viewed from the extracellular side. The inner helices form the pore, with the narrowest part corresponding to the activation gate. Each subunit is shown in a tone different from that of the neighboring subunits (built with PyMol).

(ENaC). Other family members are proteins involved in mechanoreception and neuronal degeneration. ENaC is expressed in the apical (luminal) membrane of principal cells of the collecting duct, and in epithelial cells of colon and airway epithelium. ENaC has slow kinetics, low conductance, and a high open probability. Its function is to absorb Na^+ across the apical membrane of the epithelial cells; the Na^+ is then pumped out of the cell by the Na^+,K^+-ATPase expressed in the basolateral membrane. Mammalian ENaC is a heterotrimer (α-, β-, and γ-subunits with high structural homology[12]). All three subunits are thought to contribute to the formation of the pore, but no crystal structure is available.[100]

Cl⁻ Selective Channels

The largest family of Cl^- channels is the ClC family, with nine members in mammals. ClC channels participate in cell excitability, maintenance of the resting potential, Cl^- transport in certain epithelial cells, Cl^- and H^+ transport in intracellular vesicles, and cell volume regulation. ClC genes, expressed in both prokaryotes and eukaryotes, encode both Cl^- channels and Cl^-/H^+ antiporters.[27,60] In mammals, the channels (ClC-1, ClC-2, ClC-Ka, and ClC-Kb) are expressed in the plasma membrane, whereas the antiporters (ClC-3, 4, -5, -6, and -7) are expressed in endosomal/lysosomal membranes. This is an interesting case in which members of a family of ion transport proteins include channels and carriers.[60,76]

The structure of a bacterial ClC protein[28,29] shows a double-barrel channel: homodimer with each monomer containing a pore. Each subunit has 17 transmembrane helices and Cl^- in the channel is coordinated by residues from several helices, including a highly-conserved Lys. In the membrane, ClC proteins form two hourglass-like funnels that meet in a narrow constriction near the middle of the bilayer, the anion selectivity filter.[29] Some mammalian isoforms of ClC proteins require α- and β-subunits for function.[60] The cystic fibrosis transmembrane conductance regulator (CFTR) is a Cl^- channel expressed in Cl^--secreting epithelial cells; it does not belong to the ClC family, but is a member of the ABC superfamily. ABC proteins can be either channels or pumps. CFTR is expressed in the apical membranes of airway, small intestine, pancreatic duct, biliary tree, and vas deferens epithelia. It consists of two homologous halves, each formed by six transmembrane helices followed by a nucleotide-binding domain (NBD). The two halves are joined by the regulatory or R domain, a large hydrophilic sequence located in the cytoplasm. The function of CFTR is Cl^- secretion across the apical membrane, which is the primary event for salt and water secretion by the epithelia listed above. CFTR gating is a complex process involving phosphorylation of the R domain by protein kinase A, ATP binding to the NBDs, their dimerization, and ATP hydrolysis.[15] CFTR also appears to regulate other Cl^- channels, as well as Na^+ and K^+ channels, by unclear mechanisms. CFTR is expressed in all segments of the renal tubule, but its functional role in the normal kidney is not clear; also, cystic fibrosis patients have no discernible renal phenotype.[22] In polycystic kidney disease, CFTR is abundantly expressed in the apical membranes of the cysts cells, and plays an essential role in Cl^- secretion, which drives fluid secretion and cyst growth[11] (Chapter 81).

A third group of Cl⁻ channels are Ca²⁺-activated (Ca²⁺-activated Cl⁻ channels or CaCCs). They are involved in epithelial absorption and secretion, muscle contraction, neuronal excitability, sensory transduction, cell volume regulation, and other cell functions. Several protein types have been proposed to account for CaCC currents, but very recent studies by three groups have provided solid evidence that TMEM16A (also named anoctamin-1 or ANO1) has functional characteristics consistent with CaCCs. Site-specific mutations alter channel properties, suggesting that TMEM16A is at least part of the channel. Expression of TMEM16B also results in CaCC functions, but with different biophysical properties than those associated with TMEM16A. The function(s) of other TMEM16 proteins remain unknown. TMEM16A and the nine other members of the family have a similar topology and secondary structure, with eight transmembrane helices and intracellular N- and C-termini. This protein family has been long-studied by developmental and cancer biologists. Some family members are upregulated in tumors and loss-of-function of others is conducive to defects in development (see [39] and [45] for reviews).

For a detailed discussion of ion channels, see Chapter 8. In addition, excellent treatments of ion channels in general can be found in the book by Hille,[50] and the review articles by Catterall[13] and Dawson.[18] There are also several excellent recent reviews on ion channel structure—function relationships,[24,25,42,68,69] and on ion channels in renal epithelial cells.[14,46,52,56,60] Chapters 8, 30, 31, 47, and 63 cover renal ion channels.

Carriers

Carriers are transporters that perform transmembrane translocation of solute (and perhaps water; see Chapter 4) by a sequential process thought to involve three basic steps. First, binding of the transported substrate to the carrier facing one side of the membrane; second, change in conformation of the carrier, with translocation of the substrate (and the binding site) to the opposite side of the membrane; and third, release of the substrate. It is thought that access to the binding site from either bathing solution is by diffusion (or electrodiffusion) in pore-like regions of the carrier molecule.[61] Hence, two such steps could be added to the simplified scheme above.

In carriers, there is a state in which the binding site and the substrate are inaccessible from either side of the membrane.[62] The existence of this state, called *occlusion*, is one of many arguments supporting the idea of conformational change in carrier function. Carriers behave like enzymes, in that the substrate binds to the protein; however, instead of chemical transformation of the substrate, the carrier performs its translocation. Carriers contain substrate-binding domains accessible from one side of the membrane at a time. In contrast with channels, they never form a conduit that communicates the two bathing solutions, i.e., the binding site is never accessible from both sides of the membrane. Instead, carriers undergo conformational changes that alter the "sidedness" of the substrate-binding site; the substrate binds on one side, the conformation of the carrier protein changes, the substrate is occluded, the binding site is translocated (with substrate) to the other side of the membrane, and the substrate is then released. In comparison with a channel, which has one gate, a carrier may be considered to have two gates, as illustrated in Figure 2.9.

The notion of a carrier protein as a "ferryboat" binding the substrate at a membrane—solution interface and carrying it to the other side, where the solute is released to the other solution, is inconsistent with current knowledge of the biochemistry and molecular biology of carriers. Nevertheless, kinetic schemes based on the ferryboat model remain very useful to explain carrier function at a phenomenological level.

Substrate transport by carriers is inherently slow, because each substrate molecule (or group of molecules in cases of coupled transport; see below) must undergo an independent binding reaction, followed by the conformational change of the carrier molecule. This explains the low turnover number of carriers, similar to typical rates of enzyme catalysis of 10^2-10^3 per second.[99]

Most carriers have exquisite substrate selectivity (e.g., the glucose carrier GLUT1 transports D-glucose, but not L-glucose) and can also exhibit quite specific pharmacological inhibition. At low substrate concentration, the substrate flux increases linearly with the concentration, and can be confused with simple diffusion, but at high substrate concentration it saturates, as expected from occupancy of a limited number of slowly turning binding sites. The low turnover number, high substrate selectivity and saturation of carriers, and to some extent the mechanisms of pharmacological inhibition, also support the notions of substrate binding and conformational change during the transport cycle.

Carrier-mediated transport can be classified in three types depending on the number of substrates and the transport directions (Figure 2.10). When the carrier transports only one substrate, the process is called *facilitated diffusion* or *uniport*; the carrier is a uniporter. Other carriers transport two or more substrates. When all substrates are transported in the same direction, the process is called *co-transport* or *symport*; the carrier is a *co-transporter* or *symporter*. When there is substrate transport in opposite directions, the process is called

One gate open   Both gates closed   Other gate open

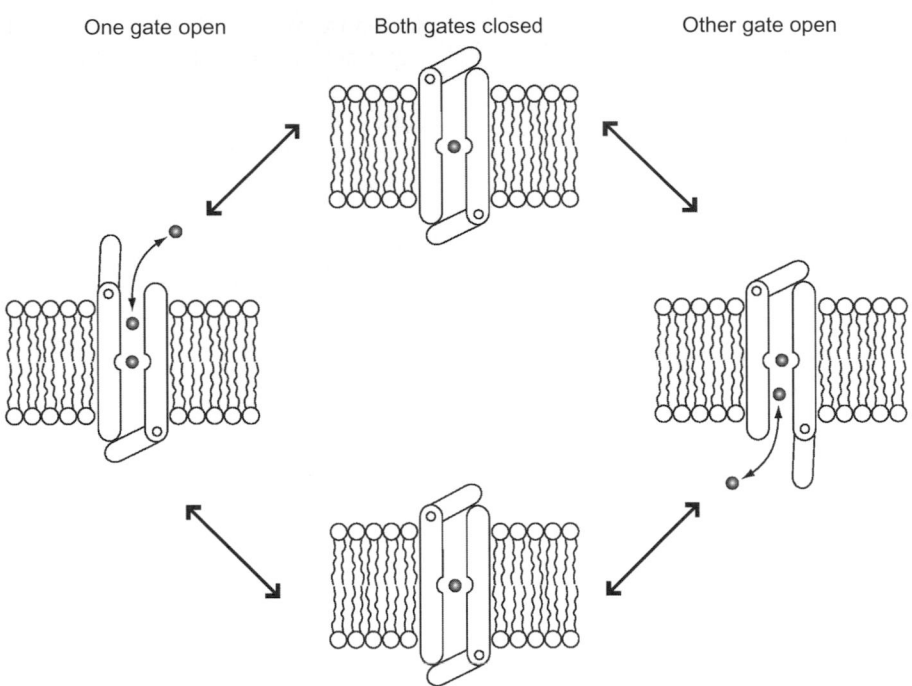

FIGURE 2.9 **Carriers.** A carrier can be understood as a membrane transport protein with two gates and one or more binding sites for the substrate. The figure depicts the transport stages for a uniporter, the simplest kind of carrier molecule. From left to right: the substrate binds to the carrier at a site available to only one side of the membrane (first gate open, second gate closed); this closes the second gate and the substrate is occluded (both gates closed); the second gate opens and the binding site and the substrate become accessible to the other side of the membrane, and the substrate is then released. The transport process is passive. The unidirectional and net fluxes are determined by the chemical or electrochemical potential difference, for uncharged and charged substrates, respectively (*modified with permission from ref. [37]*).

exchange or *antiport*; the carrier is an *exchanger* or *antiporter*. Uniporters, like channels, can only perform passive transport. The overall transport via a symporter or an antiporter is downhill. There is always passive translocation of at least one substrate, and there can be secondary active translocation of one or more additional substrates, using the energy stored in another substrate's chemical or electrochemical gradient. For example, in the case of two substrates, all the energy employed in uphill translocation of one species derives from the passive transport of the other one, so that no metabolic energy is directly used.

The largest family of secondary active transporters is the major facilitator superfamily (MFS).[87] MFS proteins are expressed from bacteria to vertebrates. They range from 400 to 600 amino acids in size, have 12 transmembrane helices, and N- and C-termini are located on the cytoplasmic side. These proteins transport numerous substrates, and may be uniporters, symporters or antiporters. The atomic structures of four bacterial members of the MFS have been solved: the H[+]-lactose co-transporter (LacY) or lac-permease,[2] the P_I/glycerol-3-phosphate antiporter (GlpT),[58] the multidrug-resistance antiporter EmrD,[117] and the fucose permease FucP.[17] In all structures the transmembrane helices

form two domains, N- and C-termini (each consisting of a six-helix bundle) with a pseudo two-fold symmetry. A large cavity open to the cytoplasm and closed to the periplasm is present in the LacY and GlpT structures, suggesting that the crystals correspond to the inward facing conformation.[2,58] The structure of the FucP shows an outward open amphipathic cavity.[17]

Of great importance for mammalian physiology in general and renal physiology in particular are the solute sodium symporters (SSS), a subset of the MFS. These constitute a large family of proteins that co-transport Na[+] with a variety of solutes, including sugars, amino acids, inorganic acids, and vitamins.[115] They are expressed in the kidney and other transport organs. The crystal structure of a bacterial Na[+]-galactose symporter was solved in 2008.[32] As predicted from earlier studies, it has 14 transmembrane helices, extracellular N- and C-termini, and a structural core formed by two clusters of five helices each, with opposite orientations. This structure is similar to that of lac-permease,[2] suggesting a common structure for sugar co-transporters. The galactose-binding site is central, and is separated from the adjacent solutions by hydrophobic amino acid residues; the Na[+]-binding site could not be identified in the crystal structure.[32] Another

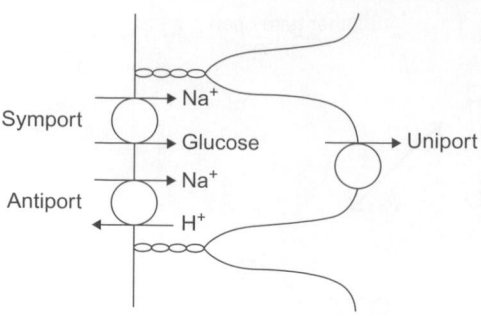

FIGURE 2.10 **Types of carrier-mediated transport.** The figure depicts an epithelial cell (e.g., renal proximal tubule) expressing different kinds of carriers, classified according to the number of substrates and the directions of the net fluxes. *Uniporter* is a carrier that transports only one substrate in a complete cycle; the process is known as facilitated diffusion or uniport, and is always passive. Shown in the figure is a glucose uniporter at the basolateral membrane. *Symporter* is a carrier that transports at least two substrates in the same direction in each cycle. The process is known as co-transport or symport; the overall transport process is downhill, but the electrochemical gradient of one substrate can be used to transport the other one actively (a form of secondary active transport). Shown in the figure is a Na^+-glucose symporter at the apical membrane. *Antiporter* is a carrier that transports at least two substrates in opposite directions in each cycle. The process is known as countertransport, exchange or antiport; the overall transport process is downhill, but again the electrochemical gradient of one substrate can be used to translocate the other one actively (secondary active transport). Shown in the figure is a Na^{++}/H^+ antiporter at the apical membrane. See also Figure 2.6.

symporter, LeuT (leucine and Na^+)[116] clearly shows leucine and Na^+ bound to a deep region of the protein (Figure 2.11). The Na^+ ions are fully dehydrated and surrounded by six oxygen atoms in one site and by five in the other. These studies represent impressive progress in a few years, but considerably more work will be needed to fully understand the function of these proteins at the atomic level.

Specific aspects of carrier-mediated transport are covered in Chapters 32, 53, 54, 55, and 73. The reader is also referred to LeFevre,[66] Schultz,[90] and Stein[99] for quantitative treatments of carrier-mediated transport. Some specific carriers are well covered in recent reviews by Abramson et al.,[1] Hediger et al.,[47] Tanner,[104] and Zachos et al.[118]

Pumps

Ion pumps are discussed in Chapter 3. Other reviews of ion pumps are Apell,[5] Brini and Carafoli,[10] Facciotti et al.,[31] Fambrough and Inesi,[33] Finbow and Harrison,[35] Horisberger,[54,55] Läuger,[65] Pedersen,[83] Sachs and Munson[85] and Toyoshima.[106]

Ion pumps can be classified according to the source of metabolic energy. Pumps in general can be driven by light, redox potential or ATP hydrolysis. Animal cell plasma membrane ATPases belong to the P type, which is characterized by the formation of a phosphorylated intermediary (Na^+,K^+-, H^+,K^+-, and Ca^{2+}-ATPase) (Figure 2.12) or to the V type (vacuolar H^+-ATPase). In intracellular membranes, there is expression of the vacuolar-type H^+ pump, as well as F-type (or F_1- or F_0- type) ATPases, the ATP synthase expressed in the inner mitochondrial membrane. ATP synthases are also expressed in purple bacteria and in green plants. Their function can be outlined as follows. Multimeric protein complexes (respiratory chain complex in mitochondria, bacteriorhodopsin in purple bacteria, photosynthetic reaction center in chloroplasts) generate an H^+ electrochemical gradient from the redox potential of NADPH (mitochondria) or light energy (others). The transmembrane H^+ electrochemical gradient is then used by ATP synthases to synthesize ATP from ADP and P_i. Hence, the function of these proteins is to synthesize ATP, dissipating the ion gradient in the process. However, they are reversible, and under appropriate conditions they will hydrolyze ATP and generate an electrochemical ion gradient. Similarly, the Na^+,K^+-ATPase normally hydrolyzes ATP to transport actively Na^+ out of the cell and K^+ into the cell, but under certain experimental conditions it can operate in a reverse mode, that is, downhill ion fluxes (Na^+ into the cell and K^+ out of the cell) coupled to the synthesis of ATP.

The ion pumps present in plasma membranes of epithelial cells are the Na^+,K^+-ATPase, Ca^{2+}-ATPase, H^+-ATPase, and H^+,K^+-ATPase. Other pumps have been suggested to exist in these tissues, but they are either unique to certain epithelia or controversial. The molecular structures of these pumps have been identified, and significant progress has been made in understanding their function, but much work remains to be done in this area. Ion occlusion is a well-known stage during the pump cycle.[40] As is the case with carrier function, occlusion denotes that the conformational change necessary for transport does change the accessibility of the substrate-binding sites to the solutions bathing the membrane.

The Na^+,K^+-, H^+,K^+-, and Ca^{2+}-ATPase are all of the P type, which is characterized by the phosphorylation of an aspartic acid residue (in the sequence DKTG) during the pump catalytic cycle. The Na^+,K^+-ATPase is a ubiquitous pump in epithelial cells. In each cycle, one ATP molecule is hydrolyzed, three Na^+ are transported from the cytoplasm to the interstitial fluid, and two K^+ are transported in the opposite direction. In each cycle there is thus a net transfer of charge across the membrane (one net positive charge is extruded), and hence the pump is electrogenic, tending to hyperpolarize the cell. Its turnover number is in the range of values for carriers less than $10^2\,s^{-1}$. The catalytic cycle of P-type ATPases is shown in Figure 2.12.

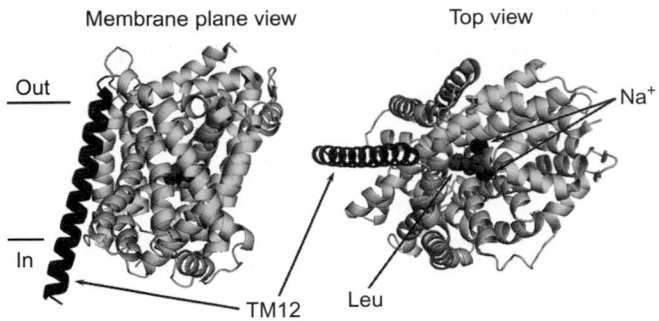

Membrane plane view **Top view**

FIGURE 2.11 **Structure of a symporter.** Side (left) and extracellular (right) views of the LeuT, a prokaryotic Leu-Na$^+$ symporter that belongs to the neurotransmitter sodium symporter family. One protomer of the dimer in the crystal structure is shown. Transmembrane helix 12 is shown in darker gray. Leu and Na$^+$ bound deep into the structure core are shown in darker gray and black, respectively (built with PyMol from PDB 2A65).

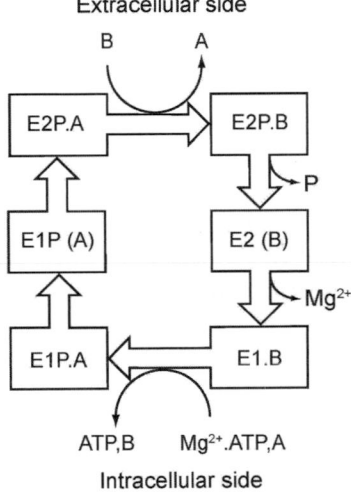

FIGURE 2.12 Catalytic cycle for P-type ATPases modeled as countertransport pumps exchanging Na$^+$ (*A*) for K$^+$ (*B*), Ca^{2+} (*A*) for H$^+$ (*B*) or H$^+$ (*A*) for K$^+$ (*B*) (Na$^+$,K$^+$-, Ca^{2+}-, and H$^+$,K$^+$-ATPase, respectively) (E1: conformation with ion-binding sites accessible from cytoplasm; E2: conformation with ion-binding sites accessible from the extracellular face; E(A) or E(B): ion "occluded" in the protein) (*modified with permission from ref. [85]*).

The Na$^+$,K$^+$-ATPase is expressed in virtually all vertebrate epithelial cells, where it is usually targeted to the basolateral membrane. In two cases, the choroid plexus and the retinal pigment epithelium, the pump is targeted to the apical membrane and epithelial cell polarity is inverted *vis-à-vis* other tissues. The pump consists of α- and β-subunits in a 1:1 stoichiometry (likely α2:β2). The α-subunit is responsible for both ion transport and ATPase activity, and contains the binding sites for Na$^+$, K$^+$, and ouabain, a specific inhibitor, as well as the phosphorylation site. The β-subunit,

previously thought to be just involved in assembly and delivery of the pump, has in addition an important role in K$^+$ binding.[93] The α-subunit has three isoforms (apparent molecular mass 120 kDa) and the β-subunit has two isoforms, with apparent molecular mass of 50 kDa. Pump isoforms are tissue-specific, change during organ development, and exhibit different pharmacological properties. The Na$^+$,K$^+$ pump was first crystallized in 2007,[79] and a higher resolution structure was obtained in 2009.[93] At this time, our understanding of the structure–function relationships is less than that for the sarcoplasmic reticulum Ca^{2+} pump (see below). The regulation of the activity of the Na$^+$,K$^+$ pump is complex, and an important regulatory mechanism in the kidney is the increase in Na$^+$ pump expression in principal cells of the collecting duct under the action of mineralocorticoids. These hormones stimulate of Na$^+$ entry via ENaC, which results in an increase in intracellular Na$^+$ concentration that appears to mediate the stimulation of pump expression.

The plasma membrane Ca^{2+} pump (PMCA pump) actively exports Ca^{2+} from the cell, exchanging it for H$^+$ (the stoichiometry appears to be 1 Ca^{2+} out:2 H$^+$ in:1 ATP molecule hydrolyzed). The pump is 120–140 kDa, with ten transmembrane helices and three substantial intracellular domains. The crystal structure of the Ca^{2+} pump from sarcoplasmic/endoplasmic reticulum (SERCA pump) was solved a decade ago.[107] It has two Ca^{2+}-binding sites from which the ions are extruded, with a stoichiometry of 2 Ca^{2+} per ATP hydrolyzed, different from that of the PMCA pump. The PMCA pump has high affinity for intracellular Ca^{2+}, in the submicromolar range. The conformational change elicited by ATP hydrolysis is thought to make the Ca^{2+} sites face the extracellular space and the affinity decrease, causing Ca^{2+} release. The function of the PMCA pump is to help maintain a low intracellular Ca^{2+} concentration. It is a high affinity, low capacity system. The PMCA pump is stimulated by calmodulin and 1,25-dihydroxyvitamin D (for a review, see [10]).

The H$^+$/K$^+$-ATPase is expressed in gastric epithelial cells (gastric isoform), colonocytes (colonic isoform), and renal collecting ducts (both isoforms). As with the Na$^+$,K$^+$-ATPase and the Ca^{2+}-ATPases, the H$^+$/K$^+$-ATPase consists of α- and β-subunits. The α-subunits of the two isoforms, are very similar in amino acid sequence to the α-subunit of the Na$^+$,K$^+$-ATPase. The function of the renal H$^+$/K$^+$-ATPase is acid secretion and K$^+$ reabsorption

In the last decade, crystal structures have been obtained for the Ca^{2+} pump from sarcoplasmic reticulum,[107,109,110] the plasma membrane Na$^+$,K$^+$-ATPase[79,80,93] and the plant plasma membrane H$^+$-ATPase.[83] Although the Ca^{2+}-ATPase from rabbit skeletal muscle sarcoplasmic reticulum (SERCA1a) is not a plasma membrane protein, it is currently the better known P-type ion transporting ATPase. The mass of SERCA1a is 110 kDa, it has 10 transmembrane helices (M1–M10), three cytoplasmic domains (A [actuator or anchor]; N [nucleotide-binding]; and P [phosphorylation]), and small SR-lumen loops. SERCA1a transports, against the electrochemical gradient across the SR membrane, two Ca^{2+} per ATP hydrolyzed, reducing $[Ca^{2+}]$ in the cytosol, and accumulating it in the SR lumen. Two or three H^+ are exchanged for the Ca^{2+} in each cycle. As is the case with other P-ATPases, primary active ion transport results from a conformational change of the pump (from E1 to E2). In E1, the Ca^{2+} ions bind with high affinity and face the cytoplasm; in E2, the affinity is low and Ca^{2+} ions face the SR lumen. The Ca^{2+} translocation would take place between E1P and E2P, two states of the phosphorylated pump. Similar states exist in the operation of the Na^+,K^+-ATPase (see Chapter 3).

The first determination of the structure of SERCA1 by X-ray crystallography in 2000[107] was followed by over 20 structures in different states that essentially cover the reaction cycle, making it the best characterized P-type ion-translocating ATPase.[106] The atomic structure, represented in Figure 2.13,[107,108] revealed that transmembrane helices 4, 5, and 6 contain the amino acid residues that bind the two Ca^{2+} ions transported per cycle. These results, combined with molecular dynamics simulations[101] have provided detailed information about the binding sites and the conformational changes underlying ion pumping.[105,106] Differences between several structures revealed that SERCA1 Ca^{2+} binding and dissociation elicit large conformational changes in the transmembrane domains, mechanically linked to similar changes in the cytoplasmic domains. Homology modeling suggests that the cation-binding sites of the Ca^{2+}- and Na^+,K^+-ATPases are virtually the same.[84] A critical movement of transmembrane helix 4 causes the release of a cation (Ca^{2+} or Na^+) and the binding of the other cation (H^+ or K^+) at a displaced position with respect to the membrane, thus preventing competition between the cations.

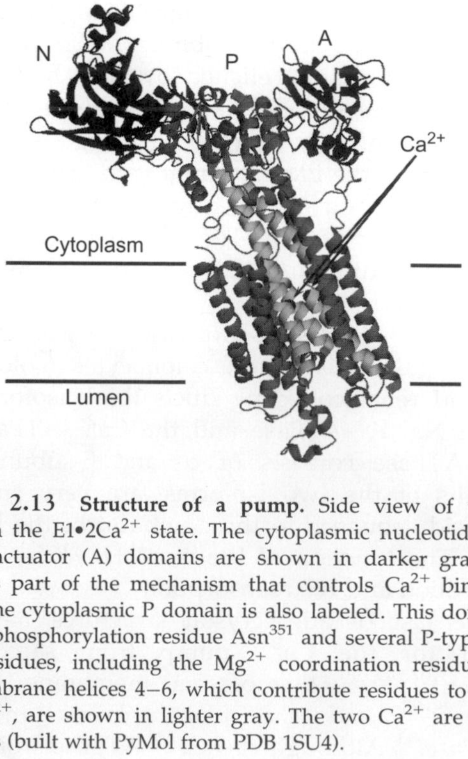

Similarities and Differences between Ion Transport Proteins

The recent progress in genomics and structural biology of membrane proteins (*ca.* 700 crystal structures, of which 250 are unique[114]), combined with increasing sophistication of biochemical and biophysical studies has began to clarify the essential similarities and differences between these proteins. We wish to make several important points in this closing section. First, there are big differences between ion channels, on the one hand, and carriers and pumps, on the other, and the differences in function are explained by the differences in structure. Second, there are families in which individuals can be either channels or carriers, or either channels or pumps, suggesting something akin to a "common ancestor." Third, there is at least one instance in which pharmacological intervention can transform a pump into a channel. We discuss briefly these three points.

1. *Channels versus carriers and pumps.* The crucial functional difference between channels, on the one hand, and carriers or pumps, on the other, is in the turnover numbers: channels conduct ions rapidly (10^6–10^8 s^{-1}), whereas carriers and pumps are much slower (10^2–10^4 s^{-1}). This difference is related to the relatively slow conformational changes that accompany solute flux in carriers and pumps, while in open channels no conformational changes occur during transport. In addition, there is a difference in access of the transported ion(s) to the critical site. As we saw in the structures of K^+ and Cl^- channels, the narrow region of the permeation pathway (selectivity filter) is short relative to the thickness of the membrane, facilitating rapid conduction. In K^+ channels, in addition, the four binding sites in single file cause repulsion between adjacent ions, also facilitating rapid conduction. In contrast, in carriers (such as LeuT) and pumps (such as the Ca^{2+}-ATPase) the ion-binding sites are located deep inside the protein, with no

FIGURE 2.13 Structure of a pump. Side view of the Ca^{2+}-ATPase in the E1•2Ca^{2+} state. The cytoplasmic nucleotide binding (N) and actuator (A) domains are shown in darker gray. The A domain is part of the mechanism that controls Ca^{2+} binding and release. The cytoplasmic P domain is also labeled. This domain contains the phosphorylation residue Asn^{351} and several P-type ATPase critical residues, including the Mg^{2+} coordination residue Asp^{703}. Transmembrane helices 4–6, which contribute residues to the binding of Ca^{2+}, are shown in lighter gray. The two Ca^{2+} are shown as black balls (built with PyMol from PDB 1SU4).

unobstructed pathway to the adjacent aqueous solutions. This feature limits the speed of ion transport, but permits occlusion, i.e., the ion pathway is never simultaneously open to both sides of the membrane. These arguments are lucidly presented by Gouaux and MacKinnon.[42]

2. *Functionally different transport proteins present in the same family.* The ClC proteins appear to be an intermediate class of ion transport proteins in between channels and carriers. Their structure is channel-like, with vestibules in series with a short selectivity filter with capacity to contain several ions. Functionally, some ClC proteins are indeed channels, whereas others are antiporters in which the Cl^- flux is coupled to flux of H^+ in the opposite direction.[3,76] A somewhat similar situation holds for the case of ABC proteins, which in most instances are pumps (ATPases), but at least one member (CFTR) is an ion channel. There is no crystal structure of CFTR yet, but from the primary and secondary structures one would not predict that the protein is a channel. It has been recently proposed that both CFTR and ClC-O are Cl^- channels evolved from transporters.[15]

3. *A pump can be transformed into a channel.* The marine toxin palitoxin (PTX) is a ~ 3000 Da molecule that consists of a chain of over 100 carbons with a complex variety of organic side groups. The mechanism of the toxic effect of PTX is to convert the Na^+,K^+-ATPase from a cation pump into a nonselective cation channel that dissipates the Na^+ and K^+ gradients between the cell and the extracellular fluid. This could be explained if the effect of PTX were to open the two gates necessary for the normal operation of the pump, thus revealing the ion translocation pathway. PTX was shown to interact with the pump in excised membrane patches, this interaction was dependent of the presence of ATP on the inside of the membrane, and was modulated by extracellular K^+, indicating that the PTX-dependent channel function shares properties of the native pump.[7,8] In other studies, the permeation pathway was mapped using the technique known as cysteine-scanning mutagenesis, in which the accessibility of amino acid sites to small hydrophilic thiol reagents is assessed after mutating those sites to Cys. Residues in transmembrane helices 4, 5, and 6 became accessible by exposure to PTX,[43,44,57] consistent with the structural studies described above.

We have presented three arguments that support the notion that ion channels, carriers, and pumps share a basic molecular architecture (see [37] and [38]). In sum, and as illustrated in Figure 2.14, the simplest ion

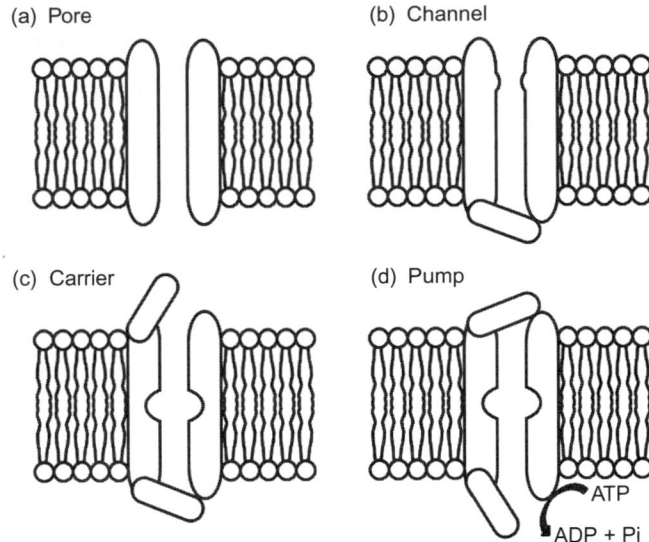

FIGURE 2.14 A simplified view of structure–function correlations in ion transport proteins. (a) Pore, the simplest ion transport protein, is a transmembrane aqueous conduit with no gates, accessible to both sides of the membrane at all times (always open). (b) Channel, a pore with a gate whose position determines whether the channel is open or closed. The open channel is accessible to both sides of the membrane. (c) Carrier, a transmembrane protein with two gates that are never open at the same time. Thus, the carrier interior may be accessible to only one side of the membrane; when both gates are closed the substrate is occluded (inaccessible to either side). (d) Pump, a carrier that is directly coupled to a metabolic energy source, e.g., hydrolysis of ATP.

transport protein would be a pore (no gate), followed by a pore with one gate (channel), a pore with two gates (carrier), and finally a pore with two gates coupled to a metabolic-energy source (pump). As more structures of membrane transport proteins become available the "missing links" might be identified.

References

[1] Abramson J, Iwata S, Kaback HR. Lactose permease as a paradigm for membrane transport proteins. Mol Membr Biol 2004;21:227–36.

[2] Abramson J, Smirnova I, Kasho V, Verner G, Kaback HR, Iwata S. Structure and mechanism of the lactose permease of *Escherichia coli*. Science 2003;301:610–5.

[3] Accardi A, Miller C. Secondary active transport mediated by a prokaryotic homologue of ClC Cl^- channels. Nature 2004;427:803–7.

[4] Aller P, Garnier N, Genest M. Transmembrane helix packing of ErB/Neu receptor in membrane environment: a molecular dynamics study. J Biomol Struct Dyn 2006;24:209–28.

[5] Apell HJ. How do P-type ATPases transport ions? Bioelectrochemistry 2004;63:149–56.

[6] Arnold WN. Yeast cell envelopes: biochemistry, biophysics, and ultrastructure. Boca Raton, FL: CRC Press; 1981.

[7] Artigas P, Gadsby DC. Na^+/K^+ pump ligands modulate gating of palytoxin-induced ion channels. Proc Natl Acad Sci USA 2003;100:501–5.

[8] Artigas P, Gadsby DC. Large diameter of palytoxin-induced Na$^+$/K$^+$ pump channels and modulation of palytoxin interaction by Na$^+$K$^+$ pump ligands. J Gen Physiol 2004;123:357–76.

[9] Behnia R, Munro S. Organelle identity and the signposts for membrane traffic. Nature 2005;438:597–604.

[10] Brini M, Carafoli E. Calcium pumps in health and disease. Physiol Rev 2009;89:1341–78.

[11] Calvet JP, Grantham JJ. The genetics and physiology of polycystic kidney disease. Semin Nephrol 2001;21:107–23.

[12] Canessa CM, Horisberger JD, Rossier BC. Epithelial sodium channel related to proteins involved in neurodegeneration. Nature 1993;361:467–70.

[13] Catterall WA. Structure and function of voltage-gated ion channels. In: Schultz SG, Andreoli TE, Brown AM, Fambrough DM, Hoffman JF, Welsh MJ, editors. Molecular biology of membrane transport disorders. New York: Plenum Press; 1996. p. 129–45.

[14] Chen TY. Structure and function of ClC channels. Annu Rev Physiol 2005;67:809–39.

[15] Chen TY, Hwang TC. CLC-0 and CFTR: chloride channels evolved from transporters. Physiol Rev 2008;88:351–87.

[16] Crane RK. Intestinal absorption of sugars. Physiol Rev 1960;40:789–825.

[17] Dang S, Sun L, Huang Y, Lu F, Liu Y, Gong H, et al. Structure of fucose transporter in an outward-open confrontation. Nature 2010;467:734–8.

[18] Dawson DC. Permeability and conductance in ion channels: a primer. In: Schultz SG, Andreoli TE, Brown AM, Fambrough DM, Hoffman JF, Welsh MJ, editors. Molecular biology of membrane transport disorders. New York: Plenum Press; 1996. p. 87–110.

[19] Dawson RJ, Locher KP. Structure of a bacterial multidrug ABC transporter. Nature 2006;443:180–5.

[20] Deisenhofer J, Epp O, Miki K, Huber R, Michel H. Structure of the protein subunits in the photosynthetic reaction centre of Rhodopseudomonas viridis at 3 Å resolution. Nature 1985;318:618–24.

[21] Delcour AH. Solute uptake through general porins. Front Biosci 2003;8:d1055–71.

[22] Devuyst O, Guggino WB. Chloride channels in the kidney: lessons learned from knockout animals. Am J Physiol Renal Physiol 2002;283:F1176–91.

[23] Dietrich B. Coordination chemistry of alkali and alkaline-earth cations with macrocyclic ligands. J Chem Educ 1985;62:954–8.

[24] Doyle DA. Molecular insights into ion channel function. Mol Membr Biol 2004;21:221–5.

[25] Doyle DA. Structural changes during ion channel gating. Trends Neurosci 2004;27:298–302.

[26] Doyle DA, Morais Cabral J, Pfuetzner RA, Kuo A, Gulbis JM, Cohen SL, et al. The structure of the potassium channel: molecular basis of K$^+$ conduction and selectivity. Science 1998;280:69–77.

[27] Duran C, Thompson CH, Xiao Q, Hartzell HC. Chloride channels: often enigmatic, rarely predictable. Annu Rev Physiol 2010;72:95–121.

[28] Dutzler R, Campbell EB, Cadene M, Chait BT, MacKinnon R. X-ray structure of a ClC chloride channel at 3.0 Å reveals the molecular basis of anion selectivity. Nature 2002;415:287–94.

[29] Dutzler R, Campbell EB, MacKinnon R. Gating the selectivity filter in ClC chloride channels. Science 2003;300:108–12.

[30] Engelman DM. Membranes are more mosaic than fluid. Nature 2005;438:578–80.

[31] Facciotti MT, Rouhani-Manshadi S, Glaeser RM. Energy transduction in transmembrane ion pumps. Trends Biochem Sci 2004;29:445–51.

[32] Faham S, Watanabe A, Besserer GM, Cascio D, Specht A, Hirayama BA, et al. The crystal structure of sodium galactose

transporter reveals mechanistic insights into Na$^+$/sugar symport. Science 2008;321:810–4.

[33] Fambrough DM, Inesi G. Cation transport ATPases. In: Schultz SG, Andreoli TE, Brown AM, Fambrough DM, Hoffman JF, Welsh MJ, editors. Molecular biology of membrane transport diseases. New York: Plenum Press; 1996. p. 223–41.

[34] Fick A. Ueber diffusion. Ann Phys Chem 1855;94:59–86.

[35] Finbow ME, Harrison MA. The vacuolar H$^+$-ATPase: a universal proton pump of eukaryotes. Biochem J 1997;324:697–712.

[36] Finkelstein A, Rosenberg PA. Single-file transport: implications for ion and water movement through gramicidin a channels. In: Stevens CF, Tsien RW, editors. Membrane transport processes. New York: Raven Press; 1979. p. 73–88.

[37] Gadsby DC. Ion transport: spot the difference. Nature 2004;427:795–7.

[38] Gadsby DC. Ion channels versus ion pumps: the principal difference, in principle. Nat Rev Mol Cell Biol 2009;10:344–52.

[39] Galietta LJ. The TMEM16 protein family: a new class of chloride channels? Biophys J 2009;97:3047–53.

[40] Glynn IM, Hoffman JF. Nucleotide requirements for sodium–sodium exchange catalysed by the sodium pump in human red cells. J Physiol 1971;218:239–56.

[41] Goldman DE. Potential, impedance, and rectification in membranes. J Gen Physiol 1943;27:37–60.

[42] Gouaux E, Mackinnon R. Principles of selective ion transport in channels and pumps. Science 2005;310:1461–5.

[43] Guennoun S, Horisberger JD. Structure of the 5th transmembrane segment of the Na, K-ATPase a subunit: a cysteine-scanning mutagenesis study. FEBS Lett 2000;482:144–8.

[44] Guennoun S, Horisberger JD. Cysteine scanning mutagenesis study of the 6th transmembrane segment of the Na, K-ATPase a subunit: a cysteine-scanning mutagenesis study. FEBS Lett 2002;513:277–88.

[45] Hartzell HC, Yu K, Xiao Q, Chien LT, Qu Z. Anoctamin/TMEM16 family members are Ca^{2+}-activated Cl$^-$ channels. J Physiol 2009;587:2127–39.

[46] Hebert SC, Desir G, Giebisch G, Wang W. Molecular diversity and regulation of renal potassium channels. Physiol Rev 2005;85:319–71.

[47] Hediger MA, Romero MF, Peng JB, Rolfs A, Takanaga H, Bruford EA. The ABCs of solute carriers: physiological, pathological and therapeutic implications of human membrane transport proteins. Pflügers Arch 2004;447:465–8.

[48] Heginbotham L, Lu Z, Abramson T, MacKinnon R. Mutations in the K$^+$ channel signature sequence. Biophys J 1994;66:1061–7.

[49] Hilgemann DW, Feng S, Nasuhoglu C. The complex and intriguing lives of PIP$_2$ with ion channels and transporters. Science-STKE 2001;111:1–8.

[50] Hille B. Ionic channels of excitable membranes. 3rd ed. Sunderland: Sinauer; 2001.

[51] Hodgkin AL, Katz B. The effect of sodium ions on the electrical activity of the giant axon of the squid. J Physiol (London) 1949;108:37–77.

[52] Hoenderop JG, Nilius B, Bindels RJ. Calcium absorption across epithelia. Physiol Rev 2005;85:373–422.

[53] Hollenstein K, Dawson R, Locher K. Structure and mechanism of ABC transporter proteins. Curr Opin Struct Biol 2007;17:412–8.

[54] Horisberger JD. The Na, K-ATPase: structure-function relationship. Boca Raton, FL: CRC Press; 1994. p. 1–20.

[55] Horisberger JD. Recent insights into the structure and mechanism of the sodium pump. Physiology (Bethesda) 2004;19:377–87.

[56] Horisberger JD, Chraibi A. Epithelial sodium channel: a ligand-gated channel? Nephron Physiol 2004;96:37–41.

[57] Horisberger JD, Kharoubi-Hess S, Guennoun S, Michielin O. The fourth transmembrane segment of the Na, K-ATPase a subunit: a systematic mutagenesis study. J Biol Chem 2004;279:29542—50.

[58] Huang Y, Lemieux MJ, Song J, Auer M, Wang DN. Structure and mechanism of the glycerol-3-phosphate transporter from *Escherichia coli*. Science 2003;301:616—20.

[59] Jacobson K, Dietrich C. Looking at lipid rafts? Trends Cell Biol 1999;9:87—91.

[60] Jentsch TJ. CLC chloride channels and transporters: from genes to protein structure, pathology and physiology. Crit Rev Biochem Mol Biol 2008;43:3—36.

[61] Krämer R. Functional principles of solute transport systems: concepts and perspectives. Biochim Biophys Acta 1994;1185:1—34.

[62] Krarup T, Jensen BS, Hoffmann EK. Occlusion of K^+ in the Na^+/K^+2Cl^- co-transporter of Ehrlich ascites tumor cells. Biochim Biophys Acta 1996;1284:97—108.

[63] Kurtzman CP, Fell JW. The yeasts: a Taxonomic study. 4th ed. Amsterdam; New York: Elsevier; 1998.

[64] Läuger P. Dynamics of ion transport systems in membranes. Physiol Rev 1987;67:1296—331.

[65] Läuger P. Electrogenic ion pumps. Sunderland: Sinauer; 1991.

[66] LeFevre PG, Bronner F, Kleinzeller A. The present state of the carrier hypothesis. Curr Top Membr Transport 1975;7:109—251.

[67] Macey RI, Moura TF. Basic principles of transport. In: Hoffman JF, Jamieson JD, editors. Handbook of physiology. Section 14: cell physiology. New York: Oxford University Press; 1997. p. 181—260.

[68] MacKinnon R. Nobel Lecture. Potassium channels and the atomic basis of selective ion conduction. Biosci Rep 2004;24:75—100.

[69] MacKinnon R. Potassium channels. FEBS Lett 2003;555:62—5.

[70] Macrez N, Mironneau J. Local $Ca^{2=}$ signals in cellular signaling. Curr Mol Med 2004;4:263—75.

[71] McIntosh TJ, Simon SA. Roles of bilayer material properties in function and distribution of membrane proteins. Annu Rev Biophys Biomol Struct 2006;35:177—98.

[72] McLaughlin S, Murray D. Plasma membrane phosphoinositide organization by protein electrostatics. Nature 2005;438:605—11.

[73] McLaughlin S, Wang J, Gambhir A, Murray D. PIP(2) and proteins: Interactions, organization, and information flow. Annu Rev Biophys Biomol Struct 2002;31:151—75.

[74] McLuskey K, Roszak AW, Zhu Y, Isaacs NW. Crystal structures of all-alpha type membrane proteins. Eur Biophys J 2010;39:723—55.

[75] Miller C. Ion Channel Reconstitution. New York: Plenum Press; 1986.

[76] Miller C. ClC chloride channels viewed through a transporter lens. Nature 2006;440:484—9.

[77] Morais-Cabral JH, Zhou Y, MacKinnon R. Energetic optimization of ion conduction rate by the K^+ selectivity filter. Nature 2001;414:37—42.

[78] Mornon J, Lehn P, Callebaut I. Molecular models of the open and closed states of the whole human CFTR protein. Cell Mol Life Sci 2009;66:3469—86.

[79] Morth JP, Pedersen BP, Toustrup-Jensen MS, Sørensen TL, Petersen J, Andersen JP, et al. Crystal structure of the sodium-potassium pump. Nature 2007;450:1043—9.

[80] Morth JP, Pedersen BP, Buch-Pedersen MJ, Andersen JP, Vilsen B, Palmgren MG, et al. A structural overview of the plasma membrane Na^+, K^+-ATPase and H^+-ATPase ion pumps. Nature Rev Mol Cell Biol 2011;12:60—70.

[81] Nernst W. Zur Kinetik der in Lösung befindlichen Körper: theorie der diffusion. Z Phys Chem 1888;2:613—37.

[82] Noury C, Grant SGN, Borg JP. PDZ domain proteins: plug and play!. Science-STKE 2003;179:1—12.

[83] Pedersen BP, Buch-Pedersen MJ, Morth JP, Palmgren MG, Nissen P. Crystal structure of the plasma membrane proton pump. Nature 2007;450:1111—4.

[84] Ogawa H, Toyoshima C. Homology modeling of the cation binding sites of the Na^+,K^+-ATPase. Proc Natl Acad Sci USA 2002;99:15977—82.

[85] Sachs G, Munson K. Mammalian phosphorylating ion motive ATPases. Curr Opin Cell Biol 1991;3:685—94.

[86] Sachs G, Shin JM, Bamberg K, Prinz C. Gastric acid secretion: the H,K-ATPase and ulcer disease. In: Schultz SG, Andreoli TE, Brown AM, Fambrough DM, Hoffman JF, Welsh MJ, editors. Molecular biology of membrane transport disorders. New York: Plenum Press; 1996. p. 469—84.

[87] Saier Jr. MH. A functional-phylogenetic classification system for transmembrane solute transporters. Microbiol Mol Biol Rev 2000;64:354—411.

[88] Sakmann B, Neher E. Single-channel recording. New York: Plenum Press; 1995.

[89] Schulz GE. The structure of bacterial outer membrane proteins. Biochim Biophys Acta 2002;1565:308—17.

[90] Schultz SG. Basic principles of membrane transport. Cambridge: Cambridge University Press; 1980.

[91] Schultz SG. Homocellular regulatory mechanisms in sodium-transporting epithelia: avoidance of extinction by "flush-through. Am J Physiol 1981;241:F579—90.

[92] Segel IH. Enzyme kinetics: behavior and analysis of rapid equilibrium and steady-state enzyme systems. New York: John Wiley & Sons, Inc.; 1975.

[93] Shinoda T, Ogawa H, Cornelius F, Toyoshima C. Crystal structure of the sodium-potassium pump at 2.4 Å resolution. Nature 2009;459:446—50.

[94] Simons K, Toomre D. Lipid rafts and signal transduction. Nat Rev Mol Cell Biol 2000;1:31—9.

[95] Singer SJ. The structure and function of membranes: a personal memoir. J Membr Biol 1992;129:3—12.

[96] Singer SJ, Nicolson GL. The fluid mosaic model of the structure of cell membranes. Science 1972;175:720—31.

[97] Skou JC. The Na-K pump. Methods Enzymol 1988;156:1—25.

[98] Skou JC, Esmann M. The Na,K-ATPase. J Bioenerg Biomembr 1992;24:249—61.

[99] Stein WD. Channels, carriers, and pumps. An introduction to membrane transport. San Diego, CA: Academic Press; 1990.

[100] Stockand JD, Staruschenko A, Pochynyuk O, Botth RE, Silverthorn DU. Insight toward epithelial Na channel mechanism revealed by the acid-sensing ion channel 1 structure. IUBMB Life 2008;60:620—8.

[101] Sugita Y, Miyashita N, Yoda T, Ikeguchi M. Structural changes in the cytoplasmic domain of phospholamban by phosphorylation at Ser16: a molecular dynamics study. Biochemistry 2006;45:11752—61.

[102] Suh BC, Hille B. PIP2 is a necessary cofactor for ion channel function: how and why? Annu Rev Biophys 2008;37:175—95.

[103] Tanford C, Reynolds JA. Membrane structure/proteins. In: Hoffman JF, Jamieson JD, editors. Handbook of physiology. Section 14: cell physiology. New York: Oxford University Press; 1997. p. 59—74.

[104] Tanner MJ. The structure and function of band 3 (AE1): recent developments. Mol Membr Biol 1997;14:155—65.

[105] Toyoshima C. Structural aspects of ion pumping by Ca^{2+}-ATPase of sarcoplasmic reticulum. Arch Biochem Biophys 2008;476:3—11.

[106] Toyoshima C. How Ca^{2+}-ATPase pumps ions across the sarcoplasmic reticulum membrane. Biochim Biophys Acta 2009;1793:941—6.

I. EPITHELIAL AND NONEPITHELIAL TRANSPORT AND REGULATION

[107] Toyoshima C, Nakasake M, Nomura H, Ogawa H. Crystal structure of the calcium pump of sarcoplasmic reticulum at 2.6 Å resolution. Nature 2000;405:647−55.

[108] Toyoshima C, Nomura H. Structural changes in the calcium pump accompanying dissociation of calcium. Nature 2002;418:605−11.

[109] Toyoshima C, Nomura H, Sugita Y. Crystal structures of Ca^{2+}-ATPase in various physiological states. Ann NY Acad Sci 2003;986:1−8.

[110] Toyoshima C, Nomura H, Sugita Y. Structural basis of ion pumping by Ca^{2+}-ATPase of sarcoplasmic reticulum. FEBS Lett 2003;555:106−10.

[111] Ussing HH. Transport of ions across cellular membranes. Physiol Rev 1949;29:127−55.

[112] Vereb G, Szöllösi J, Matkó J, Nagy P, Farkas T, Vigh L, et al. Dynamic, yet structured: the cell membrane three decades after the Singer−Nicolson model. Proc Natl Acad Sci USA 2003;100:8053−8.

[113] Ward A, Reyes CL, Yu J, Roth CB, Chang G. Flexibility in the ABC transporter MsbA: alternating access with a twist. Proc Natl Acad Sci USA 2007;104:19005−10.

[114] White S. Membrane proteins of known structure. 2010; http://blanco.biomol.uci.edu/Membrane_Proteins_xtal.html.

[115] Wright EM, Loo DD, Hirayama BA, Turk E. Surprising versatility of Na^+-glucose co-transporters: SLC5. Physiology 2004;19:370−6.

[116] Yamashita A, Singh SK, Kawate T, Jin Y, Gouaux E. Crystal structure of a bacterial homologue of Na^+/Cl^--dependent neurotransmitter transporters. Nature 2005;437:215−23.

[117] Yin Y, He X, Szewczyk P, Nguyen T, Chang G. Structure of the multidrug transporter EmrD from *Escherichia coli*. Science 2006;312:741−4.

[118] Zachos NC, Tse M, Donowitz M. Molecular physiology of intestinal Na^+/H^+ exchange. Annu Rev Physiol 2005;67:411−43.

[119] Zhou Y, MacKinnon R. The occupancy of ions in the K^+ selectivity filter: charge balance and coupling of ion binding to a protein conformational change underlie high conduction rates. J Mol Biol 2003;333:965−75.

[120] Zhou Y, Morais-Cabral JH, Kaufman A, MacKinnon R. Chemistry of ion coordination and hydration revealed by a K^+ channel-Fab complex at 2.0 Å resolution. Nature 2001;414:43−8.

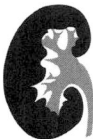

Renal Ion-Translocating ATPases

Dominique Eladari[1], Udo Hasler[2] and Eric Féraille[2]

[1]INSERM U872, Centre de Recherche des Cordeliers, Paris, France
[2]Department of Cell Physiology and Metabolism and Service of Nephrology,
University Medical Center, Geneva, Switzerland

Active transport of solutes across membranes against their concentration or electrochemical gradients requires energy. For ion-motive ATPases (F-type, V-type, and P-type), this process is an exchange between energy contained in the electrochemical gradient and chemical energy provided by ATP hydrolysis. F-type ATPases or ATP synthases are responsible for the generation of ATP using energy of the proton gradient created by the respiratory chain in mitochondria or photosynthetic complexes in chloroplasts. V-type ATPases acidify vesicles by transporting protons from the cytoplasm to the lumen of intracellular organelles (endosomes, lysosomes, vacuoles, . . .). V-ATPases are also present in the plasma membrane of some epithelial cells. Despite sharing a common general architecture and a large number of subunits, F- and V-ATPases usually work in opposite directions. P-type ATPases (also called E1-, E2-ATPases) form a third group of ion-motive ATPases that perform unidirectional or exchange transport of monovalent (H^+, Na^+, K^+) or divalent (Ca^{2+}, Cu^{2+}, Mg^{2+}, . . .) cations.

P-ATPASES

While some members of the P-ATPase family are probably active as a single polypeptide, the functional unit of others consists of several subunits. The major subunit (α- or catalytic subunit for multimeric P-ATPases) consists of a series of hairpins formed by pairs of transmembrane segments linked by short extracellular loops. Two large intracellular loops make the connection between the first, second, and third hairpins. The largest cytoplasmic loop contains the ATP-binding domain and the phosphorylation site. Transient phosphorylation of this aspartate residue

occurring during the transport cycle is a hallmark of P-ATPases (Figure 3.1).

STRUCTURE AND FUNCTION OF Ca^{2+}-ATPASES (SERCA AND PMCA)

SERCA is found in intracellular organelles related to the endoplasmic reticulum, such as the sarcoplasmic reticulum of cardiac and skeletal muscle cells. Three differently expressed genes have been identified: SERCA1 in fast-twitch skeletal muscle; SERCA2 in slow-twitch skeletal muscle, heart, and smooth muscle; and SERCA3 in blood, endothelial, and epithelial tissue. SERCA mediates uptake of Ca^{2+} from the cytoplasm into the sarcoplasmic reticulum following calcium release from intracellular stores. It therefore acts as a terminator signal in excitation—contraction coupling processes in muscle, and plays a key role in excitation—secretion coupling in neurons and other secretory cells. Extensive structure—function studies have been performed with SERCA and a high resolution (2.6 Å) structure of this protein was obtained.[1]

PMCA is expressed at the plasma membrane, where it extrudes Ca^{2+} out of the cell. Four PMCA genes are known, with multiple splicing variants for each gene, resulting in the existence of about 20 isoforms. PMCA1 and PMCA4 are ubiquitous, while PMCA2 and PMCA3 are restricted to neurons, brain, muscle, and kidney. PMCA plays an important role in tubular reabsorption of calcium.[1] The long C-terminal intracellular domain maintains PMCA in an inactive state by interacting with the catalytic site. A rise of cytosolic Ca^{2+} concentration increases Ca^{2+}—calmodulin-binding, allowing calmodulin to interact with the PMCA C-terminal domain. This releases PMCA autoinhibition, activating the pump.

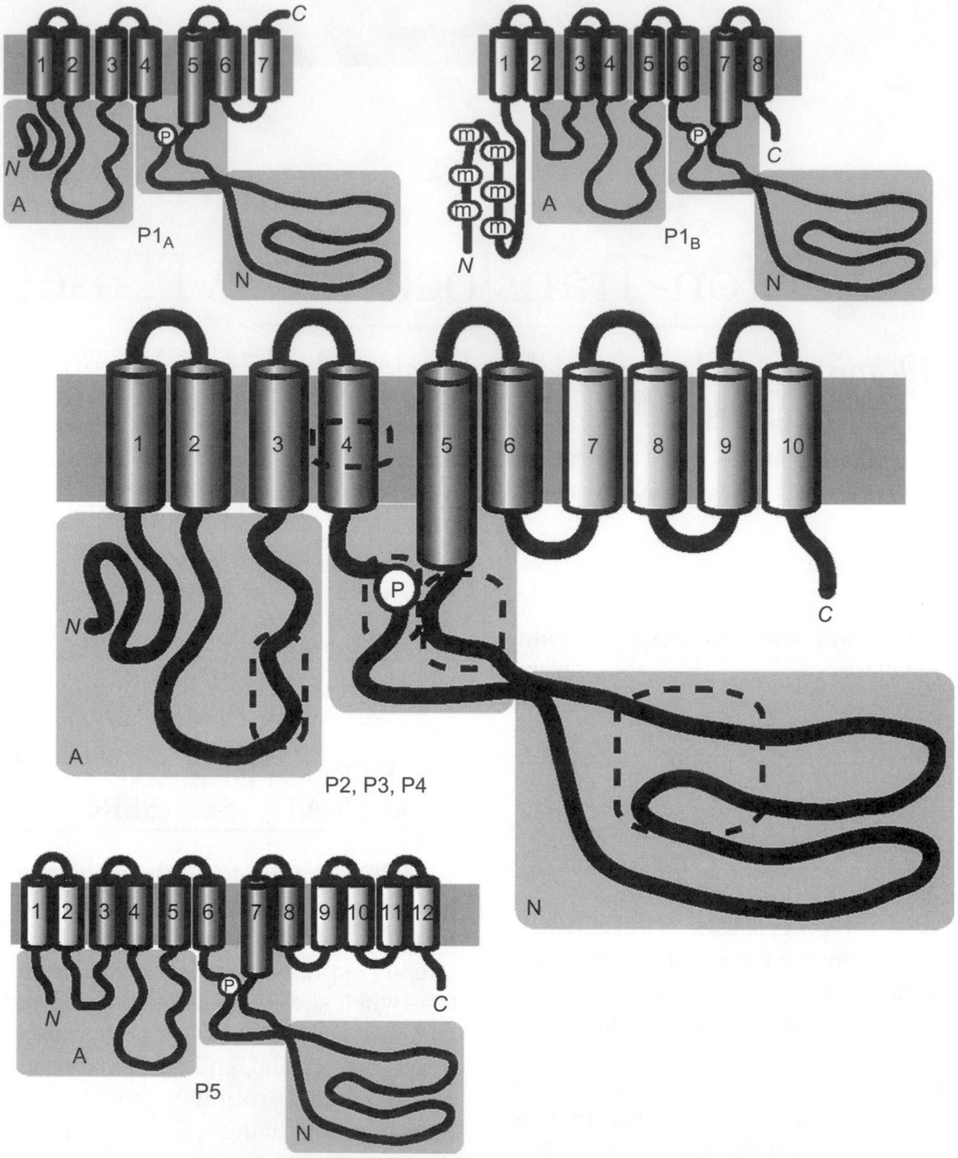

FIGURE 3.1 General structure and conserved motifs of P-ATPases. The four schemes show the general architecture of the main catalytic subunit of the large group of P-ATPases. The large scheme in the center corresponds to the common general structure of P2, P3, and P4 subfamilies. The two smaller schemes at the top illustrate the structure of bacterial KDP-B potassium transport ATPase (P1$_A$ subfamily, left) and the universal metal ion transport ATPases (P1$_B$ subfamily, right) in which the large N-terminal domain contains a number (usually 6) of cysteine-rich metal-binding domains (m). The small scheme at the bottom left illustrates the putative structure of P5-ATPase. The six transmembrane segments that are common to all P-ATPase together with the two major intracellular domains form the core of the ion translocation engine, and are shaded in a darker gray. The positions of highly conserved motives common to all P-ATPases are encircled by a dashed line. The cytoplasmic part of the protein is divided into three A, P, and N main functional domains according to Toyoshima et al.[396]. The circled P indicates the location of the phosphorylation site. The N- and C-termini are indicated by italicized N and C.

Conversely, calcium extrusion decreases cytosolic Ca^{2+} concentration, and consequently its association with calmodulin. Calmodulin release from PMCA increases PMCA auto-inhibition. Regulatory inhibition of SERCA is mediated by the small associated protein phospholamban, which plays a role equivalent to that of the PMCA C-terminal domain. Phosphorylation of phospholamban by protein kinase C releases SERCA inhibition.[1]

STRUCTURE OF Na,K-ATPASE AND H,K-ATPASE

Na,K- and H,K-ATPases are heteromeric proteins consisting of an α-subunit and a smaller glycosylated β-subunit. Na,K-ATPase hydrolytic activity, cation transport activity, and ouabain-binding properties were demonstrated by co-expression of α- and β-subunits in several expression systems (mammalian cells, *Xenopus* oocytes, baculovirus-infected insect cells, and yeast). Na- (or H-) and K-activated ATPase and cation transport activities (i.e., uphill cation transport driven by ATP hydrolysis) characteristic of Na,K- or H,K-ATPases have been demonstrated only in the presence of both α- and β-subunits. Expression of the α-subunit alone in insect cells[2] resulted in Mg^2-dependent ATPase activity that was not specifically activated by Na^+ and K^+. The exact stoichiometry of the minimal functional unit is still a matter of debate. However, Na,K-ATPase activity is associated with solublized α−β protomers,[3] and cross-linking experiments did not show evidence for a close interaction between α-subunits.[4] A third subunit, the γ-subunit, can be associated with the α−β complex (see below).

Catalytic α-Subunit

Structure

Na,K- and H,K-ATPase α-subunit peptides range in length from about 1000 to 1040 amino acids. Their primary structure is characterized by a first group of four transmembrane segments, followed by a large cytoplasmic loop, and a second group of six transmembrane segments (Figure 3.1). Crystal structures of pig[5] and shark[6] Na,K-ATPase at 3.5 and 2.4 Å resolutions, respectively, confirmed that the α-subunit has three cytoplasmic domains and 10 transmembrane helices, designated *M1* to *M10*. Two-thirds of its mass is contained in the large cytoplasmic domain, while one-third spans the lipid bilayer. Of the total mass, only a small part is extracellular.[6] Sequence homology between Na,K- and H,K-ATPases is high enough to safely predict H,K-ATPase structure, at least for the general architecture of this molecule, and for large domains where homology is highest.

Isoforms

Six different α-subunit genes have been identified in mammals: α1-4 isoforms of the Na,K-ATPase α-subunit; gastric H,K-ATPase α-subunit (αHKg); and colonic H,K-ATPase α-subunit (αHKc). Related isoforms have been identified in birds and amphibians. Na,K-ATPase sequences from *Caenorhabditis elegans* or *Drosophila melanogaster* do not show close similarity with any mammalian isoform. This suggests that the divergence between Na,K- and H,K-ATPase α-subunits precedes the divergence between mammals, amphibians and birds, and has occurred early in vertebrate evolution.

All Na,K-ATPase isoforms primarily maintain Na^+ and K^+ gradients across the cell membrane. The large inward electrochemical gradient for Na^+ is in turn used by numerous secondary active transport systems for various "housekeeping" functions: maintenance of intracellular pH via Na−H exchangers; extrusion of calcium via Na−Ca exchanger; control of cell volume via Na−K−2Cl symport and other coupled transport systems; and import of amino acids, nucleotides, and other nutrients or osmolytes through various Na^+-coupled co-transport systems. The outward electrochemical gradient for K^+ is responsible for the intracellular negative membrane potential, because K^+ flows out of the cell through K^+ selective channels that are active in most cells. In addition to these general functions, Na^+ and K^+ gradients across cell membranes are essential for specialized functions, such as the generation and propagation of action potentials in excitable cells, neurotransmitter uptake, and transcellular transport of solutes and water by epithelial cells.

The α1 isoform is the most ubiquitous and abundant α isoform, and is responsible for the maintenance of whole-cell Na^+ and K^+ gradients necessary for housekeeping functions. Because of its abundance (it is the only α isoform present in many epithelial cells, including renal cells) it provides the driving force for solute and water transepithelial transport. The α2 isoform is found in skeletal and heart muscle, and in the nervous system (neurons and glial cells). The α3 isoform is essentially neuronal, but is also found in blood cells and macrophages. The α4 isoform is mostly expressed in testes, and plays a critical role in sperm motility.[7]

αHKg is abundantly expressed in parietal cells of the gastric gland, where it plays a central role in proton secretion. Under resting conditions, it is mainly located in an intracellular tubulo−vesicular network that fuses with the apical membrane of parietal cells in response to stimuli, allowing the H,K-pump to secrete protons into the gastric gland lumen in exchange for potassium. αHKc is mainly expressed in the (rat) distal colon, but also in the kidney, uterus, and, to a lesser extent, in the heart.[8]

β-Subunit

Isoforms

As stated above, the β-subunit is an essential constituent of functional Na,K-ATPase and H,K-ATPase. Five different genes encoding similar proteins are known in mammalian genomes: β1; β2; β3; βHK; and βm ("m" emphasizes its predominant expression in skeletal muscle). β1, β2, and β3 are clearly Na,K-ATPase β-subunit isoforms, while βHK is co-expressed with gastric H,K-ATPase. Although usually described as ubiquitous, β1 appears to be absent, or at best is only a minor component, in several tissues such as liver and red blood cells. The β2 isoform was initially identified in glial cells, but is also present in other cell types, including neurons, blood cells, and epithelial cells. The β3 isoform, initially identified in nervous systems, is also widely distributed, being most abundant in testes, liver, and lungs and less so in skeletal muscle and kidney. Despite sharing sufficient sequence similarity to be classified in the same family, βm does not associate with any known mammalian α-subunit.[9]

Structure and $\alpha-\beta$ Interaction

β-subunit peptides range in length from 288 to 315 amino acids, and show a lower degree of homology (about 30%–40% identity between isoforms) than α isoforms. Crystal structures of Na,K-ATPase obtained at resolutions of 3.5 Å[5] and 2.4 Å[6] have lent detailed insight into β-subunit structure. These studies, together with experimental evidence, show that the β-subunit is a type II membrane protein consisting of a single transmembrane segment, a ~35-amino acid N-terminal domain, and a large extracellular domain containing two to seven glycosylation sites, depending on the isoform, and six cysteine residues that form three disulfide bridges (Figure 3.1).

Experimental modeling and analysis of Na,K-ATPase crystal structures has revealed complex interactions between α- and β-subunits. The transmembrane helix of the β-subunit forms several hydrogen bonds and numerous contacts with M7 and M10 transmembrane helices of the α-subunit, primarily via clusters of aromatic residues. At the extracellular side of the β-subunit, a stretch of amino acids adjacent to its transmembrane domain interacts with the αM7/M8 extracellular loop that contains a consensus sequence SYGQ.[6] Further downstream, Lys250 of the β-subunit forms a salt bridge with Glu899, located in the αM7/M8 extracellular loop.[6]

Except for gastric αHK and βHK, which are most abundantly expressed in a single cell type (parietal cells of gastric glands), there is no obvious common pattern of distribution between α isoforms and β isoforms that would define preferential physiological associations. Indeed, some cells even express as many as three α isoforms and at least two β isoforms. Unless formation of specific complexes is favored or repressed by unknown mechanisms, numerous combinations are possible, as suggested by studies using artificial expression systems. β1 is abundantly expressed in tissues in which α1 predominates, such as the kidney, strongly suggesting that α1β1 represents the predominant isozyme in these tissues. The nature of the β-subunit associated with αHKc is also a matter of debate, since all β isoforms are able to associate with αHKc, depending on the expression system used.

Functional Role

The functional interaction between α- and β-subunits has been studied and reviewed in detail.[9] By acting as a molecular chaperone, the β-subunit plays a critical role in the maturation of the α-subunit. Indeed, the α-subunit reaches a mature and functional conformation, ready to be translocated from the endoplasmic reticulum to the plasma membrane, only when associated with a β-subunit.

The β-subunit contributes to intrinsic transport properties of the whole enzyme in several expression systems by influencing its apparent K^+ and Na^+ affinities. Biochemical analysis and crystallization of Na,K-ATPase has lent some mechanistic insight as to how this is achieved. By interacting with the M7 transmembrane domain of the α-subunit, Tyr40 and Tyr44 of the β-subunit transmembrane helix help confer intrinsic transport properties of the Na,K-ATPase enzyme, as suggested by a mutagenic study.[10] Unwinding of M7 via hydrogen bonding of Tyr44 with Gly855 appears to be of central importance to K^+ binding. The role of the β-subunit ectodomain in modulating cation transport is further illustrated by the complex interactions between this domain and the αM7/M8 extracellular loop.

The role of the β-subunit in cell–cell adhesion will be discussed in the section "New Physiological Functions of Na,K-ATPase."

FXYD Proteins

Isoforms

FXYD proteins are a third component of Na,K-ATPase. There are seven isoforms in mammals, ranging from 61 to 95 amino acids in length, except for FXYD5, which consists of 178 amino acids due to an N-terminal extension. Most FXYD proteins are small type 1 membrane proteins containing an extracellular N-terminus. This family of proteins is so named since all members contain a FXYD (Phe-X-Tyr-Asp) sequence located immediately downstream of the transmembrane segment. All members also contain two conserved glycine residues in the transmembrane domain, as well as a serine residue located further downstream. As with α and β isoforms, the tissue distribution of FXYD proteins is isoform-specific.[11] FXYD1 (phospholemman) is predominately expressed in heart and skeletal muscle and, to a lesser extent, in brain, FXYD2 (γ-subunit) in kidney, FXYD3 (MAT-8) in stomach and colon, FXYD4 (CHIF) in kidney and distal colon, FXYD5 (RIC) in kidney, intestine and lung, and FXYD6 and FXYD7 in brain. In the kidney FXYD2 is mostly expressed in proximal tubule and thick ascending limb of Henle, while FXYD4 is exclusively found in the collecting duct where its expression increases from cortical to medullary portions.[12]

Function and Interaction with α- and β-Subunits

FXYD proteins were first thought to be regulators of ion channels or even to act as ion channels themselves. It has now been demonstrated that FXYD proteins interact with Na,K-ATPase. Contrary to the β-subunit, most FXYD proteins do not associate with H,K-ATPase and do not appear to act as a molecular chaperone. Rather, they regulate Na,K-ATPase functional properties. As recently reviewed,[9] analysis of FXYD-deficient mice and *in vitro* modulation of Na,K-ATPase activity by different FXYD proteins has shown that FXYD1−4, 6, and 7 all decrease Na,K-ATPase apparent affinity for Na^+ and/or K^+, with the exception of FXYD4 which has been shown to decrease apparent affinity for K^+ but increase that for Na^+. FXYD5 does not appear to influence Na,K-ATPase affinity for either Na^+ or K^+, but enhances maximal transport activity. By modulating Na,K-ATPase activity, FXYD proteins play important physiological roles, each isoform playing a different role depending on its tissue-specific distribution. For instance, FXYD1 influences myocardial contractility by modulating Na,K-ATPase activity and calcium handling, as demonstrated in FXYD1-deficient mice that display depressed cardiac contractile function and increased cardiac mass.[13] FXYD6, the only FXYD isoform expressed in the inner ear, may play an auditory and vestibular role by contributing to endolymph ionic compostion, whose production depends on Na,K-ATPase activity.[14] Reflecting altered expression levels in various types of cancer, FXYD3 may be implicated in the control of cell differentiation, proliferation, and/or apoptosis through regulation of Na,K-ATPase activity.[15] Finally, the renal tubule segment-specific distribution of FXYD2 and FXYD4 may explain, at least in part, the higher apparent Na^+ affinity of collecting duct Na,K-ATPase as compared to that of more proximal nephron segments.[16,17]

Crystallization of the Na,K-ATPase holoenzyme[5,6] has deciphered FXYD structure, and revealed how it interacts with α- and β-subunits, providing some insight into how it modulates Na,K-ATPase activity. This notably involves interaction between the transmembrane domain of FXYD proteins, particularly Gly34, with the α*M9* transmembrane domain. Hydrogen bonds between Cys31 and αGlu960 may additionally play a structural role important for FXYD functional regulation. The FXYD motif helps confer β conformational structure. This is partly achieved via Phe12, which anchors this segment to the β-subunit, and Tyr14, which forms a cluster of aromatic residues with Tyr69 of the β-subunit and Trp987 of the α*M9/M10* extracellular loop.

PROPERTIES OF Na,K-ATPase AND H,K-ATPASE

Ion Transport

Under physiological conditions, Na,K-ATPase exchanges three intracellular Na^+ for two extracellular K^+ at the expense of one ATP during each cycle, generating an outward current of one net charge per cycle. The outward current generated by the Na,K-pump tends to hyperpolarize the cell membrane to a few millivolts under steady-state conditions. The majority of the 50 to 80 mV resting-membrane potential is due to flow of K through K channels, which relies on Na, K-pump activity, since high intracellular K^+ concentration is maintained by the Na,K-pump. The apparent affinities for Na^+ and K^+ are dependent on experimental conditions, but under physiological conditions intracellular Na^+ activates the Na,K-pump with a $K^{1/2}$ of 10 to 20 mM and a Hill coefficient between 2 and 3. Extracellular K^+ has a $K^{1/2}$ of about 1 mM, with a Hill coefficient between 1 and 2.

Despite extensive studies, the difference in transport properties between Na,K-ATPase α isoforms has not been entirely resolved. Initial studies performed in native tissues indicated that α2/α3 isoforms have a higher affinity for Na^+. More recent studies comparing isoforms in the same artificial expression system revealed that α2 has a slightly lower (about 20 mM), and α3 a much lower (30−70 mM), affinity for Na.[18] However, other factors, such as the type of associated β-subunit and FXYD protein, also modulate Na,K-ATPase transport properties (see above).

The mechanism of cation translocation by Na,K-ATPase can be summarized as follows (Figure 3.2). Na,K-ATPase exists under two main conformations, E1 and E2, and transport activity is performed via a cycle in which the protein is transiently phosphorylated, and alternately adopts E1 or E2 conformations. These two conformations differ in their apparent affinities for Na^+ and K^+. The E1 conformation has high affinity sites for Na^+ exposed at the intracellular side of the membrane, while the E2 conformation has high affinity sites for K^+ exposed at the extracellular side of the membrane. Three Na^+ and two K^+ ions are alternately bound to the enzyme and then "occluded," that is, tightly bound inside the protein. This model is compatible with the reported structure of the major conformations of SERCA, and the E2-P conformation of Na,K-ATPase.[6,19]

Non-electrogenic transport is achieved by gastric H,K-ATPase, indicating that a symmetrical number of H^+ and K^+ ions are translocated across the membrane during each cycle. Transport stoichiometry depends on pH. Under conditions of high or near neutral pH, the stoichiometry is $2H,2K^+$-1ATP, and shifts to $1H,1K^+$-1ATP under physiological conditions, i.e., conditions of very low extracellular pH.[20] The transport properties of colonic H,K-ATPase and its close relatives (human ATP1AL1 and toad *Bufo marinus* bladder H,K-pump) are not yet completely defined. Artificial systems have demonstrated an inward transport of K^+, and an

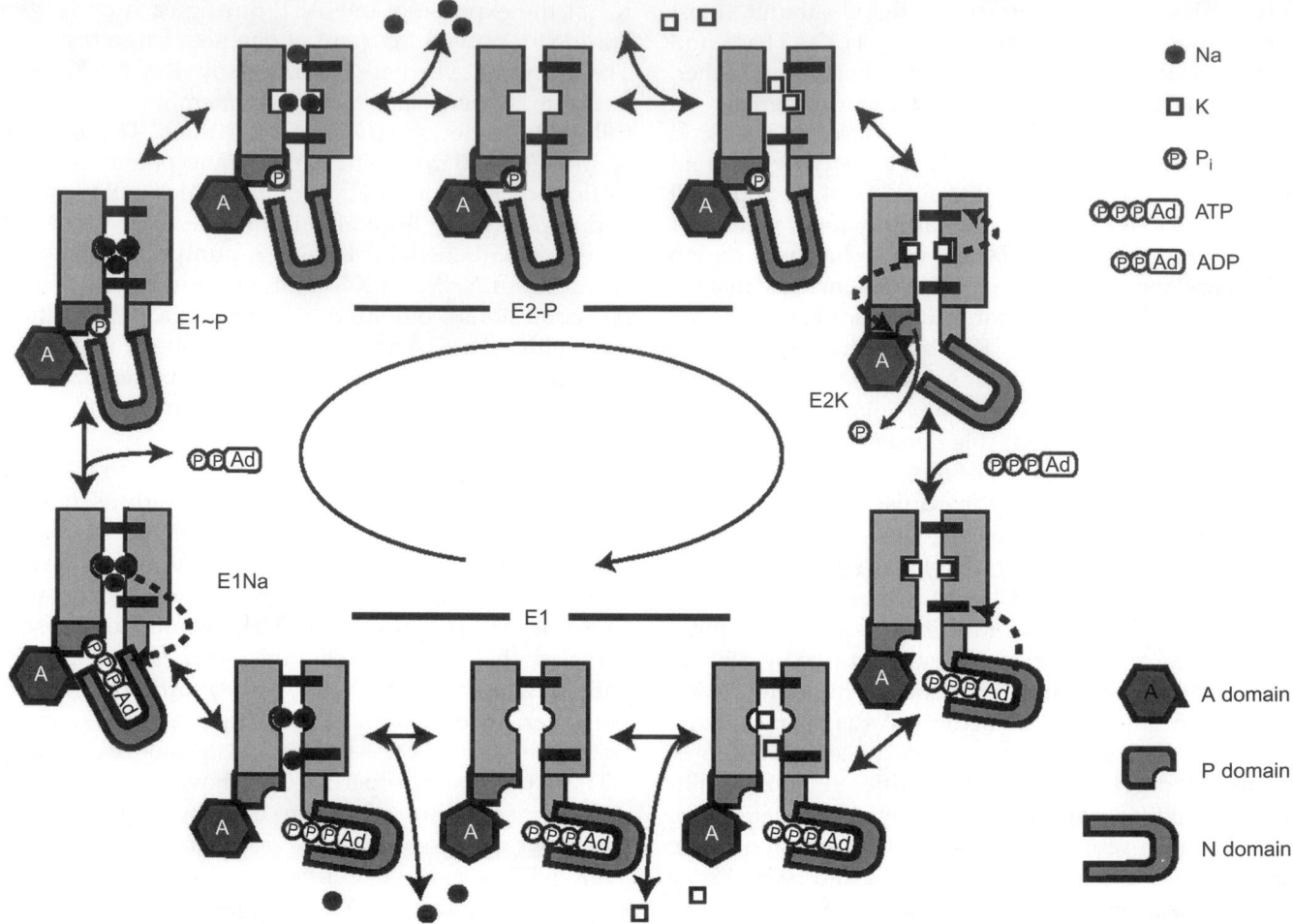

FIGURE 3.2 The Na,K-ATPase transport cycle. This cartoon illustrates the principle of the "alternating access" transport model of Na,K-ATPase. Na$^+$ ions are indicated by small, filled circles, and K$^+$ ions by small, open squares. Starting from the E$^+$ conformation where ATP is present at its binding site, three Na$^+$ ions enter from the intracellular site through an open, internal gate and reach their occlusion site (E1Na state). Na$^+$ binding induces (dotted arrow) movement of the N domain, resulting in positioning of the γ phosphate close to the phosphorylation site, phosphorylation of the α-subunit via transfer of the γ phosphate to Asp351, release of ADP and closure of the internal gate which results in the occlusion of the three Na$^+$ in the E1P state. The conformational change to the E2-P state that follows results in the opening of the extracellular gate, and a structural change of the cation-binding site, resulting in a large decrease of their affinity for Na$^+$ and an increase of their affinity for K$^+$. This leads to release of Na$^+$ to the extracellular side and loading of two K$^+$. K$^+$ binding has two major consequences (dotted arrows): first, the external gate closes, resulting in K$^+$ occlusion; and second, D$_{351}$ (E2K state) is dephosphorylated. This latter event is catalyzed by a conserved motif (TGES, small black triangle) of the A domain that is brought in contact with the phosphorylation site via rotation of this domain. The N domain also moves, allowing it to be accessible (with a low affinity) to ATP. Binding of ATP then results in opening of the intracellular gate (back to the E1 conformation), and allows release of K$^+$ ions to the intracellular side. This last step can also occur in the absence of ATP, but at a much reduced rate.

outward transport of H$^+$.[21] However, data obtained in heterologous expression systems have suggested that these enzymes may exchange Na$^+$ for K$^+$.[22]

Pharmacology

A group of natural compounds known as "cardiac steroids," so named because they contain a steroid nucleus attached to a lactone ring and are used for treatment of congestive heart failure, are potent Na,K-ATPase inhibitors. In addition, one or several endogenously related compounds may also act as hormonal

agents that participate in regulating Na,K-ATPase activity.

Cardiac steroid interaction with Na,K-ATPase, particularly ouabain, has been extensively studied. Differences of ouabain affinity between Na,K-ATPase isoforms, together with mutagenesis studies[23] and recently obtained crystal structures of ouabain bound to Na,K-ATPase,[5] all show that ouabain binds to a deep cavity formed by the transmembrane helices *M1*, *M2*, *M4*, *M5*, and *M6* at the proximity of the K$^+$-binding site. The slow kinetics of ouabain binding may be associated with partial unwinding of the *M4* helix.

Large differences in ouabain sensitivity occur among animal species. The $\alpha 1$ isoform is ouabain-resistant in rat, mouse, and toad *Bufo marinus*, but is sensitive in human, rabbit, sheep, and *Xenopus*.[23] The $\alpha 2$ and $\alpha 3$ isoforms are more sensitive than the $\alpha 1$ isoform in "resistant" species.[7] However, in humans, little difference of equilibrium binding is found among $\alpha 1$, $\alpha 2$, and $\alpha 3$ isoforms, except for a slightly higher K_I for $\alpha 2$. However, the $\alpha 2$ isoform also exhibits a faster ouabain association and dissociation rate constant than $\alpha 1$ and $\alpha 3$.[24] The "resistant" phenotype of some species is linked to charged amino acids in the first extracellular loop between *M1* and *M2*.[23] The presence of endogenous circulating inhibitors of Na,K-ATPase ("endo-ouabain") is well-demonstrated. However, their precise chemical nature needs to be clarified, their controlled synthesis and release better understood, and their specific effects more precisely described, before the hypothesis of controlled Na,K-ATPase activity by such circulating hormones can be considered as fully established.[25]

Gastric H,K-ATPase is insensitive to ouabain,[20] as demonstrated by an absence of detectable effects at millimolar concentrations of ouabain. On the other hand, non-gastric H,K-ATPases, expressed in *Xenopus* oocytes, show some sensitivity to ouabain and exhibit inhibitory constants (K_I) between 10 and 100 mM.[8] Two types of gastric H,K-pump inhibitors are known. SCH-28080 is a reversible inhibitor that competes with extracellular K^+, while substituted benzimidazole compounds irreversibly inhibit gastric H,K-ATPase by forming a covalent (disulfide) bond between the sulfonamide form of the compound (produced in very acid pH) and the thiol group of a cysteine residue exposed at the cell surface.[20]

Genetics

Gene inactivation studies have shown that Na,K-ATPase is essential for life. Absence of Na,K-ATPase $\alpha 1$ expression is embryonically lethal, even though $\alpha 1^{-/-}$ embryos develop beyond the blastocyst stage.[26] In contrast, $\alpha 2^{-/-}$ animals are born alive but die soon after birth, most likely as the result of dysfunctional neuronal circuits involved in controlled respiration.[27] $\alpha 1$ or $\alpha 2$ gene inactivation in heterozygous animal tissues leads mostly to disturbances of cardiac phenotype, supporting an important role for the $\alpha 2$ isoform in intracellular calcium homeostasis.[28,29] Only two human genetic diseases are known to be related to mutations of Na,K-ATPase α isoforms. A familial form of hemiplegic migraine has been associated with mutations in the $\alpha 2$ gene that abolish or greatly reduce enzyme activity[30,31] (OMIM #602481). Rapid onset dystonia parkinsonism has been associated with an inactivating mutation of the $\alpha 3$ gene[32] (OMIM #128235). In both cases, the mode of inheritance is dominant, suggesting that the disease is due to a haploinsufficiency of $\alpha 2$ and $\alpha 3$ isoforms, respectively. A dominant form of familial hypomagnesemia has been associated with a mutation in the FXYD2 gene.[33]

REGULATION OF Na,K-ATPASE

Obviously, the activity of an enzyme of such paramount importance for so many cellular and organ functions must be tightly regulated. Physiological regulation of Na,K-ATPase activity is complex and occurs at several levels. First, the activity of Na,K-ATPase depends on its three substrates, Na^+, K^+, and ATP. Second, for short-term regulation, the activity of Na,K-ATPase present at the cell surface can be regulated by post-translational modifications, such as phosphorylation. Third, Na,K-ATPase density at the cell surface is controlled by its rate of synthesis, at both transcriptional and post-transcriptional levels, by its degradation, and by its distribution between the cell surface and intracellular pools. Finally, there is some evidence that protein−protein interactions further regulate Na,K-ATPase activity and abundance.

Substrates

Interaction of intracellular Mg-ATP with Na,K-ATPase is complex and involves high- and low-affinity sites. Since intracellular ATP concentration is usually largely above $K_{1/2}$ values, ATP is not considered a physiological limiting factor for Na,K-ATPase activity. However, under pathological conditions, such as ischemia/hypoxia, ATP may become rate limiting. Similarly, since normal concentrations of extracellular K^+ (3.5−4.5 mM) are above $K_{1/2}$ values, physiological variations are not expected to influence Na,K-ATPase activity, although decreased activity could occur under conditions of severe hypokalemia. In contrast, intracellular Na^+ concentration is below, or close to, $K_{1/2}$ values. Considering the steep concentration−activity relationship, with a Hill coefficient between 2 and 3, a low concentration of intracellular Na^+ implies that Na,K-ATPase operates far from its maximal rate under physiological conditions. It follows that small variations in intracellular Na^+ are immediately followed by parallel variations in Na,K-ATPase activity, in order to maintain a constant intracellular Na^+ concentration.

Intracellular Na^+ and extracellular K^+ concentrations can also have a long-term effect on Na,K-pump density. The influence of extracellular K^+ on $\alpha 2$

expression was demonstrated in skeletal muscle.[34] Under conditions of hypokalemia, α2 is downregulated, allowing release of K^+ from large intracellular pools in muscle and fine regulation of K^+ homeostasis in small extracellular pools. Similarly, intracellular Na^+ modulates Na,K-ATPase expression (see "Na,K-ATPase and the Kidney").

Post-Translational Modifications

Na,K-ATPase α-subunits can be phosphorylated by several protein kinases. PKA phosphorylates a serine residue (S_{943})[35,36] located in a short intracellular loop that links the *M8* and *M9* segments, conserved in all Na,K-ATPase and H,K-ATPase isoforms. However, the functional relevance of this PKA site has been questioned, because it should be poorly accessible under native conformational states,[37] and because its mutation did not alter the effect of PKA on Na,K-ATPase activity in renal epithelial cells.[38] Activation of PKC also results in Na,K-ATPase α-subunit phosphorylation. A conserved, non-conventional PKC phosphorylation site, S_{16}, located in the intracellular N-terminal domain of the α1-subunit,[36,39] as well as two species-specific PKC sites (S_{23} in rat α1, and T_{15} in *Bufo marinus* α1) have been identified. α2- and α3-subunits are poor substrates for PKC or are not phosphorylated at all.[40] PKC phosphorylation of the α-subunit may regulate both apparent Na^+ affinity and cell surface expression of the enzyme.[41–43] More recently, tyrosine phosphorylation of α1 at Y_{10} in response to insulin,[44,45] and also at Y_{260} in response to ouabain,[46] has been described. Similarly, tyrosine phosphorylation of α2 was reported, although the phosphorylation site has not been mapped.[45] Tyrosine phosphorylation of Na,K-ATPase is functionally associated with both an increase of apparent Na^+ affinity and an increase of the enzyme's cell surface expression.[44,45] Finally, phosphorylation of α1 by ERK has been shown *in vitro* and in response to insulin in skeletal muscle. This ERK-dependent phosphorylation is associated with stimulation of Na,K-ATPase activity via increased cell surface expression.[43]

Synthesis and Degradation

Since $\alpha\beta$-subunit stoichiometry is inflexible, controlled synthesis of both subunits is expected to participate in regulating Na,K-ATPase activity. Hormonal control by glucocorticoids, mineralocorticoids, and thyroid hormones has been demonstrated. Thyroid hormones have been shown to regulate the synthesis of both subunits, but the mechanism of this regulation is complex and differs between organs.[47] For instance, glucocorticoids stimulate the transcription of mostly β-subunit mRNA in lungs, even though expression of both α and β protein is increased, indicative of complex transcriptional and post-transcriptional control.[48,49]

Regulation of Na,K-ATPase by mineralocorticoids will be discussed later in the section "Na,K-ATPase in the Kidney."

In addition to the rate of synthesis of its subunits, Na,K-ATPase abundance is dependent on its degradation rate. Recent experimental evidence obtained by pulse-chase experiments in lung alveolar[50] and renal (E. Feraille, unpublished results) epithelial cells indicates that the half-life of plasma membrane Na,K-ATPase is approximately 4 hours, while that of newly synthesized α-subunits is approximately 6 hours. Therefore, in contrast to current belief, Na,K-ATPase half-life is relatively short in epithelial cells. The majority of Na,K-ATPase is degraded by lysosomes, and ubiquitination of its α-subunit may participate in this process.[50] Regulation of Na,K-ATPase degradation in response to variations of transepithelial sodium transport will be discussed later in the section "Na,K-ATPase in the Kidney."

Membrane Trafficking

An increasing amount of experimental evidence indicates that plasma membrane Na,K-ATPase expression is controlled via regulated membrane trafficking. Regulated Na,K-ATPase endocytosis was first demonstrated in response to dopamine by atypical PKC-ζ in rat proximal tubule cells.[51] This will be discussed later in the section "Na,K-ATPase in the Kidney." The role of PKC-ζ in Na,K-ATPase endocytosis has been confirmed in alveolar lung cells in response to hypoxia.[52] Downregulation of plasma membrane Na,K-ATPase has also been demonstrated in response to ouabain in renal epithelial cells (LLCPK1 cells),[52] and to AMPK activation in response to CO_2 in lung alveolar cells.[53] Moreover, direct interaction of the Na-K-ATPase α-subunit with arrestins and spinophilin modulates its endocytotic rate in COS-7 cells.[54] It remains to be determined whether internalized Na,K-ATPase units are degraded or recycled back to the plasma membrane.

Rapid recruitment of Na,K-ATPase to the plasma membrane has first been demonstrated in response to insulin in skeletal muscle[55] and following an increase of intracellular sodium concentration in renal collecting ducts.[56] This latter event will be discussed in the section "Na,K-ATPase in the Kidney." Increased cell surface expression of Na,K-ATPase was subsequently demonstrated in response to aldosterone in renal collecting duct cells,[57] and to increased cAMP levels in both renal[58] and lung epithelial cells.[59] This process is sensitive to brefeldin A,[58] suggesting that a latent pool of Na,K-ATPase units is recruited from the trans-Golgi network. In addition, activation of PKC-β in proximal tubule cells[51] and PKC-δ−$\epsilon\delta$ in lung alveolar cells[60] increases Na,K-ATPase plasma membrane expression. Exocytosis of Na,K-ATPase is dependent on RhoA,[61] kinesin,[62] and myosin-Va[63] in lung alveolar cells. The amount of active Na,K-ATPase units at the cell surface is therefore highly regulated via both endocytotic and exocytotic processes.

Interaction with the Cytoskeleton

Na-K-ATPase interacts both directly and indirectly with the membrane cytoskeleton in several ways. Na, K-ATPase binds directly to ankyrin, which itself links Na,K-ATPase to spectrin (fodrin) and consequently to the basolateral cytoskeleton.[64,65] Ankyrin-spectrin interaction is thought to participate in specific targeting of Na-K-ATPase to the basolateral membrane of epithelial cells. Na-K-ATPase activity may also be modulated via its association with ankyrin.[66]

Na,K-ATPase and actin filaments display a complex relationship that is not fully understood. Actin filaments may directly modulate Na,K-ATPase activity[67] or indirectly control Na,K-ATPase plasma membrane expression via adducins which control actin polymerization.[68] Mutant α-adducin associated with hypertension in rats and humans was shown to decrease constitutive Na,K-ATPase endocytosis, and thereby increase the number of active Na,K-ATPase units at the cell surface.[68] Direct activation of Na,K-ATPase activity by adducin was also demonstrated.[66] In addition, Na,K-ATPase directly binds to cofilin, which modulates actin filament polymerization.[69] Na,K-ATPase basolateral targeting and modulation of its activity appears additionally to depend on its interaction with multiple cytoskeletal elements.

NEW PHYSIOLOGICAL FUNCTIONS OF Na,K-ATPASE

In addition to its well-known function, i.e., Na^+ and K^+ membrane translocation, Na,K-ATPase modulates a variety of cellular processes involved in cell growth, differentiation, and intercellular adhesion.

Cell Signaling by Na,K-ATPase

Since the pioneering work of Askari et al. which demonstrated that ouabain induces early response genes involved in cardiac hypertrophy in a Ca^{2+}-dependent manner,[70] a large body of experimental evidence collectively indicates that Na,K-ATPase behaves as a signaling platform in both mesenchymal and epithelial cells. Activation of Src and Epidermal Growth Factor (EGF) receptor tyrosine kinases, and downstream activation of MAP kinases (ERK) by ouabain at concentrations that do not alter intracellular Na^+ concentration was demonstrated in cardiac myocytes and in LLC-PK1 renal epithelial cells.[71] Ouabain induces dissociation and

activation of Src from Na,K-ATPase,[72] and subsequent transactivation of EGF receptor. This ouabain-induced signaling depends on a pool of non-functional Na,K-ATPase specifically located in caveola.[73–75] In addition to ERK activation, ouabain induces calcium oscillations via close association of phospholipase C and IP3 receptors in cell signaling microdomains.[76,77] However, these ouabain-dependent signaling events remain to be demonstrated in native tissues, and their physiological relevance is not yet established.

Role of Na,K-ATPase in Cell Adhesion

An increasing amount of experimental evidence indicates that the Na,K-ATPase β1-subunit plays a direct role in homotypic cell—cell adhesion.[78] This cell—cell adhesion function is negatively correlated with the level of complexity of β glycosylation.[79] Moreover, the transcription factor Snail, which plays a key role in epithelial-to-mesenchymal transition processes observed in poorly differentiated carcinoma cells, represses Na,K-ATPase β1-subunit transcription.[80] In addition to a direct inhibition of cell motility via increased cell—cell adhesion, Na,K-ATPase may also modulate cell migration via its interaction with the PI3-kinase p85 regulatory subunit.[81] This adhesive function of Na,K-ATPase may play important roles in organogenesis and carcinoma invasiveness.

Na,K-ATPase also modulates tight junction dynamics and permeability in cultured renal epithelial cells.[82] Indeed, both ouabain and low extracellular K^+, which inhibit Na,K-ATPase and increase intracellular Na^+, prevent tight junction recovery in calcium switch experiments performed on MDCK cells.[83] This effect is dependent on inhibition of RhoA GTPase activity by high intracellular Na^+. In addition, ouabain at concentrations that do not alter transcellular K^+ transport increases tight junction permeability via activation of Src and ERK.[84] The physiological relevance of these findings remains to be demonstrated.

Na,K-ATPASE IN THE KIDNEY

Tubular epithelial cells are characterized by their functional polarity. Na,K-ATPase is exclusively located in the basolateral membrane, the infoldings of which are closely surrounded by mitochondria which provide a constant supply of ATP. The Na^+ gradient generated by Na,K-ATPase between intra- and extracellular compartments is mainly dissipated across the apical membrane. A net reabsorption of Na^+ results from this architectural organization, and the main role of Na,K-ATPase in the kidney is to energize Na^+ reabsorption. In humans, kidneys reabsorb over 500 g of sodium per day, and utilize over 2 kg of ATP to fuel Na,K-ATPase. Although renal Na,K-ATPase also energizes secondary active transport of other solutes, its main function is related to Na^+ transport.

Measurements in microdissected segments of the mammalian renal tubule indicate that Na,K-ATPase activity is high in the thick ascending limb of Henle's loop (TAL) and the distal convoluted tubule (DCT), intermediate in the proximal tubule (PT) and the collecting duct (CD), and very low in the thin segments of Henle's loop. This distribution profile of Na,K-ATPase activity is correlated with transtubular Na^+ reabsorption capacity in various nephron segments.[85] In PT and CD, Na,K-ATPase activity declines from the kidney cortex toward the outer and inner medulla.[48] This distribution profile is confirmed by immunocytochemistry on kidney sections and by quantification of the number of pumps by ^{3}H-ouabain binding or by Western blotting of α1- and β1-subunits. Immunohistochemistry on kidney sections indicate that Na,K-ATPase expression in the collecting duct is much higher in principal than in intercalated cells. In contrast, quantification of Na,K-ATPase mRNA along the rat nephron does not confirm this axial heterogenic distribution, at least for α- and β-subunits (A. Doucet, personnal communication). This suggests the presence of segment-specific control mechanisms for Na,K-ATPase translation and/or degradation.

Regulation of Na,K-ATPase in Proximal Tubule

Na,K-ATPase activity must be tightly controlled, since the PT reabsorbs the bulk of filtrated sodium (more than 60%). Na,K-ATPase is regulated by hormones, neurotransmitters, and para/autocrine factors acting via synergistic or antagonistic signaling pathways, and one should keep in mind that the final effect, i.e., stimulation of inhibition of Na,K-ATPase activity, is not the result of activation of a single signaling pathway, but rather of a highly complex integrated response. Modulation of Na,K-ATPase cell surface expression and its affinity for Na^+ are the most important mechanisms of regulation identified in PT.

Control of Na,K-ATPase by Insulin

Stimulation of Na,K-ATPase by insulin in the PT most likely participates in stimulation of Na^+ reabsorption in this nephron segment.[86] Indeed, in isolated rat PT, insulin stimulates Na,K-ATPase transport activity in the presence of physiological concentrations of intracellular Na^+, not by changing V_{max} values, but by increasing apparent Na^+ affinity.[87] Experiments performed in isolated rat PT and in cultured OK cells (a cellular model of PT) strongly suggest that stimulation of Na,K-ATPase activity relies on phosphorylation of the α-subunit at Y_{10}.[44] However, the causal relationship

between tyrosine phosphorylation of Na,K-ATPase and increased Na^+ affinity remains to be directly demonstrated. Insulin also reduces the inhibitory effect of dopamine on Na,K-ATPase (see next section),[88] and this may also participate in its overall stimulatory effect.

Control of Na,K-ATPase by Dopamine and Parathormone

Dopamine is produced from L-dopa by PT, and its synthesis is increased by high sodium intake, making it a putative local modulator of sodium and fluid handling. Dopamine decreases fluid and sodium reabsorption in vitro in microperfused rabbit PT.[89] Accordingly, dopamine decreases Na,K-ATPase V_{max} values in rat PT,[90] as well as in OK cells.[42] Although dopamine also increases Na,K-ATPase apparent affinity for Na^+ in the PT,[90] the overall resulting effect in intact cells is Na,K-ATPase inhibition.[42] This inhibition results from activation of both dopamine DA_1- and DA_2-like receptors,[91] and is mediated by PKCζ.[51]

Within minutes, dopamine induces Na,K-ATPase endocytosis from the plasma membrane to intracellular compartments. Decreased Na,K-ATPase expression at the basolateral membrane of rat PT is associated with a sequential increase of Na,K-ATPase abundance in clathrin-coated pits (1 minute), early endosomes (2.5 minutes), and late endosomes (5 minutes).[92] Results obtained in OK cells strongly suggest that the inhibitory effect of dopamine is dependent on PKC-mediated phosphorylation of the Na,K-ATPase α-subunit on S_{23}.[42,93] Following endocytosis, the α-subunit is dephosphorylated in late endosome compartments[42] (Figure 3.3).

Dopamine-induced endocytosis of Na,K-ATPase is also associated with activation of phosphatidylinositol 3-kinase (PI3K), an enzyme critical for membrane trafficking.[94] However, dopamine-induced activation of PI3K is not secondary to its phosphorylation. Rather, S_{23} phosphorylation of the Na,K-ATPase α-subunit serves as an anchor signal for the sequential recruitment of 14-3-3 protein[95] and PI3K[96] to the membrane. Activation of PI3K in turn generates local production of phosphatidylinositol 3-phosphate, which allows binding of Na,K-ATPase with adaptor protein-2 (AP2), recruitment of clathrin, and endocytosis of Na,K-ATPase.[97] Concomitantly, dopamine activates protein phosphatase 2A which in turn dephosphorylates dynamin 2, thus allowing Na,K-ATPase recruitment at the plasma membrane.[98]

Parathormone (PTH) inhibits fluid and solute transport by PT,[99] at least in part via inhibition of Na,K-ATPase activity, as first demonstrated in PT suspensions.[100] This inhibitory effect relies partly on generation of arachidic acid metabolites via the cytochrome P450 pathway.[101] Na,K-ATPase endocytosis in response to PTH has been observed both in vitro, in OK

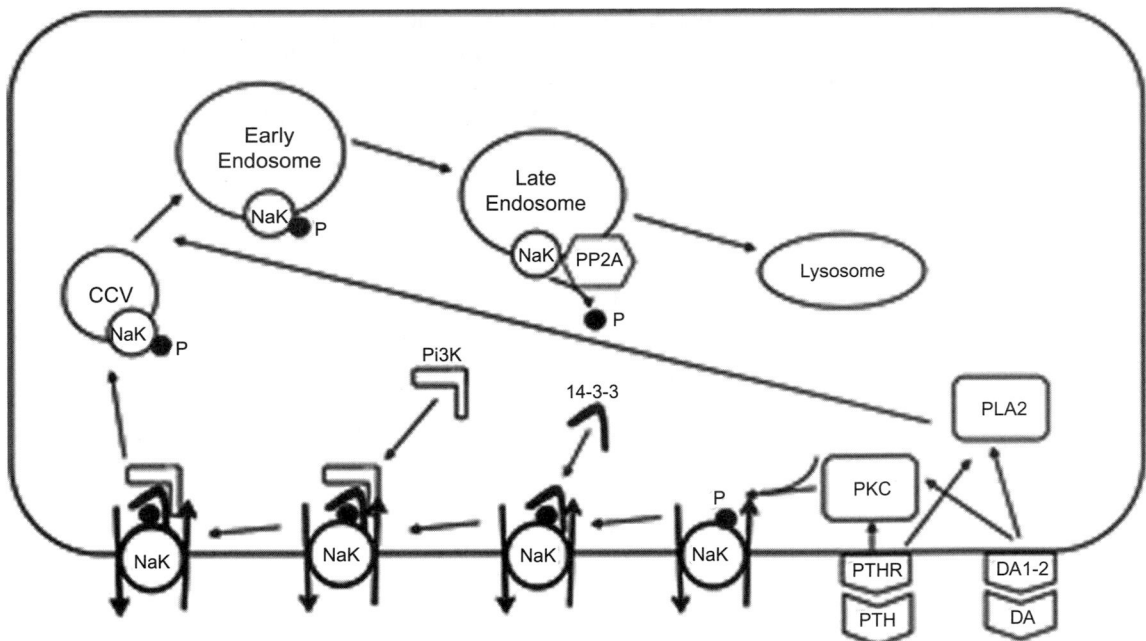

FIGURE 3.3 **Regulation of Na,K-ATPase by dopamine and parathormone (PTH) in proximal tubule.** After dopamine or PTH bind to their cognate receptor, PKC is activated leading to phosphorylation of the Na,K-ATPase α-subunit on S23, followed by binding of 14-3-3 protein and p85 subunit of the Pi3-kinase. This cascade of events leads to Na,K-ATPase endocytosis via clathrin coated vesicles (CVV). Na,K-ATPase is then dephosphorylated in endosomes by PP2A and degraded in lysosomes. Phospholipase A2 (PLA2) activation modulates Na,K-ATPase internalization.

cells,[102] and *in vivo* after infusion of PTH in normal rats,[103] and may account for the inhibitory effect of this hormone. Studies performed in the OK cell model have shown that PTH-induced endocytosis of Na,K-ATPase is ERK-dependent, requires S_{16} phosphorylation of the α-subunit and the scaffolding protein NHERF1.[102,104]

Endocytotic removal of active Na,K-ATPase from the plasma membrane therefore constitutes a major regulatory mechanism of fluid and sodium reabsorption by the PT.

Angiotensin II Exerts a Biphasic Effect on Na, K-ATPase

Angiotensin II (ANG II) controls PT Na$^+$ reabsorption from both luminal and basolateral sides. High concentrations of ANG II can be found in the PT lumen with respect to plasma circulating concentrations,[105] suggesting that the majority of luminal ANG II originates from local synthesis. Indeed, PT cells express angiotensinogen,[106] renin,[107] and angiotensin converting enzyme.[108] Only a very small fraction of ANG II is excreted in the urine, since it is almost entirely reabsorbed and degraded by PT.[109] ANG II exerts a biphasic effect. Low levels of ANG II (12^{-12} to 10^{-10} M) stimulate, while high levels of ANG II (10^{-9} to 10^{-7} M) inhibit, fluid and solute reabsorption *in vivo* in microperfused rat PT.[110] ANG II also modulates Na,K-ATPase activity in a biphasic manner in isolated PT.[111] At low concentrations, ANG II enhances

Na,K-ATPase activity via an increase in its apparent Na$^+$ affinity.[112] The mechanism by which high levels of ANG II inhibit Na,K-ATPase activity remains to be determined.

Regulation of Na,K-ATPase in Thick Ascending Limb of Henle's Loop

The TAL reabsorbs close to 15% of the filtered Na$^+$ load and is impermeable to water. As a result, fluid delivered to the distal convoluted tubule is hypotonic, NaCl concentration levels being close to 50 mM. Na$^+$ enters the luminal side of the cell via a furosemide-sensitive Na-K-2Cl-co-transporter (BSC1 or NKCC2), and Cl$^-$ leaves the cell via Cl$^-$-channels and K-Cl co-transporters. K$^+$ is recycled back to the lumen via inwardly rectifying and voltage-insensitive K$^+$-channels expressed at the apical membrane. Conductive diffusion of Cl$^-$ and K$^+$ depolarizes the basolateral membrane and hyperpolarizes the apical membrane, respectively. The combination of both diffusion potentials generates positive transepithelial voltage which provides the driving force for paracellular cation reabsorption.

Micropuncture and *in vitro* microperfusion experiments show that cAMP analogs and hormones coupled to adenylyl cyclase activation enhance NaCl reabsorption in the TAL.[48] Stimulation of Na$^+$ reabsorption by the cAMP signaling pathway is at least in part mediated by stimulation of Na,K-ATPase activity. This stimulatory effect is observed at V_{max} values, and requires sufficient amounts of oxygen and metabolic substrates. Indeed, when metabolic supply is limiting, an increase of cellular cAMP content actually inhibits Na,K-ATPase activity via generation of arachidonic acid metabolites that in turn is dependent on the cytochrome P450 pathway. Na,K-ATPase stimulation by cAMP is correlated with increased phosphorylation levels of the Na,K-ATPase α-subunit.[113] It remains to be determined whether this effect results from phosphorylation of the α-subunit by PKA or by another kinase.

The stimulatory effect of the cAMP/PKA signaling pathway is subject to negative modulation by numerous signaling pathways, including protein Gαi activation by prostaglandins,[114] cGMP generation in response to nitric oxide[115] and natriuretic peptides,[116] and PKC stimulation in response to angiotensin II,[117] bradykinin,[118] and extracellular Ca^{2+} via activation of the extracellular Ca^{2+} receptor.[119]

Control of Na,K-ATPase in Collecting Duct

Mammalian connecting tubules (CNT) and CD (cortical collecting duct: CCD, outer medullary collecting duct: OMCD, inner medullary collecting duct: IMCD) are the main sites for the fine-tuning of sodium reabsorption, crucial for the adjustment of daily urinary sodium excretion to dietary intake. In these renal tubule segments, apical sodium entry is primarily mediated by amiloride-sensitive sodium channels (ENaC),[48] and accessorily mediated by a recently identified sodium-dependent chloride/bicarbonate exchanger, SLC4A8.[120] ENaC was long thought to be the principal player for sodium transport, Na,K-ATPase activity being adapted secondarily to changes of intracellular Na^+ concentration, itself brought about by changes in ENaC activity. However, it is now clearly established that regulation of sodium transport results from the coordinated regulation of both ENaC and Na,K-ATPase.

Aldosterone Induces a Biphasic Stimulation of Na, K-ATPase

Na,K-ATPase activity (V_{max} values) is decreased by ~70% in collecting ducts[121] within 4–5 days of adrenalectomy, but is increased following administration of supraphysiological doses of mineralocorticoid. This latter effect appears after a 24-hour latency, and culminates after approximately 6 days.[85] Administration of aldosterone to adrenalectomized animals[122] or in vitro addition of aldosterone to renal tubules isolated from adrenalectomized animals[123] also increases Na,K-ATPase activity (V_{max} values) in the CD, but this effect is much more rapid than in adrenal-intact animals since it is observed after only an hour, and is maximal after only 2–3 hours. These data indicate that low levels of CCD Na,K-ATPase activity and plasma aldosterone concentration is associated with a fast stimulatory response.[124]

Short-term (2–6 hour) aldosterone challenge increases both the activity and cell surface expression of Na,K-ATPase via recruitment of a latent pool of pumps, as shown both in CD isolated from adrenalectomized rats, and in cultured mpkCCD$_{C14}$ cells, a model of CCD principal cells[57] (Figure 3.4). Although cell fractionation and cell-surface labeling studies suggest that a latent pool of Na,K-ATPase is intracellular,[58,92] its exact localization has not yet been established. Short-term stimulation of Na,K-ATPase activity occurs independently of ENaC and apical sodium entry, but does depends on de novo transcription and translation.[57] Experiments performed on Xenopus oocytes demonstrated that serum and glucocorticoid-regulated kinase-1 (SGK1), an early aldosterone-inducible gene, increased Na,K-ATPase activity and cell surface expression.[125] This suggests that aldosterone-induced recruitment of latent Na, K-ATPase units may be mediated by SGK1. Early recruitment of latent Na,K-ATPase is followed by transcriptional stimulation and synthesis of Na,K-ATPase α1- and β1-subunits.[126] In summary, after a latency period of 1 hour, aldosterone stimulates Na,K-ATPase activity in a biphasic manner. First via recruitment of an inactive Na,K-ATPase reservoir to the cell surface, and then by increased synthesis of Na,K-ATPase subunits.

Vasopressin Stimulates Na,K-ATPase

Vasopressin (AVP) is coupled to adenylyl cyclase via V_2 receptors, and stimulates the cAMP/PKA signaling pathway in CD principal cells. The major role of AVP in CD is to stimulate water reabsorption by increasing water permeability of the apical membrane of principal cells. However, in vitro microperfusion studies have shown that AVP also stimulates Na^+ reabsorption and K^+ secretion along the CD.[48] This effect of AVP on urinary Na^+ excretion has recently been confirmed in humans.[127]

Na,K-ATPase stimulation is a prerequisite for increased Na^+ reabsorption, but initial studies reported an inhibitory effect of AVP and cAMP analogs on Na,K-ATPase activity in isolated rat CCD.[128] Results from our laboratory indicate that an arachidonic acid-dependent inhibitory pathway is induced by metabolic stress related to ex vivo experimental conditions.[113] Indeed, in both well-oxygenated, isolated rat CCDs, and cultured mpkCCD$_{C14}$ cells, cAMP analogs induced a two-fold stimulation of Na,K-ATPase activity.[58,129] This stimulatory effect is rapid (5 min), and is associated with a proportional increase of Na,K-ATPase cell surface

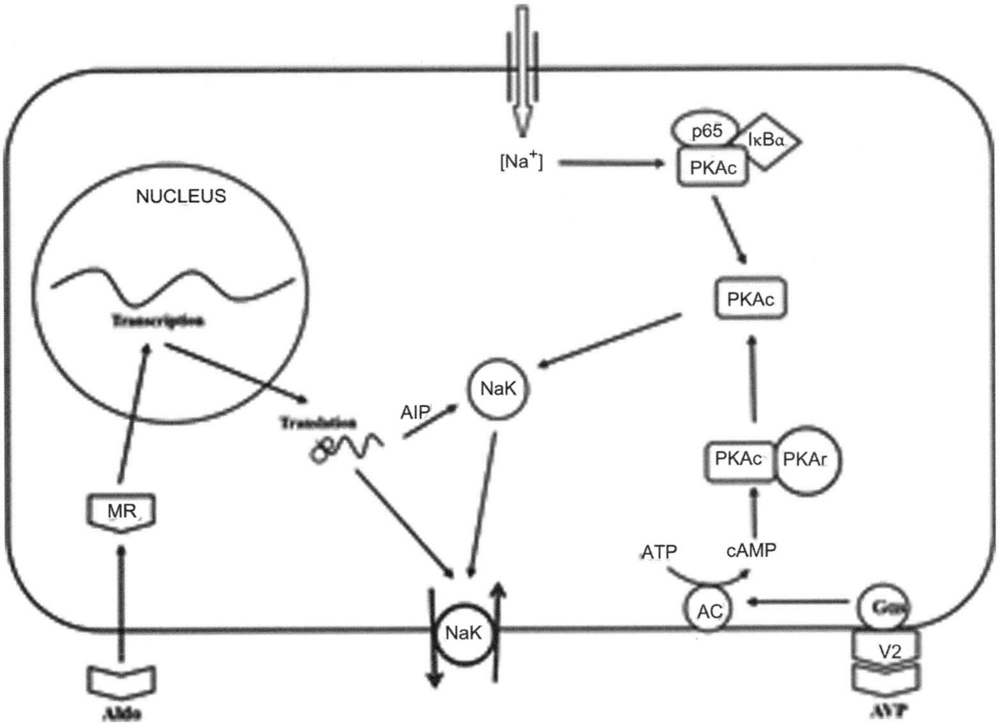

FIGURE 3.4 **Regulation of Na,K-ATPase by aldosterone, vasopressin, and Na$^+$ in the collecting duct.** Binding of aldosterone to the mineralocorticoid receptor leads to its translocation to the nucleus. This first increases the expression of early aldosterone-induced proteins (AIP), and then induces late expression of Na,K-ATPase. AIP leads to the recruitment of inactive intracellular Na,K pumps to the plasma membrane. Binding of vasopressin to its V$_2$ receptor induces cAMP synthesis, leading to dissociation of the PKA catalytic subunit (PKAc) from its regulatory subunit (PKAr). An increase of intracellular Na$^+$ leads to the dissociation of a protein complex containing p65 NF-κB, IκBα and PKAc. Free PKAc participates in the recruitment of inactive intracellular Na,K pumps to the plasma membrane.

expression in the absence of a change in whole-cell Na, K-ATPase abundance in a PKA-dependent manner[38,129] (Figure 3.4). Identification of a cAMP-responsive Na,K-ATPase pool and its relation to an aldosterone controlled reservoir remains to be determined.

Na,K-ATPase Expression is Regulated by Sodium Availability

Acute (hour) increases of intracellular Na$^+$ in CD not only activate Na,K-ATPase activity via a substrate effect, but also rapidly increase V$_{max}$ values and the number of active Na,K-ATPase units present at the cell surface.[56] This rapid stimulation occurs independently of protein synthesis, suggesting that pre-existing Na,K-ATPase units present in a latent pool are recruited to the cell surface (see above). The effect of intracellular Na$^+$ is mediated by cAMP-independent PKA activation[130] that itself results from dissociation of a complex consisting of NF-κB, IκBα and the catalytic PKA subunit.[131] This indicates that the pro-inflammatory NF-κB pathway may be part of a Na$^+$ sensing mechanism that mediates cross-talk between apical Na$^+$ entry and basolateral Na$^+$ exit (Figure 3.4). Recent experimental evidence indicates that a sustained increase of apical Na$^+$

entry also increases Na,K-ATPase expression via inhibition of Na,K-ATPase endocytosis and degradation (E. Feraille, personal communication). Such modulation of Na,K-ATPase activity by Na$^+$ load may be involved, to some extent at least, in diuretic resistance. Accordingly, chronic administration of the loop diuretic furosemide stimulates CD Na,K-ATPase activity independently of variations of circulating aldosterone.[132]

Induction of Na,K-ATPase is Associated with Sodium Retention in Nephrotic Syndrome and Liver Cirrhosis

Interstitial edema is a cardinal clinical manifestation in nephrotic syndrome. It is secondary to the accumulation of sodium in the extracellular compartment following imbalanced dietary sodium intake and urinary sodium output, and also results from alterations of fluid transfer across the capillary endothelial barrier. Mechanisms behind sodium retention have been extensively investigated using a rat model of puromycin aminonucleoside (PAN)-induced nephrotic syndrome. Both *in vivo* and *in vitro* studies demonstrated that the CCD is the main site of increased Na$^+$ reabsorption in

PAN nephrotic rats.[133,134] Na,K-ATPase hydrolytic and transport activities are increased two-fold in CCD of PAN nephrotic rats.[135] Increased Na,K-ATPase stimulation, which culminates at day 6 following PAN administration, parallels decreased urinary sodium excretion and development of a positive sodium balance.[136] Moreover, a linear inverse correlation between urinary sodium excretion and CD Na,K-ATPase activity is observed in three different experimental models of nephrotic syndrome.[136] Stimulation of Na,K-ATPase activity is paralleled by increased abundance of α and β Na,K-ATPase mRNA and basolateral protein expression.[129] Sodium retention and induction of Na,K-ATPase activity in CCD are independent of variations of circulating aldosterone.[135,137]

Interstitial edema and ascites are frequently observed in liver cirrhosis. The mechanism governing sodium retention in liver cirrhosis is under debate; however, dysregulation of CD Na,K-ATPase activity may play a key role. Indeed, in the bile duct ligation model Na,K-ATPase activity is specifically increased in mouse CCD independently of variations of circulating glucocorticoids or aldosterone.[138]

In summary, increased Na,K-ATPase activity in the CCD participates in sodium retention in both experimental nephrotic syndrome and liver cirrhosis, and may therefore play a key role in the pathogenesis of edematous diseases.

The previous paragraphs collectively outline the complexity of Na,K-ATPase regulation in the kidney. They demonstrate that: (1) hormonal triggering of intracellular signaling pathways can rapidly alter Na,K-ATPase V_{max} values and/or modulate the pump's affinity for Na^+; (2) these changes are true regulatory mechanisms that occur independently of changes in apical Na^+ entry; and (3) they are generally accompanied by a concomitant regulation of apical Na^+ entry. Thus, despite repetitive and rapid changes of Na^+ reabsorption, whole-body sodium balance and intracellular Na^+ homeostasis are maintained, at least in part, by short-term regulation of Na,K-ATPase activity. Finally, alterations of Na,K-ATPase activity are relevant to the pathophysiology of edematous diseases.

H,K-ATPASES IN KIDNEY

Kidney H,K-ATPase was first described following the discovery that it participates in primary active K^+ reabsorption, a process characterized by H,K-ATPase-like activity in the mammalian distal nephron.[139] Gastric and colonic H,K-ATPase α-subunits were subsequently cloned and mRNAs encoding these two ATPases were shown to be expressed in the kidney. We will discuss the specific inference of gastric and colonic H,K-ATPases in the kidney. Special attention will be paid to studies performed in K^+-replete and K^+-depleted animals in consideration of gastric and colonic H,K-ATPases, respectively. Indeed, kidney expression of αHKc is very low or even absent in K^+-replete animals, whereas it is markedly induced in response to K^+ depletion.

Gastric H,K-ATPase

Gastric H,K-ATPase activity, referred to as type I K-ATPase activity, was first detected as a Na^+-independent, K^+-activated ATPase activity in CD isolated from several mammalian species administered a standard diet.[139] Type I K-ATPase activity is ouabain-insensitive, and is inhibited by omeprazole and Sch 28080. This pharmacological profile fits well with that reported for gastric mucosa K-ATPase and gastric H,K-ATPase expressed in artificial systems. Moreover, Type I K-ATPase is not detected in CD of αHKg knockout mice,[21] thus demonstrating that gastric H,K-ATPase is responsible for type I K-ATPase activity. Most studies have detected moderate levels of αHKg mRNA and protein in rat and mouse CD,[140] while βHKg mRNA has been detected in rat and rabbit CD and CNT.[22] However, HKg-subunit expression remains to be demonstrated in human kidney. In situ hybridization, immunochemistry, and functional studies indicate that αHKg is mostly (if not exclusively) expressed in both α- and β-intercalated cells.[140]

In vitro microperfusion studies performed on rats have shown that HCO_3^- reabsorption is inhibited by luminal (but not peritubular) addition of Sch 28080 to OMCD, but not to CCD. However, peritubular addition of Sch 28080 reduces HCO_3^- secretion induced by in vivo CCD alkalosis. These results suggest the involvement of apical H,K-ATPase in OMCD α-intercalated cells, and in the basolateral membrane of CCD β-intercalated cells, at least during metabolic alkalosis.[141] The functional role of CD H,K-ATPase has been more extensively studied in normal rabbits. In vitro microperfusion studies performed in rabbit OMCD indicate that HCO_3^- reabsorption is markedly reduced by luminal addition of Sch 28080 and by removal of luminal K^+.[140] An Sch 28080-sensitive, K^+-dependent mechanism of H^+ extrusion has been demonstrated in CCD α- and β-intercalated cells by measuring their pH recovery following intracellular acidification.[142] However, the contribution of H,K-ATPase to K^+ reabsorption under normal conditions may be minimal, since most K^+ that enters the cytoplasm via H,K-ATPase is recycled back to the lumen via apical K^+-channels.[143]

Transgenic mice expressing βHKg containing a mutant endocytosis signal display H,K-ATPase that is constitutively expressed at the apical membrane of stomach parietal cells. This is accompanied by gastric acid hypersecretion.[144] These animals also display constitutively active renal K$^+$ reabsorption,[145] suggesting that gastric H,K-ATPase participates in K$^+$ reabsorption in mouse kidney, at least when overexpressed at the apical membrane. In contrast, transgenic mice deficient in αHKg do not display altered H$^+$ and K$^+$ renal handling.[146] Indeed, the rate of CCD K$^+$-dependent proton secretion is similar between wild-type and αHKg-deficient mice.[147] However, K$^+$-dependent H$^+$ secretion is sensitive to Sch 28080 in wild-type mice, whereas it is insensitive to Sch 28080 in αHKg-deficient mice.[147] This suggests that αHKg deficiency is functionally compensated by expression of another, yet unidentified, K$^+$-dependent H transporter.

Altogether, these studies indicate that gastric H,K-ATPase expressed in CD intercalated cells of normal rat, rabbit, and mouse kidney participates mostly in urinary acidification and/or HCO_3^- reabsorption. Its contribution to a K$^+$-reabsorption process is weak, except when artificially overexpressed.

Only a few studies evaluated how gastric H,K-ATPase adapts to disorders of acid–base balance. On the one hand, type I K-ATPase activity is increased in rat CCD and OMCD during hypercapnia-induced respiratory acidosis, whereas it is reduced by hypocapnia. On the other hand, chronic metabolic acidosis increases H,K-ATPase-mediated H$^+$ secretion by rabbit CCD that may rely on increased transcription of αHKg during the first hours of acid challenge, and thereafter on post-transcriptional mechanisms.[140,148] In contrast to acidosis, K$^+$ depletion increases neither type I K-ATPase activity, nor αHKg expression.[140] Post-transcriptional control of gastric H,K-ATPase in rat collecting ducts is demonstrated by the *in vitro* stimulatory effects of calcitonin and isoproterenol on type I K-ATPase,[149] two hormones that stimulate proton secretion and reabsorption in α- and β-intercalated cells, respectively. Stimulation of type I K-ATPase by calcitonin in α-intercalated cells is mediated by activation of ERK, by a cAMP-dependent and protein kinase A-independent mechanism, via the guanine-nucleotide exchange factor Epac 1.[150] Stimulation of type I K-ATPase by isoproterenol in β-intercalated cells is also secondary to ERK activation, occurring rather through PKA-dependent activation of the Ras/Raf1 pathway.[151]

Colonic H,K-ATPase

Type III K-ATPase activity sensitive to both Sch 28080 (IC$_{50}$ ≈ 1 μM) and ouabain (IC$_{50}$ ≈ 20 μM) is detected in CD of K$^+$-depleted, but not normal, rats.[152] Type III K-ATPase activity is absent in CD of K$^+$-depleted αHKc-deficient mice.[21] In the kidney of normal rats, αHKc mRNA is expressed at low levels along the entire distal nephron, from medullary thick ascending limb of Henle's loop to IMCD.[153] αHKc mRNA and protein expression levels are much higher in K$^+$-depleted rats than in normal rats.[140,153] Immunohistochemistry studies performed on normal rats revealed that labeling of OMCD principal cells at the apical membrane is markedly increased in K$^+$-depleted rats,[154] but that curiously K$^+$ depletion does not induce labeling of CCD principal cells, even though CCD from K$^+$-depleted rats display increased mRNA expression[153] and increased type III K-ATPase activity.[152] In normal rabbits, αHKc was detected at the apical pole of principal cells and intercalated cells in CNT and CD.[155] In transgenic mice expressing EGFP under the control of the αHKc promoter, EGFP is specifically expressed in CD principal cells.[156] Altogether, these studies demonstrate that αHKc is specifically expressed at the apical pole of CD principal cells, and that this expression is markedly increased in response to K$^+$ depletion. The site-specific localization of αHKc in principal cells is consistent with the functional localization of type III K-ATPase.[149]

Potassium depletion is a condition in which CD reabsorbs, rather than secretes, K$^+$. Because of its expression at the apical pole of principal cells, colonic H,K-ATPase was proposed to be the motor for K$^+$ reabsorption in the collecting duct that occurs during K$^+$-depletion. *In vitro* microperfusion studies provided the first evidence for H,K-ATPase-dependent reabsorption of K$^+$ and HCO_3^- in OMCD from K$^+$-deprived rabbits.[140] Sch 28080-sensitive K$^+$ reabsorption also occurs in distal tubules, accessible by *in vivo* micropuncture, in K$^+$-depleted rats, but not in normal rats.[157] In addition, part of HCO_3^- reabsorption is inhibited by both ouabain and Sch 28080 in IMCD of K$^+$-depleted rats.[158] Surprisingly, αHKc-deficient mice do not display any renal phenotype, even when fed a K$^+$-depleted diet.[159] This indicates that an alternative transport mechanism functionally compensates for colonic H,K-ATPase deficiency.

Expression of colonic H,K-ATPase in the kidney is markedly increased by dietary K$^+$ restriction.[140] Because chronic dietary K$^+$ restriction induces metabolic alkalosis, and reduces plasma aldosterone levels, the role of both of these factors in regulating CD H,K-ATPase expression was investigated. In CD of rats clamped either in the absence of circulating aldosterone or under physiological or high levels of circulating aldosterone, K$^+$ depletion increased H,K-ATPase activity to similar extents, regardless of aldosterone concentration.[160] In addition, neither adrenalectomy nor a Na$^+$-depleted diet, which increases endogenous aldosterone levels, altered αHKc mRNA expression in the rat kidney medulla.[154] Thus, aldosterone does not control H,K-ATPase expression in the CD.

Similarly, increased expression of αHKc mRNA in the kidney during K^+ depletion most likely is not related to alkalosis, since it is observed in the absence of a significant change in plasma acid–base parameters.[161]

While changes in plasma acid–base status do not alter αHKc transcription, an increase of pCO_2 results in increased H,K-ATPase-mediated potassium and bicarbonate reabsorption in the CCD of K^+-depleted rabbits,[162] demonstrating post-transcriptional regulation of colonic H,K-ATPase during acidosis. Post-transcriptional regulation of colonic H,K-ATPase also occurs in the CCD of K^+-depleted rats in response to vasopressin, which increases type III ATPase activity in a PKA-dependent manner.[149] In the long-term, cAMP also controls the expression of αHKc by binding to cAMP-responsive elements present in the αHKc promoter.[163]

In conclusion, gastric H,K-ATPase is expressed in intercalated cells of the distal nephron where, along with other systems, it participates in proton transport and helps regulate acid–base balance. Colonic H,K-ATPase is also expressed in the distal nephron, but in principal cells where it energizes potassium reabsorption, especially under conditions of dietary K^+ restriction. Neither ATPase appears to be essential for animal survival or even for the continued maintenance of acid–base and potassium balance, at least under experimental conditions studied so far. Compensatory transport systems are able to palliate the genetic absence of gastric and colonic H,K-ATPase in the kidney. Such compensatory mechanisms need to be characterized, and it remains to be determined whether their activity relies on as yet unidentified ATPases.

V-ATPase

The vacuolar H^+-ATPases (V-ATPases) are among the most broadly expressed enzymes that convert the chemical energy of ATP breakdown into electric and chemical gradients. V-ATPases share a lot of structural similarities with mitochondrial F-ATPases, probably because both complexes have subunits that arise from common ancestors.[164–167] However, F-ATPases differ from V-ATPases, in that their expression is restricted to organelles that arise from bacterial endosymbiosis such as mitochondria (or chloroplast in plants), where they serve to generate ATP at the expense of the proton motive force (pmf), whereas V-ATPases use the energy produced by ATP breakdown to pump protons across membranes. The pmf and membrane potential difference ($\Delta\psi$) that result from the primary active transport of H^+ are then used to energize a large number of secondary active transporters. V-ATPases are found in virtually all eukaryotic cell types in endomembranes of intracellular organelles from the secretory pathway. In addition, in higher organisms V-ATPases can be found at the plasma membrane of

highly specialized cells, such as the epithelial cells of the kidney, the male reproductive tract, the inner ear, and in osteoclasts. Because of this broad pattern of expression, V-ATPases play a critical role in a large number of different functions.[168] Plasma membrane V-ATPases are important for biological processes that require acidification of the extracellular space, such as bicarbonate reclamation from the urinary fluid, bone resorption, and sperm maturation, while acidification by intracellular V-ATPases of vesicles or endosomes is critical for normal endocytosis, intracellular trafficking, polypeptide processing, neurotransmitter uptake, accumulation and secretion, and for breakdown of macromolecules.

STRUCTURE AND MECHANISM OF ACTION OF V-ATPASES

Like F-ATPases, V-ATPases are integral macromolecular complexes with up to 14 different subunits. The molecular structure and the function of V-ATPases have received considerable attention, and have been the subject of excellent reviews.[168–171] V-ATPases are divided in two principal functional domains, V0, the transmembrane domain (240 kDa) that mediates the transfer of protons across the membrane and V1, the catalytic domain (900 kDa) that binds and hydrolyzes ATP. The V1 domain is always facing the cytoplasm; hence, when located in the plasma membrane, the pump always mediates extrusion of protons out of the cell, and when present in intracelullar membranes, it mediates acidification of the organelles. The V0 domain represents the proton transporting pore, and is formed by a ring of at least 6 subunits. For example, in mammals, several subunit c assembles with single subunit c", d, and e in a channel-like structure with the a subunit.[172] The V1 domain comprises at least eight different subunits (A–H), and is divided into the "catalytic unit" which binds and hydrolyzes ATP, and the "stalk" which links the hydrolytic unit to the integral V0 domain.

Studies of the prokaryotic V-Na^+-ATPase of *Enterococcus hirae*[173,174] have reached the conclusion that V-ATPase might function following the model of rotational catalysis initially proposed for F-ATPases[175,176]: the central core of the V1 stalk, consisting of subunits D and F, and the proteolipid ring of c-subunits of the V0 domain rotate, driven by the hydrolysis of ATP, while the remaining subunits of the pump are static. One proton enters the machinery through an inner hemi-channel opened at the cytosolic surface of subunit a, and reaches the binding site of one of the c-subunits in the central ring[174]; the proton is then moved by the complete rotation of the ring towards the opening of a second hemi-channel, also in the a-subunit, but open on the outer space, where it can unbind. Recently, experiments in which movements of the V1 complex of bacteriae were visualized with fluorescent actin filaments have confirmed that rotational catalysis does exist *in vivo*.[177,178] Bafilomycin and concanamycin A, which are specific inhibitors of the pump, both bind to subunit c.[179,180]

Isoforms

Multiple homologs and splice variants of the different V-ATPase subunits have been identified.[181,182] In mammals particularly, multiple variants exist for the B-, C-, E-, and G-subunits of the V1 catalytic domain, and for the a-, d-, and e-subunits of the V0 integral domain. Some of these homologs or variants, such as B2, C1, E1, G1, a1, d1, e1, have a very broad distribution, while other variants have a very restricted expression pattern. Some subunits also exhibit variable expression during development.[183] Hence, the timing and tissue specificity of V-ATPase expression, as well as the functional diversity of the pump, are thought to stem from combinations of V-ATPase subunit variants, and mutations of genes encoding for different variants of the same V-ATPase subunit can result in very different phenotypes. Furthermore, the existence of highly specific combinations of variants in one cell type or for a particular function raises the exciting possibility of developing targeted pharmacological strategies directed at one specific combination. An extended nomenclature assembly of a unique combination of the different genes and splice variants of V-ATPase subunits has been recently proposed.[182] Importantly, this work included a wide scan of published studies and sequence databases in order to provide the scientific community with the most complete catalog of function, tissue-specificity, and subcellular localization known to date for the different molecular forms of V-ATPase subunits.

Renal Isoforms of the V-ATPase

All the different subunits are necessary for the proper assembly, expression, and function of the pump, and the kidney expresses all the ubiquitous variants of V-ATPase subunits. In addition, among the different subunits with more restricted expression (for review see [184]), some variants such as B1,[185,186] C2,[187] G3,[188,189] a4,[190–192] d2,[193] and e2,[194] although not strictly "specific," are especially enriched in the kidney. In particular, the a4-subunit is expressed all along the nephron, while the B1-subunit is markedly enriched in the intercalated cells of the collecting system. The exact reason for the presence of these tissue-specific isoforms is not yet clear. It is possible that these isoforms have specific targeting or assembly motives required in a given cell type to drive the expression of the pump in a particular subcellular domain. For example, the B1-subunit differs from the B2-subunit by the presence of a COOH-terminal "DTAL" motif typical of a PDZ-interacting domain that is required for molecular interactions with the PDZ protein NHERF-1. Moreover, NHERF-1 is specifically expressed at the basolateral pole of β- but not α-intercalated cells, which raises the possibility that molecular interactions between the B1-subunit and NHERF-1 are required for the characteristic basolateral targeting of the V-ATPase in this particular cell type.[195,196] It is also possible that specific variants of the different subunits allow assembly with regulatory elements. For example, the actin cytoskeleton[197,198] or the glycolytic enzyme aldolase B[199,200] have been demonstrated to interact with the B-subunit of the V1 integral domain, and these interactions are believed to be critical for proper pump trafficking, assembly, and regulation.[201,202] An interaction between the a4-subunit and the enzyme phospho-fructokinase 1 has also been shown to be necessary for coupling the catalytic activity of the pump with its transport activity.[203] Nevertheless, the observation that inactivating mutations or disruption of genes encoding for kidney specific subunits, such as the a4- or B1-subunit, lead to a defect in proton secretion by α-Ics and to distal tubular acidosis[204–207] indicates that these tissue-specific subunits are critical for the proper functioning of the pump in the kidney. Indeed, even though under certain circumstances, such as targeted disruption of the B1-subunit in mouse, the B2-subunit can substitute partly for the B1-subunit, it cannot fully compensate for its loss.[208,209]

Multiple Functions of the V-ATPASE in the Kidney

Expression in the Kidney

The role of V-ATPase in urine acidification was first described in turtle bladder epithelium, whose characteristics are close to those of the mammalian collecting duct. In this system, H^+ secretion was shown to be an active, sodium-independent[210] process coupled to oxidative metabolism.[211,212] Final proof of a role for V-ATPase came from a very elegant study showing that reversal of H^+ fluxes induced ATP synthesis.[213] V-ATPase was subsequently purified and characterized in microsomal fractions isolated from these cells.[214] The bovine renal medulla exhibits the same V-ATPases as turtle bladder epithelium.[215] A number of subsequent studies detected the presence of V-ATPases, in both the apical plasma membrane and membranes of organelles, in almost all mammalian renal epithelial cells, including the brush border membrane of the proximal tubule,[186,216–222] and the apical membranes of the thick ascending limb[186,216,217] and distal convoluted tubule.[186,216,217] In the collecting duct, V-ATPase is present in the apical membrane and cytoplasm of α-intercalated cells and in the basolateral membrane of β-intercalated cells; low expression levels have also been reported in principal cells.[186,216,223]

Bicarbonate Absorption

Along the nephron, the role of plasma membrane V-ATPases is to excrete protons from cells into the outer space. Hence, except for β-intercalated cells in which the pump is expressed basolaterally, the pump secretes protons into the urinary fluid. Urine acidification is the primary mechanism of renal bicarbonate absorption and acid excretion, and is therefore critical for acid-base regulation. To avoid leaking bicarbonate into urine, the kidney has to reclaim virtually all the bicarbonate filtered at the glomerulus (~4300 mmol/day). Bicarbonate absorption is achieved in the proximal tubule, the ascending limb of the loop of Henle, and to lesser extent in the distal convoluted tubule. In general, protons secreted into the urinary fluid can combine with bicarbonate ions also present therein to yield carbonic acid (H_2CO_3), which is quickly dehydrated into CO_2 and H_2O by a luminal carbonic anhydrase. CO_2 diffuses back from the urinary fluid into epithelial cells down its concentration gradient. Within the cell, it is then rehydrated by a cytosolic carbonic anhydrase, and the resulting bicarbonate ion exits the cell at the basolateral side via an electrogenic Na-HCO3 co-transporter in the proximal tubule or a Cl^-/HCO_3^- exchanger in the TAL. Functional studies have shown that the main mechanism of proton secretion that drives bicarbonate absorption is Na^+/H^+ exchange,[224–226] a secondary active transport process is energized by the inward Na^+ gradient generated by the basolateral Na^+/K^+-ATPase. Molecular studies have demonstrated that this process depends on NHE3[227–229] and a Na^+-dependent amiloride-insensitive transporter[230] in the proximal tubule, and on NHE2 in the distal convoluted tubule.[228,231,232] However, a number of functional studies have also revealed the presence of bafilomycin A1-sensitive, ATP-dependent H^+ secretion that accounts for at least ~20% of proton secretion in the proximal tubule,[224–227,233,234] and that correlates with V-ATPase immunodetection in this nephron segment (see above). Moreover, pump activity appears to be stimulated by acidosis[235] or by angiotensin II[218,236] suggesting that the pump may participate significantly in bicarbonate reclamation by the proximal tubule.

Approximatively 10% of the bicarbonate filtered at the glomerulus is absorbed by the thick ascending limb of Henle's loop. As in the proximal tubule, the primary mechanism of bicarbonate absorption in the TAL is the Na^+/H^+ exchanger NHE3. Active secretion of protons with pharmacological characteristics of V-ATPases has also been detected in the TAL,[237–239] and immunoreactivity to different subunits of the pump has been shown in the apical membrane of TAL cells.[186,216,217] Even though these observations suggest that the pump might play a significant role in bicarbonate transport in the TAL, direct examination of bicarbonate transport in isolated, microperfused TAL demonstrated that all bicarbonate absorption by the TAL is sodium-dependent and sensitive to amiloride, which indicates that Na^+/H^+ exchange accounts for virtually all bicarbonate transport.[240] Thus, the role of the V-ATPase in the TAL remains unclear.

Role of the V-ATPase in Intercalated Cells

The second process that the kidney uses to keep blood bicarbonate constant is the excretion of the daily acid load generated by protein catabolism (~1 mmol/kg/j). This is achieved in the collecting system, which includes the late distal convoluted tubule, the connecting tubule, the cortical collecting duct and the medullary collecting duct. All these segments are characterized by the presence of intercalated cells (ICs), a subpopulation expressing the proton pump and characterized by the presence of the B1-subunit. At least two different sub-types of intercalated cells have been identified: the "canonical" form of type α IC secretes H^+ through the apical vacuolar H^+-ATPase and reabsorbs HCO_3^- via the basolateral $Cl^-/HCO3^-$ exchanger AE1, whereas the "canonical" form of type β IC has the opposite polarity and function.[223,241,242] There is some evidence for at least one other subtype of intercalated cells, called non-α non-β, which express both the proton pump and a $Cl^-/HCO3^-$ exchanger at the apical membrane.[242] The function of this third type remains unclear. For simplicity, the term β-IC is used in this review to refer to both canonical β and non-α non-β ICs.

Type α-intercalated cells secrete acid into a urinary fluid virtually devoid of bicarbonate, because of bicarbonate absorption in the upstream nephron segments. A fraction of protons remain free in urine and decrease urine pH. However, the amount of protons that can be freely eliminated in solution is very limited, because urine volume has to remain small and because at urine pH values below 4.4, the transepithelial gradient of H^+ overcomes the capabilities of the V-ATPase and proton secretion stops. Thus, a majority of protons secreted in the collecting system are instead titrated by urine buffers that can be weak bases (e.g., in humans, mostly creatinine and HPO_4^-) yielding titrable acids or the strong base NH_3 yielding the ammonium ion (NH_4^+). Since the different products resulting from these reactions cannot diffuse back across the collecting system epithelium, this titration serves to trap and eliminate protons in urine. In addition, because at an acidic urine pH ammonia (NH_3) is transformed into ammonium NH_4^+, the action of V-ATPase is also crucial to maintain a concentration gradient of NH_3 across the collecting duct epithelium, and V-ATPase can be viewed as the energizer of ammonium secretion.[243] Protons secreted by the V-ATPase into urine are generated, together with bicarbonate ions from CO_2 and H_2O within intercalated cells. Proton secretion is functionally coupled to basolateral bicarbonate extrusion through the Cl^-/HCO_3^- exchanger AE1, because in the absence of bicarbonate exit, accumulation of bicarbonate into the cell would limit proton secretion. Thus, the bicarbonate that has been "generated" from proton secretion by intercalated cells replaces the bicarbonate that has been consumed when buffering the metabolically produced protons.

Type β ICs have the opposite polarity of α ICs.[223,241,242] They mediate bicarbonate secretion and generate protons. They are therefore adapted to excrete bases in response to metabolic alkalosis. In intercalated cells, V-ATPase is expressed both at the plasma membrane and in intracellular vesicles that can be recruited rapidly by exocytosis when increased pump activity is required.[244] Moreover, intercalated cells are also able to reverse the polarity of the pump's expression. Induction of metabolic acidosis or alkalosis produces a profound change in the population distribution of these different cell types, with acidosis shifting the distribution towards type α with apical ATPases, and alkalosis increasing the number of canonical β-cells at the expense of α-cells. The observation that this shift from one cell type to the other occurs while the total number of ICs remains constant was interpreted as evidence that ICs can convert from one phenotype to the other.[245] Since this seminal observation, compelling evidence has shown that this interconversion can occur *in vitro* or in isolated tubules, and that it requires secretion by intercalated cells of the matrix protein hensin, and activation of a complex signaling pathway that involves integrin b1.[246−249]

The contribution of β-intercalated cells to renal NaCl balance and blood pressure regulation is an emerging aspect of intercalated cell function.[250] Studies of a mouse model with disruption of the apical Cl^-/HCO_3^- exchanger pendrin demonstrated that β ICs are the main pathway for chloride absorption across the collecting duct epithelium,[251] and disruption of pendrin impairs renal ability to conserve NaCl.[251] Conversely, disruption of Cl^- absorption by β ICs protects against mineralocorticoid-induced hypertension.[252] It has also been recently demonstrated that coupling of the sodium-independent Cl^-/HCO_3^- exchanger pendrin with the sodium-driven Cl^-/HCO_3^- exchanger NDCBE (SLC4A8) mediates thiazide-sensitive NaCl absorption.[120] Importantly, as indicated above, Cl^-/HCO_3^- exchange in intercalated cells is tightly coupled to proton transport mediated by V-ATPases. Whether the V-ATPase energizes chloride transport and thereby participates in renal NaCl handling has not yet been determined. However, it was recently shown that bafilomycin, a specific V-ATPase blocker, inhibits angiotensin II-stimulated Cl^- absorption,[253] which suggests that V-ATPases may energize part of the NaCl absorption in the distal nephron. It is noteworthy that some patients with dRTA exhibit a salt- and potassium-loosing nephropathy. Even though these features can be explained by the frequent association of dRTA with nephrocalcinosis and interstitial nephritis, the exact involvement of V-ATPase dysfunction in these disorders has not yet been directly evaluated.

Role of the V-ATPase in Endocytosis in Renal Epithelial Cells

As indicated above, V-ATPase is not exclusively present in the plasma membrane of renal cells. As in all other eukaryotic cells, V-ATPase is abundantly expressed in the membrane of intracellular organelles. In intracellular membranes, the V1 catalytic domain is located in the cytosol and therefore the pump drives the transport of protons from the cytosol into the organelles. Many cellular processes, such as endo- or exocytosis, catalytic activity into lysosomes, neurotransmitter uptake into synaptic vesicles or release from secretory granules, receptor recycling, and sorting of proteins from the golgi apparatus, are critically dependent upon proper V-ATPase activity.[168,254]

In the kidney, much attention has been paid to the link between V-ATPase-dependent acidification of endosomes and endo-exocytosis. Receptor-dependent or -independent endocytosis of filtered molecules or of apical membrane proteins is an important function achieved by proximal tubule cells. Impairment of this function leads to low molecular weight proteinuria, which is one of the most prominent features of Dent's disease,[255] a rare condition characterized by a Fanconi-like syndrome associated with nephrolithiasis or nephrocalcinosis, caused by mutations in the chloride transporter CLC5.[256−259] Because proton transport by the V-ATPase is electrogenic, intracellular organelle acidification is accompanied by the development of an inside-positive potential difference. In the absence of an electrical shunt, this membrane voltage would represent a self-limiting factor for proton pump activity. In most cells, this shunt is achieved by a chloride conductance activated by voltage. Since CLC5 co-localizes with the V-ATPase in apical endosomes,[260] it has been proposed that inactivating mutations of CLC5 inhibit endocytosis, because they prevent endosome acidification.[261–263] This paradigm, however, has been challenged by studies showing that CLC5 is not a Cl^- channel, but is rather an electrogenic Cl^-/H^+ antiporter,[264] and more recently that mutations that switch CLC5 function from Cl^-/H^+ exchange to Cl^- conductive transport are able to restore endosomal acidification, but impair endocytosis.[265] The latter study also suggests that endosomal V-ATPases control endocytosis by energizing chloride accumulation into intracellular organelles, rather than by promoting intravesicular acidification. How intravesicular chloride controls endocytosis, however, remains unsettled.

References

[1] Brini M, Carafoli E. Calcium pumps in health and disease. Physiol Rev 2009;89(4):1341–78.

[2] Blanco G, DeTomaso AW, Koster J, Xie ZJ, Mercer RW. The alpha-subunit of the Na,K-ATPase has catalytic activity independent of the beta-subunit. J Biol Chem 1994;269(38):23420–5.

[3] Ward DG, Cavieres JD. Solubilized alpha beta Na,K-ATPase remains protomeric during turnover yet shows apparent negative cooperativity toward ATP. Proc Natl Acad Sci USA 1993;90(11):5332–6.

[4] Martin DW, Sachs JR. Cross-linking of the erythrocyte Na^+,K^+-ATPase. Chemical cross-linkers induce alpha-subunit-band 3 heterodimers and do not induce alpha-subunit homodimers. J Biol Chem 1992;267(33):23922–9.

[5] Morth JP, Pedersen BP, Toustrup-Jensen MS, Sørensen TL, Petersen J, Andersen JP, et al. Crystal structure of the sodium-potassium pump. Nature 2007;450(7172):1043–9.

[6] Shinoda T, Ogawa H, Cornelius F, Toyoshima C. Crystal structure of the sodium-potassium pump at 2.4 Å resolution. Nature 2009;459(7245):446–50.

[7] Blanco G, Mercer RW. Isozymes of the Na-K-ATPase: heterogeneity in structure, diversity in function. Am J Physiol 1998;275(5 Pt 2):F633–50.

[8] DuBose Jr. TD, Gitomer J, Codina J. H^+,K^+-ATPase. Curr Opin Nephrol Hypertens 1999;8(5):597–602.

[9] Geering K. Functional roles of Na,K-ATPase subunits. Curr Opin Nephrol Hypertens 2008;17(5):526–32.

[10] Hasler U, Crambert G, Horisberger JD, Geering K. Structural and functional features of the transmembrane domain of the Na,K-ATPase beta subunit revealed by tryptophan scanning. J Biol Chem 2001;276(19):16356–64.

[11] Geering K. FXYD proteins: new regulators of Na-K-ATPase. Am J Physiol Renal Physiol 2006;290(2):F241–50.

[12] Capurro C, Coutry N, Bonvalet JP, Escoubet B, Garty H, Farman N. Cellular localization and regulation of CHIF in kidney and colon. Am J Physiol 1996;271(3 Pt 1):C753–62.

[13] Shattock MJ. Phospholemman: its role in normal cardiac physiology and potential as a druggable target in disease. Curr Opin Pharmacol 2009;9(2):160–6.

[14] Delprat B, Schaer D, Roy S, Wang J, Puel JL, Geering K. FXYD6 is a novel regulator of Na,K-ATPase expressed in the inner ear. J Biol Chem 2007;282(10):7450–6.

[15] Bibert S, Aebischer D, Desgranges F, Roy S, Schaer D, Kharoubi-Hess S, et al. A link between FXYD3 (Mat-8)-mediated Na,K-ATPase regulation and differentiation of Caco-2 intestinal epithelial cells. Mol Biol Cell 2009;20(4):1132–40.

[16] Barlet-Bas C, Cheval L, Khadouri C, Marsy S, Doucet A. Difference in the Na affinity of $Na+-K+$-ATPase along the rabbit nephron: modulation by K. Am J Physiol 1990;259(2 Pt 2):F246–50.

[17] Feraille E, Vogt B, Rousselot M, Barlet-Bas C, Cheval L, Doucet A, et al. Mechanism of enhanced Na-K-ATPase activity in cortical collecting duct from rats with nephrotic syndrome. J Clin Invest 1993;91(4):1295–300.

[18] Munzer JS, Daly SE, Jewell-Motz EA, Lingrel JB, Blostein R. Tissue- and isoform-specific kinetic behavior of the Na,K-ATPase. J Biol Chem 1994;269(24):16668–76.

[19] Toyoshima C, Inesi G. Structural basis of ion pumping by Ca^{2+}-ATPase of the sarcoplasmic reticulum. Annu Rev Biochem 2004;73:269–92.

[20] Rabon EC, Reuben MA. The mechanism and structure of the gastric H,K-ATPase. Annu Rev Physiol 1990;52:321–44.

[21] Dherbecourt O, Cheval L, Bloch-Faure M, Meneton P, Doucet A. Molecular identification of Sch28080-sensitive K-ATPase activities in the mouse kidney. Pflugers Arch 2006;451(6):769–75.

[22] Campbell-Thompson ML, Verlander JW, Curran KA, Campbell WG, Cain BD, Wingo CS, et al. In situ hybridization of H-K-ATPase beta-subunit mRNA in rat and rabbit kidney. Am J Physiol 1995;269(3 Pt 2):F345–54.

[23] Lingrel JB, Van Huysse J, O'Brien W, Jewell-Motz E, Askew R, Schultheis P. Structure–function studies of the Na,K-ATPase. Kidney Int Suppl 1994;44:S32–9.

[24] Crambert G, Hasler U, Beggah AT, Yu C, Modyanov NN, Horisberger JD, et al. Transport and pharmacological properties of nine different human Na, K-ATPase isozymes. J Biol Chem 2000;275(3):1976–86.

[25] Lingrel JB. The physiological significance of the cardiotonic steroid/ouabain-binding site of the Na,K-ATPase. Annu Rev Physiol 2010;72:395–412.

[26] Barcroft LC, Moseley AE, Lingrel JB, Watson AJ. Deletion of the Na/K-ATPase alpha1-subunit gene (Atp1a1) does not prevent cavitation of the preimplantation mouse embryo. Mech Dev 2004;121(5):417–26.

[27] Moseley AE, Lieske SP, Wetzel RK, James PF, He S, Shelly DA, et al. The Na,K-ATPase alpha 2 isoform is expressed in neurons, and its absence disrupts neuronal activity in newborn mice. J Biol Chem 2003;278(7):5317–24.

[28] Shelly DA, He S, Moseley A, Weber C, Stegemeyer M, Lynch RM, et al. Na^+ pump alpha 2-isoform specifically couples to contractility in vascular smooth muscle: evidence from gene-targeted neonatal mice. Am J Physiol Cell Physiol 2004;286(4):C813–20.

[29] Moseley AE, Huddleson JP, Bohanan CS, James PF, Lorenz JN, Aronow BJ, et al. Genetic profiling reveals global changes in multiple biological pathways in the hearts of Na, K-ATPase alpha 1 isoform haploinsufficient mice. Cell Physiol Biochem 2005;15(1-4):145–58.

[30] De Fusco M, Marconi R, Silvestri L, Atorino L, Rampoldi L, Morgante L, et al. Haploinsufficiency of ATP1A2 encoding the Na^+/K^+ pump alpha2 subunit associated with familial hemiplegic migraine type 2. Nat Genet 2003;33(2):192–6.

[31] Capendeguy O, Horisberger JD. Functional effects of Na^+,K^+-ATPase gene mutations linked to familial hemiplegic migraine. Neuromolecular Med 2004;6(2-3):105–16.

[32] de Carvalho Aguiar P, Sweadner KJ, Penniston JT, Zaremba J, Liu L, Caton M, et al. Mutations in the Na^+/K^+-ATPase alpha3 gene ATP1A3 are associated with rapid-onset dystonia parkinsonism. Neuron 2004;43(2):169–75.

[33] Meij IC, Koenderink JB, van Bokhoven H, Assink KF, Groenestege WT, de Pont JJ, et al. Dominant isolated renal magnesium loss is caused by misrouting of the Na$^+$,K$^+$-ATPase gamma-subunit. Nat Genet 2000;26(3):265—6.

[34] Thompson CB, McDonough AA. Skeletal muscle Na,K-ATPase alpha and beta subunit protein levels respond to hypokalemic challenge with isoform and muscle type specificity. J Biol Chem 1996;271(51):32653—8.

[35] Fisone G, Cheng SX, Nairn AC, Czernik AJ, Hemmings Jr. HC, Höög JO, et al. Identification of the phosphorylation site for cAMP-dependent protein kinase on Na$^+$,K$^+$-ATPase and effects of site-directed mutagenesis. J Biol Chem 1994;269 (12):9368—73.

[36] Beguin P, Beggah AT, Chibalin AV, Burgener-Kairuz P, Jaisser F, Matthews PM, et al. Phosphorylation of the Na,K-ATPase alpha-subunit by protein kinase A and C in vitro and in intact cells. Identification of a novel motif for PKC-mediated phosphorylation. J Biol Chem 1994;269(39):24437—45.

[37] Sweadner KJ, Feschenko MS. Predicted location and limited accessibility of protein kinase A phosphorylation site on Na-K-ATPase. Am J Physiol Cell Physiol 2001;280(4):C1017—26.

[38] Mordasini D, Bustamante M, Rousselot M, Martin PY, Hasler U, Feraille E. Stimulation of Na$^+$ transport by AVP is independent of PKA phosphorylation of the Na-K-ATPase in collecting duct principal cells. Am J Physiol Renal Physiol 2005;289(5): F1031—9.

[39] Logvinenko NS, Dulubova I, Fedosova N, Larsson SH, Nairn AC, Esmann M, et al. Phosphorylation by protein kinase C of serine-23 of the alpha-1 subunit of rat Na$^+$,K$^+$-ATPase affects its conformational equilibrium. Proc Natl Acad Sci U S A 1996;93 (17):9132—7.

[40] Beguin P, Peitsch MC, Geering K. alpha 1 but not alpha 2 or alpha 3 isoforms of Na,K-ATPase are efficiently phosphorylated in a novel protein kinase C motif. Biochemistry 1996;35 (45):14098—108.

[41] Feraille E, Beguin P, Carranza ML, Gonin S, Rousselot M, Martin PY, et al. Is phosphorylation of the alpha1 subunit at Ser-16 involved in the control of Na,K-ATPase activity by phorbol ester-activated protein kinase C? Mol Biol Cell 2000;11(1):39—50.

[42] Chibalin AV, Ogimoto G, Pedemonte CH, Pressley TA, Katz AI, Feraille E, et al. Dopamine-induced endocytosis of Na$^+$,K$^+$-ATPase is initiated by phosphorylation of Ser-18 in the rat alpha subunit and is responsible for the decreased activity in epithelial cells. J Biol Chem 1999;274(4):1920—7.

[43] Efendiev R, Bertorello AM, Pressley TA, Rousselot M, Feraille E, et al. Simultaneous phosphorylation of Ser11 and Ser18 in the alpha-subunit promotes the recruitment of Na$^+$, K$^+$-ATPase molecules to the plasma membrane. Biochemistry 2000;39(32):9884—92.

[44] Feraille E, Carranza ML, Gonin S, Beguin P, Pedemonte C, Rousselot M, et al. Insulin-induced stimulation of Na$^+$,K$^+$-ATPase activity in kidney proximal tubule cells depends on phosphorylation of the alpha-subunit at Tyr-10. Mol Biol Cell 1999;10(9):2847—59.

[45] Chibalin AV, Kovalenko MV, Ryder JW, Feraille E, Wallberg-Henriksson H, Zierath JR. Insulin- and glucose-induced phosphorylation of the Na$^+$,K$^+$-adenosine triphosphatase alpha-subunits in rat skeletal muscle. Endocrinology 2001;142(8): 3474—82.

[46] Holthouser KA, Mandal A, Merchant ML, Schelling JR, Delamere NA, Valdes Jr. RR, et al. Ouabain stimulates Na-K-ATPase through a sodium/hydrogen exchanger-1 (NHE-1)-dependent mechanism in human kidney proximal tubule cells. Am J Physiol Renal Physiol 2010;299(1):F77—90.

[47] Otulakowski G, O'Brodovich H. Thyroid hormone and Na$^+$-K$^+$-ATPase: more than simple transcription. Am J Physiol Lung Cell Mol Physiol 2007;292(1):L4—5.

[48] Feraille E, Doucet A. Sodium-potassium-adenosinetriphosphatase-dependent sodium transport in the kidney: hormonal control. Physiol Rev 2001;81(1):345—418.

[49] Clausen T. Na$^+$-K$^+$ pump regulation and skeletal muscle contractility. Physiol Rev 2003;83(4):1269—324.

[50] Lecuona E, Sun H, Vohwinkel C, Ciechanover A, Sznajder JI. Ubiquitination participates in the lysosomal degradation of Na, K-ATPase in steady-state conditions. Am J Respir Cell Mol Biol 2009;41(6):671—9.

[51] Efendiev R, Bertorello AM, Pedemonte CH. PKC-beta and PKC-zeta mediate opposing effects on proximal tubule Na +, K + -ATPase activity. FEBS Lett 1999;456(1):45—8.

[52] Liu J, Kesiry R, Periyasamy SM, Malhotra D, Xie Z, Shapiro JI. Ouabain induces endocytosis of plasmalemmal Na/K-ATPase in LLC-PK1 cells by a clathrin-dependent mechanism. Kidney Int 2004;66(1):227—41.

[53] Vadasz I, Dada LA, Briva A, Trejo HE, Welch LC, Chen J, et al. AMP-activated protein kinase regulates CO$_2$-induced alveolar epithelial dysfunction in rats and human cells by promoting Na,K-ATPase endocytosis. J Clin Invest 2008;118 (2):752—62.

[54] Kimura T, Allen PB, Nairn AC, Caplan MJ. Arrestins and spinophilin competitively regulate Na$^+$,K$^+$-ATPase trafficking through association with a large cytoplasmic loop of the Na$^+$, K$^+$-ATPase. Mol Biol Cell 2007;18(11):4508—18.

[55] Hundal HS, Marette A, Mitsumoto Y, Ramlal T, Blostein R, Klip A. Insulin induces translocation of the alpha 2 and beta 1 subunits of the Na$^+$/K$^+$-ATPase from intracellular compartments to the plasma membrane in mammalian skeletal muscle. J Biol Chem 1992;267(8):5040—3.

[56] Barlet-Bas C, Khadouri C, Marsy S, Doucet A. Enhanced intracellular sodium concentration in kidney cells recruits a latent pool of Na-K-ATPase whose size is modulated by corticosteroids. J Biol Chem 1990;265(14):7799—803.

[57] Summa V, Mordasini D, Roger F, Bens M, Martin PY, Vandewalle A, et al. Short term effect of aldosterone on Na,K-ATPase cell surface expression in kidney collecting duct cells. J Biol Chem 2001;276(50):47087—93.

[58] Gonin S, Deschenes G, Roger F, Bens M, Martin PY, Carpentier JL, et al. Cyclic AMP increases cell surface expression of functional Na,K-ATPase units in mammalian cortical collecting duct principal cells. Mol Biol Cell 2001;12(2):255—64.

[59] Bertorello AM, Ridge KM, Chibalin AV, Katz AI, Sznajder JI. Isoproterenol increases Na$^+$-K$^+$-ATPase activity by membrane insertion of alpha-subunits in lung alveolar cells. Am J Physiol 1999;276(1 Pt 1):L20—7.

[60] Ridgem K, Dada M, Lecuona L, Bertorello E, Katz AM, Mochly-Rosen AI, et al. J. L. Dopamine-induced exocytosis of Na,K-ATPase is dependent on activation of protein kinase C-epsilon and -delta. Mol Biol Cell 2002;13(4):1381—9.

[61] Lecuona E, Ridge K, Pesce L, Batlle D, Sznajder JI. The GTP-binding protein RhoA mediates Na,K-ATPase exocytosis in alveolar epithelial cells. Mol Biol Cell 2003;14(9):3888—97.

[62] Trejo HE, Lecuona E, Grillo D, Szleifer I, Nekrasova OE, Gelfand VI, et al. Role of kinesin light chain-2 of kinesin-1 in the traffic of Na,K-ATPase-containing vesicles in alveolar epithelial cells. FASEB J 2010;24(2):374—82.

[63] Lecuona E, Minin A, Trejo HE, Chen J, Comellas AP, Sun H, et al. Myosin-Va restrains the trafficking of Na$^+$/K$^+$-ATPase-containing vesicles in alveolar epithelial cells. J Cell Sci 2009;122(21):3915—22.

[64] Devarajan P, Scaramuzzino DA, Morrow JS. Ankyrin binds to two distinct cytoplasmic domains of Na,K-ATPase alpha subunit. Proc Natl Acad Sci USA 1994;91(8):2965—9.

[65] Nelson WJ, Hammerton RW. A membrane-cytoskeletal complex containing Na$^+$,K$^+$-ATPase, ankyrin, and fodrin in Madin—Darby canine kidney (MDCK) cells: implications for the biogenesis of epithelial cell polarity. J Cell Biol 1989;108(3): 893—902.

[66] Ferrandi M, Salardi S, Tripodi G, Barassi P, Rivera R, Manunta P, et al. Evidence for an interaction between adducin and Na$^+$K$^+$-ATPase: relation to genetic hypertension. Am J Physiol 1999;277(4 Pt 2):H1338—49.

[67] Cantiello HF. Actin filaments stimulate the Na$^+$K$^+$-ATPase. Am J Physiol 1995;269(5 Pt 2):F637—43.

[68] Torielli. L, Tivodar. S, Montella RC, Iacone R, Padoani G, Tarsini P, et al. a-adducin mutations increase Na/K pump activity in renal cells by affecting onstitutive endocytosis: implications for tubular Na reabsorption. Am J Physiol Renal Physiol 2008;295(2):F478—87.

[69] Lee K, Jung J, Kim M, Guidotti G. Interaction of the alpha subunit of Na,K-ATPase with cofilin. Biochem J 2001;353(Pt 2): 377—85.

[70] Peng M, Huang L, Xie Z, Huang WH, Askari A. Partial inhibition of Na$^+$/K$^+$-ATPase by ouabain induces the Ca^{2+}-dependent expressions of early-response genes in cardiac myocytes. J Biol Chem 1996;271(17):10372—8.

[71] Haas M, Wang H, Tian J, Xie Z. Src-mediated inter-receptor cross-talk between the Na$^+$/K$^+$-ATPase and the epidermal growth factor receptor relays the signal from ouabain to mitogen-activated protein kinases. J Biol Chem 2002;277 (21):18694—702.

[72] Tian J, Cai T, Yuan Z, Wang H, Liu L, Haas M, et al. Binding of Src to Na$^+$/K$^+$-ATPase forms a functional signaling complex. Mol Biol Cell 2006;17(1):317—26.

[73] Liang M, Tian J, Liu L, Pierre S, Liu J, Shapiro J, et al. Identification of a pool of non-pumping Na/K-ATPase. J Biol Chem 2007;282(14):10585—93.

[74] Cai T, Wang H, Chen Y, Lui L, Gunning WT, Quintas LE, et al. Regulation of caveolin-1 membrane trafficking by the Na/K-ATPase. J Cell Biol 2008;182(6):1153—69.

[75] Tian J, Li X, Liang M, Liu L, Xie JX, Ye Q, et al. Changes in sodium pump expression dictate the effects of ouabain on cell growth. J Biol Chem 2009;284(22):14921—9.

[76] Yuan Z, Cai T, Tian J, Ivanov AV, Giovannucci DR, Xie Z. Na/K-ATPase tethers phospholipase C and IP3 receptor into a calcium-regulatory complex. Mol Biol Cell 2005;16(9):4034—45.

[77] Miyakawa-Naito A, Uhlen P, Lal M, Aizman O, Mikoshiba K, Brismar H, et al. Cell signaling microdomain with Na,K-ATPase and inositol 1,4,5-trisphosphate receptor generates calcium oscillations. J Biol Chem 2003;278(50):50355—61.

[78] Padilla-Benavides T, Roldan ML, Larre I, Flores-Benitez D, Villegas-Sepulveda N, Contreras RG, et al. The polarized distribution of Na$^+$,K$^+$-ATPase: role of the interaction between b subunits. Mol Biol Cell 2010;21(13):2217—25.

[79] Liu X, Spicarova Z, Rydholm S, Li J, Brismar H, Aperia A. Ankyrin B modulates the function of Na,K-ATPase/inositol 1,4,5-trisphosphate receptor signaling microdomain. J Biol Chem 2008;283(17):11461—8.

[80] Espineda CE, Chang JH, Twiss J, Rajasekaran SA, Rajasekaran AK. Repression of Na,K-ATPase beta1-subunit by the transcription factor snail in carcinoma. Mol Biol Cell 2004;15(3):1364—73.

[81] Barwe SP, Anilkumar G, Moon SY, Zheng Y, Whitelegge JP, Rajasekaran SA, et al. Novel role for Na,K-ATPase in phosphatidylinositol 3-kinase signaling and suppression of cell motility. Mol Biol Cell 2005;16(3):1082—94.

[82] Rajasekaran AK, Rajasekaran SA. Role of Na-K-ATPase in the assembly of tight junctions. Am J Physiol Renal Physiol 2003;285(3):F388—96.

[83] Rajasekaran SA, Palmer LG, Moon SY, Peralta Soler A, Apodaca GL, Harper JF, et al. Na,K-ATPase activity is required for formation of tight junctions, desmosomes, and induction of polarity in epithelial cells. Mol Biol Cell 2001;12(12):3717—32.

[84] Mays RW, Siemers KA, Fritz BA, Lowe AW, van Meer G, Nelson WJ. Hierarchy of mechanisms involved in generating Na/K-ATPase polarity in MDCK epithelial cells. J Cell Biol 1995;130(5):1105—15.

[85] Garg LC, Knepper MA, Burg MB. Mineralocorticoid effects on Na-K-ATPase in individual nephron segments. Am J Physiol 1981;240(6):F536—44.

[86] Baum M. Insulin stimulates volume absorption in the rabbit proximal convoluted tubule. J Clin Invest 1987;79(4):1104—9.

[87] Feraille E, Carranza ML, Rousselot M, Favre H. Insulin enhances sodium sensitivity of Na-K-ATPase in isolated rat proximal convoluted tubule. Am J Physiol 1994;267(1 Pt 2): F55—62.

[88] Banday AA, Asghar M, Hussain T, Lokhandwala MF. Dopamine-mediated inhibition of renal Na,K-ATPase is reduced by insulin. Hypertension 2003;41(6):1353—8.

[89] Baum M, Quigley R. Inhibition of proximal convoluted tubule transport by dopamine. Kidney Int 1998;54(5):1593—600.

[90] Aperia A, Bertorello A, Seri I. Dopamine causes inhibition of Na$^+$K$^+$-ATPase activity in rat proximal convoluted tubule segments. Am J Physiol 1987;252(1 Pt 2):F39—45.

[91] Bertorello A, Aperia A. Inhibition of proximal tubule Na$^+$-K$^+$-ATPase activity requires simultaneous activation of DA1 and DA2 receptors. Am J Physiol 1990;259(6 Pt 2):F924—8.

[92] Chibalin AV, Katz AI, Berggren PO, Bertorello AM. Receptor-mediated inhibition of renal Na$^+$-K$^+$-ATPase is associated with endocytosis of its alpha- and beta-subunits. Am J Physiol 1997;273(5 Pt 1):C1458—65.

[93] Chibalin AV, Pedemonte CH, Katz AI, Feraille E, Berggren PO, Bertorello AM. Phosphorylation of the catalyic alpha-subunit constitutes a triggering signal for Na$^+$,K$^+$-ATPase endocytosis. J Biol Chem 1998;273(15):8814—9.

[94] Chibalin AV, Zierath JR, Katz AI, Berggren PO, Bertorello AM. Phosphatidylinositol 3-kinase-mediated endocytosis of renal Na +, K +-ATPase alpha subunit in response to dopamine. Mol Biol Cell 1998;9(5):1209—20.

[95] Efendiev R, Chen Z, Krmar RT, Uhles S, Katz AI, Pedemonte CH, et al. The 14-3-3 protein translates the Na$^+$, K$^+$-ATPase a1-subunit phosphorylation signal into binding and activation of phosphoinositide 3-kinase during endocytosis. J Biol Chem 2005;280(16):16272—7.

[96] Yudowski GA, Efendiev R, Pedemonte CH, Katz AI, Berggren PO, Bertorello AM. Phosphoinositide-3 kinase binds to a proline-rich motif in the Na$^+$, K$^+$-ATPase alpha subunit and regulates its trafficking. Proc Natl Acad Sci U S A 2000;97 (12):6556—61.

[97] Ogimoto G, Yudowski GA, Barker CJ, Kohler M, Katz AI, Feraille E, et al. G protein-coupled receptors regulate Na$^+$,K$^+$-ATPase activity and endocytosis by modulating the recruitment of adaptor protein 2 and clathrin. Proc Natl Acad Sci USA 2000;97(7):3242—7.

[98] Efendiev R, Yudowski GA, Zwiller J, Leibiger B, Katz AI, Berggren PO, et al. Relevance of dopamine signals anchoring dynamin-2 to the plasma membrane during Na$^+$,K$^+$-ATPase endocytosis. J Biol Chem 2002;277(46):44108—14.

[99] Bank N, Aynediian HS. A micropuncture study of the effect of parathyroid hormone on renal bicarbonate reabsorption. J Clin Invest 1976;58(2):336—44.

[100] Ribeiro CP, Mandel LJ. Parathyroid hormone inhibits proximal tubule Na$^+$-K$^+$-ATPase activity. Am J Physiol 1992;262(2 Pt 2): F209–16.

[101] Derrickson BH, Mandel LJ. Parathyroid hormone inhibits Na$^+$-K$^+$-ATPase through Gq/G11 and the calcium-independent phospholipase A2. Am J Physiol 1997;272(6 Pt 2): F781–8.

[102] Khundmiri SJ, Bertorello AM, Delamere NA, Lederer ED. Clathrin-mediated endocytosis of Na$^+$,K$^+$-ATPase in response to parathyroid hormone requires ERK-dependent phosphorylation of Ser-11 within the alpha1-subunit. J Biol Chem 2004;279(17):17418–27.

[103] Zhang Y, Norian JM, Magyar CE, Holstein-Rathlou NH, Mircheff AK, McDonough AA. In vivo PTH provokes apical NHE3 and NaPi2 redistribution and Na-K-ATPase inhibition. Am J Physiol 1999;276(5 Pt 2):F711–9.

[104] Lederer ED, Khundmiri SJ, Weinman EJ. Role of NHERF-1 in regulation of the activity of Na-K ATPase and sodium-phosphate co-transport in epithelial cells. J Am Soc Nephrol 2003;14 (7):1711–9.

[105] Navar LG, Harrison-Bernard LM, Imig JD, Wang CT, Cervenka L, Mitchell KD. Intrarenal angiotensin II generation and renal effects of AT1 receptor blockade. J Am Soc Nephrol 1999;10(Suppl 12):S266–72.

[106] He P, Klein J, Yun CC. Activation of Na$^+$/H$^+$ exchanger NHE3 by angiotensin II is mediated by inositol 1,4,5-triphosphate (IP3) receptor-binding protein released with IP3 (IRBIT) and Ca^{2+}/calmodulin-dependent protein kinase II. J Biol Chem 2010;285(36):27869–78.

[107] Moe OW, Ujiie K, Star RA, Miller RT, Widell J, Alpern RJ, et al. Renin expression in renal proximal tubule. J Clin Invest 1993;91(3):774–9.

[108] Bruneval P, Hinglais N, Alhenc-Gelas F, Tricottet V, Corvol P, Menard J, et al. Angiotensin I converting enzyme in human intestine and kidney. Ultrastructural immunohistochemical localization. Histochemistry 1986;85(1):73–80.

[109] Peterson DR, Oparil S, Flouret G, Carone FA. Handling of angiotensin II and oxytocin by renal tubular segments perfused in vitro. Am J Physiol 1977;232(4):F319–24.

[110] Harris PJ, Young JA. Dose-dependent stimulation and inhibition of proximal tubular sodium reabsorption by angiotensin II in the rat kidney. Pflugers Arch 1977;367(3):295–7.

[111] Bharatula M, Hussain T, Lokhandwala MF. Angiotensin II AT1 receptor/signaling mechanisms in the biphasic effect of the peptide on proximal tubular Na$^+$,K$^+$-ATPase. Clin Exp Hypertens 1998;20(4):465–80.

[112] Aperia A, Holtback U, Syren ML, Svensson LB, Fryckstedt J, Greengard P. Activation/deactivation of renal Na$^+$,K$^+$-ATPase: a final common pathway for regulation of natriuresis. FASEB J 1994;8(6):436–9.

[113] Kiroytcheva M, Cheval L, Carranza ML, Martin PY, Favre H, Doucet A, et al. Effect of cAMP on the activity and the phosphorylation of Na$^+$,K$^+$-ATPase in rat thick ascending limb of Henle. Kidney Int 1999;55(5):1819–31.

[114] Stokes JB. Effect of prostaglandin E2 on chloride transport across the rabbit thick ascending limb of Henle. Selective inhibitions of the medullary portion. J Clin Invest 1979;64 (2):495–502.

[115] Plato CF, Stoos BA, Wang D, Garvin JL. Endogenous nitric oxide inhibits chloride transport in the thick ascending limb. Am J Physiol 1999;276(1 Pt 2):F159–63.

[116] Nonoguchi H, Tomita K, Marumo F. Effects of atrial natriuretic peptide and vasopressin on chloride transport in long- and short-looped medullary thick ascending limbs. J Clin Invest 1992;90(2):349–57.

[117] Lerolle N, Bourgeois S, Leviel F, Lebrun G, Paillard M, Houillier P. Angiotensin II inhibits NaCl absorption in the rat medullary thick ascending limb. Am J Physiol Renal Physiol 2004;287(3):F404–10.

[118] Grider JS, Falcone JC, Kilpatrick EL, Ott CE, Jackson BA. P450 arachidonate metabolites mediate bradykinin-dependent inhibition of NaCl transport in the rat thick ascending limb. Can J Physiol Pharmacol 1997;75(2):91–6.

[119] De Jesus Ferreira MC, Bailly C. Extracellular Ca^{2+} decreases chloride reabsorption in rat CTAL by inhibiting cAMP pathway. Am J Physiol 1998;275(2 Pt 2):F198–203.

[120] Leviel F, Hubner CA, Houillier P, Morla L, El Moghrabi S, Brideau G, et al. The Na$^+$-dependent chloride-bicarbonate exchanger SLC4A8 mediates an electroneutral Na$^+$ reabsorption process in the renal cortical collecting ducts of mice. J Clin Invest 2010;120(5):1627–35.

[121] Doucet A, Katz AI. Short-term effect of aldosterone on Na-K-ATPase in single nephron segments. Am J Physiol 1981;241(3): F273–8.

[122] El Mernissi G, Doucet A. Short-term effect of aldosterone on renal sodium transport and tubular Na-K-ATPase in the rat. Pflugers Arch 1983;399(2):139–46.

[123] Rayson BM, Lowther SO. Steroid regulation of Na$^+$K$^+$-ATPase: differential sensitivities along the nephron. Am J Physiol 1984;246(5 Pt 2):F656–62.

[124] Hayhurst RA, O'Neil RG. Time-dependent actions of aldosterone and amiloride on Na$^+$-K$^+$-ATPase of cortical collecting duct. Am J Physiol 1988;254(5 Pt 2):F689–96.

[125] Zecevic M, Heitzmann D, Camargo SM, Verrey F. SGK1 increases Na,K-ATPase cell-surface expression and function in Xenopus laevis oocytes. Pflugers Arch 2004;448(1):29–35.

[126] Verrey F, Kraehenbuhl JP, Rossier BC. Aldosterone induces a rapid increase in the rate of Na,K-ATPase gene transcription in cultured kidney cells. Mol Endocrinol 1989;3 (9):1369–76.

[127] Bankir L, Fernandes S, Bardoux P, Bouby N, Bichet DG. Vasopressin-V2 receptor stimulation reduces sodium excretion in healthy humans. J Am Soc Nephrol 2005;16(7):1920–8.

[128] Satoh T, Cohen HT, Katz AI. Intracellular signaling in the regulation of renal Na-K-ATPase. I. Role of cyclic AMP and phospholipase A2. J Clin Invest 1992;89(5):1496–500.

[129] Deschenes G, Gonin S, Zolty E, Cheval L, Rousselot M, Martin PY, et al. Increased synthesis and avp unresponsiveness of Na, K-ATPase in collecting duct from nephrotic rats. J Am Soc Nephrol 2001;12(11):2241–52.

[130] Vinciguerra M, Deschenes G, Hasler U, Mordasini D, Rousselot M, Doucet A, et al. Intracellular Na$^+$ controls cell surface expression of Na,K-ATPase via a cAMP-independent PKA pathway in mammalian kidney collecting duct cells. Mol Biol Cell 2003;14(7):2677–88.

[131] Vinciguerra M, Hasler U, Mordasini D, Roussel M, Capovilla M, Ogier-Dennis E, et al. Cytokines and sodium induce protein kinase A-dependent cell-surface Na,K-ATPase recruitment via dissociation of NF-kappaB/IkappaB/protein kinase A catalytic subunit complex in collecting duct principal cells. J Am Soc Nephrol 2005;16(9):2576–85.

[132] Buffin-Meyer B, Younes-Ibrahim M, El Mernissi G, Cheval L, Marsy S, Grima M, et al. Differential regulation of collecting duct Na$^+$,K$^+$-ATPase and K$^+$ excretion by furosemide and piretanide: role of bradykinin. J Am Soc Nephrol 2004;15 (4):876–84.

[133] Ichikawa I, Rennke HG, Hoyer JR, Badr KF, Schor N, Troy JL, et al. Role for intrarenal mechanisms in the impaired salt excretion of experimental nephrotic syndrome. J Clin Invest 1983;71(1):91–103.

[134] Deschenes G, Wittner M, Stefano A, Jounier S, Doucet A. Collecting duct is a site of sodium retention in PAN nephrosis: a rationale for amiloride therapy. J Am Soc Nephrol 2001;12 (3):598−601.

[135] Vogt B, Favre H. Na^+,K^+-ATPase activity and hormones in single nephron segments from nephrotic rats. Clin Sci (Lond) 1991;80(6):599−604.

[136] Deschenes G, Doucet A. Collecting duct (Na^+/K^+)-ATPase activity is correlated with urinary sodium excretion in rat nephrotic syndromes. J Am Soc Nephrol 2000;11(4):604−15.

[137] Lourdel S, Loffing J, Favre G, Paulais M, Nissant A, Fakitsas P, et al. Hyperaldosteronemia and activation of the epithelial sodium channel are not required for sodium retention in puromycin-induced nephrosis. J Am Soc Nephrol 2005;16 (12):3642−50.

[138] Ackermann D, Mordasini D, Cheval L, Imbert-Teboul M, Vogt B, Doucet A. Sodium retention and ascites formation in a cholestatic mice model: role of aldosterone and mineralocorticoid receptor? Hepatology 2007;46(1):173−9.

[139] Doucet A. H^+,K^+-ATPASE in the kidney: localization and function in the nephron. Exp Nephrol 1997;5(4):271−6.

[140] Gumz ML, Lynch IJ, Greenlee MM, Cain BD, Wingo CS. The renal H^+K^+-ATPases: physiology, regulation, and structure. Am J Physiol Renal Physiol 2010;298(1):F12−21.

[141] Gifford JD, Rome L, Galla JH. H^+-K^+-ATPase activity in rat collecting duct segments. Am J Physiol 1992;262(4 Pt 2):F692−5.

[142] Silver RB, Frindt G. Functional identification of H-K-ATPase in intercalated cells of cortical collecting tubule. Am J Physiol 1993;264(2 Pt 2):F259−66.

[143] Armitage FE, Wingo CS. Luminal acidification in K-replete OMCDi: contributions of H-K-ATPase and bafilomycin-A1-sensitive H-ATPase. Am J Physiol 1994;267(3 Pt 2):F450−8.

[144] Courtois-Coutry N, Roush D, Rajendran V, McCarthy JB, Geibel J, Kashgarian M, et al. A tyrosine-based signal targets H/K-ATPase to a regulated compartment and is required for the cessation of gastric acid secretion. Cell 1997;90(3):501−10.

[145] Wang T, Courtois-Coutry N, Giebisch G, Caplan MJ. A tyrosine-based signal regulates H-K-ATPase-mediated potassium reabsorption in the kidney. Am J Physiol 1998;275(5 Pt 2): F818−26.

[146] Spicer Z, Miller ML, Andringa A, Riddle TM, Duffy JJ, Doetschman T, et al. Stomachs of mice lacking the gastric H,K-ATPase alpha-subunit have achlorhydria, abnormal parietal cells, and ciliated metaplasia. J Biol Chem 2000;275(28):21555−65.

[147] Petrovic S, Spicer Z, Greeley T, Shull GE, Soleimani M. Novel Schering and ouabain-insensitive potassium-dependent proton secretion in the mouse cortical collecting duct. Am J Physiol Renal Physiol 2002;282(1):F133−43.

[148] Silver RB, Soleimani M. H^+-K^+-ATPases: regulation and role in pathophysiological states. Am J Physiol 1999;276(6 Pt 2): F799−811.

[149] Laroche-Joubert N, Marsy S, Doucet A. Cellular origin and hormonal regulation of K^+-ATPase activities sensitive to Sch-28080 in rat collecting duct. Am J Physiol Renal Physiol 2000;279(6):F1053−9.

[150] Laroche-Joubert N, Marsy S, Michelet S, Imbert-Teboul M, Doucet A. Protein kinase A-independent activation of ERK and H,K-ATPase by cAMP in native kidney cells: role of Epac I. J Biol Chem 2002;277(21):18598−604.

[151] Laroche-Joubert N, Marsy S, Luriau S, Imbert-Teboul M, Doucet A. Mechanism of activation of ERK and H-K-ATPase by isoproterenol in rat cortical collecting duct. Am J Physiol Renal Physiol 2003;284(5):F948−54.

[152] Buffin-Meyer B, Younes-Ibrahim M, Barlet-Bas C, Cheval L, Marsy S, Doucet A. K depletion modifies the properties of Sch-28080-sensitive K-ATPase in rat collecting duct. Am J Physiol 1997;272(1 Pt 2):F124−31.

[153] Marsy S, Elalouf JM, Doucet A. Quantitative RT-PCR analysis of mRNAs encoding a colonic putative H, K-ATPase alpha subunit along the rat nephron: effect of K^+ depletion. Pflugers Arch 1996;432(3):494−500.

[154] Sangan P, Rajendran VM, Mann AS, Kashgarian M, Binder HJ. Regulation of colonic H-K-ATPase in large intestine and kidney by dietary Na depletion and dietary K depletion. Am J Physiol 1997;272(2 Pt 1):C685−96.

[155] Verlander JW, Moudy RM, Campbell WG, Cain BD, Wingo CS. Immunohistochemical localization of H-K-ATPase alpha (2c)-subunit in rabbit kidney. Am J Physiol Renal Physiol 2001;281(2):F357−65.

[156] Zhang W, Xia X, Zou L, Xu X, LeSage GD, Kone BC. In vivo expression profile of a H^+K^+-ATPase alpha2-subunit promoter-reporter transgene. Am J Physiol Renal Physiol 2004;286 (6):F1171−7.

[157] Okusa MD, Unwin RJ, Velazquez H, Giebisch G, Wright FS. Active potassium absorption by the renal distal tubule. Am J Physiol 1992;262(3 Pt 2):F488−93.

[158] Wall SM, Mehta P, DuBose Jr. TD. Dietary K^+ restriction upregulates total and Sch-28080-sensitive bicarbonate absorption in rat tIMCD. Am J Physiol 1998;275(4 Pt 2):F543−9.

[159] Meneton P, Schultheis PJ, Greeb J, Nieman ML, Liu LH, Clarke LL, et al. Increased sensitivity to K^+ deprivation in colonic H,K-ATPase-deficient mice. J Clin Invest 1998;101 (3):536−42.

[160] Eiam-Ong S, Kurtzman NA, Sabatini S. Regulation of collecting tubule adenosine triphosphatases by aldosterone and potassium. J Clin Invest 1993;91(6):2385−92.

[161] DuBose Jr. TD, Codina J, Burges A, Pressley TA. Regulation of H^+K^+-ATPase expression in kidney. Am J Physiol 1995;269(4 Pt 2):F500−7.

[162] Zhou X, Nakamura S, Xia SL, Wingo CS. Increased CO_2 stimulates K/Rb reabsorption mediated by H-K-ATPase in CCD of potassium-restricted rabbit. Am J Physiol Renal Physiol 2001;281(2):F366−73.

[163] Xu X, Zhang W, Kone BC. CREB trans-activates the murine H^+K^+-ATPase a2-subunit gene. Am J Physiol Cell Physiol 2004;287(4):C903−11.

[164] Gogarten JP, Kibak H, Dittrich P, Taiz L, Bowman BJ, Manolson MF, et al. Evolution of the vacuolar H^+-ATPase: implications for the origin of eukaryotes. Proc Natl Acad Sci USA 1989;86(17):6661−5.

[165] Bowman EJ, Tenney K, Bowman BJ. Isolation of genes encoding the Neurospora vacuolar ATPase. Analysis of vma-1 encoding the 67-kDa subunit reveals homology to other ATPases. J Biol Chem 1988;263(28):13994−4001.

[166] Bowman BJ, Allen R, Wechser MA, Bowman EJ. Isolation of genes encoding the Neurospora vacuolar ATPase. Analysis of vma-2 encoding the 57-kDa polypeptide and comparison to vma-1. J Biol Chem 1988;263(28):14002−7.

[167] Mandel M, Moriyama Y, Hulmes JD, Pan YC, Nelson H, Nelson N. cDNA sequence encoding the 16-kDa proteolipid of chromaffin granules implies gene duplication in the evolution of H^+-ATPases. Proc Natl Acad Sci U S A 1988;85(15):5521−4.

[168] Nishi T, Forgac M. The vacuolar H^+-ATPases: Nature's most versatile proton pumps. Nat Rev Mol Cell Biol 2002;3(2):94−103.

[169] Forgac M. Vacuolar ATPases: rotary proton pumps in physiology and pathophysiology. Nat Rev Mol Cell Biol 2007;8 (11):917−29.

[170] Beyenbach KW, Wieczorek H. The V-type H^+-ATPase: molecular structure and function, physiological roles and regulation. J Exp Biol 2006;209(Pt 4):577−89.

[171] Nelson N, Harvey WR. Vacuolar and plasma membrane proton-adenosinetriphosphatases. Physiol Rev 1999;79(2):361–85.

[172] Wang Y, Cipriano DJ, Forgac M. Arrangement of subunits in the proteolipid ring of the V-ATPase. J Biol Chem 2007;282 (47):34058–65.

[173] Murata T, Yamato I, Kakinuma Y, Leslie AG, Walker JE. Structure of the rotor of the V-Type Na$^+$-ATPase from *Enterococcus hirae*. Science 2005;308(5722):654–9.

[174] Murata T, Yamato I, Kakinuma Y, Shirouzo M, Walker JE, Yokoyama S, et al. Ion binding and selectivity of the rotor ring of the Na$^+$-transporting V-ATPase. Proc Natl Acad Sci USA 2008;105(25):8607–12.

[175] Noji H, Yasuda R, Yoshida M, Kinosita Jr. K. Direct observation of the rotation of F1-ATPase. Nature 1997;386 (6622):299–302.

[176] Junge W, Sielaff H, Engelbrecht S. Torque generation and elastic power transmission in the rotary F(O)F(1)-ATPase. Nature 2009;459(7245):364–70.

[177] Yokoyama K, Nakano M, Imamura H, Yoshida M, Tamakoshi M. Rotation of the proteolipid ring in the V-ATPase. J Biol Chem 2003;278(27):24255–8.

[178] Imamura H, Nakano M, Noji H, Muniyuki E, Ohkuma S, Yoshida M, et al. Evidence for rotation of V1-ATPase. Proc Natl Acad Sci USA 2003;100(5):2312–5.

[179] Bowman EJ, Siebers A, Altendorf K. Bafilomycins: a class of inhibitors of membrane ATPases from microorganisms, animal cells, and plant cells. Proc Natl Acad Sci USA 1988;85 (21):7972–6.

[180] Bowman BJ, Bowman EJ. Mutations in subunit C of the vacuolar ATPase confer resistance to bafilomycin and identify a conserved antibiotic binding site. J Biol Chem 2002;277 (6):3965–72.

[181] Smith AN, Lovering RC, Futai M, Takeda J, Brown D, Karet FE. Revised nomenclature for mammalian vacuolar-type H$^+$-ATPase subunit genes. Mol Cell 2003;12(4):801–3.

[182] Miranda KC, Karet FE, Brown D. An extended nomenclature for mammalian V-ATPase subunit genes and splice variants. PLoS One 2010;5(3):e9531.

[183] Jouret F, Auzanneau C, Debaix H, Wada GH, Pretto C, Marbaix E, et al. Ubiquitous and kidney-specific subunits of vacuolar H$^+$-ATPase are differentially expressed during nephrogenesis. J Am Soc Nephrol 2005;16(11):3235–46.

[184] Wagner CA, Finberg KE, Breton S, Marshansky V, Brown D, Geibel JP. Renal vacuolar H$^+$-ATPase. Physiol Rev 2004;84 (4):1263–314.

[185] Finberg KE, Wagner CA, Stehberger PA, Geibel JP, Lifton RP. Molecular cloning and characterization of Atp6v1b1, the murine vacuolar H$^+$-ATPase B1-subunit. Gene 2003;318:25–34.

[186] Nelson RD, Guo XL, Masood K, Brown D, Kalkbrenner M, Gluck S. Selectively amplified expression of an isoform of the vacuolar H$^+$-ATPase 56-kilodalton subunit in renal intercalated cells. Proc Natl Acad Sci USA 1992;89(8):3541–5.

[187] Sun-Wada GH, Murata Y, Namba M, Yamamoto A, Wada Y, Futai M. Mouse proton pump ATPase C subunit isoforms (C2-a and C2-b) specifically expressed in kidney and lung. J Biol Chem 2003;278(45):44843–51.

[188] Smith AN, Borthwick KJ, Karet FE. Molecular cloning and characterization of novel tissue-specific isoforms of the human vacuolar H$^+$-ATPase C, G and d subunits, and their evaluation in autosomal recessive distal renal tubular acidosis. Gene 2002;297(1-2):169–77.

[189] Sun-Wada GH, Yoshimizu T, Imai-Senga Y, Wada Y, Futai M. Diversity of mouse proton-translocating ATPase: presence of multiple isoforms of the C, d and G subunits. Gene 2003;302 (1-2):147–53.

[190] Schulz N, Dave MH, Stehberger PA, Chau T, Wagner CA. Differential localization of vacuolar H$^+$-ATPases containing a1, a2, a3, or a4 (ATP6V0A1-4) subunit isoforms along the nephron. Cell Physiol Biochem 2007;20(1-4):109–20.

[191] Kawasaki-Nishi S, Yamaguchi A, Forgac M, Nishi T. Tissue specific expression of the splice variants of the mouse vacuolar proton-translocating ATPase a4 subunit. Biochem Biophys Res Commun 2007;364(4):1032–6.

[192] Smith AN, Finberg KE, Wagner CA, Lifton RP, Devonald MA, Su Y, et al. Molecular cloning and characterization of Atp6n1b: a novel fourth murine vacuolar H$^+$-ATPase a-subunit gene. J Biol Chem 2001;276(45):42382–8.

[193] Smith AN, Jouret F, Bord S, Borthwick KJ, Al-Lamki RS, Wagner CA, et al. Vacuolar H$^+$-ATPase d2 subunit: molecular characterization, developmental regulation, and localization to specialized proton pumps in kidney and bone. J Am Soc Nephrol 2005;16(5):1245–56.

[194] Blake-Palmer KG, Su Y, Smith AN, Karet FE. Molecular cloning and characterization of a novel form of the human vacuolar H$^+$-ATPase e-subunit: an essential proton pump component. Gene 2007;393(1-2):94–100.

[195] Pushkin A, Abuladze N, Newman D, Muronets V, Sassani P, Tatischev S, et al. The COOH termini of NBC3 and the 56-kDa H + -ATPase subunit are PDZ motifs involved in their interaction. Am J Physiol Cell Physiol 2003;284(3):C667–73.

[196] Breton S, Wiederhold T, Marshansky V, Nsumu NN, Ramesh V, Broiwn D. The B1 subunit of the H$^+$ATPase is a PDZ domain-binding protein. Colocalization with NHE-RF in renal B-intercalated cells. J Biol Chem 2000;275(24):18219–24.

[197] Chen SH, Bubb MR, Yarmola EG, Zuo J, Jiang J, Lee BS, et al. Vacuolar H$^+$-ATPase binding to microfilaments: regulation in response to phosphatidylinositol 3-kinase activity and detailed characterization of the actin-binding site in subunit B. J Biol Chem 2004;279(9):7988–98.

[198] Holliday LS, Lu M, Lee BS, Nelson RD, Solivan S, Zhang L, et al. The amino-terminal domain of the B subunit of vacuolar H$^+$-ATPase contains a filamentous actin binding site. J Biol Chem 2000;275(41):32331–7.

[199] Lu M, Ammar D, Ives H, Albrecht F, Gluck SL. Physical interaction between aldolase and vacuolar H$^+$-ATPase is essential for the assembly and activity of the proton pump. J Biol Chem 2007;282(34):24495–503.

[200] Lu M, Holliday LS, Zhang L, Dunn Jr. WA, Gluck SL. Interaction between aldolase and vacuolar H$^+$-ATPase: evidence for direct coupling of glycolysis to the ATP-hydrolyzing proton pump. J Biol Chem 2001;276(32):30407–13.

[201] Beaulieu V, Da Silva N, Pastor-Soler N, Brown CR, Smith PJ, Brown D, et al. Modulation of the actin cytoskeleton via gelsolin regulates vacuolar H$^+$-ATPase recycling. J Biol Chem 2005;280(9):8452–63.

[202] Lu M, Sautin YY, Holliday LS, Gluck SL. The glycolytic enzyme aldolase mediates assembly, expression, and activity of vacuolar H$^+$-ATPase. J Biol Chem 2004;279(10):8732–9.

[203] Su Y, Blake-Palmer KG, Sorrell S, Javid B, Bowers K, Zhou A, et al. Human H$^+$ATPase a4 subunit mutations causing renal tubular acidosis reveal a role for interaction with phosphofructokinase-1. Am J Physiol Renal Physiol 2008;295(4):F950–8.

[204] Karet FE, Finberg KE, Nelson RD, Nayir A, Mocan H, Sanjad SA, et al. Mutations in the gene encoding B1 subunit of H$^+$-ATPase cause renal tubular acidosis with sensorineural deafness. Nat Genet 1999;21(1):84–90.

[205] Finberg KE, Wagner CA, Bailey MA, Paunescu TG, Breton S, Brown D, et al. The B1-subunit of the H$^+$-ATPase is required for maximal urinary acidification. Proc Natl Acad Sci USA 2005;102(38):13616–21.

[206] Stover EH, Borthwick KJ, Bavalia C, Eady N, Fritz DM, Rungroj N, et al. Novel ATP6V1B1 and ATP6V0A4 mutations in autosomal recessive distal renal tubular acidosis with new evidence for hearing loss. J Med Genet 2002;39(11):796–803.

[207] Smith AN, Skaug J, Choate KA, Navir A, Bakkaloglu A, Ozen S, et al. Mutations in ATP6N1B, encoding a new kidney vacuolar proton pump 116-kD subunit, cause recessive distal renal tubular acidosis with preserved hearing. Nat Genet 2000;26 (1):71–5.

[208] Da Silva N, Shum WW, El-Annan J, Paunescu TG, McKee M, Smith PJ, et al. Relocalization of the V-ATPase B2 subunit to the apical membrane of epididymal clear cells of mice deficient in the B1 subunit. Am J Physiol Cell Physiol 2007;293(1): C199–210.

[209] Paunescu TG, Russo LM, Da Silva N, Kovacikova J, Mohebbi N, Van Hoek AN, et al. Compensatory membrane expression of the V-ATPase B2 subunit isoform in renal medullary intercalated cells of B1-deficient mice. Am J Physiol Renal Physiol 2007;293(6):F1915–26.

[210] Al-Awqati Q, Norby LH, Mueller A, Steinmetz PR. Characteristics of stimulation of H^+ transport by aldosterone in turtle urinary bladder. J Clin Invest 1976;58(2):351–8.

[211] Beauwens R, Al-Awqati Q. Active H^+ transport in the turtle urinary bladder. Coupling of transport to glucose oxidation. J Gen Physiol 1976;68(4):421–39.

[212] Al-awqati Q, Mueller A, Steinmetz PR. Transport of H^+ against electrochemical gradients in turtle urinary bladder. Am J Physiol 1977;233(6):F502–8.

[213] Dixon TE, Al-Awqati Q. Urinary acidification in turtle bladder is due to a reversible proton-translocating ATPase. Proc Natl Acad Sci USA 1979;76(7):3135–8.

[214] Gluck S, Kelly S, Al-Awqati Q. The proton translocating ATPase responsible for urinary acidification. J Biol Chem 1982;257(16):9230–3.

[215] Gluck S, Al-Awqati Q. An electrogenic proton-translocating adenosine triphosphatase from bovine kidney medulla. J Clin Invest 1984;73(6):1704–10.

[216] Brown D, Hirsch S, Gluck S. Localization of a proton-pumping ATPase in rat kidney. J Clin Invest 1988;82(6):2114–26.

[217] Paunescu TG, Da Silva N, Marshansky V, McKee M, Breton S, Brown D. Expression of the 56-kDa B2 subunit isoform of the vacuolar H^+-ATPase in proton-secreting cells of the kidney and epididymis. Am J Physiol Cell Physiol 2004;287(1): C149–62.

[218] Wagner CA, Giebisch G, Lang F, Geibel JP. Angiotensin II stimulates vesicular H^+-ATPase in rat proximal tubular cells. Proc Natl Acad Sci U S A 1998;95(16):9665–8.

[219] Sabolic I, Haase W, Burckhardt G. ATP-dependent H^+ pump in membrane vesicles from rat kidney cortex. Am J Physiol 1985;248(6 Pt 2):F835–44.

[220] Sabolic I, Burckhardt G. Characteristics of the proton pump in rat renal cortical endocytotic vesicles. Am J Physiol 1986;250(5 Pt 2):F817–26.

[221] Jehmlich K, Sablotni J, Simon BJ, Burckhardt G. Biochemical aspects of H^+-ATPase in renal proximal tubules: inhibition by N,N′-dicyclohexylcarbodiimide, N-ethylmaleimide, and bafilomycin. Kidney Int Suppl 1991;33:S64–70.

[222] Hilden SA, Johns CA, Madias NE. $Cl^{(-)}$-dependent ATP-driven H^+ transport in rabbit renal cortical endosomes. Am J Physiol 1988;255(5 Pt 2):F885–97.

[223] Alper SL, Natale J, Gluck S, Lodish HF, Brown D. Subtypes of intercalated cells in rat kidney collecting duct defined by antibodies against erythroid band 3 and renal vacuolar H^+-ATPase. Proc Natl Acad Sci USA 1989;86(14):5429–33.

[224] Fleser A, Marshansky V, Duplain M, Noel J, Hoang A, Teledor A, et al. Cross-talk between the Na^+-K^+-ATPase and the H^+-ATPase in proximal tubules in suspension. Ren Physiol Biochem 1995;18(3):140–52.

[225] Kurtz I. Apical Na^+/H^+ antiporter and glycolysis-dependent H^+-ATPase regulate intracellular pH in the rabbit S3 proximal tubule. J Clin Invest 1987;80(4):928–35.

[226] Preisig PA, Ives HE, Cragoe Jr. EJ, Alpern RJ. Rector FC, Jr. Role of the Na^+/H^+ antiporter in rat proximal tubule bicarbonate absorption. J Clin Invest 1987;80(4):970–8.

[227] Wang T, Yang CL, Abbiati T, Schultheis PJ, Schull GE, Giebisch G, et al. Mechanism of proximal tubule bicarbonate absorption in NHE3 null mice. Am J Physiol 1999;277(2 Pt 2): F298–302.

[228] Wang T, Hropot M, Aronson PS, Giebisch G. Role of NHE isoforms in mediating bicarbonate reabsorption along the nephron. Am J Physiol Renal Physiol 2001;281(6):F1117–22.

[229] Schultheis PJ, Clarke LL, Meneton P, Miller ML, Soleimani M, Gawenis LR, et al. Renal and intestinal absorptive defects in mice lacking the NHE3 Na^+/H^+ exchanger. Nat Genet 1998;19 (3):282–5.

[230] Choi JY, Shah M, Lee MG, Schultheis PJ, Schull GE, Muallem S, et al. Novel amiloride-sensitive sodium-dependent proton secretion in the mouse proximal convoluted tubule. J Clin Invest 2000;105(8):1141–6.

[231] Bailey MA, Giebisch G, Abbiati T, Aronson PS, Gawenis LR, Schull GE, et al. NHE2-mediated bicarbonate reabsorption in the distal tubule of NHE3 null mice. J Physiol 2004;561(Pt 3):765–75.

[232] Chambrey R, Warnock DG, Podevin RA, Bruneval P, Mandet C, Belair MF, et al. Immunolocalization of the Na^+/H^+ exchanger isoform NHE2 in rat kidney. Am J Physiol 1998;275 (3 Pt 2):F379–86.

[233] Zimolo Z, Montrose MH, Murer H. H^+ extrusion by an apical vacuolar-type H^+-ATPase in rat renal proximal tubules. J Membr Biol 1992;126(1):19–26.

[234] Malnic G, Geibel JP. Cell pH and $H^{(+)}$ secretion by S3 segment of mammalian kidney: role of H^+-ATPase and Cl^-. J Membr Biol 2000;178(2):115–25.

[235] Chambrey R, Paillard M, Podevin RA. Enzymatic and functional evidence for adaptation of the vacuolar H^+-ATPase in proximal tubule apical membranes from rats with chronic metabolic acidosis. J Biol Chem 1994;269(5):3243–50.

[236] Carraro-Lacroix LR, Malnic G. Signaling pathways involved with the stimulatory effect of angiotensin II on vacuolar H^+-ATPase in proximal tubule cells. Pflugers Arch 2006;452 (6):728–36.

[237] Froissart M, Borensztein P, Houillier P, Leviel F, Poggioli J, Marty E, et al. Plasma membrane Na^+-H^+ antiporter and H^+-ATPase in the medullary thick ascending limb of rat kidney. Am J Physiol 1992;262(4 Pt 1):C963–70.

[238] Khadouri C, Marsy S, Barlet-Bas C, Cheval L, Doucet A. Effect of metabolic acidosis and alkalosis on NEM-sensitive ATPase in rat nephron segments. Am J Physiol 1992;262(4 Pt 2): F583–90.

[239] Sabatini S, Laski ME, Kurtzman NA. NEM-sensitive ATPase activity in rat nephron: effect of metabolic acidosis and alkalosis. Am J Physiol 1990;258(2 Pt 2):F297–304.

[240] Good DW, Watts III BA. Functional roles of apical membrane Na^+/H^+ exchange in rat medullary thick ascending limb. Am J Physiol 1996;270(4 Pt 2):F691–9.

[241] Brown D, Hirsch S, Gluck S. An H^+-ATPase in opposite plasma membrane domains in kidney epithelial cell subpopulations. Nature 1988;331(6157):622–4.

[242] Teng-umnuay P, Verlander JW, Yuan W, Tisher CC, Madsen KM. Identification of distinct subpopulations of intercalated cells in the mouse collecting duct. J Am Soc Nephrol 1996;7 (2):260−74.

[243] Star RA, Kurtz I, Mejia R, Burg MB, Knepper MA. Disequilibrium pH and ammonia transport in isolated perfused cortical collecting ducts. Am J Physiol 1987;253(6 Pt 2):F1232−42.

[244] Schwartz GJ, Al-Awqati Q. Carbon dioxide causes exocytosis of vesicles containing H^+ pumps in isolated perfused proximal and collecting tubules. J Clin Invest 1985;75(5):1638−44.

[245] Schwartz GJ, Barasch J, Al-Awqati Q. Plasticity of functional epithelial polarity. Nature 1985;318(6044):368−71.

[246] Takito J, Hikita C, Al-Awqati Q. Hensin, a new collecting duct protein involved in the *in vitro* plasticity of intercalated cell polarity. J Clin Invest 1996;98(10):2324−31.

[247] van Adelsberg J, Edwards JC, Takito J, Kiss B, al-Awqati Q. An induced extracellular matrix protein reverses the polarity of band 3 in intercalated epithelial cells. Cell 1994;76 (6):1053−61.

[248] Schwartz GJ, Tsuruoka S, Vijayakumar S, Petrovic S, Mian A, Al-Awqati Q. Acid incubation reverses the polarity of intercalated cell transporters, an effect mediated by hensin. J Clin Invest 2002;109(1):89−99.

[249] Vijayakumar S, Erdjument-Bromage H, Tempst P, Al-Awqati Q. Role of integrins in the assembly and function of hensin in intercalated cells. J Am Soc Nephrol 2008;19(6):1079−91.

[250] Eladari D, Chambrey R, Frische S, Vallet M, Edwards A. Pendrin as a regulator of ECF and blood pressure. Curr Opin Nephrol Hypertens 2009;18(4):356−62.

[251] Wall SM, Kim YH, Stanley L, Glapion DM, Everett LA, Green ED, et al. NaCl restriction upregulates renal Slc26a4 through subcellular redistribution: role in $Cl^−$ conservation. Hypertension 2004;44(6):982−7.

[252] Verlander JW, Hassell KA, Royaux IE, Glapion DM, Wang ME, Everett LA, et al. Deoxycorticosterone upregulates PDS (Slc26a4) in mouse kidney: role of pendrin in mineralocorticoid-induced hypertension. Hypertension 2003;42(3):356−62.

[253] Pech V, Kim YH, Weinstein AM, Everett LA, Pham TD, Wall SM. Angiotensin II increases chloride absorption in the cortical collecting duct in mice through a pendrin-dependent mechanism. Am J Physiol Renal Physiol 2007;292(3):F914−20.

[254] Marshansky V, Futai M. The V-type H^+-ATPase in vesicular trafficking: targeting, regulation and function. Curr Opin Cell Biol 2008;20(4):415−26.

[255] Wrong OM, Norden AG, Feest TG. Dent's disease: a familial proximal renal tubular syndrome with low-molecular-weight proteinuria, hypercalciuria, nephrocalcinosis, metabolic bone disease, progressive renal failure and a marked male predominance. QJM 1994;87(8):473−93.

[256] Pook MA, Wrong O, Wooding C, Norden AG, Feest TG. and Thakker, R. V. Dent's disease, a renal Fanconi syndrome with nephrocalcinosis and kidney stones, is associated with a microdeletion involving DXS255 and maps to Xp11.22. Hum Mol Genet 1993;2(12):2129−34.

[257] Fisher SE, van Bakel I, Lloyd SE, Pearce SH, Thakker RV, Craig IW. Cloning and characterization of CLCN5, the human kidney chloride channel gene implicated in Dent disease (an X-linked hereditary nephrolithiasis). Genomics 1995;29 (3):598−606.

[258] Lloyd SE, Pearce SH, Gunther W, Kawaguchi H, Igarashi T, Jentsch TJ, et al. Idiopathic low molecular weight proteinuria associated with hypercalciuric nephrocalcinosis in Japanese children is due to mutations of the renal chloride channel (CLCN5). J Clin Invest 1997;99(5):967−74.

[259] Lloyd SE, Pearce SH, Fisher SE, Steinmeyer K, Schwappach B, Scheinman SJ, et al. A common molecular basis for three inherited kidney stone diseases. Nature 1996;379 (6564):445−9.

[260] Gunther W, Luchow A, Cluzeaud F, Vandewalle A, Jentsch TJ. ClC-5, the chloride channel mutated in Dent's disease, colocalizes with the proton pump in endocytotically active kidney cells. Proc Natl Acad Sci USA 1998;95(14):8075−80.

[261] Piwon N, Gunther W, Schwake M, Bosl MR, Jentsch TJ. ClC-5 $Cl^−$-channel disruption impairs endocytosis in a mouse model for Dent's disease. Nature 2000;408(6810):369−73.

[262] Gunther W, Piwon N, Jentsch TJ. The ClC-5 chloride channel knock-out mouse − an animal model for Dent's disease. Pflugers Arch 2003;445(4):456−62.

[263] Hara-Chikuma M, Wang Y, Guggino SE, Guggino WB, Verkman AS. Impaired acidification in early endosomes of ClC-5 deficient proximal tubule. Biochem Biophys Res Commun 2005;329(3):941−6.

[264] Scheel O, Zdebik AA, Lourdel S, Jentsch TJ. Voltage-dependent electrogenic chloride/proton exchange by endosomal CLC proteins. Nature 2005;436(7049):424−7.

[265] Novarino G, Weinert S, Rickheit G, Jentsch TJ. Endosomal chloride-proton exchange rather than chloride conductance is crucial for renal endocytosis. Science 2010;328(5984):1398−401.

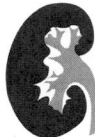

Mechanisms of Water Transport Across Cell Membranes and Epithelia

Guillermo A. Altenberg and Luis Reuss

**Department of Cell Physiology and Molecular Biophysics, and Center for Membrane Protein Research,
Texas Tech University Health Sciences Center, Lubbock, Texas, TX, USA**

INTRODUCTION

The main purpose of this chapter is to review the basic aspects of water transport mechanisms across cell membranes and epithelia. In the first section we will discuss biophysical principles and definitions, with the aim of providing a theoretical framework useful for the analysis of experimental observations. In the second section, we will address general issues pertaining to water transport across cell membranes, focusing on intracellular water, and the pathways and mechanism for osmotic water flow. In the third section, we will discuss water transport by epithelia, focusing on pathways and mechanisms, in particular the role of solute–solvent coupling. We intend this chapter to serve as both an overview and an introduction to chapters covering specific aspects of water transport (Chapters 5, 9, 41, 42, 43). The three sections of the chapter are to a certain extent independent from each other, and can be studied separately.

The field of water transport across biological membranes has made a recent major transition with the discovery and characterization of the aquaporins. Aquaporins are integral membrane proteins, most of which are highly specific water pores expressed in plants and animals from bacteria to humans. The discovery of the aquaporins confirmed a long-held prediction for the existence of these pores, emanating from biophysical studies in red blood cells[110] and renal proximal tubules.[165]

BASIC PRINCIPLES

This section is largely based on the excellent water transport treaty by Finkelstein.[34] Other sources are House,[62] Reuss and Cotton,[123] Dawson,[26] Hallows and Knauf,[50] and Macey and Moura.[91] Derivations of the equations can be found in Finkelstein's book.[34] Deliberately, this section has been kept simple, and qualitative explanations have been superimposed on a succinct quantitative analysis.

The main mechanism of *net water transport* in animal cells is osmosis, that is, net water flow driven by differences in water chemical potential, in turn dependent on differences in solute concentrations. Concerning water flow across a cell membrane, an important issue is whether water moves through the phospholipid bilayer and/or through specialized water-conducting pores. The mechanisms involved in water permeation via these two pathways constitute the main content of this first section. Hence, we start with osmosis.

Osmotic Equilibrium is a Balance of Osmotic and Hydrostatic Forces

The principle of *osmotic equilibrium* can be illustrated by considering a simple system, that is, a semipermeable membrane separating two aqueous phases: pure water and a solution that contains a nondissociating solute (Figure 4.1). The membrane is permeable to

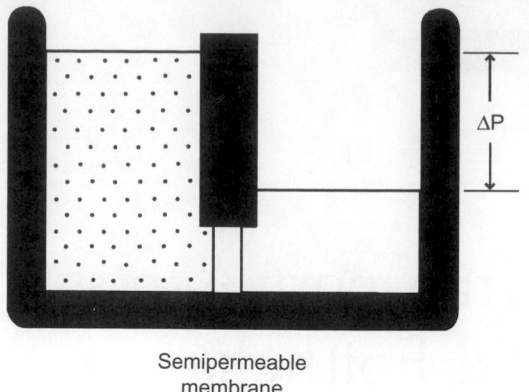

Semipermeable
membrane

FIGURE 4.1 **Osmotic equilibrium.** A semipermeable membrane (clear section of middle partition) separates two aqueous compartments: a solution containing impermeable solute (left) and pure water (right). If the heights of both compartments are initially equal, then water will flow from right to left until equilibrium is established. At equilibrium, the water flow across the membrane is zero, and is described by Eq. (4.1), that is, ΔP and $\Delta \pi$ cancel each other.

water and impermeable to the solute (hence the term *semipermeable*). At thermodynamic equilibrium, the net water flow across the membrane is zero. (In the case of water, flow can be expressed in molar terms [moles of water per unit area and unit time] or volume terms [volume of water per unit area and unit time]. For conversion to volume flow, the molar flow must be multiplied by $\overline{V}_w$ [partial molar volume, a constant equal to 18 cm^3/mole].) The equilibrium of net flows is the result of the equality of two forces: an osmotic force favoring water flow into the solution; and an opposing hydrostatic force resulting, for instance, from the difference in height of the fluid compartments generated by the osmotic water flow. For dilute solutions, osmotic equilibrium is approximately described by Van't Hoff's law[149]:

$$\Delta P = \pi = RTC_s \qquad (4.1)$$

where ΔP (atm) is the hydrostatic pressure difference between the two compartments ($P' - P''$), R (cm^3 atm mol^{-1} K^{-1}) and T [K] are the gas constant and the absolute temperature, respectively, C_s (mol cm^{-3}) is the molar concentration of the solute, and π (atm) is the *osmotic pressure* of the solution. The latter is conveniently defined as the hydrostatic pressure in the solution compartment (relative to the pressure in the water compartment) needed to abolish water flow across the membrane.

When the semipermeable membrane separates two solutions, equilibrium is described by a slightly different equation: $\Delta P = \Delta \pi = RT\Delta C_s$, where $\Delta \pi$ is the difference in osmotic pressure ($\pi' - \pi''$) and ΔC_s is the solute concentration difference ($C_s' - C_s''$).

The osmotic pressure depends on the molar concentration (C_s) and on the degree of dissociation of the solute, that is, the number of particles that each molecule yields in solution (n). Ideally, the osmolality of a solution, in osmol/kg of water, is given by $Osm = nC_s$, where C_s is in mol l^{-1}. However, the effect of solute on the activity of the solvent is generally nonideal, that is, it may depend on the nature of the solute. The correction term for this effect is the osmotic coefficient, φ_s, where the subscript denotes the solute. For physiological concentration ranges, the osmotic coefficient is closer to unity than the activity coefficient, but it can be significantly greater than 1 for macromolecules.[50] For the sake of simplicity, the osmotic coefficient will be neglected in this discussion.

A 1 Osm solution at room temperature exerts an osmotic pressure of about 24.6 atm, which is equivalent to about 18,700 mm Hg. In a mammal, a 1% change in extracellular fluid osmolality ($<$ 3 mosmol/kg) is equivalent, as a driving force for water flow, to a hydrostatic pressure of 56 mm Hg. In animal cells, changes in osmolality cause large water fluxes across the plasma membrane, whereas hydrostatic pressure changes do not. Osmolality is a measure of concentration of particles, not of osmotic pressure, but it is frequently used to denote the latter.

The generation of ΔP in the presence of impermeant solute on one side can be explained[96] on the basis of changes in the water chemical potential (μ_w), which is given by:

$$\mu_w = \mu_w^o + RT \ln X_w + P\overline{V}_w \qquad (4.2)$$

where μ_w^o is the standard chemical potential, X_w is the water mole fraction (moles of water/[moles of water + moles of solute]), and $\overline{V}_w$ is the partial molar volume of water. A solute addition to one side (at constant total volume) reduces the water chemical potential in that side (μ_w') because the water is "diluted" by the solute (and X_w falls). The difference in water chemical potential thus generated ($\Delta\mu_w' = \mu_w' - \mu_w''$) is the "driving force" for water flow toward the side of higher osmolality (and lower μ_w). If both compartments are open and of appropriate dimensions, then a ΔP will result from changes in height (Figure 4.1). If a compartment is closed, then its pressure will change in proportion to the water flux, with a proportionality constant dependent on compliance of the compartment.

Osmotic Water Flows Across Lipid and Porous Membranes have Different Properties

Near equilibrium, the volume flow is linearly related to the driving force:

$$J_v = L_p (\Delta P - \Delta \pi) \qquad (4.3)$$

where J_v is the volume flow (volume area^{-1} time^{-1}), L_p is the *hydraulic permeability coefficient* of the membrane, and ΔP and $\Delta \pi$ are the differences in hydrostatic and osmotic pressure, respectively. The L_p can be expressed in cm sec^{-1} (osmol/kg)$^{-1}$. In most cases, a *filtration* (P_f) or *osmotic permeability coefficient* (P_{os}; $P_f = P_{os}$) is used instead of L_p. The P_{os} (cm sec^{-1}) is related to L_p by $P_{os} = L_p RT / \overline{V}_w$.

The above discussion underscores the fact that ΔP and $\Delta \pi$ are equivalent as "driving forces" in causing osmotic water flow. The mechanism of this equivalence can be understood if one considers the nature of the membrane and the mechanism of osmotic water transport, as explained below.

Osmotic Water Flow Across Lipid Membranes

Osmotic water flow across lipid membranes occurs by *solubility diffusion*. Water molecules move from one aqueous solution into the lipid and then into the other solution by independent, random motion. When $\Delta P = \Delta \pi$ (0 net driving force) there are two diffusive water fluxes of equal magnitude and opposite direction, with no net water flow across the membrane. In the presence of a net driving force ($\Delta P - \Delta \pi \neq 0$), a net flux arises. To examine the mechanism of water flow, let us consider the effects of ΔC_s and ΔP on the water chemical potential in the two compartments.

A net diffusive water flow requires a difference in water chemical potential across the membrane. In a homogeneous membrane, a steady flux denotes a constant chemical potential gradient throughout the membrane thickness. If there is a difference in osmotic pressure between the two solutions, then the water mole fractions (and therefore the water concentrations) at the two sides, *just inside* the membrane must differ. It is commonly assumed that water transport across the membrane—solution interface is faster than water diffusion in the membrane itself. It follows that the water chemical potential just inside the membrane is very close to that in the adjacent layer of solution; therefore, water is near equilibrium across the interfaces. Finally, since μ_w is inversely related to C_s, a gradient of water concentration must exist across the membrane. This intramembrane gradient is the direct consequence of the differences in impermeant solute concentrations in the adjacent aqueous phases.

When $\Delta \pi = 0$, but $\Delta P \neq 0$, the chemical potentials of water in the two solutions differ (see Eq. (4.2)). If $P' > P''$, then the water flux from side ' is greater than that from side ", creating an intramembrane gradient of water concentration and chemical potential.

The osmotic water permeability coefficient of a lipid membrane is given by:

$$P_{os} = \frac{D_w^m \beta_w \overline{V}_w}{\delta_m \overline{V}_{oil}} \quad (4.4)$$

where D_w^m is the diffusion coefficient of water in the membrane, β_w is the partition coefficient of water in the membrane (oil/water), δ_w is the thickness of the membrane, and $\overline{V}_{oil}$ is the partial molar volume of the membrane lipid.

Osmotic Water Flow Across a Porous Membrane

Let us consider a membrane made of a rigid, water-impermeable material. The pore density (number of pores per unit area) is n. Each pore is a water-filled cylinder of length L and radius r, and cannot be penetrated by the solute. The mechanism of water flow in this situation depends mostly on the pore radius. In large pores there is viscous water flow that can be described by Newtonian mechanics. In pores of molecular dimensions there is no appropriate theoretical treatment, but if the pores are so small that there is single file water transport (i.e., water molecules in the pore cannot slip past each other), then there is a surprisingly simple solution.

LARGE PORES

In large pores water flow driven by a hydrostatic pressure is described by Poiseuille's law, which was derived for water flow in thin capillaries:

$$J_v = n \frac{(\varPi) r^4}{8L\eta} \Delta P \quad (4.5)$$

where η is the water viscosity and π denotes 3.1415 ... (do not confuse with π, the osmotic pressure). This law is valid for steady-state flow and neglects pore access effects. Under these conditions, the pressure gradient along the pore (dP/dL) has a constant value (Figure 4.2a). From Eq. (4.4) and the definition of P_{os}, the P_{os} for a membrane containing large homogeneous cylindrical pores is $n(\pi)r^4 RT / 8L\eta \, V_w$.

If the only driving force is osmotic, then the mechanism of water flow involves the development of a hydrostatic pressure gradient within the pore. Initially, the water concentrations in the pore and in the water-filled compartment are the same, but at the other interface the solution has lower water concentration than the pore. If water transport across the membrane interfaces is faster than within the membrane, then the water chemical potentials just inside the pore are equal to those in the adjacent solutions. At the pore end facing the water compartment there is no difference in hydrostatic pressure, but at the end facing the solution

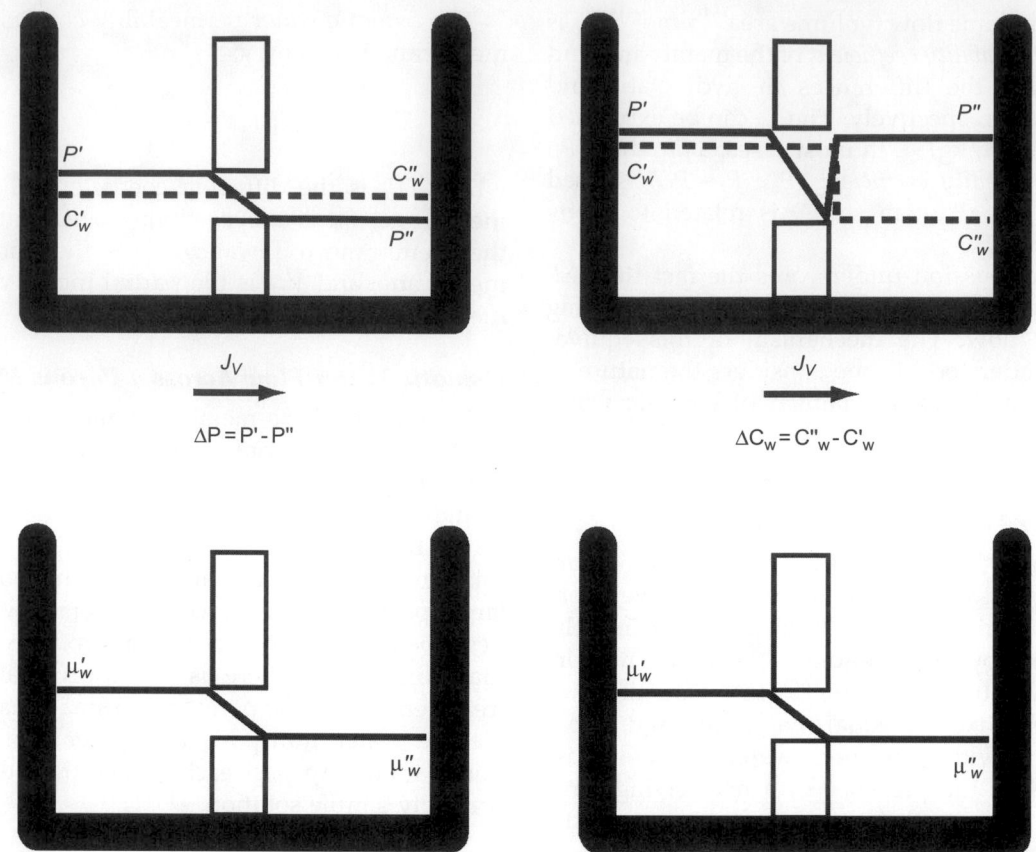

FIGURE 4.2 Water flow across a porous membrane. Top left: Driving force is a hydrostatic-pressure difference ($P' - P''$), continuous line. Same water concentrations on both sides ($C'_w - C''_w$), segmented line. Top right: Driving force is a difference in osmotic pressure. Same hydrostatic pressure on both sides, but the water concentrations differ. Bottom: The steady-state water chemical potential gradients (μ_w, proportional to the sum of hydrostatic and osmotic pressure) are the same for both conditions. *(Modified with permission from Reuss, L. (2000). General principles of water transport. In "The Kidney: Physiology and Pathophysiology," 321–340, Seldin, D. W. and Giebisch, G. (eds.). Raven Press, New York.)*

compartment the pressure inside the pore falls, because the lower water concentration in the solution elicits a water efflux from the pore. If $\Delta\mu_w$ is zero across the opening, then the difference in water concentration between solution and pore is exactly balanced by a drop in the pore pressure.[96] In the steady-state, the pressure gradient in the pore is constant (Figure 4.2, top right).

The analysis presented above holds for pores of r equal to or greater than 15 nm.[12] For pores smaller than 15 nm, several corrections have been attempted, but the underlying assumptions are questionable.[34] Regardless of the lack of a satisfactory theory, it has been suggested that Poiseuille's law is a reasonable approximation for water diffusion and convection in small pores.[86]

SINGLE-FILE PORE

The P_{os} of a single-file pore is given by[34,35]:

$$P_{os} = n\frac{\bar{v}_w kTN}{\gamma L^2} \tag{4.6}$$

where $\bar{v}_w$ is the volume of a water molecule, k is the Boltzmann constant (gas constant/molecule, equal to

R/N_A where N_A is Avogadro's number), N is the number of water molecules inside the pore, and γ is the friction coefficient per water molecule. Assuming that the water densities in the pore and in the bulk solution are equal, and recalling that $kT/\gamma = D_w$:

$$P_{os} = n\frac{(\Pi)r^2 D_w}{L} \tag{4.7}$$

which is the result expected for osmotic water flow through a single-file pore if it can be described as a diffusive flux.

Comparison of Diffusion and Osmotic Permeability Coefficients Reveals Whether Water Permeates Lipid Bilayer or Pores

Now we consider a membrane exposed to solutions of identical composition, except that water is partially replaced with tracer water at a concentration C_w (Figure 4.3). There are no other differences in composition or pressure between the two compartments.

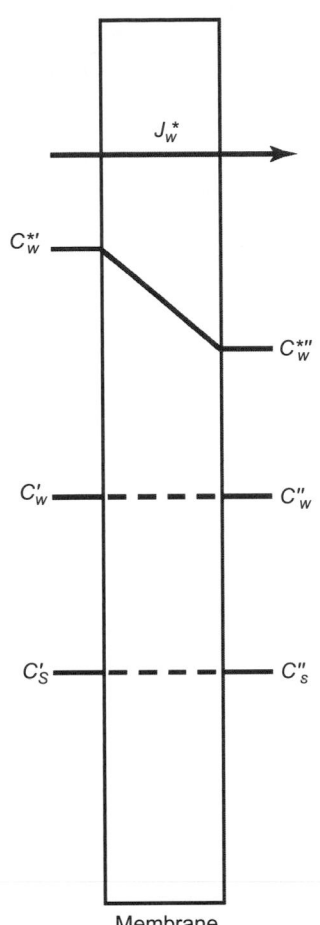

FIGURE 4.3 **Tracer water diffusion across a lipid membrane separating solutions of identical compositions** ($C'_w - C''_w$, $= C'_s - C''_s$, $= 0$, **as shown by the two lines at the bottom**). At the steady-state (constant flux, J^*_w), the tracer concentration gradient in the membrane (second line from top) is also constant. Arbitrarily, the oil/water partition coefficient (β) of tracer water is 1.0. If β were smaller, the tracer water concentrations inside the membrane would be less than in the respective solutions. *(Modified with permission from Reuss, L. (2000). General principles of water transport. In "The Kidney: Physiology and Pathophysiology," 321–340, Seldin, D. W. and Giebisch, G. (eds.). Raven Press, New York.)*

Both contain solutions of infinite volume and ideally mixed (C_w at the membrane surface $= C_w$ in the bulk solution). The tracer water flux is given by:

$$J^*_w = P_{dw}\Delta C^*_w \qquad (4.8)$$

where P_{dw} is the diffusive water permeability coefficient and ΔC^*_w is the difference in concentration of tracer water ($C^{*'}_w - C^{*''}_w$). In the case of a lipid membrane, the tracer–water flux is by solubility diffusion; hence:

$$P_{dw} = \frac{D^m_w \beta_w \overline{V}_w}{\partial_m \overline{V}_{oil}} \qquad (4.9)$$

This expression is identical to that for P_f (or P_{os}) for a lipid membrane (Eq. (4.7)). Therefore, for a lipid membrane, $P_{os} = P_{dw}$.

The case of a porous membrane is discussed below.

Porous Membrane

If the pores obey Poiseuille's law, the diffusive water flux *via* the pores is:

$$J^*_w = \frac{n(\Pi)r^2 D_w}{L}\Delta C^*_w \qquad (4.10)$$

where the pore cross-sectional area [$n(\Pi)r^2$] is available for water diffusion and is the water self-diffusion coefficient (tracer water traverses the membrane via the aqueous pores). P_{dw} is $n(\Pi)r^2 D_w/L$. Hence, the ratio between and for a porous membrane is:

$$P_{os}/P_{dw} = \frac{RT}{8\eta D_w \overline{V}_w}r^2 + 1 \qquad (4.11)$$

where the second term on the right (=1) denotes the diffusive water flow via the pores. The equivalent pore radius can be estimated from experimental values using Eq. (4.11); at 25°C, the value of [$RT/(8\eta D_w \overline{V}_w)$] is 8.04×10^{-14} cm^{-2}.

For single file pores, the diffusive water flux is $J_w = nP_{dw}\Delta n^*$, where Δn^* is the tracer-water concentration difference (molecules per unit volume). P_{dw} is given by:

$$P_{dw} = \frac{n\overline{v}_w kT}{dL^2} \qquad (4.12)$$

and the ratio P_{os}/P_{dw}, from Eqs. (4.6) and (4.12), equals the number of water molecules in the pore: $P_{os}/P_{dw} = N$.

Water movement in single file pores is not independent of the movement of neighboring water molecules: for a tracer molecule to cross the pore, other water molecules must also cross.

Unstirred Layers are a Major Source of Artifacts in Water Permeability Measurements

Unstirred layers are static layers of fluid at membrane–solution interfaces, that is, they are not mixed by convection. Unstirred-layer solute concentrations are entirely determined by diffusion, can differ from that of the bulk solutions, and are position dependent. Unstirred layers introduce errors in the experimental determination of P_{dw} and P_{os}. These errors can lead to incorrect conclusions about the existence of aqueous pores. For an excellent treatment of unstirred layers, see Barry and Diamond.[11]

Unstirred-Layer Effects on Measurement of P_{dw}

In the system illustrated in Figure 4.4, tracer water encounters three barriers to diffusion between the two

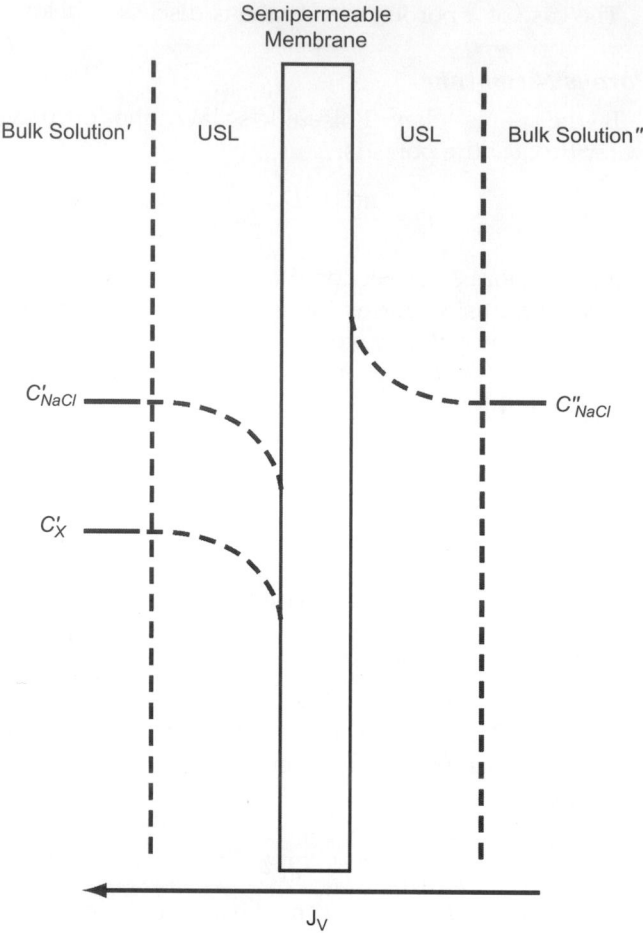

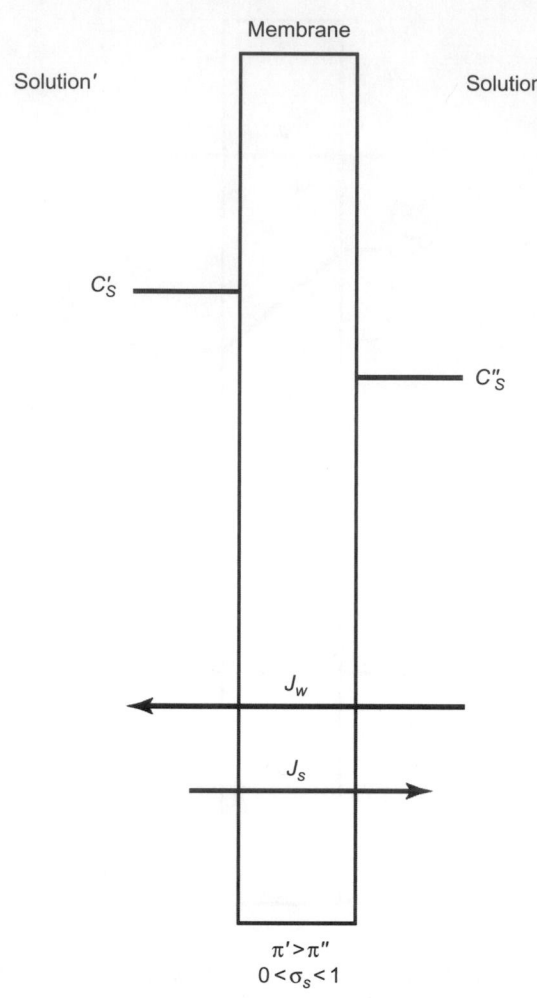

FIGURE 4.4 Unstirred-layer effects on the measurement of P_{os}, C_{NaCl} and C_x, concentrations of NaCl and the osmotic solute, respectively. Both are assumed impermeant for simplicity. The osmotic water flow ($J_w = J_v$) "dilutes" both solutes on the hyperosmotic side (solution') and "concentrates" the NaCl on the hyposmotic side (solution"). The net result is a reduction in the concentration gradient of the osmotic solute (reduced ΔC_x), and the creation of an opposing ΔC_{NaCl} at the membrane boundaries. Hence, the driving force for J_v is diminished. *(Modified with permission from Reuss, L. (2000). General principles of water transport. In "The Kidney: Physiology and Pathophysiology," 321–340, Seldin, D. W. and Giebisch, G. (eds.). Raven Press, New York.)*

FIGURE 4.5 Volume flow (J_v) between solutions containing different concentrations of a permeant solute ($0 < \sigma_s < 1$). C_s is the solute concentration. J_v is the difference between the net water flow (J_w) to the left, and the net solute flow (J_s) to the right (i.e., $J_v = J_w - J_s$). *(Modified with permission from Reuss, L. (2000). General principles of water transport. In "The Kidney: Physiology and Pathophysiology," 321–340, Seldin, D. W. and Giebisch, G. (eds.). Raven Press, New York.)*

solutions, namely the membrane and the two unstirred layers (of width Δ_1 and Δ_2, respectively). These three barriers are in series. The *observed* (experimentally determined) diffusive water permeability of the system differs from the true diffusive water permeability of the membrane (P_{dw}) according to:

$$\frac{1}{P_{dw}^o} = \frac{1}{P_{dw}} + \frac{1}{D_w/\delta_1} + \frac{1}{D_w/\delta_2} \qquad (4.13)$$

where P_{dw}^o is the observed value. Inasmuch as D_w has a finite value, P_{dw} and P_{dw}^o are equal only when $\delta_1 = \delta_2 = 0$. For typical permeability and unstirred-layer thickness values, P_{dw} can be easily underestimated by 50% or more.

Unstirred-Layer Effects on the Measurement of P_{os}

In the experiment depicted in Figure 4.5, a semipermeable membrane separates equal NaCl solutions; then, a second solute is added to one side ($C_s' > C_s''$, eliciting osmotic water flow. The NaCl concentration in the unstirred layers changes because of the water flow, rising in the right side and falling in the left side, relative to the bulk solution concentrations. The added solute qualitatively behaves like the NaCl present on the same side. Water flow tends to accentuate the changes described, whereas solute diffusion in the solution has the opposite effect. At the steady-state, the effects of osmotic water flow and solute diffusion balance each other and the unstirred-layer concentration profiles remain constant. At the surface of the membrane:

$$C_m = C_b \exp\left(\pm v\delta/D_s\right) \qquad (4.14)$$

where the sign of the exponent is $(-)$ for the left ("diluted") side and $(+)$ for the right ("concentrated") side, and denote solute concentrations (membrane surface and bulk solution, respectively), v is the water flow velocity (normal to the membrane), and D_s is the solute diffusion coefficient in water.

The ratio between P_{os}^o (observed value) and P_{os} (true value) is $-v\Delta/D_s$, that is, the magnitude of the error in estimating P_{os} is directly proportional to v and inversely proportional to D_s. In planar membranes, for small v (low water flux and flow velocity) the exponential term approaches 1. In folded membranes, where there can be water "funneling" (microvilli, lateral intercellular spaces), v can be much larger than in a planar membrane and can be seriously underestimated.[11]

The above analysis is limited to the effect of J_v on impermeant solute concentration. If permeant solutes are present as well, they must be considered, making the analysis more complex.[11]

Solute Reflection Coefficients Denote Effective Osmolality of a Solution vis-à-vis a Membrane

The situation is more complicated than the preceding analysis if the solute is permeant (Figure 4.6). In this case, J_v will be described by:

$$J_v = L_p(\Delta P - \sigma_s \Delta\pi) \qquad (4.15)$$

where σ_s is the reflection coefficient of the solute. If $\sigma_s < 1$, then J_v will be less than if the same osmotic gradient is elicited with an impermeable solute. The value of σ_s is specific for each combination of membrane and solute, and depends on both permeabilities and partial molar volumes of water and solute (see below). In general, the value of σ_s varies between 0 (solute as permeable as water) and 1 (solute impermeable).

Lipid Membrane

It can be shown that the solute reflection coefficient of a lipid membrane is[34]:

$$\sigma_s = 1 - \frac{P_{ds}\overline{V}_s}{P_{dw}\overline{V}_w} \qquad (4.16)$$

As expected, $\sigma_s = 1$ when $P_{ds} = 0$, $\sigma_s = 0$ when $P_{ds}\overline{V}_s = P_{dw}\overline{V}_w$, and $\sigma_s < 0$ when $P_{ds}\overline{V}_s > P_{dw}\overline{V}_w$. In other words, σ_s depends on the solute permeability and partial molar volume compared with those of water. If the products are the same for solute and water, then the reflection coefficient is zero: solute addition to one side

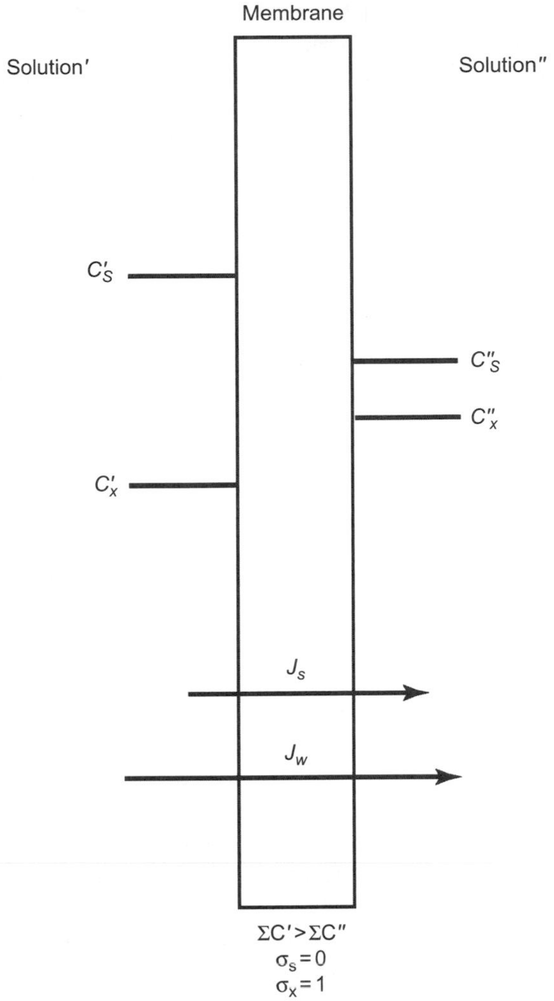

FIGURE 4.6 Volume flow (J_v) between isosmotic solutions ($\sum C' = \sum C''$). Solutes s and x gradients are of the same magnitude and opposite direction. Since the reflection coefficients differ, the effective osmolalities also differ, and there is a net J_v toward the side containing impermeant solute (i.e., $J_v = J_w + J_s$). *(Modified with permission from Reuss, L. (2000). General principles of water transport. In "The Kidney: Physiology and Pathophysiology," 321–340, Seldin, D. W. and Giebisch, G. (eds.). Raven Press, New York.)*

causes no transmembrane volume flow because the water flux toward the solute is of the same magnitude as the solute flux in the opposite direction. A solute with a negative σ_s will elicit a net volume flow in the opposite direction to the water flow ("negative osmosis").[34]

Porous Membrane

For a quantitative analysis of this complicated problem, see Anderson and Malone[3] and Finkelstein.[34] For large pores and solute particles larger than water particles, the solute is excluded from the periphery of the pore, that is, from a region slightly wider than the solute radius. In the pore axis, C_s is maximum (equal to the concentration in the bulk solution) and C_w is less than at the pore periphery (where the solute is excluded). This generates a radial water concentration gradient within the pore. At equilibrium, this gradient is balanced by a fall in hydrostatic pressure in the periphery of the pore. In addition, there is a solute concentration gradient along the pore length, because of the transmembrane difference in C_s. These two gradients combine to generate a longitudinal hydrostatic pressure gradient along the pore's periphery, which causes water flow toward the high concentration side. The thickness of the ring subjected to this regime is directly proportional to the molecular size of the solute. When the solute is so large that it cannot enter the pore, J_v is maximum and $\sigma_s = 1$. When the solute has the same size as water, its distribution within the pore is identical to that of water, no pressure gradient develops, the water and solute net fluxes are purely diffusive and of equal magnitude and opposite direction, and $J_v = 0$. When the solute is smaller than water, J_v is greater than J_w, and J_v is in the same direction as J_s. Water is largely excluded from the periphery of the pore, and the pore hydrostatic pressure gradient is opposite to that generated by the impermeant solute.

We consider now the case of single file pores; the solution is dilute enough so that the number of solute molecules inside a pore can be only 0 or 1. Two pore populations will exist at any given time: pores containing water only, through which there is water flow toward the high-C_s side, and pores containing solute, in which solute and water are transported toward the low-C_s side by single file diffusion. When both water and solute permeation are single file, σ_s is[34,87]:

$$\sigma_s = 1 - \frac{P_{ds}\overline{V}_p^s}{P_{dw}\overline{V}_p} \qquad (4.17)$$

where $\overline{V}_p$ denotes pore molar volume, solute-containing (superscript s) and solute-free (no superscript). Compare with Eq. (4.16).

In a system with more than one solute there can be net water and/or volume flows between solutions with the same total solute concentrations (and osmolalities). This will occur if the specific C_s values on the two sides of the membrane and the reflection coefficients differ. As shown in Figure 4.6, if , $\Delta C_s = -\Delta C_x$, $\sigma_s = 0$, and $\sigma_x = 1$, then there will be a net volume flow towards the right, although the solutions have equal total osmolalities. If the hydrostatic pressures are the same on both sides, then $J_v = L_pRT\ (\sigma_x\Delta C_x - \sigma_s\Delta C_s)$. Expressions such as σRTC denote "effective osmolality," in contrast with the "total osmolality" given by RTC. Effective osmolality is also referred to as *tonicity*. In epithelia, active transepithelial solute transport can generate asymmetries in the composition of the

adjacent solutions. These asymmetries may in principle drive net water transport without differences in the total osmolalities of the bulk solutions, because of differences in the solute reflection coefficients.

Solvent Drag Can Account for Uphill Solute Transport

When there is net water flow (filtration and/or osmosis) across a porous membrane and a pore-permeant solute is present, there is a solute flux in the same direction as the water flow. This flux reflects water–solute frictional interaction within the pores. In the case of large pores, if $C_s' = C_s''$, and J_v is elicited by a hydrostatic pressure gradient or an asymmetrical addition of impermeant solute, the solute flux due to solvent drag is given by:

$$J_s = J_vC_s\ (1 - \sigma_s) \qquad (4.18)$$

Uphill solute transport (i.e., transport in the absence of or against the prevailing electrochemical gradient) can be demonstrated, which is always in the same direction as the water flow. The energy is provided by the water flow, and conveyed to the solute by frictional interaction.

Demonstration of solvent drag is, in principle, a clear-cut argument for the existence of solute permeable water pores in membranes. However, many such demonstrations have been proven to be experimental artifacts. If there are unstirred layers, J_v will produce changes in solute concentrations at the membrane–solution interfaces; if the membrane is permeable to the solute, then a diffusive solute flux will occur (see Eq. (4.14)). This phenomenon is called "pseudo-solvent drag".[11] Putative demonstrations of pore-mediated water transport based on the observation of "solvent drag" must consider this possibility.

WATER TRANSPORT ACROSS THE CELL MEMBRANE

In this section we will first address some general issues pertinent to intracellular water, and then discuss in some detail the pathways and mechanisms for water transport across the cell membrane. Cell volume regulation is the subject of Chapter 5, and will not be addressed here.

Intracellular Water Behaves Similar to Water in Free Solution

The best direct assessment of the state of intracellular water was obtained from nuclear magnetic resonance (NMR) studies, which indicate that only a small fraction of cell water ($<5\%$) behaves as if it were immobilized.[137] However, indirect arguments suggest that this may be an underestimate.[50] A related issue is whether the cytosol is a near-ideal aqueous solution or a gel, as suggested by numerous observations.[85] If this is the case, its higher viscosity may have a strong effect on enzyme catalysis rates.[100] In any event, the behavior of water fluxes in cells supports the idea that most of the intracellular water behaves as water in dilute solutions.

The Osmotic Behavior of Cells is not Ideal

Consider a cell at steady-state (constant volume) in suspension; then, the external concentration of an impermeant solute (and hence the external osmolality) are suddenly changed. If the cell is permeable to water, then water will flow until its osmolality becomes equal to the new medium osmolality. Numerically, $V_0 \cdot \pi_0 = V_t \cdot \pi_t$, where V is cell water volume and π is total solute concentration (or osmolality), and the subscripts 0 and t denote steady-state values before and after the solution change. The above equation assumes that there is no change in the amount of cell solute between 0 and t, and defines the ideal ("osmometric") behavior of cells. However, not all cells behave ideally. Non-ideal behavior can result from loss or gain of solute between times 0 and t (e.g., some cell solutes are permeable) or from changes in the osmotic coefficient of intracellular solute(s) secondary to the water flux. This appears to be the case in red blood cells, because of concentration dependence of the osmotic coefficient of hemoglobin. This and other issues relevant to non-ideal osmotic behavior of cells have been discussed by Hallows and Knauf.[50]

Another important point in quantifying cell volume changes in response to alterations in extracellular osmolality is the fact that although most of the cell volume is solvent water ("osmotically sensitive"), a fraction is nonsolvent volume (also referred to as "solids"). If one considers this factor, then the above equation becomes:

$$(V_0 - b)\pi'_0 = (V_t - b)\pi'_t \qquad (4.19)$$

where b is the nonsolvent volume. This is a modified form of the Boyle–Van't Hoff equation, and is very useful to interpret changes in cell volume. The plot of Eq. (4.19) is shown in Figure 4.7.

In experimental osmotic studies, the behavior of cells or membrane vesicles may not be linear, for the reasons given above. For instance, if the amount of cell solute changes during the experiment, then the slope will not be a constant.

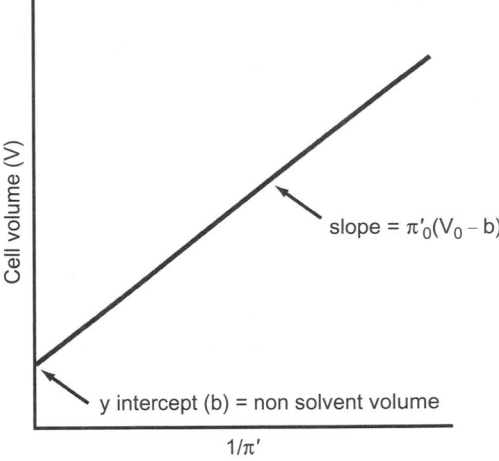

FIGURE 4.7 Boyle–Van't Hoff plot for a theoretical cell. The equation plotted is $V = (1/\pi')[\pi'_0(V_0 - b)] + b$ (see Eq. (4.19)). The y-axis intercept is b, the nonsolvent volume, and the slope is $[\pi'_0(V_0 - b)]$, that is, the amount of water-dissolved solutes in the cell. (*Copyright 1994 by CRC Press, Inc. From Hallows, K. R. and Knauf, P. A. (1994) "Principles of Cell Volume Regulation." CRC Press, Boca Raton FL. Reproduced with permission of Routledge/Taylor & Francis Group, LLC.*)

Net Water Transport Across Membranes of Animal Cells is Osmotic

In plant cells, which have rigid walls, the intracellular hydrostatic pressure can vary over a considerable range. In animal cells, which have compliant plasma membranes, hydrostatic pressure differences are small. In contrast, small differences in concentration of impermeable or low permeability solutes across the cell membrane can result in sizable water flows by osmotic mechanisms. The water flow under these conditions can be via the phospholipid bilayer (solubility diffusion), driven by the difference in water chemical potential across the membrane or via pores driven by a hydrostatic pressure gradient inside the pore. This pressure gradient is caused by the difference between the water chemical potentials inside the pore and in the external solution (see Figure 4.2). It is generally assumed that under steady-state conditions *in vivo*, the osmolalities of the intracellular and extracellular compartments are equal. There is some experimental evidence supporting this,[94] but based on rather indirect estimations of intracellular osmolality. Also, it has been argued that, in order to balance a 1 mosmol/kg difference in osmolality (cell higher), the cell hydrostatic pressure would have to be ~19 mm Hg higher than the extracellular pressure, something that a soft-tissue cell membrane is extremely unlikely to support.[93] However, mechanical support of the cell membrane by the cytoskeleton and/or the exoskeleton may allow for the maintenance of transmembrane hydrostatic pressure gradients.[50] This issue is unresolved, but it is unlikely that in the steady-state large gradients of osmotic or hydrostatic pressure exist across plasma membranes.

Quantitative treatment of water transport across the plasma membrane usually involves another assumption, namely that the cytoplasm behaves as a free solution, similar to the interstitial fluid. However, it is far more likely that the cytoplasm is a gel, as discussed above.[85] This problem is also unresolved.

The fact that animal cells lack rigid walls and do not develop sizeable transmembrane hydrostatic pressure differences determines that the only means to maintain or regulate cell volume is to change the cell content of osmotically-active solutes. This is the main theme of the next section.

Cell Volume is Determined by the Amount of Cell Solute and the Extracellular Osmolality

With the questionable exception of water co-transport (see below), net water transport between intracellular and extracellular compartments is the result of differences in effective osmotic pressure between these compartments. The effective osmotic pressure, in turn, is proportional to the total number of particles in solution, and their reflection coefficients. Hence, at the same total osmotic pressure, impermeant particles are more effective than permeant particles in generating water flow toward the side in which they are contained. This can be demonstrated experimentally by exposing cells to solutions of identical osmolalities, but different tonicities, by using solutes having different permeabilities. Depending on the relative permeabilities of the plasma membrane to water and the solute, cell volume can remain constant, increase or decrease. This phenomenon can be explained by the effect of the solute reflection coefficient on osmotic water flow.

A solution is defined as isotonic (with the cell interior) when exposure of cells to this solution results in no change in cell volume; hypertonic and hypotonic solutions elicit decreases and increases in cell volume, respectively. Therefore, a hypertonic solution has a greater effective osmolality, and a hypotonic solution a lower effective osmolality, than the isotonic solution. Because of the role of the solute reflection coefficient in determining the effective osmolality (see above), the terms hypertonic and hypotonic are not equivalent to hyperosmotic or hyposmotic; the latter expressions denote the total osmolality of the solutions, disregarding the reflection coefficients. The osmolalities of biological fluids are largely determined by their total salt concentrations, because low molecular weight salts are the solutes at highest concentrations, expressed as

number of particles relative to water mass. Hence, the extracellular fluid osmolality is largely determined by Na^+ salts (mainly sodium chloride and sodium bicarbonate), and the intracellular osmolality is mostly determined by K^+ salts.

Under most physiological and pathophysiological conditions, the intracellular and extracellular compartments can be treated as two closed compartments separated by a semipermeable membrane (i.e., a membrane permeable to water and impermeable to the solute). This simplification is valid because, in the short-term, solute gains or losses by the whole system and solute fluxes between the compartments are slow relative to potential water fluxes. It follows that: (1) the amount of solute in each compartment can be considered constant; and (2) the steady-state osmolalities of both compartments must be equal. Therefore, the amount of cell water is inextricably related to the amount of cell solute and to the extracellular osmolarity:

$$V_w^c = \frac{S^c}{Osm_{ec}} \qquad (4.20)$$

where V_w^c is the cell water volume (L), S^c is the amount of cell solute (mosmol), and Osm_{ec} is the extracellular osmolarity (mosm/L).

It follows from Eq. (4.20) that cell volume can change by two mechanisms, namely changes in the amount of cell solute or in the extracellular osmolality. From a homeostasis point of view, if pure water is added to the extracellular compartment, reducing its tonicity, then part of the water will flow across the cell membrane into the intracellular compartment, until the osmolalities are again equal. If pure water is lost from the extracellular compartment, then water will flow from the intracellular compartment until the osmolalities become equal. In contrast, if isotonic solution is added to or lost from the extracellular compartment, there will be no water flow across the cell membrane, because no osmotic pressure difference has been established, and in the body the ensuing changes in hydrostatic pressure will be very small. This analysis is rather qualitative; knowledge or assumption of the initial conditions allows for a highly quantitative analysis, essential for understanding the pathogenesis and planning the treatment of water and electrolyte disorders.

Water Permeability of the Plasma Membrane Varies Considerably Among Cell Types

Cell membranes are endowed with highly variable osmotic water permeability coefficients, ranging from practically zero (apical membrane of thick-ascending loop of Henle cells) to 400–600 µm s^{-1} in red blood cells and renal proximal tubules. Most nonepithelial cells display quite high osmotic water permeabilities. The best-studied case is that of the mammalian red blood cell, whose P_{os} is in the range of 50–400 μm s^{-1}.[39] In artificial lipid bilayers, P_{os} ranges from <1 to <100 μm s^{-1}, depending on the lipid composition. Bilayers of higher fluidity are more permeable to water, and increased bilayer cholesterol content decreases bilayer water permeability. Recent studies have shown that certain biological membranes that are highly water permeable contain water-selective pores (aquaporins).

The structural bases for the extremely low P_{os} of some cell membranes were recently discovered; others remain unknown. As detailed in Chapter 2, lipid rafts in membranes are microdomains rich in cholesterol and sphingolipids in the external leaflet and cholesterol and phospholipids with saturated fatty acids in the internal leaflet of the membrane. The surrounding bilayer is abundant in unsaturated fatty acids, and considerably more fluid than that in the raft.[71] Membrane rafts have low fluidity, and hence a low diffusional water permeability. Addition of cholesterol to liposomes formed by phosphatidylcholine produces a major decrease in water permeability.[6,7,116] In liposomes formed by mixtures of phosphatidylcholine, cholesterol, and sphingomyelin, which contain lipid microdomains similar to membrane lipid rafts, water permeability is significantly lower than that expected based on the lysis tension.[116]

Apical membranes of certain tight epithelia have an extremely low permeability to water. A case in point is the apical membrane of the urothelium, that is, the epithelium that lines the renal calices, pelvis, ureters, urinary bladder, and urethra. The apical membranes of the epithelial cells of the urothelium are covered by rigid plaques consisting of hexagonal arrays of particles.[14,57,156] The plaques contain four transmembrane domain proteins named uroplakins, of which there are four isoforms.[88,170,172] It has been suggested that uroplakins could influence the passive permeability of the apical membrane of the urothelium,[56] but evidence was lacking until the permeabilities of normal mice urinary bladders were compared to those of uroplakinIII (UPIII)-knockout mice.[64] The normal mouse bladder has high transepithelial electrical resistance, and low water permeability. The bladders from UPIII-knockout mice maintained the high transepithelial resistance, but their water permeability was 20-fold higher than in controls. These results strongly suggest that the low permeability of the tight junctions and the apical membrane to ions are preserved in the knockout mice, whereas the water permeability of the apical membrane is increased. This is the first instance in which expression of a transmembrane protein has been shown to decrease the permeability of a

biological membrane. It has been speculated that the uroplakin crystals limit plasma membrane lipid mobility, reducing fluctuations in acyl chains, decreasing water permeability through the bilayer.[73,169] However, the UPIII-knockout mice urinary bladders display significant anatomical alterations, including the presence of small hyperplastic superficial cells,[63] and therefore other mechanisms for the decrease in water permeability cannot be ruled out.

The thick ascending limb of the loop of Henle also has an extremely low permeability to water[126] necessary for the operation of the urine concentration mechanism (see Chapter 43). The biophysical reasons for this low permeability are not entirely clear. Certainly there is no expression of water pores (AQP) in the apical membrane (see Chapter 41), and its surface area is small relative to that of the basolateral membrane,[126] but whether the composition of the membrane has a role is yet to be determined.

Pathways for Water Transport Across Cell Membranes

As explained above, water transport across biological membranes can be across the lipid phase of the membrane (solubility diffusion) or across membrane proteins. The mammalian aquaporin family consists of 13 members that form water pores and are expressed in the plasma membranes of numerous cell types. Their important role in water transport across cell membranes is unquestionable. It has also been suggested that other transport proteins may transport water, in addition to their substrates. Such suggestions have been made for both ion channels and carriers. We will discuss first aquaporins and then these membrane proteins in the context of water transport across cell membranes. The accepted water transport pathways across the cell membrane are illustrated in Figure 4.8.

Water Pores Determine High Cell-Membrane Water Permeability

The existence of water pores was first deduced from biophysical studies (reviewed in Macey[90] and Verkman[150]), and then elegantly confirmed by biochemical, molecular-biological, and structural studies (reviewed in Agre[1] and King et al.[75]). Over the years, several criteria were developed to ascertain the presence of water pores in membranes. The principal ones are discussed below.

HIGH P_{os}/P_d

If the membrane contains pores, then osmotic water flow does not occur via a diffusion-like mechanism, which obeys the independence principle. Instead, it

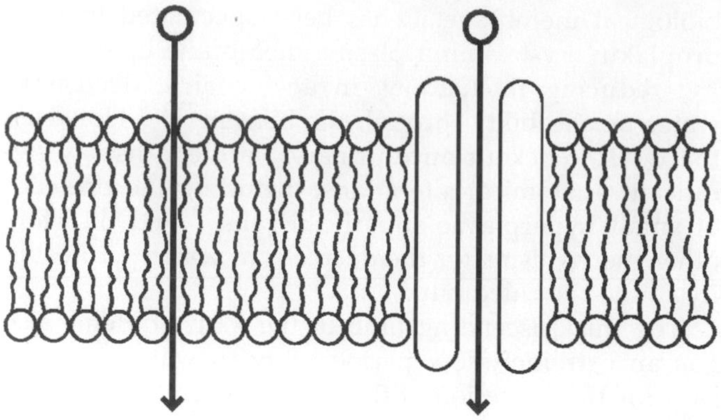

FIGURE 4.8 **Water transport pathways across plasma membranes.** Left arrow: Solubility diffusion across the phospholipid bilayer. The water permeability is directly proportional to the fluidity of the membrane. Right arrow: Permeation via pores. The water flux obeys Pouiseuille's Law in wide pores, and occurs by single-file diffusion in narrow pores such as those of aquaporins.

involves some form of interaction between water molecules, either Poiseuille-like (viscous) flow in thin capillaries or single file transport. As discussed previously, in both cases the flow of individual water molecules depends on the flow of other water molecules. It follows that the value of P_{os}/P_d is significantly greater than unity (the ratio is proportional to the square of the pore radius in case of viscous flow, and equal to the number of water molecules contained in the case of single file transport). However, unstirred-layer effects can cause a disproportionately large underestimation of P_d relative to P_{os}, with the end result of an artifactually large ratio. This error can be prevented by measuring the unstirred-layer equivalent thickness, and making appropriate corrections for P_{os} and P_d.[34] In conclusion, a correctly obtained $P_{os}/P_d > 1$ is strong evidence for water transport via pores. The value of P_{os}/P_d can denote either the pore radius or the number of water molecules in the pore. Resolving this issue requires additional experimental work, such as permeation studies with solutes of varying sizes to estimate the pore radius.

LOW ARRHENIUS ACTIVATION ENERGY

The activation energies (E_a) for water permeation via aqueous pores and for water self-diffusion are about the same (<5 kcal mol^{-1}), that is, much lower than the E_a for water permeation by solubility diffusion across a lipid membrane (<12 kcal mol^{-1}). This can be established by measuring the water permeability at different temperatures.

SENSITIVITY TO Hg

Water transport via proteinaceous pores is inhibited by HgCl$_2$ and organic mercurial compounds, an effect

suggestive of a critical SH group in the protein underlying the pore function.[91,92] This was corroborated when the protein was identified.[113] The mercury sensitivity of water transport is conferred by a specific cysteine residue (Cys189 in human AQP1),[138] located ~ 8 Å above the NPA region.[59]

FLUX INTERACTIONS

In the case of large pores with finite solute permeability, there are frictional interactions between water and solutes (see above), with the end result of solvent drag and/or electrokinetic phenomena. Although this has been demonstrated for some membrane pores, it does not seem to take place with aquaporins, the water-selective pores in animal cell membranes. This suggests that these pores are impermeable to most solutes, and hence too narrow for solvent drag or electrokinetic phenomena.

Among cell membranes from epithelia, the best studied from a water-pore viewpoint is the apical membrane of the mammalian renal proximal tubule, where the above criteria have been clearly satisfied.[167] Water pores have been identified in numerous organs and cell types, and in the renal proximal tubule they are constitutively active; in contrast, in the collecting duct under resting conditions they exist in a cytoplasmic vesicular pool, and are inserted in the apical membrane after stimulation by vasopressin.[15,16]

Cell Membrane Water Pores are Aquaporins

The existence of water pores on cell membranes was demonstrated in red blood cells and renal tubules by the biophysical approaches described above (for reviews see Macey[90] and Verkman[150]). The pores were identified by the discovery of the red cell membrane protein first named CHIP28,[29,113] and now aquaporin 1 (AQP1). When expressed in amphibian oocytes or purified and reconstituted in liposomes, AQP1 forms Hg^{2+}-sensitive water pores with low activation energy, and no ion conductance (reviewed in Agre,[2] Engel et al.,[33] Heymann,[55] King et al.[75]). Later studies have shown three important facts: (1) AQPs are expressed in plant and animal cells, in both simple and complex organisms; (2) AQPs are expressed in the plasma and intracellular membranes of most cells, not just red cells and renal epithelial cells; and (3) there are 13 AQP isoforms in mammals, which have unique cellular and subcellular distributions.[43,70,75,151] Aquaporins are present in most cell types in the body, and there is reason to suspect that they are the predominant pathway for water transport across cell membranes.[75] In this section, we will discuss aquaporins largely from a molecular point of view. Aquaporins in the kidney are treated in Chapter 41, and aquaporins in other organs by King et al.[75] For excellent recent reviews on AQPs, see Agre[1] and King et al.,[75] as well as more recent ones.[43,70,78,95,109,151,152,157] Peter Agre received the 2003 Nobel Prize in Chemistry for his work on aquaporins.

Based on their permeability properties, primary sequence, and gene structure, mammalian AQPs have been classified into three groups: Class 1, 2, and 3. Class 1 AQPs are permeated only by water (isoforms 0, 1, 2, 4, 5, 6, 8); class 2 AQPs, also known as aquaglyceroporins (isoforms 3, 7, 9, 10), are permeated by both water and small organic solutes such as glycerol; whereas class 3 AQPs are of unknown or unclear permeability properties (isoforms 11 and 12). AQPs in cell membranes are tetramers, with one subunit N-glycosylated.[72,135] Each monomer is ∼30 kD, and contains a narrow aqueous pore surrounded by α helices. AQP monomers display N- and C-termini on the same side of the membrane (intracellular for plasma membrane AQPs), and the primary and tertiary structures clearly show an inverted symmetric pattern, each formed by three bilayer-spanning α helices. In each repeat, the loops B and E (C-terminal to the transmembrane helices 2 and 5), which contain the highly conserved signature motif Asn-Pro-Ala (NPA), form short hydrophobic α helices that reach halfway through the membrane from opposite sides to end facing each other. The overall fold has been described as an hourglass consisting of the two hemipores that face each other, with wider bases and a narrow area in the membrane center, lined by the two NPA-containing loops, which contribute to the pore selectivity.[65,75,113] The hourglass model was proposed from sequence analysis,[72] and has been confirmed by cryoelectron microscopy and X-ray crystallography studies.[37,41,60,103,119,142,158,159] A schema of this structure is shown in Figure 4.9.

The class 3 AQPs, AQP11, and AQP12, are located in intracellular compartments, and are closer to the SIP plant family (Small basic Intrinsic Proteins), displaying less than 20% homology with other members of the mammalian AQP family.[95] In AQP11 and AQP12, the highly-conserved NPA motif in the AQP N-terminal half is substituted with the sequences NPC and NPT, respectively, but they still have a conserved C-terminal half NPA motif.[69] The function of AQP11 is unknown, and that of AQP12 is unclear, without evidence for water permeability in frog-oocyte studies, but displaying water permeability when reconstituted in liposomes.[69,70]

Mechanism of Water Permeation in AQPs

The high selectivity of AQPs such as AQP1 for water – excluding even proton permeation – is consistent with the minimum width of the pore (2.8 Å), which limits the size of permeant molecules. The dipole moments of the two half-helices that contain the

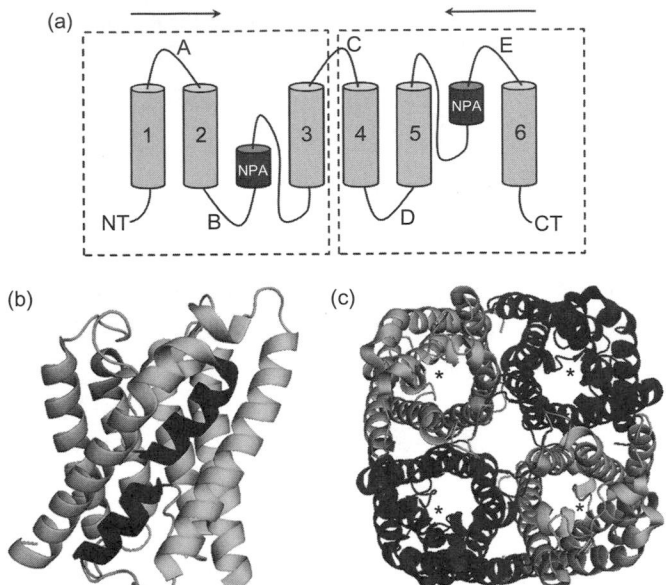

FIGURE 4.9 Membrane topology and structure of aquaporin 1 (AQP1). (a) Predicted secondary structure. AQP1 consists of two repeats of three transmembrane helices (1, 2, and 3; 4, 5, and 6). Amino and carboxy termini are on the cytoplasmic side. Loops B and E contain the Asn-Pro-Ala motifs (NPA) that form part of the water pore and are important to determine selectivity. Loop E contains Cys189, responsible for Hg^{2+} sensitivity. (b) Monomer structure (side view, ribbon representation). Transmembrane helices are shown in the same tone, whereas loops B and E, which contain the NPA sequences that meet approximately halfway into the membrane, are shown in a darker tone. (c) Tetramer structure (view from top). The monomers are functional *per se*, but AQP1 assembles into tetramers. Each monomer is shown in a tone different from that of the neighboring subunits. Asterisks denote the approximate location of the water pore in each subunit. Built with PyMol from PDB 1J4N.

NPA motifs are oriented on the center of the hydrophilic pore, creating an electrostatic barrier to H$^+$ movement, and inducing a complementary alignment of the water molecules' dipole moments as they pass the signature motif.[8,9,27,28,65,66,160] Interaction of the water molecules inside the pore with the NPA motifs dipoles prevents formation of hydrogen bonds between adjacent water molecules. In other words, similar to what happens to K$^+$ permeating K$^+$-selective channels, the water molecules in the AQP1 pore lose contact with other molecules. One could say that the water becomes "dehydrated," and permeates in single file. The lack of hydrogen bonding of water molecules inside the pore prevents proton conduction via "water wires".[142,144]

Water selectivity arises at a constriction located ∼8 Å extracellular to the NPA region, the aromatic/arginine region (ar/R), which contains a conserved arginine.[65,66,160] The ar/R region acts as a selectivity filter that limits permeation based on size and hydrophobicity.[65] This region is wider and more hydrophobic in aquaglyceroporins, allowing permeation of small

TABLE 4.1 Permeability Characteristics and Predominant Distribution for Known Mammalian Aquaporins

Isoform	Permeability	Tissue Distribution	Subcellular Distribution[a]
AQP0	Water (low)	Lens	Plasma membrane
AQP1	Water (high)[b]	Red blood cell; kidney; lung; vascular endothelium; brain; eye	Plasma membrane
AQP2	Water (high)	Kidney; vas deferens	Apical membrane; intracellular
AQP3	Water (high); glycerol (high); urea (moderate)	Kidney; skin; lung; eye; colon	Basolateral membrane
AQP4	Water (high)[b]	Brain; muscle; kidney; lung; stomach; small intestine	Basolateral membrane
AQP5	Water (high)[b]	Salivary gland; lacrimal gland; sweat gland; lung; cornea	Apical membrane
AQP6	Water (low); anions ($NO_3^- > Cl^-$)	Kidney	Plasma membrane; intracellular
AQP7	Water (high); glycerol (high); urea (high); metalloids[d]	Adipose tissue; kidney; testis	Plasma membrane
AQP8	Water (high)[c]	Testis; kidney; liver; pancreas; small intestine; colon	Plasma membrane; intracellular
AQP9	Water (low); glycerol (high); urea (high); metalloids	Liver; leukocytes; brain; testis	Plasma membrane
AQP10	Water (low); glycerol (high); urea (high)	Small intestine	Intracellular
AQP11	Water?	Testis; kidney; brain; heart; thymus; intestine; liver	Intracellular
AQP12	?	Pancreas	Intracellular

[a]Aquaporins that are present primarily in either the apical or basolateral membrane are noted as residing in one of these membranes, whereas homologs that are present in both of these membranes are described as having a plasma membrane distribution.

[b]These AQPs may be permeable to gases such as CO_2, O_2, NH_3, and/or NO.

[c]AQP8 might be permeated by water and urea.

[d]The transported species are most likely the undissociated arsenite and antimonite trioxides $As(OH)_3$ and $Sb(OH)_3$.

solutes such as glycerol.[65] In members of the AQP family such as the *Escherichia coli* GlpF channel, sequence tuning of the selectivity filter region allows permeation of small uncharged solutes.[65] In the case of GlpF, the minimum diameter of the pore is ~3.8 Å, allowing passage of glycerol. Both polarity and diameter of the selectivity filter are essential to determine the permeability properties of AQPs.[65,160]

Certain Aquaporins are Permeable to Solutes and Perhaps to Physiologic Gases

As shown in Table 4.1, five of the eleven AQP isoforms have been shown to display solute permeability, in addition to water permeability. It has also been claimed that AQP1 has ion-channel activity when stimulated by cGMP, but this is unclear at this time (see below). Class II AQPs (aquaglyceroporins, isoforms 3, 7, 9, and 10) are permeable to small, neutral, hydrophilic solutes. Of these, urea is critical for renal function (see Chapter 43). Recent observations also point to permeability to the trivalent metalloids arsenite, As (III), and antimonite, Sb(III) through aquaglyceroporins.[5] As(III) and Sb(III) are protonated at physiological

pH, with the main species in solution being the undissociated trioxides of a molecular volume slightly smaller than that of glycerol, which may explain permeation through the aquaglyceroporins.[5,114]

From the point of view of permeability properties, AQP6 differs from other AQPs in that it displays low water permeability, and behaves as an anion channel selective for anions such as nitrate over Cl^-.[67,68] Lowering pH and reaction with Hg^{2+}, a known blocker of water permeation through AQPs, increase anion conductance.[67,68,109] AQP6 has been traditionally considered an intracellular AQP present in intracellular vesicles of α-intercalated cells of the renal collecting ducts,[68,70,109] but it has been more recently identified in other tissues, including the apical membrane of parotid acinar cells, where it seems to contribute to the anionic conductance of the membrane.[67]

A very interesting issue is whether AQPs are permeable to gases, in particular CO_2 and NH_3.[21,65,104,106] It was reported that AQP1 expression in *Xenopus* oocytes elicits an almost twofold, Hg^{2+}-sensitive increase in plasma membrane CO_2 permeability,[21,106] and an even larger effect (also Hg^{2+}-sensitive) was obtained in *E. coli* membrane vesicles expressing AQP1.[112] Other aquaporins may also be permeable to gases.[104] However, the CO_2 permeabilities of red blood cells and alveolar epithelium of mice in which *Aqp1* was deleted were found to be no different from those of wild type mice.[171] The differences between these sets of studies remain unresolved (see [22,153]).

Regulation of AQP-Mediated Water Permeability

In principle, the water permeability of a cell membrane via AQP depends on the number of functional pores (N per cell or membrane surface area), the single-pore water permeability, and the pore open probability (the fraction of the time that it is water permeable). Changes in N have been clearly demonstrated to regulate AQP-mediated water permeability. The most striking example of this mechanism is the effect of vasopressin on the insertion of AQP2 in the luminal membrane of the cortical collecting duct (see Chapter 42). As discussed below, certain solutes decrease the water permeability of AQP pores, but there is no definitive evidence for a regulatory role of pore "gating" in the sense that this expression is used in ion channel function (see Chapters 2 and 8). However, there is some evidence for regulation of aquaporin opening through phosphorylation.[49,51,95,101,145]

The permeability of several AQP isoforms is modulated by the composition of the extracellular solution. The water permeability of AQP0 expressed in *Xenopus* oocytes was reported to be increased by lowering external pH and $[Ca^{2+}]$.[107] Both effects depend on the pore residue His40.[44] In another study, the water permeability of AQP3, also expressed in oocytes, was found to be reduced by external acidification, whereas AQP0, AQP1, AQP2, AQP4, and AQP5 were found to be pH-insensitive,[177] in contrast with the study quoted above. In oocytes or LLC-PK1 cells expressing heterologous AQP4, PKC agonists were reported to reduce cell membrane water permeability,[50,173] an effect abolished by deletion of Ser180.[173] However, when purified AQP4 was reconstituted in liposomes, its phosphorylation by PKC did not affect the water permeability (quoted in King et al.[75]). Finally, *Xenopus* oocytes expressing AQP1 develop an ion current after injection of cGMP, whereas this agent had no effect on oocytes expressing AQP5.[4] Further, the effect is dependent on specific charged residues in the C-terminal domain of AQP1.[13] It is not clear, however, that the pathways for water permeation and ion fluxes are the same: when the experiment was carried out with AQP1 reconstituted in planar bilayers, an organic mercurial compound inhibited water permeability, but not cGMP-induced ion conductance.[133] Further, the ratio of ion permeability to water permeability was extremely small, suggesting that only a minute fraction

of AQP1 molecules would form cGMP-activated ion channels.[133] Calmodulin binds to AQP0 and AQ6 (acidification-induced anion channel AQP), in a calcium dependent manner, and it inhibits AQP0 permeability.[107,115,118,127] The mechanism of the decrease in water permeability and functional role of the interactions of Ca^{2+}−calmodulin with AQPs have not been established. In conclusion, contrary to statements in the literature, there is no evidence that the AQP water pore is gated, that is, opens and closes stochastically as an ion channel. The available information is consistent with modulatory effects, such as by H^+ or divalent cations that could simply block the water permeation pathway. It is also clear that the finding that expression of a membrane protein results in water and ion permeability does not mean that they occur through the same pathway.

Other Membrane Proteins May Contribute to Water Transport

Water permeation through narrow ion channels has been studied by molecular-dynamics simulations based in the atomic structure of the KcsA channel[129] (see also Chapter 2). In the narrow part of the pore (selectivity filter), K^+ is transported in single file; two adjacent ions are separated by a water molecule; therefore, the molar flux ratio (K^+/water) is unity. For "near-isosmotic" water transport, the flux of 1 ion has to be coupled to that of 157 water molecules. Therefore, direct coupling between ion and water transport in narrow ion channels contributes only a minute fraction of the water flux expected to be produced by the changes in the osmolality of the solutions adjacent to the membrane that are produced by the ion flux.

One would expect that wider ion channels, in which the ions permeate in a hydrated state, would result in larger water fluxes coupled to the ion flow, and perhaps also in water permeation in the absence of a net ion flux. Although there is no direct evidence for this, it was recently shown that blocking the volume-regulated anion channel (VRAC) decreased significantly the water permeability of endothelial cells.[108] This result suggests that these channels constitute a significant pathway for osmotic water flow in these cells.

Do Co-Transporters Perform Active Water Transport?

Experiments in the choroid plexus epithelium of *Necturus maculosus*[174,175] and retinal pigment epithelium of frog[176] suggested that water transport and solute transport (KCl and lactate, respectively) are directly coupled. Under energetically favorable conditions, water would move uphill in the direction of the net ion flux and by the same pathway, implying molecular coupling (in the carrier molecule) between the solute and water fluxes. If this is correct, then the water is co-transported, that is, transported uphill by a secondary active mechanism. Several co-transporters have been suggested to perform this function when expressed in *Xenopus* oocytes: Na$^+$-glucose,[84,97,98] Na$^+$-glutamate,[89] Na$^+$-dicarboxylate,[99] and others.[80,175] The rate of water transport via these carriers would range between 40 and 600 molecules per cycle. The water/solute coupling ratio in the case of the human Na$^+$-glucose co-transporter[98] indicates that the transported fluid would be hyperosmotic, instead of near-isosmotic. Hence, near-isosmolality could result from the parallel operation of transcellular osmosis (see [175] for a recent review). The critical experimental result supporting the water co-transport hypothesis is that solute transport via a co-transporter is associated with a water flux much larger than that observed with a similar solute flux via ion channels,[83] an argument that would rule out the alternative explanation that the co-transporter-mediated solute flux increases the osmolality in the plane adjacent to the membrane, and that the resultant generated osmotic gradient is responsible for water flux across the plasma membrane,[79,80] and not necessarily the co-transporter itself. A careful study of water fluxes in *Xenopus* oocytes expressing heterologous proteins, including Na$^+$-glucose co-transporters, glucose transporters or the K$^+$-channel ROMK2, permitted another group to relate solute accumulation in the oocytes to water flow. Their conclusion is that the glucose accumulation quantitatively accounts for the water flux by simple osmosis, and therefore that there would be no need to postulate water co-transport.[20,42] A critical factor in the solute accumulation in these studies is the intracellular solute diffusion coefficient, which in the oocytes is about one-fifth of that in free solution.[19,20]

Summary and Conclusions

In conclusion, the osmotic behavior of cells is not ideal because of the presence of cell solids; water transport across the cell membrane occurs by osmosis; and the determinants of cell volume are the intracellular solute content and the extracellular osmolality. Water permeation across the plasma membrane occurs via AQP pores and/or the phospholipid bilayer. Other pathways contribute at most a small fraction of the water flow.

WATER TRANSPORT IN EPITHELIA

Two modalities of transepithelial water transport occur in renal tubules *in situ*: (1) net transport between isosmotic (or near-isosmotic) fluids (e.g., water

reabsorption in the proximal tubule); and (2) net transport in the direction of a pre-existing osmotic gradient (e.g., water reabsorption in the collecting duct). Although other mechanisms have been proposed, the dominant view is that water transport is passive and driven by osmotic forces. Pinocytosis has also been suggested, but is considered highly unlikely.[167] Solute–water co-transport, discussed in the previous section, is also unlikely given recent experimental results.[42] Electro-osmosis[132] and mechano-osmosis[130] have also been proposed, largely on the basis of neglecting the presence of unstirred layers in theoretical or experimental analyses. The reader interested in these hypotheses should consult additional references.[32,36,82,102,130,132,167]

Characteristics of Transepithelial Water Transport

The main consequence of water transport across cell membranes of epithelial cells is to contribute to transepithelial transport, that is, fluid absorption or secretion. In addition, similar to most other cells, epithelial cells are endowed with mechanisms of maintenance and regulation of their own volume. Physiologic regulation of transepithelial transport may involve changes in solute transport rate at one of the two cell membranes. This causes an instantaneous imbalance between the transport rates of apical and basolateral membranes, and therefore a change in cell solute and water content. In most epithelial cells, there is a rapid readjustment of the transport rate by a complex process called inter-membrane "cross-talk"[134,135] (see Chapter 2).

Epithelia Have Very Different Water Permeabilities

Epithelia differ widely in their osmotic water permeabilities (Table 4.2). From the points of view of magnitude and regulation of their osmotic permeability coefficient, epithelia can be classified in the following three groups:

1. *High constitutive osmotic water permeability.* In these epithelia the P_{os} is permanently high. This group includes most leaky epithelia (epithelia with high ionic paracellular permeability relative to the transcellular permeability), such as renal proximal tubule, descending limb of the loop of Henle, small intestine, gallbladder, and choroid plexus. The high value of P_{os} is in large part (or exclusively) attributable to high permeabilities of both cell membranes (apical and basolateral). The cell membranes express water pores, so that water is likely to permeate by both solubility diffusion (via the lipid bilayer) and osmosis (via the pores).

TABLE 4.2 Osmotic Water Permeability of Epithelial Cell Membranes

Epithelium	Apical	Basolateral	Transepithelial	Reference
ADH-INSENSITIVE				
Rabbit PST	4500	5000	4280	18
Necturus gallbladder	640	460	350	23
Rabbit/rat TALH	–	–	0–20[a]	117
ADH-SENSITIVE				
Rabbit CCD				
(−) ADH	70	450	–	141
(+) ADH	310	490	–	
Rabbit IMCD				38
(−) ADH	70	480	–	
(+) ADH	260	390	–	

P_f values are rounded and expressed in $\mu m\ s^{-1}$, without correction for membrane folding factors; that is, they are referred to an "idealized" epithelial surface. For P_f values considering membrane folding, see Tripathi and Boulpaep.[146]
[a]*Range of several studies.*
ADH: antidiuretic hormone (vasopressin); PST: proximal straight tubule; TALH: thick ascending limb of loop of Henle; CCD: cortical collecting duct; IMCD: inner medullary collecting duct.

It is also possible that part of the water flow is intercellular (or paracellular), as discussed below.

2. *Low constitutive osmotic water permeability.* In mammals the only epithelia with this property are the ascending limb of the loop of Henle and urinary tract epithelia. The P_{os} is extremely low and insensitive to hormonal action (vasopressin). Both the apical membranes and the junctional complexes are low permeability barriers. In the thick ascending loop of Henle, the basolateral membrane has a high water permeability, so that changes in peritubular fluid osmolality result in rapid cell volume changes, whereas changes in luminal (apical) solution osmolality are ineffective.[54,143] The transepithelial P_{os} is low, although there is a high junctional ionic permeability. This lack of correlation between permeability to ions and water is not unexpected. As discussed in the context of cell membrane water permeability, ion channels permeate little water, and their expression level is quite low, so they do not increase P_{os} by a large amount. The molecular explanations for the low P_{os} of the apical membranes and junctions of the ascending limb of loop of Henle cells are unknown. In the case of urinary tract epithelia, there appears to be a major role of apical membrane uroplakins (see previous discussion and Hu et al.[64]).

3. *Variable (regulated) water permeability.* The renal collecting duct and the anuran urinary bladder and epidermis have low baseline P_{os} values, which are elevated when plasma osmolality rises by a mechanism involving secretion of antidiuretic hormone (vasopressin) by the neurohypophysis. Vasopressin binds to the basolateral V2 receptor, and activates a signaling mechanism that involves an increase in intracellular cAMP, resulting in insertion and then retrieval of preformed water pores in the apical membrane by exocytosis and endocytosis, respectively. The cytoplasmic pool of pores is contained in subapical tubulo-vesicles.[16,38,52,53,150,154,155]

Two Types of Transepithelial Water Transport

It is not difficult to understand the mechanisms of water reabsorption in either the cortical or the medullary collecting duct (CCD and MCD, respectively) under the influence of vasopressin. The tubule fluid at the end of the distal tubule is hyposmotic to plasma (and to the renal cortex interstitial fluid). Hence, if the CCD is water permeable, then water will be reabsorbed down the osmotic gradient. A similar situation occurs in the MCD, where the entering lumen fluid is at most isosmotic to plasma and the osmolality of the surrounding interstitial fluid ranges in humans, from 300 mosmol/kg at the cortico-medullary junction to 1200 mosmol/kg at the papilla (Chapter 43). In the frog epidermis, water reabsorption occurs from the pond (osmolality <10) to the frog's extracellular fluid (200–250 mosmol/kg). Thus, in these three epithelia there is a pre-existing osmotic force, and whether water is absorbed or not depends on the P_{os} of the apical membrane of the epithelial cells. As discussed previously, P_{os} at this membrane is regulated by insertion and retrieval of AQP2 water pores in response to changes in extracellular osmolality, a process mediated by secretion of vasopressin (see also Chapters 42 and 43).

In the renal proximal tubule, small intestine, gallbladder, and other epithelia, the fluids bathing the epithelium are usually isosmotic or near-isosmotic, and transepithelial water transport can take place in the absence of a measurable driving force between the bulk solutions. Further, early experimental observations showed that water absorption can occur against the transepithelial osmotic gradient, that is, from the concentrated to the diluted solution.[25] This occurs both in small intestine and renal proximal tubule, and unquestionably demonstrates uphill water transport (see Whittembury and Hill[166] and Whittembury and Reuss[167] for detailed discussions). Of course, this does not necessarily mean that there is a "water pump" (primary or secondary active water transporter) in the system. Studies in small intestine epithelium revealed that uphill water absorption occurs only together with net solute absorption and in the same direction, suggesting some form of "coupling" between water and solute fluxes.[25,161,162,163] Over the next 50 years, these puzzling observations elicited a great deal of experimental and theoretical work, which resulted in successive proposals to explain: (1) water transport between isosmotic bulk solutions; (2) uphill water transport; and (3) the nature of the coupling between solute and water flow.

Solute—Solvent Coupling

Passive mechanisms may exist that would couple salt to water absorption or secretion. Intuitively, active salt absorption by an epithelium (see Chapter 2) will create, at both apical and basolateral membranes, differences in the concentration of salt, with the side from which the salt is transported becoming "dilute" and the side toward which the salt is transported becoming "concentrated." The magnitude of the concentration changes in the fluids adjacent to the epithelial cells will depend on whether they are mixed (by convection) with the bulk solutions, and on the rates of solute diffusion into or away from these areas. Clearly, changes in concentration must be created inside the cell, in the surfaces immediately adjacent to the membranes, where the cytosol is not well mixed and the diffusion rates are much smaller than in free solution. In addition, in the extracellular surfaces adjacent to the cell membranes the solutions are not well mixed with the bulk, for two reasons: the existence of unstirred layers (see above); and the existence of anatomic restricted spaces in which good mixing cannot occur. In the case of the basolateral cell membrane of an epithelium, the histology indicates that there cannot be good mixing with the extracellular solution because of the complex architecture of the lateral intercellular spaces, the basal membrane infoldings, and the presence of the basement membrane, which is a barrier for hydraulic flow. At the apical membrane surface, fluid mixing is easier, but is also not ideal if there are microvilli. Hence, in a fluid absorbing epithelium at the steady-state one would expect a solute concentration profile in which there are salt concentration gradients across the apical membrane, with the lumen fluid diluted with respect to the cell interior, and across the basolateral membrane, with the cell diluted with respect to the extracellular solution.

The central points in this analysis of solute—solvent coupling in epithelia will be two. First, the functional anatomy of epithelia determines the existence of compartments (i.e., spaces that are "unstirred"); in these spaces osmotic coupling occurs, explaining the relationship (coupling) between salt and water transport. Second, the water permeability of the cell membranes is so high that the osmotic gradients required for near-isosmotic coupling are very small, and detectable only under rather artificial experimental conditions. This view is not universally accepted. As we discuss the details below, we will point out criticisms and alternative explanations.

Three-Compartment Models Define the Problem

An epithelial monolayer and the surrounding fluid compartments can be modeled as a three-compartment system with two barriers. The essence of these models is that the specific properties of the barriers and the compartments can account for solute—water flux coupling and explain apparently active water transport. Two proposals were developed based on this idea, namely the three-compartment model of Curran and MacIntosh[24] and the standing-gradient hypothesis of Diamond and Bossert.[31]

In the three-compartment model, illustrated in Figure 4.10, water transport occurs from the *cis* solution (A) to the *trans* solution (B), against the osmotic pressure difference between these two solutions [C_s (B) $>$ C_s (A)]. The *cis* solution and *trans* solution are separated from the middle compartment (M) by barriers with different properties, semipermeable and porous, respectively. Active salt transport into an unstirred intraepithelial compartment renders it hyperosmotic to the *cis* solution (hyperosmotic middle compartment). Water then flows from A to M by osmosis (the membrane is semipermeable) and, as the hydrostatic pressure rises in M, solution flows from the M into B by bulk flow (the membrane is porous). The equivalent of this system in an absorptive epithelium would be as follows: the semipermeable membrane is constituted by the two cell membrane domains (apical and basolateral) in series, and the porous membrane by the distal end of the lateral intercellular spaces and the basement membrane, also in series. Compartment A is the lumen, compartment B the basolateral (interstitial) solution, and compartment M the lateral intercellular space. Water can be transported uphill (against the osmotic gradient between A and B) only while the middle compartment is hyperosmotic to the *cis* compartment. In addition, for this model to operate the absorbed fluid must be hyperosmotic to the *cis* solution. Experimental studies showed that the emerging fluid is virtually isosmotic with the *cis* solution,[30] requiring revision of the above theory. This resulted in the formulation of the standing-gradient hypothesis, explained below.

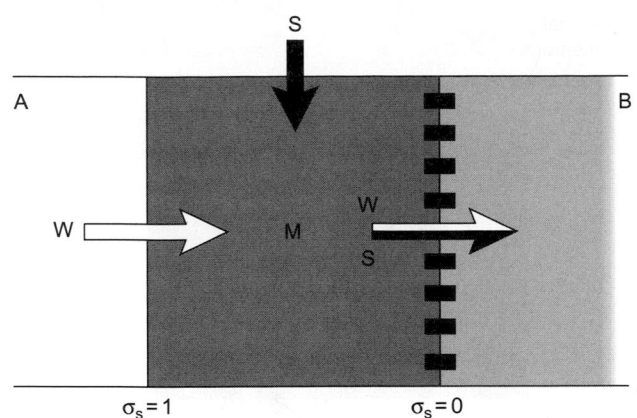

FIGURE 4.10 Three-compartment model of Curran and MacIntosh.[18] Solute entry (s, solid arrow) into the middle compartment (compartment M) causes osmotic *water* flow (w, open arrow) from compartment A to compartment M. The elevation of the hydrostatic pressure in compartment M causes *solution* flow from compartment M into compartment B (w/s open/solid arrow). Hence, there is water flux from A to B, although $C_s(B) > C_s(A)$. Darker tones in the compartment denote higher solute concentrations. See text.

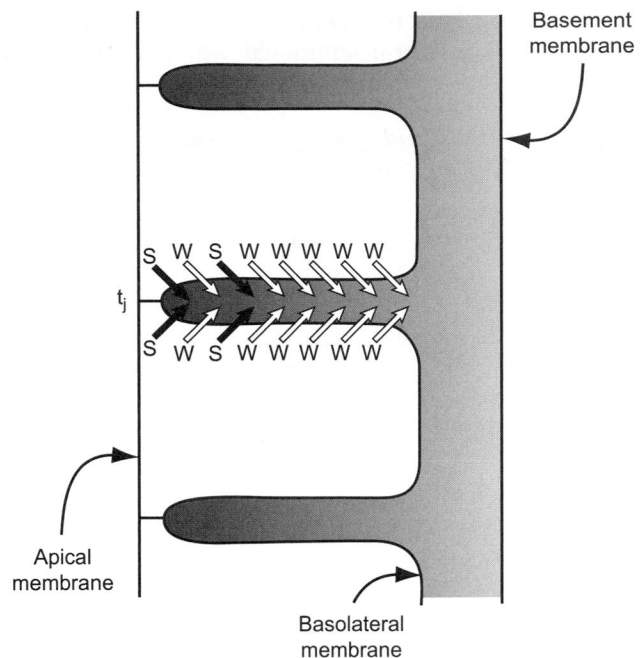

FIGURE 4.11 Standing-gradient hypothesis of Diamond and Bossert.[23] Solute transport (s, solid arrows) into the channel (lateral intercellular space) causes a local increase in osmolality; water flows osmotically across the bounding membranes (w, open arrows), "diluting" the solution in the channel. Transport toward the open end is by bulk flow and diffusion. See text.

Standing-Gradient Hypothesis Explains Near-Isosmotic Fluid Transport, but is Difficult to Reconcile with Current Experimental Knowledge

The standing-gradient hypothesis of Diamond and Bossert[31] is depicted in Figure 4.11. It is based on the following definitions and assumptions: (1) the lateral intercellular space is the hyperosmotic middle compartment; (2) the junctional complexes are impermeable to both solute and water; (3) solute transport from the cell to the *trans* solution takes place across the lateral membranes near the apical poles of the cells; (4) in contrast, secondary (osmotic) water flow occurs across the entire lateral membrane; (5) the lateral intercellular space solution is unstirred; (6) solute diffusion along the length of the lateral intercellular spaces is restricted by their geometry (the spaces are long and narrow). Under these conditions, the solution of the complicated mathematical model describing the system yields a continuously decreasing osmolality from the apical (blind) to the basolateral (open) end of the space. Also, the emerging solution is more likely to be near-isosmotic when the following conditions hold: long and narrow spaces, small solute diffusion coefficient, and high cell membrane P_{os} relative to the solute transport rate.

Direct and indirect observations demonstrated that some of the above assumptions are not correct. (1) In many instances the junctions have high permeability to ions[40,61,164,168] and perhaps to water.[165,167] (2) The Na^+, K^+-ATPase is distributed homogeneously in the lateral cell membrane,[99] not restricted to the apical region. (3) Both morphometric studies and electrophysiological computations yield short times for lateral space solute diffusion,[58,74,131,158,162] making longitudinal concentration gradients unlikely. (4) Realistic calculations based on geometry predict that the transported fluid must be hyperosmotic,[131] because the spaces are not sufficiently long and narrow. (5) The hypothesis predicted sizable hyperosmolality in the lateral intercellular spaces, but this was based on the early estimations of transepithelial P_{os}, which were in error due to unstirred-layer artifacts.[11,62] (6) Measurements of transepithelial voltage changes elicited by changes in solution osmolality revealed that the lateral intercellular spaces are in virtual osmotic equilibrium with the cell.[124,125]

An important point in this discussion is that for a constant fluid transport rate, the magnitude of the osmotic gradient and of the hyperosmolality of the transported fluid is inversely proportional to the effective P_{os} of the osmotic barriers. In fact, many of the above problems were solved with the development of methods to measure the osmotic water permeability of the cell membranes of leaky epithelia, which were demonstrated to be very large. On these bases, some of the above notions must be discarded, because they were based on incorrect experimental data and a simpler mechanism of transepithelial water transport has emerged.

Near-Isosmotic Fluid Transport Model Solves the Difficulties of Three-Compartment Models

Measurements of P_{os} in high water permeability membranes give values ranging from 100 to 400 μm s^{-1}, that is, 10- to 100-fold greater than early estimates.[167] Hence, instead of a needed osmolality difference of about 20 mosmol kg^{-1}, as predicted from the standing-gradient hypothesis, a very small difference in osmolality, of only 1–2 mosmol kg^{-1}, quantitatively accounts for the measured water transport rates.[23,111,167] As explained previously, the primary event in transepithelial water transport is active salt transport. Inasmuch as solute is removed from the *cis* side and added to the *trans* side, there must be a decrease in *cis* fluid and an increase in *trans* fluid osmolality in the immediate vicinity of the respective membranes, as well as opposite changes in osmolality at the intracellular surface of the two membranes: an increase at the apical membrane and a decrease at the basolateral membrane. The magnitude of these changes will depend on the transport rate and geometry of the systems, and can be generally expected to be quite small. Measurements in fluid samples from isolated, perfused renal tubules reveal small differences, supporting this view.[10,46] In conclusion, recent studies support the notion that so-called isosmotic transepithelial water transport is not truly isosmotic, but near-isosmotic. Further, the osmotic driving forces required to account for water transport are quite small, and hence difficult to determine *in situ*, and substantial hyperosmotic compartments or sizable longitudinal standing gradients probably do not exist[121,141,167] (see Figure 4.12).

Solute Recirculation in the Paracellular Pathway in Theory Explains Truly Isosmotic Transepithelial Fluid Transport

Truly isosmotic transepithelial water transport[147,148] may occur, in theory, if there is solute recirculation across the epithelium. In other words, it is argued that an epithelium cannot perform transepithelial truly isosmotic transport if it is bathed by identical solutions on both sides, and there are no differences in electrical potential or hydrostatic pressure, unless part of the transported solute recirculates to the solution of origin. In frog skin glands, there is transcellular Cl$^-$ secretion (secondary active uptake at the basolateral membrane, channel-mediated downhill Cl$^-$ extrusion across the apical membrane) and paracellular Na$^+$ secretion (driven by the lumen-negative transepithelial voltage generated by Cl$^-$ transport). As such, this transport

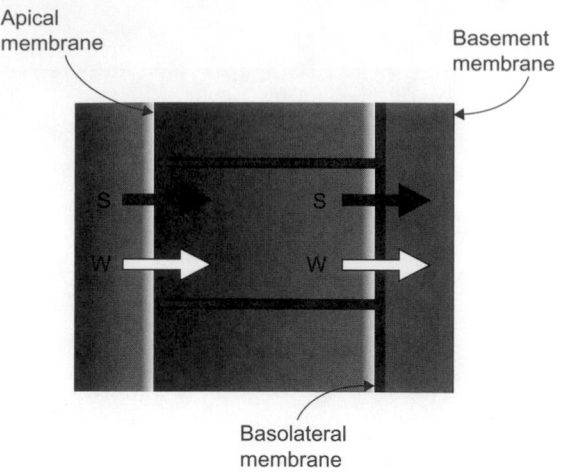

FIGURE 4.12   Near-isosmotic transport model. Because of the high osmotic water permeability of the cell membranes, the differences in solution osmolality needed to account for fluid transport are small, probably localized at epithelium—solution interfaces. Salt transport causes dilution of solution on *cis* side and concentration of the solution on *trans* side at the two cell membranes. In the case of fluid absorption, at the apical membrane the intracellular solution is hyperosmotic to the lumen solution; at the basolateral membrane, the intracellular solution is hyposmotic to the extracellular solution. These small differences in osmolality, denoted in the figure by shades of gray (hyperosmotic solution being darker), cause osmotic water flow into the cell across the apical membrane and out of the cell across the basolateral membrane. The magnitude of the paracellular water flow is uncertain. Because of the high surface area of the lateral membranes, and the small volume of the lateral intercellular spaces, the space osmolality is "clamped" by the cell osmolality, making longitudinal osmotic gradients in the spaces small at most.

mechanism would cause secretion of a hyperosmotic fluid, but it was proposed that this fluid can become truly isosmotic. Larsen and co-workers[81,82] developed an interesting mathematical model for solute recirculation in the epithelium of the small intestine. The essential points are as follows: the primary transport event is active Na$^+$ transport across the lateral cell membrane (by the Na$^+$,K$^+$-ATPase). Water follows osmotically across the lateral cell membranes and the tight junctions. With appropriate geometric and transport parameters, the solution in the lateral intercellular spaces would be hyperosmotic by a small amount. The transported fluid would become isosmotic by uptake (recirculation) of salt across the basal membrane, via Na$^+$-K$^+$-2Cl$^-$ co-transport. This model has been criticized[140] on two main grounds: the use of experimental measurements of the Cs$^+$ flux ratio to assess transcellular and paracellular Na$^+$ fluxes, and the energetic cost of recirculation, namely the fact that about half of the pump work would be wasted. However, both sides agree that the model is amenable to further experimental testing.[81,140]

In Certain Epithelia Asymmetries in Solute Composition Play Significant Roles

It is possible that factors other than the total osmolalities of the solutions on either side of the epithelium contribute to transepithelial water transport. Three possibilities should be considered (see Whittembury and Hill[166] for a more detailed discussion). First is a colloid-osmotic force: transepithelial differences in protein concentration can result in colloid-osmotic pressure differences that can be significant in the case of epithelia with high permeability to water and small solutes. In the renal proximal tubule, this factor accounts for a small portion of water reabsorption.[48] Second is a difference in the effective osmolalities of the solutions: if the epithelium is exposed to solutions containing solutes of different reflection coefficients, then there could be transepithelial effective osmolality gradients, even if the solutions have the same total osmolality. Under the conditions described there will be osmotic water flow toward the side containing the higher concentration of low permeability (high reflection coefficient) solutes.[47] This has been proposed to occur in the late renal proximal tubule because of reabsorption of organic solutes such as glucose, and preferential reabsorption of HCO_3^-. Both have been claimed to have higher reflection coefficients than Cl^-. However, the notion of low reflection coefficients in epithelial cells has been disputed, and attributed to errors caused by uncorrected unstirred-layer effects.[154] Third are hydrostatic pressure differences: under most conditions, these differences are small and hence do not contribute significantly to water flow.

Pathways for Transepithelial Water Transport are also Controversial

Is water transport transcellular and/or paracellular? Epithelial transport pathways can be in series or in parallel. The cells consist of pathways in series (apical membrane, cytoplasm, and basolateral membrane), as does the intercellular (paracellular) pathway (junction in series with lateral intercellular space). In turn, the transcellular pathway and the paracellular pathway are in parallel with each other. A major problem in the phenomenological description of transepithelial transport has been to ascertain the portions of ion and water fluxes occurring across each pathway. In the case of ions, it has been clearly shown that in some epithelia most passive permeation is paracellular (leaky epithelia); whereas in others most passive permeation is transcellular (tight epithelia) (see Reuss[123] for a review). In the case of water, there is convincing experimental evidence demonstrating transcellular transport, but paracellular transport is controversial.[122]

Transcellular Osmotic Water Transport is Supported by High Cell-Membrane P_{os}

In high water permeability epithelia (mammalian renal proximal tubule, *Necturus* gallbladder), apical and basolateral membrane P_{os} values range from <500 to 5000 μm s^{-1} (renal tubule [17,18,19,45,167]; gallbladder [23,111]). In both membrane domains, there can be considerable "amplification," by the presence of microvilli at the apical membrane and infoldings at the basolateral membrane. Hence, the P_{os} values expressed per unit surface area of membrane are much smaller than those relative to the idealized geometry of the tissue. Regardless of this, the water permeability of these epithelia is high, and attributable to the expression of water pores.

Paracellular Osmotic Water Transport is Supported by Indirect Arguments

The paracellular P_{os} can be estimated in principle from the transepithelial and cell membrane P_{os}. Given that the transcellular and paracellular pathways are in parallel:

$$P_{os}^t = P_{os}^c + P_{os}^p \qquad (4.21)$$

where P_{os} denotes osmotic permeability, and the superscripts t, c, and p refer to transepithelial, cellular, and paracellular pathways, respectively. In the proximal tubule, P_{os}^t appears to be significantly higher than P_{os}^c, suggesting that P_{os}^p is sizable.[167] The problems with these calculations are the errors involved in the measurements of transepithelial and cell membrane P_{os} values.

Paracellular water transport is also supported by quantitative assessments of the effect of organomercurial compounds, presumed to be specific pore blockers, on P_{os}^t and P_{os}^c. An agent such as pCMBS inhibits P_f^c by more than 90%, but P_{os}^t is reduced by only 50%, which strongly suggests a finite parallel water permeation pathway.[167] These calculations imply a single site of action of pCMBS and other effects are, in principle, possible.

Another argument suggesting paracellular water flow is the observation of solvent drag and electrokinetic phenomena. If osmotic water flow takes place across large pores, which are also permeable to solute, then there will be a frictional interaction between water and solute, and the water flow will cause a solute flow in the same direction. This solute flux can occur in the absence of a favorable solute electrochemical gradient between the solutions. It is usually demonstrated using hydrophilic nonelectrolytes (e.g., small sugars such as mannitol); the mannitol and water fluxes correlate linearly, as predicted by Eq. (4.18). Results suggesting solvent drag have been reported for several epithelia.[167] The simplest electrokinetic phenomenon to study is the streaming potential produced when, in the absence of a favorable electrochemical gradient, the solute is a permeant ion that flows in the same direction as water. Streaming potentials are generated if the water permeation pathway is ion-selective, that is, more permeable to that ion than to the counterion. The observation of this phenomenon has been interpreted as supportive of solute–water coupling in the paracellular pathway (reviewed in Tripathi and Boulpaep[146]).

The main problem with experiments purporting to demonstrate solvent drag or streaming potentials is the complication introduced by unstirred layers. Water transport in such a system causes changes in solute concentrations next to the membrane surfaces, raising the concentration on the *cis* side and lowering it on the *trans* side. Therefore, even if the concentrations of a given solute are the same in the bulk solution, there will be a concentration gradient at the membrane surfaces (unstirred-layer polarization), which explains the apparent solvent drag (pseudo-solvent drag). Pseudo-streaming potentials can be similarly caused by ion concentration changes elicited by the water flux. It is possible to distinguish true from apparent streaming potentials by comparing the time courses of the transepithelial voltage changes caused by the addition of nonelectrolyte or by a unilateral ionic substitution.[120,124,125] This criterion could help confirm or rule out the legitimacy of claimed true streaming potentials.

One recent approach to assess the role of the paracellular pathway in water permeation has been the use of genetic manipulation of claudins in mice and culture cells. Tight junctions are composed of several membrane proteins, including occludin and claudins.[77,136] Claudin-2 is frequently located at tight junctions of leaky epithelia that display high fluid transport rates, and seems to be responsible for the cation selectivity of the paracellular pathway in these tissues.[77,105] Recent studies have shown that expression of claudin-2 in an MDCK cell line increases water permeability,[128] and that the proximal tubules of mice deficient in claudin-2 display increased paracellular electrical resistance with loss of cation selectivity.[105] The decrease in net fluid transport in the claudin-2-deficient mice parallels the decreases in NaCl reabsorption, and cannot be unambiguously ascribed to a primary decrease in water permeability.[105,128]

In sum, the cellular pathway is certain to contribute to transepithelial osmotic water transport, and there are suggestions of a significant paracellular contribution. However, the latter is based on indirect evidence, and is questionable because of possible unstirred-layer artifacts. This problem will be definitively solved only by direct measurements of transcellular and paracellular water flows, which is a daunting task. Recent elegant fluorescence microscopy studies[76] suggest that there is no significant water flow across tight junctions of MDCK monolayers, relative to the transcellular flow. However, in these experiments the rate of transepithelial water flux was much smaller than observed in native epithelia. Sachar-Hill and Hill[130] have argued, on the basis of analyses of hydrophilic probe and water fluxes, that the paracellular water flux of several epithelia is quite high. However, the problem of unstirred layers was neglected in their analysis. Additional studies using genetic manipulations, in combination with sophisticated imaging studies, may shed light into the long-standing issue of the physiological role of water permeation through the paracellular pathway.

Summary and Conclusions

Water transport in leaky epithelia occurs in the same direction as solute transport and in near-isosmotic proportions. The available experimental evidence supports the view that the coupling between solute and water transport is not molecular, but thermodynamic, that is, osmotic. Solute transport by pumps, carriers, and/or channels elicits differences in solute concentration at the membrane surfaces, with a decrease in concentration on the *cis* side and an increase on the *trans* side. The establishment of osmotic gradients is favored because of the architecture of epithelia, which contain compartments that do not mix well with the surrounding fluids. The magnitude of the osmotic gradients is small and difficult to measure, but sufficient to account for the measured rates of fluid transport. Osmotic water flow takes place predominantly across the cell membranes, via both AQP pores and the phospholipid bilayer, with a small or nil contribution of other proteins. It is possible that part of the water flow is paracellular via the tight junctions, but this is likely to be relatively small.

References

[1] Agre P. Aquaporin water channels (Nobel Lecture). Angew Chem Int Ed Engl 2004;43:4278–90.

[2] Agre P, Preston GM, Smith BL, Jung JS, Raina S, Moon C, et al. The archetypal molecular water channel. Am J Physiol 1993;265: F463–76.

[3] Anderson JL, Malone DM. Mechanism of osmotic flow in porous membranes. Biophys J 1974;14:957–82.

[4] Anthony TL, Brooks HL, Boassa D, Leonov S, Yanochko GM, Regan JW, et al. Cloned human aquaporin-1 is a cyclic GMP-gated ion channel. Mol Pharm 2000;57:576–88.

[5] Bhattacharjee H, Rosen BP, Mukhopadhyay R. Aquaglyceroporins and metalloid transport: implications in human diseases. Handb Exp Pharmacol 2009;190:309–25.

[6] Blok MC, Van Deenen LL, De Gier J. The effect of cholesterol incorporation on the temperature dependence of water permeation through liposomal membranes prepared from phosphatidylcholines. Biochim Biophys Acta 1977;464:509—18.

[7] Bloom M, Evans E, Mouritsen OG. Physical properties of the fluid lipid-bilayer component of cell membranes: aperspective. Q Rev Biophys 1991;24:293—397.

[8] Burykin A, Warshel A. What really prevents proton transport through aquaporin? Charge self-energy versus proton wire proposals. Biophys J 2003;85:3696—706.

[9] Burykin A, Warshel A. On the origin of the electrostatic barrier for proton transport in aquaporin. FEBS Lett 2004;570: 41—6.

[10] Barfuss DW, Schafer JA. Hyperosmolarity of absorbate from isolated rabbit proximal tubules. Am J Physiol 1984;247:F130—9.

[11] Barry PH, Diamond JM. Effects of unstirred layers on membrane phenomena. Physiol Rev 1984;64:763—873.

[12] Bean CP. The physics of porous membranes—neutral pores. In: Eisenman G, editor. Membranes I. Macroscopic systems and models. New York: Dekker; 1972. p. 1—54.

[13] Boassa D, Yool AJ. Single amino acids in the carboxyl terminal domain of aquaporin-1 contribute to cGMP-dependent ion channel activation. BMC Physiol 2003;3:12.

[14] Brisson A, Wade RH. Three-dimensional structure of luminal plasma membrane protein from urinary bladder. J Mol Biol 1983;166:21—36.

[15] Brown D. Membrane recycling and epithelial cell function. Am J Physiol 1989;256:F1—12.

[16] Brown D. Structural—functional features of vasopressin-induced water flow in the kidney collecting duct. Semin Nephrol 1991;11:478—501.

[17] Carpi-Medina P, González E, Whittembury G. Cell osmotic water permeability of isolated rabbit proximal convoluted tubules. Am J Physiol 1984;244:F554—63.

[18] Carpi-Medina P, Whittembury G. Comparison of transcellular and transepithelial water osmotic permeabilities in the isolated proximal straight tubule of the rabbit kidney. Pflügers Arch 1988;412:66—74.

[19] Charron F, Lapointe JY. Slow ionic diffusion in oocytes and the water co-transport hypothesis. FASEB J 2005;19:A1156.

[20] Charron FM, Blanchard MG, Lapointe JY. Intracellular hypertonicity is responsible for water flux associated with Na^+/glucose co-transport. Biophys J 2006;90:3546—54.

[21] Cooper GJ, Boron WF. Effect of PCMBS on CO_2 permeability of Xenopus oocytes expressing aquaporin-1 or its C189S mutant. Am J Physiol 1998;275:C1481—6.

[22] Cooper GJ, Zhou Y, Bouyer P, Grichtchenko II, Boron WF. Transport of volatile solutes through AQP1. J Physiol 2002;542: 17—29.

[23] Cotton CU, Weinstein AM, Reuss L. Osmotic water permeability of Necturus gallbladder. J Gen Physiol 1989;93:649—79.

[24] Curran PF, MacIntosh JR. A model system for biological water transport. Nature (Lond) 1962;193:347—8.

[25] Curran PF, Solomon AK. Ion and water fluxes in the ileum of rats. J Gen Physiol 1957;41:143—68.

[26] Dawson DC. Water transport. In: Seldin DW, Giebisch G, editors. The Kidney: physiology and pathophysiology. New York: Raven Press; 1992. p. 301—16.

[27] de Groot BL, Frigato T, Helms V, Grubmüller H. The mechanism of proton exclusion in the aquaporin-1 water channel. J Mol Biol 2003;333:279—93.

[28] de Groot BL, Grubmüller H. The dynamics and energetics of water permeation and proton exclusion in aquaporins. Curr Opin Struct Biol 2005;15:176—83.

[29] Denker BM, Smith BL, Kuhajda FP, Agre P. Identification, purification, and partial characterization of a novel M_r 28,000 integral membrane protein from erythrocytes and renal tubule. J Biol Chem 1988;263:14634—5642.

[30] Diamond JM. The mechanism of water transport by the gallbladder. J Physiol (Lond) 1962;161:503—27.

[31] Diamond JM, Bossert WH. Standing-gradient osmotic flow: a mechanism for coupling of water and solute transport in epithelia. J Gen Physiol 1967;50:2061—83.

[32] Diecke FP, Ma L, Iserovich P, Fischbarg J. Corneal endothelium transports fluid in the absence of net solute transport. Biochim Biophys Acta 2007;1768:2043—8.

[33] Engel A, Walz T, Agre P. The aquaporin family of membrane water channels. Curr Opin Struct Biol 1994;4:545—53.

[34] Finkelstein A. Water movement through lipid bilayers, pores and plasma membranes: theory and reality. New York: John Wiley & Sons; 1986.

[35] Finkelstein A, Rosenberg PA. Single-file transport: implications for ion and water movements through gramicidin a channels. In: Stevens CF, Tsien RW, editors. Membrane transport processes, vol. 3. Copenhagen: Munksgaard; 1979. p. 107—19.

[36] Fischbarg J. Fluid transport across leaky epithelia: central role of the tightjunction and supporting role of aquaporins. Physiol Rev 2010;90:1271—90.

[37] Fischer G, Kosinska-Eriksson U, Aponte-Santamaría C, Palmgren M, Geijer C, Hedfalk K, et al. Crystal structure of a yeast aquaporin at 1.15 angstrom reveals a novel gating mechanism. PLoS Biol 2009;7:e1000130.

[38] Flamion B, Spring KR. Water permeability of apical and basolateral cell membranes of rat inner medullary collecting duct. Am J Physiol 1990;259:F986—99.

[39] Forster RE. The transport of water in erythrocytes. In: Bronner F, Kleinzeller, editors. Current topics in membranes and transport, vol. 2. New York: Academic Press; 1971. p. 41—98.

[40] Frömter E. The route of passive ion movement through the epithelium of Necturus gallbladder. J Membr Biol 1972;8: 259—301.

[41] Fu D, Libson A, Miercke LJ, Weitzman C, Nollert P, Krucinski J, et al. Structure of a glycerol-conducting channel and the basis for its selectivity. Science 2000;290:481—6.

[42] Gagnon MP, Bissonnette P, Deslandes LM, Wallendorff B, Lapointe JY. Glucose accumulation can account for the initial water flux triggered by Na^+/glucose co-transport. Biophys J 2004;86:125—33.

[43] Gomes D, Agasse A, Thiébaud P, Delrot S, Gerós H, Chaumont F. Aquaporins are multifunctional water and solute transporters highly divergent in living organisms. Biochim Biophys Acta 2009;1788:1213—28.

[44] Gonen T, Sliz P, Kistler J, Cheng Y, Walz T. Aquaporin-0 membrane junctions reveal the structure of a closed water pore. Nature 2004;429:193—7.

[45] González E, Carpi-Medina P, Whittembury G. Cell osmotic water permeability of isolated rabbit proximal straight tubules. Am J Physiol 1982;242:F321—30.

[46] Green R, Giebisch G. Luminal hypotonicity: a driving force for fluid absorption from the proximal tubule. Am J Physiol 1984;246:F167—74.

[47] Green R, Giebisch G. Reflection coefficients and water permeability in rat proximal tubule. Am J Physiol 1989;257: F658—68.

[48] Green R, Windhager EE, Giebisch G. Protein osmotic pressure effects on proximal tubule fluid movement in the rat. Am J Physiol 1974;226:267—76.

[49] Hachez C, Chaumont F. Aquaporins: a family of highly regulated multifunctional channels. Adv Exp Med Biol 2010;679: 1—17.

[50] Hallows KR, Knauf PA. Principles of cell volume regulation. In: Strange K, editor. Cellular and molecular physiology

of cell volume regulation. Boca Raton, FL: CRC Press; 1994. p. 3—29.

[51] Han H, Wax MB, Patil RV. Regulation of aquaporin-4 water channels by phorbol ester-dependent protein phosphorylation. J Biol Chem 1998;273:6001—4.

[52] Handler JS. Antidiuretic hormone moves membranes. Am J Physiol 1988;255:F375—82.

[53] Harris HW, Handler JS. The role of membrane turnover in the water permeability response to antidiuretic hormone. J Membr Biol 1988;103:207—16.

[54] Hebert SC. Hypertonic cell volume regulation in mouse thick limbs. I. ADH dependency and nephron heterogeneity. Am J Physiol 1986;250:C907—19.

[55] Heymann JB, Agre P, Engel A. Progress on the structure and function of aquaporin 1. J Struct Biol 1998;121:191—206.

[56] Hicks RM. The mammalian urinary bladder: an accommodating organ. Biol Rev Camb Philos Soc 1975;50:215—46.

[57] Hicks RM, Ketterer B. Hexagonal lattice of subunits in the thick luminal membrane of the rat urinary bladder. Nature 1969;224: 1304—5.

[58] Hill AE. Solute—solvent coupling in epithelia: a critical examination of the standing-gradient osmotic flow theory. Proc R Soc Lond Biol 1975;190:99—114.

[59] Hirano Y, Okimoto N, Kadohira I, Suematsu M, Yasuoka K, Yasui M. Molecular mechanisms of how mercury inhibits water permeation through aquaporin-1: understanding by molecular dynamics simulation. Biophys J 2010;98:1512—9.

[60] Ho JD, Yeh R, Sandstrom A, Chorny I, Harries WE, Robbins RA, et al. Crystal structure of human aquaporin 4 at 1.8 A and its mechanism of conductance. Proc Natl Acad Sci USA 2009;106: 7437—742.

[61] Hoshi T, Sakai F. A comparison of the electrical resistances of the surface cell membrane and cellular wall in the proximal tubule of the newt kidney. Jpn J Physiol 1967;17: 627—37.

[62] House CR. Water transport in cells and tissues. London: Arnold; 1974.

[63] Hu P, Deng FM, Liang FX, Hu CM, Auerbach AB, Shapiro E, et al. Ablation of uroplakin III gene results in small urothelial plaques, urothelial leakage, and vesicoureteral reflux. J Cell Biol 2000;151:961—72.

[64] Hu P, Meyers S, Liang FX, Deng FM, Kachar B, Zeidel ML, et al. Role of membrane proteins in permeability barrier function: uroplakin ablation elevates urothelial permeability. Am J Physiol Renal Physiol 2002;283:F1200—1207.

[65] Hub JS, de Groot BL. Mechanism of selectivity in aquaporins and aquaglyceroporins. Proc Natl Acad Sci USA 2008;105: 1198—203.

[66] Hub JS, Grubmüller H, de Groot BL. Dynamics and energetics of permeation through aquaporins. What do we learn from molecular dynamics simulations? Handb Exp Pharmacol 2009;190: 57—76.

[67] Ichikawa H, Shibukawa Y, Sahara Y, Tsumura M, Qi B, Satoh K, et al. Electrophysiological properties of AQP6 in mouse parotid acinar cells. J Med Invest 2009;56:347—9.

[68] Ikeda M, Beitz E, Kozono D, Guggino WB, Agre P, Yasui M. Characterization of aquaporin-6 as a nitrate channel in mammalian cells. Requirement of pore-lining residue threonine 63. J Biol Chem 2002;277:39873—9.

[69] Ishibashi K. New members of mammalian aquaporins: AQP10-AQP12. Handb Exp Pharmacol 2009;190:251—62.

[70] Ishibashi K, Hara S, Kondo S. Aquaporin water channels in mammals. Clin Exp Nephrol 2009;13:107—17.

[71] Jacobson K, Dietrich C. Looking at lipid rafts? Trends Cell Biol 1999;9:87—91.

[72] Jung JS, Preston GM, Smith BL, Guggino WB, Agre P. Molecular structure of the water channel through aquaporin CHIP: the tetrameric-hourglass model. J Biol Chem 1994;269: 14648—54.

[73] Khandelwal P, Abraham SN, Apodaca G. Cell biology and physiology of the uroepithelium. Am J Physiol Renal Physiol 2009;297:F1477—501.

[74] King-Hele JA. Approximate analytical solutions for water and solute flow in intercellular spaces with a leaky tight junction. J Theor Biol 1979;80:451—65.

[75] King LS, Kozono D, Agre P. From structure to disease: the evolving tale of aquaporin biology. Nat Rev Mol Cell Biol 2004;5:687—98.

[76] Kovbasnjuk O, Leader JP, Weinstein AM, Spring KR. Water does not flow across the tight junctions of MDCK cell epithelium. Proc Natl Acad Sci USA 1998;95:6520—6.

[77] Krause G, Winkler L, Mueller SL, Haseloff RF, Piontek J, Blasig IE. Structure and function of claudins. Biochim Biophys Acta 2008;1778:631—45.

[78] Kwon TH, Nielsen J, Møller HB, Fenton RA, Nielsen S, Frøkiaer J. Aquaporins in the kidney. Handb Exp Pharmacol 2009; 190:95—132.

[79] Lapointe Jy Gagnon M, Poirier S, Bissonnette P. The presence of local osmotic gradients can account for the water flux driven by the Na^+—glucose co-transporter. J Physiol 2002;542:61—2.

[80] Lapointe JY, Gagnon MP, Gagnon DG, Bissonnette P. Controversy regarding the secondary active water transport hypothesis. Biochem Cell Biol 2002;80:525—33.

[81] Larsen EH, Sørensen JB, Sørensen JN. Analysis of the sodium recirculation theory of solute-coupled water transport in small intestine. J Physiol 2002;542:33—50.

[82] Larsen EH, Willumsen NJ, Møbjerg N, Sørensen JN. The lateral intercellular space as osmotic coupling compartment in isotonic transport. Acta Physiol (Oxf) 2009;195:171—86.

[83] Loo DD, Wright EM, Zeuthen T. Water pumps. J Physiol 2002;542:53—60.

[84] Loo DD, Zeuthen T, Chandy G, Wright EM. Co-transport of water by the Na^+/glucose co-transporter. Proc Natl Acad Sci USA 1996;93:13367—70.

[85] Lechène C. Cellular volume and cytoplasmic gel. Biol Cell 1985;55:177—80.

[86] Levitt DG. Kinetics of diffusion and convection in 3-X pores. Exact solution by computer simulation. Biophys J 1973;13: 186—206.

[87] Levitt DG. A new theory of transport for cell membrane pores. I. General theory and application to red cell. Biochim Biophys Acta 1974;373:115—31.

[88] Lin JH, Wu XR, Kreibich G, Sun TT. Precursor sequence, processing, and urothelium-specific expression of a major 15-kDa protein subunit of asymmetric unit membrane. J Biol Chem 1994;269:1775—84.

[89] MacAulay N, Gether U, Klaerke DA, Zeuthen T. Water transport by the human Na^+coupled glutamate co-transporter expressed in Xenopus oocytes. J Physiol 2001;530:367—78.

[90] Macey RI. Transport of water and urea in red blood cells. Am J Physiol 1984;246:C195—203.

[91] Macey RI, Farmer REI. Inhibition of water and solute permeability in human red cells. Biochim Biophys Acta 1970;211: 104—6.

[92] Macey RI, Moura TF. Basic principles of transport. In: Hoffman JD, Jamieson JD, editors. Handbook of Physiology. New York: Oxford University Press; 1997. p. 181—259.

[93] Macknight ADC. Principles of cell volume regulation. Renal Physiol Biochem 1988;11:114—48.

[94] Maffly RH, Leaf A. The potential of water in mammalian tissues. J Gen Physiol 1959;42:1257—75.

[95] Maurel C, Verdoucq L, Luu DT, Santoni V. Plant aquaporins: membrane channels with multiple integrated functions. Annu Rev Plant Biol 2008;59:595—624.

[96] Mauro A. The role of negative pressure in osmotic equilibrium and osmotic flow. In: Ussing HH, Bindslev N, Lassen NA, Sten-Knudsen O, editors. Water transport across epithelia. Barriers, gradients and mechanisms. Copenhagen: Munksgaard; 1981. p. 107—19.

[97] Meinild A-K, Klaerke D, Loo DDF, Wright EM, Zeuthen T. The human Na^+/glucose co-transporter is a molecular water pump. J Physiol 1998;508:15—21.

[98] Meinild AK, Loo DD, Pajor AM, Zeuthen T, Wright EM. Water transport by the renal Na^+-dicarboxylate co-transporter. Am J Physiol Renal Physiol 2000;278:F777—83.

[99] Mills JW, DiBona DR. Distribution of Na^+ pump sites in the frog gallbladder. *Nature* (Lond) 1978;271:273—5.

[100] Minton AP, Colclasure GC, Parker JC. Model for the role of macromolecular crowding in regulation of cellular volume. Proc Natl Acad Sci USA 1992;89:10504—6.

[101] Moeller HB, Olesen ET, Fenton RA. Invited review- regulation of the water channel Aquaporin-2 by post-translational modifications. Am J Physiol Renal Physiol 2011;300:F1062—73.

[102] Montalbetti N, Fischbarg J. Frequency spectrum of transepithelial potential difference reveals transport-related oscillations. Biophys J 2009;97:1530—7.

[103] Murata K, Mitsuoka K, Hirai T, Walz T, Agre P, Heymann JB, et al. Structural determinants of water permeation through aquaporin-1. Nature 2000;407:599—605.

[104] Musa-Aziz R, Chen LM, Pelletier MF, Boron WF. Relative CO2/NH3 selectivities of AQP1, AQP4, AQP5, AmtB, and RhAG. Proc Natl Acad Sci USA 2009;106:5406—11.

[105] Muto S, Hata M, Taniguchi J, Tsuruoka S, Moriwaki K, Saitou M, et al. Claudin-2-deficient mice are defective in the leaky and cation-selective paracellular permeability properties of renal proximal tubules. Proc Natl Acad Sci USA 2010;107: 8011—6.

[106] Nakhoul NL, Davis BA, Romero MF, Boron WF. Effect of expressing the water channel aquaporin-1 on the CO_2 permeability of *Xenopus* oocytes. Am J Physiol 1988;45: C543—8.

[107] Nemeth-Cahalan KL, Hall JE. pH and calcium regulate the water permeability of aquaporin 0. J Biol Chem 2000;275: 6777—82.

[108] Nilius B. Is the volume-regulated anion channel VRAC a "water-permeable" channel? Neurochem Res 2004;29:3—8.

[109] Noda Y, Sohara E, Ohta E, Sasaki S. Aquaporins in kidney pathophysiology. Nat Rev Nephrol 2010;6:168—78.

[110] Paganelli CV, Solomon AK. The rate of exchange of tritiated water across the human red cell membrane. J Gen Physiol 1957;41:259—77.

[111] Persson BE, Spring KR. Gallbladder epithelial cell hydraulic water permeability and volume regulation. J Gen Physiol 1982;79:481—505.

[112] Prasad GV, Coury LA, Fin F, Zeidel ML. Reconstituted aquaporin 1 water channels transport CO_2 across membranes. J Biol Chem 1998;273:33123—6.

[113] Preston GM, Agre P. Isolation of the cDNA for erythrocyte integral membrane protein of 28 kilodaltons: member of an ancient channel family. Proc Natl Acad Sci USA 1991;88: 11110—4.

[114] Porquet A, Filella M. Structural evidence of the similarity of $Sb(OH)_3$ and $As(OH)_3$ with glycerol: Implications for their uptake. Chem Res Toxicol 2007;20:1269—76.

[115] Rabaud NE, Song L, Wang Y, Agre P, Yasui M, Carbrey JM. Aquaporin 6 binds calmodulin in a calcium-dependent manner. Biochem Biophys Res Commun 2009;383:54—7.

[116] Rawicz W, Smith BA, McIntosh TJ, Simon SA, Evans E. Elasticity, strength, and water permeability of bilayers that contain raft microdomain-forming lipids. Biophys J 2008;94: 4725—36.

[117] Reeves WB, Andreoli E. Sodium chloride transport in the loop of Henle. In: Seldin DW, Giebisch G, editors. The Kidney: physiology and pathophysiology. New York: Raven Press; 1992. p. 1975—2001.

[118] Reichow SL, Gonen T. Noncanonical binding of calmodulin to aquaporin-0: implications for channel regulation. Structure 2008;16:1389—98.

[119] Ren G, Reddy VS, Cheng A, Melnyk P, Mitra AK. Visualization of a water-selective pore by electron crystallography in vitreous ice. Proc Natl Acad Sci USA 2001;98:1398—403.

[120] Reuss L. Pathways for osmotic water transport in gallbladder epithelium. In: Ussing HH, Fischbarg J, Sten-Knudsen O, Larsen EH, Willumsen NJ, editors. Isotonic transport in leaky epithelia. Copenhagen: Munksgaard; 1993. p. 181—200. Alfred Benzon Symposium 34.

[121] Reuss L. Epithelial transport. In: Hoffman JE, Jamieson, editors. Handbook of physiology: cell physiology. New York: Oxford University Press; 1997. p. 309—38.

[122] Reuss L, Hirst BH. Water transport controversies-an overview. J Physiol 2002;542:1—2.

[123] Reuss L, Cotton CU. Isosmotic fluid transport across epithelia. Contemp Nephrol 1988;4:1—37.

[124] Reuss L, Simon B, Cotton CU. Pseudo-streaming potentials in *Necturus* gallbladder epithelium. II. The mechanism is a junctional diffusion potential. J Gen Physiol 1992;99:317—38.

[125] Reuss L, Simon B, Xi Z. Pseudo-streaming potentials in *Necturus* gallbladder epithelium. I. Paracellular origin of the transepithelial voltage changes. J Gen Physiol 1992;99: 297—316.

[126] Rivers R, Blanchard A, Eladari D, Leviel F, Paillard M, Podevin RA, et al. Water and solute permeabilities of medullary thick ascending limb apical and basolateral membranes. Am J Physiol 1998;274:F453—62.

[127] Rose KM, Wang Z, Magrath GN, Hazard ES, Hildebrandt JD, Schey KL. Aquaporin 0-calmodulin interaction and the effect of aquaporin 0 phosphorylation. Biochemistry 2008;47: 339—47.

[128] Rosenthal R, Milatz S, Krug SM, Oelrich B, Schulzke JD, Amasheh S, et al. Claudin-2, a component of the tight junction, forms a paracellular water channel. J Cell Sci 2010;123: 1913—21.

[129] Roux B, Schulten K. Computational studies of membrane channels. *Structure* (Camb) 2004;12:1343—51.

[130] Sachar-Hill B, Hill AE. Paracellular fluid transport by epithelia. Int Rev Cytol 2002;215:319—50.

[131] Sackin H, Boulpaep EL. Models for coupling of salt and water transport. Proximal tubular reabsorption in *Necturus* kidney. J Gen Physiol 1975;66:671—733.

[132] Sánchez JM, Li Y, Rubanshkin A, Iserovich P, Wen Q, Ruberti JW, et al. Evidence for a central role for electro-osmosis in fluid transport by corneal endothelium. J Membr Biol 2002;187: 37—50.

[133] Saparov SM, Kozono D, Rothe U, Agre P, Pohl P. Water and ion permeation of aquaporin-1 in planar lipid bilayers. J Biol Chem 2001;276:31515—20.

[134] Schultz SG. Homocellular regulatory mechanisms in sodium-transporting epithelia: avoidance of extinction by "flush-through." Am J Physiol 1981;241:F579—90.

[135] Schultz SG, Hudson RL. Biology of sodium-absorbing epithelial cells: dawning of a new era. In: Schultz SG, Field M, Frizzell RA, editors. Handbook of physiology. The gastrointestinal system. New York: Oxford University Press; 1991. p. 45—81.

[136] Shen L, Weber CR, Raleigh DR, Yu D, Turner JR. Tight junction pore and leak pathways: a dynamic duo. Annu Rev Physiol 2011;73:283—309.

[137] Shporer M, Civan MM. Structuring of water and immobilization of ions within the intracellular fluids: the contribution of NMR spectroscopy. Curr Topics Membr Trans 1977;9:1—69.

[138] Smith BL, Agre P. Erythrocyte M_r 28,000 transmembrane protein exists as a multisubunit oligomer similar to channel proteins. J Biol Chem 1991;266:6407—15.

[139] Spring KR. Routes and mechanism of fluid transport by epithelia. Annu Rev Physiol 1998;60:105—19.

[140] Spring KR. Solute recirculation. J Physiol 2002;542:51.

[141] Strange K, Spring KR. Cell membrane permeability of rabbit cortical collecting duct. J Membr Biol 1987;96:27—43.

[142] Sui H, Han BG, Lee JK, Walian P, Jap BK. Structural basis of water-specific transport through the AQP1 water channel. Nature 2001;414:872—8.

[143] Sun AM, Saltzbert SN, Kikeri D, Hebert SC. Mechanisms of cell volume regulation by the mouse medullary thick ascending limb of Henle. Kidney Int 1990;38:1019—29.

[144] Tajkhorshid E, Nollert P, Jensen MO, Miercke LJ, O'Connell J, Stroud RM, et al. Control of the selectivity of the aquaporin water channel family by global orientational tuning. Science 2002;296:525—30.

[145] Törnroth-Horsefield S, Hedfalk K, Fischer G, Lindkvist-Petersson K, Neutze R. Structural insights into eukaryotic aquaporin regulation. FEBS Lett 2010;584:2580.

[146] Tripathi S, Boulpaep EL. Mechanisms of water transport by epithelial cells. Q J Exp Physiol 1989;74:385—417.

[147] Ussing HH, Eskesen K. Mechanism of isotonic water transport in glands. Acta Physiol Scand 1989;136:443—54.

[148] Ussing HH, Lind F, Larsen EH. Ion secretion and isotonic transport in frog skin glands. J Memb Biol 1996;152:101—10.

[149] vant'Hoff JH. Die Rolle des osmotischen Druckes in der Analogie zwischen Lösungen und Gasen. Z Physik Chemie 1887;1:481—93.

[150] Verkman AS. Mechanisms and regulation of water permeability in renal epithelia. Am J Physiol 1989;257:C837—50.

[151] Verkman AS. Aquaporins: translating bench research to human disease. J Exp Biol 2009;212:1707—15.

[152] Verkman AS. Knock-out models reveal new aquaporin functions. Handb Exp Pharmacol 2009;190:359—81.

[153] Verkman AS. Does aquaporin-1 pass gas? An opposing view. J Physiol 2002;542:31.

[154] Verkman AS, van Hoek AN, Ma T, Frigeri A, Skach WR, Mitra A, et al. Water transport across mammalian cell membranes. Am J Physiol 1996;270:C12—30.

[155] Wade JB. Role of membrane traffic in the water and Na^+ responses to vasopressin. Semin Nephrol 1994;14:322—32.

[156] Walz T, Haner M, Wu XR, Henn C, Engel A, Sun TT, et al. Towards the molecular architecture of the asymmetric unit membrane of the mammalian urinary bladder epithelium: a closed "twisted ribbon" structure. J Mol Biol 1995;248:887—900.

[157] Walz T, Fujiyoshi Y, Engel A. The AQP structure and functional implications. Handb Exp Pharmacol 2009;190:31—56.

[158] Walz T, Hirai T, Murata K, Heymann JB, Mitsuoka K, Fujiyoshi Y, et al. The three-dimensional structure of aquaporin-1. Nature 1997;387:624—6.

[159] Walz T, Smith BL, Agre P, Engel A. The 3-D structure of human erythrocyte aquaporin CHIP. EMBO J 1994;13:2985—93.

[160] Wang Y, Tajkhorshid E. Molecular mechanisms of conduction and selectivity in aquaporin water channels. J Nutr 2007;137:1509S—15S.

[161] Weinstein AM, Stephenson JL. Electrolyte transport across a simple epithelium. Steady-state and transient analysis. Biophys J 1979;27:165—86.

[162] Weinstein AM, Stephenson JL. Coupled water transport in standing gradient models of the lateral intercellular space. Biophys J 1981;35:167—91.

[163] Weinstein AM, Stephenson JL. Models of coupled salt and water transport across leaky epithelia. J Membr Biol 1981;60:1—20.

[164] Whittembury G, Rawlins FA. Evidence of a paracellular pathway for ion flow in the kidney proximal tubule: electron microscopic demonstration of lanthanum precipitate in the tight junction. Pflügers Arch 1971;330:302—9.

[165] Whittembury G, Carpi-Medina P, Gonzalez E, Linares H. Effect of parachloromercuribenzene sulfonic acid and temperature on cell water osmotic permeability of proximal straight tubules. Biochim Biophys Acta 1984;775:365—73.

[166] Whittembury G, Hill A. Coupled transport of water and solute across epithelia. In: Seldin DW, Giebisch G, editors. The Kidney: physiology and pathophysiology. New York: Raven Press; 2000. p. 341—62.

[167] Whittembury G, Reuss L. Mechanisms of coupling of solute and solvent transport in epithelia. In: Seldin DW, Giebisch G, editors. The Kidney: physiology and pathophysiology. New York: Raven Press; 1992. p. 317—60.

[168] Windhager EE, Boulpaep EL, Giebisch G. Electrophysiological studies in single nephrons. In: Schreiner GE, editor. Proceedings of the third international congress on nephrology. New York: Karger; 1967. p. 35—47.

[169] Wu XR, Kong XP, Pellicer A, Kreibich G, Sun TT. Uroplakins in urothelial biology, function, and disease. Kidney Int 2009;75:1153—65.

[170] Wu XR, Manabe M, Yu J, Sun TT. Large scale purification and immunolocalization of bovine uroplakins I, II, and III. Molecular markers of urothelial differentiation. J Biol Chem 1990;265:19170—9.

[171] Yang B, Fukuda N, van Hoek A, Matthay MA, Ma T, Verkman AS. Carbon dioxide permeability of aquaporin-1 measured in erthrocytes and lung of aquaporin-1 null mice and in reconstituted liposomes. J Biol Chem 2000;275:2686—92.

[172] Yu J, Manabe M, Wu XR, Xu C, Surya B, Sun TT, et al. A 27-kD protein associated with the asymmetric unit membrane of mammalian urothelium. J Cell Biol 1990;111:1207—16.

[173] Zelenina M, Zelenin S, Bondar AA, Brismar H, Aperia A. Water permeability of aquaporin-4 is decreased by protein kinase C and dopamine. Am J Physiol 2002;283:F309—18.

[174] Zeuthen T. Co-transport of K^+, Cl^- and H_2O by membrane proteins from choroid plexus Epithelium of Necturus maculosus. J Physiol (Lond) 1994;478:203—19.

[175] Zeuthen T. Water-transporting proteins. J Membr Biol 2010;234:57—73.

[176] Zeuthen T, Hamann S, La Cour M. Co-transport of H^1, a lactate and H_2O by membrane proteins in retinal pigment epithelium of bullfrog. J Physiol 1996;497:3—17.

[177] Zeuthen T, Klaerke DA. Transport of water and glycerol in aquaporin 3 is gated by H^1. J Biol Chem 1999;274: 21631—6.

5

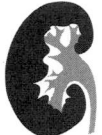

Cell Volume Control

Florian Lang

Department of Physiology, University of Tübingen, Tübingen, Germany

Cells must avoid gross alterations of volume in order to survive. Obviously, excessive cell swelling will jeopardize the integrity of the cell membrane, and both cell swelling and cell shrinkage will interfere with cytoskeletal architecture. Moreover, cellular function critically depends on the hydration of cytosolic proteins. Proteins and protein-bound water occupy a large portion of the cell interior (macromolecular crowding), leaving only a small fraction of cellular volume to free water.[1-6] Abstraction or addition of only a few percentage points of cellular water thus has profound effects on protein function and cellular performance.

In most mammalian cells, the plasma membrane is highly permeable to water,[7,8] a property in large part due to virtually ubiquitous expression of water channels in the cell membrane.[9-11] In theory, driving forces for movement of water include hydrostatic and osmotic pressure gradients. However, the cell membrane is too fragile to withstand significant hydrostatic pressure gradients, and if extension of the cell is not prevented by extracellular constraints the movement of water is governed almost exclusively by osmotic gradients.[12-15] Thus, to avoid swelling or shrinkage, a cell has to achieve osmotic equilibrium across the cell membrane (Figure 5.1). At excessive intracellular osmolarity, water will enter following its osmotic gradient, and the cell will swell. Conversely, at excessive extracellular osmolarity, water will leave, and the cell will shrink. As outlined in this chapter a wide variety of factors modify intra- or extracellular osmolarity, and thus challenge osmotic equilibrium across the cell membrane.

For maintenance of volume constancy, cells employ a number of mechanisms, including metabolism and altered transport across the cell membrane. These mechanisms may also participate in the regulation of cell function. Hormones and mediators may influence cell volume regulatory mechanisms, and thus

manipulate cell volume. Alterations of cell volume will in turn modify other cell volume-sensitive functions. The interplay among cell volume regulatory mechanisms, cell hydration, and cell function does not only contribute to physiological regulation of cellular function, but also participates in the pathophysiology of a wide variety of diseases.

In this chapter a description of cell volume regulatory mechanisms will be followed by a synopsis of factors challenging cell volume constancy, and a discussion on the impact of cell volume regulatory mechanisms on the physiology and pathophysiology of cellular function. Due to space constraints, many excellent original papers on cell volume regulation could not be cited, and the reader is referred to reviews instead. For more detailed analysis of the pertinent original literature, the reader is encouraged to consult previous reviews on cell volume regulation.[16-41]

CELL VOLUME REGULATORY MECHANISMS

Cell volume constancy is challenged by alterations of extracellular osmolarity, by intracellular metabolic generation of osmotically active solutes and by transport across the cell membrane.[31] To counteract those challenges, cells employ a variety of cell volume regulatory mechanisms.[32] Following cell swelling, these mechanisms decrease intracellular osmolarity and cell volume, thus accomplishing regulatory cell volume decrease (RVD). Upon cell shrinkage the mechanisms increase intracellular osmolarity and cell volume, thereby accomplishing regulatory cell volume increase (RVI). Upon slow changes of extracellular osmolarity, the volume regulatory mechanisms may be fast

Seldin and Giebisch's The Kidney, Fifth Edition.
DOI: http://dx.doi.org/10.1016/B978-0-12-381462-3.00005-7

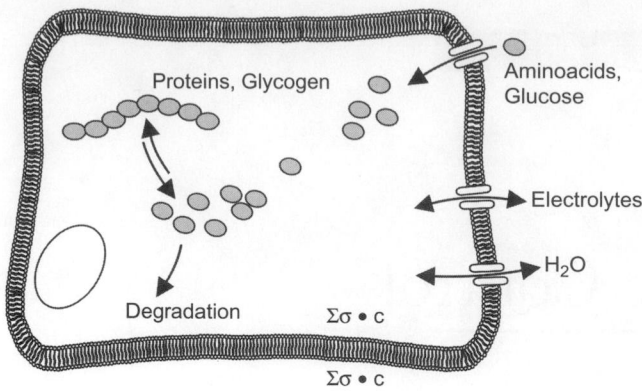

FIGURE 5.1 Determinants of cell volume. Water moves according to osmotic gradients across the cell membranes, that is, differences between intracellular and extracellular $\sum\sigma.c$, where σ is the reflection coefficient and c the concentration of each solute on either side. Even at constant extracellular $\sum\sigma.c$, an osmotic gradient is generated by transport of osmotically active solutes across the cell membrane and by metabolic generation or disposal of intracellular solutes.

enough to prevent significant alterations of cell volume, leading to isovolumetric volume regulation.[42]

The most powerful mechanisms of cell volume regulation are ion transporters in the cell membrane.[32] As outlined below, uneven ion composition of intracellular and extracellular fluid is one prerequisite for the establishment of osmotic equilibrium across the cell membrane. Furthermore, several ion transport systems in the cell membrane are modified upon alterations of cell volume. Following cell swelling they mediate cellular ion release; upon cell shrinkage they allow cellular ion accumulation to re-establish osmotic equilibrium across the cell membrane.

However, the use of ions in cellular osmoregulation is limited, since high inorganic ion concentrations interfere with the stability of proteins.[43] Beyond that, altered ion gradients across the cell membrane interfere with the function of gradient-driven transporters. For instance, an increase of intracellular Na^+ activity decreases the chemical gradient for Na^+ across the cell membrane, and reduces the driving force for Ca^{2+} extrusion via the Na^+/Ca^{2+} exchanger, which increases intracellular Ca^{2+} activity. To avoid excessive alterations of intracellular ion concentration, cells also utilize organic osmolytes for osmoregulation.[20,21,44] Moreover, cells adapt a variety of metabolic functions, and thus modify the cellular generation or disposal of osmotically active organic substances.

It should be pointed out that a single cell does not usually employ all cell volume regulatory mechanisms described in the following text. In most cases, it is not clear why a given cell selects a certain set of ion

transporters and osmolytes without using other mechanisms. Presumably, the large repertoire of cell volume regulatory transporters and osmolytes available enables any given cell to regulate its volume with relatively little impairment of its particular function.

Cell Volume Regulatory Ion Transport

To counterbalance the intracellular osmolarity due to osmotically active organic solutes, such as amino acids and carbohydrates, cell volume regulatory mechanisms need to maintain intracellular concentrations of inorganic ions below extracellular ion concentrations. In addition, cell volume regulatory ion transport systems are employed to counteract alterations of cell volume by appropriate transport of ions across the cell membrane.

Ions in Cell Volume Maintenance

To compensate for the cellular accumulation of organic solutes, cells maintain a low intracellular Cl^- concentration.[31] In most cells, Cl^- may move across the cell membrane through Cl^- channels. Cl^- movement through those channels is governed by the cell's negative potential across the cell membrane, which is built up by asymmetric cation gradients[8]: the cells extrude Na^+ in exchange for K^+ by the Na^+/K^+-ATPase. The cell membrane is, on average, less permeable to Na^+ than to K^+. K^+ tends to leave the cell through K^+ channels following its chemical gradient. The exit of K^+ generates a cell-negative potential difference across the cell membrane, and thus establishes the driving force for the exit of anions such as Cl^-. At a cell membrane potential of some $-18\,mV$, for instance, Cl^- is in equilibrium at a chemical gradient of 1:2. Accordingly, at an extracellular Cl^- concentration of 110 mmol/L, the intracellular Cl^- concentration is in electrochemical equilibrium at 55 mmol/L. In theory, such a Cl^- distribution would allow the excess accumulation of 55 mmol/L of organic solutes. In most cells the potential difference across the cell membrane is higher (more negative) than $-18\,mV$, and intracellular Cl^- is even lower than 55 mmol/L.

As long as the cell membrane is perfectly impermeable to Na^+, cell membrane potential, cytosolic Cl^- concentration, and cell volume could be maintained constant without continued expenditure of energy. Maintenance of the asymmetric cation distribution requires, however, that any Na^+ entering the cell is subsequently extruded by Na^+/K^+-ATPase, an ATP-consuming process.

Ion Release Following Cell Swelling

Ion transport is not only crucial for the establishment of osmotic equilibrium across the cell membrane, but accomplishes rapid correction of any osmotic imbalance across the cell membrane. Following cell swelling, cells must release ions to decrease their osmolarity. Most cells release ions by activation of K^+ channels and/or anion channels (Figure 5.2). Cell volume regulation requires the operation of both ion channel types, since neither K^+ nor anions can leave the cells without the respective counterion. Several cell volume regulatory ion channels have been identified at the molecular level, including the K^+ channels Kv1.3,[45] Kv1.5,[46] Kv4.2, 3,[47] IsK or KCNE1/Q1,4,5,[26,48–51] TWIK1,[52] TASK2/KCNK5,[53] TREK1/KCNK2,[26] TRAAK/KCNK4,[26] intermediate or MaxiK (Kca),[26,54] and the anion channels ClC-2,[55–59] ClC-3,[60,61] phospholemman,[62] and bestrophins.[63] The role of other ion channels in cell volume regulation, such as I_{Cln},[64–66] P-glycoprotein (MDR),[67–70] and CFTR,[71,72] has been a matter of controversy. Clearly, many different ion channels are likely to contribute to cell volume regulation in various tissues, and the molecular identity of some of those channels is still elusive. Some anion channels not only allow the exit of Cl^-, but also of HCO_3^-, organic anions, and noncharged osmolytes.[73–80]

Swelling of some cells activates unspecific cation channels, including some transient receptor potential (TRP) channels.[15,32,81–87] Since the electrochemical gradient favors entry rather than exit of cations, these channels cannot directly serve cell volume regulation. Instead, the channels allow the entry of Ca^{2+}, which in turn activates Ca^{2+}-sensitive K^+ channels and/or Cl^- channels.

Besides ion channels, the most important mechanism contributing to regulatory cell volume decrease is KCl co-transport by one of the four members of the KCC family,[88,89,90–94] which allows coupled cellular release of both ions.

Some cells release cellular KCl via parallel activation of $K^+–H^+$ exchange and $Cl^-–HCO_3^-$ exchange.[95,96] The H^+ and HCO_3^- thus taken up in exchange for KCl react via H_2CO_3 to produce CO_2, which can easily leave the cell again.

Water efflux during volume regulatory decrease could be fully accomplished by existing water channels. Nevertheless, aquaporins participate in cell volume regulation by modifying the activity of ion channels.[9]

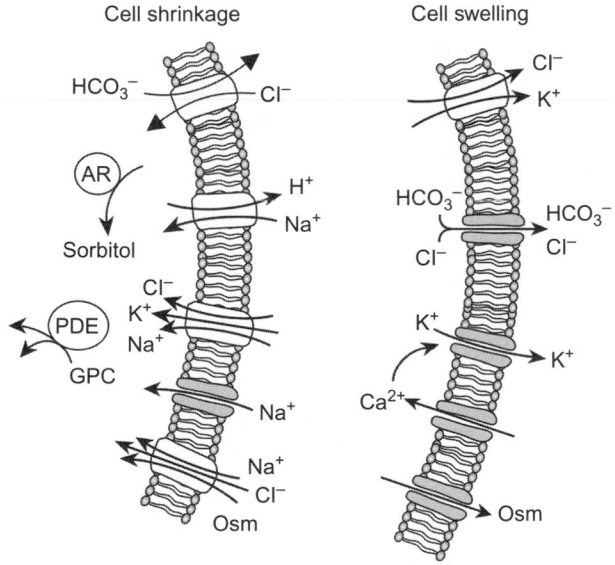

Ion Uptake upon Cell Shrinkage

Cell shrinkage activates the $Na^+–K^+–2Cl^-$ co-transporters NKCC1, and NKCC2,[97–100] and/or the Na^+/H^+ exchangers NHE1,[101] NHE2[102] or NHE4[103] parallel to the $Cl^-HCO_3^-$ exchanger AE1.[36,104,105] The parallel activation of Na^+/H^+ exchangers and Cl^-/HCO_3^- exchangers leads to uptake of NaCl, while the H^+ and HCO_3^- lost in exchange for NaCl are replenished in the cell from CO_2 via H_2CO_3 (Figure 5.2). The epithelial Na^+/H^+ exchanger NHE3 is inhibited by cell shrinkage.[106] The Na^+ ions accumulated by either $Na^+–K^+–2Cl^-$ co-transport or Na^+H^+ exchange are extruded by Na^+K^+-ATPase in exchange for K^+. Accordingly, the transporters eventually lead to cellular KCl uptake.

Several cells activate Na^+ channels or unspecific cation channels following cell shrinkage.[107–112] The channels may include some members of the transient receptor potential (TRP) channel family or ENaC.[113–116,181] The resulting depolarization drives Cl^- into the cell, so that the net effect is cellular accumulation of NaCl. Other cells inhibit K^+ and/or Cl^- channels to avoid cellular ion loss.[32]

FIGURE 5.2 **Most widely employed mechanisms of regulatory cell volume regulation.** Left: Mechanisms of regulatory cell volume decrease. Cell swelling leads to activation of KCl co-transport, anion channels, K^+ channels, cation channels, and channels releasing organic osmolytes such as sorbitol, inositol, taurine, and betaine. The cation channels do not directly serve cell volume regulatory decrease, but rather increase of cytosolic Ca^+ activity that triggers activation of Ca^{2+} sensitive K^+ channels. Right: Mechanisms of cell volume increase. Cell shrinkage leads to parallel activation of Na^+/H^+ exchanger and Cl^-/HCO_3^- exchanger, $Na^+K^+2Cl^-$ co-transport, Na^+ channels, and Na^+-coupled accumulation of inositol, taurine, and betaine. Furthermore, cell shrinkage leads to cellular accumulation of glycerophosphorylcholine by inhibition of phosphodiesterase (PDE), and of sorbitol by activation of aldosereducase (AR).

Osmolytes

The most important osmolytes are polyols such as sorbitol and myoinositol, methylamines such as betaine and glycerophosphorylcholine, as well as amino acids including taurine.[3,21,28,41,44,117,118] In contrast to inorganic ions, organic osmolytes do not destabilize proteins, but rather stabilize them. They counteract the destabilizing effects of inorganic ions, some organic ions (e.g., spermidine), and urea.[3,18] The stabilizing potency of the diverse organic osmolytes is not identical. The destabilizing effects of urea are counteracted most efficiently by betaine and glycerophosphorylcholine, and less efficiently by myoinositol.[18] The stabilizing effects of osmolytes may protect proteins against excessive ion concentrations, as well as against heat shock, freezing, desiccation, and presumably radiation.[119–123]

Osmolyte Accumulation by Metabolism

Sorbitol is generated from glucose under the catalytic action of aldose reductase.[124–126] Stimulation of the transcription rate of the aldose reductase during osmotic cell shrinkage leads to cellular accumulation of sorbitol. The expression of the protein takes many hours, and the appropriate increase of sorbitol concentration requires hours to days.[127]

Glycerophosphorylcholine (GPC) is produced from phosphatidylcholine under the catalytic action of a phospholipase A_2, which is distinct from the arachidonyl selective enzyme.[21,128] GPC is degraded by a phosphodiesterase to glycerol-phosphate and choline. Inhibition of the phosphodiesterase during cell shrinkage leads to cellular accumulation of GPC.[129]

Osmolyte Accumulation by Transport

Myoinositol (inositol),[28,130–133] betaine[134–136] and taurine[137] are taken up by specific Na^+-coupled transporters SMIT (inositol), BGT (betaine), and NCT (taurine), respectively. The carriers accumulate Na^+, the respective organic osmolyte, and in the case of BGT and NCT, Cl^- as well. Movement of excess positive charge by the carriers depolarizes the cell membrane, thus favoring entry of Cl^- via anion channels. The transporters thus mediate uptake of NaCl parallel to organic osmolytes. The transcription rate of the transporters and the cellular accumulation of the respective osmolytes are stimulated by osmotic cell shrinkage. Expression of the transporters is slow, and full adaptation requires hours to days. Moreover, volume regulation by activation of transport systems depends on the availability of osmolytes in the extracellular fluid.

Analogous to osmolytes, some amino acids are accumulated by cell volume-sensitive, Na^+-coupled transport.[138–140] In addition, amino acids could be generated by autophagic proteolysis, as discussed in the next section.

Osmolyte Release

Cell swelling stimulates the rapid release of GPC,[27,141] sorbitol,[142–144] inositol,[27,145] betaine,[27,145] and taurine.[77,146–150] The mechanisms mediating osmolyte release are still poorly understood. Clearly, several mechanisms are simultaneously operative. At least some of the release mechanisms are thought to be anion channels. As shown for taurine,[147] the osmolyte release could be triggered by oxidative stress.

Metabolic Pathways Sensitive to Cell Volume

Alterations of cell volume influence a variety of metabolic pathways. The effects of cell volume on metabolism are accomplished in part by activation and inhibition, and in part by altered expression of enzymes.[31]

Protein and Glycogen Metabolism

Cell shrinkage stimulates the breakdown of proteins to amino acids, and of glycogen to glucosephosphate.[24,151–154] Moreover, cell shrinkage inhibits protein and glycogen synthesis.[153,154] The sum of amino acids generated during proteolysis is osmotically more active than the osmolarity of the respective protein. Thus, net formation of macromolecules decreases, and net degradation of macromolecules enhances, cellular osmolarity. Cell swelling stimulates protein and glycogen synthesis, and inhibits proteolysis and glycogenolysis, thus decreasing the intracellular concentration of amino acids and glucosephosphate.

Glucose and Amino Acid Metabolism

In addition to affecting protein and glycogen metabolism, alterations of cell volume influence several pathways of glucose and amino acid metabolism.[154] Cell swelling inhibits glucose uptake and glycolysis, stimulates flux through the pentose phosphate pathway, and favors lipogenesis from glucose, effects reversed by cell shrinkage.[154–156] Transcription of phosphoenolpyruvate carboxykinase, a key enzyme for gluconeogenesis, is decreased by cell swelling. Cell swelling stimulates glycine and alanine oxidation and glutamine breakdown, as well as formation of NH_4^+ and urea from amino acids; these effects are reversed by cell shrinkage.[154]

Oxidative Metabolism

The stimulation of flux through the pentose phosphate pathway during cell swelling enhances NADPH production, which favors the formation of glutathione (GSH).[154,156] Cell shrinkage decreases NADPH production and GSH formation. Accordingly, cell swelling increases and cell shrinkage decreases cellular resistance to oxidative stress. On the other hand, cell swelling stimulates, and cell shrinkage decreases, the activity of NADPH-oxidase, thus modulating cellular O_2^- formation.[157,158] Accordingly, leukocyte oxidative burst, and thus immune response, is blunted by the high osmolarity of kidney medulla.[159,160]

Other Metabolic Pathways

Cell swelling stimulates ketoisocaproate oxidation, acetyl CoA carboxylase, and lipogenesis, and inhibits carnitine palmitoyltransferase I. It decreases cytosolic ATP and phosphocreatine concentrations, and increases respiration. Cell swelling stimulates RNA and DNA synthesis. All of these effects are reversed by cell shrinkage.[31]

Cell Volume-Sensitive Genes

Cell volume influences the transcription of a wide variety of genes,[31,44,117,161] leading to differential expression of a wide variety of proteins.[162,163] Transcription factors involved include AP1, c-FOS, cJUN, tonicity-response enhancer binding protein TONEBP, serum response factor (SRF), and myocardin related transcription factor.[26,161] Many of the cell volume-regulated genes are related to cell volume regulation. Accordingly, cell shrinkage stimulates expression of enzymes or transporters engaged in cellular formation or accumulation of osmolytes, such as aldose reductase, and the Na^+-coupled transporters for betaine (BGT), taurine (NCT), myoinositol (SMIT), and amino acids, as well as $Na^+,K^+,2Cl^-$ co-transport (see above). Moreover, cell shrinkage upregulates the expression of the ATPase α1-subunit.[164]

The products of other genes may be involved in the signaling of cell volume regulatory mechanisms, such as the kinases ERK1, ERK2, and JNK-1, which are expressed during cell swelling[165] or the serum and glucocorticoid inducible kinase SGK1[166,167] and cyclo-oxygenase-2,[168] which are preferably expressed in shrunken cells.[31]

Heat shock proteins serve to stabilize proteins, and their expression in shrunken cells may counteract the destabilizing effects of accumulated ions.[169–173] Several genes expressed in response to altered cell volume do not have obvious roles in cell volume regulation.

Cell swelling stimulates the expression of the cytoskeletal elements β-actin and tubulin, the immediate early genes c-jun and c-fos, the enzyme ornithine decarboxylase, and the cytokine TNF-α.[165,174,175]

Cell shrinkage stimulates the expression of the channels ClC-K1, the transporter P-glycoprotein, the immediate early genes Egr-1 and c-fos, the GTPase inhibitor α1-chimaerin, the CDβ antigen, the enzymes phosphoenolpyruvate carboxykinase (PEPCK), arginine succinate lyase, tyrosine aminotransferase, tyrosine hydroxylase, dopamine β-hydroxylase, matrix metalloproteinase 9, tissue plasminogen activator, as well as matrix proteins including biglycan and laminin B_2.[31] Cell shrinkage stimulates both expression and release of ADH, which serves to eliminate water and thus increase extracellular osmolarity.[176]

The mechanisms mediating the altered gene expression are beginning to be understood. The promoter region of the genes encoding aldose reductase, BGT, TAUT, and SGK1 have been ascribed to contain osmolarity responsive (ORE), tonicity responsive (TonE) or cell volume-responsive (CVE) elements, which are required for osmolarity or cell volume-sensitive expression of the respective genes.[125,177,178] TonE has been shown to bind a tonicity-responsive element-binding protein (TonEBP) for stimulation of expression.[179–186] TonEBP is regulated by ataxia teleangiectasia-mutated (ATM) kinase.[181]

Signaling of Cell Volume Regulation

The stimulation of effectors of cell volume regulation requires that alterations of cell volume or osmolarity are perceived and trigger a signaling cascade, eventually leading to stimulation of cell volume regulatory mechanisms.

Little is known about sensors of cell size and hydration. Circumstantial evidence points to the ability of cells to determine cellular protein content or macromolecular crowding.[187] It has been speculated that macromolecular crowding directly or indirectly regulates kinases which in turn influence the activity of cell volume regulatory KCl and $Na^+-K^+-2Cl^-$ co-transport (see below).[31] Alternatively, alterations of ionic strength or the concentration of individual ions such as Cl^- modify volume regulatory mechanisms.[26] Moreover, alterations of cell size are thought to impose stretch on the cytoskeleton and/or cell membrane or change the curvature of the cell membrane,[188–190] again leading directly or indirectly to activation of cell volume regulatory mechanisms.[31,191,192] Cell swelling leads to unfolding of the cell membrane and, if this does not suffice, to endomembrane insertion. Alterations of cell volume could be further sensed by cytokine[193] and Ca^{2+} sensing receptors,[194] as well as by integrins.[26]

A multitude of signaling pathways link the alterations of cell volume and cell volume regulatory mechanisms. The respective signaling varies considerably between different cells or a given cell in different functional states.

Intracellular Ca^{2+}

Cell swelling increases intracellular Ca^{2+} activity in many, but not all, cells. Ca^{2+} enters through Ca^{2+} channels in the plasma membrane, and/or is released from intracellular stores triggered by 1,4,5-inositol-trisphosphate. The channels involved include nonselective Ca^{2+} channels, Ca^{2+} permeable members of the TRP (transient receptor potential) channel family, such as TRPV4, and L-type voltage gated Ca^{2+} channels.[41,113,195,196] Ca^{2+} in turn activates some cell volume regulatory K^+ channels and Cl^- channels.[197–199] In addition to its involvement in regulatory cell volume decrease, intracellular Ca^{2+} may mediate some of the functional consequences of cell shrinkage.

Cytoskeleton

Alterations of cell volume modify the architecture of the cytoskeleton and the expression of cytoskeletal proteins.[200–204] Cell shinkage increases and cell swelling decreases actin polymerization. Both microtubules[200] and actin filaments[201] have been implicated in cell volume regulation. In several cells, disruption of actin filaments and/or the microtubule network have been shown to interfere with cell volume regulation.[31]

Protein Phosphorylation

Cell swelling and cell shrinkage have both been shown to modify the phosphorylation of a variety of proteins. Kinases reported to be activated during cell swelling include tyrosine kinases,[205–209] protein kinase-C,[210,211] phosphoinositide (PI) 3 kinase,[212] Jun-kinase, and extracellular signal-regulated kinases ERK-1 and ERK-2,[165,208,213–219] as well as focal adhesion kinase (p121^{FAK}).[212] Activation of PI3 kinase leads to stimulation of protein kinase B (Akt), and serum and glucocorticoid inducible kinase isoforms, which modify a wide variety of carriers and channels.[220] Expression of SGK1 is, however, downregulated by cell swelling, and thus SGK1 dependent signaling is disrupted.[220] In Jurkat lymphocytes, cell swelling leads to activation of the src-like kinase lck,[56] which in turn activates the cell volume regulatory Cl^- channel ORCC.[206]

Osmotic cell shrinkage stimulates WNK (with no lysine kinase) 1 and 4, which in turn activate Ste-20-related proline alanine rich kinase (SPAK) and oxidative stress responsive kinase (OSR1).[222–224] SPAK and OSR1 activate the Na^+-K^+-$2Cl^-$ co-transporters NKCC1 and NKCC2.[222,223,225] Conversely, WNK4 inhibits KCl co-transporters.[226] WNK1 activates SGK1, which in turn inhibits WNK4.[227,228] Osmotic cell shrinkage further triggers several MAP (mitogen-activated protein) kinase cascades, and activates SAPK, p38 kinase, myosin light-chain-kinase (MLCK), Jun kinase (JNK), p21-activated kinases PAKs Rho kinase, LIM kinase, and casein kinase.[193,229–239] MLCK may modulate the cytoskeleton, and thus cell volume regulatory ion transport. Moreover, the kinase cascades lead to activation of transcription factors governing expression of cell volume-regulated genes.[31] Hyperosmolarity activates the tyrosine kinase Fyn-dependent phosphorylation of caveolin,[240] which in turn inhibits volume-sensitive Cl^- channels.[241]

Phosphatidylinositol 4,5,-Bisphosphate

Cell swelling decreases and cell shrinkage increases the formation of phosphatidylinositol 4,5 bisphosphate $(PtdIns(4,5)P_2)^{242}$ by the phosphatidylinositol 4-phosphate 5-kinase beta isoform (PIP5KIbeta).[243] Among other effects, $PtdIns(4,5)P_2$ stimulates the transient receptor potential channel TRPV1, Na^+/H^+ exchanger NHE1, the Na^+/Ca^{2+} exchanger NCX, and the Na^+ channel ENaC, and inhibits the transient receptor potential channel TRPC6.[26,244] $PtdIns(4,5)P_2$ may further foster actin polymerization by inhibiting the monomer-binding protein profilin, the severing protein cofilin, the capping protein gelsolin, as well as the Wiskott–Aldrich syndrome protein (WASP).[26,245]

Phospholipase A_2 and Eicosanoids

Cell swelling activates phospholipase A_2 and subsequently stimulates the formation of the 15-lipoxygenase product hepoxilin A_3, and the 5-lipoxygenase product leukotriene LTD_4.[246] Phospholipase A2 is phosphorylated by casein kinases CK1 and CK2, protein kinase A, protein kinase C, and mitogen activated kinases.[247–249] In some cells the eicosanoids generated following ativation of phospholipase A_2 stimulate cell volume regulatory K^+, Cl^- channels, and/or taurine release.[246] Enhanced formation of leukotrienes parallels decreased formation of PGE_2, with subsequent decrease of Na^+ channel activity.[246,250] Conversely, osmotic cell shrinkage may stimulate formation of PGE_2, with subsequent activation of PGE_2-sensitive Na^+ channels.[251] In other cells PGE_2 may activate volume regulatory K^+ channels.[252] In erythrocytes, activation of phospholipase A_2 by hyperosmotic shock leads to release of platelet-activating factor PAF, which in turn activates a sphingomyelinase, thus stimulating ceramide formation.[253]

pH of Acidic Cellular Compartments

In all cells studied thus far, swelling alkalinizes and cell shrinkage acidifies acidic cellular compartments, presumably including endosomes, lysosomes, and secretory granules.[31,254] This effect is apparently mediated by the microtubules, since it is abolished by disruption of the microtubule network. The alkalinization of the acidic cellular compartments may contribute to the antiproteolytic action of cell swelling, since the pH optimum of lysosomal proteases is in the acidic range, and lysosomal alkalinization has indeed been shown to inhibit proteolysis.[255]

Others

Several G-proteins have been implicated in cell volume regulation including Rho, Rac, and Ras.[26,256,257] Hyperosmotic cell shrinkage further activates ezrin/radixin/moesin (ERM) proteins, which in turn mitigate the shrinkage-induced activation of NHE1, augment Rho activity, and presumably modify actin architecture.[258] Cell swelling may trigger release of ATP, which in turn leads to autocrine stimulation of purinergic receptors with the respective activation of cell volume regulatory ion channels.[259]

CHALLENGES AND FUNCTIONS AFFECTING CELL VOLUME

A wide variety of factors alters extracellular and/or intracellular osmolarity, and thus challenges cell volume constancy. Due to the exquisite sensitivity of cell function to even minor alterations of cell volume, those factors may modify a multitude of physiological functions and participate in several pathophysiological conditions.

Alterations of Extracellular Fluid Osmolarity and Composition

In mammals, most cells are usually bathed in well-controlled extracellular fluid. However, both extracellular osmolarity and composition could vary to an extent, challenging cell volume regulation.

Osmolarity

Excessive alterations of extracellular osmolarity are only encountered in kidney medulla, where extracellular osmolarity may approach 1400 mosmol/L in humans (see Chapter 40). Renal medullary cells are exposed to this excessive extracellular osmolarity during antidiuresis, and have to cope with rapid changes of extracellular osmolarity during transition from antidiuresis to diuresis. Blood cells passing the kidney medulla experience high medullary osmolarity and subsequent return to isoosmolarity within seconds (see Chapter 40).

During intestinal absorption, intestinal cells are exposed to anisosmotic luminal fluid, and liver cells to minor alterations of portal blood osmolarity. Other tissues are exposed to anisotonic extracellular fluid during deranged regulation of extracellular osmolarity (see Chapters 41 and 42). As Na$^+$ salts (mainly NaCl) contribute normally more than 90% to extracellular osmolarity, hypernatremia is necessarily paralleled by an increase in extracellular osmolarity (see Chapter 42). During hypernatremia, cells defend themselves against increased extracellular osmolarity by triggering regulatory cell volume increase involving cellular accumulation of osmolytes. Owing to cell volume regulation, cell volume may become normal despite enhanced extracellular osmolarity. Rapid correction of chronically enhanced osmolarity may then lead to deleterious cell swelling, since the organic osmolytes accumulated during hyperosmolarity cannot be rapidly released. The most serious consequence is cerebral edema.

Hyponatremia cannot be equated with hypoosmolarity, but may occur in isoosmolar or even hyperosmolar states, as in hyperglycemia of uncontrolled diabetes mellitus and ethanol poisoning (see Chapter 44). When hyponatremia reflects a decreased extracellular osmolarity, the cells must undergo regulatory cell volume decrease to escape cell swelling. Among other mechanisms, cells release organic osmolytes. Upon rapid correction of hyponatremia, cells are unable to rapidly accumulate the osmolytes, and the iatrogenic cell shrinkage may prove more harmful than the untreated hypoosmolarity.

Hypoosmolar hyponatremia is observed following burns, pancreatitis, and crush syndrome, which are generally paralleled by cell shrinkage.[24] In those conditions, the primary event may be cell shrinkage leading to ADH release with subsequent renal water retention and to cellular catabolism with enhanced release of organic solutes to the extracellular fluid.

Extracellular K$^+$ Concentration

The potential difference across the cell membrane is maintained by K$^+$ flux through K$^+$ channels, which in turn depends on the electrochemical driving force for K$^+$. An increase of extracellular K$^+$ concentration decreases the chemical gradient for K$^+$ ions, impedes K$^+$ efflux, depolarizes the cell membrane, and thus favors Cl$^-$ entry into the cell. The cellular accumulation of KCl eventually leads to cell swelling. Conversely, a decrease of extracellular K$^+$ may lead to cell shrinkage secondary to cellular loss of KCl.[31]

H^+ and HCO_3^- Concentration

On increase of extracellular HCO_3^- concentration, cellular HCO_3^- release through anion channels and Na^+–HCO_3^- co-transport is blunted or even reversed, and the decreased efflux of negative charge hyperpolarizes the cell membrane, and thus decreases the electrochemical gradient for K^+ efflux. As a result, the cell may swell due to accumulation of K^+ and HCO_3^-.[260]

An increasing extracellular pH favors cellular H^+ elimination through the Na^+/H^+ exchanger, and the resulting cellular Na^+ accumulation may lead to cell swelling.[261] During hyperkapnea, cellular CO_2 dissociates to form H^+, which is subsequently extruded by the Na^+/H^+ exchanger. Again, cellular Na^+ accumulation is paralleled by cell swelling. Due to sensitivity of the Na^+/H^+ exchanger to intracellular pH, cellular acidification favors cell swelling, whereas cellular alkalinization has the opposite effect.[262]

Organic Acids

Some organic anions, such as acetate, lactate, and proprionate, may enter cells as unionized acids. Intracellular dissociation of the acids then leads to intracellular acidification, stimulation of Na^+/H^+ exchange, accumulation of Na^+ and organic anions, and subsequent cell swelling.[31] Isotonic replacement of Cl^- with impermeant gluconate, on the other hand, leads to cell shrinkage due to cellular loss of Cl^-.[31]

Urea, Drugs, and Toxins

Urea readily passes cell membranes, and does not usually create osmotic gradients across them. On the other hand, it has been shown that urea destabilizes proteins, and thus shifts the cell volume regulatory set point towards smaller cell volumes. Through activation of some cell volume regulatory mechanisms, such as KCl co-transport, urea shrinks cells, as shown for erythrocytes, hepatocytes, renal cells, and vascular smooth muscle cells.[31]

Beyond these mechanisms, cell volume is influenced by a wide variety of drugs and toxins, interfering with cell volume regulatory mechanisms.[31] For instance, inhibition of K^+ channels leads to cell swelling, and inhibition of Na^+–K^+2Cl^- co-transport and/or Na^+/H^+ exchanger leads to cell shrinkage.

Functional States Affecting Cell Volume Control

Even at normal extracellular osmolarity and composition, osmotic gradients across the cell membrane could arise from unbalanced transport across the cell membrane, and from intracellular generation or disposal of osmotically active solutes. Cellular conditions and functions affecting intracellular osmolarity thus impact on cell volume control (Figure 5.3).

Energy Depletion

Impairment of Na^+/K^+-ATPase function, such as during pharmacological inhibition, energy depletion or decrease of ambient temperature, eventually leads to cell swelling due to cellular Na^+ accumulation, dissipation of the K^+ gradient, depolarization, and subsequent accumulation of Cl^-.[31] In some cells, the

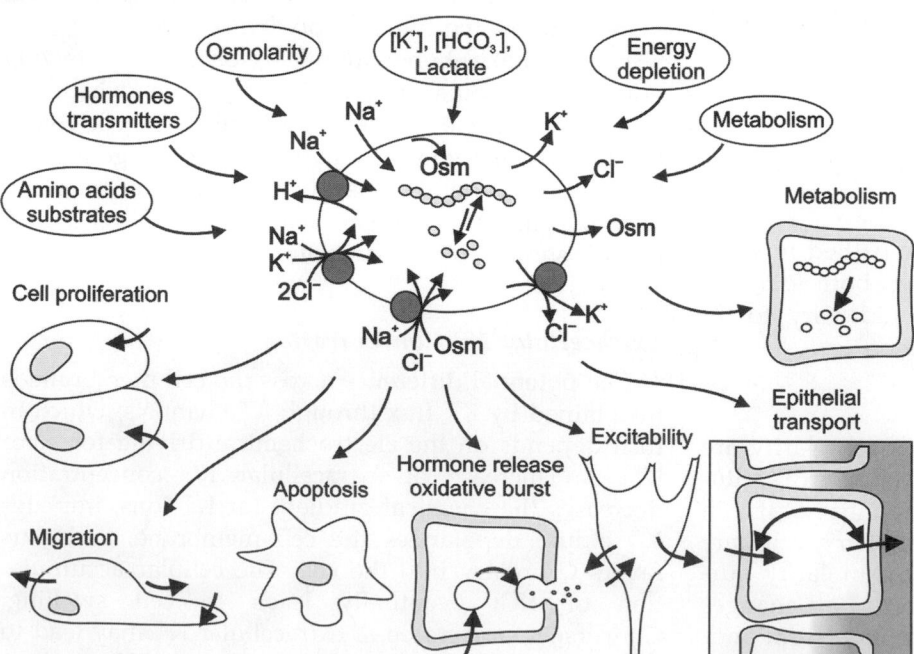

FIGURE 5.3 **Synopsis of challenges of cell volume constancy and functional significance of cell volume regulatory mechanisms.** Cell volume is altered by concentrative uptake of amino acids and additional substrates, alterations of ion transport by hormones and transmitters, changes of extracellular osmolarity, alterations of extracellular K^+, HCO_3^- and organic acid concentrations, energy depletion, and metabolic generation or disposal of osmolarity. Altered cell volume, as well as cell volume regulatory transport and metabolism, participate in the regulation of cell proliferation, migration, apoptosis, hormone release and oxidative burst, neuromuscular excitability, epithelial transport, and metabolism.

swelling is preceded by transient cell shrinkage.[263,264,265] The increase of intracellular Na^+ concentration reverses the driving force for the Na^+/Ca^{2+} exchanger; the increase of intracellular Ca^{2+} activity in turn leads to activation of Ca^{2+}-sensitive K^+ channels and/or Cl^- channels, as well as contraction of cytoskeletal elements.

Transport

Most epithelial cells are faced with large transcellular fluxes of osmotically active substances (see Chapter 2). To cope with transcellular transport, the cells have to coordinate the various transport systems at the apical and basolateral cell membranes. In both reabsorbing and secreting epithelia, cell volume participates in the coupling of those transport processes.

In proximal renal tubules[266] and intestine[267] for instance, Na^+-coupled transport of substrates such as amino acids or glucose across the luminal cell membrane leads to cellular accumulation of Na^+ and substrate. Moreover, the entry of excess positive charge leads to depolarization, impeding the exit of Cl^- and HCO_3^-, thus favoring cell swelling. In Na^+ reabsorbing epithelia, such as renal collecting duct and colon, entry of Na^+ via Na^+ channels similarly challenges cell volume constancy. Limitation of cell swelling during stimulated Na^+ transport requires the operation of cell volume regulatory mechanisms, including activation of K^+ channels, which in turn maintain the electrical driving force for Na^+ entry into the cell.[266,267] Activation of Cl^- and/or K^+ channels in several Cl^- secreting epithelia is paralleled by decrease of intracellular Cl^- activity and cell shrinkage, which in turn stimulate $Na^+-K^+-2Cl^-$ co-transport and/or Na^+H^+ exchanger with Cl^-/HCO_3^- exchanger.[268-271]

The influence of Na^+-coupled transport on cell volume is not limited to epithelial cells. In several epithelial and nonepithelial cells, concentrated uptake of substrates such as amino acids, glucose, taurine, and taurocholate increases cell volume.[31]

Deranged transport participates in disordered function of erythrocytes in sickle cell disease. In this disorder, a point mutation of hemoglobin (HbS) favors polymerization of desoxyhemoglobin, dramatically decreasing erythrocyte deformability and increasing blood viscosity.[272] The depolymerization of hemoglobin is critically dependent on cell volume. Cell shrinkage due to enhanced ambient osmolarity, activation of KCl co-transport by urea or activation of Ca^{2+}-sensitive K^+ channels by a rise in intracellular Ca^{2+} activity potentiates polymerization of HbS. The high osmolarity and urea concentration in kidney medulla thus contribute to the particular vulnerability of this tissue to ischemia in sickle cell anemia. Cell shrinkage and subsequent triggering of erythrocyte cell membrane scrambling (see below) presumably participate in accelerated erythrocyte turnover in various anemic conditions.[273]

Influence of Hormones and Transmitters on Cell Volume

A wide variety of hormones and other mediators have been shown to alter cell volume.[31] Insulin swells liver cells by activation of both Na^+/H^+ exchange and $Na^+-K^+2Cl^-$ co-transport, and glucagon shrinks hepatocytes, presumably by activation of ion channels.[274] The effect of insulin depends partially on the cell volume regulated serum and glucocorticoid inducible kinase SGK1.[275] The effect of the hormones on cell volume accounts for several of their metabolic effects (Figure 5.4). Notably, the swelling effect of insulin accounts for its antiproteolytic effect, and the shrinking effect of glucagon accounts for its proteolytic effect.[276,277]

Virtually all known growth factors increase cell volume by stimulation of Na^+/H^+ exchange, and in some cases by $Na^+K^+2Cl^-$ co-transport. As amplified below, an increase of cell volume appears to be required for cell proliferation.[35]

Several excitatory neurotransmitters, such as glutamate, activate Na^+ channels or nonselective cation channels, the entry of Na^+ and depolarization then favor cell swelling.[278-280] Other neurotransmitters, such as GABA, activate K^+ channels and/or anion channels, and thus induce cell shrinkage.[281]

Mediators and hormones regulating epithelial transport, such as ADH, adrenaline or acetylcholine, may either swell or shrink epithelial cells, depending on their effect on ion transport.[31] Stimulation of Na^+/H^+ exchange, $Na^+-K^+2Cl^-$ co-transport or Na^+ channels tends to swell epithelial cells, whereas prevailing stimulation of Cl^- and/or K^+ channels shrinks epithelial cells. Cell volume may in turn affect hormone and transmitter release. In a variety of cells, swelling stimulates and cell shrinkage inhibits the release of hormones.[282]

Neuromuscular Excitability

Cell volume could affect neuronal excitability by affecting ionic gradients, ion channel activity or cell volume regulatory release of neurotransmitters.[31] Dehydration enhances the neuronal expression of SGK1, which in turn regulates channels and transporters relevant for neuroexcitability.[283] Moreover, glial cell swelling may impede glial cell function.[284] In liver insufficiency, for instance, formation of urea is impaired, leading to accumulation of NH_3. NH_3 enters the brain and is taken up by glial cells, which then stimulates cellular formation and accumulation of glutamine, resulting eventually in glial cell swelling.[285,286] To counteract swelling, glial cells release inositol, a mechanism, however, limited by the availability of inositol.[287,288] Inhibition of glutamine synthase has indeed been shown to protect against hepatic encephalopathy.[289]

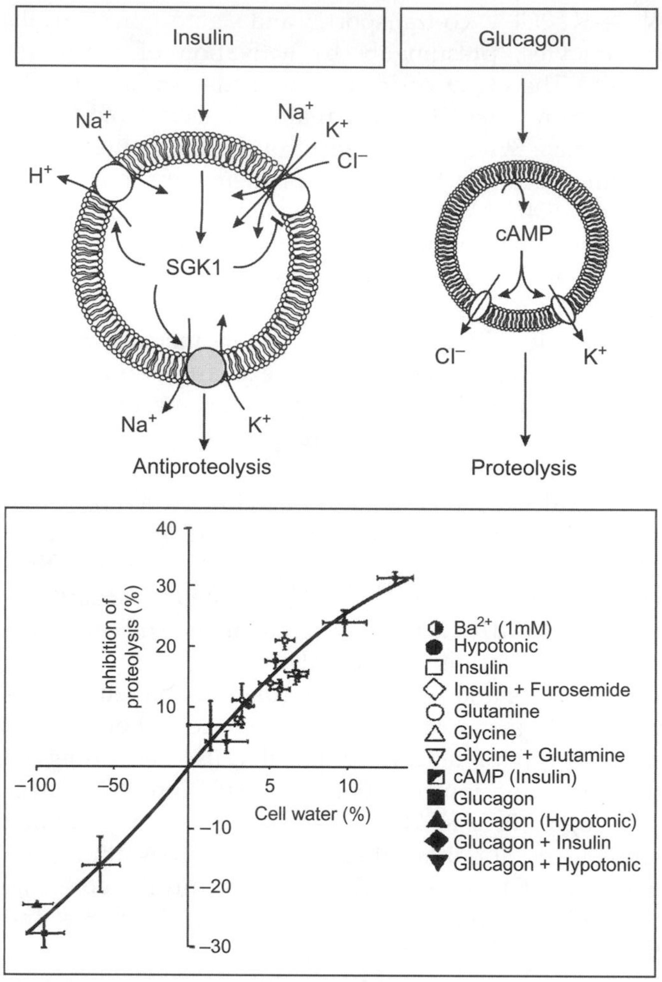

FIGURE 5.4 **Cell volume in the regulation of metabolism by hormones.** Insulin swells cells by KCl uptake via activation of Na^+/H^+ exchange, $Na^+-K^+-2Cl^-$ co-transport, and Na^+/K^+-ATPase. Glucagon shrinks cells by activation of K^+ and anion channels. The cell volume changes participate in the signaling of hormone action. Cell swelling stimulates protein synthesis, and cell shrinkage stimulates proteolysis. The diagram at the bottom illustrates the correlation between inhibition of proteolysis and hydration of hepatocytes. Cell swelling was induced by inhibition of K^+ channels (Ba^{2+}) decrease of extracellular osmolarity (hypotonic), insulin $\pm$ $Na^+-K^+2Cl^-$ co-transport inhibitor furosemide or concentrative uptake of amino acids (glutamine $\pm$ glycine). Cell swelling was counteracted or shrinkage accomplished by (additional) application of glucagon or cyclic AMP. The cell volume changes fully account for the effect of both hormones on proteolysis, and contribute to the other effects on macromolecule metabolism such as protein synthesis, as well as glycogen formation and breakdown *(modified from ref. [22]).*

Metabolism

Any reaction resulting in an increase of osmotically active solutes, such as degradation of proteins to amino acids, glycogen to glucose phosphate or triglycerides to glycerol and fatty acids, is expected to create intracellular osmolarity.[31] The degradation of the substrates to CO_2 and H_2O then decreases intracellular osmolarity.

Enhanced glycolysis, as it occurs during forced exercise for instance, leads to cellular accumulation of lactate and H^+, subsequent activation of Na^+/H^+ exchanger, and cell swelling.[290] Metabolic pathways may influence cell volume indirectly through alteration of transport across the cell membrane. A decrease of cellular ATP could activate ATP-sensitive K^+ channels, and thus shrink susceptible cells.[31] Similarly, cellular formation of peroxides may shrink cells through activation of K^+ channels, as shown for hepatocytes, pancreatic β-cells, and vascular smooth muscle cells.[31] In endothelial cells, peroxides inhibit $Na^+-K^+2Cl^-$ co-transport, an effect similarly expected to shrink the cells.[291] On the other hand, oxidation leads to inhibition of n-type K^+ channels in lymphocytes and IsK K^+ channels in a variety of tissues, effects that tend to favor cell swelling.[31]

In several hypercatabolic states, such as burns, acute pancreatitis, severe injury, and liver carcinoma, a decrease of muscle cell volume is observed that correlates with urea excretion, an indicator of protein degradation.[24] Since cell shrinkage is known to stimulate proteolysis, this correlation points to a causal role of altered cell volume in these hypercatabolic states. Conversely, hypercatabolism can be reversed by glutamine, which is known to swell cells by Na^+-coupled cellular accumulation.[24]

Diabetic ketoacidosis may be paralleled by cell swelling due to cellular accumulation of organic acids and enhanced Na^+/H^+ exchange activity in response to cellular acidosis.[221,261,292–294] Furthermore, the excessive glucose concentrations of hyperglycemia stimulate cellular formation and accumulation of sorbitol through aldose reductase.[17] As an attempt to counteract swelling, cells decrease other osmolytes such as myoinositol, an effect that can be reversed by inhibition of aldose reductase with sorbinil.[295–297] On the other hand, hyperglycemia is paralleled by hyperosmolarity, and intriguing evidence has been gathered pointing to cell shrinkage in hyperosmolar diabetes mellitus, which increases cellular Ca^{2+} concentration, and thus induces cell injury.[298,299] Obviously, more experimental information is needed to clarify the role of cell volume changes in the pathophysiology of diabetic complications.

In uremia, extracellular osmolarity is usually enhanced due to accumulation of urea, which interferes with protein stability and thus cell volume regulation (see previous discussion). The high urea concentrations in uremia stimulate the formation of methylamines, which counteract the perturbing effect of urea.[300] Rapid alterations in urea concentration such as during dialysis presumably do not allow full adjustment of osmolyte concentration, and are thus expected to disturb the balance of stabilizing osmolytes and destabilizing urea.[301] Alterations of cell volume may participate in the progression of renal failure: TGF-β1 has been postulated to accelerate renal fibrosis by inhibition of proteolysis and stimulation of protein synthesis, which both lead to enhanced deposition of matrix proteins.[299,302]

Cell Proliferation

Mitogenic factors are known to stimulate Na^+/H^+ exchange and $Na^+-K^+2Cl^-$ co-transport.[35] As shown in ras oncogene-expressing cells, activation of those carriers leads to a shift of the set point for cell volume regulation toward greater volumes (Figure 5.5). In addition, activation of Na^+/H^+ exchange leads to cellular alkalinization. Apparently, the increase of cell volume is one of the prerequisites for cell proliferation, which is impeded by pharmacological inhibition of Na^+/H^+ exchange and $Na^+-K^+2Cl^-$ co-transport, as well as osmotic cell shrinkage.[31,303] Cell volume changes parallel transition through the cell cycle,[304] and cell proliferation requires further timely activation of volume-sensitive Ca^{2+} channels, K^+ channels, and Cl^- channels.[305–307] Moreover, cell proliferation is substantially influenced by the cell volume-sensitive SGK1.[308]

Migration

Locomotion of cells requires alteration of cell shape, and thus of cytoskeletal architecture. At the leading edge actin filaments are polymerized, and at the rear they are depolymerized.[309,310] The movement of cells is paralleled by movement of water that is driven by osmotic gradients. Na^+/H^+ exchange and $Na^+-K^+2Cl^-$ co-transport drive water entry at the leading edge, and the activity of K^+ channels and anion channels drive water extrusion at the rear.[31,311–314] The respective water movement is facilitated by water channels.[315] Activation of cell volume regulatory mechanisms during migration is similar to that of cell proliferation (Figure 5.6). However, the elements are polarized, and cells undergo cell volume regulatory increase at the leading edge, and cell volume regulatory decrease at the rear.[31]

Apoptotic Cell Death

Cell shrinkage is one of the hallmarks of apoptotic cell death, and marked osmotic cell shrinkage (> 30%) has been shown to trigger this type of cell death.[193] Apoptotic cell shrinkage requires the participation of cell volume regulatory mechanisms (Figure 5.6). Apoptotic death of Jurkat T-lymphocytes following CD95 triggering is indeed paralleled by inhibition of the Na^+/H^+ exchanger, as well as activation of the anion channel ORCC and osmolyte release.[316] The release of ions, and subsequent cell shrinkage, are apparently a prerequisite for induction of apoptosis.[317–319] On the other hand, at an early stage of CD95 triggering, the cell volume-regulatory K^+ channel Kv1.3 is inhibited, and a moderate decrease of cell volume (< 30%) has been shown to blunt receptor (CD95)-triggered apoptotic cell death.[320] The cellular mechanisms triggered by moderate osmotic cell shrinkage apparently interfere with the signaling of the CD95 receptor, such as cellular O_2^--formation.

The triggering of cell death by hyperosmotic shock has been attributed to upregulation or clustering and subsequent activation of apoptosis-inducing receptors,

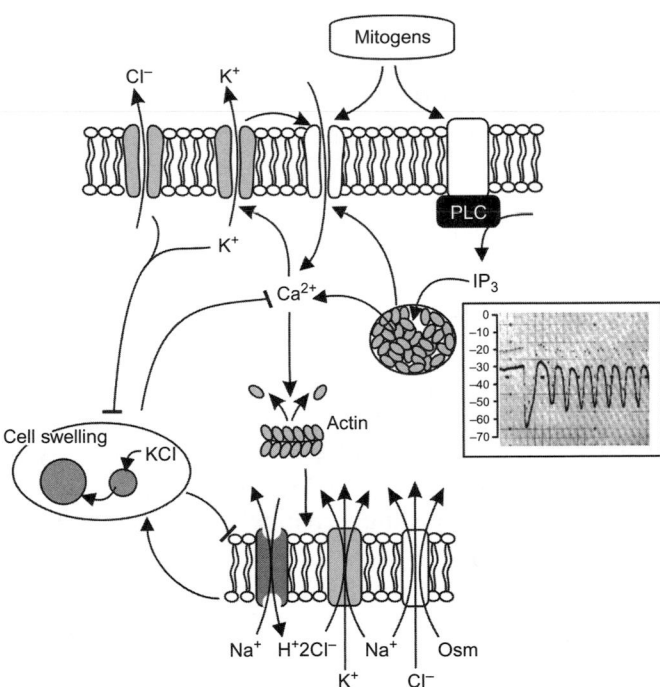

FIGURE 5.5 **Cell volume regulatory transport in regulation of cell proliferation.** The case of Ras oncogene expressing cells. Application of mitogenic factors in cells overexpressing Ras oncogene triggers intracellular Ca^+ release and Ca^+ entry, leading to oscillations of cytosolic Ca^+ activity and cell membrane potential (insert). Increased cytosolic Ca^{2+} activity stimulates Ca^{2+}-sensitive K^+ channels and triggers initial cell shrinkage. Ca^{2+} further leads to depolymerization of the microfilaments, which disinhibits the Na^+/H^+ exchanger and $Na^+-K^+-2Cl^-$ co-transporter. The activation of these carriers eventually leads to cell swelling, a prerequisite for cell proliferation (*from ref. [31]*).

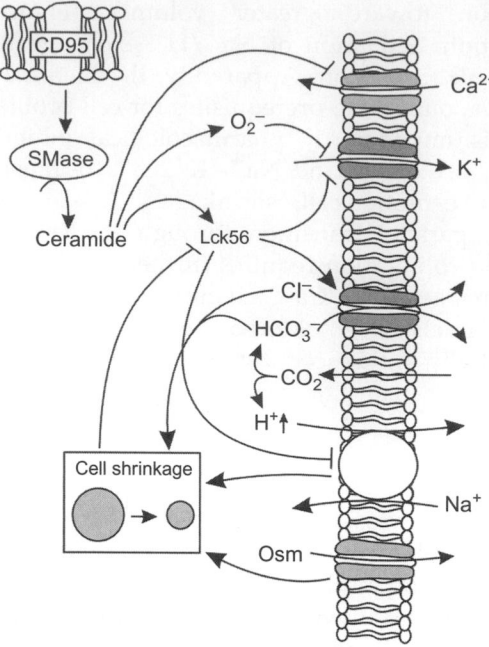

FIGURE 5.6 **Cell volume regulatory ion transport during CD95-induced apoptosis of lymphocytes.** CD95-induced apoptosis of Jurkat T-lymphocytes is paralleled by inhibition of the Na^+/H^+ exchanger, as well as activation of the anion channel ORCC and osmolyte release. The altered transport leads eventually to cytosolic acidification and cell shrinkage. Initially, CD95 stimulation leads to inhibition of the cell volume regulatory K^+ channel Kv1.3, thus preventing early cell shrinkage. At a later stage (not shown), additional activation of K^+ channels leads to apoptotic cell shrinkage. *(From Lang, F., Lepple-Wienhues, A., Paulmichi, M., Szabo, I., Siemen, D. and Gulbins, E. (1998). Ion channels, cell volume, and apoptotic cell death. Cell Physiol. Biochem. 8(6), 285–292.)*

such as CD95 or TNFα-receptor[193,321–323] or to formation of their ligands, such as TNFα.[324] Beyond that, cell shrinkage could trigger cell death more directly, by activating a signaling cascade of rac, p38 kinase, p53, and subsequent upregulation of pro-apoptotic proteins Bax/Bid.[325] Conversely, osmotic shrinkage may downregulate signaling supporting cell survival, such as the PI3 kinase pathway leading to protein kinase B-dependent phosphorylation, and thus inactivation of Bad.[236] In erythrocytes, hyperosmotic shock stimulates a phospholipase A_2 with subsequent formation of PGE_2[251] and PAF.[253] PGE_2 stimulates a cation channel, allowing the entry of Ca^{2+} and subsequent triggering of Ca^{2+}-sensitive cell membrane scrambling.[251] PAF stimulates a sphingomyelinase that leads to formation of ceramide, which sensitizes the erythrocyte for the scrambling effect of Ca^{2+}.[253] Cell membrane scrambling leads to breakdown of phosphatidylserine asymmetry and exposure of phosphatidylserine at the outer surface of the cell membrane, a typical feature of apoptotic cells (Figure 5.7).

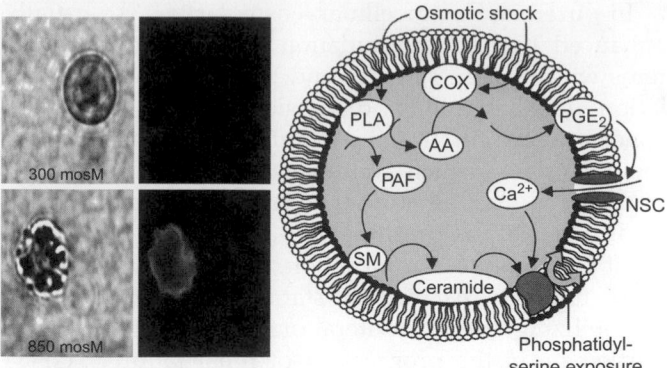

FIGURE 5.7 **Stimulation of erythrocyte death by osmotic cell shrinkage.** Osmotic shock activates a phospholipase A_2 leading to formation of platelet activating factor (PAF) on the one hand, and of arachidonic acid on the other. PAF stimulates a sphingomyelinase leading to formation of ceramide; arachidonic acid is converted by cyclooxygenase (COX) to PGE2 which activates a Ca and Na permeable cation channel. Ca entering through the cation channels activates a scramblase, leading to phosphatidylserine exposure at the cell surface (left), a typical feature of apoptotic cells. Ceramide sensitizes the scramblase for Ca, and thus contributes to the activation of this enzyme *(from ref. [273])*. See color section at back of book.

Necrotic Cell Death

As pointed out above, energy depletion impairs the function of the Na^+/K^+-ATPase, dissipates the Na^+ and K^+ gradients, depolarizes the cell membrane, and leads to cellular accumulation of Cl^-.[31] During ischemia, the cell membrane is further depolarized by increasing extracellular K^+ concentrations. Cellular Na^+ and Cl^- accumulation eventually lead to cell swelling. Moreover, the excessive formation and reduced clearance of lactate during ischemia induces cellular acidosis and enhanced Na^+/H^+ exchange activity, compounding cell swelling. In the brain, the depolarization triggers the release of glutamate, which activates unspecific cation channels and thus induces further cell swelling.[31]

References

[1] Brown GC. Total cell protein concentration as an evolutionary constraint on the metabolic control distribution in cells. J Theor Biol 1991;153:195–203.

[2] Fulton AB. How crowded is the cytoplasm? Cell 1982;30:345–7.

[3] Garner MM, Burg MB. Macromolecular crowding and confinement in cells exposed to hypertonicity. Am J Physiol 1994;266:C877–92.

[4] Minton AP. Excluded volume as a determinant of macromolecular structure and reactivity. Biopolymers 1981;20:2093–120.

[5] Minton AP. Macromolecular crowding and molecular recognition. J Mol Recognit 1993;6:211–4.

[6] Parker JC. In defense of cell volume? Am J Physiol 1993;265: C1191–200.

[7] Colombe BW, Macey RI. Effects of calcium on potassium and water transport in human erythrocyte ghosts. Biochim Biophys Acta 1974;363:226–39.

[8] Macknight AD. Principles of cell volume regulation. Ren Physiol Biochem 1988;11:114–41.

[9] Galizia L. Flamenco MP, Rivarola V, Capurro C, Ford P. Role of AQP2 in activation of calcium entry by hypotonicity: implications in cell volume regulation. Am J Physiol Renal Physiol 2008;294:F582–90.

[10] King LS, Kozono D, Agre P. From structure to disease: the evolving tale of aquaporin biology. Nat Rev Mol Cell Biol 2004;5:687–98.

[11] Liu X, Bandyopadhyay BC, Nakamoto T, Singh B, Liedtke W, Melvin JE, et al. A role for AQP5 in activation of TRPV4 by hypotonicity: concerted involvement of AQP5 and TRPV4 in regulation of cell volume recovery. J. Biol. Chem. 2006;281:15485–95.

[12] Graf J, Haddad P, Haeussinger D, Lang F. Cell volume regulation in liver. Ren Physiol Biochem 1988;11:202–20.

[13] Guharay F, Sachs F. Stretch-activated single ion channel currents in tissue-cultured embryonic chick skeletal muscle. J Physiol 1984;352:685–701.

[14] Kelly SM, Macklem PT. Direct measurement of intracellular pressure. Am J Physiol 1991;260:C652–7.

[15] Sackin H. Stretch-activated ion channels. In: Strange K, editor. Cellular and Molecular Physiology of Cell Volume Regulation. Boca Raton, FL: CRC Press; 1994. p. 215–40.

[16] Burg MB. Molecular basis of osmotic regulation. Am J Physiol 1995;268:F983–96.

[17] Burg MB, Kador PF. Sorbitol, osmoregulation, and the complications of diabetes. J Clin Invest 1988;81:635–40.

[18] Burg MB, Kwon ED, Peters EM. Glycerophosphocholine and betaine counteract the effect of urea on pyruvate kinase. Kidney Int Suppl 1996;57:S100–4.

[19] De Mello WC. Renin angiotensin system as a regulator of cell volume. Implications to myocardial ischemia. Curr Cardiol Rev 2009;5:65–8.

[20] Fisher SK, Heacock AM, Keep RF, Foster DJ. Receptor regulation of osmolyte homeostasis in neural cells. J. Physiol. 2010;288 (Pt 18):3355–64.

[21] Garcia-Perez A, Burg MB. Renal medullary organic osmolytes. Physiol Rev 1991;71:1081–115.

[22] Haussinger D, Lang F. Cell volume: a "second messenger" in the regulation of metabolism by amono acids and hormones. Cell Physiol Biochem 1991;1:121–30.

[23] Haussinger D. Osmosensing and osmosignaling in the liver. Wien Med Wochenschr 2008;158:549–52.

[24] Haussinger D, Roth E, Lang F, Gerok W. Cellular hydration state: an important determinant of protein catabolism in health and disease. Lancet 1993;341:1330–2.

[25] Hoffmann EK, Dunham PB. Membrane mechanisms and intracellular signalling in cell volume regulation. Int Rev Cytol 1995;161:173–262.

[26] Hoffmann EK, Lambert IH, Pedersen SF. Physiology of cell volume regulation in vertebrates. Physiol Rev 2009;89:193–277.

[27] Kinne RK, Czekay RP, Grunewald JM, Mooren FC, Kinne-Saffran E. Hypotonicity-evoked release of organic osmolytes from distal renal cells: systems, signals, and sidedness. Ren Physiol Biochem 1993;16:66–78.

[28] Kwon HM, Handler JS. Cell volume regulated transporters of compatible osmolytes. Curr Opin Cell Biol 1995;7:465–71.

[29] Lang F. Cell Volume Regulation. Contributions to Nephrology ed. Basel: Karger; 1998.

[30] Lang F. Mechanisms and significance of cell volume regulation. J Am Coll Nutr 2007;26:613S–23S.

[31] Lang F, Busch GL, Ritter M, Völkl H, Waldegger S, Gulbins E, et al. Functional significance of cell volume regulatory mechanisms. Physiol Rev 1998;78:247–306.

[32] Lang F, Busch GL, Volkl H. The diversity of volume regulatory mechanisms. Cell Physiol Biochem 1998;8:1–45.

[33] McManus ML, Churchwell KB, Strange K. Regulation of cell volume in health and disease. N Engl J Med 1995;333:1260–6.

[34] Pasantes-Morales H, Cruz-Rangel S. Brain volume regulation: osmolytes and aquaporin perspectives. Neuroscience 2010;168:871–84.

[35] Ritter M, Woell E. Modification of cellular ion transport by the ha-ras oncogene: steps towards malignant transformation. Cell Physiol Biochem 1996;6:245–70.

[36] Ritter M, Fuerst J, Woll E, Chwatal S, Gschwentner M, Lang F, et al. Na$^{(+)}$/H$^{(+)}$exchangers: linking osmotic dysequilibrium to modified cell function. Cell Physiol Biochem 2001;11:1–18.

[37] Schliess F, Reinehr R, Haussinger D. Osmosensing and signaling in the regulation of mammalian cell function. FEBS J 2007;274:5799–803.

[38] Strange K. Cellular and Molecular Physiology of Cell Volume Regulation. Boca Raton, FL: CRC Press; 1994.

[39] Strange K. Cellular volume homeostasis. Adv Physiol Educ 2004;28:155–9.

[40] Usher-Smith JA, Huang CL, Fraser JA. Control of cell volume in skeletal muscle. Biol Rev Camb Philos Soc 2009;84:143–59.

[41] Wehner F, Olsen H, Tinel H, Kinne-Saffran E, Kinne RK. Cell volume regulation: osmolytes, osmolyte transport, and signal transduction. Rev Physiol Biochem Pharmacol 2003;148:1–80.

[42] Lohr JW, Grantham JJ. Isovolumetric regulation of isolated S2 proximal tubules in anisotonic media. J Clin Invest 1986;78:1165–72.

[43] Minton AP. Influence of macromolecular crowding on intracellular association reactions: Possible role in volume regulation. In: Strange K, editor. Cellular and Molecular Physiology of Cell Volume Regulation. Boca Raton, FL: CRC Press; 1994. p. 181–90.

[44] Burg MB, Kwon ED, Kultz D. Osmotic regulation of gene expression. FASEB J 1996;10:1598–606.

[45] Deutsch C, Chen LQ. Heterologous expression of specific K$^+$ channels in T lymphocytes: functional consequences for volume regulation. Proc Natl Acad Sci USA 1993;90:10036–40.

[46] Felipe A, Snyders DJ, Deal KK, Tamkun MM. Influence of cloned voltage-gated K$^+$ channel expression on alanine transport, Rb$^+$ uptake, and cell volume. Am J Physiol 1993;265: C1230–8.

[47] Wang GL, Wang GX, Yamamoto S, Ye L, Baxter H, Hume JR, et al. Molecular mechanisms of regulation of fast-inactivating voltage-dependent transient outward K$^+$ current in mouse heart by cell volume changes. J Physiol 2005;568:423–43.

[48] Busch AE, Maylie J. MinK channels: a minimal channel protein with a maximal impact. Cell Physiol Biochem 1993;3:270–6.

[49] Busch AE, Varnum M, Adelman JP, North RA. Hypotonic solution increases the slowly activating potassium current IsK expressed in *Xenopus* oocytes. Biochem Biophys Res Commun 1992;184:804–10.

[50] Byfield FJ, Aranda-Espinoza H, Romanenko VG, Rothblat GH, Levitan I. Cholesterol depletion increases membrane stiffness of aortic endothelial cells. Biophys J 2004;87:3336–43.

[51] vanTol BL, Missan S, Crack J, Moser S, Baldridge WH, Linsdell P, et al. Contribution of KCNQ1 to the regulatory volume decrease in the human mammary epithelial cell line MCF-7. Am J Physiol Cell Physiol 2007;293:C1010–9.

[52] Decressac S, Franco M, Bendahhou S, Warth R, Knauer S, Barhanin J, et al. ARF6-dependent interaction of the TWIK1 K$^+$

channel with EFA6, a GDP/GTP exchange factor for ARF6. EMBO Rep 2004;5:1171–5.

[53] Barriere H, Belfodil R, Rubera I, Tauc M, Lesage F, Poujeol C, et al. Role of TASK2 potassium channels regarding volume regulation in primary cultures of mouse proximal tubules. J Gen Physiol 2003;122:177–90.

[54] Wang SX, Ikeda M, Guggino WB. The cytoplasmic tail of large conductance, voltage- and Ca^{2+}-activated K$^+$ (MaxiK) channel is necessary for its cell surface expression. J Biol Chem 2003;278:2713–22.

[55] Grunder S, Thiemann A, Pusch M, Jentsch TJ. Regions involved in the opening of ClC-2 chloride channel by voltage and cell volume. Nature 1992;360:759–62.

[56] Jentsch TJ. Molecular physiology of anion channels. Curr Opin Cell Biol 1994;6:600–6.

[57] Jentsch TJ. Chloride channels: a molecular perspective. Curr Opin Neurobiol 1996;6:303–10.

[58] Lorenz C, Pusch M, Jentsch TJ. Heteromultimeric CLC chloride channels with novel properties. Proc Natl Acad Sci USA 1996;93:13362–6.

[59] Thiemann A, Grunder S, Pusch M, Jentsch TJ. A chloride channel widely expressed in epithelial and non-epithelial cells. Nature 1992;356:57–60.

[60] Jin NG, Kim JK, Yang DK, Cho SJ, Kim JM, Koh EJ, et al. Fundamental role of ClC-3 in volume-sensitive Cl$^-$ channel function and cell volume regulation in AGS cells. Am J Physiol Gastrointest Liver Physiol 2003;285:G938–48.

[61] McCloskey DT, Doherty L, Dai YP, Miller L, Hume JR, Yamboliev IA. Hypotonic activation of short ClC3 isoform is modulated by direct interaction between its cytosolic C-terminal tail and subcortical actin filaments. J Biol Chem 2007;282:16871–7.

[62] Nilius B, Eggermont J, Voets T, Buyse G, Manolopoulos V, Droogmans G. Properties of volume-regulated anion channels in mammalian cells. Prog Biophys Mol Biol 1997;68:69–119.

[63] Chien LT, Hartzell HC. Drosophila bestrophins are dually regulated by calcium and cell volume (Abstract). J Gen Physiol 2007;130:21A–2A.

[64] Buyse G, de Greef C, Raeymaekers L, Droogmans G, Nilius B, Eggermont J. The ubiquitously expressed pICln protein forms homomeric complexes in vitro. Biochem Biophys Res Commun 1996;218:822–7.

[65] Paulmichl M, Li Y, Wickman K, Ackerman M, Peralta E, Clapham D. New mammalian chloride channel identified by expression cloning. Nature 1992;356:238–41.

[66] Ritter M, Ravasio A, Jakab M, Chwatal S, Furst J, Laich A, et al. Cell swelling stimulates cytosol to membrane transposition of ICln. J Biol Chem 2003;278:50163–74.

[67] Hardy SP, Goodfellow HR, Valverde MA, Gill DR, Sepulveda V, Higgins CF. Protein kinase C-mediated phosphorylation of the human multidrug resistance P-glycoprotein regulates cell volume-activated chloride channels. EMBO J 1995;14:68–75.

[68] Higgins CF. Volume-activated chloride currents associated with the multidrug resistance P-glycoprotein. J Physiol 1995;482:31S–6S.

[69] Jirsch J, Deeley RG, Cole SP, Stewart AJ, Fedida D. Inwardly rectifying K$^+$ channels and volume-regulated anion channels in multidrug-resistant small cell lung cancer cells. Cancer Res 1993;53:4156–60.

[70] Jirsch JD, Loe DW, Cole SP, Deeley RG, Fedida D. ATP is not required for anion current activated by cell swelling in multidrug-resistant lung cancer cells. Am J Physiol 1994;267:C688–99.

[71] Cho WK, Siegrist VJ, Zinzow W. Impaired regulatory volume decrease in freshly isolated cholangiocytes from cystic fibrosis mice: implications for cystic fibrosis transmembrane conductance regulator effect on potassium conductance. J Biol Chem 2004;279:14610–8.

[72] Valverde MA, Vazquez E, Munoz FJ, Nobles M, Delaney SJ, Wainwright BJ, et al. Murine CFTR channel and its role in regulatory volume decrease of small intestine crypts. Cell Physiol Biochem 2000;10:321–8.

[73] Chan HC, Fu WO, Chung YW, Huang SJ, Chan PS, Wong PY. Swelling-induced anion and cation conductances in human epididymal cells. J Physiol 1994;478(Pt 3):449–60.

[74] Jackson PS, Strange K. Volume-sensitive anion channels mediate swelling-activated inositol and taurine efflux. Am J Physiol 1993;265:C1489–500.

[75] Junankar PR, Kirk K. Organic osmolyte channels: a comparative view. Cell Physiol Biochem 2000;10:355–60.

[76] Kinne RK, Tinel H, Kipp H, Kinne-Saffran E. Regulation of sorbitol efflux in different renal medullary cells: similarities and diversities. Cell Physiol Biochem 2000;10:371–8.

[77] Kirk K, Ellory JC, Young JD. Transport of organic substrates via a volume-activated channel. J Biol Chem 1992;267:23475–8.

[78] Okada SF, O'Neal WK, Huang P, Nicholas RA, Ostrowski LE, Craigen WJ, et al. Voltage-dependent anion channel-1 (VDAC-1) contributes to ATP release and cell volume regulation in murine cells. J Gen Physiol 2004;124:513–26.

[79] Roy G, Banderali U. Channels for ions and amino acids in kidney cultured cells (MDCK) during volume regulation. J Exp Zool 1994;268:121–6.

[80] Strange K, Jackson PS. Swelling-activated organic osmolyte efflux: a new role for anion channels. Kidney Int 1995;48:994–1003.

[81] Nilius B, Owsianik G, Voets T, Peters JA. Transient receptor potential cation channels in disease. Physiol Rev 2007;87:165–217.

[82] Numata T, Shimizu T, Okada Y. Direct mechano-stress sensitivity of TRPM7 channel. Cell Physiol Biochem 2007;19:1–8.

[83] Numata T, Shimizu T, Okada Y. TRPM7 is a stretch- and swelling-activated cation channel involved in volume regulation in human epithelial cells. Am J Physiol Cell Physiol 2007;292:C460–7.

[84] Pedersen SF, Nilius B. Transient receptor potential channels in mechanosensing and cell volume regulation. Methods Enzymol 2007;428:183–207.

[85] Plettenberg S, Weiss EC, Lemor R, Wehner F. Subunits alpha, beta and gamma of the epithelial Na$^+$ channel (ENaC) are functionally related to the hypertonicity-induced cation channel (HICC) in rat hepatocytes. Pflugers Arch 2008;455:1089–95.

[86] Ross SB, Fuller CM, Bubien JK, Benos DJ. Amiloride-sensitive Na$^+$ channels contribute to regulatory volume increases in human glioma cells. Am J Physiol Cell Physiol 2007;293:C1181–5.

[87] Sachs F. Mechanical transduction by membrane ion channels: a mini review. Mol Cell Biochem 1991;104:57–60.

[88] Adragna NC, Lauf PK. K–Cl co-transport function and its potential contribution to cardiovascular disease. Pathophysiology 2007;14:135–46.

[89] Boettger T, Rust MB, Maier H, Seidenbecher T, Schweizer M, Keating DJ, et al. Loss of K–Cl co-transporter KCC3 causes deafness, neurodegeneration and reduced seizure threshold. EMBO J 2003;22:5422–34.

[90] Lauf PK. K:Cl co-transport: emerging molecular aspects of a ouabain-resistant, volume-responsive transport system in red blood cells. Ren Physiol Biochem 1988;11:248–59.

[91] Lauf PK, Adragna NC. K-Cl co-transport: properties and molecular mechanism. Cell Physiol Biochem 2000;10:341–54.

[92] Lauf PK, Erdmann A, Adragna NC. K-Cl co-transport, pH, and role of Mg in volume-clamped low-K sheep erythrocytes: three equilibrium states. Am J Physiol 1994;266:C95–103.

[93] Perry PB, O'Neill WC. Swelling-activated K fluxes in vascular endothelial cells: volume regulation via K-Cl co-transport and K channels. Am J Physiol 1993;265:C763–9.

[94] Thornhill WB, Laris PC. KCl loss and cell shrinkage in the Ehrlich ascites tumor cell induced by hypotonic media, 2-deoxyglucose and propranolol. Biochim Biophys Acta 1984;773:207–18.

[95] Bonanno JA. K(+)–H+ exchange, a fundamental cell acidifier in corneal epithelium. Am J Physiol 1991;260:C618–25.

[96] Cala PM. Volume regulation by *Amphiuma* red blood cells: strategies for identifying alkali metal/H+ transport. Fed Proc 1985;44:2500–7.

[97] Dunham PB, Jessen F, Hoffmann EK. Inhibition of Na-K-Cl co-transport in Ehrlich ascites cells by antiserum against purified proteins of the co-transporter. Proc Natl Acad Sci USA 1990;87:6828–32.

[98] Gamba G. Molecular physiology and pathophysiology of electroneutral cation-chloride co-transporters. Physiol Rev 2005;85:423–93.

[99] Geck P, Pfeiffer B. Na+ + K+ + 2Cl− co-transport in animal cells: its role in volume regulation. Ann NY Acad Sci 1985;456:166–82.

[100] Hebert SC, Mount DB, Gamba G. Molecular physiology of cation-coupled Cl− co-transport: the SLC12 family. Pflugers Arch 2004;447:580–93.

[101] Wakabayashi S, Shigekawa M, Pouyssegur J. Molecular physiology of vertebrate Na+/H+ exchangers. Physiol Rev 1997;77:51–74.

[102] Demaurex N, Grinstein S. Na + /H + antiport: modulation by ATP and role in cell volume regulation. J Exp Biol 1994;196:389–404.

[103] Bookstein C, Musch MW, DePaoli A, Xie Y, Villereal M, Rao MC, et al. A unique sodium-hydrogen exchange isoform (NHE-4) of the inner medulla of the rat kidney is induced by hyperosmolarity. J Biol Chem 1994;269:29704–9.

[104] Barone S, Amlal H, Xu J, Kujala M, Kere J, Petrovic S, et al. Differential regulation of basolateral Cl−. J Am Soc Nephrol 2004;15:2002–11.

[105] Grinstein S, Clarke CA, Rothstein A. Activation of Na+/H+ exchange in lymphocytes by osmotically induced volume changes and by cytoplasmic acidification. J Gen Physiol 1983;82:619–38.

[106] Good DW, Di Mari JF, Watts III BA. Hyposmolality stimulates Na(+)/H(+) exchange and HCO(3)(−) absorption in thick ascending limb via PI 3-kinase. Am J Physiol Cell Physiol 2000;279:C1443–54.

[107] Cabado AG, Vieytes MR, Botana LM. Effect of ion composition on the changes in membrane potential induced with several stimuli in rat mast cells. J Cell Physiol 1994;158:309–16.

[108] Chan HC, Nelson DJ. Chloride-dependent cation conductance activated during cellular shrinkage. Science 1992;257:669–71.

[109] Lang F, Lang KS, Wieder T, Myssina S, Birka C, Lang PA, et al. Cation channels, cell volume and the death of an erythrocyte. Pflugers Arch 2003;447:121–5.

[110] Volk T, Fromter E, Korbmacher C. Hypertonicity activates nonselective cation channels in mouse cortical collecting duct cells. Proc Natl Acad Sci USA 1995;92:8478–82.

[111] Wehner F, Bohmer C, Heinzinger H, van den BF, Tinel H. The hypertonicity-induced Na(+) conductance of rat hepatocytes: physiological significance and molecular correlate. Cell Physiol Biochem 2000;10:335–40.

[112] Wehner F, Sauer H, Kinne RK. Hypertonic stress increases the Na+ conductance of rat hepatocytes in primary culture. J Gen Physiol 1995;105:507–35.

[113] Christensen AP, Corey DP. TRP channels in mechanosensation: direct or indirect activation? Nat Rev Neurosci 2007;8:510–21.

[114] Gottlieb P, Folgering J, Maroto R, Raso A, Wood TG, Kurosky A, et al. Revisiting TRPC1 and TRPC6 mechanosensitivity. Pflugers Arch 2008;455:1097–103.

[115] Liedtke W. Transient receptor potential vanilloid channels functioning in transduction of osmotic stimuli. J Endocrinol 2006;191:515–23.

[116] Wehner F. Cell volume-regulated cation channels. Contrib Nephrol 2006;152:25–53.

[117] Burg MB, Ferraris JD, Dmitrieva NI. Cellular response to hyperosmotic stresses. Physiol Rev 2007;87:1441–74.

[118] Pasantes-Morales H, Franco R, Torres-Marquez ME, Hernandez-Fonseca K, Ortega A. Amino acid osmolytes in regulatory volume decrease and isovolumetric regulation in brain cells: contribution and mechanisms. Cell Physiol Biochem 2000;10:361–70.

[119] Back JF, Oakenfull D, Smith MB. Increased thermal stability of proteins in the presence of sugars and polyols. Biochemistry 1979;18:5191–6.

[120] Carpenter JF, Crowe JH. The mechanism of cryoprotection of proteins by solutes. Cryobiology 1988;25:244–55.

[121] Santoro MM, Liu Y, Khan SM, Hou LX, Bolen DW. Increased thermal stability of proteins in the presence of naturally occurring osmolytes. Biochemistry 1992;31:5278–83.

[122] Storey KB, Storey JM. Freeze tolerance in animals. Physiol Rev 1988;68:27–84.

[123] Taneja S, Ahmad F. Increased thermal stability of proteins in the presence of amino acids. Biochem J 1994;303(Pt 1):147–53.

[124] Bedford JJ, Bagnasco SM, Kador PF, Harris Jr. HW, Burg MB. Characterization and purification of a mammalian osmoregulatory protein, aldose reductase, induced in renal medullary cells by high extracellular NaCl. J Biol Chem 1987;262:14255–9.

[125] Ferraris JD, Williams CK, Martin BM, Burg MB, Garcia-Perez A. Cloning, genomic organization, and osmotic response of the aldose reductase gene. Proc Natl Acad Sci USA 1994;91:10742–6.

[126] Garcia-Perez A, Martin B, Murphy HR, Uchida S, Murer H, Cowley Jr. BD, et al. Molecular cloning of cDNA coding for kidney aldose reductase. Regulation of specific mRNA accumulation by NaCl-mediated osmotic stress. J Biol Chem 1989;264:16815–21.

[127] Garcia-Perez A, Ferraris JD. Aldose reductase gene expression and osmoregulation in mammalian renal cells. In: Strange K, editor. Cellular and Molecular Physiology of Cell Volume Regulation. Boca Raton, FL: CRC Press; 1994. p. 373–9.

[128] Garcia-Perez A, Burg MB. Role of organic osmolytes in adaptation of renal cells to high osmolality. J Membr Biol 1991;119:1–13.

[129] Ullrich KJ. Glycerylphosphorylcholinumsatz und Glycerylphosphorylcholindiesterase in der Säugetier-Niere. Biochem Z 1959;331:98–102.

[130] Berry GT, Mallee JJ, Kwon HM, Rim JS, Mulla WR, Muenke M, et al. The human osmoregulatory Na+/myo-inositol co-transporter gene (SLC5A3): molecular cloning and localization to chromosome 21. Genomics 1995;25:507–13.

[131] Hammerman MR, Sacktor B, Daughaday WH. Myo-inositol transport in renal brush border vesicles and its inhibition by D-glucose. Am J Physiol 1980;239:F113–20.

[132] Kwon HM, Yamauchi A, Uchida S, Preston AS, Garcia-Perez A, Burg MB, et al. Cloning of the cDNa for a Na$^+$/myo-inositol cotransporter, a hypertonicity stress protein. J Biol Chem 1992;267:6297—301.

[133] Yamauchi A, Sugiura T, Ito T, Miyai A, Horio M, Imai E, et al. Na$^+$/myo-inositol transport is regulated by basolateral tonicity in Madin—Darby canine kidney cells. J Clin Invest 1996;97:263—7.

[134] Burnham CE, Buerk B, Schmidt C, Bucuvalas JC. A liver-specific isoform of the betaine/GABA transporter in the rat: cDNA sequence and organ distribution. Biochim Biophys Acta 1996;1284:4—8.

[135] Takenaka M, Bagnasco SM, Preston AS, Uchida S, Yamauchi A, Kwon HM, et al. The canine betaine gamma-amino-n-butyric acid transporter gene: diverse mRNA isoforms are regulated by hypertonicity and are expressed in a tissue-specific manner. Proc Natl Acad Sci USA 1995;92:1072—6.

[136] Yamauchi A, Kwon HM, Uchida S, Preston AS, Handler JS. Myo-inositol and betaine transporters regulated by tonicity are basolateral in MDCK cells. Am J Physiol 1991;261:F197—202.

[137] Uchida S, Kwon HM, Yamauchi A, Preston AS, Marumo F, Handler JS. Molecular cloning of the cDNA for an MDCK cell Na($^+$)- and Cl($^-$)-dependent taurine transporter that is regulated by hypertonicity. Proc Natl Acad Sci USA 1992;89:8230—4.

[138] Chen JG, Klus LR, Steenbergen DK, Kempson SA. Hypertonic upregulation of amino acid transport system A in vascular smooth muscle cells. Am J Physiol 1994;267:C529—36.

[139] Soler C, Felipe A, Casado FJ, McGivan JD, Pastor-Anglada M. Hyperosmolarity leads to an increase in derepressed system A activity in the renal epithelial cell line NBL-1. Biochem J 1993;289(Pt 3):653—8.

[140] Yamauchi A, Miyai A, Yokoyama K, Itoh T, Kamada T, Ueda N, et al. Response to osmotic stimuli in mesangial cells: role of system A transporter. Am J Physiol 1994;267:C1493—500.

[141] Kinne RK. The role of organic osmolytes in osmoregulation: from bacteria to mammals. J Exp Zool 1993;265:346—55.

[142] Bagnasco SM, Murphy HR, Bedford JJ, Burg MB. Osmoregulation by slow changes in aldose reductase and rapid changes in sorbitol flux. Am J Physiol 1988;254:C788—92.

[143] Garty H, Furlong TJ, Ellis DE, Spring KR. Sorbitol permease: an apical membrane transporter in cultured renal papillary epithelial cells. Am J Physiol 1991;260:F650—6.

[144] Wiesinger H, Thiess U, Hamprecht B. Sorbitol pathway activity and utilization of polyols in astroglia-rich primary cultures. Glia 1990;3:277—82.

[145] Furlong TJ, Moriyama T, Spring KR. Activation of osmolyte efflux from cultured renal papillary epithelial cells. J Membr Biol 1991;123:269—77.

[146] Boese SH, Wehner F, Kinne RK. Taurine permeation through swelling-activated anion conductance in rat IMCD cells in primary culture. Am J Physiol 1996;271:F498—507.

[147] Friis MB, Vorum KG, Lambert IH. Volume-sensitive NADPH oxidase activity and taurine efflux in NIH3T3 mouse fibroblasts. Am J Physiol Cell Physiol 2008;294:C1552—65.

[148] Lambert IH. Activation and inactivation of the volume-sensitive taurine leak pathway in NIH3T3 fibroblasts and Ehrlich Lettre ascites cells. Am J Physiol Cell Physiol 2007;293: C390—400.

[149] Lambert IH, Hoffmann EK. Regulation of taurine transport in Ehrlich ascites tumor cells. J Membr Biol 1993;131:67—79.

[150] Sanchez-Olea R, Morales-Mulia M, Moran J, Pasantes-Morales H. Inhibition by polyunsaturated fatty acids of cell volume regulation and osmolyte fluxes in astrocytes. Am J Physiol 1995;269:C96—102.

[151] Berneis K, Ninnis R, Haussinger D, Keller U. Effects of hyper- and hypoosmolality on whole body protein and glucose kinetics in humans. Am J Physiol 1999;276:E188—95.

[152] Hallbrucker C, vom DS, Lang F, Haussinger D. Control of hepatic proteolysis by amino acids. The role of cell volume. Eur J Biochem 1991;197:717—24.

[153] Haussinger D, Lang F, Bauers K, Gerok W. Control of hepatic nitrogen metabolism and glutathione release by cell volume regulatory mechanisms. Eur J Biochem 1990;193:891—8.

[154] Haussinger D, Lang F, Gerok W. Regulation of cell function by the cellular hydration state. Am J Physiol 1994;267: E343—55.

[155] Gual P, Gonzalez T, Gremeaux T, Marchand-Brustel Y, Tanti JF. Osmotic regulation of cellular glucose uptake. Methods Enzymol 2007;428:343—54.

[156] Saha N, Stoll B, Lang F, Haussinger D. Effect of anisotonic cell-volume modulation on glutathione-S-conjugate release, t-butylhydroperoxide metabolism and the pentose-phosphate shunt in perfused rat liver. Eur J Biochem 1992;209:437—44.

[157] Haussinger D, Gorg B. Interaction of oxidative stress, astrocyte swelling and cerebral ammonia toxicity. Curr Opin Clin Nutr Metab Care 2010;13:87—92.

[158] Lambert IH. Reactive oxygen species regulate swelling-induced taurine efflux in NIH3T3 mouse fibroblasts. J Membr Biol 2003;192:19—32.

[159] Iyer SS, Pearson DW, Nauseef WM, Clark RA. Evidence for a readily dissociable complex of p47phox and p67phox in cytosol of unstimulated human neutrophils. J Biol Chem 1994;269:22405—11.

[160] Kataoka S, Fujita Y. [Basal experiments of active oxygen generation in urinary polymorphonuclear leukocytes]. Nippon Hinyokika Gakkai Zasshi 1991;82:16—23.

[161] Ferraris JD, Burg MB. Tonicity-regulated gene expression. Methods Enzymol 2007;428:279—96.

[162] Chen Y, Schnetz MP, Irarrazabal CE, Shen RF, Williams CK, Burg MB, et al. Proteomic identification of proteins associated with the osmoregulatory transcription factor TonEBP/OREBP: functional effects of Hsp90 and PARP-1. Am J Physiol Renal Physiol 2007;292:F981—92.

[163] Valkova N, Kultz D. Constitutive and inducible stress proteins dominate the proteome of the murine inner medullary collecting duct-3 (mIMCD3) cell line. Biochim Biophys Acta 2006;1764:1007—20.

[164] Ferrer-Martinez A, Casado FJ, Felipe A, Pastor-Anglada M. Regulation of Na$^+$,K($^+$)-ATPase and the Na$^+$/K$^+$/Cl$^-$ cotransporter in the renal epithelial cell line NBL-1 under osmotic stress. Biochem J 1996;319(Pt 2):337—42.

[165] Sadoshima J, Qiu Z, Morgan JP, Izumo S. Tyrosine kinase activation is an immediate and essential step in hypotonic cell swelling-induced ERK activation and c-fos gene expression in cardiac myocytes. EMBO J 1996;15:5535—46.

[166] Firestone GL, Giampaolo JR, O'Keeffe BA. Stimulus-dependent regulation of the serum and glucocorticoid inducible protein kinase (Sgk) transcription, subcellular localization and enzymatic activity. Cell Physiol Biochem 2003;13:1—12.

[167] Waldegger S, Barth P, Raber G, Lang F. Cloning and characterization of a putative human serine/threonine protein kinase transcriptionally modified during anisotonic and isotonic alterations of cell volume. Proc Natl Acad Sci USA 1997;94:4440—5.

[168] Zhang F, Warskulat U, Wettstein M, Schreiber R, Henninger HP, Decker K, et al. Hyperosmolarity stimulates prostaglandin synthesis and cyclooxygenase-2 expression in activated rat liver macrophages. Biochem J 1995;312(Pt 1):135—43.

[169] Alfieri R, Petronini PG, Urbani S, Borghetti AF. Activation of heat-shock transcription factor 1 by hypertonic shock in 3T3 cells. Biochem J 1996;319(Pt 2):601–6.

[170] Beck FX, Grunbein R, Lugmayr K, Neuhofer W. Heat shock proteins and the cellular response to osmotic stress. Cell Physiol Biochem 2000;10:303–6.

[171] Cohen DM, Wasserman JC, Gullans SR. Immediate early gene and HSP70 expression in hyperosmotic stress in MDCK cells. Am J Physiol 1991;261:C594–601.

[172] Sheikh-Hamad D, Garcia-Perez A, Ferraris JD, Peters EM, Burg MB. Induction of gene expression by heat shock versus osmotic stress. Am J Physiol 1994;267:F28–34.

[173] Tanaka K, Jay G, Isselbacher KJ. Expression of heat-shock and glucose-regulated genes: differential effects of glucose starvation and hypertonicity. Biochim Biophys Acta 1988;950:138–46.

[174] Finkenzeller G, Newsome W, Lang F, Haussinger D. Increase of c-jun mRNA upon hypo-osmotic cell swelling of rat hepatoma cells. FEBS Lett 1994;340:163–6.

[175] Zhang F, Warskulat U, Haussinger D. Modulation of tumor necrosis factor-alpha release by anisoosmolarity and betaine in rat liver macrophages (Küpffer cells). FEBS Lett 1996;391:293–6.

[176] Murphy D, Carter D. Vasopressin gene expression in the rodent hypothalamus: transcriptional and posttranscriptional responses to physiological stimulation. Mol Endocrinol 1990;4:1051–9.

[177] Ferraris JD, Williams CK, Jung KY. Bedford JJ, Burg MB, Garcia-Perez A. ORE, a eukaryotic minimal essential osmotic response element. The aldose reductase gene in hyperosmotic stress. J Biol Chem 1996;271:18318–21.

[178] Ruepp B, Bohren KM, Gabbay KH. Characterization of the osmotic response element of the human aldose reductase gene promoter. Proc Natl Acad Sci USA 1996;93:8624–9.

[179] Ferraris JD, Williams CK, Persaud P, Zhang Z, Chen Y, Burg MB. Activity of the TonEBP/OREBP transactivation domain varies directly with extracellular NaCl concentration. Proc Natl Acad Sci USA 2002;99:739–44.

[180] Go WY, Liu X, Roti MA, Liu F, Ho SN. NFAT5/TonEBP mutant mice define osmotic stress as a critical feature of the lymphoid microenvironment. Proc Natl Acad Sci USA 2004;101:10673–8.

[181] Irarrazabal CE, Liu JC, Burg MB, Ferraris JD. ATM a DNA damage-inducible kinase, contributes to activation by high NaCl of the transcription factor TonEBP/OREBP. Proc Natl Acad Sci USA 2004;101:8809–14.

[182] Ito T, Fujio Y, Hirata M, Takatani T, Matsuda T, Muraoka S, et al. Expression of taurine transporter is regulated through the TonE (tonicity-responsive element)/TonEBP (TonE-binding protein) pathway and contributes to cytoprotection in HepG2 cells. Biochem J 2004;382:177–82.

[183] Lam AK, Ko BC, Tam S, Morris R, Yang JY, Chung SK, et al. Osmotic response element-binding protein (OREBP) is an essential regulator of the urine concentrating mechanism. J Biol Chem 2004;279:48048–54.

[184] Lee SD, Colla E, Sheen MR, Na KY, Kwon HM. Multiple domains of TonEBP cooperate to stimulate transcription in response to hypertonicity. J Biol Chem 2003;278:47571–7.

[185] Lopez-Rodriguez C, Antos CL, Shelton JM, Richardson JA, Lin F, Novobrantseva TI, et al. Loss of NFAT5 results in renal atrophy and lack of tonicity-responsive gene expression. Proc Natl Acad Sci USA 2004;101:2392–7.

[186] Stroud JC, Lopez-Rodriguez C, Rao A, Chen L. Structure of a TonEBP-DNA complex reveals DNA encircled by a transcription factor. Nat Struct Biol 2002;9:90–4.

[187] Burg MB. Macromolecular crowding as a cell volume sensor. Cell Physiol Biochem 2000;10:251–6.

[188] Alexander RT, Malevanets A, Durkan AM, Kocinsky HS, Aronson PS, Orlowski J, et al. Membrane curvature alters the activation kinetics of the epithelial Na^+/H^+ exchanger, NHE3. J Biol Chem 2007;282:7376–84.

[189] Asaoka Y, Yoshida K, Sasaki Y, Nishizuka Y. Potential role of phospholipase A2 in HL-60 cell differentiation to macrophages induced by protein kinase C activation. Proc Natl Acad Sci USA 1993;90:4917–21.

[190] Maingret F, Patel AJ, Lesage F, Lazdunski M, Honore E. Lysophospholipids open the two-pore domain mechanogated $K^{(+)}$ channels TREK-1 and TRAAK. J Biol Chem 2000;275:10128–33.

[191] Hamill OP, Martinac B. Molecular basis of mechanotransduction in living cells. Physiol Rev 2001;81:685–740.

[192] Ingber DE. Tensegrity: the architectural basis of cellular mechanotransduction. Annu Rev Physiol 1997;59:575–99.

[193] Rosette C, Karin M. Ultraviolet light and osmotic stress: activation of the JNK cascade through multiple growth factor and cytokine receptors. Science 1996;274:1194–7.

[194] Fiol DF, Kultz D. Osmotic stress sensing and signaling in fishes. FEBS J 2007;274:5790–8.

[195] Cohen DM. TRPV4 and the mammalian kidney. Pflugers Arch 2005;451:168–75.

[196] O'Neil RG, Heller S. The mechanosensitive nature of TRPV channels. Pflugers Arch 2005;451:193–203.

[197] Chen B, Nicol G, Cho WK. Role of calcium in volume-activated chloride currents in a mouse cholangiocyte cell line. J Membr Biol 2007;215:1–13.

[198] McCarty NA, O'Neil RG. Calcium signaling in cell volume regulation. Physiol Rev 1992;72:1037–61.

[199] Tinel H, Kinne-Saffran E, Kinne RK. Calcium signalling during RVD of kidney cells. Cell Physiol Biochem 2000;10:297–302.

[200] Cornet M, Lambert IH, Hoffmann EK. Relation between cytoskeleton, hypo-osmotic treatment and volume regulation in Ehrlich ascites tumor cells. J Membr Biol 1993;131:55–66.

[201] Haussinger D, Stoll B, vom Dahl S, Theodoropoulos PA, Markogiannakis E, Gravanis A, et al. Effect of hepatocyte swelling on microtubule stability and tubulin mRNA levels. Biochem Cell Biol 1994;72:12–9.

[202] Papakonstanti EA, Vardaki EA, Stournaras C. Actin cytoskeleton: a signaling sensor in cell volume regulation. Cell Physiol Biochem 2000;10:257–64.

[203] Szaszi K, Grinstein S, Orlowski J, Kapus A. Regulation of the epithelial $Na^{(+)}/H^{(+)}$ exchanger isoform by the cytoskeleton. Cell Physiol Biochem 2000;10:265–72.

[204] Tamma G, Procino G, Svelto M, Valenti G. Hypotonicity causes actin reorganization and recruitment of the actin-binding ERM protein moesin in membrane protrusions in collecting duct principal cells. Am J Physiol Cell Physiol 2007;292:C1476–84.

[205] Feranchak AP, Kilic G, Wojtaszek PA, Qadri I, Fitz JG. Volume-sensitive tyrosine kinases regulate liver cell volume through effects on vesicular trafficking and membrane Na^+ permeability. J Biol Chem 2003;278:44632–8.

[206] Lepple-Wienhues A, Szabo I, Laun T, Kaba NK, Gulbins E, Lang F. The tyrosine kinase p56lck mediates activation of swelling-induced chloride channels in lymphocytes. J Cell Biol 1998;141:281–6.

[207] Nilius B, Eggermont J, Droogmans G. The endothelial volume-regulated anion channel, VRAC. Cell Physiol Biochem 2000;10:313–20.

[208] Tilly BC, van den BN, Tertoolen LG, Edixhoven MJ, de Jonge HR. Protein tyrosine phosphorylation is involved in osmoregulation of ionic conductances. J Biol Chem 1993;268:19919–22.

[209] van der Wijk T, Tomassen SF, de Jonge HR, Tilly BC. Signalling mechanisms involved in volume regulation of intestinal epithelial cells. Cell Physiol Biochem 2000;10:289–96.

[210] Richter EA, Cleland PJ, Rattigan S, Clark MG. Contraction-associated translocation of protein kinase C in rat skeletal muscle. FEBS Lett 1987;217:232—6.

[211] Rosales OR, Sumpio BE. Changes in cyclic strain increase inositol trisphosphate and diacylglycerol in endothelial cells. Am J Physiol 1992;262:C956—62.

[212] Tilly BC, Edixhoven MJ, Tertoolen LG, Morii N, Saitoh Y, Narumiya S, et al. Activation of the osmo-sensitive chloride conductance involves P21rho and is accompanied by a transient reorganization of the F-actin cytoskeleton. Mol Biol Cell 1996;7:1419—27.

[213] Agius L, Peak M, Beresford G, al Habori M, Thomas TH. The role of ion content and cell volume in insulin action. Biochem Soc Trans 1994;22:516—22.

[214] Belsey MJ, Davies AR, Witchel HJ, Kozlowski RZ. Inhibition of ERK and JNK decreases both osmosensitive taurine release and cell proliferation in glioma cells. Neurochem Res 2007;32:1940—9.

[215] Galcheva-Gargova Z, Derijard B, Wu IH, Davis RJ. An osmo-sensing signal transduction pathway in mammalian cells. Science 1994;265:806—8.

[216] Han J, Lee JD, Bibbs L, Ulevitch RJ. A MAP kinase targeted by endotoxin and hyperosmolarity in mammalian cells. Science 1994;265:808—11.

[217] Itoh T, Yamauchi A, Imai E, Ueda N, Kamada T. Phosphatase toward MAP kinase is regulated by osmolarity in Madin—Darby canine kidney (MDCK) cells. FEBS Lett 1995;373:123—6.

[218] Noe B, Schliess F, Wettstein M, Heinrich S, Haussinger D. Regulation of taurocholate excretion by a hypo-osmolarity-activated signal transduction pathway in rat liver. Gastroenterology 1996;110:858—65.

[219] Schliess F, Sinning R, Fischer R, Schmalenbach C, Haussinger D. Calcium-dependent activation of Erk-1 and Erk-2 after hypo-osmotic astrocyte swelling. Biochem J 1996;320(Pt 1):167—71.

[220] Lang F, Bohmer C, Palmada M, Seebohm G, Strutz-Seebohm N, Vallon V. (Patho)physiological significance of the serum- and glucocorticoid-inducible kinase isoforms. Physiol Rev 2006;86:1151—78.

[221] Clements Jr. RS, Blumenthal SA, Morrison AD, Winegrad AI. Increased cerebrospinal-fluid pressure during treatment of diabetic ketosis. Lancet 1971;2:671—5.

[222] Gagnon KB, England R, Delpire E. Characterization of SPAK and OSR1, regulatory kinases of the Na-K-2Cl co-transporter. Mol Cell Biol 2006;26:689—98.

[223] Gagnon KB, England R, Delpire E. A single binding motif is required for SPAK activation of the Na-K-2Cl co-transporter. Cell Physiol Biochem 2007;20:131—42.

[224] Zagorska A, Pozo-Guisado E, Boudeau J, Vitari AC, Rafiqi FH, Thastrup J, et al. Regulation of activity and localization of the WNK1 protein kinase by hyperosmotic stress. J Cell Biol 2007;176:89—100.

[225] Delpire E. KBSPAK Gagnon and OSR1: STE20 kinases involved in the regulation of ion homoeostasis and volume control in mammalian cells. Biochem J 2008;409:321—31.

[226] Garzon-Muvdi T, Pacheco-Alvarez D, Gagnon KB, Vazquez N, Ponce-Coria J, Moreno E, et al. WNK4 kinase is a negative regulator of K$^+$-Cl$^-$ co-transporters. Am J Physiol Renal Physiol 2007;292:F1197—207.

[227] Peng JB, Warnock DG. WNK4-mediated regulation of renal ion transport proteins. Am J Physiol Renal Physiol 2007;293:F961—73.

[228] Ring AM, Leng Q, Rinehart J, Wilson FH, Kahle KT, Hebert SC, et al. An SGK1 site in WNK4 regulates Na$^+$ channel and K$^+$ channel activity and has implications for aldosterone

[229] signaling and K$^+$ homeostasis. Proc Natl Acad Sci USA 2007;104:4025—9.

[229] Bode JG, Gatsios P, Ludwig S, Rapp UR, Haussinger D, Heinrich PC, et al. The mitogen-activated protein (MAP) kinase p38 and its upstream activator MAP kinase kinase 6 are involved in the activation of signal transducer and activator of transcription by hyperosmolarity. J Biol Chem 1999;274:30222—7.

[230] Feranchak AP, Berl T, Capasso J, Wojtaszek PA, Han J, Fitz JG. p38 MAP kinase modulates liver cell volume through inhibition of membrane Na$^+$ permeability. J Clin Invest 2001;108:1495—504.

[231] Haussinger D, Schliess F, Dombrowski F, vom Dahl S. Involvement of p38MAPK in the regulation of proteolysis by liver cell hydration. Gastroenterology 1999;116:921—35.

[232] Hilder TL, Malone MH, Johnson GL. Hyperosmotic induction of mitogen-activated protein kinase scaffolding. Methods Enzymol 2007;428:297—312.

[233] Hoffmann EK. Intracellular signalling involved in volume regulatory decrease. Cell Physiol Biochem 2000;10:273—88.

[234] Jacobsen JH, Clement CA, Friis MB, Lambert IH. Casein kinase 2 regulates the active uptake of the organic osmolyte taurine in NIH3T3 mouse fibroblasts. Pflugers Arch 2008;457:327—37.

[235] Moriguchi T, Kawasaki H, Matsuda S, Gotoh Y, Nishida E. Evidence for multiple activators for stress-activated protein kinase/c-Jun amino-terminal kinases. Existence of novel activators. J Biol Chem 1995;270:12969—72.

[236] Nielsen MB, Christensen ST, Hoffmann EK. Effects of osmotic stress on the activity of MAPKs and PDGFR-beta-mediated signal transduction in NIH-3T3 fibroblasts. Am J Physiol Cell Physiol 2008;294:C1046—55.

[237] Pan Z, Capo-Aponte JE, Zhang F, Wang Z, Pokorny KS, Reinach PS. Differential dependence of regulatory volume decrease behavior in rabbit corneal epithelial cells on MAPK superfamily activation. Exp Eye Res 2007;84:978—90.

[238] Pedersen SF, Darborg BV, Rentsch ML, Rasmussen M. Regulation of mitogen-activated protein kinase pathways by the plasma membrane Na$^+$/H$^+$ exchanger, NHE1. Arch Biochem Biophys 2007;462:195—201.

[239] Strange K, Denton J, Nehrke K. Ste20-type kinases: evolutionarily conserved regulators of ion transport and cell volume. *Physiology* (Bethesda) 2006;21:61—8.

[240] Sanguinetti AR, Cao H, Corley MC. Fyn is required for oxidative- and hyperosmotic-stress-induced tyrosine phosphorylation of caveolin-1. Biochem J 2003;376:159—68.

[241] Trouet D, Carton I, Hermans D, Droogmans G, Nilius B, Eggermont J. Inhibition of VRAC by c-Src tyrosine kinase targeted to caveolae is mediated by the Src homology domains. Am J Physiol Cell Physiol 2001;281:C248—56.

[242] Nielsen DK, Jensen AK, Harbak H, Christensen SC, Simonsen LO. Cell content of phosphatidylinositol (4,5)bisphosphate in Ehrlich mouse ascites tumour cells in response to cell volume perturbations in anisotonic and in isosmotic media. J Physiol 2007;582:1027—36.

[243] Yamamoto M, Chen MZ, Wang YJ, Sun HQ, Wei Y, Martinez M, et al. Hypertonic stress increases phosphatidylinositol 4,5-bisphosphate levels by activating PIP5KIbeta. J Biol Chem 2006;281:32630—8.

[244] Gamper N, Shapiro MS. Target-specific PIP (2) signalling: how might it work? J Physiol 2007;582:967—75.

[245] Janmey PA, Lindberg U. Cytoskeletal regulation: rich in lipids. Nat Rev Mol Cell Biol 2004;5:658—66.

[246] Lambert IH. Eicosanoids and cell volume regulation. In: Strange K, editor. Cellular and Molecular Physiology of

Cell Volume Regulation. Boca Raton, FL: CRC Press; 1994. p. 179—98.

[247] Meyer MC, McHowat J. Calcium-independent phospholipase A2-catalyzed plasmalogen hydrolysis in hypoxic human coronary artery endothelial cells. Am J Physiol Cell Physiol 2007;292:C251—8.

[248] Steer SA, Wirsig KC, Creer MH, Ford DA, McHowat J. Regulation of membrane-associated iPLA2 activity by a novel PKC isoform in ventricular myocytes. Am J Physiol Cell Physiol 2002;283:C1621—6.

[249] Tay HK, Melendez AJ. Fcgamma RI-triggered generation of arachidonic acid and eicosanoids requires iPLA2 but not cPLA2 in human monocytic cells. J Biol Chem 2004;279:22505—13.

[250] Lambert IH, Hoffmann EK, Christensen P. Role of prostaglandins and leukotrienes in volume regulation by Ehrlich ascites tumor cells. J Membr Biol 1987;98:247—56.

[251] Lang PA, Kempe DS, Myssina S, Tanneur VBC, Laufer S, Lang F, et al. PGE2 in the regulation of programmed erythrocyte death. Cell Death Diff 2005;12(5):415—28.

[252] Civan MM, Coca-Prados M, Peterson-Yantorno K. Pathways signaling the regulatory volume decrease of cultured nonpigmented ciliary epithelial cells. Invest Ophthalmol Vis Sci 1994;35:2876—86.

[253] Lang PA, Kempe DS, Tanneur V, Eisele K, Klarl BA, Myssina S, et al. Stimulation of erythrocyte ceramide formation by platelet activating factor. J. Cell Science 2005;118(Pt 6):1233—43.

[254] Busch GL, Lang HJ, Lang F. Studies on the mechanism of swelling-induced lysosomal alkalinization in vascular smooth muscle cells. Pflugers Arch 1996;431:690—6.

[255] Busch GL, Schreiber R, Dartsch PC, Volkl H, vom DS, Haussinger D, et al. Involvement of microtubules in the link between cell volume and pH of acidic cellular compartments in rat and human hepatocytes. Proc Natl Acad Sci USA 1994;91:9165—9.

[256] Malek AM, Xu C, Kim ES, Alper SL. Hypertonicity triggers RhoA-dependent assembly of myosin-containing striated polygonal actin networks in endothelial cells. Am J Physiol Cell Physiol 2007;292:C1645—59.

[257] Schneider L, Klausen TK, Stock C, Mally S, Christensen ST, Pedersen SF, et al. H-ras transformation sensitizes volume-activated anion channels and increases migratory activity of NIH3T3 fibroblasts. Pflugers Arch 2008;455:1055—62.

[258] Rasmussen M, Alexander RT, Darborg BV, Mobjerg N, Hoffmann EK, Kapus A, et al. Osmotic cell shrinkage activates ezrin/radixin/moesin (ERM) proteins: activation mechanisms and physiological implications. Am J Physiol Cell Physiol 2008;294:C197—212.

[259] Pedersen S, Pedersen SF, Nilius B, Lambert IH, Hoffmann EK. Mechanical stress induces release of ATP from Ehrlich ascites tumor cells. Biochim Biophys Acta 1999;1416:271—84.

[260] Poronnik P, Schumann SY, Cook DI. HCO3($^-$)-dependent ACh-activated Na$^+$ influx in sheep parotid secretory endpieces. Pflugers Arch 1995;429:852—8.

[261] Van der Meulen JA, Klip A, Grinstein S. Possible mechanism for cerebral oedema in diabetic ketoacidosis. Lancet 1987;2:306—8.

[262] Saltin B, Sjogaard G, Strange S, Juel C. Redistribution of K$^+$ in the human body during muscular exercise: Its role to maintain whole body homeostasis. In: Shirak KYMK, editor. Man in Stressful Environments: Thermal and Work Physiology. Springfield, IL: Thomas; 1987. p. 247—67.

[263] Chacon E, Reece JM, Nieminen AL, Zahrebelski G, Herman B, Lemasters JJ. Distribution of electrical potential, pH, free Ca^{2+}, and volume inside cultured adult rabbit cardiac myocytes during chemical hypoxia: a multiparameter digitized confocal microscopic study. Biophys J 1994;66:942—52.

[264] Faff-Michalak L, Reichenbach A, Dettmer D, Kellner K, Albrecht J. K($^+$)-, hypoosmolarity-, and NH4($^+$)-induced taurine release from cultured rabbit Muller cells: role of Na$^+$ and Cl$^-$ ions and relation to cell volume changes. Glia 1994;10:114—20.

[265] Smith TW, Rasmusson RL, Lobaugh LA, Lieberman M. Na$^+$/K$^+$ pump inhibition induces cell shrinkage in cultured chick cardiac myocytes. Basic Res Cardiol 1993;88:411—20.

[266] Lang F, Rehwald W. Potassium channels in renal epithelial transport regulation. Physiol Rev 1992;72:1—32.

[267] Schultz SG. Homocellular regulatory mechanisms in sodium-transporting epithelia: avoidance of extinction by "flush-through.". Am J Physiol 1981;241:F579—90.

[268] Foskett JK, Wong MM, Sue AQ, Robertson MA. Isosmotic modulation of cell volume and intracellular ion activities during stimulation of single exocrine cells. J Exp Zool 1994;268:104—10.

[269] Hoffmann EK, Ussing HH. Membrane mechanisms in volume regulation in vertebrate cells and epithelia. In: Giebisch GH, Schafer JA, Ussing HH, Kristensen P, editors. Membrane Transport in Biology. Heidelberg: Springer-Verlag; 1992. p. 317—99.

[270] Manganel M, Turner RJ. Agonist-induced activation of Na$^+$/H$^+$ exchange in rat parotid acinar cells is dependent on calcium but not on protein kinase C. J Biol Chem 1990;265:4284—9.

[271] Manganel M, Turner RJ. Rapid secretagogue-induced activation of Na$^+$H$^+$ exchange in rat parotid acinar cells. Possible interrelationship between volume regulation and stimulus-secretion coupling. J Biol Chem 1991;266:10182—8.

[272] Joiner CH. Cation transport and volume regulation in sickle red blood cells. Am J Physiol 1993;264:C251—70.

[273] Lang KS, Lang PA, Bauer C, Duranton C, Wieder T, Huber SM, et al. Mechanisms of suicidal erythrocyte death. Cell Physiol Biochem 2005;15:195—202.

[274] Lang F, Busch G, Völkl H, Häussinger D. Cell volume: a second message in regulation of cellular function. News Physiol Sci 1995;10:18—22.

[275] Boini KM, Graf D, Kuhl D, Haussinger D, Lang F. SGK1 dependence of insulin induced hypokalemia. Pflugers Arch 2009;457:955—61.

[276] Schliess F, Haussinger D. Cell volume and insulin signaling. Int Rev Cytol 2003;225:187—228.

[277] Schliess F, Reissmann R, Reinehr R, vom DS, Haussinger D. Involvement of integrins and Src in insulin signaling toward autophagic proteolysis in rat liver. J Biol Chem 2004;279:21294—301.

[278] Choi DW, Rothman SM. The role of glutamate neurotoxicity in hypoxic-ischemic neuronal death. Annu Rev Neurosci 1990;13:171—82.

[279] Polischuk TM, Andrew RD. Real-time imaging of intrinsic optical signals during early excitotoxicity evoked by domoic acid in the rat hippocampal slice. Can J Physiol Pharmacol 1996;74:712—22.

[280] Saransaari P, Oja SS. Excitatory amino acids evoke taurine release from cerebral cortex slices from adult and developing mice. Neuroscience 1991;45:451—9.

[281] Ballanyi K, Grafe P. Cell volume regulation in the nervous system. Ren Physiol Biochem 1988;11:142—57.

[282] Strbak V, Greer MA. Regulation of hormone secretion by acute cell volume changes: Ca($^{2+}$)-independent hormone secretion. Cell Physiol Biochem 2000;10:393—402.

[283] Bohmer C, Philippin M, Rajamanickam J, Mack A, Broer S, Palmada M, et al. Stimulation of the EAAT4 glutamate transporter by SGK protein kinase isoforms and PKB. Biochem Biophys Res Commun 2004;324:1242—8.

[284] Kimelberg HK. Current concepts of brain edema. Review of laboratory investigations. J Neurosurg 1995;83:1051—9.

[285] Cordoba J, Gottstein J, Blei AT. Glutamine, myo-inositol, and organic brain osmolytes after portocaval anastomosis in the rat: implications for ammonia-induced brain edema. Hepatology 1996;24:919—23.

[286] Norenberg MD, Bender AS. Astrocyte swelling in liver failure: role of glutamine and benzodiazepines. *Acta Neurochir Suppl* (Wien) 1994;60:24—7.

[287] Haussinger D, Laubenberger J, vom Dahl S, Ernst T, Bayer S, Langer M, et al. Proton magnetic resonance spectroscopy studies on human brain myo-inositol in hypo-osmolarity and hepatic encephalopathy. Gastroenterology 1994;107:1475—80.

[288] Kreis R, Ross BD, Farrow NA, Ackerman Z. Metabolic disorders of the brain in chronic hepatic encephalopathy detected with H-1 MR spectroscopy. Radiology 1992;182:19—27.

[289] Hawkins RA, Jessy J, Mans AM, De Joseph MR. Effect of reducing brain glutamine synthesis on metabolic symptoms of hepatic encephalopathy. J Neurochem 1993;60:1000—6.

[290] Sakai H, Kakinoki B, Diener M, Takeguchi N. Endogenous arachidonic acid inhibits hypotonically-activated Cl^- channels in isolated rat hepatocytes. Jpn J Physiol 1996;46:311—8.

[291] Elliott SJ, Schilling WP. Oxidant stress alters Na^+ pump and $Na^{(+)}$-$K^{(+)}$-Cl^- co-transporter activities in vascular endothelial cells. Am J Physiol 1992;263:H96—102.

[292] Brizzolara A, Barbieri MP, Adezati L, Viviani GL. Water distribution in insulin-dependent diabetes mellitus in various states of metabolic control. Eur J Endocrinol 1996;135:609—15.

[293] Krane EJ, Rockoff MA, Wallman JK, Wolfsdorf JI. Subclinical brain swelling in children during treatment of diabetic ketoacidosis. N Engl J Med 1985;312:1147—51.

[294] Young E, Bradley RF. Cerebral edema with irreversible coma in severe diabetic ketoacidosis. N Engl J Med 1967;276:665—9.

[295] Edmands S, Yancey PH. Effects on rat renal osmolytes of extended treatment with an aldose reductase inhibitor. Comp Biochem Physiol C 1992;103:499—502.

[296] Finegold D, Lattimer SA, Nolle S, Bernstein M, Greene DA. Polyol pathway activity and myo-inositol metabolism. A suggested relationship in the pathogenesis of diabetic neuropathy. Diabetes 1983;32:988—92.

[297] Tomlinson DR, Stevens EJ, Diemel LT. Aldose reductase inhibitors and their potential for the treatment of diabetic complications. Trends Pharmacol Sci 1994;15:293—7.

[298] Demerdash TM, Seyrek N, Smogorzewski M, Marcinkowski W, Nasser-Moadelli S, Massry SG. Pathways through which glucose induces a rise in $[Ca^{2+}]i$ of polymorphonuclear leukocytes of rats. Kidney Int 1996;50:2032—40.

[299] Lang F, Klingel K, Wagner CA, Stegen C, Warntges S, Friedrich B, et al. Deranged transcriptional regulation of cell-volume-sensitive kinase hSGK in diabetic nephropathy. Proc Natl Acad Sci USA 2000;97:8157—62.

[300] Lee JA, Lee HA, Sadler PJ. Uraemia: is urea more important than we think? Lancet 1991;338:1438—40.

[301] Friedrich B, Alexander D, Aicher WK, Duszenko M, Schaub T, Passlick-Deetjen J, et al. Influence of standard haemodialysis on transcription of human serum and glucocorticoid inducible kinase SGK1 and taurine transporter TAUT in blood leukocytes. Nephrology Dialysis Transplantation 2005;20(4): 768—74.

[302] Ling H, Vamvakas S, Busch G, Dammrich J, Schramm L, Lang F, et al. Suppressing role of transforming growth factor-beta 1 on cathepsin activity in cultured kidney tubule cells. Am J Physiol 1995;269:F911—7.

[303] Chiang Y, Chou CY, Hsu KF, Huang YF, Shen MR. EGF upregulates Na^+/H^+ exchanger NHE1 by post-translational regulation that is important for cervical cancer cell invasiveness. J Cell Physiol 2008;214:810—9.

[304] Habela CW, Sontheimer H. Cytoplasmic volume condensation is an integral part of mitosis. Cell Cycle 2007;6:1613—20.

[305] Chen LX, Zhu LY, Jacob TJ, Wang LW. Roles of volume-activated Cl^- currents and regulatory volume decrease in the cell cycle and proliferation in nasopharyngeal carcinoma cells. Cell Prolif 2007;40:253—67.

[306] Klausen TK, Bergdahl A, Hougaard C, Christophersen P, Pedersen SF, Hoffmann EK. Cell cycle-dependent activity of the volume- and Ca^{2+}-activated anion currents in Ehrlich lettre ascites cells. J Cell Physiol 2007;210:831—42.

[307] Lang F, Foller M, Lang K, Lang P, Ritter M, Vereninov A, et al. Cell volume regulatory ion channels in cell proliferation and cell death. Methods Enzymol 2007;428:209—25.

[308] Lang F, Perrotti N, Stournaras C. Colorectal carcinoma cells: regulation of survival and growth by SGK1. Int. J. Biochem. Cell Biol. 2010;42(10):1571—5.

[309] Jakab M, Ritter M. Cell volume regulatory ion transport in the regulation of cell migration. Contrib Nephrol 2006;152: 161—80.

[310] Stossel TP. On the crawling of animal cells. Science 1993;260:1086—94.

[311] Mao J, Wang L, Fan A, Wang J, Xu B, Jacob TJ, et al. Blockage of volume-activated chloride channels inhibits migration of nasopharyngeal carcinoma cells. Cell Physiol Biochem 2007;19:249—58.

[312] McFerrin MB, Sontheimer H. A role for ion channels in glioma cell invasion. Neuron Glia Biol 2006;2:39—49.

[313] Schwab A. Function and spatial distribution of ion channels and transporters in cell migration. Am J Physiol Renal Physiol 2001;280:F739—47.

[314] Schwab A, Nechyporuk-Zloy V, Fabian A, Stock C. Cells move when ions and water flow. Pflugers Arch 2007;453:421—32.

[315] Papadopoulos MC, Saadoun S, Verkman AS. Aquaporins and cell migration. Pflugers Arch 2008;456:693—700.

[316] Lang F, Gulbins E, Szabo I, Lepple-Wienhues A, Huber SM, Duranton C, et al. Cell volume and the regulation of apoptotic cell death. J Mol Recognit 2004;17:473—80.

[317] Bortner CD, Cidlowski JA. Caspase independent/dependent regulation of $K^{(+)}$, cell shrinkage, and mitochondrial membrane potential during lymphocyte apoptosis. J Biol Chem 1999;274:21953—62.

[318] Bortner CD, Hughes Jr. FM, Cidlowski JA. A primary role for K^+ and Na^+ efflux in the activation of apoptosis. J Biol Chem 1997;272:32436—42.

[319] Maeno E, Ishizaki Y, Kaneseki T, Hazama A, Okada Y. Normotonic cell shrinkage because of disordered volume regulation is an early prerequisite to apoptosis. Proc Natl Acad Sci USA 2000;97:9487—92.

[320] Gulbins E, Welsch J, Lepple-Wienhuis A, Heinle H, Lang F. Inhibition of Fas-induced apoptotic cell death by osmotic cell shrinkage. Biochem Biophys Res Commun 1997;236: 517—21.

[321] Reinehr R, Becker S, Hongen A, Haussinger D. The Src family kinase Yes triggers hyperosmotic activation of the epidermal

growth factor receptor and CD95. J Biol Chem 2004;279:23977—87.

[322] Reinehr R, Gorg B, Hongen A, Haussinger D. CD95-tyrosine nitration inhibits hyperosmotic and CD95 ligand-induced CD95 activation in rat hepatocytes. J Biol Chem 2004;279: 10364—73.

[323] Reinehr R, Haussinger D. Hyperosmotic activation of the CD95 system. Methods Enzymol 2007;428:145—60.

[324] Lang KS, Fillon S, Schneider D, Rammensee HG, Lang F. Stimulation of TNF alpha expression by hyperosmotic stress. Pflugers Arch 2002;443:798—803.

[325] Reinehr R, Schliess F, Haussinger D. Hyperosmolarity and CD95L trigger CD95/EGF receptor association and tyrosine phosphorylation of CD95 as prerequisites for CD95 membrane trafficking and DISC formation. FASEB J 2003;17: 731—3.

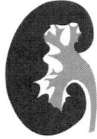 Solute Transport, Energy Consumption, and Production in the Kidney

Takashi Sekine[1] and Hitoshi Endou[2]

[1]Department of Pediatrics, Toho University School of Medicine, Ohashi Hospital, Tokyo, Japan
[2]Department of Pharmacology and Toxicology, Kyorin University School of Medicine, Tokyo, Japan

INTRODUCTION

The kidney must reabsorb more than 99% of approximately 180 liters of water and 25,000 mmoles of Na^+ daily. To do this, the kidney consumes a large amount of energy. Although the kidney is only 0.5% of the total body weight, it utilizes approximately 7% of the oxygen consumed by the body.[1] In fact, the kidney is the second only to the heart in terms of the rate of energy consumption.[1] In this chapter, first we describe the energy consuming and production processes in the kidney. Second, the mechanisms of mutual relationships between energy consumption and production will be described. Significant advances have been made with regard to this issue, and AMPK (AMP-activated kinase) is considered to be the central for the regulation of energy consuming processes. Finally, we also refer to the pathophysiological states in which renal energy production is inhibited.

ENERGY CONSUMPTION

Na Transport and Energy Consumption in the Kidney

Na+ Transport and O2 Consumption

The energy utilized in the kidney is primarily required for the active reabsorption of Na^+ from the glomerular filtrate. This seems rational considering that the amount of Na^+ reabsorbed by the kidney is much higher than that of HCO_3^- (4,000 mmole/day), Ca^{2+} (210 mmole/day), other electrolytes, and organic substances. The active Na^+ transport also energizes the reabsorption of water and other solutes by the osmotic gradient generated by Na^+ transport, and by the electrochemical gradient of Na^+ across the plasma membrane.

The data shown in Figures 6.1 and 6.2 indicate another important point. Extrapolation of the regression line to the Y ordinate indicates the basal oxygen consumption (Figure 6.1). This value is identical to the energy used for cellular functions other than Na^+ transport, and was estimated to be between 3 to 18%,[2] while other studies indicated a higher value for this basal O_2 consumption in the kidney.

With regard to energy production, the kidney generates approximately 95% of the ATP produced via aerobic mechanism,[3] while in some nephron segments anaerobic metabolism also occurs efficiently. This is reasonable because of the highly efficient ATP production by mitochondrial oxidative phosphorylation compared to anaerobic glycolysis. Thirty-six moles of ATP are generated by the mitochondrial oxidative phosphorylation of one mole of glucose, whereas only two moles of ATP are produced via glycolysis in the absence of O_2. Thus, historically, the relationship between Na transport and O_2 consumption (QO_2) in renal tissues has been extensively investigated.

Several investigators have examined Na^+/O_2 stoichiomety in the kidney.[4–6] Thurau demonstrated a linear relationship between Na^+ transport and QO_2 with a ratio of 28 Na^+/O_2 in the whole dog kidney[6] (Figure 6.1). This stoichiometry is equal to a ratio of 4.6 for Na^+/ATP, which indicates more efficient transport in the kidney compared to that in the frog skin and toad bladder. The discrepancy has been studied by many investigators and is attributed to the following.[7]

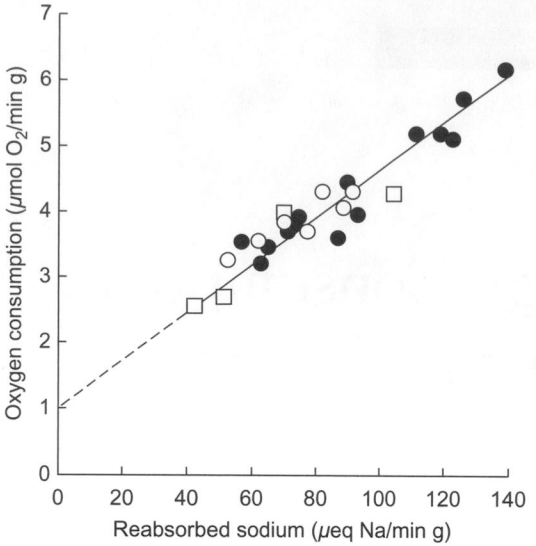

FIGURE 6.1 Oxygen consumption as a function of net sodium reabsorption in whole dog kidneys. *(Adapted from [6] with permission.)*

First, there are alternative pathways for Na^+ transport in the nephron. In the leaky epithelia, such as proximal tubule (PT), paracellular Na^+ transport occurs, while only transepithelial transport is possible in the tight epithelia in cortical collecting duct (CCD) cells. Second, coupling of Na^+ transport to that of other solutes occurs, such as bicarbonate transport in PT, and Na^+-K^+-$2Cl^-$ transport via NKCC2 in the thick ascending limb of Henle (TAL). These two mechanisms produce more efficient Na^+ transport in certain nephron segments compared to that observed in frog skin and toad bladder, where only cellular transport of Na^+ driven by Na^+,K^+-ATPase occurs. The different Na^+/O_2/ATP stoichiometry among individual nephron segments will be described below.

Heterogeneity in Na^+ Transport Efficiency among Nephron Segments

Proximal Tubule

In the PT, the Na^+/QO_2 was reported to be 24 to 30, corresponding to a Na^+/ATP ratio of 4 to 5. In the early portion of the PT (S1), preferential absorption of bicarbonate occurs,[8] resulting in a rise in the luminal Cl^- concentration, defined as axial anionic asymmetry.[9,10] In the basolateral membrane of proximal tubular cells, a Na^+-bicarbonate co-transporter (NBC) extrudes Na^+ with HCO_3^-[11] with a stoichiometry of 1:$2\sim3$.[12] The electrochemical gradient of HCO_3^- across the plasma membrane in the PT cells, which is generated by the coordinated function of carbonic anhydrase and H^+-ATPase or Na^+-H^+ exchanger, drives Na^+ efflux via NBC. Because PT is more permeable to Cl^- than to HCO_3^-, a driving force develops for isotonic

fluid transport. It was suggested that 30%[13] to 50%[14] of Na^+ transport in the PT is passive, and not directly related to ATP consumption. In addition, in the early part of the PT, glucose, amino acids, and phosphate are actively reabsorbed by the Na^+-co-transport mechanism, thereby rapidly reducing their concentration in the lumen. This luminal hypotonicity also contributes to the solvent drag which involves Na^+. Thus, in the PT, more than 3 Na^+ could be transported via the hydrolysis of one mole of ATP.

Thick Ascending Limb of Henle

In the TAL, the most efficient sodium transport occurs, with the Na^+-K^+-$2Cl^-$ co-transporter (NKCC2) playing an important role. The transport by NKCC2 is electrically neutral, and the K^+ reabsorbed by NKCC2 in the TAL is leaked back into the tubular lumen via the ROMK channel in the apical membrane. This K^+ leakage results in a positive electrical potential difference in the lumen, which drives paracellular transport of Na^+ from the lumen to the plasma (Figure 6.3). Although no direct measurement has been made of the Na^+/O_2/ATP stoichiometry in the TAL, the results obtained in the rectal gland[15] and tracheal epithelium[16] indicated that the Na^+/ATP ratio could theoretically be up to 6 in the TAL.

CCD

In the CCD, the efficiency of Na^+ transport is the lowest among the nephron segments. In this segment, the junction between the epithelia is very tight, and paracellular transport is minimal. In addition, Na^+ entry from the luminal side into CCD cells is mediated only by ENaC, which is not associated with any coupled transport other than that of Na^+. Thus, the Na^+:ATP ratio in the CCD is estimated to be 3.

Energy Cost of Primary Active Transport

The cellular transport of electrolytes and organic substances is classified into three types, namely, primary active, secondary active, and tertiary active transport. Primary active transport refers to that which directly utilizes ATP hydrolysis energy to accomplish transepithelial transport. The primary active transporter in the plasma membrane of mammalian cells is further subdivided into three subtypes, i.e., P-type-ATPase, V-type-ATPase, and ABC transporter. The secondary active transporters utilize the Na^+ gradient across the plasma membrane generated by the Na^+,K^+-ATPase. Na^+-coupled co-transporters (e.g., Na^+-glucose co-transporter, Na^+-amino acid co-transporter) transport substrates with Na^+ in the same direction, while Na^+-exchangers (e.g., NHE: the Na^+-H^+ exchanger) transport substrate

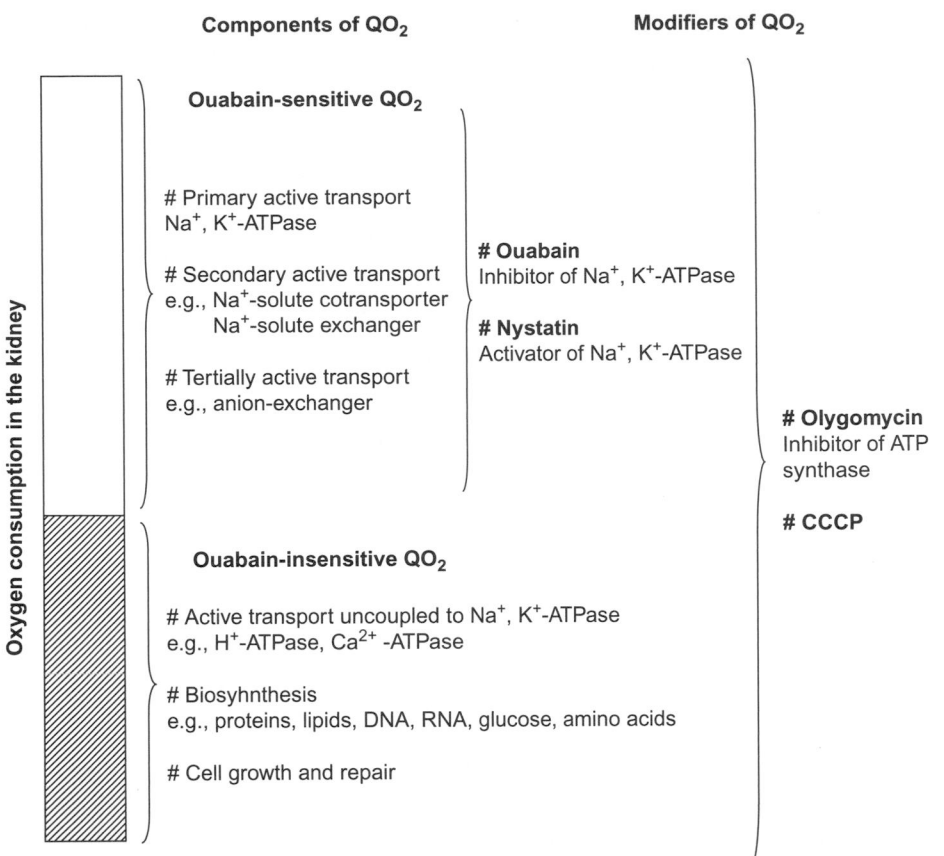

Components of QO₂

Ouabain-sensitive QO₂

Primary active transport
Na⁺, K⁺-ATPase

Secondary active transport
e.g., Na⁺-solute cotransporter
Na⁺-solute exchanger

Tertially active transport
e.g., anion-exchanger

Ouabain-insensitive QO₂

Active transport uncoupled to Na⁺, K⁺-ATPase
e.g., H⁺-ATPase, Ca²⁺-ATPase

Biosyhnthesis
e.g., proteins, lipids, DNA, RNA, glucose, amino acids

Cell growth and repair

Oxygen consumption in the kidney

Modifiers of QO₂

Ouabain
Inhibitor of Na⁺, K⁺-ATPase

Nystatin
Activator of Na⁺, K⁺-ATPase

Olygomycin
Inhibitor of ATP synthase

CCCP

FIGURE 6.2 **Cellular components of oxygen consumption (QO₂).** Cellular QO₂ is divided primarily into two components. The first is ouabain-sensitive QO₂, which is identical to the sum of Na⁺,K⁺-ATPase, secondary active and tertiary active transport coupled to the Na⁺ gradient. The other is an ouabain-insensitive portion, which is related to transport processes uncoupled to Na⁺,K⁺-ATPase (e.g., H⁺-ATPase and Ca²⁺-ATPase) and catabolic processes (e.g., biosynthesis and cell growth and repair). Ouabain-sensitive QO₂ is markedly different among nephron segments. In the PCT, 60% of QO₂ is ouabain-sensitive, whereas in OMCD, only 8% of QO₂ is ouabain-sensitive. These differences reflect the activities of Na⁺,K⁺-ATPase among nephron segments.

and Na⁺ in opposite directions. In addition, there exist the tertiary active transporters. One example of this is the anion exchangers (AE: Cl⁻/HCO₃⁻ exchanger). The proton gradient generated by the coordinated function of Na⁺,K⁺-ATPase (primary active transporter) and NHE (secondary active transporter) is used as the driving force for the exchange of Cl⁻ and HCO₃⁻ by AE (tertiary active transporter).

The energy cost for secondary and tertiary active transport processes is attributed to the active transport via Na⁺,K⁺-ATPase, which alone is accompanied by hydrolysis of ATP. Primary active transporters other than Na⁺,K⁺-ATPase are also related to the energy consumption processes in the kidney. In general, the expression level of ATPases along the nephron segments correlates well with the transport activity of each solute.

P-type-ATPases

P-type-ATPases (Figure 6.4), including Na⁺,K⁺-ATPase, H⁺,K⁺-ATPase, and Ca²⁺-ATPase, share

several common features: (1) they possess a seven amino acid motif with aspartate to which ATP binds; (2) they are transiently phosphorylated during the cation transport cycle (the term P-type derives from this transient phosphorylation); and (3) they catalyze cation transport between E_1 and E_2 conformations (P-type-ATPase was previously called E_1-E_2-ATPase). The transport activity of P-type-ATPases is commonly inhibited by vanadate.

Na⁺,K⁺-ATPase

Na⁺,K⁺-ATPase extrudes 3 Na⁺ and takes up 2 K⁺ across the plasma membranes through the hydrolysis of one ATP molecule in the presence of Mg²⁺. Na⁺,K⁺-ATPase generates an inwardly-directed Na⁺ gradient and inside a negative electrical gradient. Na⁺,K⁺-ATPase accounts for approximately half of the total Na⁺ reabsorption in the kidney.[17]

Na⁺,K⁺-ATPase is a heterodimeric integral membrane protein, with a minimal composition of α- and

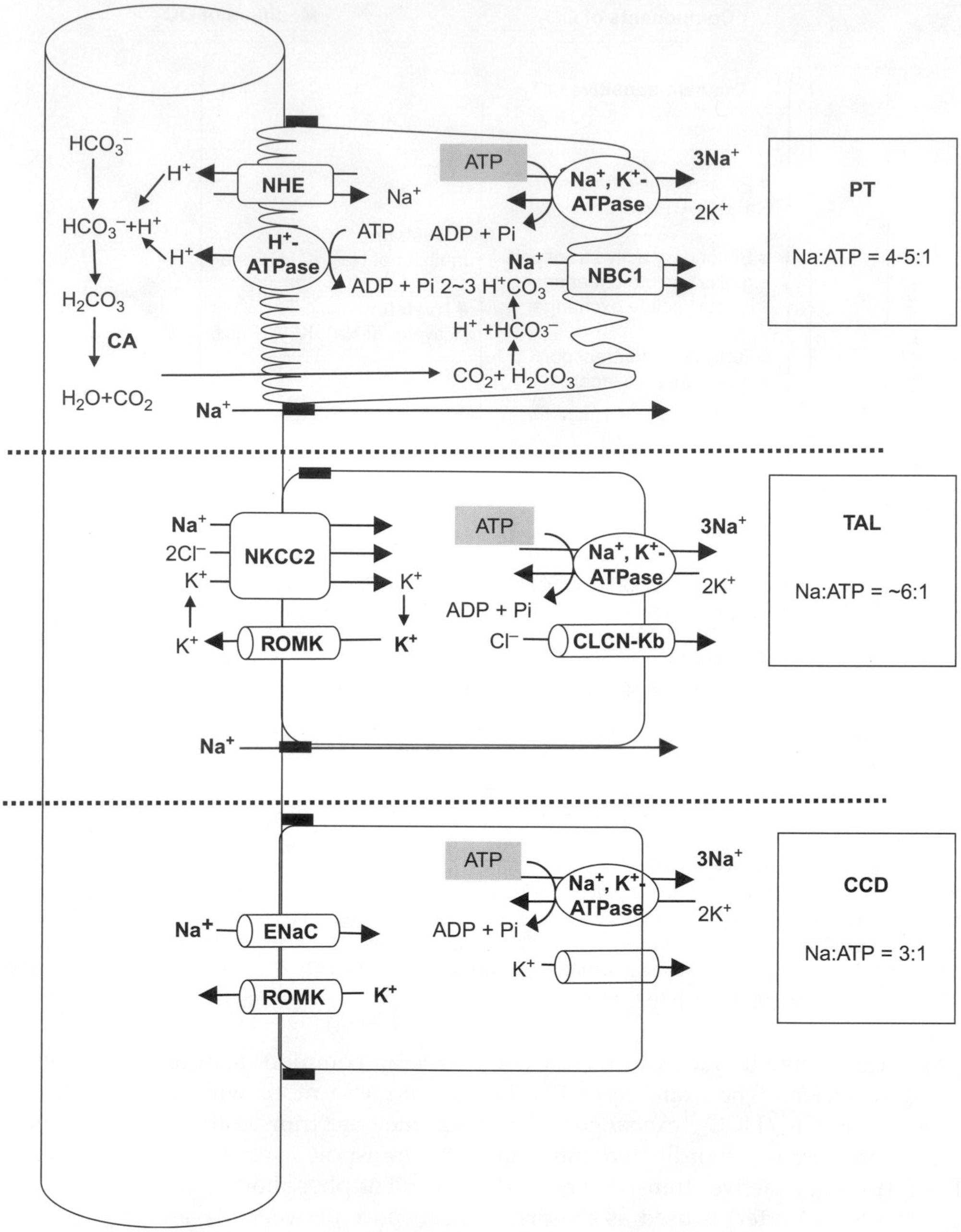

FIGURE 6.3 Heterogeneity of Na^+ transport/O_2/ATP along nephron segments.

β-subunits. The α-subunit possesses ten membrane-spanning domains with a molecular mass of approximately 100 kDa. The β-subunit is a glycosylated type II membrane protein with a molecular weight of approximately 55 kDa.[18] In mammalian genomes, four α-subunits and at least three β-subunits of Na^+,K^+-ATPase have been identified.[19,20] In addition, a γ-subunit, a member of the FXYD family of type II transmembrane proteins, constitutes an Na^+,K^+-ATPase.[21] In the kidney, two γ-subunit isoforms are expressed.[19,20] The combination of each isoform comprises a number of

Na^+,K^+-ATPase isozymes that are expressed in a tissue- and cell-specific manner to evolve distinct properties to respond to cellular requirements.[19] In the kidney, α1β1 is predominantly expressed.[20,22,23]

The α-subunit is the catalytic subunit of the Na^+, K^+-ATPase, and α1, α2, and α3 isoforms differ in their affinities for ATP, Na^+ and K^+.[24] β-subunits are suggested to facilitate the correct membrane integration and packing of the α-subunit, and β-subunits also participate in the determination of the intrinsic transport properties of Na^+,K^+-ATPase.[25] The γ-subunit was

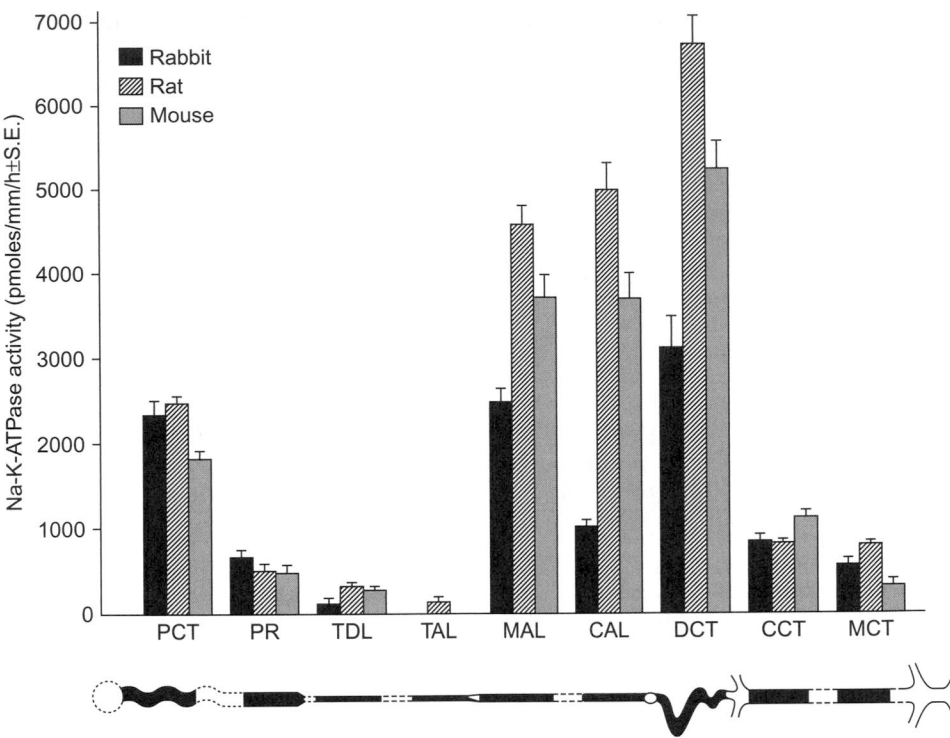

FIGURE 6.4 Na$^+$,K$^+$-ATPase activity in individual nephron segments measured using hydrolysis activity. (*Adapted from* [34] *with permission.*)

shown to be a specific regulator of renal α1β1 isozymes.[26] A putative dominant-negative mutation in the gene encoding the γ-subunit (FXYD2) which leads to defective routing of the protein in a family with dominant renal hypomagnesaemia indicates the physiological importance of the γ-subunit.[27] The overall structure of the α-subunit of Na$^+$,K$^+$-ATPase determined by electron crystallography using two-dimensional crystals is similar to the X-ray structure of Ca^{2+}-ATPase.[28,29]

The pump activity of Na$^+$,K$^+$-ATPase has been investigated using direct measurement of hydrolysis activity, and axial heterogeneity in the nephron segments was demonstrated[30–34] (Figure 6.4). Na$^+$,K$^+$-ATPase hydrolysis activity was high in the TAL, distal convoluted tubule (DCT), and proximal convoluted tubule (PCT), and low in the pars recta (PST) and collecting tubule (CT).[30–34] Ouabain binding studies show the highest density of Na$^+$,K$^+$-ATPase (20–30 fmol/mm length of tubule) in the DCT and the MTAL, intermediate density (10 fmol/ mm) in the PCT and connecting tubule (CNT), and lowest density (2–7 fmol/mm) in the PST, CTAL, and CT.[35] The pump activity was proportional to the number of catalytic units. α1β1 has a maximum turnover rate of 7,700/min.[36] The measurement of Na$^+$,K$^+$-ATPase hydrolytic activity at V$_{max}$, and initial rates of ouabain-

sensitive Rb uptake indicated that in intact cells the pump works at approximately 20–30% of its V$_{max}$.[37] Western blotting analysis,[38,39] RT-PCR using microdissected nephron segments,[39] *in situ* hybridization,[23,40] and immunohistochemical analysis[41–43] demonstrated similar intranephron heterogenetic localization of Na$^+$,K$^+$-ATPase consistent with those observed in the studies on pump activity.

Regulation of Na$^+$,K$^+$-ATPase by dexamethasone,[44] deoxycorticosterone,[45] intracellular Na concentration,[46] cAMP,[47] potassium depletion,[48] aldosterone and vasopressin[49,50] was demonstrated. Many of these modulations influence the cell surface expression of Na$^+$,K$^+$-ATPase,[49,50] while MEK1/2 inhibitors changed the intrinsic activity rather than cell surface expression.[51]

Ca^{2+}-ATPase

Renal calcium transport is comprised of two processes: a paracellular, passive process that predominates in most nephron segments; and a transcellular, energy-dependent step in the DCT. Transcellular calcium transport involves: (1) entry into the DCT cell via a Ca^{2+} channel (ECaC) across the luminal membrane; (2) intracellular Ca movement facilitated by the presence of the vitamin D-dependent calcium-binding protein (calbindin D); and (3) extrusion by the Ca^{2+}-ATPase located at the basolateral membrane.[52]

The extrusion of Ca^{2+}, the final step in the transcellular transport of Ca^{2+}, is mediated by the plasma membrane Ca^{2+}-ATPase (PMCA), which is a P-type-ATPase.

PMCA is a monomeric protein consisting of approximately 1,220 amino acids with a molecular mass of 140 kDa.[53,54] The sequence contains the calmodulin-binding domain, and two domains resembling calmodulin, one of which may play a role in the binding of Ca^{2+}.[54] There are at least four isoforms of PMCA, and isoforms 1 and 4 are more widely distributed than 2 and 3.[55-57] The activity of renal PMCA showed two saturable components: a high-affinity component with a Km of 33 μM ATP, and a low-affinity component with a Km of 0.63 mM ATP.[58] PMCA is regulated by calmodulin,[55] estrogen and dihydrotestosterone,[59] protein kinase C or A,[55] extracellular ATP,[60] and pathophysiologic states such as hypercalciuria.[61] RT-PCR,[62,63] immunohistochemical analysis,[64] and Western blot analysis[53] demonstrated high expression of PMCA in the DCT. PMCA was also detected in Madin—Darby canine kidney (MDCK) cells.[65] Doucet and co-workers examined sodium azide-insensitive plasma membrane Ca^{2+}-ATPase activity. The Ca^{2+}-ATPase was maximally activated by Ca^{2+} concentrations with an apparent Km of 0.3—0.4 μM. Ca^{2+}-ATPase activity was found in all segments of the nephron: activity was highest in the DCT and CCT, intermediate in the PCT and MTAL, and lowest in the PST, CTAL and MCT.[66]

In addition to PMCA, there exists another distinct Ca^{2+}-ATPase, the sarco/endoplasmic reticulum Ca^{2+}-ATPase (SERCA), which also belongs to the P-type-ATPase. The SERCA family includes three gene products, SERCA1 (ATP2A1), SERCA2 (ATP2A2), and SERCA 3 (ATP2A3),[67] which function in the removal of free cytosolic Ca^{2+} into the sarco/endoplasmic reticulum. Although thapsigarigin is known to be a specific inhibitor of the endoplasmic reticulum Ca^{2+}-pump,[68] no study has been reported on the relative energy consumption rate of SERCA in the kidney.

H^+,K^+-ATPase

H^+,K^+-ATPase was originally characterized in a study of gastric mucosa. The gastric H^+,K^+-ATPase is located in the apical membrane of stomach parietal cells, and mediates electroneutral exchange of K^+ and H^+. Gastric H^+,K^+-ATPase activity is independent of extracellular sodium, and is inhibited by vanadate.[69]

Molecular cloning identified two types of H^+,K^+-ATPase: gastric and colonic type H^+,K^+-ATPase. H^+,K^+-ATPase is comprised of α- and β-subunits. The catalytic α-subunit of gastric H^+,K^+-ATPase shows structural similarity to that of Na^+,K^+-ATPase, and the greatest homology occurs in the phosphorylation site

region, and domains presumably involved in nucleotide binding and energy transduction.[70] The α-subunit of colonic H^+,K^+-ATPase exhibits 63% amino acid identity to that of the gastric H^+,K^+-ATPase.[71] The β-subunit of H^+,K^+-ATPase shows 41% amino acid sequence identity to the β2-subunit of Na^+,K^+-ATPase in the rat.[72]

In the kidney, the existence of both gastric H^+,K^+-ATPase[70] and colonic H^+,K^+-ATPase[71] was demonstrated. Gastric H^+,K^+-ATPase is expressed constitutively along the length of the collecting duct, is responsible for H^+ secretion and K^+ reabsorption under normal conditions, and may be stimulated with acid—base perturbations and/or K^+ depletion.[73] The level of expression of colonic H^+,K^+-ATPase is much lower in the kidney than in the distal colon.[71]

Using in vitro microperfusion, Wingo and colleagues provided evidence of the existence of omeprazole-sensitive acidification and a K^+-absorptive mechanism in OMCD in rabbits.[74] By enzymatic analysis, Doucet[75] and Garg[76] quantified the K^+-stimulated, Na-insensitive ATPase activity in the nephron segments. K^+-stimulated ATPase activity was identified in the CNT, CCT, and MCT, although the activities were very low compared to those of other P-type-ATPases in the kidney.[76] The renal K^+-ATPase had a high affinity for K^+ (Km of approximately 0.2~0.4 mM) and was inhibited by vanadate, omeprazole, and SCH 28080, specific inhibitors of gastric H^+,K^+-ATPase, but was insensitive to ouabain.[75,76] A correlation between the magnitude of enzymatic activity and the percentage of intercalated cells in a given segment suggested that K^+-ATPase activity originates in intercalated cells.[75]

Immunohistochemical analysis revealed H^+,K^+-ATPase in intercalated cells in the CCD and OMCD. In all segments studied, except for the CCD, the percentage of H^+,K^+-ATPase-immunoreactive cells corresponded to the percentage of intercalated cells.[77] The RT-PCR technique demonstrated the gastric H^+,K^+-ATPase α-subunit in the CCD and IMCD, and a specific hybridization signal for the gastric H^+,K^+-ATPase α-subunit cDNA was demonstrated.[78] The colonic H^+,K^+-ATPase α-subunit is specifically expressed in the CCD and OMCD in K^+-depleted rats.[79] An increase in the H^+,K^+-ATPase activity,[75] and enhanced expression of gastric H^+,K^+-ATPase α-subunit[80] and colonic H^+,K^+-ATPase[73] in K^+ depletion, suggests the physiological adaptation of renal H^+,K^+-ATPase.

V-type ATPases

V-type (vacuolar) ATPases represent the second family of ATP-dependent ion pumps. Vacuolar H^+-ATPase is primarily responsible for the acidification of intracellular compartments such as endosomes, lysosomes, Golgi apparatus, and clathrin-coated vesicles.

H^+-ATPase is also expressed in the plasma membrane, and functions in acid—base transport in epithelia. In the kidney, vacuolar H^+-ATPase mediates H^+ secretion, mainly in the PT and CCD.[81,82]

H^+-ATPase is a multi-subunit complex composed of two functional domains.[83,84] The V(1) domain is a 570 kDa peripheral complex composed of eight subunits of molecular mass 73—14 kDa (subunits A—H) that is responsible for ATP hydrolysis. The V(o) domain is a 260 kDa integral complex composed of five subunits of molecular mass 100—17 kDa (subunits a, d, c, c', and c") that is responsible for proton translocation.

H^+-ATPase is insensitive to vanadate or ouabain, but inhibited by bafilomycin A, N,N'-dicyclohexylcarbodiimide (DCCD: Ki = 50 μM) and N-ethylmaleimide (NEM: Ki = 20 μM). Physiological experiments indicated the existence of H^+-ATPase in the PT. DCCD caused a fall in CO_2 absorption by 15% under eucapnia, and by 30% during acute hypercapnia in the PT.[85] In other experiments, the S_3 segment was shown to possess plasma membrane H^+-ATPase activity.[86]

The relative contribution of H^+-ATPase to ATP consumption by the kidney was examined by Noel et al. In dog proximal tubules incubated under control conditions, 81% of the respiration was directly related to oligomycin-sensitive ATP synthesis, and 29% of this amount was inhibited by bafilomycin A. In rabbit and hamster PT, the bafilomycin-sensitive ATP requirement involves only 5 and 10%, respectively, of the total ATP turnover. Thus, the metabolic cost of H^+-ATPase in PT varies significantly among species.[87]

Ait-Mohamed et al. examined the localization of NEM-sensitive ATPase in all the segments of the rat nephron; its activity was highest in the PCT; intermediate in the PST, TAL and CCT; and lowest in the OMCD.[88] Immunocytochemical analysis demonstrated localization of rat H^+-ATPase in the PCT, the initial part of the thin descending limb, TAL, DCT, and CT[89] consistent with the aforementioned H^+-ATPase activity.

Garg and co-workers examined the effect of acid-base balance[90—92] and aldosterone[93] on NEM-sensitive ATPase activity, and demonstrated the modulation of NEM-sensitive ATPase activity by metabolic acidosis and administration of aldosterone, and these effects were observed mainly in the CT.

The significance of H^+-ATPase in final urinary acidification along the collecting system has been confirmed by hereditary defects in H^+-ATPase. Mutations in the gene encoding the B1-subunit of H^+-ATPase cause distal renal tubular acidosis with sensorineural deafness, and defects in the 116 kDa subunit ATP6N1B cause recessive distal renal tubular acidosis with preserved hearing.[94—96]

ABC Superfamily

The third subgroup of primary active transporters is the ABC (ATP-binding cassette) transporter family. The prototype ABC transporter is the P-glycoprotein (P-gp) encoded by the MDR gene. P-gp was originally isolated as a drug extrusion pump in cancer cells which confers multiresistance to antineoplastic drugs.[97,98] Later, P-gp was also shown to be expressed in normal tissues such as the kidney, intestine, and brain capillary cells, where it acts as a functional barrier to xenobiotics by extruding them from the tissues. Then, a subfamily of ABC transporters, the MRP (multidrug-resistance-associated protein) family, was identified, and the number of its isoforms is expanding rapidly.[99]

The common molecular structure of ABC transporters is as follows; they possess two transmembrane (TM) domains, each with six TM segments and two nucleotide-binding domains, both of which can hydrolyze ATP.[100] The stoichiometry of two ATPs hydrolyzed per molecule of drug transported was proposed.[97]

Although the molecular properties of the members of ABC transporters, such as tissue distribution and substrate selectivity, have been extensively characterized, their significance in energy consumption in the kidney remains to be investigated, and to date no information is available.

Comparison of Ion Transporting ATPase Activities and QO₂ along the Nephron

In the upper panel of Figure 6.5 a comparison of the ion transporting ATPase activities is shown. In the lower part, relative distribution of QO_2 along the nephron segments is depicted.

METABOLIC BASIS IN THE KIDNEY

Energy Production Pathway in the Kidney

ATP synthesis in the kidney is mainly performed by mitochondrial oxidative phosphorylation, and a variety of energy fuels, such as glucose, fatty acids, and ketone bodies, are metabolized. Anaerobic glycolysis also occurs in certain nephron segments. Because of its heterogeneity in structural and functional properties, metabolic pathways and preferred substrates are distinct among the nephron. In this section, metabolic basis in the kidney and individual nephron segments are described.

Mitochondrial Oxidative Phosphorylation

Mitochondrial oxidative phosphorylation (Figures 6.6, 6.7) is comprised of the following three steps: (1)

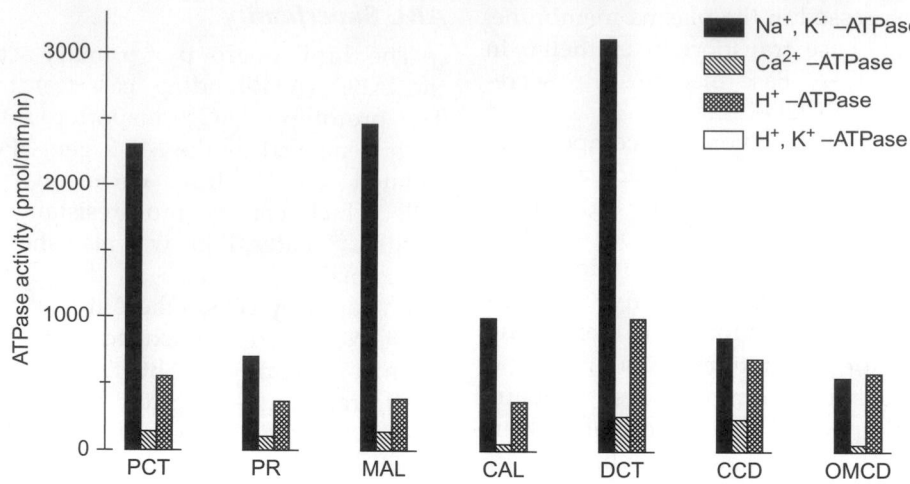

FIGURE 6.5 Comparison of ATPase activities employed from representative studies. *(Upper part adapted from [101] with permission; lower part from [102] with permission.)*

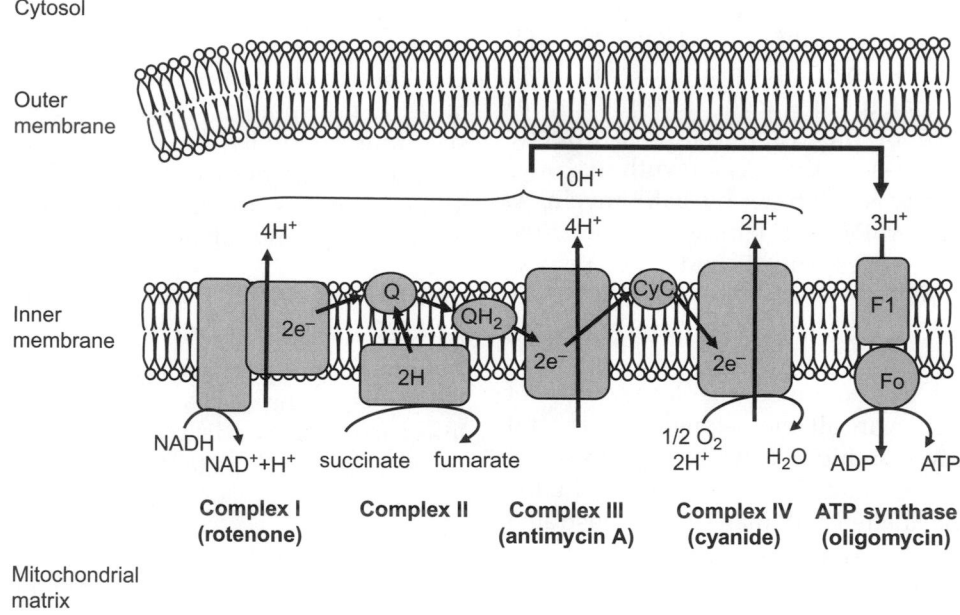

FIGURE 6.6 **Schematic representation of mitochondrial oxidative phosphorylation.** In the inner membrane of the mitochondria, four large multimeric membrane proteins complexes (complex I, II, III, and IV) catalyze electron transfer and proton extrusion. Two relatively small mobile proteins (Q and CytC) also mediate electron transport. Finally, ATP synthase produces ATP using the electrochemical gradient generated across the inner membrane of the mitochondria. Rotenone, antimycin A, cyanide, and oligomycin are representative inhibitors for the complexes I, III and IV, and ATP synthase, respectively.

production of reduced equivalents, i.e., NADH and FADH$_2$, mostly by the TCA cycle in the matrix of mitochondria; (2) electron transfer via the mitochondrial respiratory chain in the inner membrane of mitochondria, associated with proton extrusion across the inner membrane of mitochondria; and (3) ATP production by F$_0$F$_1$-ATPase using the proton gradient generated[103] (Figures 6.6 and 6.7). The mitochondrial respiratory chain catalyzes electron transfer via four large multimeric integral membrane protein complexes (complex I to IV), ATP synthase (alternatively called complex V), and two relatively small hydrophobic proteins, i.e., ubiquinone (Q: Coenzyme Q) and cytochrome c.

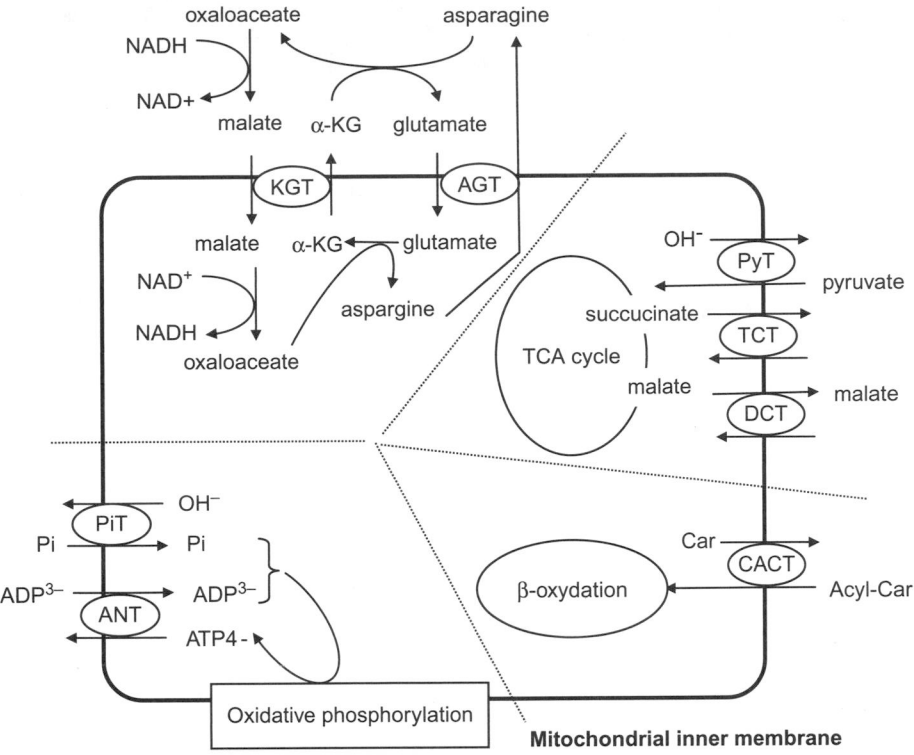

FIGURE 6.7 **Mitochondrial solute transporters located in mitochondrial inner membrane.** These transporters are divided into four groups from the functional viewpoints. The lower left part indicates the interchange of ADP, Pi, and ATP between the inner membrane by ANT and PiT. The left upper part indicates the malate-asparagine shuttle transporting the reducing potential from the cytosol to the matrix. The right upper part indicates the transport of substrates of the TCA cycle. The right lower part indicates the acyl-CoA transport to the mitochondrial matrix. Acyl-CoA is used for β-oxidation. In this figure, the ornithine transport system is not depicted.

Tricarboxylic Acid Cycle

The tricarboxylic acid (TCA) (Figure 6.8) cycle is present in all mammalian cells, except those lacking mitochondria such as mature red blood cells. The TCA cycle oxidizes acetyl CoA derived from carbohydrates, fatty acids, amino acids, and ketone bodies, and produces NADH and $FADH_2$. In addition, the TCA cycle provides intermediates that are utilized for the formation of glucose, lipids, and amino acids. Thus, the TCA cycle is central for metabolism, and is regulated to meet a variety of cellular metabolic demands.

Le Hir et al. assayed three TCA cycle enzymes, i.e., oxoglutarate dehydrogenase, citrate synthase and isocitrate dehydrogenase, in dissected rat nephron segments. The activities of the enzymes were higher in distal segments (TAL and DCT) than in the PT. The distal versus proximal ratios of activities were about 1.5, 2.5, and 2 for oxoglutarate dehydrogenase, citrate synthase, and isocitrate dehydrogenase, respectively. Oxoglutarate dehydrogenase showed the lowest activity along the entire nephron segments, and appeared to catalyze the rate-limiting step of the TCA cycle.[104] Marver et al. determined citrate synthase levels in isolated rabbit nephron segments. The order of relative citrate synthase activities in normal rabbit nephron segments (per kg of dry tissue) was as follows: DCT > PCT > CTAL > CCD > PST. The activity in CCD was regulated by aldosterone.[105]

β-Oxidation of Fatty Acids

Fatty acid is a major energy fuel in the kidney. β-Oxidation of short-, medium- and long- chain fatty acids (Figure 6.8) occurs in mitochondria, and that of very long-chain fatty acids in peroxisomes. The 3-hydroxyacyl-CoA dehydrogenase activity, which mainly represents the mitochondrial β-oxidation pathway, is similarly distributed in all cortical proximal and distal segments, and is much lower in glomeruli and collecting ducts. The peroxisomal fatty acyl-CoA oxidase is restricted to the PT, with a capacity comparable to that in liver cells.[106]

Ketone Body Metabolism

The kidney, as well as the muscle and brain, utilizes ketone bodies as metabolic fuel, while the liver cells do not. Acetoacetate and β-hydroxybutyrate are converted to acetyl CoA in the mitochondrial matrix. In this process, three enzymes, i.e., D-3-hydroxybutyrate

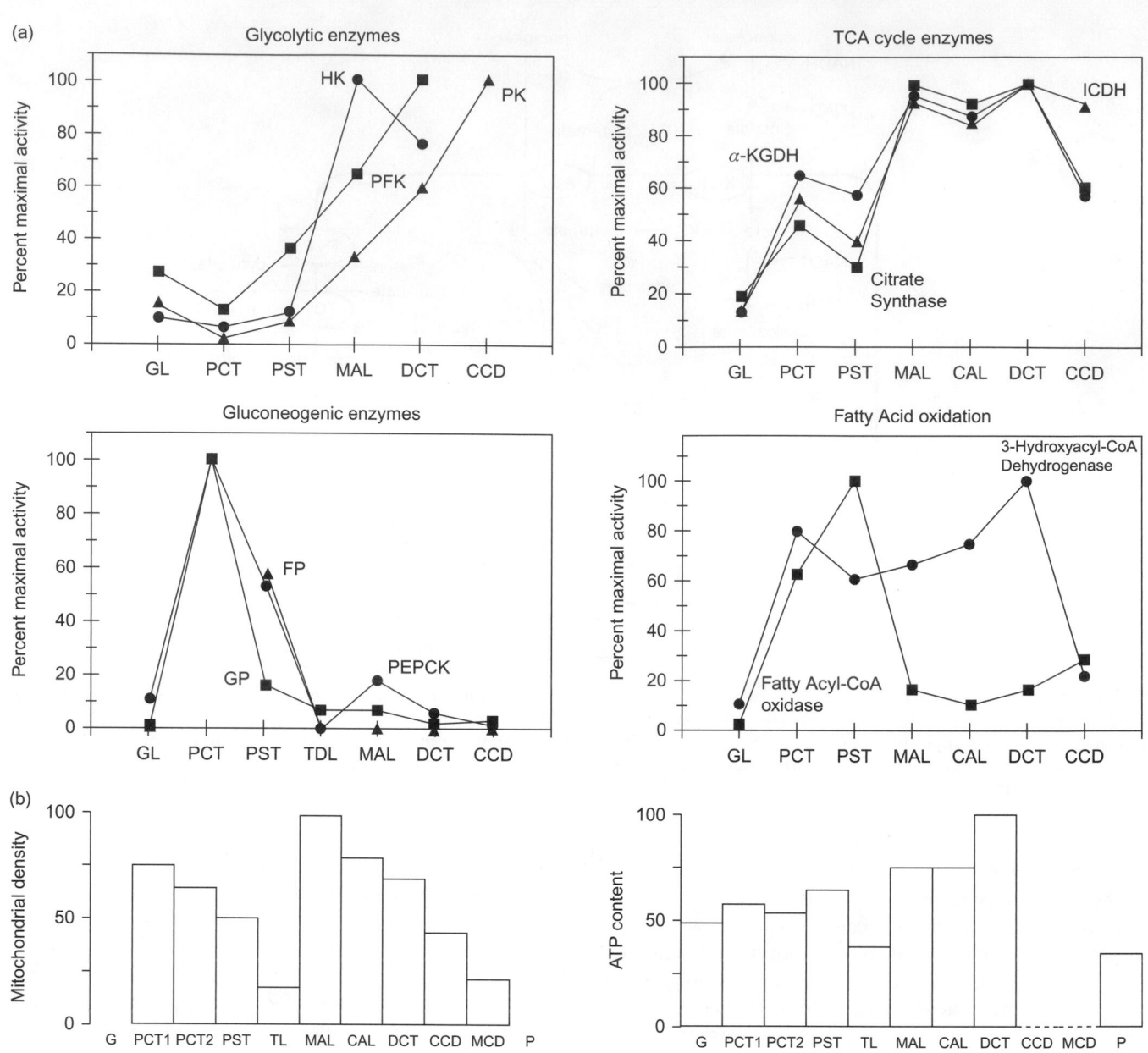

FIGURE 6.8 **(a) Distribution of enzymes involved in four major metabolic pathways:** TCA cycle, β-oxidation of fatty acids, glycolysis and gluconeogenesis. (*Adapted from* [101] *with permission.*) (b) Mitochondrial density distribution and ATP content along nephron segments. (*Adapted from* [3] *with permission.*)

dehydrogenase, 3-ketoacyl CoA transferase (3-oxoacid CoA- transferase), and acetoacetyl CoA thiorase, are involved.

Guder and co-workers measured 3-oxoacid CoA-transferase, and D-3-hydroxybutyrate dehydrogenase in mouse nephron. The activities of these enzymes were high in TAL and DCT, but decreased to nearly 20% in the CCD. In the PCT and PST, the 3-oxoacid CoA-transferase activity was almost equal, while the 3-hydroxybutyrate dehydrogenase activity was five-fold higher in PST than in PCT. In glomeruli and thin descending limbs of Henle's loop, the enzymatic

activities were markedly low. These results indicate that 3-hydroxybutyrate and acetoacetate can be metabolized in all of the mouse nephron segments with different capacities. The enzymatic activity for ketone body oxidation mirrors the distribution of mitochondria along the nephron segment.[107]

Glycolysis

The role of glycolysis (Figure 6.8) as a metabolic pathway is different among cells and the state of oxygen supply. In the kidney, glycolysis occurs primarily from glucose, since the storage of glycogen is minimal.[108] The hexokinase activity in single microdissected rabbit nephron segments was the lowest in the PCT, and increased along the nephron segments. It was the highest activity in the CNT.[109] The activities of phosphofructokinase and pyruvate kinase in the rat nephron were ten-fold higher in the distal nephron than in the proximal portion.[110] Thus, the glycolytic activity in the kidney is mostly distributed along the distal part of the nephron. Lactate production from glucose, with and without antimycin A, was investigated in the rat nephron.[111] PT produced no lactate, and the distal segments all produced lactate. Antimycin A, an inhibitor of mitochondrial oxidation, increased lactate production significantly in all of the distal segments. The increase was the largest in the MTAL (1400%), cortical (798%), and outer medullary collecting ducts (357%). Increments were smaller in CTAL (98%) and DCT (98%), and were the lowest in the IMCD (28%). Thus, anaerobic glycolysis is important, particularly in the distal segments of the nephron.

Gluconeogenesis

The capacity of the kidney to conduct gluconeogenesis (Figure 6.8) was demonstrated more than 50 years ago. Actually, the glucose synthesis rate of the kidney is higher than that of the liver when they are compared using the same tissue amount.[112] The release of glucose by the kidney has been reported to account for ~20% of all glucose released into the circulation in postabsorptive healthy humans.[113] Sustained hypoglycemia enhances the renal extraction of circulating precursors for gluconeogenesis, and stimulates renal glucose production, which may represent an important additional component of the body's defense mechanism against hypoglycemia in humans.[114,115]

Among the nephron segments, the PT is the only site where net glucose synthesis occurs.[101,116] The gluconeogenic enzyme PEPCK was exclusively found in the PT, and the PST exhibited 50% of the enzyme activity in the PCT.[109] All other renal structures exhibited only negligible PEPCK activity.[109] Thus, the activities of glycolysis and gluconeogenesis are a mirror image. Meyer et al. demonstrated that lactate is the most important precursor in renal gluconeogenesis, which exceeded the sum of renal gluconeogenesis from glycerol, glutamine, and alanine.[113] Gluconeogenesis from these substrates accounts for ~90% of renal glucose release.

Kondou et al. demonstrated that renal gluconeogenesis is stimulated by short-term ischemia.[117] They suggested that such stimulating gluconeogenesis supplies an energy fuel for further regeneration in nephron segments other than the PT.

There are several studies indicating a reciprocal relationship between Na+ transport and gluconeogenesis.

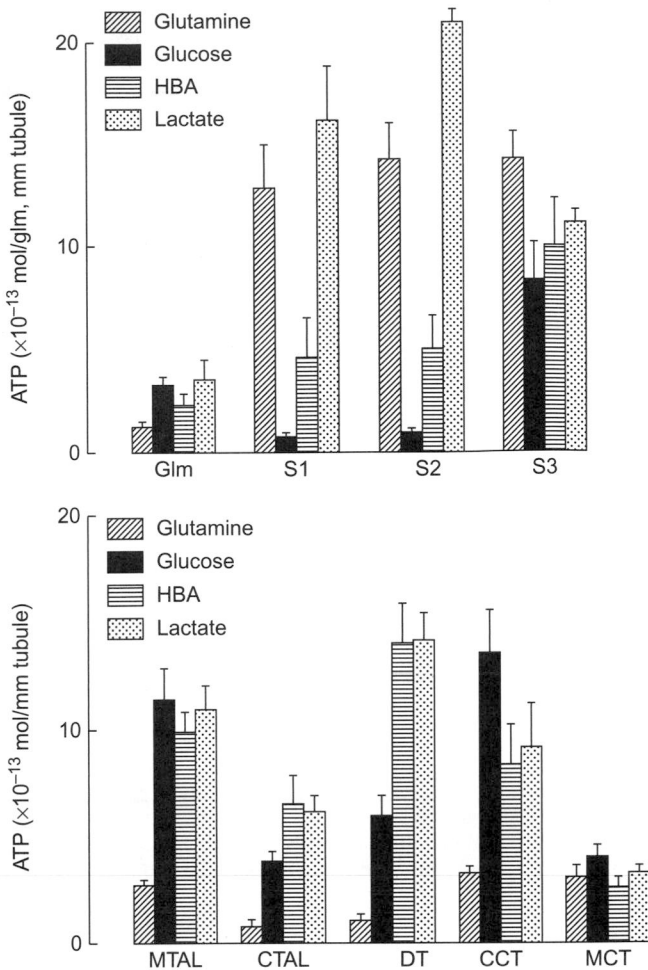

FIGURE 6.9 ATP content in nephron segments in the presence of several metabolic substrates. (*Adapted from [127] with permission.*)

The inhibition of Na+,K+-ATPase by ouabain stimulated gluconeogenesis.[118–120] In contrast, the stimulation of Na+,K+-ATPase by nystatin and monesin inhibited gluconeogenesis.[119,121] Silva et al. suggested that under certain circumstances, gluconeogenesis competes with Na+ reabsorption in an intact kidney.[122,123]

Metabolic Parameters along Nephron Segments

As described, aerobic and anaerobic metabolisms are different among the nephron segments (Figure 6.8). This difference is in good accord with the distribution of mitochondria along the nephron. Pfaller and colleagues investigated the density of mitochondrial volume (mitochondrial volume per unit volume of cytoplasm) by stereoscopic analysis, and demonstrated PCT (33%), PST (22%), thin limb (6–8%), MTAL (44%), DCT (33%), CCD (20%), and MCD (10%)[124,125] (Figure 6.8).

Intracellular ATP contents in various nephron segments were measured by several investigators.[111,126,127] Uchida and Endou demonstrated that the cellular ATP

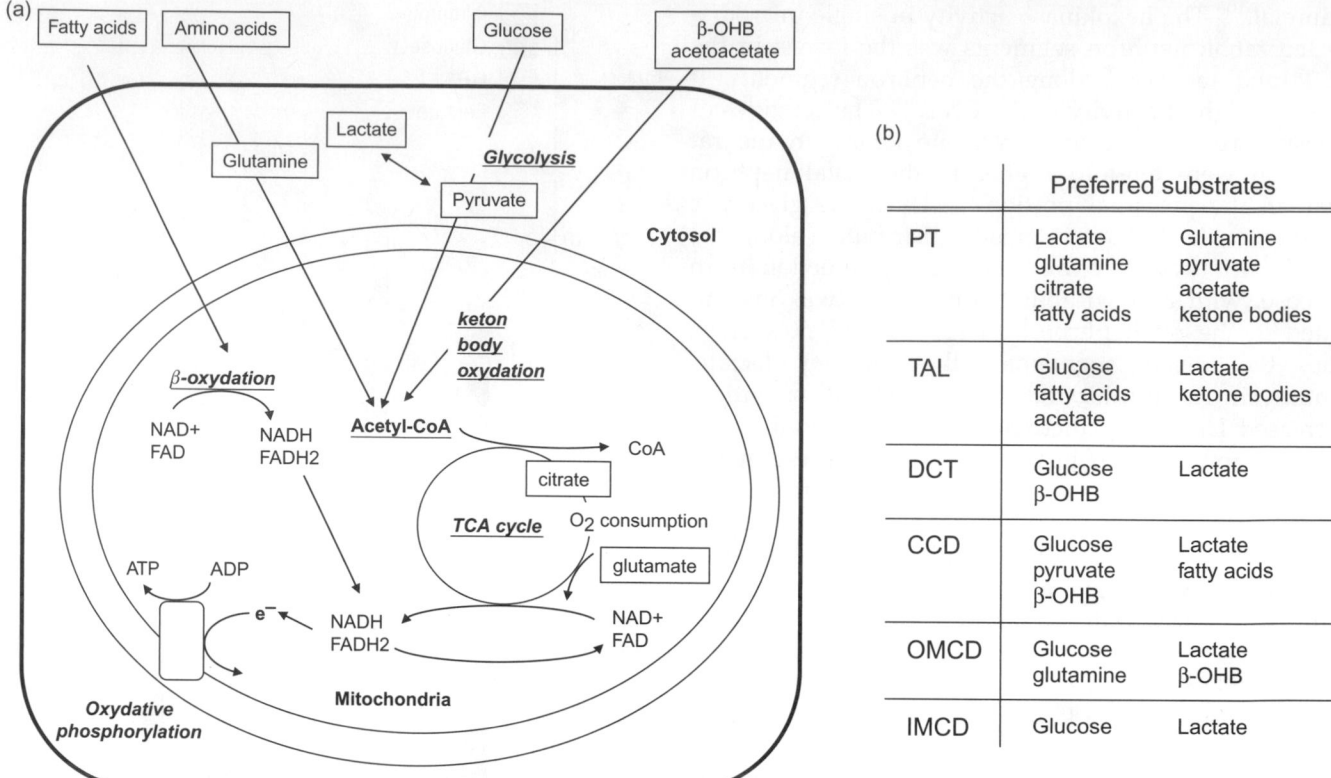

FIGURE 6.10 **Metabolic pathways and substrates used to fuel renal transport.** (a) Boxed substances are typical substrates used in nephron segments. (b) Substrate preference of each nephron segment.

content is largely dependent on the exogenous substrates available (Figure 6.9). When appropriate exogenous substrates are present, the cellular ATP content is high in the PT, MTAL DT, and CCD, whereas it is low in glomerulus, CTAL, and MCD.

Preference of Metabolic Substrates in Nephron Segments (Figure 6.10a,b)

Substrate Preference Along the Nephron Segments

Ever since Gyoergy et al. identified differences in metabolisms between the renal cortex and medulla in 1928,[128] numerous studies identified different metabolic profiles along the nephron. In the previous section, the activities of metabolic enzymes in the nephron were described. However, preferred substrates for each segment do not always correlate well with the distribution of specific enzymes. The substrate preference in a specific nephron segment depends on several factors other than the enzymatic activities, such as the cellular uptake systems for substrates, oxygen supply, hormonal stimuli, and the demand for metabolic end products.

Knowledge of the preferred substrates for each segment has accumulated, especially from studies using microdissected nephrons. The determination of $^{14}CO_2$ production from distinct labeled substrates, in conjunction with the effects of the substrate on cellular ATP level, QO_2, redox state (NADH fluorescence), and active ion transports provide evidence that a variety of metabolic fuels, such as lactate, glucose, pyruvate, fatty acids, ketone bodies, amino acids, and TCA cycle intermediates energize cellular metabolism.

In this section, we briefly summarize the data on the substrate preference in each nephron segment.

Proximal Tubule (PT)

Numerous studies examined the metabolic profiles of the PT, and consistently indicated that the PT metabolizes a variety of substrates, such as fatty acids, ketone bodies, lactate, pyruvate, glutamine, glutamate, and TCA cycle intermediates. One notable exception is glucose: the PT, especially proximal convoluted tubule (PCT), poorly metabolizes glucose.

Glucose: PT poorly metabolizes glucose, and there is a difference in the utilization of glucose between PCT and the proximal straight tubule (PST). $^{14}CO_2$ production from glucose in the PT was low,[129–131] and glucose was poorly converted to lactate under both aerobic and anaerobic conditions.[111] Uchida and

Endou measured cellular ATP contents in mouse nephron segments in the presence of several exogenous substrates. When only glucose was supplied to the PT, the cellular ATP content significantly decreased in the S1 and S2 segments, while it was sustained in the S3 segment (PST).[127] A study using rabbit PCT or PST suspensions demonstrated a similar metabolic profile for glucose: the addition of glucose to the rabbit PCT did not increase QO_2, whereas that to the rabbit PST increased it by 57%.[130] The differences in glucose utilization do not correlate with the distribution of glycolytic enzymes between the PCT and PST,[132] suggesting that a metabolic regulation mechanism other than that by glycolytic enzymes may determine the ability of each segment to utilize glucose. It should be noted that the gluconeogenic activity is high in the PT.

Fatty acids: Short-chain fatty acids are important fuels in the PT. Balaban and Mandel examined the effects of various short-chain fatty acids, carboxylic acids, and amino acids on NADH fluorescence and QO_2 in the rabbit PT.[133] The short-chain fatty acids (butyrate, valerate, and heptanoate) were the most effective in increasing NADH fluorescence and QO_2, followed by the carboxylic acids and amino acids. Butyrate supported mitochondrial respiration to a greater degree than lactate, glucose, and alanine when the Na^+,K^+-ATPase activity was maximally stimulated by nystatin.[134] Butyrate was also shown to enhance the volume regulation of the isolated nonperfused PST under hypoosmotic conditions by activating $Na^+ Cl^-$ transport.[135] Ruegg et al. demonstrated that PT exhibits maximal QO_2 and ATP content when incubated in culture medium with 2 mM heptanoate.[130] In contrast, palmitate oxidation occurs minimally in the PCT.[129] Thus, short-chain fatty acids are one of the best substrates, especially when active sodium transport is stimulated.

TCA cycle intermediates: The PCT demonstrated marked $^{14}CO_2$ production from labeled succinate, 2-oxoglutarate, glutamate, glutamine, and malate (approximately 10 to 45 pmoles/mm/hr), and moderate $^{14}CO_2$ production from citrate (approximately 3 pmoles/ml/hr).[129] Gullans et al. demonstrated that succinate stimulates gluconeogenesis, and the hyperpolarization of the plasma membrane potential, and promotes intracellular K^+ without altering Na^+,K^+-ATPase activity.[136] Since TCA cycle intermediates are highly hydrophilic substances, cellular metabolisms of TCA cycle intermediates require specific transporters in the plasma membrane. The sodium-dicarboxylate co-transporters, NaDCs encoded by the *SLC13* family, are expressed mainly in both the luminal and basolateral membrane of the PT.[137–140]

Ketone bodies: Guder et al. reported that ketone bodies, i.e., acetoacetate and β-hydroxybutyrate, are presumably the most preferred substrate as kidney fuel.[141] In a study using kidney slices, acetoacetate was estimated to support up to 80% of renal energy demands.[131] β-hydroxybutyrate supported ATP levels to the same extent as lactate and glutamine in isolated mouse S3, while S1 and S2 had a low capacity to metabolize β-hydroxybutyrate. These results correlate with the high enzyme activities for ketone bodies such as 3-hydroxybutylate dehydrogenase in this segment.[101]

Lactate: Lactate is also a preferred substrate for the PT. Goldstein et al. investigated the extraction of substrates from the blood by the rat kidney in normal, acidotic, and diabetic ketoacidotic conditions, and demonstrated that lactate accounts for 78% of the total amount of substrates extracted in normal control rats.[142] Exogenous lactate maintained the cellular ATP content in the mouse PT.[127] However, Kline et al. indicated that a negligible amount of $^{14}CO_2$ was released from the labeled lactate as well as glucose in the rat PCT.[129]

Thus, the proximal tubule metabolizes a wide range of substrates. This seems to be, at least in part, due to the existence of cellular transport systems for various substrates in the PT. PT cells possess Na-dependent transport systems for most of the nutrients across the luminal membrane. Nutrient transporters also exist in the basolateral membrane of the PT. Recent molecular studies have revealed the exclusive distribution of these transporters in the PT.

In the rat PT, preferred substrates are ketone bodies, short-chain fatty acids, lactate, and TCA cycle intermediates. However, there are species differences: the rabbit PT has a limited capacity to oxidize ketone bodies.[133]

The PT normally conducts transport work at 50 to 60% of its maximal respiratory capacity, and has significant amounts of endogenous fuels, probably neutral lipids, which support about half of the energy in the absence of exogenous substrates. Metabolism of endogenous fuel is suppressed when there is an adequate supply of exogenous substrates. The preferred substrates differ under different physiological conditions.[142]

Thin Descending Limb of the Loop of Henle (TDL)

The data available regarding the metabolic profile of the TDL is insufficient. The mitochondrial density of this segment is low, and its oxidative metabolism is limited. Jung and Endou measured the cellular ATP content in the rat short loop of TDL (SDL) and the rat long loop of TDL (LDL) in the presence of alanine, glucose, glutamine, β-HBA, lactate, and pyruvate.[143] They demonstrated that the substrate preference in SDL is pyruvate = glucose > glutamine = lactate = β-HBA

> alanine, and that in the LDL is pyruvate- = glucose = glutamine > alanine = β-HBA = lactate. They also demonstrated that ATP is depleted when the TDL is incubated in the absence of exogenous substrate, indicating a limited store of endogenous fuels in this segment.

Cortical Thick Ascending Limb of the Loop of Henle (CTAL)

In the TAL, the rate of Na^+ transport and QO_2 are high, and the mitochondria are enriched, suggesting there is active oxidative metabolism in this segment. Klein et al. measured $^{14}CO_2$ production from ^{14}C-labeled substrates in the rat MTAL and CTAL.[129] MTAL and CTAL oxidized glucose, 2-oxoglutarate, lactate, glutamate, and glutamine, but not malate, succinate, and citrate. Palmitate oxidation occurred in MTAL and CTAL.[129] Lactate production from glucose in the rat nephron indicated that the distal segments produce a significant amount of lactate from glucose, and under anaerobic conditions (with antimycin A), lactate production increased significantly in all of the distal segments. The increase was the largest in the MTAL (1400%), CCD (798%), and OMCD (357%), whereas increments were smaller in CTAL (98%) and DCT (98%), and were the lowest in the IMCD (28%).[111] Thus, CTAL possesses modest anaerobic glycolysis capacity. The ATP content in the mouse CTAL is maintained in the presence of glucose, β-OHB or lactate, but not with glutamine.[127]

Wittner et al. investigated the substrate preference by measuring the short circuit current (Isc) in the isolated rabbit CTAL perfused *in vitro*.[144] They further examined which sides, i.e., luminal or basolateral, substrates were taken up from. Isc rapidly decreased to 50% after 3 minutes and to 27% after 10 minutes without any exogenous substrates, indicating that Na^+ transport is strictly related to the presence of substrates in CTAL segments.[144] When substrates were added from the luminal side, only butyrate sustained Isc, while all other substrates tested (pyruvate, acetate, β-OHB, D-glucose, and L-lactate) showed a marked decrease in Isc. When the substrates were added from the basolateral side, D-glucose, D-mannose, butyrate, β-OHB, acetoacetate, L-lactate, acetate, and pyruvate sustained the Isc, but citrate, α-ketoglutarate, succinate, glutamate, glutamine, propionate, caprylate, and oleate did not. This study clearly indicates that the cellular uptake system is an important determinant in the substrate metabolisms in the CTAL. In the CTAL, most substrates, except for butyrate, are taken up by basolateral nutrient transporters. In fact, cytochalasin B and phloretin, inhibitors of the facilitated glucose transporter (GLUTs), inhibited the sustained Isc by glucose.[144]

Regarding fatty acids, the CTAL possesses mitochondrial β-oxidation activity (3-hydroxyacyl-CoA dehydrogenase),[106] and $^{14}CO_2$ is produced from palmitate,[129] while oleate (C-18) does not sustain Isc in the CTAL.[144] Taken together, glucose, lactate, pyruvate, ketone bodies, and fatty acids are the preferred exogenous substrates for the CTAL.

Medullary Thick Ascending Limb of the Loop of Henle (MTAL)

Chamberlin and Mandel measured QO_2 in MTAL suspensions.[145] In the absence of exogenous substrates, the control QO_2 decreased only by 15%. Torikai et al. demonstrate a similar result in the rat MTAL.[146] These results indicate that endogenous substrates support most of the energy required for the MTAL under normal conditions. However, nystatin-stimulated QO_2 was inhibited 36% in the absence of exogenous substrates, indicating that the oxidation of endogenous substrates cannot meet the ATP demand when Na^+ transport is fully stimulated. They also investigated the role of endogenous substrates in the MTAL. The inhibitors of fatty acid, carbohydrate or amino acid metabolisms further inhibited QO_2, revealing that endogenous fatty acids, glycogen, and amino acids (or proteins) contribute to energy production in the MTAL. The addition of fatty acids or acetoacetate increased QO_2 in 10 mM glucose, indicating that the MTAL oxidizes exogenous fatty acids and ketones in addition to glucose. In the MTAL, organic acids failed to enhance QO_2, possibly due to the absence of transport systems for organic acids. The rat MTAL generated $^{14}CO_2$ from glucose, lactate, palmitate, glutamate, glutamine, and α-ketoglutarate. $^{14}CO_2$ from succinate, citrate, and malate was minimal. Glucose, β-hydroxybutyrate, and lactate maintained the intracellular ATP content, whereas the effect of glutamine on the ATP content was partial.[127] The tight coupling of Na transport and QO_2 was demonstrated in the MTAL. Furosemide inhibited oxygen consumption by 43%, and ouabain inhibited it by 42%[147]; 50% of the oxygen consumption of the MTAL cells is related to the transport of Na^+ and Cl^-.[148]

In the MTAL, anaerobic glycolysis is also an important energy source.[149] Ten mimutes of anoxia led to only a 15% decrease in potassium content in the rabbit MTAL, and an anaerobic metabolism maintained 73% of cellular ATP during 10 minutes of anoxia. The exposure of anoxic tubules to iodoacetate produced a 57% decrease in ATP level, and a 33% decrease in potassium content. Lactate production was remarkably enhanced in MTAL (1400%) under anaerobic conditions with antimycin A.[111]

Distal Convoluted Tubule (DCT)

Although studies have examined the metabolic and transport properties in DCT, such as the mitochondrial density, Na^+,K^+-ATPase activity, and enzymatic activities, data regarding its substrate preference is limited. The ATP content of the DCT was maximal in the presence of β-OHB or lactate, and somewhat lower in the presence of glucose. Glutamine did not increase the ATP content in the DCT.[127] The lactate production rates from glucose under aerobic conditions were comparable to that observed in the CTAL, whereas under anoxic conditions, the glycolytic lactate production rate was increased two-fold as observed in CTAL.[111] These results indicate that DCT utilizes both oxidative metabolisms and anaerobic glycolysis.

Cortical Collecting Duct (CCD)

Torikai demonstrated that substrate deprivation for 30 minutes does not change the cellular ATP content in the rat CCD and OMCD. However, a marked decrease in the PT and medullary TDL, and a slight decrease in CTAL and MTAL were observed, suggesting that CCD and OMCD possess sufficient amount of endogenous fuels.[146] Hering-Smith et al. demonstrated the dependence of CCD on oxidative metabolisms in the Na^+ reabsorption and bicarbonate transport in the rabbit CCD.[150] There was no significant glycolysis or any difference in substrate-dependence of solute transport in the CCD. Na^+ reabsorption was optimally supported by a mixture of basolateral metabolic substrates (glucose, acetate, and fatty acid), whereas bicarbonate secretion was fully supported by either glucose or acetate. This result indicates that principal cells and intercalated cells differ not only in their morphology and function, but also in their metabolism. Alanine was not effective in the CCD. Nonaka and Stokes examined the effects of substrates on Na^+ transport in the rabbit CCD, and concluded that the majority of the energetic support of Na^+ transport appears to come from an oxidative metabolism. Glucose supports transport better than the other substrates tested, and lactate, pyruvate and some organic acids also provide near maximal support.[151]

The CCD synthesized modest amounts of lactate from glucose under aerobic conditions, which increased eight times under anaerobic conditions.[111] The addition of glucose, β-hydroxybutyrate or lactate, but not glutamine, restored the cellular ATP content, and glucose was the best substrate in CCD for maintaining the ATP level.[127] Natke showed that the rabbit nonperfused CCD regulates the cellular volume against extracellular hypertonic solution when exogenous butyrate is available,[152] although rat CCD possesses a relatively low enzymatic activity for β-oxidation.

Outer Medullary Collecting Duct (OMCD)

The OMCD cells play an important role in the final acidification of urine, which is mediated by apical H^+-ATPase.[89] The OMCD has a relatively low QO_2, which is inhibited only by 8% by ouabaine.[153] Several studies indicated the importance of anaerobic glycolysis in this segment. The ATP content in the OMCD did not significantly change with the addition of antimycin A.[146] Lactate production from glucose was significantly increased in the outer medullary collecting ducts by 357% under anaerobic conditions.[111] Under aerobic conditions, the ATP content was supported equally well by glucose, glutamine, lactate or β-hydroxybutyrate. Thus, glucose appears to be a preferred substrate for this segment, particularly under hypoxic or anoxic conditions, but other alternative substrates, such as glutamine, lactate or β-hydroxybutyrate, can be metabolized under aerobic conditions. The uptake of glucose by the OMCD, as well as that by the TAL cells, is mainly through a facilitated basolateral diffusion.[154] Studies of H^+ transport[155] and ATP content[127] also indicated the existence of a significant amount of endogenous fuel, most likely glycogen in the OMCD.

Inner Medullary Collecting Duct (IMCD)

Substrate metabolism in IMCD cells has not been sufficiently analyzed. QO_2 in IMCD is lower than that in other nephron segments.[156-158] Glycolysis under aerobic and anaerobic conditions was examined by several investigators. Addition of glucose to IMCD cells stimulates both QO_2 and lactate production, indicating that glucose can be readily metabolized to both CO_2 and lactate under aerobic conditions.[111,156,157,159] Lactate production in the IMCD under aerobic conditions was three- to five-fold greater than that in other nephron segments in the outer medulla, such as the TAL or OMCD.[111]

To evaluate the relative contributions of aerobic and anaerobic metabolism in the IMCD, the effects of specific inhibitors of mitochondrial oxidative phosphorylation and glycolysis were examined. Stokes et al. examined metabolism in rat renal papillary collecting duct cells, i.e., IMCD cells.[157] In the presence of rotenone, glycolysis increased by 56% and maintained the cellular ATP level at 65% of the control. Without any exogenous substrates, IMCD respiration was normal, and had a nearly normal ATP content, but lactate production was markedly decreased. At normal PO_2 and in the presence of D-glucose, the IMCD cells showed a substantial amount of aerobic glycolysis, although their mitochondrial respiration was not rate-limiting. In the absence of glucose, the cells acquired the majority of their energy from an endogenous substrate.[157]

Kone and co-workers showed that the addition of glucose to IMCD cells results in the accumulation of 12% more intracellular K^+, even in the presence of lactate and glutamine.[159] The data indicates that glucose is a preferred substrate in IMCD.

COUPLING OF TRANSPORT AND METABOLISM IN THE KIDNEY

As described in the section "Energy Consumption," Na transport and QO_2 show a linear relationship in the kidney. The nature of the cellular mechanism linking active transport to energy production is a fundamental physiological question. Alterations in the rate of active transport cause changes in the mitochondrial state and/or concentrations of adenine nucleotides in epithelia.[7] Conversely, the cellular respiration rate and/or ATP concentration affects active transport. This section focuses on the coupling mechanism of transport and energy production in the kidney.

The Effect of Active Transport on Metabolism

Whittam Model: Intracellular Signaling Between Transport and Energy Production

Whittam and co-workers primarily proposed a simple model indicating the coupling of active transport and mitochondrial respiration[160,161](Figure 6.11). In this model, the rate of active cation transport is a pacemaker for cellular respiration in the renal cells: increased ATP hydrolysis and elevated cytosolic levels of ADP and Pi by Na^+,K^+-ATPase activity would activate mitochondrial oxidative phosphorylation and oxygen consumption. Conversely, decreased Na^+,K^+-ATPase activity would induce the opposite result (Figure 6.11).

The validity of this model has been examined by: (1) direct measurement of ATP, ADP, Pi; and/or (2) monitoring of the mitochondrial redox state, in various states of transport. Early investigations into the intracellular nucleotide concentration failed to detect a change in the intracellular ATP levels.[162,163] This was probably due to the rapid ATP turnover in the renal cortex; the half-life of ATP in the anoxic state was estimated to be as low as 3.3 seconds.[164] Balaban and co-workers measured the cellular ATP/ADP concentrations and the QO_2 of a rabbit cortical tubule suspension under ideally designed conditions. They demonstrated that: (1) ouabain caused a 54% inhibition of QO_2 and a 30% increase in the ATP/ADP ratio; and (2) the addition of K^+ (5 mM) to K^+-depleted tubules caused an initial 127% stimulation of QO_2, followed by

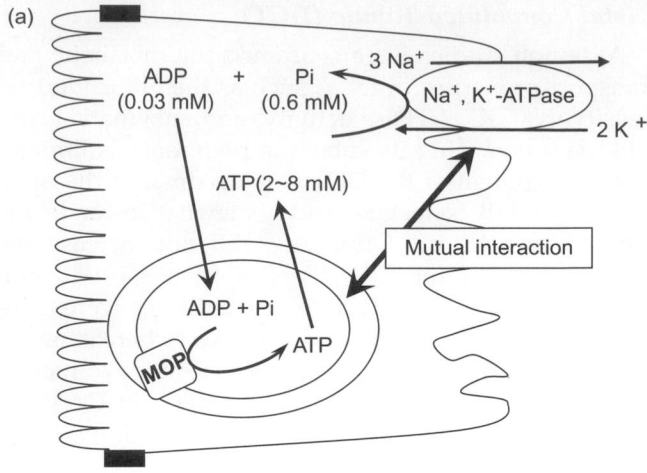

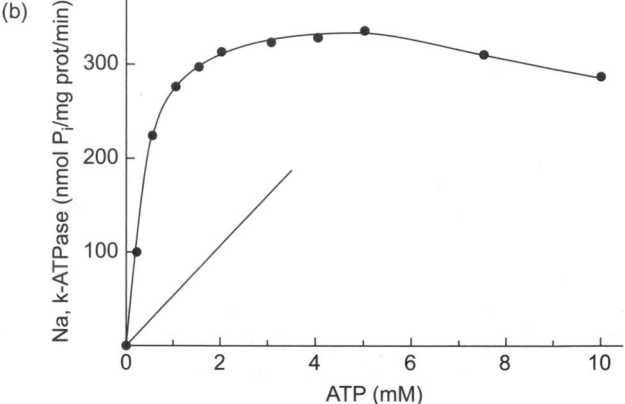

FIGURE 6.11 Schematic representation of Whittam model, and dependence of Na^+,K^+-ATPase activity on ATP concentration. (a) Schematic representation of Whittam model, MOP: mitochondrial oxidative phosphorylation; (b) Dependence of Na^+,K^+-ATPase activity of proximal tubule membranes (solid line) and that of intact proximal tubules (dashed line) on ATP concentration. (*Adapted from* [3] *with permission.*)

a new steady-state QO_2 50% above the control, and a 47% decrease in the cellular ATP/ADP ratio.[165]

The monitoring of the redox state by optical measurements also demonstrated appropriate "mitochondrial state of transition." Stimulation of Na^+,K^+-ATPase activity stimulated QO_2 and decreased NADH fluorescence (in whole kidney and proximal tubules). Inhibition of Na^+,K^+-ATPase with ouabain decreased QO_2 and increased NADH. Addition of rotenone to proximal tubules decreased QO_2, and ATP content net fluid transport with increase of NADH fluorescence.[165]

Regulation of Mitochondrial Respiration

The precise mechanism by which the rate of mitochondrial oxidative phosphorylation is regulated is of major interest in the field. There is much evidence suggesting the importance of cytosolic ADP concentration. Chance and Williams first proposed that the availability of ADP determines the mitochondrial respiration rate.[166–168] The respiratory state of mitochondria was classified into five states according to the supply of ADP, Pi, substrates, and O_2.[7,166] The addition of ADP to the mitochondria with a sufficient amount of substrates and O_2 induces the maximal rate of respiration, called "state 3 (active)" respiration. When all of the ADP is phosphorylated to ATP, QO_2 and ATP production decrease (the phase called "state 4 resting" respiration). The ratio of QO_2 in state 3 and state 4 is termed the *"respiratory control index."* This change in respiration was also demonstrated in proximal tubules permeabilized to ADP by digitonin, in which QO_2 was stimulated by four- to five-fold by the addition of ADP.[169] Nevertheless, the predominant parameter, (e.g., only [ADP] itself, [ATP]/[ADP] ratio or [ATP]/[ADP][Pi] ratio), should be determined by further studies using mitochondria, and two conflicting hypotheses on mitochondrial phosphorylation have been proposed.

The first hypothesis indicated that the [ATP]/[ADP] ratio is the rate-limiting step in oxidative phosphorylation.[170] This hypothesis is founded on kinetic considerations of adenine nucleotide translocase. Addition of atractyloside, an inhibitor of ATP/ADP translocase, caused inhibition of ADP influx into the mitochondrial matrix and oxidative respiration.[171] However, the data from intact tissues with high oxidative phosphorylation capacities, i.e., heart, brain, and kidney, indicated that the cytosolic concentration of ADP and Pi do not change significantly with work.[172]

The second hypothesis, called the "near-equilibrium theory," stated that oxidative phosphorylation is dependent on the phosphorylation potential.[173,174] This hypothesis suggested that oxidative phosphorylation is regulated thermodynamically by four factors: (1) [ATP]/[ADP][Pi] ratio; (2) intramitochondrial [NAD⁺]/[NADH] ratio; (3) respiratory chain components, especially cytochrome c oxidase; and (4) oxygen concentration. This theory was partially correct, however, oxidative phosphorylation is not always close to equilibrium, at least in isolated mitochondria.[175]

Furthermore, both of these hypotheses should be re-evaluated by the determination of the cytosolic concentration of ATP, ADP, and Pi by nuclear magnetic resonance (NMR) spectroscopy. NMR spectroscopy is a method by which the radiofrequency signal of specific molecules (P, N, C, and H) in a strong magnetic field can be recorded and quantified. There are particular features of this technology which can be applied to the measurement of biological events as follows: (1) the ability to define the chemical nature of phosphorus-containing molecules and follow their transition in time; (2) completely nondestructive and repeated determination is possible; (3) rapid determination over a few seconds; and (4) wide application from isolated mitochondria to intact kidney *in vivo*.[176,177] Freeman and colleagues quantified inorganic phosphate (Pi) and high-energy phosphates in the isolated, functioning perfused rat kidney. Compared with enzymatic analysis, 100% of ATP, but only 25% of ADP and 27% of Pi were visible by NMR spectroscopy,[178] indicating that a large proportion of both ADP and Pi are bound to proteins in the intact kidney. The data obtained by NMR spectroscopy, in conjunction with biochemical assays, estimated the free concentration of cytosolic ADP as approximately 30 μM[178,179] and Pi as 0.6 mM.[178] As a consequence, the [ATP]/[ADP][Pi] ratio (phosphorylation potential) and [ATP]/[ADP] ratio should be at least one order of magnitude higher than previously estimated values.

There are several other theories on the regulation of mitochondrial respiration. One claimed that the interplay of all aspects of oxidative phosphorylation affects respiration control.[180] Another new hypothesis implies the regulation of respiration and ATP synthesis via allosteric modification of respiratory chain complexes, in particular of cytochrome c oxidase by metabolites, cofactors, ions, hormones, and the membrane potential.[181,182] At the moment, there seems no simple answer to the question "what controls respiration?" The answer varies with: (1) the size of the system examined (mitochondria, cells or organs); (2) the conditions (rate of ATP use, level of hormonal stimulation); and (3) the particular organ examined.[175]

The Effect of Metabolism on Active Transport

Intracellular ATP and Cation Transport

The intracellular ATP content was reported 2~8 mM,[165,183–187] and the Km value of α-subunits for ATP was estimated to be 0.1 to 0.4 mM.[188] Therefore, Na^+,K^+-ATPase should be saturated for ATP under physiological conditions. However, intact renal cells normally function at almost half of their maximal respiratory capacity.[189] Harris measured cellular QO_2 during stimulation and inhibition of the Na^+,K^+-ATPase in mitochondria released from the rabbit renal tubules by digitonin shock. In the presence of NADH-linked substrates and fats, isolated renal cells respired at 50 to 60% of the maximum occurring in state 3 respiration, and addition of ouabain resulted in a decline in respiration to 25 to 30%. Stimulation of Na^+,K^+-ATPase by nystatin resulted in increased respiration with increased oxygen consumption.[134] Gullans and colleagues demonstrated that partial inhibition of oxidative metabolism with rotenone caused proportional reduction in QO_2, ATP content, and absorption rates of fluid and phosphate.[190] The effect of inhibition of oxidative metabolism on transport systems was also

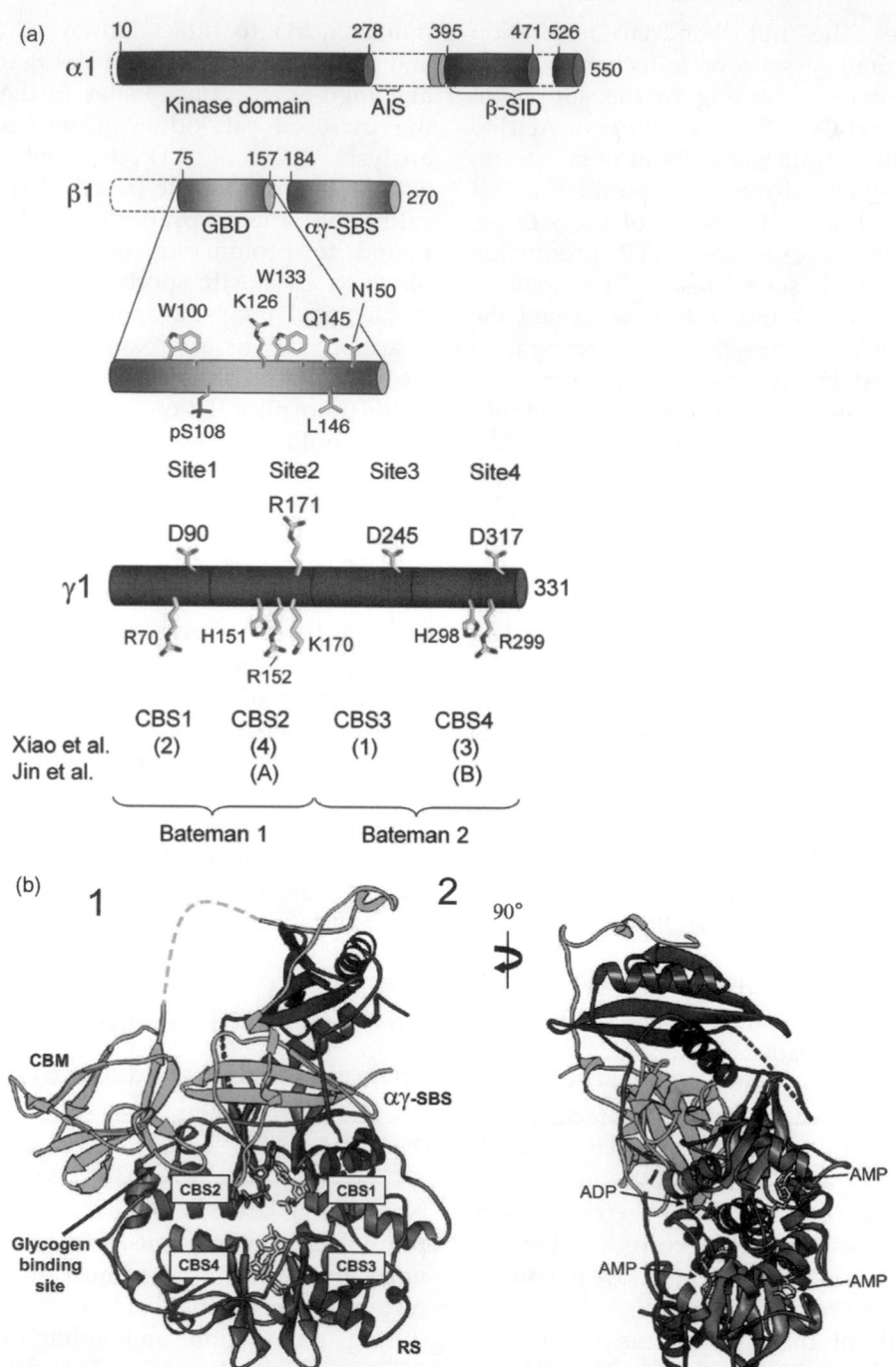

FIGURE 6.12   Structure and function of AMPK. (a) AMPK subunit composition. Details are described in the text. (b) Tertiary structure of AMPK. *(Adapted from [195] with permission).*

demonstrated using arsenate, which uncouples oxidative phosphorylation.[191]

This inconsistency was explained through a study by Soltoff and Mandel. In the membrane fraction of the PT, Na$^+$,K$^+$-ATPase hydrolytic activity showed saturated kinetics with a Km value of 0.4 mM for ATP. In contrast, Na$^+$,K$^+$-ATPase activity was demonstrated to have a linear, nonsaturating dependence on the ATP concentration in the intact proximal cells (Figure 6.11).[186] The authors speculated that unknown cytosolic factors in the intact renal cell, such as local concentration of ADP, Pi, and Mg in the vicinity of Na$^+$,K$^+$-ATPase may be different, which might account for the discrepancy between the two measurements. In contrast to Na^+,K^+-ATPase, decreased concentration of cytosolic ATP does not significantly alter the Ca^{2+}-ATPase activity, probably due to its relatively high affinity for ATP.[192]

AMPK-Activated Protein Kinase (AMPK): A Regulator of Energy Consumption and Generation

For the last decade, numerous experimental data have indicated the significant role of AMP-activated kinase (AMPK) in the regulation of the energy consuming and producing process in the living cells. AMPK appears to be the molecular entity which Whittam had proposed as "the pacemaker of respiration." AMPK has been extensively analyzed in the regulation of metabolism of carbohydrate, lipid, protein, and other cellular functions, such as cell polarity and growth; several studies have demonstrated its critical roles in solute transport in the kidney. In this section, we will review AMPK, and thereafter describe its role in the kidney.

AMP-Activated Protein Kinase (AMPK)

The AMP-activated protein kinase is an evolutionarily conserved heterotrimeric kinase acting as an ultrasensitive cellular energy sensor.[193–195] AMPK is activated by increased levels of cytoplasmic AMP, and controls various energy-dependent cellular processes. Recent studies have shown that the activities of membrane proteins, such as epithelial Na^+ channel (ENaC), Na^+-K^+-$2Cl^-$ co-transporter (NKCC2), cystic fibrosis transmembrane conductance regulator (CFTR), and vacuolar H^+-ATPase, are regulated by AMPK.[193] This evidence strongly suggests that energy sensing by AMPK would be a physiologically relevant mechanism by which renal tubular cells maintain tight coupling between energy metabolism and tubular transport.[193] AMPK appears to be the molecule which couples cellular respiration and solute transport proposed by Whittam and colleagues (Figure 6.11). In this section the biological basis of AMPK is briefly reviewed, and the current information on AMPK in solute transport in the kidney will be described.

Discovery of AMPK as an Ultrasensitive Cellular Energy Sensor

In 1980, Yeh et al. demonstrated that the rate of phosphorylation and inactivation of rat liver acetyl-CoA carboxylase (ACC) was stimulated by AMP and inhibited by high levels of ATP[196]. In 1988, Munday and colleagues demonstrated that the enzyme formerly called acetyl-CoA carboxylase kinase-3 (ACC kinase-3)

reduces the maximum velocity of ACC, and they proposed the name of AMP-activated protein kinase for ACC kinase-3.[197] Mammalian AMPK was first purified and sequenced by two groups from porcine or rat liver.[198,199] Subsequent studies revealed that AMPK acts to balance energy status by stimulating pathways leading to ATP synthesis and inhibiting those leading to ATP consumption.

One of the best characterized pathways and substrates regulated by AMPK is 3-hydroxy-3-methylglutaryl (HMG)-CoA reductase, the rate-limiting enzyme for cholesterol synthesis.[195] Other than enzymatic activities, diverse biological processes have been reported to be regulated by AMPK, such as cellular nutrient uptake, protein synthesis, gene transcription, inflammation, autophagy, cellular polarity, and nitric oxide synthesis.[195] In addition to these metabolic processes, recent studies have indicated that solute transport is also regulated by AMPK.[193]

Structure and Regulation of AMPK

Mammalian AMPK is a heterotrimeric protein that comprises of two α-subunits, two regulatory β-subunits, and three regulatory γ-subunits allowing for the generation of 12 different heterotrimeric complexes[193,195,200] (Figure 6.13). γ-Subunits have several spliced variants.[193] The AMPK α1- and α2-subunits are approximately 550 residue proteins, and comprise an N-terminal kinase domain, followed by an auto-inhibitory sequence (AIS), and a β-subunit interacting domain. Phosphorylation at Thr^{271} in the α-subunit kinase domain is essential for activation of AMPK, and significantly increases its kinase activity.[201] β-Subunits have a carbohydrate-binding domain (CBM) in their central region, which binds glycogen and regulates AMPK activity. The C-terminus of β-subunits is necessary for the formation of αβγ AMPK heteromer. γ-Subunits possess the binding sites for AMP, which is the key process for the regulation of AMPK activity. In the c-terminus of γ-subunits, there are four cystathione-β-synthase (CBS) domains, and two CBS domains form one Bateman domain which bind AMP or ATP.[202] The Bateman domain has higher affinity for AMP than ATP, and the Kd for ATP is 3.3-fold higher than that for AMP.[202] The activity of AMPK is regulated by the concentration of AMP and an increase in the AMP/ATP ratio. As AMP levels rise, there is a resulting AMP binding to the Bateman domain of the regulatory γ-subunit.[202]

When ATP is utilized and its intacellular level decreased, cellular concentrations of AMP increase drastically, which leads to activation of AMPK, and activated AMPK regulates the energy homeostasis by

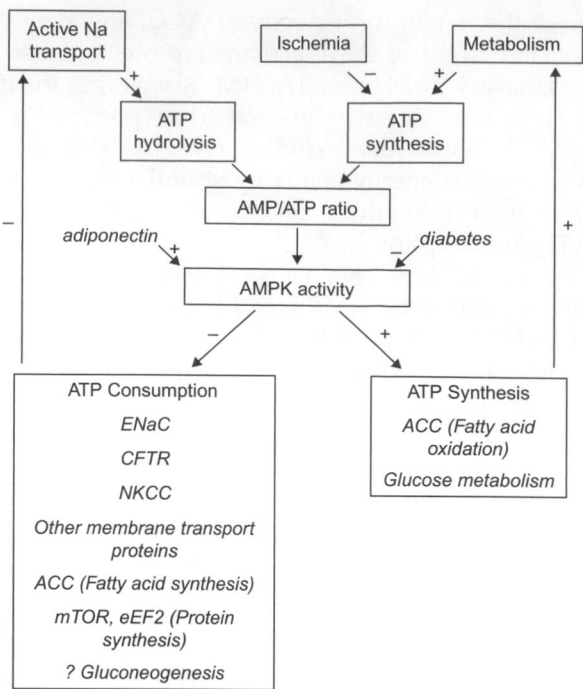

FIGURE 6.13 Proposed role for AMPK. Deduced role of AMPK in the kidney. Catabolic pathway requiring ATP hydrolysis (primarily sodium transport) and metabolic pathways leading to ATP synthesis (primarily fatty acid and glucose oxidation) are depicted. (*Adapted from* [193] *with permission.*)

stimulating energy production and minimizing energy consumption. AMPK activity is regulated by three mechanisms.[194] First, AMP allosterically activates AMPK complex in mammalian cells.[194] Second, AMP binding to the Betaman domain of the γ-subunit activates phosphorylation of Thr[271] by upstream AMPK kinases. The third is that AMP binding to AMPK significantly reduces the dephosphorylation of Thr[172] by 2Cα dephosphorylation phosphatase.[200] These three mechanisms make AMPK very sensitive to energy status, i.e., changes of cellular AMP and ATP concentration.

So far, three physiological kinases upstream of AMPK have been identified, namely LKB1, CaMKKβ (Ca²⁺/calmodulin-dependent protein kinase kinase β), and TAK1 (a member of the mitogen-activated protein kinase kinase family).[200]

Expression of AMPK in the Kidney and Localization along the Nephron Segment

Expression of the AMPK catalytic α-subunit and its enzymatic activity was examined in various tissues.[203] In the rat, mRNA of the α1-subunit of AMPK was ubiquitously expressed among tissues including heart, brain, spleen, lung, liver skeletal muscle, and kidney,

whereas the α2-subunit is strongly expressed in the heart, liver, and skeletal muscle, but its expression was comparatively weak in the brain, lung and kidney. Expression of α1- and α2-subunit protein showed similar patterns to those of mRNA: mRNA of the α2-subunit in the kidney was very weak. In terms of kinase activity, AMPK activity was highest in the kidney, followed by liver, lung, heart, and brain. Taken together, the kidney possesses very high AMPK activity, and its main α-subunit is α1.

Localization of AMPK subunits along the nephron segments has been investigated in the rat.[204,205] Immunoprecipitation and Western blot of protein lysates from whole rat kidney showed that the α1 catalytic subunit is expressed in the kidney, associated with the β2- and either γ1- or γ2-subunits. Phospho-Thr[172] AMPK (pThr[172]) was expressed on the apical surface of the cortical thick ascending limb of the loop of Henle, including the macula densa, and some parts of the distal convoluted tubule. α1-pThr[172] AMPK was also expressed on the basolateral surface of the cortical and medullary collecting ducts, as well as some portions of the distal convoluted tubules.[204] In another study, AMPK catalytic α2-subunits were expressed in the isolated distal tubule.[205] There seems some species difference as to which isoform(s) of each subunit are predominantly expressed in the nephron segment.[193] At the moment, there is limited information on the expression of AMPK isoforms in the kidney. Further studies are required to elucidate the significance of AMPK in the kidney, because there are remarkable differences in the metabolic profile among the nephron segments, as described in this chapter.

Regulation of Solute Transport by AMPK

Recently, regulation of renal solute transport by AMPK has been examined in several important transport and channel proteins. Low sodium and low chloride conditions activate AMPK in the murine macula densa cells indicating a potential role of AMPK in salt homeostasis in the body.[204] As is been expected, AMPK regulates the solute transport in accordance with the energy status in the kidney cells.

NA⁺,K⁺-ATPASE

Considering the relationship between the cellular energy status and solute transport activity, Na⁺,K⁺-ATPase is the membrane protein whose regulation by AMPK should first be elucidated in the kidney. So far, no definite information on this relationship in the kidney has been reported, while it was examined in the lung cells. Woollhead and colleagues examined the effect of AMPK on Na$^+$,K$^+$-ATPase using H441 lung cells.[206,207] H441 human lung epithelial cells express α1 and α2 catalytic subunits of AMPK, and additional activators of AMPK, phenformin and 5-aminoimidazole-4-carboxamide-1-beta-D-ribofuranoside (AICAR), to H441 cells increased AMPK activity in a dose-dependent fashion. Both agents significantly decreased basal ion transport (measured as short circuit current) across H441 monolayers by approximately 50% compared with that of controls. Phenformin and AICAR significantly reduced amiloride-sensitive transepithelial Na$^+$ transport compared with controls. This was a result of both decreased Na$^+$, K$^+$-ATPase activity and amiloride-sensitive apical Na$^+$ conductance.

Vadász et al. examined the mechanisms regulating CO$_2$-induced Na$^+$,K$^+$-ATPase endocytosis in alveolar epithelial cells (AECs).[208] They showed that elevated CO$_2$ levels are sensed by AECs, and that AMPK mediates CO$_2$-induced Na$^+$,K$^+$-ATPase endocytosis. Elevated CO$_2$ levels caused a rapid activation of AMPK in AECs. Activation of AMPK was mediated by a CO$_2$-triggered increase in intracellular Ca^{2+} concentration and Ca^{2+}/calmodulin-dependent kinase kinase-β (CaMKK-β). Chelating intracellular Ca^{2+} or abrogating CaMKK-β function prevented the CO$_2$-induced AMPK activation in AECs. Activation of AMPK or overexpression of constitutively active AMPK was sufficient to activate PKC-zeta and promote Na$^+$,K$^+$-ATPase endocytosis. Inhibition or downregulation of AMPK using dominant-negative AMPK-α1 prevented CO$_2$-induced Na$^+$,K$^+$-ATPase endocytosis.

The Epithelial Na$^+$ Channel (ENaC)

Oocytes microinjected with mouse ENaC (mENaC) with either active AMPK protein or an AMPK activator inhibited mENaC currents relative to controls, as measured by two-electrode voltage-clamp studies.[209] In addition, pharmacological AMPK activation or overexpression of an activating AMPK mutant in mpkCCD (c14) cells inhibited amiloride-sensitive short circuit currents via ENaC. However, AMPK did not bind ENaC or phosphorylate ENaC *in vitro*.[209] Furthermore, they demonstrated that AMPK promotes ENaC-Nedd4-2 interaction, thereby inhibiting ENaC by increasing Nedd4-2-dependent ENaC retrieval from the plasma membrane. The results indicated that AMPK-dependent ENaC inhibition is mediated through a decrease in the number of active channels at the plasma membrane, presumably due to enhanced Nedd4-2-dependent ENaC endocytosis. This regulation

of ENaC by AMPK was confirmed by AMPK α1-KO mice.[210] Almaça et al. demonstrated AMPK-α1 KO mice showed enhanced electrogenic Na$^+$ absorption, and that AMPK uses the ubiquitin ligase Nedd4-2 to inhibit ENaC by increasing ubiquitination and endocytosis of ENaC, leading to the enhanced expression of ENaC detected in the colon, airways, and kidney of AMPK-α1 KO mice.

Bhalla et al. examined the effects of AMPK activation on ENaC currents in *Xenopus* oocytes co-expressing ENaC and wild-type (WT) or mutant forms of Nedd4-2. ENaC inhibition by AMPK was blocked in oocytes expressing either a dominant-negative or constitutively active Nedd4-2 mutant, suggesting that AMPK-dependent modulation of Nedd4-2 function is involved.[211] Moreover, cellular AMPK activation significantly enhanced the interaction of the β-EnaC-subunit with Nedd4-2, as measured by co-immunoprecipitation assays in HEK-293 cells.

Na$^+$-K$^+$-2Cl$^-$ Co-transporter 2 (NKCC2)

It has been known that renal-specific NKCC2 (Na$^+$-K$^+$-2Cl$^-$ co-transporter 2) is regulated by changes in phosphorylation state, however, the phosphorylation sites and kinases responsible have not been fully elucidated. Fraser et al. demonstrated a physical association between AMPK and the N-terminal cytoplasmic domain of NKCC2 by immunoprecipitation experiments.[212] Activation of AMPK in the mouse macula densa-derived 1 cell line resulted in an increase in Ser126 phosphorylation of NKCC *in situ*, suggesting that AMPK may phosphorylate NKCC2 *in vivo*. When exogenously expressed in *Xenopus laevis* oocytes, S126A mutated NKCC showed a marked reduction in co-transporter activity. Thus, Ser^{126} in the N-terminus of NKCC2 was identified as a novel activating phosphorylation site by AMPK.

The Vacuolar H$^+$-ATPase (V-ATPase)

V-ATPase subcellular localization in intercalated cells by PKA and AMPK was examined in rat kidney tissue slices *ex vivo*.[213] Immunofluorescence labeling of kidney slices revealed that the PKA activator induced V-ATPase apical membrane accumulation in collecting duct intercalated cells. Pre-incubation of kidney slices with an AMPK activator blocked V-ATPase apical membrane accumulation induced by PKA activator, suggesting that AMPK antagonizes cAMP/PKA effects on V-ATPase distribution.

The Cystic Fibrosis Transmembrane Conductance Regulator (CFTR)

The cystic fibrosis transmembrane conductance regulator is an ATP-gated Cl$^-$ channel that regulates other epithelial transport proteins. Using a yeast two-hybrid screening technique, the α1- and α2-subunit of AMPK was identified as a novel interacting protein. AMPK phosphorylated full-length CFTR *in vitro*, and AMPK co-expression with CFTR in *Xenopus* oocytes inhibited cAMP-activated CFTR whole-cell Cl$^-$ conductance by approximately 35—50%.[214]

Other Transport Proteins and Channels Regulated by AMPK

Other than the above-mentioned transporters and channels, several membrane proteins have been reported to be regulated by AMPK. These include a Na$^+$-coupled glucose carrier SGLT1[215] and an ATP-sensitive K$^+$ (K$_{ATP}$) channel.[216]

Other Factors Linking Transport and Cellular Metabolism

ATP-Sensitive Cation Channels

ATP-sensitive K$^+$-channels (K$^+$-ATP channels), the activity of which are inhibited by micromolar to millimolar concentrations of ATP, contribute to the potassium balance by coupling cellular metabolism with K$^+$ transport.[217–219] Tsuchiya of the Welling laboratory identified K$^+$-ATP channel activity at the basolateral membrane in the PT, which is a major determinant of the macroscopic K conductance.[220] The open probability of K$^+$-ATP channel determined by the intracellular ATP concentration altered the extent of K recycling: a decrease in intracellular ATP by stimulation of Na$^+$, K$^+$-ATPase activity increased the macroscopic K conductance, and intracellular ATP loading uncoupled the response. Wang and Giebisch demonstrated the effect of ATP on the small-conductance potassium channel in the apical membrane of CCD using the patch-clamp technique.[221] A dual effect of ATP was observed: low concentrations of ATP (0.05—0.1 mM) restored channel activity in the presence of cAMP-dependent PKA, while high concentrations of ATP (1 mM) and ADP (1.2 mM) blocked it completely. The dual effect of ATP was explained by assuming: (1) ATP-dependent PKA-mediated phosphorylation of the potassium channel under physiological conditions; and (2) direct inhibitory action of high concentrations of ATP on the channel activity. ATP-sensitive K$^+$ channels, the open probability of which was downregulated by ATP concentrations greater than 0.1 mmol/l, were also identified in the TAL.[222] These studies indicate that ATP acts as a coupling modulator between cellular metabolism and K$^+$-ATP channel activity, and regulates the transepithelial transport of K$^+$. Tsuboi and co-workers investigated the molecular effect of ATP on a Kir6.2, a K$^+$-ATP channel. ATP inhibits the channel activity by binding to a specific site formed by the N- and C-termini of the pore-forming subunit. The structural changes associated with the interaction of ATP with Kir6.2 were as follows: (1) the interaction between the N- and C-terminal domains was altered; (2) both intra-subunit and intersubunit interactions were probably involved; (3) ligand binding and not channel gating was affected; and (4) these effects occurred in intact cells when subplasmalemmal ATP concentrations changed in the millimolar range.[223]

The regulation of cation transport by intracellular ATP was also identified in a stretch-activated nonselective cation channel in the basolateral membrane of the PT.[224] This cation channel is primarily regulated by stretching (membrane deformation), depolarization, and hypotonic swelling. In addition, intracellular ATP reversibly blocks this cation channel (Ki approximately 0.48 mM). Thus, this cation channel activity is coupled to the metabolic state of the cell, particularly when intracellular ATP is depleted, as occurs during increased transepithelial transport or ischemia.

Purinergic Receptors

ATP and its metabolites, ADP, UTP, and UDP, act as extracellular signaling molecules via purinergic P2 receptors.[225–227] ATP is readily released from epithelial cells across their luminal membrane when the cells are damaged by ischemia or the toxic effects of exogenous compounds. ATP released from the cells is metabolized by ecto-nucleotidases, and thereby acts on the epithelial cells as paracrine and autocrine regulators. Mammalian P2 receptors are subdivided into P2Y (G-protein-coupled) and P2X (ligand-gated channels). In the kidneys, P2 receptors are expressed both in the basolateral and luminal membranes, and induce a variety of biological effects. In the distal nephron, luminal nucleotides inhibit Ca^{2+} and Na$^+$ absorption and K$^+$ secretion via the P2Y$_2$ receptor. In steroid-sensitive cells, luminal ATP/UTP inhibits epithelial Na$^+$ channel-mediated Na$^+$ absorption. Adenosine generated by ecto-nucleotidases may introduce further effects on ion transport, often opposite to those caused by ATP. Bailey demonstrated that activation of the P2Y$_1$ receptor impairs acidification in the PT through inhibiting the reabsorption of bicarbonate.[228] As well as having effects on solute transport, P2 receptors also modulate cellular metabolism. Cha and Endou demonstrated that renal gluconeogenesis was increased via P2Y stimulation.[229] The suggested functions of luminal P2 receptors include: (1) an epithelial "secretory" defense; (2) the regulation of cell volume when transcellular solute transport is out of balance; and (3) autocrine/paracrine regulators mediating cellular protection and regeneration after ischemic cell damage.[225]

Nephrons are also equipped with adenosine/P1 receptors, which have been further subdivided into four subtypes, A1, A2A, A2B, and A3, all of which couple to G-proteins.[226] Adenosine is produced by biochemical reactions, and by the extracellular cAMP-adenosine pathway, in which cAMP effluxed from cells is converted to adenosine by the serial actions of ecto-phosphodiesterase and ecto-5′-nucleotidase.[230] Adenosine modulates Na^+,K^+-ATPase via A1 and A2 adenosine receptors.[231]

Nitric oxide (NO)

In the kidney, nitric oxide participates in several regulatory processes, including those for the glomerular and medullary hemodynamics, the tubuloglomerular feedback, renin release, and the extracellular fluid volume.[232,233] NO is formed from L-arginine by NO synthases (NOSs), a family of related enzymes encoded by separate unlinked genes. Three isoforms of NOS, i.e., nNOS (or NOS I), eNOS (or NOS III), and iNOS (or NOS III) were shown to be expressed in the kidney with distinct localization.[232,234] NO affects transporters and channels, such as Na^+,K^+-ATPase, NHE3, NKCC2, H^+-ATPase, and K^+-channels, in a segment-specific manner.[233] For examples, NO inhibited Na^+,K^+-ATPase in PT cells, while it did not change Na^+,K^+-ATPase activity in the TAL and CCD.[233] NO also affects mitochondrial QO_2. Granger and Lehninger initially observed an inhibition of mitochondrial electron transport in a murine cell line exposed to endotoxin-stimulated macrophages,[235] and subsequently NO was suggested to mediate this phenomenon.[236] NO inhibits QO_2,[237] and conversely nitro-L-arginine, a NO synthesis inhibitor, increases QO_2.[238] The inhibitory effect of NO on QO_2 appears to occur reversibly through the direct inhibition of the mitochondrial electron transport chain.[239,240] Adler et al. investigated the effects of renal NO production on QO_2 using eNOS KO mice.[241] Basal QO_2 in the renal cortex was higher in eNOS KO mice than in the heterozygous control mice. NO production stimulated by bradykinin or ramiprilat decreased QO_2 to a lesser extent in eNOS KO mice than in the control mice. These results indicate that NO production via eNOS regulates the renal QO_2. Laycock and colleagues indicated that NO plays a role in maintaining a balance between QO_2 and sodium reabsorption in the dog.[242] The administration of nitro-L-arginine decreased sodium reabsorption, and increased renal QO_2.

PATHOPHYSIOLOGICAL STATES IN ENERGY PRODUCTION IN THE KIDNEY

Pathophysiological states, in which energy production is inhibited, lead to significant alterations in renal function. In this final section, we focus on these pathophysiological states.

Mitochondrial Cytopathies

Mitochondrial cytopathies are metabolic diseases caused by mutations in nuclear DNA or mitochondrial DNA encoding the proteins involved in the mitochondrial oxidative chain. These genetic lesions alter mitochondrial oxidative phosphorylation, with a reduction in energy produced for cell activity.[243] The manifestation of mitochondrial cytopathies occurs in tissues where energy requirement is high, such as skeletal muscle and brain. Given the high energy utilization in the kidney, it is not surprising that mitochondrial cytopathies cause dysfunction of renal transport, and various renal involvements in mitochondrial diseases have been reported.

In most cases of Fanconi syndrome, a generalized dysfunction of proximal tubular cells results in glucosuria, aminoaciduria, and phosphaturia.[244–249] In patients manifesting Fanconi syndrome, defects in complex IV (CCO) activities are most commonly detected.[247] Bartter syndrome,[250] acute renal failure,[251] chronic renal failure,[252] and chronic tubulointerstitial nephritis[253,254] were also reported. The renal tubule in patients with mitochondrial disease may be susceptible to renal hypoxic injury and acute renal failure. In the renal tissues of patients with mitochondrial cytopathies, giant and degenerated mitochondria are observed by electron microscopy.[255,256] Glomerular involvement was occasionally reported.[245,257–261]

Renal Ischemia

Ischemia-induced renal dysfunction involves multifactorial events, and there are two effects regarding tubular damage due to ischemia: effects that occur during ischemia; and those occurring during reperfusion (reoxygenation), although these two factors are not always separable.[262] If the ischemic damage is severe, tubular cells undergo necrosis and/or apoptosis.

Necrosis is characterized by the progressive loss of cytoplasmic membrane integrity, rapid influx of Na^+, Ca^{2+}, and water due to the disturbance of several ATP-dependent ion channels, which results in cytoplasmic swelling, the disruption of the actin cytoskeleton, nuclear pyknosis, and eventual collapse of the cells.[263,264] Necrosis is considered to be mediated by ATP depletion,[265] the redistribution of Na^+,K^+-ATPase,[266] an increase in free cytosolic Ca^{2+},[267] reactive oxygen species generation,[268] and activation of several enzymes, such as proteases, phospholipases, and endonucleases. Apoptosis is a highly coordinated process mediated by active intrinsic mechanism or extrinsic factors.[264]

Both apoptosis and necrosis occur simultaneously in acute renal failure (ARF),[269] and the relative contribution of the two mechanisms depends on the severity of the injury and the cell type.[270] Lieberthal et al. investigated the effect of graded ATP depletion ranging from 2 to 70% of control levels induced by either antimycin or 2-deoxyglucose in mouse PT cells.[271] The cells subjected to ATP depletion to less than 15% of the control level developed necrosis uniformly. In contrast, the cells subjected to ATP depletion to between 25 and 70% of control levels developed apoptosis. A narrow range of ATP depletion exists (15 to 25% of control level), representing a threshold that determines whether cells die by necrosis or apoptosis. The degree of cellular GTP depletion plays also a crucial role in determining the mode of cell death.[272]

ATP Depletion during Acute Ischemia and its Consequence

After one minute of ischemia, whole kidney ATP content decreased by 70%,[273] and after 10 minutes renal ischemia ATP levels fall quickly to less than 10% of control values.[274] During ischemia, tubular cells should maintain ATP content by anaerobic metabolisms, and the vulnerability of each nephron segment depends partly on the glycolytic properties. The S3 (PST) segment of the PT is extremely susceptible to ischemic injury, because of its low glycolytic capacity, and severe ATP depletion leads to necrotic cell death in this segment. In the rabbit PT, hypoxia (1% O_2) induced lactate production, whereas anoxia (0% O_2) failed to stimulate glycolysis. The addition of ouabain during rotenone treatment reduced lactate production by 50%, indicating that glycolytic ATP can be used to fuel the Na^+,K^+-ATPase when mitochondrial ATP production is inhibited. In addition, this study suggested that mitochondrial inhibition is not obligatorily linked to the activation of glycolysis.[275]

Weinberg and colleagues investigated anaerobic metabolism other than glycolysis in the PT during ischemia.[276,277] A severe mitochondrial energy deficit in the PT subjected to hypoxia/reoxygenation was prevented, and reversed by supplementation with α-ketoglutarate (α-KG) and aspartate. The anaerobic metabolism of α-KG and aspartate generated ATP, and maintained the mitochondrial membrane potential. Malate and fumarate were also effective singly or in combination with α-KG, while succinate showed a protective effect only during reoxygenation. In other studies, Weinberg and co-workers further demonstrated that the events upstream of complex I are important for the energetic deficit in the PT during hypoxia.[278]

The TAL possesses a relatively greater glycolytic capacity than the PT, and is less vulnerable to ischemic injury.[279,280] In a suspension of rabbit MTAL under anoxic conditions, anaerobic metabolism maintained 73% of cellular ATP during 10 minutes of anoxia, and exposure of anoxic tubules to iodoacetate, an inhibitor of glycolysis, resulted in a 57% decline in ATP levels, indicating that glycolysis is an important pathway in supplying energy during anaerobiosis in MTAL.[149] The cellular damage of the TAL by ischemia is influenced by cellular transport. The TAL develops a specific structural lesion during perfusion of the isolated rat kidney. The fraction of the TAL showing severe damage was reduced by furosemide, but not by acetazolamide, and the lesion was also eliminated by perfusion with ouabain or by preventing glomerular filtration.[281]

Mitochondrial Injury during Reperfusion

It is known that cell death following ischemia-reperfusion is closely related to functional changes in the mitochondria. Liu et al. revealed that apoptotic programmed death is associated with the release of cytochrome c (cyt c) due to caspase (cysteinyl aspartate-specific proteinase) activity.[282] Cyt c release is dependent on the site and the type of mitochondrial injury. Isolated mouse PT was subjected to mitochondrial oxidative phosphorylation inhibitors, rotenone and antimycin A or hypoxia. Antimycin A caused a significantly higher level of cyt c release from the PT than rotenone or hypoxia.[283] The efflux of cyt c and other apoptosis-related compounds, such as apotosis-inducing factor (AIF) and pro-caspases-2, -3, and -9, is mediated by the disrupted mitochondrial membrane or MPT (mitochondrial permeability transition).[284] Although the precise molecular mechanism of MPT remains to be elucidated, MPT occurs by a multiprotein channel composed of a voltage-dependent anion channel (VDAC), which comprises a nonselective channel for any substances with a molecular mass less than 15 kDa,[285] and adenine nucleotide translocase (ANT).

ATP depletion causes an increase in cellular free Ca^{2+},[286,287,288] and this phenomenon causes mitochondrial injury and apoptosis in renal tubular cells. Tanaka and colleagues demonstrated that voltage-dependent Ca^{2+} channels are involved in cellular and mitochondrial accumulation of Ca^{2+} due to ATP depletion.[289]

Chronic Ischemia

Recently, accumulating evidence has emphasized the effects of chronic hypoxia on renal structure and function.[290] In the advanced stage of renal dysfunction with tubulointerstitial damage, peritubular capillaries are lost, and the development of interstitial fibrosis decreases oxygen diffusion to tubules. As a consequence, nephron segments are exposed to chronic hypoxia, and this in turn exacerbates renal insufficiency. Diffuse cortical hypoxia was demonstrated in the puromycin aminonucleoside-induced nephrotic syndrome and focal and segmental hypoxia in a remnant kidney model.[291]

When cells are exposed to hypoxia, the activation of hypoxia-inducible factor-1 (HIF-1) occurs, which is a primary defensive mechanism against hypoxia.[292,293] HIF-1 transcriptionally regulates many factors associated with hypoxia, such as the increased expression of VDGF,[294] erythropoietin,[295] a glucose transporter (Glut-1),[296] and PGK,[297] thereby chronic hypoxia alters the cellular transport and metabolism via HIF-1 activation. It is suggested that the induction of the HIF signal, which adapts the renal cells to hypoxia, may be a therapeutic option against the development of renal dysfunction.

Nephrotoxicants

Several nephrotoxic drugs, such as certain cephalosporins,[298] tacrolimus and sirolimus,[299] cadmium metallothionein,[300] probenecid,[301] prednisolone and azathioprine,[302] and cyclosporine A,[303] were shown to impair mitochondria and cellular metabolism. Ochratoxin A, a mycotoxin, also inhibits mitochondrial oxidative phosphorylation in the PT.[304] In contrast, enalapril and losartan attenuate mitochondrial dysfunction.[305]

A Novel Technology Analyzing Renal Blood Oxygenation

Recently, a novel technique called the Blood Oxygen Level-Dependent (BOLD) MRI method has been applied to renal physiology. The BOLD MRI method measures blood deoxyhemoglobin, and indirectly estimates intrarenal oxygenation in a noninvasive fashion, allowing sequential measurements in humans as well as animals in response to a variety of physiological or pharmacological stimuli with high reproducibility.[306,307] The effects of diuretics on renal oxygenation were investigated using the BOLD method. Furosemide, but not acetazolamide, increased medullary oxygenation by inhibiting active transport and QO_2 in the medullary thick ascending limb, consistent with their separate sites of action in the nephron.[308] The effect of furosemide on medullary oxygenation was absent or slight in an elderly human population.[309] Moreover, the BOLD method was applied to changes in intrarenal oxygenation in a variety of pathophysiological states, such as an acute reduction in RBF,[310] the diabetic state,[311] and the administration of NO synthase inhibitor.[312] BOLD-contrast imaging appears to predict the tissue at risk from ischemia by revealing information on the balance between tubular workload and delivery of oxygen.[311] Refined methods with improved visualization and more precise quantification have been developed.[313]

CONCLUSIONS

Most of the energy produced in the kidney is primarily utilized for the active reabsorption of Na+, which further drives the cellular and paracellular transport of water and solutes. Renal metabolism for energy production is regulated by transport activity, and conversely, transport is affected by the cellular energy status. The intracellular adenine nucleotide level is an important regulatory factor for metabolism and transport; however, the interactions of these two processes are diverse and complex. For the last decade, AMPK was identified as the critical molecule for the regulator of cell metabolisms in various cells. Although the current information on its importance in the kidney is not abundant, emerging evidence has demonstrated its significance in the kidney, especially in energy metabolism in several solute transports. Other regulators, such as ATP-sensitive cation channels, NO, and purinergic receptors, should play some roles. Futher studies are required to elucidate the fine regulatory mechanisms for renal transport and cellular metabolisms. A novel methodology, BOLD MRI, will provide some progress in this field.

From pathophysiological viewpoints, the susceptibility of the kidney to ischemia and agents affecting energy production are critical clinical issues. Not only the role of acute ischemia, but also that of chronic ischemia in the kidney is now beginning to be a novel research subject.

References

[1] Valtin H. Renal function: mechanisms preserving fluid and solute balance in health. 2nd ed. Boston: Little, Brown; 1983.

[2] Cohen JJ, Kamm DE. Renal metabolism: relation to renal function. In: Brenner BM, Rector FC, editors. The kidney. Philadelphia: Saunders; 1976.

[3] Soltoff S. ATP and the regulation of renal cell function. Annu Rev Physiol 1986;48:9–31.

[4] Deetjen P. Measurement of metabolism during renal work. Int J Biochem 1980;12:243–4.

[5] Kiil F, Aukland K, Refsum HE. Renal sodium transport and oxygen consumption. Am J Physiol 1961;201:511–6.

[6] Thurau K. Renal Na-reabsorption and O_2-uptake in dogs during hypoxia and hydrochlorothiazide infusion. Proc Soc Exp Biol Med 1961;106:714–7.

[7] Mandel LJ, Balaban RS. Stoichiometry and coupling of active transport to oxidative metabolism in epithelial tissues. Am J Physiol 1981;240:F357–371.

[8] Gottschalk CW, Mylle M. Micropuncture study of the mammalian urinary concentrating mechanism: evidence for the countercurrent hypothesis. Am J Physiol 1959;196:927–36.

[9] Andreoli TE, Schafer JA. Effective luminal hypotonicity: the driving force for isotonic proximal tubular fluid absorption. Am J Physiol 1979;236:F89–96.

[10] Schafer JA, Patlak CS, Andreoli TE. Fluid absorption and active and passive ion flows in the rabbit superficial pars recta. Am J Physiol 1977;233:F154–167.

[11] Soleimani M, Burnham CE. Na+:HCO(3-) co-transporters (NBC): cloning and characterization. J Membr Biol 2001;183:71–84.

[12] Gross E, Hawkins K, Pushkin A, Sassani P, Dukkipati R, Abuladze N, et al. Phosphorylation of Ser(982) in the sodium bicarbonate co-transporter KNBC1 shifts the HCO(3)(−): Na (+) stoichiometry from 3: 1 to 2: 1 in murine proximal tubule cells. J Physiol 2001;537:659–65.

[13] Kiil F, Sejersted OM, Steen PA. Energetics and specificity of transcellular NaCl transport in the dog kidney. Int J Biochem 1980;12:245–50.

[14] Fromter E, Rumrich G, Ullrich KJ. Phenomenologic description of Na$^+$, Cl$^-$ and HCO$_3^-$ absorption from proximal tubules of rat kidney. Pflugers Arch 1973;343:189–220.

[15] Silva P, Myers MA. Stoichiometry of sodium chloride transport by rectal gland of *Squalus acanthias*. Am J Physiol 1986;250: F516–519.

[16] Welsh MJ. Energetics of chloride secretion in canine tracheal epithelium. comparison of the metabolic cost of chloride transport with the metabolic cost of sodium transport. J Clin Invest 1984;74:262–8.

[17] Ross B, Leaf A, Silva P, Epstein FH. Na-K-ATPase in sodium transport by the perfused rat kidney. Am J Physiol 1974;226:624–9.

[18] Kaplan JH. Biochemistry of Na,K-ATPase. Annu Rev Biochem 2002;71:511–35.

[19] Blanco G, Mercer RW. Isozymes of the Na-K-ATPase: heterogeneity in structure, diversity in function. Am J Physiol 1998;275: F633–650.

[20] Jorgensen PL. Aspects of gene structure and functional regulation of the isozymes of Na,K-ATPase. *Cell Mol Biol* (Noisy-le-grand) 2001;47:231–8.

[21] Sweadner KJ, Rael E. The FXYD gene family of small ion transport regulators or channels: cDNA sequence, protein signature sequence, and expression. Genomics 2000;68:41–56.

[22] Barlet-Bas C, Arystarkhova E, Cheval L, Marsy S, Sweadner K, Modyanov N, et al. Are there several isoforms of Na,K-ATPase alpha subunit in the rabbit kidney? J Biol Chem 1993;268:11512–5.

[23] Farman N, Corthesy-Theulaz I, Bonvalet JP, Rossier BC. Localization of alpha-isoforms of Na(+)-K(+)-ATPase in rat kidney by *in situ* hybridization. Am J Physio 1991;260: C468–474.

[24] Segall L, Daly SE, Blostein R. Mechanistic basis for kinetic differences between the rat Alpha 1, Alpha 2, and Alpha 3 isoforms of the Na,K-ATPase. J Biol Chem 2001;276:31535–41.

[25] Geering K. The functional role of beta subunits in oligomeric P-type ATPases. J Bioenerg Biomembr 2001;33:425–38.

[26] Geering K, Beguin P, Garty H, Karlisch S, Füzesi M, Horisberger JD, et al. FXYD proteins: new tissue- and isoform-specific regulators of Na,K-ATPase. Ann N Y Acad Sci 2003;986:388–94.

[27] Meij IC, Koenderink JB, van Bokhoven H, Assink KF, Groenestege WT, de Pont JJ, et al. Dominant isolated renal magnesium loss is caused by misrouting of the Na(+),K (+)-ATPase gamma-subunit. Nat Genet 2000;26:265–6.

[28] Hebert H, Purhonen P, Thomsen K, Vorum H, Maunsbach AB. Renal Na,K-ATPase structure from cryo-electron microscopy of two-dimensional crystals. Ann NY Acad Sci 2003;986:9–16.

[29] Jorgensen PL, Hakansson KO, Karlish SJ. Structure and mechanism of Na,K-ATPase: functional sites and their interactions. Annu Rev Physiol 2003;65:817–49.

[30] Doucet A. Function and control of Na-K-ATPase in single nephron segments of the mammalian kidney. Kidney Int 1988;34:749–60.

[31] Doucet A, Morel F, Katz AI. Microdetermination of Na-K-ATPase in single tubules: its application for the localization of physiologic processes in the nephron. Int J Biochem 1980;12:47–52.

[32] Garg LC, Knepper MA, Burg MB. Mineralocorticoid effects on Na-K-ATPase in individual nephron segments. Am J Physiol 1981;240:F536–544.

[33] Katz AI. Distribution and function of classes of ATPases along the nephron. Kidney Int 1986;29:21–31.

[34] Katz AI, Doucet A, Morel F. Na-K-ATPase activity along the rabbit, rat, and mouse nephron. Am J Physiol 1979;237: F114–120.

[35] El Mernissi G, Doucet A. Quantitation of [3h]ouabain binding and turnover of Na-K-ATPase along the rabbit nephron. Am J Physiol 1984;247:F158–167.

[36] Jorgensen PL. Structure, function and regulation of Na,K-ATPase in the kidney. Kidney Int 1986;29:10–20.

[37] Cheval L, Doucet A. Measurement of Na-K-ATPase-mediated rubidium influx in single segments of rat nephron. Am J Physiol 1990;259:F111–121.

[38] McDonough AA, Magyar CE, Komatsu Y. Expression of Na (+)-K(+)-ATPase alpha- and beta-subunits along rat nephron: isoform specificity and response to hypokalemia. Am J Physiol 1994;267:C901–908.

[39] Tumlin JA, Hoban CA, Medford RM, Sands JM. Expression of Na-K-ATPase alpha- and beta-subunit mRNA and protein isoforms in the rat nephron. Am J Physiol 1994;266:F240–245.

[40] Ahn KY, Madsen KM, Tisher CC, Kone BC. Differential expression and cellular distribution of mRNAs encoding alpha- and beta-isoforms of Na$^{(+)}$-K$^{(+)}$-ATPase in rat kidney. Am J Physiol 1993;265:F792–801.

[41] Kashgarian M, Biemesderfer D, Caplan M, Forbush III B. Monoclonal antibody to Na,K-ATPase: immunocytochemical localization along nephron segments. Kidney Int 1985;28:899–913.

[42] Piepenhagen PA, Peters LL, Lux SE, Nelson WJ. Differential expression of Na(+)-K(+)-ATPase, ankyrin, fodrin, and e-cadherin along the kidney nephron. Am J Physiol 1995;269: C1417–1432.

[43] Wetzel RK, Sweadner KJ. Immunocytochemical localization of Na-K-ATPase alpha- and gamma-subunits in rat kidney. Am J Physiol Renal Physiol 2001;281:F531–545.

[44] Doucet A, Hus-Citharel A, Morel F. *In vitro* stimulation of Na-K-ATPase in rat thick ascending limb by dexamethasone. Am J Physiol 1986;251:F851–857.

[45] Terada Y, Knepper MA. Na$^+$-K$^+$-ATPase activities in renal tubule segments of rat inner medulla. Am J Physiol 1989;256: F218–223.

[46] Vinciguerra M, Deschenes G, Hasler U, Mordasini D, Rousselot M, Doucet A, et al. Intracellular Na$^+$ controls cell surface expression of Na,K-ATPase via a camp-independent PKA

pathway in mammalian kidney collecting duct cells. Mol Biol Cell 2003;14:2677—88.

[47] Kiroytcheva M, Cheval L, Carranza ML, Martin PY, Favre H, Doucet A, et al. Effect of Camp on the activity and the phosphorylation of Na$^+$,K($+$)-ATPase in rat thick ascending limb of Henle. Kidney Int 1999;55:1819—31.

[48] Buffin-Meyer B, Verbavatz JM, Cheval L, Marsy S, Younes-Ibrahim M, Le Moal C, et al. Regulation of Na $+$, K($+$)-ATPase in the rat outer medullary collecting duct during potassium depletion. J Am Soc Nephrol 1998;9:538—50.

[49] Feraille E, Doucet A. Sodium-potassium-adenosinetriphosphatase-dependent sodium transport in the kidney: hormonal control. Physiol Rev 2001;81:345—418.

[50] Feraille E, Mordasini D, Gonin S, Deschênes G, Vinciguerra M, Doucet A, et al. Mechanism of control of Na,K-ATPase in principal cells of the mammalian collecting duct. Ann NY Acad Sci 2003;986:570—8.

[51] Michlig S, Mercier A, Doucet A, Schild L, Horisberger JD, Rossier BC, et al. ERK1/2 controls Na,K-ATPase activity and transepithelial sodium transport in the principal cell of the cortical collecting duct of the mouse kidney. J Biol Chem 2004;279:51002—12.

[52] Bronner F. Renal calcium transport: mechanisms and regulation—an overview. Am J Physiol 1989;257:F707—711.

[53] Magyar CE, White KE, Rojas R, Apodaca G, Friedman PA. Plasma membrane Ca^{2+}-ATPase and NCX1 Na$^+$/Ca^{2+} exchanger expression in distal convoluted tubule cells. Am J Physiol Renal Physiol 2002;283:F29—40.

[54] Verma AK, Filoteo AG, Stanford DR, Wieben ED, Penniston JD, Strehler EE, et al. Complete primary structure of a human plasma membrane Ca^{2+} pump. J Biol Chem 1988;263:14152—9.

[55] Penniston JT, Enyedi A. Modulation of the plasma membrane Ca^{2+} pump. J Membr Biol 1998;165:101—9.

[56] Stauffer TP, Guerini D, Carafoli E. Tissue distribution of the four gene products of the plasma membrane Ca^{2+} pump. A study using specific antibodies. J Biol Chem 1995;270:12184—90.

[57] Stauffer TP, Hilfiker H, Carafoli E, Strehler EE. Quantitative analysis of alternative splicing options of human plasma membrane calcium pump genes. J Biol Chem 1993;268:25993—6003.

[58] Brunette MG, Mailloux J, Chan M, Ramachandran C. Characterization of the high and low affinity components of the renal Ca2($+$)-Mg2$+$ ATPase. Can J Physiol Pharmacol 1990;68:718—26.

[59] Dick IM, Liu J, Glendenning P, Prince RL. Estrogen and androgen regulation of plasma membrane calcium pump activity in immortalized distal tubule kidney cells. Mol Cell Endocrinol 2003;212:11—8.

[60] Qi Z, Murase K, Obata S, Sokabe M. Extracellular ATP-dependent activation of plasma membrane Ca(2$+$) pump in HEK-293 cells. Br J Pharmacol 2000;131:370—4.

[61] Caride AJ, Chini EN, Penniston JT, Dousa TP. Selective decrease of mRNAs encoding plasma membrane calcium pump isoforms 2 and 3 in rat kidney. Kidney Int 1999;56:1818—25.

[62] Caride AJ, Chini EN, Homma S, Penniston JT, Dousa TP. mRNA encoding four isoforms of the plasma membrane calcium pump and their variants in rat kidney and nephron segments. J Lab Clin Med 1998;132:149—56.

[63] Magosci M, Yamaki M, Penniston JT, Dousa TP. Localization of mRNAs coding for isozymes of plasma membrane Ca($^{2+}$)-ATPase pump in rat kidney. Am J Physiol 1992;263:F7—14.

[64] Loffing J, Loffing-Cueni D, Valderrabano V, Kläusli L, Hebert SC, Rossier BC, et al. Distribution of transcellular calcium and sodium transport pathways along mouse distal nephron. Am J Physiol Renal Physiol 2001;281:F1021—1027.

[65] Kip SN, Strehler EE. Characterization of PMCA isoforms and their contribution to transcellular Ca^{2+} flux in MDCK cells. Am J Physiol Renal Physiol 2003;284:F122—132.

[66] Doucet A, Katz AI. High-affinity Ca-Mg-ATPase along the rabbit nephron. Am J Physiol 1982;242:F346—352.

[67] Martin V, Bredoux R, Corvazier E, Van Gorp R, Kovacs T, Gelebart P, et al. Three novel sarco/endoplasmic reticulum Ca^{2+}-ATPase (SERCA) 3 isoforms. Expression, regulation, and function of the membranes of the SERCA3 family. J Biol Chem 2002;277:24442—52.

[68] Thastrup O, Cullen PJ, Drobak BK, Hanley MR, Dawson AP. Thapsigargin, a tumor promoter, discharges intracellular Ca^{2+} stores by specific inhibition of the endoplasmic reticulum Ca2($+$)-ATPase. Proc Natl Acad Sci USA 1990;87:2466—70.

[69] Doucet AH. K($+$)-ATPase in the kidney: localization and function in the nephron. Exp Nephrol 1997;5:271—6.

[70] Shull GE, Lingrel JB. Molecular cloning of the rat stomach (H$^+$ $+$ K$^+$)-ATPase. J Biol Chem 1986;261:16788—91.

[71] Crowson MS, Shull GE. Isolation and characterization of a cDNA encoding the putative distal colon H$^+$,K($+$)-Atpase. Similarity of deduced amino acid sequence to gastric H$^+$,K ($+$)-ATPase and Na$^+$,K($+$)-ATPase and mRNA expression in distal colon, kidney, and uterus. J Biol Chem 1992;267:13740—8.

[72] Canfield VA, Okamoto CT, Chow D, Dorfman J, Gros P, Forte JG, et al. Cloning of the H,K-ATPase beta subunit. Tissue-specific expression, chromosomal assignment, and relationship to Na,K-ATPase beta subunits. J Biol Chem 1990;265:19878—84.

[73] Silver RB, Soleimani H. H$^+$-K$^+$-ATPases: regulation and role in pathophysiological states. Am J Physiol 1999;276:F799—811.

[74] Wingo CS. Active proton secretion and potassium absorption in the rabbit outer medullary collecting duct. Functional evidence for proton-potassium-activated adenosine triphosphatase. J Clin Invest 1989;84:361—5.

[75] Doucet A, Marsy S. Characterization of K-ATPase activity in distal nephron: stimulation by potassium depletion. Am J Physiol 1987;253:F418—423.

[76] Garg LC, Narang N. Ouabain-insensitive K-adenosine triphosphatase in distal nephron segments of the rabbit. J Clin Invest 1988;81:1204—8.

[77] Wingo CS, Madsen KM, Smolka A, Tisher CC. H-K-ATPase immunoreactivity in cortical and outer medullary collecting duct. Kidney Int 1990;38:985—90.

[78] Ahn KY, Kone BC. Expression and cellular localization of mRNA encoding the "gastric" isoform of H($^+$)-K($^+$)-ATPase alpha-subunit in rat kidney. Am J Physiol 1995;268:F99—109.

[79] Marsy S, Elalouf JM, Doucet A. Quantitative Rt-Pcr analysis of mRNAs encoding a colonic putative H, K-ATPase alpha subunit along the rat nephron: effect of K$^+$ depletion. Pflugers Arch 1996;432:494—500.

[80] Ahn KY, Turner PB, Madsen KM, Kone BC. Effects of chronic hypokalemia on renal expression of the "gastric" H($^+$)-K ($^+$)-ATPase alpha-subunit gene. Am J Physiol 1996;270: F557—566.

[81] Gluck SL, Underhill DM, Iyori M, Holliday LS, Kostrominova TY, Lee BS. Physiology and biochemistry of the kidney vacuolar H$^+$-ATPase. Annu Rev Physiol 1996;58:427—45.

[82] Wagner CA, Finberg KE, Breton S, Marshansky V, Brown D, Geibel JP. Renal vacuolar H$^+$-ATPase. Physiol Rev 2004;84:1263—314.

[83] Forgac M. Structure, mechanism and regulation of the clathrin-coated vesicle and yeast vacuolar H($+$)-ATPases. J Exp Biol 2000;203:71—80.

[84] Gruber G. Introduction: a close look at the vacuolar ATPase. J Bioenerg Biomembr 2003;35:277—80.

[85] Bank N, Aynedjian HS, Mutz BF. Evidence for a DCCD-sensitive component of proximal bicarbonate reabsorption. Am J Physiol 1985;249:F636—644.

[86] Kurtz I. Apical Na⁺/H⁺ antiporter and glycolysis-dependent H⁺-ATPase regulate intracellular Ph in the rabbit S3 proximal tubule. J Clin Invest 1987;80:928—35.

[87] Noel J, Vinay P, Tejedor A, Fleser A, Laprade R. Metabolic cost of bafilomycin-sensitive H⁺ pump in intact dog, rabbit, and hamster proximal tubules. Am J Physiol 1993;264:F655—661.

[88] Ait-Mohamed AK, Marsy S, Barlet C, Khadouri C, Doucet A. Characterization of N-ethylmaleimide-sensitive proton pump in the rat kidney. Localization along the nephron. J Biol Chem 1986;261:12526—33.

[89] Brown D, Hirsch S, Gluck S. Localization of a proton-pumping ATPase in rat kidney. J Clin Invest 1988;82:2114—26.

[90] Garg LC, Narang N. Changes in H-ATPase activity in the distal nephron segments of the rat during metabolic acidosis and alkalosis. Contrib Nephrol 1991;92:39—45.

[91] Garg LC, Narang N. Decrease in N-ethylmaleimide-sensitive ATPase activity in collecting duct by metabolic alkalosis. Can J Physiol Pharmacol 1990;68:1119—23.

[92] Garg LC, Narang N. Stimulation of an N-ethylmaleimide-sensitive ATPase in the collecting duct segments of the rat nephron by metabolic acidosis. Can J Physiol Pharmacol 1985;63:1291—6.

[93] Garg LC, Narang N. Effects of aldosterone on Nem—sensitive ATPase in rabbit nephron segments. Kidney Int 1988;34:13—7.

[94] Karet FE, Finberg KE, Nelson RD, Nayir A, Mocan H, Sanjad SA, et al. Mutations in the gene encoding B1 subunit of H⁺-ATPase cause renal tubular acidosis with sensorineural deafness. Nat Genet 1999;21:84—90.

[95] Smith AN, Skaug J, Choate KA, Nayir A, Bakkaloglu A, Ozen S, et al. Mutations in ATP6N1B, encoding a new kidney vacuolar proton pump 116-Kd subunit, cause recessive distal renal tubular acidosis with preserved hearing. Nat Genet 2000;26:71—5.

[96] Stover EH, Borthwick KJ, Bavalia C, Eady N, Fritz DM, Rungroj N, et al. Novel ATP6V1B1 and ATP6V0A4 mutations in autosomal recessive distal renal tubular acidosis with new evidence for hearing loss. J Med Genet 2002;39:796—803.

[97] Ambudkar SV, Kimchi-Sarfaty C, Sauna ZE, Gottesman MM. P-glycoprotein: from genomics to mechanism. Oncogene 2003;22:7468—85.

[98] Gottesman MM, Fojo T, Bates SE. Multidrug resistance in cancer: role of ATP-dependent transporters. Nat Rev Cancer 2002;2:48—58.

[99] Haimeur A, Conseil G, Deeley RG, Cole SP. The MRP-related and BCRP/ABCG2 multidrug resistance proteins: biology, substrate specificity and regulation. Curr Drug Metab 2004;5:21—53.

[100] Hrycyna CA, Ramachandra M, Ambudkar SV, Ko YH, Pedersen PL, Pastan I, et al. Mechanism of action of human P-glycoprotein ATPase activity. Photochemical cleavage during a catalytic transition state using orthovanadate reveals cross-talk between the two ATP sites. J Biol Chem 1998;273:16631—4.

[101] Gullans SR, Mandel LJ. In: Seldin, Giebisch G, editors. The kidney: physiology & pathophysiology. 3rd ed Williams & Wilkins; 2000.

[102] Kone BC, The metabolic basis of solute transport. Brenner BM, editor. The Kidney; 2004.

[103] Hatefi Y. The mitochondrial electron transport and oxidative phosphorylation system. Annu Rev Biochem 1985;54:1015—69.

[104] Le Hir M, Dubach UC. Activities of enzymes of the tricarboxylic acid cycle in segments of the rat nephron. Pflugers Arch 1982;395:239—43.

[105] Marver D, Schwartz MJ. Identification of mineralocorticoid target sites in the isolated rabbit cortical nephron. Proc Natl Acad Sci USA 1980;77:3672—6.

[106] Le Hir M, Dubach UC. Peroxisomal and mitochondrial beta-oxidation in the rat kidney: distribution of fatty acyl-coenzyme a oxidase and 3-hydroxyacyl-coenzyme a dehydrogenase activities along the nephron. J Histochem Cytochem 1982;30:441—4.

[107] Guder WG, Purschel S, Wirthensohn G. Renal ketone body metabolism. Distribution of 3-Oxoacid Coa-Transferase and 3-hydroxybutyrate dehydrogenase along the mouse nephron. Hoppe Seylers Z Physiol Chem 1983;364:1727—37.

[108] Schlender KK. Regulation of renal glycogen synthase. interconversion of two forms in vitro. Biochim Biophys Acta 1973;297:384—98.

[109] Vandewalle A, Wirthensohn G, Heidrich HG, Guder WG. Distribution of hexokinase and phosphoenolpyruvate carboxykinase along the rabbit nephron. Am J Physiol 1981;240:F492—500.

[110] Schmid H, Mall A, Scholz M, Schmidt U. Unchanged glycolytic capacity in rat kidney under conditions of stimulated gluconeogenesis. Determination of phosphofructokinase and pyruvate kinase in microdissected nephron segments of fasted and acidotic animals. Hoppe Seylers Z Physiol Chem 1980;361:819—27.

[111] Bagnasco S, Good D, Balaban R, Burg M. Lactate production in isolated segments of the rat nephron. Am J Physiol 1985;248:F522—526.

[112] Krebs HA. Renal gluconeogenesis. Adv Enzyme Regul 1963;17:385—400.

[113] Meyer C, Stumvoll M, Dostou J, Welle S, Haymond M, Gerich J. Renal substrate exchange and gluconeogenesis in normal postabsorptive humans. Am J Physiol Endocrinol Metab 2002;282:E428—434.

[114] Cersosimo E, Garlick P, Ferretti J. Renal glucose production during insulin-induced hypoglycemia in humans. Diabetes 1999;48:261—6.

[115] Cersosimo E, Garlick P, Ferretti J. Renal substrate metabolism and gluconeogenesis during hypoglycemia in humans. Diabetes 2000;49:1186—93.

[116] Maleque A, Endou H, Koseki C, Sakai F. Nephron heterogeneity: gluconeogenesis from pyruvate in rabbit nephron. FEBS Lett 1980;116:154—6.

[117] Kondou I, Nakada J, Hishinuma H, Masuda F, Machida T, Endou H. Alterations of gluconeogenesis by ischemic renal injury in rats. Ren Fail 1992;14:479—83.

[118] Friedrichs D, Schoner W. Stimulation of renal gluconeogenesis by inhibition of the sodium pump. Biochim Biophys Acta 1973;304:142—60.

[119] Gullans SR, Brazy PC, Dennis VW, Mandel LJ. Interactions between gluconeogenesis and sodium transport in rabbit proximal tubule. Am J Physiol 1984;246:F859—869.

[120] Nagami GT, Lee P. Effect of luminal perfusion on glucose production by isolated proximal tubules. Am J Physiol 1989;256:F120—127.

[121] Veiga JA, Carpenter CA, Saggerson ED. Effect of the Na⁺ ionophore monensin on basal and noradrenaline stimulated gluconeogenesis in rat renal tubule fragments. FEBS Lett 1981;134:183—4.

[122] Silva P, Hallac R, Spokes K, Epstein FH. Relationship among gluconeogenesis, QO₂, and Na⁺ transport in the perfused rat kidney. Am J Physiol 1982;242:F508—513.

[123] Silva P, Ross B, Spokes K. Competition between sodium reabsorption and gluconeogenesis in kidneys of steroid-treated rats. Am J Physiol 1980;238:F290–295.

[124] Pfaller W. Structure function correlation on rat kidney. Quantitative correlation of structure and function in the normal and injured rat kidney. Adv Anat Embryol Cell Biol 1982;70:1–106.

[125] Pfaller W, Rittinger M. Quantitative morphology of the rat kidney. Int J Biochem 1980;12:17–22.

[126] Burch HB, Choi S, Dence CN, Alvey TR, Cole BR, Lowry OH. Metabolic effects of large fructose loads in different parts of the rat nephron. J Biol Chem 1980;255:8239–44.

[127] Uchida S, Endou H. Substrate specificity to maintain cellular ATP along the mouse nephron. Am J Physiol 1988;255: F977–983.

[128] Gyoergy P, Keller W, Brehme TH. Nierestoffwechsel und nierenentwicklung. Biochem Zeitschr 1928;200:356–66.

[129] Klein KL, Wang MS, Torikai S, Davidson WD, Kurokaqwa K. Substrate oxidation by isolated single nephron segments of the rat. Kidney Int 1981;20:29–35.

[130] Ruegg CE, Mandel LJ. Bulk isolation of renal Pct and Pst. Ii. Differential responses to anoxia or hypoxia. Am J Physiol 1990;259:F176–185.

[131] Weidemann MJ, Krebs HA. The fuel of respiration of rat kidney cortex. Biochem J 1969;112:149–66.

[132] Guder WG, Ross BD. Enzyme distribution along the nephron. Kidney Int 1984;26:101–11.

[133] Balaban RS, Mandel LJ. Metabolic substrate utilization by rabbit proximal tubule. An NADH fluorescence study. Am J Physiol 1988;254:F407–416.

[134] Harris SI, Balaban RS, Barrett L, Mandel LJ. Mitochondrial respiratory capacity and Na^+- and K^+-dependent adenosine triphosphatase-mediated ion transport in the intact renal cell. J Biol Chem 1981;256:10319–28.

[135] Rome L, Grantham J, Savin V, Lohr J, Lechene C. Proximal tubule volume regulation in hyperosmotic media: intracellular K^+, Na^+, and Cl. Am J Physiol 1989;257:C1093–1100.

[136] Gullans SR, Harris SI, Mandel LJ. Glucose-dependent respiration in suspensions of rabbit cortical tubules. J Membr Biol 1984;78:257–62.

[137] Markovich D, Murer H. The Slc13 gene family of sodium sulphate/carboxylate co-transporters. Pflugers Arch 2004;447:594–602.

[138] Pajor AM. Sodium-coupled transporters for Krebs Cycle intermediates. Annu Rev Physiol 1999;61:663–82.

[139] Sekine T, Cha SH, Hosoyamada M, Kanai Y, Watanabe N, Furuta Y, et al. Cloning, functional characterization, and localization of a rat renal Na^+-dicarboxylate transporter. Am J Physiol 1998;275:F298–305.

[140] Unwin RJ, Capasso G, Shirley DG. An overview of divalent cation and citrate handling by the kidney. Nephron Physiol 2004;98:p15–20.

[141] Guder WG, Wagner S, Wirthensohn G. Metabolic fuels along the nephron: pathways and intracellular mechanisms of interaction. Kidney Int 1986;29:41–5.

[142] Goldstein L. Renal substrate utilization in normal and acidotic rats. Am J Physiol 1987;253:F351–357.

[143] Jung KY, Endou H. Cellular adenosine triphosphate production and consumption in the descending thin limb of Henle's loop in the rat. Ren Physiol Biochem 1990;13:248–58.

[144] Wittner M, Weidtke C, Schlatter E, di Stefano A, Greger R. Substrate utilization in the isolated perfused cortical thick ascending limb of rabbit nephron. Pflugers Arch 1984;402:52–62.

[145] Chamberlin ME, Mandel LJ. Substrate support of medullary thick ascending limb oxygen consumption. Am J Physiol 1986;251:F758–763.

[146] Torikai S. Dependency of microdissected nephron segments upon oxidative phosphorylation and exogenous substrates: a relationship between tubular anatomical location in the kidney and metabolic activity. *Clin Sci* (Lond) 1989;77: 287–95.

[147] Chamberlin ME, LeFurgey A, Mandel LJ. Suspension of medullary thick ascending limb tubules from the rabbit kidney. *Am J Physiol* 1984;247:F955–964.

[148] Eveloff J, Bayerdorffer E, Silva P, Kinne R. Sodium-chloride transport in the thick ascending limb of Henle's loop. Oxygen consumption studies in isolated cells. Pflugers Arch 1981;389:263–70.

[149] Chamberlin ME, Mandel LJ. Na^+-K^+-ATPase activity in medullary thick ascending limb during short-term anoxia. Am J Physiol 1987;252:F838–843.

[150] Hering-Smith KS, Hamm LL. Metabolic support of collecting duct transport. Kidney Int 1998;53:408–15.

[151] Nonaka T, Stokes JB. Metabolic support of Na^+ transport by the rabbit CCD: analysis of the use of equivalent current. Kidney Int 1994;45:743–52.

[152] Natke Jr. E. Cell volume regulation of rabbit cortical collecting tubule in anisotonic media. Am J Physiol 1990;258: F1657–1665.

[153] Zeidel ML, Seifter JL, Lear S, Brenner BM, Silva P. Atrial peptides inhibit oxygen consumption in kidney medullary collecting duct cells. Am J Physiol 1986;251:F379–383.

[154] Vinay P, Senecal J, Noel J, Chirinian C, Vinay MC, Ammann H, et al. Basolateral glucose transport in distal segments of the dog nephron. Can J Physiol Pharmacol 1991;69:964–77.

[155] Zeidel ML, Silva P, Seifter JL. Intracellular pH regulation in rabbit renal medullary collecting duct cells. Role of chloride-bicarbonate exchange. J Clin Invest 1986;77:1682–8.

[156] Grunewald RW, Kinne RK. Sugar transport in isolated rat kidney papillary collecting duct cells. Pflugers Arch 1988;413:32–7.

[157] Stokes JB, Grupp C, Kinne RK. Purification of rat papillary collecting duct cells: functional and metabolic assessment. Am J Physiol 1987;253:F251–262.

[158] Zeidel ML. Hormonal regulation of inner medullary collecting duct sodium transport. Am J Physiol 1993;265:F159–173.

[159] Kone BC, Kikeri D, Zeidel ML, Gullans SR. Cellular pathways of potassium transport in renal inner medullary collecting duct. Am J Physiol 1989;256:C823–830.

[160] Blond DM, Whittam R. The regulation of kidney respiration by sodium and potassium ions. Biochem J 1964;92:158–67.

[161] Whittam R. Active cation transport as a pace-maker of respiration. Nature 1961;191:603–4.

[162] Rea C, Segal S. ATP content of rat kidney cortex slices: relation to alpha-aminoisobutyric acid uptake. Kidney Int 1972;2:101–6.

[163] Urbaitis BK, Kessler RH. Actions of inhibitor compounds on adenine nucleotides of renal cortex and sodium excretion. Am J Physiol 1971;220:1116–23.

[164] Needleman P, Passonneau JV, Lowry OH. Distribution of glucose and related metabolites in rat kidney. Am J Physiol 1968;215:655–9.

[165] Balaban RS, Mandel LJ, Soltoff SP, Storey JM. Coupling of active ion transport and aerobic respiratory rate in isolated renal tubules. Proc Natl Acad Sci USA 1980;77:447–51.

[166] Chance BG, Williams R. The respiratory chain and oxidative phosphorylation. Adv Enzymol Relat Subj Biochem 1956;17:65–134.

[167] Jacobus WE, Moreadith RW, Vandegaer KM. Mitochondrial respiratory control. evidence against the regulation of respiration by extramitochondrial phosphorylation potentials or by [Atp]/[Adp] Ratios. J Biol Chem 1982;257:2397–402.

[168] Lardy HA, Wellman H. Oxidative phosphorylations: role of inorganic phosphate and acceptor systems in control of metabolic rates. J Biol Chem 1952;195:215–24.

[169] Harris SI, Balaban RS, Mandel LJ. Oxygen consumption and cellular ion transport: evidence for adenosine triphosphate to O_2 ratio near 6 in intact cell. Science 1980;208:1148–50.

[170] Slater EC, Rosing J, Mol A. The phosphorylation potential generated by respiring mitochondria. Biochim Biophys Acta 1973;292:534–53.

[171] Lemasters JJ, Sowers AE. Phosphate dependence and atractyloside inhibition of mitochondrial oxidative phosphorylation. The ADP-ATP carrier is rate-limiting. J Biol Chem 1979;254:1248–51.

[172] Balaban RS. Regulation of oxidative phosphorylation in the mammalian cell. Am J Physiol 1990;258:C377–389.

[173] Erecinska M, Wilson DF. Regulation of cellular energy metabolism. J Membr Biol 1982;70:1–14.

[174] Erecinska M, Wilson DF, Nishiki K. Homeostatic regulation of cellular energy metabolism: experimental characterization in vivo and fit to a model. Am J Physiol 1978;234:C82–89.

[175] Brown GC. Control of respiration and ATP synthesis in mammalian mitochondria and cells. Biochem J 1992;284(Pt 1):1–13.

[176] Foxall PJ, Nicholson JK. Nuclear magnetic resonance spectroscopy: a non-invasive probe of kidney metabolism and function. Exp Nephrol 1998;6 1998;:409–14.

[177] Wong GG, Ross BD. Application of phosphorus nuclear magnetic resonance to problems of renal physiology and metabolism. Miner Electrolyte Metab 1983;9:282–9.

[178] Freeman D, Bartlett S, Radda G, Ross B. Energetics of sodium transport in the kidney. Saturation transfer 31P-NMR. Biochim Biophys Acta 1983;762:325–36.

[179] Veech RL, Lawson JW, Cornell NW, Krebs HA. Cytosolic phosphorylation potential. J Biol Chem 1979;254:6538–47.

[180] Brand MD, Murphy MP. Control of electron flux through the respiratory chain in mitochondria and cells. Biol Rev Camb Philos Soc 1987;62:141–93.

[181] Kadenbach B. Intrinsic and extrinsic uncoupling of oxidative phosphorylation. Biochim Biophys Acta 2003;1604:77–94.

[182] Kadenbach B. Regulation of respiration and ATP synthesis in higher organisms: hypothesis. J Bioenerg Biomembr 1986;18:39–54.

[183] Akerboom TP, Bookelman H, Tager JM. Control of ATP transport across the mitochondrial membrane in isolated rat-liver cells. FEBS Lett 1977;74:50–4.

[184] Pfaller W, Guder WG, Gstraunthaler G, Kotanko P, Jehart I, Pürschel S. Compartmentation of ATP within renal proximal tubular cells. Biochim Biophys Acta 1984;805:152–7.

[185] Schwenke WD, Soboll S, Seitz HJ, Sies H. Mitochondrial and cytosolic ATP/ADP ratios in rat liver in vivo. Biochem J 1981;200:405–8.

[186] Soltoff SP, Mandel LJ. Active ion transport in the renal proximal tubule. III. The ATP dependence of the Na pump. J Gen Physiol 1984;84:643–62.

[187] Urbaitis BK, Kessler RH. Concentration of adenine nucleotide compounds in renal cortex and medulla. Nephron 1969;6:217–34.

[188] Daly SE, Lane LK, Blostein R. Functional consequences of amino-terminal diversity of the catalytic subunit of the Na,K-ATPase. J Biol Chem 1994;269:23944–8.

[189] Mandel LJ. Primary active sodium transport, oxygen consumption, and ATP: coupling and regulation. Kidney Int 1986;29:3–9.

[190] Gullans SR, Brazy PC, Soltoff SP, Dennis VW, Mandel LJ. Metabolic inhibitors: effects on metabolism and transport in the proximal tubule. Am J Physiol 1982;243:F133–140.

[191] Brazy PC, Balaban RS, Gullans SR, Mandel LJ, Dennis VW. Inhibition of renal metabolism. relative effects of arsenate on sodium, phosphate, and glucose transport by the rabbit proximal tubule. J Clin Invest 1980;66:1211–21.

[192] Goligorsky MS, Hruska KA. Hormonal modulation of cytoplasmic calcium concentration in renal tubular epithelium. Miner Electrolyte Metab 1988;14:58–70.

[193] Hallows K, Mount P, Pastor-Soler N, Power DA. Role of the energy sensor AMP-activated protein kinase in renal physiology and disease. Am J Physiol Renal Physiol 2010;298:F1067–1077.

[194] Kahn B, Alquier T, Carling D, Hardie DG. AMP-activated protein kinase: ancient energy gauge provides clues to modern understanding of metabolism. Cell Metab 2005;1:15–25.

[195] Steinberg G, Kemp B. AMPK in health and disease. Physiol Rev 2009;89:1025–78.

[196] Yehm L, Lee K, Kim K. Regulation of rat liver acetyl-coa carboxylase. regulation of phosphorylation and inactivation of acetyl-coa carboxylase by the adenylate energy charge. J Biol Chem 1980;255:2308–14.

[197] Munday M, Campbell D, Carling D, Hardie DG. Identification by amino acid sequencing of three major regulatory phosphorylation sites on rat acetyl-CoA carboxylase. Eur J Biochem 1988;175:331–8.

[198] Carling D, Aguan K, Woods A, Verhoeven AJ, Beri RK, Brennan CH, et al. Mammalian AMP-activated protein kinase is homologous to yeast and plant protein kinases involved in the regulation of carbon metabolism. J Biol Chem 1994;269:11442–8.

[199] Mitchelhill K, Stapleton D, Gao G, House C, Michell B, Katsis F, et al. Mammalian AMP-activated protein kinase shares structural and functional homology with the catalytic domain of yeast SNF1 protein kinase. J Biol Chem 1994;269:2361–4.

[200] Sanders M, Grondin P, Hegarty B, Snowden MA, Carling D. Investigating the mechanism for AMP activation of the AMP-activated protein kinase cascade. Biochem J 2007;403:139–48.

[201] Hawley S, Selbert M, Goldstein E, Edelman AM, Carling D, Hardie DG. 5′-AMP activates the AMP-activated protein kinase cascade, and Ca^{2+}/calmodulin activates the calmodulin-dependent protein kinase I cascade, via three independent mechanisms. J Biol Chem 1995;270:27186–91.

[202] Scott J, Hawley S, Green K, Anis M, Stewart G, Scullion GA, et al. CBS domains form energy-sensing modules whose binding of adenosine ligands is disrupted by disease mutations. J Clin Invest 2004;113:182–4.

[203] Stapleton D, Mitchelhill K, Gao G, Widmer J, Michell BJ, Teh T, et al. Mammalian AMP-activated protein kinase subfamily. J Biol Chem 1996;271:611–4.

[204] Fraser S, Mount P, Hill R, Levidiotis V, Katsis F, Stapleton D, et al. Regulation of the energy sensor AMP-activated protein kinase in the kidney by dietary salt intake and osmolality. Am J Physiol Renal Physiol 2005;288:F578–586.

[205] Cammisotto P, Londono I, Gingras D, Bendayan M. Control of glycogen synthase through ADIPOR1-AMPK pathway in renal distal tubules of normal and diabetic rats. Am J Physiol Renal Physiol 2008;294:F881–889.

[206] Woollhead A, Scott J, Hardie D, Baines DL. Phenformin and 5-aminoimidazole-4-carboxamide-1-beta-D-ribofuranoside (Aicar) activation of amp-activated protein kinase inhibits

transepithelial Na$^+$ transport across H441 lung cells. J Physiol 2005;566:781—92.

[207] Woollhead A, Sivagnanasundaram J, Kalsi K, Pucovsky V, Pellatt LJ, Scott JW, et al. Pharmacological activators of amp-activated protein kinase have different effects on Na + transport processes across human lung epithelial cells. Br J Pharmacol 2007;151:1204—15.

[208] Vadász I, Dada L, Briva A, Trejo HE, Welch LC, Chen J, et al. AMP-activated protein kinase regulates CO$_2$-induced alveolar epithelial dysfunction in rats and human cells by promoting Na,K-ATPase endocytosis. J Clin Invest 2008;118:752—62.

[209] Carattino M, Edinger R, Grieser H, Wise R, Neumann D, Schlattner U, et al. Epithelial sodium channel inhibition by AMP-activated protein kinase in oocytes and polarized renal epithelial cells. J Biol Chem 2005;280:17608—16.

[210] Almaça J, Kongsuphol P, Hieke B, Ousingsawat J, Viollet B, Schreiber R, et al. AMPK controls epithelial Na$^{(+)}$ channels through Nedd4-2 and causes an epithelial phenotype when mutated. Pflugers Arch 2009;458:713—21.

[211] Bhalla V, Oyster N, Fitch A, Wijngaarden MA, Neumann D, Schlattner U, et al. AMP-activated kinase inhibits the epithelial Na + channel through functional regulation of the ubiquitin ligase Nedd4-2. J Biol Chem 2006;281:26159—69.

[212] Fraser S, Gimenez I, Cook N, Jennings I, Katerelos M, Katsis F, et al. Regulation of the renal-specific Na$^+$-K$^+$-2Cl$^-$ co-transporter NKCC2 by amp-activated protein kinase (AMPK). Biochem J 2007;405:85—93.

[213] Gong F, Alzamora R, Smolak C, Li H, Naveed S, Neumann D, et al. Vacuolar H$^+$-ATPase apical accumulation in kidney intercalated cells is regulated by PKA and AMP-activated protein kinase. Am J Physiol Renal Physiol 2010; epub ahead of print.

[214] Hallows K, Raghuram V, Kemp B, Witters LA, Foskett JK. Inhibition of cystic fibrosis transmembrane conductance regulator by novel interaction with the metabolic sensor AMP-activated protein kinase. J Clin Invest 2000;105:1711—21.

[215] Sopjani M, Bhavsar S, Fraser S, Kemp BE, Föller M, Lang F. Regulation of Na$^+$-coupled glucose carrier SGLT1 by AMP-activated protein kinase. Mol Membr Biol 2010;27:137—44.

[216] Sukhodub A, Jovanović S, Du Q, Budas G, Clelland AK, Shen M, et al. AMP-activated protein kinase mediates preconditioning in cardiomyocytes by regulating activity and trafficking of sarcolemmal ATP-sensitive K(+) channels. J Cell Physiol 2007;210:224—36.

[217] Hebert SC, Desir G, Giebisch G, Wang W. Molecular diversity and regulation of renal potassium channels. Physiol Rev 2005;85:319—71.

[218] Misler S, Giebisch G. ATP-sensitive potassium channels in physiology, pathophysiology, and pharmacology. Curr Opin Nephrol Hypertens 1992;1:21—33.

[219] Wang W. Renal potassium channels: recent developments. Curr Opin Nephrol Hypertens 2004;13:549—55.

[220] Tsuchiya K, Wang W, Giebisch G, Welling PA. ATP is a coupling modulator of parallel Na,K-ATPase-K-channel activity in the renal proximal tubule. Proc Natl Acad Sci USA 1992;89:6418—22.

[221] Wang W, Giebisch G. Dual effect of adenosine triphosphate on the apical small conductance K$^+$ channel of the rat cortical collecting duct. J Gen Physiol 1991;98:35—61.

[222] Bleich M, Schlatter E, Greger R. The luminal K$^+$ channel of the thick ascending limb of Henle's loop. Pflugers Arch 1990;415:449—60.

[223] Tsuboi T, Lippiat JD, Ashcroft FM, Rutter GA. ATP-dependent interaction of the cytosolic domains of the inwardly rectifying

K$^+$ channel KIR6.2 revealed by fluorescence resonance energy transfer. Proc Natl Acad Sci USA 2004;101:76—81.

[224] Hurwitz CG, Hu VY, Segal AS. A mechanogated nonselective cation channel in proximal tubule that is ATP sensitive. Am J Physiol Renal Physiol 2002;283:F93—104.

[225] Leipziger J. Control of epithelial transport via luminal P2 receptors. Am J Physiol Renal Physiol 2003;284:F419—432.

[226] Ralevic V, Burnstock G. Receptors for purines and pyrimidines. Pharmacol Rev 1998;50:413—92.

[227] Unwin RJ, Bailey MA, Burnstock G. Purinergic signaling along the renal tubule: the current state of play. News Physiol Sci 2003;18:237—41.

[228] Bailey MA. Inhibition of bicarbonate reabsorption in the rat proximal tubule by activation of luminal P2y1 receptors. Am J Physiol Renal Physiol 2004;287:F789—796.

[229] Cha SH, Jung KY, Endou H. Effect of P2y-purinoceptor stimulation on renal gluconeogenesis in rats. Biochem Biophys Res Commun 1995;211:454—61.

[230] Jackson EK, Raghvendra DK. The extracellular cyclic AMP-adenosine pathway in renal physiology. Annu Rev Physiol 2004;66:571—99.

[231] Wengert M, Berto Jr. C, Kaufman J, Leão-Ferreira LR, Paes-de-Carvalho R, Lopes AG, et al. Stimulation of the proximal tubule Na$^+$-ATPase activity by adenosine A(2a) receptor. Int J Biochem Cell Biol 2005;37:155—65.

[232] Kone BC. Nitric oxide in renal health and disease. Am J Kidney Dis 1997;30:311—33.

[233] Ortiz PA, Garvin JL. Role of nitric oxide in the regulation of nephron transport. Am J Physiol Renal Physiol 2002;282:F777—784.

[234] Terada Y, Tomita K, Nonoguchi H, Marumo F. Polymerase chain reaction localization of constitutive nitric oxide synthase and soluble guanylate cyclase messenger RNAs in microdissected rat nephron segments. J Clin Invest 1992;90:659—65.

[235] Granger DL, Lehninger AL. Sites of inhibition of mitochondrial electron transport in macrophage-injured neoplastic cells. J Cell Biol 1982;95:527—35.

[236] Stuehr DJ, Nathan CF. Nitric oxide. A macrophage product responsible for cytostasis and respiratory inhibition in tumor target cells. J Exp Med 1989;169:1543—55.

[237] Shen W, Hintze TH, Wolin MS. Nitric oxide. An important signaling mechanism between vascular endothelium and parenchymal cells in the regulation of oxygen consumption. Circulation 1995;92:3505—12.

[238] Shen W, Xu X, Ochoa M, Zhao G, Wolin MS, Hintze TH. Role of nitric oxide in the regulation of oxygen consumption in conscious dogs. Circ Res 1994;75:1086—95.

[239] Brown GC. Nitric oxide regulates mitochondrial respiration and cell functions by inhibiting cytochrome oxidase. FEBS Lett 1995;369:136—9.

[240] Brown GC, Cooper CE. Nanmolar concentrations of nitric oxide reversibly inhibit synaptosomal respiration by competing with oxygen at cytochrome oxidase. FEBS Lett 1994;356:295—8.

[241] Adler S, Huang H, Loke KE, Xu X, Tada H, Laumas A, et al. Endothelial nitric oxide synthase plays an essential role in regulation of renal oxygen consumption by NO. Am J Physio l Renal Physiol 2001;280:F838—843.

[242] Laycock SK, Vogel T, Forfia PR, Tuzman J, Xu X, Ochoa M, et al. Role of nitric oxide in the control of renal oxygen consumption and the regulation of chemical work in the kidney. Circ Res 1998;82:1263—71.

[243] Buemi M, Allegra A, Rotig A, Gubler MC, Aloisi C, Corica F, et al. Renal failure from mitochondrial cytopathies. Nephron 1997;76:249—53.

[244] Kuwertz-Broking E, Koch HG, Marquardt T, Rossi R, Helmchen U, Müller-Höcker J, et al. Renal Fanconi syndrome: first sign of partial respiratory chain complex IV deficiency. Pediatr Nephrol 2000;14:495−8.

[245] Mochizuki H, Joh K, Kawame H, Imadachi A, Nozaki H, Ohashi T, et al. Mitochondrial encephalomyopathies preceded by De-Toni-Debre-Fanconi syndrome or focal segmental glomerulosclerosis. Clin Nephrol 1996;46:347−52.

[246] Niaudet P. Mitochondrial disorders and the kidney. Arch Dis Child 1998;78:387−90.

[247] Niaudet P, Rotig A. Renal involvement in mitochondrial cytopathies. Pediatr Nephrol 1996;10:368−73.

[248] Rotig A. Renal disease and mitochondrial genetics. J Nephrol 2003;16:286−92.

[249] Wang LC, Lee WT, Tsai WY, Tsau YK, Shen YZ. Mitochondrial cytopathy combined with Fanconi's syndrome. Pediatr Neurol 2000;22:403−6.

[250] Goto Y, Itami N, Kajii N, Tochimaru H, Endo M, Horai S. Renal tubular involvement mimicking bartter syndrome in a patient with Kearns−Sayre syndrome. J Pediatr 1990;116:904−10.

[251] Hsieh F, Gohh R, Dworkin L. Acute renal failure and the Melas syndrome, a mitochondrial encephalomyopathy. J Am Soc Nephrol 1996;7:647−52.

[252] Yanagihara C, Oyama A, Tanaka M, Nakaji K, Nishimura Y. An autopsy case of mitochondrial encephalomyopathy with lactic acidosis and stroke-like episodes syndrome with chronic renal failure. Intern Med 2001;40:662−5.

[253] Rotig A, Goutieres F, Niaudet P, Rustin P, Chretien D, Guest G, et al. Deletion of mitochondrial DNA in patient with chronic tubulointerstitial nephritis. J Pediatr 1995;126:597−601.

[254] Szabolcs MJ, Seigle R, Shanske S, Bonilla E, DiMauro S, D'Agati V. Mitochondrial DNA deletion: a cause of chronic tubulointerstitial nephropathy. Kidney Int 1994;45:1388−96.

[255] Gilbert RD, Emms M. Pearson's syndrome presenting with Fanconi syndrome. Ultrastruct Pathol 1996;20:473−5.

[256] Zsurka G, Ormos J, Ivanyi B, Turi S, Endreffy E, Magyari M, et al. Mitochondrial mutation as a probable causative factor in familial progressive tubulointerstitial nephritis. Hum Genet 1997;99:484−7.

[257] Cheong HI, Chae JH, Kim JS, Park HW, Ha IS, Hwang YS, et al. Hereditary glomerulopathy associated with a mitochondrial tRNA(Leu) gene mutation. Pediatr Nephrol 1999;13:477−80.

[258] Doleris LM, Hill GS, Chedin P, Nochy D, Bellanne-Chantelot C, Hanslik T, et al. Focal segmental glomerulosclerosis associated with mitochondrial cytopathy. zz 2000;58:1851−8.

[259] Jansen JJ, Maassen JA, van der Woude FJ, Lemmink HA, van den Ouweland JM, t' Hart LM, et al. Mutation in mitochondrial tRNA(Leu(UUR)) gene associated with progressive kidney disease. J Am Soc Nephrol 1997;8:1118−24.

[260] Kurogouchi F, Oguchi T, Mawatari E, Yamaura S, Hora K, Takei M, et al. A case of mitochondrial cytopathy with a typical point mutation for Melas, presenting with severe focal-segmental glomerulosclerosis as main clinical manifestation. Am J Nephrol 1998;18:551−6.

[261] Scaglia F, Vogel H, Hawkins EP, Vladutiu GD, Liu LL, Wong LJ. Novel homoplasmic mutation in the mitochondrial tRNA Tyr gene associated with atypical mitochondrial cytopathy presenting with focal segmental glomerulosclerosis. Am J Med Genet A 2003;123:172−8.

[262] Dickman KG, Jacobs WR, Mandel LJ. Renal metabolism and acute renal failure. Pediatr Nephrol 1987;1:359−66.

[263] Barros LF, Hermosilla T, Castro J. Necrotic volume increase and the early physiology of necrosis. Comp Biochem Physiol A Mol Integr Physiol 2001;130:401−9.

[264] Padanilam BJ. Cell death induced by acute renal injury: a perspective on the contributions of apoptosis and necrosis. Am J Physiol Renal Physiol 2003;284:F608−627.

[265] Lieberthal W, Nigam SK. Acute renal failure. I. Relative importance of proximal vs. distal tubular injury. Am J Physiol 1998;275:F623−631.

[266] Molitoris BA. Na(+)-K(+)-ATPase that redistributes to apical membrane during ATP depletion remains functional. Am J Physiol 1993;265:F693−697.

[267] Edelstein CL, Ling H, Schrier RW. The nature of renal cell injury. Kidney Int 1997;51:1341−51.

[268] Thadhani R, Pascual M, Bonventre JV. Acute renal failure. N Engl J Med 1996;334:1448−60.

[269] De Broe ME. Apoptosis in acute renal failure. Nephrol Dial Transplant 2001;16(Suppl 6):23−6.

[270] Lieberthal W, Levine JS. Mechanisms of apoptosis and its potential role in renal tubular epithelial cell injury. Am J Physiol 1996;271:F477−488.

[271] Lieberthal W, Menza SA, Levine JS. Graded ATP depletion can cause necrosis or apoptosis of cultured mouse proximal tubular cells. Am J Physiol 1998;274:F315−327.

[272] Lieberthal W, Koh JS, Levine JS. Necrosis and apoptosis in acute renal failure. Semin Nephrol 1998;18:505−18.

[273] Hems DA, Brosnan JT. Effects of ischaemia on content of metabolites in rat liver and kidney in vivo. Biochem J 1970;120:105−11.

[274] Siegel NJ, Avison MJ, Reilly HF, Alger JR, Schulman RG. Enhanced recovery of renal Atp with postischemic infusion of ATP-MgCl2 determined by 31P-NMR. Am J Physiol 1983;245:F530−534.

[275] Dickman KG, Mandel LJ. Differential effects of respiratory inhibitors on glycolysis in proximal tubules. Am J Physiol 1990;258:F1608−1615.

[276] Weinberg JM, Venkatachalam MA, Roeser NF, Nissim I. Mitochondrial dysfunction during hypoxia/reoxygenation and its correction by anaerobic metabolism of citric acid cycle intermediates. Proc Natl Acad Sci USA 2000;97:2826−31.

[277] Weinberg JM, Venkatachalam MA, Roeser NF, Saikumar P, Dong Z, Senter RA, et al. Anaerobic and aerobic pathways for salvage of proximal tubules from hypoxia-induced mitochondrial injury. Am J Physiol Renal Physiol 2000;279:F927−943.

[278] Feldkamp T, Kribben A, Roeser NF, Senter RA, Kemner S, Venkatachalam MA, et al. Preservation of complex i function during hypoxia-reoxygenation-induced mitochondrial injury in proximal tubules. Am J Physiol Renal Physiol 2004;286:F749−759.

[279] Bonventre JV. Mechanisms of ischemic acute renal failure. Kidney Int 1993;43:1160−78.

[280] Bonventre JV, Weinberg JM. Recent advances in the pathophysiology of ischemic acute renal failure. J Am Soc Nephrol 2003;14:2199−210.

[281] Brezis M, Rosen S, Silva P, Epstein FH. Transport activity modifies thick ascending limb damage in the isolated perfused kidney. Kidney Int 1984;25:65−72.

[282] Liu X, Kim CN, Yang J, Jemmerson R, Wang X. Induction of apoptotic program in cell-free extracts: requirement for dATP and cytochrome c. Cell 1996;86:147−57.

[283] Zager RA, Johnson AC, Hanson SY. Proximal tubular cytochrome C efflux: determinant, and potential marker, of mitochondrial injury. Kidney Int 2004;65:2123−34.

[284] Kowaltowski AJ, Castilho RF, Vercesi AE. Mitochondrial permeability transition and oxidative stress. FEBS Lett 2001;495:12−5.

[285] Tatton WG, Olanow CW. Apoptosis in neurodegenerative diseases: the role of mitochondria. Biochim Biophys Acta 1999;1410:195−213.

[286] McCoy CE, Selvaggio AM, Alexander EA, Schwartz JH. Adenosine triphosphate depletion induces a rise in cytosolic free calcium in canine renal epithelial cells. J Clin Invest 1988;82:1326−32.

[287] Snowdowne KW, Freudenrich CC, Borle AB. The effects of anoxia on cytosolic free calcium, calcium fluxes, and cellular ATP levels in cultured kidney cells. J Biol Chem 1985;260:11619−26.

[288] Weinberg JM, Davis JA, Trivedi B. Calcium compartmentation in isolated renal tubules in suspension. Biochem Med Metab Biol 1988;39:234−45.

[289] Tanaka T, Nangaku M, Miyata T, Inagi R, Ohse T, Ingelfinger JR, et al. Blockade of calcium influx through L-type calcium channels attenuates mitochondrial injury and apoptosis in hypoxic renal tubular cells. J Am Soc Nephrol 2004;15:2320−33.

[290] Eckardt K, Rosenberger C, Jürgensen J, Wiesener MS. Role of hypoxia in the pathogenesis of renal disease. Blood Purif 2003;21:253−7.

[291] Tanaka T, Miyata T, Inagi R, Fujita T, Nangaku M. Hypoxia in renal disease with proteinuria and/or glomerular hypertension. Am J Pathol 2004;165:1979−92.

[292] Maxwell P. HIF-1: an oxygen response system with special relevance to the kidney. J Am Soc Nephrol 2003;14:2712−22.

[293] Manotham K, Tanaka T, Ohse T, Kojima I, Miyata T, Inagi R, et al. A biologic role of HIF-1 in the renal medulla. Kidney Int 2005;67:1428−39.

[294] Bernaudin M, Tang Y, Reilly M, Petit E, Sharp FR. Brain genomic response following hypoxia and re-oxygenation in the neonatal rat. Identification of genes that might contribute to hypoxia-induced ischemic tolerance. J Biol Chem 2002;277:39728−38.

[295] Bernaudin M, Marti HH, Roussel S, Divoux D, Nouvelot A, MacKenzie ET, et al. A potential role for erythropoietin in focal permanent cerebral ischemia in mice. J Cereb Blood Flow Metab 1999;19:643−51.

[296] Ebert BL, Firth JD, Ratcliffe PJ. Hypoxia and mitochondrial inhibitors regulate expression of glucose transporter-1 via distinct cis-acting sequences. J Biol Chem 1995;270:29083−9.

[297] Rodriguez H, Drouin R, Holmquist GP, Akman SA. A hot spot for hydrogen peroxide-induced damage in the human hypoxia-inducible factor 1 binding site of the PGK 1 gene. Arch Biochem Biophys 1997;338:207−12.

[298] Tune BM, Hsu CY. Toxicity of cephalosporins to fatty acid metabolism in rabbit renal cortical mitochondria. Biochem Pharmacol 1995;49:727−34.

[299] Simon N, Morin C, Urien S, Tillement JP, Bruquerolle B. Tacrolimus and sirolimus decrease oxidative phosphorylation of isolated rat kidney mitochondria. Br J Pharmacol 2003;138:369−76.

[300] Tang W, Shaikh ZA. Renal cortical mitochondrial dysfunction upon cadmium metallothionein administration to Sprague-Dawley rats. J Toxicol Environ Health A 2001;63:221−35.

[301] Masereeuw R, van Pelt AP, van Os SH, Willems PH, Smits P, Russel FG. Probenecid interferes with renal oxidative metabolism: a potential pitfall in its use as an inhibitor of drug transport. Br J Pharmacol 2000;131:57−62.

[302] Simon N, Zini R, Morin C, Bree F, Tillement JP. Prednisolone and azathioprine worsen the cyclosporine A-induced oxidative phosphorylation decrease of kidney mitochondria. Life Sci 1997;61:659−66.

[303] Justo P, Lorz C, Sanz A, Egido J, Ortiz A. Intracellular mechanisms of cyclosporin A-induced tubular cell apoptosis. J Am Soc Nephrol 2003;14:3072−80.

[304] Jung KY, Endou H. Nephrotoxicity assessment by measuring cellular ATP Content. II. Intranephron site of ochratoxin a nephrotoxicity. Toxicol Appl Pharmacol 1989;100: 383−90.

[305] de Cavanagh EM, Piotrkowski B, Basso N, Stella I, Inserra F, Ferder L, et al. Enalapril and losartan attenuate mitochondrial dysfunction in aged rats. Faseb J 2003;17:1096−8.

[306] Li LP, Storey P, Pierchala L, Li W, Polzin J, Prasad P. Evaluation of the reproducibility of intrarenal R2* and Deltar2* measurements following administration of furosemide and during waterload. J Magn Reson Imaging 2004;19:610−6.

[307] Prasad PV, Priatna A. Functional imaging of the kidneys with Fast MRI techniques. Eur J Radiol 1999;29:133−48.

[308] Prasad PV, Edelman RR, Epstein FH. Noninvasive evaluation of intrarenal oxygenation with BOLD MRI. Circulation 1996;94:3271−5.

[309] Epstein FH, Prasad P. Effects of furosemide on medullary oxygenation in younger and older subjects. Kidney Int 2000;57:2080−3.

[310] Juillard L, Lerman LO, Kruger DG, Haas JA, Rucker BC, Polzin JA, et al. Blood oxygen level-dependent measurement of acute intra-renal ischemia. Kidney Int 2004;65:944−50.

[311] Ries M, Basseau F, Tyndal B, Jones R, Deminière C, Catargi B, et al. Renal diffusion and BOLD MRI in experimental diabetic nephropathy. Blood oxygen level-dependent. J Magn Reson Imaging 2003;17:104−13.

[312] Li L, Storey P, Kim D, Prasad P. Kidneys in hypertensive rats show reduced response to nitric oxide synthase inhibition as evaluated by BOLD MRI. J Magn Reson Imaging 2003;17:671−5.

[313] Zuo CS, Rofsky NM, Mahallati H, Yu J, Zhang M, Gilbert S, et al. Visualization and quantification of renal R2* changes during water diuresis. J Magn Reson Imaging 2003;17:676−82.

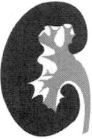

Electrophysiological Analysis of Transepithelial Transport

Henry Sackin[1] and Lawrence G. Palmer[2]

[1]Department of Physiology & Biophysics, Rosalind Franklin University/The Chicago Medical School,
North Chicago, IL, USA

[2]Department of Physiology & Biophysics, Weill Medical College of Cornell University, New York City, NY, USA

INTRODUCTION

In this chapter we discuss electrophysiological approaches to the study of renal function. The purpose is to provide an overview of the available techniques, with particular emphasis on what can be learned using the latest methods. However, the chapter is neither a technical manual nor a comprehensive review of the literature. For this, we refer the reader to other sections of the book which deal with specific nephron segments and transport mechanisms. Finally, we will not derive mathematical equations from first principles. Those equations that are essential to the text are provided in the main body of the chapter, while the more detailed formulae are described in the appendices.

We have arbitrarily divided the field of epithelial electrophysiology into three major sections. The first describes measurements of transepithelial electrical properties. The second section focuses on the use of intracellular microelectrodes to discriminate apical and basolateral membrane properties. The final section deals with the technique of patch clamping to investigate the functional characteristics of individual ion channels, and in some cases their molecular identification.

The interpretation of electrical signals from epithelia is complicated by the geometry of the tissues. At least three structures within an epithelium contribute to its electrical properties: the apical plasma membrane; the basolateral plasma membrane; and the paracellular pathway. The individual cell membrane properties will, in turn, be determined by various conductive pathways, including those of passive or dissipative pathways, through which ions flow driven by their own electrochemical potential differences, and active transport, which can use metabolic energy to drive ions against these potential differences. The paracellular pathway, in turn, consists of the tight junctions connecting the epithelial cells and the lateral interspaces between the cells.

The electrical properties of this complex structure can be most easily understood in terms of equivalent circuits. A comprehensive equivalent circuit of a generic reabsorbing epithelium is illustrated in Figure 7.1. Electrolyte diffusion across the apical membrane can be separated into its constituent ionic pathways, as shown by the expanded view of the apical membrane in Figure 7.1. Each ionic pathway is associated with an electromotive force (EMF) or battery representing the chemical potential for each ion. Electrogenic carriers such as the Na-glucose co-transporter can also be represented by an additional resistor (R_{glu}) and EMF (E_{glu}) in parallel with the diffusional elements. All of the batteries and resistors can be lumped respectively into a single apical EMF (E_{ap}) and a single resistance R_{ap} as shown in the center diagram. The basal membrane has a similar set of elements: R_b and E_b which represent a dissipative ion pathway in parallel with an active transport pathway, represented by a resistor (R_{ap}) and an EMF (E_p). Thus:

$$E_x = -\frac{RT}{z_i F} Ln \frac{[X_1]}{[X_2]} \tag{7.1}$$

where $[X_1]$ and $[X_2]$ are the concentrations of ion X on the two sides of the membrane, and z_i is the charge on the

Seldin and Giebisch's The Kidney, Fifth Edition.
DOI: http://dx.doi.org/10.1016/B978-0-12-381462-3.00007-0

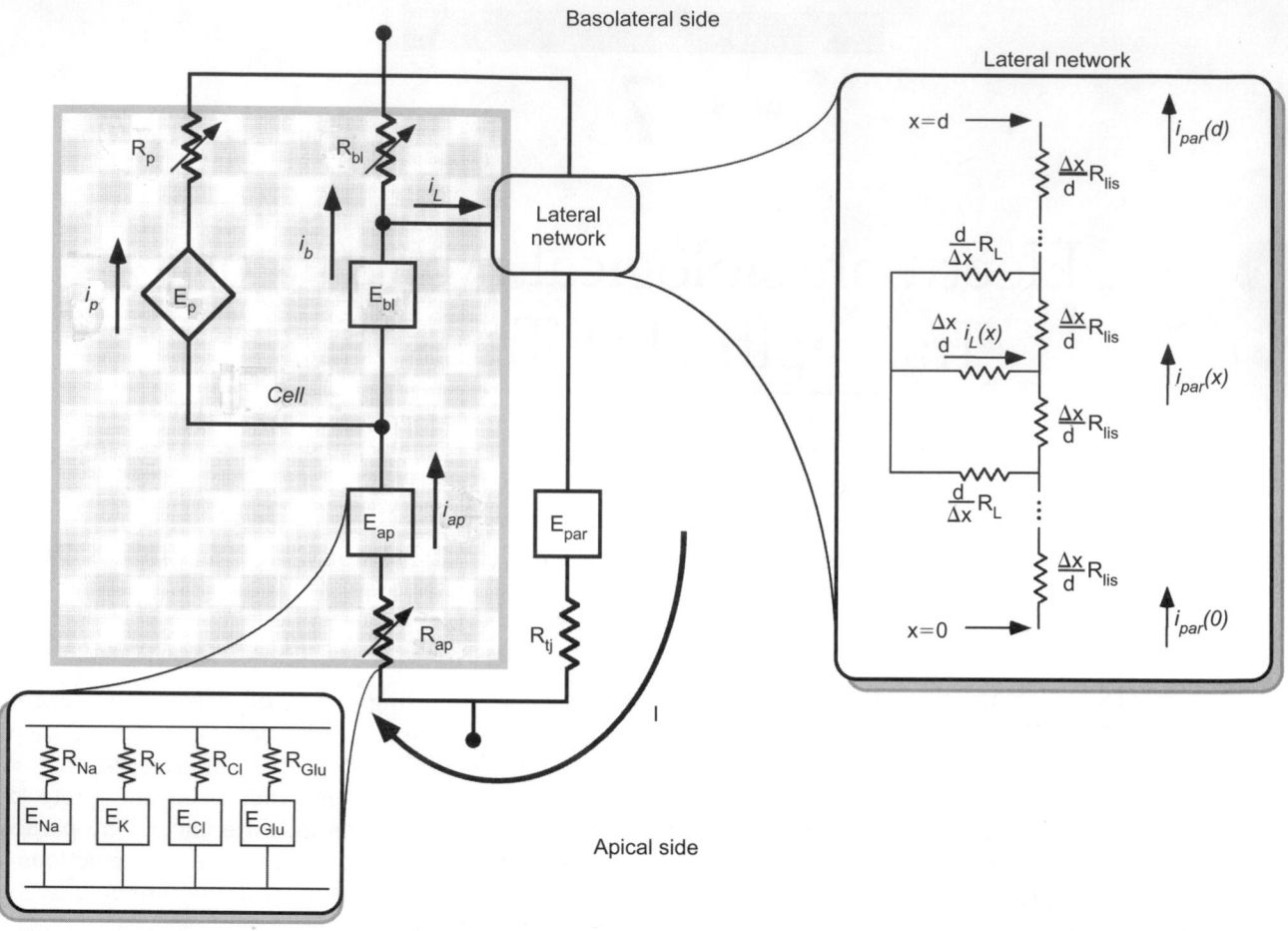

FIGURE 7.1   Electrical equivalent circuit for a general epithelium. Each membrane or barrier is associated with an electromotive force (**E**) that represents the weighted average of the ionic diffusion potentials at that barrier. Electrogenic carriers (such as the apical Na-glucose co-transporter) and electrogenic pumps (such as the basolateral Na,K-ATPase) can also be formally represented by a series resistor and an associated EMF. The lateral network takes into account the nonzero electrical resistance of the lateral intercellular spaces.

ion. The weighting factor for each ion is the transference number, t_x, which expresses the fraction of membrane conductance that is attributable to that particular ion:

$$t_x = \frac{g_x}{g_{tot}} \tag{7.2}$$

where g represents the conductance of the individual ion pathways and g_{tot} is the total ionic conductance of the membrane. In most cases g_{tot} will simply be the sum of the Na, K, and Cl conductances of the barrier. Hence, the total EMF can be generally expressed by the equation:

$$E = t_{Na}E_{Na} + t_K E_K + t_{Cl}E_{Cl}$$
$$= -\frac{RT}{F} \sum_{x=Na,K,Cl} \frac{t_x}{z_x} Ln \frac{[X_1]}{[X_2]} \tag{7.3}$$

The overall goal of classical electrophysiology, described in the first two sections of this chapter, is to evaluate the different elements of this equivalent

circuit, to quantify the various resistances and EMFs, and to describe the extent to which they change during regulation. To this end, it has often been desirable to use reductions of the main equivalent circuit of Figure 7.1, and to work under conditions in which these reduced circuits are applicable. Such simplifications are discussed in more detail in the sections entitled, "Transepithelial Measurements" and "Intracellular Measurements." Finally, the section entitled, "Measurements of Individual Ion Channels" describes application of the patch clamp technique to epithelia, and permits a description of ion transport in more molecular terms.

The rationale for representing the pump by a resistance and an EMF is discussed further in the section entitled "Intracellular Measurements." Briefly, the E_p represents the maximum amount of energy that the pump derives from splitting ATP or, alternatively, the maximum electrochemical potential difference against which the pump can operate. The pump pathway must also include a non-zero internal resistance. The magnitude of this internal resistance is determined by the actual current—voltage relation for the membrane bound Na-K-ATPase. To maintain generality, all membrane resistances are shown as variable resistors to include the possibility of intrinsic or extrinsic regulation of ion channels.

Although the paracellular pathway is not a membrane barrier, it can also be modeled by resistive (R_{tj}) and electromotive elements (E_{par}). A lateral network (indicated to the right of the main circuit) is also included in the model. This network takes into consideration the finite resistance of fluid in the lateral spaces. This aspect of the circuit becomes important for calculation of individual membrane resistances from voltage deflection experiments (see Section entitled "Intracellular Measurements").

TRANSEPITHELIAL MEASUREMENTS

Measurements of transepithelial electrical properties are by far the simplest to perform, and the most difficult to interpret. They are easy to carry out because they are non-invasive; only extracellular electrodes are employed. They are difficult to interpret because the parameters which can be measured reflect, in most cases, a combination of many of the circuit elements shown in Figure 7.1. In this chapter we will describe how transepithelial techniques are used to measure three basic parameters that characterize an epithelium: transepithelial voltage; transepithelial resistance; and short-circuit current. We will then discuss a number of special extracellular approaches which have been employed to gain additional insights into epithelial properties.

Measurement of Transepithelial Voltage

Methods of measuring transepithelial voltage (V_{te}) are conceptually simple. In principle, the potential difference between two electrodes placed on either side of the epithelium is simply determined with an appropriate electrometer. With flat epithelia that can be mounted in Ussing chambers, the transepithelial electrodes are placed in the two bathing compartments.[1] In cylindrical epithelia such as the renal nephron, classical measurements of transepithelial potential have been performed in vivo using micropuncture techniques. In this technique, a pipette filled with electrolyte is introduced into the lumen of the tubule, and voltage is measured relative to another electrode placed in a capillary. Here, the presumption is that the voltage reflects the properties of the impaled tubule, and is not greatly influenced by those of neighboring segments. Under most conditions this should be a reasonable

assumption. For a lumen of 10 μm diameter and an iso-osmotic saline solution with a resistivity of around 60 Ω•cm, the axial resistance of the tubule will be about 8×10^7 Ω/cm. This is much larger than the value of the transepithelial resistance of around 100 Ω•cm^2 (Table 7.1), which for the same 10 μm lumen is equivalent to 3×10^4 Ω/cm. Thus, each part of the nephron will be effectively electrically isolated from other parts of the high resistance of the luminal pathway. If the nephron segment can be isolated and perfused in vitro, the perfusion and/or collection pipette can be used to monitor the intraluminal voltage with respect to the bath potential. This is illustrated in Figure 7.2.

Measurement of Transepithelial Resistance

For measurements of transepithelial resistance (R_{te}), current must be injected across the epithelium to perturb V_{te}. This is most easily accomplished when the epithelium can be mounted in Ussing chambers, where current flow and voltage changes are assumed to be uniform in the plane of the tissue. Resistance can then be computed from Ohms law as the ratio of the change in V_{te} to the amount of current passed:

$$R_{te} = \frac{\Delta V_{te}}{\Delta I} \qquad (7.4)$$

Epithelia can be studied in open-circuited or voltage-clamped conditions. In open circuit the tissue is allowed to maintain its spontaneous transepithelial voltage. In this case the resistance is determined from the change in voltage produced by passing a known amount of current. Under voltage-clamp conditions a current is passed across the epithelium to maintain the transepithelial voltage at a predetermined level. In the case where this level is zero, so that the transepithelial voltage is abolished, it is called the "short-circuited" state. If the epithelium is voltage-clamped, resistance is determined from the change in current produced by a controlled voltage step. In open-circuited tubular epithelia, transepithelial current flow is not constant along the length of the tubule. In this case, cable analysis must be used to estimate the transepithelial resistance (see below).

Measurement of Transepithelial Resistance in Open Circuited Renal Tubules

The measurement of overall transepithelial resistance, R_{te}, in renal tubules under open circuit conditions is best carried out with a double-barreled perfusion pipette system similar to the one illustrated in Figure 7.2. In this technique, the tubule is cannulated at both the perfusion and collection ends. The

TABLE 7.1   Transepithelial Properties of Renal Epithelia

Tissue	V_{te} (mV)	R_{te} (Ωcm^2)	R_{par} (Ωcm^2)	P_{Na}/P_{Cl}	Reference
Amphibians					
Proximal tubule (*Ambystoma*)	−10	70	70	0.25	4
Diluting segment (*Amphiuma*, frog)	+10	290	306	4 to 5	135
Collecting duct (*Amphiuma*)	−24	160	200	0.84	136
Urinary bladder (Toad)	−94	8,900	50,000	−	22
Mammals					
Proximal tubule (rabbit)	−2 to +2	5	5		13
TALH[a] (rabbit)	+3 to +10	10 to 35	10 to 50	2 to 4	12
CCD[a] (rabbit)	0 to −60	110	160	0.8	137
OMCD[a] (rabbit)	−2 to −11	233			138
IMCD[a] (rabbit)	−2 to 0	73			139
Urinary bladder (rabbit)	−20 to −75	13,000 to 23,000	>78,000	−	140

[a]*TALH, thick ascending limb of Henle's loop; CCD, cortical collecting duct; OMCD, outer medullary collecting duct; IMCD, inner medullary collecting duct.*

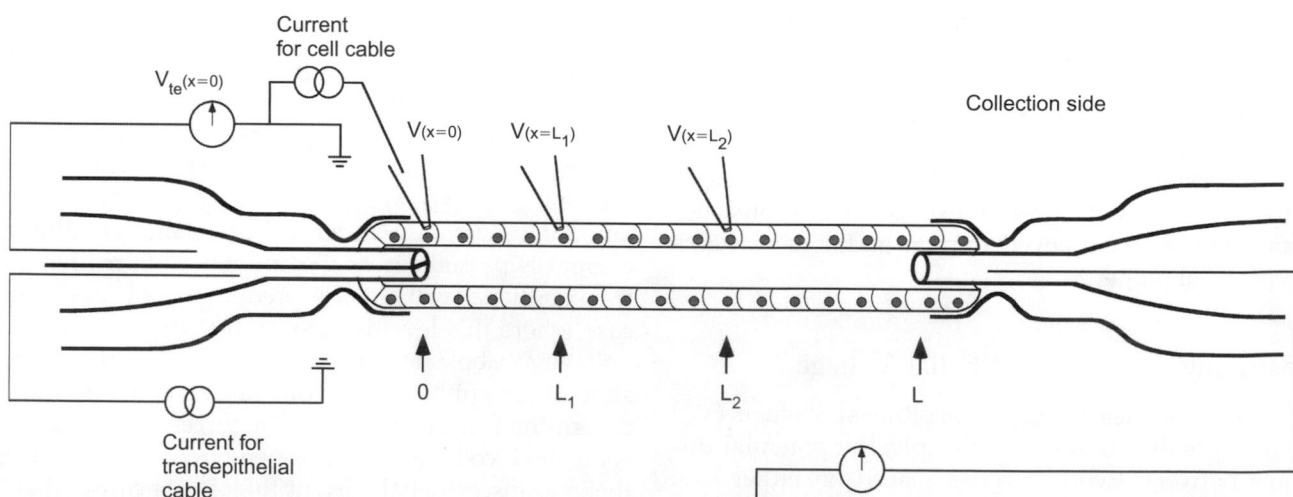

FIGURE 7.2   Experimental apparatus for determining electrophysiological properties of renal epithelia. The segment of isolated renal tubule is held at both ends by constriction pipettes. The tubule perfusion pipette is fabricated from "theta" glass and has separate pathways for both current injection and transepithelial measurement, $V_{te}(x = 0)$. The transepithelial potential, $V_{te}(x = L)$, can also be determined at the collection side of the tubule. For determination of cell membrane resistance, current is passed into the cell layer via the microelectrode at location $x = 0$ and the resultant voltage deflections are measured by intracellular microelectrodes at locations $x = 0$, L_1, and L_2.

double-barreled perfusion pipette, fabricated from *theta* glass[2−4] creates separate pathways for current flow and voltage recording. An alternative technique uses the same single-barreled pipette for both current injection and voltage measurement. This is not nearly as accurate as the double-barreled technique, because the voltage deflection arising from the internal resistance of the perfusion pipette must be nulled with a bridge circuit. The microelectrodes in Figure 7.2 are for evaluation of individual cell membrane resistances. This will be discussed in the section entitled, "Intracellular Measurements."

A thin fluid-exchange tubing (not shown) can be inserted into one barrel of the perfusion pipette of Figure 7.2 to permit rapid exchange of the perfusion solution while measuring the transepithelial potential $V_{te}(x = 0)$. Current is passed from a chlorided silver wire glued into the other barrel of the pipette. The transepithelial length constant of the tubule λ_{te} is determined from the voltage deflections at the perfusion, $\Delta V_{te}(x = 0)$, and collection, $\Delta V_{te}(x = L)$, sides of the tubule, resulting from a transepithelial current pulse, I_{te}, through the current side of the perfusion pipette. For a doubly cannulated, isolated tubule of length L, λ_{te} is given by Eq. (7.5) from Sackin and Boulpaep[5]:

$$\frac{L}{\lambda_{te}} = cosh^{-1}\left[\frac{\Delta V_{te}(x = 0)}{\Delta V_{te}(x = L)}\right] \qquad (7.5)$$

The transepithelial resistance R_{te} in Ωcm^2 is given by Eq. (7.6):

$$R_{te} = 2\sqrt{\pi \lambda_{te}^3 R_{in} R_i} \sqrt{tanh(L/\lambda_{te})} \qquad (7.6)$$

In the above equation, R_{in} is the input resistance measured in ohms (Ω). It is operationally defined as the voltage deflection at the perfusion end $\Delta V_{te}(x = 0)$ divided by the total injected current I_{te}. Typical injected currents for proximal tubules are 100 nA pulses of 1 to 5 seconds duration. Ideally, none of the current injected into the lumen from the perfusion pipette enters the compressed region of tubule within the holding pipette, which presumably acts like an electrical insulator when compared to the relatively low resistance of the tubule. However, artifacts may still arise from current leaks at either the perfusion or collection ends of the tubule. These can be detected by a "mismatch" between the calculated electrical radius (r_e) of the tubule and its measured optical radius (r_o).

$$r_e = \frac{2 R_i \lambda_{te}^2}{R_{te}} \qquad (7.7)$$

Use of a double-barreled perfusion pipette (Figure 7.2) eliminates much of the uncertainty in R_{in}. Double-barreled perfusion pipettes have the additional advantage that R_{te} can be measured during changes in the perfusion solution. This is practically impossible with a single-barreled perfusion pipette, because the bridge circuit is unstable during solution changes. Finally, the term R_i ($\Omega \bullet cm$) is the volume resistivity of the perfusion solution, as measured with a standard conductivity meter.

Measurement of Transepithelial Resistance in Voltage Clamped Renal Tubules

There have been a number of early attempts to elucidate the electrical properties of renal tubules using voltage clamp techniques similar to those originally developed for flat epithelia. The basis of these methods is to isolate a segment of tubule (usually with oil droplets) that is short enough to permit a uniform current distribution across the epithelium. To accomplish this, metallic axial electrodes are directly inserted into the lumen of the tubule.[6] These axial electrodes can also be used for AC impedance analysis.[7,50] However, one important problem with metal electrodes is the release of ions into a restricted space during continuous current flow.

An alternative technique employs segments of isolated, perfused tubules that have been shortened to such an extent that the current distribution within the lumen is virtually homogeneous.[8] In this case R_{te} is essentially determined from the input resistance according to Eq. (7.8):

$$R_{te} = 2\pi r_o L \cdot R_i \qquad (7.8)$$

where r_o is the optical radius, and R_{te} has units of $\Omega \bullet cm^2$.

Typical Results

Measurements of V_{te} and R_{te} in some representative epithelia are shown in Table 7.1. The range of both these parameters is large, with values of V_{te} ranging from ± 2 mV in the proximal tubule to as much as -60 to -80 mV in the CCT. R_{te} values vary from less than 10 Ωcm^2 in proximal tubule to more than 5000 Ωcm^2 in urinary bladder. Despite the range of values observed, the transepithelial voltages in all cases reflect two factors: the conductance of the epithelium to the major ions and the active transport of ions. In general, a high value of V_{te} indicates that active transport is taking place across a high resistance epithelium, whereas low values of V_{te} can reflect either a low R_{te} or a low rate of active transport.

Traditionally, epithelia have been divided into the categories "tight" and "leaky," according to their transepithelial resistances. In leaky epithelia the low value of R_{te} is thought to largely reflect the low resistance of the tight junctions which constitute the major electrical resistance of the paracellular pathway between the epithelial cells.[9] In tight epithelia the tight junctional resistance, and therefore the transepithelial resistance, is much higher. However, the resistance above which an epithelium is considered "tight" is not precisely defined.[10] Even though the amphibian proximal tubule and the mammalian collecting duct have similar absolute values of paracellular resistance, the proximal tubule is considered a leaky epithelium, whereas the collecting duct is usually referred to as "tight." Thus, a better definition of a leaky epithelium is one in which the paracellular resistance is low relative to that of the cell membranes. For example, in Table 7.1 it can be seen that in leaky proximal tubules R_{te} is virtually equal to R_{par}, which is small compared to the parallel transcellular resistance R_c. In tight epithelia R_{par} is significantly larger than R_{te}. This implies that R_{par} is of the same order of magnitude as R_c or even much larger in the case of the urinary bladder. Another feature of a tight epithelium is its ability to separate two fluid compartments with very different ion compositions. High resistance tight junctions slow the "backleak" of ions and other solutes down their concentration gradients. Thus, in a tight epithelium it is harder to dissipate the ion gradients established by active transport processes.

Interpretation of Measurements of V_{te} and R_{te}

As discussed above, transepithelial measurements of voltage and resistance are difficult to interpret because they lump together information from many different electrical pathways arranged in parallel. To analyze such data, it is often useful to use a simplified equivalent electrical circuit.

The terms R_c and E_c represent the resistance and electromotive forces across the transcellular pathway, whereas R_{ti} and E_{par} are respectively the resistance and electromotive forces across the paracellular pathway. If the potential differences V_{te}, E_c, and E_{par} are all defined with respect to the bath or serosal side, the overall measured transepithelial values R_{te} and V_{te} are related to this circuit by Eqs (7.9) and (7.10):

$$R_{te} = \frac{R_{tj}R_c}{R_{tj} + R_c} \tag{7.9}$$

$$V_{te} = \frac{E_cR_{tj} + E_{par}R_c}{R_{tj} + R_c} \tag{7.10}$$

The dissection of the measured parameters into the appropriate contributions from cellular and paracellular pathways can sometimes be accomplished by using maneuvers that affect only one of the pathways or cause one pathway to dominate the other. Some of these perturbations and special conditions will be discussed below.

Contribution of Active Transport to V_{te}

The major effect of the pump is to establish transmembrane ionic gradients, i.e., to keep cell Na low and cell K high. As was first pointed out by Koefoed-Johnsen and Ussing in their classic paper of 1958,[11] the permeability properties of the apical and basolateral membranes of the frog skin are quite different. Since the apical membrane is selectively permeable to Na, and the driving force for this ion is inward, the entry of Na will tend to make the cell

voltage positive with respect to the mucosal solution. Conversely, the basolateral membrane is selectively permeable to K. This ion will tend to flow out of the cell, making the cell voltage negative with respect to that of the serosal fluid. The EMFs E_{ap} ($=RT/F$ Δln [Na]) and E_{bl} ($=RT/F$ Δln[K]) will be in the same direction with respect to the epithelium and the transepithelial EMF, and hence V_{te}, will reflect their sum (Figure 7.4).

Although the Na-K-ATPase is ultimately responsible for the transepithelial potential in many Na-reabsorptive epithelia, the magnitude of V_{te} does not correlate with the magnitude of active transport when different tissues are compared. In general, the effect of active ion transport will be shunted by the paracellular resistance. This shunting is least in the tight epithelia such as frog skin and toad urinary bladder, where V_{te} can be over 100 mV. In leaky epithelia such as the proximal tubule the shunting is considerable, and the values of V_{te} are much lower.

In leaky epithelia, E_{par} will be much smaller than E_c (Figure 7.3), since ion gradients across the tight junction are relatively small. In tight epithelia where ion gradients can be significant, $R_{tj} > R_c$ so that the term $E_{par}R_c$ will be small compared to E_cR_{tj}, and Eq. (7.10) becomes:

$$V_{te} = \frac{E_c}{1 + R_c/R_{tj}} \tag{7.11}$$

The implication of Eq. (7.11) is that if $R_{tj} >> R_c$, V_{te} will approach E_c, a quantity which is limited by the EMF of the Na-pump. In general, V_{te} will be reduced according to the ratio R_c/R_{tj}. The contribution of active transport to cell membrane potential is discussed in the section entitled, "Estimation of renal Na,K pump current and electrogenic potential."

The mammalian TALH, and its amphibian counterpart the diluting segment, have lumen-positive V_{te} despite the fact that they are also Na-reabsorbing epithelia (Table 7.1, Figure 7.4). This turns out to be the exception that proves the rule. As discussed in detail by Greger,[12] Na does not enter the TALH cell through a conductive mechanism, as in the frog skin and other epithelia, but through an

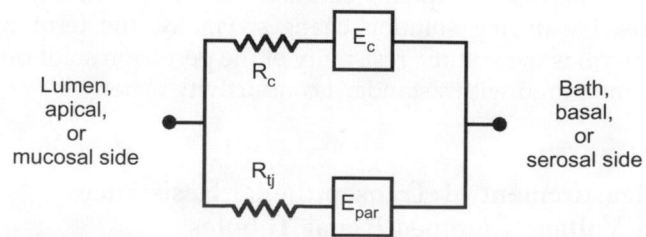

FIGURE 7.3 Simplified equivalent electrical circuit for an epithelium.

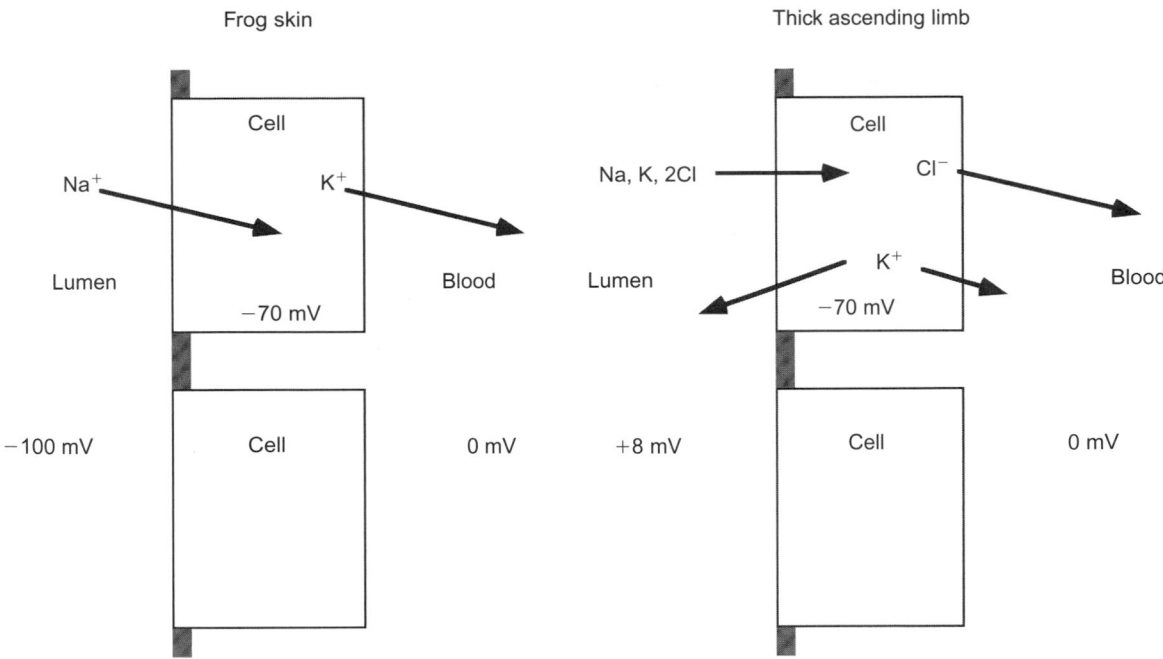

FIGURE 7.4 Contribution of transcellular potentials to the transepithelial potential. On the left is a tight epithelium such as the frog skin or cortical collecting duct (CCD). Influx of Na across the apical membrane and efflux of K across the basolateral membrane create a lumen-negative voltage which is not significantly shunted because of the high tight-junctional resistance. Consequently, most of the transepithelial potential arises from diffusion potentials for Na and K that are established across the cell membranes by active transport, and by the different ion-selectivities of the apical and basolateral membranes. The figure on the right is a model of a TALH cell. Here Na entry across the luminal membrane is electrically silent. The dominant electrodiffusive ion movements are K efflux across both apical and basolateral membranes, and Cl efflux across the basolateral membrane. The basolateral Cl conductance makes the cell less negative relative to interstitial fluid versus luminal fluid.

electrically neutral co-transport system along with K and Cl. Thus, Na entry does not contribute to a lumen-negative voltage, and in fact the membrane is more permeable to K than to Na. Furthermore, the basolateral membrane has a rather high permeability to Cl. This makes the lumped EMF E_{ap} less negative than E_{bl}, and the potential difference between the cell and the blood side is less negative than the potential difference between the cell and the lumen. Hence, the mechanism for the lumen-positive potential in the TALH is accounted for by the different permeability properties of the two membranes, just as in the frog skin.

Contribution of Diffusion Potentials to V_{te}

Paracellular diffusion potentials can contribute significantly to the overall transepithelial potential, especially when V_{te} is small. For example, in the mammalian proximal tubule the early portion of the segment has a lumen-negative V_{te} *in vivo*, which is thought to reflect active Na reabsorption. Farther down the nephron, however, the lumen becomes positive with respect to the blood. Preferential luminal reabsorption of HCO_3^- relative to Cl^- establishes opposing gradients for Cl^- and HCO_3^- across the tight junction (Figure 7.5). This results in a

lumen-positive potential since Cl^- diffuses more rapidly across the junctions than HCO_3^-.[13]

Diffusion potentials may also contribute to the normal lumen-positive V_{te} in the mammalian TALH (Table 7.1). In this segment NaCl is reabsorbed but water is not, leading to a dilution of the luminal fluid. Since the tight junctions of the mammalian TALH are cation-selective, Na diffuses back more rapidly than the Cl, contributing to a lumen-positive diffusion potential[12] (Figure 7.5).

Contribution of Circulating Current to V_{te}

The different equivalent EMFs at the apical and basolateral sides of the cell produce a circulating current (*I*) which traverses both cell membranes in series, and returns via the paracellular shunt (Figure 7.1). The magnitude of this current depends on the relative resistances of paracellular versus cell pathways, as well as the active transport rate for the particular epithelium.[14,15] For example, in renal proximal tubules, the low shunt resistance (compared to transcellular resistance) characterizes this nephron segment as a leaky epithelia with large circulating current.[13,16] On the other hand, tight epithelia like the urinary bladder or the frog skin have shunt resistances comparable to or larger

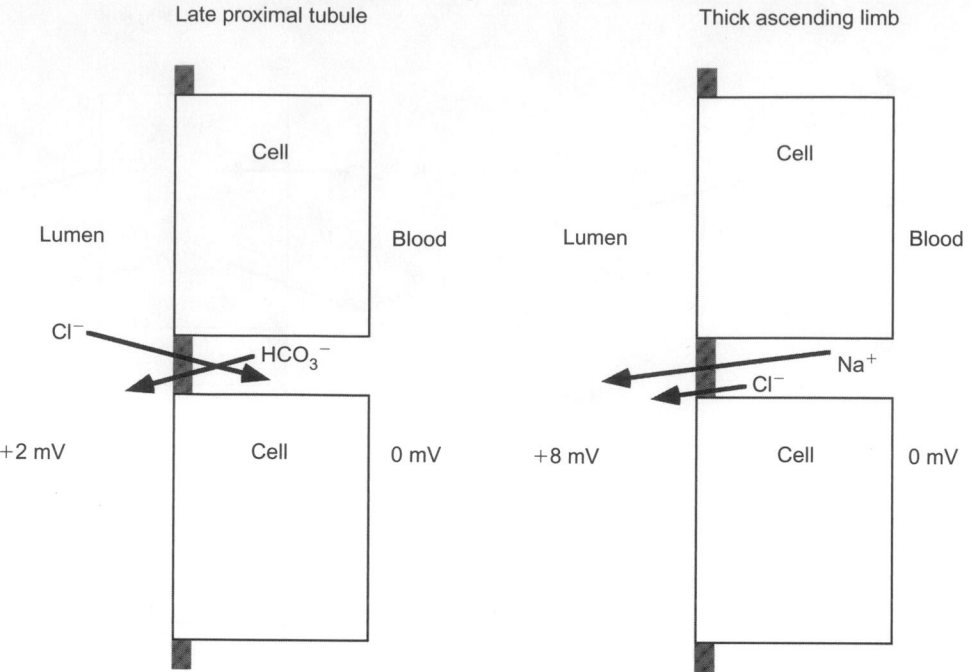

FIGURE 7.5   Contribution of paracellular potentials to the transepithelial potential. The figure on the left corresponds to the late proximal tubule. Preferential reabsorption of HCO_3^- in the early proximal tubule produces opposite gradients for Cl^- and HCO_3^- across the tight junction of late proximal tubule. Since the junctions are more permeable to Cl^- than to HCO_3^-, a lumen-positive diffusion potential develops. The paracellular contribution in the TALH is illustrated on the right. Here, reabsorption of NaCl across the water-impermeable epithelium results in an accumulation of NaCl within the interspaces between the cells, producing a similar gradient for both Na^+ and Cl^- across the tight junction. Since the junctions in this epithelium are more permeable to Na^+ than to Cl^-, a lumen-positive diffusion potential develops.

than the transcellular resistance, so that the circulating current is small in comparison with proximal tubule.[17]

The effect of circulating current on renal trans-epithelial potentials can be understood qualitatively by considering the electrical profiles depicted in Figure 7.6. In this figure, the serosal or blood side of the epithelium is considered at ground and the voltage at any point is displayed as a function of distance from mucosa to serosa. For the sake of simplicity, we have assumed that the apical membrane is primarily selective to sodium, the basolateral membrane is primarily selective to potassium, and the interior of the cell is isopotential. Therefore, in the absence of circulating current, there is a "staircase" voltage profile through the epithelium determined by the respective diffusion potentials across the mucosal (or apical) membrane and across the serosal (or basolateral) membrane (Figure 7.6a). Under these conditions the measured V_{te} (mucosa minus serosa) would actually be more negative than the basolateral cell membrane potential (E_K).

In most epithelia the diffusion potential steps of Figure 7.6a would be modified by the effect of circulating current (I) across the resistance of the mucosal and serosal barriers. Specifically, the mucosal to cell step will be raised by an amount: $I \bullet R_{ap}$ due to the circulating current crossing the mucosal membrane

resistance (Figure 7.6b). The same current crossing the basolateral side of the cell will decrease the size of the cell-to-serosal step by $I \bullet R_{bl}^*$, where R_{bl}^* is the effective basolateral resistance. The final values of V_{te} and V_{bl} can be calculated by considering the complete equivalent circuit (Appendix 7.1).

In most epithelia, the resistance of the apical membrane is larger than the resistance of the basolateral membrane, and the effect of the circulating current is to transform the staircase potential (Figure 7.6a) into a "well-type" potential (Figure 7.6c), where the intracellular region is the most negative space and V_{te} is directly dependent on the magnitude of the current and the tightness of the epithelial cell layer. In some tight epithelia (*Necturus* urinary bladder) with high paracellular resistance and low circulating current, the "staircase" potential profile is still maintained despite "IR drops" at both membranes.[18]

Short-Circuit Current

It is also possible to measure transepithelial currents while controlling the transepithelial voltage. A special case of this voltage-clamp approach is the short-circuit current technique[1] in which V_{te} is maintained at zero.

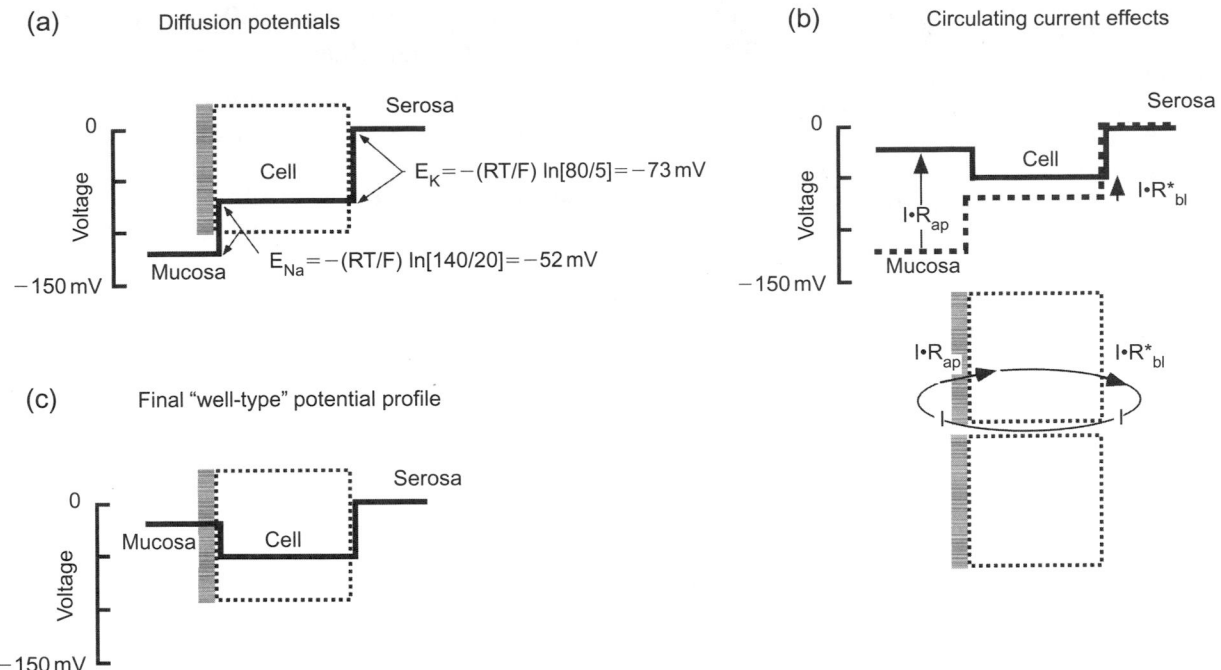

FIGURE 7.6 Electrical potential profiles across a simple epithelium. (a) In the absence of circulating currents, the electrical potential from serosal to mucosal sides would be largely determined by the Na diffusion potential at the apical membrane, and the K diffusion potential at the serosal membrane. (b) Circulating currents that arise from a net (open-circuit) EMF produce additional voltage drops across both the apical membrane ($=I \cdot R_{ap}$) and across the basolateral membrane ($=I \cdot R_{bl}$). (c) This changes the "staircase" potential profile to a "well-type" potential, where the cell is more negative than either the mucosal or serosal sides.

If the solutions on both sides of the epithelium are identical, there is no net movement of ions through the paracellular spaces, since both electrical and chemical driving forces are reduced to zero. The current across the tissue, which must also pass through the external circuit and can thus be readily measured, results only from active transport processes (defined as those which take place against an electrochemical activity gradient). Thus this current (called the short-circuit current), will equal the sum of all active ion transport processes.

The particular ion being actively transported can be identified rigorously by measuring net fluxes at the same time as the short circuit current. For some cases, such as the frog skin and toad bladder,[19,20] the short-circuit current can be accounted for by the active transport of only one ion species, namely Na (Table 7.2). In general, the short-circuit current will represent the sum of the net transport of Na, K, H, Cl, and HCO_3. Another way to identify actively transported ions is to eliminate them from the bathing media and measure the resulting effects on short-circuit current. This approach is often experimentally much simpler, but it is less rigorous since the apical and basolateral solutions will not be identical. Furthermore, changing the external environment of the tissue can lead to secondary changes in cell composition and volume. In any case, once the transported species have been identified,

TABLE 7.2 Equivalence of Net Na + Fluxes and Short-Circuit Current in Model Epithelia, Transepithelial fluxes (nEq/cm²/min)

Type of Epithelium	Mucosal to Serosal	Serosal to Mucosal	Net	Short-circuit Current
Frog skin	24.6	1.5	23.1	23.6
Toad urinary bladder	35.7	9.5	26.2	26.8

Data are from [1] for frog skin and from [19] for toad bladder.

the technique becomes a very convenient way to analyze the regulation of the active transport systems.

An important limitation of the short-circuit current technique is that it often requires unphysiological conditions. For example, short-circuiting high resistance epithelia like frog skin will reduce the normally large V_{te} to values near zero. This will necessarily affect the transmembrane voltage of one or both cell membranes, which may in turn affect the ionic conductances of those membranes.

The short-circuit technique also involves bathing the apical side of the tissue with a solution that has an electrolyte composition close to that of the blood. This is a highly unphysiological condition for many tight epithelia like the frog skin, which is normally in contact with pond water, and the toad bladder, which is normally in contact with dilute urine. Another important problem with short-circuit experiments is that short-circuited tissues do not have to maintain the electroneutrality of the transported species. For example, in Na-transporting epithelia, such as the frog skin, Na ions can be reabsorbed only if another cation (e.g., K, H) is secreted or if an anion (Cl) is also reabsorbed. Under physiological conditions these other ionic pathways can be rate-limiting for Na reabsorption.

Finally, the uniform current distribution required by the short-circuit technique has largely restricted its use to flat epithelia which can be mounted in Ussing chambers. However, in some cases it has been possible to voltage-clamp large-diameter amphibian tubules.[21] Attempts have also been made to circumvent these technical problems by defining an "equivalent short-circuit current" for renal epithelia. In this method, the current at $V_{te} = 0$ is estimated by dividing the spontaneous value of V_{te} by the transepithelial resistance R_{te}. This approach assumes that R_{te} is constant; i.e., that the current voltage relation of the epithelium is linear. Even when this condition is satisfied, it is not always possible to attribute the equivalent short-circuit current to specific ion species, since net fluxes of the ions must be measured under true short-circuited conditions.

Technical Problems

For epithelia that can be studied as flat sheets *in vitro*, the major technical problem with transepithelial measurements is avoiding edge damage to the tissues, particularly when these tissues are mounted in Ussing chambers.[22,23] On the other hand, for renal micropuncture experiments performed *in situ*, the major technical problem is localization of the microelectrode tip within the tubular lumen.[13]

The most important general problem in the measurement of transepithelial resistance is the choice of the magnitude and duration of the applied perturbations. Currents (or voltage changes) which are too large can result in changes in the electrical properties of the membranes due to voltage-dependent ion conductances. Perturbations which are either too large or too long can lead to redistribution of ions across the cell membranes, which can also alter electrical properties. For example, in toad urinary bladder modest changes in V_{te} in the order of 10 mV under voltage-clamp conditions can result in time-dependent changes in the tissue resistance.[24] On the other hand, if perturbations are too small they are difficult to measure accurately, and if they are applied for too short a time the capacitative, as well as the resistive, properties of the epithelium will affect the response. There are no generally accepted rules for determining the size and duration of the perturbations.

Estimation of Membrane Parameters from Transepithelial Measurements

Measurement of transepithelial electrical properties does not, in general, give any direct, quantitative information about the circuit elements of greatest interest, namely the conductances of individual membranes to specific ions. As emphasized throughout this section, R_{te} is a lumped parameter determined by R_{ap}, R_b, R_{tj}, and in some cases R_{lis} (see Figure 7.1). V_{te} is determined by all the R_s and EMFs in the circuit. Clearly, measuring two parameters is insufficient to determine seven or eight unknowns.

However, in some cases it has been possible to either use conditions which simplify the equivalent circuit or to use experimental perturbations that selectively change only one electrical parameter. These methods have provided a good deal of information about epithelial properties from purely transepithelial measurements. Some examples are given below.

Paracellular Resistance and Selectivity

When the paracellular (tight junction) resistance is low compared to the transcellular resistance, the transepithelial resistance is dominated by the resistance of the paracellular pathway. This happens in a leaky epithelium like the proximal tubule. This condition can also be produced in some tight epithelia by blocking the major conductive pathways at the apical membrane. The most frequently used blockers are amiloride, for the Na conductance, and Ba, for the K conductance. In both of these cases the paracellular resistance can then be estimated from transepithelial measurements (Table 7.1), although intracellular recordings are usually required to prove that the transcellular resistance is high.

The ion selectivity of the paracellular pathway can also be evaluated under these circumstances. This involves measurement of the transference numbers for various ions across the tight junction (see Eq. (7.12)). The most important ions in this case are Na and Cl, and their transference numbers can be estimated by reducing the concentration of NaCl on one side of the junction by diluting one of the bathing solutions. If the transcellular resistance is sufficiently high (i.e., $R_{ap} \gg R_{tj}$, see Eq. (A2.3) in Appendix 2) and is unaffected by the dilution, the measured change in V_{te} will approximately reflect the change in E_{par} where:

$$\Delta E_{par} = -\frac{RT}{F}(t_{Na} - t_{Cl}) Ln \frac{[NaCl]_1}{[NaCl]_2} \qquad (7.12)$$

If sodium and chloride are the only conducting ions in the external solutions, the absolute transference numbers can be calculated from Eq. (7.12) and the requirement that $t_{Na} + t_{Cl} = 1$. Some measurements of paracellular selectivity in renal epithelia are listed in Table 7.1. This parameter is of considerable physiological interest. The results range from a significant selectivity for anions (Cl) over cations (Na) in the amphibian proximal tubule, to a cation selectivity in the thick ascending limb of Henle's loop or its counterpart, the diluting segment, in the amphibian kidney. If ions moved through the tight junctions as if they were in free solution, a permeability ratio P_{Na}/P_{Cl} of 0.8 would be expected. The variations in selectivity result from differences in the expression of specific members of the tight-junction proteins claudins.[25]

Membrane Selectivity

If the paracellular or tight junction resistance is much greater than the transcellular resistance, it is possible to determine the ion selectivity of the individual cell membranes. Specifically, if R_{tj} is very large compared to $R_{ap} + R_{bl}$, there will be negligible current through either the paracellular pathway or the cell pathway under open-circuit conditions. Under these conditions, the circuit of Figure 7.1 predicts that changes in E_{ap} will parallel changes in V_{ap} which, in turn, can be estimated from the measured changes in transepithelial potential ΔV_{te} (see Equations (A1.8) and (A1.11)–(A1.13) of Appendix 7.1). Such a situation was studied by Koefoed-Johnsen and Ussing[11] in their classic paper on the frog skin, where pre-treatment of the skins with low concentrations of Cu^{+2} produced very high values of R_{te} and V_{te}.

This permits evaluation of individual membrane selectivities from transepithelial measurements alone if the concentration of just one ion on one side of the epithelium is replaced with an impermeant species, and the conditions associated with Eq. (A1.13) (Appendix 7.1) are satisfied. If this is the case and Na is partially replaced on the apical side, then:

$$\Delta V_{te} = \Delta E_{ap} = -\frac{RT}{F} t_{Na} Ln \frac{[Na]_{ap}^{exp}}{[Na]_{ap}^{con}} \; for \; R_{tj} \gg R_{ap} + R_{bl}^*$$

(7.13)

where the change in potential is measured as experimental minus control. $[Na]^{exp}$ and $[Na]^{con}$ represent the concentrations of Na under experimental and control conditions, i.e., after and before the solution change.

Koefoed-Johnsen and Ussing[11] found that changes in mucosal Na produced changes in V_{te} close to those which would be expected if $t_{Na} = 1$. From this they inferred that the apical membrane was primarily conductive to Na ions. Similarly, changes in serosal K concentration produced changes consistent with the idea that the basolateral membrane conducted only K. The

elegant conclusions of this study depended upon the rather unusual conditions achieved, namely a very high paracellular resistance and the absence of other "leak" pathways due to other cell types. Except for the case of the urinary bladder, such conditions are difficult to achieve in renal epithelia where paracellular pathways are usually leakier than in the frog skin.

Selectivity of the epithelial basolateral membrane has also been studied by using pore-forming polyene antibiotics to reduce apical membrane resistance[26] so that V_{te} becomes a reasonable estimate of the basolateral potential V_{bl} (see Equation A1.16 of Appendix 7.1). For example, in the turtle colon, Germann et al.[27] were able to characterize two different conductances for K across the basolateral membrane using the amphotericin-B permeabilized epithelium. This approach has also been used mostly in flat epithelia rather than renal tubules.

Impedance Analysis

Impedance analysis permits estimation of the electrical properties of individual membranes using transepithelial measurements.[28] In principle, transepithelial impedance can be measured from the time-course of the response to any electrical perturbation. In practice, it is usually obtained either under "current-clamp" conditions, using sine wave current perturbations at different frequencies or under voltage-clamp conditions by applying voltage perturbations. Since the apical and basolateral membranes will each have an associated complex impedance that depends on frequency, it is possible to distinguish contributions from the two membranes if they have very different time constants ($\tau = RC$, where R is the resistance and C the capacitance).

Typically four parameters (consisting of the amplitudes and time-constants of the two membrane components) are measured to fit a circuit with five parameters (resistance and capacitance of apical and basolateral membranes and the paracellular resistance). To fully solve the system one model parameter (e.g., the paracellular resistance) usually must be determined independently.

Impedance analysis has also been used to derive detailed information about the paracellular pathway, including the distribution of resistance across tight junctions and along intercellular spaces. In this regard, it has been used to estimate individual resistances and capacitances of the apical and basolateral membranes of flat epithelial sheets obtained from frog skin, amphibian and mammalian urinary bladder, colon, and cultured epithelial cells.[29–32] The elegance of the technique is that it is non-invasive, yielding information about individual membranes without the need for intracellular probes or electrodes. Because of the requirement of uniform currents or voltage fields, its application to renal tubules has been very limited.[7,33]

CONCLUSIONS

Many important epithelial properties can be determined from transepithelial measurements alone. In fact, the original Koefoed-Johnsen/Ussing model for Na transport by the frog skin was based entirely on transepithelial electrical and flux measurements, and the ingenious use of special simplifying conditions. Thus, a number of important physical and thermodynamic properties of epithelia are still estimated from transepithelial measurements, particularly in renal tissues. These include the magnitude and selectivity of the paracellular shunt pathway, the ion selectivity of cell membranes (qualitatively in most instances), and the currents and EMF's associated with active transepithelial transport. On the other hand, the quantitative description of membrane properties requires detailed intracellular measurements to specifically characterize the apical and basolateral membrane components, as well as the contribution of the paracellular pathway. These measurements will be discussed in the next section.

INTRACELLULAR MEASUREMENTS

Intracellular measurements with voltage-sensitive and ion-sensitive microelectrodes permit a more detailed evaluation of individual membrane parameters than transepithelial measurements. This has been essential to our understanding of ion transport in epithelia. Three important membrane characteristics that are amenable to study with intracellular techniques are: (1) ionic selectivity; (2) membrane conductance; and (3) estimation of pump current. Although there are significant differences in the methodology of these measurements depending on the particular tissue involved, much of the underlying theory is similar in both flat epithelia and renal tubules. The emphasis of this section will be on describing the simplest and most straightforward methods for evaluation of single-membrane parameters with emphasis on renal epithelia, although much of the theory is applicable to flat epithelia as well.

Cell Membrane Potentials in Epithelia

An epithelium is a sheet of polarized cells joined together to function as a selective barrier between two compartments. Epithelia not only structurally define two compartments, but also maintain the composition

of those compartments via the specific transport of electrolytes, non-electrolytes, and water. The electrical voltage measured across either the apical or basolateral membrane of an epithelium is the sum of the ionic diffusion potentials across the membrane, and the voltage drops arising from current flow across the resistance of that membrane. This current flow (depicted by the thick arrow in Figure 7.1) arises in part from the differences in membrane ionic diffusion potentials and the sum of epithelial barrier electrical resistances (Appendix 7.1).

In practice, cell membrane potentials are determined by impaling the cell with fine tipped glass microelectrodes, filled with a highly conductive electrolyte solution (1 M or 3 M KCl). Uniform filling is often accomplished by starting with glass tubing that contains a thin glass filament, allowing solution to flow smoothly from the back to the tip of the finished electrode. The microelectrode is then mounted on a stable micromanipulator. Given the elasticity of most cell membranes, impalement usually requires a rapid forward movement of the tip that can be accomplished either mechanically or with piezoelectric headstage. Sometimes a high frequency alternating current is briefly applied to the tip to permit entry into the cell with minimum damage.

A major technical problem with microelectrode measurements is the damage to the cell that may be produced by impalement. For a discussion of this topic see Higgins et al.[18] and Nelson et al..[34] Cell damage can be minimized by utilizing epithelia with large cells (e.g., *Necturus*; *Amphiuma*), and by recording from the basolateral rather than the apical membrane. This will result in less electrical shunting of the membrane potential, since in many cases the basolateral membrane has a much lower resistance than the apical membrane and an additional leak conductance at the basal side will have a smaller overall effect.[18] Furthermore, epithelia like the proximal tubule, whose cells are electrically coupled, are less sensitive to impalement artifacts, since the effective cell membrane area is larger. Finally, the use of very fine-tipped micropipettes can minimize membrane damage during intracellular measurements. However, such pipettes are more likely to produce artifacts due to changes in the liquid-junction potentials ("tip potentials") when the tip enters the cytoplasm.

Use of microelectrodes to measure cell potential may result in KCl leakage into the cell. Although these tips are extremely small ($< 0.2 \, \mu m$), the use of concentrated KCl in the electrode to minimize liquid junction potentials can lead to KCl influx into the cell, alterations in cell composition, and cell swelling.[34] Thus, the choice of a filling solution is a trade-off between a concentrated KCl solution, which yields low tip potentials but possible KCl leakage, versus a low salt pipette solution, which results in higher tip potentials but less salt leakage into the cytoplasm.

Intracellular potential can also be measured with relatively large diameter patch-clamp pipettes. In a "whole-cell clamp" experiment, a high resistance seal is formed between the pipette and the cell membrane. This permits direct electrical contact between the recording electrode and the cell interior with negligible impalement damage. If the amplifier is used in the voltage-clamp mode, the holding potential that reduces the membrane current to zero becomes a good measure of the cell potential. One disadvantage of using the whole-cell clamp to measure cell potential is that the cell is dialyzed with the pipette solution.[35] The exchange of vital cell constituents with the pipette solution may alter the intracellular ion composition, as well as change the normal cell membrane permeabilities through the loss of regulatory factors. The latter effect can be minimized by using the "perforated-patch" technique, in which the patch is permeabilized by the addition of pore-forming substances such as nystatin to the pipette solution.[36]

Evaluation of Individual Membrane Resistances from an Equivalent Circuit Analysis

The simplest technique for determining individual cell membrane resistance is to measure intracellular and transepithelial potential during an experimental maneuver that produces only a single perturbation in the parameters of the equivalent circuit. These techniques have been particularly useful in mammalian proximal tubules where multiple microelectrode impalements are difficult or in nephron segments that are not electrically coupled.

When only one microelectrode is used, the circuit of Figure 7.1 must be simplified to permit an indirect evaluation of the cell membrane resistances. This type of reduction is illustrated in Figure 7.7, and is permissible when most of the paracellular resistance is contributed by the tight junction resistance (i.e., when $R_{par} \approx R_{tj}$), which is equivalent to the assumption that R_{tj} is $>>$ lateral interspace resistance ($=R_{lis}$). This is particularly appropriate for mammalian proximal tubule, where basal interdigitations of adjacent cells greatly reduce the lateral space resistance, and most of the paracellular resistance is contributed by the tight junction resistance.

The circuit of Figure 7.7a can be further reduced to the simpler form of Figure 7.7b by defining an effective basolateral EMF (E_{bl}^*) and an effective basolateral resistance (R_{bl}^*), as described in Appendix 7.1. Although the electromotive forces or EMFs (E_{ap}, E_{bl}, E_{par}) in the circuit cannot be measured directly, the potential differences across each barrier can be measured with intracellular or transepithelial electrodes. These are defined as transepithelial potential (lumen-bath) $= V_{te}$, apical cell membrane potential (lumen-cell) $= V_{ap}$, and basolateral potential (cell-bath) $= V_{bl}$.

An important consequence of the circulating epithelial current in Figure 7.7 is that alterations in any of the electrical parameters on one side of the cell will produce changes in the measured electrical potentials on the contralateral side. This actually provides an indirect method for evaluating those resistances that remain constant during a change in loop current, I. Individual cell membrane resistances R_{bl}^* and R_{ap} can be evaluated by any experimental maneuver that changes only the parameters at one membrane. For example, rapid addition of amiloride or glucose to the apical solution presumably alters only the resistance and/or the EMF of the apical membrane by blocking Na channels or stimulating Na-glucose co-transport, respectively.

Amiloride causes a hyperpolarization of V_{bl} by both increasing the measured apical resistance (R_{ap}) and decreasing the contribution of the Na gradient to the value of E_{ap} (see Appendix 7.1, Eq. (A1.7)). On the other hand, addition of glucose to the luminal solution depolarizes V_{bl} by stimulating Na-glucose co-transport, which effectively increases both the apical Na conductance and the relative contribution of the Na gradient to the apical diffusion potential. Since the primary effect of both amiloride and glucose occurs at the apical membrane, the ratio of basolateral to apical resistance is directly related to the measured ratio of basolateral to transepithelial voltage deflections according to Eq. (7.14), which applies for addition of either apical-side amiloride or apical-side glucose:

$$\frac{R_{bl}^*}{R_{tj}} = -\frac{\Delta V_{bl}}{\Delta V_{te}} = \beta \qquad (7.14)$$

This equation implicitly assumes that neither glucose nor amiloride affect the paracellular pathway, and that the potential measurements can be performed before any changes in cell composition have occurred that would affect E_{ap}, E_{bl}, and R_{bl}.

Similarly, measurement of the ratio of apical to transepithelial potential change following addition of barium to the basolateral solution permits estimation of the apical membrane resistance via Eq. (7.15):

$$\frac{R_{ap}}{R_{tj}} = -\frac{\Delta V_{ap}}{\Delta V_{te}} = \frac{\Delta V_{bl}}{\Delta V_{te}} - 1 = \alpha \qquad (7.15)$$

Again, it has been assumed that basolateral application of barium has no effect on the paracellular pathway, and that the measurement can be performed rapidly enough to avoid changes in cell composition.

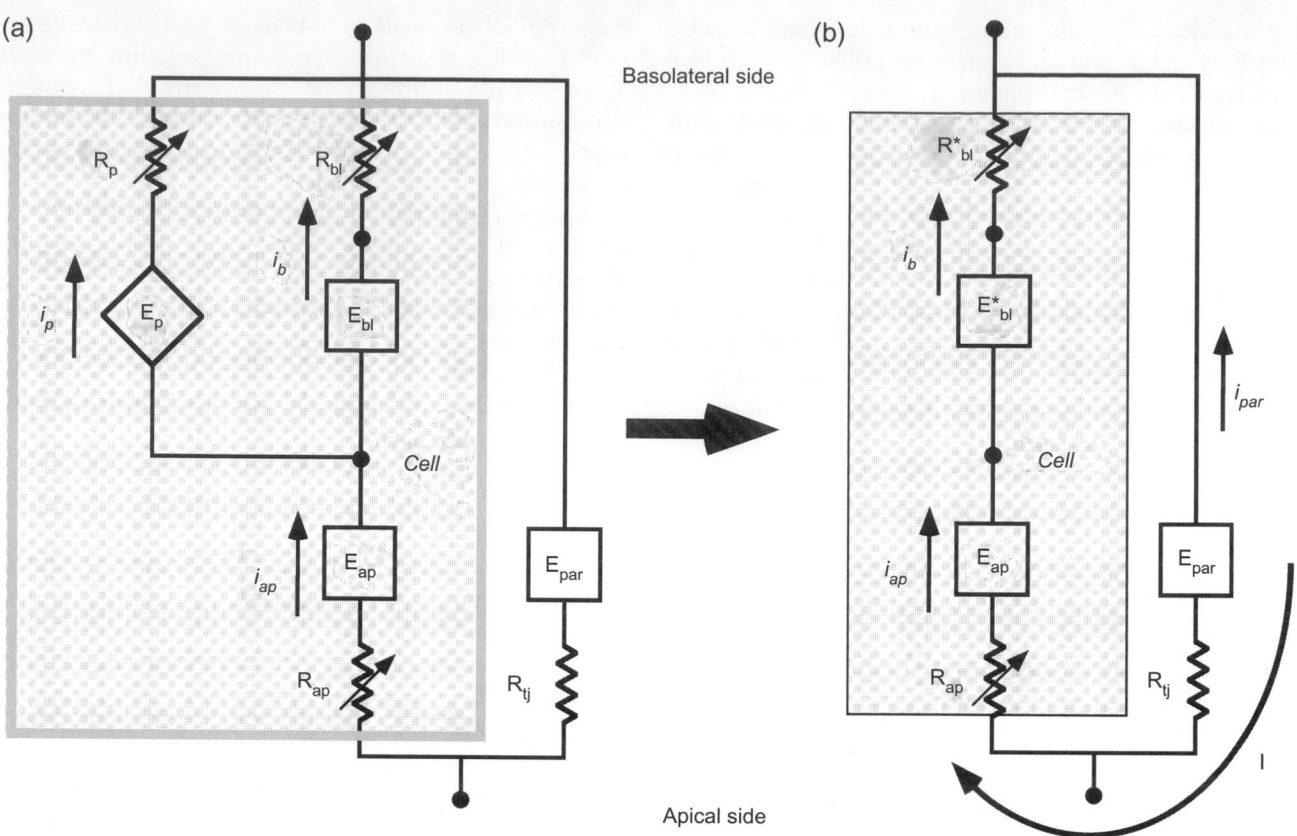

FIGURE 7.7 (a) Reduced form of the general equivalent circuit, where the lateral resistive network has been neglected because most of the paracellular resistance is assumed to reside at the tight junction (i.e., $R_{tj} \gg R_{lis}$). This situation applies in a number of epithelia and greatly simplifies the equivalent circuit. (b) Reduced circuit in which the parallel diffusive and active transport paths across the basolateral membrane have been combined into an effective basolateral EMF (E_{bl}^*) and an effective basolateral resistance (R_{bl}^*). "I" denotes direction of positive net circulating current under open-circuit conditions.

Finally, in cases where it is feasible to make changes on only one side of the epithelium, the voltage divider ratio can be used instead of either Eq. (7.14) or Eq. (7.15). When current is injected into the tubule lumen via the perfusion pipette, a certain fraction of that current will cross the apical and basolateral cell membrane in series, producing voltage deflections ΔV_{ap} and ΔV_{bl}. If the lateral and basal resistances of Figure 7.1 are combined into a single effective resistance R_{bl}^* (defined in Appendix 7.1, Eq. (A1.4)) the ratio of apical to basolateral resistance during transepithelial injection of current is given by Eq. (7.16):

$$\gamma = \frac{R_{ap}}{R_{bl}^*} = \frac{\Delta V_{ap}}{\Delta V_{bl}} = \frac{\Delta V_{te}}{\Delta V_{bl}} - 1 \qquad (7.16)$$

The term "γ" is sometimes referred to as the voltage divider ratio. An alternative to Eq. (7.16) is to define the "fractional resistance" of either the apical (fR_{ap}) or basolateral membranes (fR_{bl}), according to Eqs. (7.17a), (7.17b):

$$fR_{ap} = \frac{R_{ap}}{R_{ap} + R_{bl}^*} = 1 - \frac{\Delta V_{bl}}{\Delta V_{te}} \qquad (7.17a)$$

$$fR_{bl}^* = \frac{R_{bl}^*}{R_{ap} + R_{bl}^*} = \frac{\Delta V_{bl}}{\Delta V_{te}} \qquad (7.17b)$$

Since γ, α, β, and R_{te} are all measured quantities, the individual resistances: R_{bl}^*, R_{ap}, R_{tj}, can be evaluated by using any three of the four equations Eqs. (7.14), (7.15), (7.16), and Eq. (A1.5).

An example of these methods is illustrated by the experiment depicted in Figure 7.8.[37] In this experiment, changes in transepithelial (V_{te}) and basolateral potential (V_{bl}) are shown during addition of 1 mM barium to the bath (Figure 7.8a), followed by addition of 8 mM glucose to the lumen (Figure 7.8b). The superimposed smaller deflections are due to periodic current injection for evaluating "γ" from Eq. (7.16).

In both these experiments, ΔV_{bl} and ΔV_{te} were taken as the initial changes in voltage resulting from a particular maneuver. For example, in the barium experiment, only changes in V_{bl} and R_{bl}^* were presumed to occur, and ΔV_{bl} was taken as the difference between the baseline V_{bl} and the V_{bl} at the inflection point (asterisk). The origin of the slow secondary depolarization of V_{bl} in Figure 7.8a is not known.

The above methods have been used to determine individual cell membrane resistance in mammalian proximal tubule. Some of these results are summarized in Table 7.3. Although there are some differences in the absolute values of cell resistances, there is general agreement that in proximal tubule the resistance of the cellular pathway is between 20 and 30 times higher than the resistance of the shunt pathway. This factor is even higher in amphibian proximal tubule.

Determination of individual membrane parameters from Eqs. (7.14)–(7.16) involves certain practical problems. These methods require measurement of ΔV_{te} and ΔV_{bl} in the same tubule at the same axial distance along its length. As indicated in Figure 7.8, the small magnitude of the change in transepithelial potential renders the two ratios α and β in Eqs. (7.14) and (7.15) particularly susceptible to errors in ΔV_{te}. Measurements of ΔV_{te} obtained by advancing a microelectrode into the lumen are unreliable, because damage to the epithelium can produce artificially low values of ΔV_{te}. Since transepithelial potential is measured only at the perfusion or collection ends of the tubule, the value of ΔV_{te} must be calculated from the electrotonic voltage spread along the tubule using a terminated cable analysis (see section entitled, "Transepithelial Measurements").

Evaluation of Individual Membrane Resistances Using Multiple Intracellular Recordings

In the relatively large cells of amphibian proximal tubule (30 μm diameter), direct electrical measurement of cell membrane resistance is possible. Exploiting the property of electrical coupling between adjacent proximal cells,[16] it is possible to pass current from an intracellular microelectrode through an annular syncytium, with an outer specific resistance of R_{bl}^* and an inner specific resistance of R_{ap}. This cannot be done in nephron segments like the collecting duct, where adjacent cells are not electrically coupled.[38]

The use of cellular cable analysis to evaluate the individual resistances R_{bl}^*, R_{ap}, and R_{tj} still depends on the definition of transepithelial resistance (Eq. (A1.5)) and the "voltage-divider" ratio (Eq. (7.16)) that were discussed in the section entitled, "Cell Membrane Potentials in Epithelia." However, instead of relying on the ratio $\Delta V_{bl}/\Delta V_{te}$, obtained during application of barium or amiloride, the parallel resistance of the cell layer (R_z) is computed directly from the electrotonic voltage spread along the double core cable, where R_z is defined by Eq. (7.18).

$$1/R_z = 1/R_{ap} + 1/R_{bl}^* \qquad (7.18)$$

In practice, R_z is evaluated by injecting current I_o into the cell layer at x = 0 via a microelectrode and

measuring the voltage deflection ΔV_x at two or more locations "x," downstream from the injection site. The arrangement of microelectrodes is illustrated in Figure 7.2. If x is at least twice the diameter of the tubule, the electrotonic voltage spread along the cable will be given by Eq. (7.19), where λ_c is the cellular length constant of the tubule[5]:

$$Ln[\Delta V_x] = Ln\left[\frac{R_z I_o}{4\pi r \lambda_c}\right] - \frac{1}{\lambda_c}x \qquad (7.19)$$

The best fit for the two unknown parameters λ_c and R_z is determined by evaluating Eq. (7.19) at a number of locations along the tubule. The radius of the tubule, r_o, is measured with an optical micrometer. Combining Eqs. (7.16), (7.18), (7.19), and (A1.5), the individual membrane resistances R_{ap}, R_{bl}^*, and R_{tj} are uniquely determined by the two parameters R_z, γ, and the measured value of R_{te} according to Eqs. (7.20)–(7.22):

$$R_{ap} = R_z[1 + \gamma] \qquad (7.20)$$

$$R_{bl}^* = R_z\left[1 + \frac{1}{\gamma}\right] \qquad (7.21)$$

$$R_{ti} = \frac{R_{te}[R_{bl}^* + R_{ap}]}{R_{ap} + R_{bl}^* - R_{te}} \qquad (7.22)$$

The transepithelial resistance of the tubule, R_{te}, is determined by passing current and measuring voltage through a doubled-barreled perfusion pipette according to the methods described in the section entitled, "Transepithelial Measurements" and Figure 7.2.

In amphibian proximal tubule, most measurements of individual cell resistances have been performed using a cellular cable analysis with two or more intracellular microelectrodes. On the other hand in mammalian tubules, the method of relative voltage deflections (Eqs. (7.14) and (7.15)) have been used exclusively. However, in *Ambystoma* proximal tubule, a direct comparison of the two methods has been made under similar conditions. These results are summarized in the first two rows of Table 7.4. As indicated, the absolute values of resistance are quite close considering the propagation of errors that occur with both types of measurements. The remaining rows of Table 7.4 summarize additional resistance measurements in amphibian renal epithelia.

As with the mammalian proximal tubule, the ratio of shunt to cell resistance clearly establishes the amphibian proximal tubule as a "leaky" epithelium. In contrast, the *Necturus* urinary bladder (a "tight" epithelium) possesses a shunt resistance that is several times larger than the cell resistance pathway. Neither the diluting segment nor the collecting tubule of the *Amphiuma* fall neatly into the "tight" or "leaky" category, since both of these segments have cellular

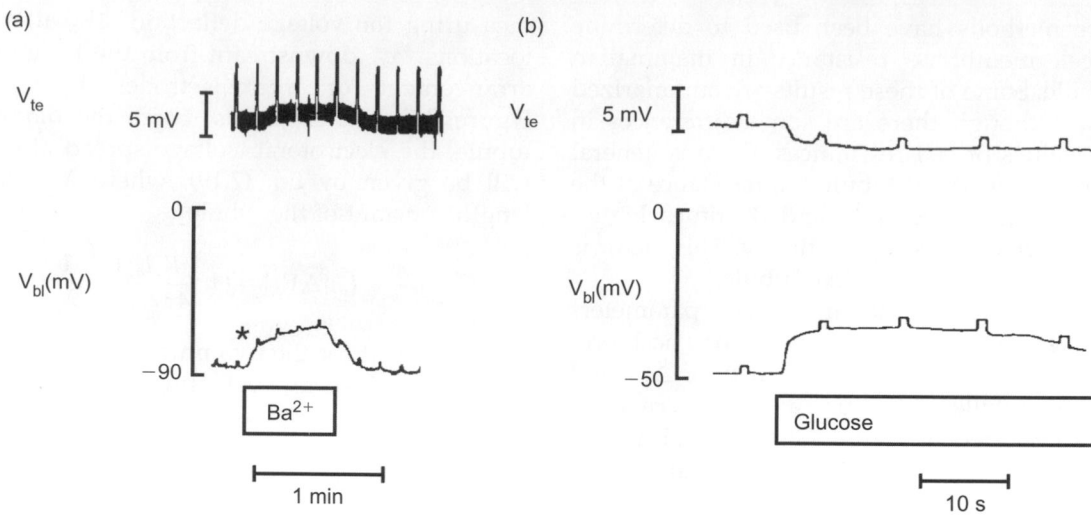

FIGURE 7.8 Effect of barium and glucose on membrane voltages in rabbit proximal convoluted tubule (from [37]). (a) Reversible depolarization of both the transepithelial (V_{te}) and the basolateral membrane potential (V_{bl}) produced by addition of barium to the basolateral side of isolated proximal tubules. (b) Simultaneous depolarization of the transepithelial (V_{te}), and hyperpolarization of the basolateral membrane potential (V_{bl}) produced by addition of glucose to the apical side of isolated proximal tubules. In both panels the superimposed periodic voltage deflections were produced by current pulses injected through the perfusion pipette.

TABLE 7.3 Cell Membrane Resistances in Mammalian Tubules (Ωcm^2 Epithelium)

Segment	Apical Resistance	Basolateral Resistance	Shunt Resistance	Method	Species	Reference
PCT	238	68	16	Apical glucose	Rabbit (PCT)	37
				Basal Ba[21]		
				Voltage divider		
PCT	118	39	8	Apical glucose	Rabbit (PCT)	141
				Voltage divider		
PCT	255	92	5	Apical glucose	Rat	142
				Voltage divider		
TALH	88	47	47	Apical high K^+, Ba^{2+}	Rabbit	41
				Voltage divider		
TALH	57	21	37	Apical Ba^{2+}	Mouse	12
				Voltage divider		
CCD	149	123	166	Apical Ba^{2+}	Rabbit	143
				Voltage divider		
CCD	57	80	230	Apical amiloride, Ba^{2+} +	Rabbit	144
				Voltage divider		
OMCD	707	176	393	Apical glucose	Rabbit	138,145
				Voltage divider		
Urinary bladder	3700 to 154,000	5000 to 10,300	6500 to 38,000	Apical amiloride		146
				Voltage divider	Rabbit	
				Cell cable		

Adapted from ref. [145]. TALH, thick ascending limb of Henle's loop; CCD, cortical collecting duct; OMCD, outer medullary collecting duct; PCT, proximal convoluted tubule.

and paracellular resistances that are in the same order of magnitude. Interestingly, both the diluting segment and collecting duct have higher shunt resistances and lower cellular resistances than the corresponding membrane of the proximal tubule. Mammalian collecting ducts and diluting segments also have higher shunt resistances than mammalian proximal tubules, although differences in cell resistance are less dramatic along the mammalian nephron.

The resistances quoted for the *Amphiuma* diluting segment in Table 7.4 assumed a single cell type throughout the cable analysis.[39] This greatly simplified the calculation of membrane resistance. Unfortunately, subsequent experiments indicated that this nephron segment actually consists of two different cell types with dissimilar conductive properties.[40] One cell type has a high basal K and Cl conductance (HBC), whereas the other cell type (LBC) has a low basolateral conductance for both ions.[40] There is also some evidence that mammalian TALH may exhibit a certain amount of cell heterogeneity as well.[41] Since it is unlikely that different cell types in the same nephron segment are directly coupled to each other, a unique value of cell membrane resistance cannot be determined from cable analysis on these nephron segments unless all recordings are made from the same cell type.

The cellular cable equations (Eqs. (7.18) and (7.19)) were originally derived for *in situ* proximal tubules, in which the cables are effectively infinite in length.[16] However, they should be reasonably valid for isolated perfused tubules as long as the voltage recording microelectrodes are several tubule diameters from either end of the tubule. Under these conditions the electrotonic voltage spread would be effectively the same as for an infinite cable. The problem of "cross-talk" or interactions between the transepithelial and cellular cables has been suggested as a source of error in these measurements.[42] The complication of cable–cable interactions would only be significant if current injected into the cell layer leaks into the lumen and then re-enters the cell layer at the some point downstream. A thorough analysis by Guggino et al.[16] for *Necturus* proximal tubule suggests that cross-talk will be negligible if intracellular voltage deflections ΔV_x are recorded at locations $x > \lambda_c$.

Evaluation of cell membrane resistance via Eqs. (7.14)–(7.16) is only as accurate as the equivalent circuit of Figure 7.7. An important aspect of this electrical model is the assumption that the tight junction constitutes the principal resistance of the paracellular pathway, or $R_{par} \approx R_{tj}$. This is probably true in tight epithelia like the urinary bladder, where the lateral intercellular space has a negligible resistance compared to that of the tight junction. However, the low transepithelial resistance of the proximal tubule raises the possibility

that the resistivity of free solution in the lateral space contributes significantly to overall shunt resistance. In this case, evaluation of the divider ratio is complicated by the lateral resistive network shown in Figure 7.1. Current flow through a distributed network of this kind will cause the measured value of $\Delta V_{ap}/\Delta V_{bl}$ to *underestimate* the actual value of R_{ap}/R_{bl}^* by an amount that depends on the ratio of lateral space resistance, R_{lis}, to paracellular resistance R_{par} (see Figure 7.9).

As illustrated in Figure 7.9, the larger the contribution of the fluid-filled interspace to the total paracellular resistance (i.e., the larger the ratio R_{lis}/R_{par}), the more the measured voltage ratio will underestimate the actual resistance ratio, γ. In epithelia where the paracellular resistance is essentially determined by the resistance of the tight junction and $R_{lis}/R_{par} < 0.01$, the resistance ratio (γ) will be correctly given by Eq. (7.16). On the other hand, if the lateral interspace is long and narrow and constitutes a non-negligible electrical resistance, R_{par} will be related to R_{te} according to a complicated function (see Eqs. (31–40)) of reference[6] with $R_3 = R_{par}$). As can be seen in the figure, significant deviations from Eq. (7.16) occur even if R_{lis} is as little as 10% of R_{par}. A detailed analysis regarding the effect of lateral resistive networks on measurement of cell membrane resistance has also been presented by Weber and Frömter.[43]

Determination of individual cell membrane resistances involves a number of technical difficulties. In addition to those indicated above, positioning of the intracellular electrodes is particularly tedious. If the first cell voltage electrode is within one cell length constant of the cell current electrode there may be significant cross-talk between cell and luminal cables. If the second cell voltage electrode is too far from the current injection electrode, the size of the deflection will be immeasurably small. Use of a third voltage recording electrode gives a better definition of the electrotonic voltage spread, but is often impractical. If sequential voltage impalements are used, the first recording should be made at the farthest distance from the current electrode. In this manner, intracellular recording at $x = L_1$ will be insignificantly affected by cell damage at $x = L_2$, as long as $L_2 > L_1$, and the current electrode is maintained at $x = 0$ (see Figure 7.2).

A significant source of error in cellular cable measurements arises from voltage-dependent membrane conductances. These can result from asymmetry of the electrolyte composition on the two sides of the membrane ("Goldman rectification"). Furthermore, patch-clamp experiments have indicated that a number of renal channels are voltage-gated. The specific magnitude and type of gating varies with each nephron segment. Since the current injections used for determination of cell membrane resistance often

TABLE 7.4   Cell Membrane Resistances in Amphibian Tubules (Ωcm^2 Epithelium)

Segment	Apical Resistance	Basolateral Resistance	Shunt Resistance	Method	Species	Reference
Proximal tubule	2509	683	71	Apical glucose Basal barium Voltage divider	*Ambystoma*	37
Proximal tubule	2305	591	53	2 electrode Cable analysis	*Ambystoma*	5,147
Proximal tubule	6957	2399	267	2 electrode Cable analysis	*Necturus*	16
Proximal tubule	2700	1900	—	2 electrode Cable analysis	Frog	148
Proximal tubule	1350	2100	166	2 electrode Cable analysis	*Triturus*	149
Dilute segment[a]	550	219	306	2 electrode Cable analysis	*Amphiuma*	39
Collecting tubule	154	192[b]	454	Voltage clamp Voltage divider	*Amphiuma*	53,150
Urinary bladder	9000–65,000	1000–7000	100,000	Apical amiloride Voltage divider	*Necturus*	151

[a] *These measurements assumed that the Amphiuma diluting segment has only one cell type.*
[b] *The basolateral conductance of this segment is strongly inward rectifying and quoted value applies only at a membrane potential of −60 mV.*

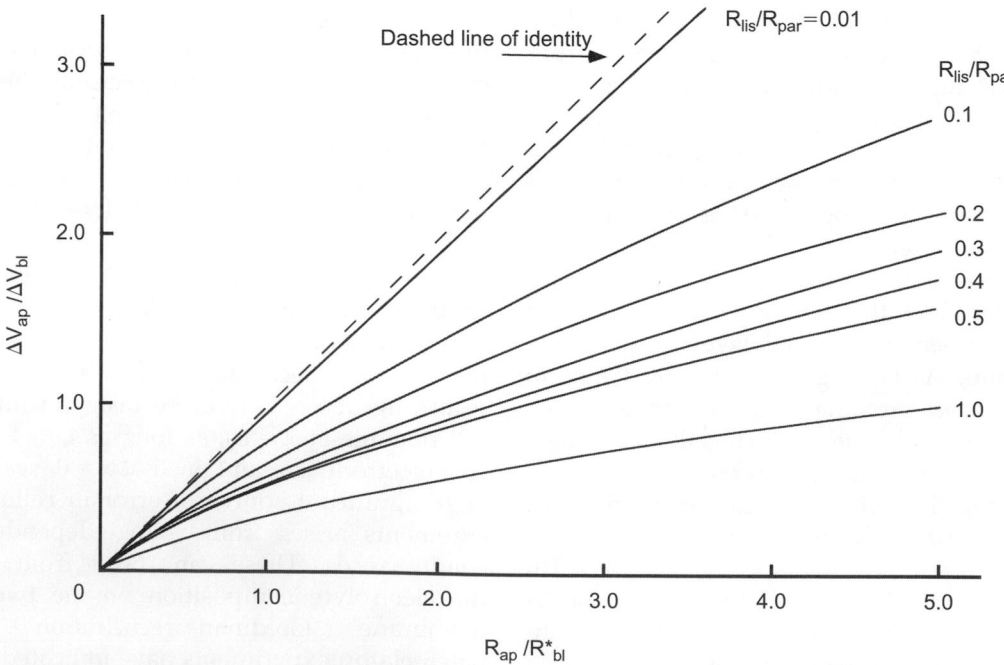

FIGURE 7.9   **Relationship between the measured voltage divider ratio ($\Delta V_{ap}/\Delta V_{bl}$) and the actual ratio of apical to basolateral resistance (R_{ap}/R_{bl}) at different values of fractional interspace resistance (R_{lis}/R_{par}).** Negligible values of R_{lis} result in the voltage divider ratio being a good measure of R_{ap}/R_{bl} (line of identity). In epithelia where R_{lis} is a significant fraction of the paracellular resistance, the voltage divider ratio is not a good measure of the apical to basal resistance ratio.[179]

produce 10 to 15 mV voltage deflections across the basolateral membrane, the conductance could be affected by the process of measurement. One solution to this difficulty has been to take the average value of ΔV_{bl} determined from both positive and negative going currents.

Evaluation of Ion Selectivities from Ion Substitution Experiments

One of the most important membrane properties that can be determined from electrophysiological measurements is membrane selectivity. The basic equation that defines the transference number of the membrane for ion x is obtained by rearranging Eq. (7.3) to yield Eq. (7.23) below:

$$t_x = - \frac{\Delta E}{\frac{RT}{z_x F} Ln \left[\frac{[X^{expt}]}{[X^{con}]} \right]}$$ (7.23)

Eq. (7.23) can then be used to evaluate the ion selectivity of the individual epithelial membranes from changes in the total EMF ΔE (expt − control) produced by replacement of a specific *apical* ion X by an impermeant ion. In Eq. (7.23), X^{expt} and X^{con} respectively refer to the extracellular ion concentration of the apical solution under experimental (expt) or control (con) conditions. If ΔE is produced by a change in *basolateral* composition, the transference numbers would be calculated from the negative of Eq. (7.23). As indicated in Figure 7.7b, the circulating current, I, prevents a simple equivalence between the measured change in potential difference (ΔV) and the actual change in the EMF of the membrane (ΔE). The effects of circular current flow on the actual changes in EMF resulting from ion substitution, ΔE, are described in detail in Appendix 7.2. These equations are essential for evaluating membrane selectivities from ion substitution experiments.

The partial conductance of the membrane for any ion "x" (G_x) can be determined from the transference number for the membrane and the total ionic conductance of that membrane (G_{tot}), according to Eq. (7.24):

$$G_x = t_x \cdot G_{tot}$$ (7.24)

There is no simple relation between the partial ionic *conductance* and the *permeability* of the membrane to a particular ion. However, it is possible to develop a general relation between the conductance and the permeability of a particular ion (X). This is given by Eq. (7.25), where $\langle X \rangle$ is a weighted average of the concentrations of X on both sides of the membrane. Its value depends on the particular assumptions about ion permeation across the membrane.

$$G_x \approx P_x \frac{z^2 F^2}{RT} \langle X \rangle$$ (7.25)

In the constant field assumption, $\langle X \rangle$ is a complicated function of both the membrane potential and the ion concentrations on both sides of the membrane. Explicit forms of Eq. (7.25) are discussed in Appendix 7.3. However, if the membrane is assumed to be permeant to only three ions: Na, K, and Cl, the permeability ratios P_{Na}/P_K and P_{Cl}/P_K can be evaluated from a two parameter fit to the general form of the Goldman−Hodgkin−Katz equation.[44] This procedure has not been used extensively for renal epithelia because of uncertainties in a simultaneous evaluation of P_{Na}/P_K and P_{Cl}/P_K.

On the other hand, if the membrane is primarily selective to two rather than three ions, a closed form expression can be obtained for the permeability ratio:

$$\frac{P_K}{P_{Na}} = \frac{[Na]_o - [Na]_i \exp\left(\frac{E_{rev}}{RT/F}\right)}{[K]_i \exp\left(\frac{E_{rev}}{RT/F}\right) - [K]_o}$$ (7.26)

In Eq. (7.26) the term, E_{rev}, is the potential difference, inside (i) minus outside (o), associated with zero current across the membrane. The principle disadvantage of Eq. (7.26) for kidney tubules is that determination of E_{rev} requires voltage-clamping the individual cell membranes of the epithelium. So far this has really only been accomplished for the *Amphiuma* collecting tubule.[21]

Since the specific conductance of a membrane for ion X is generally a function of the concentration of that ion (Eq. (7.25)), the values of t_x obtained from Eq. (7.23) only apply to the concentration range over which the ion replacement is actually performed. Consequently, any determination of normal transference numbers requires that the ionic replacement: $X^{con} - X^{expt}$ be as small as possible, but still produce a measurable ΔE. On the other hand, the permeability ratio of Eq. (7.26) should (in theory) be less dependent on external ion concentrations.

Estimation of Renal Na-K Pump Current and Electrogenic Potential

The 3Na/2K stoichiometry and electrogenic nature of the Na/K pump has been demonstrated in a number of non-epithelial tissues.[45,46] Most studies on red cells,[47,48] squid axon,[49] and Purkinje fibers[50] indicate a fairly consistent Na/K coupling ratio of 3/2 for the Na-K-ATPase. This electrogenicity not only causes the pump to contribute to total membrane potential, but also requires that the pump itself be dependent on membrane potential.

Mullins and Noda[51] and Ascher (cited in [52]) have derived an expression for the electrogenic contribution to the membrane potential of nerve and muscle cells which predicts a steady-state contribution of no larger than about 11 mV. This theory depends on the observation that electroneutrality conditions on symmetric cells require that there be no net macroscopic current under open-circuit, steady-state conditions. The estimate of 11 mV maximal electrogenic hyperpolarization also depends on the assumption that the membrane permeabilities are voltage independent, which is somewhat of an approximation, even for non-excitable tissues.

In epithelial tissues, where current circulates around a cellular and paracellular path (see Figure 7.7), the electrogenic contribution to the membrane potential may be larger than in symmetric cells, but it is also more difficult to quantify. Early estimates of pump current and electrogenic potential in epithelial tissues were determined by comparing the observed change in basolateral potential ΔV_{bl} to the potential changes predicted from the measured ion gradients and electrical resistances, during rapid return of K to the basolateral solution[5] or application of cardiac glycosides.[21,53] These experiments clearly demonstrated net transfer of charge by the pump, but uncertainty about the potassium concentration in unstirred layers outside the cell made it difficult to determine pump stoichiometry from these types of experiments.

In general, the calculation of the electrogenic potential in epithelial tissues requires explicit knowledge of both membrane and pump resistances, which may themselves be a function of pump activity (see Appendix 7.4). This significantly complicates the situation, and the electrogenicity of the pump is better characterized by evaluating its I−V relation than by evaluating its contribution to the open-circuit potential.

Since electrogenicity requires that pump current be sensitive to membrane potential, the I−V relation for the pump must intersect the voltage axis at some reversal potential E_p. The reversal potential of the pump should correspond to the membrane potential against which the pump can no longer translocate a net charge (i.e., 3Na for 2 K). The value of E_p can be calculated from Eq. (7.27) using estimates of the free energy of ATP hydrolysis (E_{ATP}) and the concentration work involved in moving "m" sodium ions (mE_{Na}) and "n" potassium ions (nE_K) per molecule of ATP split.[54]

$$E_p = EMF_{pump} = \frac{E_{ATP} + mE_{Na} - nE_K}{m - n} \qquad (7.27)$$

where E_{ATP} is the free energy of ATP hydrolysis (about −600 mV for m − n = 1, from ref [14]), and E_{Na}, E_K, are respectively the Na and K Nernst potentials across the membrane. For amphibian tubules, E_{Na} is about 55 mV and E_K is about −80 mV at room temperature. According to Eq. (7.27), the predicted value of E_p is about −275 mV for a net translocation of one (m − n) positive charge. This value of E_p corresponds to the reversal potential of the current−voltage relation for the pump.

The existence of a pump reversal potential defined by Eq. (7.27) provides no information about the sensitivity of pump current to membrane voltage. This sensitivity is determined by the specific shape of the current−voltage (I−V) relation of the pump. For example, if the pump I−V relation exhibits a low angle slope in the region of normal membrane potential, the pump would be best represented as a (Norton equivalent) constant current source. On the other hand, if the I−V relation is linear between zero voltage and the pump reversal potential, the pump would be best represented as a (Thevenin equivalent) constant voltage source (Figures 7.1 and 7.7). Four examples of I−V relations for the Na,K-ATPase are illustrated in Figure 7.10.

These pump, current−voltage relations were determined by measuring either the strophanthidin (a, c) or the ouabain (b, d)-sensitive currents at different voltages. Figure 7.10a and 7.10b are I−V relations from symmetric cell preparations, whereas Figure 7.10c and 7.10d were measured in renal epithelia. In both isolated guinea-pig ventricular myocytes[55] and *Xenopus* oocytes,[56] pump current is linearly dependent on membrane voltage with a reversal potential of at least −150 mV. Saturation of current, with decreasing slope, was only evident at positive membrane potentials.

On the other hand, voltage-clamp studies in amphibian (*Amphiuma*) collecting tubules[21] indicate a curvilinear I−V relation (Figure 7.10c), which would imply that (in this tissue) the Na,K pump behaves as a constant current source at normal membrane potentials (− 20 mV to −75 mV). Differences in the I−V curves of Figures 7.10a, 7.10b, and 7.10c may indicate true distinctions between Na pumps of different preparations or may simply reflect differences in experimental technique. The final I−V relation (Figure 7.10d)[57] indicates that the pump current in the mammalian CCD, like that of symmetric cells, is sensitive to voltage in the physiological range.

The variability in the shape of the I−V relations for the Na,K-ATPase (Figure 7.10) implies some uncertainty as to whether the Na pump of a particular tissue behaves more like a constant current or a constant voltage source. Nonetheless, we have chosen to represent the Na pump in the equivalent circuits of Figures 7.1 and 7.7 as a voltage source (E_p) in series with an internal resistance (R_p), because this is a somewhat more general form than a constant-current source.

CONCLUSIONS

With the use of microelectrodes to record intracellular voltages and voltage changes, it has been possible to characterize renal epithelia according to the equivalent circuit in Figure 7.1. Overall conductances of apical and basolateral membranes can be computed, and the contribution of various ions to these conductances can be estimated. Our understanding of the major nephron segments at this level is fairly secure. In the next section we discuss how measurements at the single-channel level have yielded a more detailed description of renal ion transport processes.

Patch-Clamp and Single-Channel Analysis

Defining a Channel

The ability to measure currents through individual ion channels in small "patches" of biological membranes has, over the course of the last 25 years, increased enormously the type of information that can be gleaned about ion channels and the details of our knowledge of how these transport proteins work. With this technique we can find out how many different types of channels there are in a membrane, and how many of each type is present, without the need for specific pharmacological agents. It is possible to determine what gene produces a given membrane conductance by comparing the properties of the channels in that membrane with those of the gene product when it is heterologously expressed in another cells type. In other cases a gene can be specifically deleted using genetic techniques, and the disappearance of a channel type from the membrane can be followed. The patch-clamp technique can also be very useful to determine what agents or second messengers directly or indirectly regulate ion channels.

An ion channel is defined in physical terms as a membrane protein which forms a continuous pathway for the diffusion of an ion from one side of the membrane to the other. In contrast to active transporters, the direction of movement of the ion is determined by the electrochemical energy difference across the membrane. Unlike more complex "carriers" (including facilitated transporters and co- and counter-transporters) a conformation change in the channel protein is not required for the translocation of the ions. This permits ions to move quite quickly through the channels. While co-transporters or exchangers generally have maximal turnover rates of about 10^5/sec, and metabolically driven pumps are even slower, channels can achieve rates of 10^8/sec or more through individual units.[58]

Most channels exhibit gating; they switch between distinct open and closed states, producing abrupt transitions in current under voltage-clamp conditions. Patch-clamp recording can generally resolve currents of around 10^6/sec or 0.15 pA. Thus, the ability to see an individual transport unit using the patch-clamp is a reasonably good operating definition of a channel. Although the appearance of current transitions is a good operational definition of channel activity, this is actually too restrictive since some channels may have a low turnover rate. Nevertheless the definition is a useful one, and most channels that we know about have currents large enough — at least under optimal conditions — to be seen by patch-clamp.

Most biologically important channels will also have a density high enough to be observed frequently. For a moderate membrane conductance of 1 mS/cm^2, a single channel conductance of 40 pS and an open probability of 0.5, the density of channels will be 5×10^7/cm^2 or 0.5/μm^2. If a patch contains 5 μm^2 it will have on the average 2 to 3 channels. This simple calculation illustrates that a patch pipette of average diameter will usually contain at least one channel, making this technique a highly efficient method for studying the characteristics of individual ion channels.

High resolution patch-clamp recording was developed in the early 1980s by Neher, Sackmann, and colleagues.[35] The patch methodology consists of four major configurations, three of which can be used to study single channels. As illustrated in Figure 7.11, the cell-attached patch consists simply of forming a seal on the surface of a cell, and studying the resulting piece of membrane *in situ*. This is obviously the most physiological condition. The same patch can be excised from the cell membrane, forming an inside-out patch in which the cytoplasmic surface of the membrane now faces the bathing medium. This is useful for studying the effects of second messengers and other cytoplasmic components which can be added back to the medium to test for their ability to regulate the channels. A cell-attached patch can also be broken with suction, to form a whole-cell voltage-clamp. This is a very convenient method for studying the total current from the entire cell membrane. It is usually not possible to resolve single-channel events in this configuration, although noise analysis of whole-cell recordings can give information about single-channel properties (see below). Finally, withdrawing the pipette from the cell under the whole-cell condition often gives rise to the outside-out configuration, in which a new patch is formed with the former extracellular surface of the membrane facing the bath. This can be used to study the effects of hormones, drugs, and other ligands which interact with the external face of the channel.

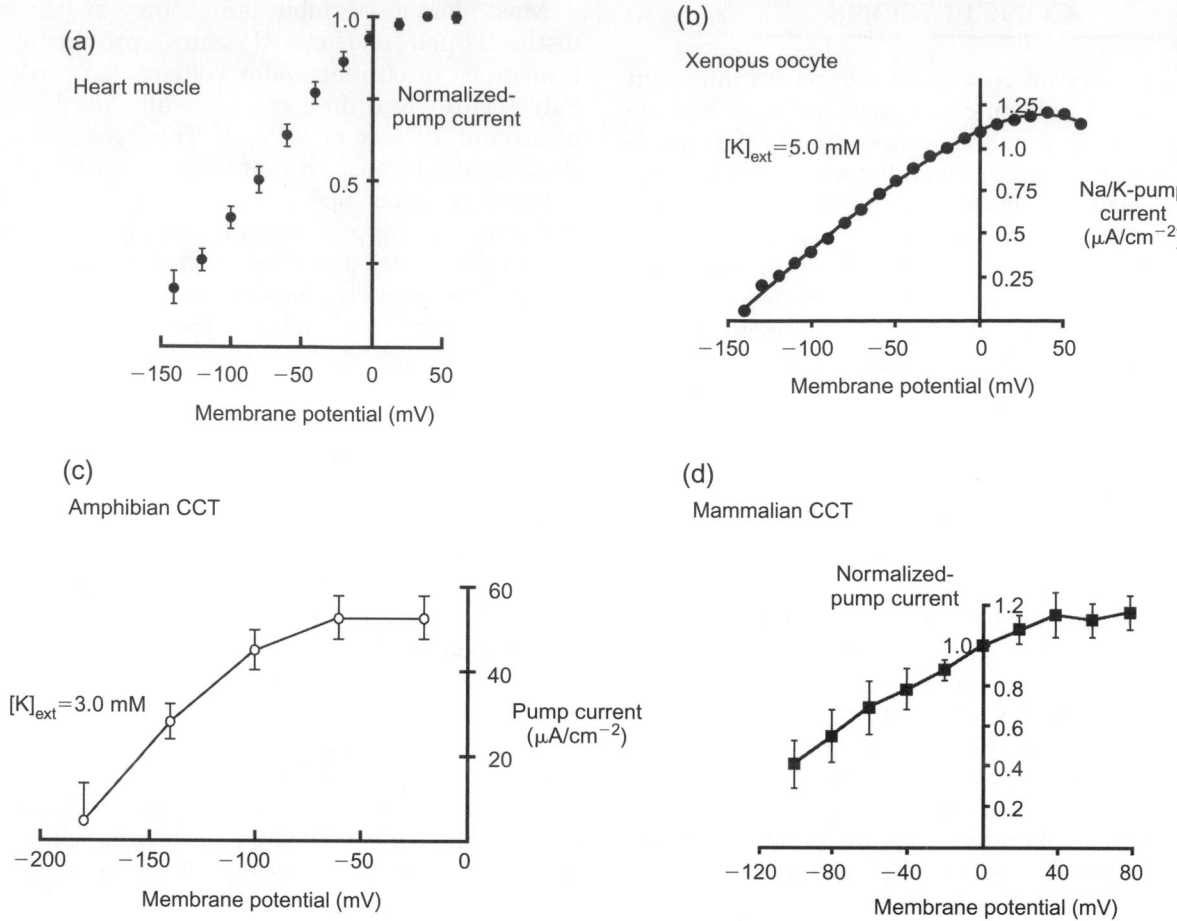

FIGURE 7.10 (a) Current-voltage relation of the cardiac Na-K-ATPase as determined from the strophanthidin-sensitive pump current in a whole-cell recording from a single isolated ventricular myocyte. Dissipative current pathways were blocked with Cs, Cd, TEA, and Ba (from [55]). (b) Current-voltage relation for the Na/K pump of *Xenopus* oocytes, bathed in a 90 mM Na, 5 mM K solution. Pump current was determined as the difference between current measured at 5 mM external K and current measured in K-free solutions (from [180]). (c) Current-voltage relation of the basolateral Na pump of *Amphiuma* collecting tubule as determined from the strophanthidin-sensitive current in short segments of voltage-clamped tubules (from [150]). (d) Current-voltage relation of the rat principal cell Na-K-ATPase. Ouabain-sensitive currents were normalized to their values at zero mV (from [57]).

PARAMETERS MEASURED ON SINGLE CHANNELS

Single-Channel Current

The simplest measure of channel electrical activity is the single-channel current (Figure 7.12). This is the change in current under voltage-clamp conditions which occurs when a channel opens or closes. It is generally quite reproducible for a given set of conditions, but varies with ion concentration, temperature, and voltage. It is common to characterize channels by their single-channel conductance. This is defined as the slope of the current versus the voltage relationship. For some channels this conductance is roughly independent of voltage. Many others, however, have highly non-linear current-voltage relationships. In the latter case, the voltage at which the conductance was measured must always be specified.

Normally, the lowest single channel conductance that can be reliably measured is in the neighborhood of 1 pS. This would correspond to measuring a 0.1 pA current at an electrical driving force of 100 mV. Most channels can conduct much larger currents; an upper limit of about 33 pA has been estimated from limitations of diffusion rates.[58] Eukaryotes have channels with conductances up to about 400 pS.

Some channels have more than one conducting state. Usually the largest one is chosen as the characteristic conductance, and smaller ones are referred to as "sub-conductance" states. Presumably these reflect different conformations of the channel protein. In one special case of the Cl channel CLC-0, the channel has two conductance states, with one being precisely half of the

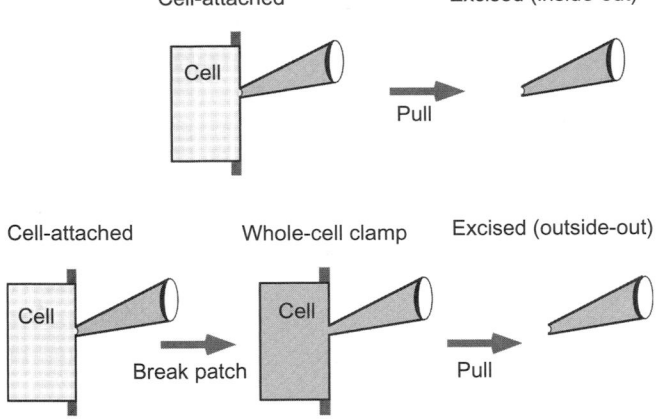

Cell-attached   Excised (inside-out)

Cell

Pull

Cell-attached   Whole-cell clamp   Excised (outside-out)

Cell

Cell

Break patch

Pull

FIGURE 7.11 **Schematic of the patch-clamp technique, applied to the apical membrane of an epithelium.** Patch-clamping the basolateral membrane involves a similar procedure. In a cell-attached recording, the cell retains its original composition. Formation of a (conventional) whole-cell clamp causes most of the cell contents to be replaced by pipette solution. Withdrawal of the pipette from the whole-cell configuration often produces an excised, outside-out patch.

other.[59] The interpretation of these results was that two identical conducting pores are linked together such that they can close either separately or together. The "full" conductance state represents both pores conducting simultaneously, and the "sub" conductance state reflects the opening of just one of them. In general, the structural basis of subconductance states — which can have any fraction of the full conductance — is not well-understood.

Channel Selectivity

In addition to conductance, the ionic selectivity of the channel can also be determined from single-channel i-V plots under appropriate conditions. As in the case of macroscopic currents discussed in the last section, the selectivity of an individual ion channel can be defined and measured in different ways. Inside-out and outside-out patches are particularly well suited for measurements of permeability ratios, since the ions on both sides of the membrane can be set to known concentrations.

The ionic transference numbers for a channel can be evaluated using the same relationships discussed previously (see Eq. (7.23)). However, instead of perturbing the concentration of an ion across the membrane, it is simpler in a patch-clamp experiment to change the transmembrane voltage (see Eq. (7.26)). The reversal potential (E_{rev}) is then defined as the voltage at which current flow through the channel changes direction. Measurement of E_{rev} is easiest to interpret in excised patches, where ionic concentrations can be precisely controlled. For measurement of cation versus anion

selectivity, dilution conditions are normally used, with a single salt at different concentrations (S1 and S2) on both sides of the membrane. For the case of a monovalent salt:

$$E_{rev} = (t_+ - t_-)\frac{RT}{F}Ln\frac{S_1}{S_2} \qquad (7.28)$$

where t_+ and t_- are the transference numbers for ion movement through the individual pore, and S_1 and S_2 are the salt concentrations on either side of the membrane. This is equivalent to Eq. (7.12). Thus, if a channel has perfect selectivity for cations (or for anions) the reversal potential will shift by 59 mV for a 10-fold concentration gradient (at 25°C).

The permeability ratio is a common measure of the selectivity among ions of the same charge. In general, the permeability ratio can be computed from a constant-field equation similar to Eq. (7.26). This equation reduces to a particularly simple and useful form under bi-ionic conditions, with two different salts at the same concentration on either side of the membrane (e.g., NaCl and KCl for an exclusively cation-selective channel):

$$E_{rev} = \frac{RT}{F}Ln\frac{P_x}{P_y} \qquad (7.29)$$

where P_x and P_y represent the permeabilities of the two ions x and y. A selectivity (permeability ratio) of 10 will give rise to a reversal potential of 59 mV at 25°C. Notice that Eq. (7.29) does not involve the actual salt concentration, as long as the concentration of salt X on one side is the same as the concentration of salt Y on the other side.

The relative permeability of a channel to different ions can be measured in cell-attached patches, even when the intracellular ion composition is not precisely known, from changes in the single-channel reversal potential associated with different patch pipette solutions. When the highly selective renal K channel, ROMK2, is expressed in K-depolarized *Xenopus* oocytes, the single-channel (cell-attached) i-V curve intersects the origin at a reversal potential of zero (solid line, Figure 7.13). When the same experiment is performed with Rb (rather than K) in the patch pipette, the single channel i-V relation becomes less steep, and the reversal potential shifts in a negative direction by 14 mV (dashed line, Figure 7.13). Using Eq. (7.29), this change in reversal potential implies a permeability ratio, $P_{Rb}/P_K = 0.63$ for ROMK2, expressed in *Xenopus* oocytes.

Ionic selectivity can also be estimated from single-channel conductance ratios determined under different ionic conditions. These can be compared with selectivity ratios derived from the permeability ratios described above. In general, the conductance ratio will

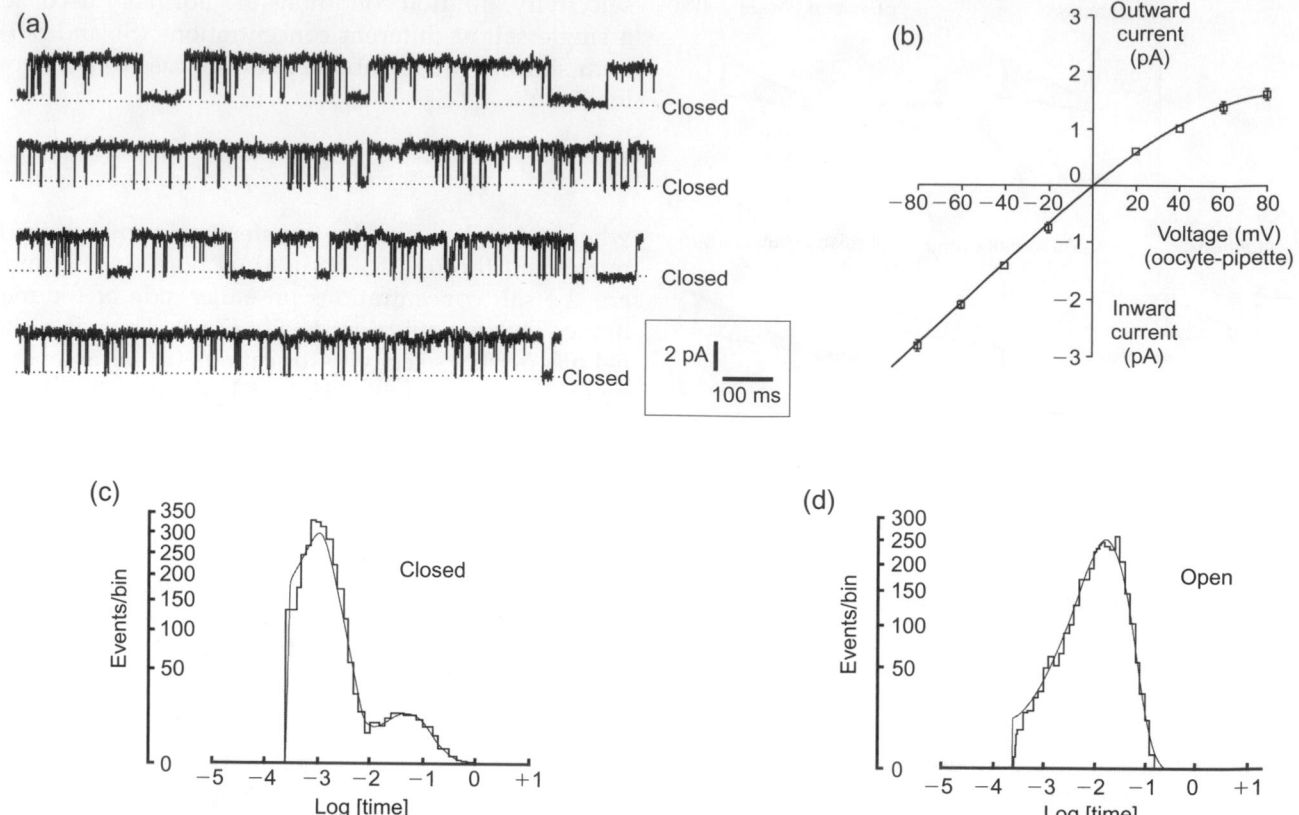

FIGURE 7.12 Example of single-channel current records and associated analysis. ROMK2 was expressed in *Xenopus* oocytes, and currents were recorded from a single channel in a cell-attached patch. The oocyte membrane potential was reduced close to zero by 100 mM KCl in the bath. The patch pipette also contained 100 mM KCl. Neither divalent ions nor specific chelating agents like EDTA were added to the pipette. (a) Currents recorded with the membrane potential clamped at -80 mV (cytoplasm relative to pipette). Upward deflections from the closed state correspond to inward K currents. (b) Current voltage relation for ROMK2, constructed by recording currents at different (clamped) membrane potentials. (c) Closed time distribution at -80 mV, showing two discrete closed states with time constants of 1.2 msec and 47 msec. (d) Open time distribution at -80 mV, with mean open time of 19 msec (from [60]).

differ from the permeability ratio, derived from reversal potentials and Eq. (7.29). For example, using the data of Figure 7.13, the ratio of inward Rb conductance to inward K conductances is $g_{Rb}/g_K = 0.36$. This differs significantly from the permeability ratio, $P_{Rb}/P_K = 0.63$ determined from reversal potentials. The discrepancy is even larger when the selectivity of K versus NH_4 is considered. Here the shift in reversal potential implies $P_{NH4}/P_K = 0.1$. However, the conductance to NH_4 at large negative potentials is equal to or higher than that to K at voltages driving inward currents, giving $g_{NH4}/g_K \geq 1$.[60,61] Discrepancies of this kind may indicate an interaction between the permeant ions and the channel. Rb may bind tightly a particular site within the pore, thus passing slowly through the channel. However, this binding will displace K from the channel, also reducing K conductance. The permeability ratio will reflect the relative affinity of the binding site for the two ions. Conversely, NH_4 may bind less tightly than K within the conduction pathway.

Open Probability

A second fundamental parameter of an ion channel that can be measured directly using single-channel recording is the open probability (P_o) or the fraction of time the channel spends in the open state. If there is only a single channel in the patch, P_o is determined by dividing the amount of time spent in the open state by the total recording time. P_o can also be measured in patches with more than one channel, provided that the number of channels (N) is known. This requires identification of the states with all channels open and with all channels closed, as discussed below.

A useful measure of overall channel activity in multichannel patches is the mean number of open channels, defined by Eq. (7.30):

$$NP_o = \sum_{n=1}^{N} nP_n \qquad (7.30)$$

where P_n equals (the dwell time with n channels open)/(total time); and N is the total number of

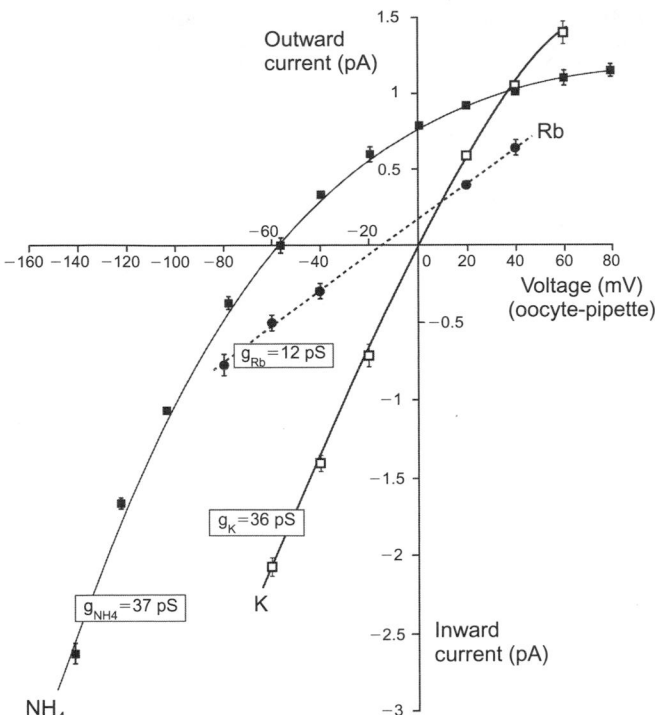

FIGURE 7.13 Differences between relative conductances and relative permeabilities. When R_b replaces K as the permeating cation of ROMK2, there is a shift in both the reversal potential (x intercept) and single-channel conductance (slope) of the i-V relation. The Rb/K permeability ratio calculated from the change in reversal potential was 0.63, which is significantly larger than the Rb/K conductance ratio of 0.36 determined from the inward slopes of the i-V curves. Similarly, the NH_4/K permeability ratio calculated from the change in reversal potential was 0.12, compared to a NH_4/K inward conductance ratio of unity (from [60]).

channels in the patch. Single-channel open probability (P_o) can be readily determined from Eq. (7.30), if the number (N) of channels in the patch is known. One caveat is that channels whose kinetics are very slow relative to the recording time may not be counted by Eq. (7.30).

An alternative method for estimating open probability is to compare the total macroscopic current (I) resulting from N channels to the single channel current (i), using Eq. (7.31), assuming that the number of channel proteins (N^*) can be measured independently. Under these conditions, the open probability would be given by (P^*_o):

$$P^*_o = I/N^*i \qquad (7.31)$$

In *Xenopus* oocytes expressing ENaC channels, P^*_o was estimated to be 0.05 with Eq. (7.31) (Table 7.5). This is an order of magnitude lower than the P_o of about 0.5 that was determined by conventional electrical methods.[62] Presumably, this difference reflects a large number of silent channels, which are electrically invisible and therefore do not contribute to patch-clamp determinations of P_o. Equations (7.30) and (7.31) yield comparable estimates of P_o only for the special case where all channels in the membrane are active during the electrical measurements.

NUMBER OF CHANNELS

The number of channels in a patch (N) divided by the area of the patch will reflect, on average, the density of channels in the membrane. In principle, N can be observed. In practice, not all the possible current levels will be visited during the lifetime of the recording. This is particularly problematic when the P_o of the channels is either very low or very high. Sometimes this difficulty can be mitigated by maximally activating or deactivating channels at the end of a recording by applying voltage or chemical regulators.

If the properties of all channels are identical and are independent of each other, then the percentage of time spent in each state (e.g., 1 channel open, 2 channels open, etc.) should follow the binomial distribution. Fitting the measured distribution of times with a binomial function can then be used to estimate channel number.[63] This method is less biased than that of counting current levels, as the latter will always be an underestimate. However, the assumption that channels have identical kinetics is probably not always valid.

In some cases the kinetics of the channels can be used to estimate N. If all channels have a high P_o such that the state with all channels open is clearly defined, and a reproducible mean open time t_{open} (see below), then the mean time that an ensemble of N channels will stay in the all-open state will be t_{open}/N. Thus, N can be estimated even if the current level with all channels closed is never directly identified.[64] A similar procedure can be used on channels with a low P_o if the mean closed time is reproducible. This procedure works only if the channels have a single open (or closed) state (see below).

The area of patches is also difficult to quantify precisely. When the membrane patch can be seen in the light microscope, it often appears to be drawn a considerable distance into the patch-clamp pipette by the process of seal formation.[65,66] A typical patch geometry might correspond to a membrane area of about 5 μm^2. Areas estimated from electrical capacitance measurements varied from about 1 μm^2 to over 15 μm^2.[65] The area will depend on both the size of the micropipette and the cell type. Perhaps the surest way of estimating single-channel density is to combine single-channel measurements with a macroscopic measurement. For example, the number of Na channels in the apical membrane of the rat CCD has been estimated from the whole-cell, amiloride-sensitive conductance, and the

TABLE 7.5 Open Probability of Na Channels Expressed in *Xenopus* Oocytes[a]

Direct measurement: $P_o = 0.42$	Patch-clamp
Macroscopic current: $I = 0.94\,\mu A$ (100 mV)	TEVC
Single-channel current: $i = 0.60$ (-100 mV)	Patch-clamp
Channel number $N^* = 1.7 \times 10^8/$cell	Ab binding (assume 4 subunits/channel)
Open probability: $P_o{}^* = I/N^*i = 0.04$	

[a]Data from [62].

TABLE 7.6 Computation of Na-Channel Density in Rat[a]

Macroscopic conductance: $I_{Na} = 510\,pA/cell$ ($V_m = -100$ mV)	Whole-cell clamp
Apical membrane area: $A = 185\,\mu m^2/cell$	Morphological studies
Single channel conductance: $i_{Na} = 0.81\,pA$ ($V_m = -100$ mV)	Patch-clamp
Open probability: $P_o = 0.5$	Patch-clamp
Channel density $N = I_{Na}/[A \cdot i_{Na} \cdot P_o]$	
$N = 1260/cell = 6.8\,\mu m^2$	

[a]Data from [152–154].

average single-channel conductance and open probability measured under similar conditions (Table 7.6).

OPEN AND CLOSED TIMES

All channels that open and close can be characterized, not only by the percent time in the open state (P_o), but also by the mean times spent in these states or, equivalently, the rates of transition between them. The mean lifetimes of the open and closed states can range from less than 1 msec to more than 1 second. The lifetimes of a given state are presumed to be exponentially distributed, similar to those of radioactive isotopes. The transition rates can be estimated by plotting the number of open (or closed) events of a given duration as a function of that duration.

In the simplest kinetic scheme, a channel that has just one open and one closed state can be diagrammed as follows:

```
Open  ⟷  Closed
```

This will result in open- and closed-time histograms which are monotonically decreasing functions of interval length, and which can be fitted by a single exponential decay curve.

In practice, the kinetic parameters of a particular channel are usually estimated by fitting the open and closed dwell time distributions with multiple exponential components. In this regard, it has proved most useful to generate event histograms with a logarithmic time axis and a square root transformation of the ordinate.[67] This greatly simplifies interpretation and fitting of distributions that contain multiple exponential components. Examples of two such fitted distributions are shown in Figure 7.12c and Figure 7.12d, respectively, for the closed and open times of single ROMK2 channels expressed in

Xenopus oocytes. In this type of representation, the peaks of each of the skewed, bell-shaped curves correspond to time constants for the open and closed states of the channel.

Even after the number and duration of closed and open states have been determined, the exact kinetic scheme for the channel may still be ambiguous. Both of the models depicted below are consistent with two closed states and one open state. The first model corresponds to transitions between a single open state and a long-lived closed state (closed 2) that can only be reached by passage through a short-lived closed state (closed 1). In the second model, both the short and long-lived closed states are accessible from the open state. Even with this modest degree of complexity these two patterns cannot readily be distinguished, and the rate constants among the states cannot always be unequivocally derived.

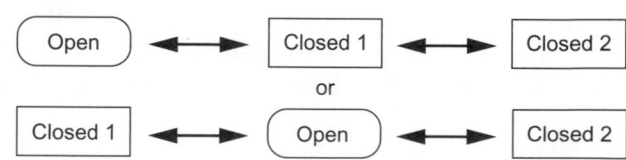

Channels can have multiple open states as well as multiple closed states. In Ca-activated BK channels, for example, models with 50 different states are required to portray channel kinetics.[68] As the number of possible open and closed states increases, the difficulty of the analysis increases as well, making it difficult to assign values to individual rate constants or to distinguish alternative kinetic schemes.

The situation can be even more complicated if the channel exhibits bursts of activity that are themselves part of a larger pattern of activity. This behavior requires even more states. Alternatively, a kinetic scheme based on fractals has been proposed[69] on the basis that a burst within a burst pattern will continue to be observed as the time domain over which measurements are made becomes smaller or larger. The relative merits of fractal models as opposed to the more conventional discrete-state models are discussed in detail elsewhere.[70–72] Although the fractal approach is mathematically elegant, it is rarely used in practice since discrete-state models more closely correspond to the simple physical picture of a channel protein having several alternative conformations. It emphasizes, however, that the kinetic models are based on measurable time scales determined by technical limitations. Events of <0.1 msec duration are difficult to resolve with current instrumentation. On the other side of the spectrum, it is difficult to record a sufficient number of events of duration >10 sec to analyze accurately.

In some cases multiple gating "modes" have been distinguished from different kinetic states.[73,74] Here a channel will shift abruptly from one pattern of gating to another. This can be thought of as preserving the same open and closed states, but changing the rate constants for moving from one state to another. In some cases, changes in gating mode could reflect a chemical modification of a channel, such as a change in the phosphorylation state. However, reversible mode switches have also been observed with channels reconstituted into planar lipid bilayers.[75] In these cases the modes must be intrinsic to the channel proteins themselves.

Channel Pharmacology

Another defining characteristic of a channel type is its response to pharmacological agents, usually those which block the channel. If a specific blocker can be identified, it is also quite useful to compare single-channel data with macroscopic currents, similar to what was shown above for estimation of channel density. Amiloride is a commonly used blocker for epithelial Na channels, whereas Ba, TEA or Cs, block K channels. The dihydropyridines and certain divalent cations such as Cd^{+2} block Ca-selective channels, disulfonic stilbenes as well as a variety of organic anions block Cl channels, and gadolinium inhibits stretch-activated cation channels. A variety of naturally produced toxins work by blocking ion channels; most are directed against voltage-gated channels in excitable epithelia. However, tertiapin, a component of honey-bee venom, is a potent and fairly selective blocker of the renal K channel ROMK.[76,77] In addition, high-throughput screening has been used to identify novel inhibiters of specific ion channels. This approach has identified small-molecule blockers of ROMK channels that may be useful for *in vivo* or clinical applications.[78]

Channel blockers can affect either the open probability of the channel or its (apparent) single-channel conductance. The effect depends on the rates of association and dissociation of the blocker with the channel. In particular, if the off-rate is *slow* relative to the bandwidth of the recording device and the duration of the spontaneous open and closed states, the blocking action will be revealed as a new long-lived closed state. Block of the maxi-K channel by Ba^{+2} on the cytoplasmic side is an example of this type of interaction (Figure 7.14a). On the other hand, if the blocking action is *fast* relative to the bandwidth, it will show up as a decrease in the apparent single-channel conductance. Block of the maxi-K channel by extracellular TEA is a good example (Figure 7.14b).

Often the on-rates for blocking ions are diffusion-limited, i.e., very roughly in the range of $10^8 \, sec^{-1} \, M^{-1}$. In this case, the rates of unblocking are inversely related to the affinities of block. For blockers with affinities in the nM range, the off-rate will be $10^{-1}/sec$. This is a slow block, with a mean lifetime of the blocked state of 10 sec. For blockers with affinities in the μM range the mean lifetime could be 10 msec, corresponding to an intermediate blocking speed in which the blocking events are readily observed in patch-clamp recordings. For blockers with affinities in the mM range, the mean lifetime of the closed state would be 10 μsec, too fast to be resolved under most conditions.

There are at least two basic mechanisms of block, regardless of the blocking kinetics. In one, the blocker enters the pore part way, and sticks there by binding to a site within the pore. This type of block is usually voltage-dependent, particularly if the blocker is charged, since the transmembrane electric field will tend to either pull it into the pore or push it out. Voltage dependence may also arise if the blocker displaces permeant ions from the electric field. Examples of this type of block include those of Mg^{+2} and polyamines in inward-rectifier channels,[79] Ba^{+2} on several types of K channels,[80] and amiloride on the epithelial Na channel.[81] Another type of block involves an allosteric interaction with the channel protein. This changes the conformation of the protein to one in which the pore is closed or stabilizing a spontaneously occurring closed conformation. A well-studied example of this type of block is that of dihydropyridines on voltage-dependent Ca-channels.[73] The second type of block may be voltage-independent. However, a voltage-dependence could arise if the conformational change involves a movement of charge on the channel protein with respect to the electric field across the membrane.

(a)

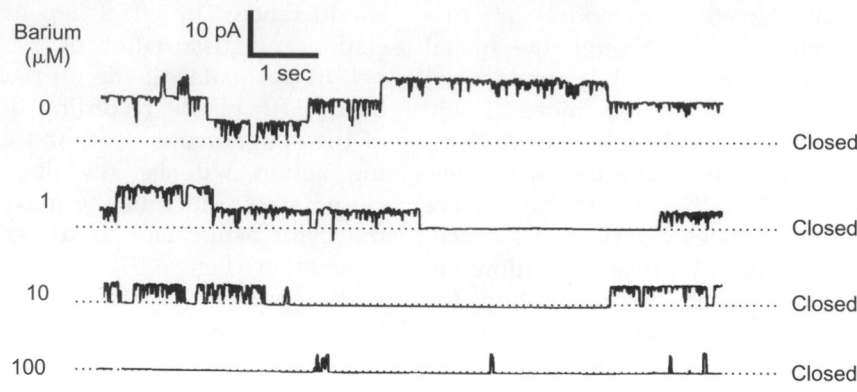

(b)

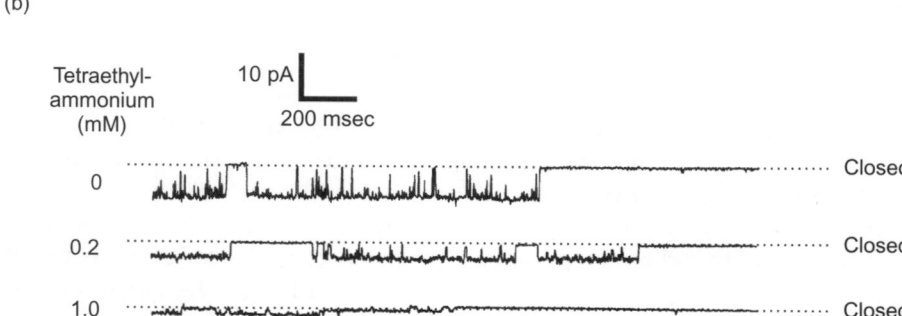

FIGURE 7.14 Comparison of (a) block of maxi-K channels by a slow blocker, Ba, which is effective at micromolar concentrations and reduces the open probability, with (b) block by tetraethyl ammonium, which is effective at mM concentrations and reduces the apparent single channel conductance (from [181]).

APPLICATION TO EPITHELIA

One of the major difficulties in the application of the patch-clamp technique to renal epithelia has been gaining access to the plasma membranes. Different methods have been used for both apical and basolateral membranes.

Apical Membranes

One successful approach to gaining access to the apical membrane is to split the tubules mechanically and flatten them onto their basolateral surfaces.[82,83] The use of a transparent, non-toxic, molluscan adhesive (Cell-Tak, Becton-Dickinson, Bedford, MA) has greatly improved attachment of the basement membrane to the bottom of the chamber and increased the stability of the patch-clamp recording.[82,84] An example of a split, flattened proximal tubule from *Necturus*

maculosus is shown in Figure 7.15. Absence of staining with Trypan blue, except around the edge of the tissue, indicates viability of most of the hexagonal cells. Gigaohm seals can be formed on the apical surface of this preparation (shadow of a patch pipette can be seen near the center of the field). Although splitting individual nephron segments works best in large, amphibian tubules,[82,84–86] it has also been successfully used in mammalian CCD and TALH.[83,87,88]

A second approach to patch-clamping the apical surface of renal tubules has been to insert a micropipette into the open lumen of a perfused tubule.[89] This has the advantage of maintaining the tubule in the perfused state, and theoretically permits independent control of the solution on both sides of the tubule. However, this technique significantly increases the complexity of the patch-clamp procedure and decreases cell visibility, making it difficult or impossible to be absolutely sure which cell type is actually being studied within a given nephron segment.

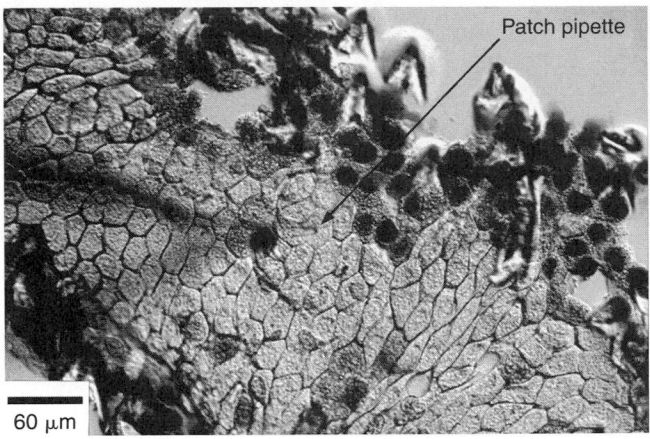

Patch pipette

60 μm

FIGURE 7.15 **Light micrograph of split-open *Necturus* proximal tubule (apical side up), viewed from below with modulation contrast optics.** The tissue was attached with Cell-Tak. Nuclei of damaged cells at the periphery are readily identified by their uptake of Trypan blue. Undamaged cells are approximately hexagonal in shape and exhibit well-defined boundaries with a diagonal diameter of about 30 μm. The tip and shadow of a patch pipette are visible at the left of the figure.

Another technique that preserves the separation of apical and basolateral solutions entails the eversion of the entire tubule, which can then be perfused with the luminal surface on the outside.[90–92] This approach has the advantage of maintaining the integrity of the entire tubule, but is technically demanding.

Finally, renal cells can be studied in culture, taking advantage of the tendency of epithelial cells to attach to a suitable substrate with their basolateral side down, leaving the apical membranes facing up and accessible for patch-clamping. Both continuous cell lines[93–95] and primary cultures of renal tubules[34,84,86,96–98] have been used. A problem with this approach is the difficulty of preserving the properties of the original cells in culture. One cell line which does appear to closely resemble native epithelial cells from the distal nephron is the A6 line from *Xenopus* kidney.[99] This has been a particularly useful preparation for studying epithelial Na channels.[93,100–102] A mammalian cell line that also preserves a distal nephron phenotype and has been used for patch-clamp is the mouse line mpkCCDc14.[95,103]

Basolateral Membranes

Basolateral channels are difficult to study because the basal surface is covered with a basement membrane that must be removed to allow access to the plasma membrane. With isolated amphibian tubules it has been possible to gain access to the basolateral membrane by manually removing a small segment of basement membrane.[84,104] This process has also been applied to the mammalian collecting tubule.[105] However, most patch-clamp studies on mammalian basolateral membranes have used pre-treatment of the

tubules with a collagenase solution to remove enough of the basement membrane to permit formation of a high resistance patch-clamp seal.[105–109]

In an effort to circumvent the possible problems associated with enzymatic digestion, the lateral cell membranes of mammalian nephron segments have been patch-clamped either on the open end of a perfused tubule[89] or by mechanically removing an adjacent cell in an otherwise intact epithelium. The latter method was used to study basolateral channels on the lateral membrane of principal cells of rat CCD.[110] Here, a suction pipette is used to remove an entire intercalated cell from a split-open rat collecting tubule. This exposes a clean, lateral surface of an adjacent principal cell on which a high resistance seal can be formed with a standard patch pipette (Figure 7.16).

Isolated Cells

Another way of gaining access to either the apical or basolateral cell membranes is to use isolated, polarized cells, derived by a brief collagenase or trypsin treatment of the epithelium. This weakens the basement membrane sufficiently so that individual, undamaged cells can be obtained by moderate mechanical agitation. A number of studies have been carried out using isolated cell preparations of proximal tubules, since these cells often retain their polarity for extended periods.[111–115] Detailed cytochemical studies on isolated cells of this type have confirmed the stability of markers normally associated with either the apical or basolateral membranes of intact epithelia.[115] An example of an isolated amphibian proximal tubule cell is illustrated in Figure 7.16.[112,115] These cells maintain their polarity by assuming a bi-spherical,

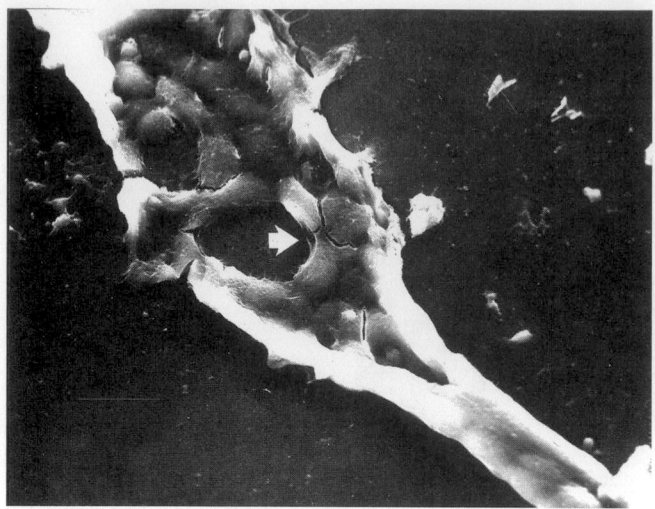

FIGURE 7.16　Scanning electron micrograph of split open CCD. Arrow shows lateral membrane of a principal cell. The intercalated cell adjacent to the principal cell was removed by mechanical suction, leaving the principal cell intact (from [110]).

minimum energy configuration. In this picture the apical surface, with brush border, is clearly visible as the smaller hemisphere, whereas the larger spherical surface consists of basolateral membrane.

NOISE ANALYSIS

Noise or fluctuation analysis provides an alternative approach to obtaining information at the level of single channels. In this technique the mean current level, as well as the variations about the mean, is used to infer single-channel properties. The principle behind the measurement is that random openings and closures of channels within a population will give rise to appreciable fluctuations in the overall number of open channels. The amplitudes of the fluctuations depend on the number channels, their open probability, and the single-channel current (see below). For a given mean current level, the fluctuations will be larger for a small number of channels (with large single-channel currents) than for a large number of channels (with smaller single-channel currents), since opening or closing one channel will produce a larger change in the mean current. A major disadvantage of this approach versus that of patch-clamp is that the single-channel events are not observed directly, but need to be extracted from the data using kinetic models, Fourier transforms, and curve fitting. A second drawback is that information on variations in channel behavior may be lost, and only the mean properties of an ensemble of the channels are obtained. This loss of information can sometimes be a blessing in disguise, particularly when the

overall performance of the whole population of channels needs to be assessed, by focusing attention on the quantitatively important aspects of channel function. Another advantage is that the sampling of channel properties is not biased by those of a few "good" patches which may be easy to analyze, but are not necessarily representative. A third advantage of noise analysis over direct recording of single-channel events is that it can resolve smaller single-channel currents. For example, the inward-rectifier K channel Kir7.1 has a single-channel conductance of $\sim 50 \, fS$ estimated from noise analysis.[116] Single-channel openings and closings associated with this conductance would be impossible to see using patch-clamp recordings.

Like single-channel recordings, noise analysis depends on abrupt changes in currents which occur when channels open or close, giving rise to fluctuations. Although it is possible to analyze noise due to spontaneous opening and closing, in practice most uses of noise analysis in epithelia have made use of blocker-induced noise in which the fluctuations are promoted by addition of blocking ions to the medium. This has two advantages. First, if the blockers interact with the channel through a first-order process, the kinetic scheme is particularly simple:

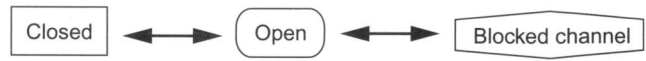

In the frequency domain, such a scheme predicts fluctuations which follow the form of a simple Lorentzian equation[117]:

$$S = S_o/[1 + (f/f_c)^2] \qquad (7.32)$$

Where S is the power associated with a given frequency f, S_o is the plateau power approached at low frequencies, and f_c is a constant called the corner frequency, and is the frequency at which the power is reduced to half that of the plateau (Figure 7.17). Furthermore, f_c is determined by the kinetics of the blocking interaction:

$$2\pi f_c = [B]k_{on} + k_{off} \qquad (7.33)$$

where [B] is the blocker concentration, and k_{on} and k_{off} are the on and off rate constants, respectively for the blocking reaction.

A second advantage of studying blocker-induced noise is that both the blocker and its concentration can be chosen to optimize the frequency of the fluctuations. This is important because technical problems can often limit the frequencies over which the noise can be reliably measured. For example, although amiloride-induced noise was originally used to study properties of epithelial Na channels,[117] recordings could be improved by using a lower affinity analog which produced fluctuations at higher frequencies.[118]

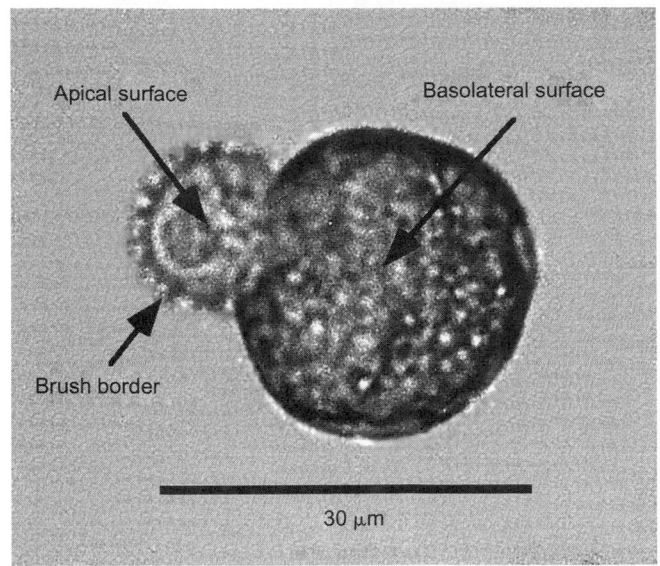

FIGURE 7.17 Isolated *Necturus* proximal tubule cell. The cell is bi-spherical in shape and about 30 microns in diameter. Evidence of a brush border is apparent on the smaller apical sphere. The larger spherical side of the cell consists of basolateral membrane. Isolated amphibian proximal tubule cells retain their polarity much longer than mammalian isolated epithelial cells. Patch-clamp recordings from both apical and basal surfaces indicate channel types similar to those found in native tubules.

The simplest piece of information that can be extracted from the noise analysis is the single-channel current[117]:

$$i = S_o 2\pi f_c / 4IF_B \tag{7.34}$$

Where F_B represents the fraction of blocked channels and I is the total (mean) current through the ensemble of channels measured in the presence of the blocker. F_B can be determined from the ratio of k_{on}/k_{off}, noting that $F_B = 1/(1 + k_{off}/k_{on} \cdot [B])$. F_B can also be estimated from the macroscopic dose-response curve (Figure 7.18a), although this may give different results if the blocker increases the number of channels contributing to the noise. The quantity N_o (=mean number of open + blocked channels) can be calculated from:

$$N_o = I/[i(1 - F_B)] \tag{7.35}$$

In general, N_o will be smaller than the total number of active channels N, since closed channels are not included. Helman and colleagues have made use of this discrepancy, and the finding that N_o increases as the concentration of blocker is increased, to assess P_o, the open probability of unblocked channels. This was analyzed in terms of a three-state model [118]:

Open + Blocker ⟷ Blocked channel

Assuming that closed channels cannot be blocked, the number of open + blocked channels is

increased by the blocker through the principal of mass action.

A second approach to estimate P_o is to measure the fluctuations associated with the spontaneous opening and closing.[119] Again a simple model is assumed:

Closed ⟷ Open

In which the variance (σ^2) of the current is given by[58]:

$$\sigma^2 = Ni^2P_o(1 - P_o) = I(1 - P_o)i \tag{7.36}$$

Therefore, the three measurements of blocker-induced noise, mean current, and variance in the absence of blocker can be used to estimate the three variables i, N, and P_o.

Most noise analysis studies have used flat epithelia in which the transepithelial voltage is clamped. Both native tissues[44,117,120,121] and cultured cells[118,122] have been successfully studied. In these instances blockers have been added to the apical side of the epithelia to measure properties of Na channels (using amiloride or its analogs as blockers) or K channels (using Ba^{+2}). More recently, fluctuation analysis has been applied to whole-cell recordings of renal epithelia, particularly the CCD, where the cells are not electrically coupled to each other.[38] Na channel fluctuations similar to those of flat epithelial can be measured in this way.[119] Another application involved characterization of basolateral K channels which, as described above, are difficult to study directly.[123] Similar techniques were also used to examine cell-attached patches in which channel density was too high to resolve single-channel events directly.[124]

Molecular Identification of Channels

Detailed information about channel properties obtained from patch-clamp analysis can, in some cases, be used to establish the molecular identity of the channels. Ideally this identification is corroborated using biochemical and genetic techniques. Table 7.7 provides a list of such channels for the mammalian nephron.

ROMK (Kir1.1), the apical K^+ channel of the TAL and CNT/CCD, provides a good example of this process. The channel was observed characterized in both of these segments[125,126] before the cDNA encoding it was cloned.[127] Subsequent detailed comparison of the biophysical properties of the native and cloned channels made it highly likely that the two were identical.[61] This was supported by immunocytochemical evidence demonstrating expression of the channel protein in the luminal membrane of the appropriate segments of the rat kidney.[128–130] Finally, genetic deletion of ROMK

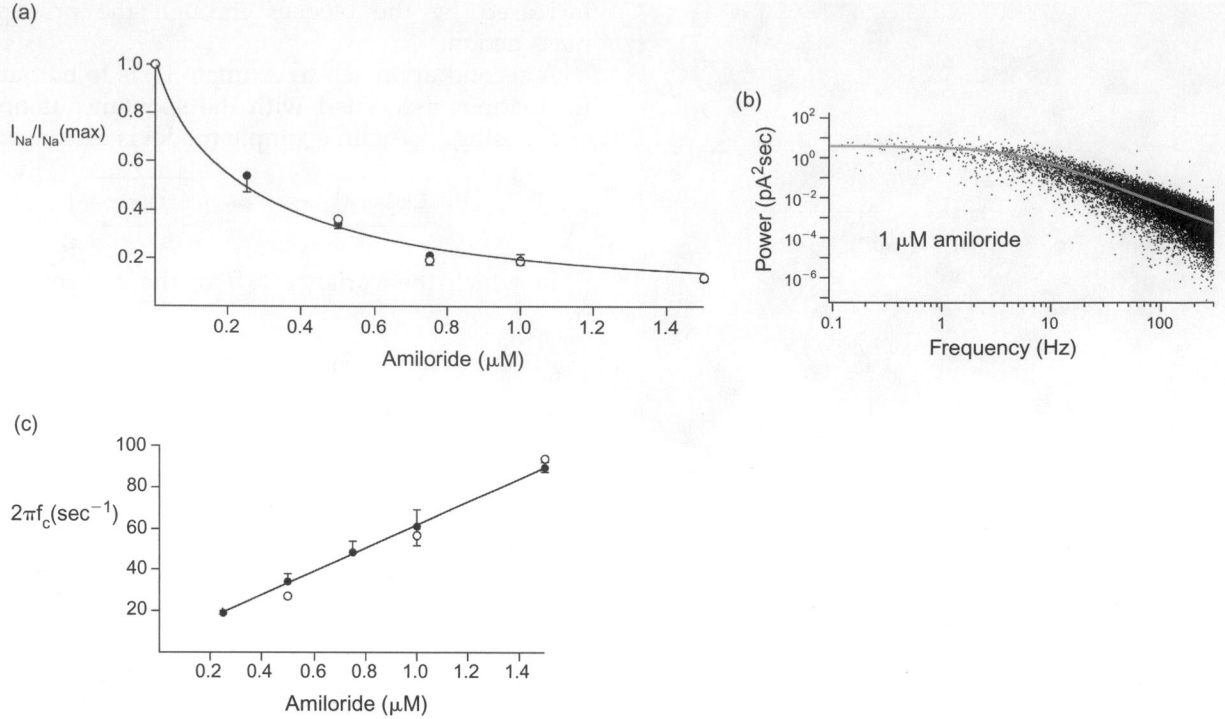

FIGURE 7.18 Noise analysis of whole-cell currents in a principal cell of the mouse CCD. The power density spectrum was obtained with 1 μM amiloride in the bath. The line represents a fit to a Lorentzian function with So = 3.06 pA^2 sec and f$_c$ = 3.8 Hz (from [119]).

in the mouse led to the disappearance of the channels from the apical membranes of both the CCD and TALH.[131]

Although few channels have been examined as fully as ROMK, the list of fully and partially identified conductances is growing. In some cases, the genetic identification cited in Table 7.7 entails the analysis of phenotypes of human mutations such Bartter's[132] and SESAME/EAST[133,134] syndromes rather than a knock-out line. This is a less direct approach, but one that increases the pathophysiological relevance of the channel.

CONCLUSIONS

The patch-clamp approach has made it possible to study renal ion channels one molecule at a time. Insights into ion transport mechanisms that have emerged from these studies have greatly expanded the information that was previously available from equivalent circuit analysis. Although single-channel measurements provide details about how ion *channels* work, they do not provide complete information about how an *epithelium* works. Achieving this goal requires measurements of transepithelial, intracellular, and single channel properties.

APPENDIX 1. THE BASIC EQUATIONS FOR THE GENERAL EQUIVALENT CIRCUIT

The lateral resistive network in the circuit of Figure 7.1 makes it difficult to obtain a closed form solution for the electrical parameters of interest. However, if the lateral network is neglected, Figure 7.1 reduces to the simpler circuit of Figure 7.7a, which can be evaluated as follows.

Since the pump and diffusional EMFs are in parallel, the effective electromotive force of the cellular pathway is the sum of the individual EMFs weighted by their relative conductances:

$$E_{bl}^* = \frac{R_{bl}}{R_p + R_{bl}} E_p + \frac{R_p}{R_p + R_{bl}} E_{bl} \qquad (A1.1)$$

where E$_p$ is the reversal potential of the pump and E$_{bl}$ is the total ionic diffusion potential across the basolateral membrane, as given either by the mosaic membrane equation (Eq. (A1.2)) or the constant field equation (Eq. (A1.3)):

$$E_{bl} = -\frac{RT}{F} \left[t_{Na} Ln \frac{[Na]_c}{[Na]_b} + t_K Ln \frac{[K]_c}{[K]_b} + t_{Cl} Ln \frac{[Cl]_b}{[Cl]_c} \right]$$

$$(A1.2)$$

TABLE 7.7 Molecular Identification of Ion Channels in Renal Tubules

Channel		Identification		
	Function	Protein	Genetic
PROXIMAL TUBULE				
Basolateral	K: K$_{ATP}$ (Kir6?)	106, 107, 109, 155	–	–
TALH				
Apical	K: Kir1.1 (ROMK)	126	128, 130, 156	131
Basolateral	Cl: CLCK1(A)/2(B)	108, 157	158-160	132, 161
DCT				
Basolateral	K: Kir4.1/5.1	162	163, 164	133, 134
	Cl: CLCK2(B)	165, 166	159	–
CNT/CD PRINCIPAL CELL				
Apical	Na: ENaC	87, 167	168, 169	170
	K: Kir1.1 (ROMK)	125, 171	128, 130, 156	131
	K: mSlo (BK)	83, 172	–	–
Basolateral	K: Kir4.1/5.1	173	173	–
	K: Kir4.1	110, 123	173	–
	Cl: CLCK2(B)	174	159	–
CNT/CD INTERCALATED CELL				
Apical	K: mSlo (BK)	175, 176	177	–
Basolateral	Cl: CLCK2(B)	174, 178	158, 159	–

$$E_{bl} = -\frac{RT}{F} Ln \frac{P_{Na}[Na]_c + P_K[K]_c + P_{Cl}[Cl]_b}{P_{Na}[Na]_b + P_K[K]_b + P_{Cl}[Cl]_c} \quad (A1.3)$$

The effective basolateral resistance R_{bl}^* is the parallel sum of pump resistance (R_p) and the passive resistive elements of the membrane (R_{bl}):

$$R_{bl}^* = \frac{R_p \cdot R_{bl}}{R_p + R_{bl}} \quad (A1.4)$$

Transepithelial resistance (R_{te}) is a function of the other resistances in the network as defined by:

$$\frac{1}{R_{te}} = \frac{1}{R_{tj}} + \frac{1}{R_{ap} + R_{bl}^*} \quad (A1.5)$$

Considering the circuit of Figure 7.7b, the total circulating current (I) can be calculated from the total EMF of the circuit divided by the total resistance according to the equation:

$$I = \frac{-E_{bl}^* - E_{ap} + E_{par}}{R_{bl}^* + R_{ap} + R_{tj}} \quad \text{where } E_{bl}^* \text{ and } E_{ap} < 0 \quad (A1.6)$$

Under these conditions, the measured basolateral potential will be given by:

$$V_{bl} = E_{bl}^* + I \cdot R_{bl}^* = \frac{E_{bl}^*(R_{ap} + R_{tj}) + R_{bl}^*(E_{par} - E_{ap})}{R_{bl}^* + R_{ap} + R_{tj}} \quad (A1.7)$$

The measured apical membrane potential will be given by:

$$V_{ap} = E_{ap} + I \cdot R_{ap} = \frac{E_{ap}(R_{bl}^* + R_{tj}) + R_{ap}(E_{par} - E_{bl}^*)}{R_{bl}^* + R_{ap} + R_{tj}} \quad (A1.8)$$

and the measured transepithelial potential will be given by:

$$V_{te} = E_{par} - I \cdot R_{par} = \frac{E_{par}(R_{ap} + R_{bl}^*) + R_{tj}(E_{ap} + E_{bl}^*)}{R_{bl}^* + R_{ap} + R_{tj}} \quad (A1.9)$$

Equations (A1.7)–(A1.9) can be evaluated for the limiting cases of very tight and very leaky epithelia. In the case where the cell (rather than the interspace) is the primary conductive pathway:

$$Lim \ V_{bl} = E_{bl}^* \quad \text{for } R_{tj} \gg R_{ap} + R_{bl}^* \quad (A1.10)$$
$$\text{(very tight epithelium)}$$

and:

$$Lim \ V_{ap} = E_{ap} \quad \text{for } R_{tj} \gg R_{ap} + R_{bl}^* \quad (A1.11)$$
$$\text{(very tight epithelium)}$$

If perturbations are confined to the apical membrane, the additional limiting case is sometimes useful when only transepithelial measurements can be performed:

$$Lim \ \Delta V_{ap} = \Delta E_{ap} = \Delta V_{te} \qquad \text{for } R_{tj} \gg R_{ap} + R_{bl}^*$$

$$\text{(very tight epithelium)}$$

$$(A1.12)$$

since:

$$Lim \ V_{te} = E_{ap} + E_{bl}^* \qquad \text{for } R_{tj} \gg R_{ap} + R_{bl}^*$$

$$\text{(very tight epithelium)}$$

$$(A1.13)$$

At the other extreme, if the paracellular pathway has a much higher conductance than the cellular pathway:

$$Lim \ V_{te} = E_{par} \qquad \text{for } R_{ap} + R_{bl}^* \gg R_{tj}$$

$$\text{(very leaky epithelium)} \qquad (A1.14)$$

Finally, two other limiting cases of the general circuit equations permit determination of cell membrane properties from transepithelial measurements under special conditions. First, application of a high K solution to the serosal side of an epithelium having a predominantly K selective basolateral membrane reduces both R_{bl}^* and E_{bl}^* to values close to zero. Under these conditions, Eqs. (A1.8) and (A1.9) imply the following simple relation between V_{ap} and V_{te}.

$$V_{ap} = V_{te} = \frac{R_{tj}}{R_{ap} + R_{tj}} E_{ap} + \frac{R_{ap}}{R_{ap} + R_{tj}} E_{par}$$

$$(A1.15)$$

(K depolarized tissue)

Second, protocols that involve selective permeabilization of the apical membrane reduce both R_{ap} and E_{ap} to values near zero, and Eqs. (A1.7) and (A1.9) imply a simple relation between V_{bl} and V_{te}:

$$V_{bl} = V_{te} = \frac{R_{tj}}{R_{bl}^* + R_{tj}} E_{bl}^* + \frac{R_{bl}^*}{R_{bl}^* + R_{tj}} E_{par}$$

$$(A1.16)$$

(permeabilized apical membrane)

APPENDIX 2. RELATION BETWEEN THE REAL CHANGE IN EMF AND THE MEASURED CHANGE IN POTENTIAL

Circular current flow in polarized epithelial cells produces important discrepancies between the real change in EMF at a particular barrier, ΔE, and the change in voltage, ΔV, that can actually be measured with electrodes (see Figure 7.7). In order to evaluate individual ion selectivities, some assumption must be made about the equivalent circuit of the epithelium. In the simple model of Figure 7.7a, luminal replacement of Na, K or Cl with an impermeant ion will produce changes in the measured basolateral ΔV_{bl} and transepithelial potentials ΔV_{te} that are related to the change in apical membrane EMF according to:

$$\Delta E_{ap} = \Delta V_{te} - \Delta V_{bl} \left[1 + \frac{R_{ap}}{R_p} + \frac{R_{ap}}{R_{bl}} \right] \qquad (A2.1)$$

where R_{ap}, R_{bl}, and R_p respectively refer to the apical membrane resistance, the lumped basolateral membrane resistance, and the intrinsic resistance of the basolateral Na-K pump. In Eqs. (A2.1)–(A2.3), it is assumed that the external ion replacements are performed rapidly enough so that the resistance ratios (R_{ap}/R_p, R_{ap}/R_{bl}) are constant, and the ion composition of the cell is essentially unchanged. The equations were derived by noting that the total current entering the cell across the apical membrane must equal the total current leaving the cell across the basolateral membrane.

Basolateral replacement of Na, K or Cl with an impermeant ion yields an analogous expression for the relation between the change in basolateral EMF and the measured potentials ΔV:

$$\Delta E_{bl} = \Delta V_{bl} \left[1 + \frac{R_{bl}}{R_p} + \frac{R_{bl}}{R_{ap}} \right] - \frac{R_{bl}}{R_{ap}} \Delta V_{te} \qquad (A2.2)$$

Finally, the paracellular EMF would be given by Eq. (A2.3) for experiments involving basolateral replacement of Na, K or Cl by an impermeant ion.

$$\Delta E_{par} = \Delta V_{te} \left[1 + \frac{R_{tj}}{R_{ap}} \right] - \frac{R_{tj}}{R_{ap}} \Delta V_{bl} \qquad (A2.3)$$

Equations (A2.1)–(A2.3) would be used together with Eq. (7.23) of the text to evaluate the ionic transference numbers of the apical, basolateral, and paracellular barriers.

APPENDIX 3. EQUATIONS FOR PARTIAL IONIC CONDUCTANCE

Specific expressions for the partial conductance G_x can be obtained by differentiating the Goldman–Hodgkin–Katz flux equation with respect to voltage:

$$G_x = \frac{\partial I_x}{\partial V}$$

$$= \frac{\partial}{\partial V} \left\{ P_x \frac{z^2 F^2}{RT} V \cdot \left[\frac{[X]_o - [X]_i e^{zFV/RT}}{(1 - e^{zFV/RT})} \right] \right\} \qquad (A3.1)$$

In the limiting case of zero membrane potential, the complicated form of Eq. (A3.1) reduces to the arithmetic average of the concentrations on both sides of the membrane. This equation does not depend on the ion being distributed near its electrochemical equilibrium:

$$G_x \approx P_x \frac{z^2 F^2}{RT} \frac{1}{2}(X_o + X_i) \tag{A3.2}$$

At large negative membrane potentials, positive ions will be driven from outside to inside, and the limiting conductance will be:

$$G_x \approx P_x \frac{z^2 F^2}{RT} X_o \tag{A3.3}$$

Conversely, at large positive potentials, negative ions will be driven from inside to outside, and the limiting conductance will be:

$$G_x \approx P_x \frac{z^2 F^2}{RT} X_i \tag{A3.4}$$

Although the above relations reduce the complicated general equation (Eq. (A3.1)) to a manageable form, neither the assumption of zero membrane potential (Eq. (A3.2)) nor the assumption of very large membrane potentials (Eqs. (A3.3), (A3.4)) are terribly physiological.

For ions like K and Cl, which are often distributed close to their electrochemical equilibrium, it is possible to simplify the algebraic form of the 'X' term in Eq. (7.25) of the text. Under these conditions, the conductance would be given by the equation:

$$G_x \approx P_x \frac{z_x^2 F^2}{RT} \left(\frac{[X]_i [X]_o}{[X]_o - [X]_i} \right) \text{Ln} \frac{[X]_o}{[X]_i} \tag{A3.5}$$

If more than one ion (X and Y) is distributed close to equilibrium across the membrane, the ratios of transference numbers, conductances and permeabilities are given by the equation:

$$\frac{t_x}{t_y} = \frac{G_x}{G_y} \approx \frac{P_x}{P_y} \cdot \frac{[X]_o}{[Y]_i} = \frac{P_x}{P_y} \cdot \frac{[X]_i}{[Y]_o} \tag{A3.6}$$

APPENDIX 4. CONTRIBUTION OF THE ELECTROGENIC Na-K PUMP TO THE MEMBRANE POTENTIAL

The contribution of the Na-K pump to the cell membrane potential of epithelial tissues is different than its contribution to the membrane potential of symmetric cells. The existence of circulating currents in the open-circuited state places a different set of constraints on the magnitude of the cell potential. This can be derived from the reduced equivalent circuit of Figure 7.7b. In this circuit, the electrogenic and diffusive ion pathways are combined into an effective EMF of the basolateral membrane (E_{bl}^*), and an effective basolateral resistance (R_{bl}^*). These lumped quantities are directly related to the individual parameters of the pump and the basolateral diffusion potential according to standard equations of linear circuit theory:

$$R_{bl}^* = \frac{R_{bl} \cdot R_p}{R_{bl} + R_p} \tag{A4.1}$$

$$E_{bl}^* = \frac{R_{bl}}{R_{bl} + R_p} E_p + \frac{R_p}{R_{bl} + R_p} E_{bl} \tag{A4.2}$$

If the circulating currents of Figure 7.7b are also considered, the measured membrane potential (V_{bl}) can be described by Eq. (A4.3), which indicates the specific contribution of the electrogenic pump (E_p), the ionic diffusion potential (E_{bl}), and the apical and paracellular diffusion potentials (E_{ap}, E_{par}).

$$V_{bl} = f \left[\frac{R_{bl}}{R_{bl} + R_p} \right] E_p$$

$$+ f \left[\frac{R_p}{R_{bl} + R_p} \right] E_{bl} + g \left[E_{par} - E_{ap} \right] \tag{A4.3}$$

where the factors "f" and "g" arise from the circulating current "I" in the model of Figure 7.7b:

$$f = \frac{R_{ap} + R_{tj}}{R_{bl}^* + R_{ap} + R_{tj}} \tag{A4.4}$$

$$g = \frac{R_{bl}^*}{R_{bl}^* + R_{ap} + R_{tj}} \tag{A4.5}$$

Equations (A4.3)−(A4.5) are the general equations for the relative contributions of the electrogenic pump (denoted by E_p), ionic diffusion (denoted by E_{bl}), and circulating current (denoted by $E_{par} - E_{ap}$) to the observed basolateral membrane potential (V_{bl}). As indicated by Eq. (A4.3), the membrane potential depends critically on the relative magnitude of the pump resistance (R_p) versus the diffusion resistance of the membrane R_{bl}.

The term R_{bl}^* can be determined from cable analysis (as described in the text). This value can then be used to calculate R_{bl} from Eq. (A4.1), assuming that the internal resistance of the pump (R_p) can be estimated from its I−V relation (see Figure 7.10).

If the internal pump resistance (R_p) is high compared to the ionic resistance (R_{bl}), the ratio $R_{bl}/(R_{bl} + R_p)$ will be low, and the measured membrane potential V_{bl} (given by Eq. (A4.3)) will be dominated by the diffusional EMF term involving E_{bl}. Conversely, if the internal pump resistance is low, V_{bl} will be dominated by the pump term involving E_p.

References

[1] Ussing HH, Zerahn K. Active transport of sodium as the source of electric current in the short-circuited isolated frog skin. Acta Physiol Scand 1951;23:110–27.

[2] Greger R. Cation selectivity of the isolated perfused cortical thick ascending limb of Henle's loop of rabbit kidney. Pflügers Arch 1981;390:30–7.

[3] Hebert SC, Andreoli TE. Control of NaCl transport in the thick ascending limb. Am J Physiol 1984;246:F745–56.

[4] Sackin H, Boulpaep EL. Isolated perfused salamander proximal tubule: methods, electrophysiology, and transport. Am J Physiol 1981;241:F39–52.

[5] Sackin H, Boulpaep EL. Rheogenic transport in the renal proximal tubule. J Gen Physiol 1983;82:819–51.

[6] Spring K. Insertion of an axial electrode into renal proximal tubule. Yale J Biol Med 1972;45:426.

[7] Hegel U, Boulpaep EL. Studies of electrical impedence of kidney proximal tubular epithelium in *Necturus*. Abstr 6th Intern Congr Nephr 1975;45.

[8] Horisberger J-D, Giebisch G. Voltage dependence of the basolateral membrane conductance in the *Amphiuma* collecting tubule. J Membr Biol 1988;105:257–63.

[9] Frömter E. The route of passive ion movement through the epithelium of *Necturus* gallbladder. J Membr Biol 1972;8:259–301.

[10] Frömter E, Diamond JM. Route of passive ion permeation in epithelia. Nature New Biol 1972;235:9–13.

[11] Koefoed-Johnsen V, Ussing HH. On the nature of the frog skin potential. Acta Physiol Scand 1958;42:298–308.

[12] Greger R. Ion transport mechanisms in thick ascending limb of Henle's loop of mammalian nephron. Physiol Rev 1985;65:760–97.

[13] Frömter E. Viewing the kidney through microelectrodes. Am J Physiol 1984;247:F695–705.

[14] Boulpaep E. Electrical phenomena in the nephron. Kidney Int 1976;9:88–102.

[15] Boulpaep EL, Sackin H. Equivalent electrical circuit analysis and rheogenic pumps in epithelia. Federation Proc 1979;38:2030–6.

[16] Guggino WB, Windhager EE, Boulpaep EL, Giebisch G. Cellular and paracellular resistances of the *Necturus* proximal tubule. J Membrane Biol 1982;67:143–54.

[17] Wills NK, Eaton D, Lewis SA, Ifshin M. Current-voltage relationship of the basolateral membrane of a tight epithelium. Biochim Biophys Acta 1979;555:519–23.

[18] Higgins JT, Gebler B, Frömter E. Electrical properties of amphibian urinary bladder epithelia II. The cell potential profile in *Necturus* maculosus. Pflügers Arch 1977;371:87–97.

[19] Leaf A, Anderson J, Page LB. Active sodium transport by the isolated toad bladder. J Gen Physiol 1958;41:657–68.

[20] Ussing HH, Windhager EE. Nature of shunt path and active sodium transport path through frog skin epithelium. Acta Physiol Scand 1964;61:484–504.

[21] Horisberger J-D, Giebisch G. Na/K pump currents in the *Amphiuma* collecting tubule. J Gen Physiol 1989;94:493–510.

[22] Erlij D. Basic electrical properties of tight epithelia determined with a simple method. Pflügers Archiv 1976;364:91–3.

[23] Helman SI, Miller DA. *In vitro* techniques for avoiding edge damage in studies of the frog skin. Science 1971;173:146–8.

[24] Weinstein FC, Rosowski JJ, Peterson K, Delalic Z, Civan MM. Relationship of transient electrical properties to active sodium transport by toad urinary bladder. J Membrane Biol 1980;52:25–35.

[25] Van Itallie CM, Anderson JM. Claudins and epithelial paracellular transport. Annu Rev Physiol 2006;68:403–29.

[26] Lewis SA, Eaton DC, Clausen C, Diamond JM. Nystatin as a probe for investigating the electrical properties of a tight epithelium. J Gen Physiol 1977;70:427–40.

[27] Germann WJ, Lowy ME, Ernst SA, Dawson DC. Differentiation of two distinct K conductances in the basolateral membrane of turtle colon. J Gen Physiol 1986;88:237–51.

[28] Clausen C, Wills NK. Impedance analysis in epithelia. In: Schultz SG, editor. Ion Transport by Epithelia: Recent Advances. New York: Raven Press; 1981. p. 79–92.

[29] Awayda M, Van Driessche W, Helman SI. Frequency-dependent capacitance of the apical membrane of frog skin: Dielectric relaxation processes. Biophysical Journal 1999;76:219–32.

[30] Clausen C, Lewis SA, Diamond JM. Impedance analysis of a tight epithelium using a distributed resistance model. Biophys J 1979;26:291–317.

[31] Van-Driessche W, Erlij D. Cyclic AMP increases electrical capacitance of apical membrane of toad urinary bladder. Arch Int Physiol Biochim Biophys 1991;99(6):409–11.

[32] Wills NK, Purcell RK, Clausen C. Na$^+$ transport and impedance properties of cultured renal (A6 and 2F3) epithelia. J Membr Biol 1992;125(3):273–85.

[33] Spring KR. Current-induced voltage transients in *Necturus* proximal tubule. J Membr Biol 1973;13:299–322.

[34] Nelson DJ, Ehrenfeld J, Lindemann B. Volume changes and potential artifacts of epithelial cells of frog skin following impalement with microelectrodes filled with 3M KCl. J Membrane Biol 1978;40(Special Issue):91–119.

[35] Hamill OP, Marty A, Neher E, Sakmann B, Sigworth FJ. Improved patch clamp techniques for high resolution current recording from cells and cell-free membrane patches. Pflügers Arch 1981;391:85–100.

[36] Horn R, Marty A. Muscarinic activation of ionic currents measured by a new whole-cell recording method. J Gen Physiol 1988;92(2):145–59.

[37] Bello-Reuss E. Cell membrane and paracellular resistances in isolated renal proximal tubules from rabbit and *Ambystoma*. J Physiol 1986;370:25–38.

[38] Frindt G, Sackin H, Palmer LG. Whole-cell currents in rat cortical collecting tubule: Low-Na diet increases amiloride-sensitive conductance. Am J Physiol 1990;258:F562–7.

[39] Oberleithner H, Guggino W, Giebisch G. Resistance properties of the diluting segment of *Amphiuma* kidney: influence of K adaptation. J Membr Biol 1985;88:139–47.

[40] Guggino WB. Functional heterogeneity in the early distal tubule of the *Amphiuma* kidney: evidence for two modes of Cl and K transport across the basolateral cell membrane. Am J Physiol 1986;250:F430–40.

[41] Greger R, Schlatter E. Properties of the lumen membrane of the cortical thick ascending limb of Henle's loop of rabbit kidney: a model for secondary active chloride transport. Pflügers Arch 1983;396:315–24.

[42] Anagnostopoulos T, Velu E. Electrical resistance of cell membranes in *Necturus* kidney. Pflügers Arch 1974;346:327–39.

[43] Weber GH, Frömter E. Influence of lateral intercellular spaces on current propagation in tubular epithelia as estimated by a multi-cable model. Pflügers Arch 1988;411:153–9.

[44] Wills NK, Alles WP, Sandle GI, Binder HJ. Apical membrane properties and amiloride binding kinetics of the human descending colon. Am J Physiol 1984;247:G749–57.

[45] DeWeer P. Electrogenic pumps: theoretical and practical considerations. In: Blaustein M, Lieberman M, editors. Electrogenic transport: Fundamental Principles and Physiological Implications. New York: Raven Press; 1984.

[46] Glynn IM. The electrogenic sodium pump. In: Blaustein MP, Lieberman M, editors. Electrogenic Transport: Fundamental Principles and Physiological Implications, 38. New York: Raven Press; 1984. p. 33–48.

[47] Garrahan PJ, Glynn IM. The stoichiometry of the sodium pump. J Physiol (Lond) 1967;192:217–35.

[48] Post RL, Jolly PC. The linkage of sodium, potassium and ammonium active transport across the human erthrocyte membrane. Biochim Biophys Acta 1957;25:118–28.

[49] Rakowski RF, Gadsby DC, DeWeer P. Stoichiometry and voltage dependence of the sodium pump in voltage-clamped, internally dialyzed squid giant axon. J Gen Physiol 1989;93:903–41.

[50] Eisner DA, Lederer WJ, Vaughan-Jones RD. The dependence of sodium pumping and tension on intracellular sodium activity in voltage-clamped sheep Purkinje fibres. J Physiol (Lond) 1981;317:163–87.

[51] Mullins LJ, Noda K. The influence of sodium-free solutions on the membrane potential of frog muscle fibers. J Gen Physiol 1963;47:117–39.

[52] Thomas RC. Electrogenic sodium pump in nerve and muscle cells. Physiol Rev 1972;52:563–94.

[53] Horisberger JD, Giebisch G. Voltage dependence of the basolateral membrane conductance in the *Amphiuma* collecting tubule. J Membrane Biol 1988;105:257–63.

[54] DeWeer P. Cellular sodium–potassium transport. In: Seldin DW, Giebisch G, editors. The Kidney: Physiology and Pathophysiology. New York: Raven Press; 1985.

[55] Gadsby D, Nakao M. The steady-state current-voltage relationship of the Na/K pump in guinea pig ventricular myocytes. J Gen Physiol 1989;94:511–37.

[56] Rakowski. Charge movement by the Na/K pump in *Xenopus* oocytes. J Gen Physiol 1993;101:117–44.

[57] Palmer LG, Antonian L, Frindt G. Regulation of the Na-K pump of the rat cortical collecting tubule by aldosterone. J Gen Physiol 1993;102(1):43–57.

[58] Hille B. Ionic channels of excitable membranes. *3rd ed.* Sunderland, Massachusetts: Sinauer Associates; 2001.

[59] Miller C. Open-state substructure of single chloride channels from *Torpedo* electroplax. Phil Trans R Soc Lond B 1982;299:401–11.

[60] Chepilko S, Zhou H, Sackin H, Palmer LG. Permeation and gating properties of a cloned renal K^+ channel. Am J Physiol 1995;268:C389–401.

[61] Palmer LG, Choe H, Frindt G. Is the secretory K channel in the rat CCT ROMK? Am J Physiol 1997;273:F404–10.

[62] Firsov D, Schild L, Gautschi I, Merillat AM, Schneeberger E, Rossier BC. Cell surface expression of the epithelial Na channel and a mutant causing Liddle syndrome: a quantitative approach. Proc Natl Acad Sci USA 1996;93(26):15370–5.

[63] Palmer LG, Frindt G. Conductance and gating of epithelial Na channels from rat cortical collecting tubule. Effects of Na and Li. J Gen Physiol 1988;92:121–38.

[64] Palmer LG, Frindt G. Regulation of apical K channels in rat cortical collecting tubule during changes in dietary K intake. Am J Physiol 1999;277:F805–12.

[65] Sakmann B, Neher E. Single-Channel Recording. 2nd ed. New York: Plenum Press; 1995.

[66] Sokabe M, Sachs F. The structure and dynamics of patch-clamped membranes: a study using differential interference contrast light microscopy. J Cell Biol 1990;111:599–606.

[67] Sigworth FJ, Sine SM. Data transformations for improved display and fitting of single-channel dwell time histograms. Biophys J 1987;52:1047–54.

[68] Cox DH, Aldrich RW. Role of the beta1 subunit in large-conductance Ca^{2+}-activated K^+ channel gating energetics.

Mechanisms of enhanced Ca^{2+} sensitivity. J Gen Physiol 2000;116:411–32.

[69] Liebovitz LS, Fischbarg J, Koniarek JP. Ion channel kinetics: a model based on fractal scaling rather than multistate Markov processes. Math Biosci 1987;84:37–68.

[70] Korn SJ, Horn R. Statistical discrimination of fractal and Markov models of single-channel gating. Biophys J 1988;54:871–7.

[71] McManus OB, Weiss DS, Spivak CE, Blatz AL, Magleby KL. Fractal models are inadequate for the kintics of four different ion channels. Biophys J 1988;45:859–70.

[72] Millhauser GL, Salpeter EE, Oswald RE. Diffusion models of ion-channel gating and the origin of power-law distributions from single channel recordings. Proc Natl Acad Sci 1988;85:1503–7.

[73] Hess P, Lansman JB, Tsien RW. Different modes of Ca channel gating behaviour favored by dihydropyridine Ca agonists and antagonists. Nature 1984;311:538–44.

[74] Horn R, Vandenbert C, Lange K. Statistical analysis of single sodium channels. Effects of N-bromoacetamide. Biophys J 1984;45:323–35.

[75] O'Connell A.M. *Modal gating behavior of batrachotoxin-modified sodium channels* [Ph.D. thesis], Cornell University Medical College; 1992.

[76] Jin W, Klem AM, Lewis JH, Lu Z. Mechanisms of inward-rectifier K^+ channel inhibition by tertiapin-Q. Biochemistry 1999;38:14294–301.

[77] Jin W, Lu Z. A novel high-affinity inhibitor for inward-rectifier K^+ channels. Biochemistry 1998;37:13291–9.

[78] Lewis LM, Bhave G, Chauder BA, Banerjee S, Lornsen KA, Redha R, et al. High-throughput screening reveals a small-molecule inhibitor of the renal outer medullary potassium channel and Kir7.1. Mol Pharmacol 2009;76(5):1094–103.

[79] Lopatin AN, Makhina EN, Nichols CG. The mechanism of inward rectification of potassium channels: "Long-pore plugging" by cytoplasmic polyamines. J Gen Physiol 1995;106:923–56.

[80] Latorre R, Miller C. Conduction and selectivity in potassium channels. J Membr Biol 1983;71:11–30.

[81] Palmer LG. Voltage-dependent block by amiloride and other monovalent cations of apical Na channels in the toad urinary bladder. J Membrane Biol 1984;80:153–65.

[82] Filipovic D, Sackin H. A calcium-permeable stretch-activated cation channel in renal proximal tubule. Am J Physiol 1991;260:F119–29.

[83] Hunter M, Lopes AG, Boulpaep E, Giebisch G. Single channel recordings of calcium-activated potassium channels in the apical membrane of rabbit cortical collecting tubule. Proc Natl Acad Sci USA 1984;81:4237–9.

[84] Sackin H, Palmer LG. Basolateral potassium channels in renal proximal tubule. Am J Physiol 1987;253:F476–87.

[85] Sackin H. Stretch-activated potassium channel in renal proximal tubule. Am J Physiol 1987;253:F1253–62.

[86] Sackin H. A stretch-activated K^+ channel sensitive to cell volume. Proc Natl Acad Sci USA 1989;86:1731–5.

[87] Palmer LG, Frindt G. Amiloride-sensitive Na channels from the apical membrane of the rat cortical collecting tubule. Proc Natl Acad Sci U S A 1986;83:2767–70.

[88] Wang W, White S, Geibel J, Giebisch G. A potassium channel in the apical membrane of rabbit thick ascending limb of Henle's loop. Am J Physiol 1990;258:F244–53.

[89] Gögelein H, Greger R. Single channel recordings from basolateral and apical membranes of renal proximal tubules. Pflügers Archiv 1984;401:424–6.

[90] Engbretson BG, Beyenbach KW, Stoner LC. The everted renal tubule: a methodology for direct assessment of apical membrane function. Am J Physiol 1988;255:F1276−80.

[91] Stoner LC, Engbretson BG, Viggiano SC, Benos DJ, Smith PR. Amiloride-sensitive apical membrane sodium channels of everted *Ambystoma* collecting tubule. J Membr Biol 1995;144 (2):147−56.

[92] Stoner LC, Morley GE. Effect of basolateral or apical hyposmolarity on apical maxi K channels of everted rat collecting tubule. Am J Physiol 1995;268(4 Pt 2):F569−580.

[93] Hamilton KL, Eaton DC. Single-channel recordings from amiloride-sensitive epithelial sodium channel. Am J Physiol 1985;249:C200−7.

[94] Lang F, Friedrich F, Paulmilch M, Schobersberger W, Jungwirth A, Ritter M, et al. Ion channels in Madin−Darby canine kidney cells. Renal Physiol Biochem 1990;13:82−93.

[95] Staruschenko A, Pochynyuk O, Vandewalle A, Bugaj V, Stockand JD. Acute regulation of the epithelial Na$^+$ channel by phosphatidylinositide 3-OH kinase signaling in native collecting duct principal cells. J Am Soc Nephrol 2007;18 (6):1652−61.

[96] Gitter AH, Beyenbach KW. Christine C, Gross P, Minuth WW, Frömter E. High conductance K$^+$ channel in apical membranes of principal cells cultured from rabbit renal cortical collecting duct anlagen. Pflügers Arch 1987;408:282−90.

[97] Light DB, McCann FV, Keller TM, Stanton BA. Amiloride-sensitive cation channel in apical membrane of inner medullary collecting duct. Am J Physiol 1988;255:F278−86.

[98] Ling BN, Hinton CF, Eaton DC. Amiloride-sensitive sodium channels in rabbit cortical collecting tubule primary cultures. Am J Physiol 1991;261:F933−44.

[99] Handler JS, Perkins FM, Johnson JP. Hormone effects on transport in cultured epithelia with high electrical resistance. Am J Physiol 1981;240:C103−5.

[100] Ma HP, Li L, Zhou ZH, Eaton DC, Warnock DG. ATP masks stretch activation of epithelial sodium channels in A6 distal nephron cells. Am J Physiol 2002;282:F501−5.

[101] Marunaka Y, Eaton DC. Effects of vasopressin and cAMP on single amiloride-blockable Na channels. Am J Physiol 1991;260:C1071−84.

[102] Ohara A, Matsunaga H, Eaton DC. G protein activation inhibits amiloride-blockable highly selective sodium channels in A6 cells. Am J Physiol 1993;:.

[103] Duong Van Huyen J, Bens M, Vandewalle A. Differential effects of aldosterone and vasopressin on chloride fluxes in transimmortalized mouse cortical collecting duct cells. J Membr Biol 1998;164(1):79−90.

[104] Kawahara K, Hunter M, Giebisch G. Potassium channels in *Necturus* proximal tubule. Am J Physiol 1987;253:F488−94.

[105] Sansom SC, La BQ, Carosi SL. Double-barrelled choride channels of collecting duct basolateral membrane. Am J Physiol 1990;259:F46−52.

[106] Hurst AM, Beck J, Laprade R, Lapointe J-Y. Na pump inhibition downregulates an ATP-sensitive K channel in rabbit proximal tubule. Am J Physiol 1993;264:F760−4.

[107] Parent L, Cardinal J, Sauvé R. Single-channel analysis of a K channel at basolateral membrane of rabbit proximal convoluted tubule. Am J Physiol 1988;254:F105−13.

[108] Paulais M, Teulon J. cAMP-activated chloride channel in the basolateral membrane of the thick ascending limb of the mouse kidney. J Membr Biol 1990;113(3):253−60.

[109] Tsuchiya K, Wang W, Giebisch G, Welling PA. ATP is a coupling modulator of parallel Na/K ATPase K channel activity in the renal proximal tubule. Proc Natl Acad Sci USA 1992;89:6418−22.

[110] Wang W-H, McNicholas CM, Segal AS, Giebisch G. A novel approach allows identification of K channels in the lateral membrane of rat CCD. Am J Physiol 1994;266:F813−22.

[111] Cemerikic D, Sackin H. Substrate activation of mechanosensitive, whole cell currents in renal proximal tubule. Am J Physiol 1993;264:F707−14.

[112] Filipovic D, Sackin H. Stretch- and volume-activated channels in isolated tubule cells. Am J Physiol 1992;262:F857−70.

[113] Kawahara K. A stretch-activated K$^+$ channel in the basolateral membrane of *Xenopus* kidney proximal tubule cells. Pflügers Arch 1990;415:624−9.

[114] Robson L, Hunter M. Volume regulatory responses in frog isolated proximal tubules. Pflügers Arch 1994;428:60−8.

[115] Segal A, Boulpaep EL, Maunsbach AB. A novel preparation of dissociated renal proximal tubule cells that maintain epithelial polarity in suspension. Am J Physiol (Cell) 1996;270: C1843−63.

[116] Krapininsky G, Medina I, Eng L, Krapivinsky L, Yang Y, Clapham D. A novel inward rectifier K$^+$ channel with unique pore properties. Neuron 1998;20:995−1005.

[117] Lindemann B, Van Driessche W. Sodium specific membrane channels of frog skin are pores: Current fluctuations reveal high turnover. Science 1977;195:292−4.

[118] Helman SI, Baxendale LM. Blocker-related changes of channel density. Analysis of a three-state model for apical Na channels of frog skin. J Gen Physiol 1990;95:647−78.

[119] Dahlmann A, Pradervand S, Hummler E, Rossier BC, Frindt G, Palmer LG. Mineralocorticoid regulation of epithelial Na$^+$ channels is maintained in a mouse model of Liddle's syndrome. Am J Physiol 2003;285:F310−8.

[120] Li H-Y, Palmer LG, Edelman IS, Lindemann B. The role of Na channel density in the natriferic response of the toad urinary bladder to an antidiuretic hormone. J Membr Biol 1982; 64:77−89.

[121] Van Driessche W, Zeiske W. Ba^{2+}-induced conductance fluctuations of spontaneously fluctuating K$^+$ channels in the apical membrane of frog skin (*Rana temporaria*). J Membr Biol 1980;56:31−42.

[122] Blazer-Yost BL, Helman SI. The amiloride-sensitive epithelial Na$^+$ channel: Binding sites and channel densities. Am J Physiol 1997;272(3):C761−9.

[123] Gray DA, Frindt G, Zhang YY, Palmer LG. Basolateral K$^+$ conductance in principal cells of rat CCD. Am J Physiol Renal Physiol 2005;288(3):F493−504.

[124] Frindt G, Silver RB, Windhager EE, Palmer LG. Feedback regulation of Na channels in rat CCT. III. Response to cAMP. Am J Physiol 1995;268:F480−9.

[125] Frindt G, Palmer LG. Low-conductance K channels in apical membrane of rat cortical collecting tubule. Am J Physiol 1989;256:F143−51.

[126] Wang W, White S, Geibel J, Giebisch G. A potassium channel in the apical membrane of rabbit thick ascending limb of Henle's loop. Am J Physiol 1990;258:F244−53.

[127] Ho KH, Nichols CG, Lederer WJ, Lytton J, Vassilev PM, Kanazirska MV, et al. Cloning and expression of an inwardly rectifying ATP-regulated potassium channel. Nature 1993;362:31−7.

[128] Kohda Y, Ding W, Phan E, Housini I, Wang J, Star RA, et al. Localization of the ROMK potassium channel to the apical membrane of distal nephron in rat kidney. Kidney Int 1998;54:1214−23.

[129] Mennitt PA, Wade JB, Ecelbarger CA, Palmer LG, Frindt G. Localization of ROMK channels in the rat kidney. J Am Soc Nephrol 1997;8:1823−30.

[130] Xu JZ, Hall AE, Peterson LN, Bienkowski MJ, Eesalu TB, Hebert SC. Localization of the ROMK protein on apical

membranes of rat kidney nephron segments. Am J Physiol 1997;273:F739−48.

[131] Lu M, Wang T, Yan Q, Yang X, Dong K, Knepper MA, et al. Absence of small conductance K$^+$ channel (SK) activity in apical membranes of thick ascending limb and cortical collecting duct in ROMK (Barrter's) knockout mice. J Biol Chem 2002;277:37881−7.

[132] Simon DB, Bindra RS, Mansfield TA, Nelson-Williams C, Mendonca E, Stone R, et al. Mutations in the chloride channel gene, CLCNKB, cause Bartter's syndrome type III. Nat Genet 1997;17(2):171−8.

[133] Bockenhauer D, Feather S, Stanescu HC, Bandulik S, Zdebik AA, Reichold M, et al. Epilepsy, ataxia, sensorineural deafness, tubulopathy, and KCNJ10 mutations. N Engl J Med 2009;360(19):1960−70.

[134] Scholl UI, Choi M, Liu T, Ramaekers VT, Hausler MG, Grimmer J, et al. Seizures, sensorineural deafness, ataxia, mental retardation, and electrolyte imbalance (SeSAME syndrome) caused by mutations in KCNJ10. Proc Natl Acad Sci USA 2009;106(14):5842−7.

[135] Guggino WB, Oberleithner H, Giebisch G. The amphibian diluting segment. Am J Physiol 1988;254:F615−27.

[136] Hunter M, Horisberger J-D, Stanton BA, Giebisch G. The collecting tubule of Amphiuma I. Electrophysiological characterization. Am J Physiol 1987;253:1263−72.

[137] Koeppen BM, Biagi BA, Giebisch G. Intracellular microelectrode characterization of the rabbit cortical collecting duct. Am J Physiol 1983;244:F35−47.

[138] Koeppen BM. Conductive properties of the rabbit outer medullary collecting duct: Outer stripe. Am J Physiol 1986;250: F70−6.

[139] Stanton BA. Characterization of apical and basolateral membrane conductances of rat inner medullary collecting duct. Am J Physiol 1989;256:F862−8.

[140] Lewis SA, Diamond JM. Na$^+$ transport by rabbit urinary bladder, a tight epithelium. J Membrane Biol 1976;28:1−40.

[141] Lapointe JY, Laprade R. Cardinal J. Transepithelial and cell membrane electrical resistances of the rabbit proximal convoluted tubule. Am J Physiol 1984;247:F637−49.

[142] Frömter E. Electrophysiological analysis of rat renal sugar and amino acid transport. I. Basic phenomena. Pflügers Arch 1982;393:179−89.

[143] O'Neil RG, Sansom SC. Electrophysiological properties of cellular and paracellular conductive pathways of the rabbit cortical collecting duct. J Membr Biol 1984;82:281−95.

[144] Koeppen B, Giebisch G. Cellular electrophysiology of potassium transport in the mammalian cortical collecting tubule. Pflügers Arch 1985;405(Suppl 1):S143−6.

[145] Koeppen B. Electrophysiology of ion transport in renal tubule epithelia. Semin Nephrol 1987;7:37−47.

[146] Lewis SA, Eaton DC, Diamond JM. The mechanism of Na$^+$ transport by rabbit urinary bladder. J Memb Biol 1976;28:41−70.

[147] Maunsbach AB, Boulpaep EL. Quantitative ultrastructure and functional correlates in proximal tubules of Ambystoma and Necturus. Am J Physiol 1984;246:F710−24.

[148] Messner G, Wang W, Paulmichl M, Oberleithner H, Lang F. Ouabain decreases apparent potassium-conductance in proximal tubules of the amphibian kidney. Pflügers Arch 1985;404:131−7.

[149] Hoshi T, Kawahara K, Yokoyama R, Suenga K. Change in membrane resistances of renal proximal tubule induced by cotransport of sodium and organic solutes. In: Takacs L, editor. Adv Physiol. Sci (Kidney and Body Fluids), 11. Budapest: Pergamon Press and Akademiai Kiado; 1981.

[150] Horisberger JD, Giebisch G. Intracellular Na and K activities and membrane conductances in the collecting tubule of Amphiuma. J Gen Physiol 1988;92:643−65.

[151] Frömter E, Gebler B. Electrical properties of amphibian urinary bladder epithelia III. The cell membrane resistances and the effect of amiloride. Pflügers Arch 1977; 371:99−108.

[152] Frindt G, Masilamani S, Knepper MA, Palmer LG. Activation of epithelial Na channels during short-term Na deprivation. Am J Physiol 2001;280:F112−8.

[153] Pácha J, Frindt G, Antonian L, Silver R, Palmer LG. Regulation of Na channels of the rat cortical collecting tubule by aldosterone. J Gen Physiol 1993;102:25−42.

[154] Palmer LG, Sackin H, Frindt G. Regulation of Na channels by luminal Na in rat cortical collecting tubule. J Physiol (London) 1998;509:151−62.

[155] Gögelein H, Greger R. Properties of single K channels in the basolateral membrane of rabbit proximal straight tubules. Pflügers Archiv 1987;410:288−95.

[156] Mennitt PA, Frindt G, Silver RB, Palmer. Potassium restriction downregulates ROMK expression in rat kidney. Am J. Physiol (Renal) 2000;278:F916−24.

[157] Reeves WB, Winters CJ, Filipovic DM, Andreoli TE. Cl$^-$ channels in basolateral renal medullary vesicles. IX. Channels from mouse MTAL cell patches and medullary vesicles. Am J Physiol 1995;269(5 Pt 2):F621−627.

[158] Estevez R, Boettger T, Stein V, Birkenhager R, Otto E, Hildebrandt F, et al. Barttin is a Cl$^-$ channel beta-subunit crucial for renal Cl$^-$ reabsorption and inner ear K$^+$ secretion. Nature 2001;414(6863):558−61.

[159] Kobayashi K, Uchida S, Mizutani S, Sasaki S, Marumo F. Intrarenal and cellular localization of CLC-K2 protein in the mouse kidney. J Am Soc Nephrol 2001;12(7):1327−34.

[160] Vandewalle A, Cluzeaud F, Bens M, Kieferle S, Steinmeyer K, Jentsch TJ. Localization and induction by dehydration of ClC-K chloride channels in the rat kidney. Am J Physiol 1997;272(5 Pt 2):F678−688.

[161] Zimniak L, Winters CJ, Reeves WB, Andreoli TE. Cl$^-$ channels in basolateral renal medullary vesicles XI. rbClC-Ka cDNA encodes basolateral MTAL Cl$^-$ channels. Am J Physiol 1996;270(6 Pt 2):F1066−1072.

[162] Lourdel S, Paulais M, Cluzeaud F, Bens M, Tanemoto M, Kurachi Y, et al. An inward rectifier K(+) channel at the basolateral membrane of the mouse distal convoluted tubule: similarities with Kir4-Kir5.1 heteromeric channels. J Physiol 2002;538(Pt 2):391−404.

[163] Ito M, Inanobe A, Horio Y, Hibino H, Isomoto S, Ito H, et al. Immunolocalization of an inwardly rectifying K$^+$ channel, K (AB)-2 (Kir4.1), in the basolateral membrane of renal distal tubular epithelia. FEBS Lett 1996;388(1):11−5.

[164] Tucker SJ, Imbrici P, Salvatore L, D'Adamo MC, Pessia M. pH dependence of the inwardly rectifying potassium channel, Kir5.1, and localization in renal tubular epithelia. J Biol Chem 2000;275(22):16404−7.

[165] Lourdel S, Paulais M, Marvao P, Nissant A, Teulon J. A chloride channel at the basolateral membrane of the distal-convoluted tubule: a candidate ClC-K channel. J Gen Physiol 2003;121(4):287−300.

[166] Nissant A, Lourdel S, Baillet S, Paulais M, Marvao P, Teulon J, et al. Heterogeneous distribution of chloride channels along the distal convoluted tubule probed by single-cell RT-PCR and patch clamp. Am J Physiol Renal Physiol 2004;287(6): F1233−1243.

[167] Frindt G, Palmer LG. Na channels in the rat connecting tubule. Am J Physiol 2004;286:F669−74.

[168] Duc C, Farman N, Canessa C, Bonvalet J-P, Rossier B. Cell-specific expression of epithelial sodium channel α, β and γ subunits in aldosterone-responsive epithelia from the rat: localization by *in situ* hybridization and immunocytochemistry. J Cell Biol 1994;127:1907–21.

[169] Loffing J, Pietri L, Aregger F, Bloch-Faure M, Ziegler U, Meneton P, et al. Differential subcellular localization of ENaC subunits in mouse kidney in response to high- and low-Na diets. Am J Physiol Renal Physiol 2000;279(2):F252–258.

[170] Rubera I, Loffing J, Palmer LG, Frindt G, Fowler-Jaeger N, Sauter D, et al. Collecting duct specific gene inactivation of αENaC in the mouse kidney does not impair sodium and potassium balance. J Clin Invest 2003;112:554–65.

[171] Wang W, Schwab A, Giebisch G. Regulation of small conductance K channel in apical membrane of rat cortical collecting tubule. Am J Physiol 1990;259:F494–502.

[172] Bailey MA, Cantone A, Yan Q, MacGregor GG, Leng Q, Amorim JB, et al. Maxi-K channels contribute to urinary potassium excretion in the ROMK-deficient mouse model of Type II Bartter's syndrome and in adaptation to a high-K diet. Kidney Int 2006;70(1):51–9.

[173] Lachheb S, Cluzeaud F, Bens M, Genete M, Hibino H, Lourdel S, et al. Kir4.1/Kir5.1 channel forms the major K$^+$ channel in the basolateral membrane of mouse renal collecting duct principal cells. Am J Physiol Renal Physiol 2008;294(6):F1398–1407.

[174] Palmer LG, Frindt G. Cl$^-$ channels of the distal nephron. Am J Physiol Renal Physiol 2006;:.

[175] Pácha J, Frindt G, Sackin H, Palmer LG. Apical maxi K channels in intercalated cells of CCT. Am J Physiol 1991;261: F696–705.

[176] Palmer LG, Frindt G. High-conductance K channels in intercalated cells of the rat distal nephron. Am J Physiol Renal Physiol 2007;292(3):F966–973.

[177] Najjar F, Zhou H, Morimoto T, Bruns JB, Li HS, Liu W, et al. Dietary K$^+$ regulates apical membrane expression of maxi-K channels in rabbit cortical collecting duct. Am J Physiol Renal Physiol 2005;289(4):F922–932.

[178] Nissant A, Paulais M, Lachheb S, Lourdel S, Teulon J. Similar chloride channels in the connecting tubule and cortical collecting duct of the mouse kidney. Am J Physiol Renal Physiol 2006;290(6):F1421–1429.

[179] Boulpaep EL, Sackin H. Electrical analysis of intraepithelial barriers. Curr Top Membr Transp 1980;13:169–97.

[180] Rakowski RF, Vasilets LA, LaTona J, Schwarz W. A negative slope in the current-voltage relationship of the Na/K pump in *Xenopus* oocytes produced by reduction of external [K]. J Membr Biol 1991;121:177–87.

[181] Frindt G, Palmer LG. Ca-activated K channels in apical membrane of mammalian CCT, and their role in K secretion. Am J Physiol 1987;252:F458–67.

Renal Ion Channels, Electrophysiology of Transport, and Channelopathies

James D. Stockand

Department of Physiology, University of Texas Health Science Center, San Antonio, TX, USA

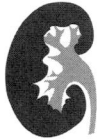

The purposes of this chapter are to explain what an ion channel is and how it works, provide an overview of the contribution ion channel proteins make to renal transport, and suggest how changes in the structure and biophysical properties of renal ion channels cause disease. Emphasis is placed on recent information gained from the latest techniques. This chapter is neither a technical manual nor a comprehensive review. Its goal, rather, is to demonstrate how appreciation of renal physiology is expanded by considering the structure and biophysical properties of ion channels. Important equations are provided only in their simplest forms to demonstrate how the understanding of channel biophysics informs us about the role played by these proteins in the kidney. The goals of this chapter necessitate coverage of a wide subject matter. Several topics are introduced here in brief but are covered in more depth in other chapters of this book and elsewhere.[1,2,3] This chapter is about how we move from understanding channel biophysics and structure to understanding how changes in them cause disease.

Ion channels are central to renal transport. A diverse group of ion channels, including Ca^{2+}, Cl^-, K^+, Mg^{2+}, Na^+, and non-selective cation channels, are expressed along the length of the renal tubule and collecting duct system. Figure 8.1 and Table 8.1 report the expression profile for ion channels in the kidney at sites where their functions have been firmly established. Channels act as selective and regulated gateways, conducting ions down electrochemical gradients via restrictive diffusion. This enables channel proteins to serve as physical conduits for the movement of ions across epithelial cell membranes. In addition to functioning as gateways during transport, channel activity sets the electrical and chemical forces driving the movement of ions and coupled molecules, such as water and glucose, through and between renal epithelial cells. As such, the activities of renal ion channels often serve as the final arbiters of the electrolyte content of urine and plasma. This is true for Ca^{2+}, K^+, Mg^{2+}, and Na^+. Ion channels in the kidney, consequently, are targets for hormones and pharmacological agents to affect plasma ion content and volume. Aberrant regulation of renal ion channels or dysfunction of these proteins, moreover, cause kidney disease with compromised tubule transport. For instance, renal Mg^{2+} excretion is fine-tuned in the early distal convoluted tubule (DCT). Inactivating mutations in the Mg^{2+}-selective transient receptor potential (TRP) channel, TRPM6, causes hypomagnesemia with secondary hypocalcemia (HSH). This is a familial form of an autosomal recessive renal Mg^{2+}- and Ca^{2+}-wasting tubulopathy that ultimately leads to neurological damage and dysfunction.[4,5,6,7,8,9] Figure 8.2 shows models of epithelial cells in different segments of the nephron, and emphasizes the location of transport proteins and ion channels.

Renal ion channels also play important roles in cell signaling. They set membrane potential that modulates intracellular signaling. They also allow access to the ions involved in cell signaling, as typified by Ca^{2+}. Involvement of renal channels in cell signaling is highlighted by the role played by TRPC6 channels in podocytes of Bowman's capsule. Here, gain-of-function mutations in TRPC6 facilitate Ca^{2+} entry, leading to prolonged changes in the dynamics of Ca^{2+} signaling ultimately causing a familial form of focal segmental glomerulosclerosis (FSGS[10,11,12,13]).

Over the last few decades, the application of contemporary molecular genetics and gene knockout technology to cell biology and physiological questions

Seldin and Giebisch's The Kidney, Fifth Edition.
DOI: http://dx.doi.org/10.1016/B978-0-12-381462-3.00008-2

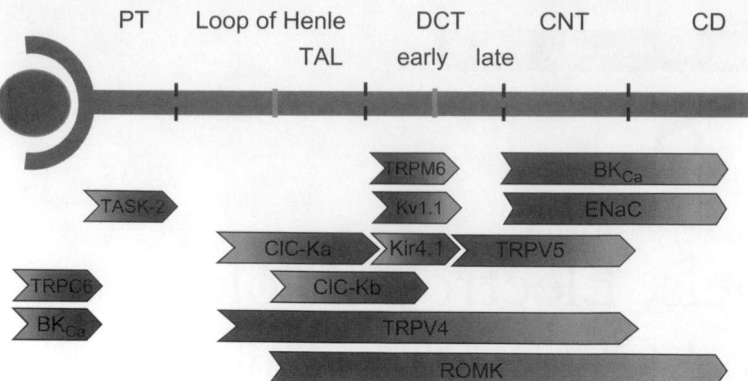

FIGURE 8.1 **Functional expression of ion channels in the nephron.** Expression in the apical membrane is indicated by a darker to lighter gray scale. Expression in the basolateral membrane is indicated by a lighter to darker gray scale.

has revealed much about the roles played by renal ion channels, and the diseases caused by their dysfunction. An improvement in electrophysiological methods has allowed the detailed study of single ion channel proteins. Furthermore, the resolution of the crystal structures for several different channels has contributed greatly to determining the mechanisms by which channels gate and are regulated, facilitating our understanding at the atomic level of structure—function relations in these proteins. This allows the rationalization of how mutations in the genes encoding renal channels and channel regulators lead to disease, and how agents used in the clinic to modulate renal channel activity exert their pharmacological actions. For instance, it is recognized now that the renal phenotype resulting from decreased activity of the luminal Na^+,K^+,Cl^--co-transporter (NKCC2) in the thick ascending limb (TAL) shares many common features with those arising from inactivation of the luminal renal outer medullary K^+ (ROMK) channel responsible for K^+ recycling across the apical membrane of TAL epithelial cells and serosal ClC-Kb channels responsible for Cl^- exit from these cells, in that they all cause Bartter syndrome (BS) with hallmark NaCl wasting and compromised urine-concentrating ability.[14,15,16,17,18] Smilar salt- and water-wasting stems from the inhibition of NKCC2 in the TAL by furosemide and bumetenide loop diuretics. Both are important clinical tools used in the treatment of high blood pressure and heart failure.

As stated above, this chapter applies understanding of channel biophysics to the understanding of physiology, focusing on the role played by channels in renal transport, and rationalizes how compromises in channel properties cause channelopathies and tubulopathy. Important concepts are reinforced with specific examples. To facilitate discussion, a general appreciation of the structure and functional properties of the renal epithelium to include routes of transport, types of transport proteins common to epithelial cell membranes and forces driving transport are first developed. These are covered in greater detail in Chapters 1 and

2. What an ion channel is, and the biophysical explanation and atomic origins of gating, selectivity, and permeation are also addressed. Again, this material has some overlap with that presented in Chapter 7. The rich understanding of renal ion channels that has emerged over the last two decades makes it reasonable to describe briefly the roles played by these channels in transport and disease, and to discuss how the biophysical properties of renal channels determine their function in the kidney (see also Chapters 30, 31, 47, 62 and 80). The number of crystal structures now available for different types of channels makes it feasible to include a brief review of channel structure, and to discuss how this determines channel properties. Examples then can be examined where known changes in the biophysical properties of specific renal channels cause tubulopathies.

STRUCTURE—FUNCTION OF TUBULE EPITHELIUM

The renal tubule is a single epithelial cell thick. It is linear with ultrafiltrate and pro-urine separated from interstitial fluid by epithelial cells coupled together with tight junctions to form the epithelium. Fluid flows down the tubule in one direction from Bowman's space to the collecting duct system, ultimately into the ureter. Fluid flows down the tubule driven by hydrostatic pressure renewed by constant filtration at the glomerulus.

The Tubule is a Barrier

The structure of the tubule provides a barrier function separating fluid compartments; pro-urine from interstitial fluid. The electrical properties of the tubule and transport across the tubule can be understood in terms of equivalent circuits, such that ions cross a resistive barrier driven by electrochemical forces

TABLE 8.1 Renal Ion Channels with Recognized Function

Channel	Alternative Names	Expression	Gene Pore/ Accessory	Chromosome Location	Function	References
CALCIUM						
TRPC3	TRP3	podocyte + CD (ubiquitous)	*TRPC3*	4, 123.02-123.09	Receptor operated Ca^{2+} entry pathway in podocytes.	10, 11, 12
TRPC6	FSGS2, TRP6	podocyte + CD	*TRPC6*	11, 101.32-101.45	Receptor operated Ca^{2+} entry pathway in podocytes; role in CD less clear but may be involved in mechanosensation.	10, 11, 12
TRPP2	PCL, PKD2L, PKDL	TAL + DCT	*PKD2L1*	10, 102.04-102.08	See chapter 80	
TRPV4	OTRPC4, TRP12 VRL-2, VROAC,	AtL + TAL + DCT + CNT	*TRPV4*	12, 108.71-108.76	Molecular osmoreceptor.	12
TRPV5	ECaC1, CAT2, OTRPC3	late DCT + CNT	*TRPV5*	7, 142.32-142.34	Apical entry pathway for Ca^{2+} in the late DCT.	84, 85, 12, 49
CHLORIDE						
ClC-Ka[a]	ClC-K1	AtL, TAL	*CLCNKA + BSND* (Barttin)	1, 16.22-16.23 1, 55.24-55.25	Basolateral Cl^- exit pathway.	79, 59, 71, 60
ClC-Kb[a]	ClC-K2	TAL + early DCT	*CLCNKB + BSND* (Barttin)	1, 16.24-16.26 1, 55.24-55.25	Basolateral Cl^- exit pathway.	79, 59, 71, 60
POTASSIUM						
BK$_{Ca}$	maxi K$^+$, Slo	podocytes, CNT + CCD	α, *KCNMα1* + β1, *KCNMβ1*, β4, *KCNMβ4*	10, 78.31-79.07 5, 169.74-169.75 12, 69.05-69.11	Stabilizes membrane potential in podocytes to facilitate Ca^{2+} entry via TRPC6; flow-sensitive K^+ secretion in the distal nephron.	10, 11, 12
Kir4.1[a]	BIRK-10, KCNJ13-PEN, Kir1.2	DCT + CNT	*KCNJ10*	1, 158.27-158.31	Allows basolateral K^+ recycling facilitating Mg^{2+} reabsorption via TRPM6/TRPM7.	96, 92, 97, 98
Kv1.1	HUK1, RBK1, AEMK, HBK1, MK1	DCT	*KCNA1*	12, 4.89-4.9	Hyperpolarizes the luminal membrane to facilitate Mg^{2+} influx thru TRPM6/TRPM7.	20, 92
ROMK1	ROMK, K$_{ir}$1.1	TAL + DCT + CNT + CD	*KCNJ1*	11, 128.21-128.24	Apical K^+ recycling in the TAL; aldosterone and plasma K^+-sensitive K^+ secretion from principal cells in the CNT + CD	14, 23, 31, 33
TASK-2[a]	K$_{2P}$5.1	PT	*KCNK5*	6, 39.26-39.31	Functions as a hyperpolarizing influence to maintain favorable conditions across the basolateral membrane for electrogenic HCO_3^- reabsorption.	80, 99
MAGNESIUM						
TRPM6	CHAK2, HMGX, HSH, HOMG	early DCT	*TRPM6*	9, 76.53-76.69	Apcial entry pathway for Mg^{2+} in the early DCT.	10, 20, 12, 24, 9
TRPM7	CHAK1, TRP-PLIK	ubiquitous	*TRPM7*	15, 48.64-48.77	Apical entry pathway for Mg^{2+} in the early DCT.	10, 20, 12, 24, 9
SODIUM						
ENaC		CNT + CCD	α, *SCNN1A* β, *SCNN1B* γ, *SCNN1C*	12, 6.33-6.35 16, 23.22-23.3 16, 23.1-23.14	Apical entry pathway for Na^+ in CNT and CD principal cells.	41, 83

[a]*Expressed in the basolateral membrane.*

I. EPITHELIAL AND NONEPITHELIAL TRANSPORT AND REGULATION

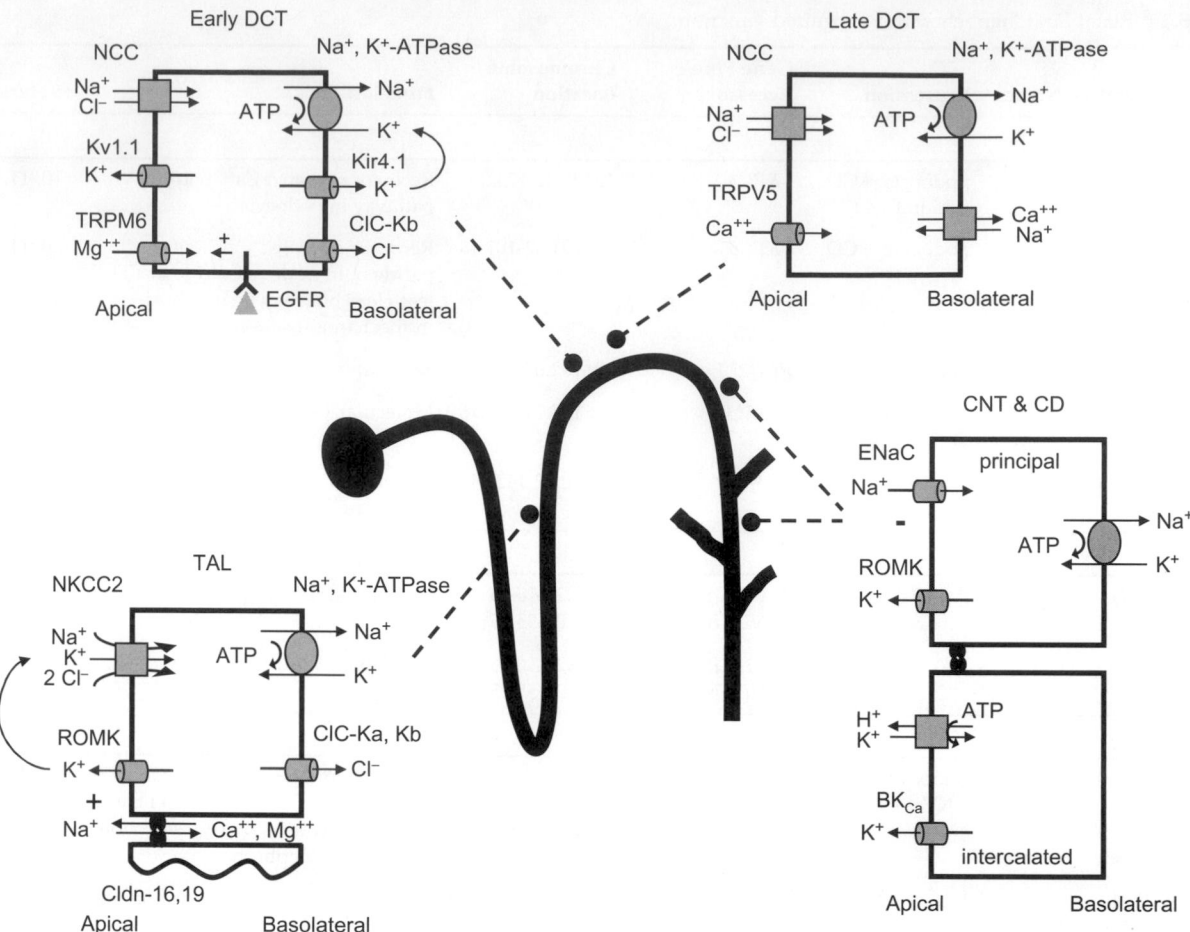

FIGURE 8.2   Models of renal epithelial cells lining the tubule emphasizing the location of transport proteins and ion channels.

through conductive pathways. Figure 8.3 shows a simplified equivalent circuit representing tubule epithelium. In this regard, ion channels and tight junctions serve as conductive pathways across epithelial cell membranes and the epithelial barrier, respectively, with voltage and concentration gradients existing across these membranes and the barrier. Because channels, which are gated, make a significant contribution to membrane resistance, epithelial cell membranes are best described as variable resistors. Accordingly, channels affect the resistance of the epithelial cell membrane and electrochemical driving forces across these membranes and the epithelium.

Routes of Transport across the Tubule

Two different routes of transit from one fluid compartment to the other exist across the renal epithelial barrier. Movement through the epithelial cell is termed transcellular, and between epithelial cells across tight junctions is termed paracellular. Transcellular

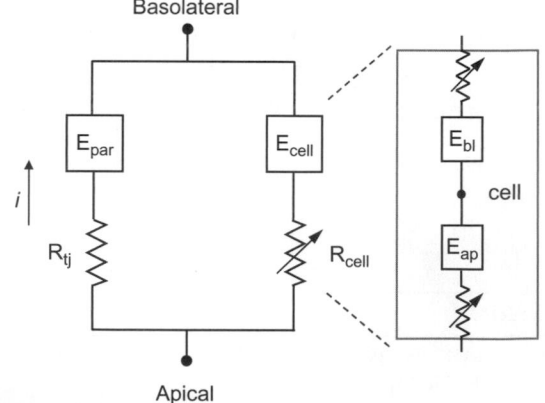

FIGURE 8.3   Tubule epithelium can be represented by an equivalent circuit. (Abbreviations: ap: apical; bl: basolateral; par: paracellular; tj: tight junction.)

movement, as depicted in the simple equivalent circuit shown in Figure 8.3, includes crossing both the apical and basolateral membranes. Channels facilitate the crossing of these membranes by ions. Tight junctions serve a similar function for paracellular movement across the epithelium. Tight junctions, like channels, are selectively permeable. Nothing to date, though, suggests that tight junctions act in a gated manner; rather, they function as doorways of fixed resistance that are selective in what they let pass. Diffusion through tight junctions is passive, driven by electrochemical gradients.

Epithelial Cells are Polarized

Tubule epithelial cells, and thus the tubule epithelium, are polarized with distinct membranes facing the pro-urine, the apical membrane, and the interstitial fluid, the basolateral membrane. These distinct membranes have different protein profiles, including the expression of ion channels. The net result is that each cell membrane has different capability, selectivity, and capacity for moving ions and other molecules. This, combined with the barrier function of the epithelium, provides epithelial cells with the ability to transport in a directional manner. This process is often termed vectoral transport.

Types of Transport and Transporters

Epithelial transport and specific transport proteins are covered in more detail in Chapters 1 and 2. In brief, transport across an epithelial cell can be divided into those that do not require a protein, and those that are protein-mediated. The former is termed simple diffusion and is passive, being dependent on the concentration gradient and surface area. If a molecule is capable of permeating the cell membrane, it will cross according to its chemical gradient. Molecules that move using this form of transport are exclusively small and non-polar, and are capable of crossing a lipid bilayer. Simple diffusion cannot be saturated and is

not regulated. The movement of NH_3 in parts of the tubule is a good example of this form of transport. Mediated transport, in contrast, is capable of being saturated, and is dependent on the presence of specific proteins. Moreover, it often is regulated by cell signaling. Figure 8.4 shows models representative of the different classes of transport proteins common to renal epithelial cells. Forces driving protein-mediated transport are discussed in more detail below, but they can include the concentration difference of the molecule to be transported across the membrane or barrier, electrical potential differences, and the activity of transport proteins.

Facilitative diffusion, similar to simple diffusion, is passive, allowing molecules to move down concentration gradients. Facilitative transporters translocate molecules across membranes. An example of a facilitative transport protein in the kidney is the proximal tubule glucose transporter, GLUT2.

Ion channels allow restrictive diffusion, a unique form of passive transport. Channels form selective pores in the membrane, allowing ions to cross the membrane through permeation rather than being translocated across the membrane. Restrictive diffusion through ion channels is driven by electrochemical gradients.

The two remaining types of transport proteins allow active transport: the active movement of molecules against gradients. This type of transport is directly, in the case of primary active transport, and indirectly, in the case of secondary active transport, tied to the consumption of energy. Primary active transporters require ATP to transport molecules against their concentration gradients. As discussed below, this ultimately energizes all transport across the renal tubule. The Na^+,K^+-ATPase is a notable primary active transporter in the tubule and

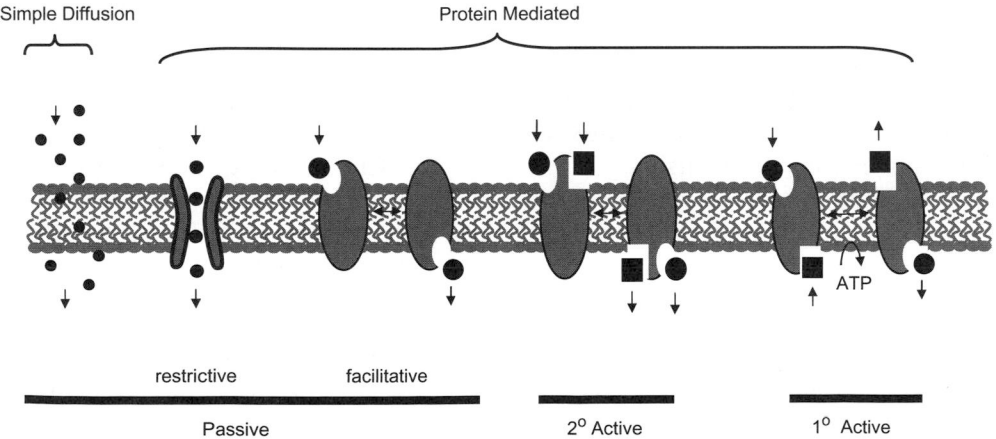

FIGURE 8.4 **Representative models of the different types of renal transport proteins.**

collecting duct system. Secondary active transporters use gradients established by primary active transporters. They couple the movement of one molecule against its gradient to the movement of another molecule down its gradient. NKCC2 in the TAL and the thiazide-sensitive Na^+,Cl^--co-transporter (NCC) in the DCT are prominent secondary active transporters in the kidney. The latter couples the inward movement of Cl^- into the cell against its gradient to the inward movement of Na^+ into the cell with its gradient. Thus, Na^+ entering the cell downhill on this transporter pulls Cl^- uphill with it.

Forces Driving Transport across the Tubule: The Importance of Disequilibrium

Filtration at the glomerulus, as discussed in Chapter 21, is governed by Starling forces. The difference in hydrostatic pressure between plasma in the glomerular capillary and ultrafiltrate in Bowman's space, the beginning of the tubule, drives filtration. The difference in oncotic pressure between these fluids impedes filtration. The net result of filtration is that ultrafiltrate entering the renal tubule is similar in content to plasma minus blood cells and proteins. Electrolytes or other small molecules, therefore, have little gradient initially to cross the epithelial barrier, leaving pro-urine for interstitial fluid or *vice versa*. The activity of the Na^+,K^+-ATPase pump localized to the basolateral membrane of all tubule epithelial cells changes this by providing the motivation, ultimately, for all transport. This protein consumes ATP to generate disequilibrium for Na^+ and K^+ across cell membranes. Because epithelial cell membranes are effective at separating fluid compartments, this disequilibrium can be maintained and converted into voltage differences and differences in ion concentrations by the activities of ion channels, other transport proteins, and the capacitive nature of cell membranes. Similarly, because epithelial cells, coupled together by tight junctions, effectively separate fluid compartments, disequilibrium across the tubule epithelium is maintained. Urine flowing in only one direction down the tubule also helps maintain disequilibrium, by moving processed fluid too quickly for equilibrium to be reached. Ion channels and other transport proteins tap these electrochemical gradients to transport molecules across the epithelium. Thus, disequilibrium enables modification of urine by tubule epithelial cells. Renal transport ultimately, then, is the movement of molecules through channels and other transporters, tending towards an equilibrium that is kept beyond reach by the continuous activity of the Na^+,K^+-ATPase.

The Tubule Epithelium has Emergent Properties

The importance of the structure of the epithelial barrier and state of disequilibrium maintained across this barrier to transport is apparent when considering the similar Ca^{2+}- and Mg^{2+}-wasting phenotypes arising from inactivation in the TAL of NKCC2, ROMK, claudin-16, and claudin-19.[19,20,21,22,23,24] Dysfunction of claudin-16 and -19 cause familial hypomagnesemia, with hypercalciuria and nephrocalcinosis (FHHNC[25,26,27,28]). These claudins are critical components of the tight junction in the TAL, where they provide cation-selectivity, allowing Na^+ back-flux into tubular fluid more rapidly than Cl^-, contributing to a lumen-positive diffusion potential. The lumen-positive potential that results from the combination of this Na^+ back-flux with apical K^+ recycling mediated by the coordinated activities of luminal ROMK channels and NKCC2 drives paracellular Mg^{2+} and Ca^{2+} transport. Claudin dysfunction, like dysfunction of ROMK or NKCC2, then compromises the electrochemical gradient responsible for divalent cation reabsorption in the TAL. This illustrates that a break in function of any of several components of the whole leads to the same disease. This is an important concept: epithelial cells and epithelial barriers have emergent properties that are dependent on the proper functioning of each component part, including ion channels.

Urine Flows down the Tubule

An additional point important to recognize about renal transport is that urine flows in the tubule in one direction; what happens upstream affects transport downstream. This is so because the modification of urine in upstream segments determines the constituents of urine in downstream segments. For instance, inhibition of NKCC2 in the TAL by loop diuretics, in addition to compromising urine-concentrating ability by destroying the axial corticomedullary hyperosmotic gradient, also leads to an increase in K^+ secretion at the collecting duct (CD), and ultimately to K^+ excretion by the kidney. This is due to increased urine flow and Na^+ delivery to the CD. Increased urine delivery to the CD promotes flow-induced K^+ secretion by BK_{Ca} channels, which are activated by mechanical stimuli.[29,30] Increased Na^+ delivery drives increased Na^+ reabsorption via the epithelial Na^+ channel (ENaC) across principal cells of the CD, due to a change in the electrochemical gradient for Na^+ across the apical membrane. This increase in Na^+ reabsorption in turn affects the electrochemical gradient across the apical membrane, driving additional K^+ secretion through ROMK channels.[31,32] For the same reasons, any inactivating mutation in a TAL transport protein involved in NaCl reabsorption, including NKCC2, ClC-Kb, and ROMK channels, causes the renal K$^+$ wasting associated with Bartter syndrome.[15,16,17,18] Moreover, disease resulting from inactivation of NCC and the ClC chloride channel beta subunit barttin, and diuretics such as thiazide inhibitors of the NCC co-transporter that decrease NaCl reabsorption in the DCT, also cause renal K$^+$ wasting by this common mechanism.

Transport does not Happen in a "Vacuum"

Another concept emerging from the above discussion is that the transport of one type of ion through renal ion channels influences the movement of different ions through other distinct channels. This coupling is a manifestation of ion channel activity influencing electrochemical driving forces. An example of this, as discussed above, is the electrogenic Na$^+$ reabsorption via ENaC influencing ROMK-mediated K$^+$ secretion in the CD. This will be touched upon again in more detail below. Similarly, as mentioned earlier, Mg^{2+} and Ca^{2+} reabsorption in the TAL are positively coupled to NaCl reabsorption with K$^+$ recycling across the luminal membrane via ROMK channels and paracellular Na$^+$-back flux via claudin proteins, setting the electrochemical driving forces moving these divalent cations.[21,22,26,31,33]

ION CHANNELS: BIOPHYSICAL PROPERTIES

An ion channel is an integral membrane protein or protein complex that forms a continuous conductive pore through a membrane. The pore spans the entirety of the membrane with the conduction pathway perpendicular to the plane of the lipid bilayer. The mouths of an ion channel pore are in contact with the aqueous solutions on both sides of the bilayer. As ions enter the permeation pathway of a channel pore and reach the selectivity-filter, they become partially dehydrated, moving through the channel only after losing surrounding water molecules. Binding sites within the pore then mimic solvation by water as ions permeate across the membrane through the channel.

Channel pores are selective and gated. The basis of selectivity is usually a defined sequence of residues at the narrowest part of the pore. Residues in the selectivity-filter are highly conserved across a channel family, and generally across a class of channels. Most, if not all, K$^+$-selective channels, for instance, share the common signature selectivity sequence TXGYG.[32,34,35,36] Moreover, all known

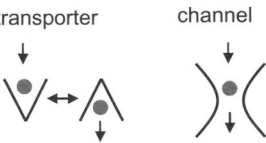

FIGURE 8.5 **Simplified modes of transport used by transporters versus ion channels.** Translocation of molecules across the membrane by transporters entails relatively large changes in conformation compared to ion permeation across the membrane through ion channels.

K$^+$ channels with this selectivity-filter use a common mechanism of permeation to conduct K$^+$ through the pore, as discussed in greater detail below.

Ion Channels Provide a Unique Form of Passive Diffusion

As emphasized in the simplified forms of transport shown in Figure 8.5, ion channels differ from other transport proteins, in that they form a physical hole through the membrane. No other type of transport protein does this. Rather, the molecule to be translocated by transport proteins other than ion channels interacts with a binding site on one face of the protein, but does not actually move across the membrane until a change in conformation takes place where the initial entry site closes as the exit site opens to allow the bound molecule to be released and egress out across the opposite face of the protein from which it entered. Ion channels also contain binding sites for permeant ions. Ions transiently bind to these sites during permeation, with the electrochemical gradient driving the direction of transport. In conjunction with properties of the pore and charge repulsion between permeant ions, this gradient determines the magnitude of ion flow.[36,37,38] Because channels are pores that allow ions to permeate through the membrane, they facilitate crossing of the membrane with relatively little change in overall conformation. Transporters, in comparison, typically require greater relative changes in conformation to translocate molecules across the membrane. The result is that single-channel proteins move a far greater number of molecules per unit of time (10^7 to 10^8 ions/second) compared to any other single-transport protein.

Recording Ion Channel Activity with Patch-Clamp Electrophysiology

When open, a channel conducts the movement of ions across the cell membrane. This manifests as a decrease in resistance the membrane has to the permeant ion. Current through an ion channel is dependent on the electrochemical driving force, whether

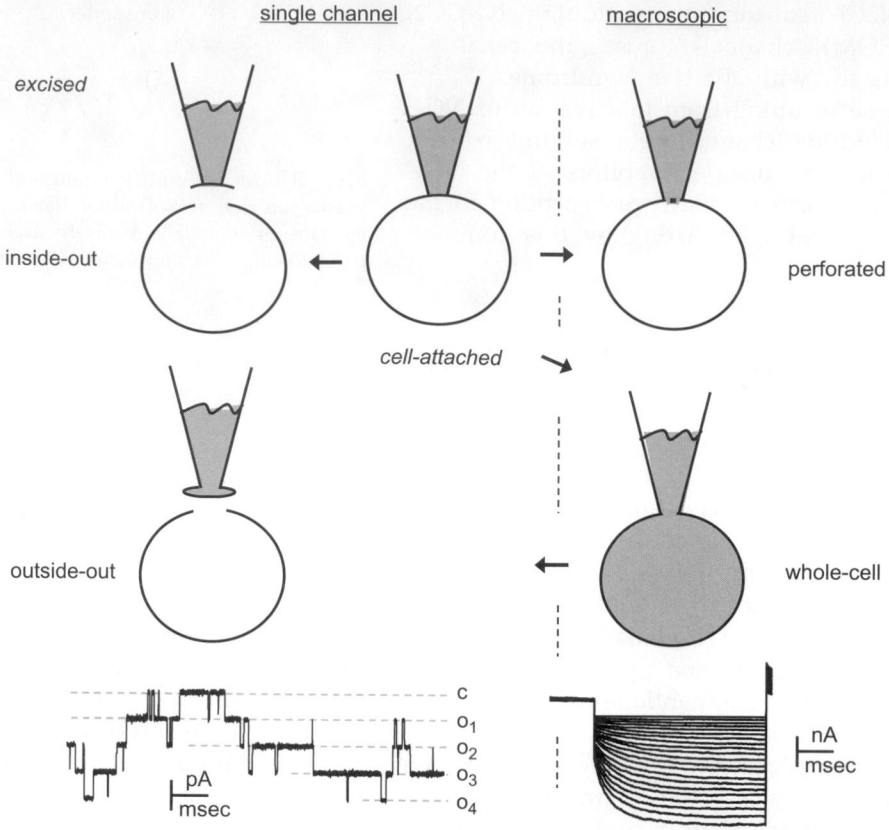

FIGURE 8.6   **Patch-clamp configurations.** This illustration depicts the five different seal configurations available for patch-clamp analysis: three are amenable to single channel recording, cell-attached, excised inside-out and excised outside-out; and two for macroscopic current recording, perforated and whole-cell. In this figure, the cell is represented as a circle and the recording pipette as a V. Gray shading defines continuity between the solution in the recording pipette and intracellular solution. Arrows represent transition steps during seal formation taken to establish the distinct types of seals. Shown below are representative current data from configurations with single channel (left) and macroscopic (right) resolutions. Closed (C) and open (O) states are noted in the single channel trace. *(Data from J.D. Stockand or published previously in ref. [39].)*

the channel is open or closed and the selectivity of the channel, and how well a certain ion moves through, or rather permeates through, the conduction pathway. The activity and biophysical properties of ion channels can be assayed in experiments with electrophysiological tools, including sharp electrodes and two-electrode voltage clamping. The most sophisticated tool used to probe the biophysical properties of channels is patch-clamp electrophysiology. Erwin Neher and Bert Sakmann were awarded the Nobel Prize in Physiology or Medicine in 1991, in part for this development.[3] Patch-clamp electrophysiology enables the study of both macroscopic and single-channel currents. It has a high degree of precision and fidelity, allowing the resolution of the activity of a single protein in real-time. Figure 8.6 shows the different patch configurations available for the study of ion channels, and sample data from experiments investigating the single-channel properties of wild-type ENaC (left) and macroscopic currents from a mutant form of ENaC (right) that activates upon

hyperpolarization due to the voltage-dependent block of the pore by intracellular Na^+.[39]

Adaptation of Ohm's Law to Biological Systems: Explaining Current Carried by Ion Channels

Current flow in an electrical circuit obeys Ohm's Law which, when reordered, states $I = gE$, where current (I) equals the product of the conductance (g) and voltage difference (E) across the conductor, which in biological systems is an ion channel protein. This simple formula was adapted to $I_x = g_x (E - E_x)$ by Hodgkin and Huxley, in their seminal electrophysiological studies (as explained by Hille and Cole in their books[2,40]) to fit biological reality better where current through an ion channel crosses a capacitive membrane that separates fluid compartments of different ionic activities. The gradient across the membrane acts like a battery represented by an equivalent circuit with an

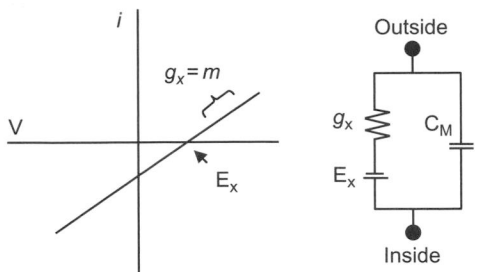

FIGURE 8.7 An idealized I−V relation and equivalent circuit describing a channel obeying Ohm's Law. Conductance (g) is equal to the slope of the I−V line. E_x is the reversal potential, and C_M is membrane capacitance.

electromotive force, E_x, in series with a channel resistor, g_x. This conductive branch is in parallel with the capacitor representing the membrane. In this modified equation, E remains voltage across the membrane, and the net driving force on ion X is now $E - E_x$. Thus, current in biological systems is driven by an electrochemical gradient rather than by voltage alone.

Figure 8.7 shows a graphical representation of an idealized current−voltage relation for an equivalent circuit describing an open ion channel obeying this modified Ohm's Law. When voltage, E, is equal to E_x, no net current flows through the channel. When $E < E_x$, current flows into the cell. If this represents a cation channel, for instance ENaC, and extracellular $[Na^+]$ is greater than intracellular $[Na^+]$, as is the normal case in physiological systems, this inward current flow would be carried by Na^+ entering the cell through ENaC. This represents the normal conditions under which ENaC functions in CD principal cells, allowing Na^+ to enter the cell across the apical membrane during electrogenic Na^+ reabsorption.[41,42] The typical concentration of ions in urine and intracellular fluid combined with the activities of K^+ channels in the apical and basolateral membranes set the potential (E) across the apical membrane lower than E_{Na}. This facilitates Na^+ influx through ENaC. In contrast, when $E > E_x$ current flows outwards, Na^+ exits the cell. This explains the consequences of the electrochemical gradient driving Na^+ through ENaC. Sodium movement through ENaC across the membrane, in turn, influences electrochemical gradients. If no other parameter changed, Na^+ moving through ENaC would dissipate the $E - E_{Na}$ difference, eventually arriving at equilibrium where E and E_{Na} are equalized. Restated, net flux through a channel occurs only as long as the system is out of electrochemical equilibrium. This is where the Na^+, K^+-ATPase and separation of fluid compartments with different ionic activities by cell membranes come into play. They enable epithelial cells to remain out of equilibrium.

The Nernst Equation

In the above description, E_x is the equilibrium potential (or reversal potential) for ion X, a state where the tendency for further change vanishes, and all existing forces on X are in balance. This would be where voltage across the membrane containing the channel permeable to ion X equals the diffusion potential developed by the ionic gradient for ion X across this membrane. Mathematically, as noted above, this is where $E = E_x$. Equilibrium potentials are easily measured in the laboratory with electrophysiology. Moreover, they can be calculated empirically using a formula developed by Nernst in 1888.[40,43] This led to the equilibrium potential sometimes being referred to as the Nernst potential. The Nernst equation states $E_x = (RT/zF)\ln([X]_o/[X]_i)$, where R and F are physical constants having the usual meanings of Universal Gas constant and Faraday's constant, T is temperature in kelvin, z accounts for the charge and valence of ion X, ln indicates natural logarithm, and $[X]_o$ and $[X]_i$ are the concentrations of ion X outside and inside the cell, respectively. Accordingly, the equilibrium potential falls to zero in the absence of a gradient, reverses signs as the direction of the gradient is reversed (e.g., that for Na^+ compared to K^+) and as the charge of the ion is reversed, for example Na^+ versus Cl^-. Equilibrium potentials across cell membranes for ions common to physiological solutions are ~ 130, -98 and 67 mV, respectively, for Ca^{2+}, K^+, and Na^{+} [2]. The equilibrium potential for Cl^- is more variable, because $[Cl^-]_i$ varies more widely with cell type, but it usually is close to the resting membrane potential of the cell, often being slightly above or below that level. Calculating equilibrium potential across tubular epithelial cell membranes is complicated by the luminal and serosal membranes facing different solutions. The apical membrane may have a different equilibrium potential for Na^+ as compared to that across the basolateral membrane, because the concentration of this ion in urine may be greater or less than that of plasma, depending on Na^+ and water transport along the length of the nephron.

The Goldman−Hodgkin−Katz Voltage Equation

Work performed by Hodgkin, Huxley, and Goldman and others led to the realization that cell membrane potential reflects the equilibrium potentials of all permeant ions at a given time, and that this can be mathematically represented.[2,40] When calculating membrane potential (E_{mem}), the magnitude of ion movement through any given class of channel, for example K^+ versus Na^+ channels, is accounted for by using weighted averages of each ion's equilibrium potential. These weighted averages convey the relative

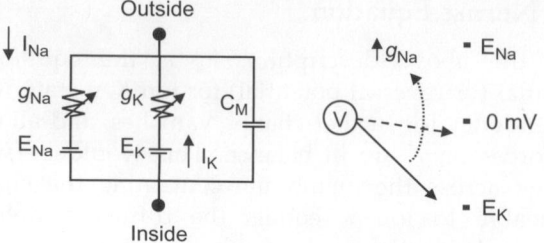

FIGURE 8.8   A simplified equivalent circuit of a cell containing Na⁺ and K⁺ channels contributing to membrane potential. Shown to the right is the change in membrane potential resulting from activation of Na⁺ channels.

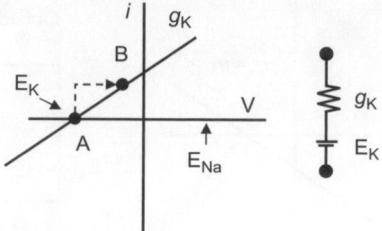

FIGURE 8.9   Changes in membrane potential influence current through open channels. Shown are an idealized I–V relation (left), and associated equivalent circuit (right) for a K⁺ channel. Movement from point A to B notes the effect on current through this channel as the membrane becomes depolarized in response to the activation of Na⁺ channels.

permeability (P_x) of each ion to total ion permeability (P_{tot}). By using the simplified condition of only considering flux of monovalent cations through channels, which is not too distant from reality, the Goldman–Hodgkin–Katz (GHK) equation is $E_{mem} = (P_K/P_{tot})E_K + (P_{Na}/P_{tot})E_{Na}$. Figure 8.8 shows an equivalent circuit representing the cell membrane and individual ionic conductances contributing to this membrane potential. Because K⁺ channel activity predominates at rest with P_K approaching P_{tot}, membrane potential is closest to E_K. An increase in the activity of Na⁺ channels, which increases the relative permeability of this ion, causes the membrane to become more depolarized, as represented by the volt meter in Figure 8.8 moving E_{mem} towards E_{Na} as ENaC becomes active.

What do Ohm's Law, the Nernst Equation, and the GHK Equation Tell us About Transport?

Reconsidering now Figure 8.7 and the scenario described earlier, inward Na⁺ flow through ENaC depolarizes the apical membrane, moving E_{mem} towards E_{Na}. Because the ionic gradient for K⁺ across the apical membrane is the reverse of that for Na⁺, depolarizing the apical membrane would move E_{mem} further away from E_K, driving more K⁺ out of the cell through apical K⁺ channels, for instance, through ROMK channels in the apical membrane of principal cells.[32] Figure 8.9 shows an idealized current–voltage relation for an open K⁺ channel, and notes the influence of membrane depolarization (moving from A to B) on K⁺ current through this channel as the apical membrane is depolarized by Na⁺ reabsorption through ENaC, activated perhaps by the addition of aldosterone. There is greater outward K⁺ current and greater K⁺ secretion. The idealized graphs of cumulative K⁺ secretion, membrane voltage, and relative K⁺ and Na⁺ permeability shown in Figure 8.10 expand on this concept. Basolateral leak K⁺ channels, which provide the majority of ion permeability at rest, sets E_{mem} of CD principal

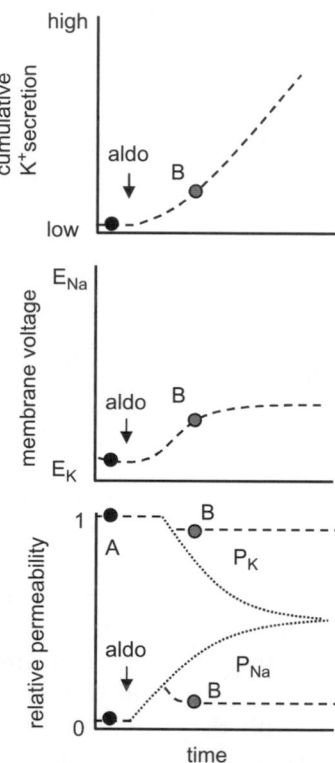

FIGURE 8.10   Activation of ENaC depolarizes the apical membrane driving K⁺ secretion through ROMK. Shown are idealized graphs representing changes in K⁺ secretion (top); apical membrane potential (middle); and relative permeability (bottom) as ENaC becomes activated by aldosterone to drive K secretion through ROMK, moving from point A to point B.

cells to near E_K. There is little electrochemical force, therefore, for K⁺ to exit the cell through ROMK under these conditions. This resting condition is time A, with little K⁺ secretion across the apical membrane. The introduction of aldosterone to the system activates ENaC, increasing the relative permeability of Na⁺ and allowing this ion to enter the cell down its electrochemical gradient. This begins to depolarize the apical membrane, as E_{mem} moves towards E_{Na}. As E_{mem} moves towards E_{Na}, K^+ exits the cell at an increased rate across apical ROMK channels. This is time B.

Another consequence of ENaC opening is that the relative permeability of K^+ begins to fall as that of Na^+ rises; however, as K^+ exits the cell through ROMK, a new steady-state is reached where membrane potential has increased, and P_{Na} and P_K have stabilized with constant K^+ secretion. Neither the K^+ nor Na^+ concentration gradients change substantially across the apical membrane, due to the constant activity of the Na^+,K^+-ATPase pump. These gradients are also protected by the constant flow of urine, bringing Na^+ to the cell and washing away K^+ that has been secreted through ROMK. This scenario is simplified compared to the real-life situation, but it shows how the equations described above can be used to understand the role played by renal ion channels better. This simplified description, moreover, reveals the mechanistic underpinnings of why K^+ secretion from CD principal cells is tied in a positive manner to Na^+ reabsorption by these cells, as initially raised in earlier sections. In addition, it explains why diuretics, such as amiloride and triemterene, which block ENaC, also have K^+-sparing action.[41,44] They retard the development of the normal electrochemical driving forces favoring K^+ secretion from the CD, because they block the entry of Na^+ across the apical membrane necessary to drive K^+ from the cell. Because the CD is the final site along the nephron where urinary $[K^+]$ is fine-tuned, decreased secretion here leads to K^+ retention in plasma.

Channels are Selective

Ion channels need to be selective to perform their role of converting chemical disequilibrium into electrical signals. In epithelial cells, moreover, they need to be selective to facilitate vectoral transport. The chemistry of selectivity (often called the selectivity sequence), for a channel can also be empirically determined using the GHK Voltage Equation discussed above. The extended equation is $E_{rev} = (RT/F) \ln \{(P_K[K]_o + P_{Na}[Na]_o + P_{Cl}[Cl]_i)/(P_K[K]_i + P_{Na}[Na]_i + P_{Cl}[Cl]_o)\}$.[2] This equation allows one to calculate permeability ratios by measuring reversal potential, but it does not allow the determination of absolute permeabilities. Bi-ionic conditions, where only one permeant ion is presented to either side of the channel, are the simplest when testing selectivity. Under such conditions, the equation reduces to $E_{rev} = (RT/zF) \ln \{(P_x[X]_o)/(P_y[Y]_i)\}$. Figure 8.11 shows predicted results from a hypothetical excised inside-out patch-clamp experiment with bi-ionic conditions used to determine that the channel within the patched membrane is selective for Na^+ over K^+. With Na^+ in

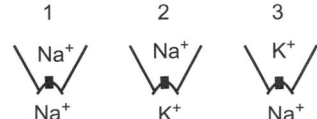

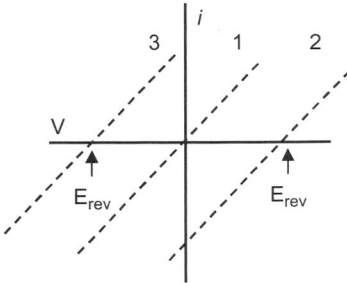

FIGURE 8.11 A channel's selectivity sequence can be experimentally determined by quantifying how different ionic gradients influence reversal potential. Shown at top are three different experimental conditions with distinct Na^+ and K^+ concentrations in the bath and pipette solutions for an excised inside-out patch containing an ion channel. Below is the predicted I−V relation for a Na^+ channel in this patched membrane under the three conditions.

the bath and recording pipette, there is no gradient across the membrane, and reversal potential is 0 mV (condition 1). Next, when the bath contains K^+ as the sole cation, condition 2, the reversal potential moves to E_{Na}, which is ~ 70 mV. Similarly, when the cations in the pipette and bath are reversed, the equilibrium potential again moves to E_{Na}, which is ~ -70 mV with condition 3.

What provides a channel with selectivity? In the simplest sense, it is how capable binding sites within the pore are at coordinating an ion permeating through the pore. If we view a channel pore as a tunnel with consecutive constrictions followed by recesses, as shown in Figure 8.12a, then the selectivity-filter is the tightest constriction. A pore can also be understood by considering thermodynamics. As shown in Figure 8.12b, there would be energy wells followed by energy barriers along the length of the pore. The selectivity-filter then is the greatest barrier that a permeant ion must cross to move through the channel. Using equivalent circuits to describe ion channels, as shown in Figure 8.12c, a change in selectivity would be observed as a change in the electromotive force driving current across the channel upon ion substitution.

The physical basis of selectivity is set by the selectivity-filter defining an internal diameter within the pore, which prohibits molecules larger than this diameter from crossing. This represents the idea that ion channel pores are sieves, selecting on size. With such a description, a selectivity-filter that passes large ions, presumably, would also pass smaller ions, but clearly this is not the case. There are, obviously, other

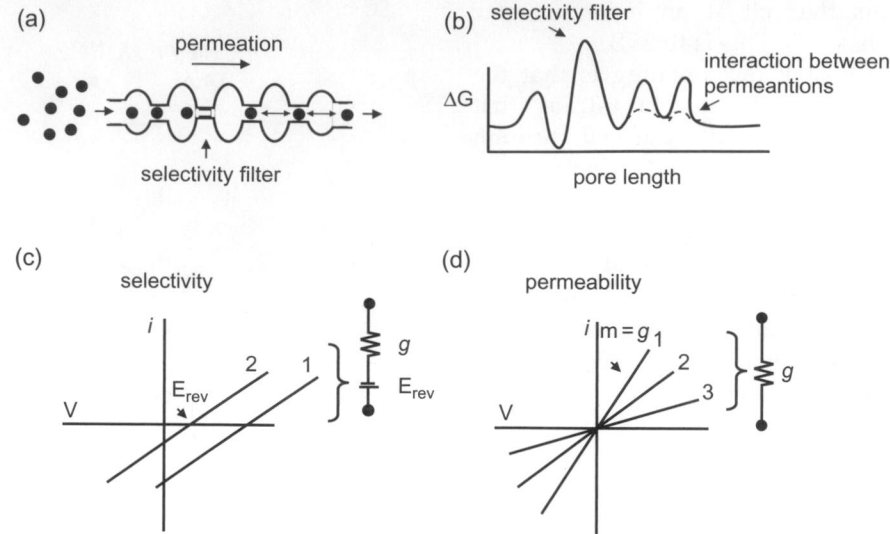

FIGURE 8.12 **Selectivity and permeation.** Shown in (a) is an illustration of a channel pore acting as a filter selecting on size. Ions permeating through the channel pore are shown as black balls. Shown in (b) is a representation of a channel pore as understood by thermodynamics. The I−V relation and equivalent circuit shown in (c) emphasize that selectivity is calculated experimentally by measuring changes in reversal potential resulting from changes in ionic gradients. The I−V relation and equivalent circuit shown in (d) emphasize that permeation is measured in experiments by calculating conductance in the presence of different permeant ions. The two-headed arrows in (a) indicate charge repulsion between permeant ions within the pore. The dashed lines in (b) show decreases in energy barriers along the pore and also indicate the effects of charge repulsion on permeation.

factors contributing to selectivity. Ions move through channel-selectivity filters only after they shed their layer of surrounding water.[35,36,37,45,46] So, it is the dehydrated diameter of an ion, and its ability to shed surrounding water molecules, that are important when moving through a selectivity-filter. Moreover, selectivity-filters also select on the basis of charge: side chains of amino acids defining or near the selectivity-filter present as a charge barrier. The side chains and backbone carbons of residues within or near the selectivity-filter also form transient bonds with the permeant ion and, thus, there is a chemical component to selectivity. Selectivity, then, is a culmination of several factors, including size and charge, and the ability to shed solvating water molecules and interact with residues at or near the selectivity-filter. The precision of selectivity among ion channels varies widely from ENaC having a $P_{Na}/P_K > 100$ being at the highly selective end of the spectrum, to some TRP channels with $P_{Na}/P_K \approx 1$ being at the other end of the spectrum of non-selective channels.[11,47,48,49]

It is easiest to view selectivity as fixed and immutable. However, this is not exactly the case. Channel selectivity can be influenced by experimental conditions, and even the presence or absence of permeant ions in the pore.[50,51] Moreover, the selectivity-filter can be involved in channel gating, as it is in ROMK and ClC channels.[32,52,53,54,55] Gating is discussed in more detail below.

Ions Permeate Through Channels

Selectivity and permeation are related, but they are not exactly the same thing. Selectivity, as emphasized in Figures 8.12a and 8.12b, is set by the physical properties of ion-binding sites within the pore, and how well they coordinate permeant ions when bound. Permeation refers to how fast or rather how many ions move through the pore per unit of time, and speaks of how well an ion surmounts energy barriers within the pore. Stated another way, selectivity can be viewed as a filter with certain physical properties, and permeation is how well molecules cross this filter. Experimentally, as shown in Figure 8.12d, permeation is measured as conductance, where a channel passing a more permeant ion has a higher conductance relative to when it passes a less permeant ion. Ions permeate through the narrowest portions of a channel pore in a single-file manner.[34,35,36,45,56] One then might expect a channel that is less selective to have a higher conductance compared to a highly selective channel. In general, this rule is only loosely obeyed. The reasons for this are discussed below. One might also expect that the ion for which a channel is most selective would permeate through the channel best. This is most often the case, but it is not absolute.

Permeation is a result of how easily an ion surmounts every energy barrier within the pore, as well as interactions between permeant ions with each other when occupying the pore. Ions occupying the pore can exert a pushing effect on each other, impeding and propelling progression depending on the relative order of these ions within the pore and opposing energy barriers each ion is facing. Repulsion between ions within a pore is indicated in Figures 8.12a and 8.12b with two-headed arrows and decreases in the size of energy barriers, respectively. Such repulsion contributes to highly selective channels passing large numbers of ions per second. For instance, charge repulsion between the Cl^- ions occupying the pore of ClC channels makes a significant contribution to the conductance of these channels.[53,57] In addition, most channels have large aqueous vestibules lined by polar residues at the extracellular and intracellular mouths of their pores.[36,37,45,46,58] The vestibules act as reservoirs concentrating the permeant ion, increasing conductance.

The pores of ClC and ENaC channels contain three binding sites for permeant ions.[37,52,55,58] In ENaC, sites immediately adjacent likely are not occupied simultaneously, due to charge repulsion between permeant ions within the pore. This is also the case for K^+ channels, such as Kv and Kir, which use a single-file mode of multiple ion permeation with four pause/binding sites within the pore.[35,36,45,56] As illustrated in Figure 8.13, only two sites are occupied at any one time, with the occupied pairs always separated by an empty site filled with water.[35,36,45,56]

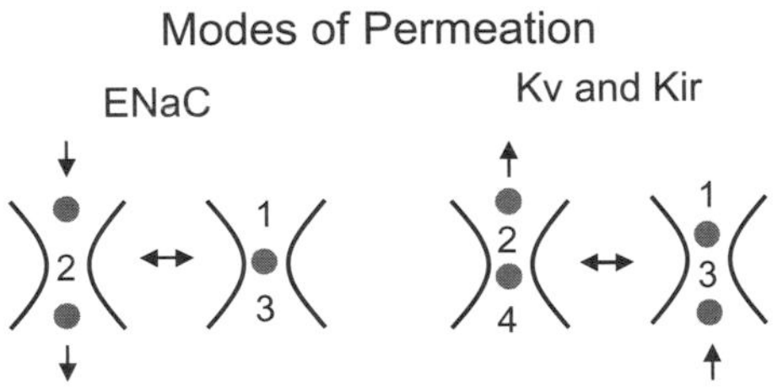

Channels Gate

Channels transition between closed and open states as they gate.[2,3] By definition, no current flows through a closed channel. Upon opening, current flows through the channel obeying $i = g_x(E - E_x)$. The open current level of a single channel then is a determinant of its conductance, which is measured by taking the slope of $i-V$ curves for single-channel currents captured with a voltage-clamp recording (see Figure 8.12d). Current flow through a channel, as shown in Figure 8.14, is an all-or-nothing event: with no change in driving force, the channel transitions from closed to open and back again, always the same as defined by a normally distributed Gaussian curve unitary step in single-channel current.

Channels gate in a stochastic manner: a new and random pattern of openings is observed for each trial period.[2] The stochastic nature of gating makes it possible to describe gating in terms of probabilities, where the sum of the probability of a channel being in either the open (P_o) or closed (P_c) state is equal to 1. Channel open probability is calculated from single-channel activity (NP_o) defined as $NP_o = \sum(t_1 + 2t_2 + \ldots nt_n)$, where N and P_o are the number of channels in a patch and the mean P_o of these channels, and t_n is the fractional open time spent at each of the observed current levels. P_o is calculated by dividing NP_o by the number of active channels (N) within a patch, as defined by all-point amplitude histograms. Another common way of representing this is:

$$NP_o = \sum_{i=0}^{N_A} \frac{it_i}{T}$$

where T is the total recording time, N_A is the observable number of current levels corresponding to channel number as established with all-point histograms, i is the number of channels open, and t_i is the time during which i channels are open. P_o can be calculated as above, by dividing NP_o by the channel number.

Modes of Permeation

ENaC   Kv and Kir

FIGURE 8.13 Modes of permeation. Shown here are representative modes of ion (represented by gray balls) permeation through ENaC (left); and Kv and Kir (right) channels. Ions permeate through channel pores in a single-file manner with several ions occupying different binding/pause sites along the length of the pore at any one time. However, charge repulsion often precludes neighboring sites from being occupied by permeant ions simultaneously. Such mechanisms of permeation allow highly selective channels to have large conductance.

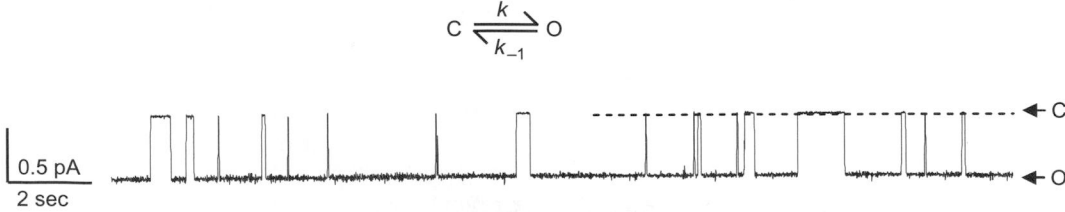

FIGURE 8.14 Channels gate in a stochastic manner. Shown here is a typical single-channel current trace for ENaC in an excised outside-out patch containing a single channel. Open and closed states are indicated with O and C, respectively. Shown above is a kinetic scheme describing gating. At a fixed driving force, the channel opening is always to the same unitary current level, and gating is stochastic.

Macroscopic channel current is related to unitary current by $I = i\mathrm{NP_o}$, where i is unitary single-channel current at a given voltage. Similarly, macroscopic conductance is $G = g\mathrm{NP_o}$. This provides another means for estimating $\mathrm{NP_o}$ from experimental data where $\mathrm{NP_o}$ can be estimated as I/i. This latter estimation is often used in experiments where N cannot be fixed with certainty, but i can be or when N and I (and i) are measured independently of each other.

All channels have inherent gating activity: with time, they transition between open and closed states in a random manner driven by thermal energy. So, all channels have at least one gate. The physical nature of a channel gate, though, may be different among different kinds of channels. Moreover, channels often have more than one distinct gate. This seems to be the rule rather than the exception. For example, ClC channels are double-barreled channels containing two proto-pores, each having an independent gate.[53,57,59,60] Both proto-pores, moreover, are also covered by a common gate. For the channel to be open, both the gate of the proto-pore and the common gate must be open. Similarly, Kir channels, such as ROMK, have fast and slow gating, showing the effects of at least two different gates.[32,34,35,45,56]

Types of Gates

We typically think of a channel gate as a domain or residue that occludes or covers the pore in a dynamic manner. This may be the case for gates in many types of channels typified by the regulated gate in Kv channels, the slow-gate in Kir, and the common gate in ClC channels.[37,52,61] The crystal structures of many ion channels have recently advanced the understanding of gates. As depicted in Figure 8.15, at least two types of gates are now known to exist. Several channels contain both types of gates, as typified by the fast and slow gates in Kir channels.[32] These two types of gates share some properties, such as they both prevent further permeation of the conductance pathway, but also have important differences albeit sometimes subtle. In addition to a physical gating particle that may obstruct the pore, collapse of the pore around a permeant ion prohibiting further permeation has also been identified as a means of gating.[32,35,36] During pore-gating, the channel is open when the pore is open, and closed when the pore is collapsed. So, there is no true gate with a pore-gating mechanism, rather the physical diameter of the pore is the gate.

In the pore-gating model, the selectivity-filter or another portion of the pore is the working part. This is the case for the fast gating seen in the ROMK channel, where K^+ occupancy of the pore has a profound

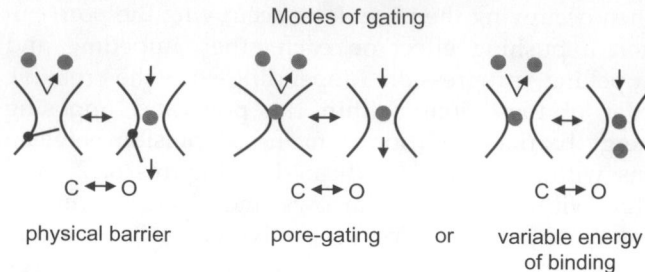

Modes of gating

physical barrier   pore-gating   or   variable energy
                                                of binding

FIGURE 8.15 Two different general types of gates are known to exist in channels. Illustrated are the two different types of channel gates identified to date. The left shows a representation of a physical barrier functioning as a gate where the barrier is a side chain, residue or domain of the channel (represented by a black line connected to a small black circle on the wall of the pore) that occludes the pore in the closed state. The regulated common gate and slow gate in ClC and Kir channels, respectively, are this type of gate. The middle and right illustrations represent two different understandings of a pore-gate where the pore collapses around a permeant ion (middle) or the permeant ion sticks to a binding site within the pore (right) to occlude the pore in the closed state. Fast gating of Kir channels and fast gating of proto-pores in ClC channels represent gating of this type. Closed-to-open transitions are shown below, and movement of the permeant ion (gray ball) through the pore is indicated by arrows.

influence on the structure of the selectivity-filter.[32] Fast gating is characterized by the rapid transition between the open and shortest-lived closed states. The role of pore-gating and the selectivity-filter in this fast-gating process was noticed because the rate of entering the shortest-lived closed state varies as a function of K^+ concentration, and is proportional to current amplitude.[50,51,62–64] The crystal structures of bacterial Kir channels, sharing structure with ROMK as discussed below, provides additional support for this mechanism, showing how a pore may collapse around a permeant ion to gate the channel. A similar relation between extracellular Cl^- and gating of ClC channels has also been noticed.[65–68] This has led to speculation that the proto-pores of ClC channels may also use a pore-gating mechanism. This is supported by the crystal structure of ClC channels.[37,46,53,57]

An alternative to mechanical collapse of the pore/selectivity-filter around the permeant ion to explain pore-gating is a variable energy-of-binding model. Simply put, in some instances, such as that during the shortest-lived closed state of ROMK channels, K^+ may be bound so tightly to the pore that it briefly plugs the permeation pathway.[63] This latter mechanism shares similarities with a traditional gate, in that it is a manifestation of a particle physically clogging the pore to prevent further permeation, but here the gating particle is also the permeant ion rather than a distinct part of the channel. It is different from a pore-collapse mechanism, in that the pore remains in an open state in the variable energy-of-binding model, merely being clogged. Both the mechanical pore collapse and variable energy-of-binding modes of gating result from interactions between the ion permeating the pore and pore residues.

Regulation of Gating

The inherent activities of gates can be influenced by factors that change the kinetics and equilibrium between the closed and open states. This change can be reversible or irreversible. Only the former is involved in the dynamic regulation of channel activity. The latter permanently changes the gating state. Factors that influence gating assume many forms. They can be extracellular and intracellular ligands that bind the channel, for instance Ca^{2+} binding to calcium bowls and RCK domains in the intracellular portions of BK_{Ca} channels.[69,70] They can be enzymes, for instance kinases and proteases, which chemically modify channels or change channel structure. For instance, ROMK is activated and maintained in a high-P_o state by PKA phosphorylation, and inhibited by intracellular acidification.[32] Voltage also can influence the gating of some channels. This represents a special case as discussed below in the section titled "Some Channels Rectify." Channel oligomerization and association with accessory subunits can also influence gating. Barttin plays such a role for ClC-Ka and ClC-Kb channels.[71] As shown in Figure 8.16, the presence of barttin reverses the voltage-dependence of the rat ClC-Ka ortholog, ClC-K1, switching it from being activated by membrane depolarization to being activated by membrane hyperpolarization. Such regulation of gating allows ClC-Ka and ClC-Kb channels to be active under physiological conditions, facilitating NaCl reabsorption in both the TAL and DCT.[72,73]

Many factors that influence gating to change P_o work through an allosteric mechanism, using a binding or effector site that is away from the pore. With such a mechanism, the effector molecule or influence of voltage affects an allosteric site where the free energy of interaction at this site is translated into a change in conformation that alters gating kinetics, equilibrium or both. As discussed further below, channel subunits in the Kv channel family have a core structure containing six transmembrane domains with an extracellular pore-forming loop between S5 and S6. In these channels, S4 is the voltage-sensor. This transmembrane domain contains conserved positive charged residues that sense voltage and move the S4 domain in response to a voltage-change across the membrane. In this sense, S4 is a molecular voltmeter. Movement of S4 is conveyed to the gate to change its position. BK_{Ca} channels contain intracellular Ca^{2+}-binding sites that also act as allosteric regulators of gating.[69,70] Occupancy of these sites by Ca^{2+} increases P_o by making it more likely that the channel will be in an open state.

Pore-gates, like those in ClC channels, can also be influenced by modulators to change gating. For instance, ClC channels are also voltage-dependent (see Figure 8.16). Because of the nature of the gate in these channels, regulation of ClC gating by voltage, though, is not allosteric. Rather, voltage directly influences the interaction of Cl^- with residues in the pore.[37,46,61]

The Consequences of Regulation of Gating

Regulation of gating determines how active a channel is, and the magnitude of the current through the channel. For instance, the regulation of gating, as noted above, enables ClC channels to be active under physiological conditions. Because gating can be regulated, channels act as variable resistors in equivalent circuits: their mode of gating can change, which causes P_o to be able to be changed in a dynamic manner. Recall that $I = iNP_o$ and $G = gNP_o$. In experiments quantifying macroscopic current, like the idealized results shown in

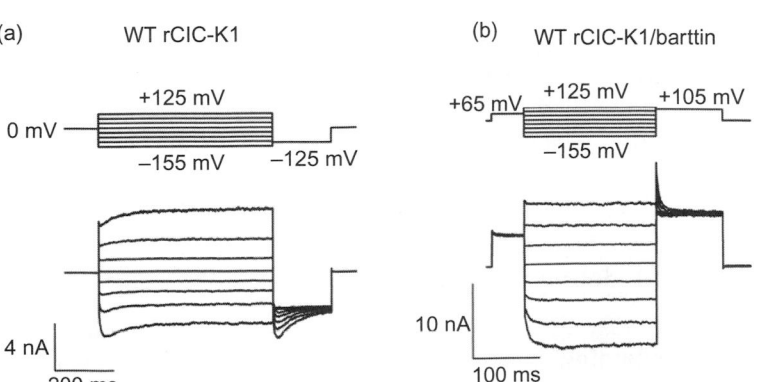

(a) WT rClC-K1

(b) WT rClC-K1/barttin

FIGURE 8.16 The regulatory subunit, barttin, reverses the voltage-dependence of ClC-K channels, allowing them to be active under physiological conditions. (*Adapted from Figure 1 in [72].*) Voltage-step protocols and representative current responses for cells expressing rat ClC-K1 alone (a) or together with barttin (b).

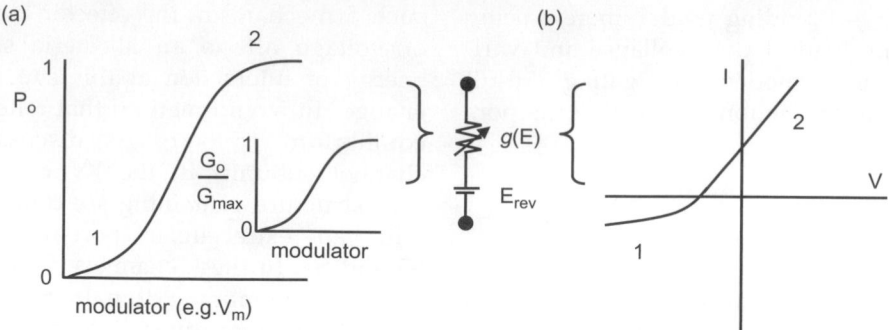

FIGURE 8.17 Changes in gating influence channel activity. The idealized graph in (a) shows P_o as a function of the effects of a modulator of gating, which changes the resistance of the channel shown in the idealized equivalent circuit shown to the right. (The inset in (a) shows the effects of a gating modulator on channel conductance.) The I−V relation in (b) shows the effects of the gating modulator changing P_o on macroscopic current, with point 1 being when the channel has low P_o and point 2 when P_o is approaching 1.

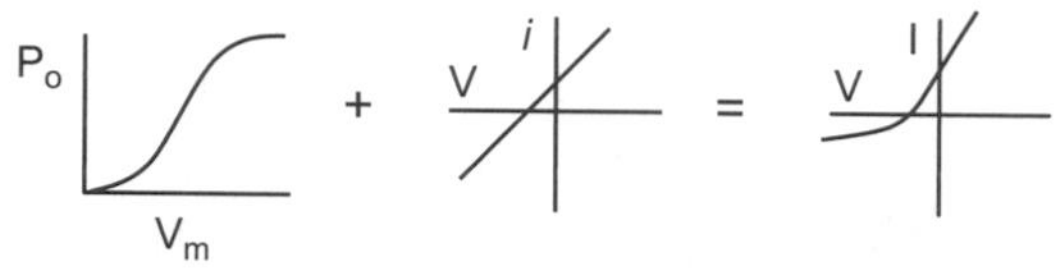

FIGURE 8.18 A channel's macroscopic I−V relation is a determinant of the effects of gating modulators on P_o and its single-channel i−V relation.

Figure 8.17, conductance changes as P_o changes, as a result of effectors influencing gating. The importance of this to physiology is clear when considering that voltage-dependent activation of BK_{Ca} channels enables them to conduct more current at depolarizing potentials, which in turn prevents further membrane depolarization by driving the membrane potential toward E_K. As noted previously, feedback activation of BK_{Ca} channels is critical to nearby TRPC6 channels functioning as Ca^{2+} entry pathways in podocytes.[11]

Some Channels Rectify

Rectification is when the macroscopic I−V relation of a channel deviates from strictly obeying Ohm's Law.[2] A macroscopic I−V relation, as detailed in Figure 8.18, is the sum of the single-channel i−V relation, and effects of gating modulators on channel P_o. Our discussion of ion channels has been simplified, in that we have presumed that they all rigorously follow Ohm's Law. This is not actually the case. As the concentration gradient of the permeant ion across the membrane increases, and as the concentration of the permeant ion approaches 0, all channels show some degree of rectification. This is referred to as Goldman rectification, and is a manifestation of the asymmetrical distribution of permeant ions across the membrane.[2] As such, it can be described by the GHK current equation. Further discussion of this, though, is beyond the scope of our discourse. Rectification that is of relevance here is

that caused by voltage-dependent gating, because it can influence (as discussed immediately above) how active a channel is under physiological conditions.

Modulation of gating by voltage represents a special case. In this case, voltage has two affects. It influences P_o and the unitary current i of the channel. As such, macroscopic I−V relations for voltage-gated channels show rectification. Channels that rectify exhibit greater conductance at either positive or negative potentials applied across the membrane, meaning that they facilitate the movement of ions in a particular direction (into the cell or out of the cell). Macroscopic I−V relations for such channels are illustrated in Figures 8.17 and 8.18. The voltage-dependence of gating is routinely described with a Boltzmann function where $P_o = 1/[1 + e^{-V-V1/2zF/RT}]$.[2] All symbols in this equation have their usual meaning as described in previous sections, and $V_{1/2}$ is the voltage at which P_o is 0.5 or, if used to describe macroscopic conductance, the voltage at which conductance is half of the maximum. In most cases, when fitting the voltage-dependence of macroscopic conductance, G is normalized to maximum conductance (G_{max}), giving $G = G_{max}/[1 + e^{-V-V1/2zF/RT}]$. Fitting with a Boltzmann function provides two important pieces of information describing the effects of voltage on gating. It provides the voltage at which half the channels are open, telling us about the threshold for activation by voltage. It also describes the degree to which a channel responds to voltage. This is the slope of the fit, and informs us about the range over which the channel responds to voltage and how tightly channel gating is linked to changes in voltage: a steeper slope indicates a tighter association.

Modeling Channel Gating

Gating of an ion channel is akin to an enzyme transitioning between an unbound and substrate-bound active state, with rate constants determining the state

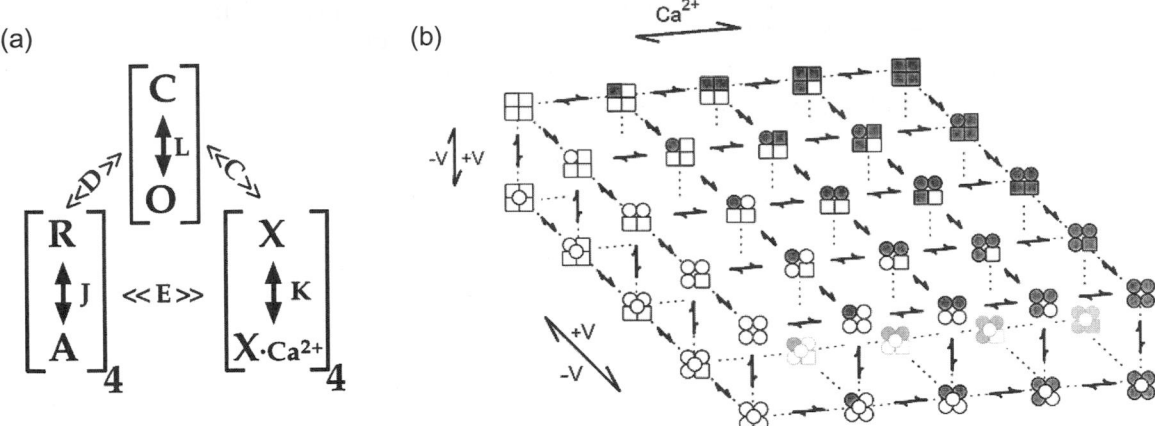

FIGURE 8.19 Channel gating can be described with kinetic models and state diagrams. The kinetic model (a) and state diagram (b) describing BK_{Ca} channel gating are from [69] and [70], respectively. The gating mechanism involves an allosteric interaction between channel opening (C–O) and voltage sensor activation (R–A). L is the C–O equilibrium constant when all voltage sensors are in the resting (R) state. J is the R–A equilibrium constant when channels are closed. D is the allosteric interaction factor where the C–O equilibrium constant increases D-fold for each voltage sensor activated, and the R–A equilibrium constant increases D-fold when the channel opens. Subscripts for closed and open states denote 0–4 activated voltage sensors of the tetrameric channel. The Ca^{2+}-binding transition (X–XCa) for each subunit has an equilibrium constant $K = [Ca^{2+}]/K_D$ when channels are closed and voltage sensors are not activated. Allosteric interactions of Ca^{2+}-binding with channel opening and voltage sensor activation are determined by the allosteric factors C and E, respectively. In the state diagram, a change in subunit conformation is indicated by the square-to-circle transition. The effects of voltage and Ca^{2+} are noted on the axes, with Ca^{2+}-binding indicated with gray shading. The open channel state is noted by a white circle in the center of the tetramer.

occupied. This allows gating to be viewed as a biochemical reaction, where standard analysis of reaction rates and kinetics can be used to describe the gating process. The simplest mode of gating is one containing forward and backward transitions between a single closed and open state. Such a gating scheme with associated kinetic constants is shown above the current trace in Figure 8.14.

Kinetic models and state diagrams have explained much about how factors influence gating. As we learn more about the biophysical properties of channels, these models have been becoming more complex, but also they are better at explaining the features and caveats of how channels transition and gate. Figure 8.19 shows a kinetic model and state diagram explaining the effects of voltage and Ca^{2+} on BK_{Ca} channel gating. Both models assume allosteric interaction between the voltage-sensor and Ca^{2+}-binding site(s) with the channel gate. When expanded, these models contain at least 50 different states. The kinetic model originated from the investigation of macroscopic currents under extreme conditions used to isolate specific effects of voltage and Ca^{2+} away from intrinsic gating events.[69] The state diagram was derived from single-channel data, including the analysis of single-channel gating kinetics.[70] These models have common features, and do a good job of predicting the voltage- and Ca^{2+}-dependence of BK_{Ca}-channel gating over a range of $[Ca^{2+}]$ and voltages, justifying their continued use for explaining BK_{Ca}-channel activity and regulation.

Such models have important ramifications for how we think about renal ion channels and understand their role in physiology. BK_{Ca} channels are critical to protecting membrane potential in podocytes during TRPC6-mediated Ca^{2+} influx, and are involved in K^+ secretion from the CD.[10,11,12] A detailed understanding of how BK_{Ca} channels gate in response to voltage and Ca^{2+} then is critical to appreciating these processes.

Pore Block

Although not a true change in gating in that the gate is not affected, a block of the pore by a factor other than the permeant ion or gating particle may also alter single-channel and macroscopic currents. For instance, the blocking of the ENaC pore by amiloride decreases the mean P_o these channels have with channels spending briefer periods in the open state.[47,48,74,75] In experiments, this appears as frequent transitions between the open and open-blocked state, with the latter appearing as a closed state. Block of a pore can also be voltage-sensitive if the blocker interacts with the blocking site in a voltage-dependent manner. For instance, rectification of Kir channels results from voltage-dependent block of the pore by Mg^{2+} and polyamines. This appears as an effect on gating.[43,76,77] Because such factors influence P_o and the time channels spend in the open state, their actions can also be assessed with standard kinetic analysis and measurements of voltage-dependence.

FUNCTION OF RENAL ION CHANNELS

Interpreting experimental results from a biophysical perspective, as developed above, has been instrumental in defining the roles of many channels in the kidney. In the next section, expression patterns are discussed in terms of where function has been established with some degree of certainty from experimental results (see Figures 8.1 and 8.2 and Table 8.1). Two channel proteins in the ClC transporter/channel family are expressed in the kidney: ClC-Ka in the basolateral membrane of ascending thin limb (ATL) and TAL cells, and CLC-Kb in the basolateral membrane of TAL and DCT cells.[60,78,79] Barttin, a regulatory subunit obligatory for ClC-Ka and ClC-Kb activity, is expressed along with these channel proteins in the nephron.[71,72,73] K^+ channels from at least four different families are functionally expressed in the kidney. The inward rectifiers Kir1.1 and 4.1 are expressed in the apical membranes of TAL, DCT, CNT and CD, and the basolateral membrane of DCT cells, respectively.[20] BK_{Ca} channels are expressed in podocytes and the apical membranes of CD cells.[11,19,29,30,31,33] Proximal tubule epithelial cells express the TWIK-related acid-sensitive K^+-2 (TASK-2) channel, a member of the two-pore K^+ channel family, in their basolateral membranes.[80] Kv1.1 is expressed in the luminal membrane of DCT cells.[20] A single type of Na^+ channel, ENaC, is expressed in the kidney in the apical membrane of CD principal cells.[41,81,82,83] Several members of the TRP channel family are expressed in the kidney. TRPC6 is expressed in podocytes.[11,13] The nonselective TRPV4 channel is expressed in the apical membranes of cells lining the water-impermeable segments of the tubule, including the ATL, TAL, and DCT.[12] TRPP2 is expressed in the apical membranes of TAL and DCT cells, as well as in other segments of the nephron.[12] Inactivating mutations in the gene encoding this channel protein cause autosomal dominant polycystic kidney disease. Coverage of this area of research is broad and beyond the scope of the current chapter. Chapter 80 discusses polycystic kidney disease, and TRPP2. The Mg^{2+}-selective TRPM6 channel is expressed in the apical membrane of early DCT cells.[9,10,19,20] The epithelial Ca^{2+} channel, TRPV5, is expressed in the apical membrane of late DCT and CNT cells.[49,84,85,86]

CLC (CLCN) Channels and Barttin (BSND)

The ClC proteins are members of a large family of Cl^- transport proteins that serve diverse functions (Chapter 31).[59,60] These proteins are widely expressed in every animal and most, if not all, bacteria. The ClC family is divided into two branches depending on function; three if sequence identity is the discriminator. Members of one branch (two if using identity) function as electrogenic anti-porters, moving $2Cl^-$ and H^+ in opposite directions in a secondary-active manner. This branch is likely to be the older for most, if not all, ClC proteins identified in bacteria belong to it. The younger branch contains proteins that have lost their need for H^+ to move Cl^- in a coupled manner, and now function as voltage-gated ion channels with anions moving through the ClC channel pore via restrictive diffusion.

ClC-Ka and ClC-Kb proteins form anion channels selective for Cl^- with similar biophysical properties. ClC-Ka and ClC-Kb have overlapping, but not identical, function in the kidney. This was revealed by the different tubulopathies arising from the inactivation of ClC-Ka (diabetes insipidus) versus ClC-Kb (Bartter's syndrome type III), and the realization that inactivation of barttin (BS type IV with sensorineural deafness) recapitulates the entirety of the phenotype resulting from loss of both ClC channels.[14,18,71,87] In the TAL, ClC-Ka and ClC-Kb serve as basolateral exit pathways for Cl^- brought into the cell along with Na^+ and K^+ by apical NKCC2. ClC-Kb, but not ClC-Ka, serves a similar function in the DCT, with the caveat that Cl^- enters these cells along with Na^+ across the apical membrane on NCC. Because ClC-Kb functions as a basolateral Cl^- exit gateway in both the TAL and DCT, inactivating mutations in this gene sometimes can appear to result in a mixed Bartter–Gitleman's phenotype.[14,18,88] Moreover, because both ClC-Ka and ClC-Kb are expressed in the TAL, the phenotype resulting from inactivation of ClC-Kb is not as severe as that seen with inactivation of barttin (BS type IV) or NKCC2 (BS type I).

Barttin, as indicated above, is required for ClC-Ka and ClC-Kb activity, making mutations in this accessory subunit also capable of causing disease.[72,73] The effect of barttin on ClC-K channels is complex and not fully-understood. What is clear is that ClC-K channels are the only members of the ClC family not to contain the critical E166 gating moiety at the extracellular mouth of the pore. Rather, these channels have a Val residue here.[46,57,61,72] This may contribute in part to why these channels are not functional in the absence of barttin, for this gating moiety enables other ClC channels to sense and respond to voltage with activation. Mutagenesis studies have shown that the transmembrane core of barttin is necessary and sufficient to promote ClC-K trafficking to the plasma membrane, a short cytoplasmic segment following the second transmembrane domain modifies the unitary conductance of ClC-K channels, and the entire COOH-terminal cytoplasmic domain is involved in affecting channel P_o.[73] The biophysical mechanism whereby barttin affects ClC-K channel P_o involves locking the common gate covering the two proto-pores open: in the presence of barttin, ClC-Ka and ClC-Kb channels can reach full activity with their proto-pore gates primarily modulating P_o.[72] The physiological importance of this is clear. Without barttin, there is no ClC-K channel activity, concomitant K^+ recycling across the apical membrane of TAL cells or dependent NaCl reabsorption, resulting in the compromise of the axial corticomedullary hypertonic gradient necessary to concentrate urine.

KCNA (Kv) Channels

The Kv1.1 channel is expressed in the luminal membrane of DCT cells.[20] Kv1.1 is best known as the first cloned mammalian fast delayed rectifier channel belonging to the Shaker subfamily, named so because flies lacking the Shaker channel shake their legs while under ether anesthesia.[89,90,91] There is little difference between the intracellular and extracellular concentrations of ionized Mg^{2+} in the renal tubule. The electrochemical force driving cell entry of Mg^{2+} as a consequence is mostly a result of the apical membrane being hyperpolarized. Kv1.1 is K^+-selective and voltage-gated, rapidly activating upon membrane depolarization. Activation of Kv1.1 stabilizes the potential across the luminal membrane hyperpolarized near E_K. This function makes Kv1.1 well-qualified to facilitate Mg^{2+} reabsorption in the DCT. Inactivation of Kv1.1 leads to autosomal dominant hypomagnesaemia resulting from decreases in Mg^{2+} reabsorption in the DCT.[20,92]

KCNM (BK$_{Ca}$) Channels

BK$_{Ca}$ channels are expressed in both podocytes and the apical membrane of CD epithelial cells. In podocytes, BK$_{Ca}$ channels co-localize with TRPC6 channels, where they serve in a feedback capacity to facilitate and fine-tune receptor-operated Ca^{2+} influx mediated by TRPC6.[11] The Ca^{2+} and voltage-sensitivity of BK$_{Ca}$ channels, as well as their selectivity and the influence that activating these channels have on membrane potential, makes them well-suited for such a task. This function, though, is not definitive; rather it is extrapolated from co-localization with TRPC6, and the biophysical properties of BK$_{Ca}$ and TRPC6 channels. It has not been determined yet whether BK$_{Ca}$ channel mutation causes any type of proteinuric glomerulopathy akin to the FSGS arising from the mutation of TRPC6.[13]

BK$_{Ca}$ channels are also expressed in the apical membrane of CD epithelial cells. Here, they function

as one of two discrete apical exit gateways for K^+ secretion in the distal nephron.[23,29,31,33] ROMK, as discussed below, serves a similar function in the parallel secretory pathway. Although both pathways mediating K^+ secretion in the distal nephron coexist and provide some redundancy and protection, they do not have a complete overlap of function. The ability of BK$_{Ca}$ channels to respond to mechanical stimuli with changes in gating and P_o makes them particularly well-suited to mediate flow-induced K^+ secretion.[29,30] In comparison, ROMK activity is not sensitive to flow. Decreases in K^+ excretion in electrolyte-balance studies during states of high K^+ intake in animals with compromised BK$_{Ca}$ channel activity resulting from gene deletion of the critical $\beta 1$ regulatory subunit recapitulate findings testing the actions of BK$_{Ca}$ channel blockers on K^+ secretion in isolated perfused tubules.[93]

KCNJ (Kir) Channels

ROMK (Kir1.1) is the founding member of the inward-rectifying K^+ channel family.[94] Inward-rectifying K^+ channels exhibit a non-linear I–V relation characterized by a larger inward current than outward current. ROMK, though, is only weakly inwardly rectified. ROMK is active at physiological potentials with electrochemical gradient, rectification, and other regulatory factors fine-tuning the amount of outward current carried by this channel. Under normal conditions, activated ROMK is well-suited for K^+ secretion, having a P_o approaching 0.9.

ROMK channels serve a dual role in the kidney. In the TAL, ROMK channels provide the majority of apical membrane K^+ conductance. This activity enables K^+ recycling across the apical membrane, to facilitate NaCl entry along with K^+ on the NKCC2 driving NaCl reabsorption by this segment of the tubule and, ultimately, creation of the axial corticomedullary hyperosmotic gradient necessary for concentrating urine.[31,32,33] This function of ROMK was revealed upon discovery of the genetic basis of Bartter syndrome.

ROMK is also an essential component of one of two parallel K^+ secretory pathways in the CNT and CD.[31,32,33,95] As discussed above, BK$_{Ca}$ channels replace ROMK in the ROMK-independent K^+ secretory pathway. This explains how K^+-wasting can happen in BS type II, even in the absence of ROMK. In the same way, upregulation of ROMK channels preserves K^+ secretion in BK$_{Ca}$ channel knockout mice. It has been speculated that this redundancy is a protective mechanism to ensure high-capacity K^+ excretion to guard against fatal hyperkalemia.[32]

Kir4.1 is another member of the inward rectifier family of K^+ channels expressed in the kidney.[92,96,97,98] Compared to ROMK, less is known about the function of this channel in the kidney, but emerging evidence supports that it acts as an important basolateral K^+ exit pathway in DCT cells. Potassium exiting through this channel contributes to the extracellular pool of K^+ immediately available to serosal Na^+,K^+-ATPases. This is necessary for Mg^{2+} reabsorption in the DCT, because Mg^{2+} entry across the apical membrane is intimately tied to membrane potential and NaCl reabsorption where maximal Na^+,K^+-ATPase activity is required to maintain the electrochemical gradients driving Mg^{2+} across the luminal membrane. Proper Kir4.1 function in the DCT is critical, in that the loss of this channel's function causes disease, SeSAME, with notable renal Mg^{2+}-wasting.[92,96,97,98] Clearly, the unique biophysical properties this channel provides to the basolateral membrane of DCT cells cannot be compensated for by the presence of other K^+ channels.

KCNK (K_{2P}) Channels

TASK-2 is a member of the alkaline-activated TALK sub-family within the larger two-pore K^+ channel family.[80] TASK-2 is expressed in the basolateral membrane of PT epithelial cells. As revealed in TASK-2 $-/-$ mice, this channel functions as an alkali-activated counterbalance to the depolarizing influence of the electrogenic Na^+,3-HCO_3^--co-transporter also in the basolateral membrane of PT cells.[80,99] Outward K^+ conductance through TASK-2 counteracts the depolarizing effects of this co-transporter by hyperpolarizing membrane potential back towards E_K. This function makes TASK-2 a key component of a positive feedback pathway maximizing HCO_3^- reabsorption in the PT. Loss of TASK-2 function causes metabolic acidosis, as expected but also modestly increases Na^+ and water excretion by the kidney.[99,100] These effects on pH and renal salt and water handling are akin to those seen with diuretic inhibitors of carbonic anydrase, which promote a weak diuresis by decreasing bulk fluid reabsorption in the PT due to decreased $NaHCO_3^-$ reabsorption. Although the role of TASK-2 in the mouse is clear, it remains to be determined whether mutations in this channel account for familial forms of proximal renal tubule acidosis in humans.

SCNN (ENaC) Channels

ENaC is a member of the ENaC/Degenerin channel family.[101-103] Acid-sensing ion channels (ASIC) are also in this family. ENaC/Deg channels are widely distributed in epithelial and nervous tissues. These channels are Na^+- or non-selective cation channels. Some of the non-selective ENaC/Deg channels also conduct Ca^{2+}. ENaC, which is highly selective for Na^+, though, does not.[41,83,104,141] The activity of ENaC in the CNT and CD is limiting for electrogenic transcellular Na^+ reabsorption here.[41,82,83] This reabsorption fine-tunes urine and plasma Na^+ content. Consequently, ENaC is a physiologically important target for hormones that control blood pressure through feedback regulation of systemic Na^+ and water levels, including those in the renin—angiotensin—aldosterone system. As such, ENaC mutation resulting in gain- and loss-of-function cause improper Na^+ retention and excretion, respectively, leading to increases and decreases in blood pressure.[83,106,107] The prior is Liddle's syndrome, and the latter is pseudohypoaldosteronism (PHA) type-I. Because the electrochemical gradients driving Na^+ reabsorption and K^+ secretion across the apical membrane of CD principal cells are intimately tied to each other, factors that change ENaC activity, including the steroid hormone aldosterone, also affect renal K^+ excretion.

TRP Channels

The TRP protein family is a diverse group of cation channels that participate in a wide range of physiological processes. The mono- and divalent cation conductance of TRP channels enables them to influence both membrane potential and intracellular Ca^{2+} signaling, allowing them to function as important signal transduction switches and gateways for Ca^{2+} and Mg^{2+} entry into the cell during transcellular transport. Mammalian TRP proteins are organized into six subfamilies based on sequence identity. These are C (Canonical, TRPC1-TRPC7 with TRPC2 being a pseudogene in humans), V (Vanilloid, TRPV1-TRPV6), M (Melastatin, TRPM1-TRPM8), A (Ankyrin, TRPA1), P (Polycystin, TRPP1-TRPP3), and ML (Mucolipin, TRPML1-TRPML3).

TRPC6

TRPC6 is a non-selective cation channel with finite Ca^{2+} permeability.[10-12] This channel is expressed in the foot processes of podocytes of Bowman's capsule in the vicinity of the slit diaphragm, as well as in the cell body and major processes of these cells. TRPC6, possibly oligomerized with TRPC3, functions as a receptor-operated Ca^{2+} entry channel in podocytes, where activation leads to cell entry of Ca^{2+} capable of modulating a host of secondary cascades. TRPC6 is only Ca^{2+} permeable under hyperpolarizing conditions. During depolarization Ca^{2+} binds to an inhibitory site within the pore. Binding to this site results in the block of the pore, with a dependent decrease in P_o and inward rectification of macroscopic TRPC6 currents.[108,109,110] Pore block of TRPC6 by a permeant ion is accurately described by a standard single binding site, two-barrier pore model, where the binding site has a two-fold higher affinity for Ca^{2+} than it does for monovalent cations.[108] Consequently, binding to the inhibitory site impedes Ca^{2+} permeation, causing a relative increase in permeation of monovalent cations. The result is that, in the presence of membrane depolarization, TRPC6 converts from a Ca^{2+} entry channel that affects cell signaling to a channel that depolarizes the membrane. BK_{Ca} channels co-localize with TRPC6 channels in the foot processes and other major structures of podocytes.[11] This suggests a tight relation between the function of these channels with TRPC6 allowing Ca^{2+} to enter the cell, which in turn activates nearby BK_{Ca} channels to facilitate or fine-tune further Ca^{2+} entry through TRPC6 channels. Gain-of-function mutations in TRPC6, leading to increased activity and plasma membrane expression, cause familial forms of FSGS.[10,11,12,13] Mutation of other proteins in the podocyte, including nephron and podocin, that interact with TRPC6 also cause FSGS-like proteinuric glomerulopathies.[10,11] Similarly, the mutation of PLC-ε, an important regulator of DAG-sensitive TRPC6 channel activity, causes an FSGS-like disease.[10]

TRPM6

TRPM6 functions as a Mg^{2+}-selective channel in the apical membrane of early DCT cells.[4,19,20,24] TRPM6 may possibly oligomerize with the more widely-expressed TRPM7 to perform this function. Nevertheless, it is clear that TRPM6 brings a unique component to the channel for inactivating mutations in the gene encoding TRPM6 leading to HSH and, thus, TRPM7 does not fully recapitulate the properties of TRPM6.[4,10,12,19,20,24] Macroscopic current through channels containing TRPM6 is both outwardly and inwardly rectified, and activated by deceases in intracellular Mg^{2+}. This activation serves as a feedback mechanism favoring Mg^{2+} reabsorption. In addition to inactivating mutations in TRPM6, mutations in the genes encoding regulators of this channel cause hypomagnesemia.

Inactivation of the gene encoding pro-epidermal growth factor (EGF), for instance, causes isolated autosomal-recessive hypomagnesemia.[9,10,19,20,24] EGF is a magnesiotropic factor that controls the expression of TRPM6 in the apical membrane of DCT cells. Cetuximab, which is an inactivating monoclonal antibody inhibitor of the EGF receptor used in the treatment of colorectal cancer, causes pronounced renal Mg^{2+}-wasting, also resulting from decreased TRPM6 expression, an acquired form of isolated renal

hypomagnesemia.[20,111,112] Magnesium reabsorption via TRPM6 is dependent on NaCl reabsorption and membrane potential in the DCT mediated by the coordinated activities of the apical membrane thiazide-sensitive NCC co-transporter and basolateral Na^+,K^+-ATPase. Mutation of the *FXYD2* gene, which encodes the γb splice variant of the Na^+,K^+-ATPase γ-subunit expressed in this segment of the tubule, causes isolated dominant hypomagnesemia.[9,19,20] Similarly, one component of the complex renal salt-wasting phenotype arising from the inactivation of NCC (Gitleman's syndrome) is Mg^{2+}-wasting.[9,12,19,20,88]

TRPV4

TRPV4 was originally described as an osmotically-responsive monovalent cation-selective cation channel/current with the different names of OTRPC4, VR-OAC, TRP12, and VRL-2.[12] This channel is activated by hypotonic stimuli, resulting in an increase in $[Ca^{2+}]_i$. Increases in Ca^{2+} are secondary to membrane depolarization, rather than Ca^{2+} flux through the channel. TRPV4 is expressed in the water-impermeable segments of the nephron and circumventricular nuclei of the CNS, which governs vasopressin release. The osmotic sensitivity of this channel and its expression in the part of the CNS controlling AVP release led to the idea that TRPV4 contributes to the sensing of osmotic stress and plasma osmolarity. Such a function is supported by findings that AVP release is dysregulated in TRPV4 knockout mice.[113,114] The expression pattern of this channel in the kidney is also consistent with it acting as a cellular-level osmoreceptor that enables epithelial cells to adapt and respond to changes in osmolarity with a change in NaCl transport. Again, findings in the knockout animal are consistent with this.[114,115]

TRPV5

The activity of TRPV5 is voltage- and Ca^{2+}-dependent. This channel is active at physiological potentials and $[Ca^{2+}]_i$ concentrations, but quickly inactivates in response to feedback regulation from intracellular Ca^{2+}.[12,49,84,85] TRPV5 is permeable to Ca^{2+}, and is selective for this divalent cation over monovalent cations. The relative permeability of Ca^{2+} versus Na^+ for channels containing TRPV5 is greater than 100. This is fairly unique for TRP channels, with TRPV6 being the only other TRP channel to share this preference for Ca^{2+}. The selectivity and activity of TRPV5 allows it to function as the apical gateway for Ca^{2+} entry into late DCT and CNT epithelial cells. As such, TRPV5 activity is rate-limiting for Ca^{2+} reabsorption in the nephron beyond the Loop of Henle, where urine and plasma $[Ca^{2+}]$ are fine-tuned. Inactivating mutations of TRPV5 or proteins that regulate the activity of this channel, such as Klotho, cause hypercalcuria and renal Ca^{2+}-wasting in mice.[12,49,84] It has not been established yet if mutations in human TRPV5 cause a similar renal phenotype.

ION CHANNEL STRUCTURE

Ion channels are multimeric, made of component subunits. There are two general types of channel subunits: those that form the pore, termed pore-forming or α-subunits, and those that do not directly contribute to the pore, but rather modify the properties of the channel proper or pore-forming subunits; these routinely are labeled accessory or β-subunits, but also have been called auxiliary and regulatory subunits. Pore-forming subunits must span the lipid bilayer to create the conductive pore. As depicted in the idealized models of the different subunits making renal channels shown in Figure 8.20, pore-forming subunits contain two or more membrane-spanning domains. Many, but not all, accessory subunits are also integral membrane proteins. (These are not represented in Figure 8.20.) The presence or absence of an accessory subunit has significant consequence to the biophysical and physiological function of a channel. For instance, the activities and properties of the human ClC channels,

ClC-Ka and ClC-Kb, are greatly changed by interaction with their β-subunit, barttin.[71,72,73]

Families of pore-forming channel subunits are comprised of homologous proteins that share amino acid identity. The degree of similarity determines how much overlapping function members within a family have. The consequence of a channel family being composed of homologous subunits is that they often differentially assemble into homomeric and heteromeric channels containing a single type of subunit or one with many different but related subunits. The biophysical ramifications of this ability to assemble differentially are profound, leading to differences in channel gating, expression, and regulation to name just a few. This greatly broadens the functional range of channels within the same family. It also can impact the ability to use redundancy to circumvent pathological consequences when one subunit is compromised. Moreover, it can confound the understanding of the specific role played by a particular channel protein within a channel family.

Pore-forming subunits oligomerize into one of three general quaternary structures, as represented in Figure 8.20. ClC family members dimerize into channels containing two subunits, with each subunit encompassing an independent pore.[53,57,116] Most often, as is the case for the renal ClC-Ka and ClC-Kb channels, these dimers are made of identical subunits,

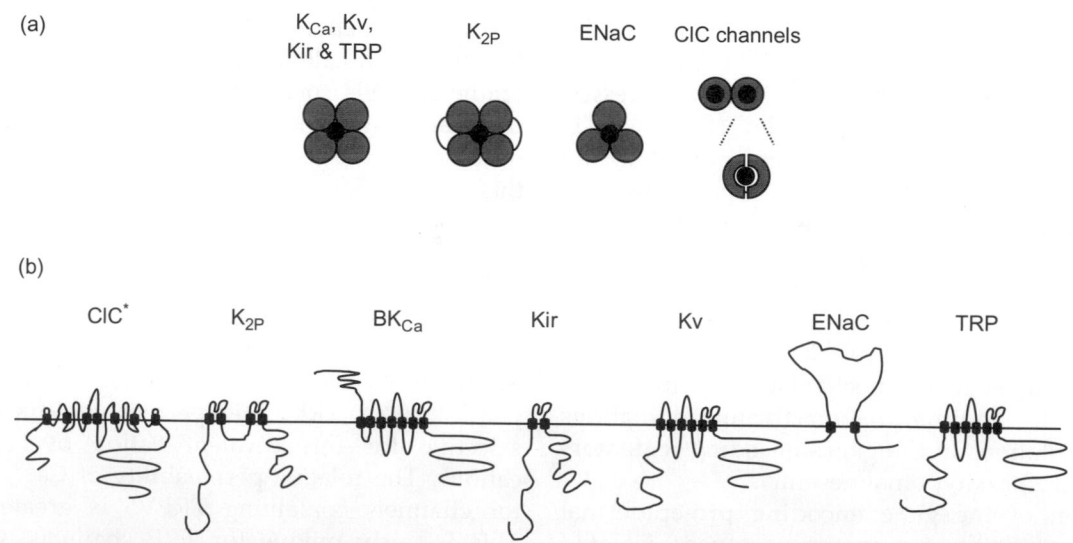

FIGURE 8.20 Channel structure. The idealized illustrations in (a) indicate how renal ion channel subunits assemble to form pores. Subunits are indicated by gray circles or half circles with black lines representing the connection between the two subdomains within each monomer of dimeric K_{2P} and ClC channels. The position of the pore is represented by a black circle. Views are parallel to the plane of the membrane. The idealized illustrations in (b) represent the topology of pore-forming subunits of renal ion channels. These views are perpendicular to the plane of the membrane, which is represented by a solid black horizontal line. Transmembrane domains are represented by small black barrels. Extracellular and cytoplasmic portions of these channel subunits are shown above and below the line representing the plasma membrane, respectively, and only loosely correspond to the real structure of these domains. It is difficult to represent the structure of ClC subunits faithfully using such a diagram, as many intra-membrane helices in this channel do not fully span the membrane. Refer to Figures 8.21 and 8.23 for a better understanding of the secondary and tertiary structure of transmembrane helices in ClC channel subunits.

being homodimers. ENaC is an obligatory heterotrimeric channel containing one α-, β-, and γ-subunit surrounding a central pore.[117,118] (The Greek letters referring to the subunits in ENaC are not indicative of whether they contribute to formation of the pore or not for they all do; rather, they reflect the order of cloning.) In comparison, K⁺-channel subunits and TRP subunits assemble into tetramers with identical or like subunits forming homotetramic and heterotetramic channels with a central pore. K₂P channels are a slight variation on this theme. These channels are homodimers, with each component subunit containing two pore-forming domains that contribute to a central pore that has four-fold symmetry.[119] Thus, K₂P subunits oligomerize into a channel with structure that is reminiscent of that formed by Kir channel subunits. Because good structural information exists for ClC, ENaC, and Kir channels or channels closely related to them, discussion in the next section focuses on these channels as representative of the three types of general structure renal channels assume.

The Architecture of ClC Channels

Every ClC protein, including both transporters and channels, shares a conserved molecular architecture consisting of a complex transmembrane transport domain and soluble regulatory domain. Representative crystal structures for both domains are available: the transmembrane domains of two bacteria ClC homologs, ClC-ec1 and ClC-st1, and a cyanobacterial ClC protein, ClC-sy1, and the regulatory domains of three eukaryote family members, ClC-0, ClC-Ka, and ClC-5.[53,57,116,120–122] ClC channels are unique for ion channel proteins, probably reflecting their evolutionary roots as transporters, in that many of their intramembrane helices are of unequal size not completely crossing the membrane. This places several intramembrane helices of ClC proteins at acute angles, rather than right angles as is more common for channels, to the plane of the lipid bilayer. This is clear in the crystal structure for ClC-ec1 shown in Figure 8.21.[52]

Also clear in this structure is that the assembled ClC channel is a homodimer containing two similar

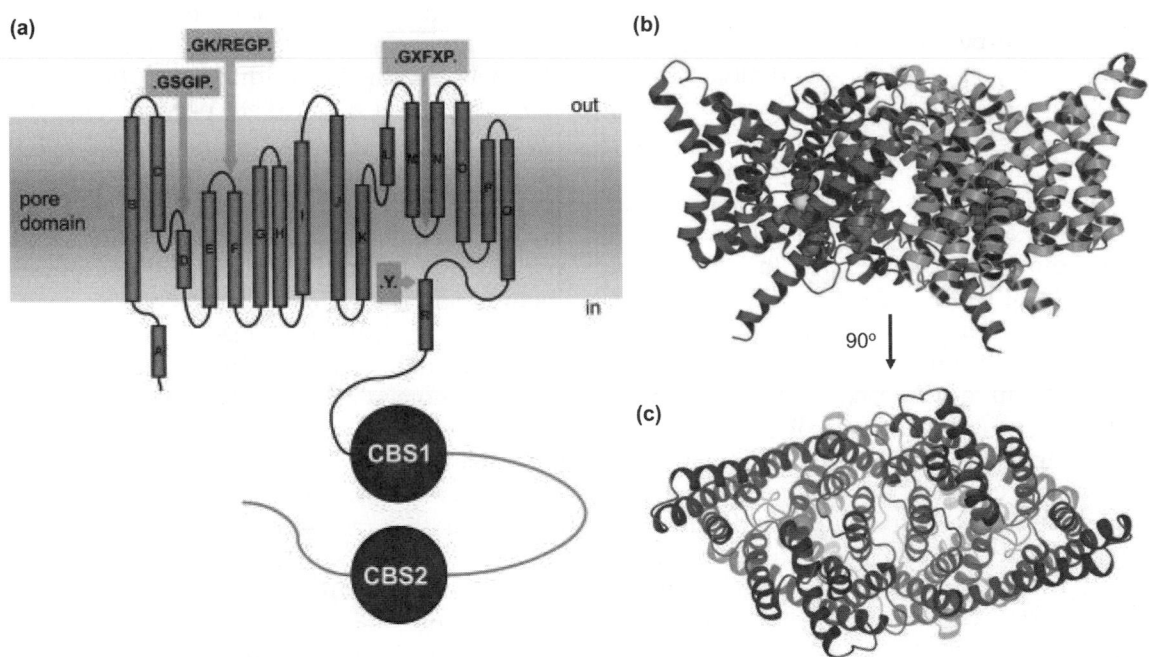

FIGURE 8.21 Topology and structure of ClC proteins. (a) *(Figure from [52].)* Schematic representation of ClC channel proteins with topology inferred from the known structure of the bacterial homolog ClC-ec1. The 18 α-helices in these proteins are labeled A–R. The two similar halves within the transmembrane domain (α-helices B–I and J–Q), which have anti-parallel orientation, are colored in green and cyan, respectively. The sequence and position of conserved residues that contribute to the Cl⁻ selectivity filter are noted with arrows and peach highlighting. The two cytoplasmic CBS domains are shown as red and blue spheres. (b) *(Figure from [79].)* Crystal structure of the *Salmonella enterica* serovar *typhimurium* ClC protein viewed parallel to the plane of the lipid bilayer. One subunit of the dimeric protein is shown in blue and the other green. Cl⁻ ions in the pore are shown as yellow spheres. Residues comprising the selectivity filter (S106, E1148, and Y445) are shown as red spheres. (c) *(Figure from [52].)* Structure of the *Escherichia coli* ClC protein, ClC-ec1, viewed from the extracellular side. The two subunits of the homodimer are colored red and blue, with ions in the selectivity filter of each subunit represented as green spheres. See color section at the back of the book.

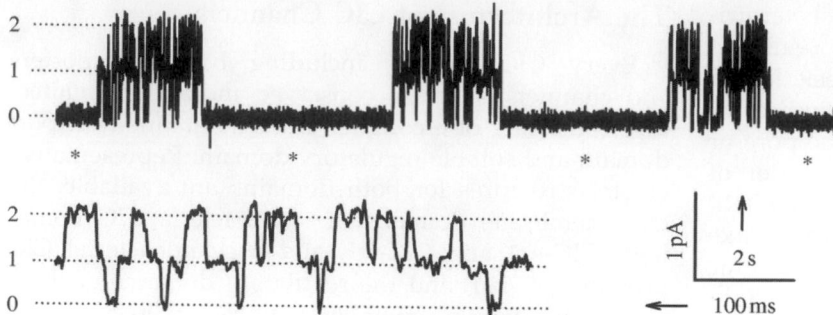

FIGURE 8.22 ClC subunits form double-barreled Cl⁻ channels. *(Figure from [61].)* Shown here is a representative single-channel current trace of a ClC-0 channel. Slow gating by the common gate is noted by asterisks. Fast gating of the proto-pore gates occurs between slow-gate closures: conductance level 0, both pores closed; conductance level 1, one pore closed, one pore open; conductance level 2, both pores open. Below is part of the current trace shown with an expanded timescale.

monomers, each having two topologically related halves, which span the membrane in opposite directions in an antiparallel arrangement. Despite their similarity in structure, the two antiparallel halves of each monomer share only weak conservation at the 1° amino acid sequence level. The two monomers within the channel are structurally related by an axis of two-fold symmetry perpendicular to the membrane plane. When viewed looking down on the plane of the extracellular leaflet of the membrane, the two monomers appear triangular, with a subunit interface at the bases of these triangles. A pore is completely contained within the center of each triangular subunit. That the assembled ClC homodimeric channel contains two independent pores with separate but identical ion permeation pathways has led to these channels being referred to as double-barreled channels. This is consistent with early electrophysiological work on the ClC-0 channel predicting this double-barreled architecture.[52,61,79] Each pore, sometimes termed proto-pore, has its own gate that functions independently gating in a fast manner. Both pores also are covered by a common gate that gates, in comparison, slower. These types of gating are clear in the representative single-channel current trace of homodimeric ClC-0 shown in Figure 8.22. In comparison to this fully assembled channel, the limiting functional unit of a ClC pore, as recently proven by Jayaram and colleagues using a molecularly "designed" ClC-ec1 protein mutating it from a transporter to channel, is a monomer containing the two antiparallel halves capable of conducting Cl⁻ through a single pore.[123] Experiments on this designed ClC-ec1 channel, moreover, addressed the line separating ClC channels from ClC transporters: it was shown to be thin, involving replacement of only two amino acids. Although the limiting functional unit is a monomer, binding sites critical to regulation of gating, for instance that for Ca²⁺, are formed at the interface between the two monomers of the homodimer.[124]

The Cl⁻ Permeation Pathway in ClC Channels: The Molecular Basis of Selectivity

All known ClC channel subunits use a conserved permeation pathway through the protein and common binding sites to conduct Cl⁻.[37,46] This vestigal pathway is also present and used in ClC anti-porters to translocate Cl⁻. The permeation pathway for anions was unexpectedly revealed by the presence of Cl⁻ ions bound within each pore in the first crystal structures of bacterial ClC transporters.[53,57] As recognized now from this early work, and reflected in the ribbon structures shown in Figure 8.23, the permeation pathway contains three Cl⁻-binding sites: an external binding site, S_{ext}; a central binding site, S_{cen}; and an internal binding site, S_{int}. The external binding site can be occupied by Cl⁻ or the side chain of a conserved Glu residue, E148 in bacterial ClC homologs.[46,52,79] This observation generated many of the initial hypotheses regarding the molecular basis of fast gating in ClC channels. This will be addressed further below.

Formation of a complete permeation pathway containing a selectivity-filter with three Cl⁻-binding sites, as depicted in Figure 8.23, is possible because the two structurally related antiparallel halves of a monomer are arranged in opposite directions, giving rise to a pseudo two-fold axis of symmetry in the center of the membrane. This makes it possible to bring together loops at the end of helices from different parts of the structure to form the pore in the center of the triangular monomer. Moreover, in this arrangement, the positive ends of the helix dipole point toward the ions entering the pore and stabilize them by electrostatic interactions. Interestingly, nature seems to have conserved this means of pore formation, because an antiparallel architecture also forms the pore of the unrelated aquaporins.[125,126]

Although scattered across the entire subunit, the signature sequences defining the three Cl⁻-binding sites, as noted in Figure 8.21, are conserved throughout all ClC proteins.[46–52] This speaks to the functional importance of conserving key residues at critical sites in the three-dimensional structure of the protein. The pore of ClC channels is hourglass in shape, bound by aqueous vestibules on the extracellular and intracellular end narrowing in the middle at the selectivity-filter. The intracellular Cl⁻-binding site is located at the interface between the intracellular vestibule and

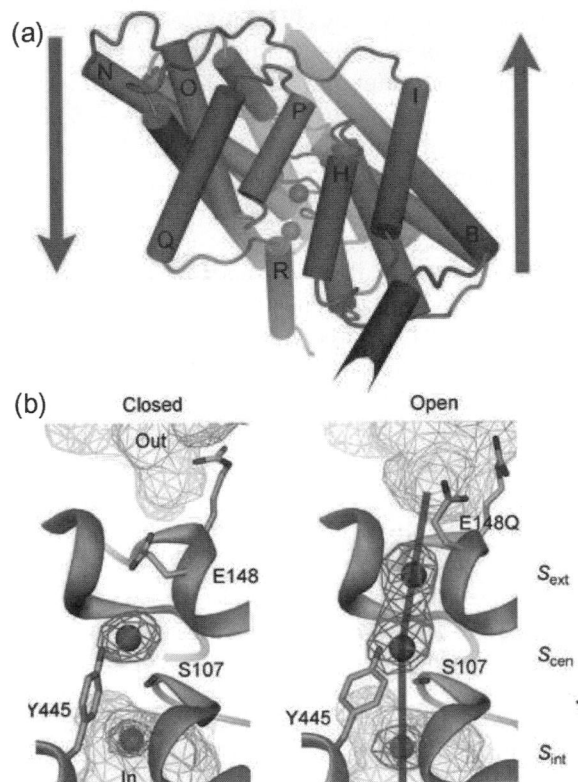

FIGURE 8.23 The selectivity filter of ClC channels. (a) (*Figure from* [52].) View of an EcClC monomer parallel to the plane of the membrane. The two anti-parallel halves of the monomer are colored blue and green. Their orientation in the membrane is indicated by arrows and helices are labeled. Ions in the pore are shown as red spheres. Regions of the protein contributing to the selectivity filter are colored red. (b) (*Figure from* [55].) The selectivity filter of wild-type EcClC (closed) and the EcClC mutant E148Q (open) viewed parallel to the plane of the lipid bilayer. The protein backbone is shown as a ribbon with NH_2-terminal ends of α-helices colored cyan. Selected residues are shown as sticks. Ions in the pore are represented as red spheres. The contoured (at 6σ) Br^- anomalous difference density is shown superimposed (red). Aqueous cavities from the extracellular (out) and intracellular (in) solutions are shown as cyan mesh. Ion-binding sites in the pore are labeled. See color section at the back of the book.

negative charge is also placed within 4 Å of the Cl^- ion occupying S_{cen}. This provides two alternatives to explain gating: a physical occlusion of the pore and a repulsion mechanism involving pore-gating. When the channel is conducting, E148 has moved from S_{ext}, opening this binding site to the Cl^- ion. Supporting this are findings showing that, upon substituting E148 with either an Ala or a Gln, a Cl^- ion is bound to this site coordinated by free backbone amide NH groups of residues in the NH_2-termini of the N and F helices.[37,46,57]

ClC Channel Gating

The gating of ClC channels is complex and incompletely understood. More is understood about the mechanisms underpinning fast gating of proto-pores, as compared to gating by the common gate. Gating of both the fast and common gates is inextricably linked to ion permeation.[37,61,127] In addition to being modulated by extracellular $[Cl^-]$ where increases in $[Cl^-]_{ex}$ increase P_o, fast gating (and also slow gating) is modulated in a positive manner by depolarizing voltages and decreases in pH.[61,67,128,129] Dependence on pH is thought to be a remnant from its days as a transporter. Compelling evidence has emerged that E148 mediates the effects of pH on the fast gate. There is a real possibility also, as supported by experimental evidence, that the effects of voltage on the fast gate are felt by the permeant Cl^- ion and/or modulatory H^+.[61,130] This likely arises from the fact that proto-pores use some form of a pore-gating mechanism, with the interaction between the permeant ion and permeation pathway doing the "gating." Working in combination with this is the charged side chain of E148, which also may be sensitive to voltage or even extracellular $[Cl^-]$ and pH in a voltage-dependent manner.

An important point to note is that ClC-Ka and ClC-Kb do not have a Glu at the position corresponding to 148, which is 166 in ClC-Kb, but rather have a Val at this site, yet both channels show fast gating.[46,79,131] This suggests that, while E148 and the corresponding Glu residues in other ClC channels may be involved in gating, it is not functioning in isolation. In addition, ClC-K1 channels are voltage-sensitive where interaction with the accessory subunit barttin reverses the voltage-activation profile (see Figure 8.16[72,73]). Chimeras of ClC-K1 and ClC-Kb retain this barttin-dependent switch in voltage-sensitivity, suggesting that ClC-Kb channels are also voltage-sensitive in the absence of barttin and E148. The importance of E148 to gating in most ClC channels, though, is not trivial for mutation of the homologous residues in ClC-0, ClC-1, and ClC-2 to neutral residues abolishes voltage-dependent gating.[57,132,133]

selectivity-filter. The Cl^- ion occupying S_{int} is only partly desolvated, and still hydrated where it is exposed to the aqueous environment of the vestibule. The desolvated surface of this Cl^- ion is coordinated by backbone amide groups on the loop preceding the D helix. The Cl^- ion at S_{cen} has completely shed its water shell, and is now coordinated by partial positive charges from backbone amide nitrogen groups in residues preceding the N helix. In addition, key interactions are made here with selectivity-filter side chain hydroxyls of S107 in the conserved GSGIP sequence and of Y445 located at the beginning of the R helix. When S_{ext} is occupied by E148, not only is the pore physically blocked by the residue side-chain, but a

The Architecture of ENaC/Deg Channels

The three-dimensional structure of ENaC awaits elucidation, but much can be inferred with a degree of certainty from the known structure of chicken ASIC1.[58,117] As discussed below, we can make predictions about the selectivity-filter and permeation pathway of ENaC and how the channel gates, which are supported by electrophysiology studies.[104,105,134–136]

Subunits forming ENaC/Deg channels share a common topology, which is shown in Figure 8.24, containing a large extracellular domain with much secondary structure bound by two transmembrane (TM) domains, TM1 and TM2, with intracellular NH_2- and COOH-termini.[58,117] As noted above, ENaC is an obligatory heterotrimer containing one α-, one β-, and one γ-subunit contributing to a central pore.[118] These

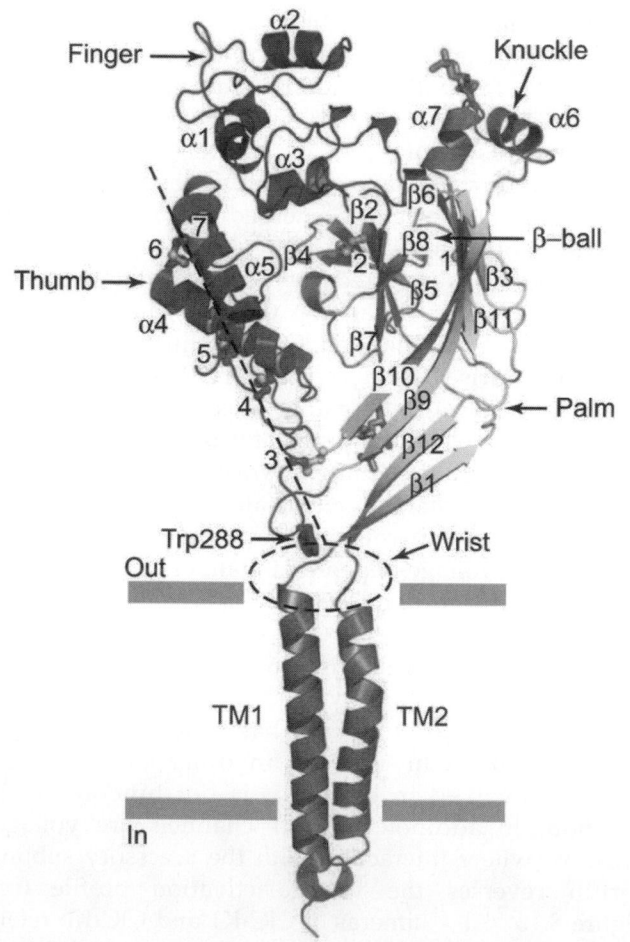

FIGURE 8.24 The topology of ENaC/Deg channel subunits. *(Figure from [117].)* This cartoon shows the topology of a monomer within the homotrimeric cASIC1 channel, as defined by the crystal structure. The view is perpendicular to the plane of the membrane. Transmembrane helices (TM1 and TM2) are shown in red. Location of intra-subunit disulphide bridges are labelled 1–7. See color section at the back of the book.

orthologs are encoded by different genes.[101,102] The relative order of subunits within ENaC has yet to be determined. Oligomerized ENaC likely appears as a "chalice," similar to that shown in Figure 8.25, with extracellular domains forming the cup, the transmembrane domains the stem, and intracellular domains the base.[117,137] In comparison to K^+ channels, the ENaC/Deg pore and selectivity-filter, as defined by the cASIC1 crystal, are not made of P-loops diving back into the membrane, but rather are formed by the TM2 domains of the three component subunits as they run in a linear manner through the membrane. The pore as defined by TM2 domains is "hourglass" in shape, with wide extracellular and intracellular facing vestibules and a narrowing in the middle. The extracellular mouth of the pore is coupled to the extracellular domain by short linker sequences in the wrist of the channel. TM1 domains lie just outside TM2 domains within the same subunit as they run the length of the pore sheltering TM2 residues, with TM1 making most of the contact with the lipid bilayer. There are extensive interactions between residues in the adjacent TM1 and TM2 helices within the same subunit, and also between TM domains in neighboring subunits.

The Permeation Pathway in ENaC/Deg Channels: Selectivity and Ion-Binding Sites

Similar to cASIC1, the ENaC pore likely has pseudo three-fold symmetry around the central axis of the pore, perpendicular to the plane of the lipid bilayer. Ions enter the extracellular mouth of the pore proper through a large vestibule that has profound negative electrostatic potential where the lower half of this molecular "basket" sits within the membrane plane. The negative electrostatic potential of the vestibule allows it to act as a cation reservoir, concentrating cations around the mouth of the pore, contributing to robust channel conductance.[58] The bottom of this vestibule in cASIC1 is defined by D433 corresponding to N530 in γ-ENaC, which when substituted as discussed below causes disease.[58,138] D433 has been proposed to contribute to the desensitization gate in cASIC1 in response to H^+.[58] The cytoplasmic mouth of the pore, similarly, is bound by a large vestibule, shaped like an inverted cone. This vestibule is lined by residues with negatively charged side chains, again possibly allowing the vestibule to act as a cation reservoir. Substitution leading to charge neutralization of these negatively charged residues in ENaC eliminates conductance through the channel.[136]

Figure 8.26 shows the three-dimensional structure of cASIC1, including the radius of a possible conduction pathway along the three-fold axis. The cASIC1 pore, and likely that in ENaC, contains three Na^+-

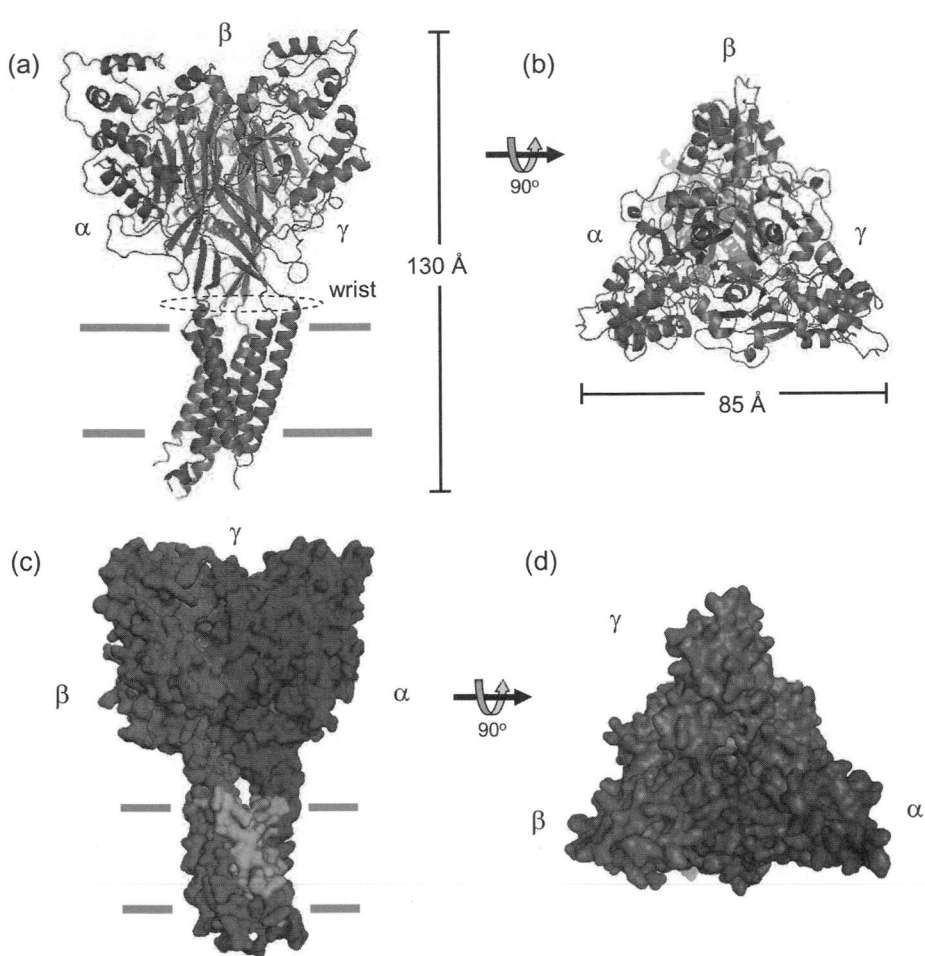

FIGURE 8.25 **Predicted structure of ENaC.** *(Figure adapted from Figure 3 in [137].)* View of the predicted ribbon and space-filled structure of heterotrimeric ENaC perpendicular (a and c) and parallel (b and d), from the extracellular side, to the molecular three-fold axis. ENaC subunits, α- (red), β- (yellow), and γ- (blue), modeled using the 2QTS structural coordinates for the A, B, and C subunits of the cASIC1 homotrimer.[117] See color section at the back of the book.

binding sites that are occupied during permeation. Adjacent sites are unlikely to be occupied at the same time due to charge repulsion (see Figure 8.15[58]). In open cASIC1, main chain carbonyl oxygen atoms from the symmetry-related G436, G439, and G443 residues coordinate Na^+ permeating through the pore. As shown in Figure 8.27, permeant ions are bound by six ligands arranged in a trigonal antiprism geometry arising from the three ligands on the upper triangular plane being staggered in comparison to those in the lower triangular plane. This geometry provides the appropriate number of partial negative charges for coordination of a Na^+ ion, while perfectly accommodating the underlying molecular symmetry of the trimeric channel.

Several of the coordinating Gly residues in cASIC1 are replaced by Ser residues in ENaC subunits (see Figure 8.27a). ENaC is about 10-fold more selective for Na^+ than ASIC.[47,48,58,139] Although Gly and Ser are structurally similar, the latter is larger, containing an extra carbon and hydroxyl moiety. Thus, Ser occupies a larger volume. Perhaps this larger volume introduces a steric constraint that allows better accommodation

of Na^+ in the permeation pathway over other cations. This awaits experimental testing. Nevertheless, the geometry and atomic volumes of the pore in cASIC1 suggest that Na^+ sheds its hydration shell to permeate through the channel. Electrophysiology findings for ENaC support this. Mutations in and near the ENaC selectivity-filter reduce both the Na^+ conductance and Na^+ to K^+ selectivity, possibly because of a perturbation of precise channel-ion hydration geometry.[104,105,140]

The trigonal antiprism coordination of Na^+ in the pore of ENaC/Deg channels, as exemplified by cASIC1, has been proposed to be the archetypal molecular basis of permeation through cation-selective ion channels containing three component subunits.[58] The crystal structure of the P2X4 channel, which also was recently solved, agrees with this position.[58,141] The P2X4 channel is cation-selective, and has 2°, 3°, and 4° structures similar to those in ENaC/Deg channels, but little 1° amino acid sequence identity. Yet, both use identical modes and means of permeation and coordination of permeant ions. The ideal ion-to-ligand distance in the trigonal antiprism arrangement in

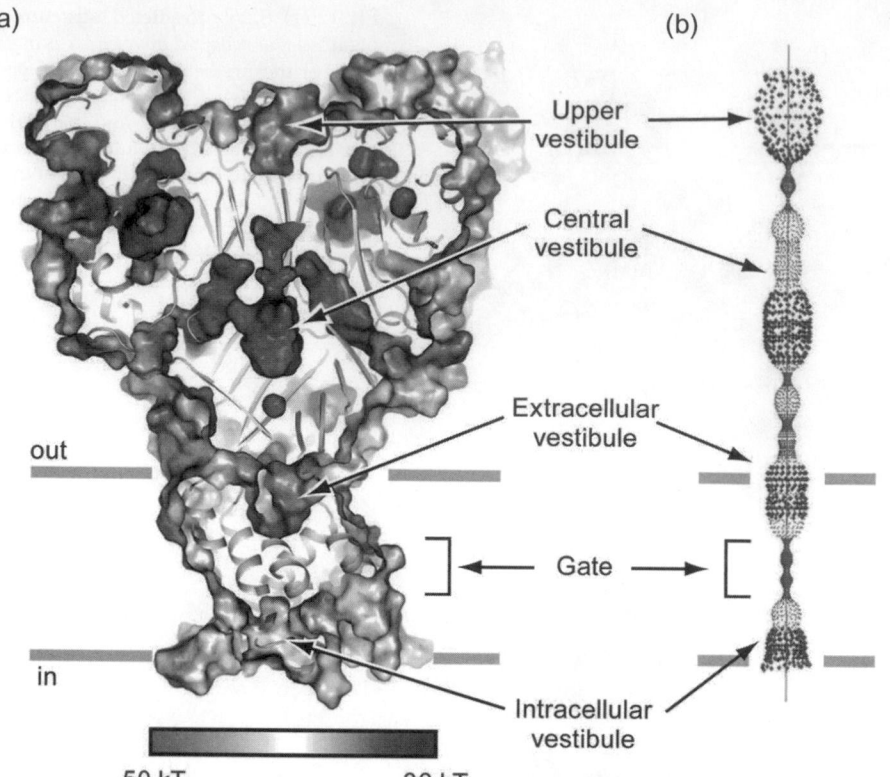

FIGURE 8.26 The structure of ASIC. *(Figure from [58].)* (a) An electrostatic potential surface and cartoon representation of cASIC1 viewed along the molecular three-fold axis of symmetry. Color is based on electrostatic potential, ranging from −50 kT (red) to +30 kT (blue). White is 0 kT. (b) Illustration of the radius of possible pathways along the three-fold axis of cASIC1 where red <1.4 Å <green <2.3 Å < purple. See color section at the back of the book.

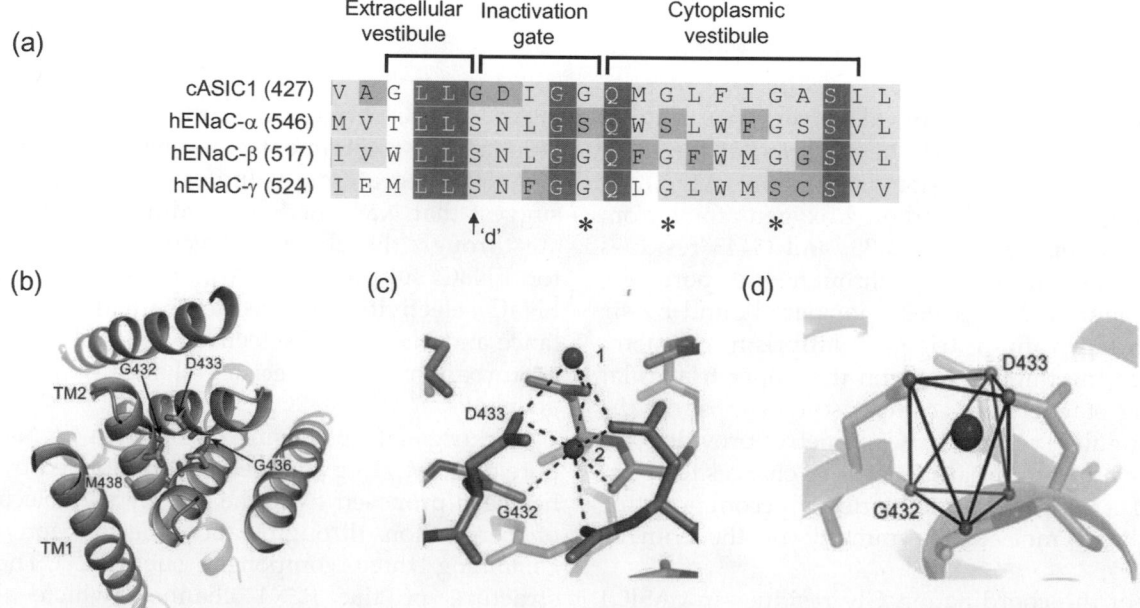

FIGURE 8.27 The pore of ENaC/Deg channels. *(Figures adapted from Figures 4 and 5 in [58].)* (a) Sequence alignment of pore lining residues in TM2 of cASIC1 and human ENaC subunits. Identity indicated with red, conservative substitutions yellow, and similarity light-blue coloring. Asterisks indicate residues thought to contribute to binding sites within the permeation pathway of the pore. "d" indicates the degenrin site.[144,145] (b) View of the cASIC pore from the extracellular side of the membrane, with the position of selected side chain residues shown. (c) Key interactions between Cs⁺ ions, shown as purple balls, in the cASIC1 pore with main chain and side chain oxygen atoms of Gly 432 and Asp 433, respectively. (d) Trigonal antiprism coordination of a Cs⁺ ion in the cASIC1 pore by the symmetry related Gly 432 carbonyl and Asp 433 carboxyl oxygens in the three momomers. Oxygen atoms are shown as red spheres. See color section at the back of the book.

ENaC/Deg channels, where six partial-charge ligands coordinate cation binding, is stereochemically analogous to the eight-fold square antiprism coordination of larger K^+ ions in K^+ channels containing four subunits.[36,58] In both ENaC/Deg and K^+ channels, the symmetry of the pore and number of subunits contributing to the pore are matched to the optimal coordination requirements of the permeant ion.[142,143] Moreover, although the linear pore of ENaC/Deg channels lined by the three TM2 domains of component subunits differs in general construction from the pore of K^+ channels, which is formed by the four-component P-loops dipping back into the membrane, the basic chemistry and physical tenets underpinning the coordination of permeant ions within these pores are conserved. This speaks to conservation by nature of a workable blueprint.

The Gate in ENaC/Deg Channels

Compared to ASIC channels, which activate and inactivate in response to H^+ binding to an extracellular allosteric site, ENaC is held to gate in a constitutive manner, with gating modulated by regulatory factors.[41,58,81,117] In cASIC1, a constriction formed by the crossing of TM2 domains at D433 occludes the pore acting as an inactivation gate. The channel is thought to open by TM domains untwisting around the central axis of the pore perpendicular to the plane of the lipid bilayer, partially uncrossing TM2 domains and relieving obstruction of the pore by the inactivation gate. The *degenerin* mutation that constitutively activates ENaC/Deg channels by locking them in long-lived open states is at 432 in cASIC1, one position upstream of the crossing site of TM2 domains.[144,145] Placement of an amino acid larger than Gly at this site sterically clashes with symmetry-related TM2 domains, providing a mechanism whereby mutations at the *degenerin* site perturb gating.

It is interesting that Asn residues, as clear in the alignment shown in Figure 8.27, occupy the positions in ENaC subunits homologous to D433 in cASIC1. This appears to be a signature feature of ENaC, as most other non-ENaC subunits in the ENaC/Deg family have Asp at this position. Moreover, it is likely to be of biophysical importance, for Asn is the uncharged derivative of Asp. This may explain why ENaC constitutively gates and does not inactivate. In ENaC, TM2 crossing at this Asn, for instance, may not be as stable as that in cASIC1 and, thus, transient or it may not obstruct the pore. In addition to an inactivation gate, the crystal structure of cASIC1 suggested that ENaC/Deg channels use a pore-gating mechanism.[58] This possibly explains constitutive gating of ENaC.

The Architecture of K^+ Channels and TRP Channels: ROMK as a Representative

Subunits that form K^+ channels have either two, four, six or six-plus-one transmembrane domains, as typified by Kir-, K_{2P}-, Kv-, and BK_{Ca}-subunits, respectively (see Figure 8.20). Whereas at first glance the apparently different $2°$ and $3°$ structures of these subunits may suggest that they assemble into channels of different $4°$ structure, the fact is they do not, but rather all form channels having a similar core structure surrounding a central pore with four-fold symmetry.[35,36,45,56,146,147] The canonical K^+ channel pore is formed by transmembrane domains and the P-loop, as defined by the two transmembrane domains of Kir channels. The crystal structures of the bacterial KvAP, MthK, KirBac1.1, KirBac3.1, and KcsA channels (and chimeras of KcsA-Kv1.3 and Kir3.1-prokaryotic Kir channel) show slight variations of a common K^+ channel pore, informing on the molecular basis of selectivity, permeation, and gating.[35,36,45,56,146,147] Segments defining this core pore structure are repeated as a pair in the four transmembrane domains of K_{2P} channels. This explains why these channel subunits form a dimeric channel with a central pore that has four-fold symmetry.[80] Moreover, this core pore-forming structure is retained in Kv and BK_{Ca} channels as the S5-P-loop-S6 domains.[2] BK_{Ca} channels mirror the general structure of Kv channels, with the exception that they have one additional transmembrane domain placing their NH_2-terminus outside the cell. TRP channels are also thought to assume this basic structure, often being modeled on the six transmembrane Kv channel.[2,119] The formal structure of TRP channels, however, awaits crystallization studies.

To facilitate discussion of the molecular basis of selectivity, permeation, and gating of the common K^+ channel pore, we focus on ROMK. The reason for this is that the ROMK channel is made of subunits having two transmembrane domains containing all the components comprising the core K^+ channel pore and a regulated gate.

The ROMK Channel Pore: Selectivity and Permeation

Welling and Ho,[32] in a recent review article, reported a compelling atomic model for ROMK based on known Kir channel structures, including regions defined in the crystal structures of the bacterial KirBac1.1 channel, a chimeric Kir3.1-prokaryotic Kir channel, the pore region of the mammalian GIRK1 channel, and the cytoplasmic domains of Kir2.1 and Kir3.1.[35,56,146,147] This model is shown in Figure 8.28.[32] ROMK contains the canonical transmembrane pore common to all K^+ channels, but also a unique central

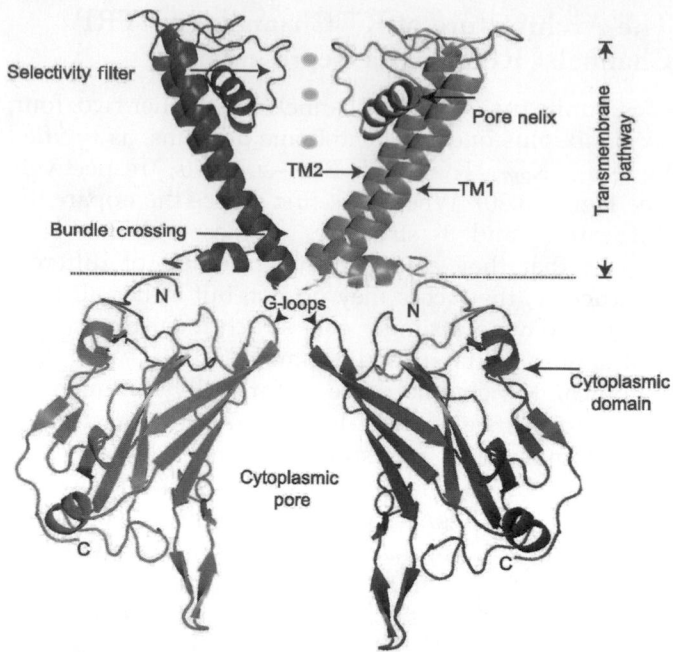

FIGURE 8.28   Predicted structure of ROMK. *(Figure from [32].)* An atomic model of ROMK was developed from known K_{ir} channel structures and an iterative optimization algorithm. Shown are two subunits, one green and the other blue, of the tetrameric channel. See color section at the back of the book.

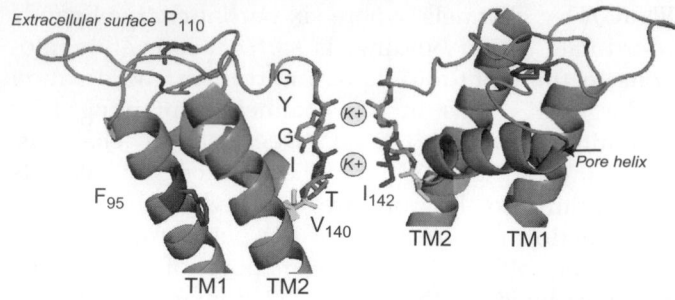

FIGURE 8.29   The selectivity filter of ROMK. *(Figure from [32].)* Backbone carbonyl oxygens of selectivity-filter residues $T_{141}IGYG$ point into the pore, mimicking the hydration shell of potassium. Rapid conformational movement of $T_{141}I_{142}$ likely underpins fast gating in ROMK. Residues in red are mutated in Bartter's syndrome type II. See color section at the back of the book.

cavity contained by a large cytoplasmic domain, which is characteristic of Kir channels.[148,149]

The four component subunits of ROMK assemble around a central pore that has four-fold symmetry. The helices of TM2 domains span the membrane at a tilt, narrowing at the intracellular base of the pore. The four TM2 helices of the component subunits frame the pore as it spans the membrane, with TM1 domains running along but outside TM2 domains of the same subunit. The narrowest part of the open conduction pathway is defined by P-loops of the four subunits. These P-loops are linker regions that connect TM1 to TM2 and contain short helical domains that dip back into the mouth of the pore. The symmetry related linkers contain the conserved K^+-selectivity sequence, T[V/I]GYG.[35,36,45,56,146] This motif adopts a strand conformation, as depicted in Figure 8.29, where the NH_2-terminal end is deepest in the pore and COOH-terminal end at the mouth of the pore. The backbone carbonyl oxygen of these T[V/I]GYG residues projects into the central axis of the open pore. Similar to all K^+ channels, the carbonyl oxygen of residues in this selectivity sequence from each symmetry-related subunit form four equally spaced K^+-binding sites in the pore. Four oxygen atoms at the top and bottom of each binding site cage a K^+ ion with eight-fold square antiprism coordination. Such coordination is similar to the way water molecules surround K^+ ions in

solution.[36,142,143] This mimicry of water solvation at the selectivity-filter creates an energetically favorable means for K^+ to diffuse into binding sites as they shed their surrounding water shell. Because the volume and ion coordination of these binding sites do not accommodate smaller ions in a dehydrated state, like Na^+, this molecular structure provides high-fidelity K^+-selectivity.

The sequential arrangement of the four equally spaced K^+-binding sites in the linear ROMK pore facilitates a single-file multiple-ion conduction mechanism in agreement with findings from early biophysical measurements.[150–152] As revealed in the crystal structure of the KcsA channel, K^+ ions are simultaneously absorbed to two binding sites at a time, with an empty site positioned between the two occupied sites due to electrostatic charge repulsion between permeant ions.[36,45,151,152] Conduction by K^+ channels then, as depicted in Figure 8.13, is the rapid jumping of K^+ ions in a pair-wise manner from one to the other paired-binding sites within the pore. Such movement involves several rounds of dehydration and rehydration, as the K^+ ion moves into the pore and is absorbed and released from each binding site, and as it exits the pore. The energetics of this sequential dehydration and rehydration as counterbalanced by electrochemical driving forces and electrostatic repulsion between ions within the pore sets conductance. Such a structure enables K^+ ions to move through the pore with high-throughput, but yet with remarkable selectivity.[151,153]

Molecular Basis of Rectification in ROMK Channels

A unique feature of ROMK and other inward rectifier K^+ channels, as their name suggests, is that they have larger inward currents compared to outward currents.[32] The molecular basis of this rectification involves a pore-block mechanism, where Mg^{2+} and polyamines enter the pore at depolarizing voltages through the intracellular mouth of the channel.[76,77] Once in the pore, Mg^{2+} and polyamines interact with a binding site near the selectivity-filter, plugging the pore. This gives rise to inward rectification, which actually is a decrease in P_o as a function of a voltage-dependent block of the pore where channel P_o is higher at hyperpolarizing potentials compared to depolarizing potentials, allowing greater inward as compared to outward current flow. The degree of rectification is different between distinct members of the Kir channel family, depending on subtle differences in the binding sites for blocking Mg^{2+} and polyamines. ROMK only marginally rectifies. This rectification phenotype is largely a factor of N171 in the pore lining TM2 domain of ROMK or its equivalent in other Kir channels. This is supported by the observation that the N171D substitution in ROMK produces strong rectification. The reverse mutation, D172N, in the strong inward-rectifying Kir2.1 channel weakens rectification, making it more akin to that of ROMK.[154] Figure 8.30 reports the relative position of N171 in ROMK showing that its side chain projects into the aqueous environment of the pore, a position consistent with it being involved in an intra-pore binding site for large blocking cations like Mg^{2+} and polyamines.

Molecular Basis of ROMK Gating

ROMK channels have, at least, two different types of gates. The fast gating of ROMK, as discussed above, involves a pore-gating mechanism. Potassium in the pore of ROMK has profound influence on the structure of the selectivity-filter and pore-binding sites.[151,152] As K^+ binds to a particular position in the selectivity-filter of ROMK (as seen in Figure 8.29), the energetics of binding to this site cause a conformational change at T141-I142, briefly shuttling the channel into a non-conducting conformation.[50,51] An alternative to this

physical mechanism, as mentioned above, is a chemical mechanism where the pore does not change conformation but rather K^+ binding affects the energy of binding where the permeant ion is briefly stuck and is unable to move along the pore.[63]

In addition to using a pore-gating mechanism for fast gating, ROMK channels also use a distinct type of gating mechanism that is slower and is regulated. As shown in Figure 8.30, the side chain of L179 in the TM2 domain of ROMK subunits projects into the mouth of the pore and obstructs permeation. It is widely held that regulated K^+ channel opening involves the movement of the pore helices (TM2) away from the bundle-crossings (with TM1) at the intracellular base of the pore, with extracellular G167 and G176 or their equivalents acting as flexible "hinges" allowing this opening pivot. This movement carries the putative L179 gate at the base of TM2 away from the pore, physically removing this obstruction. Replacement of L179 with small or charged residues stabilizes the open state, just as would be predicted if this residue acts as a regulated gate to obstruct the conduction pathway during the closed state.[155,156] Moreover, such a gating movement is consistent with the differences identified in the crystal structure "snap-shots" of KirBac3.1 in the open and closed state.[35] Figure 8.31 shows these structures. The Y132 gating residue in KirBac3.1 corresponds to L179 in ROMK.

The regulated gate is actually a larger structure involving complex interactions between residues in TM2 and TM1, where an ε-nitrogen of K80 in TM1 forms a hydrogen bond with the backbone carbonyl oxygen of A177 to control the energetics of gating as performed by L179. Such a gating structure provides the molecular basis for regulation, with information arising from conformational changes in intracellular domains translated to the gate via K80. K80 sits at the base of TM1 at the bundle-crossing, which is positioned immediately above the G-loops of the cytoplasmic domains. The idea is that allosteric sites in the

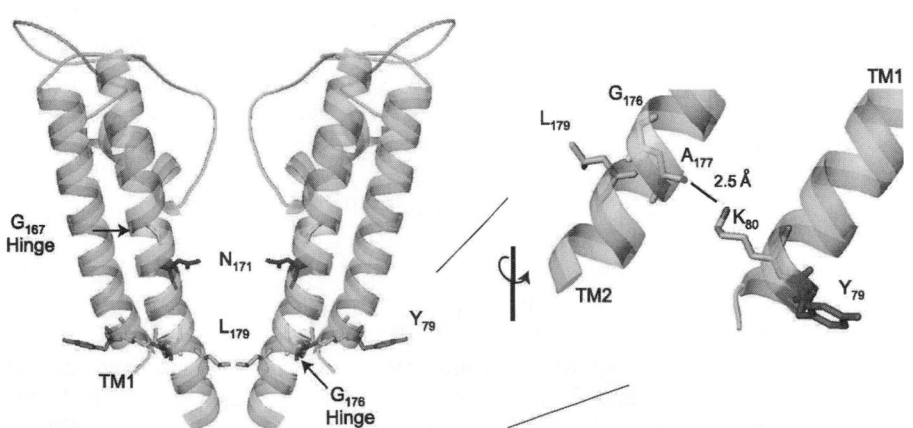

FIGURE 8.30 The molecular determinants of regulated gating and rectification of ROMK. *(Figure from* [32].*)* ROMK gating is thought to involve the twisting of membrane helices pulling L179, the putative gate, out of the pore. Hydrogen bonds between K80 at the base of TM1, and A177, in TM2 stabilizes the gate. Y79 is mutated in Bartter's syndrome. The side chain of N171 projects into the pore and is a key determinant of inward rectification.

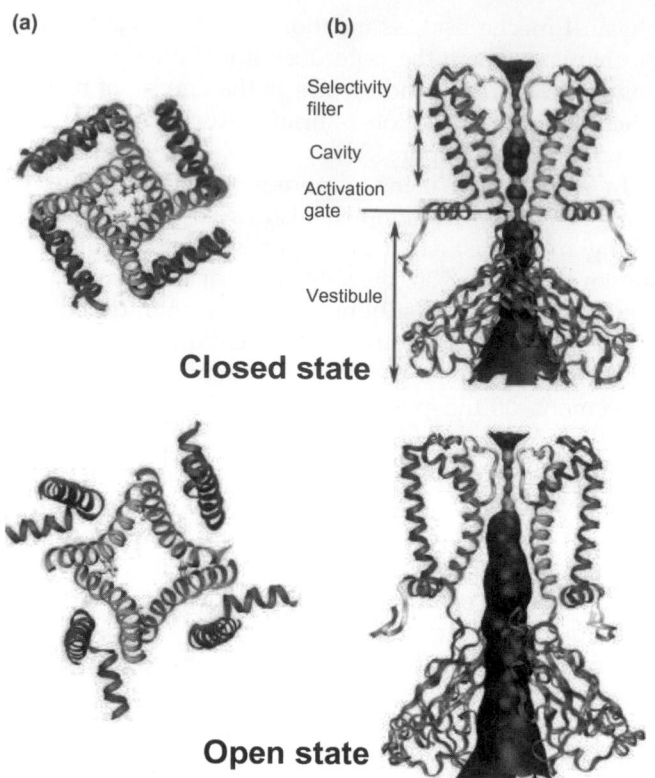

Closed state

Open state

FIGURE 8.31 *"Snap-shots" of KirBac3.1 in the closed and open state. (Figure from* [35].) (a) View of the transmembrane section of KirBac from the extracellular side of the membrane in a closed (top) and open (bottom) conformation. Helices are shown as ribbons with outer helices, purple; inner helices, green; and the slide helices, red. The activation gate is displayed as yellow sticks. (b) Two monomers of the closed (top) and open (bottom) channel are shown superimposed on a representation of the diameter of the central ion conduction pathway. Structural elements are colored as in (a). Red coloring in the central conduction pathway indicates that there is not enough space to allow a water molecule to pass; green shows where one or two water molecules could fit; and blue where many water molecules can fit. See color section at the back of the book.

intracellular portion of the channel communicate to the gate through the G-loop positioned just below the intracellular mouth of the pore, although this remains an open question.[32]

The cytoplasmic domains of ROMK assemble just below the canonical transmembrane pore to form a long water-filled cavity extending the length of the conduction pathway. The characteristics of secondary structures and position of side chains of residues lining this water-filled cavity are consistent with it being a pathway for permeation. For instance, this intracellular pore is lined by residues that provide an electrostatic environment favorable for efficient K^+ transport and cation-blocker binding.[157] In addition, there is a high degree of concordance between residues contributing to the electrostatic field, favoring transport and binding with residues known from mutagenesis

studies to affect cation block and single-channel conductance.[43] Moreover, studies on the chimeric ROMK-Kir2.1 channel, in addition to other mutagenesis studies, revealed that residues lining the inner wall of this intracellular pore, with N259 in ROMK playing the most significant role, directly influence single-channel conductance. This effect is independent of structures in the transmembrane selectivity-filter, suggesting that the symmetry related cytoplasmic domains provide additional energy barriers to the flow of K^+ through the channel.[157–159] The putative gate for this intracellular pore is thought to be at the narrowing created by the four G-loops as they coalesce just below the mouth of the membrane-spanning pore. This gate is believed to create a flexible diffusion barrier between the cytoplasmic and transmembrane pores. Supporting this are findings that mutations in this region of Kir2.1 and Kir3.1 alter channel gating and inward rectification.[160]

TUBULOPATHIES RESULTING FROM CHANGES IN CHANNEL BIOPHYSICAL PROPERTIES

The majority of channelopathies, including those causing tubulopathy, result from loss of expression or changes in the expression level of functional channels at the membrane. These are not covered here. Less common are channelopathies resulting from mutations that affect the biophysical properties of an ion channel. The latter are informative about residues and structures critical to function. Such mutations, as listed in Table 8.2, are a focus of this discussion.

ClC-Kb: Barrter Syndrome Type III

Mutations in the gene *CLCNKB* encoding the ClC-Kb Cl^- channel cause Bartter syndrome type III, characterized by hypokalaemic metabolic alkalosis, renal salt-wasting, and hyper-reninaemic hyperaldosteronism.[14,18,161] The root cause of BS type III is abberant transport in the TAL and DCT, stemming from pathological changes in membrane voltage and diffusion potentials resulting from loss of the basolateral exit pathway for Cl^-. Although several missense mutations resulting in amino acid substitutions in ClC-Kb are known to cause BS type III, the effects of these mutations on the biophysical properties of this channel are largely unexplored. The R351W Bartter mutation in ClC-Kb is an exception.[162]

Homodimeric ClC-Ka and ClC-Kb channels contain extracellular regulatory Ca^{2+}- and H^+-binding sites at inter-subunit interfaces.[124] Increases in extracellular $[Ca^{2+}]$ and extracellular alkalinization increase ClC-K

TABLE 8.2 Renal Channelopathies Caused by Changes in Biophysical Properties

Channel	Disease Causing Mutation[a]	Result	Disease	References
ENaC	G37S in β-ENaC	Decreased activity due to voltage-dependent block of the pore by a permeant ion.	PHA-I	174, 134
	S562P in α-ENaC	Likely to affect ENaC selectivity or permeation.	PHA-I	107, 181
	N530S in γ-ENaC	Likely to lock the channel in a high P_o state.	Liddle's syndrome	138
ROMK	Y79H, A177T	Disrupts the regulated gating-structure at the bundle-crossing in ROMK.	BS-II	15, 189
	T332*fs*	Disrupts domains involved in sensing or conveying pH-dependent effects to the regulated gate.	BS-II	195, 148, 185, 186
	A306T	Disrupts the gate in the cytosolic domain of the channel.	BS-II	15
	C49Y, I51T, A214V and L220F[b]	Disrupts PIP_2-regulation of gating.	BS-II	15, 194, 186
	S219R and S313C	Disrupts PKA phosphorylation sites essential for modulating the effects of gating factors.	BS-II	194, 186
	R311Q/W[b]	Disrupts a critical salt bridge.	BS-II	15, 194
	I142T	Disrupts K^+ selectivity filter sequence decreasing K^+ conductance.	BS-II	185
	A198T, Y314C and V315G[b]	Decreased activity due to entering a long closed/inactive state.	BS-II	198, 185, 15
	W99C, A103V, P110L and N124K	Loss-of-function with dominant negative effect.	BS-II	185
	T71M, F95S, A156V and R324L	Loss-of-function where the molecular mechanism is undefined, but channels make it to the membrane in some systems.	BS-II	15
ClC-Kb	R351W	Decreases activation by extracellular Ca^{2+} and alkaline pH.	BS-III	162
	A77T, L139P, A204, S297R, S337F, A349D, H357Q, R438C, R438H, R438L and R538P	Loss-of-function where the molecular mechanism, as yet, is undefined.	BS-III	161, 165, 166
	K560M and S573Y	Substitutions within the first CBS domain of ClC-Kb possibly affecting regulation of gating.	BS-III	79, 161
	P124L and Y432H	Substitution near a Cl^- binding site within the permeation pathway possibly affecting permeabiton, gating or selectivity.	BS-III	46, 79, 161, 165, 166
Barttin	R8L, R8W and G10S	Inactivating mutants in BSND causing loss of function of membrane ClC-Ka and ClC-Kb channels.	BS-IV	71, 173, 73
	G47R	Decreased interaction with ClC-K channels leading to a milder decrease in function and a milder phenotype.	BS-IV	71, 173
TRPM6	P1017R	Decreases activity of membrane resident TRPM6/TRPM7 channels.	HSH	4

[a]*Positions noted for human sequences.*
[b]*These mutations may also be involved in coupling to/from PKA phosphorylation sites or the state of phosphorylation — fs = frameshift.*

channel activity: Ca^{2+} binding is stimulatory, whereas H^+ binding is inhibitory.

The R351W substitution in ClC-Kb abolishes sensitivity to extracellular $[Ca^{2+}]$, and markedly reduces activation by alkaline pH.[162] The consequence of these changes in biophysical properties is that mutant ClC-Kb is less active under physiological conditions. The mechanism whereby mutation of R351 affects Ca^{2+}- and pH-regulated gating has not been determined. R351 is positioned at the COOH-terminal end of the linker coupling helices K and L. This positions the residue near the extracellular surface of the channel. Perhaps R351 plays a role in coupling Ca^{2+}- and H^+-binding to the channel gate or it is an essential component of an allosteric regulatory binding site, or integral to the structure of the gate itself. The importance of this position to ClC channel function is underscored by the fact that mutations in this region of ClC-1, for instance F413C and A415V corresponding to two and four positions downstream from R351 in ClC-Kb, cause myotonia.[163,164]

In addition to R351W, a host of other point mutations, as listed in Table 8.2, decrease ClC-Kb channel activity to cause BS type III.[161,165] As yet, no experimental information is avaliable about how these Bartter mutations cause ClC-Kb dysfunction. There is circumstantial evidence, though, that some may affect the biophysical properties of the channel, for they involve nonconservative substitutions of residues highly conserved across paralogs and orthologs. For instance, L139 is conserved in most ClC proteins across species ranging from *C. elegans* to man, and S297 and S337 are conserved in all mammalian ClC-K channels. The P124L substitution changes a conserved residue in the first Cl^--binding site in the permeation pathway, predicting a change in conductance, selectivity or even gating, considering ClC channels use a pore-gating mechanism.[55,161,166] The S123P mutation in this region of the ClC-0 channel, that corresponds to three residues upstream of P124 in ClC-Kb, increases nitrate permeability.[167] Moreover, covalent modification by sulfhydryl reagents of a P126C mutant in ClC-0, which corresponds to P124 in ClC-Kb, markedly reduces P_o.[168] The Y432H mutation, similarly, is four positions downstream of residues forming the third Cl^--binding site, suggesting that it may also impact permeation. Additional support comes from the fact that several Bartter mutations in ClC-Kb occupy the same sites or are near residues in ClC-1 that when mutated, cause myotonia. For instance, the A349D mutation in ClC-Kb is two positions downstream of the F413C, and homologous with the A415V myotonia causing mutations.[161,163,164] The Bartter mutation H357Q is one position upstream of the myotonia mutation I424M. Futher investigation of these Bartter mutations is of importance, moreover, for they cause disease with varying degrees of severity, and several of them, as typified by mutation of R438 and the P124L substituion, appear in unrelated families of different ethnic origin in different geographical locations.[161,165]

The cytoplasmic COOH-terminal domains of all mammalian ClC proteins contain two interacting cystathionine-β-synthase CBS domains that form intrasubunit dimers.[121,122] CBS domains regulate ClC channel gating. For instance, ATP binding is coordinated at the CBS1/CBS2 interface, as shown in the ClC-5 crystal structure,[169] and ATP is known to modulate gating of ClC-1 and ClC-2 channels.[170,171,172] The Bartter mutations K560M and S573Y substitutions in ClC-Kb are within the first CBS domain, predicting that they may influence regulated gating.[121]

Barttin: Bartter Syndrome Type IV

Barttin is an obligatory accessory subunit for human ClC-K channel activity.[71] Inactivating mutations in barttin cause corresponding loss of ClC-K channel function, leading to BS type IV.[18,71,173] This form of Bartter syndrome has the hallmark renal salt-wasting phenotype, but also a sensorineural deafness phenotype. The reason for the additional phenotype in BS type IV is that, similar to their roles in renal epithelial cells, ClC-K channels also serve as Cl^- exit pathways in strial marginal cells.[87] Barttin is required for this activity, which in turn is required for active K^+ secretion into endolymph. In the ear, loss of ClC-Ka or ClC-Kb individually can be compensated for by the presence of the other protein; however, the loss of both channel proteins or of barttin cannot be.[87] Compensation also explains why loss of ClC-Kb, but not ClC-Ka, causes BS type III without accompanying deafness.[14,87] Although ROMK mediates apical K^+ secretion in TAL epithelial cells, KCNQ1 oligomerized with KCNE1 mediates apical K^+ secretion in marginal cells.[87] This explains why BS type II, which results from loss-of-function of ROMK, as discussed below, is not associated with deafness.

Several missense mutations causing substitutions in barttin change the biophysical properties of ClC-K channels to cause disease. The Bartter mutations R8L, R8W, and G10S in barttin eliminate ClC-Ka and ClC-Kb function, as shown in Figure 8.32, but they do not prevent channel insertion into the membrane (not shown[71,173]). This identifies changes in either channel gating or permeation as the disease-causing defects. It is not clear yet which of these two alternatives is correct. However, investigation of chimeric hClC1-ClC-Kb channels, as shown in Figure 8.33, revealed that these mutations influence voltage-dependent activation, with channels containing mutant barttin having less activity at hyperpolarizing potentials. This is most consistent with an effect on gating.

The Bartter's mutation G47R in barttin produces a mild renal phenotype.[71,173] The G47 residue is at the intracellular COOH-terminus of the second transmembrane domain of barttin. This position, and the fact that barttin containing the G47R substitution interacts less effectively with ClC-Kb, suggests that association of the accessory subunit with the pore-forming subunit is compromised in some manner. Such interpretation is consistent with the recent finding that the

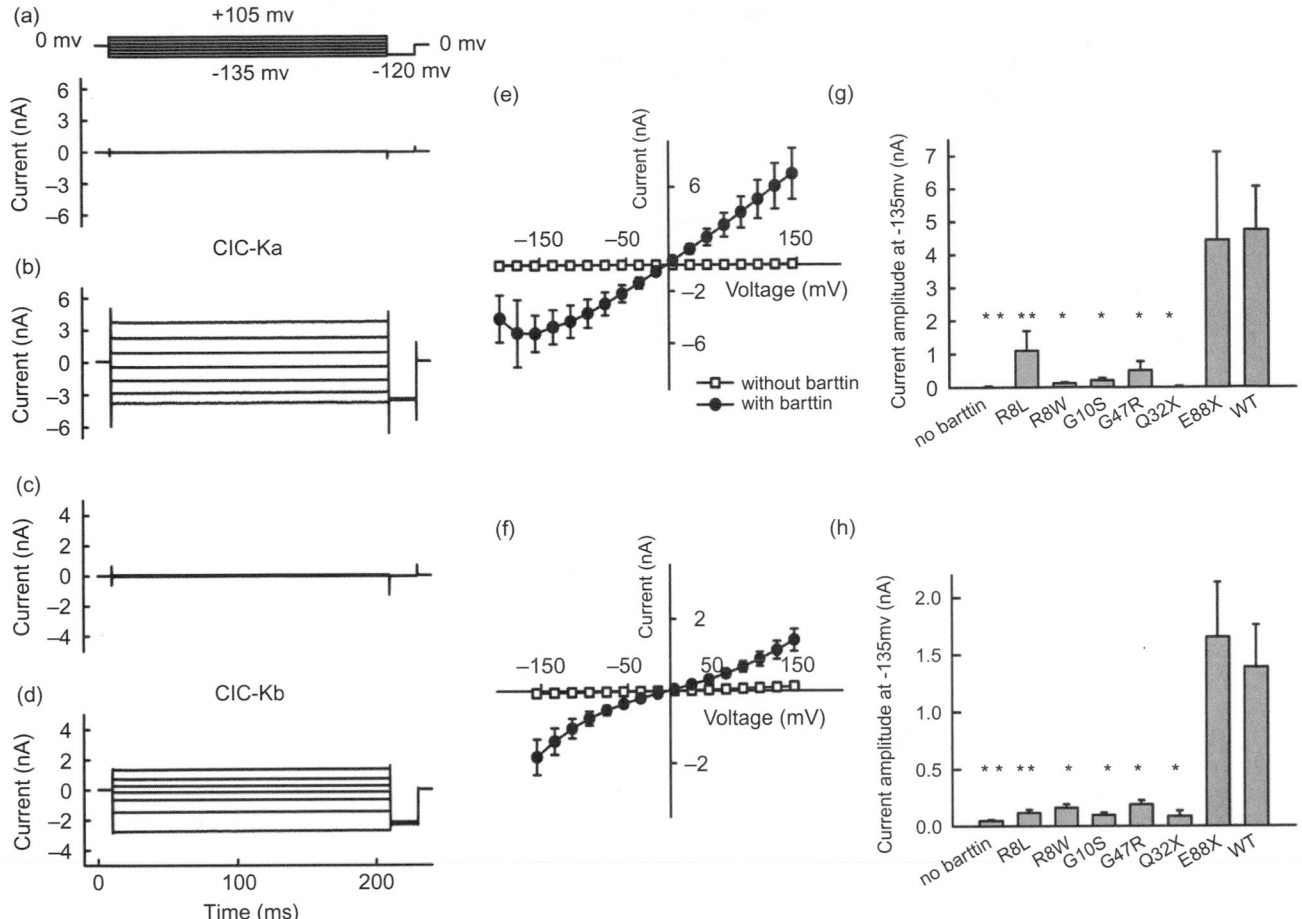

FIGURE 8.32 **Some disease-causing mutations in barttin decrease ClC-Ka and ClC-Kb channel activity.** *(Figure from[173].)* (a)–(d) Representative macroscopic ClC-Ka ((a) and (b)) and ClC-Kb ((c) and (d)) currents with ((b) and (d)) and without ((a) and (c)) barttin. Corresponding I–V relations for ClC-Ka and ClC-Kb with and without barttin are shown in (e) and (f), respectively. Steady-state currents at −135 mV for ClC-Ka and ClC-Kb expressed with wild-type and barttin containing Bartter mutations are shown in g and h, respectively.

transmembrane core of barttin is necessary and sufficient to promote ClC-K channel trafficking.[73] Moreover, the fact that the G47R phenotype is milder compared to that seen with complete loss or inactivation of barttin demonstrates that the physiological effects of barttin can be titrated, indicating that there is some finite threshold at which the loss of barttin activity causes disease.

ENaC

ENaC activity, as mentioned above, is the final arbiter of renal Na^+ reabsorption setting urinary and plasma $[Na^+]$[82,83,106]. This function makes ENaC an important end-effector of feedback systems controlling blood pressure. As such, ENaC activity is a critical determinant of blood pressure in all mammals, including humans. Loss- and gain-of-function mutations in ENaC and modulators of this channel then cause a host of diseases having pathological changes in renal Na^+ handling and blood pressure.

PHA-I: Loss of ENaC Function

Pseudohypoaldosteronism is a group of rare genetic diseases presenting with hallmark hyperkalemia and renal Na^+ wasting in the presence of high aldosterone.[107,174] Renal Na^+ wasting is a consequence of decreased Na^+ reabsorption in the CNT and CD. Such a phenotype represents end-organ resistance, identifying ENaC or cellular regulators of this channel as dysfunctional.

Compared to ROMK, less is known about the structure of the cytoplasmic portions of ENaC. Therefore, we do not have precise structural information to guide the interpretation of recent electrophysiology findings relevant to PHA. The missense mutation, G37S, in human β-ENaC nonetheless causes PHA type-I.[134,174] This Gly residue is in an absolutely conserved HG motif located in the intracellular NH_2-terminal portions of all

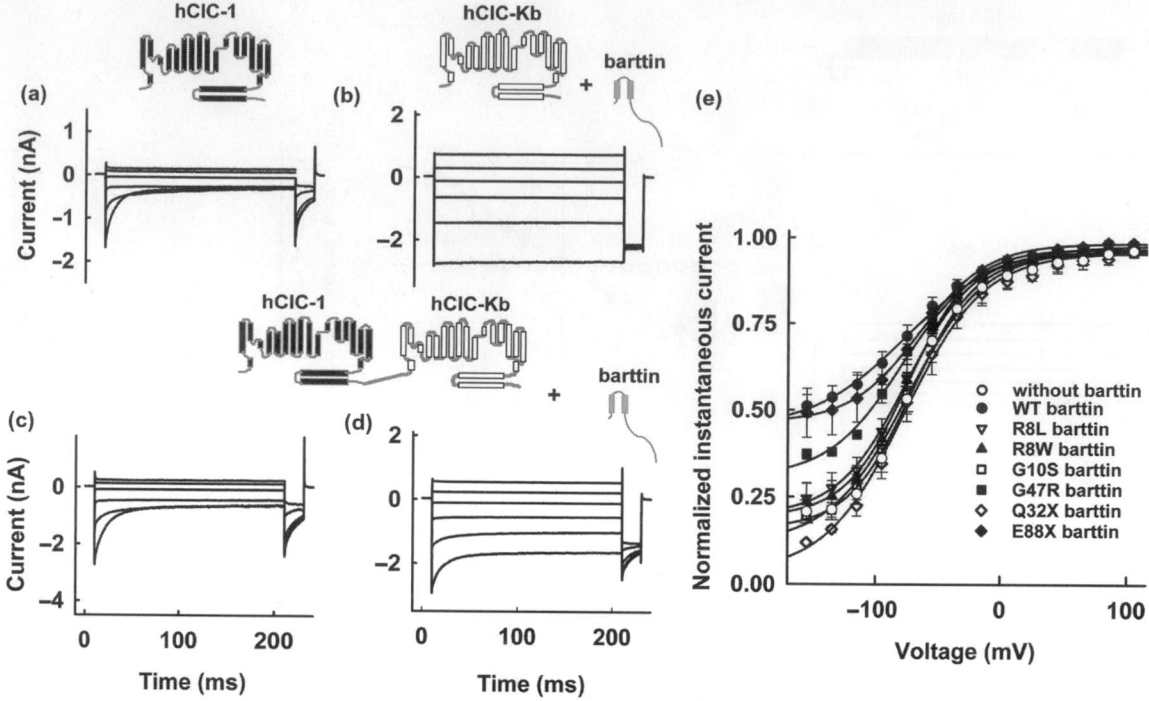

FIGURE 8.33 **Some disease-causing mutations in barttin affect ClC-K channel gating.** *(Figure from [173].)* (a)–(d) Representative macroscopic currents from human ClC-1 alone (a), ClC-Kb with barttin (b), and concatameric hClC-1-ClC-Kb without barttin (c), and with barttin (d). (e) Normalized instantaneous macroscopic currents as a function of voltage for hClC-1-ClC-Kb concatamers alone and together with wild-type and mutant barttin. The action of voltage on normalized current indicates that these mutations in barttin affect ClC-K channel gating.

ENaC/Deg subunits. The HG motif is required for normal gating.[134,135,174] The molecular mechanism whereby the HG motif influences the gate is unknown, but in the primary sequence of ENaC, the motif is in the NH_2-terminal cytoplasmic domain just preceding TM1. As shown by the results in Figure 8.34 from whole-cell and outside-out single-channel patch-clamp experiments probing the effects on gating, substituting either the H or G residue decreases P_o to where ENaC is not active under physiological conditions.[175] Decreases in P_o, as supported by results shown in Figure 8.35, arise from the voltage-dependent block of the pore by the permeant ion where the block is from the intracellular side and relieved by hyperpolarization.[39] A possible explanation for this is that ENaC gates through a pore-gating mechanism, and mutation of the HG motif destabilizes the pore to where Na^+ sometimes sticks to a binding site in the permeation pathway or the pore collapses around a Na^+ ion moving through the pore. More study is needed to determine if this is the case, but the crystal structure of cASIC1 is consistent with ENaC/Deg channels using a pore-gating mechanism.[58] Moreover, the biophysical consequences of substituting a Trp residue (W112 in α-mENaC) at the base of TM1 mimic the effects of substituting HG motif residues.[39] Like the HG motif, this Trp is conserved in all

ENaC/Deg subunits. It is unknown at this time if mutation of this key Trp also causes PHA-I.

Many ion channels contain similar interfacial Trp residues at the intracellular bases of transmembrane domains.[176–178] Such Trp residues often modulate gating. In cASIC1, the side chain of the homologous Trp at the base of TM1 projects into the aqueous environment of the pore.[58] Interestingly, M_2 proton channels also contain a critical Trp residue at the intracellular base of the transmembrane domain lining the pore. The side chain of this Trp, akin to that in ENaC/Deg channels, projects into the aqueous mouth of the pore. Through Pi-bond interactions with a nearby His, the critical Trp in a M_2 proton channel stabilizes the gating state.[176,179,180] Perhaps the homologous Trp in ENaC interacting with the His in the HG motif serves a similar function. This possibility seems to reconcile the parallel findings that substitution of the HG motif and interfacial Trp residues cause identical changes in ENaC biophysical properties. Although further research is required to clarify the structure–function relation between the conserved HG motif and interfacial Trp in ENaC if there is any, it is clear that a pathological consequence of mutating the HG motif is that ENaC gating becomes voltage-dependent, with P_o being extremely low at physiological voltages.

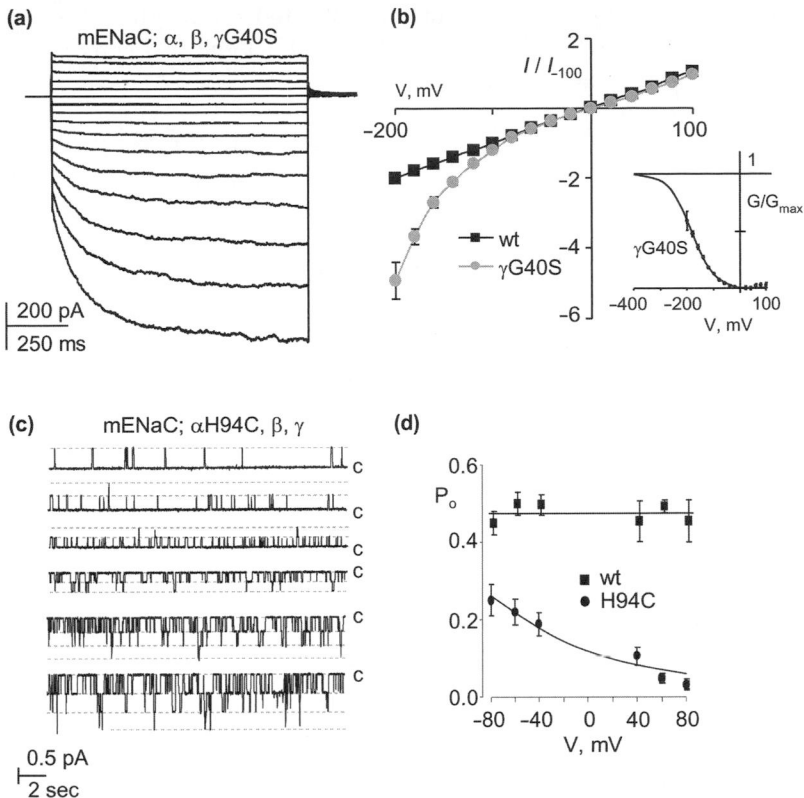

FIGURE 8.34 Some disease-causing PHA-I mutations in ENaC affect channel gating. *(Figure from [175].)* (a) Representative macroscopic Na$^+$ currents for a mouse ENaC channel containing the γG40S PHA-I mutation. (b) Macroscopic current-voltage (*I–V*) relations for CHO cells expressing wild-type (black lines) and mutant mENaC (gray lines) containing the γG40S mutation. For presentation, current normalized to current at −100 mV. The inset shows the G−V relation for mutant ENaC. (c) Representative single channel current traces for mouse ENaC harboring a αH94C substitution in outside-out patches stepped from 80 mV to −80 mV. Inward Na$^+$ current is downwards and closed states noted with (c). (d) Plot showing ENaC open probability (P$_o$) as a function of voltage for wild-type (black squares) and mutant mENaC containing αH94C. Data fit with a Boltzman function.

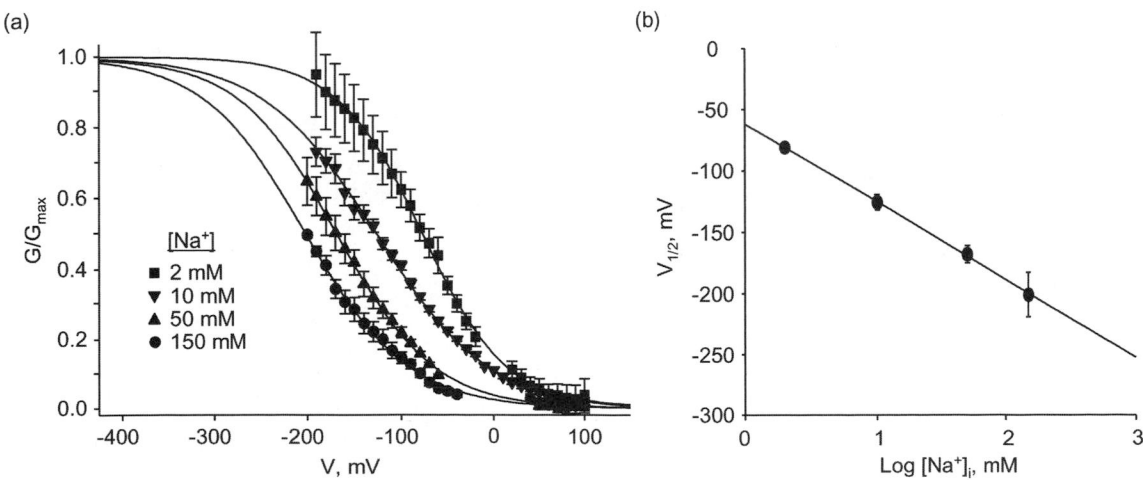

FIGURE 8.35 Intracellular Na$^+$ can block mutant ENaC in a voltage-dependent manner to decrease macroscopic conductance. *(Figure from [39].)* (a) Summary G−V curves for steady-state currents from mutant ENaC, containing the αW112C mutation, acquired in symmetrical 150, 50, 10, and 2 mm [Na$^+$]. (b) Summary graph showing the voltage resulting in half-maximal activity at steady-state, as established from G−V curves, for mutant ENaC as a function of [Na$^+$]$_i$.

Decreased ENaC P_o, then, is the biophysical cause of this form of PHA-I.

A missense mutation, S562P, in α-ENaC also causes familial PHA-I.[181] S562 occupies the third position in the selectivity-filter, GSS, sequence.[104,105,136] Little electrophysiology information is available for this mutant, but understanding that channel function is determined by its structural and biophysical properties makes it reasonable to predict that the S562P substitution disrupts permeation, resulting in a disease-causing loss-of-function.

Liddle's Syndrome: Gain of ENaC Function

Gain-of-function mutations in ENaC cause an inheritable form of hypertension, Liddle's syndrome, marked by high blood pressure in the presence of low plasma renin and aldosterone, and uncontrolled Na^+ reabsorption in the distal nephron.[106] This also represents end-organ resistance, where ENaC activity is inappropriately high in the presence of low aldosterone. Amiloride, an inhibitor of ENaC, reverses the high blood pressure and renal phenotype of Liddle's syndrome. The majority of mutations in ENaC that cause Liddle's syndrome retard retrieval of the channel from the apical membrane of CNT and CD principal cells.[182–184] An exception to this common mechanism is the Liddle mutation N530S in γ-ENaC, which increases channel activity but not membrane expression level.[138] Detailed biophysical experiments have yet to be performed on this mutant. Its position in the channel when considering the three-dimensional structure of cASIC1,[58] and previous findings from the study of the activating *Degenerin* mutation in *C. elegans* homologs,[144,145] though, are informative. N530 is one position downstream of the *Deg* position in the primary structure of ENaC (see Figure 8.27). This places it at the extracellular apex of the TM2 pore-lining transmembrane domain. This region of ENaC/Deg channels is thought to be important for ion permeation and gating. It is widely held that the *Deg* mutation locks open ENaC/Deg channels, because it occupies such a position. Perhaps the N530S Liddle mutation does the same thing in ENaC. ENaC locked in an open state would maximize Na^+ reabsorption in the distal nephron, moving it beyond the control of feedback regulation, explaining the salt-sensitive hypertension in this form of Liddle's syndrome even in the presence of low aldosterone. Supporting such a role are findings that covalent modification by sulfhydryl reagents of a N530C mutant in γ-ENaC and modification of Cys substitutions of the corresponding residues in α- and β-subunits increase activity of ENaC within the membrane.[140] In fact, this region of ENaC is particularly sensitive to alteration. Modification of cysteines substituted for residues throughout this region consistently affect channel activity.[105,136,140]

ROMK: Bartter Syndrome Type II

A constellation of mutations in *KCNJ1* leading to loss-of-function of ROMK causes BS type II.[14,15,23,185,186] Several of these mutations, as listed in Table 8.2, affect channel gating and conductance. It is possible, with our current understanding of ROMK structure and biophysical properties, to rationalize how these Bartter mutations affect channel function to change physiology and cause disease. Bartter mutations in ROMK that change biophysical properties can be placed into several groups. First are those that immediately disturb the gate based around the interaction of K80 at the intracellular base of TM1 with A177 at the intracellular base of TM2 as it couples to the putative L179 gate. This structure is held to be the regulated gate responsive to pH, PKA phosphorylation, and PIP_2-binding.[32] The remaining types of Bartter mutations that change the biophysical properties of ROMK interrupt regions in cytoplasmic domains to affect gating. They include those that disrupt PIP_2 binding sites, critical PKA phosphorylation sites, domains important for a response to pH, and inter- and intra-subunit salt-bridges required for normal structure. In addition to these are Bartter mutations that affect a distinct gate in the cytosolic portion of the channel, and one that affects a key residue in the selectivity-filter.

Mutation of the Regulated Gating Structure at the Bundle-Crossing

A hallmark feature of ROMK, as emphasized in Figure 8.36, is its sensitivity to intracellular pH, where P_o

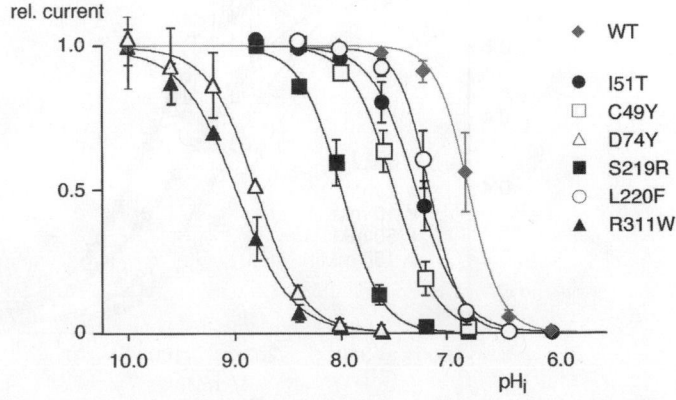

FIGURE 8.36 ROMK gates in a pH-dependent manner with some Bartter mutations changing the apparent pK_a of activation. (*Figure from* [194].) Current-pH_i relations are shown for wild-type ROMK and channels containing Bartter mutations.

increases as a function of increasing pH_i with intracellular acidification inducing a long-lived closed-state.[187,188] Residues and domains in ROMK involved in sensing pH are yet to be identified. Nevertheless, sensitivity to pH is routinely measured using titration experiments plotting relative current as a function of pH, and fitting the data with a modified Hill equation, such as $I/I_{max} = 1/(1 + ([H^+]/K_a)^{n_H})$, where K_a is the half-maximal inhibitory proton concentration and n_H is the Hill coefficient.[148] As noted above, the influence of pH on gating is manifested by the regulated L179-gate coupled to A177 and K80.[32,148] The A177T Bartter mutation disrupts this interaction, and causes a marked alkaline-shift in the pH sensitivity of ROMK gating effectively turning the channel off at physiological pH_i.[15,189] The biophysical and physiological consequences are that, although the driving force remains for K^+ efflux across the apical membrane of TAL cells through ROMK, it cannot be harnessed, with the result that NKCC2 cannot run at full capacity. This compromises NaCl reabsorption in the loop of Henle, and breaks down the axial corticomedullary hyperosmotic gradient, causing a pathological decrease in the ability to concentrate urine. Substitution of K80 with residues unable to form an H-bond with A177, in addition, alters gating in a similar manner.[190] Additional support for this mechanism of pathology is the finding that the Bartter mutation Y79H also disrupts regulated gating.[15] The side chain of Y79 projects into the lipid bilayer, possibly stabilizing the interaction of K80 with A177 and ultimately the L179 gate. Interestingly, mutations in comparable residues in the Kir6.2 K_{ATP} channel alter ATP-dependent gating, and cause neonatal diabetes.[191] Such results summate to suggest that the energetics of regulated K^+ channel opening are strongly influenced by H-bonds formed between residues at the base of TM1 and TM2, and between interactions of residues in TM1 with the inner leaflet. Disruption of this gating structure, then, is one cause of ROMK channel dysfunction in BS type II.

Mutation Leading to Loss of pH-Sensitivity

ROMK gates in a high P_o state at normal intracellular pH_i, with a pK_a near neutral pH making the channel especially susceptible to pathological changes in pH_i. Interestingly, the pK_a for activation of ROMK is under physiological control, and can be dynamically changed by PIP_2 binding and PKA phosphorylation of the channel.[192,193] Bartter mutations disrupting the normal regulation of pK_a shift the pH_i of activation.[194] Moreover, a Bartter mutation causing a frameshift at T332 interrupts pH-dependent gating, moving the apparent pK_a at which ROMK opens markedly in the alkaline direction outside the physiological range.[148,186,185] The biophysical consequence of this is that the channel enters long-closed states for prolonged periods of time, greatly decreasing K^+ exit across the apical membrane. The structural basis for this effect remains to be determined, but clearly, this mutation involves changes in the intracellular domains of ROMK likely resulting in destruction or uncoupling of allosteric sites from the regulated gate.

Mutation of the Intracellular Gating Structure

The narrowing at the apex of the cytoplasmic pore of ROMK where G-loops coalesce is also involved in gating.[32] The Bartter mutation A306T disrupts K^+ conductance by ROMK.[15] This residue is located in the G-loop, possibly affecting the intracellular gate. Underscoring the importance of this intracellular resistance barrier to channel structure and function are findings that disease (Andersen−Tawil syndrome)-causing mutations in other Kir channels cluster in G-loops.[196,197] The Y314C, V315G, and A198T Bartter mutations, as discussed below, may also affect gating that involves the interactions of intracellular domains of the channel with the bundle-crossing.[15,185,198]

Mutation of the PIP_2-Binding Site

Phosphoinositide 4,5-bisphosphate (PIP_2) is an important physiological regulator of Kir channel gating, including ROMK, which it stabilizes in a high P_o state.[32,199,200,201] A comprehensive investigation of ROMK mutants and mutants of its homolog, Kir2.1, combined with the study of Kir1.1-Kir2.1 chimeric channel proteins, identified several basic amino acids corresponding to R48, K181, K184, K186, R188, R217, K218, and R311 in ROMK that are required for PIP_2-dependent gating.[201−203] Substitution that neutralizes these charged residues reduces channel activity. That the side chains of these residues carry a positive charge is consistent with them contributing to a bona fide allosteric PIP_2-binding site. This was reinforced by findings that a portion of ROMK containing four of these basic residues (aa. 183−221) has the capacity in solution to bind PIP_2.[204] Although these four basic residues are in a portion of Kir for which structure has not been resolved, their position in the linear sequence suggests that they reside at the apex of the cytoplasmic domains near the intracellular face of the lipid bilayer.[32] Moreover, modeling clusters R48, R217, and R218 at the top of the cytoplasmic domain where they are predicted to face the inner lipid leaflet. Considering findings from functional studies and lipid-binding studies, this position is consistent with these residues having the capacity to interact in a direct manner with membrane phospholipids. That ROMK and other Kir channels contain a PIP_2-binding site capable of signaling to a gate becomes important when recognizing that a group of Bartter mutations, C49Y, I51T, A214V, and L220F, disrupt PIP_2-dependent gating.[15,186,194] In three-dimensional ROMK models, all of these residues cluster on the membrane-facing surface of the cytoplasmic domain near the putative PIP_2-binding pocket, suggesting that they modulate binding to this site or transduction of information from this site to the gate. Importantly, similar observations made for Kir2.1, which when dysfunctional causes the familial Andersen—Tawil form of long QT syndrome, have been interpreted to indicate that the disruption of PIP_2-binding underlies many Kir channelopathies.[200,201,205]

Mutation of Salt-Bridges Critical to Structure

The cytoplasmic domain of ROMK is stabilized by inter- (R311—E302) and intrasubunit (R41—E318) salt-bridges. Compromise of these bridges uncouples ligand binding in cytoplasmic domains from the regulated gate.[15,194] This is underscored by the dramatic alkaline-shift in apparent pK_a of activation for ROMK containing the R311W or R311Q Bartter mutation. A shift in pK_a leads to these channels being in a prolonged closed state at physiological pH_i.

Mutation of PKA Phosphorylation Sites

Similar to the secretory channel in native tissue, ROMK in heterologous expression systems is also responsive to PKA phosphorylation.[206,207] In concert with physiological pH_i and PIP_2 levels, PKA phosphorylation sets ROMK to a high P_o state.[32] Biochemical studies identified three discrete PKA phosphorylation sites in the cytoplasmic NH_2- and COOH-termini of ROMK: S44, S219, and S313.[208,209,210] Each of these must be phosphorylated for full channel function. The site in the NH_2-terminus is an absolute requirement for expression at the membrane. Those in the COOH-terminus are necessary for the high P_o state, modulating regulated-gating in response to pH, PIP_2, and ATP.[192,211] These latter two phosphorylation sites are strategically positioned in the channel to modulate the effects of regulators of gating. S219 is positioned between a PIP_2-binding site, the G-loop, and an intersubunit (E311—E302) salt-bridge. In comparison, S313 is sandwiched between an intrasubunit (R41—E318) and intersubunit (E311—E302) salt-bridge. Such positions provide a structural explanation for how phosphorylation may be involved in the functional coupling of gating factors. As such, phosphorylation of S219 and S313 provoke an acidic shift in the apparent pK_a activating ROMK at physiological pH_i.[192] The Bartter mutations S219R and S313C remove these critical phosphorylation sites; consequently, ROMK containing these mutations has decreased activity, being in a low P_o state under physiological

conditions.[186,194] Two other Bartter mutations, Y314C and V315G, are one and two positions downstream of the critical Ser at 313.[198] It is not clear yet, but the Bartter mutations L220F and R311W may also influence the phosphorylation state or be involved in coupling PIP_2 binding and PKA phosphorylation. These are reasonable expansions on the possibility that the L220F mutation impacts PIP_2 binding and R311W is critical to salt-bridge formation, and is also possibly involved in PIP_2 binding as discussed above.

Mutation of a Selectivity-Filter Residue

ROMK channels, similar to all K^+ channels, contain the signature K^+-selectivity sequence T[V/I]GYG in the P-loop linking TM1 to TM2 (see Figure 8.29). The Bartter mutation I142T substitutes the critical second residue in this selectivity sequence, disrupting K^+ permeation significantly and decreasing conductance.[15] I142 is also involved in pore-gating of ROMK channels, as discussed above.[50,51] Therefore, this mutation may also affect gating. Regardless, as a result of this mutation, the ability to reabsorb NaCl in the TAL is compromised, destroying the axial corticomedullary hyperosmotic gradient necessary to concentrate urine.

Loss-of-Function Mutations with Undefined Mechanism

There are several other mutations in ROMK that also possibly change the channel's biophysical properties to cause disease. For instance, the Bartter mutations W99C, A103V, P110L, and N124K act in a dominant negative manner. When co-expressed with wild-type subunits, these mutant subunits decrease channel activity.[185] This is consistent with channels containing both wild-type and mutant subunits making it to the membrane, but having abnormal biophysical properties. Similarly, ROMK channels containing the T71M, F95S, A156V, and R324L Bartter mutations also traffic in a normal manner to the plasma membrane in some expression systems, but have decreased activity.[15] Again, this points to a change in biophysical properties as the disease-causing mechanism.

TRPM6: Hypomagnesemia with Secondary Hypocalcemia

Genetic studies in patients with hereditary HSH identified disease-causing mutations in TRPM6.[9,10,19,20,24] The missense substitution, P1017R, in TRPM6 is one such mutation.[4,10] Although a crystal structure for TRP channels is currently not available, it is accepted that these channels contain six transmembrane domains and assume a tetrameric structure similar to voltage-gated K^+ channels, with extracellular P-loops diving into the membrane to form the pore. Using the structural coordinates of the KvAP channel to model the putative S5-S6 segment of TRPM6, including the putative P-loop, places P1017 in the predicted pore region of the channel.[4,212] A recent study by Chubanov and colleagues showed that co-expression of wild-type TRPM6 with TRPM7 significantly increases current through the channel.[4] In contrast, co-expression of TRPM6 containing the P1017R mutation with wild-type TRPM7 suppresses channel activity. Consistent with this dominant-negative effect, co-expression of TRPM7 containing a homologous P-to-R mutation decreases wild-type TRPM6 activity. This action is restricted to changes in the biophysical properties of the channel, for the P1017R mutation has no effect on channel assembly or trafficking. These results strongly suggest that the P1017R mutation affects either permeation through the channel or channel gating to decrease activity. Decreases in TRPM6 channel activity would reduce Mg^{2+} reabsorption by the kidney, leading to the disease phenotype.

Acknowledgments

I thank Drs. John Johnson (Dept. Physiology, UTHSCSA), Kishore Kamaraju (Dept. Physiology, UTHSCSA), Volodymyr Kucher (Dept. Physiology, UTHSCSA), Steve Sansom (Dept. Cellular and Integrative Physiology, UNMC), and Bin Wang (Dept. Physiology, UTHSCSA) for critically reading this chapter.

References

[1] Ashcroft FM. Ion channels and disease. Oxford: Academic Press; 2000.

[2] Hille B. Ion channels of excitable membranes. Sinauer Associates, Inc; 2001.

[3] Sackin H, Nanazashvili M, Palmer LG, Krambis M, Walters DE. Structural locus of the pH gate in the Kir1.1 inward rectifier channel. Biophys J 2005;88:2597—606.

[4] Chubanov V, Schlingmann KP, Waring J, Heinzinger J, Kaske S, Waldegger S, et al. Hypomagnesemia with secondary hypocalcemia due to a missense mutation in the putative pore-forming region of TRPM6. J Biol Chem 2007;282:7656—67.

[5] Schlingmann KP, Konrad M, Jeck N, Waldegger P, Reinalter SC, Holder M, et al. Salt wasting and deafness resulting from mutations in two chloride channels. N Engl J Med 2004;350:1314—9.

[6] Tseng PY, Bennetts B, Chen TY. Cytoplasmic ATP inhibition of CLC-1 is enhanced by low pH. J Gen Physiol 2007;130:217—21.

[7] Waldegger S, Jentsch TJ. Functional and structural analysis of ClC-K chloride channels involved in renal disease. J Biol Chem 2000;275:24527—33.

[8] Walder RY, Landau D, Meyer P, Shalev H, Tsolia M, Borochowitz Z, et al. Mutation of TRPM6 causes familial hypomagnesemia with secondary hypocalcemia. Nat Genet 2002;31:171—4.

[9] Woda CB, Bragin A, Kleyman TR, Satlin LM. Flow-dependent K^+ secretion in the cortical collecting duct is mediated by a maxi-K channel. Am J Physiol Renal Physiol 2001;280:F786—93.

[10] Dietrich A, Chubanov V, Gudermann T. Renal TRPathies. J Am Soc Nephrol 2010;21:736—44.

[11] Dryer SE, Reiser J. TRPC6 channels and their binding partners in podocytes: role in glomerular filtration and pathophysiology. Am J Physiol Renal Physiol 2010;299:F689—701.

[12] Hsu YJ, Hoenderop JG, Bindels RJ. TRP channels in kidney disease. Biochim Biophys Acta 2007;1772:928—36.

[13] Williamson IM, Alvis SJ, East JM, Lee AG. The potassium channel KcsA and its interaction with the lipid bilayer. Cell Mol Life Sci 2003;60:1581—90.

[14] Hebert SC. Bartter syndrome. Curr Opin Nephrol Hypertens 2003;12:527—32.

[15] Pegan S, Arrabit C, Zhou W, Kwiatkowski W, Collins A, Slesinger PA, et al. Cytoplasmic domain structures of Kir2.1 and Kir3.1 show sites for modulating gating and rectification. Nat Neurosci 2005;8:279—87.

[16] Pochynyuk O, Kucher V, Boiko N, Mironova E, Staruschenko A, Karpushev AV, et al. Intrinsic voltage dependence of the epithelial Na^+ channel is masked by a conserved transmembrane domain tryptophan. J Biol Chem 2009;284:25512—21.

[17] Schlanger LE, Kleyman TR, Ling BN. K^+-sparing diuretic actions of trimethoprim: inhibition of Na^+ channels in A6 distal nephron cells. Kidney Int 1994;45:1070—6.

[18] Schwalbe RA, Bianchi L, Accili EA, Brown AM. Functional consequences of ROMK mutants linked to antenatal Bartter's syndrome and implications for treatment. Hum Mol Genet 1998;7:975—80.

[19] Dimke H, Hoenderop JG, Bindels RJ. Hereditary tubular transport disorders: implications for renal handling of Ca^{2+} and Mg^{2+}. Clin Sci (Lond) 2010;118:1—18.

[20] Glaudemans B, Knoers NV, Hoenderop JG, Bindels RJ. New molecular players facilitating Mg(2+) reabsorption in the distal convoluted tubule. Kidney Int 2010;77:17—22.

[21] Hou J, Goodenough DA. Claudin-16 and claudin-19 function in the thick ascending limb. Curr Opin Nephrol Hypertens 2010;19:483—8.

[22] Hou J, Renigunta A, Konrad M, Gomes AS, Schneeberger EE, Paul DL, et al. Claudin-16 and claudin-19 interact and form a cation-selective tight junction complex. J Clin Invest 2008;118:619—28.

[23] Landau D. Potassium-related inherited tubulopathies. Cell Mol Life Sci 2006;63:1962—8.

[24] Voets T, Nilius B, Hoefs S, van der Kemp AW, Droogmans G, Bindels RJ, et al. TRPM6 forms the Mg^{2+} influx channel involved in intestinal and renal Mg^{2+} absorption. J Biol Chem 2004;279:19—25.

[25] Hou J, Renigunta A, Gomes AS, Hou M, Paul DL, Waldegger S, et al. Claudin-16 and claudin-19 interaction is required for their assembly into tight junctions and for renal reabsorption of magnesium. Proc Natl Acad Sci USA 2009;106:15350—5.

[26] Konrad M, Hou J, Weber S, Dotsch J, Kari JA, Seeman T, et al. CLDN16 genotype predicts renal decline in familial hypomagnesemia with hypercalciuria and nephrocalcinosis. J Am Soc Nephrol 2008;19:171—81.

[27] Konrad M, Schaller A, Seelow D, Pandey AV, Waldegger S, Lesslauer A, et al. Mutations in the tight-junction gene claudin 19 (CLDN19) are associated with renal magnesium wasting, renal failure, and severe ocular involvement. Am J Hum Genet 2006;79:949—57.

[28] Simon DB, Bindra RS, Mansfield TA, Nelson-Williams C, Mendonca E, Stone R, et al. Mutations in the chloride channel gene, CLCNKB, cause Bartter's syndrome type III. Nat Genet 1997;17:171—8.

[29] Richard EA, Miller C. Steady-state coupling of ion-channel conformations to a transmembrane ion gradient. Science 1990;247:1208—10.

[30] Winn MP, Conlon PJ, Lynn KL, Farrington MK, Creazzo T, Hawkins AF, et al. A mutation in the TRPC6 cation channel causes familial focal segmental glomerulosclerosis. Science 2005;308:1801–4.

[31] Murata K, Mitsuoka K, Hirai T, Walz T, Agre P, Heymann JB, et al. Structural determinants of water permeation through aquaporin-1. Nature 2000;407:599–605.

[32] Warth R, Barriere H, Meneton P, Bloch M, Thomas J, Tauc M, et al. Proximal renal tubular acidosis in TASK2 K^+ channel-deficient mice reveals a mechanism for stabilizing bicarbonate transport. Proc Natl Acad Sci USA 2004;101:8215–20.

[33] Wang W, Giebisch G. Dual modulation of renal ATP-sensitive K^+ channel by protein kinases A and C. Proc Natl Acad Sci USA 1991;88:9722–5.

[34] Boiteux C, Kraszewski S, Ramseyer C, Girardet C. Ion conductance vs. pore gating and selectivity in KcsA channel: modeling achievements and perspectives. J Mol Model 2007;13:699–713.

[35] Kuo A, Domene C, Johnson LN, Doyle DA, Venien-Bryan C. Two different conformational states of the KirBac3.1 potassium channel revealed by electron crystallography. Structure 2005;13:1463–72.

[36] Zhang YY, Robertson JL, Gray DA, Palmer LG. Carboxy-terminal determinants of conductance in inward-rectifier K channels. J Gen Physiol 2004;124:729–39.

[37] Dutzler R. Structural basis for ion conduction and gating in ClC chloride channels. FEBS Lett 2004;564:229–33.

[38] Krapivinsky G, Gordon EA, Wickman K, Velimirovic B, Krapivinsky L, Clapham DE. The G-protein-gated atrial K^+ channel IKACh is a heteromultimer of two inwardly rectifying K(+)-channel proteins. Nature 1995;374:135–41.

[39] Pluznick JL, Wei P, Grimm PR, Sansom SC. BK-{beta}1 subunit: immunolocalization in the mammalian connecting tubule and its role in the kaliuretic response to volume expansion. Am J Physiol Renal Physiol 2005;288:F846–54.

[40] Cole KS. Membranes, ions and impulses: a chapter of classical biophysics. Berkely: University of California Press; 1968.

[41] Kellenberger S, Schild L. Epithelial sodium channel/degenerin family of ion channels: a variety of functions for a shared structure. Physiol Rev 2002;82:735–67.

[42] Nishida M, MacKinnon R. Structural basis of inward rectification: cytoplasmic pore of the G protein-gated inward rectifier GIRK1 at 1.8 Å resolution. Cell 2002;111:957–65.

[43] Kurata HT, Marton LJ, Nichols CG. The polyamine binding site in inward rectifier K^+ channels. J Gen Physiol 2006;127:467–80.

[44] Schild L. The epithelial sodium channel and the control of sodium balance. Biochim Biophys Acta 2010;1802:1159–65.

[45] Doyle DA, Morais CJ, Pfuetzner RA, Kuo A, Gulbis JM, Cohen SL, et al. The structure of the potassium channel: molecular basis of K^+ conduction and selectivity. Science 1998;280:69–77.

[46] Dutzler R. The structural basis of ClC chloride channel function. Trends Neurosci 2004;27:315–20.

[47] Hamilton KL, Eaton DC. Single-channel recordings from two types of amiloride-sensitive epithelial Na^+ channels. Membr Biochem 1986;6:149–71.

[48] Hinton CF, Eaton DC. Expression of amiloride-blockable sodium channels in Xenopus oocytes. Am J Physiol 1989;257(Pt 1):C825–829.

[49] McNicholas CM, Wang W, Ho K, Hebert SC, Giebisch G. Regulation of ROMK1 K^+ channel activity involves phosphorylation processes. Proc Natl Acad Sci USA 1994;91:8077–81.

[50] Berneche S, Roux B. A gate in the selectivity filter of potassium channels. Structure 2005;13:591–600.

[51] Domene C, Klein ML, Branduardi D, Gervasio FL, Parrinello M. Conformational changes and gating at the selectivity filter of potassium channels. J Am Chem Soc 2008;130:9474–80.

[52] Dutzler R. A structural perspective on ClC channel and transporter function. FEBS Lett 2007;581:2839–44.

[53] Dutzler R, Campbell EB, Cadene M, Chait BT, MacKinnon R. X-ray structure of a ClC chloride channel at 3.0 Å reveals the molecular basis of anion selectivity. Nature 2002;415:287–94.

[54] Hierholzer K, and Lange S. Kidney and urinary tract Physiology. 1995.

[55] Lobet S, Dutzler R. Ion-binding properties of the ClC chloride selectivity filter. EMBO J 2006;25:24–33.

[56] Kuo A, Gulbis JM, Antcliff JF, Rahman T, Lowe ED, Zimmer J, et al. Crystal structure of the potassium channel KirBac1.1 in the closed state. Science 2003;300:1922–6.

[57] Dutzler R, Campbell EB, MacKinnon R. Gating the selectivity filter in ClC chloride channels. Science 2003;300:108–12.

[58] Gonzales EB, Kawate T, Gouaux E. Pore architecture and ion sites in acid-sensing ion channels and P2X receptors. Nature 2009;460:599–604.

[59] Dutzler R. The ClC family of chloride channels and transporters. Curr Opin Struct Biol 2006;16:439–46.

[60] Jentsch TJ, Neagoe I, Scheel O. CLC chloride channels and transporters. Curr Opin Neurobiol 2005;15:319–25.

[61] Lisal J, Maduke M. Review. Proton-coupled gating in chloride channels. Philos Trans R Soc Lond B Biol Sci 2009;364:181–7.

[62] Choe H, Palmer LG, Sackin H. Structural determinants of gating in inward-rectifier K^+ channels. Biophys J 1999;76:1988–2003.

[63] Choe H, Sackin H, Palmer LG. Permeation and gating of an inwardly rectifying potassium channel. Evidence for a variable energy well. J Gen Physiol 1998;112:433–46.

[64] Choe H, Sackin H, Palmer LG. Gating properties of inward-rectifier potassium channels: effects of permeant ions. J Membr Biol 2001;184:81–9.

[65] Pusch M. Myotonia caused by mutations in the muscle chloride channel gene CLCN1. Hum Mutat 2002;19:423–34.

[66] Pusch M. Structural insights into chloride and proton-mediated gating of CLC chloride channels. Biochemistry 2004;43:1135–44.

[67] Pusch M, Ludewig U, Jentsch TJ. Temperature dependence of fast and slow gating relaxations of ClC-0 chloride channels. J Gen Physiol 1997;109:105–16.

[68] Rychkov GY, Pusch M, Astill DS, Roberts ML, Jentsch TJ, Bretag AH. Concentration and pH dependence of skeletal muscle chloride channel ClC-1. J Physiol 1996;497(Pt 2):423–35.

[69] Horrigan FT, Aldrich RW. Coupling between voltage sensor activation, Ca^{2+} binding and channel opening in large conductance (BK) potassium channels. J Gen Physiol 2002;120:267–305.

[70] Rohacs T, Chen J, Prestwich GD, Logothetis DE. Distinct specificities of inwardly rectifying K(+) channels for phosphoinositides. J Biol Chem 1999;274:36065–72.

[71] Estevez R, Boettger T, Stein V, Birkenhager R, Otto E, Hildebrandt F, et al. Barttin is a Cl^- channel beta-subunit crucial for renal Cl^- reabsorption and inner ear K^+ secretion. Nature 2001;414:558–61.

[72] Fischer M, Janssen AG, Fahlke C. Barttin activates ClC-K channel function by modulating gating. J Am Soc Nephrol 2010;21:1281–9.

[73] Schnell JR, Chou JJ. Structure and mechanism of the M2 proton channel of influenza A virus. Nature 2008;451:591–5.

[74] Palmer LG. Epithelial Na channels: function and diversity. Annu Rev Physiol 1992;54:51–6.

[75] Palmer LG, Andersen OS. Interactions of amiloride and small monovalent cations with the epithelial sodium channel. Inferences about the nature of the channel pore. Biophys J 1989;55:779–87.

[76] Lopatin AN, Nichols CG. Internal Na^+ and Mg^{2+} blockade of DRK1 (Kv2.1) potassium channels expressed in *Xenopus* oocytes. Inward rectification of a delayed rectifier. J Gen Physiol 1994;103:203—16.

[77] Lu Z, MacKinnon R. Electrostatic tuning of Mg^{2+} affinity in an inward-rectifier K^+ channel. Nature 1994;371:243—6.

[78] Accardi A, Picollo A. CLC channels and transporters: proteins with borderline personalities. Biochim Biophys Acta 2010;1798:1457—64.

[79] Duran C, Thompson CH, Xiao Q, Hartzell HC. Chloride channels: often enigmatic, rarely predictable. Annu Rev Physiol 2010;72:95—121.

[80] Bayliss DA, Barrett PQ. Emerging roles for two-pore-domain potassium channels and their potential therapeutic impact. Trends Pharmacol Sci 2008;29:566—75.

[81] Benos DJ, Stanton BA. Functional domains within the degenerin/epithelial sodium channel (Deg/ENaC) superfamily of ion channels. J Physiol (Lond) 1999;520(Pt 3):631—44.

[82] Loffing J, Korbmacher C. Regulated sodium transport in the renal connecting tubule (CNT) via the epithelial sodium channel (ENaC). Pflugers Arch 2009;458:111—35.

[83] Sakmann B, Neher E. Single-Channel recording. New York: Plenum Press; 1983.

[84] Boros S, Bindels RJ, Hoenderop JG. Active Ca(2+) reabsorption in the connecting tubule. Pflugers Arch 2009;458:99—109.

[85] de GT, Bindels RJ, Hoenderop JG. TRPV5: an ingeniously controlled calcium channel. Kidney Int 2008;74:1241—6.

[86] Dimke H, Hoenderop JG, Bindels RJ. Molecular basis of epithelial Ca^{2+} and Mg^{2+} transport: insights from the TRP channel family. J. Physiol. 2011;589(Pt 7):1535—42.

[87] Lang F, Vallon V, Knipper M, Wangemann P. Functional significance of channels and transporters expressed in the inner ear and kidney. Am J Physiol Cell Physiol 2007;293: C1187—208.

[88] Knoers NV, Levtchenko EN. Gitelman syndrome. Orphanet J Rare Dis 2008;3:22.

[89] Gan L, Kaczmarek LK. When, where, and how much? Expression of the Kv3.1 potassium channel in high-frequency firing neurons. J Neurobiol 1998;37:69—79.

[90] Kamb A, Iverson LE, Tanouye MA. Molecular characterization of Shaker, a *Drosophila* gene that encodes a potassium channel. Cell 1987;50:405—13.

[91] Tejpar S, Piessevaux H, Claes K, Piront P, Hoenderop JG, Verslype C, et al. Magnesium wasting associated with epidermal-growth-factor receptor-targeting antibodies in colorectal cancer: a prospective study. Lancet Oncol 2007;8:387—94.

[92] Glaudemans B, van der WJ, Scola RH, Lorenzoni PJ, Heister A, van der Kemp AW, et al. A missense mutation in the Kv1.1 voltage-gated potassium channel-encoding gene KCNA1 is linked to human autosomal dominant hypomagnesemia. J Clin Invest 2009;119:936—42.

[93] Plaster NM, Tawil R, Tristani-Firouzi M, Canun S, Bendahhou S, Tsunoda A, et al. Mutations in Kir2.1 cause the developmental and episodic electrical phenotypes of Andersen's syndrome. Cell 2001;105:511—9.

[94] Ho K, Nichols CG, Lederer WJ, Lytton J, Vassilev PM, Kanazirska MV, et al. Cloning and expression of an inwardly rectifying ATP-regulated potassium channel. Nature 1993;362:31—8.

[95] Wang WH, Giebisch G. Regulation of potassium (K) handling in the renal collecting duct. Pflugers Arch 2009;458:157—68.

[96] Bockenhauer D, Feather S, Stanescu HC, Bandulik S, Zdebik AA, Reichold M, et al. Epilepsy, ataxia, sensorineural deafness, tubulopathy, and KCNJ10 mutations. N Engl J Med 2009;360:1960—70.

[97] Scholl U, Hebeisen S, Janssen AG, Muller-Newen G, Alekov A, Fahlke C. Barttin modulates trafficking and function of ClC-K channels. Proc Natl Acad Sci USA 2006;103:11411—6.

[98] Tempel BL, Papazian DM, Schwarz TL, Jan YN, Jan LY. Sequence of a probable potassium channel component encoded at Shaker locus of *Drosophila*. Science 1987;237:770—5.

[99] Wang WH, Yue P, Sun P, Lin DH. Regulation and function of potassium channels in aldosterone-sensitive distal nephron. Curr. Opin. Nephrol. Hypertens. 2010;19(5):463—70.

[100] Rychkov GY, Pusch M, Roberts ML, Jentsch TJ, Bretag AH. Permeation and block of the skeletal muscle chloride channel, ClC-1, by foreign anions. J Gen Physiol 1998;111:653—65.

[101] Canessa CM, Horisberger JD, Rossier BC. Epithelial sodium channel related to proteins involved in neurodegeneration. Nature 1993;361:467—70.

[102] Canessa CM, Schild L, Buell G, Thorens B, Gautschi I, Horisberger JD, et al. Amiloride-sensitive epithelial Na channel is made of three homologous subunits. Nature 1994;367:463—7.

[103] Lingueglia E, Voilley N, Waldmann R, Lazdunski M, Barbry P. Expression cloning of an epithelial amiloride-sensitive Na^+ channel. A new channel type with homologies to Caenorhabditis elegans degenerins. FEBS Lett 1993;318:95—9.

[104] Kellenberger S, Gautschi I, Schild L. A single point mutation in the pore region of the epithelial Na^+ channel changes ion selectivity by modifying molecular sieving. Proc Natl Acad Sci USA 1999;96:4170—5.

[105] Kellenberger S, Hoffmann-Pochon N, Gautschi I, Schneeberger E, Schild L. On the molecular basis of ion permeation in the epithelial Na^+ channel. J Gen Physiol 1999;114:13—30.

[106] Lifton RP, Gharavi AG, Geller DS. Molecular mechanisms of human hypertension. Cell 2001;104:545—56.

[107] Rieg T, Vallon V, Sausbier M, Sausbier U, Kaissling B, Ruth P, et al. The role of the BK channel in potassium homeostasis and flow-induced renal potassium excretion. Kidney Int 2007;72:566—73.

[108] Estacion M, Sinkins WG, Jones SW, Applegate MA, Schilling WP. Human TRPC6 expressed in HEK 293 cells forms non-selective cation channels with limited Ca^{2+} permeability. J Physiol 2006;572:359—77.

[109] Inoue R, Okada T, Onoue H, Hara Y, Shimizu S, Naitoh S, et al. The transient receptor potential protein homologue TRP6 is the essential component of vascular alpha(1)-adrenoceptor-activated Ca(2+)-permeable cation channel. Circ Res 2001;88:325—32.

[110] Sheng S, McNulty KA, Harvey JM, Kleyman TR. Second transmembrane domains of ENaC subunits contribute to ion permeation and selectivity. J Biol Chem 2001;276:44091—8.

[111] Scholl UI, Choi M, Liu T, Ramaekers VT, Hausler MG, Grimmer J, et al. Seizures, sensorineural deafness, ataxia, mental retardation, and electrolyte imbalance (SeSAME syndrome) caused by mutations in KCNJ10. Proc Natl Acad Sci USA 2009;106:5842—7.

[112] Tang Y, Zaitseva F, Lamb RA, Pinto LH. The gate of the influenza virus M2 proton channel is formed by a single tryptophan residue. J Biol Chem 2002;277:39880—6.

[113] Liedtke W, Choe Y, Marti-Renom MA, Bell AM, Denis CS, Sali A, et al. Vanilloid receptor-related osmotically activated channel (VR-OAC), a candidate vertebrate osmoreceptor. Cell 2000;103:525—35.

[114] Liedtke W, Friedman JM. Abnormal osmotic regulation in trpv4−/− mice. Proc Natl Acad Sci USA 2003;100:13698—703.

[115] Meyer S, Savaresi S, Forster IC, Dutzler R. Nucleotide recognition by the cytoplasmic domain of the human chloride transporter ClC-5. Nat Struct Mol Biol 2007;14:60—7.

[116] Jayaram H, Robertson JL, Wu F, Williams C, Miller C. Structure of a slow CLC Cl/H + antiporter from a cyanobacterium. Biochemistry 2011;50:788–94.

[117] Jasti J, Furukawa H, Gonzales EB, Gouaux E. Structure of acid-sensing ion channel 1 at 1.9 Å resolution and low pH. Nature 2007;449:316–23.

[118] Snyder PM, Price MP, McDonald FJ, Adams CM, Volk KA, Zeiher BG, et al. Mechanism by which Liddle's syndrome mutations increase activity of a human epithelial Na$^+$ channel. Cell 1995;83:969–78.

[119] Kollewe A, Lau AY, Sullivan A, Roux B, Goldstein SA. A structural model for K2P potassium channels based on 23 pairs of interacting sites and continuum electrostatics. J Gen Physiol 2009;134:53–68.

[120] Alioth S, Meyer S, Dutzler R, Pervushin K. The cytoplasmic domain of the chloride channel ClC-0: structural and dynamic characterization of flexible regions. J Mol Biol 2007;369:1163–9.

[121] MacKinnon R. Nobel Lecture. Potassium channels and the atomic basis of selective ion conduction. Biosci Rep 2004;24:75–100.

[122] Mensenkamp AR, Hoenderop JG, Bindels RJ. TRPV5, the gateway to Ca^{2+} homeostasis. Handb Exp Pharmacol 2007;:207–20.

[123] Jayaram H, Accardi A, Wu F, Williams C, Miller C. Ion permeation through a Cl$^-$-selective channel designed from a CLC Cl$^-$/H$^+$ exchanger. Proc Natl Acad Sci USA 2008;105:11194–9.

[124] Gradogna A, Babini E, Picollo A, Pusch M. A regulatory calcium-binding site at the subunit interface of CLC-K kidney chloride channels. J Gen Physiol 2010;136:311–23.

[125] Mizuno A, Matsumoto N, Imai M, Suzuki M. Impaired osmotic sensation in mice lacking TRPV4. Am J Physiol Cell Physiol 2003;285:C96–101.

[126] Waldmann R, Champigny G, Voilley N, Lauritzen I, Lazdunski M. The mammalian degenerin MDEG, an amiloride-sensitive cation channel activated by mutations causing neurodegeneration in *Caenorhabditis elegans*. J Biol Chem 1996;271:10433–6.

[127] Rapedius M, Haider S, Browne KF, Shang L, Sansom MS, Baukrowitz T, et al. Structural and functional analysis of the putative pH sensor in the Kir1.1 (ROMK) potassium channel. EMBO Rep 2006;7:611–6.

[128] Chen TY, Miller C. Nonequilibrium gating and voltage dependence of the ClC-0 Cl$^-$ channel. J Gen Physiol 1996;108:237–50.

[129] Hanke W, Miller C. Single chloride channels from *Torpedo electroplax*. Activation by protons. J Gen Physiol 1983;82:25–45.

[130] Roux B, MacKinnon R. The cavity and pore helices in the KcsA K$^+$ channel: electrostatic stabilization of monovalent cations. Science 1999;285:100–2.

[131] Capaldi RA. Membrane proteins. New York, New York: Marcel Dekker Inc; 1995.

[132] Fahlke C, Yu HT, Beck CL, Rhodes TH, George Jr. AL. Pore-forming segments in voltage-gated chloride channels. Nature 1997;390:529–32.

[133] Thompson DA, Feather S, Stanescu HC, Freudenthal B, Zdebik AA, Warth R, et al. Altered electroretinograms in patients with KCNJ10 mutations and EAST syndrome. J. Physiol. 2011;589(Pt 7):1681–9.

[134] Grunder S, Firsov D, Chang SS, Jaeger NF, Gautschi I, Schild L, et al. A mutation causing pseudohypoaldosteronism type 1 identifies a conserved glycine that is involved in the gating of the epithelial sodium channel. EMBO J 1997;16:899–907.

[135] Grunder S, Jaeger NF, Gautschi I, Schild L, Rossier BC. Identification of a highly conserved sequence at the N-terminus of the epithelial Na$^+$ channel alpha subunit involved in gating. Pflugers Arch 1999;438:709–15.

[136] Seyberth HW. An improved terminology and classification of Bartter-like syndromes. Nat Clin Pract Nephrol 2008;4:560–7.

[137] Staub O, Dho S, Henry P, Correa J, Ishikawa T, McGlade J, et al. domains of Nedd4 bind to the proline-rich PY motifs in the epithelial Na$^+$ channel deleted in Liddle's syndrome. EMBO J 1996;15:2371–80.

[138] Hiltunen TP, Hannila-Handelberg T, Petajaniemi N, Kantola I, Tikkanen I, Virtamo J, et al. Liddle's syndrome associated with a point mutation in the extracellular domain of the epithelial sodium channel gamma subunit. J Hypertens 2002;20:2383–90.

[139] Yu Y, Xu C, Pan X, Ren H, Wang W, Meng X, et al. Identification and functional analysis of novel mutations of the CLCNKB gene in Chinese patients with classic Bartter syndrome. Clin Genet 2010;77:155–62.

[140] Simon DB, Lu Y, Choate KA, Velazquez H, Al-Sabban E, Praga M, et al. Paracellin-1, a renal tight junction protein required for paracellular Mg^{2+} resorption. Science 1999;285:103–6.

[141] Kawate T, Michel JC, Birdsong WT, Gouaux E. Crystal structure of the ATP-gated P2X(4) ion channel in the closed state. Nature 2009;460:592–8.

[142] Harding MM. Metal-ligand geometry relevant to proteins and in proteins: sodium and potassium. Acta Crystallogr D Biol Crystallogr 2002;58:872–4.

[143] Harding MM. The architecture of metal coordination groups in proteins. Acta Crystallogr D Biol Crystallogr 2004;60:849–59.

[144] Goodman MB, Ernstrom GG, Chelur DS, O'Hagan R, Yao CA, Chalfie M. MEC-2 regulates *C. elegans* DEG/ENaC channels needed for mechanosensation. Nature 2002;415:1039–42.

[145] Walder RY, Shalev H, Brennan TM, Carmi R, Elbedour K, Scott DA, et al. Familial hypomagnesemia maps to chromosome 9q, not to the X chromosome: genetic linkage mapping and analysis of a balanced translocation breakpoint. Hum Mol Genet 1997;6:1491–7.

[146] Nanazashvili M, Li H, Palmer LG, Walters DE, Sackin H. Moving the pH gate of the Kir1.1 inward rectifier channel. Channels (Austin) 2007;1:21–8.

[147] Nishida M, Cadene M, Chait BT, MacKinnon R. Crystal structure of a Kir3.1-prokaryotic Kir channel chimera. EMBO J 2007;26:4005–15.

[148] Flagg TP, Yoo D, Sciortino CM, Tate M, Romero MF, Welling PA. Molecular mechanism of a COOH-terminal gating determinant in the ROMK channel revealed by a Bartter's disease mutation. J Physiol 2002;544:351–62.

[149] Stouffer AL, Acharya R, Salom D, Levine AS, Di CL, Soto CS, et al. Structural basis for the function and inhibition of an influenza virus proton channel. Nature 2008;451:596–9.

[150] Lu Z, MacKinnon R. A conductance maximum observed in an inward-rectifier potassium channel. J Gen Physiol 1994;104:477–86.

[151] Macgregor GG, Xu JZ, McNicholas CM, Giebisch G, Hebert SC. Partially active channels produced by PKA site mutation of the cloned renal K$^+$ channel, ROMK2 (kir1.2). Am J Physiol 1998;275:F415–22.

[152] Rothberg BS, Magleby KL. Voltage and Ca^{2+} activation of single large-conductance Ca^{2+}-activated K$^+$ channels described by a two-tiered allosteric gating mechanism. J Gen Physiol 2000;116:75–99.

[153] Berneche S, Roux B. Energetics of ion conduction through the K$^+$ channel. Nature 2001;414:73–7.

[154] Welling PA, Ho K. A comprehensive guide to the ROMK potassium channel: form and function in health and disease. Am J Physiol Renal Physiol 2009;297:F849–63.

[155] Muto S. Potassium transport in the mammalian collecting duct. Physiol Rev 2001;81:85–116.

[156] Sachs F, Qin F. Gated, ion-selective channels observed with patch pipettes in the absence of membranes: novel properties of a gigaseal. Biophys J 1993;65:1101–7.

[157] Riepe FG, van Bemmelen MX, Cachat F, Plendl H, Gautschi I, Krone N, et al. Revealing a subclinical salt-losing phenotype in heterozygous carriers of the novel S562P mutation in the alpha subunit of the epithelial sodium channel. Clin Endocrinol (Oxf) 2009;70:252–8.

[158] Choe H, Sackin H, Palmer LG. Permeation properties of inward-rectifier potassium channels and their molecular determinants. J Gen Physiol 2000;115:391–404.

[159] Zhang P, Canessa CM. Single-channel properties of recombinant acid-sensitive ion channels formed by the subunits ASIC2 and ASIC3 from dorsal root ganglion neurons expressed in Xenopus oocytes. J Gen Physiol 2001;117:563–72.

[160] Pegan S, Arrabit C, Slesinger PA, Choe S. Andersen's syndrome mutation effects on the structure and assembly of the cytoplasmic domains of Kir2.1. Biochemistry 2006;45:8599–606.

[161] Konrad M, Vollmer M, Lemmink HH, van den Heuvel LP, Jeck N, Vargas-Poussou R, et al. Mutations in the chloride channel gene CLCNKB as a cause of classic Bartter syndrome. J Am Soc Nephrol 2000;11:1449–59.

[162] Yoo D, Kim BY, Campo C, Nance L, King A, Maouyo D, et al. Cell surface expression of the ROMK (Kir 1.1) channel is regulated by the aldosterone-induced kinase, SGK-1, and protein kinase A. J Biol Chem 2003;278:23066–75.

[163] Kubisch C, Schmidt-Rose T, Fontaine B, Bretag AH, Jentsch TJ. ClC-1 chloride channel mutations in myotonia congenita: variable penetrance of mutations shifting the voltage dependence. Hum Mol Genet 1998;7:1753–60.

[164] Pressler CA, Heinzinger J, Jeck N, Waldegger P, Pechmann U, Reinalter S, et al. Late-onset manifestation of antenatal Bartter syndrome as a result of residual function of the mutated renal Na$^+$-K$^+$-2Cl$^-$ co-transporter. J Am Soc Nephrol 2006;17:2136–42.

[165] Shi J, Mori E, Mori Y, Mori M, Li J, Ito Y, et al. Multiple regulation by calcium of murine homologues of transient receptor potential proteins TRPC6 and TRPC7 expressed in HEK293 cells. J Physiol 2004;561:415–32.

[166] Wagner CA. Disorders of renal magnesium handling explain renal magnesium transport. J Nephrol 2007;20:507–10.

[167] Bergsdorf EY, Zdebik AA, Jentsch TJ. Residues important for nitrate/proton coupling in plant and mammalian CLC transporters. J Biol Chem 2009;284:11184–93.

[168] Engh AM, Maduke M. Cysteine accessibility in ClC-0 supports conservation of the ClC intracellular vestibule. J Gen Physiol 2005;125:601–17.

[169] Meyer S, Dutzler R. Crystal structure of the cytoplasmic domain of the chloride channel ClC-0. Structure 2006;14:299–307.

[170] Bennetts B, Rychkov GY, Ng HL, Morton CJ, Stapleton D, Parker MW, et al. Cytoplasmic ATP-sensing domains regulate gating of skeletal muscle ClC-1 chloride channels. J Biol Chem 2005;280:32452–8.

[171] Traverso S, Elia L, Pusch M. Gating competence of constitutively open CLC-0 mutants revealed by the interaction with a small organic Inhibitor. J Gen Physiol 2003;122:295–306.

[172] Zhou Y, Morais-Cabral JH, Kaufman A, MacKinnon R. Chemistry of ion coordination and hydration revealed by a K$^+$ channel-Fab complex at 2.0 Å resolution. Nature 2001;414:43–8.

[173] Janssen AG, Scholl U, Domeyer C, Nothmann D, Leinenweber A, Fahlke C. Disease-causing dysfunctions of barttin in Bartter syndrome type IV. J Am Soc Nephrol 2009;20:145–53.

[174] Chang SS, Grunder S, Hanukoglu A, Rosler A, Mathew PM, Hanukoglu I, et al. Mutations in subunits of the epithelial sodium channel causes salt wasting with hyperkalaemic acidosis, pseudohypoaldosteronism type 1. Nature Genet 1996;12:248–53.

[175] Kucher V, Boiko N, Pochynyuk O, Stockand JD. Voltage-dependent gating underlies loss of ENaC function in pseudo-hypoaldosteronis type 1. Biophys. J. 2011;100(8):1930–9.

[176] Tammaro P, Flanagan SE, Zadek B, Srinivasan S, Woodhead H, Hameed S, et al. Kir6.2 mutation causing severe functional effects in vitro produces neonatal diabetes without the expected neurological complications. Diabetologia 2008;51:802–10.

[177] Wible BA, Taglialatela M, Ficker E, Brown AM. Gating of inwardly rectifying K$^+$ channels localized to a single negatively charged residue. Nature 1994;371:246–9.

[178] Xu ZC, Yang Y, Hebert SC. Phosphorylation of the ATP-sensitive, inwardly rectifying K$^+$ channel, ROMK, by cyclic AMP-dependent protein kinase. J Biol Chem 1996;271: 9313–9.

[179] Schlingmann KP, Weber S, Peters M, Niemann NL, Vitzthum H, Klingel K, et al. Hypomagnesemia with secondary hypocalcemia is caused by mutations in TRPM6, a new member of the TRPM gene family. Nat Genet 2002;31:166–70.

[180] Stockand JD, Staruschenko A, Pochynyuk O, Booth RE, Silverthorn DU. Insight toward epithelial Na$^+$ channel mechanism revealed by the acid-sensing ion channel 1 structure. IUBMB Life 2008;60:620–8.

[181] Riepe FG. Clinical and molecular features of type 1 pseudohypoaldosteronism. Horm Res 2009;72:1–9.

[182] Goulet CC, Volk KA, Adams CM, Prince LS, Stokes JB, Snyder PM. Inhibition of the epithelial Na$^+$ channel by interaction of Nedd4 with a PY motif deleted in Liddle's syndrome. J Biol Chem 1998;273:30012–7.

[183] Snyder PM, Olson DR, Bucher DB. A pore segment in DEG/ENaC Na(+) channels. J Biol Chem 1999;274:28484–90.

[184] Staruschenko A, Adams E, Booth RE, Stockand JD. Epithelial Na$^+$ channel subunit stoichiometry. Biophys J 2005;88:3966–75.

[185] Jeck N, Derst C, Wischmeyer E, Ott H, Weber S, Rudin C, et al. Functional heterogeneity of ROMK mutations linked to hyperprostaglandin E syndrome. Kidney Int 2001;59: 1803–11.

[186] Schulte U, Hahn H, Konrad M, Jeck N, Derst C, Wild K, et al. pH gating of ROMK (K(ir)1.1) channels: control by an Arg-Lys-Arg triad disrupted in antenatal Bartter syndrome. Proc Natl Acad Sci USA 1999;96:15298–303.

[187] Choe H, Zhou H, Palmer LG, Sackin H. A conserved cytoplasmic region of ROMK modulates pH sensitivity, conductance, and gating. Am J Physiol 1997;273:F516–29.

[188] Markovic S, Dutzler R. The structure of the cytoplasmic domain of the chloride channel ClC-Ka reveals a conserved interaction interface. Structure 2007;15:715–25.

[189] Rapedius M, Fowler PW, Shang L, Sansom MS, Tucker SJ, Baukrowitz T. H bonding at the helix-bundle crossing controls gating in Kir potassium channels. Neuron 2007;55:602–14.

[190] Pusch M, Ludewig U, Rehfeldt A, Jentsch TJ. Gating of the voltage-dependent chloride channel ClC-O by the permeant anion. Nature 1995;373:527–31.

[191] Hattersley AT, Ashcroft FM. Activating mutations in Kir6.2 and neonatal diabetes: new clinical syndromes, new scientific insights, and new therapy. Diabetes 2005;54:2503–13.

[192] Leipziger J, Macgregor GG, Cooper GJ, Xu J, Hebert SC, Giebisch G. PKA site mutations of ROMK2 channels shift the pH dependence to more alkaline values. Am J Physiol Renal Physiol 2000;279:F919–26.

[193] Leung YM, Zeng WZ, Liou HH, Solaro CR, Huang CL. Phosphatidylinositol 4,5-bisphosphate and intracellular pH

regulate the ROMK1 potassium channel via separate but interrelated mechanisms. J Biol Chem 2000;275:10182−9.

[194] Schrag D, Chung KY, Flombaum C, Saltz L. Cetuximab therapy and symptomatic hypomagnesemia. J Natl Cancer Inst 2005;97:1221−4.

[195] Flagg TP, Tate M, Merot J, Welling PA. A mutation linked with Bartter's syndrome locks Kir 1.1a (ROMK1) channels in a closed state. J Gen Physiol 1999;114:685−700.

[196] Ma D, Tang XD, Rogers TB, Welling PA. An Andersen−Tawil syndrome mutation in Kir2.1 (V302M) alters the G-loop cytoplasmic K^+ conduction pathway 1. J Biol Chem 2007;282: 5781−9.

[197] Palmer LG, Frindt G. Amiloride-sensitive Na channels from the apical membrane of the rat cortical collecting tubule. Proc Natl Acad Sci USA 1986;83:2767−70.

[198] Fallen K, Banerjee S, Sheehan J, Addison D, Lewis LM, Meiler J, et al. The Kir channel immunoglobulin domain is essential for Kir1.1 (ROMK) thermodynamic stability, trafficking and gating. Channels (Austin) 2009;3:57−68.

[199] Cheng WW, D'Avanzo N, Doyle DA, Nichols CG. Dual-mode phospholipid regulation of human inward rectifying potassium channels. Biophys J 2011;100:620−8.

[200] D'Avanzo N, Cheng WW, Doyle DA, Nichols CG. Direct and specific activation of human inward rectifier K^+ channels by membrane phosphatidylinositol 4,5-bisphosphate. J Biol Chem 2010;285:37129−32.

[201] Lopes C, Zhang H, Rohacs T, Jin T, Logothetis D. Alterations in conserved Kir channel-PIP2 interactions underlie channelopathies. Neuron 2002;34:933−44.

[202] Robertson JL, Palmer LG, Roux B. Long-pore electrostatics in inward-rectifier potassium channels. J Gen Physiol 2008;132: 613−32.

[203] Rohacs T, Lopes C, Jin T, Ramdya P, Molnar Z, Logothetis D. Specificity of activation by phosphoinositides determines lipid regulation of Kir channels. PNAS 2003;100:745−50.

[204] Peters M, Ermert S, Jeck N, Derst C, Pechmann U, Weber S, et al. Classification and rescue of ROMK mutations underlying hyperprostaglandin E syndrome/antenatal Bartter syndrome. Kidney Int 2003;64:923−32.

[205] McNicholas CM, Macgregor GG, Islas LD, Yang Y, Hebert SC, Giebisch G. pH-dependent modulation of the cloned renal K^+ channel, ROMK. Am J Physiol 1998;275:F972−81.

[206] Walz T, Hirai T, Murata K, Heymann JB, Mitsuoka K, Fujiyoshi Y, et al. The three-dimensional structure of aquaporin-1. Nature 1997;387:624−7.

[207] MacGregor G, Dong K, Vanoye C, Tang L, Giebisch G, Hebert S. Nucleotides and phospholipids compete for binding to the C terminus of K-ATP channels. PNAS 2002;99:2726−31.

[208] Xi Q, Hoenderop JG, Bindels RJ. Regulation of magnesium reabsorption in DCT. Pflugers Arch 2009;458:89−98.

[209] Yau WM, Wimley WC, Gawrisch K, White SH. The preference of tryptophan for membrane interfaces. Biochemistry 1998;37:14713−8.

[210] Liou HH, Zhou SS, Huang CL. Regulation of ROMK1 channel by protein kinase A via a phosphatidylinositol 4,5-bisphosphate-dependent mechanism. Proc Natl Acad Sci USA 1999;96:5820−5.

[211] Jiang Y, Lee A, Chen J, Ruta V, Cadene M, Chait BT, et al. X-ray structure of a voltage-dependent K^+ channel. Nature 2003;423:33−41.

[212] Zifarelli G, Pusch M. The muscle chloride channel ClC-1 is not directly regulated by intracellular ATP. J Gen Physiol 2008;131:109−16.

Microvascular Permeability and the Exchange of Water and Solutes Across Microvascular Walls

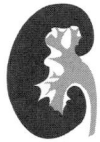

C. Charles Michel

Department of Bioengineering, Imperial College, London, UK

INTRODUCTION

Exchange through microvascular walls is both the initial and the final step of transport of materials by the circulation. In most tissues, microvascular exchange is a passive process, driven by differences in hydrostatic pressure and solute concentration between the circulating plasma and the interstitial fluid that flank microvessel walls. Lipophilic molecules and small water-soluble molecules and ions can exchange rapidly in most vascular beds, but microvascular walls are a barrier to macromolecules, severely impeding their exchange. The consequent differences in macromolecular concentration across microvascular walls are responsible for differences in osmotic pressure, which were identified over a century ago to play an essential role in the balance of fluid between the circulating blood and the tissues.[121]

Although small hydrophilic molecules can exchange rapidly between the blood and the tissues, it is wrong to assume that microvascular walls are no barrier to them. The rate at which changes of concentration of a solute in the blood can be reflected as changes in interstitial fluid (ISF) concentration depends both on the blood flow to the capillary beds, and on the permeability of the capillary walls to the solute. It is often assumed that for small molecules only blood flow is important, but once flow has exceeded a certain minimum range of values, the rate of equilibration of blood and ISF becomes limited by permeability.

Microvascular exchange and microvascular permeability are sometimes regarded as synonymous but this in incorrect and it is important to distinguish between them. Microvascular permeability to a substance is the conductivity of the microvessel wall and the permeability coefficients which describe permeability in functional terms are determined by the structure and properties of the pathways through which its molecules traverse the vessel wall. Microvascular exchange rates and net transport through microvascular walls for a particular substance are determined by microvascular permeability to that substance and also by the value and direction of net fluid flow through the vessel wall and by differences in concentration of the substance between plasma and ISF. The difference between microvascular exchange and microvascular permeability is important when interpreting methods that claim to demonstrate changes in permeability. Many of these methods involve the measurement of changes in net transport of macromolecules between blood and tissues, without controlling the transcapillary differences in hydrostatic pressure and macromolecular concentration. We shall consider the potential errors later in this chapter.

First, we consider microvascular permeability, and then microvascular exchange. Not included in this chapter is a consideration of transport through the walls of microvessels of the central nervous system. The low permeabilities of these vessels and the specialized transport mechanisms for certain solutes constituting the

Seldin and Giebisch's The Kidney, Fifth Edition.
DOI: http://dx.doi.org/10.1016/B978-0-12-381462-3.00009-4

blood—brain barrier are atypical of other microvessels, and resemble those of tight epithelia.

MICROVASCULAR PERMEABILITY

Microvascular Ultrastructure

Capillary walls consist of a single layer of flattened endothelial cells, the endothelia, and these cells constitute the barrier between the blood and the ISF. Electron microscopy has revealed that endothelial cells in different tissues are of two distinct types: "continuous" and "fenestrated" (Figure 9.1). Continuous endothelium is found in microvessels of skin, muscle, lung, and connective tissues. Here, the endothelial cells are joined together by tight junctions to form a continuous layer surrounded by a continuous basement membrane. The plasmalemmal membranes of the continuous endothelia retain their integrity; even in areas where the cells are flattened, reducing their thickness to less than 0.1 μm, the distinct luminal and abluminal membranes are separated by a thin layer of cytoplasm.

Fenestrated endothelium is found in microvessels associated with secretory and absorptive epithelia, e.g., the capillaries of the intestinal mucosae, glomerular, and peri-tubular capillaries of the kidney. The walls of fenestrated microvessels are also made of a single continuous layer of endothelial cells joined by tight junctions and surrounded by a continuous basement membrane, but in these vessels attenuated areas of cells appear to be penetrated by circular openings 40 to 70 nm in diameter. These are the fenestrae (or fenestrations), and in most cases the fenestrations are closed by a thin electron-dense diaphragm, which appears to be arranged as a series of broad spokes with central "hub"[14] (Figure 9.2).

Covering the luminal surface of endothelial cells is a layer of glycoprotein called the glycocalyx or endocapillary layer (ECL). First identified by Luft in 1966[68] using ruthenium red staining, its importance has only come to be widely appreciated in the past 15 years. Although both continuous and fenestrated endothelia have been found to contain the various inclusions common to most cells (e.g., mitochondria, rough and smooth endoplasmic reticulum) the dominating ultrastructural feature seen in transmission electron micrographs is the large number of small endoplasmic vesicles (Figure 9.3). The majority of vesicles are arranged in fused clusters that communicate with each other and with flask like pits on either the luminal or abluminal surfaces of the cells called the caveolae

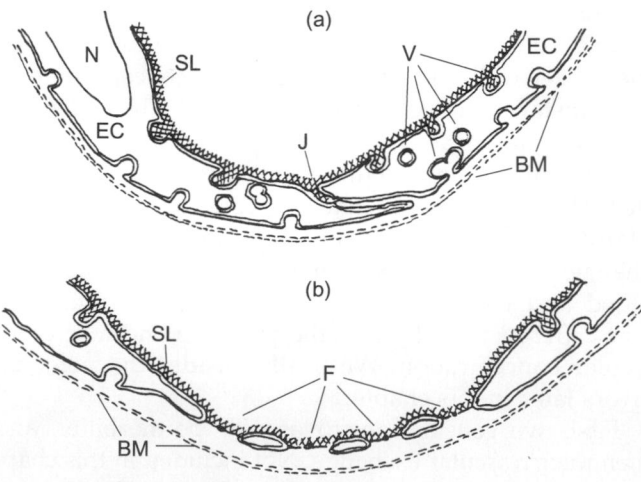

FIGURE 9.1 **Diagrams showing the ultrastuctural features of microvascular walls in transverse section: (a) Vessel with continuous endothelium; (b) Vessel with fenestrated endothelium**. The basement membrane (BM) forms a continuous layer around the outside of both vessel types and the luminal surfaces of both endothelia are covered with a negatively charged glycocalyx (SL) (EC: endothelial cell; J: junction; F: fenestration (fenestra); N: endothelial cell nucleus).

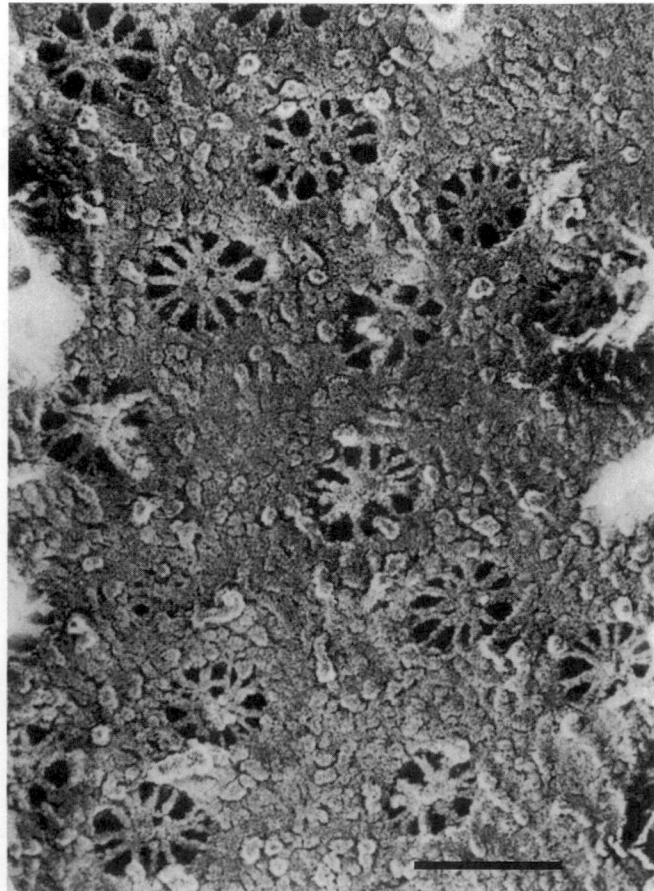

FIGURE 9.2 *En face* **view of fenestrated endothelium of peri-tubular capillary of the kidney in a rapid freeze deep etch preparation**. Scale bar = 0.1 μm. *(From ref. [14].)*

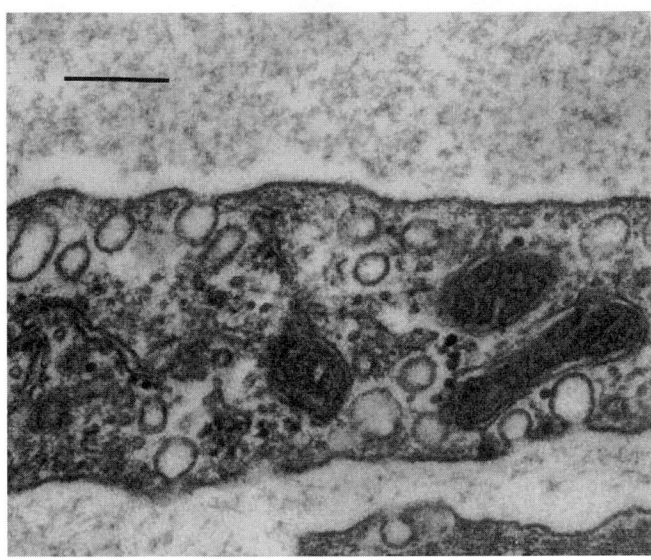

FIGURE 9.3 **Electron micrograph of microvascular endothelium of frog.** There are three mitochondria in the central part of the cell and large numbers of plasmalemmel vesicles. Scale bar = 0.2 μm. (*Electron micrograph by H.Moffitt.*)

intracellulares. Chains of fused vesicles forming channels that pass through endothelial cells[119] appear to be relatively rare occurrences in unstimulated endothelium, but are a feature of endothelium activated by certain mediators.[34,35]

The intercellular clefts of continuous endothelia, the fenestrae of fenestrated endothelia, and the small vesicles have all been implicated as pathways through the endothelia as a result of experiments using electron-dense tracers. Controversy surrounded the interpretation of many of these experiments, but progress has been made over the past 20 years as physiological evidence clarified their interpretation. For this reason, the ultrastructural basis of permeability is considered after we have defined the permeability coefficients by considering the principles of passive transport and have discussed their values in different endothelia to different types of molecules.

Passive Transport and Permeability Coefficients of Porous Membranes

The mechanisms of transport are convection and diffusion. Convection is equivalent to bulk flow of solutions and the solutes within them. Thus, if a solution flows from a reservoir A at a high pressure to a second reservoir, B, at a lower pressure, there is bulk flow of the solution and transport of the solutes by convection. If J_V ml sec^{-1} is the rate at which the solution flows from A to B, it is proportional to the difference in hydrostatic pressure, ΔP, between A and B as follows:

$$J_V = K\Delta P \qquad (9.1)$$

where K is the conductance of the system between A and B.

If A and B are separated by a porous membrane, K is proportional to the area of the membrane, A_m, through which fluid can flow. Thus:

$$J_V = L_P A_m \Delta P$$

and

$$L_P = (J_V/A_m\Delta P) \qquad (9.2)$$

where L_P is the hydraulic conductivity or hydraulic permeability of the membrane. L_P is one of several membrane permeability coefficients. It describes the ease with which fluid flows through a unit area of membrane when driven by a unit difference in pressure. It can be thought of as describing the frictional interactions between the membrane molecules and the molecules of the solution (principally water), and like the other permeability coefficients its value depends on the structure of the membrane. If small water-filled pores penetrate the membrane, L_P is proportional to the number of pores per unit area of membrane, to the fluid viscosity, and to a function of the dimensions of the pores. This function depends on the size and shape of the pores and the nature of flow through them.

Equation (9.2) describes the flow of a solution through a membrane only if the solute molecules can pass through the membrane as easily as the water molecules. If movement of solute is hindered to a greater extent than the water, filtration of the solution leads to the development of a solute concentration difference across the membrane as water enters compartment B faster than solute. The difference in solute concentration gives rise to a difference in osmotic pressure which opposes filtration of the solution across the membrane. The force driving solution through the membrane is no longer just ΔP, but ΔP minus the effective osmotic pressure between the solutions in A and B. The magnitude of this osmotic pressure difference is related not only to the concentration difference itself, but also to the degree to which the membrane hinders the movement of solute relative to water. This is described by a second membrane coefficient, σ_d, referred to as the osmotic reflection coefficient. If the channels in the membrane are permeable to water but not solute molecules, filtration of a solution of this solute through the membrane will separate the solute from the water, with pure water leaving the membrane and concentration of the solution upstream. Since all the solute molecules are reflected at the membrane, σ_d has a value of 1.0. The osmotic pressure exerted by differences in its concentration across this particular membrane should be close to that calculated from Van't Hoff's law, i.e., $\Delta\Pi = RT\Delta C$, depending on the "ideality" of the solution. If, alternatively the solute molecules are able to pass through the membrane as easily as the water molecules, σ_d has a value of 0, as none of the solute molecules are reflected. If the solute passes the membrane more easily than water, σ_d has a negative value. If only a fraction of the solute molecules are "reflected" during ultrafiltration of the solution, σ_d has a value between zero and one.

Only those molecules that are reflected at the membrane during ultrafiltration can exert an osmotic pressure across it. Thus, the osmotic pressure difference, $\Delta\Pi$, is related to the concentration difference, ΔC, through the universal gas constant, R, and the absolute temperature, T:

$$\Delta\Pi = \sigma_d\, RT\Delta C$$

and

$$\sigma_d = \frac{\Delta\Pi}{RT\Delta C} \qquad (9.3)$$

At microvascular walls, macromolecules such as plasma proteins have high values of σ_d and σ_f (0.8–0.999), whereas small ions (e.g., Na^+, K^+, Cl^-) and small hydrophilic molecules (e.g., glucose, lactic acid, amino acids, urea) have values of σ less than 0.2 in most vessels.

Net fluid flow through microvascular walls carries dissolved solutes by convection. The rate of solute transport by convection from A to B depends on J_V, and also upon the value of σ for the particular solute at the membrane. If σ has a value of zero, then J_S is equal to J_VC (in moles per second), where C is the solute concentration in the solution (in moles per ml), i.e., the solution flowing out of the membrane into B has the same concentration as that entering the membrane from A. If, however, σ has a value between zero and one, then the solution emerging from the membrane into B will have a lower solute concentration than that entering the membrane at A. Convective transport of solute through the membrane is now described by the relation:

$$J_S = J_V(1 - \sigma_f)C \qquad (9.4)$$

where C now refers to the concentration entering the membrane from A. Note that in Eq. (9.4) σ is written as σ_f, whereas in describing the effective osmotic pressure σ is written as σ_d. For "an ideal solute" $\sigma_f = \sigma_d$, but solutions of macromolecules deviate from "ideal" behavior and σ_d is often measurably greater than σ_f. Rearrangement of Eq. (9.3) provides a definition of σ_f:

$$\sigma_f = 1 - \frac{J_S}{J_VC} \qquad (9.5)$$

If the only pathway for both water and solutes through the membrane is a population of equally sized channels, σ_d and σ_f are determined only by the ratio of the dimensions of the solute molecules to those of the channels, and are independent of the number of channels per unit area of membrane.

A second mechanism of transport through porous membranes is diffusion. This is most important for the transport of small molecules across microvascular walls. In contrast to the stately progression of molecules by convection, diffusion results from the random jostling of all molecules in a solution that represents their thermal energy. Diffusion is a mixing process, and where there are differences in concentration in a solution diffusion is responsible for the spontaneous net transport of solute from regions of high to regions of low concentration. On a macroscopic scale, Fick's first law of diffusion describes net transport of solute by diffusion:

$$J_S = DA\left(\frac{-dC}{dx}\right) \qquad (9.6)$$

where D is the diffusion coefficient of the solute in the solution, A is the area through which diffusion occurs, and the derivative $(-dC/dx)$ is the concentration gradient of solute down which diffusion occurs. The negative sign of the derivative is to indicate that diffusion occurs from a region of high concentration (low value of x) to a region of lower concentration (higher value of x), i.e., the diffusion of a solute is directed down its concentration gradient.

Diffusion coefficients of solutes in aqueous solutions reflect the ability of solute molecules to slip past adjacent molecules of water. They are measured and defined in terms of net movements of solute under conditions in which there is no overall movement of the solution. Thus, diffusion in solution is a displacement process whereby the displacement of a solute molecule in one direction is accompanied by the displacement of an equal volume of water in the opposite direction. Because the rate at which displacement occurs is dependent on the thermal energy of the solution, the diffusion coefficient is directly proportional to temperature. It is also inversely proportional to the frictional interactions between the solute and water molecules.

When diffusion of a solute occurs through a thin porous membrane, the diffusional permeability of the membrane to the solute, P_d, is defined in terms of the net solute flux, J_S, the solute concentration difference across the membrane, ΔC, and the membrane area, A_m, under conditions where there is no volume flow through the membrane. Thus:

$$P_d = \left(\frac{J_S}{A_m \Delta C}\right)_{J_V = 0} \quad (9.7)$$

P_d has units of velocity (cm sec^{-1}), and like L_P and σ_f, it has meaning in terms of the interactions between the solute molecules, the molecules of the membrane, and the water within the membrane. Such interactions depend critically upon the ultrastructure of the pathways for solute and water through the membrane, particularly when the width of the pathways is comparable to the diameter of the diffusing molecules.

Diffusional permeability coefficients are defined under conditions where there is no net volume flow through the membrane. In measuring P_d of microvascular walls, it is often convenient to use radioactive isotopes or fluorescent tracers, because their fluxes can be detected when their concentration differences are in the micromolar range. Larger differences in concentration may set up significant differences in osmotic pressure, which may complicate the estimation of P_d by giving rise to net fluid flows in the opposite direction to those of the diffusing molecules.

Permeability to Lipophilic Solutes

Solutes that can dissolve to a significant extent in lipids have high cell membrane permeabilities, and very high microvascular permeabilities. It is assumed that these molecules diffuse directly through the entire microvascular wall. This group of solutes includes gas molecules, including O_2 and CO_2, as well as N_2, the inert gases, and molecules of general anesthetics, although recent evidence suggests CO_2 and NH_3 may cross membranes additionally through specialized channels.[15]

So rapidly can small lipophilic solutes cross microvascular walls that, under physiological conditions, their transport between the blood and the tissues is always limited by their rate of delivery or clearance by blood flow through the microcirculation, and it has been impossible to estimate their microvascular permeability coefficients with accuracy with values for some greater than 10^{-2} cm.sec^{-1}.

Microvascular permeability to lipophilic molecules is, however, sensitive to temperature. Renkin[101] showed that antipyrene, which is fat-soluble at body temperature, could exert substantial osmotic pressures across the walls of capillaries in cat hind limbs when the tissue was cooled to 15°C, but not when the tissue was at 37°C. A similar phenomenon has been demonstrated by Curry[25] in single mesenteric capillaries.

Permeability Coefficients to Small Hydrophilic Molecules

Microvascular permeability to macromolecules is usually considered separately from permeability to hydrophilic molecules smaller than serum albumin, as different mechanisms of transport appear to be involved. Evidence for this emerged in 1956 from studies on the passage of a range of dextran polymers between plasma and lymph.[45] Some of the original data are shown in Figure 9.4, where it is seen that the steady-state concentrations of the smaller dextrans in the lymph draining hind limb tissues of anesthetized dogs relative to the plasma levels fall rapidly as their molecular radii increase up to 4—5 nm; for the larger molecules the decline of lymph concentration with molecular size is so small as to appear barely significant in these data.

This two-component relation between P_d and molecular diameter is seen in nearly all microvascular beds, suggesting that small molecules use different mechanisms or pathways to cross microvascular walls from those used by macromolecules.[78,108,123]

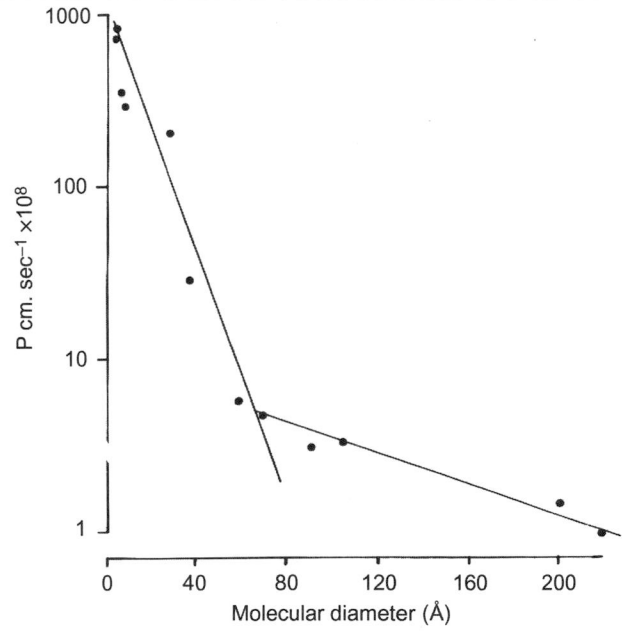

FIGURE 9.4 Relations between permeability (P) of dog hind limb microvessels to hydrophilic solutes and the molecular diameter of the solutes. The endothelium of these vessels is continuous and P has been calculated assuming they have a surface area for exchange of 7000 cm^2 100g^{-1} of tissue. Note that P, which has been plotted on a logarithmic scale, declines sharply as molecular diameter increases up to 70 Å (7 nm), which is approximately the diameter of serum albumin. A less steep relation is seen for larger molecules. (From ref. [78]. With permission)

Permeability Coefficients to Small Hydrophilic Molecules

In Figure 9.5, the values of P_d measured in microvascular beds of skeletal muscle and single mesenteric microvessels to some small water soluble solutes have been plotted against solute molecular radius. In mesenteric capillaries, values for P_d to the smallest molecules and ions (e.g., Na^+, K^+, urea) are ten times greater than values of P_d for the same solutes in muscle capillaries. To make the comparison easier, both the P_d values and values for molecular radius are shown on logarithmic scales. The decline of P_d with molecular radius for both types of microvessel is much greater than the decline of diffusion coefficient (D) for the same molecules in open aqueous solution. The more rapid decline of P_d can be accounted for if molecules were diffusing through water-filled channels whose widths were comparable to their own diameters.[94] The smooth curves, which have been fitted to the data, converge as molecular radius increases. If the channels were cylindrical pores, the convergence implies that the radii of the pores is very similar in mesenteric and muscle capillaries, but there are ten times more pores penetrating per unit area of the walls of mesenteric capillaries than of muscle capillaries. The value of molecular radius at which the curves intersect provides an estimate of the pore radius – in this case between 3.5 and 4 nm.

This pattern of declining P_d to small hydrophilic solutes with increasing molecular diameter is seen in all microvessels where it has been sought, and curves based on the theory of diffusion through pores of radii between 3.5 nm–5 nm can be fitted to these data.

The values of P_d to a particular small hydrophilic solute (e.g., Na^+, K^+, sucrose, and inulin) in different microvascular beds correlate with the values of hydraulic permeability (L_P). This is shown in Figure 9.6, where each point represents the mean value of L_P plotted against the mean value of P_d to Na^+ or K^+ in the same microvessel or microvascular bed, different points representing values for vessels in different tissues. The data have been plotted on logarithmic scales so that values covering two orders of magnitude can be compared. The slope that has been drawn through the points has been given a value of unity, to indicate that direct proportionality is a reasonable description of the relationship. The correlation is strong circumstantial evidence for believing that the same pathways through the endothelium serve both for the rapid exchange of small hydrophilic solutes, and for most net fluid movements. Furthermore, because Na^+ ions are likely to follow an extracellular route, it seems likely that this shared pathway is extracellular. This line of reasoning is greatly strengthened by the demonstration of similar linear correlations between L_P and P_d values for other extracellular solutes, such as sucrose and inulin[81] in different microvascular beds.

Although the exchange of small hydrophilic molecules occurs through the same channels that account for most of L_P, some water may also cross microvascular walls of continuous endothelium by channels not available to solutes. This additional route has been

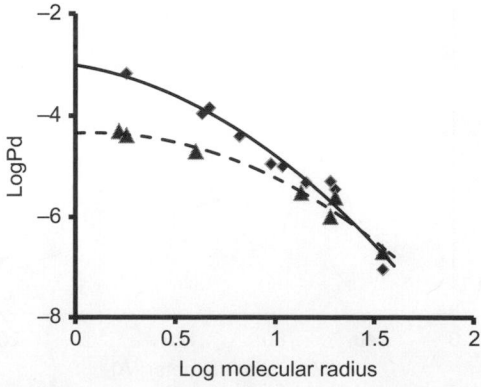

FIGURE 9.5 Relations between the logarithms of P_d and molecular radius for small to intermediate sized hydrophilic solutes in capillaries of frog mesentery (filled circles) and cat skeletal muscle (filled triangles). Data for frog obtained from measurements made in single perfused microvessels *in situ*. Data from cat based on measurements on perfused vascular bed. Both types of vessel have continuous endothelium. Note whereas P_d for the smallest solutes is 10 times greater in mesentery than in muscle (1 $\log_{10}$ unit = 10×), values for P_d converge as molecular size increases.

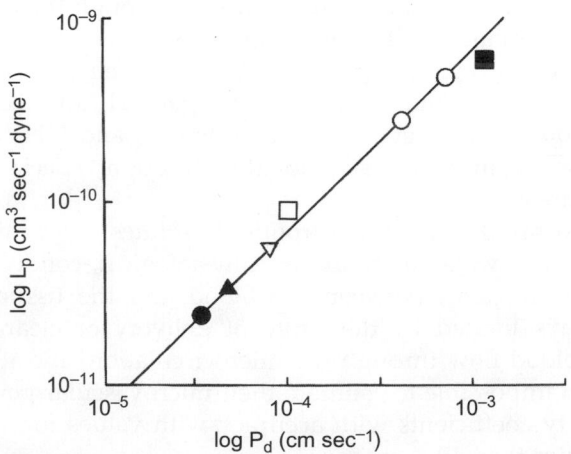

FIGURE 9.6 Variations in L_P and P_d to small ions (Na^+ and K^+) in different microvascular beds. The scales are logarithmic to include values covering two orders of magnitude, and the line has a slope of 1.0, indicating direct proportionality. Each point represents the value for L_P and P_d for one vascular bed; where several values of P_d are available the largest has been used to minimize errors resulting from flow-limited transport. ○, frog mesentery; ∇, frog muscle; ●, mammalian skeletal muscle; ϒ, mammalian heart muscle; ▲, dog lung; ■, cat salivary gland. *(From ref. [74]. With permission)*

identified by Pallone et al.[92] as channels formed by the membrane protein aquaporin-1, AQP-1.[6] The first real evidence for a "water only" pathway was indicated by Yudilevich and Alvarez from measurements of the rates of diffusion of triated water and Na^+ through dog heart capillaries. From measurements of σ to small hydrophilic solutes, Curry and colleagues[29] estimated that in single perfused capillaries between 5 and 10% of the pathways responsible for L_P were available only to water, and not to small solutes. More recently, Turner and Pallone[126] have shown that "water only" channels account for a similar proportion of the L_P of descending vasa recta of rat kidney. It is worth emphasizing that although fluid movements through AQP-1 channels of the descending vasa recta are of physiological importance, the channels contribute no more than 5 to 10% to the total L_P of these vessels. Although it has been suggested that AQP-1 channels might contribute to as much as 30% of the L_P of skeletal muscle capillaries,[137] the strong correlation between P_d and L_P shown in Figure 9.6 indicates that the contribution of AQP-1 channels to the L_P of most exchange vessels is small.

Although absolute values of L_P and P_d to small hydrophilic solutes vary greatly from one microvascular bed to another, the reflection coefficient to large molecules are remarkably similar in different vessels when the tissues are undamaged (or unstimulated). This is shown in Figure 9.7, where the mean values of

σ to serum albumin have been plotted against the mean value of L_P for various tissues. Whereas L_P varies over three orders of magnitude, σ to albumin is usually in the range of 0.8 to 1.0. There is no trend in the relation between $\sigma_{albumin}$ and L_P. Vessels with high values of L_P have mean values of $\sigma_{albumin}$ that are as high, if not higher, than in vessels with low values of L_P. This means that the channels or pores that are largely responsible for the L_P of vessels in different tissues all restrict the passage of albumin to a similar extent. Thus, both the variations of P_d with molecular size and the variations in $\sigma_{albumin}$ and L_P in different capillary beds lead to the same conclusion: individual channels for exchange of water and small hydrophilic solutes are similar in different capillary types, but the density of these channels in vessel walls varies considerably.

Permeability Coefficients to Macromolecules

Apart from the sinusoids of the liver and spleen, microvascular walls have high reflection coefficients and low permeabilities to macromolecules. These permeability properties are essential if the circulating blood is to be retained within the vascular system. Although their permeabilities are low, macromolecules do cross the walls of all microvessels at slow but finite rates. Table 9.1 compares estimates of σ and P_d made from the transport of macromolecules between blood and lymph in the dog paw and the cat intestine.[106] Although it is possible that the values given in this table are actually overestimates of the permeability coefficient of macromolecules, there are three important points to note here. First, the values of P_d for serum albumin are more than 3000 times less than the permeabilities of the same vessels to Na^+ and urea. The diffusion coefficient of albumin in aqueous solutions is only 20 times less than those of Na^+ and urea. This means that the diffusion of albumin molecules through microvascular walls is hindered 150 times more than the diffusion of Na^+ ions or urea molecules. Second, compared with the changes seen for small molecules, there is a relatively small decrease in P_d and rise in σ with increases in molecular size. The third point is the similarity of the values of P_d to the same macromolecule at the predominantly continuous endothelium of the dog paw capillaries, and also at the predominantly fenestrated endothelium of vessels in the small intestine. The values of L_P and P_d to small hydrophilic solutes in these two microvascular beds differ by nearly two orders of magnitude. This would seem to be further evidence supporting the belief that the transport pathways through microvascular walls are different for macromolecules from those responsible for water small hydrophilic solutes.

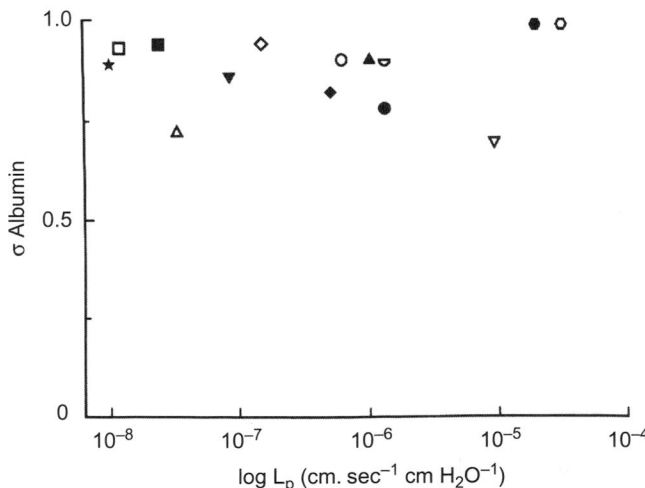

FIGURE 9.7 Relation between the reflection coefficient to serum albumin (σ) and the L_P in different microvascular beds. Each point represents a mean value for one vascular bed: * dog paw; □ dog skeletal muscle; ■ rat skeletal muscle; △ dog lung; ▼ rabbit heart muscle; rat mesentery; □ frog mesentery; ○ cat vary gland; ▲ rat descending vasa recta; ▽ cat small intestine; ● rabbit synovium; ▽ rat ascending vasa recta; ● dog renal glomerulus; ○ rat renal glomerulus. (With permission from ref. [74].)

TABLE 9.1   Reflection Coefficients (σ) and Permeability Coefficients (P_d) to Macromolecules of Selected Molecular Radii (a_{ES}, nm) in Microvascular Beds of Dog Paw and Cat Ileum

			Dog Paw		Cat Ileum
Molecule	a_{ES} (nm)	σ	$P_d \times 10^8$ (cm sec^{-1})	σ	$P_d \times 10^8$ (cm sec^{-1})
Serum albumin	3.55	0.89	1.0–4.7	0.9	3.0
Transferrin	4.3	0.89	6.3	–	–
Haptoglobin	4.6	0.91	3.1	–	1.4
Immunoglobulin	5.6	0.91	3.3	0.95	–
Fibrinogen	10.0	0.94	1.6	0.98	0.7

Renkin, E. M. (1988). Transport pathways and processes. In "Endothelial Cell Biology," 51–68, Simionescu, N., and Simionescu, M., (eds.) Plenum Publishing, New York.[104]

It is possible that some of the values for P_d in Table 9.1 are overestimates and those for σ are underestimates because, in calculating vascular permeability coefficients from plasma to lymph transport, it is assumed that a steady-state has been established between the newly formed filtrate surrounding the microvessels and the ISF entering the lymph. Simple calculations suggest that in some tissues the time taken to reach a steady-state after a change in microvascular filtration rate can be many hours.[78] This can be understood by considering the events that follow an increase in microvascular filtration. A rise in filtration rate is accompanied by a rise in lymph flow and a fall in the concentrations of macromolecules in the newly formed interstitial fluid. It may, however, take several hours before the lymph has the same composition as this new filtrate, and if the lymph is sampled prematurely its concentration of macromolecules will be greater than that in the ultrafiltrate. The lymph flow, however, may reach its new steady-state level before the lymph concentration of macromolecules, and if flux of macromolecules is estimated from values for the product of lymph flow and lymph concentration of macromolecules at this stage, its value will exceed the real rate of transport into the tissue. Not only is macromolecular transport overestimated, but the mean concentration differences across the microvascular walls are also underestimated.[107]

Since 1990, much work has been conducted on the passage of macromolecules through monolayers of culture endothelial cells. In many of these studies, changes in permeability to macromolecules have been investigated, and relative rather than absolute values of permeability coefficients have been reported. In most but not all studies, absolute values for P_d of monolayers of cultured endothelial cells to albumin lie in the range of 10^{-6} cm sec^{-1}, about 100 times greater than the values of P_d to albumin at microvascular walls *in situ*.[9] In a few laboratories, values in the range of 10^{-7} to 10^{-6} cm sec^{-1} have been reported, but even these values are at the very high end of the range

found in microvessel walls *in vivo*. The reasons for this difference are not understood at present. Although studies on cultured endothelial cells have provided essential information of intracellular processes, conclusions from them relating to macromolecular permeability should be viewed with caution.

Like smaller hydrophilic molecules, the microvascular permeability coefficients to macromolecules decrease as molecular size increases, although the decline is considerably less steep. Molecular charge is also more important as molecular size increases. Evidence for the charge-selective nature of ultrafiltration in the renal glomerular capillaries is well-known, but in other microvessels, charge selectivity has been investigated in less detail. Areekul[8] first provided evidence for charge selectivity in systemic capillaries. Working on the isolated perfused rabbit ear, he showed that σ_d to sulfated dextran (which is negatively charged) was always greater than σ_d to neutral dextran of the same molecular weight. Work on single perfused capillaries[2] and on microvascular beds in rat hind limbs also supported the view of microvascular walls as a negatively-charged barrier.

This picture was temporarily confused by studies on the transport of charged macromolecules between plasma and lymph. Negatively-charged macromolecules appeared more rapidly in the lymph and at higher concentration than positively-charged molecules, suggesting a positively-charged barrier. It was then appreciated that the large number of fixed anionic sites in the interstitium (see [49]) would reduce the volume of distribution of the negatively-charged molecules relative to cationic or neutral molecules of the same molecular size. Parker and co-workers[95] showed that the greater volume of distribution of neutral and cationic molecules increased the time for these molecules to reach a steady-state concentration in the ISF. This delay accounted for the apparently more rapid transport of the anionic molecules, a conclusion reinforced by the recent study of

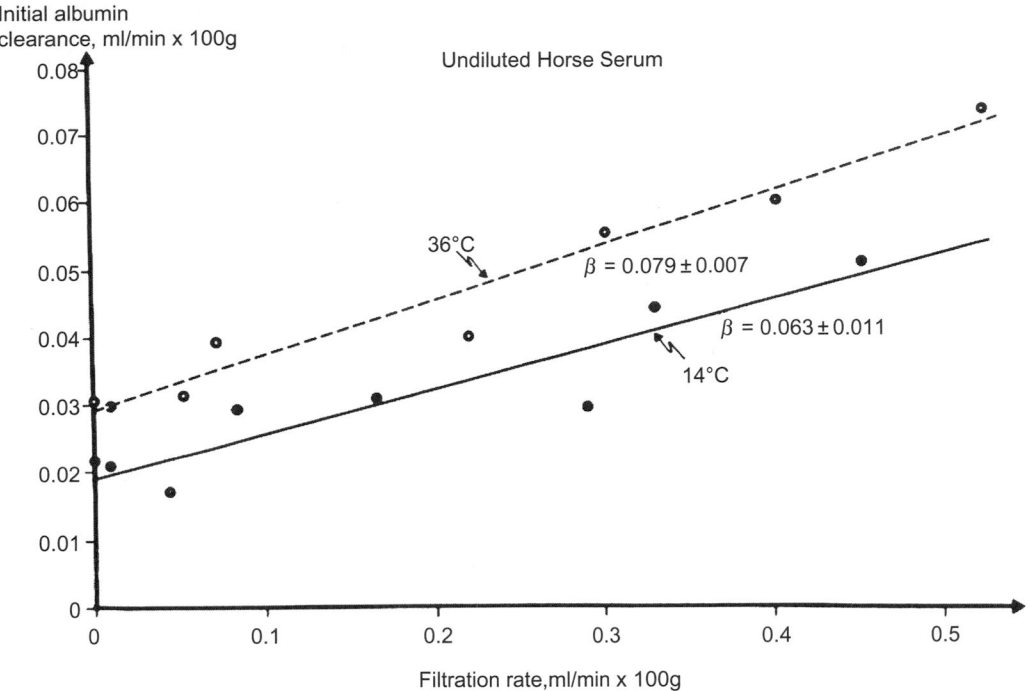

FIGURE 9.8 The clearance of serum albumin from perfusate into tissues of rat skeletal muscle at different filtration rates in experiments conducted at 36°C and 13–15°C. β is the slope of the relation. *(From ref. [107]. With permission.)*

Gyenge and her co-workers[49] on albumin distribution in skin and muscle tissue. With this point clarified, the evidence once again supports the concept of a negatively-charged barrier at microvascular walls hindering the transport of negatively-charged macromolecules greater than 3.0 nm in diameter.

The decline of P_d (and an increase in σ) with an increase in molecular size led to the suggestion that macromolecules cross the endothelium through a system of large pores with radii in the range of 20–40 nm. These pores would be few in number compared with the small pores that act as a pathway for small hydrophilic solutes.[45] Calculations suggest that individual capillaries in skeletal muscle may have an average of only three large pores[81] and with the usual variation between microvessels this indicates that many vessels will have no large pores at all. In a comprehensive review, Taylor and Granger[123] showed that microvascular permeability to macromolecules in different tissues could be described by transport through a population of small pores (radii 3.5–5 nm) and a set of large pores (15–30 nm radii). If large pores do exist, then transport of macromolecules through them will be largely convective, sensitive to microvascular pressure, and increase with fluid filtration rate. Experiments by Rippe and his colleagues[109] showed that this is the case for the transport of labelled albumin from capillaries in skeletal muscle of an isolated

perfused rat limb preparation. Defining the clearance of tracer from the blood into the tissue as the rate of its accumulation divided by the perfusate concentration, they not only showed that clearance of albumin increased linearly with fluid filtration into the tissues, but also that cooling the tissue from 36° to 14°C reduced albumin clearance by only 40%. This was similar to the reduction of the apparent hydraulic permeability of the microvessels. The results of this classic experiment are shown in Figure 9.8. A 40% reduction in L_P would be expected because the filtrate flow through the water-filled channels through the vessel walls is inversely proportional to fluid viscosity, and the viscosity of water at 36°C is approximately 60% of that at 14°C. Because albumin transported is proportional to filtration rate and is reduced in parallel to J_V as the viscosity of water is increased, Rippe and his colleagues[109] concluded that albumin is transport through water-filled channels in the microvascular walls. Figure 9.8 shows that the clearance of albumin from plasma to tissue is significant when fluid filtration is zero. Rippe and his colleagues[109] accounted for this by pointing out that, because the hydrostatic pressure difference across microvascular walls is greater than zero under these conditions, there would still be fluid filtration through the large pores, and consequent transport of albumin because σ_d to plasma proteins here is low. This filtration through the large pores would not be detected in whole tissue, because it would be balanced by an equal and opposite uptake of fluid through the "small pores" where σ_d to plasma proteins is high. As we shall see, the steady uptake of fluid from tissues into capillary blood may peter out and become a low level of filtration in tissues such as muscle.

Ultrastructural Basis of Permeability

Small Hydrophilic Solutes and Water

If the molecular sieving properties of microvascular endothelia are determined by pores or channels of similar dimensions, one might expect to find common structural features in all endothelia that are more frequent in the more permeable vessels. Unfortunately, electron micrographs of endothelia do not reveal an obvious structure that might fill this role.

The endothelia of the vessels with the four highest values of L_P in Figure 9.9 are fenestrated, while those with the seven lowest L_P values are continuous. In some others (e.g., small intestine) values of L_P and σ represent those of a microvascular bed where there are both fenestrated and non-fenestrated vessels. In a quantitative analysis of permeability of fenestrated vessels, Levick and Smaje[66] found that variations in L_P and P_d to small hydrophilic solutes in fenestrated vessels can be correlated with the number of fenestrations per unit area of endothelium. From their analysis they estimated the mean hydraulic conductance per unit increment of area for fenestrations in a variety of microvascular beds as $0.38 \, \mu m.sec^{-1} \, mmHg^{-1}$ ($2.8 \times 10^{-5} \, cm.sec^{-1} \, cmH_2O^{-1}$). This means that the addition of a single fenestration (diameter = 60 nm) to one μm^2 of the endothelium of a skeletal muscle

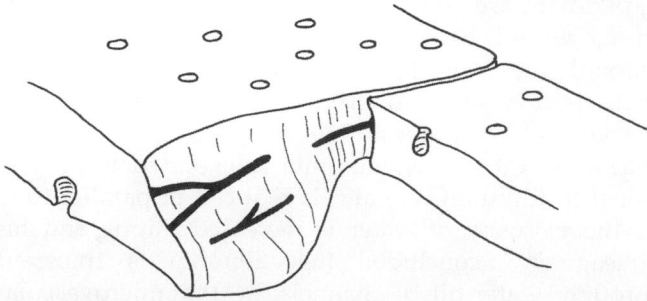

FIGURE 9.9 Diagram of the ultra-structure of an intercellular cleft based on reconstructions from serial ultrathin sections (A&M). Part of the cell in the foreground has been removed to expose the interior of the cleft showing the junctional strands (heavy lines), which correspond to points of close apposition between the cells (tight junctions) in single sections. Lanthanum ions cannot diffuse through the junctional strands, but pass through breaks in the strands. Because there is usually only one continuous strand in the junctions of mesenteric microvessels, each break provides a direct pathway through the cleft.

microvessel increases the L_P of that area approximately 2.6 times. Although fenestrations appear as large pores passing through the endothelium, the fenestrations themselves are much too large to account for molecular sieving and their high reflection coefficients to macromolecules. Molecular sieving is now thought to be achieved by the endothelial glycocalyx, with significant contributions to the hydraulic resistance from the fenestral diaphragms and the basement membrane.

The luminal glycocalyx was proposed by Curry and Michel[30] as the structure responsible for molecular sieving in microvessels with continuous endothelia. Its wide acceptance came after direct observations of the exclusion of macromolecules from the luminal surface of living microvessels had been demonstrated 16 years later by Vink and Duling.[129] Whereas variations in L_P of fenestrated vessels results from variations in the number of fenestrae per unit area of vessel wall, the variations in L_P and P_d to small hydrophilic molecules in vessels with continuous endothelia appears to correlate with the numbers of breaks and complexity of the junctional strands of the intercellular clefts. Although evidence for this concept was available in 1978 from the work of Wissig and Williams,[136] progress was hindered by the beliefs that: (1) the molecular sieve consisted of pores or narrow openings in the tight junction strands; and (2) that the breaks forming a pathway through the junctional strands were too few in number to account for permeability to water and small hydrophilic solutes. Thus, Bundgaard[19] reconstructed the intercellular clefts of rat heart capillaries from ultrathin serial sections and confirmed the presence of a tortuous pathway through the cleft, but rejected this as the route taken by water and small hydrophilic solutes on the grounds that the dimensions of the openings through the junctional strands were too great to filter plasma proteins, and the number of breaks per unit length of junction were too few to account for water and small solute permeabilities.

The question was clarified by Adamson and Michel.[4] Working on frog mesenteric capillaries *in situ*, they perfused single capillaries briefly with solutions containing lanthanum ions, before the tissues were fixed for electron microscopy. Micrographs of serial sections of the walls of the perfused vessels demonstrated that lanthanum ions were only able to pass through the intercellular clefts at breaks in the junctional strands. In a second series of experiments, they measured L_P in individual capillaries *in situ* before fixing the tissue for electron microscopy (EM). The three-dimensional structures of the intercellular clefts of that capillary were then reconstructed from long runs of ultrathin sections of the vessel. Although the breaks only represented 3–10% of the length of the strands, Adamson and Michel[4] used a mathematical model of Parker and colleagues to show that this was more than sufficient to account for permeabilities that were three times greater than those they had measured. The mathematical model provided a rigorous argument for believing that a small break in the junctional strands has a much greater effect upon L_P than its size might suggest. The pressure gradient driving fluid flow through the intercellular cleft is steepest across the tiny distance through the break in the strand, and is much greater than that calculated for the entire cleft. More detailed mathematical models have been developed by Weinbaum and his colleagues[38,55,133] and more recently, Adamson et al.[3] have shown that the fine structure of the tight junction in intercellular clefts of rat mesenteric venules is very similar to that seen in frog vessels.

The L_P of mesenteric vessels is approximately three times greater than the L_P of heart muscle capillaries, which is approximately three times greater than the L_P of capillaries in skeletal muscle. These differences in permeability appear to correlate with the complexity of the pathway through the tight junction in these different types of capillary. This is illustrated in Figure 9.10 for pathways through the intercellular clefts of mesenteric, cardiac, and skeletal muscle capillaries. It seems most probable that the wide variations in permeability to fluid and small hydrophilic solutes that is found in microvessels with continuous endothelium are determined by the complexity of the tight junctional architecture within the intercellular clefts.

As mentioned earlier, the glycocalyx on the luminal surface of the endothelium that covers the entrances to intercellular clefts and fenestrae is now considered to be the barrier to macromolecules. When this was first proposed[30] there was indirect evidence to support it, and more evidence of this kind accumulated during the 1980s.[81] In 1990, Adamson[1] showed that the L_P of single vessels was doubled by brief perfusions of pronase that disrupt the glycocalyx without having any other detectable effects on endothelial ultrastructure

when electron micrographs of the same vessels were inspected. General recognition of the concept of the glycocalyx barrier resulted from some remarkable *in vivo* observations of Vink, Duling, and their colleagues.[52,128,129] Using confocal microscopy to visualize capillaries in rat cremaster muscle, these authors observed that FITC dextrans were excluded from the endothelial cell membranes by a distance of $0.5 \mu m$. The exclusion layer was diminished or even abolished by prolonged exposure to UV light and after perfusion with hyaluronidase. Observations of this kind continue to bolster the view of the glycocalyx as a barrier.

Direct evidence for how its structure acts as a molecular filter comes from the analysis of electron micrographs of glycocalyx.[9,120] Examining very differently prepared specimens, including some made by the rapid freeze-deep etch technique in the absence of chemical fixatives, Squire et al.[120] have concluded that the glycocalyx may be regarded as a regular cubic lattice with side length of 20 nm and a cubic internal space of side length 8 nm (see Figure 9.11). Since serum albumin molecules have diameter of 7–7.2 nm, the dimensions of this internal space are consistent with the glycocalyx acting as the molecular filter in microvascular walls. The initial observations were all made on the glycocalyx of continuous endothelia of the frog, but more recent work has revealed very similar structural features to the glycocalyx covering both continuous and fenestrated endothelia, including that over fenestrae in mammalian microvessels in a wide range of tissues.[9]

In summary, the main permeability pathways through microvascular walls to water and small hydrophilic solutes are located in the fenestrations of fenestrated endothelium, and through the intercellular clefts in vessels with continuous endothelium. In both types of endothelia, the molecular filter that forms the barrier to macromolecules at most microvascular walls is in the luminal glycocalyx of the endothelial cells.

Macromolecules

Just how macromolecules cross the walls of small blood vessels remains a controversial subject. Two apparently conflicting hypotheses emerged from very different lines of evidence more than 40 years ago, and the question of which is more correct has not been finally resolved. As summarized earlier, a purely functional approach has led to the proposal that microvascular walls were penetrated by a small number of "large pores" (30–80 nm in diameter) through which macromolecules pass from plasma to interstitial fluid (ISF).[45] The large pores are estimated to occur so infrequently that their contribution to the P_d of small hydrophilic solutes would be negligible, although they might make a 5 to 10% contribution to L_P. The large pores, however, would be entirely responsible for the permeability of

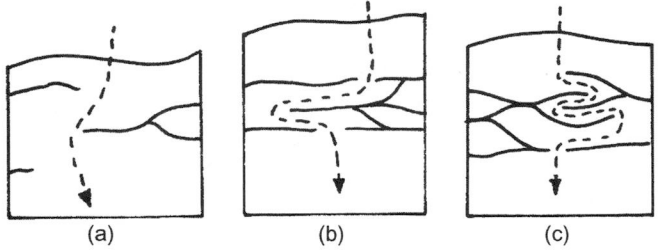

(a)   (b)   (c)

FIGURE 9.10 Variations in the complexity of arrangement of junctional strands in intercellular clefts of microvessels with different hydraulic permeabilities. The dashed lines with arrows indicate potential pathways through the breaks in the strands. (a) Mesenteric capillary (based on [4] and [5]); (b) Cardiac muscle capillary (based on [19]); (c) Skeletal muscle capillary (based on [136]).

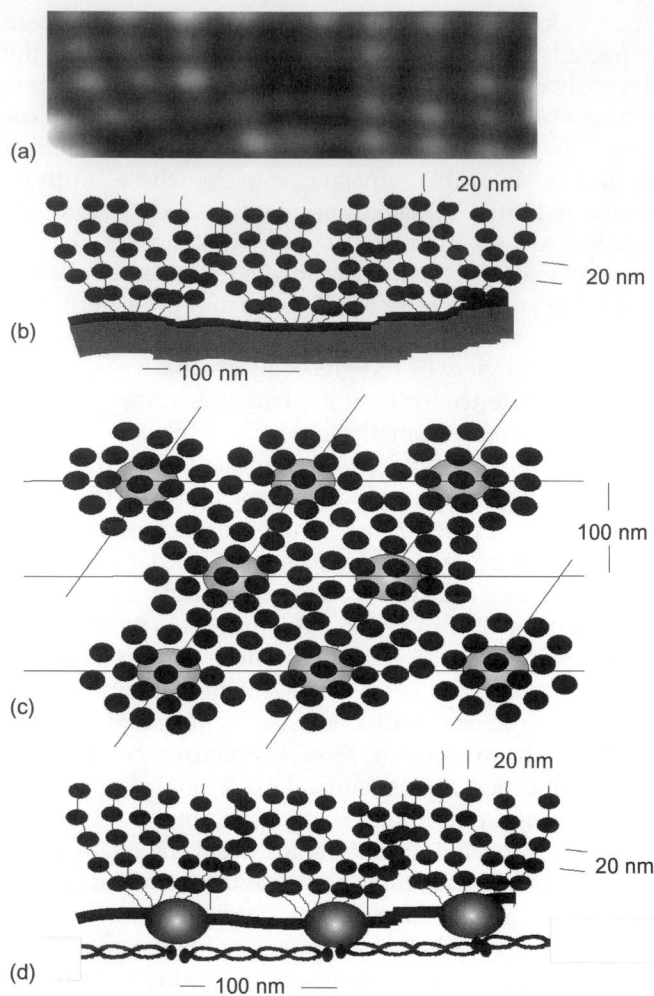

FIGURE 9.11 Models of glycocalyx based on image analysis of electron micrographs. (a) An autocorrelation function of the glycocalyx indicating the underlying regularity of structure with a periodicity of approximately 20 nm both parallel and perpendicular to the cell membrane. (b) A molecular interpretation of (a). It consists of clusters of fibrous strands projecting perpendicular to the luminal cell membrane with periodicity along the strand provided by equally spaced globular proteins. It is suggested that adjacent clusters are separated by approximately 100 nm (consistent with a longer range periodicity) where they linked to the cortical cytoskeleton of the cell. Figures 9.11(c) and (d) show luminal surface and saggital views of the proposed structure. (*From ref. [118].*)

macromolecules, and transport through them would be largely by convection.

The alternative arises from electron microscopy, and proposes that macromolecules cross endothelial cells by transcytosis via the small vesicles.[17,18] After their injection into the blood, electron-dense macromolecules have been found labeling caveolae and small vesicles of the endothelia. Initially it was suggested that the vesicles acted as ferries, equilibrating with

plasma when they opened as caveolae at the luminal surface, then budding off as small vesicles to travel across the cell where they fused with the abluminal surface of the endothelium and equilibrated with the ISF. In the absence of evidence for active transport of macromolecules through microvascular walls, it was suggested that equal fluxes of vesicles occurred in opposite directions across the cells, and the vesicles moved as a result of Brownian motion.[22] The size dependence of macromolecular permeability arises in vesicular transport from volume exclusion of the macromolecules by the walls of the vesicles.[103] The exclusion effect is considerably enhanced if the caveolae and small vesicles are lined with glycocalyx.[67,118]

A detailed examination of the labeling of vesicles with ferritin molecules led to a more complicated model, in which neighboring vesicles periodically fused transiently for long enough for their contents to equilibrate.[23] It was also shown that cooling the tissue inhibited the labeling of vesicles with ferritin.[24] This fusion—fission hypothesis was consistent with the detailed structural analysis showing the vesicles to be arranged in fused clusters communicating with caveolae at either the luminal or the abluminal cell membranes.[20,36] One extreme form of the fusion—fission hypothesis is for the joined vesicles to form channels through the endothelium. Evidence for such vesicular channels has been reported,[119] and these could act as large pores.

Direct evidence for transport by vesicles through normal endothelium has been reported by Wagner and Chen,[130] who demonstrated caveolae emptying terbium label at the abluminal endothelial surface at points distant from intercellular clefts. The demonstration of membrane binding sites for transferrin,[56] insulin,[59] ceruloplasmin,[122] and albumin[42] on endothelia suggested that the vesicle pathway might be involved in receptor mediated transport. A series of papers by Schnitzer and colleagues[113–117] seemed to bolster the idea of vesicular shuttling or fusion—fission as an important mechanism of macromolecular transport through endothelium. The cholesterol scavenger, filipin, removes caveolae in cultured endothelial cells and in rat lung microvessels, and was also reported to reduce the clearance of albumin from perfusate to tissue in the isolated perfused rat lung.[113] It was also reported that N-ethylmaleimide (NEM), which inhibits fusion processes of vesicles and vacuoles in yeast, in synaptic vesicles, and in transport vesicles operating between the Golgi stacks and the endoplasmic reticulum, inhibited transendothelial transport of macromolecules in microvessels of mouse heart and rat lung.[114] Schnitzer and colleagues[117] have reported that endothelial caveolae from rat lung capillaries can bud away from their anchorage in the presence of GTP and extracts of cytosol. Critical studies by Rippe and his colleagues, however, have cast serious doubt on the relevance of these findings to macromolecular permeability.[21,111] They found that both filipin and NEM increased albumin transport in the isolated perfused rat lung. NEM was found to reduce σ to albumin. Reducing the tissue temperature from 35° to 22°C, however, lowered both albumin clearance and $L_P S$ in rough proportion to increased water viscosity. NEM also increased both albumin clearance and $L_P S$ in the microcirculation of rat muscle,[21] and increased pre-capillary vascular resistance in both rat lung and rat muscle. The authors suggested that increased resistance would reduce microvascular perfusion, and this could account for the earlier studies where NEM appeared to reduce albumin clearance. Rippe and colleagues have recently reviewed the controversy,[110] and provided further less direct evidence against endothelial transcytosis of macromolecules from studies of peritoneal dialysis.[112]

Rippe's arguments for convective transport of macromolecules via large pores are convincing. At present it seems that whereas there is strong evidence favoring convective transport of macromolecules (i.e., the large pore hypothesis), evidence that transcytosis makes a significant contribution to transendothelial transport of macromolecules is lacking. It is possible that the caveolae/small vesicle system is important for the transport of specific molecules. The blood–tissue transport of insulin, for example, appears to be anomalous for a protein of its size,[53] and is more consistent with receptor-mediated transport.[59] As mentioned already, the large pores carrying most macromolecules could be trans-endothelial channels formed by the fusion of vesicles. At normal tissue temperatures they might be continually forming and re-forming, accounting for the progressive labeling of the vesicle system with tracer macromolecules. On cooling the tissues, the open channels would remain open, but no new channels would form, consistent with both the effects of cooling on albumin transport, and the reduced vesicle labeling reported by electron microscopists.

The question of whether macromolecules are transported mainly by convection through large pores in the walls of microvessels in normal healthy tissue has implications for our understanding of fluid exchange between the blood and the tissues.

THE EXCHANGE OF FLUID AND SOLUTES BY CONVECTION AND DIFFUSION THROUGH MICROVASCULAR WALLS

Coupling of Fluid and Solute Transport during Ultrafiltration

In most tissues, ISF is formed by the ultrafiltration of plasma, a process that is driven by the greater hydrostatic pressure inside the microvessels than in the surrounding tissues. As fluid begins to be filtered through the vessel walls, its composition is determined by the rates at which the different plasma solutes can move with the filtrate by convection and diffusion. If one considers the transport of a solute past a point at a distance x cm along a pathway within the microvascular wall, and of cross-sectional area, A, the net flux of solute, J_S, can be described by adding together the contributions of convection and diffusion. Thus from Eqs. (9.4)–(9.6):

Total transport = Convective transport + Diffusive transport

$$J_S = J_V(1 - \sigma_f)C + D'A(-dC/dx) \tag{9.8}$$

where C is the solute concentration of the solute at x, D' is solute diffusion coefficient, and $(-)$ is the direction of the concentration gradient (from plasma to ISF). The first term on the right hand side of Eq. (9.8) is the convective component of transport, and the second term is the diffusive component. The concentration gradient that is responsible for net transport by diffusion is equal to the solute concentration difference between the plasma and the ISF, divided by the length of the pathway through the wall only when fluid filtration is zero and there is no convection of solute. When net fluid movements are present they distort the concentration gradients in the channels within the vessel walls. Once a steady-state is established so the solute flux, J_S, is the same at all points along the diffusion pathway (i.e., the rate of solute entry equals the rate of its exit from the channels), then the extent of the distortion can be inferred by integrating Eq. (9.8). This leads to a form of the Patlak expression[96] which here relates J_S through an area of vessel wall, A_m, to the plasma concentration of solute, C_p, and the concentration emerging from the vessel walls into the peri-capillary ISF, C_i:

$$\frac{J_S}{A_m} = \frac{J_V}{A_m}(1 - \sigma_f)\frac{(C_p - C_i e^{-Pe})}{(1 - e^{-Pe})} \tag{9.9}$$

where

$$Pe = \frac{J_V(1 - \sigma_f)}{P_d A_m}$$

Pe is a dimensionless number, called the Péclet number, which expresses the ratio of solute velocities by convection and diffusion, P_d being the diffusional permeability coefficient. Curry[26] has recast Eq. (9.9) in a form that allows the convective and diffusive components of transport to be recognized:

$$\frac{J_S}{A_m} = \frac{J_V}{A_m}(1 - \sigma_f)C_p + P_d(C_p - C_i)\left(\frac{Pe}{e^{Pe} - 1}\right) \tag{9.10}$$

Equation (9.10) is analogous to Eq. (9.8), with the first term on the right-hand-side describing convective transport, and the second term describing diffusion. The expression $Pe/(e^{Pe} - 1)$ describes the effects of solute convection upon the mean concentration gradient within the diffusion pathway by convective flow in the same direction as net diffusion.

Earlier it was noted that ultrafiltration through microvascular walls is driven by the hydrostatic pressure difference, ΔP, between the plasma inside the vessels and the surrounding ISF. If, initially, all the solutes were at the same concentration in plasma and ISF, the filtration rate per unit area of vessel wall (J_V) is $L_P A_m \Delta P$, as in Eq. (9.2). The process of ultrafiltration, however, soon leads to differences in solute concentration between the plasma and the newly formed ISF, as a consequence of the differences in σ and the Péclet numbers of the different solutes. These concentration differences give rise to osmotic pressure differences that oppose ΔP. In this way, the rate of fluid filtration per unit area of vessel wall becomes the product of L_P and the difference between ΔP and the sum of all the osmotic pressures opposing it. Thus:

$$\frac{J_V}{A} = L_P\left(\Delta P - \sum_n \sigma_{d_n}\Delta\Pi_n\right) \qquad (9.11)$$

where $\sigma_{dn}\Delta\Pi_n$ is the effective osmotic pressure set up across the vessel wall by the nth solute.

Equation (9.9) can be used to calculate the contribution of different plasma solutes to the osmotic term in Eq. (9.11). When the filtration rate is steady, C_i becomes equal to the ratio of the rate of solute transport to the filtration rate i.e., $C_i = J_S/J_V$. Combining this relation with Eq. (9.9) leads to the following expressions for C_i and $\Delta C = C_p - C_i$:

$$C_i = \frac{J_S}{J_V} = C_P \frac{(1 - \sigma_f)}{(1 - \sigma_f e^{-Pe})} \qquad (9.12)$$

and:

$$\Delta C = C_p - C_i = C_p\sigma_f \frac{(1 - e^{-Pe})}{(1 - \sigma_f e^{-Pe})} \qquad (9.13)$$

Differences in concentration (and hence differences in osmotic pressure) can only be sustained for those solutes that have low permeabilities. If permeability is high, concentration gradients are dissipated by diffusion, and for differences of concentration and osmotic pressure to be maintained both reflection coefficient and Péclet number of the solute must be high. The implication of this is that when Pe is zero (e.g., when $J_V = 0$) the concentration differences will dissipate, even for those solutes that have very low permeabilities.[75]

The message of Eq. (9.13) can be appreciated by evaluating Pe for urea and serum albumin during slow filtration (at a rate of $2 \times 10^{-7} \text{cm}^{-2}\text{sec}^{-1}$) through the walls of skeletal muscle capillaries.[75] For urea, P_d is 2.7×10^{-5} cm sec^{-1} and σ is 0.1, so that Pe is 0.0074; for serum albumin with P_d at 10^{-8} cm sec^{-1} and σ at 0.95, Pe is 1. Thus, C_i would be more than 99.9% C_p for urea, and ΔC is therefore 0.1% C_p, so that urea makes a negligible contribution to $\sigma_{ds}\Delta\Pi$ (about 0.1 cmH$_2$O). For serum albumin, however, C_i is only 7.6% of C_p and ΔC is 92.4% C_p accounting for the major contribution of albumin to $\sigma_{ds}\Delta\Pi$ (about 19 cmH$_2$O). Similar calculations can be made for microvessels in most other tissues (the exception being those of the brain), and it is therefore the osmotic pressure of the macromolecules that constitute the osmotic pressure difference that acts as a break on fluid filtration and holds the plasma in the vascular system. The osmotic pressure of the macromolecules of plasma and other body fluids is often referred to as the *oncotic pressure*.

Equations (9.12) and (9.13) indicate the close coupling between microvascular fluid exchange and microvascular solute permeability. The concentration of plasma proteins in the ISF (and hence the ISF oncotic pressure) is almost an inverse function of ultrafiltration rate. This relation is of considerable significance in interpreting microvascular fluid exchange, and its consequences are discussed further below.

Fluid Movements through Microvascular Walls

General Approximation: Starling Forces

The principle that fluid is held in the vascular system by a balance of hydrostatic and oncotic pressures across capillary walls was recognized over a century ago by Ernest Starling.[121] Since then it has been demonstrated to apply in a large number of vascular beds in different animals, including humans, using a variety of techniques. It remains the basis for understanding fluid exchange between the blood and the tissues.[65,77,79,81,83]

For most purposes, Eq. (9.11) can be written in a simplified form, in which the effective osmotic pressure term becomes the effective oncotic pressure difference across microvascular walls, $\sigma_m(\Pi_c - \Pi_i)$, i.e.:

$$\frac{J_V}{A} = L_P(\Delta P - \sigma_m\Delta\Pi) = L_P[(P_c - P_i) - \sigma_m(\Pi_c - \Pi_i)]$$

$$(9.14)$$

The reflection coefficient, σ_m, refers to the mean (or effective) reflection coefficient of microvascular walls to macromolecules and the pressures, P_c, P_i, Π_c, and Π_i are often referred to as the *Starling pressures*.

Equation (9.14) is a clear statement of Starling's principle of fluid movement between the plasma and the ISF. Under suitable experimental conditions it is possible to compare fluid movements through microvascular walls when ΔP is varied as $\Delta \Pi$ is held constant. This has been achieved most unambiguously in single perfused microvessels (e.g., Figure 9.12). Essentially similar results have been obtained by less direct methods in perfused vascular beds[93]; see [79] for review).

Experiments such as that shown in Figure 9.12 reveal several general features of the permeability of microvascular walls.[74] The linearity of the relation between fluid flux and pressure suggests that the pathways conducting fluid through the vessel walls are not stretched or deformed over this range of pressures. If the channels were stretched and widened, their conductivity, L_P, would be raised and this would be seen as an increase in the slope of the relation between J_V/A and ΔP (which is L_P) with increasing pressure. Furthermore, the value of L_P is the same during fluid absorption (negative values of J_V/A) as it is during filtration, indicating that there is no significant rectification of flow within the conducting channels. (With less careful experimental design, however, rectification of flow may appear to occur.) A third feature of importance is the effect of changing the concentration of macromolecules in the perfusate. The consequent change in oncotic pressure results in a parallel shift of the relation between J_V/A and fluid pressure. The magnitude of the displacement is equivalent to 70% of the perfusate oncotic pressure, as measured in a membrane osmometer. This indicates that σ_d is greater than or at least equal to 0.7 in this vessel. Overall, the experiment reveals that the permeability coefficients L_P and σ_m, can be regarded as independent of the Starling forces. Although permeability can be modulated, a background of constant permeability provides a basis to discuss fluid movements that occur physiologically as a result of changes in the Starling pressures.

Changes in Microvascular Pressure

Although textbooks so often say that P_c has a mean value that approximates to plasma oncotic pressure, this is true only for systemic microvessels of small mammals, and for systemic pressures at heart level in larger mammals. In the pulmonary microcirculation of all mammals investigated, mean P_c is more often closer to a third of the value of plasma oncotic pressure. In larger mammals, such as humans, mean P_c varies with the vertical height between the vessel and the heart. When a human subject lies horizontally, mean P_c in most systemic microcirculations may approximate to plasma oncotic pressure, but as soon as the subject sits or stands, P_c in vessels below the heart increases, and that in vessels above the heart decreases. The changes in P_c above and below the heart are not symmetrical; the decrease in P_c in vessels in the upper parts of the body is checked as the local venous pressure falls below atmospheric and the veins collapse. Measurements of P_c in skin suggest that once this happens, P_c becomes independent of position.[60] Below the heart, arterial and venous pressures increase in proportion to their vertical distance beneath the heart providing the subject remains still, and mean P_c in the feet also increases but to a lesser extent than arterial and venous pressures (see Figure 9.13). Movements of the legs increase venous return from the feet, reducing the local venous pressures and P_c.

The smaller increase in P_c than arterial and venous pressure in tissues below heart level (see Figure 9.13) suggests how P_c may be regulated. For blood to flow through a vascular bed there must be a lower pressure in the veins than in the capillaries, and in the capillaries than in the arteries. The fall in pressure from arteries to capillaries, $P_a - P_c$, is the product of the blood flow from arteries to capillaries, and the resistance of the vessels between them (i.e., the pre-capillary resistance, r_a). Similarly, the fall in pressure between the capillaries to the veins, $P_c - P_v$, is the product of the blood flow and the post-capillary resistance, r_v. Providing the blood flows into and out of the circulation are equal, P_c can be related to P_a and P_v through r_a and r_v:

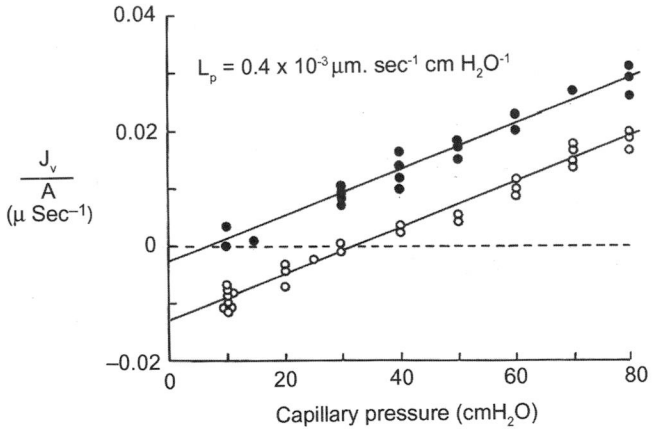

FIGURE 9.12 **Relation between net fluid movement per unit area of microvascular wall (JV/A) and capillary pressure in a single frog mesenteric capillary perfused with Ringer's solution containing high (o) and low (●) concentrations of serum albumin.** Positive values of JV/A indicate fluid filtration from vessel to tissue and negative values show movement from tissue into vessel. (*From ref. [72]. With permission.*)

$$\frac{(P_a - P_a)}{(P_c - P_v)} = \frac{r_a}{r_v}$$

which can be rearranged in the form derived by Pappenheimer and Soto-Rivera[93]:

$$P_c = \frac{P_a + P_v(r_a/r_v)}{1 + r_a/r_v} \qquad (9.15)$$

Equation (9.15) reveals how the value of P_c between P_a and P_v is determined by the ratio of r_a/r_v, and since local blood flow is regulated in most vascular beds by alterations in r_a, it also suggests how P_c might be regulated. Even if P_a and P_v remain constant, arteriolar vasodilatation, which reduces r_a/r_v, increases P_c and enhances fluid filtration. Arteriolar vasoconstriction, which increases r_a/r_v, reduces P_c consequently promoting fluid absorption from the tissues. A sudden loss of a substantial volume of blood (e.g., by hemorrhage or blood donation) is followed by intensive vasoconstriction, increasing r_a/r_v and leading to a shift of fluid from ISF to plasma (largely in skin and muscle).

It is seen as a fall in hematocrit, and is usually complete within 30 minutes of the cessation of bleeding.[91]

In most tissues a local increase in P_v is associated with constriction of the local arterioles, increasing r_a/r_v and tending to minimize the increase in P_c. This phenomenon has been called the veno-arteriolar response, and appears to be a local response dependent on the presence, but not the central connections, of the sympathetic nerves.[51] It is largely responsible for the smaller increase in P_c than either P_a or P_v in the skin of the human foot as the subject moves from a supine to a standing position (Figure 9.13). Although P_c has to remain above P_v, it approaches P_v very closely when the subject is standing still. As soon as the subject moves, P_v falls. With an efficient muscle pump acting on the veins in the leg, P_v may be reduced from 120 to 130 cmH$_2$O when the person is standing still, to less than 30 cmH$_2$O in within a few seconds of starting to walk, and P_c presumably is reduced.

Landis[61] argued that P_c was the most variable of the Starling pressures in human subjects, drawing attention to the large changes in its value that followed changes in posture. P_c is also the one Starling pressure that can be regulated quickly in parallel with the local blood flow, inducing fluid shifts between the circulation and the ISF that appear to improve the chances of the organism's survival.

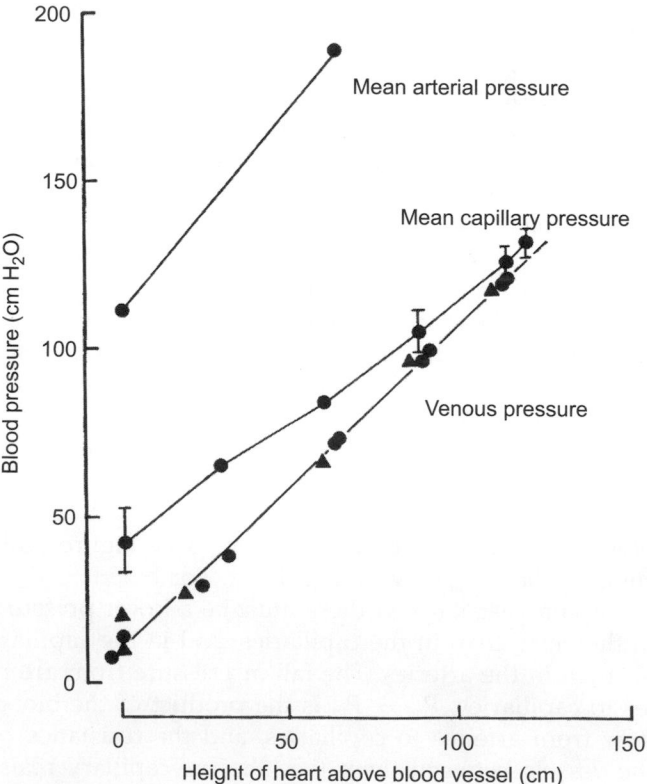

FIGURE 9.13 Relation between the local blood pressure in the feet and the height of the heart above the feet in two normal subjects in supine, sitting, and standing positions. Mean values for capillary pressure were based on direct measurements (by micropuncture) of capillary loops in the nail fold of the great toe. *(From ref. [62]. With permission.)*

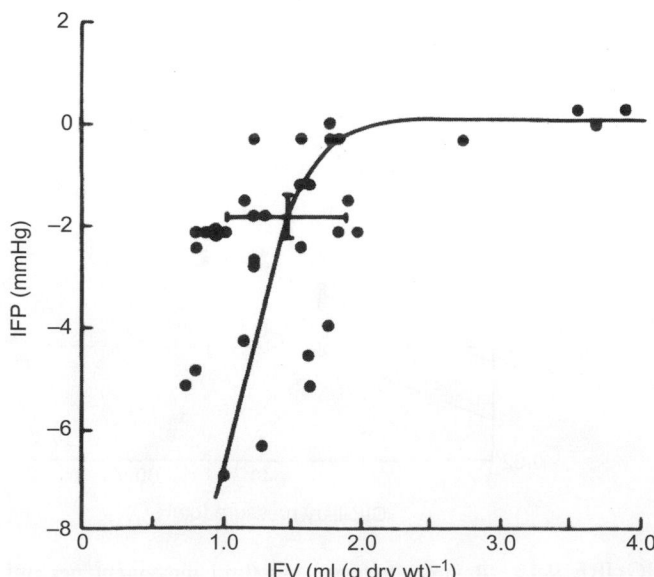

FIGURE 9.14 The effects of changes in interstitial fluid volume (IFV) upon the interstitial fluid pressure (IFP) in cat skin. Mean and standard deviations represent control values. IFV was varied by intravenous infusion of saline or by peritoneal dialysis. *(From ref. [131]. With permission.)*

Plasma Oncotic Pressure

Although reduced levels of circulating plasma proteins may be associated with edema, the steady-state relations between edema formation and plasma protein concentration are complicated by adjustments of microvascular pressures, and of ISF hydrostatic and oncotic pressures.[90] There is evidence to suggest that the oncotic pressure difference may be adjusted by atrial natriuretic peptide regulating the transport of proteins from plasma to ISF.[31,127]

In normal healthy subjects, oncotic pressure of the arterial plasma may be regarded as constant in the short-term. The plasma oncotic pressure, however, may increase considerably as blood flows through the microcirculation under conditions where the filtration rate becomes a significant fraction of the plasma flow. In most microvascular beds, L_P is too low for this to be significant, but it does occur in the renal glomerular capillaries, where L_P is very high,[16] and in the microcirculation of the feet of human subjects during prolonged standing or sitting, where P_c is high and plasma flow is very low.[40,87,89] In the glomerular capillaries it underlies the dependence of glomerular filtration rate upon renal blood flow (see Chapter on Glomerular Filtration).

Interstitial Hydrostatic Pressure

Before 1963, P_i was believed to approximate to atmospheric pressure in non-edematous tissues and steady fluid filtration, which expanded ISF volume, was thought to increase P_i proportionately. In this way, the increase in P_i would reduce the difference in hydrostatic pressure across microvascular walls, and so limit the rate of filtration protecting the tissues from edema.

The pioneering work of Guyton and colleagues showed that P_i of subcutaneous tissues and many others was 4 to 7 mmHg below atmospheric pressure.[46,47,48] After much controversy, sub-atmospheric or negative values for P_i in non-edematous tissues have been confirmed using a series of different techniques. There is some variation from tissue to tissue, most negative values being found in the lung and positive values being found in the kidney with the subcutaneous tissues of many mammals being in the range of -0.5 to -2.0 mmHg.[10,99]

At an early stage in his investigations, Guyton[47] showed that expansion of the ISF by filtration from the microvasculature quickly raised P_i to atmospheric pressure. Further expansion of the ISF volume, however, was accompanied by little change of P_i in most tissues. These relations between P_i and ISF volume have been extended and confirmed by others (see Figure 9.14 and [134]). Whereas there have been minor differences in some of the absolute values reported by different investigators, the general picture of a steep relation between P_i and ISF volume (low interstitial compliance) at normal and at low ISF volumes, and a flat relation between P_i and ISF volume (high compliance) when ISF volume is slightly expanded and P_i has risen to atmospheric pressure, has been widely confirmed (see Figure 9.14). The renal interstitium appears to be an exception to this general pattern. In the kidney, P_i is $+4$ to $+6$ mmHg, and increases and decreases linearly with ISF volume.[41] It has been argued that, in the kidney, P_i does fulfill the role of limiting the expansion of ISF volume, and promotes the uptake of fluid and solutes (including macromolecules) by the microcirculation.[10,69,70] For a more detailed discussion of the role of P_i in trans-capillary fluid exchange the reader is referred to the recent review of Reed and Rubin.[100]

Interstitial Oncotic Pressure

Measurements of ISF oncotic pressure are usually global values for a particular tissue. The values of importance for microvascular fluid exchange, however, are those for the newly formed ISF in contact with the abluminal surface of the ultrafilter within walls of the microvessels. Here, we have to be guided by theory. Equations (9.12) and (9.13) argue that if microvascular permeability of a solute is finite, the concentration of that solute in the ISF ultimately depends on its permeability and the rate of fluid filtration through the microvascular walls. If the Péclet number is zero (net filtration = 0), the concentration of a protein such as serum albumin in the interstitial fluid, C_i, will rise until it equals its plasma concentration. In the presence of net filtration from plasma to ISF, the concentration of plasma protein in the newly formed ISF will fall, reaching a plateau when C_i approximates to $C_p(1 - \sigma_f)$, as shown in the upper panel of Figure 9.15. The effective osmotic pressure difference exerted by albumin (and other large plasma protein molecules) across microvascular walls ($\sigma \Delta \Pi$) under conditions of steady fluid filtration varies with the filtration rate. This variation is shown in the lower panel of Figure 9.15. It can be estimated as follows:

$$\sigma \Delta \Pi = \sigma(\Pi_c - \Pi_i) = \sigma_d RT(\gamma_c C_c - \gamma_i C_i) \qquad (9.16)$$

The symbols γ_c and γ_i are the osmotic coefficients of albumin at its concentrations in capillary plasma and ISF. If they are approximated by a single value γ, Eq. (9.16) can be developed using Eq. (9.13)[75]:

$$\sigma_d \Delta \Pi = \sigma_d RT \gamma(C_c - C_i) = \sigma_d \sigma_f RTC_c \left(\frac{1 - e^{-Pe}}{1 - \sigma_f e^{-Pe}} \right)$$

$$(9.17)$$

Equation (9.17) provides an explicit statement of the effective osmotic pressure difference exerted by a plasma protein across microvascular walls in terms of the filtration rate and through the Péclet number, the permeability coefficients P_d and σ_f of the vessel walls to the protein. Increases in J_V increase Pe and as e^{-Pe} approaches zero, $\sigma_d \Delta\Pi$ approaches a limit of $\sigma_d \sigma_f \Pi_c$, or approximately $\sigma^2 \Pi_c$.

Both P_i and π_i change[75] with fluid filtration rate, and since they themselves influence J_V, after a step change in P_c, an initial change of J_V is likely to be followed by a further changes as P_i and Π_i adjust to their new steady-state values. Thus, we should expect there to be differences between the initial transient changes in J_V and the steady-state values, and we shall consider these differences next.

Transient and Steady-State Fluid Movements through Microvascular Walls

Figure 9.16 shows the results of an experiment on a single mesenteric capillary perfused with a Ringer solution containing serum albumin and the macromolecule Ficoll 70.[84] Both the immediate (transient) and steady-state values of fluid filtration were measured following step changes in capillary pressure. The transient changes (open circles) were measured after the vessel had been perfused at high pressure (35–50 cmH$_2$O) for several minutes, and then the pressure lowered to a predetermined value. The steady-state measurements (solid circles) were made after the vessel had been perfused for several minutes at that pressure, and preliminary measurement suggested a steady-state had been achieved. The transient values of J_V/A are related to P_c in the same linear fashion predicted by the standard Starling equation (Eq. (9.14)), and as shown by a similar experiment in Figure 9.12. This is the expected relation between ΔP and J_V/A when ΔP is varied and $\sigma_d \Delta\Pi$ remains constant. The steady-state measurements (solid circles) can be described by a non-linear (hockey stick) curve which can be predicted using Eq. (9.17) to calculate $\sigma_d \Delta\Pi$.

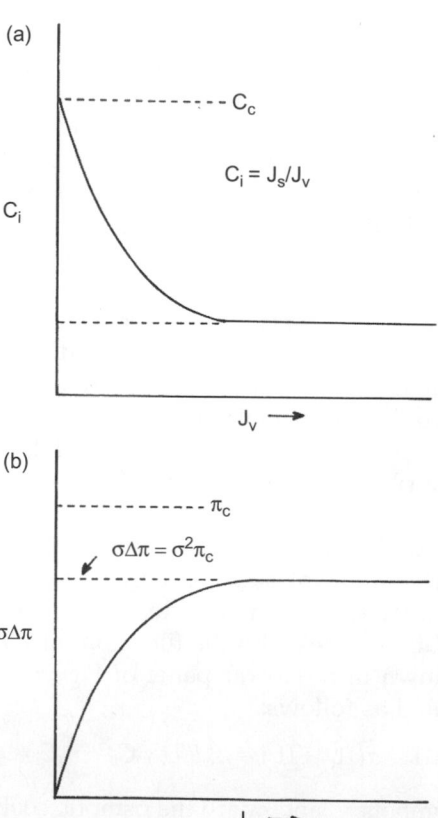

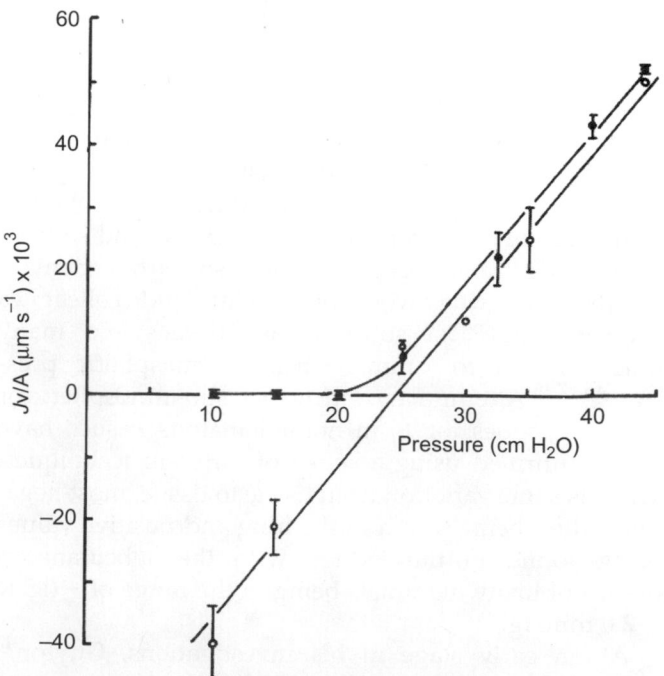

FIGURE 9.15   (a) Steady-state relations between the concentration of proteins (C_i) in capillary ultrafiltrate and the capillary filtration rate, J_V. The limiting value of C_i is $C_c(1 - \sigma)$ where C_c is the concentration of protein in the capillary. (b) Steady-state relations between the effective oncotic pressure across the walls of the microvessel ($\sigma\Delta\Pi$) consequent to changes in C_i and J_V. The oncotic pressure of the plasma, Π_c, is indicated as is the maximum value of $\sigma\Delta\Pi$. *(From [77]. With permission.)*

FIGURE 9.16   The relations between fluid filtration and absorption (J_V/A) and microvascular pressure in a single frog mesenteric microvessel under transient (o) and steady-state (●) conditions. Perfusate oncotic pressure was 32 cmH$_2$O. The oncotic pressure difference was the same at all values of J_V/A under transient conditions, but varied with J_V/A in the steady-state in the way indicated in Figure 9.15b. Note that absorption of fluid from the tissues is seen only under transient conditions. *(From ref. [82]. With permission.)*

Here, Π_c is constant, but Π_i varies with J_V, which changes Pe.

When P_c is greater than the effective osmotic pressure opposing filtration, both transient and steady-state values lie close together, and the linear portion of the steady-state relation at these higher values of ΔP has a slope of L_P, and is described by the following expression:

$$\frac{J_V}{A} = L_P(\Delta P - \sigma_m^2 \Pi_c) \qquad (9.18)$$

At low values of P_c the transient and steady-state values of J_V/A deviate considerably with no fluid uptake from the tissue occurring under steady-state conditions. Not only are these results consistent with the theoretical picture, but analysis of the steady-state data also allows estimates to be made for both σ_m and P_d (the macromolecular permeability), which agree quantitatively with other determinations.[84] One surprising observation made during the measurement of the steady-state relations on single mesenteric capillaries was the relatively short time (2–5 minutes) required for a new steady-state to be established after capillary pressure had been changed.[84] This drew attention to the importance of the value of Π_i in the small volume of ISF in contact microvessel, and the relative lack of importance of the value of Π_i for the ISF of the entire tissue.

Figure 9.17 summarizes the transient and steady-state changes in fluid filtration and absorption in a microvessel of constant permeability, perfused at a rate sufficient to keep the plasma oncotic pressure

constant. The dashed lines are drawn with a slope = L_P for the vessel. The solid line indicates the steady-state relations between J_V/A and ΔP. If P_c initially has a value, A, which is less than the plasma oncotic pressure, and remains constant for long enough for a steady-state to be established (at point T), a subsequent increase in P_c from A to B leads to a rapid increase in filtration (T→W). J_V then attenuates (to X), as Π_i is reduced and P_i increases. If P_c is then returned to A, fluid uptake from the tissues occurs (X→S), and the rate of absorption diminishes as Π_i increases returning J_V to its initial level of T.

In the pulmonary microcirculation, mean values of P_c are usually well below Π_c, and fluid movements fluctuate around a point half-way along the flat part of the steady-state relationship. Small changes in P_c lead to changes in filtration or absorption that are rapidly checked as a new steady-state is established. So long as $P_c - P_i$ is greater than $\Pi_c - \Pi_i$, there is a low level of fluid filtration into the tissues that is balanced by lymph drainage.

The steady-state analysis predicts that when the exchange vessels are finitely permeable to macromolecules, and there is no source of ISF other than the ultrafiltrate from these vessels, fluid absorption from the tissues is transient, and low levels of fluid filtration from blood to the tissues maintain the differences in oncotic pressures between the plasma and the ISF. The sustained levels of fluid filtration are matched by lymphatic drainage from the tissue, so that ISF volume remains approximately constant. Providing that the time-averaged mean P_c in most tissues approximates to the plasma oncotic pressure, this picture is consistent with blood–tissue fluid balance. It is not consistent, however, with the popular representation of the Starling Principle, which depicts fluid being filtered into the tissues from the arterial end of a capillary and absorbed from the tissues at its venous end. Quite apart from the lack of evidence for this picture, the steady-state analysis predicts that rising concentrations of macromolecules around the venular regions of the vessel would bring absorption to a halt. The experimental and theoretical arguments against this textbook picture of the filtering-absorbing capillary have been forcefully expressed in a series of publications by Levick.[62,63]

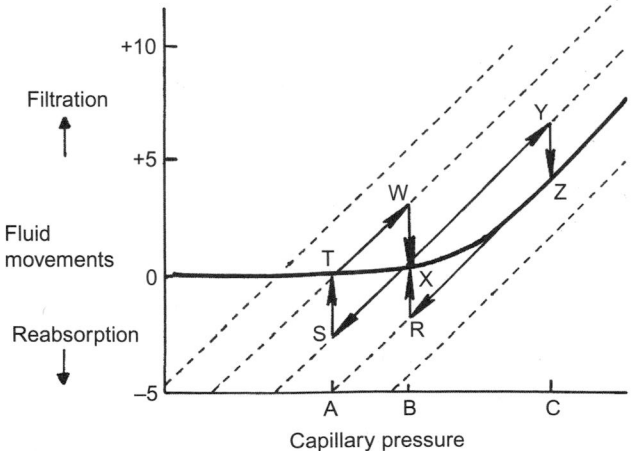

FIGURE 9.17 Transient and steady-state relations between fluid movements and microvascular (capillary) pressure. The dashed lines have slopes equal to L_P. The arrowed straight lines show transient changes in fluid movements with changes in pressure. The OTXZ (heavy line) represents the steady-state relation between J_V/A and capillary pressure. (*From ref. [81]. With permission.*)

Steady-State Fluid Uptake into Microvessels Associated with Absorptive Epithelia

Continuous uptake of fluid into the microcirculation does occur in tissues such as intestinal mucosa, the post-glomerular capillaries of the renal cortex, and the ascending vasa recta of the renal medulla. Here, however, the bulk of the ISF is not formed by filtration from the capillaries, but by the secretion of protein free fluid from the adjacent epithelia. In intestinal mucosa and in renal cortex, the large fluid uptake from the ISF into the blood capillaries is accompanied by a very much smaller flow of ISF into the lymphatics.[43,44] Although only a fraction of the fluid is absorbed from the ISF, the lymph flow is sufficient to clear proteins and keep their ISF concentrations low.

The renal medulla, however, has no lymphatics and special mechanisms appear to operate here. The continuous addition of protein free fluid into the medullary ISF is matched by the uptake of fluid into the ascending vasa recta (AVR). The AVR have relatively low σ to plasma proteins (0.7 to albumin). This allows the absorbed fluid to carry protein from the ISF into the blood. The uptake of labeled proteins from medullary ISF into the blood has been demonstrated directly,[125] and estimates of P_c, P_i, Π_c, and Π_i in and around the AVR indicate that these favor fluid uptake.[70] Theoretical studies have supported this "bootstrap" mechanism, whereby plasma proteins are carried up their own concentration gradient by the osmotic flow that arises from that same gradient.[70,131,138] In addition, unusual structural features of the ascending vasa recta, and the low compliance of the renal interstitium, ensure that fluid uptake is maintained even if Π_i increases. The low compliance means that P_i is high, and rises if ISF volume expands to levels that may equal or even exceed the pressure in the ascending vasa recta. When this occurs the vessels do not collapse as there are fine projections from their endothelial cells, which are inserted into the basal laminae of neighboring vessels and tubules, holding them open.[69] Because L_P of these fenestrated vessels is very high, an increment of P_i over P_c of only 1.0 to 2.5 cm H_2O is sufficient to account for the clearance of all fluid entering the medullary ISF from the loops of Henle and collecting ducts.[69] A more detailed discussion of the special features of the extra-glomerular renal microcirculation is given elsewhere in this volume.

Starling Pressures and Local Lymph Flow

In most tissues, ISF volume is maintained by a low level of filtration from the microcirculation being matched by an equal efflux of fluid from the tissue in the lymph. From this, one would anticipate that the magnitude of the lymph flow from a tissue could be estimated from the mean Starling pressures, the L_P, and the exchange surface area of the microcirculation. In an incisive review, Levick[62] pointed out that where the mean Starling pressures have been measured, they predict much greater filtration rates

than the lymph flow and the lymph protein concentration would indicate. From 15 sets of data, he estimated P_0, the net pressure opposing filtration from the following relation:

$$P_0 = \sigma_m(\Pi_c - \Pi_i) + P_i \qquad (9.19)$$

When values of P_0 are compared with direct measurements of pressure in post-capillary venules, P_{Vc}, it is found that P_{Vc} is nearly always greater than P_0, and in several cases P_{Vc} exceeds P_0 by 5 to 10 mmHg (Table 9.2). Net driving pressures for filtration of this magnitude would be expected to result in high lymph flows, but in most of the tissues concerned (e.g., subcutaneous tissue, muscle, and mesentery), the basal lymph flows are so low that they are difficult to measure.

To account for these discrepancies, Levick[62] suggested that vasomotion, the spontaneous contraction and relaxation of arteriolar smooth muscle, might be responsible for large variations in P_c, and that P_c measurements tended to be made in vessels where there was brisk flow and a higher than average P_c. The few direct estimates of P_c during vasomotion, however, suggest that the fluctuations are relatively small.

An alternative hypothesis was put forward by Michel[79] and Weinbaum.[132] Independently, they both realized that if the filtrate leaving the "small pores" was uncontaminated by fluid containing the higher concentration of macromolecules, the effective $\sigma\Delta\Pi$ opposing filtration may approximate to that across the small pores. This would be considerably greater than that calculated from global values of Π_i, and would increase the force opposing filtration (P_0), reducing filtration rates to levels consistent with basal rates of lymph flow. The significant deviations between P_0 and P_{Vc} reported by Levick[62] are found in microvessels with continuous endothelium, where the small pores are the interstices of the glycocalyx lying above the intercellular clefts. The downstream side of the

TABLE 9.2 Starling Pressures in Muscle, Mesentery, and Subcutaneous Tissues at Heart Level

Species and Tissue	Π_c	Π_i	P_i	P_o	P_c	$P_c - P_o$
Dog, skeletal muscle	26.0	11.0	−2.0	13.0	12−20	−1 + 7
Cat, mesentery	19.1	6.1	0	13.0	23.5	10.5
Human, chest subcutis	26.8	15.6	−1.5	9.7	>15.0	>5.3

P_o is calculated from Eq. (9.17) assuming that $\sigma = 1$ and thus is an overestimate. P_c is based on direct measurements in venules or venular capillaries, and is therefore an underestimate of mean P_c. The difference $(P_c - P_o)$ is consequently the minimum difference based on available data. From Levick, J. R. (1991). Capillary filtration–absorption balance reconsidered in light of dynamic extravascular factors. *Exp. Physiol.* **76**, 825−85.[60]

microvascular ultrafilter is therefore the abluminal surface of the glycocalyx, which is separated from the ISF immediately outside the microvessel by the intercellular cleft with its tortuous pathway through the tight junctions. The pathway for macromolecules (the large pores) is either through the endothelial cell vesicles (via channels or by a fission—fusion mechanism) or by the very occasional leaky intercellular cleft. For the high protein concentration of this large pore filtrate to mix with that emerging from the small pores, protein molecules would have to diffuse back through the intercellular clefts to the site of ultrafiltration at the glycocalyx. Although this pathway is short, diffusion has to occur against the flow of fluid from the vessel lumen. The velocity of this filtrate is increased ten-fold or more as it passes through the breaks in the tight junctions. Rough calculations[79] and a detailed mathematical model[55] both indicate that, even with filtration rates driven by pressure differences across the glycocalyx as small as 1—2 cm H_2O, the fluid velocity through the breaks in the tight junctions impose a major barrier to the diffusion of proteins through the clefts in the luminal direction. These levels of filtration, nevertheless, are consistent with basal rates of lymph flow.

The hypothesis has been examined experimentally in single frog mesenteric capillaries[54] and in rat mesenteric venules.[3] In these studies, it was found that even when the interstitial concentration of serum albumin in contact with the outside wall of a vessel was the same as that in the perfusate, fluid movements through the vessel wall were opposed by oncotic pressures much greater than those estimated from global values of Π_i. The authors concluded that these observations were consistent with the oncotic pressures opposing fluid filtration from continuous (non-fenestrated) capillaries are developed across the glycocalyx, and that global values of Π_i do not determine fluid exchange directly. Some of their data are shown in Figure 9.18.

Transient and steady-state fluid exchange and their relations to local lymph flow have been reviewed recently by Levick and Michel.[64]

Microvascular Blood Flow and Solute Transport

The rate of delivery of molecules, and the rate of their clearance to and from a tissue, depends on both microvascular blood flow and microvascular permeability. Where permeability is very high, transport depends on blood flow alone and is said to be "flow limited." Where solute permeability is low, increasing blood flow increases transport to a progressively smaller extent, and when further increases in blood flow no longer increase transport, transport is said to be *"diffusion limited"* or *"permeability limited."* Renkin set out the general principles of blood—tissue exchange in a series of papers between 1955 and 1970.[101,102,104,105] Figure 9.19 is taken from Renkin's work, to illustrate *flow limited* transport of antipyrene and *permeability limited* transport of urea between the microcirculation of skeletal muscle tissue. Both solutes are usually considered to have high permeabilities, but it is seen that as flow increases, the transport of urea becomes independent of flow. This maximum level of transport is determined by the product of P_d to urea and the surface area of the exchange vessels. Antipyrene is lipid soluble and has a much higher permeability than urea. Its transport remains proportional to flow over the range investigated.

Insight into the relations between blood flow and solute transport can be gained by considering the plasma or blood concentrations of a diffusible solute as it flows along an exchange vessel. If the Péclet number for the solute is low (as it is for most small solutes), its unidirectional transport through the vessel wall from a small volume of plasma, ΔV, flowing along the vessel is proportional to the product of its concentration, C, in that volume and its permeability, P_d (Figure 9.20). It is also proportional to the surface area, ΔS, with which ΔV makes contact as it flows along the vessel.

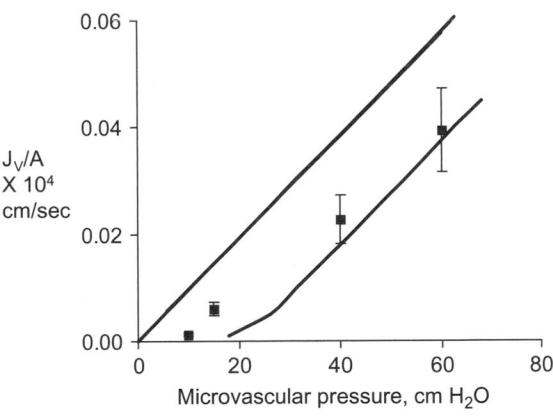

FIGURE 9.18 **Steady-state relations between microvascular filtration (J_V/A) and pressure in rat microvessels when the interstitial oncotic pressure is varied by superfusion.** The vessel is perfused with a 5% serum albumin solution ($\Pi_c = 21.25$ cmH$_2$O). The points are mean values from four experiments in which the ISF concentration of albumin in contact with the outside of the vessel was equal to the perfusate concentration. The curve on the left is the relation predicted when the interstitial concentration of albumin in contact with vessel is the same as the perfusate concentration; that on the right shows the relations when no albumin is added to the superfusate. Note that at high P_c, J_V/A has values comparable with those expected with no albumin present outside the vessel. Only at low J_V/A, when P_c is less than Π_c, does Π_i appear to influence the steady-state. *(From ref. [3].)*

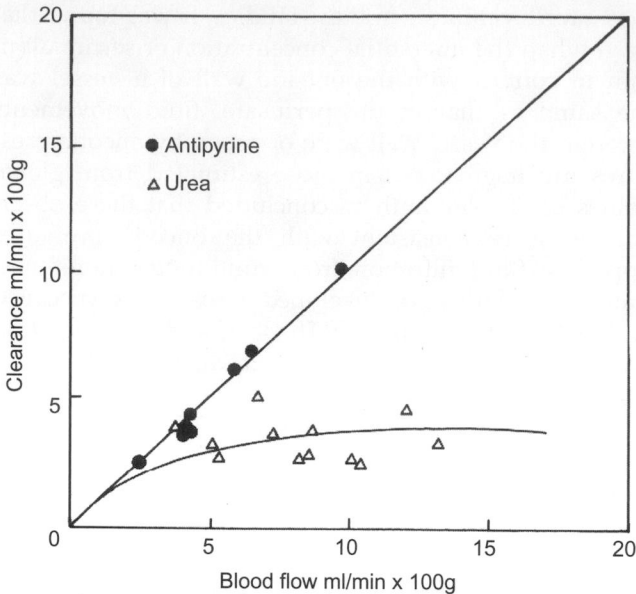

FIGURE 9.19 Relations between blood–tissue clearance and blood flow for a small lipid soluble solute (antipyrene) and a small hydrophilic solute (urea) in skeletal muscle. Whereas the clearance of antipyrene is limited only by blood flow over the range of flows investigated, clearance of urea is limited by its microvascular permeability, and is independent of flow when this exceeds 5 ml min − 1 100 g − 1 tissue. *(Re-plotted from ref. [102]. With permission.)*

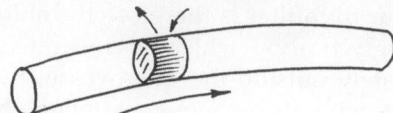

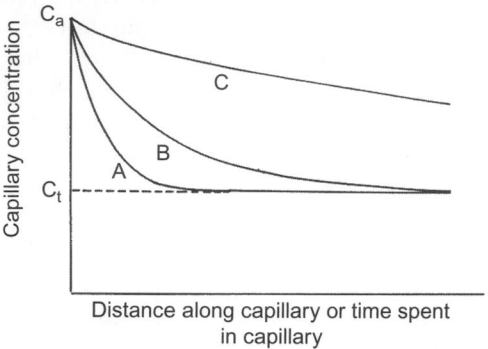

FIGURE 9.20   Model illustrating the principles of diffusion and flow in microvascular exchange. Exchange of solute is considered to occur from a small volume as it flows along a cylindrical microvessel.

FIGURE 9.21   Decrease in plasma concentration of three solutes as they equilibrate with the tissues during their passage along a microvessel. The vessel is more permeable to A than to B, and more permeable to B than to C. Because equilibration is achieved for A and B before the blood leaves the vessel, net transport for these substances can only be increased by increasing the flow (cf. curve for antipyrene in Figure 9.20). Substance C does not equilibrate, and its transport is said to be permeability- or diffusion-limited (cf. with curve for urea in Figure 9.20). *(From ref. [71]. With permission.)*

The changes in C resulting from unidirectional loss of solute from ΔV are given by the following equation:

$$-\Delta V \frac{dC}{dt} = P_d \Delta A.C \qquad (9.20)$$

For a cylindrical vessel, the ratio of $\Delta A/\Delta V$ is constant and is equal to the ratio of surface area to volume for the entire vessel, A/V. Thus:

$$C_{(t)} = C_0 \exp\left(\frac{-P_d A.t}{V}\right) \qquad (9.21)$$

where $C_0 = C$ at time $= 0$, that is the concentration of solute at the point of entry to the vessel, and this would usually be the arterial concentration, C_a. When $t = \tau$, the transit time through the vessel, $C = C_v$, the venous concentration of the solute. Furthermore, V/τ is equivalent to the flow through the vessel, F, so that Eq. (9.19) can be rewritten as:

$$C_V = C_a e^{-P_d A/F} \qquad (9.22)$$

The net transport of solute from blood to tissue is equal to J_S:

$$J_S = F(C_a - C_v) = FC_a(1 - e^{-P_d A/F}) \qquad (9.23)$$

Since the clearance of solute from blood to tissue is J_S/C_a, clearance becomes:

$$Clearance = F(1 - e^{-P_d A/F}) \qquad (9.24)$$

Renkin used expressions such as Eq. (9.24) to describe data such as those shown in Figure 9.19.

Equation (9.21) can be used to give additional insight into the nature of flow-limited and permeability limited transport. In Figure 9.21, Eq. (9.21) has been used to calculate the changes in concentration that occur in a bolus of blood flowing along a single vessel. The three curves represent the concentrations for three solutes that have different values of P_d. It is assumed that the flow is constant, so that distance and time are directly proportional to one another. The three curves start from the same value of C_a and finish at three different points, the venous concentrations. From Eq. (9.23), the net transport of solute from blood to tissue, J_S, for each solute is $F(C_a - C_v)$. F varies inversely with τ so that if F is doubled, τ is halved. Because solute A reaches its end capillary concentration before it has spent half its residence time in the vessel, doubling F will not change $(C_a - C_v)$. Doubling F will therefore double J_S and the relation between clearance and blood flow is linear so that transport is flow-limited over this range of flows, and will resemble that for antipyrene in Figure 9.19. By contrast, for solute C, halving τ almost halves $(C_a - C_v)$, so that the product, $F(C_a - C_v)$ remains almost constant as flow is increased. Transport is now "permeability-limited," and the relation between clearance and flow resembles that shown for urea at high blood flows in Figure 9.19. In theory, the transport of all solutes is limited by permeability if blood flow is high enough. In practice, the permeability of microvascular walls to some substances is so high that transport is always flow-limited.

Although so far we have discussed only solute transport from blood to tissue, equivalent expressions describe the clearance of substances from tissues to blood, so long as the barrier to diffusion through microvascular walls is greater than the resistance to diffusion through the tissues. The latter is certainly not true when the clearance of highly diffusible lipid soluble solutes is being considered. For these molecules, transport between blood and tissues is determined more by the gradients of their concentration in the tissues.

The Renkin expressions (e.g., Eqs. (9.22) and (9.24)) have provided the basis of understanding blood tissue exchange, but Renkin himself has drawn attention to their limitations.[105] Considerations of heterogeneity of microvascular flow and permeability in different vessels in a microvascular bed have led to sophisticated models for the analysis of blood tissue exchange in intact tissues.[13,105] These models may well have to be revised in the light of observations on the relations between flow and transport of small hydrophilic solutes in single capillaries in situ. Indications that P_d may itself vary with flow have been confirmed, and greatly extended in a series of measurements on single microvessels of frogs and rats.[57,58,86] The increase in P_d with flow can be inhibited in rat vessels with NO-synthase blockers, and by procedures that raise intracellular cAMP levels. The effects of flow P_d are largest for small ions and hydrophilic molecules. They appear to involve a pathway more selective than the traditional small pores, and therefore make little contribution to fluid exchange.[86]

The implications of these findings for blood–tissue transport in the intact animal have yet to be assessed, but it could mean that increases in P_dA that, in the past, have been interpreted as the consequence of increases in A, are the result of changes in P_d, and a common set of control mechanisms regulate the permeability and the perfusion of the microcirculation.

Increased Microvascular Permeability

Over 50 years ago Majno and Palade[71] demonstrated that the classical mediators of acute inflammation (e.g., histamine, serotonin) increased vascular permeability by inducing openings in the endothelia of the post-capillary venules. The openings were believed to lie between the endothelial cells, and Majno[72] suggested that they were formed by the contraction of adjacent endothelial cells away from each other. This view, however, was controversial, and continues to be so.[5]

Two groups working in the mid-1990s, reconstructed openings in endothelium from electron micrographs of ultrathin serial sections of venules exposed to a range of mediators to increase their permeability. Whereas with some stimuli (e.g., substance P and PAF), the openings were predominantly paracellular with other stimuli (e.g., VEGF and A23187), they passed through the body of one cell close to the intercellular cleft, but clearly separate from it.[35,88] It seems that transcellular openings may be derived from vesicles or vacuoles in the endothelium.[88] Dvorak and her colleagues identified fused clusters of vesicles and vacuoles, the vacuolar-vesicular organelles (VVOs) in the highly permeable vessels of tumors as transcellular pathways.[33] Subsequent work revealed that VVOs were present in normal (healthy) vessels, but did not form a pathway for macromolecules until the tissues were stimulated by mediators, when they develop into transcellular openings.[34]

Considerable progress has been made unraveling the signaling events that follow the binding of an agonist with its receptor on the venular endothelial cell and the appearance of openings in the vessel wall.[27,28] From studies both in cultured endothelial cells and in intact vessels, it is clear that the early stages of signaling involve a steep rise in the intracellular activity of free Ca^{2+}. The agonist molecules, such as histamine and ATP, bind to endothelial cell membrane receptors linked to G-proteins, which then activate phospholipases (particularly β and γ isoforms of phospholipase-C) that release inositol tri-phosphate (IP$_3$) and di-acyl glyceric acid (DAG) from the membrane lipids. IP$_3$ releases Ca^{2+} from the intracellular Ca^{2+} stores, and this in turn leads to the opening of Ca^{2+} channels in the cell membrane so that the Ca^{2+} activity of the cytosol is rapidly raised by the combined influx of Ca^{2+} from both the stores and ISF (for review see [28]). Agonists such as VEGF bind to a tyrosine kinase receptor that phophorylates PLC-γ, and activate a DAG signal that opens membrane Ca^{2+} channels directly.[11,97] With VEGF, the rise in cytostolic Ca^{2+} is achieved entirely by influx from the ISF, and is independent of its release from the intracellular Ca^{2+} stores.

The sequence of events that follows the rise of cytostolic Ca^{2+} activity remains less clear, and this is particularly true of the final stages when the endothelial openings are formed. Several different studies have shown that, in intact venules, there is cascade involving NO and cGMP downstream from the initial peak of intracellular Ca^{2+} activity.[12,27] The effects of PAF and VEGF on permeability are prevented or greatly attenuated if the enzymes of the NO-synthase — cGMP cascade are blocked.[50,135] The details of other events are continually changing as new investigations are published, and the reader is referred to a recent review of Curry and Adamson,[28] and other contributors to the same issue of *Cardiovascular Research*.

Measuring Increases in Vascular Permeability

To assess the role of different molecules in signaling or in the mechanics of increased permeability, it is necessary to have trustworthy methods for measuring permeability. Earlier we have seen that the permeability coefficients, L_P, σ, and P_d provide quantitative estimates of the permeability properties of microvascular walls. Figure 9.22 shows the results of an experiment on a single rat venule where values of J_V/A were measured at two different microvascular pressures before and after exposure to histamine.[82] From this experiment, the values of L_P and σ can be estimated and interpreted in terms of endothelial openings forming and closing.

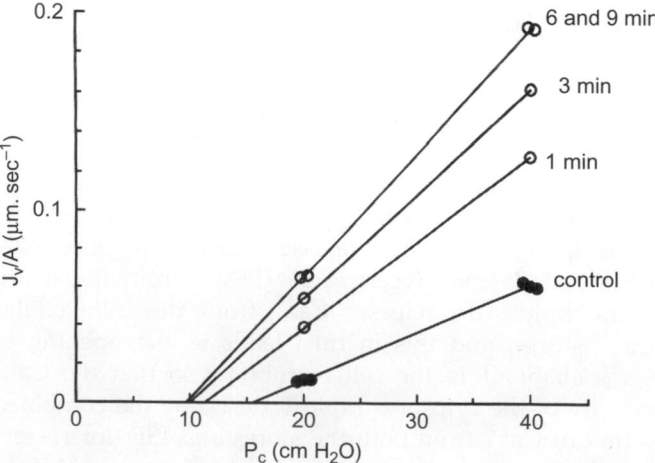

FIGURE 9.22 **Relations between fluid filtration (J_V/A) and microvascular pressure (P_c) before and following addition of histamine to the solution washing a single venule in rat mesentery.** Note how the slope of the relation between J_V/A and P_c (L_P) increases rapidly and the intercept with the P_c axis ($\sigma\Delta\Pi$) falls over the first 6min of exposure to histamine. *(From ref. [80].)*

While this practice of measuring permeability coefficients to chart increases in vascular permeability is used by some investigators, and provides reliable information, the great majority of reports of increased permeability are based on estimates of the rates of transport of macromolecules through endothelia. In the latter case the results should be viewed critically until the reader is satisfied that changes in permeability really have been demonstrated. In this final section, we discuss how results from two frequently used assays of changes in permeability can be easily misinterpreted.

A comparison of the rates of labeled serum albumin transport through monolayers of cultured endothelium *in vitro* in the absence and presence of various concentrations of a potential mediator are frequently used to assay the latter's potency in increasing permeability. The most important question to ask of these studies is the absolute value of the permeability of the monolayer under control conditions. This is often unavailable, as authors have expressed their results as relative increases in permeability. The reason for questioning these assays is that most published control values of P_d for endothelial monolayers to serum albumin are high[7] ($> 10^{-6}$ cm.sec^{-1}). This leads one to suspect that endothelial monolayers form leaky barriers to macromolecules. Strengthening this criticism is the finding that thrombin, which increases permeability of endothelial monolayers by inducing large openings between the cells, has no effects on unstimulated microvascular endothelium *in vivo*.[1] Thrombin will increase permeability in microvessels that are already in a pre-inflammatory state.[32]

Other studies compare transport rates of labeled macromolecules into tissues *in vivo*. Many of these derive from the method described by Miles and Miles[85] in 1952. Here, labeled protein is injected into the circulation of an experimental animal (rat, mouse, guinea pig or rabbit) in which a relatively large area of its dorsal skin has been shaved. Small volumes of varying concentrations of a potential mediator, suitably diluted in physiological salt solution, are injected into the skin. To act as a control, a similar volume of the physiological salt solution containing no mediator is also injected. If the potential mediator does increase vascular permeability to macromolecules, label will accumulate in the area where the injections have been made, and these are then compared with the accumulation of label at the control site over the same period. Initially the labels used were blue dyes that bound to plasma proteins, and the degree of accumulation was estimated from the mean diameter of blue area around the injection site. Later, the technique was made more quantitative by extracting the dye from the tissue or by using radioactive agents. A further refinement was measurement of the plasma concentration of labeled macromolecule during the period that it was accumulating in the tissue. From these data it was possible to estimate the clearance of label from the plasma in the test and control areas.

Although methods such as these are very widely used, the belief that changes in the flux of macromolecules from blood to tissues reflect changes in permeability quantitatively is only valid when all other factors determining the flux rate are constant. It is apparent from Eq. (9.10) that net transport has a convective component, and while an increase in L_P and a fall in σ might both be responsible for increasing J_V, the increase will only be proportional to the permeability change if $P_c - P_i$ is unchanged. Many of the molecules that increase permeability also cause vasodilatation of the arterioles, so that by reducing r_a/r_v they will also raise P_c (see Eq. (9.15)). A vasodilator might also open previously unperfused microvessels, increasing the area available for exchange in Eq. (9.10). In these ways, changes in local blood flow compromise the quantitative relation between changes in net macromolecular flux from blood to tissue and changes in permeability, and mean that permeability assays based macromolecular leakage can only be used as qualitative guides of changes in permeability unless additional evidence is available. Sometimes molecules that are vasodilators and have no action on vascular permeability are erroneously reported as amplifying or potentiating increased permeability. This error was exposed in experiments by Williams and Peck,[135] who showed that the effects of prostaglandins E_1 and E_2 in enhancing protein leakage in inflammation were due to its action as a vasodilator. Not only did the effectiveness of the prostaglandins to enhance protein leakage correlate with their potency as vasodilators, but similar enhancement of protein leakage could be produced by other vasodilators not associated with inflammation. Finally, it is worth emphasizing that if σ to a macromolecule is high in non-stimulated endothelium, quite a modest fall in its value can have a large effect on the convective transport to that macromolecule. For example, if under control conditions σ to serum albumin at the wall of a venule is 0.98, and after exposure to a possible mediator σ falls to 0.80 (a reduction of σ of less than 20%), the convective component of albumin transport increases ten-fold in the presence of the mediator, even if P_c and L_P (and hence J_V) are unchanged. This is because the convective component is proportional to $(1 - \sigma)$, which increases from 0.02 to 0.2.

In conclusion, large changes in the net flux of macromolecules from blood to tissues usually indicate increased vascular permeability, but information obtained in this way is qualitative and should be treated as such unless strict control of J_V has been maintained. If one wants to measure changes in vascular permeability one should measure the changes in the permeability coefficients, for these are the functional measures of the properties of the endothelial barrier.

References

[1] Adamson RH. Permeability of frog mesenteric capillaries after partial pronase digestion of the endothelial glycocalyx. J Physiol 1990;428:1−13.

[2] Adamson RH, Huxley VH, Curry FE. Single capillary permeability to proteins having similar size but different charge. Am J Physiol 1988;254:H304−12.

[3] Adamson RH, Lenz JF, Zhang X, Adamson GN, Weinbaum S, Curry FE. Oncotic pressures opposing filtration across non-fenestrated rat microvessels. J Physiol 2004;557:889−907.

[4] Adamson RH, Michel CC. Pathways through the intercellular clefts of frog mesenteric capillaries (Appendix by Parker KH, Phillips CG, Wang W) J Physiol 1993;466:303−27.

[5] Adamson RH, Zeng M, Adamson GN, Lenz JF, Curry FE. PAF- and bradykinin-induced hyperpermeability of rat venules is independent of actin myosin contraction. Am J Physiol 2003;285:H406−17.

[6] Agre P, Brown D, Nielsen S. Aquaporin water channels: unanswered questions and unresolved controversies. Curr Opin Cell Biol 1995;7(472):483.

[7] Albelda SM, Sampson PM, Haselton FR, McNiff JM, Meuller SM, Williams SK, et al. Permeability characteristics of cultured endothelial cell monolayers. J Appl Physiol 1988;64:308−22.

[8] Areekul S. Reflection coefficients of neutral and sulphate-substituted dextran molecules in capillaries of the isolated perfused ear. Acta Societatis Medicorum Uppsaliensis 1969;74:129−38.

[9] Arkill KP, Knupp C, Michel CC, Neal CR, Qvortrup K, Rostgaard J, et al. Similar endothelial glycocalyx structures in microvessels from a range of mammalian tissues: evidence for a common filtering mechanism. Biophysical Journal 2011;101:1046−56.

[10] Aukland K, Bogufsky RT, Renkin EM. Renal cortical interstitium and fluid absorption by peritubular capillaries. Am J Physiol 1994;266:F175−84.

[11] Bates DO. Vascular endothelial growth factors and vascular permeability. Cardiovasc Res 2010;87:262−71.

[12] Bates DO, Curry FE. Vascular endothelial growth factor increases microvascular permeability via Ca^{2+}-dependent pathway. Am J Physiol 1997;273:H687−94.

[13] Bass L. Flow dependence of first-order uptake of substances by heterogeneous perfused organs. J Theor Biol 1980;86:365−76.

[14] Bearer EL, Orci L. Endothelial fenestral diaphragms: a quick freeze, deep etch study. J Cell Biol 1985;100:418−28.

[15] Boron WF. Sharpey-Schafer Lecture: gas Channels. Exp. Physiol. 2010;95:1107−30.

[16] Brenner BM, Baylis C, Deen WM. Transport of molecules across renal glomerular capillaries. Physiol Rev 1976;56:502−34.

[17] Bruns RR, Palade GE. Studies on blood capillaries. I. General organization of blood capillaries in muscle. J Cell Biol 1968;37 (2):244−76.

[18] Bruns RR, Palade GE. Studies on blood capillaries. II. Transport of ferritin molecules across the wall of muscle capillaries. J Cell Biol 1968;37(2):277−99.

[19] Bundgaard M. The three dimensional organization of tight junctions in a capillary endothelium as revealed by serial section electron microscopy. J Ultrastruct Res 1984;88:1−17.

[20] Bundgaard M, Frokjaer-Jensen J, Crone C. Endothelial plasma-lemmal vesicles as elements in a system of branching invaginations from the cell surface. Proc Natl Acad Sci 1979;76:6439–42.

[21] Carlsson O, Rosengren B-I, Rippe B. Transcytosis inhibitor N-ethylmaleimide increases microvascular permeability in rat muscle. Am J Physiol 2001;281:H1728–33.

[22] Casley-Smith JR. The Brownian movements of pinocytotic vesicles. J Microscopy 1963;82:257.

[23] Clough G, Michel CC. The role of vesicles in the transport of ferritin across frog endothelium. J Physiol 1981;315:127–42.

[24] Clough G, Michel CC. The effects of temperature on ferritin transport by endothelial cell vesicles in capillaries of frog mesentery. Int J Microcirc Clin Exp 1982;1:29–39.

[25] Curry FE. Antipyrine and aminopyrine permeability of individually perfused frog capillaries. Am J Physiol 1981;240:H597–605.

[26] Curry FE. Mechanics and thermodynamics of transcapillary exchange Sec 2 In: Renkin EM, Michel CC, editors. Handbook of Physiology, vol IV. Washington DC: American Physiological Society; 1984. p. 309–74.

[27] Curry FE. Modulation of venular microvessel permeability by calcium influx into endothelial cells. FASEB J 1992;6:2456–66.

[28] Curry FE, Adamson RH. Vascular permeability modulation at the cell. Microvessel, or whole organ level: Towards closing gaps in our knowledge. Cardiovasc Res 2010;87:218–29.

[29] Curry FE, Mason JC, Michel CC. Osmotic reflection coefficients of capillary walls to low molecular weight hydrophilic solutes measured in single perfused capillaries of the frog mesentery. J Physiol 1976;261:319–36.

[30] Curry FE, Michel CC. A fiber matrix model of capillary permeability. Microvasc Res 1980;20:96–9.

[31] Curry FE, Rygh CB, Karlsen T, Wiig H, Adamson RH, Clark JF, et al. Atrial natriuretic peptide modulation of albumin clearance and contrast agent permeability in mouse skeletal muscle and skin: Role in regulation of plasma volume. J Physiol 2010;588:325–39.

[32] Curry FE, Zeng M, Adamson RH. Thrombin increases permeability only in venules exposed in inflammatory conditions. Am J Physiol 2003;285:H2446–53.

[33] Dvorak AM, Kohn S, Morgan ES, Fox P, Nagy JA, Dvorak HF. The vesiculo-vacuolar organelle (VVO): A distinct endothelial cell structure that provides a transcellular pathway for macromolecular extravasation. J Leukoc Biol 1996;59:100–15.

[34] Feng D, Nagy JA, Hipp J, Dvorak HF, Dvorak AM. Vesiculo-vacuolar organelles and the regulation of venule permeability to macromolecules by vascular permeability factor, histamine and serotonin. J Exp Med 1996;183:1981–6.

[35] Feng D, Nagy JA, Hipp J, Pine K, Dvorak HF, Dvorak AM. Reinterpretation of endothelial cell gaps induced by vasoactive mediators in guinea pig, mouse and rat: Many are transcellular pores. J Physiol 1997;504:747–61.

[36] Frøkjaer-Jensen J. Three dimensional organization of plasmalemmal vesicles in endothelial cell: An analysis based on serial sectioning of frog mesenteric capillaries. J Ultrastruct Res 1980;73:9–20.

[37] Fu BM, Weinbaum S, Tsay RY, Curry FE. A junction-orifice-fiber entrance layer model for capillary permeability: application to frog mesenteric capillaries. J Biomechan Eng 1994;116:502–13.

[38] Gamble J, Christ F, Gartside IB. The effect of passive tilting on microvascular parameters in the human calf: a strain gauge plethysmographic study. J Physiol 1997;498:541–52.

[39] Garcia-Estan J, Roman RJ. Role of interstitial hydrostatic pressure in the pressure diuresis response. Am J Physiol 1989;256:F63–70.

[40] Ghitescu L, Fixman M, Simionescu M, Simionescu N. Specific binding sites for albumin restricted to plasmalemmal vesicles of continuous capillary endothelium: receptor mediated transcytosis. J Cell Biol 1986;102:1304–11.

[41] Gore R, Bohlen HG. Microvascular pressures in rat intestinal smooth muscle and mucosal villi. Am J Physiol 1978;233:H685–93.

[42] Granger DN, Kvietys PR, Premen AJ. Microcirculation of the intestinal mucosa section 6, The Gastrointestinal System In: Schultz SG, Woods JD, editors. Handbook of Physiology, vol 1. Bethesda MD: American Physiological Society; 1989. p. 1405–74.

[43] Grotte G. Passage of dextran molecules across the blood–lymph barrier. Acta Chir Scand Suppl 1956;211:1–84.

[44] Guyton AC. A concept of negative interstitial pressure based on pressures in implanted perforated capsules. Circ Res 1963;12:399–415.

[45] Guyton AC. Interstitial fluid pressure. II: pressure volumes curves of the interstitial space. Circ Res 1965;16:452–60.

[46] Guyton AC, Granger HJ, Taylor AE. Interstitial fluid pressure. Physiol Rev 1971;51:527–63.

[47] Gyenge CC, Tenstad O, Wiig H. In vivo determination of steric and electrostatic exclusion of albumin in rat skin and skeletal muscle. J Physiol 2003;552:907–16.

[48] He P, Zeng M, Curry FE. cGMP modulates basal and activated microvascular permeability independently of $[Ca^{2+}]_i$. Am J Physiol 1998;274:H1865–74.

[49] Henriksen O. Local sympathetic reflex mechanism in regulation of blood flow in human subcutaneous adipose tissue. Acta Physiol Scand 1977;(Suppl. 450):7–48.

[50] Henry CBS, Duling BR. Permeation of the luminal capillary glycocalyx is determined by hyaluronan. Am J Physiol 1999;277:H508–14.

[51] Holmang A, Björntorp P, Rippe B. Tissue uptake of insulin and inulin in red and white skeletal muscle in vivo. Am J Physiol 1992;263:H1170–6.

[52] Hu X, Adamson RH, Lui B, Curry FE, Weinbaum S. Starling forces that oppose filtration after tissue oncotic pressure is increased. Am J Physiol 2000;279:H1724–36.

[53] Hu X, Weinbaum S. A new view of Starling's hypothesis at the microstructural level. Microvasc Res 1999;58:281–304.

[54] Jeffries W, Brandon M, Hunt S, Williams AF, Gatter KC, Mason DY. Transferrin receptor on endothelium of brain capillaries. Nature 1984;312:162–3.

[55] Kajimura M, Head SD, Michel CC. The effects of flow on the transport of potassium ions through the walls of single perfused frog mesenteric capillaries. J Physiol 1998;511:707–18.

[56] Kajimura M, Michel CC. Flow modulates the transport of K^+ through the walls of single perfused mesenteric venules in anaesthetized rats. J Physiol 1999;521:665–7.

[57] King G, Johnson S. Receptor mediated transport of insulin across endothelial cells. Science 1985;227:1583–6.

[58] Landis EM. Micro-injection studies of capillary blood pressure in human skin. Heart 1930;15:209–28.

[59] Landis EM. Capillary pressure and capillary permeability. Physiol Rev 1934;14:404–81.

[60] Levick JR. Capillary filtration-absorption balance reconsidered in the light of extravascular factors. Exp Physiol 1991;76:825–57.

[61] Levick JR. An introduction to cardiovascular physiology. Fifth edition London: Hodder Arnold; 2010:170-198 [Chapter 11].

[62] Levick JR, Michel CC. The effects of position and skin temperature on the capillary pressure in the fingers and toes. J Physiol 1978;274:97–109.

[63] Levick JR, Michel CC. Microvascular fluid exchange and revised Starling principle. Cardiovasc Res 2010;87:198–210.

[64] Levick JR, Smaje LH. An analysis of the permeability of a fenestra. Microvasc Res 1987;33:233–56.

[65] Loudon MF, Michel CC, White IF. The labeling of vesicles on frog endothelial cells with ferritin. J Physiol 1979;296:97–112.

[66] Luft JH. Fine structure of the capillary and endo-capillary layer as revealed by ruthenium red. Fed Proc 1966;25:1773–83.

[67] Macphee PJ, Michel CC. Sub-atmospheric closing pressures in individual microvessels of rats and frogs. J Physiol 1995;486:183–7.

[68] Macphee PJ, Michel CC. Fluid uptake from the renal medulla into the ascending vasa recta of anaesthetized rats. J Physiol 1995;487:169–83.

[69] Majno G, Palade GE. Studies on inflammation. I. The effects of histamine and serotonin on vascular permeability. An electron microscopic study. J Biophy Biochem Cytol 1961;11:571–605.

[70] Majno G, Shea S, Leventhal M. Endothelial contraction induced by histamine type mediators. An electron microscopic study. J Cell Biol 1969;42:647–72.

[71] Michel CC. Flows across the capillary wall. In: Bergel DH, editor. *Cardiovascular fluid dynamics 2*. New York: Academic Press; 1972. p. 241–98.

[72] Michel CC. The flow of water through the capillary wall. In: Ussing HH, Bindslev N, Lassen NA, et al., editors. *Water transport across epithelia*. Copenhagen: Munksgaard; 1981. p. 268–79.

[73] Michel CC. Fluid movements through capillary walls Section 2, Microcirculation In: Renkin EM, Michel CC, editors. *Handbook of Physiology*, vol 4. Bethesda MD: American Physiological Society; 1984. p. 375–409.

[74] Michel CC. Review lecture: capillary permeability and how it may change. J Physiol 1988;404:1–29.

[75] Michel CC. One hundred years of Starling's hypothesis. News in Physiol Sci 1996;11:229–37.

[76] Michel CC. Transport of macromolecules through microvascular walls. Cardiovasc Res 1996;32:644–53.

[77] Michel CC. Starling: the formulation of his hypothesis of microvascular fluid exchange and its significance after 100 years. Exp Physiol 1997;82:1–30.

[78] Michel CC, Clough GF. Capillary permeability and transvascular fluid balance. In: Sleight P, Vann Jones J, editors. Scientific foundations of cardiology. London: Heineman; 1983. p. 25–30.

[79] Michel CC, Curry FE. Microvascular permeability. Physiol Rev 1999;79:703–61.

[80] Michel CC, Kendall S. Differing effects of histamine and serotonin on microvascular permeability in anaesthetized rats. J Physiol 1997;501:657–62.

[81] Michel CC, Moyses C. The measurement of fluid filtration in human limbs. In: Tooke JE, Smaje LH, editors. Clinical investigation of the microcirculation. Boston: Martinus Nijhoff; 1986.

[82] Michel CC, Phillips ME. Steady-state filtration at different capillary pressures in perfused frog mesenteric capillaries. J Physiol 1987;:421–35.

[83] Miles AA, Miles EM. Vascular reactions to histamine, histamine liberator and leukotaxine in skin of guinea pigs. J Physiol 1952;118:228–57.

[84] Montermini D, Winlove CP, Michel CC. Effects of perfusion rate on permeability of frog and rat microvessels to sodium fluorescein. J Physiol 2002;543:959–75.

[85] Moyses C, Cederholm-Williams SA, Michel CC. Haemoconcentration and accumulation of white cells in the feet during venous stasis. Int J Microcirc Clin Exp 1987;5:311–20.

[86] Neal CR, Michel CC. Transcellular gaps in microvascular walls of frog and rat when permeability is increased by perfusion with the ionophore A23187. J Physiol 1995;488:427–37.

[87] Noddeland H, Aukland K, Nicolaysen G. Plasma colloid osmotic pressure in venous blood from the human foot in orthostasis. Acta Physiol Scand 1981;113:447–54.

[88] Noddeland H, Riisnes SM, Fadnes HO. Interstitial fluid colloid osmotic pressure and hydrostatic pressure in subcutaneous tissue of patients with nephritic syndrome. Scand J Clin Lab Invest 1982;42:139–46.

[89] Öberg B. Effects of cardiovascular reflexes on net capillary fluid transfer. Acta Physiol Scand 1964;62(Suppl):229.

[90] Pallone TL, Kishore BK, Nielsen S, Agre P, Knepper MA. Evidence that aquaporin-1 mediates NaCl induced water flux across the descending vasa recta. Am J Physiol 1997;272:F587–96.

[91] Pappenheimer JR, Soto-Rivera A. Effective osmotic pressure of the plasma proteins and other quantities associated with the capillary circulation in the hind limbs of cats and dogs. Am J Physiol 1948;152:471–91.

[92] Pappenheimer JR, Renkin EM, Borrero LM. Filtration, diffusion and molecular sieving through peripheral capillary membranes. A contribution to the pore theory of capillary permeability. Am J Physiol 1951;167:13–46.

[93] Parker JC, Gilchrist S, Cartledge JT. Plasma-lymph exchange and interstitial distribution volumes of charged macromolecules in the lung. Am J Physiol 1985;59:1128–36.

[94] Patlak CS, Goldstein DA, Hoffman JF. The flow of solute and solvent across a two-membrane system. J Theoret Biol 1963;5:426–42.

[95] Pocock TM, Foster RR, Bates DO. Evidence for a role for TRPC channels in VEGF-mediated increased vascular permeability *in vivo*. Am J Physiol 2004;286:H1015–26.

[96] Reed RK. Transcapillary albumin extravasation in rat skin and muscle: Effect of increased venous pressure. Acta Physiol Scand 1988;134:375–82.

[97] Reed RK. Interstitial fluid pressure. In: Reed RK, McHale NG, Bert JL, et al., editors. *Interstitium, connective tissue and lymphatics*. London: Portland Press; 1995. p. 85–100.

[98] Reed RK, Rubin K. Transcapillary exchange: role and importance of the interstitial fluid pressure and extracellular matrix. Cardiovasc Res 2010;87:211–7.

[99] Renkin EM. Capillary permeability to lipid soluble molecules. Am J Physiol 1952;168:538–45.

[100] Renkin EM. Transport of potassium-42 from blood to tissue in isolated mammalian skeletal muscle. Am J Physiol 1959;197:125–1210.

[101] Renkin EM. Transport of large molecules across capillary walls. Physiologist 1964;7:13–28.

[102] Renkin EM. Blood flow and transcapillary exchange in skeletal and cardiac muscle. In: Marchetti G, Taccardi B, editors. International symposium on coronary circulation. Basel: Karger; 1967. p. 18–30.

[103] Renkin EM. Control of microcirculation and blood tissue exchange. In: Renkin EM, Michel CC, editors. Handbook of physiology. the cardiovascular system. microcirculation, vol IV. Washington DC: American Physiological Society; 1984: 627–87.

[104] Renkin EM. Transport pathways and processes. In: Simionescu N, Simionescu M, editors. *Endothelial cell biology*. New York: Plenum Publishing; 1988.

[105] Renkin EM, Tucker VL. Measurements of microvascular transport parameters of macromolecules in tissues and organs of intact animals. Microcirculation 1998;5:139–52.

[106] Rippe B, Haraldsson B. Transport of macromolecules across microvascular walls: two pore theory. Physiol Rev 1994;74:163–219.

[107] Rippe B, Kamiya A, Folkow B. Transcapillary passage of albumin, effects of tissue cooling and of increases in filtration and plasma colloid osmotic pressure. Acta Physiol Scand 1979;105:171–87.

I. EPITHELIAL AND NONEPITHELIAL TRANSPORT AND REGULATION

[108] Rippe B, Rosengren B-I, Carlsson O, Venturoli D. Transendothelial transport: the vesicle controversy. J Vasc Res 2002;39:375—90.

[109] Rippe B, Taylor AE. NEM and filipin increase albumin transport in lung microvessels. Am J Physiol 2001;280:H34—41.

[110] Rosengren B-I, Rippe A, Rippe C, Venturoli D, Swärd K, Rippe B. Transvascular protein transport in mice lacking caveolae. Am J Physiol 2006;291:H1371—7.

[111] Schnitzer J, Oh P, Pinney E, Allard J. Filipin sensitive caveolae-mediated transport in endothelium: reduced transcytosis, scavenger endocytosis and capillary permeability of select macromolecules. J Cell Biol 1994;127:1217—32.

[112] Schnitzer J, Allard J, Oh P. NEM inhibits transcytosis, endocytosis and capillary permeability: Implication of caveolae fusion in endothelia. Am J Physiol 1995;37:H48—55.

[113] Schnitzer J, Oh P, Jacobson BS, Dvorak AM. Caveolae from luminal plasmalemma of rat lung endothelium: Microdomains enriched in caveolin, Ca^{2+}-ATPase and IP3 receptor. Proc Natl Acad Sci USA 1995;92:1759—63.

[114] Schnitzer J, Lui J, Oh P. Endothelial caveolae have the molecular transport machinery for vesicle budding, docking and fusion including VAMP, NSF, SNAP, annexins and GTPases. J Biol Chem 1995;270:14399—404.

[115] Schnitzer J, Oh P, McIntosh DP. Role of GTP hydrolysis in fission of caveolae directly from plasma membranes. Science 1996;274:239—42.

[116] Shirahama T, Cohen AS. The role of mucopolysaccharides in vesicle architecture and endothelial transport. J Cell Biol 1972;52:198—205.

[117] Simionescu N, Simionescu M, Palade GE. Permeability of muscle capillaries to small hemepeptides. J Cell Biol 1975;64:586—607.

[118] Squire JM, Chew M, Nneji G, Neal C, Barry J, Michel C. Quasi-periodic substructure in the microvessel endothelial glycocalyx: a possible explanation for molecular filtering? J Struct Biol 2001;136:239—55.

[119] Starling EH. On the absorption of fluids from connective tissue spaces. J Physiol 1896;19:312—26.

[120] Tavassoli M, Kishimoto T, Kataoka M. Liver endothelium mediates the hepatocyte's uptake of ceruloplasmin. J Cell Biol 1986;102:1298—303.

[121] Taylor AE, Granger DN. Exchange of macromolecules across the microcirculation. In: Renkin EM, Michel CC, editors. Handbook of physiology. microcirculation, vol IV. Washington: American Physiological Society; 1984. p. 467—520.

[122] Tenstad O, Heyeraas KJ, Wiig H, Aukland K. Drainage of plasma proteins from the renal medullary interstitium in rats. J Physiol 2001;:533—9.

[123] Turner MR, Pallone TL. Hydraulic and diffusional permeabilities of isolated outer medullary descending vasa recta from the rat. Am J Physiol 1997;272:H392—400.

[124] Tucker VL, Simanok KE, Renkin EM. Tissue specific effects of physiological ANP infusion on blood tissue albumin transport. Am J Physiol 1992;63:R945—53.

[125] Van Haaren PMA, VanBavel E, Vink H, Spaan JAE. Localization of the permeability barrier to solutes in isolated arteries by confocal microscopy. Am J Physiol 2003;285:H2848—56.

[126] Vink H, Duling BR. Identification of distinct luminal domains for macromolecules, erythrocytes and leukocytes within mammalian capillaries. Circ Res 1996;79:581—9.

[127] Wagner RC, Chen SC. Transcapillary transport of solute by the endothelial vesicular system: Evidence from serial section analysis. Microvasc Res 1991;42:139—50.

[128] Wang W, Michel CC. Modeling exchange of plasma proteins between microcirculation and interstitium of renal medulla. Am J Physiol 2000;279:F334—44.

[129] Weinbaum S. Distinguished lecture. Models to solve the mysteries in biomechanics at a cellular level. A new view of fiber matrix layers. Ann Biomed Eng 1998;26:627—43.

[130] Weinbaum S, Tsay R, Curry FE. A three-dimensional junction-pore matrix model for capillary permeability. Microvasc Res 1992;44:85—111.

[131] Wiig H, Reed RK. Interstitial compliance and transcapillary pressures in cat skin and skeletal muscle. Am J Physiol 1985;248:H666—73.

[132] Williams TJ, Peck MJ. Role of prostaglandin-mediated vasodilatation in inflammation. Nature 1977;270:530—2.

[133] Wissig S, Williams MC. The permeability of muscle capillaries to microperoxidase. J Cell Biol 1978;76:341—59.

[134] Wolf MB, Watson PD. Measurement of osmotic reflection coefficient for small molecules in cat hind limbs. Am J Physiol 1989;256:H282—90.

[135] Wu HM, Huang Q, Yuan Y, Granger HJ. VEGF induces NO-dependent hyperpermeability in coronary venules. Am J Physiol 1996;271:H2735—9.

[136] Yuan Y, Granger HJ, Zawieja DC, Chilian WM. Flow modulates coronary venular permeability by a nitric oxide related mechanism. *Am J Physiol* 1992; 263 1992;:H641—6.

[137] Yudilevich DL, Alvarez OA. Water, sodium and thiourea transcapillary diffusion in the dog heart. Am J Physiol 1967;213:308—14.

[138] Zhang W, Edwards A. Transport of plasma proteins across vasa recta in the renal medulla. Am J Physiol 2001;281:F478—92.

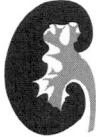

External Balance of Electrolytes and Acids and Alkali

Man S. Oh

State University of New York, Downstate Medical Center, Brooklyn, NY, USA

This chapter will cover discussions on principles of external balance for electrolytes, and for acids and bases. The first section will deal with discussions on principles of electrolyte balance in general, and the second section discusses the acid—base balance.

PRINCIPLES OF ELECTROLYTE BALANCE

Introduction

Prolonged imbalance between input and output of most quantifiable elements in a living organism is incompatible with life. The duration of imbalance varies, but eventually balance must be restored for maintenance of survival. This rule applies to all quantifiable elements *in vivo* as well as *in vitro*. Red cell destruction equals red cell production. Oxygen uptake equals oxygen utilization. Sodium intake must equal sodium output, and water input must match water loss. Yet transient discrepancies occur regularly in living organisms, but balance is ultimately achieved. The same rule applies to the balance of any quantifiable elements in nature. The duration of imbalance is usually quite short in living organisms, because protracted imbalance results in death. However, not limited by survival, the duration of imbalance in nature could be more protracted.

The main aim of this chapter is to describe the underlying principles for eventual restoration of balance in nature, and then to extrapolate these principles to the understanding of human physiology, particularly the principles of fluid and electrolyte balance.

WHY IS BALANCE ALWAYS RESTORED?

The underlying mechanism that allows eventual restoration of balance is perfect and foolproof. As an example, the kidney is a central player in the restoration and achievement of fluid and electrolyte balance in living organisms, but the smartness of the kidney is not the reason for perfect balance. The kidney merely accelerates the process by utilizing a principle ubiquitous in nature, but it does not determine its ultimate outcome. The most crucial element of the control system that restores ultimate balance is that a discrepancy between intake and output inevitably leads to a change in total content of the element in the system, and the uncorrected imbalance is cumulative. When input is greater than output the content increases, and the continued imbalance keeps increasing the content. When output is greater than input the content decreases, and the continuing imbalance keeps decreasing the content. In a system with a limited capacity, a change in content of a substance alters its concentration; this invariably affects output, and sometimes also input. The key points here are: (1) an uncorrected balance invariably leads to a change in content; (2) a change in content leads to a change in concentration; (3) an altered concentration affects output or input; and (4) these effects are cumulative.

IS THE CAPACITY OF ANY SYSTEM ALWAYS LIMITED?

Is the capacity of any system always limited? The answer is yes. We often say: the sky has no limit. Yet

Seldin and Giebisch's The Kidney, Fifth Edition.
DOI: http://dx.doi.org/10.1016/B978-0-12-381462-3.00010-0

there is a limit even to the capacity of atmospheric air volume. The apparent air volume is about 4.08×10^{21} liters. (The apparent air volume is calculated considering that air is denser at sea level, and density declines progressively with rising altitude until there are no more air molecules. Thus, the apparent air volume is the theoretical volume that would be required if all the gases in the air were contained at the same concentrations as those at sea level at a pressure of 760 mmHg when the 1 mole of gas is contained in 22.4 liters.)

In recent years, the rising CO_2 concentration of the atmosphere and its impact on global warming is the source of a great deal of public concern. The rising CO_2 concentration implies that the amount of CO_2 added to the atmosphere is more than the amount eliminated from the atmosphere. However, the discrepancy will not and cannot remain permanent, because the CO_2 concentration in the atmosphere has a positive influence on the rate of its removal from the atmosphere. The main source of CO_2 addition to the air is the burning of fossil fuels (oil, gas, and coal). The total amount of CO_2 added is about 30 billion tons per year.[1] This amount added to the air volume of 4.08×10^{21} liters would increase atmospheric CO_2 concentration by about 3.74 ppm per year. Currently, the actual rise in CO_2 concentration is about 2 ppm per year. The difference, 1.74 ppm, is absorbed by the oceans, mostly by direct diffusion and some by diffusion into rain water entering the ocean. In the ocean, CO_2 is in equilibrium with bicarbonate and carbonate.[2] As the atmospheric CO_2 concentration increases, the amount entering the ocean would increase progressively. Since the industrial revolution, the atmospheric CO_2 level has been rising rapidly, because the rate of CO_2 addition has been increasing rapidly with the progressively greater consumption of fossil fuel worldwide. Once the rate of fossil fuel consumption stops increasing further, the rate of CO_2 removal will eventually equal the rate of CO_2 addition. Of course, it is quite likely that at the time of new balance, the earth could be much warmer and the ocean much more acidic, with major ecological changes. Nevertheless, imbalance does not last forever, because imbalance always leads to a new balance.

Many substances in the human body utilize the same principles to reach a state of balance. For example, if creatinine production is doubled in the absence of any change in GFR, serum creatinine would exactly double, at which point the renal excretion of creatinine would also double. At this point a new balance is reached between production and excretion. For some substances, a new balance is accelerated by physiological control mechanisms. For example, if sodium intake is doubled, renal sodium excretion will also double, but doubling of renal sodium excretion does not require doubling of serum sodium or total body sodium content, only a slight increase in sodium content of the body, because of the excellent renal regulation of sodium balance. By the same token, a reduction in sodium intake to 1/10 of the usual amount does not require sodium content of the body to decrease to 1/10 of normal when the balance is restored.

In the human body, the capacity for most substances is quite limited, and daily variations for most electrolytes are quite large in relation to total body content. Furthermore, there is a limit to which the organism can tolerate a deviation in the content of these substances. Therefore, survival of the organism demands the existence of certain physiological mechanisms to accelerate the compensation processes, to prevent a deviation from occurring to a lethal level.

Following is the sequence of events in the control system: a certain amount of an element is contained in a compartment, if input of the element into the compartment exceeds its output, the content will increase. The higher content influences the control mechanisms to reduce input or to increase output. As long as the discrepancy remains, the content will keep increasing, because the consequence of discrepancy is cumulative; the higher the content, the greater the effect on input or output. A cumulative change stops only when input equals output. When input is less than output, the opposite sequence of events restores the balance (Figure 10.1).

Restoration of salt balance will be used as an example. A person in a state of sodium balance has been ingesting 10 g of salt per day, and excreting 10 g of salt per day. Now, assume that a diuretic is given to this person. On the first day of diuretic therapy, salt output is 20 g per day, with net loss of 10 g of salt. The next day, although the diuretic dosage remains unchanged, salt excretion has to be less, for example, 15 g a day, because the reduction in effective vascular volume caused by the previous day's salt loss has activated salt-retaining mechanisms, and has reduced salt losing hormones. Still, the overall result is an additional negative balance of 5 g of salt. Although the negative balance is less on the second day, the cumulative loss (15 g) is greater on the second day than on the first, and the effective vascular volume is even lower on the second day than the first. The lower effective volume reduces salt output further to 12 g per day on the third day, with an additional negative balance of 2 g. The overall cumulative loss is now 17 g, resulting in a further decrease in effective vascular volume. As long as the salt output remains greater than salt intake, cumulative salt loss becomes larger and larger, albeit less steeply than before. Cumulative salt loss stops only when salt output equals salt intake. Indefinite net salt loss is theoretically impossible, because continued salt loss will ultimately cause such severe volume depletion that the

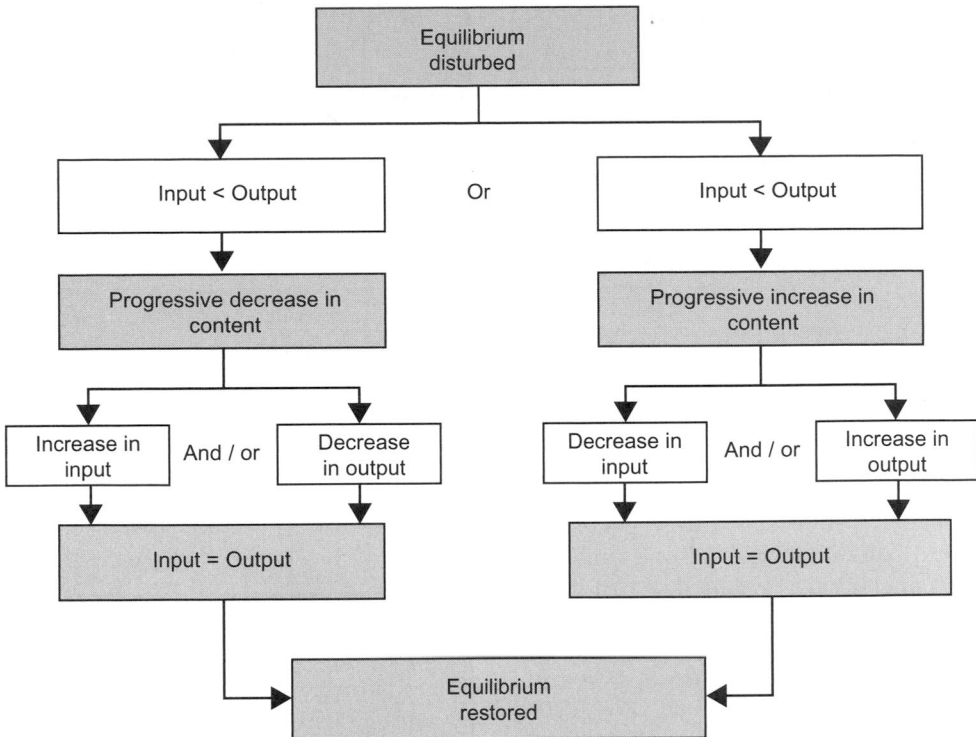

FIGURE 10.1 Mechanisms by which balance is restored.

person will become hypotensive, and salt excretion would stop completely. Of course, long before reaching such an extreme state, renal excretion of salt would decrease to a level equaling intake.

In the example given, what causes restoration of balance is not the smartness of the kidney or the cleverness of humoral mechanisms, but the principle of balance restoration, which is ubiquitous in nature. For example, sodium balance in a person on chronic diuretic therapy would still be restored in the absence of aldosterone, in which case the person could be quite sick with dehydration when balance is attained.

The same control mechanism explains why urinary excretion of potassium does not remain greater than intake in patients with primary hyperaldosteronism. With increased aldosterone, K output will initially exceed K intake. The resulting negative K balance causes hypokalemia, which in turn reduces urine K excretion. As long as K excretion exceeds K intake, serum K will decrease progressively until K excretion equals K intake. Occasionally, a patient dies of a cardiac arrhythmia before balance is attained. In the vast majority of cases, balance is achieved before the patient dies.

SPEED OF BALANCE RESTORATION

In a living organism, the speed of restoration of balance is teleologically determined. If an organism can tolerate protracted imbalance of a particular element without death or severe disability, balance need not be restored promptly. If quick restoration of balance is vital for survival, a mechanism for rapid restoration of balance is necessarily acquired in the process of evolution. Thus, the acceptable duration of discrepancy or alternatively speed with which restoration of balance is achieved, depends on the importance of maintaining the content of an element within a narrow range, in order to prevent the demise or serious disability of the organism. Four main factors influence the speed of balance restoration (Table 10.1).

For example, an adult of average size has about 40 liters of total body water, and daily intake and output of water is about 2 liters. Obviously, water output exceeding water intake by one liter a day would lead to fatal dehydration in 10 days to two weeks. Conversely, water intake exceeding water output by the same magnitude would lead to water intoxication and death. An opposite example is calcium balance. The total body calcium content of an average adult man is about 1,200,000 mg (60,000 mEq), and net daily external flux is about 150 mg (7.5 mEq). A daily negative balance of calcium of 100 mg for one year would reduce total body calcium by mere 36,500 mg; 3% of total body calcium content. Obviously, a negative calcium balance of such a magnitude, even for a protracted period, is not incompatible with life. Indeed, during the period of development of osteoporosis,

TABLE 10.1 Factors Influencing the Speed of Balance Restoration

1. Magnitude of flux.
2. Basal store.
3. Capacity for additional storage.
4. The physiological limit for deviation of the body content.

TABLE 10.2 Major Elements of Human Body: Total Body Content, Daily Turnover Rate, and Days Required for 50% Turnover

Body Elements	Total Body Content	Usual Daily Turnover	Days for 50% Turnover
Na	3500 mEq	4%	12
K	3000 mEq	2.3%	22
Ca	60,000 mEq	0.01%	2700
Mg	2000 mEq	0.5%	100
P	18,000 mmol	0.17%	290
Water	40 L	5%	10
Alkali	28,000 mEq	0.2%	250
Calories	130,000 kcal	1.5%	33
Creatinine	400 mg	400%	0.12
Urea-N	4000 mg	250%	0.2

a substantial negative balance of calcium for 10 years or longer is a common occurrence. Similarly, a positive caloric balance of 500 calories a day for a year will result in a total positive balance of 182,500 calories ($500 \times 365 = 182,500$). This amount would result in an increase in adipose tissue weight of about 50 lbs, an undesirable situation, but with no immediate effect on survival.

A large storage capacity does not guarantee a protracted imbalance. A quantitative analysis must be applied before that conclusion is reached. Once it was widely accepted that a large store of alkali of the bone was responsible for the maintenance of stable serum bicarbonate concentrations in chronic renal failure, despite a substantial daily positive balance of acid.[3,4] However, this conclusion was reached without quantitative analysis. The bone content of alkali is indeed very large, but it is not sufficiently large to provide 19 mEq of alkali per day for six years in chronic renal failure. Since the total content of acid in the bone is about 25,000 mEq, a quick calculation would indicate that at a rate of consumption at 19 mEq per day, the entire bone content of alkali would be gone in about 3.6 years. Clearly, uremic patients with metabolic acidosis are in states of good or near acid–base balance, i.e., acid production equals acid excretion.

The cumulative net loss of a substance from the body cannot exceed the total amount of that substance contained in the body (Table 10.2). For example, one can conclude with certainty that a person who has total body sodium content of 3500 mEq could not have been in daily negative balance of sodium by 10 mEq per day for one year, since the total loss of 3650 mEq ($10 \times 365 = 3650$) would exceed the total body store of sodium. Even before exceeding the total body content, one cannot exceed a physiological limit of deficit for the substance. For example, potassium loss in excess of a third of the body store (3000 mEq) is usually fatal. Hence, you would reject a claim that a patient with Conn's tumor has been losing 20 mEq of potassium daily for three months, since loss of such an amount ($20 \times 30 \times 3 = 1800$ mEq) would certainly be lethal. In contrast, the body can tolerate a greater fraction of sodium loss. A person who loses half of the body's sodium would be gravely ill, but still alive.

While the total stored amount sets the absolute upper limit on losses, the amount that can be gained depends on the additional storage capacity, which varies widely with electrolytes. In the case of sodium, the storage capacity for additional Na^+ in the body is enormous. In certain edema-forming states, the Na^+ content may increase by 300% of the basal amount. Caloric balance is another example. In a normally-built adult, the total stored in fat and protein is about 130,000 calories. At the caloric consumption rate of 1200 calories per day, about 50% of the stored calories would be consumed in 55 days. In contrast, a person can gain as much as 500 lbs of fat, which are equal to 4,500,000 calories, about 35 times the normal caloric storage.

MECHANISM OF BALANCE RESTORATION

All control mechanisms are activated by the introduction of a new influence into a system that causes imbalance between input and output of an element, and this leads to an alteration in a parameter of the element in the system. In biological systems, parameters that are most often disturbed are concentrations of elements in the plasma. Other disturbed parameters include pressure, volume, temperature, and body weight. Alterations in a parameter affect either input or output, which in turn affects the parameter directly or indirectly. Examples of an element that is directly responsible for a change in a parameter are balance of potassium (element) affecting plasma potassium concentration (parameter), and balance of magnesium (element) affecting the plasma magnesium concentration (parameter). Examples of an element that is indirectly responsible for a change in parameter include the balance of sodium (element) affecting the effective vascular volume (parameter), and the balance of calories (element) affecting body weight (parameter).

The effectiveness of the compensation mechanism determines the degree of deviation of a parameter from the baseline value when the balance is restored. A poor compensation mechanism restores balance with the parameter greatly deviated from the baseline value. An example of a poor compensation mechanism is a change in plasma urea concentration with a change in the rate of urea production. When urea production doubles, the renal excretion will eventually also double and equal the increased production rate. However, at equilibrium the plasma urea concentration will be twice the baseline value. An example of a good compensation mechanism is a change in a sodium content of the body in response to a change in sodium intake. When salt intake is doubled, renal excretion of salt will eventually double; at this point the total body sodium content would be very slightly greater than the baseline value.

MODELS OF EXTERNAL BALANCE

The pattern of restoration of new balance for control of various elements in the human body is broadly classified into three models. The main source of input for most electrolytes in our body is oral intake and the main output the renal excretion, with some additional output through the GI tract.

Model A

This model is depicted in Figure 10.2 as a cylinder filled with water. Water enters from a faucet into the cylinder, and leaves through a hole at the bottom. The height of the water column depends on water input and water output, and water output in turn depends on the size of the hole at the bottom and the hydrostatic pressure. The hydrostatic pressure in turn depends on the height of water column. Under these conditions, only two factors can change the height of the water column permanently; the rate of water input and the size of the hole. If the rate of water input is doubled while the size of the outlet hole is kept constant, water output will also double when the balance is restored.

With the same size outlet hole, doubling of water output would require doubling of hydrostatic pressure, which in turn requires doubling of the water column height. Before balance is restored, the water column height rises, because water input exceeds water output. The rise in the water column height gradually increases the hydrostatic pressure, and

therefore the water output. Hence the discrepancy between the water input and the water output gradually lessens. However, as long as water input remains greater than water output, the water level will keep rising, and the rise will stop only when the water output equals the water input; this occurs when the water column height is exactly doubled.

Conversely, decreasing the size of the outlet hole to double the resistance to water flow, with an unchanged rate in the water input, would initially reduce the water output to half. The ensuing imbalance between the water output and the water input would cause a rise in the water column height. A higher hydrostatic pressure resulting from the rise in the water column would allow more water to come out through a narrower hole. Thus, in this example, doubling of the water column height will restore the water output to the baseline value.

The main characteristic of this type of compensation is that the alteration in content or concentration caused by a disturbance is directly or inversely proportionate to the magnitude of the alteration in input or output function. For example, if the input of a substance is doubled, the content or concentration of the substance will be doubled when balance is restored. If input is increased three-fold, the content or concentration will be tripled. Similarly, if the output function is halved, the content or concentration will be doubled when balance is restored. If the output function is reduced to one tenth of the baseline, the content or concentration will be increased ten-fold when balance is restored.

Many substances in the body follow this pattern of compensation mechanism in order to achieve a new balance. When a substance follows this pattern of compensation, the body must have a high degree of tolerance for a large deviation in the body content or concentration for the substance. For example, if creatinine clearance diminishes to half of the baseline value with an unchanged creatinine production rate, serum creatinine concentration will double in order to achieve the same rate. Similarly, if creatinine production is reduced to half of the baseline value with the same renal creatinine clearance, serum creatinine concentration will be half of the original value. Likewise, if urea production is doubled, with unchanged kidney function, serum urea concentration is doubled when balance is restored.

Model B

In this model, the cylinder has a wedge-shaped slit on its side instead of a hole at the bottom (Figure 10.3). Water enters the cylinder from a faucet, and leaves through the slit. As in model A, water output depends on the height of the water column. But, because of the

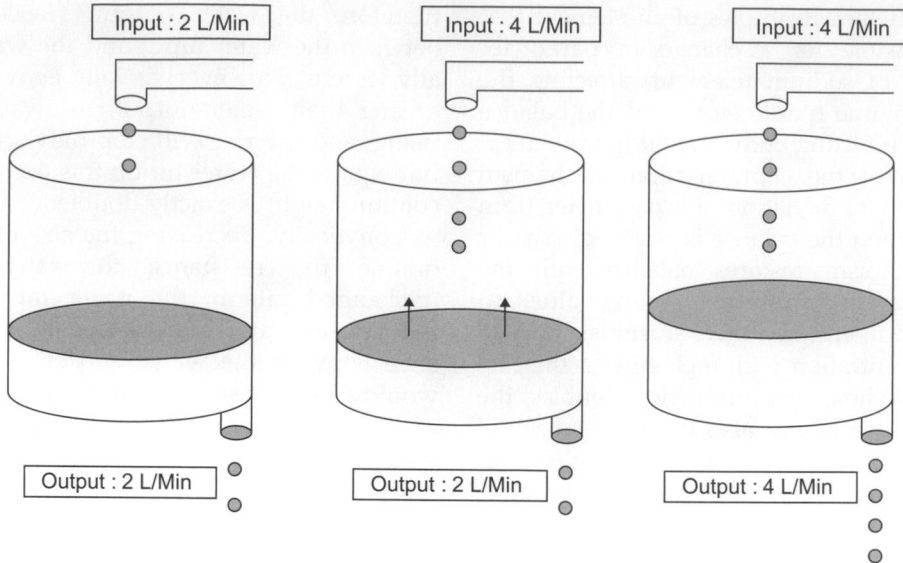

FIGURE 10.2   Model A. The input and output determines the balance, but the output changes in proportion to the height of the water column. When the water input doubles while the size of the output hole remains unchanged, the only way for the output to increase to the same level as the input is to double the height of the water column. At this point, a new balance is struck between input and output. For example, if creatinine production doubled while creatinine clearance remained unchanged, serum creatinine concentration will be doubled when a new balance is achieved between creatinine production and creatinine excretion

wedge shaped slit, the effect of a rise in water level on water output is exponential. Therefore, when water intake doubles, doubling of water output does not require doubling of the water column height. Depending on the shape of the slit, the water level may rise only slightly before a new balance is restored. In other words, an increase in water output in response to a change in the height of water column is magnified in this system. Furthermore, unlike model A, when the water level drops below the lowest part of the slit, water output stops altogether.

The regulation of the body content or plasma concentration of most electrolytes and other essential body elements utilizes this type of compensation. For example, when potassium intake is increased five-fold, plasma potassium concentration does not increase five-fold when balance is restored. In the presence of normal renal function and normal aldosterone response, plasma potassium concentration will increase only slightly. Likewise, a five-fold increase in sodium intake causes only a slight increase in body sodium content or plasma sodium concentration; when sodium intake is greatly reduced, the body sodium content decreases only slightly before renal sodium excretion ceases.

Model C

The pattern of water excretion in model C (Figure 10.4) is similar to model A, but in this model two cylinders, one big (A) and the other small (B), are connected at the bottom. Water enters only into cylinder A, but once it enters, it equilibrates with cylinder B. Ordinarily, because cylinder A has a bigger hole than cylinder B, the water output is determined primarily by the size of hole A. However, as the size of hole A decreases, the role of hole B increases. When water input is doubled, the height of the water column will have to be doubled in order to permit establishment of a new steady-state. On the other hand, when the resistance to flow through hole A is doubled, the height of the water column will be less than doubled when balance is restored, provided that the size of hole B is unchanged.

When the excretion rate through hole A decreases, the excretion through hole B becomes more important. The regulation of plasma concentration of uric acid follows the pattern in model C. Uric acid is cleared by the kidney, and is also cleared metabolically by colonic bacteria. The renal clearance of uric acid is normally about 8 liters per day, and the colonic clearance is about 4 liters per day. Thus, 2/3 of the uric acid produced is cleared by the kidney and 1/3 by the colon.[5] If the plasma concentration of uric acid is 5 mg/dl (50 mg/L), renal excretion of uric acid would be 400 mg per day (uric acid clearance of 8 liters per day), and the amount cleared by the colonic bacteria would be 200 mg, with a total uric acid removal rate of 600 mg per day. If chronic renal disease reduces the renal clearance of uric acid to 4 L a day (half of normal), total uric acid clearance would now be 8 liters

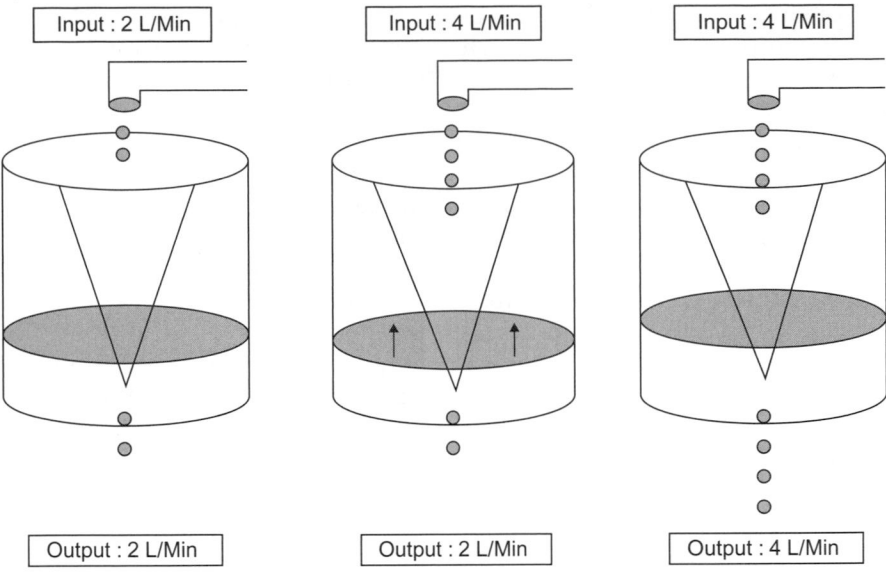

FIGURE 10.3 **Model B.** As in model A, input and output determines the balance, and output depends on the height of water column. However, unlike model A, a change in water output by the change in the height of water column is magnified. When the height of water column increases slightly, water output increases greatly, and a decrease in its height reduces water output markedly. Furthermore, when the height of the water column decreases below a certain level, output ceases completely. Thus, doubling of input from 2 liters per minute to 4 liters per minute requires increases in water level only slightly before output also increased to 4 liters a minute.

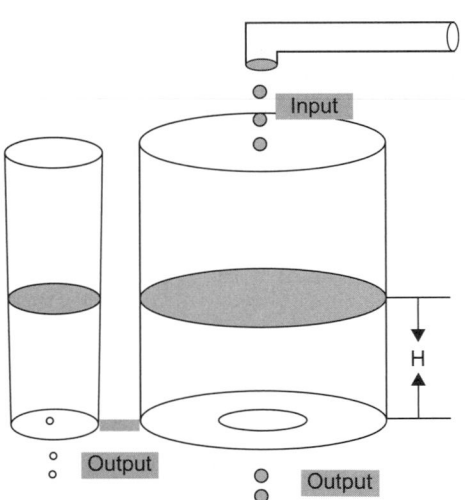

FIGURE 10.4 **Model C.** Two compartments A and B are connected to each other, and each has an outlet hole. Water output from both compartments depends on the height of water column. Because hole A is much larger than hole B, the bulk of water output occurs through hole A. When hole A becomes smaller, output through hole B plays a greater role in water output.

per day, if the colonic clearance remained unchanged at 4 liters per day. If the rate of production remained the same (600 mg/day), plasma uric acid concentration would not double to 10 mg/dl, but would increase to 7.5 mg/dl, because total body uric acid clearance would be 8 liters per day (4 + 4 = 8 liters); at this concentration, the total amount of uric acid cleared would be 600 mg/day (75 mg/L × 8 L/day = 600 mg/day).

The regulation of plasma creatinine concentration follows the same type of compensation as shown in model C. Normally, creatinine is cleared mainly by the kidney, with a daily clearance of about 180 liters, but the colonic bacteria also remove a small amount of creatinine, providing about 3 liters of creatinine clearance per day.[6] Thus, normally the colonic clearance, which constitutes less than 2% of the total creatinine clearance, has little impact on the plasma concentration of creatinine. However, in the presence of advanced renal failure, which does not diminish the colonic clearance of creatinine, it could have a substantial impact on plasma concentration of creatinine. For example, in a person who has 5 ml/min of renal creatinine clearance (7.2 liters per day), 3 liters of colonic clearance would now represent about 30% of the total creatinine clearance. For these reasons, the rate of rise in serum creatinine in advanced renal failure is not exactly inversely proportionate to the reduction in renal clearance of creatinine.

INFINITE GAIN CONTROL MECHANISM

The ultimate aim of all compensation mechanisms is restoration of balance between input and output, after balance is disturbed by introduction of an abnormality. In most instances restoration of balance is possible only when the abnormality persists. For example, increased renal excretion of potassium by primary hyperaldoteronism will result in imbalance between input and output, with output exceeding input. Development of hypokalemia is needed for output to decrease to match input, and hypokalemia is the price that must paid in order to restore balance. Similarly, an increase salt intake would result in chronic volume expansion, in order for salt excretion to increase to equal the increased intake. The infinite gain control mechanism, to be discussed below, is unique in that the abnormality is corrected completely when a balance is restored.

This principle is well illustrated in Figure 10.5. In this model system, water enters the tank from a faucet at the top, and leaves the tank through a hole at the bottom. The input is independently regulated, but the water output depends on two factors, the size of the outlet hole and the hydrostatic pressure. The hydrostatic pressure in turn depends on the water level, which is determined by the balance between the water input and water output. At equilibrium, the water input is equal to the water output. What would happen if the capacity of the tank is suddenly altered at this point by, for example, placing a brick in the tank, without a change in the water input or the size of outlet hole (i.e., output function)? Initially, the water level would rise and hydrostatic pressure at the bottom of the tank would be increased. The higher pressure with the same size outlet hole would cause the output of water to exceed water input. The consequent imbalance between the input and output would cause a gradual decline in the water level. But, as long as the water level is higher, even slightly, than the baseline value, the water output will exceed the water input. Only when the water level decreases to the original level, will the water input equal the water output. A sudden increase in the capacity of the tank, for example by creating a pouch on the tank, would cause an imbalance between the water input and the water output because of the initial reduction in the water level and the hydrostatic pressure, but the discrepancy would be only transient. At equilibrium, the water level will return to the original level.

This type of compensation mechanism is ubiquitous in various physiological and pathological states in the human body, but the importance of this mechanism was first recognized by Guyton, who presented the concept in his discussion of the regulation of arterial blood pressure.[7-10] He boldly predicted that in the absence of an altered function of renal excretion of salt, no abnormality will sustain hypertension chronically. This prediction was made on the basis of the observation that the arterial blood pressure is normally a powerful regulator of renal salt excretion, and that a minute increase in blood pressure results in a large increase in salt excretion, and salt excretion in excess of salt intake will continue until the blood pressure returns to normal[9].

Suppose hypertension develops as a result of increased systemic vascular resistance, while the responsiveness of the kidney to changes in blood pressure to influence salt output (i.e., renal function curve in response to blood pressure) remains unchanged; the higher the pressure, the higher the renal salt output. Increased salt output caused by a higher blood pressure in the absence of commensurate increase in salt intake would lead to a negative salt balance. The negative salt balance would reduce effective vascular volume, circulating blood volume, and eventually cardiac output. A lower cardiac output will reduce blood pressure to a lower level, but as long as the blood pressure is still higher than the baseline, salt output will remain greater than the basal salt output. The salt output in excess of salt intake progressively reduces the salt content of the body. Only when blood pressure returns to the original value will the renal salt output return to the baseline value. At this point, balance is restored between salt intake and salt output, and the abnormality in blood pressure is completely dissipated.

In Guyton's use, the term "gain" is defined as the fraction of abnormality that has been corrected divided by the fraction yet to be corrected.[8] For example, if an abnormality causes an increase in blood pressure, and a control system brings it back halfway to the original value, the feedback gain is one ($0.5/0.5 = 1$). Gain is zero if a control system does not correct at all ($0/1 = 0$). Gain is infinite if the abnormality is almost all corrected completely with virtually nothing left to be corrected, because division of a number with an infinitely small number results in an infinitely large number.

What is the reason why an abnormality disappears completely in the infinite gain control mechanism, but not in other control mechanisms? The main difference is in the nature of the influence that causes disturbances in the system. When the disturbance affects either input or responsiveness of the system to change in a parameter for the output (i.e., output function), the abnormality will not be corrected completely, and the compensation mechanism does not involve the infinite gain control mechanism. On the other hand, when the disturbance introduced is not one of these two kinds, the compensation mechanism is an infinite gain control mechanism.

COMMON MISCONCEPTIONS AND NEW INSIGHTS

A series of topics discussed in the following section deals with widespread misconceptions regarding principles related to restoration of balance states.

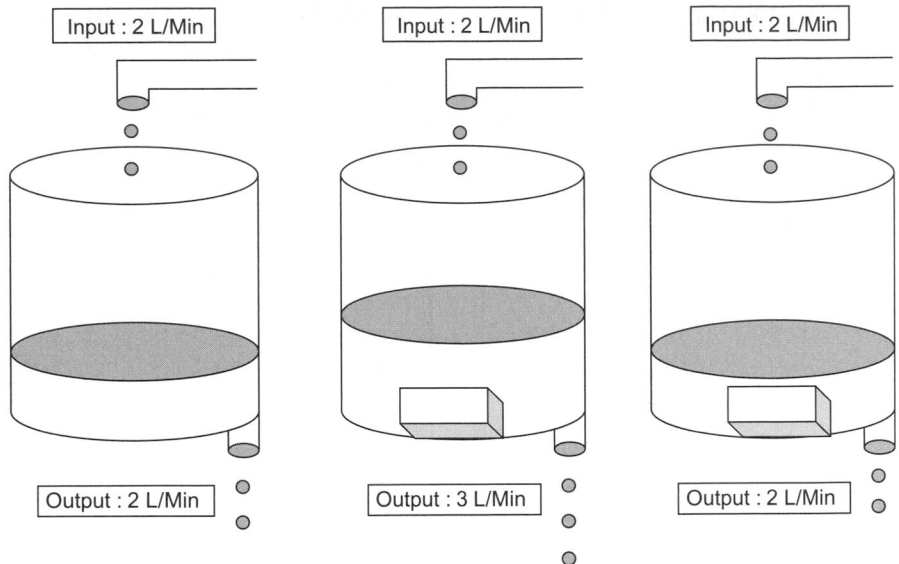

FIGURE 10.5   An example of infinite gain control mechanism. Water input and water output determine the balance, but water output is determined by the size of the hole at the bottom and the height of the water column. If water input and the size of the hole at the bottom remain unchanged, any change in the capacity of the tank will alter the height of water column only temporarily. For example, putting a brick into the tank reduces the capacity of the tank. This will increase the water column height only transiently. A higher level of water column with the same size of outlet hole will increase water output. Water output in excess of water input gradually decreases the height of the water column. Only when the height of the water column returns to the original level, is a balance restored between input and output.

There is no Set Point for Renal Salt Excretion

Hollenberg, citing the earlier writing on the same subject by Straus and colleagues[11] proposed a hypothesis for the existence of a set point for the regulation of body sodium content by the kidney. The set point is defined in his writings as the level of sodium content in the body that the kidney tries to maintain as the normal and desirable level. Henceforth, this hypothesis will be called the *set point hypothesis*. The evidence for the set point hypothesis follows.

First, when sodium intake is suddenly reduced, the rate of decrease in urine sodium excretion is exponential. The authors of the hypothesis consider the exponential decline thermodynamically unsound. If the decline were in response to progressive volume depletion, the authors argued, the decline should be accelerating, not declining exponentially. Second, when patients in sodium balance on a low sodium diet (10 mEq/day) were given a small amount of extra sodium (e.g., 30 mEq), the extra sodium was promptly excreted. It is further argued that if the patient had been volume depleted at the time, he should not have excreted the extra sodium. Finally, when a patient who was volume depleted by chronic diuretic therapy was given sodium, no sodium diuresis occurred until the body sodium content was brought back to the level that was achieved on zero sodium intake.

On the basis of these observations, the set point for renal sodium excretion was defined as the amount of

sodium in the body when the subject is in balance on a salt-free diet. Accordingly, most humans are in a state of sodium excess, and hence the unloading of excess sodium diminishes the stimulus for sodium diuresis, producing an exponential decrease in renal sodium excretion. It was further argued that the absence of a set point would lead to chaos, and a control system without a reference point is unimaginable. The possibility of a set point being higher or lower than the level defined above was dismissed; the exponential decrease in sodium excretion on a salt-free diet is considered to be evidence against a higher set point, whereas the absence of sodium diuresis upon salt administration in patients pretreated with a diuretic was thought to be evidence against the existence of a lower set point. The set point hypothesis has been debated in the public forum previously[12,13] - but the uniqueness of the current argument against the hypothesis is that it is advanced by the use of counter examples (three counter examples follow).

1. When water intake is suddenly stopped after a period of normal water intake, the pattern of urine water output follows the same pattern as the renal salt output after sudden curtailment of salt intake. With increasing water deficit on a zero water intake, urine output declines exponentially, not accelerating, despite progressive water deficit and progressive activation of the water-conserving mechanism. Clearly, the water content of the body

on zero water intake cannot be the desirable water content.

2. When a patient is on a potassium-free diet, urinary excretion of potassium declines exponentially, not accelerating, despite a progressive increase in potassium deficit. Again, no one would argue that the potassium content of the body on zero potassium intake is the desirable body potassium content.

3. The arterial pCO_2 declines exponentially with increasing severity of metabolic acidosis, despite metabolic acidosis becoming more and more severe.

These counter examples indicate that the finding that urinary sodium declines exponentially neither supports nor argues against the existence of a set point, as previously defined. When sodium intake is stopped, urine sodium decreases progressively because effective vascular volume declines progressively, and as a result sodium reabsorption mechanisms in the kidney are activated progressively. Whether the body sodium content at usual sodium intake is normal or excessive is not a question that can be decided by the pattern of renal sodium excretion, just as we cannot decide the normal plasma potassium concentration by the pattern of renal potassium output in response to a change in potassium intake.

In an attempt to define a normal value in the set point hypothesis, a special meaning has been attached to the pattern of renal sodium excretion. However, normalcy of any physiological values must ultimately be decided by their relation to morbidity and mortality. Given the well-known effects of the body salt content on blood pressure, it may be more advantageous to have a salt content that is achieved on a near salt-free diet than the content attained on the current usual salt intake. The fact that the body's sodium content attained on a near salt free diet is more advantageous to human health is, in my opinion, pure chance, but may have contributed to the set point hypothesis. At different times in human history, a slight excess in sodium content might have been beneficial to survival, when salt was not readily available in many parts of the world and salt loss was a common occurrence from gastroenteritis and sweating. This scenario seems more plausible when one realizes that the main adverse effect of excess salt content in the body is increase in blood pressure, and hypertension was not the main cause of death when the average lifespan was 30 to 40 years. Normally, urine sodium excretion decreases when effective vascular volume declines. Thus, the relationship between effective vascular volume and renal sodium excretion can be summed up in one sentence: the lower the effective vascular volume, the lower the renal sodium output, and the higher the effective vascular volume, the higher the renal sodium output.

As explained in model B (Figure 10.3), the relationship between renal sodium excretion and effective vascular volume is not continuous; below a certain level of effective vascular volume, renal sodium output virtually disappears, and this happens before any overt signs of clinical dehydration. When effective vascular volume decreases further, renal sodium excretion cannot decrease further because renal sodium excretion cannot be a negative number, even though the sodium retaining mechanisms are even more activated. Administration of sodium in such a state would not cause sodium diuresis until effective vascular volume increases to a higher level. The proponent of the set point hypothesis asks the question: "if a subject is volume depleted on 10 mEq per day sodium diet, why would he excrete the administered sodium?" The simple answer would be "because he is less volume depleted now."

It is the central core of the set point hypothesis that the kidney stops excreting sodium at the set point, i.e., the salt content attained at near zero sodium intake, in order to preserve the most desirable value of body sodium content. However, that is not the consistent behavior of the kidney. Urine output never becomes zero until the kidney is completely shut off, despite progressive water deficit and clear clinical evidence of dehydration. Likewise, renal potassium output does not cease on a zero potassium intake, despite clinically evident hypokalemia.[14]

Renal Salt Output Does Not Exceed Salt Intake in Salt Losing Nephropathy

An often-cited diagnostic criterion for salt losing nephropathy is urine sodium excretion in excess of sodium intake.[15] This is obviously impossible on a chronic basis, just as chronic diuretic therapy cannot produce persistent net sodium loss. Salt intake must equal salt output in the long run, but transient imbalance often occurs. Salt output exceeds intake while volume depletion develops, but the reverse occurs when volume depletion is being corrected. If a patient with salt-losing nephropathy who had been on a high-salt diet reduces salt intake because of an illness, the patient will develop volume depletion, and during this period urine salt output exceeds salt intake, and hence a negative salt balance occurs. On the other hand, when the same patient resumes his usual salt intake or receives intravenous fluid, salt balance will be positive during the period of recovery. The diagnosis of salt losing nephropathy requires documentation of inappropriate urinary salt excretion in the presence of volume depletion.

Mechanism of Low Urea Nitrogen Concentration in Liver Disease

It is often stated that serum urea nitrogen level is very low in chronic liver disease because urea is produced in the liver, and the diseased liver cannot produce urea at the normal rate.[16] It is obvious that a low serum urea concentration without increased urea clearance must be due to reduced production, but impaired liver function is not the reason for reduced production. Once ingested protein is broken down to individual amino acids, and is absorbed into the bloodstream, it has three metabolic pathways: (1) metabolism to urea to be excreted in urine; (2) metabolism to non-urea nitrogen compounds to be excreted in urine; and (3) protein synthesis. Patients with chronic liver disease are not in a state of net protein synthesis, i.e., an anabolic state. Major non-urea nitrogen compounds normally excreted in urine include ammonia, amino acids, creatinine, and uric acid, and urinary excretion of these compounds is not increased in chronic liver disease. One might suggest that nitrogen could accumulate as ammonia in the blood as metabolic conversion of ammonia to urea is impaired in liver disease. In severe liver disease, ammonia concentration in plasma is indeed increased, but the total amount of nitrogen that can accumulate in the body in the form of ammonia without fatal consequences is extremely small. The concentrations of ammonia in plasma are expressed in micrograms per dl, whereas those of urea are in milligrams per dl. Accumulation of only 10% of ingested nitrogen as ammonia instead of its conversion to urea would lead to fatal hyper-ammonemia within hours.

The only logical explanation for low urea production, therefore, is reduced protein intake. Chronic alcoholics often have persistently low protein ingestion, and they have low plasma urea nitrogen. However, any normal person ingesting a low protein diet will also have low urea nitrogen production, and therefore low plasma urea nitrogen. A strict vegetarian often has a low urea nitrogen concentration, for these reasons. When a patient with a liver disease has a G-I hemorrhage, serum urea nitrogen concentration rises promptly, indicating that the diseased liver can produce urea rapidly when substrate is available. If a person with severe liver disease ingests a normal amount of protein, urea production will be normal, but plasma ammonia will be higher.

It is a general rule that an impaired metabolic pathway does not reduce the output of its metabolic product unless there is another pathway to which the precursor of the product can be shunted. In the absence of another pathway, at equilibrium the concentration of the precursor will be increased, and the rate of output of the metabolic product will return to the baseline. The situation is analogous to the quantity of creatinine excretion in chronic renal failure. When the kidney function is impaired, the amount of creatinine excreted in the urine does not decrease, as long as creatinine production remains unchanged. The amount excreted will decrease at the onset of renal failure, but at equilibrium it will return to baseline. One does not measure the rate of urinary creatinine excretion as a means of determining renal function; one looks at serum creatinine concentration instead. Likewise, the rate of production of urea by the liver does not offer any clue to the level of liver function, but serum ammonia level does.

Sodium Intake and Sodium Balance are Poor Predictors of Effective Vascular Volume

The assessment of effective vascular volume by urinary sodium excretion is a widely used and useful clinical tool. Most physicians, however, believe that knowledge of both sodium intake and urine sodium output provides a better clue to the status of effective vascular volume. The following example explains why this reasoning is flawed.

Question: Two subjects, A and B, have been admitted to the hospital with unknown status of their effective vascular volume. Subject A is given a diet containing 100 mEq of sodium per day, and subject B gets a sodium intake of 20 mEq a day. In the next 24 hours, subject A excretes 60 mEq of sodium per day, and subject B excretes 40 mEq of sodium per day. On the basis of this information, which subject do you believe has a higher effective vascular volume? You should assume that neither subject has any renal or hormonal disorder that would affect renal sodium excretion.

Answer and discussion: The most common answer is that A has a lower effective vascular volume than B. The reasoning for the answer: person A is in positive sodium balance because the "smart kidney," sensing volume depletion, retains sodium, whereas person B is in negative sodium balance because the "smart kidney," sensing the volume expansion, compels him to excrete the excess sodium. It is true that the balance data indicates that A is in a state of sodium retention and B in a state of sodium loss. However, sodium retention need not indicate the presence of volume depletion, and sodium loss not does prove the state of expanded volume. The following examples will make these points obvious.

A person in salt balance while ingesting 100 mEq of sodium per day suddenly increased sodium intake to 200 mEq per day. Salt excretion will eventually increase to the same level as intake, but not on the first day. If adjustment in salt excretion matched intake immediately, there would be no retention of sodium, and there would be no harmful effect of a high salt intake. Instead, there would be some sodium retention. On the first day he may excrete only 150 mEq, causing net retention of 50 mEq of sodium. The positive sodium balance in this instance is due to increased intake, not to reduced excretion. Furthermore, a positive sodium balance increases the effective vascular volume to a higher level than the previous day, and the higher effective vascular volume is indeed the reason for the greater urinary sodium excretion. Clearly, positive sodium balance does not necessarily mean low effective vascular volume.

In another example, a patient with intractable heart failure is ingesting 50 mEq of sodium per day and excretes only 10 mEq per day. He is retaining sodium avidly, and hence the term renal sodium retention would be appropriate in this setting, as positive sodium balance in this instance is due to low effective vascular volume. Frustrated by relentless sodium retention, the physician prescribes a salt-free diet, and urine sodium drops further to 5 mEq per day. At this point, however, his overall sodium balance is −5 mEq per day. Can we say, then, that his effective vascular volume is no longer diminished, since he is no longer retaining sodium?

Sodium intake itself has no direct effect on renal sodium output. Any influence of sodium intake on renal sodium output is always mediated through effective vascular volume, because balance between sodium intake and sodium output influences effective vascular volume. If we think of renal sodium output in terms of model B (Figure 10.3), the height of the water column represents effective vascular volume. Just as the only factor that influences water output in model B is the height of water column, the only factor that influences renal sodium excretion directly is effective vascular volume. The higher the effective vascular volume, the higher is the urine sodium; the lower the effective vascular volume, the lower is the urine sodium. Once this relationship is understood, the question regarding subjects A and B is easy; subject A has higher effective vascular volume, because he is excreting more sodium in urine than subject B.

The reason for the widespread belief that sodium intake and output is a better predictor of effective vascular volume is likely to be due to the misuse of the term renal sodium retention. The train of logic goes as follows. First, sodium intake in excess of sodium output represents sodium retention. Second, sodium retention in most clinical situations is due to reduced renal excretion of sodium. Third, reduced renal excretion of sodium is most often due to low effective vascular volume. Fourth, therefore sodium retention is

most often due to low effective vascular volume. Finally, any sodium retention, i.e., positive sodium balance, signifies low effective vascular volume. Although the fatal error in reasoning is in the final step, the major mistake occurred in the thinking that sodium retention is always due to reduced renal sodium output, instead of thinking that it is *usually* due to reduced renal sodium output.[17]

Does Overflow Mechanism Explain Ascites Formation?

The overflow theory of ascites formation states that an important mechanism of sodium retention in ascites formation in cirrhosis of the liver is primary renal sodium retention due to a diseased liver. The argument is based on the data from drug-induced cirrhosis of the liver in dogs, which developed ascites and salt retention in the absence of signs of reduced effective vascular volume, such as elevated PRA and plasma aldosterone concentration. On the basis of these observations, the authors of the study concluded that renal sodium retention could not have been a response to volume depletion caused by loss of fluid to the peritoneal cavity (i.e., under-filling), and therefore renal salt retention was a primary event that led to increased effective vascular volume resulting in the ascites formation (i.e., overflow).[18,19] Two major errors were made in this line of thinking.

The first error is the assumption that the proof of salt retention (i.e., positive salt balance) due to the under-filling mechanism requires the presence of overt volume depletion. The following example will demonstrate how effective vascular volume could remain "normal" during the period of positive salt balance by an under-filling mechanism. Assume that a person, who has been in salt balance while ingesting 15 g of salt a day and excreting 15 g a day, develops chronic diarrhea and loses 5 g of salt in the stool daily. The net GI absorption of salt after subtracting the amount lost in the stool would then be 10 g per day, and he would excrete 10 g of salt in the urine per day. His effective vascular volume during diarrhea will be lower than it was before the start of diarrhea, but not lower than that of a person ingesting only 10 g of salt per day without diarrhea. Likewise, if a person ingesting 15 g of salt per day develops ascites slowly, and sequesters 5 g of salt daily in the peritoneal space, his effective vascular volume would not be lower than a person who ingests 10 g of salt a day without development of ascites. In both cases, ingestion of 15 g of salt, in the absence of abnormal salt loss, would have resulted in excretion of 15 g of salt. With ascites formation or diarrhea, the kidney excretes 10 g instead of 15 g, because the effective vascular volume is slightly lower than in a person without ascites formation or diarrhea. In both cases, the reduction in renal sodium output clearly was in response to "under-filling," even though there would be no discernible volume depletion. In both examples, effective vascular volume was maintained sufficiently high to allow renal excretion of 10 g of salt a day. If plasma renin activity were measured during the period of sodium retention in these examples, it would have been normal. The absence of apparent volume depletion in any edema-forming conditions does not prove that the kidney did not retain sodium in response to a volume stimulus.

The second error is the failure to recognize that the infinite gain control mechanism operates in ascites formation by the under-filling mechanism. If the salt intake and the function curve for renal salt output remain unchanged, effective vascular volume would return to the baseline when steady-state is achieved. The sequence of events would be as follows. Ascites formation by the transudation of fluid from the vascular space into the peritoneal cavity would reduce effective vascular volume, which reduces renal salt output. The normal salt intake with reduced renal salt output causes salt retention, which would tend to increase effective vascular volume. However, as long as effective vascular volume remains lower than the baseline value, renal salt output will remain lower than the baseline, and the positive salt balance will continue. Only when effective vascular volume returns to the baseline, will renal salt output return to the baseline, and the salt retention will stop. Thus, at equilibrium, effective vascular volume in any patient with ascites would be normal, unless he is treated with a low-salt diet or a diuretic.

Main Mechanism of Nephrotic Edema: Low Oncotic Pressure versus Primary Renal Salt Retention

It has been suggested that primary renal salt retention plays a more important role in the formation of nephrotic edema than low oncotic pressure which would cause secondary renal salt retention.[20] This belief is based on the observation that in untreated subjects with nephrotic syndrome, plasma renin activity is often reduced. The reasoning goes this way: if low oncotic pressure is the primary cause of edema formation, transudation of fluid from the vascular space into the interstitial space would reduce effective vascular volume, which is expected to increase plasma renin activity; the suppressed plasma renin activity, therefore, is the evidence for primacy of primary salt retention in the pathogenesis of nephrotic edema.

The flaw of this reasoning lies in the faulty assumption that edema due to low oncotic pressure must be accompanied by low effective vascular volume. The truth is that nephrotic edema entirely due to low oncotic pressure would not maintain low effective vascular volume, unless the patient is treated with salt restriction or a diuretic. The compensation mechanism against a low effective vascular volume in such situations would be the infinite gain control mechanism.

Imagine a patient in a third world country develops nephrotic syndrome. The patient is not treated with a diuretic, and he does not know the value of a low-salt diet in treating edema. He continues to ingest a diet that contains the usual amount of salt. Yet almost invariably, his renal salt output returns to the baseline and salt retention stops. Otherwise, the patient will develop relentless sodium retention and progressive edema, and will die in a relatively short period with massive edema. Since a slight reduction in effective vascular volume diminishes renal sodium excretion to virtually zero, restoration of renal sodium excretion to a usual normal value is proof that effective vascular volume has been restored to normal. Plasma renin activity at this point would be normal.

If a patient now develops a renal disease that results in primary renal salt retention, edema will be worse and effective vascular volume will be greater than the usual value, which would cause suppression of plasma renin activity. When the natriuretic effect of the increased effective vascular volume is sufficient to counterbalance the sodium retaining effect of the renal disease, renal sodium output will increase further to achieve a new balance. At this point, edema will not progress any further. The presence of suppressed plasma renin activity in a patient with nephrotic syndrome is a strong indication for the presence of primary renal sodium retention, but it does not prove that low oncotic pressure is not the main cause of edema formation. Indeed, primary renal Na retention alone, e.g., acute glomerulonephritis, rarely causes as severe edema as a non-nephrotic cause of low oncotic pressure, such as severe protein malnutrition.

CLINICAL APPLICATION OF EXTERNAL BALANCE

A serious topic discussed below utilizes the principles of external balance to explain physiological concepts and clinical manifestations of certain disorders of fluid and electrolyte balance.

Determinants of Sodium Delivery to the Cortical Collecting Duct and Renal K Excretion

According to the principles outlined at the beginning of this chapter, in the steady-state, sodium output is equal to sodium intake, including all salt-retaining and salt-wasting conditions, such as hyperaldosteronism and hypoaldosteronism. One might therefore conclude that sodium delivery to the cortical collecting duct cannot remain chronically abnormal unless intake is altered. However, the principles discussed in earlier sections predict that total sodium output will eventually equal intake; it does not predict that sodium delivery to any particular nephron site cannot remain chronically altered.

In the steady-state, a patient receiving chronic diuretic therapy or one with primary hyperaldosteronism will excrete the same amount of sodium as before the abnormalities developed, if the intake remains the same. In both states, however, a greater amount of sodium would be reabsorbed at the collecting duct because of the increased aldosterone effect, but the amount excreted in the final urine cannot be more or less than the intake. To satisfy both conditions, sodium delivery to the collecting duct at the time of balance restoration must be increased in hyperaldosteronism, and decreased in hypoaldosteronism. Primary hyperaldosteronism will be used as an example to explain this.

The initial abnormality in primary hyperaldosteronism is increased salt reabsorption, mainly at the cortical collecting duct, resulting in reduced salt output. The consequent positive salt balance increases effective vascular volume, which inhibits the proximal tubular salt reabsorption, resulting in increased delivery of salt to the cortical collecting duct. With the increased delivery of salt, the amount of salt that escapes into the urine is more now than at the beginning, but still less than intake because of increased salt reabsorption in the collecting duct. As long as urinary excretion of salt is less than intake, net positive salt retention continues, causing further increase in effective vascular volume. A higher effective vascular volume further inhibits proximal tubular salt reabsorption, causing even greater increase in the distal delivery of salt. The process will continue, with progressive increase in effective vascular volume and further increase in salt excretion. Only when excretion of salt is equal to intake will positive salt balance stop. At equilibrium, salt output equals salt intake, but the quantity of salt delivered to the collecting duct remains increased.

In the case of therapy with a loop diuretic or a thiazide diuretic, initially salt delivery to the collecting duct would be greatly increased; during this period salt balance will be negative. The ensuing volume depletion activates salt-retaining mechanisms at the proximal tubule, and also stimulates aldosterone secretion causing increased reabsorption of salt in the cortical collecting duct. One might predict that in a steady-state, sodium delivery to the collecting duct would be normalized as the two opposing effects cancel out each other's effect. However, as long as the increased aldosterone secretion caused by volume depletion increases reabsorption of Na in the cortical collecting duct, Na delivery to the collecting duct must remain increased, in order to have a normal amount of Na excretion in the final urine. In other words, the combined effect of increased proximal Na reabsorption and decreased Na reabsorption by the diuretics would be chronic increase in Na delivery to the cortical collecting duct. Normal delivery of sodium accompanied by increased reabsorption of sodium at the cortical collecting duct would result in reduced excretion of sodium in the final urine; this is impossible.

For the same reasons, sodium delivery to the cortical collecting duct remains reduced chronically in states of hypoaldosteronism, such as Addison's disease. Because the Na reabsorption at the cortical collecting duct is reduced, the only way to have the same normal amount of Na excretion in the final urine is to have reduced delivery of Na to the collecting duct.

Two most important factors that influence renal K excretion are the amount of Na delivery to the cortical collecting duct and aldosterone concentration. Most clinical states that cause increased renal excretion of K are accompanied by increased Na delivery and increased aldosterone, whereas conditions characterized by reduced renal K excretion are accompanied by reduced Na delivery and a low plasma aldosterone or an impaired aldosterone effect. Renal K excretion is unaffected when these two factors are altered in opposite directions. In a high-salt diet sodium delivery to the cortical collecting duct is increased, but aldosterone secretion is reduced, resulting in a normal K excretion. A salt restriction reduces sodium delivery to the cortical collecting duct, but the aldosterone secretion is increased, resulting in a normal K excretion (Table 10.3).

Enigma of Pendred Syndrome

Pendred syndrome is a genetic disorder characterized by goiter and sensorineural hearing loss, responsible for about 7.5% of congenital hearing loss. The disease is named after Vaughan Pendred, an English physician who first described the condition in 1896.[21] The mechanism of the disease is a defect in an anion exchanger pendrin, which is located in the inner ear, thyroid gland, and the cortical collecting duct. The exchanger, located on the luminal membrane of beta-intercalated cells, appears to play an important role in the reabsorption of chloride, and therefore indirectly of sodium.[22]

Despite the common belief that chloride reabsorption in the collecting tubule duct depends mainly on

TABLE 10.3 Na Delivery to Cortical Collecting Duct (CCD) and Aldosterone Affecting Urine K

Clinical States	Na Delivery to CCD	Aldosterone Effect	Urine K Excretion
Hyperaldosteronism	Increased	Increased	Increased
Diuretics	Increased	Increased	Increased
Hypoaldosteronism	Decreased	Decreased	Decreased
K sparing diuretics	Decreased	Decreased	Decreased
Pendred syndrome	Decreased	Increased	Normal
High-salt diet	Increased	Decreased	Normal
Low-salt diet	Decreased	Increased	Normal

the paracellular chloride channel, supportive evidence is not very strong. For example, in severe volume depletion states, urine chloride concentration is as low as 2 mEq/L.[23] The Nernst Equation would predict that such a low chloride concentration, to be explained entirely by a passive mechanism through the paracellular pathway, would require the transepithelial voltage of over 100 mV. The highest transepithelial voltage observed in states of high aldosterone effect is about 60 mV. It is likely that other mechanisms exist for reabsorption of chloride in the cortical collecting duct, and the most likely one is pendrin-mediated chloride reabsorption.[22] If pendrin were such an important transporter for reabsorption of chloride in the cortical collecting duct, why isn't a pendrin defect associated with any electrolyte abnormality? Indeed, the apparent absence of electrolyte abnormalities is one of the reasons why Pendred syndrome, well-known among specialists of ENT, is not widely appreciated among nephrologists.

The most common and apparent electrolyte abnormality associated with impaired renal salt transport is hypokalemia, but Pendred syndrome is not known to be associated with hypokalemia. The following is the likely scenario. A pendrin defect would reduce the overall reabsorption of NaCl in the cortical collecting duct, and the ensuing volume depletion would stimulate renin and hence aldosterone. However, unlike defects in salt transport caused by impaired salt reabsorption in the distal convoluted tubule (Gitelman's syndrome) or the thick ascending limb of Henle (Bartter's syndrome), both of which are characterized by increased salt delivery to the cortical collecting duct, the delivery of salt to the cortical collecting duct in Pendred syndrome would be reduced. That is because the site of defect in salt transport is the cortical collecting duct itself. According to the principle of external balance, in the long run salt intake must equal

salt output, no matter what and where defects in renal salt transport may be. Thus, a patient with Pendred syndrome would be excreting the normal amount of salt in the final urine. The excretion of the normal amount of salt and the reduced salt reabsorption at the cortical collecting duct is possible if the amount delivered to the cortical collecting duct is reduced. The end result is that patients with Pendred syndrome would have hyperaldosteronism, but reduced delivery of salt to the collecting duct. There has been no measurement of plasma aldosterone in patients with Pendred syndrome, but effective vascular volume is likely to be reduced and plasma aldosterone is likely to be increased. As supportive evidence, in a study of 21 patients with Pendred syndrome, not a single subject was shown to have hypertension.[24]

Is it possible that salt reabsorption at the cortical collecting duct is not reduced in Pendred syndrome because of the two opposite influences, a high aldosterone state increasing salt reabsorption and a defective pendrin impairing salt reabsorption? That is unlikely because reduced salt delivery with normal salt reabsorption at the cortical collecting duct would mean reduced salt excretion. Remember that in a steady-state final urine sodium excretion is always normal. Is it possible that salt delivery to the cortical collecting duct is normalized in a steady-state? Again, it is unlikely, because normal salt delivery would mean normal effective vascular volume, and then aldosterone secretion cannot be increased. In the end, in a steady-state in Pendred syndrome, there must be some volume depletion accompanied by hyperaldosteronism. At equilibrium renal K excretion in Pendred syndrome would be normal, because two main regulators of renal K excretion are altered in opposite directions; aldosterone is increased and Na delivery to the cortical collecting duct is reduced. The situation would be analogous to a person on a low-salt diet, in which aldosterone is increased but sodium delivery is reduced (Table 10.3). Thus, the patient with Pendred syndrome would be normotensive (low normal blood pressure) and normokalemic, and have no apparent electrolyte abnormalities.

In a recent case report,[25] a patient with Pendred syndrome treated with a thiazide diuretic developed severe hypokalemia (serum K 2.2 mEq/L) and signs of profound volume depletion. The likely explanation for severe potassium depletion is that the patient has impaired salt transport in both the distal convoluted tubule and collecting duct. Severe renal K-wasting occurred because sodium delivery to the cortical collecting duct was increased by a thiazide diuretic in the setting of high aldosterone. In another report, a patient with Pendred syndrome developed life-threatening metabolic alkalosis during intercurrent illnesses, indicating the importance in chloride reabsorption.[26]

Hypoxemia is necessary to restore balance between oxygen supply and oxygen demand

While the principle of external balance is most useful in explaining homeostatic mechanisms of fluid and electrolyte balance, the same principle applies to restoration of balances in other homeostatic mechanisms. The following example illustrates the mechanism by which a patient with severe lung disease can maintain the normal supply of oxygen necessary to sustain life.

The basal oxygen consumption of a person with advanced lung disease is no less, perhaps slightly greater because of the increased work of breathing, than that of a healthy individual. This means that the diseased lung somehow takes up a normal amount of oxygen. How does this happen? Here is the explanation. A normal person who has alveolar ventilation of 4 liters a minute needs an uptake of 200 ml of oxygen per minute at the basal state. The oxygen content of one liter of inspired air at an atmospheric pO_2 of 150 mmHg is 200 ml, and the oxygen content the expired air is about 150 ml per liter with the pO_2 at 110 mmHg. With an alveolar–arterial pO_2 gradient of 10 mmHg, the arterial pO_2 would be about 100 mmHg. This means that each liter of ventilated air has resulted in uptake of 50 ml of oxygen or total of 200 ml of oxygen by 4 liters of alveolar ventilation. When alveolar ventilation is reduced to 2 liters per minute, how is it possible to extract the same 200 ml of oxygen? A quick calculation will indicate that, in order to extract the same 200 ml of oxygen, each of 2 liters of alveolar ventilation must result in an uptake of 100 ml of oxygen. Since the inspired air has still the same oxygen content at pO_2 150 mmHg, the expired air must have a pO_2 of 70 mmHg. This requires alveolar pO_2 to decrease to 70 mmHg. Since arterial pO_2 is about 10 mmHg lower, it must decrease to 60 mmHg. In other words, hypoxemia is a necessary condition for restoring oxygen uptake to normal.

How does the body know to reduce the arterial pO_2 precisely to the right level to restore oxygen balance? The body does not know, but the general principle of external balance allows automatic restoration of balance. Let us suppose that alveolar ventilation drops to half that of normal. Initially there will be a discrepancy between the body's demand for oxygen and oxygen supply. The reduced supply in the face of unchanged demand will decrease arterial pO_2. A lower arterial pO_2 means a lower alveolar pO_2, which permits greater uptake of oxygen for a given volume of alveolar ventilation. As long as oxygen uptake is less than oxygen demand, arterial pO_2 will keep decreasing, with further reduction in alveolar pO_2. Only when the alveolar pO_2 decreases sufficiently to allow oxygen uptake to meet oxygen demand, is a new balance achieved between oxygen demand and oxygen uptake.

Will this mechanism of external balance restore oxygen uptake at any severity of lung disease? The answer is no. What would happen if the alveolar ventilation decreased to 1 liter per minute? In order to have an uptake of 200 ml of oxygen by 1 liter of alveolar ventilation, each liter now extracts the entire oxygen content of the inspired air, since the total content of oxygen at pO_2 of 150 mmHg is 200 ml. This would mean that alveolar pO_2 must be 0 mmHg, clearly an impossible situation, since arterial pO2, always lower than alveolar pO2, must be a negative number. Long before the alveolar pO_2 drops to 0 mmHg, the person will die of severe hypoxia.

Mechanism of Volume Expansion in SIADH

Ample evidence exists that patients with SIADH with chronic hyponatremia are volume expanded. Evidence for expanded volume includes low plasma creatinine, low plasma urea, and low plasma uric acid,[27,28] all caused by increased renal clearances. However, persistence of chronic volume expansion in SIADH would seem paradoxical. In the absence of disorders that cause primary renal Na retention, such as renal diseases and primary hyperaldosteronism, would the normal kidney not promptly eliminate the excess Na until the volume is restored to normal?

The explanation for the persistence of volume expansion in SIADH lies in the antinatriuretic effect of hyponatremia.[29,30] The sequence of events is as follows. Initially, water retention causes hyponatremia and volume expansion. Volume expansion causes sodium diuresis, resulting in further reduction in serum sodium. But as serum sodium declines, the antinatriuretic effect of hyponatremia opposes the natriuretic effect of volume expansion. When these two opposing effects are equal, renal Na excretion returns to the baseline value, and a new balance is established, with renal Na excretion equaling salt intake. In other words, when renal Na excretion returns to the baseline, the effective vascular volume must be expanded.

Mechanism of Volume Depletion in Chronic Hypernatremia

In the presence of normal renal function, chronic hypernatremia is always accompanied by reduced effective vascular volume, and the degree of reduction in effective vascular volume is proportionate to the level of serum sodium.[31,32] Exceptions are chronic hypernatremia in renal failure or hypernatremia that develops as a result of chronic administration of a large amount of sodium. Even in the latter condition, the effective vascular volume would be lower with high serum sodium than with normal serum sodium for the same amount of sodium administered. Although some authors postulate that the effective vascular volume is normal in essential hypernatremia,[31] this rule applies to all hypernatremic states including essential hypernatremia. The following analysis will elaborate on the mechanism.

As hyponatremia is antinatriuretic, hypernatremia is natriuretic.[33,34] For this reason, renal sodium excretion would be increased in normovolemic hypernatremia, as long as the kidney function is normal. Increased renal sodium excretion with the usual intake of sodium would reduce effective vascular volume. Volume depletion would reduce renal sodium excretion and oppose the natriuretic effect of hypernatremia. As long as renal sodium excretion exceeds sodium intake, volume depletion will become progressively greater. Only when volume depletion is sufficiently great to exactly oppose the natriuretic effect of hypernatremia, does renal sodium excretion return to the baseline, equaling the intake. At this point, a new sodium balance is struck between sodium intake and output, but at the expense of volume depletion. Since the natriuretic effect of hypernatremia is proportionate to the degree of hypernatremia, the magnitude of volume depletion needed to counterbalance the natriuretic effect of hypernatremia must also be proportionately great, to match the degree of hypernatremia when the new sodium balance is achieved. In other words, the more severe the hypernatremia, the greater is the volume depletion in a steady-state.

It has been suggested that patients with essential hypernatremia are euvolemic, because hypernatremia in this condition is a result of the resetting of the osmostat.[31] Resetting means that the osmostat is regulated normally, but at higher than usual serum sodium concentrations. More recent evidence indicates that essential hypernatremia is caused by defects in the osmoreceptors, not the resetting.[35] However, regardless of its pathogenetic mechanism, chronic volume depletion is inevitable in essential hypernatremia if renal function is normal. Mild volume depletion can escape detection even by careful physical examination. For example, a small amount of a diuretic, e.g., 50 mg hydrochlorothiazide, can reduce effective vascular volume sufficiently for the kidney to sense a reduction in volume, and thereby reduce clearances of urea, creatinine, and uric acid. Yet a careful physical examination by an astute physician will not detect signs of dehydration without the help of laboratory tests, e.g., a higher serum urate. Indeed, it has been shown that most patients with essential hypernatremia have laboratory evidence of volume depletion when the data are carefully analyzed.[32]

EXTERNAL BALANCE OF PROTONS

Determination of external balance of most univalent ions such as sodium, potassium, and chloride is straightforward; intestinal absorption is complete and they are eventually eliminated from the body since none is metabolized. Balance of polyvalent inorganic ions such as calcium, magnesium and phosphate is more complicated, because of incomplete intestinal absorption. External balance of acids and bases is even more complicated than that of polyvalent ions, because of uncertainties in their intestinal absorption and variations in their metabolism after absorption.

In the steady-state, hydrogen ions enter the body through ingestion of acid or are created endogenously through metabolism. The pH of food offers little guidance to its character as a donor of acid or alkali. Most fruit juices have low pH because of the organic acids in them, but overall they are contributors of alkali, because organic acid is metabolized to CO_2, while organic anions are metabolized to bicarbonate. Sulfur-containing amino acids are mostly metabolized to produce sulfuric acid, but not all sulfur is metabolized to sulfuric acid.

Under steady-state conditions, net acid production must equal net acid excretion, and the traditional view of the external balance of acid–base has been as follows. Acids are produced from three main sources: sulfuric acid derived from the metabolism of sulfur-containing amino acids; incompletely metabolized organic acids; and acid (or alkali) from the diet absorbed in the intestine.[36–38] Acids are excreted either in the form of ammonium or titratable acid, while a small amount of alkali is lost in the urine as bicarbonate. Hence, the total acid excretion measured as the sum of urine ammonium and titratable acid minus bicarbonate is called net acid excretion. However, this traditional view of the acid–base balance must be re-evaluated in light of conceptual uncertainties of this approach, and methodological limitations in the measurement of parameters of acid–base balance by conventional techniques.[38] The following discussion will shed some light on these uncertainties and limitations.

MEASUREMENT OF NET ACID EXCRETION

The concept of titratable acid is straightforward. The pH of urine following glomerular ultrafiltration is the same as that of plasma, but decreases progressively with addition of H^+ by tubular secretion. Most of the secreted H^+ is buffered by HCO_3^-, and this represents indirect reabsorption of HCO_3^-. As urine pH falls further with tubular secretion of H^+, other urinary buffers are titrated to retard a fall in urine pH. Addition of alkali to the urine until its pH is the same as that of the plasma measures the titratable acid. This back-titration of urine releases all the H^+ titrated by non-bicarbonate buffers except those in the form of NH_4^+, which is not titrated because of its high pK (9.2), and therefore is measured separately.

However, the measurement of titratable acid, ammonium, and bicarbonate does not accurately reflect net acid excretion by the kidney, for the following reasons. First, there is a technical problem with the measurement of titratable acid.[39] Addition of alkali to the urine causes partial precipitation of some urine calcium with HPO_4^{2-}. Selective depletion of HPO_4^{2-} causes conversion of $H_2PO_4^-$ to HPO_4^{2-} with liberation of protons, leading to overestimation of titratable acid. Furthermore, titration of urine to the plasma pH results in titration of 1/64th of urinary ammonium (calculated with the pKa of ammonium of 9.2), resulting in further overestimation of titratable acid; this error is usually negligible, but would be substantial when urine contains a large amount of ammonium.

A potentially more serious source of error is the presence of buffers other than ammonium that are not titrated when urine pH is increased to 7.4.[40] The original assumption that ammonium is the only urinary buffer that escapes titration during the measurement of titratable acid has not been fully proven. Normal urine contains various amines such as ethanolamine, phosphoethanolamine, methylamine, and dimethylamine. Urinary excretion of these substances would represent acid excretion, as does the excretion of ammonium. However, titration of urine to pH 7.4 would not detect the presence of such substances. The individual urine concentration of each of these substances appears to be quite low individually, but the amount might be substantial collectively.

SOURCES OF ACID

Sulfuric Acid

The metabolism of sulfur-containing amino acids produces sulfuric acid:

$$RN - S \rightarrow CO_2 + UREA + H_2SO_4.$$

The resulting H_2SO_4 is buffered by the body alkali, mainly HCO_3^-. Previously it was assumed that virtually all urinary sulfates originate from sulfur-containing amino acids. However, this assumption is wrong, since soft drinks regularly contain sulfate as a preservative, and persons consuming large quantities of soft drinks could acquire a substantial amount of sulfate. In one such study, the average amount of urinary sulfate originating from soft drinks was estimated to be 15 mEq/day.[41] Furthermore, the metabolism of sulfur-containing amino acids does not always result in production of sulfuric acid,[42,43] because some of the sulfur is excreted in a neutral form, such as cystine, taurine or sulfate conjugate.[44-46] Each mmol of sulfur metabolized to H_2SO_4 produces 2 mEq of protons in the following reaction:

$$H_2SO_4 \rightarrow SO_4^= + 2H^+$$

On the other hand, the sulfate conjugation reaction consumes a proton; the result is net production of only 1 mEq of proton for each mole of sulfur oxidized when the final product is sulfate conjugate.

$$R - OH + SO_4^= + H^+ \rightarrow R - O - SO_3^-$$

Sulfate conjugation reaction is an important detoxicification mechanism, and the reactions are regulated by various enzymes, such as phenol sulfotransferase.[44-46] The rate of sulfate conjugation reaction seems to depend, in part, on the availability of inorganic sulfate. For these reasons, the fraction of sulfur contained in amino acids that is oxidized to sulfuric acid might vary with individuals, and also with the amount of protein intake. In one study, urinary sulfate recovered following ingestion of methionine was shown to be 85–90% of the sulfur content of the ingested amino acid.[43] On the other hand, urinary excretion of sulfate esters is shown to be as much as 17% of total urinary sulfur excretion,[47] and the amount might be higher in certain situations such as renal insufficiency, in which plasma sulfate concentrations are much higher.[48,49] Another common pathway for sulfate conjugation is the formation of sulfated glycosaminoglycans, such as chondroitin sulfate and heparin (Table 10.4).

The sulfur content of proteins of different food sources varies greatly, and depends on the content of methionine and cysteine.[50] For example, the sulfur content of human milk protein is only half of that of most cereal proteins. The sulfur content of beef is less than that of pork or lamb. In general, with the exception of grains, proteins of vegetable origin have lower sulfur content than proteins from animal sources.[50] The rate of excretion of sulfate in patients on CAPD was shown to be much less than in normal subjects,[48] suggesting the possibility that a greater fraction of sulfur is excreted as sulfate conjugate and other organic sulfur compounds.

In conclusion, the proper method for determining the contribution of sulfur-containing amino acids to the endogenous acid production would require the measurement of sulfate, sulfate esters, and neutral sulfur in the urine. In addition, the dietary intake of sulfate from soft drinks must be known.[41]

Organic Acid

Production of organic acid results in consumption of HCO_3^- in the reaction:

$$RH + HCO_3^- \rightarrow R^- + H_2CO_3$$

If the organic anion is retained in the body, and subsequently metabolized to HCO_3^-, there is no net loss of alkali. When the organic anion is not metabolized, is not metabolizable (e.g., urate) or escapes metabolism because it is excreted in the urine (e.g., citrate), this represents a net loss of alkali. The nature of many of these organic anions excreted in the urine is not known,[51-53] and therefore total organic acid production cannot be determined by measuring individual components. Instead, they are measured collectively by titration of urine. However, the titration method used most widely, the van Slyke and Palmer method,[54] contains many potential sources of error, some of which result in underestimation and some in overestimation.[55,56]

When a metabolizable organic anion cannot be excreted because of renal failure, it is eventually metabolized. Hence, renal function is an important consideration in the overall contribution of organic acids to total acid production. In the absence of renal excretion, only non-metabolizable organic acids would accumulate. It is not known what fraction of organic acids normally excreted in urine is metabolizable. To the extent that metabolizable organic anions are not excreted, patients in renal failure would have reduced net acid production, as shown in patients treated with maintenance hemodialysis.[57] On the other hand, net organic acid production is greatly increased during hemodialysis procedures, as a large quantity of organic anions are lost into the dialysate during dialysis.[57]

Net organic acid production is also regulated by the blood pH.[58-60] The regulation of net production of organic acids occurs in two ways. One way is the regulation of its production, which is pH-dependent; acidic systemic pH decreases production of both ketoacids and lactic acid, while alkaline pH promotes their production.[60] Another mechanism is regulation of their renal excretion. This effect is mediated mainly by the proximal tubular cell pH. An acidic pH of the proximal tubular cell increases reabsorption of organic anions, and thereby reduces urinary excretion, while an alkaline pH has the opposite effect.[58] Usually the proximal cell pH parallels the blood pH, but sometimes the two are dissociated. In proximal (type II) renal tubular acidosis (RTA) and type IV RTA, the systemic pH is low, but the proximal tubular cell pH is not, and hence organic anion excretion remains normal. On the other hand, in

TABLE 10.4 Major Sulfated Glycosaminoglycan in Human Body

Chondroitin sulfate
Keratan sulfate
Dermatan sulfate
Heparin sulfate
Heparan sulfate

K^+ depletion, the tubular cell pH tends to be low (as H^+ enters the cell in exchange for K^+), and therefore organic anion loss is reduced, contributing to the pathogenesis of metabolic alkalosis.

Phosphoric Acid

Phosphate is ingested as inorganic phosphate and organic phosphate. Phosphates in milk and other dairy products are mostly inorganic. Inorganic phosphates in food usually exist at neutral pH, and hence their influence on the acid—base balance depends mainly on the absorption of phosphate relative to its accompanying cation, calcium and magnesium.[61] To the extent that phosphate absorption exceeds calcium absorption, it will add acid to the body.

Organic phosphates are ingested in food as components of intracellular organic compounds. These include creatine phosphate, ATP, ADP, AMP, cyclic AMP, phospholipids in the cell membrane and intracellular organelles, nucleic acids in DNA and RNA, and phosphoproteins. Their eventual fate either as acid or alkali depends on the number of non-metabolizable cations that balance the phosphate anions. If the total number of non-metabolizable cations in mEq is equal to 1.8 times the number of phosphate in mM, the compound is neutral upon complete metabolism. This prediction is based on the fact the average balance of phosphate at pH 7.4 is 1.8. When the number is greater than 1.8 times phosphate, the compound is an alkali, and when it is less than 1.8, it would be an acid. For example, each molecule of ATP has three molecules of phosphate (which has 5.4 negative charge equivalents when metabolized completely) balanced by four cationic charges, two of which are usually provided by magnesium. Hence, metabolic breakdown of each mole of ATP to adenosine and phosphate results in production of 1.4 mEq of acid. Likewise, metabolism of ADP (3 cationic charges against anionic charges of 3.6 P) and cyclic AMP (1 cationic charge against anionic charges of 1.8 P) produce acid, while breakdown of AMP (2 cationic charges against 1.8 P) would produce alkali (Table 10.5).

Conversion of ATP to ADP during exercise therefore represents an acid releasing process, as the net acid value of 1.4 (ATP) is reduced to the net acid value of 0.6 (ADP). Conversely, conversion of ADP to ATP represents an alkali releasing process. On the other hand, breakdown of creatine-P to creatine and phosphate represents an alkali releasing process by a slight extent, as it consumes 0.2 mEq of proton for each mmol of creatine-P broken down.

It must be realized, however, that these calculations are based on the mean valence of phosphate of 1.8, which is the value at pH of 7.4. The value will change at different pH values. For example, at the usual pH of the cell, 7.1, the mean valence of phosphate is 1.67, and at a pH of 6.8, the mean phosphate valence is 1.5. Thus, at pH 6.8 (the likely muscle cell pH during exercise), metabolism of each mole of ATP would yield 0.5 mole of acid and that of ADP would result in zero acid production; the conversion of one mole of ATP to ADP would produce 0.5 mole of acid.

Metabolism of phospholipids and nucleic acids in DNA and RNA produces acid, whereas metabolism of phosphoproteins and creatine phosphate produces alkali (Table 10.5). The type of phosphate in the diet is a factor determining the magnitude of intestinal absorption. Phosphate present in phytic acid is poorly absorbable, because the human body lacks the enzyme phytase.[62] However, its GI absoption is greatly increased when phytic acid is broken down by bacterial phytase in the colon.

Another way of determining the fate of phosphate as a generator of acid or alkali is to examine the number of ester bonds. Phosphate has a total of three anionic charges when it is fully dissociated. As phosphate forms an ester bond with an organic substance, the number of anionic charges is reduced, and hence the requirement for the number of non-metabolizable cations such as potassium to balance the anion is also reduced. Thus, when phosphate forms two ester bonds (di-ester bonds) it has only one anionic charge remaining to be balanced by a cation. Phosphates in ATP, ADP, nucleic acids in the DNA and RNA, and phospholipids all form di-ester bonds. This explains why metabolism of AMP results in production of alkali, whereas metabolism of cyclic AMP and cyclic GMP (both are di-esters) result in production of acid. In the case of ATP, first two phosphates form di-ester bonds, and the third phosphate has a mono-ester bond. When phosphate contains tri-ester bonds, it has no metabolizable alkali, and its acid content is equal to the molal content of phosphate × 1.8.

The effect of phosphate in the diet on acid–base balance depends on the extent of GI absorption. The fraction of phosphate absorbed depends greatly on the type of cation that accompanies phosphate. When phosphate is ingested from the usual diet, about 2/3 is absorbed because food contains calcium, and calcium binds phosphate to form brushite ($CaHPO_4$), which is rapidly precipitated and excreted in stools. On the other hand, phosphate ingested as Na or K

TABLE 10.5 Alkali Value of Phosphate Compounds after Complete Breakdown to Inorganic Phosphate at pH 7.4

ATP^{4-}: 3 P and 4 negative charges: $4 - (3 \times 1.8) = -1.4$ (net acid)
ADP^{3-}: 2 P and 3 negative charges: $3 - (2 \times 1.8) = -0.6$ (net acid)
AMP^{2-}: 1 P and 2 negative charges: $2 - (1 \times 1.8) = 0.2$ (net alkali)
GMP^{2-}: 1 P and 2 negative charges: $2 - (1 \times 1.8) = 0.2$ (net alkali)
Cyclic AMP^-: 1 P and 1 negative charge: $1 - (1 \times 1.8) = -0.8$ (net acid)
Cyclic GMP^-: 1 P and 1 negative charge: $1 - (1 \times 1.8) = -0.8$ (net acid)
Creatine-P^{2-}: 1 P and 2 negative charges: $2 - (1 \times 1.8) = 0.2$ (net alkali)
DNA: 1 P and 1 negative charge: $1 - (1 \times 1.8) = -0.8$ (net acid).
RNA: 1 P and 1 negative charge: $1 - (1 \times 1.8) = -0.8$ (net acid)

phosphate is nearly completely absorbed along with sodium and potassium, as long as the amount ingested does not exceed the capacity of the sodium–phosphate transporter.[63–65] When a large amount of sodium phosphate is ingested, the excess amount causes diarrhea. In summary, the contribution of phosphate to net acid production cannot be determined from dietary intake or urinary excretion of phosphate, but is included as part of net GI alkali absorption, which will be discussed separately later in this chapter.

Conversion of Creatine-P to ATP

During anaerobic metabolism, creatine-P is converted to ATP, which results in the generation of one mole of alkali for each mole of such conversion. The actual chemical reaction that occurs can be summarized as follows: creatine-P + ADP + $H^+ \rightarrow$ ATP + creatine. In other words, conversion of creatine-P to creatine with the simultaneous conversion of ADP to ATP results in the consumption of a proton. This reaction can also be summarized this way. Each molecule of creatine-P has two negative charges, each molecule of ADP has three negative charges, but ATP has four negative charges. Hence, one anionic charge must be buffered by the consumption of H^+. In other words, transfer of P from creatine-P to ADP to form ATP is a hydrogen ion-consuming process. If these reactions occurred at pH 6.8, conversion of 1 mmol of ADP to ATP would lead to production of 0.5 mmol of alkali, and the metabolism of creatine-P to creatine and phosphate would result in the additional production of 0.5 mmol of alkali. A hypothesis has been proposed to explain hyperkalemia during vigorous exercise as a response to the initial increase in intracellular pH caused by these reactions. According to this hypothesis, at the start of vigorous muscle exercise, a fall in ATP concentration causes a conversion of creatine-P in the muscle to ATP, and this is accompanied by an increase in intracellular pH.[66] There are several flaws to this hypothesis, for many reasons.

First, the actual gain in alkali by these reactions is much less, because the overall reaction assumes gain of ATP at the expense of creatine-P. However, if the primary driving force of the reaction is low ATP, there must be net conversion of ATP to ADP, which is an acid-producing process. Second, the authors assumed that creatine-P exists as a trivalent anion, resulting in overestimation of alkali production upon conversion of creatine-P to creatine and phosphate. Finally, the consumption of creatine-P and ADP to produce creatine and ATP during vigorous exercise is not mediated by low ATP, but by low intracellular pH.[67] There is very little change in ATP concentration in the early stages of muscular exercise, but a huge decrease in pH during vigorous exercise. The initial intracellular shift of hydrogen ion during the early stages of exercise may be due to an extracellular shift of K, which in turn is caused by repeated depolarization of muscle cells during exercise. This, indeed, has been the traditional explanation for exercise-induced hyperkalemia.[68]

Amino acids

Proteins are potential sources of acid, based mainly on their sulfur content, which has already been discussed. Acidity or alkalinity of proteins also depends on the relative content of basic and acidic amino acids. Metabolism of cationic amino acids, arginine and lysine, produces acid:

$$Arginine^+Cl^- \rightarrow urea + CO_2 + HCl.$$

On the other hand, metabolism of aspartic acid and glutamic acid results in production of alkali:

$$Na^+glutamate^- + H_2CO_3 \rightarrow NaHCO_3 + CO_2 + urea.$$

However, the net content of acid and base of proteins cannot simply be determined from the total amounts of basic amino acids relative to the total content of acidic amino acids. We can understand this from plasma albumin. The total number of glutamate and aspartate in a molecule of albumin is 99, and the total number of arginine and lysine is 81, and the net excess of acidic amino acid over basic amino acid would be 18. The molecular weight of albumin is 66,5000 Da, and at a plasma concentration of albumin of 4 g/dL, the concentration of albumin in molarity is about 0.6 mmol/L. If each mole contains 18 negative charges, the net negative charge would be 10.8 mmol/L. In addition, albumin also contains 16 histidine molecules, and some of these will be in a cationic form, and therefore net negative charge should be less than 10.8 mmol/L. The actual measured net negative charge

of albumin is about 12 mmol/L,[69] and the greater net negative charges may be explained by the reaction of cationic amino acids with various organic compounds. For example, N-acetylation and glycosylation of amino acids would reduce cationic charges and increase net anionic charges. Furthermore, some of the cationic charges of the amino groups of lysine are no longer cationic at pH 7.4.

The imidazole group of histidine is present in either of two forms: neutral or cationic. Metabolism of the cationic histidine results in the production of acid, whereas metabolism of neutral histidine has no effect on acid balance. The ratio of the neutral histidine to cationic histidine depends on the pK of the imidazole group in the molecule, and the pH of the solution in which histidine is dissolved. The pK of histidine varies widely between 5 and 8, depending on the nature of the molecule with which histidine is associated.[70] The pK is 6. 1 in histidine, but carnosine, a dipeptide composed of beta-alanine and histidine, an important intracellular buffer in the muscle of many vertebrates, has a pK of 6.83.[71] When histidine is part of a protein molecule or peptide molecule, its pK depends on the adjacent amino acid. Next to an acidic group, the pK of histidine rises, and next to a basic group, the pK decreases. Each of 16 histidine molecules in albumin has different pK values because of the differing influences of neighboring amino acids.[72]

The histidine content of hemoglobin is particularly high (38 per molecule of hemoglobin), this fact and a very high concentration of hemoglobin (about 7 times that of plasma albumin) explain the excellent buffering capacity of hemoglobin.[73] Oxygenation of hemoglobin at the lung reduces the pK of the imidazole group, i.e., it becomes a stronger acid. The acid reacts with bicarbonate to create more CO_2, which is eliminated by ventilation.

Even in the case of the basic and acidic amino acids, their eventual acidity or alkalinity depends on the nature of the counter-ions balancing the respective amino or carboxyl groups; when these groups are balanced by non-combustible ions such as Na^+, K^+, Cl^- or phosphate, their metabolism results in a net gain of acid or alkali. If the counter-ions are organic ions, the metabolism of the amino acid does not result in a net gain of acid or alkali. In most foods the total number of non-metabolizable cations exceeds that of non-metabolizable anions,[74] and therefore, apart from the contribution of sulfuric acid production, their metabolism would produce alkali.

Organic Acids in Meat

A substantial amount of organic anions, especially lactate, has been found in meat, and it has been suggested that in the overall calculation of dietary net acid production a role for lactic acid be included.[75] However, most of lactate present in meat is produced after the death of the animal. Initially, lactic acid is formed and reacts with cellular alkali. When meat is digested and absorbed, during the process of lactate metabolism, exactly the same amount of protons is consumed as were released during the production of lactic acid. In the end, the net alkali or acid content of the body is unaffected by the production of lactic acid. By analogy, addition of acetic acid in the form of vinegar to food would produce acetate, but would not alter the net acid or alkali value of the food. As long as the content of non-combustible cations and anions remains the same, the net acid or alkali of meat would not change.

GI ABSORPTION OF ACIDS AND ALKALI

The normal diet contains large quantities of alkali, potential alkali, acids, and potential acids, but their ultimate impact on the body's acid–base balance depends primarily on their absorption. The pattern of absorption depends not only on the nature of the substance, but also on its interaction with other chemicals, both endogenous and exogenous.[76,77] In general, the amount absorbed is nearly equal to the amount ingested, if the substance is soluble and is readily absorbed. The examples include $NaHCO_3$, Na^+ citrate, K^+ citrate, and NH_4Cl. An insoluble substance such as $CaCO_3$ must react with gastric acid or acid in food to become soluble and absorbable. In some cases, only the anionic part is absorbable (e.g., Cl^- in cholestyramine chloride); in other cases, only the cationic part (e.g., Na^+ sodium polystyrene sulfonate) is absorbable. The overall effects of these substances on the body's acid–base balance are complex, and are often unrelated to the acidity or alkalinity of the substance. The following section describes two major categories of chemical substances, and the effects of their ingestion on acid–base balance.

Ingestion of a Poorly- or Non-Absorbable Cation Accompanied by an Absorbable Anion

Intravenous $CaCl_2$ is neutral, but ingested $CaCl_2$ is an acidifying agent. When ingested, virtually all of the Cl^-, but only a fraction of the Ca^{2+}, is absorbed. The excess Ca^{2+} remaining in the gut is excreted in the stool after combining with $CO_3^=$, organic anions or $HPO_4^=$. The type of anionic exchange determines the effect on acid–base balance. Typically, ingested $CaCl_2$ reacts with $NaHCO_3$:

$$CaCl_2 + 2NaHCO_3 \rightarrow 2NaCl + CaCO_3 + H_2CO_3$$

$NaCl$ is absorbed and the insoluble $CaCO_3$ is excreted in the stool, resulting in net loss of $NaHCO_3$. Thus, the net effect of oral ingestion of $CaCl_2$ that results in formation and fecal excretion of $CaCO_3$ is loss of two moles of alkali for each mole of Ca ingested. On the other hand, when $CaCl_2$ reacts with Na_2HPO_4, $NaCl$ is absorbed and $CaHPO_4$ is excreted in the stool:

$$CaCl_2 + Na_2HPO_4 \rightarrow 2NaCl + CaHPO_4$$

The loss of one mole of Na_2HPO_4 changes the ratio of Na_2HPO_4/NaH_2PO_4 from 4:1 to 3:1. In order to re-establish the ratio of Na_2HPO_4/NaH_2PO_4 at 4:1, 0.2 mole of NaH_2PO_4 must be converted to 0.2 mole of Na_2HPO_4, which would release of 0.2 mole of H^+. The new ratio would be 3.2 $(3 + 0.2)/0.8$ $(1 - 0.2)$, the same 4:1 ratio. Thus, the net effect is the gain of 0.2 mole of acid for each mole of $CaCl_2$ ingested. $CaCl_2$, if absorbed, would have no effect on the acid–base balance.

Since $SO_4^=$ is more readily absorbed than Mg^{2+}, the overall effect of $MgSO_4$ ingestion would be similar to that of ingestion of $CaCl_2$. Similarly, $FeSO_4$ could result in a net gain of acid, to the extent that more SO_4^{2-} than Fe^{2+} is absorbed.

When a person ingests salts consisting of a non-absorbable or poorly absorbable cation, accompanied by an absorbable and metabolizable anion, for example, $CaCO_3$, $Al(OH)_3$, Ca acetate, and Ca citrate, the amount of alkali gained depends on the absorption of anions, either with the accompanying cations or in exchange for non-metabolizable anions, such as phosphate. Absorption of $CaCO_3$ is facilitated when it reacts with HCl in the stomach or acid in food, because $CaCO_3$ is poorly soluble. The reaction in the stomach will be:

$$CaCO_3 + 2HCl \rightarrow CaCl_2 + H_2CO_3.$$

The fate of $CaCl_2$ formed will be the same as that of $CaCl_2$ ingested. Absorption of Ca as $CaCO_3$ or $CaCl_2$ represents a gain of alkali. Absorption of $CO_3^=$ in exchange for $HPO_4^=$ also represents a gain of alkali. Loss of $CaCO_3$ in the stool has no effect on the acid–base balance. Ingestion of organic salts of calcium, such as calcium citrate, calcium lactate, calcium gluconate, and calcium acetate also result in a similar gain of alkali. As with calcium carbonate, alkali gain occurs when these organic anions are absorbed either with calcium or in exchange with phosphate. The overall alkalinizing effect of various calcium antacids depends more on the ability of calcium to bind phosphate than on the absorption of calcium, because the amount of Ca^{2+} absorbed is usually much less than the amount bound to phosphate to be excreted in the stool. The phosphate-binding ability depends in part on availability of soluble calcium.[78] This might explain why the amount of phosphate bound by calcium when calcium is ingested as $CaCl_2$ is comparable to that bound by aluminum ingested as $Al(OH)_3$,[79] whereas calcium carbonate salt removes only half as much phosphate for the same amount of calcium, because of its poor solubility. Despite poor absorption of aluminum, net gain of alkali is greater with $Al(OH)_3$ than with $CaCO_3$, because aluminum is a more effective binder of phosphate than calcium.[80]

Anion exchange resins are other examples of non-reabsorbable cations accompanied by absorbable anions.[79] As with calcium salts, they have either an acidifying or alkalinizing effect, depending on whether the accompanying anion is metabolizable or not. When the counter-ion is non-metabolizable, such as chloride (e.g., cholestyramine), its absorption in exchange for organic anions, carbonate or bicarbonate represent loss of alkali. When chloride is exchanged for phosphate, it represents 0.2 mEq of alkali loss for each mmol of phosphate lost as HPO_4. When the counter-ion is metabolizable (e.g., acetate), a net gain of alkali occurs when the metabolizable anion is absorbed in exchange for chloride or phosphate. An exchange of a metabolizable anion with organic anions, carbonate or bicarbonate is a neutral process (Table 10.6).

Ingestion of a Poorly- or Non-Absorbable Anion Accompanied by an Absorbable Cation

An example is ingestion of Na^+ or K^+ phosphate. Intestinal absorption of Na^+ and K^+ is nearly complete as long as the accompanying anion can also be readily absorbed. Absorption of phosphate, on the other hand, is limited for two reasons. First, absorption of phosphate is achieved by sodium–phosphate co-transporters,[63–65] which have a limited capacity. When the intake of phosphate is in excess of the transporter capacity, unabsorbed phosphate is excreted in the stool. This explains why an excessive amount of sodium phosphate causes diarrhea. Second, some of the ingested phosphate can form an insoluble complex with calcium, which is precipitated and excreted in the stool. Na^+ or K^+ will then be balanced by the anion that is left behind, and the precipitated calcium will be absorbed. If the anion that is absorbed with sodium or potassium is an organic anion or carbonate, the result will be net gain of alkali:

$$Na_2HPO_4 + CaCO_3 \rightarrow Na_2CO_3 \text{ (absorbed after conversion to } NaHCO_3 \text{)} + CaPO_4 \text{ (excreted in stool)}$$

TABLE 10.6 Effect on Acid–Base Balance of Anion Exchange Resins (AER), Depending on its Accompanying Anion and Type of Anion in the Gut to be Exchanged

- Resin with metabolizable anion, exchanged for non-metabolizable anion: Gain of alkali
- Resin with metabolizable anion, exchanged for metabolizable anion: Neutral
- Resin with non-metabolizable anion, exchanged for metabolizable anion: Gain of Acid
- Resin with non-metabolizable anion, exchange for non-metabolizable anion: Neutral

Ingestion of a Cation-Exchange Resin Results in Net Gain of Alkali by a Similar Mechanism

The unabsorbable polyanion in a cation exchange resin is usually sulfonate attached to a polystyrene skeleton balanced by an exchangeable and absorbable cation, e.g., Na^+ in sodium polystyrene sulfonate (Kayexalate). When Na^+ exchanges for K^+, it has no effect on acid–base balance. An exchange of Na^+ for NH_4^+ or H^+ results in gain of alkali. When it exchanges with Ca^{2+}, the net effect is also gain of alkali, because normally the bulk of Ca^{2+} excreted in the stool is insoluble calcium carbonate, which represents loss of alkali.[80,81] When Ca^{2+} in calcium carbonate is exchanged for Na^+ in sodium polystyrene sulfonate (PSS), Na_2CO_3 is formed and then absorbed; at physiological pH, Na_2CO_3 will react with H_2CO_3, and two molecules of $NaHCO_3$ will form, and then be absorbed. This effect is more pronounced when the resin is administered with calcium salts,[80,81] aluminum salts or magnesium salts. Exchange between Na^+ and Al^{3+} or between Na^+ and Mg^{2+} results in formation of NaOH or Na^+ carbonate, which is readily absorbable directly or indirectly.

$$Na_2 - PSS + CaCO_3 \rightarrow Ca - PSS \text{ (excreted in stool)} + Na_2CO_3 \text{ (absorbed after conversion to } NaHCO_3\text{).}$$

If sodium polystyrene sulfonate (PSS) is ingested along with $Al(OH)_3$, the following reaction will occur:

$$Na_3 - PSS + Al(OH)_3 \rightarrow Al - PSS \text{ (excreted in stool)} + 3NaOH \text{ (absorbed after conversion to } 3NaHCO_3\text{).}$$

Calculation of Net Alkali in a Complex System

Ingestion of, for example, 20 mmol of K^+ citrate, which is completely absorbable and metabolized to $KHCO_3$ in the body, would result in net gain of

20 mEq of alkali. Ingestion of 10 mmol of arginine Cl would result in net gain of 10 mEq of acid. If a food contained both, the net gain of alkali would be 10 mEq. The food contains numerous chemicals, and their absorption depends not only on the type of chemicals ingested, but also on interactions with gastric acid and other chemicals in simultaneously ingested food or drugs. Thus, prediction of the effect of food ingestion on acid–base balance is nearly impossible. Measurements are made, instead, by analyzing net alkali content of food and feces. The difference between these two represents net alkali absorbed.

Net alkali content of food and feces is estimated by the electrolyte balance technique, i.e., the sum of non-combustible cations ($Na^+ + K^+ + Ca^{2+} + Mg^{2+}$) minus the sum of non-combustible anions ($Cl^- + 1.8$ P).[36] The assumption here is that when non-metabolizable cations are accompanied by metabolizable anions, the subsequent absorption and metabolism of their anions would result in gain of alkali, and that ingestion and absorption of non-metabolizable anions accompanied by metabolizable cations would lead to gain of acid. Hence, the difference between the two represents a net gain of alkali or acid. The concentrations of all of the electrolytes are expressed in mEq, except phosphate, which is expressed in mmol and then multiplied by the factor 1.8, the average valence of phosphate at pH 7.4. The pH of food or feces is not a determinant in the calculation of valency of phosphate, since that pH is relevant only in reference to blood pH.

For the calculation of net alkali content of food and feces, the only non-metabolizable ions presumed to be present are Na^+, K^+, Ca^{2+}, Mg^{2+}, Cl^-, and P, because no other ions in food are present in significant amounts. Urinary excretion of sulfate is substantial, but it is assumed to originate almost exclusively from sulfur-containing amino acids, and is measured separately.[43] This assumption does not appear valid any longer, because of ingestion of inorganic sulfates that are contained in substantial amounts in soft drinks. According to one estimate, an average amount of sulfate ingested per day in USA is about 15 mEq/day.[41] Thus, the presence of inorganic sulfate in the diet would lead to the estimation of a falsely increased amount of net GI alkali content. On the other hand, the inclusion of sulfate that originates from inorganic sulfate in soft drinks in the calculation of endogenous acid production would falsely increase its estimation. Thus, these two errors would cancel each other out.

Some organic anions found in food, e.g., tartarate, are poorly metabolized by the human body, and such anions would also result in a falsely increased estimation of net GI alkali absorption. On the other hand, all organic anions excreted in the urine estimated by the titration method are assumed to originate from organic acids produced in the body, and this assumption results in a falsely increased measurement of organic acid generation by the presence of substances such as tartarate in urine. These two errors would cancel each other out. Furthermore, it has been shown that the bulk of ingested tartarate in humans is actually metabolized by colonic bacteria, and only about 14% of ingested tartarate appear in urine unchanged.[82] Choline is an example of an incompletely metabolizable cation, but choline is also mostly metabolized by colonic bacteria.[83]

The measurement of GI absorption of alkali by the analysis of food and feces is difficult and prone to inaccuracies for obvious technical reasons. Measurements can be made only in inpatient settings with controlled diet, and consequently no study has measured net GI absorption of alkali on a normal diet in an outpatient setting. In a simplified technique, net GI absorption of alkali is estimated as urinary non-combustible cations minus urinary non-combustible anions:[84]

$$Net\ GI\ Alkali\ absorption = Urine\,(Na^+ + K^+ + Ca^{2+} +$$
$$Mg^{2+}) - Urine\,(Cl^- + P \times 1.8).$$

The method is based on the assumption that the difference between the amounts of non-combustible cations and non-combustible anions absorbed from the gut equal the difference between the amounts excreted in the urine under stable conditions. The validity of this assumption is supported by empirical, as well as theoretical, evidence. Theoretically, the amount of non-metabolizable ions absorbed must equal the amount excreted, for the following reasons. The total extracellular content of divalent ions is small (about 45 mEq of Ca^{2+}, 30 mEq of Mg^{2+}, and 30 mEq of P), and their daily net flux with bone is negligible.[38] Hence, the amount of divalent ions excreted in the urine must be quite close to the amount absorbed from the GI tract. For univalent ions, Na^+, K^+, and Cl^-, their GI absorption is nearly complete. Consequently, the amount excreted in the urine would closely reflect the amount absorbed from the GI tract in states of acid–base balance. In a non-steady-state with a net gain of acid by the kidney, there would be excess excretion of Na and K. In a non-steady-state with a net gain of alkali by the kidney, there would be excess excretion of Cl.

Empirically, the measurement of net alkali absorption from the GI tract measured by the analysis of diet and stool showed near perfect correlation with the measurement made by urine electrolytes.[84] The amount of net alkali absorbed on a usual diet by the latter technique is about 30 mEq/day.[38]

BONE BUFFERING IN METABOLIC ACIDOSIS

Bone Buffering in Chronic Metabolic Acidosis

It was once widely believed that bone was very important in maintaining stable serum HCO_3^- in chronic renal acidosis. Studies have shown that patients with chronic renal acidosis are able to maintain a stable serum HCO_3^-, despite retention of 12—19 mEq of acid daily, with the average duration of acidosis of six years. Because bone is known to have a large alkali reserve, the maintenance of a stable serum HCO_3^- in such settings has been attributed to the sustained release of alkali from bone.[3,4]

However, there has been little direct evidence for substantial bone buffering of acids in chronic acidosis of such long duration. The best evidence against a substantial role of bone in chronic renal acidosis is the lack of significant calciuria.[85] Addition of alkali to the body from Ca^{2+} release by bone occurs only when Ca^{2+} is excreted in urine. Re-deposition of Ca^{2+} salts in tissues or excretion in the stool as alkaline Ca^{2+} salts would reclaim alkali released from bone.[86] If the released calcium is lost in the stool as $CaCO_3$, it would actually result in net loss of alkali. Each mmol of Ca hydroxyapatite releases 10 mmol of Ca and 9.2 mEq of alkali. Loss of 10 mmols of calcium as calcium carbonate excreted in the stool removes 20 mmols of alkali from the body. Hence, the net alkali loss would be 10.8 mmols. If calcium from bone is released as $CaCO_3$, and excreted in the stool as $CaCO_3$, there will be no loss or gain of alkali. Release of calcium from hydroxy apatite with subsequent deposition as hydroxy apatite represents no gain or loss of alkali.

Furthermore, the total amount of alkali reserve in bone is insufficient to account for the buffering of acid for such a protracted period. Assuming total bone content of Ca^{2+} at 60,000 mEq, the total alkali content of bone is estimated to be about 25,000 mEq. At the rate of 19 mEq of acid buffering per day, the bone alkali store would be exhausted in 3.6 years.[38,87]

Bone Buffering in Acute Metabolic Acidosis

It is also widely believed that bone plays an important role in buffering in super-acute acidosis, but the available evidence is not convincing. Fraley and Adler showed that rats and dogs with total thyroparathyroidectomy developed a much more severe metabolic acidosis than those with intact organs.[88] The authors concluded that without intact parathyroid glands, non-extracellular buffers were responsible for titrating only 3 and 22% of the administered acid in rats and dogs, respectively. They concluded that the difference in buffering capacity was due to a difference in bone buffering. Arruda et al. concurred with Fraley and Adler that PTH significantly affected the overall buffering,[89] but the data of Madias et al. did not show any difference in buffering capacity.[90] Buffering of acid by bone could occur in three different ways: (1) release of cations such as Na^+, K^+, Ca^{2+}, and Mg^{2+} accompanied by carbonate, hydroxide or phosphate; (2) exchange of bone carbonate for extracellular phosphate; and (3) deposition of extracellular non-metabolizable anion such as Cl^- along with an H^+.

The third mechanism has not been shown to exist. For the first mechanism to operate, a cation must be released from bone. Mg^{2+} does not participate in acid buffering of bone. Release of bone K^+ cannot play a quantitatively significant role, because the entire bone content of K^+ in adult humans is a mere 20 mEq.[91] Evidence for Na^+ release from bone exists in acute metabolic acidosis, but the magnitude is a not very substantial. Bettice and Gamble showed that the bone content of exchangeable Na^+ decreased by about 5% in 5 hours following acute acid loading in dogs.[92] The bone Na^+ content is about 1200 mEq, and about 40% of this, 480 mEq, is exchangeable. Thus, 5% of 480 mEq represents a mere 24 mEq ($480 \times 0.05 = 24$). In conclusion, it seems highly improbable that bone contributes substantially to the buffering in super-acute metabolic acidosis (acidosis within a few hours).

Release of Ca^{2+} from bone is an important mechanism of bone buffering in acute metabolic acidosis. Urinary excretion of Ca^{2+} can increase by 80 mEq per day. If the entire amount came from Ca^{2+} carbonate, that amount of calcium release would release 80 mEq of alkali. If the same amount of Ca^{2+} originated from hydroxyapatite, alkali released is 36.8 mEq. Increased excretion of Ca^{2+} in metabolic acidosis reaches a maximal value a few days after the start of acid load.[93]

The likely explanation for the appearance of impaired buffering in animals with thyroparathyroidectomy is tissue under-perfusion due to circulatory shock. Since the blood flow to the muscle in humans is only about 700 ml per minute, it is obvious that buffering by skeletal muscle would not be complete in 30 minutes in a resting state. Reduced blood flow by circulatory shock would further delay the buffering by both intra- and extracellular fluid of the muscle, and could have given the impression that cell buffering was virtually absent in this setting.

In conclusion, bone is quantitatively an unimportant source of alkali in chronic metabolic acidosis of several years' duration. In acute acidosis, contribution of bone to acid buffering could be substantial, but its contribution in super-acute acidosis (that of several hours duration) appears negligible.

References

[1] Pearson PN, Palmer MR. Atmospheric carbon dioxide concentrations over the past 60 million years. Nature 2000;406:695–9.

[2] Canadell JG, Le Quéré C, Raupach MR, Field CB, Buetenhuis ET, Ciais P, et al. Contributions to accelerating atmospheric CO_2 growth from economic activity, carbon intensity, and efficiency of natural sinks. Proc Natl Acad Sci 2007;104:18866–70.

[3] Lemann Jr J, Litzow JR, Lennon EJ. The effects of chronic acid loads in normal man: further evidence for the participation of bone mineral in the defense against chronic metabolic acidosis. J Clin Invest 1966;45:1608–14.

[4] Goodman AD, Lemann Jr J, Lennon EJ, Relman AS. Production, excretion and net balance of fixed acid in patients with renal acidosis. J Clin Invest 1965;44:495–506.

[5] Vaziri ND, Freel RW, Hatch M. Effect of chronic experimental renal insufficiency on urate metabolism. J Am Soc Nephrol 1995;6:1313–7.

[6] Costello JF, Smith M, Stolarski C, Sadovnic MJ. Extrarenal clearance of oxalate increases with progression of renal failure in the rat. J Am Soc Nephrol 1992;3:1098–104.

[7] Guyton A. Control of blood pressure. Am J Med 1972;52:484–92.

[8] Guyton AC, Hall JE, Lohmeier TE, Jackson TE, Kastner PR. Blood pressure regulation: basic concepts. Fed Proc 1981;4:2252–6.

[9] Guyton AC. Abnormal renal function and autoregulation in essential hypertension. Hypertension 1991;18(Suppl. 3):49–53.

[10] Guyton AC. The surprising kidney-fluid mechanism for pressure control: its infinite gain!. Hypertension 1990;16:725–30.

[11] Hollenberg NK. Set point for sodium homeostasis: surfeit, deficit and their implications. Kidney Int 1980;17:423–9.

[12] Walser M. Phenomenological analysis of sodium and potassium homeostasis. Kidney Int 1985;217:837–41.

[13] Bonventre JV, Leaf A. Sodium homeostasis: steady states without a set point. Kidney Int 1982;21:880–3.

[14] Squires RD, Huth EJ. Experimental potassium depletion in normal human subjects. Relation of ion intake to the renal conservation of potassium. J Clin Invest 1959;38:1134–48.

[15] Uribarri J, Oh MS, Carroll HJ. Salt-losing nephropathy. Clinical presentation and mechanisms. Am J Nephrol 1983;3:193–8.

[16] Lum G, Leal-Khouri S. Significance of low serum urea nitrogen concentrations. Clin Chem 1989;35:639–40.

[17] Oh MS, Carroll HJ. Salt output in relation to salt intake vs. salt output alone: which is a better predictor of effective vascular volume? Nephron 1992;61:7–9.

[18] Levy M, Wexler MJ. Renal sodium retention and ascites formation in dogs with experimental cirrhosis but with portal hypertension or increased splanchnic vascular capacity. J Lab Clin Med 1978;91:520.

[19] Cardenas A, Arroyo V. Mechanisms of water and sodium retention in cirrhosis and the pathogenesis of ascites. Best Pract Res Clin Endocrinol Metab 2003;17:607–22.

[20] Dorhout EJ, Roos JC, Boer P, Yoe EH, Simatupang TA. Observations on edema formation in the nephrotic syndrome in adults with minimal lesions. Am J Med 1979;67:378–84.

[21] Pendred V. Deaf-mutism and goitre. Lancet 1896;2:532.

[22] Eladari D, Chambrey R, Frische S, Vallet M, Edwards A. Pendrin as a regulator of ECF and blood pressure. Curr Opin Nephrol Hypertens 2009;18:356–62.

[23] Kamel KS, Magner PO, Ethier JH, Halperin ML. Urine electrolytes in the assessment of extracellular fluid volume contraction. Am J Nephrol 1989;9:344–7.

[24] Madeo AC, Manichaikul A, Pryor SP, Griffith AJ. Do mutations of the Pendred syndrome gene, SLC26A4, confer resistance to asthma and hypertension? J Med Genet 2009;46:405–6.

[25] Bigozzi M, Bianchi B. Profound hypokalemia and hypochloremic metabolic alkalosis during thiazide therapy in a child with Pendred syndrome. Clin Nephrol 2008;69:450–3.

[26] Kandasamy N, Fugazzola L, Evans M, Chatterjee K, Karret F. Life-threatening metabolic alkalosis in Pendred syndrome. Eur J Endocrinol 2011;165:167–70.

[27] Decaux G, Genette F, Mokel J. Hyponatremia in the syndrome of inappropriate ADH secretion. Ann Intern Med 1980;93:716–22.

[28] Jaenike JR, Waterhouse C. The renal response to sustained administration of water and vasopressin in man. J Clin Endocrinol Metab 1961;21:231.

[29] Boonjaren S, Stein J, Baehler R, Osgood RW, Hsueh W, Cohen S, et al. Effect of plasma sodium concentration on diluting segment sodium reabsorption. Kidney Int 1974;5:1.

[30] Schrier RW, Fein FL, McNeil TS, Cirksena WJ. Influence of interstitial fluid volume expansion and plasma sodium concentration on the natriuresis response to volume expansion in dogs. Clin Sci 1969;36:371.

[31] Oh MS, Carroll HJ. Essential hypernatremia: is there such a thing? Nephron 1994;67:144–7.

[32] Alford FP, Scoggins BA, Wharton C. Symptomatic essential hypernatremia. Am J Med 1973;54:359.

[33] Kamm DE, Levinsky NG. Inhibition of renal tubular sodium reabsorption by hypernatremia. J Clin Invest 1965;44:1144.

[34] Bresler EH, Nielson KT, Miller III MC, Stoud MR. Renal tubular reabsorptive response to hypernatremia. Am J Physiol 1976;231:642.

[35] Robertson GL, Aycinena P, Zerbe RL. Neurogenic disorders of osmoregulation. Am J Med 1982;72:339–53.

[36] Relman AS, Lennon EJ, Lemann Jr. J. Endogenous production of fixed acid and the measurement of the net balance of acid in normal subjects. J Clin Invest 1961;40:1621–30.

[37] Lennon EJ, Lemann Jr J, Litzow JR. The effects of diet and stool composition on the net external acid balance of normal subjects. J Clin Invest 1966;45:1601–7.

[38] Oh MS, Carroll HJ. Whole body acid-base balance. In: Berlyne G, editor. The kidney today. Selected topics in renal science. Contrib Nephrol 1992;100:89–104

[39] Lemann Jr J, Lennon EJ, Brock J. A potential error in the measurement of urinary titratable acid. J Lab Clin Med 1966;67:906–13.

[40] Oh MS, Kim MJ, Tan C, et al. Untitrated titratable acid in urine. Proc Am Soc Nephrol 1992;3:328.

[41] Magee EA, Curno R, Edmond LM, Cummings JH. Contribution of dietary protein and inorganic sulfur to urinary sulfate toward a biomarker of inorganic sulfur intake. Am J Clin Nutr 2004;80:137–42.

[42] Lemann Jr J, Relman AS. The relation of sulfur metabolism to acid–base balance and electrolyte excretion: the effects of DL-methionine in normal man. J Clin Invest 1959;38:2215–23.

[43] Hunt JN. The influence of dietary sulphur on the urinary output of acid in man. Clin Sci 1956;15:119–34.

[44] Banoglu E. Current status of the cytosolic sulfotransferases in the metabolic activation of promutagens and procarcinogens. Curr Drug Metab 2000;1:1–30.

[45] Kauffman FC. Sulfonation in pharmacology and toxicology. Drug Metab Rev 2004;36:823–43.

[46] Glatt H. Sulfotransferases in the bioactivation of xenobiotics. Chem Biol Interact 2000;1(129):141–70.

[47] Baldetorp L, Martensson J. Urinary excretion of inorganic sulfate, ester sulfate, total sulfur and taurine in cancer patients. Acta Med Scand 1980;208:293–5.

[48] Uribarri J, Buquing J, Oh MS. Acid–base balance in chronic peritoneal dialysis patients. Kidney Int 1995;47:269–73.

[49] Uribarri J, Zia M, Mahmood J, Marcus RA, Oh MS. Acid production in chronic hemodialysis patients. J Am Soc Nephrol 1998;9:114–20.

[50] Lenter C. Ed. Composition of foods. In Geigy Scientific Tables. vol. 1. Units of measurement, body fluids, composition of the body, nutrition. Basel, Switzerland: Ciba-Geigy Ltd, Basel; 1981 p. 241–66

[51] Chalmers RA, Healy MJ, Lawson AM, Hart JT, Watts RW. Urinary organic acids in man. III. Quantitative ranges and patterns of excretion in a normal population. Clin Chem 1976;22:1292–8.

[52] Chalmers RA, Healy MJ, Lawson AM, Watts RW. Urinary organic acids in man. II. Effects of individual variation and diet on the urinary excretion of acidic metabolites. Clin Chem 1976;22:1288–91.

[53] Lawson AM, Chalmers RA, Watts RW. Urinary organic acids in man. I. Normal patterns. Clin Chem 1976;22:1283–7.

[54] Van Slyke DD, Palmer WW. Studies of acidosis. XVI. Titration of organic acids in urine. J Biol Chem 1920;41:567–9.

[55] Oh MS, Rakesh V, Carroll HJ. A new method for measurement of organic anions in urine. Proc Amer Soc Nephrol 1993;:38 Boston

[56] Dawson J, Dempsey E, Bartter F, Leaf A, Albright F. Evidence for the presence of an amphoteric electrolyte in the urine of patients with "renal tubular acidosis.". Metabolism 1953;2:225–37.

[57] Uribarri J, Douyon H, Oh MS. A re-evaluation of the urinary parameters of acid production and excretion in patients with chronic renal acidosis. Kidney Int 1995;47:624–7.

[58] Kaufman AM, Brod-Miller C, Kahn T. Role of citrate excretion in acid–base balance in diuretic-induced alkalosis in the rat. Am J Physiol 1985;248:F796–803.

[59] Brown JC, Packer RK, Knepper MA. Role of organic anions in renal response to dietary acid and base loads. Am J Physiol 1989;257:F170–176.

[60] Hood VL, Tannen RL. Protection of acid-base balance by pH regulation of acid production. N Engl J Med 1998;339:819–26.

[61] Lennon EJ, Lemann Jr J, Relman AS. The effects of phosphoproteins on acid balance in normal subjects. J Clin Invest 1962;41:637–45.

[62] Hubert W, Lopez HW, Coudray C, et al. Mineral utilization in rats. J Clin Nutri 1998;128:1192–8.

[63] Quamme GA, Shapiro RJ. Membrane controls of epithelial phosphate transport. Can J Physiol Pharmacol 1987;65:275–86.

[64] Murer H, Forster I, Biber J. The sodium phosphate cotransporter family SLC34. Pflugers Arch 2004;447:763–7.

[65] Murer H, Hernando N, Forster L, Biber J. Molecular mechanisms in proximal tubular and small intestinal phosphate reabsorption. Mol Membr Biol 2001;18:3–11.

[66] Wasserman K, Stringer WW, Caserburi R. The mechanism of exercise hyperkalemia: an alternative hypothesis. J Appl Physiol 1997;8:631–43.

[67] Sahlin K, Harris RC, Hultman E. Creatine kinase equilibrium and lactate compared with muscle pH in tissue obtained after isometric exercise. Biochem J 1975;152:173–80.

[68] Lindinger JI, McKelvie RS, Heigenhauser JF. K^+ and Lac^- distribution in humans during exercise during and after high intensity exercise. J Appl Physiol 1995;78:765–77.

[69] Watson PD. Modeling the effects of proteins on pH in plasma. J Appl Physiol 1999;86:1421–7.

[70] Hochachka PW, Somero GN. Biochemical adaptations. Princeton, New Jersey: Princeton University Press; 1984. p. 337–48

[71] Bate-Smith EC. The buffering of muscle in rigor: protein, phosphate and carnosine. J Physiol 1938;92:336–43.

[72] Figge J, Mydosh T, Fencl V. Serum protein and acid–base equilibria: a follow-up. J Lab Clin Med 1992;120:713–9.

[73] Riggs A. The amino acid composition of some mammalian hemoglobins. J Biol Chem 1963;238:2983–7.

[74] Halperin ML, Jungas RL. Metabolic production and renal disposal of hydrogen ions. Kidney Int 1983;24:709–13.

[75] Berlyne GM, Adler AJ, Barth RH. Perspectives on acid–base balance in advanced chronic renal failure. In: Berlyne G, editor. The kidney today. Selected topics in renal science. Contrib Nephrol 1992;100:105–17

[76] de Strihou C, van Y. Importance of endogenous acid production in the regulation of acid–base equilibrium: the role of the digestive tract. Adv Nephrol 1980;9:367–85.

[77] Lennon EJ, Lemann Jr J, Litzow JR. The effects of diet and stool composition on the net external acid balance of normal subjects. J Clin Invest 1966;45:1601–7.

[78] Sheikh MS, Maguire JA, Emmett M, Santa Ana CA, Nicar MJ, Schiller LR, et al. Reduction of dietary phosphorus absorption by phosphorus binders. a theoretical, *in vitro*, and *in vivo* study. J Clin Invest 1989;83:66–73.

[79] Hurst PE, Morrison RB, Timoneer J, Metcalfe-Gibson A, Wrong O. The effect of oral anion exchange resins on faecal anions. Comparison with calcium salts and aluminium hydroxide. Clin Sci 1963;24:187–200.

[80] Schroeder ET. Alkalosis resulting from combined administration of a "nonsystemic" antacid and a cation-exchange resin. Gastroenterology 1969;56:868–74.

[81] Madias NE, Levey AS. Metabolic alkalosis due to absorption of "nonabsorbable" antacids. Am J Med 1983;74:155–8.

[82] Chadwick VS, Vince A, Killingley M, Wrong OM. The metabolism of tartrate in man and the rat. Clin Sci Mol Med 1978;54:273–81.

[83] De La Huerga J, Gyorgy P, Waldstein D, Katz R, Popper H. The effects of antimicrobial agents upon choline degradation in the intestinal tract. J Clin Invest 1953;32:1117–20.

[84] Oh MS, Carroll HJ. A new method for the measurement of net GI absorption of alkali. Kidney Int 1989;36:915–7.

[85] Litzow JR, Lemann Jr J, Lennon EJ. The effect of treatment of acidosis on calcium balance in patients with chronic azotemic renal disease. J Clin Invest 1967;46:280–6.

[86] Contiguglia SR, Alfrey AC, Miller NL, Runnells DE, Le Geros RZ. Nature of soft tissue calcification in uremia. Kidney Int 1973;4:229–35.

[87] Oh MS. Irrelevance of bone buffering to acid–base homeostasis in chronic metabolic acidosis. Nephron 1991;59:7–10.

[88] Fraley DS, Adler S. An extrarenal role for parathyroid hormone in the disposal of acute acid loads in rats and dogs. J Clin Invest 1979;63:985–97.

[89] Arruda JA, Alla V, Rubinstein H, Cruz-Soto M, Sabatini S, Battle DC, et al. Metabolic and hormonal factors influencing extrarenal buffering of an acute acid load. Miner Electrolyte Metab 1982;:36–43.

[90] Madias NE, Johns CA, Homer SM. Independence of the acute acid-buffering response from endogenous parathyroid hormone. Am J Physiol 1982;243:F141–149.

[91] Pellegrino ED, Biltz RM. The composition of human bone in uremia. Observations on the reservoir functions of bone and demonstration of a labile fraction of bone carbonate. Medicine (Baltimore) 1965;44:397–418.

[92] Bettice JA, Gamble Jr. JL. Skeletal buffering of acute metabolic acidosis. Am J Physiol 1975;229:1618–24.

[93] Leman J, John R, Litzow JR, Lennon EJ. Studies of the mechanism by which chronic metabolic acidosis augments urinary calcium excretion in man. J Clin Invest 1967;46:1318–28.

11

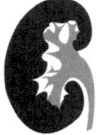

Renal Cilia Structure, Function, and Physiology

Jay N. Pieczynski and Bradley K. Yoder

Department of Cell Biology, University of Alabama at Birmingham, Birmingham, AL, USA

INTRODUCTION

The first descriptions of the cilium are generally attributed to Leeuwenhoek (as translated in [1]). Cilia were thought to be analogous to the flagellum used by single cell organisms for motility. It soon became obvious that motile cilia also have a function in multiple human tissues; motile cilia found in the respiratory track are involved in clearance of mucus and debris, cerebral spinal fluid movement is assisted by motile cilia on ependymal cells lining the brain ventricles, and flagella function to propel sperm through the reproductive tract for fertilization. In fact, the first human disease associated with cilia dysfunction was Primary Ciliary Dyskinesia ("primary" here referring to the fact that impaired movement of cilia was the cause of the disease (PCD)[2,3]). These patients suffer from chronic rhinitis, bronchiectasis, infertility, and abnormal left−right body axis specification caused by defects in cilia motility.

Most cell types in the mammalian body do not have motile cilia; they possess a single immotile cilium (referred to as the *primary cilium*). The functional importance of the primary cilium remained enigmatic, and the primary cilium was often considered vestigial. It wasn't until the mid-1990s and early 2000s that a number of essential observations were made linking the primary cilium to disease phenotypes, largely through studies in model organisms. One of the initial breakthroughs came from a large-scale insertional mutagenesis project conducted on mice in the laboratory of Dr. Rick Woychik at the Oak Ridge National Laboratories. This screen resulted in the identification of the Oak Ridge Polycystic Kidney (*orpk*) mouse,[4] a genetic model for autosomal recessive polycystic kidney disease (ARPKD, OMIM# 263200). *orpk* mutants have multi-organ defects, including cystic lesions in the kidney, liver, and pancreas, hydrocephalus, anosmia, retinal degeneration, skin and hair abnormalities, brain malformation, and skeletal defects.[5] Many of the phenotypes observed in the *orpk* mutants have also been reported in human disorders caused by mutations in proteins associated with the cilium (Table 11.1). These disorders are collectively referred to as "*ciliopathies*," and the *orpk* mutant mouse has become an important mammalian model system for studying ciliary dysfunction and disease. The transgene insertion in *orpk* mutant mice caused a hypomorphic mutation in a gene called "*Tg737*" that encodes the protein Polaris.[4,6,7] Polaris localizes to the cilium, and in the *orpk* mutants both motile and primary cilia were stunted and malformed, although the function of the protein remained unknown.[8]

Another major advance came from the proteomic analysis of flagella isolated from the green alga *Chlamydomonas reinhardt*.[9] This study identified several components of the intraflagellar transport (IFT) particle that included intraflagellar protein 88 (*Ift88*), the homolog of Polaris in *Chlamydomonas*.[10] IFT is an evolutionarily conserved transport system that mediates bidirectional movement of proteins between the base and tip of the cilia/flagella, and is essential for the construction and maintenance of cilia/flagella (Figure 11.1; Table 11.2; see section "Intraflagellar Transport (IFT) and IFT Motors").[11] In agreement with a role in IFT, further studies in *Caenorhabditis elegans* (*C. elegans*) on OSM-5, the IFT88/Polaris homolog, revealed that mutations disrupting this protein also cause severe defects in cilia assembly.[12]

TABLE 11.1 Ciliopathy Genes that Cause Known Renal Phenotypes[a]

Gene Name	Gene Location	Protein Name	Aliases	Overlapping Loci	Associated Ciliopathies	Protein Characteristics	Subcellular Localization
BBS1	11q13.2	BBS1	BBS2L2		BBS	BBSome component	Basal body; cilium
BBS2	16q12.2	BBS2	—		BBS	BBSome component	Basal body; cilium
ARL6	3q11.2	Arl6	—		BBS	GTPase	Basal body; cilium
BBS4	15q24.1	BBS4	—		BBS	BBSome component	Basal body; cilium
BBS5	2q31.1	BBS5	—		BBS	BBSome component	Basal body; cilium
MKKS	20p12.2	BBS6	—		BBS	Chaperonin-like	Basal body
BBS7	4q27	BBS7	BBS2L1, FLJ10715		BBS	BBSome component	Basal body; cilium
TTC8	14q31.3	BBS8	—		BBS	BBSome component	Basal body; cilium
PTHB1	7p14.3	BBS9	—		BBS	BBSome component	Basal body; cilium
BBS10	12q21.2	BBS10	—		BBS	Chaperonin-like	Basal body
TRIM32	9q33.1	BBS11	HT2A		BBS	E3 ubiquitin ligase motif; RING zinc finger	Cytosol; nucleus
BBS12	4q27	BBS12	FLJ35630		BBS	Chaperonin-like	Basal body
WDPCP	2p15	BBS15	Fritz		BBS	WD40 domains	Cytosol
INPP5E	9q34.3	INPP5E	CORS1, MORMS		JBTS	Inositol polyphosphate-5-phosphatase	Cilium
AHI1	6q23.3	AHI1	Jouberin		JBTS	SH3 domain; W40 repeats; coiled-coil domain	Cilium
ARL13B	3q11.1	ARL13B	ARL2L1		JBTS	GTPase	Basal body; cilium
ACLS	15q26.1	Klf7	KIF7, Costal2		JBTS	Kinesin-family protein	Cilium
TCTN1	12q24.11	Tectonic	TECT-1, Tectonic 1		JBTS, MKS?	Transmembrane domain	Transition zone
MKS1	17q22	MKS1	MKS	BBS13	MKS, BBS	B9 domain	Transition zone
TMEM216	11q12.2	MKS2	JBTSB, CORS2	JBTS2	MKS, JBTS	Transmembrane domain	Transition zone
TMEM67	8q22.1	MKS3	Meckelin	JBTS6, NPHP11	MKS, JBTS, NPHP	7-pass transmembrane domain protein	Transition zone
CEP290	12q21.32	Cep290	—	NPHP6, BBS14, JBTS5, SLSN6	MKS, BBS, NPHP, JBTS, SLSN	Coiled-coil domains/ bipartite NLS	Basal body/ centrosome
RPGR1P1L	16q12.2	MKS5	NPHP8	NPHP8, JBTS7	MKS, NPHP, JBTS	C2 domains, coiled-coil domains, bipartite NLS	Transition zone
CC2D2A	4p15.32	MKS6	—	JBTS9	MKS, JBTS	C2 domains, coiled-coil domains	Transition zone
TCTN2	12q24.31	Tectonic-2			MKS	Transmembrane domain	Transition zone
B9D1	17p11.2	B9D1			MKS	B9 domain	Transition zone
B9D2	19q13.2	B9D2			MKS	B9 domain	Transition zone
NPHP1	2q13	NPHP1		JBTS4, SLSN1	NPHP, JBTS, SLSN	SH3 domain/coiled-coil domain	Transition zone, adherens junctions
INVS	9q31.1	Inversin	NPHP2		NPHP	IQ calmodulin-binding domain/ankyrin repeats	Inversin domain, cilium

(Continued)

TABLE 11.1 (Continued)

Gene Name	Gene Location	Protein Name	Aliases	Overlapping Loci	Associated Ciliopathies	Protein Characteristics	Subcellular Localization
NPHP3	3q22.1	NPHP3	Nephrocystin-3, NPH3	MKS7, SLSN3	NPHP, MKS, SLSN	IQ calmodulin-binding domain	Cilium
NPHP4	1p36.31	NPHP4	Nephroretinin	SLSN4	NPHP, SLSN	SH3 domain	Transition zone, adherens junctions
IQCB1	3q13.33	NPHP5	PIQ	SLSN5	NPHP, SLSN	IQ calmodulin-binding domain	Inversin domain, cilium
GLIS2	15p13.3	Glis2	—		NPHP	Kruppel-like zinc finger	Cilium
NEK8	17q11.2	Nek8	NPHP9, JCK		NPHP	NIMA kinase	Inversin domain, cilium
SDCCAG8	1q43	SDCCAG8	NPHP10, CCCAP	SLSN7	NPHP, SLSN	Coiled-coil domains, colon cancer auto-antigen	Basal body/centrosome
XPNPEP3	22q13.2	NPHP-1L	APP3		NPHP	Peptidase	Mitochondria
ATD	15q13	ATD1	ATD		ATD	Unknown	Cilium?
IFT80	3q25.33	IFT80	WDR56		ATD	IFT-B complex, WD40 domains	Cilium
DYNC2H1	11q22.3	Dync2H1	DHC2, DHC1B		ATD	Cytoplasmic dyenin component	Cilium, cytosol
TTC21B	2q24.3	IFT139	THM1	JBTS11, NPHP12	ATD, NPHP, JBTS	IFT-A complex, TPR repeats	Cilium
IFT122	3q21.3−q22.1	IFT122	WDR10		CED	IFT-A complex, WD40 domains	Cilium
WDR35	2p24.1	IFT121	TULP4, Naofen		CED	IFT-A complex, WD40 domains	Cilium
IFT43	14q24.3	IFT43	—		CED	IFT-A complex	Cilium
OFD1	Xp22.2	Ofd1	—	JBTS10	OFD, JBTS	Coiled-coil domains	Basal body/centrosome
ΛLSM1	2p13.1	ΛLSM	ΛLSS		ALMS	Trafficking protein?	Cytosol
ATXN10	22q13.31	Ataxin 10	E46L, SCA10		MKS?	ATTCT repeats	Perinuclear

*a*Genes are categorized by ciliopathy based on Online Mendelian Inheritance in Man (OMIM, http://www.ncbi.nlm.nih.gov/omim) entries at time of writing.

Thus, the function IFT88 is highly conserved across diverse species.

One of the most significant breakthroughs connecting cilia dysfunction to human diseases came from studies in *C. elegans* by Barr et al. They conducted a genetic screen to identify genes involved in male mating behavior and uncovered mutations in *lov-1* and *pkd-2*, the homologs of human polycystin-1 (PC-1) and polycystin-2 (PC-2), respectively.[13] Importantly, mutations in these two genes cause human autosomal dominant polycystic kidney disease (ADPKD OMIM# 601313, # 173910); a disorder that affects nearly 1 in 1000 individuals and is a leading cause of end-stage renal disease. In *C. elegans*, both *lov-1* and *pkd-2* proteins localize to the cilium of male sensory neurons.[14] Subsequently, the mammalian proteins were also localized in the cilium of renal epithelium[15,16] leading to a paradigm shift in the understanding of the possible mechanisms involved in human PKD. Multiple cystic kidney disease genes in mice, rats, and humans have now been identified and in nearly every case, the affected proteins encoded by these genes are associated with the cilium (reviewed in [17-20]).

These initial observations in model systems ushered in a renewed interest into the functions and clinical importance of the primary cilium. Even though research into the role of primary cilia has now extended to almost every tissue in the body, the involvement of the cilium in the kidney has garnered particular focus. In part this may reflect the morbidity and mortality associated with PKD, as well as the high incidence of PKD.

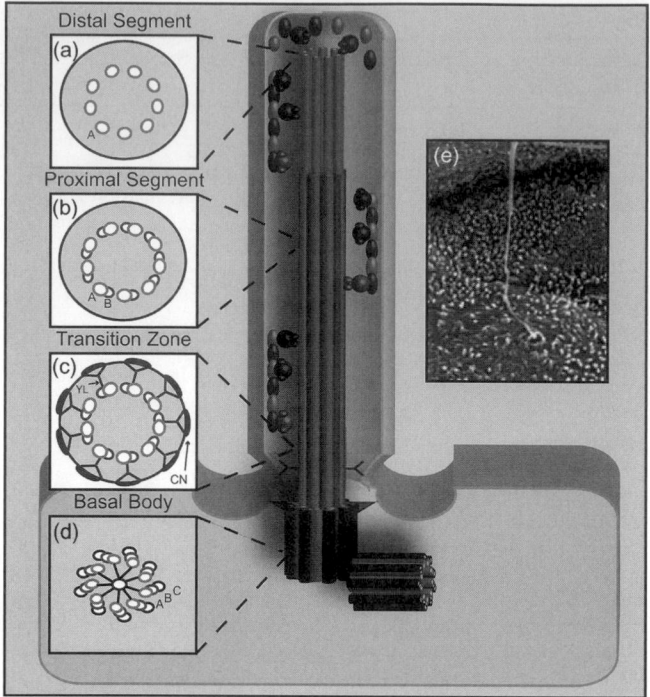

FIGURE 11.1 **Ultrastructure of the primary cilium**. A microtubule-based axoneme nucleates from the basal body and extends the length of the cilium. IFT-A (maroon) and IFT-B (light blue) complexes form IFT-A/B particle trains and travel along the axoneme via IFT with their associated cargoes. Anterograde IFT (left side of axoneme) occurs via Kinesin-2 (dark blue) and Kif-17 (purple) motor proteins. IFT-A/B particle trains are disassembled and reassembled at the ciliary tip. Retrograde IFT (right side of the axoneme) removes IFT-A/B particles and associated proteins from the cilium via the cytoplasmic dynein-1 retrograde motor protein (red). Insets (a–d) illustrate cross-sections of ciliary microtubule structure. (a) Distal segment with 9 + 0 "A" axonemal microtuble singlets; (b) Proximal segment with 9 + 0 "A/B" axonemal doublets; (c) transition zone with Y-links (YL) and ciliary necklace (CN) respectively; (d) basal body with "A/B/C" microtubule triplets; (e) scanning electron micrograph of the primary cilium. *(Image adapted from Alvaro, D. et al. (2008). Am. J. Pathol. Feb; **172**(2), 321–332, with permission.)* See color section at the end of the book.

CILIA ULTRASTRUCTURE AND COMPONENTS

The primary cilium on renal epithelial cells is a small, membranous, hair-like extension protruding from the surface of the cell into the lumen of the nephron tubule. This simple description, however, disguises the high level of complexity that is necessary for the cilium to function as an intricate signaling and sensory organelle (Figure 11.1). Below the membranous covering of the cilium lies a precisely ordered series of axoneme microtubules. At the base of the cilium, the axoneme microtubules are anchored to the cell and cell membrane by a series of specialized structural components including transition fibers, the transition zone,

ciliary necklace, and a modified centriole termed the *basal body*. These structures are further defined below.

Centrosomes and Basal Bodies

Centrosomes are comprised of a pair of centrioles, an older mother centriole and a daughter centriole, surrounded by a proteinaceous matrix. Mother–daughter centrioles are aligned orthogonally, with the mother centriole aligned towards the cell surface. The mother centriole becomes the basal body, which acts as a microtubule-organizing center (MTOC) for axonemal nucleation at the base of the extending cilium. Basal bodies are comprised of a nine-ring helix of triplet microtubules that contain γ-tubulin, in addition to α- and β-tubulins (Figure 11.1d). Axoneme microtubule polymerization is initiated by nucleation of γ-tubulin-containing microtubules of the basal body.

In addition to their microtubule cores, basal bodies are also comprised of numerous associated proteinaceous appendages that facilitate ciliogenesis. Although the basal body appears symmetrical, the distribution of centriolar appendages gives the basal body asymmetry with respect to its proximal–distal axis. The basal foot (also called sub-distal appendages) and the transition fibers (also called distal appendages) extend from the more distal end of the basal body. The formation of transition fibers on the basal body is a distinct process from that of ciliogenesis, yet it has been demonstrated that transition fibers are necessary for cilia to form.[21,22] Transition fibers appear necessary for tethering the basal body to the membrane (see section "Transition Fibers" and [23]), thus establishing the basis for cilia anchorage.

The proteinaceous matrix surrounding the basal body is termed the *pericentriolar material* and contains centriolar components. Although the pericentriolar material does not form the structure of the centriole/basal body, these proteins are necessary for centriolar organization and control of mitosis. Puncta of proteins surrounding centrioles (centriolar satellites) will often be dynamically associated with the centrosome depending on cell cycle stage.[24]

Ciliary Axoneme

The core of both motile and primary cilium is an organized microtubule-based axoneme extending from the basal body. Axonemal microtubules have (+) ends, localized at the ciliary tip, and (−) ends anchored to the basal body. These microtubules serve as tracks for molecular motor protein transport of cargo along the cilium (Table 11.2 and see section "Intraflagellar Transport (IFT) and IFT Motors").

TABLE 11.2 Intraflagellar Transport (IFT) Complex Proteins and Motors (Known Disease Genes are Annotated)

IFTA-Complex	IFTB-Complex	IFT Anterograde Motors	IFT Retrograde Motors
IFT43[*]	IFT20	KIF3A	Cytoplasmic dynenin2[^]
IFT121[*]	IFT22	KIF3B	
IFT122[*]	IFT25	KAP3	
IFT139[^]	IFT27		
IFT140	IFT46		
IFT144	IFT52		
	IFT54		
	IFT57		
	IFT70		
	IFT74		
	IFT80[^]		
	IFT81		
	IFT88		
	IFT172		

[*]Mutated in CED.
[^]Mutated in ATD.

Axonemal microtubules are arranged in a ring of nine doublets (Figure 11.1b). Cryo-electron tomography imaging of cilia axoneme microtubules by Sui and Downing[25] illustrate that each doublet is comprised of a larger A-tubule, and a smaller incomplete B-tubule. Both A and B tubules of the axoneme microtubules are comprised of α- and β-tubulin protofilaments similar to the cytoplasmic microtubules. The axonemal microtubule doublet may either extend the entire length of the cilium or terminate into a mircotubule singlet that continues into the distal cilium (Figure 11.1a). Most motile forms of cilia also contain additional structures used in generating motility. These include a central pair of microtubules, in addition to their nine-ring doublet, radial spokes, inner and outer dynein arms, and nexin links.[26] The incorporation of a central pair of microtubules in motile cilia is referred to as a *9 + 2 arrangement*. However, not all *9 + 2* cilia are motile, as revealed by olfactory sensory neuron cilia. Immotile primary cilia, such as those found in renal epithelia, lack the central microtubule pair and many of the motility components.[27] Lack of a central microtubule pair is referred to as a *9 + 0 axonemal* microtubule arrangement (Figure 11.1).

The Transition Zone

The cilium is not a simple extension of the cell membrane or cytosol, but rather it has a distinct complement of proteins necessary for its construction, signaling, and sensory functions. The specialization is established by structures located at the base of the cilium that function to separate the ciliary compartment from the rest of the cell.

At the proximal end of the cilium nearest the basal body, the cilia membrane is closely associated with the axoneme microtubules. This region is known as the *transition zone*. Ultrastructurally, the transition zone (Figure 11.1c) is comprised of a radial array of Y-shaped links, with the bottom of the "Y" attaching to each axonemal microtubule doublet and top of the "Y" likely forming attachments with the nearby cilia membrane.[28] The molecular composition of the Y-links are unknown, however, centrosomal protein 290 (CEP290)[29] and the protein p210[30] were shown to localize to the distal end of the basal body in the area of the transition zone Y-links in *Chlamydomonas*. The transition zone appears to be an important domain, as many proteins associated with Meckel-Gruber Syndrome (MKS, OMIM# 249000) and Nephronophthisis (NPHP, OMIM# 256100) function as part of genetically and biochemically interacting complexes that also localize in this region.[31,32] In *C. elegans*, mutations disrupting the interactions between the transition zone proteins involved in NPHP and MKS cause the loss of Y-links, detachment of the ciliary membrane from the axoneme, abnormalities in regulating protein entry into the cilium, and defects in cilia positioning, orientation, and assembly.[32] It is not currently known whether the MKS and NPHP proteins are a direct component of the Y-links or whether the loss of the Y-links in *nphp* and *mks* mutants is a secondary consequence.

The Ciliary Necklace

At the position where the Y-links attach to the inside of the ciliary membrane, the outside of the membrane is decorated with electron-dense proteinaceous nodules.[28] These decorations are collectively referred to as the *"ciliary necklace"* (Figure 11.1d; denoted "CN"). When observed by electron microscopy, the ciliary necklace appears to restrict around the axoneme, and somewhat resemble tight junctions in epithelial cells. As such, the ciliary necklace, along with the Y-links, may function as a barrier machinery that is selective for ciliary transmembrane and membrane associated proteins. The composition of the ciliary necklace remains to be defined, and the mechanisms by which this region may function as ciliary barrier is a major focus of ongoing studies.

Transition Fibers

Through electron microscopy studies, it is apparent that there are electron-dense fiber-like structures extending from the distal end of the basal body that tether the basal body to the base of the ciliary membrane.[23] These structures are known as transition fibers (Figure 11.1). Nine transition zone fibers extend at an angle from the distal tip of the basal body and connect with membrane creating an elaborate pinwheel-like conformation.[23] Space filling models reconstructed from electron micrographs suggest that the space between transition fibers could accommodate particles up to 60 nm,[23] suggesting that this region could act as part of a ciliary gating or barrier mechanism preventing soluble cytosolic protein from entering the cilia. It has therefore been hypothesized that there must be other, active mechanisms for ciliary entry that are localized to this region.[33] Data obtained from studies in *C. elegans* suggest that the transition fibers are docking sites for the IFT particles (see section "Cilia Transport and Trafficking"), and that the transition fibers function in loading and unloading of ciliary cargo onto the IFT particles for transport.[34] Relatively few transition fiber proteins have been identified. One candidate is Cep164, which localizes in the region of the transition fibers and is necessary for ciliogenesis.[21]

Cilia Membrane

The cilium has a distinct composition with regards to both protein and lipid content.[35,36] Identifying the composition of the primary cilia in mammalian cells has been technically challenging, as the surface area of the cilia membrane comprises a small fraction of the total cell membrane. Initial analyses indicate that the cilia membrane contains a high concentration of sterols relative to phosphinostitides when compared to plasma membrane.[37] The high levels of sterols in cilia have led some to speculate that cilia are enriched in lipid rafts, which also have high sterol content. In fact, several ciliary and cystic kidney disease proteins, such as cystin, associate with lipid raft components, and inhibiting this association can impair their transport to the cilium.[38]

Information regarding the protein composition of the cilium has been obtained through proteomic and genetic studies in model systems, as well as comparing the genomes of ciliated and non-ciliated organisms.[39] Although proteomic analysis has been performed on motile cilia and photoreceptor cilia isolated from mammalian cells, currently the most complete information regarding the protein composition of the cilium/flagellum come from *Chlamydomonas*.[40] This is in part due to the ease with which deflagellation can be induced in this organism, allowing for purification and proteomic analyses.

Proteomic data revealed that the cilium contains a large number of transmembrane and membrane associated proteins that in many cases are not found in other regions of the cell. These proteins must be specifically targeted to the cilium (see section "Cilia Transport and Trafficking"). The localization of proteins in the cilia membrane is necessary for normal cilia mediated sensory functions and signaling activities (see section "Cilia Signaling in the Nephron"). This has important implications in common renal disorders, since transmembrane proteins, such as PC-1 and PC-2[15,16] localize in the cilium (see Chapter 81 for a detailed description). Other cystic kidney disease transmembrane proteins found in the cilium include fibrocystin/polyductin, and the Meckel–Gruber syndrome proteins 2[41] and 3[42] (MKS2 and MKS3 respectively) that localize to the transition zone region (see section "Transition Fibers").

CILIA TRANSPORT AND TRAFFICKING

For the cilium to function as a sensory and signaling center, it requires the specific targeting and transport of proteins into and out of the cilium. Although the mechanism of ciliary targeting and protein transport remain poorly understood, great advances have come from seminal studies in model organisms and human ciliopathy patients. We now know many of the core components of the cilia trafficking machinery. Machinery involved in cilia trafficking include the microtubule motor driven intraflagellar transport (IFT) proteins originally defined in *Chlamydomonas*, and the BBSome, a complex of proteins disrupted in Bardet–Biedl syndrome (BBS, OMIM# 209900), that function in cilia membrane protein trafficking and vesicular transport. It has become evident that ciliary trafficking machinery often utilizes canonical endocytic pathways involving the Rab-family of proteins (reviewed in [43]). Understanding how ciliary trafficking falls into conventional trafficking modules is the focus of many ongoing studies.

Intraflagellar Transport (IFT) and IFT Motors

The axoneme provides the cilium structure, and also serves an important role in building the organelle and trafficking proteins through the cilium. Axonemal microtubules are used for trafficking components in both anterograde (toward the cilia tip) and retrograde (toward the basal body) directions in a process known as *intraflagellar transport* (IFT).[11] Coordinated, bidirectional IFT movement is localized between the outer doublet microtubules and the ciliary membrane.

IFT is required to build and maintain the primary cilium through the movement of two interacting macromolecule complexes, IFT-A and IFT-B (summarized in Table 11.2 and reviewed in [44,45]). IFT-A and IFT-B interact to form a large IFT-A/B particle chain that moves together in both anterograde and retrograde IFT. It has been documented that mutations in IFT complex proteins can cause human ciliopathies. Both Jeune Asphixiating Thoracic Dystrophy (ATD, OMIM# 208500) and Sensenbrenner syndrome (CED, OMIM# 218330) are caused by mutations in IFT genes (Tables 11.1 and 11.2, and see sections "Jeune Asphyxiating Thoracic Dystrophy (ATD)" and "Sensenbrenner Syndrome (Cranionectodermal Dysplasia, CED)." In general, the mutations in IFT proteins identified in human patients are thus far hypomorphic, suggesting that complete loss of IFT function is not viable.

In addition to the proteins that make up IFT complexes A and B proper, there is emerging evidence for IFT associated proteins that are important for ciliary protein trafficking and ciliary function. For example, IFT20 is associated with trafficking of proteins from the Golgi to the cilia base.[46] Also, IFT27 (Rabl4) and IFTA-2 (Rabl5) are both Rab-like proteins that associate with the IFT-A/B complex.[47,48] The function of these proteins is poorly understood; however, in the absence of *Rabl5* in *C. elegans*, cilia regulated signaling pathways are affected even though *Rabl5* is not required for ciliogenesis.[48] Thus, the current hypothesis is that *Rabls5* and other IFT associated proteins may function to connect specific cargo with the IFT complex or in more subtle regulation of cilia signaling and sensory activities.

Specific motor proteins mediate IFT bidirectional movement in the cilium (Table 11.2). Kinesin-2 associates with the IFT-A/B complex to move the IFT particle in the anterograde direction toward the cilia distal segment.[49,50] A second kinesin, Kif17, specifically associates with the IFT-B complex, and appears to function largely in movement of the IFT-A/B particle along the distal segment of the cilium.[51] The retrograde motor, cytoplasmic dynein-2, mediates movement of the IFT-A/B particle with its associated cargo in the retrograde direction toward the basal body.[52] It should be noted that most of the data concerning motor-microtubule specificity is largely based on studies using homologs of cilia motor proteins in *C. elegans* and *Chlamydomonas*.

IFT builds and maintains its primary cilium by shuttling tubulin subunits to the growing (+) end of the axoneme microtubules at the ciliary tip by anterograde IFT, while cilia microtubules are cleared from the cilia by retrograde IFT. This can be demonstrated both *in vivo* and *in vitro*, where mutations in Kinesin-2 proteins (anterograde motor) lead to the absence of cilia,[53,54] while mutations in cytoplasmic dynein-2

(retrograde motor) lead to bulbous, stumpy cilia caused by an accumulation of IFT particles and other ciliary proteins.[52,55-57]

Mechanisms of Cilia Protein Entry

The correct function of the primary cilium is dependent on the localization or enrichment of receptors, channels, and effectors in this specialized compartment. As such, the mechanisms restricting or facilitating protein entry into the cilium remain an area of intense research.

A ciliary barrier or gate, which is likely found at the base of the cilium, could function to restrict entry of non-ciliary proteins and/or impair exit of proteins from the cilium. As indicated above, one of the current models is that the transition zone, transition fibers, and ciliary necklace constitute the barrier machinery (Figure 11.1). Evidence supporting a diffusion barrier at the base of the cilium comes from studies using a glycosylphosphatidylinositol-anchored fluorescent protein that is targeted to the apical plasma membrane.[36] This protein diffuses rapidly across the apical surface, but is restricted from the cilium and a region around the base of the cilium called the *periciliary membrane domain*. Similarly, other membrane proteins localized to the apical plasma membrane are not found in the cilium.

Although there is evidence for a cilia barrier, there are also data indicating that cilia access may in part be determined by protein size and governed by diffusion. GFP is a 27 kDal protein that rapidly equilibrates between the cilium and cytosol. However, larger proteins do not accumulate freely in the cilium, and are dependent on IFT. This has led to the hypothesis that the ciliary barrier may be analogous to nuclear pore complex. Passage through the nuclear pore involves the association of a protein containing a nuclear localization signal (NLS) binding to an importin-family protein for movement into the nucleus catalyzed by Ran GTPase activity. Intriguingly, importin-β2 has been localized to the basal body/transition zone in cultured cells, and knockdown of importin-β2 inhibits cilia localization of retinitis pigmentosa 2.[58] Likewise, Ran is found in the cilium, and experiments using mutated Ran have shown that ciliary entry is mediated through a Ran-GTP gradient.[59] The question remains as to whether there are specific cilia localization signals (CLS) similar to the putative NLS sequence. Indeed, NLS-like sequences have been reported in cilia proteins, such the kinesin KIF17, and disruption of this NLS motif inhibits Kif17 cilia localization.[59] A sequence, V-x-P, necessary for ciliary localization[60] has also been identified in the transmembrane proteins

PC-2 and CNGB1b, and in several G-protein coupled receptors (SSTR3, 5HT6, DRD1, Rhodopsin, and MCHR1); however, the mechanism by which this motif targets these proteins to the cilium is variable, and is most likely protein-specific. Most other cilia transmembrane proteins do not have this signature, indicating there is no universal sequence directing proteins into the cilium.

An alternate hypothesis for ciliary enrichment was proposed by Hu et al. and involves inhibition of lateral diffusion. Ciliary proteins were highly mobile within the cilium, but there was limited exchange between the plasma membrane and the cilium. These data suggest a barrier-impeded diffusion. Hu et al. demonstrated that septin-2 is located around the base of the cilium, and may function as this barrier.[61] Septins were originally identified as a family of guanosine triphosphatases with diffusion barrier function. Knockdown of septin-2 in embryonic fibroblasts and renal epithelium resulted in a marked increase in diffusion and exchange between cell and ciliary membranes, defects in ciliogenesis, and inhibition of cilia dependent signaling (e.g., Sonic Hedgehog (Shh) pathway, see section "Renal Cilia and Hedgehog Signaling").[61] Thus, one possible mechanism is that ciliary transmembrane proteins are continually transported into the cilium and accumulate there as a consequence of slow outward diffusion.

Recently, another model for ciliary membrane protein entry was proposed from the laboratory of Ira Mellman.[62] Francis et al. analyzed gp135/podocalyxin, which is a transmembrane protein localized to the apical surface of renal epithelial cells that is also restricted from the cilium and the periciliary membrane region around the cilia base. gp135 is anchored to the cortical actin cytoskeleton through its PDZ domain. When this motif was disrupted, gp135 was now present ectopically in the cilium. Conversely, proteins that normally enter the cilia could be inhibited from doing so if the gp135 PDZ domain was incorporated into the protein. These data suggested that ciliary exclusion was dependent on attachment of membrane proteins to the cytoskeletal network, rather than the presence of a diffusion barrier. This model is hard to reconcile with the septin-2 data from Hu et al.,[61] the evidence for the BBSome in cilia membrane trafficking of specific GPCRs (see section "Ciliary Targeting and the BBSome" and [60,63,64]), and the presence of multiple membrane proteins that are freely diffusible and have not been detected in the cilium.[36] Further, lipid content in the cilium has been reported to be distinct from that of cell membrane (reviewed in [65]). In the absence of a barrier, one would expect an equilibration between the two compartments.

Vesicular Trafficking of Transmembrane Proteins to the Cilium

Transmembrane proteins destined for the cilia are dependent on the activity of Rab-GTPases. One of the initial Rabs shown to be involved in ciliary targeting was Rab8. Inhibition of Rab8 leads to accumulation of vesicles at the base of the cilium, while Rab8 constitutive activation causes elongated cilia.[66] Rab8 utilizes the ciliary localized exocyst complex and activity from its guanine nucleotide exchange factor (GEF) Rabin8 to dock and fuse vesicles at the cilia base. Although the process of targeting transmembrane proteins to the ciliary base is still being fully deduced, one of the most widely accepted models involves polarized exocytosis through a Rab11-associated trafficking pathway. Through this pathway, transmembrane proteins are shuttled from a Rab11 positive compartment to a Rab8 positive vesicle, dependent on Rab11 activation of Rabin8. Transmembrane proteins in these Rab8 positive vesicles are then transported to the cilia base, and inserted directly into the periciliary membrane domain.[67,68] Importantly, although some vesicular structures have been reported in olfactory and chondrocyte cilia,[69,70] vesicles are not commonly seen in most other cilia or flagella. These data indicate that if polarized exocytosis occurs, the fusion of the vesicles with the cilia membrane likely occurs at the base. In support of this are ultrastructural studies showing numerous vesicles containing putative ciliary-targeted proteins located around the base of cilia and flagella actively fusing with the membrane.[71,72] How these proteins then get across a ciliary barrier, if it exists, is unknown.

It is also possible that the initial targeting of ciliary transmembrane proteins is to the plasma membrane. The ciliary protein would then translocate into the cilium by either lateral diffusion or through an endocytic pathway. This is best understood in the case of Smoothened (Smo), the transmembrane effector protein of the Sonic hedgehog-signaling pathway (Shh). In response to Shh stimulation, Smo translocates from the cell membrane into the cilium. This translocation is not inhibited by expression of a dominant negative form of dynamin,[73] a GTPase required for scission of vesicles during endocytosis in eukaryotic cells. Thus, the data indicate that at least in this case, ciliary targeting is likely mediated through lateral diffusion, and does not require endocytosis of vesicles from the plasma membrane.

Ciliary Targeting and the BBSome

The BBSome is a protein complex involved in trafficking of specific cilia membrane proteins.[64,66]

Mutations affecting this complex of proteins cause Bardet–Biedl Syndrome (BBS). BBS is a rare human ciliopathy characterized by obesity, sensory defects, and cystic kidney disease (see section "Bardet-Biedl Syndrom (BBS)"). The assembled BBSome shares structural similarities with the COP/clatherin family of coat proteins, suggesting the BBSome functions as a coat for ciliary cargos. The BBSome coat associates with the GTPase Arl6 (also known as BBS3) when Arl6 is in its GTP–bound, active state. The BBSome/Arl6 complex recognizes the ciliary localization sequence (CLS) in proteins such as SSTR3, and then escorts the protein into the cilium. The BBSome may also function for removal of proteins from the cilium. This is evidenced by the abnormal accumulation of specific transmembrane proteins in the cilium of *bbs* mutant mice.[63]

CILIOGENESIS

Cilia are complex structures that require continual maintenance[74] and must be dissembled and subsequently reassembled at the beginning and end of each cell cycle. The process of building a cilium (ciliogenesis) requires the coordination of centriolar modification/maturation to form a basal body, the motor driven process of IFT to build the cilia axoneme, and carefully timed transcriptional events. These processes are synchronized with cell cycle progression, as cilia are assembled on quiescent cells.[75] Likewise, during mitosis the centrioles must be released from their position below the cilia, and migrate to opposite spindle poles for proper cell division. Ciliogenesis can also be regulated by other factors, such as cell confluence, fluid flow, mechanical stimuli, and injury.[76]

Transcriptional Control of Ciliogenesis

Cilia are extremely dynamic structures that grow and reabsorb depending on physiological conditions. Ciliogenesis is in part regulated through transcriptional control. This is demonstrated in *Chlamydomonas*, where experimentally induced deflagellation results in a large increase in the expression of flagellar genes, including the IFT proteins.[39,40,72,77–79] In addition, in *C. elegans* and mammalian systems, transcription factors of the RFX (regulatory factor X) family have been shown to coordinately control expression of several IFT genes through a motif called the X-box located in their promoters.[80] This process is evolutionarily conserved, and was first reported in *C. elegans*. The RFX transcription factor DAF-19 was needed for expression of several IFT proteins, as well as a few proteins known to be involved in human syndromes with cystic kidney disease phenotypes.[81,82] This includes transition zone proteins such as the NPHP genes *nphp-1* and *nphp-4*, and the MKS genes *mks-1*, *b9d1(mksr1)*, and *b9d2(mksr2)*, as well as multiple BBS genes including *bbs-1*, *bbs-2*, *bbs-5*, *bbs-8*, and *bbs-9* (reviewed in [83]).

Cilia and the Cell Cycle

The basal body (see section "Centrosomes and Basal Bodies") is generated from the centrioles that are also components of mitotic machinery. Therefore, cell division, cell differentiation, and ciliogenesis are inherently linked. As cells exit mitosis, ciliogenesis is initiated in the G_1 or G_0 phase of the cell cycle. This can be modeled *in vitro*, as cells will become increasingly ciliated as they reach confluence. Additionally, ciliogenesis can be induced precociously in subconfluent cells when cultured in serum-free medium. These data indicate that cilia formation and mitosis are intertwined, and has led to the proposal that the presence of the cilium may act as a G_0 checkpoint and thus as a tumor suppressor.[84] In addition, rapid or aberrantly dividing cells, such as some tumor cells, frequently do not have a cilium.[85,86] Despite this connection, increased tumor rates are uncommon in human ciliopathy patients or mouse cilia mutants. An exception to this was recently shown in the skin of cilia mutant mouse models in tumors associated with Shh signaling, where cilia have a direct role in pathway regulation.[87]

As cells re-enter the cell cycle, cilia begin to be dismantled. This usually occurs by the G2 phase. Deconstruction of the cilium can occur by either cilia severing or resorbtion.[75] These mechanism(s) regulating deciliation are still poorly understood. Work from *Chlamydomonas* suggests that katanin, a microtubule-severing protein, cleaves microtubules at the junction between the axoneme and the basal body to facilitate cilia release.[88] In *Chlamydomonas*, the kinase activity of Nek8 (NPHP9) is required for deflagellation.[89] In mammalian systems, HEF1 (human enhancer of filamentation 1) in association with Aurora A kinase and the tubule deacetylase (HDAC6) reduce axoneme microtubule stability and induce deciliation.[90]

Cilia Extension

At the initiation of ciliogenesis, the centriole migrates towards the cell surface and proteins required for ciliogenesis, including the IFT proteins, begin to aggregate at a *preciliary patch*. There appear to be at least two mechanisms in which cilia initially form. The first method requires the formation of a ciliary vesicle (CV),[91] a Golgi-derived structure that forms at the distal tip of the mother centriole. As the CV-mother centriole nears the cell surface, the cilium axoneme extends into the CV. The CV fuses with the plasma membrane, allowing the cilium to extend from the cell surface and emerge into the extracellular space. As a consequence, the basal body and the cilium remain in a small depression in the cell called the *ciliary pocket*.[92,93] The functional importance of the pocket is not certain, but it closely resembles the flagella pocket present in some protists. In these organisms, the pocket serves as a critical sight for vesicular trafficking and endo- and exocytic activity. In the second method, the cell forgoes forming a CV, and the centrosome complex migrates to the cell surface. It is at the cell surface that the mother centriole recruits materials to begin forming the cilia from plasma membrane components.

Post Ciliogenesis Growth Control

Cilia length is an actively controlled process, and is important for normal function (reviewed in [44]). In motile cilia, the increase in cilia length alters beating frequency and pattern, and thus disrupts fluid movement. In primary cilia, it is less clear how changes in length may influence many of the signaling activities. Normal control of cilia length is important, as both excessively short or elongated cilia in the kidney have been shown to cause cysts.[94-97]

Cilia length control is best understood from studies in *Chlamydomonas*, where genetic mutants have been isolated that produce either short or long flagella. Several genes involved in this process have been identified and encode kinases, such as cyclin-dependant kinase,[98] and a mitogen-activated protein kinase (MAPK) member.[99] The homologs for these proteins are present in mammals, suggesting evolutionarily conserved pathways; however, the targets of the kinases are not known.

One of the initial functions assigned to primary cilia in the kidney and several other tissues is that of a mechanosensor (see section "Renal Cilia and Mechanosensation"). Thus, cilia length could greatly influence the response or sensitivity of the cell to mechanical stimuli. As in some ciliated protists, mammalian cells are also able to modulate cilia length. Recent studies have revealed that decreased Ca^{2+} or increased levels of cAMP can cause a marked increase in cilia length.[100,101] This length increase is in part dependent on protein kinase A (PKA), and is associated with increased rate of anterograde IFT. Shear stress across the surface of many cell types is able to reduce cilia length. This was also shown to decrease cAMP levels. Importantly, this adaptive response to shear stress was not observed in cells that lack the polycystins.[102] Thus, it has been proposed that dynamic regulation of cilia length is an important regulatory process that controls sensitivity to extracellular stimuli, and that in PKD this has been disconnected.

In addition, cilia length in the kidney, pancreas, and other tissues can be influenced by injury.[103,104] Since renal injury causes rapid cyst formation in the inducible adult cilia mutant mice but not their controls,[105,106] it is tempting to speculate that the cilium may have a function in regulating a pathway involved in a tissue repair process.

Other studies have revealed that cilia length can be influenced by changes in the actin and microtubule cytoskeleton. In a genomic screen for modulators of cilia length, Gleeson and colleagues identified numerous genes required for ciliogenesis, as well as for the maintenance of cilia length.[107] Among these were genes involved in actin dynamics and organization. This included ARP3, a protein necessary for actin polymerization at filament branches, that when knocked-down caused cilia elongation. This effect was further demonstrated using the actin polymerization inhibitor cytochalasin D. These effects on actin are believed to interrupt vesicular docking and stabilization of the periciliary membrane domain at the ciliary base. Further, Sharma et al. demonstrated that actin disruption leads to a concurrent increase in the levels of soluble tubulin that can now be incorporated into the elongating ciliary axoneme. This cilia elongation was inhibited by pretreatment with the microtubule-stabilizing drug paclitaxel.[101] This phenomenon is further supported by data showing that low levels of nocodazole, a microtubule-depolymerizing agent, could recapitulate the effects observed with actin destabilization.

CILIA SIGNALING IN THE NEPHRON

The spectrum of processes regulated by the renal cilium is not fully known. There are a large number of receptors and channels that have now been localized or enriched in the cilium.[15,60,102,108-110] For several of these proteins, their localization in the cilium has great importance to their function. In many cases, loss of ciliary signaling leads to the formation of renal cysts. Therefore, much of our understanding of cilia signaling in the kidney comes from the study of cystic kidney disease models. This section discusses some of the major signaling pathways involved in renal development and physiology in which the cilium is required for efficient signal transduction, and how disruption of these signals results in cyst formation.

Renal Cilia and Mechanosensation

Data indicating that renal cilium function as a mechanosensor came from studies in Ken Spring's laboratory.[111–113] Fluid-flow induced deflection of the cilium causes a transient increase in cytosolic calcium (Figure 11.2). Furthermore, studies by Liu et al.[114] demonstrated that in perfused tubules from the *orpk* mutants, where cilia are severely truncated, this calcium signal is abrogated. The proteins involved in this signal are believed to be polycystin-1 (PC-1) and polycystin-2 (PC-2), both of which localize to the primary cilium. PC-2 is a transient receptor potential (TRP)-like cation channel known to mediate calcium signals. PC-1, which binds to PC-2, is suspected to be a regulator of the channel. Mutations in PC-1 or PC-2 disrupt this calcium signal, even in the presence of a fully formed cilium.[102] This led to a model of cystogenesis where the loss of a cilia-mediated mechanical signal was a driving force responsible for the development of renal cysts.

Recently, data from inducible cilia and *PKD1* mutant mice have raised concern about the cilia mechanosensory model of cyst formation.[106] Disruption of *IFT88* or *PKD1* using conditional alleles and tamoxifen inducible Cre-deletor lines revealed that cilia dysfunction induced prior to postnatal day 12 (P12) caused a rapid onset of the cystic kidney phenotype.[115–117] However, cyst formation is very protracted if induction of cilia loss occurred after P12. It is difficult to reconcile how cyst development could be delayed in the adult induced cilia mutants if cysts arose due simply to the loss of a mechanosensory signal.

Renal Cilia and Jak/STAT Signaling

The loss of the mechanosensory-based increase in transient cellular Ca^{2+} levels alone is not enough to induce the formation of renal cysts, as revealed by the large delay in cyst formation observed when cilia dysfunction is induced in adult mice. Recently, it has been demonstrated that in addition to regulating PC-2 channel activity, PC-1 also plays a role in transducing a flow-induced signal in the renal cilium through either the Jak/STAT pathway or mTOR signaling (see section "Renal Cilia and mTOR"). PC-1 activates the STAT-family of transcription factors via dual mechanisms (Figure 11.3a,b),[118] depending on the proteolytic processing and nuclear translocation of the PC-1 C-terminal tail (PC-1 CTT).[119,120] In a direct activation pathway, PC-1 resides in the cilium and is able to bind the Jak2 kinase.[118] When luminal flow is lost, Jak2 kinase phosphorylates and activates STAT3, which translocates to the nucleus (Figure 11.3b). Importantly, this process requires the PC-1 CTT to remain membrane-bound to activate STAT3.[118] Also, when fluid flow is lost in the nephron and PC1 is cleaved to release the PC-1 CTT, the PC-1 CTT can bind and activate both P100 and STAT6, which can be found in the cilium or at the basal body (Figure 11.3a).[120] This complex then enters the nucleus to influence gene expression. Alternatively, the PC-1-CTT has been shown to translocate directly into the nucleus, where it enhances the activity of cytokine activated STAT1 and/or STAT3.[118]

The Jak/STAT pathway is canonically described in the human immune response, driving differentiation and proliferation in response to cytokines. So what is the function of the Jak/Stat pathway in the cilium, and how does this relate to cyst growth? Under loss of flow conditions, such as injury, obstruction or cyst formation, the kidney undergoes an inflammatory response, which includes an increase in cytokine levels,[121,122] and infiltration of macrophages.[123–125] The increased cytokine levels trigger the upregulation of the Jak/STAT pathway in the cilium, possibly through association of PC-1 acting as a pseudo-cytokine receptor for Jak2 kinase.[118] This in turn begins the Jak/STAT signaling cascade, where the PC-1 CTT is eventually cleaved and enters the nucleus leading to proliferation. Indeed, high levels of nuclear PC-1 CTT have been observed in the metanephric mesenchyme, developing tubules,[119] and in cyst lining cells[120] where proliferation levels are high.

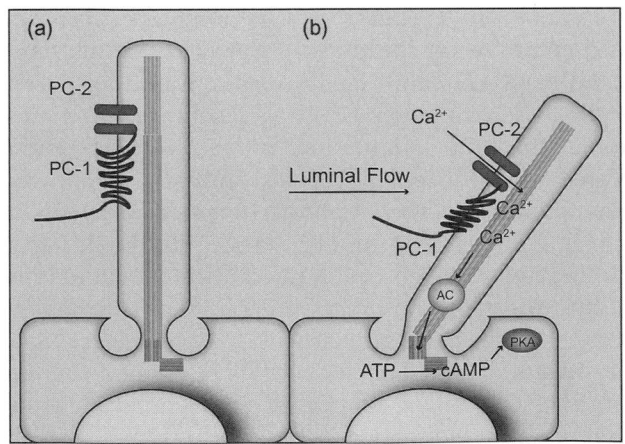

FIGURE 11.2 Cilia and mechanosensation. In low flow conditions (a), the TRP-like cation channel, polycystin-2 (PC-2, red) localizes to the cilium and is regulated by polcysitin-1 (PC-1, maroon). Under flow conditions (b), deflection of the primary results in an opening of the PC-2 channel, allowing Ca^{2+} ions to enter the cell, and increasing cytosolic Ca^{2+} levels. As a result of increased Ca^{2+} concentration, adenylyl cyclase (AC, orange) becomes activated, converts free ATP to cAMP, and cAMP activates protein kinase A (PKA) which phosphorylates multiple downstream targets. See color section at the end of the book.

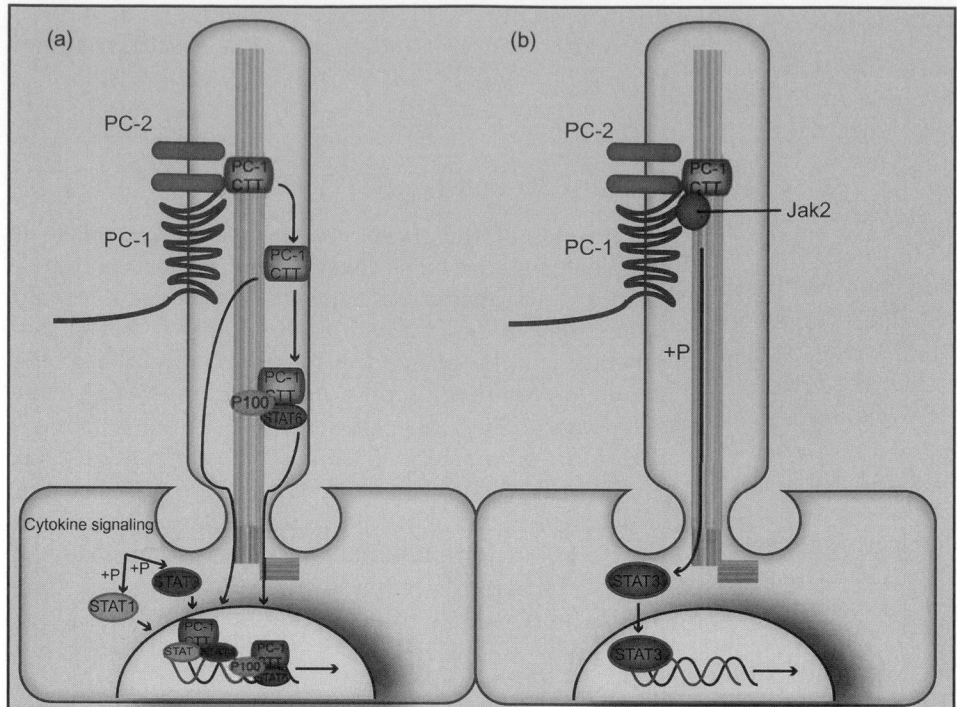

FIGURE 11.3 Cilia and Jak/STAT signaling. (a) When luminal flow is lost, the polycystin-1 C-terminal tail (PC-1 CTT, maroon) is cleaved and regulates the nuclear localization and activity of STAT6 (gray) and p100 (green). The PC1-CTT may also translocate into the nucleus to enhance activity of nuclear STAT1 (orange) and STAT3 (blue). (b) Membrane-associated polycystin-1 also directly interacts with Jak2 kinase (purple) to activate STAT3 under low flow conditions. See color section at the end of the book.

Further evidence to support the model of inflammation-based cyst growth has been demonstrated by monitoring macrophage infiltration in renal ischemic injury. The macrophage infiltrate found in ischemic reperfusion injury mice are pro-proliferation instead of pro-inflammatory.[124] Furthermore, Karihaloo and colleagues demonstrated that depleting macrophages in *PKD1* mutant mice lowered cystic growth significantly.[123] Continued work on the contribution of the immune response is needed to fully understand the role of Jak/STAT- and cilia-regulated signaling in the kidney.

Renal Cilia and Non-Canonical Wnt/Planar Cell Polarity (PCP) Signaling

Non-canonical Wnt signaling (Figure 11.4b) is best known for regulating planar cell polarity (PCP). PCP is the ability of cells to position and orient themselves along the plane of the tissue (Figure 11.5). This is accomplished by modulating the cytoskeleton via the Rho-kinase family, positioning of basal bodies, and the asymmetric distribution of proteins to establish cell orientation. Evidence from model organisms demonstrates a role for cilia in controlling the PCP response, most likely due to the close association of the cilium with the basal body and cell cytoskeleton. Morpholino knockdown of cilia or BBS genes in zebrafish give defects in body axis elongation typical of altered convergent extension during gastrulation.[126] Similarly, *bbs*

and *ift88* mutant mice have inner ear abnormalities typical of PCP defects.[126,127] Collectively, these findings led to a model where cilia function to modulate the strength and spatial activity of the non-canonical Wnt pathway.

In the developing kidney, PCP likely has a role in controlling orientated cell division, and for convergent extension like movements that occur in the early developing nephron.[128] Therefore, loss of cilia-regulated oriented cell division could cause defects in development of the nephron, and lead to cyst formation. Using mouse and rat models of PKD, Fischer et al. demonstrated that the orientation of the mitotic spindle became randomized in cystic animals, rather than being parallel to the nephron lumen as seen in the control kidneys (Figure 11.5[129]). Similarly, the cystic kidney phenotype observed in conditional cilia mutant mice or mice with mutations in PCP genes, such as the proto-cadherin Fat4, are associated with misorientated cell division.[130–134] The above data suggested that parallel divisions to the long axis of the nephron would drive nephron elongation, whereas division perpendicular to the long axis would result in tubule diameter expansion and eventual cyst development. One proposed model was that cilia function in establishing the position of the mitotic spindle through a mechanical signal, such as fluid flow. Loss of the signal resulting from cilia dysfunction would then alter orientation of cell division and eventually lead to cyst formation.

The connection between changes in orientation of cell division and cyst formation must be considered

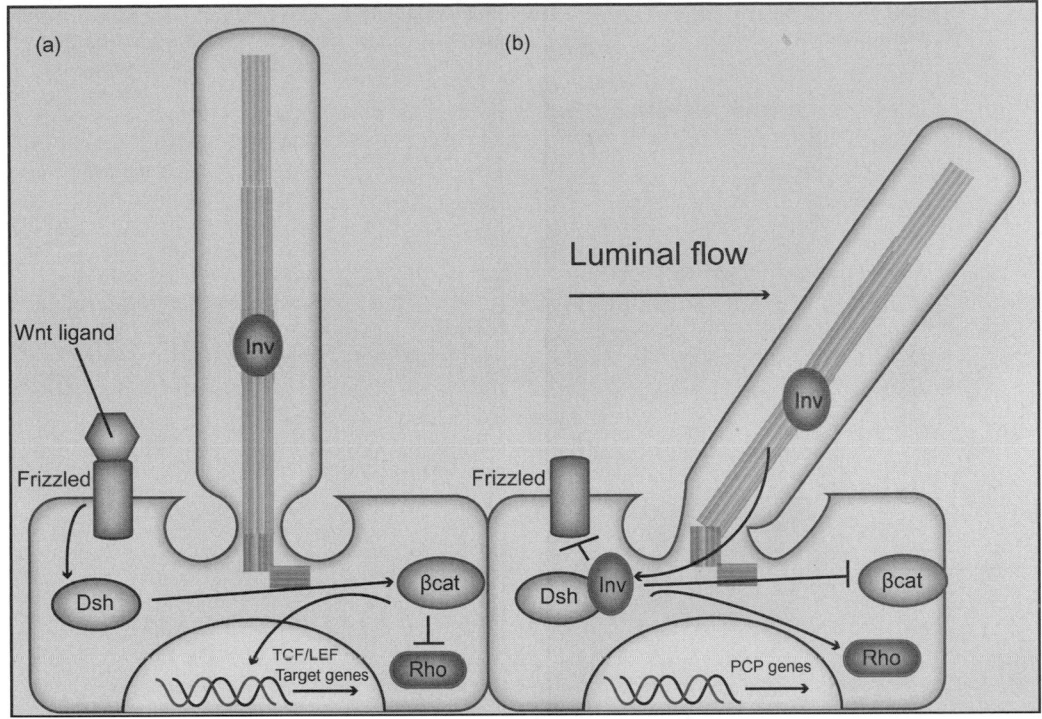

FIGURE 11.4 Wnt signaling in the cilium. In the canonical Wnt pathway (a), Wnt ligands (gray) bind the Frizzled receptor (green). Frizzled activates Disheveled (Dsh, blue) which in turn activates β-catenin (βcat, orange). βcat translocates to the nucleus (yellow), resulting in transcription of TCF/LEF target genes. (b) In the presence of fluid flow, cilia bending causes Inversin/NPHP2 (Inv, red) to translocate from the cilium to inhibit Dsh activation of the non-canonical Wnt pathway. Without Dsh activation, βcat is not activated and degraded. Rho-family kinases and PCP genes then become activated. See color section at the end of the book.

in the context of proliferation rate in the developing tubule. As noted in "Renal Cilia and Mechanosensation" there is a dramatic shift in the rate of cyst progression in mouse cilia mutant kidneys after day P12–13.[115–117] Importantly, in mice there is a dramatic drop in proliferation that occurs in a wild-type kidney as part of its maturation process around P12. Thus, it has been proposed that a combination of a highly proliferative environment, along with misorientated cell division that occurs in cilia or PCP mutants, leads to rapid cyst formation. The possible effect of proliferation on cyst initiation and progression was further analyzed using renal injury models. Through either ischemia reperfusion or nephrotoxin induced injury in the adult induced cilia mutants, several groups have shown that insult and subsequent proliferation induced by the repair process reinitiates a program of rapid cyst development, similar to that seen in the young (≤P12) cilia mutants.[105,135,136] This injury model data must be viewed with caution, as the injury also causes significant inflammation, apoptosis, and dedifferentiation of the nephron segments as a part of the repair process. The contribution of these factors to the rate of cyst formation after injury is not known, and could also contribute to cystogenic mechanisms.

The connection between cilia, cyst development, and oriented cell division was recently brought into question as a result of analysis in the *pkhd1* mutants. *PKHD1* mutations in humans cause ARPKD. In the *pkhd1* mouse mutants the orientation of cell division in the nephron was abnormal, yet they do not develop renal cysts.[137] These data indicate that changes in orientation of cell division are not sufficient to cause cystic disease.

Renal Cilia and Canonical Wnt Signaling

In the canonical Wnt pathway, a Wnt ligand binds to and activates a Frizzled-family receptor that stabilizes β-catenin (Figure 11.4a). β-catenin then translocates into the nucleus, where it combines with TCF/LEF to activate transcription of target genes. One of the initial studies establishing a cilia-Wnt connection came from analysis of *nephrocystin-2* (NPHP2, *Inv*) a gene disrupted in human patients with NPHP (see [138] and section "Nephronophthisis (NPHP)"). NPHP2 localizes to cilia and antagonizes Disheveled, a Wnt pathway component regulating β-catenin stability. NPHP2 expression was able to inhibit the ability of Disheveled to activate Wnt signaling. Simmons et al. have demonstrated a link

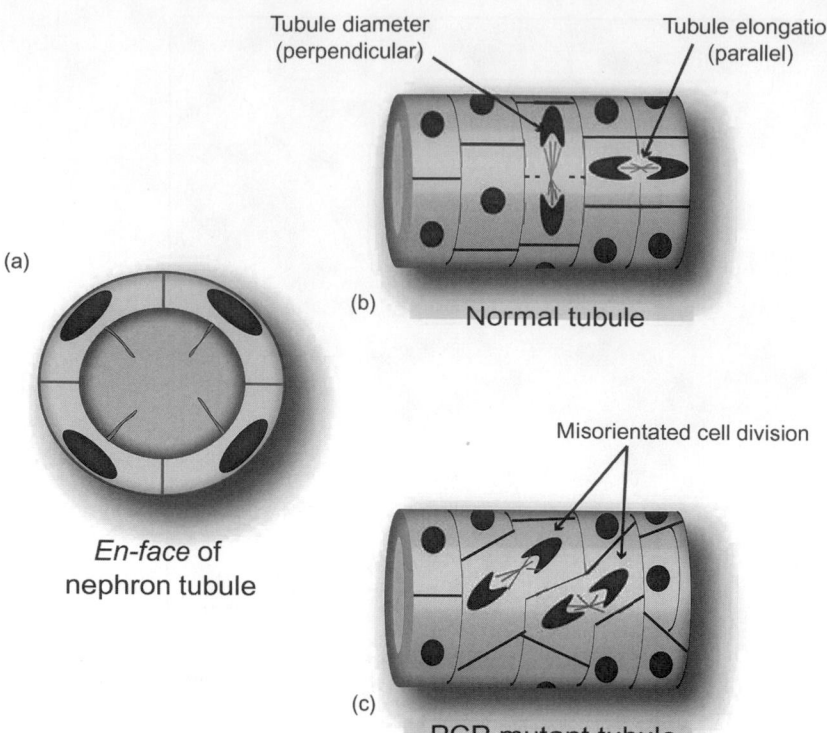

(b) Normal tubule

Tubule diameter (perpendicular)

Tubule elongation (parallel)

(a) En-face of nephron tubule

Misorientated cell division

(c) PCP mutant tubule

FIGURE 11.5 **Cilia influence planar cell polarity (PCP).** (a) Cilia (light blue) extend from the apical surface (red) into the lumen of the nephron tubule. Under normal conditions (b) cilia may modulate signals controlling cell division, either parallel to the long axis of the tubule to increase tubular length or perpendicular to the long axis of the tubule to increase tubule diameter. In some cilia mutants, a PCP-like pathway is disrupted (c) and cell division becomes random and disorientated with respect to the axis of the tubule. See color section at the end of the book.

between fluid flow through the renal tubules and a switch between canonical and non-canonical Wnt signaling pathways.[139] In this process, NPHP2 modulates the balance between the two different Wnt signaling pathways. Additionally, knockdown studies of the BBS genes lead to an increase in canonical Wnt response, and also inhibited non-canonical Wnts from repressing the canonical response in cultured cells.[140] Furthermore, genetic mutations in the IFT genes *kif3a*, *ift88* or *ahi1*, a cilia gene involved in Joubert Syndrome (JBTS, OMIM# 21330), caused an increase in canonical Wnt activity *in vivo*.[141,142] *Ahi1* mutant mice have vermis-midline fusion defects, and these defects could be partially restored by the canonical Wnt agonist lithium chloride.[142]

In contrast, several studies have argued against any direct role for cilia in Wnt signaling (see [143]). This is supported by the lack of clear canonical phenotypes in most tissues of cilia mutant mice, and in zebrafish maternal zygotic mutants in the *ift88* (*oval*) gene. These studies also analyzed Wnt signaling in mutant fibroblasts, and in direct contrast to the previous data did not find changes in Wnt signaling.[144]

Renal Cilia and mTOR

The renal cilium has also been shown to be a regulator of the mammalian target of Rapamycin (mTOR).

mTOR integrates multiple upstream signals to regulate cell processes such as translation, cell growth, proliferation, and protein synthesis. In several of the cystic kidney disease mouse models the mTOR pathway is aberrantly activated.[145–147] Intriguingly, mTOR activation was also shown to be downstream of PC-1 proteolytic processing in the cilium (Figure 11.6a). Dere et al. demonstrated that the C-terminal tail of PC-1 undergoes cleavage in the absence of flow. This regulates the localization of tuberous sclerosis complex 2 (TSC2) to the cell membrane. Importantly, TSC2 is an inhibitor of mTOR, and TSC2 inhibitor activity is controlled by its membrane localization.[148] Therefore, in the absence of PC-1, the PC-1 tail does not undergo processing, which in turn affects the ability of TSC2 membrane association and inhibition of mTOR signaling.

Additional studies indicated that renal cells without a cilium were markedly larger than cells with a cilium when placed in fluid flow conditions. This was also associated with changes in activity of the mTOR pathway. The effect of flow on cell size could be inhibited by treating cells with Rapamycin or inactivating Raptor, a key component of the mTOR pathway.[146] Surprisingly, this fluid flow/cell-size correlation was not dependent on calcium signal mediated by PC-2 or PC-1 cleavage, but rather the tumor suppressor kinase LKB1. LKB1 localizes to the cilium, and has increased activity in response to flow conditions (Figure 11.6b). LKB1 inhibits the mTOR pathway through AMP-

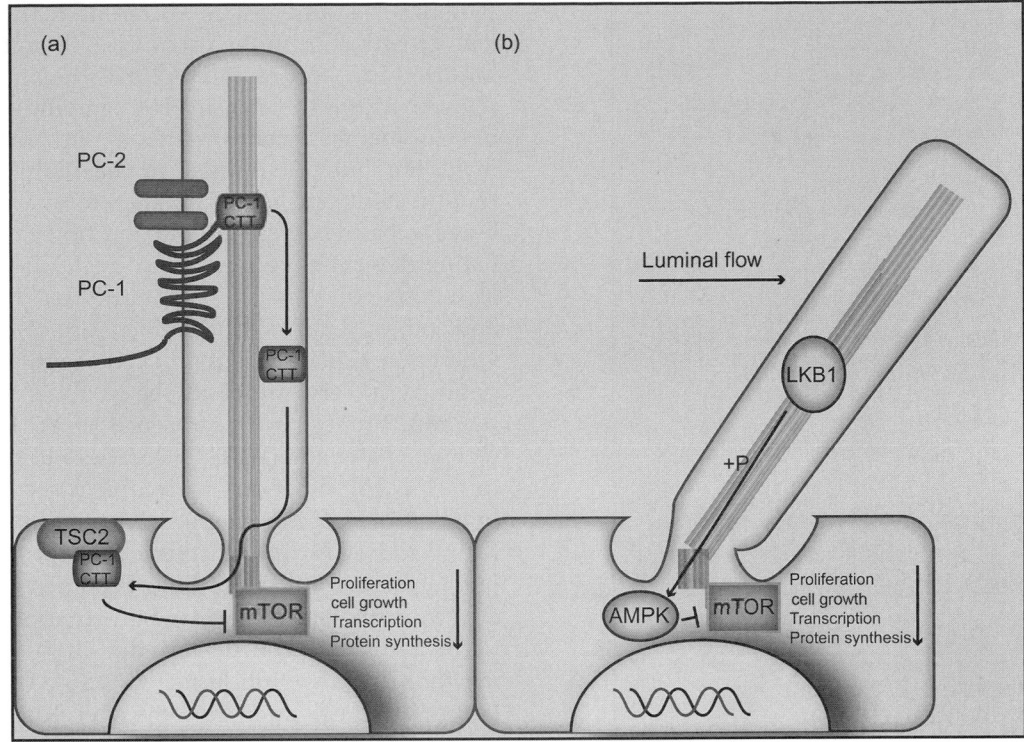

FIGURE 11.6   Cilia and mTOR signaling under no flow and flow conditions. Under static conditions (a), TSC2 (orange) is associated with the plasma membrane and functions to inhibit mTOR (green) signaling. The polycystin-1 C-terminal tail (PC-1 CTT, maroon) undergoes proteolytic cleavage by an unknown mechanism. The PC-1 CTT leaves the cilium, binds TSC2, and retains it at the plasma membrane, thus enhancing the ability of TSC2 to inhibit mTOR signaling. Under flow conditions (b), the ciliary kinase LKB1 (blue) phosphorylates and activates AMP-activated protein kinase (AMPK, tan). AMPK in turn phosphorylates and restrains mTOR activity. See color section at the end of the book.

activated protein kinase (AMPK). Thus, the cell size decrease induced by flow appeared to be regulated by cilia deflection that promotes LKB1 activity to phosphorylate AMPK at the basal body to restrain mTOR signaling.

Another connection between mTOR and the renal cilium was reported by Bell et al., using the adult induced cilia mutant mouse model and unilateral nephrectomy.[145] In contrast to the renal damage and the complex repair process that occurs in the ischemia reperfusion/nephrotoxin injury model, unilateral nephrectomy predominantly leads to a hypertrophic signal in the remaining kidney. In control mice, nephrectomy caused normal activation of mTOR, and produced appropriate structural and functional hypertrophy in the absence of cyst formation. In contrast, in cilia mutant mice there was an exaggerated and prolonged activation of mTOR, increased renal hypertrophy, and accelerated cystogenesis.

The increase in mTOR activity reported in multiple cystic kidney diseases, and its disregulation in cilia mutants, suggested that mTOR inhibition was a potential common site for therapeutic intervention. This was demonstrated in several cystic kidney mouse models

where Rapamycin treatment was shown to be a potent inhibitor of cyst formation.[149,150] However, initial clinical trials of mTOR inhibitors in human PKD patients have not been overly encouraging (see [149] for a summary of results).

Renal Cilia and Vasopressin Signaling

Vasopressin (ADH) is the major hormone responsible for regulating water homeostasis throughout the body. The vasopressin type-2 receptor (V2R) localizes to the primary renal cilium (Figure 11.7), in addition to its normal basolateral localization in renal collecting duct epithelia. *In vitro* assays confirmed that V2R in the cilium is a functional G-protein coupled receptor (GPCR) activating G_s.[109] The G_s subunit in turn activates adenyl cylclase (AC) in the presence of ADH. AC initiates the conversion of ATP to cAMP, and cAMP ultimately activates protein kinase-A (PKA). PKA is responsible for the phosphorylation of the water channel Aquaporin-2 (AQP2).[151] The phosphorylation of AQP2 by PKA causes trafficking of the AQP2 to the apical (luminal) surface to facilitate water

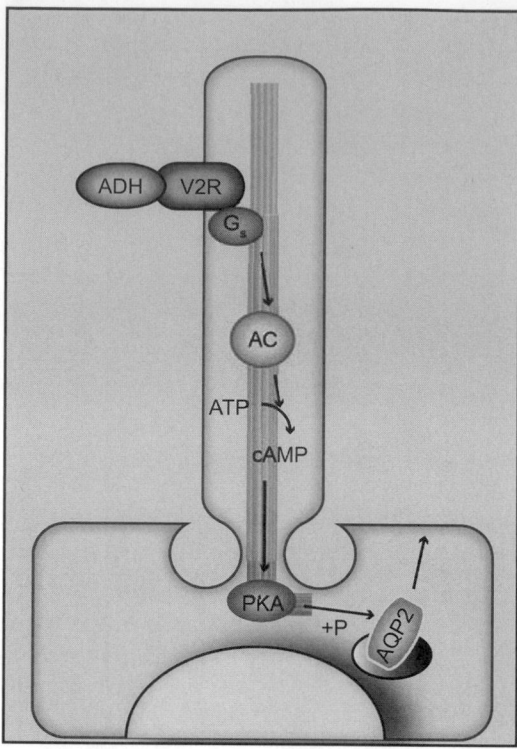

FIGURE 11.7 Proposed mechanism for the cilium in vasopressin (ADH) signaling. Luminal ADH signaling is believed to utilize the primary renal cilium. Luminal vasopressin receptor (V2R, purple) localizes to the primary cilium and binds ADH (gray). Binding of ADH triggers the canonical-ADH signaling pathway where G_s activates adenylyl cyclase (AC, orange), causing an increase in cellular cAMP levels. cAMP activates PKA which phosphorylates internalized aquaporin-2 (AQP2, blue), and causes AQP2 trafficking to the apical membrane and water uptake by the renal epithelium. See color section at the end of the book.

uptake and ultimately produce more concentrated urine. As a consequence of V2R signaling and corresponding downstream activation of cAMP, *AQP2* gene transcription is increased to further enhance cellular response to dehydration.

Interestingly, mice with cilia dysfunction often have defects in urine concentrating ability that may be associated with altered V2R activity.[152] Also, nearly all cystic kidney mutant mice and human cystic patients have marked elevation of intracellular cAMP levels (reviewed in [153]). The most recent therapeutic strategies have targeted these elevated levels of cAMP using V2R antagonists.[110,154,155] In mouse models, this approach has been remarkably successful in correcting the cystic phenotype,[110] and clinical trials in human patients are currently underway.[156]

Renal Cilia and Hedgehog Signaling

During development, the Hedgehog (Hh) signaling pathway is necessary for the establishment of body pattern, cell and tissue differentiation, proliferation, and growth. Components of the Hh signaling cascade localize to, and function in, the primary cilium (Figure 11.8). Defects in Hh signaling cause severe developmental malformations in many systems, including but not limited to the brain, skeleton, and renal system, and in adults altered Hh signaling contributes to basal cell carcinoma and other tumors. Hh signaling defects have not been directly implicated in the formation of renal cysts, although hydronephrosis and other renal abnormalities are present in mice where Hh signaling is disrupted. Regulation of the Hh pathway is very complex (see [157] for a recent in-depth review). Briefly, in the absence of an Hh ligand, the receptor Patched1 (PTCH1) localizes to the primary cilium. PTCH1 functions to inhibit a second transmembrane protein Smoothened (Smo). Binding of an Hh ligand to PTCH1 in the cilium induces its translocation out of the cilium, while Smo becomes enriched in the ciliary compartment. Additional components of the Hh pathway have also been reported in the cilium, including the Gli transcription factors (Gli1-3), Suppressor of Fussed (SuFu), and the kinesins Kif7/Kif27. When Smo is activated, which appears to require the cilium,[158] it induces the pathway leading to the activation of the Gli proteins. The activated Gli transcription factors enter the nucleus and induce expression of the downstream target genes. In the absence of the Hh ligand, the Gli proteins (Gli3 in particular) are proteolytically processed to a smaller Gli3 repressor (Gli3R) to keep the pathway off. The processing of the Gli proteins into their repressor forms, as well as the initial activating step are both dependent on the presence of the cilium.[159,160] Thus, in the absence of the cilium neither the Gli activator nor repressor proteins are formed, leading to a deregulated pathway.

Multiple Hh signaling components are expressed in the developing and adult kidney. Sonic Hedgehog (Shh) is expressed in the embryonic distal epithelium of the ureter and medulary collecting ducts, and mutations in Shh cause renal aplasia.[161] This in turn influences nephron number[162] and renal patterning[163] during continued development. *Glis2* (NPHP7), a Gli-like protein, transduces an Hh signal in the kidney, and *Glis2* mutant mice have severe renal fibrosis and renal atrophy.[164] Multiple syndromes associated with Hh signaling defects have been identified in humans, and in several cases these syndromes are associated with renal malformation. For example, Pallister—Hall syndrome (PHS) is caused by a mutation in the DNA binding domain of Gli3R, and causes renal dysplasia, hypoplasia, hydroureter, and hydronephrosis (see,[165] and reviewed in [166]). These data suggest an important role for Hh signaling and the primary renal cilium during normal kidney development.

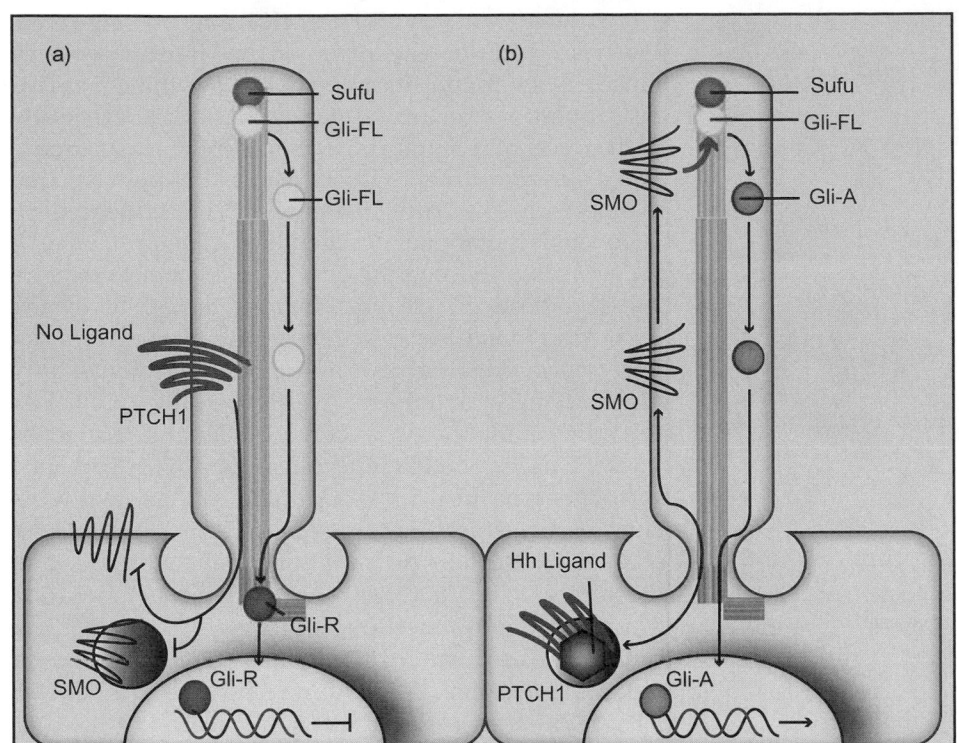

FIGURE 11.8 Cilia and hedgehog signaling. In the absence of Hh ligand (a), ciliary Patched-1 (PTCH1, blue) inhibits Smoothened (SMO, purple). Without SMO activation, Supressor of Fused (Sufu, orange) is in association with full-length Gli (Gli-FL, yellow) at the ciliary tip, where SuFu protects Gli-GL from degradation. In an unknown mechanism, Gli-FL is processed to Gli-repressor (Gli-R, red). Gli-R enters the nucleus and silences transcription of Gli-target genes. In the presence of Hh ligand (b), PTCH1 no longer inhibits SMO. PTCH1 translocates from the cilium to the cytosol and SMO enters the cilium. Ciliary SMO activates Gli-FL (red arrow) at the ciliary tip converting Gli-FL to activated Gli (Gli-A, green). Gli-A then translocates out of the cilium and enters the nucleus to transcribe Gli-target genes. See color section at the end of the book.

MODEL SYSTEMS FOR THE STUDY OF CILIOGENESIS AND CILIA DISEASE

Cilia are ancient organelles that have high levels of evolutionary conservation from invertebrates to humans. This high degree of conservation has allowed for the extensive use of model systems to identify molecular mechanisms of ciliogenesis, and has facilitated the analysis of how cilia function as specialized signaling centers. Despite the fact that many of these model systems do not have organs analogous to mammals, they have contributed enormously to the identification of novel ciliopathy genes and the characterization of disease causing alleles. In this section, we discuss some common model systems to study cilia/flagella, and provide a brief description of how these models are contributing to our understanding of cilia function and cystic kidney disease.

Chlamydomonas reinhardtii

Chlamydomonas reinhardtii are single-celled, fresh water, biflagellate alga (Figure 11.9a). One of the most significant contributions to our understanding of cilia biology from *Chlamydomonas* was the initial description of the intraflagellar transport (IFT) system.[11] The ease with which flagella can be isolated from *Chlamydomonas* then led to the isolation of the IFT complex, the identification of individual IFT protein components, and subsequently to the characterization of the entire flagella proteome. Work by Pazour et al. revealed that one of the IFT proteins in *Chlamydomonas* was the homolog of a gene identified in the Oak Ridge Polycystic Kidney (*orpk*) disease mouse model,[10] and is one of the seminal studies establishing the ciliary hypothesis of cystic kidney disease. Importantly, many of the proteins involved in human ciliopathies are present in the proteome of the *Chlamydomonas* flagella. This database of flagella/cilia proteins (http://labs.umassmed.edu/chlamyfp/) continues to be a major resource available to basic and clinical scientists to prioritize candidate genes involved in human disorders thought to be related to ciliary dysfunction.

Caenorhabditis elegans

C. elegans is a transparent soil nematode that provides a powerful genetic model for analysis of the cilium (Figure 11.9b). Unlike mammalian systems, where most cell types contain a cilium, *C. elegans* only have cilia on a subset of sensory neurons. Several of these cilia extend through small pores in the worm cuticle and are exposed to the environment, where they mediate sensory activities involved in chemotaxis and repulsion. These cilia also allow males to locate hermaphrodites and detect the vulva during mating,

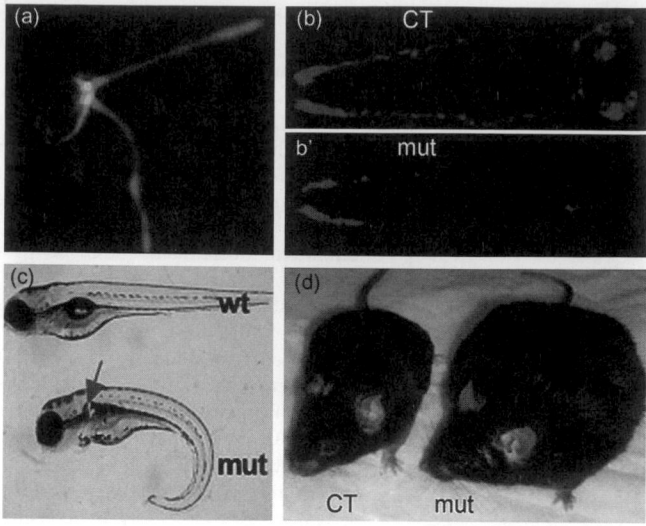

FIGURE 11.9 **Model systems to study cilia structure and function.** (a). *Chlamydomonas reinhardtii* expressing acetylated tubulin (green) in the flagella and IFT72/74 (red) in the cell body and basal bodies. (Adapted from Pedersen et al. (2005). *Curr Biol.* Feb 8; **15**(3), 262–266. With permission.) (b) Dye filling of Control (CT) and (b′) cilia double mutant (mut) *Caenorhabditis elegans*. Note the dye-filling defective (dyf) phenotype of the mutant strain. (Image: J. Pieczynski, unpublished.) (c) Wild-type (top) and *seahorse* mutant *Dario reno* (zebrafish). The *seahorse* gene product, Lrrc6l, modulates Wnt and non-canonical Wnt signaling in zebrafish, and when mutated results in a cystic pronephros phenotype (red arrow). (Image adapted with permission from Kishimoto et al. (2008). *Dev. Cell* Jun; **14**(6), 954–961.) (d) Control (CT, left) and BBS mutant (mut, right) mice (*Mus musculus*). Note the obesity phenotype found in BBS mutants. *(Image from Sharma et al. (2008). Curr. Top. Dev. Biol. **85**, 371–427, with permission.)* See color section at the end of the book.

and to assess food status and population density. Exposed sensory cilia able absorb fluorescent based dyes and worms with cilia abnormalities are often dye-filling defective (*Dyf*). Thus, *C. elegans* provides easily quantifiable traits to probe behavioral defects and structural phenotypes associated with cilia genes.

Even though *C. elegans* does not have the equivalent of the mammalian kidney, this model system has been responsible for another of the initial breakthroughs connecting cilia to cystic kidney disease. This came from a genetic screen by Barr et al. looking for mutations that cause male mating defects. Two of the mutations identified were in the gene *lov-1* (Location Of Vulva defective) and *pkd-2*, which are the homolog of human PC-1 and PC-2.[13] *lov-1* and *pkd-2* were placed genetically in the same signaling pathway in *C. elegans*, and the localization of these proteins in the cilium was first reported in this model.[14]

Recently the *Dyf* phenotype has been utilized as a means to analyze genetic interactions between mutations in ciliopathy genes associated with cystic kidney phenotypes.[32] Ciliopathies (see "The Human Renal

Ciliopathies") such as NPHP, MKS, and BBS are recessive disorders; however, in many human patients mutations are found in only one copy of the gene. This raises questions regarding genetic causality, especially in the case of polymorphisms resulting in missense changes in the protein. This led to the hypothesis that phenotype in ciliopathy patients can be influenced by the overall mutational load in the cilia proteome.[167] *C. elegans* is providing an important system to explore this hypothesis. Single homozygous mutations in any of the known *nphp* or *mks* genes in *C. elegans* does not cause major cilia structural defects and have only minor changes in cilia signaling activity. However, combining mutations between an *nphp* and *mks* genes caused a near complete *Dyf* phenotype. This synthetic *Dyf* phenotype in *nphp;mks* double mutant worms is amiable to chemical mutagenesis screens that will lead to the identification of mutations in genetic loci that interact with either an *nphp* or *mks* mutation (Masyukova and Yoder, in prep).

Another area in which *C. elegans* is providing important insights is in assessing the pathogenic potential of missense mutations that were identified in human ciliopathy patients. This is becoming a major issue as a consequence of NextGen sequencing efforts that have uncovered a large number of missense changes in suspected ciliopathy patients. The contribution of these polymorphisms to disease pathogenesis requires functional assessment. Since *C. elegans* has easily quantifiable phenotypes associated with cilia dysfunction, these phenotypes can be used to assay the pathogenic outcome of these mutations. This has recently been demonstrated for heterozygous missense changes identified in NPHP4 in human NPHP patients.[168] Several of these missense changes altered NPHP4 protein localization/function, enhanced phenotypes in the presence of other ciliopathy gene mutations, and disrupted cilia mediated signaling, and thus are likely to have pathogenic effects.

Danio rerio

Danio rerio, (zebrafish) has become one of the primary vertebrate model systems for analyzing cilia and cilia related diseases (Figure 11.9c). A large number of mutations affecting cilia proteins have now been identified in zebrafish. Unlike *C. elegans* and *Chlamydomonas*, zebrafish contains most of the same basic organ systems as the human body. Thus, these cilia mutants develop many of the same multi-organ phenotypes as observed in human ciliopathy patients, such as hydrocephalus, retinal degeneration, left–right body axis defects, and cystic kidney disease. This is true particularly in the zebrafish kidney, which contains a highly simplified pronephros consisting of a central glomerulus connected to two pronephric ducts that extend along the body empting through the cloaca. This pronephric tubule consists of epithelial cells with multiple motile cilia and single cilia. The function of these cilia and the consequences of their dysfunction have been well-characterized by Iain Drummond and co-workers.[169] The presence of similar multiciliated cells is not observed in the normal mammalian kidney; however, they have been reported in human diseased kidneys, as well as in distended renal tubules from the $pkhd1^{-/-}$ mutant rat.[170] The formation of these motile multiciliated cells in mammals is associated with the induction of the transcription factor FoxJ1 in response to tissue damage.[171]

Zebrafish has become a primary model system for analysis of cilia, in part due to the ease of genetic manipulation and the ability to conduct live, *in vivo* imaging in embryos or high-resolution analysis in fixed tissue. Cilia can easily be visualized with fluorescent tagged proteins using transgenic lines that allow cilia orientation and beat to be evaluated through high-speed video microscopy. Additionally, one of the major uses of the zebrafish model is the ability to conduct morpholino (MO) antisense oligonucleotide knockdown studies utilizing high-throughput approaches. This permits rapid analysis of gene function, and the analysis of the pathogenic effect of missense mutations associated with ciliopathy patients. These studies are done utilizing MO knockdowns to disrupt the function of the endogenous gene, followed by assessing whether expression of the human gene containing the specific missense mutation is able to rescue the ciliary phenotypes. Using these techniques, Nicolas Katsanis and co-workers have demonstrated genetic interactions between ciliopathy genes involved in BBS and assessed mutational load on disease presentation.[172] These studies have also demonstrated a connection between cilia and regulation of canonical and non-canonical Wnt signaling (see sections "Renal Cilia and Jak/STAT Signaling" and "Renal Cilia and Non-Canonical Wnt/Planar Cell Polarity (PCP) Signaling") during convergent extension movements and body axis elongation that may involve the planar cell polarity pathway (reviewed in [173]).

Mus musculus

The mouse (Figure 11.9d) has played a seminal role as the *in vivo* model to assess ciliopathy phenotypes, and was a key factor establishing the initial connection between cilia dysfunction and renal cystic disorders (reviewed in [5]). As described earlier in this chapter, this came from the *orpk* mutant mouse that had a hypmorphic mutation in the *IFT88* gene.[4,174] The *orpk* mouse develops cystic kidney disease, along with other ciliopathy phenotypes including biliary and pancreatic duct cysts, hepatic and pancreatic fibrosis, hydrocephlalus, skeletal patterning and osteogenic abnormalities, retinal degeneration, anosmia, along with skin, hair, and other ectodermal defects.[5] Left—right body axis defects were subsequently observed in mice with null mutations in *IFT88*[6] and *pkd2* mutant mice.[175] The numerous conditional alleles generated in cilia related genes, along with specificity of Cre-deletor lines, are now providing the means to assess cilia function in different developmental stages, specific tissues, and in defined cell types.

THE HUMAN RENAL CILIOPATHIES

The renal ciliopathies are a complex group of oligogenic disorders that now include Polycystic Kidney Disease (PKD, OMIM# 173900, described in Chapter 81), Nephronophthisis (NPHP, OMIM# 256100), Joubert Syndrome (JBTS, OMIM# 21330), Meckel—Gruber Syndrome (MKS, OMIM# 249000), Bardet—Biedl Syndrome (BBS, OMIM# 209900), Alstrom syndrome (ALMS, OMIM# 203800), Orofaciodigital Syndrome Type 1 (OFD1, OMIM# 311200), Jeune Asphyxiating Thoracic Dystrophy (ATD, OMIM# 208500), and Sensenbrenner Syndrome (Cranioectodermal Dysplasia, CED, OMIM# 218330). The phenotypes associated with the ciliopathies can include renal, hepatic, and pancreatic cysts (Figure 11.10a), mental retardation, obesity (Figure 11.10b), neural tube closure and patterning abnormalities, oculomotor apraxia, polydactyly and other skeletal malformations (Figure 11.10c), retinal degeneration, hypotonia, ataxia and cereberellar hypoplasia (Figure 11.10d), hydrocephalus, and cardiovascular defects. Other ciliopathies such as Leber Congenital Amaurosis (LCA, OMIM# 611755) or Senior—Loken syndrome (SLSN, OMIM# 266900), represent variations of the above syndromes (including renal phenotypes) and are not discussed below.

More than 45 human renal ciliopathy disease genes have been identified (Table 11.1); however, in most patients the underlying genetic defect remains unknown. The pace with which ciliopathy mutations are being identified is increasing rapidly due to advances in whole genome sequencing and the availability of cilia/flagella proteome databases. Surprisingly, ciliopathy syndromes share loci (Figure 11.11) despite having very distinct clinical presentations. It is thought that these disorders represent a spectrum of related phenotypes, determined in part by the gene affected and the nature of the mutation. For example, missense mutations may lead to non-lethal ciliopathies, such as NPHP or SLSN, while truncating mutations or null deletions in the same gene cause the lethal MKS. This genotype—phenotype

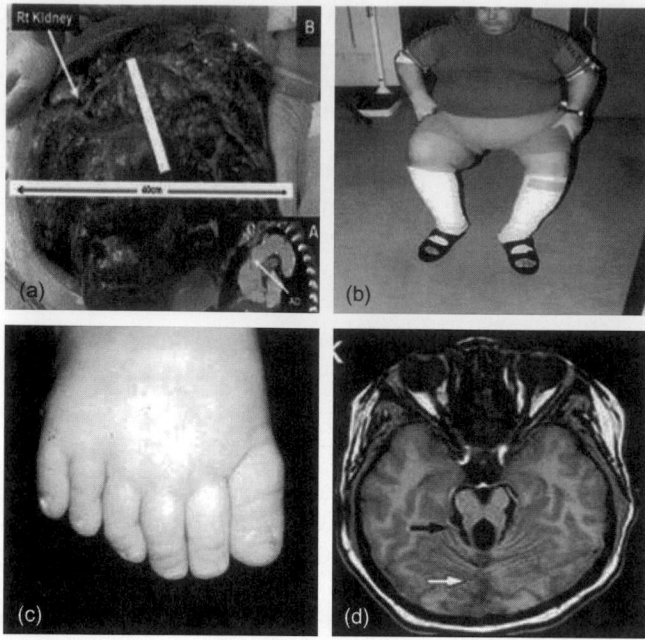

FIGURE 11.10   Common phenotypes associated with cilia dysfunction. (a) Cystic kidneys are a common phenotype to many ciliopathies. *(Image adapted from Menon et al. (2011). Ann. Thorac. Surg. Mar; 91 (3), 919–920. With permission.)* (b) Obese BBS patient. *(Image adapted from Iannello et al. (2002). Obes. Rev. May; 3(2), 123–135. With permission.)* (c) Polydactyly associated with in an intra-familiar BBS patient. *(Image adapted from Riise et al. (1997). Br. J. Ophthalmol. May; 81(5), 378–385. With permission.)* (d) Molar tooth malforma- tion (MTM) found in the cerebral vermis of a JBTS patient. *(Image adapted from Gunay-Aygunetal. (2009). J. Pediatr. Sep; 155(3), 386–392, with permission.)* See color plate section at the back of the book.

correlation, however, has not held up in many ciliopathy patients, leading to the possibility that strong genetic interactions or modifier effects will ultimately determine a phenotype based on the combination of different ciliopathy mutations in the patient's background (reviewed in [167]). The contribution that mutational load has on disease phenotypes will be addressed in the near future through next-generation sequencing of ciliopathy patients, the identification of the full complement of ciliopathy genes, and the generation of informative animal models.

Polycystic Kidney Disease (PKD)

PKD is one of the most common and widely studied ciliopathies. Nearly 1 in 1000 individuals are afflicted with PKD. Most forms of PKD result from mutations in three genes. Autosomal dominant PKD (ADPKD) is caused by mutations in either *PKD1* or *PKD2*, which code for the proteins PC-1 and PC-2 respectively. Autosomal recessive PKD (ARPKD) results from mutations in *PKHD1*, the gene for fibrocystin/polyductin. PC-1, PC-2, and fibrocystin/polyductin localize in the cilium, and

have been shown to be involved in the cilia mechanosory signal (see section "Renal Cilia and Mechanosensation").

Nephronophthisis (NPHP)

NPHP is an autosomal recessive cystic kidney disease associated with mutations in at least 13 loci (*NPHP1-12* and *NPHP1L*; Table 11.1 and Figure 11.11). The most frequent mutation occurs in the gene NPHP1 (20%) with mutations in the other known genes (NPHP2-NPHP12, and NPHP1L) accounting for approximately 3% of the cases.[176] In most patients (~70%), the causative mutation is still unknown.

NPHP is the leading cause of heritable end-stage renal failure (ESRF) in children and adolescents, and depending of the genetic mutation,[177] ESRF occurs in infantile, juvenile or adolescent life. All NPHP cases involve renal defects, but approximately 15% of NPHP patients also experience extra-renal phenotypes including mental retardation, retinal degeneration (characterized as SLSN; Figure 11.11), brainstem malformation, situs inversus, cerebellar vermis aplasia (JBTS, see section "Joubert Syndrome (JBTS)"), oculomotor apraxia (Cogan Syndrome), and hepatic and pancreatic fibrosis. Unlike cysts associated with PKD, renal cysts in NPHP patients are located in the corticomedullary junction of the kidney, and the kidney remains normal size or even reduced in size.[178,179]

NPHP proteins localize to the transition zone, centrosome or in some cases cell–cell junctions, where they may have scaffolding functions (reviewed extensively in [20]). Physical interactions link NPHP proteins into functional complexes[31] with several other ciliopathy diseases proteins, such as TCTN1 (Tectonic, see section "Joubert Syndrome (JBTS)"), MKS5, and B9D1 (see section "Meckel-Gruber Syndrome (MKS)"). In general, mutations in NPHP proteins do not cause ciliogenesis defects, and the phenotype in human NPHP patients is thought to be due to abnormal cilia mediated signaling or sensory function. However, stunted cilia were reported in some NPHP shRNA knockdown studies.[180] Also, in *nphp4* mutant mice there is retinal degeneration and male sterility due to photoreceptor cilia defects and loss of sperm flagella, although no cysts are evident in the kidney.[181] Mutations in either *nphp2* or *nphp3* cause more severe instances of NPHP, often associated with extra-renal developmental phenotypes (situs inversus, cardiac ventricular septal defects), and are involved in modulating Wnt signaling (see sections "Renal Cilia and Jak/STAT Signaling" and "Renal Cilia and Non-Canonical Wnt/Planar Cell Polarity (PCP) Signaling" and [139]). For a comprehensive review of NPHP the reader is referred to Wolf and Hildebrandt.[20]

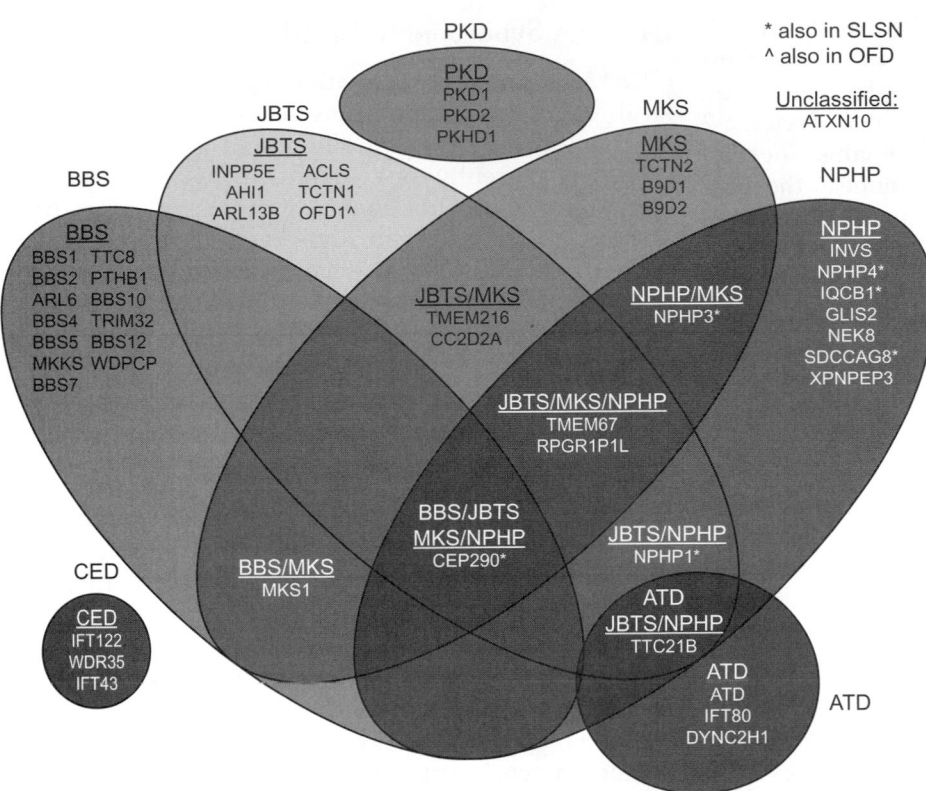

FIGURE 11.11 Overlapping genes of ciliopathies. A four-way Venn diagram showing the overlapping causative genes behind renal ciliopathies, creating a spectrum of disease phenotypes that include the kidney but may extend to other organs.

Joubert Syndrome (JBTS)

JBTS is a highly variable disorder with renal phenotypes similar to juvenile NPHP patients (i.e., as small cysts at the cortico-medullary junction and a potential delay in ESRF). Additional phenotypes include vermis hypoplasia, polydactyly, mental retardation, ataxia, retinal degeneration, hypotonia, abnormal breathing pattern, and oculomotor apraxia. The presence of distinct defects in the cerebellar vermis gives JBTS an indicative Molar Tooth Malformation (MTM) that can be clearly distinguished via MRI. There is significant overlap of genetic loci between JBTS patients and those loci associated with other ciliopathies (Table 11.1, Figure 11.11), perhaps explaining why JBTS displays such heterogeneous phenotypes. For this reason, JBTS is often categorized as Joubert Syndrome Related Disorders or JSRD.

There are currently 13 identified JBTS loci (Table 11.1), with *INPP5E* (JBTS1), *AHI1* (JBTS3), *ARL13B* (JBTS8), and *TCTN1* (JBTS13) being identified solely in JBTS. INPP5E is involved in regulating phosphatidyl inostitol signaling,[182] furthering the hypothesis that the primary cilium function as complex signaling centers. Consistent with signaling in cilia, ARL13B (JBTS8) is a Ras-family GTPase localized to the cilia that causes Shh mutant-like phenotypes and lethality when mutated in mice.[183,184] AHI1 interacts with Rab8[185] and with NPHP1,[186] demonstrating a

physical linkage between NPHP and JBTS proteins, and possibly explaining the similarity of phenotypes between the syndromes. Likewise, TCTN1 is a transmembrane protein with physical interactions to NPHP and MKS proteins.[31] *TCTN1* mutant mice also have Hh signaling defects[187] consistent with a role for JBTS proteins in cilia signaling.

Meckel–Gruber Syndrome (MKS)

MKS is a prenatal lethal ciliopathy that displays severe developmental defects, including occipital encephalocole, postaxial polydactyly, and cystic kidneys. Other common traits include CNS malformation, underdeveloped genitals, oral/facial abnormalities, and hepatic cysts. There are 10 identified MKS loci that include both cytosolic and tramsmembrane proteins (Table 11.1). A comprehensive review of MKS can be found in.[188]

Many of the known the MKS proteins share similar C2 (MKS5 and MKS6) and B9 (MKS1, B9D1, and B9D2) domains thought to mediate calcium-dependent lipid binding. In *C. elegans*, the B9/C2 domain proteins form a complex (MKS complex) at the transition zone. This complex was shown to genetically interact with several genes encoding NPHP proteins to regulate cilia formation, positioning, and cilia protein composition.[189]

Since these MKS proteins co-localize in the transition zone, it has been hypothesized that they are components of the ciliary necklace and Y-links (see section "The Transition Zone"). MKS2, MKS3, and Tectonic-2 (TCTN2) all contain transmembrane domains, suggesting they may be the anchors that connect the cilia membrane to the microtubule axoneme. This hypothesis is strengthened by data on Cep290 (MKS4) in *Chlamydomonas* showing that it localizes to the Y-links in the transition zone, and that in its absence the Y-links are disrupted.[29]

Bardet—Biedl Syndrome (BBS)

BBS is a ciliopathy with extensive pleiotropy. Phenotypes include hypertension, mental retardation, obesity, retinopathy, hypogonadism, polydactyly, anosmia, and renal malformations. Renal phenotypes of BBS vary, and can include the formation of renal cysts, urine acidification, and reduced filtration rate with difficulties concentrating urine being the most common phenotype.[190,191] Renal mass, localization of cysts, and tubule size can vary widely between BBS patients. It has been demonstrated that ESRD often occurs in BBS patients, and is a significant contributing factor towards mortality. For a comprehensive review of BBS the reader is referred to Zaghloul et al.[192]

BBS has been linked to at least 15 identified genetic loci (Table 11.1). BBS1, BBS2, BBS4, BBS5, BBS7, BBS8, and BBS9 are components of a complex called the BBSome. The BBSome has important functions in regulating cilia membrane composition, possibly as coat proteins on vesicular structures, and for the transport of specific transmembrane proteins into or out of the cilium[64,66] (see section "Ciliary Targeting and the BBSome").

Interestingly, a comparative histological analysis of the renal phenotypes between *bbs2* and *bbs4* null mice showed that although these two genes code for components of the BBSome, they produce different BBS associated renal phenotypes.[193] Differences in renal phenotypes between *bbs2* and *bbs4* mice argue that BBS proteins may have tissue specific functions that contribute to pleiotropy of the disease.[193] Other BBS proteins such as BBS6, BBS10, and BBS12 are not components of the BBSome, and are believed to have chaperone activity facilitating the formation of the BBSome complex.[194] *In vitro* analysis of BBS6, BBS10, and BBS12 knockdown cell lines suggests that these BBS proteins are essential for ciliogenesis, and that dilute urine found in BBS patients could be attributed to the inability to target V2R to the cilium.[152]

Alstrom Syndrome (ALMS)

ALMS is a rare ciliopathy highly related to BBS, with the main distinguishing feature being later onset of symptoms than typically found in BBS patients. There is currently one identified ALMS locus. The majority of mutations in *ALMS1* result in severe truncations of the protein, however the protein still appears to maintain partial function. Interestingly, mutant mouse models of *ALMS* have no cilia structural defects, yet *in vitro* knockdown studies show defects in ciliogenesis.[195]

Orofaciodigital Syndrome Type 1 (OFD1)

OFD1 is a ciliopathy affecting the development of the craniofacial region, central nervous system, and limbs, in the form of postaxial polydactyl. In a few cases of OFD1, patients presented cystic kidneys. The OFD1 protein is expressed in the metanephric mesenchyme during development,[196] and localizes to the basal body[24] where it is required for ciliogenesis.[197] Ablation of the *OFD1* gene in the kidney in mice results in renal cyst formation, and cells lining these cysts fail to form cilia.[147] The cystic phenotype in *OFD1* animals was further associated with an upregulation of the mTOR pathway (see section "Renal Cilia and Canonical Wnt Signaling"), suggesting a mechanism of cyst growth.[147]

Jeune Asphyxiating Thoracic Dystrophy (ATD)

ATD is a ciliopathy classified in the category of autosomal recessive chondrodysplasias. Commonly associated bone defects in ATD include a shortening of long bones, polydactyly, and constriction of the thoracic rib cage. Approximately 30% of documented ATD patients also display renal phenotypes consistent with the loss or dysfunction of cilia.[198] Causative genes of ATD include *IFT80*,[199] *DYNC2H1*,[200] and *TTC21B* (*IFT139*).[201] Importantly, ATD represents one of the first human ciliopathies with identified mutations in IFT genes. These mutations are largely hypomorphic, thus potentially explaining the phenotypic variability found in ATD patients. The identity of genes mutated in ATD suggests that ATD is related to defects in retrograde IFT. Evidence that mutations in *TTC21B* and *DYNC2H1* cause defects in Hh signaling, possibly related to the inability to translocate Hh components (see section "Renal Cilia and Hedgehog Signaling") from the cilia,[57,199,202] are consistent with this hypothesis. Recently, an ATD patient with a *TTC21B* mutation and associated NPHP was uncovered.[201] This study demonstrated genetic interactions between *TTC21B* and other ciliopathy genes, and further extends the hypothesis of the oligogenic nature of ciliopathies.

Sensenbrenner Syndrome (Cranionectodermal Dysplasia, CED)

CED is a ciliopathy highly related to ATD, with craniosynostosis being the distinguishing feature in CED.[202] Patients may also develop renal phenotypes similar to NPHP. As with ATD, CED represents a ciliopathy with mutations in IFT genes. All currently known CED loci are IFT-A components: *IFT43*,[203] *IFT122*,[204] and *WDR35 (TULP4/IFT121)*,[202] and are likely hypomorphic mutations. At the cellular level, CED appears to be correlated with Shh signaling (see section "Renal Cilia and Hedgehog Signaling") defects that arise from improper IFT[203,204] similar to ATD.

CONCLUDING REMARKS

The primary cilium is an evolutionarily conserved organelle, in terms of structure and its capacity to act as a complex signaling and sensory center for the cell. In the past 15–20 years, there have been remarkable advances in our understanding of the role of primary cilium in signaling and development. This is due, in large part, to the multiple model systems available to study the relationship between cilia structure and function. Importantly, since the initial publication of the *orpk* mouse model, the kidney has remained at the forefront of cilia related research. Much of our understanding of cilia biology is due to the use of renal cystic disease models that clearly demonstrate the developmental consequences of cilia dysfunction. Current advances in sequencing, proteomics, microscopy, and molecular genetics will only serve to further our understanding of cilia biology in the kidney and beyond.

References

[1] Dobell C, Leeuwenhoek Av. Antony van Leeuwenhoek and his "Little animals;" being some account of the father of protozoology & bacteriology and his multifarious discoveries in these disciplines. New York: Russell & Russell; 1958.

[2] Kartagener M. Zur pathogenese der Bronchiectasien. I Mitteilung: Bronchiectasien bei situs viscerum inversus. Betr Klin Tuberk 1933;83:498–501.

[3] Siewert A. Uber einem fall von Bronchiectasie bei einem patienten mit situs inversusviscerum. Berliner klinische Wochenschrift 1904;41:139–41.

[4] Moyer JH, Lee-Tischler MJ, Kwon HY, Schrick JJ, Avner ED, Sweeney WE, et al. Candidate gene associated with a mutation causing recessive polycystic kidney disease in mice. Science 1994;264(5163):1329–33.

[5] Lehman JM, Michaud EJ, Schoeb TR, Aydin-Son Y, Miller M, Yoder BK. The oak ridge polycystic Kidney mouse: modeling ciliopathies of mice and men. Dev Dyn 2008;237(8):1960–71.

[6] Murcia NS, Richards WG, Yoder BK, Mucenski ML, Dunlap JR, Woychik RP. The oak ridge polycystic Kidney (orpk) disease gene is required for left–right axis determination. Development 2000;127(11):2347–55.

[7] Taulman PD, Haycraft CJ, Balkovetz DF, Yoder BK. Polaris, a protein involved in left–right axis patterning, localizes to basal bodies and cilia. Mol Biol Cell 2001;12(3):589–99.

[8] Yoder BK, Tousson A, Millican L, Wu JH, Bugg Jr. CE, Schafer JA, et al. Polaris, a protein disrupted in orpk mutant mice, is required for assembly of renal cilium. Am J Physiol Renal Physiol 2002;282(3):F541–552.

[9] Cole DG, Diener DR, Himelblau AL, Beech PL, Fuster JC, Rosenbaum JL. *Chlamydomonas* kinesin-II-dependent intraflagellar transport (IFT): IFT particles contain proteins required for ciliary assembly in *Caenorhabditis elegans* sensory neurons. J Cell Biol 1998;141(4):993–1008.

[10] Pazour GJ, Dickert BL, Vucica Y, Seeley ES, Rosenbaum JL, Witman GB, et al. *Chlamydomonas* IFT88 and its mouse homologue, polycystic kidney disease gene tg737, are required for assembly of cilia and flagella. J Cell Biol 2000;151(3): 709–18.

[11] Kozminski KG, Johnson KA, Forscher P, Rosenbaum JL. A motility in the eukaryotic flagellum unrelated to flagellar beating. Proc Natl Acad Sci USA 1993;90(12):5519–23.

[12] Haycraft CJ, Swoboda P, Taulman PD, Thomas JH, Yoder BK. The *C. elegans* homolog of the murine cystic kidney disease gene Tg737 functions in a ciliogenic pathway and is disrupted in osm-5 mutant worms. Development 2001;128(9):1493–505.

[13] Barr MM, Sternberg PW. A polycystic kidney-disease gene homologue required for male mating behaviour in *C. elegans*. Nature 1999;401(6751):386–9.

[14] Barr MM, DeModena J, Braun D, Nguyen CQ, Hall DH, Sternberg PW. The *Caenorhabditis elegans* autosomal dominant polycystic kidney disease gene homologs lov-1 and pkd-2 act in the same pathway. Curr Biol 2001;11(17):1341–6.

[15] Pazour GJ, San Agustin JT, Follit JA, Rosenbaum JL, Witman GB. Polycystin-2 localizes to kidney cilia and the ciliary level is elevated in orpk mice with polycystic kidney disease. Curr Biol 2002;12(11):R378–380.

[16] Yoder BK, Hou X, Guay-Woodford LM. The polycystic kidney disease proteins, polycystin-1, polycystin-2, polaris, and cystin, are co-localized in renal cilia. J Am Soc Nephrol 2002;13(10): 2508–16.

[17] Badano JL, Mitsuma N, Beales PL, Katsanis N. The ciliopathies: an emerging class of human genetic disorders. Annu Rev Genomics Hum Genet 2006;7:125–48.

[18] Brancati F, Dallapiccola B, Valente EM. Joubert syndrome and related disorders. Orphanet J Rare Dis 2010;5:20.

[19] Sharma N, Berbari NF, Yoder BK. Ciliary dysfunction in developmental abnormalities and diseases. Curr Top Dev Biol 2008;85:371–427.

[20] Wolf MT, Hildebrandt F. Nephronophthisis. Pediatr Nephrol Feb 2011;26(2):181–94.

[21] Graser S, Stierhof YD, Lavoie SB, Gassner OS, Lamla S, Le Clech M, et al. Cep164, a novel centriole appendage protein required for primary cilium formation. J Cell Biol 2007;179(2): 321–30.

[22] Ishikawa H, Kubo A, Tsukita S. Odf2-deficient mother centrioles lack distal/subdistal appendages and the ability to generate primary cilia. Nat Cell Biol 2005;7(5):517–24.

[23] Anderson RG. The three-dimensional structure of the basal body from the rhesus monkey oviduct. J Cell Biol. 1972;54(2): 246–65.

[24] Lopes CA, Prosser SL, Romio L, Hirst RA, O'Callaghan C, Woolf AS, et al. Centriolar satellites are assembly points for proteins implicated in human ciliopathies, including oral-facial-digital syndrome 1. J Cell Sci. 2011;124(Pt 4):600—12.

[25] Sui H, Downing KH. Molecular architecture of axonemal microtubule doublets revealed by cryo-electron tomography. Nature 2006;442(7101):475—8.

[26] Sanchez T, Welch D, Nicastro D, Dogic Z. Cilia-like beating of active microtubule bundles. Science 2011;333(6041):456—9.

[27] Andrews PM, Porter KR. A scanning electron microscopic study of the nephron. Am J Anat 1974;140(1):81—115.

[28] Gilula NB, Satir P. The ciliary necklace. A ciliary membrane specialization. J Cell Biol 1972;53(2):494—509.

[29] Craige B, Tsao CC, Diener DR, Hou Y, Lechtreck KF, Rosenbaum JL, et al. CEP290 tethers flagellar transition zone microtubules to the membrane and regulates flagellar protein content. J Cell Biol 2010;190(5):927—40.

[30] Lechtreck KF, Teltenkotter A, Grunow A. A 210 kDa protein is located in a membrane-microtubule linker at the distal end of mature and nascent basal bodies. J Cell Sci 1999;112(Pt 11):1633—44.

[31] Sang L, Miller JJ, Corbit KC, Giles RH, Brauer MJ, Otto EA, et al. Mapping the NPHP-JBTS-MKS protein network reveals ciliopathy disease genes and pathways. Cell 2011;145(4):513—28.

[32] Williams CL, Li C, Kida K, Inglis PN, Mohan S, Semenec L, et al. MKS and NPHP modules cooperate to establish basal body/transition zone membrane associations and ciliary gate function during ciliogenesis. J Cell Biol 2011;192(6):1023—41.

[33] Satir P, Christensen ST. Overview of structure and function of mammalian cilia. Annu Rev Physiol 2007;69:377—400.

[34] Deane JA, Cole DG, Seeley ES, Diener DR, Rosenbaum JL. Localization of intraflagellar transport protein IFT52 identifies basal body transitional fibers as the docking site for IFT particles. Curr Biol 2001;11(20):1586—90.

[35] Janich P, Corbeil D. GM1 and GM3 gangliosides highlight distinct lipid microdomains within the apical domain of epithelial cells. FEBS Lett 2007;581(9):1783—7.

[36] Vieira OV, Gaus K, Verkade P, Fullekrug J, Vaz WL, Simons K. FAPP2, cilium formation, and compartmentalization of the apical membrane in polarized Madin—Darby canine kidney (MDCK) cells. Proc Natl Acad Sci USA 2006;103(49):18556—61.

[37] Montesano R. Inhomogeneous distribution of filipin-sterol complexes in the ciliary membrane of rat tracheal epithelium. Am J Anat. 1979;156(1):139—45.

[38] Tao B, Bu S, Yang Z, Siroky B, Kappes JC, Kispert A, et al. Cystin localizes to primary cilia via membrane microdomains and a targeting motif. J Am Soc Nephrol 2009;20(12):2570—80.

[39] Li JB, Gerdes JM, Haycraft CJ, Fan Y, Teslovich TM, May-Simera H, et al. Comparative genomics identifies a flagellar and basal body proteome that includes the BBS5 human disease gene. Cell 2004;117(4):541—52.

[40] Pazour GJ, Agrin N, Leszyk J, Witman GB. Proteomic analysis of a eukaryotic cilium. J Cell Biol 2005;170(1):103—13.

[41] Valente EM, Logan CV, Mougou-Zerelli S, Lee JH, Silhavy JL, Brancati F, et al. Mutations in TMEM216 perturb ciliogenesis and cause Joubert, Meckel and related syndromes. Nat Genet 2010;42(7):619—25.

[42] Smith UM, Consugar M, Tee LJ, McKee BM, Maina EN, Whelan S, et al. The transmembrane protein meckelin (MKS3) is mutated in Meckel—Gruber syndrome and the wpk rat. Nat Genet 2006;38(2):191—6.

[43] Lim YS, Chua CE, Tang BL. Rabs and other small GTPases in ciliary transport. Biol Cell 2011;103(5):209—21.

[44] Ishikawa H, Marshall WF. Ciliogenesis: building the cell's antenna. Nat Rev Mol Cell Biol. 2011;12(4):222—34.

[45] Silverman MA, Leroux MR. Intraflagellar transport and the generation of dynamic, structurally and functionally diverse cilia. Trends Cell Biol 2009;19(7):306—16.

[46] Follit JA, Tuft RA, Fogarty KE, Pazour GJ. The intraflagellar transport protein IFT20 is associated with the Golgi complex and is required for cilia assembly. Mol Biol Cell. 2006;17(9):3781—92.

[47] Qin H, Wang Z, Diener D, Rosenbaum J. Intraflagellar transport protein 27 is a small G protein involved in cell-cycle control. Curr Biol 2007;17(3):193—202.

[48] Schafer JC, Winkelbauer ME, Williams CL, Haycraft CJ, Desmond RA, Yoder BK. IFTA-2 is a conserved cilia protein involved in pathways regulating longevity and dauer formation in Caenorhabditis elegans. J Cell Sci 2006;119(Pt 19):4088—100.

[49] Ou G, Blacque OE, Snow JJ, Leroux MR, Scholey JM. Functional coordination of intraflagellar transport motors. Nature 2005;436(7050):583—7.

[50] Pan X, Ou G, Civelekoglu-Scholey G, Blacque OE, Endres NF, Tao L, et al. Mechanism of transport of IFT particles in C. elegans cilia by the concerted action of kinesin-II and OSM-3 motors. J Cell Biol 2006;174(7):1035—45.

[51] Snow JJ, Ou G, Gunnarson AL, Walker MR, Zhou HM, Brust-Mascher I, et al. Two anterograde intraflagellar transport motors cooperate to build sensory cilia on C. elegans neurons. Nat Cell Biol. 2004;6(11):1109—13.

[52] Pazour GJ, Wilkerson CG, Witman GB. A dynein light chain is essential for the retrograde particle movement of intraflagellar transport (IFT). J Cell Biol 1998;141(4):979—92.

[53] Kozminski KG, Beech PL, Rosenbaum JL. The Chlamydomonas kinesin-like protein FLA10 is involved in motility associated with the flagellar membrane. J Cell Biol 1995;131(6 Pt 1):1517—27.

[54] Lin F, Hiesberger T, Cordes K, Sinclair AM, Goldstein LS, Somlo S, et al. Kidney-specific inactivation of the KIF3A subunit of kinesin-II inhibits renal ciliogenesis and produces polycystic kidney disease. Proc Natl Acad Sci USA 2003;100(9):5286—91.

[55] Pazour GJ, Dickert BL, Witman GB. The DHC1b (DHC2) isoform of cytoplasmic dynein is required for flagellar assembly. J Cell Biol 1999;144(3):473—81.

[56] Schafer JC, Haycraft CJ, Thomas JH, Yoder BK, Swoboda P. XBX-1 encodes a dynein light intermediate chain required for retrograde intraflagellar transport and cilia assembly in Caenorhabditis elegans. Mol Biol Cell 2003;14(5):2057—70.

[57] Tran PV, Haycraft CJ, Besschetnova TY, Turbe-Doan A, Stottmann RW, Herron BJ, et al. THM1 negatively modulates mouse sonic hedgehog signal transduction and affects retrograde intraflagellar transport in cilia. Nat Genet 2008;40(4):403—10.

[58] Hurd TW, Fan S, Margolis BL. Localization of retinitis pigmentosa 2 to cilia is regulated by Importin beta2. J Cell Sci 2011;124(Pt 5):718—26.

[59] Dishinger JF, Kee HL, Jenkins PM, Fan S, Hurd TW, Hammond JW, et al. Ciliary entry of the kinesin-2 motor KIF17 is regulated by importin-beta2 and RanGTP. Nat Cell Biol 2010;12(7):703—10.

[60] Berbari NF, Johnson AD, Lewis JS, Askwith CC, Mykytyn K. Identification of ciliary localization sequences within the third intracellular loop of G protein-coupled receptors. Mol Biol Cell. 2008;19(4):1540—7.

[61] Hu Q, Milenkovic L, Jin H, Scott MP, Nachury MV, Spiliotis ET, et al. A septin diffusion barrier at the base of the primary

cilium maintains ciliary membrane protein distribution. Science 2010;329(5990):436—9.

[62] Francis SS, Sfakianos J, Lo B, Mellman I. A hierarchy of signals regulates entry of membrane proteins into the ciliary membrane domain in epithelial cells. J Cell Biol 2011;193(1): 219—33.

[63] Domire JS, Green JA, Lee KG, Johnson AD, Askwith CC, Mykytyn K. Dopamine receptor 1 localizes to neuronal cilia in a dynamic process that requires the Bardet—Biedl syndrome proteins. Cell Mol Life Sci 2011;68(17):2951—60.

[64] Jin H, White SR, Shida T, Schulz S, Aguiar M, Gygi SP, et al. The conserved Bardet—Biedl syndrome proteins assemble a coat that traffics membrane proteins to cilia. Cell 2010;141(7): 1208—19.

[65] Emmer BT, Maric D, Engman DM. Molecular mechanisms of protein and lipid targeting to ciliary membranes. J Cell Sci 2010;123(Pt 4):529—36.

[66] Nachury MV, Loktev AV, Zhang Q, Westlake CJ, Peranen J, Merdes A, et al. A core complex of BBS proteins cooperates with the GTPase Rab8 to promote ciliary membrane biogenesis. Cell 2007;129(6):1201—13.

[67] Knodler A, Feng S, Zhang J, Zhang X, Das A, Peranen J, et al. Coordination of Rab8 and Rab11 in primary ciliogenesis. Proc Natl Acad Sci USA 2010;107(14):6346—51.

[68] Westlake CJ, Baye LM, Nachury MV, Wright KJ, Ervin KE, Phu L, et al. Primary cilia membrane assembly is initiated by Rab11 and transport protein particle II (TRAPPII) complex-dependent trafficking of Rabin8 to the centrosome. Proc Natl Acad Sci USA 2011;108(7):2759—64.

[69] Poole CA, Flint MH, Beaumont BW. Analysis of the morphology and function of primary cilia in connective tissues: a cellular cybernetic probe? Cell Motil 1985;5(3):175—93.

[70] Reese TS. Olfactory cilia in the frog. J Cell Biol 1965;25(2): 209—30.

[71] Baldari CT, Rosenbaum J. Intraflagellar transport: It's not just for cilia anymore. Curr Opin Cell Biol 2010;22(1):75—80.

[72] Perrone CA, Tritschler D, Taulman P, Bower R, Yoder BK, Porter ME. A novel dynein light intermediate chain colocalizes with the retrograde motor for intraflagellar transport at sites of axoneme assembly in chlamydomonas and mammalian cells. Mol Biol Cell 2003;14(5):2041—56.

[73] Milenkovic L, Scott MP, Rohatgi R. Lateral transport of Smoothened from the plasma membrane to the membrane of the cilium. J Cell Biol 2009;187(3):365—74.

[74] Berbari NF, O'Connor AK, Haycraft CJ, Yoder BK. The primary cilium as a complex signaling center. Curr Biol 2009;19(13): R526—535.

[75] Quarmby LM, Parker JD. Cilia and the cell cycle? J Cell Biol 2005;169(5):707—10.

[76] Jain R, Pan J, Driscoll JA, Wisner JW, Huang T, Gunsten SP, et al. Temporal relationship between primary and motile ciliogenesis in airway epithelial cells. Am J Respir Cell Mol Biol 2010;43(6): 731—9.

[77] Lefebvre PA, Silflow CD, Wieben ED, Rosenbaum JL. Increased levels of mRNAs for tubulin and other flagellar proteins after amputation or shortening of Chlamydomonas flagella. Cell 1980;20(2):469—77.

[78] Remillard SP, Witman GB. Synthesis, transport, and utilization of specific flagellar proteins during flagellar regeneration in Chlamydomonas. J Cell Biol 1982;93(3):615—31.

[79] Stolc V, Samanta MP, Tongprasit W, Marshall WF. Genome-wide transcriptional analysis of flagellar regeneration in Chlamydomonas reinhardtii identifies orthologs of ciliary disease genes. Proc Natl Acad Sci USA 2005;102(10):3703—7.

[80] Efimenko E, Bubb K, Mak HY, Holzman T, Leroux MR, Ruvkun G, et al. Analysis of xbx genes in C. elegans. Development 2005;132(8):1923—34.

[81] Swoboda P, Adler HT, Thomas JH. The RFX-type transcription factor DAF-19 regulates sensory neuron cilium formation in C. elegans. Mol Cell. 2000;5(3):411—21.

[82] Winkelbauer ME, Schafer JC, Haycraft CJ, Swoboda P, Yoder BK. The C. elegans homologs of nephrocystin-1 and nephrocystin-4 are cilia transition zone proteins involved in chemosensory perception. J Cell Sci 2005;118(Pt 23):5575—87.

[83] Thomas J, Morle L, Soulavie F, Laurencon A, Sagnol S, Durand B. Transcriptional control of genes involved in ciliogenesis: a first step in making cilia. Biol Cell 2010;102(9):499—513.

[84] Michaud EJ, Yoder BK. The primary cilium in cell signaling and cancer. Cancer Res. 2006;66(13):6463—7.

[85] Kobayashi T, Dynlacht BD. Regulating the transition from centriole to basal body. J Cell Biol 2011;193(3):435—44.

[86] Seeley ES, Carriere C, Goetze T, Longnecker DS, Korc M. Pancreatic cancer and precursor pancreatic intraepithelial neoplasia lesions are devoid of primary cilia. Cancer Res 2009;69(2): 422—30.

[87] Wong SY, Seol AD, So PL, Ermilov AN, Bichakjian CK, Epstein Jr. EH, et al. Primary cilia can both mediate and suppress Hedgehog pathway-dependent tumorigenesis. Nat Med 2009;15(9):1055—61.

[88] Rasi MQ, Parker JD, Feldman JL, Marshall WF, Quarmby LM. Katanin knockdown supports a role for microtubule severing in release of basal bodies before mitosis in Chlamydomonas. Mol Biol Cell 2009;20(1):379—88.

[89] Mahjoub MR, Qasim Rasi M, Quarmby LMA. NIMA-related kinase, Fa2p, localizes to a novel site in the proximal cilia of Chlamydomonas and mouse kidney cells. Mol Biol Cell 2004; 15(11):5172—86.

[90] Pugacheva EN, Jablonski SA, Hartman TR, Henske EP, Golemis EA. HEF1-dependent Aurora A activation induces disassembly of the primary cilium. Cell 2007;129(7):1351—63.

[91] Sorokin S. Centrioles and the formation of rudimentary cilia by fibroblasts and smooth muscle cells. J Cell Biol 1962;15:363—77.

[92] Ghossoub R, Molla-Herman A, Bastin P, Benmerah A. The ciliary pocket: a once-forgotten membrane domain at the base of cilia. Biol Cell 2011;103(3):131—44.

[93] Molla-Herman A, Ghossoub R, Blisnick T, Meunier A, Serres C, Silbermann F, et al. The ciliary pocket: an endocytic membrane domain at the base of primary and motile cilia. J Cell Sci 2010;123(Pt 10):1785—95.

[94] Bonnet CS, Aldred M, von Ruhland C, Harris R, Sandford R, Cheadle JP. Defects in cell polarity underlie TSC and ADPKD-associated cystogenesis. Hum Mol Genet 2009;18(12):2166—76.

[95] DiBella LM, Park A, Sun Z. Zebrafish Tsc1 reveals functional interactions between the cilium and the TOR pathway. Hum Mol Genet 2009;18(4):595—606.

[96] Smith LA, Bukanov NO, Husson H, Russo RJ, Barry TC, Taylor AL, et al. Development of polycystic kidney disease in juvenile cystic kidney mice: insights into pathogenesis, ciliary abnormalities, and common features with human disease. J Am Soc Nephrol 2006;17(10):2821—31.

[97] Tammachote R, Hommerding CJ, Sinders RM, Miller CA, Czarnecki PG, Leightner AC, et al. Ciliary and centrosomal defects associated with mutation and depletion of the Meckel syndrome genes MKS1 and MKS3. Hum Mol Genet 2009;18(17): 3311—23.

[98] Tam LW, Wilson NF, Lefebvre PAA. CDK-related kinase regulates the length and assembly of flagella in Chlamydomonas. J Cell Biol 2007;176(6):819—29.

[99] Berman SA, Wilson NF, Haas NA, Lefebvre PA. A novel MAP kinase regulates flagellar length in *Chlamydomonas*. Curr Biol 2003;13(13):1145–9.

[100] Besschetnova TY, Kolpakova-Hart E, Guan Y, Zhou J, Olsen BR, Shah JV. Identification of signaling pathways regulating primary cilium length and flow-mediated adaptation. Curr Biol 2010;20(2):182–7.

[101] Sharma N, Kosan ZA, Stallworth JE, Berbari NF, Yoder BK. Soluble levels of cytosolic tubulin regulate ciliary length control. Mol Biol Cell 2011;22(6):806–16.

[102] Nauli SM, Alenghat FJ, Luo Y, Williams E, Vassilev P, Li X, et al. Polycystins 1 and 2 mediate mechanosensation in the primary cilium of kidney cells. Nat Genet 2003;33(2):129–37.

[103] Verghese E, Ricardo SD, Weidenfeld R, Zhuang J, Hill PA, Langham RG, et al. Renal primary cilia lengthen after acute tubular necrosis. J Am Soc Nephrol 2009;20(10):2147–53.

[104] Verghese E, Weidenfeld R, Bertram JF, Ricardo SD, Deane JA. Renal cilia display length alterations following tubular injury and are present early in epithelial repair. Nephrol Dial Transplant 2008;23(3):834–41.

[105] Patel V, Li L, Cobo-Stark P, Shao X, Somlo S, Lin F, et al. Acute kidney injury and aberrant planar cell polarity induce cyst formation in mice lacking renal cilia. Hum Mol Genet 2008;17(11):1578–90.

[106] Takakura A, Contrino L, Zhou X, Bonventre JV, Sun Y, Humphreys BD, et al. Renal injury is a third hit promoting rapid development of adult polycystic kidney disease. Hum Mol Genet 2009;18(14):2523–31.

[107] Kim J, Lee JE, Heynen-Genel S, Suyama E, Ono K, Lee K, et al. Functional genomic screen for modulators of ciliogenesis and cilium length. Nature 2010;464(7291):1048–51.

[108] Berbari NF, Lewis JS, Bishop GA, Askwith CC, Mykytyn K. Bardet–Biedl syndrome proteins are required for the localization of G protein-coupled receptors to primary cilia. Proc Natl Acad Sci USA 2008;105(11):4242–6.

[109] Raychowdhury MK, Ramos AJ, Zhang P, McLaughin M, Dai XQ, Chen XZ, et al. Vasopressin receptor-mediated functional signaling pathway in primary cilia of renal epithelial cells. Am J Physiol Renal Physiol 2009;296(1):F87–97.

[110] Wang X, Wu Y, Ward CJ, Harris PC, Torres VE. Vasopressin directly regulates cyst growth in polycystic kidney disease. J Am Soc Nephrol 2008;19(1):102–8.

[111] Praetorius HA, Frokiaer J, Nielsen S, Spring KR. Bending the primary cilium opens Ca^{2+}-sensitive intermediate-conductance K$^+$ channels in MDCK cells. J Membr Biol 2003;191(3):193–200.

[112] Praetorius HA, Spring KR. Removal of the MDCK cell primary cilium abolishes flow sensing. J Membr Biol 2003;191(1):69–76.

[113] Praetorius HA, Spring KR. The renal cell primary cilium functions as a flow sensor. Curr Opin Nephrol Hypertens 2003;12(5):517–20.

[114] Liu W. Mechanoregulation of intracellular Ca^{2+} concentration is attenuated in collecting duct of monocilium-impaired orpk mice. Am J Physiol Renal Physiol 2005;289(5):F978–988.

[115] Davenport JR, Watts AJ, Roper VC, Croyle MJ, van Groen T, Wyss JM, et al. Disruption of intraflagellar transport in adult mice leads to obesity and slow-onset cystic kidney disease. Curr Biol 2007;17(18):1586–94.

[116] Lantinga-van Leeuwen IS, Leonhard WN, van der Wal A, Breuning MH, de Heer E, Peters DJ. Kidney-specific inactivation of the Pkd1 gene induces rapid cyst formation in developing kidneys and a slow onset of disease in adult mice. Hum Mol Genet 2007;16(24):3188–96.

[117] Piontek K, Menezes LF, Garcia-Gonzalez MA, Huso DL, Germino GG. A critical developmental switch defines the

[118] Talbot JJ, Shillingford JM, Vasanth S, Doerr N, Mukherjee S, Kinter MT, et al. Polycystin-1 regulates STAT activity by a dual mechanism. Proc Natl Acad Sci USA 2011;108(19):7985–90.

[119] Chauvet V, Tian X, Husson H, Grimm DH, Wang T, Hiesberger T, et al. Mechanical stimuli induce cleavage and nuclear translocation of the polycystin-1 C terminus. J Clin Invest 2004;114(10):1433–43.

[120] Low SH, Vasanth S, Larson CH, Mukherjee S, Sharma N, Kinter MT, et al. STAT6, and P100 function in a pathway that transduces ciliary mechanosensation and is activated in polycystic kidney disease. Dev Cell 2006;10(1):57–69.

[121] Gardner Jr. KD, Burnside JS, Elzinga LW, Locksley RM. Cytokines in fluids from polycystic kidneys. Kidney Int 1991;39(4):718–24.

[122] Mrug M, Zhou J, Woo Y, Cui X, Szalai AJ, Novak J, et al. Overexpression of innate immune response genes in a model of recessive polycystic kidney disease. Kidney Int 2008;73(1):63–76.

[123] Karihaloo A, Koraishy F, Huen SC, Lee Y, Merrick D, Caplan MJ, et al. Macrophages promote cyst growth in polycystic kidney disease. J Am Soc Nephrol 2011;22(10):1809–14.

[124] Lee S, Huen S, Nishio H, Nishio S, Lee HK, Choi BS, et al. Distinct macrophage phenotypes contribute to kidney injury and repair. J Am Soc Nephrol 2011;22(2):317–26.

[125] Zhou J, Ouyang X, Cui X, Schoeb TR, Smythies LE, Johnson MR, et al. Renal CD14 expression correlates with the progression of cystic kidney disease. Kidney Int 2010;78(6):550–60.

[126] Ross AJ, May-Simera H, Eichers ER, Kai M, Hill J. Disruption of Bardet–Biedl syndrome ciliary proteins perturbs planar cell polarity in vertebrates. Nat Genet 2005;37(10):1135–40.

[127] Jones C, Roper VC, Foucher I, Qian D, Banizs B, Petit C, et al. Ciliary proteins link basal body polarization to planar cell polarity regulation. Nat Genet 2008;40(1):69–77.

[128] Karner CM, Chirumamilla R, Aoki S, Igarashi P, Wallingford JB, Carroll TJ. Wnt9b signaling regulates planar cell polarity and kidney tubule morphogenesis. Nat Genet 2009;41(7):793–9.

[129] Fischer E, Legue E, Doyen A, Nato F, Nicolas JF, Torres V, et al. Defective planar cell polarity in polycystic kidney disease. Nat Genet 2006;38(1):21–3.

[130] Delaval B, Bright A, Lawson ND, Doxsey S. The cilia protein IFT88 is required for spindle orientation in mitosis. Nat Cell Biol 2011;13(4):461–8.

[131] Jonassen JA, San Agustin J, Follit JA, Pazour GJ. Deletion of IFT20 in the mouse kidney causes misorientation of the mitotic spindle and cystic kidney disease. J Cell Biol 2008;183(3):377–84.

[132] Rawls AS, Guinto JB, Wolff T. The cadherins fat and dachsous regulate dorsal/ventral signaling in the *Drosophila* eye. Curr Biol 2002;12(12):1021–6.

[133] Saburi S, Hester I, Fischer E, Pontoglio M, Eremina V, Gessler M, et al. Loss of Fat4 disrupts PCP signaling and oriented cell division and leads to cystic kidney disease. Nat Genet 2008;40(8):1010–5.

[134] Yang CH, Axelrod JD, Simon MA. Regulation of Frizzled by fat-like cadherins during planar polarity signaling in the *Drosophila* compound eye. Cell 2002;108(5):675–88.

[135] Happe H, Leonhard WN, van der Wal A, van de Water B, Lantinga-van Leeuwen IS, Breuning MH, et al. Toxic tubular injury in kidneys from Pkd1-deletion mice accelerates cystogenesis accompanied by dysregulated planar cell polarity

and canonical Wnt signaling pathways. Hum Mol Genet 2009;18(14):2532—42.

[136] Verdeguer F, Le Corre S, Fischer E, Callens C, Garbay S, Doyen A, et al. A mitotic transcriptional switch in polycystic kidney disease. Nat Med 2010;16(1):106—10.

[137] Nishio S, Tian X, Gallagher AR, Yu Z, Patel V, Igarashi P, et al. Loss of oriented cell division does not initiate cyst formation. J Am Soc Nephrol 2010;21(2):295—302.

[138] Otto EA, Schermer B, Obara T, O'Toole JF, Hiller KS, Mueller AM, et al. Mutations in INVS encoding inversin cause nephronophthisis type 2, linking renal cystic disease to the function of primary cilia and left—right axis determination. Nat Genet 2003;34(4):413—20.

[139] Simons M, Gloy J, Ganner A, Bullerkotte A, Bashkurov M, Kronig C, et al. Inversin, the gene product mutated in nephronophthisis type II, functions as a molecular switch between Wnt signaling pathways. Nat Genet 2005;37(5): 537—43.

[140] Wiens CJ, Tong Y, Esmail MA, Oh E, Gerdes JM, Wang J, et al. Bardet—Biedl syndrome-associated small GTPase ARL6 (BBS3) functions at or near the ciliary gate and modulates Wnt signaling. J Biol Chem 2010;285(21):16218—30.

[141] Corbit KC, Shyer AE, Dowdle WE, Gaulden J, Singla V, Chen MH, et al. Kif3a constrains beta-catenin-dependent Wnt signalling through dual ciliary and non-ciliary mechanisms. Nat Cell Biol 2008;10(1):70—6.

[142] Lancaster MA, Gopal DJ, Kim J, Saleem SN, Silhavy JL, Louie CM, et al. Defective Wnt-dependent cerebellar midline fusion in a mouse model of Joubert syndrome. Nat Med 2011;17(6): 726—31.

[143] Sugiyama N, Tsukiyama T, Yamaguchi TP, Yokoyama T. The canonical Wnt signaling pathway is not involved in renal cyst development in the kidneys of inv mutant mice. Kidney Int 2011;79(9):957—65.

[144] Ocbina PJ, Tuson M, Anderson KV. Primary cilia are not required for normal canonical Wnt signaling in the mouse embryo. PLoS One 2009;4(8):e6839.

[145] Bell PD, Fitzgibbon W, Sas K, Stenbit AE, Amria M, Houston A, et al. Loss of primary cilia upregulates renal hypertrophic signaling and promotes cystogenesis. J Am Soc Nephrol 2011;22(5):839—48.

[146] Boehlke C, Kotsis F, Patel V, Braeg S, Voelker H, Bredt S, et al. Primary cilia regulate mTORC1 activity and cell size through Lkb1. Nat Cell Biol 2010;12(11):1115—22.

[147] Zullo A, Iaconis D, Barra A, Cantone A, Messaddeq N, Capasso G, et al. Kidney-specific inactivation of Ofd1 leads to renal cystic disease associated with upregulation of the mTOR pathway. Hum Mol Genet 2010;19(14):2792—803.

[148] Dere R, Wilson PD, Sandford RN, Walker CL. Carboxy terminal tail of polycystin-1 regulates localization of TSC2 to repress mTOR. PLoS One 2010;5(2):e9239.

[149] Huber TB, Walz G, Kuehn EW. mTOR and rapamycin in the kidney: signaling and therapeutic implications beyond immunosuppression. Kidney Int 2011;79(5):502—11.

[150] Shillingford JM, Piontek KB, Germino GG, Weimbs T. Rapamycin ameliorates PKD resulting from conditional inactivation of Pkd1. J Am Soc Nephrol 2010;21(3):489—97.

[151] Nishimoto G, Zelenina M, Li D, Yasui M, Aperia A, Nielsen S, et al. Arginine vasopressin stimulates phosphorylation of aquaporin-2 in rat renal tissue. Am J Physiol 1999;276(2 Pt 2): F254—259.

[152] Marion V, Schlicht D, Mockel A, Caillard S, Imhoff O, Stoetzel C, et al. Bardet—Biedl syndrome highlights the major role of the primary cilium in efficient water reabsorption. Kidney Int 2011;79(9):1013—25.

[153] Calvet JP. Strategies to inhibit cyst formation in ADPKD. Clin J Am Soc Nephrol 2008;3(4):1205—11.

[154] Chen NX, Moe SM, Eggleston-Gulyas T, Chen X, Hoffmeyer WD, Bacallao RL, et al. Calcimimetics inhibit renal pathology in rodent nephronophthisis. Kidney Int 2011;80(6):612—9.

[155] Torres VE. Role of vasopressin antagonists. Clin J Am Soc Nephrol 2008;3(4):1212—8.

[156] Patel V, Chowdhury R, Igarashi P. Advances in the pathogenesis and treatment of polycystic kidney disease. Curr Opin Nephrol Hypertens 2009;18(2):99—106.

[157] Ingham PW, Nakano Y, Seger C. Mechanisms and functions of Hedgehog signalling across the metazoa. Nat Rev Genet 2011;12(6):393—406.

[158] Corbit KC, Aanstad P, Singla V, Norman AR, Stainier DY, Reiter JF. Vertebrate smoothened functions at the primary cilium. Nature 2005;437(7061):1018—21.

[159] Haycraft CJ, Banizs B, Aydin-Son Y, Zhang Q, Michaud EJ, Yoder BK. Gli2 and Gli3 localize to cilia and require the intraflagellar transport protein polaris for processing and function. PLoS Genet 2005;1(4):e53.

[160] Huangfu D, Anderson KV. Cilia and Hedgehog responsiveness in the mouse. Proc Natl Acad Sci USA 2005;102(32): 11325—30.

[161] Yu J, Carroll TJ, McMahon AP. Sonic hedgehog regulates proliferation and differentiation of mesenchymal cells in the mouse metanephric kidney. Development 2002;129(22): 5301—12.

[162] Hu MC, Mo R, Bhella S, Wilson CW, Chuang PT, Hui CC, et al. GLI3-dependent transcriptional repression of Gli1, Gli2 and kidney patterning genes disrupts renal morphogenesis. Development 2006;133(3):569—78.

[163] Cain JE, Islam E, Haxho F, Chen L, Bridgewater D, Nieuwenhuis E, et al. GLI3 repressor controls nephron number via regulation of Wnt11 and Ret in ureteric tip cells. PLoS One 2009;4(10):e7313.

[164] Attanasio M, Uhlenhaut NH, Sousa VH, O'Toole JF, Otto E, Anlag K, et al. Loss of GLIS2 causes nephronophthisis in humans and mice by increased apoptosis and fibrosis. Nat Genet 2007;39(8):1018—24.

[165] Cain JE, Islam E, Haxho F, Blake J, Rosenblum ND. GLI3 repressor controls functional development of the mouse ureter. J Clin Invest 2011;121(3):1199—206.

[166] Cain JE, Rosenblum ND. Control of mammalian kidney development by the Hedgehog signaling pathway. Pediatr Nephrol 2011;26(9):1365—71.

[167] Zaghloul NA, Katsanis N. Functional modules, mutational load and human genetic disease. Trends Genet 2010;26(4): 168—76.

[168] Masyukova SV, Winkelbauer ME, Williams CL, Pieczynski JN, Yoder BK. Assessing the pathogenic potential of human Nephronophthisis disease-associated NPHP-4 missense mutations in C. elegans. Hum Mol Genet 2011;20(15):2942—54.

[169] Drummond IA. Kidney development and disease in the zebrafish. J Am Soc Nephrol 2005;16(2):299—304.

[170] Woollard JR, Punyashtiti R, Richardson S, Masyuk TV, Whelan S, Huang BQ, et al. A mouse model of autosomal recessive polycystic kidney disease with biliary duct and proximal tubule dilatation. Kidney Int 2007;72(3):328—36.

[171] Hellman NE, Liu Y, Merkel E, Austin C, Le Corre S, Beier DR, et al. The zebrafish foxj1a transcription factor regulates cilia function in response to injury and epithelial stretch. Proc Natl Acad Sci USA 2010;107(43):18499—504.

[172] Zaghloul NA, Liu Y, Gerdes JM, Gascue C, Oh EC, Leitch CC, et al. Functional analyses of variants reveal a significant role for dominant negative and common alleles in oligogenic

Bardet—Biedl syndrome. Proc Natl Acad Sci USA 2010;107 (23):10602—7.

[173] Wallingford JB, Mitchell B. Strange as it may seem: the many links between Wnt signaling, planar cell polarity, and cilia. Genes Dev 2011;25(3):201—13.

[174] Yoder BK, Richards WG, Sweeney WE, Wilkinson JE, Avener ED, Woychik RP. Insertional mutagenesis and molecular analysis of a new gene associated with polycystic kidney disease. Proc Assoc Am Physicians 1995;107(3):314—23.

[175] Bataille S, Demoulin N, Devuyst O, Audrezet MP, Dahan K, Godin M, et al. Association of PKD2 (Polycystin 2) mutations with left—right laterality defects. Am J Kidney Dis 2011;58(3): 456—60.

[176] Hildebrandt F, Otto E, Rensing C, Nothwang HG, Vollmer M, Adolphs J, et al. A novel gene encoding an SH3 domain protein is mutated in nephronophthisis type 1. Nat Genet 1997;17(2): 149—53.

[177] Hildebrandt F, Otto E. Cilia and centrosomes: a unifying pathogenic concept for cystic kidney disease? Nat Rev Genet 2005;6(12):928—40.

[178] Waldherr R, Lennert T, Weber HP, Fodisch HJ, Scharer K. The nephronophthisis complex. A clinicopathologic study in children. Virchows Arch A Pathol Anat Histol 1982;394(3):235—54.

[179] Zollinger HU, Mihatsch MJ, Edefonti A, Gaboardi F, Imbasciati E, Lennert T. Nephronophthisis (medullary cystic disease of the kidney). A study using electron microscopy, immunofluorescence, and a review of the morphological findings. Helv Paediatr Acta 1980;35(6):509—30.

[180] Delous M, Hellman NE, Gaude HM, Silbermann F, Le Bivic A, Salomon R, et al. Nephrocystin-1 and nephrocystin-4 are required for epithelial morphogenesis and associate with PALS1/PATJ and Par6. Hum Mol Genet 2009;18(24):4711—23.

[181] Won J, Marin de Evsikova C, Smith RS, Hicks WL, Edwards MM, Longo-Guess C, et al. NPHP4 is necessary for normal photoreceptor ribbon synapse maintenance and outer segment formation, and for sperm development. Hum Mol Genet 2011;20(3):482—96.

[182] Bielas SL, Silhavy JL, Brancati F, Kisseleva MV, Al-Gazali L, Sztriha L, et al. Mutations in INPP5E, encoding inositol polyphosphate-5-phosphatase E, link phosphatidyl inositol signaling to the ciliopathies. Nat Genet 2009;41(9):1032—6.

[183] Caspary T, Larkins CE, Anderson KV. The graded response to Sonic Hedgehog depends on cilia architecture. Dev Cell 2007; 12(5):767—78.

[184] Horner VL, Caspary T. Disrupted dorsal neural tube BMP signaling in the cilia mutant Arl13b hnn stems from abnormal Shh signaling. Dev Biol 2011;355(1):43—54.

[185] Hsiao YC, Tong ZJ, Westfall JE, Ault JG, Page-McCaw PS, Ferland RJ. Ahi1, whose human ortholog is mutated in Joubert syndrome, is required for Rab8a localization, ciliogenesis and vesicle trafficking. Hum Mol Genet 2009;18(20):3926—41.

[186] Eley L, Gabrielides C, Adams M, Johnson CA, Hildebrandt F, Sayer JA. Jouberin localizes to collecting ducts and interacts with nephrocystin-1. Kidney Int 2008;74(9):1139—49.

[187] Reiter JF, Skarnes WC. Tectonic, a novel regulator of the Hedgehog pathway required for both activation and inhibition. Genes Dev 2006;20(1):22—7.

[188] Alexiev BA, Lin X, Sun CC, Brenner DS. Meckel—Gruber syndrome: pathologic manifestations, minimal diagnostic criteria, and differential diagnosis. Arch Pathol Lab Med 2006;130(8): 1236—8.

[189] Williams CL, Winkelbauer ME, Schafer JC, Michaud EJ, Yoder BK. Functional redundancy of the B9 proteins and nephrocystins in Caenorhabditis elegans ciliogenesis. Mol Biol Cell 2008;19(5):2154—68.

[190] Fralick RA, Leichter HE, Sheth KJ. Early diagnosis of Bardet—Biedl syndrome. Pediatr Nephrol 1990;4(3):264—5.

[191] Harnett JD, Green JS, Cramer BC, Johnson G, Chafe L, McManamon P, et al. The spectrum of renal disease in Laurence—Moon—Biedl syndrome. N Engl J Med 1988;319(10): 615—8.

[192] Zaghloul NA, Katsanis N. Mechanistic insights into Bardet—Biedl syndrome, a model ciliopathy. J Clin Invest 2009;119(3):428—37.

[193] Guo DF, Beyer AM, Yang B, Nishimura DY, Sheffield VC, Rahmouni K. Inactivation of Bardet—Biedl syndrome genes causes kidney defects. Am J Physiol Renal Physiol 2011;300(2): F574—580.

[194] Seo S, Baye LM, Schulz NP, Beck JS, Zhang Q, Slusarski DC, et al. BBS10, and BBS12 form a complex with CCT/TRiC family chaperonins and mediate BBSome assembly. Proc Natl Acad Sci USA 2010;107(4):1488—93.

[195] Li G, Vega R, Nelms K, Gekakis N, Goodnow C, McNamara P, et al. A role for Alstrom syndrome protein, alms1, in kidney ciliogenesis and cellular quiescence. PLoS Genet 2007;3(1):e8.

[196] Romio L, Wright V, Price K, Winyard PJ, Donnai D, Porteous ME, et al. OFD1, the gene mutated in oral—facial—digital syndrome type 1, is expressed in the metanephros and in human embryonic renal mesenchymal cells. J Am Soc Nephrol 2003;14(3):680—9.

[197] Singla V, Romaguera-Ros M, Garcia-Verdugo JM, Reiter JF. Ofd1, a human disease gene, regulates the length and distal structure of centrioles. Dev Cell 2010;18(3):410—24.

[198] Keppler-Noreuil KM, Adam MP, Welch J, Muilenburg A, Willing MC. Clinical insights gained from eight new cases and review of reported cases with Jeune syndrome (asphyxiating thoracic dystrophy). Am J Med Genet A 2011;155A(5): 1021—32.

[199] Rix S, Calmont A, Scambler PJ, Beales PL. An Ift80 mouse model of short rib polydactyly syndromes shows defects in hedgehog signalling without loss or malformation of cilia. Hum Mol Genet 2011;20(7):1306—14.

[200] Dagoneau N, Goulet M, Genevieve D, Sznajer Y, Martinovic J, Smithson S, et al. DYNC2H1 mutations cause asphyxiating thoracic dystrophy and short rib-polydactyly syndrome, type III. Am J Hum Genet 2009;84(5):706—11.

[201] Davis EE, Zhang Q, Liu Q, Diplas BH, Davey LM, Hartley J, et al. TTC21B contributes both causal and modifying alleles across the ciliopathy spectrum. Nat Genet 2011;43(3):189—96.

[202] Gilissen C, Arts HH, Hoischen A, Spruijt L, Mans DA, Arts P, et al. Exome sequencing identifies WDR35 variants involved in Sensenbrenner syndrome. Am J Hum Genet 2010;87(3): 418—23.

[203] Arts HH, Bongers EM, Mans DA, van Beersum SE, Oud MM, Bolat E, et al. C14ORF179 encoding IFT43 is mutated in Sensenbrenner syndrome. J Med Genet 2011;48(6):390—5.

[204] Walczak-Sztulpa J, Eggenschwiler J, Osborn D, Brown DA, Emma F, Klingenberg C, et al. Cranioectodermal dysplasia, sensenbrenner syndrome, is a ciliopathy caused by mutations in the IFT122 gene. Am J Hum Genet 2010;86(6):949—56.

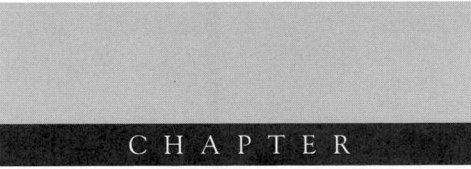

CHAPTER

12

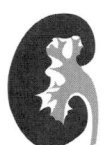

Intercellular Junctions

Alan S. L. Yu[1], Fiona Hanner[2,3] and János Peti-Peterdi[2,3]

[1]Division of Nephrology, and Hypertension, and The Kidney Institute, University of Kansas Medical Center,
Kansas City, KS, USA

[2]Department of Physiology and Biophysics, University of Southern California Keck School of Medicine,
Los Angeles, CA, USA

[3]Zilkha Neurogenetic Institute, University of Southern California Keck School of Medicine, Los Angeles, CA, USA

TIGHT JUNCTIONS

Structure

General Structure

The tight junction is the most apical component of the junctional complex (Figure 12.1). It is located at the boundary between the apical and lateral membranes, and encircles the cells to form a continuous belt-like attachment. By transmission electron microscopy, it appears morphologically as a series of appositions or "kisses" between the lateral membranes of adjacent cells (Figure 12.2a). The outer leaflet of the lipid bilayers approach each other so closely that they appear to be fused. In the technique of freeze-fracture electron microscopy, the hydrophobic phospholipid interior of the lipid bilayer is cleaved, allowing the tight junctions to be visualized within the plane of the lateral membrane. By this means, tight junctions appear as a series of continuous, anastomosing intramembranous strands on the protoplasmic or P-face, with complementary grooves on the exoplasmic or E-face (Figure 12.5). It is believed that these strands associate in pairs from neighboring cells and obliterate the intercellular space, thus accounting for the kissing points seen by transmission electron microscopy (Figure 12.2b).

Early models of the tight junction posited that it was composed purely of lipid organized into inverted cylindrical micelles, that constituted the tight junction strands.[2,3] There now exist three lines of evidence that refute this. First, tight junction strands were found to be resistant to deoyxcholate, an ionic detergent that should solubilize lipids.[4] Second, the lipid model

predicts that the outer leaflets of the bilayers of adjacent cells are continuous, yet no transfer of glycolipid or a fluorescent probe could be demonstrated.[5-7] Finally, the discovery of integral membrane proteins within the tight junction now supports a model in which tight junction strands are composed of proteins embedded in the lipid membrane (see below).

Regional Differences in Structure

The structure of the tight junction varies considerably in different regions of the kidney. This is summarized briefly below. For further details, the reader is referred to comprehensive surveys by Orci, Brown, and colleagues.[8,9]

GLOMERULUS

The parietal epithelium of Bowman's capsule is constituted of squamous cells whose extensions overlap obliquely (Figure 12.3). Their tight junctions consist of networks of two to four anastomosing strands with many discontinuities.[10,11] The mature visceral epithelial cell (podocyte) forms a specialized intercellular junction, the slit diaphragm (Chapter 23). Short elements of incomplete tight junctions can sometimes also be seen between the foot processes of adjacent podocytes. True tight junctions do form between immature podocytes in the fetal glomerulus and are of uncertain functional significance.[12,13] These disappear during development, but can reappear during nephrotic states, coincident with effacement of the foot processes and obliteration of the slit pore[14-16] (Figure 12.4).

Seldin and Giebisch's The Kidney, Fifth Edition.
DOI: http://dx.doi.org/10.1016/B978-0-12-381462-3.00012-4

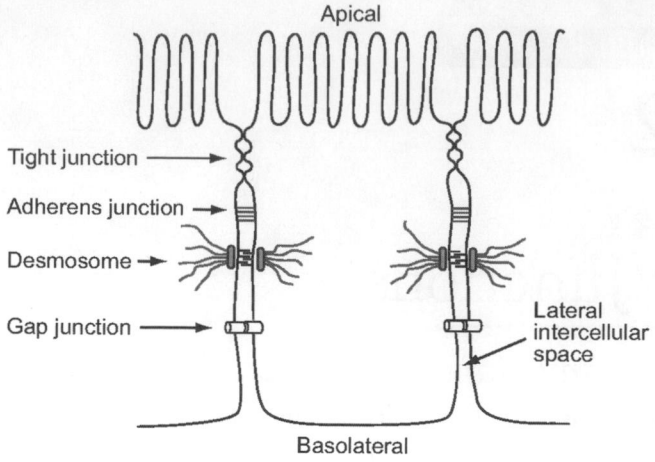

FIGURE 12.1 Organization of the junctional complex in a typical monolayer of epithelial cells.

RENAL TUBULE

Tight junctions are found between the epithelial cells of all tubules, but they vary considerably in their morphology in different tubule segments (Figure 12.5 and Table 12.1). In general, the more proximal segments tend to have simpler junctions, with fewer strands and more discontinuities, correlating with a leaky paracellular pathway, as judged by transepithelial resistance (TER). By contrast, more distal segments tend to have greater numbers of strands, with more continuity and complex anastomosing patterns, loosely correlating with higher TER. Indeed, Claude proposed a model in which TER is dependent primarily on strand number.[17] However, as discussed below, we now know that the TER is also highly dependent on the composition of the tight junction.

Physiological Functions

Gate Function

The gate function refers to the ability to regulate the paracellular permeability. This determines the rate of passive diffusion of extracellular solutes and water between the apical and basolateral aqueous compartments. Early studies, using extracellular macromolecules and lanthanum as electron-dense markers, clearly established the tight junction as the site of the paracellular gate.[1,18,19]

In epithelia that mediate active, uphill transcellular transport, such as the collecting duct of the kidney, this gate must act predominantly as a barrier to prevent backleak of solute gradients that have been generated. To do so, these so-called "tight" epithelia must have very low paracellular permeability and conductance (typical transepithelial resistances (TER) range from $1-2 \, \text{k}'\Omega.\text{cm}^2$ for the renal collecting duct[20] to $\sim 8 \, \text{k}'\Omega.\text{cm}^2$ for amphibian skin[21]).

In contrast, in epithelia that mediate bulk transport of solutes via the paracellular pathway, the gate is predominantly open. For example, in the late proximal tubule of the kidney about one-third of NaCl reabsorption occurs by the paracellular route,[22] and in the thick ascending limb of Henle, Ca^{2+} and Mg^{2+} are exclusively reabsorbed via the paracellular pathway.[23] Characterization of the properties of leaky epithelia have indicated that there must be paracellular aqueous pores.[24,25] Fromter and Diamond were the first to prove that the paracellular leak is physically located at the intercellular junction.[26] Thus, the tight junction is not always a complete barrier, but must also have pores that pass through it.

Fence Function

In epithelia, the lipid and protein components of the plasma membrane are separated into distinct apical and basolateral domains at the tight junction, and this polarity is critical for functions such as vectorial transport. Apical–basolateral polarity is initially established by the Par/aPKC, Crumbs, and Scribble complexes,[27,28] while the tight junction is primarily responsible for maintenance of this polarity. Specifically, the tight junction behaves like a fence, preventing diffusion within the plane of the lipid bilayer. Interestingly, markers that are confined to the exocytoplasmic leaflet cannot pass across the tight junction, but markers that can flip-flop across the bilayer freely diffuse across it,[6,29] suggesting that the fence is located in the exocytoplasmic half of the plasma membrane. Several manipulations can dissociate the barrier and fence functions of the tight junction. Transient ATP depletion[30,31] and depolymerization of the cortical actin network[32] disrupt the paracellular barrier while preserving fence function. This suggests that the fence function of the tight junction is mechanistically independent of its gate function.

Biochemical Composition

The first tight junction-associated protein to be identified was ZO-1, in 1986.[33] Since then, it has become clear that the tight junction is actually a complex of many different proteins. These fall into one of four categories: transmembrane proteins; scaffolding proteins; signaling molecules; and transcriptional regulators. These molecules are associated, through multiple protein–protein interactions, with the scaffolding proteins serving to anchor the complex to the cortical actin cytoskeleton. Table 12.2 lists the known molecules in each category. Here, we focus solely on the transmembrane proteins. These are important because their transmembrane domains traverse the lipid bilayer, while their extracellular domains protrude into the paracellular space. Thus, tight junction membrane proteins are the leading candidates to mediate both gate and fence functions.

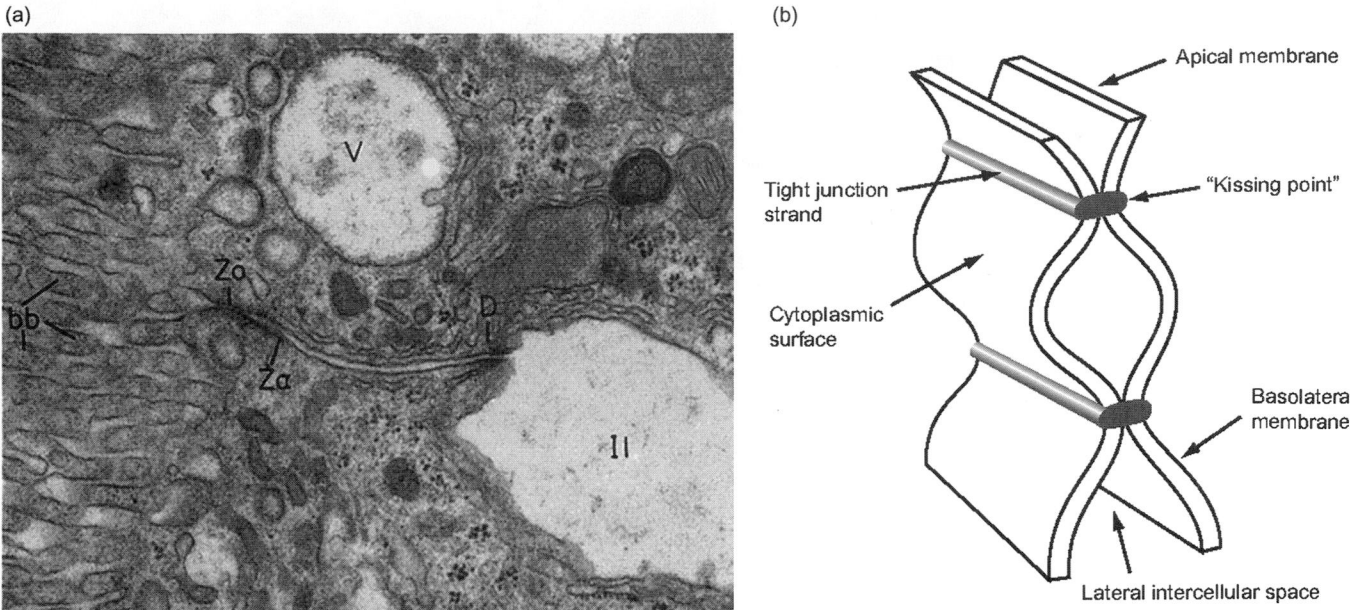

FIGURE 12.2 **Structure of the tight junction.** (a) Transmission electron micrograph of the junctional complex in the epithelium of the rat proximal convoluted tubule (Zo: zonula occludens (tight junction); Za: zonula adherens (adherens junction); D: desmosome; bb: brush border; Il: lateral intercellular space). (b) Three-dimensional depiction of the tight junction. Tight junction strands of neighboring cells associate in a pairwise manner at points where the lateral membranes are closely apposed, obliterating the intercellular space ("kissing points"). (©*The Rockefeller University Press. The Journal of Cell Biology, (1963). 17, 375–412.*[1])

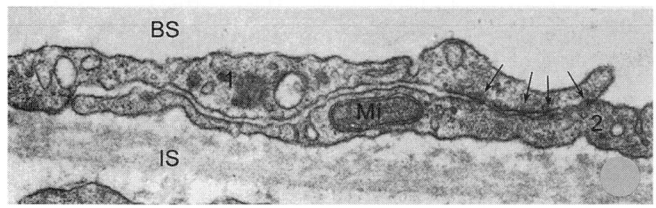

FIGURE 12.3 **Section through Bowman's capsule of rat kidney showing two adjacent parietal epithelial cells (labeled 1 and 2).** The cells are flat, so that their extensions overlap obliquely to form the tight junction. Arrows indicate points of close apposition between their lateral membranes (BS: Bowman's space; IS: interstitial space; Mi: mitochondrion; × 40,000). (*Reproduced with permission from Taugner et al. (1976). Cell Tissue Res. 172(4), 431–446.*[10])

Occludin

Occludin was the first integral tight junction membrane protein to be identified.[34] It has four transmembrane domains with intracellular N- and C-termini. Occludin is ubiquitously expressed in epithelial cells, localizing predominantly at bicellular junctions (junctions where two cells meet). Its role is poorly understood. Overexpression of a C-terminally truncated occludin protein increases TER, but paradoxically increases mannitol flux, and also disrupts tight junction fence function.[35,36] However, after knockdown or knockout of occludin, cells can still form normally appearing tight junction strands.[37,38] In fibroblasts that do not have tight junctions,

occludin cannot reform tight junction networks, but it does co-polymerize into strands with claudin-1.[39] Knockdown of occludin in MDCK cells causes only a slight increase in permeability to small inorganic and organic cations.[38] Interestingly, occludin null mice have assorted unexplained abnormalities, including retarded postnatal growth, male sterility, and chronic inflammation and epithelial hyperplasia in the gastric mucosa.[40] Importantly, though, epithelial barrier function is normal in these mice.[41] Thus, occludin is neither necessary nor sufficient to form tight junction strands and perform barrier, pore or fence functions. However, occludin can incorporate into claudin-based strands, in which case dominant-negative occludin constructs are presumably able to disrupt normal tight junction function.

Tricellulin

Tricellulin is a homolog of occludin that is localized to tricellular junctions (junctions at the confluence of three cells).[42] It is clearly important for barrier function, because knockdown of tricellulin increases paracellular conductance and permeability to uncharged macromolecules,[42] and its overexpression reduces macromolecular permeability.[43] Mutations in tricellulin cause a form of non-syndromic hereditary deafness, indicating that it plays a critical role in inner ear function,[44] but its role in the kidney has not been explored.

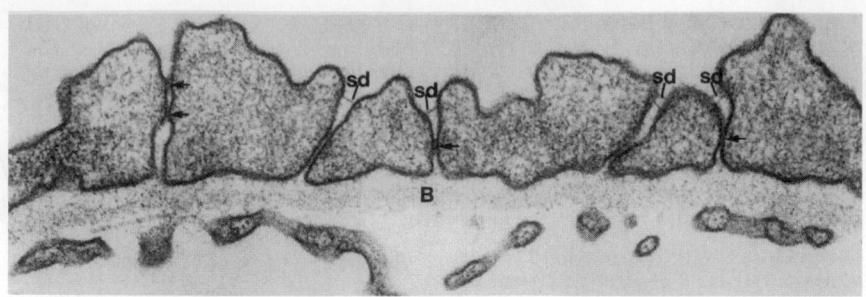

FIGURE 12.4　Morphologic changes in glomerular podocytes in the puromycin aminonucleoside nephrotic rat kidney. The membranes of the foot processes appear to come into close apposition or to be fused (arrows), forming tight junction-like structures between neighboring processes. The slit diaphragms (sd), which are normally located above the basement membrane (B), are found above the newly formed junctions between the podocytes ($\times$ 74,000). (*Reprinted from* Am. J. Pathol. (1992), **141**, 805–816.[226] *With permission from the American Society for Investigative Pathology.*)

Claudins

Claudins were discovered by Tsukita and colleagues.[45] They are members of a multigene family of ~20–24 kDa tight junction proteins with four predicted transmembrane segments and two extracellular domains (see refs [46–48] for several recent reviews). When expressed in claudin-deficient cells such as fibroblasts, claudins can form tight junction-like networks of strands, indicating that they polymerize in *cis* (within the same cell membrane), and can mediate intercellular adhesion, indicating the ability to interact in *trans* (across two lateral membranes of adjacent cells).[39,49] Thus, claudins have all the properties expected for a structural component of the paracellular barrier. In 1999, Lifton's group identified the culprit gene mutated in familial hypercalciuric hypomagnesemia, an inherited disorder thought to be due to failure of paracellular reabsorption of divalent cations in the thick ascending limb of the renal tubule. This gene, which was initially named paracellin, turned out to be a claudin (claudin-16),[50] and its involvement in this disease strongly suggested that claudins play a role in regulating paracellular transport. This is now supported by numerous studies demonstrating that overexpressing or ablating expression of various claudin isoforms in cultured cell lines or in mice affects both the degree of paracellular permeability, and its selectivity (reviewed in ref [51]). Moreover, Colegio et al. have convincingly shown that the net charge on residues in the first extracellular domain of claudins determines the charge selectivity of paracellular conductance.[52,53] This suggests fairly strongly that the first extracellular domain of claudins actually forms the lining of the paracellular pore. The permeability properties of different claudin isoforms, as inferred from *in vitro* overexpression and knockdown studies, are summarized in Table 12.3.

FUNCTIONAL DOMAINS OF CLAUDIN

The functions of several of the domains within the claudin protein have been determined (Figure 12.6). The first extracellular loop of claudin forms the lining of the paracellular pore. Chimera studies have shown that exchanging the first extracellular loop between different claudin isoforms confers different pore selectivity characteristics.[53] Furthermore, point mutations that reverse the charge on residues in the first extracellular loop alter the charge selectivity of the paracellular pore, as would be expected if this domain faced the pore lumen.[52] In claudin-2, a cation-selective pore, this loop specifically contains an aspartate residue (Asp-65) that acts as a Na^+-binding site.[54] Several other residues in this domain have also been mapped by cysteine-scanning mutagenesis.[55]

The second extracellular loop of claudin is postulated to participate in *trans*-intermolecular interactions, acting as the adhesion receptor between neighboring cells. This is based on the finding that mutations of selected residues in the second extracellular loop of claudin-5 abolish its ability to concentrate at cell contact sites when expressed in HEK cells.[56]

Claudins all have a long cytoplasmic C-terminal tail that appears to be involved in protein trafficking and degradation. Deletion of this tail in claudin-5 and -6 leads to accumulation of the protein in the cytoplasm.[57,58] This domain also affects protein stability, since swapping it between different claudins confers different protein half-lives.[59] The terminal dipeptide motif in claudins (tyrosine-valine in the majority) binds to PDZ domains on the scaffolding proteins, ZO-1, 2, and 3,[60] and MUPP1.[61,62] However, deletion of this motif does not seem to affect normal trafficking of claudins to the tight junction.[57,63]

The cytoplasmic C-terminal tail in all claudin isoforms also contains multiple potential

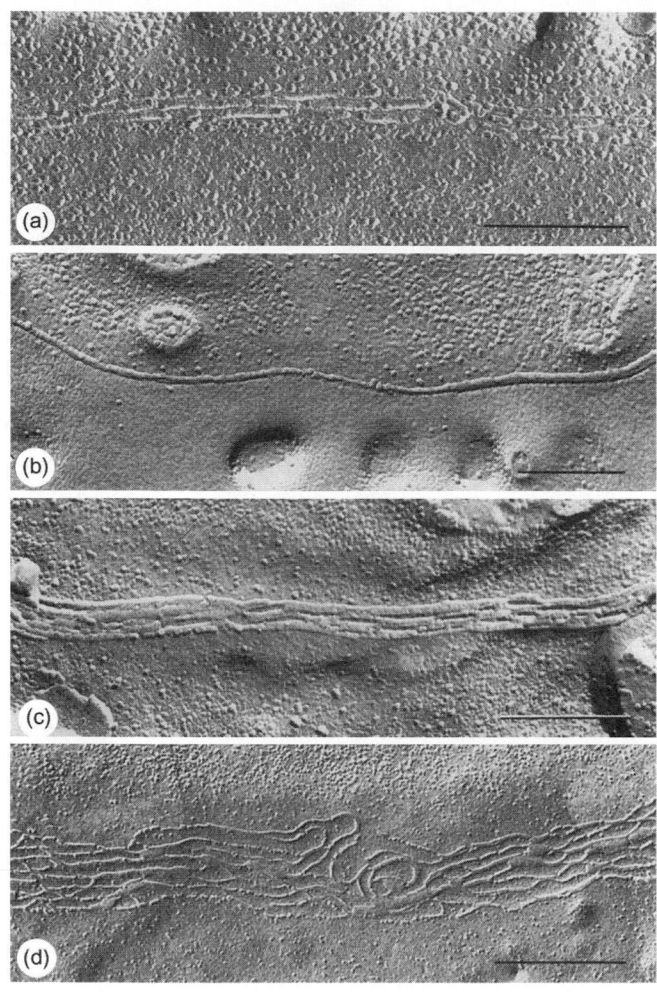

FIGURE 12.5 Freeze-fracture morphology of tight junctions on the P-faces of four regions of the urinary tubule. The tight junctions of the proximal convoluted tubule (a) are characterized by fibrils that are often ill-defined and discontinuous. In the ascending thin limb of Henle (b), the tight junctions usually appear as one continuous strand or two closely apposed strands that are covered with fragments of E-face from the adjacent cell, giving the impression of a single, thick strand. In the distal tubule (c), the junctions are composed of several parallel elements. In the collecting duct (d), the tight junctions are the most complex in the entire urinary tubule, and are formed of multiple, branching fibrils (a–c: bar = 0.25 μm; d: bar = 0.5 μm). (*Reproduced with permission from Orci et al. (1981). Int. Rev. Cytol. 73, 183–242.[9]*)

TABLE 12.1 Morphology of the Tight Junctions Compared with Transepithelial Resistance in Different Nephron Segments of the Rat Renal Tubule[a]

Tubular segment	Transepithelial resistance ('Ω.cm²)[b]	Number of junctional strands (typical range)
Proximal	5–7	1–2
Thin descending limb of Henle	700[c]	1
Thick ascending limb of Henle	10–35	5–6[d]
Distal convoluted tubule	350	
Collecting duct	867	8–9

[a]Table adapted with permission from Pricam et al.[158]
[b]Values from references.[218–222]
[c]Values measured in the rabbit.
[d]Values from both thick ascending limb and distal convoluted tubule.

TABLE 12.2 Composition of the Tight Junction Protein Complex

Transmembrane proteins	Scaffolding proteins	Signaling proteins	Transcriptional regulators
Occludin	ZO-1, 2, 3	aPKC	ZONAB
Claudins	Par-3, 6	GEF-H1	Symplekin
Tricellulin	Pals1	Gαi-2, αo, α12	AP-1
MarvelD3	PATJ	Rab13, 3B	
JAM	MUPP1	c-Yes	
CAR	MAGI-2, 3	WNK3, 4	
	JACOP/ paracinguilin	CDK4	
	Cingulin		
	AF-6		

been shown to be palmitoylated, and this seems to be required for efficient localization to the tight junction.[71]

Physiology of the Tight Junction in Different Nephron Segments

Different nephron segments exhibit different tight junction permeability characteristics that are important for their specific function. These paracellular permeability characteristics are likely a function both of the general structure of the tight junction (discussed above), and of the properties of the specific claudin isoforms expressed in that segment. The nephron

phosphorylation sites for a variety of protein kinases (see ref [64] for a comprehensive review). The most common outcome of phosphorylation by protein kinases in this domain is increased assembly at the tight junction,[65,66] but there are examples of phosphorylation leading to decreased assembly at the tight junction,[67] and also to changes in paracellular permeability.[68–70]

Finally, all claudins have two pairs of conserved cysteines immediately following the second and fourth transmembrane domains. In claudin-14, these have

TABLE 12.3 Putative Ion Permeability Characteristics of Claudin Isoforms[a]

Pore-forming claudins[b]	Refs	Barrier-forming claudins	Refs
Cation-selective pore		**Cation barrier**	
Claudin-2	54,86,87	Claudin-1	36,74
Claudin-10b	90	Claudin-3	114
Claudin-16	109–111	Claudin-4[c]	115,125
Anion-selective pore		Claudin-5	223
Claudin-4[c]	125	Claudin-6[d]	93
Claudin-10a	90	Claudin-8	116,224
Claudin-11[c]	88	Claudin-9[d]	93
Claudin-17	108	Claudin-11[c]	88
		Claudin-14	117
		Claudin-18	118
	Anion barrier		
		Claudin-15	52,88
		Claudin-19[e]	112

[a]Based on in vitro overexpression or knockdown studies in cultured cell lines. We assume that permeability and selectivity are properties intrinsic to individual claudin isoforms, and ignore the possible confounding effect of heteromeric interactions between isoforms. Claudin-7 is omitted because conflicting data exist suggesting that it is either a Cl-barrier[124,225] or a Na-barrier/Cl-pore.[125]

[b]Pore-forming claudins refer to those that predominantly decrease TER or increase solute permeability, while barrier-forming claudins refer to those that predominantly increase TER or decrease solute permeability. The distinction is somewhat arbitrary, since most claudins probably have some finite permeability to most solutes, and the observable phenotype is highly dependent on the properties of the host cell line.[87,222]

[c]Acts as a Na barrier in MDCK II cells, but as a Cl pore in LLC-PK1 cells.

[d]Net flux studies suggest that claudin-6 and -9 may also act as Cl-barriers.[93]

[e]Conflicting data also exists suggesting claudin-19 can act as a Na barrier.[105]

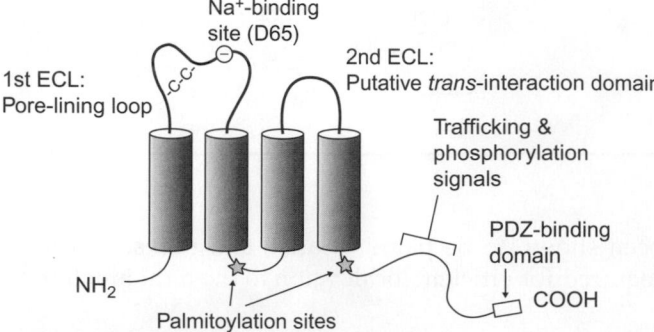

FIGURE 12.6 Functional domains that have been mapped in claudins. The Na$^+$-binding site at D65 has been demonstrated in claudin-2 (ECL: extracellular loop).

segment localization of different claudin isoforms is summarized in Figure 12.7.

Bowman's Capsule

The function of the parietal epithelium of Bowman's capsule is poorly understood, but one might assume that it needs to act primarily as a barrier to contain the glomerular filtrate, and direct flow into the proximal tubule. The tight junction of parietal epithelial squamous cells is unique among cells of the nephron in expressing claudin-1,[72,73] an isoform that has been shown to act as a barrier to ion conductance, and to permeation of 4–40 kDa dextran.[36,74] Claudin-2, a cation- and water-permeable claudin isoform predominantly expressed in the proximal tubule (see below), has also been reported to be expressed in the parietal epithelium.[72,73] However, it is well-known that the parietal epithelium at the urinary pole is constituted of columnar cells that are distinct from the squamous parietal epithelial cells, and morphologically and functionally resemble proximal tubule cells.[75,76] These columnar cells can cover a substantial surface area of Bowman's capsule, for example, one-third of it in male mice, and it is probably just these cells that express claudin-2 (see, for example, Fig. 3A in ref [77]).

Ohse recently showed that the parietal epithelium in mice functions as a barrier to macromolecules, as detected with 3 kDa dextran and 45 kDa ovalbumin as tracers.[78] After experimental induction of glomerulonephritis, this barrier is disrupted and the macromolecule tracers can be observed leaking into the space between the parietal epithelium and the underlying basement membrane of Bowman's capsule, as well as the extraglomerular space.

Proximal Tubule

The primary role of the proximal tubule is bulk reclamation of solutes that evade the glomerular filter, such as Na, K, Ca, Cl, HCO$_3$, phosphate, glucose, and water. Since the free concentration of these solutes in the glomerular filtrate is similar to that of the peritubular fluid, relatively little energy expenditure should be needed to transport them across the epithelium. To achieve this sort of energy efficiency, the proximal tubule uses a two-step process. In the first step, ATP consumed by the Na-K-ATPase is used to generate a transmembrane Na gradient that drives secondary and tertiary active transcellular reabsorption of Na and other solutes. The stoichiometry of the Na-K-ATPase dictates that the hydrolysis of each ATP molecule in this step should be coupled to the direct transport of three Na ions. In the second step, the transepithelial electrochemical gradients generated by transcellular transport then provide the driving force for passive diffusion of solutes across the paracellular pathway. Measurements of whole kidney oxygen consumption have been used to estimate that five Na ions are transported per ATP molecule,[79,80] demonstrating that paracellular transport greatly enhances the metabolic efficiency of the proximal tubule.

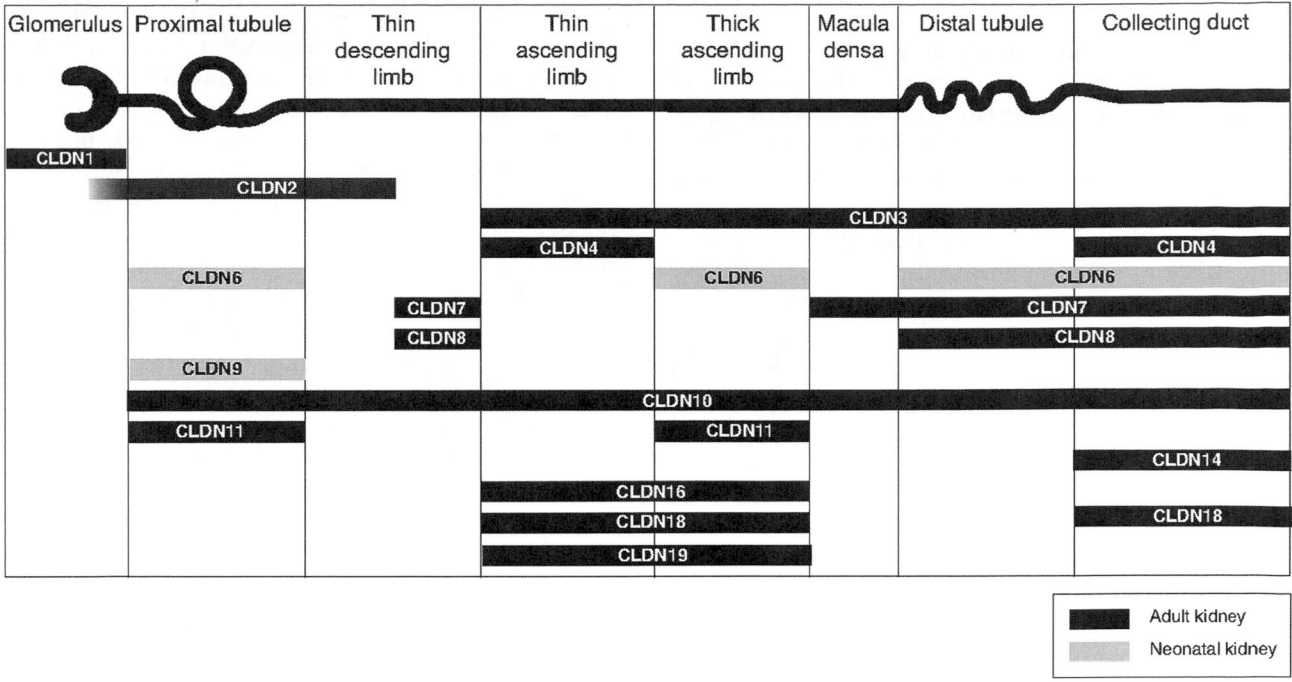

FIGURE 12.7 **Localization of claudin proteins in rodent kidney.** Localization data were collated from the following studies: claudins 1, 3, and 4,[72] claudin-2,[77] claudin-6,[92] claudins 7 and 8,[227] claudin-9,[92] claudin-10,[90] claudin-14,[108] claudin-16,[106] claudin-17,[85] claudin-18,[107] and claudin-19.[105,106] Macula densa claudin expression is from our own unpublished results. Tubule expression of claudins 6 and 9 are only found in neonatal kidney.[92] Localization of claudins in human kidney are essentially identical,[50,228] except that claudin-1 is found in collecting duct and distal tubule, claudin-10 is not found in the distal nephron, and claudin-14 is reportedly in the distal convoluted tubule.[228] Many of these claudins have not been rigorously examined in all nephron segments so the data shown are not comprehensive. Claudins 5 and 15 are confined to endothelial cells of the vasculature and glomeruli,[72] and so are not shown. Claudins 12, 18 and 20–24 have not yet been examined. *(Figure modified from Angelow, S. and Yu, A. S. (2007). Claudins and paracellular transport: an update. Curr. Opin. Nephrol. Hypertens. **16**, 459–464. Copyright Lippincott, Williams & Wilkins, 2007.)*

NaCL REABSORPTION

The underlying mechanism for paracellular NaCl reabsorption in the proximal tubule was first proposed by Rector.[22,81] In this model, transcellular Na reabsorption in the early proximal convoluted tubule is coupled primarily to reabsorption of most of the organic solutes and significant amounts of bicarbonate, and followed by isosmotic reabsorption of water. This leads to a luminal fluid that is high in chloride, but low in bicarbonate. The late proximal tubule has a very high passive permeability (presumably due to the paracellular pathway) both to Na and to Cl, but much less so to HCO_3.[82–84] Thus, Cl is reabsorbed paracellularly, driven by its concentration gradient. This in turn generates a lumen-positive electrical potential which then drives concomitant reabsorption of Na.

The claudin isoforms that are known to be expressed in the proximal tubule are claudin-2, -10, and -17.[72,77,85] Claudin-2 behaves *in vitro* as a cation-selective paracellular pore.[54,86–88] Knockout of claudin-2 in mice led to an approximately two-fold reduction in transepithelial conductance, P_{Na}/P_{Cl}, and passive flux of Na, Cl, and water in perfused S2 segments, and an exaggerated natriuretic response to a NaCl challenge.[89] Thus, claudin-2 seems to be the primary route for paracellular Na reabsorption. Claudin-10 exists in two splice variants that differ in their first extracellular domain, and hence charge selectivity.[90] Claudin-10a behaves as a Cl-selective pore, while claudin-10b is Na-selective. The 10a splice variant is uniquely expressed in the kidney, and by *in situ* hybridization appears to be predominantly in the cortex, although tubule localization could not be ascertained. Studies of claudin-17 overexpression in MDCK-C7 cells and knockdown in LLC-PK1 cells indicate that it functions as a Cl pore.[85] Thus, either claudin-10a or -17 could potentially mediate paracellular Cl reabsorption in the proximal tubule.

The neonate proximal tubule has a lower chloride permeability than the adult, which may predispose it to salt-wasting and dehydration.[91] Claudins 6 and 9 are predominantly expressed in the neonatal proximal tubule,[92] but the published functional data are somewhat conflicting as to whether they primarily act as Cl-barriers (which would be consistent with the tubule physiology) or Na-barriers.[93]

WATER REABSORPTION

A substantial amount of water is reabsorbed in the proximal tubule. It is now clear that the majority of water transport is transcellular and mediated by aquaporins. Nevertheless, knockout of AQP1 in mice only reduces proximal tubule water transport by 80%, suggesting that an alternative pathway for water transport exists and is either active under normal conditions or is upregulated to compensate for loss of AQP1.[94] Weinstein has argued that the low reflection coefficient for NaCl (~ 0.7)[95] suggests the existence of a paracellular shunt pathway for water.[96] However, Preisig and Berry measured the permeability of the proximal tubule to mannitol and sucrose and, assuming that they were only transported paracellularly, modeled the pore size with the Renkin equation to predict the paracellular water permeability and concluded that it was <2% of transepithelial water permeability.[97] Moreover, Spring measured water flow in the lateral intercellular spaces of MDCK cells (admittedly not necessarily a proximal tubule model cell line) by an optical technique, and concluded that water transport in these cells was entirely transcellular.[98] Thus, the existence of paracellular water reabsorption in the proximal tubule has been quite controversial. Recently, Rosenthal et al. reported that transfection of claudin-2 increases transepithelial osmotic water permeability.[99] Interestingly, they found that when they imposed a transepithelial Na^+ concentration gradient, not only was Na^+ transported vectorially, but water flowed in the same direction, suggesting that Na^+ and water movement are in some way "coupled," and therefore that they probably flow through the same pore.

REABSORPTION OF OTHER CATIONS

A substantial proportion of the filtered load of K, Ca, and Mg are reabsorbed in the proximal tubule, largely by the paracellular pathway. The driving force in each case is probably both an increased concentration of the cation in the lumen due to water reabsorption, and the lumen-positive voltage in the mid-to-late proximal tubule. Claudin-2 is permeable to both K and Ca (Mg has not been tested),[54] and therefore likely mediates their reabsorption by diffusion down their electrochemical gradients.

Thick Ascending Limb of Henle

The thick ascending limb of Henle is a quantitatively important site for paracellular reabsorption of the divalent cations, Ca and Mg.[100] In addition, some of the Na reabsorbed in this nephron segment is also thought to occur paracellularly, thus enhancing the metabolic efficiency of transcellular Na reabsorption, just as in the proximal tubule. The driving force for

paracellular reabsorption of each of these cations is a lumen-positive electrical potential difference. This voltage is generated by two distinct and additive mechanisms: (1) transcellular reabsorption of NaCl through the apical Na-K-2Cl co-transporter and basolateral Na-K-ATPase and ClC-K chloride transporter occurs concomitantly with apical recycling of K through the apical K channel, ROMK, giving rise to a net movement of positive charge apically; this generates a 3−9 mV lumen-positive transepithelial potential difference[101]; (2) because the paracellular pathway of the thick ascending limb is highly cation-selective (P_{Na}/$P_{Cl} = 2-6$),[101,102] accumulation of a high concentration of reabsorbed NaCl basolaterally generates a diffusion potential, adding another 10−15 mV to the transepithelial voltage.[103] The paracellular pathway of the thick ascending limb is well adapted for this purpose. It is characterized by a low TER ($11-34 \ \Omega.cm^2$),[104] high selectivity for Na over Cl, and high permeability to divalent cations.[23]

The thick ascending limb is known to express claudins 3, 10, 11, 14, 16, 18, and 19.[50,72,90,105−108] Claudin-16 (also known as paracellin) and claudin-19 are of particular interest, because mutations in these genes cause familial hypercalciuric hypomagnesemia with nephrocalcinosis (FHHNC), an autosomal recessive disorder characterized by renal Ca and Mg wasting.[50,106] There are two prevailing hypotheses as to the physiological role of claudins 16 and 19. The first hypothesis, initially suggested by Simon et al.,[50] is that they are divalent cation-permeable paracellular pore proteins. In this model, Ca and Mg normally diffuse through these claudins, driven by the lumen-positive potential, but in FHHNC this pathway is abolished. Consistent with this, Ikari et al. found that overexpression of claudin-16 increased Ca permeability, and that this could be competitively inhibited by Mg, while TER was paradoxically increased.[109] Similarly, Kausalya et al. found that claudin-16 increased Mg permeability, but did not affect P_{Na}/P_{Cl}.[110] The second hypothesis is that claudin-16 and -19 together form a pore that is highly selective for Na over Cl, and therefore facilitates the component of the lumen-positive potential generated by the NaCl concentration gradient (component (2) above). In other words, claudin-16 and -19 are involved in creating the driving force for Ca and Mg reabsorption, rather than being part of the permeation pathway. This second hypothesis is supported predominantly by the work of Hou, Goodenough, and colleagues. In their hands, claudin-16 acts like a cation pore that is not selective between monovalent and divalent cations,[111] and claudin-19 acts like an anion barrier.[112] Hou et al. showed that the two isoforms physically interact with each other, and have additive effects to increase P_{Na}/P_{Cl} when co-expressed together.[112] Indeed, knockdown of both isoforms in mice recapitulated the main features of FHHNC, and was associated with decreased P_{Na}/P_{Cl} as measured in isolated, perfused thick ascending limbs.[107,113]

Claudin-14 appears to act as a negative regulator that binds to claudin-16 to reduce the PNa/PCl of this complex.[108] Importantly, claudin-14 expression is upregulated in response to high extracellular calcium or a high-calcium diet, which stimulate the Ca-sensing receptor in the thick ascending limb and thereby downregulate two micro-RNAs that normally suppress claudin-14 expression. This provides an elegant homeostatic mechanism to increase renal calcium excretion in the setting of calcium excess. The role of the other claudins in this segment is not known at this time.

Aldosterone-Sensitive Distal Nephron

The aldosterone-sensitive distal nephron (ASDN) encompasses the distal convoluted tubule, connecting segment, and collecting duct. This is the last section of the nephron, and is responsible for fine-tuning urinary composition. The remaining excess Na in the tubular fluid has to be reabsorbed here, and K and H^+ secreted. These are active, highly energy-consuming processes, because they need to drive transport uphill against steep electrochemical gradients, utilizing transcellular pathways. Transtubular concentration gradients for Na, K, and H^+ (lumen:blood) of 1:3, 20:1, and 1000:1, respectively, are often achieved by the end of the collecting duct. Thus, the major role of the tight junction in the ASDN is to act as a very tight paracellular cation barrier to prevent dissipation of these transtubular cation gradients. Consistent with this, the ASDN (or at least the collecting duct) expresses five claudins that function primarily as cation barriers: claudins 3, 4, 8, 14, and 18.[114-118] For claudin-8 and -18, the ability to act as a barrier to acid permeation has also been demonstrated.[118,119]

In the connecting segment and collecting duct, Na is reabsorbed primarily electrogenically through epithelial Na channels (ENaC), as distinct from the distal convoluted tubule, which mediates electroneutral, NaCl reabsorption. Thus, Cl in the connecting segment and collecting duct must be reabsorbed either through an independent transcellular pathway (e.g., via the Na-driven Cl-bicarbonate exchanger and pendrin in β-intercalated cells[120,121]) or paracellularly. Consistent with a role in paracellular Cl transport, the cortical collecting duct has been shown to have a substantial paracellular permeability to Cl.[122] A recent study suggests that this paracellular Cl permeability may be mediated by claudin-4 and -8, perhaps interacting with each other to form a heteromeric pore.[123]

Claudin-7 is expressed in the ASDN. When overexpressed in LLC-PK cells, it appeared to reduce Cl permeability (i.e., acted as a Cl barrier).[124] However, knockdown of its expression paradoxically also decreased Cl permeability, suggesting that claudin-7 might normally behave as a Cl pore, and might be responsible for the paracellular Cl conductance in the ASDN.[125] Importantly, mice that had claudin-7 knocked-out by gene targeting exhibited severe renal salt-wasting, hypovolemia, and acute renal failure,[126] which is consistent with a role for claudin-7 in ASDN Cl reabsorption.

REGULATION BY ALDOSTERONE AND WNK KINASES

NaCl reabsorption in the ASDN is stimulated by mineralocorticoids. This is achieved in part by stimulating transcellular Na transport. In addition, aldosterone and other mineralocorticoids regulate paracellular permeability. For example, mineralocorticoids reduce Na permeability in the inner medullary collecting duct.[127-129] This would serve to limit paracellular backleak of Na, and thereby enhance the efficiency of Na reabsorption. Mineralocorticoids have also been shown to reduce paracellular Cl permeability in the collecting duct,[129,130] but the physiological significance of this is less clear. Interestingly, Le Moellic et al. found that in a rat cortical collecting duct cell line, very brief (<1 hour) aldosterone exposure actually increased paracellular anion permeability.[69] This correlated temporally with phosphorylation of claudin-4 at a threonine residue, although a causal relationship was not established.

NaCl reabsorption in the ASDN is also regulated by WNK1 and WNK4. These are protein kinases that, when mutated, cause pseudohypoaldosteronism, type II (PHAII), a genetic disorder characterized by salt-sensitive hypertension and hyperkalemia.[131] The normal physiological function of the WNKs is quite controversial, but it is clear that PHAII mutations in WNK4 lead to enhanced NaCl reabsorption in the ASDN. This is partly transcellular and mediated by stimulation of the thiazide-sensitive NaCl co-transporter, NCC.[132,133] However, there is also evidence that WNK4 regulates paracellular Cl permeability. WNK4 is localized to the tight junction in vivo.[131] When overexpressed in cell lines, WNK4 (particularly the PHAII mutant) stimulates paracellular Cl conductance.[68,70,134] The exact mechanism is unclear. There is evidence both for[68,70] and against[135] direct phosphorylation by WNK4 of several claudin isoforms, including claudins 4 and 7, that are normally expressed in the ASDN.

Tight Junction Dysfunction in Ischemic Acute Kidney Injury

Ischemic injury to the kidney causes reversible disruption of renal tubule epithelial barrier function and polarity. Renal ischemia or ATP depletion in humans, animal models, and cultured cells cause disruption of the tight junction,[30,136] with internalization of occludin, ZO-1 and -2, and cingulin.[137,138] Similar findings have been demonstrated in renal allografts with post-ischemic injury.[139] One consequence of this is loss of the epithelial barrier and backleak of filtrate into the interstitium,[139,140] which can partly explain the oliguria seen in severe acute kidney injury. Renal ischemia also impairs tight junction fence function, and disrupts epithelial polarity, including mislocalization of the Na-K-ATPase,[141,142] which would be predicted to impair transcellular tubular Na reabsorption. This probably contributes to the inappropriately elevated fractional excretion of Na (F_ENa) commonly observed clinically in ATN, and may also stimulate tubuloglomerular feedback, and thereby contribute to the reduction in GFR.

GAP JUNCTIONS AND CONNEXIN HEMICHANNELS

Structure and Biochemical Composition

Gap junctions are non-selective channels located in the plasma membranes of adjacent cells, and are critical to intercellular communication in most cell types. Functionally, they serve to couple non-excitable cells by allowing the passage of small molecules (less than 1 kDa in size), such as inorganic ions and secondary messengers, between the two cells.[143] Gap junction channels exhibit open and closed configurations, and this gating can be regulated by intracellular molecule concentration, mechanical stress, metabolic inhibition, and transjunctional voltage.[144−146]

Each half of the gap junction, known as a connexon, is composed of six transmembrane proteins from the connexin (Cx) family. There are 21 known human Cx isoforms, all of which present the same topology: intracellular N- and C-termini; four transmembrane domains; two extracellular loops with three cysteine residues; and a single intracellular loop. The N-terminus and position of the cysteine residues are conserved. Variability among the Cx isoforms is found in the intracellular loop and C-terminus. Consequently, these regions appear to be responsible for differences that exist in charge and size discrimination among isoforms.[143] Two styles of nomenclature identifying these isoforms are used. Cxs are most commonly identified by their molecular weight in kiloDaltons (e.g., Cx45), which presents a problem when discussing Cx expression in different species, as molecular weight of the same isoform can vary. Alternatively, Cx isoforms are sorted by class (alpha, beta, gamma), and assigned a number (e.g., Gja1).[147] For simplicity, we will adhere to the first naming convention throughout the chapter.

Connexons may be composed of a single isoform (homomeric) or a mix of Cxs (heteromeric), and their trafficking can occur by two pathways. The first involves formation of the connexon at the endoplasmic reticulum, with trafficking through the Golgi apparatus to the plasma membrane. Alternatively, Cx proteins may bypass the Golgi, and form the hexamer once in the plasma membrane. In either case, the transmembrane domains appear to be involved in the oligomerization process. Within the plasma membrane, connexons tend to group together to form a gap junction plaque. The plaque is a highly dynamic body, with gap junction protein half-life in the order of 2−5 hours. This allows for rapid regulation of the composition of Cxs within the plaque in response to cellular demands.[143] Docking of the connexons in adjacent cells creates the intercellular channel, and connexons of different Cx isoforms can couple to form heterotypic gap junctions. Since different Cx isoforms exhibit variation in terms of gating, regulation, and interaction, the modular and combinatorial nature of gap junctions allows a diversity of function within one type of channel.[148,149]

Beyond the typical intercellular gap junction structure, there is evidence that Cxs can regulate intercellular communication without directly coupling cells. Uncoupled connexons form transmembrane pores known as hemichannels, and these Cx hemichannels serve as a conduit between the intra- and extracellular environments, facilitating the transport of signaling molecules such as ATP.[150,151] They are gated, since a constitutively open channel would be lethal to the cell, and are regulated by the same factors as gap junctions.[146,152] Cx hemichannels are thought to conduct intercellular communication via calcium wave propagation. In this model, mechanical or chemical stimulation triggers the opening of Cx hemichannels in a cell which allows ATP to passively move through the hemichannel into the extracellular environment. The newly released ATP binds to purinergic receptors on local cells, triggering an increase in intracellular calcium levels in these cells, thereby propagating the calcium signal. The functionality of Cx hemichannels, however, remains controversial and it is difficult to prove their existence with certainty.[151]

Gap junctions play a vital role in many cellular processes in nearly every cell type in the body, facilitating normal development, physiology, and apoptosis. Consequently, Cx mutations are associated with pathophysiological conditions including Charcot Marie Tooth disease, congenital deafness, and the skin disease erythrokeratoderma variabilis.[147] Outside of hereditary conditions, complex diseases including diabetes and hypertension have been linked to changes in the expression of Cxs.[153−155]

Renal Localization

Renal intercellular channels were first identified in afferent arteriole vascular smooth muscle cells (VSMC) in the 1970s.[156] Electron microscopy images later provided evidence of gap junction channels in the renal tubules, as well as in the renal vasculature.[157,158] Specification of the Cx isoforms that made up renal gap junctions came later, with mRNA expression studies.[159–164] Localization of Cx proteins in the kidney has been limited by the availability of specific antibodies, and by variation among species. As a result, different studies present divergent results. More recently, the development of Cx knockout and reporter mouse models have provided new insight into the expression of Cxs within the nephron, as well as suggesting their significance in renal physiology.[165–170] Table 12.4 summarizes the renal localization of connexin isoforms.

Vasculature

The renal vasculature expresses Cxs37, 40, 43, and 45, which are found in all vascular systems.[159,166,171,172] Within vessels, gap junction coupling occurs between endothelial cells, between the smooth muscle cells, and at the myoendothelial junctions. Cx expression is best defined in endothelial cells. In rodents, Cx40 is abundantly expressed in the afferent arteriole endothelium, with lower levels of Cx37 and 43 also detected.[159,164,173] In the endothelial cells of the efferent arteriole, Cx37 is expressed in rat, while mice express Cx43.[172,173] Beyond the juxtaglomerular apparatus (JGA), all three isoforms are expressed in the vasa recta and vascular bundles.[173] Cx43 is also expressed in the peritubular capillaries and renal veins.[171,173]

The identity of the vascular smooth muscle Cx(s) is less clear. Cx37 was detected in the VSMCs of murine arcuate and interlobular arteries,[173] but not in rats.[159,174] Likewise, one study found evidence of Cx43 in the preglomular media,[161] but later reports have failed to confirm this.[159,164,174] Cx45, which is commonly expressed in smooth muscle cells in other vascular systems,[175] appears to exhibit the same characteristic localization in the kidney. Several studies have shown Cx45 expression in VSMCs of the interlobular, afferent, and efferent arterioles, both by immunohistochemistry and reporter gene mouse methods.[166,171,176] A lack of Cx40 expression in renal VSMCs has been shown in all studies.[159,164,173]

Glomerulus and Juxtaglomerular Apparatus

Both the glomerulus and juxtaglomerular apparatus (JGA) express gap junction proteins abundantly. Podocytes, endothelial cells, mesangial cells, and the renin-producing JG cells are all characterized by gap

TABLE 12.4 Summary of the Localization of Connexin Isoforms in the Kidney

Cx	Renal Localization	Cell Type	Species
26	Proximal tubule*	Epithelial	Mouse
30	Distal nephron	Epithelial	Rat
	Cortical CD, CNT	Intercalated	Mouse, rabbit, rat
30.3	ATL	Epithelial	Mouse, rabbit, rat
	Cortical CD	Intercalated	Mouse, rabbit, rat
32	Proximal tubule*	Epithelial	Mouse
37	Arcuate artery; IA*	VSMC	Mouse
	RA; AA, EA	Endothelial	Mouse, rat
	Vasa recta	Pericytes	Rat
	Vascular bundles	Endothelial	Mouse
	JGA*	Granular, mesangial	Mouse, rat
	Proximal tubule, TAL, DCT	Epithelial	Mouse, rat
	CNT, CD	Principal > Intercalated	Mouse, rat
40	RA; Arcuate artery; IA; AA	Endothelial	Mouse, rat
	Vasa recta	Endothelial	Rat
	Vascular bundles	Endothelial	Mouse
	Glomerulus	Endothelial*, mesangial	Mouse
	JGA	Endothelial*, granular, mesangial	Mouse, rat
43	RA, AA, EA	Endothelial, VSMC*	Mouse, rat
	Peritubular capillaries	Endothelial	Mouse
	Vascular bundles, vasa recta	Endothelial	Rat
	Renal veins	Endothelial	Mouse
	Glomerulus	Podocytes	Human
	Proximal tubule	Epithelial	Human
	Inner medullary CD*	Epithelial	Rat
45	IA, AA, EA	VSMC	Mouse
	Glomerulus	Mesangial, podocytes	Mouse
	JGA	Granular*, mesangial	Mouse

*indicates conflicting localization data; > indicates stronger than. (Table modified with permission from Hanner, F., Sorensen, C. M., Holstein-Rathlou, N. H. and Peti-Peterdi, J. (2010). Connexins and the kidney. Am. J. Physiol. Regul. Integr. Comp. Physiol. 298, R1143–1155. Copyright American Physiological Society).
ATL: Ascending thin limb of the loop of Henle; AA: afferent arteriole; CD: Collecting duct; CNT: connecting tubule; DCT: Distal convoluted tubule; EA: efferent arteriole; IA: interlobular artery. JGA: juxtaglomerular apparatus; RA: renal artery; TAL: thick ascending limb of the loop of Henle; VSMC: vascular smooth muscle cell.

junction coupling. In addition, the different cell types that constitute the JGA appear to be interconnected by gap junctions. The macula densa cells, however, are exclusive of gap junctions.[157,177] Again, Cx isoform localization has been primarily determined by antibody-based localization techniques, and as a result many studies present differing data. In podocytes, Cx43 is primarily expressed, although Cx45 has been detected in these cells as well.[178] Glomerular endothelial cells showed expression of Cx40 in one study,[164] but another report was unable to reproduce this finding.[173] Cx40 is, however, prominently expressed in the intra- and extraglomerular mesangium, as well as the renin-producing JG cells.[159,171–173] Cx37 follows a similar, if weaker, pattern of expression as Cx40. Expression in the intraglomerular mesangium is limited to the vascular pole, and lower levels of Cx37 staining are found in the extraglomerular mesangium and JG cells.[172,173] The glomerulus also appears to be positive for Cx45, and studies using reporter gene mouse models indicated Cx45 expression was localized to the mesangial cells. These studies also showed Cx45-positive cells expressing renin, leading to the conclusion that the JG cells express Cx45 alongside Cx40.[166] This study conflicts with antibody-based approaches, where Cx45 labeling is only evident in JG cells during embryogenesis.[171] Finally, the endothelial cells of the afferent and efferent arterioles closest to the glomerulus lack any Cx protein expression or structural evidence of gap junction coupling.[164]

Tubules

Despite the recognition of gap junction channels in the proximal tubules,[179] attempts to localize Cx isoforms along the nephron present a complex picture, with different techniques and species again producing varying expression patterns. In the proximal tubules, Cxs26, 37, and 43 have been detected in epithelial cells; however, proximal tubule Cx expression appears weak at best.[180,181] The distal tubules present much stronger levels of gap junction protein expression, but lack any signs of gap junction coupling by freeze-fracture microscopy.[182] While no Cx isoforms have been found in the descending limb of the loop of Henle, the ascending portion expresses Cxs30 and 30.3 in the apical membrane of the thin limb, and Cx37 in the basolateral membrane of the thick limb.[170,180,183] Continuing the pattern seen in Henle's loop Cx30, 30.3, and 37 are expressed along the connecting segment and collecting duct, and are similarly localized to the apical or basolateral membranes. Both Cx30 and Cx30.3 were detected in the intercalated, but not the principal, cells of connecting segment and cortical collecting duct.[170,180,183] The absence of gap junction coupling between epithelial cells, as well as their

subcellular localization to apical or basolateral membranes, suggests these Cx proteins may form hemichannels in this region of the nephron. This hypothesis appears to be supported by a study of primary proximal tubular cells that expressed Cx43 and demonstrated hemichannel activity.[182]

Physiological Function in the Kidney

As is the case with the localization of renal connexins, the physiological significance of gap junction proteins in the kidney is still emerging, and current research does not always present a consistent story. To study the functional roles of gap junction proteins in the kidney, both specific methods and non-specific inhibitors are used. In the latter category are chemical gap junction uncouplers and blockers, such as heptanol and carbenoxolone, that inhibit channel activity without regard to their component proteins.[184–186] More specific approaches focus on the Cx isoforms involved, and include the use of knockout mice and gap mimetic peptides.[187–190] These peptides mimic the extracellular loop sequence of Cx isoforms and block gap junction channels through an unknown mechanism.

Vascular Conduction and Myoendothelial Communication

One key area where gap junction coupling influences renal vascular physiology is in the propagation of a vasomotor response, either dilatory or constrictive, along vessels in response to local stimulation. In rat preglomerular arteries and vasa recta, vascular conducted responses are inhibited by the gap junction uncouplers carbenoxolone and 18α-glycyrrhetinic acid.[185,186] Interestingly, vasodilation and vasoconstriction responses appear to involve gap junctions via independent mechanisms. Studies with Cx40 knockout mice and Cx40 mimetic peptides both demonstrated an inhibitory effect of Cx40 loss on vasodilation in mesenteric arteries.[188,190] Conversely, Cx37, but not Cx40, knockout mice have reduced vasoconstriction responses.[190]

Vasomotor stimulation may also spread between the endothelium and the smooth muscle cells of renal vessels via myoendothelial gap junctions. Vasodilation of smooth muscle occurs in response to the hyperpolarization of endothelial cells, and this response can be inhibited by non-specific gap junction blockers in rabbit renal arteries.[184] A similar effect was observed with Cx40 and Cx43 mimetic peptides; however, the inhibition appears to be dependent on the agonist used.[187,189]

Tubuloglomerular Feedback and Renin Secretion

The JGA regulates renal hemodynamics through the mechanism of tubuloglomerular feedback (TGF), whereby variations in tubular fluid flow and composition in the cortical thick ascending limb are detected by the macula densa cells, and trigger changes in afferent arteriole diameter and renin secretion in response (see also Chapter 24). The TGF mechanism involves a calcium wave (Figure 12.8) which propagates through the JGA.[191] The regulation of calcium signaling by Cxs is well-established in other systems,[143] and given the extensive gap junction coupling in the JGA it appears that this calcium wave is similarly controlled. The gap junction uncoupler 18α-glycyrrhetinic acid and heptanol inhibit the spread of calcium in the JGA in response to an increase in flow.[191] Two possible pathways explain how gap junction proteins coordinate calcium signaling in the JGA. Calcium may spread in coupled cells directly via intercellular gap junction communication. Alternatively, the calcium wave may propagate indirectly via purinergic signaling. In this model, increased intracellular calcium triggers the opening of Cx hemichannels and the release of ATP/ UTP to the extracellular environment, which subsequently binds purinergic receptors on neighboring cells, increasing intracellular $[Ca^{2+}]$.[192] Several

observations point to the latter mechanism. Removal of direct contact between cells did not inhibit calcium signaling, and stimulation of cells led to the release of ATP, as measured by a biosensor cell technique. The use of purinergic receptor blockers and ATP scavengers also inhibited the JGA calcium wave.[191,193] Both Cx40 and Cx45 appear to function in the JGA calcium wave. Cx40 siRNA reduced calcium signaling in glomerular endothelial cells, while VSMCs isolated from a conditional Cx45 knockout mouse model or treated with a Cx45 gap mimetic peptide showed reduced propagation speed.[166,193]

Renin secretion regulation and control of systemic blood pressure also require gap junction protein expression. Cx40 knockout mice have high blood pressure and high plasma renin, due primarily to the lack of negative feedback control of renin secretion by blood pressure and angiotensin II. Regulation of renin by beta adrenergic receptor stimulation and dietary salt is not affected.[194,195] These mice also show aberrant expression of renin in the preglomerular interstitium, extraglomerular mesangium, and glomerular tuft, while the afferent arteriole VSMCs are entirely devoid of renin. Cx45-deficient mice, which lack Cx45 in afferent and efferent VSMCs, renin-producing granular cells, and mesangium have a similar phenotype as the Cx40 knockout mouse.[166] Replacement of Cx40 by Cx45 (Cx40KI45) results in a reduction of blood pressure and the return of renin regulation. Normal renin cell recruitment in response to a low-salt diet is not restored.[176] These results indicate that cell–cell communication via Cx channels is critical to renin secretion, and that specifically Cx40 is required for renin expression. Cx37 knockout mice have normal renin regulation, while Cx43 knockout models are lethal. Replacement of Cx43 by Cx32 (Cx43KI32) resulted in reduced plasma renin content, loss of renin regulation, and *de novo* renin expression in endothelial cells.[196] An endothelial-specific Cx43 knockout model, however, does not show any changes to renin secretion.[197]

Tubule Function

The role of Cxs in tubular function remains largely unclear despite the expression of Cx proteins along the nephron and gap junction coupling in the proximal tubules. The expression of Cxs 30 and 37 is regulated by dietary salt, with high salt increasing Cx30 expression at the apical membrane of medullary collecting ducts, and low salt increasing cortical expression of Cx37, presumably along basolateral membranes.[180,183] It is hypothesized that Cx hemichannels regulate epithelial transport along the nephron via purinergic signaling (Figure 12.9). Activation of P2 purinergic receptors in the nephron is known to regulate renal transporters, modulating sodium, potassium, and

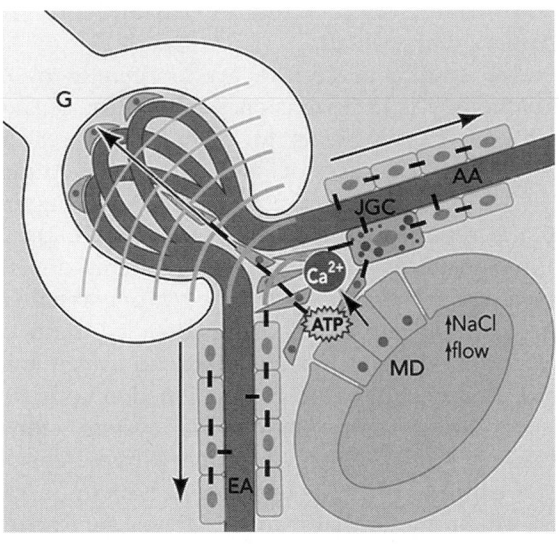

FIGURE 12.8 Role of gap junctions in the juxtaglomerular apparatus. Components of the TGF calcium wave include ATP release from macula densa (MD) cells in response to elevations in tubular NaCl and/or flow rate, and paracrine, purinergic calcium signaling. Extracellular ATP-induced elevations in mesangial, vascular smooth muscle (VSMC), and renin-producing juxtaglomerular cell (JGC) $[Ca^{2+}]_i$ are then propagated via gap junctions to distant cells of the afferent arteriole (AA), efferent arteriole (EA), and glomerulus (G) away from the MD region, causing cell contractions. All cell types of the JGA are abundant in gap junctions (−), except for the cells of the MD. Vascular endothelial cells in the AA, EA, and G are also connected with each other and JGCs and VSMCs via gap junctions, and are involved in the calcium wave of TGF. *(Figure modified from Peti-Peterdi, J., Toma, I., Sipos, A. and Vargas, S. L. (2009). Multiphoton imaging of renal regulatory mechanisms. Physiology (Bethesda)* **24***, 88–96. Copyright American Physiological Society.)*

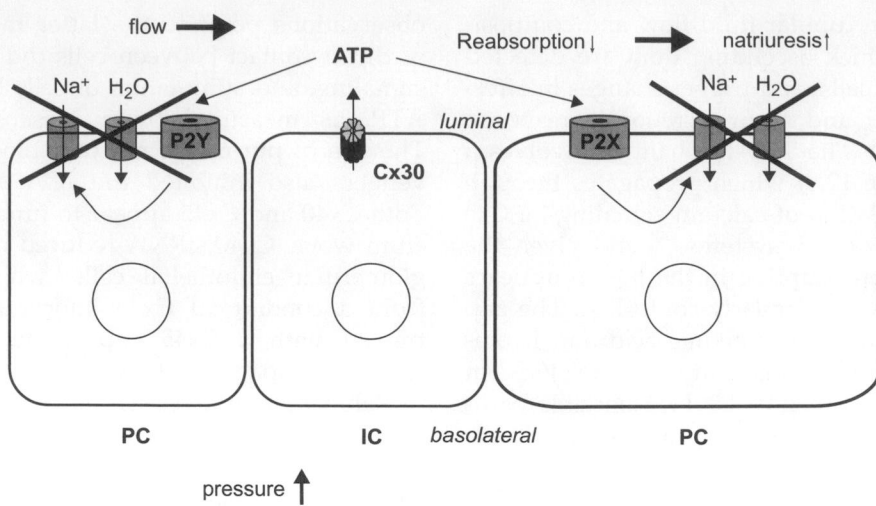

FIGURE 12.9 **Schematic illustration of mechanically induced, Cx30 hemichannel-mediated ATP release into the tubular lumen in the cortical collecting duct (CCD), and its paracrine effects on salt and water reabsorption, natriuresis, and diuresis.** Increases in intra-renal pressure and/or tubular flow rate that accompany blood pressure elevations result in the opening of Cx30 hemichannels at the luminal membrane of CCD intercalated cells (IC), and the release of ATP. Stimulation of luminal purinergic receptors (mainly P_2Y_2) in adjacent principal cells (PC) results in the inhibition of salt and water reabsorption, and increased natriuresis and diuresis. This inhibitory mechanism is absent in $Cx30^{-/-}$ mice, resulting in a salt retention phenotype. *(Reproduced with permission from Sipos et al. (2009). J. Am. Soc. Nephrol. **20**(8), 1724–1732.[10])*

water reabsorption.[198–200] The close proximity of ecto-nucleotidases and purinergic receptors in the tubular lumen implies local release of ATP.[199,201] Supporting this hypothesis is recent data which shows that Cx30 knockout mice have an impaired pressure natriuresis response, and that at the cellular level, isolated cortical collecting ducts from these mice release less ATP in response to stimulation than their wild-type counterparts. Based on these findings, the study presented a model suggesting a mechanism by which Cx30 plays a role in pressure natriuresis. Increased pressure/flow in the collecting ducts induces the opening of Cx30 hemichannels, allowing ATP to enter the local extracellular environment and bind local P2 receptors. Activation of these receptors inhibits salt and water reabsorption, resulting in homeostasis.[167]

Roles in Renal Pathology

In the kidney, the role that Cxs plays in pathology is relatively unknown and mostly hypothetical. Human mutations in gap junction genes are linked to a variety of diseases, with altered expression of Cxs leading to the pathophysiology observed. Moreover, primary diseases can result in changes to the levels and localization of gap junction proteins. Global genetic knockouts of several Cx genes are embryonically lethal, indicating their importance during development.[147] Despite the widespread expression of gap junctions in the kidney, mutations in Cx genes have only minor effects on renal organogenesis.[202] As described above, Cx40 knockout

mice show defects in JGA renin localization, but this is only apparent after birth.[168]

In adult mutant mice, the predominantly observed renal pathology is hypertension. Genetic loss of Cx40 or Cx45 in the kidney leads to high blood pressure in mice, as does the use of gap mimetic peptides in rats.[166,172,194,195] Knockin mice in which the coding region of Cx43 is replaced by that of Cx32 (Cx43KI32) have a protective phenotype, failing to develop renin-dependent hypertension in response to clipping one renal artery (two-kidney, one-clip model).[196] As detailed in the previous section, it appears that the effect on systemic blood pressure is due to the loss of gap junction communication, preventing renin–angiotensin system signaling. There is no known effect of primary hypertension on renal Cx expression in rats or mice. In humans, a variant in the Cx40 promoter that results in lower gene activity is associated with increased risk of high blood pressure, but it is unclear what mechanism drives this correlation.[203]

An increase in vascular intercellular communication and changes in renal Cx expression are also associated with diabetes.[204,205] In diabetic mice, endothelial cells express Cx40 in place of Cx37, and Cx43 is expressed in renin-producing cells *de novo*. The link between Cx expression and diabetes appears to be the nitric oxide (NO) pathway. Diabetes is associated with increased NO availability, and when diabetes was induced in endothelial nitric oxide synthase (eNOS) knockout mice, no changes in Cx expression were observed. Overexpression of eNOS caused changes in renal Cx expression which mimic the pattern seen in diabetes.[173]

ADHERENS JUNCTIONS AND DESMOSOMES

The adherens junction and desmosome are considered together here, because they share a similar function—to maintain the physical association between cells—and similar arrangements of their molecular components. These junctions are found in all epithelia, and there is little about them that is unique to the kidney, so we summarize here the general features of adherens junctions and desmosomes, and refer the reader to several recent reviews for more in-depth discussions.[206,207]

Structure and Localization of the Adherens Junction

The adherens junction in epithelia spans the lateral plasma membranes of adjacent cells at a distance of 10—20 nm, and forms a continuous belt around the circumference of each cell (the "zonula adherens")[206] (Figure 12.2a). The calcium-dependent component is formed by a classical (Type I) cadherin (such as E-cadherin or N-cadherin), a transmembrane protein whose extracellular domain undergoes homophilic adhesion in the presence of calcium, and whose cytoplasmic domain binds to p120-catenin and either β- or γ-catenin (plakoglobin) (Figure 12.10a). These catenins in turn associate with a number of other cytosolic proteins (e.g., α-catenin), some of which are responsible for anchoring the adherens junction to the actin cytoskeleton. In addition, there is a calcium-independent component to the adherens junction, which is formed by members of the nectin family of transmembrane proteins. Nectins, like cadherins, interact via their extracellular domains, although preferentially in a heterotypic manner. Their cytoplasmic terminal has a PDZ-binding motif that associates with afadin (AF6), which can either bind actin directly or indirectly via α-catenin and its partners.

As alluded to in the introduction to this chapter, the mature glomerular slit diaphragm expresses several adherens junction proteins,[208] including P-cadherin, FAT,[209] α-, β-, and γ-catenin, and so it has been proposed to represent a modified adherens junction.[208] In the adult renal tubule, there is differential localization of classical cadherins. The proximal tubule predominantly expresses N-cadherin; the thick ascending limb, distal tubule, and collecting duct predominantly express E-cadherin; and Bowman's capsule and the thin limbs of Henle express both isoforms.[210–212] However, the functional significance of this is unknown. In contrast, the cytoplasmic catenins are ubiquitously expressed in all tubule segments.[213]

Structure and Localization of Desmosomes

Desmosomes are specialized anchoring junctions that serve as tethers for cytoplasmic intermediate filaments.[207] While they are particularly important for maintaining the integrity of tissues subject to mechanical stress, such as the epidermis and myocardium, they are also present in all epithelia and are thought to play roles in tissue morphogenesis. Desmosomes appear as

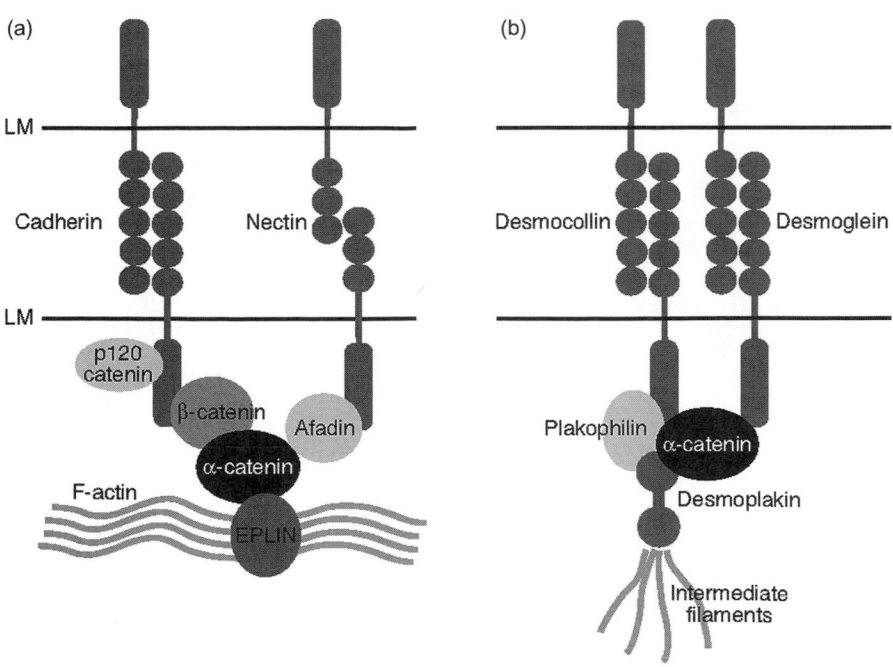

FIGURE 12.10 Molecular components of the adherens junction (a) and desmosome (b). LM: lateral plasma membrane.

pairs of dense, disc-shaped plaques on opposing lateral membranes of adjacent cells (Figure 12.2a). The desmosomal cadherins, desmoglein and desmocollin, mediate cell—cell adhesion via their extracellular domains (Figure 12.10b). The armadillo proteins, plakoglobin/γ-catenin, and plakophilin act as adaptor proteins that link the cytoplasmic domain of the desmosomal cadherins to desmoplakin, which in turn links the desmosomal plaque to the intermediate filament cytoskeleton.

In mice, desmoplakin and plakoglobin are expressed at highest levels in the distal tubule, connecting tubule, and collecting duct,[211] whereas in humans, plakoglobin, like other catenins, is expressed along the entire nephron.[213]

Adherens and Desmosomal Junctions in Kidney Disease

In ischemic acute kidney injury, as discussed earlier, there is disruption of the tight junction. This is also associated with degradation of E-cadherin, and dissolution of the adherens junction complex.[139,214] Polycystin-1, the product of the gene PKD1 that is mutated in autosomal dominant polycystic kidney disease (ADPKD), is localized to adherens junctions and desmosomes in renal epithelia, and participates in cell—cell adhesion.[215] In ADPKD, both adherens and desmosomal junctions are abnormal in morphology.[216] Most of the cysts are of distal tubule origin, yet they lack E-cadherin at the adherens junction, and N-cadherin is expressed in its place.[217]

References

[1] Farquhar MG, Palade GE. Junctional complexes in various epithelia. J Cell Biol 1963;17:375—412.

[2] Kachar B, Reese TS. Evidence for the lipidic nature of tight junction strands. Nature 1982;296(5856):464—6.

[3] Pinto da Silva P, Kachar B. On tight-junction structure. Cell 1982;28(3):441—50.

[4] Stevenson BR, Goodenough DA. Zonulae occludentes in junctional complex-enriched fractions from mouse liver: preliminary morphological and biochemical characterization. J Cell Biol 1984;98(4):1209—21.

[5] van Meer G, Gumbiner B, Simons K. The tight junction does not allow lipid molecules to diffuse from one epithelial cell to the next. Nature 1986;322(6080):639—41.

[6] van Meer G, Simons K. The function of tight junctions in maintaining differences in lipid composition between the apical and the basolateral cell surface domains of MDCK cells. EMBO J 1986;5(7):1455—64.

[7] Nichols GE, Borgman CA, Young Jr. WW. On tight junction structure: Forssman glycolipid does not flow between MDCK cells in an intact epithelial monolayer. Biochem Biophys Res Commun 1986;138(3):1163—9.

[8] Brown D, Orci L. Junctional complexes and cell polarity in the urinary tubule. J Electron Microsc Tech 1988;9(2):145—70.

[9] Orci L, Humbert F, Brown D, Perrelet A. Membrane ultrastructure in urinary tubules. Int Rev Cytol 1981;73:183—242.

[10] Taugner R, Boll U, Zahn P, Forssmann WG. Cell junctions in the epithelium of Bowman's capsule. Cell Tissue Res 1976;172(4):431—46.

[11] Kuhn K, Reale E, Wermbter G. The glomeruli of the human and the rat kidney studied by freeze-fracturing. Cell Tissue Res 1975;160(2):177—91.

[12] Humbert F, Montesano R, Perrelet A, Orci L. Junctions in developing human and rat kidney: a freeze-fracture study. J Ultrastruct Res 1976;56(2):202—14.

[13] Reeves W, Caulfield JP, Farquhar MG. Differentiation of epithelial foot processes and filtration slits: sequential appearance of occluding junctions, epithelial polyanion, and slit membranes in developing glomeruli. Lab Invest 1978;39(2):90—100.

[14] Caulfield JP, Reid JJ, Farquhar MG. Alterations of the glomerular epithelium in acute aminonucleoside nephrosis. Evidence for formation of occluding junctions and epithelial cell detachment. Lab Invest 1976;34(1):43—59.

[15] Ryan GB, Leventhal M, Karnovsky MJ. A freeze-fracture study of the junctions between glomerular epithelial cells in aminonucleoside nephrosis. Lab Invest 1975;32(3):397—403.

[16] Pricam C, Humbert F, Perrelet A, Amherdt M, Orci L. Intercellular junctions in podocytes of the nephrotic glomerulus as seen with freeze-fracture. Lab Invest 1975;33(3):209—18.

[17] Claude P. Morphological factors influencing transepithelial permeability: a model for the resistance of the zonula occludens. J Membr Biol 1978;39:219—32.

[18] Kaye GI, Pappas GD. Studies on the cornea. I. The fine structure of the rabbit cornea and the uptake and transport of colloidal particles by the cornea in vivo. J Cell Biol 1962;12:457—79.

[19] Martinez-Palomo A, Erlij D, Bracho H. Localization of permeability barriers in the frog skin epithelium. J Cell Biol 1971;50(2):277—87.

[20] Rau WS, Fromter E. Electrical properties of the medullary collecting ducts of the golden hamster kidney. II. The transepithelial resistance. Pflugers Arch 1974;351(2):113—31.

[21] Isaacson LC. Resolution of parameters in the equivalent electrical circuit of the sodium transport mechanism across toad skin. J Membr Biol 1977;30(4):301—17.

[22] Rector Jr FC, Martinez-Maldonado M, Brunner FP, Seldin DW. Evidence for passive reabsorption of NaCl in proximal tubule of rat kidney. J Clin Invest 1966;45:1060—70.

[23] Bourdeau JE, Burg MB. Voltage dependence of calcium transport in the thick ascending limb of Henle's loop. Am J Physiol 1979;236:F357—64.

[24] Barry PH, Diamond JM, Wright EM. The mechanism of cation permeation in the rabbit gallbladder: dilution potentials and biionic potentials. J Membr Biol 1971;4:358—94.

[25] Wright EM, Barry PH, Diamond JM. The mechanism of cation permeation in the rabbit gallbladder: conductances, the current—voltage relation, the concentration dependence of anion—cation discrimination, and the calcium competition effect. J Membr Biol 1971;4:331—57.

[26] Fromter E, Diamond J. Route of passive ion permeation in epithelia. Nat New Biol 1972;235(53):9—13.

[27] Wang Q, Margolis B. Apical junctional complexes and cell polarity. Kidney Int 2007;72(12):1448—58.

[28] Goldstein B, Macara IG. The PAR proteins: fundamental players in animal cell polarization. Dev Cell 2007;13(5):609—22.

[29] Dragsten PR, Blumenthal R, Handler JS. Membrane asymmetry in epithelia: Is the tight junction a barrier to diffusion in the plasma membrane? Nature 1981;294(5843):718—22.

[30] Bacallao R, Garfinkel A, Monke S, Zampighi G, Mandel LJ. ATP depletion: a novel method to study junctional properties

in epithelial tissues. I. Rearrangement of the actin cytoskeleton. J Cell Sci 1994;107(Pt 12):3301—13.

[31] Mandel LJ, Bacallao R, Zampighi G. Uncoupling of the molecular "fence" and paracellular "gate" functions in epithelial tight junctions. Nature 1993;361(6412):552—5.

[32] Takakuwa R, Kokai Y, Kojima T, Akatsuta T, Tobioka H, Sawada N, et al. Uncoupling of gate and fence functions of MDCK cells by the actin-depolymerizing reagent mycalolide B. Exp Cell Res 2000;257(2):238—44.

[33] Stevenson BR, Siliciano JD, Mooseker MS, Goodenough DA. Identification of ZO-1: a high molecular weight polypeptide associated with the tight junction (zonula occludens) in a variety of epithelia. J Cell Biol 1986;103(3):755—66.

[34] Furuse M, Hirase T, Itoh M, Nagafuchi A, Yonemura S, Tsukita S, et al. Occludin: a novel integral membrane protein localizing at tight junctions [see comments]. J Cell Biol 1993;123(6 Pt 2):1777—88.

[35] Balda MS, Whitney JA, Flores C, Gonzalez S, Cereijido M, Matter K. Functional dissociation of paracellular permeability and transepithelial electrical resistance and disruption of the apical—basolateral intramembrane diffusion barrier by expression of a mutant tight junction membrane protein. J Cell Biol 1996;134(4):1031—49.

[36] McCarthy KM, Francis SA, McCormack JM, Lai J, Rogers RA, Skare IB, et al. Inducible expression of claudin-1-myc but not occludin-VSV-G results in aberrant tight junction strand formation in MDCK cells. J Cell Sci 2000;113:3387—98.

[37] Saitou M, Fujimoto K, Doi Y, Itoh M, Fujimoto T, Furuse M, et al. Occludin-deficient embryonic stem cells can differentiate into polarized epithelial cells bearing tight junctions. J Cell Biol 1998;141(2):397—408.

[38] Yu AS, McCarthy KM, Francis SA, McCormack JM, Lai J, Rogers RA, et al. Knockdown of occludin expression leads to diverse phenotypic alterations in epithelial cells. Am J Physiol Cell Physiol 2005;288(6):C1231—1241.

[39] Furuse M, Sasaki H, Fujimoto K, Tsukita S. A single gene product, claudin-1 or -2, reconstitutes tight junction strands and recruits occludin in fibroblasts. J Cell Biol 1998;143(2):391—401.

[40] Saitou M, Furuse M, Sasaki H, Schulzke JD, Fromm M, Takano H, et al. Complex phenotype of mice lacking occludin, a component of tight junction strands. Mol Biol Cell 2000;11(12):4131—42.

[41] Schulzke JD, Gitter AH, Mankertz J, Speigel S, Siedler U, Amashe S, et al. Epithelial transport and barrier function in occludin-deficient mice. Biochim Biophys Acta 2005;1669 (1):34—42.

[42] Ikenouchi J, Furuse M, Furuse K, Sasaki H, Tsukita S. Tricellulin constitutes a novel barrier at tricellular contacts of epithelial cells. J Cell Biol 2005;171(6):939—45.

[43] Krug SM, Amasheh S, Richter JF, Milatz S, Gunzel D, Westphal JK, et al. Tricellulin forms a barrier to macromolecules in tricellular tight junctions without affecting ion permeability. Mol Biol Cell 2009;20(16):3713—24.

[44] Riazuddin S, Ahmed ZM, Fanning AS, Lagzeil A, Kitajiri S, Ramzan K, et al. Tricellulin is a tight-junction protein necessary for hearing. Am J Hum Genet 2006;79(6):1040—51.

[45] Furuse M, Fujita K, Hiiragi T, Fujimoto K, Tsukita S. Claudin-1 and -2: novel integral membrane proteins localizing at tight junctions with no sequence similarity to occludin. J Cell Biol 1998;141(7):1539—50.

[46] Furuse M, Tsukita S. Claudins in occluding junctions of humans and flies. Trends Cell Biol 2006;16(4):181—8.

[47] Van Itallie CM, Anderson JM. Claudins and epithelial paracellular transport. Annu Rev Physiol 2006;68:403—29.

[48] Angelow S, Ahlstrom R, Yu AS. Biology of claudins. Am J Physiol Renal Physiol 2008;295(4):F867—876.

[49] Kubota K, Furuse M, Sasaki H, Sonoda N, Fujita K, Nagafuchi A, et al. Ca(2 +)-independent cell-adhesion activity of claudins, a family of integral membrane proteins localized at tight junctions. Curr Biol 1999;9(18):1035—8.

[50] Simon DB, Lu Y, Choate KA, Velazquez H, El-Sabban E, Praga M, et al. Paracellin-1, a renal tight junction protein required for paracellular Mg^{2+} resorption. Science 1999;285:103—6.

[51] Van Itallie CM, Anderson JM. Claudins and epithelial paracellular transport. Annu Rev Physiol 2005.

[52] Colegio OR, Van Itallie CM, McCrea HJ, Rahner C, Anderson JM. Claudins create charge-selective channels in the paracellular pathway between epithelial cells. Am J Physiol Cell Physiol 2002;283(1):C142—147.

[53] Colegio OR, Van Itallie C, Rahner C, Anderson JM. Claudin extracellular domains determine paracellular charge selectivity and resistance but not tight junction fibril architecture. Am J Physiol Cell Physiol 2003;284(6):C1346—1354.

[54] Yu AS, Cheng MH, Angelow S, Gunzel D, Kanzawa SA, Schneeberger EE, et al. Molecular basis for cation selectivity in claudin-2-based paracellular pores: identification of an electrostatic interaction site. J Gen Physiol 2009;133(1):111—27.

[55] Angelow S, Yu AS. Structure—function studies of claudin extracellular domains by cysteine-scanning mutagenesis. J Biol Chem 2009;284(42):29205—17.

[56] Piontek J, Winkler L, Wolburg H, Muller SL, Zuleger N, Piehl C, et al. Formation of tight junction: determinants of homophilic interaction between classic claudins. Faseb J 2008;22(1):146—58.

[57] Ruffer C, Gerke V. The C-terminal cytoplasmic tail of claudins 1 and 5 but not its PDZ-binding motif is required for apical localization at epithelial and endothelial tight junctions. Eur J Cell Biol 2004;83(4):135—44.

[58] Arabzadeh A, Troy TC, Turksen K. Role of the Cldn6 cytoplasmic tail domain in membrane targeting and epidermal differentiation in vivo. Mol Cell Biol 2006;26(15):5876—87.

[59] Van Itallie CM, Colegio OR, Anderson JM. The cytoplasmic tails of claudins can influence tight junction barrier properties through effects on protein stability. J Membr Biol 2004;199(1):29—38.

[60] Itoh M, Furuse M, Morita K, Kubota K, Saitou M, Tsukita S. Direct binding of three tight junction-associated MAGUKs, ZO-1, ZO-2, and ZO-3, with the COOH termini of claudins. J Cell Biol 1999;147(6):1351—63.

[61] Hamazaki Y, Itoh M, Sasaki H, Furuse M, Tsukita S. Multi-PDZ domain protein 1 (MUPP1) is concentrated at tight junctions through its possible interaction with claudin-1 and junctional adhesion molecule. J Biol Chem 2002;277(1):455—61.

[62] Jeansonne B, Lu Q, Goodenough DA, Chen YH. Claudin-8 interacts with multi-PDZ domain protein 1 (MUPP1) and reduces paracellular conductance in epithelial cells. Cell Mol Biol (Noisy-le-grand) 2003;49(1):13—21.

[63] Kobayashi J, Inai T, Shibata Y. Formation of tight junction strands by expression of claudin-1 mutants in their ZO-1 binding site in MDCK cells. Histochem Cell Biol 2002;117(1):29—39.

[64] González-Mariscal L, Garay E, Quirós M. Regulation of claudins by post-translational modifications and cell signaling cascades. In: Yu AS, editor. Claudins, vol 65. Philadelphia, PA: Elsevier; 2010. p. 113—50.

[65] Ishizaki T, Chiba H, Kojima T, Fujibe M, Soma T, Miyajima H, et al. Cyclic AMP induces phosphorylation of claudin-5 immunoprecipitates and expression of claudin-5 gene in blood—brain-barrier endothelial cells via protein kinase A-dependent and -independent pathways. Exp Cell Res 2003;290(2):275—88.

[66] Ikari A, Matsumoto S, Harada H, Takagi K, Hayashi H, Suzuki Y, et al. Phosphorylation of paracellin-1 at Ser217 by protein kinase A is essential for localization in tight junctions. J Cell Sci 2006;119(Pt 9):1781–9.

[67] Tanaka M, Kamata R, Sakai R. EphA2 phosphorylates the cytoplasmic tail of Claudin-4 and mediates paracellular permeability. J Biol Chem 2005;280(51):42375–82.

[68] Yamauchi K, Rai T, Kobayashi K, Sohara E, Suzuki T, Itoh T, et al. Disease-causing mutant WNK4 increases paracellular chloride permeability and phosphorylates claudins. Proc Natl Acad Sci USA 2004;101(13):4690–4.

[69] Le Moellic C, Boulkroun S, Gonzalez-Nunez D, Dublineau I, Cluzead F, Fay M, et al. Aldosterone and tight junctions: modulation of claudin-4 phosphorylation in renal collecting duct cells. Am J Physiol Cell Physiol 2005;289(6): C1513–1521.

[70] Tatum R, Zhang Y, Lu Q, Kim K, Jeansonne BG, Chen YH. WNK4 phosphorylates ser(206) of claudin-7 and promotes paracellular Cl(−) permeability. FEBS Lett 2007;581 (20):3887–91.

[71] Van Itallie CM, Gambling TM, Carson JL, Anderson JM. Palmitoylation of claudins is required for efficient tight-junction localization. J Cell Sci 2005;118(Pt 7):1427–36.

[72] Kiuchi-Saishin Y, Gotoh S, Furuse M, Takasuga A, Tano Y, Tsukita S. Differential expression patterns of claudins, tight junction membrane proteins, in mouse nephron segments. J Am Soc Nephrol 2002;13(4):875–86.

[73] Ohse T, Pippin JW, Vaughan MR, Brinkkoetter PT, Krofft RD, Shankland SJ. Establishment of conditionally immortalized mouse glomerular parietal epithelial cells in culture. J Am Soc Nephrol 2008;19(10):1879–90.

[74] Inai T, Kobayashi J, Shibata Y. Claudin-1 contributes to the epithelial barrier function in MDCK cells. Eur J Cell Biol 1999;78(12):849–55.

[75] Crabtree C. Sex differences in the structure of Bowman's capsule in the mouse. Science 1940;91(2360):299.

[76] Dietert SC. The columnar cells occurring in the parietal layer of Bowman's capsule. Cellular fine structure and protein transport. J Cell Biol 1967;35(2):435–44.

[77] Enck AH, Berger UV, Yu AS. Claudin-2 is selectively expressed in proximal nephron in mouse kidney. Am J Physiol Renal Physiol 2001;281(5):F966–974.

[78] Ohse T, Chang AM, Pippin JW, Jarad G, Hudkins KL, Alpers CE, et al. A new function for parietal epithelial cells: a second glomerular barrier. Am J Physiol Renal Physiol 2009;297(6):F1566–1574.

[79] Torelli G, Milla E, Faelli A, Costantini S. Energy requirement for sodium reabsorption in the in vivo rabbit kidney. Am J Physiol 1966;211(3):576–80.

[80] Knox FG, Fleming JS, Rennie DW. Effects of osmotic diuresis on sodium reabsorption and oxygen consumption of kidney. Am J Physiol 1966;210(4):751–9.

[81] Berry CA, Rector Jr. FC. Mechanism of proximal NaCl reabsorption in the proximal tubule of the mammalian kidney. Semin Nephrol 1991;11(2):86–97.

[82] Kokko JP, Burg MB, Orloff J. Characteristics of NaCl and water transport in the renal proximal tubule. J Clin Invest 1971;50(1):69–76.

[83] Schafer JA, Troutman SL, Andreoli TE. Volume reabsorption, transepithelial potential differences, and ionic permeability properties in mammalian superficial proximal straight tubules. J Gen Physiol 1974;64(5):582–607.

[84] Neumann KH, Rector Jr. FC. Mechanism of NaCl and water reabsorption in the proximal convoluted tubule of rat kidney. J Clin Invest 1976;58(5):1110–1.

[85] Krug SM, Gunzel D, Conrad MP, et al. Claudin-17 forms tight junction channels with distinct anion selectivity. Cell Mol Life Sci 2012;69(20):2765–78.

[86] Furuse M, Furuse K, Sasaki H, Tsukita S. Conversion of zonulae occludentes from tight to leaky strand type by introducing claudin-2 into Madin–Darby canine kidney I cells. J Cell Biol 2001;153(2):263–72.

[87] Amasheh S, Meiri N, Gitter AH, Schoneberg T, Mankertz J, Schulzke JD, et al. Claudin-2 expression induces cation-selective channels in tight junctions of epithelial cells. J Cell Sci 2002;115(Pt 24):4969–76.

[88] Van Itallie C, Fanning AS, Anderson JM. Reversal of charge selectivity in cation or anion selective epithelial lines by expression of different claudins. Am J Physiol Cell Physiol 2003;286:F1078–1084.

[89] Muto S, Hata M, Taniguchi J, Tsururoka S, Moriwaki K, Saitou M, et al. Claudin-2-deficient mice are defective in the leaky and cation-selective paracellular permeability properties of renal proximal tubules. Proc Natl Acad Sci USA 2010;107(17):8011–6.

[90] Van Itallie CM, Rogan S, Yu AS, Seminario-Vidal L, Holmes J, Anderson JM. Two splice variants of claudin-10 in the kidney create paracellular pores with different ion selectivities. Am J Physiol Renal Physiol 2006;291:F1288–1299.

[91] Quigley R, Baum M. Developmental changes in rabbit proximal straight tubule paracellular permeability. Am J Physiol Renal Physiol 2002;283(3):F525–531.

[92] Abuazza G, Becker A, Williams SS, Chakravarty S, Truong HT, Lin F, et al. Claudins 6, 9, and 13 are developmentally expressed renal tight junction proteins. Am J Physiol Renal Physiol 2006;291:F1132–1141.

[93] Sas D, Hu M, Moe OW, Baum M. Effect of claudins 6 and 9 on paracellular permeability in MDCK II cells. Am J Physiol Regul Integr Comp Physiol 2008;295(5):R1713–1719.

[94] Schnermann J, Chou CL, Ma T, Traynor T, Knepper MA, Verkman AS. Defective proximal tubular fluid reabsorption in transgenic aquaporin-1 null mice. Proc Natl Acad Sci USA 1998;95(16):9660–4.

[95] Ullrich KJ, Rumrich G, Schmidt-Nielsen B. Reflection coefficient of different nonelectrolytes in the proximal convolution of the rat kidney. Federation Proc 1967;26:375.

[96] Weinstein AM. Transport by epithelia with compliant lateral intercellular spaces: asymmetric oncotic effects across the rat proximal tubule. Am J Physiol 1984;247(5 Pt 2):F848–862.

[97] Preisig PA, Berry CA. Evidence for transcellular osmotic water flow in rat proximal tubules. Am J Physiol 1985;249(1 Pt 2): F124–131.

[98] Kovbasnjuk O, Leader JP, Weinstein AM, Spring KR. Water does not flow across the tight junctions of MDCK cell epithelium. Proc Natl Acad Sci USA 1998;95(11):6526–30.

[99] Rosenthal R, Milatz S, Krug SM. et al. The tight junction protein claudin-2 forms a paracellular water channel. (Abstr); New Orleans 2009 [Paper presented at: Experimental Biology Annual Meeting].

[100] Gunzel D, Yu AS. Function and regulation of claudins in the thick ascending limb of Henle. Pflugers Arch 2009;458 (1):77–88.

[101] Burg MB, Green N. Function of the thick ascending limb of Henle's loop. Am J Physiol 1973;224(3):659–68.

[102] Greger R. Cation selectivity of the isolated perfused cortical thick ascending limb of Henle's loop of rabbit kidney. Pflugers Arch 1981;390(1):30–7.

[103] Greger R. Chloride reabsorption in the rabbit cortical thick ascending limb of the loop of Henle. A sodium dependent process. Pflugers Arch 1981;390(1):38–43.

[104] Burg M, Good D. Sodium chloride coupled transport in mammalian nephrons. Annu Rev Physiol 1983;45:533—47.

[105] Angelow S, El-Husseini R, Kanzawa SA, Yu AS. Renal localization and function of the tight junction protein, claudin-19. Am J Physiol Renal Physiol 2007;293(1):F166—177.

[106] Konrad M, Schaller A, Seelow D, et al. Mutations in the tight-junction gene claudin 19 (CLDN19) are associated with renal magnesium wasting, renal failure, and severe ocular involvement. Am J Hum Genet 2006;79(5):949—57.

[107] Hou J, Renigunta A, Gomes AS, Hou M, Paul DL, Waldegger S, et al. Claudin-16 and claudin-19 interaction is required for their assembly into tight junctions and for renal reabsorption of magnesium. Proc Natl Acad Sci USA 2009;106(36):15350—5.

[108] Gong Y, Renigunta V, Himmerkus N, et al. Claudin-14 regulates renal Ca(++) transport in response to CaSR signalling via a novel microRNA pathway. The EMBO journal. 2012;31(8):1999—2012.

[109] Ikari A, Hirai N, Shiroma M, Harada H, Sakai H, Hayashi H, et al. Association of paracellin-1 with ZO-1 augments the reabsorption of divalent cations in renal epithelial cells. J Biol Chem 2004;279(52):54826—32.

[110] Kausalya PJ, Amasheh S, Gunzel D, Wurps H, Muller D, Fromm M, et al. Disease-associated mutations affect intracellular traffic and paracellular Mg^{2+} transport function of Claudin-16. J Clin Invest 2006;116(4):878—91.

[111] Hou J, Paul DL, Goodenough DA. Paracellin-1 and the modulation of ion selectivity of tight junctions. J Cell Sci 2005;118(Pt 21):5109—18.

[112] Hou J, Renigunta A, Konrad M, Gomes AS, Schneeberger EE, Paul DL, et al. Claudin-16 and claudin-19 interact and form a cation-selective tight junction complex. J Clin Invest 2008;118(2):619—28.

[113] Hou J, Shan Q, Wang T, Gomes AS, Yan Q, Paul DL, et al. Transgenic RNAi depletion of claudin-16 and the renal handling of magnesium. J Biol Chem 2007;282(23):17114—22.

[114] Milatz S, Krug SM, Rosenthal R, Gunzel D, Muller D, Schulzke JD, et al. Claudin-3 acts as a sealing component of the tight junction for ions of either charge and uncharged solutes. Biochim Biophys Acta 2010;1798(11):2048—57.

[115] Van Itallie C, Rahner C, Anderson JM. Regulated expression of claudin-4 decreases paracellular conductance through a selective decrease in sodium permeability. J Clin Invest 2001;107(10):1319—27.

[116] Yu AS, Enck AH, Lencer WI, Schneeberger EE. Claudin-8 expression in MDCK cells augments the paracellular barrier to cation permeation. J Biol Chem 2003;278:17350—9.

[117] Ben-Yosef T, Belyantseva IA, Saunders TL, et al. Claudin 14 knockout mice, a model for autosomal recessive deafness DFNB29, are deaf due to cochlear hair cell degeneration. Hum Mol Genet 2003;12(16):2049—61.

[118] Jovov B, Van Itallie CM, Shaheen NJ, Carson JL, Gambling TM, Anderson JM, et al. Claudin-18: a dominant tight junction protein in Barrett's esophagus and likely contributor to its acid resistance. Am J Physiol Gastrointest Liver Physiol 2007;293(6):G1106—1113.

[119] Angelow S, Kim KJ, Yu AS. Claudin-8 modulates paracellular permeability to acidic and basic ions in MDCK II cells. J Physiol 2006;571:15—26.

[120] Pech V, Kim YH, Weinstein AM, Everett LA, Pham TD, Wall SM. Angiotensin II increases chloride absorption in the cortical collecting duct in mice through a pendrin-dependent mechanism. Am J Physiol Renal Physiol 2007;292(3):F914—920.

[121] Leviel F, Hubner CA, Houillier P, et al. The Na^+-dependent chloride-bicarbonate exchanger SLC4A8 mediates an electroneutral Na^+ reabsorption process in the renal cortical collecting ducts of mice. J Clin Invest 2010;120(5):1627—35.

[122] Sansom SC, Weinman EJ, O'Neil RG. Microelectrode assessment of chloride-conductive properties of cortical collecting duct. Am J Physiol 1984;247(2 Pt 2):F291—302.

[123] Hou J, Renigunta A, Yang J, Waldegger S. Claudin-4 forms paracellular chloride channel in the kidney and requires claudin-8 for tight junction localization. Proc Natl Acad Sci USA 2010;107(42):18010—5.

[124] Alexandre MD, Lu Q, Chen YH. Overexpression of claudin-7 decreases the paracellular Cl^- conductance and increases the paracellular Na^+ conductance in LLC-PK1 cells. J Cell Sci 2005;118:2683—93.

[125] Hou J, Gomes AS, Paul DL, Goodenough DA. Study of claudin function by RNA interference. J Biol Chem 2006;281(47):36117—23.

[126] Tatum R, Zhang Y, Salleng K, Lu Z, Lin JJ, Lu Q, et al. Renal salt wasting and chronic dehydration in claudin-7-deficient mice. Am J Physiol Renal Physiol 2010;298(1):F24—34.

[127] Uhlich E, Baldamus CA, Ullrich KJ. [Effect of aldosterone on sodium transport in the collecting ducts of the mammalian kidney]. Pflugers Arch 1969;308(2):111—26.

[128] Uhlich E, Halbach R, Ullrich KJ. [Influence of aldosterone on 24Na-efflux in collecting ducts of rats]. Pflugers Arch 1970;320(3):261—4.

[129] Sands JM, Nonoguchi H, Knepper MA. Hormone effects on NaCl permeability of rat inner medullary collecting duct. Am J Physiol 1988;255(3 Pt 2):F421—428.

[130] O'Neil RG, Helman SI. Transport characteristics of renal collecting tubules: influences of DOCA and diet. Am J Physiol 1977;233(6):F544—558.

[131] Wilson FH, Disse-Nicodeme S, Choate KA, et al. Human hypertension caused by mutations in WNK kinases. Science 2001;293(5532):1107—12.

[132] Wilson FH, Kahle KT, Sabath E, Lalioti MD, Rapson AK, Hoover RS, et al. Molecular pathogenesis of inherited hypertension with hyperkalemia: The Na-Cl co-transporter is inhibited by wild-type but not mutant WNK4. Proc Natl Acad Sci USA 2003;100(2):680—4.

[133] Yang CL, Angell J, Mitchell R, Ellison DH. WNK kinases regulate thiazide-sensitive Na-Cl co-transport. J Clin Invest 2003;111(7):1039—45.

[134] Kahle KT, Macgregor GG, Wilson FH, et al. Paracellular Cl^- permeability is regulated by WNK4 kinase: insight into normal physiology and hypertension. Proc Natl Acad Sci USA 2004;101(41):14877—82.

[135] Vitari AC, Deak M, Morrice NA, Alessi DR. The WNK1 and WNK4 protein kinases that are mutated in Gordon's hypertension syndrome phosphorylate and activate SPAK and OSR1 protein kinases. Biochem J 2005;391(Pt 1):17—24.

[136] Molitoris BA, Falk SA, Dahl RH. Ischemia-induced loss of epithelial polarity. Role of the tight junction. J Clin Invest 1989;84(4):1334—9.

[137] Gopalakrishnan S, Raman N, Atkinson SJ, Marrs JA. Rho GTPase signaling regulates tight junction assembly and protects tight junctions during ATP depletion. Am J Physiol 1998;275(3 Pt 1):C798—809.

[138] Tsukamoto T, Nigam SK. Tight junction proteins form large complexes and associate with the cytoskeleton in an ATP depletion model for reversible junction assembly. J Biol Chem 1997;272(26):16133—9.

[139] Kwon O, Nelson WJ, Sibley R, Huie P, Scandling JD, Dafoe D, et al. Backleak, tight junctions, and cell—cell adhesion in post-ischemic injury to the renal allograft. J Clin Invest 1998;101 (10):2054—64.

[140] Moran SM, Myers BD. Pathophysiology of protracted acute renal failure in man. J Clin Invest 1985;76(4):1440—8.

[141] Mandel LJ, Doctor RB, Bacallao R. ATP depletion: a novel method to study junctional properties in epithelial tissues. II. Internalization of Na + ,K(+)-ATPase and E-cadherin. J Cell Sci 1994;107(Pt 12):3315—24.

[142] Kwon O, Corrigan G, Myers BD, Sibley R, Scandling JD, Dafoe D, et al. Sodium reabsorption and distribution of Na$^+$/K$^+$-ATPase during postischemic injury to the renal allograft. Kidney Int 1999;55(3):963—75.

[143] Evans WH, Martin PE. Gap junctions: structure and function (Review). Mol Membr Biol 2002;19(2):121—36.

[144] Bao L, Sachs F, Dahl G. Connexins are mechanosensitive. Am J Physiol Cell Physiol 2004;287(5):C1389—1395.

[145] Qu Y, Dahl G. Function of the voltage gate of gap junction channels: selective exclusion of molecules. Proc Natl Acad Sci USA 2002;99(2):697—702.

[146] Contreras JE, Sanchez HA, Eugenin EA, Speidel D, Theis M, Willecke K, et al. Metabolic inhibition induces opening of unapposed connexin 43 gap junction hemichannels and reduces gap junctional communication in cortical astrocytes in culture. Proc Natl Acad Sci USA 2002;99(1):495—500.

[147] Willecke K, Eiberger J, Degen J, Eckardt D, Romualdi A, Güldenagel M, et al. Structural and functional diversity of connexin genes in the mouse and human genome. Biol Chem 2002;383(5):725—37.

[148] Rackauskas M, Kreuzberg MM, Pranevicius M, Willecke K, Verselis VK, Bukauskas FF. Gating properties of heterotypic gap junction channels formed of connexins 40, 43, and 45. Biophys J 2007;92(6):1952—65.

[149] Bukauskas FF, Angele AB, Verselis VK, Bennett MV. Coupling asymmetry of heterotypic connexin 45/connexin 43-EGFP gap junctions: properties of fast and slow gating mechanisms. Proc Natl Acad Sci USA 2002;99(10):7113—8.

[150] Ebihara L. New roles for connexons. News Physiol Sci 2003;18:100—3.

[151] Spray DC, Ye ZC, Ransom BR. Functional connexin "hemichannels:" a critical appraisal. Glia 2006;54(7):758—73.

[152] Paul DL, Ebihara L, Takemoto LJ, Swenson KI, Goodenough DA. Connexin46, a novel lens gap junction protein, induces voltage-gated currents in nonjunctional plasma membrane of Xenopus oocytes. J Cell Biol 1991;115(4):1077—89.

[153] Figueroa XF, Duling BR. Gap junctions in the control of vascular function. Antioxid Redox Signal 2009;11(2):251—66.

[154] Hamelin R, Allagnat F, Haefliger JA, Meda P. Connexins diabetes and the metabolic syndrome. Curr Protein Pept Sci 2009;10(1):18—29.

[155] Haefliger JA, Demotz S, Braissant O, Suter E, Waeber B, Nicod P, et al. Connexins 40 and 43 are differentially regulated within the kidneys of rats with renovascular hypertension. Kidney Int 2001;60(1):190—201.

[156] Biava C, West M. Fine structure of normal human juxtaglomerular cells. I. General structure and intercellular relationships. Am J Pathol 1966;49(4):679—721.

[157] Taugner R, Schiller A, Kaissling B, Kriz W. Gap junctional coupling between the JGA and the glomerular tuft. Cell Tissue Res 1978;186(2):279—85.

[158] Pricam C, Humbert F, Perrelet A, Orci L. A freeze-etch study of the tight junctions of the rat kidney tubules. Lab Invest 1974;30(3):286—91.

[159] Arensbak B, Mikkelsen HB, Gustafsson F, Christensen T, Holstein-Rathlou NH. Expression of connexin 37, 40, and 43 mRNA and protein in renal preglomerular arterioles. Histochem Cell Biol 2001;115(6):479—87.

[160] Guo R, Liu L, Barajas L. RT-PCR study of the distribution of connexin 43 mRNA in the glomerulus and renal tubular segments. Am J Physiol 1998;275(2 Pt 2):R439—447.

[161] Barajas L, Liu L, Tucker M. Localization of connexin43 in rat kidney. Kidney Int 1994;46(3):621—6.

[162] Haefliger JA, Bruzzone R, Jenkins NA, Gilbert DJ, Copeland NG, Paul DL. Four novel members of the connexin family of gap junction proteins. Molecular cloning, expression, and chromosome mapping. J Biol Chem 1992;267(3):2057—64.

[163] Hillis GS, Duthie LA, Mlynski R, McKay NG, Mistry S, Macleod AM, et al. The expression of connexin 43 in human kidney and cultured renal cells. Nephron 1997;75(4):458—63.

[164] Hwan Seul K, Beyer EC. Heterogeneous localization of connexin40 in the renal vasculature. Microvasc Res 2000;59 (1):140—8.

[165] de Wit C, Roos F, Bolz SS, Kirchoff S, Krüger O, Willecke K, et al. Impaired conduction of vasodilation along arterioles in connexin40-deficient mice. Circ Res 2000;86(6):649—55.

[166] Hanner F, von Maltzahn J, Maxeiner S, Toma I, Sipos A, Krüger O, et al. Connexin45 is expressed in the juxtaglomerular apparatus and is involved in the regulation of renin secretion and blood pressure. Am J Physiol Regul Integr Comp Physiol 2008;295(2):R371—380.

[167] Sipos A, Vargas SL, Toma I, Hanner F, Willecke K, Peti-Peterdi J. Connexin 30 deficiency impairs renal tubular ATP release and pressure natriuresis. J Am Soc Nephrol 2009;20 (8):1724—32.

[168] Kurtz L, Schweda F, de Wit C, Kriz W, Witzgall R, Warth R, et al. Lack of connexin 40 causes displacement of renin-producing cells from afferent arterioles to the extraglomerular mesangium. J Am Soc Nephrol 2007;18(4):1103—11.

[169] Kruger O, Maxeiner S, Kim JS, van Rijen HV, de Bakker JM, Eckhardt D, et al. Cardiac morphogenetic defects and conduction abnormalities in mice homozygously deficient for connexin40 and heterozygously deficient for connexin45. J Mol Cell Cardiol 2006;41(5):787—97.

[170] Hanner F, Schnichels M, Zheng-Fischhofer Q, Yang LE, Toma I, Willecke K, et al. Connexin 30.3 is expressed in the kidney but not regulated by dietary salt or high blood pressure. Cell Commun Adhes 2008;15(1):219—30.

[171] Kurtz L, Janssen-Bienhold U, Kurtz A, Wagner C. Connexin expression in renin-producing cells. J Am Soc Nephrol 2009;20 (3):506—12.

[172] Takenaka T, Inoue T, Kanno Y, Okada H, Meaney KR, Hill CE, et al. Expression and role of connexins in the rat renal vasculature. Kidney Int 2008;73(4):415—22.

[173] Zhang J, Hill CE. Differential connexin expression in preglomerular and postglomerular vasculature: accentuation during diabetes. Kidney Int 2005;68(3):1171—85.

[174] Gustafsson F, Mikkelsen HB, Arensbak B, Thuneberg L, Neve S, Jensen LJ, et al. Expression of connexin 37, 40 and 43 in rat mesenteric arterioles and resistance arteries. Histochem Cell Biol 2003;119(2):139—48.

[175] Rummery NM, Hill CE. Vascular gap junctions and implications for hypertension. Clin Exp Pharmacol Physiol 2004;31 (10):659—67.

[176] Schweda F, Kurtz L, de Wit C, Janssen-Bienhold U, Kurtz A, Wagner C. Substitution of connexin40 with connexin45 prevents hyperreninemia and attenuates hypertension. Kidney Int 2009;75(5):482—9.

[177] Taugner R, Kirchheim H, Forssmann WG. Myoendothelial contacts in glomerular arterioles and in renal interlobular arteries of rat, mouse and *Tupaia belangeri*. Cell Tissue Res 1984;235(2):319—25.

[178] Sawai K, Mukoyama M, Mori K, et al. Redistribution of connexin43 expression in glomerular podocytes predicts poor renal prognosis in patients with type 2 diabetes and overt nephropathy. Nephrol Dial Transplant 2006;21 (9):2472—7.

[179] Kuhn K, Reale E. Junctional complexes of the tubular cells in the human kidney as revealed with freeze-fracture. Cell Tissue Res 1975;160(2):193—205.

[180] Stoessel A, Himmerkus N, Bleich M, Bachmann S, Theilig F. Connexin 37 is localized in renal epithelia and responds to changes in dietary salt intake. Am J Physiol Renal Physiol 2010;298(1):F216—223.

[181] Butterweck A, Gergs U, Elfgang C, Willecke K, Traub O. Immunochemical characterization of the gap junction protein connexin45 in mouse kidney and transfected human HeLa cells. J Membr Biol 1994;141(3):247—56.

[182] Vergara L, Bao X, Bello-Reuss E, Reuss L. Do connexin 43 gap-junctional hemichannels activate and cause cell damage during ATP depletion of renal-tubule cells? Acta Physiol Scand 2003;179(1):33—8.

[183] McCulloch F, Chambrey R, Eladari D, Peti-Peterdi J. Localization of connexin 30 in the luminal membrane of cells in the distal nephron. Am J Physiol Renal Physiol 2005;289(6): F1304—1312.

[184] Kagota S, Yamaguchi Y, Nakamura K, Kunitomo M. Characterization of nitric oxide- and prostaglandin-independent relaxation in response to acetylcholine in rabbit renal artery. Clin Exp Pharmacol Physiol 1999;26 (10):790—6.

[185] Sorensen CM, Salomonsson M, Braunstein TH, Nielsen MS, Holstein-Rathlou NH. Connexin mimetic peptides fail to inhibit vascular conducted calcium responses in renal arterioles. Am J Physiol Regul Integr Comp Physiol 2008;295(3): R840—847.

[186] Zhang Q, Cao C, Mangano M, Zhang Z, Silldorf EP, Lee-Kwon W, et al. Descending vasa recta endothelium is an electrical syncytium. Am J Physiol Regul Integr Comp Physiol 2006;291(6):R1688—1699.

[187] De Vriese AS, Van de Voorde J, Lameire NH. Effects of connexin-mimetic peptides on nitric oxide synthase- and cyclooxygenase-independent renal vasodilation. Kidney Int 2002;61 (1):177—85.

[188] de Wit C, Roos F, Bolz SS, Pohl U. Lack of vascular connexin 40 is associated with hypertension and irregular arteriolar vasomotion. Physiol Genomics 2003;13(2):169—77.

[189] Karagiannis J, Rand M, Li CG. Role of gap junctions in endothelium-derived hyperpolarizing factor-mediated vasodilatation in rat renal artery. Acta Pharmacol Sin 2004;25 (8):1031—7.

[190] McKinnon RL, Lidington D, Bolon M, Ouellette Y, Kidder GM, Tyml K. Reduced arteriolar conducted vasoconstriction in septic mouse cremaster muscle is mediated by nNOS-derived NO. Cardiovasc Res 2006;69(1):236—44.

[191] Peti-Peterdi J. Calcium wave of tubuloglomerular feedback. Am J Physiol Renal Physiol 2006;291(2):F473—480.

[192] Cotrina ML, Lin JH, Alves-Rodrigues A, Liu S, Li J, Azmi-Ghadimi H, et al. Connexins regulate calcium signaling by controlling ATP release. Proc Natl Acad Sci USA 1998;95 (26):15735—40.

[193] Toma I, Kang JJ, Sipos A, Vargas S, Bansal E, Hanner F, et al. Succinate receptor GPR91 provides a direct link between high glucose levels and renin release in murine and rabbit kidney. J Clin Invest 2008;118(7):2526—34.

[194] Krattinger N, Capponi A, Mazzolai L, Aubert JF, Caille D, Nicod P, et al. Connexin40 regulates renin production and blood pressure. Kidney Int 2007;72(7):814—22.

[195] Wagner C, de Wit C, Kurtz L, Grunberger C, Kurtz A, Schweda F. Connexin40 is essential for the pressure control of renin synthesis and secretion. Circ Res 2007;100 (4):556—63.

[196] Haefliger JA, Krattinger N, Martin D, Pedrazzini T, Capponi A, Döring B, et al. Connexin43-dependent mechanism modulates renin secretion and hypertension. J Clin Invest 2006;116 (2):405—13.

[197] Liao Y, Day KH, Damon DN, Duling BR. Endothelial cell-specific knockout of connexin 43 causes hypotension and bradycardia in mice. Proc Natl Acad Sci USA 2001;98 (17):9989—94.

[198] Schwiebert EM, Kishore BK. Extracellular nucleotide signaling along the renal epithelium. Am J Physiol Renal Physiol 2001;280(6):F945—963.

[199] Vallon V. P2 receptors in the regulation of renal transport mechanisms. Am J Physiol Renal Physiol 2008;294(1):F10—27.

[200] Praetorius HA, Leipziger J. Intrarenal purinergic signaling in the control of renal tubular transport. Annu Rev Physiol 2010;72:377—93.

[201] Le Hir M, Kaissling B. Distribution and regulation of renal ecto-5′-nucleotidase: implications for physiological functions of adenosine. Am J Physiol 1993;264(3 Pt 2):F377—387.

[202] Willecke K, Kirchhoff S, Plum A, Temme A, Thonnissen E, Ott T. Biological functions of connexin genes revealed by human genetic defects, dominant negative approaches and targeted deletions in the mouse. Novartis Found Symp 1999;219:76—88 discussion 88-96

[203] Firouzi M, Kok B, Spiering W, et al. Polymorphisms in human connexin40 gene promoter are associated with increased risk of hypertension in men. J Hypertens 2006;24(2):325—30.

[204] Kuroki T, Inoguchi T, Umeda F, Ueda F, Nawata H. High glucose induces alteration of gap junction permeability and phosphorylation of connexin-43 in cultured aortic smooth muscle cells. Diabetes 1998;47(6):931—6.

[205] Inoguchi T, Ueda F, Umeda F, Yamashita T, Nawata H. Inhibition of intercellular communication via gap junction in cultured aortic endothelial cells by elevated glucose and phorbol ester. Biochem Biophys Res Commun 1995;208(2):492—7.

[206] Meng W, Takeichi M. Adherens junction: molecular architecture and regulation. Cold Spring Harb Perspect Biol 2009;1(6): a002899.

[207] Huber O. Structure and function of desmosomal proteins and their role in development and disease. Cell Mol Life Sci 2003;60(9):1872—90.

[208] Reiser J, Kriz W, Kretzler M, Mundel P. The glomerular slit diaphragm is a modified adherens junction. J Am Soc Nephrol 2000;11(1):1—8.

[209] Inoue T, Yaoita E, Kurihara H, et al. FAT is a component of glomerular slit diaphragms. Kidney Int 2001;59(3):1003—12.

[210] Nouwen EJ, Dauwe S, van der Biest I, De Broe ME. Stage- and segment-specific expression of cell-adhesion molecules N-CAM, A-CAM, and L-CAM in the kidney. Kidney Int 1993;44(1):147—58.

[211] Piepenhagen PA, Peters LL, Lux SE, Nelson WJ. Differential expression of Na(+)-K(+)-ATPase, ankyrin, fodrin, and E-cadherin along the kidney nephron. Am J Physiol 1995;269(6 Pt 1):C1417—1432.

[212] Tani T, Laitinen L, Kangas L, Lehto VP, Virtanen I. Expression of E- and N-cadherin in renal cell carcinomas, in renal cell

carcinoma cell lines *in vitro* and in their xenografts. Int J Cancer 1995;64(6):407—14.

[213] Kwon O, Myers BD, Sibley R, Dafoe D, Alfrey E, Nelson WJ. Distribution of cell membrane-associated proteins along the human nephron. J Histochem Cytochem 1998;46(12):1423—34.

[214] Bush KT, Tsukamoto T, Nigam SK. Selective degradation of E-cadherin and dissolution of E-cadherin- catenin complexes in epithelial ischemia. Am J Physiol Renal Physiol 2000;278(5): F847—852.

[215] Streets AJ, Newby LJ, O'Hare MJ, Bukanov NO, Ibraghimov-Beskrovnaya O, Ong AC. Functional analysis of PKD1 transgenic lines reveals a direct role for polycystin-1 in mediating cell-cell adhesion. J Am Soc Nephrol 2003;14(7):1804—15.

[216] Russo RJ, Husson H, Joly D, Bukanov NO, Patey N, Knebelmann B, et al. Impaired formation of desmosomal junctions in ADPKD epithelia. Histochem Cell Biol 2005;124 (6):487—97.

[217] Roitbak T, Ward CJ, Harris PC, Bacallao R, Ness SA, Wandinger-Ness A. A polycystin-1 multiprotein complex is disrupted in polycystic kidney disease cells. Mol Biol Cell 2004;15(3):1334—46.

[218] Abramow M, Orci L. On the "tightness" of the rabbit descending limb of the loop of Henle: physiological and morphological evidence. Int J Biochem 1980;12(1-2):23—7.

[219] Hegel U, Fromter E, Wick T. [Transmural electrical resistance of the proximal convoluted rat kidney tubule]. Pflugers Arch Gesamte Physiol Menschen Tiere 1967;294(4):274—90.

[220] Greger R. Ion transport mechanisms in thick ascending limb of Henle's loop of mammalian nephron. Physiol Rev 1985;65 (3):760—97.

[221] Malnic G, Giebisch G. Some electrical properties of distal tubular epithelium in the rat. Am J Physiol 1972;223 (4):797—808.

[222] Helman SI, Grantham JJ, Burg MB. Effect of vasopressin on electrical resistance of renal cortical collecting tubules. Am J Physiol 1971;220(6):1825—32.

[223] Wen H, Watry DD, Marcondes MC, Fox HS. Selective decrease in paracellular conductance of tight junctions: role of the first extracellular domain of claudin-5. Mol Cell Biol 2004;24 (19):8408—17.

[224] Angelow S, Schneeberger EE, Yu AS. Claudin-8 expression in renal epithelial cells augments the paracellular barrier by replacing endogenous claudin-2. J Membr Biol 2007;215(2-3):147—59.

[225] Alexandre MD, Jeansonne BG, Renegar RH, Tatum R, Chen YH. The first extracellular domain of claudin-7 affects paracellular Cl$^-$ permeability. Biochem Biophys Res Commun 2007;357 (1):87—91.

[226] Kurihara H, Anderson JM, Kerjaschki D, Farquhar MG. The altered glomerular filtration slits seen in puromycin aminonucleoside nephrosis and protamine sulfate-treated rats contain the tight junction protein ZO-1. Am J Pathol 1992;141 (4):805—16.

[227] Li WY, Huey CL, Yu AS. Expression of claudin-7 and -8 along the mouse nephron. Am J Physiol Renal Physiol 2004;286(6): F1063—1071.

[228] Kirk A, Campbell S, Bass P, Mason J, Collins J. Differential expression of claudin tight junction proteins in the human cortical nephron. *Nephrol Dial Transplant* 2010;25(7):2107—19.

13

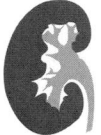

Principles of Cell Signaling

Lloyd Cantley

Yale University School of Medicine, New Haven, CT, USA

INTRODUCTION

The successful transition from single cells to complex multicellular organisms has required the development of mechanisms for cells to communicate with each other, so as to act in concert during processes such as nutrient acquisition, motility, and defense. The most fundamental of these are cell—cell junctions that serve as structural organizers, but also provide information that individual cells can utilize to orient themselves in relation to the remainder of the organism. In larger species that contain multiple organs and cell types, the need to communicate information over long distances has led to the development of diffusible factors that are secreted by one cell and travel to distant cells. These factors can be delivered locally, via the circulation (e.g., hormones and cytokines) or via the nervous system (e.g., neurotransmitters), and are recognized by the appropriate cell surface receptor on the recipient cell. The complex nature of the numerous signals presented to the cell at any given point in time has led to the development of an intricate array of receptor-activated intracellular second messengers that, by undergoing a coordinated series of interactions and enzymatic alterations, can transduce the information presented on the cell surface to effector molecules that mediate the appropriate cellular response.

The kidney serves to protect the internal milieu of higher organisms from perturbations due to the accumulation of metabolic products, as well as those resulting from fluctuations in the intake or loss of water and various salts. To regulate this intricate function, the body must continuously monitor the composition and quantity of the extracellular fluid, and then signal the nephron to appropriately regulate glomerular filtration and tubular cell function in response to changes in these parameters. Regulation of these exquisitely precise events requires that the cells of the kidney are able to respond to signals emanating from distant sites, and

then efficiently communicate in an intercellular and intracellular manner to coordinate the response. This chapter will provide an overview of several of the most common receptors and intracellular second messenger pathways that are utilized in this process.

CELL SURFACE RECEPTORS

In the best studied pathway of cell signaling, a first messenger is secreted by one group of cells and travels either to distant cells (endocrine factors) or to local cells (autocrine or paracrine factors), where it binds to a specific receptor. The first messengers in these classic pathways are generally either proteins (growth factors, cytokines), catecholamines (epinephrine, dopamine) or steroids (mineralocorticoids, sex hormones), although receptors have been identified for multiple circulating factors including lipids (e.g., lysophosphatidic acid), ions (e.g., calcium), eicosanoids (e.g., prostaglandin E_2), sugars (e.g., glucose), nucleosides (e.g., ATP), and gases (e.g., nitric oxide). Most of these receptors are located on the cell surface and have an extracellular region (domain) that recognizes and binds to the specific ligand. This ligand-binding domain is connected via one or more transmembrane segments to the intracellular (cytosolic) domain that undergoes a change in conformation or activity in response to ligand binding, and thus initiates the activation and/or modification of intracellular second messengers. In contrast to these cell surface receptors, steroid receptors, which are discussed later in this chapter, are typically located in the cytoplasm. The lipophilic steroid ligands are capable of crossing the cell membrane and binding the receptor, which then initiates signaling events by translocating into the nucleus where the ligand—receptor complex can regulate gene transcription.

Seldin and Giebisch's The Kidney, Fifth Edition.
DOI: http://dx.doi.org/10.1016/B978-0-12-381462-3.00013-6

Based on their structure, the type of ligand that they bind, and the principle second messengers that are activated, classical cell surface receptors can be grouped into G-protein coupled receptors, receptor tyrosine kinases (RTKs), serine/threonine kinase receptors, and receptor-like phosphatases. However, it has become increasingly clear that other surface proteins serve as signaling initiators to transduce information about the environment surrounding the cell. Thus, cell–cell and cell–matrix adhesion molecules initiate signaling cascades that regulate cell shape, differentiation, proliferation, and survival. The following section will provide a brief overview of these various signaling initiators, focused on those presently considered to be important in regulating normal renal development and maintaining adult kidney homeostasis.

G-Protein Coupled Receptors

The receptor sub-type that is responsible for mediating the signaling responses of the greatest number of ligands in the kidney is probably the G-protein-coupled receptor (GPCR). GPCRs make up the largest family of cell surface receptors, with over 800 members predicted from the sequence of the human genome (reviewed in [1]) (Figure 13.1). GPCRs are transmembrane proteins with their amino terminus on the cell exterior, seven transmembrane α helical segments, and the carboxyl terminus in the cell interior. This arrangement results in three extracellular loops and three intracellular loops joining the transmembrane segments. They bind to extracellular ligands such as epinephrine, dopamine, angiotensin II, adenosine, vasopressin, calcium, and parathyroid hormone, and mediate their intracellular actions.

The extracellular loops serve as the primary binding site for the specific GPCR ligand, with the amino terminus also contributing to the binding site for some ligands. The intracellular loops, most critically the 5–6 loop, serve as the binding site for the principal GPCR intracellular effectors, the heterotrimeric G-proteins. These small GDP/GTP-binding protein complexes are made up of α-, β-, and γ-subunits, with the α-subunit serving as the GDP/GTP-binding site, and the $\beta\gamma$-subunits acting both as regulators of α-subunit localization, and independently as intracellular signaling effectors. The existence of multiple different α-, β-, and γ-subunits allows for hundreds of potential combinations of heterotrimeric G-proteins, and thus imparts specificity of response to the individual GPCR and its ligand.

In the absence of receptor activation, the α-subunit is bound to GDP, and associates with the $\beta\gamma$-subunits at the membrane. However, following ligand binding to the extracellular surface of the GPCR, a conformational change of the receptor results in disassociation of GDP, and binding of GTP to the α-subunit. The binding of GTP stimulates disassociation of the α-subunit from the $\beta\gamma$-subunits and the receptor. The GTP-loaded α-subunit can then associate with its intermediary effectors (such as adenylyl cyclase and phospholipase), while the $\beta\gamma$-subunits can associate with and regulate independent effectors, such as ion channels and the β adrenergic receptor kinase (βARK) (reviewed in [2,3]).

The protein products of the 16 mammalian genes encoding Gα-subunits have been grouped into four classes, the $G_{s\alpha}$ (stimulatory for adenylyl cyclase), $G_{i\alpha}$ (inhibitory for adenylyl cyclase), $G_{q/11\alpha}$ (regulators of phospholipase Cβ (PLCβ)), and $G_{12\alpha}$ (regulators of RhoGEF). Binding of the appropriate GTP-loaded Gα-subunit to its primary effector results in the

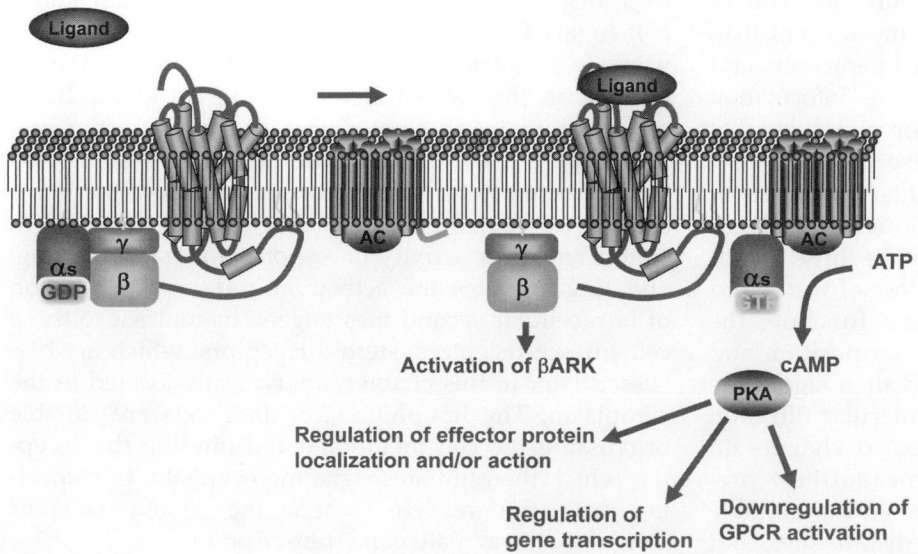

FIGURE 13.1 GPCR signaling through adenylate cyclase. Binding of the extracellular ligand to the GPCR results in the exchange of GTP for GDP on Gα, and its disassociation from the $\alpha\beta\gamma$ heterotrimer. $\beta\gamma$ can then associate with and activate downstream effectors such as the β-adregeneric receptor kinase (BARK), while the GTP-loaded α-subunit can bind and regulate effectors including adenylate cyclase (AC). In the example shown, Gsα activates AC to convert ATP to cAMP, and thus stimulates downstream PKA signaling.

activation or inhibition of effector function; for example, adenylyl cyclase catalyzes the cyclation of ATP to form 3′,5′-cyclic AMP (cAMP), an intracellular second messenger that can bind and activate downstream signaling proteins such as protein kinase A (PKA). This reaction is activated by GTP-$G_{s\alpha}$ binding to adenylyl cyclase and inhibited by GTP-$G_{i\alpha}$ binding. In addition, $\beta\gamma$ binding to adenylyl cyclase can augment its activation by GTP-$G_{s\alpha}$.

An important concept in all forms of signal transduction is the ability of the cell to carefully control the location, amplitude, and duration of the signal. Signal amplification is the process whereby the cell can regulate the amplitude of the signal. For example, a single GPCR can generate between tens and hundreds of GTP-coupled $G\alpha$-subunits, which can subsequently bind to and activate similar numbers of adenylyl cyclase enzymes, which in turn generate multiple copies of cAMP. The number and availability of the intracellular effector enzymes and substrates thus determines the level of signal amplification following the activation of relatively few receptors on the cell surface.

Just as important as signal amplification is the ability of the cell to downregulate the signaling pathway once the desired response has been initiated. For GPCRs, this occurs in several ways. First, the α-subunit is itself a GTPase, meaning that it hydrolyzes GTP to form GDP and inorganic phosphate. This hydrolysis occurs spontaneously following GTP binding to $G\alpha$, but can be augmented by the association of specific RGS proteins (regulators of G-protein signaling) with the GDP/$G\alpha$ complex, as this interaction stabilizes the inactivated state. Once the $G\alpha$-subunit is in the GDP-bound state, it can associate again with the $\beta\gamma$-subunit to regenerate the inactive heterotrimeric G-protein.

In addition, many GPCRs are themselves inactivated by a process called homologous desensitization. As has been noted above, the $\beta\gamma$-subunits can associate with the cytosolic protein βARK. βARK, also known as GRK2, is a member of the G-protein-coupled receptor kinases (GRKs) that, following association with $G_{\beta\gamma}$, phosphorylate the intracellular loops and/or C terminus of ligand-associated GPCRs on serine and/or threonine residues. This phosphorylation results in the association of β-arrestin with the receptor, mediating the uncoupling of the ligand–receptor complex from the heterotrimeric G-proteins, and thus diminishing its activity. Binding of β-arrestin has also been shown to target the receptor–ligand complexes to clathrin-coated pits on the cell surface, followed by internalization and either lysosomal degradation or recycling of the inactivated receptor to the cell surface.[4]

The downstream GPCR effector adenylyl cyclase is also subject to phosphorylation-dependent inhibition.

As noted above, activated adenylyl cyclase catalyzes the formation of cAMP, which in turn associates with and activates PKA. This enzyme, an intracellular serine/threonine kinase, has multiple phosphorylation substrates within the cell. Phosphorylation of these substrates can regulate their activity, cellular localization, and/or their interaction with other proteins. One phosphorylation substrate is adenylyl cyclase itself, resulting in inhibition of cAMP production. A second substrate is the GPCR. In a process known as heterologous desensitization, activation of PKA by a non-GPCR signal can result in phosphorylation of the GPCR and subsequent inhibition of ligand-mediated GPCR activation.[5]

Receptors for Dopamine and AVP are GPCRs that Regulate Adenylyl Cyclase

A prototypic family of GPCRs in the kidney is the dopamine receptors. There are five dopamine receptors presently described ($D_1–D_5$), and they are further sub-classified into D_1-like (D_1 and D_5) or D_2-like ($D_2–D_4$). The D_1-like receptors are associated with $G_{s\alpha}$, and therefore activate adenylyl cyclase, whereas the D_2-like receptors inhibit adenylyl cyclase activity (reviewed in [6,7]). In the kidney, D_1-like and D_2-like receptors are expressed throughout the tubules. The net effect of activating these receptors is the induction of a salt and water diuresis, although by different mechanisms in the different tubular segments. Dopamine-mediated activation of D_1 receptors in the proximal tubule results in activation of adenylyl cyclase, leading to cAMP-dependent inhibition of the activity of NHE-3, NaPi-2, and the Na,K-ATPase, thus inhibiting proximal sodium reabsorption. In contrast, activation of the D_2-like receptor D_4 in the cortical collecting duct leads to a water diuresis by preventing vasopressin-stimulated adenylyl cyclase activation. Dopamine receptors also mediate renal vasodilation, and appear to regulate renin secretion. Due to these effects, defects in dopamine receptor function in mice are associated with salt retention, vasoconstriction, and increased blood pressure.[8–10]

Arginine vasopressin (AVP, also known as antidiuretic hormone (ADH)) binds to three GPCRs, the $G_{q/11\alpha}$-linked V1a and V1b receptors, and the $G_{s\alpha}$-linked V2 receptor. V1 receptors are located on several cell types, including smooth muscle cells of blood vessels, where they mediate the vasoconstrictive ("pressor") response of vasopressin, while V2 receptors are located on epithelial cells in the collecting duct and mediate water reabsorption. Binding of vasopressin to the V2 receptor stimulates adenylyl cyclase-mediated cAMP production, which in turn causes insertion of vesicles containing the water channel aquaporin-2 into the apical membrane of collecting duct cells. By inhibiting adenylyl cyclase activation in these cells, dopamine can partially counteract this water-reabsorptive effect of vasopressin.

GPCRs Can also Signal through Phospholipase C and MAPK

An example of a GPCR that is coupled to PLCβ signaling is the type 1 receptor for angiotensin II (AT_1R). Angiotensin II is the eight amino acid peptide product of the angiotensin converting enzyme (ACE)-mediated cleavage of angiotensin I. Angiotensin II is capable of binding to and activating two distinct G-protein coupled receptors, the type 1 receptor (AT_1R) and the type 2 receptor (AT_2R). The predominant actions of angiotensin in the kidney and adrenal gland are mediated by the AT_1R, including vasoconstriction, smooth muscle hypertrophy, sodium retention, and aldosterone secretion. Most data presently support the idea that the AT_2R receptor acts as an antagonist to AT_1R signaling,[11] although exactly how the AT_2R signals has been much less apparent. The topology of the AT_2R is consistent with a seven transmembrane G-protein coupled receptor, yet it has been controversial as to whether AT_2R in fact signals via traditional G-proteins. There have been several reports that AT_2R can signal via $G_{i\alpha}$, although this has not been universally accepted (reviewed in [12]). Other groups have suggested that AT_2R signaling is pertussis-toxin insensitive (i.e., not dependent on $G_{i\alpha}$), and is instead mediated by production of cyclic GMP.[13] It remains unclear whether the generation of cGMP is a direct result of AT_2R activation or is mediated in an autocrine/paracrine fashion by AT_2R-stimulated bradykinin production.[14]

The AT_1R is in the $G_{q/11\alpha}$ family of GPCRs, meaning that binding of angiotensin II to the receptor stimulates GTP-loading of $G_{q\alpha}$ which in turn associates with and activates phospholipase Cβ (PLCβ) (Figure 13.2). The active form of PLCβ mediates the hydrolysis of phosphotidylinositol 4,5 bisphosphate ($PI_{4,5}P_2$) in the membrane to produce diacylglycerol (DAG) and inositol trisphosphate (IP_3). IP_3 is hydrophilic and enters the cytoplasm where it activates the IP_3 receptor on the surface of the endoplasmic reticulum, thereby stimulating calcium release from internal stores. The simultaneous production of DAG at the membrane, and local release of stored calcium, leads to the recruitment and activation of the classic, calcium-dependent protein kinases C (PKCs). Activation of PKC appears to be required for angiotensin II-mediated renal efferent arteriole vasoconstriction,[15] Na,K-ATPase recruitment to the membrane in proximal tubule cells (resulting in increased proximal sodium reabsorption),[16,17] and stimulation of aldosterone secretion by adrenal zona glomerulosa cells.[18]

In addition to activation of PLCβ, a second signaling pathway that is activated by the AT_1R is the mitogen activated protein kinase (MAPK) pathway. As mentioned earlier, phosphorylation of GPCRs by βARK results in the recruitment of β-arrestin to the receptor complex, and subsequent receptor internalization. β-arrestin has been found to act as a binding scaffold for the core components of the MAPK pathway, including Raf, MEK, and ERK (see "Intracellular Signaling Pathways," below; reviewed in [19]), resulting in the activation of this pathway that mediates cell growth and proliferation.[20-22] This scaffolding function of β-arrestin appears to be both cell type and receptor specific, and can mediate activation of additional intracellular signaling pathways, including the phosphoinositide 3-kinase (PI 3-K) pathway that will be discussed later in this chapter.[23] Activation of these signaling pathways appears to play an important role during kidney development, since newborn mice null for the type I angiotensin receptor or in which angiotensin signaling has been inhibited, have significant renal developmental abnormalities, including renal arterial hypertrophy and papillary atrophy.[24,25]

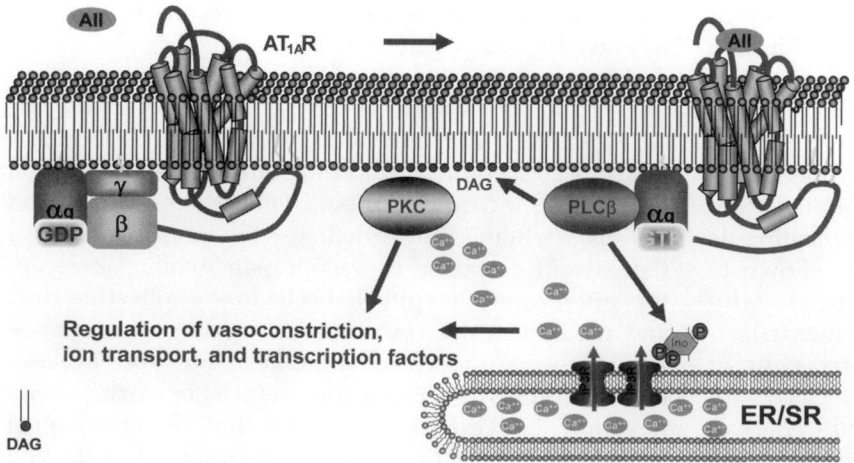

FIGURE 13.2 Signaling by the angiotensin II (AII) receptor. Binding of AII results in GTP-loading of the associated Gqα-subunit of the αβγ heterotrimer, which in turn activates phospholipase C β (PLCβ). Activated PLCβ stimulates the hydrolysis of $PI_{4,5}P_2$ in the membrane to form IP3 and diacylglycerol (DAG). IP3 can then bind to its receptor on the endoplasmic or sarcoplasmic reticulum, activating calcium release. The increase in cytosolic calcium can stimulate multiple cellular responses, including activation of PKC (which associates with DAG at the membrane), influx of extracellular calcium via channels at the cell surface, and contraction via actin—myosin coupling.

Regulation of vasoconstriction, ion transport, and transcription factors

A second means by which GPCRs can activate MAPK signaling was discovered when the levels of β-arrestin were depleted using RNA interference (RNAi). Under these conditions, angiotensin II was still able to activate MAPK, although to a lesser degree. These experiments uncovered a β-arrestin-independent pathway of angiotensin II-dependent MAPK stimulation that occurs via activation of a second cell surface receptor, a process known as receptor transactivation. As noted above, stimulation of $G_{q\alpha}$ by the $AT_{1A}R$ leads to activation of PKC. PKC, in addition to regulating processes such as ion transport, can activate a cell surface protein called heparin-binding epidermal growth factor (HB-EGF). HB-EGF is one of the ligands for a separate cell surface receptor, the epidermal growth factor receptor (EGFR), and binding of HB-EGF to the EGFR results in the stimulation of multiple signaling events, including MAPK activation (see "Intracellular Signaling Pathways").[18]

Localization and Timing of Pathway Activation Promotes Diverse Cell type Specific Responses

These two independent pathways for activating MAPK signaling provide an example of how scaffolding proteins can compartmentalize signaling within the cell. The β-arrestin-mediated ERK activation is sustained for several hours and occurs in the cytoplasm, whereas the $G_{q\alpha}$/PKC-dependent ERK activation appears to be more transient and primarily within the nucleus. This ability to localize activated ERK in different cellular compartments allows the cell to differentially regulate specific effector proteins, and thus direct distinct cellular outcomes. In the heart, for example, AT_1R-mediated $G_{q\alpha}$/PKC-dependent transactivation of the EGFR, and ultimately MAPK nuclear signaling, is believed to at least partially mediate angiotensin-stimulated cardiac hypertrophy.[26,27]

Many GPCRs can activate multiple Gα-subunits, depending on cellular location and availability. For example, the parathyroid hormone (PTH) receptor can potentially activate $G_{s\alpha}$ (thus activating adenylate cyclase and PKA), $G_{q\alpha}$ (activating PLCβ and PKC), and G_i (inhibiting adenylate cyclase). PTH is an 84 amino acid peptide hormone secreted by the parathyroid gland that acts on bone to increase calcium and phosphate release into the circulation, as well as on the proximal and distal tubules of the kidney to inhibit phosphate reabsorption and stimulate calcium reabsorption, respectively. PTH is proteolytically processed to generate multiple fragments which can bind to and activate the PTH receptor, a class B GPCR (defined by the six conserved cysteine residues that form disulfide bonds in the large extracellular amino terminal domain).[28] Expression of a mutant form of the receptor that selectively fails to activate

$G_{q\alpha}$-dependent PLCβ signaling in mice results in abnormalities in bone ossification without a change in serum calcium.[29] The normal serum calcium in these animals suggests that renal tubular calcium handling in these mice is dependent on $G_{s\alpha}$- or G_i-regulated adenylate cyclase signaling, while bone ossification appears to require $G_{q\alpha}$-PLCβ signaling. In support of this hypothesis, complete loss of PTH receptor signaling results in hypocalcemia in addition to bone abnormalities.[30,31] In humans, this is recapitulated by an autosomal recessive mutation in the receptor in patients with Blomstrand chondrodysplasia, a lethal disorder characterized by excessive bone maturation and mineralization.[32]

As noted previously, receptor internalization mediated by β-arrestin is frequently a means by which GPCR are uncoupled from their ligands and signaling is downregulated. For example, PTH related protein (PTHrP) can bind and activate the PTH receptor, leading to GTP-loading of $G_{s\alpha}$ and a transient increase in cAMP followed by receptor desensitization. In contrast, PTH receptor ligands such as PTH_{1-34} (the first 34 amino acids of PTH) can induce a more sustained increase in adenylyl cyclase activation and cAMP levels, leading to systemic responses such as increased vitamin D hydroxylation and higher serum calcium levels. Investigation into the mechanism of this difference has demonstrated that binding of PTH_{1-34} to the PTH receptor leads to internalization of the active receptor−ligand complex in endosomes that also contain adenylyl cyclase, leading to sustained signaling from this intracellular site.[33] These structures, referred to as signaling endosomes, have been shown to mediate signaling via multiple receptor types in addition to GPCR, and to regulate complex cellular responses such as migration, differentiation, and asymmetric division.[34,35]

Kinase Receptors

A second class of transmembrane receptors is the kinase receptors. These proteins typically contain an extracellular ligand-binding domain at the amino terminus, a single membrane-spanning domain, and an intracellular carboxy terminus that includes the kinase domain. In most cases, binding of the ligand to the receptor results in homodimerization of two receptor molecules, bringing the intracellular kinase domains into close proximity where they phosphorylate substrate residues on the adjacent receptor. This phosphorylation step generates binding sites for the recruitment of intracellular signaling molecules, as well as further activating the kinase domain so that non-receptor substrates recruited to the complex can also be phosphorylated.

Tyrosine Kinase Receptors

The largest class of kinase receptors is the tyrosine kinase receptors, also known as receptor tyrosine kinases (RTKs) (Figure 13.3). These molecules frequently serve as receptors for extracellular growth factors, circulating proteins that stimulate cell growth and division. Examples of ligand–receptor combinations in this family include epidermal growth factor (EGF) and its receptors ErbB1 (or EGFR) and ErbB2; platelet-derived growth factor (PDGF) and the PDGF receptor; insulin and the insulin receptor; and vascular endothelial growth factor and its major receptors VEGFR1 and VEGFR2 (also called Flt1 and Flk1).

Once the growth factor has bound to and activated the receptor, newly phosphorylated tyrosine residues on the intracellular carboxy terminus of the receptor serve as binding sites for cytosolic or membrane-associated proteins that contain phosphotyrosine-binding domains. The best characterized of these domains are the src-homology 2 (SH2) domains that share characteristic features first described in the phosphotyrosine-binding region of the cytosolic tyrosine kinase Src. SH2 domains are approximately 100 amino acids in length, and provide specificity of interaction in two ways. First, the interaction of the binding pocket of the SH2 domain and the tyrosine residue is only stabilized when the tyrosine residue is phosphorylated. Second, the amino acids immediately flanking the phosphorylated tyrosine residue determine which SH2 domain interaction is preferred. For example, the SH2 domain on the p85 adaptor protein, α-subunit of the lipid enzyme phosphoinositide 3-kinase (PI 3-K, see "Intracellular Signaling Pathways," below), strongly prefers to bind to phosphotyrosine with a methionine residue at the +3 position.[36]

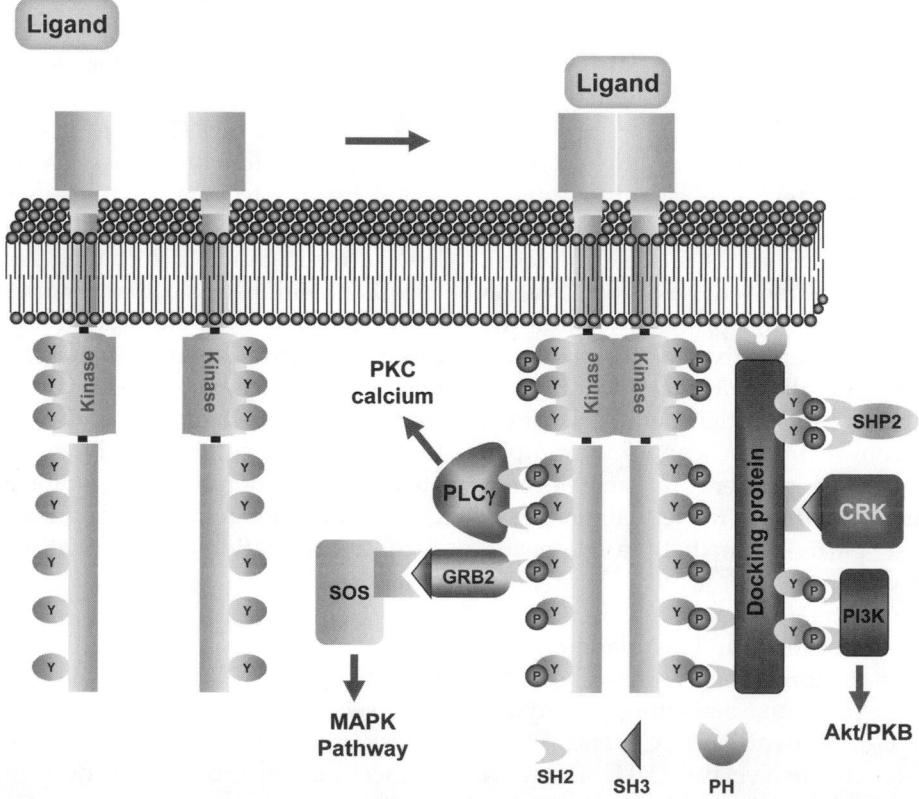

FIGURE 13.3   Schematic view of a receptor tyrosine kinase (RTK). In the inactive state, the receptor is primarily in the monomeric form. Following binding of the extracellular ligand, the receptor dimerizes, bringing the kinase domains in close proximity where they cross-phosphorylate each other. This enhances the kinase activity and leads to phosphorylation of tyrosine residues outside of the kinase domain, which in turn become binding sites for proteins that contain SH2 domains. In this manner, downstream signaling pathways can be regulated by recruitment to the receptor. This recruitment can occur via direct association of the effector protein with the receptor (as is the case for phospholipase Cγ (PLCγ)), via association with small adaptor proteins such as Grb2 (as is the case for the guanine exchange factor Sos) or via association with a larger docking protein such as Gab1 or Nck that mediates the association of multiple proteins with the receptor (as can be seen with the phosphoinositide 3-kinase (PI 3K) or the tyrosine phosphatase SHP2). Some docking proteins are additionally stabilized at the membrane via lipid binding domains, such as the pleckstrin homology (PH) domain on Gab1. In addition to SH2 domain interactions, multiple other protein–protein interactions occur and regulate the recruitment of proteins into the complex, including interactions between SH3 domains and proline-rich regions in interacting partners. In this manner, multiple signaling effectors are brought into close proximity where they can interact with each other, be phosphorylated or dephosphorylated (thereby altering their activity or interacting partners) or regulate processes at the cell membrane.

Thus, receptors containing the sequence pTyr-X-X-Met (where X can be almost any amino acid) specifically recruit and activate the PI 3-K.

In the kidney, tyrosine kinase receptors have been implicated in controlling development, mediating hypertrophy, regulating the balance between repair and fibrosis after injury, and promoting the growth of renal carcinomas. During development, glial derived neurotrophic factor (Gdnf) is made by the embryonic metanephric mesenchyme and activates the c-Ret tyrosine kinase receptor that is expressed on the epithelial cells of the adjacent Wolffian duct. The activation of Ret is somewhat unusual, since Gdnf does not directly bind to Ret, but rather binds to a third membrane protein, Gfrα, that mediates dimerization of Ret in response to association with Gdnf (reviewed in [37]). Activation of Ret in this manner results in the activation of multiple intracellular signaling pathways, including the Erk-MAPK pathway, the PI 3-K pathway, members of the Src family of non-receptor tyrosine kinases, and phospholipase Cγ (PLCγ). Activation of the MAPK and Src pathways (see "Intracellular Signaling Pathways") have been found to be critical for the outgrowth and branching of the ureteric bud from the Wolffian duct, the first step in the formation of the metanephric kidney.[38]

Signaling by several other tyrosine kinase receptors has been implicated in kidney development, including the fibroblast growth factor (FGF) receptors, hepatocyte growth factor receptor (Met), and the epidermal growth factor receptor.[39,40] FGF signaling is a complex process that includes 18 known ligands and 4 distinct tyrosine kinase receptors (FGFR1-4) (reviewed in [41]). Like many receptor ligands, FGFs are secreted glycoproteins that are concentrated in proximity to their cell surface receptor by binding to heparan sulfate proteoglycans on the cell and/or nearby matrix components. The interaction between FGFs and their receptors can be further regulated by cell- or tissue-specific expression of FGF co-receptors such as Klotho.[42] Intracellular signaling by the FGFR is regulated in part by the cytosolic adaptor protein FGFR substrate 2 (FRS2), which is phosphorylated by the FGFR kinase domain, leading to the recruitment and activation of downstream MAPK and PI 3-K signaling. In the developing kidney, FGF7 and FGF10, signaling via the IIIb isoform of FGFR2,[43] have been shown to be critical for normal branching and extension of the collecting system,[44] while FGF8 appears to be required for nephrogenesis by the adjacent metanephric mesenchyme.[45]

Many growth factor receptors are expressed in the mature kidney, and are believed to be critical for maintenance of normal tubule architecture and for regulating the cellular response to injury. Renal tubular epithelial cells express EGF receptors as well as Met,

the receptor for hepatocyte growth factor (HGF). These tyrosine kinase receptors directly bind their respective ligands via their extracellular amino terminal domains, followed by homodimerization and activation of intracellular signaling. A major mediator of the intracellular signaling mediated by EGF and HGF is the Gab1 docking protein, which functions in a manner similar to that of FRS2 for the FGFR.[46] Recruitment of Gab1 to Met or the EGFR results in its phosphorylation on multiple tyrosine residues and subsequent association with p85, PLCγ, Grb2, a second adaptor protein known as Crk, and the protein tyrosine phosphatase SHP2.[47] Following acute kidney injury, the level of HGF increases in the kidney, resulting in activation of Met, mediating MAPK, PI 3-K, and PLC signaling.[48,49] These pathways in turn are believed to be important for inhibition of apoptosis (the PI 3-K pathway), and stimulation of cell migration and proliferation during the repair process (PI 3-K, MAPK, and PLC pathways).[50–52]

Serine-Threonine Kinase Receptors

A second group of transmembrane kinase receptors are the serine-threonine kinase receptors. Like the non-receptor kinases PKA and PKC, these receptors catalyze the phosphorylation of serine or threonine residues in their substrate molecules. Perhaps the best studied of these receptors in the kidney is the receptor for transforming growth factor β (TGFβ), a member of the TGFβ superfamily of secreted factors that also includes the bone morphogenic proteins (BMPs) and activin.[53] TGFβ-like proteins signal into the cell via a heterotetrameric complex comprised of two subclasses of serine-threonine kinase receptors, the type I receptor and the type II receptor.[54] Like the tyrosine kinase receptors, these proteins have an extracellular ligand recognition domain, a single transmembrane spanning domain, and an intracellular kinase domain. The different TGFβ-like ligands utilize distinct type I and II receptor combinations. For example, TGFβ1-3 signals via the combination of the type II receptor TβR-II and the type I receptors activin receptor-like kinase 1 (ALK-1) or ALK-5,[55,56] while BMPs signal through the type II receptors ActR-II or BMPR-II and the type I receptors ALK-2, ALK-3 or ALK-6.[57]

TGFβ receptor signaling begins when the ligand binds to the extracellular domain of its cognate type II receptor (Figure 13.4). The kinase domain of type II receptors is constitutively active, and binding to the extracellular ligand results in the recruitment of the appropriate type I receptor to the complex, where it is phosphorylated and activated by the type II receptor. In this manner, the TGFβ1-dependent association of ALK-5 with TβR-II allows the constitutively active TβR-II to phosphorylate ALK-5 and activate its intracellular

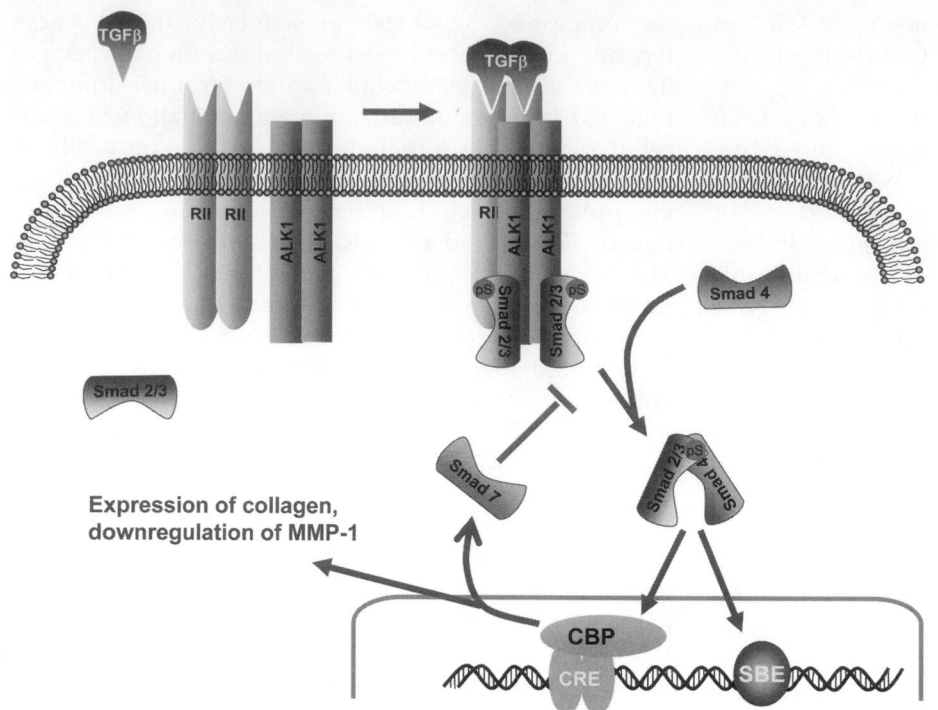

FIGURE 13.4 Signaling by the TGFβ family of serine-threonine kinase receptors. Binding of the TGF ligand to the constitutively active type II receptor results in association of RII with the appropriate type I receptor (in this case ALK-1), which is phosphorylated and activated. The activated type I receptor can then phosphorylate the appropriate Smad protein, which then disassociates from the receptor complex, associates with Smad 4, and translocates into the nucleus. In the nucleus the Smad complex can regulate RNA transcription by binding directly to the appropriate DNA Smad-binding elements (SBE) or by binding to and regulating transcriptional regulators such as the cAMP response element (CRE) binding protein (CBP). One of the DNA targets induced by Smad activation is the inhibitory Smad, Smad7. Increased expression of Smad7 inhibits further TβR signaling, providing negative feedback to prevent sustained activation of the pathway.

serine-threonine kinase domain. The specificity of signaling by TGFβ family members is further regulated by the presence in many cells of the accessory receptors betaglycan and endoglin. These transmembrane proteins lack intracellular kinase domains, and appear to regulate the affinity of TGFβ proteins for the various type II receptors, as well as modifying intracellular signaling by the ligand−receptor complex.[58,59]

As opposed to tyrosine kinase receptors that signal primarily via recruitment of SH2 domain containing proteins to activate pathways such as MAPK and PI 3-K, TGFβ receptors signal primarily via a distinct signaling pathway, the Smad proteins. Smads are small cytoplasmic proteins that contain a DNA-binding domain and a TβR-I/Smad4-interacting domain. Based on their structure and function, Smads have been divided into three groups, the receptor activated Smads (Smad1, 2, 3, 5, 8), a regulatory Smad (Smad4), and the inhibitory Smads (Smad6, 7). Upon activation of TβR-I, the appropriate receptor activated Smads (e.g., Smad2 and 3 for ALK-5) are phosphorylated on regulatory serine residues in the TβR-I/Smad4 interacting domain, resulting in their disassociation from the receptor and association with Smad4. This Smad2−Smad4 complex then translocates to the nucleus, where the Smad DNA-binding domain can mediate direct association with Smad-binding elements (SBE) in the DNA of the promotor region of target genes, as well as association with other transcriptional regulators.

One of the transcriptional targets that is regulated by Smad2−4 signaling is another member of the Smad family, Smad7. Smad7 is an inhibitory Smad that can bind to TβR-I, and prevent Smad2 or Smad3 from associating and being activated. In this manner, TGFβ stimulation of Smad7 transcription provides a negative feedback loop that acts to prevent sustained Smad2 and Smad3 activation by the TGFβ receptor.[60]

TGFβ Signaling in the Kidney

Studies in mice that have undergone genetic inactivation of various TGFβ family members demonstrate that Bmp2 and Bmp4 have important roles in normal kidney development (reviewed in [57]). In the mouse embryo, Bmp4 is expressed in the metanephric mesenchyme surrounding the Wolffian duct and adjacent to the ureteric bud (the epithelial structure that will branch to form the entire collecting system of the kidney), while Bmp2 is expressed in the condensing mesenchyme at the tips of the ureteric bud (the region that will differentiate into the glomerulus and proximal portions of the nephron through the connecting segment). The Bmp receptors Alk3 and Alk6 are expressed on the invading urteric bud itself.[61] While complete loss of Bmp2 or Bmp4 results in embryonic lethality prior to kidney development,[62] mice that are heterozygous for loss of Bmp4 expression exhibit multiple defects in the collecting system of the kidney, including doubling of the collecting system, hydroureter, and dysplastic kidneys,[61] and Bmp2 heterozygotes demonstrate exaggerated uretic bud branching.[63]

Thus, it appears that Bmps normally act to inhibit ureteric bud outgrowth and branching during development.

In addition to their role in kidney development, TGFβ proteins have been shown to play a major role in regulating fibrotic responses of the adult kidney by both increasing new matrix deposition and inhibiting matrix degradation.[53,64] *In vitro* studies have shown that TGFβ-dependent Smad3—Smad4 nuclear signaling can induce the expression of multiple collagen isoforms, along with their cellular binding partner β1 integrin,[65-67] and activated Smad3 has been found to mediate decreased transcription of the gene for matrix metalloproteinase-1 (*MMP-1*)[68]. In support of an important role for the TGFβ-Smad signaling pathway in the development and progression of renal fibrosis *in vivo*, genetic overexpression of TGFβ in the rat has been shown to induce glomerulosclerosis due to increased extracellular matrix deposition,[69] while mice lacking Smad3 demonstrate less fibrosis following ureteral obstruction.[70]

Receptor-Like Phosphatases

Much attention has been focused in the field of signal transduction on the role of substrate phosphorylation by receptor kinases in regulating protein—protein interactions or altering the activity of effector proteins. However, a second class of proteins, the phosphatases, is emerging as equally important signaling regulators in determining cellular responses. Similar to kinases, phosphatases can be grouped into transmembrane receptor-like phosphatases and intracellular (cytosolic) phosphatases (to be discussed below). The receptor-like phosphatases that have been identified to date are protein tyrosine phosphatases (PTPs) with an extracellular domain, single transmembrane spanning segment, and intracellular phosphatase domain.

The first receptor-like PTP to be cloned and sequenced was the neutrophil antigen CD45. This protein was found to be necessary for both T-cell development and T-cell activation following engagement of the T-cell receptor (reviewed in [71]). Although there has been no activating ligand identified for CD45, binding to extracellular galectin-1 inhibits CD45 phosphatase activity, resulting in T-cell death.[72] Several intracellular substrates for CD45 have been identified, including members of the Src and JAK kinase families. One critical substrate of CD45 in T-cell signaling is the cytosolic tyrosine kinase Lck[73](Figure 13.5). Lck, like the related tyrosine kinase Src, is normally maintained in the inactive state by the association of phosphotyrosine 505 near the carboxy terminus with its own SH2 domain closer to the amino terminus of the protein.[74] This interaction results in folding of Lck, and thereby prevents the intervening tyrosine kinase domain from recognizing or phosphorylating its substrates. Dephosphorylation of phosphotyrosine 505 by CD45 following antigen presentation by a nearby dendritic cell allows Lck to unfold, and activates the kinase domain.[75] The resultant phosphorylation of the ζ-chain of the T-cell receptor by activated Lck is necessary for recruitment of a second cytosolic tyrosine kinase, ZAP70, to the complex, and subsequent T-cell activation.[76] The administration of monoclonal antibodies that prevent activation of CD45 has been shown to markedly diminish the occurrence of acute rejection in a rodent model of kidney transplantation.[77]

In contrast to CD45, the receptor-like protein tyrosine phosphatase PTPζ/β is expressed on epithelial cells, and has been found to bind to several putative extracellular ligands, including contactin, neural cell adhesion molecule (NCAM), and pleiotrophin.[78,79] Rather than activating PTPζ/β, as is typical of most ligand—receptor interactions, the association of pleiotrophin with PTPζ/β inhibits the phosphatase activity of PTPζ/β.[80] In the kidney, pleiotrophin has been shown to markedly increase branching by the explanted ureteric bud, and thus is believed to play a significant role in determining the number of nephrons that form during kidney development.[81] One substrate for PTPζ/β is the cytosolic protein Git1,[82] a multifunctional adaptor protein that can regulate the signaling pathways that control actin cytoskeletal rearrangement.[83] Dephosphorylation of Git1 by PTPζ/β is therefore proposed to play an important role in the regulation of cell adhesion and migration, as well as cytosolic vesicle trafficking.[84]

Receptors Activated by Proteolytic Cleavage

The previously described receptors bind to their respective ligands and then signal into the cell via activation of substrate protein phosphorylation or dephosphorylation, thus regulating cytosolic signaling pathways that in turn mediate the activation or inhibition of downstream effectors. In contrast, cleavage-activated receptors such as Notch signal directly to the nucleus to regulate gene transcriptional events. Notch is a cell surface protein that contains an extracellular ligand-binding domain, a single transmembrane spanning segment, and an intracellular domain capable of binding and activating nuclear transcriptional factors (reviewed in [85]). The classic Notch ligands, Jagged and Delta, are also transmembrane proteins that contain extracellular EGF-like repeats and a unique domain for binding Notch. When Jagged on one cell engages Notch on an adjacent cell, a cleavage

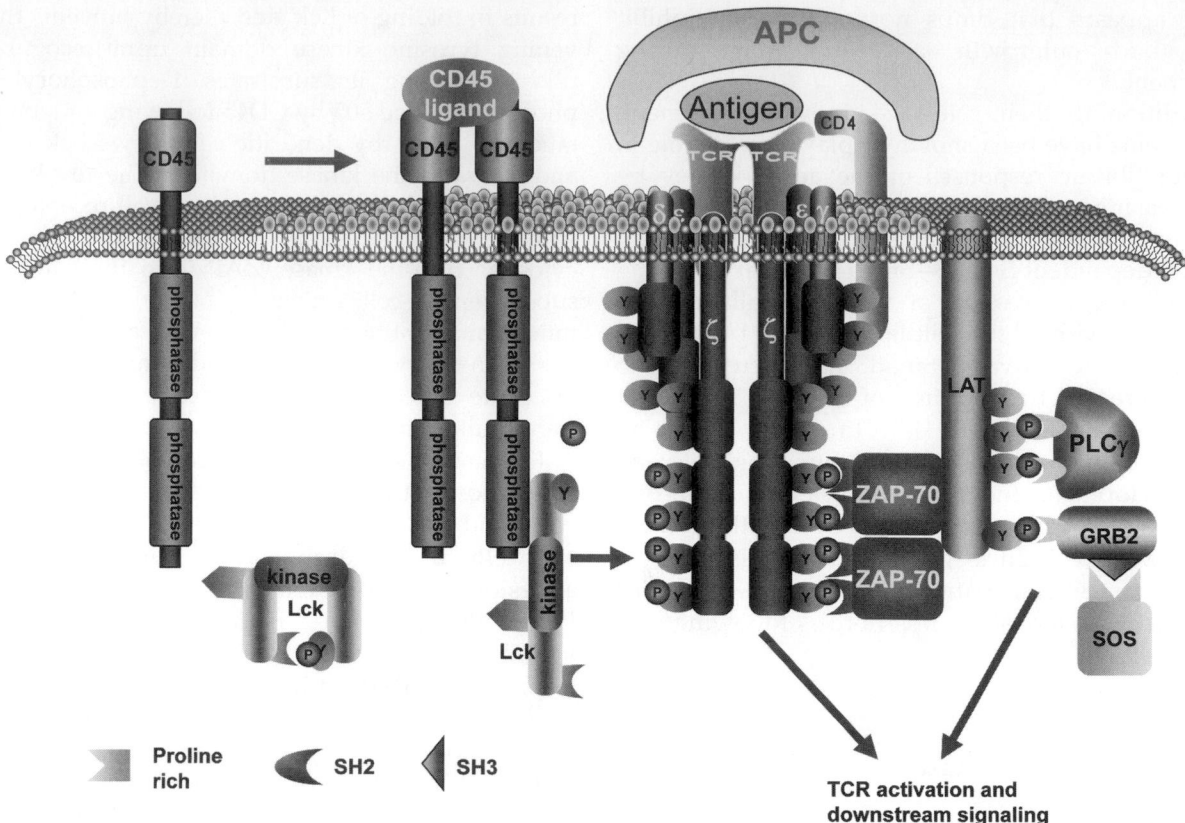

FIGURE 13.5   Signaling by the CD45 receptor phosphatase. CD45 is a single membrane spanning receptor phosphatase that is activated by an unknown extracellular ligand. Ligand binding activates the intracellular phosphatase domains, possibly by clustering of the receptors, which dephosphorylate the carboxy terminal tyrosine residue on the cytosolic non-receptor tyrosine kinase Lck. This allows a conformational change in Lck that exposes the kinase domain and facilitates phosphorylation of the ζ chain of the multimeric T-cell receptor. In conjunction with antigen presentation by an antigen presenting cell (APC) to the extracellular domain of the TCR, Lck phosphorylation of the TCR results in recruitment of a second tyrosine kinase, Zap70, to the complex via binding of the Zap70 SH2 domains to the phosphorylated receptor. Zap70 recruitment and activation are required for normal TCR activation, and for phosphorylation of the adaptor protein, Linker for Activation of T cells (LAT). LAT in turn serves as the site for recruitment of multiple signaling pathways involved in the T-cell immune response, including PLCγ (for activation of PKC and calcium signaling) and Grb2-Sos (for MAPK signaling).

site is exposed on the extracellular side of Notch near the membrane, and Notch is cleaved by a member of the A Disintegrin And Metalloproteinase (ADAM) family of proteases.[86] The remaining transmembrane/intracellular portion of Notch then becomes a target for further cleavage by presenilin (a member of the γ-secretase complex) at a conserved site in the intramembranous domain of Notch.[87] Cumulatively, this process is termed regulated intramembranous proteolysis (RIP) (Figure 13.6).

This final cleavage event releases the cytosolic domain of Notch (called the Notch intracellular domain (NICD)) that translocates to the nucleus where it can directly bind and regulate transcription factors. In mammals, Notch controls transcriptional regulation by interacting with the DNA-binding protein CSL (also called RBP-J), which in turn regulates transcriptional expression of members of the Hairy and Enhancer of Split (HES), and Hairy-Related Transcription factor (HRT) family of transcription factors. These nuclear proteins control the expression of genes that are critical for regulating normal development.

In the kidney, activation of Notch signaling has been implicated in the specification of the proximal tubule and glomerular podocytes during development.[88,89] The cleaved form of Notch is present in the developing S-shaped body that ultimately differentiates into the nephron, and inhibition of γ-secretase in organ culture leads to the loss of the proximal nephron, even though the distal nephron still develops and fuses to the collecting duct.[90] Genetic interruption of Notch expression has revealed that nuclear signaling by Notch2, rather than Notch1, is required for this proximal specification.[91] In the mature kidney, Notch expression is normally downregulated. However, in disease states such as diabetic nephropathy, re-expression of Notch can activate the transcription of cell cycle genes, leading to increased cell proliferation and ultimately exaggerated fibrosis.[92]

More recently, it has become clear that receptor activation by regulated cleavage plays a role in

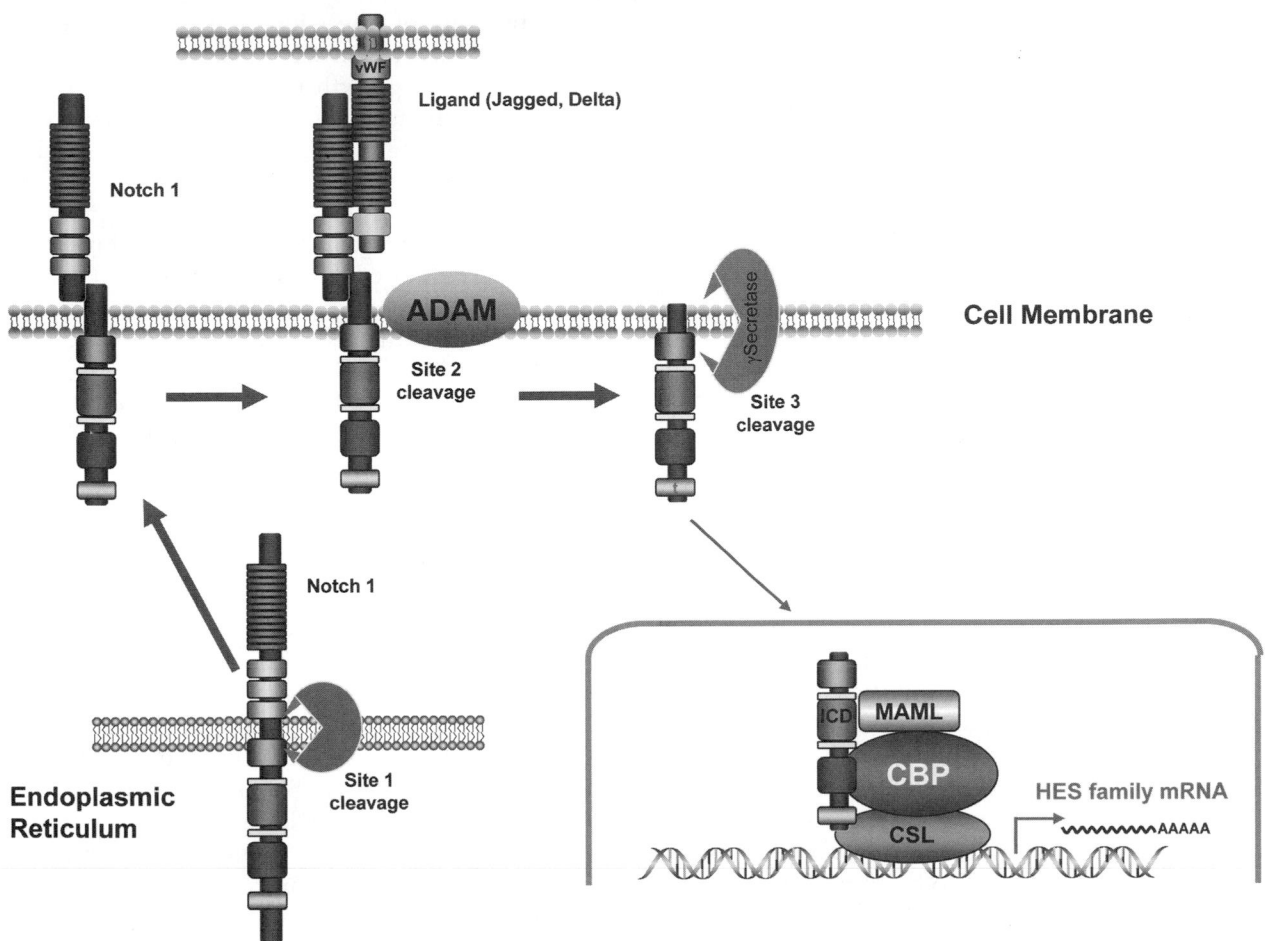

FIGURE 13.6 Notch signaling as an example of regulated intramembranous proteolysis (RIP). It is believed that Notch is proteolytically processed in the ER (site 1 cleavage), and expressed on the cell surface as a disulfide-linked dimer of the extracellular domain and the transmembrane-intracellular domain. Binding of the extracellular domain to a Notch ligand (such as Jagged-1) on an adjacent cell exposes a juxtamembrane cleavage site (site 2) for a member of the ADAM family of extracellular proteases. This second cleavage allows the γ-secretase complex (containing presenilin) to cleave the remaining carboxy-terminus at a site within the membrane (site 3 cleavage), releasing the intracellular domain (ICD) which translocates to the nucleus. In the nucleus, the ICD of Notch can bind to members of the CSL family of transcriptional repressors, and in the presence of CSL-binding protein (CBP) and mastermind like protein-1 (MAML), activate transcription of the HES family of genes.

signaling by other cell surface proteins. For example, the γ-secretase complex has been shown to cleave the EGF tyrosine kinase receptor ErbB4 and the adherens junction protein E-cadherin.[93] In the case of ErbB4, this cleavage event is required for the normal proapoptotic effects of receptor activation, arguing that some cell outcomes previously ascribed to activation of tyrosine kinase cascades may in fact be due to receptor cleavage, and subsequent direct regulation of nuclear transcriptional events.[94] While the nuclear targets of some of these cleaved receptors remain to be determined, the likely importance of this pathway in normal cell signaling is emphasized by the finding that the HGF receptor c-Met undergoes a similar cleavage event that regulates cell survival signaling.[95]

Recently recognized targets of regulated intramembrane proteolysis in the kidney include the proximal tubule scavenger receptor megalin, as well as polycystin-1. In the proximal tubule, megalin can undergo ligand-dependent γ-secretase mediated cleavage,[96] leading to release of the megalin intracellular domain that in turn downregulates mRNA expression for both megalin itself and the Na^+/H^+ exchanger 3 (NHE3).[97] Polycystin-1, the protein product of the PKD1 gene that is defective in the majority of patients with autosomal dominant polycystic kidney disease (ADPKD), has also been shown to undergo RIP, releasing an intracellular carboxy-terminal tail (CTT) that is believed to traffic to the nucleus, where it can regulate gene expression.[98,99] γ-Secretase-mediated cleavage of polycystin-1 to generate the CTT appears to be dependent on the presence of polycystin-2, as well as mechanical stimuli such as those that might occur with urinary flow.[100]

Receptors that Signal Cell Location

One of the most important roles of cell signaling is to organize when a given cell should undergo differentiation toward a highly specialized function (such as the increase in sodium transporters in the brush border of a proximal tubule cell in response to angiotensin II signals mediated by volume depletion[101]) or should revert to more basic processes such as cell division and migration (e.g., during development of the embryonic kidney or recovery of the adult kidney from acute kidney injury). While these widely divergent responses are primarily mediated by receptor–ligand interactions such as those mentioned above, cells also have surface proteins that provide important clues regarding cell location and density, and thus establish their level of differentiation, polarity, and responsiveness to outside signals.

Cell–Matrix Interactions can Signal Cell Location

The cells of the nephron reside on a complex basement membrane that provides specific clues regarding cell location. In the glomerulus this structure is highly specialized to not only support epithelial cell attachment (the podocyte), but also endothelial cell attachment, and to serve as a significant component of the glomerular filtration barrier. The basement membrane of the kidney has been shown to be composed of multiple matrix proteins, including collagen, laminin, perlecan, nidogen, nephronectin, and entactin. The specific isoforms and relative contributions of these proteins vary during the course of renal development, as well as along the length of the adult nephron (reviewed in [102]). These matrix proteins interact with members of a large family of specific cell surface receptors, the heterodimeric α/β integrins.

In the kidney, $\alpha_1\beta_1$, $\alpha_2\beta_1$, $\alpha_3\beta_1$, $\alpha_6\beta_4$, $\alpha_8\beta_1$, and $\alpha_V\beta_3$ have been found to be highly expressed in developing and/or adult renal tubular cells (reviewed in [103]). The binding of the heterodimeric integrin complex to its matrix ligand in the basement membrane ($\alpha_1\beta_1$ integrin and type IV collagen, for example) results in clustering of the integrins on the basal surface of the cell at contact sites known as focal contacts or adhesions, and the concomitant accumulation of a large group of intracellular signaling proteins at these sites known as the focal adhesion complex. This complex typically includes the focal adhesion scaffolding proteins paxillin and HEF1, the non-receptor kinases Src, PI 3-K, integrin-linked kinase (ILK) and focal adhesion kinase (FAK), the small G-protein regulated signaling proteins PIX and PAK, and actin-binding proteins such as vinculin, talin, and actopaxin (reviewed in [104,105]). Signaling through this complex can occur in a traditional "outside-in" manner, in which integrin binding to matrix results in formation and activation of the signaling complex or in an "inside-out" manner, in which signals from other sites, such as activated growth factor receptors, can regulate the affinity of the integrin complex for its matrix ligand, for example during growth factor-stimulated cell adhesion and/or migration.

Signals emanating from focal adhesions provide critical clues regarding cell location, establishment of cell polarity, regulation of cell proliferation, and determination of cell differentiation. The recruitment of actin-binding proteins into the focal adhesion complex provides important clues for cell polarity, while the regulation of small G-proteins such as Rac and Cdc42 is critical for regulating cell differentiation and directed migration.[106] Focal adhesion signaling through Src, FAK, and the P I3-K are required to normally activate the ERK MAPK pathway in response to proliferative growth factor stimuli, and thus promote entry into the cell cycle and subsequent cell proliferation.[107] In the event that cell–matrix adhesion is lost, such as can occur in proximal tubule cells following ischemic renal injury, growth factor signaling is muted, the cells enter cell cycle arrest and eventually undergo anoikis (programmed cell death induced by cell detachment) due to activation of the JNK MAPK pathway (see "Intracellular Signaling Pathways").[108]

The importance of providing the right matrix environment for normal kidney development and function has been demonstrated in mice lacking specific matrix proteins and/or integrin receptors. For example, failure to express laminin-10 results in severe abnormalities in glomerular development, as does loss of expression of the laminin-10 receptor $\alpha_3\beta_1$ integrin,[109,110] while loss of $\beta1$ integrin severely impairs branching of the ureteric bud.[111] In contrast, mice lacking integrin α_1 expression demonstrate normal kidney development,[112] but have increased fibrosis after glomerular injury, due to an increase in reactive oxygen species (ROS) generation[113] (Figure 13.7).

Cell–Cell Interactions such as Adherens Junctions and Gap Junctions can Signal Cell Density and allow Cells to act in Concert

A second means by which cells obtain clues about their immediate environment is via cell–cell interactions. Of the many types of cell–cell interactions, at least three, adherens junctions, tight junctions, and the gap junctions, play important roles in cell signaling. Adherens junctions form at the lateral border of adjacent cells due to the intercellular interactions of cadherins, a family of cell type specific transmembrane proteins (reviewed in [114]). There are multiple cadherin family members, including the classic epithelial cell member E-cadherin, the endothelial cell cadherin VE-cadherin, and the renal tubule associated cadherin Ksp-cadherin.[115] The extracellular portion of cadherins

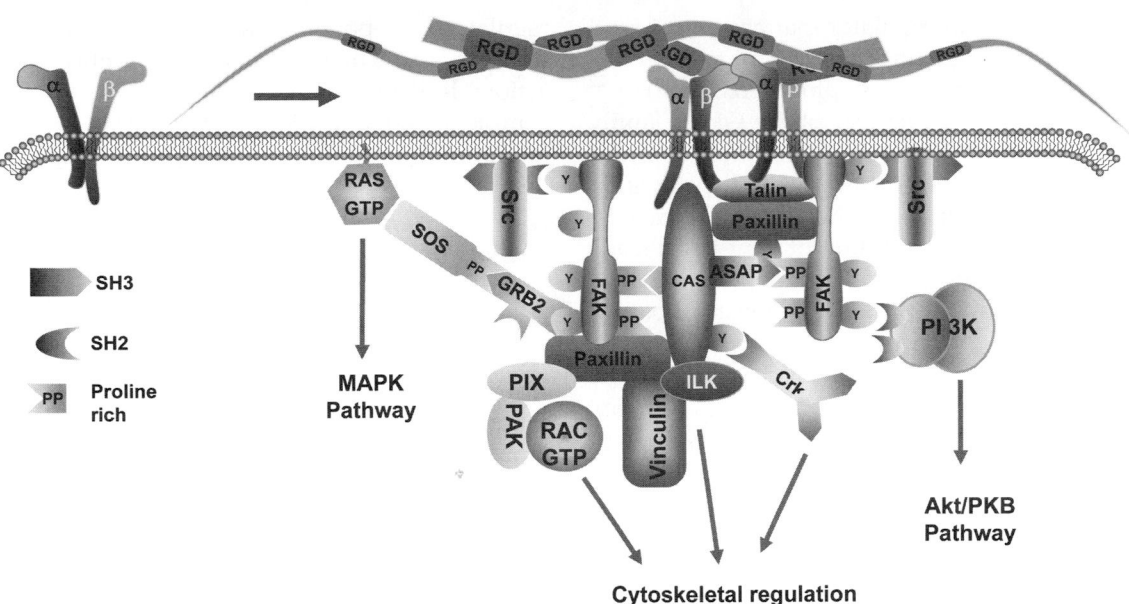

FIGURE 13.7 **Integrin signaling at the cell—matrix interface.** The αβ integrin heterodimers on the cell surface bind to specific sequences in the subcellular matrix (RGD domains in collagen for example), triggering a conformational change in the integrin, and the subsequent recruitment of a large number of cytosolic and membrane-associated proteins (the focal adhesion complex). These proteins include the adaptor and scaffolding proteins p130Cas, Paxillin, Crk, and Grb2. These adaptor proteins in turn mediate the interaction of large numbers of signaling proteins, including tyrosine kinases such as Src, which can phosphorylate and activate other proteins in the complex (including the EGF receptor), and FAK, which activates turnover of the focal adhesion so that cells can migrate. The formation of this complex also activates cell survival and proliferation signals, including the PI 3-kinase and MAPK pathways, and regulators of the actin cytoskeleton such as vinculin, talin, integrin-linked kinase (ILK), and Rac.

contains five repeat sequences (known as EC repeats), that can interact in a homophilic, calcium-dependent manner with the EC repeats present on cadherins in adjacent cells. This interaction is important for providing cell sorting signals during tissue development.[116]

The intracellular domain of the cadherins associates with a group of cytoplasmic proteins known as the catenins. One of these proteins, β-catenin, has a dual role in the cell. It directly binds to cadherins, and thus participates in the formation of cell—cell junctions, but it can also disassociate from adherens junctions and translocate to the nucleus, where it regulates signaling events involved in cell differentiation and proliferation. Originally it was believed that the direct interaction of cadherins with β-catenin created a stable binding site for the actin-binding protein α-catenin, thus generating a static site for lateral attachment of the actin cytoskeleton. However, more recent studies have demonstrated that this protein complex is a dynamic structure that can support actin filament rearrangement during the movement of cells, while maintaining cell—cell junctional integrity.[117]

β-Catenin Signaling can Regulate Cell Differentiation and Proliferation

As noted, β-catenin can leave the adherens junction and enter the nucleus, where it acts as a transcriptional regulator by binding to the TCF/Lef transcriptional complex.[118] Genes that are induced downstream of β-catenin typically lead to increased cell proliferation and regulation of differentiation, events that are important during normal development, but that are typically downregulated in the adult.[119] This transcriptional activity of β-catenin is tightly regulated by controlling the free cytosolic pool of β-catenin that is available for translocation into the nucleus. In the adult renal tubule, the extensive array of intercellular adherens junctions that forms in the confluent monolayer of epithelial cells results in sequestration of the majority of β-catenin with cadherin. To further ensure that free β-catenin levels remain low in the cytosol, a serine-threonine kinase, glycogen synthase kinase-3β (GSK-3β), phosphorylates cytosolic β-catenin and targets it for degradation by the proteosomal pathway.[120] GSK-3β is associated with the adenomatous polyposis coli (APC) protein, and mutations in this complex that prevent β-catenin phosphorylation and degradation lead to increased nuclear β-catenin signaling, cell proliferation, and subsequent tumor formation.[121]

During organ development, and following some types of organ injury, β-catenin nuclear signaling is activated by destabilization of adherens junctions (thereby releasing β-catenin into the cytoplasm) and coincident inhibition of GSK-3β kinase activity.

The classic developmental regulator that has been found to activate β-catenin signaling in this manner is the growth factor Wnt and its receptor Frizzled (Fz)[122] (Figure 13.8). Frizzled is a member of the GPCR family of seven membrane spanning cell surface receptors, and has been proposed to signal, at least in part, by activation of heterotrimeric G-proteins.[123] However, in the canonical Wnt signaling pathway, binding of Wnt to Fz leads to the GSK-3β-dependent phosphorylation of a second membrane spanning protein, the Low-density lipoprotein Receptor-related Proteins 5 and/or 6 (LRP5/6), which in turn mediate the recruitment/activation of the cytosolic protein dishevelled (Dsh).[124] This complex appears to inhibit GSK-3β-dependent phosphorylation of β-catenin and other substrates in the cytosol by sequestering GSK-3β into multivesicular endosomes, thus preventing β-catenin degradation.[125,126]

During kidney development, Wnt4 and Wnt9b, acting at least in part via activation of β-catenin, have been shown to be required for both maintenance of the nephron progenitor pool and normal differentiation of these progenitor cells to form the nephron, suggesting that careful titration of the level of activation of canonical Wnt signaling is critical during mesenchymal-to-epithelial differentiation.[127–129] In addition, multiple Wnts are upregulated following kidney injury, where they appear to play a role in normal repair, as well as in the promotion of fibrosis.[130,131]

Podocyte Slit Diaphragms are Highly Specialized Tight Junctions that Signal to the Cystoskeleton

Tight junctions are cell—cell junctions that are typically located at the interface of the apical and basolateral membranes of epithelial cells, where they serve to regulate the composition of the fluid that moves between cells into the interstitial space. In glomerular podocytes, tight junctions have evolved into elaborate structures that support the extensive interdigitation of adjacent cells along the glomerular basement membrane, and thus constitute a critical component of the glomerular filtration barrier. These cell—cell junctions are termed slit diaphragms, and form when Ig-like domains in the extracellular portion of the transmembrane proteins nephrin and Neph1 form homotypic and heterotypic interactions with nephrin/Neph1 molecules in the adjacent podocyte.[132] Dynamic regulation of these interactions is critical for maintaining the integrity of the slit diaphragm, which is achieved by signaling from the slit diaphragm to the actin cytoskeleton (reviewed in [133,134]). This signaling involves phosphorylation of the intracellular domain of nephrin by the Src-family kinase Fyn, followed by recruitment of a signaling complex including the adaptor proteins Nck1/2, Grb2, and p85, which in turn mediate recruitment/activation of cytoskeletal regulatory proteins including WASP, Pak, and Rac that regulate actin polymerization/depolymerization in the foot process. Mutations that alter nephrin/NEPH interactions lead to disruption of this intracellular signaling complex, destabilization of the actin cytoskeleton and foot process retraction/fusion.

Gap Junctions Promote Rapid Signaling Between Groups of Cells

A second type of cell—cell interaction that is important for cell signaling is the gap junction. These junctions are formed by the alignment of hemichannels on the lateral borders of two adjacent cells to establish a direct cytoplasmic link between the cells, thus allowing the rapid movement of small molecules and electrical charge through multiple cells within a specified region of the organ.[135] Gap junctions are primarily composed of a family of proteins known as connexins, and have traditionally been studied for their ability to rapidly transmit contraction signals through muscles. Investigation of gap junction function within the kidney has demonstrated that mesangial cells contain large numbers of gap junctions comprised of connexin 43 (Cx43), and that these are critical for mediating intercellular calcium-dependent coordinated mesangial contraction.[136] In addition, tubular epithelial cells maintain intercellular gap junctions that can be regulated by growth factors, as well as by ischemic injury,[137,138] although the precise role of these channels in normal tubule function is presently not well-understood.

The Cilia as a Signaling Structure

Many cells of the body, including renal epithelial cells, have a surface structure known as the primary cilium. Cilia are elongated membrane protrusions that surround a central core of microtubules arising from a microtubule organizing center known as the basal body (reviewed in [139,140]). Cells that express cilia with a microtubular arrangement of 9 + 2 (9 microtubule doublets arranged in a cylinder around a core of 2 microtubule singlets), such as those lining the trachea, are motile and can act to facilitate directional movement of fluid (reviewed in [141]). In other cells, such as those lining the renal tubules, cilia have a 9 + 0 arrangement, are non-motile, and were previously believed to be rudimentary structures. However, the finding that genetic mutations that interrupt cilia formation can result in cystic kidney diseases in rodents,[142,143] along with the recent discovery that the two predominant gene products known to cause human autosomal dominant polycystic kidney disease, polycystin-1 (Pc-1) and polycystin-2 (Pc-2), localize to cilia, has resulted in intense investigations into the role of non-motile cilia as renal epithelial mechanosensors.[143,144]

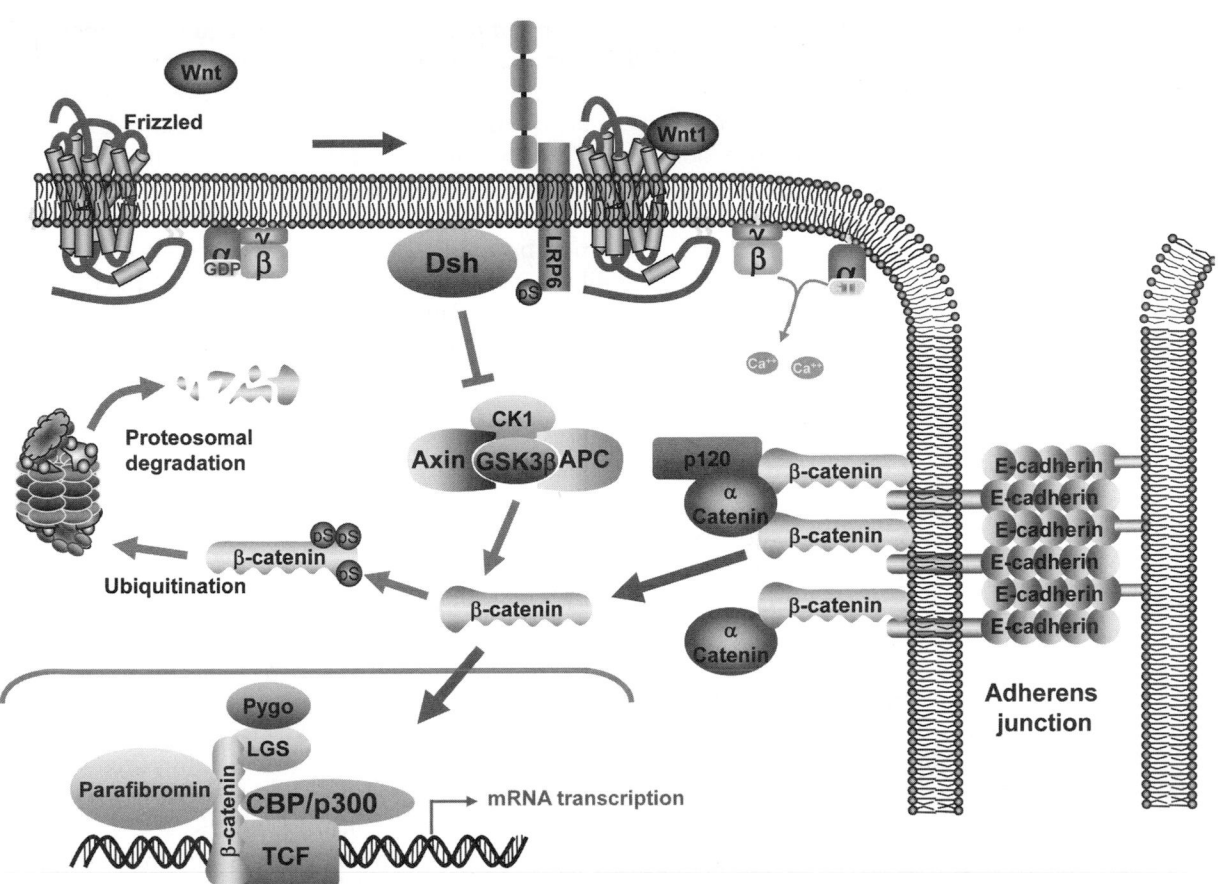

FIGURE 13.8 Wnt/β-catenin signaling. Formation of stable cell—cell adherens junctions in mature epithelia occurs due to the lateral interactions of cadherins on adjacent cells. This results in the formation of an intracellular complex of proteins comprised of β-catenin, α-catenin, and p120. α-Catenin can interact with the actin cytoskeleton and the adherens junction complex in a dynamic manner, and thus serve as a nidus for actin cytoskeletal arrangement along the lateral border of the cell. β-catenin can either be sequestered in the adherens junction or released into the cytosol where it is capable of translocating to the nucleus and activating the transcription of multiple genes involved in cell proliferation and dedifferentiation. In mature, non-proliferating cells, free cytosolic β-catenin is rapidly degraded, because phosphorylation by GSK-3β targets β-catenin for ubiquitination and degradation in the proteosome. GSK-3β is found in a complex that includes the regulatory/targeting proteins axin and APC. The kinase activity of GSK-3β can be inhibited following activation of several growth factor receptors. In the best studied pathway, stimulation of the Wnt receptor Frizzled leads to phosphorylation of the membrane spanning protein Lrp6, which in turn activates the Dishevelled (Dsh)-dependent sequestration and inhibition of GSK-3β. The resultant increase in free cytosolic β-catenin leads to its nuclear translocation, where it serves as a scaffold for the association of a complex of proteins that bind and activate RNA polymerase II, leading to gene transcription. There is data supporting a second signaling pathway downstream of Frizzled in which GTP-loading of the Gαi-subunit of the heterotrimeric G-protein results in release of the βγ-subunit, which in turn activates phosphoinositide hydrolysis and downstream calcium release.

These studies have demonstrated that Pc-2 acts as a cation channel, and that regulation of this channel activity can be mediated by its interaction with Pc-1.[145–147] *In vitro* studies have demonstrated that Pc-1 and Pc-2 co-localize on the primary cilium of the apical cell membrane in renal epithelial cells, and that physiological levels of fluid shear stress, such as that created by urine flow in the renal tubule, may be sufficient to stimulate cilia-dependent Pc-1/Pc-2-mediated calcium signaling.[143,148,149] It is presently hypothesized that failure of this signaling pathway can result in abnormalities in both the rate and organization of cell proliferation, and thus can lead to cyst formation.[150]

INTRACELLULAR SIGNALING PATHWAYS

As is clear from the preceding section, activation of cell surface receptors results in the regulation of multiple intracellular signaling pathways. Although numerous studies from the past decade have emphasized the vast amount of cross-talk between the proteins involved in these pathways, it remains useful to identify core signaling cascades that can transduce signals from the receptor to effector proteins that mediate specific cellular responses. Several of these signaling cascades, including the heterotrimeric G-protein-adenylate cyclase-cAMP-PKA pathway, the TGFβ-Smad pathway, and the Wnt-Fz-Dsh-Gsk3β-β-catenin pathways, have been described in some detail in the section "Cell Surface Receptors." This section will focus on several other signaling cascades that are believed to be fundamental regulators of cell survival and function in the kidney, including the PLC-Ca-PKC pathway, the MAPK pathway, and the PI 3-kinase pathway.

The Phospholipase C Pathway Regulates Intracellular Calcium Release and Activates PKC Signaling

Phospholipase C (PLC) is an enzyme that catalyzes the hydrolysis of the membrane lipid phosphoinositide 4,5 bisphosphate ($PI_{4,5}P_2$) to generate diacylglycerol (DAG) in the membrane and release inositol trisphosphate (IP_3) into the cytoplasm (reviewed in [151]). DAG provides a binding site to recruit protein kinase C (PKC) to the membrane, while IP_3 binds to its receptor on the endoplasmic reticulum that mediates the intracellular release of stored calcium. Thus, activation of PLC regulates both PKC-dependent and calcium-dependent intracellular signaling.

In mammals, there are four known families of phospholipases C, PLCβ, PLCγ, PLCδ, and PLCε. While all four groups share the catalytic X and Y lipase domains, the regulatory domains are widely divergent, allowing activation by distinct upstream receptors. For example, PLCβ is activated following stimulation of certain GPCRs, because it has a carboxy terminal domain that recognizes and binds GTP-loaded $G_{q\alpha}$, as well as the free βγ heterodimer[152,153] (see section "G-protein coupled receptors"). Activation of PLCδ and PLCε are less well-understood, although each appears to be mediated by interaction with small GTP-binding proteins. PLCδ can be activated by associating with the GTPase Ral, whereas PLCε has a Ras-binding domain and can be activated by associating with GTP-loaded Ras.[154–157]

In contrast, PLCγ family members lack the Gα- and βγ-binding regions, but instead encode two SH2 domains and one SH3 domain that mediate their recruitment and activation by receptor tyrosine kinases (RTKs) such as the PDGF receptor, vascular endothelial growth factor (VEGF) receptor, and HGF receptor.[158] Interestingly, PLCγ can also be phosphorylated and activated by non-receptor protein tyrosine kinases, such as Src family members. In this manner, PLCγ can be secondarily activated in immune cells downstream of T-cell receptor activation (see Figure 13.5), as well as following activation of certain GPCRs, such as the angiotensin II receptor.[159]

For PLC to hydrolyze $PI_{4,5}P_2$, it must be recruited to the membrane. Members of both the PLCβ and PLCγ families have pleckstrin homology (PH) domains at their amino termini that promote membrane association by binding to select membrane phospholipids, such as $PI_{4,5}P_2$ and $PI_{3,4,5}P_3$.[160] PLCβ family members are further stabilized at the membrane because their PH domain can also interact with the membrane bound βγ G-protein heterodimer, while the SH2 domains of PLCγ proteins enhance membrane association by mediating recruitment to cell surface receptors. In this manner, PLC is recruited to specific sites at the membrane in the vicinity of the activating receptor, allowing the cell to selectively upregulate DAG and IP_3 production in that area.

PLC-dependent generation of DAG provides a membrane binding site for recruitment and activation of several members of the protein kinase C (PKC) family of non-receptor serine-threonine kinases (Figure 13.9). PKCs are a large group of proteins that are subdivided into the conventional PKCs, novel PKCs, and atypical PKCs. The conventional PKCs (PKCα, PKCβ, PKCγ) are activated in a calcium-dependent fashion following recruitment to the cell membrane by binding to DAG and phospholipids such as phosphatidylserine (PS). The novel PKCs (PKCδ, PKCε, PKCη, and PKCθ) are also recruited to the membrane by binding to DAG and membrane phospholipids, but do not require calcium for activation. The atypical PKCs (PKCλ, PKCζ, PKCμ, and PKCι) lack both the DAG and calcium binding sites, and instead appear to be associated with the membrane and activated solely via their association with membrane phospholipids (reviewed in [161]). In addition to PS, it has been found that the 3-phosphorylated lipid products of the PI 3-K (such as $PI_{3,4}P_2$ and $PI_{3,4,5}P_3$) can bind and activate both novel and atypical PKCs.[162]

Once activated, PKCs have multiple potential phosphorylation targets in the cell. The determination of which targets are phosphorylated is dependent on cell type, the isoform of PKC that is activated, and targeting proteins that specify subcellular localization of the activated PKC. Proteins that are not phosphorylation substrates of PKC, but serve only to target specific PKCs to select sites in the cell, are collectively termed RACKs (receptors of activated C kinase). For example, the cell polarity proteins Par3 and Par6 associate with atypical PKCs, such as PKCζ, and specifically target them to epithelial tight junctions on renal tubular cells.[163] In this location, PKCζ has been shown to regulate both tight junction assembly and disassembly, although the exact phosphorylation targets of PKCζ have yet to be identified.[164,165]

Recent studies have demonstrated that PKC localization to the basolateral membrane can regulate Na,K-ATPase activity in the renal tubule as well. Several phosphorylation sites for classical PKCs (such as PKCα) have been identified in the amino terminus of the Na,K-ATPase α-subunit, and phosphorylation of

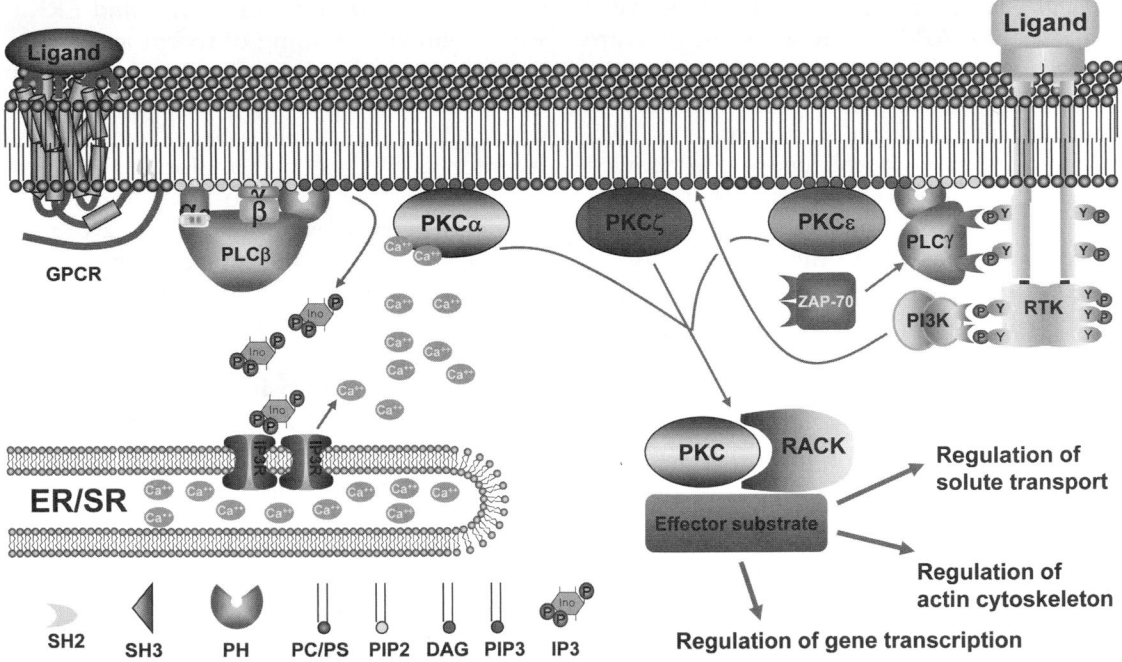

FIGURE 13.9 **Phospholipase C-protein kinase C signaling.** Activation of GPCRs coupled to Gαq can recruit PLCβ to the membrane and activate its phospholipase activity via interactions with the GTP-loaded α-subunit, as well as the free βγ-subunit. PLCγ is classically activated via binding of its SH2 domains to phosphotyrosine residues on RTKs, although PLCγ can also be activated by the non-receptor tyrosine kinase Zap-70. Both PLCβ and PLCγ are stabilized at the membrane via their lipid-binding PH domain, where they hydrolyze PI4,5P2 (PIP2) to generate DAG and IP3. DAG serves as a binding site at the membrane for both conventional PKCs (such as PKCα) and novel PKCs (such as PKCε). While novel PKCs are activated as a consequence of this membrane recruitment, conventional PKCs also require calcium-binding for full activation. This calcium signal comes from IP3-mediated calcium release from intracellular stores. A third family of PKCs, the atypical PKCs such as PKCζ, lack the DAG-binding domain, and are recruited to the membrane and activated by binding to phosphatidyl serine (PS) as well as the lipid product of the PI3K, $PI_{3,4,5}P_3$ (PIP3). Specificity of signaling for this diverse family of serine-threonine kinases is provided by association with receptors of activated C kinase (RACKs) which target the activated PKC isoform to the correct effector protein (such as the α-subunit of the Na,K-ATPase in renal tubular cells).

these sites appears to increase cellular sodium pump activity by increasing membrane localization of the enzyme.[166,167] Interestingly, activation of PKC downstream of the D_1-type dopamine receptors appears to have the opposite effect, inhibiting sodium pump activity as part of the overall effect of the D_1 receptor in inhibiting tubular sodium reabsorption.[168] Exploration of this response has demonstrated that novel PKCs such as PKCθ and PKCε are likely to mediate this Na,K-ATPase inhibitory effect.[169] It is unknown whether these PKCs phosphorylate different sites on the sodium pump than PKCα or act indirectly via phosphorylation of intermediate proteins such as the sodium hydrogen regulatory factor Nherf-1.[170]

Another group of PKC regulatory targets are transcription factors. PKC isoforms such as PKCδ, PKCε, and PKCθ have been found to regulate the activity of multiple transcription factors, including NF-κB (involved in immune and inflammatory responses), signal transducers and activators of transcription (STATs, regulators of inflammatory responses, cell proliferation, and differentiation), and Jun N-terminal kinase (JNK, involved in cell stress response and survival) (reviewed in [171]). By acting upstream of JNK as well as the Raf-MEK-ERK pathway (see below), PKC isoforms can cooperate to mediate increased activity of the immediate early response genes Jun and Fos.[172]

An interesting example of convergence of PKC with other signaling pathways is seen during the activation of T-cells. The rise in intracellular calcium following T-cell stimulation results in the activation of calmodulin and binding of the calcium—calmodulin complex to the non-receptor serine-threonine phosphatase calcineurin (also known as protein phosphatase 2B or PP2B). Activated calcineurin dephosphorylates and activates the nuclear translocation of another protein, nuclear factor of activated T-cells or NFAT (reviewed in [173,174]). While originally described in T-cells, NFATs are expressed in multiple cell types and control the expression of genes such as Il-2, GM-CSF, interferon-γ, TNFα, and Cox2 that regulate processes as diverse as T- and B-cell proliferation in response to antigen stimulation, cardiac myocyte differentiation and hypertrophy, and sodium channel expression (reviewed in [175,176]).

However, the DNA-binding sites of many of these gene targets contain nearby AP-1 promoter sites, and are only upregulated in an efficient manner following the concerted actions of NFAT and the AP-1 binding elements Jun and Fos. Thus, concerted activation of PKC (to activate Jun and Fos) and calcineurin (to activate NFAT) leads to maximal gene expression and cellular response. The importance of calcineurin in mediating immune cell activation has led to the extensive use of calcineurin inhibitors, such as cyclosporine and tacrolimus, for the prevention of transplant rejection.

The Mitogen Activated Protein Kinase (MAPK) Pathway Regulates Cell Survival, Proliferation, and Morphology

The MAPK pathway provides an excellent example of the way in which different extracellular signals can converge on the regulation of a single intracellular signaling pathway, and demonstrates how targeting of that pathway to specific sites in the cell via scaffolding proteins can determine which effector proteins are regulated, and what cell responses are affected. As the name implies, this protein cascade was originally identified based on its activation downstream of pro-proliferative growth factors such as insulin and EGF.[177] In the classic MAPK cascade, binding of the growth factor to its receptor tyrosine kinase (RTK) initiates a series of protein–protein interactions that ultimately result in activation of the cytosolic serine-threonine kinase ERK, which can phosphorylate and regulate diverse effector substrates including transcription factors in the nucleus, focal adhesion proteins at the cell surface, and contractile proteins in the cytosol.[178–180]

The core proteins of this classic MAPK cascade are three kinases, Raf, MEK, and ERK. Raf-1 (also called MEK kinase (MEKK) or MAPK kinase kinase (MAPKKK)) is a serine-threonine kinase that phosphorylates and activates two closely related MEK isoforms, MEK1 and 2. MEK1/2 are dual specificity (tyrosine as well as serine/threonine) kinases that phosphorylate ERK1 and 2 on a highly conserved amino acid motif, Thr-Glu-Tyr, contained in the activation loop of the protein.[181] The efficient activation of ERK in this cascade requires that the three proteins (Raf, MEK, and ERK) are brought into close proximity on a single scaffolding protein. Present studies indicate that several different proteins can serve this scaffolding function, including β-arrestin, IQGAP, kinase suppressor of Ras (KSR), and paxillin.[20,182–184] The location of the scaffolding protein and the regulation of Raf/MEK/ERK association determines which effector proteins are likely to be regulated (reviewed in [185]).

The core module of Raf, MEK, and ERK can be activated following binding of receptor tyrosine kinases to their extracellular ligands. The initial step in RTK-mediated MAPK activation is the recruitment of the GRB2 adaptor protein to the tyrosine phosphorylated receptor. GRB2 is a small molecule that is composed of one SH2 domain and two SH3 domains.[186] As noted previously, proteins containing SH2 domains interact with other proteins that contain phosphorylated tyrosine residues flanked by the appropriate amino acids. The GRB2 SH2 domain preferentially binds to phosphotyrosine residues with an asparagine at the +2 position, such as tyrosine 1096 in the activated c-Ret receptor (pYA$\underline{N}$W) or tyrosine 1356 in activated c-Met (pYV$\underline{N}$V). In contrast, SH3 domains typically mediate constitutive association with short proline-rich sequences in target proteins. The guanine nucleotide exchange factor (GEF) Sos contains such a sequence, and associates with the GRB2 SH3 domain in a constitutive fashion. Sos acts as a GEF for the membrane-associated small GTP-binding protein Ras.[187]

Ras is structurally similar to the α-subunit of the αβγ heterotrimer that associates with GPCRs. However, Ras is activated by non-GPCR GEFs such as Sos and, in the GTP-bound state, associates with and activates Raf rather than adenylyl cylase. This activation step appears to involve the Ras-dependent dephosphorylation of Raf by PP2A, a non-receptor protein phosphatase.[188] Thus, RTK activation results in recruitment of the GRB2-Sos complex to the membrane where it mediates GTP-loading of Ras, and activation of the Raf-MEK-ERK signaling pathway (Figure 13.10).

In addition to this classic model of GRB2-Sos-Ras-dependent MAPK activation mediated by RTKs, several alternative mechanisms of MAPK pathway activation have now been elucidated. For example, as described in the section "G-protein coupled receptors," the recruitment of β-arrestin to activated GPCRs can result in β-arrestin-dependent scaffolding of Raf, MEK, and ERK, and thus can facilitate ERK activation (reviewed in [189]). Another pathway of MAPK activation is that of PKC-mediated Raf activation. As noted previously, PKCs are activated downstream of GPCRs, RTKs, and non-receptor kinases (such as the PI 3-K) by associating with DAG and/or phospholipids at the cell membrane. Once activated, one of the PKC phosphorylation targets is Raf,[190] leading to Raf activation and the downstream activation of MEK and ERK, even in the absence of GTP-loaded Ras.[191]

ERK Activation is Regulated by the Cross-Talk of Multiple Signaling Pathways

Classically, activated ERK has been shown to regulate gene transcription factors involved in promoting cell survival and inducing cell proliferation. Careful

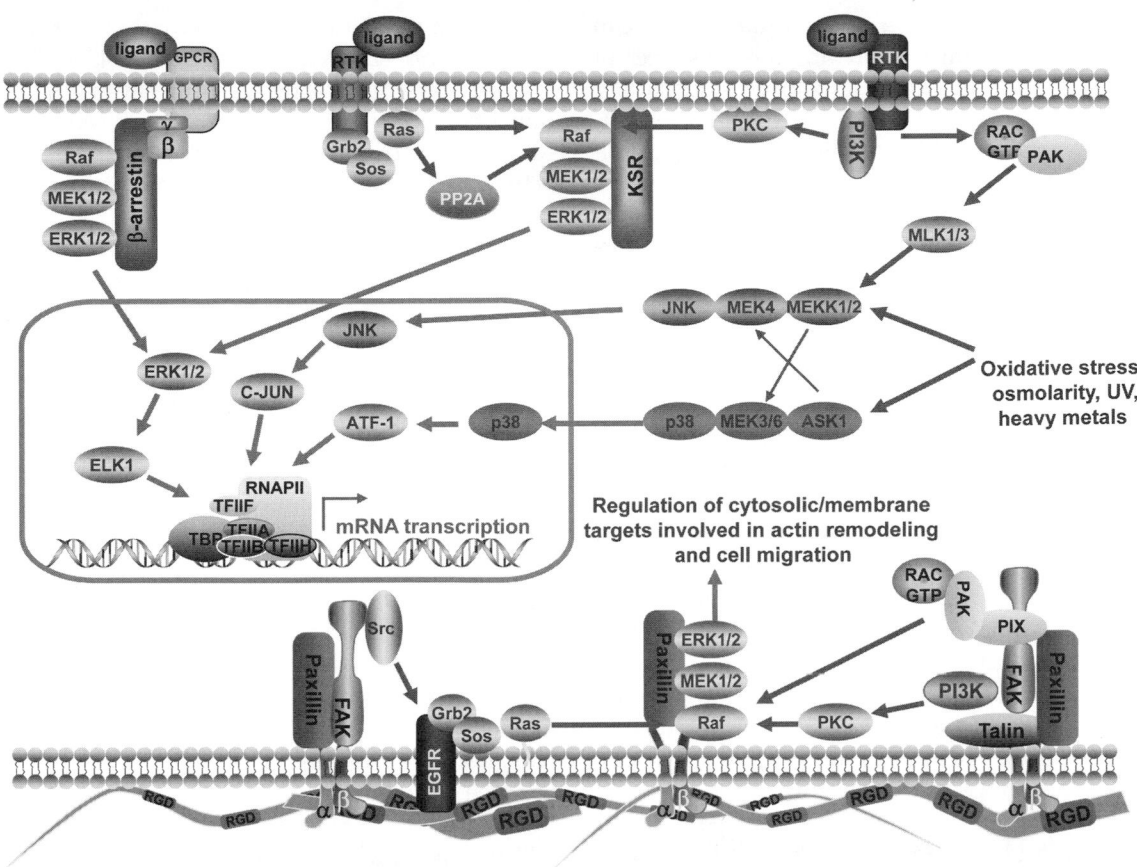

FIGURE 13.10 MAPK signaling. The prototypic MAPK pathway involves the growth factor stimulated activation of the small G-protein Ras at the membrane, followed by Ras binding and activation of the serine-threonine kinase Raf (a MAPK kinase kinase or MAPKKK). This process involves dephosphorylation of Raf at an inhibitory site by the serine-threonine phosphatase PP2A. In addition, Raf can be activated by PKC-dependent phosphorylation or by recruitment to the GPCR scaffolding protein β-arrestin. The MAPK pathway can also be activated in a growth factor-independent fashion via focal adhesion signaling when cells attach to the basement membrane. Activation of Raf results in phosphorylation and activation of the downstream kinases MEK and ERK. Depending on the site of ERK activation, it can translocate to the nucleus where it phosphorylates and activates transcription factors such as Elk1 or it can remain in the cytoplasm where it phosphorylates and regulates proteins involved in actin cytoskeletal rearrangement and cell migration, such as Myosin Light Chain Kinase (MLCK) and paxillin. Two other MAPK pathways present in most cells are the stress-activated protein kinases (SAPK) p38 and JNK. Multiple factors have been shown to activate p38 and JNK, including oxidative or osmolar stress, heavy metals, cytokines, and growth factors such as EGF and TGFβ. These stimuli induce the activation of a group of MAPKKKs including apoptosis signal-regulating kinase 1 (ASK1) and MEKK1/2. Activation of the MAPKKK results in phosphorylation of the appropriate dual specificity MAPKK (MEK) such as MEK3, MEK4, and MEK6, which in turn phosphorylate and activate JNK and p38. Small G-proteins such as Rac and Cdc42 can also activate the p38 and JNK pathways via binding and activating intermediate kinases such as the Mixed Lineage Kinase (MLK) family of serine-threonine kinases. There is considerable cross-talk between these pathways, resulting in simultaneous activation of JNK and p38 under many conditions. Like ERK, activated JNK and p38 translocate into the nucleus, where they phosphorylate regulatory transcription factors such as c-Jun, ATF-1, Elk-1, and Sap1. These in turn regulate the RNA polymerase transcription initiation complex to activate the transcription of multiple genes including pro-survival and pro-apoptotic factors, matrix proteins, heat shock factors, etc.

control of these events is fundamental to normal organ physiology, so it is not surprising that ERK activation is regulated by a complex series of signals derived from extracellular stimuli, such as growth factors and cell—matrix interactions. It has long been known that adherent cells, such as endothelial cells and epithelial cells, can proliferate when attached to the proper basement membrane, but undergo anoikis when they lose their attachment. This type of cell death is common in detached tubular epithelial cells following acute renal

injury, and it is believed that the loss of anoikis contributes to the metastatic spread of tumor cells.[192–194] As described earlier, the sites of cell attachment to the basement membrane, focal adhesions, provide the nidus for the aggregation of multiple signaling proteins on the cytosolic face of the attachment. Among the many proteins involved in this complex are the MAPK scaffolding protein paxillin, the Rac-activated protein p21 associated kinase (PAK), the EGF receptor, and the non-receptor tyrosine kinases Src and FAK.

Attachment of the cell to a subcellular matrix can activate MAPK signaling, even in the absence of extracellular growth factor or cytokine stimulation. One mechanism for this activation is that attachment-dependent activation of FAK results in the recruitment and activation of the PI 3-kinase, which leads to the local production of $PI_{3,4,5}P_3$. As noted earlier, $PI_{3,4,5}P_3$ binds and activates PKC, which in turn can phosphorylate and activate Raf.[195] Furthermore, the EGF receptor localizes to focal adhesions in adherent cells, and can be phosphorylated and transactivated by the non-receptor tyrosine kinase Src even in the absence of extracellular EGF, thus mediating ERK activation via the classical Grb2-Sos-Ras pathway. In addition to the ability of focal adhesions to directly activate MAPK signaling, these signaling structures are also required for growth factors to efficiently stimulate MAPK signaling.[196] Although the mechanism of this is not entirely understood, recent studies suggest that activation of the focal adhesion associated serine-threonine kinase PAK leads to phosphorylation of Raf that is required for the efficient activation of Raf by GTP-Ras.[197] Thus, focal adhesions serve as sites to directly activate ERK, as well as supporting ERK activation downstream of proliferative stimuli.

ERK Regulates both Nuclear and Cytosolic Protein Actions

Translocation of activated ERK to the nucleus has been found to signal both pro-proliferative and anti-apoptotic responses. In the nucleus, ERK phosphorylates and activates transcription factors such as Elk-1 and RUNX2, which in turn regulate the mRNA expression of the cell cycle proteins cyclin D1 and $p21^{WAF1}$,[198–200] (reviewed in [201]). Furthermore, ERK activation can downregulate the expression of pro-apoptotic proteins such as Bim1, a process that is believed to be critical for ERK-dependent inhibition of anoikis.[202] These effects of ERK depend on both the amplitude and the duration of ERK activation. For example, transient high level ERK activation in renal tubular cells treated with the growth factor HGF results in activation of focal complex signaling and Rac-dependent cell migration, but does not result in significant cell proliferation.[183] In contrast, sustained low level ERK activation appears to be required for cell cycle entry (leading to proliferation) and the anti-apoptotic effects of ERK.[203–205] For this reason, the degree of ERK activation is tightly regulated by a series of phosphorylation and dephosphorylation steps at the level of Raf.[188]

Activation of ERK can also lead to the phosphorylation of substrate proteins in the cytoplasm. ERK has been shown to phosphorylate and activate myosin light chain kinase (MLCK), resulting in stimulation of cell motility.[180] In addition, ERK activation at focal adhesions

in renal epithelial cells can mediate phosphorylation of paxillin, and subsequent FAK and PI 3-K activation.[52] This process plays a regulatory role in the local activation of another family of small GTP-binding proteins, Rho, Rac, and Cdc42. These proteins are regulators of actin cytoskeletal remodeling, and by binding to their respective effector proteins (such as the Rho-kinase for Rho), mediate the cytoskeletal changes required for cell spreading, lamellipodia formation, and migration (reviewed in [206]). Besides activation downstream of ERK and the PI 3-K, focal adhesion signaling can also activate Rho family members by stimulating the guanine nucleotide exchange factors Vav and/or PIX (reviewed in [207]). In the kidney, regulated activation of Rac and Rho are fundamental for the morphogenic changes involved in developmental tubulogenesis,[208] and Rho activation appears to be required for angiotensin II-dependent regulation of glomerular arteriolar tone.[209]

In addition to the classic ERK MAPK pathway, two other well-conserved MAPK pathways, the JNK and p38 pathways, have been extensively studied and found to play important roles in regulating cell survival (reviewed in [210,211]). Similar to the ERK pathway, p38 and JNK signaling are mediated by a core complex of three proteins, including a MEK kinase which phosphorylates a MEK family member (MEK3 or 6 in the p38 pathway, MEK4 or 7 in the JNK pathway), which in turn phosphorylates the effector kinase p38 or JNK, respectively. Activated p38 or JNK can then translocate to the nucleus, where they phosphorylate and regulate transcription factors such as ATF-1, ATF-2, c-Jun, and STAT-3.

Activation of the p38 and JNK signaling cascades occurs in response to cell stress signals, including UV irradiation, ischemia, and hypoxia, as well as following cytokine stimulation (IL-1 and TNFα) and certain growth factors (EGF, TGFβ).[212,213] Based on in vitro studies demonstrating increased extracellular matrix production following p38 activation, it has been proposed that p38 may play an important role in the development of renal fibrosis following injury (reviewed in [214]). In support of this, in vivo studies using p38 inhibitors in rodents have demonstrated that activation of p38 stimulates the progressive renal tubular fibrosis seen in models of chronic ureteral obstruction.[215] Similarly, mice that overexpress TGFβ exhibit p38-dependent glomerular podocyte apoptosis, an early component of the progression to glomerulosclerosis,[213] and p38 activation may be required for the development of proteinuria following acute glomerular injury.[216] Activation of the ERK, p38, and JNK pathways occurs during the oxidative stress of renal ischemia/reperfusion. Under these conditions, JNK activation appears to mediate the tubular cell apoptotic response, while ERK activation can be protective.[217–219]

The Phosphoinositide 3-Kinase Pathway Regulates Diverse Events Including Glucose Metabolism, Cell Migration, Cell Survival, and Proliferation

Another major intracellular signaling pathway is regulated by a lipid kinase known as the phosphoinositide 3-kinase (PI 3-K).[220] This enzyme is composed of two subunits, the p85 adapter protein and the p110 catalytic-subunit. Recruitment of the p85/p110 complex to the membrane occurs when p85 binds via its SH2 domains to tyrosine phosphorylated receptors (such as the PDGF receptor) or docking proteins (such as the EGF receptor associated protein Gab1 or the insulin receptor associated protein IRS-1). The p110 enzymatic-subunit is activated by this translocation and phosphorylates target lipids, such as $PI_{4,5}P_2$ (PIP2), to form the 3-phosphorylated derivative $PI_{3,4,5}P_3$ (PIP3). PIP3 then serves as a membrane-binding site for multiple proteins that contain lipid-binding domains, such as the pleckstrin homology (PH) domain, the PTB domain, and FYVE domains (reviewed in [221]).

As described previously, several PKC family members are recruited to the membrane and activated by binding to PIP3, as are the docking protein DOCK180 and the guanine nucleotide exchange factor Vav.[222,223] However, the best described targets of PIP3 are the PH-domain containing proteins 3-phosphoinositide dependent kinase-1 (PDK1) and its major substrate enzyme Akt (also known as protein kinase B (PKB)). The generation of PIP3 at the membrane results in recruitment and activation of PDK1, which in turn phosphorylates and activates Akt.[224] In addition to Akt, activated PDK1 can phosphorylate and activate IKK, the upstream regulator of NF-κB, as well as the p70 and p90 ribosomal S6 kinases, and several PKC isoforms.[225,226]

Akt is a serine-threonine kinase that regulates multiple intracellular events, including protein ubiquitination/degradation, glucose metabolism, nitric oxide generation, cell survival, and cell proliferation. To regulate these disparate processes, Akt associates with and phosphorylates multiple cytosolic protein targets (reviewed in [227]). One of these targets is the constitutively active cytosolic enzyme glycogen synthase kinase-3β (GSK-3β), described earlier for its role as a regulator of β-catenin ubiquitination and degradation downstream of the Wnt signaling pathway.[228,229] Phosphorylation of serine 9 at the N-terminus of GSK-3β by Akt causes the kinase domain of GSK-3β to recognize this region as a pseudosubstrate, leading to autoinhibition of the GSK-3β kinase activity and an increase in free cytosolic β-catenin levels.[230,231] β-catenin can then translocate into the nucleus, where it regulates the transcriptional expression of genes involved in stimulating cell proliferation and dedifferentiation. In addition to β-catenin, GSK-3β has also been shown to phosphorylate several other cellular substrates that regulate cell proliferation as well as cell survival. For example, GSK-3β can enter the nucleus where it phosphorylates the cell cycle protein cyclin D1, thus targeting it for rapid degradation.[232] In addition, phosphorylation of translation initiation factor eIF2B by GSK-3β inhibits protein translation, leading to initiation of apoptosis and ultimately cell death.[233] Thus, activation of the PI 3-K/Akt pathway by inhibiting GSK-3β results in increased cyclin D1 levels and eIF2B activation, promoting entry into the cell cycle and preventing apoptotis.

Besides these indirect effects of Akt in preventing cell apoptosis, Akt activation directly inhibits apoptotic responses by phosphorylating and inhibiting the pro-apoptotic factors BAD and caspase 9, as well as the forkhead transcription factor FKHRL1.[234] In addition, Akt activation can stimulate protein synthesis and cell growth via its effects on mTOR, the mammalian target of rapamycin (reviewed in [235]). mTOR is a serine-threonine kinase that phosphorylates and activates the ribosomal protein translation initiators S6 kinase and 4EBP, leading to increased protein translation and promoting cell growth and division. Rapamycin, by inhibiting mTOR, prevents protein translation and inhibits cell division, leading to its use to suppress tumor growth, and as an immune suppressant (due to inhibition of T- and B-cell expansion).

The kinase activity of mTOR is activated by binding to the small GTP-binding protein Rheb. Like Ras, Rac, and Gα, Rheb is active when in the GTP-bound state, and inactive when in the GDP-bound state. Conversion of GTP-Rheb to GDP-Rheb is mediated by a GTPase complex made up of two proteins, tuberin and hammartin. The GTPase activity of these proteins, which are mutated in many patients with tuberous sclerosis, is in turn negatively regulated by phosphorylation of tuberin by activated Akt.[236] In this manner, activation of Akt downstream of the PI 3-K results in stabilization of Rheb in the GTP-bound state, thereby activating mTOR and accelerating cell growth and division (Figure 13.11).

In addition to its fundamental role in regulating cell survival and proliferation, another major physiologic process regulated by the PI 3-K/Akt pathway is insulin-dependent glucose metabolism (reviewed in [237]). Binding of insulin to its receptor tyrosine kinase results in the tyrosine phosphorylation of a docking protein, insulin receptor substrate (IRS-1), which in turn activates multiple intracellular signaling pathways including the PI 3-K. Activation of the PI 3-K has been shown to regulate insulin-dependent glucose uptake, glycogen synthesis, and lipolysis. Glucose uptake is

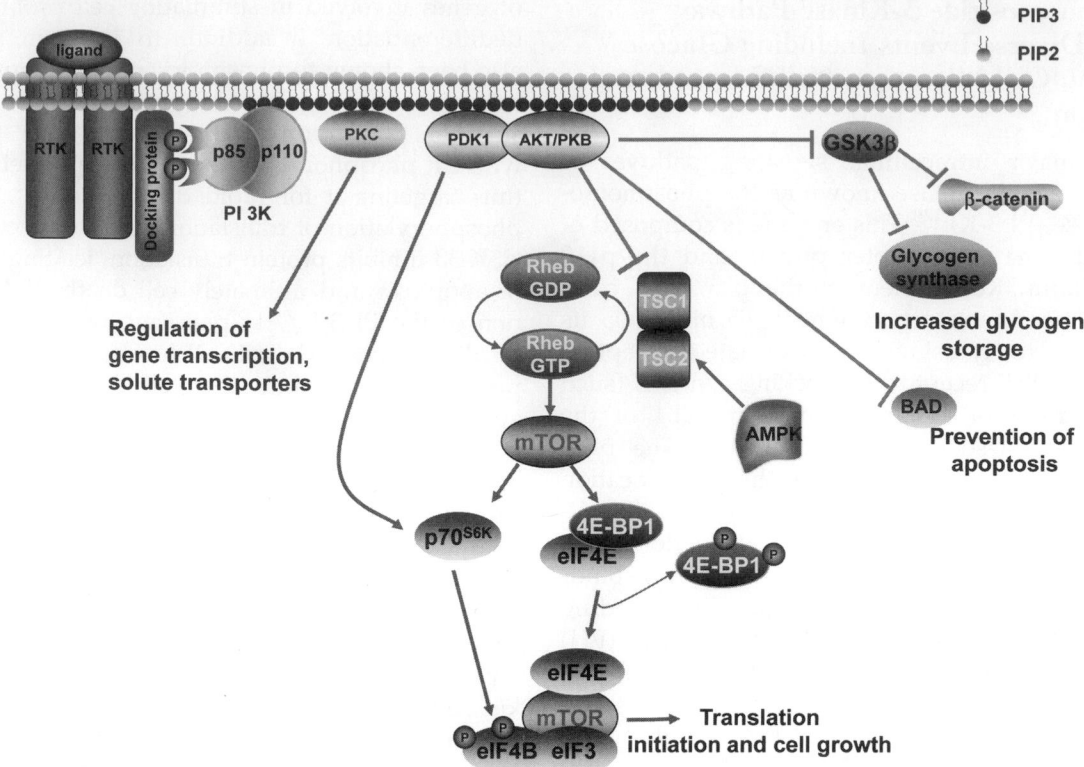

FIGURE 13.11   Signaling through the PI 3-kinase/Akt pathway. The activation of growth factor receptors results in the recruitment of the p85/p110 PI 3-kinase heterodimer to the membrane via binding of the SH2 domains of p85 to phosphotyrosine residues on the receptor or an associated docking protein such as IRS-1. Activation of the lipid kinase activity of p110 occurs, resulting in generation of $PI_{3,4,5}P_3$ (PIP3) at the inner leaflet of the membrane. PIP3 serves as a binding site for proteins that contain lipid-binding domains, including several PKC family members, docking proteins, and the serine-threonine kinase phosphoinositide-dependent kinase (PDK1). PDK1 has several targets in the cell, including the protein translation activator p70 S6kinase and the cytosolic serine-threonine kinase protein kinase B (PKB), also known as Akt. Akt phosphorylates multiple substrates in the cell (typically resulting in inhibition of their action) that promote cell growth and survival. Thus, phosphorylation of the tuberosis sclerosis complex (TSC1 and TSC2) inhibits their GTPase activity, leading to accumulation of GTP Rheb and activation of mTOR. mTOR in turn activates p70 S6kinase and phosphorylates 4E-BP, resulting in its disassociation from eukaryotic initiation factor 4E (eIF4E), and cumulatively stimulating increased protein translation. During times of ATP depletion and AMP accumulation, mTOR activity is inhibited by the AMP activated kinase AMPK. AMPK phosphorylates and activates the TSC complex, thus converting GTP Rheb to GDP Rheb and inactivating mTOR. Activated Akt also phosphorylates and inhibits pro-apoptotic factors such as BAD and caspase 9, and inhibits degradation of intracellular proteins, such as glycogen synthase, by phosphorylating and inhibiting GSK-3β.

mediated by the transport protein GLUT4. In the absence of insulin, GLUT4 is located in intracellular vesicles, but fuses with the plasma membrane following insulin stimulation. This translocation of GLUT4-containing vesicles to the membrane is mediated by $PI_{3,4,5}P_3$-dependent activation of both PKCζ and Akt (reviewed in [238]).

Once glucose enters the cell, it is rapidly sequestered by conversion into glycogen via the actions of the enzyme glycogen synthase. In quiescent cells, the constitutively active form of GSK-3β normally phosphorylates glycogen synthase, keeping it in the inactive state. By stimulating the PI 3-kinase, insulin can increase Akt activation, thereby inhibiting GSK-3β activity and increasing glycogen synthase-dependent incorporation of glucose into glycogen.[239]

EXAMPLES OF SIGNALING EFFECTORS IN THE KIDNEY

The extraordinarily complex interactions that initiate, regulate, and terminate intracellular second messenger pathways, such as those described above, ultimately lead to the change in location, function or amount of effector proteins that actually mediate the cellular response to the initial signal. These effector proteins regulate fundamental cellular events such as division, programmed cell death, migration, and differentiation that are required for the development, maintenance, and repair of all tissues. In the kidney, signaling pathways are also critical for the precise regulation of glomerular filtration and for alteration of tubular cell channel function in response to changes in the internal milieu. While more detailed descriptions of these regulatory events are presented in the appropriate chapters of this book, examples of several specific effector proteins are presented here in order to provide general paradigms of the ways in which signaling pathways can regulate effector protein function in the kidney.

Angiotensin II Signaling in Glomerular Vascular Smooth Muscle

Maintenance of GFR in the face of falling renal perfusion is achieved by the independent regulation of afferent and efferent vascular tone, which is in part determined by the arteriolar smooth muscle response to locally produced angiotensin II. In the efferent arteriole of the glomerulus, stimulation of smooth muscle contraction by angiotensin II requires the coordinated regulation of both myosin light chain kinase (MLCK) and myosin light chain phosphatase (MLCP, reviewed in [240,241]). Activation of the AT1 receptor on the efferent arteriole results in activation of $G_{\alpha q}$ and the downstream second messenger PLCβ. As noted previously, the hydrolysis of PIP2 by PLCβ results in the formation of DAG and the release of IP₃. In smooth muscle cells, IP3 binds to its receptor on the sarcoplasmic reticulum, stimulating intracellular calcium release, which in turn activates calcium entry from outside the cell. The resultant rise in intracellular calcium leads to calmodulin-dependent activation of MLCK, which in turn phosphorylates and activates the regulatory light chain of smooth muscle myosin II, leading to actin—myosin coupling and muscle contraction.

The phosphorylation sites on myosin II are targets for subsequent dephosphorylation by MLCP (also known as myosin phosphatase). In concert with its activation of MLCK, activation of the AT1 receptor stimulates two pathways that lead to inhibition of MLCP (reviewed in [242]). First, the formation of DAG in the membrane, coupled with the rise in intracellular calcium, leads to recruitment and activation of both conventional and novel PKCs. One of the phosphorylation targets of activated PKC in the smooth muscle cell is CPI-17, and in the phosphorylated state CPI-17 associates with and inhibits MLCP via binding to the PP1Cδ catalytic-subunit.

A second group of proteins phosphorylated by PKC are the matrix metalloproteinases.[243] These proteins are involved in cleaving and shedding cell surface proteins, including the cell attached growth factor HB-EGF. Shedding of HB-EGF leads to activation of the EGF receptor, with stimulation of downstream signaling including the PI 3-kinase. This process of GPCR-dependent activation of a nearby growth factor receptor is termed transactivation. In smooth muscle cells, one target of the activated PI 3-kinase is a Rho GEF named leukemia-associated Rho guanine nucleotide exchange factor (LARG).[244] Activation of LARG converts Rho to the GTP-bound state, mediating its association with Rho kinase. This activation of Rho kinase can inhibit MLCP activity, both by direct phosphorylation of MLCP at an inhibitory site, and via phosphorylation of CPI-17 in conjunction with PKC. By simultaneously increasing the phosphorylation of the light chain of myosin II via activation of MLCK and inhibiting its dephosphorylation via inactivation of MLCP, angiotensin II can greatly augment myosin II coupling with actin and subsequent smooth muscle contraction. In addition to stimulating smooth muscle contraction, sustained angiotensin II-dependent increases in intracellular calcium can lead to calmodulin—calcineurin interactions and subsequent activation of NFAT, which in turn activates the transcription of genes involved in promoting muscle cell hypertrophy (reviewed in [245]) (Figure 13.12).

Regulation of Ion Transport Channels

The regulation of GFR by controlling afferent and efferent vascular tone must be coordinated with appropriate changes in solute reabsorption along the nephron. Typically this regulation occurs in one of three ways: regulation of the amount of the transporter in the cell; regulation of the location of the transporter; or regulation of the active state of the transporter at the membrane. In most cases, more than one of these regulatory steps is utilized, allowing both short- and long-term regulation of transporter function.

Sodium Reabsorption in the Collecting Duct can be Regulated by Controlling Cellular Levels of ENaC

The epithelial sodium channel ENaC is expressed on the apical membrane of principal cells of the collecting duct. Regulation of ENaC function is one of the major ways in which the kidney controls the amount of sodium that is excreted in the urine each day. ENaC is comprised of three subunits that are synthesized in the ER and then transported to the Golgi for proteolytic cleavage and activation, followed by trafficking to the apical membrane. ENaC channels present in the membrane can then be internalized where they are either degraded or maintained in a submembranous pool available for rapid recycling back to the membrane. The principal factors that regulate the synthesis, location, and degradation of ENaC are aldosterone and, to a lesser degree, AVP.

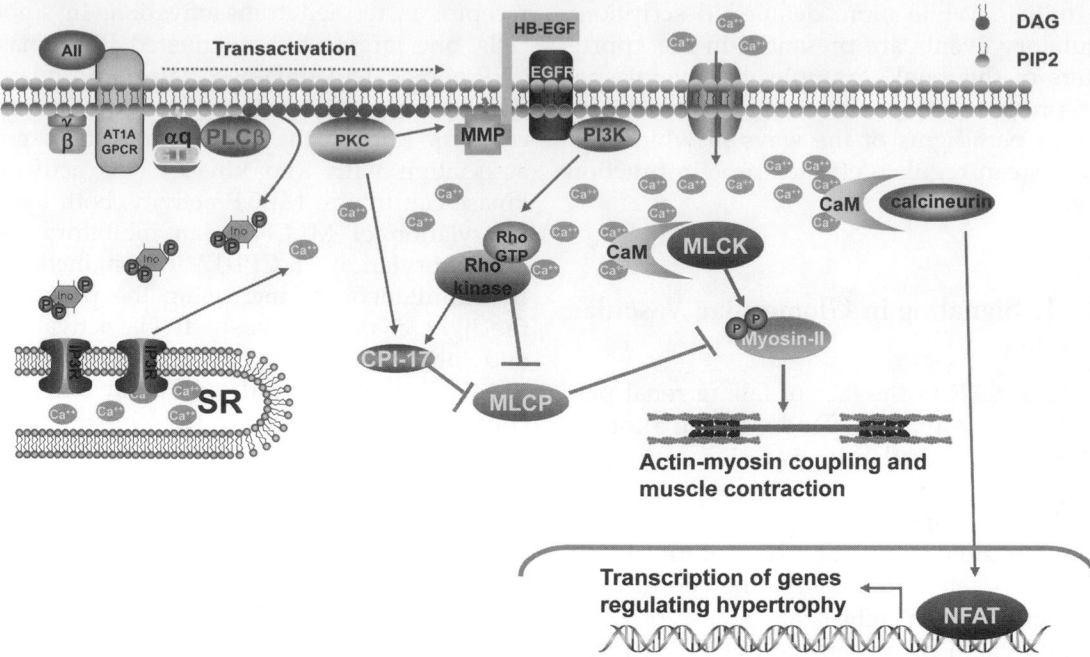

FIGURE 13.12 **Angiotensin II regulation of vascular smooth muscle contraction.** Binding of angiotensin II to the AT1A receptor results in activation of PLCβ, and subsequent generation of IP3 and DAG. DAG production at the membrane can mediate the recruitment and activation of PKC, while IP3 binding to the IP3 receptor in the sarcoplasmic reticulum stimulates calcium release. Angiotensin II may also stimulate extracellular calcium entry via cell surface calcium channels. Binding of the calcium to calmodulin (CaM) results in calmodulin-dependent activation of myosin light chain kinase (MLCK), which phosphorylates myosin II to initiate actin—myosin contraction. Myosin II is dephosphorylated by myosin light chain phosphatase (MLCP) to end the contraction. However, during the period immediately after AT1A stimulation, myosin II phosphorylation is maximized, because MLCP is inhibited by PKC-dependent phosphorylation of the MLCP inhibitory binding protein CPI-17. In addition, GPCR activation can stimulate transactivation of nearby growth factor receptors (such as the EGFR) which in turn can activate the PI 3-K. One mechanism of transactivation is the PKC-dependent activation of matrix metalloproteinases (MMP) which cause shedding of the cell attached protein HB-EGF, which binds and activates the EGFR. The resultant PI 3-K activation mediates GTP loading of the small G-protein Rho, and subsequent activation of Rho kinase. Rho kinase can directly phosphorylate MLCP at an inhibitory site, and can phosphorylate CPI-17 and thus increase its inhibitory effect on MLCP. Sustained contractile stimuli result in the calmodulin-dependent activation of calcineurin. Calcineurin is a phosphatase that binds to and dephosphorylates the nuclear factor of activated T-cells (NFAT), resulting in NFAT-dependent transcriptional regulation of genes involved in smooth muscle cell hypertrophy.

Steroid Hormones such as Aldosterone Bind to Cytoplasmic Receptors and Regulate Nuclear Transcription Events

Aldosterone is a steroid hormone that binds to and activates the mineralocorticoid receptor (MR), which is present in the principal cell, but also in other cell types including intestinal epithelial cells, neuronal cells, and cardiac myocytes. The MR is a member of the steroid/thyroid family of ligand-inducible transcription factors that includes the vitamin D receptor, glucocorticoid receptor, thyroid receptor, and retinoic acid receptor (reviewed in [246]). Unlike the transmembrane receptors discussed in the section "Cell Surface Receptors," these receptors reside in the cytoplasm. The ligand, such as thyroid hormone or aldosterone, can cross the cell membrane, bind the cytosolic receptor, and then translocate as a ligand—receptor complex into the nucleus and bind to specific DNA sequences known as steroid response elements (SRE). In the case of aldosterone, these regulatory sequences are found in the promoter regions of target genes such as *SCNN1A* (the ENaC α-subunit gene) and *SGK-1* (encodes SGK, serum, and glucocorticoid-induced kinase).

In the principal cell, the β- and γ-subunits of ENaC are produced in excess, but do not traffic efficiently to the cell surface until the α-subunit is made (reviewed in [247]). The increase in ENaC α-subunit protein expression that occurs following stimulation with aldosterone leads to ER assembly of αβγ in a complex with the predicted stoichiometry of 2α:β:γ, and its subsequent proteolytic activation in the Golgi. In this manner, aldosterone directly increases the total number of active ENaC transporters available in the cell, leading to an increase in sodium reabsorptive capacity.

A second way in which aldosterone can increase the number of ENaC channels available to reabsorb sodium is by inhibiting ENaC degradation. This is mediated by the transcriptional regulation of SGK expression.[248] SGK is a serine-threonine kinase that phosphorylates and inactivates Nedd4-2, a ubiquitin—protein ligase that can associate with ENaC and stimulate its internalization and degradation[249] (Figure 13.13). By increasing SGK expression, aldosterone inhibits Nedd4-2-mediated ENaC degradation, and thereby increases the amount of ENaC present on the cell surface. Mutations in ENaC that prevent its association with Nedd4-2 lead to sustained increases in sodium reabsorption due to increased ENaC expression, resulting in the progressive hypertension seen in Liddle's syndrome.[250]

Regulation of Water Reabsorption in the Collecting Duct is Achieved by Trafficking of Aquaporin-2.

The regulation of channel amount by altering rates of synthesis and/or degradation is a relatively slow process that typically takes hours to days to accomplish, and is believed to be most relevant in the adaptive responses to long-standing volume depletion or

volume excess. In contrast, regulation of channel location provides a way to rapidly alter channel function in the cell. Aquaporins, transmembrane channels that provide a conduit for water movement across cell membranes, are one of many proteins that can be regulated in this fashion. In the kidney, aquaporin-2 (AQP2) is expressed in cells of the collecting duct, and its ability to mediate water movement is regulated by AVP (reviewed in [251]). In contrast, AQP1 (present in the proximal tubule and thin descending limb[252]) and AQP3 (present on the basolateral side of collecting duct cells[253]) are relatively insensitive to AVP.

In the absence of AVP, AQP2 is present primarily in submembranous vesicles in the collecting duct. Stimulation of V2 receptors by AVP results in the fusion of these vesicles with the apical membrane of the collecting duct cell. Mutations in either the V2

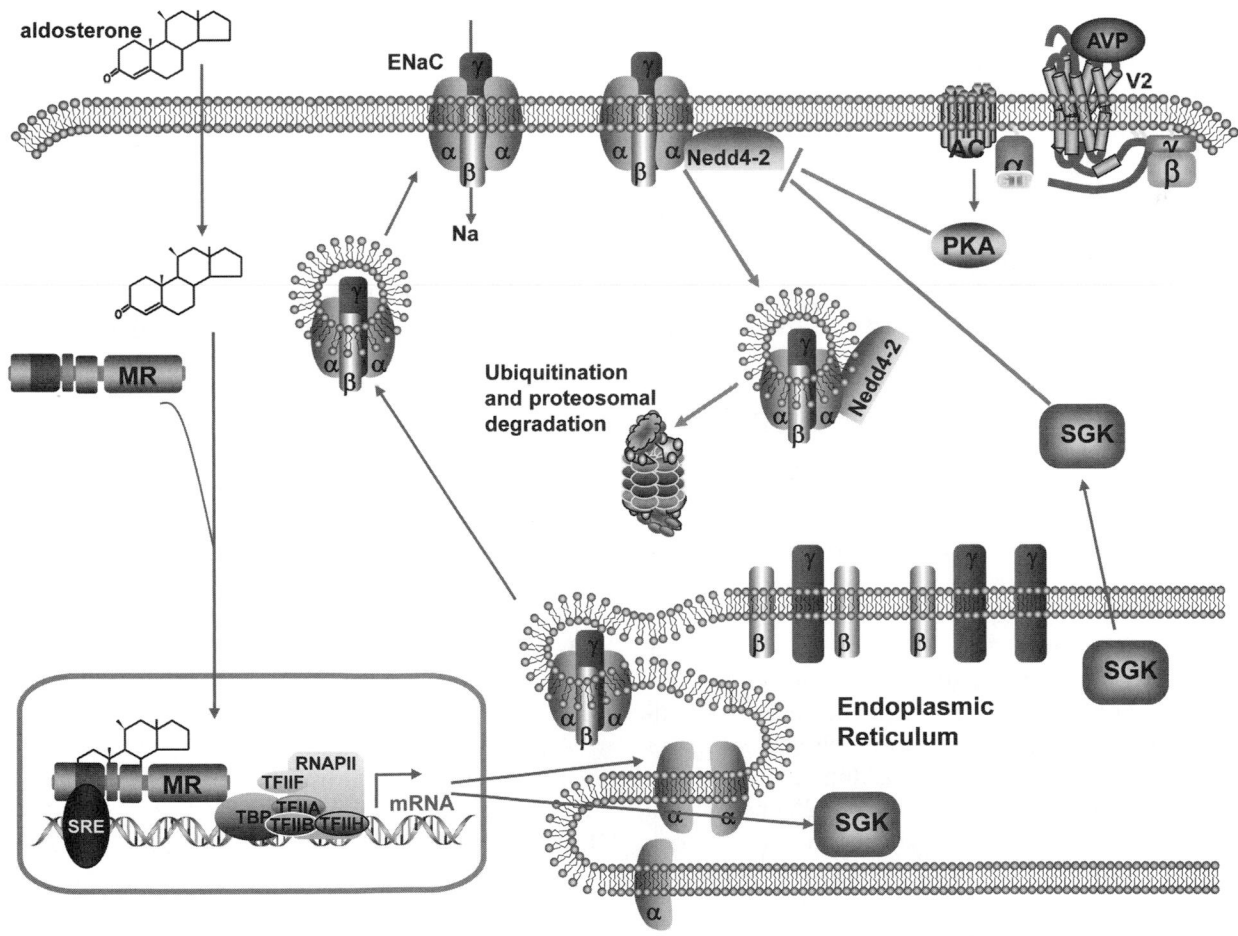

FIGURE 13.13 Regulation of ENaC. Aldosterone is a steroid hormone that can cross the cell membrane and bind to the mineralocorticoid receptor (MR) in the cell cytoplasm. The aldosterone—MR complex translocates into the nucleus, where it binds to steroid response elements in genes such as *SCNN1A* encoding the α-subunit of ENaC and *SGK-1* encoding a cytosolic serine threonine kinase. Synthesis of the α-subunit of ENaC promotes formation of the complete ENaC multimer in the ER and its translocation to the cell surface. At the membrane, the ubiquitin ligase Nedd4-2 can bind to ENaC, targeting it for internalization and proteosomal degradation. Nedd4-2 function is inhibited following phosphorylation by SGK, further increasing ENaC expression at the cell membrane, and therefore sodium reabsorptive capacity. Vasopressin (AVP), acting through the V2 GPCR, can also increase collecting duct sodium reabsorption. V2 activation leads to cAMP production and subsequent PKA activation. Like SGK, PKA can phosphorylate and inhibit Nedd4-2.

receptor or AQP2 itself result in nephrogenic diabetes insipidus, due to the failure of the collecting duct to increase water reabsorption in response to AVP. The translocation of AQP2 vesicles to the cell membrane is dependent on AVP-stimulated production of cAMP, and the subsequent activation of PKA. Activated PKA is targeted to AQP2-containing vesicles via association with A kinase anchoring proteins (AKAPs). AKAPs comprise a large family of proteins that localize activated PKA to specific sites within the cell, thus providing specificity and compartmentalization of PKA signaling. AKAP18δ, PKA, and AQP2 can be co-purified from vesicles isolated from the cytosol of inner medullary collecting duct cells, suggesting that this AKAP may be important for facilitating the recruitment of PKA to AQP2-containing vesicles.[254]

Activated PKA directly phosphorylates serine 256 in the carboxy terminus of AQP2, stimulating membrane translocation of the AQP2-containing vesicles.[255] How phosphorylation of serine-256 in AQP2 mediates vesicle fusion with the membrane is not yet fully-understood (reviewed in [256]). Based on present studies, it appears that membrane targeting involves the actin cytoskeletal-dependent association of SNARE proteins (such as syntaxin-3 and -4) on the AQP2-containing vesicles with SNAP23 at the cell membrane.[257,258]

The vesicles that mediate AQP2 translocation to the membrane also carry signals for downregulation of the pathway. Recently it has been found that these vesicles contain cAMP-specific phosphodiesterase-4D (PDE4D), an enzyme that can degrade cAMP, leading to inactivation of PKA.[259] In the presence of the AKAP18δ scaffold, PKA can phosphorylate and activate PDE4D, leading to decreased cAMP, loss of PKA activation, and prevention of AQP2 phosphorylation and translocation. In addition, the serine-threonine phosphatase PP2B is present in these vesicles, and is capable of dephosphorylating AQP2, thereby potentially inhibiting channel translocation.[260]

AQP2 function can be regulated by mechanisms in addition to membrane trafficking. In the setting of continuous stimulation by AVP, total cellular levels of AQP2 message and protein increase, demonstrating that AVP can induce transcription of the AQP2 gene. In vitro experiments have suggested that this is due to transcriptional activation of AQP2 mRNA expression via a cyclic AMP response element (CRE) in the AQP2 promotor.[261] Activation of multiple intracellular serine-threonine kinases, including PKA, can stimulate phosphorylation and activation of the CRE-binding protein (CREB), which in turn binds CRE and activates transcription of the appropriate target gene, in this case AQP2. Sustained exposure to hypertonicity can also increase AQP2 mRNA expression in cultured collecting duct cells, independent of AVP-mediated PKA activation.[262]

In addition to its ability to regulate AQP2-mediated water absorption, AVP has been shown to regulate ENaC-mediated salt absorption (see Figure 13.13). Nedd4-2, the ubiquitin ligase that is inactivated by SGK-mediated phosphorylation, can be phosphorylated at the same sites by AVP-activated PKA, leading to inhibition of the Nedd4-2/ENaC association and increased ENaC protein stability.[263] In addition, the cAMP-stimulated activation of PKA by AVP can promote the translocation of ENaC from a pool of internalized channels to the membrane, similar to its effects on AQP2.[264,265] The increase in ENaC surface expression resulting from these signaling events is believed to partially mediate the observed increase in sodium reabsorption following AVP treatment[266] (reviewed in [267]).

Transporters such as ROMK can be Regulated by Changes in their Active State

A third way in which transporters can be regulated is via alteration of the active state of the protein. For membrane channels this typically means a change in the open probability (P_o) of the channel (the time that the channel spends in the open configuration). ROMK (also known as Kir1.1) is an apical membrane potassium channel in thick ascending limb cells and principal cells that is required for potassium recycling in the TAL, and potassium secretion in the collecting duct (reviewed in [268]). One of the major determinants of P_o for ROMK is the concentration of PIP_2 in the membrane in the vicinity of the channel, an effect that appears to be due to an extensive series of interactions between the basic amino acids in the carboxy terminus of ROMK and the negatively charged head groups of the membrane phospholipids (reviewed in [269]). PIP_2 is produced by lipid kinases such as the $PI(4)P_5$ kinase, and degraded by phospholipases such as PLA_2 and PLC (reviewed in [270,271]). Thus, it is speculated that signals that enhance PIP_2 production or inhibit its degradation will increase ROMK activity at the membrane, whereas pathways that reduce PIP_2 levels, such as activation of PKC, will inhibit its activity.

Alterations in the P_o for ROMK have also been found to be due to direct phosphorylation of the channel by PKA (reviewed in [269]). In vitro studies have demonstrated three PKA phosphorylation sites in ROMK, and phosphorylation of two of those sites (serine 219 and 313) causes an increase in P_o for the channel, without changing the number of channels at the membrane. As with other PKA effectors, the presence of the appropriate AKAP is required to target activated PKA to ROMK at the membrane. Although the precise mechanism by which PKA phosphorylation regulates P_o in ROMK has yet to be determined, it appears that at least part of the effect is due to an increased affinity of ROMK for PIP_2, thus reducing the concentration of PIP_2 needed to support the channel in the open state.[272] Based on these studies, it is presently believed that the AVP-stimulated increase in thick ascending limb potassium recycling is due to V2-dependent activation of PKA, and subsequent phosphorylation and activation of ROMK.[273]

Similar to the regulation of aquaporin-2 and ENaC, ROMK can also be regulated by altering channel location or synthesis. Several kinases have been implicated in regulating the trafficking of ROMK, including PKA, SGK, and a recently described kinase WNK (with no K (lysine)). As noted above, there are three PKA phosphorylation sites on ROMK. While two of the sites directly regulate channel open probability, phosphorylation of the third residue (serine 44) increases the number of channels present on the cell membrane. In addition to PKA, SGK can phosphorylate ROMK on serine 44 and increase channel activity in the oocyte expression system.[274] This appears to occur in concert with a scaffolding protein, NHERF2, which increases trafficking of ROMK to the membrane via its interaction with the carboxy terminal PDZ-binding motif.[275] Thus, the increased expression of SGK following aldosterone stimulation can lead to sustained increases in ROMK-dependent potassium excretion via increased numbers of channels on the cell membrane.

Recently, another family of serine/threonine kinases, the WNKs, have been found to play an important role in regulating the activity of diverse ion channels in the kidney (reviewed in [276]). To date there have been four WNK kinases described in humans, all sharing the unusual substitution of a cysteine residue for the more typical lysine in β strand 3 of the kinase domain.[277] Of these four, WNK1, WNK3, and WNK4 have been directly implicated in regulation of tubular ion transport, including the sodium-potassium-chloride co-transporter in the TAL (NKCC2), the sodium-chloride co-transporter in the distal convoluted tubule (NCC), ROMK, EnaC, and the tight junctional proteins claudin1-4 that regulate paracellular chloride flux,([278−280] reviewed in [281]). Mutations of WNK1 and WNK4 have been shown to cause pseudohypoaldosteronism II (PHAII), a syndrome consisting of hypertension with increased sodium reabsorption and hyperkalemia.[282]

The mechanisms by which WNKs regulate ROMK and NCC depend on distinct aspects of WNK function. Mutations in WNK1 and WNK4 that cause PHAII result in decreased ROMK at the membrane, and therefore hyperkalemia due to decreased K secretion.[280,283] It has been shown that ROMK associates with a complex including WNK1, WNK4, and the scaffolding protein intersectin, and that intersectin is required for the endocytosis of ROMK in clathrin-coated vesicles.[284] The formation of this complex is independent of WNK kinase activity, and instead requires the association of proline-rich regions of WNK1 and WNK4 with the SH3 domain of intersectin. Mutations in WNK4 that cause PHAII appear to increase the association of the ROMK−WNK1−WNK4 complex with intersectin, thereby augmenting ROMK internalization and impairing potassium secretion.[285]

WNK kinases regulate sodium uptake by determining both the surface availability and activation state of NCC. This process is complex and not yet fully elucidated, but appears to involve a balance between WNK4-dependent degradation of NCC and WNK1-dependent activation of NCC that is present on the cell surface (reviewed in [276]). In the presence of active WNK4, newly synthesized NCC is targeted via sortilin for lysosomal degradation rather than cell surface expression, thus reducing the pool of NCC available for sodium transport.[286,287] In contrast, WNK1 and WNK3 activate the sodium transport function of NCC that is on the cell surface by phosphorylating the intracellular kinase SPAK, which then phosphorylates and activates NCC. A second phosphorylation target of WNK3 is WNK4 itself, resulting in inhibition of the WNK4-mediated NCC degradation, and thus increasing NCC surface expression. Mutations in WNK4 that cause PHAII result in increased sodium reabsorption at least in part due to increased NCC on the cell surface.[288]

References

[1] Miura S, Saku K, Karnik SS. Molecular analysis of the structure and function of the angiotensin II type 1 receptor. Hypertens Res 2003;26:937.

[2] Malbon CC. G proteins in development. Nat Rev Mol Cell Biol 2005;6:689.

[3] Strock J, Diverse-Pierluissi MA. Ca²⁺ channels as integrators of G protein-mediated signaling in neurons. Mol Pharmacol 2004;66:1071.

[4] Krasel C, Bunemann M, Lorenz K, Lohse MJ. Beta-arrestin binding to the beta2-adrenergic receptor requires both receptor phosphorylation and receptor activation. J Biol Chem 2005;280:9528.

[5] Tran TM, Friedman J, Quniabi E, Baameur F, Moore RH, Clark RB. Characterization of agonist stimulation of cAMP-dependent protein kinase and G protein-coupled receptor kinase phosphorylation of the beta2-adrenergic receptor using phosphoserine-specific antibodies. Mol Pharmacol 2004;65:196.

[6] Jose PA, Eisner GM, Felder RA. Renal dopamine and sodium homeostasis. Curr Hypertens Rep 2000;2:174.

[7] Beaulieu JM, Gainetdinov RR. The physiology, signaling, and pharmacology of dopamine receptors. Pharmacol Rev 2011;63:182.

[8] Jose PA, Eisner GM, Felder RA. Role of dopamine receptors in the kidney in the regulation of blood pressure. Curr Opin Nephrol Hypertens 2002;11:87.

[9] Yang Z, Sibley DR, Jose PA. D5 dopamine receptor knockout mice and hypertension. J Recept Signal Transduct Res 2004;24:149.

[10] Banday AA, Lokhandwala MF. Dopamine receptors and hypertension. Curr Hypertens Rep 2008;10:268.

[11] Carey RM. Update on the role of the AT2 receptor. Curr Opin Nephrol Hypertens 2005;14:67.

[12] Porrello ER, Delbridge LM, Thomas WG. The angiotensin II type 2 (AT2) receptor: an enigmatic seven transmembrane receptor. Front Biosci 2009;14:958.

[13] Siragy HM, Carey RM. The subtype-2 (AT2) angiotensin receptor regulates renal cyclic guanosine 3′, 5′-monophosphate and AT1 receptor-mediated prostaglandin E2 production in conscious rats. J Clin Invest 1996;97:1978.

[14] Tsutsumi Y, Matsubara H, Masaki H, Kurihara H, Murusawa S, Takai S, et al. Angiotensin II type 2 receptor overexpression activates the vascular kinin system and causes vasodilation. J Clin Invest 1999;104:925.

[15] Nagahama T, Hayashi K, Ozawa Y, Takenaka T, Saruta T. Role of protein kinase C in angiotensin II-induced constriction of renal microvessels. Kidney Int 2000;57:215.

[16] Rangel LB, Caruso-Neves C, Lara LS, Lopes AG. Angiotensin II stimulates renal proximal tubule Na(+)-ATPase activity through the activation of protein kinase C. Biochim Biophys Acta 2002;1564:310.

[17] Efendiev R, Budu CE, Cinelli AR, Bertorello AM, Pedemonte CH. Intracellular Na$^+$ regulates dopamine and angiotensin II receptors availability at the plasma membrane and their cellular responses in renal epithelia. J Biol Chem 2003;278:28719.

[18] Foster RH. Reciprocal influences between the signalling pathways regulating proliferation and steroidogenesis in adrenal glomerulosa cells. J Mol Endocrinol 2004;32:893.

[19] DeFea KA. Beta-arrestins as regulators of signal termination and transduction: how do they determine what to scaffold? Cell Signal 2011;23:621.

[20] Wei H, Ahn S, Shenoy SK, Karnik SS, Hunyady L, Luttrell MM, et al. Independent beta-arrestin 2 and G protein-mediated pathways for angiotensin II activation of extracellular signal-regulated kinases 1 and 2. Proc Natl Acad Sci USA 2003;100:10782.

[21] Kim J, Ahn S, Ren XR, Whalen EJ, Reiter E, Wei H, et al. Functional antagonism of different G protein-coupled receptor kinases for beta-arrestin-mediated angiotensin II receptor signaling. Proc Natl Acad Sci USA 2005;102:1442.

[22] Meng D, Lynch MJ, Huston E, Beyermann M, Eichorst J, Adams DR, et al. MEK1 binds directly to betaarrestin1, influencing both its phosphorylation by ERK and the timing of its isoprenaline-stimulated internalization. J Biol Chem 2009;284:11425.

[23] Reiter E, Ahn S, Shukla AK, Lefkowitz RJ. Molecular mechanism of β-arrestin-biased agonism at seven-transmembrane receptors. Annu Rev Pharmacol Toxicol 2012;52:179−97.

[24] Tsuchida S, Matsusaka T, Chen X, Okubo S, Nijmura F, Nishimura H, et al. Murine double nullizygotes of the angiotensin type 1A and 1B receptor genes duplicate severe abnormal phenotypes of angiotensinogen nullizygotes. J Clin Invest 1998;101:755.

[25] Chen Y, Lasaitiene D, Friberg P. The renin−angiotensin system in kidney development. Acta Physiol Scand 2004;181:529.

[26] Eguchi S, Numaguchi K, Iwasaki H, Matsumoto T, Yamakawa T, Utsunomiya H, et al. Calcium-dependent epidermal growth factor receptor transactivation mediates the angiotensin II-induced mitogen-activated protein kinase activation in vascular smooth muscle cells. J Biol Chem 1998;273:8890.

[27] Thomas WG, Brandenburger Y, Autelitano DJ, Pham T, Qian H, Hannan RD. Adenoviral-directed expression of the type 1A angiotensin receptor promotes cardiomyocyte hypertrophy via transactivation of the epidermal growth factor receptor. Circ Res 2002;90:135.

[28] Gensure RC, Gardella TJ, Juppner H. Parathyroid hormone and parathyroid hormone-related peptide, and their receptors. Biochem Biophys Res Commun 2005;328:666.

[29] Guo J, Chung UI, Kondo H, Bringhurst FR, Kronenberg HM. The PTH/PTHrP receptor can delay chondrocyte hypertrophy in vivo without activating phospholipase C. Dev Cell 2002;3:183.

[30] Kovacs CS, Lanske B, Hunzelman JL, Guo J, Karaplis AC, Kronenberg HM. Parathyroid hormone-related peptide (PTHrP) regulates fetal-placental calcium transport through a receptor distinct from the PTH/PTHrP receptor. Proc Natl Acad Sci USA 1996;93:15233.

[31] Lanske B, Karaplis AC, Lee K, Luz A, Vortkamp A, Pirro A, et al. PTH/PTHrP receptor in early development and Indian hedgehog-regulated bone growth. Science 1996;273:663.

[32] Jobert AS, Zhang P, Couvineau A, Bonaventure J, Roume J, Le Merrer M, et al. Absence of functional receptors for parathyroid hormone and parathyroid hormone-related peptide in Blomstrand chondrodysplasia. J Clin Invest 1998;102:34−40.

[33] Ferrandon S, Feinstein TN, Castro M, Wang B, Bouley R, Potts JT, et al. Sustained cyclic AMP production by parathyroid hormone receptor endocytosis. Nat Chem Biol 2009;5:734−42.

[34] Miaczynska M, Bar-Sagi D. Signaling endosomes: seeing is believing. Curr Opin Cell Biol 2010;22:535.

[35] Schiefermeier N, Teis D, Huber LA. Endosomal signaling and cell migration. Curr Opin Cell Biol 2011.

[36] Songyang Z, Blechner S, Hoagland N, Hoekstra MF, Piwinica-Worms H, cantley LC. Use of an oriented peptide library to determine the optimal substrates of protein kinases. Curr Biol 1994;4:973−82.

[37] Sariola H, Saarma M. Novel functions and signalling pathways for GDNF. J Cell Sci 2003;116:3855.

[38] Degl'Innocenti D, Arighi E, Popsueva A, Sangregorio R, Alberti L, Rizzetti MG, et al. Differential requirement of Tyr1062 multidocking site by RET isoforms to promote neural cell scattering and epithelial cell branching. Oncogene 2004;23:7297−309.

[39] Bates CM. Role of fibroblast growth factor receptor signaling in kidney development. Pediatr Nephrol 2007;22:343.

[40] Ishibe S, Karihaloo A, Ma H, Zhang J, Marlier A, Mitobe M, et al. Met and the epidermal growth factor receptor act cooperatively to regulate final nephron number and maintain collecting duct morphology. Development 2009;136:337−45.

[41] Turner N, Grose R. Fibroblast growth factor signalling: from development to cancer. Nat Rev Cancer 2010;10:116.

[42] Kurosu H, Kuro OM. The Klotho gene family as a regulator of endocrine fibroblast growth factors. Mol Cell Endocrinol 2009;299:72.

[43] Revest JM, Spencer-Dene B, Kerr K, De Moerlooze L, Rosewall I, Dickson C. Fibroblast growth factor receptor 2-IIIb acts upstream of Shh and Fgf4 and is required for limb bud maintenance but not for the induction of Fgf8, Fgf10, Msx1, or Bmp4. Dev Biol 2001;231:47−62.

[44] Qiao J, Uzzo R, Obara-Ishihara T, Degenstein L, Fuchs E, Herzlinger D. FGF-7 modulates ureteric bud growth and nephron number in the developing kidney. Development 1999;126:547−54.

[45] Grieshammer U, Cebrián C, Ilagan R, Meyers E, Herzlinger D, Martin GR. FGF8 is required for cell survival at distinct stages of nephrogenesis and for regulation of gene expression in nascent nephrons. Development 2005;132:3847−57.

[46] Holgado-Madruga M, Emlet DR, Moscatello DK, Godwin AK, Wong AJ. A Grb2-associated docking protein in EGF- and insulin-receptor signalling. Nature 1996;379:560.

[47] Weidner KM, Di Cesare S, Sacks M, Brinkmann V, Behrens J, Birchmeier W. Interaction between Gab1 and the c-Met receptor tyrosine kinase is responsible for epithelial morphogenesis. Nature 1996;384:173−6.

[48] Ishibashi K, Sasaki S, Sakamoto H, Hoshino Y, Nakamura T, Marumo F. Expressions of receptor gene for hepatocyte growth

factor in kidney after unilateral nephrectomy and renal injury. Biochem Biophys Res Commun 1992;187:1454–9.

[49] Joannidis M, Spokes K, Nakamura T, Faletto D, Cantley LG. Regional expression of hepatocyte growth factor/c-met in experimental renal hypertrophy and hyperplasia. Am J Physiol 1994;267:F231.

[50] Miller SB, Martin DR, Kissane J, Hammerman MR. Hepatocyte growth factor accelerates recovery from acute ischemic renal injury in rats. Am J Physiol 1994;266:F129.

[51] Maroun CR, Naujokas MA, Holgado-Madruga M, Wong AJ, Park M. The tyrosine phosphatase SHP-2 is required for sustained activation of extracellular signal-regulated kinase and epithelial morphogenesis downstream from the met receptor tyrosine kinase. Mol Cell Biol 2000;20:8513.

[52] Ishibe S, Joly D, Liu ZX, Cantley LG. Paxillin serves as an ERK-regulated scaffold for coordinating FAK and Rac activation in epithelial morphogenesis. Mol Cell 2004;16:257.

[53] Wang W, Koka V, Lan HY. Transforming growth factor-beta and Smad signalling in kidney diseases. Nephrology (Carlton) 2005;10:48.

[54] Luo K, Lodish HF. Signaling by chimeric erythropoietin-TGF-beta receptors: homodimerization of the cytoplasmic domain of the type I TGF-beta receptor and heterodimerization with the type II receptor are both required for intracellular signal transduction. Embo J 1996;15:4485.

[55] Oh SP, Seki T, Goss KA, Imamura T, Yi Y, Donahoe PK, et al. Activin receptor-like kinase 1 modulates transforming growth factor-beta 1 signaling in the regulation of angiogenesis. Proc Natl Acad Sci USA 2000;97:2626–31.

[56] Schnaper HW, Hayashida T, Hubchak SC, Poncelet AC. TGF-beta signal transduction and mesangial cell fibrogenesis. Am J Physiol Renal Physiol 2003;284:F243.

[57] Cain JE, Hartwig S, Bertram JF, Rosenblum ND. Bone morphogenetic protein signaling in the developing kidney: present and future. Differentiation 2008;76:831.

[58] Sankar S, Mahooti-Brooks N, Centrella M, McCarthy TL, Madri JA. Expression of transforming growth factor type III receptor in vascular endothelial cells increases their responsiveness to transforming growth factor beta 2. J Biol Chem 1995;270:13567.

[59] Letamendia A, Lastres P, Botella LM, Raab U, Langa C, Velasco B, et al. Role of endoglin in cellular responses to transforming growth factor-beta. A comparative study with betaglycan. J Biol Chem 1998;273:33011–9.

[60] Nakao A, Afrahkte M, Moren A, Nakayama T, Christian JL, Heuchel R, et al. Identification of Smad7, a TGFbeta-inducible antagonist of TGF-beta signalling. Nature 1997;389:631–5.

[61] Miyazaki Y, Oshima K, Fogo A, Hogan BL, Ichikawa I. Bone morphogenetic protein 4 regulates the budding site and elongation of the mouse ureter. J Clin Invest 2000;105:863.

[62] Lawson KA, Dunn NR, Roelen BA, Zeinstra LM, Davis AM, Wright CV, et al. Bmp4 is required for the generation of primordial germ cells in the mouse embryo. Genes Dev 1999;13:424–36.

[63] Hartwig S, Hu MC, Cella C, Pisicone T, Filmus J, Rosenblum ND. Glypican-3 modulates inhibitory Bmp2-Smad signaling to control renal development in vivo. Mech Dev 2005;122:928–38.

[64] Border WA, Noble NA. TGF-beta in kidney fibrosis: a target for gene therapy. Kidney Int 1997;51:1388.

[65] Verrecchia F, Chu ML, Mauviel A. Identification of novel TGF-beta/Smad gene targets in dermal fibroblasts using a combined cDNA microarray/promoter transactivation approach. J Biol Chem 2001;276:17058.

[66] Basu RK, Hubchak S, Hayashida T, Runyan CE, Schumacker PT, Schnaper HW. Interdependence of HIF-1alpha and TGF-beta/Smad3 signaling in normoxic and hypoxic renal epithelial

cell collagen expression. Am J Physiol Renal Physiol 2011;300: F898–905.

[67] Yeh YC, Wei WC, Wang YK, Lin SDC, Sung JM, Tang MJ. Transforming growth factor-{beta}1 induces Smad3-dependent {beta}1 integrin gene expression in epithelial-to-mesenchymal transition during chronic tubulointerstitial fibrosis. Am J Pathol 2010;177:1743–54.

[68] Hall MC, Young DA, Waters JG, Rowan AD, Chantry A, Edwards DR, et al. The comparative role of activator protein 1 and Smad factors in the regulation of Timp-1 and MMP-1 gene expression by transforming growth factor-beta 1. J Biol Chem 2003;278:10304–13.

[69] Isaka Y, Fujiwara Y, Ueda N, Kaneda Y, Kamada T, Imai E. Glomerulosclerosis induced by in vivo transfection of transforming growth factor-beta or platelet-derived growth factor gene into the rat kidney. J Clin Invest 1993;92:2597–601.

[70] Sato M, Muragaki Y, Saika S, Roberts AB, Ooshima A. Targeted disruption of TGF-beta1/Smad3 signaling protects against renal tubulointerstitial fibrosis induced by unilateral ureteral obstruction. J Clin Invest 2003;112:1486.

[71] Saunders AE, Johnson P. Modulation of immune cell signalling by the leukocyte common tyrosine phosphatase, CD45. Cell Signal 2010;22:339.

[72] Earl LA, Bi S, Baum LG. N- and O-glycans modulate galectin-1 binding, CD45 signaling, and T cell death. J Biol Chem 2010;285:2232.

[73] Grigorian A, Torossian S, Demetriou M. T-cell growth, cell surface organization, and the galectin-glycoprotein lattice. Immunol Rev 2009;230:232.

[74] Yamaguchi H, Hendrickson WA. Structural basis for activation of human lymphocyte kinase Lck upon tyrosine phosphorylation. Nature 1996;384:484.

[75] Mustelin T, Coggeshall KM, Altman A. Rapid activation of the T-cell tyrosine protein kinase pp56lck by the CD45 phosphotyrosine phosphatase. Proc Natl Acad Sci USA 1989;86:6302.

[76] Iwashima M, Irving BA, van Oers NS, Chan AC, Weiss A. Sequential interactions of the TCR with two distinct cytoplasmic tyrosine kinases. Science 1994;263:1136.

[77] Lazarovits AI, Poppema S, Zhang Z, Khandaker M, Le Feuvre CE, Singhal SK, et al. Prevention and reversal of renal allograft rejection by antibody against CD45RB. Nature 1996;380:717–20.

[78] Peles E, Nativ M, Campbell PL, Sakuri T, Martinez R, Lev S, et al. The carbonic anhydrase domain of receptor tyrosine phosphatase beta is a functional ligand for the axonal cell recognition molecule contactin. Cell 1995;82:251–60.

[79] Maeda N, Nishiwaki T, Shintani T, Hamanaka H, Noda M. 6B4 proteoglycan/phosphacan, an extracellular variant of receptor-like protein-tyrosine phosphatase zeta/RPTPbeta, binds pleiotrophin/heparin-binding growth-associated molecule (HB-GAM). J Biol Chem 1996;271:21446.

[80] Meng K, Rodriguez-Pena A, Dimitrov T, Chen W, Yamin M, Noda M, et al. Pleiotrophin signals increased tyrosine phosphorylation of beta beta-catenin through inactivation of the intrinsic catalytic activity of the receptor-type protein tyrosine phosphatase beta/zeta. Proc Natl Acad Sci USA 2000;97:2603–8.

[81] Sakurai H, Bush KT, Nigam SK. Identification of pleiotrophin as a mesenchymal factor involved in ureteric bud branching morphogenesis. Development 2001;128:3283.

[82] Kawachi H, Fujikawa A, Maeda N, Noda M. Identification of GIT1/Cat-1 as a substrate molecule of protein tyrosine phosphatase zeta /beta by the yeast substrate-trapping system. Proc Natl Acad Sci USA 2001;98:6593.

[83] Manabe R, Kovalenko M, Webb DJ, Horwitz AR. GIT1 functions in a motile, multi-molecular signaling complex that

regulates protrusive activity and cell migration. J Cell Sci 2002;115:1497.

[84] Fujikawa A, et al. Mice deficient in protein tyrosine phosphatase receptor type Z are resistant to gastric ulcer induction by VacA of *Helicobacter pylori*. Nat Genet 2003;33:375.

[85] Andersson ER, Sandberg R, Lendahl U. Notch signaling: simplicity in design, versatility in function. Development 2011;138:3593.

[86] Brou C, Logeat F, Gupta N, Bessia C, LeBail O, Doedens JR, et al. A novel proteolytic cleavage involved in Notch signaling: the role of the disintegrin-metalloprotease TACE. Mol Cell 2000;5:207—16.

[87] De Strooper B, et al. A presenilin-1-dependent gamma-secretase-like protease mediates release of Notch intracellular domain. Nature 1999;398:518—22.

[88] Cheng HT, Kopan R. The role of Notch signaling in specification of podocyte and proximal tubules within the developing mouse kidney. Kidney Int 2005;68:1951.

[89] Kopan R, Cheng HT, Surendran K. Molecular insights into segmentation along the proximal—distal axis of the nephron. J Am Soc Nephrol 2007;18:2014.

[90] Cheng HT, Miner JH, Lin M, Tansey MG, Roth. K, Kopan R. Gamma-secretase activity is dispensable for mesenchyme-to-epithelium transition but required for podocyte and proximal tubule formation in developing mouse kidney. Development 2003;130:5031—42.

[91] Cheng HT, Kim M, Valerius MT, Surendran K, Schuster-Gossler K, Gossler A, et al. Notch2, but not Notch1, is required for proximal fate acquisition in the mammalian nephron. Development 2007;134:801—11.

[92] Bielesz B, Sirin Y, Si H, Niranjan T, Gruenwald A, Ahn S, et al. Epithelial Notch signaling regulates interstitial fibrosis development in the kidneys of mice and humans. J Clin Invest 2010;120:4040—54.

[93] Ni CY, Murphy MP, Golde TE, Carpenter G. gamma-Secretase cleavage and nuclear localization of ErbB-4 receptor tyrosine kinase. Science 2001;294:2179.

[94] Vidal GA, Naresh A, Marrero L, Jones FE. Presenilin-dependent gamma-secretase processing regulates multiple ERBB4/HER4 activities. J Biol Chem 2005;280:19777.

[95] Tulasne D, et al. Proapoptotic function of the MET tyrosine kinase receptor through caspase cleavage. Mol Cell Biol 2004;24:10328.

[96] Zou Z, Chung B, Nguyen T, Mentone S, Thomson B, Beimesderfer D. Linking receptor-mediated endocytosis and cell signaling: evidence for regulated intramembrane proteolysis of megalin in proximal tubule. J Biol Chem 2004;279:34302—10.

[97] Li Y, Cong R, Biemesderfer D. The COOH terminus of megalin regulates gene expression in opossum kidney proximal tubule cells. Am J Physiol Cell Physiol 2008;295:C529.

[98] Chauvet V, et al. Mechanical stimuli induce cleavage and nuclear translocation of the polycystin-1 C terminus. J Clin Invest 2004;114:1433.

[99] Low SH, Vansanth S, Larson CH, Mukherjee S, Sharma N, Kinter MT, et al. Polycystin-1, STAT6, and P100 function in a pathway that transduces ciliary mechanosensation and is activated in polycystic kidney disease. Dev Cell 2006;10:57—69.

[100] Bertuccio CA, Chapin HC, Cai Y, Mistry K, Chauvet V, Somlo S, et al. Polycystin-1 C-terminal cleavage is modulated by polycystin-2 expression. J Biol Chem 2009;284:21011—26.

[101] Kwon TH, Nielsen J, Kim YH, Knepper MA, Frokaier J, Nielsen S. Regulation of sodium transporters in the thick ascending limb of rat kidney: response to angiotensin II. Am J Physiol Renal Physiol 2003;285:F152—165.

[102] Miner JH. Renal basement membrane components. Kidney Int 1999;56:2016.

[103] Pozzi A, Zent R. Integrins: sensors of extracellular matrix and modulators of cell function. Nephron Exp Nephrol 2003;94:e77.

[104] Turner CE. Paxillin and focal adhesion signalling. Nat Cell Biol 2000;2:E231.

[105] Zheng M, McKeown-Longo PJ. Regulation of HEF1 expression and phosphorylation by TGF-beta 1 and cell adhesion. J Biol Chem 2002;277:39599.

[106] Cox EA, Sastry SK, Huttenlocher A. Integrin-mediated adhesion regulates cell polarity and membrane protrusion through the Rho family of GTPases. Mol Biol Cell 2001;12:265.

[107] Schwartz MA, Assoian RK. Integrins and cell proliferation: regulation of cyclin-dependent kinases via cytoplasmic signaling pathways. J Cell Sci 2001;114:2553.

[108] Frisch SM, Vuori K, Kelaita D, Sicks S. A role for Jun-N-terminal kinase in anoikis; suppression by bcl-2 and crmA. J Cell Biol 1996;135:1377.

[109] Miner JH, Li C. Defective glomerulogenesis in the absence of laminin alpha5 demonstrates a developmental role for the kidney glomerular basement membrane. Dev Biol 2000;217:278.

[110] Kreidberg JA, Donovan MJ, Goldstein SL, Rennke H, Shepherd K, Jones RC, et al. Alpha 3 beta 1 integrin has a crucial role in kidney and lung organogenesis. Development 1996;122:3537—47.

[111] Zhang X, et al. beta1 integrin is necessary for ureteric bud branching morphogenesis and maintenance of collecting duct structural integrity. Development 2009;136:3357.

[112] Gardner H, Kreidberg J, Koteliansky V, Jaenisch R. Deletion of integrin alpha 1 by homologous recombination permits normal murine development but gives rise to a specific deficit in cell adhesion. Dev Biol 1996;175:301.

[113] Chen X, Moeckel G, Morrow JD, Cosgrove D, Harris RC, Fogo AB, et al. Lack of integrin alpha1beta1 leads to severe glomerulosclerosis after glomerular injury. Am J Pathol 2004;165:617—30.

[114] Gumbiner BM. Regulation of cadherin-mediated adhesion in morphogenesis. Nat Rev Mol Cell Biol 2005;6:622.

[115] Thomson RB, Igarashi P, Biemesderfer D, Kim R, Abu-Alfa A, Soleimani M, et al. Isolation and cDNA cloning of Ksp-cadherin, a novel kidney-specific member of the cadherin multigene family. J Biol Chem 1995;270:17594—601.

[116] Steinberg MS, Takeichi M. Experimental specification of cell sorting, tissue spreading, and specific spatial patterning by quantitative differences in cadherin expression. Proc Natl Acad Sci USA 1994;91:206.

[117] Drees F, Pokutta S, Yamada S, Nelson WJ, Weis WI. Alpha-catenin is a molecular switch that binds E-cadherin-beta-catenin and regulates actin-filament assembly. Cell 2005;123:903.

[118] Molenaar M, et al. XTcf-3 transcription factor mediates beta-catenin-induced axis formation in *Xenopus* embryos. Cell 1996;86:391.

[119] Nelson WJ, Nusse R. Convergence of Wnt, beta-catenin, and cadherin pathways. Science 2004;136:3357.

[120] Fagotto F, Guger K, Gumbiner BM. Induction of the primary dorsalizing center in *Xenopus* by the Wnt/GSK/beta-catenin signaling pathway, but not by Vg1, Activin or Noggin. Development 1997;124:453.

[121] Korinek V, Barker N, Morin PJ, van Wichen D, de Weger R, Kinzler KW, et al. Constitutive transcriptional activation by a beta-catenin-Tcf complex in APC − / − colon carcinoma. Science 1997;275:1784—7.

[122] Wodarz A, Nusse R. Mechanisms of Wnt signaling in development. Annu Rev Cell Dev Biol 1998;14:59.

[123] Slusarski DC, Corces VG, Moon RT. Interaction of Wnt and a Frizzled homologue triggers G-protein-linked phosphatidylinositol signalling. Nature 1997;390:410.

[124] Zeng X, Tamai K, Doble B, Li S, Huang H, Habas R, et al. A dual-kinase mechanism for Wnt co-receptor phosphorylation and activation. Nature 2005;438:873–7.

[125] Wallingford JB, Habas R. The developmental biology of Dishevelled: an enigmatic protein governing cell fate and cell polarity. Development 2005;132:4421.

[126] Taelman VF, et al. Wnt signaling requires sequestration of glycogen synthase kinase 3 inside multivesicular endosomes. Cell 2010;143:1136.

[127] Kuure S, Popsueva A, Jakobson M, Sainio K, Sariola H. Glycogen synthase kinase-3 inactivation and stabilization of beta-catenin induce nephron differentiation in isolated mouse and rat kidney mesenchymes. J Am Soc Nephrol 2007;18:1130.

[128] Park JS, Valerius MT, McMahon AP. Wnt/beta-catenin signaling regulates nephron induction during mouse kidney development. Development 2007;134:2533.

[129] Schmidt-Ott KM, Barasch J. WNT/beta-catenin signaling in nephron progenitors and their epithelial progeny. Kidney Int 2008;74:1004.

[130] Lin SL, et al. Macrophage Wnt7b is critical for kidney repair and regeneration. Proc Natl Acad Sci USA 2010;107:4194.

[131] He W, Dai C, Li Y, Zeng G, Monga SP, Liu Y. Wnt/beta-catenin signaling promotes renal interstitial fibrosis. J Am Soc Nephrol 2009;20:765–76.

[132] Patrakka J, Tryggvason K. Nephrin: a unique structural and signaling protein of the kidney filter. Trends Mol Med 2007;13:396.

[133] Machuca E, Benoit G, Antignac C. Genetics of nephrotic syndrome: connecting molecular genetics to podocyte physiology. Hum Mol Genet 2009;18:R185.

[134] Schermer B, Benzing T. Lipid–protein interactions along the slit diaphragm of podocytes. J Am Soc Nephrology: JASN 2009;20:473.

[135] Li H, Liu TF, Lazrak A, Peracchia C, Goldberg GS, Lampe PD, et al. Properties and regulation of gap junctional hemichannels in the plasma membranes of cultured cells. J Cell Biol 1996;134:1019–30.

[136] Yao J, Morioka T, Li B, Oite T. Coordination of mesangial cell contraction by gap junction-mediated intercellular Ca(2 +) wave. J Am Soc Nephrol 2002;13:2018.

[137] Vikhamar G, Rivedal E, Mollerup S, Sanner T. Role of Cx43 phosphorylation and MAP kinase activation in EGF induced enhancement of cell communication in human kidney epithelial cells. Cell Adhes Commun 1998;5:451.

[138] Vergara L, Bao X, Cooper M, Bello-Reuss E, Reuss L. Gap-junctional hemichannels are activated by ATP depletion in human renal proximal tubule cells. J Membr Biol 2003;196:173.

[139] Davenport JR, Yoder BK. An incredible decade for the primary cilium: a look at a once-forgotten organelle. Am J Physiol Renal Physiol 2005;289:F1159.

[140] Praetorius HA, Spring KR. A physiological view of the primary cilium. Annu Rev Physiol 2005;67:515.

[141] Afzelius BA. Cilia-related diseases. J Pathol 2004;204:470.

[142] Taulman PD, Haycraft CJ, Balkovetz DF, Yoder BK. Polaris, a protein involved in left–right axis patterning, localizes to basal bodies and cilia. Mol Biol Cell 2001;12:589.

[143] Yoder BK, Hou X, Guay-Woodford LM. The polycystic kidney disease proteins, polycystin-1, polycystin-2, polaris, and cystin, are co-localized in renal cilia. J Am Soc Nephrol 2002;13:2508.

[144] Nauli SM, Zhou J. Polycystins and mechanosensation in renal and nodal cilia. Bioessays 2004;26:844.

[145] Cai Y, et al. Identification and characterization of polycystin-2, the PKD2 gene product. J Biol Chem 1999;274:28557.

[146] Hanaoka K, et al. Co-assembly of polycystin-1 and -2 produces unique cation-permeable currents. Nature 2000;408:990.

[147] Gonzalez-Perrett S, et al. Polycystin-2, the protein mutated in autosomal dominant polycystic kidney disease (ADPKD), is a Ca^{2+}-permeable nonselective cation channel. Proc Natl Acad Sci USA 2001;98:1182.

[148] Nauli SM, et al. Polycystins 1 and 2 mediate mechanosensation in the primary cilium of kidney cells. Nat Genet 2003;33:129.

[149] Liu W, Murcia NS, Duan Y, Weinbaum S, Yoder BK, Schweibert E, et al. Mechanoregulation of intracellular Ca2 + concentration is attenuated in collecting duct of monocilium-impaired orpk mice. Am J Physiol Renal Physiol 2005;289: F978–988.

[150] Gallagher AR, Germino GG, Somlo S. Molecular advances in autosomal dominant polycystic kidney disease. Adv Chronic Kidney Dis 2010;17:118.

[151] Rhee SG. Regulation of phosphoinositide-specific phospholipase C. Annu Rev Biochem 2001;70:281.

[152] Park D, Jhon DY, Lee CW, Ryu SH, Rhee SG. Removal of the carboxyl-terminal region of phospholipase C-beta 1 by calpain abolishes activation by G alpha q. J Biol Chem 1993;268:3710.

[153] Park D, Jhon DY, Lee CW, Lee KH, Rhee SG. Activation of phospholipase C isozymes by G protein beta gamma-subunits. J Biol Chem 1993;268:4573.

[154] Sidhu RS, Clough RR, Bhullar RP. Regulation of phospholipase C-delta1 through direct interactions with the small GTPase Ral and calmodulin. J Biol Chem 2005;280:21933.

[155] Allen V, Swigart P, Cheung R, Cockcroft S, Katan M. Regulation of inositol lipid-specific phospholipase cdelta by changes in Ca^{2+} ion concentrations. Biochem J 1997;327:545.

[156] Kelley GG, Reks SE, Ondrako JM, Smrcka AV. Phospholipase C (epsilon): a novel Ras effector. Embo J 2001;20:743.

[157] Bunney TD, Katan M. Phospholipase C epsilon: linking second messengers and small GTPases. Trends Cell Biol 2006;16:640.

[158] Van Lint J, Ni Y, Valius M, Merlevede W, Vandenheede JR. Platelet-derived growth factor stimulates protein kinase D through the activation of phospholipase Cgamma and protein kinase C. J Biol Chem 1998;273:7038.

[159] Haendeler J, et al. GIT1 mediates Src-dependent activation of phospholipase Cgamma by angiotensin II and epidermal growth factor. J Biol Chem 2003;278:49936.

[160] Bae YS, Cantley LG, Chen CS, Kim SR, Kwon KS, Rhee SG. Activation of phospholipase C-gamma by phosphatidylinositol 3,4,5-trisphosphate. J Biol Chem 1998;273:4465–9.

[161] Ron D, Kazanietz MG. New insights into the regulation of protein kinase C and novel phorbol ester receptors. Faseb J 1999;13:1658.

[162] Toker A, Meyer M, Reddy KK, Falck JR, Aneja R, Aneja S, et al. Activation of protein kinase C family members by the novel polyphosphoinositides PtdIns-3,4-P2 and PtdIns-3,4,5-P3. J Biol Chem 1994;269:32358–67.

[163] Joberty G, Petersen C, Gao L, Macara IG. The cell-polarity protein Par6 links Par3 and atypical protein kinase C to Cdc42. Nat Cell Biol 2000;2:531.

[164] Gao L, Joberty G, Macara IG. Assembly of epithelial tight junctions is negatively regulated by Par6. Curr Biol 2002;12:221.

[165] Togawa A, Sfakianos J, Ishibe S, Suzuki S, Fujigaki Y, Kitagawa M, et al. Hepatocyte Growth Factor stimulated cell scattering requires ERK and Cdc42-dependent tight junction disassembly. Biochem Biophys Res Commun 2010;400:271–7.

[166] Pedemonte CH, Pressley TA, Lokhandwala MF, Cinelli AR. Regulation of Na,K-ATPase transport activity by protein kinase C. J Membr Biol 1997;155:219.

[167] Efendiev R, Bertorello AM, Pressley TA, Rousselot M, Feraille E, Pedemonte CH. Simultaneous phosphorylation of Ser11 and Ser18 in the alpha-subunit promotes the recruitment of Na(+),K(+)-ATPase molecules to the plasma membrane. Biochemistry 2000;39:9884—92.

[168] Gomes P, Soares-da-Silva P. Role of cAMP-PKA-PLC signaling cascade on dopamine-induced PKC-mediated inhibition of renal Na(+)-K(+)-ATPase activity. Am J Physiol Renal Physiol 2002;282:F1084.

[169] Yao LP, Li XX, Yu PY, Xu J, Ascio LD, Jose PA. Dopamine D1 receptor and protein kinase C isoforms in spontaneously hypertensive rats. Hypertension 1998;32:1049—53.

[170] Salyer S, Lesousky N, Weinman EJ, Clark BJ, Lederer ED, Khundmiri SJ. Dopamine regulation of Na^+K^+-ATPase requires the PDZ-2 domain of sodium hydrogen regulatory factor-1 (NHERF-1) in opossum kidney cells. Am J Physiol Cell Physiol 2011;300:C425—434.

[171] Steinberg SF. Distinctive activation mechanisms and functions for protein kinase Cdelta. Biochem J 2004;384:449.

[172] Soh JW, Lee EH, Prywes R, Weinstein IB. Novel roles of specific isoforms of protein kinase C in activation of the c-fos serum response element. Mol Cell Biol 1999;19:1313.

[173] Isakov N, Altman A. Protein kinase C(theta) in T cell activation. Annu Rev Immunol 2002;20:761.

[174] Schulz RA, Yutzey KE. Calcineurin signaling and NFAT activation in cardiovascular and skeletal muscle development. Dev Biol 2004;266:1.

[175] Macian F, Lopez-Rodriguez C, Rao A. Partners in transcription: NFAT and AP-1. Oncogene 2001;20:2476.

[176] Kobayashi H, Shiraishi S, Yanagita T, Yokoo H, Yamamoto R, Minami S, et al. Regulation of voltage-dependent sodium channel expression in adrenal chromaffin cells: Iinvolvement of multiple calcium signaling pathways. Ann NY Acad Sci 2002;971:127—34.

[177] Boulton TG, Yancopoulos GD, Gregory JS, Slaughter C, Moomaw C, Hsu J, et al. An insulin-stimulated protein kinase similar to yeast kinases involved in cell cycle control. Science 1990;249:64—7.

[178] Whitmarsh AJ, Shore P, Sharrocks AD, Davis RJ. Integration of MAP kinase signal transduction pathways at the serum response element. Science 1995;269:403.

[179] Liu ZX, Yu CF, Nickel C, Thomas S, Cantley LG. Hepatocyte growth factor induces ERK-dependent paxillin phosphorylation and regulates paxillin-focal adhesion kinase association. J Biol Chem 2002;277:10452.

[180] Klemke RL, Cai S, Giannini AL, Gallagher PJ, de Lanerolle P, Cheresh DA. Regulation of cell motility by mitogen-activated protein kinase. J Cell Biol 1997;137:481—92.

[181] Crews CM, Alessandrini A, Erikson RL. The primary structure of MEK, a protein kinase that phosphorylates the ERK gene product. Science 1992;258:478.

[182] Nguyen A, et al. Kinase suppressor of Ras (KSR) is a scaffold which facilitates mitogen-activated protein kinase activation in vivo. Mol Cell Biol 2002;22:3035.

[183] Ishibe S, Joly D, Zhu X, Cantley LG. Phosphorylation-dependent paxillin-ERK association mediates hepatocyte growth factor-stimulated epithelial morphogenesis. Mol Cell 2003;12:1275.

[184] Roy M, Li Z, Sacks DB. IQGAP1 is a scaffold for mitogen-activated protein kinase signaling. Mol Cell Biol 2005;25:7940.

[185] Kolch W. Coordinating ERK/MAPK signalling through scaffolds and inhibitors. Nat Rev Mol Cell Biol 2005;6:827.

[186] Lowenstein EJ, et al. The SH2 and SH3 domain-containing protein GRB2 links receptor tyrosine kinases to ras signaling. Cell 1992;70:431.

[187] Bonfini L, Karlovich CA, Dasgupta C, Banerjee U. The Son of sevenless gene product: a putative activator of Ras. Science 1992;255:603.

[188] Dougherty MK, et al. Regulation of Raf-1 by direct feedback phosphorylation. Mol Cell 2005;17:215.

[189] Kovacs JJ, Hara MR, Davenport CL, Kim J, Lefkowitz RJ. Arrestin development: emerging roles for beta-arrestins in developmental signaling pathways. Developmental Cell 2009;17:443.

[190] Siegel JN, Klausner RD, Rapp UR, Samelson LE. T cell antigen receptor engagement stimulates c-raf phosphorylation and induces c-raf-associated kinase activity via a protein kinase C-dependent pathway. J Biol Chem 1990;265:18472.

[191] Kolch W, Hiedecker G, Kochs G, Hummel R, Vahidi H, Mischak H, et al. Protein kinase C alpha activates RAF-1 by direct phosphorylation. Nature 1993;364:249—52.

[192] Racusen LC, Fivush BA, Li YL, Slatnik I, Solez K. Dissociation of tubular cell detachment and tubular cell death in clinical and experimental "acute tubular necrosis.". Lab Invest 1991;64:546.

[193] Park MY, Lee RH, Lee SH, Jung JS. Apoptosis induced by inhibition of contact with extracellular matrix in mouse collecting duct cells. Nephron 1999;83:341.

[194] Nony PA, Schnellmann RG. Mechanisms of renal cell repair and regeneration after acute renal failure. J Pharmacol Exp Ther 2003;304:905.

[195] Subauste MC, Pertz O, Adamson ED, Turner CE, Junger S, Hahn KM. Vinculin modulation of paxillin-FAK interactions regulates ERK to control survival and motility. J Cell Biol 2004;165:371—81.

[196] Aplin AE, Juliano RL. Integrin and cytoskeletal regulation of growth factor signaling to the MAP kinase pathway. J Cell Sci 1999;112(Pt 5):695.

[197] Edin ML, Juliano RL. Raf-1 serine 338 phosphorylation plays a key role in adhesion-dependent activation of extracellular signal-regulated kinase by epidermal growth factor. Mol Cell Biol 2005;25:4466.

[198] Gille H, Kortenjaan M, Thomae O, Moomaw C, Slaughter C, Cobb MH, et al. ERK phosphorylation potentiates Elk-1-mediated ternary complex formation and transactivation. Embo J 1995;14:951—62.

[199] Talarmin H, et al. The mitogen-activated protein kinase kinase/extracellular signal-regulated kinase cascade activation is a key signalling pathway involved in the regulation of G(1) phase progression in proliferating hepatocytes. Mol Cell Biol 1999;19:6003.

[200] Qiao M, Shapiro P, Kumar R, Passaniti A. Insulin-like growth factor-1 regulates endogenous RUNX2 activity in endothelial cells through a phosphatidylinositol 3-kinase/ERK-dependent and Akt-independent signaling pathway. J Biol Chem 2004;279:42709.

[201] Roovers K, Assoian RK. Integrating the MAP kinase signal into the G1 phase cell cycle machinery. Bioessays 2000;22:818.

[202] Reginato MJ, Mills KR, Paulus JK, Lynch DK, Sjroi DC, Debnath J, et al. Integrins and EGFR coordinately regulate the pro-apoptotic protein Bim to prevent anoikis. Nat Cell Biol 2003;5:733—40.

[203] Marshall CJ. Specificity of receptor tyrosine kinase signaling: transient versus sustained extracellular signal-regulated kinase activation. Cell 1995;80:179.

[204] Thrane EV, Schwarze PE, Thoresen GH, Lag M, Refsnes M. Persistent versus transient map kinase (ERK) activation in the

proliferation of lung epithelial type 2 cells. Exp Lung Res 2001;27:387.

[205] Collins NL, Reginato MG, Paulus JK, Sgroi DC, Labaer J, Brugge JS. G1/S cell cycle arrest provides anoikis resistance through Erk-mediated Bim suppression. Mol Cell Biol 2005;25:5282–91.

[206] Heasman SJ, Ridley AJ. Mammalian Rho GTPases: new insights into their functions from *in vivo* studies. Nat Rev Mol Cell Biol 2008;9:690.

[207] DeMali KA, Wennerberg K, Burridge K. Integrin signaling to the actin cytoskeleton. Curr Opin Cell Biol 2003;15:572.

[208] Rogers KK, Jou TS, Guo W, Lipschutz JH. The Rho family of small GTPases is involved in epithelial cystogenesis and tubulogenesis. Kidney Int 2003;63:1632.

[209] Nakamura A, Hayashi K, Ozawa Y, Fujiwara K, Okubo K, Kanda T, et al. Vessel- and vasoconstrictor-dependent role of rho/rho-kinase in renal microvascular tone. J Vasc Res 2003;40:244–51.

[210] Zarubin T, Han J. Activation and signaling of the p38 MAP kinase pathway. Cell Res 2005;15:11.

[211] Roux PP, Blenis J. ERK and p38 MAPK-activated protein kinases: a family of protein kinases with diverse biological functions. Microbiol Mol Biol Rev 2004;68:320.

[212] Chen Z, et al. MAP kinases. Chem Rev 2001;101:2449.

[213] Schiffer M, Bitzer M, Roberts IS, Koop JB, ten Dijke P, Mundel P, et al. Apoptosis in podocytes induced by TGF-beta and Smad7. J Clin Invest 2001;108:807–16.

[214] Ma FY, Sachchithananthan M, Flanc RS, Nikolic-Paterson DJ. Mitogen activated protein kinases in renal fibrosis. Front Biosci (Schol Ed) 2009;1:171.

[215] Stambe C, Atkins RC, Tesch GH, Masaki T, Schreiner GF, Nikolic-Paterson DJ. The role of p38alpha mitogen-activated protein kinase activation in renal fibrosis. J Am Soc Nephrol 2004;15:370–9.

[216] Koshikawa M, et al. Role of p38 mitogen-activated protein kinase activation in podocyte injury and proteinuria in experimental Nephrotic syndrome. J Am Soc Nephrol 2005;16:2690.

[217] Park KM, Kramers C, Vayssier-Taussat M, Chen A, Bonventre JV. Prevention of kidney ischemia/reperfusion-induced functional injury, MAPK and MAPK kinase activation, and inflammation by remote transient ureteral obstruction. J Biol Chem 2002;277:2040.

[218] Hung CC, Ichimura T, Stevens JL, Bonventre JV. Protection of renal epithelial cells against oxidative injury by endoplasmic reticulum stress preconditioning is mediated by ERK1/2 activation. J Biol Chem 2003;278:29317.

[219] Arany I, Megyesi JK, Kaneto H, Tanaka S, Safirstein RL. Activation of ERK or inhibition of JNK ameliorates $H_{(2)}O_{(2)}$ cytotoxicity in mouse renal proximal tubule cells. Kidney Int 2004;65:1231.

[220] Auger KR, Serunian LA, Soltoff SP, Libby P, Cantley LC. PDGF-dependent tyrosine phosphorylation stimulates production of novel polyphosphoinositides in intact cells. Cell 1989;57:167.

[221] Balla T. Inositol-lipid binding motifs: signal integrators through protein–lipid and protein–protein interactions. J Cell Sci 2005;118:2093.

[222] Kobayashi S, Shirai T, Kiyokawa E, Mochizuki N, Matsuda M, Fukui Y. Membrane recruitment of DOCK180 by binding to PtdIns(3,4,5)P3. Biochem J 2001;354:73–8.

[223] Palmby TR, Abe K, Der CJ. Critical role of the pleckstrin homology and cysteine-rich domains in Vav signaling and transforming activity. J Biol Chem 2002;277:39350.

[224] Andjelkovic M, Maira SM, Cron P, Parker PJ, Hemmings BA. Domain swapping used to investigate the mechanism of protein kinase B regulation by 3-phosphoinositide-dependent protein kinase 1 and Ser473 kinase. Mol Cell Biol 1999;19:5061.

[225] Alessi DR, Kozlowski MT, Weng QP, Morrice N, Avruch J. 3-Phosphoinositide-dependent protein kinase 1 (PDK1) phosphorylates and activates the p70 S6 kinase *in vivo* and *in vitro*. Curr Biol 1998;8:69.

[226] Tanaka H, Fujita N, Tsuruo T. 3-Phosphoinositide-dependent protein kinase-1-mediated IkappaB kinase beta (IkkB) phosphorylation activates NF-kappaB signaling. J Biol Chem 2005;280:40965.

[227] Woodgett JR. Recent advances in the protein kinase B signaling pathway. Curr Opin Cell Biol 2005;17:150.

[228] Cross DA, Alessi DR, Cohen P, Andjelkovich M, Hemmings BA. Inhibition of glycogen synthase kinase-3 by insulin mediated by protein kinase B. Nature 1995;378:785.

[229] Rubinfeld B, Albert I, Porfiri E, Fiol C, Munemitsu S, Polakis P. Binding of GSK3beta to the APC-beta-catenin complex and regulation of complex assembly. Science 1996;272:1023–6.

[230] Ilouz R, Pietrokovski S, Eisenstein M, Eldar-Finkelman H. New insights into the autoinhibition mechanism of glycogen synthase kinase-3beta. J Mol Biol 2008;383:999.

[231] Ishibe S, Haydu JE, Togawa A, Marlier A, Cantley LG. Cell confluence regulates hepatocyte growth factor-stimulated cell morphogenesis in a beta-catenin-dependent manner. Mol Cell Biol 2006;26:9232.

[232] Diehl JA, Cheng M, Roussel MF, Sherr CJ. Glycogen synthase kinase-3beta regulates cyclin D1 proteolysis and subcellular localization. Genes Dev 1998;12:3499.

[233] Pap M, Cooper GM. Role of translation initiation factor 2B in control of cell survival by the phosphatidylinositol 3-kinase/ Akt/glycogen synthase kinase 3beta signaling pathway. Mol Cell Biol 2002;22:578.

[234] Brunet A, Bonni A, Zigmond MJ, Lin MZ, Juo P, Hu LS, et al. Akt promotes cell survival by phosphorylating and inhibiting a Forkhead transcription factor. Cell 1999;96:857–68.

[235] Fingar DC, Blenis J. Target of rapamycin (TOR): an integrator of nutrient and growth factor signals and coordinator of cell growth and cell cycle progression. Oncogene 2004;23:3151.

[236] Manning BD, Cantley LC. United at last: the tuberous sclerosis complex gene products connect the phosphoinositide 3-kinase/Akt pathway to mammalian target of rapamycin (mTOR) signalling. Biochem Soc Trans 2003;31:573.

[237] Katso R, Okkenhaug K, Ahmadi K, White S, Timms J, Waterfield MD. Cellular function of phosphoinositide 3-kinases: implications for development, homeostasis, and cancer. Annu Rev Cell Dev Biol 2001;17:615–75.

[238] Ishiki M, Klip A. Minireview: recent developments in the regulation of glucose transporter-4 traffic: new signals, locations, and partners. Endocrinology 2005;146:5071.

[239] Summers SA, Kao AW, Kohn AD, Backus GS, Roth RA, Pessin JE, et al. The role of glycogen synthase kinase 3beta in insulin-stimulated glucose metabolism. J Biol Chem 1999;274:17934–40.

[240] Kanaide H, Ichiki T, Nishimura J, Hirano K. Cellular mechanism of vasoconstriction induced by angiotensin II: it remains to be determined. Circ Res 2003;93:1015.

[241] Woodsome TP, Polzin A, Kitazawa K, Eto M, Kitazawa T. Agonist- and depolarization-induced signals for myosin light chain phosphorylation and force generation of cultured vascular smooth muscle cells. J Cell Sci 2006;119:1769.

[242] Ito M, Nakano T, Erdodi F, Hartshorne DJ. Myosin phosphatase: structure, regulation and function. Mol Cell Biochem 2004;259:197.

[243] Flannery PJ, Spurney RF. Transactivation of the epidermal growth factor receptor by angiotensin II in glomerular podocytes. Nephron Exp Nephrol 2006;103:e109.

[244] Ying Z, Jin L, Palmer T, Webb RC. Angiotensin II up-regulates leukemia-associated rho guanine nucleotide exchange factor (LARG), a RGS domain containing RhoGEF, in vascular smooth muscle cells. Mol Pharmacol 2005;14:14.

[245] Im SH, Rao A. Activation and deactivation of gene expression by Ca^{2+}/calcineurin-NFAT-mediated signaling. Mol Cells 2004;18:1.

[246] Rogerson FM, Brennan FE, Fuller PJ. Mineralocorticoid receptor binding, structure and function. Mol Cell Endocrinol 2004;217:203.

[247] Snyder PM. Minireview: regulation of epithelial Na^+ channel trafficking. Endocrinology 2005;146:5079.

[248] Naray-Fejes-Toth A, Fejes-Toth G. The sgk, an aldosterone-induced gene in mineralocorticoid target cells, regulates the epithelial sodium channel. Kidney Int 2000;57:1290.

[249] Snyder PM, Olson DR, Thomas BC. Serum and glucocorticoid-regulated kinase modulates Nedd4-2-mediated inhibition of the epithelial Na^+ channel. J Biol Chem 2002;277:5.

[250] Hansson JH, et al. Hypertension caused by a truncated epithelial sodium channel gamma-subunit: genetic heterogeneity of Liddle syndrome. Nat Genet 1995;11:76.

[251] Valenti G, Procino G, Tamma G, Carmosino M, Svelto M. Minireview: aquaporin 2 trafficking. Endocrinology 2005;146:5063.

[252] Sabolic I, Valenti G, Verbavatz JM, Van Hoek AN, Verkman AS, Ausiello DA, et al. Localization of the CHIP28 water channel in rat kidney. Am J Physiol 1992;263:C1225–1233.

[253] Ishibashi K, et al. Molecular cloning and expression of a member of the aquaporin family with permeability to glycerol and urea in addition to water expressed at the basolateral membrane of kidney collecting duct cells. Proc Natl Acad Sci USA 1994;91:6269.

[254] Henn V, et al. Identification of a novel A-kinase anchoring protein 18 isoform and evidence for its role in the vasopressin-induced aquaporin-2 shuttle in renal principal cells. J Biol Chem 2004;279:26654.

[255] Kuwahara M, Fushimi K, Terada Y, Bai L, Marumo F, Sasaki S. cAMP-dependent phosphorylation stimulates water permeability of aquaporin-collecting duct water channel protein expressed in *Xenopus* oocytes. J Biol Chem 1995;270:10384–7.

[256] Nedvetsky PI, Tamma G, Beulshausen S, Valenti G, Rosenthal W, Klussmann E. Regulation of aquaporin-2 trafficking. Handb Exp Pharmacol 2009;190:133–57.

[257] Gouraud S, et al. Functional involvement of VAMP/synaptobrevin-2 in cAMP-stimulated aquaporin 2 translocation in renal collecting duct cells. J Cell Sci 2002;115:3667–74.

[258] Mistry AC, Mallick R, Klein JD, Weimbs T, Sands JM, Frölich O. Syntaxin specificity of aquaporins in the inner medullary collecting duct. Am J Physiol Renal Physiol 2009;297:F292–300.

[259] Stefan E, et al. Compartmentalization of cAMP-dependent signaling by phosphodiesterase-4D is involved in the regulation of vasopressin-mediated water reabsorption in renal principal cells. J Am Soc Nephrol: JASN 2007;18:199.

[260] Jo I, Ward DT, Baum MA, Scott JD, Coghlan VM, Hammond TG, et al. AQP2 is a substrate for endogenous PP2B activity within an inner medullary AKAP-signaling complex. Am J Physiol Renal Physiol 2001;281:F958–965.

[261] Yasui M, Zelenin SM, Celsi G, Aperia A. Adenylate cyclase-coupled vasopressin receptor activates AQP2 promoter via a dual effect on CRE and AP1 elements. Am J Physiol 1997;272: F443.

[262] Hasler U, Vinciguerra M, Vandewalle A, Martin PY, Feraille E. Dual effects of hypertonicity on aquaporin-2 expression in cultured renal collecting duct principal cells. J Am Soc Nephrol 2005;16:1571.

[263] Snyder PM, Olson DR, Kabra R, Zhou R, Steines JC. cAMP and serum and glucocorticoid-inducible kinase (SGK) regulate the epithelial Na(+) channel through convergent phosphorylation of Nedd4-2. J Biol Chem 2004;279:45753.

[264] Snyder PM. Liddle's syndrome mutations disrupt cAMP-mediated translocation of the epithelial Na(+) channel to the cell surface. J Clin Invest 2000;105:45.

[265] Butterworth MB, Edinger RS, Johnson JP, Frizzell RA. Acute ENaC stimulation by cAMP in a kidney cell line is mediated by exocytic insertion from a recycling channel pool. J Gen Physiol 2005;125:81.

[266] Schnizler M, Mastroberardino L, Reifarth F, Weber WM, Verrey F, Clauss W. cAMP sensitivity conferred to the epithelial Na^+ channel by alpha-subunit cloned from guinea-pig colon. Pflugers Arch 2000;439:579–87.

[267] Stockand JD. Vasopressin regulation of renal sodium excretion. Kidney international 2010;78:849.

[268] Welling PA, Ho K. A comprehensive guide to the ROMK potassium channel: form and function in health and disease. Am J Physiol Renal Physiol 2009;297:F849.

[269] Hebert SC, Desir G, Giebisch G, Wang W. Molecular diversity and regulation of renal potassium channels. Physiol Rev 2005;85:319.

[270] Heath CM, Stahl PD, Barbieri MA. Lipid kinases play crucial and multiple roles in membrane trafficking and signaling. Histol Histopathol 2003;18:989.

[271] Doughman RL, Firestone AJ, Anderson RA. Phosphatidylinositol phosphate kinases put PI4,5P(2) in its place. J Membr Biol 2003;194:77.

[272] Liou HH, Zhou SS, Huang CL. Regulation of ROMK1 channel by protein kinase A via a phosphatidylinositol 4,5-bisphosphate-dependent mechanism. Proc Natl Acad Sci USA 1999;96:5820.

[273] Reeves WB, McDonald GA, Mehta P, Andreoli TE. Activation of K^+ channels in renal medullary vesicles by cAMP-dependent protein kinase. J Membr Biol 1989;109:65.

[274] Yoo D, Kim BY, Campo C, Nance L, King A, Mauoyo D, et al. Cell surface expression of the ROMK (Kir 1.1) channel is regulated by the aldosterone-induced kinase, SGK-1, and protein kinase A. J Biol Chem 2003;278:23066–75.

[275] Yoo D, Flagg TP, Ohlson O, Raghuram V, Foskett JK, Welling PA. Assembly and trafficking of a multiprotein ROMK (Kir 1.1) channel complex by PDZ interactions. J Biol Chem 2004;279:6863–73.

[276] Hoorn EJ, Nelson JH, McCormick JA, Ellison DH. The WNK kinase network regulating sodium, potassium, and blood pressure. J Am Soc Nephrol: JASN 2011;22:605.

[277] Verissimo F, Jordan P. WNK kinases, a novel protein kinase subfamily in multi-cellular organisms. Oncogene 2001;20:5562.

[278] Leng Q, Kahle KT, Rinehart J, MacGregor GG, Wilson FH, Canessa CM, et al. WNK3, a kinase related to genes mutated in hereditary hypertension with hyperkalemia, regulates the K^+ channel ROMK1 (Kir1.1). J Physiol 2005;15:15.

[279] Rinehart J, et al. WNK3 kinase is a positive regulator of NKCC2 and NCC, renal cation-Cl^- cotransporters required for normal blood pressure homeostasis. Proc Natl Acad Sci USA 2005;102:16777.

[280] Lazrak A, Liu Z, Huang CL. Antagonistic regulation of ROMK by long and kidney-specific WNK1 isoforms. Proc Natl Acad Sci USA 2006;103:1615.

[281] Kahle KT, Wilson FH, Lifton RP. Regulation of diverse ion transport pathways by WNK4 kinase: a novel molecular switch. Trends Endocrinol Metab 2005;16:98.

[282] Wilson FH, et al. Human hypertension caused by mutations in WNK kinases. Science 2001;293:1107.

[283] Kahle KT, Gimenez I, Hassan H, Wilson FH, Wong RD, Forbush B, et al. WNK4 regulates apical and basolateral Cl⁻ flux in extrarenal epithelia. Proc Natl Acad Sci USA 2004;101:2064—9.

[284] Huang CL, Yang SS, Lin SH. Mechanism of regulation of renal ion transport by WNK kinases. Curr Opin Nephrol Hypertens 2008;17:519.

[285] He G, Wang HR, Huang SK, Huang CL. Intersectin links WNK kinases to endocytosis of ROMK1. J Clin Invest 2007;117:1078.

[286] Subramanya AR, Liu J, Ellison DH, Wade JB, Welling PA. WNK4 diverts the thiazide-sensitive NaCl cotransporter to the lysosome and stimulates AP-3 interaction. J Biol Chem 2009;284:18471.

[287] Zhou B, Zhuang J, Gu D, Wang H, Cebotaru L, Guggino WB, et al. WNK4 enhances the degradation of NCC through a sortilin-mediated lysosomal pathway. J Am Soc Nephrol:JASN 2010;21:82—92.

[288] Lalioti MD, et al. Wnk4 controls blood pressure and potassium homeostasis via regulation of mass and activity of the distal convoluted tubule. Nat Genet 2006;38:1124.

14

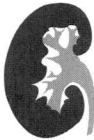

Scaffolding Proteins in Transport Regulation

Paul A. Welling

Department of Physiology, University of Maryland School of Medicine, Baltimore, MD, USA

PDZ-PROTEINS

PDZ domains (also known as DHR domains or GLGF repeats) are ~90 amino acid, protein—protein interaction modules that bind short amino-acid motifs (4—5 residues) generally found at the extreme COOH-terminus of target proteins.[1] More rarely, PDZ domains recognize internal sequences that mimic the COOH-terminal binding motif.[2,3] The term PDZ is derived from the names of the three proteins that the structure was originally identified from (PSD 95, a post synaptic density protein), Dlg (Dropsophila Disc large tumor suppressor), and ZO-1 (zona occludens, the tight junction protein). Since its discovery as a region of sequence homology in these few proteins,[4] the PDZ domain has become recognized as one of the most common interaction modules. The human genome contains over 250 PDZ domains in nearly 100 human proteins. The structure is evolutionarily conserved, emerging largely in metazoans, perhaps to accommodate the increased signaling needs of multicellular organisms.[5]

PDZ domain containing proteins usually possess multiple protein—protein recognition modules. Because the domains act independently and allow concurrent recruitment of different binding targets, PDZ proteins function as molecular scaffolds. Indeed, PDZ proteins facilitate multi-protein complex formation, and organize expression of target proteins on specific membrane domains for a wide range of physiological processes. A growing body of work has strongly implicated PDZ proteins in targeting and clustering various receptors, channels, transporters, and signal transduction elements at specific plasma membrane domains in different cell types, including neurons,[6] muscle,[7] and the visual system.[8] PDZ proteins play especially important roles in epithelial transport processes.

CLASSES OF PDZ DOMAINS

PDZ domains have been traditionally divided into three different classes, categorized by the nature of their ligands.[1] The different ligand classes are distinguished by differences in the binding residues found at the extreme COOH of target proteins (Figure 14.1). Type I domains recognize the sequence, X-S/T-X-Φ* (where X = any amino acid; Φ = hydrophobic amino acid; * = COOH terminus). Type II domains bind to ligands with the sequence X-Φ-X-Φ*. Type III domains interact with X-D/E-X-Φ* sequences.[9,10] Binding specificity within each domain class can be conferred by the variant (X) residues, as well as residues outside the canonical binding motif, especially at the -3 and -4 positions (where 0 position is the C-terminal residue). Moreover, a few PDZ domains do not fall into any of these specific classes.[5]

Based on large-scale proteomic analysis of PDZ-ligand interactions, it has been suggested the traditional three-class definition be extended to include 16 distinct binding classes.[11] Such a classification has been proposed to predict specific interaction partners of known PDZ domains with greater fidelity than the traditional scheme.

STRUCTURAL BASIS FOR PDZ INTERACTION

In recent years, the structures of over 20 different PDZ domains have been solved at atomic resolution. Like many protein—protein recognition modules, PDZ domains are small globular structures. Comprised of six β-strands (βA-βF) and two alpha helices (αA and

Seldin and Giebisch's The Kidney, Fifth Edition.
DOI: http://dx.doi.org/10.1016/B978-0-12-381462-3.00014-8

(a)

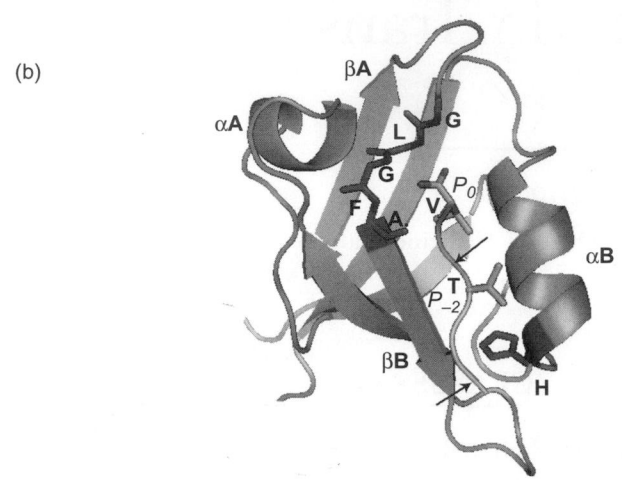

	$(X - P_{-2} - X - P_0)$
Type I	$X - S/T - X - \Phi - COOH$
Type II	$X - \Phi - X - \Phi - COOH$
Type III	$X - D/E - X - \Phi - COOH$

(b)

FIGURE 14.1 PDZ-binding classes and structures. (a) PDZ-binding motifs of the three different PDZ ligand classes are shown (X: any amino acid; Φ: hydrophobic amino acid). Residues in PDZ ligands are conventionally numbered from the final amino acid at the extreme COOH terminus, the so-called P0 position. (b) Structure of a type I PDZ domain with its ligand (third PDZ domain of PSD-95 is shown (PDB,1BFE) Doyle). The conserved GLGF motif in βA-βB linker provides a cradle of main chain amides for interaction with the terminal carboxylate group of the P0 residue. A hydrophobic pocket accommodates the hydrophobic P0 side chain. The first residue of the αB helix, a conserved histidine, forms hydrogen bonds with the P-2 threonine residue in the target protein.

αB), PDZ domains fold into a six stranded beta sandwich[12,13] (Figure 14.1). The peptide ligand inserts into a binding cleft, created by the βB strand and the αB helix, effectively forming an additional antiparallel beta strand. An extensive network of hydrogen bonds and hydrophobic interactions stabilizes binding of the peptide. For instance, the conserved glycine-leucine-glycine-phenylalanine-alanine (GLGF) motif contained within a βA-βB linker provides a cradle of main chain amides, and confers recognition of the terminal carboxylate group of the peptide.[13] A hydrophobic pocket accommodates the hydrophobic COOH-terminal residue, thereby accounting for preferential interaction with proteins ending with a hydrophobic residue (the so-called P0 position).

Binding specificity among the different binding classes is determined partly by an interaction between the P-2 residue of the target protein and the first residue of the PDZ domain αB-helix.[13] In Class I PDZ domains, a conserved histidine residue forms hydrogen bonds with the invariant P-2 serine or threonine residue in the target protein. In class II PDZ domains, this position of the PDZ domain and the P-2 residue of the target protein are usually occupied by a hydrophobic amino acid.[14]

Binding specificity within each domain class is also observed. At least three factors account for this. First, unique residues within or adjacent to the peptide-binding groove in the PDZ domain can interact with the target at sites other than the P-2 and P0 residues.[13,15–17] For example, the side chain of the P-1 target protein residue usually points away from the invariant interaction surface but, in some cases, it can bond with residues that are distinct to a particular PDZ domain.[15,17] Likewise, the P-3 side chain can make contact with unique residues in the interaction groove. Sites proximal to the archetypal, four amino acid-binding motif can also interact with regions outside the canonical-binding site, and thereby also contribute to binding specificity and affinity.[17,18] Second, because interacting residues in PDZ domains can undergo large ligand-dependent conformational changes,[19,20] variations in binding pocket flexibility may contribute to binding specificity. Such a mechanism has been proposed to explain the different binding specificity of the two highly homologous PDZ domains in NHERF1.[21] Finally, genome-wide analysis of PDZ domain binding suggests that PDZ domain selectivity is also achieved by the cellular and subcellular context of the interaction, and this may actually play a more important role than inherent binding specificity.[22]

REGULATION OF PDZ BINDING

PDZ interactions can be dynamically regulated to control the composition and stoichiometry of different multimeric complexes. Phosphorylation of the binding target is the most common mechanism. This is explained by the fact the P-2 serine or threonine in canonical type I PDZ targets can be a substrate for phosphorylation. In these cases, phosphorylation of the residue creates an energetically unfavorable PDZ ligand. For example, phosphorylation of the COOH-terminal site in the Kir 2.3 channel by Protein Kinase A inhibits its interaction with the synaptic PDZ protein, PSD-95,[23] to regulate the channel.[24] Likewise, phosphorylation of the P-2 serine in the $\beta 2$ adrenergic receptor uncouples the receptor from the NHERF1 PDZ protein, and disrupts receptor recycling in the post-endocytic pathway.[25]

Phosphorylation of sites within PDZ proteins is emerging as an additional mechanism for modulating PDZ binding. Evidence for this was first provided by observations that the interaction of a PDZ protein, NHERF1 (see below), with CFTR is negatively regulated by phosphorylation of a residue in the second PDZ domain.[26] Phosphorylation of sites in or near the first PDZ domain of NHERF1 also disrupt interaction with the Na-phosphate co-transporter, Npt2a.[27−29] Phosphorylation of sites that are involved in PDZ−PDZ protein oligomerization has also been observed.[30] This is believed to modulate the extent to which some PDZ proteins can form higher order scaffolding complexes.[31,32]

Finally, switching interactions with different PDZ proteins can differently regulate the activity and localization of target proteins. This occurs when the target has the capacity to bind to several PDZ proteins that have different properties. For example, TIP-1, a protein that consists of a single PDZ domain and lacks other protein−protein interaction modules, binds to certain target proteins to antagonize the scaffolding functions of canonical PDZ proteins.[33]

POLARIZED EXPRESSION OF PDZ PROTEINS IN EPITHELIAL CELLS

A number of PDZ proteins are preferentially expressed at polarized membrane domains or within critical sorting compartments (Figure 14.2), where they perform retention/sorting operations and organize local signaling complexes at polarized locales.[34] Examples of PDZ proteins that predominately reside at the basolateral membrane of certain intestinal and renal epithelia include syntrophin[35] (see "Dystrophin-Associated Protein Complex," below), Lin-7[36,37] (see "Lin-7/CASK/SAP97," below), the ErbB interacting protein, ERBIN,[38] and certain members of the membrane associated guanylate kinase family of PDZ proteins, such as CASK,[39] PSD-93,[40] and SAP97 (aka Discs large homolog 1[41]). Other PDZ proteins, including the sodium hydrogen exchange regulator factors (see "NHERF," below), Shank2E,[42] and PSD-95,[40] are chiefly expressed on or near the apical membrane. Some PDZ proteins, such as

zonula occludens, PALS1 (Stardust), and PATJ (Disc lost),[43] play important roles in the generation and maintenance of the tight junction.[44] Still others, like CAL, which is primarily located in the Golgi[45] or SNX27,[46] and syntenin,[47,48] which are found in endosomes, reside in biosynthetic or endocytotic sorting compartments.

A PDZ-binding motif can serve as a polarized sorting[49] or retention signal.[50] One of the first examples evolved from studies with the GABA transporters or GATs[51]; deletion of the PDZ-binding motif from the apical isoform GAT-3 caused the transporter to localize randomly to both apical and basolateral membranes.[52] Basolateral membrane expression of several membrane proteins has also been found to require a PDZ-binding motif. For instance ERBB receptors, which play crucial roles in morphogenesis and oncogenesis, interact with a basolateral PDZ protein, called ERBIN, and require a PDZ-binding motif for basolateral membrane expression.[38] ERBIN is targeted to the basolateral membrane by its leucine-rich repeat domain.[53] Efficient basolateral membrane expression of a number of transporters that interact with the basolateral PDZ protein Lin-7 also require an intact PDZ-binding site (see below).

MAGUKS, THE ARCHETYPAL PDZ SCAFFOLDS

Members of the MAGUK (membrane associated guanylate kinase) family of PDZ proteins are the archetypal PDZ scaffolds. MAGUK proteins are equipped to assemble large molecular complexes, having one to three PDZ domains, a SRC homology 3 domain (SH3), and a catalytically inactive guanylate kinase-like (GK) domain. In addition to the PDZ domains, the GK and the SH3 domains function as independent protein−protein interaction modules; GK domains recruit scaffold adaptor molecules called guanylate kinase-associated proteins or GKAPs,[54] while SH3 domains have been shown to coordinate interaction with at least one non-

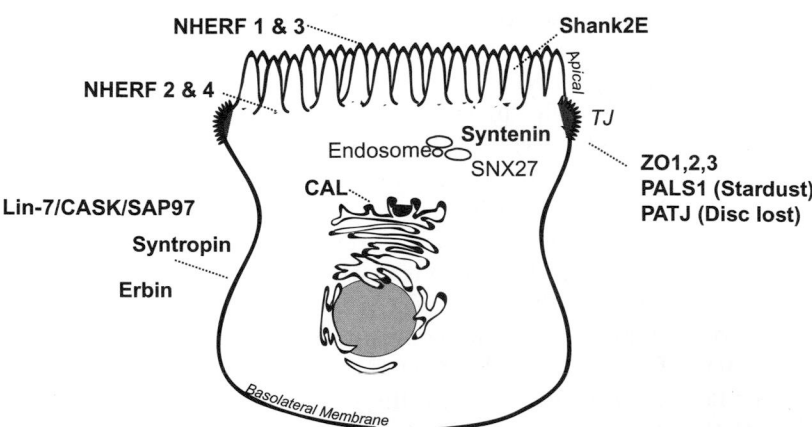

FIGURE 14.2 Major PDZ proteins in epithelial cells. PDZ domain containing proteins differentially localize to epithelial cell brush borders, subapical domains, endosomes, tight junctions, and basolateral membranes.

receptor tyrosine kinase.[55] The SH3 and GK domains can also interact with one another, forming a composite SH3–GK structure[56,57] that acts as an additional inter-molecular protein–protein interaction domain with a binding specificity that is distinct from either SH3 or GK domains.[58]

The PSD-95 family, encoded by four genes (PSD-95/SAP90, PSD-93/Chapsyn-110, SAP102, and SAP97), exemplifies MAGUK proteins. Two of these, PSD-93[40] and SAP97 (see below), are expressed in renal epithelial cells. However, the best characterized member, PSD-95, is largely expressed in excitable tissues, and plays central roles in maintaining and modulating the strength and structure of glutamatergic synapses.[59] Generally, its properties and functions are likely to be applicable to the other MAGUKs, including those expressed in the kidney.

Like many scaffolds, PSD-95 not only contains multiple protein–protein interaction modules, it also assembles into multimers, creating an extended platform for efficient scaffolding.[60,61] These qualities, combined with palmitoylation-dependent membrane tethering and synaptic localization signals,[62] make PSD-95 ideally designed to cluster ion channels, receptors, trafficking proteins, and signal transduction machinery at the post-synaptic membrane. In doing so, PSD-95 influences trafficking, endocytosis, and activities of target proteins at the synapse.[59] Organizing local signaling complexes is one of the most important clustering functions of PSD-95. For example, the PDZ domains in PSD-95 independently interact with the calcium/calmodulin-activated nitric oxide synthase, nNOS, and NMDA (N-methyl-D-aspartate) receptors to form a ternary complex.[63,64] The organization is thought to be important for regulated synthesis of nitric oxide. Because NMDA receptors are permeable to calcium, the physical linkage of nNOS with the excitatory receptors is believed to allow nitric oxide production to be efficiently coupled to receptor activation, calcium influx, and local changes in intracellular calcium.[65] Significantly, disruption of NMDAR interaction with PSD-95 dissociates the receptors from downstream neurotoxic signaling, without blocking synaptic activity or calcium influx.[66]

Local signaling complexes that control the production of NOS in the kidney have been proposed.[67] One may involve PSD-93, the predominate MAGUK in renal epithelial cells.[40] Similar to PSD-95, PSD-93 associates with the plasmalemma via palmitoylation-dependent tethering signals,[68] where it recruits and clusters various target proteins, including nNOS.[69] In the kidney, PSD-93 is largely expressed along the basolateral membrane of the thick ascending limb, macula densa cells and the distal nephron.[40] In the macula densa, PSD-93 colocalizes with the pool of nNOS that is associated with intracellular vesicles and the basolateral membrane.[40] It remains to be tested if PSD-93 interaction with nNOS in the macula densa coordinates regulated NO production in the manner that is observed with PSD-95 at the excitatory synapse.

FORM AND FUNCTION OF PDZ PROTEIN FAMILIES IN THE KIDNEY

Apical Membrane PDZ Protein Complexes

NHERF

The Na/H exchange regulator factor PDZ proteins, NHERF, are highly expressed in the kidney and small intestine where they act as molecular scaffolds, associating with a number of transporters, channels, signaling proteins, transcription factors, and receptors to regulate apical membrane transport processes.[70,71] There is a family of four related NHERF proteins encoded by separate genes[72,73] (Figure 14.3). Originally known by many names, a unifying nomenclature has been proposed,[72,73] designating the genes as NHERF-1[74,75] (also known as Ezrin Binding Protein-50, EBP-50[76]); NHERF-2 (also known as NHE-3 kinase A (E3KARP)[77]; tyrosine kinase activator-1 (TKA) and sex-determining region of the Y chromosome (SRY-1)-interacting protein[78]; NHERF-3 (also called PDZK1,[79] Cap70,[80] DiPHOR or NaPi-Cap1[81]); and NHERF-4 (also called IKEPP,[82] DIPHOR-2, and NaPi-Cap 2[81]). Each member of the NHERF family of proteins is believed to play important roles in the regulation of transport processes within the proximal tubule, as well as other sites along the nephron, acting by three different but not mutually exclusive mechanisms. Present evidence indicates that the NHERFs function to: (1) organize local signaling complexes; (2) control apical membrane trafficking; and (3) couple apical membrane transport proteins with other PDZ-binding targets. In this way, NHERFs modulate transporter activity and/or apical abundance of transporters, channels, and receptors. Importantly, each NHERF isoform appears to have unique regulatory properties that are manifested in cell-specific manners.[83] Studies in NHERF isoform knockout-mice have begun to clarify their different physiologic roles in the renal proximal tubule, small intestine, and other epithelia.

Like other scaffolding proteins, the functions of the NHERFs are made possible by the presence of their multiple protein–protein interaction domains. NHERF-1 and NHERF-2 contain two PDZ domains and a COOH-terminal Ezrin/Radixin/Mosein/Merlin (ERM)-binding domain. The latter coordinates interaction with the ERM family of actin binding and A-kinase anchoring proteins to direct linkage with the actin cytoskeleton[84] and signal transduction machinery.[85] By contrast, NHERF-3 and

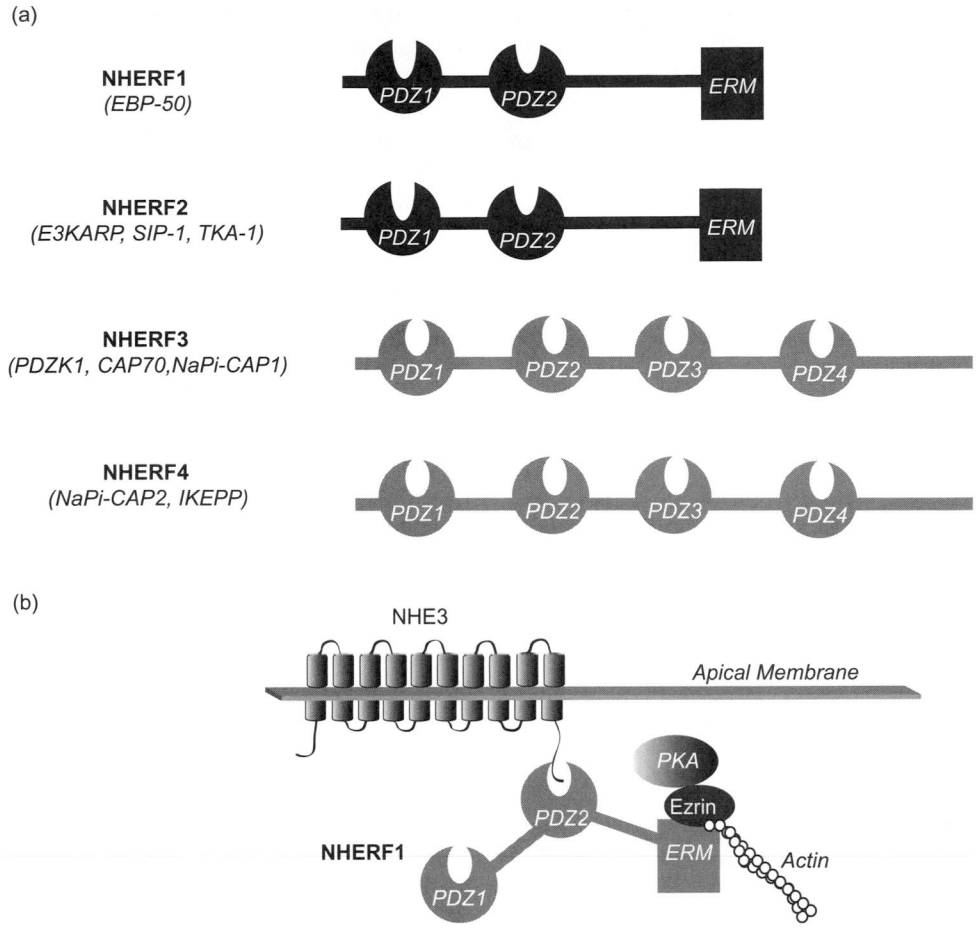

FIGURE 14.3   NHERF. (a) Domain architecture of NHERF family members. NHERF 1 and NHERF 2 contain two PDZ domains and an ERM-binding domain. NHERF 3 and NHERF 4 contain four PDZ domains, but no ERM-binding domain. (b) The protein–protein interaction modules in NHERF1 allow it to assemble multi-protein complexes, consisting of PDZ-binding targets (such as NHE3, shown), ezrin, and PKA.

NHERF-4 contain four PDZ domains, but no ERM domain (Figure 14.3).

NHERF proteins can also interact with one another, forming higher order protein networks. Indeed, NHERF1 and NHERF2 associate as homodimers and heterodimers.[30,86–88] Interestingly, oligomerization of NHERF-1, but not NHERF-2, is highly regulated by association with other proteins and by phosphorylation.[30] NHERF3 has been reported to interact with NHERF1 and NHERF2 to form an extensive heteromeric complex.[87] Interaction between NHERF1 and NHERF3 and ezrin is corroborative, providing a mechanism to regulate formation of a ternary scaffolding complex that contributes to the organization microvilli.[31,89,90]

NHERF in Epithelial Transport

A growing body of evidence indicates each NHERF isoform has individual and specialized activities in the kidney. It some cases, specific roles of several NHERF proteins may converge and act cooperatively to regulate target proteins. Here we review the state of knowledge about each NHERF isoform.

NHERF1 was originally discovered as a co-factor necessary for cAMP-kinase dependent phosphorylation and inhibition of NHE3, a brush border Na^+/H^+ exchanger.[74,75] Biochemical studies and work in heterologous expression systems established a likely mechanism whereby NHERF1 organizes a local PKA signaling complex, using its PDZ domains and the ERM-binding domain (Figure 14.3b). The second PDZ domain of NHERF1 directly interacts with NHE3,[91] while the ERM-binding domain simultaneously engages ezrin.[92] By acting as an A-kinase anchor protein (AKAP, see below),[85] ezrin recruits the regulatory subunit of PKA II[92] to the NHERF1 complex. Consequently, NHERF1 juxtaposes PKA with NHE3 for efficient phosphorylation of the transporter and inhibition of Na^+/H^+ exchange. Consistent with the model, removal of the ERM-binding domain in NHERF1 disrupts formation of NHERF1−ezrin signal complex and attenuates the inhibitory effect of cAMP on NHE3 activity.[93] EPAC (the exchange protein directly activated by cAMP) also participates in the NHERF1-dependent inhibitory response in the proximal tubule, but it is not presently understood how NHERF couples EPAC to NHE3.[94]

Direct evidence that the NHERF1 signal complex is required for phospho-regulation of NHE3 has been provided by studies in NHERF1 gene knockout mice.[95] In this model, activation of PKA fails to phosphorylate and inhibit NHE3 activity in the proximal tubule.[96] The response appears to be specific to NHERF1 removal, in that other proximal tubule NHERF isoforms are not affected by NHERF1 gene ablation. Moreover, the inhibitory effect of PKA can be completely restored in NHERF1-null proximal tubule cells upon adenoviral-mediated delivery of wild-type NHERF1.[97]

The PKA coupling function of NHERF1 is believed to be widespread, with a body of work indicating that the NHERF1 can act as a nexus of signaling complex assembly for efficient phosphorylation and regulation of a variety of transporters, channels, and receptors (reviewed in [98]). For example, NHERF1 (as well as NHERF2[99]) binds to CFTR[100,101] through a PDZ interaction to potentiate PKA phosphorylation-dependent CFTR Cl(−) currents[102] in an ezrin-AKAP dependent manner.

Simultaneous PDZ-dependent recruitment of G-protein coupled receptors by NHERF proteins can further focus local signaling around NHE3 and other transport proteins.[71] For instance, studies in heterologous systems reveal that NHERF binds to the β2-adrenergic receptor (BAR2) by means of a PDZ domain-mediated interaction to recruit NHE3 and the receptor into a local signaling complex for efficient receptor-mediated regulation of sodium−hydrogen exchange. Removal of the PDZ interaction motif in the BAR2 disrupts receptor interaction with NHERF1, and markedly reduces β2-adenergic receptor-mediated regulation of NHE3 without altering activation of adenylyl cyclase.[103] Likewise, NHERF1 facilitates the assembly of a complex containing the β2-adenergic receptor, ezrin, PKA, and CFTR at the apical membrane of epithelial cells for compartmentalized and specific signaling of the channel.[104] Other examples have recently been extensively reviewed.[71]

The tandem PDZ domains in NHERF1 also provide a structural framework to link PDZ-binding transport proteins with PDZ-binding signal transduction machinery. Indeed, several different kinases,[105,106] phospholipase C isoforms,[107] and the receptor for activated C kinase, RACK,[108] have been identified as NHERF1 PDZ-binding targets. Characterization of consensus binding sequences of isolated NHERF-1 PDZ domains by phage-display, affinity selection techniques revealed that the two PDZ domains have different ligand-binding specificities, with distinct preferences for residues at the 0, −1 and −3 positions of type I PDZ ligands.[101] Thus, NHERF1 has a biochemical capacity to tether different PDZ-binding targets together. In addition, because NHERF1 interacts with itself and links with the actin cytoskeleton, formation of an extended network of NHERF1 molecules may join different PDZ-interacting proteins to the same locale. Such a mechanism has been proposed to explain NHERF1-dependent coupling of phospholipase C with the TRP4 channel.[107]

In some cases, the PDZ domains in NHERF1 can support simultaneous interaction of two identical proteins. The best-characterized example is CFTR, which interacts with both PDZ domains in NHERF1, albeit with different binding affinities.[109] In this case, NHERF1 has been reported to induce a high open probability conformation of CFTR by cross-linking the C-terminal tails of a CFTR dimer. Because CFTR binds to the two PDZ domains with different kinetics and affinities, channel gating is profoundly sensitive to alterations in NHERF1 abundance. Moreover, the composition and stoichiometry of NHERF-CFTR interactions can be dynamically regulated. Phosphorylation of NHERF1 has been found to specifically disrupt CFTR interaction with the second PDZ domain, uncoupling the tethered C-terminal tails and inducing a low open-probability conformation.[26] A similar PDZ-dependent cross-linking mechanism has been described with NHERF3.[80]

NHERF1-Dependent Apical Membrane Trafficking

In addition to co-localizing key components of signal transduction pathways, NHERF1 can also regulate cell surface expression and localization of some of its binding targets. It appears to function by controlling trafficking operations in the post-endocytic recycling pathway,[25,110] as well as by anchoring target proteins on the plasma membrane,[100,111] likely by interactions with the cytoskeleton.

Regulation of the Na-dependent phosphate transporter, Npt2a, in the proximal tubule provides a salient example. It is well-known that factors which regulate proximal tubule Pi reabsorption and Pi homeostasis do so by altering the density of Npt2a at the apical membrane. NHERF1 plays an important role in this process. Indeed, NHERF1 gene ablation causes diminished expression of Npt2a at the apical membrane and renal phosphate-wasting.[95] In the NHERF1 knockout model, the Npt2a transporter is misrouted into a subapical, intracellular compartment,[95,112] indicative of a trafficking defect.

Studies in model systems have begun to cast light on the underlying mechanism. Npt2a binds to the first PDZ domain of NHERF1 via a type 1 interaction, requiring the last three amino acids of the co-transporter.[81] These residues are also necessary for efficient apical expression of Npt2a,[111,113,114] suggesting that apical targeting and/or anchoring is specified by direct NHERF1 interaction. Apical localization of the co-transporter can be blocked by ectopic expression of truncated NHERF1 proteins, which contain the first PDZ domain and are able to interact with the transporter, but lack the ERM-binding domain. Thus, it is likely that NHERF1 coordinates localization of the co-transporter by tethering Npt2a with the actin cytoskeleton through the ERM-binding domain.[111]

Exciting recent studies reveal that PTH induced internalization and lysosomal degradation of Npt2a in the proximal tubule are coincident with phosphorylation of NHERF1, and disruption of Npt2a/NHERF1 interaction.[115] These observations strongly suggest that Npt2a—NHERF1 interactions are physiologically regulated to control Npt2a apical surface density for maintenance of calcium and phosphate metabolism. Recent live-cell imaging studies indicate NHERF1 regulates apical expression of Npt2a by a brush border retention mechanism.[116,117] A similar process controls the localization of the PTH receptor.[118] In other proteins, such as CFTR[110] and certain G-protein coupled receptors,[25,119] NHERF1 maintains surface expression by driving recycling to the cell surface after internalization.

Although NHERF1 effectively anchors NHE3 and Npt2a within the microvilli by directly interacting with the transporters and engaging the underlying microvillar cytoskeleton, the transporters have different fates in the renal proximal tubule when they disassociate from NHERF1. In NHERF1 knockout mice, localization of NHE3 is maintained within the microvilli, but Npt2a is targeted to the lysosome. By contrast, when interaction with NHERF1 become severed by physiological signaling processes (e.g., PTH-dependent), a myosin VI driven translocation process moves NHE3 and Npt2a out of the microvilli.[120–123] Because NHE3 selectively assimilates with lipid rafts, the translocated NHE3 molecules are effectively excluded from clathrin-coated pits and consequently are retained at the base of the microvilli.[121] By contrast, Npt2a transporters do not partition into rafts, and are free to be internalized once its ties with the microvillar anchor are broken.

Direct phosphorylation of NHERF1 is emerging as an important mechanism for negatively regulating PDZ-dependent binding interactions in the proximal tubule. Two residues, threonine 95 and serine 77, within the first PDZ domain are phosphorylated in response to PTH and dopamine treatment in the renal proximal tubule. This decreases the binding affinity for the Npt2a transporter, and likely contributes to the hormonal suppression of renal phosphate transport.[27–29] Additional phosphorylation-dependent mechanisms have been reported to control binding at the second PDZ domain in ways that are important for regulating microvilli assembly.[31]

NHERF2

NHERF2 appears to have different functions than NHERF1 in the kidney,[72,124] even though the two PDZ proteins share a common domain structure and NHERF2 is equally effective as NHERF1 in mediating cAMP inhibition of NHE3 in heterologous systems.[77] Unlike NHERF1, which is exclusively expressed in the human, rat, and mouse proximal tubule, expression of NHERF2 in the proximal tubule is species-specific. Found only in the mouse proximal tubule, NHERF2 predominantly localizes to a subapical, intermicrovillar compartment that is distinct from NHERF1 in the brush border.[125] Importantly, NHERF2 does not support phosphorylation-dependent inhibition of NHE3 or apical localization of Npt2a in the NHERF1 knockout model, indicating that NHERF2 does not share physiologically redundant functions with NHERF1 in the proximal tubule.[124]

The functions of NHERF2 are, in fact, better understood at sites outside the proximal tubule. In the kidney, NHERF2 is predominately expressed in the glomerulus, vas recta, and the collecting duct.[126] Physiologically important PDZ-binding partners have been identified in each of these locales. In the glomerulus, NHERF2 interacts with podocalyxin, possibly functioning to retain podocalyxin at the apical surface of the podocyte and provide a mechanism for linking this important surface sialomucin to the actin cytoskeleton.[127] NHERF2 associates with the TRPC4 channel in the descending vasa recta, where it has been suggested to control Ca^{2+} signaling[128] in a similar way that the INAD PDZ protein controls TRP in the *Drosophila* eye.[129] In the collecting duct, NHERF2 co-localizes and interacts with the ROMK channel. Studies in heterologous expression systems indicate that NHERF2 couples accessory proteins and signal transduction machinery to ROMK for efficient channel regulation and trafficking.[130]

The PDZ-binding specificity of NHERF2 also undoubtedly contributes to its unique functions as compared to NHERF1. While NHERF2 shares many of the same PDZ-binding partners as NHERF1, with nearly 60 having been identified,[70] it also interacts with several proteins that NHERF1 does not react with. These include alpha-actinin-4[131]; cGMP kinase I and II[132]; a putative Cl/HCO_3 exchanger downregulated in adenoma[133]; podocalyxin[127]; human Y-linked testis determining gene-binding factor[78]; serum gluco-corticoid stimulated kinase, SGK-1[134]; and transcriptional co-activation with PDZ-binding motif, TAZ.[135]

By organizing these unique partners into protein complexes, NHERF2 can affect functions that are distinct from NHERF1. NHERF isoform-specific regulation of NHE3 in heterologous systems provides an excellent illustration. NHERF2 uniquely confers Ca^{2+}-dependent inhibition on NHE3[136] by scaffolding the exchanger to PKCα and alpha-actinin-4.[72] NHERF1 does not support this activity, presumably because it is not capable of interacting with alpha-actinin-4. Likewise, by acting as a unique protein kinase G-anchoring protein, NHERF2 specifically confers cGMP inhibition on NHE3.[83,132] Finally, activation of NHE3 by dexamethasone requires NHERF2 rather than NHERF1.[134] In this case, the first PDZ domain of NHERF2 uniquely recruits the serum- and glucocorticoid-induced protein kinase, SGK1, into a complex with NHE3 to phosphorylate and enhance exchanger activity. Such a mechanism has been suggested to offer an explanation for glucocorticoid stimulation of sodium absorption in ileum, proximal colon, and renal proximal tubule.[134]

NHERF2-dependent scaffolding of SGK1 may also play an important role in the collecting duct for the regulation of the potassium secretory channel, ROMK.[137,138] It has been reported that NHERF2 can synergize with SGK1 to augment cell surface expression of ROMK in oocyte expression experiments.[138] Biochemical studies indicate that NHERF2 has the capacity to recruit ROMK and SGK-1 into a ternary complex by preferentially binding to the channel with the first PDZ domain,[130] while simultaneously recruiting the kinase by preferred interaction with the second PDZ domain.[134] Formation of such a complex would allow efficient phosphorylation of a residue that is required for delivery of the channel to the cell surface. Indeed, SGK1 directly phosphorylates serine 44[137] in ROMK1, creating a forward trafficking signal[139] that overrides an endoplasmic reticulum localization signal.[140,139] Together the observations suggest a potential molecular mechanism for the regulation of ROMK density by dietary potassium, whereby the NHERF2 scaffold juxtaposes the SGK-1 with ROMK for efficient phosphorylation-dependent trafficking to the apical membrane.

NHERF3

NHERF3 was first discovered as PDZK1, a PDZ domain-containing protein that is upregulated in carcinomas, and abundantly expressed in the proximal tubule brush border.[79,87,141] Significantly, the four PDZ domains of NHERF3 support interaction with many proximal tubule apical membrane transporter proteins, including Npt2a, the solute carrier SLC17A1 (NaPi-I),

NHE3, the organic cation transporter (OCTN1), chloride-formate exchanger (CFEX), and the urate-anion exchanger (URAT1),[87] as well as a protein kinase A anchoring protein, D-AKAP2.[142] Based on these observations and findings that NHERF1 can interact with NHERF3, it has been suggested that NHERF3 and NHERF1 may form an extended scaffolding network in brush borders of proximal tubular cells for the regulation of transport.

Although the NHERF3-NHERF1 scaffolding network concept is an attractive hypothesis, it should be pointed out that targeted disruption of the NHERF3 gene by homologous recombination does not[143] cause global alterations in the expression or localization of most of its interacting transport proteins in the proximal tubule.[144,145] Instead, the major effects of NHERF3 gene disruption presently appear to be very specific, confined only to two interacting proteins. A selective reduction in the abundance and functional activity of the chloride-formate exchanger, CFEX, at the proximal tubule brush border is observed in NHERF3-null animals.[145] Physiologic stimulation of the NaPi-IIc isoform by dietary phosphate restriction is also impaired in NHERF3-null animals. A minor role of NHERF3 in Npt2a regulation can be provoked by physiological perturbations; while NHERF3 null animals on a normal or low phosphate diet do not exhibit alterations in Npt2a abundance or function, high dietary phosphate unmasks a modest attenuation of Npt2a levels at the proximal tubule brush border.[146] Differences in affinities of the NaPi-II isoforms for NHERF1(Npt2a) and NHERF3 (Npt2c) have been proposed to account for this behavior.[147]

NHERF4

This member of the NHERF family was originally identified in independent screens for PDZ-binding partners of the Npt2a transporter[81] and the receptor guanylyl cyclase.[82] First dubbed as NaPi Cap-2 or IKEPP (Intestinal and Kidney-Enriched PDZ Protein), it was subsequently reclassified as NHERF4 based on sequence homology modeling.[73] In the proximal tubule where it is abundantly expressed, NHERF4 localizes to a subapical region, like NHERF2, that is distinct from the brush border and NHERF1.[81] Little is known about the function of NHERF4 except that it inhibits heat stable toxin induced cGMP synthesis,[82] by a mechanism suggested to involve PDZ-dependent recruitment of inhibitory factors.[73] Roles in regulating the TRPV5 and TRPV6 calcium channels have also been described.[203] Based on its structural similarities with other NHERF forms and the site of expression in the kidney,[73] it seems likely that NHERF4 also modulates apical membrane transport and cell signaling in the proximal tubule.

Shank (SH3 Domain and Ankyrin Repeating Proteins, A.K.A Proline-Rich Synapse-Associated Protein-1/Cortactin-Binding Protein 1 (ProSAP1/CortBP1))

In addition to the established role as master scaffolds at the postsynaptic density,[148] members of the Shank (SH3 domain and ankyrin repeating proteins) family of proteins play roles as apical membrane-associated scaffolds in epithelial cells. The three known Shank genes (Shank1, Shank2, and Shank3) are expressed in a tissue-specific manner. Shank 1 is almost exclusively expressed in the brain, products of the Shank2 gene are found in brain, kidney, and liver, whereas Shank 3 is most abundantly expressed in the heart.[149] The prototypical Shank, Shank1, is a relatively large protein ($>$ 200 KDa) containing multiple ankyrin repeats,[150] a SH3 domain, a PDZ domain, and a long proline repeat domain. A self-oligomerization domain, called a sterile alpha motif (SAM), assembles the scaffolds into head-to-tail helical sheets, forming an extensive Shank network for protein complex assembly.[151] In neurons, Shank forms a polymeric structure with another protein, Homer, to serve as a platform for assembling postsynaptic density proteins.[152] Multiple splice variants of each gene have been identified that contain different combinations of protein—protein interaction domains (Figure 14.4). For example, Shank2E, a form that is predominantly expressed in epithelial cells,[42] contains ankyrin repeats whereas the Shank2 splice form found in the brain does not.

Extensive studies in the brain provide models for Shank function in epithelial cells. It is well-established that Shank family members localize to the postsynaptic density of excitatory synapses, where they act as master scaffolds along with Homer and PSD-95.[148] Here, the Shanks physically couple the two major receptor complexes, N-methyl-d-aspartate receptors (NMDAR) and metabotropic glutamate receptors (mGluR), and recruit associated signaling proteins. They do so by concurrently engaging two different adaptors through distinct protein—protein interaction domains. The Shank PDZ domain associates with the GUK-associated protein, GKAP which, in turn, interacts with the PSD-95 complex, containing NMDA receptors.[148] At the same time, the proline rich domain of Shank interacts with another adaptor protein, Homer, to link with metabotropic glutamate receptors. Proline rich domains often serve as binding sites for SH3 (SrC homology), WW (conserved two-tryptophan domain), and EVH1 domains (enabled/vasodilator-stimulated phosphoprotein homology 1).[153] A single EVH1 domain in Homer directly interacts with a PPXXF motif in the Shank proline-rich domain, as well as with similar proline motifs in group 1 mGluR and other proteins, such as the IP3 receptor.[154] Because Homer proteins self-associate in a head-to-tail fashion, two EVH1 domains per dimer are available to bridge Shank with group 1 mGluRs. Consequently, Shank cross-links Homer and PSD-95 complexes in the PSD, presumably to couple signaling transduction pathways emanating from NMDAR and mGluR. Disruption in this synaptic scaffolding mechanism may be responsible for human disease, as mutations in SPAK2 have been associated with autism and mental retardation.[155]

More recently, Shank2 forms have been implicated in the modulation of apical membrane transport

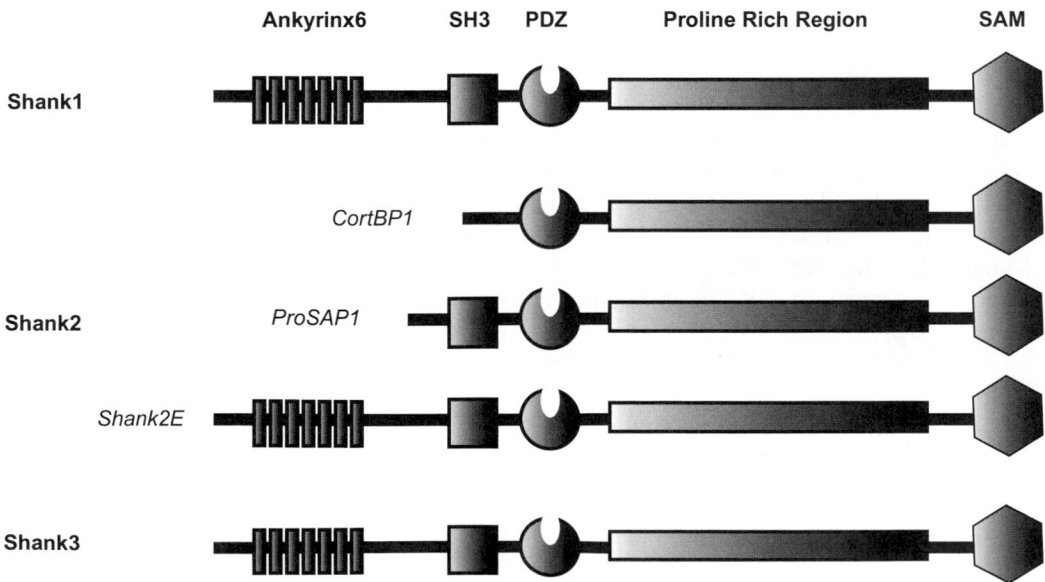

FIGURE 14.4   Shank family members. Domain architectures of Shank1, 2, 3, and Shank2 splice variants are shown. The major epithelial form, Shank2E, contains six ankyrin repeats, a SH3 domain, a PDZ domain, a proline rich domain, and a self-oligomerization region called a SAM domain.

processes. In the kidney, Shank2E is concentrated at the apical membrane of proximal tubule cells were it interacts with NHE3 and Npt2a, similar to NHERF1. Present evidence indicates that Shank2 and NHERF may control the activity of these transport proteins in divergent manners. Studies with NHE3 in heterologous expression systems, for example, revealed that Shank2 positively regulates NHE3 membrane expression and blunts the cAMP-dependent inhibition of NHE3, in part by antagonizing the action of NHERF1. Likewise, in pancreatic duct cells, Shank2E associates with CFTR at the apical membrane and inhibits Cl channel activity,[156] contrasting the positive effects of NHERF1 and NHERF2 on CFTR (see above). Shank2 also positively regulates NHE3 by recruiting BetaPix, a guanine nucleotide exchange factor for the Rho-GTPase.[157] Because retention and targeting of NHE3 in the apical microvilli depends on the sustained activity of Rho-GTPases,[158] the interaction between NHE3 and the Shank2-BetaPix complex may allow NHE3 trafficking to be linked to the maintenance of the microvilliar actin cytoskeleton.

Shank2E appears to regulate Npt2a in a different manner than NHERF1. In the proximal tubule, increased extracellular Pi triggers internalization and degradation of Shank2E and Npt2a in parallel, but has no effect on NHERF1 localization or abundance.[159] Combined with observations that regulated endocytosis of Npt2a is associated with disruption of Npt2a/NHERF1 interaction at the brush border,[115] one might speculate that internalization of Npt2a involves a NHERF1-to-Shank2E interaction switch. Importantly, Shank redistributes with Npt2a during regulated endocytosis,[160] and interacts with dynamin II, a GTPase that is critical for endocytic vesicle formation, via proline-rich domain interaction.[161] Thus, Shank2E is especially poised to facilitate Npt2a endocytosis and/or lysosomal trafficking, in contrast to the apparent membrane-retention and/or recycling function of NHERF1. The molecular mechanisms underlying the function of Shank2E in the proximal tubule remain to be firmly established, however. It will be interesting to learn if the activities of Shank2E in the kidney depend on scaffold adaptors, such as Homer and GKAP, as has been shown in excitatory synapses.

BASOLATERAL MEMBRANE PDZ PROTEIN COMPLEXES

The Lin-7/CASK/PSD-97 System

Lin-7 and CASK (Lin-2) are components of an evolutionarily conserved basolateral membrane scaffolding complex, important for polarized targeting and controlling cell surface density of their PDZ-binding partners.

They were discovered along with another PDZ protein, Lin-10 (Lin, from abnormal cell lineage), in a genetic screen for components of the LET-23 receptor tyrosine kinase signaling pathway in *C. Elegans* vulva progenitor cells (VPC).[162] These molecules form a tripartite protein complex in VPC that interacts with a receptor tyrosine kinase, LET-23, to coordinate receptor expression on the basolateral membrane.[162–164] Importantly, null mutations in Lin-7, Lin-2 or Lin-10 cause the Let-23 receptor to become mislocalized to the apical membrane, and consequently disrupt LET-23 signaling and VPC development.

Orthologs of the *C. elegans* PDZ protein complex have been identified in mammalian tissues (Lin-7 = mLin7/Veli/MALS; Lin-2 = CASK; Lin-10 = Mint-1/X11).[37,165–167] In the mammalian kidney, a partially conserved complex, consisting of mLin-7 and CASK but not Lin-10,[19] localizes to the basolateral membrane[36,37] where it coordinates polarized expression of mLin-7-binding partners (Figure 14.5). It has been implicated in basolateral expression of the epithelial GABA transporter, BGT-1,[168] the strong inward-rectifying potassium channels, Kir 2.X,[167,169,170] the EGF-like receptor, ErbB-2/Her2,[171] and the insulin receptor substrate, p53.[172] Present evidence suggests that the mLin-7/CASK complex may offer a general mechanism for polarized expression of basolateral membrane proteins containing Type I PDZ-binding motifs.

Lin-7 acts as the upstream scaffolding molecule. It binds directly to target molecules through a Type I PDZ interaction while simultaneously engaging CASK via another protein—protein interaction module,[37,173] called a L27 domain (from Lin-2, Lin-7).[174] L27 domains, which present a number of related PDZ proteins (see PALS, below), are helical bundle structures[175,176] that mediate heterotypic assembly, important for polymerization of different scaffolds. In fact, basolateral membrane localization of Lin-7 and its PDZ-binding partners is afforded by the L27 domain and CASK interaction.[37,177,178]

CASK associates with the basolateral membrane through a web of interactions to function as the master basolateral membrane attachment factor. As a member of the MAGUK family (see above), CASK contains multiple protein—protein interactions sites, allowing it to simultaneously bind to Lin-7, extracellular matrix receptors, adhesion molecules, the actin cytoskeleton 4.1-binding proteins,[39] and another MAGUK protein, SAP-97.[173] The mLin-7 and SAP-97 L27 domains separately assemble with two L27 domains of CASK, possibly as a dimer of L27 heterodimers,[175,176] to form a mLin-7/SAP97/CASK complex.[170,173] By linking extracellular matrix receptors and the cytoskeleton, the Lin-7/CASK/SAP97 complex has the capacity to act as a stable anchor to retain Lin-7 interacting proteins on the basolateral membrane.

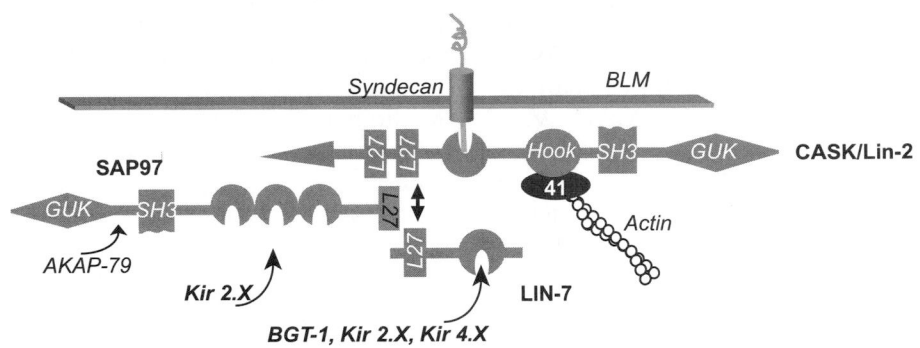

FIGURE 14.5 **Lin-7/CASK/SAP-97 complex at the basolateral membrane (BLM).** Lin-7 recruits PDZ-binding targets, such as the BGT-1 transporter and the inwardly rectifying potassium channels, Kir 2.X and Kir 4.X, to the basolateral membrane by interacting with CASK through a L27 domain interaction. CASK acts as the master anchor; it not only interacts with Lin-7, it also binds to extracellular matrix receptors, such as syndecan, through a type II PDZ interaction, while simultaneously engaging the actin cytoskeleton through a hook domain interaction with 4.1 proteins. CASK also recruits SAP-97 to the basolateral membrane through an L27 interaction. SAP-97 has the capacity to recruit PDZ-binding targets, as well as proteins that interact with the guanylate kinase (GK) and SH3 domains, such as AKAP-79.

The mammalian counterpart of Lin-10 is actually encoded by a family of proteins called the Mints or X11s.[179] Although all three members of the Mint family share C-terminal PDZ and PTB domains, only Mint-1 contains a CASK interaction domain.[165] In neuronal tissues and the heart, which express the complete Lin-7/CASK/Mint-1 complex, Mint-1 has been suggested to provide an additional membrane trafficking function. Mint-1 interacts with microtubule motors, and has been reported to transport N-methyl-D-aspartate (NMDA)-type receptor vesicles along microtubules.[180] In addition, Mint-1 interacts with Munc-18 docking machinery.[165,166,181] Importantly, mammalian epithelial cells do not express Mint-1. In its absence, the Lin-2/CASK system loses the obvious link to microtubule-mediated trafficking and fusion, suggesting that Lin-7/CASK plays a major role in retention rather than directed-delivery in renal epithelia.

Consistent with this notion, present evidence indicates that Lin-7/CASK primarily functions to retain target proteins at the basolateral membrane of mammalian epithelia. For example, Perego et al. found that removing the PDZ ligand in BGT-1 disrupted Lin-7 association in MCDK cells and dramatically increased the internalization of the transporter from the plasmalemma.[168] The retention function of Lin-7 depends on its L27 domain, which directs interaction with a cognate L27 domain in CASK.[170,177] In this way, Lin-7 acts as a PDZ-to-L27 adapter, mediating indirect association of its PDZ-binding target proteins with the larger basolateral membrane scaffold, CASK.

Although Lin-7 primarily operates as a component of a basolateral membrane retention machine in mammalian epithelial cells, it should be pointed out that disruption of Lin-7 interactions can produce a wide range of mis-localization phenotypes, depending on the Lin-7-binding partner and the types of sorting signals

embedded within them. For instance, mutant BGT transporters, lacking their PDZ-binding motif, are predominately localized on the basolateral membrane. In this case, BGT-1 transporters are presumably directed to the basolateral membrane by non-PDZ-dependent sorting signals.[182] On the other hand, mutant Kir2.3 channels, lacking the PDZ-binding motif, are largely directed to an endosomal compartment, rather than the basolateral membrane,[167,177] consistent with strong endosomal targeting signals. An apical-missorting phenotype is produced by removing the PDZ-binding site from a chimeric LET-23/nerve growth factor receptor protein.[183] In this case, Lin-7 interaction may stabilize the receptor on the basolateral membrane or limit post-endocytic trafficking in such a way that it prevents transcytosis to the apical membrane.

At present, it is not known if the Lin-7/CASK/SAP97 scaffold also participates in signal complex localization and organization at the basal membrane in the way that has been described for the NHERF proteins at the apical membrane. SAP97 has been shown to recruit AKAP proteins to related PDZ protein complexes in neurons,[58] and the *Drosophila* CASK ortholog protein, Camguk, functionally modulates Ether-a-go-go potassium channels by a phosphorylation-dependent mechanism.[184] Interestingly, CASK contains an unusual CAM-kinase like domain, which can phosphorylate interacting proteins at the synapse.[185] However, it remains to be established if similar mechanisms are in place at the basolateral membrane of renal epithelial cells, which express the Lin-7/CASK/SAP97 complex.

Lin 7 Isoforms (Veli/MALS) and PALS (Partners of Lin7) in the Kidney

Three different Lin-7 isoforms, encoded by separate genes, have been identified. In mammalian systems, these are often called Veli/MALS 1,2,3 (Vertebrate Lin-7 or Mammalian Lin Seven). Each of the MALS/Veli isoforms are expressed in the kidney, but each are differentially localized along the nephron.[36] MALS/Veli 1 is predominately expressed in the glomerulus, thick ascending limb of Henle's loop (TAL), and the distal convoluted tubule (DCT). MALS/Veli 2 is exclusively expressed in the vasa recta. MALS/Veli 3 is largely located in the proximal tubule, DCT, and collecting duct. The subcellular localization of MALS/Veli proteins can vary, depending on the isoform and the cell type. In contrast to the predominate basolateral location of MALS/Veli 1 in the TAL and DCT and MALS/Veli 3 in the DCT, MALS/Veli 1 is found diffusely throughout the cytosol of intercalated cells. In the collecting duct, MALS/Veli 3 is chiefly located on the basal membrane. Collectively, these results suggest that different MALS/Veli isoforms may carry out cell type-specific functions. MALS/Veli 1 and 2 isoforms in the thick ascending limb and distal segments appear to have the most significant capacity for a basolateral membrane targeting mechanism. MAL3/Veli 3 has been implicated in generation of polarity in the proximal tubule.[186]

The disparate subcellular localization patterns of MALS/Veli isoforms are likely to arise from at least two different factors. First, differences in the primary structures provide reason to suspect that the MALS/Velis may have specific binding preferences. In contrast to the nearly identical PDZ domains amongst the MALS/Veli isoforms, the extreme NH$_2$- and COOH-termini are highly divergent. Most importantly, the region believed to direct MALS/Veli subcellular localization, the L27 interaction module, exhibits only 57% amino acid identity between isoforms, raising the possibility that different isoforms preferentially bind to different L27 domain proteins. Second, cell-specific expression of Lin-7-binding partners may account for differences in isoform localization in different nephron segments and cell-types. A group of CASK-like MAUGK proteins, called PALS (Partners of Lin-7), that contain L27 hetero-oligomerization domains, have been identified as potential partners of Lin-7.[187] The different PALS might substitute for CASK under certain circumstances, forming MALS/Veli complexes with different subcellular locations and disparate functions. For instance, PALS1 targets Lin-7 to the tight junction,[188] in contrast to the basolateral membrane location of the CASK/Lin-7 complex.

Dystrophin-Associated Protein Complex

The dystrophin-associated protein complex (DPC) is a transmembrane scaffolding machine that is expressed in a variety of tissues. Extensive studies in skeletal muscle revealed the DPC serves structural and signaling functions.[189] In epithelia, the DPC localizes to the basolateral membrane (Figure 14.6), where it is organized in a manner similar to the skeletal muscle complex, functioning to compartmentalize and tether signaling and transport proteins.

In the sarcolemma, the DPC is nucleated by dystrophin, a flexible rod-like cytoplasmic protein containing multiple spectrin-like repeats. Dystrophin directly interacts with the transmembrane protein, β-dystroglycan, via a C-terminal cysteine-rich region, and connects the complex to lammin through α-dystroglycan (Figure 14.6). Because dystrophin also binds actin, it effectively links the extracellular matrix with the cytoskeleton, offering an architecture that protects the sarcolemma from shearing forces of contraction. This point is underscored by the link to disease. Specific mutations in the X-linked dystrophin have been identified that disrupt dystrophin and consequently destabilize DGC elements at the sarcolemma, producing Duchenne muscular dystrophy, the milder Becker muscular dystrophy, and X-linked dilated cardiomyopathy (reviewed in [189]).

Dystrophin also interacts with the scaffolding molecules dystrobrevin, and three isoforms of syntrophin (α1, β1 and β2), to organize local signaling complexes in muscle. The syntrophrins contain several protein–protein interaction domains, including two pleckstrin homology domains and a PDZ domain. The PDZ domains recruit a variety of proteins to the DPC, including voltage-gated sodium channels[190,191] and nNOS.[2] α-Dystrobrevin directly interacts with dystrophin via coiled-coil domains, while simultaneously binding to the syntrophins through an independent binding site.[192]

The basolateral membrane associated DRC in renal epithelial cells exhibits the same basic design as in skeletal muscle, but differs somewhat in molecular composition.[193,194] An autosomal homolog of dystrophin, called utrophin, along with less abundant C-terminal dystrophin isoforms, Dp71 and Dp140,[189] takes the place of the longer muscle-specific dystrophin in renal epithelia. In addition, differential expression of dystrobrevin and three syntrophin isoforms along the nephron give rise to nephron segment-specific DPCs with distinct molecular properties.[193] In the connecting segment and the cortical collecting duct where the DPC is especially enriched, the DPC includes utrophin, β1-/β2 syntrophin, dystrobrevin, and β-dystroglycan.[193]

Like dystrophin in muscle, utrophin directly interacts with the actin cytoskeleton in epithelial cells,[195] while associating with laminin in the extracellular matrix via the basolateral dystroglycans[196] (Figure 14.6). Thus,

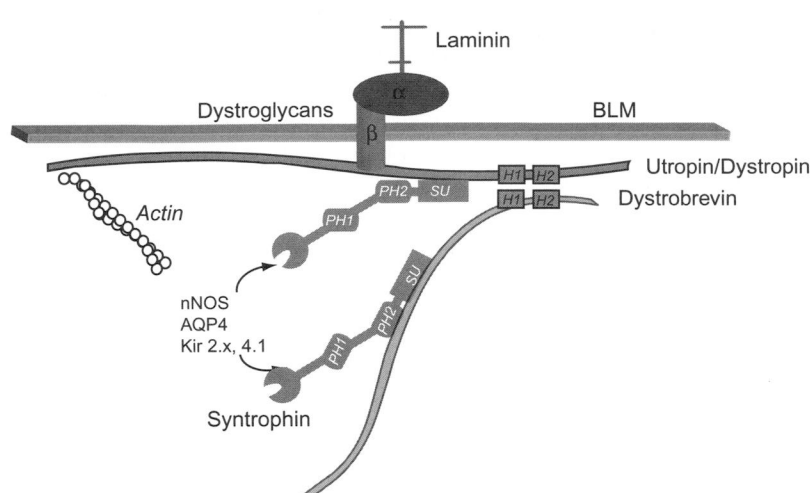

Laminin

FIGURE 14.6 **The dystrophin-associated protein complex (DPC) at the basolateral membrane.** The PDZ protein, syntrophin, is recruited to the basolateral membrane via its interaction with utropin and possibly dystrobrevin, requiring one of its pleckstrin homology (PH2) domains and the syntrophin unique (SU) domain. This leaves the syntrophin PDZ domain free to recruit basolateral membrane proteins, such as the AQP4 water channel, potassium channels, Kir 2.X and Kir 4.X, as well as nNOS. Utropin/dystropin interacts with actin via N-terminal spectrin repeats, with β-dystroglycan via a C-terminal cysteine-rich region and with dystrobrevin via coiled-coiled domains (H1, H2).

utrophin is poised to provide a secure anchoring point for polarized expression of syntrophin. Consistent with this notion, it has been reported that basolateral membrane localization of β2-syntrophin depends on its utrophin-binding activity, requiring one of its pleckstrin homology domains and the syntrophin unique (SU) domain.[35] Moreover, utrophin knockout mice exhibit a selective reduction of β2-syntrophin at renal epithelial basolateral membrane domains.[193] Syntrophins also interact with dystrobrevin via the PH and SU domains, allowing recruitment of additional syntrophin molecules to the same DPC.[197]

Importantly, the association of syntrophin with dystrobrevin, utrophin, and the basolateral membrane occurs independently of the syntrophin PDZ domain.[35] This leaves the Type I PDZ domain free to interact with proteins containing a syntrophin PDZ recognition motif. Basolateral membrane proteins, such as the inward rectifying channel proteins Kir 2.X[169] and Kir 4. X,[198] the AQP4 water channel,[199] as well as nNOS, have been shown to interact with the syntrophin PDZ-binding domain. At present, the functional relevance of these interactions in the kidney is not well-understood.

Several clues about the roles of transport protein interaction with syntrophin and the DPC are provided by studies in other tissues. In astrocytes, for example, α-syntrophin is required for the polarized expression of AQP4[199] and Kir 4.1[198] at end-feet membranes adjacent to blood vessels for efficient water and potassium siphoning.[200,201] It will be interesting to learn if genetic ablation of β2 syntrophin, the prevalent form in the kidney, has similar effects on AQP4 in the proximal straight tubule[202] and Kir 4.1 in the distal nephron.[203]

Utrophin knockout animals have been generated.[204] Unfortunately, expression of the shorter C-terminal dystrophin forms in the kidney compensate for the utrophin ablation, making it difficult to precisely define the functional role of the renal DPC by a genetic approach. Double utrophin/dystrophin knockout mice exhibit a fragile phenotype with complete disintegration of the DPC and premature death.[193] It will be important to determine how much of the phenotype can be attributed to impaired kidney function.

AKAP

AKAPs (A-kinase anchoring proteins) are a diverse group of molecules that function as cell signaling scaffolds. Specifically, AKAPs organize and juxtapose protein kinase A (PKA) with specific substrates and other signaling machinery at specific cellular locales. In doing so, AKAP proteins can precisely control where and when second-messengers will act on select cellular effectors. Since the first discovery of an AKAP, a microtubule anchoring protein that binds to the regulatory subunit of PKA with high affinity,[205] nearly 50 AKAP proteins have been identified. Many of them control phosphorylation of channels, receptors, and membrane transport proteins.[206] Several are suspected of modulating renal tubule transport processes.

COMMON PROPERTIES OF AKAP PROTEINS

AKAP proteins are structurally diverse, related only by general signaling functions and three common properties. First, classification as an AKAP protein requires the presence of a PKA-anchoring domain. Second, AKAPs contain cellular localization signals that provide a means to spatially organize second-messenger cascades at specific subcellular compartments. Third, AKAPs possess other protein—protein interaction domains, which specify interaction with select effectors and/or other signaling molecules. While all AKAPs have these common properties, they each have distinct targeting signals and different scaffolding motifs. Consequently, they have specialized functions, modulating distinct intracellular signaling events.

AKAPs bind PKA by means of a small anchoring domain, comprised of a short (13–18 amino acid), amphipathic α-helix. NMR solution structures reveal that the hydrophobic side of the amphipathic helix makes numerous hydrophobic contacts within a hydrophobic surface of a four-helix bundle formed by the N-terminal domains of the PKA regulatory subunit homodimer.[208–210] Consequently, the AKAP–PKA interaction occurs with relatively high affinity (∼1–10 nM). While most AKAPs interact with the RII isotypes of the PKA regulatory subunit, several AKAPs have been identified, D-AKAP1[211] and D-AKAP2,[211] which can interact with both RI and RII forms. Sphingosine kinase interacting protein (SKIP), an AKAP that is enriched in the inner mitochondrial membrane, exclusively interacts with RI.[212] Importantly, AKAP function can be disrupted by exogenous expression of a peptide mimic of the amphipathic helix.[213] Regulatory subunit isotype specific competitors have been developed.[214]

Specialized targeting sequences on anchoring proteins compartmentalize different AKAPs to distinct subcellular compartments, including plasma membrane microdomains, intracellular vesicles, nuclei, mitochondria, microtubules, and the actin cytoskeleton.[215] Certain AKAPs contain polarized trafficking signals that direct asymmetric localization in epithelial cells. AKAP2 (AKAP-KL), for example, is compartmentalized on the apical membrane[216] by its PDZ-binding motif, which specifies interaction with NHERF3.[81] Similarly ezrin, a low RII affinity AKAP, localizes to the apical membrane through a protein–protein recognition domain that directs interaction with NHERF1.[217] In many cases, different splice products of the same AKAP gene can be differentially targeted to different compartments. Splice forms of the AKAP18 gene, for instance, are expressed on opposite plasma membrane domains in epithelial cells; AKAP18-α is targeted to basolateral membranes, whereas AKAP18-β localizes to the apical membrane. In this case, a unique 23 amino acid insert in AKAP18-β acts as an apical membrane targeting determinant.[218]

As multivalent scaffolds, AKAPs can juxtapose the right combination of enzymes with their substrates. Consequently, AKAPs not only synchronize signal transduction processes, but they can also orchestrate signal termination events. The archetypal example is provided by the AKAP75/150 family, which influences the phosphorylation state of several different channels and transporters, including the Npt2a co-transporter,[219] L-type calcium channels,[220] M-type potassium channels,[221] and AMPA-type glutamate receptors.[222,223] AKAP75 not only contains a binding

site for PKA, it also directly interacts with PKC and the calcium-calmodulin-dependent phosphatase, PP2B (calcineurin).[224,225] Consequently, the same AKAP scaffold can coordinate signal transduction processes by phosphorylation as well as dephosphorylation. Thus, AKAPs can influence the balance of signal transduction and termination by differentially tethering different signaling components and effectors.[226]

Function of AKAPS in Kidney Transport Processes

AKAP-Dependent AQP2 Water Channel Shuttling

A critical role for AKAPs in water channel trafficking is strongly suggested by observations that cAMP-dependent AQP2 translocation to the cell surface can be inhibited with a synthetic peptide mimic of the AKAP amphipathic helix, which prevents binding of AKAPs to the PKA RII subunit.[227] Several different AKAPs appear to be associated with endosomal structures containing AQP2. Biochemical characterization of inner medullary collecting duct (IMCD) heavy endosomes, containing AQP2, revealed the presence of an associated multiprotein-signaling complex, composed of a 90 kD AKAP, PKA, and protein phosphatase 2a.[228] While the precise molecular identity of the 90 kD AKAP is still not certain, a smaller anchoring protein, AKAP18-δ, was subsequently discovered.[229] In the kidney, AKAP18-δ is mainly expressed in IMCD principal cells, where it appears to be confined to intracellular vesicles containing AQP2 and PKA. Observations that vasopressin recruits AKAP18-δ with AQP2 to the plasma membrane suggest that this AKAP is specifically involved in the PKA phosphorylation-dependent AQP2 translocation process. Reminiscent of the multifactoral roles of AKAP75 (see above), the AKAP-signaling complex in IMCD endosomes also contains PP2B[228] and phosphodiesterases.[230] Thus, the endosomal AKAPs in the collecting duct are also likely to participate in maintaining AQP2 in a quiescent dephosphorylated conformation in water diuresis.

AKAPs in the Proximal Tubule Apical Membrane Scaffolding Complex

Two different AKAPs, D-AKAP2 and AKPA79, have been implicated in the modulation of proximal tubule sodium phosphate transport. AKAP2 has been shown to interact with a PDZ scaffolding protein, NHERF3, at the apical membrane where it has been suggested to play an important role in the parathyroid hormone (PTH)-mediated regulation of Npt2a, involving PKA compartmentalization.[142] In a proximal tubule model, OK cells, PTH-dependent regulation of Npt2a can be uncoupled with a synthetic peptide mimic of the AKAP amphipathic helix, indicating that an AKAP is required for PKA-dependent modulation of Npt2a regulation. In this system, AKAP79 was shown to associate with the Npt2a transporter, PKA, and the parathyroid hormone receptor.[219] Because AKAP 79 also has the capacity to interact with PDZ proteins in neuronal systems,[58] it may interact with the Npt2a co-transporter and the PTH receptor through its interaction with the apical NHERF complex.

AKAP Control of the Potassium Secretory Channel ROMK (Kir 1.1)

Studies of the renal potassium secretory channel, ROMK, in heterologous expression systems have suggested a potential role for AKAPs in the physiological regulation of potassium secretion. Because open channel gating and cell surface expression of the ROMK require direct phosphorylation by PKA[231,232] and other kinases,[137] a critical role of an AKAP has been an attractive idea. In fact, it has been reported that maximal activation of ROMK in *Xenopus* oocytes by forskolin and/or 8-bromo-cAMP-dependent kinase requires co-expression of an AKAP.[233] High basal phosphorylation of the channel in this expression system makes the effects of AKAPs modest. Nevertheless, the response appears to be AKAP specific, being dependent on AKAP-75 but not AKAP18, AKAP-2 (KL).[234] AKAP-75 is not expressed with ROMK in the thick ascending limb or collecting duct, however, so the AKAP in the kidney that interacts with ROMK still remains to be determined. Given observations that ROMK interacts with NHERF1 and 2 (see above), the ERM proteins[85] are obvious AKAP candidates.

CONCLUSION

Exciting discoveries in recent years have cast light onto the molecular mechanisms of epithelial transport modulation. The discovery of proteins that bring together physiologically appropriate assemblages of cell signaling and trafficking proteins with transport molecules for efficient regulation has been especially insightful. The molecular identities and functions of many of these scaffolding molecules in the kidney have now begun to come into focus. Still, there is much more to be learned. For example, observations that some transport proteins such as NHE1, the housekeeping sodium-hydrogen exchanger,[207] NHE3,[235] and the Na/K ATPase,[236,237] might twilight as scaffolding proteins is emerging as an intriguing possibility that we certainly will hear more about in the future. Also, with the application of powerful new tools in cell biology, genomics, and proteomics, it is likely that more scaffolding candidates will be identified. As they are,

it will be important not only to continue probing into the mechanistic basis of function in model systems, but also to rigorously explore how these fascinating molecules work in their native cellular environments.

References

[1] Songyang Z, Fanning AS, Fu C, Xu J, Marfatia SM, Chishti AH, et al. Recognition of unique carboxyl-terminal motifs by distinct PDZ domains. Science 1997;275:73–7.

[2] Hillier BJ, Christopherson KS, Prehoda KE, Bredt DS, Lim WA. Unexpected modes of PDZ domain scaffolding revealed by structure of nNOS-syntrophin complex. Science 1999;284:812–85.

[3] Harris BZ, Hillier BJ, Lim WA. Energetic determinants of internal motif recognition by PDZ domains. Biochim Biophys Acta 2001;40:5530–921.

[4] Cho KO, Hunt CA, Kennedy MB. The rat brain postsynaptic density fraction contains a homolog of the *Drosophila* discs-large tumor suppressor protein. Neuron 1992;9:929–42.

[5] Harris BZ, Lim WA. Mechanism and role of PDZ domains in signaling complex assembly. J Cell Sci 2001;114:3219–31.

[6] Sheng M, Sala C. PDZ domains and the organization of supramolecular complexes. Annual Review of Neuroscience 2001;24:1–29.

[7] Adams ME, Mueller HA, Froehner SC. *In vivo* requirement of the alpha-syntrophin PDZ domain for the sarcolemmal localization of nNOS and aquaporin-4. J Cell Biol 2001;155:113–22.

[8] Xu XZ, Choudhury A, Li X, Montell C. Coordination of an array of signaling proteins through homo- and heteromeric interactions between PDZ domains and target proteins. J Cell Biol 1998;142:545–55.

[9] Borrell-Pages M, Fernandez-Larrea J, Borroto A, Rojo F, Baselga J, Arribas J. The carboxy-terminal cysteine of the tetraspanin L6 antigen is required for its interaction with SITAC, a novel PDZ protein. Mol Biol Cell 2000;11:4217–425.

[10] Maximov A, Sudhof TC, Bezprozvanny I. Association of neuronal calcium channels with modular adaptor proteins. J Biol Chem 1999;274:24453–6.

[11] Tonikian R, Zhang Y, Sazinsky SL, Currell B, Yeh JH, Reva B, et al. A specificity map for the PDZ domain family. PLoS Biol 2008;6:e239.

[12] Cabral JH, Petosa C, Sutcliffe MJ, Raza S, Byron O, Poy F, et al. Crystal structure of a PDZ domain. Nature 1996;382:649–52.

[13] Doyle DA, Lee A, Lewis J, Kim E, Sheng M, MacKinnon R. Crystal structures of a complexed and peptide-free membrane protein-binding domain: Molecular basis of peptide recognition by PDZ. Cell 1996;85:1067–76.

[14] Daniels DL, Cohen AR, Anderson JM, Brunger AT. Crystal structure of the hCASK PDZ domain reveals the structural basis of class II PDZ domain target recognition. Nat Struct Biol 1998;5:317–25.

[15] Karthikeyan S, Leung T, Ladias JA. Structural basis of the Na^+/H^+ exchanger regulatory factor PDZ1 interaction with the carboxyl-terminal region of the cystic fibrosis transmembrane conductance regulator. J Biol Chem 2001;276:11966–9683.

[16] Tochio H, Zhang Q, Mandal P, Li M, Zhang M. Solution structure of the extended neuronal nitric oxide synthase PDZ domain complexed with an associated peptide. Nat Struct Biol 1999;6:417–21.

[17] Zhang Y, Yeh S, Appleton BA, Held HA, Kausalya PJ, Phua DC, et al. Convergent and divergent ligand specificity among PDZ domains of the LAP and zonula occludens (ZO) families. J Biol Chem 2006;281:22299–311.

[18] Birrane G, Chung J, Ladias JA. Novel mode of ligand recognition by the Erbin PDZ domain. J Biol Chem 2003;278:1399−402.

[19] Elkins JM, Gileadi C, Shrestha L, Phillips C, Wang J, Muniz JR, et al. Unusual binding interactions in PDZ domain crystal structures help explain binding mechanisms. Protein Sci 2010;19:731−41.

[20] Karthikeyan S, Leung T, Ladias JA. Structural determinants of the Na^+/H^+ exchanger regulatory factor interaction with the beta 2 adrenergic and platelet-derived growth factor receptors. J Biol Chem 2002;277:18973−8.

[21] Ladias JA. Structural insights into the CFTR-NHERF interaction. J Mol Biol 2003;192:79−88.

[22] te Velthuis AJ, Sakalis PA, Fowler DA, Bagowski CP. Genome-wide analysis of PDZ domain binding reveals inherent functional overlap within the PDZ interaction network. PLoS One 2011;6:e16047.

[23] Cohen NA, Brenman JE, Snyder SH, Bredt DS. Binding of the inward rectifier K channel Kir2.3 to PSD-95 is regulated by protein kinase A phosphorylation. Neuron 1996;17:759−67.

[24] Horio Y, Hibino H, Inanobe A, Yamada M, Ishii M, Tada Y, et al. Clustering and enhanced activity of an inwardly rectifying potassium channel, Kir4.1, by an anchoring protein, PSD-95/SAP90. J Biol Chem 1997;272:12885−8.

[25] Cao TT, Deacon HW, Reczek D, Bretscher A, von Zastrow M. A kinase-regulated PDZ-domain interaction controls endocytic sorting of the beta2-adrenergic receptor. Nature 1999;401:286−90.

[26] Raghuram V, Hormuth H, Foskett JK. A kinase-regulated mechanism controls CFTR channel gating by disrupting bivalent PDZ domain interactions. Proc Natl Acad Sci USA 2003;100:9620−5.

[27] Voltz JW, Brush M, Sikes S, Steplock D, Weinman EJ, Shenolikar S. Phosphorylation of PDZ1 domain attenuates NHERF-1 binding to cellular targets. J Biol Chem 2007;282:33879−87.

[28] Weinman EJ, Biswas RS, Peng G, Shen L, Turner CL, E Xiaofei, et al. Parathyroid hormone inhibits renal phosphate transport by phosphorylation of serine 77 of sodium-hydrogen exchanger regulatory factor-1. J Clin Invest 2007;117:3412−20.

[29] Weinman EJ, Steplock D, Zhang Y, Biswas R, Bloch RJ, Shenolikar S. Cooperativity between the phosphorylation of Thr95 and Ser77 of NHERF-1 in the hormonal regulation of renal phosphate transport. J Biol Chem 2010;285:25134−8.

[30] Lau AG, Hall RA. Oligomerization of NHERF-1 and NHERF-2 PDZ domains: Differential regulation by association with receptor carboxyl-termini and by phosphorylation. Biochemistry 2001;40:8572−80.

[31] Garbett D, LaLonde DP, Bretscher A. The scaffolding protein EBP50 regulates microvillar assembly in a phosphorylation-dependent manner. J Cell Biol 2010;191:397−413.

[32] Li J, Poulikakos PI, Dai Z, Testa JR, Callaway DJ, Bu Z. Protein kinase C phosphorylation disrupts Na^+/H^+ exchanger regulatory factor 1 autoinhibition and promotes cystic fibrosis transmembrane conductance regulator macromolecular assembly. J Biol Chem 2007;282:27086−99.

[33] Alewine C, Olsen O, Wade JB, Welling PA. TIP-1 has PDZ scaffold antagonist activity. Mol Biol Cell 2006;17:4200−11.

[34] Campo C, Mason A, Maouyo D, Olsen O, Yoo D, Welling PA. Molecular mechanisms of membrane polarity in renal epithelial cells. Rev Physiol Biochem Pharmacol 2005;153:47−99.

[35] Kachinsky AM, Froehner SC, Milgram SL. A PDZ-containing scaffold related to the dystrophin complex at the basolateral membrane of epithelial cells. J Cell Biol 1999;145:391−402.

[36] Olsen O, Wade JB, Morin N, Bredt DS, Welling PA. Differential localization of mammalian Lin-7 (MALS/Veli) PDZ proteins in the kidney. Am J Physiol Renal Physiol 2005;288:F345−352.

[37] Straight SW, Karnak D, Borg JP, Kamberov E, Dare H, Margolis B, et al. mLin-7 is localized to the basolateral surface of renal epithelia via its NH(2) terminus. Am J Physiol Renal Physiol 2000;278:F464−75.

[38] Borg JP, Marchetto S, Le Bivic A, Ollendorff V, Jaulin-Bastard F, Saito H, et al. ERBIN: A basolateral PDZ protein that interacts with the mammalian ERBB2/HER2 receptor. Nat Cell Biol 2000;2:407−14.

[39] Cohen AR, Woods DF, Marfatia SM, Walther Z, Chishti AH, Anderson JM, et al. Human CASK/LIN-2 binds syndecan-2 and protein 4.1 and localizes to the basolateral membrane of epithelial cells [published erratum appears in J Cell Biol 1998 Aug 24;142(4): following 1156]. J Cell Biol 1998;142:129−38.

[40] Tojo A, Bredt DS, Wilcox CS. Distribution of postsynaptic density proteins in rat kidney: relationship to neuronal nitric oxide synthase. Kidney Int 1999;55:1384−94.

[41] Wu H, Reuver SM, Kuhlendahl S, Chung WJ, Garner CC. Subcellular targeting and cytoskeletal attachment of SAP97 to the epithelial lateral membrane. J Cell Sci 1998;111:2365−76.

[42] McWilliams RR, Gidey E, Fouassier L, Weed SA. and Doctor RB. Characterization of an ankyrin repeat-containing Shank2 isoform (Shank2E) in liver epithelial cells. Biochem J 2004;380:181−91.

[43] Roh MH, Margolis B. Composition and function of PDZ protein complexes during cell polarization. Am J Physiol Renal Physiol 2003;285:F377−387.

[44] Pieczynski J, Margolis B. Protein complexes that control renal epithelial polarity. Am J Physiol Renal Physiol 2011;300:F589−601.

[45] Cheng J, Moyer BD, Milewski M, Loffing J, Ikeda M, Mickle JE, et al. Golgi-associated PDZ domain protein modulates cystic fibrosis transmembrane regulator plasma membrane expression. J Biol Chem 2002;277:3520−9.

[46] Joubert L, Hanson B, Barthet G, Sebben M, Claeysen S, Hong W, et al. New sorting nexin (SNX27) and NHERF specifically interact with the 5-HT4a receptor splice variant: Roles in receptor targeting. J Cell Sci 2004;117:5367−79.

[47] Fialka I, Steinlein P, Ahorn H, Bock G, Burbelo PD, Haberfellner M, et al. Identification of syntenin as a protein of the apical early endocytic compartment in Madin-Darby canine kidney cells. J Biol Chem 1999;274:26233−9.

[48] Simonsen A, Gaullier JM, D'Arrigo A, Stenmark H. The Rab5 effector EEA1 interacts directly with syntaxin-6. J Biol Chem 1999;274:28857−60.

[49] Maday S, Anderson E, Chang HC, Shorter J, Satoh A, Sfakianos J, et al. PDZ-binding motif controls basolateral targeting of syndecan-1 along the biosynthetic pathway in polarized epithelial cells. Traffic 2008;9:1915−24.

[50] Straight SW, Pieczynski JN, Whiteman EL, Liu CJ, Margolis B. Mammalian lin-7 stabilizes polarity protein complexes. J Biol Chem 2006;281:37738−47.

[51] Ahn J, Mundigl O, Muth TR, Rudnick G, Caplan MJ. Polarized expression of GABA transporters in Madin-Darby canine kidney cells and cultured hippocampal neurons. J Biol Chem 1996;271:6917−24.

[52] Muth TR, Ahn J, Caplan MJ. Identification of sorting determinants in the C-terminal cytoplasmic tails of the gamma-aminobutyric acid transporters GAT-2 and GAT-3. J Biol Chem 1998;273:25616−27.

[53] Legouis R, Jaulin-Bastard F, Schott S, Navarro C, Borg JP, Labouesse M. Basolateral targeting by leucine-rich repeat domains in epithelial cells. EMBO Rep 2003;4:1096−102.

[54] Kim E, Naisbitt S, Hsueh YP, Rao A, Rothschild A, Craig AM, et al. GKAP, a novel synaptic protein that interacts with the guanylate kinase-like domain of the PSD-95/SAP90 family of channel clustering molecules. J Cell Biol 1997;136:669−78.

[55] Seabold GK, Burette A, Lim IA, Weinberg RJ, Hell JW. Interaction of the tyrosine kinase Pyk2 with the N-methyl-D-aspartate receptor complex via the Src homology 3 domains of PSD-95 and SAP102. J Biol Chem 2003;278:15040–8.

[56] McGee AW, Dakoji SR, Olsen O, Bredt DS, Lim WA, Prehoda KE. Structure of the SH3-guanylate kinase module from PSD-95 suggests a mechanism for regulated assembly of MAGUK scaffolding proteins. Mol Cell 2001;8:1291–301.

[57] Tavares GA, Panepucci EH, Brunger AT. Structural characterization of the intramolecular interaction between the SH3 and guanylate kinase domains of PSD-95. Mol Cell 2001;8:1313–25.

[58] Colledge M, Dean RA, Scott GK, Langeberg LK, Huganir RL, Scott JD. Targeting of PKA to glutamate receptors through a MAGUK-AKAP complex. Neuron 2000;27:107–19.

[59] Kim E, Sheng M. PDZ domain proteins of synapses. Nat Rev Neurosci 2004;5:771–81.

[60] Christopherson KS, Sweeney NT, Craven SE, Kang R, El-Husseini AD, Bredt DS. Lipid- and protein-mediated multimerization of PSD-95: Implications for receptor clustering and assembly of synaptic protein networks. J Cell Sci 2003;116:3213–9.

[61] Hsueh YP, Kim E, Sheng M. Disulfide-linked head-to-head multimerization in the mechanism of ion channel clustering by PSD-95. Neuron 1997;18:803–14.

[62] El-Husseini AE, Craven SE, Chetkovich DM, Firestein BL, Schnell E, Aoki C, et al. Dual palmitoylation of PSD-95 mediates its vesiculotubular sorting, postsynaptic targeting, and ion channel clustering. J Cell Biol 2000;148:159–72.

[63] Brenman JE, Chao DS, Gee SH, McGee AW, Craven SE, Santillano DR, et al. Interaction of nitric oxide synthase with the postsynaptic density protein PSD-95 and alpha-1 syntrophin mediated by PDZ motifs. Cell 1996;84:757–67.

[64] Christopherson KS, Hillier BJ, Lim WA, Bredt DS. PSD-95 assembles a ternary complex with the N-methyl-D-aspartic acid receptor and a bivalent neuronal NO synthase PDZ domain. J Biol Chem 1999;274:27467–73.

[65] McGee AW, Bredt DS. Assembly and plasticity of the glutamatergic postsynaptic specialization. Curr Opin Neurobiol 2003;13:111–8.

[66] Aarts M, Liu Y, Liu L, Besshoh S, Arundine M, Gurd JW, et al. Treatment of ischemic brain damage by perturbing NMDA receptor- PSD-95 protein interactions. Science 2002;298:846–50.

[67] Kone BC, Kuncewicz T, Zhang W, Yu ZY. Protein interactions with nitric oxide synthases: controlling the right time, the right place, and the right amount of nitric oxide. Am J Physiol Renal Physiol 2003;285:F178–190.

[68] El-Husseini AE, Topinka JR, Lehrer-Graiwer JE, Firestein BL, Craven SE, Aoki C, et al. Ion channel clustering by membrane-associated guanylate kinases. Differential regulation by N-terminal lipid and metal binding motifs. J Biol Chem 2000;275:23904–10.

[69] Brenman JE, Christopherson KS, Craven SE, McGee AW, Bredt DS. Cloning and characterization of postsynaptic density 93, a nitric oxide synthase interacting protein. J Neurosci 1996;16:7407–15.

[70] Shenolikar S, Weinman EJ. NHERF: Targeting and trafficking membrane proteins. Am J Physiol Renal Physiol 2001;280:F389–95.

[71] Weinman EJ, Hall RA, Friedman PA, Liu-Chen LY, Shenolikar S. The association of NHERF adaptor proteins with G protein-coupled receptors and receptor tyrosine kinases. Annu Rev Physiol 2006;68:491–505.

[72] Donowitz M, Cha B, Zachos NC, Brett CL, Sharma A, Tse CM, et al. NHERF family and NHE3 regulation. J Physiol 2005;567:3–11.

[73] Thelin WR, Hodson CA, Milgram SL. Beyond the brush border: NHERF4 blazes new NHERF turf. J Physiol 2005;567:13–9.

[74] Weinman EJ, Steplock D, Shenolikar S. CAMP-mediated inhibition of the renal brush border membrane Na$^+$-H$^+$ exchanger requires a dissociable phosphoprotein cofactor. J Clin Invest 1993;92:1781–6.

[75] Weinman EJ, Steplock D, Wang Y, Shenolikar S. Characterization of a protein cofactor that mediates protein kinase a regulation of the renal brush border membrane Na($^+$)-H$^+$ exchanger. J Clin Invest 1995;95:2143–219.

[76] Reczek D, Berryman M, Bretscher A. Identification of EBP50: A PDZ-containing phosphoprotein that associates with members of the ezrin-radixin-moesin family. J Cell Biol 1997;139:169–79.

[77] Yun CH, Oh S, Zizak M, Steplock D, Tsao S, Tse CM, et al. cAMP-mediated inhibition of the epithelial brush border Na$^+$/H$^+$ exchanger, NHE3, requires an associated regulatory protein. Proc Natl Acad Sci USA 1997;94:3010–5.

[78] Poulat F, Barbara PS, Desclozeaux M, Soullier S, Moniot B, Bonneaud N, et al. The human testis determining factor SRY binds a nuclear factor containing PDZ protein interaction domains. J Biol Chem 1997;272:7167–72.

[79] Kocher O, Comella N, Gilchrist A, Pal R, Tognazzi K, Brown LF, et al. PDZK1, a novel PDZ domain-containing protein up-regulated in carcinomas and mapped to chromosome 1q21, interacts with cMOAT (MRP2), the multidrug resistance-associated protein. Lab Invest 1999;79:1161–70.

[80] Wang S, Yue H, Derin RB, Guggino WB, Li M. Accessory protein facilitated CFTR-CFTR interaction, a molecular mechanism to potentiate the chloride channel activity. Cell 2001;103:169–79.

[81] Gisler SM, Stagljar I, Traebert M, Bacic D, Biber J, Murer H. Interaction of the type IIa Na/Pi co-transporter with PDZ proteins. J Biol Chem 2001;276:9206–913.

[82] Scott RO, Thelin WR, Milgram SL. A novel PDZ protein regulates the activity of guanylyl cyclase C, the heat-stable enterotoxin receptor. J Biol Chem 2002;277:22934–41.

[83] Sarker R, Valkhoff VE, Zachos NC, Lin R, Cha B, Chen TE, et al. NHERF1 and NHERF2 are necessary for multiple but usually separate aspects of basal and acute regulation of NHE3 activity. Am J Physiol Cell Physiol 2011;300:C771–782.

[84] Bretscher A, Edwards K, Fehon RG. ERM proteins and merlin: Integrators at the cell cortex. Nat Rev Mol Cell Biol 2002;3:586–99.

[85] Dransfield DT, Bradford AJ, Smith J, Martin M, Roy C, Mangeat PH, et al. Ezrin is a cyclic AMP-dependent protein kinase anchoring protein. EMBO J 1997;16:35–43.

[86] Fouassier L, Yun CC, Fitz JG, Doctor RB. Evidence for ezrin-radixin-moesin-binding phosphoprotein 50 (EBP50) self-association through PDZ-PDZ interactions. J Biol Chem 2000;275:25039–45.

[87] Gisler SM, Pribanic S, Bacic D, Forrer P, Gantenbein A, Sabourin LA, et al. PDZK1: I. A major scaffolder in brush borders of proximal tubular cells. Kidney Int 2003;64:1733–45.

[88] Shenolikar S, Minkoff CM, Steplock DA, Evangelista C, Liu M, Weinman EJ. N-terminal PDZ domain is required for NHERF dimerization. FEBS Lett 2001;489:233–6.

[89] LaLonde DP, Bretscher A. The scaffold protein PDZK1 undergoes a head-to-tail intramolecular association that negatively regulates its interaction with EBP50. Biochemistry 2009;48:2261–71.

[90] LaLonde DP, Garbett D, Bretscher A. A regulated complex of the scaffolding proteins PDZK1 and EBP50 with ezrin contribute to microvillar organization. Mol Biol Cell 2010;21:1519–29.

[91] Weinman EJ, Wang Y, Wang F, Greer C, Steplock D, Shenolikar SA. C-terminal PDZ motif in NHE3 binds NHERF-1 and enhances cAMP inhibition of sodium–hydrogen exchange. Biochemistry 2003;42:12662–8.

[92] Lamprecht G, Weinman EJ, Yun CH. The role of NHERF and E3KARP in the cAMP-mediated inhibition of NHE3. J Biol Chem 1998;273:29972−8.

[93] Weinman EJ, Steplock D, Wade JB, Shenolikar S. Ezrin binding domain-deficient NHERF attenuates cAMP-mediated inhibition of Na$^{(+)}$/H$^{(+)}$ exchange in OK cells. Am J Physiol Renal Physiol 2001;281:F374−380.

[94] Murtazina R, Kovbasnjuk O, Zachos NC, Li X, Chen Y, Hubbard A, et al. Tissue-specific regulation of sodium/proton exchanger isoform 3 activity in Na$^{(+)}$/H$^{(+)}$ exchanger regulatory factor 1 (NHERF1) null mice. cAMP inhibition is differentially dependent on NHERF1 and exchange protein directly activated by cAMP in ileum versus proximal tubule. J Biol Chem 2007;282:25141−51.

[95] Shenolikar S, Voltz JW, Minkoff CM, Wade JB, Weinman EJ. Targeted disruption of the mouse NHERF-1 gene promotes internalization of proximal tubule sodium-phosphate co-transporter type IIa and renal phosphate wasting. Proc Natl Acad Sci USA 2002;99:11470−5.

[96] Weinman EJ, Steplock D, Shenolikar S. NHERF-1 uniquely transduces the cAMP signals that inhibit sodium−hydrogen exchange in mouse renal apical membranes. FEBS Lett 2003;536:141−4.

[97] Cunningham R, Steplock D, Wang F, Huang H, X E, Shenolikar S, et al. Defective parathyroid hormone regulation of NHE3 activity and phosphate adaptation in cultured NHERF-1$^{-/-}$ renal proximal tubule cells. J Biol Chem 2004;279:37815−21.

[98] Weinman EJ. New functions for the NHERF family of proteins. J Clin Invest 2001;108:185−6.

[99] Hall RA, Ostedgaard LS, Premont RT, Blitzer JT, Rahman N, Welsh MJ, et al. C-terminal motif found in the beta2-adrenergic receptor, P2Y1 receptor and cystic fibrosis transmembrane conductance regulator determines binding to the Na$^+$/H$^+$ exchanger regulatory factor family of PDZ proteins. Proc Natl Acad Sci USA 1998;95:8496−501.

[100] Short DB, Trotter KW, Reczek D, Kreda SM, Bretscher A, Boucher RC, et al. An apical PDZ protein anchors the cystic fibrosis transmembrane conductance regulator to the cytoskeleton. J Biol Chem 1998;273:19797−801.

[101] Wang S, Raab RW, Schatz PJ, Guggino WB, Li M. Peptide binding Consensus of the NHE-RF-PDZ1 doamin matches the C-terminal sequence of CFTR. FEBS Letters 1998;427:103−8.

[102] Sun F, Hug MJ, Lewarchik CM, Yun CH, Bradbury NA, Frizzell RA. E3KARP mediates the association of ezrin and protein kinase A with the cystic fibrosis transmembrane conductance regulator in airway cells. J Biol Chem 2002;275:29539−46.

[103] Hall RA, Premont RT, Chow CW, Blitzer JT, Pitcher JA, Claing A, et al. The beta2-adrenergic receptor interacts with the Na$^+$/H$^+$-exchanger regulatory factor to control Na$^+$/H$^+$ exchange. Nature 1998;392:626−30.

[104] Naren AP, Cobb B, Li C, Roy K, Nelson D, Heda GD, et al. A macromolecular complex of beta 2 adrenergic receptor, CFTR, and ezrin/radixin/moesin-binding phosphoprotein 50 is regulated by PKA. Proc Natl Acad Sci USA 2003;100:342−6.

[105] Hall RA, Spurney RF, Premont RT, Rahman N, Blitzer JT, Pitcher JA, et al. G protein-coupled receptor kinase 6A phosphorylates the Na$^{(+)}$/H$^{(+)}$ exchanger regulatory factor via a PDZ domain-mediated interaction. J Biol Chem 1999;274:24328−34.

[106] Mohler PJ, Kreda SM, Boucher RC, Sudol M, Stutts MJ, Milgram SL. Yes-associated protein 65 localizes p62(c-Yes) to the apical compartment of airway epithelia by association with EBP50. J Cell Biol 1999;147:879−90.

[107] Tang Y, Tang J, Chen Z, Trost C, Flockerzi V, Li M, et al. Association of mammalian trp4 and phospholipase C isozymes with a PDZ domain-containing protein, NHER. J Biol Chem 2000;275:37559−64.

[108] Liedtke CM, Yun CH, Kyle N, Wang D. Protein kinase C epsilon-dependent regulation of cystic fibrosis transmembrane regulator involves binding to a receptor for activated C kinase (RACK1) and RACK1 binding to Na$^+$/H$^+$ exchange regulatory factor. J Biol Chem 2002;277:22925−33.

[109] Raghuram V, Mak DD, Foskett JK. Regulation of cystic fibrosis transmembrane conductance regulator single-channel gating by bivalent PDZ-domain-mediated interaction. Proc Natl Acad Sci USA 2001;98:1300−5.

[110] Swiatecka-Urban A, Duhaime M, Coutermarsh B, Karlson KH, Collawn J, Milewski M, et al. PDZ domain interaction controls the endocytic recycling of the cystic fibrosis transmembrane conductance regulator. J Biol Chem 2002;277:40099−105.

[111] Hernando N, Deliot N, Gisler SM, Lederer E, Weinman EJ, Biber J, et al. PDZ-domain interactions and apical expression of type IIa Na/P(i) co-transporters. Proc Natl Acad Sci USA 2002;99:11957−62.

[112] Weinman EJ, Boddeti A, Cunningham R, Akom M, Wang F, Wang Y, et al. NHERF-1 is required for renal adaptation to a low-phosphate diet. Am J Physiol Renal Physiol 2003;285:F1225−32.

[113] Hernando N, Karim-Jimenez Z, Biber J, Murer H. Molecular determinants for apical expression and regulatory membrane retrieval of the type IIa Na/Pi co-transporter. Pflug Archiv - Eur J Physiol 2001;60:431−45.

[114] Karim-Jimenez Z, Hernando N, Biber J, Murer H. Molecular determinants for apical expression of the renal type IIa Na$^+$/Pi-co-transporter. Pflug Archiv - Eur J Physiol 2001;442:782−90.

[115] Deliot N, Hernando N, Horst-Liu Z, Gisler SM, Capuano P, Wagner CA, et al. Parathyroid hormone treatment induces dissociation of type IIa Na$^+$-P(i) co-transporter-Na$^+$/H$^+$ exchanger regulatory factor-1 complexes. Am J Physiol Cell Physiol 2005;289:C159−167.

[116] Weinman EJ, Steplock D, Cha B, Kovbasnjuk O, Frost NA, Cunningham R, et al. PTH transiently increases the percent mobile fraction of Npt2a in OK cells as determined by FRAP. Am J Physiol Renal Physiol 2009;297:F1560−1565.

[117] Weinman EJ, Steplock D, Shenolikar S, Blanpied TA. Dynamics of PTH-induced disassembly of Npt2a/NHERF-1 complexes in living OK cells. Am J Physiol Renal Physiol 2011;300:F231−235.

[118] Wang B, Bisello A, Yang Y, Romero GG, Friedman PA. NHERF1 regulates parathyroid hormone receptor membrane retention without affecting recycling. J Biol Chem 2007;282:36214−22.

[119] Sneddon WB, Syme CA, Bisello A, Magyar CE, Rochdi MD, Parent JL, et al. Activation-independent parathyroid hormone receptor internalization is regulated by NHERF1 (EBP50). J Biol Chem 2003;278:43787−96.

[120] Blaine J, Okamura K, Giral H, Breusegem S, Caldas Y, Millard A, et al. PTH-induced internalization of apical membrane NaPi2a: role of actin and myosin VI. Am J Physiol Cell Physiol 2009;297:C1339−1346.

[121] Riquier AD, Lee DH, McDonough AA. Renal NHE3 and NaPi2 partition into distinct membrane domains. Am J Physiol Cell Physiol 2009;296:C900−910.

[122] Riquier-Brison AD, Leong PK, Pihakaski-Maunsbach K, McDonough AA. Angiotensin II stimulates trafficking of NHE3, NaPi2, and associated proteins into the proximal tubule microvilli. Am J Physiol Renal Physiol 2010;298:F177−186.

[123] Yang LE, Maunsbach AB, Leong PK, McDonough AA. Redistribution of myosin VI from top to base of proximal tubule microvilli during acute hypertension. J Am Soc Nephrol 2005;16:2890–6.

[124] Weinman EJ, Cunningham R, Wade JB, Shenolikar S. The role of NHERF-1 in the regulation of renal proximal tubule sodium-hydrogen exchanger 3 and sodium-dependent phosphate co-transporter 2a. J Physiol 2005;567:27–32.

[125] Wade JB, Liu J, Coleman RA, Cunningham R, Steplock DA, Lee-Kwon W, et al. Localization and interaction of NHERF isoforms in the renal proximal tubule of the mouse. Am J Physiol Cell Physiol 2003;285:C1494–1503.

[126] Wade JB, Welling PA, Donowitz M, Shenolikar S, Weinman EJ. Differential renal distribution of NHERF isoforms and their colocalization with NHE3, ezrin, and ROMK. Am J Physiol Cell Physiol 2001;280:C192–8.

[127] Li Y, Li J, Straight SW, Kershaw DB. PDZ domain-mediated interaction of rabbit podocalyxin and Na$(^+)$/H$(^+)$ exchange regulatory factor-2. Am J Physiol Renal Physiol 2004;282:F1129–39.

[128] Lee-Kwon W, Wade JB, Zhang Z, Pallone TL, Weinman EJ. Expression of TRPC4 channel protein that interacts with NHERF-2 in rat descending vasa recta. Am J Physiol Cell Physiol 2005;288:C942–949.

[129] Montell C. TRP trapped in fly signaling web. Curr Opin Neurobiol 1998;8:389–97.

[130] Yoo D, Flagg TP, Olsen O, Raghuram V, Foskett JK, Welling PA. Assembly and trafficking of a multiprotein ROMK (Kir 1.1) channel complex by PDZ interactions. J Biol Chem 2004;279:6863–73.

[131] Kim JH, Lee-Kwon W, Park JB, Ryu SH, Yun CH, Donowitz M. Ca$(^{2+})$-dependent inhibition of Na$^+$/H$^+$ exchanger 3 (NHE3) requires an NHE3-E3KARP-alpha-actinin-4 complex for oligomerization and endocytosis. J Biol Chem 2002;277:23714–24.

[132] Cha B, Kim JH, Hut H, Hogema BM, Nadarja J, Zizak M, et al. cGMP inhibition of Na$^+$/H$^+$ antiporter 3 (NHE3) requires PDZ domain adapter NHERF2, a broad specificity protein kinase G-anchoring protein. J Biol Chem 2005;280:16642–50.

[133] Lamprecht G, Heil A, Baisch S, Lin-Wu E, Yun CC, Kalbacher H, et al. The down regulated in adenoma (dra) gene product binds to the second PDZ domain of the NHE3 kinase A regulatory protein (E3KARP), potentially linking intestinal Cl$^-$/HCO$_3^-$ exchange to Na$^+$/H$^+$ exchange. Biochemistry 2002;41:12336–42.

[134] Yun CC, Chen Y, Lang F. Glucocorticoid activation of Na$(^+)$/H$(^+)$ exchanger isoform 3 revisited. The roles of SGK1 and NHERF2. J Biol Chem 2002;277:7676–783.

[135] Kanai F, Marignani PA, Sarbassova D, Yagi R, Hall RA, Donowitz M, et al. TAZ: a novel transcriptional co-activator regulated by interactions with 14-3-3 and PDZ domain proteins. Embo J 2000;19:6778–91.

[136] Lee-Kwon W, Kim JH, Choi JW, Kawano K, Cha B, Dartt DA, et al. Ca^{2+}-dependent inhibition of NHE3 requires PKC alpha which binds to E3KARP to decrease surface NHE3 containing plasma membrane complexes. Am J Physiol Cell Physiol 2003;285:C1527–1536.

[137] Yoo D, Kim BY, Campo C, Nance L, King A, Maouyo D, et al. Cell surface expression of the ROMK (Kir 1.1) channel is regulated by the aldosterone-induced kinase, SGK-1, and protein kinase A. J Biol Chem 2003;278:23066–75.

[138] Yun CC, Palmada M, Embark HM, Fedorenko O, Feng Y, Henke G, et al. The serum and glucocorticoid-inducible kinase SGK1 and the Na$(^+)$/H$(^+)$ exchange regulating factor NHERF2 synergize to stimulate the renal outer medullary K$(^+)$ channel ROMK1. J Am Soc Nephrol 2002;13:2823–30.

[139] Yoo D, Fang L, Mason A, Kim BY, Welling PA. A phosphorylation-dependent export structure in ROMK (Kir 1.1) channel overrides an endoplasmic reticulum localization signal. J Biol Chem 2005;280:35281–9.

[140] O'Connell AD, Leng Q, Dong K, MacGregor GG, Giebisch G, Hebert SC. Phosphorylation-regulated endoplasmic reticulum retention signal in the renal outer-medullary K$^+$ channel (ROMK). Proc Natl Acad Sci USA 2005;102:9954–9.

[141] Kocher O, Comella N, Tognazzi K, Brown LF. Identification and partial characterization of PDZK1: A novel protein containing PDZ interaction domains. Lab Invest 1998;78:117–25.

[142] Gisler SM, Madjdpour C, Bacic D, Pribanic S, Taylor SS, Biber J, et al. PDZK1: II. An anchoring site for the PKA-binding protein D-AKAP2 in renal proximal tubular cells. Kidney Int 2003;64:1746–54.

[143] van de Graaf SF, Hoenderop JG, van der Kemp AW, Gisler SM, Bindels RJ. Interaction of the epithelial Ca^{2+} channels TRPV5 and TRPV6 with the intestine- and kidney-enriched PDZ protein NHERF4. Pflugers Arch 2006;452:407–17.

[144] Kocher O, Pal R, Roberts M, Cirovic C, Gilchrist A. Targeted disruption of the PDZK1 gene by homologous recombination. Mol Cell Biol 2003;23:1175–80.

[145] Thomson RB, Wang T, Thomson BR, Tarrats L, Girardi A, Mentone S, et al. Role of PDZK1 in membrane expression of renal brush border ion exchangers. Proc Natl Acad Sci USA 2005;102:13331–6.

[146] Capuano P, Bacic D, Stange G, Hernando N, Kaissling B, Pal R, et al. Expression and regulation of the renal Na/phosphate co-transporter NaPi-IIa in a mouse model deficient for the PDZ protein PDZK1. Pflugers Arch 2005;449:392–402.

[147] Lanzano L, Lei T, Okamura K, Giral H, Caldas Y, Masihzadeh O, et al. Differential modulation of the molecular dynamics of the type IIa and IIc sodium phosphate co-transporters by parathyroid hormone. Am J Physiol Cell Physiol 2011;301:C850–861.

[148] Sheng M, Kim E. The Shank family of scaffold proteins. J Cell Sci 2000;113(Pt 11):1851–6.

[149] Lim S, Naisbitt S, Yoon J, Hwang JI, Suh PG, Sheng M, et al. Characterization of the Shank family of synaptic proteins. Multiple genes, alternative splicing, and differential expression in brain and development. J Biol Chem 1999;274:29510–8.

[150] Mosavi LK, Cammett TJ, Desrosiers DC, Peng ZY. The ankyrin repeat as molecular architecture for protein recognition. Protein Sci 2004;13:1435–48.

[151] Baron MK, Boeckers TM, Vaida B, Faham S, Gingery M, Sawaya MR, et al. An architectural framework that may lie at the core of the postsynaptic density. Science 2006;311:531–5.

[152] Hayashi MK, Tang C, Verpelli C, Narayanan R, Stearns MH, Xu RM, et al. The postsynaptic density proteins Homer and Shank form a polymeric network structure. Cell 2009;137:159–71.

[153] Kay BK, Williamson MP, Sudol M. The importance of being proline: The interaction of proline-rich motifs in signaling proteins with their cognate domains. FASEB Journal 2000;14:231–41.

[154] Xiao B, Tu JC, Worley PF. Homer: a link between neural activity and glutamate receptor function. Curr Opin Neurobiol, 10. 2000.

[155] Berkel S, Marshall CR, Weiss B, Howe J, Roeth R, Moog U, et al. Mutations in the SHANK2 synaptic scaffolding gene in autism spectrum disorder and mental retardation. Nat Genet 2010;42:489–91.

[156] Kim JY, Han W, Namkung W, Lee JH, Kim KH, Shin H, et al. Inhibitory regulation of cystic fibrosis transmembrane conductance regulator anion-transporting activities by Shank2. J Biol Chem 2004;279:10389–96.

[157] Lee JS, Lee YM, Kim JY, Park HW, Grinstein S, Orlowski J, et al. BetaPix up-regulates Na$^+$/H$^+$ exchanger 3 through a Shank2-mediated protein–protein interaction. J Biol Chem 2010;285:8104–13.

[158] Alexander RT, Furuya W, Szaszi K, Orlowski J, Grinstein S. Rho GTPases dictate the mobility of the Na/H exchanger NHE3 in epithelia: Role in apical retention and targeting. Proc Natl Acad Sci USA 2005;102:12253–8.

[159] McWilliams RR, Breusegem SY, Brodsky KF, Kim E, Levi M, Doctor RB. Shank2E binds NaP(i) co-transporter at the apical membrane of proximal tubule cells. Am J Physiol Cell Physiol 2005;289:C1042–1051.

[160] Dobrinskikh E, Giral H, Caldas YA, Levi M, Doctor RB. Shank2 redistributes with NaPilla during regulated endocytosis. Am J Physiol Cell Physiol 2010;299:C1324–1334.

[161] Okamoto PM, Gamby C, Wells D, Fallon J, Vallee RB. Dynamin isoform-specific interaction with the shank/ProSAP scaffolding proteins of the postsynaptic density and actin cytoskeleton. J Biol Chem 2001;276:48458–65.

[162] Kaech SM, Whitfield CW, Kim SK. The LIN-2/LIN-7/LIN-10 complex mediates basolateral membrane localization of the C. elegans EGF receptor LET-23 in vulval epithelial cells. Cell 1998;94:761–71.

[163] Rongo C, Whitfield CW, Rodal A, Kim SK, Kaplan JM. LIN-10 is a shared component of the polarized protein localization pathways in neurons and epithelia. Cell 1998;94:751–9.

[164] Simske JS, Kaech SM, Harp SA, Kim SK. LET-23 receptor localization by the cell junction protein LIN-7 during C. elegans vulval induction. Cell 1996;85:195–204.

[165] Borg JP, Straight SW, Kaech SM, de Taddeo-Borg M, Kroon DE, Karnak D, et al. Identification of an evolutionarily conserved heterotrimeric protein complex involved in protein targeting. J Biol Chem 1998;273:31633–6.

[166] Butz S, Okamoto M, Sudhof TC. A tripartite protein complex with the potential to couple synaptic vesicle exocytosis to cell adhesion in brain. Cell 1998;94:773–82.

[167] Olsen O, Liu H, Wade JB, Merot J, Welling PA. Basolateral membrane expression of the Kir 2.3 channel is coordinated by PDZ interaction with Lin-7/CASK complex. Am J Physiol Cell Physiol 2002;282:C183–95.

[168] Perego C, Vanoni C, Villa A, Longhi R, Kaech SM, Frohli E, et al. PDZ-mediated interactions retain the epithelial GABA transporter on the basolateral surface of polarized epithelial cells. EMBO J 1999;18:2384–93.

[169] Leonoudakis D, Conti LR, Anderson S, Radeke CM, McGuire LM, Adams ME, et al. Protein trafficking and anchoring complexes revealed by proteomic analysis of inward rectifier potassium channel (Kir2.x)-associated proteins. J Biol Chem 2004;279:22331–46.

[170] Leonoudakis D, Conti LR, Radeke CM, McGuire LM, Vandenberg CA. A multiprotein trafficking complex composed of SAP97, CASK, Veli, and Mint1 is associated with inward rectifier Kir2 potassium channels. J Biol Chem 2004;279:19051–63.

[171] Shelly M, Mosesson Y, Citri A, Lavi S, Zwang Y, Melamed-Book N, et al. Polar expression of ErbB-2/HER2 in epithelia. Bimodal regulation by Lin-7. 2003;5: 475–86.

[172] Massari S, Perego C, Padovano V, D'Amico A, Raimondi A, Francolini M, et al. LIN7 mediates the recruitment of IRSp53 to tight junctions. Traffic 2009;10:246–57.

[173] Lee S, Fan S, Makarova O, Straight S, Margolis B. A novel and conserved protein–protein interaction domain of mammalian Lin-2/CASK binds and recruits SAP97 to the lateral surface of epithelia. Mol Cell Biol 2002;22:1778–91.

[174] Doerks T, Bork P, Kamberov E, Makarova O, Muecke S, Margolis B. L27, a novel heterodimerization domain in receptor targeting proteins Lin-2 and Lin-7. Trends Biochem Sci 2000;25:317–38.

[175] Feng W, Long JF, Fan JS, Suetake T, Zhang M. The tetrameric L27 domain complex as an organization platform for supramolecular assemblies. Nat Struct Mol Biol 2004;11:475–80.

[176] Li Y, Karnak D, Demeler B, Margolis B, Lavie A. Structural basis for L27 domain-mediated assembly of signaling and cell polarity complexes. Embo J 2004;23:2723–33.

[177] Alewine C, Kim BY, Hegde V, Welling PA. Lin-7 targets the Kir 2.3 channel on the basolateral membrane via a L27 domain interaction with CASK. Am J Physiol Cell Physiol 2007;293: C1733–1741.

[178] Lozovatsky L, Abayasekara N, Piawah S, Walther Z. CASK deletion in intestinal epithelia causes mislocalization of LIN7C and the DLG1/Scrib polarity complex without affecting cell polarity. Mol Biol Cell 2009;20:4489–99.

[179] Okamoto M, Sudhof TC. Mints, Munc18-interacting proteins in synaptic vesicle exocytosis. J Biol Chem 1997;272:31459–64.

[180] Setou M, Nakagawa T, Seog DH, Hirokawa N. Kinesin superfamily motor protein KIF17 and mLin-10 in NMDA receptor-containing vesicle transport. Science 2000;288:1796–802.

[181] Hata Y, Slaughter CA, Sudhof TC. Synaptic vesicle fusion complex contains unc-18 homologue bound to syntaxin. Nature 1993;366:347–51.

[182] Perego C, Bulbarelli A, Longhi R, Caimi M, Villa A, Caplan MJ. Sorting of two polytopic proteins, the gamma-aminobutyric acid and betaine transporters, in polarized epithelial cells. J Biol Chem 1997;272:6584–92.

[183] Straight SW, Chen L, Karnak D, Margolis B. Interaction with mLin-7 alters the targeting of endocytosed transmembrane proteins in mammalian epithelial cells. Mol Biol Cell 2001;12:1329–40.

[184] Marble DD, Hegle AP, Snyder 2nd ED, Dimitratos S, Bryant PJ, Wilson GF. Camguk/CASK enhances Ether-a-go-go potassium current by a phosphorylation-dependent mechanism. J Neurosci 2005;25:4898–907.

[185] Mukherjee K, Sharma M, Urlaub H, Bourenkov GP, Jahn R, Sudhof TC, et al. CASK functions as an Mg^{2+}-independent neurexin kinase. Cell 2008;133:328–39.

[186] Olsen O, Funke L, Long JF, Fukata M, Kazuta T, Trinidad JC, et al. Renal defects associated with improper polarization of the CRB and DLG polarity complexes in MALS-3 knockout mice. J Cell Biol 2007;179:151–64.

[187] Kamberov E, Makarova O, Roh M, Liu A, Karnak D, Straight S, et al. Molecular cloning and characterization of Pals, proteins associated with mLin-7. J Biol Chem 2000;275:11425–31.

[188] Roh MH, Makarova O, Liu CJ, Shin K, Lee S, Laurinec S, et al. The Maguk protein, Pals1, functions as an adapter, linking mammalian homologues of Crumbs and Discs Lost. J Cell Biol 2002;157:161–72.

[189] Lapidos KA, Kakkar R, McNally EM. The dystrophin glycoprotein complex: Signaling strength and integrity for the sarcolemma. Circ Res 2004;94:1023–31.

[190] Gee SH, Madhavan R, Levinson SR, Caldwell JH, Sealock R, Froehner SC. Interaction of muscle and brain sodium channels with multiple members of the syntrophin family of dystrophin-associated proteins. J Neurosci 1998;18:128–37.

[191] Schultz J, Hoffmuller U, Krause G, Ashurst J, Macias MJ, Schmieder P, et al. Specific interactions between the syntrophin PDZ domain and voltage-gated sodium channels. Nat Struct Biol 1998;5:19–24.

[192] Grady RM, Grange RW, Lau KS, Maimone MM, Nichol MC, et al. Role for alpha-dystrobrevin in the pathogenesis of dystrophin-dependent muscular dystrophies. Nat Cell Biol 1999;1:215—20.

[193] Haenggi T, Schaub MC, Fritschy JM. Molecular heterogeneity of the dystrophin-associated protein complex in the mouse kidney nephron: differential alterations in the absence of utrophin and dystrophin. Cell Tissue Res 2005;319:299—313.

[194] Loh NY, Newey SE, Davies KE, Blake DJ. Assembly of multiple dystrobrevin-containing complexes in the kidney. J Cell Sci 2000;113(Pt 15):2715—24.

[195] Keep NH, Winder SJ, Moores CA, Walke S, Norwood FL, Kendrick-Jones J. Crystal structure of the actin-binding region of utrophin reveals a head-to-tail dimer. Structure 1999;7:1539—46.

[196] James M, Nuttall A, Ilsley JL, Ottersbach K, Tinsley JM, Sudol M, et al. Adhesion-dependent tyrosine phosphorylation of (beta)-dystroglycan regulates its interaction with utrophin. J Cell Sci 2000;113(Pt 10):1717—26.

[197] Newey SE, Benson MA, Ponting CP, Davies KE, Blake DJ. Alternative splicing of dystrobrevin regulates the stoichiometry of syntrophin binding to the dystrophin protein complex. Curr Biol 2000;10:1295—8.

[198] Connors NC, Adams ME, Froehner SC, Kofuji P. The potassium channel Kir4.1 associates with the dystrophin—glycoprotein complex via alpha-syntrophin in glia. J Biol Chem 2004;279:28387—92.

[199] Neely JD, Amiry-Moghaddam M, Ottersen OP, Froehner SC, Agre P, Adams ME. Syntrophin-dependent expression and localization of Aquaporin-4 water channel protein. Proc Natl Acad Sci USA 2001;98:14108—13.

[200] Amiry-Moghaddam M, Otsuka T, Hurn PD, Traystman RJ, Haug FM, Froehner SC, et al. An alpha-syntrophin-dependent pool of AQP4 in astroglial end-feet confers bidirectional water flow between blood and brain. Proc Natl Acad Sci USA 2003;100:2106—11.

[201] Amiry-Moghaddam M, Williamson A, Palomba M, Eid T, de Lanerolle NC, Nagelhus EA, et al. Delayed K$^+$ clearance associated with aquaporin-4 mislocalization: Phenotypic defects in brains of alpha-syntrophin-null mice. Proc Natl Acad Sci USA 2003;100:13615—20.

[202] Nielsen S, Frokiaer J, Marples D, Kwon TH, Agre P, Knepper MA. Aquaporins in the kidney: From molecules to medicine. Physiol Rev 2002;82:205—44.

[203] Ito M, Inanobe A, Horio Y, Hibino H, Isomoto S, Ito H, et al. Immunolocalization of an inwardly rectifying K$^+$ channel, K (AB)-2 (Kir4.1), in the basolateral membrane of renal distal tubular epithelia. FEBS Letters 1996;388:11—5.

[204] Deconinck AE, Potter AC, Tinsley JM, Wood SJ, Vater R, Young C, et al. Postsynaptic abnormalities at the neuromuscular junctions of utrophin-deficient mice. J Cell Biol 1997;136:883—94.

[205] Lohmann SM, DeCamilli P, Einig I, Walter U. High-affinity binding of the regulatory subunit (RII) of cAMP-dependent protein kinase to microtubule-associated and other cellular proteins. Proc Natl Acad Sci USA 1984;81:6723—7.

[206] Fraser ID, Scott JD. Modulation of ion channels: a "current" view of AKAPs. Neuron 1999;23:423—6.

[207] Baumgartner M, Patel H, Barber DL. Na($^+$)/H($^+$) exchanger NHE1 as plasma membrane scaffold in the assembly of signaling complexes. Am J Physiol Cell Physiol 2004;287:C844—850.

[208] Banky P, Newlon MG, Roy M, Garrod S, Taylor SS, Jennings PA. Isoform-specific differences between the type Ialpha and IIalpha cyclic AMP-dependent protein kinase anchoring domains revealed by solution NMR. J Biol Chem 2000;275:35146—52.

[209] Newlon MG, Roy M, Morikis D, Carr DW, Westphal R, Scott JD, et al. A novel mechanism of PKA anchoring revealed by solution structures of anchoring complexes. Embo J 2001;20:1651—62.

[210] Newlon MG, Roy M, Morikis D, Hausken ZE, Coghlan V, Scott JD, et al. The molecular basis for protein kinase A anchoring revealed by solution NMR. Nat Struct Biol 1999;6:222—7.

[211] Huang LJ, Wang L, Ma Y, Durick K, Perkins G, Deerinck TJ, et al. NH2-Terminal targeting motifs direct dual specificity A-kinase-anchoring protein 1 (D-AKAP1) to either mitochondria or endoplasmic reticulum. J Cell Biol 1999;145:951—9.

[212] Means CK, Lygren B, Langeberg LK, Jain A, Dixon RE, Vega AL, et al. An entirely specific type I A-kinase anchoring protein that can sequester two molecules of protein kinase A at mitochondria. Proc Natl Acad Sci USA 2011;108:E1227—1235.

[213] Alto NM, Soderling SH, Hoshi N, Langeberg LK, Fayos R, Jennings PA, et al. Bioinformatic design of A-kinase anchoring protein-in silico: A potent and selective peptide antagonist of type II protein kinase A anchoring. Proc Natl Acad Sci USA 2003;100:4445—50.

[214] Burns-Hamuro LL, Ma Y, Kammerer S, Reineke U, Self C, Cook C, et al. Designing isoform-specific peptide disruptors of protein kinase A localization. Proc Natl Acad Sci USA 2003;100:4072—7.

[215] Wong W, Scott JD. AKAP signalling complexes: Focal points in space and time. Nat Rev Mol Cell Biol 2004;5:959—70.

[216] Dong F, Feldmesser M, Casadevall A, Rubin CS. Molecular characterization of a cDNA that encodes six isoforms of a novel murine A kinase anchor protein. J Biol Chem 1998;273:6533—41.

[217] Morales FC, Takahashi Y, Kreimann EL, Georgescu MM. Ezrin-radixin-moesin (ERM)-binding phosphoprotein 50 organizes ERM proteins at the apical membrane of polarized epithelia. Proc Natl Acad Sci USA 2004;101:17705—10.

[218] Trotter KW, Fraser ID, Scott GK, Stutts MJ, Scott JD, Milgram SL. Alternative splicing regulates the subcellular localization of A-kinase anchoring protein 18 isoforms. J Cell Biol 1999;147:1481—92.

[219] Khundmiri SJ, Rane MJ, Lederer ED. Parathyroid hormone regulation of type II sodium-phosphate co-transporters is dependent on an A kinase anchoring protein. J Biol Chem 2003;278:10134—41.

[220] Gao T, Yatani A, Dell'Acqua ML, Sako H, Green SA, Dascal N, et al. cAMP-dependent regulation of cardiac L-type Ca^{2+} channels requires membrane targeting of PKA and phosphorylation of channel subunits. Neuron 1997;19:185—96.

[221] Hoshi N, Zhang JS, Omaki M, Takeuchi T, Yokoyama S, Wanaverbecq N, et al. AKAP150 signaling complex promotes suppression of the M-current by muscarinic agonists. Nat Neurosci 2003;6:564—71.

[222] Carr DW, Stofko-Hahn RE, Fraser ID, Bishop SM, Acott TS, Brennan RG, et al. Interaction of the regulatory subunit (RII) of cAMP-dependent protein kinase with RII-anchoring proteins occurs through an amphipathic helix binding motif. J Biol Chem 1991;266:14188—92.

[223] Rosenmund C, Carr DW, Bergeson SE, Nilaver G, Scott JD, Westbrook GL. Anchoring of protein kinase A is required for modulation of AMPA/kainate receptors on hippocampal neurons. Nature 1994;368:853—6.

[224] Coghlan VM, Perrino BA, Howard M, Langeberg LK, Hicks JB, Gallatin WM, et al. Association of protein kinase A

and protein phosphatase 2B with a common anchoring protein. Science 1995;267:108—11.

[225] Klauck TM, Faux MC, Labudda K, Langeberg LK, Jaken S, Scott JD. Coordination of three signaling enzymes by AKAP79, a mammalian scaffold protein. Science 1996;271:1589—92.

[226] Hoshi N, Langeberg LK, Scott JD. Distinct enzyme combinations in AKAP signalling complexes permit functional diversity. Nat Cell Biol 2005;7:1066—73.

[227] Klussmann E, Maric K, Wiesner B, Beyermann M, Rosenthal W. Protein kinase A anchoring proteins are required for vasopressin-mediated translocation of aquaporin-2 into cell membranes of renal principal cells. J Biol Chem 1999;274:4934—8.

[228] Jo I, Ward DT, Baum MA, Scott JD, Coghlan VM, Hammond TG, et al. AQP2 is a substrate for endogenous PP2B activity within an inner medullary AKAP-signaling complex. Am J Physiol Renal Physiol 2001;281:F958—965.

[229] Henn V, Edemir B, Stefan E, Wiesner B, Lorenz D, Theilig F, et al. Identification of a novel A-kinase anchoring protein 18 isoform and evidence for its role in the vasopressin-induced aquaporin-2 shuttle in renal principal cells. J Biol Chem 2004;279:26654—65.

[230] McSorley T, Stefan E, Henn V, Wiesner B, Baillie GS, Houslay MD, et al. Spatial organisation of AKAP18 and PDE4 isoforms in renal collecting duct principal cells. Eur J Cell Biol 2006;85:673—8.

[231] MacGregor GG, Xu JZ, McNicholas CM, Giebisch G, Hebert SC. Partially active channels produced by PKA site mutation of the cloned renal K^+ channel, ROMK2 (kir1.2). Am J Physiol 1998;275:F415—22.

[232] Xu ZC, Yang Y, Hebert SC. Phosphorylation of the ATP-sensitive, inwardly rectifying K^+ channel, ROMK, by cyclic AMP-dependent protein kinase. J Biol Chem 1996;271:9313—9.

[233] Ali S, Chen X, Lu M, Xu JZ, Lerea KM, Hebert SC, et al. The A kinase anchoring protein is required for mediating the effect of protein kinase A on ROMK1 channels. Proc Natl Acad Sci USA 1998;95:10274—1028.

[234] Ali S, Wei Y, Lerea KM, Becker L, Rubin CS, Wang W. PKA-induced stimulation of ROMK1 channel activity is governed by both tethering and non-tethering domains of an A kinase anchor protein. Cell Physiol Biochem 2001;11:135—42.

[235] Donowitz M, Mohan S, Zhu CX, Chen TE, Lin R, Cha B, et al. NHE3 regulatory complexes. J Exp Biol 2009;212:1638—46.

[236] Xie Z. Molecular mechanisms of Na/K-ATPase-mediated signal transduction. Ann NY Acad Sci 2003;986:497—503.

[237] Yuan Z, Cai T, Tian J, Ivanov AV, Giovannucci DR, Xie Z. Na/K-ATPase tethers phospholipase C and IP3 receptor into a calcium-regulatory complex. Mol Biol Cell 2005;16:4034—45.

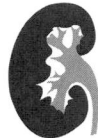

CHAPTER

15

The Renin–Angiotensin System

Thu H. Le[1], Steven D. Crowley[2], Susan B. Gurley[2] and Thomas M. Coffman[2,3]

[1]Division of Nephrology, Department of Medicine, University of Virginia, Charlottesville, VA, USA
[2]Division of Nephrology, Department of Medicine, Duke University and Durham VA Medical Centers, Durham, North Carolina, USA
[3]Cardiovascular and Metabolic Disorders Research Program, Duke-NUS, Singapore

Highly conserved through phylogeny, the renin–angiotensin system (RAS) is an essential regulator of blood pressure and fluid balance. This biological system is a multi-enzymatic cascade in which angiotensinogen, its major substrate, is processed in a two-step reaction by renin- and angiotensin-converting enzyme (ACE), resulting in the sequential generation of angiotensin I and angiotensin II. Along with its importance in maintaining normal circulatory homeostasis, abnormal activation of the RAS can contribute to the development of hypertension and target organ damage.

The importance of the RAS in clinical medicine is highlighted by two sets of observations. First are associations between polymorphisms of genes encoding RAS components and cardiovascular disease.[1–6] Second, and perhaps more compelling, is the impressive efficacy of pharmacological agents that inhibit the synthesis or activity of angiotensin II. For example, angiotensin converting enzyme (ACE) inhibitors are very effective and well-tolerated anti-hypertensive agents.[7] Along with their ability to lower blood pressure, these agents also effectively prevent or ameliorate morbidity and mortality associated with cardiovascular diseases. In this regard, large clinical trials have demonstrated that ACE inhibitors improve survival in patients with congestive heart failure,[8,9] and in patients with risk factors for coronary artery disease.[10] They also slow the progression of a variety of kidney diseases, including diabetic nephropathy.[11] Angiotensin receptor blockers (ARBs), which block AT_1 receptors, are similarly effective for treating these disorders.[12–14] The purpose of this chapter is to provide an overview of the major physiological features of the RAS, focusing on its role in the kidney.

THE COMPONENTS OF THE RENIN–ANGIOTENSIN SYSTEM

Renin

The aspartyl protease renin was first isolated from the kidney by Tigerstedt more than a century ago. Renin is synthesized as a precursor protein, pro-renin, containing an additional 43 amino acids at the N-terminus that block the enzyme's active site.[15] Active renin is generated by removal of this N-terminal peptide fragment, presumably by proteases in the juxtaglomerular cells of the kidney. Whether intact pro-renin has a distinct physiological role remains to be determined; however, there is accumulating evidence suggesting specific contributions of the pro-renin molecule in some normal and disease states.[16–19]

Active renin specifically cleaves the 10 amino acids from the N-terminus of angiotensinogen to form angiotensin I. A substantial excess of angiotensinogen is present in serum, and ACE is ubiquitous in the endothelium and plasma.[20] Accordingly, in the bloodstream, the amount of renin is the rate-limiting step determining the level of angiotensin II, and thus the activity of the system. The primary source of renin in the circulation is the kidney, where its expression and secretion are tightly regulated at the juxtaglomerular apparatus by two distinct mechanisms: a renal baroreceptor[21,22] and sodium chloride delivery to the macula densa.[23–25] Through these sensing mechanisms, levels of renin in plasma can be incrementally titrated in response to changes in blood pressure and salt balance. These regulatory principles provide a basis for many of the physiological characteristics of the RAS, and regulation of renin release in the kidney will be discussed in detail below.

Seldin and Giebisch's The Kidney, Fifth Edition.
DOI: http://dx.doi.org/10.1016/B978-0-12-381462-3.00015-X

In addition to its protease activity, renin may also bind specifically to other proteins or putative receptors.[19,26–28] This binding may induce physiologically significant intracellular signaling.[27] It has been suggested that the mannose-6-phosphate receptor (M6P-R), also known as insulin-like growth factor II receptor, binds renin and pro-renin, leading to internalization and degradation.[26] Nguyen et al. reported cloning a receptor from human kidney expression library that binds renin and pro-renin specifically and with high affinity, termed the (pro)renin receptor (PRR). Binding of PRR causes a conformational change of renin that leads to increased renin catalytic activity. Similarly, binding of PRR to pro-renin causes a conformational change, resulting in an ezymatically active pro-renin without the requirement for cleavage of the pro-segment. Furthermore, binding of renin to this receptor induces a rapid and sustained activation of ERK1/ERK2, without affecting concentrations of calcium or cAMP.[27] It has been suggested that it may mediate angiotensin II-independent effects of renin, and might also indicate a functional role of pro-renin.[29] Although the physiological significance of PRR remains unclear, recent studies suggest PRR may have a role in blood pressure regulation. Transgenic rats overexpressing human PRR selectively in vascular smooth muscle cells display elevated blood pressure and heart rate.[30,31] In addition, human PRR gene polymorphism has been shown to be associated with ambulatory blood pressure in Japanese men.[32] PRR may also play a role in development. Deletion of PRR in mice results in early embryonic lethality.[33] In a family with X-linked mental retardation and epilepsy, linkage analysis identified an exonic splice enhancer in the PRR gene as the only mutation, and this resulted in the loss of the capacity of renin to phosphorylate ERK1/2.[34]

The pro-renin receptor appears to have other functions independent of the renin–angiotensin system. For example, it is found as part of a complex required for the normal function of V-ATPase in several cell lineages, including cardiac myocytes.[35] The pro-renin receptor acts as an adaptor between the Wnt receptor and V-ATPase in a Wnt/β-catenin signaling complex required for normal CNS development.[36] Thus, deletion of the pro-renin receptor gene causes a lethal phenotype at a very early embryonic stage, which contrasts significantly with the phenotype of renin knockouts,[37] indicating important functions of the receptor that are independent of its actions in the RAS. Two groups have recently described studies of mouse lines in which the pro-renin receptor was deleted specifically from podocytes. In both cases, there was a similar, dramatic phenotype characterized by disruption of the glomerular filtration barrier, with marked proteinuria and abnormal podocyte structure, perhaps due to dysregulated autophagy.[38,39] Thus, while this molecule appears to play a critical role in the kidney, much remains to be learned about its functions in normal kidney physiology and disease, including the extent to which these functions are influenced by renin or pro-renin binding.

Angiotensinogen

Angiotensinogen, the substrate for renin, is the source of all angiotensin peptides. Angiotensinogen in the circulation is derived primarily from synthesis in the liver. In humans, plasma concentrations of angiotensinogen are typically near the Km for renin,[40] so that changes in plasma concentration may influence the rate of angiotensin I generation at any given level of renin. In human hypertensive siblings, Jeunemaitre et al.[2] showed that a specific variant of the human angiotensinogen gene, M235T, was linked to hypertension, and was also associated with a modestly elevated plasma angiotensinogen concentration, about 120% of normal. They proposed that this variant of the AGT gene leads to an increase in plasma angiotensinogen levels and thereby eventually to increased blood pressure. However, because amino acid 235 is in a non-conserved portion of the angiotensinogen protein and variation of this amino acid does not affect protein stability, a mechanism to explain the physiological consequences of the mutation was not clear. An apparent explanation came later, when the M235T variant was found to be in linkage disequilibrium with another variant in the 5′ untranslated region of the AGT gene.[41] This second variant, a single nucleotide substitution in the promoter of the AGT gene, was associated with increased transcriptional activity of the gene.[41] Higher levels of AGT mRNA were found in patients carrying the variant allele.[41] The causal capacity of alterations in plasma angiotensinogen level to affect blood pressure was demonstrated in studies of mice engineered to carry from 0 to 4 copies of the AGT gene.[42] In these animals, there was a positive correlation between the number of AGT gene copies, plasma levels of angiotensinogen, and blood pressure.

In addition to its synthesis by the liver, angiotensinogen is also produced by other tissues including the brain, the immune system, and the kidney.[43] In the kidney, synthesis of angiotensinogen in proximal tubules has been well-documented,[44] and proximal tubule synthesis may be regulated in part by the end-product, angiotensin II.[45] Along with angiotensinogen, the kidney expresses all of the other components of the RAS. Accordingly, it has been suggested that regulation and functioning of autonomous "tissue" renin–angiotensin systems in the kidney, as well as other organs, may contribute to the physiological functions of the system, especially in disease states.[46] This hypothesis has been used to explain additional complexity of the system, whereby the apparent activity of the RAS is not reflected by measured plasma levels of it major components. For example, in the broad population of patients with hypertension, diabetes, and cardiovascular disease, pharmacological antagonists of the RAS lower blood pressure and prevent end-organ damage, even in the absence of overt elevation of plasma renin levels. However, the precise nature and physiological contributions of these tissue systems has been difficult to define experimentally.

Angiotensin Converting Enzyme

Angiotensin converting enzyme (ACE) is a carboxypeptidase that generates the vasoactive peptide angiotensin II by cleaving two amino acids from the c-terminus of the inactive precursor angiotensin I.[47] There are two distinct forms of ACE, somatic and testicular, both generated by alternative splicing of a single gene.[48–50] Somatic ACE is expressed as an ectoenzyme on the surface of endothelial cells throughout the body, and is particularly abundant in lung, intestine, choroid plexus, placenta, and on brush border membranes in the kidney. A soluble form of ACE that circulates in plasma is formed by enzymatic cleavage of tissue-bound ACE at its transmembrane domain.[51] As with other components of the RAS, molecular variants of *ACE* have been proposed as candidate genes in hypertension, cardiovascular, and kidney diseases.[52] Insertion (I) and deletion (D) polymorphisms of the human *ACE* gene are common, and have been associated with altered levels of ACE in plasma.[53,54] In some cohorts, but not others, these *ACE* gene variants have been linked to differing susceptibilities to hypertension, cardiovascular, and renal diseases.[52,55]

In addition to angiotensin I, other biologically active peptides are substrates for ACE. Perhaps the most important of these is bradykinin.[56] ACE degrades bradykinin into an inactive peptide, representing a significant biological pathway for bradykinin metabolism *in vivo*[57]; in older literature, ACE was referred to as kininase II. Since bradykinin has vasodilator and natriuretic properties,[56] it has been suggested that one mechanism of blood pressure reduction with ACE inhibition is blockade of this kininase activity. This was clearly demonstrated by Brown and associates, who showed that the anti-hypertensive efficacy of ACE inhibitors is attenuated by simultaneous administration of a bradykinin receptor antagonist.[58]

Using genome-based strategies, homologs of ACE have been identified.[59–61] One of these, ACE2, exhibits more than 40% identity at the protein level with the catalytic domain of ACE.[59,60] Similar to ACE, ACE2 is expressed on the surface of certain endothelial cell populations. However, compared to the ubiquitous distribution of ACE, the expression pattern of ACE2 is more limited, with most abundant expression in kidney followed by heart and testis.[59,60] Their substrate specificities also differ; ACE2 hydrolyzes angiotensin II with high efficiency, but has much lower activity against angiotensin I.[59,62] Hydrolysis of angiotensin II by ACE2 generates another peptide with putative biological actions: angiotensin 1-7.[62] Accumulating evidence indicates that this peptide causes vasodilation, natriuresis, and may promote reduced blood pressures[63] via the Mas receptor.[64] It has been further suggested that ACE2 may be a major pathway for synthesis of angiotensin 1-7.[65] Thus, the functions of ACE2 may be determined by its distinct actions to metabolize angiotensin II and to generate angiotensin 1-7.

Although the precise physiological role of ACE2 is not clear, it was originally identified and cloned from a cDNA library prepared from ventricular tissue of a patient with heart failure.[59] Initial studies in ACE2-deficient mice have suggested a role for ACE2 in cardiac function[364,365] and in blood pressure regulation.[66] More recent work by many groups has demonstrated roles for ACE2 in renal diseases, such as diabetic and non-diabetic kidney disease,[67–70] and hypertension[67,71,72] in both experimental models and human cohorts.

A third member of the ACE gene family, collectrin, was identified as a gene that is upregulated in the subtotal nephrectomy model of chronic kidney disease.[73] Collectrin is highly homologous to the transmembrane portion of ACE2, but lacks the carboxypeptidase domain.[61] Its physiological functions are emerging[74,75] and appear to regulate amino acid transport by the kidney.

Angiotensin Receptors

The biological actions of angiotensin II are mediated by cell surface receptors that belong to the large family of 7 transmembrane receptors.[7,76] The angiotensin receptors can be divided into two pharmacological classes, type 1 (AT_1) and type 2 (AT_2), based on their different affinities for various non-peptide antagonists (Figure 15.1). Studies using these antagonists suggested that most of the classically recognized functions of the RAS are mediated by AT_1 receptors.[76] Gene targeting studies have confirmed these conclusions.[77]

AT_1 receptors from a number of species have been cloned[78–80] and two subtypes, designated AT_{1A} and

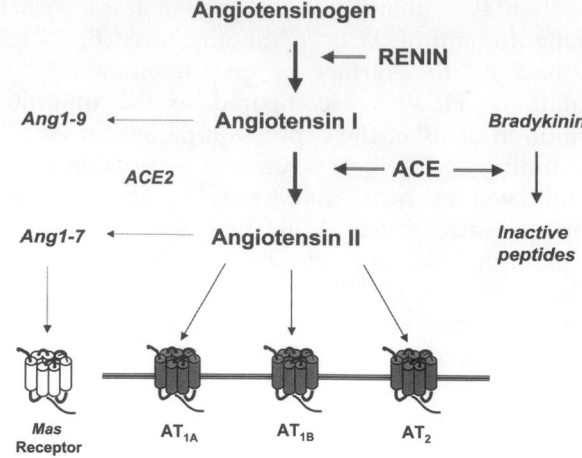

FIGURE 15.1 Angiotensinogen is cleaved by renin to form angiotensin I, which is then cleaved by angiotensin-converting enzyme (ACE) to form angiontesin II, the major effector molecule of the RAS. The biological effects of angiotensin II are mediated by the G-protein-coupled seven-transmembrane cell surface receptors AT1 and AT2. Angiotensin II is hydrolyzed by angiotensin-converting enzyme 2 (ACE2), a homologue of ACE. This hydrolysis results in the generation of the angiotensin 1–7 peptide, the actions of which are mediated by the *Mas* receptor. After: *Le, TH and Coffman TM. Targeting genes in the renin-angiotensin system. Current Opinion in Nephrology and Hypertension 2008, 17:57-63. Lippincott Williams & Wilkins.*

AT_{1B}, have been identified in rat[81–83] and mouse.[84] In the classical view, AT_1 receptors signal through $G_{\alpha q}$-linked signaling pathways involving phospholipase C, IP3, and increases in intracellular calcium.[85] However, the AT_1 receptor has also been linked to JAK/STAT activation,[86] as well as β-arrestin-dependent pathways linked to ERK activation.[87–89] In addition, recent studies have shown that the AT1 receptor has the capacity to transactivate the EGF receptor, which may be independent of ligand.[90,91] This pathway may contribute to chronic kidney injury.[92]

The murine AT_1 receptors are products of separate genes and share substantial sequence homology.[83,93,94] AT_{1A} receptors predominate in most organs, except the adrenal gland and regions of the CNS, where AT_{1B} expression may be more prominent.[93,95,96] A single report has suggested that AT_{1B} receptors might also exist in man,[97] but this has not been confirmed in the unpublished work of several independent groups, and the consensus view is that there is no human counterpart to the murine AT_{1B} receptor. Thus, the AT_{1A} receptor is considered the closest murine homolog to the single human AT_1 receptor.

The binding signatures of the AT_{1A} and AT_{1B} receptors are virtually identical,[98] and it was difficult to discriminate their *in vivo* functions pharmacologically. Experiments using gene targeting have provided insights into the discrete functions of the two AT_1

receptor genes.[99,100] Although the AT_{1B} receptor has a unique role to mediate thirst responses in the CNS,[101] AT_{1A} receptors have the predominant role in determining the level of blood pressure,[102–104] and in mediating vasoconstrictor responses.[99,102] The phenotype of markedly reduced blood pressures and profound sodium sensitivity in mice lacking the AT_{1A} receptor[102,105] underscores its importance in blood pressure control.

Pharmacological and genetic studies have confirmed that virtually all of the classically recognized functions of the RAS are mediated by AT_1 receptors. Until recently, little was known about the physiological role of AT_2 receptors. AT_2 receptors are found in abundance during fetal development,[106,107] but their expression generally falls after birth. However, persistent AT_2 receptor expression can be detected in several adult tissues including the kidney, adrenal gland and the brain, and absolute levels of AT_2 receptor expression may be modulated by angiotensin II and certain growth factors.[108] AT_2 receptors appear to signal by coupling to $G_{\alpha i2}$ and $G_{\alpha i3}$ proteins.[109] Using site-directed mutagenesis, the intermediate portion of the third intracellular loop of the AT_2 receptor was found to be necessary for normal receptor signaling.[110,111] Moreover, it has been suggested that activation of AT_2 receptors stimulates bradykinin, nitric oxide, and guanosine cyclic 3′,5′-monophosphate (cGMP),[112,113] and these pathways may mediate actions of the receptor to promote natriuresis and blood pressure lowering. Finally, there is also evidence to support HETEs as second messengers for AT_2 receptors in the kidney, leading to ERK1/2 phosphorylation.[114]

Targeted disruption of the mouse *Agtr2* gene did not cause a dramatically abnormal phenotype. These animals clearly manifest increased sensitivity to the pressor actions of angiotensin II.[115,116] One of the AT_2 deficient lines manifested increased baseline blood pressure and heart rate.[115] Interestingly, behavioral changes were also observed in AT_2-deficient mice. They had decreased spontaneous movements and rearing activity,[115,116] and impaired drinking response to water deprivation.[116] Transgenic mice that overexpress the AT_2 receptor gene under control of a cardiac-specific promoter have decreased sensitivity to AT_1-mediated pressor and chronotropic actions.[117] Moreover, the pressor actions of angiotensin II are significantly attenuated in these transgenic mice. This attenuation was completely reversed following pretreatment with a specific AT_2 receptor antagonist. Taken together, these data suggest that a primary function of the AT_2 receptor may be to negatively modulate the actions of the AT_1 receptor. Along similar lines, the recently described non-peptide agonist, compound 21, has been used to uncover additional functions of the AT_2 receptor, which appear quite diverse. Studies with this agonist regarding blood pressure have been variable, but it appears to have minimal effect on blood pressure in normal situations; the potential to affect blood pressure in disease states may be different.[118]

Aldosterone

Aldosterone is a steroid hormone synthesized in the zona glomerulosa (ZG) of the adrenal gland. The two dominant regulators of aldosterone synthesis and release are angiotensin II and the level of serum potassium.[119] The RAS-dependent component of aldosterone regulation is triggered by binding of angiotensin II to AT_1 receptors in the ZG.[119] Stimulation of aldosterone release by angiotensin II contributes to enhanced sodium reabsorption and anti-natriuresis. Independently of angiotensin II, hyperkalemia can control the release of aldosterone through a process that involves the membrane depolarization of ZG cells.[120,121] In addition, adrenocorticotropic hormone (ACTH) can stimulate aldosterone via its G-protein coupled receptor.[121] Elevations in ACTH influence aldosterone production only during short-term stress, as this response is attenuated with persistent exposure to ACTH. In contrast, angiotensin II and potassium can both exert a chronic, sustained stimulation of aldosterone generation by the zona glomerulosa.[122]

The classically recognized effects of aldosterone to influence sodium handling in the distal nephron are mediated by aldosterone binding to the mineralocorticoid receptor (MR). The MR is a 107 kD protein that acts as a transcription factor to regulate gene expression in target tissues. The molecular mechanisms used by the MR to drive epithelial sodium channel (ENaC) function in the collecting tubule have been reviewed recently.[123] Cortisol actually exhibits a higher affinity for the mineralocorticoid receptor than aldosterone, but locally expressed 11ß-hydroxysteroid dehydrogenase type 2 "protects" the MR by converting cortisol to cortisone, which does not activate the MR.[124] The binding of aldosterone to the MR in the principal cell of the collecting tubule epithelium induces transcription of the α-subunit, the multimeric coupling of the α-, β-, and γ-subunits of the EnaC, and the translocation of the ENaC complex to the luminal surface of the tubule.[125,126] Aldosterone-induced expression of the αENaC-subunit, in particular, follows a diurnal variation pattern that depends on the circadian transcription factor Period1.[127]

Aldosterone stimulates ENaC transcription and activity largely through the upregulation of serum- and glucocorticoid-regulated kinase 1 (sgk1).[128–130] At the transcriptional level, Sgk1 phosphorylates ALL1-fused gene from chromosome 9 (Af9), which in turn blocks the repressor effects of the histone H3 Lys79 methyltransferase disruptor of telomeric silencing alternative splice variant a (Dot1a) on αENaC gene transcription.[131] At the post-translational level, Sgk1 phosphorylates Nedd4-2, causing ENaC proteins to remain in the apical membrane of the principal cell.[132,133] Once inserted into the luminal membrane of the principal cell, ENaC permits cellular uptake of intraluminal sodium, generating an electronegative potential in the distal tubular lumen which favors secretion of potassium from the principal cell into the urinary filtrate via the renal outer medullary potassium channel (ROMK). Sgk1 may also phosphorylate ROMK, similarly increasing its apical density, further facilitating the kaliuresis induced by aldosterone.[134] In addition, aldosterone appears to directly increase ROMK expression.[135] Finally, aldosterone modulates sodium transport in the distal nephron independently of ENaC by enhancing expression and activity of the thiazide-sensitive Na-Cl co-transporter (NCC). Sgk-1 mediates this effect by phosphorylating serine/threonine kinase with-no-lysine 4 (WNK4), thereby diminishing the inhibitory effects of WNK4 on NCC activity.[136] Through these pathways, the MR regulates sodium and potassium transport within the mineralocorticoid-responsive segments of the distal nephron.

Recent human phenotyping studies and animal studies using gene-targeting strategies have confirmed the contribution of the MR to tubular function and salt balance. For example, in humans with a mutation leading to a constitutively active MR, early onset hypertension develops,[137] whereas heterozygosity for an inactivating mutation of the MR leads to salt-wasting, hypotension, metabolic acidosis, and hyperkalemia.[138] Mice genetically deficient for the MR similarly develop severe salt-wasting that leads to neonatal death,[139] whereas mice with genetic deletion of the MR restricted to the principal cell waste salt and lose body weight only when exposed to a low-sodium diet,[140] suggesting that at baseline the late distal convoluted tubule and early connecting tubule may be able to compensate for a lack of ENaC activity in the distal nephron. Alternatively, the discrepancy in phenotypes between the global and conditional knockout mice may be due to discrete functions of aldosterone to modulate solute transport in the proximal tubule[141,142] and/or medullary thick ascending limb.[143] Mutations that activate the ENaC may cause hypertension,[144–146] whereas global inactivation of the subunits of the ENaC in mice causes sodium-wasting, potassium retention, and early mortality, and in humans pseudohypoaldosteronism type 1 with severe salt-wasting.[147] In contrast, inactivation of the α-ENaC gene only in the collecting duct does not impair sodium and potassium balance,[148] again indicating that the regulation by aldosterone of ENaC in the latter regions of the distal convoluted tubule and/or the connecting tubule may also contribute to sodium and fluid homeostasis.[149]

In addition to its physiologic effects on renal solute handling, aldosterone has the capacity to mediate direct cellular injury in the kidney.[150] In this regard, pathologic functions of aldosterone in non-tubular renal compartments become increasingly relevant. For example, aldosterone impairs vascular reactivity by diminishing expression of glucose-6-phosphate in the endothelium[151] and mediates direct vascular injury via a placental growth factor-dependent pathway.[152] In mesangial cells, aldosterone activates sgk-1, NF-kB, and MAP kinases, leading to cellular proliferation, generation of oxidative stress, and connective tissue growth factor expression.[153–155] Emerging evidence suggest aldosterone may also promote oxidative stress and apoptosis directly within podocytes.[156,157] Consistent with these pathologic effects of aldosterone in several cell lineages of the kidney glomerulus, human studies have now demonstrated a role for aldosterone blockade in ameliorating the progression of proteinuric kidney disease.[158]

Integrated Actions of the RAS in the Kidney

The important role of the kidney in regulation of blood pressure has been long recognized,[159] and the relationship between alterations in systemic blood pressure and changes in renal sodium excretion is well-documented.[160] For example, an elevation in perfusion pressure in the renal artery results in a rapid increase in sodium and water excretion by the kidney, so-called "pressure natriuresis".[160] Based on such observations, Guyton and co-workers suggested that whenever arterial pressure is elevated, activation of this pressure-natriuresis mechanism will cause sufficient excretion of sodium and water to return systemic pressures to normal.[161] They further hypothesized that the substantial capacity for sodium excretion by the kidney provides a compensatory system of virtually infinite gain to oppose processes, including increases in peripheral vascular resistance, which would tend to increase blood pressure. It follows that defects in renal excretory function would therefore be a pre-requisite for sustaining a chronic increase in intra-arterial pressure.

The RAS has potent actions to modulate pressure-natriuresis relationships in the kidney[162,163] and these actions shape the characteristics of RAS-dependent blood pressure regulation in normal physiology and in disease states. For example, as depicted in Figure 15.2, chronic infusion of angiotensin II causes a shift of the pressure natriuresis curve to the right, suggesting that when the RAS is activated, higher pressures are required to excrete an equivalent sodium load[164] (Figure 15.2). Conversely, administration of ACE inhibitors or ARBs shifts the curve to the left, meaning that natriuresis is facilitated at lower levels of blood pressure (Figure 15.2). The basic features of endogenous control of the RAS are consistent with these homeostatic functions. As shown in Figure 15.2, the system is activated at low levels of salt intake, stimulating renal sodium reabsorption and conservation of body fluid volumes and blood pressure. In contrast, with high sodium intake, the system is suppressed, facilitating natriuresis.

REGULATION OF RENIN

As discussed above, the concentration of renin in plasma is the rate-limiting step in the production of angiotensin II. Accordingly, the activity of the RAS in the circulation is largely determined by the factors that regulate renin. The kidney is the major source of renin, where its generation and secretion are primarily controlled by renal perfusion pressure and by the luminal delivery of sodium chloride to the macula densa in the distal nephron. The major features of these regulatory processes are described in the sections that follow.

Sources of Renin

The major source of renin in the circulation is the kidney. Following bilateral nephrectomy, plasma levels of renin and angiotensin II fall precipitously.[165] In the kidney, the location of renin-expressing cells varies from development through adulthood, and in response to homeostatic challenges. During embryonic development, renin-expressing cells are found in the undifferentiated metanephric mesenchyme.[166] In the fetal kidney, these cells are present in the large intrarenal arteries, glomeruli, and interstitium.[166] In the adult kidney, renin expression is primarily restricted to granular cells which are modified smooth muscle cells within the juxtaglomerular apparatus (JGA). The JGA is located in the region where the afferent arteriole enters the glomerulus.[167,168] As shown in Figure 15.3, the JGA is a highly organized structure composed of three distinct anatomical parts: granular cells, the macula densa, and the extraglomerular mesangial cells.[169] The macula densa is a specialized tubular area that marks the transition from the ascending loop of Henle to the distal tubule lying in direct contact with the vascular pole of the glomerulus from which it originated.[169] By light microscopy, the unique characteristics of the macula densa epithelial cells can be discerned by their narrow, columnar shape and apparent

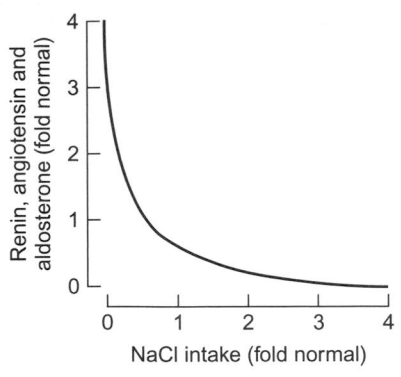

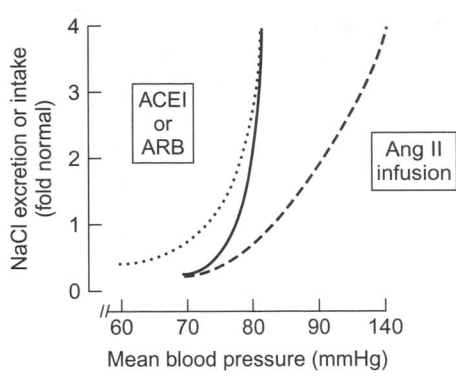

FIGURE 15.2 Chronic infusion of angiotensin II causes a shift of the pressure natriuresis curve to the right. Conversely, administration of ACE inhibitors or ARBs shifts the curve to the left. After: *Guyton, AC et al. In: Hypertension, Pathophysiology, Diagnosis and Management. Laragh, JH and Brenner, BM (Eds). Raven Press, NY (Publ). pp 1311-1326, 1995.*

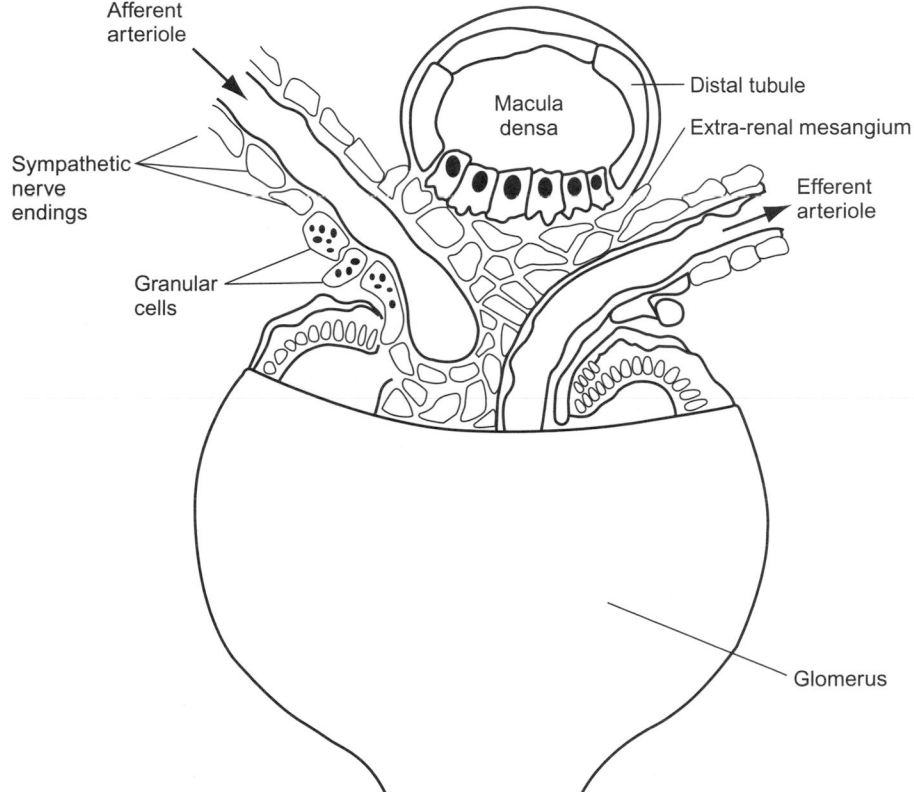

FIGURE 15.3 The juxtaglomerular apparatus (JGA). Integration of the regulated secretion of renin is carried out at the JGA. There are three major pathways regulating the secretion of renin by granular cells at the JGA: the baroreceptor, the macula densa mechanism, and direct stimulation by the sympathetic nervous system. The renal baroreceptor monitors renal perfusion pressure and signals an increase in renin when renal perfusion pressure falls. In the macula densa mechanism, macula densa cells sense the decrease in chloride ions in the filtrate in the distal tubule, thereby stimulating release of renin. Increased activity of renal sympathetic nerves directly stimulates renin release via activation of adrenergic receptors. Sympathetic innervation also modulates both the baroreceptor and macula densa mechanisms. After: *Francois H and Coffman TM. Prostanoids and blood pressure: which way is up? J Clin Invest. 2004; 114(6):757-759. American Society for Clinical Investigation.*

accumulation of nuclei, distinguishing them from cells in the adjacent parts of the distal tubule.[167] By electron microscopy, the basement membrane of the macula densa appears to be fused with the vacular component, and continuous with the basement membranes surrounding the granular and agranular cells in the extraglomerular mesangium.[167] As described below, the macula densa acts as a sensor of chloride concentration in the distal tubule, providing signals that are important for control of renin.[169] The anatomical organization of the JGA facilitates the regulation of renin secretion in response to critical environmental cues.

Although JG cells are clearly the primary source of renin in the adult kidney, studies by Gomez and associates suggest that renin-expressing cells are not terminally differentiated, but can be recruited during periods of homeostatic pertubations such as dehydration and hypotension. For example, in angiotensinogen-deficient mice, renin is expressed extensively along the entire length of the afferent arteriole and intrarenal arteries.[170] Similarly, in mice subjected to a low-sodium diet combined with captopril treatment, renin-expressing cells can be found throughout the length of the afferent arteriole, in the glomerular and extraglomerular messangium, and in the glomerular capsule.[170] Studies by Lalouel and associates suggest that renin is also present in the connecting tubule, at least in the mouse kidney. Moreover, their studies indicate that renin expression in the connecting tubule may be regulated by sodium intake.[171] Although its physiological role is unclear, it has been suggested that renin expressed in the distal nephron may contribute to regulation of angiotensin peptide concentrations in the tubular lumen.

Expression of renin outside the kidney has also been documented. Levi and associates have recently shown that mast cells express renin mRNA and contain large quantities of renin protein, apparently within the secretory granules.[172] Mast cell-derived renin can efficiently convert angiotensinogen to angiotensin I after mast cell degranulation.[172] Moreover, release of renin by cardiac mast cells can be triggered by ischemia, producing pathophysiologic consequences such as release of norepinephrine and generation of cardiac arrhythmias.[173] Taken together, this work has suggested that resident mast cells in the heart and perhaps other organs, upon appropriate stimulation, are capable of generating ample quantities of renin to activate the RAS locally, and thereby affect organ function. Furthermore, it appears the factors controlling renin release from mast cells will be quite different from those that regulate JG cells, and are likely to involve signals associated with inflammation and injury.[174] Nonetheless, it remains to be determined whether this alternative pathway for RAS activation plays any major role in physiology or disease pathogenesis.

Baroreceptor Regulation of Renin Release

The baroreceptor theory was developed to explain observations that renin secretion is directly stimulated by reduced renal perfusion. This theory was first developed in the context of experimental observations that granularity of the JG cells was inversely correlated with the magnitude of renal perfusion pressure.[175] Since then, numerous studies have shown that renin secretion is inversely related to renal perfusion pressure or pulse amplitude.[21,176–179] This relationship is preserved in denervated kidneys[180,181] and in isolated perfused kidneys with a non-functioning macula densa mechanism.[182–184] Thus, the baroreceptor is an independent mechanism for controlling renin, residing within the kidney and clearly separate from regulation by the sympathetic nervous system.[179] In renovascular hypertension, the baroreceptor is the primary mechanism for stimulating renin release. In the presence of a critical stenosis of the renal artery, renal perfusion pressure drops, stimulating renin and generating hypertension.[185]

While the independent nature of the baroreceptor mechanism and its localization to the kidney has been clearly established, identification of its precise nature has been elusive. Various models have been proposed to explain the mechanism for pressure sensing and consequent signal transduction, including direct stretch of the JG cells due to transmural pressure across the afferent arteriole[22,186] or indirect pathways involving secondary release of autocoids.[187] Some of these candidate soluble factors include nitric oxide[188–190] and prostanoids,[191,192] which are stimulatory or endothelins, which are inhibitory.[193]

Gene-targeting in the mouse has been utilized to examine the role of some of these mediators in the baroreceptor response. In one study, genetic deletion of endothelial nitric oxide synthase (eNOS) had no effect on renin release in response to change in renal perfusion pressure, suggesting that eNOS-derived nitric oxide is not a mediator of the baroreceptor–renin coupling.[194] On the other hand, the absence of the IP receptor, the single known receptor for PGI_2 (prostacyclin), conferred substantial resistance to hypertension and hyperreninemia after unilateral renal artery stenosis.[195] This suggests an absolute requirement for PGI_2 in triggering renin release after baroreceptor activation. A number of questions remain concerning the mechanism and cell lineages controlling synthesis of key mediators such as prostacyclin, and the cellular targets for these mediators affecting renin release.[196]

Over the past 40 years, much deliberation has been rendered regarding the existence and location of a baroreceptor for renin release. The mechanism by which renal perfusion pressure regulates renin secretion remains poorly understood. However, this mechanism appears to be dependent on extracellular calcium concentration. Kurtz and colleagues demonstrated that when the extracellular level of calcium is lowered, the inhibitory effect of renal perfusion pressure on renin release is abolished.[197] A potential mediator in this process may involve connexin proteins that form gap junctions between JG cells and adjacent endothelial cells. Disruption of connexin40 (Cx40) in the mouse, either through gene deletion or point mutation, results in hyperreninemia and hypertension, and loss of pressure control of renin release[198,366-368]; similar to the effect observed with the lowering of extracellular calcium concentration.[197] Other connexin proteins have been demonstrated to also play a role in renin release. Connexin45, another gap junction protein, can replace the function of connexin40, since genetic substitution of the coding region of connexin40 by connexin45 resulted in the attenuation of hypertension and near normalization of the pressure control of renin secretion.[200] Replacement of connexin43 by connexin32 in the mouse resulted in decreased renin levels that did not change in response to a high-salt diet and protection from hypertension induced by a 2-kidney-1clip model.[201] A consensus remains to be established regarding whether connexin proteins (and which one (s)), are indeed the elusive baroreceptor, but the evidence suggests that connexins play an essential role in the regulation of renin release in response to change in perfusion pressure. Future studies are required to determine whether these connexins interact in coordination with other mediators mentioned above in the baroreceptor response.

Macula Densa Mechanism for Renin Regulation

The second major pathway for physiological regulation of renin is the so-called macula densa mechanism, whereby cells at the macula densa sense a reduction in chloride ions in the filtrate of the distal tubule, triggering renin release.[25] In this circumstance, release of renin and the consequent generation of angiotensin II are believed to serve as a mechanism for enhancing renal sodium reabsorption in states of fluid volume depletion. The anatomical association of the macula densa with the JG cells stimulated the first speculation by Goormaghtigh of its physiological function.[202] As mentioned above, the macula densa is made up of specialized epithelial cells at the terminal portion of the thick ascending limb. Their basolateral membrane is in contact with glomerular mesangial cells which, in turn, are contiguous with granular cells in the JGA.[24] The role of the macula densa in renin regulation was initially hypothesized by Vander in 1967,[169] and there is now general consensus that this mechanism provides a control of renin secretion that is directly determined by sodium chloride delivery to the distal nephron.[203,204] Moreover, several studies indicate that chloride flux through the Na-K-2Cl transporter (NKCC2) regulates the signaling pathways linked to renin secretion.[205,206] Increased chloride delivery to the MD inhibits, whereas reduced chloride delivery stimulates, renin release.[23,197,207]

In addition to the well-studied NKCC2 transporter, the Na^+/H^+ exchanger isoform 2 (NHE2) expressed on the apical surface of the macula densa also plays a role in renin release, perhaps through its effect on macula densa cell volume. A recent study by Peti-Peterdi and colleagues demonstrated that NHE2-deficient mice have significant mechanisms responsible for increased renin levels which are macula-densa specific,[208] since these mice have been characterized to have normal blood pressure.[209]

Several candidate signaling pathways linking distal tubule solute concentration to control of renin have been proposed. These include adenosine, nitric oxide, and prostanoids.[210] The most compelling current evidence suggests that MD stimulation of renin involves activation of cyclo-oxygenase (COX)-2[211] constitutively expressed at high levels in the macula densa, generating the prostanoid PGE_2.[212,213] PGE_2 then activates an EP receptor on granular cells in the JGA to stimulate renin release.[214] The EP4 receptor is likely the major EP receptor that mediates the actions of PGE2 in this process. Facemire et al. demonstrated that EP4 receptor-deficient mice display a ~70% reduction in renal renin expression and plasma renin concentration compared to wild-type mice after treatment with furosemide.[215] In contrast, deletion of EP2 receptors in the mice has no effect on renin stimulation by furosemide. Interestingly, this study also suggested that the source of PGE2 in this pathway is not dependent on microsomal PGE synthases 1 and 2 (mPGES1, mPGES2). The capacity for prostaglandins to directly stimulate renin secretion has been long recognized.[216,217] Moreover, studies using specific inhibitors and COX-2 deficient mice have clearly demonstrated the importance of COX-2 in the macula densa pathway.[218,219] In addition, the activity of various components of this system has been demonstrated in the isolated perfused macula densa segments[220] and JG cell lines.[221] However, at least one study[195] has failed to confirm a non-redundant role for individual EP receptors for PGE_2 in furosemide-stimulated renin release in vivo.

Initial evidence suggesting a role for adenosine in MD signaling came from studies using the selective A1AR antagonist 8-cyclopentyl-1,3-dipropylxanthine. The major effect of the inhibitor was to attenuate the actions of increasing luminal NaCl concentrations to inhibit renin release.[222] Later studies using A1AR-deficient mice confirmed that the role of adenosine is primarily restricted to the arm mediating inhibition of renin release. In A1AR-deficient mice, renin-inhibitory actions of enhanced sodium chloride delivery to the macula densa are blocked, whereas stimulation of renin secretion caused by reduced sodium chloride transport at the macula densa is unaffected.[223]

Macula densa cells express high levels of neuronal nitric oxide synthase (nNOS).[224,225] The role of NO in regulation of renin was first tested using nonselective inhibitors of nitric oxide synthesis, which attenuated renin release stimulated by reduced luminal sodium chloride concentrations.[226,227] The specific roles of the individual NOS isoforms have been examined using mice with targeted deletion of nNOS or eNOS. In these studies, activation of the macula densa pathway was achieved by administration of NKCC2 blocking loop diuretics in vivo and in isolated perfused mouse kidneys. Deficiency of either nNOS or eNOS alone did not significantly affect macula densa-dependent renin secretion,[228] while nonspecific NOS blockade attenuated renin stimulation by loop diuretics. This suggests that nitric oxide plays a permissive, rather than a

Short Loop Feedback: Regulation of Renin by Angiotensin II

Angiotensin II also contributes to the regulatory pathways for renin and may control its own synthesis by activating AT_1 receptors, highly expressed at the JGA, thereby suppressing renin release.[229,230] Evidence supporting the existence of this so-called short-loop feedback mechanism includes studies in the isolated perfused kidney, where infusion of angiotensin II suppresses renin release.[179] Administration of ACE inhibitors and angiotensin receptor blockers increases renin mRNA expression and causes JGA hypertrophy.[231] Similarly, mice lacking AT_{1A} receptors also develop marked JGA hypertrophy.[103,230] However, in $Agtr1a^{-/-}$ chimeric mice,[103] and in kidney cross-transplantation experiments,[232] JGA hypertrophy correlated with blood pressure, but not with the absence of AT_1 receptors at the JGA, indicating a significant role for baroreceptor mechanisms in this response. Nonetheless, a role for the short-loop feedback mechanism to alter the sensitivity of baroreceptor or MD mechanisms would be consistent with current data.

Role of Sympathetic Nerve Activity

The capacity for sympathetic nerve activation to stimulate renin has been long recognized. For example, β-adrenoceptors are abundant in the JGA of kidneys from various species.[233] Furthermore, numerous studies have demonstrated that β-adrenergic agonists stimulate renin release.[234] Chronic renal nerve activation also stimulates renin,[235,236] along with its affects to modulate renal blood flow and tubular function. In experiments controlling for these factors, a clear relationship between increasing renal sympathetic nerve activity and renin secretion is maintained.[237,238] However, as discussed above, renal denervation does not abolish the capacity of the baroreceptor[181,239] or macula densa mechanisms to stimulate renin.[182–184] Accordingly, it appears likely that β-sympathetic tone has a modulatory, rather than primary, role in regulation of renin. Recently, a randomized controlled clinical trial demonstrated that renal sympathetic denervation is more effective than medical management alone in patients with resistant hypertension.[240] The original report did not mention any measurement of renin, but it will be of significant interest to determine the effect of the procedure on plasma renin levels in patients who did or did not have a significant reduction in blood pressure.

Regulation of Cellular Release of Renin

At the JGA, renin is stored in cytoplasmic granules within granular cells. In response to activating stimuli, renin is released into the circulation by exocytosis. This process of renin secretion is carried out by fusion events between the secretory granules and cell membrane of afferent arterioles.[241] Furthermore, the extent of secretory activity or exocytosis can be assessed using electrophysiological techniques that directly measure cell membrane capacitance of single mouse JG cells.[242] The control mechanisms for renin, described above, act by triggering this exocytotic pathway. Compared to the relative wealth of available information about physiological regulation of renin, much less is known about the precise intracellular pathways involved in renin secretion, and how these mechanisms are controlled in the granular cell. The general consensus is that the environmental signals regulating renin act through a limited number of intracellular second messengers, including calcium and cyclic AMP.[214,243]

The cyclic AMP pathway appears to be the major trigger for cellular release of renin. In a variety of experimental models, maneuvers causing an elevation of intracellular concentrations of cyclic AMP cause rapid stimulation of renin secretion.[243,244] In this regard, most of the documented secretagogues for renin, including PGE_2, PGI_2, dopamine, and β-adrenoreceptor, act via 7 transmembrane receptors linked to G_s-proteins that increase cyclic AMP levels in JG cells.[244] The specific biochemical pathways by which cyclic AMP acts to stimulate renin secretion are unclear, but likely involve protein kinase A, since inhibition of protein kinase A attenuates the stimulatory effect of β-adrenoreceptors on renin secretion.[190]

By contrast, increases in intracellular calcium levels may inhibit renin release. For example, experimental maneuvers that reduce intracellular calcium concentration stimulate renin release.[243] Moreover, several mediators with putative actions to inhibit renin release, such as angiotensin II, α-receptor agonists, vasopressin, and endothelins, have receptors that couple to G_q-proteins, and activation of these receptors by ligand increases intracellular calcium concentrations in JG cells.[214,243] The inhibitory effect of calcium on renin release appears to be mediated by protein kinase C, since stimulation of protein kinase C inhibits renin secretion,[245–247] whereas blockade of protein kinase C attenuates the inhibitory effect on renin secretion.[245–247] There is also evidence that the effects of calcium on renin release are mediated in part by a calmodulin-dependent process, since inhibition of calmodulin activity stimulates renin secretion.[248,249] Antagonistic interactions between the cyclic AMP and intracellular calcium may ultimately determine the final consequences of extracellular signals on renin release.[243,250]

Regulation of Renin Gene Expression

The steady-state activity of the RAS is generally reflected by renin mRNA levels in the kidney. During chronic stimulation of the RAS, for example, upregulation of renin gene expression is required to sustain over time the enhanced release of renin protein by the JGA. Understanding of tissue-specific control of renin gene expression has been complicated by the difficulty of developing tractable cell culture preparations derived from JG cells. Thus, transgenic mice have been used extensively to assess *in vivo* regulation of renin gene expression.[251,252] Using this approach, minimal segments of the human renin gene sufficient to recapitulate temporal- and cell-specific patterns of gene expression have been identified.[251,252]

There is strong sequence conservation of 5′ proximal promoter regions between the renin genes of the human, rat, and mouse.[253] This region contains a cyclic AMP (cAMP) response element (CRE),[254–256] which is required for cAMP stimulation of transcription.[254,257] In addition, there are at least seven transcription factor-binding sites within the proximal promoter, including a binding site for HOX proteins that play critical roles in specifying positional information along embryonic axes.[253] The renin promoter is relatively weak in isolation,[254,257,258] but is strengthened up to 80-fold by a distal enhancer element.[259,260] This enhancer contains at least eleven transcription factor-binding sites responsive to a variety of signal transduction pathways.[261] Inhibitory factors, including endothelin-1, angiotensin II, mechanical stretch, and inflammatory cytokines, may act through target sequences within the enhancer.[261]

Post-transcriptional mechanisms also play a key role in determining steady-state renin mRNA levels. cAMP appears to be a critical mediator in this process. For example, in cell systems, cAMP has only a modest effect in inducing renin gene transcription of the renin gene, but nonetheless it causes marked induction of renin mRNA levels.[262] This augmentation is associated with enhanced stability of renin mRNA.[263] cAMP also increases levels of RNA-binding proteins targeting the 3′UTR of the human renin gene,[264] suggesting a potential mechanism for its effects to promote renin mRNA stability.

Control of Renal Hemodynamics by the RAS

Angiotensin II, acting via its AT_1 receptor, is a potent vasoconstrictor. Stimulation of AT_1 receptors in vascular smooth muscle cells initiates a signaling cascade including increased intracellular calcium concentration and alterations in cytoskeleton, inducing contraction with consequent increases in vascular resistance.[265] Studies in mice deficient in both the AT_{1A} and AT_{1B} receptor isoforms have confirmed the importance of AT_1 receptors in this response.[102,100] The pressor response to acute angiotensin II infusion is completely abolished in these double-knockout animals[100]; whereas response to another pressor agent, epinephrine, is not affected. These vasoconstrictor actions of angiotensin II play a central role in maintaining circulatory homeostasis in a number of tissues, including the kidney. In the kidney, the hemodynamic actions of angiotensin II impact renal blood flow, glomerular filtration rate, excretion of salt and water, and progression of renal damage in disease states.

Glomerular Microcirculation

The coordinated regulation of resistances in the afferent and efferent arterioles plays a critical role in determining and maintaining the glomerular filtration rate (GFR). The RAS has potent effects on glomerular hemodynamics. Angiotensin II causes constriction of both the afferent and efferent arterioles. However, the effect of high levels of angiotensin II is to induce a more profound constriction of the efferent arteriole.[266–268] The reasons for this disproportionate effect of angiotensin II on the efferent arteriole are not clear, but may include differences in levels of AT_1 receptor expression,[269] modulating actions of vasodilators such as prostaglandins and nitric oxide on preglomerular vessels[270,271] or differences in calcium responses to angiotensin II in the afferent versus efferent arterioles.[272–274] In mice, the AT_{1A} and AT_{1B} receptor isoforms have distinct actions in the glomerular circulation. Both AT_{1A} and AT_{1B} receptors contribute to the afferent arteriolar response to angiotensin II, whereas the efferent arteriolar response is mediated exclusively by AT_{1A} receptors.[275]

The overall effect of angiotensin II on glomerular hemodyamics is a predominant increase in post-glomerular resistance, resulting in an increase in glomerular hydrostatic pressure. These actions serve to protect GFR in states of intravascular volume depletion. Because angiotensin II also simultaneously reduces renal blood flow, there will be a coincident increase in filtration fraction, and a decrease in peritubular capillary pressure[276] promoting an increase in sodium reabsorption in the proximal tubule.[277,278] The importance of angiotensin II in maintaining GFR when renal perfusion is threatened is illustrated by the effect of ACE inhibitors in patients with critical bilateral renal artery stenosis or critical stenosis in the renal artery of a single functioning kidney. When blood pressures in such patients are reduced to equivalent levels with a non-specific vasodilator, such as nitroprusside, compared to an ACE inhibitor, the ACE inhibitor causes a much more marked deterioration in GFR.[279,280]

The glomerular hemodynamic responses to angiotensin II may be modified significantly by other circulating factors. For example, the vasoconstrictor actions of angiotensin II may be substantially augmented in the presence of elevated adenosine levels.[281–285] This can occur in pathologic states including malignant hypertension, renal artery stenosis, and in some experimental models of renal ischemia.[286–288] When both angiotensin II and adenosine are present at high concentrations, there is a dramatic increase in preglomerular resistance that does not occur with either agent alone. Other mediators, such as prostanoids[289] and nitric oxide, may also modulate the actions of angiotensin II in the glomerular microcirculation, particularly in disease states such as diabetes.[290] In angiotensin II-induced hypertension, for example, nitric oxide attenuates afferent arteriolar constriction.[291]

In kidney disease, abnormal activation of the RAS and coincident increases in glomerular hydrostatic pressure have been suggested to contribute to progressive renal injury.[292,293] For example, in the remnant kidney model of chronic kidney disease, post-glomerular resistances are increased, and this is associated with increased glomerular hydrostatic pressures.[294,295] This abnormal glomerular hemodynamic pattern is reversed with RAS blockade. These observations formed the basis of the rationale for using ACE inhibitors or angiotensin receptor blockers in chronic kidney diseases. Reduction of glomerular hemodynamic pressure may be a key mechanism explaining the renoprotective effects of these agents in diseases such as diabetic nephropathy.[11,13,14]

Renal Medullary Circulation

Along with its effects on the glomerular circulation angiotensin II, acting through AT_1 receptors, has important regulatory functions in the renal circulation in general. In the mouse, regulation of renal blood flow by angiotensin II is primarily mediated by AT_{1A} receptors.[296] Moreover, effects of AT_1 receptors to modulate blood flow in the medulla significantly impact the kidney's excretory capacity for sodium.[297] In this regard, it has been suggested that regulation of medullary blood flow by angiotensin II represents a critical pathway for modulating the pressure-natriuresis response discussed earlier in the chapter.[161,276] Thus, regulation of medullary blood flow by the RAS is likely to be a key pathway used by the kidney to maintain blood pressure homeostasis.

The mechanisms controlling medullary blood flow in the kidney are complex. As in the glomerulus, vasodilator effects of mediators such as nitric oxide and prostanoids act to counterbalance the actions of angiotensin II. For example, a subpressor dose of angiotensin II, which by itself has a negligible effect on the medullary circulation, significantly reduces medullary blood flow when combined with the NO inhibitor L-NAME.[298] Cortical blood flow is unaffected in this circumstance. Nitric oxide also protects medullary blood flow during chronic infusion of angiotensin II.[299] In the outer medulla, angiotensin II stimulates NO production by tubular epithelium, potentially as a compensatory mechanism, and this may be an example of "tubulo-vascular cross-talk," whereby the effects of angiotensin II on tubular epithelium may modify its vasoconstrictor actions.[300] Similarly, renal prostaglandins also appear to modulate pressure natriuresis by altering renal medullary hemodynamics.[301] These hemodynamic changes from the inhibition of prostaglandin production lead to increased chloride reabsorption in the loop of Henle and collecting duct.[302,303]

Alterations in the balance of angiotensin II and NO in the medulla may have significant consequences on systemic blood pressure regulation. For example, angiotensin II-stimulated NO production is impaired in Dahl-sensitive hypertensive rats,[263,304,305] and attenuated generation of NO in kidneys of these animals is associated with reduced medullary blood flow.[306,307] Furthermore, delivery of L-NAME directly into the renal medulla of Dahl salt-sensitive rats reverses the hypertensive actions of angiotensin II,[305] as does intravenous infusion of L-arginine.[308]

RENAL EPITHELIAL ACTIONS OF THE RAS

Along with its hemodynamic actions, angiotensin II may modulate fluid and solute excretion through two distinct pathways: (1) an indirect pathway involving stimulation of aldosterone release from the adrenal gland; and (2) through direct effects of AT_1 receptors expressed by renal epithelia.[162]

In the adrenal cortex, activation of AT_1 receptors stimulates the release of aldosterone[119] which in turn promotes sodium reabsorption by binding to mineralocorticoid receptors in the mineralocorticoid-responsive segments of the distal nephron.[125] The biology of the aldosterone system is described elsewhere, and historically was thought to be the major effector system used by the RAS to control renal sodium handling.[123] Direct actions of angiotensin II in the kidney were defined later using isolated perfused tubules[309–314] and micropuncture studies.[315–318] Using these approaches, renal epithelial responses to angiotensin II were documented in several nephron segments. However, it has been difficult, in the intact animal, to separate the effects of AT_1 receptors in renal epithelium from other renal and systemic effects of angiotenson II, and to determine their contribution to integrated control of blood pressure. Nonetheless, recent studies using renal cross-transplantation and regional genetic deletion clearly indicate significant, non-redundant contributions of AT_1 receptors within the kidney to determining the level of blood pressure.[232,319] Activation of AT_1 receptors in the nephron can have physiologic or pathophysiologic effects depending on the clinical context. For example, stimulation of AT_1 receptors in the proximal tubules helps to prevent circulatory collapse at baseline by promoting sodium retention,[319] whereas the accumulated stimulation of AT_1 receptors on tubular cells that occurs over the span of a normal lifetime downregulates pro-survival genes including sirtuin 3, such that AT_1 receptor deficiency is associated with enhanced longevity in mice.[320] In the next section, we will provide an overview of tubular actions of the RAS.

Tubular Effects of Angiotensin II

Proximal Tubule

Direct actions of angiotensin II in the proximal tubule are perhaps the best characterized. These actions were first implied in whole animal studies,[321–323] and then were specifically defined using *in vitro* perfused proximal tubules[313] and micropuncture studies.[317] Taken together, these studies suggest that angiotensin II, acting through AT_1 receptors on the basolateral surface of proximal tubules, promotes sodium reabsorption by coordinately stimulating the sodium-proton anti-porter on the luminal membrane along with the sodium-potassium-ATPase on the basolateral surface.[310,313,317] These actions result in enhanced basolateral sodium bicarbonate flux.[310] In addition, although angiotensin II is thought to regulate renal water handling primarily through actions in the collecting tubule (discussed below), data are emerging to suggest that AT_1 receptor activation also modulates proximal tubular expression of the aquaporin 1 channel, heretofore considered to be constitutively expressed.[324]

The capacity for proximal tubular actions of the RAS to influence blood pressure was first demonstrated in elegant experiments by Sigmund and associates.[325] In these studies, isolated co-expression of human renin and angiotensinogen in the proximal tubule caused hypertension without any detectable increase in circulating angiotensin II levels. In more recent work from this group, overexpression of the type AT_1 receptor in the proximal tubule raised baseline blood pressure levels.[326] Inversely, Gurley and colleagues showed that deletion of AT_1 receptors selectively from the proximal tubular epithelium using a Cre/loxp approach reduces the baseline level of blood pressure by diminishing fluid reabsorption from the proximal tubule, and protects from angiotensin II-induced hypertension by mitigating sodium reabsorption.[319] These studies also illustrated that angiotensin II regulates the abundance of key apical membrane sodium transporters, as AT_1 receptor deletion in the proximal tubule allowed the downregulation of the NHE3 exchanger and the NaPi2 co-transporter, thereby facilitating hypertension-induced natriuresis.[319] Complementary studies in a rat model demonstrated that angotensin II directs these transporters to redistribute within the luminal membrane microvilli of the proximal tubular cell to promote sodium and water reabsorption.[327]

AT_1 receptors are also present on the luminal brush border of the proximal tubular epithelium.[328–330] Moreover, angiotensin II is secreted into, and endocytosed from, the proximal tubular lumen where its levels may not correlate with plasma angiotensin II levels.[331–333] It has been suggested that control of angiotensin II generation in this luminal compartment might provide separate regulation of epithelial function that is independent of the systemic RAS.[334] Moreover, activation of AT_1 receptors on the luminal membrane of the proximal tubular cell can promote sodium reabsorption, in part through a G_i-protein-mediated reduction in cyclic AMP.[313,317,333] There is some evidence for an independent regulation of luminal concentrations of angiotensin II. For example, although both whole kidney and proximal tubular angiotensin II levels are elevated in response to reduced renal perfusion,[335] angiotensin II levels in proximal tubular fluid are not suppressed with acute volume expansion, and may even increase in this setting.[335,336]

The net effect of angiotensin II on bicarbonate handling in the proximal tubule appears to be neutral. Coordinating with its stimulation of the apical membrane sodium-proton exchanger, angiotensin II enhances the activity of the sodium-bicarbonate co-transporter on the basolateral surface of the early proximal tubule.[310,313] As such, angiotensin II acts as a potent stimulus for proximal acidification, coupled to reclamation of bicarbonate from the early proximal tubule.[310,337,338] Nevertheless, the resulting reduction in delivery of bicarbonate to the late proximal tubule leads to less bicarbonate reabsorption in that segment. Moreover, at higher concentrations, angiotensin II paradoxically inhibits sodium-bicarbonate transporter activity,[339] such that overall the bicarbonate concentration in the urinary filtrate reaching the distal convoluted tubule is not altered by angiotensin II stimulation.[340] Thus, the contribution of the RAS to acid–base regulation is primarily mediated by aldosterone in the distal nephron.[341–345]

Loop of Henle

Compared to the proximal tubule, the functions of angiotensin II in the medullary thick ascending limb (MTAL) are not as well-characterized. AT_1 receptors are expressed on both the luminal and basolateral membranes of the MTAL epithelium.[346,347] In vitro studies addressing the role of angiotensin II in MTAL ion transport suggest that cellular responses may differ, depending on the local concentrations of angiotensin II.[348,349] At lower concentrations of angiotensin II, inhibition of the sodium-potassium-chloride co-transporter (NKCC2) may be seen,[348,349] whereas stimulation of NKCC2 can be seen at higher concentrations.[348] In vivo microperfusion experiments have also demonstrated physiological consequences of angiotensin II in the MTAL, including increased bicarbonate transport out of the urinary filtrate.[350] This heightened bicarbonate flux is likely due to an increase in sodium–hydrogen exchange, as has been observed in the proximal tubule, suggesting that angiotensin II increases sodium reabsorption from the MTAL. These data are consistent with the finding that in vivo administration of angiotensin II leads to heightened expression of both the NHE3 sodium-hydrogen exchanger and NKCC2 in the MTAL.[351]

Distal Nephron

SOLUTE TRANSPORT

Although angiotensin II indirectly influences distal and collecting tubular function through the generation of aldosterone, more recent studies have demonstrated that angiotensin II also has direct effects in modulating ion flux along the distal nephron. As in other nephron segments, all the elements of the RAS are present along the distal nephron, and relatively high concentrations of angiotensin II can be detected in the tubular fluid of these segments.[171,330,332] Angiotensin II, acting via AT_1 receptors, stimulates sodium–hydrogen exchange in the cortical and outer medullary collecting tubule by increasing the density of the vacuolar sodium-hydrogen-ATPase in the apical membrane of the type A intercalated cell, which in turn leads to an increase in bicarbonate reabsorption.[315,316,352,353] On the apical membrane of the principal cells in the cortical collecting duct (CCD), luminal angiotensin II stimulates amiloride-sensitive sodium transport by increasing activity of the epithelial sodium channel (ENaC) through an AT_1 receptor-dependent mechanism.[312,318] Furthermore, activation of AT_1 receptors on the basolateral membrane of CCD cells stimulates the activity of potassium channels via a nitric oxide-dependent pathway.[354] As the distal nephron ultimately determines urine flow and composition, actions of angiotensin II to modulate sodium handling at this site may impact blood pressure homeostasis.[164,312]

WATER HANDLING

Recent studies suggest a role for the RAS in the control of urinary concentrating mechanisms and free water handling. For example, the complete absence of angiotensinogen, ACE or AT_{1A}/AT_{1B} receptors in mice is associated with atrophy of the renal papilla and a marked urinary concentrating defect.[230,355,356] Mice lacking AT_{1A} receptors are also unable to generate maximally concentrated urine, despite having apparently normal renal papillae.[357] These animals generate vasopressin normally in response to water restriction, but are resistant to dDAVP.[357] Administration of an AT_1 receptor-antagonist to wild-type mice, and even selective deletion of AT_1 receptors from the collecting duct using a Cre/loxp approach, recapitulates this urinary concentrating defect.[357,358] Similarly, AT_1 receptor blockade also blunts the maximal urine concentrating capacity in DDAVP-challenged rats, and this effect is associated with reduced expression of aquaporins-1 and -2.[359] In the medullary collecting duct, angiotensin II upregulates gene expression for the V_2 vasopressin receptor, and the expression and apical membrane targeting of the aquaporin-2 channel.[360–363] These effects are mediated through a protein kinase A-dependent pathway.[360] Thus, direct effects of angiotensin II on expression of water channels and perhaps vasopressin receptors may contribute to its actions on renal water handling.

References

[1] Tiret L, Bonnardeaux A, Poirier O, Ricard S, Marques-Vidal P, Evans A, et al. Synergistic effects of angiotensin converting enzyme and angiotensin II type I receptor polymorphisms on risk of myocardial infarction. Lancet 1994;344:910–3.

[2] Jeunemaitre X, Soubrier F, Kotelevtsev YV, Lifton RP, Williams CS, Charru A, et al. Molecular basis of human hypertension: role of angiotensinogen. Cell 1992;71(1):169–80.

[3] Bonnardeaux A, Davies E, Jeunemaitre X, Féry I, Charru A, Clauser E, et al. Angiotensin II type 1 receptor gene polymorphisms in human essential hypertension. Hypertension 1994;24:63–9.

[4] Benetos A, Gautier S, Ricard S, Topouchian J, Asmar R, Poirier O, et al. Angiotensin-converting enzyme inhibitors: influence of angiotensin-converting enzyme and angiotensin II type 1 receptor gene polymorphisms on aortic stiffness in normotensive and hypertensive patients. Circulation 1996;94:698–703.

[5] Wang J, Staessen J. Genetic polymorphisms in the renin–angiotensin system: relevance for susceptibility to cardiovascular disease. Eur J Pharmacol 2000;410:289–302.

[6] Yoshida H, Kon V, Ichikawa I. Polymorphisms of the renin–angiotensin system genes in progressive renal diseases. Kidney Int 1996;50:732–44.

[7] Husain A, Drugs Graham R. Enzymes and Receptors of the Renin-Angiotensin System: Celebrating a Century of Discovery. Sidney: Harwood Academic; 2000.

[8] Investigators TS. Effect of enalapril on survival in patients with reduced left ventricular ejection fractions and congestive heart failure. The SOLVD Investigators. N Engl J Med 1991;325:293–302.

[9] Investigators TS. Effect of enalapril on mortality and the development of heart failure in asymptomatic patients with reduced left ventricular ejection fractions. The SOLVD Investigators. N Engl J Med 1992;327:725–7.

[10] Yusuf S, Sleight P, Pogue J, Bosch J, Davies R, Dagenais G. Effects of an angiotensin-converting-enzyme inhibitor, ramipril, on cardiovascular events in high-risk patients. The Heart Outcomes Prevention Evaluation Study Investigators. N Engl J Med 2000;342(3):145–53.

[11] Lewis EJ, Hunsicker LG, Bain RP, Rohde RD. The effect of angiotensin-converting-enzyme inhibition on diabetic nephropathy. The Collaborative Study Group. N Engl J Med 1993;329 (20):1456–62.

[12] Dahlof B, Devereux RB, Kjeldsen SE, Julius S, Beevers G, de Faire U, et al. Cardiovascular morbidity and mortality in the Losartan Intervention For Endpoint reduction in hypertension study (LIFE): a randomised trial against atenolol. Lancet 2002;359(9311):995–1003.

[13] Lewis EJ, Hunsicker LG, Clarke WR, Berl T, Pohl MA, Lewis JB, et al. Renoprotective effect of the angiotensin-receptor antagonist irbesartan in patients with nephropathy due to type 2 diabetes. N Engl J Med 2001;345(12):851–60.

[14] Brenner BM, Cooper ME, de Zeeuw D, Keane WF, Mitch WE, Parving HH, et al. Effects of losartan on renal and cardiovascular outcomes in patients with type 2 diabetes and nephropathy. N Engl J Med 2001;345(12):861–9.

[15] Danser AH, Deinum J. Renin, pro-renin and the putative (pro) renin receptor. Hypertension 2005;46(5):1069–76.

[16] Luetscher JA, Kraemer FB, Wilson DM, Schwartz HC, Bryer-Ash M. Increased plasma inactive renin in diabetes mellitus. A marker of microvascular complications. N Engl J Med 1985;312(22):1412–7.

[17] Deinum J, Ronn B, Mathiesen E, Derkx FH, Hop WC, Schalekamp MA. Increase in serum pro-renin precedes onset of microalbuminuria in patients with insulin-dependent diabetes mellitus. Diabetologia 1999;42(8):1006–10.

[18] Veniant M, Menard J, Bruneval P, Morley S, Gonzales MF, Mullins J. Vascular damage without hypertension in transgenic rats expressing pro-renin exclusively in the liver. J Clin Invest 1996;98(9):1966–70.

[19] Peters J, Farrenkopf R, Clausmeyer S, Zimmer J, Kantachuvesiri S, Sharp MG, et al. Functional significance of pro-renin internalization in the rat heart. Circ Res 2002;90(10):1135–41.

[20] Peach MJ. Renin–angiotensin system: Biochemistry and mechanisms of action. Physiol Rev 1977;57(2):313–70.

[21] Bock HA, Hermle M, Brunner FP, Thiel G. Pressure dependent modulation of renin release in isolated perfused glomeruli. Kidney Int 1992;41(2):275–80.

[22] Carey RM, McGrath HE, Pentz ES, Gomez RA, Barrett PQ. Biomechanical coupling in renin-releasing cells. J Clin Invest 1997;100(6):1566–74.

[23] Lorenz JN, Weihprecht H, Schnermann J, Skott O, Briggs JP. Renin release from isolated juxtaglomerular apparatus depends on macula densa chloride transport. Am J Physiol 1991;260(4 Pt 2):F486–493.

[24] Bell PD, Lapointe JY, Sabirov R, Hayashi S, Peti-Peterdi J, Manabe K, et al. Macula densa cell signaling involves ATP release through a maxi anion channel. Proc Natl Acad Sci USA 2003;100(7):4322–7.

[25] Lorenz JN, Weihprecht H, He XR, Skott O, Briggs JP, Schnermann J. Effects of adenosine and angiotensin on macula densa-stimulated renin secretion. Am J Physiol 1993;265(2 Pt 2): F187–194.

[26] Admiraal PJ, van Kesteren CA, Danser AH, Derkx FH, Sluiter W, Schalekamp MA. Uptake and proteolytic activation of pro-renin by cultured human endothelial cells. J Hypertens 1999;17(5):621–9.

[27] Nguyen G, Delarue F, Burckle C, Bouzhir L, Giller T, Sraer JD. Pivotal role of the renin/pro-renin receptor in angiotensin II production and cellular responses to renin. J Clin Invest 2002;109(11):1417–27.

[28] van Kesteren CA, Danser AH, Derkx FH, Dekkers DH, Lamers JM, Saxena PR, et al. Mannose 6-phosphate receptor–mediated internalization and activation of pro-renin by cardiac cells. Hypertension 1997;30(6):1389–96.

[29] Nguyen G. Renin/pro-renin receptors. Kidney Int 2006;69 (9):1503–6.

[30] Burckle C, Bader M. Pro-renin and its ancient receptor. Hypertension 2006;48(4):549–51.

[31] Burckle CA, Jan Danser AH, Muller DN, Garrelds IM, Gasc JM, Popova E, et al. Elevated blood pressure and heart rate in human renin receptor transgenic rats. Hypertension 2006;47 (3):552–6.

[32] Hirose T, Hashimoto M, Totsune K, Metoki H, Asayama K, Kikuya M, et al. Association of (pro)renin receptor gene polymorphism with blood pressure in Japanese men: the Ohasama study. Am J Hypertens 2009;22(3):294–9.

[33] Nguyen G, Muller DN. The biology of the (pro)renin receptor. J Am Soc Nephrol 2010;21(1):18–23.

[34] Ramser J, Abidi FE, Burckle CA, Lenski C, Toriello H, Wen G, et al. A unique exonic splice enhancer mutation in a family with X-linked mental retardation and epilepsy points to a novel role of the renin receptor. Hum Mol Genet 2005;14(8):1019–27.

[35] Kinouchi K, Ichihara A, Sano M, Sun-Wada GH, Wada Y, Kurauchi-Mito A, et al. The (pro)renin receptor/ATP6AP2 is essential for vacuolar H^+-ATPase assembly in murine cardiomyocytes. Circ Res 2010;107(1):30–4.

[36] Cruciat CM, Ohkawara B, Acebron SP, Karaulanov E, Reinhard C, Ingelfinger D, et al. Requirement of pro-renin receptor and vacuolar H^+-ATPase-mediated acidification for Wnt signaling. *Science* 2010;327(5964):459–63.

[37] Yanai K, Saito T, Kakinuma Y, Kon Y, Hirota K, Taniguchi-Yanai K, et al. Renin-dependent cardiovascular functions and renin-independent blood–brain barrier functions revealed by renin-deficient mice. J Biol Chem 2000;275(1):5–8.

[38] Oshima Y, Kinouchi K, Ichihara A, Sakoda M, Kurauchi-Mito A, Bokuda K, et al. Pro-renin receptor is essential for normal podocyte structure and function. *J Am Soc Nephrol* 2011;22 (12):2203–12.

[39] Riediger F, Quack I, Qadri F, Hartleben B, Park JK, Potthoff SA, et al. Pro-renin receptor is essential for podocyte autophagy and survival. *J Am Soc Nephrol* 2011;22(12):2193–202.

[40] Gould AB, Green D. Kinetics of the human renin and human substrate reaction. Cardiovasc Res 1971;5(1):86–9.

[41] Inoue I, Nakajima T, Williams CS, Quackenbush J, Puryear R, Powers M, et al. A nucleotide substitution in the promoter of human angiotensinogen is associated with essential hypertension and affects basal transcription *in vitro*. J Clin Invest 1997;99 (7):1786–97.

[42] Kim HS, Krege JH, Kluckman KD, Hagaman JR, Hodgin JB, Best CF, et al. Genetic control of blood pressure and the

angiotensinogen locus. Proc Natl Acad Sci USA 1995;92 (7):2735–9.

[43] Dickson ME, Sigmund CD. Genetic basis of hypertension: revisiting angiotensinogen. Hypertension 2006;48(1):14–20.

[44] Ingelfinger JR, Zuo WM, Fon EA, Ellison KE, Dzau VJ. In situ hybridization evidence for angiotensinogen messenger RNA in the rat proximal tubule. An hypothesis for the intrarenal renin angiotensin system. J Clin Invest 1990;85(2):417–23.

[45] Kobori H, Harrison-Bernard LM, Navar LG. Expression of angiotensinogen mRNA and protein in angiotensin II-dependent hypertension. J Am Soc Nephrol 2001;12(3):431–9.

[46] Dzau VJ, Ellison KE, Brody T, Ingelfinger J, Pratt RE. A comparative study of the distributions of renin and angiotensinogen messenger ribonucleic acids in rat and mouse tissues. Endocrinology 1987;120(6):2334–8.

[47] Corvol P, Williams TA, Soubrier F. Peptidyl dipeptidase A: Angiotensin I-converting enzyme. Methods Enzymol 1995;248:283–305.

[48] Ehlers MR, Fox EA, Strydom DJ, Riordan JF. Molecular cloning of human testicular angiotensin-converting enzyme: the testis isozyme is identical to the C-terminal half of endothelial angiotensin-converting enzyme. Proc Natl Acad Sci USA 1989;86 (20):7741–5.

[49] Hubert C, Houot AM, Corvol P, Soubrier F. Structure of the angiotensin I-converting enzyme gene. Two alternate promoters correspond to evolutionary steps of a duplicated gene. J Biol Chem 1991;266(23):15377–83.

[50] Langford KG, Shai SY, Howard TE, Kovac MJ, Overbeek PA, Bernstein KE. Transgenic mice demonstrate a testis-specific promoter for angiotensin-converting enzyme. J Biol Chem 1991;266 (24):15559–62.

[51] Beldent V, Michaud A, Wei L, Chauvet MT, Corvol P. Proteolytic release of human angiotensin-converting enzyme. Localization of the cleavage site. J Biol Chem 1993;268 (35):26428–34.

[52] Sayed-Tabatabaei FA, Oostra BA, Isaacs A, van Duijn CM, Witteman JC. ACE polymorphisms. Circ Res 2006;98(9):1123–33.

[53] Rigat B, Hubert C, Alhenc-Gelas F, Cambien F, Corvol P, Soubrier F. An insertion/deletion polymorphism in the angiotensin I-converting enzyme gene accounting for half the variance of serum enzyme levels. J Clin Invest 1990;86(4):1343–6.

[54] Villard E, Tiret L, Visvikis S, Rakotovao R, Cambien F, Soubrier F. Identification of new polymorphisms of the angiotensin I-converting enzyme (ACE) gene, and study of their relationship to plasma ACE levels by two-QTL segregation-linkage analysis. Am J Hum Genet 1996;58(6):1268–78.

[55] Takahashi N, Smithies O. Human genetics, animal models and computer simulations for studying hypertension. Trends Genet 2004;20(3):136–45.

[56] Margolius HS. Kallikreins and kinins. Molecular characteristics and cellular and tissue responses. Diabetes 1996;45(Suppl 1): S14–19.

[57] Campbell DJ, Alexiou T, Xiao HD, Fuchs S, McKinley MJ, Corvol P, et al. Effect of reduced angiotensin-converting enzyme gene expression and angiotensin-converting enzyme inhibition on angiotensin and bradykinin peptide levels in mice. Hypertension 2004;43(4):854–9.

[58] Gainer JV, Morrow JD, Loveland A, King DJ, Brown NJ. Effect of bradykinin-receptor blockade on the response to angiotensin-converting-enzyme inhibitor in normotensive and hypertensive subjects. N Engl J Med 1998;339(18):1285–92.

[59] Donoghue M, Hsieh F, Baronas E, Godbout K, Gosselin M, Stagliano N, et al. A novel angiotensin-converting enzyme-related carboxypeptidase (ACE2) converts angiotensin I to angiotensin 1-9. Circ Res 2000;87(5):E1–9.

[60] Tipnis SR, Hooper NM, Hyde R, Karran E, Christie G, Turner AJ. A human homolog of angiotensin-converting enzyme. Cloning and functional expression as a captopril-insensitive carboxypeptidase. J Biol Chem 2000;275(43):33238–43.

[61] Zhang H, Wada J, Hida K, Tsuchiyama Y, Hiragushiet K, Shikata K, et al. Collectrin, a collecting duct-specific transmembrane glycoprotein, is a novel homolog of ACE2 and is developmentally regulated in embryonic kidneys. J Biol Chem 2001;276(20):17132–9.

[62] Vickers C, Hales P, Kaushik V, Dick L, Gavin J, Tang J, et al. Hydrolysis of biological peptides by human angiotensin-converting enzyme-related carboxypeptidase. J Biol Chem 2002;277 (17):14838–43.

[63] Ferrario C, Brosnihan K, Diz D, Jaiswal N, Khosla MC, Milsted A, et al. Angiotensin-(1-7): a new hormone of the angiotensin system. Hypertension 1991;18: [III-126-133]

[64] Santos RA, Simoes e Silva AC, Maric C, Silva DM, Machado RP, de Buhr I, et al. Angiotensin-(1-7) is an endogenous ligand for the G protein-coupled receptor Mas. Proc Natl Acad Sci USA 2003;100(14):8258–63.

[65] Ferrario CM, Trask AJ, Jessup JA. Advances in biochemical and functional roles of angiotensin-converting enzyme 2 and angiotensin-(1-7) in regulation of cardiovascular function. Am J Physiol Heart Circ Physiol 2005;289(6):H2281–2290.

[66] Gurley SB, Allred A, Le TH, Griffiths R, Mao L, Philip N, et al. Altered blood pressure responses and normal cardiac phenotype in ACE2-null mice. J Clin Invest 2006;116 (8):2218–25.

[67] Oudit GY, Herzenberg AM, Kassiri Z, Wong D, Reich H, Khokha R, et al. Loss of angiotensin-converting enzyme-2 leads to the late development of angiotensin II-dependent glomerulosclerosis. Am J Pathol 2006;168(6):1808–20.

[68] Oudit GY, Liu GC, Zhong J, Basu R, Chow FL, Zhou J, et al. Human recombinant ACE2 reduces the progression of diabetic nephropathy. Diabetes 2009;59(2):529–38.

[69] Wong DW, Oudit GY, Reich H, Kassiri Z, Zhou J, Liu QC, et al. Loss of angiotensin-converting enzyme-2 (Ace2) accelerates diabetic kidney injury. Am J Pathol 2007;171(2):438–51.

[70] Wysocki J, Ye M, Soler MJ, Gurley SB, Xiao HD, Bernstein KE, et al. ACE and ACE2 activity in diabetic mice. Diabetes 2006;55 (7):2132–9.

[71] Gurley SB, Coffman TM. Angiotensin-converting enzyme 2 gene targeting studies in mice: mixed messages. Exp Physiol 2008;93(5):538–42.

[72] Zhong J, Guo D, Chen CB, Wang W, Schuster M, Loibner H, et al. Prevention of angiotensin II-mediated renal oxidative stress, inflammation, and fibrosis by angiotensin-converting enzyme 2. Hypertension 2010;57(2):314–22.

[73] Zhang H, Wada J, Kanwar YS, Tsuchiyama Y, Hiragushi K, Hida K, et al. Screening for genes upregulated in 5/6 nephrectomized mouse kidney. Kidney Int 1999;56(2):549–58.

[74] Malakauskas SM, Quan H, Fields TA, McCall SJ, Yu MJ, Kourany WM, et al. Aminoaciduria and altered renal expression of luminal amino acid transporters in mice lacking novel gene collectrin. Am J Physiol Renal Physiol 2007;292(2): F533–544.

[75] Danilczyk U, Sarao R, Remy C, Benabbas C, Stange G, Richter A, et al. Essential role for collectrin in renal amino acid transport. Nature 2006;444(7122):1088–91.

[76] Timmermans PB, Wong PC, Chiu AT, Herblin WF, Benfield P, Carini DJ, et al. Angiotensin II receptors and angiotensin II receptor antagonists. Pharmacol Rev 1993;45(2):205–51.

[77] Tharaux P-L, Coffman TM. Transgenic mice as a tool to study the renin–angiotensin system. Contrib Nephrol 2001;135:72–91.

[78] Murphy TJ, Alexander RW, Griendling KK, Runge MS, Bernstein KE. Isolation of a cDNA encoding the vascular type-1 angiotensin II receptor. Nature 1991;351(6323):233–6.

[79] Sasaki K, Yamano Y, Bardhan S, Iwai N, Murray JJ, Hasegawa M, et al. Cloning and expression of a complementary DNA encoding a bovine adrenal angiotensin II type-1 receptor. Nature 1991;351(6323):230–3.

[80] Inagami T, Iwai N, Sasaki K, Yamamo Y, Bardhan S, Chaki S, et al. Cloning, expression and regulation of angiotensin II receptors. J Hypertens 1992;10(8):713–6.

[81] Sandberg K, Ji H, Clark AJ, Shapira H, Catt KJ. Cloning and expression of a novel angiotensin II receptor subtype. J Biol Chem 1992;267(14):9455–8.

[82] Iwai N, Inagami T. Identification of two subtypes in the rat type I angiotensin receptor. FEBS Letts 1992;298:257–60.

[83] Kakar S, Riel K, Neill J. Differential expression of angiotensin II receptor subtype mRNAs (AT-1A and AT-1B) in the brain. Biochem Biophys Res Comm 1992;185:688–92.

[84] Sasamura H, Hein L, Krieger JE, Pratt RE, Kobilka BK, Dzau VJ. Cloning, characterization, and expression of two angiotensin receptor (AT-1) isoforms from the mouse genome. Biochem Biophys Res Commun 1992;185(1):253–9.

[85] de Gasparo M, Catt KJ, Inagami T, Wright JW, Unger T. International union of pharmacology. XXIII. The angiotensin II receptors. Pharmacol Rev 2000;52(3):415–72.

[86] Marrero M, Schieffer B, Paxton W, Heerdt L, Berk BC, Delafontaine P, et al. Direct stimulation of Jak/STAT pathway by the angiotensin II AT$_1$ receptor. Nature 1995;375:247–50.

[87] Rakesh K,, Yoo B,, Kim IM,, Salazar N,, Kim KS,, Rockman HA. beta-Arrestin-biased agonism of the angiotensin receptor induced by mechanical stress. *Sci Signal*.3(125):ra46.

[88] Shenoy SK, Lefkowitz RJ. Angiotensin II-stimulated signaling through G proteins and beta-arrestin. Sci STKE 2005;(311):cm14.

[89] Ahn D, Ge Y, Stricklett PK, Gill P, Taylor D, Hughes AK, et al. Collecting duct-specific knockout of endothelin-1 causes hypertension and sodium retention. J Clin Invest 2004;114(4):504–11.

[90] Yasuda N,, Akazawa H,, Ito K,, Shimizu I,, Kudo-Sakamoto Y,, Yabumoto C,, et al. Agonist-independent constitutive activity of angiotensin II receptor promotes cardiac remodeling in mice. *Hypertension*. March;59(3):627-633.

[91] Eguchi S, Numaguchi K, Iwasaki H, Matsumoto T, Yamakawa T, Utsunomiya H, et al. Calcium-dependent epidermal growth factor receptor transactivation mediates the angiotensin II-induced mitogen-activated protein kinase activation in vascular smooth muscle cells. J Biol Chem 1998;273(15):8890–6.

[92] Lautrette A, Li S, Alili R, Sunnarborg SW, Burtin M, Lee DC, et al. Angiotensin II and EGF receptor cross-talk in chronic kidney diseases: a new therapeutic approach. Nat Med 2005;11(8):867–74.

[93] Burson JM, Aguilera G, Gross KW, Sigmund CD. Differential expression of angiotensin receptor 1A and 1B in mouse. Am J Physiol 1994;267(2 Pt 1):E260–267.

[94] Iwai N, Inagami T, Ohmichi N, Nakamura Y, Saeki Y, Kinoshita M. Differential regulation of rat AT1a and AT1b receptor mRNA. Biochem Biophys Res Commun 1992;188(1):298–303.

[95] Gasc JM, Shanmugam S, Sibony M, Corvol P. Tissue-specific expression of type 1 angiotensin II receptor subtypes. An *in situ* hybridization study. Hypertension 1994;24(5):531–7.

[96] Llorens-Cortes C, Greenberg B, Huang H, Corvol P. Tissular expression and regulation of type 1 angiotensin II receptor subtypes by quantitative reverse transcriptase-polymerase chain reaction analysis. Hypertension 1994;24(5):538–48.

[97] Konishi H, Kuroda S, Inada Y, Fujisawa Y. Novel subtype of human angiotensin II type 1 receptor: cDNA cloning and expression. Biochem Biophys Res Commun 1994;199(2):467–74.

[98] Chiu A, Dunscomb J, McCall D, Benfield P, Baubonis W, Sauer B. Characterization of angiotensin AT1A receptor isoform by it ligand binding signature. Regul Pept 1993;44:141–7.

[99] Oliverio MI, Best CF, Kim HS, Arendshorst WJ, Smithies O, Coffman TM. Angiotensin II responses in AT1A receptor-deficient mice: a role for AT1B receptors in blood pressure regulation. Am J Physiol 1997;272(4 Pt 2):F515–520.

[100] Oliverio MI, Kim HS, Ito M, Le T, Audoly L, Best CF, et al. Reduced growth, abnormal kidney structure, and type 2 (AT2) angiotensin receptor-mediated blood pressure regulation in mice lacking both AT1A and AT1B receptors for angiotensin II. Proc Natl Acad Sci USA 1998;95(26):15496–501.

[101] Davisson RL, Oliverio MI, Coffman TM, Sigmund CD. Divergent functions of angiotensin II receptor isoforms in the brain. J Clin Invest 2000;106(1):103–6.

[102] Ito M, Oliverio MI, Mannon PJ, Best CF, Maeda N, Smithies O, et al. Regulation of blood pressure by the type 1A angiotensin II receptor gene. Proc Natl Acad Sci USA 1995;92(8):3521–6.

[103] Matsusaka T, Nishimura H, Utsunomiya H, Kakuchi J, Nijmura F, Inagami T, et al. Chimeric mice carrying "regional" targeted deletion of the angiotensin type 1A receptor gene. Evidence against the role for local angiotensin in the *in vivo* feedback regulation of renin synthesis in juxtaglomerular cells. J Clin Invest 1996;98(8):1867–77.

[104] Sugaya T, Nishimatsu S, Tanimoto K, Takimoto E, Yamagishi T, Imamura K, et al. Angiotensin II type 1a receptor-deficient mice with hypotension and hyperreninemia. J Biol Chem 1995;270(32):18719–22.

[105] Oliverio MI, Best CF, Smithies O, Coffman TM. Regulation of sodium balance and blood pressure by the AT(1A) receptor for angiotensin II. Hypertension 2000;35(2):550–4.

[106] Grady E, Sechi L, Griffn C, Schambelan M, Kalinyak J. Expression of AT2 receptors in the developing rat fetus. J Clin Invest 1991;88:921–33.

[107] Millan M, Carvallo P, Izumi S-I, Zemel S, Catt K, Aguilera G. Novel sites of expression of functional angiotensin II receptors in the late gestation fetus. Science 1989;244:1340–2.

[108] Ichiki T, Kambayashi Y, Inagami T. Multiple growth factors modulate mRNA expression of angiotensin II type-2 receptor in R3T3 cells. Circ Res 1995;77(6):1070–6.

[109] Berry C, Touyz R, Dominiczak AF, Webb RC, Johns DG. Angiotensin receptors: Signaling, vascular pathophysiology, and interactions with ceramide. Am J Physiol Heart Circ Physiol 2001;281(6):H2337–2365.

[110] Hayashida W, Horiuchi M, Dzau VJ. Intracellular third loop domain of angiotensin II type-2 receptor. Role in mediating signal transduction and cellular function. J Biol Chem 1996;271(36):21985–92.

[111] Lehtonen JY, Daviet L, Nahmias C, Horiuchi M, Dzau VJ. Analysis of functional domains of angiotensin II type 2 receptor involved in apoptosis. Mol Endocrinol 1999;13(7):1051–60.

[112] Carey RM, Wang ZQ, Siragy HM. Role of the angiotensin type 2 receptor in the regulation of blood pressure and renal function. Hypertension 2000;35(1 Pt 2):155–63.

[113] Siragy HM, Carey RM. The subtype-2 (AT2) angiotensin receptor regulates renal cyclic guanosine 3′,5′-monophosphate and AT1 receptor-mediated prostaglandin E2 production in conscious rats. J Clin Invest 1996;97(8):1978–82.

[114] Dulin NO, Alexander LD, Harwalkar S, Falck JR, Douglas JG. Phospholipase A2-mediated activation of mitogen-activated

protein kinase by angiotensin II. Proc Natl Acad Sci USA 1998;95(14):8098–102.

[115] Hein L, Barsh GS, Pratt RE, Dzau VJ, Kobilka BK. Behavioural and cardiovascular effects of disrupting the angiotensin II type-2 receptor in mice. Nature 1995;377(6551):744–7.

[116] Ichiki T, Labosky PA, Shiota C, Okuyama S, Imagawa Y, Fogo A, et al. Effects on blood pressure and exploratory behaviour of mice lacking angiotensin II type-2 receptor. Nature 1995;377(6551):748–50.

[117] Masaki H, Kurihara T, Yamaki A, Inomata N, Nozawa Y, Mori Y, et al. Cardiac-specific overexpression of angiotensin II AT2 receptor causes attenuated response to AT1 receptor-mediated pressor and chronotropic effects. J Clin Invest 1998;101(3):527–35.

[118] Steckelings UM, Larhed M, Hallberg A, Widdop RE, Jones ES, Wallinder C, et al. Non-peptide AT2-receptor agonists. Curr Opin Pharmacol 2011;11(2):187–92.

[119] Aguilera G. Role of angiotensin II receptor subtypes on the regulation of aldosterone secretion in the adrenal glomerulosa zone in the rat. Mol Cell Endocrinol 1992;90(1):53–60.

[120] Okubo S, Niimura F, Nishimura H, Takemoto F, Fogo A, Matsusaka T, et al. Angiotensin-independent mechanism for aldosterone synthesis during chronic extracellular fluid volume depletion. J Clin Invest 1997;99(5):855–60.

[121] Quinn SJ, Williams GH. Regulation of aldosterone secretion. Annu Rev Physiol 1988;50:409–26.

[122] Aguilera G. Factors controlling steroid biosynthesis in the zona glomerulosa of the adrenal. J Steroid Biochem Mol Biol 1993;45(1-3):147–51.

[123] Fuller PJ, Young MJ. Mechanisms of mineralocorticoid action. Hypertension 2005;46(6):1227–35.

[124] Rogerson FM, Fuller PJ. Mineralocorticoid action. Steroids 2000;65(2):61–73.

[125] Masilamani S, Kim GH, Mitchell C, Wade JB, Knepper MA. Aldosterone-mediated regulation of ENaC alpha, beta, and gamma subunit proteins in rat kidney. J Clin Invest 1999;104 (7):R19–23.

[126] Asher C, Wald H, Rossier BC, Garty H. Aldosterone-induced increase in the abundance of Na+ channel subunits. Am J Physiol 1996;271(2 Pt 1):C605–611.

[127] Gumz ML, Stow LR, Lynch IJ, Greenlee MM, Rudin A, Cain BD, et al. The circadian clock protein Period 1 regulates expression of the renal epithelial sodium channel in mice. J Clin Invest 2009;119(8):2423–34.

[128] Naray-Fejes-Toth A. Sgk: a new player (star?) in the early action of aldosterone. News Physiol Sci 1999;14:274–5.

[129] Brennan FE, Fuller PJ. Rapid upregulation of serum and glucocorticoid-regulated kinase (sgk) gene expression by corticosteroids in vivo. Mol Cell Endocrinol 2000;166(2):129–36.

[130] Bhargava A, Fullerton MJ, Myles K, Purdy TM, Funder JW, Pearce D, et al. The serum- and glucocorticoid-induced kinase is a physiological mediator of aldosterone action. Endocrinology 2001;142(4):1587–94.

[131] Zhang W, Xia X, Reisenauer MR, Rieg T, Lang F, Kuhl D, et al. Aldosterone-induced Sgk1 relieves Dot1a-Af9-mediated transcriptional repression of epithelial Na+ channel alpha. J Clin Invest 2007;117(3):773–83.

[132] McCormick JA, Bhalla V, Pao AC, Pearce D. SGK1: a rapid aldosterone-induced regulator of renal sodium reabsorption. Physiology (Bethesda) 2005;20:134–9.

[133] Vallon V, Wulff P, Huang DY, Loffing J, Völkl H, Kuhl D, et al. Role of Sgk1 in salt and potassium homeostasis. Am J Physiol Regul Integr Comp Physiol 2005;288(1):R4–10.

[134] Yoo D, Kim BY, Campo C, Nance L, King A, Maouyo D, et al. Cell surface expression of the ROMK (Kir 1.1) channel is regulated by the aldosterone-induced kinase, SGK-1, and protein kinase A. J Biol Chem 2003;278(25):23066–75.

[135] Beesley AH, Hornby D, White SJ. Regulation of distal nephron K+ channels (ROMK) mRNA expression by aldosterone in rat kidney. J Physiol 1998;509(Pt 3):629–34.

[136] Rozansky DJ. Cornwall T, Subramanya AR, Rogers S, Yang YF, David LL, Zhu X, Yang CL, Ellison DH. Aldosterone mediates activation of the thiazide-sensitive Na-Cl co-transporter through an SGK1 and WNK4 signaling pathway. J Clin Invest 2009;119(9):2601–12.

[137] Geller DS, Farhi A, Pinkerton N, Fradley M, Moritz M, Spitzer A, et al. Activating mineralocorticoid receptor mutation in hypertension exacerbated by pregnancy. Science 2000;289(5476):119–23.

[138] Geller DS, Rodriguez-Soriano J, Vallo Boado A, Schifter S, Bayer M, Chang SS, et al. Mutations in the mineralocorticoid receptor gene cause autosomal dominant pseudohypoaldosteronism type I. Nat Genet 1998;19(3):279–81.

[139] Berger S, Bleich M, Schmid W, Cole TJ, Peters J, Watanabe H, et al. Mineralocorticoid receptor knockout mice: Pathophysiology of Na+ metabolism. PNAS 1998;95(16):9424–9.

[140] Ronzaud C, Loffing J, Bleich M, Gretz N, Grone HJ, Schutz G, et al. Impairment of sodium balance in mice deficient in renal principal cell mineralocorticoid receptor. J Am Soc Nephrol 2007;18(6):1679–87.

[141] Pergher PS, Leite-Dellova D, de Mello-Aires M. Direct action of aldosterone on bicarbonate reabsorption in in vivo cortical proximal tubule. Am J Physiol Renal Physiol 2009;296(5): F1185–1193.

[142] Leite-Dellova DC, Oliveira-Souza M, Malnic G, Mello-Aires M. Genomic and nongenomic dose-dependent biphasic effect of aldosterone on Na+/H+ exchanger in proximal S3 segment: role of cytosolic calcium. Am J Physiol Renal Physiol 2008;295 (5):F1342–1352.

[143] Watts 3rd BA, George T, Good DW. Aldosterone inhibits apical NHE3 and HCO3− absorption via a nongenomic ERK-dependent pathway in medullary thick ascending limb. Am J Physiol Renal Physiol 2006;291(5):F1005–1013.

[144] Lifton R. Genetic determinants of human hypertension. PNAS 1995;92(19):8545–51.

[145] Firsov D, Schild L, Gautschi I, Merillat A-M, Schneeberger E, Rossier Bernard C. Cell surface expression of the epithelial Na channel and a mutant causing Liddle syndrome: a quantitative approach. PNAS 1996;93(26):15370–5.

[146] Tamura H, Schild L, Enomoto N, Matsui N, Marumo F, Rossier BC. Liddle disease caused by a missense mutation of beta subunit of the epithelial sodium channel gene. J Clin Invest 1996;97(7):1780–4.

[147] Rossier BC, Pradervand S, Schild L, Hummler E. Epithelial sodium channel and the control of sodium balance: interaction between genetic and environmental factors. Annu Rev Physiol 2002;64:877–97.

[148] Rubera I, Loffing J, Palmer LG, Frindt G, Fowler-Jaeger N, Sauter D, et al. Collecting duct-specific gene inactivation of alphaENaC in the mouse kidney does not impair sodium and potassium balance. J Clin Invest 2003;112(4):554–65.

[149] Biner HL, Arpin-Bott MP, Loffing J, Wang X, Knepper M, Hebert SC, et al. Human cortical distal nephron: distribution of electrolyte and water transport pathways. J Am Soc Nephrol 2002;13(4):836–47.

[150] Greene EL, Kren S, Hostetter TH. Role of aldosterone in the remnant kidney model in the rat. J Clin Invest 1996;98 (4):1063–8.

[151] Leopold JA, Dam A, Maron BA, Scribner AW, Liao R, Handy DE, et al. Aldosterone impairs vascular reactivity by

decreasing glucose-6-phosphate dehydrogenase activity. Nat Med 2007;13(2):189—97.

[152] Jaffe IZ, Newfell BG, Aronovitz M, Mohammad NN, McGraw AP, Perreault RE, et al. Placental growth factor mediates aldosterone-dependent vascular injury in mice. J Clin Invest 2010;120(11):3891—900.

[153] Terada Y, Kobayashi T, Kuwana H, Tanaka H, Inoshita S, Kuwahara M, et al. Aldosterone stimulates proliferation of mesangial cells by activating mitogen-activated protein kinase 1/2, cyclin D1, and cyclin A. J Am Soc Nephrol 2005;16(8):2296—305.

[154] Miyata K, Rahman M, Shokoji T, Nagai Y, Zhang GX, Sun GP, et al. Aldosterone stimulates reactive oxygen species production through activation of NADPH oxidase in rat mesangial cells. J Am Soc Nephrol 2005;16(10):2906—12.

[155] Terada Y, Kuwana H, Kobayashi T, Okado T, Suzuki N, Yoshimoto T, et al. Aldosterone-stimulated SGK1 activity mediates profibrotic signaling in the mesangium. J Am Soc Nephrol 2008;19(2):298—309.

[156] Shibata S, Nagase M, Yoshida S, Kawachi H, Fujita T. Podocyte as the target for aldosterone: roles of oxidative stress and Sgk1. Hypertension 2007;49(2):355—64.

[157] Lee SH, Yoo TH, Nam BY, Kim DK, Li JJ, Jung DS, et al. Activation of local aldosterone system within podocytes is involved in apoptosis under diabetic conditions. Am J Physiol Renal Physiol 2009;297(5):F1381—1390.

[158] Chrysostomou A, Pedagogos E, MacGregor L, Becker GJ. Double-blind, placebo-controlled study on the effect of the aldosterone receptor antagonist spironolactone in patients who have persistent proteinuria and are on long-term angiotensin-converting enzyme inhibitor therapy, with or without an angiotensin II receptor blocker. Clin J Am Soc Nephrol 2006;1(2):256—62.

[159] Cowley Jr. AW, Roman RJ. The role of the kidney in hypertension. Jama 1996;275(20):1581—9.

[160] Aperia AC, Broberger CG, Soderlund S. Relationship between renal artery perfusion pressure and tubular sodium reabsorption. Am J Physiol 1971;220(5):1205—12.

[161] Guyton AC, Coleman TG, Cowley Jr. AV, Scheel KW, Manning Jr. RD, Norman Jr. RA. Arterial pressure regulation. Overriding dominance of the kidneys in long-term regulation and in hypertension. Am J Med 1972;52(5):584—94.

[162] Hall JE, Brands MW, Henegar JR. Angiotensin II and long-term arterial pressure regulation: the overriding dominance of the kidney. J Am Soc Nephrol 1999;10(Suppl 12):S258—265.

[163] Hall JE, Granger JP. Adenosine alters glomerular filtration control by angiotensin II. Am J Physiol 1986;250(5 Pt 2):F917—923.

[164] Hall JE. Control of sodium excretion by angiotensin II: Intrarenal mechanisms and blood pressure regulation. Am J Physiol 1986;250(6 Pt 2):R960—972.

[165] Campbell DJ. Extrarenal renin and blood pressure regulation. An alternative viewpoint. Am J Hypertens 1989;2(4):266—75.

[166] Sequeira Lopez ML, Pentz ES, Robert B, Abrahamson DR, Gomez RA. Embryonic origin and lineage of juxtaglomerular cells. Am J Physiol Renal Physiol 2001;281(2):F345—356.

[167] Barajas L. Anatomy of the juxtaglomerular apparatus. Am J Physiol 1979;237(5):F333—343.

[168] Taugner C, Poulsen K, Hackenthal E, Taugner R. Immunocytochemical localization of renin in mouse kidney. Histochemistry 1979;62(1):19—27.

[169] Vander AJ. Control of renin release. Physiological Review 1967;47(3):359—82.

[170] Sequeira Lopez ML, Gomez RA. The role of angiotensin II in kidney embryogenesis and kidney abnormalities. Curr Opin Nephrol Hypertens 2004;13(1):117—22.

[171] Rohrwasser A, Morgan T, Dillon HF, Zhao L, Callaway CW, Hillas E, et al. Elements of a paracrine tubular renin-angiotensin system along the entire nephron. Hypertension 1999;34(6):1265—74.

[172] Silver RB, Reid AC, Mackins CJ, Askwith T, Schaefer U, Herzlinger D, et al. Mast cells: a unique source of renin. Proc Natl Acad Sci USA 2004;101(37):13607—12.

[173] Mackins CJ, Kano S, Seyedi N, Schafer U, Reid AC, Machida T, et al. Cardiac mast cell-derived renin promotes local angiotensin formation, norepinephrine release, and arrhythmias in ischemia/reperfusion. J Clin Invest 2006;116(4):1063—70.

[174] Le TH, Coffman TM. A new cardiac MASTer switch for the renin—angiotensin system. J Clin Invest 2006;116(4):866—9.

[175] Tobian L, Tomboulian A, Janecek J. The effect of high perfusion pressures on the granulation of juxtaglomerular cells in an isolated kidney. J Clin Invest 1959;38(4):605—10.

[176] Skinner SL, McCubbin JW, Page IH. Control of renin secretion. Circ Res 1964;15:64—76.

[177] Kirchheim H, Ehmke H, Persson P. Physiology of the renal baroreceptor mechanism of renin release and its role in congestive heart failure. Am J Cardiol 1988;62(8):68E—71E.

[178] Nobiling R, Munter K, Buhrle CP, Hackenthal E. Influence of pulsatile perfusion upon renin release from the isolated perfused rat kidney. Pflugers Arch 1990;415(6):713—7.

[179] Hackenthal E, Paul M, Ganten D, Taugner R. Morphology, physiology, and molecular biology of renin secretion. Physiol Rev 1990;70(4):1067—116.

[180] Blaine EH, Davis JO, Witty RT. Renin release after hemorrhage and after suprarenal aortic constriction in dogs without sodium delivery to the macula densa. Circ Res 1970;27(6):1081—9.

[181] Blaine EH, Davis JO, Prewitt RL. Evidence for a renal vascular receptor in control of renin secretion. Am J Physiol 1971;220(6):1593—7.

[182] Fray JC. Stretch receptor model for renin release with evidence from perfused rat kidney. Am J Physiol 1976;231(3):936—44.

[183] Hofbauer KG, Zschiedrich H, Hackenthal E, Gross F. Function of the renin—angiotensin system in the isolated perfused rat kidney. Circ Res 1974;:I193—202.

[184] Tokumori Y, Kurahashi A, Murakami J, Mokuda GO, Ikeda T, Takeda A, et al. Biphasic renin release from perfused rat kidney. Horm Metab Res 1983;15(6):310—1.

[185] Romero JC, Feldstein AE, Rodriguez-Porcel MG, Cases-Amenos A. New insights into the pathophysiology of renovascular hypertension. Mayo Clin Proc 1997;72(3):251—60.

[186] Fray JC. Regulation of renin secretion by calcium and chemiosmotic forces: (Patho) physiological considerations. Biochim Biophys Acta 1991;1097(4):243—62.

[187] Osborn JL, Kopp UC, Thames MD, DiBona GF. Interactions among renal nerves, prostaglandins, and renal arterial pressure in the regulation of renin release. Am J Physiol 1984;247(5 Pt 2):F706—713.

[188] Knoblich PR, Freeman RH, Villarreal D. Pressure-dependent renin release during chronic blockade of nitric oxide synthase. Hypertension 1996;28(5):738—42.

[189] Persson PB, Baumann JE, Ehmke H, Hackenthal E, Kirchheim HR, Nafz B. Endothelium-derived NO stimulates pressure-dependent renin release in conscious dogs. Am J Physiol 1993;264(6 Pt 2):F943—947.

[190] Kurtz A, Wagner C. Role of nitric oxide in the control of renin secretion. Am J Physiol 1998;275(6 Pt 2):F849—862.

[191] Data JL, Gerber JG, Crump WJ, Frolich JC, Hollifield JW, Nies AS. The prostaglandin system. A role in canine baroreceptor control of renin release. Circ Res 1978;42(4):454—8.

[192] Gerber JG, Keller RT, Nies AS. Prostaglandins and renin release: the effect of PGI2, PGE2, and 13,14-dihydro PGE2 on the baroreceptor mechanism of renin release in the dog. Circ Res 1979;44(6):796–9.

[193] Munter K, Hackenthal E. The effects of endothelin on renovascular resistance and renin release. J Hypertens Suppl 1989;7(6): S276–277.

[194] Beierwaltes WH, Potter DL, Shesely EG. Renal baroreceptor-stimulated renin in the eNOS knockout mouse. Am J Physiol Renal Physiol 2002;282(1):F59–64.

[195] Fujino T, Nakagawa N, Yuhki K, Hara A, Yamada T, Takayama K, et al. Decreased susceptibility to renovascular hypertension in mice lacking the prostaglandin I2 receptor IP. J Clin Invest 2004;114(6):805–12.

[196] Francois H, Coffman TM. Prostanoids and blood pressure: which way is up? J Clin Invest 2004;114(6):757–9.

[197] Scholz H, Gotz KH, Hamann M, Kurtz A. Differential effects of extracellular anions on renin secretion from isolated perfused rat kidneys. Am J Physiol 1994;267(6 Pt 2):F1076–1081.

[198] Krattinger N, Capponi A, Mazzolai L, Aubert JF, Caille D, Nicod P, et al. Connexin40 regulates renin production and blood pressure. Kidney Int 2007;72(7):814–22.

[199] Wagner C, de Wit C, Kurtz L, Grunberger C, Kurtz A, Schweda F. Connexin40 is essential for the pressure control of renin synthesis and secretion. Circ Res 2007;100(4):556–63.

[200] Schweda F, Kurtz L, de Wit C, Janssen-Bienhold U, Kurtz A, Wagner C. Substitution of connexin40 with connexin45 prevents hyperreninemia and attenuates hypertension. Kidney Int 2009;75(5):482–9.

[201] Haefliger JA, Krattinger N, Martin D, Pedrazzini T, Capponi A, Doring B, et al. Connexin43-dependent mechanism modulates renin secretion and hypertension. J Clin Invest 2006;116 (2):405–13.

[202] Goormaghtigh N. Fact in favor of an endocrine function of the renal arterioles. J. Pathol Bacteriol 1945;57:392–404.

[203] Thurau K, Schnermann J, Nagel W, Horster M, Wahl M. Composition of tubular fluid in the macula densa segment as a factor regulating the function of the juxtaglomerular apparatus. Circ Res 1967;21((1):Suppl 2):79–90.

[204] Skott O, Briggs JP. Direct demonstration of macula densa-mediated renin secretion. Science 1987;237(4822):1618–20.

[205] Schlatter E, Salomonsson M, Persson AE, Greger R. Macula densa cells sense luminal NaCl concentration via furosemide sensitive $Na^+2Cl^-K^+$ co-transport. Pflugers Arch 1989;414 (3):286–90.

[206] Martinez-Maldonado M, Gely R, Tapia E, Benabe JE. Role of macula densa in diuretics-induced renin release. Hypertension 1990;16(3):261–8.

[207] Kotchen TA, Galla JH, Luke RG. Failure of $NaHCO_3$ and $KHCO_3$ to inhibit renin in the rat. Am J Physiol 1976;231 (4):1050–6.

[208] Hanner F, Chambrey R, Bourgeois S, Meer E, Mucsi I, Rosivall L, et al. Increased renal renin content in mice lacking the Na^+/H^+ exchanger NHE2. Am J Physiol Renal Physiol 2008;294(4):F937–944.

[209] Ledoussal C, Lorenz JN, Nieman ML, Soleimani M, Schultheis PJ, Shull GE. Renal salt wasting in mice lacking NHE3 Na^+/H^+ exchanger but not in mice lacking NHE2. Am J Physiol Renal Physiol 2001;281(4):F718–727.

[210] Churchill PC, Churchill MC. A1 and A2 adenosine receptor activation inhibits and stimulates renin secretion of rat renal cortical slices. J Pharmacol Exp Ther 1985;232(3):589–94.

[211] Harris RC, Breyer MD. Physiological regulation of cyclooxygenase-2 in the kidney. Am J Physiol Renal Physiol 2001;281 (1):F1–11.

[212] Schweda F, Klar J, Narumiya S, Nusing RM, Kurtz A. Stimulation of renin release by prostaglandin E2 is mediated by EP2 and EP4 receptors in mouse kidneys. Am J Physiol Renal Physiol 2004;287(3):F427–433.

[213] Schnermann J, Homer W. Smith Award lecture. The juxtaglomerular apparatus: from anatomical peculiarity to physiological relevance. J Am Soc Nephrol 2003;14(6):1681–94.

[214] Schweda F, Kurtz A. Cellular mechanism of renin release. Acta Physiol Scand 2004;181(4):383–90.

[215] Facemire CS, Nguyen M, Jania L, Beierwaltes WH, Kim HS, Koller BH, et al. A major role for the EP4 receptor in regulation of renin. Am J Physiol Renal Physiol 2011;301(5): F1035–1041.

[216] Beierwaltes WH, Schryver S, Sanders E, Strand J, Romero JC. Renin release selectively stimulated by prostaglandin I2 in isolated rat glomeruli. Am J Physiol 1982;243(3):F276–283.

[217] Webber PC, Larsson C, Anggard E, Hamberg M, Corey EJ, Nicolaou KC, et al. Stimulation of renin release from rabbit renal cortex by arachidonic acid and prostaglandin endoperoxides. Circ Res 1976;39(6):868–74.

[218] Harding P, Sigmon DH, Alfie ME, Huang PL, Fishman MC, Beierwaltes WH, et al. Cyclooxygenase-2 mediates increased renal renin content induced by low-sodium diet. Hypertension 1997;29(1 Pt 2):297–302.

[219] Cheng H, Harris R. Angiotensin converting enzyme inhibitor-mediated increases in renal renin expression are not seen in cyclooxygenase-2 knockout mice. J Am Soc Nephrol 1999;10:343A.

[220] Peti-Peterdi J, Komlosi P, Fuson AL, Guan Y, Schneider A, Qi Z, et al. Luminal NaCl delivery regulates basolateral PGE2 release from macula densa cells. J Clin Invest 2003;112(1):76–82.

[221] Yang T, Endo Y, Huang YG, Smart A, Briggs JP, Schnermann J. Renin expression in COX-2-knockout mice on normal or low-salt diets. Am J Physiol Renal Physiol 2000;279(5): F819–825.

[222] Weihprecht H, Lorenz JN, Schnermann J, Skott O, Briggs JP. Effect of adenosine1-receptor blockade on renin release from rabbit isolated perfused juxtaglomerular apparatus. J Clin Invest 1990;85(5):1622–8.

[223] Kim SM, Mizel D, Huang YG, Briggs JP, Schnermann J. Adenosine as a mediator of macula densa-dependent inhibition of renin secretion. Am J Physiol Renal Physiol 2006;290(5): F1016–1023.

[224] Mundel P, Bachmann S, Bader M, Fischer A, Kummer W, Mayer B, et al. Expression of nitric oxide synthase in kidney macula densa cells. Kidney Int 1992;42(4):1017–9.

[225] Wilcox CS, Welch WJ. Macula densa nitric oxide synthase: expression, regulation, and function. Kidney Int Suppl 1998;67:S53–57.

[226] He XR, Greenberg SG, Briggs JP, Schnermann JB. Effect of nitric oxide on renin secretion. II. Studies in the perfused juxtaglomerular apparatus. Am J Physiol 1995;268(5 Pt 2): F953–959.

[227] Tharaux PL, Dussaule JC, Pauti MD, Vassitch Y, Ardaillou R, Chatziantoniou C. Activation of renin synthesis is dependent on intact nitric oxide production. Kidney Int 1997;51 (6):1780–7.

[228] Castrop H, Schweda F, Mizel D, Huang Y, Briggs J, Kurtz A, et al. Permissive role of nitric oxide in macula densa control of renin secretion. Am J Physiol Renal Physiol 2004;286(5): F848–857.

[229] Shricker K, Holmer S, Kramer BK, Riegger GA, Kurtz A. The role of angiotensin II in the feedback control of renin gene expression. Pflugers Arch 1997;434(2):166–72.

[230] Oliverio MI, Madsen K, Best CF, Ito M, Maeda N, Smithies O, et al. Renal growth and development in mice lacking AT1A receptors for angiotensin II. Am J Physiol 1998;274(1 Pt 2): F43–50.

[231] Gomez RA, Chevalier RL, Everett AD, Elwood JP, Peach MJ, Lynch KR, et al. Recruitment of renin gene-expressing cells in adult rat kidneys. Am J Physiol 1990;259(4 Pt 2):F660–665.

[232] Crowley SD, Gurley SB, Oliverio MI, Pazmino AK, Griffiths R, Flannery PJ, et al. Distinct roles for the kidney and systemic tissues in blood pressure regulation by the renin–angiotensin system. J Clin Invest 2005;115(4):1092–9.

[233] Lew R, Summers RJ. The distribution of beta-adrenoceptors in dog kidney: an autoradiographic analysis. Eur J Pharmacol 1987;140(1):1–11.

[234] Keeton TK, Campbell WB. The pharmacologic alteration of renin release. Pharmacol Rev 1980;32(2):81–227.

[235] Holdaas H, DiBona GF, Kiil F. Effect of low-level renal nerve stimulation on renin release from nonfiltering kidneys. Am J Physiol 1981;241(2):F156–161.

[236] Holdaas H, Langard O, Eide I, Kiil F. Mechanism of renin release during renal nerve stimulation in dogs. Scand J Clin Lab Invest 1981;41(7):617–25.

[237] DiBona GF. Neural regulation of renal tubular sodium reabsorption and renin secretion. Fed Proc 1985;44(13):2816–22.

[238] Kirchheim HR, Gross R, Hackenberg HM, Hackenthal E, Huber J. Autoregulation of renin release and its modification by renal sympathetic nerves in conscious dogs. Kidney Inst 1981;20:152.

[239] Blaine EH, Davis JO. Evidence for a renal vascular mechanism in renin release: new observations with graded stimulation by aortic constriction. Circ Res 1971;28((5):Suppl 2):118–26.

[240] Esler MD, Krum H, Sobotka PA, Schlaich MP, Schmieder RE, Bohm M. Renal sympathetic denervation in patients with treatment-resistant hypertension (The Symplicity HTN-2 Trial): a randomised controlled trial. *Lancet* 2010;376 (9756):1903–9.

[241] Friis UG, Jensen BL, Hansen PB, Andreasen D, Skott O. Exocytosis and endocytosis in juxtaglomerular cells. Acta Physiol Scand 2000;168(1):95–9.

[242] Friis UG, Jensen BL, Aas JK, Skott O. Direct demonstration of exocytosis and endocytosis in single mouse juxtaglomerular cells. Circ Res 1999;84(8):929–36.

[243] Churchill PC. Second messengers in renin secretion. Am J Physiol Renal Physiol 1985;249(2):F175–184.

[244] Kurtz A, Wagner C. Cellular control of renin secretion. J Exp Biol 1999;202(Pt 3):219–25.

[245] Kurtz A, Pfeilschifter J, Hutter A, Buhrle C, Nobiling R, Taugner R, et al. Role of protein kinase C in inhibition of renin release caused by vasoconstrictors. Am J Physiol 1986;250(4 Pt 1):C563–571.

[246] Churchill MC, Churchill PC. 12-0-Tetradecanoylphorbol 13-acetate inhibits renin secretion of rat renal cortical slices. Journal of Hypertension 1984;2(1):25–8.

[247] Churchill PC, Rossi NF, Churchill MC, Ellis VR. Effect of melittin on renin and prostaglandin E2 release from rat renal cortical slices. J Physiol 1990;428:233–41.

[248] Park CS, Honeyman TW, Chung ES, Lee JS, Sigmon DH, Fray JC. Involvement of calmodulin in mediating inhibitory action of intracellular Ca^{2+} on renin secretion. Am J Physiol 1986;251 (6 Pt 2):F1055–1062.

[249] Della Bruna R, Pinet F, Corvol P, Kurtz A. Calmodulin antagonists stimulate renin secretion and inhibit renin synthesis *in vitro*. Am J Physiol 1992;262(3 Pt 2):F397–402.

[250] Rasmussen H, Barrett PQ. Calcium messenger system: an integrated view. Physiol Rev 1984;64(3):938–84.

[251] Sigmund CD, Jones CA, Kane CM, Wu C, Lang JA, Gross KW. Regulated tissue- and cell-specific expression of the human renin gene in transgenic mice. Circ Res 1992;70 (5):1070–9.

[252] Fukamizu A, Hatae T, Kon Y, Sugimura M, Hasegawa T, Yokoyama M, et al. Human renin in transgenic mouse kidney is localized to juxtaglomerular cells. Biochem J 1991;278(Pt 2):601–3.

[253] Pan L, Wang Y, Jones CA, Glenn ST, Baumann H, Gross KW. Enhancer-dependent inhibition of mouse renin transcription by inflammatory cytokines. Am J Physiol Renal Physiol 2005;288(1):F117–124.

[254] Borensztein P, Germain S, Fuchs S, Philippe J, Corvol P, Pinet F. cis-Regulatory elements and trans-acting factors directing basal and cAMP-stimulated human renin gene expression in chorionic cells. Circ Res 1994;74(5):764–73.

[255] Smith DL, Morris BJ, Do YS, Law RE, Shaw KJ, Hseuh WA. Identification of cyclic AMP response element in the human renin gene. Biochem Biophys Res Commun 1994;200 (1):320–9.

[256] Paul M, Burt DW, Krieger JE, Nakamura N, Dzau VJ. Tissue specificity of renin promoter activity and regulation in mice. Am J Physiol 1992;262(5 Pt 1):E644–650.

[257] Morris BJ, Smith DL, Law RE, Do YS, Shaw KJ, Hsueh WA. Function of human renin proximal promoter DNA. Kidney Int 1994;46(6):1516–21.

[258] Ying L, Morris BJ, Sigmund CD. Transactivation of the human renin promoter by the cyclic AMP/protein kinase A pathway is mediated by both cAMP-responsive element binding protein-1 (CREB)-dependent and CREB-independent mechanisms in Calu-6 cells. J Biol Chem 1997;272(4):2412–20.

[259] Petrovic N, Black TA, Fabian JR, Kane C, Jones CA, Loudon JA, et al. Role of proximal promoter elements in regulation of renin gene transcription. J Biol Chem 1996;271(37):22499–505.

[260] Germain S, Bonnet F, Philippe J, Fuchs S, Corvol P, Pinet F. A novel distal enhancer confers chorionic expression on the human renin gene. J Biol Chem 1998;273(39):25292–300.

[261] Pan L, Gross KW. Transcriptional regulation of renin: an update. Hypertension 2005;45(1):3–8.

[262] Lang JA, Ying LH, Morris BJ, Sigmund CD. Transcriptional and posttranscriptional mechanisms regulate human renin gene expression in Calu-6 cells. Am J Physiol 1996;271(1 Pt 2): F94–100.

[263] Chen M, Schnermann J, Smart AM, Brosius FC, Killen PD, Briggs JP. Cyclic AMP selectively increases renin mRNA stability in cultured juxtaglomerular granular cells. J Biol Chem 1993;268(32):24138–44.

[264] Morris BJ, Adams DJ, Beveridge DJ, van der Weyden L, Mangs H, Leedman PJ. cAMP controls human renin mRNA stability via specific RNA-binding proteins. Acta Physiol Scand 2004;181(4):369–73.

[265] Griendling KK, Ushio-Fukai M, Lassegue B, Alexander RW. Angiotensin II signaling in vascular smooth muscle. New concepts. Hypertension 1997;29(1 Pt 2):366–73.

[266] Blantz RC, Konnen KS, Tucker BJ. Angiotensin II effects upon the glomerular microcirculation and ultrafiltration coefficient of the rat. J Clin Invest 1976;57(2):419–34.

[267] Dworkin LD, Ichikawa I, Brenner BM. Hormonal modulation of glomerular function. Am J Physiol 1983;244(2):F95–104.

[268] Navar LG, Inscho EW, Majid SA, Imig JD, Harrison-Bernard LM, Mitchell KD. Paracrine regulation of the renal microcirculation. Physiol Rev 1996;76(2):425–536.

[269] Mendelsohn F, Dunbar M, Allen A, Chou S, Millan M, Aguilera G. Angiotensin II receptors in the kidney. Fed Proc 1986;45:1420–5.

[270] Ito S, Johnson CS, Carretero OA. Modulation of angiotensin II-induced vasoconstriction by endothelium-derived relaxing factor in the isolated microperfused rabbit afferent arteriole. J Clin Invest 1991;87(5):1656–63.

[271] Olsen ME, Hall JE, Montani JP, Cornell JE. Interaction between renal prostaglandins and angiotensin II in controlling glomerular filtration in the dog. Clin Sci (Lond) 1987;72(4):429–36.

[272] Fleming JT, Parekh N, Steinhausen M. Calcium antagonists preferentially dilate preglomerular vessels of hydronephrotic kidney. Am J Physiol 1987;253(6 Pt 2):F1157–1163.

[273] Carmines PK, Morrison TK, Navar LG. Angiotensin II effects on microvascular diameters of in vitro blood-perfused juxtamedullary nephrons. Am J Physiol 1986;251(4 Pt 2):F610–618.

[274] Carmines PK, Navar LG. Disparate effects of Ca channel blockade on afferent and efferent arteriolar responses to ANG II. Am J Physiol 1989;256(6 Pt 2):F1015–1020.

[275] Harrison-Bernard LM, Monjure CJ, Bivona BJ. Efferent arterioles exclusively express the subtype 1A angiotensin receptor: functional insights from genetic mouse models. Am J Physiol Renal Physiol 2006;290(5):F1177–1186.

[276] Cowley AW, Roman RJ, Fenoy FJ, Mattson DL. Effect of renal medullary circulation on arterial pressure. J Hypertens Suppl 1992;10(7):S187–193.

[277] Earley LE, Friedler RM. Changes in renal blood flow and possibly the intrarenal distribution of blood during the natriuresis accompanying saline loading in the dog. J Clin Invest 1965;44:929–41.

[278] Earley LE, Friedler RM. The effects of combined renal vasodilatation and pressor agents on renal hemodynamics and the tubular reabsorption of sodium. J Clin Invest 1966;45(4):542–51.

[279] Hricik DE. Captopril-induced renal insufficiency and the role of sodium balance. Ann Intern Med 1985;103(2):222–3.

[280] Textor SC, Tarazi RC, Novick AC, Bravo EL, Fouad FM. Regulation of renal hemodynamics and glomerular filtration in patients with renovascular hypertension during converting enzyme inhibition with captopril. Am J Med 1984;76(5B):29–37.

[281] Miller WL, Thomas RA, Berne RM, Rubio R. Adenosine production in the ischemic kidney. Circ Res 1978;43(3):390–7.

[282] Haddy FJ, Scott JB. Metabolically linked vasoactive chemicals in local regulation of blood flow. Physiol Rev 1968;48(4):688–707.

[283] Spielman WS, Thompson CI. A proposed role for adenosine in the regulation of renal hemodynamics and renin release. Am J Physiol 1982;242(5):F423–435.

[284] Woodcock EA, Loxley R, Leung E, Johnston CI. Demonstration of RA-adenosine receptors in rat renal papillae. Biochem Biophys Res Commun 1984;121(2):434–40.

[285] Miyamoto M, Yagil Y, Larson T, Robertson C, Jamison RL. Effects of intrarenal adenosine on renal function and medullary blood flow in the rat. Am J Physiol 1988;255(6 Pt 2):F1230–1234.

[286] Mason J. The pathophysiology of ischaemic acute renal failure. A new hypothesis about the initiation phase. Ren Physiol 1986;9(3):129–47.

[287] Osswald H, Schmitz HJ, Kemper R. Tissue content of adenosine, inosine and hypoxanthine in the rat kidney after ischemia and postischemic recirculation. Pflugers Arch 1977;371(1-2):45–9.

[288] Yagil Y, Miyamoto M, Jamison RL. Inner medullary blood flow in postischemic acute renal failure in the rat. Am J Physiol 1989;256(3 Pt 2):F456–461.

[289] Purdy KE, Arendshorst WJ. Prostaglandins buffer ANG II-mediated increases in cytosolic calcium in preglomerular VSMC. Am J Physiol 1999;277(6 Pt 2):F850–858.

[290] Jaimes EA, Hua P, Tian RX, Raij L. Human glomerular endothelium: interplay among glucose, free fatty acids, angiotensin II, and oxidative stress. Am J Physiol Renal Physiol 2010;298(1):F125–132.

[291] Ichihara A, Imig JD, Inscho EW, Navar LG. Interactive nitric oxide-angiotensin II influences on renal microcirculation in angiotensin II-induced hypertension. Hypertension 1998;31(6):1255–60.

[292] Zatz R, Dunn B, Anderson S, Rennke H, Brenner B. Prevention of diabetic glomerulopathy by pharmacological amelioration of glomerular capillary hypertension. J Clin Invest 1986;77:1925–30.

[293] Meyer TW, Anderson S, Rennke HG, Brenner BM. Reversing glomerular hypertension stabilizes established glomerular injury. Kidney Int 1987;31(3):752–9.

[294] Anderson S, Meyer T, Rennke H, Brenner B. Control of glomerular hypertension limits renal injury in rats with reduced renal mass. J Clin Invest 1985;76:612–9.

[295] Simons JL, Provoost AP, De Keijzer MH, Anderson S, Rennke HG, Brenner BM. Pathogenesis of glomerular injury in the fawn-hooded rat: effect of unilateral nephrectomy. J Am Soc Nephrol 1993;4(6):1362–70.

[296] Ruan X, Oliverio MI, Coffman TM, Arendshorst WJ. Renal vascular reactivity in mice: AngII-induced vasoconstriction in AT1A receptor null mice. J Am Soc Nephrol 1999;10(12):2620–30.

[297] Faubert PF, Chou SY, Porush JG. Regulation of papillary plasma flow by angiotensin II. Kidney Int 1987;32(4):472–8.

[298] Zou AP, Wu F, Cowley Jr. AW. Protective effect of angiotensin II-induced increase in nitric oxide in the renal medullary circulation. Hypertension 1998;31(1 Pt 2):271–6.

[299] Szentivanyi Jr. M, Maeda CY, Cowley Jr. AW. Local renal medullary L-NAME infusion enhances the effect of long-term angiotensin II treatment. Hypertension 1999;33(1 Pt 2):440–5.

[300] Dickhout JG, Mori T, Cowley Jr. AW. Tubulovascular nitric oxide crosstalk: buffering of angiotensin II-induced medullary vasoconstriction. Circ Res 2002;91(6):487–93.

[301] Roman RJ, Lianos E. Influence of prostaglandins on papillary blood flow and pressure-natriuretic response. Hypertension 1990;15(1):29–35.

[302] Roman RJ, Kauker ML. Renal effect of prostaglandin synthetase inhibition in rats: Micropuncture studies. Am J Physiol 1978;235(2):F111–118.

[303] Higashihara E, Stokes JB, Kokko JP, Campbell WB, DuBose Jr. TD. Cortical and papillary micropuncture examination of chloride transport in segments of the rat kidney during inhibition of prostaglandin production. Possible role for prostaglandins in the chloruresis of acute volume expansion. J Clin Invest 1979;64(5):1277–87.

[304] Chen PY, Sanders PW. L-arginine abrogates salt-sensitive hypertension in Dahl/Rapp rats. J Clin Invest 1991;88(5):1559–67.

[305] Szentivanyi Jr. M, Zou AP, Mattson DL, Soares P, Moreno C, Roman RJ, et al. Renal medullary nitric oxide deficit of Dahl S rats enhances hypertensive actions of angiotensin II. Am J Physiol Regul Integr Comp Physiol 2002;283(1):R266–272.

[306] He H, Kimura S, Fujisawa Y, Tomohiro A, Kiyomoto K, Aki Y, et al. Dietary L-arginine supplementation normalizes regional blood flow in Dahl-Iwai salt-sensitive rats. Am J Hypertens 1997;10(5 Pt 2):89S–93S.

[307] Hu L, Manning Jr. RD. Role of nitric oxide in regulation of long-term pressure-natriuresis relationship in Dahl rats. Am J Physiol 1995;268(6 Pt 2):H2375−2383.

[308] Rajapakse NW, Mattson DL. Role of L-arginine uptake mechanisms in renal blood flow responses to angiotensin II in rats. Acta Physiol (Oxf) 2011;203(3):391−400.

[309] Weiner I, New A, Milton A, Tisher C. Regulation of luminal alkalinization and acidification in the cortical collecting duct by angiotensin II. Am J Physiol 1995;38:F730−8.

[310] Geibel J, Giebisch G, Boron WF. Angiotensin II stimulates both Na$^{(+)}$-H$^+$ exchange and Na$^+$/HCO$_3^-$ co-transport in the rabbit proximal tubule. Proc Natl Acad Sci USA 1990;87 (20):7917−20.

[311] Komlosi P, Fuson A, Fintha A, Peti-Peterdi J, Rosivall L, Warnock DG, et al. Angiotensin I conversion to angiotensin II stimulates cortical collecting duct sodium transport. Hypertension 2003;42:195−9.

[312] Peti-Peterdi J, Warnock DG, Bell PD. Angiotensin II directly stimulates ENaC activity in the cortical collecting duct via AT (1) receptors. J Am Soc Nephrol 2002;13(5):1131−5.

[313] Schuster VL, Kokko JP, Jacobson HR. Angiotensin II directly stimulates sodium transport in rabbit proximal convoluted tubules. J Clin Invest 1984;73(2):507−15.

[314] Tojo A, Tisher CC, Madsen KM. Angiotensin II regulates H ($^+$)-ATPase activity in rat cortical collecting duct. Am J Physiol 1994;267(6 Pt 2):F1045−1051.

[315] Barreto-Chaves ML, Mello-Aires M. Effect of luminal angiotensin II and ANP on early and late cortical distal tubule HCO$_3^-$ reabsorption. Am J Physiol 1996;271(5 Pt 2):F977−984.

[316] Levine DZ, Iacovitti M, Buckman S, Burns KD. Role of angiotensin II in dietary modulation of rat late distal tubule bicarbonate flux in vivo. J Clin Invest 1996;97(1):120−5.

[317] Cogan MG. Angiotensin II: a powerful controller of sodium transport in the early proximal tubule. Hypertension 1990;15 (5):451−8.

[318] Wang T, Giebisch G. Effects of angiotensin II on electrolyte transport in the early and late distal tubule in rat kidney. Am J Physiol 1996;271(1 Pt 2):F143−149.

[319] Gurley SB, Riquier-Brison AD, Schnermann J, Sparks MA, Allen AM, Haase VH, et al. AT1A angiotensin receptors in the renal proximal tubule regulate blood pressure. Cell Metab 2011;13(4):469−75.

[320] Benigni A, Corna D, Zoja C, Sonzogni A, Latini R, Salio M, et al. Disruption of the Ang II type 1 receptor promotes longevity in mice. J Clin Invest 2009;119(3):524−30.

[321] Olsen ME, Hall JE, Montani JP, Guyton AC, Langford HG, Cornell JE. Mechanisms of angiotensin II natriuresis and antinatriuresis. Am J Physiol 1985;249(2 Pt 2):F299−307.

[322] Hall JE, Guyton AC, Smith Jr MJ, Coleman TG. Blood pressure and renal function during chronic changes in sodium intake: role of angiotensin. Am J Physiol Renal Physiol 1980;239(3): F271−280.

[323] Hall JE, Guyton AC, Jackson TE, Coleman TG, Lohmeier TE, Trippodo NC. Control of glomerular filtration rate by renin−angiotensin system. Am J Physiol 1977;233(5):F366−372.

[324] Bouley R, Palomino Z, Tang SS, Nunes P, Kobori H, Lu HA, et al. Angiotensin II and hypertonicity modulate proximal tubular aquaporin 1 expression. Am J Physiol Renal Physiol 2009;297(6):F1575−1586.

[325] Davisson R, Ding Y, Stec D, Catterall J, Sigmund C. Novel mechanism of hypertension revealed by cell-specific targeting of human angiotensinogen in transgenic mice. Physiol Genomics 1999;1:3−9.

[326] Li H, Weatherford ET, Davis DR, Keen HL, Grobe JL, Daugherty A, et al. Renal proximal tubule angiotensin AT1A receptors regulate blood pressure. Am J Physiol Regul Integr Comp Physiol 2011;301(4):R1067−1077.

[327] Riquier-Brison AD, Leong PK, Pihakaski-Maunsbach K, McDonough AA. Angiotensin II stimulates trafficking of NHE3, NaPi2, and associated proteins into the proximal tubule microvilli. Am J Physiol Renal Physiol 2010;298(1): F177−186.

[328] Brown GP, Douglas JG. Angiotensin II binding sites on isolated rat renal brush border membranes. Endocrinology 1982;111(6):1830−6.

[329] Brown GP, Douglas JG. Angiotensin II-binding sites in rat and primate isolated renal tubular basolateral membranes. Endocrinology 1983;112(6):2007−14.

[330] Harrison-Bernard LM, Navar LG, Ho MM, Vinson GP, el-Dahr SS. Immunohistochemical localization of ANG II AT1 receptor in adult rat kidney using a monoclonal antibody. Am J Physiol 1997;273(1 Pt 2):F170−177.

[331] Braam B, Mitchell KD, Fox J, Navar LG. Proximal tubular secretion of angiotensin II in rats. Am J Physiol 1993;264(5 Pt 2):F891−898.

[332] Navar LG, Lewis L, Hymel A, Braam B, Mitchell KD. Tubular fluid concentrations and kidney contents of angiotensins I and II in anesthetized rats. J Am Soc Nephrol 1994;5(4):1153−8.

[333] Li XC, Hopfer U, Zhuo JL. AT1 receptor-mediated uptake of angiotensin II and NHE-3 expression in proximal tubule cells through a microtubule-dependent endocytic pathway. Am J Physiol Renal Physiol 2009;297(5):F1342−1352.

[334] Quan A, Baum M. Endogenous production of angiotensin II modulates rat proximal tubule transport. J Clin Invest 1996;97 (12):2878−82.

[335] Boer WH, Braam B, Fransen R, Boer P, Koomans HA. Effects of reduced renal perfusion pressure and acute volume expansion on proximal tubule and whole kidney angiotensin II content in the rat. Kidney Int 1997;51(1):44−9.

[336] Thomson SC, Deng A, Wead L, Richter K, Blantz RC, Vallon V. An unexpected role for angiotensin II in the link between dietary salt and proximal reabsorption. J Clin Invest 2006;116 (4):1110−6.

[337] Liu FY, Cogan MG. Angiotensin II: a potent regulator of acidification in the rat early proximal convoluted tubule. J Clin Invest 1987;80(1):272−5.

[338] Liu FY, Cogan MG. Angiotensin II stimulation of hydrogen ion secretion in the rat early proximal tubule. Modes of action, mechanism, and kinetics. J Clin Invest 1988;82(2):601−7.

[339] Li Y, Yamada H, Kita Y, Kunimi M, Horita S, Suzuki M, et al. Roles of ERK and cPLA2 in the angiotensin II-mediated biphasic regulation of Na$^+$-HCO$_3$($^-$) transport. J Am Soc Nephrol 2008;19(2):252−9.

[340] Liu FY, Cogan MG. Role of angiotensin II in glomerulotubular balance. Am J Physiol 1990;259(1 Pt 2):F72−79.

[341] Stone DK, Seldin DW, Kokko JP, Jacobson HR. Mineralocorticoid modulation of rabbit medullary collecting duct acidification. A sodium-independent effect. J Clin Invest 1983;72(1):77−83.

[342] Weiner ID, Hamm LL. Regulation of intracellular pH in the rabbit cortical collecting tubule. J Clin Invest 1990;85(1):274−81.

[343] Hays SR. Mineralocorticoid modulation of apical and basolateral membrane H$^+$/OH$^-$/HCO$_3^-$ transport processes in the rabbit inner stripe of outer medullary collecting duct. J Clin Invest 1992;90(1):180−7.

[344] Harrington JT, Hulter HN, Cohen JJ, Madias NE. Mineralocorticoid-stimulated renal acidification: the critical role of dietary sodium. Kidney Int 1986;30(1):43−8.

[345] Batlle DC. Segmental characterization of defects in collecting tubule acidification. Kidney Int 1986;30(4):546−54.

[346] Paxton WG, Runge M, Horaist C, Cohen C, Alexander RW, Bernstein KE. Immunohistochemical localization of rat angiotensin II AT1 receptor. Am J Physiol 1993;264(6 Pt 2): F989–995.

[347] Poumarat JS, Houillier P, Rismondo C, Rogues B, Lazar G, Paillard M, et al. The luminal membrane of rat thick limb expresses AT1 receptor and aminopeptidase activities. Kidney Int 2002;62(2):434–45.

[348] Amlal H, LeGoff C, Vernimmen C, Soleimani M, Paillard M, Bichara M. ANG II controls $Na^{(+)}$-K^{+}(NH_4^{+})-$2Cl^{-}$ co-transport via 20-HETE and PKC in medullary thick ascending limb. Am J Physiol 1998;274(4 Pt 1):C1047–1056.

[349] Lerolle N, Bourgeois S, Leviel F, Lebrun G, Paillard M, Houillier P. Angiotensin II inhibits NaCl absorption in the rat medullary thick ascending limb. Am J Physiol Renal Physiol 2004;287(3):F404–410.

[350] Capasso G, Unwin R, Ciani F, De Santo NG, De Tommaso G, Russo F, et al. Bicarbonate transport along the loop of Henle. II. Effects of acid–base, dietary, and neurohumoral determinants. J Clin Invest 1994;94(2):830–8.

[351] Kwon TH, Nielsen J, Kim YH, Knepper MA, Frokiaer J, Nielsen S. Regulation of sodium transporters in the thick ascending limb of rat kidney: response to angiotensin II. Am J Physiol Renal Physiol 2003;285(1):F152–165.

[352] Rothenberger F, Velic A, Stehberger PA, Kovacikova J, Wagner CA. Angiotensin II stimulates vacuolar H^{+}-ATPase activity in renal acid-secretory intercalated cells from the outer medullary collecting duct. J Am Soc Nephrol 2007;18 (7):2085–93.

[353] Pech V, Zheng W, Pham TD, Verlander JW, Wall SM. Angiotensin II activates H^{+}-ATPase in type A intercalated cells. J Am Soc Nephrol 2008;19(1):84–91.

[354] Wei Y, Wang W. Angiotensin II stimulates basolateral K channels in rat cortical collecting ducts. Am J Physiol Renal Physiol 2003;284(1):F175–181.

[355] Esther C, Howard T, Marino E, Goddard J, Capecchi M, Bernstein K. Mice lacking angiotensin converting enzyme have low blood pressure, renal pathology, and reduced male fertility. Lab Invest 1996;74:953–65.

[356] Kihara M,, Umemura S,, Sumida Y,, Yokoyama M,, Yabana M,, Nyui N,, et al. Genetic deficiency of angiotensinogen produces an impaired urine concentrating ability in mice. 1998;53(3):548.

[357] Oliverio MI, Delnomdedieu M, Best CF, Li P, Morris M, Callahan MF, et al. Abnormal water metabolism in mice lacking the type 1A receptor for ANG II. Am J Physiol Renal Physiol 2000;278(1):F75–82.

[358] Sparks MA, Parsons KK, Stegbauer J, Gurley SB, Vivekanandan-Giri A, Fortner CN, et al. Angiotensin II type 1A receptors in vascular smooth muscle cells do not influence aortic remodeling in hypertension. *Hypertension* 2011;57(3):577–85.

[359] Kwon T-H, Nielsen J, Knepper MA, Frokiaer J, Nielsen S. Angiotensin II AT1 receptor blockade decreases vasopressin-induced water reabsorption and AQP2 levels in NaCl- restricted rats. Am J Physiol Renal Physiol 2005;288(4):F673–684.

[360] Wong NL, Tsui JK. Angiotensin II upregulates the expression of vasopressin V2 mRNA in the inner medullary collecting duct of the rat. Metabolism 2003;52(3):290–5.

[361] Wang W, Li C, Summer S, Falk S, Schrier RW. Interaction between vasopressin and angiotensin II *in vivo* and *in vitro*: effect on aquaporins and urine concentration. Am J Physiol Renal Physiol 2010;299(3):F577–584.

[362] Li C, Wang W, Rivard CJ, Lanaspa MA, Summer S, Schrier RW. Molecular mechanisms of angiotensin II stimulation on aquaporin-2 expression and trafficking. Am J Physiol Renal Physiol 2011;300(5):F1255–1261.

[363] Stegbauer J, Gurley SB, Sparks MA, Woznowski M, Kohan DE, Yan M, et al. AT1 receptors in the collecting duct directly modulate the concentration of urine. *J Am Soc Nephrol* 2011;22 (12):2237–46.

[364] Crackower MA, Sarao R, Oudit GY, et al. Angiotensin-converting enzyme 2 is an essential regulator of heart function. Nature 2002;417(6891):822–8.

[365] Yamamoto K, Ohishi M, Katsuya T, et al. Deletion of angiotensin-converting enzyme 2 accelerates pressure overload-induced cardiac dysfunction by increasing local angiotensin II. Hypertension 2006;47(4):718–26.

[366] Krattinger N, Capponi A, Mazzolai L, et al. Connexin40 regulates renin production and blood pressure. Kidney Int 2007;72 (7):814–22.

[367] Lubkemeier I, Machura K, Kurtz L, et al. The connexin 40 A96S mutation causes renin-dependent hypertension. J Am Soc Nephrol 2011;22(6):1031–40.

[368] Wagner C, de Wit C, Kurtz L, Grunberger C, Kurtz A, Schweda F. Connexin40 is essential for the pressure control of renin synthesis and secretion. Circ Res 2007;100(4):556–63.

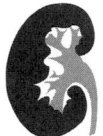

Neural Control of Renal Function

Edward J. Johns[1] *and Ulla C. Kopp*[2]

[1]Department of Physiology, University College Cork, Cork, Republic of Ireland
[2]Departments of Internal Medicine & Pharmacology, University of Iowa Carver College of Medicine,
Iowa City, IA, USA

RENAL SYMPATHETIC NERVES

Introduction

One of the first observations of a potential neural control of kidney function was made by Claude Bernard in the middle of the 19th century, who reported a unilateral diuresis following section of the greater splanchnic nerve of the anesthetized dog.[17] However, the critical role of the sympathetic nervous system in the control of renal function was long questioned due to the views of Homer Smith,[244] who regarded the renal innervation to be of little importance in determining the function of the kidney. It was not until the 1960s that the innervation of the kidney and its regulation of renal function came under detailed scrutiny. Over the following three-to-four decades a wealth of information has been generated and concepts developed which have provided the foundation for how the renal sympathetic nerves regulate all aspects of vascular, tubular, and secretory functions of the kidney, both normally and in pathophysiological states of cardiovascular diseases. A number of major reviews have brought together the most significant pieces of information about the renal sympathetic nerves over this period.[51,52,58,189] This knowledge is now being translated into therapeutic approaches in man, particularly in relation to hypertension, heart failure, and renal disease.[53,234] The recent reports by Esler and co-workers[76,172,173,234] that bilateral renal denervation in patients with resistant hypertension resulted in a profound and sustained ($\geq$2 years) reduction in blood pressure reinforces the important contribution of the autonomic control of the kidney in determining cardiovascular homeostasis and how it

may be involved in pathophysiological states. These findings are set to reinforce the drive to gain knowledge of both the efferent and afferent innervations of the kidney, and to stimulate the development of further therapeutic avenues to modulate the neural control of the kidney.

NEUROANATOMY, PHARMACOLOGY, AND PHYSIOLOGY

Extrinsic Innervation

The efferent innervation of the kidney comprises pre-ganglionic fibers which arise from spinal segments $T_{11}-L_3$, and traverse to both pre-vertebral (thoraco-lumbar sympathetic chain) and para-vertebral ganglia (aortico-renal, splanchnic, coeliac, superior mesenteric ganglia) which give rise to the post-ganglionic fibers. There is great species variation in the overall contribution from the various ganglia, for example, with 80% arising from the ipsilateral para-vertebral ganglia ($T_{11}-L_2$) in the rat and hamster, but only 50% for the cat and monkey ($T_{11}-L_3$).[58] Figure 16.1 gives a brief outline of these different neural pathways. Tracer studies with horseradish peroxidase and herpes virus have been used to demonstrate the neural pathways for the sympathetic innervation. The pre-ganglionic sympathetic nerve fibers in the rat are primarily located in the intermediolateral column of the spinal cord, from T_9-T_{13}, suggesting that they descend three to four segments before exiting the spinal column at $T_{11}-L_3$. A number of nuclei within the central nervous system project to these intermediolateral areas of the spinal cord, including the raphe nuclei, rostral

Seldin and Giebisch's The Kidney, Fifth Edition.
DOI: http://dx.doi.org/10.1016/B978-0-12-381462-3.00016-1

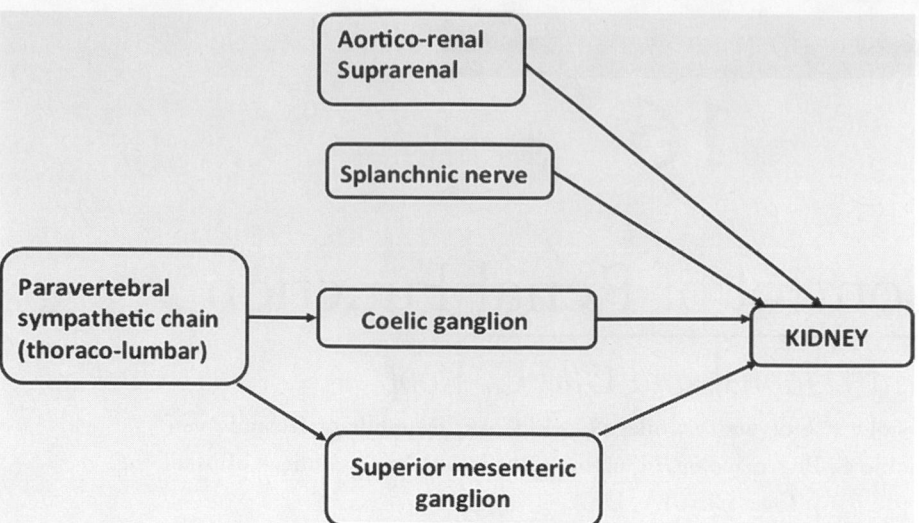

FIGURE 16.1 This shows the main ganglia providing the sympathetic post-ganglionic fibers which innervate the kidney.

venterolateral medulla, an A5 group, and the paraventricular hypothalamic nucleus.[42] Together, there is a view that descending projections from the supra-spinal systems are the primary regulators of sympathetic outflow to the kidney.

There has been a continuing evaluation of the size and type of nerves forming the efferent innervation of the kidney. Analyses performed in the rabbit utilizing electron microscopy have demonstrated two types of nerve fibers with different diameters in the renal cortex,[49,183] suggesting that different functionalities may exist within these different nerve populations. Detailed counts of fiber number and diameter in the rat[67,233] have found that the majority of the fibers are unmyelinated (96%) with the remainder being myelinated. The average diameter of the unmyelinated fibers was approximately 1.3 μm, and while DiBona and colleagues[67] reported a bimodal distribution, this was not observed in the report of Sato and co-workers.[233] More recently, Fazan and colleagues[81] investigated the situation in the mouse and found that, although the nerve fibers had a similar mean diameter, 0.76 ± 0.02 μm, compared to the rat, the distribution was clearly unimodal. Together, these observations provide no consistent support for the argument that different nerve fibers are directed towards the innervation of specific cell types (vascular, epithelial or granular) in order to control selected functions.

Intrinsic Innervation

The sympathetic nerves generally traverse from the ganglia, running alongside the renal artery, and enter the hilus of the kidney where they begin to divide, with smaller nerve bundles approximately following the

major divisions of the blood vessels. The sympathetic nerves begin to divide into smaller bundles which penetrate and form a network throughout the cortical and juxta-medullary areas. Early studies by Barajas and co-workers[9,10] demonstrated discrete neuro-effector junctions present at the afferent and efferent arterioles, the granular cells of the juxtaglomerular apparatus, the proximal and distal tubules, and the thick limb of the ascending limb of the loop of Henle. This group of investigators, utilizing electron microscopy, went on to show that the sympathetic nerves were typical autonomic fibers having varacosities associated with the neuro-effector junctions that contained dense cored vesicles. Using a tritiated noradrenaline radiographic approach they[9,10] clearly showed the presence of noradrenaline, and although there was a suggestion that acetylcholine esterase was present, there was no indication that the fibers were cholinergic. Later, more detailed studies indicated that there was a variation in the number of neuro-effector junctions along the nephron, with the greatest number being at the proximal tubule, fewer at the thick ascending limb of the loop of Henle, and the smallest number at the distal tubules and collecting duct.[58] Interestingly, when calculated as the density of neuro-effector junctions per unit length, the density was found to be greatest in the thick ascending limb of the loop of Henle and progressively less in the distal and proximal tubules.[9,10] There is also a regional variation, with the innervation being greatest along the cortico-medullary border and becoming less in the outer cortex and deeper regions of the medulla. This regional variation in innervation density is paralleled in both the vascular and tubular structures. Figure 16.2 illustrates the cell types where neuro-effector junctions have been described and the functions they may regulate.

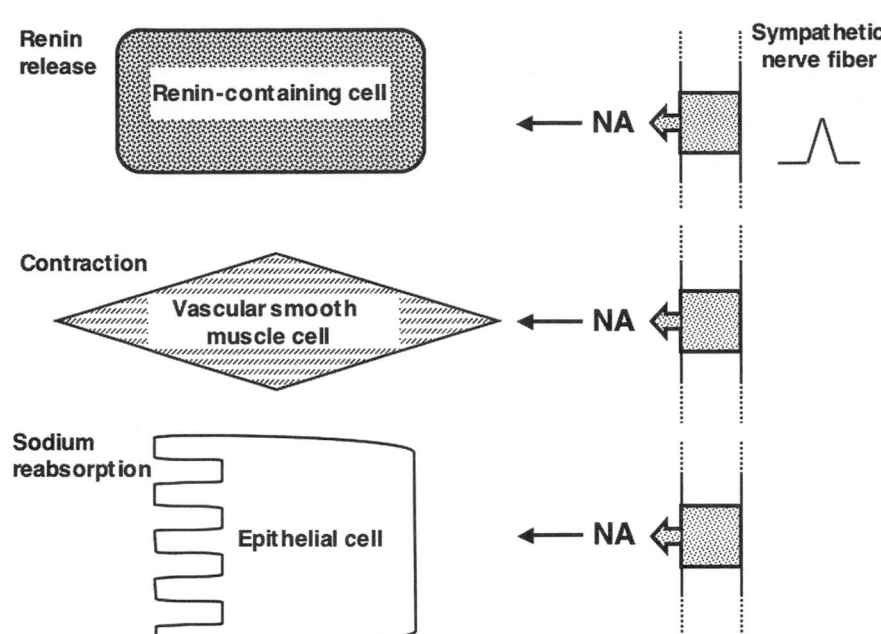

FIGURE 16.2 Neuro-effector junctions are formed at the renin-containing cells, the vascular smooth muscle cells (interlobular arteries, afferent, and efferent arterioles) and the epithelial cells of the proximal tubule, thick ascending limb of the loop of Henle, and the distal tubule. Noradrenaline (NA) is contained in granules within varicosities which are exocytosed following passage of an action potential.

Pharmacology

Neurotransmitters

A large body of evidence from biochemical and pharmacological studies indicates that the primary neurotransmitter arising from the sympathetic innervation is noradrenaline. Functional studies have shown that renal denervation, in the initial stages, is associated with a marked decrease in noradrenaline content of some 95%,[58] while activation of the renal sympathetic nerves results in an elevation in noradrenaline production or spillover into the renal venous blood.[75,76] The role of dopamine and potential dopaminergic nerve-mediated influences remains unclear, as all adrenergic nerve varicosities contain dopamine as an intermediary in noradrenaline biosynthesis, but there is little evidence that dopamine acts as a neurotransmitter[58] in the neural regulation of either renal hemodynamic function, renin release or fluid reabsorption.

Adrenoceptors

Multiple types of adrenoceptors are present within the kidney mediating the actions of noradrenaline released from the nerve varicosities, and a range of α_1- and α_2-adrenoceptors subtypes exist along the renal vasculature and nephrons. At a functional level, stimulation of the α-adrenoceptors causes a vasoconstriction of vascular smooth muscle and reabsorption of fluid at tubular epithelial cells. Stimulation of β-adrenoceptors increases renin release at the juxtaglomerular granular cells. A number of molecular biological and cloning investigations have defined α_1-adrenoceptors into α_{1A}-, α_{1B}-, and α_{1D}-subtypes, α_2-adrenoceptors into α_{2A}-, α_{2B}-, and α_{2C}-subtypes, and β-adrenoceptors as β_1-, β_2-, and

β_3-subtypes, all of which are G-protein coupled receptors comprising a superfamily of membrane proteins that signal the actions of adrenaline and noradrenaline.[251] The α_1-adrenoceptors utilize a range of signaling pathways including activation of phospholipases A and C, mobilization of intracellular calcium stores, as well as opening of voltage-dependent and independent calcium channels[225] which results in a rapid vascular smooth muscle contraction. Interestingly, noradrenaline binding to α_1-adrenoceptors also activates the MAP kinase pathways which, in the longer term, are responsible for regulating growth and hypertrophy of the vascular smooth muscle.[263] There are reports that α_{1A}- and α_{1B}-adrenoceptors are present to a similar degree in the cortex and outer stripe of the medulla, while in the inner stripe of the medulla the α_{1B}-adrenoceptor subtype appears to predominate.[83] However, in terms of hemodynamic functionality, α_{1A}-adrenoceptors are more effective than the α_{1B}-adrenoceptor subtypes in causing renal vasoconstriction.

α-Adrenoceptors are also present on the epithelial cells of the nephron, where they modulate fluid reabsorption. There is evidence, at least in the proximal tubule, that α_1-adrenoceptor stimulation engages both the phospholipase C and MAP kinase[264] pathways, but these signal to different end-points, that is to the sodium/hydrogen exchanger, isoforms-1 (NHE1) and isoform-3 (NHE3), respectively.[179] At the more distal sections of the nephron, the distal tubule and collecting duct, α_2-adrenoceptors are the primary subtype, and in this segment their activation results in a decrease in cAMP which blunts the action of other factors signaling through this pathway. A key example is AVP,[223] which stimulates both water reabsorption and ENaC insertion in this region where these actions are blunted by α_2-adrenoceptor agonists.[8] β_1-adrenoceptors are found primarily on the granular renin-containing cells of the afferent arteriole, and their activation stimulates adenylyl cyclase which increases intracellular levels of cAMP. The β_2-adrenoceptors found on the tubules, primarily collecting duct, also utilize cAMP production as the signaling molecule, but their function at this site has not been resolved.

PHYSIOLOGY

Activation of the various signaling pathways via ligand binding to the adrenoceptors increases fluid reabsorption at the level of the proximal tubule. In the proximal tubule, the catecholamines stimulate Na/K-ATPase at the basolateral membrane,[4] resulting in increased sodium reabsorption from the tubular lumen across the apical membrane. There is evidence from micropuncture studies,[212] as well as in vitro studies,[180] that the sodium−hydrogen exchanger is activated, particularly isoform 3 (NHE3), the isoform primarily responsible for the regulation of sodium entry into the epithelial cells at the proximal tubule.[179,180] The NHE3 protein in the proximal tubule appears to be present in the microvillae, either incorporated into the plasma membrane[273] where it is likely to be active or internally in the subapical vesicles, where it is considered to be inactive in terms of a transporting protein. The mechanisms involved in the translocation of the NHE3 from the plasma membrane into the subapical vesicles are complex[197] and require the interaction of a number of proteins (NHERF1, myosin VI, ezrin, raft, non-raft, and myosin). McDonough[197] has recently reviewed the evidence showing that when blood pressure is elevated acutely[273] or when the sympathetic nervous system is reflexly activated there is increased movement of NHE3 into the subapical compartment where the transporter is inactive. McDonough and co-workers have put forward the concept that translocation of the NHE3 into the subapical regions is a key element whereby sodium reabsorption may be regulated by catecholamines, both in the short-term as well as over a longer timeframe, thereby contributing to cardiovascular homeostasis.[197,198]

Autocrine and Paracrine Influences on Neurotransmission

The interstitium of the kidney contains a complex milieu of hormones and factors which may vary across the cortex and medulla, but can determine the level of functions of all cell types, vascular smooth muscle,

renin containing, and epithelial cells. There are modulator influences at the neuro-effector junction which can come into play and influence the amount of noradrenaline released in response to depolarization caused by the passage of an action potential. An outline of potential interactions with various agents is illustrated in Figure 16.3.

Adrenoceptors

At an early stage it was recognized that pre-synaptic α_2-adrenoceptors were able to act in an auto-inhibitory fashion, whereby when activated by noradenaline released into the neuro-effector junction, they decreased neurotransmitter release caused by subsequent depolarizations. There is evidence that this situation pertains at the kidney. α_2-adrenoceptors are present in the kidney,[18,19] and their blockade enhances noradrenaline release and renal nerve induced vasoconstriction in the dog.[113] In the rabbit[109] blockade of α_2-adrenoceptors peripherally has little effect on renal nerve-induced vasoconstrictions, but potentiates the renal nerve-mediated antidiuresis and antinatriuresis.

Angiotensin II

A second important neuro-modulator is angiotensin II, which is present in the renal interstitium at high levels in conditions of increased endogenous angiotensin II production.[122,211,243] Activation of pre-synaptic AT-1 receptors facilitates the release of noradrenaline. This was first reported by Boke and Malik[21] using the isolated perfused rat kidney. They found that renal nerve-induced catacholamine release into the renal vein was facilitated when angiotensin II was added to the perfusate. At a functional level, studies in the anaesthetized rat using both direct and reflex activation of the renal nerves, at levels which had little or no effect on renal hemodynamics, caused decreases in fluid excretion which were blocked in the presence of an angiotensin-converting enzyme inhibitor,[102] and restored following administration of exogenous angiotensin II.[129] Similar observations were reported by Veelken and colleagues[258] in the conscious rat, where administration of the AT1-receptor antagonist ZD 7155 blunted the renal nerve-dependent antidiuresis and antinatriuresis in response to an air-jet stress test. Together, these findings support the view that at both renal vascular and epithelial cell neuro-effector junctions occupation of pre-synaptic AT1 receptors enhances neurotransmission. It would seem that these receptors are fully occupied, even at low endogenous levels of angiotensin II[256,258] and under normal conditions the facilitation is maximal but when production is prevented, then neurotransmission will be blunted. There may be other interactions at the post-synaptic membranes of the epithelial cells. Quan and colleagues[228,229] demonstrated that the ability of angiotensin II

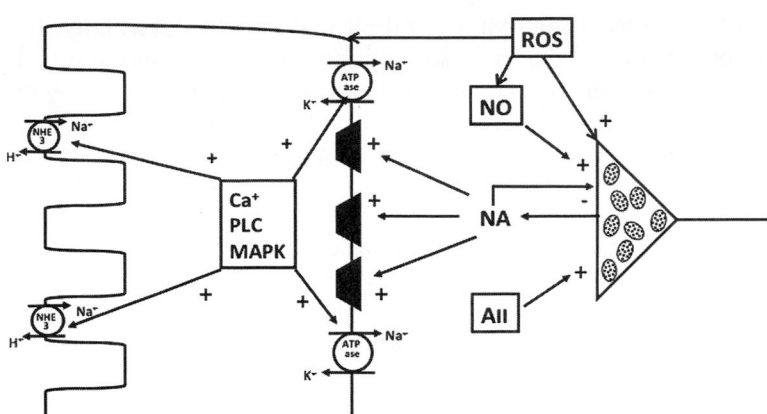

FIGURE 16.3 Noradrenaline (NA) acts on the epithelial cells to activate phospholipase C, increases intracellular calcium (Ca^+) which initiates MAP kinase signaling pathways stimulating both the apical sodium—hydrogen exchanger isoform 3 (NHE3) and the basolateral sodium/potassium-ATPase. Noradrenaline exerts an auto-inhibitory feedback action on further release (−) while nitric oxide (NO) and angiotensin II (AII) exert an action (+) to increase the amount of noradrenaline release on passage of each action potential. Reactive oxygen species (ROS) appear to directly facilitate noradrenaline release and indirectly to modulate the action of NO.

to stimulate proximal tubule fluid reabsorption was blunted following acute renal denervation, but augmented if the renal sympathetic nerves were stimulated at low levels not affecting filtration rate. A comparable interaction was reported by Abdulla and co-workers,[1,2] who found that the renal vasoconstriction caused by close renal arterial infusion of angiotensin II was blunted following acute renal denervation. Thus, these observations demonstrate that angiotensin II has modulatory activities at the neuro-effector junction, both pre-synaptically and post-synaptically, which determine the effectiveness of the neural control of renin release, fluid reabsorption, and vascular tone in the kidney.

Nitric Oxide

A third potentially important factor determining noradrenaline release, and hence its impact on functional end-points, is nitric oxide (NO). All isoforms of nitric oxide synthase (NOS), endothelial (eNOS), neuronal (nNOS), and inducible (iNOS) are present in the kidney. eNOS has been found along the vasculature and glomerular capillaries,[7,194] nNOS is present in the renal nerves,[156,181] at low concentrations along the tubules[24] and high concentrations in the macula densa,[7] while iNOS is expressed constitutively in the medulla.[142] It is possible that in the environment of the neuro-effector junction, NO may have both pre-synaptic and post-synaptic actions, and this probably contributes to the conflicting findings which have been reported. Thus, in the anaesthetized dog, the low level renal nerve stimulated noradrenaline output was enhanced following NOS inhibition and suppressed in the presence of an NO donor, consistent with an inhibitory pre-synaptic action.[71,188] In contrast in the rat, NOS blockade suppressed renal nerve mediated noradrenaline output and neurally induced renal vasoconstriction.[253,259] In terms of the influence of NO on renal nerve stimulated increases in sodium reabsorption, there is a lack of consistency. It is evident that NOS inhibition increases, and exogenous NO decreases, proximal tubule fluid

reabsorption,[72,213] suggesting an inhibitory action of NO on reabsorptive processes. Importantly, this action of NO is only evident if the renal nerves are intact.[266] In an apparent conflict with these studies are the findings that renal nerve-induced increases in fluid reabsorption are prevented by NOS blockade, consistent with a facilitating action of NO.[268] In attempting to clarify these differing reports, it is possible that NO could act in two ways, directly within the post-synaptic cell, either vasculature or epithelial cells, where it may blunt the neurally controlled cell function, or indirectly by facilitating neurotransmitter release. The differing balances between these two sites of action may simply reflect how the NO generating systems may be activated by the various experimental conditions of the investigations.

Reactive Oxygen Species

The generation of cellular energy results in the production of reactive oxygen species which comprise radicals that can damage both nuclear and cytoplasmic proteins and phospholipids. A raised output of reactive oxygen species is recognized as a state of oxidative stress that is associated with a range of metabolic and cardiovascular diseases. Reactive oxygen species comprise superoxide anions, H_2O_2, and other reactive radicals which are able to influence both neurotransmission and the responsiveness of the target cells to the neurotransmitter. The actions of the reactive oxygen species may be either direct or indirect, as a consequence of their ability to reduce the bioavailability of NO. There are reports that systemic infusion of tempol, a synthetic diffusible superoxide dismutase mimetic which scavenges superoxide anions,[239,272] reduced blood pressure and renal sympathetic nerve activity to the same extent before and following NOS blockade. These findings would be compatible with the argument that in states of oxidative stress, for example hypertension, increased production of superoxide anions could enhance the activity of the sympathetic nervous system, and hence the level at which it influences kidney function. The enzymes NAD(P)H and superoxide dismutase are present in both the cortex and medulla of the kidney,[133] with the level of the latter being somewhat higher in the medulla. This group[133] demonstrated that oxidative stress increased the activity of NAD(P)H, but not superoxide dismutase, in the cortex but not the medulla. This would suggest that in renal oxidative stress whereas superoxide anion generation would increase, the level of scavenging would remain unaltered, implying greater activity of the reactive oxygen species. This is important in terms of renal sympathetic nerve activity, as Shokoji et al.[239] demonstrated that direct application of tempol or DETC, a blocker of superoxide dismutase, directly onto renal sympathetic nerve fibers decreased and increased nerve traffic, respectively. These findings imply that oxidative stress in the kidney can itself alter the level of reactive oxygen species in the local environment, which may directly affect the level of renal sympathetic nerve activity and renal nerve-dependent function.

CONTROL OF THE RENAL CIRCULATION

Activation of Renal Sympathetic Nerves

The earliest studies by Cohnheim and Roy[38] using a renal plethysmograph, demonstrated that renal volume was decreased following asphyxia or when the cut ends of the renal nerves were stimulated. Indeed, these early plethysmographic studies also identified the spinal origin of the vasoconstrictor fibers. The advent of the modern flowmeters to measure renal blood flow dynamically allowed studies in anaesthetized dogs, cats, rabbits, and rats[58] which convincingly demonstrated that direct electrical stimulation of the renal nerves caused frequency related reductions in renal blood flow. Furthermore, reflex activation of the renal sympathetic nerves, either as a consequence of activation of the baroreceptor reflex by reduction in carotid sinus pressure[54,69] or activation of the somatosensory system[45,255] resulted in a renal nerve-mediated reduction in renal blood flow. Together, these reports indicate that renal nerves cause contraction of the vascular smooth muscle of the resistance vessels, thereby reducing blood flow. While the innervation of the afferent arteriole would cause a reduction in renal blood flow because it is the major resistance bed within the kidney, the impact and relative importance of a neurally induced vasoconstriction at the efferent arteriole is less clear cut in terms of its overall contribution to the reduction in renal blood flow. Luff and co-workers[49,183] were able to identify at the ultrastructural level two types of fibers in the rabbit that were differentially distributed, one type solely innervating the afferent arteriole and a second type evenly distributed to both afferent and efferent arterioles, which they argued enabled an independent regulation of the two resistance vasculatures. However, an alternative view is that because of the differing wall thicknesses and lengths of the afferent and efferent arterioles, even if both vessels constricted to a similar degree, the efferent arteriolar constriction would have a greater impact on glomerular filtration pressure,[48,50] and hence filtration rate.

A number of studies have reported a disparity in the magnitudes of the reduction in renal blood flow and glomerular filtration rate produced by renal nerve stimulation. Studies in the anaesthetized rabbit,[108] cat,[131] and rat[102] demonstrated that modest neurally induced reductions in renal blood flow (of 15–20%) were accompanied by either no change or a small 2–5% reduction in glomerular filtration. However, if angiotensin II activity was reduced by converting enzyme inhibitors, angiotensin II type 1 (AT-1) receptor blocking drugs or β-adrenoceptor antagonists, the neural impact on glomerular filtration rate became greater, with the magnitude of reductions in glomerular filtration rate becoming roughly proportionate with renal blood flow.[128] These reports gave rise to the important concept that the renal nerves, indirectly via locally produced angiotensin II acting at the efferent arteriole, could ensure that over a modest range of variation in renal blood flow, the glomerular filtration rate, and hence filtered load presented to the nephrons, was maintained at a relatively constant level.

Renal Denervation

An important question is whether under basal, unstressed conditions the renal sympathetic nerves have a tonic influence on basal blood flow through the kidney. The reasons for this uncertainty reside in the manner of the experimental studies, whether anaesthetized or conscious preparations were used, the degree of surgical stress and type of anaesthesia used, and, to a degree, the species under study. Thus, in a number of reports in the anaesthetized rat, there was very little change in renal blood flow following acute renal denervation.[58] However, in these studies there was often a relatively long period of time between basal measurements, the surgical manipulation and denervation of the kidney, and the post-surgery measurements, with the result that it was difficult to determine whether changes had taken place. In an attempt to resolve this issue, Kompanowska-Jezierska and colleagues[141] inserted an electro-cautery wire around the bulk of the nerves, and instantaneous denervation occurred when a current was passed to destroy the neural tissue. Under these conditions, it was found that over the first 10 to 20 minutes an increase of some 20% in blood perfusing the outer cortex occurred when measured by laser Doppler flowmetry, suggesting there was sufficient activity within the renal nerves to decrease basal renal blood flow. This view was to a degree supported by the conscious rabbit reports of Malpas and co-workers,[190] who found that seven days after renal denervation, renal blood flow was some 55% to 65% higher in the denervated compared to the innervated kidney, the large difference most likely indicative of greater basal sympathetic outflow in the rabbit.

The studies of Miki and co-workers[277] using the conscious rat showed that while basal renal blood flow in the groups of animals with either intact or denervated kidneys could not be distinguished, an increase in renal sympathetic nerve activity during grooming and movement caused a proportionate decrease in blood flow to the intact kidneys of some 15%, whereas that to the denervated kidneys tended to increase in line with blood pressure. The relationship between renal blood flow and stress-induced activation of the sympathetic nervous system was the basis of the study undertaken by Brod and co-workers.[25] They demonstrated in man that, in the unstressed state, administration of an adrenergic blocking drug, dibenamine, had no effect on para aminohippurate (PAH) clearance (effective renal plasma flow), but if the patients were tense, anxious, and stressed, the dibenamine administration was associated with a rise in PAH clearance compatible with the view that there was a tonic renal nerve-induced reduction in renal blood flow. Thus, the degree of tonic influence of the renal sympathetic nerves on basal hemodynamics is dependent on the level of stress impinging on the subjects, and in the normal conscious state the renal sympathetic nerves have relatively little impact.

Neural Regulation of Intra-Renal Hemodynamics

Measurement of Intra-Renal Hemodynamics

The measurement of blood flow through the cortical and medullary regions of the kidney is difficult and fraught with technical limitations. Videomicroscopic techniques have been used to evaluate blood flow through single vasa recta vessels.[41] The limitation of many techniques used such as the Rhubidium-86 methodology is single estimations from one kidney,[107] the H_2-washout method is the accuracy of curve fitting of the data,[5,6] and the trapping of labeled microspheres in glomerular is only two to three measurements per kidney.[37] More recently, there has been greater use of laser-Doppler technology, which allows continuous measurements of blood perfusion through the cortex and medulla of the same kidney. The limitations of this technique are that the values recorded are not flow, but are a flux measurement derived from the product of the velocity as well as the number of red cells moving through the volume of tissue illuminated by the laser. Consequently, the values arising from this technique represent qualitative rather than quantitative evaluations of blood flow.

Activation of the Renal Nerves

There have been a series of investigations addressing how and whether the renal sympathetic nerves may differentially regulate blood flow through the cortex and medulla. Early studies in this area applying the H_2-washout approach in the anaesthetized dog[5,6] indicated that adrenergically-mediated decreases in flow were of comparable magnitude in both cortical and medullary regions. Similar findings were reported using the Rhubidium-86 methodology,[107] in that stimulation of the renal sympathetic nerves caused equivalent decreases in flow through both cortex and medulla. By contrast in later reports, Rudenstam et al.[231] used laser-Doppler flowmetry in the rat and observed a relative resistance of medullary perfusion to decrease in response to renal sympathetic nerve stimulation. Evans and co-workers,[74,97,177] using the same technique in the anaesthetized rabbit, demonstrated smaller reductions of the perfusion in the medulla than in the cortex or total renal blood flow. Further studies in rabbits[96] showed that the magnitude of reduction was similar across the medullary region, irrespective of the depth at which measurements were made (inner or outer medulla). This, to a degree, contrasts with the findings in the anaesthetized rat,[259] where the inner medullary perfusion was less responsive than the outer medullary area to renal nerve stimulation. The reasons underlying the differences reported in the sensitivity of the two vascular regions (cortex versus medulla) to adrenergic stimulation are unclear, but they may reside in the differing characteristics of the afferent and efferent arterioles (which may also vary between outer and inner cortical regions), possible variations in innervation density, species variation or the mix of paracrine and autocrine factors residing in the interstitium in these different regions. The potential interactions of all these factors have been considered in detail in recent reviews.[78,79]

CONTROL OF RENAL TUBULAR SOLUTE AND WATER TRANSPORT

Renal Denervation

Claude Bernard[17] first noted that section of the splanchnic nerve of the anaesthetized dog caused an increase in urine flow. Questions arising from this finding were whether the raised fluid excretion was due indirectly to an increase in glomerular filtration rate, whether it was the result of a direct action on the tubular reabsorptive processes of the epithelial cells or a combination of these mechanisms. This problem was addressed by Bonjour and co-workers[22] using the anaesthetized dog, who convincingly demonstrated that the elevated urine flow and sodium excretion subsequent to the section of the renal sympathetic nerves was independent of any changes in glomerular filtration rate. They concluded that the raised fluid excretion reflected a direct influence of the nerves on tubular function. Thereafter, this view was supported by a series of reports using micropuncture techniques which directly examined reabsorptive rates along accessible segments of the nephron. Bello-Reuss and colleagues[14,15] observed in the anaesthetized rat that section of the splanchnic nerves had a minimal effect on single nephron glomerular filtration rate, but was associated with significant decreases in both absolute and fractional sodium and water reabsorption at the proximal tubule. These conclusions were supported by other investigators at that time, using comparable techniques to directly measure tubular function.[252,267,268]

Renal Nerve Stimulation

The removal of the influence of the renal sympathetic nerves represents only one way of illustrating their action, and to fully appreciate their influence a corresponding series of studies were necessary in which the renal nerves were activated. In a ground-breaking study, LaGrange and co-workers,[175] using the anaesthetized dog, found that direct electrical stimulation of the nerves at levels that were sub-threshold for changing either renal blood flow or glomerular filtration rate, caused a 30—40% fall in water and sodium excretion, which was interpreted as a direct action of the renal nerves on tubular fluid reabsorption. A similar situation was found to exist in the rabbit[108] and rat,[132] in that electrical stimulation of the renal nerves at levels subthreshold for decreasing renal blood flow, decreased both urine flow and sodium excretion. These observations were supported by micropuncture studies which more directly evaluated the tubular actions of the nerves. These studies[16] demonstrated that the absolute and fractional sodium and water reabsorption of the proximal tubule was increased by low frequency direct electrical stimulation of the renal nerves which was without effect on single nephron filtration rate. Moreover, DiBona and Sawin[62] found in the anaesthetized rat that low frequency stimulation of the renal nerves, at rates which did not alter renal blood flow or glomerular filtration rate, also increased fluid reabsorption at the thick limb of the ascending loop of Henle.

Thus, there is a large body of information which substantiates the view that the renal sympathetic nerves, when activated at low rates which have minimal effects on renal hemodynamics, have a direct action on the transport processes of the epithelial cells of the proximal tubule and the thick ascending limb of the loop of Henle. The situation regarding the distal tubule and the collecting duct has not been investigated in depth, primarily because of the technical hurdles required to evaluate reabsorption in these segments *in vivo*. Interestingly, Bankir and colleagues[8] have reviewed evidence for the concept that activation of vasopressin V2 receptors along the collecting duct not only increases water abstraction, but also activates epithelial sodium channels (ENaC) in the principal cells of this nephron segment. The EnaC-mediated antinatriuresis takes place in association with V2-induced increases in cAMP, and occurs at high plasma levels of vasopressin typically seen in pathophysiological states. The possibility arises that activation of α_2-adrenoceptors along this nephron segment,[222,223] which are known to suppress cAMP, could interact with vasopressin to determine the level not only of water retention, but also of the sodium due to ENaC insertion. The relationship between vasopressin and adrenoceptor activation at this nephron segment remains a source of investigation.

NEURAL CONTROL OF RENIN RELEASE

Renin Containing Cells

Renin Production

The granular cells of the juxtaglomerular apparatus contain renin. These cells are found in the afferent arterioles at increasing density as the vessel approaches the glomerulus.[98] The origin of these cells has been examined in a study by Sequeira-Lopez et al.[236] using single cell PCR and double immunostaining combined with lineage markers. By transplanting embryonic kidneys between genetically lineage marked mice containing cells for renin, smooth muscle, and endothelial cells with wild-type mice, they showed two distinct populations of cells expressing either renin or smooth muscle cell markers, but never both in the same cell. During the course of maturation, the renin cell began to express the smooth muscle cell markers, suggesting that renin cells could progress into smooth muscle cells and, if required, back into renin cells. Importantly, it appears that the transformation the other way round cannot happen, that is, the smooth muscle cells do not transform into renin cells.[220,236] The situation seems to be that when demand for renin is high, for example as a consequence of reduced renal perfusion pressure or following a low dietary sodium intake, some smooth muscles will transform back into renin producing cells. Expression of the renin gene generates a specific mRNA which translates into a large protein, pre-pro-renin, which then undergoes processing to generate pro-renin.[98] The pro-renin then undergoes one of two fates, it can be secreted constitutively in an unchanged form, which represents "inactive" renin or it is incorporated into the secretory granules, where it undergoes further modification into mature renin. The secretion of renin occurs when exocytosis of the granules is stimulated. The exocytosis of the granular cells is regulated by two main intracellular signaling molecules, cAMP which stimulates renin release and intracellular calcium ion concentration (Ca^{2+}) which inhibits renin secretion.

Renin Cell Electrophysiology

The membrane potential of the granular cells is determined by a variety of ion channels influenced by cAMP and Ca^{2+}. Large conductance calcium-sensitive voltage-activated channels (BKa) are opened by increased intracellular cAMP, resulting in hyperpolarization. L-type voltage-dependent calcium channels ($Ca_v1.2$) which inhibit cAMP-mediated exocytosis.[85,86] The normal physiological process is one where the cAMP stimulation of renin granule exocytosis is protected against activation of L-type calcium channel by the hyperpolarization that results from the cAMP induced opening of the BKa. In this way, renin secretion can occur in a regulated manner independent of intracellular Ca^{2+}. These relationships and interactions are illustrated in Figure 16.4.

There are three primary intracellular signaling pathways which interact to determine the rate of renin secretion: cAMP; cGMP; and cytosolic calcium. Good

evidence exists[13] that cAMP is the key signaling molecule. In mice with deletion of the G-protein $G_{s\alpha}$ in juxtaglomerular cells,[30] plasma renin is low and the mice are unresponsive to stimuli such as β_1-adrenoceptor stimulation which utilize cAMP. On the other hand in intact mice, challenges that stimulate adenyl cyclase or suppress phosphodiesterase enzymes result in increased renin release. The role of intracellular calcium in the regulation of renin secretion is only now becoming clear.[235] Angiotensin II-, endothelin-, and ADH- receptor-mediated increases in intracellular calcium suppress the exocytosis of the renin granules. Indeed, the intracellular calcium levels are inversely proportional to those of cAMP, that is, as intracellular calcium decreases there is an increase in cAMP and renin release, and *vice versa*.[98,221] It would seem that adenylyl cyclase isoforms 5/6 are inhibited by increased intracellular calcium, thereby determining the rate of cAMP generation. Taken together, the scenario put forward[235] is that cAMP is the primary intracellular signaling molecule eliciting renin release, and this occurs through activation of β_1-adrenoceptors. The other factors and mechanisms, which exert their actions via changes in calcium entry into the granular cells and therefore the activity of adenyl cyclase 5/6, will serve to modulate the sensitivity of the cAMP-dependent pathways for renin secretion.

Activation of the Renal Nerves

The stimulation of renal secretion and the exocytosis of the granules are regulated through three main routes, the renal baroreceptor mechanism, the macula densa and the renal sympathetic nerves. Many of the early investigations utilized either electrical stimulation or reflex activation of the renal sympathetic nerves, and showed that plasma renin activity or renin

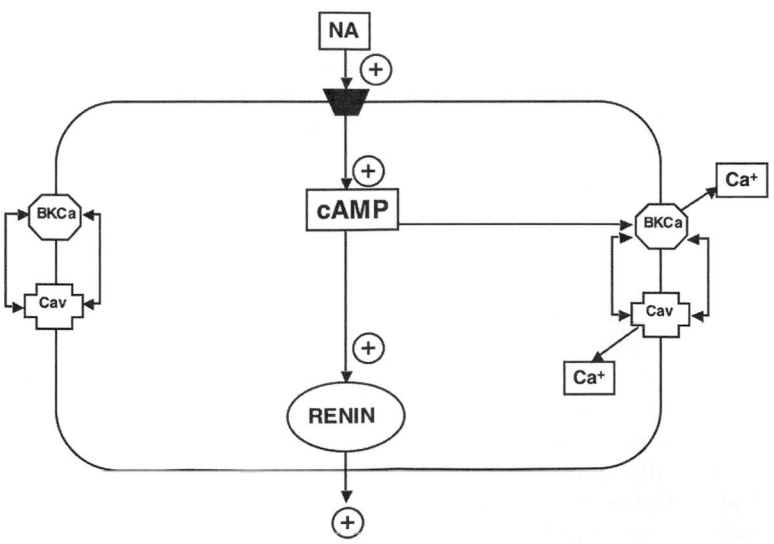

FIGURE 16.4 Noradrenaline-adrenoceptor on a renin-containing cell to increase (NA) stimulates intracellular cAMP which then initiates exocytosis of renin-containing granules, releasing renin. At the same time, cAMP acts at the BKCa channel to cause a hyperpolarization which to a degree suppresses the CaV channel offsetting calcium entry, an effect tending to inhibit renin secretion.

secretion was increased[58,143] which could be prevented by administration of β-adrenoceptor antagonists. Often interpretation of these findings was complicated by the concomitant reductions in renal blood flow and glomerular filtration rate which could have also contributed to the rise in renin release. The reports by Kopp et al.[143] and Osborn et al.[215] demonstrated that electrical stimulation of the renal sympathetic nerves at low frequencies producing no or small decreases in renal blood flow resulted in increases in renin release that were prevented by administration of a β$_1$-adrenoceptor antagonist in anesthetized dogs. This view of renin release from the granular cells being due to a direct action of neurally released noradrenaline has been supported by comparable observations in the rabbit and rat, as well as man.[128,269]

It is now clear that the neurally-induced renin release is associated with a rise in renal renin mRNA. This effect becomes measurable at relatively high levels of renal nerve stimulation over an extended period of time, of approximately an hour, causing large increases in plasma renin activity.[207] Interestingly, a number of reports have indicated that cAMP stimulates renin gene expression by binding to an enhancer region upstream of the gene,[218,240] as well as increasing the stability of renin mRNA.[221,242,261] The mechanisms involve cAMP-dependent phosphorylation mediated by ERK kinases.[98] Thus, the nerve-mediated increase in cAMP may act in several ways, first to cause an immediate release of renin as a result of exocytosis of the granules; second to increase renin gene expression; and third to cause a stabilization and prolongation of the action of renin mRNA, all actions to ensure that sufficient renin is available and stores are replenished.

Neural and Non-Neural Interactions and Renin Release

A number of early observations gave rise to the concept that a background level of renal nerve activity was necessary to allow the differing renin releasing mechanisms to operate normally. It was the initial studies of Stella et al.[248] in the anaesthetized cat that demonstrated that increased renin secretion as a result of reductions in renal perfusion pressure or renal blood flow were blunted in the denervated compared to the innervated kidneys. Furthermore, Johns[130] demonstrated that during reflex activation of the sympathetic nervous system following reduction of perfusion pressure at the carotid sinus, the magnitude of renin release when renal perfusion pressure was reduced was greater in the innervated than denervated kidneys. These findings were extended by Holdaas

et al.[114] and Osborn et al.[216] using the anaesthetized dog, who found that furosemide-induced renin release was enhanced when the renal sympathetic nerves were intact compared to that obtained when the kidneys were denervated. Indeed, Kopp and DiBona[160] clearly demonstrated in the dog that the relationship between the magnitude of renin released in response to a particular level of electrical stimulation of the renal nerves was dependent on the prevailing level of renal perfusion pressure. The mechanisms involved at the cellular level remain undefined.

INTEGRATION OF RENAL NERVE ACTIVITY AND FUNCTION

Recruitment of Functionalities

An important consideration after having defined the exact mechanisms by which the renal nerves exert their influence on the different end-points of kidney function, renin release, fluid reabsorption, and renal hemodynamics, is the relationship between the recruitment of these functionalities under normal conditions. At low levels of renal nerve stimulation, which is sub-threshold for changing fluid reabsorption and renal hemodynamics, there is an increase in renin secretion. At somewhat higher levels of renal nerve activation, but again sub-threshold for impacting on renal hemodynamics, not only are there larger increases in renin secretion, but there is also an antidiuresis and antinatriuresis which has been demonstrated in the anaesthetized dog, rabbit, and rat.[58] It is clear that the renal nerve-induced sodium and water retention under these conditions reflects a direct action on proximal tubule reabsorptive processes, as described in micropuncture studies using the anaesthetized rat.[16,266,267] At high levels of renal nerve stimulation, the raised renin release and fluid retention is enhanced, but is now accompanied by a reduction in renal blood flow and, depending on the actual level of stimulation, a decrease in glomerular filtration rate.[58] Indeed, this progressive recruitment of renal functionalities has been shown to occur in man in an elegant study by Wurzner et al.[269] who used lower body negative pressure (LBNP) to reflexly activate the sympathetic nervous system. They found that as LBNP was progressively reduced, there were associated proportionate increases in plasma noradrenaline and plasma renin activity, while sodium excretion was only reduced at the lowest LBNP used. During these challenges neither renal blood flow nor glomerular filtration rate were changed. The way in which these functionalities are recruited is illustrated in Figure 16.5.

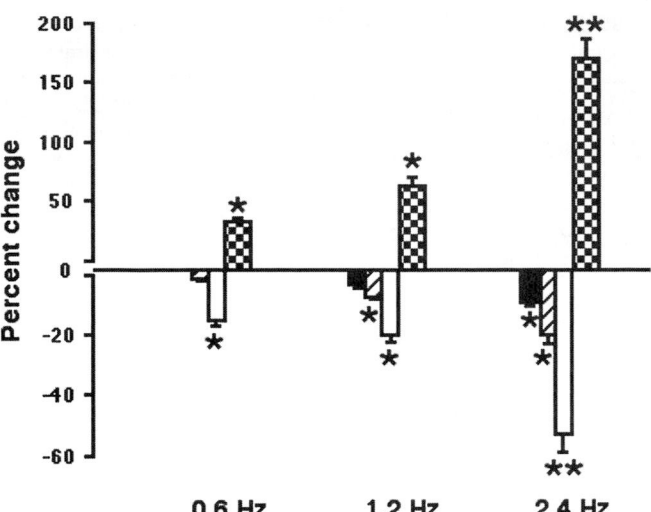

FIGURE 16.5 **At the lowest level of renal nerve stimulation (0.6 Hz), there are significant increases in plasma renin activity (stippled bars) and decreases in sodium excretion (open bars), but no effect on either renal blood flow (hatched bars) or glomerular filtration rate (filled bars).** As the frequency of stimulation is increased there are larger increases in all variables, particularly the decreases in renal hemodynamics which become significant. Importantly the frequency–response relationships are much steeper for plasma renin activity and sodium excretion than for renal blood flow or glomerular filtration rate. *(Modified from ref. [109].)*

There are two important considerations which arise from this pattern of responses. At low levels of renal sympathetic nerve activity, the major impact will be on renin release and sodium and water reabsorption. At these low levels of activity there will only be small increases in circulating renin (50–70%) and reductions in sodium excretion of some 20–40%. However, if these effects persist over a long timeframe, they could have a profound impact on extracellular fluid volume, and thereby on the level at which blood pressure is set. Again, it is worth reiterating that these renin releasing and sodium retaining responses can occur with little evidence of major reductions in renal hemodynamics.

By contrast, when renal sympathetic nerve activity is raised to higher levels by major stressors (for example emotional challenges, severe exercise), then blood flow through the kidney will be markedly reduced. However, it is important to emphasize that these are short acting events, and therefore they are likely to have only minor influences on overall cardiovascular homeostasis.

Patterns of Electrical Stimulation of the Renal Nerves

Patterns of Efferent Activity

The concepts of how the renal nerves influence kidney function have been based largely on experiments in which the sympathetic nerves to the kidney have been dissected out, placed on electrodes, and stimulated using square wave pulses of defined width and voltage at increasing frequencies and constant current delivery. It has been recognized that this pattern of stimulation bears no relation to that passing down the nerves naturally to reach the kidney. Indeed, multifiber nerve recordings have shown the signal to be composed of a bursting nature where larger or smaller numbers of fibers fire together in a coordinated or disparate fashion, with the result that complex patterns are generated. The issue is whether the effectiveness or impact of the nerves on one or more functions might be different if they were stimulated in a way more representative of that occurring under natural conditions.

Lacroix et al.[176] and Nilsson et al.,[210] using isolated mesenteric and nasal vessels, demonstrated that larger sympathetically-mediated vasoconstrictions were produced using high frequency bursts of impulses compared to the delivery of the same number of impulses as a continuous train. This was to a degree reinforced by the observations of Hardebo,[103] who found that the high frequency bursting pattern caused a greater release of noradrenaline from cerebral vessels than that achieved with the same number of impulses delivered as a continuous stream. Thus, the amount of neurotransmitter released can be influenced by the exact pattern of stimulation used.

Electrical Activation with Frequency Enriched Stimuli

HEMODYNAMICS AND FUNCTION

The question therefore arises as to whether the effectiveness or impact of the renal sympathetic nerves could be influenced by the pattern of the stimulation parameters. This was investigated by DiBona and Sawin[66] in the anaesthetized rat using a complex computer generated stimulus pattern basically of a sine wave, within which was embedded a randomly generated white noise signal. The patterned stimulus was designed to approximate that which the kidney might normally be expected to receive. The authors used two levels of intensities, one impacting on renal hemodynamics and one at a lower level which only influenced excretory function. Importantly, they showed that for the same integrated voltage applied to the nerves, the magnitude of reduction in renal blood flow was greater with the sinusoidal patterned stimulus than with the square wave stimulus at all frequencies tested. This data is presented in Figure 16.6, where there is a clear shift of the frequency–response curve to the left with the sinusoidal stimuli compared to the square wave stimuli. In a similar way, application of sub-threshold stimuli for changing renal hemodynamics had no effect

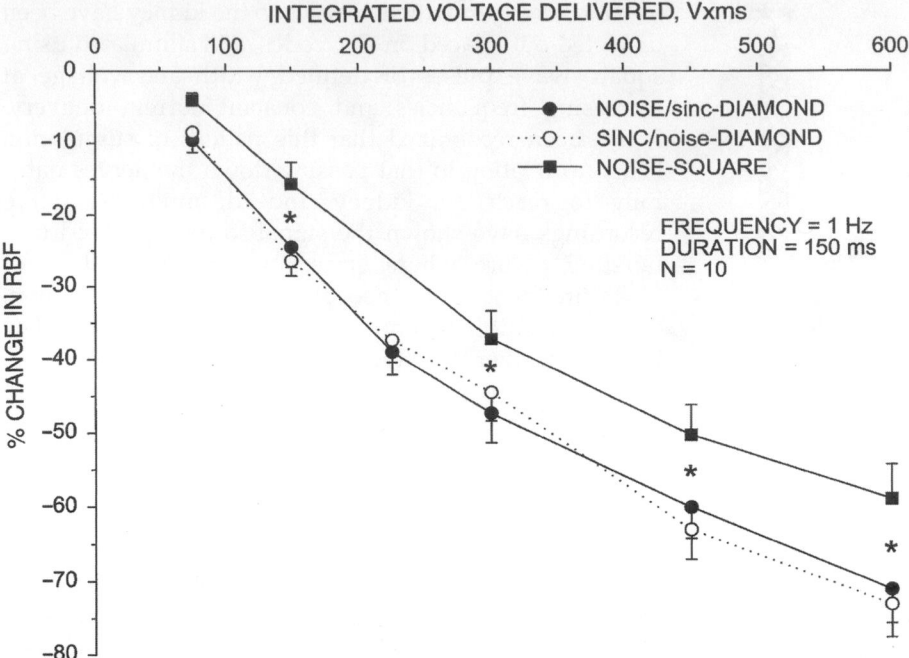

FIGURE 16.6 This figure *(taken from ref. [66] with permission)* demonstrates that delivery of an electrical stimulus as a square wave pulse (NOISE-SQUARE) is less efficient in decreasing renal blood flow (RBF) at every integrated voltage step compared with stimuli delivered as a sinusoidal wave containing either noise (NOISE/SINC-DIAMOND) or fixed frequency within the sinusoidal wave (SINC/NOISE-DIAMOND).

on sodium excretion if delivered in a square wave form, but did cause an antidiuresis and antinatriuresis at the same integrated voltage if the sinusoidal signal was used, and this is illustrated in Figure 16.7. Thus, together these reports serve to emphasize that the way in which the neural signals are delivered into the kidney can determine the impact on end-organ function.

HEMODYNAMICS

Malpas and colleagues,[95,191,192] using the anaesthetized rabbit, investigated whether the bursting pattern of naturally occurring renal nerve activity could in any way determine the dynamic regulation of renal blood flow. Utilizing a similar patterned stimulus, i.e., a sine wave of varying voltage within which square wave pulses were embedded, as against steady square wave pulses, they showed that the frequency of the sine wave could determine the degree of reduction in renal blood flow, even though the total current delivered was the same.[191] The authors proposed that the low frequency pulses in renal sympathetic nerve activity were likely to result in an enhanced dynamic gain to allow the renal blood flow to respond rapidly to normal everyday variations in blood pressure. Interestingly, this hypothesis was not supported by an investigation in the rat[63] in which the renal nerves were similarly stimulated with sine wave modulation with embedded high frequency pulses. These investigators found that there were reductions in renal blood flow with superimposed low frequency oscillations, but that the magnitude of these vasoconstrictor responses were not altered when basal tone was increased by exogenous administration of

noradrenaline or angiotensin II. The reasons why there is a disparity between these reports are unclear, but may reflect a fundamental difference in the regulation of the renal vasculature in the rabbit versus the rat.

Analysis of Renal Nerve Activity

The central mechanisms involved in the generation, regulation, and analysis of the sympathetic outflow have been reviewed in detail by Malpas.[189] It has become possible to resolve the frequency and amplitude components, phase relationships, and coherence between renal sympathetic nerve activity, renal blood flow, and blood pressure. These techniques have been applied to gain insight into how low levels of renal sympathetic nerve activity may influence renal function. It is evident that renal sympathetic nerve activity is at a level which tonically reduces renal blood flow, at least, in the rabbit.[96,190] Moreover, following power spectral analysis of the renal blood flow signal it has become apparent that at a spectral frequency range above 0.6 Hz in the renal sympathetic nerve signal, the nerves exert a tonic vasoconstrictor action on the renal vasculature.[191] However, the lower frequency power spectral peaks, below 0.6 Hz, cause slow cycles of vasoconstriction and vasodilation which, it has been argued, may enhance the responsiveness of the vasculature to other stimuli to allow renal blood flow and glomerular filtration rate to dynamically adapt to ensure constancy of filtered load, and hence fluid processing by the nephron.[192] Indeed, it has been emphasized that this role of the renal nerves is integral to the maintenance of cardiovascular homeostasis.[12]

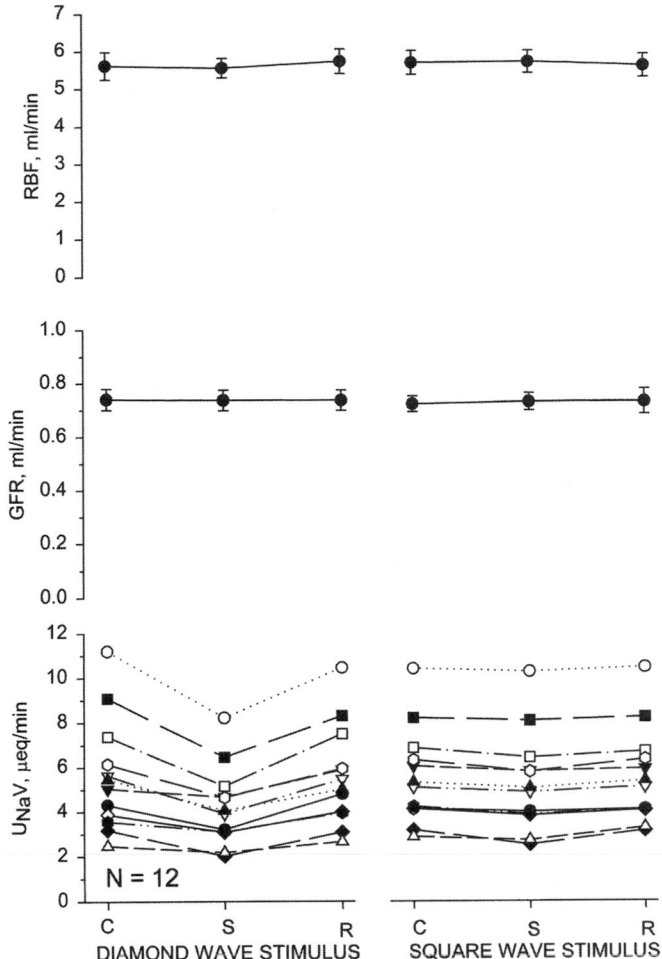

FIGURE 16.7 Electrical stimulation of the renal sympathetic nerves with the diamond wave stimulus, which had no effect on either renal blood flow (RBF) or glomerular filtration rate, (GFR) significantly decreased sodium excretive (UNAV), whereas delivery of the same integrated voltage as a square wave stimulus was without effect on any of the measured variables. *(Taken with permission from ref. [66].)*

They found that acute denervation had little impact on the overall pattern of transfer function gain over the whole frequency range.[61] In contrast, in two pathophysiological states, congestive heart failure and in the spontaneously hypertensive rat where basal renal sympathetic nerve activity is elevated, transfer function gain was suppressed over both these frequency ranges, but was relatively normalized following acute renal denervation.[63] The authors concluded that in the rats with elevated renal nerve activity, the coupling between blood pressure and renal blood flow was overridden such that autoregulation of renal blood flow was impaired. These authors went on to show that this effect was mediated via angiotensin II, as blockade of angiotensin AT1 receptors with losartan depressed the transfer function gain in rats fed on low or normal dietary sodium intake, but not a high dietary sodium intake.[59,63] Indeed, the outcome of these studies indicated that the renin—angiotensin system enhanced the tubuloglomerular feedback component of autoregulation, but not the myogenic component, and that the elevated angiotensin II increased the efficiency of transfer of the neural signal to control the renal vasculature.

Reflex Regulation of the Renal Nerves

Activity within the renal sympathetic nerves represents an integration of a number of sensory inputs arising from different regions of the body by the central nervous system. Malpas has recently reviewed the central mechanisms regulating sympathetic outflow to the periphery, including that to the kidney.[189] The changing output of renal sympathetic nerve activity represents a means by which renal functionalities, that is, renin release, sodium reabsorption, and renal hemodynamics are regulated at an appropriate level. The different sensory systems sending information into the central nervous system are shown in Figure 16.8.

Cardiovascular Baroreceptors

HIGH PRESSURE BARORECEPTORS

A number of early studies demonstrated that the high pressure baroreceptors in the carotid sinuses exerted an important influence on the neural regulation of the kidney. Studies undertaken in anaesthetized and conscious dogs in which carotid sinus pressure was reduced mechanically[94,278] or as a consequence of periods of head up tilt[54,201,202] increased renal nerve activity, renin secretion, and caused a renal nerve-dependent antidiuresis and antinatriuresis with relatively little change in renal hemodynamics. This means that during everyday activity, the baroreflex control of blood pressure will impact on kidney function; renin

The situation in the rat appears somewhat different, as many reports[58] demonstrate that under basal conditions the renal sympathetic nerves have a much smaller, if any, influence on basal renal blood flow. DiBona and Sawin[61,65] evaluated the transfer function gain between blood pressure and renal blood flow under a variety of conditions where renal sympathetic nerve activity was removed or enhanced. There was a characteristic pattern to the transfer function gain under basal conditions. The transfer function gain decreased below zero over the frequency range 0.02 and 0.06 Hz, which was taken to represent a slower tubuloglomerular feedback mechanism of autoregulation, and increased above zero with a plateau region over the higher frequency range 0.1 to 0.2 Hz, which was taken to reflect the myogenic component of autoregulation.

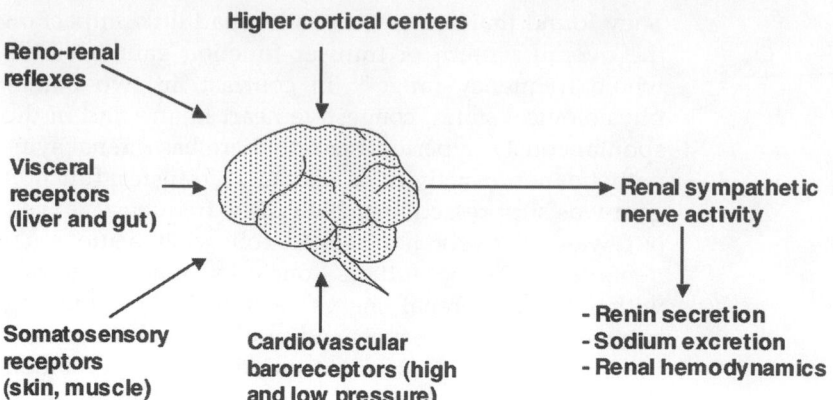

release and sodium and water retention to a greater degree than vasomotor tone. However, what has become evident from the conscious rat studies of Miki and colleagues, is that the baroreflex control of renal sympathetic nerve activity is shifted towards a higher blood pressure as muscle activity increases, for example during grooming and exercise on a treadmill.[204,206,277]

LOW PRESSURE BARORECEPTORS

The low pressure baroreceptors are contained in the cardiopulmonary areas, and are mechanosensitive nerves embedded in the atria and great veins (superior and inferior venae cavae and pulmonary vein) which respond to stretch. Activation of these sensory nerves by inflation of balloons in the left atria results in a reflex decrease in renal sympathetic nerve activity associated with a rise in water and sodium excretion.[90,178] While many of these studies were undertaken in anaesthetized preparations, DiBona and Sawin[68] demonstrated in the conscious rat that volume expansion decreased and volume depletion increased renal sympathetic nerve activity. These observations correlated with a key report by Miki et al.[201] in the conscious dog showing that head-out total body water immersion, a maneuver that shifts fluid into the more central compartments of the cardiovascular system, caused a reflex renal sympatho-inhibition associated with a diuresis and natriuresis. The cardiopulmonary receptors were demonstrated to be essential in this reflex, as following chronic cardiac denervation both the renal sympatho-inhibition and excretory responses were markedly blunted when these dogs were subjected to the water immersion challenge.[202]

Somatosensory System

There are mechanosensory nerve fibers in the joints and tendons, chemosensitive nerves within the muscle tissue itself depolarized by metabolites.[127,128] The skin contains nociceptors and thermoreceptors. Each of these classes of sensory nerves sends important afferent information into the central nervous system to be integrated. At the level of the kidney, an early study by Thames and Abboud[255] demonstrated that sciatic nerve stimulation caused profound reductions in renal blood flow. In the anaesthetized rat, electrical stimulation of the brachial nerves, application of capsaicin subcutaneously to depolarize afferent nerve endings or inhalation of noxious fumes[45,46,279] caused increases in renal sympathetic nerve activity and a renal nerve-mediated antidiuresis and antinatriuresis with little change in renal hemodynamics. Interestingly, the magnitude of the renal sympathetic nerve activity responses is under tonic inhibitory control by the cardiopulmonary receptors, as suggested by studies showing that activation of the cardiopulmonary receptors blunts the sympatho-excitatory and antinatriuretic responses to capsaisin-induced activation of the afferent nerves.[279] These studies illustrate the point that the somatosensory system does provide an important input to the brain, but its impact is modulated by input from the cardiovascular baroreceptors.

Visceral System

Less well-studied, but nonetheless important, are the chemo- and mechano sensory nerves in the visceral system. In early studies, Weaver and co-workers[262] demonstrated that activation of chemosensitive nerve fibers in the small intestine of the cat, by bradykinin, caused a reflex activation of the renal sympathetic nerves. Furthermore, they demonstrated that the effectiveness of this sensory input from the gut was under a tonic inhibitory influence from both the low and high pressure cardiovascular baroreceptor.

Chemo- and mechanosensory nerves are also present within the liver, where they modulate renal sympathetic nerve activity and renal nerve mediated fluid excretion.[110,111,171,205] A reduction in plasma sodium concentration in the hepatic portal vein, but not hepatic artery, resulted in increased adrenaline secretion, indicative of a sympatho-excitation, which was blocked by denervation of the hepatic portal vein.[110,111] Moreover, infusion of a hypertonic solution in the hepatic portal vein[205] caused a renal sympatho-inhibition and a renal nerve-dependent increase in sodium and water excretion. Taken together, these observations lay the foundation of important reflexes whereby food and fluid absorption from the gut initiates an appropriate neural regulation of kidney function to ensure that sodium and water homeostasis is maintained.

The spleen has also been found to be a source of sensory information which can modulate renal sympathetic nerve activity and its functional end-points. Hamza and Kaufman[99–101] reported that an increase in splenic venous pressure resulted in small rises in blood pressure and reductions in renal blood flow, with the latter being prevented following surgical section of the renal sympathetic nerves. It can be speculated that this relationship becomes important in portal hypertension and liver cirrhosis in eliciting a reflex renal sympatho-excitation which will contribute to the sodium retention associated with these disease states.

Higher Cortical Centers

The role of psychological stress in regulating renal sympathetic nerve outflow and renal function is less clear-cut and far more difficult to study. Nonetheless, chronically instrumented rats have been used and subjected to a range of challenges to engage the higher cortical centers. An arousal stimulus of an air jet stress has been found to reflexly increase renal sympathetic nerve activity along with a renal nerve-dependent antinatriuresis and antidiuresis.[64,258] However, studies to determine potential control by the cardiovascular baroreceptors of physiological stresses have been difficult to achieve in conscious studies. Nonetheless, the recent observations of Miki and his group have revealed a number of important findings. First, it was apparent that renal sympathetic nerve activity was lower during rapid eye movement sleep than in non-rapid eye movement sleep and became higher as the level of physical activity rose, from quiet awake to grooming.[277] At the same time, there was an adaptation of the baroreflex to function over a higher blood pressure range as the activity of the animal increased.[277] Second, during treadmill exercise,[204] there was an increased sensitivity of the baroreflex relationship, which they interpreted as important in buffering the raised blood pressure under conditions of increased muscular activity. This group has also evaluated the cardiovascular changes induced during "freezing" behavior, when conscious rats are exposed to a high level of white noise.[203,276] Under these conditions, there was a minimal change in blood pressure, but heart rate decreased while renal sympathetic nerve activity increased, and lumbar sympathetic nerve activity did not change. The alterations in renal sympathetic nerve activity and heart rate during the freezing behavior were largely prevented by prior sino-aortic denervation, which indicated their important contribution to this pattern of responses. Thus, the cardiovascular and sympathetically-mediated responses during the freezing behavior prepare the animal for an active response to the threatening situation. Taken together, it is apparent that in all these different behavioral states central command exerts an important differential regulatory influence on the baroreflex control of sympathetic outflow to many organs, including that to the kidney.

Reflex Control of Selective Functions

Attention has been focused on whether the renal innervation could selectively regulate either renal hemodynamics or tubular fluid reabsorption or renin secretion. The findings of Luff et al. in the rabbit[183] and DiBona and Sawin in the rat[67] demonstrated that two types of structurally different nerve fibers exist within the nerve bundles and within the kidney itself. Evidence has been produced in the rabbit, where glomerular capillary pressure was measured as an indirect estimate of pre- and post-glomerular resistances.[48–50] Using an angiotensin II clamp, to remove any confounding influences of changes in endogenous angiotensin II levels, a hypoxic challenge increased glomerular filtration pressure. The authors' interpreted these observations as reflecting a selective neural regulation post-glomerular vascular resistance, possibly via one of the subtypes of nerve fiber, independent of the renin–angiotensin system.

DiBona and colleagues[51,67] using the rat analyzed the strength-duration relationship during direct electrical renal nerve stimulation in relation to renal blood flow, urine flow, and sodium excretion. They found a higher stimulation threshold for the nerve fibers involved in regulating renal blood flow than for those involved in regulating fluid excretion. Moreover, activity in single sympathetic fibers innervating the kidney could be selectively modified by different reflexes. Thus, stimulation of arterial baroreceptors, central chemoreceptors, and thermoreceptors activated a large proportion (88%) of spontaneously active fibers, whereas thermoreceptors only increased the firing rate of those fibers which had no spontaneous activity. In a different series of studies, examining patterns of renal sympathetic nerve activity by evaluating the peaks of activity and time between peaks, DiBona and co-workers were able to show that although somatosensory (pinch) and heat stimuli resulted in similar increases in total renal sympathetic nerve activity, it was only the heat stimulus that caused a decrease in renal blood flow. The authors took these responses to indicate that two different stimuli could result in a distinctly different control of sympathetic outflow regulating renal hemodynamics.

It would seem that there is a small, but persuasive, body of evidence for the view that there may be a degree of selectivity of functional control in the neural control of the kidney. There is a need for more investigation of this particular topic.

Central Nervous System

Central Processing

The processing of this sensory information within the central nervous system to generate an appropriate level of sympathetic outflow, not only to the kidney but to other organs, is complex and attention has been directed towards the cardiovascular baroreceptors which exert a major influence on autonomic control.[44] The sensory information from both the high and low pressure baroreceptors pass to the nucleus tractus solitarius (NTS) for initial processing, and subsequently via multiple pathways to the caudal and rostral ventrolateral medulla (CVLM and RVLM) where a complex interaction takes place before the pre-ganglionic fibers are stimulated. The way in which the major sensory inputs feed into these pathways is illustrated and summarized in Figure 16.9.

The situation regarding the somatosensory and visceral systems and their inputs to the areas regulating the autonomic nervous system are much less defined. The somatosensory system appears to have a direct input at three levels, NTS, CVLM, and RVLM,[42] but the actions exerted at each of these sites, whether excitatory or inhibitory, and the neurotransmitters involved, have not been resolved.

There is now a body of evidence that autonomic control is organized in a patterned manner. Micro-injection of glutamate onto the RVLM elicited an increase in cardiac, splenic, and renal sympathetic nerve activities that were very different in magnitude.[195,196] In conscious rat studies there is a relatively low degree of autonomic control of lumbar sympathetic nerve activity during treadmill exercise or in the freezing behavior,[203,204,276] whereas there are large dynamic responses in renal sympathetic nerve activity. There is also a clear differential control of cardiac and renal sympathetic outflow in the conscious sheep. Thus, following an infusion of hypertonic saline icv, renal sympathetic nerve activity markedly decreased, whereas cardiac sympathetic nerve activity did not change.[195] By contrast, in a model of pacing-induced heart failure, there was a large elevation in cardiac sympathetic, but not renal sympathetic, nerve activity. It was also reported in conscious rats[275] that icv infusion of angiotensin II reduced renal, but not lumbar, sympathetic nerve activity. A fuller analysis of the

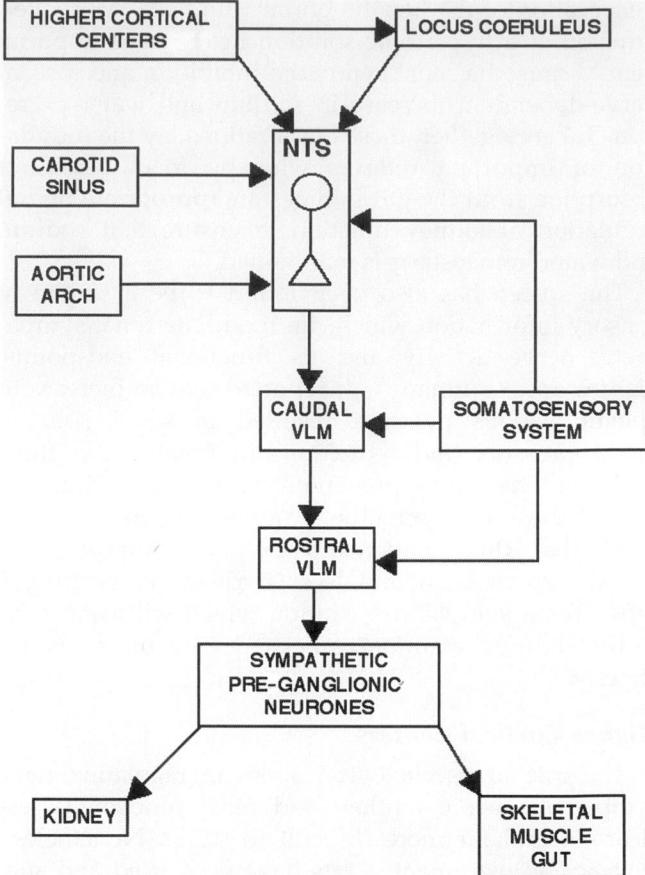

FIGURE 16.9 This illustration indicates how input from the baroreceptors, somatosensory system, and higher cortical centers act at the nucleus tractus solitarus (NTS), which feeds into the caudal and rostal venterolateral medulla (CVLM and RVLM). This determines the level of excitability of pre-ganglionic neurones and thereby sympathetic outflow to the kidney and other vascular beds.

evidence has been presented by Malpas[189] in a recent review. The exact way in which information from each sensory system is integrated to provide an appropriate output of renal sympathetic nerve activity and neural control of renal function in order to ensure cardiovascular homeostasis remains to be explored.

Brain Angiotensin II

ANGIOTENSIN II AND AUTONOMIC PATHWAYS

There is accumulating evidence that the renin—angiotensin system and angiotensin II can influence the reflex responses in sympathetic nerve activity generated by the central nervous system. This can arise in two ways, either via circulating angiotensin II or by means of angiotensin II generated locally within the brain at specific nuclei. Moreover, angiotensin II receptors have been demonstrated in many regions of the brain, and particularly at those nuclei involved with cardiovascular control.[3] It is now accepted that in the areas of the circumventricular organs the blood–brain barrier is leaky,[200] enabling angiotensin II to act on nuclei within this region which have been shown to contain a high density of angiotensin II receptors. At these sites the peptide is able to influence fluid balance; it stimulates drinking, induces ADH release, and causes increased sodium reabsorption and renin release.[199] The second route whereby angiotensin II may influence autonomic control is that generated within the brain itself, as all components of the renin–angiotensin system are present, that is renin, angiotensinogen, converting enzyme, and angiotensin II receptors.[265] It is also necessary to emphasize that immunocytochemical, in situ hybridization studies, and mRNA measurements of angiotensin II receptors and angiotensinogen have shown them to be present or their genes expressed at those nuclei involved with autonomic control, that is the NTS, RVLM, and CVLM, and the paraventricular nucleus (PVN),[199] as well as those other nuclei of the subfornical organ and the area postrema which are most likely subject to the action of circulating angiotensin II. Neurophysiological studies have shown that local administration of angiotensin II onto the NTS and RVLM is excitatory and produces a sympathetically-mediated pressor response, but when applied to the CVLM it causes a sympatho-inhibition[43,105]; thus, angiotensin II may have different actions and consequences depending on its site of production and action.

BRAIN ANGIOTENSIN II AND NEURAL CONTROL OF THE KIDNEY

The functional role played by angiotensin II within the brain in modulating autonomic control, both normally and in pathophysiological states, is only now being elucidated. There are now a number of reports showing that the baroreflex control of renal sympathetic nerve activity was suppressed by angiotensin II in conscious normotensive Wistar rats,[120] and enhanced in the spontaneously hypertensive rat (SHR).[117,174] In terms of the somatosensory reflex, angiotensin II within the central nervous system is important, in that losartan given icv blocked the renal nerve-mediated antinatriuresis and antidiuresis resulting from nociceptor stimulation[118] and angiotensin II icv restored the renal nerve-dependent functional responses[119] which could be correlated with marked changes in the pattern with which energy was distributed within the renal nerve signal.[127,279] The central issue which arises is to understand which factors could affect the level of angiotensin II within the central nervous system which would then impact on the degree of autonomic control exerted peripherally and particularly at the kidney. Indeed, it is important to distinguish between acute bolus administration of angiotensin II administered systemically and the application of the peptide as an icv infusion which

may be associated with increases in blood pressure and a renal sympatho-excitation.

The level of dietary sodium intake can modulate this very important link between the autonomic control of the cardiovascular system and brain angiotensin II. An early report by Huang and Leenen[117] demonstrated that raised levels of dietary sodium intake in normotensive rats from four to eight weeks-of-age, led to an increase in baroreflex gain associated with a resetting to a higher pressure for renal nerve activity, but not for heart rate. The importance of dietary sodium intake during development has been reinforced by the studies of Osborn and his group,[27,214] who showed that in rats fed a high-salt diet from four to eight weeks-of-age, low dose infusion of angiotensin II into the brain (icv) over five days caused a sustained increase in blood pressure associated with a renal nerve-dependent antinatriuresis. This was not observed in rats fed a normal or low-salt diet. Further evidence for this role of the renal sympathetic nerves was reported by Houghton and co-workers[115,116] who found that a bolus injection of angiotensin II icv had vasopressor and renal sympatho-excitatory actions, the magnitudes of which were enhanced in rats fed a high-sodium diet over the period of growth and development that was in part mediated by vasopressin release both systemically and within the spinal cord.

This influence of dietary sodium intake on the contribution of angiotensin II in the brain on central pathways regulating renal sympathetic nerve activity has received some attention. DiBona and co-workers[56,57] using rats subjected to a low, normal or high dietary sodium intake for two weeks, microinjected an AT-1 receptor antagonist onto the RVLM, and observed a decreased blood pressure and a shift in the baroreflex gain curve for renal nerve activity to a lower pressure in the animals fed a low-sodium diet, but not in those animals fed the normal or high-sodium intakes. Furthermore, it was evident that administration of an AT-1 receptor antagonist to the RVLM blunted the increases in blood pressure, heart rate, and renal sympathetic nerve activity produced by bicuculline, a GABA receptor antagonist, injected onto the PVN. Importantly, the renal sympathetic nerve responses to the bicuculline administration into the PVN were enhanced in the rats subjected to the low-sodium diet, but blunted in those fed the high salt intake.[55]

Together, these findings highlight the importance of the brain renin–angiotensin system and the significance of angiotensin II in determining the sensitivity of neural pathways regulating sympathetic outflow to the kidney. They also emphasize how alterations in dietary sodium intake may impact on these neural control pathways, which may reset kidney function to a level which could predispose the individual to a hypertensive state.

Neural Regulation of the Kidney in Man

Knowledge of the sympathetic nerve control of the kidney in experimental animals under normal physiological conditions is now extensive in relation to the regulation of renal hemodynamics, renin secretion, and tubular sodium reabsorption. Indeed, although not touched upon in this chapter, there is an extensive body of work in relation to the role of the renal sympathetic nerves in pathophysiological states.[53,58,124,189] However, knowledge of the importance and significance of the renal sympathetic nerves in man remains a relatively unexplored area, although their contribution to cardiovascular and renal diseases is increasingly recognized and alluded to above in different sections. The most striking demonstration of their importance in man has come in a report by Krum et al.,[172,173] who utilized an angioplasty catheter inserted into the renal arteries with a probe at the tip which emitted radiofrequencies with sufficient intensity to disrupt the renal nerves passing alongside the renal artery. In a group of patients with hypertension that was resistant to conventional drug based therapy, bilateral ablation of the renal nerves in this way resulted in a reduction in systolic blood pressure of some 30 mmHg which was maintained for at least 24 months after the manoeuvre. Currently, these initial observations are being further investigated in randomized multicenter trials. DiBona and Esler[53] have emphasized that the knowledge gained from the experimental studies is now being successfully translated into therapeutic approaches, and that the role of the renal sympathetic nerves in heart failure, renal failure, and metabolic diseases of diabetes and obesity will now be explored.

AFFERENT RENAL SENSORY NERVES

Introduction

Not much focus has previously been placed on the afferent sensory innervation of the kidney and its physiological importance in the cardiovascular regulation compared to the efferent renal sympathetic innervation of the kidney. However, recent studies in man showing long-term depressor effects following renal nerve ablation which reduces both efferent and afferent renal nerve activity have highlighted a possible role for the afferent renal nerves in hypertension.[53] As will be discussed in more detail below, in healthy animals activation of the afferent renal sensory nerves elicits an inhibitory renorenal reflex response consisting of increases in afferent renal nerve activity, the nerve signals going from the kidney to the neuraxis, causing decreases in efferent renal sympathetic nerve activity which in turn result in a natriuresis (Figure 16.10). Available evidence would suggest that in many pathological conditions the nature of the renorenal reflexes is switched from being of an inhibitory to an excitatory nature (*vide infra*).

NEUROANATOMY

In the kidney, the majority of the afferent renal nerves containing substance P and calcitonin gene-related peptide (CGRP) are located in the renal pelvic wall,[147,156,182] where their circumferential orientation make them ideally suitable for sensing stretch (Figure 16.11). The majority of the renal sensory nerves are unmyelinated.[139]

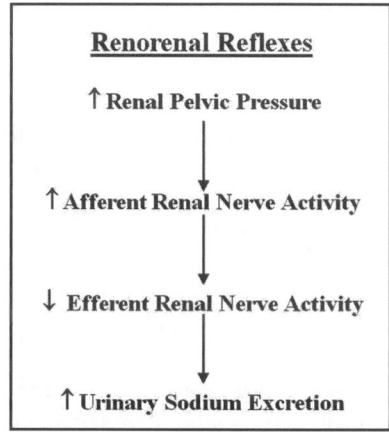

FIGURE 16.10 Increasing renal pelvic pressure ≥ 3 mmHg stretches the renal pelvic wall, leading to activation of the afferent renal mechanosensory nerves. The increase in afferent renal nerve activity leads to decreases in efferent renal nerve activity, which in turn increases urinary sodium excretion, i.e., a renorenal reflex mechanism.

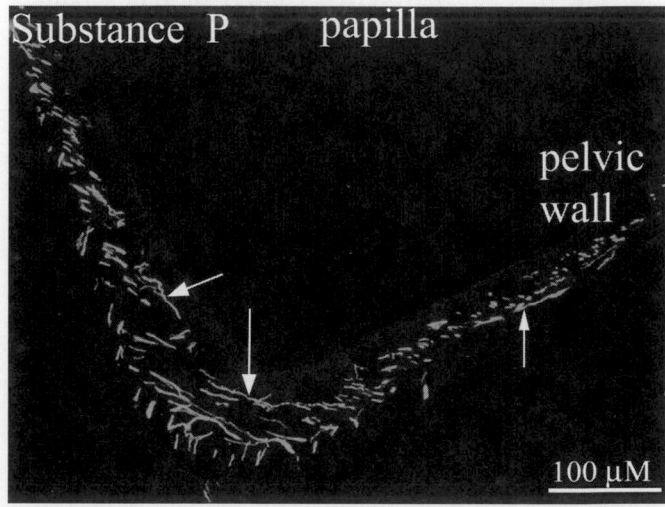

FIGURE 16.11 In the kidney, the majority of the substance P containing nerve fibers (arrows) is located in the muscular layer of the renal pelvic wall.

Depending on the species, the cell bodies of the afferent renal nerves are located in ipsilateral dorsal root ganglia (DRG) from T_6-L_4, with predominance in $T_{12}-L_3$.[58] Viral tracing studies combined with dorsal rhizotomy (DRX) at $T_{10}-T_{13}$ have provided evidence for the afferent renal nerves projecting from the DRG to the ipsilateral dorsal horn mainly in Laminae I, III−V,[36] where they synapse with interneurons projecting to sites within the central nervous system which are associated with cardiovascular regulation, including nucleus tractus solitarius, rostral ventrolateral medulla, subfornical organ, and paraventricular nucleus of hypothalamus.[247] There is also evidence for a monosynaptic projection of the afferent renal nerves to areas within the brainstem.[270]

Stimulation of the afferent renal nerves may activate spinal and supraspinal pathways.[29,35,138,241] Electrical stimulation of the afferent renal nerves results in widespread decreases in efferent renal sympathetic nerve activity, including renal, cervical, and cardiac nerves, in association with decreases in arterial pressure.[232] A majority of the neurons in the ventral lateral medulla that decrease their activity in response to afferent renal nerve stimulation also respond to stimulation of the central portion of the aortic nerves, with a decrease in efferent renal sympathetic nerve activity.[232] These neurons are also responsive to inputs from the carotid sinus nerves.[254] In addition, activation of the afferent renal nerves alters the activity of vasopressin and oxytocin neurons in the paraventricular nucleus of hypothalamus in rats,[35] resulting in increases in arterial pressure and plasma vasopressin and oxytocin concentrations. These effects are abolished by prior denervation of the stimulated kidney.

The convergence of the afferent signals from the renal and carotid sinus nerves on neurons in several brain areas involved in cardiovascular control[26,82,247] provides an anatomical basis for possible interactions among the afferent signals deriving from various organs, including the kidney.

Two classes of renal sensory nerves have been identified neurophysiologically: renal mechanosensory nerves responding to stretch of the renal pelvic wall; and renal chemosensory nerves responding to renal ischemia and/or changes in the chemical environment of the renal interstitium. The electrophysiology of the renal sensory nerves has previously been reviewed extensively.[58,249] Isotonic saline volume expansion results in a differential activation of renal mechano- and chemosensitive nerves.[33] Whereas volume expansion increased the activity of mechanosensitive nerves, it decreased the activity of the chemosensitive nerves, type R2 chemoreceptors. Stretch is associated with an increase in muscle spindle cell membrane sodium permeability, resulting in an inward flux of sodium and depolarization.[121,217] The afferent renal nerve activity responses to increased renal pelvic pressure are reduced by renal pelvic administration of amiloride and lidocaine,[165,169] agents known to reduce sodium influx by different mechanisms. Conversely, inhibition of Na^+-K^+-ATPase by ouabain increases the afferent renal nerve activity response to increased renal pelvic pressure.[170] These studies suggest that changes in intracellular sodium concentration may modulate the responsiveness of renal pelvic mechanosensitive nerves.

RENORENAL REFLEXES

The identification of a reflex originating in one kidney and affecting contralateral renal function was first demonstrated in the early 1980s. In healthy normotensive animals, the afferent renal nerves were activated by increases in renal pelvic pressure of a magnitude ≥ 3 mmHg, commonly seen during high urine flow rate,[33,88,151] suggesting that the afferent renal nerves were tonically active in conditions of high-sodium diet and/or volume expansion. Supporting this argument were studies in anesthetized volume expanded rats showing that increases in ipsilateral urinary sodium excretion produced by total, i.e., efferent plus afferent, unilateral renal denervation were accompanied by decreases in contralateral urinary sodium excretion. The contralateral antinatriuresis was caused by increases in contralateral efferent renal sympathetic nerve activity; this is called a renorenal reflex response[39,60] (Figure 16.12). Because unilateral renal denervation results in an ipsilateral diuresis and natriuresis, total (ipsilateral plus contralateral) urine flow rate and urinary sodium excretion are unchanged. Thus, the afferent renal nerves exert tonic inhibitory effects on contralateral efferent renal sympathetic nerve activity.

Selective Afferent Renal Denervation: Dorsal Rhizotomy

The overall importance of the natriuretic inhibitory renorenal reflexes can be evaluated by selective bilateral afferent renal denervation produced by dorsal rhizotomy (DRX) at T_9-L_1. Cutting the dorsal roots from T_9-L_1 interrupts the afferent renal neural input to the central nervous system.[70] Both DRX and sham-DRX rats are able to establish external sodium balance on both a normal dietary sodium intake and a four-fold higher dietary sodium intake. However, this is achieved at markedly different levels of arterial pressure.[150] On a normal or low-sodium diet, the levels of mean arterial pressure are similar in DRX and sham-DRX rats.[126,150] However, the process of achieving external sodium balance while consuming an increased dietary sodium intake resulted in a mean arterial pressure in DRX rats

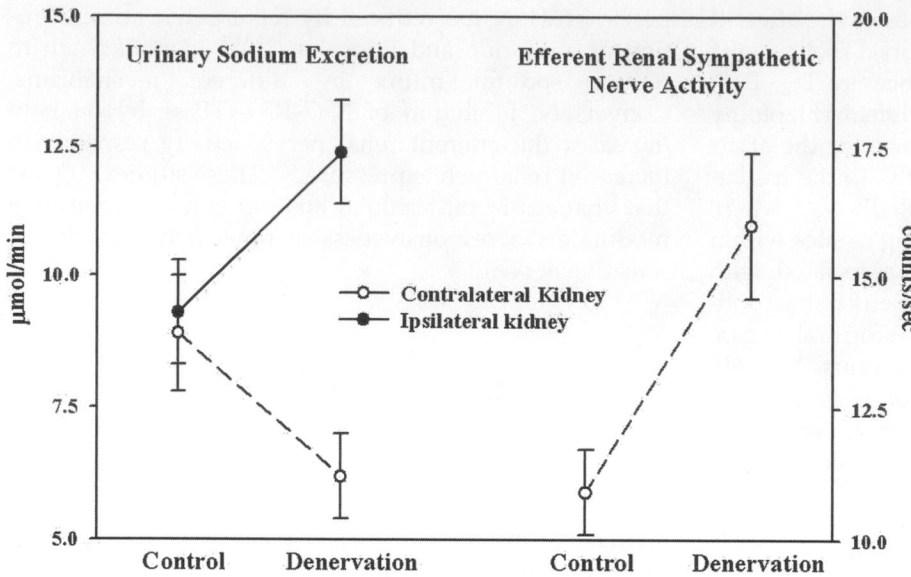

FIGURE 16.12 In normotensive healthy rats, denervation of one kidney (ipsilateral kidney) results in increases in ipsilateral urinary sodium excretion, and decreases in contralateral urinary sodium excretion. The decreases in contralateral urinary sodium excretion are the result of increases in contralateral efferent renal sympathetic nerve activity, i.e., the afferent renal nerves exert a tonic inhibition of sympathetic nerve activity to the contralateral kidney. (Modified from ref. [58].)

that was some 30 mmHg greater than that in sham-DRX rats[150] (Figure 16.13). These findings support the view that the afferent renal nerves are tonically active in high-sodium dietary conditions.[151] Thus, the afferent renal nerves are essential for achieving sodium balance during increased dietary sodium intake. Rats lacking intact afferent renal innervation can only achieve sodium balance at the cost of increased mean arterial pressure. Thus, afferent renal denervation leads to salt-sensitive hypertension. Among the mechanisms contributing to the development of salt-sensitive hypertension in DRX rats are increased efferent renal sympathetic nerve activity and increased responsiveness of efferent renal sympathetic nerves to various sympathetic stimuli due, at least in part, to impairment of the arterial baroreflex function.[164]

Wang and co-workers have presented evidence for salt-sensitive hypertension in rats neonatally treated with capsaicin to destroy the sensory innervation of all organs.[260] The salt-sensitive hypertension in DRX rats would suggest that the lack of intact afferent renal innervation in the capsaicin treated rats may contribute to the increased arterial pressure in these rats when fed a high-sodium diet.

Activation of Renal Mechanosensory Nerves: Physiological Conditions

The inhibitory nature of the afferent renal nerves in healthy normal rats has been further demonstrated in studies examining the functional responses to activation of the afferent renal nerves. The renal mechanosensory nerves respond to stretch of the smooth muscle layer in which many of the sensory nerves are embedded. Studies in cats showed that the increased

urine flow rate produced by volume expansion resulted in parallel increases in renal pelvic pressure and afferent renal nerve activity.[88] Importantly, the activation threshold of the mechanosensory nerves was <5 mmHg above baseline pelvic pressure, suggesting that the renal pelvic mechanosensory nerves are activated by increases in renal pelvic pressure within the physiological range and below that required for sensation of pain. Studies to examine the mechanisms involved in the activation of the renal sensory nerves in the absence of changes in the renal circulation utilized a fluid-filled ureteral catheter elevated to different levels above the kidney. These studies, performed in rats, showed that graded increases in renal pelvic pressure resulted in graded increases in afferent renal nerve activity, with the activation threshold being between 3 to 5 mmHg,[170] i.e., a similar activation threshold as that produced by volume expansion. The increase in afferent renal nerve activity produced bilateral decreases in efferent renal sympathetic nerve activity and increases in urinary sodium excretion[166,169,187] (Figure 16.10). Ipsilateral renal denervation blocks the increases in urinary sodium excretion, demonstrating that stimulation of renal mechanosensory nerves activates an inhibitory bilateral renorenal reflex mechanism. The afferent renal nerves are not responsive to NaCl concentrations within the physiological range, as shown by lack of increases in afferent renal nerve activity in response to renal pelvic perfusion with NaCl at <900 mM.[170]

The natriuretic nature of the renorenal reflexes would suggest that this reflex mechanism contributes to total body sodium and fluid volume balance by assisting in the excretion of sodium and water. In this case, it would be expected that this reflex mechanism would be enhanced or upregulated during conditions

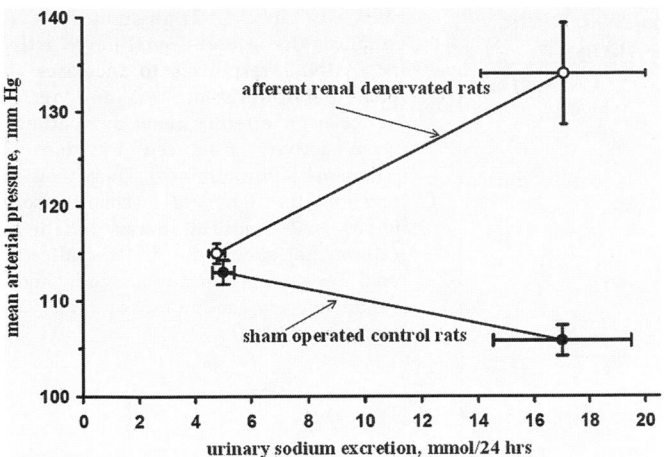

FIGURE 16.13 Recording mean arterial pressure in conscious rats fed either normal or high-sodium diet for three weeks following dorsal rhizotomy at T_9-L_1 to remove the afferent renal innervation showed markedly elevated mean arterial pressure in the afferent renal denervated rats fed a high-sodium diet compared to the sham-operated litter mates. Mean arterial pressure was similar in the two groups of rats fed normal sodium diet. Thus, afferent renal denervated rats are characterized by salt-sensitive hypertension. *(Modified from references [53,152]).*

of sodium and volume-loading. Indeed, studies examining the responsiveness of the renal mechanosensory nerves in rats fed various sodium diets showed that, in comparison to low-sodium dietary intake, high-sodium dietary intake enhances the renorenal reflex responses.[151] At every level of renal pelvic pressure, the increases in both afferent renal nerve activity and urinary sodium excretion were greater in rats fed high-sodium diet compared to rats fed low-sodium diet (Figure 16.14). Importantly, in rats fed high-sodium diet, the threshold of activation of the renal mechanosensory nerves was 2–3 mmHg, suggesting that the afferent renal nerves are tonically active in high-sodium dietary conditions.

Interaction between Efferent and Afferent Renal Nerve Activity

Not only is the renal pelvic wall innervated by afferent sensory nerves, but it is also innervated by efferent sympathetic nerves which are in close contact with the sensory nerves in the renal pelvic wall[157] (Figure 16.15). These findings provide anatomical support for a functional interaction between the efferent and afferent renal nerves. As discussed above in normotensive rats, activation of the afferent renal sensory nerves leads to decreases in efferent renal sympathetic nerve activity and natriuresis, an inhibitory renorenal reflex response.[166] However, not only do increases in afferent renal nerve activity decrease efferent renal sympathetic nerve activity, but increases in efferent

renal sympathetic nerve activity increase afferent renal nerve activity[157,163,158] (Figure 16.16). The increased afferent renal nerve activity will, in turn, decrease efferent renal sympathetic nerve activity via activation of the renorenal reflexes, a negative feedback mechanism, to maintain low-level efferent renal sympathetic nerve activity (Figure 16.17). Similar to the responsiveness of the renal mechanosensory nerves being modulated by dietary sodium, the interaction between efferent renal sympathetic nerve activity and afferent renal nerve activity is also modulated by dietary sodium. Reflex increases in efferent renal sympathetic nerve activity results in much larger increases in afferent renal nerve activity in rats fed high-sodium diet than in rats fed low-sodium diet (Figure 16.14).

Thus, in high-sodium dietary conditions, the enhanced afferent renal nerve activity responses to increases in efferent renal sympathetic nerve activity and/or increases in renal pelvic pressure would lead to enhanced inhibitory renorenal reflex control of efferent renal sympathetic nerve activity to minimize sodium retention. Conversely, in low-sodium dietary conditions, the suppressed afferent renal nerve activity responses to increases in efferent renal sympathetic nerve activity and/or increases in renal pelvic pressure would result in little or no inhibition of efferent renal sympathetic nerve activity, which eventually would lead to sodium retention. It is important to note that these are physiologically appropriate responses to changes in dietary sodium in the overall goal of maintaining sodium balance.

Mechanisms Involved in Activation of Renal Mechanosensory Nerves

SUBSTANCE P

Substance P is produced in the neural cell bodies in the dorsal root ganglia and transported along the afferent nerves towards the peripheral nerve endings, where it is stored in vesicles and released in response to various stimuli. The presence of substance P-containing sensory nerves in the renal pelvic wall[156] (Figure 16.11) suggested a role for this neuropeptide in the activation of the renal sensory nerves. Single unit recordings of afferent renal nerve activity showed that the same single nerve fiber could be activated by increases in renal pelvic pressure and substance P administered directly into the renal pelvic area, suggesting an important role for substance P in the inhibitory renorenal reflex responses to increased renal pelvic pressure.[185] Substance P is released from the renal pelvic sensory nerves by a calcium (Ca^{2+})-dependent mechanism requiring influx of Ca_i^{2+} via N-type Ca_i^{2+} channels in response to prostaglandin E_2 (PGE_2),[146] a known activator of sensory neurons.[31,112,257]

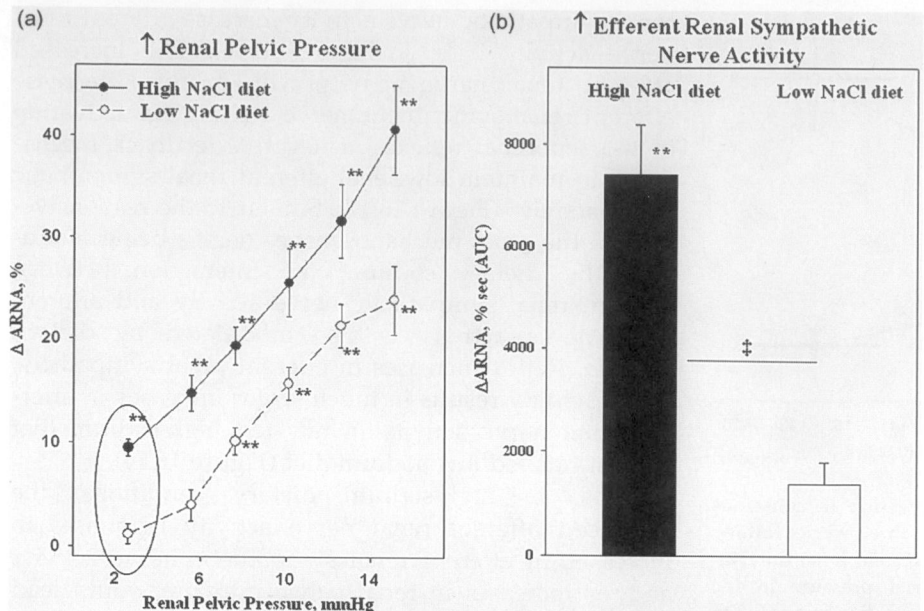

FIGURE 16.14 High-sodium diet enhances the afferent renal nerve activity (ARNA) responses to increases in renal pelvic pressure **(a)** and reflex increases in efferent renal sympathetic nerve activity produced by thermal cutaneous stimulation **(b).** The activation threshold for the renal mechanosensory nerves is 2–3 mmHg in rats fed high-sodium diet suggesting that the afferent renal nerves are tonically active in high-sodium dietary conditions. *(Modified from references [151,158].)*

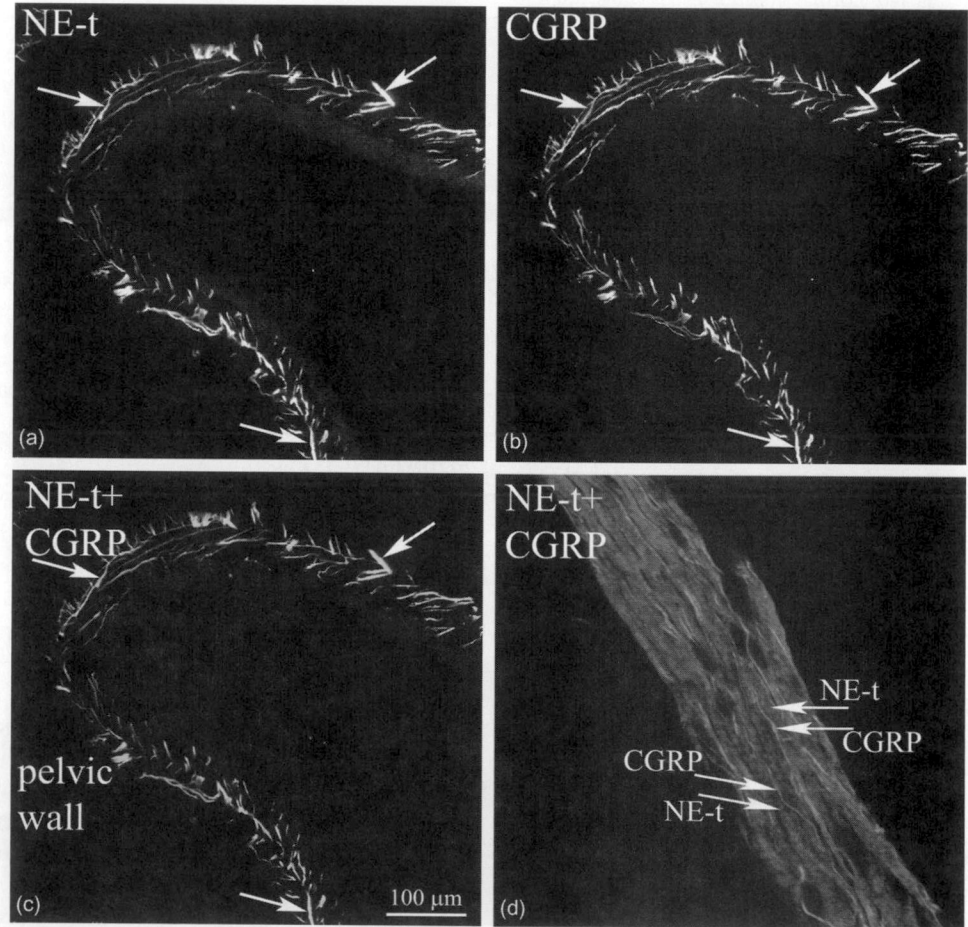

FIGURE 16.15 Applying antibodies against the norepinephrine transporter (NE-t) and the neuropeptide calcitonin gene-related peptide (CGRP) to kidney tissue to identify sympathetic and sensory nerve fibers, respectively (arrows) showed that the sympathetic nerves in the renal pelvic wall (a); are in close contact with the sensory nerves (b); as indicated by the color yellow (c). Higher magnification showed that the sympathetic and sensory nerves are separate fibers in close contact in the same nerve bundle (d). *(Modified from reference [157].)* See color section at the back of the book.

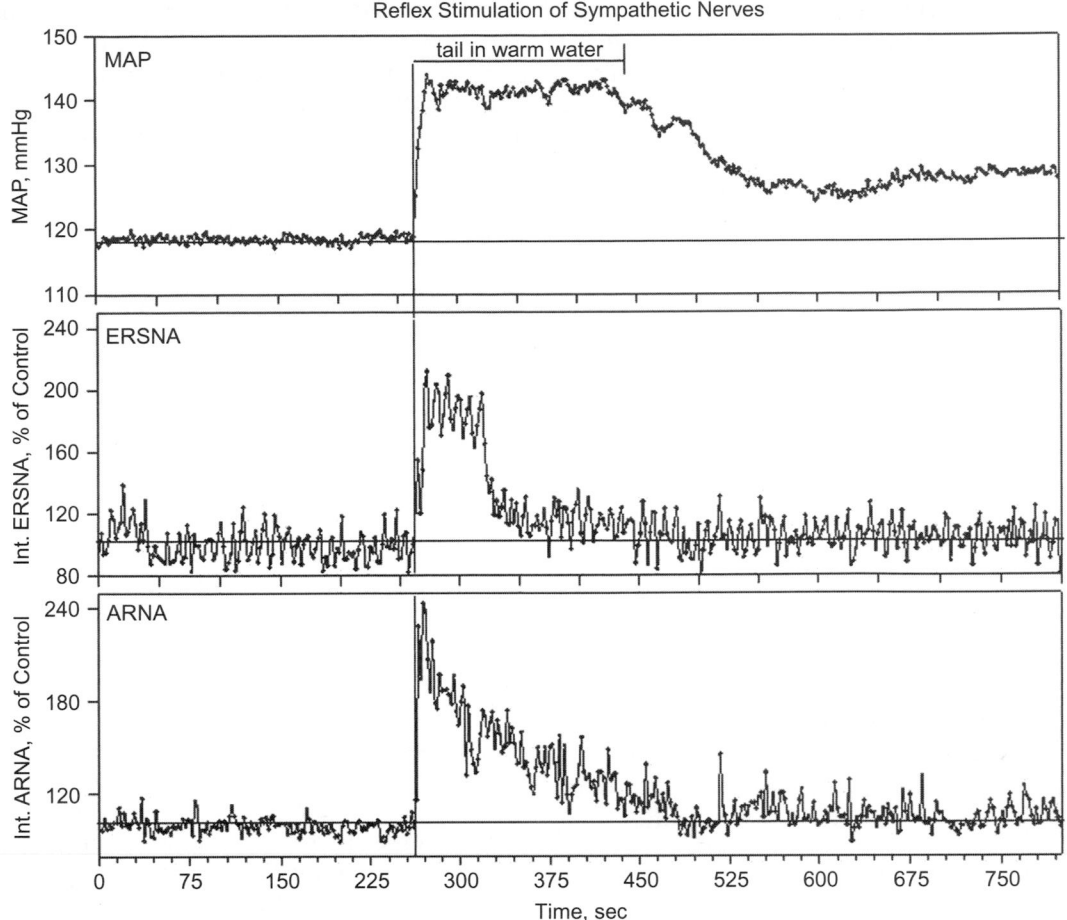

FIGURE 16.16 Thermal cutaneous stimulation by placing the rat's tail in 47°C water results in a general increase in sympathetic nerve activity, as indicated by the increases in mean arterial pressure (MAP) and efferent renal sympathetic nerve activity (ERSNA). The increases in ERSNA produced the increases in afferent renal nerve activity (ARNA), see text for further details. *(Modified from reference [157].)*

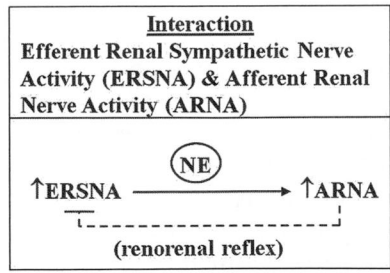

FIGURE 16.17 There is a reciprocal interaction between efferent renal sympathetic nerve activity (ERSNA) and afferent renal nerve activity (ARNA). Increases in ERSNA increase ARNA, the increase in ARNA would in turn decrease ERSNA via activation of the inhibitory renorenal reflexes in the overall goal of maintaining low ERSNA to minimize sodium retention. Norepinephrine (NE) is involved in the ERSNA-induced increase in ARNA.

Functional support for a role of substance P in the activation of renal pelvic sensory nerves is derived from *in vivo* studies showing that activation of renal mechanosensory nerves results in renal pelvic release of substance P.[155,161,162] Renal pelvic administration of substance P receptor antagonists abolishes the renorenal reflex responses to increased renal pelvic pressure.[167]

On the other hand, the role of CGRP in the activation of renal sensory nerves is unclear. Although CGRP is colocalized with substance P in the majority of the sensory nerves in the renal pelvic wall and released in response to stimuli that also release substance P,[154,156] blocking CGRP receptors does not reduce the responsiveness of the afferent renal nerves to various stimuli. Rather, available evidence would indicate that CGRP plays a role in delaying the catabolism of substance P, thereby prolonging the effects of neurally released substance P.[92,93]

There is considerable evidence for the transient receptor potential vanilloid type 1 (TRPV1) channels in the renal pelvic wall which, upon activation, elicits a similar inhibitory renorenal reflex response as activation of renal mechanosensory nerves. The TRPV1 channels are nonselective cation channels that can be activated by capsaicin, resiniferatoxin, noxious heat or a low pH. In the kidney, activation of the TRPV1 channels by capsaicin or a capsaicin analog activates renal mechanosensory nerves resulting in increases in substance P release, afferent renal nerve activity, and a contralateral natriuresis. The physiological importance of the TRPV1 channels is currently not known, although it has been proposed that they serve as an integral part of the mechanosensory nerve complex.[84,280]

PROSTAGLANDIN E₂ (PGE₂)

There is considerable evidence for prostaglandins (PGs) enhancing the responsiveness of various sensory nerve fibers.[208,219] The kidney, especially the renal medulla, is an active PG-producing tissue.[23] A role for PGs in renal sensory receptor activation by reduced renal perfusion pressure was demonstrated by the finding that PG synthesis inhibition reduced the afferent renal nerve activity and reflex pressor responses to reduction in renal blood flow.[11,80]

Stretching the renal pelvic wall leads to activation of protein kinase C (PKC) via activation of bradykinin 2 (B2) receptors (*vide infra*) and induction of cyclooxygenase-2 (COX-2) mRNA in the renal pelvic wall, with a resultant increase in renal pelvic release of PGE₂[146,147,154,162] (Figure 16.18). PGE receptors have been classified into four general subtypes, EP1, EP2,

EP3, and EP4, based on cloning and pharmacological interventions.[20] Immunohistochemical studies together with functional studies have provided evidence for a role of EP4 receptors in the activation of renal pelvic mechanosensory nerves.[147] It is well-established that PGE₂ activates the cAMP-protein kinase A (PKA) transduction cascade in DRG neurons, leading to depolarization of the cell membrane and a release of substance P and CGRP.[73,209,245] Using various activators and inhibitors of cAMP and PKA it was shown that PGE₂ increased the release of substance P and stimulated renal mechanosensory nerves by activating the cAMP/PKA transduction cascade in renal pelvic tissue.[154]

ANGIOTENSIN II

In normal rats, low-sodium diet reduces the responsiveness of renal mechanosensory nerves,[151] i.e., similar to the well-known reduced responsiveness of carotid baroreceptors in healthy low-sodium diet rats.[57,117] The reduced afferent renal nerve activity response to increased renal pelvic pressure in low-sodium diet rats was associated with impaired PGE₂-mediated release of substance P from the isolated renal pelvic wall preparation. These data suggested that the reduced responsiveness of the renal sensory nerves was, at least in part, due to a mechanism at the peripheral sensory nerve endings.

A low-sodium diet is characterized by increased activity of the renin–angiotensin system.[56–58] Angiotensin II present in the renal pelvic wall is modulated by dietary sodium.[149] Renal pelvic administration of angiotensin II reduces, and renal pelvic administration of the AT1 receptor antagonist losartan enhances, the PGE₂-mediated release of substance P and activation of renal mechanosensory nerves.[151] Because the effects of losartan on the PGE₂-mediated release of substance P were observed in response to acute administration of losartan to an isolated renal pelvic wall preparation, these data suggest that endogenous angiotensin II exerts its inhibitory effect on renal mechanosensory nerves by a mechanism at the peripheral renal sensory nerve endings. Further studies showed that endogenous angiotensin II in the renal pelvic tissue reduces the responsiveness of the renal sensory nerves by suppressing the PGE₂-mediated activation of cAMP by a pertussis toxin sensitive mechanism[149] (Figure 16.18).

ALPHA-ADRENOCEPTORS

The increases in afferent renal nerve activity produced by reflex increases in efferent renal sympathetic nerve activity are reduced by renal pelvic administration of prazosin, an α_1-adrenoceptor antagonist, and enhanced by rauwolscine, an α_2-adrenoceptor antagonist[157] in rats fed normal-sodium diet, demonstrating that changes in

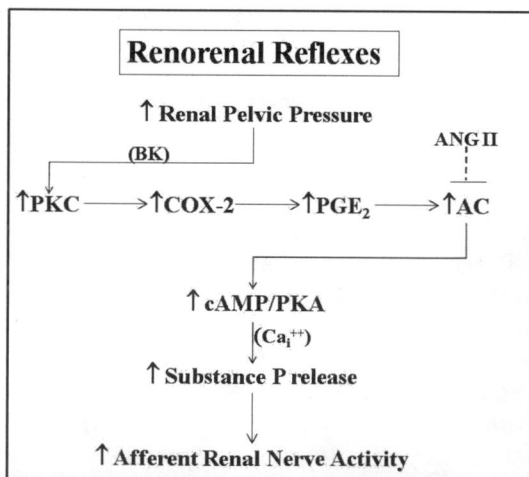

FIGURE 16.18 Mechanisms involved in the activation of renal mechanosensory nerves. Stretching the renal pelvic wall by increasing renal pelvic pressure activates bradykinin (BK) 2 receptors, leading to activation of protein kinase C (PKC) and induction of cyclooxygenase-2 (COX-2) with a resultant increase in renal pelvic release of PGE₂. PGE₂ activates EP4 receptors on/close to the renal sensory nerves which leads to activation of adenylyl cyclase (AC)/cAMP/protein kinase A (PKA) transduction pathway, resulting in a calcium-dependent release of substance P and increases in afferent renal nerve activity. In conditions of increased endogenous angiotensin (ANG) II activity, e.g., low-sodium diet, the responsiveness of the renal mechanosensory nerves is suppressed due to ANG II reducing the PGE₂-mediated activation of AC by a pertussis toxin sensitive mechanism. (*Data derived from references [146,147,151,154,162].*)

efferent renal sympathetic nerve activity modulate afferent renal nerve activity by the release of norepinephrine (Figure 16.17). The presence of α_1-adrenoceptors on the renal sensory nerves modulating their activation was demonstrated in an isolated renal pelvic wall preparation. These studies showed that norepinephrine resulted in a release of substance P that was blocked by prazosin and dependent on intact renal PG synthesis. Prazosin reduced the norepinephrine-induced release of PGE_2. Taken together these findings suggest that increases in efferent renal sympathetic nerve activity increases the release of norepinephrine which activates α_1-adrenoceptors on or close to the renal sensory nerves, resulting in increases in PGE_2 synthesis leading to release of substance P and increases in afferent renal nerve activity.

Similar to the responsiveness of the renal mechanosensory nerves being modulated by dietary sodium, the interaction between efferent renal sympathetic nerve activity and afferent renal nerve activity is also modulated by dietary sodium. Examining the mechanisms involved in the reduced responsiveness of the renal sensory nerves to increases in efferent renal sympathetic nerve activity in rats fed low-sodium diet it became clear that renal pelvic administration of losartan alone failed to enhance the efferent renal sympathetic nerve activity-induced increase in afferent renal nerve activity or the norepinephrine-induced increase in substance P. These findings suggested that the impaired responsiveness of the renal sensory nerves to increases in efferent renal sympathetic nerve activity may involve additional mechanisms upstream of PGE_2. Because activation of renal pelvic α_2-adrenoceptors reduces the activation of renal sensory nerves in rats fed normal-sodium diet,[157] one of the mechanisms contributing to the suppressed responsiveness of the renal sensory nerves in low-sodium diet rats likely involved increased activation of renal α_2-adrenoceptors. The involvement of α_2-adrenoceptors in the central nervous system in the cardiovascular regulation has long been known.[224,226] Of the three subtypes of α_2-adrenoceptors, the α^2_A- and α^2_C-adrenoceptors are expressed on primary afferent neurons in the spinal cord and DRG.[237,238] Whether α_{2B}-adrenoceptors are also expressed on DRG is not clear.[34,91,238] In the kidney, α_{2A}- and α_{2C}-adrenoceptors are localized on or close to sensory nerve fibers in the renal pelvic wall[158] (Figure 16.19). A role for increased activation of these receptors in the suppressed responsiveness of the renal sensory nerves to increases in efferent renal sympathetic nerve activity was subsequently shown by studies which showed that a combination of losartan plus rauwolscine enhanced the responsiveness of the renal sensory nerves to norepinephrine towards that seen in high-sodium diet rats.[158] Importantly, rauwolscine has no effect in rats fed a high-sodium diet.

Taken together in low-sodium dietary conditions, increased activation of α_2-adrenoceptors together with increased endogenous angiotensin II activity suppress the norepinephrine-mediated activation of the renal sensory nerves. The consequence is decreased PG synthesis and reduced PGE_2-mediated activation of the adenylyl cyclase/cAMP/PKA transduction pathway, leading to little or no increase in substance P release, and afferent renal nerve activity, and thereby no inhibition of efferent renal sympathetic nerve activity. In high-sodium dietary conditions, the enhanced norepinephrine-mediated activation of renal sensory nerves is due, at least in part, to little or no activation of renal α_2-adrenoceptors and very low endogenous angiotensin II opposing the norepinephrine-mediated increase in afferent renal nerve activity which will eventually lead to renorenal reflex decreases in efferent renal sympathetic nerve activity (Figure 16.20).

BRADYKININ

Among the various mechanisms involved in the release of substance P and activation of renal mechanosensory nerves is bradykinin (*vide supra*). Bradykinin is a well-known activator of sensory nerve fibers.[89] Bradykinin receptors have been localized on sensory nerve fibers[250] and in the lamina propria of the tissue lining the pelvis.[193] Bradykinin increases afferent renal nerve activity when administered into the renal pelvis in association with an increased renal pelvic release of PGE_2 and substance P, and a contralateral natriuresis. B2 receptor antagonists block the renorenal reflex responses to either bradykinin *per se* or increases in renal pelvic pressure.[161,162] Interestingly, the responses to bradykinin are dependent on the route of administration. In contrast to the inhibitory reflex response elicited by renal pelvic administration of bradykinin,[161,162] administration of bradykinin into the renal artery (i.r.a.) elicits an excitatory reflex which includes activation of neurosecretory vasopressin cells in the supraoptic nucleus,[47] increases in plasma ADH concentration, and increased arterial pressure and vascular resistance in most circulatory beds.[246] The sympatho-excitatory effects of i.r.a. bradykinin were due to activation of afferent renal nerves since they were abolished by denervation of the infused kidney. This reflex has been suggested to be of importance during renal ischemia, which is likely to be associated with increased release of bradykinin.

These findings suggest that bradykinin activates different reflex pathways, one excitatory and one inhibitory, when administered into the renal artery and pelvis, respectively. The physiological or pathophysiological significance of these different reflexes is currently not known.

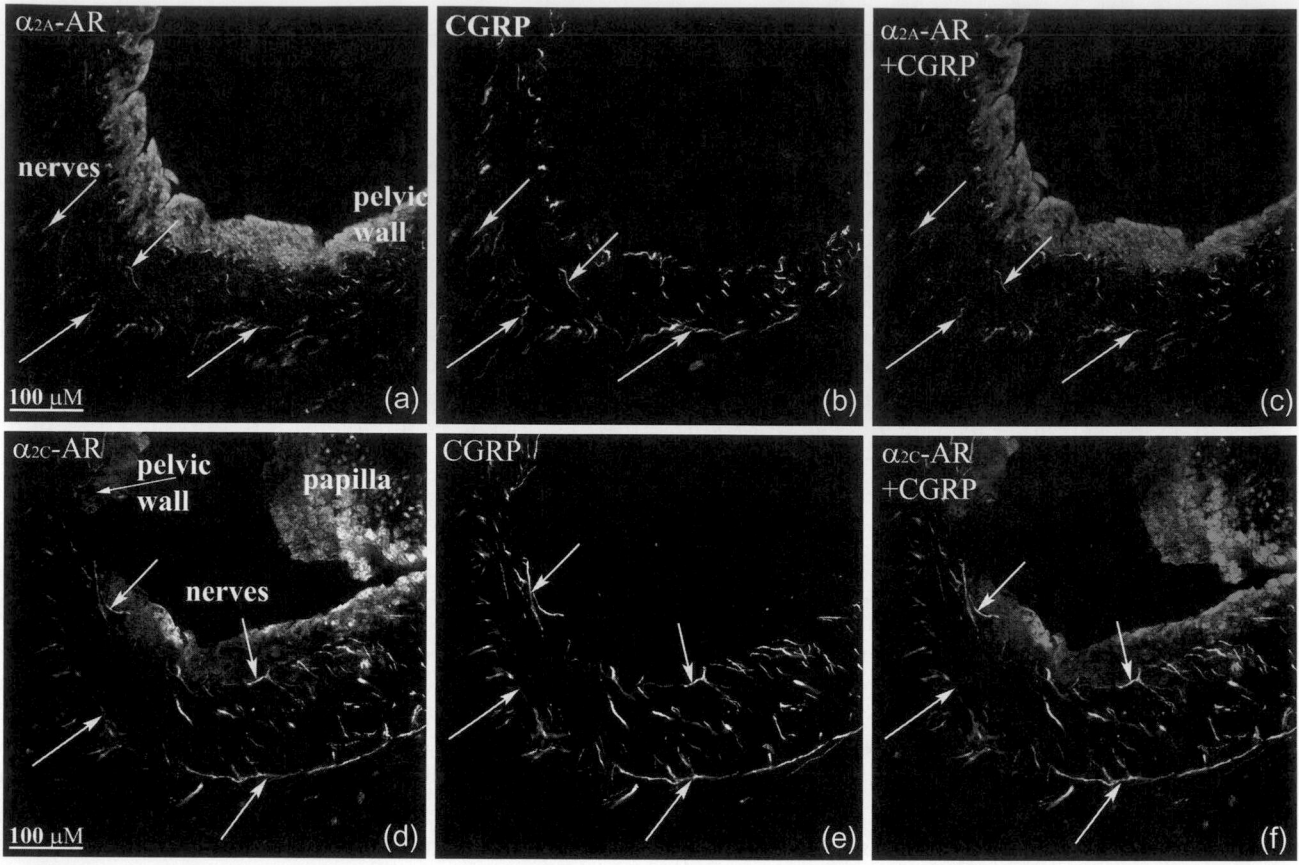

FIGURE 16.19   Applying antibodies against α_{2A}-adrenoceptors (AR) (a) and α_{2C}-(AR) (d) labels nerve fibers (arrows) in the renal pelvic wall that are also labeled with an antibody against CGRP, a marker for sensory nerve fibers (b,e) as shown by the color yellow in (c) and (f). *(Reference [158].)* See color section at the back of the book.

ENDOTHELIN

Endothelin is abundantly expressed throughout the body, including the brain and the kidney.[106] Endothelin exerts its effects by activating two G-protein coupled receptors, endothelin-A (ETA) and endothelin-B (ETB) receptors.[230] Both ETA and ETB receptors are localized in the renal pelvic wall, the ETA receptors on smooth muscle cells and the ETB receptors on or close to the afferent renal sensory nerves,[163] suggesting a role for endothelin in modulating the activation of afferent renal sensory nerves. Studies examining the role of endothelin in the activation of afferent renal sensory nerves by increased renal pelvic pressure or reflex increases in efferent renal sympathetic nerve activity suggested an important role for endothelin in modulating the responsiveness of the renal sensory nerves. The nature of the endothelin-induced activation of the afferent renal sensory nerves is dependent on dietary sodium intake.[163] In low-sodium dietary conditions, activation of ETA-receptors contributes to the suppressed responsiveness of the renal sensory nerves, whereas in high-sodium dietary conditions activation of ETB-receptors plays a major

role in the enhanced responsiveness of the renal sensory nerves. These findings are of interest in view of the well-documented hypertension in ETB-receptor deficient rats and mice fed high-sodium diets.[87,227] Together, these studies may suggest that impairment of the inhibitory renorenal reflexes contributes to the salt-sensitive hypertension in conditions of renal ETB-receptor deficiency. Further support for this hypothesis is derived from studies in rats treated neonatally with capsaicin to destroy all sensory nerves.[274] These rats develop salt-sensitive hypertension which is reduced by ETA receptor antagonists in a similar fashion to that seen in ETB receptor deficient rats.[87,227]

The similar effects of an ETA-receptor antagonist and an AT1-receptor antagonist in low-sodium diet rats to restore the suppressed activation of renal sensory nerves towards that seen in rats fed normal-sodium diet[151,163] suggested an interaction between angiotensin II and endothelin. Comparing the effects of inhibitors of ETA-receptors and AT-1 receptors on the responses to activation of the renal mechanosensory nerves showed that ETA receptors play an important contributory role to the angiotensin II-induced

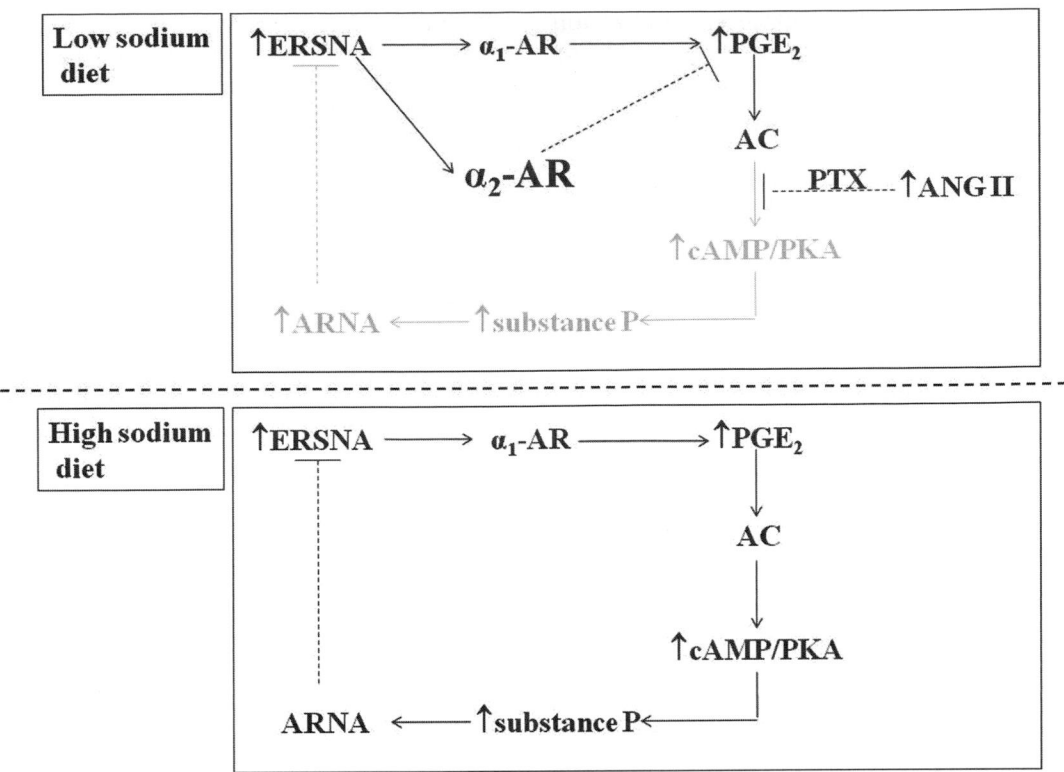

FIGURE 16.20 In low-sodium dietary conditions, increased activation of α_2-adrenoceptor (AR) together with increased endogenous angiotensin (ANG) II activity suppresses the norepinephrine-mediated activation of the renal sensory nerves by decreasing PG synthesis, leading to reduced PGE_2-mediated activation of adenylyl/cAMP/PKA transduction pathway resulting in little or no increase in substance P release and increase in afferent renal nerve activity, and thereby no inhibition of efferent renal sympathetic nerve activity (ERSNA). In high-sodium dietary conditions, the enhanced norepinephrine-mediated activation of renal sensory nerves is due, at least in part, to little or no activation of renal α_2-AR and very low endogenous ANG II activity opposing the norepinephrine-mediated increase in PGE_2 synthesis, substance P release, and increase in afferent renal nerve activity, leading to renorenal reflex decreases in ERSNA. Modulation of the interaction between efferent and afferent renal nerve activity is an appropriate physiological response to changes in dietary sodium intake in the overall goal of maintaining water and sodium balance.

suppression of the responsiveness of the afferent renal mechanosensory nerves[148] in low-sodium diet rats. These findings are supported by the considerable evidence showing that angiotensin II increases the expression of preproendothelin-1 mRNA in various tissues, including the kidney and urinary bladder,[123] increases endothelin-1 protein expression and secretion in vascular smooth muscle cells, cardiomyocytes and mesangial cells,[125,140,271] and increases ETA expression in cardiomyocytes.[125]

Activation of Renal Mechanosensory Nerves: Pathophysiological Conditions

Impairment of the Inhibitory Renorenal Reflexes in Various Diseases

Activation of the renal mechanosensory nerves is impaired in various pathological conditions of increased efferent renal sympathetic nerve activity and sodium retention, including congestive heart failure, spontaneous

hypertension, diabetes type I, ischemia-induced acute renal failure, obstructive nephropathy, cirrhosis, and chronic hypoxia.[32,33,145,152,153,159,168,185–187] Impairment of the inhibitory renorenal reflexes in pathological conditions would aggravate and/or contribute to further increases in efferent renal sympathetic nerve activity and sodium retention. Many of these pathological conditions are characterized by increased angiotensin II activity. Importantly, renal pelvic administration of an AT-1 receptor antagonist has been shown to markedly improve the responsiveness of the renal mechanosensory nerves in rats with congestive heart failure, hypertension, and diabetes type I.[145,153,159] The marked enhancement of the renorenal reflex mechanism produced by AT1 receptor antagonists may contribute to the well-known beneficial effects of inhibiting the renin—angiotensin system in heart failure and hypertension.

In addition to the impaired responsiveness of the renal mechanosensory nerves in spontaneous hypertensive rats, the interaction between efferent renal sympathetic nerve activity and afferent renal nerve activity is also impaired. The impaired interaction between efferent renal sympathetic nerve activity and afferent renal nerve activity is related to increased activation of renal pelvic α_2-adrenoceptors, in addition to increased activation of AT-1 receptors,[152] i.e., similar mechanisms as those contributing to the suppressed responsiveness of the renal sensory nerves in low-sodium diet rats.

Excitatory Reflexes Originating in Injured/Diseased Kidneys

The depressor effects of (T_9-L_1)DRX observed in rats with one-kidney, one-clip hypertension,[137] 5/6 nephrectomy,[28] and in rats exposed to i.v. infusion of cyclosporine[184] would appear to contradict the notion of the afferent renal nerves exerting a tonic inhibitory effect on efferent renal sympathetic nerve activity. However, it is likely that different mechanisms are involved in the activation of renal sensory nerves in normal and diseased kidneys. Whereas in normal kidneys activation of renal sensory nerves elicits inhibitory renorenal reflexes (*vide supra*), in diseased kidneys when the inhibitory renorenal reflexes are impaired, activation of renal sensory nerves may result in excitatory reflexes. Studies in 2-kidney 1-clip rats would support this notion. The responsiveness of the renal mechanosensory nerves in the clipped ischemic kidney is impaired.[144] Interestingly, renal denervation of the clipped kidney increased urinary sodium excretion from both the clipped and the contralateral non-clipped kidney, which is in contrast to the findings in normal healthy rats in which unilateral renal denervation decreases contralateral urinary sodium excretion.[39,60] In 2-kidney 1-clip rats, the contralateral natriuretic response was associated with decreases in contralateral efferent renal sympathetic nerve activity, suggesting that the balance between inhibitory and excitatory reflexes originating in the kidney was shifted from mainly being of an inhibitory nature to being of an excitatory nature in ischemic kidneys.[144] Thus, these data suggest that the afferent renal nerves in the ischemic kidney exert an excitatory influence on the sympathetic nervous system, in contrast to the inhibitory reflexes originating from normal healthy kidneys.[39,60] Further support for excitatory reflexes originating in an ischemic kidney derives from long-term blood pressure recordings in conscious rats following the onset of hypertension in 2-kidney 1-clip hypertension rats. Whereas renal denervation of the clipped kidney (six weeks after renal artery clipping) reduced arterial pressure almost to the same level as removing the clip from the renal artery, denervation of the contralateral non-clipped kidney had no effect on arterial pressure.[136] Further studies suggested an important role for adenosine in the excitatory reflexes originating in the ischemic kidneys. Intrarenal administration of adenosine deaminase reduced arterial pressure in 1-kidney 1-clip hypertensive rats, but had no effect in healthy normal rats.[134] Also, administration of adenosine into one renal artery resulted in increases in contralateral efferent renal sympathetic nerve activity and arterial pressure which were abolished by renal denervation of the infused kidney in healthy dogs.[135] Taken together, these studies suggest that excitatory reflexes originating in ischemic kidneys involve adenosine activating chemosensitive afferent renal nerves.

Further evidence for excitatory reflexes originating in diseased/injured kidneys is derived from studies in humans and rats with renal failure. Comparing arterial blood pressure and muscle sympathetic nerve activity in hemodialysis patients with and without their native diseased kidneys intact showed markedly reduced arterial pressure and muscle sympathetic nerve activity in patients with bilateral nephrectomy compared with patients who had their kidneys intact.[40] These findings were subsequently confirmed and extended in studies comparing arterial pressure and muscle sympathetic nerve activity in patients with kidney transplants, with and without their native kidneys intact.[104] None of the patients were uremic, thus they all had well-functioning renal grafts. However, muscle sympathetic nerve activity was increased in all patients versus healthy controls, except in the patients in which bilateral nephrectomy had been performed. In a subgroup of transplant patients, muscle sympathetic nerve activity was measured before and after the second kidney was removed, and was found to be reduced following removal of the second diseased kidney. Thus, these studies provide strong evidence for the diseased kidneys exerting an excitatory effect on sympathetic nerve activity. Studies in rats with chronic renal failure would support the notion that excitatory effects exerted by the diseased kidneys are related to activation of the afferent renal nerves in the diseased/injured kidney.[28] These rat studies showed that chronic renal failure increased arterial pressure and norepinephrine turnover in posterior hypothalamus and locus coeruleus. Importantly, prior dorsal rhizotomy to remove the afferent renal innervation prevented the increases in arterial pressure and norepinephrine turnover in the various brain regions.

Thus, local renal injury may result in sympathoexcitatory reflexes involving afferent renal nerves, central cardiovascular regulatory areas, and efferent systemic and renal sympathetic nerve activity, eventually leading to hypertension.

The notion of excitatory reflexes originating in diseased/injured kidney may provide an explanation to the marked prolonged decrease in arterial pressure in drug-resistant hypertensive patients following the one-time renal denervation procedure.[53,77,173] The reduction in arterial pressure following renal denervation is associated with reduction in whole body norepinephrine spillover and reduction in muscle sympathetic nerve activity, indicative of removal of excitatory reflexes originating in the kidneys.

SUMMARY

The efferent renal sympathetic and afferent renal nerves constitute a significant control system for the physiological regulation of renal function. Efferent renal sympathetic nerve activity is governed by a centrally-based reflex control system which responds to diverse peripheral and central afferent inputs. The kidney is densely innervated by sympathetic nerves, including the renal vasculature, the nephron, the juxtaglomerular cells, and the renal pelvic wall, enabling the renal nerves to contribute to one of the major tasks of the kidney, the homeostatic regulation of body fluid volume.

Activation of the afferent renal nerves located in the renal pelvic wall leads to decreases in efferent renal sympathetic nerve activity and increases in urinary sodium excretion, a renorenal reflex response. Changes in efferent renal sympathetic nerve activity modulate the responsiveness of the renal sensory nerves. Increases in efferent renal sympathetic nerve activity increase afferent renal nerve activity. The increased afferent renal nerve activity will, in turn, decrease efferent renal sympathetic nerve activity via activation of the renorenal reflexes, a negative feedback mechanism, to maintain low-level efferent renal sympathetic nerve activity. Thus, there is an interaction between efferent renal sympathetic nerve activity and afferent renal nerve activity in the renal neural control of body fluid and sodium homeostasis wherein activation of the afferent renal nerves buffers the antinatriuretic effects of increases in efferent renal sympathetic nerve activity. This is most clearly evident in conditions of high-sodium dietary intake, when the afferent renal nerves are tonically active to suppress efferent renal sympathetic nerve activity to minimize sodium retention. Conversely, in low-sodium dietary conditions when increased efferent renal sympathetic nerve activity is essential for maintaining sodium balance, the activity of the afferent renal nerves are suppressed.

In pathophysiological sodium-retaining states, efferent renal sympathetic nerve activity is inappropriately increased in the presence of sodium retention. It has long been known that impairment of the aortic and arterial baroreflexes contributes to the inappropriately increased efferent renal sympathetic nerve activity in these pathological conditions. What has previously been overlooked is an impairment of reflexes originating in the kidneys, *per se*. However, there is now convincing evidence that impairment of the inhibitory renorenal reflexes contributes to the increased efferent renal sympathetic nerve activity and sodium retention prevalent in hypertension and various disease models of sodium retention. In conditions of renal injury/disease, available data would suggest that there is a shift from inhibitory to excitatory renorenal reflexes which would contribute to the increased efferent renal sympathetic nerve activity, leading to increased sodium retention and arterial pressure prevalent in these pathophysiological conditions.

Acknowledgments

The work performed in the authors' laboratories was supported by the National Institutes of Health, Heart, Lung and Blood Institute, RO1 HL66068, and by research grants from the Department of Veterans Affairs and the American Heart Association (Kopp), The British Heart Foundation (Johns), Wellcome Trust (Johns), Health Research Board (Johns), and Science Foundation Ireland (Johns).

References

[1] Abdulla MH, Sattar MA, Abdul Hye Khan M, Abdullah NA, Johns EJ. Influence of sympathetic and AT(1)-receptor blockade on angiotensin II and adrenergic agonists-induced renal vasoconstrictions in spontaneously hypertensive rats. Acta Physiol 2008;195:397−404.

[2] Abdulla MH, Sattar MA, Khan MA, Abdullah NA, Johns EJ. Influence of sympathetic and AT-receptor blockade on angiotensin II and adrenergic agonist-induced renal vasoconstrictions in spontaneously hypertensive rats. Acta Physiol (Oxf) 2009;195:397−404.

[3] Allen AM, Moeller I, Jenkins TA, Zhuo J, Aldred GP, Chai SY, et al. Angiotensin receptors in the nervous system. Brain Res Bull 1998;47:17−28.

[4] Aperia A, Ibarra F, Svensson LB, Klee C, Greengard P. Calcineurin mediates alpha-adrenergic stimulation of Na^+, K^+-ATPase activity in renal tubule cells. Proc Natl Acad Sci USA 1992;89:7394−7.

[5] Aukland K. Hydrogen polarography in measurement of local blood flow; theoretical and empirical basis. Acta Neurol Scand Suppl 1965;14:42−5.

[6] Aukland K, Bower BF. Berliner RW. Measurement of local blood flow with hydrogen gas. Circ Res 1964;14:164−87.

[7] Bachmann S, Bosse HM, Mundel P. Topography of nitric oxide synthesis by localizing constitutive NO synthases in mammalian kidney. Am J Physiol 1995;268:F885−898.

[8] Bankir L, Bichet DG, Bouby N. Vasopressin V2 receptors, ENaC, and sodium reabsorption: a risk factor for hypertension? Am J Physiol 2010;299:F917−928.

[9] Barajas L, Liu L, Powers K. Anatomy of the renal innervation: intrarenal aspects and ganglia of origin. Can J Physiol Pharmacol 1992;70:735−49.

[10] Barajas L, Powers K, Wang P. Innervation of the renal cortical tubules: a quantitative study. Am J Physiol 1984;247:F50−60.

[11] Barber JD, Moss NG. Reduced renal perfusion pressure causes prostaglandin-dependent excitation of R2 chemoreceptors in rats. Am J Physiol 1990;259:R1243−9.

[12] Barrett CJ, Navakatikyan MA, Malpas SC. Long-term control of renal blood flow: what is the role of the renal nerves? Am J Physiol 2001;280:R1534−1545.

[13] Beierwaltes WH. The role of calcium in the regulation of renin secretion. Am J Physiol 2010;298:F1−11.

[14] Bello-Reuss E, Colindres RE, Pastoriza-Munoz E, Mueller RA, Gottschalk CW. Effects of acute unilateral renal denervation in the rat. J Clin Invest 1975;56:208–17.

[15] Bello-Reuss E, Pastoriza-Munoz E, Colindres RE. Acute unilateral renal denervation in rats with extracellular volume expansion. Am J Physiol 1977;232:F26–32.

[16] Bello-Reuss E, Trevino DL, Gottschalk CW. Effect of renal sympathetic nerve stimulation on proximal water and sodium reabsorption. J Clin Invest 1976;57:1104–7.

[17] Bernard C. Lecons sur les Proprietes Physiologique et les Alterations Pathoogique des Liquides de l'Organisme. Paris: Bailleère et Fils 1859;2:170–1.

[18] Bohmann C, Schollmeyer P, Rump LC. Alpha 2-autoreceptor subclassification in rat isolated kidney by use of short trains of electrical stimulation. Br J Pharmacol 1993;108:262–8.

[19] Bohmann C, Schollmeyer P, Rump LC. Effects of imidazolines on noradrenaline release in rat isolated kidney. Naunyn Schmiedebergs Arch Pharmacol 1994;349:118–24.

[20] Boie Y, Stocco R, Sawyer N, Slipetz DM, Ungrin MD, Neuschafer-Rube F, et al. Molecular cloning and characterization of the four rat prostaglandin E2 prostanoid receptor subtypes. Eur J Pharmacol 1997;340:227–41.

[21] Boke T, Malik KU. Enhancement by locally generated angiotensin II of release of the adrenergic transmitter in the isolated rat kidney. J Pharmacol Exp Ther 1983;226:900–7.

[22] Bonjour JP, Churchill PC, Malvin RL. Change of tubular reabsorption of sodium and water after renal denervation in the dog. J Physiol 1969;204:571–82.

[23] Bonvalet JP, Pradelles P, Farman N. Segmental synthesis and actions of prostaglandins along the nephron. Am J Physiol 1987;253:F377–87.

[24] Bosse HM, Bohm R, Resch S, Bachmann S. Parallel regulation of constitutive NO synthase and renin at JGA of rat kidney under various stimuli. Am J Physiol 1995;269:F793–805.

[25] Brod J. [Regulation of renal function.]. Chekh Fiziol 1952;1:274–300.

[26] Calaresu FR, Ciriello J. Renal afferent nerves affect discharge rate of medullary and hypothalamic single units in the cat. J Auton Nerv Syst 1981;3:311–20.

[27] Camara AK, Osborn JL. AT1 receptors mediate chronic central nervous system AII hypertension in rats fed high sodium chloride diet from weaning. J Auton Nerv Syst 1998;72:16–23.

[28] Campese VM, Kogosov E. Renal afferent denervation prevents hypertension in rats with chronic renal failure. Hypertension 1995;25:878–82.

[29] Caverson MM, Ciriello J. Effect of stimulation of afferent renal nerves on plasma levels of vasopressin. Am J Physiol 1987;252:R801–7.

[30] Chen L, Kim SM, Oppermann M, Faulhaber-Walter R, Huang Y, Mizel D, et al. Regulation of renin in mice with Cre recombinase-mediated deletion of G protein Gsalpha in juxtaglomerular cells. Am J Physiol 2007;292:F27–37.

[31] Chen HI, Chapleau MW, McDowell TS, Abboud FM. Prostaglandins contribute to activation of baroreceptors in rabbits. Possible paracrine influence of endothelium. Circ Res 1990;67:1394–404.

[32] Chien CT, Chien HF, Cheng YJ, Chen CF, Hsu SM. Renal afferent signaling diuretic response is impaired in streptozotocin-induced diabetic rats. Kidney Int 2000;57:203–14.

[33] Chien CT, Fu TC, Wu MS, Chen CF. Attenuated response of renal mechanoreceptors to volume expansion in chronically hypoxic rats. Am J Physiol 1997;273:F712–7.

[34] Cho HJ, Kim DS, Lee NH, Kim JK, Lee KM, Han KS, et al. Changes in the alpha 2-adrenergic receptor subtypes gene expression in rat dorsal root ganglion in an experimental model of neuropathic pain. Neuroreport 1997;8:3119–22.

[35] Ciriello J. Afferent renal inputs to paraventricular nucleus vasopressin and oxytocin neurosecretory neurons. Am J Physiol 1998;275:R1745–54.

[36] Ciriello J, Calaresu FR. Central projections of afferent renal fibers in the rat an antegrade transport study of horseradish peroxidase. J Auton Nerv Syst 1983;8:273–85.

[37] Clausen G, Tyssebotn I, Kirkebo A, Ofjord ES, Aukland K. Distribution of blood flow in the dog kidney. III. Local uptake of 10 mum and 15 mum microspheres during renal vasodilation and constriction. Acta Physiol Scand 1981;113:471–9.

[38] Cohnhein J, Roy S. Untersuchungen uber die Zirkulation in den Nieren. Virchows Arch Path Anat Physiol 1883;93:424–57.

[39] Colindres RE, Spielman WS, Moss NG, Harrington WW, Gottschalk CW. Functional evidence for renorenal reflexes in the rat. Am J Physiol 1980;239:F265–70.

[40] Converse Jr RL, Jacobsen TN, Toto RD, Jost CM, Cosentino F, Fouad-Tarazi F, et al. Sympathetic overactivity in patients with chronic renal failure. N Engl J Med 1992;327:1912–8.

[41] Cupples WA, Marsh DJ. Autoregulation of blood flow in renal medulla of the rat: no role for angiotensin II. Can J Physiol Pharmacol 1988;66:833–6.

[42] Dampney RA. Functional organization of central pathways regulating the cardiovascular system. Physiol Rev 1994;74:323–64.

[43] Dampney RA, Fontes MA, Hirooka Y, Horiuchi J, Potts PD, Tagawa T. Role of angiotensin II receptors in the regulation of vasomotor neurons in the ventrolateral medulla. Clin Exp Pharmacol Physiol 2002;29:467–72.

[44] Dampney RA, Horiuchi J, Tagawa T, Fontes MA, Potts PD, Polson JW. Medullary and supramedullary mechanisms regulating sympathetic vasomotor tone. Acta Physiol Scand 2003;177:209–18.

[45] Davis G, Johns EJ. Effect of somatic nerve stimulation on the kidney in intact, vagotomized and carotid sinus-denervated rats. J Physiol 1991;432:573–84.

[46] Davis G, Johns EJ. Somatosensory regulation of renal function in the stroke-prone spontaneously hypertensive rat. J Physiol 1994;481(Pt 3):753–9.

[47] Day TA, Ciriello J. Effects of renal receptor activation on neurosecretory vasopressin cells. Am J Physiol 1987;253:R234–41.

[48] Denton KM, Fennessy PA, Alcorn D, Anderson WP. Morphometric analysis of the actions of angiotensin II on renal arterioles and glomeruli. Am J Physiol 1992;262:F367–372.

[49] Denton KM, Luff SE, Shweta A, Anderson WP. Differential neural control of glomerular ultrafiltration. Clin Exp Pharmacol Physiol 2004;31:380–6.

[50] Denton KM, Shweta A, Flower RL, Anderson WP. Predominant postglomerular vascular resistance response to reflex renal sympathetic nerve activation during ANG II clamp in rabbits. Am J Physiol 2004;287:R780–786.

[51] DiBona GF. Nervous kidney. Interaction between renal sympathetic nerves and the renin–angiotensin system in the control of renal function. Hypertension 2000;36:1083–8.

[52] DiBona GF. Peripheral and central interactions between the renin–angiotensin system and the renal sympathetic nerves in control of renal function. Ann N Y Acad Sci 2001;940:395–406.

[53] DiBona GF, Esler M. Translational medicine: the antihypertensive effect of renal denervation. Am J Physiol 2010;298:R245–253.

[54] DiBona GF, Johns EJ. A study of the role of renal nerves in the renal responses to 60 degree head-up tilt in the anaesthetized dog. J Physiol 1980;299:117–26.

[55] DiBona GF, Jones SY. Effect of dietary sodium intake on the responses to bicuculline in the paraventricular nucleus of rats. Hypertension 2001;38:192–7.

[56] DiBona GF, Jones SY. Sodium intake influences hemodynamic and neural responses to angiotensin receptor blockade in rostral ventrolateral medulla. Hypertension 2001;37:1114—23.

[57] DiBona GF, Jones SY, Sawin LL. Effect of endogenous angiotensin II on renal nerve activity and its arterial baroreflex regulation. Am J Physiol 1996;271:R361—367.

[58] DiBona GF, Kopp UC. Neural control of renal function. Physiol Rev 1997;77:75—197.

[59] Dibona GF, Sawin LL. Effect of endogenous angiotensin II on the frequency response of the renal vasculature. Am J Physiol 2004;287:F1171—1178.

[60] DiBona GF, Rios LL. Renal nerves in compensatory renal response to contralateral renal denervation. Am J Physiol 1980;238:F26—30.

[61] DiBona GF, Sawin LL. Effect of renal denervation on dynamic autoregulation of renal blood flow. Am J Physiol 2004;286:F1209—1218.

[62] DiBona GF, Sawin LL. Effect of renal nerve stimulation on NaCl and H$_2$O transport in Henle's loop of the rat. Am J Physiol 1982;243:F576—580.

[63] DiBona GF, Sawin LL. Effect of renal nerve stimulation on responsiveness of the rat renal vasculature. Am J Physiol 2002;283:F1056—1065.

[64] DiBona GF, Sawin LL. Exaggerated natriuresis in experimental hypertension. Proc Soc Exp Biol Med 1986;182:43—51.

[65] DiBona GF, Sawin LL. Frequency response of the renal vasculature in congestive heart failure. Circulation 2003;107:2159—64.

[66] Dibona GF, Sawin LL. Functional significance of the pattern of renal sympathetic nerve activation. Am J Physiol 1999;277:R346—353.

[67] DiBona GF, Sawin LL. Renal hemodynamic effects of activation of specific renal sympathetic nerve fiber groups. Am J Physiol 1999;276:R539—549.

[68] DiBona GF, Sawin LL. Renal nerve activity in conscious rats during volume expansion and depletion. Am J Physiol 1985;248:F15—23.

[69] DiBona GF, Zambraski EJ, Aguilera AJ, Kaloyanides GJ. Neurogenic control of renal tubular sodium reabsorption in the dog: a brief review and preliminary report concerning possible humoral mediation. Circ Res 1977;40:I127—130.

[70] Donovan MK, Wyss JM, Winternitz SR. Localization of renal sensory neurons using the fluorescent dye technique. Brain Res 1983;259:119—22.

[71] Egi Y, Matsumura Y, Murata S, Umekawa T, Hisaki K, Takaoka M, et al. The effects of NG-nitro-L-arginine, a nitric oxide synthase inhibitor, on norepinephrine overflow and antidiuresis induced by stimulation of renal nerves in anesthetized dogs. J Pharmacol Exp Ther 1994;269:529—35.

[72] Eitle E, Hiranyachattada S, Wang H, Harris PJ. Inhibition of proximal tubular fluid absorption by nitric oxide and atrial natriuretic peptide in rat kidney. Am J Physiol 1998;274:C1075—1080.

[73] England S, Bevan S, Docherty RJ. PGE2 modulates the tetrodotoxin-resistant sodium current in neonatal rat dorsal root ganglion neurones via the cyclic AMP-protein kinase A cascade. J Physiol 1996;495(Pt 2):429—40.

[74] Eppel GA, Malpas SC, Denton KM, Evans RG. Neural control of renal medullary perfusion. Clin Exp Pharmacol Physiol 2004;31:387—96.

[75] Esler M. The sympathetic system and hypertension. Am J Hypertens 2000;13:99S—105S.

[76] Esler M, Rumantir M, Kaye D, Jennings G, Hastings J, Socratous F, et al. Sympathetic nerve biology in essential hypertension. Clin Exp Pharmacol Physiol 2001;28:986—9.

[77] Esler MD, Krum H, Sobotka PA, Schlaich MP, Schmieder RE, Bohm M. Renal sympathetic denervation in patients with treatment-resistant hypertension (The Symplicity HTN-2 Trial): a randomised controlled trial. Lancet 2010;376:1903—9.

[78] Evans RG, Eppel GA, Anderson WP, Denton KM. Mechanisms underlying the differential control of blood flow in the renal medulla and cortex. J Hypertension 2004;22:1439—51.

[79] Evans RG, Head GA, Eppel GA, Burke SL, Rajapakse NW. Angiotensin II and neurohumoral control of the renal medullary circulation. Clin Exp Pharmacol Physiol 2010;37:e58—69.

[80] Faber JE. Role of prostaglandins and kinins in the renal pressor reflex. Hypertension 1987;10:522—32.

[81] Fazan VP, Ma X, Chapleau MW, Barreira AA. Qualitative and quantitative morphology of renal nerves in C57BL/6J mice. Anat Rec 2002;268:399—404.

[82] Felder RB. Excitatory and inhibitory interactions among renal and cardiovascular afferent nerves in dorsomedial medulla. Am J Physiol 1986;250:R580—8.

[83] Feng F, Pettinger WA, Abel PW, Jeffries WB. Regional distribution of alpha 1-adrenoceptor subtypes in rat kidney. J Pharmacol Exp Ther 1991;258:263—8.

[84] Feng N-H, Lee H-H, Shiang J-C, Ma M-C. Transient receptor potential vanilloid type 1 channels act as mechanoreceptors and cause substance P release and sensory activation in rat kidneys. Am J Physiol 2008;294:F316—25.

[85] Friis UG, Jensen BL, Sethi S, Andreasen D, Hansen PB, Skott O. Control of renin secretion from rat juxtaglomerular cells by cAMP-specific phosphodiesterases. Circ Res 2002;90:996—1003.

[86] Friis UG, Jorgensen F, Andreasen D, Jensen BL, Skott O. Membrane potential and cation channels in rat juxtaglomerular cells. Acta Physiol Scand 2004;181:391—6.

[87] Gariepy CE, Ohuchi T, Williams C, Richardson JA, Yanagisawa M. Salt-sensitive hypertension in endothelin-B receptor-deficient rats. J Clin Invest 2000;105:925—33.

[88] Genovesi S, Pieruzzi F, Wijnmaalen P, Centonza L, Golin R, Zanchetti A, et al. Renal afferents signaling diuretic activity in the cat. Circ Res 1993;73:906—13.

[89] Geppetti P. Sensory neuropeptide release by bradykinin: mechanisms and pathophysiological implications. Regul Pept 1993;47:1—23.

[90] Gilmore JP, Echtenkamp S, Wesley CR, Zucker IH. Atrial receptor modulation of renal nerve activity in the nonhuman primate. Am J Physiol 1982;242:F592—598.

[91] Gold MS, Dastmalchi S, Levine JD. Alpha 2 adrenergic receptor subtypes in rat dorsal root and superior cervical ganglion neurons. Pain 1997;69:179—90.

[92] Gontijo RJ, Kopp UC. Renal sensory receptor activation by calcitonin gene-related peptide. Hypertension 1994;23(Part 2):1063—7.

[93] Gontijo JR, Smith LA, Kopp UC. CGRP activates renal pelvic substance P receptors by retarding substance P metabolism. Hypertension 1999;33:493—8.

[94] Gross R, Ruffmann K, Kirchheim H. The separate and combined influences of common carotid occlusion and nonhypotensive hemorrhage on kidney blood flow. Pflügers Arch 1979;379:81—8.

[95] Guild SJ, Austin PC, Navakatikyan M, Ringwood JV, Malpas SC. Dynamic relationship between sympathetic nerve activity and renal blood flow: a frequency domain approach. Am J Physiol 2001;281:R206—212.

[96] Guild SJ, Barrett CJ, Evans RG, Malpas SC. Interactions between neural and hormonal mediators of renal vascular tone in anaesthetized rabbits. Exp Physiol 2003;88:229—41.

[97] Guild SJ, Eppel GA, Malpas SC, Rajapakse NW, Stewart A, Evans RG. Regional responsiveness of renal perfusion to activation of the renal nerves. Am J Physiol 2002;283:R1177—1186.

1. EPITHELIAL AND NONEPITHELIAL TRANSPORT AND REGULATION

[98] Hackenthal E, Paul M, Ganten D, Taugner R. Morphology, physiology, and molecular biology of renin secretion. Physiol Rev 1990;70:1067–116.

[99] Hamza SM, Kaufman S. Effect of mesenteric vascular congestion on reflex control of renal blood flow. Am J Physiol 2007;293:R1917–1922.

[100] Hamza SM, Kaufman S. Role of spleen in integrated control of splanchnic vascular tone: physiology and pathophysiology. Can J Physiol Pharmacol 2009;87:1–7.

[101] Hamza SM, Kaufman S. Splenorenal reflex modulates renal blood flow in the rat. J Physiol 2004;558:277–82.

[102] Handa RK, Johns EJ. Interaction of the renin–angiotensin system and the renal nerves in the regulation of rat kidney function. J Physiol 1985;369:311–21.

[103] Hardebo JE. Influence of impulse pattern on noradrenaline release from sympathetic nerves in cerebral and some peripheral vessels. Acta Physiol Scand 1992;144:333–9.

[104] Hausberg M, Kosch M, Harmelink P, Barenbrock M, Hohage H, Kisters K, et al. Sympathetic nerve activity in end-stage renal disease. Circulation 2002;106:1974–9.

[105] Head GA. Role of AT1 receptors in the central control of sympathetic vasomotor function. Clin Exp Pharmacol Physiol Suppl 1996;3:S93–98.

[106] Hemsen A, Lundberg JM. Presence of endothelin-1 and endothelin-3 in peripheral tissues and central nervous system of pig. Reg Peptides 1991;36:71–83.

[107] Hermansson K, Kallskog O, Wolgast M. Effect of renal nerve stimulation on the activity of the tubuloglomerular feedback mechanism. Acta Physiol Scand 1984;120:381–5.

[108] Hesse IF, Johns EJ. The effect of graded renal nerve stimulation on renal function in the anaesthetized rabbit. Comp Biochem Physiol A 1984;79:409–14.

[109] Hesse IF, Johns EJ. The subtype of alpha-adrenoceptor involved in the neural control of renal tubular sodium reabsorption in the rabbit. J Physiol 1984;352:527–38.

[110] Hevener AL, Bergman RN, Donovan CM. Hypoglycemic detection does not occur in the hepatic artery or liver: findings consistent with a portal vein glucosensor locus. Diabetes 2001;50:399–403.

[111] Hevener AL, Bergman RN, Donovan CM. Portal vein afferents are critical for the sympathoadrenal response to hypoglycemia. Diabetes 2000;49:8–12.

[112] Hintze TH, Kaley G. Ventricular receptors activated following myocardial prostaglandin synthesis initiate reflex hypotension, reduction in heart rate, and redistribution of cardiac output in the dog. Circ Res 1984;54:239–47.

[113] Hisa H, Araki S, Tomura Y, Hayashi Y, Satoh S. Effects of alpha adrenoceptor blockade on renal nerve stimulation-induced norepinephrine release and vasoconstriction in the dog kidney. J Pharmacol Exp Ther 1989;248:752–7.

[114] Holdaas H, DiBona GF, Kiil F. Effect of low-level renal nerve stimulation on renin release from nonfiltering kidneys. Am J Physiol 1981;241:F156–161.

[115] Houghton BL, Huang C, Johns EJ. Influence of dietary sodium on the blood pressure and renal sympathetic nerve activity responses to intracerebroventricular angiotensin II and angiotensin III in anaesthetized rats. Exp Physiol 2010;95:282–95.

[116] Houghton BL, Johns EJ. The pressor and renal sympathetic nerve responses to vascular and spinal V1 receptor activation after manipulation of dietary sodium intake. J Hypertens 2011.

[117] Huang BS, Leenen FH. Dietary Na and baroreflex modulation of blood pressure and RSNA in normotensive vs. spontaneously hypertensive rats. Am J Physiol 1994;266:H496–502.

[118] Huang C, Johns EJ. Role of ANG II in mediating somatosensory-induced renal nerve-dependent antinatriuresis in the rat. Am J Physiol 1998;275:R194–202.

[119] Huang C, Johns EJ. Role of brain angiotensin II in the somatosensory induced antinatriuresis in the anaesthetized rat. Clin Exp Pharmacol Physiol 2000;27:191–6.

[120] Huang C, Yoshimoto M, Miki K, Johns EJ. The contribution of brain angiotensin II to the baroreflex regulation of renal sympathetic nerve activity in conscious normotensive and hypertensive rats. J Physiol 2006;574:597–604.

[121] Hunt CC, Wilkinson RS, Fukami Y. Ionic basis of the receptor potential in primary endings of mammalian muscle spindles. J Gen Physiol 1978;71:683–98.

[122] Ichihara A, Kobori H, Nishiyama A, Navar LG. Renal renin–angiotensin system. Contrib Nephrol 2004;143:117–30.

[123] Imai T, Hirata Y, Emori T, Yanagisawa M, Masaki T, Marumo F. Induction of endothelin-1 gene by angiotensin and vasopressin in endothelial cells. Hypertension 1992;19:753–7.

[124] Ishii M, Ikeda T, Takagi M, Sugimoto T, Atarashi K, Igari T, et al. Elevated plasma catecholamines in hypertensives with primary glomerular diseases. Hypertension 1983;5:545–51.

[125] Ito H, Hirata Y, Adachi S, Tanaka M, Tsujino M, Koike A, et al. Endothelin-1 is an autocrine/paracrine factor in the mechanism of angiotensin II-induced hypertrophy in cultured rat cardiomyocytes. J Clin Invest 1993;92:398–403.

[126] Janssen BJ, Struijker Boudier HA, Smits JF. Role of afferent renal nerves in renal adaptation to sodium restriction in uninephrectomized rats. Acta Physiol Scand 1994;151:395–402.

[127] Johns EJ. The autonomic nervous system and pressure-natriuresis in cardiovascular–renal interactions in response to salt. Clin Auton Res 2002;12:256–63.

[128] Johns EJ. Role of angiotensin II and the sympathetic nervous system in the control of renal function. J Hypertension 1989;7:695–701.

[129] Johns EJ. The role of angiotensin II in the antidiuresis and antinatriuresis induced by stimulation of the sympathetic nerves to the rat kidney. J Auton Pharmacol 1987;7:205–14.

[130] Johns EJ. Role of the renal nerves in modulating renin release during pressure reduction at the feline kidney. Clin Sci (Lond) 1985;69:185–95.

[131] Johns EJ, Lewis BA, Singer B. The sodium-retaining effect of renal nerve activity in the cat: role of angiotensin formation. Clin Sci Mol Med 1976;51:93–102.

[132] Johns EJ, Manitius J. An investigation into the neural regulation of calcium excretion by the rat kidney. J Physiol 1987;383:745–55.

[133] Johns EJ, O'Shaughnessy B, O'Neill S, Lane B, Healy V. Impact of elevated dietary sodium intake on NAD(P)H oxidase and SOD in the cortex and medulla of the rat kidney. Am J Physiol 2010;299:R234–240.

[134] Katholi RE, McCann WP, Woods WT. Intrarenal adenosine produces hypertension via renal nerves in the one-kidney, one-clip rat. Hypertension 1985;7(Pt 2):I88–93.

[135] Katholi RE, Whitlow PL, Hageman GR, Woods WT. Intrarenal adenosine produces hypertension by activating the sympathetic nervous system via the renal nerves in the dog. J Hypertension 1984;2:349–59.

[136] Katholi RE, Whitlow PL, Winternitz SR, Oparil S. Importance of the renal nerves in established two-kidney, one-clip Goldblatt hypertension. Hypertension 1982;4(suppl II):II-166–74.

[137] Katholi RE, Woods WT. Afferent renal nerves and hypertension. Clin Exp Hypertens A 1987;9(Suppl 1):211–26.

[138] Knuepfer MM, Akeyson EW, Schramm LP. Spinal projections of renal afferent nerves in the rat. Brain Res 1988;446:17–25.

[139] Knuepfer M, Schramm LP. The conduction velocities and spinal projections of single renal afferent fibers in the rat. Brain Res 1987;435:167—73.

[140] Kohno M, Horio T, Ikeda M, Yokokawa K, Fukui T, Yasanari K, et al. Angiotensin II stimulates endothelin-1 secretion in cultured rat mesangial cells. Kid Int 1992;42:860—6.

[141] Kompanowska-Jezierska E, Walkowska A, Johns EJ, Sadowski J. Early effects of renal denervation in the anaesthetised rat: natriuresis and increased cortical blood flow. J Physiol 2001;531:527—34.

[142] Kone BC, Baylis C. Biosynthesis and homeostatic roles of nitric oxide in the normal kidney. Am J Physiol 1997;272:F561—578.

[143] Kopp U, Aurell M, Nilsson IM, Ablad B. The role of beta-1-adrenoceptors in the renin release response to graded renal sympathetic nerve stimulation. Pflugers Arch 1980;387:107—13.

[144] Kopp UC, Buckley-Bleiler RL. Impaired renorenal reflexes in two-kidney, one-clip hypertensive rats. Hypertension 1989;14:445—52.

[145] Kopp UC, Cicha MZ. Impaired substance P release from renal sensory nerves in SHR involves a pertussis toxin-sensitive mechanism. Am J Physiol 2004;286:R326—33.

[146] Kopp UC, Cicha MZ. PGE_2 increases substance P release from pelvis sensory nerves via activation of N-type calcium channels. Am J Physiol 1999;276:R1241—8.

[147] Kopp UC, Cicha MZ, Nakamura K, Nusing RM, Smith LA, Hökfelt T. Activation of EP4 receptors contributes to prostaglandin E2-mediated stimulation of renal sensory nerves. Am J Physiol 2004;287:F1269—82.

[148] Kopp UC, Cicha MZ, Smith LA. Activation of endothelin-A receptors contributes to angiotensin-induced suppression of renal sensory nerve activation. Hypertension 2007;49:141—7.

[149] Kopp UC, Cicha MZ, Smith LA. Angiotensin blocks substance P release from renal sensory nerves by inhibiting PGE_2-mediated activation of cAMP. Am J Physiol 2003;285:F472—83.

[150] Kopp UC, Cicha MZ, Smith LA. Dietary sodium loading increases arterial pressure in afferent renal-denervated rats. Hypertension 2003;42:968—73.

[151] Kopp UC, Cicha MZ, Smith LA. Endogenous angiotensin modulates PGE_2-mediated release of substance P from renal mechanosensory nerve fibers. Am J Physiol 2002;282:R19—30.

[152] Kopp UC, Cicha MZ, Smith LA. Impaired interaction between efferent and afferent renal nerve activity in SHR involves increased activation of α_2-adrenoceptors. Hypertension 2011;57(part 2):640—7.

[153] Kopp UC, Cicha MZ, Smith LA. Impaired responsiveness of renal mechanosensory nerves in heart failure: role of endogenous angiotensin. Am J Physiol 2003;284:R116—24.

[154] Kopp UC, Cicha MZ, Smith LA. PGE_2 increases release of substance P from renal sensory nerves by activating the cAMP-PKA transduction cascade. Am J Physiol 2002;282:R1618—27.

[155] Kopp UC, Cicha MZ, Smith LA, Haeggstrom JZ, Samuelsson B, Hokfelt T. Cyclooxygenase-2 involved in stimulation of renal mechanosensitive neurons. Hypertension 2000;35:373—8.

[156] Kopp UC, Cicha MZ, Smith LA, Hokfelt T. Nitric oxide modulates renal sensory nerve fibers by mechanisms related to substance P receptor activation. Am J Physiol 2001;281: R279—90.

[157] Kopp UC, Cicha MZ, Smith LA, Mulder J, Hökfelt T. Renal sympathetic nerve activity modulates afferent renal nerve activity by PGE2-dependent activation of alpha1- and alpha2-adrenoceptors on renal sensory nerve fibers. Am J Physiol 2007;293:R1561—1572.

[158] Kopp UC, Cicha MZ, Smith LA, Ruohonen S, Scheinin M, Fritz N, et al. Dietary sodium modulates the interaction between efferent and afferent renal nerve activity by altering activation of α_2-adrenoceptors on renal sensory nerves. Am. J. Physiol 2011;300:R298—310.

[159] Kopp UC, Cicha MZ, Yorek MA. Impaired responsiveness of renal sensory nerves in streptozotocin-treated rats and obese Zucker diabetic fatty rats: role of angiotensin. Am J Physiol 2008;294:R858—66.

[160] Kopp UC, DiBona GF. Interaction between neural and nonneural mechanisms controlling renin secretion rate. Am J Physiol 1984;246:F620—626.

[161] Kopp UC, Farley DM, Cicha MZ, Smith LA. Activation of renal mechanosensitive neurons involves bradykinin, protein kinase C, PGE2, and substance P. Am J Physiol 2000;278: R937—46.

[162] Kopp UC, Farley DM, Smith LA. Bradykinin-mediated activation of renal sensory neurons due to prostaglandin-dependent release of substance P. Am J Physiol 1997;272:R2009—16.

[163] Kopp UC, Grisk O, Cicha MZ, Smith A, Steinbach A, Schlüter T, et al. Dietary sodium modulates the interaction between efferent renal sympathetic nerve activity and afferent renal nerve activity: role of endothelin. Am J Physiol 2009;297:R337—51.

[164] Kopp UC, Jones SY, DiBona GF. Afferent renal denervation impairs baroreflex control of efferent renal sympathetic nerve activity. Am J Physiol 2008;295:R1882—90.

[165] Kopp UC, Matsushita K, Sigmund RD, Smith LA, Watanabe S, Stokes JB. Amiloride-sensitive Na^+ channels in pelvic uroepithelium involved in renal sensory receptor activation. Am J Physiol 1998;275:R1780—92.

[166] Kopp UC, Olson LA, DiBona GF. Renorenal reflex responses to mechano- and chemoreceptor stimulation in the dog and rat. Am J Physiol 1984;246:F67—77.

[167] Kopp UC, Smith LA. Effects of the substance P receptor antagonist CP-96,345 on renal sensory receptor activation. Am J Physiol 1993;264:R647—53.

[168] Kopp UC, Smith LA, DiBona GF. Impaired renorenal reflexes in spontaneously hypertensive rats. Hypertension 1987;9:69—75.

[169] Kopp UC, Smith LA, DiBona GF. Renorenal reflexes: neural components of ipsilateral and contralateral renal responses. Am J Physiol 1985;249:F507—17.

[170] Kopp UC, Smith LA, Pence AL. Na^+-K^+-ATPase inhibition sensitizes renal mechanoreceptors activated by increases in renal pelvic pressure. Am J Physiol 1994;267:R1109—17.

[171] Kostreva DR, Castaner A, Kampine JP. Reflex effects of hepatic baroreceptors on renal and cardiac sympathetic nerve activity. Am J Physiol 1980;238:R390—394.

[172] Krum H, Schlaich M, Whitbourn R, Sobotka PA, Sadowski J, Bartus K, et al. Catheter-based renal sympathetic denervation for resistant hypertension: a multicentre safety and proof-of-principle cohort study. Lancet 2009;373:1275—81.

[173] Krum H, Barman N, Schlaich M, Sobotka P, Esler M, Mahfoud F, et al. (Simplicity HTN-1 Investigators). Catheter-based renal sympathetic denervation for resistant hypertension: durability of blood pressure reduction out to 24 months. Hypertension 2011;57:911—7.

[174] Kumagai H, Averill DB, Ferrario CM. Renal nerve activity in rats with spontaneous hypertension: effect of converting enzyme inhibitor. Am J Physiol 1992;263:R109—115.

[175] La Grange RG, Sloop CH, Schmid HE. Selective stimulation of renal nerves in the anesthetized dog. Effect on renin release during controlled changes in renal hemodynamics. Circ Res 1973;33:704—12.

[176] Lacroix JS, Stjarne P, Anggard A, Lundberg JM. Sympathetic vascular control of the pig nasal mucosa: (I). Increased resistance and capacitance vessel responses upon stimulation with irregular bursts compared to continuous impulses. Acta Physiol Scand 1988;132:83—90.

[177] Leonard BL, Evans RG, Navakatikyan MA, Malpas SC. Differential neural control of intrarenal blood flow. Am J Physiol 2000;279:R907–916.

[178] Linden RJ, Mary DA, Weatherill D. The nature of the atrial receptors responsible for a reflex decrease in activity in renal nerves in the dog. J Physiol 1980;300:31–40.

[179] Liu F, Gesek FA. alpha(1)-Adrenergic receptors activate NHE1 and NHE3 through distinct signaling pathways in epithelial cells. Am J Physiol 2001;280:F415–425.

[180] Liu F, Nesbitt T, Drezner MK, Friedman PA, Gesek FA. Proximal nephron Na$^+$/H$^+$ exchange is regulated by alpha$_{1A}$- and alpha$_{1B}$-adrenergic receptor subtypes. Mol Pharmacol 1997;52:1010–8.

[181] Liu GL, Liu L, Barajas L. Development of NOS-containing neuronal somata in the rat kidney. J Auton Nerv Syst 1996;58:81–8.

[182] Liu L, Barajas L. The rat renal nerves during development. Anat Embryol (Berl) 1993;188:345–61.

[183] Luff SE, Hengstberger SG, McLachlan EM, Anderson WP. Two types of sympathetic axon innervating the juxtaglomerular arterioles of the rabbit and rat kidney differ structurally from those supplying other arteries. J Neurocytol 1991;20:781–95.

[184] Lyson T, McMullan DM, Ermel LD, Morgan BJ, Victor RG. Mechanism of cyclosporine-induced sympathetic activation and acute hypertension in rats. Hypertension 1994;23:667–75.

[185] Ma MC, Huang HS, Chen CF. Impaired renal sensory responses after unilateral urseteral obstruction in the rat. J Am Soc Nephrol 2002;13:1008–16.

[186] Ma MC, Huang HS, Chien CT, Wu MS, Chen CF. Temporal decrease in renal sensory responses in rats after chronic ligation of the bile duct. Am J Physiol 2002;283:F164–72.

[187] Ma MC, Huang HS, Wu MS, Chien CT, Chen CF. Impaired renal sensory responses after renal ischemia in the rat. J Am Soc Nephrol 2002;13:1872–83.

[188] Maekawa H, Matsumura Y, Matsuo G, Morimoto S. Effect of sodium nitroprusside on norepinephrine overflow and antidiuresis induced by stimulation of renal nerves in anesthetized dogs. J Cardiovasc Pharmacol 1996;27:211–7.

[189] Malpas SC. Sympathetic nervous system overactivity and its role in the development of cardiovascular disease. Physiol Rev 2010;90:513–57.

[190] Malpas SC, Evans RG. Do different levels and patterns of sympathetic activation all provoke renal vasoconstriction? J Auton Nerv Syst 1998;69:72–82.

[191] Malpas SC, Hore TA, Navakatikyan M, Lukoshkova EV, Nguang SK, Austin PC. Resonance in the renal vasculature evoked by activation of the sympathetic nerves. Am J Physiol 1999;276:R1311–1319.

[192] Malpas SC, Leonard BL. Neural regulation of renal blood flow: a re-examination. Clin Exp Pharmacol Physiol 2000;27:956–64.

[193] Manning DC, Snyder SH. Bradykinin receptors localized by quantitative autoradiography in kidney, ureter, and bladder. Am J Physiol 1989;256:F909–15.

[194] Mattson DL, Wu F. Nitric oxide synthase activity and isoforms in rat renal vasculature. Hypertension 2000;35:337–41.

[195] May CN, Frithiof R, Hood SG, McAllen RM, McKinley MJ, Ramchandra R. Specific control of sympathetic nerve activity to the mammalian heart and kidney. Exp Physiol 2010;95:34–40.

[196] McAllen RM, May CN. Differential drives from rostral ventrolateral medullary neurons to three identified sympathetic outflows. Am J Physiol 1994;267:R935–944.

[197] McDonough AA. Mechanisms of proximal tubule sodium transport regulation that link extracellular fluid volume and blood pressure. Am J Physiol 2010;298:R851–861.

[198] McDonough AA, Leong PK, Yang LE. Mechanisms of pressure natriuresis: how blood pressure regulates renal sodium transport. Ann NY Acad Sci 2003;986:669–77.

[199] McKinley MJ, Albiston AL, Allen AM, Mathai ML, May CN, McAllen RM, et al. The brain renin–angiotensin system: location and physiological roles. Int J Biochem Cell Biol 2003;35:901–18.

[200] McKinley MJ, Pennington GL, Oldfield BJ. Anteroventral wall of the third ventricle and dorsal lamina terminalis: headquarters for control of body fluid homeostasis? Clin Exp Pharmacol Physiol 1996;23:271–81.

[201] Miki K, Hayashida Y, Sagawa S, Shiraki K. Renal sympathetic nerve activity and natriuresis during water immersion in conscious dogs. Am J Physiol 1989;256:R299–305.

[202] Miki K, Hayashida Y, Shiraki K. Role of cardiac-renal neural reflex in regulating sodium excretion during water immersion in conscious dogs. J Physiol 2002;545:305–12.

[203] Miki K, Yoshimoto M. Role of differential changes in sympathetic nerve activity in the preparatory adjustments of cardiovascular functions during freezing behaviour in rats. Exp Physiol 2010;95:56–60.

[204] Miki K, Yoshimoto M, Tanimizu M. Acute shifts of baroreflex control of renal sympathetic nerve activity induced by treadmill exercise in rats. J Physiol 2003;548:313–22.

[205] Morita H, Nishida Y, Hosomi H. Neural control of urinary sodium excretion during hypertonic NaCl load in conscious rabbits: role of renal and hepatic nerves and baroreceptors. J Auton Nerv Syst 1991;34:157–69.

[206] Nagura S, Sakagami T, Kakiichi A, Yoshimoto M, Miki K. Acute shifts in baroreflex control of renal sympathetic nerve activity induced by REM sleep and grooming in rats. J Physiol 2004;558:975–83.

[207] Nakamura A, Johns EJ. Effect of renal nerves on expression of renin and angiotensinogen genes in rat kidneys. Am J Physiol 1994;266:E230–241.

[208] Nicol GD, Cui M. Enhancement by prostaglandin E$_2$ of bradykinin activation of embryonic rat sensory neurones. J Physiol 1994;480(Pt 3):485–92.

[209] Nicol GD, Klingberg DK, Vasko MR. Prostaglandin E$_2$ increases calcium conductance and stimulates release of substance P in avian sensory neurons. J Neurosci 1992;12:1917–27.

[210] Nilsson H, Ljung B, Sjoblom N, Wallin BG. The influence of the sympathetic impulse pattern on contractile responses of rat mesenteric arteries and veins. Acta Physiol Scand 1985;123:303–9.

[211] Nishiyama A, Seth DM, Navar LG. Angiotensin II type 1 receptor-mediated augmentation of renal interstitial fluid angiotensin II in angiotensin II-induced hypertension. J Hypertension 2003;21:1897–903.

[212] Nord EP, Howard MJ, Hafezi A, Moradeshagi P, Vaystub S, Insel PA. Alpha 2 adrenergic agonists stimulate Na$^+$-H$^+$ antiport activity in the rabbit renal proximal tubule. J Clin Invest 1987;80:1755–62.

[213] Ortiz PA, Garvin JL. Role of nitric oxide in the regulation of nephron transport. Am J Physiol 2002;282:F777–784.

[214] Osborn JL, Camara AK. Renal neurogenic mediation of intracerebroventricular angiotensin II hypertension in rats raised on high sodium chloride diet. Hypertension 1997;30:331–6.

[215] Osborn JL, DiBona GF, Thames MD. Beta-1 receptor mediation of renin secretion elicited by low-frequency renal nerve stimulation. J Pharmacol Exp Ther 1981;216:265–9.

[216] Osborn JL, Thames MD, DiBona GF. Role of macula densa in renal nerve modulation of renin secretion. Am J Physiol 1982;242:R367–371.

[217] Ottoson D, Shepherd GM. Transducer characteristics of the muscle spindle as revealed by its receptor potential. Acta Physiol Scand 1971;82:545–54.

[218] Pan L, Black TA, Shi Q, Jones CA, Petrovic N, Loudon J, et al. Critical roles of a cyclic AMP responsive element and an E-box in regulation of mouse renin gene expression. J Biol Chem 2001;276:45530–8.

[219] Pateromichelakis S, Rood JP. Prostaglandin E1-induced sensitization of A delta moderate pressure mechanoreceptors. Brain Res 1982;232:89–96.

[220] Persson PB. Renin: origin, secretion and synthesis. J Physiol 2003;552:667–71.

[221] Persson PB, Skalweit A, Thiele BJ. Controlling the release and production of renin. Acta Physiol Scand 2004;181:375–81.

[222] Pettinger WA, Smyth DD, Umemura S. Renal alpha 2-adrenoceptors, their locations and effects on sodium excretion. J Cardiovasc Pharmacol 1985;7(Suppl 8):S24–27.

[223] Pettinger WA, Umemura S, Smyth DD, Jeffries WB. Renal alpha 2-adrenoceptors and the adenylate cyclase-cAMP system: biochemical and physiological interactions. Am J Physiol 1987;252:F199–208.

[224] Philipp M, Brede M, Hein L. Physiological significance of α_2-adrenergic receptor subtype diversity: one receptor is not enough. Am J Physiol 2002;283:R287–95.

[225] Piascik MT, Perez DM. Alpha1-adrenergic receptors: new insights and directions. J Pharmacol Exp Ther 2001;298:403–10.

[226] Pohjanoksa K, Jansson CC, Luomala K, Marjamäki A, Savola JM, Scheinin M. α_2-adrenoceptor regulation of adenylyl cyclase in CHO cells: dependence on receptor density, receptor subtype and current activity of adenylyl cyclase. Eur J Pharmacol 1997;335:53–63.

[227] Pollock DM, Pollock JS. Evidence for endothelin involvement in the response to high salt. Am J Physiol 2001;281:F144–50.

[228] Quan A, Baum M. Renal nerve stimulation augments effect of intraluminal angiotensin II on proximal tubule transport. Am J Physiol 2002;282:F1043–1048.

[229] Quan A, Baum M. The renal nerve is required for regulation of proximal tubule transport by intraluminally produced ANG II. Am J Physiol 2001;280:F524–529.

[230] Rubanyi GM, Polokoff MA. Endothelins: molecular biology, biochemistry, pharmacology, physiology and pathophysiology. Pharmacol Rev 1994;46:325–415.

[231] Rudenstam J, Bergstrom G, Taghipour K, Gothberg G, Karlstrom G. Efferent renal sympathetic nerve stimulation in vivo. Effects on regional renal haemodynamics in the Wistar rat, studied by laser-Doppler technique. Acta Physiol Scand 1995;154:387–94.

[232] Saeki Y, Terui N, Kumada M. Physiological characterization of the renal-sympathetic reflex in rabbits. Jap J Physiol 1988;38:251–66.

[233] Sato KL, do Carmo JM, Fazan VP. Ultrastructural anatomy of the renal nerves in rats. Brain Res 2006;1119:94–100.

[234] Schlaich MP, Krum H, Esler MD. New therapeutic approaches to resistant hypertension. Curr Hypertension Rep 2010;12:296–302.

[235] Schweda F, Friis U, Wagner C, Skott O, Kurtz A. Renin release. Physiology (Bethesda) 2007;22:310–9.

[236] Sequeira Lopez ML, Pentz ES, Robert B, Abrahamson DR, Gomez RA. Embryonic origin and lineage of juxtaglomerular cells. Am J Physiol 2001;281:F345–356.

[237] Shi TS, Winzer-Serhan U, Leslie F, Hökfelt T. Distribution and regulation of α_2-adrenoceptors in rat dorsal root ganglia. Pain 2000;84:319–30.

[238] Shi TS, Winzer-Serhan U, Leslie F, Hökfelt T. Distribution of α_2-adrenoceptor mRNAs in the rat lumbar spinal cord in normal and axotomized rats. NeuroReport 1999;10:2835–9.

[239] Shokoji T, Fujisawa Y, Kimura S, Rahman M, Kiyomoto H, Matsubara K, et al. Effects of local administrations of tempol and diethyldithio-carbamic on peripheral nerve activity. Hypertension 2004;44:236–43.

[240] Sigmund CD, Jones CA, Fabian JR, Mullins JJ, Gross KW. Tissue and cell specific expression of a renin promoter-reporter gene construct in transgenic mice. Biochem Biophys Res Commun 1990;170:344–50.

[241] Simon JK, Ciriello J. Contribution of afferent renal nerves to the metabolic activity of central structures involved in the control of the circulation. Can J Physiol Pharmacol 1989;67:1130–9.

[242] Sinn PL, Sigmund CD. Human renin mRNA stability is increased in response to cAMP in Calu-6 cells. Hypertension 1999;33:900–5.

[243] Siragy HM, Howell NL, Ragsdale NV, Carey RM. Renal interstitial fluid angiotensin. Modulation by anesthesia, epinephrine, sodium depletion, and renin inhibition. Hypertension 1995;25:1021–4.

[244] Smith H. The kidney: Structure and Function in Health and Disease. New York: Oxford University Press; 1951.

[245] Smith JA, Davis CL, Burgess GM. Prostaglandin E$_2$-induced sensitization of bradykinin-evoked responses in rat dorsal root ganglion neurons is mediated by cAMP-dependent protein kinase A. Eur J Neurosci 2000;12:3250–8.

[246] Smits JF, Brody MJ. Activation of afferent renal nerves by intrarenal bradykinin in conscious rats. Am J Physiol 1984;247: R1003–8.

[247] Solano-Flores LP, Rosa-Arellano MP, Ciriello J. Fos induction in central structures after afferent renal stimulation. Brain Res 1997;753:102–19.

[248] Stella A, Calaresu F, Zanchetti A. Neural factors contributing to renin release during reduction in renal perfusion pressure and blood flow in cats. Clin Sci Mol Med 1976;51:453–61.

[249] Stella A, Zanchetti A. Functional role of renal afferents. Physiol Rev 1991;71:659–82.

[250] Steranka LR, Manning DC, DeHaas CJ, Ferkany JW, Borosky SA, Connor JR, et al. Bradykinin as a pain mediator: receptors are localized to sensory neurons, and antagonists have analgesic actions. Proc Natl Acad Sci USA 1988;85:3245–9.

[251] Summers RJ, Broxton N, Hutchinson DS, Evans BA. The Janus faces of adrenoceptors: factors controlling the coupling of adrenoceptors to multiple signal transduction pathways. Clin Exp Pharmacol Physiol 2004;31:822–7.

[252] Szenasi G, Bencsath P, Takacs L. Proximal tubular transport and urinary excretion of sodium after renal denervation in sodium depleted rats. Pflugers Arch 1985;403:146–50.

[253] Tanioka H, Nakamura K, Fujimura S, Yoshida M, Suzuki-Kusaba M, Hisa H, et al. Facilitatory role of NO in neural norepinephrine release in the rat kidney. Am J Physiol 2002;282: R1436–1442.

[254] Terui N, Saeki Y, Kumuda M. Barosensory neurons in the ventrolateral medulla in rabbits and their responses to various afferent inputs from peripheral and central sources. Jap J Physiol 1986;36:1141–64.

[255] Thames MD, Abboud FM. Interaction of somatic and cardiopulmonary receptors in control of renal circulation. Am J Physiol 1979;237:H560–565.

[256] Tobian L, MacNeill D, Johnson MA, Ganguli MC, Iwai J. Potassium protects against renal tubule lesions in NaCl-fed hypertensive Dahl S rats. Trans Assoc Am Physicians 1983;96:417–25.

[257] Vasko MR, Campbell WB, Waite KJ. Prostaglandin E2 enhances bradykinin-stimulated release of neuropeptides from rat sensory neurons in culture. J Neurosci 1994;14:4987–97.

[258] Veelken R, Hilgers KF, Stetter A, Siebert HG, Schmieder RE, Mann JF. Nerve-mediated antidiuresis and antinatriuresis after

air-jet stress is modulated by angiotensin II. Hypertension 1996;28:825—32.

[259] Walkowska A, Badzynska B, Kompanowska-Jezierska E, Johns EJ, Sadowski J. Effects of renal nerve stimulation on intrarenal blood flow in rats with intact or inactivated NO synthases. Acta Physiol Scand 2005;183:99—105.

[260] Wang DH, Li J, Qiu J. Salt-sensitive hypertension induced by sensory denervation: introduction of a new model. Hypertension 1998;32:649—53.

[261] Wang J, Rose JC. Developmental changes in renal renin mRNA half-life and responses to stimulation in fetal lambs. Am J Physiol 1999;277:R1130—1135.

[262] Weaver LC, Genovesi S, Stella A, Zanchetti A. Neural, hemodynamic, and renal responses to stimulation of intestinal receptors. Am J Physiol 1987;253:H1167—1176.

[263] Widmann C, Gibson S, Jarpe MB, Johnson GL. Mitogen-activated protein kinase: conservation of a three-kinase module from yeast to human. Physiol Rev 1999;79:143—80.

[264] Williams NG, Zhong H, Minneman KP. Differential coupling of alpha1-, alpha2-, and beta-adrenergic receptors to mitogen-activated protein kinase pathways and differentiation in transfected PC12 cells. J Biol Chem 1998;273:24624—32.

[265] Wright JW, Harding JW. Important role for angiotensin III and IV in the brain renin—angiotensin system. Brain Res Brain Res Rev 1997;25:96—124.

[266] Wu XC, Harris PJ, Johns EJ. Nitric oxide and renal nerve-mediated proximal tubular reabsorption in normotensive and hypertensive rats. Am J Physiol 1999;277:F560—566.

[267] Wu XC, Johns EJ. Interactions between nitric oxide and super-oxide on the neural regulation of proximal fluid reabsorption in hypertensive rats. Exp Physiol 2004;89:255—61.

[268] Wu XC, Johns EJ. Nitric oxide modulation of neurally induced proximal tubular fluid reabsorption in the rat. Hypertension 2002;39:790—3.

[269] Wurzner G, Chiolero A, Maillard M, Nussberger J, Hayoz D, Brunner HR, et al. Renal and neurohormonal responses to increasing levels of lower body negative pressure in men. Kidney Int 2001;60:1469—76.

[270] Wyss JM, Donovan K. A direct projection from the kidney to the brainstem. Brain Res 1984;298:130—4.

[271] Xia Y, Karmazyn M. Obligatory role for endogenous endothelin in mediating the hypertrophic effects of phenylephrine and angiotensin II in neonatal rat ventricular myocytes: evidence for two distinct mechanisms for endothelin regulation. J Pharmacol Exp Ther 2004;310:43—51.

[272] Xu H, Fink GD, Galligan JJ. Tempol lowers blood pressure and sympathetic nerve activity but not vascular O_2^- in DOCA-salt rats. Hypertension 2004;43:329—34.

[273] Yang L, Leong PK, Chen JO, Patel N, Hamm-Alvarez SF, McDonough AA. Acute hypertension provokes internalization of proximal tubule NHE3 without inhibition of transport activity. Am J Physiol 2002;282:F730—740.

[274] Ye DZ, Wang DH. Function and regulation of endothelin-1 and its receptors in salt sensitive hypertension induced by sensory nerve degeneration. Hypertension 2002;39:673—8.

[275] Yoshimoto M, Miki K, Fink GD, King A, Osborn JW. Chronic angiotensin II infusion causes differential responses in regional sympathetic nerve activity in rats. Hypertension 2010;55:644—51.

[276] Yoshimoto M, Nagata K, Miki K. Differential control of renal and lumbar sympathetic nerve activity during freezing behavior in conscious rats. Am J Physiol 2010;299:R1114—1120.

[277] Yoshimoto M, Sakagami T, Nagura S, Miki K. Relationship between renal sympathetic nerve activity and renal blood flow during natural behavior in rats. Am J Physiol 2004;286:R881—887.

[278] Zambraski EJ, Dibona GF, Kaloyanides GJ. Effect of sympathetic blocking agents on the antinatriuresis of reflex renal nerve stimulation. J Pharmacol Exp Ther 1976;198:464—72.

[279] Zhang T, Johns EJ. Somatosensory influences on renal sympathetic nerve activity in anesthetized Wistar and hypertensive rats. Am J Physiol 1997;272:R982—990.

[280] Zhu Y, Wang Y, Wang DH. Diuresis and natriuresis caused by activation of VR1-positive sensory nerves in renal pelvis of rats. Hypertension 2005;46:992—7.

Eicosanoids and Renal Function

Matthew D. Breyer[1], Raymond C Harris[2] and Richard M. Breyer[2]

[1]Biotechnology Discovery Research Eli Lilly and Company Indianapolis, IN, USA
[2]Division of Nephrology, Department of Medicine, Vanderbilt University, Nashville, TN, USA

Perhaps nothing underscores the special relationship between the kidney and the eicosanoids better than the profound clinical effects non-steroidal anti-inflammatory drugs (NSAIDS) have on kidney function. NSAIDs are widely used to treat pain and inflammatory diseases, and work by blocking the enzymatic synthesis of prostaglandins, a type of eicosanoid, from arachidonic acid. However, chronic NSAID use is often complicated by major side effects, including renal sodium retention, resulting in edema, hypertension, and congestive heart failure.[1,2] Conversely, in the sodium depleted state, NSAIDs can reduce renal blood flow, glomerular filtration rate, and cause acute renal failure.[3–5] These observations underscore the critical role cyclooxygenase-derived arachidonic acid metabolites play in maintaining normal kidney function — particularly in the setting of physiological stress.

CELLULAR ORIGIN OF EICOSANOIDS

Eicosanoids are a family of biologically active, oxygenated metabolites derived from arachidonic acid (AA). AA is comprised of 20 carbon atoms configured as a polyunsaturated fatty acid chain with four double bonds (C20:4). Mammals lack the enzymatic machinery to synthesize AA *de novo*, instead it must be formed from dietary linoleic acid (C18:2) by addition of two carbons and further desaturation.[6,7] Essential fatty acid (EFA) deficiency occurs in the absence of dietary linoleic and other fatty acid AA precursors, depleting the hormone-responsive pool of AA metabolite products.[8,9] Of the approximate 10 gm of linoleic acid ingested per day, only about 1 mg/day is eliminated as end products of AA metabolism.[10–12] Following its formation, AA is esterified into cell membrane phospholipids, principally at the 2 position of the phosphatidylinositol fraction (i.e., sn-2 esterified AA). This source comprises the major hormone-sensitive pool of AA that is susceptible to release by phospholipases.

Phospholipase-Mediated Arachidonic Acid Release

Multiple stimuli lead to release of membrane-phospholipid esterified AA via activation of cellular phospholipases, principally phospholipase A2s (PLA$_2$).[13,14] This cleavage step is rate-limiting in the production of arachidonate metabolites. Activation of phospholipase C or PLD, on the other hand, releases AA via the sequential action of the phospholipase C-mediated production of diacylglycerol (DAG), with subsequent release of AA from DAG by DAG lipase.[15] The physiological significance of AA release by these other phospholipases remains uncertain since, at least in the setting of inflammation, phospholipase A$_2$ action appears to be essential for the generation of biologically active AA metabolites.[16] Cellular levels of free arachidonic acid available for eicosanoid production are primarily controlled by phospholipase A2 (PLA2).[16–18] So far, more than 30 enzymes with PLA$_2$ activity have been identified, and have been classified into four groups: secretory PLA$_2$ (sPLA2); cytosolic PLA2 (cPLA2); calcium-independent PLA2 (iPLA2); and PAF acetylhydrolases (PAF-AH).[14,19] The activity of cPLA2 is regulated by diverse cell membrane receptors, including the EGF receptor, and transmembrane guanine-nucleotide protein coupled (GPCRs) including adrenergic receptors, angiotensin II receptors, and purinergic receptors.[20–25] These receptors activate guanine nucleotide-binding (G) proteins, leading to PLA$_2$-mediated release of AA from membrane phospholipids.[20,26,27] Alternatively, these receptors may activate $cPLA_2$ via mitogen-activated protein kinases (MAPK), protein kinase C (PKC), and Ca^{2+}-calmodulin-dependent kinases.

Ambient physical conditions in the kidney including hypoxia, oxidative stress, and mechanical stretch can also activate PLA_2 activity.[28–32] Dysregulated renal PLA_2 activity with attendant change in AA release results in altered substrate availability for the production of downstream metabolic products. This activation is believed to contribute to pathologic processes including acute kidney injury, diabetic nephropathy, and inflammatory glomerulonephritis.[33–35] Some snake and bee venoms are imbued with high levels of secretory PLA_2 activity and, in part through this activity, can induce acute renal failure[36,37]. A role for secretory PLA_2 in the pathogenesis of acute ischemic-reperfusion renal injury has also been supported by studies showing that $sPLA_2$ neutralizing antibodies protect rats from this form of injury.[36,38]

Phospholipase A2 Receptors

Recently, an important role for a transmembrane cell surface secretory PLA_2 receptor (PLA_2R) has been recognized in the pathogenesis of human idiopathic membranous nephropathy.[39] Auto-antibodies to PLA_2R are detected in $\sim 70\%$ of cases of human idiopathic membranous nephropathy.[39] The antigen appears to be selectively expressed in podocytes[39]; however, the mechanism by which the auto-antibodies induce proteinuria and how these auto-antibodies arise remains to be determined. PLA_2R is a type I transmembrane receptor and one of four mammalian members of the mannose-receptor family.[40] PLA_2R was initially identified as a binding protein for secreted phospholipase A_2 (PLA_2) that now has been expanded to a PLA_2R family that exhibit different affinities for the secreted PLA_2.[41] New studies suggest these receptors could play additional transmembrane signaling roles, and may promote terminal cell differentiation and mitotic arrest.[42]

Arachidonic Acid Metabolism

Following its release from membrane phospholipids, AA is usually rapidly re-esterified into the membrane or avidly bound by intracellular proteins, becoming unavailable for further metabolism. Should AA escape re-esterification and protein binding, it may be metabolized through one of three major enzymatic transformations, the common result of which is the incorporation of oxygen atoms at various sites of the fatty acid backbone, with accompanying changes in its molecular structure (such as ring formation). This results in the formation of biologically active molecules, collectively referred to as "eicosanoids." The specific nature of the products generated is a function of the initial stimuli for AA release, as well as the metabolic enzymes available, as determined by the cell type involved.[43,44]

Enyzmes capable of mediating AA metabolism through all three known pathways are present in the kidney, including cyclooxygenases 1 and 2, lipoxygenases, and cytochrome P450s (Figure 17.1). Cyclooxygenase (COX, also called Prostaglandin H2 synthase or PGHS)-mediated AA metabolism comprises the first committed step in the formation of prostaglandins (PGs), prostacyclin, and thromboxane.[45] The lipoxygenase pathway mediates the formation of mono-, di-, and trihydroxyeicosatetraenoic acids (HETEs), leukotrienes (LTs), and lipoxins (LXs),[46,47] and the cytochrome P450-dependent oxygenation of AA mediates the formation of epoxyeicosatrienoic acids (EETs), their corresponding diols, HETEs, and monooxygenated AA derivatives.[48–50] Fish oil diets, rich in n-3 polyunsaturated fatty acids (n-3 fatty acids are those in which the double bond is three carbons from the terminal, i.e., n carbon, that is furthest from the carboxy-group atom, AA is thus an n-6 fatty acid) interfere with metabolism via all three pathways by competing with AA oxygenation, resulting in the formation of biologically inactive end-products.[51,52] Interference with the production of pro-inflammatory lipids has been hypothesized to underlie the beneficial effects of fish-oil in IgA nephropathy, membranous nephropathy, and other cardiovascular diseases.[7,53,54]

CYCLOOXYGENASE DERIVED PROSTANOIDS

Prostanoids, including the prostaglandins PGE_2, $PGF_{2\alpha}$, and PGD_2, as well as the non-prostaglandin molecules thromboxane A_2 (TxA2) and prostacyclin (PGI_2), are derived from arachidonic acid via its dioxygenation by cyclooxygenases 1 and 2 (COX1 and COX2).[52] Cyclooxygenases exist as homodimers that are physically associated with, but do not pass through, the intracellular endoplasmic reticular membrane.[55–57] Cyclooxygenases mediate a two-step reaction, initially converting free arachidonic acid to the unstable intermediate PGG_2 via a bis-oxygenase activity. PGG_2 is converted to PGH_2 via the peroxidase activity of COX.[52,58–63] PGH_2 is subsequently metabolized to more stable primary biologically active prostanoids PGE_2, $PGF_{2\alpha}$, PGD_2, PGI_2, and TxA_2 by distinct enzymatic prostanoid synthases. These prostanoids exit the cell through uncharacterized mechanisms, where they exert paracrine or autocrine activity on specific and distinct cell surface G-protein coupled receptor(s).[64,65] There is also less definitive evidence that prostanoids may provide physiologically relevant

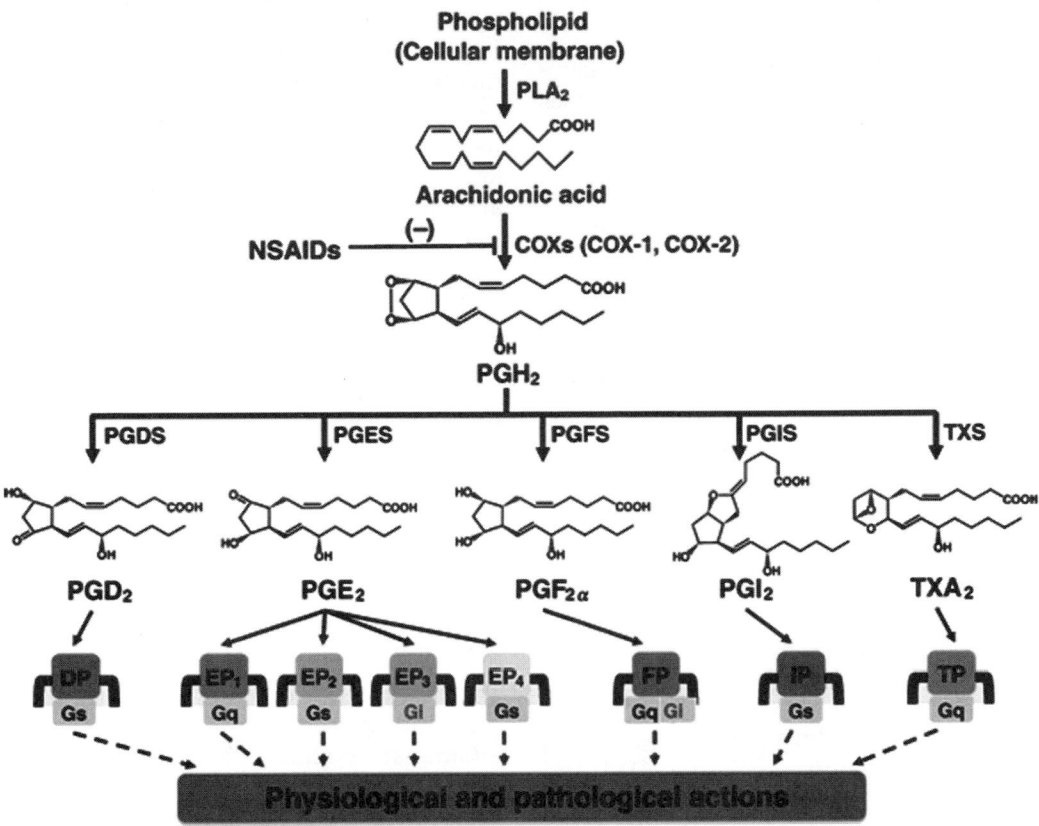

FIGURE 17.1 **Prostaglandin synthesis and the family of G-protein coupled receptors that mediate their functional effects.** *(With permission from Yuhki et al.*[348]*.)*

ligands for nuclear hormone receptors, including peroxisome proliferator activated receptors.[66–68]

Two isoforms of COX have been identified, designated COX1 and COX2.[69–71] Based on transcriptional elements in its 5′ upstream sequence, COX1 is believed to serve a constitutive housekeeping role, responsible for maintaining basic physiological function such as cytoprotection of the gastric mucosa, and control of platelet aggregation.[72,73] Conversely, COX2 upstream promoter region has NF-κB, NFAT, and its expression is potently induced by inflammatory mediators and mitogens, consistent with its role in pathophysiologic processes including angiogenesis, inflammation, and tumorigenesis.[74–77]

The major phenotype of COX2 knockout mice is renal dysgenesis,[78–80] underscoring the special role COX2 plays in the kidney. This defect is characterized by a structurally normal medulla, but hypotrophic renal cortical development with small glomerular size,[79] due to a defect occurring relatively late in parturition.[79] The mechanism is undetermined, but may be related to the particular expression pattern of COX2 in the kidney since normally it is focally expressed adjacent to the glomerulus in the macula densa and the surrounding thick ascending limb cells.[81–83] As in other organs, the housekeeping gene is COX1, which is also constitutively expressed at high levels in the kidney but in cellular compartments distinct from COX2, especially in the collecting duct and glomerular parietal epithelium.[84,85] Low levels of COX1 are also detected in medullary interstitial cells,[81,86,87] but these cells are also uniquely characterized by high endogenous levels of COX2.[81,88,89]

Clinical pharmacologic studies are also consistent with a critical role of COX2 for maintaining cardiovascular homeostasis and normal renal function.[90–92] Indeed, most of the clinically observed side effects associated with the use of non-selective NSAIDs, including edema, hypertension, increased congestive heart failure, hyperkalemia, and acute renal failure, have also been observed with COX2 selective inhibitors.[3] COX2-dependent PGE_2 production is inversely related to luminal chloride concentration delivered to the macula densa,[93] so that in volume depleted states high PGE_2 production rates may exert a vasodilator effect on the afferent arteriole, contributing to maintenance of glomerular blood flow. Impairment of renal function is presumed due to loss of specific prostanoids, derived from the metabolism of the common cyclooxygenase product PGH_2.

Prostanoid Function

Once formed, the COX-derived arachidonate metabolite PGH_2 is further metabolized by prostanoid synthases into at least five primary biologically active prostanoids. Prostanoid synthases include PGE_2 synthase (PGES), prostacyclin synthase (PGIS), PGD synthase (PGDS), PGF synthase (PGFS), and thromboxane synthase, responsible for PGE2, PGI2, PGD2, PGF2α, and TxA2 biosynthesis respectively.[77,94,95]

Most prostanoids are short lived, being highly susceptible to enzymatic inactivation, thereby limiting their effect to the immediate vicinity of their synthesis. The paracrine and autocrine biologic effects of COX-derived prostanoids are diverse and complex, depending on which prostanoid is produced and which receptor is available.[96,97] Thus, the effects of prostanoids on kidney function rely on distinct enzymatic machinery that couples phospholipase and COX to specific prostanoid synthase in specific cells, yielding a specific prostanoid which acts locally through specific G-protein coupled receptors, exerting its particular effect.[96]

At steady-state PGE_2 is the most abundant prostanoid in the mouse kidney, followed by PGI_2, $PGF_{2\alpha}$, and TxA_2.[98] Under basal conditions, both COX1 and COX2 pathways are responsible for the biosynthesis of these prostanoids.[98] Similarly, PGE2 is the most abundant prostanoid in human urine, and under basal, non-stressed conditions is produced by both COX1 and COX.[99,100] In contrast, COX2 primarily contributes to angiotensin II-induced PGE_2 and PGI2 generation in the kidney,[98] and under conditions of low-sodium diet in humans.[101] The intrarenal cellular sites where COX1 and COX2 prostanoids are synthesized remain to be fully defined.

Following their synthesis, these prostanoids become available to exert their biological effects via a diverse family of membrane spanning G-protein coupled prostanoid receptors. These include the DP, EP, FP, IP, and TP receptors, each of which is selectively activated by a specific ligand – PGD_2, PGE_2, $PGF_{2\alpha}$, PGI_2 or TXA_2, respectively.[97,102] PGE2 receptors, designated EP receptors, are unique in that they are encoded by four distinct genes encoding the proteins for EP1, EP2, EP3, and EP4 receptors.[102,103] Each prostanoid receptor activates a distinct G-protein coupled signaling pathway. The IP, DP1, EP2, and EP4 receptors are coupled to the stimulatory G-protein (Gs) and signal by increasing intracellular cAMP levels, whereas the TP, FP, and EP1 receptors induce calcium mobilization.[96,97] The FP, DP2, and EP3 receptors can couple to an inhibitory G-protein (Gi) and reduce cAMP synthesis.[97,102,104]

Restricted cellular expression of prostanoid receptors provides an important mechanism by which a COX-derived prostanoid can exert differential actions in physiological and pathophysiological processes. In the kidney the EP receptors map to distinct segments of the nephron.[96,105] Similarly, all four EP receptors have been described in major inflammatory cells including T-lymphocytes, B-lymphocytes, macrophage, and mast cells[106]; however, whether these receptors are simultaneously expressed in individual cells is uncertain. It has been proposed that activation of different receptors on different cells at different stages of inflammation may account for the pro- or anti-inflammatory action of PGE_2.[107,108]

Prostaglandin E2

PGE_2 is synthesized by at least three forms of PGE synthases, including microsomal PGE synthase 1 (mPGES1), microsomal PGE synthase 2 (mPGES2), and cytosolic PGE synthase (cPGES1).[109–111] The two membrane associated PGE_2 synthases are 33 kDa and 16 kDa enzymes designated mPGES1 and mPGES2, respectively. Microsomal PGES1 displays a higher catalytic activity relative to other PGE synthases and, like COX2, its expression can be induced by cytokines and inflammatory stimuli.[109] In contrast, the expression of cPGES and mPGES2 do not seem to be inducible and may play housekeeping functions.

Genetic disruption confirms that mPGES1$^{-/-}$ mice exhibit a marked reduction in inflammatory responses compared with mPGES1$^{+/+}$ mice,[112] and indicates that mPGES1 is critical for the induction of inflammatory fever.[113] It has been proposed that mPGES1 couples primarily to the inducible COX2 in inflammatory cells.[114] In contrast, intrarenal expression of mPGES1 maps to cells of the collecting duct that primarily express COX1 with lower expression in medullary interstitial cells and macula densa that express COX2[84,115–117] (Figure 17.2). Thus, in the kidney mPGE1 co-localizes with both cyclooxygenase 1 and 2.

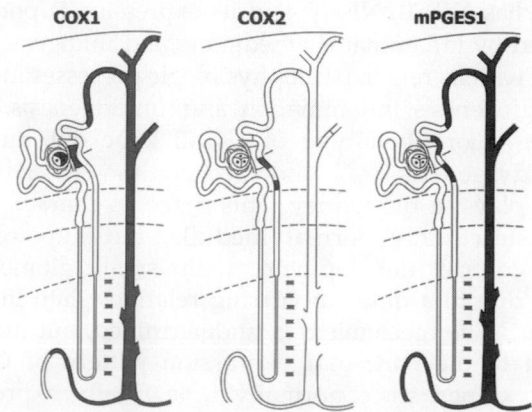

FIGURE 17.2 Expression of COX1, COX2, and microsomal prostaglandin E synthase 1 in the kidney. *(With permission from ref.* [84].*)*

The renal phenotype of the mPGE1 knockout mouse is relatively subtle, and is characterized by increased blood pressure sensitivity to high-sodium diet and mineralocorticoids, as well as increased vascular reactivity to angiotensin-II,[118,119] although not all investigators have seen these effects.[120] These results are consistent with a role for mPGES1-derived PGE_2 in buffering physiologic stresses that tend to increase blood pressure. Notably, the kidneys of mPGES1$^{-/-}$ mice are normal and do not exhibit the renal dysgenesis observed in COX2$^{-/-}$ mice.[78,80] Nor do these mice exhibit perinatal death from patent ductus arteriosus observed with the prostaglandin EP4 receptor knockout mouse,[121] suggesting other sources of PGE2 production are sufficient to provide adequate receptor activation. These sources could include cPGES and mPGES2.[122] Both cPGES and mPGES2 are expressed in the kidney[123]; however, their intrarenal role(s) have not yet been elucidated. In addition, several cytosolic glutathione-S-transferases have the capacity to convert PGH_2 to PGE_2; however, their physiologic role in this process remains uncertain.[122]

E-Prostanoid Receptors

All four E-Prostanoid receptors (EP receptors) are expressed in the kidney (Figure 17.3). Each exhibits a distinct mRNA expression profile along the nephron. The EP4 receptor predominates in the glomerulus, while the EP3 and EP1 receptors are primarily detected in the thick limb and collecting duct.[105,124] The EP2 receptor is expressed at lower levels in the renal vaculature and stroma.[125,126] Each receptor plays a distinct role in these regions, mediating many of the well-defined physiologic actions of PGE_2 that have been identified over the past several decades.

EP₁ Receptor

The EP1 receptor was originally identified pharmacologically via its smooth muscle constrictor activity in guinea pig ileum, and its unique profile of response to a series of prostanoid analogs.[127–130] The EP1 receptor cDNA has been cloned from numerous species, including human, dog, mouse, rat, and rabbit.[131–135] The human EP1 receptor cDNA encodes a 402 amino acid polypeptide with a predicted molecular mass of 41,858 kDa.[131] This receptor signals via a mechanism linked to increased cell Ca^{2+}, and is accompanied by modest increases in IP_3 generation.

Studies of EP1 receptors have taken advantage of several relatively selective antagonists that block their activation, including SC-19220, SC-53122,[136,137] and ONO-8130.[138–141] A significant impetus behind the development of clinically active EP1 receptor antagonists derives from evidence that the EP₁ receptor plays an important role in prostaglandin-mediated pain,[140,142,143] and that EP1 receptor antagonists have EP1 properties.[136,137,139,144,145] These antagonists provide useful tools to study EP₁ receptor physiology *in vivo*.

The EP1 receptor is highly expressed in the kidney, where it primarily localizes to the collecting duct with an increasing mRNA expression gradient from the cortical to the medullary collecting duct.[105,132,146] In the collecting duct, activation of the EP1 receptor inhibits Na^+ and water reabsorption via a Ca^{2+}-coupled mechanism.[132] These results suggest that renal EP₁ receptor activation contributes to PGE_2-dependent natriuresis by inhibiting Na^+ transport in the collecting duct. Despite this *in vitro* demonstration, these natriuretic effects have been difficult to demonstrate *in vivo*.[132,143]

Genetic disruption of the EP1 receptor does not lead to a significant impairment of sodium excretion; however, EP1 knockout mice do exhibit increased renin and aldosterone levels, consistent with maintenance of normotension at the expense of activation of the renin–angiotensin system.[132,143] EP1 receptor knockout mice not only exhibit reduced blood pressure on normal chow, but also impaired pressor response to angiotensin II.[145] These studies identified EP1 mRNA expression in small resistance vessels of mice including the afferent arterioles of the glomerulus, and are

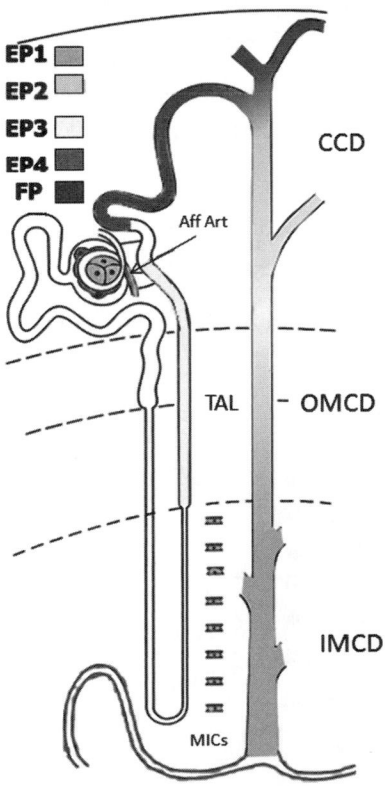

FIGURE 17.3 Distribution of EP1, 2, 3, 4, and FP receptors in the kidney.

consistent with more recent studies suggesting Ang II-stimulated vasoconstriction may in part be mediated by activation of vascular EP1 receptors.[147] EP1 receptors have also been identified in glomerular mesangial cells, where they may contribute to mesangial contraction. Inhibition of the EP1 receptor slows the progression of mesangial expansion in experimental models of diabetic nephropathy.[139] EP1 receptor knockout mice are resistant to the pressor effects of angiotensin II, and EP1 receptor antagonists can also block the Ang II pressor activity.[145,147–149] It is instructive to consider the role of PGE2 as a vasoconstrictor through its actions on the EP1 receptor, as opposed to its classically characterized role as a vasodilator/vasodepressor. This underscores the capacity of PGE2 to serve as a physiological buffer of blood pressure, either in support or reduction of blood pressure (see below).

EP2 Receptors

In contrast to the smooth muscle constrictor activity of the EP1 receptor, the EP2 receptor was originally defined by its relaxant activity in smooth muscle.[128] The human EP2 receptor cDNA encodes a 358 amino acid polypeptide, which signals through increased cAMP and is selectively activated by butaprost.[150] The EP2 receptor may be distinguished from the EP4 receptor, the other major cAMP stimulating and vasorelaxant EP receptor, by its selective activation by butaprost and relative insensitivity to the EP4 agonist PGE1-OH.[150] Literature prior to 1995 may be confusing regarding the EP2receptor, because before the human EP2 receptor was cloned, the previously cloned EP4 receptor was classified as the EP2 receptor.[150,151]

The physiological processes mediated by the EP2 receptor include important roles in reproduction and blood pressure regulation. The precise tissue distribution of the EP2 receptor has only been characterized by Northern blot analysis of mRNA distribution. This reveals a major mRNA species of ~3.1 kb that is most abundant in the uterus, lung, and spleen, exhibiting only low levels of expression in the kidney.[135,150,152] EP2 knockout mice exhibit a fertility defect and the development of hypertension on a high NaCl diet (these latter effects are significantly influenced by the genetic background of the mouse strain).[153,154] In the kidney, despite incomplete histological characterization, a preponderance of functional and mRNA expression evidence suggests the EP2 receptor is expressed in stromal cells of the kidney, including renal medullary interstitial cells,[125] vascular pericytes along the vasa recta,[126,155,156] and glomerular arterioles where it contributes to afferent arteriolar dilation (Figure 17.4).[126,157] Evidence suggests that deletion of the EP2 receptor in renal medullary interstitial cells,[158] combined with the absence of its systemic vasodilator activity, contributes to salt-sensitive hypertension in the EP2 knockout mouse.

EP3 Receptor

In smooth muscle the EP3 receptor generally acts as a constrictor.[159,160] This receptor is unique, in that at least seven alternatively spliced variants defined by unique COOH-terminal cytoplasmic tails exist in humans alone, and over 22 unique variants have been observed in rats, rabbits, mice, cows, and humans.[161–164] These splice variants encode proteins of a predicted molecular mass between 40 and 45 kDa.[161–164] All the EP3 splice variants bind PGE2 and the EP3 specific prostanoid analogs with similar affinity, and inhibit cAMP generation via a pertussis toxin-sensitive G_i-coupled mechanism; however, additional signaling mechanisms may be differentially activated by the different COOH-terminal tails.[165]

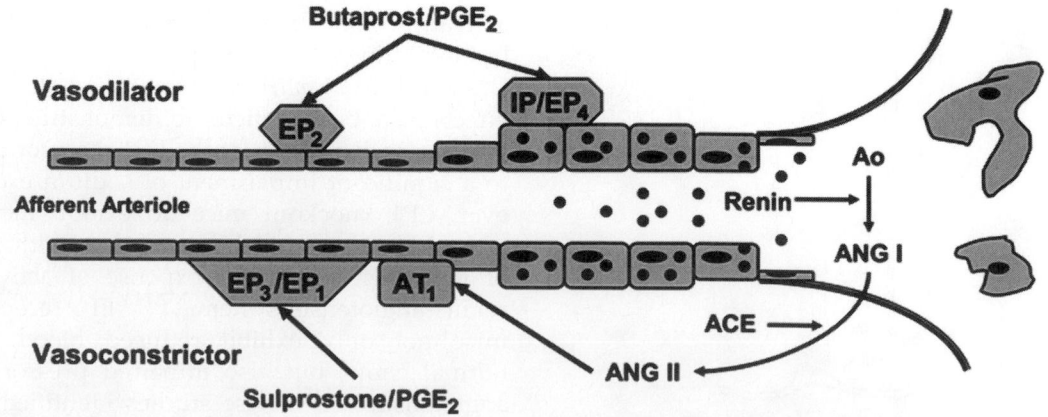

FIGURE 17.4 Schematic of prostanoid receptor action at the afferent arteriole including EP1, EP2, EP3, EP4, and IP receptors. *(From ref. [157], with permission from Am J. Physiol.)*

Mice with targeted deletion of the EP_3 receptor exhibit an impaired febrile response to lipopolysaccaride and PGE_2, suggesting that the EP_3 receptor antagonists could be effective antipyretic agents.[166] In the kidney the EP_3 receptor is highly expressed in the cortical and outer medullary collecting duct, where it antagonizes vasopressin-stimulated water absorption via pertussis toxin-sensitive inhibition of cAMP generation.[167,168] Despite relatively high levels of EP_3 receptor in the kidney collecting duct, mice with targeted disruption of this receptor only display a subtle alteration with altered urinary concentrating ability in mice treated with NSAIDs.[169] These findings raise the possibility that prostaglandin receptors other than the EP_3 receptor exert overlapping effects that also (such as the EP1 and FP receptor) modulate the urinary concentration and dilution by this segment of the nephron.

EP_4 Receptor

The EP_4 receptor can be distinguished from the EP_1 and EP_3 receptors by its insensitivity to sulprostone, and from EP_2 receptors by its insensitivity to butaprost and relatively selective activation by PGE_1-OH.[129,150,170,171] The human EP_4 receptor cDNA encodes a 488 amino acid polypeptide with a predicted molecular mass of ~53 kDa.[171] Like the EP_2 receptor, EP_4 signals through increased cAMP, but may also engage other signaling mechanisms including PI3K activation.[172,173] EP_4 receptor mRNA is relatively highly expressed compared with the EP_2 receptor and widely distributed, with a major species of ~3.8 kb detected by Northern analysis in thymus, ileum, lung, spleen, adrenal gland, and kidney.[133,174,175] In contrast to other EP receptor knockouts, EP4 receptor knockout mice exhibit a profound perinatal lethal phenotype due to impaired closure of the ductus arteriosus,[121,176] consistent with its robust expression in this vessel.

In the kidney, EP4 receptor mRNA is predominantly expressed in the glomerulus[105,124,126] where it modulates glomerular hemodynamics through opposing direct vasodilator activity,[157,177] and an indirect vasoconstrictor activity via stimulation of renin release (Figure 17.4).[178] The ability of PGE_2 to increase renin release is well-established[178–181] and of clinical relevance, since NSAID blockade of prostaglandin synthesis can be associated with hyporeninemic hypoaldosteronism,[182] and COX2 inhibitors can block the hyper-reninemia associated with volume depletion or Bartter's syndrome.[101,183,184] Accumulating evidence supports a role for COX2-mediated PGE_2 production, and subsequent activation of juxtaglomerular EP4 receptor in mediating renin release.[93,181]

As mPGES-specific inhibitors and EP4 receptor antagonists become increasingly available it will be important to determine the relative contribution of PGE2-dependent renin release versus prostacyclin-dependent effects (see below).

In volume depletion,[185] congestive heart failure,[186] and shock, intrarenal PGE_2 production helps maintain glomerular perfusion via afferent arteriolar vasodilator EP2 receptors[157] (Figure 17.4), while simultaneously maintaining systemic blood pressure by stimulating renin release through EP4 receptors.[187,188] Genetic deletion of the EP4 receptor or EP4 inhibitors impairs renin release in mice following furosemide-induced volume depletion.[181] Inhibition of PGE_2 synthesis using NSAIDs or COX2 inhibition in these settings can actually drop blood pressure by inhibiting renin release,[189] and lead to acute renal failure due to decreased glomerular perfusion.[190–192]

The EP4 receptor is also abundant in glomerular podocytes.[124,193,194] In podocytes EP4 receptor activation may impair their ability to withstand mechanical stress, since podocyte selective overexpression of EP4 receptors accelerates renal injury in a mouse renal ablation model of kidney disease.[195]

Other roles for the EP4 receptor in controlling blood pressure have been suggested, including the ability to stimulate aldosterone release from zona glomerulosa cells.[196] It remains to be determined whether the adrenal EP4 receptor plays any role in hyperkalemia and hyporeninemic hypoaldosteronism associated with NSAID blockade of prostaglandin synthesis[182,197,198] or whether this is primarily due to hyporeninemia.[199] Important vasodilator effects of EP_4 receptor activation in venous and arterial beds have been described.[130,200] Roles for EP4 receptors in immune cell activation and osteoblast function have also been reported.[201–203]

Prostaglandin F Synthesis

$PGF_{2\alpha}$ may derive either directly from PGH_2 via a PGF synthase[204] or via a NADPH-dependent 9 keto-reductase, which converts PGE_2 into $PGF_{2\alpha}$. This enzymatic activity is typically cytosolic,[204] and may be detected in homogenates from renal cortex, medulla or papilla.[204,205] Another more obscure pathway for PGF formation is by the action of a PGD_2 ketoreductase, yielding a stereoisomer of $PGF_{2\alpha}$, $9\alpha,11\beta$-PGF_2 (11epi-$PGF_{2\alpha}$).[204] This reaction, and conversion of PGD_2 into the biologically active metabolite ($9\alpha,11\beta$-$PGF_{2\alpha}$) has been documented *in vivo*.[206] This $PGF_{2\alpha}$ isomer can also ligate and activate the FP receptor.[207] The physiologically relevant enzymes responsible for $PGF_{2\alpha}$ formation in the kidney remain incompletely characterized.

Prostaglandin 9-Ketoreductase (PG9KR) and PGF$_{2\alpha}$ Synthesis

Prostaglandin F synthase activity may be mediated via several distinct, and incompletely defined, enzymes. One major synthetic pathway appears to occur via a member of the aldo-ketoreductase 1C family.[208] Renal PGE$_2$ 9-ketoreductase also exhibits 20α-hydroxyl-steroid reductase activity that may be involved in steroid metabolism.[204] PG9KR activity appears to be particularly robust in suspensions from the thick ascending limb of Henle (TALH).

Interestingly, some studies suggest activity of a 9-ketoreductase may be modulated by salt intake and the angiotensin AT2 receptor.[209] This activity may play a role in the development of salt-sensitive hypertension.[210] AT2 receptor knockout mice exhibit salt-sensitive hypertension associated with increased PGE$_2$ production and reduced production of PGF$_{2\alpha}$,[209] consistent with decreased 9-ketoreductase activity. Other studies suggest increased dietary potassium intake may also enhance the activity of conversion from PGE$_2$ to PGF$_{2\alpha}$.[211] The intrarenal sites of expression of this enzymatic activity remain to be characterized.

F-Prostanoid Receptors

Once formed, PGF$_{2\alpha}$ is available to interact with the intrarenal FP receptors. The human FP receptor mRNA is predicted to encode 359 amino acid residues with a molecular mass of ~ 40 kDa.[212] In fibroblasts and smooth muscle the FP receptor signals through increased cellular calcium, and its activation is associated with muscle contraction.[213–215] The FP receptor is highly expressed in the ovarian corpus luteum, and mice lacking the FP receptor exhibit a major reproductive defect due to failure of partuition because of impaired reduction of progesterone at term.[216] FP receptor antagonists have been developed, and their use proposed as a means of delaying pre-term delivery.[217,218] The FP receptor is highly expressed in the ocular ciliary body and FP selective agonists including travaprost, latanoprost, and bimatoprost are in use for clinical treatment of glaucoma d.[214,219] In the kidney, the FP receptor is highly expressed in the distal convoluted tubule, connecting tubule, and cortical collecting duct, where it inhibits vasopressin-stimulated renal water transport[104,220] consistent with recent studies that the FP receptor knockout mice exhibit mild polyuria and polydipsia.[221] Interestingly, in the rabbit cortical collecting duct epithelium the FP receptor appears to signal through a pertussis toxin-sensitive G$_i$-coupled mechanism, rather than the classical Ca^{2+}-coupled signaling mechanism observed in smooth muscle cells.[104]

Vascular expression of FP receptor in pre-glomerular arterioles and other resistance vessels has also been demonstrated, and studies in FP receptor knockout mice show they are relatively hypotensive.[221] These studies also provide evidence that renal JGA FP receptor activation directly stimulates renin release.[221]

Prostaglandin D$_2$ is derived from PGH$_2$ via the action of specific enzymes designated PGD synthases. Two major enzymes are capable of transforming PGH$_2$ to PGD$_2$ — a lipocalin type PGD synthase and a hematopoietic type PGDS.[222,223] RT-PCR showed that L-PGDS is strongly expressed in kidney cortex and outer medulla, including in nearly all segments of the nephron,[224] while H-PGDS mRNA is only detected in microdissected outer medullary collecting duct.[224]

Lipocalin PGD synthase (L-PGDS) is a multifunctional molecule, and on addition to prostaglandin H2 it binds a variety of small lipophilic molecules including bilirubin and biliverdin.[225] Mice lacking the lipocalin D synthase gene exhibit pain sensation.[226] LPGDS-mediated PGD2 synthesis also appears to play an important role in the sleep/wake cycle,[225] but its role in renal PGD2 synthesis has not been studied. Urinary levels of L-PGDS, also known as beta-trace protein, have been increasingly studied as a biomarker of acute and chronic renal injury.[227–230] LPDGS knockout mice appear to be more susceptible to diabetic nephropathy.[231]

PGD$_2$ is the major prostanoid released from mast cells following challenge with IgE, and this synthesis appears to be mediated by the hematopoietic form of PGDS.[223,232,233] The precise role of hematopoietic PGDS in the kidney remains uncertain, as does the significance of its reported localization in the outer medullary collecting duct.[224]

D-Prostanoid Receptors

Once synthesized, PGD$_2$ is available to interact with either the DP1 or DP2 (originally identified as CRTH2) receptors or undergo further metabolism to a PGF$_2$-like compound that can interact with the FP receptor (see above). The human DP1 receptor is a cAMP-coupled GPCR with a predicted molecular mass similar to other prostanoid receptors (~ 40 kDa).[234,235] It exhibits a relatively selective tissue distribution, with particularly high expression in retina and small intestine, where it appears to be highly expressed in mucus secreting goblet cells.[235] The DP2 receptor is a GPCR that is also activated by PGD2, but it is unrelated in sequence to the classic prostanoid receptor family, being more closely related to members of the N-formyl peptide receptor (FPR) subfamily.[236,237] DP2 is selectively expressed in Th2 cells, cytotoxic T-cells, eosinophils, and basophils. DP and DP2 receptors are intimately involved in the immune allergic response.[236,238] Neither DP1 receptors nor DP2 receptors appear to be highly expressed in the kidney, and while infusion of a DP1 selective agonist lowers blood pressure these effects appear to be primarily due to peripheral vasodilation and not by directly affecting renal blood flow.[239]

Prostacyclin (PGI$_2$)

The biological effects of prostacyclin are numerous and include nocioception, anti-thrombosis, and vasodilator actions, which have been targeted therapeutically to treat pulmonary hypertension.[240] Prostacyclin (PGI$_2$) is derived from the enzymatic conversion of PGH$_2$ via prostacyclin synthase (PGIS) to PGI$_2$. The PGIS cDNA is comprised of a 1500 bp open reading frame that encodes a 500 amino acid protein of approximately 56 kDa.[241] Northern blot analysis shows prostacyclin synthase mRNA is widely expressed in human tissues and is particularly abundant in ovary, heart, skeletal muscle, lung, and prostate. PGI synthase expression exhibits segmental expression in the kidney, especially in kidney inner medulla tubules and interstitial cells.[224,242]

PGI$_2$ synthase-null mice exhibit a profound renal phenotype with nephrosclerosis and areas of renal infarction.[243] PGI$_2$ levels in the plasma, kidneys, and lungs were reduced, documenting the role of this enzyme as an *in vivo* source of PGI$_2$. Blood pressure and blood urea nitrogen and creatinine in the PGIS knockout mice were significantly increased, and renal pathological findings included surface irregularity, fibrosis, cysts, arterial sclerosis, and hypertrophy of vessel walls. Thickening of the thoracic aortic media and adventitia were observed in aged PGIS-null mice.[243] Interestingly, this is a phenotype different from that reported for the IP receptor knockout mouse,[244] which failed to exhibit abnormal kidney morphology. These differences suggests the presence of additional IP receptor independent PGI$_2$ activated signaling pathways — possibly through nuclear receptors such as PPARdelta.[245,246] Regardless, these findings demonstrate the importance of PGI$_2$ in the maintenance of blood vessels and to the kidney.

IP Receptor

The IP receptor mRNA is highly expressed in the afferent arteriole, where it may combine with the effects of EP2 and EP4 receptors to dilate renal arterioles and stimulate renin release.[247,248] IP receptor deficient mice exhibit reduced renin and are resistant to the development of hypertension following unilateral renal artery stenosis, consistent with an impaired IP receptor-mediated renin release.[249] COX2-derived prostacyclin from the endothelium also appears to serve an atheroprotective role in mice, and its loss could contribute to the cardiovascular risks associated with the use of COX2 inhibitors.[250] Conversely, thromboxane receptors may counteract the effects of these protective effects of prostacyclin and accelerate atherosclerotic lesions, as well as increasing vascular resistance.

Thromboxane A2

Thromboxane A$_2$ (TxA$_2$) is produced from PGH$_2$ by thromboxane synthase (TxAS), a microsomal protein of 533 amino acids with a predicted molecular weight of ~ 60 kDa. The human gene is located on chromosome 7q, and the enzyme exhibits homology to the cytochrome P450s and is now classified as CYP5A1.[251] TxAS mRNA is highly expressed in hematopoietic cells, including platelets, macrophages, and leukocytes, as well as thymus, kidney, lung, spleen, prostate, and placenta.[252,253] Immunolocalization of TxA synthase demonstrates high expression in the dendritic cells of the interstitium, with lower expression in glomerular podocytes of human kidney.[254] In the kidney, thromboxane synthase is mainly detected in the glomeruli.[224] TxA$_2$ synthase expression is regulated by dietary salt intake.[255] Furthermore, experimental use of ridogrel, a specific thromboxane synthase inhibitor, reduced blood pressure in spontaneously hypertensive rats.[256] The clinical use of TxA$_2$ synthase inhibitors is complicated by the fact that its endoperoxide precursors (PGG$_2$/PGH$_2$) are also capable of activating its downstream target, the TP receptor,[257] so thromboxane receptor antagonists would be expected to more definitively interfere with this pathway.

TP Receptor

The thromboxane receptor (TP) was the first member of the prostanoid receptor family cloned.[258] This GPCR has a predicted molecular mass ~ 37.5 kDa, and is highly expressed in platelets and vascular tissue where its activation increases intracellular calcium.[258] In the kidney TP receptor mRNA is predominantly expressed in the glomerulus and vascular tissue,[224,259] where it contributes to vasoconstrictor activity following Ang II infusion[260] and following renal injury.[261–263]

Prostaglandin Transport

One of the major areas of uncertainty in eicosanoid research is precisely how prostanoids, synthesized inside the cell, transit the cell membrane to become available to interact with cell surface receptors.

Recent studies have identified several transmembrane proteins capable of facilitated transport of prostaglandins across cell membranes.[264] Schuster's group identified a lactate/PGE_2 exchanger they designated prostaglandin transporter or PGT.[265] The importance of PGT in mediating the *in vivo* effects of PGE_2 has been substantially bolstered by studies showing genetic disruption of the PGT gene is associated with perinatal death due to persistence of a patent ductus arteriosus[266] recapitulating the phenotype of the EP4 receptor knockout.[121,176] Although this prostaglandin transporter appears poised primarily to provide a PGE2 re-uptake mechanism, it is notable that the transporter is expressed in renal cells that are major sites of prostaglandin synthesis,[267] rather than those renal cells involved in PGE_2 inactivation.[264] These findings are consistent with the possibility that PGT plays an important role in directing vectorial PGE_2 release. Nevertheless, it seems unlikely that this protein comprises the pathway mediating PGE_2 release. More recent evidence supports a role for the multi-drug resistance protein 4 (MRP4) as a potential PGE_2 efflux mechanism.[268] MRP4 knockout mice exhibit low levels of circulating PGE_2 and reduced inflammatory pain,[269] consistent with a role in PGE2 extrusion.

Prostaglandins and the Pathogenesis of Kidney Disease

Renal Inflammation

Increased glomerular COX1 or COX2 expression has been reported in patients with nephritis, and in animal models of nephritis.[270,271] Glomerular expression of COX2 is upregulated in patients with active lupus nephritis and in lupus nephritis animal models.[270,272] COX2 inhibition has shown beneficial effects on passive Heymann nephritis (PHN), a model of membranous nephropathy.[273] Cell culture studies show that thromboxane A2 contributes to complement-induced cytotoxicity of glomerular epithelial cells.[273] In contrast, in anti-Thy1.1 glomerulonephritis model, an animal model of mesangioproliferative glomerulonephritis (MPGN) that is characterized by endothelial injury, COX2 inhibition is associated with increased mesangiolysis, albuminuria, and delayed recovery from glomerular injury.[274] Further studies suggest that healing of injured glomerular capillary endothelium in this model may depend on COX2-derived prostanoids, and COX2 inhibition may lead to impaired capillary endothelium healing.[274] The role of COX-derived prostanoids in autoimmune and inflammatory disease has been well-documented.[275,276] COX2 expression and prostanoid biosynthesis can be induced in macrophages and dendritic cells by inflammatory agents, such as LPS, IL-1ß, and interferon.[74,75] PGDS expression or activity has been described in dendritic cells, macrophage, eosinophil, neutrophil, and mast cells.[106] Prostanoids, particularly PGE2 and PGI2, have been shown to enhance inflammatory reactions.[106] Conversely prostanoids also exert anti-inflammatory effects. The pro- or anti-inflammatory effect of prostanoids is dependent on specific prostanoid, receptor subtype, cell population, and context of activation.[106] Additional studies are required to define the precise roles of prostanoids in different forms of glomerulonephritis.

Renal COX-Derived Prostanoids and Diabetic Nephropathy

Diabetic nephropathy is characterized by microalbuminuria, glomerular hypertrophy, mesangial expansion with glomerular basement membrane thickening, arteriolar hyalinosis, and global glomerular sclerosis, which ultimately lead to the progression to proteinuria and renal failure.[277,278] Supra-normal GFR (hyperfiltration) typifies the early stages of diabetic nephropathy.[279–282] Studies in diabetic humans and streptozotocin (STZ)-induced type I diabetic rats show increased renal PGE2, PGI2, and TxB2 levels.[282–285] COX2 expression is increased in the thick ascending limb and macula densa in diabetic humans and rodents.[286–288] Selective COX2 inhibition reduces glomerular hyperfiltration in streptozotocin-induced diabetic rats, consistent with COX2-derived prostanoids increasing renal blood flow in the diabetic kidney.[288] The identity of the specific COX2-derived prostanoids and their cognate receptors involved in pathogenesis of diabetic hyperfiltration has not been completely characterized. EP1 receptor antagonist treatment ameliorates renal and glomerular hypertrophy, and decreases mesangial expansion.[139] A thromboxane receptor (TP) antagonist has also been reported to attenuate proteinuria and ameliorate histological changes of diabetic nephropathy in diabetic apolipoprotein E-deficient mice.[289] It has not been determined whether similar beneficial effects might be observed in human diabetic nephropathy.

Prostaglandins and Progression of Kidney Disease

COX-derived prostanoids may also modify renal function and glomerular damage in non-diabetic chronic renal disease.[290,291] After subtotal renal ablation, renal cortical COX2 expression is increased, predominantly in the macula densa and surrounding cTAL.[291,292] Selective COX2 inhibition decreases proteinuria and inhibits the development of glomerular sclerosis.[291,292] These studies are consistent with a role of COX2-derived prostanoids in the pathogenesis of structural and functional deterioration of kidney in chronic kidney disease.

LIPOXYGENASE DERIVED EICOSANOIDS: 5-, 12-, AND 15-HETES AND LEUKOTRIENES

Arachidonic acid may be metabolized to form leukotrienes and hydroxyeicosatetraenoic acids (HETEs) by a family of enzymes designated lipoxygenases[293,294] (Figure 17.5). Leukotriene arachidonic acid metabolites play a major role in inflammatory disease, especially asthma and other inflammatory pulmonary diseases where cysteinyl leukotriene receptor antagonists have found a place as a standard of care.[295,296] In contrast to the prostaglandins, it has been difficult to demonstrate a major role for leukotrienes in the normal kidney.

Lipoxygenases (LOX) are comprised of non-heme iron containing enzymes that insert molecular oxygen into polyunsaturated fatty acids such as arachidonic acid and linoleic acid.[294,297] Six functional human lipoxygenases have been cloned: 5-lipoxygenase (gene name: ALOX5); platelet-type 12-lipoxygenase (gene name: ALOX12); 12/15-lipoxygenase (leukocyte-type 12-LO for mice, 15-LO type 1 for human, gene name: ALOX15); epidermal-type 12-lipoxgenase (gene name: ALOXE3); 12(R)-lipoxygenase (gene name: ALOX12B); and 15-lipoxygenase type 2 (gene name: ALOX15B, 8-lipoxygenase in mice).[293,297]

5-Lipoxygenase is the key enzyme in leukotriene biosynthesis.[293,296,297] In the presence of 5-LO-activating protein (FLAP)[298] 5-lipoxygenase catalyzes the generation of leukotriene A4 (LTA4). LTA4, in turn, is converted by LTA4 hydrolase to LTB4, capable of activating LTB4 receptors. LTB4 is a potent chemotactic substance, and increases polymorphonuclear leukocytes (PMN) aggregation and adhesion to the endothelium.[299,300] Alternatively, LTA4 can be converted to cysteinyl (cys) leukotrienes (LTC4, LTD4, and LTE4) through leukotriene C4 synthase.[297] LTC4 and LTD4 contract vascular smooth muscle cells and increase vascular permeability.[301–304] These leukotrienes are usually released locally by leukocytes. Mice with 5-LO gene disruption exhibit a reduced inflammatory reaction,[305–307] supporting the pro-inflammatory action of 5-LO-derived metabolites. Recently, increased expression of leukotriene C4 synthase and formation of cysteinyl-leukotrienes have been reported in human abdominal aortic aneurysm.[308]

As might be predicted from its expression in inflammatory cells, 5-LO-derived products appear to play an important role in glomerular immune injury.[309–311] 5-LO mRNA and 5-LOX-activating protein (FLAP) mRNA are detected in the glomeruli and vasa recta.[312] Both leukotriene receptor B4 and the cysteinyl leukotriene receptor type 1 are selectively expressed in the

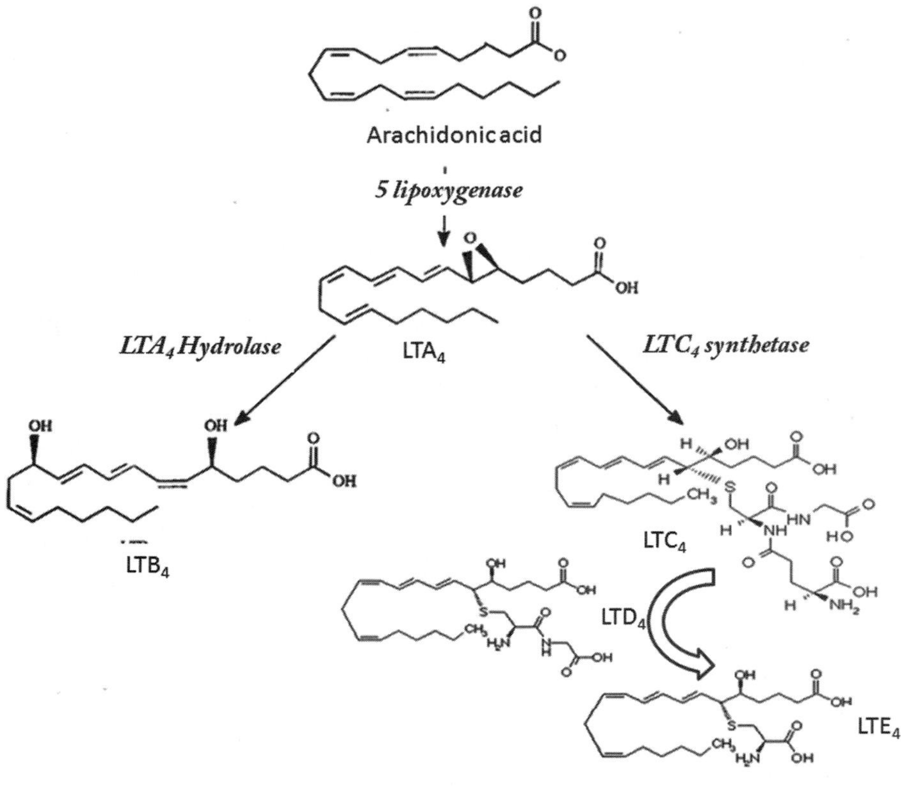

FIGURE 17.5 Leukotriene synthetic pathway.

glomerulus,[312] suggesting 5-LO products are involved in glomerular function. Glomerular synthesis of LTB4 and LTC4/LTD4 is markedly enhanced in both human disease and experimental glomerular immune injury.[313–315] LTD4 may contribute to the reduction of GFR in the acute phase of injury by virtue of its potent vasoconstrictor action and contraction of mesangial cells.[314] LTD4 may also increase intraglomerular pressure, contributing to proteinuria.[315] LTB4, a potent promoter of PMN attraction, participates in glomerular damage by amplifying PMN-dependent mechanisms of injury.[314]

The biological functions of the other members of the lipoxygenase family are more obscure. The 12-LO, catalyzes the formation of oxidized lipids 12(S)-hydroxyeicosatetraenoic acid [12(S)-HETE]. Human 15-LO type 1 shares high homology with rodent leukocyte-type 12-LO; both can mediate the formation of 12(S)-HETE and 15(S)-HETE from arachidonic acid, and are thus classified as 12/15-LO.[293,297,316] Some evidence suggests that 12(S)-HETE and 15(S)-HETE play important roles in systemic homeostasis and renal–cardiovascular pathology[317,318]; however, specific receptors for these products have not yet been identified. A recent study implicates ALOX15 as playing a role in bone mineralization.[319] 12/15-Lipoxygenase products also appear to be involved in the pathogenesis of atherosclerosis.[320]

12/15-Lipoxygenase-derived products may contribute to the pathogenesis of diabetic complications, including diabetic nephropathy.[321,322] 12/15-LO is detected in renal microvessels, glomeruli, and mesangial cells.[312,323,324] 12/15-LO levels are increased in the glomeruli of experimental diabetic animals.[321,325] The 12/15 LO pathway has been shown to be a critical mediator of TGFβ and angiotensin II (ANG II)-induced mesangial cell hypertrophy and extracellular matrix accumulation.[322,326,327] These studies also suggest that ANG II-induced mesangial cell hypertrophy and extracellular matrix synthesis in cultured rat mesangial cells can be blocked by an LO inhibitor or targeted 12/15 LO gene deletion.

CYTOCHROME P450 MONOOXYGENASE-DERIVED EICOSANOIDS: 20-HETE AND EETS

Free arachidonic acid can also be metabolized by the cytochrome P450 monooxygenases (CYP450) to produce hydroxy- and epoxy-arachidonic acid derivatives.[328,329] The major CYP450-catalyzed reactions in most tissues are mediated by epoxygenase and ω-hydroxylase activities of the CYP450 family, which are responsible for biosynthesis of epoxyeicosatrienoic acids (EETs) and 20-hydroxyeicosatetraenoic acid (20-HETE), respectively[328,329] (Figure 17.6). These metabolites have been shown to possess biological activity, but the mechanisms mediating these biological effects remain obscure since specific receptors have not been identified.[48,330,331]

Members of the P450 *CYP2C*, and *2J* subfamilies have been identified as functionally relevant epoxygenases, while members of 4A and 4F are ω-hydroxylases, respectively.[48,331–333] 20-HETE is a potent vasoconstrictor.[334–336] EETs are produced in the vascular endothelium, and are potent vasodilators.[337,338] EETs are also produced in tubules, including the proximal tubule and collecting ducts in the rodent kidney.[335,339] EETs have been shown to inhibit ENaC activity,[339,340] which may contribute to their natriuretic effect. EETs have also been shown to mediate the natriuretic effect of angiotensin II.[339,341] Studies of knockout mice have supported a role for CYP450 metabolism in the regulation of blood pressure, but the mechanisms of these effects remain incompletely understood. Genetic disruption of CYP2J8 was associated with hypertension in females, but it is uncertain whether this effect is related to its arachidonate epoxygenase activity in mice or an effect on estrogen metabolism.[342] Genetic disruption of cyp4a10 and 4a14 are also associated with hypertension,[343,344] adding to uncertainty regarding the distinct roles of epoxygenase and ω-hydroxylase activity of arachidonic acid in regulating vascular tone and blood pressure.

Role of Renal CYP450-Derived Arachidonate Metabolites in Renal Damage

Increased EET formation has been reported in the kidney of rats with liver cirrhosis. While it is well-documented that renal vasoconstriction leading to impaired renal function occurs during cirrhosis, this result suggests increased EET synthesis may be a homeostatic response to help preserve renal perfusion.[345] Reduced CYP arachidonate hydroxyglase activity and 20-HETE levels have been reported in the kidney following ischemia and reperfusion. Reduced CYP4A protein expression and enzyme activity in ischemia/reperfusion was suggested as an adaptive mechanism to preserve renal vasculature from excessive vasoconstriction.[346] Other studies suggest that the CYP hydroxylase-derived product 20-HETE plays an important role in the maintenance of the glomerular protein permeability barrier.[347] An *in vitro* glomerular albumin permeability study using isolated rat glomeruli shows that puromycin aminonucleoside (PAN) significantly increases glomerular albumin permeability.[347] 20-HETE treatment blocks PAN-induced increase in albumin permeability.[347]

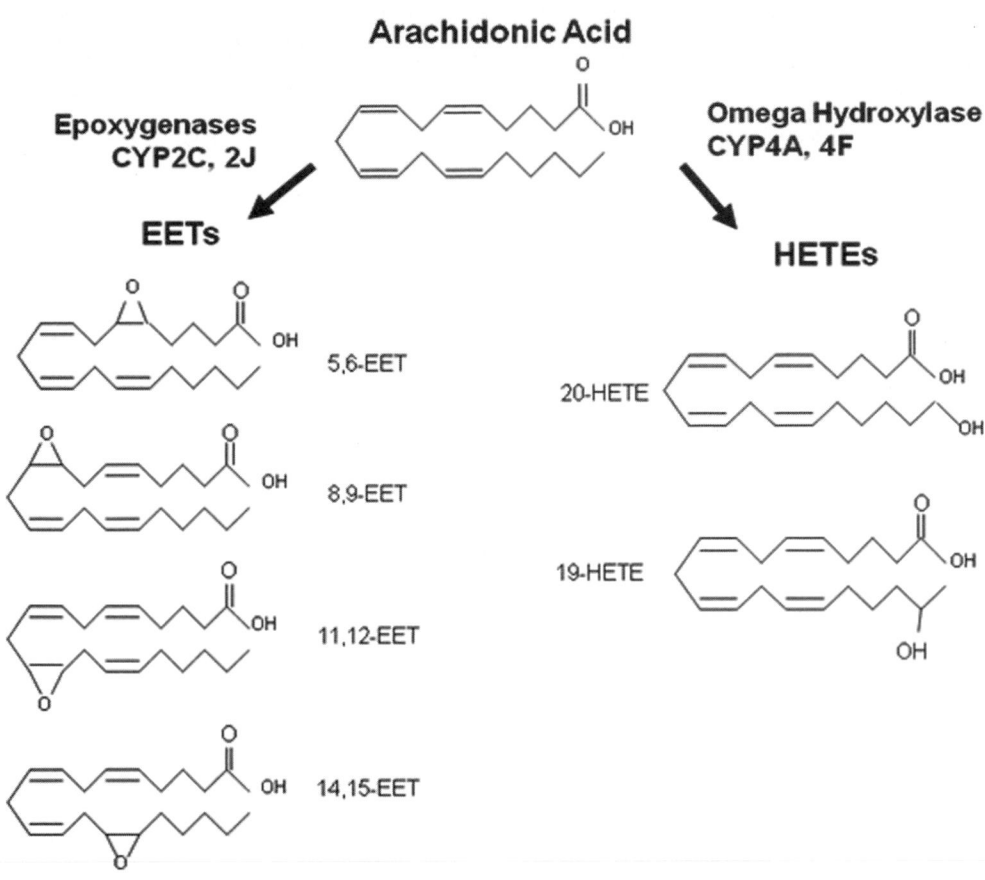

FIGURE 17.6 Products of cytochrome P450-mediated metabolism of arachidonic acid.

SUMMARY

Eicosanoids exert diverse and sometimes self-opposing functions. The specific effect of each eicosanoid depends on sequential enzymatic machinery in a specific cell, yielding a specific eicosanoid, exerting its distinct function. The biosynthesis of each eicosanoid is regulated at multiple levels from phospholipase A2 that catalyzes the release of arachidonic acid to specific enzymes that catalyze the formation of bioactive eicosanoids. Arachidonate-derived eicosanoids including prostanoids, leukotrienes, 12/15-HETEs, EETs, and HETEs, and sphingomyelin-derived ceramide play important roles in maintaining normal renal function. They are also involved in the pathophysiology of diabetic nephropathy, and inflammatory or toxic glomerular injury. Those signaling pathways should provide a fruitful area to identify targets for intervention in the pharmacologic treatment of renal disease.

References

[1] Page J, Henry D. Consumption of NSAIDs and the development of congestive heart failure in elderly patients: an underrecognized public health problem. Arch Intern Med 2000;160:777–84.

[2] White WB. Cardiovascular risk, hypertension, and NSAIDs. Curr Rheumatol Rep 2007;9:36–43.

[3] Breyer MD, Harris RC. Cyclooxygenase 2 and the kidney. Curr Opin Nephrol Hypertens 2001;10:89–98.

[4] Eras J, Perazella MA. NSAIDs and the kidney revisited: are selective cyclooxygenase-2 inhibitors safe? Am J Med Sci 2001; 321:181–90.

[5] Winkelmayer WC, Waikar SS, Mogun H, Solomon DH. Nonselective and cyclooxygenase-2-selective NSAIDs and acute kidney injury. Am J Med 2008;121:1092–8.

[6] Hansen AE, Burr GO. Essential fatty acids and human nutrition. J Am Med Assoc 1946;132:855–9.

[7] De Caterina R. n-3 Fatty acids in cardiovascular disease. N Engl J Med 2011;364:2439–50.

[8] Burr GO, Burr MM. Nutrition classics from The Journal of Biological Chemistry 82:345-67, 192[9] A new deficiency disease produced by the rigid exclusion of fat from the diet. Nutr Rev 1973;31:248–9.

[9] Lands WE. The biosynthesis and metabolism of prostaglandins. Annu Rev Physiol 1979;41:633–52.

[10] Dunham EW, Balasingam M, Privett OS, Nickell EC. Effects of essential fatty acid deficiency on prostaglandin synthesis and fatty acid composition in rat renal medulla. Lipids 1978;13:892–7.

[11] Moussa M, Garcia J, Ghisolfi J, Periquet B, Thouvenot JP. Dietary essential fatty acid deficiency differentially affects tissues of rats. J Nutr 1996;126:3040–5.

[12] Soares AF, Santiago RC, Alessio ML, Descomps B, de Castro-Chaves C. Biochemical, functional, and histochemical effects of

essential fatty acid deficiency in rat kidney. Lipids 2005; 40:1125—33.

[13] Boyanovsky BB, Webb NR. Biology of secretory phospholipase A2. Cardiovasc Drugs Ther 2009;23:61—72.

[14] Burke JE, Dennis EA. Phospholipase A2 structure/function, mechanism, and signaling. J Lipid Res 2009;50:S237—42.

[15] Boulven I, Palmier B, Robin P, Vacher M, Harbon S, Leiber D. Platelet-derived growth factor stimulates phospholipase C-gamma 1, extracellular signal-regulated kinase, and arachidonic acid release in rat myometrial cells: contribution to cyclic 3′,5′-adenosine monophosphate production and effect on cell proliferation. Biol Reprod 2001;65:496—506.

[16] Fujishima H, Sanchez Mejia RO, Bingham III CO, Lam BK, Sapirstein A, Bonventre JV, et al. Cytosolic phospholipase A2 is essential for both the immediate and the delayed phases of eicosanoid generation in mouse bone marrow-derived mast cells. Proc Natl Acad Sci USA 1999;96:4803—7.

[17] Samad TA, Moore KA, Sapirstein A, Billet S, Allchorne A, Poole S, et al. Interleukin-1beta-mediated induction of Cox-2 in the CNS contributes to inflammatory pain hypersensitivity. Nature 2001;410:471—5.

[18] Sapirstein A, Bonventre JV. Specific physiological roles of cytosolic phospholipase A(2) as defined by gene knockouts. Biochim Biophys Acta 2000;1488:139—48.

[19] Kudo I, Murakami M. Phospholipase A2 enzymes. Prostag Oth Lipid M 2002;68-69:3—58.

[20] Mangat H, Peterson LN, Burns KD. Hypercalcemia stimulates expression of intrarenal phospholipase A2 and prostaglandin H synthase-2 in rats. Role of angiotensin II AT1 receptors. J Clin Invest 1997;100:1941—50.

[21] Pavoine C, Behforouz N, Gauthier C, Le Gouvello S, Roudot-Thoraval F, Martin CR, et al. beta2-Adrenergic signaling in human heart: shift from the cyclic AMP to the arachidonic acid pathway. Mol Pharmacol 2003;64:1117—25.

[22] Xing M, Insel PA. Protein kinase C-dependent activation of cytosolic phospholipase A2 and mitogen-activated protein kinase by alpha 1-adrenergic receptors in Madin—Darby canine kidney cells. J Clin Invest 1996;97:1302—10.

[23] Jiao H, Cui XL, Torti M, Chang CH, Alexander LD, Lapetina EG, et al. Arachidonic acid mediates angiotensin II effects on p21ras in renal proximal tubular cells via the tyrosine kinase-Shc-Grb2-Sos pathway. Proc Natl Acad Sci USA 1998; 95:7417—21.

[24] Marin Castano ME, Schanstra JP, Hirtz C, Pesquero JB, Pecher C, Girolami JP, et al. B2 kinin receptor upregulation by cAMP is associated with BK-induced PGE2 production in rat mesangial cells. Am J Physiol 1998;274:F532—40.

[25] Murakami M, Kambe T, Shimbara S, Kudo I. Functional coupling between various phospholipase A2s and cyclooxygenases in immediate and delayed prostanoid biosynthetic pathways. J Biol Chem 1999;274:3103—15.

[26] Jacobs LS, Douglas JG. Angiotensin II type 2 receptor subtype mediates phospholipase A2-dependent signaling in rabbit proximal tubular epithelial cells. Hypertension 1996;28:663—8.

[27] Slivka SR, Insel PA. Alpha 1-adrenergic receptor-mediated phosphoinositide hydrolysis and prostaglandin E2 formation in Madin—Darby canine kidney cells. Possible parallel activation of phospholipase C and phospholipase A2. J Biol Chem 1987; 262:4200—7.

[28] Choi KH, Edelstein CL, Gengaro P, Schrier RW, Nemenoff RA. Hypoxia induces changes in phospholipase A2 in rat proximal tubules: evidence for multiple forms. Am J Physiol 1995;269: F846—53.

[29] Osada-Oka M, Takahashi M, Akiba S, Sato T. Involvement of Ca^{2+}-independent phospholipase A2 in the translocation of

hypoxia-inducible factor-1alpha to the nucleus under hypoxic conditions. Eur J Pharmacol 2006;549:58—62.

[30] Petry C, Huwiler A, Eberhardt W, Kaszkin M, Pfeilschifter J. Hypoxia increases group IIA phospholipase A(2) expression under inflammatory conditions in rat renal mesangial cells. J Am Soc Nephrol 2005;16:2897—905.

[31] Goto S, Nakamura H, Morooka H, Terao Y, Shibata O, Sumikawa K. Role of reactive oxygen in phospholipase A2 activation by ischemia/reperfusion of the rat kidney. J Anesth 1999;13:90—3.

[32] Alexander LD, Alagarsamy S, Douglas JG. Cyclic stretch-induced cPLA2 mediates ERK 1/2 signaling in rabbit proximal tubule cells. Kidney Int 2004;65:551—63.

[33] Bonventre JV. The 85-kD cytosolic phospholipase A2 knockout mouse: a new tool for physiology and cell biology. J Am Soc Nephrol 1999;10:404—12.

[34] DeRubertis FR, Craven PA. Eicosanoids in the pathogenesis of the functional and structural alterations of the kidney in diabetes. Am J Kidney Dis 1993;22:727—35.

[35] Beck S, Beck G, Ostendorf T, Floege J, Lambeau G, Nevalainen T, et al. Upregulation of group IB secreted phospholipase A(2) and its M-type receptor in rat ANTI-THY-1 glomerulonephritis. Kidney Int 2006;70:1251—60.

[36] Zager RA, Schimpf BA, Gmur DJ, Burke TJ. Phospholipase A2 activity can protect renal tubules from oxygen deprivation injury. Proc Natl Acad Sci USA 1993;90:8297—301.

[37] dos Reis MA, Costa RS, Coimbra TM, Teixeira VP. Acute renal failure in experimental envenomation with Africanized bee venom. Ren Fail 1998;20:39—51.

[38] Takasaki J, Kawauchi Y, Urasaki T, Tanaka H, Usuda S, Masuho Y. Antibodies against type II phospholipase A2 prevent renal injury due to ischemia and reperfusion in rats. FEBS Lett 1998;440:377—81.

[39] Beck Jr. LH, Bonegio RG, Lambeau G, Beck DM, Powell DW, Cummins TD, et al. M-type phospholipase A2 receptor as target antigen in idiopathic membranous nephropathy. N Engl J Med 2009;361:11—21.

[40] Lambeau G, Lazdunski M. Receptors for a growing family of secreted phospholipases A2. Trends Pharmacol Sci 1999; 20:162—70.

[41] Rouault M, Le Calvez C, Boilard E, Surrel F, Singer A, Ghomashchi F, et al. Recombinant production and properties of binding of the full set of mouse secreted phospholipases A2 to the mouse M-type receptor. Biochemistry 2007;46: 1647—62.

[42] Augert A, Payre C, de Launoit Y, Gil J, Lambeau G, Bernard D. The M-type receptor PLA2R regulates senescence through the p53 pathway. EMBO Rep 2009;10:271—7.

[43] Fitzpatrick FA, Soberman R. Regulated formation of eicosanoids. J Clin Invest 2001;107:1347—51.

[44] FitzGerald GA, Loll P. COX in a crystal ball: current status and future promise of prostaglandin research. J Clin Invest 2001; 107:1335—7.

[45] Smith WL, DeWitt DL, Garavito RM. Cyclooxygenases: structural, cellular, and molecular biology. Annu Rev Biochem 2000; 69:145—82.

[46] Funk CD. Prostaglandins and leukotrienes: advances in eicosanoid biology. Science 2001;294:1871—5.

[47] Murphy RC, Gijon MA. Biosynthesis and metabolism of leukotrienes. Biochem J 2007;405:379—95.

[48] Capdevila JH. Regulation of ion transport and blood pressure by cytochrome p450 monooxygenases. Curr Opin Nephrol Hypertens 2007;16:465—70.

[49] Fleming I. Epoxyeicosatrienoic acids, cell signaling and angiogenesis. Prostaglandins Other Lipid Mediat 2007;82:60—7.

[50] Zeldin DC. Epoxygenase pathways of arachidonic acid metabolism. J Biol Chem 2001;276:36059—62.

[51] Hansen RA, Ogilvie GK, Davenport DJ, Gross KL, Walton JA, Richardson KL, et al. Duration of effects of dietary fish oil supplementation on serum eicosapentaenoic acid and docosahexaenoic acid concentrations in dogs. Am J Vet Res 1998; 59:864—8.

[52] Smith WL. Nutritionally essential fatty acids and biologically indispensable cyclooxygenases. Trends Biochem Sci 2008;33: 27—37.

[53] De Caterina R, Caprioli R, Giannessi D, Sicari R, Galli C, Lazzerini G, et al. n-3 Fatty acids reduce proteinuria in patients with chronic glomerular disease. Kidney Int 1993;44:843—50.

[54] Grande JP, Donadio Jr. JV. Dietary fish oil supplementation in IgA nephropathy: a therapy in search of a mechanism? Nutrition 1998;14:240—2.

[55] Garavito MR, Malkowski MG, DeWitt DL. The structures of prostaglandin endoperoxide H synthases-1 and -2. Prostag Oth Lipid M 2002;68-69:129—52.

[56] Kiefer JR, Pawlitz JL, Moreland KT, Stegeman RA, Hood WF, Gierse JK, et al. Structural insights into the stereochemistry of the cyclooxygenase reaction. Nature 2000;405:97—101.

[57] Picot D, Loll PJ, Garavito RM. The X-ray crystal structure of the membrane protein prostaglandin H2 synthase-1. Nature 1994; 367:243—9.

[58] Yuan C, Sidhu RS, Kuklev DV, Kado Y, Wada M, Song I, et al. Cyclooxygenase allosterism, fatty acid-mediated cross-talk between monomers of cyclooxygenase homodimers. J Biol Chem 2009;284:10046—55.

[59] Yuan C, Rieke CJ, Rimon G, Wingerd BA, Smith WL. Partnering between monomers of cyclooxygenase-2 homodimers. PNAS 2006;103:6142—7.

[60] Mbonye UR, Wada M, Rieke CJ, Tang HY, Dewitt DL, Smith WL. The 19-amino acid cassette of cyclooxygenase-2 mediates entry of the protein into the endoplasmic reticulum-associated degradation system. J Biol Chem 2006;281:35770—8.

[61] Sidhu, R. S., Lee, J. Y., Yuan, C., and Smith, W. L. Comparison of cyclooxygenase-1 crystal structures: cross-talk between monomers comprising cyclooxygenase-1 homodimers. *Biochemistry* 49:7069—7079.

[62] Rimon, G., Sidhu, R. S., Lauver, D. A., Lee, J. Y., Sharma, N. P., Yuan, C., et al. Coxibs interfere with the action of aspirin by binding tightly to one monomer of cyclooxygenase-1. *Proc Natl Acad Sci USA* 107:28—33.

[63] Dong L, Vecchio AJ, Sharma NP, Jurban BJ, Malkowski MG, Smith WL. Human cyclooxygenase-2 is a sequence homodimer that functions as a conformational heterodimer. J Biol Chem 2011;286:19035—46.

[64] Kobayashi T, Narumiya S. Function of prostanoid receptors: studies on knockout mice. Prostaglandins Other Lipid Mediat 2002;68-69:557—73.

[65] Narumiya S, Sugimoto Y, Ushikubi F. Prostanoid receptors: structures, properties, and functions. Physiol Rev 1999;79:1193—226.

[66] Kliewer S, Lenhard J, Wilson T, Patel I, Morris D, Lehmann J. A prostaglandin J_2 metabolite binds peroxisome proliferator-activated receptor gamma and promotes adipocyte differentiation. Cell 1995;83:813—9.

[67] Narumiya S, Ohno K, Fujiwara M, Fukushima M. Site and mechanism of growth inhibition by prostaglandins. II. Temperature-dependent transfer of a cyclopentenone prostaglandin to nuclei. J Pharmacol Exp Ther 1986;239:506—11.

[68] Reginato MJ, Krakow SL, Bailey ST, Lazar MA. Prostaglandins promote and block adipogenesis through opposing effects on peroxisome proliferator-activated receptor gamma. J Biol Chem 1998;273:1855—8.

[69] Hla T, Neilson K. Human cyclooxygenase-2 cDNA. Proc Natl Acad Sci USA 1992;89:7384—8.

[70] Kujubu DA, Fletcher BS, Varnum BC, Lim RW, Herschman HR. TIS10, a phorbol ester tumor promoter-inducible mRNA from Swiss 3T3 cells, encodes a novel prostaglandin synthase/ cyclooxygenase homologue. J Biol Chem 1991;266:12866—72.

[71] Kujubu DA, Herschman HR. Dexamethasone inhibits mitogen induction of the TIS10 prostaglandin synthase/cyclooxygenase gene. J Biol Chem 1992;267:7991—4.

[72] Tanabe T, Tohnai N. Cyclooxygenase isozymes and their gene structures and expression. Prostaglandins Other Lipid Mediat 2002;68-69:95—114.

[73] Cheng Y, Wang M, Yu Y, Lawson J, Funk CD, Fitzgerald GA. Cyclooxygenases, microsomal prostaglandin E synthase-1, and cardiovascular function. J Clin Invest 2006;116:1391—9.

[74] Hla T, Bishop-Bailey D, Liu CH, Schaefers HJ, Trifan OC. Cyclooxygenase-1 and -2 isoenzymes. Int J Biochem Cell Biol 1999;31:551—7.

[75] Herschman HR. Prostaglandin synthase 2. Bba-Lipid Lipid Metab 1996;1299:125—40.

[76] Smith WL. Prostanoid biosynthesis and mechanisms of action. Am J Physiol 1992;263:F181—91.

[77] Smith WL, Langenbach R. Why there are two cyclooxygenase isozymes? J Clin Invest 2001;107:1491—5.

[78] Dinchuk JE, Car BD, Focht RJ, Johnston JJ, Jaffee BD, Covington MB, et al. Renal abnormalities and an altered inflammatory response in mice lacking cyclooxygenase II. Nature 1995;378:406—9.

[79] Komhoff M, Wang JL, Cheng HF, Langenbach R, McKanna JA, Harris RC, et al. Cyclooxygenase-2-selective inhibitors impair glomerulogenesis and renal cortical development. Kidney Int 2000;57:414—22.

[80] Morham SG, Langenbach R, Loftin CD, Tiano HF, Vouloumanos N, Jennette JC, et al. Prostaglandin synthase 2 gene disruption causes severe renal pathology in the mouse. Cell 1995;83:473—82.

[81] Harris RC, McKanna JA, Akai Y, Jacobson HR, Dubois RN, Breyer MD. Cyclooxygenase-2 is associated with the macula densa of rat kidney and increases with salt restriction. J Clin Invest 1994;94:2504—10.

[82] Komhoff M, Jeck ND, Seyberth HW, Grone HJ, Nusing RM, Breyer MD. Cyclooxygenase-2 expression is associated with the renal macula densa of patients with Bartter-like syndrome. Kidney Int 2000;58:2420—4.

[83] Vio CP, An SJ, Cespedes C, McGiff JC, Ferreri NR. Induction of cyclooxygenase-2 in thick ascending limb cells by adrenalectomy. J Am Soc Nephrol 2001;12:649—58.

[84] Campean V, Theilig F, Paliege A, Breyer M, Bachmann S. Key enzymes for renal prostaglandin synthesis: site-specific expression in rodent kidney (rat, mouse). Am J Physiol Renal Physiol 2003;285:F19—32.

[85] Smith WL, Bell TG. Immunohistochemical localization of the prostaglandin-forming cyclooxygenase in renal cortex. Am J Physiol 1978;235:F451—7.

[86] Yang T, Singh I, Pham H, Sun D, Smart A, Schnermann JB, et al. Regulation of cyclooxygenase expression in the kidney by dietary salt intake. Am J Physiol 1998;274:F481—9.

[87] Castrop H, Schweda F, Schumacher K, Wolf K, Kurtz A. Role of renocortical cyclooxygenase-2 for renal vascular resistance and macula densa control of renin secretion. J Am Soc Nephrol 2001;12:867—74.

[88] Guan Y, Chang M, Cho W, Zhang Y, Redha R, Davis L, et al. Cloning, expression, and regulation of rabbit cyclooxygenase-2 in renal medullary interstitial cells. Am J Physiol 1997;273: F18—26.

[89] Hao CM, Komhoff M, Guan Y, Redha R, Breyer MD. Selective targeting of cyclooxygenase-2 reveals its role in renal medullary interstitial cell survival. Am J Physiol 1999; 277:F352—9.

[90] Bresalier RS, Sandler RS, Quan H, Bolognese JA, Oxenius B, Horgan K, et al. Cardiovascular events associated with rofecoxib in a colorectal adenoma chemoprevention trial. N Engl J Med 2005;352:1092—102.

[91] Zewde T, Mattson DL. Inhibition of cyclooxygenase-2 in the rat renal medulla leads to sodium-sensitive hypertension. Hypertension 2004;44:424—8.

[92] Zhang MZ, Yao B, Cheng HF, Wang SW, Inagami T, Harris RC. Renal cortical cyclooxygenase 2 expression is differentially regulated by angiotensin II AT(1) and AT(2) receptors. Proc Natl Acad Sci USA 2006;103:16045—50.

[93] Peti-Peterdi J, Komlosi P, Fuson AL, Guan Y, Schneider A, Qi Z, et al. Luminal NaCl delivery regulates basolateral PGE2 release from macula densa cells. J Clin Invest 2003;112:76—82.

[94] Helliwell RJ, Adams LF, Mitchell MD. Prostaglandin synthases: recent developments and a novel hypothesis. Prostaglandins Leukot Essent Fatty Acids 2004;70:101—13.

[95] Urade Y, Watanabe K, Hayaishi O. Prostaglandin D, E, and F synthases. J Lipid Mediat Cell Signal 1995;12:257—73.

[96] Breyer MD, Breyer RM. Prostaglandin E receptors and the kidney. Am J Physiol Renal Physiol 2000;279:F12—23.

[97] Narumiya S, FitzGerald GA. Genetic and pharmacological analysis of prostanoid receptor function. J Clin Invest 2001; 108:25—30.

[98] Qi Z, Cai H, Morrow JD, Breyer MD. Differentiation of cyclooxygenase 1- and 2-derived prostanoids in mouse kidney and aorta. Hypertension 2006;48:323—8.

[99] Murphey LJ, Williams MK, Sanchez SC, Byrne LM, Csiki I, Oates JA, et al. Quantification of the major urinary metabolite of PGE2 by a liquid chromatographic/mass spectrometric assay: Determination of cyclooxygenase-specific PGE2 synthesis in healthy humans and those with lung cancer. Anal Biochem 2004;334:266—75.

[100] Whelton A, Schulman G, Wallemark C, Drower EJ, Isakson PC, Verburg KM, et al. Effects of celecoxib and naproxen on renal function in the elderly. Arch Intern Med 2000; 160:1465—70.

[101] Kammerl MC, Nusing RM, Schweda F, Endemann D, Stubanus M, Kees F, et al. Low sodium and furosemide-induced stimulation of the renin system in man is mediated by cyclooxygenase 2. Clin Pharmacol Ther 2001;70:468—74.

[102] Breyer RM, Kennedy CR, Zhang Y, Breyer MD. Structure—function analyses of eicosanoid receptors. Physiologic and therapeutic implications. Ann NY Acad Sci 2000;905:221—31.

[103] Sugimoto Y, Narumiya S. Prostaglandin E receptors. J Biol Chem 2007;282:11613—7.

[104] Hebert RL, Carmosino M, Saito O, Yang G, Jackson CM, Qi Z, et al. Characterization of a rabbit PGF2alpha (FP) receptor exhibiting Gi-restricted signaling and that inhibits water absorption in renal collecting duct. J Biol Chem 2005;280: 35028—37.

[105] Breyer MD, Davis L, Jacobson HR, Breyer RM. Differential localization of prostaglandin E receptor subtypes in human kidney. Am J Physiol 1996;270:F912—8.

[106] Tilley SL, Coffman TM, Koller BH. Mixed messages: modulation of inflammation and immune responses by prostaglandins and thromboxanes. J Clin Invest 2001;108:15—23.

[107] Cronstein BN, Weissmann G. Targets for antiinflammatory drugs. Annu Rev Pharmacol Toxicol 1995;35:449—62.

[108] Honda T, Tokura Y, Miyachi Y, Kabashima K. Prostanoid receptors as possible targets for anti-allergic drugs: recent advances in prostanoids on allergy and immunology. Curr Drug Targets 2010;11:1605—13.

[109] Jakobsson PJ, Thoren S, Morgenstern R, Samuelsson B. Identification of human prostaglandin E synthase: a microsomal, glutathione-dependent, inducible enzyme, constituting a potential novel drug target. Proc Natl Acad Sci USA 1999; 96:7220—5.

[110] Tanioka T, Nakatani Y, Semmyo N, Murakami M, Kudo I. Molecular identification of cytosolic prostaglandin E2 synthase that is functionally coupled with cyclooxygenase-1 in immediate prostaglandin E2 biosynthesis. J Biol Chem 2000;275: 32775—82.

[111] Tanikawa N, Ohmiya Y, Ohkubo H, Hashimoto K, Kangawa K, Kojima M, et al. Identification and characterization of a novel type of membrane-associated prostaglandin E synthase. Biochem Biophys Res Commun 2002;291:884—9.

[112] Trebino CE, Stock JL, Gibbons CP, Naiman BM, Wachtmann TS, Umland JP, et al. Impaired inflammatory and pain responses in mice lacking an inducible prostaglandin E synthase. Proc Natl Acad Sci USA 2003;100:9044—9.

[113] Engblom D, Saha S, Engstrom L, Westman M, Audoly LP, Jakobsson P -J, et al. Microsomal prostaglandin E synthase-1 is the central switch during immune-induced pyresis. Nat Neurosci 2003;6:1137—8.

[114] Uematsu S, Matsumoto M, Takeda K, Akira S. Lipopolysaccharide-dependent prostaglandin E(2) production is regulated by the glutathione-dependent prostaglandin E(2) synthase gene induced by the Toll-like receptor 4/MyD88/NF-IL6 pathway. J Immunol 2002;168:5811—6.

[115] Schneider A, Zhang Y, Zhang M, Lu WJ, Rao R, Fan X, et al. Membrane-associated PGE synthase-1 (mPGES-1) is coexpressed with both COX-1 and COX-2 in the kidney. Kidney Int 2004;65:1205—13.

[116] Guan Y, Zhang Y, Schneider A, Riendeau D, Mancini JA, Davis L, et al. Urogenital distribution of a mouse membrane-associated prostaglandin E(2) synthase. Am J Physiol Renal Physiol 2001;281:F1173—7.

[117] Ouellet M, Falgueyret JP, Hien Ear P, Pen A, Mancini JA, Riendeau D, et al. Purification and characterization of recombinant microsomal prostaglandin E synthase-1. Protein Expr Purif 2002;26:489—95.

[118] Jia Z, Aoyagi T, Yang T. mPGES-1 protects against DOCA-salt hypertension via inhibition of oxidative stress or stimulation of NO/cGMP. Hypertension 2010;55:539—46.

[119] Jia Z, Guo X, Zhang H, Wang MH, Dong Z, Yang T. Microsomal prostaglandin synthase-1-derived prostaglandin E2 protects against angiotensin II-induced hypertension via inhibition of oxidative stress. Hypertension 2008;52:952—9.

[120] Francois H, Facemire C, Kumar A, Audoly L, Koller B, Coffman T. Role of microsomal prostaglandin E synthase 1 in the kidney. J Am Soc Nephrol 2007;18:1466—75.

[121] Nguyen M, Camenisch T, Snouwaert JN, Hicks E, Coffman TM, Anderson PA, et al. The prostaglandin receptor EP4 triggers remodelling of the cardiovascular system at birth. Nature 1997;390:78—81.

[122] Murakami M, Nakatani Y, Tanioka T, Kudo I. Prostaglandin E synthase. Prostaglandins Other Lipid Mediat 2002;68-69: 383—99.

[123] Zhang Y, Schneider A, Rao R, Lu WJ, Fan X, Davis L, et al. Genomic structure and genitourinary expression of mouse cytosolic prostaglandin E(2) synthase gene. Biochim Biophys Acta 2003;1634:15—23.

[124] Breyer RM, Davis LS, Nian C, Redha R, Stillman B, Jacobson HR, et al. Cloning and expression of the rabbit prostaglandin EP4 receptor. Am J Physiol 1996;270:F485—93.

[125] Guan Y, Stillman BA, Zhang Y, Schneider A, Saito O, Davis LS, et al. Cloning and expression of the rabbit prostaglandin EP2 receptor. BMC Pharmacol 2002;2:14.

[126] Jensen BL, Stubbe J, Hansen PB, Andreasen D, Skott O. Localization of prostaglandin E(2) EP2 and EP4 receptors in the rat kidney. Am J Physiol Renal Physiol 2001;280:F1001−9.

[127] Sheldrick R, Coleman R, Lumley P. Iloprost-A potent EP1- and IP- receptor agonist. Br J Pharmacol 1987;: xxx: 334p

[128] Coleman RA, Kennedy I, Humphrey PPA, Bunce K, Lumley P. Prostanoids and their Receptors. In: Emmet JC, editor. Comprehensive Medicinal Chemistry. Oxford: Pergammon Press; 1990. p. 643−714.

[129] Coleman RA, Smith WL, Narumiya S. VIII. International union of pharmacology classification of prostanoid receptors: properties, distribution, and structure of the receptors and their subtypes. Pharmacol Rev 1994;46:205−29.

[130] Lawrence RA, Jones RL, Wilson NH. Characterization of receptors involved in the direct and indirect actions of prostaglandins E and I on the guinea-pig ileum. Br J Pharmacol 1992;105:271−8.

[131] Funk C, Furchi L, FitzGerald G, Grygorczyk R, Rochette C, Bayne MA, et al. Cloning and expression of a cDNA for the human prostaglandin E receptor EP_1 subtype. J Biol Chem 1993;268:26767−72.

[132] Guan Y, Zhang Y, Breyer RM, Fowler B, Davis L, Hebert RL, et al. Prostaglandin E2 inhibits renal collecting duct Na^+ absorption by activating the EP1 receptor. J Clin Invest 1998;102:194−201.

[133] Hibbs TA, Lu B, Smock SL, Vestergaard P, Pan LC, Owen TA. Molecular cloning and characterization of the canine prostaglandin E receptor EP2 subtype. Prostaglandins Other Lipid Mediat 1999;57:133−47.

[134] Watabe A, Sugimoto Y, Honda A, Irie A, Namba T, Negishi M, et al. Cloning and expression of cDNA for a mouse EP1 subtype of prostaglandin E receptor. J Biol Chem 1993;268: 20175−8.

[135] Boie Y, Stocco R, Sawyer N, Slipetz DM, Ungrin MD, Neuschafer-Rube F, et al. Molecular cloning and characterization of the four rat prostaglandin E2 prostanoid receptor subtypes. Eur J Pharmacol 1997;340:227−41.

[136] Hallinan EA, Hagen TJ, Tsymbalov S, Husa RK, Lee AC, Stapelfeld A, et al. Aminoacetyl moiety as a potential surrogate for diacylhydrazine group of SC-51089, a potent PGE2 antagonist, and its analogs. J Med Chem 1996;39:609−13.

[137] Hallinan EA, Hagen TJ, Tsymbalov S, Stapelfeld A, Savage MA. 2,4-Disubstituted oxazoles and thiazoles as latent pharmacophores for diacylhydrazine of SC-51089, a potent PGE2 antagonist. Bioorg Med Chem 2001;9:1−6.

[138] Hall A, Atkinson S, Brown SH, Chessell IP, Chowdhury A, Giblin GM, et al. Discovery of novel, non-acidic 1,5-biaryl pyrrole EP1 receptor antagonists. Bioorg Med Chem Lett 2007;17: 1200−5.

[139] Makino H, Tanaka I, Mukoyama M, Sugawara A, Mori K, Muro S, et al. Prevention of diabetic nephropathy in rats by prostaglandin E receptor EP1-selective antagonist. J Am Soc Nephrol 2002;13:1757−65.

[140] Miki T, Matsunami M, Nakamura S, Okada H, Matsuya H, Kawabata A. ONO-8130, a selective prostanoid EP1 receptor antagonist, relieves bladder pain in mice with cyclophosphamide-induced cystitis. Pain 2011;152:1373−81.

[141] Naganawa A, Matsui T, Ima M, Saito T, Murota M, Aratani Y, et al. Further optimization of sulfonamide analogs as EP1 receptor antagonists: synthesis and evaluation of bioisosteres for the carboxylic acid group. Bioorg Med Chem 2006;14: 7121−37.

[142] Johansson T, Narumiya S, Zeilhofer HU. Contribution of peripheral versus central EP1 prostaglandin receptors to inflammatory pain. Neurosci Lett 2011;495:98−101.

[143] Stock JL, Shinjo K, Burkhardt J, Roach M, Taniguchi K, Ishikawa T, et al. The prostaglandin E2 EP1 receptor mediates pain perception and regulates blood pressure. J Clin Invest 2001;107:325−31.

[144] Biswas S, Bhattacherjee P, Paterson CA, Maruyama T, Narumiya S. Modulation of ocular inflammatory responses by EP1 receptors in mice. Exp Eye Res 2007;84:39−43.

[145] Guan Y, Zhang Y, Wu J, Qi Z, Yang G, Dou D, et al. Antihypertensive effects of selective prostaglandin E2 receptor subtype 1 targeting. J Clin Invest 2007;117:2496−505.

[146] Sugimoto Y, Namba T, Shigemoto R, Negishi M, Ichikawa A, Narumiya S. Distinct cellular localization of mRNAs for three subtypes of prostaglandin E receptor in kidney. Am J Physiol 1994;266:F823−8.

[147] Capone C, Faraco G, Anrather J, Zhou P, Iadecola C. Cyclooxygenase 1-derived prostaglandin E2 and EP1 receptors are required for the cerebrovascular dysfunction induced by angiotensin II. Hypertension 2010;55:911−7.

[148] Pena-Silva RA, Heistad DD. EP1c times for angiotensin: EP1 receptors facilitate angiotensin II-induced vascular dysfunction. Hypertension 2010;55:846−8.

[149] Rutkai I, Feher A, Erdei N, Henrion D, Papp Z, Edes I, et al. Activation of prostaglandin E2 EP1 receptor increases arteriolar tone and blood pressure in mice with type 2 diabetes. Cardiovascular Research 2009;83:148−54.

[150] Regan JW, Bailey TJ, Pepperl DJ, Pierce KL, Bogardus AM, Donello JE, et al. Cloning of a novel human prostaglandin receptor with characteristics of the pharmacologically defined EP2 subtype. Mol Pharmacol 1994;46:213−20.

[151] Nishigaki N, Negishi M, Honda A, Sugimoto Y, Namba T, Narumiya S, et al. Identification of prostaglandin E receptor 'EP2 cloned from mastocytoma cells as EP4 subtype. FEBS Letters 1995;364:339−41.

[152] Katsuyama M, Nishigaki N, Sugimoto Y, Morimoto K, Negishi M, Narumiya S, et al. The mouse prostaglandin E receptor EP2 subtype: cloning, expression, and Northern blot analysis. FEBS Lett 1995;372:151−6.

[153] Kennedy CR, Zhang Y, Brandon S, Guan Y, Coffee K, Funk CD, et al. Salt-sensitive hypertension and reduced fertility in mice lacking the prostaglandin EP2 receptor. Nat Med 1999;5: 217−20.

[154] Tilley SL, Audoly LP, Hicks EH, Kim HS, Flannery PJ, Coffman TM, et al. Reproductive failure and reduced blood pressure in mice lacking the EP2 prostaglandin E2 receptor. J Clin Invest 1999;103:1539−45.

[155] Pallone T. Vasoconstriction of outer medullary vasa recta by angiotensin II is modulated by prostaglandin E2. Am J Physiol 1994;266:F850−7.

[156] Pallone TL, Silldorff EP. Pericyte regulation of renal medullary blood flow. Exp Nephrol 2001;9:165−70.

[157] Imig JD, Breyer MD, Breyer RM. Contribution of prostaglandin EP(2) receptors to renal microvascular reactivity in mice. Am J Physiol Renal Physiol 2002;283:F415−22.

[158] Chen J, Zhao M, He W, Milne GL, Howard JR, Morrow J, et al. Increased dietary NaCl induces renal medullary PGE2 production and natriuresis via the EP2 receptor. Am J Physiol Renal Physiol 2008;295:F818−25.

[159] Savage MA, Moummi C, Karabatsos PJ, Lanthorn TH. SC-46275: a potent and highly selective agonist at the EP3 receptor. Prostaglandins Leukot Essent Fatty Acids 1993;49:939−43.

[160] van Rodijnen WF, Korstjens IJ, Legerstee N, Ter Wee PM, Tangelder GJ. Direct vasoconstrictor effect of prostaglandin E2

on renal interlobular arteries: role of the EP3 receptor. Am J Physiol Renal Physiol 2007;292:F1094—101.

[161] Breyer RM, Emeson RB, Tarng JL, Breyer MD, Davis LS, Abromson RM, et al. Alternative splicing generates multiple isoforms of a rabbit prostaglandin E2 receptor. J Biol Chem 1994;269:6163—9.

[162] Irie A, Segi E, Sugimoto Y, Ichikawa A, Negishi M. Mouse prostaglandin E receptor EP3 subtype mediates calcium signals via Gi in cDNA-transfected Chinese hamster ovary cells. Biochem Biophys Res Commun 1994;204:303—9.

[163] Pierce KL, Regan JW. Prostanoid receptor heterogeneity through alternative mRNA splicing. Life Sci 1998;62:1479—83.

[164] Schmid A, Thierauch KH, Schleuning WD, Dinter H. Splice variants of the human EP3 receptor for prostaglandin E2. Eur J Biochem 1995;228:23—30.

[165] Namba T, Sugimoto Y, Negishi M, Irie A, Ushikubi F, Kakizuka A, et al. Alternative splicing of C-terminal tail of prostaglandin E receptor subtype EP3 determines G-protein specificity. Nature 1993;365:166—70.

[166] Ushikubi F, Segi E, Sugimoto Y, Murata T, Matsuoka T, Kobayashi T, et al. Impaired febrile response in mice lacking the prostaglandin E receptor subtype EP3. Nature 1998;395: 281—4.

[167] Hébert, R, Jacobson, H, Breyer, M. PGE2 inhibits AVP induced water flow in cortical collecting ducts by protein kinase C activation. Am J Physiol 1990;259:F318—5.

[168] Sonnenburg, WK, Zhu, J, Smith, WL. A prostglandin E receptor coupled to a pertussis toxin-sensitive guanine nucleotide regulatory protein in rabbit cortical collecting tubule cells. J Biol Chem 1990;265:8479—83.

[169] Fleming E, Athirakul K, Oliverio M, Key M, Goulet J, Koller B, et al. Urinary concentrating function in mice lacking the EP3 receptors for prostaglandin E2. Am J Physiol 1998;275:F955—61.

[170] Abramovitz M, Adam M, Boie Y, Carriere M, Denis D, Godbout C, et al. The utilization of recombinant prostanoid receptors to determine the affinities and selectivities of prostaglandins and related analogs. Biochim Biophys Acta 2000; 1483:285—93.

[171] Bastien L, Sawyer N, Grygorczyk R, Metters KM, Adam M. Cloning, functional expression, and characterization of the human prostaglandin E2 receptor EP2 subtype. J Biol Chem 1994;269:11873—7.

[172] Fujino H, Salvi S, Regan JW. Differential regulation of phosphorylation of the cAMP response element-binding protein after activation of EP2 and EP4 prostanoid receptors by prostaglandin E2. Mol Pharmacol 2005;68:251—9.

[173] Fujino H, West KA, Regan JW. Phosphorylation of glycogen synthase kinase-3 and stimulation of T-cell factor signaling following activation of EP2 and EP4 prostanoid receptors by prostaglandin E2. J Biol Chem 2002;277:2614—9.

[174] Bastien L, Sawyer N, Grygorczyk R, Metters K, Adam M. Cloning, functional expression, and characterization of the human prostaglandin E_2 receptor EP_2 subtype. J Biol Chem 1994;269:11873—7.

[175] Narko K, Saukkonen K, Ketola I, Butzow R, Heikinheimo M, Ristimaki A. Regulated expression of prostaglandin E(2) receptors EP2 and EP4 in human ovarian granulosa-luteal cells. J Clin Endocrinol Metab 2001;86:1765—8.

[176] Segi E, Sugimoto Y, Yamasaki A, Aze Y, Oida H, Nishimura T, et al. Patent ductus arteriosus and neonatal death in prostaglandin receptor EP4-deficient mice. Biochem Biophys Res Commun 1998;246:7—12.

[177] Lawrence RA, Jones RL. Investigation of the prostaglandin E (EP-) receptor subtype mediating relaxation of the rabbit jugular vein. Br J Pharmacol 1992;105:817—24.

[178] Schweda F, Klar J, Narumiya S, Nusing RM, Kurtz A. Stimulation of renin release by prostaglandin E2 is mediated by EP2 and EP4 receptors in mouse kidneys. Am J Physiol Renal Physiol 2004;287:F427—33.

[179] Bugge JF, Stokke ES, Vikse A, Kiil F. Stimulation of renin release by PGE2 and PGI2 infusion in the dog: enhancing effect of ureteral occlusion or administration of ethacrynic acid. Acta Physiol Scand 1990;138:193—201.

[180] Ito S, Carretero OA, Abe K, Beierwaltes WH, Yoshinaga K. Effect of prostanoids on renin release from rabbit afferent arterioles with and without macula densa. Kidney Int 1989; 35:1138—44.

[181] Nusing RM, Treude A, Weissenberger C, Jensen B, Bek M, Wagner C, et al. Dominant role of prostaglandin E2 EP4 receptor in furosemide-induced salt-losing tubulopathy: a model for hyperprostaglandin E syndrome/antenatal Bartter syndrome. J Am Soc Nephrol 2005;16:2354—62.

[182] Tan SY, Shapiro R, Franco R, Stockard H, Mulrow PJ. Indomethacin-induced prostaglandin inhibition with hyperkalemia. A reversible cause of hyporeninemic hypoaldosteronism. Ann Intern Med 1979;90:783—5.

[183] Kammerl MC, Nusing RM, Richthammer W, Kramer BK, Kurtz A. Inhibition of COX-2 counteracts the effects of diuretics in rats. Kidney Int 2001;60:1684—91.

[184] Reinalter SC, Jeck N, Brochhausen C, Watzer B, Nusing RM, Seyberth HW, et al. Role of cyclooxygenase-2 in hyperprostaglandin E syndrome/antenatal Bartter syndrome. Kidney Int 2002;62:253—60.

[185] Harding P, Sigmon DH, Alfie ME, Huang PL, Fishman MC, Beierwaltes WH, et al. Cyclooxygenase-2 mediates increased renal renin content induced by low-sodium diet. Hypertension 1997;29:297—302.

[186] Blackshear JL, Davidman M, Stillman MT. Identification of risk for renal insufficiency from nonsteroidal anti-inflammatory drugs. Arch Intern Med 1983;143:1130—4.

[187] Hockel G, Cowley A. Prostaglandin E2-induced hypertension in conscious dogs. Am J Physiol 1979;237:H449—54.

[188] Oliver JA, Pinto J, Sciacca RR, Cannon PJ. Increased renal secretion of norepinephrine and prostaglandin E2 during sodium depletion in the dog. J Clin Invest 1980;66:748—56.

[189] Hartner A, Cordasic N, Goppelt-Struebe M, Veelken R, Hilgers KF. Role of macula densa cyclooxygenase-2 in renovascular hypertension. Am J Physiol Renal Physiol 2002;:.

[190] Ahmad SR, Kortepeter C, Brinker A, Chen M, Beitz J. Renal failure associated with the use of celecoxib and rofecoxib. Drug Saf 2002;25:537—44.

[191] Perneger TV, Whelton PK, Klag MJ. Risk of kidney failure associated with the use of acetaminophen, aspirin, and nonsteroidal antiinflammatory drugs. N Engl J Med 1994;331: 1675—9.

[192] Yussim E, Schwartz E, Sidi Y, Ehrenfeld M. Acute renal failure precipitated by non-steroidal anti-inflammatory drugs (NSAIDs) in multiple myeloma. Am J Hematol 1998;58:142—4.

[193] Bek MJ, Wahle S, Muller B, Benzing T, Huber TB, Kretzler M, et al. Stra13, a prostaglandin E2-induced gene, regulates the cellular redox state of podocytes. Faseb J 2003;17:682—4.

[194] Martineau LC, McVeigh LI, Jasmin BJ, Kennedy CR. p38 MAP kinase mediates mechanically induced COX-2 and PG EP4 receptor expression in podocytes: implications for the actin cytoskeleton. Am J Physiol Renal Physiol 2004;286:F693—701.

[195] Stitt-Cavanagh EM, Faour WH, Takami K, Carter A, Vanderhyden B, Guan Y, et al. A maladaptive role for EP4 receptors in podocytes. J Am Soc Nephrol 2010;21:1678—90.

[196] Muro S, Tanaka I, Usui T, Kotani M, Koide S, Mukoyama M, et al. Expression of prostaglandin E receptor EP4 subtype in

rat adrenal zona glomerulosa: involvement in aldosterone release. Endocr J 2000;47:429−36.

[197] Galler M, Folkert VW, Schlondorff D. Reversible acute renal insufficiency and hyperkalemia following indomethacin therapy. JAMA 1981;246:154−5.

[198] Miller KP, Lazar EJ, Fotino S. Severe hyperkalemia during piroxicam therapy. Arch Intern Med 1984;144:2414−5.

[199] Inada M, Iwasaki K, Imai C, Hashimoto S. Hyperpotassemia and bradycardia in a bedridden elderly woman with selective hypoaldosteronism associated with low renin activity. Intern Med 2010;49:307−13.

[200] Baxter GS, Clayton JK, Coleman RA, Marshall K, Sangha R, Senior J. Characterization of the prostanoid receptors mediating constriction and relaxation of human isolated uterine artery. Br J Pharmacol 1995;116:1692−6.

[201] Kabashima K, Sakata D, Nagamachi M, Miyachi Y, Inaba K, Narumiya S. Prostaglandin E(2)-EP4 signaling initiates skin immune responses by promoting migration and maturation of Langerhans cells. Nat Med 2003;9:744−9.

[202] Miyaura C, Inada M, Suzawa T, Sugimoto Y, Ushikubi F, Ichikawa A, et al. Impaired bone resorption to prostaglandin E2 in prostaglandin E receptor EP4-knockout mice. J Biol Chem 2000;275:19819−23.

[203] Yoshida K, Oida H, Kobayashi T, Maruyama T, Tanaka M, Katayama T, et al. Stimulation of bone formation and prevention of bone loss by prostaglandin E EP4 receptor activation. Proc Natl Acad Sci USA 2002;99:4580−5.

[204] Watanabe K. Prostaglandin F synthase. Prostaglandins Other Lipid Mediat 2002;68-69:401−7.

[205] Lee SC, Levine L. Purification and regulatory properties of chicken heart prostaglandin E 9-ketoreductase. J Biol Chem 1975;250:4549−55.

[206] Roberts II LJ, Seibert K, Liston TE, Tantengco MV, Robertson RM. PGD2 is transformed by human coronary arteries to 9 alpha, 11 beta-PGF2, which contracts human coronary artery rings. Adv Prostaglandin Thromboxane Leukot Res 1987;17A:427−9.

[207] Sharif NA, Xu SX, Williams GW, Crider JY, Griffin BW, Davis TL. Pharmacology of [3H]prostaglandin E1/[3H]prostaglandin E2 and [3H]prostaglandin F2alpha binding to EP3 and FP prostaglandin receptor binding sites in bovine corpus luteum: characterization and correlation with functional data. J Pharmacol Exp Ther 1998;286:1094−102.

[208] Wallner EI, Wada J, Tramonti G, Lin S, Srivastava SK, Kanwar YS. Relevance of aldo-keto reductase family members to the pathobiology of diabetic nephropathy and renal development. Ren Fail 2001;23:311−20.

[209] Siragy HM, Senbonmatsu T, Ichiki T, Inagami T, Carey RM. Increased renal vasodilator prostanoids prevent hypertension in mice lacking the angiotensin subtype-2 receptor. J Clin Invest 1999;104:181−8.

[210] Siragy HM, Inagami T, Ichiki T, Carey RM. Sustained hypersensitivity to angiotensin II and its mechanism in mice lacking the subtype-2 (AT2) angiotensin receptor. Proc Natl Acad Sci USA 1999;96:6506−10.

[211] Siragy HM, Carey RM. The subtype 2 angiotensin receptor regulates renal prostaglandin F2 alpha formation in conscious rats. Am J Physiol 1997;273:R1103−7.

[212] Abramovitz M, Boie Y, Nguyen T, Rushmore TH, Bayne MA, Metters KM, et al. Cloning and expression of a cDNA for the human prostanoid FP receptor. J Biol Chem 1994;269: 2632−6.

[213] Griffin BW, Williams GW, Crider JY, Sharif NA. FP prostaglandin receptors mediating inositol phosphates generation and calcium mobilization in Swiss 3T3 cells: a pharmacological study. J Pharmacol Exp Ther 1997;281:845−54.

[214] Kelly CR, Williams GW, Sharif NA. Real-time intracellular Ca^{2+} mobilization by travoprost acid, bimatoprost, unoprostone, and other analogs via endogenous mouse, rat, and cloned human FP prostaglandin receptors. J Pharmacol Exp Ther 2003;304:238−45.

[215] Woodward DF, Lawrence RA. Identification of a single (FP) receptor associated with prostanoid-induced Ca^{2+} signals in Swiss 3T3 cells. Biochem Pharmacol 1994;47:1567−74.

[216] Sugimoto Y, Yamasaki A, Segi E, Tsuboi K, Aze Y, Nishimura T, et al. Failure of parturition in mice lacking the prostaglandin F receptor. Science 1997;277:681−3.

[217] Chollet A, Tos EG, Cirillo R. Tocolytic effect of a selective FP receptor antagonist in rodent models reveals an innovative approach to the treatment of preterm labor. BMC Pregnancy Childbirth 2007;7(Suppl. 1):S16.

[218] Griffin BW, Klimko P, Crider JY, Sharif NA. AL-8810: a novel prostaglandin F2 alpha analog with selective antagonist effects at the prostaglandin F2 alpha (FP) receptor. J Pharmacol Exp Ther 1999;290:1278−84.

[219] Sharif NA, Kelly CR, Crider JY. Agonist activity of bimatoprost, travoprost, latanoprost, unoprostone isopropyl ester and other prostaglandin analogs at the cloned human ciliary body FP prostaglandin receptor. J Ocul Pharmacol Ther 2002;18:313−24.

[220] Saito O, Guan Y, Qi Z, Davis LS, Komhoff M, Sugimoto Y, et al. Expression of the prostaglandin F receptor (FP) gene along the mouse genitourinary tract. Am J Physiol Renal Physiol 2003;284: F1164−70.

[221] Yu Y, Lucitt MB, Stubbe J, Cheng Y, Friis UG, Hansen PB, et al. Prostaglandin F2alpha elevates blood pressure and promotes atherosclerosis. Proc Natl Acad Sci USA 2009;106:7985−90.

[222] Urade Y, Eguchi N. Lipocalin-type and hematopoietic prostaglandin D synthases as a novel example of functional convergence. Prostaglandins & Other Lipid Mediators 2002;68-69:375−82.

[223] Shimura C, Satoh T, Igawa K, Aritake K, Urade Y, Nakamura M, et al. Dendritic cells express hematopoietic prostaglandin D synthase and function as a source of prostaglandin D2 in the skin. Am J Pathol 2010;176:227−37.

[224] Vitzthum H, Abt I, Einhellig S, Kurtz A. Gene expression of prostanoid forming enzymes along the rat nephron. Kidney Int 2002;62:1570−81.

[225] Qu WM, Huang ZL, Xu XH, Aritake K, Eguchi N, Nambu F, et al. Lipocalin-type prostaglandin D synthase produces prostaglandin D2 involved in regulation of physiological sleep. Proc Natl Acad Sci USA 2006;103:17949−54.

[226] Eguchi N, Minami T, Shirafuji N, Kanaoka Y, Tanaka T, Nagata A, et al. Lack of tactile pain (allodynia) in lipocalin-type prostaglandin D synthase-deficient mice. Proc Natl Acad Sci USA 1999;96:726−30.

[227] Nakayama H, Echizen H, Gomi T, Shibuya Y, Nakamura Y, Nakano K, et al. Urinary lipocalin-type prostaglandin D synthase: a potential marker for early gentamicin-induced renal damage? Ther Drug Monit 2009;31:126−30.

[228] Uehara Y, Makino H, Seiki K, Urade Y. Urinary excretions of lipocalin-type prostaglandin D synthase predict renal injury in type-2 diabetes: a cross-sectional and prospective multicentre study. Nephrol Dial Transplant 2009;24:475−82.

[229] Ogawa M, Hirawa N, Tsuchida T, Eguchi N, Kawabata Y, Numabe A, et al. Urinary excretions of lipocalin-type prostaglandin D2 synthase predict the development of proteinuria and renal injury in OLETF rats. Nephrol Dial Transplant 2006; 21:924−34.

[230] Tsuchida T, Eguchi N, Eguchi Y, Numabe A, Nakajima H, Oda H, et al. Lipocalin-type prostaglandin D synthase in urine in adriamycin-induced nephropathy of mice. Nephron Physiol 2004;96:p42−51.

[231] Ragolia L, Palaia T, Hall CE, Maesaka JK, Eguchi N, Urade Y. Accelerated glucose intolerance, nephropathy, and atherosclerosis in prostaglandin D2 synthase knock-out mice. J Biol Chem 2005;280:29946—55.

[232] Kanaoka Y, Ago H, Inagaki E, Nanayama T, Miyano M, Kikuno R, et al. Cloning and crystal structure of hematopoietic prostaglandin D synthase. Cell 1997;90:1085—95.

[233] Kanaoka Y, Urade Y. Hematopoietic prostaglandin D synthase. Prostaglandins Leukot Essent Fatty Acids 2003;69:163—7.

[234] Boie Y, Sawyer N, Slipetz DM, Metters KM, Abramovitz M. Molecular cloning and characterization of the human prostanoid DP receptor. J Biol Chem 1995;270:18910—6.

[235] Wright DH, Nantel F, Metters KM, Ford-Hutchinson AW. A novel biological role for prostaglandin D2 is suggested by distribution studies of the rat DP prostanoid receptor. Eur J Pharmacol 1999;377:101—15.

[236] Hirai H, Tanaka K, Yoshie O, Ogawa K, Kenmotsu K, Takamori Y, et al. Prostaglandin D2 selectively induces chemotaxis in T helper type 2 cells, eosinophils, and basophils via seven-transmembrane receptor CRTH2. J Exp Med 2001;193:255—62.

[237] Toh H, Ichikawa A, Narumiya S. Molecular evolution of receptors for eicosanoids. FEBS Letters 1995;361:17—21.

[238] Kabashima K, Narumiya S. The DP receptor, allergic inflammation and asthma. Prostaglandins Leukot Essent Fatty Acids 2003;69:187—94.

[239] Koch KA, Wessale JL, Moreland R, Reinhart GA, Cox BF. Effects of BW245C, a prostaglandin dp receptor agonist, on systemic and regional haemodynamics in the anaesthetized rat. Clin Exp Pharmacol Physiol 2005;32:931—5.

[240] Hoeper MM, Schwarze M, Ehlerding S, Adler-Schuermeyer A, Spiekerkoetter E, Niedermeyer J, et al. Long-term treatment of primary pulmonary hypertension with aerosolized iloprost, a prostacyclin analogue. N Engl J Med 2000;342:1866—70.

[241] Yokoyama C, Yabuki T, Inoue H, Tone Y, Hara S, Hatae T, et al. Human gene encoding prostacyclin synthase (PTGIS): Genomic organization, chromosomal localization, and promoter activity. Genomics 1996;36:296—304.

[242] Tone Y, Inoue H, Hara S, Yokoyama C, Hatae T, Oida H, et al. The regional distribution and cellular localization of mRNA encoding rat prostacyclin synthase. Eur J Cell Biol 1997;72:268—77.

[243] Yokoyama C, Yabuki T, Shimonishi M, Wada M, Hatae T, Ohkawara S, et al. Prostacyclin-deficient mice develop ischemic renal disorders, including nephrosclerosis and renal infarction. Circulation 2002;106:2397—403.

[244] Murata T, Ushikubi F, Matsuoka T, Hirata M, Yamasaki A, Sugimoto Y, et al. Altered pain perception and inflammatory response in mice lacking prostacyclin receptor. Nature 1997;388:678—82.

[245] Hao CM, Redha R, Morrow J, Breyer MD. Peroxisome proliferator-activated receptor delta activation promotes cell survival following hypertonic stress. J Biol Chem 2002;277:21341—5.

[246] Lim H, Gupta RA, Ma WG, Paria BC, Moller DE, Morrow JD, et al. Cyclo-oxygenase-2-derived prostacyclin mediates embryo implantation in the mouse via PPARdelta. Genes Dev 1999;13:1561—74.

[247] Namba T, Oida H, Sugimoto Y, Kakizuka A, Negishi M, Ichikawa A, et al. cDNA cloning of a mouse prostacyclin receptor: multiple signaling pathways and expression in thymic medulla. J Biol Chem 1994;269:9986—92.

[248] Oida H, Namba T, Sugimoto Y, Ushikubi F, Ohishi H, Ichikawa A, et al. In situ hybridization studies on prostacyclin receptor mRNA expression in various mouse organs. Br J Pharmacol 1995;116:2828—37.

[249] Fujino T, Nakagawa N, Yuhki K, Hara A, Yamada T, Takayama K, et al. Decreased susceptibility to renovascular hypertension in mice lacking the prostaglandin I2 receptor IP. J Clin Invest 2004;114:805—12.

[250] Egan KM, Lawson JA, Fries S, Koller B, Rader DJ, Smyth EM, et al. COX-2-derived prostacyclin confers atheroprotection on female mice. Science 2004;306:1954—7.

[251] Chevalier D, Lo-Guidice JM, Sergent E, Allorge D, Debuysere H, Ferrari N, et al. Identification of genetic variants in the human thromboxane synthase gene (CYP5A1). Mutat Res 2001;432:61—7.

[252] Miyata A, Yokoyama C, Ihara H, Bandoh S, Takeda O, Takahashi E, et al. Characterization of the human gene (TBXAS1) encoding thromboxane synthase. Eur J Biochem 1994;224:273—9.

[253] Zhang LQ, Chase MB, Shen RF. Molecular cloning and expression of murine thromboxane synthase. Biochem Biophys Res Commun 1993;194:741—8.

[254] Nusing R, Fehr PM, Gudat F, Kemeny E, Mihatsch MJ, Ullrich V. The localization of thromboxane synthase in normal and pathological human kidney tissue using a monoclonal antibody Tu 300. Virchows Arch 1994;424:69—74.

[255] Wilcox CS, Welch WJ. Thromboxane synthase and TP receptor mRNA in rat kidney and brain: effects of salt intake and ANG II. Am J Physiol Renal Physiol 2003;284:F525—31.

[256] Quest DW, Wilson TW. Effects of ridogrel, a thromboxane synthase inhibitor and receptor antagonist, on blood pressure in the spontaneously hypertensive rat. Jpn J Pharmacol 1998;78:479—86.

[257] Vezza R, Mezzasoma AM, Venditti G, Gresele P. Prostaglandin endoperoxides and thromboxane A2 activate the same receptor isoforms in human platelets. Thromb Haemost 2002;87:114—21.

[258] Hirata M, Hayashi Y, Ushikubi F, Yokota Y, Kageyama R, Nakanishi S, et al. Cloning and expression of cDNA for a human thromboxane A2 receptor. Nature 1991;349:617—20.

[259] Abe T, Takeuchi K, Takahashi N, Tsutsumi E, Taniyama Y, Abe K. Rat kidney thromboxane receptor: molecular cloning, signal transduction, and intrarenal expression localization. J Clin Invest 1995;96:657—64.

[260] Francois H, Athirakul K, Mao L, Rockman H, Coffman TM. Role for thromboxane receptors in angiotensin-II-induced hypertension. Hypertension 2004;43:364—9.

[261] Boffa JJ, Just A, Coffman TM, Arendshorst WJ. Thromboxane receptor mediates renal vasoconstriction and contributes to acute renal failure in endotoxemic mice. J Am Soc Nephrol 2004;15:2358—65.

[262] Schnermann J, Traynor T, Pohl H, Thomas DW, Coffman TM, Briggs JP. Vasoconstrictor responses in thromboxane receptor knockout mice: Tubuloglomerular feedback and ureteral obstruction. Acta Physiol Scand 2000;168:201—7.

[263] Snoeijs MG, Hoogland PR, Boonen B, Coffman TM, Peutz-Kootstra CJ, Buurman WA, et al. Thromboxane receptor signalling in renal ischemia reperfusion injury. Free Radic Res 2011;45:699—706.

[264] Schuster VL. Prostaglandin transport. Prostaglandins Other Lipid Mediat 2002;68-69:633—47.

[265] Kanai N, Lu R, Satriano JA, Bao Y, Wolkoff AW, Schuster VL. Identification and characterization of a prostaglandin transporter. Science 1995;268:866—9.

[266] Chang HY, Locker J, Lu R, Schuster VL. Failure of postnatal ductus arteriosus closure in prostaglandin transporter-deficient mice. Circulation 2010;121:529—36.

[267] Bao Y, Pucci ML, Chan BS, Lu R, Ito S, Schuster VL. Prostaglandin transporter PGT is expressed in cell types that

synthesize and release prostanoids. Am J Physiol Renal Physiol 2002;282:F1103–10.

[268] Reid G, Wielinga P, Zelcer N, van der Heijden I, Kuil A, de Haas M, et al. The human multidrug resistance protein MRP4 functions as a prostaglandin efflux transporter and is inhibited by nonsteroidal antiinflammatory drugs. Proceedings of the National Academy of Sciences 2003;100:9244–9.

[269] Lin ZP, Zhu Y -L, Johnson DR, Rice KP, Nottoli T, Hains BC, et al. Disruption of cAMP and prostaglandin E2 transport by multidrug resistance protein 4 deficiency alters cAMP-mediated signaling and nociceptive response. Mol Pharmacol 2008; 73:243–51.

[270] Tomasoni S, Zappella S, Gotti E, Casiraghi F, Bonazzola S, Benigni A, et al. Upregulation of renal and systemic cyclooxygenase-2 in patients with active lupus nephritis. J Am Soc Nephrol 1998;9:1202–12.

[271] Schneider A, Harendza S, Zahner G, Jocks T, Wenzel U, Wolf G, et al. Cyclooxygenase metabolites mediate glomerular monocyte chemoattractant protein-1 formation and monocyte recruitment in experimental glomerulonephritis [see comments]. Kidney Int 1999;55:430–41.

[272] Zoja C, Benigni A, Verroust P, Ronco P, Bertani T, Remuzzi G. Indomethacin reduces proteinuria in passive Heymann nephritis in rats. Kidney Int 1987;31:1335–43.

[273] Takano T, Cybulsky AV, Cupples WA, Ajikobi DO, Papillon J, Aoudjit L. Inhibition of cyclooxygenases reduces complement-induced glomerular epithelial cell injury and proteinuria in passive Heymann nephritis. J Pharmacol Exp Ther 2003; 305:240–9.

[274] Kitahara M, Eitner F, Ostendorf T, Kunter U, Janssen U, Westenfeld R, et al. Selective cyclooxygenase-2 inhibition impairs glomerular capillary healing in experimental glomerulonephritis. J Am Soc Nephrol 2002;13:1261–70.

[275] Anderson GD, Hauser SD, McGarity KL, Bremer ME, Isakson PC, Gregory SA. Selective inhibition of cyclooxygenase (COX)-2 reverses inflammation and expression of COX-2 and interleukin 6 in rat adjuvant arthritis. J Clin Invest 1996;97:2672–9.

[276] Simon LS. Role and regulation of cyclooxygenase-2 during inflammation. Am J Med 1999;106:37S–42S.

[277] Mauer SM, Steffes MW, Ellis EN, Sutherland DE, Brown DM, Goetz FC. Structural–functional relationships in diabetic nephropathy. J Clin Invest 1984;74:1143–55.

[278] Najafian B, Alpers CE, Fogo AB. Pathology of human diabetic nephropathy. Contrib Nephrol 2011;170:36–47.

[279] Ciavarella A, Galuppi V, Forlani G, Vannini P. The prevalence of glomerular hyperfiltration in type 1 (insulin-dependent) diabetes mellitus. Diabete Metab 1988;14:73–4.

[280] Levine DZ, Iacovitti M, Robertson SJ, Mokhtar GA. Modulation of single-nephron GFR in the db/db mouse model of type 2 diabetes mellitus. Am J Physiol Regul Integr Comp Physiol 2006;290:R975–81.

[281] Qi Z, Fujita H, Jin J, Davis LS, Wang Y, Fogo AB, et al. Characterization of susceptibility of inbred mouse strains to diabetic nephropathy. Diabetes 2005;54:2628–37.

[282] Viberti GC, Benigni A, Bognetti E, Remuzzi G, Wiseman MJ. Glomerular hyperfiltration and urinary prostaglandins in type 1 diabetes mellitus. Diabet Med 1989;6:219–23.

[283] Craven PA, Caines MA, DeRubertis FR. Sequential alterations in glomerular prostaglandin and thromboxane synthesis in diabetic rats: relationship to the hyperfiltration of early diabetes. Metabolism 1987;36:95–103.

[284] Mathiesen ER, Hommel E, Olsen UB, Parving HH. Elevated urinary prostaglandin excretion and the effect of indomethacin on renal function in incipient diabetic nephropathy. Diabet Med 1988;5:145–9.

[285] Moel DI, Safirstein RL, McEvoy RC, Hsueh W. Effect of aspirin on experimental diabetic nephropathy. J Lab Clin Med 1987; 110:300–7.

[286] Cheng HF, Wang CJ, Moeckel GW, Zhang MZ, McKanna JA, Harris RC. Cyclooxygenase-2 inhibitor blocks expression of mediators of renal injury in a model of diabetes and hypertension. Kidney Int 2002;62:929–39.

[287] Khan KN, Stanfield KM, Harris RK, Baron DA. Expression of cyclooxygenase-2 in the macula densa of human kidney in hypertension, congestive heart failure, and diabetic nephropathy. Ren Fail 2001;23:321–30.

[288] Komers R, Lindsley JN, Oyama TT, Schutzer WE, Reed JF, Mader SL, et al. Immunohistochemical and functional correlations of renal cyclooxygenase-2 in experimental diabetes. J Clin Invest 2001;107:889–98.

[289] Xu S, Jiang B, Maitland KA, Bayat H, Gu J, Nadler JL, et al. The thromboxane receptor antagonist S18886 attenuates renal oxidant stress and proteinuria in diabetic apolipoprotein E-deficient mice. Diabetes 2006;55:110–9.

[290] Pelayo JC, Shanley PF. Glomerular and tubular adaptive responses to acute nephron loss in the rat. Effect of prostaglandin synthesis inhibition. J Clin Invest 1990;85:1761–9.

[291] Wang JL, Cheng HF, Shappell S, Harris RC. A selective cyclooxygenase-2 inhibitor decreases proteinuria and retards progressive renal injury in rats. Kidney Int 2000;57:2334–42.

[292] Cheng H, Zhang M, Moeckel GW, Zhao Y, Wang S, Qi Z, et al. Expression of mediators of renal injury in the remnant kidney of ROP mice is attenuated by cyclooxygenase-2 inhibition. Nephron Exp Nephrol 2005;101:e75–85.

[293] Funk CD, Chen X -S, Johnson EN, Zhao L. Lipoxygenase genes and their targeted disruption. Prostaglandins & Other Lipid Mediators 2002;68-69:303–12.

[294] Brash AR. Lipoxygenases: occurrence, functions, catalysis, and acquisition of substrate. J Biol Chem 1999;274:23679–82.

[295] Duroudier NP, Tulah AS, Sayers I. Leukotriene pathway genetics and pharmacogenetics in allergy. Allergy 2009;64: 823–39.

[296] Peters-Golden M, Henderson Jr. WR. Leukotrienes. N Engl J Med 2007;357:1841–54.

[297] Rinaldo-Matthis A, Haeggstrom JZ. Structures and mechanisms of enzymes in the leukotriene cascade. Biochimie 2010; 92:676–81.

[298] Jawien J, Gajda M, Rudling M, Mateuszuk L, Olszanecki R, Guzik TJ, et al. Inhibition of five lipoxygenase activating protein (FLAP) by MK-886 decreases atherosclerosis in apoE/LDLR-double knockout mice. Eur J Clin Invest 2006;36: 141–6.

[299] Samuelsson B, Funk CD. Enzymes involved in the biosynthesis of leukotriene B4. J Biol Chem 1989;264:19469–72.

[300] Shimizu T, Yokomizo T, Izumi T. Leukotriene-B4 receptor and signal transduction. Ernst Schering Res Found Workshop 2000;:125–41.

[301] Kolaczkowska E, Shahzidi S, Seljelid R, van Rooijen N, Plytycz B. Early vascular permeability in murine experimental peritonitis is co-mediated by resident peritoneal macrophages and mast cells: crucial involvement of macrophage-derived cysteinyl-leukotrienes. Inflammation 2002;26:61–71.

[302] Porreca E, Di Febbo C, Di Sciullo A, Angelucci D, Nasuti M, Vitullo P, et al. Cysteinyl leukotriene D4 induced vascular smooth muscle cell proliferation: a possible role in myointimal hyperplasia. Thromb Haemost 1996;76:99–104.

[303] Farrukh IS, Sciuto AM, Spannhake EW, Gurtner GH, Michael JR. Leukotriene D4 increases pulmonary vascular permeability and pressure by different mechanisms in the rabbit. Am Rev Respir Dis 1986;134:229–32.

[304] Fiedler VB, Mardin M, Abram TS. Leukotriene D4-induced vasoconstriction of coronary arteries in anaesthetized dogs. Eur Heart J 1984;5:253—60.

[305] Collin M, Rossi A, Cuzzocrea S, Patel NS, Di Paola R, Hadley J, et al. Reduction of the multiple organ injury and dysfunction caused by endotoxemia in 5-lipoxygenase knockout mice and by the 5-lipoxygenase inhibitor zileuton. J Leukoc Biol 2004; 76:961—70.

[306] Patel NS, Cuzzocrea S, Chatterjee PK, Di Paola R, Sautebin L, Britti D, et al. Reduction of renal ischemia-reperfusion injury in 5-lipoxygenase knockout mice and by the 5-lipoxygenase inhibitor zileuton. Mol Pharmacol 2004;66:220—7.

[307] Kitagawa K, Matsumoto M, Hori M. Cerebral ischemia in 5-lipoxygenase knockout mice. Brain Res 2004;1004:198—202.

[308] Di Gennaro A, Wågsäter D, Mäyränpää MI, Gabrielsen A, Swedenborg J, Hamsten A, et al. Increased expression of leukotriene C4 synthase and predominant formation of cysteinyl-leukotrienes in human abdominal aortic aneurysm. Proc Natl Acad Sci 2010;107:21093—7.

[309] Ardaillou R, Baud L, Sraer J. Leukotrienes and other lipoxygenase products of arachidonic acid synthesized in the kidney. Am J Med 1986;81:12—22.

[310] Badr KF. 15-Lipoxygenase products as leukotriene antagonists: Therapeutic potential in glomerulonephritis. Kidney Int Suppl 1992;38:S101—8.

[311] Kawasaki Y, Tanji M, Takano K, Fukuda Y, Isome M, Nozawa R, et al. The leukotriene B4 receptor antagonist ONO-4057 inhibits mesangioproliferative changes in anti-Thy-1 nephritis. Nephrology Dialysis Transplantation 2005;20:2697—703.

[312] Reinhold SW, Vitzthum H, Filbeck T, Wolf K, Lattas C, Riegger GA, et al. Gene expression of 5-, 12-, and 15-lipoxygenases and leukotriene receptors along the rat nephron. Am J Physiol Renal Physiol 2006;290:F864—72.

[313] Menegatti E, Roccatello D, Fadden K, Piccoli G, De Rosa G, Sena LM, et al. Gene expression of 5-lipoxygenase and LTA4 hydrolase in renal tissue of nephrotic syndrome patients. Clin Exp Immunol 1999;116:347—53.

[314] Badr KF. Five-lipoxygenase products in glomerular immune injury. J Am Soc Nephrol 1992;3:907—15.

[315] Katoh T, Lianos EA, Fukunaga M, Takahashi K, Badr KF. Leukotriene D4 is a mediator of proteinuria and glomerular hemodynamic abnormalities in passive Heymann nephritis. J Clin Invest 1993;91:1507—15.

[316] Natarajan R, Nadler JL. Lipid inflammatory mediators in diabetic vascular disease. Arterioscler Thromb Vasc Biol 2004; 24:1542—8.

[317] Dailey LA, Imming P. 12-Lipoxygenase: classification, possible therapeutic benefits from inhibition, and inhibitors. Curr Med Chem 1999;6:389—98.

[318] Zhao L, Moos MP, Grabner R, Pedrono F, Fan J, Kaiser B, et al. The 5-lipoxygenase pathway promotes pathogenesis of hyperlipidemia-dependent aortic aneurysm. Nat Med 2004; 10:966—73.

[319] Klein RF, Allard J, Avnur Z, Nikolcheva T, Rotstein D, Carlos AS, et al. Regulation of bone mass in mice by the lipoxygenase gene Alox15. Science 2004;303:229—32.

[320] Poeckel D, Funk CD. The 5-lipoxygenase/leukotriene pathway in preclinical models of cardiovascular disease. Cardiovasc Res 2010;86:243—53.

[321] Kang SW, Natarajan R, Shahed A, Nast CC, LaPage J, Mundel P, et al. Role of 12-lipoxygenase in the stimulation of p38 mitogen-activated protein kinase and collagen alpha5(IV) in experimental diabetic nephropathy and in glucose-stimulated podocytes. J Am Soc Nephrol 2003;14:3178—87.

[322] Kim YS, Xu ZG, Reddy MA, Li SL, Lanting L, Sharma K, et al. Novel interactions between TGF-{beta}1 actions and the 12/15-lipoxygenase pathway in mesangial cells. J Am Soc Nephrol 2005;16:352—62.

[323] Xu ZG, Li SL, Lanting L, Kim YS, Shanmugam N, Reddy MA, et al. Relationship between 12/15-lipoxygenase and COX-2 in mesangial cells: potential role in diabetic nephropathy. Kidney Int 2006;69:512—9.

[324] Gonzalez-Nunez D, Sole M, Natarajan R, Poch E. 12-Lipoxygenase metabolism in mouse distal convoluted tubule cells. Kidney Int 2005;67:178—86.

[325] Kang SW, Adler SG, Nast CC, LaPage J, Gu JL, Nadler JL, et al. 12-lipoxygenase is increased in glucose-stimulated mesangial cells and in experimental diabetic nephropathy. Kidney Int 2001;59:1354—62.

[326] Guo QY, Miao LN, Li B, Ma FZ, Liu N, Cai L, et al. Role of 12-lipoxygenase in decreasing P-cadherin and increasing angiotensin II type 1 receptor expression according to glomerular size in type 2 diabetic rats. Am J Physiol Endocrinol Metab 2011;300:E708—16.

[327] Xu ZG, Miao LN, Cui YC, Jia Y, Yuan H, Wu M. Angiotensin II type 1 receptor expression is increased via 12-lipoxygenase in high glucose-stimulated glomerular cells and type 2 diabetic glomeruli. Nephrol Dial Transplant 2009;24:1744—52.

[328] Capdevila JH, Harris RC, Falck JR. Microsomal cytochrome P450 and eicosanoid metabolism. Cell Mol Life Sci 2002; 59:780—9.

[329] McGiff JC. Cytochrome P-450 metabolism of arachidonic acid. Annu Rev Pharmacol Toxicol 1991;31:339—69.

[330] Camara NO, Martins JO, Landgraf RG, Jancar S. Emerging roles for eicosanoids in renal diseases. Curr Opin Nephrol Hypertens 2009;18:21—7.

[331] Spector AA. Arachidonic acid cytochrome P450 epoxygenase pathway. J Lipid Res 2009;50(Suppl.):S52—6.

[332] Kroetz DL, Zeldin DC. Cytochrome P450 pathways of arachidonic acid metabolism. Curr Opin Lipidol 2002;13:273—83.

[333] Scarborough PE, Ma J, Qu W, Zeldin DC. P450 subfamily CYP2J and their role in the bioactivation of arachidonic acid in extrahepatic tissues. Drug Metab Rev 1999;31:205—34.

[334] Lasker JM, Chen WB, Wolf I, Bloswick BP, Wilson PD, Powell PK. Formation of 20-hydroxyeicosatetraenoic acid, a vasoactive and natriuretic eicosanoid, in human kidney. Role of Cyp4F2 and Cyp4A11. J Biol Chem 2000;275:4118—26.

[335] Roman RJ. P-450 Metabolites of arachidonic acid in the control of cardiovascular function. Physiol Rev 2002;82:131—85.

[336] Imig J, Gebremedhin D, Zou A, Stec D, Harder D, Falck J, et al. Formation and actions of 20-hydroxyeicosatetraenoic acid in the renal microcirculation. Am J Physiol 1996;270:R217—27.

[337] Larsen BT, Gutterman DD, Hatoum OA. Emerging role of epoxyeicosatrienoic acids in coronary vascular function. Eur J Clin Invest 2006;36:293—300.

[338] Oltman CL, Weintraub NL, VanRollins M, Dellsperger KC. Epoxyeicosatrienoic acids and dihydroxyeicosatrienoic acids are potent vasodilators in the canine coronary microcirculation. Circ Res 1998;83:932—9.

[339] Wei Y, Lin DH, Kemp R, Yaddanapudi GS, Nasjletti A, Falck JR, et al. Arachidonic acid inhibits epithelial Na channel via cytochrome P450 (CYP) epoxygenase-dependent metabolic pathways. J Gen Physiol 2004;124:719—27.

[340] Wang S, Meng F, Xu J, Gu Y. Effects of lipids on ENaC activity in cultured mouse cortical collecting duct cells. J Membr Biol 2009;227:77—85.

[341] Sun P, Lin DH, Yue P, Jiang H, Gotlinger KH, Schwartzman ML, et al. High potassium intake enhances the inhibitory effect of 11,12-EET on ENaC. J Am Soc Nephrol 2010;21:1667—77.

[342] Athirakul K, Bradbury JA, Graves JP, DeGraff LM, Ma J, Zhao Y, et al. Increased blood pressure in mice lacking cytochrome P450 2J5. FASEB J 2008;22:4096—108.

[343] Holla VR, Adas F, Imig JD, Zhao X, Price Jr. E, Olsen N, et al. Alterations in the regulation of androgen-sensitive Cyp 4a monooxygenases cause hypertension. Proc Natl Acad Sci USA 2001;98:5211—6.

[344] Nakagawa K, Holla VR, Wei Y, Wang WH, Gatica A, Wei S, et al. Salt-sensitive hypertension is associated with dysfunctional Cyp4a10 gene and kidney epithelial sodium channel. J Clin Invest 2006;116:1696—702.

[345] Miyazono M, Zhu D, Nemenoff R, Jacobs ER, Carter EP. Increased epoxyeicosatrienoic acid formation in the rat kidney during liver cirrhosis. J Am Soc Nephrol 2003;14:1766—75.

[346] Hercule H, Oyekan A. Renal cytochrome p450 oxygenases and preglomerular vascular response to arachidonic acid and endothelin-1 following ischemia/reperfusion. J Pharmacol Exp Ther 2002;302:717—24.

[347] McCarthy ET, Sharma R, Sharma M. Protective effect of 20-hydroxyeicosatetraenoic acid (20-HETE) on glomerular protein permeability barrier. Kidney Int 2005;67:152—6.

[348] Yuhki K -I, Kojima F, Kashiwagi H, Kawabe J -I, Fujino T, Narumiya S, et al. Roles of prostanoids in the pathogenesis of cardiovascular diseases: novel insights from knockout mouse studies. Pharm Therap 2011;129:195—205.

18

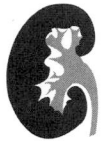

Extracellular Nucleotides and Renal Function

David G. Shirley[1], Matthew A. Bailey[2], Scott S. P. Wildman[3],
Frederick W. K. Tam[4] and Robert J. Unwin[1]

[1]UCL Centre for Nephrology, University College London Medical School, UK
[2]British Heart Foundation Centre for Cardiovascular Science, University of Edinburgh, UK
[3]Medway School of Pharmacy, The Universities of Kent and Greenwich at Medway, UK
[4]Kidney and Transplant Institute, Imperial College School of Medicine, UK

Historically, the control of renal vascular and tubular function has been attributed solely to neural and endocrine regulation. However, in addition to these extrinsic factors, it is now recognized that several complex humoral control systems exist *within* the kidney that act in an autocrine and/or paracrine manner. One of these is the extracellular nucleotide/P2 receptor system.

Although physiological actions of extracellular adenine nucleotides were reported as long ago as 1929,[34] it was not until many years later (1972) that the importance of ATP as a transmitter for non-adrenergic, non-cholinergic neurones of the autonomic nervous system was proposed by Geoffrey Burnstock.[13] Since then it has become apparent that the function of extracellular nucleotides is not confined to neurones: rather, they are ubiquitous autocrine/paracrine agents regulating diverse physiological processes in almost every tissue in the body. Information on their roles in the kidneys has only really begun to emerge in the last decade.

P2 RECEPTORS

Extracellular nucleotides exert their effects by binding to and activating cell surface located receptors; P2 receptors. These are subdivided into P2X receptors, of which seven mammalian subunits have been cloned (P2X$_{1-7}$), and P2Y receptors, of which eight mammalian subtypes are currently recognized, P2Y$_{1, 2, 4, 6}$, and P2Y$_{11-14}$.[14]

P2X Receptors

P2X receptor subunits are proteins with two transmembrane-spanning regions, the N- and C-termini being within the cell.[114] Three P2X subunits assemble to form a P2X receptor ion channel that, when activated, is permeable to small cations (Na$^+$, K$^+$, Ca^{2+}). Each of the seven P2X subunits can make homomeric ion channels, and can also form heteromeric assemblies involving more than one type of subunit. Until recently it had been thought that P2X$_7$ subunits could only make homomeric assemblies, but a P2X$_{4/7}$ heteromer has now been described.[51] As well as a non-selective ion channel, the P2X$_7$ receptor can form a larger membrane pore, and initiate cell death by necrosis or apoptosis.

The principal natural ligand for all P2X subunits is ATP. The P2X$_1$ subunit is the most sensitive (requiring sub-micromolar concentrations of ATP); P2X$_{2-6}$ subunits require micromolar concentrations, while the P2X$_7$ subunit is easily the least sensitive, requiring almost millimolar concentrations.

P2Y Receptors

P2Y receptors are G-protein-coupled receptors with seven transmembrane-spanning regions; the C-terminus is inside the cell and the N-terminus extracellular. In rodents, ATP is probably the principal natural ligand for P2Y$_{2, 4}$ and P2Y$_{11}$ subtypes and, at sufficiently high dose and/or receptor density, can activate P2Y$_{1, 12}$ and P2Y$_{13}$

subtypes. However, the natural ligand for P2Y$_{1, 12,}$ and P2Y$_{13}$ subtypes is ADP. Although P2Y$_6$ receptors can also be activated by ADP, UDP is much more potent. In rodents, UTP activates P2Y$_2$ and P2Y$_4$ subtypes with similar potency to ATP, an observation often used in physiological studies as an initial pointer to receptor identity. Human P2Y$_4$ receptors, however, are activated primarily by UTP (50-fold more potent than ATP[178]). This is a particularly striking example of species differences, serving to highlight the need for caution before extrapolating from findings in one species to another. The P2Y$_{14}$ receptor is exceptional in that its natural ligand is UDP-glucose; although originally believed to be unaffected by unglycosylated purine- or pyrimidine-based nucleotides, it is now known that UDP is also a full agonist at rat and human P2Y$_{14}$ receptors.[55]

P2Y receptors are coupled to either G$_q$ or G$_i$ signaling proteins. P2Y$_{1, 2, 4, 6,}$ and P2Y$_{11}$ subtypes are coupled to G$_q$/G$_{11}$, resulting in PLC-β activation and increased [Ca^{2+}]$_i$, while P2Y$_{12-14}$ are coupled to G$_i$/G$_o$, resulting in adenylyl cyclase inhibition and reduced cAMP levels. The P2Y$_{11}$ subtype is unusual, in that it can couple to both G$_q$ and G$_s$, resulting in both PLC-β and adenylyl cyclase activation, causing increased cAMP levels.[172]

Heterodimeric Receptors and Dinucleotide Receptors

A further layer of complexity has been added to the picture with the finding that adenosine A1 receptors can be co-expressed with P2Y$_1$ or P2Y$_2$ receptors (and possibly other P2Y subtypes) as a discrete receptor type, at least in non-renal cells. The chimeric nature of such receptors is reflected in their mixed pharmacological and signaling properties.[200,201] The possible functional significance of these heterodimeric P1/P2Y receptors with regard to the kidneys is currently unknown.

Finally, a number of dinucleotides, in which the 5′-carbon positions of two nucleosides are linked by a polyphosphate chain, occur naturally in the body. These dinucleotides can be symmetrical (e.g., Ap$_4$A, where two adenosine moieties are linked by a chain of four phosphates) or asymmetrical (e.g., Up$_4$A, where a uridine moiety and an adenosine moiety are similarly linked). Dinucleotides can have both vascular and tubular effects within the kidneys (*vide infra*), but the receptors responsible are unknown; evidence for dinucleotide-specific receptors has been provided in other tissues, but several P2Y receptors (P2Y$_{1, 2, 4,}$ and P2Y$_6$) and P2X receptors (P2X$_{1-5}$) are known to be dinucleotide-sensitive.[81,143]

It is likely that both adenine-based and uracil-based nucleotides are released from most cells in the body (including renal cells); moreover, ecto-enzymes that metabolize nucleotides, either inactivating them or converting them to molecular forms that can stimulate different P2 receptor subtypes, are ubiquitous (*vide infra*). Figure 18.1 shows the molecular structures of some of the principal nucleotides involved, and Figure 18.2 provides a simplified overview of nucleotide release, degradation, and purinoceptor (i.e., P1 (adenosine) receptor and P2 receptor) activation.

Synthetic Agonists and Antagonists of P2 Receptors

Agonists

An ever-increasing range of synthetic nucleotide analogs and non-nucleotide agonists is being developed in an attempt to find agents that, unlike naturally occurring nucleotides, are not subject to degradation by ectonucleotidases, and can act as selective agonists for given receptor subtypes. Such exclusivity is rarely achieved, although substantial progress is now being made. Unfortunately, many of the initial observations on P2 receptor stimulation and renal function were made at a time when information on the selectivity of agonists was incomplete, and the agonists used were often more promiscuous than was appreciated, giving rise to misleading interpretations. Thus, although 2 meSADP, for example, has been used as an agonist for P2Y$_1$ receptors, it also activates P2Y$_{12}$ and P2Y$_{13}$ subtypes; the same applies to 2 meSATP which, additionally, can stimulate a number of P2X receptors, while ATPγS, originally used as a P2Y$_2$ and/or P2Y$_4$ agonist, is now known as a broad-spectrum agonist, being effective in a range of P2Y and P2X receptors. Another ATP analog, 2′3′-O-(4-benzoylbenzoyl)ATP (BzATP), has often been used as a "selective" P2X$_7$ agonist, given that it is more potent than ATP at this receptor subunit, but it is also effective at P2X$_{1, 3}$ and P2Y$_5$ subunits, so it is in reality only a nonselective P2X agonist. Furthermore, BzATP has been shown to act as an antagonist at P2Y$_4$ receptors.[185]

As our knowledge of truly selective P2 agonists expands, future investigations should provide more precise information about the purinoceptor subtype(s) involved in a given physiological response. That knowledge, however, is still limited. The *N*-methanocarba-ADP derivative MRS2365 is selective for P2Y$_1$ receptors; MRS2698 and INS365 (Up$_4$U or "diquafosol") are selective P2Y$_2$ agonists; and UDPβS, INS48823, and MRS2693 are selective P2Y$_6$ agonists.[14,72,178] At the time of writing, a selective agonist for P2Y$_4$ receptors has not been identified. Similarly, a truly selective agonist for any of the P2X subunits is still lacking.

Antagonists

As with agonists, nucleotide receptor-selective antagonists are something of a rarity. Probably the compound

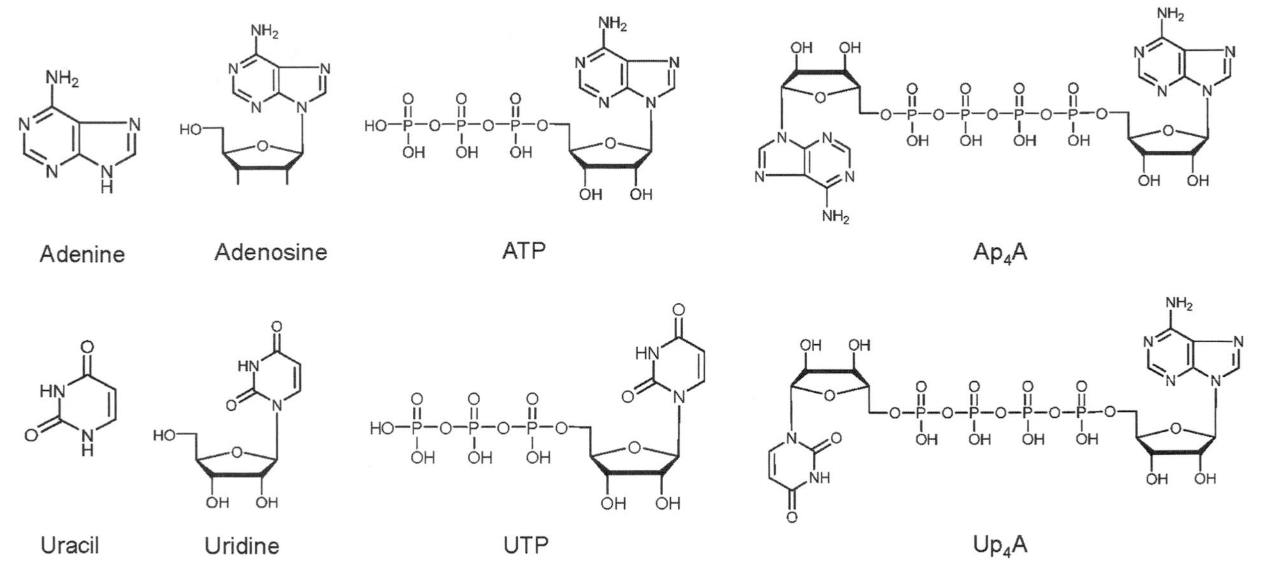

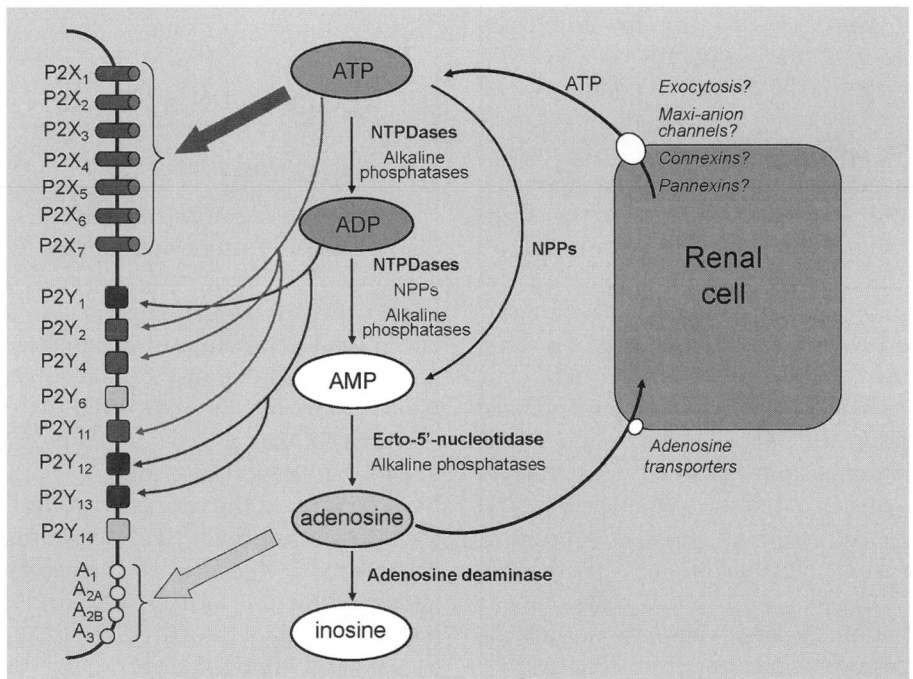

FIGURE 18.1 Molecular structures of some of the principal nucleotides and their parent nucleosides and purine/pyrimidine bases.

FIGURE 18.2 **The renal purinoceptor system and its modulation by the major renal ectonucleotidases.** The mechanism of ATP release from renal cells is still a matter of debate (see text for details). It is important to note that nucleotides derived from other bases are also likely to be secreted and are also hydrolyzed/synthesized by ectonucleotidases, but have been omitted for clarity. Uracil-based nucleotides are particularly significant: UTP is a potent agonist of $P2Y_2$ and $P2Y_4$ subtypes, and its derivative UDP is the major naturally occurring agonist of the $P2Y_6$ subtype.

most commonly used to inhibit P2 receptors is suramin, although it also affects a variety of other cellular processes. In sufficient concentration, suramin antagonizes practically every P2 receptor subtype, be it P2Y or P2X. The same comment applies to PPADS (pyridoxal-5-phosphate-6-azophenyl 2′,4′-disulphonic acid) and, to a lesser extent, reactive blue 2 (RB-2). However, a clutch of selective and potent antagonists is now available. Thus, the ADP derivatives MRS2179, MRS2279, and MRS2500 are selective $P2Y_1$ antagonists; AR-C126313 and AR-C118925 are selective $P2Y_2$ antagonists; MRS2578 is a selective $P2Y_6$ antagonist; INS49266, INS50589, and AZD6140 are selective $P2Y_{12}$ antagonists; and MRS2211 is a selective $P2Y_{13}$ antagonist.[14,72,178]

I. EPITHELIAL AND NONEPITHELIAL TRANSPORT AND REGULATION

For P2X subunits, the list is shorter. Ip$_5$I is a selective P2X$_1$ antagonist,[14] and A-740003 and A-438079 are selective P2X$_7$ antagonists.[33] Trinitrophenyl-ATP (TNP-ATP) "selectively" antagonizes P2X$_{1-5}$ subunits without affecting P2Y receptors.

Assignment of Physiological Responses to Specific P2 Receptor Subtypes

The plasma membranes of any renal cell, be it vascular or tubular, can contain a variety of P2 receptor subtypes. Moreover, epithelial cells can have different (as well as the same) subtypes on their apical and basolateral membranes. This raises the question of how to attribute a given functional response to a particular subtype. A number of approaches can be used. First, it is useful to identify immunologically the subtypes present in the region of interest (although this, of course, depends on the availability of suitable antibodies) and, if possible, to localize the receptor to apical and/or basolateral membrane. In some cases, instead of the immunohisto-chemical approach, determination of mRNA has been used, although this obviously does not guarantee the presence of the receptor protein itself. Second, it is possible to try to mimic the effect of the naturally occurring nucleotide using "selective" agonists and antagonists. However, as indicated above, only a few of these are truly selective (although the situation is improving). Consequently, it is usually necessary to compare the individual responses to a variety of agonists (both natural and synthetic) to provide a pharmacological profile from which tentative conclusions can be drawn, but even then their effects will depend not only on agonist/antagonist concentration, but also on the number and distribution of receptor subtypes. Moreover, naturally occurring agonists are degraded by ectonucleotidases, making it difficult to control their absolute concentrations at the receptor site. A further limitation is the use of intracellular Ca^{2+} transients to assess responses to direct application of agonists, since these are not invariably associated with recognizable functional changes.

A completely different, and superficially more attractive, approach is to use "knockout" mice in which the gene encoding the receptor of interest has been deleted. However, this is not without its own potential problems. Life-long, global deletion of a receptor subtype that performs a vital function is likely to lead to compensatory changes in several organ systems. The P2 receptor profile within the kidney may then change in order to restore overall excretion rates, which could then lead to misleading conclusions about the role of the receptor. The Cre-loxP system adds a degree of refinement to the gene-targeting approach, permitting tissue- or cell-type-specific deletion. Nevertheless, compensatory changes in up- or downstream nephron segments cannot be excluded, and this approach is further complicated by incomplete (knockdown rather than knockout) and off-target deletion. Furthermore, genetically-engineered deletions have so far been restricted to mice, where P2Y$_2$ receptors seem to predominate in the renal tubule. There are important differences in the distributions of receptor subtypes between mice and rats — and presumably between mice and other species. Thus, for the foreseeable future it seems that we will need to continue to rely on a combination of approaches; as yet, there is no "silver bullet" when it comes to defining P2 receptor function.

Finally, to obviate the need for working with complex renal tubules, many investigators have made use of simpler systems: immortalized cell lines originally derived from renal-like tissue (e.g., Madin–Darby canine kidney (MDCK) cells). Unfortunately, these cell lines often express membrane proteins that differ from those found in native tissue. Consequently, in this chapter we will avoid deductions based solely on observations concerning P2 receptors in non-native renal tissue.

P2 RECEPTORS AND RENAL FUNCTION

The Renal Vasculature

Figure 18.3 summarizes current knowledge about the distribution of P2 receptors in renal vascular and tubular structures. P2 receptors are expressed widely in the renal vasculature, in the glomerulus, and in the extraglomerular mesangium. Immunohistochemical and Western analyses indicate that P2X$_1$ receptors are present in the vascular smooth muscle of the rat renal artery, arcuate and interlobular arteries, and the afferent arteriole, but not in the efferent arteriole.[19,171] Functional approaches have confirmed the expression of a P2X$_1$-like receptor in the afferent arteriole.[70] P2X$_2$ subunits have been immunolocalized in the smooth muscle of larger arteries and veins within the kidney,[66,171] and molecular evidence has recently been provided for P2X$_4$ subunits, at least in arcuate and interlobular arteries.[56] Of the P2Y receptors, P2Y$_1$ has an extensive distribution, being expressed in the endothelium of the large arteries, and both afferent and efferent arterioles.[171]

Most information concerning P2 receptor expression in the glomerulus comes from cell culture systems. On the basis of mRNA detection and/or agonist profiling, P2Y$_{1,2,4}$ and P2Y$_6$ subtypes and P2X$_{2,3,4,5}$ and P2Y$_7$ subunits have been identified in glomerular mesangial cells[53,65,132,151]; P2Y$_{1,2}$ and P2Y$_6$ subtypes in podocytes[41]; and P2Y$_1$ and P2Y$_2$ subtypes in glomerular endothelial cells.[12] Studies performed on RNA extracted from pools of intact glomeruli from rats found messages encoding P2Y$_{1,2,4}$ and P2Y$_6$

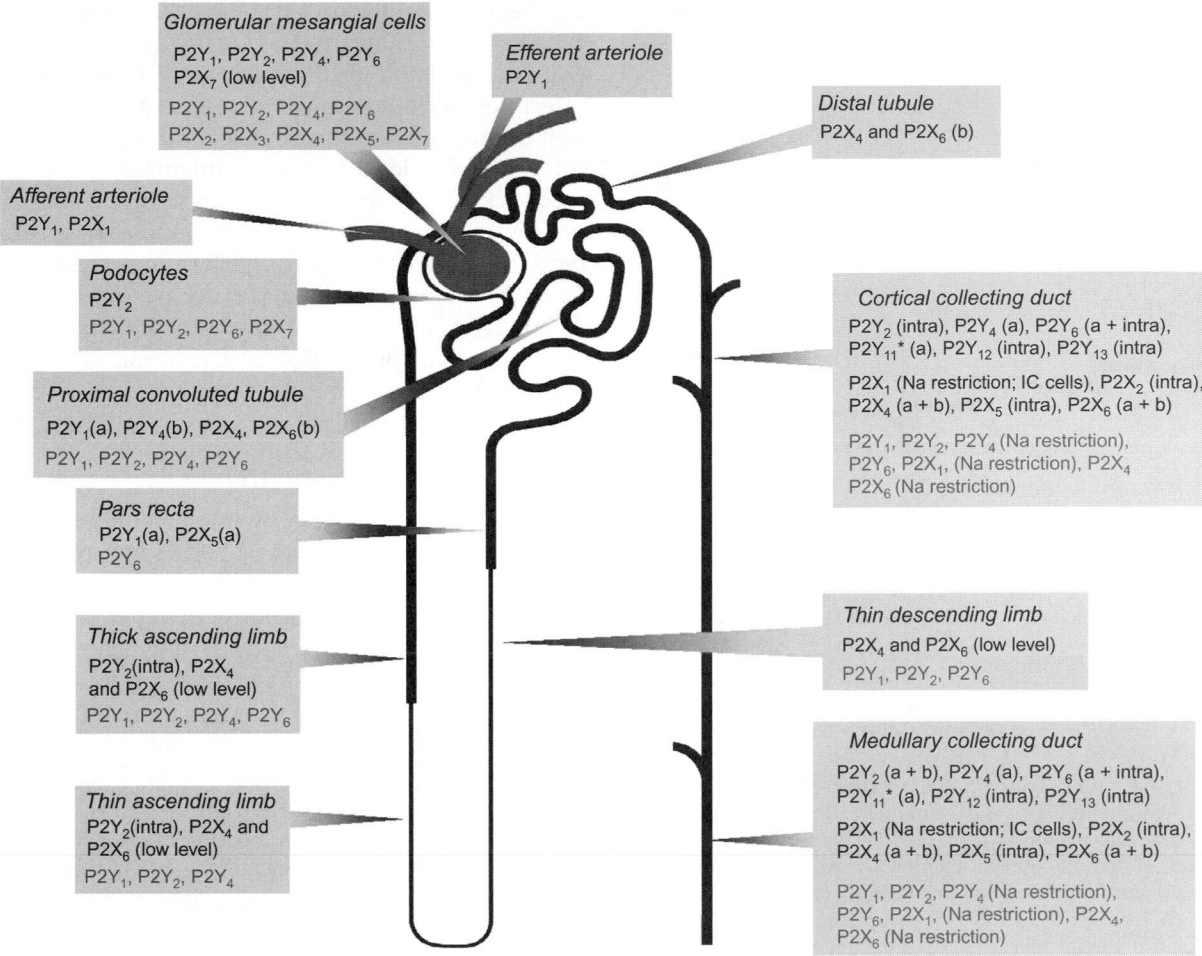

FIGURE 18.3 P2 receptors in the vasculature and tubules of the rat kidney. Those receptors in the rat kidney for which firm evidence from immunohistochemical studies and/or Western blotting has been obtained are shown in black. Those receptors for which expression of mRNA has been documented are shown in red. Where possible, apical (a), basolateral (b) or intracellular (intra) location is indicated. *The antibody used to detect $P2Y_{11}$ was raised against an epitope of human, not rat, $P2Y_{11}$ receptors. Information is taken from ref. 4–7,19,41,53,83,132,151,171,187,203

subtypes[7]; the expression of other P2Y receptors was not assessed. Immunohistochemical analysis and measurements of agonist-induced phosphoinositide production confirmed the presence $P2Y_1$ and $P2Y_2$ subtypes in the rat glomerulus. On the basis of co-localization with cell-specific markers, $P2Y_1$ receptors were localized in mesangial cells and $P2Y_2$ receptors in podocytes[7,171]; expression of $P2Y_4$ and $P2Y_6$ receptor protein could not be confirmed, either functionally or immunologically. Of the P2X subtypes, only a low and variable expression of $P2X_7$ immunoreactivity was found in the rat glomerulus.[171]

Physiological Responses

Infusion of ATP into the renal artery has long been known to alter renal vascular resistance, although the nature and magnitude of the response are dependent upon species, basal vascular tone, and to some extent the experimental approach.[67] The larger renal arteries

serve principally as conductance vessels,[202] and renal vascular resistance (and therefore renal blood flow) is regulated primarily through pressure-dependent vasoactivity of the preglomerular arterioles[153] and, to a lesser extent, the small interlobular arteries.[58] The responsiveness to ATP of the arcuate and interlobular arteries and the glomerular arterioles has been evaluated in rats using the isolated perfused kidney preparation.[70] The preglomerular arteries were relatively insensitive to ATP, with micromolar concentrations evoking transient vasoconstriction (Figure 18.4). In contrast, the afferent arteriole underwent sustained contraction at concentrations in the submicromolar range, whereas the efferent arteriole was unresponsive to extracellular ATP. Thus, in the isolated perfused rat kidney, intrarenal administration of ATP is normally vasoconstrictive. This vasoconstriction can be potentiated by inhibition of nitric oxide (NO) synthesis.[37] However, when baseline renal vascular resistance is

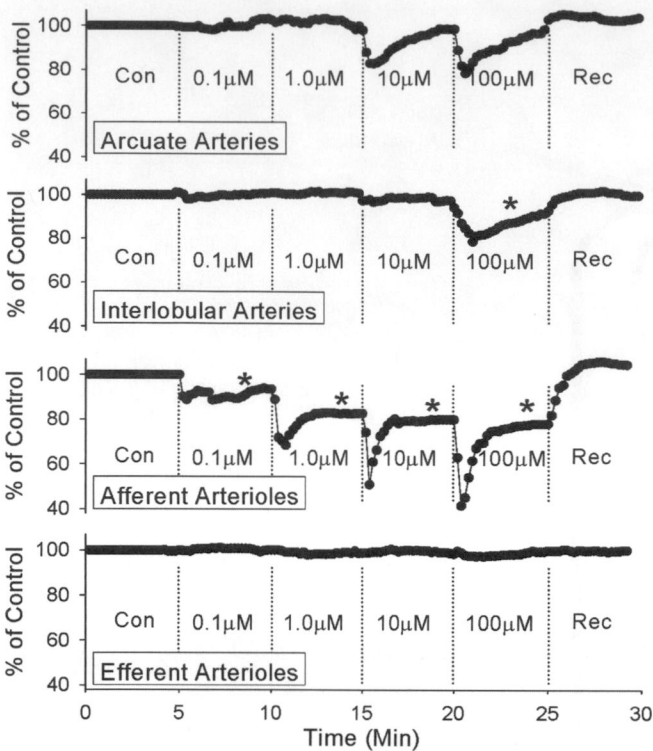

FIGURE 18.4   ATP concentration–response relationships for pre- and post-glomerular vasculature. The figure shows average segmental diameter responses evoked by ATP applied to the adventitial surface of arcuate arteries, interlobular arteries, afferent arterioles, and efferent arterioles of rat juxtamedullary vascular segments. After the control period (Con), increasing concentrations of ATP were applied at 5 min intervals; each protocol ended with a 5 min recovery period (Rec). Each data point is normalized as a percentage of the control diameter *(from ref. [67]).*

high, ATP induces *vasodilatation*, due to P2Y-mediated production of NO.[40] Thus, P2 receptor "tone" can influence renal vascular resistance, with P2Y/NO-mediated vasodilatation exerting a counterbalancing influence on P2X$_1$-mediated vasoconstriction. The dominant receptor pool, as well as the source and local concentration of extracellular nucleotide, will therefore influence the net physiological response to extracellular nucleotides. ATP released from renal nerve terminals, for example, will act directly on the vascular smooth muscle, promoting P2X$_1$-mediated vasoconstriction.[139,162] Conversely, release of ATP in the vicinity of the endothelial P2Y receptors would be expected to promote NO synthesis and vasodilatation.

Renal Autoregulation

The majority of vascular beds stabilize blood flow in the face of fluctuating blood pressure. This autoregulation of blood flow is an intrinsic property of the vasculature, and in the kidney it is highly efficient: over the physiological range, renal blood flow can be effectively independent of blood pressure.[26] Whole-kidney autoregulation is governed through the combined influence of at least two mechanisms, tubuloglomerular feedback (TGF) and the intrinsic myogenic response of the vascular smooth muscle; these regulatory systems have different, but overlapping, operational frequencies. Computational analysis of the dynamic frequencies of the two systems indicates a degree of interaction; constriction of the terminal afferent arteriole by TGF increases pressure in the upstream vasculature and the myogenic response is enhanced.[180]

Myogenic Responses to Altered Perfusion Pressure

Of the two major components, only the intrinsic myogenic response to altered perfusion pressure is both necessary and sufficient for full, whole kidney autoregulation.[26] The myogenic response operates along the preglomerular vascular tree, reacting to increased transmural pressure by channel-mediated calcium influx and reflex vasoconstriction of the vascular smooth muscle. The exact signaling mechanisms are not defined, but local release of ATP is implicated. In the afferent arteriole, pressure-mediated vasoconstriction is markedly blunted by PPADS or suramin, or by the saturation and subsequent desensitization of the P2 receptor system.[69] The central role of the P2 system is further underscored by experiments in P2X$_1$-deficient mice, in which pressure-induced reductions in afferent arteriole diameter are abolished[68] (Figure 18.5). Similarly, pharmacological[119] or pathological[50] maneuvers that impair P2X$_1$ receptor signaling significantly attenuate whole kidney autoregulation of blood flow both *in vivo* and *in vitro*. Furthermore, mice with a targeted deletion of the ecto-nucleotidase NTPDase1 (thereby prolonging the half-life of extracellular ATP — *vide infra*) exhibit enhanced pressure-induced vasocontriction in the mesenteric artery,[78] consistent with a key role for local nucleotide signaling in the general myogenic response.

Tubuloglomerular Feedback and the Juxtaglomerular Apparatus

Tubuloglomerular feedback (TGF) is a dynamic process whereby changes in the concentration of NaCl in the fluid emerging from the loop of Henle elicit inverse changes in the glomerular filtration rate of the nephron of origin. TGF is mediated by the juxtaglomerular apparatus (JGA), which includes a sensor, the macula densa, and an effector, the granulated cells of the afferent arteriole; other components of the JGA (e.g., mesangial cells) also play a role.

Bell and colleagues demonstrated the release of ATP across the basolateral membrane of the macula

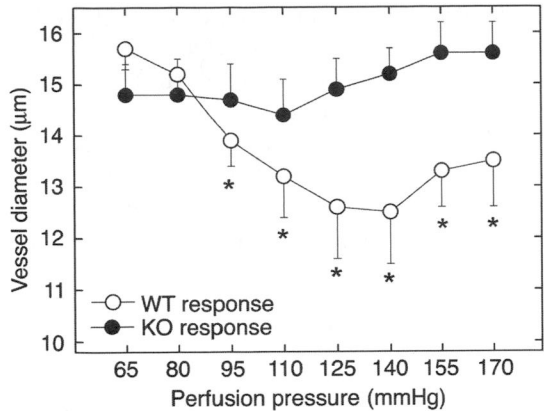

FIGURE 18.5 Autoregulatory responses in P2X1 knockout (KO) mice versus wild-type (WT) mice. The normal autoregulatory vasoconstrictor response to increases in perfusion pressure is absent in the KO mice. *(from ref. [68]).*

densa plaque in response to altered luminal NaCl concentration within the physiological range,[11,87] and the concentration of ATP in the cortical interstitium was shown to respond appropriately to inhibition or activation of TGF *in vivo*.[112] This compelling evidence suggests that ATP is the primary signaling molecule for TGF, the effects of which might well be modulated by other paracrine agents produced in the macula densa cell, such as nNOS- (NOS1-) derived NO and COX2-derived prostaglandin E_2.[10] Gene-targeting experiments, however, suggest that ATP may not be the ultimate signal through which TGF causes constriction of the afferent arteriole; hydrolysis of ATP to adenosine appears to be critical. *In vivo* TGF responses are attenuated in mice lacking either adenosine A_1 receptors[157] or ecto-5′-nucleotidase, the enzyme catalyzing the final stage of the degradation of ATP to adenosine.[15] This proposition is supported by a recent *in vivo* study in which the TGF response in mice (as assessed by changes in stop-flow pressure in the proximal tubule) was unaffected during intravenous infusion of PPADS or suramin.[136]

It would be rash, however, to conclude that the P2 receptor system has no role in TGF. Desensitization of this system inhibits TGF in rats,[113] and it is notable that *in vivo* manipulations of TGF affect the interstitial concentration of ATP, but not of adenosine.[67] Furthermore, an anatomical consideration argues strongly for involvement of the P2 receptor system in the TGF response: the ATP released from macula densa cells cannot directly activate P2 receptors in the afferent arteriole, being physically separated in most species by the extraglomerular mesangium. An intact mesangium is required for TGF responses,[129] and Peti-Peterdi has demonstrated that TGF activation

causes a wave of increased cytosolic calcium to pass through the mesangium, to the granulated cells of the afferent arteriole and into the glomerular podocytes.[121] Propagation of this calcium wave was abolished by suramin, but not by adenosine receptor antagonism. The P2 receptor response was later shown to be dependent on gap junctional coupling, being inhibited by specific antagonists against connexins 37 and 40[159] (*vide infra* for discussion of connexins).

The basolateral membrane of macula densa cells expresses a $P2Y_2$-like receptor, the function of which is not yet known.[10] It is possible that this provides a negative feedback loop for TGF signaling or a mechanism through which ATP release can be coupled to production.

Glomerular and Medullary Microcirculation

Infusions of nucleotide analogs into the renal artery exert powerful effects on regional blood flow, which can be measured by laser-Doppler flow probes inserted into specific regions of the kidney. In the rabbit, ATP evokes a biphasic response, with vasoconstriction of the medullary blood flow being followed by hyperemia.[39] On the basis of relative agonist potency, the vasoconstriction was attributed to $P2X_1$ receptors; the secondary vasodilatation, which was independent of NO, was partially mediated by adenosine receptors. In the rat, the net effect of ATP is influenced by sodium status. In sodium-restricted rats, ATP increased medullary blood flow in a nitric oxide-dependent manner.[32] In rats fed a high-salt diet, ATP caused vasoconstriction in the outer medulla, without affecting inner medullary flow. The authors' speculated that the inner medullary vasodilatation reflected an effect of nucleotides on vasa recta pericytes. However, preliminary data from Peppiatt-Wildman's laboratory, obtained in slices of rat kidney, suggest that P2 receptor activation promotes vasoconstriction in this setting.[79]

Renin Release

The renin–angiotensin system is influenced by many factors, the final pathways of which converge at the level of altered $[Ca^{2+}]_i$ in the granular cell; renin secretion is inversely related to $[Ca^{2+}]_i$. The combined use of receptor-selective agonists and antagonists has demonstrated that A_1 receptors exert a tonic inhibitory effect on renin secretion at the level of the granular cell.[110] However, the adenosine receptor system is not vital for the control of renin secretion, since A_1 receptor knockout mice are able to raise their secretion appropriately in response to a low-salt diet,[140] a regimen that increases two-fold the sensitivity to luminal NaCl of ATP release by the macula densa.[87]

The role of the P2 receptor system in the regulation of renin release is not entirely clear, and is to some extent contradictory. Purinoceptor signaling is a prerequisite for synchronization of the intercellular calcium wave that controls renin secretion in the JGA,[198] and infusion of ATP into the isolated perfused rat kidney causes profound inhibition of renin secretion.[198] On the other hand, activation of an ADP-selective receptor, thought to be P2Y$_1$, was shown to stimulate renin secretion in rat renal cortical slices via a nitric oxide-dependent mechanism.[21] Resolution of this issue awaits further investigation.

Proximal Tubule

Immunohistochemical studies have identified apical expression of P2Y$_1$ and P2X$_5$ receptors in the S3 segment of the rat pars recta, and basolateral expression of P2Y$_4$ and P2X$_6$ receptors in the proximal convoluted tubule (PCT); low-level expression of P2X$_4$ protein was also seen in the PCT, although the membrane domain was not identified.[171] Western blot analysis has additionally shown the presence of P2Y$_1$ receptors in brush-border membrane vesicles from the S2 segment of rat PCT[6] (see Figure 18.3). Messenger RNA expression has been assessed for only four P2 receptor subtypes: P2Y$_{1, 2, 4}$ and P2Y$_6$ are all present in rat proximal tubule.[4,5] In terms of Ca^{2+} transients following application of P2 receptor agonists of varying selectivity, supportive evidence has been provided for apical P2Y$_1$-like receptors in an immortalized cell line with a proximal phenotype,[76] and for basolateral P2Y$_1$ receptors in native rat PCT[4,17]; Bailey and colleagues[5] also reported that basolateral UDP was effective in increasing [Ca^{2+}]$_i$, corroborating the presence of P2Y$_6$ receptors. Finally, ATP and UTP were equally effective in stimulating Ca^{2+} transients when applied to rat or rabbit basolateral membranes,[4,196] implying mediation by P2Y$_2$ or P2Y$_4$ receptors; the immunohistochemical evidence in rats favors P2Y$_4$ receptors.[171]

Using a stationary microperfusion technique in rat PCT in vivo, Bailey[2] showed that addition of adenosine nucleotides to the lumen inhibited bicarbonate reabsorption. ADP was more effective than ATP, implicating P2Y$_1$ receptors; this was supported by the observation that the P2Y$_1$ agonist 2 meSADP also had a potent inhibitory effect, which was blocked by the P2Y$_1$-selective antagonist MRS2179. (When the tubule was perfused with MRS2179 alone, a small increase in bicarbonate reabsorption was seen, suggesting a tonic inhibitory effect of endogenous nucleotides acting via P2Y$_1$ receptors.) The P2Y$_1$-mediated effect on bicarbonate reabsorption involved inhibition of the Na$^+$/H$^+$ exchanger NHE3, since it was not additive to that of EIPA. The effect was blocked by either U73122 or H89, indicating involvement of phospholipase C and

protein kinase A. In apparent contrast to these findings from intraluminal perfusions, Diaz-Silvester et al.[31] found that addition of ATP to peritubular capillaries perfused in vivo caused an increase in transepithelial bicarbonate reabsorption in rat PCT. Conceivably, given the presence of ectonucleotidases in peritubular capillaries and the peritubular space (vide infra), degradation of ATP through to the nucleoside adenosine (which stimulates proximal tubular bicarbonate reabsorption[29]) could not be ruled out. However, increasing the viscosity of the peritubular perfusate also stimulated bicarbonate reabsorption, and this effect was blocked by peritubular suramin, suggesting P2 receptor mediation. (Shear stress was proposed as the activating factor.) Interestingly, the increase in bicarbonate reabsorption induced by ATP or by raised viscosity could be blocked by a nitric oxide synthase inhibitor.

In a preliminary study of membrane transporters in the tubules of P2Y$_2$ receptor knockout mice, Listhrop et al.[99] reported increased expression of NaPT2 protein in the proximal tubule (but no change in NHE3 abundance). In line with this, ATP has been shown to inhibit phosphate uptake (and mRNA for NaPT2) in primary cultures of rabbit PCTs.[94] Interestingly, in the same preparation, ATP stimulates sodium-glucose co-transport by increasing both SGLT1 and SGLT2 protein expression.[93]

A renal clearance study in rats, using lithium clearance as an index of end-proximal tubular fluid delivery,[165] reported remarkable effects of the naturally occurring diadenosine polyphosphate Ap$_4$A. When infused intravenously, Ap$_4$A increased lithium clearance almost two-fold, despite a fall in GFR, indicating a profound reduction in fractional proximal tubular reabsorption.[154] Although a fascinating observation, it is debatable whether intravenous infusion of relatively high-dose exogenous nucleotide provides physiologically useful information about normal autocrine/paracrine control by endogenous agents. It is also difficult to know which P2 receptor(s) is/are involved, since Ap$_4$A can stimulate a number of subtypes, including P2Y$_1$ and P2Y$_4$ receptors,[143,185] which are both expressed in the rat proximal tubule (P2Y$_1$ apically, P2Y$_4$ basolaterally); intravenous delivery of the agonist does not allow differentiation between these possibilities.

In addition to effects on proximal tubular transport, both adenine-based and uracil-based nucleotides can stimulate gluconeogenesis, an important metabolic function of this nephron segment.[16,109] Diadenosine polyphosphates also have this effect.[35] As these experiments were performed using tubule suspensions or isolated tubules, the agonists will presumably have gained access to both apical and basolateral membranes; moreover, ectonucleotidase-mediated metabolism of the nucleotides is a possibility, hindering identification of the receptor subtype(s) responsible. However, ATP and UTP were equipotent in stimulating gluconeogenesis, implicating $P2Y_2$ or $P2Y_4$ receptors.[109] Although these authors plumped for $P2Y_2$ mediation, the fact that $P2Y_2$ receptors have not been found in rat proximal tubules, whereas $P2Y_4$ receptors have (vide supra), makes a basolateral $P2Y_4$-mediated effect more likely.

Loop of Henle

The pars recta (also called the thick descending limb of Henle), has been dealt with in the preceding section. In the rat thin descending limb there is some immunohistochemical evidence for $P2X_4$ and $P2X_6$ receptors (membrane domain not stated[171]), and indications, from measurements of $[Ca^{2+}]_i$ transients during superfusion of isolated segments with various agonists, of a basolateral pyrimidine receptor,[4] although no $P2Y_2$ or $P2Y_4$ protein has yet been identified. Messenger RNA is expressed for $P2Y_1$ and $P2Y_6$,[4,5] but again immunohistochemical evidence of receptor protein is lacking. In the rat thin ascending limb, similar evidence for a basolateral pyrimidine receptor[4] is in this case accompanied by immunohistochemical confirmation of (intracellular) $P2Y_2$ receptor protein; low-level $P2X_4$ and $P2X_6$ protein expression has also been reported.[171] Hardly surprisingly, given the paucity of information regarding normal transport processes in these nephron segments, the functional significance of P2 receptors in the thin limbs is unknown.

Consideration of P2 receptors in the thick ascending limb (TAL) of the loop of Henle must take account of species differences between rat and mouse. In the rat TAL, binding sites for $ATP\gamma S$ are present on the basolateral membrane[3]; this agonist stimulates several P2Y and most P2X subtypes. Immunohistochemistry has identified $P2Y_2$ (intracellularly), $P2X_4$, and $P2X_6$ (membrane domain not stated) receptor proteins.[171] In addition, mRNA is expressed for $P2Y_{1,2,4}$, and $P2Y_6$ subtypes.[4,5,83] It has been reported that rat TAL segments are poorly responsive to basolateral application of nucleotides, at least in terms of Ca^{2+} transients,[4,5] which is in marked contrast to the situation in mice, where basolateral ATP and UTP were each found to evoke large Ca^{2+} transients, consistent with activation of $P2Y_2$ receptors.[3,120] A major role for $P2Y_2$ receptors in mice was supported by Jensen et al.[75] who showed, in mouse medullary TAL (mTAL) perfused in vitro, that luminal application of ATP or UTP caused almost identical increases in Ca^{2+}_i and, importantly, that these increases were absent in $P2Y_2$ knockout mice. In the same study, however, significantly different results were obtained when the nucleotides were applied basolaterally: both ATP and UTP caused an initial

peak in $[Ca^{2+}]_i$ followed by a sustained plateau, but whereas both phases were virtually abolished in mTAL from $P2Y_2$ knockout mice treated with UTP, the plateau phase in mTAL from $P2Y_2$ knockout mice treated with ATP persisted, suggesting the presence of an additional basolateral P2 receptor. Since the plateau phase was dependent on extracellular Ca^{2+}, the authors proposed a Ca^{2+}-permeable P2X receptor.[75]

Some information, albeit circumstantial, on the effects of $P2Y_2$ receptors on transport processes in the TAL has come from a comprehensive study of the renal phenotype of $P2Y_2$ knockout mice by Vallon's group. These animals were shown to exhibit increased expression of the apical $Na^+K^+2Cl^-$ co-transporter (NKCC-2) in mTAL, associated with an increased natriuretic response to furosemide.[130] The obvious implication is that nucleotide activation of $P2Y_2$ receptors inhibits NaCl transport in mouse TAL.

During the last decade, in a series of meticulously controlled experiments using cell suspensions or nephron segments perfused in vitro, Garvin's group has begun to piece together evidence for a functional role of ATP on TAL function in the rat. Using suspensions of rat mTAL, Silva et al.[146] showed that ATP increased intracellular NO production in a concentration-dependent manner, and that the response was significantly inhibited by suramin. Although the EC_{50} value for the NO response to ATP was high, at $37\ \mu M$, prevention of ATP hydrolysis by administration of the ectonucleotidase inhibitor ARL67156 reduced the EC_{50} to $0.8\ \mu M$. On the basis that the ATP analog $\beta\gamma meATP$ caused an increase in NO production, it was argued that the response was mediated primarily by P2X receptors, although it was noted that UTP also had a weak effect. A recent study from the same group[148] has provided some insight into the signaling cascade involved in ATP-stimulated NO production. Confirmation that endothelial nitric oxide synthase (eNOS; or NOS3) is the enzyme responsible came from the finding that ATP was unable to stimulate NO production in TAL cells from NOS3 knockout mice, whereas a normal response was seen in wild-type mice given NOS1- or NOS2-selective inhibitors. The PI_3 kinase inhibitor LY294002 caused a major reduction in the response to ATP, and a similar reduction was seen in the presence of an Akt-selective inhibitor. This finding, together with the observation that ATP stimulated Akt1 (serine threonine kinase; also called protein kinase B) phosphorylation, whereas phosphorylation of Akt2 and Akt3 was either unchanged or reduced, led the authors to conclude that ATP increases NOS3-derived NO via activation of Akt1. A possible functional link between the recently observed effect of increased flow on nucleotide release in the TAL[75]; (vide infra) and the production of NO can be drawn from an earlier study by

Ortiz et al.,[118] in which increasing flow (in the physiological range) in isolated perfused TALs from rat caused markedly increased NO production (which was all but blocked by the NOS inhibitor L-NAME). Notably, increasing luminal flow caused a redistribution of NOS3 within the TAL cells, with translocation towards the apical membrane. It was already known that NO (and presumably therefore ATP) can reduce TAL transport by inhibiting NKCC-2 activity[117] and (to a lesser extent) Na^+/H^+ exchange,[45] but a recent study from this group explored the possibility that ATP might have a primary effect in reducing basolateral Na^+K^+-ATPase activity, and thereby Na^+ extrusion from the TAL cell.[149] Using rat mTAL suspensions, it was found that ATP reduced oxygen consumption in a dose-dependent manner and that this was blocked by suramin, but not by the adenosine receptor antagonist theophylline; it was also blocked by the NOS inhibitor L-NAME. The "2P2X-selective" agonist βγmeATP also reduced oxygen consumption concentration-dependently, while the "P2X-selective" antagonist NF023 blocked ATPs action. (However, as with nucleotide-stimulated NO production, it was found that UTP had a (weak) inhibitory effect on oxygen consumption, suggesting some P2Y involvement.) When NKCC-2 and Na^+/H^+ exchange were blocked with a combination of furosemide and dimethyl amiloride, oxygen consumption fell, and was no longer affected by ATP; while the Na^+ ionophore nystatin increased oxygen consumption to a similar extent in TALs treated with ATP or vehicle alone. These experiments provide powerful confirmatory evidence that ATP, by increasing NO production, can inhibit Na^+ transport in the rat TAL, not by inhibiting basolateral Na^+K^+-ATPase activity, but principally by reducing apical Na^+ entry, particularly via the $Na^+K^+2Cl^-$ co-transporter. Whilst this series of *in vitro* findings is strongly suggestive of a physiological role for nucleotides in autocrine/paracrine control of TAL function (a putative schema is shown in Figure 18.6), a full assessment awaits a comprehensive investigation of electrolyte transport in the loop of Henle *in vivo*.

Distal Tubule

Little is known about P2 receptor distribution in this nephron segment (which, here, we arbitrarily define as distal convoluted tubule (DCT) plus connecting tubule (CNT); the final segment of the properly defined distal tubule — the initial collecting tubule — will be included under "Cortical Collecting Duct"). Immunohistochemical studies have identified $P2X_4$ and $P2X_6$ receptors on the basolateral membrane in rat distal tubule[171] (although it is not clear which region of the distal tubule was involved, as no markers of cell types were used in this study), and basolateral application of ATP to

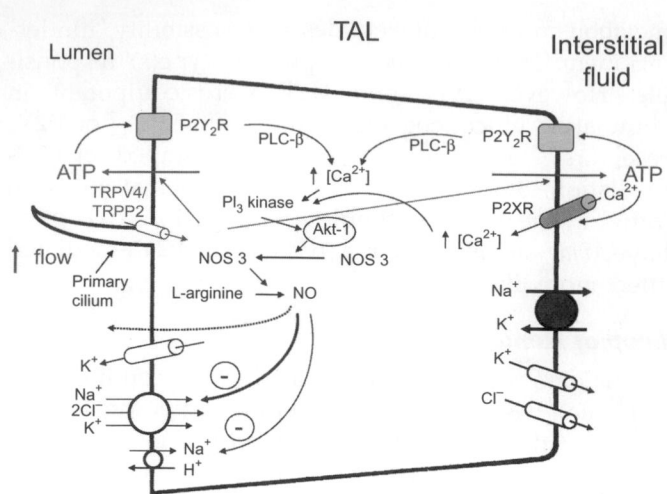

FIGURE 18.6 Putative effects of flow-induced stimulation of ATP release in thick ascending limb of Henle (TAL). According to this hypothesis, an increase in tubular flow is most likely detected by the primary cilium, and the consequent increase in Ca^{2+} influx stimulates ATP release. ATP, acting on apical and basolateral P2 receptors, stimulates (via intracellular 2nd messengers) PI_3 kinase which, in turn, phosphorylates Akt1. This kinase phosphorylates NOS3 (which itself may be translocated towards the apical membrane); thus activated, the enzyme stimulates the production of nitric oxide, which inhibits apical sodium entry into the cell via the $Na^+K^+2Cl^-$ co-transporter and the Na^+/H^+ exchanger, thereby inhibiting net Na^+ reabsorption. Information compiled from references [44,45,64,75,118,127,146,148,149]. $P2Y_2R$, $P2Y_2$ receptor; P2XR, P2X receptor; NO, nitric oxide; NOS3, nitric oxide synthase 3.

microdissected rat DCTs resulted in (weak) Ca^{2+} transients,[4] but no corresponding investigations have been made in other species or in CNT. Furthermore, no direct studies of distal tubular transport function have been made in native tissue, either *in vitro* or *in vivo*; the only information we have from whole-animal studies is that thiazide-sensitive sodium excretion is unaffected in $P2Y_2$ knockout mice, corresponding with a lack of change in Na^+-Cl^- co-transporter (NCC) abundance.[99,130] Consequently, our knowledge of the role of P2 receptors in these nephron segments is fragmentary and largely restricted to findings from studies of primary cultures of native cells or immortalized distal or "distal-like" cell lines.

Considerable evidence exists for the expression of a number of P2 receptor subtypes and for a range of P2-mediated actions in *Xenopus* A6 cells and Madin–Darby canine kidney (MDCK) cells, both widely used as "distal-like" cell lines. However, as indicated above, for reasons of physiological relevance it will not be considered here, as such cell lines often express membrane proteins different from those found in native tissue. Similar considerations may apply to immortalized cell lines derived from DCT: activation of apical receptors, characterized pharmacologically as $P2Y_2$ subtype, in immortalized rabbit DCT was shown to increase apical chloride conductance[134]; while activation of receptors (membrane domain not stated) characterized pharmacologically as P2X, rather than P2Y, in immortalized mouse DCT was shown to inhibit magnesium reabsorption.[27] Finally, cultured cells from rabbit CNTs responded to extracellular ATP with an increase in $[Ca^{2+}]_i$ and inhibition of sodium and calcium absorption, although these inhibitory effects were not dependent on the Ca^{2+} transient.[88,173] Either apical or basolateral application of ATP was effective and, when ATP was added to both compartments, the inhibitory effects were additive. On the basis of pharmacological profiling, $P2Y_2$ receptors were implicated.[88]

It is difficult to build a coherent picture from these disparate findings. As with the loop of Henle, a comprehensive *in vivo* assessment of distal tubular function is required.

Collecting Duct

A large array of P2 receptor subtypes has been reported in rat collecting duct (CD) (Figure 18.3). Immunohistochemistry has indicated the expression of $P2Y_2$, $P2Y_4$, $P2Y_6$, $P2Y_{11}$, $P2Y_{12}$, and $P2Y_{13}$ subtypes, and $P2X_1$ (sodium-restricted rats only, intercalated cells only), $P2X_2$, $P2X_4$, $P2X_5$, and $P2X_6$ subunits[83,171,187] with, in some cases, differential expression in the different subsegments of the CD. With respect to membrane localization in principal cells, $P2Y_{4,6}$, and $P2Y_{11}$ were reported to be exclusive to the apical membrane, whereas $P2Y_2$ and $P2X_4$ and $P2X_6$ were found in both apical and basolateral membranes; staining for $P2Y_{12}$ and $P2Y_{13}$ subtypes and $P2X_2$ and $P2X_5$ subunits was designated "intracellular".[187] In the mouse, immunohistochemistry has localized $P2X_1$ and $P2X_4$ subunits to the apical membrane of medullary CD cells.[97]

Expression of P2 receptor mRNA in the rat kidney broadly agrees with the immunohistochemical findings — at least in the one study in which both methodologies were used.[187] Messenger RNA has been identified for $P2Y_{1,2,4}$, and $P2Y_6$ subtypes, and $P2X_4$ subunits in cortical (CCD) and outer medullary CD (OMCD),[4,5,187] and for $P2Y_{1,2,4}$ and $P2Y_6$ subtypes in inner medullary CD (IMCD).[83,203] Additionally, mRNA for $P2X_1$ and $P2X_6$ receptors has been reported in CCD and OMCD following dietary sodium restriction.[187] Messenger RNA levels for $P2Y_{11,12,13}$, and $P2Y_{14}$ receptors have not yet been investigated. Studies using mice have so far focused on P2X receptors, and have identified mRNA for $P2X_{1,4,5,6}$, and $P2X_7$ subunits in CCD and OMCD,[46,97] suggesting a species difference. As far as the human kidney is concerned, the only published information we have comes from a heroic study by Charbardès-Garonne and co-workers, in which the transcriptome from human kidneys was characterized using serial analysis of gene expression (SAGE). They found that, of tags for 258 genes

conferring transport properties, the only P2X receptor detected in significant amounts in the CD was $P2X_4$.[18]

A complex picture is beginning to emerge concerning the role of P2 receptors in the CD. A combination of approaches has demonstrated that extracellular nucleotides, acting from both apical and basolateral sides, can have significant effects on water and electrolyte handling in this important nephron segment — the final site of regulation of urinary output.

Water

In the mid-1990s it was shown that activation of basolateral P2 receptors in rabbit CCD and rat IMCD, perfused *in vitro*, reversibly inhibited vasopressin-stimulated osmotic water permeability.[82,133] On the basis that UTP and ATP were equipotent, whereas other nucleotides were without effect, the inhibition found in the rat was attributed to basolateral $P2Y_2$ receptors[82]; this P2 receptor-mediated inhibition has been found to be PKC-dependent, and to result from decreased intracellular cAMP and increased PGE_2 levels.[181] The inhibitory action (at least in IMCD) appeared to be mediated only by basolateral receptors, since luminal application of ATP was without effect in this nephron segment.[36] Enhanced expression of $P2Y_2$ mRNA, and of the receptor protein itself, in the inner medulla of hydrated versus dehydrated rats, has provided additional evidence for a regulatory role for $P2Y_2$ receptors in modulating CD water reabsorption,[85] and this view is supported by the observation that chronic vasopressin V_2 receptor stimulation with dDAVP reduces inner medullary $P2Y_2$ mRNA and protein expression.[158] Gene deletion studies further substantiate a role for the $P2Y_2$ receptor in ATP-evoked inhibition of AVP-stimulated osmotic water permeability in the CD. Under basal conditions, $P2Y_2^{-/-}$ mice concentrated their urine to a greater degree, and their renal medullary aquaporin-2 (AQP2) abundance was significantly higher, compared with values in wild-type mice, despite almost identical plasma vasopressin levels,[130,205] and following chronic dDAVP treatment, inner medullary AQP2 expression was increased to a markedly greater extent in the $P2Y_2$ knockout animals.[205] In summary, the overall picture is that $P2Y_2$ receptor activation inhibits vasopressin-stimulated, AQP2-mediated water transport in the CD, and this results from decreased intracellular cAMP and increased intracellular PGE_2; the latter, in turn, can reduce cAMP levels and effect the retrieval of AQP2 from the apical membrane.[86]

A recent study from our laboratory, albeit in a cultured, immortalized mouse CCD cell line (mpkCCDc14), has provided additional evidence that P2 receptor activation may exert its inhibitory effect on water transport via altered AQP2 trafficking. Application of dDAVP to the basolateral membrane for four days resulted in marked AQP2 immunofluorescence in the apical membrane, but when ATP or ATPγS was then added to the medium, either apically or basolaterally, the AQP2 was internalized.[186] Treatment with dDAVP induced gene expression of P2X$_1$ in the apical domain, and led to translocation of P2X$_2$ and P2Y$_2$ to the apical and basolateral membranes, respectively. When these three subtypes were co-expressed with AQP2 in *Xenopus* oocytes, their activation reduced cell membrane AQP2 abundance and consequently reduced water permeability.[186] These findings suggest that: (1) in addition to basolateral P2Y$_2$ receptors, apically located P2 receptors can contribute to the downregulation of AQP2-stimulated water transport; (2) altered trafficking of AQP2 is involved; and (3) vasopressin itself can increase membrane abundance of P2 receptors (c.f. [158]). However, it must be stressed that the observations were confined to *in vitro* systems using a mouse CD-derived cell line and *Xenopus* oocytes. As such, they must be viewed with caution.

Potassium

Although early studies in MDCK cells reported that ATP activates K$^+$ channels,[42] evidence in native CD suggests that K$^+$ secretion by principal cells is *inhibited* by nucleotides. A patch-clamp investigation of split-open mouse CCDs (allowing access to the apical membrane) demonstrated that ATP reversibly inhibits the activity of the small-conductance K$^+$ (SK; also called ROMK) channels, which are believed to mediate most potassium secretion in the distal nephron.[104] On the basis of equipotency of ATP and UTP, and the absence of effect of $\alpha\beta$meATP and 2 meSATP, it was concluded that apical P2Y$_2$ receptors were responsible. That P2Y$_2$ knockout mice maintain a robust potassium excretion despite mild hypokalemia is consistent with this hypothesis.[130] It is worth noting that the inhibitory effect of ATP on SK channel activity observed by Lu and colleagues[104] could be blocked by the NOS inhibitor L-NAME, which implies that the NO-dependency of nucleotide-induced physiological actions may not be confined to the TAL (*vide supra*).

K$^+$ secretion in the distal nephron is generally enhanced when tubular flow rates are increased. This flow-induced increase in K$^+$ secretion is now thought to be mediated not by SK channels, but by large-conductance, maxi-K (big K; BK) channels.[191] Activation of BK channels is through increased [Ca^{2+}]$_i$,[100] and there is good evidence for a causal link between increased tubular flow rate, increased tubular nucleotide secretion, and increased [Ca^{2+}]$_i$ (*vide infra*). Although highly speculative at this stage, one implication of these various observations is that nucleotides may have conflicting effects on SK and BK channels.

Sodium

Studies into the effects of extracellular nucleotides on CD Na$^+$ transport have generally used sensitivity to amiloride as a basis for identifying ENaC-mediated transport; although occasionally sensitivity to benzamil — a more selective inhibitor of ENaC — has been employed. Koster and colleagues were the first to report that benzamil-sensitive transcellular Na$^+$ transport is inhibited by nucleotide activation of P2 receptors.[88] Using primary cultures of rabbit CD (and CNT) cells grown to confluence, they demonstrated that apically or basolaterally applied ATP inhibited benzamil-sensitive short circuit current (SCC; used as an index of Na$^+$ transport) across cell monolayers; the mechanism involved activation of PKC and/or PLC. The P2 receptor responsible for this inhibition was equally sensitive to ATP and UTP, but was insensitive to ADP. On this basis, the inhibition of ENaC was attributed to activation of P2Y$_2$ receptors. Subsequent studies using the mouse M1 cell line reported similar findings, except that the mechanism did not involve PKC.[25,164] Another CD cell model, the mouse mIMCD-K2, responded similarly to apical (but not basolateral) nucleotides, although in this case, on the basis of pharmacological profiling and mRNA expression, P2X receptors (P2X$_3$ and P2X$_4$) as well as P2Y receptors (P2Y$_1$ and P2Y$_2$) were thought to be responsible.[107] A more recent study, using the mouse IMCD-3 cell line, provided an exception to the "rule" of nucleotide-induced inhibition of CD transport: apical application of ATP induced an *increase* in SSC,[97] although sensitivity to amiloride or benzamil was not tested. Since this effect could be reproduced by the P2X agonist BzATP, it was inferred that the receptors responsible were P2X$_1$ and/or P2X$_4$, as located in native medullary collecting duct (*vide supra*), although UTP was able to increase SCC to some extent, implying a contribution from P2Y receptors.

Investigations of nucleotide effects on CD sodium transport are not limited to cell cultures: nucleotide-induced inhibition of Na$^+$ reabsorption in the CD has also been reported in native tissue. In mouse CCD perfused *in vitro*, ATP and UTP, applied either luminally or basolaterally, caused an increase in [Ca^{2+}]$_i$ (and subsequent activation of PKC), and inhibition of amiloride-sensitive SCC, an effect attributed to P2Y$_2$ receptor activation.[28,95] Subsequent single-channel patch-clamp experiments, using both rat and mouse CCD, showed that activation of apical P2 receptors with ATP decreased ENaC open probability (P$_o$), via PLC-dependent breakdown of PIP$_2$.[123] Although not tested in rats, it was found that in mice UTP was able to reduce P$_o$ to the same extent as ATP. Further pharmacological profiling led to the conclusion that P2Y$_2$ receptors were responsible (at least in mice). The fact that in $P2Y_2^{-/-}$ mice the effect of ATP on ENaC P_o was severely blunted provided strong support for this conclusion,[123] although a residual effect was still evident, suggesting partial involvement of other P2 receptors. A follow-up study from the same laboratory showed that increased dietary sodium causes a lowering of ENaC P_o in wild-type mice, but not in $P2Y_2$ knockout mice, implying a central role for $P2Y_2$ receptors in the CD response to changes in sodium intake.[124] More recently, the same group has extended this conclusion to implicate $P2Y_2$ receptors in the phenomenon of aldosterone escape — the restoration of normal sodium excretion rates in the face of chronically raised mineralocorticoid levels. Hitherto, aldosterone escape had been thought to rely on compensatory changes in more proximal segments of the nephron delivering an increased sodium load to the aldosterone-sensitive sites. However, Stockand and colleagues found that whereas wild-type mice on a high-sodium diet excreted appropriately high levels of sodium in the face of three days of deoxycorticosterone acetate treatment, owing partly to reduced ENaC activity, in $P2Y_2^{-/-}$ mice the reduction in ENaC activity was much less pronounced, and the natriuresis correspondingly compromised.[155]

At the time of writing, only one study of the effect of nucleotides on CD Na^+ reabsorption *in vivo* has been published.[144] Late distal tubules of rats were microperfused with artificial tubular fluid containing ^{22}Na, the urinary recovery of which was recorded. In animals fed a low-sodium diet (to upregulate ENaC activity), addition of ATPγS to the luminal perfusate was found to inhibit CD ^{22}Na reabsorption. Despite firm evidence from *in vitro* studies in mice for $P2Y_2$ mediation, "selective" $P2Y_2/P2Y_4$ agonists were ineffective *in vivo* in rats, and a P2X heteromer-mediated effect was suggested.[144] A recent patch-clamp investigation of split-open rat CCD (allowing access to the apical membrane) has provided evidence that both apical P2X and P2Y receptors can affect ENaC activity.[187] Activation of P2Y receptors, molecularly and pharmacologically characterized as $P2Y_2$ and/or $P2Y_4$ subtypes, inhibited ENaC activity by a PLC-dependent mechanism. Notably, activation of P2X receptors, characterized as $P2X_4$ and/or $P2X_{4/6}$ receptors, either inhibited or potentiated ENaC activity, depending on the luminal concentration of sodium. When luminal sodium was 145 mM (which is the concentration typically used in this type of *in vitro* experiment), $P2X_4$ and/or $P2X_{4/6}$ activation with 2 meSATP inhibited ENaC activity, whereas when luminal sodium concentration was 50 mM (which mimics the normal sodium concentration of fluid entering the CD *in vivo*), $P2X_4$ and/or $P2X_{4/6}$ activation with 2 meSATP potentiated ENaC activity (Figure 18.7). These findings led us to propose that $P2X_4$ and/or $P2X_{4/6}$ receptors might act as apically expressed

sodium sensors for the local regulation of ENaC activity in the rat CD.[187] The situation is almost certainly more complex, since preliminary data from our laboratory, using the same electrophysiological techniques, have demonstrated that $P2X_4$ and $P2X_{4/6}$, and $P2Y_2$ and $P2Y_4$ receptor-mediated regulation of ENaC is also dependent on nucleotide concentration, duration of exposure to nucleotide, and tubular pH: higher nucleotide concentrations and prolonged exposure favor P2Y-mediated inhibition, while reducing tubular fluid acidity favors P2X-mediated increases in ENaC activity.[183] Staying with the $P2X_4$ theme, a causal link has been established between P2X activation, the apical insertion of ENaC, and enhancement of sodium transport, albeit in a "distal-like" cell line; activation of a basolateral $P2X_4$-like receptor in *Xenopus* A6 cells alters cell shape by a rearrangement of the cytoskeleton, which results in increased Na^+ transport[204] brought about by the unruffling of the apical membrane and insertion of ENaC.[49]

Gene deletion studies have so far concentrated on murine $P2Y_2$ knockout models, although studies using the $P2X_4^{-/-}$ mouse (which, like the $P2Y_2$ knockout, is hypertensive[197]) are afoot. Unsurprisingly (on the basis of the studies cited above), $P2Y_2$ gene deletion was found to result in facilitated Na^+ reabsorption in the kidney but, unexpectedly, this appeared to stem from increased expression of the $Na^+K^+2Cl^-$ co-transporter in the TAL (*vide supra*); expression of α-ENaC was *reduced*, while no overall change in amiloride-sensitive sodium transport was seen.[130] Subsequent studies using the $P2Y_2^{-/-}$ mouse have proposed that the $P2Y_2$ receptor tonically regulates ENaC activity by reducing ENaC P_o.[124] It has been suggested that in $P2Y_2$ knockout mice, the increase in ENaC P_o is compensated for in the longer-term by suppression of the renin—angiotensin—aldosterone system, resulting in downregulation of ENaC expression.[172]

In summary, a variety of approaches leaves little room for doubt that apical and basolateral nucleotides can alter ENaC-mediated Na^+ reabsorption in the CD, and more than likely play a role in blood pressure regulation. In simplistic terms, it appears that activation of $P2Y_2$ receptors inhibits ENaC activity, and activation of $P2X_4$ receptors stimulates ENaC activity. In reality, however, P2 receptor and ENaC interactions in the CD are complex, with an interplay between P2X and P2Y receptors dependent on a variety of factors yet to be unraveled.

Secretion of Nucleotides

As indicated earlier, it is thought that virtually all cells are able to release nucleotides,[127] renal vascular and epithelial cells included. Initial support for the

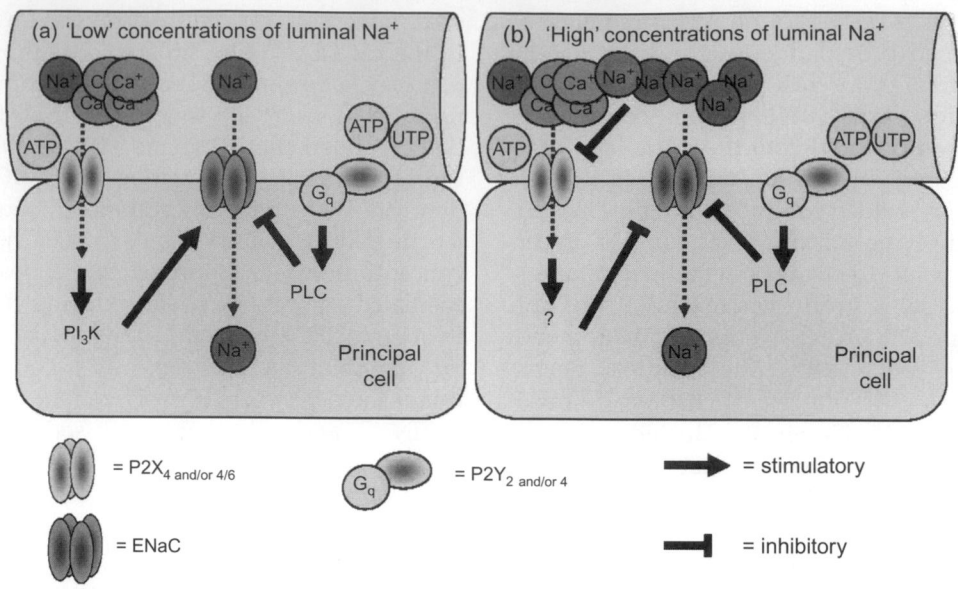

FIGURE 18.7 Proposed regulation of ENaC activity by P2 receptors in principal cells of rat CD. The hypothesis is that ENaC activity in the rat CD is differentially regulated by P2X$_4$ and/or P2X$_{4/6}$ receptors, depending on the concentration of luminal Na$^+$; i.e., that P2X$_4$ and/or P2X$_{4/6}$ receptors act as Na$^+$ sensors. Real time-PCR and immunohistochemistry suggest that levels of P2Y$_4$ and P2X$_4$ and/or P2X$_{4/6}$ are increased when ENaC is expressed. (a) When the concentration of luminal Na$^+$ is low (i.e., at 50 mM in our experiments), activation of apically expressed P2X$_4$ and/or P2X$_{4/6}$ receptors (which are highly permeable to Ca^{2+} and to a lesser extent to Na$^+$) increases ENaC activity through the activation of PI3K. In contrast, activation of apically expressed P2Y$_2$ and/or P2Y$_4$ receptors inhibits ENaC activity through the activation of PLC. N.B. The overall effect of P2 receptor activation (i.e., both P2X and P2Y, by using ATP) is a small degree of ENaC inhibition. (b) When the concentration of luminal Na$^+$ is high (i.e., at 145 mM in our experiments), activation of P2X$_4$ and/or P2X$_{4/6}$ receptors results in inhibition of ENaC activity by an unidentified mechanism, possibly involving an influx of Na$^+$. As before, activation of apically expressed P2Y$_2$ and/or P2Y$_4$ receptors inhibits ENaC activity through activation of PLC. The overall effect of P2 receptor activation (i.e., both P2X and P2Y, by using ATP) is a much larger degree of ENaC inhibition. *(from ref. [187]).*

latter came from studies using epithelial cultures and cell lines,[141,142,174] but clear evidence now exists that native renal tubules are also able to secrete ATP. (Cellular secretion of UTP and diadenosine polyphosphates also occurs,[74,199] but has not yet been firmly established in renal tubules.) The question of whether nucleotide release from renal tubular epithelia is constitutive (raising the concept of "purinergic tone"[127]) or is triggered by mechanical or agonist-induced stimuli, now appears to be resolved: both are likely.

Vekaria et al.[176] reported intraluminal ATP concentrations in rat PCTs *in vivo* of 200–300 nmol/l; these concentrations were markedly higher than those in the glomerular filtrate, suggesting secretion of ATP by PCT cells. Intraluminal concentrations in distal tubules were only ~30 nmol/l; the possibility that this ATP was merely flushed downstream, rather than secreted by distal tubular cells, could not be discounted. Using mouse medullary thick ascending limbs (mTALs) perfused *in vitro*, Leipziger's group demonstrated spontaneous oscillatory increases in [Ca^{2+}]$_i$ that appeared to require tubular nucleotide release.[47] An increase in intraluminal pressure from 10 to 80 cm H$_2$O also resulted in elevations in [Ca^{2+}]$_i$.[75] Convincing evidence was provided that this flow-induced Ca^{2+} transient

was itself dependent on nucleotide release, being prevented by luminal or basolateral application of either apyrase (an ATP scavenger) or the P2 receptor blocker suramin. Moreover, both the oscillatory and flow-induced increases in [Ca^{2+}]$_i$ were greatly reduced in P2Y$_2$ receptor knockout mice. In an elegant follow-up study, the same group assessed agonist-induced, rather than flow-induced, nucleotide release in mouse mTAL, and made use of 132-1N1 astrocyte cells transfected with human P2Y$_2$ receptors, positioned at the outflow of perfused mTAL to act as biosensors for ATP[116]; these transfected cells respond dose-dependently to extracellular ATP by increasing their [Ca^{2+}]$_i$. Using this preparation, spontaneous nucleotide secretion was documented, while intraluminal vasopressin or dDAVP (10 nM) triggered [Ca^{2+}]$_i$ bursts. Since the 132-1N1 cells' response was mediated by P2Y$_2$ receptors, it was impossible to distinguish between ATP and UTP as the nucleotide in question, but calibration of the response to vasopressin revealed peak intraluminal nucleotide concentrations of 200–300 nmol/l, remarkably similar to *in vivo* ATP concentrations in the PCT.[176] In the same study, Odgaard et al.[116] found that vasopressin also triggered nucleotide secretion from mouse CCD perfused *in vitro*; intraluminal ATP/UTP concentrations again reached values approaching 300 nmol/l. Unfortunately, no parallel studies in $P2Y_2$ knockout mice were reported.

It is open to debate whether the nucleotide concentrations measured intraluminally in the above studies reflect those in the vicinity of the P2 receptors in the cell membrane. Membrane-bound and soluble ectonucleotidases (*vide infra*) will rapidly metabolize secreted nucleotides, and it has been estimated that bulk-phase measurements could underestimate concentrations at the cell membrane by more than 20-fold, at least in astrocytes.[77]

Role of Primary Cilium in Flow-Induced Nucleotide Release

A discussion of nucleotide secretion in the tubule would be incomplete without reference to the possible role of the primary cilium. Most renal cells possess a primary cilium protruding from the centriole into the lumen; in the absence of fluid flow it is perpendicular to the cell membrane, but flow causes the cilium to bend, with a consequent increase in $[Ca^{2+}]_i$ in the relevant cell.[128] The question is whether this increase in $[Ca^{2+}]_i$ is triggered by nucleotide release. *In vitro* studies using a cell line (MDCK cells) provided support for nucleotide involvement, as ciliated cells released ATP (detected by biosensor cells downstream) in response to an increase in flow, whereas cells deciliated by means of chloral hydrate did not; apical apyrase or suramin also abolished the response.[127] It is thought that the link between the bending of the cilium and the release of ATP involves a member of the transient receptor potential vanilloid (TRPV) channels — TRPV4 — which is expressed along the TAL and all subsequent nephron segments.[166] Silva and Garvin[147] provided strong evidence that secretion of ATP by cell suspensions of mTAL in response to reduced tonicity depends on activation of TRPV4 channels: the response was reduced by ~75% after blockade of TRPV4 with ruthenium red, while treatment with siRNA against TRPV4 had a similar inhibitory effect. In MDCK cells, ruthenium red also inhibited flow-stimulated Ca^{2+} transients,[89] and it was noted that in these cells TRPV4 co-localizes in cilia with TRPP2 (polycystin 2), an ion channel that is required for cilia-mediated Ca^{2+} transients, but has no mechanosensitive properties. When these two channels were co-expressed in *Xenopus* oocytes, hypotonicity-induced cell swelling was found to cause a bigger increase in membrane currents than that seen when TRPV4 was expressed alone (no currents were sustained by TRPP2 alone).[89] The implication is that TRPV4 and TRPP2 form a sensory channel complex in the primary cilium,

which mediates Ca^{2+} influx when the cilium is bent, thereby triggering the release of nucleotides into the surrounding extracellular space which, in turn, activate P2 receptors and cause a more general increase in $[Ca^{2+}]_i$.[127]

Further support for a role of the primary cilium came from a study of collecting duct principal cells derived from the Oak Ridge polycystic kidney (*orpk*) mouse model. These cells lack a well-formed apical cilium; however, they can be genetically rescued with the wild-type *orpk* gene. Constitutive ATP release under basal conditions was not different in mutant versus rescued monolayers of cells, but hypotonicity or increased flow rate induced markedly greater responses from the rescued cells than from those lacking primary cilia.[64]

The evidence thus far, then, favors a crucial role for the primary cilium, but the key question is whether it is equally important in native tissue. In this connection, Woda et al.[192] found comparable flow-induced increases in $[Ca^{2+}]_i$ in principal and intercalated cells of rabbit CCD, despite the fact that intercalated cells in rabbit CCDs do not have cilia.[101] However, the increases in $[Ca^{2+}]_i$ did not appear to depend on nucleotide secretion, since they were unaffected by suramin. It might be, therefore, that rabbits are a special case.

Mechanism of Nucleotide Release

The mechanism of secretion of nucleotides from renal tubular cells is not yet resolved. A large intracellular pool of ATP is available, but the exit route for the nucleotide is controversial, and it may well differ from segment to segment. In neurones and neuroendocrine cells, exocytosis of vesicles containing ATP is well-established, and circumstantial evidence has been provided for a similar mechanism in a proximal tubular cell line,[174] but confirmation is lacking. A variety of channels/transporters has been implicated in nucleotide release. A notable example is the ATP transport across the basolateral membrane of macula densa cells in response to increased NaCl delivery to this nephron site, which is mediated by maxi-anion channels (*vide supra*[10]). Speculation that CFTR channels can also mediate ATP release in the kidney[152] has not received firm support.[126]

In recent years, attention has focused on the possible role of connexin hemichannels in ATP release from renal cells. Connexins (Cxs) are a family of transmembrane proteins comprising approximately 20 members. Messenger RNA and immunohistochemistry studies indicate that several members of the connexin family are expressed in the renal vasculature and tubules.[52] When six connexins assemble, either as homomers or heteromers, they form a connexon. When two connexons from neighboring cells dock, they form a gap junction; a channel with a central pore. Undocked connexons ("hemichannels") can also function independently as transmembrane channels. Although their functional role, if any, in the tubule remains to be clarified, it has been shown that dietary sodium intake can influence Cx30 and Cx37 expression in tubular cells,[108,156] and evidence is beginning to accumulate for involvement of connexin hemichannels in tubular ATP secretion, as has already been established in other cell types.[24] Evidence for such a role in the distal nephron has come from a recent study using Cx30 knockout mice.[150] Partially split-open CCDs were microperfused *in vitro* and PC12 cells (expressing P2X$_2$ receptors and used as ATP biosensors) were placed in direct contact with the apical membranes of principal cells and intercalated cells. In wild-type mice, increases in tubular flow or reductions in osmolality of the bathing solution evoked increases in $[Ca^{2+}]_i$ in the PC12 cells. Interestingly, these increases were much greater in PC12 cells placed in the vicinity of intercalated cells than in those placed in the vicinity of principal cells, which correlates with the observation that in the mouse distal nephron, immunohistochemical labeling for Cx30 is restricted to the apical membrane of intercalated cells.[108] Also notable was the calculated ATP concentration of $10-50\,\mu mol/l$, far in excess of concentrations measured in the bulk phase,[116] thus corroborating the view that bulk-phase measurements may be wide of the physiological mark. Responses were abolished by preincubation of the PC12 cells with suramin, and were almost absent in Cx30 knockout mice. These observations in themselves were striking enough, but the same study went on to assess their physiological significance by comparing pressure—natriuresis curves in wild-type and Cx30 knockout mice. While both groups responded to an imposed increase in renal perfusion pressure (to ~150 mmHg) by a natriuresis, the response in knockout mice was significantly blunted, despite almost identical GFRs in the two groups.[150]

There can be little doubt that these findings provide powerful evidence not only for a crucial role of Cx30 in ATP release in the CCD, but also for an important autocrine/paracrine function of nucleotides in the tubular response to elevations in blood pressure, at least under the conditions of the study. However, a cautionary note should be sounded concerning the physiological significance of the observations: the perfusion rates employed *in vitro* ($2-20$ nl/min) were far in excess of those found in mouse CCD *in vivo*, and it is clear that the authors used tubular flow rates in the rat, rather than in the mouse, as their reference point. Furthermore, connexin hemichannels appear to open only under non-physiological conditions, such as removal of extracellular divalent cations or major membrane depolarization.[127] In contrast, another group of proteins — the pannexins, which are structurally homologous to connexins and can also form hemichannels[8,135] — is permeable to ATP and can be activated by membrane depolarizations in the physiological range.[102] Further studies will be needed to determine their physiological or pathophysiological role in the kidney.

Ectonucleotidases

As indicated above, the nucleotides that are released from the renal vasculature and from apical and basolateral membranes of renal epithelial cells elicit a variety of autocrine/paracrine actions via P2 receptors. However, these nucleotides are rapidly degraded by surface-located and soluble enzymes (ectonucleotidases) to other nucleotides or nucleosides. Four families of ectonucleotidases, with differing but partly overlapping properties, exist: ectonucleoside triphosphate diphosphohydrolases (NTPDases); ectonucleotide pyrophosphatase phosphodiesterases (NPPs); ecto-5′-nucleotidase; and alkaline phosphatases. Members of all four families have been identified in the kidney,[145] where they will have a profound influence on the stimulation of purinoceptors, not only because the availability of nucleotide agonists is regulated by their hydrolysis, but also because the generation of other nucleotides (e.g., ADP) preferentially targets different P2 receptor subtypes, while the nucleoside derivative adenosine targets P1 (adenosine) receptors (Figure 18.2).

In addition to enzymes that break down nucleotides, two families of phosphorylating enzymes exist: nucleoside diphosphate kinases, which catalyze the transfer of the terminal phosphate of nucleoside 5′-triphosphates to nucleoside 5′-diphosphates (e.g., $ATP + GDP \rightleftharpoons ADP + GTP$), and adenylate kinases, which catalyze the production of ADP from ATP and AMP or *vice versa*, depending on the concentrations of the respective nucleotides ($ATP + AMP \rightleftharpoons 2ADP$). Although initially believed to be restricted to the cell cytosol, there is evidence that nucleoside diphosphate kinases are also present in the cell membrane[199]; mRNA and protein for these enzymes have been identified in rat kidney,[80] but their distribution is unknown. Adenylate kinases are also largely intracellular but, again, ecto-adenylate kinase activity has also been identified.[199] Adenylate kinase enzyme action has been documented along the nephron,[22] although the relative contributions of intracellular and extracellular activity could not be differentiated.

The principal catalytic activities of the ectonucleotidases and phosphorylating enzymes expressed in the kidney are summarized in Table 18.1. Since no

TABLE 18.1 Catalytic Activities of the Ectonucleotidases and Phosphorylating Enzymes Expressed in the Kidney

Enzyme	Hydrolysis Pathways
NTPDases	
NTPDase1	$ATP \rightarrow ADP + Pi \rightarrow AMP + 2P_i$
	$ADP \rightarrow AMP + P_i$
NTPDase2	$ATP \rightarrow ADP + P_i$
	$ADP \rightarrow AMP + P_i$
NTPDase3	$ATP \rightarrow ADP + P_i$
NTPDase8	$ADP \rightarrow AMP + P_i$
NPPs	
NPP1	$ATP \rightarrow AMP + PP_i$
NPP3	$ADP \rightarrow AMP + P_i$
	$3',5'\text{-cAMP} \rightarrow AMP$
	$Ap_nA \rightarrow AMP + Ap_{n-1}$
NPP2	$ATP \rightarrow AMP + PP_i$
	$ADP \rightarrow AMP + P_i$
	$3',5'\text{-cAMP} \rightarrow AMP$
	$Ap_nA \rightarrow AMP + Ap_{n-1}$
Ecto-5'-nucleotidase	$AMP \rightarrow adenosine + P_i$
Alkaline phosphatases	$ATP \rightarrow ADP + P_i$
	$ADP \rightarrow AMP + P_i$
	$AMP \rightarrow adenosine + P_i$
Nucleotide diphosphate kinases	$ADP + NTP \rightleftharpoons ATP + NDP$
Adenylate kinases	$ATP + AMP \rightleftharpoons 2ADP$

(Adapted from ref. [145].)

Major pathways are shown in black, others in gray. NB: In many cases, nucleotides derived from other bases (UTP, GTP, TTP, CTP, UDP, GDP, TDP, and CDP) can also act as substrates (NDP: nucleoside diphosphate; NTP: nucleoside triphosphate).

information is yet available on the possible functional relevance of the phosphorylating enzymes, in the account below we will restrict ourselves to ectonucleotidases. More detailed information can be found in recent reviews.[145,199]

Although the NTPDase family comprises eight members, only four of these (NTPDases 1, 2, 3, and 8) hydrolyze extracellular nucleotides. NTPDase1 hydrolyzes ATP and ADP with almost equal preference, whereas NTPDase2 has a much greater preference for ATP, therefore causing accumulation of ADP; NTPDases 3 and 8 are intermediate in their preference.[145] The possible functional consequence is that if NTPDase1 is present, P2 receptor stimulation will be abruptly terminated, whereas if NTPDase2 (and to some extent NTPDases 3 and 8) is expressed in the absence of NTPDase1 (or of NPPs), local production and accumulation of ADP would be expected to stimulate $P2Y_1$ (and $P2Y_{12}$ and $P2Y_{13}$) receptors.[172] In rats and mice, NTPDase1 is prominent throughout most of the renal vasculature (interlobular arteries, afferent arterioles, glomeruli, mesangial cells, peritubular capillaries) and is also present in the thin ascending limb of Henle and medullary CD.[84,175] NTPDase2 has been immunolocalized to Bowman's capsules and to most nephron segments beyond the proximal tubule[84,175]; the intrarenal expression of NTPDase3 has been investigated only in the rat where, like NTPDase2, it was found in TAL, distal tubule and CD.[175] Information on NTPDase8 is confined to porcine kidney and is incomplete.

The NPP family comprises seven members, but only NPPs 1–3 are able to hydrolyze nucleotides. NPPs can hydrolyze not only ATP and ADP to AMP, but also dinucleoside polyphosphates (again to AMP; see Table 18.1). Information on the intrarenal distribution of NPPs is limited. Staining for NPP1 protein has been identified in mouse proximal tubules and (more strongly) in basolateral membranes of distal tubules,[54] while prominent staining for NPP3 has been found in rat glomeruli and in the apical membrane of the pars recta, but not in more distal segments.[175]

Ecto-5'-nucleotidase catalyzes the final stage of nucleotide hydrolysis to nucleoside (e.g., $AMP \rightarrow adenosine + P_i$). It has a high level of expression in the kidney; it is found in apical membranes of rat PCT and in intercalated cells throughout the distal nephron, as well as the peritubular space.[43,92,175]

An alkaline phosphatase has been identified in the apical membrane of PCT and pars recta of rat kidney.[9] Although alkaline phosphatases have broad substrate specificity, capable of breaking down ATP right through to adenosine, the K_m values for adenine nucleotides are in the low millimolar range, raising questions about the physiological significance of this enzyme, at least in relation to nucleotide degradation.

A summary of existing knowledge of the distribution of ectonucleotidases in the kidney is shown in Figure 18.8.

Given that our knowledge of ectonucleotidase location is incomplete, we can only make a limited number of speculations concerning their possible function in the kidney. The NTPDase1 located in the renal vasculature seems likely to fulfill an important function of that found elsewhere in the body: termination of the platelet aggregation response to extracellular ADP.[38] This enzyme may also terminate the vasoconstrictive action of locally produced ATP on $P2X_1$ receptors in afferent arterioles (*vide supra*) and, along with glomerular NPP3, may modulate the action of ATP on mesangial cells,[73] thereby influencing the ultrafiltration

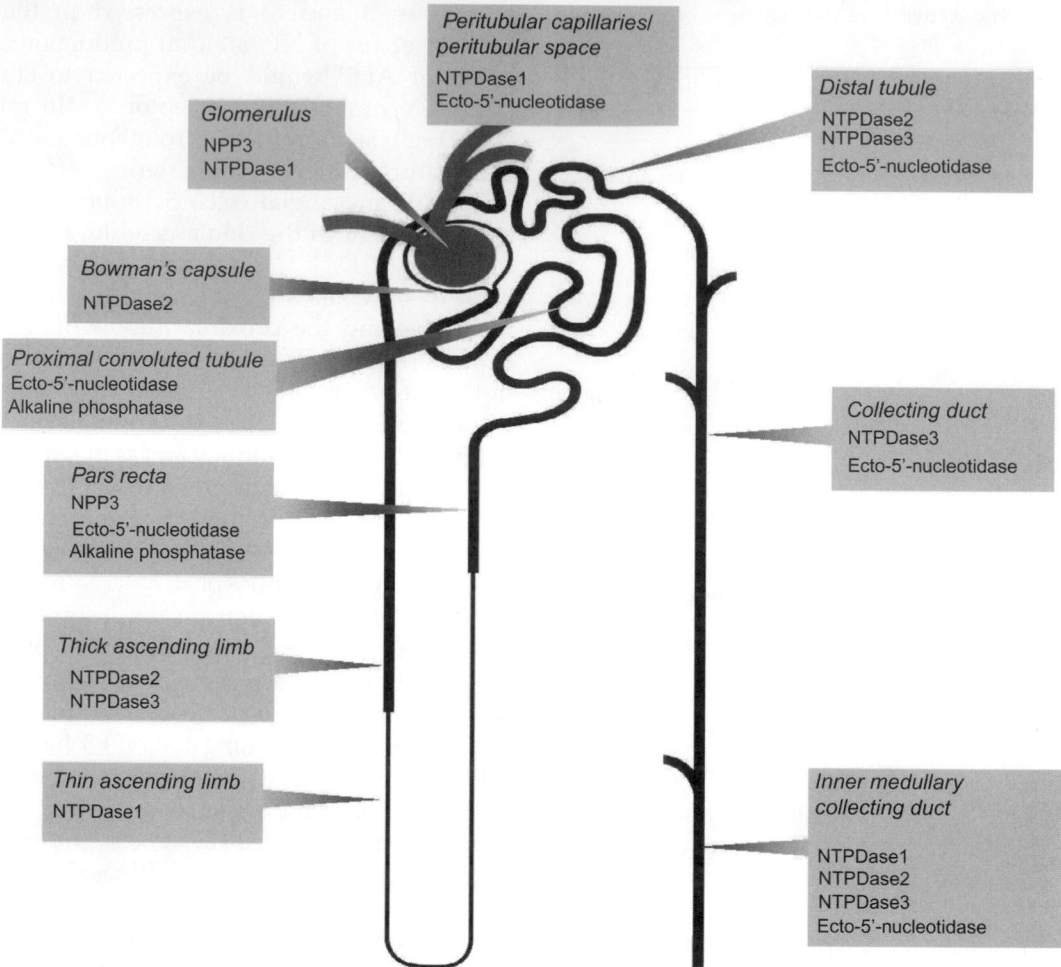

FIGURE 18.8 **Distribution of ectonucleotidases along the rat nephron.** Information compiled from [22,43,84,92,175]. N.B. No information is yet available concerning NPPs 1 and 2 in the rat. (*Adapted from ref. [145]*).

coefficient. The possible roles of ATP and adenosine in mediating TGF have already been discussed. In this context, NTPDase1, expressed in the peritubular space, and/or NPP1, present in basolateral membranes of mouse distal tubule, together with ecto-5′-nucleotidase, also expressed in the peritubular space, are available for the conversion of ATP to adenosine.

As yet, no enzymes that initiate the degradation of ATP have been identified in the PCT (although it should be noted that no suitable antibodies to rat NPP1 or NPP2 are available) and, as already indicated, it is unlikely that proximal tubular alkaline phosphatase could effect ATP degradation at the normal physiological concentrations of the nucleotide. However, it is worth noting that ATPase and ADPase activities have been described in porcine PCT apical membranes.[96] Any AMP produced in the proximal tubule will be converted rapidly to adenosine by the apical ecto-5′-nucleotidase present throughout this part of the nephron. The adenosine could then either activate

adenosine A_1 receptors, increasing proximal tubular fluid reabsorption,[182] be converted to inosine or be transported into proximal tubular cells for reuse.[106] Finally, given the effects of extracellular nucleotides on solute and water transport in the distal nephron (*vide supra*), and the inhibitory effect of A_1 receptor activation on sodium reabsorption in the medullary collecting duct,[195] the NTPDases and ecto-5′-nucleotidase present throughout the distal nephron are likely to be of considerable functional significance.

In conclusion, although our knowledge of the intrarenal location of ectonucleotidases is still incomplete, it seems clear that their distribution varies along the nephron, and this provides scope for the rapid termination of the actions of locally produced ATP and/or initiation of ADP-mediated or adenosine-mediated effects.

Role of P2 Receptors in Renal Pathophysiology

The well-documented release of ATP from injured and dying cells at sites of injury and inflammation, and from red cells and platelets during thrombus formation, suggests that the P2 receptor system could be involved in the pathophysiology of renal disease.[20] As well as producing changes in vascular tone and in fluid and electrolyte reabsorption or secretion (*vide supra*), stimulation of P2 receptors can influence renal cell growth[53,71,138] and — especially in the case of the P2X$_7$ receptor — can also result in cell death and promote inflammation.[59,137]

The published work supporting a pathophysiological role for P2 receptors in the kidney is still limited and remains somewhat speculative. Two disease models have been the main focus of interest: (1) renal cystic disease; and (2) glomerular injury and inflammation. The first stems from work on P2 receptors in secretory epithelia,[91] in particular the airway epithelium in cystic fibrosis,[115] and has been extrapolated to a potential role for these receptors in renal cyst growth in polycystic kidney disease.[142] The second concerns the broadly pro-proliferative effect of stimulating various P2Y receptor subtypes,[132] and the pro-apoptotic effect of activating the P2X$_7$ receptor, particularly when expressed by renal glomerular cells,[179] inflammatory macrophages,[167] and interstitial fibroblasts.[125]

Polycystic Kidney Disease

Mutations in polycystin 1, a membrane receptor, or polycystin 2, a putative Ca^{2+} channel (*vide supra*), give rise to polycystic kidney disease (PKD), a condition associated with uncontrolled proliferation of renal epithelial cells and disordered fluid transport, leading to tubular dilatation and formation and expansion of fluid-filled cysts, which eventually compress and destroy adjacent normal tissue.[189] Cyst-lining cells are thought to exhibit: (1) disordered regulation of proliferation and apoptosis; (2) abnormal secretion of fluid and electrolytes; and (3) disturbed polarity of membrane transport proteins and receptors, which is also believed to relate to a defect in mechanosensation (including detection of the flow of tubular fluid) due to mislocalization and dysfunction of the epithelial cell primary cilium.[193]

In culture, human PKD cells have been shown to release more ATP than normal proximal tubular cells, predominantly from their apical surface.[190] The cysts themselves accumulate and concentrate ATP (0.5–10 μM) and their ecto-ATPase activity appears to be diminished.[142] This extracellular ATP, acting on P2Y (and possibly P2X) receptors on cyst-lining cells, may not only promote cell growth and fluid secretion, but also, by activating the P2X$_7$ receptor, increase cell loss by apoptosis as part of the remodeling necessary for progressive cyst expansion (Figure 18.9); in this regard it is worth noting that inhibition of caspase-mediated apoptosis slows PKD progression.[161] However, much of the evidence in support of this appealing hypothesis is indirect and circumstantial. Schwiebert and

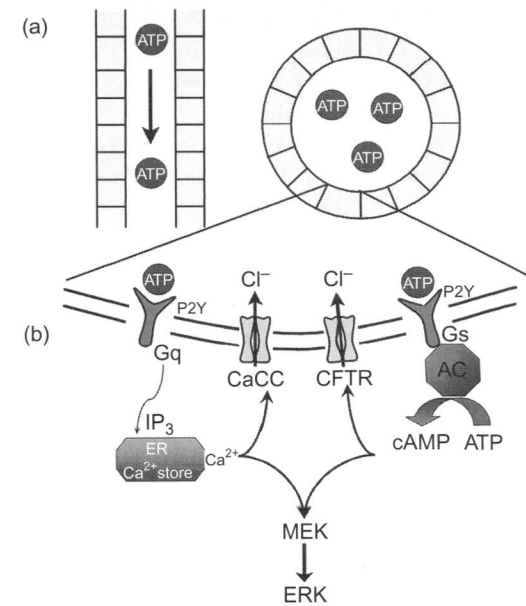

FIGURE 18.9 Proposed role of P2 receptor signaling in cyst growth. (a) Remodeling of the normal renal tubule (top left) into an enclosed cyst (top right) allows ATP to accumulate. Reduced nucleotidase activity, coupled with the large representation of P2 receptor subtypes likely to be present in these cyst lining epithelial cells, would allow an amplifying loop of autocrine signaling to occur that might promote osmotically driven fluid accumulation and cellular proliferation. (b) Exploded view of the apical cell membrane lining a hypothetical renal cyst. G-protein-coupled P2Y receptor activation triggers release of Ca^{2+} from the endoplasmic reticulum or production of cAMP via adenylyl cyclase (AC) and subsequent activation of calcium-sensitive chloride channels (CaCC) or CFTR, respectively. The facilitated transcellular transport of Cl^- creates a solute gradient that promotes the osmotic flow of water into the cyst lumen. The increase in $[Ca^{2+}]_i$ and cAMP can modulate the ERK pathway and consequently cellular proliferation. (*from ref. [167]*).

colleagues performed an *in vitro* analysis of P2 receptor signaling in cyst-derived epithelial cells. They confirmed ATP release and P2 receptor-mediated stimulation of SCC (Cl^- secretion), and they also documented mRNA expression for several P2Y and P2X receptor subtypes.[142] At the same time Hillman and co-workers demonstrated expression of the P2X$_7$ receptor (at mRNA and protein levels) in the cystic epithelium of the *cpk/cpk* mouse model of autosomal recessive PKD.[60] Using cells isolated from the *cpk/cpk* mouse, a three-dimensional (3D) suspension model of cyst development was used to study the effects of P2X$_7$ receptor activation on cyst development. The widely used P2X receptor agonist BzATP *reduced* cyst number, but not cyst size, in this model[61] (although BzATP is not selective for P2X$_7$ and can act as an antagonist at some P2Y receptors). In another 3D model of cyst formation using MDCK cells, cyst expansion was inhibited by BzATP; however, this appeared to depend on P2Y, rather than P2X, stimulation.[168] In a rat model (Han-SPRD) of autosomal dominant PKD, although the P2X$_7$ subtype was detected in cyst-lining cells and its mRNA level increased, other P2X and P2Y receptors were also detected, with particular increases in P2Y$_{2, 4,}$ and P2Y$_6$ subtypes.[169] All this suggests a complex interplay of P2 receptor subtypes in PKD, with perhaps differing effects on cyst number and cyst size.

More mechanistically, expression of a C-terminal polycystin 1 construct, fused to a membrane expression cassette in a mouse CD cell line (M1), upregulated ATP-stimulated Cl$^-$ secretion, which was associated with a rise in [Ca^{2+}]$_i$ due to an increase in Ca^{2+} entry.[63,184] However, more recent studies of cultured human PKD cells have described a loss of flow-mediated ATP release and the flow-dependent rise in [Ca^{2+}]$_i$, and this was attributed to reduced P2X$_7$ expression and function.[193,194] In this same model, expression of the ectonucleotidase NTPDase1 was also reduced, which would be expected to lead to an increase in local ATP levels. These human PKD cells have also been shown to have defective cilia, which are presumed to be the sensors for flow-activated cell signaling; in ciliated airway epithelia, cilial motion is increased by ATP and these cilia express a P2X receptor that is probably a heteromer of P2X$_{4/7}$,[105] P2X subtypes that are also found in PKD cells. However, although tantalizing, these findings provide more questions than answers, and the exact role of P2 receptors in PKD pathogenesis is still unclear.

The P2X$_7$ Receptor and Renal Inflammation

As already indicated, P2X$_7$ receptor expression is barely detectable in normal healthy kidney. However, its expression is increased in rodent models of glomerular injury, diabetes mellitus, and renin-dependent hypertension.[179] As well as the ability to form a non-selective cation channel or a larger membrane pore leading to cell death by necrosis or apoptosis, the P2X$_7$ receptor can mediate an inflammatory response by causing release of interleukin (IL)-1β (Figure 18.10).[30] Factors that determine whether P2X$_7$ receptor stimulation will cause cell necrosis or apoptosis, and/or inflammatory cytokine release, include the cell type, the concentration of ATP and duration of exposure to the nucleotide, as well as the level of P2X$_7$ receptor surface expression. In cultured human embryonic kidney cells expressing P2X7 receptors, membrane blebbing and microvesiculation are seen within seconds-to-minutes of receptor stimulation, which is associated with cell death by apoptosis.[188] More prolonged receptor stimulation leads to formation of a large membrane pore that permits leakage of vital intracellular components (including ATP) and loss of membrane potential, ultimately leading to cell death and necrosis[114]; somewhat paradoxically, lower

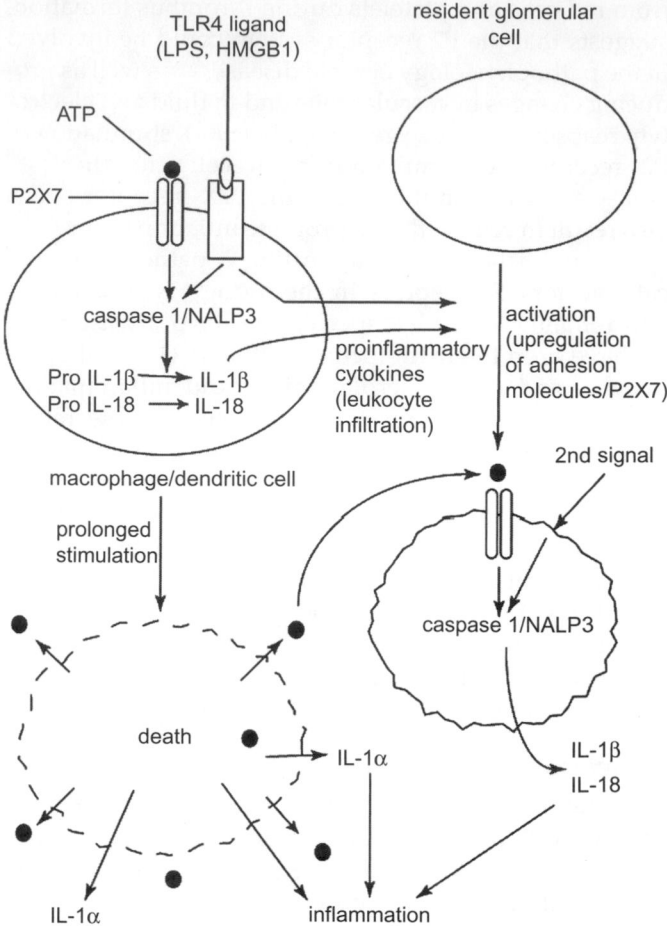

FIGURE 18.10 Putative role of the P2X7 receptor in inflammatory glomerular disease. Following initial injury to the kidney, ATP released from damaged cells, possibly together with endogenous Toll-like receptor 4 (TLR4) ligands such as High Mobility Group Box 1 (HMGB1) and lipopolysaccharide (LPS), stimulates the NALP3 inflammasome. Inflammasome activation leads to the maturation of caspase 1, which in turn promotes cleavage, maturation, and release of IL-1β and IL-18 from resident macrophages. Released cytokines promote leukocyte influx and stimulate upregulation of P2X$_7$ on intrinsic renal cells. Prolonged P2X$_7$ stimulation results in cell death with release of intracellular pro-inflammatory mediators such as ATP, IL-1α, and HMGB1, resulting in further rounds of P2X$_7$ stimulation. *(from ref. [167]).*

concentrations of ATP (and perhaps tonic stimulation of P2X7) in at least some cell types seem to be able to enhance cell proliferation, rather than cause cell death.[1]

Activation of the P2X$_7$ receptor promotes release of mature IL-1β, IL-6, and IL-18 from activated macrophages, and both interferon-γ and tumor necrosis factor-α (TNF-α) can increase expression of P2X$_7$ receptors,[53,90,98,177] suggesting that this receptor can both regulate, and is regulated by, inflammatory cytokine processing and release. Moreover, we have observed a marked increase in glomerular expression of P2X$_7$ receptors in a rodent model of proliferative glomerulonephritis, reaching a peak that coincides with the onset of proteinuria.[170] Macrophage infiltration and release of inflammatory cytokines are characteristic features of glomerular damage in many forms of glomerulonephritis.[160] P2X$_7$ receptor gene knockout or treatment with a P2X$_7$ receptor antagonist significantly reduced the severity of proliferative glomerulonephritis in mouse and rat models, respectively, as shown by reduced renal expression of CC chemokine ligand 2 (CCL2; monocyte chemoattractant-1 (MCP-1)), reductions in glomerular macrophage infiltration, glomerular capillary thrombosis and proteinuria, and a smaller rise in serum creatinine concentration.[163] In the rat diabetic model, both glomerular epithelial (podocytes) and mesangial cells express P2X$_7$ receptors[179]; damaged podocytes have been shown to release IL-13[111]; and both IL-13 and TNF-α are increased in diabetic glomeruli.[57] Thus, ATP, acting via the P2X$_7$ receptor, could interact with, and control, the inflammatory response, eventually leading to cell death, perhaps as a mechanism for deleting damaged cells without dispersal of their potentially toxic contents. Two auto-inflammatory rheumatic diseases, SAPHO and Schnitzler's syndrome, involve an enhanced interaction and dysregulation of the P2X$_7$ receptor with the inflammasome, leading to excessive IL-1β production and release,[23,122] which suggests a wider and more fundamental role for this receptor in tissue inflammation.

Fibrosis often follows inflammation, and it has always been a major goal to determine which factors during inflammation determine its resolution and repair, and which ones lead to chronicity and progressive fibrosis. The potential role of the P2X$_7$ receptor in renal fibrosis has been investigated in a mouse model of unilateral ureteric obstruction. Transient expression of P2X$_7$ receptors was detected in tubular epithelial cells following ureteric obstruction, and the severity of tubulo-interstitial macrophage infiltration, and expression of TGF-β and fibrosis, were reduced in P2X$_7$ receptor knockout mice.[48] In the kidney, interstitial fibroblasts are important in normal repair, and their P2X$_7$-mediated loss might contribute to post-injury fibrosis and scarring in this model.[125] A similar protective effect of P2X$_7$ gene deletion has been reported recently in a model of lung fibrosis.[131]

In another model of proliferative glomerulonephritis, the P2Y$_1$ receptor has been implicated.[62] Interestingly, the acute injury was similar in P2Y$_1$ knockout and wild-type mice (cf. P2X$_7$), but there was less glomerular capillary loss and fibrosis in the P2Y$_1$ knockouts at later time points (10 and 28 days). It would clearly be useful to explore the relationship and possible interaction between P2Y$_1$ and P2X$_7$ receptors in this and related models of acute glomerulonephritis, and whether there might be synergy in targeting therapeutically both receptors.

Finally, P2 receptor activation has also been implicated in the renal injury resulting from ischaemia-reperfusion (IR), a major cause of clinical acute renal failure. Such injury can result from a wide variety of insults, including transplantation, and a common unifying mechanism is therefore difficult to define. Nevertheless, the broad-spectrum P2 inhibitor suramin was found to attenuate the renal infiltration of leukocytes and tubular cell apopotosis that usually follows IR injury.[206] Furthermore, gene deletion of ecto-5′-nucleotidase also ameliorated IR-induced apoptotic and histological renal damage, while deletion of NTPDase1 aggravated it.[103]

CONCLUDING REMARKS

For extracellular nucleotides to be effective autocrine/paracrine agents, there are three fundamental requirements: release of nucleotides from cells; controlled degradation of the nucleotides once released; and the presence of specific nucleotide receptors that can initiate transduction of the signal to a functional response. In the fourth edition of this textbook it was established that these conditions were met, both in the vasculature and the tubule. Since then, significant advances have been made in all three areas, and the many and varied functions of nucleotides in the kidneys have received increased attention. Consequently, in some areas the situation is becoming clearer. For example, nucleotide-induced NO synthesis can account for an inhibitory effect on transport in the TALH; and, given NOs putative actions in the proximal tubule and CD, this might provide a unifying hypothesis to explain nucleotide-induced effects in these segments. On the other hand, several areas continue to defy understanding — for example, the mechanism(s) of release of nucleotides and the apparently differential effects of P2Y and P2X receptors on ENaC activity. As more and more sophisticated techniques are brought to bear, it is to be hoped that ongoing research will solve even the most intransigent problems. Furthermore, although much of the work on renal pathophysiology remains at a descriptive stage, altered P2 receptor signaling is strongly implicated, and the potential for novel therapeutic targets is high.

Acknowledgments

Work in the authors' laboratories was supported by the Wellcome Trust, the Medical Research Council, Kidney Research UK, the British Heart Foundation, the Biotechnology and Biological Sciences Research Council, the Diamond Fund (Imperial College Healthcare Charity) and St Peter's Trust for Kidney, Bladder & Prostate Research.

References

[1] Adinolfi E, Callegari MG, Cirillo M, Pinton P, Giorgi C, Cavagna D, et al. Expression of the $P2X_7$ receptor increases the Ca^{2+} content of the endoplasmic reticulum, activates NFATc1, and protects from apoptosis. J Biol Chem 2009;284:10120–8.

[2] Bailey MA. Inhibition of bicarbonate reabsorption in the rat proximal tubule by activation of luminal $P2Y_1$ receptors. Am J Physiol Renal Physiol 2004;287:F789–96.

[3] Bailey MA, Hillman KA, Unwin RJ. P2 receptors in the kidney. J Auton Nerv Syst 2000;81:264–70.

[4] Bailey MA, Imbert-Teboul M, Turner C, Marsy S, Srai K, Burnstock G, et al. Axial distribution and characterization of basolateral P2Y receptors along the rat renal tubule. Kidney Int 2000;58:1893–901.

[5] Bailey MA, Imbert-Teboul M, Turner C, Srai K, Burnstock G, Unwin RJ. Evidence for basolateral $P2Y_6$ receptors along the rat proximal tubule: functional and molecular characterization. J Am Soc Nephrol 2001;12:1640–7.

[6] Bailey MA, Shirley DG. Effects of extracellular nucleotides on renal tubular solute transport. Purinergic Signal 2009;5:473–80.

[7] Bailey MA, Turner CM, Hus-Citharel A, Marchetti J, Imbert-Teboul M, Milner P, et al. P2Y receptors present in the native and isolated rat glomerulus. Nephron Physiol 2004;96:p79–90.

[8] Barbe MT, Monyer H, Bruzzone R. Cell–cell communication beyond connexins: the pannexin channels. Physiology (Bethesda) 2006;21:103–14.

[9] Beliveau R, Brunette MG, Strevey J. Characterization of phosphate binding by alkaline phosphatase in rat kidney brush border membrane. Pflügers Arch 1983;398:227–32.

[10] Bell PD, Komlosi P, Zhang Z-R. ATP as a mediator of macula densa cell signaling. Purinergic Signal 2009;5:461–71.

[11] Bell PD, Lapointe JY, Sabirov R, Hayashi S, Peti-Peterdi J, Manabe K, et al. Macula densa cell signaling involves ATP release through a maxi anion channel. Proc Natl Acad Sci USA 2003;100:4322–7.

[12] Briner VA, Kern F. ATP stimulates Ca^{2+} mobilization by a nucleotide receptor in glomerular endothelial cells. Am J Physiol 1994;266:F210–7.

[13] Burnstock G. Purinergic nerves. Pharmacol Rev 1972;24:509–81.

[14] Burnstock G. Purine and pyrimidine receptors. Cell Mol Life Sci 2007;64:1471–83.

[15] Castrop H, Huang Y, Hashimoto S, Mizel D, Hansen P, Theilig F, et al. Impairment of tubuloglomerular feedback regulation of GFR in ecto-5′-nucleotidase/CD73-deficient mice. J Clin Invest 2004;114:634–42.

[16] Cha SH, Jung KY, Endou H. Effect of P2Y-purinoceptor stimulation on renal gluconeogenesis in rats. Biochem Biophys Res Commun 1995;211:454–61.

[17] Cha SH, Sekine T, Endou H. P2 purinoceptor localization along rat nephron and evidence suggesting existence of subtypes $P2Y_1$ and $P2Y_2$. Am J Physiol 1998;274:F1006–14.

[18] Chabardès-Garonne D, Méjean A, Aude J-C, et al. A panoramic view of gene expression in the human kidney. Proc Natl Acad Sci USA 2003;100:13710–5.

[19] Chan CM, Unwin RJ, Bardini M, Oglesby IB, Ford AP, Townsend-Nicholson A, et al. Localization of $P2X_1$ purinoceptors by autoradiography and immunohistochemistry in rat kidneys. Am J Physiol 1998;274:F799–804.

[20] Chan CM, Unwin RJ, Burnstock G. Potential functional roles of extracellular ATP in kidney and urinary tract. Exp Nephrol 1998;6:200–7.

[21] Churchill PC, Ellis VR. Purinergic P2y receptors stimulate renin secretion by rat renal cortical slices. J Pharmacol Exp Ther 1993;266:160–3.

[22] Cole BR, Hays AE, Boylan JG, Burch HB, Lowry OH. Distribution of enzymes of adenylate and guanylate nucleotide metabolism in rat nephron. Am J Physiol 1982;243:F349–55.

[23] Colina M, Pizzirani C, Khodeir M, Falzoni S, Bruschi M, Trotta F, et al. Dysregulation of $P2X_7$ receptor-inflammasome axis in SAPHO syndrome: successful treatment with anakinra. Rheumatology (Oxford) 2010;49:1416–8.

[24] Cotrina ML, Lin JH, Alves-Rodrigues A, Liu S, Li J, Azmi-Ghadimi H, et al. Connexins regulate calcium signaling by controlling ATP release. Proc Natl Acad Sci USA 1998;95:15735–40.

[25] Cuffe JE, Bielfeld-Ackermann A, Thomas J, Leipziger J, Korbmacher C. ATP stimulates Cl^- secretion and reduces amiloride-sensitive Na^+ absorption in M-1 mouse cortical collecting duct cells. J Physiol 2000;524:77–90.

[26] Cupples WA, Braam B. Assessment of renal autoregulation. Am J Physiol Renal Physiol 2007;292:F1105–23.

[27] Dai L-J, Kang HS, Kerstan D, Ritchie G, Quamme GA. ATP inhibits Mg^{2+} uptake in MDCT cells via P2X purinoceptors. Am J Physiol Renal Physiol 2001;281:F833–40.

[28] Deetjen P, Thomas J, Lehrmann H, Kim SJ, Leipziger J. The luminal P2Y receptor in the isolated perfused mouse cortical collecting duct. J Am Soc Nephrol 2000;11:1798–806.

[29] Di Sole F. Adenosine and renal tubular function. Curr Opin Nephrol Hypertens 2008;17:399–407.

[30] Di Virgilio F. Liaisons dangereuses: $P2X_7$ and the inflammasome. Trends Pharmacol Sci 2007;28:465–72.

[31] Diaz-Sylvester P, Mac Laughlin M, Amorena C. Peritubular fluid viscosity modulates H^+ flux in proximal tubules through NO release. Am J Physiol Renal Physiol 2001;280:F239–43.

[32] Dobrowolski L, Walkowska A, Kompanowska-Jezierska E, Kuczeriszka M, Sadowski J. Effects of ATP on rat renal haemodynamics and excretion: role of sodium intake, nitric oxide and cytochrome P450. Acta Physiol (Oxford) 2007;189:77–85.

[33] Donnelly-Roberts DL, Jarvis MF. Discovery of $P2X_7$ receptor-selective antagonists offers new insights into $P2X_7$ receptor function and indicates a role in chronic pain states. Br J Pharmacol 2007;151:571–9.

[34] Drury AN, Szent-Gyorgyi A. The physiological activity of adenine compounds with special reference to their action upon the mammalian heart. J Physiol 1929;68:213–37.

[35] Edgecombe M, Craddock HS, Smith DC, McLennan AG, Fisher MJ. Diadenosine polyphosphate-stimulated gluconeogenesis in isolated rat proximal tubules. Biochem J 1997;323:451–6.

[36] Edwards RM. Basolateral, but not apical, ATP inhibits vasopressin action in rat inner medullary collecting duct. Eur J Pharmacol 2002;438:179–81.

[37] Eltze M, Ullrich B. Characterization of vascular P2 purinoceptors in the rat isolated perfused kidney. Eur J Pharmacol 1996;306:139–52.

[38] Enjyoji K, Sévigny J, Lin Y, et al. Targeted disruption of cd39/ATP diphosphohydrolase results in disordered hemostasis and thromboregulation. Nat Med 1999;5:1010–7.

[39] Eppel GA, Ventura S, Evans RG. Regional vascular responses to ATP and ATP analogues in the rabbit kidney in vivo: roles for adenosine receptors and prostanoids. Br J Pharmacol 2006;149:523–31.

[40] Fernández O, Wangensteen R, Osuna A, Vargas F. Renal vascular reactivity to P2-purinoceptor activation in spontaneously hypertensive rats. Pharmacology 2000;60:47–50.

[41] Fischer KG, Saueressig U, Jacobshagen C, Wichelmann A, Pavenstadt H. Extracellular nucleotides regulate cellular functions of podocytes in culture. Am J Physiol Renal Physiol 2001;281:F1075–81.

[42] Friedrich F, Weiss H, Paulmichl M, Woll E, Waldegger S, Lang F. Further analysis of ATP-mediated activation of K^+ channels in renal epithelioid Madin−Darby canine kidney (MDCK) cells. Pflügers Arch 1991;418:551−5.

[43] Gandhi R, Le Hir M, Kaissling B. Immunolocalization of ecto-5′-nucleotidase in the kidney by a monoclonal antibody. Histochemistry 1990;95:165−74.

[44] Garvin JL, Herrera M, Ortiz PA. Regulation of renal NaCl transport by nitric oxide, endothelin, and ATP: clinical implications. Annu Rev Physiol 2011;:73.

[45] Garvin JL, Hong NJ. Nitric oxide inhibits sodium/hydrogen exchange activity in the thick ascending limb. Am J Physiol Renal Physiol 1999;277:F377−82.

[46] George SN, Kennedy-Lydon T, Callaghan H, et al. Decreased $P2X_7$ receptor mRNA expression in the CCD of the $P2X_4^{-/-}$ mouse: a clue to the identity of the P2X luminal sodium sensor? J Am Soc Nephrol 2010; F-PO1611 (Abstract)

[47] Geyti CS, Odgaard E, Overgaard MT, Jensen ME, Leipziger J, Praetorious HA. Slow spontaneous $[Ca^{2+}]_i$ oscillations reflect nucleotide release from renal epithelia. Pflügers Arch 2008;455:1105−17.

[48] Goncalves RG, Gabrich L, Rosario Jr. A, Takiya CM, Ferreira ML, Chiarini LB, et al. The role of purinergic $P2X_7$ receptors in the inflammation and fibrosis of unilateral ureteral obstruction in mice. Kidney Int 2006;70:1599−606.

[49] Gorelik J, Zhang Y, Sanchez D, Shevchuk A, Frolenkov G, Lab M, et al. Aldosterone acts via an ATP autocrine/paracrine system: the Edelman ATP hypothesis revisited. Proc Natl Acad Sci USA 2005;102:15000−5.

[50] Guan Z, Fuller BS, Yamamoto T, Cook AK, Pollock JS, Inscho EW. Pentosan polysulfate treatment preserves renal autoregulation in Ang II-Infused hypertensive rats via normalization of $P2X_1$ receptor activation. Am J Physiol Renal Physiol 2011; in press.

[51] Guo C, Masin M, Qureshi OS, Murrell-Lagnado RD. Evidence for functional $P2X_4$/$P2X_7$ heteromeric receptors. Mol Pharmacol 2007;72:1447−56.

[52] Hanner F, Sorensen CM, Holstein-Rathlou N-H, Peti-Peterdi J. Connexins and the kidney. Am J Physiol Regul Integr Comp Physiol 2010;298:R1143−55.

[53] Harada H, Chan CM, Loesch A, Unwin R, Burnstock G. Induction of proliferation and apoptotic cell death via P2Y and P2X receptors, respectively, in rat glomerular mesangial cells. Kidney Int 2000;57:949−58.

[54] Harahap AR, Goding JW. Distribution of the murine plasma cell antigen PC-1 in non-lymphoid tissues. J Immunol 1988;141:2317−20.

[55] Harden TK, Sesma JI, Fricks IP, Lazarowski ER. Signaling and pharmacological properties of the $P2Y_{14}$ receptor. Acta Physiol (Oxford) 2010;199:149−60.

[56] Harhun MI, Povstyan OV, Gordienko DV. Purinoreceptor-mediated current in myocytes from renal resistance arteries. Br J Pharmacol 2010;160:987−97.

[57] Hasegawa G, Nakano K, Sawada M, Uno K, Shibayama Y, Ienaga K, et al. Possible role of tumor necrosis factor and interleukin-1 in the development of diabetic nephropathy. Kidney Int 1991;40:1007−12.

[58] Heyeraas KJ, Aukland K. Interlobular arterial resistance: influence of renal arterial pressure and angiotensin II. Kidney Int 1987;31:1291−8.

[59] Hillman KA, Burnstock G, Unwin RJ. The $P2X_7$ receptor in the kidney: a matter of life or death?. Nephron Exp Nephrol 2005;101:e24−30.

[60] Hillman KA, Johnson TM, Winyard PJ, Burnstock G, Unwin RJ, Woolf AS. $P2X_7$ receptors are expressed during mouse nephrogenesis and in collecting duct cysts of the cpk/cpk mouse. Exp Nephrol 2002;10:34−42.

[61] Hillman KA, Woolf AS, Johnson TM, Wade A, Unwin RJ, Winyard PJ. The $P2X_7$ ATP receptor modulates renal cyst development in vitro. Biochem Biophys Res Commun 2004;322:434−9.

[62] Hohenstein B, Renk S, Lang K, Daniel C, Freund M, Leon C, et al. $P2Y_1$ gene deficiency protects from renal disease progression and capillary rarefaction during passive crescentic glomerulonephritis. J Am Soc Nephrol 2007;18:494−505.

[63] Hooper KM, Unwin RJ, Sutters M. The isolated C-terminus of polycystin-1 promotes increased ATP-stimulated chloride secretion in a collecting duct cell line. Clin Sci (Lond) 2003;104:217−21.

[64] Hovater MB, Olteanu D, Hanson EL, et al. Loss of apical monocilia on collecting duct principal cells impairs ATP secretion across the apical cell surface and ATP-dependent and flow-induced calcium signals. Purinergic Signal 2008;4:155−70.

[65] Huwiler A, Wartmann M, van den Bosch H, Pfeilschifter J. Extracellular nucleotides activate the p38-stress-activated protein kinase cascade in glomerular mesangial cells. Br J Pharmacol 2000;129:612−8.

[66] Inscho EW. Renal microvascular effects of P2 receptor stimulation. Clin Exp Pharmacol Physiol 2001;28:332−9.

[67] Inscho EW. ATP, P2 receptors and the renal microcirculation. Purinergic Signal 2009;5:447−60.

[68] Inscho EW, Cook AK, Imig JD, Vial C, Evans RJ. Physiological role for $P2X_1$ receptors in renal microvascular autoregulatory behavior. J Clin Invest 2003;112:1895−905.

[69] Inscho EW, Cook AK, Navar LG. Pressure-mediated vasoconstriction of juxtamedullary afferent arterioles involves P2-purinoceptor activation. Am J Physiol 1996;271:F1077−85.

[70] Inscho EW, Ohishi K, Navar LG. Effects of ATP on pre- and postglomerular juxtamedullary microvasculature. Am J Physiol Renal Physiol 1992;263:F886−93.

[71] Ishikawa S, Higashiyama M, Kusaka I, Saito T, Nagasaka S, Fukuda S, et al. Extracellular ATP promotes cellular growth of renal inner medullary collecting duct cells mediated via P2u receptors. Nephron 1997;76:208−14.

[72] Jacobson KA, Ivanov AA, de Castro S, Harden TK, Ko H. Development of selective agonists and antagonists of P2Y receptors. Purinergic Signal 2009;5:75−89.

[73] Jankowski M, Szczepanska-Konkel M, Kalinowski L, Angielski S. The role of P2Y-receptors in the regulation of glomerular volume. Med Sci Monit 2001;7:340−635.

[74] Jankowski V, Karadogan S, Vanholder R, et al. Paracrine stimulation of vascular smooth muscle proliferation by diadenosine polyphosphates released from proximal tubule epithelial cells. Kidney Int 2007;71:994−1000.

[75] Jensen ME, Odgaard E, Christensen MH, Praetorius HA, Leipziger J. Flow-induced $[Ca^{2+}]_i$ increase depends on nucleotide release and subsequent purinergic signaling in the intact nephron. J Am Soc Nephrol 2007;18:2062−70.

[76] Jin W, Hopfer U. Purinergic-mediated inhibition of Na^+-K^+-ATPase in proximal tubule cells: elevated cytosolic Ca^{2+} is not required. Am J Physiol 1997;272:C1169−77.

[77] Joseph SM, Buchakjian MR, Dubyak GR. Colocalization of ATP release sites and ecto-ATPase activity at the extracellular surface of human astrocytes. J Biol Chem 2003;278:23331−42.

[78] Kauffenstein G, Drouin A, Thorin-Trescases N, Bachelard H, Robaye B, D'Orleans-Juste P, et al. Dase1 (CD39) controls nucleotide-dependent vasoconstriction in mouse. Cardiovasc Res 2010;85:204−13.

[79] Kennedy-Lydon T, Callaghan H, Sprott C, et al. P2 receptor-mediated changes in vasa recta diameter by *in situ* pericytes: evidence for tubular/vascular cross-talk?. J Am Soc Nephrol 2010; F-PO1742 (Abstract)

[80] Kimura N, Shimada N, Nomura K, Watanabe K. Isolation and characterization of a cDNA clone encoding rat nucleoside diphosphate kinase. J Biol Chem 1990;265:15744–9.

[81] King BF, Townsend-Nicholson A. Nucleotide and nucleoside receptors. Tocris Rev 2003;23:1–11.

[82] Kishore BK, Chou CL, Knepper MA. Extracellular nucleotide receptor inhibits AVP-stimulated water permeability in inner medullary collecting duct. Am J Physiol 1995;269:F863–9.

[83] Kishore BK, Ginns SM, Krane CM, Nielsen S, Knepper MA. Cellular localization of P_2Y_2 purinoceptor in rat renal inner medulla and lung. Am J Physiol Renal Physiol 2000;278: F43–51.

[84] Kishore BK, Isaac J, Fausther M, Tripp SR, Shi H, Gill PS, et al. Expression of NTPDase1 and NTPDase2 in murine kidney: Relevance to regulation of P2 receptor signaling. Am J Physiol Renal Physiol 2005;288:F1032–43.

[85] Kishore BK, Krane CM, Miller RL, Shi H, Zhang P, Hemmert A, et al. P_2Y_2 receptor mRNA and protein expression is altered in inner medullas of hydrated and dehydrated rats: relevance to AVP-independent regulation of IMCD function. Am J Physiol Renal Physiol 2005;288:F1164–72.

[86] Kishore BK, Nelson RD, Miller RL, et al. P_2Y_2 receptors and water transport in the kidney. Purinergic Signal 2009;5:491–9.

[87] Komlosi P, Peti-Peterdi J, Fuson AL, Fintha A, Rosivall L, Bell PD. Macula densa basolateral ATP release is regulated by luminal [NaCl] and dietary salt intake. Am J Physiol Renal Physiol 2004;286:F1054–8.

[88] Koster HPG, Hartog A, van Os CH, Bindels RJ. Inhibition of Na^+ and Ca^{2+} reabsorption by P2u purinoceptors requires PKC but not Ca^{2+} signaling. Am J Physiol 1996;270:F53–60.

[89] Köttgen M, Buchholz B, Garcia-Gonzalez MA, et al. TRPP2 and TRPV4 form a polymodal sensory channel complex. J Cell Biol 2008;182:437–47.

[90] Labasi JM, Petrushova N, Donovan C, McCurdy S, Lira P, Payette MM, et al. Absence of the $P2X_7$ receptor alters leukocyte function and attenuates an inflammatory response. J Immunol 2002;168:6436–45.

[91] Lazarowski ER, Boucher RC. UTP as an extracellular signaling molecule. News Physiol Sci 2001;16:1–5.

[92] Le Hir M, Kaissling B. Distribution of 5′-nucleotidase in the renal interstitium of the rat. Cell Tissue Res 1989;258:177–82.

[93] Lee YJ, Park SH, Han HJ. ATP stimulates Na^+-glucose co-transporter activity via cAMP and p38 MAPK in renal proximal tubule cells. Am J Physiol Cell Physiol 2005;289:C1268–1276.

[94] Lee YJ, Park SH, Jeung TO, Kim KW, Lee JH, Han HJ. Effect of adenosine triphosphate on phosphate uptake in renal proximal tubule cells: involvement of PKC and p38 MAP. J Cell Physiol 2005;205:68–76.

[95] Lehrmann H, Thomas J, Kim SJ, Jacobi C, Leipziger J. Luminal P_2Y_2 receptor-mediated inhibition of Na^+ absorption in isolated perfused mouse CCD. J Am Soc Nephrol 2002;13:10–8.

[96] Lemmens R, Kupers L, Sévigny J, Beaudoin AR, Grondin G, Kittel A, et al. Purification, characterization, and localization of an ATP diphosphohydrolase in porcine kidney. Am J Physiol Renal Physiol 2000;278:F978–88.

[97] Li L, Lynch IJ, Zheng W, Cash MN, Teng X, Wingo CS, et al. Apical P2XR contribute to $[Ca^{2+}]_i$ signaling and Isc in mouse renal MCD. Biochem Biophys Res Commun 2007;359:438–44.

[98] Lister MF, Sharkey J, Sawatzky DA, Hodgkiss JP, Davidson DJ, Rossi AG, et al. The role of the purinergic $P2X_7$ receptor in inflammation. J Inflamm 2007;4:5.

[99] Listhrop R, Nelson R, Ecelbarger CA, et al. Genetic deletion of P_2Y_2 receptor (P2Y2-R) alters the protein abundances of renal sodium transporters and channels. FASEB J 2007;21(937):4 (Abstract).

[100] Liu W, Morimoto T, Woda C, Kleyman TR, Satlin LM. Ca^{2+} dependence of flow-stimulated K secretion in the mammalian cortical collecting duct. Am J Physiol Renal Physiol 2007;293: F227–35.

[101] Liu W, Xu S, Woda C. Effect of flow and stretch on the $[Ca^{2+}]_i$ response of principal and intercalated cells in cortical collecting duct. Am J Physiol Renal Physiol 2003;285: F998–1012.

[102] Locovei S, Bao L, Dahl G. Pannexin 1 in erythrocytes: function without a gap. Proc Natl Acad Sci USA 2006;103:7655–9.

[103] Lu B, Rajakumar SV, Robson SC, Lee EK, Crikis S, d'Apice AJ, et al. The impact of purinergic signaling on renal ischemia-reperfusion injury. Transplantation 2008;86:1707–12.

[104] Lu M, MacGregor GG, Wang W, Giebisch G. Extracellular ATP inhibits the small-conductance K channel on the apical membrane of the cortical collecting duct from mouse kidney. J Gen Physiol 2000;116:299–310.

[105] Ma W, Korngreen A, Weil S, Cohen EB, Priel A, Kuzin L, et al. Pore properties and pharmacological features of the P2X receptor channel in airway ciliated cells. J Physiol 2006;571:503–17.

[106] Mangravite LM, Xiao G, Giacomini KM. Localization of human equilibrative nucleoside transporters, hENT1 and hENT2, in renal epithelial cells. Am J Physiol Renal Physiol 2003;284:F902–10.

[107] McCoy DE, Taylor AL, Kudlow BA, Karlson K, Slattery MJ, Schwiebert LM, et al. Nucleotides regulate NaCl transport in mIMCD-K2 cells via P2X and P2Y purinergic receptors. Am J Physiol 1999;277:F552–9.

[108] McCulloch F, Chambrey R, Eladari D, Peti-Peterdi J. Localization of connexin 30 in the luminal membrane of cells in the distal nephron. Am J Physiol Renal Physiol 2005;289: F1304–12.

[109] Mo J, Fisher MJ. Uridine nucleotide-induced stimulation of gluconeogenesis in isolated rat proximal tubules. Naunyn Schmiedebergs Arch Pharmacol 2002;366:151–7.

[110] Modlinger PS, Welch WJ. Adenosine A_1 receptor antagonists and the kidney. Curr Opin Nephrol Hypertens 2003;12:497–502.

[111] Niemir ZI, Stein H, Dworacki G, Mundel P, Koehl N, Koch B, et al. Podocytes are the major source of IL-1 alpha and IL-1 beta in human glomerulonephritides. Kidney Int 1997;52: 393–403.

[112] Nishiyama A, Majid DS, Walker III M, Miyatake A, Navar LG. Renal interstitial ATP responses to changes in arterial pressure during alterations in tubuloglomerular feedback activity. Hypertension 2001;37:753–9.

[113] Nishiyama A, Navar LG. ATP mediates tubuloglomerular feedback. Am J Physiol Regul Integr Comp Physiol 2002;283: R273–5 discussion R278-R279.

[114] North RA. Molecular physiology of P2X receptors. Physiol Rev 2002;82:1013–67.

[115] Novak I. ATP as a signaling molecule: the exocrine focus. News Physiol Sci 2003;18:12–7.

[116] Odgaard E, Praetorius HA, Leipziger J. AVP-stimulated nucleotide secretion in perfused mouse medullary thick ascending limb and cortical collecting duct. Am J Physiol Renal Physiol 2009;297:F341–9.

[117] Ortiz PA, Hong NJ, Garvin JL. NO decreases thick ascending limb chloride absorption by reducing $Na^+K^+2Cl^-$ co-transporter activity. Am J Physiol Renal Physiol 2001;281: F819–25.

[118] Ortiz PA, Hong NJ, Garvin JL. Luminal flow induces eNOS activation and translocation in the rat thick ascending limb. Am J Physiol Renal Physiol 2004;287:F274—80.

[119] Osmond DA, Inscho EW. P2X$_1$ receptor blockade inhibits whole kidney autoregulation of renal blood flow *in vivo*. Am J Physiol Renal Physiol 2010;298:F1360—8.

[120] Paulais M, Bandouin-Legros M, Teulon J. Extracellular ATP and UTP trigger calcium entry in mouse cortical thick ascending limb. Am J Physiol 1995;268:F496—502.

[121] Peti-Peterdi J. Calcium wave of tubuloglomerular feedback. Am J Physiol Renal Physiol 2006;291:F473—80.

[122] Pizzirani C, Falzoni S, Govoni M, et al. Dysfunctional inflammasome in Schnitzler's syndrome. Rheumatology (Oxford) 2009;48:1304—8.

[123] Pochynyuk O, Bugaj V, Rieg T, Insel PA, Mironova E, Vallon V, et al. Paracrine regulation of the epithelial Na$^+$ channel in the mammalian collecting duct by purinergic P2Y$_2$ receptor tone. J Biol Chem 2008;283:36599—607.

[124] Pochynyuk O, Rieg T, Bugaj V, Schroth J, Fridman A, Boss GR, et al. Dietary Na$^+$ inhibits the open probability of the epithelial sodium channel in the kidney by enhancing apical P2Y$_2$-receptor tone. FASEB J 2010;24:2056—65.

[125] Ponnusamy M, Ma L, Gong R, Pang M, Chin YE, Zhuang S. P2X$_7$ receptors mediate deleterious renal epithelial-fibroblast cross talk. Am J Physiol Renal Physiol 2011;300: F62—70.

[126] Praetorius HA, Leipziger J. ATP release from non-excitable cells. Purinergic Signal 2009;5:433—46.

[127] Praetorius HA, Leipziger J. Intrarenal purinergic signaling in the control of renal tubular transport. Annu Rev Physiol 2010;72:377—93.

[128] Praetorius HA, Spring KR. A physiological view of the primary cilium. Annu Rev Physiol 2005;67:515—29.

[129] Ren Y, Carretero OA, Garvin JL. Role of mesangial cells and gap junctions in tubuloglomerular feedback. Kidney Int 2002;62:525—31.

[130] Rieg T, Bundey RA, Chen Y, Deschenes G, Junger W, Insel PA, et al. Mice lacking P2Y$_2$ receptors have salt-resistant hypertension and facilitated renal Na$^+$ and water reabsorption. FASEB J 2007;21:3717—26.

[131] Riteau N, Gasse P, Fauconnier L, et al. Extracellular ATP is a danger signal activating P2X$_7$ receptor in lung inflammation and fibrosis. Am J Respir Crit Care Med 2010;182: 774—83.

[132] Rost S, Daniel C, Schulze-Lohoff E, Baumert HG, Lambrecht G, Hugo C. P2 receptor antagonist PPADS inhibits mesangial cell proliferation in experimental mesangial proliferative glomerulonephritis. Kidney Int 2002;62:1659—71.

[133] Rouse D, Leite M, Suki WN. ATP inhibits the hydrosmotic effect of AVP in rabbit CCT: evidence for a nucleotide P2u receptor. Am J Physiol 1994;267:F289—95.

[134] Rubera I, Tauc M, Bidet M, Verheecke-Mauze C, De Renzis G, Poujeol C, et al. Extracellular ATP increases [Ca^{2+}]$_i$ in distal tubule cells. II. Activation of a Ca^{2+}-dependent Cl$^-$ conductance. Am J Physiol Renal Physiol 2000;279:F102—11.

[135] Scemes E, Spray DC, Meda P. Connexins, pannexins, innexins: novel roles of 'hemi-channels'. Pflügers Arch 2009;457:1207—26.

[136] Schnermann J. Maintained tubuloglomerular feedback responses during acute inhibition of P2 purinergic receptors in mice. Am J Physiol Renal Physiol 2011 in press.

[137] Schulze-Lohoff E, Hugo C, Rost S, Arnold S, Gruber A, Brune B, et al. Extracellular ATP causes apoptosis and necrosis of cultured mesangial cells via P2Z/P2X$_7$ receptors. Am J Physiol 1998;275:F962—71.

[138] Schulze-Lohoff E, Ogilvie A, Sterzel RB. Extracellular nucleotides as signaling molecules for renal mesangial cells. J Auton Pharmacol 1996;16:381—4.

[139] Schwartz DD, Malik KU. Renal periarterial nerve stimulation-induced vasoconstriction at low frequencies is primarily due to release of a purinergic transmitter in the rat. J Pharmacol Exp Ther 1989;250:764—71.

[140] Schweda F, Wagner C, Kramer BK, Schnermann J, Kurtz A. Preserved macula densa-dependent renin secretion in A$_1$ adenosine receptor knockout mice. Am J Physiol Renal Physiol 2003;284:F770—7.

[141] Schwiebert EM, Kishore BK. Extracellular nucleotide signaling along the renal epithelium. Am J Physiol Renal Physiol 2001;280:F945—63.

[142] Schwiebert EM, Wallace DP, Braunstein GM, King SR, Peti-Peterdi J, Hanaoka K, et al. Autocrine extracellular purinergic signaling in epithelial cells derived from polycystic kidneys. Am J Physiol Renal Physiol 2002;282:F763—75.

[143] Shaver SR, Rideout JL, Pendergast W, Douglass JG, Brown EG, Boyer JL, et al. Structure-activity relationships of dinucleotides: potent and selective agonists of P2Y receptors. Purinergic Signal 2005;1:183—91.

[144] Shirley DG, Bailey MA, Unwin RJ. *In vivo* stimulation of apical P2 receptors in collecting ducts: evidence for inhibition of sodium reabsorption. Am J Physiol Renal Physiol 2005;288: F1243—8.

[145] Shirley DG, Vekaria RM, Sévigny J. Ectonucleotidases in the kidney. Purinergic Signal 2009;5:501—11.

[146] Silva G, Beierwaltes WH, Garvin JL. Extracellular ATP stimulates NO production in rat thick ascending limb. Hypertension 2006;47:563—7.

[147] Silva GB, Garvin JL. TRPV4 mediates hypotonicity-induced ATP release by the thick ascending limb. Am J Physiol Renal Physiol 2008;295:F1090—5.

[148] Silva GB, Garvin JL. Akt1 mediates purinergic-dependent NOS3 activation in thick ascending limbs. Am J Physiol Renal Physiol 2009;297:F646—52.

[149] Silva GB, Garvin JL. Extracellular ATP inhibits transport in medullary thick ascending limbs: role of P2X receptors. Am J Physiol Renal Physiol 2009;297:F1168—73.

[150] Sipos A, Vargas SL, Toma I, Hanner F, Willecke K, Peti-Peterdi J. Connexin 30 deficiency impairs renal tubular ATP release and pressure natriuresis. J Am Soc Nephrol 2009;20:1724—32.

[151] Solini A, Iacobini C, Ricci C, Chiozzi P, Amadio L, Pricci F, et al. Purinergic modulation of mesangial extracellular matrix production: role in diabetic and other glomerular diseases. Kidney Int 2005;67:875—85.

[152] Souza-Menezes J, Morales MM. CFTR structure and function: is there a role in the kidney? Biophys Rev 2009;1:3—12.

[153] Steinhausen M, Blum M, Fleming JT, Holz FG, Parekh N, Wiegman DL. Visualization of renal autoregulation in the split hydronephrotic kidney of rats. Kidney Int 1989;35: 1151—60.

[154] Stiepanow-Trzeciak A, Jankowski M, Angielski S, Szczepanska-Konkel M. P^1,P^4-diadenosine tetraphosphate (Ap$_4$A) inhibits proximal tubular reabsorption of sodium in rats. Nephron Physiol 2007;106:p13—18.

[155] Stockand JD, Mironova E, Bugaj V, Rieg T, Insel PA, Vallon V, et al. Purinergic inhibition of ENaC produces aldosterone escape. J Am Soc Nephrol 2010;21:1903—11.

[156] Stoessel A, Himmerkus N, Bleich M, Bachmann S, Theilig F. Connexin 37 is localized in renal epithelia and responds to changes in dietary salt intake. Am J Physiol Renal Physiol 2010;298:F216—23.

I. EPITHELIAL AND NONEPITHELIAL TRANSPORT AND REGULATION

[157] Sun D, Samuelson LC, Yang T, Huang Y, Paliege A, Saunders T, et al. Mediation of tubuloglomerular feedback by adenosine: evidence from mice lacking adenosine 1 receptors. Proc Natl Acad Sci USA 2001;98:9983–8.

[158] Sun R, Miller RL, Hemmert AC, Zhang P, Shi H, Nelson RD, et al. Chronic dDAVP infusion in rats decreases the expression of P_2Y_2 receptor in inner medulla and P_2Y_2 receptor-mediated PGE_2 release by IMC. Am J Physiol Renal Physiol 2005;289: F768–76.

[159] Takenaka T, Inoue T, Kanno Y, Okada H, Hill CE, Suzuki H. Connexins 37 and 40 transduce purinergic signals mediating renal autoregulation. Am J Physiol Regul Integr Comp Physiol 2008;294:R1–11.

[160] Tam FWK. Current pharmacotherapy for the treatment of crescentic glomerulonephritis. Expert Opin Investig Drugs 2006;15:1353–69.

[161] Tao Y, Kim J, Faubel S, Wu JC, Falk SA, Schrier RW, et al. Caspase inhibition reduces tubular apoptosis and proliferation and slows disease progression in polycystic kidney disease. Proc Natl Acad Sci USA 2005;102:6954–9.

[162] Tarasova O, Sjöblom-Widfeldt N, Nilsson H. Transmitter characteristics of cutaneous, renal and skeletal muscle small arteries in the rat. Acta Physiol Scand 2003;177:157–66.

[163] Taylor SR, Turner CM, Elliott JI, et al. $P2X_7$ deficiency attenuates renal injury in experimental glomerulonephritis. J Am Soc Nephrol 2009;20:1275–81.

[164] Thomas J, Deetjen P, Ko WH, Jacobi C, Leipziger J. P_2Y_2 receptor-mediated inhibition of amiloride-sensitive short circuit current in M-1 mouse cortical collecting duct cells. J Membr Biol 2001;183:115–24.

[165] Thomsen K, Shirley DG. The validity of lithium clearance as an index of sodium and water delivery from the proximal tubules. Nephron 1997;77:125–38.

[166] Tian W, Salanova M, Xu H, Lindsley JN, Oyama TT, Anderson S, et al. Renal expression of osmotically responsive cation channel TRPV4 is restricted to water-impermeant nephron segments. Am J Physiol Renal Physiol 2004;287:F17–24.

[167] Turner CM, Elliot JI, Tam FWK. P2 receptors in renal pathophysiology. Purinergic Signal 2009;5:513–20.

[168] Turner CM, King BF, Srai KS, Unwin RJ. Antagonism of endogenous putative P2Y receptors reduces the growth of MDCK-derived cysts cultured in vitro. Am J Physiol Renal Physiol 2007;292:F15–25.

[169] Turner CM, Ramesh B, Srai SK, Burnstock G, Unwin RJ. Altered ATP-sensitive P2 receptor subtype expression in the Han:SPRD cy/ + rat, a model of autosomal dominant polycystic kidney disease. Cells Tissues Organs 2004;178:168–79.

[170] Turner CM, Tam FWK, Lai PC, Tarzi RM, Burnstock G, Pusey CD, et al. Increased expression of the pro-apoptotic ATP-sensitive $P2X_7$ receptor in experimental and human glomerulonephritis. Nephrol Dial Transplant 2007;22:386–95.

[171] Turner CM, Vonend O, Chan C, Burnstock G, Unwin RJ. The pattern of distribution of selected ATP-sensitive P2 receptor subtypes in normal rat kidney: an immunohistological study. Cells Tissues Organs 2003;175:105–17.

[172] Vallon V. P2 receptors in the regulation of renal transport mechanisms. Am J Physiol Renal Physiol 2008;294:F10–27.

[173] van Baal J, Hoenderop JGJ, Groenendijk M, van Os CH, Bindels RJ, Willems PH, et al. Am J Physiol 1999;277: F899–906.

[174] Vekaria RM. Vesicular storage and release of ATP in a rat proximal tubule cell line. J Physiol 2004;560P:C17 (Abstract)

[175] Vekaria RM, Shirley DG, Sévigny J, Unwin RJ. Immunolocalization of ectonucleotidases along the rat nephron. Am J Physiol Renal Physiol 2006;290:F550–60.

[176] Vekaria RM, Unwin RJ, Shirley DG. Intraluminal ATP concentrations in rat renal tubules. J Am Soc Nephrol 2006;17:1841–7.

[177] Verhoef PA, Estacion M, Schilling W, Dubyak GR. $P2X_7$ receptor-dependent blebbing and the activation of Rho-effector kinases, caspases, and IL-1 beta release. J Immunol 2003;170:5728–38.

[178] von Kugelgen I. Pharmacological profiles of cloned mammalian P2Y-receptor subtypes. Pharmacol Ther 2006;110:415–32.

[179] Vonend O, Turner CM, Chan CM, Loesch A, Dell'Anna GC, Srai KS, et al. Glomerular expression of the ATP-sensitive P2X receptor in diabetic and hypertensive rat models. Kidney Int 2004;66:157–66.

[180] Walker III M, Harrison-Bernard LM, Cook AK, Navar LG. Dynamic interaction between myogenic and TGF mechanisms in afferent arteriolar blood flow autoregulation. Am J Physiol Renal Physiol 2000;279:F858–65.

[181] Welch BD, Carlson NG, Shi H, Myatt L, Kishore BK. $P2Y_2$ receptor-stimulated release of prostaglandin E_2 by rat inner medullary collecting duct preparations. Am J Physiol Renal Physiol 2003;285:F711–21.

[182] Wilcox CS, Welch WJ, Schreiner GF, Belardinelli L. Natriuretic and diuretic actions of a highly selective adenosine A_1 receptor antagonist. J Am Soc Nephrol 1999;10:714–20.

[183] Wildman SS, Brown SG. The complex nature of P2 receptor-mediated regulation of ENaC: dependence on Na concentration, nucleotide concentration and exposure time, and tubular pH. J Am Soc Nephrol 2010;: F-PO1610 (Abstract)

[184] Wildman SS, Hooper KM, Turner CM, Sham JS, Lakatta EG, King BF, et al. The isolated polycystin-1 cytoplasmic COOH terminus prolongs ATP-stimulated Cl^- conductance through increased Ca^{2+} entry. Am J Physiol Renal Physiol 2003;285: F1168–78.

[185] Wildman SS, Unwin RJ, King BF. Extended pharmacological profiles of rat $P2Y_2$ and rat $P2Y_4$ receptors and their sensitivity to extracellular H^+ and Zn^{2+} ions. Br J Pharmacol 2003;140:1177–86.

[186] Wildman SSP, Boone M, Peppiatt-Wildman CM, Contreras-Sanz A, King BF, Shirley DG, et al. Nucleotides downregulate aquaporin 2 via activation of apical P2 receptors. J Am Soc Nephrol 2009;20:1480–90.

[187] Wildman SSP, Marks J, Turner CM, Yew-Booth L, Peppiatt-Wildman CM, King BF, et al. Sodium-dependent regulation of renal amiloride-sensitive currents by apical P2 receptors. J Am Soc Nephrol 2008;19:731–42.

[188] Wilson HL, Wilson SA, Surprenant A, North RA. Epithelial membrane proteins induce membrane blebbing and interact with the $P2X_7$ receptor C terminus. J Biol Chem 2002;277: 34017–23.

[189] Wilson PD. Polycystic kidney disease. N Engl J Med 2004;350:151–64.

[190] Wilson PD, Hovater JS, Casey CC, Fortenberry JA, Schwiebert EM. ATP release mechanisms in primary cultures of epithelia derived from the cysts of polycystic kidneys. J Am Soc Nephrol 1999;10:218–29.

[191] Woda CB, Bragin A, Kleyman TR, Satlin LM. Flow-dependent K^+ secretion in the cortical collecting duct is mediated by a maxi-K channel. Am J Physiol Renal Physiol 2001;280: F786–93.

[192] Woda CB, Leite Jr M, Rohatgi R, Satlin LM. Effects of luminal flow and nucleotides on $[Ca^{2+}]_i$ in rabbit cortical collecting duct. Am J Physiol Renal Physiol 2002;283:F437–46.

[193] Xu C, Rossetti S, Jiang L, Harris PC, Brown-Glaberman U, Wandinger-Ness A, et al. Human ADPKD primary cyst

epithelial cells with a novel, single codon deletion in the PKD1 gene exhibit defective ciliary polycystin localization and loss of flow-induced Ca^{2+} signaling. Am J Physiol Renal Physiol 2007;292:F930—45.

[194] Xu C, Shmukler BE, Nishimura K, Kaczmarek E, Rossetti S, Harris PC, et al. Attenuated, flow-induced ATP release contributes to absence of flow-sensitive, purinergic Ca_i^{2+} signaling in human ADPKD cyst epithelial cells. Am J Physiol Renal Physiol 2009;296:F1464—76.

[195] Yagil C, Katni G, Yagil Y. The effects of adenosine on transepithelial resistance and sodium uptake in the inner medullary collecting duct. Pflügers Arch 1994;427:225—32.

[196] Yamada H, Seki G, Taniguchi S, Uwatoko S, Suzuki K, Kurokawa K. Mechanism of $[Ca^{2+}]_i$ increase by extracellular ATP in isolated rabbit renal proximal tubules. Am J Physiol 1996;270:C1096—104.

[197] Yamamoto K, Sokabe T, Matsumoto T, et al. Impaired flow-dependent control of vascular tone and remodeling in $P2X_4$-deficient mice. Nat Med 2006;12:133—7.

[198] Yao J, Suwa M, Li B, Kawamura K, Morioka T, Oite T. ATP-dependent mechanism for coordination of intercellular Ca^{2+} signaling and renin secretion in rat juxtaglomerular cells. Circ Res 2003;93:338—45.

[199] Yegutkin GG. Nucleotide- and nucleoside-converting ectoenzymes: important modulators of purinergic signaling cascade. Biochim Biophys Acta 2008;1783:673—94.

[200] Yoshioka K, Saitoh O, Nakata H. Heteromeric association creates a P2Y-like adenosine receptor. Proc Natl Acad Sci USA 2001;98:7617—22.

[201] Yoshioka K, Saitoh O, Nakata H. Agonist-promoted heteromeric oligomerization between adenosine A_1 and $P2Y_1$ receptors in living cells. FEBS Lett 2002;523:147—51.

[202] Zamir M, Phipps S. Morphometric analysis of the distributing vessels of the kidney. Can J Physiol Pharmacol 1987;65:2433—40.

[203] Zhang Y, Kohan DE, Nelson RD, Carlson NG, Kishore BK. Potential involvement of P_2Y_2 receptor in diuresis of postobstructive uropathy in rats. Am J Physiol Renal Physiol 2010;298:F634—42.

[204] Zhang Y, Sanchez D, Gorelik J, Klenerman D, Lab M, Edwards C, et al. Basolateral $P2X_4$-like receptors regulate the extracellular ATP-stimulated epithelial Na^+ channel activity in renal epithelia. Am J Physiol Renal Physiol 2007;292: F1734—40.

[205] Zhang Y, Sands JM, Kohan DE, Nelson RD, Martin CF, Carlson NG, et al. Potential role of purinergic signaling in urinary concentration in inner medulla: insights from P_2Y_2 receptor gene knockout mice. Am J Physiol Renal Physiol 2008;295: F1715—24.

[206] Zhuang S, Lu B, Daubert RA, Chavin KD, Wang L, Schnellmann RG. Suramin promotes recovery from renal ischemia/reperfusion injury in mice. Kidney Int 2009;75:304—11.

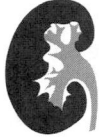

Paracrine Regulation of Renal Function by Dopamine

Pedro A. Jose[1], Robin A. Felder[2] and Gilbert M. Eisner[3]

[1]Division of Nephrology, Department of Medicine, University of Maryland School of Medicine, USA
[2]University of Virginia Health Sciences Center, USA
[3]Georgetown University Medical Center, USA

HISTORICAL PERSPECTIVE

Classical transmitter ligands evolved about 1000 million years ago.[1] The role of dopamine as a neurotransmitter has evolved with time. In primordial and plant cells, dopamine is present, even though catecholamine signaling is not used. In invertebrate neural systems, dopamine is the pre-eminent catecholamine. In vertebrates, the catecholamine pathway terminates in norepinephrine and epinephrine.[2] Endogenous dopamine was mainly recognized as a precursor to norepinephrine and epinephrine[3] until the late 1950s, when Carlsson demonstrated that dopamine itself had a transmitter role.[4] This finding, for which he was awarded the Nobel Prize in Physiology or Medicine 2000, was revolutionary for the understanding of various central functions of the brain, including memory, learning, drug abuse, cognition, and attention; it has also enlightened us regarding the pathogenesis and treatment of various psychiatric and neurological disorders.

Since 1910, dopamine has been known to be a vasoconstrictor, but less potent than norepinephrine and epinephrine. However, in 1942 Holtz et al. reported that dopamine, via its oxidized form, decreases blood pressure in the guinea pig and rabbit.[5] In 1958, Hornykiewicz reported that the vasodepressor effect of dopamine is due to dopamine *per se*.[6] Goldberg et al. confirmed the depressor effect of low doses of dopamine in 1959, and demonstrated a direct negative effect of dopamine on vascular resistance in 1962.[7,8] The same group reported that dopamine increased renal blood flow, glomerular filtration rate, and sodium excretion in dogs and humans. In 1977, Lokhandwala and Buckley subsequently reported that presynaptic dopamine receptors may be responsible for the dopaminergic inhibition of renal neurogenic vasoconstriction.[10] In 1981, Morgunov and Baines demonstrated a positive relationship between renal sodium and dopamine excretion that was independent of renal nerves,[11] indicating that the kidney can synthesize dopamine. Dopamine had been shown to increase cAMP production in the canine renal artery in 1973,[12] and in renal particulate preparations containing tubules, glomeruli, and blood vessels in 1977.[13] In 1980 Nakajima and Kuruma reported that renal particulate preparations had two binding sites to a radio-labeled dopamine receptor antagonist, indicating two types of dopamine receptors.[14] In 1984, Felder et al. reported that renal tubules and glomeruli express D_1-like and D_2-like receptors, respectively.[15] That dopamine can directly inhibit sodium transport in the renal proximal tubule was demonstrated by Bello-Reuss et al. in 1982[16]; Aperia et al. in 1987[17] showed that this occurs, in part, by inhibition of Na^+,K^+-ATPase activity. Subsequently, renal endogenous dopamine was shown to be important in the regulation of renal sodium excretion[18–20] in normotensive rats, but not in spontaneously hypertensive rats (SHRs).[21] In mice, deletion of any of the dopamine receptor gene subtypes produces hypertension, the mechanism of which is specific to the particular dopamine receptor subtype deleted.[22–27]

OVERVIEW

Pharmacological doses of dopamine, such as those administered intravenously to increase blood pressure, achieve concentrations that stimulate other G-protein-coupled receptors (GPCRs) (e.g., α- and β-adrenergic receptors) in addition to dopamine receptors. In this dose range, the vasoconstrictor action of α-adrenergic receptors completely overcomes any vasodilatory effect of dopamine. Normal circulating concentrations of dopamine (picomolar range) are not sufficiently high to activate vascular dopamine receptors, but high nanomolar to low micromolar concentrations can be attained in dopamine-producing tissues.[10,28–32] The Ki of dopamine for its receptors may be as low as 5 nM[33] and as high as 2.5 μM.[34]

Dopamine is important in the regulation of water and electrolyte balance, and blood pressure,[29–31] partly by regulation of the secretion/release of hormones and humoral agents that affect water and electrolyte balance. Dopamine also modulates water and electrolyte intake via the "appetite" centers in the brain,[35] and regulates ion and water transport in the kidney[29–31] and gastrointestinal tract.[32] Physiological concentrations of locally produced dopamine, acting in an autocrine or paracrine manner, inhibit ion transporter/channel/pump activity directly by actions on enzyme or channel kinetics, and indirectly by regulating their protein expression and cellular distribution. The physiological effects of dopamine occur by occupation of its specific receptors, as well as via synergistic interaction with natriuretic agents/receptors such as atrial natriuretic peptide (ANP)/ANPA,[36] eicosanoids,[37,38] endothelin/ETBR,[39] nitric oxide,[40] prolactin,[41] urodilatin,[36] angiotensin III/AT$_2$R,[42] and negative interaction with antinatriuretic agents/receptors such as insulin,[43] renin,[44] angiotensin II/AT$_1$R,[45,46] and aldosterone.[37,47,48] In general, under normal conditions and especially when extracellular fluid volume is moderately expanded, dopamine impedes ion and water transport and facilitates their excretion. During normal or moderately increased NaCl intake, inhibition of D$_1$-like receptors decreases sodium chloride excretion by about 60%.[18–22,29–31,49] Dopamine, however, is not important in natriuresis with marked volume expansion with isotonic saline[20,49] or even moderate volume expansion with albumin[50] or hypotonic saline.[51] With volume deficit renal dopamine production decreases[52–54]; this may allow sodium retaining mechanisms to work more effectively. The decrease in renal dopamine production during volume depletion has been related to a decrease in angiotensin II-mediated renal tubular uptake of dopamine,[55] and an increase in renal MAO activity and dopamine turnover, without altering COMT activity.[52,55] Indeed, during volume deficit, exogenous dopamine may actually decrease sodium excretion, apparently caused by an increase in sodium reabsorption in the distal nephron.[56]

RENAL DOPAMINE PRODUCTION

Plasma dopamine is freely filtered through the glomerulus, but the concentration of free dopamine in the plasma is normally too low (below 1 nmol/L)[57] to account for any significant contribution to urinary dopamine, which is in the high nanomolar to low micromolar range.[23,32,58–63] Renal deconjugation of circulating conjugated dopamine probably does not occur and, therefore, cannot account for the free dopamine in the urine.[64] Intact afferent vagal pathways have been shown to mediate the increase in renal dopamine production during acute volume expansion with isotonic saline.[65] However, renal dopaminergic nerves[66] contribute less than 30% of renal dopamine production.[11,30,31] Moreover, renal denervation does not prevent the dopaminergic-mediated increase in sodium excretion associated with volume expansion with isotonic saline.[67]

The synthesis of dopamine differs between renal tubular and neural cells. Neural cells express tyrosine hydroxylase (TH), which converts tyrosine to L-3,4-dihydroxyphenylalanine (L-DOPA) that is subsequently decarboxylated to dopamine by aromatic acid decarboxylase (AADC). Non-neural tissues, such as the renal tubules (Figure 19.1), do not express TH,[68] and therefore cannot synthesize L-DOPA. Rather, L-DOPA is taken up intracellularly by renal tubule cells and converted to dopamine by AADC, which is expressed in many non-neuronal tissues, such as immune cells,[69] kidney,[68,70,71] liver,[72] adrenal,[72] spleen,[72] pancreas,[73] and thyroid,[74] among others. There is sexual dimorphism in the levels of AADC in mice; AADC protein expression and activity are higher in the kidneys of females than in males, while the converse is true in the intestines.[71]

Renal dopamine production is regulated by several factors, including the availability and renal tubular uptake of L-DOPA, activity of AADC, transport of dopamine from inside the proximal tubule cell into the tubular lumen and perivascular space, and metabolism of dopamine. However, sodium intake and intracellular sodium are probably the major stimuli in the renal tubular synthesis/release of dopamine in normal adults.[23,54,63,75]

Sources of L-DOPA

As previously mentioned, the major source of renal dopamine production is the renal tubular

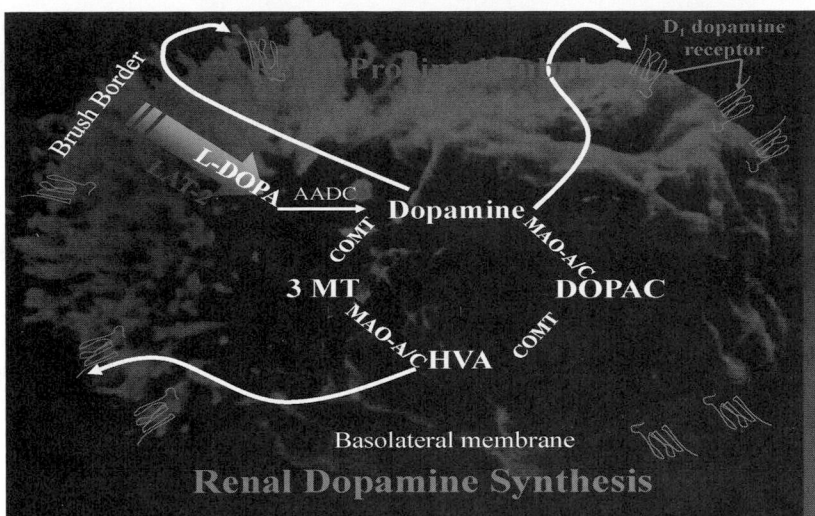

FIGURE 19.1 **Dopamine synthesis inside a renal proximal tubule cell (scanning electron microscopy).** The principal source of renal dopamine is from circulating L-dihydroxyphenylalanine (L-DOPA) which is found in the general circulation and is freely filtered by the glomerulus. Dopamine is produced in renal tubules following uptake by a sodium-independent and pH-sensitive L-type amino acid transporter (LAT2) and rBAT (related to Bo amino acid transporter and other transporters, including ASCT2, B0AT1, among others.), which is rate-limiting of the renal tubular dopamine synthesis. Renal proximal tubules convert L-DOPA to dopamine, via L-aromatic amino acid decarboxylase (AADC). In renal tubules, dopamine is produced from tyrosine and not converted to norepinephrine, because unlike neural tissue renal tubules do not express tyrosine hydroxylase or dopamine β-hydroxylase (COMT: catechol-O-methyl transferase; MAO: monoamine oxidase; 3MT: 3 methoxytyramine; HVA: homovanillic acid; DOPAC: 3,4 dihydroxymandelic acid). See color plate section at the back of the book.

decarboxylation of L-DOPA taken up by renal tubule cells from the glomerular filtrate and circulation.[76] Plasma L-DOPA, which is about 2 μM, reflects catecholamine turnover from sympathetically innervated tissues, such as skeletal muscle, heart, adrenal gland, and gut.[75,76] There are non-neuronal sources of plasma L-DOPA, because patients with pure autonomic failure have normal plasma levels of L-DOPA.[77] Indeed, L-DOPA is produced by non-neuronal cells that express TH in mesenteric organs (gastrointestinal tract, spleen, and pancreas[78]). Plasma L-DOPA sulfate levels increase after meals, possibly related to the amount of DOPA in the food.[79–83] Inhibition of the decarboxylation of L-DOPA during a protein meal doubles its plasma levels, indicating that normally a protein meal-induced increase in plasma L-DOPA is immediately decarboxylated.[82] Tyrosinase activation,[83] decreased degradation of L-DOPA, and renal demethylation of 3-O-methyl DOPA may be additional sources of urinary dopamine.[84–86]

segment,[68,90] although AADC is also present in more distal nephron segments.[90–92] L-DOPA is taken up by the renal tubules via organic cation transporters[87,93] located at both apical and basolateral membranes.[94] These include sodium-dependent amino acid transporters, L-amino acid transporter-2 (LAT-2), and related to b0,+ amino acid transporter (rBAT), sodium-dependent L-amino acid transporters, ASCT2 and B0AT1, and as yet unidentified transporters.[95,96] rBAT is predominantly expressed at the apical membrane, while LAT-2 is expressed at both apical and basolateral membranes. In normotensive rats, LAT-2 and rBAT may account for more than 50% of the L-DOPA uptake in renal proximal tubules, while ASCT2 and B0AT1 may account for the rest.[95,96] In contrast in SHRs, 50% of L-DOPA uptake occurs via LAT-1, 25% via LAT-2, and 25% via ASCT2 and B0AT1.[95,97] Aging is associated with a decreased tubular uptake of L-DOPA resulting in a decrease in urinary dopamine production, the mechanism of which has not been determined.[98]

Renal Tubular Uptake of L-DOPA

As already indicated, the rate-limiting step in the synthesis of dopamine by the kidney is the uptake of L-DOPA by renal tubule cells from the circulation and glomerular filtrate.[76,87] The conversion of L-DOPA to dopamine[66,88,89] occurs mainly in the proximal tubule, since AADC activity is highest in this nephron

Aromatic Amino Acid Decarboxylase (AADC) Activity

Renal AADC activity is dependent on L-DOPA concentration and not on its Km. However, the increase in urinary dopamine in sodium-replete states may be caused, in part, by increased AADC activity.[89,99,100]

Patients with AADC deficiency have normal or increased levels of urinary dopamine that may be explained, in part, via tyramine hydroxylation by renal CYP2D6.[101] Hypertonic saline can increase the expression of AADC, that is mediated, in part, by TonEBP.

Dopamine Transporters

The accumulation of monoamines from the cytoplasm to storage organelles and their secretion are dependent on vesicular monoamine transporters 1 and 2 (VMAT-1, VMAT-2). VMAT-2 is expressed in neurons and certain neuroendocrine cells, while VMAT-1 is expressed in endocrine and rat renal proximal tubule cells.[60] VMAT-1 may participate in the dopaminergic regulation of renal ion transport, because renal tubular VMAT-1 mRNA and protein expression are increased by a high sodium diet.[60] However, dopamine synthesized in renal tubules is not stored, but is transported both to the basolateral membrane and into the tubular lumen, where it acts on its receptors locally.[31] Dopamine is secreted into the basolateral space via organic acid cationic transporters,[102] while dopamine probably diffuses into the lumen where it is concentrated, reaching high nanomolar to low micromolar concentrations (see above), as a result of water reabsorption and can stimulate its receptors in more distal nephron segments.[28–31]

Dopamine Metabolism

Dopamine that is synthesized in the renal tubule cells is probably not converted to norepinephrine or epinephrine. Dopamine β-hydroxylase (DBH) mRNA is not expressed in bovine or rat kidneys.[103] However, DBH is expressed in adrenergic nerves supplying the kidney, and inhibition of DBH increases renal dopamine concentration three-fold.[104] In tissues expressing phenylethanolamine-N-methyl transferase (PNMT) (e.g., adrenal medulla, heart, and some areas of the brain) norepinephrine is converted to epinephrine (Figure 19.1). PNMT is also not expressed in human renal proximal tubules, but is expressed in glomeruli, renal distal tubules, and endothelial cells.[105] Non-specific NMT, which is expressed in non-neuronal tissues including the kidney, enables the synthesis of epinephrine even after denervation.[106] More recent studies have also shown that TH and DBH are expressed in mesangial and renal proximal tubule cells in culture, in a pig renal tubular cell line (LLCPK) with proximal tubule and distal tubule characteristics,[107] in a canine distal tubular cell line, MDCK, and mouse inner medullary collecting duct cells.[91] Because TH is not expressed in renal proximal tubules,[68] the presence of TH in LLCPK could be indicative of its distal tubular characteristics.[107] Although dopamine may have access

to non-specific NMT,[106] the increase in urinary dopamine with salt loading is not accompanied by an increase in urinary norepinephrine or epinephrine.[23,25,51,58]

In renal tubules, dopamine is degraded both by deamination via monoamine oxidase (MAO) to 3,4-dihydroxyphenylacetic acid (DOPAC), and by methylation via COMT to 3-methoxytyramine. Newly formed dopamine is metabolized predominantly by MAO-A rather than MAO-B, especially in the proximal tubule.[108] In contrast, dopamine is metabolized by COMT in more distal nephron segments.[109,110] A novel flavin adenine dinucleotide-dependent amine oxidase named renalase or MAO-C has been identified in the kidney, but its role in the intrarenal metabolism of renal dopamine is unknown.[111] Acute inhibition of COMT activity may be more important than MAO in the short-term,[112] while the converse is true for chronic inhibition.[110] The inhibition of dopamine degrading enzymes can increase its concentration. However, the increase in urinary dopamine with high salt intake is probably not related to any decrease in dopamine degradation.[62,99]

Dietary Influence Including Salt Intake

Feeding increases urinary dopamine that have been related to the amount of sodium in the diet. Most studies have shown that a low sodium intake is associated with low urinary dopamine, while the converse occurs with a high sodium diet.[31,50,53,58,62–65,92,113–117] This could be due to an increased spillover of L-DOPA into the arterial blood,[53,61] as ingestion of food/protein which contains sodium causes an increase in circulating L-DOPA.[80–84] However, plasma L-DOPA levels may not be increased by a high sodium diet.[32] Even if circulating L-DOPA is not increased by salt intake, the increase in urinary dopamine with salt loading is associated with an increase in urinary excretion of L-DOPA.[61] Therefore, the increase in urinary excretion of dopamine appears to be secondary to an increase in the uptake of L-DOPA by renal proximal tubules, presumably from the glomerular filtrate and circulation.[61,88,93–99,118–120] There may also be a mechanism by which L-DOPA is delivered to the kidney independent of circulating L-DOPA (e.g., via the adrenal gland).[121,122]

Chloride may be more important than sodium in the regulation of renal dopamine production, because an increase in the intake of chloride without sodium increases urinary dopamine, while sodium bicarbonate does not.[115] An increase in the intake of phosphate[112] or calcium[115,123] also increases renal dopamine production. Blockade of N-type, but not L-type, calcium channels can decrease urinary dopamine excretion.[124,125]

An important factor in the increase in urinary dopamine caused by sodium loading is the preferential egress of dopamine into the renal tubular lumen, rather than into the interstitium.[62,126] In LLC-PK1 cells dopamine egresses at the apical surface by a non--saturable process, while its egress at the basolateral surface is saturable, with the latter 5–7-fold higher than the former.[94] The egress of dopamine in LLC-PK1 is probably not related to VMAT-1, because the egress of dopamine is not inhibited by dopamine transporter inhibitors.[94] However, chronic sodium loading increases the expression of the VMAT-1 in the renal proximal tubule, which may contribute to the modification of the polarity of dopamine secretion during sodium loading.[60] Inhibition of sodium hydrogen exchanger (NHE) activity decreases efflux of dopamine into the peritubular space, which presumably favors luminal outflow. Thus, dopamine, by inhibiting proximal tubular luminal NHE activity,[127–133] may facilitate its own egress into the tubular lumen. The preferential luminal efflux and tubular fluid reabsorption result in high nanomolar to low micromolar concentrations[31,134] of dopamine in the tubular lumen, concentrations that approach the EC_{50} of dopamine and D_1-like receptor agonists to stimulate adenylyl cyclase and phospholipase C activity.[127,131,135–143] This mechanism, and the fact that dopamine can also be synthesized in more distal nephron segments, albeit to a lower extent relative to the proximal tubule, enables dopamine to stimulate its receptors in more distal nephron segments.

There may not always be a relationship among dietary sodium, urinary dopamine, and sodium excretion.[143–153] Mühlbauer and colleagues have claimed that food intake rather than sodium is responsible for the increase in urinary dopamine.[145–147] However, all the acute saline loading studies were performed in rats in which food, but not water, was withheld for 24 hours.[20,21,49,117] Differences in the amount[49,117] and duration[116,148–150] of the sodium load in the food, as well as differences in the strains of rats studied (see below) are possible explanations. In humans, increasing sodium intake from 20 to >200 mmol/day increases renal dopamine production that peaks by the second day, followed by a gradual decline to 50% of the peak value by the 5th day.[116] In rats, sodium chloride loading maximally increases dopamine excretion on the first few days, with the excretion decreasing close to control levels at 1 week, only to gradually increase again from 2 to 4 weeks.[148,149] Renal dopamine concentrations are not higher in non-salt loaded rats than in rats loaded with salt for 6 weeks.[150] There may also be an interaction between sodium and other substances in food, e.g., protein. Ingestion of food with very low sodium content (<0.02% sodium) is not associated with an increase in sodium excretion (unpublished data).

The renal production of dopamine is strain-dependent in rodents. Urine dopamine is lower in Sprague-Dawley than in Dahl salt-sensitive or -resistant rats[61] or in WKY and SHRs.[151] A strain of WKY rat increases urinary dopamine after 24 hours of salt loading at 4 weeks, but not at 12 weeks of age.[61] Uninephrectomy increases urinary dopamine in Wistar-Han from Harlan, but not from Charles-Rivers or WKY rats from Harlan.[97,152] The increase in urinary dopamine with chronic sodium chloride loading is less in the salt-sensitive C57BL/6 than the salt-resistant SJL mice from Jackson Laboratory.[153]

The renal production of dopamine is also age-dependent. Renal dopamine synthesis increases with development.[92] However, in contrast to the stimulatory effect of sodium intake on dopamine excretion in normal adult humans,[53,58,113,115,116] in pre-term infants sodium supplementation prevents, while sodium restriction increases, urinary dopamine[154]; the significance of this in terms of sodium balance remains to be determined. The stimulatory effect of increased dietary sodium on renal dopamine production and ability to excrete salt load are diminished with aging.[98,100,155–157] Urinary dopamine excretion is also decreased in patients with chronic renal failure, but due to loss of nephron number rather than an inability to synthesize dopamine.[158]

Gender may influence the urinary dopaminergic response to a sodium load. For example, sodium loading has been reported to increase urinary dopamine excretion in Chinese females, but not Chinese males.[159] Ethnic differences in the relationship between urine dopamine and sodium have been reported.[160–162] The blunted increase in urinary dopamine in response to acute volume expansion in blacks may be caused by reduced decarboxylation of L-DOPA.[125]

Patients with type 1 or type 2 diabetes have decreased basal urinary dopamine,[163,164] as well as a deficient response to high sodium chloride diet[165] or infusion.[166] Decreased dopamine production in human adults[164,167] and children[168] with type 2 diabetes[169] may affect the ability to excrete a sodium load. Rats with type 1 diabetes also have decreased renal dopamine production.[170]

Patients with salt-sensitive, low renin or non-modulating hypertension, and some with normal renin hypertension[161,171–174] have a blunted increase in urinary dopamine in response to salt loading, despite higher rates of L-DOPA excretion.[173] Protein intake[171] or high dietary sodium intake may not increase urinary dopamine in essential hypertensive patients or even normotensive subjects with a family history of hypertension.[159,165,172,175–177] However, salt-sensitive[173] and normal renin essential hypertensives[178] have normal basal urinary dopamine. Mild exercise has been reported to increase renal dopamine production in Stage 1 hypertensive subjects.[179] Borderline and young hypertensives[180,181] have higher basal urinary dopamine than control subjects or stable hypertensive patients,[181,182] suggesting that the renal dopaminergic system may act as an early defense against hypertension that fails during its progression.[183]

There are also abnormalities in renal dopamine production in animal models of genetic hypertension. Renal dopamine production may be decreased in adult spontaneously hypertensive and Dahl salt-sensitive rats relative to their normotensive controls, the WKY and Dahl salt-resistant rat, respectively.[63,184] However, urinary free dopamine and renal tissue dopamine are actually increased in young SHRs in comparison with WKY rats,[184,185] but the difference disappears at age 16 weeks. In the young Dahl salt-sensitive rat, urinary dopamine is normal and increases with salt intake, as in Dahl salt-resistant rats,[63,186] although kidney levels of dopamine are lower in Dahl salt-sensitive than in salt-resistant rats on a high salt diet.[186] In adult Dahl salt-sensitive rats, the urinary excretion of dopamine is not increased or may even be decreased in response to acute volume expansion or salt loading.[185,187] Mice deficient of D_2 dopamine receptors have salt-sensitive hypertension and decreased renal dopamine production.[23,24]

Dopamine Receptor Subtypes

Dopamine receptors probably evolved from a common ancient ancestor over 750 million years ago, before the divergence of vertebrates and invertebrates.[188] Dopamine receptors belong to the α group of the rhodopsin-like family of GPCRs,[29–31,189–193] characterized by seven transmembrane domains. Based on their ability to stimulate or inhibit adenylyl cyclase, dopamine receptors have been classified into two families (Table 19.1): D_1-like receptors stimulate adenylyl cyclases, while D_2-like receptors inhibit adenylyl cyclases.[29–31,189–193] There are two D_1-like receptors in eutherian mammals, D_{1A} and D_{1B}, also known as D_1 and D_5 in humans; archosaurs have four D_1-like receptors, D_{1A}, D_{1B}, D_{1C}, and D_{1D}; all other jawed vertebrates have three D1-like receptors, D_{1A}, D_{1B}, and D_{1C}.[194] The D_2-like receptors include D_2 (D_2R), D_3 (D_3R), and D_4 (D_4R).[29–31,189–193] The rank order affinity of dopamine to its receptors is: $D_3R \geq D_4R > D_5R \geq D_2R > D_1R$.[195]

Based on site-directed mutagenesis and protein modeling of some GPCRs, including D_2R, the binding of their respective agonist has been suggested to occur at the hydrophobic transmembrane domains, i.e., aspartate residues in transmembrane domains II and III, two serine residues in transmembrane V, and a phenylalanine residue in transmembrane VI.[190] Dopamine receptors have not been crystallized, but studies of the crystallized β2-adrenergic receptor suggest that agonist binding occurs at the extracellular ends of helices III, IV, V, and VII, with the cytosolic ends mediating G-protein activation.[196] Nuclear magnetic resonance spectroscopy has revealed three distinct conformations of the β2AR: unliganded receptor or neutral antagonist, inverse agonist, and agonist.[197] The binding pocket of the A_{2A} adenosine receptor is slightly different, with the binding pocket closer to helices VI and VII, suggesting GPCR specificity.[198]

Dopamine Receptor Signaling

Receptor activation, at least for rhodopsin, occurs by a disruption of the Arg135/Glu134 ionic bond in transmembrane VI resulting in the formation of a new Arg135/Tyr223 interaction in transmembrane V261. This causes the GPCR to function as a guanine nucleotide exchange factor promoting the exchange of GDP with GTP on the Gα-subunit, resulting in the dissociation and release of the Gα-subunit from the Gβγ-subunit.[189,199] The dissociated G-protein-subunits then initiate the activation or inhibition of downstream effectors. Hydrolysis of GTP by the intrinsic GTPase activity of Gα promotes the reassociation of the G-protein-subunits. RGS (regulators of G-protein signaling) acting as a GTPase-activating protein (GAP), stimulate the hydrolysis of GTP and, therefore, the reassociation of the G-protein-subunits. RGS act as a GAP for GαS, Gαi and Gαq. While a primary function of RGS is to suppress G-protein signaling via GAP activity, RGS have non GAP actions such as direct antagonism of Gα and binding of Gβ/γ. Specific RGS have been reported to regulate dopamine receptors. For example, RGS7 with Gβ5 can regulate dopamine receptor signaling[200] and RGS9-2, but not RGS4, inhibits D_2R internalization,[201] while RGS19 inhibits D_2R signaling.[202] RGS4 may be involved in D_1R signaling.[203] In contrast, RGS2 may be regulated by both D_1R and D_2R.[204]

In some instances, agonist specific ligand binding does not cause dissociation of the protein subunits, but rather a conformational change.[205] Heterotrimeric G-proteins can also interact with proteins other than GPCRs to regulate physiological processes.[206] These include activators of G-protein signaling (AGS) which promote guanine nucleotide exchange independent of GPCRs and activate or inhibit adenylyl cyclase or phospholipase C. Dopamine receptors have been reported to decrease AGS1 expression.[207] In addition, GPCR signaling can be independent of G-protein-subunits.[208] For example, the inotropic effect of angiotensin II with occupation of $AT_{1a}R$ in cardiomyocytes occurs via a Gαq/PKC-independent, but GRK6/β-arrestin 2-dependent, mechanism.[209]

Both D_1-like receptors, D_1R and D_5R couple to $Gα_S$[29–31,189–193] and $Gα_q$.[135,136,138–142] There are also differences in G-protein linkage between D_1R and D_5R. For example, the D_1R, but not D_5R, also couples to Go[210] and $G\alpha_{Olf}$,[211] which is expressed in renal tubules and macula densa.[212] In contrast, D_5R, but not D_1R, couples to Gz and $G\alpha_{12/13}$.[211,213] $G\alpha_{12/13}$ proteins may have functions different from those ascribed to GPCR activation, including cell movement, actin cytoskeleton, and protein phosphatase 2A activity.[214] Because the recycling of D_1R is partly under the control of protein phosphatase 2A or a protein phosphatase 2-like enzyme,[215,216] this may be a mechanism for D_5R and D_1R cross-talk.

The linkage of G-protein-subunits to the specific D_1-like receptor may be tissue-specific. This apparently discordant linkage of D_1-like receptors to G-protein-subunits can be explained by recent observations that a specific ligand acting on the same receptor recruits specific signaling proteins that elicit a specific phenotype.[217] For example, most D_1-like receptor agonists stimulate both adenylyl cyclase and phospholipase C. However, there are exceptions; SKF83822 stimulates adenylyl cyclase but not phospholipase C,[218] whereas SKF83959 stimulates phospholipase C but actually inhibits adenylyl cyclase.[219]

Adenylyl Cyclase and Protein Kinase A (PKA)

As indicated above, D_1-like receptors are linked to stimulation of adenylyl cyclase which leads to the formation of cAMP. There are at least 10 isoforms of adenylyl cyclase (adenylyl cyclases I-IX and adenylyl cyclase short). In the neostriatum, the D_1R is linked to adenylyl cyclase V.[191] However, adenylyl cyclase V is not expressed in the rat renal proximal tubules[220] (but may be expressed in humans, unpublished observations). In kidney tubule cells, D_1R is linked to adenylyl cyclase VI, while D_5R is linked to adenylyl cyclase IV.[221] cAMP binds to the regulatory subunits of PKA resulting in the activation (disinhibition) of its catalytic subunits. There are two PKA isoforms, but D_1-like receptors, specifically D_1R, may utilize PKA II rather than PKA I.[222,223] There are several PKA substrates, among which are dopamine and cAMP-regulated 32 kDa phosphoprotein (DARPP-32) which inhibits protein phosphatase 1.[224] In contrast to the stimulatory effect of the D_1R/PKA pathway on DARPP-32, the D_1R/phospholipase C pathway inhibits DARPP-32.[225] The roles of PKA, DARPP-32, and protein-phosphatases in renal sodium transport are discussed below.

Phospholipase C

Phospholipase C catalyzes the formation of diacylglycerol and inositol phosphates. D_1-like receptors are linked to phospholipase C, via $G\alpha q$, independent of adenylyl cyclase, a phenomenon that was initially described in renal cortical tubules.[135,136,138–142] There are several isoforms of phospholipase C; the D_1R directly stimulates phospholipase $C\beta1$ in renal cortical[140] but not in medullary membranes, and indirectly stimulates phospholipase $C\gamma$ via PKA and PKC, in fibroblasts.[139]

In neuroblastoma cells, the D_1R is not linked to G_q[210] and in neurons, D_1R-mediated stimulation of phospholipase C may require the presence of D_2R[226] while D_5R, by itself, can increase phospholipase C-mediated calcium mobilization that is inhibited by D_2R.[227] However, in a pituitary adenoma rat cell line (GH4C1) transfected with the D_5R, the D_5R activation actually decreases inositol phosphate production.[228] The report that D_1-like receptor-stimulated phospholipase C persists in $D_1^{-/-}$ mice[229] has been taken to indicate that there is a D_1-like receptor other than D_1R that can stimulate phospholipase C. This is indeed the case, as the D_5R is also linked to phospholipase C activation in neural tissue (hippocampus, cortex, and striatum).[230]

Phospholipase D

Phospholipase D (PLD) hydrolyzes phospholipids, such as phosphatidylcholine, to form phosphatidic acid and the free polar head group of the phospholipid substrate. Phosphatidic acid can be cleaved by phosphatidic acid phosphohydrolase to produce diacylglycerol; both are important second messengers in the "late" response of cells to certain stimuli.[231] The two mammalian isoforms of PLD (PLD1 and PLD2) have ~50% identity, and are distributed widely in mammalian tissues and cells. They are believed to play an important role in the regulation of cell function and cell fate by a variety of extracellular signals.[231] D_5R inhibits PLD2 activity in renal proximal tubule cells,[232] while both D_1R and D_5R can inhibit phospholipase D activity in vascular smooth muscle cells.[233] These actions lead to inhibition of the production of reactive oxygen species (ROS).[232–234] The D_3R heterologously expressed in HEK293 cells has been reported to activate PLD, via Rho and independent of Gi/Go.[235] The relationship between PLD and endogenously expressed D_3R remains to be determined.

Protein Kinase C

Protein kinase C (PKC) isoforms are classified into three groups: (1) conventional PKCs (cPKC-α, -βI, -βII, and -γ); (2) novel PKCs (nPKC-δ, -ϵ, -θ, and -η/G); and (3) atypical PKCs (aPKC-λ(ι) and -ξ) and PKCμ, also called PKD which consists of PKD1, PKD2, and

PKD3.[236] In renal tubule cells, D_1-like receptors can stimulate PKCθ[237] and PKCξ,[237,238] and inhibit PKCδ.[237] The D_1R increases the phosphorylation of PKCθ[S676] in human embryonic kidney (HEK293) cells.[239] D_1-like receptors can also translocate specific PKC isoforms. Thus, D_1-like receptors translocate conventional (α, β) and novel (ε) PKCs from renal tubule cytosol into membranes,[240,241] and the novel PKC-δ from membranes to cytosol.[240] Some studies have shown that the stimulation of PKC by dopamine may be secondary to PKA activation.[139,242]

While PKA and PKC mediate the actions of D_1R, both can also regulate D_1R signaling. PKC activation can produce differential D_1R and D_5R signaling. PKC can increase the membrane expression of D_1R in vascular smooth muscle cells.[243] In HEK293 cells, novel PKC isoforms stimulate D_1R signaling, but inhibit D_5R signaling.[244] However, in HEK293T cells, PKCα, β1, γ, δ, and ε constitutively phosphorylate and dampen D_1R signaling.[245] Ethanol enhances D_1R signaling by inhibiting PKCγ and PKCδ.[246] PKA and PKC have been reported to phosphorylate D_1R, modulating the rate of agonist-induced D_1R desensitization and intracellular trafficking.[243–248] RanBP9 and RanBP10 interact with both PKCδ/γ to increase the phosphorylation and desensitization of D_1R in neural and renal proximal tubule cells.[248] RanBP9 and RanBP10 may function as scaffolding proteins to regulate the spatial and temporal organization of D_1R and PKC. In renal proximal tubule cells, NHERF-1 is necessary for the D_1R-mediated stimulation of cAMP accumulation and PKC activity.[249]

D_2-Like Receptors

The D_2-like receptors couple to G-proteins $Gα_i$ and G_o, and inhibit adenylyl cyclases.[29–31,189–193]

There are two isoforms of D_2R; postsynaptic D_2R effects are mediated by the long isoform, $D_{2L}R$, while the presynaptic D_2R effects are mediated by the short isoform, $D_{2S}R$.[192,250] The $D_{2S}R$ is localized at the plasma membrane, while the $D_{2L}R$ is localized in the perinuclear region in several cell lines heterologously expressing $D_{2S}R$ and $D_{2L}R$.[251] However, in renal proximal tubule cells that express the $D_{2L}R$ rather than the $D_{2S}R$, the $D_{2L}R$ is expressed mainly at the plasma membrane.[252] The particular G-protein-subunit that interacts specifically with either D_2R isoform is not clear.[253] The D_2R can couple to the same extent to $Gα_i$ ($Gα_i2$ and $Gα_i3$) and Gz,[253] but $Gα_o$ may be the major G-protein that is activated by $D_{2S}R$ and $D_{2L}R$[254]; neither $D_{2S}R$ nor $D_{2L}R$ subtype is linked to Gq11 or $Gα_{12/13}$. A splice variant of $Gα_i2$, $sGα_{i2}$, is important in the intracellular localization of D_2R, and its

dissociation from D_2R following D_2R agonist stimulation increases cell surface D_2R expression.[254]

The D_4R, like the D_2R, couples to $Gα_i$ ($Gα_{i2}$ and $Gα_{i3}$), $Gα_o$, Gz, and $Gα_t2$.[191,255] Different numbers of 16 amino acid repeats in the third cytoplasmic loop cause several human D_4R isoforms (e.g., D4-2, D4-4, and D4-7).[256] The role of these D_4R isoforms in cell function remains to be determined. However, the D_4R long (at least one 7 to 10 repeat) has been reported to be associated with higher diastolic and systolic blood pressure.[257]

The D_3R linkage to $Gα_i$ is not robust, in contrast to that observed for D_2R and D_4R.[258] In rat renal proximal tubule cells the D_3R stimulation of phospholipase C is via $Gα_{i3}$.[259] The signaling of D_3R, like the D_2R and D_4R, may be mediated by $Gα_o$.[191] The utilization of G-proteins in D_2R and D_3R-mediated stimulation of extracellular signal-regulated kinase differs, D_2R utilizes $Gα_i$ while D_3R utilizes $Gα/o$ and the βγ-subunit of G_i.[260] The D_3R also couples to Gz and, in the presence of pertussis toxin, the D_3R can also couple to $Gα_s$.[253] The D_3R can also couple to Gq11.[259] The linkage of the D_3R to other effectors, such as inhibition of K^+ and Ca^{2+}, may be more sensitive than its weak linkage to G-proteins.[258] The D_3R is also insensitive to GTP, relative to the other dopamine receptor subtypes.[191] There could be seven distinct alternatively spliced D_3R variants.[261] The full-length D_3R and a shorter receptor isoform, the D_3S, bind to dopamine. The five other alternatively spliced D_3R variants do not bind dopamine, but one of them, D_3Rnf, regulates receptor dimerization.

Adenylyl Cyclase

Although D_2-like receptors inhibit adenylyl cyclase activity, in many cell lines heterologously expressing the D_3R, its linkage to $Gα_i$ is not robust.[258] However, the D_3R robustly inhibits adenylyl cyclase isoform V,[258] but because this adenylyl cyclase isoform is not expressed in the rat renal proximal tubule,[220] it is expressed in human renal proximal tubule cells (unpublished data). D_3R action in this rat nephron segment is not due to $Gα_i$ signaling. Because D_3R can couple to $Gα_s$ in the presence of pertussis toxin,[253] the D_3R could increase adenylyl cyclase activity in this nephron segment in the rat. This has not been directly tested, but D_1R and D_3R dimerization increases the ability of dopamine to stimulate adenylyl cyclase activity.[262] In contrast, the co-expression of D_2R with D_3R increases the ability of D_2-like agonists to inhibit adenylyl cyclase activity.[263] This becomes a conundrum in cells expressing these dopamine receptor subtypes, but at least in renal proximal tubules there is no evidence of D_1R and D_2R or D_2R and D_3R heterodimerization (unpublished data). However, in the kidney and vascular smooth muscle D_1R and D_3R do interact, and this interaction probably predominates over the other possible D_1-like and D_2-like interactions.[264–266] While D_2R, by itself, stimulates Na^+K^+-ATPase activity,[267] simultaneous stimulation of D_1-like and other D_2-like receptors inhibits Na^+K^+-ATPase activity.[268] Furthermore, $D_{2L}R$ and $D_{4.4}R$ can potentiate PKC-stimulated adenylyl cyclase II activity through the release of β/γ-subunits,[269] and $D_{2L}R$ can sensitize adenylyl cyclase VI.[270] Although these adenylyl cyclase isoforms are expressed in renal proximal tubule cells, this interaction probably does not occur in renal proximal tubule cells because quinpirole, a D_2-like receptor agonist with preference for the D_3R and D_4R over the D_2R, does not stimulate adenylyl cyclase activity (unpublished studies). As stated above, there are species differences because adenylyl cyclase V is expressed in the human (unpublished data) but not in the rat renal proximal tubule.[220]

Phospholipase C

In neural cells, D_2R, via $G\beta/\gamma$, stimulates phospholipase C[191] and specifically phospholipase $C\beta4$ in the intermediate lobe of the pituitary gland[271]. D_1R and D_2R can interact to stimulate phospholipase C in neural cells,[226] but as stated above there is no evidence for D_2R and D_3R interaction in renal proximal tubule cells. D_2R and D_5R can also heterodimerize to stimulate phospholipase C in neural tissue and HEK-293 cells.[227] The $D_{2S}R$ can also stimulate phospholipase D,[272] but the latter enzyme is inhibited by D_5R.[232] These effects need not be counter-regulatory, because as previously mentioned the $D_{2S}R$ is presynaptic, while the D_5R inhibition of phospholipase D is postsynaptic in renal proximal tubule cells (in particular). In addition, presynaptic inhibition of adrenergic neurotransmitters by $D_{2S}R$ facilitates the inhibitory effects of dopamine on ion transport.

Dopamine Regulation of Ion Channels

D_1-like receptors inhibit voltage-gated K^+ channels and G-protein-regulated inward rectifying channels, but stimulate L-type Ca^{2+} channels.[191] D_1-like receptors inhibit G-protein-dependent inward rectifier K-like channels in medial prefrontal cortex via PKC.[273] In contrast, D_2-like receptors stimulate voltage-gated K^+ channels and G-protein-regulated inward rectifying channels, but inhibit L-type Ca^{2+} channels. Both D_1-like and D_2-like receptors inhibit N-, P-, and Q-type Ca^{2+} channels and transient sodium channels, but stimulate persistent P sodium channels.[191] We have reported that the D_3R-mediated vasorelaxation of rat mesenteric arteries is due to stimulation of small- and/or large-Ca^{2+}-activated K^+ channels.[264] In human coronary vascular smooth muscle cells, D_5R stimulates Ca^{2+}-activated big K^+ channel,[274] via cAMP-mediated stimulation of PKG.

Dopamine Regulation of Mitogen-Activated Protein (MAP) Kinase and other Kinases

D_1-like receptors may activate MAP kinases, including p38MAP kinase, and c-jun amino-terminal kinase.[191] In the brain, D_1-like receptors can also activate ERK,[275] but ERK1/2 is actually inhibited by D_5R but not by D_1R in human renal proximal tubule cells.[276] D_2-like receptors can also activate MAP kinase via $G\beta/\gamma$.[277] D_2-like receptor-mediated stimulation of $Na^+ K^+$-ATPase in the kidney is linked to the p44/42 MAP kinase pathway.[278] Aberrant D_1R activation of ERK1/2/MAP kinase has been reported in D_1R supersensitivity.[279] However, in the kidney, MAP kinase reduces D_1R affinity and G-protein coupling.[280]

Dopamine inhibits DNA synthesis of cultured human mesangial cells.[281] In rat vascular smooth muscle cells, D_1R or D_3R does not affect vascular smooth muscle cell proliferation, but inhibits the proliferative effect of insulin and norepinephrine.[282,283] D_2R, via inhibition of MAP kinase, inhibits angiotensin II-induced hypertrophy of cultured neonatal rat ventricular myocytes.[284] However, dopamine increases the phosphorylation of and activates p44/42 MAP kinases in rabbit renal proximal tubule cells in primary culture.[285] In human renal proximal tubule cells and Chinese hamster ovary cells, the D_3R promotes mitogenesis or cell proliferation through the activation of MAP kinases.[191,286,287] The variable effects of dopamine on MAP kinase in smooth muscle and epithelial cells may be related to tissue- or cell-specificity.

DARPP-32

As stated above, DARPP-32 was identified initially as a major target for dopamine-activated adenylyl cyclase in striatum.[224] Since the mid-1980s, DARPP-32 has been acknowledged as a crucial mediator of the biochemical, electrophysiological, transcriptional, and behavioral effects of dopamine.[288] The state of DARPP-32 phosphorylation has been shown to provide a mechanism for integrating information arriving at dopaminoceptive neurons, in multiple brain regions, via a variety of neurotransmitters, neuromodulators, neuropeptides, and steroid hormones. Activation of PKA or PKG stimulates DARPP-32 phosphorylation at Thr,[34] and thereby converts DARPP-32 into a potent inhibitor of protein phosphatase-1 (PP1). Protein phosphatase-2B (PP2B) is the most effective protein phosphatase in dephosphorylating DARPP-32 at Thr.[34] Thus, DARPP-32 acts as an amplifier of PKA and PKG-mediated signaling when it is phosphorylated on Thr,[34] which converts it into an inhibitor of PP1. The role of DARPP-32 in signaling has turned out to be very complex. Under basal conditions, DARPP-32 is phosphorylated at Thr[75] and inhibits PKA. Thus, DARPP-32 has the unique property of acting either as an inhibitor of PP1 or an inhibitor of PKA. However, under hyperdopaminergic conditions, the phosphorylated state of Thr[75] is reduced, allowing increased phosphorylation at Thr.[34] This positive feedback loop acts as a switch to potentiate dopaminergic signaling. Cdk5, a cyclin-dependent kinase family member, also phosphorylates DARPP-32 at Thr.[75] Furthermore, protein phosphatase 2A dephosphorylates DARPP-32 both at Thr[34] and Thr,[75] and the state of phosphorylation of DARPP-32 at Thr[34] depends on the phosphorylation state of two serine residues, Ser[102] and Ser.[137] DARPP-32 has been demonstrated with biochemical, immunohistochemical, and *in situ* hybridization techniques to have an anatomical distribution similar to that of dopaminoceptive cells possessing D_1Rs in the central nervous system.[289–291] DARPP-32 is also expressed in several peripheral tissues, including brown fat cells, parathyroid, retina, and renal tissue.[289,291–293] The ability of D_1R to stimulate protein phosphatase 2A[215,294] may serve as a negative feedback in the D_1R and DARPP-32 relationship, and prevent the inhibitory effect of DARPP-32 on PKA.

Regulation of Dopamine Receptor Function

Effect of Sodium on Dopamine Receptor Expression

While acute sodium loading generally increases renal dopamine production,[31,50,53,58,62–65,92,99,113,114,119] it may decrease brain[295] and renal D_1-like and D_2-like receptor density.[296,297] However, the decrease in renal D_1-like receptor expression occurs after 7–28 days of increased sodium intake during peak renal dopamine production.[148,149] In C57BL/6 mice, increasing NaCl diet to 6% for 5–7 days decreases renal D_1R expression, but increases renal D_3R expression without affecting the renal expression of D_2R, D_4R or D_5R (unpublished observations).

Dopamine Receptor Recycling

As with other GPCRs, dopamine receptor signal transduction is precisely regulated.[189–193,195,298,299] In the basal state, in human renal tubules, human D_1Rs exist as homo-oligomers in lipid raft microdomains.[300] Occupation of D_1Rs increases the amount of D_1R monomers associated with a transient increase in D_1R function, as a result of the recruitment of D_1R from an intracellular pool of D_1R to the lipid rafts of plasma membranes.[215,300–304] Following the transduction of the GPCR signals, there is a transient loss of receptor responsiveness (desensitization). This mechanism dampens short-term agonist effects following repeated agonist exposure. At least three families of regulatory molecules contribute to GPCR desensitization: second messenger-dependent protein kinase; G-protein-coupled receptor kinases (GRKs); and arrestins.[141,189–191,195,280,286,298,299,305–308] Homologous desensitization, in response to agonist stimulation, occurs via action of a member(s) of the GRK family. Heterologous desensitization, mediated by second messenger-dependent kinases, occurs when a decrease in receptor responsiveness is induced by a ligand other than its own specific ligand. The phosphorylation of GPCRs, including the D_1R, leads to the binding of a member(s) of the arrestin family, uncoupling of the receptor from its G-protein complex, and a decrease in its functional response. Desensitization of GPCRs involves phosphorylation, sequestration/internalization, and degradation of receptors. The D_1R (but not D_5R), expressed endogenously in renal proximal tubule cells,[288,299–307] is regulated to a lesser extent by GRK2 and to a greater extent by GRK4 in human kidneys,[299] but the converse may be true in rat kidneys.[305] Moreover, GRK4 may constitutively phosphorylate D_1R.[307] GRK3 regulates rat D_1R overexpressed in HEK293 cells.[308] It is not clear whether or not GRK5 regulates the rat D_1R.[308] GRK6 is not important in the regulation of D_1R in the kidney (unpublished), but it is important in the desensitization of the D_1R in intestinal crypt cells,[309] emphasizing the importance of cell type in D_1R regulation. The desensitization of D_5R, in contrast, does not involve GRKs, but rather sorting nexin 1.[310] Similarly, GRK is not involved in the first 20 minutes of D_1R desensitization in human renal proximal tubule cells,[299] but could be related to sorting nexins (unpublished data). It has also been suggested that GRK2 may negatively regulate D_2R signaling by a phosphorylation-independent mechanism.[311]

Heterologously expressed D_1Rs, after ligand stimulation, rapidly (but not completely) internalize (5–12 minutes) in cell lines (HEK-293 and Neuro2A neuroblastoma cells).[307] In HEK-293 cells heterologously expressing rat D_1R, 15 minutes of agonist stimulation does not completely desensitize D_1R.[307] Presumably, the internalized D_1R continues to function until it is completely desensitized.[312] Phosphorylation, desensitization, and internalization cannot be directly equated.[216,298,299] GPCR desensitization cannot be completely explained by phosphorylation; ubiquitination may also play a role.[46,313] AT_1R,[46] D_1R, and D_5R (unpublished data) are ubiquitinated within the first 15 minutes following ligand stimulation; AT_1R and D_5R,[46] but not D_1R, are targeted for degradation following ligand occupation. Thus, desensitization may also occur at the plasma membrane.[216] Cell membrane invagination and endocytosis are important in D_1R trafficking; prevention of endocytosis with hypertonic sucrose abrogates ligand-induced D_1R desensitization in human renal proximal tubule cells.[314] The phosphorylated GPCR/β-arrestin complex undergoes endocytosis/internalization via clathrin-coated pits into a series of endosomal units, where it is dephosphorylated and recycled back to the plasma membrane or degraded. Dopamine receptors belong to Class A receptors that are rapidly recycled to the plasma membrane. In contrast, AT_1R receptors belong to Class B receptors that are slowly recycled to the plasma membrane, and some are actually degraded.[315] Protein phosphatases are involved in the resensitization of GPCRs in endosomes[316] and at the plasma membrane.[216] Protein phosphatases, including protein phosphatase 2A (PP2A),[215,294,317,318] a GPCR phosphatase,[216] and PP2B (calcineurin)[319] have been reported to resensitize D_1R, but PP2A is probably the major protein phosphatase involved in D_1R function and/or resensitization in renal tubule cells.[215,294,317]

The D_2R, like some GPCRs, is not desensitized by phosphorylation but rather by association with β-arrestin, but phosphorylation is required for its recycling.[256,311,320] The GRK regulating D_2R in renal tubule cells is not known, but D_2R in other cells is regulated by GRK2, GRK3, GRK5, and GRK6,[256,287,311,320] and constitutively desensitized by GRK2. GRK2 and GRK3 preferentially sequester $D_{2S}R$ over $D_{2L}R$, while β-arrestin 2 has the converse effect.[256] GRK2 or GRK3, but not GRK5 or GRK6, is involved in the desensitization of the calcium signal mediated by the interaction of D_1R/D_2R heterologously expressed in HEK293TSA cells.[321] The desensitization of D_3R is weakly regulated by GRK2 and GRK3,[322] but robustly by GRK4 (GRK4γ > GRK4α); GRK4 and D_3R colocalize and interact in human renal proximal tubule cells.[286] D_4R, like some GPCRs, e.g., AT_2R and β$_1$R, may not undergo internalization and is resistant to desensitization.[256,323] The GRK regulating D_4R is not clear, but does not seem to involve either GRK2 or GRK3. The GRK regulating D_5R is also not clear, but does not seem to involve GRK4.

Membrane Microdomains

Cholesterol rich domains in membranes are called lipid rafts and the rest are called non-lipid rafts.[324,325] Lipid rafts serve as signaling platforms for several signaling molecules such as G-protein-subunits, enzymes, and adaptor proteins. Lipid rafts can affect the function of GPCRs by inducing a conformational change and/or alteration of the physical properties of the membrane in which the GPCR is embedded. We have reported that angiotensin II does not affect the differential expression of AT_1R in lipid and non-lipid rafts in renal proximal tubule cells from normotensive rats, but increases the amount of glycosylated AT_1R in lipid rafts in renal proximal tubule cells from SHRs; this may lead to an increased ability of angiotensin II to stimulate the Cl^-/HCO_3^- exchanger.[326] D_1-like receptors also regulate NADPH oxidase activity and subunit expression in lipid microdomains of renal proximal tubule cells.[327] The D_2-like receptor antagonist, haloperidol, has been reported to disrupt lipid rafts.[328] Interestingly, high doses of simvastatin, a cholesterol depleting reagent, increase dopamine receptor expression in the rat prefrontal cortex.[329] In human renal tubule cells, heterologously or endogenously expressed D_1R exists as homo-oligomers; agonist stimulation increases the amount of D_1R monomers[300,330,331] consistent with other GPCRs.[332–334] D_1R oligomers exist in caveolae-like microdomains; decreasing caveolin expression or depleting cholesterol impairs D_1R-mediated generation of cAMP and oligomer formation.[300] Renal inhibition of caveolin-1 expression, an important component of lipid rafts, via caveolin-1 siRNA in the kidney impairs D_1-like receptor-mediated natriuresis in salt-loaded rats and produces hypertension.[335] Thus, the function of GPCRs, including dopamine receptors, can be regulated by cholesterol membrane microdomains.

Regulation of GPCR Membrane Expression

Plasma membrane expression of GPCRs requires proper folding that is aided by chaperones.[336] Homodimerization has been suggested to help in GPCR folding. Indeed, folding efficiency has been suggested to regulate the expression of D_4R.[337] A proper amount of calnexin, an endoplasmic reticulum chaperone, is important in the proper trafficking of both D_1R and D_2R to the plasma membrane.[338]

D_1R

Dopamine receptor interacting protein 78 (DRiP78) is an endoplasmic reticulum protein that regulates the transport of D_1R and other GPCRs, including AT_1R, and the assembly of G-protein β- and γ-subunits.[339] Increased expression of DRiP78 impairs the transport of D_1R from the endoplasmic reticulum to the plasma membrane.[340] In contrast, DRiP78 increases the plasma membrane expression of AT_1R,[341] another example of how certain proteins have contrasting effects on AT_1R, and dopamine receptor trafficking and expression.[45,46,342,343] Neurofilament-M specifically decreases the cell surface membrane expression of D_1R (not with D_2-like receptors and weakly with D_5R).[344] Calcyon is another D_1R interacting protein that may be important in D_1R-calcium-mediated signaling in neural tissue.[345] Whether these proteins regulate D_1R endogenously expressed in renal tissue remains to be determined. However, RanBP9/10 which colocalizes with D_1R in renal and neural tissues, phosphorylates and impairs D_1R function.[248]

D_2R

Cbl-interacting protein of 85 kDa (CIN85) may be important in the trafficking of D_2R, at least in striatal tissue.[346] Absence of striatal CIN85 is associated with decreased endocytosis of D_2R and implicated in the hyperactivity of CIN85-deficient mice. A Ca^{2+}-binding protein, S100B, increases the ability of D_2R to inhibit adenylyl cyclase and stimulate ERK activity.[347] Two D_2R interacting proteins decrease the expression and/or function of D_2R, including neuronal calcium sensor 1[348] and protein kinase Cξ-interacting protein.[349] In neural cells, a spliced variant of the $G\alpha i2$ may also be important in the plasma membrane expression of the D_2R[350] and protein 4.1N for both D_2R and D_3R.[351]

D_3R

The D_3R has been reported to interact with proteins that affect plasma membrane localization. Filamin-A interacts with D_2R and D_3R, linking them to the cytoskeleton and increasing their plasma membrane localization.[322,352] In contrast, paralemmin specifically interacts with the D_3R decreasing its localization to the plasma membrane.[353] The role of these interacting proteins on D_3R function in renal proximal tubules or blood vessels remains to be determined.

D_4R

KLHL12, which can act as a ubiquitin ligase, interacts with the D_4R, but its ubiquitination does not result in its degradation.[354] Indeed, the D_4R is resistant to agonist-induced internalization and degradation.[323]

D_5R

The D_5R, but not the D_1R, requires N-glycosylation for membrane localization in transfected HEK-293 cells. However, it does not contribute to the radioligand-binding properties of D_5R.[355]

Renal Distribution of Dopamine Receptors

The expression of the dopamine receptors in the kidney (Table 19.1) of several mammals has been reported.

Tubular Distribution

The dopamine receptor subtypes are differentially expressed along the mammalian nephron.[213,252,356–365]

However, their expression in the medulla is species-dependent. In the rat, the D_2R and D_4R are expressed in the inner medulla[357,365] (Table 19.1). The mouse kidney has no dopamine receptors in the inner medulla[360] (unpublished observations). High concentration of dopamine (100 μM) stimulates prostaglandin E2 production in the inner medulla and thin limb of Henle.[358] The dopamine receptor subtype expressed in the thin limb of Henle is not known, although dopamine (100 μM) stimulates prostaglandin E2 production in rat thin ascending limb cells[366].

Immunohistochemical studies in human and rodent kidneys have shown expression of D_1R in the apical and basolateral membranes, as well as in the cytoplasm of proximal tubules (mouse:S3 > S1 = S2), distal convoluted tubules, medullary thick ascending limb (mTAL) of Henle, macula densa, and cortical collecting duct.[356,361,364,365] The presence of D_1R in the rat outer or inner medulla has not been shown consistently using immunohistochemistry[356,361,362,365] or *in situ* mRNA amplification,[367] and dopamine does not stimulate cAMP production via dopamine receptors,[368,369] in this nephron segment. Moreover, there is no D_1-like receptor radioligand-binding in the rat inner or outer medulla.[370,371] The human[372] and mouse kidney[360] (unpublished observations), do not express dopamine receptors in the inner medulla.

$D_{2L}R$ mRNA is expressed in the rat cortex, and outer and inner medulla.[252] Immunoreactive D_2R is present in rat[357] and human (unpublished observations) proximal tubule (mouse:S2 > S1/S3), distal convoluted tubule, and cortical and outer medullary collecting duct. The D_2R is expressed in the intercalated cells of the medullary collecting duct in the rat,[357] but not in the mouse (unpublished data). D_2R protein is also expressed in the OK cell, an opossum proximal tubule cell line that also exhibits distal tubular cell characteristics.[373]

D_3R mRNA is expressed in the rat cortex, and outer medulla and inner medulla.[252] Immunoreactive D_3R is expressed in rat apical and subapical areas, but not in the basolateral membrane of proximal tubules (S1 >> S2/S3) in three reports[357,373,375]; one study also showed immunoreactive D_3R in the distal convoluted tubule,[375] and two studies showed D_3R protein in the cortical collecting duct.[357,375] One[357] of three reports[374,375] found D_3R immunostaining in the inner medulla. Immunoreactive D_3R is present in mouse proximal tubule, thick ascending limb of Henle, and distal convoluted tubule, but not in the cortical collecting or outer and inner medullary collecting ducts (Table 19.1).

D_4R is present in the rat proximal tubule (S1 > S2 > S3), distal convoluted tubule, and especially in the cortical[357,376] and outer and inner medullary collecting ducts, where it is more abundant at the luminal than at the basolateral areas.[365] In the mouse, D_4R is present in the proximal convoluted tubule (but not proximal straight tubule), thick ascending limb of Henle, and cortical and outer medullary collecting duct (unpublished observations). D_4R mRNA is expressed in the human kidney, but its expression along the nephron has not been reported.[377]

D_5R is expressed in the rat and mouse proximal tubule (S1 > S2/S3), thick ascending limb, and distal convoluted tubule and cortical and outer medullary collecting duct.[213,360,364] The expression of D_5R protein has not been reported in human kidney, but is expressed in human renal proximal tubule cells in culture,[46,276] and D_5R may be expressed preferentially over the D_1R in the thick ascending limb of Henle and the cortical collecting duct, while the D_1R is preferentially expressed in the proximal tubule[378] (unpublished data).

VASCULAR RECEPTORS

D_1-Like Receptors

The D_5R may have chemo- and mechano sensory roles in primary cilia of mouse vascular endothelial cells.[379] D_1Rs, and to a greater extent D_5Rs, are expressed in the tunica media of rat mesenteric, pial, and renal arteries.[361,380,381] They are mainly located postjunctionally, which has been confirmed by insensitivity to chemical sympathectomy.[381] In the rat kidney, D_1R mRNA is also found in smooth muscle cells of large and small arteries, and afferent and efferent arterioles.[367] In humans D_1R protein is also present in vascular smooth muscle cells in the large intrarenal arteries, but not in renal veins.[372]

D_2-Like Receptors

The D_2-like receptors are expressed in the adventitia and adventitia—media border of arteries. D_2R and D_4R, but not D_3R, are expressed in rat mesenteric and pial arteries. Rat renal arterial branches express D_2R and D_3R.[380] Although renal arteries and arterioles in Wistar rats were not found to express D_4R,[380] a subsequent study in Sprague-Dawley rats showed expression of D_4R in large segmental, arcuate, interlobar, interlobular, and afferent and efferent arterioles.[376] Bilateral superior cervical ganglionectomy and renal denervation confirmed the prejunctional localization of the D_2-like receptors, and the location of D_2-like receptors in the renal artery suggest their prejunctional localization.[376,380] However, we have reported that D_3R stimulation relaxes mesenteric arterial rings, independent of the endothelium.[264] The failure of the endothelium to influence the vasorelaxant effect of D_3R stimulation is in agreement with the absence of D_2-like receptor expression in the intima.[380] One study could not find D_3R expression in renal vessels,[374] although another study found D_3R immunostaining in medial and adventitial layers of renal arteries[378] in agreement with the report of D_3R mRNA in renal microvessels.[252]

GLOMERULAR RECEPTORS

Radioligand binding and autoradiographic studies using D_1-like receptor ligands that recognize both D_1R and D_5R have failed to detect specific binding in rat and human glomeruli.[370,371,381,382] D_1R mRNA studied by in situ mRNA amplification is not detected in rat renal glomeruli[367] (Table 19.1). Immunoreactive D_1R[361,372] or D_5R[360,364] has not been demonstrated in rat or human glomeruli. In rat glomeruli isolated by sieving, two[383,384] of three[15] studies showed that dopamine, via an uncharacterized dopamine receptor, increased cAMP production. Dopamine increases cGMP, but not cAMP production in isolated dog glomeruli, also obtained by sieving.[385] However, because afferent and efferent arterioles express D_1R and D_5R (Table 19.1) it is possible that glomerular preparations that contain arterial vessels may confound the results. Nevertheless, rat glomerular mesangial cells[386] and mouse glomerular podocytes,[387] in culture, express D_1-like receptors, assessed by an increase in cAMP production in response to dopamine or D_1-like receptor agonist. Rat glomerular epithelial cells in culture do not increase cAMP production in response to dopamine.[386]

D_2-like receptors, $D_{2L}R$, D_3R, and D_4R, are present in rat glomeruli[252,357,375,381,388] (Table 19.1). Specifically, immunoreactive D_2R and D_3R have been reported in rat mesangial cells in one study[357] and in podocytes in another study.[375] However, there are three reports of the absence of D_4R receptors in rat glomeruli.[357,365,376] D_2-like receptor stimulation decreases cAMP production in rat glomeruli.[15] Dopamine attenuates the contractile response to angiotensin II in rat isolated glomeruli, but the receptor mediating this effect is not known.[389]

Receptors in Juxtaglomerular Apparatus

Rat[361,390] and mouse (unpublished observations) but not human[372] juxtaglomerular cells, in situ, and rat juxtaglomerular cells in culture[390] express D_1R (Table 19.1). Rat[361] and mouse (unpublished studies) but not human[372] macula densa cells express D_1R. Rat[364] but not mouse[360] juxtaglomerular or macula cells express

D_5R. Rat[361] but not mouse (unpublished studies) macula densa cells express D_1R. D_5R expression in human juxtaglomerular or macula cells has not been reported.

Rat, mouse, and human (unpublished studies) juxtaglomerular cells, *in situ*, do not express D_2R. Mouse juxtaglomerular cells, *in situ*, express D_3R (Table 19.1). In contrast, rat juxtaglomerular cells, *in situ*, also do not express D_3R[374,375] or D_4R,[365,376] but express D_3R and D_4R in culture.[391] Rat macula densa cells were found to express D_3R in one[375] of two reports.[374] Mouse macula densa cells express D_3R and D_4R (unpublished studies). D_2R is not expressed in human or mouse macula densa cells, but is expressed in rat macula densa (unpublished studies; Table 19.1); D_3R and D_4R expression has not been studied in human macula densa.

DOPAMINE AND RENAL HEMODYNAMICS

D_1-Like Receptors

Dopamine, administered in low doses intravenously or directly into the renal artery, increases renal blood flow and decreases renal vascular resistance.[9,392,393] The renal vasodilatory effect of dopamine is mimicked by D_1-like receptor agonists and blocked by the D_1-like receptor antagonists.[394–397] The contribution of D_1R and D_5R in this action remains to be determined. Dopamine and D_1-like receptor agonists dilate afferent and efferent arterioles to the same extent.[398,399] However, afferent arterioles are preferentially dilated in the hydronephrotic kidney.[400] Dopamine induces a greater vasodilatory effect in the renal artery than in the coronary artery,[401] mesenteric,[402] in agreement with the receptor density data.[403]

cAMP/PKA[12,404–406] is the primary signaling pathway of the renal vasodilatory effect of dopamine via D_1-like receptors. However, a dopamine-mediated stimulation of PKC is associated with increased expression of D_1-like receptors that enhances cAMP production in renal vascular smooth muscle cells.[243] However, as stated earlier in HEK293 cells, novel PKC isoforms stimulate D_1R[244] but inhibit D_5R signaling, while conventional PKCs and two of the novel PKCs (δ and ε) impair D_1R signaling.[245] In coronary arteries, the vasorelaxant effect of D_1-like receptors has also been attributed to PKA/PKG-dependent activation of K^+-ATP, calcium-, and voltage-activated K^+ channels.[274] Prostacyclins may also contribute to dopamine- and D_1-like receptor-mediated renal vasodilation.[407]

The effect of D_1-like receptors in the rat aorta and tail artery is complex. Dopamine has been reported to decrease both sodium influx and efflux by inhibition of NHE and Na^+/K^+-ATPase activity, respectively, in part via PKA, in rat aorta smooth muscle cells.[408] A predominant inhibitory effect on NHE activity would result in a decrease in intracellular sodium and a decrease in vessel tone, while a predominant inhibitory effect on Na^+/K^+-ATPase activity would result in an increase in intracellular sodium and an increase in vascular tone. The latter situation may explain the apparent vasoconstrictor action of a D_1-like receptor agonist in the rat tail artery.[409] In the rat tail artery, dopamine and SKF 38393, a D_1-like receptor agonist, inhibited Na^+/K^+-ATPase and increased vascular tone, an effect that was associated with activation of phospholipase C.[409] Since the effects were abolished by pertussis toxin, the D_1-like receptor in the rat tail artery is must be different from the D_1-like receptor in renal proximal tubules, because in this tissue phospholipase C is pertussis-toxin resistant and linked to G_q.[142,410] When phospholipase $C\beta1$ is not expressed, D_1-like agonists can be indirectly linked to phospholipase $C\gamma1$ via PKA.[139] The effect of dopamine in resistance vessels may not be the same as that in conduit vessels (e.g., aorta) and in the rat tail artery, which may subserve a thermoregulatory function.

D_2-Like Receptors

Both the $D_{2S}R$ and $D_{2L}R$ may act as autoreceptors in certain nerves (GABA transmission), while the $D_{2S}R$ but not the $D_{2L}R$ regulates glutamate release.[411] However, the $D_{2S}R$ but not the $D_{2L}R$ is involved in presynaptic dopamine transmission, while postsynaptic dopamine transmission is via the $D_{2L}R$.[412] The D_3R[413] but not the D_4R[414] can also function as an autoreceptor (presumably located in prejunctional areas) and inhibit catecholamine release. Prejunctional D_2-like receptors in the kidney inhibit norepinephrine release.[415,416] This effect may explain the ability of bromocriptine (D_2R and D_3R agonist), but also with D_1-like antagonistic properties, to increase renal blood flow in the anesthetized rat,[417,418] and the renal vasodilatory effect of endogenous dopamine in humans on a low-sodium diet.[419]

The effect of postjunctional D_2-like receptors on the renal vasculature is inconsistent. When both α- and β-adrenergic receptors are blocked in the dog kidney, the renal vasodilatory effect of dopamine is antagonized by D_1-like but not by D_2-like receptor blockade.[395] However, in a similar preparation, bromocriptine has been reported to decrease renal blood flow.[420] In the conscious, chronically instrumented dog on a moderate sodium intake (40 mmol/day), low (picomolar) concentrations of quinpirole, a D_2-like receptor agonist with selectivity for the D_3R and D_4R over the D_2R, also produces vasoconstriction.[421] This result agrees with the report that D_3R stimulation constricts renal vessels in volume-loaded rats.[422] In humans, D_2-like receptor blockade with L-sulpiride does not affect renal plasma flow but potentiates the renal vasoconstrictor effect of NO inhibition with L-NAME.[423] D_4R stimulation also enhances the contractile response of guinea pig vas deferens.[424]

In contrast to the above observations that D_2-like receptors induce vasoconstriction, in the preconstricted isolated perfused rat kidney bromocriptine (D_2R/D_3R agonist) induces vasodilation via postjunctional D_2-like receptors.[425] In the norepinephrine- or high-potassium-preconstricted rat mesenteric arterial rings, D_3R stimulation induces vasorelaxation.[264,426] The vasodilatory effect of D_3R is caused by activation of potassium channels (small- and/or large-conductance calcium-activated potassium channels).[264,426] Although the D_3R is present in the intima, the vasodilatory effects of the D_1R and D_3R agonists are endothelium independent; D_1R is not expressed in the intima.[264,426] In humans, the renal vasodilatory effect of D_2-like receptors is reduced during sodium loading and increased during sodium restriction.[419] This is in contrast to the lack of effect of sodium loading on the renal vasodilatory effect of D_1-like receptors.[427]

The D_3R can augment the vasodilatory effect of the D_1R by mechanisms independent of signal transduction. In embryonic thoracic aortic smooth muscle cells and coronary artery smooth muscle cells, stimulation of the D_1R increases D_1R and D_3R expression.[264,426] However, the additive vasorelaxant effects of D_1R and D_3R could not be explained by the increased expression of those two receptors, because the vasorelaxant effect occurs within minutes following agonist stimulation. Rather, the D_1R and D_3R may acutely and physically interact with each other; D_1R and D_3R co-immunoprecipitate within minutes after agonist stimulation, consistent with the timeframe of the additive vasodilation effect of D_1R and D_3R.[264]

The published studies show that D_1-like receptors cause renal vasodilation. Stimulation of pre-junctional D_2-like receptors should cause vasorelaxation, while stimulation of post-junctional D_2-like receptors can result in either vasodilation or vasoconstriction. With chronic sodium chloride loading, basal reactivity of renal vessels may be enhanced by an increase in levels of endogenous Na^+/K^+-ATPase inhibitor, e.g., ouabain, and an increase in intracellular sodium and calcium.[428] Ouabain, *per se*, can decrease renal D_1R expression and function.[429] Under these conditions, dopamine can further increase intracellular sodium by stimulating NHE1 activity via D_2-like receptors.[430] The increase in intracellular sodium increases sodium calcium exchanger activity. The increase in intracellular calcium increases vascular reactivity and, thus, dopamine, via D_2-like receptors which can then elicit

vasoconstriction. When renal nerve activity is increased, as seen in renal nerve stimulation, low-sodium diet, hypovolemia or during anesthesia, the vasodilator effect of dopamine occurs via prejunctional D_2-like receptors,[415,416] presumably of the D_3R subtype.[264,426] In addition, when renal vascular resistance is increased, the D_2-like receptor effect at postjunctional sites would be that of vasodilation, since D_2-like receptors inhibit Ca^{2+} channels and stimulate K^+ channels, both of which can lead to vasorelaxation. Under these conditions, a synergistic effect between D_1- and D_2-like receptors may become evident.[264,394,398,426] The effect of dopamine on vascular tone may differ between conduit (e.g., aorta) and resistance (e.g., mesenteric and renal arterioles) vessels. The increase in vascular tone produced by D_1-like receptor agonists in conduit vessels may serve to increase perfusion in downstream vessels dilated by D_1-like receptors.

Glomerular Filtration

Although low concentrations (nM) of dopamine consistently increase renal blood flow, this is not the case for glomerular filtration rate.[427,431,432] Normally, low concentrations of dopamine dilate afferent and efferent arterioles to the same degree, and therefore transglomerular pressure remains unchanged.[368] However, dopamine can ameliorate the reduced glomerular filtration rate caused by amphotericin B,[433] radiocontrast material, and hypovolemic states.[434] This could be a direct effect on glomerular cells, since dopamine can attenuate the contractile effect of angiotensin II in isolated glomeruli.[389] This effect is probably exerted via D_2-like receptors, because D_1-like receptors are not expressed in glomerular mesangial cells, *in situ*.[15,360,361,364,367,370-372,381,382] It is only after culture that glomeruli express D_1-like receptors and their stimulation increases cAMP production.[383,384,386,387] In isolated dog glomeruli, dopamine increases cGMP formation[385] and in isolated rat glomeruli, dopamine decreases adenylyl activity,[15] in keeping with the presence of D_2-like receptors[252,357,376,381,388] (Table 19.1). *In vivo*, D_2-like receptors can decrease or increase glomerular filtration rate, depending upon the state of renal vascular D_2-like receptor activation. When the interaction of D_1- and D_2-like receptors results in a greater vasodilatory effect on afferent than efferent arterioles, glomerular filtration rate can increase.[435] D_2-like receptors are involved in the increase in glomerular filtration rate associated with amino acid infusion, an effect that is mediated by renal nerves.[436] The D_2-like receptor-mediated decrease in renal blood flow is associated with greater constriction of afferent than efferent arterioles, resulting in a greater decrease in glomerular filtration rate than renal blood flow and, therefore, a fall in filtration fraction.[421,437]

Tubuloglomerular Feedback

Tubuloglomerular feedback describes a mechanism by which changes in distal tubular sodium chloride delivery induce changes in afferent glomerular arteriolar resistance mediated by the adenosine A_1 receptor.[438–441] Tubuloglomerular feedback is initiated by transport of sodium via sodium potassium 2 chloride transporters type A (NKCC2A) and type B (NKCC2B) at the macula densa.[441] Because dopamine stimulates NKCC2 activity,[442] it would be expected that dopamine should promote the tubuloglomerular feedback. However, dopamine inhibits tubuloglomerular feedback[443] by occupation of luminal D_1R but not D_2R on macula densa cells that may be more evident during sodium surfeit.[444] How can this be done when D_1R stimulates NKCC2?[442] There are several possible explanations. D_1-like receptors counteract the effect of adenosine A_1 receptors on the tubuloglomerular feedback.[134] The heterodimerization of the D_1R and adenosine A_1 receptor[445] and D_2-like and adenosine A_{2A} receptors[446] inhibit dopamine receptor function (see adenosine and dopamine receptor interaction). Adenosine A_{2A} receptors counteract the effect of adenosine A_1 receptors on tubuloglomerular feedback[447] and dopamine (probably via D_2-like receptors) counters the effects of adenosine A_{2A} receptors.[446] Superoxide anion activates 5′-nucleotidase, thereby increasing adenosine generation in the kidney. Dopamine also induces ecto-5′nucleotidase in glomeruli[448] and because ecto-5′-nucleotidase catalyzes the formation of adenosine, dopamine should enhance tubuloglomerular feedback.[438,440] However, the ability of dopamine receptors to inhibit ROS production[449] may also play a role, because ROS is also involved in tubuloglomerular feedback.[439] These counteracting effects of dopamine on adenosine formation, adenosine receptor action, NKCC2, and ROS may explain the variable effect of dopamine on tubuloglomerular feedback.

RENIN, ANGIOTENSINOGEN, AND ALDOSTERONE SECRETION

Dopamine can increase, decrease or have no effect on renin secretion, *in vivo*.[44] Dopamine can alter renin secretion directly or indirectly by effects on blood pressure and renal tubular ion transport. As indicated above, rat and mouse juxtaglomerular cells express the D_1R[361,367,390] (Table 19.1). The D_1R stimulates secretion of renin in rat primary cultured cells.[390,450] In pithed rats and anesthetized dogs, dopamine and D_1-like

receptor agonists increase renin release.[451,452] However, in non-pithed rats, dopamine or a D_1-like receptor agonist inhibits renin secretion on a low or normal salt diet, by inhibiting cyclooxygenase 2 expression.[44] However, when cyclooxygenase 2 expression[44] is already inhibited, as is the case with salt-loading, D_1-like receptor stimulation increases renin secretion.[44] In humans on low or high sodium (300 mmol/day) intake D_1-like receptor stimulation does not affect renin secretion,[427] in agreement with the absence of D_1R in human juxtaglomerular cells.[372] D_1-like receptor stimulation also does not affect plasma renin activity in subjects with mild essential hypertension on an unmonitored sodium intake,[453] but increases it in hypertensive humans on a high (150 mmol Na)[454] or normal sodium intake.[455] The role of D_5R on renin secretion in the rat remains to be determined; D_5R is expressed in rat[364] but not in mouse[360] juxtaglomerular cells and deletion of *Drd5* does not affect plasma or renal renin levels.[360]

In salt replete humans, D_2-like receptor blockade with metoclopramide does not affect plasma renin activity[456] but another D_2-like receptor antagonist, domperidone, inhibits the fall in plasma renin activity induced by intravenous γ-L-glutamyl-L-dopa in humans on an unmonitored salt intake.[457] Disruption of the *Drd3* in mice leads to increased renin release and renin-dependent hypertension.[25] In contrast, deletion of *Drd4* does not affect plasma or renal renin levels.[26] D_2R also probably do not play a role in renin secretion, because they are not expressed in the juxtaglomerular cell in rat,[357] mouse or human kidney (unpublished observations). Whether or not the reported effects of dopamine and D_1-like and D_2-like receptors on renin secretion are exerted at the macula densa remains to be confirmed, but all the dopamine receptor subtypes have been found in macula densa cells, albeit with species variability (Table 19.1). These studies would suggest that in humans, the predominant effect of dopamine receptors on renin secretion is inhibitory, via D_2-like receptors. A stimulatory effect could occur in hypertensive humans (see above), similar to that suggested in Sprague-Dawley rats[44], which are salt-sensitive.

D_1R is expressed in the zona glomerulosa of rat adrenal glands[458] and increases aldosterone secretion in isolated and cultured rat adrenal glomerulosa cells.[459] In humans, dopamine does not affect aldosterone secretion in the salt-replete state[460] but dopamine[461] inhibits angiotensin II-induced aldosterone secretion. This would be in keeping with the attenuation of angiotensin II-induced aldosterone secretion by bromocriptine (D_2R/D_3R agonist) in human adrenal cortical and adenocarcinoma cells.[462] These observations are confounded by the report that stimulation of D_4R enhances[463] angiotensin II-stimulated aldosterone

TABLE 19.1 Renal Dopamine Receptor Subtype Expression (Normal Sodium Intake)

Dopamine Receptor Subtype	Species	Glomerulus		Proximal Tubule		TDL, ATL	TAL	DCT	Collecting Duct			Juxtaglomerular Apparatus		Arterial Vessel
		MC	Podocytes	PCT	PST				CCD	OMCD	IMCD	JGC	MD	
D_1R														
mRNA	mouse													
	rat	No[367]	No[367]	Yes[a,367]	No[367]	No[367]	Yes[367]	Yes[365,367]	No[367]	No[367]	Yes[367,390]	No[367]	Yes[367]	No[367]
	human													
Protein	mouse	Yes[b]	Yes[387*]		Yes[b]	No[b]	Yes[b]	Yes[b]	Yes[b]	Yes[b]	No[b]	Yes[b]	Yes[b]	Yes[b]
	rat	Yes[356c] No[361,364,365, 381,382]	No[356,361,364,365]	Yes[356,361,364]		No[361]	No[361] Yes[364]	Yes[361, 364]	Yes[356, 361,364d]	No[361] Yes[364d]	No[361] Yes[356]	Yes[a, 361]	Yes[361]	Yes[361]
	human	No[372, 381,382]	No[372,381,382]	Yes[372]			Yes[372]	Yes[372]	Yes[372]	Yes[372d]		No[372]	No[372]	Yes[372]
D_2R														
mRNA	mouse													
	rat	Yes[252]		Yes[252]						Yes[252]				Yes[252]
	human													
Protein	mouse	No[b]	No[b]	Yes[b]	Yes[b]	No[b]	Yes[b]	Yes[b]	Yes[b]	No[b]	No[b]	No[b]	No[b]	No[b]
	rat	Yes[357]	No[357]	Yes[357]	Yes[b]	No[357]	Yes[b]	Yes[b]	Yes[357]	Yes[b]	Yes[357,f]	No[b]	Yes[b]	Yes[b]
	human	No[b]	Yes[b]	Yes[b]	No[b]	No[b]	Yes[b]	Yes[b]	Yes[b]	Yes[b]	No[b]	No[b]	No[b]	Yes[b]
D_3R														
mRNA	mouse													
	rat	Yes[252,388]		Yes[252,388]	Yes[252,388]				Yes[252,388]					Yes[252]
	human													
Protein	mouse	Yes[b]	Yes[b]	Yes[b]	Yes[b]		Yes[b]	Yes[b]	No[b]	No[b]	No[b]	Yes[b]	Yes[b]	
	rat	Yes[357g,375] No[374]	Yes[375] No[374]	Yes[374,375]	No[374]	No[374]	No[374]	Yes[357,375] No[374]	Yes[357, 375] No[374]	No[374, 375]	Yes[357] No[374,375]	No[374, 375] Yes[391,i]	Yes[375] No[374]	Yes[375] No[374]
	human													

(Continued)

TABLE 19.1 (Continued)

Dopamine Receptor Subtype	Species	Glomerulus		Proximal Tubule		TDL, ATL	TAL	DCT	Collecting Duct			Juxtaglomerular Apparatus		Arterial Vessel
		MC	Podocytes	PCT	PST				CCD	OMCD	IMCD	JGC	MD	
D4R														
mRNA	mouse													
	rat								Yes[365]					
	human													
Protein	mouse	Yes[b]		Yes[b]	No[b]	No[b]	Yes[b]	Yes[b]	Yes[b]	Yes[b]	No[b]		Yes[b]	Yes[b]
	rat	No[357,365,376]		Yes[357,376]		No	No[376]	Yes[376]	Yes[357,365,376]	Yes[365,376]	Yes[357,365,376]	No[365,376]	No[365,376]	Yes[376h]
	human													
D5R														
mRNA	mouse		Yes[387*]											
	rat			Yes[b]			Yes[b]	Yes[b]	Yes[b]					
	human													
Protein	mouse	No[360]	No[360]	Yes[360]	Yes[360]	No[360]	Yes[360]	Yes[360]	Yes[360]	Yes[360]	No[360]	No[360]	No[360]	Yes[360]
	rat	No[364]		Yes[213,364]			Yes[364]	Yes[364]	Yes[364d]	Yes[364d]		Yes[364]	Yes[b]	Yes[b]
	human													

*did not distinguish D1R from D5R

[a] Yamaguchi I, Jose PA, Mouradian MM, et al. Expression of dopamine D1A receptor gene in proximal tubule of rat kidneys. Am J Physiol. 1993 Feb;264(2 Pt 2):F280–5.

[b] Unpublished data.

[c] Not universally expressed in the WKY rat, not expressed in the SHR.[356]

[d] Not indicated as to location in outer or inner medulla.

[e] Expressed in the WKY, not expressed in the SHR.[357]

[f] Expressed in intercalated cells.

[g] More in SHR than in WKY.[357]

[h] Disappeared with renal denervation.

[i] In culture.

The renal expression of dopamine receptor subtypes is species dependent. In the rat, all the dopamine receptors except the D5R are expressed in the outer and inner medulla[213,252,356-365]. The mouse kidney has no dopamine receptors in the inner medulla[360] (unpublished observations).

Abbreviations: Glom: glomerulus; MC: mesangial cell; PCT: proximal convoluted tubule; PST: proximal straight tubule; TDL: thin descending limb; ATL: ascending thin limb; TAL: thick ascending limb; DCT: distal convoluted tubule, CCD: cortical collecting duct, OMCD: outer medullary collecting duct; IMCD: inner medullary collecting duct; JGC: Juxtaglomerular cell; MD: Macula densa.

secretion in the same human adrenal cortical and adenocarcinoma cells. However, in hypertensive subjects, the D_2-like receptor agonist bromocriptine (D_2R/D_3R agonist) decreased renin and aldosterone secretion which was reversed by metoclopramide, a non-selective D_2-like receptor antagonist.[464] Metoclopramide did not affect aldosterone levels in saline-loaded normal and heart failure subjects.[465] Because saline loading normally decreases aldosterone levels, this study suggests that dopamine does not normally stimulate aldosterone secretion.[465] However, the inhibitory effect of D_2R on aldosterone secretion is consistent with the increase in urinary aldosterone in $D_2^{-/-}$ mice.[47] In contrast, urinary aldosterone is not different between $D_4^{-/-}$ and $D_4^{+/+}$ mice, $D_3^{-/-}$ and $D_3^{+/+}$ mice (unpublished studies) or $D_5^{-/-}$ and $D_5^{+/+}$ mice.[360] Thus, dopamine probably normally is inhibitory of aldosterone secretion, mainly via the D_2R.

Autocrine/Paracrine Regulation of Renal Function by Dopamine

The autocrine/paracrine regulation of renal tubular sodium transport, via D_1-like receptors, is mediated by tubular and not by hemodynamic mechanisms[18–21,371,466,467] (also see below). Systemically administered dopaminergic drugs may not mimic the autocrine/paracrine function of dopamine. The quantitative contribution of each dopamine receptor subtype on renal sodium transport remains to be determined. However, the D_1R is responsible for $\approx 80\%$ of D_1-like receptor activity in renal proximal tubule cells[468]; D_5R may be more important in the distal nephron,[360] while the D_3R may regulate glomerular dynamics.[422] Each of the dopamine receptor subtypes, alone or via interaction with the other dopamine receptor subtypes or other GPCRs, regulates sodium transport in a unique fashion.[30] Indeed, disruption of any of the dopamine receptor genes results in hypertension, the pathogenesis of which is specific for each subtype.[22–27]

REGULATION OF ION AND WATER TRANSPORT

Ion Transport

Euvolemia and Moderate Volume Expansion

Dopamine and its receptors are important in the regulation of ion transport during euvolemia or moderate volume expansion, but have a minor role under marked volume expansion.[49,117] Inhibition of renal dopamine production by pharmacological inhibition of DOPA decarboxylase activity[469] or silencing of *Ddc* in mouse proximal tubule[470] impairs the ability to excrete a sodium load. In contrast, inhibition of the breakdown of renal tubular dopamine by inhibition of COMT but not MAO activity increases sodium excretion.[471] Deletion of *Comt* in mice, however, decreases the natriuretic response to an acute sodium load, apparently because in these mice, basal renal dopamine production is increased and is not futher increased by saline loading.[472] The increase in ion excretion caused by dopamine or D_1-like receptor agonists cannot be entirely ascribed to its ability to increase renal blood flow or glomerular filtration rate.[21,371,427,431,432,466,467,473] Reduction in renal blood flow to control values decreases but does not abolish the natriuretic effect of the D_1-like receptor agonist fenoldopam administered into the renal artery.[396] Rather, dopamine can directly inhibit renal tubular ion transport by inhibition of ion transporters, sodium channels, and sodium pump activity.[18–21,28–31] The short-term inhibition of ion transport by dopamine involves alteration in enzyme kinetics[89,474] and internalization of ion transporters/pump.[132,242,249,301,302,475–482] The long-term inhibition of sodium transport by dopamine may involve regulation of protein expression by decreasing gene transcription and translation, and increasing their degradation.[360]

The inhibitory effect of dopamine on ion transport is not simply a direct effect, but is modulated by its regulation of the release or secretion of other hormones/humoral substances. Hormones which directly inhibit ion transport interact with dopamine to increase (e.g., angiotensin III/AT_2R,[43] ANP/ANPA,[36,483–485] eicosanoids,[37,38,358,486] nitric oxide,[41,423,487,488] prolactin,[42,489] and urodilatin[36]) their inhibition of ion and water transport. In addition, dopamine negatively interacts with hormones that increase ion transport (e.g., angiotensin II,[45,46,490–494] insulin,[495,496] renin,[44] angiotensin II/AT_1R,[45,46] and aldosterone[37,47,48,461,463]) and water transport (e.g., vasopressin[51,365,497–499]). The natriuretic effect of D_1-like receptor stimulation persists even after renal denervation.[67]

The inhibitory effects of dopamine, via D_1-like receptors, on renal ion transport *in vivo* is well-established (*vide infra*). In contrast, the effect of D_2-like receptor agonists on ion transport *in vivo* has not been consistent; reports have found no effect,[395,418] a decrease[421,437,500] or an increase in sodium excretion.[24,419,501,502] The effect of blockade of D_2-like receptors may not become evident unless the nitric oxide mechanism is impaired.[423] The D_2R and D_2-like receptors have been reported to stimulate Na^+K^+-ATPase.[267,278,503,504] The D_2R/D_3R agonist, bromocriptine, transiently increases basolateral chloride transport in the isolated mTAL.[505] However, D_2-like receptor stimulation inhibits the stimulatory effect of angiotensin II on Na^+K^+-ATPase.[493]

Stimulation of D_3R also inhibits NHE3 activity.[506] The apparent discrepancies in these studies may be related, in part, to the status of the extracellular fluid volume.[24,419] For example, a two-day administration of quinpirole, a D_2R/D_3R agonist, increased while a D_2R antagonist decreased sodium excretion in $D_2^{+/+}$ mice fed high but not normal sodium diet.[24] Because D_1-like receptor effect is increased with moderate sodium loading,[18–22,29–31,49,466,507] this would indicate the need of D_1-like receptors for D_2-like receptors to inhibit Na^+ transport.[268,473,508,509] A selective D_3R agonist, 7-OH-DPAT, increases sodium excretion in rats on a normal and high salt diet.[501] The natriuresis in rats with strepto-zotocin-induced diabetes is decreased by D_3R antago-nist.[502] However, the natriuretic effect of another D_3R agonist, pramipexole, is blocked by a D_1-like receptor antagonist.[266] The natriuretic effect of dopamine has also been shown to depend on the activation of both D_1-like and D_2-like receptors.[508] Therefore, the inhibitory effect of D_2-like receptors on sodium transport may not be observed, unless the animals are salt-loaded, a state that enhances the natriuretic effect of D_1-like receptors.

In hypovolemic or euvolemic states where vasopres-sin levels are elevated, the ability of D_2-like receptor agonists, probably acting via the D_4R, to inhibit the effects of vasopressin[498,510] may obscure any stimula-tory effect of D_2-like receptors, probably via the D_2R, on water and ion transport in more proximal parts of the nephron. However, preliminary studies suggest that D_4R stimulation inhibits NCC activity in mouse renal distal convoluted tubule cells.[511]

Dopamine inhibits ion and water transport in the proximal and distal nephron,[427,512–514] as estimated from lithium clearance studies. It must be noted that the renal tubular site of action of endogenous dopa-mine and its agonists on ion transport may not always match that given exogenously. Most of the renal dopa-mine is produced in the proximal tubule, and so its effects in the distal nephron could be limited while exogenously administered dopamine would reach all nephron segments equally.

Luminal Membrane

Proximal Tubule

As stated earlier, all the dopamine receptor subtypes are expressed in the proximal tubule. The stimulation of D_1-like receptors decreases the activity of several ion transporters, including the sodium hydrogen exchanger 3 (NHE3, SLC9A3),[22,127–133,515] sodium phosphate co-transporter (NaPi-IIa/SLC34A1 and NaPi-IIc/SLC34A3)[242,476,482,516–519] and Cl^-/HCO_3^- exchanger (SLC26A6)[520] at the luminal membrane. G-protein-dependent, cAMP/PKA-, PKC-, NHERF-1-, and phos-phatase-dependent and -independent mechanisms are involved in the dopamine or D_1-like receptor inhibition

of NHE3, $Na^+/Pi2$, Na^+/HCO_3, and Cl^-/HCO_3^- exchanger activity, including their translocation out of the brush border membranes into the cytosol.[127,130–133,249,476–482,515,518] The signaling path-ways by which D_1-like receptors inhibit NHE3 activity may be species-specific, involving PKA only in rat and human renal proximal tubule cells (Figure 19.2), but involving both PKA and PKC in renal opossum kidney cells.[521] Specific PDZ domains of Pals-associated tight junction protein (PDZ 2, 4 or 5) or NHERF-1 (PDZ 2) may be important in organizing the signaling pathways by which dopamine inhibits sodium transporter/pump activity.[249,477–480,518,522] In contrast, NHERF3/4 regu-lates the internalization of NaPiIIa.[482]

The D_3R[506] and D_4R may also regulate NHE3 (Table 19.2) because its expression is increased in $D_3^{-/-}$ and $D_4^{-/-}$ mice on normal salt intake.[523] However, the inhibitory effect of the D_3R on NHE3 activity in renal proximal tubules is not linked to $G\alpha s$ because pretreatment of the cells with cholera toxin did not prevent the D_3R effect. Rather, the D_3R-medi-ated inhibition of NHE3 activity in renal proximal tubules is related to $G\alpha_{i3}$, stimulation of PKC, and modulation of intracellular calcium.[259] The effect of the D_3R, in the rat, is probably independent of changes in intracellular cAMP because renal proximal tubules do not express adenylyl cyclase V.[220] In mesenteric arteries, D_3R causes vasodilation that is mediated by inhibition of Ca^{2+} channels and modula-tion of K^+ channels,[264] in agreement with the sugges-tion that the linkage of the D_3R to other effectors, such as inhibition of K^+ and Ca^{2+} may be more sensi-tive than the weak linkage to G-proteins.[258]

Loop of Henle

The mTAL expresses the D_1R, D_3R (in the mouse but not in the rat), D_4R, and D_5R. D_1-like and D_2-like receptor agonists administered to the apical membrane of the rat mTAL do not affect chloride transport. However, their application to the basolateral mem-brane decreases chloride transport via D_1-like recep-tors[505] that is unrelated to PKA or PKC, but rather to PLA2-mediated formation of 20-HETE.[524] Incubation of mTAL suspensions with dopamine increases sodium potassium 2 chloride co-transporter (NKCC2, SLC12A1) activity.[442] Indeed, NKCC2 activity is stimu-lated by PKA and PKC, but inhibited by 20-HETE.[525] The PKA-mediated stimulation of Na^+/K^+-ATPase activity is observed only under oxygenated conditions, but is overridden by PLA2 inhibitory pathways under hypoxic conditions.[526] Therefore, overall ion transport is inhibited, probably because of inhibition of basolat-eral chloride[505] transport and Na^+/K^+-ATPase activ-ity.[442,527] The D_1-like receptor-mediated stimulation of

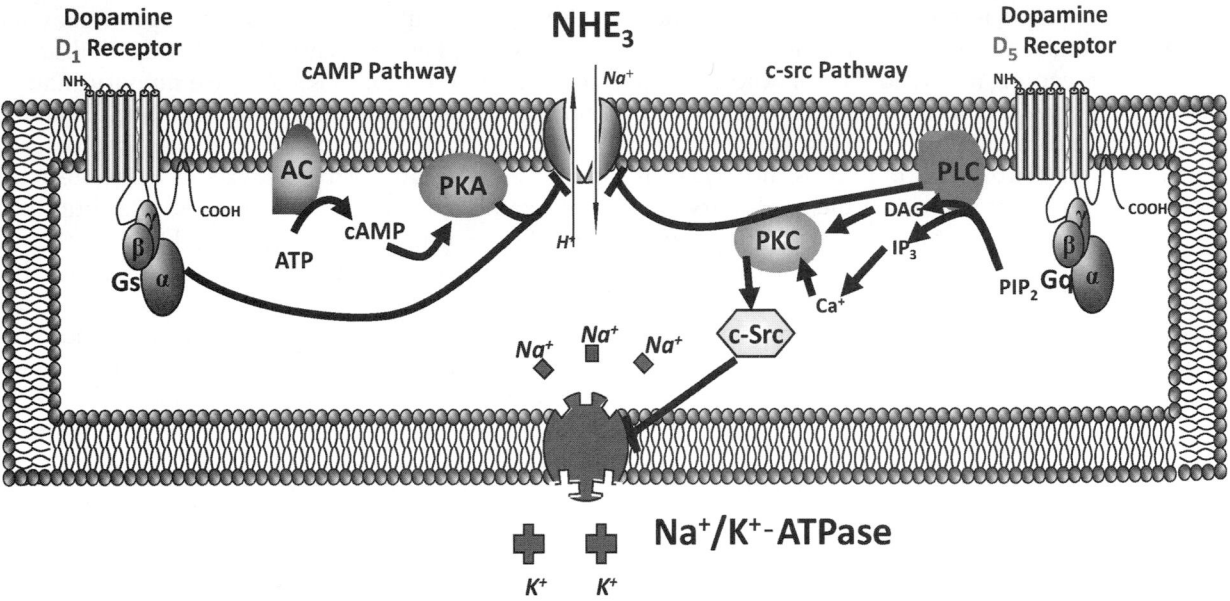

FIGURE 19.2 **Schematic model of the intracellular 2nd messenger pathways known for the dopamine-1 and dopamine-5 receptors (D_1R, D_5R) in the human renal proximal tubule cell.** The D_1R is coupled through Gas to stimulate adenylyl cyclase activity which converts ATP to cAMP. cAMP dependent protein kinase A (PKA) then inhibits the sodium hydrogen exchanger type 3 (NHE3); GaS can also directly inhibit NHE3. The D_5R interacts with Gaq to stimulate phospholipase C (PLC)[230] which converts phosphatidylinositol 4,5-bisphosphate (PIP₂) to diacylglycerol (DAG) and inositol 1,4,5-trisphosphate (IP₃) (The co-activation of D_1R and D_2R can also increase PLC activity.[226]) DAG and IP₃, through its release of intracellular calcium (Ca^{2+}), stimulate protein kinase C (PKC). Na^+/K^+-ATPase is then inhibited via a c-Src-mediated pathway. The inhibitory effect of D_1-like receptors on Na^+/K^+-ATPase also involves PKA in the distal convoluted tubule and cortical collecting duct, while eicosanoids are involved in all nephron segments, including the mTAL[241,522,530,539,540–544]; PKC may also be involved in the inhibition of Na^+/K^+-ATPase in the mTAL.[527] *(The authors acknowledge Robby Van Sciver for producing this diagram.)*

NKCC2 may be important in K^+ recycling in the mTAL.[442] Bromocriptine (D_2R/D_3R agonist) increases chloride transport, albeit transiently,[505] reminiscent of the ability of this agonist to increase Na^+/K^+-ATPase activity in renal proximal tubules.[267] However, the D_4R and D_5R may negatively regulate NKCC2 expression because its expression is increased in $D_4^{-/-}$ (unpublished) and $D_5^{-/-}$ mice.[360] NKCC2 expression is not altered in $D_2^{-/-}$ and $D_3^{-/-}$ mice and has not been reported in $D_1^{-/-}$ mice (Table 19.2).

Distal Convoluted Tubule

The distal convoluted tubule expresses all the dopamine receptor subtypes, but their effect on ion transport in this nephron segment has not been reported, except for D_4R which inhibits NCC.[511] However, the D_2R, D_3R, D_4R, and D_5R may regulate NCC because its expression is increased in $D_2^{-/-}$, $D_3^{-/-}$, $D_4^{-/-}$ and $D_5^{-/-}$ mice[360,528] (unpublished data). NCC expression has not been reported in $D_1^{-/-}$ mice (Table 19.2).

Cortical Collecting Duct

D_1-like receptor stimulation of the rabbit cortical collecting duct depolarizes the luminal membrane and increases cAMP production.[363,530] D_5R may regulate ENaC because α- and γ-subunit expressions are increased in $D_5^{-/-}$ mice[360]; sodium transporters in $D_1^{-/-}$ mice have not yet been quantified. Dopamine, via D_4R, at the basolateral membrane decreases sodium transport in the rabbit cortical collecting duct.[529] The D_4R may also inhibit the increase in sodium transport mediated by vasopressin, via a decrease in cAMP.[365,498] αENaC is increased in $D_4^{-/-}$ mice but only following a high salt diet (unpublished observations). ENaC expression is not altered in $D_2^{-/-}$ and $D_3^{-/-}$ mice. ENaC expression has not been reported in $D_1^{-/-}$ mice (Table 19.2).

Medullary Collecting Duct

The D_1R is expressed in the collecting duct or in the outer but probably not in the inner medulla, while the D_5R is also expressed in the outer but not in the inner medullary collecting duct in the mouse kidney.[360,528] Indeed, dopamine does not stimulate cAMP production in the rat inner medullary collecting duct.[369] D_2-like receptors are expressed in the medullary collecting duct; the D_2R is expressed in the intercalated cells,[357] while D_3R and D_4R are not differentially expressed between intercalated and principal cells.[357,528] A D_2-like receptor has been shown to stimulate PGE2 production in rat inner medullary collecting duct cells.[358,359] The specific D_2-like receptor involved is not known, but only the D_4R is expressed in the inner medullary collecting duct; the expression of the D_2R has not been consistently shown (Table 19.2).[528] It is not clear if dopamine regulates ion transport in the medullary collecting duct. Indeed, the inhibitory effect of dopamine on vasopressin-induced water permeability and cAMP accumulation in the rat inner medullary collecting duct is mediated by the α_2 adrenergic receptor.[368]

Basolateral Membrane

D_1-like receptors inhibit the electrogenic Na^+/HCO_3^- co-transporter (NBCe1A, SLC4A4) expressed in the basolateral membrane of the proximal tubule[481] and Na^+/K^+-ATPase expressed at the basolateral membrane in all nephron segments studied (proximal tubule, thick ascending limb of Henle, cortical collecting duct).[17,38,89,268,293,301,304,318,319,477−480,495,522,526−543]

Although stimulation of D_2-like receptors may increase Na^+/K^+-ATPase activity,[267,373,503] the inhibitory effect of dopamine on Na^+/K^+-ATPase activity may require simultaneous stimulation of D_1-like and D_2-like receptors,[268] and could result in a potentially greater inhibition of the sodium pump caused by D_1-like receptors. For example, in the rat proximal tubule (but not in the mTAL or cortical collecting duct) D_2-like receptors act in conjunction with D_1-like receptors to inhibit Na^+/K^+-ATPase activity and decrease sodium transport, similar to that proposed for NaPiII[545] and NHE3.[546] Under normal circumstances, dopamine receptors probably do not regulate the expression of the α-subunit of Na^+/K^+ATPase, because its expression is not altered in $D_2^{-/-}$, $D_3^{-/-}$, $D_4^{-/-}$, and $D_5^{-/-}$ mice on a normal salt intake[360,523,528] although this has not been studied in $D_1^{-/-}$ mice.

The inhibitory effect of D_1-like receptors on Na^+/K^+-ATPase is mediated by cAMP/PKA, certain PKC isoforms, and 20-HETE. The overall consequence of D_1-like receptor stimulation is internalization of $Na^+/$

TABLE 19.2 Characteristics of Mice With Knockout of Dopamine Receptor Subtype Gene (Normal Sodium Intake Unless Indicated)

Variable	$D_1^{-/-}$	$D_2^{-/-}$	$D_3^{-/-}$	$D_4^{-/-}$	$D_5^{-/-}$
Blood Pressure	High[22]	High[23,47]	High[25], Normal[560]*	High[26]	High[27,232,234]
Salt Sensitivity (chronic NaCl load)	Yes#	BP increased only with sodium load[24]	Yes#, No[560]*	Yes#	Yes[234,360]
Increased Na^+ transporter/ exchanger, channel	ND	NHE3, NCC#	NHE3, NCC#	NHE3, NKCC2, NCC#	NKCC2, NCC, α & β ENaC subunits[360]
Na^+K^+ATPase, a subunit	ND	Low activity[23] and protein#	Normal#	High#	Normal[360]
GPCR (kidney)	ND	Normal AT_1R#, normal response to ARB, increased ETBR[23]	High AT_1R[342],	High AT_1R[26]	High AT_1R[a,46, 360]
Renin-Angiotensin	ND	ND	High[25]	Normal[26]	Normal[360]
Aldosterone	ND	High[47]	Normal#	Normal#	Normal[360]
Reactive Oxygen Species	ND	High[47]	Normal#	Normal#	High[a, 234]
Inflammation	ND	High#	Normal	Normal#	ND
Body Weight	Low [22,561]	Normal[23,24,47], Low[b]	Normal[25,560], Fat load increases body weight in males; increased body fat in males and females[c]	Normal[26]	Normal[360]

ND = not determined, # unpublished, *chronic administration of D_3R antagonist causes salt-dependent hypertension in rats.[501] Please read text for important details.

a. Asico L, Zhang X, Jiang J, et al. Lack of renal dopamine D5 receptors promotes hypertension. J Am Soc Nephrol. 20;22(1):82−89.

b. Kim KS, Yoon YR, Lee HJ, et al. Enhanced hypothalamic leptin signaling in mice lacking dopamine D2 receptors. J Biol Chem. 2010;285 (12):8905−8917.

c. McQuade JA, Benoit SC, Xu M, Woods SC, Seeley RJ. High-fat diet induced adiposity in mice with targeted disruption of the dopamine-3 receptor gene. 2004;151(1−2):313−319.

K^+-ATPase subunits.[301,477–480,533–536,540] The inhibitory effect of D_1-like receptors on Na^+/K^+-ATPase involves PKC in the proximal convoluted tubule (Figure 19.2) and PKA in the distal convoluted tubule and cortical collecting duct, while the eicosanoids are involved in all nephron segments, including the mTAL,[241,522,530,539,540,544] PKC may also be involved in the inhibition of Na^+/K^+-ATPase in the mTAL.[527] 20-HETE is important in the ability of dopamine to inhibit Na^+/K^+-ATPase activity in rat renal cortex, because it overrides the stimulatory effect of PKA.[38,544] In the renal medulla, but not in the renal cortex, PKA[544] and phosphatase inhibition also contribute to the inhibition of Na^+,K^+-ATPase activity that may be related to DARPP-32 inhibition of PP-1,[293,317,543] in the case of dopamine.

The effect of dopamine on Na^+/K^+-ATPase is tissue-specific. As stated above, dopamine inhibits Na^+/K^+-ATPase activity in renal cortical and medullary tubules.[17,38,89,268,293,301,304,318,319,477–480,495,522,526–543] However, the regulation of the phosphorylation of Na^+/K^+-ATPase at Ser-23 is different between the proximal convoluted tubule and thick ascending limb of Henle; PKC phosphorylates Na^+/K^+-ATPase at Ser-23 in the proximal tubule but not in the mTAL.[527] D_1-like receptors may actually stimulate Na^+/K^+-ATPase activity in human ciliary nonpigmented epithelial[547] and pulmonary alveolar cells.[548] $D_{2L}R$ also stimulates Na^+/K^+-ATPase in murine fibroblasts.[503] D_1R and D_2R, on the one hand, and Na^+/K^+-ATPase, on the other, can also negatively regulate each other in HEK293T cell by direct protein–protein interaction.[549] While the inhibition of Na^+/K^+-ATPase in the kidney by dopamine under conditions of sodium chloride excess is beneficial, inhibition of Na^+/K^+-ATPase activity in neuronal cells by high concentrations of dopamine can lead to cell death.[550] Inhibition of Na^+/K^+-ATPase activity in vascular smooth muscle cells would increase vascular resistance, as has been reported in the rat tail.[409] Low concentrations of dopamine, however, decrease systemic vascular resistance probably by mechanisms other than via regulation of sodium transporter or pump activity,[264,551,552] e.g., opening of potassium channels[274,553–555] (vide supra, "Dopamine and Renal Hemodynamics").

Water Transport

Dopamine may also regulate water transport.[497] Dopamine inhibits arginine vasopressin-mediated increase in water transport,[510] via the D_4R in the rat cortical collecting duct.[498] Dopamine has been reported also to inhibit vasopressin-stimulated increase in water permeability in inner medullary collecting duct cells.[368] Although it has been claimed to be exerted at

a_2-adrenergic receptors, the effect could be[498] inhibited by clozapine, a D_4R antagonist. The dopamine-mediated reversal of vasopressin-mediated increase in water transport has been related to a decrease in expression, and increase in phosphorylation, of aquaporin 2 at the apical plasma membrane.[499] In addition, dopamine, via D_4R, increases the ubiquitin-mediated degradation of aquaporin 2 in lysosomes and decreases the aquaporin 2 transcription by decreasing vasopressin-induced increase in cAMP production.[497] D_1-like receptors probably do not play a role in the vasopressin-mediated transport, at least in the rat inner medullary collecting duct, because dopamine does not increase cAMP levels in this nephron segment.[369] Aquaporin 4-mediated increase in basolateral permeability is also impaired by dopamine, via a yet to be determined receptor subtype that is linked to PKC.[556] The D_2R can regulate aquaporin 4 in glial cells,[557] but is probably not the dopamine receptor involved in the medullary collecting duct because the D_2R is not expressed in principal cells of this nephron segment.[357] The diuresis associated with hypotonic saline loading has been related to the ability of D_1-like receptor antagonist to decrease vasopressin release.[51] However, dopamine is known to increase vasopressin secretion from the hypophysis.[558] This discrepancy could be taken to indicate that the dopamine-mediated release of vasopressin may be influenced by the state of volume expansion.

Hypovolemia

In contrast to the natriuretic effect of endogenous renal dopamine in euvolemic and in moderately volume-expanded states, in sodium-depleted states the D_1-like agonist, fenoldopam, does not affect sodium excretion,[427] while dopamine actually decreases sodium excretion.[56] A limited number of studies have assessed the dopamine receptor subtype that may increase renal sodium reabsorption in hypovolemic states. In conscious, chronically instrumented dogs on a sodium intake of 40 mmol/day, quinpirole (D_3R and D_4R agonist) decreased sodium excretion as a consequence of both a decrease in renal blood flow and an increase in tubular sodium reabsorption.[421] Dopamine has also been reported to stimulate NHE3 and Na^+/K^+-ATPase activity in rabbit renal proximal tubule cells[559] and NKCC2 in mTAL[442]; bromocriptine (D_2R/D_3R agonist) stimulates Na^+/K^+-ATPase activity in rat renal proximal tubule cells[267] and increases chloride transport in the mTAL.[505] Stimulation of the $D_{2S}R$ or $D_{2L}R$ heterologously expressed in murine LTK-cells increased Na^+/K^+-ATPase[503] and NHE1[430] activity. These may be the mechanisms by which dopamine increases sodium transport during hypovolemia.[56]

Dopamine Receptor Subtype Mutant Mice

The deletion of dopamine receptor subtype in mice has helped to determine the role of each dopamine receptor subtype in the regulation of renal function and blood pressure.[22–27,30,232,234,360,511,523,528,560] Each dopamine receptor subtype participates in the regulation of blood pressure by mechanisms specific for the subtype. As described above, some receptors influence epithelial transport. Others, as described below, regulate blood pressure by influencing the central and/or peripheral nervous system and regulating the secretion and receptors of several humoral agents (Table 19.2).

D_1R Mutant Mice

$D_1^{-/-}$ mice are growth retarded without obvious neurological defects, but exhibit a decrease in rearing behavior.[561] The low survival after weaning is caused by decreased feeding ability. $D_1^{-/-}$ mice and $D_1^{-/+}$ mice (C57BL/6 background) on a normal NaCl diet have higher systolic and diastolic blood pressures than D_1R wild-type ($D_1^{+/+}$) mice.[22] Homozygous $D_1^{-/-}$ mice do not increase renal tubular cAMP accumulation in response to dopamine stimulation, but the response to parathyroid hormone is intact. These data indicate D_1R specificity in the increased blood pressure in mice.[22] However, it is not clear why the other D_1-like receptor, D_5R, is unable to compensate for the lack of D_1R; D_5R expression is not altered in $D_1^{-/-}$ mice[193,229] and D_1R expression is not altered in $D_5^{-/-}$ mice.[27] The hypertension of $D_1^{-/-}$ mice is aggravated by an increase in salt intake (Table 19.2). The hypertension of $D_1^{-/-}$ mice is aggravated by an increase in salt intake (Table 19.2).

D_2R Mutant Mice

$D_2^{-/-}$ mice in C57BL/6J background have decreased motor activity but rotarod performance is not impaired.[192] D_1-like receptor binding may be decreased, while D_3R is transiently increased after birth in $D_2^{-/-}$ mice.[192] $D_2^{-/-}$ and $D_2^{-/+}$ mice (C57BL/6J) on a normal NaCl diet have higher systolic and diastolic blood pressures than D_2 wild-type ($D_2^{+/+}$) mice.[23] α-Adrenergic blockade decreases blood pressure to a greater extent in $D_2^{-/-}$ mice than in $D_2^{+/+}$ mice, but acute adrenalectomy decreases blood pressure to a similar level in $D_2^{-/-}$ and $D_2^{+/+}$ mice. ETB receptor expression is greater in $D_2^{-/-}$ mice than in $D_2^{+/+}$ mice, and ETB receptor blocker decreases blood pressure in $D_2^{-/-}$ mice but not $D_2^{+/+}$ mice. $D_2^{-/-}$ mice also have increased production of ROS; increasing antioxidant activity with hemin normalizes the increased blood pressure.[47] These data indicate that $D_2^{-/-}$ mice may have enhanced vascular reactivity caused by increased sympathetic and ETB

receptor activities, and oxidative stress.[47] The $D_2^{-/-}$ mice also have increased production of aldosterone, and treatment with a mineralocorticoid receptor blocker normalizes blood pressure but not the increased oxidative stress in these mice,[47] indicating that the increased mineralocorticoid activity is distal to the increased oxidative stress. In an unspecified strain of $D_2^{-/-}$ mice, blood pressure is increased only when the mice are fed a high-salt diet; this is associated with a decrease in renal AADC activity and renal dopamine production. Sympathetic activity is not increased in these $D_2^{-/-}$ mice.[24] The differences between the two strains of $D_2^{-/-}$ mice could be related to differences in the genetic background,[153] similar to the differences in behavior of $D_2^{-/-}$ mice from different genetic backgrounds.[192,193]

D_3R Mutant Mice

The locomotor phenotype of $D_3^{-/-}$ mice does not resemble that of $D_2^{-/-}$ mice. $D_3^{-/-}$ mice may show a transient locomotor hyperactivity in a novel environment.[562] The D_3R may be involved in seeking behavior for natural reinforcers such as food in rodent models of obesity[563]; $D_3^{-/-}$ mice fed a high fat diet become obese.[564] $D_3^{-/-}$ and $D_3^{-/+}$ mice (C57BL/6J) on a normal NaCl diet have both higher systolic and diastolic blood pressure than their wild-type ($D_3^{+/+}$) littermates.[25] These $D_3^{-/-}$ and $D_3^{-/+}$ mice have increased renal renin production, but sustained decrease in blood pressure with AT_1R blockade is observed in the $D_3^{-/-}$ but not $D_3^{-/+}$ or $D_3^{+/+}$ mice.[25] An unspecified strain of $D_3^{-/-}$ mice has normal blood pressure regardless of salt intake.[560] Nevertheless, these two strains (C57BL/6 and an unspecified strain) of $D_3^{-/-}$ mice have decreased sodium excretion after an acute or chronic sodium chloride load. Differences in phenotypes can occur depending on the genetic background, and even the same mouse strain from different commercial sources. For example, the blood pressure of C57BL/6 from Jackson Laboratories is salt-sensitive while the blood pressure of C57BL/6 mice from Taconic is salt-resistant.[153] The salt-sensitive hypertensive phenotype of human G-protein-coupled receptor kinase type 4 (GRK4) 486V transgenic mice is dependent on the percentage of genetic background from salt-resistant SJL mice.[565]

D_4R Mutant Mice

D_4R deficient ($D_4^{-/-}$) mice have impaired photoreceptor response, reduced response to novelty, but attenuated locomotor response to amphetamine, but not to methylphenidate or cocaine.[192] Congenic $D_4^{-/-}$[26] but not $D_4^{-/+}$ (Table 19.2) mice have increased systolic and diastolic blood pressures. The blood pressure is increased further with increased sodium intake in

$D_4^{-/-}$ mice (Table 19.2) but the effect of sodium intake on blood pressure in $D_4^{-/+}$ has not been tested. $D_4^{-/-}$ mice do not have altered circulating or renal renin or aldosterone levels.[26] Renal and brain, but not cardiac, AT_1R expression is increased in $D_4^{-/-}$ mice. The hypotensive effect of a bolus intravenous injection of the angiotensin type 1 receptor blocker, losartan, persists longer in $D_4^{-/-}$ than in $D_4^{+/+}$ mice. Thus, the hypertension brought about by the absence of the D_4R is mediated, in part, by increased AT_1R expression , similar seen in $D_3^{-/-}$ and $D_5^{-/-}$ (vide infra).[26]

D_5R Mutant Mice

$D_5^{-/-}$ mice have no impairment in learning and memory.[27,192] $D_5^{-/-}$ mice have normal expression of the other dopamine receptors, including the D_1R, a feature found in the other dopamine receptor subtype knockout mice except for the $D_2^{-/-}$ mice.[192] $D_5^{-/-}$[27] and $D_5^{-/+}$ mice are hypertensive. As with the $D_4^{-/-}$ mice (Table 19.2), the blood pressure is increased further with increased sodium intake in $D_5^{-/-}$ mice.[360] Epinephrine/norepinephrine ratio and the hypotensive response to the acute administration of an α-adrenergic blocker are greater in $D_5^{-/-}$ mice than their $D_5^{+/+}$ littermates, indicating that increased sympathetic activity plays a role in the elevated blood pressure observed with deletion of the Drd5 gene.[27] Central nervous system pathways involving glutaminergic, oxytocin, vasopressin, and adrenergic receptors are important in the pathogenesis of hypertension in $D_5^{-/-}$ mice.[27] Besides these central nervous system mechanisms, renal AT_1R[46,567] and increased production of ROS are also involved[232,234] in the hypertension of $D_5^{-/-}$ mice.

DOPAMINE RECEPTOR INTERACTIONS

Interaction among the Dopamine Receptors and with Other GPCRs in the Regulation of Renal Function and Blood Pressure

Dopamine Receptor Subtype Interaction

D_1-like and D_2-like receptors[266,473,508,509] interact to enhance the natriuretic effect of dopamine in sodium-replete states. In sodium-replete states, the synergistic interaction between D_1-like and D_2-like receptors to increase sodium excretion occurs by inhibiting NHE3[546] and Na^+/K^+-ATPase[38,268,362] activity, as stated above.

D_1R and D_3R

D_1R and D_3R synergistically interact to decrease sodium transport in renal proximal tubule cells[265,266,426] and to relax vascular smooth muscle cells.[264,283] D_1R and D_3R reciprocally regulate each

other's function and trafficking in HEK293 cells heterologously expresses tagged D_1R and D_3R, but not D_5R.[262] This has to be reconciled to the fact that $G\alpha_S$, which by itself decreases NHE3 activity independently of PKA,[130] is linked to both D_1R[30,183–193,687] and D_3R.[253] $G\alpha q/11$, involved in the D_1-like receptor inhibition of Na^+/K^+-ATPase,[410] can also be linked to D_3R.[568] The natriuretic action of the D_3R agonist pramipexole is partially blocked by a D_1-like receptor antagonist.[266] The D_3R co-localizes with D_1R in renal proximal tubule cells of WKY rats and in these cells, stimulation of D_3R increases both the co-immunoprecipitation of D_1R with D_3R, and the protein expression of D_1R.[265] The individual inhibitory effect of either D_1-like receptors or the D_3R on transporters is not 100%, not always on the same transporter or in the same nephron segment, and thus, additive or even synergistic effects are possible with co-stimulation. In mouse brain, the ALG-2 interacting protein 1 may be important in the interaction between D_1R and D_3R.[569] Whether or not this protein is also important in D_1R and D_2R interaction in the kidney remains to be determined.

The D_3R promotes natriuresis, in the short-term, alone[388,501,502] and by interacting with the D_1R.[266] In the long-term, the D_3R increases the expression of D_1R.[426] The interaction between D_1R and D_3R receptors is absent or impaired in hypertension, and results in defective inhibition of sodium transport and relaxation of vascular smooth muscles and ultimately in the development or maintenance of high blood pressure.[264,265,283,426]

D_2R and D_3R

In HEK293 cells, activation of heterologous D_2R inhibits both adenylyl cyclases V and VI, while activation of D_3R inhibits only adenylyl cyclase V and does not affect the activity of adenylyl cyclase VI.[258] However, when D_2R and D_3R are co-expressed in a monkey kidney cell line, lower concentrations of a D_2-like receptor agonist are needed to induce inhibition of adenylyl cyclase VI than those needed in cells expressing only the D_2R.[263] This suggests that the D_2R/D_3R heterodimer may enable the G-protein coupling of the D_3R to adenylyl cyclase VI. The D_3R, however, cannot inhibit adenylyl cyclase V in the rat renal proximal tubule, because this isoform is not expressed in this rat nephron segment.[220]

D_1R, D_5R, and D_2R

D_1R and D_2R heterodimerize in expression systems[570] and neural tissues,[571] and the degree of receptor protein−protein interaction is significantly enhanced by concomitant addition of D_1R and D_2R receptor subtype-specific agonists.[570] The physical interaction between D_1R and D_2R is increased by the chaperone, calnexin.[338] The co-activation of D_1R and D_2R increases phospholipase C products[571] and eicosanoids[572] which inhibit sodium transport. In the brain striatum, the D_1R and D_2R complex activates calcium—calmodulin-dependent protein kinase 2α.[573] The D_1R can inhibit the cellular sequestration of D_2R and could explain the synergy between these two dopamine receptor subtypes.[256] The D_2R also hetero-oligomerizes with D_5R, which causes a decrease in D_5R-mediated increase in intracellular calcium levels.[227] However, there is no evidence of a D_1R and D_2R or D_5R and D_2R heterodimerization in renal tubule cells. It remains to be determined whether or not D_1R and D_5R interact to regulate renal ion.

D_4R and Other Dopamine Receptor Subtypes

A direct interaction between D_4R and the other dopamine receptor subtypes has not been reported. However, the dopaminergic regulation of glutamate N-methyl-D-aspartate receptor activity in the amygdala may be due to a functional interaction between D_1R and D_4R.[574] Gene—gene interaction between D_2R and D_4R is associated with the development of conduct disorder and adult antisocial behavior in males.[575]

Dopamine Interaction with Other GPCRs

The dopamine receptor subtypes interact with several GPCRs, e.g., D_1R and μ opioid receptor,[576] and N-methyl-D-aspartic acid glutamate receptor.[577–579] Only those receptors that have been shown to be involved or have the potential to be involved in the regulation of renal function are included in this review.

Adenosine Receptors

Stimulation of renal adenosine receptors lowers glomerular filtration rate by constricting afferent arterioles, and exerts differential effects on NaCl transport along the nephron, depending upon the adenosine receptor subtype; the adenosine type 2 receptor decreases (adenosine A_{2b} promotes chloride secretion), while the adenosine A_1 receptor increases sodium transport. Adenosine antagonizes some effects of dopamine. The dopamine-mediated inhibition of tubuloglomerular feedback is antagonized by adenosine via the regulation of adenylyl cyclase activity in the macula densa.[134] In opossum kidney cells, low concentrations of an adenosine analog, via the adenosine A_1 receptor, stimulate NHE3 activity and attenuate dopamine-mediated inhibition of NHE3.[580] Adenosine A_1 receptor modulates D_1R; co-administration of adenosine A_1R receptor and D_1R agonists in HEK293 cells stably expressing both receptors

potentiate the D_1R-mediated desensitization of D_1R.[581] Interestingly, adenosine A_1 receptor and D_1R have been shown to physically interact in the central nervous system, with the formation of a heteromeric complex that leads to the uncoupling of the D_1R from its Gs-like protein complex.[445,581] However, in COS-7 cells and fibroblasts heterologously expressing adenosine A_1 receptor, D_1R, and D_5R, activation of adenosine A_1 receptor blocks the desensitization of D_1R but not D_5R,[582] another instance of cell-specific effects or related gene overexpression. In contrast, in HEK293 cells heterologously expressing adenosine A_1 receptor, D_1R, activation of adenosine A_1 receptor desensitizes the D_1R.[581] These studies illustrate the importance of studying receptor function in cells where such GPCRs are endogenously expressed.

The adenosine A_2 receptor isoform, A_{2A} receptor, heterodimerizes with D_2R in striatal membranes and reduces the high affinity state of D_2Rs, especially the high-affinity agonists.[583] The heterodimerization of adenosine A_{2A} receptor and D_3R or D_4R also results in an impairment of D_3R and D_4R function.[584]

Adrenergic Receptors

β-Adrenergic receptor agonists interact with dopamine in the regulation of Na^+/K^+-ATPase activity in the rat kidney. Activation of β-receptors with isoproterenol increases D_1R translocation from the cytosol to the membranes and D_1R-mediated inhibition of Na^+/K^+-ATPase activity in renal proximal tubule cells.[585] However, as stated above, stimulation of β_2Rs reduces the uptake of L-DOPA and the production of dopamine.[586] Thus, endogenous renal β-adrenergic receptors may not always enhance the dopaminergic inhibition of sodium transport.

Dopamine receptors may counter-regulate the actions of α-adrenergic receptors on renal sodium transport (unpublished data) and vascular proliferation. Stimulation of α_1Rs increases proliferation of vascular smooth muscle cells. However, in the presence of D_1-like or D_3R agonists, the proliferative effect of norepinephrine, via α_1Rs, is inhibited, although D_1-like or D_3R agonists have no effect by themselves. Moreover, co-stimulation of D_1-like or D_3R has an additive inhibitory effect on norepinephrine-mediated vascular smooth muscle cell contraction and proliferation.[264] The failure of dopamine to induce natriuresis in sodium-depleted states may be a consequence of increased sympathomimetic activity.[56]

Angiotensin II and Angiotensin Receptors

AT_1R and Dopamine Receptors

There are several areas of interaction between the dopamine and the renin—angiotensin system (RAS).

The D_3R, D_4, and D_5R D_4R and D_5R or D_2R (Table 19.2), but not D_1R, decrease AT_1R expression in the kidney.[26,46,276] In contrast, the D_2R may negatively regulate the expression of AT_1R,[587] and angiotensin II may increase D_2R expression in neural cells.[588]

Angiotensin II inhibits the uptake of dopamine by rat renal tubule cells[589] and the intravenous infusion of angiotensin II in humans reduces urinary dopamine.[590] Angiotensin II, via AT_1R, causes renal vasoconstriction while at low concentrations of dopamine, D_1-like receptors cause vasodilation.[405,591] Activation of the RAS may cause the development of tolerance to the hypotensive action of D_1-like receptor agonists.[592] In the rat, dopamine attenuates the glomerular mesangial contractile response to angiotensin II independently of eicosanoids.[389] D_1-like receptor agonists block angiotensin II-induced afferent and efferent arteriolar constriction.[399,591] Blockade of AT_1R normalizes the impaired renal vasodilator effect of D_1-like receptor stimulation in the SHR.[492] The increased vasodilatory effect of a D_3R/D_4R agonist (quinpirole) after renal denervation may also depend on decreased activity of the RAS).[593]

Activation of the RAS has been suggested to cause attenuation of the natriuretic effect of the D_1-like receptor agonist, fenoldopam, in sodium-deplete states.[427] When angiotensin II generation is inhibited or AT_1Rs are blocked, the natriuretic effect of dopaminergic drugs is enhanced.[490,491,492] In humans, this effect is seen mainly in subjects on a low salt diet (Natarajan et al., unpublished studies). D_1- and D_2-like receptor agonists also antagonize the stimulatory effect of angiotensin II, acting on AT_1R, on renal proximal tubule sodium transport.[45,397,493,494,589] These counterbalancing effects of dopamine and angiotensin II on sodium transport occur by the regulation of sodium transporter/channel/pump activity in the short-term, and the regulation of receptor expression in the long-term.[477,534,528] The short-term counteracting actions may occur by differential cell membrane trafficking. Thus, angiotensin II, via the AT_1R, in renal proximal tubule cells, induces recruitment of Na^+/K^+-ATPase to the plasma membrane. At an intracellular concentration of sodium of 9 mM, angiotensin II increases Na^+/K^+-ATPase activity[534]; dopamine is without effect. Increasing intracellular sodium to 19 mM is associated with an increasing inhibition of Na^+/K^+-ATPase activity by dopamine and blunting of the stimulatory effect of angiotensin II. This is associated with the recruitment of D_1R to the plasma membrane and a reduction in plasma membrane AT_1R.[534]

The mechanism by which dopamine receptors interact with the angiotensin receptors is receptor subtype-specific. The D_1R[45,343] and the D_3R[342] inhibit angiotensin II effects via physical interaction (heterodimerization) with the AT_1R. In contrast, the D_5R and AT_1R can also heterodimerize but negatively regulate each other's expression. In renal proximal tubule cells, the D_5R (not the D_1R) decreases AT_1R expression and AT_1R-mediated extracellular signal-regulated kinase phosphorylation. The D_1-like receptor-induced decrease in AT_1R expression is reversed by tyrosine-kinase inhibition and proteasome inhibitor, demonstrating that the D_5R-mediated decrease in total cell AT_1R expression is a result of a c-Src- and proteasome-dependent process.[45,46,276,567] Dopamine has also been reported to decrease AT_1R mRNA expression in renal proximal tubules.[594] The D_4R also negatively regulates AT_1R expression, but the mechanism remains to be determined.[26]

AT_2R and Dopamine Receptors

In the rat striatum, AT_2R stimulation decreases dopamine synthesis.[595] However, stimulation of D_1-like receptors induces an AT_2R-dependent natriuresis.[596] Selective intrarenal activation of D_1-like receptors induces sustained natriuresis and diuresis in sodium-loaded Sprague-Dawley rats that is abolished by intrarenal AT_2R inhibition. D_1-like receptor-mediated natriuresis is accompanied by recruitment of both D_1Rs and AT_2Rs to the plasma membrane of renal proximal tubular cells. These observations suggest that D_1-like receptor-induced natriuresis and diuresis are modulated by functional AT_2Rs that are translocated from intracellular compartments to the plasma membrane of renal proximal tubule cells in response to D_1-like receptor activation, and that dopamine-induced natriuresis requires AT_2R activation.[596] Therefore, in the normotensive state, dopaminergic stimulation favors natriuresis not only via specific dopamine receptor subtype mechanisms, but also by enhancing AT_2R function[596]; D_1R increases AT_2R expression. In addition, dopamine impairs AT_1R function by decreasing AT_1R expression via D_3R,[342] D_4R,[27] and D_5R,[46,276,567] and a negative interaction of AT_1R with D_1R,[45,343] D_3R, and D_5R.[46,276,567]

Atrial Natriuretic Peptide (ANP)

The inhibition of dopamine synthesis or uptake impairs the ability of ANP to inhibit renal tubular Na^+K^+-ATPase activity.[597] The inhibitory effect of ANP on NHE3 activity becomes manifest in the presence of dopamine.[598] However, the ability of carbidopa to affect sodium excretion or the natriuretic effect of ANP in humans has not been consistent.[599−603] This could be related to the state of hydration.[599−603] The renal dopaminergic system is not responsible for the natriuresis caused by marked volume expansion,[49,117] and dopamine does not affect sodium excretion in subjects fed a low salt diet[427] and may actually decrease sodium excretion during hypovolemia.[56] The natriuretic effects of dopamine and ANP are additive in humans.[604] Carbidopa or dopamine receptor blockade, especially by D_1-like receptor blocker, attenuates the natriuretic effect of ANP in rats[605–608] and the natriuretic effect of ANP is abolished in mice lacking *Ppp1r1b*, which is also involved in D_1R signaling.[224,225,288–293] The potentiation of the natriuretic effect of dopamine by ANP may be due to its ability to recruit D_1R to the plasma membrane.[609] The conflicting effects of carbidopa on the natriuretic effect of ANP may also be related to the fact that ANP can increase or decrease renal tubular dopamine synthesis.[597,610]

Cholecystokinin Receptors

There are two cholecystokinin receptors, namely, cholecystokinin type A receptor (CCKAR) and cholecystokinin type B receptor (CCKBR). Cholecystokinin modulates dopamine release in the nucleus accumbens through CCKAR. Cholecystokinin may also modulate D_2R expression in the nucleus accumbens; D_2R expression is higher in CCKAR$^{-/-}$ and lower in CCKBR$^{-/-}$ mice than in wild-type controls.[611] Also, activation of CCKBR reduces the affinity of the D_2R in the brain.[612,613] Cholecystokinin at low concentrations activates Na^+/K^+-ATPase activity via the CCKAR.[614] CCKBR is expressed in the kidney, and the postprandial increase in sodium excretion may be mediated by an increase in serum gastrin acting at CCKBR in the kidney to decrease Na^+/K^+-ATPase activity.[615]

Endothelin Receptors

There are two endothelin receptors, endothelin A receptor (ETAR) and endothelin B receptor (ETBR).[616] In the brain striatum, stimulation of the ETBR increases dopamine release, but dopamine does not increase endothelin-1 levels.[617] The ETB and dopamine receptors can interact to regulate renal function and blood pressure. Stimulation of the D_3R increases ETBR protein expression and D_3R/ETB receptor co-immunoprecipitation and co-localization in renal proximal tubules.[39,618] The interaction between D_3R and ETBR has physiological significance, because pretreatment with a D_3R agonist increases the ETBR-mediated inhibitory effect on Na^+/K^+-ATPase activity in renal proximal tubule cells from WKY rats.[39,618] Conversely, stimulation of ETBR increases D_3R expression and function in renal proximal tubule cells from WKY rats (unpublished data). The natriuretic effect of D_3R may be, in part, mediated by ETBR, because the natriuretic effect is attenuated in WKY rats when the renal ETBR is blocked.[39,618] In renal proximal tubule cells, the ability of D_3R to stimulate ETB expression is blocked by an L-type calcium channel blocker.[39]

The D_2R may also regulate ETB receptor expression. $D_2R^{-/-}$ mice have increased ETBR expression and an ETBR blocker normalized blood pressure in these mice, but did not affect blood pressure of D_2R wild-type littermates.[23] GPR37, a parkin-associated endothelin-like receptor, can associate with D_2R in HEK-293 cells.[619] In rat lactotrophs, D_2-like receptor stimulation antagonizes the ETAR-mediated activation of large-conductance K^+ channels.[620] The functional consequences of D_2R and ETBR interaction on renal ion transport remain to be determined.

Insulin and Insulin Receptors

Insulin and dopamine have opposite effects on Na^+/K^+-ATPase activity in renal proximal tubule cells, and may counter-regulate each other. Chronic exposure of renal proximal tubule cells to insulin causes a reduction in D_1R abundance and uncoupling from G-proteins, resulting in impairment of the inhibitory effect of dopamine on Na^+/K^+-ATPase.[621] This suggests a direct role of insulin in D_1R regulation.[495,622] Insulin causes renal D_1R desensitization via GRK2-mediated receptor phosphorylation (*vide infra*) involving PI3 kinase and PKC.[305] Hyperinsulinemic animals and patients with type 2 diabetes have a defective renal dopaminergic system.[623] In obese Zucker rats, a model of type 2 diabetes or in insulin-induced hypertension, renal D_1Rs are downregulated and dopamine fails to produce diuresis and natriuresis.[621] Treatment with an insulin sensitizer, rosiglitazone, decreases plasma insulin levels and restores D_1R function in obese Zucker rats.[622,624] Insulin has also been shown to increase the expression of the D_5R in renal proximal tubular cells from WKY rats, probably a compensatory response. In HEK293 cells heterologously expressing the D_5R, pretreatment with insulin increases the D_5R-mediated inhibition of Na^+/K^+-ATPase.[496] Both PKC and PI3 kinase are involved in the signaling pathway leading to increased D_5R expression.

Dopaminergic activity may influence insulin secretion, and *vice versa*. Insulin has been reported to increase renal proximal tubule uptake of L-DOPA, which should increase dopamine synthesis,[625] but this could be an attempt to compensate for the ability of insulin to decrease and uncouple D_1R.[621] The D_1-like receptor agonist fenoldopam improves peripheral insulin sensitivity and renal function in streptozotocin-induced type 2 diabetes in rats.[626] Normalizing blood sugar levels with insulin also normalizes renal D_1R expression and function in rats with sreptozotocin-induced diabetes.[627] D_2-like receptors in pancreatic β-cells inhibit[628] or stimulate glucose-stimulated insulin secretion, depending on dopamine concentration; an inhibitory effect occurs at higher dopamine concentration (10^{-7}–10^{-4} M), while the effect is stimulatory at lower dopamine concentrations ($<10^{-8}$ M).[629] Bromocriptine (D_2R/D_3R agonist) decreases insulin levels and ameliorates several metabolic features in obese women.[630] The counter-regulatory actions of the insulin and dopamine receptors extend to their effects on vascular proliferation. Bromocriptine (D_2R/D_3R agonist) inhibits the insulin-like growth factor-mediated proliferation in rat vascular smooth muscle cells (A7r5) and human aortic smooth muscle cells.[631] Stimulation of D_1-like receptors or D_3R inhibits insulin receptor expression and insulin-mediated proliferative effects in vascular smooth muscle cells, showing an interaction between dopamine (D_1-like and D_3R) and insulin receptors.[40,632] A D_3R antagonist was found to be protective of renal injury in hypertensive type II diabetic SHR/Ncp rats.[633] In these rats, a D_3R antagonist ameliorated glomerulosclerosis and prevented mesangial cell proliferation. These apparent contradictory interactions between D_3R and insulin may be related to the biphasic effect of dopamine on insulin secretion.

Dopamine and Mineralocorticoid Receptor

Aldosterone increases catecholamine production in a pheochromocytoma cell line.[634] In the rabbit cortical collecting duct D_2-like, but not D_1-like, receptor stimulation at the basolateral surface depolarizes transepithelial voltage and decreases sodium transport.[529] It is possible that this effect is related to D_4-like negative interaction with the non-genomic effects of aldosterone.[48]

Dopamine and Prolactin

D_2R inhibits prolactin secretion by the pituitary gland.[189,193] However, prolactin is also expressed in the renal cortex and induces a natriuresis that requires an intact renal dopaminergic system. Prolactin recruits D_1Rs to the plasma membrane in renal proximal tubules which inhibits Na^+K^+-ATPase activity that involves activation of PKA, PKC, and PI-3 kinase.[42]

Dopamine and Prostaglandins

Earlier studies have suggested that the renal vasodilatory effect of dopamine is independent of prostaglandins because indomethacin, an inhibitor of prostaglandin synthase, did not affect the renal vasodilatory effect of dopamine or the D_1-like receptor agonist fenoldopam in the dog, rat[635] or humans.[636] The intrarenal arterial infusion of the D_1-like receptor agonist fenoldopam is also not associated with an increase in urinary prostaglandin E2 (PGE2) and $F_2\alpha$ in the dog.[396] Subsequent studies in normotensive humans revealed that the renal vasodilatory effect of dopamine was also not associated with an increase in urinary excretion of PGE2, but rather with 6-keto-PGF1α, a stable metabolite of prostacyclin. The effect of dopamine was blocked by metoclopramide or domperidone, D_2-like receptor antagonists, and two cyclooxygenase inhibitors.[407] These studies suggest that the dopamine and prostaglandin communication is via the D_2-like rather than D_1-like receptors. D_2-like but not D_1-like receptors may also regulate PGE2 synthesis in rat inner medullary collecting cells.[358] Dopamine stimulates medullary prostaglandin production, and may be involved in the attenuation of deoxycorticosterone acetate/high salt-induced increase in blood pressure.[37] Eicosanoids may act synergistically with D_1-like receptors to inhibit Na^+/K^+-ATPase activity in the proximal tubule, mTAL, and cortical collecting duct.[38,524,530,539,541] Moreover, the renal cortical expression of COX-2 is tonically suppressed by the renal D_1-like receptors secondary to inhibition of proximal tubular reabsorption.[44,637]

Regulation of Reactive Oxygen Species (ROS)

Dopamine regulates ROS production, stimulating production at high concentrations ($\geq 10\,\mu M$) but physiological concentrations of dopamine decrease ROS production via D_1-like receptors.[233,638,639] All the dopamine receptor subtypes are capable of decreasing ROS production. However, deletion of $Drd2$ or $Drd5$ but not $Drd3$ or $Drd4$ in mice is associated with increased ROS production. The D_1R inhibits NADPH oxidase activity via PKA and PKC cross-talk[239]; the D_5R inhibits NADPH oxidase directly and also indirectly, by inhibiting phospholipase D activity and independent of cAMP.[232,234] The D_5R may also positively regulate antioxidants such as heme oxygenase 1 (HO-1).[640] Plasma thiobarbituric acid-reactive substances (TBARS), an index of systemic oxidative stress, and PLD and NADPH oxidase subunit expression and activity are higher in $D_5R^{-/-}$ mice than in $D_5R^{+/+}$ mice[232,234] (Table 19.2). Chronic administration of apocynin, an NADPH inhibitor, normalizes blood pressure, plasma TBARs, and NADPH oxidase activity in the brain and kidney of $D_5R^{-/-}$ mice, suggesting that the D_5R keeps blood pressure in the normal range by preventing excessive ROS production.[234] The redox status of the $D_1R^{-/-}$ mice remains to be determined. ROS impair the function of renal D_1-like receptor. Rat renal proximal tubules treated with hydrogen peroxide, and those from streptozotocin-treated or old rats, have increased oxidative stress and impaired D_1-like receptor function.[449,641–643] Oxidative stress causes the nuclear translocation of NFκB and subsequent activation of PKC and GRK2, which in turn increases D_1R phosphorylation, impairing its activity.[641,642]

The D_2R has also antioxidant activity. The neuroprotective effect of D_2R may be related to its ability to decrease ROS production by the mitochondria.[644] D_2R, similar to the D_1-like receptors, decreases oxidative stress by inhibition of NADPH oxidase and stimulation of HO-2,[47] $D_2^{-/-}$ mice are hypertensive and have increased urinary excretion of 8-isoprostane, a parameter of oxidative stress, as well as increased activity and expression of NADPH oxidase and decreased expression of the antioxidant enzyme HO-2 in the kidney. Apocynin (an NADPH inhibitor) or hemin (an inducer of HO) normalizes blood pressure in $D_2^{-/-}$ mice. Spironolactone normalizes the blood pressure in $D_2^{-/-}$ mice, but does not normalize the renal expression of NADPH oxidase, indicating that the increased ROS production is proximal to the increased aldosterone secretion in $D_2^{-/-}$ mice.[47]

The effect of D_3R receptors on ROS production is controversial. The D_3R has been reported to increase a dopamine autotrophic factor that has an antioxidant action, and thus the D_3R has antioxidant effect, albeit indirectly.[645] The selective D_3R agonist pramipexole inhibits lipid peroxidation,[646] increases the activity of antioxidant enzymes (glutathione peroxidase and catalase), and inhibits the production of ROS by the mitochondria, but this effect is not related to its dopamine agonist properties.[647] Moreover, the D_3R has been reported to stimulate PLD activity in HEK293 cells heterologously expressing the human D_3R.[235] The D_3R and D_4R may also have neuroprotective effects by inhibition of ROS production.[648,649]

Regulation of Inflammation

Lymphocytes can synthesize catecholamines, including dopamine.[650] All the dopamine receptor subtypes are expressed in normal human leukocytes, with the highest expression in B-lymphocytes and natural killer cells, followed by neutrophils and eosinophils, with least expression in T-lymphocytes and monocytes.[650–653] Dopamine, D_1- and D_2-like receptor subtype agonists can regulate the immune response and inhibit the inflammatory reaction,[654–657] the extent of their involvement is tissue-dependent. Dopamine inhibits the release of pro-inflammatory cytokines (e.g., interleukin-2 (IL-2), interferon (IFN)γ, IL-4,[657] but stimulates the production of the anti-inflammatory IL-10 in immune cells.[658] The D_1-like receptors and D_3R but not D_2R or D_4R can also stimulate TNFα secretion.[658] Indeed, the D_2R may actually decrease lipopolysaccharide-induced release of TNFα.[659] Dopamine or bromocriptine (D_2R/D_3R agonist), inhibits lymphocyte proliferation,[660] decreases the antigen-induced macrophage activation and the secretion of IL-2, IL-4 and IFNγ.[661]

Renal tubule cells produce pro-inflammatory cytokines and chemokines (e.g., IL-1, TNFα, IL-6, IL-8, IL-12, and macrophage chemoattractant protein (MCP)-1), as well as anti-inflammatory cytokines (e.g., IL-10).[662–664] Both pro-inflammatory and anti-inflammatory cytokines are secreted by tubular cells across their apical or basolateral membranes.[664] The pro-inflammatory cytokines contribute to the development and progression of glomerular and tubular injury.[662–664] Lipopolysaccharide causes dysfunction of renal D_1R and salt-sensitive hypertension,[665] but the D_2R may protect the kidney from the adverse effects of inflammation.[666] Silencing the D_2R in renal proximal tubule cells increases the expression of TNFα and MCP-1; expression of TNFα, MCP-1, IL-6, and IL-10 are increased in the renal cortex of $D_2^{-/-}$ mice. These mice show renal injury and increased urinary albumin, suggesting that impaired D_2R function results in renal inflammation and injury.[666] The role of the other dopamine receptor subtypes in inflammation remains to be determined.

Dopamine and Essential Hypertension

About 50% of human essential hypertension is thought to be heritable, but the genetic causes of essential hypertension have been difficult to identify.[667] More than one gene is undoubtedly involved, because Mendelian dominant and recessive traits are not readily discernible in hypertensive subjects, except in those with monogenic forms of hypertension. Indeed, recent genome-wide association studies (GWAS) have been able to identify 2% of genetic factors believed to influence blood pressure.[668–674] However, the GWAS were not designed to identify predisposing genes engaged in a complex network of gene–gene and gene/environment interactions.[675] One example is salt sensitivity, a dietary sodium-induced increase in blood pressure that may or may not produce elevation in the hypertensive range. Several criteria have been suggested to link gene (s) to complex diseases such as hypertension and salt sensitivity, but the definitive evidence is swapping one phenotype for another (i.e., transgenic studies).[676] Many genes have been proposed to be causal of hypertension; however, their gene variants, including those identified in the GWAS, have not been shown to produce hypertension in mice. Many gene overexpression and deletion studies are performed in mice without taking into account the salt sensitivity of the strain. C57BL/6 mice from Jackson Laboratories have an impaired ability to excrete a salt (NaCl) load with a resultant increase in blood pressure, while others are salt-resistant (e.g., SJL mice).[153]

GRK4 regulates renal D_1R[298] and D_3R.[286] Renal D_1-like receptor function is impaired in C57BL/6 Jackson mice, and is associated with increased expression of GRK4 upon salt loading.[153] Deletion of the *Grk4* gene in C57BL/6 mice prevents the development of salt-sensitive hypertension.[677] Renal cortical silencing of *Grk4* attenuates the increase in blood pressure with age in SHRs, but not in normotensive WKY rats.[306] Aging and obesity are associated with decreased D_1-like receptor dysfunction.[100,532,542] In obese rats, the D_1-like receptor dysfunction is acquired and has been related to increased GRK4 expression and membrane translocation of GRK2 due to insulin resistance.[624]

The GRK4 locus on human chromosome 4p16.3 is linked with hypertension.[678,679] Interestingly, adolescents with GRK4 65L, 142V, and A486 haplotype have a greater increase in blood pressure with age than those with the wild-type GRK4 haplotype.[680] GRK4 gene variants (65L, 142V, and 486V) are associated with essential hypertension in several ethnic groups: Caucasians, Chinese, Ghanaians, and Japanese.[681-686] In salt-sensitive hypertensive Japanese, the presence of three GRK4 variants impaired the natriuretic effect of a dopaminergic drug and predicted salt-sensitive hypertension correctly in 94% of cases.[683] In Ghanaians, the combination of angiotensin-converting enzyme insertion/deletion polymorphism and GRK4 65L has an estimated predictive accuracy for hypertension of 70%.[685,686] A meta-analysis revealed a significant association of GRK4 486V with hypertension with an odds ratio of 1.5 (95% CI: 1.2 to 1.9).[687] A re-analysis of a negative study in Han Chinese[688] found an association of GRK4 486V and other genes (GNB3A-350G) with essential hypertension.[682] One study, however, did not find an association of GRK4 486V with the top fifth percentile of diastolic blood pressure of subjects with white European ancestry; however, the authors did not test the association of GRK4 gene variants with hypertension.[689] Another study did not find an association between GRK4 142V and hypertension, but did find an association between variants of the promoter region of D_1R and hypertension.[690] The discordance of this report in European Caucasians[690] with other populations may be the influence of ethnicity in the phenotypic expression of a quantitative trait such as essential hypertension. Interestingly, low-renin hypertension is less frequent in Caucasians (15–20%)[708] than in other ethic groups (e.g., 40–60% in Japanese).[709] In the Japanese, the single best genetic model for low-renin hypertension

included only GRK4 A142V, by itself, or GRK4 A142V and aldosterone synthase gene, CYP11B2, with an estimated predictive accuracy of 78%.[683] Ethnicity may also explain some of the discordances. GRK4 65L and GRK4 142V are less frequent, while GRK4 486V is more frequent in Asians than in African-Americans. GRK4 486V is also more frequent in Hispanic and non-Hispanic whites than in African-Americans.[710] The recent GWAS did not identify GRK4 as associated with hypertension.[669-673] This is probably because salt sensitivity was not taken into account and because previous studies have shown that it was critical to assess the role of GRK4 in conjunction with other single nucleotide polymorphisms and genes, e.g., ACE with GRK4 65L,[685,686] and *ADRB2* and *TH* with *GRK4 486V*.[682] While GRK4γ142V transgenic mice are hypertensive even on a normal salt diet,[298,691] GRK4γ486V transgenic mice develop hypertension only when stressed by a high salt diet.[692] Depending upon the genetic background of the mouse, overexpression of human GRK4γ wild-type converts a salt-sensitive phenotype to a salt-resistant phenotype, while overexpression of human GRK4γ486V converts a salt-resistant phenotype to a salt-sensitive phenotype.[692]

Polymorphisms in the non-coding region of the human D_1R gene are associated with decreased[690,693] and increased blood pressure.[694] However, D_1R and D_3R expression is not always decreased in hypertension.[29,30,141,298,343,426,695] Polymorphisms in the coding region of D_1R and D_3R genes[690,694,696] have also not been associated with essential hypertension. A D_2R variant may be associated with salt-sensitive human essential hypertension (unpublished studies). The D_4R long (at least one 7 to 10 repeat) has been reported to be associated with higher diastolic and systolic blood pressure.[697] There are inactivating mutations of D_5R,[698] but their association with hypertension has not been studied. D_1-like and D_2-like receptor functions are impaired in other rodent models of human essential hypertension, such as in the spontaneously hypertensive rat (SHR) and the Dahl salt-sensitive rat (DSS). As indicated earlier, deletion of any of the dopamine receptor genes causes hypertension,[22-27] and dopamine receptor dysfunction is found in several animal models of hypertension.[29,30]

Dopamine and Blood Pressure Regulation: Peripheral versus Central Nervous System

The effect of dopamine in the regulation of blood pressure differs in the kidney from that in the central nervous system. Overactivity of the dopaminergic system in the brain, e.g., the amygdala, is associated with hypertension.[699] Hypertension induced in rats by decreasing blood flow to one kidney is also associated with increased levels of dopamine and dopamine metabolites in the brain striatum.[700] However, monkeys made hypertensive by constricting the aorta have decreased D_1-like receptor binding in the pre-frontal cortex,[701] and decreased post-synaptic dopaminergic and cholinergic functions in the ventrolateral striatum of SHR,[702] reinforcing the similarities and differences in the regulation of blood pressure between the dopaminergic system inside and outside the central nervous system.

Dopamine Pharmacogenetics and Hypertension

Current treatment of essential hypertension is empirical. It is not based on the molecular mechanisms of essential hypertension. Theoretically, drugs prescribed based on one's genetic make-up would be more effective, with fewer and lesser side-effects than empirical treatment. In African-American men with early hypertensive nephrosclerosis, GRK4 65L and 142V are associated with a poor response to β-adrenergic blockers, while GRK4 142V is associated with a good response to a β-adrenergic blocker.[703] In another study in two cohorts, GRK4 142V, but not GRK4 486V, was also associated with a blood pressure response to a β-adrenergic blocker.[704] There are at least two mechanisms by which β-adrenergic blockers may be beneficial in hypertensive subjects with GRK4 142V polymorphisms. The activity of GRK4, which decreases plasma membrane β-adrenergic receptor expression, can be blocked by β-adrenergic receptor antagonists.[705] As indicated above, normally the D_3R may be important in the negative regulation of renin secretion, at least in mice,[25] and because GRK4 142V can impair D_3R function, this may provide an explanation for the good response of subjects to β-adrenergic blockers. In an African hypertensive population, GRK4 142V is associated with a poor response to reduction in sodium intake,[706] in agreement with the report that human GRK4142V transgenic mice develop hypertension even on a normal salt intake.[298,691] In a Japanese population with essential hypertension (n = 881, unpublished data), carriers of the GRK4 142V allele had a larger drop in systolic blood pressure than non-carriers in response to angiotensin receptor blockade.[707] The addition of a diuretic to the non-responders (n = 94) decreased blood pressure which was associated with GRK4A486V,[707] in agreement with the reports that human GRK4γ 486V transgenic mice develop salt sensitivity that is dependent on genetic background.[692] Japanese with at least three GRK4 polymorphisms have salt-sensitive hypertension.[683]

CONCLUSION

Dopamine, one of the oldest hormones in phylogeny, serves not only as a precursor to norepinephrine and epinephrine, but also as a neurotransmitter. However, in non-neural cells, dopamine acts independently of the other catecholamines. Dopamine controls water and electrolyte balance and blood pressure by regulating the secretion/release of hormones and humoral agents that affect water and electrolyte balance, salt "appetite" centers in the brain, and ion and water transport in the kidney and gastrointestinal tract. Independent of innervation, the kidney and intestines synthesize dopamine from circulating or filtered L-DOPA (kidney only) that is not metabolized to norepinephrine or epinephrine. Sodium intake and intracellular sodium are probably the major determinants of the renal tubular synthesis/release of dopamine. In mammals, the actions of dopamine occur by occupation of two families of cell surface receptors, D_1-like receptors (D_1R and D_5R), and D_2-like receptors (D_2R, D_3R, and D_4R). The dopamine receptor subtypes interact among themselves, resulting in new signaling pathways. They also interact extensively with other GPCR, hormones, and humoral agents. D_1-like receptors are linked to vasodilation, while the effect of D_2-like receptors on the renal vasculature is probably dependent upon the state of renal nerve activity. The dopamine-induced increase in renal blood flow is not consistently associated with an increase in glomerular filtration rate. The autocrine/paracrine regulation of renal tubular sodium transport, mainly via D_1-like receptors, is mediated by tubular and not by hemodynamic mechanisms. The dopamine receptor subtypes are differentially expressed along the nephron and species-specific; all the five dopamine receptor subtypes are expressed in the proximal tubule, mTAL distal convoluted tubule, and cortical collecting duct, and only D_4R in the cortical TAL, D_1R, D_2R, D_4R, and D_5R in the outer medullary collecting duct, and only the D_2-like receptors, D_2R, D_3R, and D_4R in the inner medullary collecting duct. Dopamine inhibits ion transport in the proximal and distal nephron. D_1-like receptors inhibit NHE3, NaPi2 co-transporter, Cl^-/HCO_3^- exchanger, and ENaC at the apical membrane, and the electrogenic Na^+/HCO_3^- co-transporter and Na^+/K^+-ATPase at the basolateral membrane. Dopamine may also inhibit NCC but stimulates NKCC2, the latter effect for K^+ recycling. The inhibitory effects of dopamine and its receptors on ion transport are important under conditions of euvolemia and moderate volume expansion, but play a minor role under marked volume expansion. D_2-like receptors also participate in the inhibition of ion transport during conditions of euvolemia and moderate volume expansion, but may increase ion transport in hypovolemic states. Dopamine also controls sodium transport and blood pressure by regulating the production of ROS and the inflammatory response. Aging, obesity, metabolic syndrome, and essential hypertension are associated with abnormalities in dopamine production, and receptor number, post-translational modification, and function.

Acknowledgment

This work was supported in part by grants from the National Institutes of Health, HL023081, DK039308, HL074940, HL068686, and HL092196.

References

[1] Walker RJ, Brooks HL, Holden-Dye L. Evolution and overview of classical transmitter molecules and their receptors. Parasitology 1996;113(Suppl.):S3–33.

[2] Stefano GB, Kream RM. Endogenous morphine synthetic pathway preceded and gave rise to catecholamine synthesis in evolution (Review). Int J Mol Med 2007;20(6):837–41.

[3] Shepherd DM, West GB. Hydroxytyramine and the adrenal medulla. J Physiol 1953;120(1-2):15–9.

[4] Carlsson A, Lindqvist M, Magnusson T, Waldeck B. On the presence of 3-hydroxy-tyramine in brain. Science 1958; 127(3296):471.

[5] Holtz P, Credner K, Koepp W. Die enzymatische entstehung von oxytyramin im organismus und die physiologische bedeutung der dopadecarboxylase. Naunyn Schmiedebergs Arch Exp Pathol Pharmakol 1942;200(2-5):356–88.

[6] Hornykiewicz O. The action of dopamine on the arterial blood pressure of the guinea-pig. Br J Pharmacol 1958;13(1):91–4.

[7] Goldberg LI, Sjoerdsma A. Effects of several monoamine oxidase inhibitors on the cardiovascular actions of naturally occurring amines in the dog. J Pharmacol Exp Ther 1959;127(3):212–8.

[8] Goldberg LI, Horwitz D, Sjoerdsma A. Attenuation of cardiovascular responses to exercise as a possible basis for effectiveness of monoamine oxidase inhibitors in angina pectoris. J Pharmacol Exp Ther 1962;137(1):39–46.

[9] McDonald Jr RH, Goldberg LI, McNay JL, Tuttle Jr EP. Effects of dopamine in man: augmentation of sodium excretion, glomerular filtration rate and renal plasma flow. J Clin Invest 1964;43(6):1116–24.

[10] Lokhandwala MF, Buckley JP. Presynaptic dopamine receptors as mediators of dopamine-induced inhibition of neurogenic vasoconstriction. Eur J Pharmacol 1977;45(3):305–9.

[11] Morgunov N, Baines AD. Renal nerves and catecholamine excretion. Am J Physiol 1981;240(1):F75–81.

[12] Murthy VV, Gilbert JC, Goldberg LI, Kuo JF. Dopamine-sensitive adenylate cyclase in canine renal artery. J Pharm Pharmacol 1976;28(7):567–71.

[13] Nakajima T, Naitoh F, Kuruma I. Dopamine-sensitive adenylate cyclase in the rat kidney particulate preparation. Eur J Pharmacol 1977;41(2):163–9.

[14] Nakajima T, Kuruma I. Characterization with 3H-haloperidol of the dopamine receptor in the rat kidney particulate preparation. Jpn J Pharmacol 1980;30(6):891–8.

[15] Felder RA, Blecher M, Eisner GM, Jose PA. Cortical tubular and glomerular dopamine receptors in the rat kidney. Am J Physiol 1984;246(5 Pt 2):F557–68.

[16] Bello-Reuss E, Higashi Y, Kaneda Y. Dopamine decreases fluid reabsorption in straight portions of rabbit proximal tubule. Am J Physiol 1982;242(6):F634–40.

[17] Aperia A, Bertorello A, Seri I. Dopamine causes inhibition of Na^+-K^+-ATPase activity in rat proximal convoluted tubule segments. Am J Physiol 1987;252(1 Pt 2):F39–45.

[18] Siragy HM, Felder RA, Howell NE, Chevalier RL, Peach MJ, Carey RM. Intrarenal dopamine acts at the dopamine-1 receptor to control renal function. J Hypertens Suppl 1988;6(4):S479–81.

[19] Felder RA, Robillard J, Eisner GM, Jose PA. Role of endogenous dopamine on renal sodium excretion. Semin Nephrol 1989; 9(1):91–3.

[20] Hegde SS, Jadhav AL, Lokhandwala MF. Role of kidney dopamine in the natriuretic response to volume expansion in rats. Hypertension 1989;13(6 Pt 2):828–34.

[21] Felder RA, Seikaly MG, Cody P, Eisner GM, Jose PA. Attenuated renal response to dopaminergic drugs in spontaneously hypertensive rats. Hypertension 1990;15(6 Pt 1):560–9.

[22] Albrecht FE, Drago J, Felder RA, Printz MP, Eisner GM, Robillard JE, et al. Role of the D_{1A} dopamine receptor in the pathogenesis of genetic hypertension. J Clin Invest 1996;97 (10):2283–8 Erratum in: J Clin Invest 1996;97(12):following 2925

[23] Li XX, Bek M, Asico LD, Yang Z, Grandy DK, Goldstein DS, et al. Adrenergic and endothelin B receptor-dependent hypertension in dopamine receptor type-2 knockout mice. Hypertension 2001;38 (3):303–8.

[24] Ueda A, Ozono R, Oshima T, Yano A, Kambe M, Teransihi Y, et al. Disruption of the type 2 dopamine receptor gene causes a sodium-dependent increase in blood pressure in mice. Am J Hypertens 2003;16(10):853–8.

[25] Asico LD, Ladines C, Fuchs S, Accili D, Carey RM, Semeraro C, et al. Disruption of the dopamine D3 receptor gene produces renin-dependent hypertension. J Clin Invest 1998;102(3):493–8.

[26] Bek MJ, Wang X, Asico LD, Jones JE, Zheng S, Li X, et al. Angiotensin-II type 1 receptor-mediated hypertension in D4 dopamine receptor-deficient mice. Hypertension 2006;47 (2):288–95 Erratum in: Hypertension. 2006;47(5):e[23]

[27] Hollon TR, Bek MJ, Lachowicz JE, et al. Mice lacking D5 dopamine receptors have increased sympathetic tone and are hypertensive. J Neurosci 2002;22(24):10801–10.

[28] Aperia AC. Intrarenal dopamine: a key signal in the interactive regulation of sodium metabolism. Annu Rev Physiol 2000;62:621–47.

[29] Banday AA, Lokhandwala MF. Dopamine receptors and hypertension. Curr Hypertens Rep 2008;10(4):268–75.

[30] Zeng C, Armando I, Luo Y, Eisner GM, Felder RA, Jose PA. Dysregulation of dopamine-dependent mechanisms as a determinant of hypertension: studies in dopamine receptor knockout mice. Am J Physiol Heart Circ Physiol 2008;294(2):H551–69.

[31] Wang ZQ, Siragy HM, Felder RA, Carey RM. Intrarenal dopamine production and distribution in the rat. Physiological control of sodium excretion. Hypertension 1997;29(1 Pt 2):228–34.

[32] Lucas-Teixeira VA, Hussain T, Serrão P, Soares-da-Silva P, Lokhandwala MF. Intestinal dopaminergic activity in obese and lean Zucker rats: response to high salt intake. Clin Exp Hypertens 2002;24(5):383–96.

[33] List SJ, Seeman P. [3H]dopamine labeling of D3 dopaminergic sites in human, rat, and calf brain. J Neurochem 1982;39(5):1363–73.

[34] Sunahara RK, Guan HC, O'Dowd BF, Seeman P, Laurier LG, Ng G, et al. Cloning of the gene for a human dopamine D5 receptor with higher affinity for dopamine than D1. Nature 1991;350(6319):614–9.

[35] Fulton S. Appetite and reward. Front Neuroendocrinol. 2010;31 (1):85–103.

[36] Citarella MR, Choi MR, Gironacci MM, Medici C, Correa AH, Fernández BE. Urodilatin and dopamine: a new interaction in the kidney. Regul Pept 2009;153(1-3):19–24.

[37] Yao B, Harris RC, Zhang MZ. Intrarenal dopamine attenuates deoxycorticosterone acetate/high salt-induced blood pressure elevation in part through activation of a medullary cyclooxygenase 2 pathway. Hypertension 2009;54(5):1077–83.

[38] Kirchheimer C, Mendez CF, Acquier A, Nowicki S. Role of 20-HETE in D1/D2 dopamine receptor synergism resulting in the inhibition of Na^+-K^+-ATPase activity in the proximal tubule. Am J Physiol Renal Physiol 2007;292(5):F1435–42.

[39] Yu C, Yang Z, Ren H, et al. D3 dopamine receptor regulation of ETB receptors in renal proximal tubule cells from WKY and SHRs. Am J Hypertens 2009;22(8):877–83.

[40] Venkatakrishnan U, Chen C, Lokhandwala MF. The role of intrarenal nitric oxide in the natriuretic response to dopamine-receptor activation. Clin Exp Hypertens 2000;22(3):309–24.

[41] Crambert S, Sjöberg A, Eklöf AC, Ibarra F, Holtbäck U. Prolactin and dopamine 1-like receptor interaction in renal proximal tubular cells. Am J Physiol Renal Physiol 2010;299(1):F49–54.

[42] Padia SH, Kemp BA, Howell NL, Fournie-Zaluski MC, Roques BP, Carey RM. Conversion of renal angiotensin II to angiotensin III is critical for AT2 receptor-mediated natriuresis in rats. Hypertension 2008;51(2):460–5.

[43] Muhammad AB, Lokhandwala MF, Banday AA. Exercise reduces oxidative stress but does not alleviate hyperinsulinemia or renal dopamine D1 receptor dysfunction in obese rats. Am J Physiol Renal Physiol 2011;300(1):F98–104.

[44] Zhang MZ, Yao B, Fang X, Wang S, Smith JP, Harris RC. Intrarenal dopaminergic system regulates renin expression. Hypertension 2009;53(3):564–70.

[45] Khan F, Spicarová Z, Zelenin S, Holtbäck U, Scott L, Aperia A. Negative reciprocity between angiotensin II type 1 and dopamine D1 receptors in rat renal proximal tubule cells. Am J Physiol Renal Physiol 2008;295(4):F1110–6.

[46] Li H, Armando I, Yu P, et al. Dopamine 5 receptor mediates Ang II type 1 receptor degradation via a ubiquitin-proteasome pathway in mice and human cells. J Clin Invest 2008;118(6):2180–9 Erratum in:* J Clin Invest. 2008 Aug;118(8):2986 Gildea, John J [added].

[47] Armando I, Wang X, Villar VA, Jones JE, Asico LD, Escano C, et al. Reactive oxygen species-dependent hypertension in dopamine D2 receptor-deficient mice. Hypertension 2007;49(3):672–8.

[48] Schafer JA, Li L, Sun D. The collecting duct, dopamine and vasopressin-dependent hypertension. Acta Physiol Scand 2000;168(1):239–44.

[49] Hansell P, Fasching A. The effect of dopamine receptor blockade on natriuresis is dependent on the degree of hypervolemia. Kidney Int 1991;39(2):253–8.

[50] Faucheux B, Buu NT, Kuchel O. Effects of saline and albumin on plasma and urinary catecholamines in dogs. Am J Physiol 1977;232(2):F123–7.

[51] Angchanpen P, Marin-Grez M, Schnermann J. Effect of dopamine antagonists on the urine flow of rats infused with hypotonic saline. Br J Pharmacol 1988;93(1):151–5.

[52] De Luca Sarobe V, Nowicki S, Carranza A, Levin G, Barontini M, Arrizurieta E, et al. Low sodium intake induces an increase in renal monoamine oxidase activity in the rat. Involvement of an angiotensin II dependent mechanism. Acta Physiol Scand 2005;185(2):161–7.

[53] Goldstein DS, Stull R, Eisenhofer G, Gill Jr JR. Urinary excretion of dihydroxyphenylalanine and dopamine during alterations of dietary salt intake in humans. Clin Sci (Lond) 1989;76(5):517–22.

[54] Carey RM, Van Loon GR, Baines AD, Ortt EM. Decreased plasma and urinary dopamine during dietary sodium depletion in man. J Clin Endocrinol Metab 1981;52(5):903–9.

[55] Choi MR, Lee BM, Medici C, Correa AH, Fernández BE. Effects of angiotensin II on renal dopamine metabolism: synthesis, release, catabolism and turnover. Nephron Physiol 2010;115(1):1–7.

[56] Agnoli GC, Cacciari M, Garutti C, Ikonomu E, Lenzi P, Marchetti G. Effects of extracellular fluid volume changes on renal response to low-dose dopamine infusion in normal women. Clin Physiol 1987;7(6):465–79.

[57] Puyó AM, Levin GM, Armando I, Barontini MB. Free and conjugated plasma catecholamines in pheochromocytoma patients with and without sustained hypertension. Acta Endocrinol (Copenh) 1996;113(1):111–7.

[58] Alexander RW, Gill Jr JR, Yamabe H, Lovenberg W, Keiser HR. Effects of dietary sodium and of acute saline infusion on the interrelationship between dopamine excretion and adrenergic activity in man. J Clin Invest 1974;54(1):194–200.

[59] Chen N, Reith ME. Interaction between dopamine and its transporter: role of intracellular sodium ions and membrane potential. J Neurochem 2004;89(3):750–65.

[60] Maurel A, Spreux-Varoquaux O, Amenta F, Tayebati SK, Tomassoni D, Sequelas MH, et al. Vesicular monoamine transporter 1 mediates dopamine secretion in rat proximal tubular cells. Am J Physiol Renal Physiol 2007;292(5):F1592–8.

[61] Pinho MJ, Serrão MP, Soares-da-Silva P. High-salt intake and the renal expression of amino acid transporters in spontaneously hypertensive rats. Am J Physiol Renal Physiol 2007;292(5):F1452–63.

[62] Baines AD. Effects of salt intake and renal denervation on catecholamine catabolism and excretion. Kidney Int 1982;21(2):316–22.

[63] Grossman E, Hoffman A, Tamrat M, Armando I, Keiser HR, Goldstein DS. Endogenous dopa and dopamine responses to dietary salt loading in salt-sensitive rats. J Hypertens 1991;9(3):259–63.

[64] Unger T, Buu NT, Kuchel O, Schürch W. Conjugated dopamine: peripheral origin, distribution, and response to acute stress in the dog. Can J Physiol Pharmacol 1980;58(1):22–7.

[65] Morgunov N, Baines AD. Vagal afferent activity and renal nerve release of dopamine. Can J Physiol Pharmacol 1985;63(6):636–41.

[66] Dinerstein RJ, Vannice J, Henderson RC, Roth LJ, Goldberg LI, Hoffmann PC. Histofluorescence techniques provide evidence for dopamine-containing neuronal elements in canine kidney. Science 1979;205(4405):497–9.

[67] Jose PA, Felder RA, Holloway RR, Eisner GM. Dopamine receptors modulate sodium excretion in denervated kidney. Am J Physiol 1986;250(6 Pt 2):F1033–8.

[68] Bertorello A, Hökfelt T, Goldstein M, Aperia A. Proximal tubule Na^+-K^+-ATPase activity is inhibited during high-salt diet: evidence for DA-mediated effect. Am J Physiol 1988;254(6 Pt 2):F795–801.

[69] Kokkinou I, Nikolouzou E, Hatzimanolis A, Fragoulis EG, Vassilacopoulou D. Expression of enzymatically active L-DOPA decarboxylase in human peripheral leukocytes. Blood Cells Mol Dis 2009;42(1):92–8.

[70] Soares Da Silva P, Pestana M, Fernandes MH. Involvement of tubular sodium in the formation of dopamine in the human renal cortex. J Am Soc Nephrol 1993;3(9):1591–9.

[71] López-Contreras AJ, Galindo JD, López-García C, Castells MT, Cremades A, Peñafiel R. Opposite sexual dimorphism of 3,4-

dihydroxyphenylalanine decarboxylase in the kidney and small intestine of mice. J Endocrinol 2008;196(3):615–24.

[72] Kubovcakova L, Krizanova O, Kvetnansky R. Identification of the aromatic L-amino acid decarboxylase gene expression in various mice tissues and its modulation by immobilization stress in stellate ganglia. Neuroscience 2004;126 (2):375–80.

[73] Borelli MI, Villar MJ, Orezzoli A, Gagliardino JJ. Presence of DOPA decarboxylase and its localisation in adult rat pancreatic islet cells. Diabetes Metab 1997;23(2):161–3.

[74] Maayan ML, Sellitto RV, Volpert EM. Dopamine and L-dopa: inhibition of thyrotropin-stimulated thyroidal thyroxine release. Endocrinology 1986;118(2):632–6.

[75] Grossman E, Hoffman A, Armando I, Abassi Z, Kopin IJ, Goldstein DS. Sympathoadrenal contribution to plasma dopa (3,4-dihydroxyphenylalanine) in rats. Clin Sci (Lond) 1992; 83(1):65–74.

[76] Goldstein DS, Udelsman R, Eisenhofer G, Stull R, Keiser HR, Kopin IJ. Neuronal source of plasma dihydroxyphenylalanine. J Clin Endocrinol Metab 1987;64(4):856–61.

[77] Goldstein DS, Polinsky RJ, Garty M, Robertson D, Brown RT, Biaggioni I, et al. Patterns of plasma levels of catechols in neurogenic orthostatic hypotension. Ann Neurol 1989;26 (4):558–63.

[78] Esplugues JV, Caramona MM, Moura D, Soares-da-Silva P. Effects of chemical sympathectomy on dopamine and noradrenaline content of the dog gastrointestinal tract. Auton Pharmacol 1985;5(3):189–95.

[79] Goldstein DS, Swoboda KJ, Miles JM, Coppack SW, Aneman A, Holmes C, et al. Sources and physiological significance of plasma dopamine sulfate. J Clin Endocrinol Metab 1999; 84(7):2523–31.

[80] Eldrup E, Moller SE, Andreasen J, Christensen NJ. Effects of ordinary meals on plasma concentrations of 3,4-dihydroxyphenylalanine, dopamine sulphate and 3,4-dihydroxyphenylacetic acid. Clin Sci (Lond) 1997;92(4):423–30.

[81] Eisenhofer G, Coughtrie MW, Goldstein DS. Dopamine sulphate: an enigma resolved. Clin Exp Pharmacol Physiol Suppl 1999;26:S41–53.

[82] Banwart B, Miller TD, Jones JD, Tyce GM. Plasma dopa and feeding. Proc Soc Exp Biol Med 1989;191(4):357–61.

[83] Williams M, Young JB, Rosa RM, Gunn S, Epstein FH, Landsberg L. Effect of protein ingestion on urinary dopamine excretion. Evidence for the functional importance of renal decarboxylation of circulating 3,4-dihydroxyphenylalanine in man. J Clin Invest 1986;78(6):1687–93.

[84] Rios M, Habecker B, Sasaoka T, Eisenhofer G, Tian H, Landis S, et al. Catecholamine synthesis is mediated by tyrosinase in the absence of tyrosine hydroxylase. J Neurosci 1999; 19(9):3519–26.

[85] Ibarra FR, Aguirre J, Nowicki S, Barontini M, Arrizurieta EE, Armando I. Demethylation of 3-O-methyldopa in the kidney: a possible source for dopamine in urine. Am J Physiol 1996;270(5 Pt 2):F862–8.

[86] Helkamaa T, Männistö PT, Rauhala P, Cheng ZJ, Finckenberg P, Huotari M, et al. Resistance to salt-induced hypertension in catechol-O-methyltransferase-gene-disrupted mice. J Hypertens 2003;21(12):2365–74.

[87] Soares-da-Silva P, Serrão MP. High- and low-affinity transport of L-leucine and L-DOPA by the hetero amino acid exchangers LAT1 and LAT2 in LLC-PK1 renal cells. Am J Physiol Renal Physiol 2004;287(2):F252–61.

[88] Baines AD, Chan W. Production of urine free dopamine from DOPA: a micropuncture study. Life Sci 1980;26 (4):253–9.

[89] Seri I, Kone BC, Gullans SR, Aperia A, Brenner BM, Ballermann BJ. Influence of Na^+ intake on dopamine-induced inhibition of renal cortical Na^+-K^+-ATPase. Am J Physiol 1990;258(1 Pt 2):F52–60.

[90] Hayashi M, Yamaji Y, Kitajima W, Saruta T. Aromatic L-amino acid decarboxylase activity along the rat nephron. Am J Physiol 1990;258(1 Pt 2):F28–33.

[91] Di Marco GS, Vio CP, Dos Santos OF, Schor N, Casarini DE. Catecholamine production along the nephron. Cell Physiol Biochem 2007;20(6):919–24.

[92] Meister B, Fried G, Holgert H, Aperia A, Hökfelt T. Ontogeny of aromatic L-amino acid decarboxylase-containing tubule cells in rat kidney. Kidney Int 1992;42(3):617–23.

[93] Gomes P, Serrão MP, Viera-Coelho MA, Soares-da-Silva P. Opossum kidney cells take up L-DOPA through an organic cation potential-dependent and proton-independent transporter. Cell Biol Int 1997;21(4):249–55.

[94] Soares-Da-Silva P, Serrão MP, Vieira-Coelho MA. Apical and basolateral uptake and intracellular fate of dopamine precursor L-dopa in LLC-PK1 cells. Am J Physiol 1998;274(2 Pt 2): F243–51.

[95] Pinho MJ, Serrão MP, Gomes P, Hopfer U, Jose PA, Soares-da-Silva P. Over-expression of renal LAT1 and LAT2 and enhanced L-DOPA uptake in SHR immortalized renal proximal tubular cells. Kidney Int 2004;66(1):216–26.

[96] Quiñones H, Collazo R, Moe OW. The dopamine precursor L-dihydroxyphenylalanine is transported by the amino acid transporters rBAT and LAT2 in renal cortex. Am J Physiol Renal Physiol 2004;287(1):F74–80.

[97] Pinho MJ, Serrão MP, José PA, Soares-da-Silva P. Organ specific underexpression renal of Na^+-dependent B^0AT1 in the SHR correlates positively with overexpression of NHE3 and salt intake. Mol Cell Biochem 2007;306(1-2):9–18.

[98] Armando I, Nowicki S, Aguirre J, Barontini M. A decreased tubular uptake of dopa results in defective renal dopamine production in aged rats. Am J Physiol 1995;268(6 Pt 2): F1087–92.

[99] Hayashi M, Yamaji Y, Kitajima W, Saruta T. Effects of high salt intake on dopamine production in rat kidney. Am J Physiol 1991;260(5):E675–9.

[100] Vieira-Coelho MA, Hussain T, Kansra V, Serrao MP, Guimaraes JT, Pestana M, et al. Aging, high salt intake, and renal dopaminergic activity in Fischer 344 rats. Hypertension 1999;34(4 Pt 1):666–72.

[101] Wassenberg T, Willemsen MA, Geurtz PB, Lammens M, Verrijp K, Wilmer M, et al. Urinary dopamine in aromatic L-amino acid decarboxylase deficiency: the unsolved paradox. Mol Genet Metab 2010;101(4):349–56.

[102] Wu X, Huang W, Ganapathy ME, Wang H, Kekuda R, Conway SJ, et al. Structure, function, and regional distribution of the organic cation transporter OCT3 in the kidney. Am J Physiol Renal Physiol 2000;279(3):F449–58.

[103] Hartman BK. Immunofluorescence of dopamine-β-hydroxylase. Application of improved methodology to the localization of the peripheral and central noradrenergic nervous system. J Histochem Cytochem 1973;21(4):312–32.

[104] Kinoshita S, Ohlstein EH, Felder RA. Dopamine-1 receptors in rat proximal convoluted tubule: regulation by intrarenal dopamine. Am J Physiol 1990;258(4 Pt 2):F1068–74.

[105] Kennedy B, Bigby TD, Ziegler MG. Nonadrenal epinephrine-forming enzymes in humans. Characteristics, distribution, regulation, and relationship to epinephrine levels. J Clin Invest 1995;95(6):2896–902.

[106] Ziegler MG, Kennedy B, Elayan H. Rat renal epinephrine synthesis. J Clin Invest 1989;84(4):1130–3.

I. EPITHELIAL AND NONEPITHELIAL TRANSPORT AND REGULATION

[107] Jans DA, Hemmings BA. cAMP-dependent protein kinase activation affects vasopressin V2-receptor number and internalization in LLC-PK1 renal epithelial cells. FEBS Lett 1991;281 (1-2):267–71.

[108] Fernandes MH, Soares-da-Silva P. Role of monoamine oxidase and catechol-O-methyltransferase in the metabolism of renal dopamine. J Neural Transm Suppl 1994;41:101–16.

[109] Ibarra FR, Armando I, Nowicki S, Carranza A, De Luca Sarobe V, Azzurieta EE, et al. Dopamine is metabolised by different enzymes along the rat nephron. Pflugers Arch 2005;450(3):185–91.

[110] Wang Y, Berndt TJ, Gross JM, Peterson MA, So MJ, Knox FG. Effect of inhibition of MAO and COMT on intrarenal dopamine and serotonin and on renal function. Am J Physiol Regul Integr Comp Physiol 2001;280(1):R248–54.

[111] Xu J, Li G, Wang P, Velasquez H, Yao X, Li Y, et al. Renalase is a novel, soluble monoamine oxidase that regulates cardiac function and blood pressure. J Clin Invest 2005; 115(5):1275–80.

[112] Isaac J, Berndt TJ, Chinnow SL, Tyce GM, Dousa TP, Knox FG. Dopamine enhances the phosphaturic response to parathyroid hormone in phosphate-deprived rats. J Am Soc Nephrol 1992;2 (9):1423–9.

[113] Clark BA, Rosa RM, Epstein FH, Young JB, Landsberg L. Altered dopaminergic responses in hypertension. Hypertension 1992; 19(6 Pt 1):589–94.

[114] Akpaffiong MJ, Redfern PH, Woodward B. Factors affecting the release and excretion of dopamine in the rat. J Pharm Pharmacol 1980;32(12):839–43.

[115] Ball SG, Oats NS, Lee MR. Urinary dopamine in man and rat: effects of inorganic salts on dopamine excretion. Clin Sci Mol Med 1978;55(2):167–73.

[116] Oates NS, Ball SG, Perkins CM, Lee MR. Plasma and urine dopamine in man given sodium chloride in the diet. Clin Sci (Lond) 1979;56(3):261–4.

[117] Chen CJ, Lokhandwala MF. Role of endogenous dopamine in the natriuretic response to various degrees of iso-osmotic volume expansion in rats. Clin Exp Hypertens A. 1991;13(6-7):1117–26.

[118] Ball SG, Gunn IG, Douglas IH. Renal handling of dopa, dopamine, norepinephrine, and epinephrine in the dog. Am J Physiol 1982;242(1):F56–62.

[119] Boren DR, Henry DP, Selkurt EE, Weinberger MH. Renal modulation of urinary catecholamine excretion during volume expansion in the dog. Hypertension 1980;2(4):383–9.

[120] Chan YL. Cellular mechanisms of renal tubular transport of L-dopa and its derivatives in the rat: microperfusion studies. J Pharmacol Exp Ther 1976;199(1):17–24.

[121] Okubo M, Kaku K, Kaneko T, Yanaihara N. Effects of bombesin and gastrin releasing peptide on catecholamine secretion from rat adrenal gland, in vitro. Endocrinol Jpn 1985; 32(1):21–7.

[122] Abramczyk P, Ziecina R, Lisiecka A, Papierski K, Przybylski J. The adrenal renal vascular connection plays an essential role in the pathogenesis of renovascular hypertension in the rat. J Physiol Pharmacol 2000;51(1):35–40.

[123] Sutoo D, Akiyama K. Effect of dopamine receptor antagonists on the calcium-dependent central function that reduces blood pressure in spontaneously hypertensive rats. Neurosci Lett 1999;269(3):133–6.

[124] Takeda S, Ueshiba H, Hattori Y, Irie M. Cilnidipine, the N- and L-type calcium channel antagonist, reduced on 24-h urinary catecholamines and C-peptide in hypertensive non-insulin-dependent diabetes mellitus. Diabetes Res Clin Pract 1999;44(3):197–205.

[125] Damasceno A, Santos A, Pestana M, Serrao P, Caupers P, Soares-da-Silva P, et al. Acute hypotensive, natriuretic,

and hormonal effects of nifedipine in salt-sensitive and salt-resistant black normotensive and hypertensive subjects. J Cardiovasc Pharmacol 1999;34(3):346–53.

[126] Wang ZQ, Siragy HM, Felder RA, Carey RM. Preferential release of renal dopamine into the tubule lumen: effect of chronic sodium loading. Clin Exp Hypertens 1997;19(1-2):107–16.

[127] Felder CC, Campbell T, Albrecht F, Jose PA. Dopamine inhibits Na$^+$-H$^+$ exchanger activity in renal BBMV by stimulation of adenylate cyclase. Am J Physiol 1990;259(2 Pt 2):F297–303.

[128] Gesek FA, Schoolwerth AC. Hormone responses of proximal Na$^+$-H$^+$ exchanger in spontaneously hypertensive rats. Am J Physiol 1991;261(3 Pt 2):F526–36.

[129] Jadhav AL, Liu Q. DA1 receptor mediated regulation of Na$^+$-H$^+$ antiport activity in rat renal cortical brush border membrane vesicles. Clin Exp Hypertens A. 1992;14(4):653–66.

[130] Felder CC, Albrecht FE, Campbell T, Eisner GM, Jose PA. Cyclic AMP- independent, G protein-linked inhibition of Na$^+$/H$^+$ exchange in renal brush border by D1 dopamine agonists. Am J Physiol 1993;264(6 Pt 2):F1032–7.

[131] Albrecht FE, Xu J, Moe OW, Hopfer U, Simonds WF, Orlowski J, et al. Regulation of NHE3 activity by G protein subunits in renal brush-border membranes. Am J Physiol Regul Integr Comp Physiol 2000;278(4):R1064–73.

[132] Bacic D, Kaissling B, McLeroy P, Zou L, Baum M, Moe OW. Dopamine acutely decreases apical membrane Na/H exchanger NHE3 protein in mouse renal proximal tubule. Kidney Int 2003;64(6):2133–41.

[133] Bobulescu IA, Quiñones H, Gisler SM, Di Sole F, Hu MC, Shi M, et al. Acute regulation of renal Na$^+$/H$^+$ exchanger NHE3 by dopamine: role of protein phosphatase 2A. Am J Physiol Renal Physiol 2010;298(5):F1205–13.

[134] Häberle DA, Königbauer B, Kawabata M, Ushiogi Y. Renal blood flow control by tubuloglomerular feedback (TGF) in normal and spontaneously hypertensive rats—a role for dopamine and adenosine. Klin Wochenschr 1991; 69(13):587–956.

[135] Felder CC, Blecher M, Jose PA. Dopamine-1-mediated stimulation of phospholipase C activity in rat renal cortical membranes. J Biol Chem 1989;264(15):8739–45.

[136] Gomes P, Soares-da-Silva P. Role of cAMP-PKA-PLC signaling cascade on dopamine-induced PKC-mediated inhibition of renal Na$^+$-K$^+$-ATPase activity. Am J Physiol Renal Physiol 2002;282(6):F1084–96.

[137] Felder RA, Kinoshita S, Ohbu K, Mouradian MM, Sibley DR, Monsma Jr FJ, et al. Organ specificity of the dopamine1 receptor/adenylyl cyclase coupling defect in spontaneously hypertensive rats. Am J Physiol 1993;264(4 Pt 2):R726–32.

[138] Vyas SJ, Eichberg J, Lokhandwala MF. Characterization of receptors involved in dopamine-induced activation of phospholipase-C in rat renal cortex. J Pharmacol Exp Ther 1992;260 (1):134–9.

[139] Yu PY, Eisner GM, Yamaguchi I, Mouradian MM, Felder RA, Jose PA. Dopamine D1A receptor regulation of phospholipase C isoform. J Biol Chem 1996;271(32):19503–8.

[140] Yu PY, Asico LD, Eisner GM, Jose PA. Differential regulation of renal phospholipase C isoforms by catecholamines. J Clin Invest 1995;95(1):304–8.

[141] Banday AA, Lokhandwala MF. Oxidative stress reduces renal dopamine D1 receptor-Gq/11α G protein-phospholipase C signaling involving G protein-coupled receptor kinase 2. Am J Physiol Renal Physiol 2007;293(1):F306–15.

[142] Felder CC, Jose PA, Axelrod J. The dopamine-1 agonist, SKF 82526, stimulates phospholipase C activity independent of adenylate cyclase. J Pharmacol Exp Ther 1989;248(1):171–5.

[143] Barendregt JN, Muizert Y, van Nispen tot Pannerden LL, Chang PC. Intrarenal production of dopamine and natriuresis following DOPA and saline infusions in healthy human volunteers. J Hum Hypertens 1995;9(3):187−94.

[144] Vieira-Coelho MA, Pestana M, Soares-da-Silva P. High sodium intake increases the urinary excretion of L-3,4-dihydroxyphenylalanine but fails to alter the urinary excretion of dopamine and amine metabolites in Wistar rats. Gen Pharmacol 1996; 27(8):1421−7.

[145] Luippold G, Benöhr P, Piesch C, Heyne N, Mühlbauer B. Urinary dopamine excretion in healthy volunteers: effect of sodium diet and acute water load. Pflugers Arch 2000;440 (1):28−33.

[146] Mühlbauer B, Osswald H. Feeding but not salt loading is the dominant factor controlling urinary dopamine excretion in conscious rats. Naunyn Schmiedebergs Arch Pharmacol 1992;346(4):469−71.

[147] Mühlbauer B, Osswald H. Feeding-induced increase in urinary dopamine excretion is independent of renal innervation and sodium intake. Am J Physiol 1994;266(4 Pt 2): F563−7.

[148] Jadhav AL, Lokhandwala MF. Dietary sodium-induced changes in renal noradrenergic and dopaminergic responses in rats. J Hum Hypertens 1990;4(2):163−4.

[149] Yoshimura M, Yamazaki H, Takashina R, Kambara S, Iyoda I, Sasaki S, et al. The significance of duration of salt loading on cardiovascular response and urinary excretion of catecholamine in rats. Endocrinol Jpn 1986;33(2):169−75.

[150] Petrovic T, Bell C. Catecholamines in kidneys of normotensive and genetically hypertensive rats. Effects of salt load. Hypertension 1986;8(2):122−7.

[151] Dantonello TM, Küster E, Mühlbauer B. Urinary dopamine and renal handling of L-DOPA in fasted spontaneously hypertensive rats. Kidney Blood Press Res 1998;21(6): 438−44.

[152] Sampaio-Maia B, Serrão P, Vieira-Coelho MA, Pestana M. Differences in the renal dopaminergic system activity between Wistar rats from two suppliers. Acta Physiol Scand 2003; 178(1):83−9.

[153] Escano CS, Armando I, Wang X, Asico LD, Pascua A, Yang Y, et al. Renal dopaminergic defect in C57BL/6J mice. Am J Physiol Regul Integr Comp Physiol 297(6):R1660-R1669.

[154] Sulyok E. Dopaminergic control of neonatal salt and water metabolism. Pediatr Nephrol 1988;2(1):163−5.

[155] Young JB, Troisi RJ, Weiss ST, Parker DR, Sparrow D, Landsberg L. Relationship of catecholamine excretion to body size, obesity, and nutrient intake in middle-aged and elderly men. Am J Clin Nutr 1992;56(5):827−34.

[156] Ferreira A, Bettencourt P, Pestana M, Correia F, Serrão P, Martins L, et al. Heart failure, aging, and renal synthesis of dopamine. Am J Kidney Dis 2001;38(3):502−9.

[157] Soares-Da-Silva P, Fernandes MH. A study on the renal synthesis of dopamine in aged rats. Acta Physiol Scand 1991;143 (3):287−93.

[158] Pestana M, Jardim H, Correia F, Vieira-Coelho MA, Soares-da-Silva P. Renal dopaminergic mechanisms in renal parenchymal diseases and hypertension. Nephrol Dial Transplant 2001;16(Suppl. 1):53−9.

[159] Chan TY, Critchley JA, Ho CS, Chan JC, Tomlinson B. Urinary dopamine and noradrenaline outputs during oral salt loading in healthy Chinese subjects with a family history of hypertension. J Auton Pharmacol 1996;16(1):1−6.

[160] Sowers JR, Zemel MB, Zemel P, Beck FW, Walsh MF, Zawada ET. Salt sensitivity in blacks. Salt intake and natriuretic substances. Hypertension 1988;12(5):485−90.

[161] Damasceno A, Santos A, Serrão P, Caupers P, Soares-da-Silva P, Polónia J. Deficiency of renal dopaminergic-dependent natriuretic response to acute sodium load in black salt-sensitive subjects in contrast to salt-resistant subjects. J Hypertens 1999; 17(12 Pt 2):1995−2001.

[162] Weder AB, Gleiberman L, Sachdeva A. Urinary dopamine excretion and renal responses to fenoldopam infusion in blacks and whites. J Clin Hypertens (Greenwich) 2009; 11(12):707−12.

[163] Gerdts E, Svarstad E, Myking OL, Lund-Johansen P, Omvik P. Salt sensitivity in hypertensive type-1 diabetes mellitus. Blood Press 1996;5(2):78−85.

[164] Segers O, Anckaert E, Gerlo E, Dupont AG, Somers G. Dopamine-sodium relationship in type 2 diabetic patients. Diabetes Res Clin Pract 1996;34(2):89−98.

[165] Rudberg S, Lemne C, Persson B, Krekula A, de Faire U, Aperia A. The dopaminuric response to high salt diet in insulin-dependent diabetes mellitus and in family history of hypertension. Pediatr Nephrol 1997;11(2):169−73.

[166] Stenvinkel P, Saggar-Malik AK, Wahrenberg H, Diczfalusy U, Bolinder J, Alvestrand A. Impaired intrarenal dopamine production following intravenous sodium chloride infusion in type 1 (insulin-dependent) diabetes mellitus. Diabetologia 1991;34(2):114−8.

[167] Shigetomi S, Yamada ZO, Ishii H, Sanada H, Watanabe H, Fukuchi S. Dopaminergic activity and endorenal dopamine synthesis in non-insulin dependent diabetes mellitus. Hypertens Res 1995;18(Suppl. 1):S125−30.

[168] Madácsy L, Sulyok E, Klujber L, Vámosi I, Barkai L, Baranyai Z. Decreased urinary excretion of dopamine and sodium in diabetic children with incipient nephropathy. Padiatr Padol 1991;26(6):253−6.

[169] Murabayashi S, Baba T, Tomiyama T, Takebe K. Urinary dopamine, noradrenaline and adrenaline in type 2 diabetic patients with and without nephropathy. Horm Metab Res 1989; 21(1):27−32.

[170] Carranza A, Karabatas L, Barontini M, Armando I. Decreased tubular uptake of L-3,4-dihydroxyphenylalanine in streptozotocin-induced diabetic rats. Horm Res 2001;55(6):282−7.

[171] Kuchel O, Buu NT, Unger T, Lis M, Genest J. Free and conjugated plasma and urinary dopamine in human hypertension. J Clin Endocrinol Metab 1979;48(3):425−9.

[172] Shikuma R, Yoshimura M, Kambara S, Yamazaki H, Takashina R, Takahashi H, et al. Dopaminergic modulation of salt sensitivity in patients with essential hypertension. Life Sci 1986;38(10):915−21.

[173] Gill Jr JR, Grossman E, Goldstein DS. High urinary dopa and low urinary dopamine-to-dopa ratio in salt-sensitive hypertension. Hypertension 1991;18(5):614−21.

[174] Gordon MS, Steunkel CA, Conlin PR, Hollenberg NK, Williams GH. The role of dopamine in nonmodulating hypertension. J Clin Endocrinol Metab 1989;69(2):426−32.

[175] Iimura O, Shimamoto K. Salt and hypertension: water-sodium handling in essential hypertension. Ann N Y Acad Sci 1993;676:105−21.

[176] Harvey JN, Casson IF, Clayden AD, Cope GF, Perkins CM, Lee MR. A paradoxical fall in urine dopamine output when patients with essential hypertension are given added dietary salt. Clin Sci (Lond) 1984;67(1):83−8.

[177] Saito I, Takeshita E, Saruta T, Nagano S, Sekihara T. Urinary dopamine excretion in normotensive subjects with or without family history of hypertension. J Hypertens 1986;4(1):57−60.

[178] Gill Jr JR, Gullner G, Lake CR, Lakatua DJ, Lan G. Plasma and urinary catecholamines in salt-sensitive idiopathic hypertension. Hypertension 1988;11(4):312−9.

I. EPITHELIAL AND NONEPITHELIAL TRANSPORT AND REGULATION

[179] Sakai T, Ideishi M, Miura S, Maeda H, Tashiro E, Koga M, et al. Mild exercise activates renal dopamine system in mild hypertensives. J Hum Hypertens 1998;12(6):355−62.

[180] Saito I, Itsuji S, Takeshita E, Kawabe H, Nishino M, Wainai H, et al. Increased urinary dopamine excretion in young patients with essential hypertension. Clin Exp Hypertens 1994;16 (1):29−39.

[181] Castellano M, Beschi M, Agabiti-Rossi E, Muiesan ML, Romanelli G, Falo F, et al. Renal noradrenergic and dopaminergic activity in patients with borderline essential hypertension. J Cardiovasc Pharmacol 1986;8(Suppl. 5):S116−8.

[182] Kuchel O, Cuche JL, Buu NT, Genest J. An increase in urinary catecholamines of renal origin in patients with "borderline" hypertension. Am J Med Sci 1976;272(3):263−8.

[183] Kuchel O. Peripheral dopamine in essential hypertension. An early defense against hypertension failing during its progression? Am J Hypertens 1990;3(6 Pt 2):104S−7S.

[184] Sanada H, Watanabe H, Shigetomi S, Fukuchi S. Gene expression of aromatic L-amino acid decarboxylase mRNA in the kidney of normotensive and hypertensive rats. Hypertens Res 1995;18(Suppl. 1):S179−81.

[185] Kuchel O, Racz K, Debinski W, Falardeau P, Buu NT. Contrasting dopaminergic patterns in two forms of genetic hypertension. Clin Exp Hypertens A. 1987;9(5-6):987−1008.

[186] DeFeo ML, Jadhav AL, Lokhandwala MF. Dietary sodium intake and urinary dopamine and sodium excretion during the course of blood pressure development in Dahl salt-sensitive and salt-resistant rats. Clin Exp Hypertens A. 1987; 9(12):2049−60.

[187] Moller B, Hansell P. Sodium and dopamine excretion in prehypertensive Dahl rats during severe hypervolaemia. Acta Physiol Scand 1995;155(2):165−71.

[188] Cravchik A, Goldman D. Neurochemical individuality: Genetic diversity among human dopamine and serotonin receptors and transporters. Arch Gen Psychiatry 2000; 57(12):1105−14.

[189] Beaulieu JM, Gainetdinov RR. The physiology, signaling, and pharmacology of dopamine receptors. Pharmacol Rev. 2011; 63(1):182−217.

[190] Premont RT, Gainetdinov RR. Physiological roles of G protein-coupled receptor kinases and arrestins. Annu Rev Physiol 2007;69:511−34.

[191] Neve KA, Seamans JK, Trantham-Davidson H. Dopamine receptor signaling. J Recept Signal Transduct Res 2004; 24(3):165−205.

[192] Holmes A, Lachowicz JE, Sibley DR. Phenotypic analysis of dopamine receptor knockout mice; recent insights into the functional specificity of dopamine receptor subtypes. Neuropharmacology 2004;47(8):1117−34.

[193] Sibley DR. New insights into dopaminergic receptor function using antisense and genetically altered animals. Annu Rev Pharmacol Toxicol 1999;39:313−41.

[194] Kapsimali M, Dumond H, Le Crom S, Coudouel S, Vincent JD, Vernier P. [Evolution and development of dopaminergic neurotransmitter systems in vertebrates] [Article in French]. J Soc Biol 2000;194(2):87−93.

[195] Rondou P, Haegeman G, Van Craenenbroeck K. The dopamine D4 receptor: biochemical and signalling properties. Cell Mol Life Sci 2010;67(12):1971−86.

[196] Rosenbaum DM, Cherezov V, Hanson MA, Rasmussen SG, Thian FS, Kobilka TS, et al. GPCR engineering yields high-resolution structural insights into β_2-adrenergic receptor function. Science 2007;318(5854):1266−73.

[197] Bokoch MP, Zou Y, Rasmussen SG, Liu CW, et al. Ligand-specific regulation of the extracellular surface of a G-protein-coupled receptor. Nature 2010;463(7277):108−12.

[198] Jaakola VP, Griffith MT, Hanson MA, Cherezov V, Chien EY, Lane JR, et al. The 2.6 angstrom crystal structure of a human A2A adenosine receptor bound to an antagonist. Science 2008;322(5905):1211−7.

[199] Scheerer P, Park JH, Hildebrand PW, Kim YJ, Krauss N, Choe HW, et al. Crystal structure of opsin in its G protein interacting conformation. Nature 2008;455(7212):497−502.

[200] Anderson GR, Lujan R, Martemyanov KA. Changes in striatal signaling induce remodeling of RGS complexes containing Gbeta5 and R7BP subunits. Mol Cell Biol 2009;29(11):3033−44.

[201] Celver J, Sharma M, Kovoor A. RGS9-2 mediates specific inhibition of agonist-induced internalization of D2-dopamine receptors. J Neurochem 2010;114(3):739−49.

[202] Jeanneteau F, Guillin O, Diaz J, Griffon N, Sokoloff P. GIPC recruits GAIP (RGS19) to attenuate dopamine D2 receptor signaling. Mol Biol Cell 2004;15(11):4926−37.

[203] Stanwood GD, Parlaman JP, Levitt P. Genetic or pharmacological inactivation of the dopamine D1 receptor differentially alters the expression of regulator of G-protein signaling (Rgs) transcripts. Eur J Neurosci 2006;24(3):806−18.

[204] Taymans JM, Kia HK, Claes R, Cruz C, Leysen J, Langlois X. Dopamine receptor-mediated regulation of RGS2 and RGS4 mRNA differentially depends on ascending dopamine projections and time. Eur J Neurosci 2004;19(8):2249−6220.

[205] Zürn A, Zabel U, Vilardaga JP, Schindelin H, Lohse MJ, Hoffmann C. Fluorescence resonance energy transfer analysis of α_{2a}-adrenergic receptor activation reveals distinct agonist-specific conformational changes. Mol Pharmacol 2009; 75(3):534−41.

[206] Marty C, Ye RD. Heterotrimeric G protein signaling outside the realm of seven transmembrane domain receptors. Mol Pharmacol 2010;78(1):12−8.

[207] Schwendt M, McGinty JF. Amphetamine up-regulates activator of G-protein signaling 1 mRNA and protein levels in rat frontal cortex: The role of dopamine and glucocorticoid receptors. Neuroscience 2010;168(1):96−107.

[208] Rajagopal K, Lefkowitz RJ, Rockman HA. When 7 transmembrane receptors are not G protein-coupled receptors. J Clin Invest 2005;115(11):2971−4.

[209] Rajagopal K, Whalen EJ, Violin JD, Stilber JA, Rosenberg PB, Premont RT, et al. β-arrestin2-mediated inotropic effects of the angiotensin II type 1A receptor in isolated cardiac myocytes. Proc Natl Acad Sci USA 2006;103(44):16284−9.

[210] Kimura K, White BH, Sidhu A. Coupling of human D-1 dopamine receptors to different guanine nucleotide binding proteins: evidence that D-1 dopamine receptors can couple to both Gs and Go. J Biol Chem 1995;270(24):14672−8.

[211] Corvol JC, Studler JM, Schonn JS, Girault JA, Hervé D. $G\alpha_{olf}$ is necessary for coupling D1 and A2a receptors to adenylyl cyclase in the striatum. J Neurochem 2001;76(5):1585−8.

[212] Pluznick JL, Zou DJ, Zhang X, Yan Q, Rodriguez-Gil DJ, Eisner C, et al. Functional expression of the olfactory signaling system in the kidney. Proc Natl Acad Sci USA 2009; 106(6):2059−64.

[213] Zheng S, Yu P, Zeng C, Wang Z, Yang Z, Andrews PM, et al. $G\alpha_{12}$- and $G\alpha_{13}$-protein subunit linkage of D5 dopamine receptors in the nephron. Hypertension 2003;41(3):604−10.

[214] Yamaguchi Y, Katoh H, Mori K, Negishi MG. $G\alpha_{12}$ and $G\alpha_{13}$ interact with Ser/Thr protein phosphatase type 5 and stimulate its phosphatase activity. Curr Biol 2002;12(15):1353−8.

[215] Yu P, Asico LD, Luo Y, Andrews P, Eisner GM, Hopfer U, et al. D1 dopamine receptor hyperphosphorylation in renal proximal tubules in hypertension. Kidney Int 2006;70(6):1072—9.

[216] Gardner B, Liu ZF, Jiang D, Sibley DR. The role of phosphorylation/dephosphorylation in agonist-induced desensitization of D1 dopamine receptor function: evidence for a novel pathway for receptor dephosphorylation. Mol Pharmacol 2001; 59(2):310—21.

[217] Millar RP, Newton CL. The year in G protein-coupled receptor research. Mol Endocrinol 2010;24(1):261—74.

[218] O'Sullivan GJ, Roth BL, Kinsella A, Waddington JL. SK&F 83822 distinguishes adenylyl cyclase from phospholipase C-coupled dopamine D1-like receptors: behavioural topography. Eur J Pharmacol 2004;486(3):273—80.

[219] Jin LQ, Goswami S, Cai G, Zhen X, Friedman E. SKF83959 selectively regulates phosphatidylinositol-linked D1 dopamine receptors in rat brain. J Neurochem 2003;85(2):378—86.

[220] Bek MJ, Zheng S, Xu J, Yamaguchi I, Asico LD, Sun XG, et al. Differential expression of adenylyl cyclases in the rat nephron. Kidney Int 2001;60(3):890—9.

[221] Yu P, Zhang Y, Jose PA. Differential regulation of adenylyl cyclases in lipid rafts in human kidney cells. J Am Soc Nephrol 2010;21: 370A—370A.

[222] Dmitrieva RI, Lalli E, Doris PA. Regulation of adrenocortical cardiotonic steroid production by dopamine and PKA signaling. Front Biosci 2005;10:2489—95.

[223] Ventura AL, Sibley DR. Altered regulation of the D1 dopamine receptor in mutant Chinese hamster ovary cells deficient in cyclic AMP-dependent protein kinase activity. J Pharmacol Exp Ther 2000;293(2):426—34.

[224] Hemmings Jr HC, Greengard P, Tung HY, Cohen P. DARPP-32, a dopamine-regulated neuronal phosphoprotein, is a potent inhibitor of protein phosphatase-1. Nature 1984; 310(5977):503—5.

[225] Kuroiwa M, Bateup HS, Shuto T, Higashi H, Tanaka M, Nishi A. Regulation of DARPP-32 phosphorylation by three distinct dopamine D1-like receptor signaling pathways in the neostriatum. J Neurochem 2008;107(4):1014—26.

[226] Pollack A. Coactivation of D1 and D2 dopamine receptors: in marriage, a case of his, hers, and theirs. Sci STKE 2004; 2004(255):pe50.

[227] So CH, Verma V, Alijaniaram M, Cheng R, Rashid AJ, O'Dowd BF, et al. Calcium signaling by dopamine D5 receptor and D5-D2 receptor hetero-oligomers occurs by a mechanism distinct from that for dopamine D1-D2 receptor hetero-oligomers. Mol Pharmacol 2009;75(4):843—5.

[228] Sidhu A, Kimura K, Uh M, White BH, Patel S. Multiple coupling of human D5 dopamine receptors to guanine nucleotide binding proteins G_s and G_z. J Neurochem 1998;70(6):2459—67.

[229] Friedman E, Jin LQ, Cai GP, Hollon TR, Drago J, Sibley DR, et al. D_1-like dopaminergic activation of phosphoinositide hydrolysis is independent of D_{1A} dopamine receptors: evidence from D_{1A} knockout mice. Mol Pharmacol 1997;51(1):6—11.

[230] Sahu A, Tyeryar KR, Vongtau HO, Sibley DR, Undieh AS. D_5 dopamine receptors are required for dopaminergic activation of phospholipase C. Mol Pharmacol 2009;75 (3):447—53.

[231] Gomez-Cambronero J, Keire P. Phospholipase D: a novel major player in signal transduction. Cell Signal 1998;10(6):387—97.

[232] Yang Z, Asico LD, Yu P, Wang Z, Jones JE, Bai RK, et al. D5 dopamine receptor regulation of phospholipase D. Am J Physiol Heart Circ Physiol 2005;288(1):H55—61.

[233] Yasunari K, Kohno M, Kano H, Minami M, Yoshikawa J. Dopamine as a novel antioxidative agent for rat vascular smooth muscle cells through dopamine D1-like receptors. Circulation 2000;101(19):2302—8.

[234] Yang Z, Asico LD, Yu P, Wang Z, Jones JE, Escano CS, et al. D_5 dopamine receptor regulation of reactive oxygen species production, NADPH oxidase, and blood pressure. Am J Physiol Regul Integr Comp Physiol 2006;290(1): R96—104.

[235] Everett PB, Senogles SE. D3 dopamine receptor signals to activation of phospholipase D through a complex with Rho. J Neurochem 2010;112(4):963—71.

[236] Guo J, Gertsberg Z, Ozgen N, Sabri A, Steinberg SF. Protein kinase D isoforms are activated in an agonist-specific manner in cardiomyocytes. J Biol Chem 2011;286(8):6500—9.

[237] Yao LP, Li XX, Yu PY, Xu J, Asico LD, Jose PA. Dopamine D1 receptor and protein kinase C isoforms in spontaneously hypertensive rats. Hypertension 1998;32(6):1049—53.

[238] Efendiev R, Bertorello AM, Pedemonte CH. PKC-β and PKC-ζ mediate opposing effects on proximal tubule Na^+,K^+-ATPase activity. FEBS Lett 1999;456(1):45—8.

[239] Yu P, Han W, Villar VA, Li H, Arnaldo FB, Concepcion GP, et al. Dopamine D1 receptor-mediated inhibition of NADPH oxidase activity in human kidney cells occurs via protein kinase A-protein kinase C cross talk. Free Radic Biol Med 2011;50(7):832—40.

[240] Asghar M, Hussain T, Lokhandwala MF. Overexpression of PKCβ I and -δ contributes to higher PKC activity in the proximal tubules of old Fischer 344 rats. Am J Physiol Renal Physiol 2003;285(6):F1100—7.

[241] Nowicki S, Kruse MS, Brismar H, Aperia A. Dopamine-induced translocation of protein kinase C isoforms visualized in renal epithelial cells. Am J Physiol Cell Physiol 2000;279(6): C1812—8.

[242] Cunningham R, Biswas R, Brazie M, Steplock D, Shenolikar S, Weinman EJ. Signaling pathways utilized by PTH and dopamine to inhibit phosphate transport in mouse renal proximal tubule cells. Am J Physiol Renal Physiol 2009;296 (2):F355—61.

[243] Yasunari K, Kohno M, Murakawa K, Yokokawa K, Horio T, Takeda T. Interaction between a phorbol ester and dopamine DA1 receptors on vascular smooth muscle. Am J Physiol 1993;264(1 Pt 2):F24—30.

[244] Jackson A, Sedaghat K, Minerds K, James C, Tiberi M. Opposing effects of phorbol-12-myristate-13-acetate, an activator of protein kinase C, on the signaling of structurally related human dopamine D1 and D5 receptors. J Neurochem 2005;95 (5):1387—400.

[245] Rankin ML, Sibley DR. Constitutive phosphorylation by protein kinase C regulates D1 dopamine receptor signaling. J Neurochem 2010;115(6):1655—67.

[246] Rex EB, Rankin ML, Ariano MA, Sibley DR. Ethanol regulation of D1 dopamine deceptor signaling is mediated by protein kinase C in an isozyme-specific manner. Neuropsychopharmacology 2008; 33(12):2900—11.

[247] Mason JN, Kozell LB, Neve KA. Regulation of dopamine D_1 receptor trafficking by protein kinase A-dependent phosphorylation. Mol Pharmacol 2002;61(4):806—16.

[248] Rex EB, Rankin ML, Yang Y, Lu Q, Gerfen CR, Jose PA, et al. Identification of RanBP 9/10 as interacting partners for protein kinase C (PKC) γ/δ and the D1 dopamine receptor: regulation of PKC-mediated receptor phosphorylation. Mol Pharmacol 2010;78(1):69—80.

[249] Weinman EJ, Biswas R, Steplock D, Douglass TS, Cunningham R, Shenolikar S. Sodium-hydrogen exchanger regulatory factor 1 (NHERF-1) transduces signals that mediate dopamine inhibition of sodium-phosphate co-transport in mouse kidney. J Biol Chem 2010;285(18):13454—60.

[250] Centonze D, Usiello A, Gubellini P, Pisani A, Borrelli E, Bernardi G, et al. Dopamine D2 receptor-mediated inhibition of dopaminergic neurons in mice lacking D2L receptors. Neuropsychopharmacology 2002;27(5):723−6.

[251] Prou D, Gu WJ, Le Crom S, Vincent JD, Salamero J, Vernier P. Intracellular retention of the two isoforms of the D2 dopamine receptor promotes endoplasmic reticulum disruption. J Cell Sci 2001;114(Pt 19):3517−27.

[252] Gao DQ, Canessa LM, Mouradian MM, Jose PA. Expression of the D2 subfamily of dopamine receptor genes in kidney. Am J Physiol 1994;266(4 Pt 2):F646−50.

[253] Obadiah J, Avidor-Reiss T, Fishburn CS, Carmon S, Bayewitch M, Vogel Z, et al. Adenylyl cyclase interaction with the D2 dopamine receptor family; differential coupling to Gi, Gz, and Gs. Cell Mol Neurobiol 1999;19(5):653−64.

[254] Gazi L, Nickolls SA, Strange PG. Functional coupling of the human dopamine D_2 receptor with $G\alpha_{i1}$, $G\alpha_{i2}$, $G\alpha_{i3}$ and $G\alpha_o$ G proteins: evidence for agonist regulation of G protein selectivity. Br J Pharmacol 2003;138(5):775−86.

[255] Yamaguchi I, Harmon SK, Todd RD, O'Malley KL. The rat D4 dopamine receptor couples to cone transducin ($G\alpha t2$) to inhibit forskolin-stimulated cAMP accumulation. J Biol Chem 1997;272(26):16599−602.

[256] Cho DI, Beom S, Van Tol HH, Caron MG, Kim KM. Characterization of the desensitization properties of five dopamine receptor subtypes and alternatively spliced variants of dopamine D2 and D4 receptors. Biochem Biophys Res Commun 2006;350(3):634−40.

[257] Sen S, Nesse R, Sheng L, Stoltenberg SF, Gleiberman L, Burmeister M, et al. Association between a dopamine-4 receptor polymorphism and blood pressure. Am J Hypertens 2005;18(9 Pt 1):1206−10.

[258] Robinson SW, Caron MG. Selective inhibition of adenylyl cyclase type V by the dopamine D_3 receptor. Mol Pharmacol 1997;52(3):508−14.

[259] Pedrosa R, Gomes P, Hopfer U, Jose PA, Soares-da-Silva P. $Gi\alpha3$ protein-coupled dopamine D_3 receptor-mediated inhibition of renal NHE3 activity in SHR proximal tubular cells is a PLC-PKC-mediated event. Am J Physiol Renal Physiol 2004;287(5):F1059−66.

[260] Beom S, Cheong D, Torres G, Caron MG, Kim KM. Comparative studies of molecular mechanisms of dopamine D_2 and D_3 receptors for the activation of extracellular signal-regulated kinase. J Biol Chem 2004; 279(27):28304−14.

[261] Richtand NM. Behavioral sensitization, alternative splicing, and D3 dopamine receptor-mediated inhibitory function. Neuropsychopharmacology 2006;31(11):2368−75.

[262] Fiorentini C, Busi C, Gorruso E, Gotti C, Spano P, Missale C. Reciprocal regulation of dopamine D_1 and D_3 receptor function and trafficking by heterodimerization. Mol Pharmacol 2008;74(1):59−69.

[263] Scarselli M, Novi F, Schallmach E, Lin R, Baragli A, Colzi A, et al. D_2/D_3 dopamine receptor heterodimers exhibit unique functional properties. J Biol Chem 2001;276(32):30308−14.

[264] Zeng C, Wang D, Yang Z, Wang Z, Asico LD, Wilcox CS, et al. Dopamine D_1 receptor augmentation of D_3 receptor action in rat aortic or mesenteric vascular smooth muscles. Hypertension 2004;43(3):673−9.

[265] Zeng C, Wang Z, Li H, Yu P, Zheng S, Wu L, et al. D_3 dopamine receptor directly interacts with D_1 dopamine receptor in immortalized renal proximal tubule cells. Hypertension 2006;47(3):573−9.

[266] Kaneko S, Albrecht F, Asico LD, Eisner GM, Robillard JE, Jose PA. Ontogeny of DA1 receptor-mediated natriuresis in

the rat: In vivo and in vitro correlations. Am J Physiol 1992;263(3 Pt 2):R631−8.

[267] Hussain T, Abdul-Wahab R, Lokhandwala MF. Bromocriptine stimulates Na^+, K^+-ATPase in renal proximal tubules via the cAMP pathway. Eur J Pharmacol 1997;321(2):259−63.

[268] Bertorello A, Aperia A. Inhibition of proximal tubule Na^+-K^+-ATPase activity requires simultaneous activation of DA1 and DA2 receptors. Am J Physiol 1990;259(6 Pt 2):F924−8.

[269] Watts VJ, Neve KA. Activation of type II adenylate cyclase by D_2 and D_4 but not D_3 dopamine receptors. Mol Pharmacol 1997;52(2):181−6.

[270] Beazely MA, Watts VJ. Activation of a novel PKC isoform synergistically enhances D_{2L} dopamine receptor-mediated sensitization of adenylate cyclase type 6. Cell Signal 2005; 17(5):647−53.

[271] Hozumi Y, Watanabe M, Goto K. signaling cascade of diacylglycerol kinase β in the pituitary intermediate lobe: Dopamine D2 receptor/phospholipase $C\beta4$/diacylglycerol kinase β/protein kinase $C\alpha$. J Histochem Cytochem 2010;58(2):119−29.

[272] Senogles SE. D2s dopamine receptor mediates phospholipase D and antiproliferation. Mol Cell Endocrinol 2003;209(1-2):61−9.

[273] Witkowski G, Szulczyk B, Rola R, Szulczyk P. D_1 dopaminergic control of G protein-dependent inward rectifier K^+ (GIRK)-like channel current in pyramidal neurons of the medial prefrontal cortex. Neuroscience 2008;155(1):53−63.

[274] Natarajan A, Han G, Chen SY, Yu P, White R, Jose P. The D_5 dopamine receptor mediates large-conductance, calcium- and voltage-activated potassium channel activation in human coronary artery smooth muscle cells. J Pharmacol Exp Ther 2010;332(2):640−9.

[275] Acquas E, Vinci S, Ibba F, Spiga S, De Luca MA, Di Chiara G. Role of dopamine D_1 receptors in caffeine-mediated ERK phosphorylation in the rat brain. Synapse 2010;64(5):341−9.

[276] Gildea JJ, Wang X, Jose PA, Felder RA. Differential D_1 and D_5 receptor regulation and degradation of the angiotensin type 1 receptor. Hypertension 2008;51(2):360−6.

[277] Choi EY, Jeong D, Park KW, Baik JH. G protein-mediated mitogen activated protein kinase activation by two dopamine D2 receptors. Biochem Biophys Res Commun 1999; 256(1):33−40.

[278] Narkar V, Hussain T, Lokhandwala M. Role of tyrosine kinase and p44/42 MAPK in D_2-like receptor-mediated stimulation of Na^+, K^+-ATPase in kidney. Am J Physiol Renal Physiol 2002;282(4):F697−702.

[279] Gerfen CR, Miyachi S, Paletzki R, Brown P. D1 dopamine receptor supersensitivity in the dopamine depleted striatum results from a switch in the regulation of ERK1/2/MAP kinase. J Neurosci 2002;22(12):5042−54.

[280] Banday AA, Fazili FR, Marwaha A, Lokhandwala MF. Mitogen-activated protein kinase upregulation reduces renal D1 receptor affinity and G-protein coupling in obese rats. Kidney Int 2007;71(5):397−406.

[281] Vlahović P, Stefanović V. Effect of dopamine on ecto-5′-nucleotidase expression in human glomerular mesangial cells. Arch Int Physiol Biochim Biophys 1994;102(3):171−3.

[282] Zeng C, Han Y, Huang H, Yu C, Ren H, Shi W, et al. D_1-like receptors inhibit insulin-induced vascular smooth muscle cell proliferation via down-regulation of insulin receptor expression. J Hypertens 2009;27(5):1033−41.

[283] Li Z, Yu C, Han Y, Ren H, Shi W, Fu C, et al. Inhibitory effect of D_1-like and D_3 dopamine receptors on norepinephrine-induced proliferation in vascular smooth muscle cells. Am J Physiol Heart Circ Physiol 2008;294(6):H2761−8.

[284] Li H, Shi S, Sun YH, Zhao YJ, Li QF, Li HZ, et al. Dopamine D2R receptor stimulation inhibits angiotensin II-induced

hypertrophy in cultured neonatal rat ventricular myocytes. Clin Exp Pharmacol Physiol 2009;36(3):312−8.

[285] Han JY, Heo JS, Lee YJ, Lee JH, Taub M, Han HJ. Dopamine stimulates $^{45}Ca^{2+}$ uptake through cAMP, PLC/PKC, and MAPKs in renal proximal tubule cells. J Cell Physiol 2007; 211(2):486−94.

[286] Villar VA, Jones JE, Armando I, Palmes-Saloma C, Yu P, Pascua AM, et al. G protein-coupled receptor kinase 4 (GRK4) regulates the phosphorylation and function of the dopamine D_3 receptor. J Biol Chem 2009;284(32):21425−34.

[287] Cho DI, Zheng M, Kim KM. Current perspectives on the selective regulation of dopamine D_2 and D_3 receptors. Arch Pharm Res 2010;33(10):1521−38.

[288] Svenningsson P, Nishi A, Fisone G, Girault JA, Nairn AC, Greengard P. DARPP-32: An integrator of neurotransmission. Annu Rev Pharmacol Toxicol. 2004;44:269−96.

[289] Meister B, Arvidsson U, Hemmings Jr HC, Greengard P, Hökfelt T. Dopamine- and adenosine-3':5'-monophosphate (cAMP)-regulated phospho-protein of Mr 32,000 (DARPP-32) in the retina of cat, monkey and human. Neurosci Lett 1991;131(1):66−70.

[290] Ouimet CC, Miller PE, Hemmings Jr HC, Walaas SI, Greengard P. DARPP-32, a dopamine- and adenosine 3':5'-monophosphate-regulated phosphoprotein enriched in dopamine-innervated brain regions. III. Immunocytochemical localization. J Neurosci 1984;4(1):111−24.

[291] Walaas SI, Greengard P. DARPP-32, a dopamine- and adenosine3':5'-monophosphate-reglated phosphoprotein enriched in dopamine-innervated brain regions. I. Regional and cellular distribution in the brain. J Neurosci 1984; 4(1):84−98.

[292] Meister B, Askergren J, Tunevall G, Hemmings Jr HC, Greengard P. Identification of a dopamine- and 3'5'-cyclic adenosine monophosphate-regulated phosphoprotein of 32 kD (DARPP-32) in the parathyroid hormone-producing cells of the human parathyroid gland. J Endocrinol Invest 1991; 14(8):655−61.

[293] Meister B, Fryckstedt J, Schalling M, Cortes R, Hokfelt T, Aperia A, et al. Dopamine- and cAMP-regulated phosphoprotein (DARPP-32) and dopamine DA1 agonist-sensitive Na +, K + -ATPase in renal tubule cells. Proc Natl Acad Sci USA 1989;86(20):8068−72.

[294] Yu P, Asico LD, Eisner GM, Hopfer U, Felder RA, Jose PA. Renal protein phosphatase 2A activity and spontaneous hypertension in rats. Hypertension 2000;36(6):1053−8.

[295] Sharif NA, Nunes JL, Rosenkranz RP, Whiting RL, Eglen RM. Quantitative autoradiography demonstrates selective modulation of rat brain regional dopamine (D1 and D2) receptor subtypes after chronic manipulation of dietary salt. Neurochem Res 1995;20(2):121−8.

[296] Jadhav AL, Ricci A, Amenta F, Lokhandwala MF. Renal dopamine and changes in dopamine receptor ligand binding during high sodium intake. Clin. Exp. Hypertens. [A] 1991; 13(8):1371−81.

[297] Sharif NA, Nunes JL, Lake KD, McClelland DL, Corkins SF, Lakatos I, et al. Chronic manipulation of dietary salt modulates renal physiology and kidney dopamine receptor subtypes: functional and autoradiographic studies. Gen Pharmacol 1995;26(4):727−35.

[298] Felder RA, Sanada H, Xu J, Yu PY, Wang Z, Watanabe H, et al. G protein-coupled receptor kinase 4 gene variants in human essential hypertension. Proc Natl Acad Sci USA 2002;99 (6):3872−7.

[299] Watanabe H, Xu J, Bengra C, Jose PA, Felder RA. Desensitization of human renal D1 dopamine receptors by G

[300] Yu P, Yang Z, Jones JE, Wang Z, Owens SA, Mueller SC, et al. D1 dopamine receptor signaling involves caveolin-2 in HEK-293 cells. Kidney Int 2004;66(6):2167−8.

[301] Gildea JJ, Israel JA, Johnson AK, Zhang J, Jose PA, Felder RA. Caveolin-1 and dopamine-mediated internalization of NaKATPase in human renal proximal tubule cells. Hypertension 2009;54(5):1070−6.

[302] Adachi S, Scott L, Holtbäck U, Greengard P, Aperia A, Brismar H. Recruitment of renal dopamine 1 receptors requires an intact microtubulin network. Pflugers Arch 2003;445(5):534−9.

[303] Brismar H, Asghar M, Carey RM, Greengard P, Aperia A. Dopamine-induced recruitment of dopamine D1 receptors to the plasma membrane. Proc Natl Acad Sci USA 1998;95 (10):5573−8.

[304] Trivedi M, Narkar VA, Hussain T, Lokhandwala MF. Dopamine recruits D1A receptors to Na-K-ATPase-rich caveolar plasma membranes in rat renal proximal tubules. Am J Physiol Renal Physiol 2004;287(5):F921−31.

[305] Banday AA, Fazili FR, Lokhandwala MF. Insulin causes renal dopamine D1 receptor desensitization via GRK2-mediated receptor phosphorylation involving phosphatidylinositol 3-kinase and protein kinase C. Am J Physiol Renal Physiol 2007;293(3):F877−84.

[306] Sanada H, Yatabe J, Midorikawa S, Katoh H, Hashimoto S, Watanabe T, et al. Amelioration of genetic hypertension by suppression of renal G protein-coupled receptor kinase type 4 expression. Hypertension 2006;47(6):1131−9.

[307] Rankin ML, Marinec PS, Cabrera DM, Wang Z, Jose PA, Sibley DR. The D_1 dopamine receptor is constitutively phosphorylated by G protein-coupled receptor kinase 4. Mol Pharmacol 2006;69(3):759−69.

[308] Tiberi M, Nash SR, Bertrand L, Lefkowitz RJ, Caron MG. Differential regulation of dopamine D1A receptor responsiveness by various G protein-coupled receptor kinases. J Biol Chem 1996;271(7):3771−8.

[309] Fraga S, Jose PA, Soares-da-Silva P. Involvement of G protein-coupled receptor kinase 4 and 6 in rapid desensitization of dopamine D1 receptor in rat IEC-6 intestinal epithelial cells. Am J Physiol Regul Integr Comp Physiol 2004;287(4):R772−9.

[310] Heydorn A, Søndergaard BP, Hadrup N, Holst B, Haft CR, Schwartz TW. Distinct in vitro interaction pattern of dopamine receptor subtypes with adaptor proteins involved in post-endocytotic receptor targeting. FEBS Lett 2004;556(1-3):276−80.

[311] Namkung Y, Dipace C, Javitch JA, Sibley DR. G protein-coupled receptor kinase-2 constitutively regulates D2 dopamine receptor expression and signaling independently of receptor phosphorylation. J Biol Chem 2009;284(49):34103−15.

[312] Miaczynska M, Pelkmans L, Zerial M. Not just a sink: endosomes in control of signal transduction. Curr Opin Cell Biol 2004;16(4):400−6.

[313] Wojcikiewicz RJ. Regulated ubiquitination of proteins in GPCR-initiated signaling pathways. Trends Pharmacol Sci 2004;25(1):35−41.

[314] Zeng C, Watanabe H, Hopfer U, Felder RA, Jose PA. Desensitization of renal D1 dopamine receptor involves formation of endocytic vesicles. FASEB J 2005;19(5): A1137−A1137.

[315] Oakley RH, Laporte SA, Holt JA, Caron MG, Barak LS. Differential affinities of visual arrestin, βarrestin1, and βarrestin2 for G protein-coupled receptors delineate two major classes of receptors. J Biol Chem 2000;275(22):17201−10.

[316] Pitcher JA, Payne ES, Csortos C, DePaoli-Roach AA, Lefkowitz RJ. The G-protein-coupled receptor phosphatase: a protein

protein-coupled receptor kinase 4. Kidney Int 2002; 62(3):790−8.

phosphatase type 2A with a distinct subcellular distribution and substrate specificity. Proc Natl Acad Sci USA 1995; 92(18):8343—7.

[317] Slobodyansky E, Aoki Y, Gaznabi AK, Aviles DH, Fildes RD, Jose PA. Dopamine and protein phosphatase activity in renal proximal tubules. Am J Physiol 1995;268(2 Pt 2):F279—84.

[318] Efendiev R, Yudowski GA, Zwiller J, Leibiger B, Katz AL, Berggren PO, et al. Relevance of dopamine signals anchoring dynamin-2 to the plasma membrane during Na^+,K^+-ATPase endocytosis. J Biol Chem 2002;277(46):44108—14.

[319] Aperia A, Fryckstedt J, Svensson L, Hemmings Jr HC, Nairn AC, Greengard P. Phosphorylated Mr 32,000 dopamine- and cAMP-regulated phosphoprotein inhibits Na +,K + -ATPase activity in renal tubule cells. Proc Natl Acad Sci USA 1991; 88(7):2798—801.

[320] Iwata K, Ito K, Fukuzaki A, Inaki K, Haga T. Dynamin and rab5 regulate GRK2-dependent internalization of dopamine D2 receptors. Eur J Biochem 1999;263(2):596—602.

[321] So CH, Verma V, O'Dowd BF, George SR. Desensitization of the dopamine D_1 and D_2 receptor hetero-oligomer mediated calcium signal by agonist occupancy of either receptor. Mol Pharmacol 2007;72(2):450—62.

[322] Kim KM, Gainetdinov RR, Laporte SA, Caron MG, Barak LS. G protein-coupled receptor kinase regulates dopamine D_3 receptor signaling by modulating the stability of a receptor-filamin-β-arrestin complex. A case of autoreceptor regulation. J Biol Chem 2005;280(13):12774—80.

[323] Spooren A, Rondou P, Debowska K, Lintermans B, Vermeulen L, Samyn B, et al. Resistance of the dopamine D4 receptor to agonist-induced internalization and degradation. Cell Signal 2010;22(4):600—9.

[324] Lingwood D, Simons K. Lipid rafts as a membrane-organizing principle. Science 2010;327(5961):46—50.

[325] Insel PA, Head BP, Ostrom RS, Patel HH, Swaney JS, Tang CM, et al. Caveolae and lipid rafts: G protein-coupled receptor signaling microdomains in cardiac myocytes. Ann N Y Acad Sci 2005;1047:166—72.

[326] Pedrosa R, Villar VA, Pascua AM, Simao S, Hopfer U, Jose PA, et al. H2O2 stimulation of the Cl^-/HCO_3^- exchanger by angiotensin II and angiotensin II type 1 receptor distribution in membrane microdomains. Hypertension 2008;51(5):1332—8.

[327] Li H, Han W, Villar VA, Keever LB, Lu Q, Hopfer U, et al. D_1-like receptors regulate NADPH oxidase activity and sub-unit expression in lipid raft microdomains of renal proximal tubule cells. Hypertension 2009;53(6):1054—61.

[328] Sánchez-Wandelmer J, Dávalos A, de la Peña G, Cano S, Giera M, Canfran-Duque A, et al. Haloperidol disrupts lipid rafts and impairs insulin signaling in SH-SY5Y cells. Neuroscience 2010;167(1):143—53.

[329] Wang Q, Ting WL, Yang H, Wong PT. High doses of simva-statin upregulate dopamine D_1 and D_2 receptor expression in the rat prefrontal cortex: possible involvement of endothelial nitric oxide synthase. Br J Pharmacol 2005;144(7):933—9.

[330] Han W, Li H, Villar VA, Pascua AM, Dajani MI, Wang X, et al. Lipid rafts keep NADPH oxidase in the inactive state in human renal proximal tubule cells. Hypertension 2008; 51(2):481—748.

[331] O'Dowd BF, Ji X, Alijaniaram M, Rajaram RD, Kong MM, Rashid A, et al. Dopamine receptor oligomerization visualized in living cells. J Biol Chem 2005;280(44):37225—35.

[332] Bulenger S, Marullo S, Bouvier M. Emerging role of homo- and heterodimerization in G-protein-coupled receptor bio-synthesis and maturation. Trends Pharmacol Sci 2005;26 (3):131—7.

[333] Simpson LM, Taddese B, Wall ID, Reynolds CA. Bioinformatics and molecular modelling approaches to GPCR oligomerization. Curr Opin Pharmacol 2010;10(1):30—7.

[334] Milligan G. G protein-coupled receptor hetero-dimerization: contribution to pharmacology and function. Br J Pharmacol 2009;158(1):5—14.

[335] Gildea JJ, Kemp BA, Howell NL, Van Sciver RE, Carey RM, Felder RA. Inhibition of renal caveolin-1 reduces natriuresis and produces hypertension in sodium-loaded rats. Am J Physiol Renal Physiol 2011;300(4):F914—20.

[336] Achour L, Labbé-Jullié C, Scott MG, Marullo S. An escort for GPCRs: implications for regulation of receptor density at the cell surface. Trends Pharmacol Sci 2008;29(10):528—35 41

[337] Van Craenenbroeck K, Clark SD, Cox MJ, Oak JN, Liu F, Van Tol HH. Folding efficiency is rate-limiting in dopamine D_4 receptor biogenesis. J Biol Chem 2005;280(19):19350—7.

[338] Free RB, Hazelwood LA, Cabrera DM, Spadling HN, Namkung Y, Rankin ML, et al. D_1 and D_2 dopamine receptor expression is regulated by direct interaction with the chaperone protein calnexin. J Biol Chem 2007; 282(29):21285—300.

[339] Dupré DJ, Robitaille M, Richer M, Ethier N, Mamarbachi AM, Hébert TE. Dopamine receptor-interacting protein 78 acts as a molecular chaperone for Gγ subunits before assembly with Gβ. J Biol Chem 2007;282(18):13703—15.

[340] Bermak JC, Li M, Bullock C, Zhou QY. Regulation of transport of the dopamine D1 receptor by a new membrane-associated ER protein. Nat Cell Biol 2001;3(5):492—8.

[341] Leclerc PC, Auger-Messier M, Lanctot PM, Escher E, Leduc R, Guillemette G. A polyaromatic caveolin-binding-like motif in the cytoplasmic tail of the type 1 receptor for angiotensin II plays an important role in receptor trafficking and signaling. Endocrinology 2002;143(12):4702—10.

[342] Zeng C, Liu Y, Wang Z, He D, Huang L, Yu P, et al. Activation of D3 dopamine receptor decreases angiotensin II type 1 receptor expression in rat renal proximal tubule cells. Circ Res 2006;99(5):494—500.

[343] Zeng C, Wang Z, Hopfer U, et al. Rat strain effects of AT1 receptor activation on D1 dopamine receptors in immortalized renal proximal tubule cells. Hypertension 2005;46(4):799—805.

[344] Kim OJ, Ariano MA, Lazzarini RA, Levine MS, Sibley DR. Neurofilament-M interacts with the D_1 dopamine receptor to regulate cell surface expression and desensitization. J Neurosci 2002;22(14):5920—30.

[345] Bai J, He F, Novikova SI, Undie AS, Dracheva S, Haroutunian V, et al. Abnormalities in the dopamine system in schizophre-nia may lie in altered levels of dopamine receptor-interacting proteins. Biol Psychiatry 2004;56(6):427—40.

[346] Shimokawa N, Haglund K, Hölter SM, et al. CIN85 regulates dopamine receptor endocytosis and governs behaviour in mice. EMBO J 2010;29(14):2421—32.

[347] Liu Y, Buck DC, Neve KA. Novel interaction of the dopamine D_2 receptor and the Ca^{2+} binding protein S100B: role in D_2 receptor function. Mol Pharmacol 2008;74(2):371—8.

[348] Negyessy L, Goldman-Rakic PS. Subcellular localization of the dopamine D_2 receptor and coexistence with the calcium-binding protein neuronal calcium sensor-1 in the primate prefrontal cortex. J Comp Neurol 2005;488(4):464—75.

[349] Kim OJ, Ariano MA, Namkung Y, Marinec P, Kim E, Han J, et al. D_2 dopamine receptor expression and trafficking is regulated through direct interactions with ZIP. J Neurochem 2008; 106(1):83—95.

[350] Tirotta E, Fontaine V, Picetti R. Signaling by dopamine regu-lates D2 receptors trafficking at the membrane. Cell Cycle 2008;7(14):2241—8.

[351] Binda AV, Kabbani N, Lin R, Levenson R. D_2 and D_3 dopamine receptor cell surface localization mediated by interaction with protein 4.1N. Mol Pharmacol 2002;62(3):507—13.

[352] Lin R, Karpa K, Kabbani N, Goldman-Rakic P, Levenson R. Dopamine D_2 and D_3 receptors are linked to the actin cytoskeleton via interaction with filamin A. Proc Natl Acad Sci USA 2001;98(9):5258—63.

[353] Basile M, Lin R, Kabbani N, Karpa K, Kilimann M, Simpson I, et al. Paralemmin interacts with D3 dopamine receptors: implications for membrane localization and cAMP signaling. Arch Biochem Biophys 2006;446(1):60—8.

[354] Rondou P, Skieterska K, Packeu A, Lintermans B, Vanhoenacker P, Vauquelin G, et al. KLHL12-mediated ubiquitination of the dopamine D4 receptor does not target the receptor for degradation. Cell Signal 2010;22(6):900—13.

[355] Karpa KD, Lidow MS, Pickering MT, Levenson R, Bergson C. N-linked glycosylation is required for plasma membrane localization of D_5, but not D_1, dopamine receptors in transfected mammalian cells. Mol Pharmacol 1999;56(5):1071—8.

[356] Sidhu A, Kumar U, Uh M, Patel S. Diminished expression of renal dopamine D1A receptors in the kidney inner medulla of the spontaneously hypertensive rat. J Hypertens 1998;16(5):601—8.

[357] Shin Y, Kumar U, Patel Y, Patel SC, Sidhu A. Differential expression of D2-like dopamine receptors in the kidney of the spontaneously hypertensive rat. J Hypertens 2003;21(1):199—207.

[358] Huo TL, Healy DP. Prostaglandin E2 production in rat IMCD cells. I. Stimulation by dopamine. Am J Physiol 1991;261(4 Pt 2):F647—f654.

[359] Huo T, Ye MQ, Healy DP. Characterization of a dopamine receptor (DA2K) in the kidney inner medulla. Proc Natl Acad Sci USA 1991;88(8):3170—4.

[360] Wang X, Luo Y, Escano CS, Yang Z, Asico LD, Li H, et al. Upregulation of renal sodium transporters in D5 dopamine receptor-deficient mice. Hypertension 2010;55(6):1431—7.

[361] O'Connell DP, Botkin SJ, Ramos SI, Sibley DR, Ariano MA, Felder RA, et al. Localization of dopamine D1A receptor protein in rat kidneys. Am J Physiol 1995;268(6 Pt 2):F1185—97.

[362] Takemoto F, Satoh T, Cohen HT, Katz AI. Localization of dopamine-1 receptors along the microdissected rat nephron. Pflugers Arch 1991;419(3-4):243—8.

[363] Ohbu K, Felder RA. DA1 dopamine receptors in renal cortical collecting duct. Am J Physiol 1991;261(5 Pt 2):F890—5.

[364] Amenta F, Barili P, Bronzetti E, Ricci A. Dopamine D1-like receptor subtypes in the rat kidney: a microanatomical study. Clin Exp Hypertens 1999;21(1-2):17—23.

[365] Sun D, Wilborn TW, Schafer JA. Dopamine D4 receptor isoform mRNA and protein are expressed in the rat cortical collecting duct. Am J Physiol 1998;275(5 Pt 2):F742—51.

[366] Grupp C, Begher M, Cohen D, Raghunath M, Franz HE, Müller GA. Isolation and characterization of the lower portion of the thin limb of Henle in primary culture. Am J Physiol 1998;274(4 Pt 2):F775—82.

[367] O'Connell DP, Aherne AM, Lane E, Felder RA, Carey RM. Detection of dopamine receptor D1A subtype-specific mRNA in rat kidney by in situ amplification. Am J Physiol 1998;274(1 Pt 2):F232—41.

[368] Edwards RM, Brooks DP. Dopamine inhibits vasopressin action in the rat inner medullary collecting duct via α_2-adrenoceptors. J Pharmacol Exp Ther 2001;298(3):1001—6.

[369] Maeda Y, Terada Y, Nonoguchi H, Knepper MA. Hormone and autacoid regulation of cAMP production in rat IMCD subsegments. Am J Physiol 1992;263(2 Pt 2):F319—27.

[370] Felder RA, Jose PA. Dopamine1 receptors in rat kidneys identified with 1251-Sch 23982. Am. J. Physiol. (Renal Fluid Electrolyte Physiol.) 1988;255(4):F970—6.

[371] Hedge SS, Ricci A, Amenta F, Lokhandwala MF. Evidence from functional and autoradiographic studies for the presence of tubular dopamine-1 receptors and their involvement in the renal effects of fenoldopam. J Pharmacol Exp Ther 1989;251(3):1237—45.

[372] Ozono R, O'Connell DP, Wang ZQ, Moore AF, Sanada H, Felder RA, et al. Localization of the dopamine D1 receptor protein in the human heart and kidney. Hypertension 1997;30(3 Pt 2):725—9.

[373] Narkar VA, Hussain T, Pedemonte C, Lokhandwala MF. Dopamine D2 receptor activation causes mitogenesis via p44/42 mitogen-activated protein kinase in opossum kidney cells. J Am Soc Nephrol 2001;12(9):1844—52.

[374] Nurnberger A, Rabiger M, Mack A, Diaz J, Sokoloff P, Muhlbauer B, et al. Subapical localization of the dopamine D3 receptor in proximal tubules of the rat kidney. J Histochem Cytochem 2004;52(12):1647—55.

[375] O'Connell DP, Vaughan CJ, Aherne AM, Botkin SJ, Wang ZQ, Felder RA, et al. Expression of the dopamine D3 receptor protein in the rat kidney. Hypertension 1998;32(5):886—95.

[376] Ricci A, Marchal-Victorion S, Bronzetti E, Parini A, Amenta F, Tayebati SK. Dopamine D4 receptor expression in rat kidney: evidence for pre- and postjunctional localization. J Histochem Cytochem 2002;50(8):1091—6.

[377] Matsumoto M, Hidaka K, Tada S, Tasaki Y, Yamaguchi T. Full-length cDNA cloning and distribution of human dopamine D4 receptor. Brain Res Mol Brain Res 1995;29(1):157—62.

[378] Amenta F. Light microscope autoradiography of peripheral dopamine receptor subtypes. Clin Exp Hypertens 1997;19(1-2):27—41.

[379] Abdul-Majeed S, Nauli SM. Dopamine receptor type 5 in the primary cilia has dual chemo- and mechano-sensory roles. Hypertension 2011;58(2):325—31.

[380] Amenta F, Barili P, Bronzetti E, Felici L, Mignini F, Ricci A. Localization of dopamine receptor subtypes in systemic arteries. Clin Exp Hypertens 2000;22(3):277—88.

[381] Amenta F. Density and distribution of dopamine receptors in the cardiovascular system and in the kidney. J Auton Pharmacol 1990;10(Suppl. 1):s11—8.

[382] Ricci A, Escaf S, Vega JA, Amenta F. Autoradiographic localization of dopamine D1 receptors in the human kidney. J Pharmacol Exp Ther 1993;264(1):431—7.

[383] Dousa TP, Shah SV, Abboud HE. Potential role of cyclic nucleotides in glomerular pathophysiology. Adv Cyclic Nucleotide Res 1980;12:285—99.

[384] Kotake C, Hoffmann PC, Goldberg LI, Cannon JG. Comparison of the effects of dopamine and beta-adrenergic agonists on adenylate cyclase of renal glomeruli and striatum. Mol Pharmacol 1981;20(2):429—34.

[385] Wargo AA, Slotkoff LM, Jose PA, Pelayo JC, Eisner GM. Cyclic nucleotide response to stimulation in isolated glomeruli from dog kidney. Nephron 1982;32(2):165—9.

[386] Shultz PJ, Sedor JR, Abboud HE. Dopaminergic stimulation of cAMP accumulation in cultured rat mesangial cells. Am J Physiol 1987;253(2 Pt 2):H358—64.

[387] Bek M, Fischer KG, Greiber S, Hupfer C, Mundel P, Pavenstädt H. Dopamine depolarizes podocytes via a D1-like receptor. Nephrol Dial Transplant 1999;14(3):581−7.

[388] Luippold G, Küster E, Joos TO, Mühlbauer B. Dopamine D3 receptor activation modulates renal function in anesthetized rats. Naunyn Schmiedebergs Arch Pharmacol 1998;358(6):690−3.

[389] Barnett R, Singhal PC, Scharschmidt LA, Schlondorff D. Dopamine attenuates the contractile response to angiotensin II in isolated rat glomeruli and cultured mesangial cells. Circ Res 1986;59(5):529−33.

[390] Yamaguchi I, Yao L, Sanada H, et al. Characterization of dopamine D_{1A} receptors in rat juxtaglomerular cells. Hypertension 1997;29(4):962−8.

[391] Sanada H, Yao L, Jose PA, Carey RM, Felder RA. Dopamine D3 receptors in rat juxtaglomerular cells. Clin Exp Hypertens 1997;19(1-2):93−105.

[392] Olsen NV, Lund J, Jensen PF, Espersen K, Kanstrup IL, Plum I, et al. Dopamine, dobutamine, and dopexamine. A comparison of renal effects in unanesthetized human volunteers. Anesthesiology 1993;79(4):685−94.

[393] Smit AJ, Meijer S, Wesseling H, Donker AJ, Reitsma WD. Effect of metoclopramide on dopamine-induced changes in renal function in healthy controls and in patients with renal disease. Clin Sci (Lond) 1988;75(4):421−8.

[394] Hahn RA, Wardell Jr. JR. Renal vascular activity of SK&F 38393 and dopamine in anesthetized dogs. J Cardiovasc Pharmacol 1980;2(5):583−93.

[395] Frederickson ED, Bradley T, Goldberg LI. Blockade of renal effects of dopamine in the dog by the DA1 antagonist SCH 23390. Am J Physiol 1985;249(2 Pt 2):F236−40.

[396] Jose PA, Eisner GM, Robillard JE. Renal hemodynamics and natriuresis induced by the dopamine-1 agonist, SKF 82526. Am J Med Sci 1987;294(3):181−6.

[397] Yatsu T, Arai Y, Takizawa K, Kasai-Nakagawa C, Takanashi M, Uchida W, et al. Renal effect of YM435, a new dopamine D1 receptor agonist, in anesthetized dogs. Eur J Pharmacol 1997;322(1):45−53.

[398] Edwards RM. Comparison of the effects of fenoldopam, SK & F R-87516 and dopamine on renal arterioles in vitro. Eur J Pharmacol 1986;126(1-2):167−70.

[399] Takenaka T, Forster H, Epstein M. Characterization of the renal microvascular actions of a new dopaminergic (DA1) agonist, YM435. J Pharmacol Exp Ther 1993;264(3):1154−9.

[400] Steinhausen M, Weis S, Fleming J, Dussel R, Parekh N. Responses of in vivo renal microvessels to dopamine. Kidney Int 1986;30(3):361−70.

[401] Lang WJ, Woodman OL. Comparison of the vasodilator action of dopamine and dopamine agonists in the renal and coronary beds of the dog. Br J Pharmacol 1982;77(1):23−82.

[402] van Kesteren RG, van Alphen MM, Charbon GA. Effects of dopamine on intestinal vessels in anesthetized dogs. Circ Shock 1988;25(1):41−51.

[403] Jin XH, Wang WZ, Zhao RR. Comparison of the characteristics and density of dopamine-1 receptors in membranes from different arteries using [^{3}H]SCH23390 binding. Methods Find Exp Clin Pharmacol 1995;17(7):455−61.

[404] Alkadhi KA, Sabouni MH, Ansari AF, Lokhandwala MF. Activation of DA1 receptors by dopamine or fenoldopam increases cyclic AMP levels in the renal artery but not in the superior cervical ganglion of the rat. J Pharmacol Exp Ther 1986;238(2):547−53.

[405] Chatziantoniou C, Ruan X, Arendshorst WJ. Defective G protein activation of the cAMP pathway in rat kidney during genetic hypertension. Proc Natl Acad Sci USA 1995;92(7):2924−8.

[406] Tamaki T, Hura CE, Kunau Jr. RT. Dopamine stimulates cAMP production in canine afferent arterioles via DA1 receptors. Am J Physiol 1989;256(3 Pt 2):H626−9.

[407] Manoogian C, Nadler J, Ehrlich L, Horton R. The renal vasodilating effect of dopamine is mediated by calcium flux and prostacyclin release in man. J Clin Endocrinol Metab 1988;66(4):678−83.

[408] Borin ML. Dual inhibitory effects of dopamine on Na^+ homeostasis in rat aorta smooth muscle cells. Am J Physiol 1997;272(2 Pt 1):C428−38.

[409] Rashed SM, Songu-Mize E. Regulation of Na^+-pump activity by dopamine in rat tail arteries. Eur J Pharmacol 1995;284(3):289−97.

[410] Hussain T, Lokhandwala MF. Renal dopamine DA1 receptor coupling with G_S and $G_{q/11}$ proteins in spontaneously hypertensive rats. Am J Physiol 1997;272(3 Pt 2):F339−f346.

[411] Centonze D, Gubellini P, Usiello A, Rossi S, Tscherter A, Bracci E, et al. Differential contribution of dopamine D2S and D2L receptors in the modulation of glutamate and GABA transmission in the striatum. Neuroscience 2004;129(1):157−66.

[412] Lindgren N, Usiello A, Goiny M, Haycock J, Erbs E, Greengard P, et al. Distinct roles of dopamine D2L and D2S receptor isoforms in the regulation of protein phosphorylation at presynaptic and postsynaptic sites. Proc Natl Acad Sci USA 2003;100(7):4305−9.

[413] Chen PC, Lao CL, Chen JC. The D_3 dopamine receptor inhibits dopamine release in PC-12/hD3 cells by autoreceptor signaling via PP-2B, CK1, and Cdk-5. J Neurochem 2009;110(4):1180−90.

[414] Tang L, Todd RD, O'Malley KL. Dopamine D2 and D3 receptors inhibit dopamine release. J Pharmacol Exp Ther 1994;270(2):475−9.

[415] Lokhandwala MF, Steenberg ML. Selective activation by LY-141865 and apomorphine of presynaptic dopamine receptors in the rat kidney and influence of stimulation parameters in the action of dopamine. J Pharmacol Exp Ther 1984;228(1):161−7.

[416] Rump LC, Schwertfeger E, Schuster MJ, Schaible U, Frankenschmidt A, Schollmeyer PJ. Dopamine DA2-receptor activation inhibits noradrenaline release in human kidney slices. Kidney Int 1993;43(1):197−204.

[417] Seri I, Eklöf AC, Aperia A. Role of dopamine2-receptors in mediating renal vascular response to low dose dopamine infusion in the rat. Acta Physiol Scand 1987;130(4):563−9.

[418] Stier Jr CT, Cowden EA, Allison ME. Effects of bromocriptine on single nephron and whole-kidney function in rats. J Pharmacol Exp Ther 1982;220(2):366−3670.

[419] Bughi S, Jost-Vu E, Antonipillai I, Nadler J, Horton R. Effect of dopamine2 blockade on renal function under varied sodium intake. J Clin Endocrinol Metab 1994;78(5):1079−84.

[420] Horn PT, Kohli JD. Absence of postsynaptic DA2 dopamine receptors in the dog renal vasculature. Eur J Pharmacol 1991;197(2-3):125−30.

[421] Siragy HM, Felder RA, Peach MJ, Carey RM. Intrarenal DA2 dopamine receptor stimulation in the conscious dog. Am J Physiol 1992;262(6 Pt 2):F932−8.

[422] Luippold G, Schneider S, Vallon V, Osswald H, Mühlbauer B. Postglomerular vasoconstriction induced by dopamine D_3 receptor activation in anesthetized rats. Am J Physiol Renal Physiol 2000;278(4):F570−5.

[423] Montanari A, Tateo E, Fasoli E, Donatini A, Cimolato B, Perinotto P, et al. Dopamine-2 receptor blockade potentiates

the renal effects of nitric oxide inhibition in humans. Hypertension 1998;31(1 Pt 2):277–82.

[424] Morishita H, Katsuragi T. Existence and pharmacological properties of dopamine D4 receptors in guinea pig vas deferens. Eur J Pharmacol 1999;374(2):255–61.

[425] Woodman OL, Rechtman MP, Lang WJ. A comparison of the responses to some dopamine-receptor agonists and antagonists in the isolated perfused rat kidney. Arch Int Pharmacodyn Ther 1980;248(2):203–11.

[426] Zeng C, Wang D, Asico LD, Welch WJ, Wilcox CS, Hopfer U, et al. Aberrant D1 and D3 dopamine receptor transregulation in hypertension. Hypertension 2004;43(3):654–60.

[427] Ragsdale NV, Lynd M, Chevalier RL, Felder RA, Peach MJ, Carey RM. Selective peripheral dopamine-1 receptor stimulation. Differential responses to sodium loading and depletion in humans. Hypertension 1990;15(6 Pt 2):914–21.

[428] Blaustein MP, Hamlyn JM. Signaling mechanisms that link salt retention to hypertension: endogenous ouabain, the Na^+ pump, the Na^+/Ca^{2+} exchanger and TRPC proteins. Biochim Biophys Acta 2010;1802(12):1219–29.

[429] Zhang Y, Yuan Z, Ge H, Ren Y. Effects of long-term ouabain treatment on blood pressure, sodium excretion, and renal dopamine D_1 receptor levels in rats. J Comp Physiol B 2010;180(1):117–24.

[430] Neve KA, Kozlowski MR, Rosser MP. Dopamine D2 receptor stimulation of Na^+/H^+ exchange assessed by quantification of extracellular acidification. J Biol Chem 1992;267(36):25748–53.

[431] O'Connell DP, Ragsdale NV, Boyd DG, Felder RA, Carey RM. Differential human renal tubular responses to dopamine type 1 receptor stimulation are determined by blood pressure status. Hypertension 1997;29(1 Pt 1):115–22.

[432] Pollock DM, Arendshorst WJ. Tubuloglomerular feedback and blood flow autoregulation during DA1-induced renal vasodilation. Am J Physiol 1990;258(3 Pt 2):F627–35.

[433] Reiner NE, Thompson WL. Dopamine and saralasin antagonism of renal vasoconstriction and oliguria caused by amphotericin B in dogs. J Infect Dis 1979;140(4):564–75.

[434] ter Wee PM, Donker AJ. Pharmacologic manipulation of glomerular function. Kidney Int 1994;45(2):417–24.

[435] Seri I, Aperia A. Contribution of dopamine 2 receptors to dopamine-induced increase in glomerular filtration rate. Am J Physiol 1988;254(2 Pt 2):F196–201.

[436] Mühlbauer B, Spöhr F, Schmidt R, Osswald H. Role of renal nerves and endogenous dopamine in amino acid-induced glomerular hyperfiltration. Am J Physiol 1997;273(1 Pt 2):F144–9.

[437] Siragy HM, Felder RA, Howell NL, Chevalier RL, Peach MJ, Carey RM. Evidence that dopamine-2 mechanisms control renal function. Am J Physiol 1990;259(5 Pt 2):F793–800.

[438] Vallon V. Tubuloglomerular feedback and the control of glomerular filtration rate. News Physiol Sci 2003;18:169–714.

[439] Wilcox CS. Redox regulation of the afferent arteriole and tubuloglomerular feedback. Acta Physiol Scand 2003;179(3):217–23.

[440] Satriano J, Wead L, Cardus A, Deng A, Boss GR, Thomson SC, Blantz RC. Regulation of ecto-5'-nucleotidase by NaCl and nitric oxide: potential roles in tubuloglomerular feedback and adaptation. Am J Physiol Renal Physiol 2006;291(5):F1078–82.

[441] Castrop H, Schnermann J. Isoforms of renal Na-K-2Cl cotransporter NKCC2: Expression and functional significance. Am J Physiol Renal Physiol 2008;295(4):F859–66.

[442] Aoki Y, Albrecht FE, Bergman KR, Jose PA. Stimulation of Na^+-K^+-$2Cl^-$ co-transport in rat medullary thick ascending limb by dopamine. Am J Physiol 1996;271(6 Pt 2):R1561–1567.

[443] Schnermann J, Todd KM, Briggs JP. Effect of dopamine on the tubuloglomerular feedback mechanism. Am J Physiol 1990;258 (4 Pt 2):F790–8.

[444] Häberle DA, Königbauer B. Inhibition of tubuloglomerular feedback by the D1 agonist fenoldopam in chronically salt-loaded rats. J Physiol 1991;441:23–34.

[445] Fuxe K, Marcellino D, Borroto-Escuela DO, Guescini M, Fernandez-Duenas V, Tanganelli S, et al. Adenosine-dopamine interactions in the pathophysiology and treatment of CNS disorders. CNS Neurosci Ther 2010;16(3):e18–42.

[446] Trincavelli ML, Cuboni S, Catena Dell'osso M, Maggio R, Klotz KN, Novi F, et al. Receptor crosstalk: haloperidol treatment enhances A_{2A} adenosine receptor functioning in a transfected cell model. Purinergic Signal 2010;6(4):373–81.

[447] Carlström M, Wilcox CS, Welch WJ. Adenosine A2A receptor activation attenuates tubuloglomerular feedback responses by stimulation of endothelial nitric oxide synthase. Am J Physiol Renal Physiol 2011;300(2):F457–64.

[448] Vlahović P, Stefanović V. Effect of dopamine on ecto-5'-nucleotidase expression in human glomerular mesangial cells. Arch Int Physiol Biochim Biophys 1994;102(3):171–3.

[449] Zeng C, Villar VA, Yu P, Zhou L, Jose PA. Reactive oxygen species and dopamine receptor function in essential hypertension. Clin Exp Hypertens 2009;31(2):156–78.

[450] Kurtz A, Della Bruna R, Pratz J, Cavero I. Rat juxtaglomerular cells are endowed with DA-1 dopamine receptors mediating renin release. J Cardiovasc Pharmacol 1988;12(6):658–63.

[451] Imbs JL, Schmidt M, Schwartz J. Effect of dopamine on renin secretion in the anesthetized dog. Eur J Pharmacol 1975;33(1):151–7.

[452] Mizoguchi H, Dzau VJ, Siwek LG, Barger AC. Effect of intrarenal administration of dopamine on renin release in conscious dogs. Am J Physiol 1983;244(1):H39–45.

[453] Ventura HO, Messerli FH, Frohlich ED, Kobrin I, Oigman W, Dunn FG, et al. Immediate hemodynamic effects of a dopamine-receptor agonist (fenoldopam) in patients with essential hypertension. Circulation 1984;69(6):1142–5.

[454] Carey RM, Stote RM, Dubb JW, Townsend LH, Rose Jr CE, Kaiser DL. Selective peripheral dopamine-1 receptor stimulation with fenoldopam in human essential hypertension. J Clin Invest 1984;74(6):2198–207.

[455] Glück Z, Jossen L, Weidmann P, Gnädinger MP, Peheim E. Cardiovascular and renal profile of acute peripheral dopamine1-receptor agonism with fenoldopam. Hypertension 1987;10(1):43–54.

[456] Carey RM, Thorner MO, Ortt EM. Effects of metoclopramide and bromocriptine on the renin–angiotensin–aldosterone system in man. Dopaminergic control of aldosterone. J Clin Invest 1979;63(4):727–35.

[457] Worth DP, Harvey JN, Brown J, Worral A, Lee MR. Domperidone treatment in man inhibits the fall in plasma renin activity induced by intravenous γ-L-glutamyl-L-dopa. Br J Clin Pharmacol 1986;21(5):497–502.

[458] Aherne AM, Vaughan CJ, Carey RM, O'Connell DP. Localization of dopamine D1A receptor protein and messenger ribonucleic acid in rat adrenal cortex. Endocrinology 1997;138(3):1282–8.

[459] Gallo-Payet N, Chouinard L, Balestre MN, Guillon G. Mechanisms involved in the interaction of dopamine with angiotensin II on aldosterone secretion in isolated and cultured rat adrenal glomerulosa cells. Mol Cell Endocrinol 1991;81(1-3):11–23.

[460] Drake Jr CR, Ragsdale NV, Kaiser DL, Carey RM. Dopaminergic suppression of angiotensin II-induced

aldosterone secretion in man: differential responses during sodium loading and depletion. Metabolism 1984;33 (8):696–702.

[461] Drake Jr CR, Carey RM. Dopamine modulates sodium-dependent aldosterone responses to angiotensin II in humans. Hypertension 1984;6(2 Pt 2):I119–23.

[462] Chang HW, Chu TS, Huang HY, Chueh SC, Wu VC, Chen YM, et al. Down-regulation of D2 dopamine receptor and increased protein kinase Cμ phosphorylation in aldosterone-producing adenoma play roles in aldosterone overproduction. J Clin Endocrinol Metab 2007;92(5):1863–70.

[463] Chang HW, Wu VC, Huang CY, Huang HY, Chen YM, Chu TS, et al. dopamine receptor enhances angiotensin II-stimulated aldosterone secretion through PKC-ε and calcium signaling. Am J Physiol Endocrinol Metab 2008;294(3): E622–629.

[464] Luchsinger A, Grilli M, Forte P, Morales E, Velasco M. Metoclopramide blocks bromocriptine induced antihypertensive effect in hypertensive patients. Int J Clin Pharmacol Ther 1995;33(9):509–12.

[465] Alvelos M, Ferreira A, Bettencourt P, Pimenta J, Azevedo A, Serrao P, et al. Effect of saline load and metoclopramide on the renal dopaminergic system in patients with heart failure and healthy controls. J Cardiovasc Pharmacol 2005; 45(3):197–203.

[466] Siragy HM, Felder RA, Howell NL, Chevalier RL, Peach MJ, Carey RM. Evidence that intrarenal dopamine acts as a paracrine substance at the renal tubule. Am J Physiol 1989;257(3 Pt 2): F469–77.

[467] Pelayo JC, Fildes RD, Eisner GM, Jose PA. Effects of dopamine blockade on renal sodium excretion. Am J Physiol 1983;245(2): F247–53.

[468] Sanada H, Xu J, Watanabe H, Jose PA, Felder RA. Differential expression and regulation of dopamine-1 (D-1) and dopamine-5 (D-5) receptor function in human kidney. Am J Hypertens 2000;13: 156A-156A

[469] Ball SG, Lee MR. The effect of carbidopa administration on urinary sodium excretion in man.Is dopamine an intrarenal natriuretic hormone? Br J Clin Pharmacol 1977;4(2):115–9.

[470] Zhang MZ, Yao B, Wang S, Fan X, Wu G, Yang H, et al. Intrarenal dopamine deficiency leads to hypertension and decreased longevity in mice. J Clin Invest 2011;121 (7):2845–54.

[471] Odlind C, Fasching A, Liss P, Palm F, Hansell P. Changing dopaminergic activity through different pathways: consequences for renal sodium excretion, regional blood flow and oxygen tension in the rat. Acta Physiol Scand 2001;172 (3):219–26.

[472] Odlind C, Reenilä I, Männistö PT, Juvonen R, Uhlen S, Gogos JA, et al. Reduced natriuretic response to acute sodium loading in COMT gene deleted mice. BMC Physiol 2002;2:14.

[473] Ladines CA, Zeng C, Asico LD, et al. Impaired renal D1-like and D2-like dopamine receptor interaction in the spontaneously hypertensive rat. Am J Physiol Regul Integr Comp Physiol 2001;281(4):R1071–8.

[474] Gomes P, Soares-da-Silva P. Dopamine acutely decreases type 3 Na+/H+ exchanger activity in renal OK cells through the activation of protein kinases A and C signalling cascades. Eur J Pharmacol 2004;488(1-3):51–9.

[475] Amaral JS, Pinho MJ, Soares-da-Silva P. Regulation of amino acid transporters in the rat remnant kidney. Nephrol Dial Transplant 2009;24(7):2058–67.

[476] Bacic D, Capuano P, Baum M, Zhang J, Stange G, Biber J, et al. Activation of dopamine D1-like receptors induces acute internalization of the renal Na+/phosphate co-transporter NaPi-IIa

in mouse kidney and OK cells. Am J Physiol Renal Physiol 2005;288(4):F740–7.

[477] Chen Z, Leibiger I, Katz AI, Bertorello AM. Pals-associated tight junction protein functionally links dopamine and angiotensin II to the regulation of sodium transport in renal epithelial cells. Br J Pharmacol 2009;158(2):486–93.

[478] Cinelli AR, Efendiev R, Pedemonte CH. Trafficking of Na-K-ATPase and dopamine receptor molecules induced by changes in intracellular sodium concentration of renal epithelial cells. Am J Physiol Renal Physiol 2008;295(4): F1117–25.

[479] Gomes P, Soares-da-Silva P. Dopamine-induced inhibition of Na+-K+-ATPase activity requires integrity of actin cytoskeleton in opossum kidney cells. Acta Physiol Scand 2002; 175(2):93–101.

[480] Khundmiri SJ, Weinman EJ, Steplock D, Cole J, Ahmad A, Baumann PD, et al. Parathyroid hormone regulation of Na+, K+ -ATPase requires the PDZ 1 domain of sodium hydrogen exchanger regulatory factor-1 in opossum kidney cells. J Am Soc Nephrol 2005;16(9):2598–607.

[481] Kunimi M, Seki G, Hara C, Taniguchi S, Uwatoko S, Goto A, et al. Dopamine inhibits renal Na+:HCO3− co-transporter in rabbits and normotensive rats but not in spontaneously hypertensive rats. Kidney Int 2000;57(2):534–43.

[482] Lanaspa MA, Giral H, Breusegem SY, Halaihel N, Baile G, Catalan J, et al. Interaction of MAP17 with NHERF3/4 induces translocation of the renal Na/Pi IIa transporter to the trans-Golgi. Am J Physiol Renal Physiol 2007;292(1):F230–42.

[483] Correa AH, Choi MR, Gironacci M, Aprile F, Fernández BE. Atrial natriuretic factor decreases renal dopamine turnover and catabolism without modifying its release. Regul Pept 2008;146(1-3):238–42.

[484] Marin-Grez M, Angchanpen P, Gambaro G, Schnermann J, Schubert G, Briggs JP. Evidence for an involvement of dopamine receptors in the natriuretic response to atrial natriuretic peptide. Klin Wochenschr 1987;65(Suppl. 8):97–102.

[485] Hegde SS, Chen CJ, Lokhandwala MF. Involvement of endogenous dopamine and DA-1 receptors in the renal effects of atrial natriuretic factor in rats. Clin Exp Hypertens A 1991; 13(3):357–69.

[486] Bughi S, Horton R, Antonipillai I, Manoogian C, Ehrlich L, Nadler J. Comparison of dopamine and fenoldopam effects on renal blood flow and prostacyclin excretion in normal and essential hypertensive subjects. J Clin Endocrinol Metab 1989;69(6):1116–21.

[487] Costa MA, Elesgaray R, Loria A, Balaszczuk AM, Arranz C. Vascular and renal effects of dopamine during extracellular volume expansion: role of nitric oxide pathway. Life Sci 2006;78(14):1543–9.

[488] Venkatakrishnan U, Chen C, Lokhandwala MF. The role of intrarenal nitric oxide in the natriuretic response to dopamine-receptor activation. Clin Exp Hypertens 2000;22 (3):309–24.

[489] Ibarra F, Crambert S, Eklöf AC, Lundquist A, Hansell P, Holtbäck U. Prolactin, a natriuretic hormone, interacting with the renal dopamine system. Kidney Int 2005;68(4): 1700–7.

[490] Chen C, Lokhandwala MF. Potentiation by enalaprilat of fenoldopam-evoked natriuresis is due to blockade of intrarenal production of angiotensin-II in rats. Naunyn Schmiedebergs Arch Pharmacol 1995;352(2):194–200.

[491] Clark KL, Hilditch A, Robertson MJ, Drew GM. Effects of dopamine DA1-receptor blockade and angiotensin converting enzyme inhibition on the renal actions of fenoldopam in the anaesthetized dog. J Hypertens 1991;9(12):1143–50.

[492] de Vries PA, de Zeeuw D, de Jong PE, Navis G. The abnormal renal vasodilator response to D1-like receptor stimulation in conscious SHR can be normalized by AT1 blockade. J Cardiovasc Pharmacol 2004;44(5):571–6.

[493] Hussain T, Abdul-Wahab R, Kotak DK, Lokhandwala MF. Bromocriptine regulates angiotensin II response on sodium pump in proximal tubules. Hypertension 1998;32(6):1054–9.

[494] Sheikh-Hamad D, Wang YP, Jo OD, Yanagawa N. Dopamine antagonizes the actions of angiotensin II in renal brush-border membrane. Am J Physiol 1993;264(4 Pt 2):F737–43.

[495] Banday AA, Asghar M, Hussain T, Lokhandwala MF. Dopamine-mediated inhibition of renal Na,K-ATPase is reduced by insulin. Hypertension 2003;41(6):1353–8.

[496] Yang J, Cui Z, He D, Ren H, Han Y, Yu C, et al. Insulin increases D_5 dopamine receptor expression and function in renal proximal tubule cells fromWistar-Kyoto rats. Am J Hypertens 2009;22(7):770–6.

[497] Boone M, Kortenoeven ML, Robben JH, Tamma G, Deen PM. Counteracting vasopressin-mediated water reabsorption by ATP, dopamine, and phorbol esters: mechanisms of action. Am J Physiol Renal Physiol 2011;300(3):F761–71.

[498] Sun D, Schafer JA. Dopamine inhibits AVP-dependent Na^+ transport and water permeability in rat CCD via a D_4-like receptor. Am J Physiol 1996;271(2 Pt 2):F391–400.

[499] Nejsum LN, Zelenina M, Aperia A, Frøkiaer J, Nielsen S. Bidirectional regulation of AQP2 trafficking and recycling: Involvement of AQP2-S256 phosphorylation. Am J Physiol Renal Physiol 2005;288(5):F930–8.

[500] Bennett ED, Tighe D, Wegg W. Abolition, by dopamine blockade, of the natriuretic response produced by lower body positive pressure. Clin Sci (Lond) 1982;63(4):361–6.

[501] Luippold G, Zimmermann C, Mai M, Kloor D, Starck D, Gross G, et al. Dopamine D_3 receptors and salt-dependent hypertension. J Am Soc Nephrol 2001;12(11):2272–9.

[502] Luippold G, Beilharz M, Wehrmann M, Unger L, Gross G, Mühlbauer B. Effect of dopamine D3 receptor blockade on renal function and glomerular size in diabetic rats. Naunyn Schmiedebergs Arch Pharmacol 2005;371(5):420–7.

[503] Yamaguchi I, Walk SF, Jose PA, Felder RA. Dopamine D2L receptors stimulate Na^+/K^+-ATPase activity in murine LTK-cells. Mol Pharmacol 1996;49(2):373–8.

[504] Narkar VA, Hussain T, Lokhandwala MF. Activation of D_2-like receptors causes recruitment of tyrosine-phosphorylated NKA α1-subunits in kidney. Am J Physiol Renal Physiol 2002;283(6):F1290–5.

[505] Grider J, Kilpatrick E, Ott C, Jackson B. Effect of dopamine on NaCl transport in the medullary thick ascending limb of the rat. Eur J Pharmacol 1998;342(2-3):281–4.

[506] Pedrosa R, Gomes P, Hopfer U, Jose PA, Soares-da-Silva P. Giα3 protein-coupled dopamine D_3 receptor-mediated inhibition of renal NHE3 activity in SHR proximal tubular cells is a PLC-PKC-mediated event. Am J Physiol Renal Physiol 2004;287(5):F1059–1066.

[507] Chen CJ, Lokhandwala MF. An impairment of renal tubular DA-1 receptor function as the causative factor for diminished natriuresis to volume expansion in spontaneously hypertensive rats. Clin Exp Hypertens A. 1992;14(4):615–28.

[508] Eklöf AC. The natriuretic response to a dopamine DA1 agonist requires endogenous activation of dopamine DA2 receptors. Acta Physiol Scand 1997;160(4):311–4.

[509] Jose PA, Asico LD, Eisner GM, Pocchiari F, Semeraro C, Felder RA. Effects of costimulation of dopamine D_1- and D_2-like receptors on renal function. Am J Physiol 1998;275(4 Pt 2): R986–94.

[510] Muto S, Tabei K, Asano Y, Imai M. Dopaminergic inhibition of the action of vasopressin on the cortical collecting tubule. Eur J Pharmacol 1985;114(3):393–7.

[511] Upadhyay K, Jose P, Wang X. Inhibitory effect of dopamine 4 receptor on sodium chloride co-transporter in the renal distal convoluted tubule. Annual Meeting Pediatric Academic Societies 2011;: Abstract 3750.1

[512] Leyssac PP, Karlsen FM, Holstein-Rathlou NH, Skøtt O. On determinants of glomerular filtration rate after inhibition of proximal tubular reabsorption. Am J Physiol 1994;266(5 Pt 2): R1544–50.

[513] Nielsen CB, Pedersen EB. Abnormal distal tubular sodium reabsorption during dopamine infusion in patients with essential hypertension evaluated by the lithium clearance methods. Clin Nephrol 1997;47(5):304–9.

[514] Olsen NV, Olsen MH, Bonde J, Kanstrup IL, Plum I, Strandgaard S, et al. Dopamine natriuresis in salt-repleted, water-loaded humans: a dose–response study. Br J Clin Pharmacol 1997;43(5):509–20.

[515] Hu MC, Fan L, Crowder LA, Karim-Jimenez Z, Murer H, Moe OW. Dopamine acutely stimulates Na^+/H^+ exchanger (NHE3) endocytosis via clathrin-coated vesicles: dependence on protein kinase A-mediated NHE3 phosphorylation. J Biol Chem 2001;276(29):26906–15.

[516] Debska-Slizien A, Ho P, Drangova R, Baines AD. Endogenous renal dopamine production regulates phosphate excretion. Am J Physiol 1994;266(6 Pt 2):F858–67.

[517] Ba J, Brown D, Friedman PA. Calcium-sensing receptor regulation of PTH-inhibitable proximal tubule phosphate transport. Am J Physiol Renal Physiol 2003;285(6):F1233–43.

[518] Khundmiri SJ, Ahmad A, Bennett RE, Weinman EJ, Steplock D, Cole J, et al. Novel regulatory function for NHERF-1 in Npt2a transcription. Am J Physiol Renal Physiol 2008;294(4):F840–9.

[519] Weinman EJ, Biswas R, Steplock D, Wang P, Lau YS, Desir GV, et al. Increased renal dopamine and acute renal adaptation to a high-phosphate diet. Am J Physiol Renal Physiol 2011;300(5):F1123–9.

[520] Pedrosa R, Jose PA, Soares-da-Silva P. Defective D_1-like receptor-mediated inhibition of the Cl^-/HCO_3^- exchanger in immortalized SHR proximal tubular epithelial cells. Am J Physiol Renal Physiol 2004;286(6):F1120–6.

[521] Pedrosa R, Gomes P, Soares-da-Silva P. Distinct signalling cascades downstream to Gsα coupled dopamine D_1-like NHE3 inhibition in rat and opossum renal epithelial cells. Cell Physiol Biochem 2004;14(1-2):91–100.

[522] Salyer S, Lesousky N, Weinman EJ, Clark BJ, Lederer ED, Khundmiri SJ. Dopamine regulation of Na^+-K^+-ATPase requires the PDZ-2 domain of sodium hydrogen regulatory factor-1 (NHERF-1) in opossum kidney cells. Am J Physiol Cell Physiol 2011;300(3):C425–34.

[523] Wang X, Luo Y, Asico L, Jones JE, Escano CS, Jose PA. Increased renal sodium transporters are associated with hypertension in D4 dopamine receptor deficient mice. FASEB J 2007;21: A1366-A1366.

[524] Grider JS, Ott CE, Jackson BA. Dopamine D1 receptor-dependent inhibition of NaCl transport in the rat thick ascending limb: Mechanism of action. Eur J Pharmacol 2003;473(2-3):185–90.

[525] Amlal H, Legoff C, Vernimmen C, Paillard M, Bichara M. Na^+-K^+($NH4^+$)-$2Cl^-$ co-transport in medullary thick ascending limb: Control by PKA, PKC, and 20-HETE. Am J Physiol 1996;271(2 Pt 1):C455–63.

[526] Kiroytcheva M, Cheval L, Carranza ML, Martin PY, Favre H, Doucet A, et al. Effect of cAMP on the activity and the

phosphorylation of Na^+,K^+-ATPase in rat thick ascending limb of Henle. Kidney Int 1999;55(5):1819–31.

[527] Bertuccio CA, Cheng SX, Arrizurieta EE, Martín RS, Ibarra FR. Mechanisms of Na^+-K^+-ATPase phosphorylation by PKC in the medullary thick ascending limb of Henle in the rat. Pflugers Arch 2003;447(1):87–96.

[528] Wang X, Villar VM, Armando I, Eisner GM, Felder RA, Jose PA. Dopamine, kidney and hypertension: studies in dopamine receptor knockout mice. Pediatr Nephrol 2008;23 (12):2131–46.

[529] Saito O, Ando Y, Kusano E, Asano Y. Functional characterization of basolateral and luminal dopamine receptors in rabbit CCD. Am J Physiol Renal Physiol 2001;281(1):F114–22.

[530] Satoh T, Cohen HT, Katz AI. Different mechanisms of renal Na-K-ATPase regulation by protein kinases in proximal and distal nephron. Am J Physiol 1993;265(3 Pt 2):F399–405.

[531] Asghar M, Kansra V, Hussain T, Lokhandwala MF. Hyperphosphorylation of Na-pump contributes to defective renal dopamine response in old rats. J Am Soc Nephrol 2001;12(2):226–32.

[532] Banday AA, Hussain T, Lokhandwala MF. Renal dopamine D_1 receptor dysfunction is acquired and not inherited in obese Zucker rats. Am J Physiol Renal Physiol 2004;287(1):F109–16.

[533] Bertorello AM, Komarova Y, Smith K, Leibiger IB, Efendiev R, Pedemonte CH, et al. Analysis of Na^+,K^+-ATPase motion and incorporation into the plasma membrane in response to G protein-coupled receptor signals in living cells. Mol Biol Cell 2003;14(3):1149–57.

[534] Efendiev R, Budu CE, Cinelli AR, Bertorello AM, Pedemonte CH. Intracellular Na^+ regulates dopamine and angiotensin II receptors availability at the plasma membrane and their cellular responses in renal epithelia. J Biol Chem 2003;278(31): 28719–26.

[535] Efendiev R, Chen Z, Krmar RT, Uhles S, Katz AI, Pedemonte CH, et al. The 14-3-3 protein translates the Na^+,K^+-ATPase α1-subunit phosphorylation signal into binding and activation of phosphoinositide 3-kinase during endocytosis. J Biol Chem 2005;280(16):16272–7.

[536] Efendiev R, Cinelli AR, Leibiger IB, Bertorello AM, Pedemonte CH. FRET analysis reveals a critical conformational change within the Na,K-ATPase α1 subunit N-terminus during GPCR-dependent endocytosis. FEBS Lett 2006;580(21):5067–70.

[537] Eklöf AC, Holtbäck U, Sundelöf M, Chen S, Aperia A. Inhibition of COMT induces dopamine-dependent natriuresis and inhibition of proximal tubular Na^+,K^+-ATPase. Kidney Int 1997;52(3):742–7.

[538] Nishi A, Eklöf AC, Bertorello AM, Aperia A. Dopamine regulation of renal Na^+,K^+-ATPase activity is lacking in Dahl salt-sensitive rats. Hypertension 1993;21(6 Pt 1):767–71.

[539] Satoh T, Cohen HT, Katz AI. Intracellular signaling in the regulation of renal Na-K-ATPase. II. Role of eicosanoids. J Clin Invest 1993;91(2):409–15.

[540] Doné SC, Leibiger IB, Efendiev R, Katz AI, Leibiger B, Berggren PO, et al. Tyrosine 537 within the Na^+,K^+-ATPase alpha-subunit is essential for AP-2 binding and clathrin-dependent endocytosis. J Biol Chem 2002;277(19):17108–11.

[541] Ominato M, Satoh T, Katz AI. Regulation of Na-K-ATPase activity in the proximal tubule: role of the protein kinase C pathway and of eicosanoids. J Membr Biol 1996;152(3):235–43.

[542] Asghar M, George L, Lokhandwala MF. Exercise decreases oxidative stress and inflammation and restores renal dopamine D1 receptor function in old rats. Am J Physiol Renal Physiol 2007;293(3):F914–9.

[543] Li D, Aperia A, Celsi G, da Cruz e Silva EF, Greengard P, Meister B. Protein phosphatase-1 in the kidney: evidence for a

[role in the regulation of medullary Na^+-K^+-ATPase. Am J Physiol 1995;269(5 Pt 2):F673–80.

[544] Bełtowski J, Marciniak A, Wójcicka G, Górny D. The opposite effects of cyclic AMP-protein kinase a signal transduction pathway on renal cortical and medullary Na^+,K^+-ATPase activity. J Physiol Pharmacol 2002;53(2):211–31.

[545] Perrichot R, Garcia-Ocaña A, Couette S, Comoy E, Amiel C, Friedlander G. Locally formed dopamine modulates renal Na-Pi co-transport through DA1 and DA2 receptors. Biochem J. 1995;312(Pt 2):433–7.

[546] Wiederkehr MR, Di Sole F, Collazo R, Quinones H, Fan L, Murer H, et al. Characterization of acute inhibition of Na exchanger NHE-3 by dopamine in opossum kidney cells. Kidney Int 2001;59(1):197–209.

[547] Riese K, Beyer AT, Lui GM, Crook RB. Dopamine D1 stimulation of Na^+,K^+,Cl^- co-transport in human NPE cells: effects of multiple hormones. Invest Ophthalmol Vis Sci 1998;39 (8):1444–52.

[548] Bertorello AM, Sznajder JI. The dopamine paradox in lung and kidney epithelia: sharing the same target but operating different signaling networks. Am J Respir Cell Mol Biol 2005;33(5):432–7.

[549] Hazelwood LA, Free RB, Cabrera DM, Skinbjerg M, Sibley DR. Reciprocal modulation of function between the D_1 and D_2 dopamine receptors and the Na^+,K^+-ATPase. J Biol Chem 2008;283(52):36441–53.

[550] Bagh MB, Maiti AK, Jana S, Banerjee K, Roy A, Chakrabarti S. Quinone and oxyradical scavenging properties of N-acetylcysteine prevent dopamine mediated inhibition of Na^+, K^+-ATPase and mitochondrial electron transport chain activity in rat brain: implications in the neuroprotective therapy of Parkinson's disease. Free Radic Res 2008;42(6):574–81.

[551] Okamura T, Toda N. Comparison of the effect of dopamine in primate arteries and veins. Hypertens Res 1995;18(Suppl. 1): S35–7.

[552] Polakowski JS, Segreti JA, Cox BF, Hsieh GC, Kolasa T, Moreland RB, et al. Effects of selective dopamine receptor subtype agonists on cardiac contractility and regional haemodynamics in rats. Clin Exp Pharmacol Physiol 2004;31 (12):837–41.

[553] Han G, Kryman JP, McMillin PJ, White RE, Carrier GO. A novel transduction mechanism mediating dopamine-induced vascular relaxation: opening of BKCa channels by cyclic AMP-induced stimulation of the cyclic GMP-dependent protein kinase. J Cardiovasc Pharmacol 1999;34(5):619–27.

[554] Kawano H, Kawano T, Tanaka K, Eguchi S, Takahashi A, Nakaya A, et al. Effects of dopamine on ATP-sensitive potassium channels in porcine coronary artery smooth-muscle cells. J Cardiovasc Pharmacol 2008;51(2):196–201.

[555] White RE, Kryman JP, El-Mowafy AM, Han G, Carrier GO. cAMP-dependent vasodilators cross-activate the cGMP-dependent protein kinase to stimulate BK_{Ca} channel activity in coronary artery smooth muscle cells. Circ Res 2000;86(8):897–905.

[556] Zelenina M, Zelenin S, Bondar AA, Brismar H, Aperia A. Water permeability of aquaporin-4 is decreased by protein kinase C and dopamine. Am J Physiol Renal Physiol 2002; 283(2):F309–18.

[557] Pannicke T, Iandiev I, Uckermann O, Biedermann B, Kutzera F, Wiedemann P, et al. A potassium channel-linked mechanism of glial cell swelling in the postischemic retina. Mol Cell Neurosci 2004;26(4):493–502.

[558] Gálfi M, Baláspiri L, Tóth R, Pávó I, László F, Morschl E, et al. Inhibitory effect of galanin on dopamine-induced enhanced vasopressin secretion in rat neurohypophyseal tissue cultures. Regul Pept 2002;110(1):17–23.

I. EPITHELIAL AND NONEPITHELIAL TRANSPORT AND REGULATION

[559] Laradi A, Sakhrani LM, Massry SG. Effect of dopamine on sodium uptake by renal proximal tubule cells of rabbit. Miner Electrolyte Metab 1986;12(5-6):303–7.

[560] Staudacher T, Pech B, Tappe M, Gross G, Mühlbauer B, Luippold G. Arterial blood pressure and renal sodium excretion in dopamine D_3 receptor knockout mice. Hypertens Res 2007;30(1):93–101.

[561] Drago J, Gerfen CR, Lachowicz JE, Steiner H, Hollon TR, Love PE, et al. Altered striatal function in a mutant mouse lacking D_{1A} dopamine receptors. Proc Natl Acad Sci USA 1994;91(26):12564–8.

[562] Accili D, Fishburn CS, Drago J, Steiner H, Lachowicz JE, Park BH, et al. A targeted mutation of the D_3 dopamine receptor gene is associated with hyperactivity in mice. Proc Natl Acad Sci USA 1996;93(5):1945–9.

[563] Thanos PK, Michaelides M, Ho CW, Wang GJ, Newman AH, Heidbreder CA, et al. The effects of two highly selective dopamine D_3 receptor antagonists (SB-277011A and NGB-2904) on food self-administration in a rodent model of obesity. Pharmacol Biochem Behav 2008;89(4):499–507.

[564] McQuade JA, Benoit SC, Xu M, Woods SC, Seeley RJ. High-fat diet induced adiposity in mice with targeted disruption of the dopamine-3 receptor gene. Behavioural Behav Brain Res 2004;151(1-2):313–9.

[565] Wang Z, Asico LD, Escano CS, Felder RA, Jose PA. Human G protein-coupled receptor kinase type 4 (hGRK4 γ) wild-type prevents salt sensitivity while its variant, hGRK4γ 486V, promotes salt sensitivity in transgenic mice: role of genetic background [Abstract]. Hypertension 2006;48:e27.

[566] Thanos PK, Bermeo C, Rubinstein M, Suchland KL, Wang GJ, Grandy DK, Volkow ND. Conditioned place preference and locomotor activity in response to methylphenidate, amphetamine and cocaine in mice lacking dopamine D4 receptors. J Psychopharmacol 2010;24(6):897–904.

[567] Zeng C, Yang Z, Wang Z, Jones J, Wang X, Altea J, et al. Interaction of angiotensin II type 1 and D_5 dopamine receptors in renal proximal tubule cells. Hypertension 2005;45(4):804–10.

[568] Newman-Tancredi A, Cussac D, Audinot V, Pasteau V, Gavaudan S, Millan MJ. G protein activation by human dopamine D_3 receptors in high-expressing Chinese hamster ovary cells: a guanosine-5′-O-(3-[^{35}S]thio)- triphosphate binding and antibody study. Mol Pharmacol 1999;55(3):564–74.

[569] Zhan L, Liu B, Jose-Lafuente M, Chibalina MV, Grierson A, Maclean A, et al. ALG-2 interacting protein AIP1: a novel link between D1 and D3 signalling. Eur J Neurosci 2008;27(7):1626–33.

[570] Dziedzicka-Wasylewska M, Faron-Górecka A, Andrecka J, Polit A, Kuśmider M, Wasylewski Z. Fluorescence studies reveal heterodimerization of dopamine D1 and D2 receptors in the plasma membrane. Biochemistry 2006;45(29):8751–9.

[571] Lee SP, So CH, Rashid AJ, Varghese G, Cheng R, Lanca AJ, et al. Dopamine D_1 and D_2 receptor co-activation generates a novel phospholipase C-mediated calcium signal. J Biol Chem 2004;279(34):35671–8.

[572] Kitaoka S, Furuyashiki T, Nishi A, Shuto T, Koyasu S, Matsuoka T, et al. Prostaglandin E_2 acts on EP1 receptor and amplifies both dopamine D_1 and D_2 receptor signaling in the striatum. J Neurosci 2007;27(47):12900–7.

[573] Ng J, Rashid AJ, So CH, O'Dowd BF, George SR. Activation of calcium/calmodulin-dependent protein kinase IIa in the striatum by the heteromeric D1-D2 dopamine receptor complex. Neuroscience 2010;165(2):535–41.

[574] Martina M, Bergeron R. D1 and D4 dopaminergic receptor interplay mediates coincident G protein-independent and

[575] Beaver KM, Wright JP, DeLisi M, Walsh A, Vaughn MG, Boisvert D, et al. A gene × gene interaction between DRD2 and DRD4 is associated with conduct disorder and antisocial behavior in males. Behav Brain Funct 2007;3:30.

[576] Juhasz JR, Hasbi A, Rashid AJ, So CH, George SR, O'Dowd BF. Mu-opioid receptor heterooligomer formation with the dopamine D1 receptor as directly visualized in living cells. Eur J Pharmacol 2008;581(3):235–43.

[577] Guo Y, Wang HL, Xiang XH, Zhao Y. The role of glutamate and its receptors in mesocorticolimbic dopaminergic regions in opioid addiction. Neurosci Biobehav Rev 2009;33(6):864–73.

[578] Lee FJ, Xue S, Pei L, Vukusic B, Chery N, Wang Y, et al. Dual regulation of NMDA receptor functions by direct protein-protein interactions with the dopamine D1 receptor. Cell 2002;111(2):219–30.

[579] Scott L, Aperia A. Interaction between N-methyl-D-aspartic acid receptors and D1 dopamine receptors: an important mechanism for brain plasticity. Neuroscience 2009;158(1):62–6.

[580] Di Sole F, Cerull R, Petzke S, Casavola V, Burckhardt G, Helmle-Kolb C. Bimodal acute effects of A_1 adenosine receptor activation on Na^+/H^+ exchanger 3 in opossum kidney cells. J Am Soc Nephrol 2003;14(7):1720–30.

[581] Cao Y, Xie KQ, Zhu XZ. The enhancement of dopamine D_1 receptor desensitization by adenosine A_1 receptor activation. Eur J Pharmacol 2007;562(1-2):34–8.

[582] Le Crom S, Prou D, Vernier P. Autocrine activation of adenosine A_1 receptors blocks D_{1A} but not D_{1B} dopamine receptor desensitization. J Neurochem 2002;82(6):1549–52.

[583] Ferre S, von Euler G, Johansson B, Fredholm BB, Fuxe K. Stimulation of high-affinity adenosine A_2 receptors decreases the affinity of dopamine D_2 receptors in rat striatal membranes. Proc Natl Acad Sci USA 1991;88(16):7238–41.

[584] Torvinen M, Marcellino D, Canals M, Agnati LF, Lluis C, Franco R, et al. Adenosine A_{2A} receptor and dopamine D_3 receptor interactions: evidence of functional A_{2A}/D_3 heteromeric complexes. Mol Pharmacol 2005;67(2):400–7.

[585] Brismar H, Agren M, Holtback U. β-Adrenoceptor agonist sensitizes the dopamine-1 receptor in renal tubular cells. Acta Physiol Scand 2002;175(4):333–40.

[586] Carranza A, Nowicki S, Barontini M, Armando I. L-Dopa uptake and dopamine production in proximal tubular cells are regulated by $β_2$-adrenergic receptors. Am J Physiol Renal Physiol 2000;279(1):F77–83.

[587] Jenkins TA, Chai SY, Mendelsohn FA. Upregulation of angiotensin II AT1 receptors in the mouse nucleus accumbens by chronic haloperidol treatment. Brain Res 1997;748(1-2):137–42.

[588] Moore R, Krstew EV, Kirchhoff J, Davisson RL, Lawrence AJ. Central overexpression of angiotensin AT_{1A} receptors prevents dopamine D_2 receptor regulation of alcohol consumption in mice. Alcohol Clin Exp Res 2007;31(7):1128–37.

[589] Choi MR, Medici C, Gironacci MM, Correa AH, Fernández BE. Angiotensin II regulation of renal dopamine uptake and Na^+,K^+-ATPase activity. Nephron Physiol 2009;111(4):53–8.

[590] Eadington DW, Swainson CP, Frier BM, Johnston N, Samson RR, Lee MR. Urinary dopamine response to angiotensin II is not abnormal in type 1 (insulin-dependent diabetes mellitus. Nephrol Dial Transplant 1993;8(1):36–40.

[591] Chatziantoniou C, Ruan X, Arendshorst WJ. Interactions of cAMPmediated vasodilators with angiotensin II in rat kidney during hypertension. Am J Physiol 1993;265(6 Pt 2):F845–52.

[592] Lefèvre-Borg F, Lorrain J, Lechaire J, Thiry C, Hicks PE, Cavero I. Studies on the mechanisms of the development of

tolerance to the hypotensive effects of fenoldopam in rats. J Cardiovasc Pharmacol 1988;11(4):444—55.

[593] Luippold G, Max A, Albinus M, Osswald H, Mühlbauer B. Role of the renin-angiotensin system in the compensation of quinpirole-induced blood pressure decrease. Naunyn Schmiedebergs Arch Pharmacol 2003;367(5):427—33.

[594] Cheng HF, Becker BN, Harris RC. Dopamine decreases expression of type-1 angiotensin II receptors in renal proximal tubule. J Clin Invest 1996;97(12):2745—52.

[595] Mertens B, Vanderheyden P, Michotte Y, Sarre S. Direct angiotensin II type 2 receptor stimulation decreases dopamine synthesis in the rat striatum. Neuropharmacology 2010;58 (7):1038—44.

[596] Salomone LJ, Howell NL, McGrath HE, Kemp BA, Keller SR, Gildea JJ, et al. Intrarenal dopamine D_1-like receptor stimulation induces natriuresis via an angiotensin type-2 receptormechanism. Hypertension 2007;49(1):155—61.

[597] Correa AH, Choi MR, Gironacci M, Valera MS, Fernández BE. Signaling pathways involved in atrial natriuretic factor and dopamine regulation of renal Na^+, K^+ -ATPase activity. Regul Pept 2007;138(1):26—31.

[598] Winaver J, Burnett JC, Tyce GM, Dousa TP. ANP inhibits Na^+-H^+ antiport in proximal tubular brush border membrane: role of dopamine. Kidney Int 1990;38(6):1133—40.

[599] Castellano M, Beschi M, Agabiti-Rosei E, Rizzoni D, Rossini P, Poiesi C, et al. Renal and hemodynamic effects of atrial natriuretic peptide infusion are not mediated by peripheral dopaminergic mechanisms. Am J Hypertens 1991;4(4 Pt 1): 385—8.

[600] Stokes GS, Monaghan JC, Pillai DN. Effects of carbidopa and of intravenous saline infusion into normal and hypertensive subjects on urinary free and conjugated dopamine. J Hypertens 1997;15(7):761—8.

[601] Lucarini AR, Arrighi P, Favilla S, Simonini N, Salvetti A. The influence of dopamine-1 receptor blockade on the humoral and renal effects of low-dose atrial natriuretic factor in human hypertensives. J Hypertens Suppl 1989;7(6):S230—1.

[602] Kageyama S, Brown J, Causon R, O'Flynn M, Aber V. DOPA decarboxylase inhibition does not influence the diuretic and natriuretic response to exogenous alpha-atrial natriuretic peptide in man. Eur J Clin Pharmacol 1990;38(3):223—7.

[603] Lewis HM, Wilkins MR, Kendall MJ, Lee MR. Carbidopa does not affect the renal response to atrial natriuretic factor in man. Clin Sci (Lond) 1989;77(3):281—5.

[604] Hirata Y, Fukui K, Hayakawa H, et al. Renal effects of atrial natriuretic peptide during dopamine infusion. Am J Hypertens 1990;3(11):866—9.

[605] Webb RL, Della Puca R, Manniello J, Robson RD, Zimmerman MB, Ghai RD. Dopaminergic mediation of the diuretic and natriuretic effects of ANF in the rat. Life Sci 1986;38(25):2319—27.

[606] Hansell P, Fasching A, Sjoquist M, Anden NE, Ulfendahl HR. The dopamine receptor antagonist haloperidol blocks natriuretic but not hypotensive effects of the atrial natriuretic factor. Acta Physiol Scand 1987;130(3):401—7.

[607] Katoh T, Sophasan S, Kurokawa K. Permissive role of dopamine in renal action of ANP in volume-expanded rats. Am J Physiol 1989;257(2 Pt 2):F300—9.

[608] Ortola FV, Seri I, Downes S, Brenner BM, Ballermann BJ. Dopamine1-receptor blockade inhibits ANP-induced phosphaturia and calciuria in rats. Am J Physiol 1990;259(1 Pt 2): F138—46.

[609] Holtbäck U, Brismar H, DiBona GF, Fu M, Greengard P, Aperia A. Receptor recruitment: a mechanism for interactions between G protein-coupled receptors. Proc Natl Acad Sci USA 1999;96(13):7271—5.

[610] Soares-da-Silva P, Fernandes MH. Effect of α-human atrial natriuretic peptide on the synthesis of dopamine in the rat kidney. Br J Pharmacol 1992;105(4):869—74.

[611] Miyasaka K, Hosoya H, Takano S, Ohta M, Sekime A, Kanai S, et al. Differences in ethanol ingestion between cholecystokinin-A receptor deficient and -B receptor deficient mice. Alcohol Alcohol 2005;40(3):176—80.

[612] Li XM, Hedlund PB, Fuxe K. Cholecystokinin octapeptide in vitro and ex vivo strongly modulates striatal dopamine D2 receptors in rat forebrain sections. Eur J Neurosci 1995; 7(5):962—71.

[613] Dasgupta S, Li XM, Jansson A, Finnman UB, Matsui T, Rinken A, et al. Regulation of dopamine D_2 receptor affinity by cholecystokinin octapeptide in fibroblast cells cotransfected with human CCK_B and D_2L receptor cDNAs. Brain Res Mol Brain Res 1996;36(2):292—9.

[614] Roots K, Kairane C, Salum T, Koks S, Karelson E, Vasar E, et al. Very low levels of cholecystokinin octapeptide activate Na-pump in the cerebral cortex of CCK2 receptor-deficient mice. Int J Dev Neurosci 2006;24(6):395—400.

[615] Pisegna JR, Tarasova NI, Kopp JA, et al. Cholecystokinin type B receptors (CCKBRs) in the rat kidney mediate gastrin-stimulated urinary sodium excretion through inositol phosphate turnover (IP) and inhibition of Na^+/K^+ ATPase. Gastroenterology 2000;118(4): A301-A301

[616] Pollock JS, Pollock DM. Endothelin and NOS1/nitric oxide signaling and regulation of sodium homeostasis. Curr Opin Nephrol Hypertens 2008;17(1):70—5.

[617] Van Den Buuse M, Webber KM. Endothelin and dopamine release. Prog Neurobiol 2000;60(4):385—405.

[618] Zeng C, Asico LD, Yu C, Villar VA, Shi W, Luo Y, et al. Renal D_3 dopamine receptor stimulation induces natriuresis by endothelin B receptor interactions. Kidney Int 2008; 74(6):750—9.

[619] Dunham JH, Meyer RC, Garcia EL, Hall RA. GPR37 surface expression enhancement via N-terminal truncation or protein—protein interactions. Biochemistry 2009;48(43):10286—97.

[620] Kanyicska B, Freeman ME, Dryer SE. Endothelin activates large conductance K^+ channels in rat lactotrophs: Reversal by long-term exposure to dopamine agonist. Endocrinology 1997;138(8):3141—53.

[621] Hussain T, Beheray SA, Lokhandwala MF. Defective dopamine receptor function in proximal tubules of obese zucker rats. Hypertension 1999;34(5):1091—6.

[622] Umrani DN, Banday AA, Hussain T, Lokhandwala MF. Rosiglitazone treatment restores renal dopamine receptor function in obese Zucker rats. Hypertension 2002; 40(6):880—5.

[623] Tsuchida H, Imai G, Shima Y, Satoh T, Owada S. Mechanism of sodium load-induced hypertension in non-insulin dependent diabetes mellitus model rats: defective dopaminergic system to inhibit Na-K-ATPase activity in renal epithelial cells. Hypertens Res 2001;24(2):127—35.

[624] Trivedi M, Lokhandwala MF. Rosiglitazone restores renal D_{1A} receptor-G_s protein coupling by reducing receptor hyperphosphorylation in obese rats. Am J Physiol Renal Physiol 2005;289(2):F298—304.

[625] Carranza A, Musolino PL, Villar M, Nowicki S. Signaling cascade of insulin-induced stimulation of L-dopa uptake in renal proximal tubule cells. Am J Physiol Cell Physiol 2008;295(6): C1602—9.

[626] Umrani DN, Goyal RK. Fenoldopam treatment improves peripheral insulin sensitivity and renal function in STZ-induced type 2 diabetic rats. Clin Exp Hypertens 2003; 25(4):221—33.

[627] Moreira-Rodrigues M, Quelhas-Santos J, Serrão P, Fernandes-Cerqueira C, Sampaio-Maia B, Pestana M. Glycaemic control with insulin prevents the reduced renal dopamine D_1 receptor expression and function in streptozotocin-induced diabetes. Nephrol Dial Transplant 2010;25(9):2945−53.

[628] Rubı B, Ljubicic S, Pournourmohammadi S, Carrobio S, Armanet M, Bartley C, et al. Dopamine D_2-like receptors are expressed in pancreatic beta cells and mediate inhibition of insulin secretion. J Biol Chem 2005;280(44):36824−32.

[629] Shankar E, Santhosh KT, Paulose CS. Dopaminergic regulation of glucose-induced insulin secretion through dopamine D2 receptors in the pancreatic islets in vitro. IUBMB Life 2006; 58(3):157−63.

[630] Kok P, Roelfsema F, Frolich M, van Pelt J, Stokkel MP, Meinders AE, et al. Activation of dopamine D2 receptors simultaneously ameliorates various metabolic features of obese women. Am J Physiol Endocrinol Metab 2006;291(5): E1038−43.

[631] Zhang Y, Cincotta AH. Inhibitory effects of bromocriptine on vascular smooth muscle cell proliferation. Atherosclerosis 1997;133(1):37−44.

[632] Huang H, Han Y, Wang X, Chen C, Yu C, He D, et al. Inhibitory effect of the D_3 dopamine receptor on insulin receptor expression and function in vascular smooth muscle cells. Am J Hypertens 2011;24(6):654−60.

[633] Gross ML, Koch A, Mühlbauer B, Adamczak M, Ziebart H, Drescher K, et al. Renoprotective effect of a dopamine D3 receptor antagonist in experimental type II diabetes. Lab Invest 2006;86(3):262−74.

[634] Goto J, Otsuka F, Yamashita M, Suzuki J, Otani H, Takahashi H, et al. Enhancement of aldosterone-induced catecholamine production by bone morphogenetic protein-4 through activating Rho and SAPK/JNK pathway in adrenomedullar cells. Am J Physiol Endocrinol Metab 2009;296(4):E904−16.

[635] Robertson MJ, Horn NM, Chapman BJ. The depressor and renal vasodilator responses to dopamine in the rat do not depend on prostaglandin biosynthesis. J Pharm Pharmacol 1980;32(11):782−5.

[636] Glück Z, Jossen L, Weidmann P, Gnädinger MP, Peheim E. Cardiovascular and renal profile of acute peripheral dopamine1-receptor agonism with fenoldopam. Hypertension 1987;10(1):43−54.

[637] Zhang MZ, Yao B, McKanna JA, Harris RC. Cross talk between the intrarenal dopaminergic and cyclooxygenase-2 systems. Am J Physiol Renal Physiol 2005;288(4):F840−5.

[638] Grima G, Benz B, Parpura V, Cuénod M, Do KQ. Dopamine-induced oxidative stress in neurons with glutathione deficit: implication for schizophrenia. Schizophr Res 2003;62(3):213−24.

[639] Cosentino M, Rasini E, Colombo C, Marino F, Blandini F, Ferrari M, et al. Dopaminergic modulation of oxidative stress and apoptosis in human peripheral blood lymphocytes: evidence for a D1-like receptor-dependent protective effect. Free Radic Biol Med 2004;36(10):1233−40.

[640] Lu Q, Asico LD, Jones JE, et al. Impaired heme oxygenase activity, increased reactive oxygen species, and high blood pressure in D5 dopamine receptor deficient mice. J Am Soc Nephrol 2005;16: 163A-163A.

[641] Banday AA, Fazili FR, Lokhandwala MF. Oxidative stress causes renal dopamine D_1 receptor dysfunction and hypertension via mechanisms that involve nuclear factor-κB and protein kinase C. J Am Soc Nephrol 2007;18(5):1446−57.

[642] Asghar M, Banday AA, Fardoun RZ, Lokhandwala MF. Hydrogen peroxide causes uncoupling of dopamine D1-like receptors from G proteins via a mechanism involving protein kinase C and G-protein-coupled receptor kinase 2. Free Radic Biol Med 2006;40(1):13−20.

[643] Chugh G, Lokhandwala MF, Asghar M. Oxidative stress alters renal D1 and AT1 receptor functions and increases blood pressure in old rats. Am J Physiol Renal Physiol 2011;300(1): F133−8.

[644] Parvez S, Winkler-Stuck K, Hertel S, Schönfeld P, Siemen D. The dopamine-D2-receptor agonist ropinirole dose-dependently blocks the Ca^{2+}-triggered permeability transition of mitochondria. Biochim Biophys Acta 2010;1797(6-7):1245−50.

[645] Carvey PM, McGuire SO, Ling ZD. Neuroprotective effects of D3 dopamine receptor agonists. Parkinsonism Relat Disord 2001;7(3):213−23.

[646] Zou L, Xu J, Jankovic J, He Y, Appel SH, Le W. Pramipexole inhibits lipid peroxidation and reduces injury in the substantia nigra induced by the dopaminergic neurotoxin 1-methyl-4-phenyl-1,2,3,6-tetrahydropyridine in C57BL/6 mice. Neurosci Lett 2000;281(2-3):167−70.

[647] Le WD, Jankovic J, Xie W, Appel SH. Antioxidant property of pramipexole independent of dopamine receptor activation in neuroprotection. J Neural Transm 2000;107(10):1165−73.

[648] Gribkoff VK, Bozik ME. KNS-760704 [(6R)-4,5,6,7-tetrahydro-N6-propyl-2, 6-benzothiazole-diamine dihydrochloride monohydrate] for the treatment of amyotrophic lateral sclerosis. CNS Neurosci Ther 2008;14(3):215−26.

[649] Ishige K, Chen Q, Sagara Y, Schubert D. The activation of dopamine D4 receptors inhibits oxidative stress-induced nerve cell death. J Neurosci 2001;21(16):6069−76.

[650] Cosentino M, Fietta AM, Ferrari M, Rasini E, Bombelli R, Carcano E, et al. Human $CD4^+CD25^+$ regulatory T cells selectively express tyrosine hydroxylase and contain endogenous catecholamines subserving an autocrine/paracrine inhibitory functional loop. Blood 2007;109(2):632−42.

[651] Sarkar C, Basu B, Chakroborty D, Dasgupta PS, Basu S. The immunoregulatory role of dopamine: an update. Brain Behav Immun 2010;24(4):525−8.

[652] Ricci A, Bronzetti E, Mignini F, Tayebati SK, Zaccheo D, Amenta F. Dopamine D1-like receptor subtypes in human peripheral blood lymphocytes. J Neuroimmunol 1999;96 (2):234−40.

[653] McKenna F, McLaughlin PJ, Lewis BJ, Sibbring GC, Cummerson JA, Bowen-Jones D, et al. Dopamine receptor expression on human T- and B-lymphocytes, monocytes, neutrophils, eosinophils and NK cells: a flow cytometric study. J Neuroimmunol 2002;132(1-2):34−40.

[654] Nakano K, Yamaoka K, Hanami K, Saito K, Sasaguri Y, Yanagihara N, et al. Dopamine induces IL-6-dependent IL-17 production via D1-like receptor on CD4 naive T cells and D1-like receptor antagonist SCH-23390 inhibits cartilage destruction in a human rheumatoid arthritis/SCID mouse chimera model. J Immunol 2011;186(6):3745−52.

[655] Huang Y, Qiu AW, Peng YP, Liu Y, Huang HW, Qiu YH. Roles of dopamine receptor subtypes in mediating modulation of T lymphocyte function. Neuro Endocrinol Lett 2010;31 (6):782−91.

[656] Gomez F, Ruiz P, Briceño F, Rivera C, Lopez R. Macrophage Fcgamma receptors expression is altered by treatment with dopaminergic drugs. Clin Immunol 1999;90(3):375−87.

[657] Ghosh MC, Mondal AC, Basu S, Banerjee S, Majumder J, Bhattacharya D, et al. Dopamine inhibits cytokine release and expression of tyrosine kinases, Lck and Fyn in activated T cells. Int Immunopharmacol 2003;3(7):1019−26.

[658] Besser MJ, Ganor Y, Levite M. Dopamine by itself activates either D2, D3 or D1/D5 dopaminergic receptors in normal human T-cells and triggers the selective secretion

of either IL-10, TNFα or both. J Neuroimmunol 2005;169 (1-2):161−71.

[659] Haskó G, Szabó C, Merkel K, Bencsics A, Zingarelli B, Kvetan V, et al. Modulation of lipopolysaccharide-induced tumor necrosis factor-alpha and nitric oxide production by dopamine receptor agonists and antagonists in mice. Immunol Lett 1996;49(3):143−7.

[660] Morikawa K, Oseko F, Morikawa S. Immunosuppressive activity of bromocriptine on human T lymphocyte function in vitro. Clin Exp Immunol 1994;95(3):514−8.

[661] Ghosh MC, Mondal AC, Basu S, Banerjee S, Majumder J, Bhattacharya D, et al. Dopamine inhibits cytokine release and expression of tyrosine kinases, Lck and Fyn in activated T cells. Int Immunopharmacol 2003;3(7):1019−26.

[662] Godet C, Goujon JM, Petit I, Lecron JC, Hauet T, Mauco G, et al. Endotoxin tolerance enhances interleukin-10 renal expression and decreases ischemia-reperfusion renal injury in rats. Shock 2006;25(4):384−8.

[663] de Haij S, Woltman AM, Bakker AC, Daha MR, van Kooten C. Production of inflammatory mediators by renal epithelial cells is insensitive to glucocorticoids. Br J Pharmacol 2002;137 (2):197−204.

[664] Wang Y, Tay YC, Harris DC. Proximal tubule cells stimulated by lipopolysaccharide inhibit macrophage activation. Kidney Int 2004;66(2):655−62.

[665] Asghar M, Chugh G, Lokhandwala MF. Inflammation compromises renal dopamine D1 receptor function in rats. Am J Physiol Renal Physiol 2009;297(6):F1543−9.

[666] Zhang Y, Cuevas S, Asico LD, Escano C, Yang Y, Pascua AM, Wang LX, Jones JE, Grandy D, Eisner G, Jose PA, Armando I. Deficient dopamine D2 receptor function causes renal inflammation independently of high blood pressure. PLoS One 2012;7(6):e38745.

[667] Rafiq S, Anand S, Roberts R. Genome-wide association studies of hypertension: have they been fruitful? Cardiovasc Transl Res 2010;3(3):189−96.

[668] Harrap SB. Blood pressure genetics: time to focus. J Am Soc Hypertens 2009;3(4):231−7.

[669] Adeyemo A, Gerry N, Chen G, Herbert A, Doumatey A, Huang H, et al. A genome wide association study of hypertension and blood pressure in African-Americans. PLoS Genet 2009;5(7):e1000564.

[670] Cho YS, Go MJ, Kim YJ, Heo JY, Oh JH, Ban HJ, et al. A large-scale genome-wide association study of Asian populations uncovers genetic factors influencing eight quantitative traits. Nat Genet 2009;41(5):527−34.

[671] Johnson AD, Newton-Cheh C, Chasman DI, Ehret GB, Johnson T, Rose L, et al. Association of hypertension drug target genes with blood pressure and hypertension in 86 588 individuals. Hypertension 2011;57(5):903−10.

[672] Levy D, Ehret GB, Rice K. Genome-wide association study of blood pressure and hypertension. Nat Genet 2009;41(6):677−87.

[673] Newton-Cheh C, Johnson T, Gateva V, Tobin MD, Bochud M, Coin L, et al. Genome-wide association study identifies eight loci associated with blood pressure. Nat Genet 2009; 41(6):666−76.

[674] Wang Y, O'Connell JR, McArdle PF, Wade JB, Dorff SE, Shah SJ, et al. Whole-genome association study identifies STK39 as a hypertension susceptibility gene. Proc Natl Acad Sci USA 2009;106(1):226−321.

[675] Moore JH, Williams SM. New strategies for identifying gene-gene interactions in hypertension. Ann Med 2002;34(2):88−95.

[676] Glazier AM, Nadeau JH, Aitman TJ. Finding genes that underlie complex traits. Science 2002;298(5602):2345−9.

[677] Armando I, Jones JE, EscanoC, Asico L, Premont RT, Jose PA. Deletion of the GRK4 gene decreases blood pressure and reverses salt sensitivity. Proc Am Soc Hypertens 2008;:P-194.

[678] Allayee H, de Bruin TW, Michelle Dominguez K, Cheng LS, Ipp E, Cantor RM, et al. Genome scan for blood pressure in Dutch dyslipidemic families reveals linkage to a locus on chromosome 4p. Hypertension. 2001;38(4):773−8.

[679] Chen W, Li S, Srinivasan SR, Boerwinkle E, Berenson GS. Autosomal genome scan for loci linked to blood pressure levels and trends since childhood: the Bogalusa Heart Study. Hypertension 2005;45(5):954−9.

[680] Zhu H, Lu Y, Wang X, Treiber FA, Harshfield GA, Snieder H, et al. The G protein-coupled receptor kinase 4 gene affects blood pressure in young normotensive twins. Am J Hypertens 2006;19(1):61−6.

[681] Bengra C, Mifflin TE, Khripin Y, Manunta P, Williams SM, Jose PA, et al. Genotyping of essential hypertension single-nucleotide polymorphisms by a homogeneous PCR method with universal energy transfer primers. Clin Chem 2002;48 (12):2131−40.

[682] Gu D, Su S, Ge D, Chen S, Huang J, Li B, et al. Association study with 33 single-nucleotide polymorphisms in 11 candidate genes for hypertension in Chinese. Hypertension 2006;47 (6):1147−54.

[683] Sanada H, Yatabe J, Midorikawa S, Hashimoto S, Watanabe T, Moore JH, et al. Single-nucleotide polymorphisms for diagnosis of salt-sensitive hypertension. Clin Chem 2006; 52(3):352−60.

[684] Speirs HJ, Katyk K, Kumar NN, Benjafield AV, Wang WY, Morris BJ. Association of G-protein-coupled receptor kinase 4 haplotypes, but not HSD3B1 or PTP1B polymorphisms, with essential hypertension. J Hypertens 2004;22(5):931−6.

[685] Williams SM, Ritchie MD, Phillips III JA, Dawson E, Prince M, Dzhura E, et al. Multilocus analysis of hypertension: a hierarchical approach. Hum Hered 2004;57(1):28−38.

[686] Williams SM, Addy JH, Phillips 3rd JA, Dai M, Kpodonu J, Afful J, et al. Combinations of variations in multiple genes are associated with hypertension. Hypertension 2000;36(1):2−6.

[687] Zeng C, Villar VA, Eisner GM, Williams SM, Felder RA, Jose PA. G protein-coupled receptor kinase 4: Role in blood pressure regulation. Hypertension 2008;51(6):1449−55.

[688] Wang Y, Li B, Zhao W, Liu P, Zhao Q, Chen S, et al. Association study of G protein-coupled receptor kinase 4 gene variants with essential hypertension in northern Han Chinese. Ann Hum Genet 2006;70(Pt 6):778−83.

[689] Rana BK, Insel PA, Payne SH, Abel K, Beutler E, Ziegler MG, et al. Population-based sample reveals gene-gender interactions in blood pressure in White Americans. Hypertension 2007;49(1):96−106.

[690] Staessen JA, Kuznetsova T, Zhang H, Maillard M, Bochud M, Hasenkamp S, et al. Blood pressure and renal sodium handling in relation to genetic variation in the DRD1 promoter and GRK4. Hypertension 2008;51(6):1643−50.

[691] Wang Z, Armando I, Asico LD, Escano C, Wang X, Lu Q, et al. The elevated blood pressure of human GRK4γ A142V transgenic mice is not associated with increased ROS production. Am J Physiol Heart Circ Physiol 2007;292(5):H2083−92.

[692] Wang Z, Asico LD, Escano CS, Felder RA, Jose PA. Human G protein coupled receptor kinase type 4 (hGRK4 γ) wild-type prevents salt sensitivity while its variant, hGRK4γ 486V, promotes salt sensitivity in transgenic mice: role of genetic background [Abstract]. Hypertension 2006;48:e27.

[693] Doris PA. Promoting regulatory gene variation in sodium reabsorption. Hypertension 2008;52(4):623−4.

[694] Sato M, Soma M, Nakayama T, Kanmatsuse K. Dopamine D1 receptor gene polymorphism is associated with essential hypertension. Hypertension 2000;36(2):183—6.

[695] Sanada H, Jose PA, Hazen-Martin D, Yu PY, Xu J, Bruns DE, et al. Dopamine-1 receptor coupling defect in renal proximal tubule cells in hypertension. Hypertension 1999;33(4):1036—42.

[696] Soma M, Nakayama K, Rahmutula D, Uwabo J, Sato M, Kunimoto M, et al. Ser9Gly polymorphism in the dopamine D3 receptor gene is not associated with essential hypertension in the Japanese. Med Sci Monit 2002;8(1):CR1—4.

[697] Sen S, Nesse R, Sheng L, Stoltenberg SF, Gleiberman L, Burmeister M, et al. Association between a dopamine-4 receptor polymorphism and blood pressure. Am J Hypertens 2005;18(9 Pt 1):1206—10.

[698] Cravchik A, Gejman PV. Functional analysis of the human D5 dopamine receptor missense and nonsense variants: differences in dopamine binding affinities. Pharmacogenetics 1999; 9(2):199—206.

[699] De Brito Gariepy H, Carayon P, Ferrari B, Couture R. Contribution of the central dopaminergic system in the anti-hypertensive effect of kinin B1 receptor antagonists in two rat models of hypertension. Neuropeptides 2010; 44(2):191—8.

[700] Sawamura T, Nakada T. Role of dopamine in the striatum, renin—angiotensin system and renal sympathetic nerve on the development of two-kidney, one-clip Goldblatt hypertension. J Urol 1996;155(3):1108—11.

[701] Moore TL, Killiany RJ, Rosene DL, Prusty S, Hollander W, Moss MB. Hypertension-induced changes in monoamine receptors in the prefrontal cortex of rhesus monkeys. Neuroscience 2003;120(1):177—89.

[702] Fujita S, Adachi K, Lee J, Uchida T, Koshikawa N, Cools AR. Decreased postsynaptic dopaminergic and cholinergic functions in the ventrolateral striatum of spontaneously hypertensive rat. Eur J Pharmacol 2004;484(1):75—82.

[703] Bhatnagar V, O'Connor DT, Brophy VH, Schork NJ, Richard E, Salem RM, et al. G-protein-coupled receptor kinase 4 polymorphisms and blood pressure response to metoprolol among African Americans: sex-specificity and interactions. Am J Hypertens 2009;22(3):332—8.

[704] Vandell AG, Lobmeyer MT, Gawronski BE, Langaee TY, Gong Y, Gums JG, et al. G protein receptor kinase 4 polymorphisms: β-Blocker Pharmacogenetics and treatment-related outcomes in Hypertension. Hypertension 2012;60(4):957—64.

[705] Leineweber K, Rohe P, Beilfuss A, Wolf C, Sporkmann H, Bruck H, et al. G-protein-coupled receptor kinase activity in human heart failure: effects of β-adrenoceptor blockade. Cardiovasc Res 2005;66(3):512—9.

[706] Rayner B, Ramesar R, Steyn K, Levitt N, Lombard C, Charlton K. G-protein-coupled receptor kinase 4 polymorphisms predict blood pressure response to dietary modification in Black patients with mild-to-moderate hypertension. J Hum Hypertens 2011; 26(5):334—9.

[707] Sanada H, Yatabe J, Yatabe MS, et al. G Protein-coupled receptor type 4 gene variants and response to antihypertensive medication. Circulation 2009;120(18):S1087 (Abstract 5413)

[708] Grant FD, Romero JR, Jeunemaitre X, Hunt SC, Hopkins PN, Hollenberg NH, Williams GH. Low-renin hypertension, altered sodium homeostasis, and an α-adducin polymorphism. Hypertension 2002;39(2):191—6.

[709] Sugimoto K, Hozawa A, Katsuya T, Matsubara M, Ohkubo T, Tsuji I, et al. α-Adducin Gly460Trp polymorphism is associated with low renin hypertension in younger subjects in the Ohasama study. J Hypertens 2002;20(9):1779—84.

[710] Lohmueller KE, Wong LJ, Mauney MM, Jiang L, Felder RA, Jose PA, Williams SM. Patterns of genetic variation in the hypertension candidate gene GRK4: ethnic variation and haplotype structure. Ann Hum Genet 2006;70(Pt 1): 27—41.

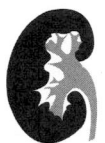

STRUCTURAL AND FUNCTIONAL ORGANIZATION OF THE KIDNEY

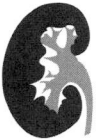

Structural Organization of the Mammalian Kidney

Wilhelm Kriz[1] *and Brigitte Kaissling*[2]

[1]Department of Anatomy and Developmental Biology, Medical Faculty Mannheim, University of Heidelberg, Mannheim, Germany

[2]Institute for Anatomy, University of Zürich, Switzerland

KIDNEY TYPES AND RENAL PELVIS

The mammalian kidney is multiform. The basic architecture is best understood in the unipapillary kidney, which is common in all small species. A coronal section of this kidney shows the main structural parts (Figure 20.1a). The renal cortex, as a whole, is cup-shaped with inverted margins, and surrounds the renal medulla. The medulla can be roughly compared to a pyramid; its top portion, the papilla, projects into the renal pelvis. The pelvis is located within the renal sinus, which opens through the renal hilum to the medial surface of the kidney.

The cortical parenchyma is divided into the cortical labyrinth and the medullary rays. The uppermost part of the cortex, a continuous layer that covers the tops of the medullary rays, is called the cortex corticis. The medulla is divided into an outer medulla (subdivided into outer and inner stripes) and an inner medulla. The innermost part of the inner medulla generally forms the papilla.

The unipapillary kidney is the most simple kidney type; in comparative anatomy, such a kidney as a whole corresponds to a renculus. All other kidney types may be regarded as adaptations to larger body sizes. The crest kidney and the kidney with tubi maximi are magnifications of a one-reniculus unit. The multipapillary kidney (Figure 20.2) and the reniculus kidney multiply this unit.[1,2,3] The human kidney is a multipapillary kidney; however, it is particular because a variable number of papillae are generally fused, forming compound papillae.[4]

The renal pelvis (Figures 20.1a and b) or the renal calyces (Figure 20.2) are anchored to the renal parenchyma by connective and smooth-muscle tissues that follow the intrarenal arteries. The cavity of the pelvis and calyx surrounds the renal papilla (or its equivalent in other kidney types). In many species the pelvic cavity forms different kinds of pelvic extensions (Figure 20.1b).[5,6] Leaf-like extensions called "specialized fornices" accompany the large vessels for some distance along their entry into the renal parenchyma. Secondary pouches protrude toward the hilus, communicating with the primary pelvic cavity only above the free semi-lunar borders of the pelvic septa. These extensions increase the contact area between the pelvic cavity and the renal medulla, especially the outer medulla.[7]

RENAL VASCULATURE

Close to the renal hilum and afterwards within the renal sinus the renal artery undergoes several divisions, finally establishing the interlobar arteries which then enter the renal tissue at the border between the cortex and medulla (Figures 20.1a and 20.2). From there they follow an arc-like course and are therefore called arcuate arteries. They give rise to the cortical radial arteries, which ascend radially within the cortical labyrinth. The cortex is very densely penetrated by arteries; in contrast, no arteries enter the medulla. The renal veins (cortical radial (interlobular) veins, arcuate veins) accompany the corresponding arteries. In some species (cat, dog, man) the venous blood from the outer

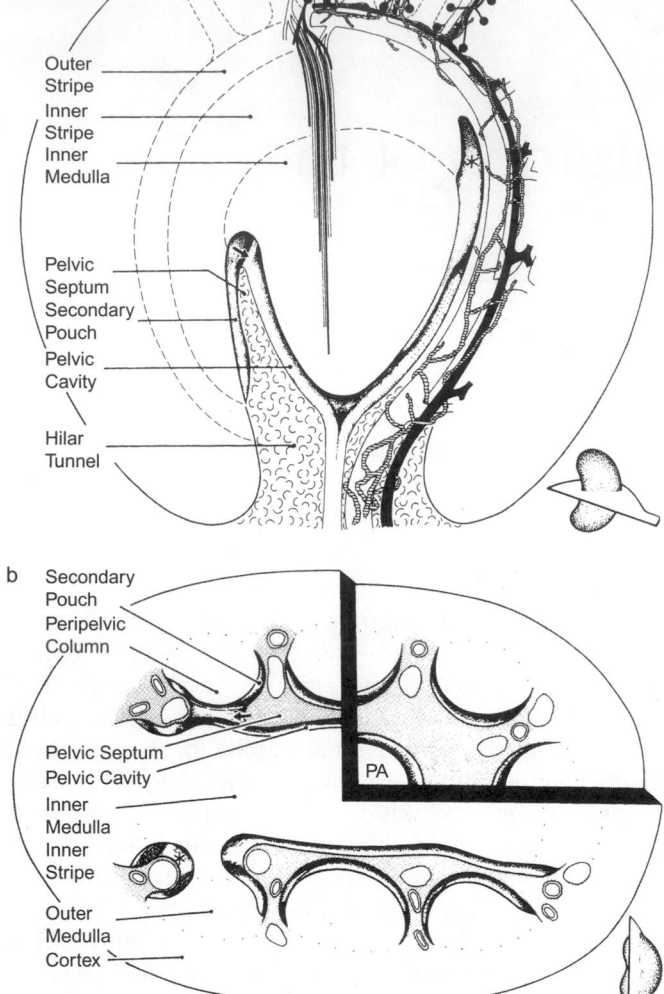

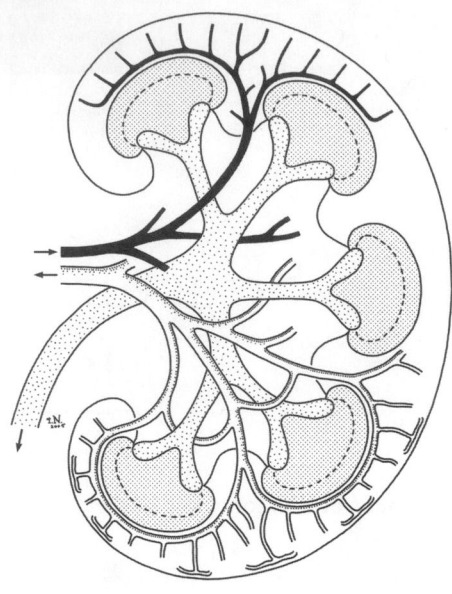

FIGURE 20.2   Schematic illustration of a compound multipapillary kidney (coronal section) similar to the human kidney. The renal cortex as a whole encloses several papillae; fused papillae typical for the human kidney are not shown. The central region, the renal sinus, contains the calyces and the pelvis (stippled), the pattern of branching arteries (black), and joining veins (white). The arcuate arteries, running at the cortico-medullary border, do not form true arches, but rather represent end-arteries. In contrast, the veins do form anastomoses at the level of the arcuate and interlobar veins. In the human kidney there are two types of cortical radial veins (interlobular veins); one group starting as stellate veins drains the most superficial cortex, the second group starts at deeper levels in the cortex; both drain into arcuate veins.

FIGURE 20.1   Schematics of a coronal and two transverse (b) sections through the rabbit kidney. The inset in the right lower corner indicates the section plane. The general architecture of the kidney and the renal pelvis is demonstrated. (a) Arterial vessels, including glomeruli and descending vasa recta, are shown in black, venous vessels are gray, and lymphatics are hatched. (b) The section plane of the main drawing runs through the middle part of the inner medulla; a deeper section through the papilla (PA) is shown in the upper right quarter. The cross-sectioned pelvic septa are stippled. The leaf-like extensions of the pelvic cavity are marked by a star, the free semilunar edges of the main pelvic septa by an arrow (in a and b). *(Adapted from Kaissling, B., and Kriz, W. (1979). Structured analysis of the rabbit kidney. Adv. Anat. Embryol. Cell Biol. **56**, 1–123, with permission.)*

cortex drains into veins on the renal surface (in man called "stellate veins") which are connected by additional cortical radial veins (interlobular veins) to arcuate veins. Such additional veins are not accompanied by arteries.[8]

The microvasculature pattern of the kidney appears to be very similar among mamma*lian species; a basic pattern can be described (Figures 20.3 and 20.4a).[9–11] The afferent arterioles arise from the cortical radial arteries (a minor portion from the arcuate arteries) and supply the glomerular tufts of the renal corpuscles. The efferent arterioles drain the glomeruli. Several types of efferent arterioles have been described.[11,12] Basically, a distinction between superficial, midcortical, and juxtamedullary renal corpuscles is essential (Figures 20.3 and 20.5). The efferent arterioles of juxtamedullary glomeruli turn toward the medulla; they supply the medulla. Juxtamedullary glomeruli are best defined by this type of efferent arteriole. The superficial efferent arterioles extend to the kidney surface before dividing. Again, superficial glomeruli are best defined because of the typical pattern of their efferent arterioles. The efferent arterioles of midcortical nephrons (defined by exclusion) vary in length between those that branch abruptly near the glomerulus and others that extend to a medullary ray before splitting off into capillaries. All the efferent arterioles together (superficial, midcortical, and also small

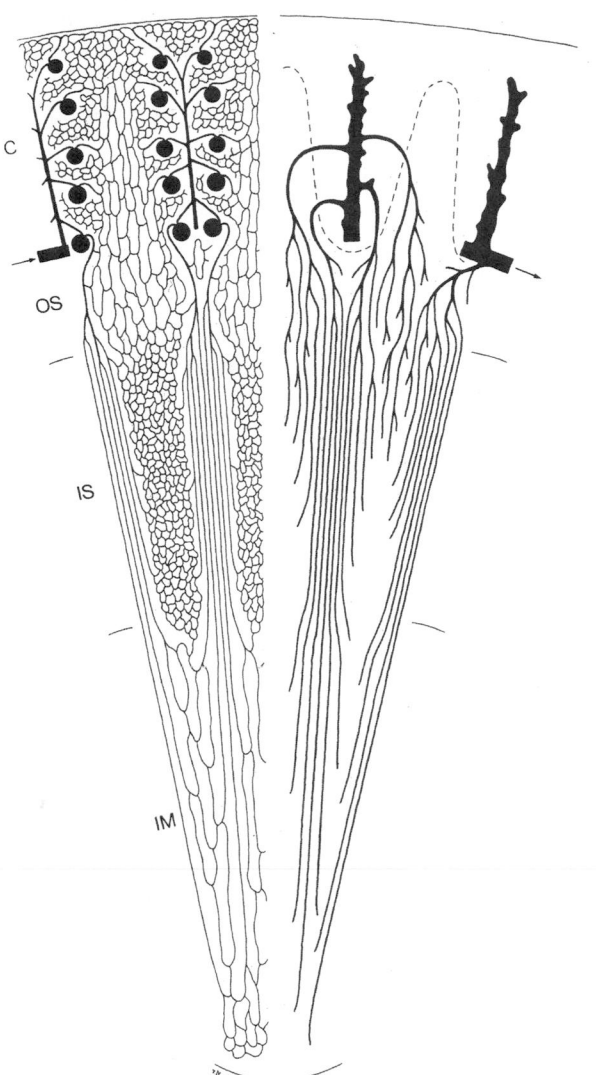

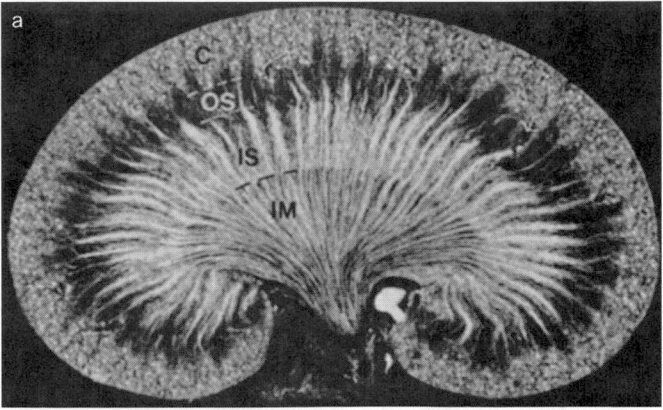

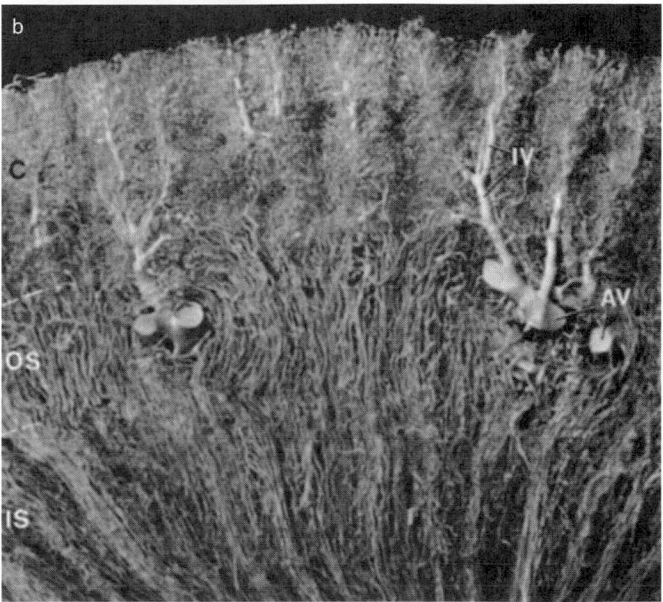

FIGURE 20.3 Schematic of the microvasculature of the rat kidney (C: cortex; OS: outer stripe; IS: inner stripe; IM: inner medulla). The left panel shows the arterial vessels and capillaries. An arcuate artery (arrow) gives rise to a cortical radial (interlobular) artery, from which afferent arterioles originate to supply the glomeruli. The efferent arterioles of the juxtamedullary glomeruli descend into the medulla and divide into the descending vasa recta, which, together with ascending vasa recta, form the vascular bundles of the renal medulla. At intervals, descending vasa recta leave the bundles to feed the adjacent capillaries. The right panel shows the venous vessels. The interlobular veins start in the superficial cortex. In the inner cortex they, together with the arcuate veins, receive the ascending vasa recta from the medulla. The vasa recta ascending from the inner medulla all traverse the inner stripe within the vascular bundles, whereas most of the vasa recta from the inner stripe ascend outside the bundles. Both of these types of ascending vasa recta traverse the outer stripe as wide, tortuous channels. (*Adapted from Kriz, W., and Lever, A. F. (1969). Renal countercurrent mechanisms: Structure and function. Am. Heart J.* **78**(1), *101–118 and Rollhaeuser, H., and Kriz, W. (1964). The vascular system of the rat kidney. Z. Zellforsch. Mikrosk. Anat.* **64**, *381–403, with permission.*)

FIGURE 20.4 Microvasculature. (a) Rat kidney; silicon rubber (Microfil) filling of the arterial vessels. Cortex (C), outer stripe (OS), inner stripe (IS), and inner medulla (IM) are clearly distinguishable by their vessel patterns. The vascular bundles take shape along the OS and are best developed within the IS. Only a minor part of the descending vasa recta of each bundle enter the IM, where they gradually decrease in number toward the papilla. Note the scantiness of capillaries in the OS (×8). (b) Rabbit kidney; silicon rubber filling of the venous vessels. The interlobular veins (IV) accept the cortical capillaries and a major part of the ascending vasa recta. Note the density of ascending vasa recta within the OS. In the IS, ascending vasa recta are found within the bundles (mostly originating from the IM) and between the vascular bundles (draining the interbundle regions of the IS) (AV: arcuate vein; ×14). (*In cooperation with L. Bankir.*)

branches of the juxtamedullary efferent arterioles) supply the cortical peritubular capillaries. Direct aglomerular arterial supplies to the peritubular capillaries or to the medulla are sparse[13] and have frequently been shown to be the result of degeneration of the corresponding glomeruli.[14]

Within the capillary network of the cortex (Figures 20.3 and 20.4), a differentiation between two parts is necessary: namely, the dense, round-meshed

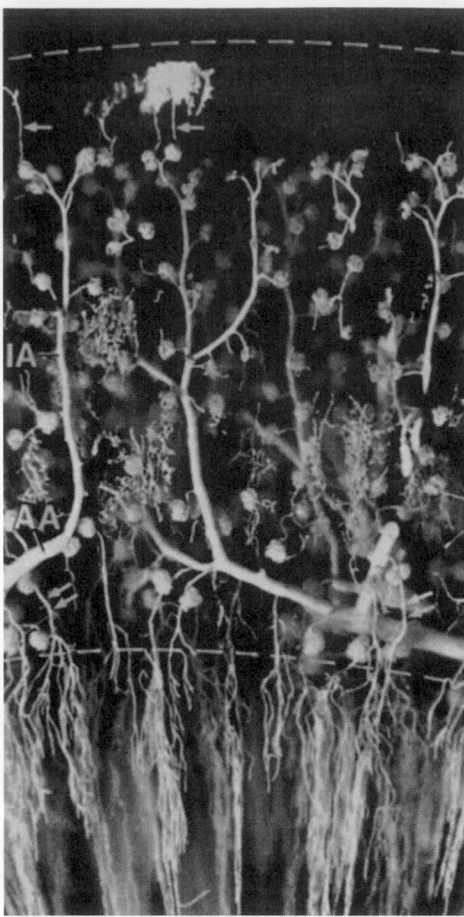

FIGURE 20.5 Arterial vessels after filling with silicone rubber; rabbit kidney. The broken lines show the renal surface and the cortico-medullary border. Arcuate arteries (AA) give rise to cortical radial arteries which split into the afferent arterioles. The efferent arterioles of superficial glomeruli (arrow) ascend unbranched to the kidney surface before splitting into capillaries. The efferent arterioles of juxtamedullary nephrons (arrowheads) descend into the outer stripe and devide into the descending vasa recta (×80). *(From ref. [5].)*

capillary plexus of the cortical labyrinth (including the cortex corticis); and the less dense, long-meshed plexus of the medullary rays, both associated with the course of the tubules. Functionally these two plexuses are different with respect to their drainage. The blood from the medullary ray plexus has to pass the plexus of the cortical labyrinth to gain access to the interlobular veins. Therefore, the blood that has perfused the straight tubules within the medullary rays mixes with the blood that perfuses the convoluted tubules of the cortical labyrinth.

The medulla (Figures 20.3, 20.4, and 20.5) is exclusively supplied by the efferent arterioles of the juxtamedullary glomeruli.[5,8,10,11,15,16] These efferent arterioles descend through the outer stripe and divide into the descending vasa recta. In addition, the efferent arteriole and its first divisions give rise to small side branches that supply the sparse capillary plexus of the outer stripe of the outer medulla. This plexus is continuous with the cortical capillary plexus above and the capillary plexus of the inner stripe below. The descending vasa recta then penetrate the inner stripe of the outer medulla in cone-shaped vascular bundles. At intervals, descending vasa recta leave the bundles to join the capillary plexus at the adjacent medullary level, most leaving the bundle within the inner stripe. Only a small portion of the descending vasa recta penetrate the inner medulla, and even fewer reach the tip of the papilla.

The capillary plexuses of the renal medulla (Figures 20.3 and 20.4a) differ in the three regions. That of the outer stripe is sparse. In contrast, the capillary plexus of the inner stripe is very dense and characteristically round-meshed in appearance. In the inner medulla the capillary plexus is less dense and long-meshed.

The ascending vasa recta are the draining vessels of the renal medulla (Figures 20.3 and 20.4b). In the inner medulla they arise at every level and ascend as unbranched vessels to the border between the inner and outer medulla. At this point, they join the vascular bundles and traverse the inner stripe of the outer medulla within the vascular bundles. The ascending vasa recta, which drain the inner stripe, behave differently. Those of the lowermost part of the inner stripe (and therefore probably a minor portion) join the bundles as they pass through this region. Those from the middle and upper part (and thus probably the majority) do not join the bundles, but ascend directly within the interbundle regions to the outer stripe. There are, however, interspecies differences; in the sand rat (*Psammomys obesus*), all ascending vasa recta that drain the inner stripe ascend directly to the outer stripe without joining the bundles.[17]

Within the outer stripe, the vasa recta ascending within the bundles spread out and, together with the directly ascending vasa recta, traverse the outer stripe as individual tortuous channels with wide lumina (Figure 20.4b). They contact the tubules like true capillaries, and because the true capillaries which are derived from direct branches of efferent arterioles are few in the outer stripe (Figure 20.3a), they mainly affect the blood supply to the tubules in this region. At the corticomedullary border, the ascending venous vessels of the medulla empty into the arcuate veins or into the basal parts of interlobular veins. In some species, such as rat, guinea pig, and especially the sand rat (*Psammomys obesus*) some of the venous medullary vessels continue to ascend within the medullary rays of the cortex and finally empty into middle or even upper parts of interlobular veins.

Wall Structure of Intrarenal Vessels

The intrarenal arteries and the proximal portions of the afferent arterioles appear to be similar to arteries and arterioles of the same size elsewhere in the body. The terminal portions of the afferent arterioles are unique because of the occurrence of granular cells (renin producing cells) which replace ordinary smooth muscle cells in their wall.[18] It is generally agreed that granular cells are modified smooth muscle cells. Compared to proper smooth muscle cells, granular cells contain less myofilaments; thus, the contractile capacity of the very last portion of the afferent arteriole appears to be considerably decreased.[19] The endocrine function of granular cells will be considered later in the context of the juxtaglomerular apparatus. The glomerular capillaries will be described together with the glomerulus.

Efferent arterioles are already established inside the glomerular tuft. Thus, in contrast to afferent arterioles, efferent arterioles have an intraglomerular segment which passes through the glomerular stalk[20,21] (Figure 20.6a). After this, efferent arterioles have a segment which is narrowly associated with the extraglomerular mesangium (details will be given later in the context of the glomerulus). Thereafter, the efferent arterioles are established as arterioles with a proper media made up of smooth muscle cells.

Efferent arterioles from juxtamedullary glomeruli differ considerably from those of cortical (midcortical and superficial) glomeruli (compare Figures 20.6b and 20.6c). Juxtamedullary efferent arterioles are larger in diameter than cortical efferent arterioles; their size even exceeds that of their corresponding afferent arterioles. In the rabbit, the diameters of afferent arterioles throughout the cortex average approximately 20 μm; juxtamedullary efferent arterioles average 28 μm, and cortical efferent arterioles average only 12 μm.[22] Similar differences have been found in dog,[12] rat,[23] and human[24] kidneys.

Cortical efferent arterioles (Figure 20.6b) are only sparsely equipped with smooth muscle cells (generally not more than one layer). A striking feature of efferent arterioles (including those from juxtamedullary glomeruli) is the thick, irregular basement membrane. In contrast to the usual appearance of a basement membrane, basement membrane-like material fills the wide and irregular spaces between the endothelium and the muscle layer. The juxtamedullary efferent arterioles (Figure 20.6c) are surrounded by two to four layers of smooth muscle cells. Their endothelium is composed of a strikingly large number of longitudinally arranged cells; up to 30 individual cells may be found in cross-sections.[23,25]

In the descending vasa recta (Figure 20.6d) the smooth muscle cells are gradually replaced by

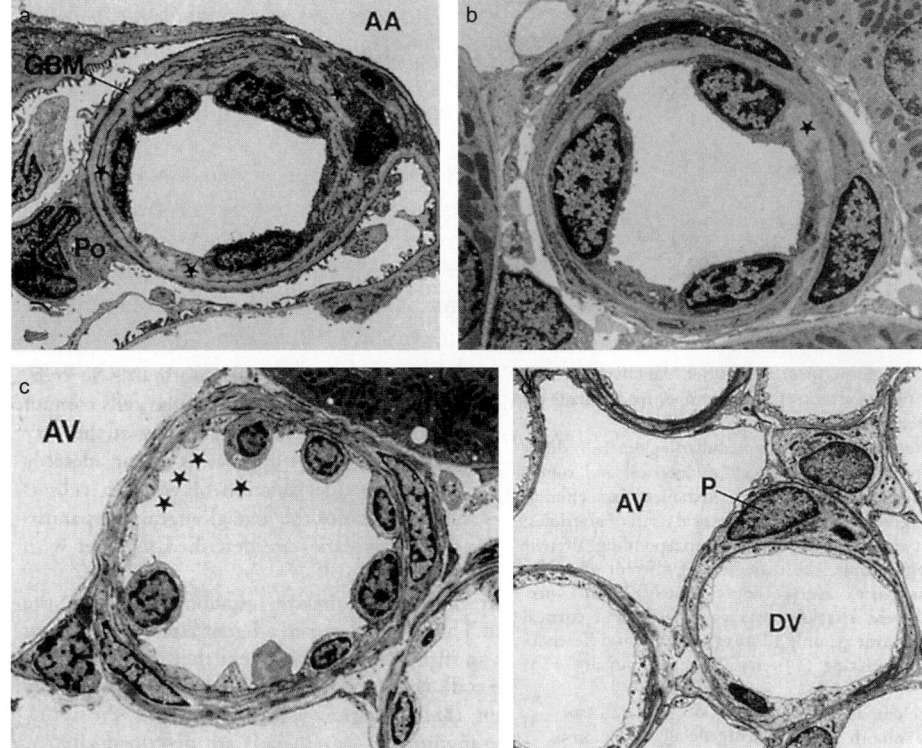

FIGURE 20.6 Efferent arteriole. (a) Intraglomerular segment of the efferent arteriole. Between the basement membrane (GBM) and the endothelium a mesangial layer is interposed. Note the intimate relationships of the afferent arteriole (AA) to the mesangium. PO: podocyte (Rat; TEM ×∼4600). (b) Efferent arteriole of a superficial glomerulus. Note the irregular basement membrane-like material beneath the endothelium (*). One to two layers of smooth muscle cells (SM) are encountered (Rabbit; TEM ×∼3400). (c) Efferent arteriole of a juxtamedullary glomerulus. Note the many profiles of endothelial cells (*); the tight junctions between them are shallow (Rat; TEM ×∼2450). (d) Descending (DV) and ascending (AV) vasa recta of a vascular bundle are shown. The continuous endothelium of the descending vas rectum is surrounded by a pericyte (P). The endothelium of the ascending vas rectum is highly fenestrated (arrows) (Rabbit; TEM ×∼2400).

pericytes, which form an incomplete layer around the vessel trunk. Pericytes should be regarded as contractile cells. The pattern of these cells, which encircle the endothelial tube-like hoops, and their dense assemblys of microfilaments strongly imply that they have a contractile function. In contrast to smooth muscle cells, they are not contacted by nerve terminals. The descending vasa recta finally lose their pericytes, and the concurrent appearance of endothelial fenestrations marks their gradual transformation into medullary capillaries.

The ultrastructure of the capillaries in the kidney is similar in both the cortex and the medulla (with the exception of glomerular capillaries; *vide infra*). The capillaries of the kidney are of the fenestrated type (Figure 20.7). The capillary wall consists of an extremely flat endothelium surrounded by a thin basement membrane. In non-nuclear regions the endothelial cells contain densely and regularly arranged fenestrations that (in contrast to the glomerular capillaries) are bridged by a thin diaphragm. An estimated 50% of the capillary circumference is composed of these fenestration-bearing areas.[23] The fenestrations themselves are of rather complex structure. In normal TEM sections the diaphragm appears as a very thin (5–6 nm) single-layered proteinaceous membrane provided with a central knob. Deep-etch freezing techniques have revealed

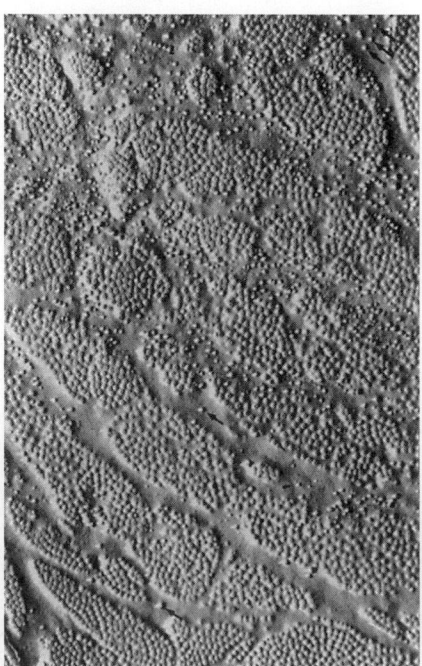

FIGURE 20.7 Freeze-fracture electron micrograph demonstrating the dense arrangement of fenestrations within the wall of a peritubular capillary (rabbit). Pinocytotic vesicles (arrows) are found within areas of thicker cytoplasm, which connect the perikaryon and the more voluminous areas along the cell borders (not shown) (×7600). (*In cooperation with A. Schiller and R. Taugner.*)

a composition of radial fibrils converging to the central knob.[26] So far only one protein, PV1, a caveolar transmembrane protein, has been attributed to the diaphragm.[27] The diaphragm is considered to be permeable to water and small water-soluble substances.

The wall structure of the ascending vasa recta (Figure 20.6d) is similar to that of the capillaries. These draining vessels, with wide lumina, are bound for their entire length by an extremely flat endothelium with extensive fenestrations. The same structure is found in the large veins of the cortex and at the corticomedullary border (Figures 20.8 and 20.15). The interlobular and arcuate veins are not veins in the classic sense, but they have a wall structure fundamentally the same as that of the renal capillaries.[9,23] This wall consists solely of an extremely flattened, partly fenestrated endothelium that rests on a basement membrane.

NEPHRONS AND COLLECTING DUCT SYSTEM

The specific structural units of the kidney are the nephrons. In the rat, each kidney contains 30,000 to 35,000 nephrons[28]; each human kidney has an estimated 1 million,[29] but great interindividual differences exist.[30,31]

The nephron consists of a renal corpuscle connected to a complicated and twisted tube that finally drains into a collecting duct. Based on the location of the renal corpuscles within the cortex, three types of nephrons are distinguished: superficial; midcortical; and juxtamedullary nephrons. Exact definitions of these types, grounded on more than arbitrary decisions, can be based on the different patterns of the efferent arterioles (*vide supra*).

The tubular part of the nephron consists of a proximal and a distal portion connected by a loop of Henle. For details of subdivisions, see Figures 20.9 and 20.10.

According to the lengths of the loops of Henle, two types of nephrons are distinguished (Figure 20.9): those with long loops and those with short loops (including those with cortical loops). Short loops turn back in the outer medulla. In many species (rat, rabbit), the bends of the short loops are all located roughly at the same level of the inner stripe, namely, near the junction to the inner medulla. In other species (pig and human), short loops may form their bends at any level of the outer medulla, and even in the cortex (cortical loops).

The long loops turn back at successive levels of the inner medulla, many at its start; others reach intermediate levels, and only a few reach the tip of the papilla. Thus, the number of loops is successively reduced along the inner medulla toward the papilla. This decrease is paralleled by a decrease in collecting ducts

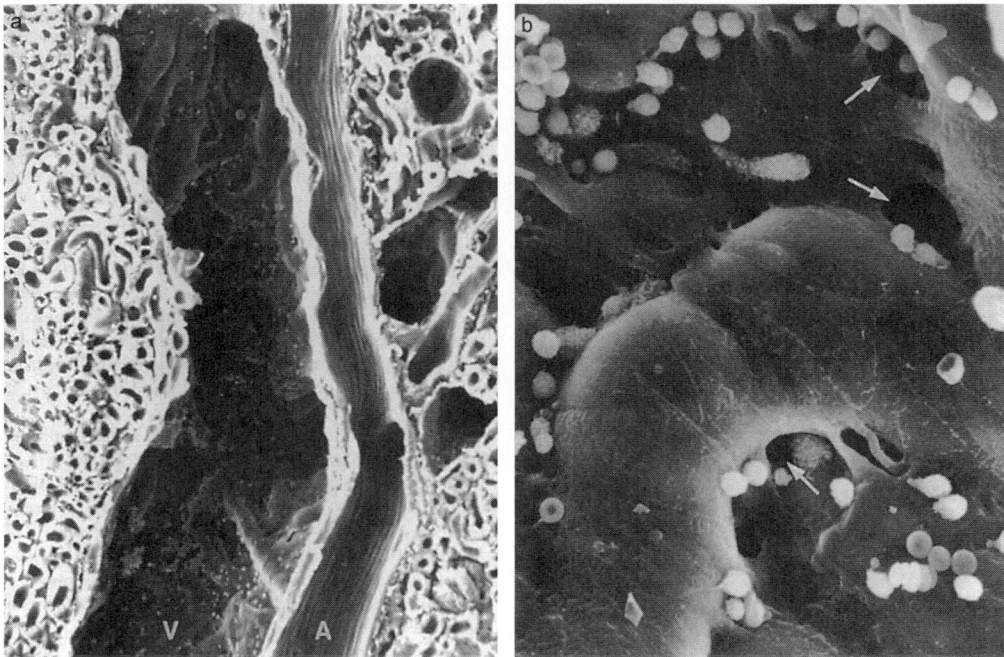

FIGURE 20.8 **Scanning electron micrographs of the inner surface of an arcuate artery and vein (Rat).** (a) The tubules underneath the venous wall are clearly discernible through the endothelium, which covers the tubules as a thin coat. (b) Higher magnification of the venous endothelium. The openings in the endothelial wall (arrows) mark the positions where venous vasa recta and capillaries empty into the vein. (a) × ~120; (b) × ~1900. *(From Frank, M., and Kriz, W. (1988). The luminal aspect of intrarenal arteries and veins in the rat as revealed by scanning electron microscopy. Anat. Embryol. (Berl) **177**(4), 371−376, with permission.)*

and vasa recta, leading to the characteristic form of the inner medulla, which in all species tapers from a broad basis to a papilla (or crest).

The division of nephrons according to the position of their corpuscles in the cortex does not coincide with the division based on the length of their loops. Among species, all three types of renal corpuscles may be attached to both short and long loops. However, within a given species (with short and long loops), the long loops always belong to the deeper renal corpuscles (i.e., juxtamedullary and deep midcortical) and the short loops to the more superficially situated corpuscles.

The number of short and long loops varies among species. Some species have only short loops (mountain beaver, muskrat), and consequently lack an inner medulla, which results in a poor ability to concentrate urine.[6] Only two species, cat and dog, are known to have just long loops. In comparison with other species, their urine concentrating ability is considered to be average. In the cat, however, many long loops penetrate into the inner medulla for a very short distance (less than 0.5 μm. Defining a loop by ultrastructural criteria (*vide infra*), a feline kidney does contain many loops resembling the short loops in other species. The formerly held presumption that rodent species with the most powerful ability to concentrate urine, like *Psammomys* or *Meriones*, have only long loops has been proved incorrect.[32] Most species have short and long

loops whose ratio varies from species to species. A correlation between the ratio of short and long loops and urine concentrating ability is not obvious. Most rodent species that have a high urine concentrating ability (rat, mouse, golden hamster, *Psammomys*, *Meriones*) have more short loops than long loops.[32−34]

The collecting ducts are formed in the renal cortex by the joining of several nephrons (Figures 20.9 and 20.10). The location of the exact border between a nephron and a collecting duct is disputed. According to cytological criteria, a connecting tubule is interposed between a nephron and a cortical collecting duct. Whether this connecting tubule derives from the nephrogenic blastema, and therefore must be considered as a part of the nephron, or from the ureteral bud, and therefore is part of the collecting ducts, remains an open question.

Microanatomically, the connecting tubules of deep and superficial nephrons differ (Figure 20.9). The connecting tubules of deep nephrons generally join to form an arcade before draining into a collecting duct; superficial nephrons drain via an individual connecting tubule. The numerical ratio between nephrons draining through an arcade and those draining individually varies greatly among species. In rat, rabbit, and pig, the majority of nephrons drain via arcades; as Sperber[3] observed, some arcades probably exist in all mammalian kidneys. An arcade ascends within the cortical labyrinth before

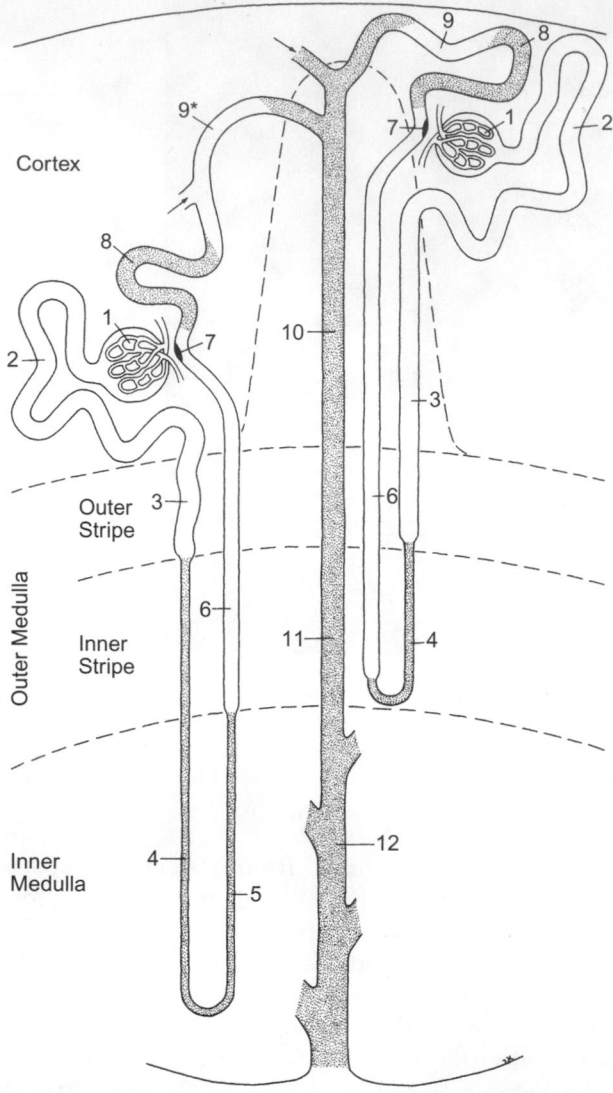

FIGURE 20.9   Schematic of nephrons and collecting duct. This scheme depicts a short-looped and a long-looped nephron, together with the collecting system. Not drawn to scale. Within the cortex a medullary ray is delineated by a dashed line. (*From Kriz, W., and Bankir, L. (1988). A standard nomenclature for structures of the kidney. The Renal Commission of the International Union of Physiological Sciences (IUPS). Kidney Int, 33, 1–7, with permission.*) 1: Renal corpuscle including Bowman's capsule and the glomerulus (glomerular tuft); 2: Proximal convoluted tubule; 3: Proximal straight tubule; 4: Descending thin limb; 5: Ascending thin limb; 6: Distal straight tubule (thick ascending limb); 7: Macula densa located within the final portion of the thick ascending limb; 8: Distal convoluted tubule; 9: Connecting tubule; 9*: Connecting tubule of the juxtamedullary nephron that forms an arcade; 10: Cortical collecting duct; 11: Outer medullary collecting duct; 12: Inner medullary collecting duct.

draining into a cortical collecting duct (Figure 20.9). Functionally, an arcade appears to serve as a device that prevents the addition of dilute distal urine to collecting ducts at the corticomedullary junction.[35]

The cortical collecting ducts descend within the medullary rays of the cortex and then, as unbranched tubes,

traverse the outer medulla (outer medullary collecting ducts). On entering the inner medulla (inner medullary collecting ducts), they fuse successively. In the human kidney, an average of eight fusions has been found,[36] a number that may also be a good approximation for other species.[37] Because a cortical collecting duct in the human kidney accepts 11 nephrons on average, it can be calculated that a papillary duct (opening into the renal pelvis) drains a total of 2750 nephrons. In the rabbit kidney, which has only 6 nephron tributaries to a cortical collecting duct,[5] approximately 1000 nephrons are drained by a terminal collecting duct. It must be emphasized that an inner medullary collecting duct is not a single unbranched tube, but rather is a system of tubules that fuse successively.

INTERSTITIUM

Definition, Volume Fraction

The space between the basement membranes of the renal epithelia and the peritubular capillaries (Figure 20.11) is called the *"interstitial space."* Cells and extracellular matrix within this space constitute the *"interstitium."* The fractional volume of the interstitium in the cortex in healthy kidneys has been estimated between 4 to 9%,[38–41] in the outer stripe of the outer medulla and in the vascular bundle compartment ~3–5%. In the interbundle compartment of the inner stripe the fractional volume amounts to 10% in rat,[42,41] and in the inner zone the relative interstitial volume continuously increases from the base (10–15% fractional volume in rat, 20–25% in rabbit) to the tip of the papilla (~30% in rat; more than 40% in rabbit[42,43]). Reabsorption and secretion of fluid and solutes, as well as the transport for many regulatory substances from their site of production to their target site, implies a transit across the interstitial compartment.[44] In the cortex only about 26%[39] or 42%[40] of the total outer tubular surfaces are directly apposed to capillaries.

Cellular Constituents

The majority of cells in the interstitium of healthy kidneys are *interstitial fibroblasts* and *dendritic cells* (Figure 20.12). Other cell types (*macrophages* and *lymphocytes*) are scarce in healthy kidneys,[45] but they invade the interstitial spaces under inflammatory conditions.[46]

Interstitial Fibroblasts

Interstitial fibroblasts provide the scaffolding of the tissue, take part in the modeling of the extracellular matrix, and play a role in the production of regulatory

FIGURE 20.10 Segmentation of the renal tubule.

Microanatomical terms	Main divisions	Subdivisions	Segmentation	Abbreviation	Cell types	Other frequently used denominations
Proximal convolution	PROXIMAL TUBULE	pars convoluta or convoluted part	Proximal Convoluted Tubule, S 1 - segment	PCT	S 1 cells	P 1 segment — PT
			S 2 - segment			
		pars recta or straight part	Proximal Straight Tubule, S 2 - segment	PST	S 2 cells	P 2 segment
			S 3 - segment		S 3 cells	P 3 segment — PR
Loop of Henle	INTERMEDIATE TUBULE	pars descendens or descending part	Descending Thin Limb, of short loops	DTL	DTL cells Type 1	Short Descending Thin Limb of Henle's loop (SDL)
			of long loops, upper part		Type 2	Long Descending Thin Limb, upper part (LDLu)
			lower part		Type 3	Long Descending Thin Limb, lower part (LDLl)
			pre-bend segment			
		pars ascendens or ascending part	Ascending Thin Limb	ATL	ATL cells Type 4	TAL — Thin Ascending Limb (of long loops only)
	DISTAL TUBULE	pars recta or straight part	Distal Straight Tubule or Thick Ascending Limb, Medullary straight part	MTAL (DST or TAL)	DST or TAL cells	MAL, mTALH — Thick Ascending Limb of Henle's Loop, Medullary Thick Limb
			Cortical straight part	CTAL		CAL, cTALH — Cortical Thick Limb (incl. Macula Densa)
			Macula Densa	MD	MD cells	MD
			postmacular segment			
Distal convolution		pars convoluta or convoluted part	Distal Convoluted Tubule	DCT	DCT cells (+ IC cells)	DCTa* early distal tubule; DCTb* Distal Tubule
	COLLECTING SYSTEM		Connecting Tubule	CNT	CNT cells + IC cells	DCTg* CCTg* late distal tubule — Connecting Segment
Collecting duct		Collecting Duct	Cortical Collecting Duct	CCD	CD cells = principal cells = light cells + IC cells = intercalated cells = mitochondria-rich cells = carboanhydrase-rich cells = dark cells	DCTl* CCTl* Cortical Collecting Tubule (CCT); Initial Collecting Tubule (CCTi)
			Outer Medullary Collecting Duct	OMCD		Outer Medullary Collecting Tubule (OMCT)
			Inner Medullary Collecting Duct	IMCD	CD cells = principal cells	Inner Medullary Collecting Tubule (IMCT); Papillary Collecting Duct (PCD) or Ducts of Bellini

FIGURE 20.10 Segmentation of the renal tubule. This table summarizes the nomenclature of segments and cells of the renal tubule. A continuous serpentine arrow means that the transition between the two structures is gradual. An interrupted serpentine arrow means that the transition is gradual in some species, abrupt in others. Abbreviations marked by a star were introduced by Morel and co-workers: *Functional segmentation of the rabbit distal tubule by microdetermination of hormone-dependent adenylate cyclase activity. Kidney Int. 1976; 9, 264–277* (DCTa: Distal convoluted tubule, initial portion; DCTb: Distal convoluted tubule, bright portion; DCTg: Distal convoluted tubule, granular portion; DCTl: Distal convoluted tubule, light portion; CCTg: Cortical collecting tubule, granular portion; CCTl: Cortical collecting tubule, light portion). (From ref. [542].)

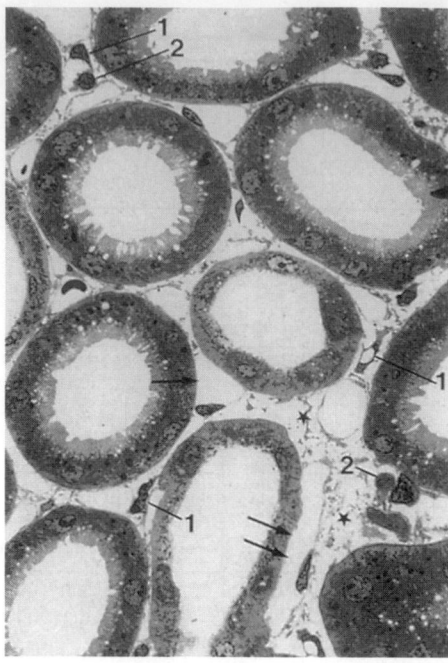

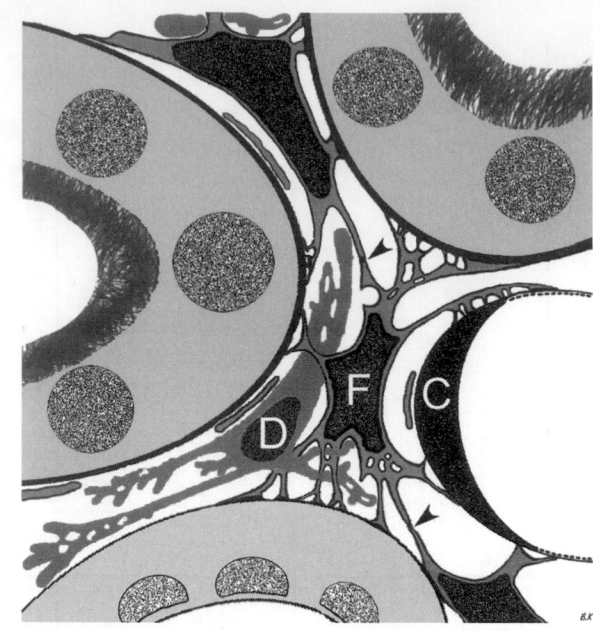

FIGURE 20.11   Peritubular interstitium of the renal cortex with narrow (arrows) and wide (stars) portions. Interstitial cells are resident fibroblasts (1) and temporarily sojourning dendritic/mononuclear cells (2) (rat kidney; TEM × ~720).

FIGURE 20.12   Schematic representation of cortical interstitial fibroblast (F) and dendritic cell (D) in the cortical interstitial space of a healthy kidney. The dark outline of fibroblasts indicates the f-actin layer under the plasma membrane (except for nuclei no cell organelles are shown); the fibroblasts are affixed to tubules and capillaries (C); the arrow heads indicate interconnection of fibroblasts by adhering junctions; the extensions of dendritic cells are narrowly intermingled with fibroblast cell processes. See color plate section at the back of the book.

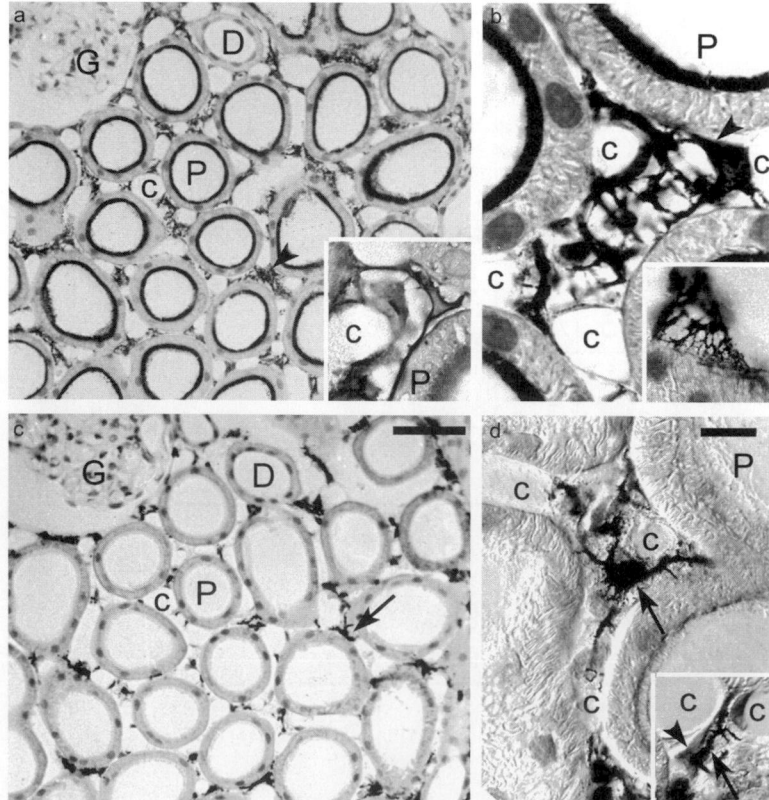

FIGURE 20.13   Interstitial cells, labeled by immunogold staining for ecto-5′-nucleotidase (a,b) and MHC class II (c,d) on consecutive (a,c) cryostat sections. P: Proximal tubule; D: Distal convoluted tubule; G: Glomerulus; C: Capillary; Arrowheads: Fibroblasts; Arrows: Dendritic cells. (a) 5′NT labeling highlights the abundance of interstitial fibroblasts (arrow) and the brush border of proximal tubules. Insert: Higher magnification of a fibroblast, labeled for 5′NT by enzyme-histochemistry, demonstrating the far extending processes within the interstitial space. (b) Fibroblasts (arrowheads) bridge the interstitial space between the basement membranes of tubules and capillaries. Insert: Detail of the attachment of a fibroblast process to a tubular basement membrane. (c) Dendritic cells (arrow) labeled for MHC class II, share the interstitial space with fibroblasts. (d) and insert: Differential interference contrast shows the narrow contact of dendritic cells and their extensions (arrow) to fibroblasts (arrowhead) (a,c × ~340; b,d × ~1200; Bars a,c ~50 μm; b,d ~10 μm).

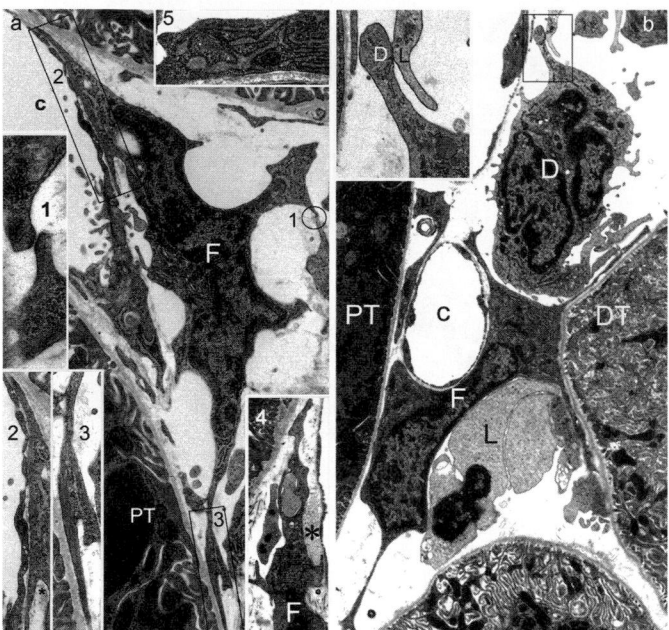

FIGURE 20.14 (a) Fibroblast with sharply outlined pericaryon in the cortical interstitium of a rat kidney; a filiform processes (1) is interconnected with another fibroblast by intermediate junctions (Insert 1); pedicle-like processes of the same fibroblast adhere to the basement membrane of a capillary (c) (2; Insert 2) and of a proximal tubule (PT) (3; Insert 3; Star: Extracellular matrix) with pedicle-like processes that reveal dense stress-fiber-like F-actin filaments; (Insert 4): collagen fibrils (asterisk) closely associated with a fibroblast extension (F) which encloses part of a dendritic cell (D); (Insert 5) the broad cytoplasmic extensions show abundant cisterns of rough endoplasmic reticulum (TEM ×~11,800; Inserts: 1 ×~50,000; 2,3 ×~23,000; 4 ×~11,800; 5 ×~23,000). (b) Fibroblast (F) in focal peritubular inflammation, caused by a lesion in a distal tubule; the fibroblast bridges the space between a healthy proximal tubule (PT), and a diseased distal tubule (DT), extends with thin processes closely along the basement membrane of the DT, partially encloses a profile of a peritubular capillary (C), and has close contact to migrating cells of the immune system (L: lymphocyte; D: dendritic cell; Insert: Higher magnification of the contact ("kiss") of the extension of the dendritic cell and a lymphocyte; TEM ×~6000; Insert ×~23,000).

substances. Interstitial fibroblasts bridge the interstitial space (Figures 20.12, 20.13 and 20.14). They are physically affixed to the basement membranes of tubules, renal corpuscles, and peritubular capillaries, they are interconnected by adhering junctions[44,45,47–49] (Figures 20.12 and 20.14), and narrowly contact all types of migrating cells within the interstitial space (Figures 20.12 and 20.13).

Cortical Interstitial Fibroblasts

In transmission electron microscopic (TEM) images (Figure 20.14), cortical interstitial fibroblasts display a heterochromatin-rich angular nucleus which is surrounded by a narrow organelle-free cytoplasmic rim.

Filiform and leaf-like, perforated and filiform processes spread from the cell body, traverse the interstitial space and are affixed to the basement membranes of tubules, enveloping glomerular arterioles and cells of the immune system.[50] Characteristic for fibroblasts is the dense layer of f-actin filaments immediately under the plasmalemma (Figures 20.12 and 20.14). In the filiform processes and the pedicle- or spine-like attachments to the basement membranes, the f-actin is markedly dense[48] (Figures 20.12 and 20.14).

The anchorage of fibroblasts to tubular and capillary basement membranes and their interconnections suggests the possibility that each configurational change of tubules or capillaries (e.g., related with tubular/capillary growth, tubular/capillary dilatation or collapse) exerts mechanical forces on the f-actin frame of the fibroblasts and induces signaling pathways.[51,52] In concert with chemokines and other factors[53] the mechanical forces might be essential components in the cross-talk between fibroblasts and epi- or endothelia,

The production of *extracellular matrix* is another distinguishing characteristic of fibroblasts. The morphological correlate for matrix production is the prominent apparatus for protein synthesis, i.e., abundant large profiles of rough endoplasmic reticulum filled with flocculent, rather electron-dense material, as well as several sets of Golgi-fields. These organelles, including mitochondria, are predominantly located in the peripheral thicker parts of the leaf-like processes, close to the sites of release of matrix and collagen fibrils into the interstitial space (Figure 20.14).[47,48]

The *extracellular matrix* of the interstitium is composed of a network of fibers, proteoglycans, glycoproteins, and interstitial fluid.[44,54] Several types of fibers are found, among them typical interstitial collagen fibers (type 1, type 3, and type 6).[55] Microfibrils (collagen type 1) are found throughout the renal interstitium. Type 3 fibers correspond to the reticular fibers which form a network enveloping individual tubules. Proteoglycans are an important component of the interstitial matrix in the kidney.[56] As elsewhere in the body, various glycoproteins (fibronectin, laminin, and others) are found associated with tubular basement membranes, as well as with fibrillar structures. All these substances contribute to the scaffolding function of the interstitium. Furthermore, they are important substrates for migrating immune cells in the interstitial space.

Fibroblasts can accumulate *lipid droplets*. These are not common in cortical fibroblasts (in contrast to medullary fibroblasts, see below) of healthy kidneys; yet, they may also appear in cortical fibroblasts under specific functional conditions (e.g., anemia[38]). Lysosomal bodies are rarely observed under control conditions.

Cortical interstitial fibroblasts play important roles in the adaptive response to local and systemic hypoxia.

The cleavage of AMP by ecto-5′-nucleotidase (5′NT) on the plasmalemma of cortical fibroblasts generates *extra-cellular adenosine (ADO)* in the cortical interstitium.[57] ADO has been widely implicated in adaptive responses to local hypoxia[58] and in regulating local hemodynamics.[59] The particularly narrow sheathing of glomerular arterioles by 5′NT-positive fibroblasts[48,60] suggests a role of ADO in the regulation of glomerular blood flow and glomerular filtration rate. Indeed, purinergic receptors in afferent and efferent glomerular arterioles are implicated in the regulation of renal functions and hypertension.[61] Studies on 5′NT-deficient mice have confirmed that ADO mediates the vascular response elicited by changes in NaCl concentration at the macula densa.[62] Cortical fibroblasts also exhibit soluble guanylyl cyclase (sGC),[63] and a *b*-type cytochrome 558.[64]

Interstitial fibroblasts in the deep cortex are the source of renal erythropoietin.[65−67] The hypoxia-inducible factor (HIF Hif-2), which has also been located to 5′NT-positve fibroblasts,[68,69] mediates regulation of transcription of erythropoietin following changes in oxygen supply.[70] In conditions of anemia[38] and hypoxia, cortical interstitial fibroblasts from all cortical regions are rapidly recruited for EPO-synthesis.[71]

Extensive phenotypical modulations of cortical peritubular fibroblasts *in vivo* occur under the concerted action of inflammatory cytokines and growth factors.[72−74] Under these conditions, the interstitial fibroblasts proliferate and transform into *myofibroblasts*.[75] Morphologically myofibroblasts differ from interstitial fibroblasts of the healthy renal interstitium, having rounded, euchromatin-rich nuclei and large irregularly-shaped cellular extensions containing dramatically expanded cisterns of rER,[75] and by increased junctional coupling.[76] Differing from healthy interstitial fibroblasts, myofibroblasts express αSMA and vimentin, and 5′NT is internalized from the plasma membrane into the cytoplasm. Functionally, myofibroblasts have an increased capacity for quantitatively and qualitatively different matrix production,[72−74] and a reduced potential for erythropoietin gene expression.[70]

Medullary Interstitial Fibroblasts

The phenotype of fibroblasts in the medulla is basically the same as in the cortex, yet their three-dimensional configuration[50] changes in correlation with the change in tubular arrangement, from convolutions in the cortex to the strictly parallel course of tubules and vessels in the inner zone. The longitudinal axis of the pericaryon of inner medullary fibroblasts is oriented perpendicularly to the longitudinal axis of tubules and vessels (Figure 20.15), and in two-dimensional microscopic images they appear like "rungs of a ladder".[44]

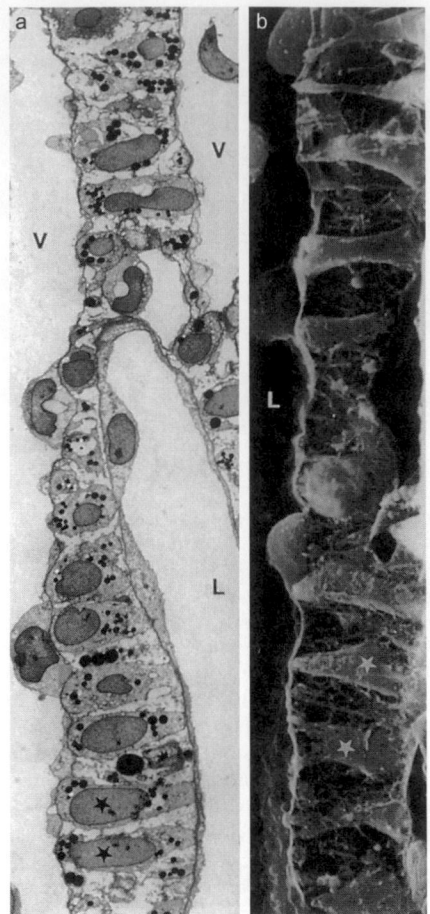

FIGURE 20.15 Interstitial fibroblasts of the inner medulla, demonstrated in longitudinal sections. The fibroblasts (asterisks) are arranged like the rungs of a ladder between parallel running tubules or vessels. The fibroblasts contain numerous lipid granules (black) of different sizes (visible in a). (L: loop limb; V: vessel; (a) *Psammomys*; TEM ×∼1350; (b) Rat; SEM ×∼3400). (*In cooperation with J. M. Barrett.*)

One noticeable change in the ultrastructure of medullary fibroblasts is the progressive increase in cytoskeletal elements towards the deep inner zone; actin filaments form a very prominent layer under the plasma membrane of the pericaryon (Figure 20.16) and the processes. The latter may be interconnected by a composite type of intercellular junction.[49] The increase in cytoskeletal elements in the cells in the inner zone most probably contributes to withstanding the increasing osmotic pressure towards the papillary tip. Furthermore, the occurrence of lipid granules increases progressively from the outer medulla towards the inner medulla where they may be so prominent that the cells were designated as "lipid-laden cells." However, inner medullary fibroblasts may also lack lipid droplets.[44] *In vitro* studies have revealed that the

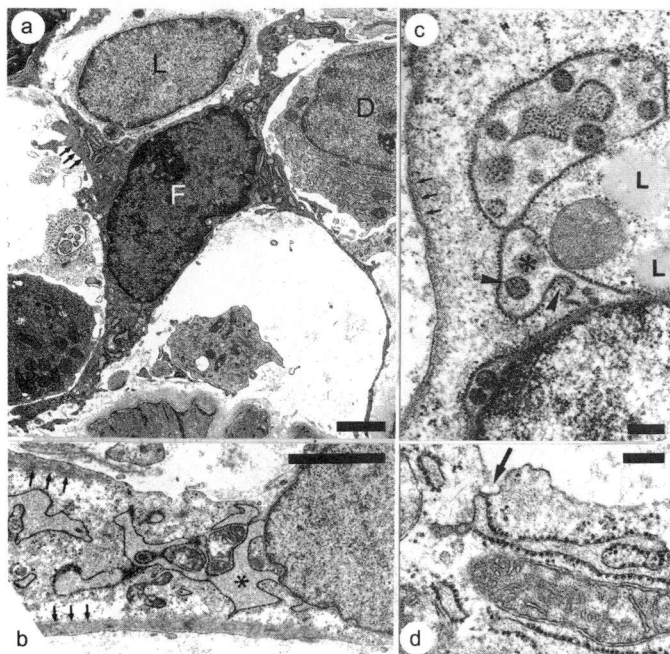

FIGURE 20.16 Medullary fibroblasts, (a, b, d) human fibroblasts from a renal biopsy; (c) fibroblast from a perfusion-fixed rat kidney. (a) Human fibroblast at the cortico-medullary border; stellate pericaryon and microfilament-rich cell processes (small arrows), extending between immune cells. (b) Part of a human fibroblast in the inner stripe of the outer medulla; the cisterns of the rough endoplasmic reticulum are widened and filled with flocculent material (Asterisk: Dilated perinuclear cistern; Small arrows: Accumulations of microfilaments along the plasma membrane). (c) Rat fibroblast from the inner medulla showing dilated perinuclear and endoplasmic reticulum cisterns (asterisk); infoldings of the ER into the cistern (arrow head) (L: Lipid droplets). (d) Fibroblast in the outer stripe of the outer medulla; a profile of rough endoplasmic reticulum in direct contact with the plasma membrane (arrow) (TEM (a): × ~4760; (b): × ~8500; (c) × ~37,400; (d) × ~33,150; Bars: (a,b): ~2 mm; (c,d): ~0.2 mm). *(From ref. [47].)*

occurrence and amount of lipid droplets in the inner medullary fibroblasts depends on the specific environment of the cells, conditioned by the presence of inner medullary collecting duct cells, and that inner medullary fibroblasts can transform to myofibroblasts with upregulation of alpha smooth muscle actin and desmin.[77] In medullary fibroblasts the cisterns of rough endoplasmic reticulum, including the perinuclear cistern, are often strikingly enlarged and they may narrowly enclose mitochondria (Figure 20.16). Occasionally the rER membranes are in direct contact with the plasma membrane (Figure 20.16). The functional interpretation of these particular features, only rarely observed in cortical fibroblasts, is still to be resolved.

The medullary fibroblasts do not display 5'NT or mRNA for EPO. A role of medullary interstitial cells has been proposed in the regulation of urinary osmolarity. *Glycosaminoglycans* are particularly abundant in the inner medullary interstitium,[78] and condensed hyaluronate-proteoglycan aggregates are associated with basement membranes, with collagen fibers, as well as with diffuse reticular structures.

The inner medulla has the greatest capacity for *renal prostaglandin* (PG) synthesis.[79,80] *Cyclooxygenase* (COX) isoforms, rate-limiting enzymes in PG biosynthesis, are expressed at substantially higher levels in the inner medulla than in the renal cortex.[81–84] COX-2 is found predominantly in inner medullary interstitial fibroblasts, and its expression increases under chronic salt loading.[84]

Dendritic Cells

Dendritic cells (DC) belong to the mononuclear phagocyte system and constitute the major antigen-presenting cell population in the healthy kidney.[85] Interstitial DCs continually probe the surrounding environment through dendrite extensions, and readily respond to insults to the parenchyma.[86–88] DCs have been recognized by their expression of MHC class II (Figures 20.12 and 20.13) and CD11c. In the healthy kidney DCs are present in their immature phenotype with comparatively low levels of MHC class II and of co-stimulatory proteins,[89] but with a high capacity for uptake of antigens.[86]

Similar to fibroblasts, DCs form an organ-spanning network,[88] located in very close contact with fibroblasts (Figures 20.12, 20.13 and 20.14).[45,47] DCs are constantly moving. Unlike fibroblasts, the pericaryon of DCs is large and confines the often rounded or elongated nucleus together with most cell organelles. The rER profiles of dendritic cells are narrow and less abundant than in fibroblasts. The intermediate filament protein vimentin is regularly present in the pericaryon of DCs, whereas it is absent in fibroblasts in the healthy renal cortex. Dendritic cells have, in comparison to macrophages and lymphocytes, more mitochondria, more rER, and a large Golgi apparatus. Lysosomes are less apparent than in macrophages. The so-called Birbeck granules, which are characteristic for dendritic cells, are a special formation of the endocytotic compartment serving as a loading compartment and/or reservoir of antigens before DC maturation.[90]

The ramified "veil-like" and perforated cellular extensions (Figure 20.12) lack the prominent stuffing with f-actin filaments, and are largely devoid of cell organelles, in marked contrast to fibroblasts. The long filiform processes of DCs have approximately the same diameter as the filiform fibroblast processes, but due to the lack of f-actin filaments are much less electron-dense (Figure 20.14). In contrast to fibroblasts, DCs have no junctional connections among each other or with tubules or vessels. However, frequently the plasma membranes of dendritic cells and of fibroblasts or dendritic cells and lymphocytes form points of membrane adhesion, so-called "kisses" (Figure 20.14). Parts of dendritic cells are often nestled into the hollows of the pericaryon or the processes of fibroblasts. The narrow intermingling of both cell types (Figures 20.12, 20.13 and 20.14) suggests the possibility of extensive cross-talk between them.

Dendritic cells are abundant in the inner stripe in the outer medulla and, as in the cortex, are narrowly associated with fibroblasts. Accumulations of dendritic cells are particularly striking around collecting ducts and thick ascending limbs.

In the inner medulla the pericaryon of dendritic cells is often situated in the spaces between the "ladder rungs" formed by the fibroblasts, and their processes may extend over several "ladder rungs." In the lower two-thirds of the inner medulla bone marrow-derived cells are not detected in the healthy kidney.[45,47]

Macrophages and Lymphocytes

Macrophages and lymphocytes are rarely found in the healthy renal interstitium, but they massively invade the interstitial spaces under inflammatory conditions.[46] A large proportion of the invading mononuclear cells display the established "marker proteins" (CD 45, CD3, CD4, CD 8; ED1, ED2, CD44, etc.) and the protein S100A4.[35,91] Neutrophil granulocytes are found occasionally, basophil and eosinophil granulocytes and plasma cells are rare in the healthy cortical renal interstitium.

PERIARTERIAL CONNECTIVE TISSUE AND LYMPHATICS

The periarterial tissue is a sheath of loose connective tissue, surrounding the intrarenal arteries (arcuate arteries, cortical radial arteries). The considerable thickness of the periarterial sheath is apparent in quick-frozen specimens,[92] and in perfusion fixed tissue. It attenuates towards the end of the cortical radial arteries and terminates along the afferent arteriole at the vascular pole of the glomerulus (Figures 20.17, 20.18 and 20.19). The periarterial sheath is continuous with the peritubular interstitium and with the connective tissue underlying the epithelium of the renal pelvis and ureter at all sites. The renal veins are apposed to the periarterial sheath.[92]

The periarterial sheath constitutes wide meshes of the extremely attenuated processes of 5'NT-negative, but weakly alpha-smooth muscle actin- and vimentin-positive fibroblasts.[47] The meshes are filled with thick

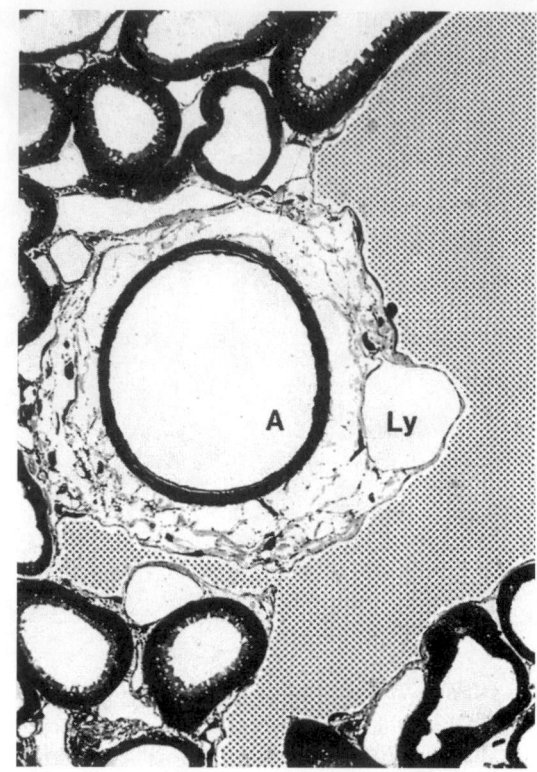

FIGURE 20.17   Cross-section through the deep cortex (rat). The cortical radial artery (A) is surrounded by a layer of loose connective tissue that contains the lymphatics (L_Y). The cortical radial vein is only partly shown; its lumen and those of direct tributaries have been highlighted by a dotted pattern. Note the intimate relationships of the artery, vein, and lymphatic, mediated by the periarterial loose connective tissue (TEM: $\times \sim 360$).

bundles of collageneous fibers and interstitial fluid and regularly confine some macrophages and dendritic cells.

The periarterial connective tissue sheath provides the path for renal nerves (see below) and for *renal lymphatics*.[92] Lymphatics start in the vicinity of the glomerular vascular pole[25] or at a more proximal level of the afferent arteriole, depending on the species, and travel along the branches of the renal arteries towards the renal hilum (Figures 20.17 and 20.18). Their recognition and distinction from blood capillaries at light microscopic levels is facilitated by their specific expression of podoplanin.[93] Also, 5'NT labels in rat and mice lymphatics, but not in blood vessels. Lymphatic endothelial cells secrete chemokines that attract dendritic cells. An increase in lymphatic microvessels has been observed, e.g., in tubulointerstitial fibrosis and progression to end-stage renal failure in remnant kidney.[93]

Regulatory substances that are released into the peritubular interstitium might access the systemic blood circulation via the lymphatics in the periarterial sheath. This suggestion has been made for renin,[92] and it may

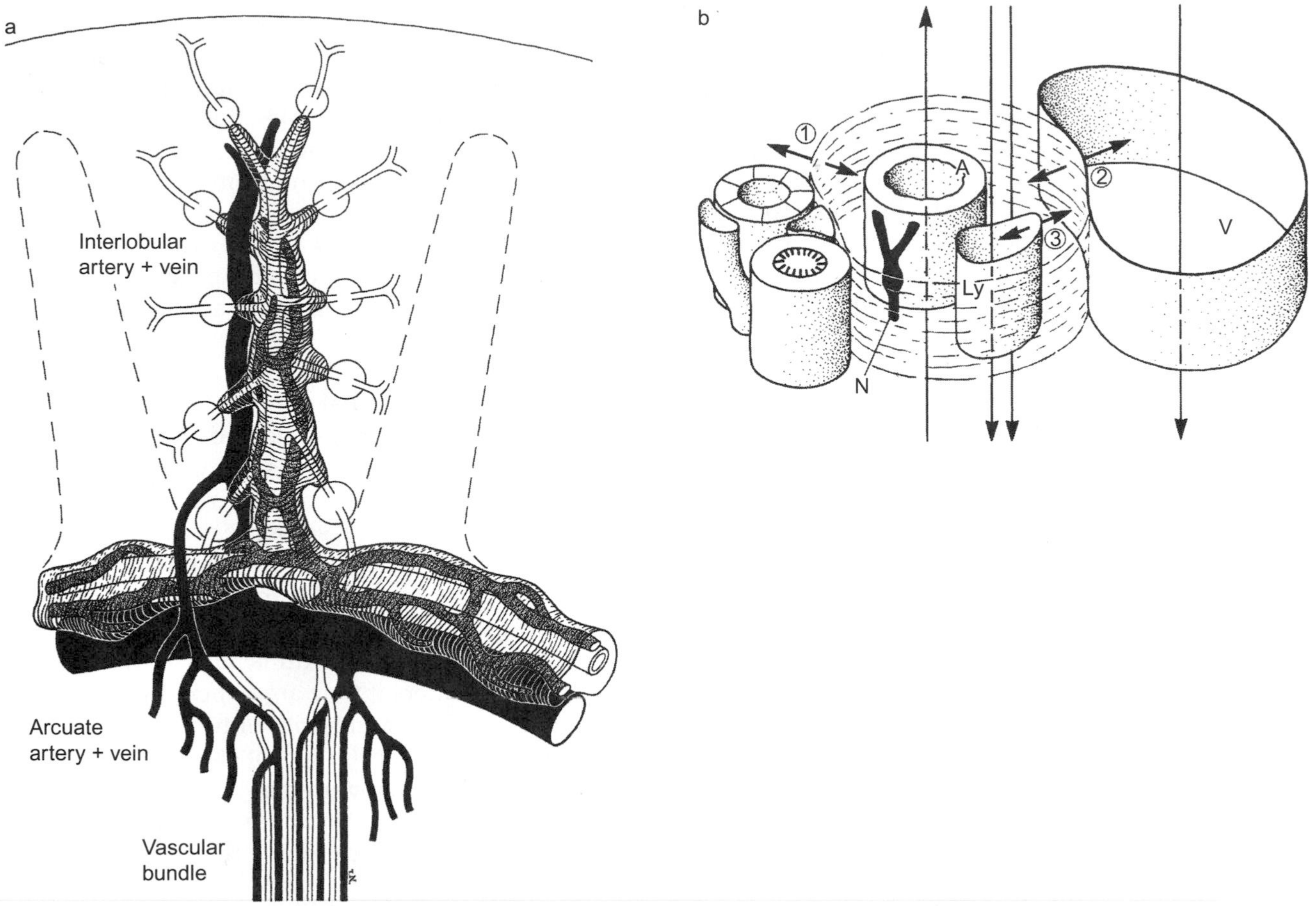

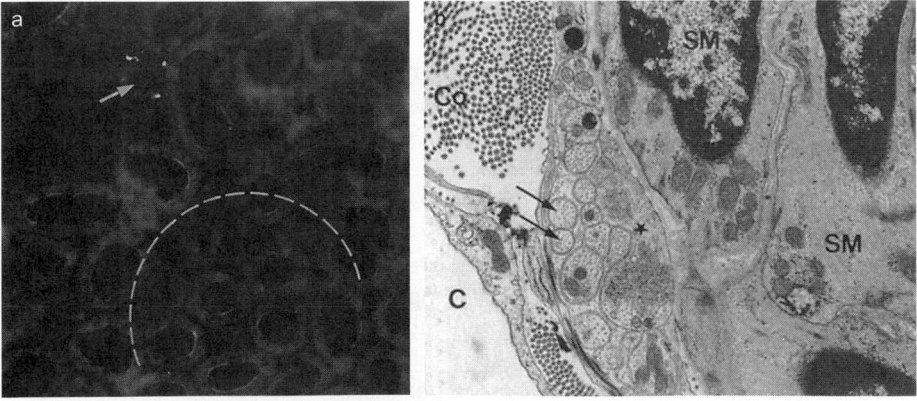

FIGURE 20.18 Schematics to show (a) the distribution, and (b) the topographical relationships of the periarterial connective tissue sheath. Not drawn to scale. (a) The periarterial sheath is schematically indicated as a wide "stocking" drawn over the intrarenal arteries and lymphatics. In reality this stocking has no limiting tissue that separates the interior from the surroundings. An arcuate artery transforms into a cortical radial artery, which gives rise to afferent arterioles. These segments are surrounded by the periarterial connective tissue sheath. The efferent arterioles, as well as the veins (drawn in black), are not included. The lymphatics (stippled) originate and travel within the periarterial sheath. Note there are no lymphatics coming up from the medulla. Within the cortex, medullary rays are indicated by a broken line. In (b) a transverse section through an cortical radial artery (A) shows the relationships of the periarterial sheath and the possibilities for functional exchanges (double-headed arrows) with surrounding structures: (1) with the peritubular interstitium; (2) with the accompanying vein (V); and (3) with lymphatics (Ly). The single-headed arrows indicate the flow of the respective fluid. Note the nerves (N) traveling through the periarterial tissue. In addition, two neighboring tubules, including an arcade and a proximal tubule, together with peritubular capillaries, are drawn. *(From ref. [92], with permission.)*

FIGURE 20.19 The renal nerves accompany (a) the intrarenal arteries. A cortical radial artery (arrow) is seen which is associated with three nerve bundles, identified by staining with a monoclonal antibody against protein gene product 9.5 (PGP 9.5) which is a universal marker for vertebrate neurons. Among the tubules no nerves are found. A medullary ray is delineated by a hatched line (Rat; LM ×∼240). *(In cooperation with M. Siry, W. Kummer and S. Bachmann).* (b) A large terminal nerve accompanying an afferent arteriole. Several axons (arrows) and a varicosity (star) with synaptic vesicles are seen (SM: Smooth muscle cell; CO: Collagen; C: Capillary; Rabbit kidney: TEM ×∼12,000).

apply to other protein hormones such as erythropoietin. The periarterial tissue sheaths have been interpreted as a mixing chamber for a variety of vasoactive substances, ultimately determining the contractile status of the renal resistance vessels. In addition to the lymphatics, the periarterial tissue itself constitutes a pathway for interstitial fluid drainage. Indeed, a tracer injected under the renal capsule can be followed within the periarterial tissue, as well as within the lymphatics.

While a fraction of cortical interstitial fluid gains access to the periarterial tissue, and eventually to lymphatics, there is no direct pathway for regulatory substances released in the cortical interstitium to reach medullary targets. It has been proposed that the intimate relationships between cortical radial arteries and veins permits countercurrent exchange of O_2, being responsible — at least in part — for the low partial pressure of O_2 in the superficial cortex.[94,95]

NERVES

The efferent nerves of the kidney are composed of sympathetic nerves and terminal axons, which accompany the intrarenal arteries, and the afferent and efferent arterioles (Figures 20.18 and 20.19).[96] The nerve fibers are monoaminergic. Norepinephrine[97–99] and dopamine have been identified.[100] In addition, several neuropeptides are co-localized with norepinephrine in renal nerves.[101] The presence of acetylcholinesterase in renal nerves cannot be taken to indicate cholinergic nerves, but rather that monoaminergic nerves obviously possess acetylcholinesterase activity.[97]

The nerve fibers run in the loose connective tissue around the arteries and arterioles. The descending vasa recta within the medulla are also innervated by adrenergic nerve terminals as far as they are enveloped by smooth muscle cells.[102,103] A dense assembly of nerves and terminal axons is found around the juxtaglomerular apparatus[99] which is described in more detail along with the JGA.

Tubules have direct relationships to terminal axons only when they are located around the arteries or arterioles.[96,99] Tubules adjacent to the juxtaglomerular apparatus (terminal portion of the cortical thick ascending limb) are more frequently touched by terminal axons than at other sites.[99] The density of nerve contacts to convoluted proximal tubules (located in the cortical labyrinth) is low[104]; nerve contacts to straight proximal tubules (located in the medullary rays and the outer stripe) have never been encountered. The overwhelming majority of tubular portions have no direct relationships to nerve terminals.

Consequently, morphologists are left with the question of how the neuronal influence on tubular function[105] is mediated. In addition to a systemic distribution of catecholamines, a more specific, but also indirect, mode seems possible for certain tubular segments.[5] Because nerve fibers do pass along the vascular pole of each glomerulus from afferent to efferent arterioles, the distribution of nerves in the renal cortex is dense. Catecholamines (and other transmitters) released from nerve terminals at the vascular poles and at the efferent arterioles may gain access to peritubular capillaries, and in this way may perfuse the convoluted tubules of the cortical labyrinth. Tubules arranged around the cortical radial arteries would be reached most easily by transmitters released from periarterially located nerve terminals. This may be of relevance with respect to arcades (connecting tubules), which have been shown to be sensitive to isoproterenol.[106] Exposure of the straight tubules within the medullary rays of the cortex to neural transmitters reaching them directly by diffusion from nerve terminal is improbable.

Tubules in the outer medulla may only be reached by neurotransmitters if they are either situated adjacent to vascular bundles (a minority of tubules) or secondarily, by a capillary distribution of the transmitters from nerve terminals accompanying the vascular bundles. The tubules of the inner medulla cannot be reached by neurotransmitters directly delivered from nerve terminals in the medulla.

Little is known about the afferent nerves of the kidney; they are commonly believed to be sparse, but the issue remains unresolved.[102,105,107–110]

TOPOGRAPHICAL RELATIONSHIPS

Cortex

The architectural pattern of the renal cortex is best understood when viewing a cross-section through the midcortex (Figures 20.20 and 20.21). Two portions within the cortical parenchyma, the labyrinth and the medullary rays, are distinguishable. Within the cortical labyrinth, the vascular axes, which consist of the cortical radial (interlobular) artery, vein, and a lymphatic, are regularly distributed. The renal corpuscles and the corresponding convoluted tubules (proximal and distal) are situated around each vascular axis. Barriers separating the population of renal corpuscles and convoluted tubules belonging to another vascular axis are not discernible. Thus, the cortical labyrinth is a continuous parenchymal layer that contains the vascular axes of the cortex and the medullary rays in a regular pattern. The straight tubules (proximal and distal), together with the collecting ducts, are located within the medullary rays. Because the number of straight tubules increases

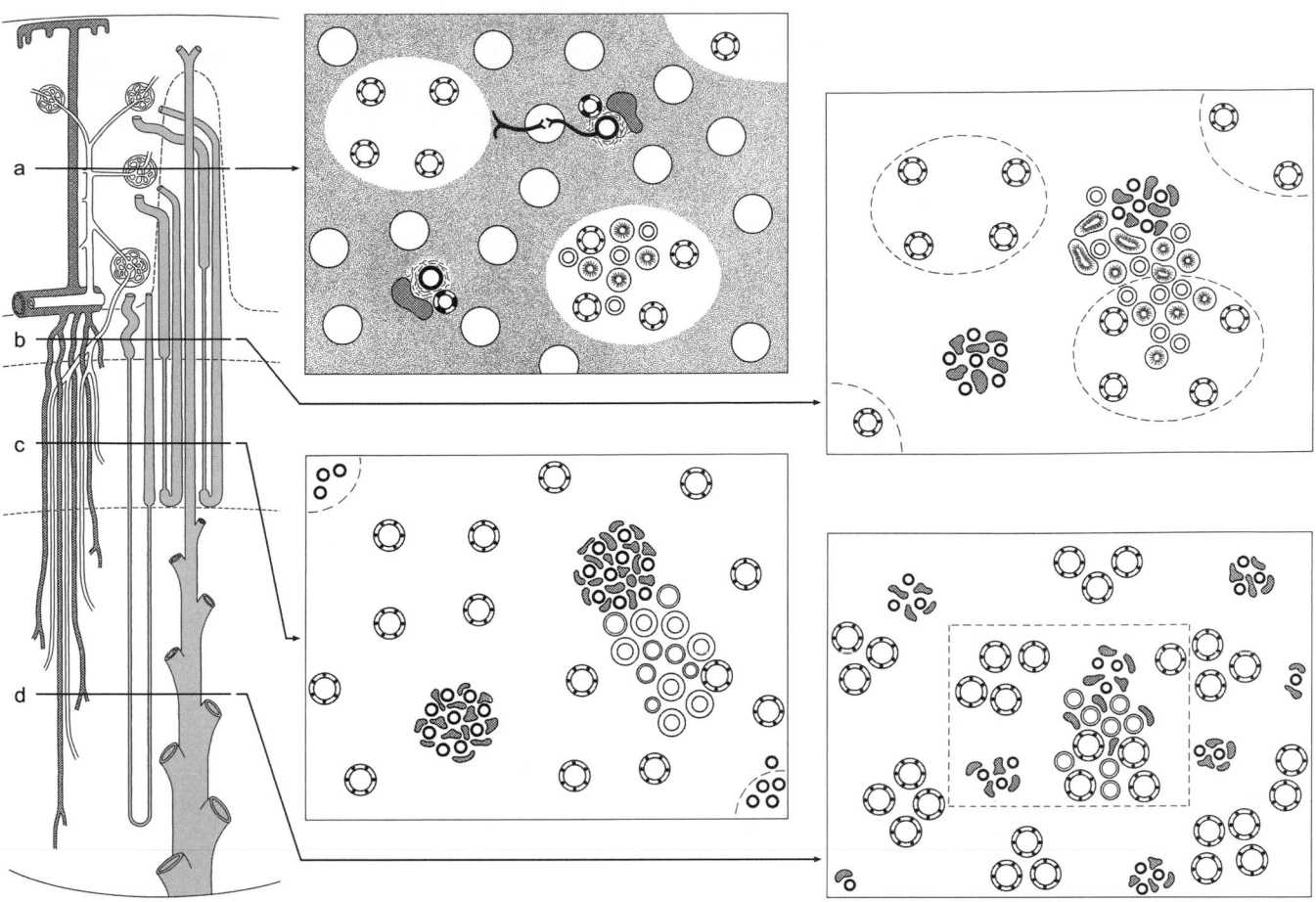

FIGURE 20.20 **Schematics of histotopography.** Histotopography of the kidney as revealed by four successive cross-sections through: (a) cortex; (b) outer stripe; (c) inner stripe; and (d) inner medulla. The simple type of the medulla (rabbit, man) is shown. (*From Koushanpour, E., and Kriz, W. (1986). In "Renal Physiology. Principles, Structure and Function." Springer-Verlag, New York, with permission.*) In the cortex the cortical labyrinth (shaded area) and the medullary rays (white) are shown. The labyrinth contains the cortical radial (interlobular) blood vessels, glomeruli, and the convoluted tubular portions (the latter are not shown). The arcades accompany the interlobular vessels. The medullary rays contain the collecting ducts and the straight proximal and distal tubules. Note the typical grouping of collecting ducts within a medullary ray. In the outer stripe, vascular bundles replace the interlobular vessel axis of the cortex. The continuations of the medullary rays are surrounded by hatched lines. Within these areas the collecting ducts and the loop limbs of superficial and midcortical nephrons are found. The loop limbs of juxtamedullary nephrons are situated around the vascular bundles. In the inner stripe, the vascular bundles are fully developed. Like in the outer stripe, the loop limbs of juxtamedullary nephrons are situated near the bundles, and those from superficial and midcortical nephrons together with the collecting ducts are located distant from the bundles. Note the heterogeneity of the thin limbs: Those of juxtamedullary nephrons lie near the bundles and are thicker in diameter, whereas those of the superficial nephrons lie distant from the bundles. Inner medulla. The area defined by the dashed rectangle corresponds to the entire area shown in section (c). This reduction in size is because short loops and many vasa recta have turned back in the inner stripe. Note the grouping of collecting ducts reflecting their medullary ray arrangement in the cortex. Thin limbs (both descending and ascending) are associated with vasa recta or collecting ducts.

toward the corticomedullary border, the medullary rays increase in width toward the outer stripe.

A regular pattern of the convoluted tubules within the labyrinth is not apparent. Proximal and distal convoluted tubules (the latter constitute only a minor portion of profiles in comparison with proximal tubules) are equally embedded in the dense capillary plexus of this region. A strikingly constant position is occupied by the arcades (if they are present). They ascend within the cortical labyrinth and are grouped immediately around the vascular axes. The topographical

relationships within the juxtaglomerular apparatus will be described later.

Within the medullary rays the straight tubules of superficial nephrons (proximal and distal) generally occupy a central position, and those of midcortical nephrons occupy a peripheral position. The collecting ducts are situated between the two groups, and therefore are situated neither in the center nor at the very border of a medullary ray. Efferent arterioles do not enter the medullary rays, but frequently break off into capillaries just at the border between the labyrinth and

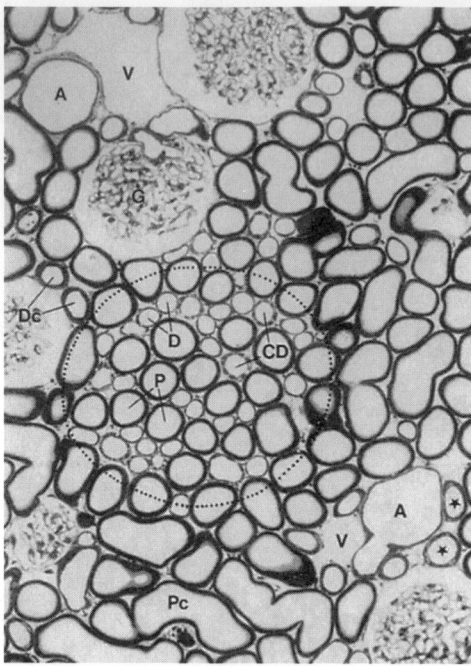

FIGURE 20.21 Renal cortex of the rat; 1 μm cross-section. The architectural pattern of the cortex is demonstrated. A medullary ray is delineated by a dashed line. It contains the straight proximal tubules (P), the straight distal tubules (thick ascending limb; asterisks), and the collecting ducts (C). The cortical radial vessels (A: Artery; V: Vein), glomeruli (G), and convoluted proximal (Pc) and distal (D) tubules establish the cortical labyrinth. Arcades (stars) ascend close to the cortical radial vessels (×∼200).

the medullary rays. As a result, the blood supply of the medullary ray tubules is as direct as that of the tubules within the cortical labyrinth. However, blood that perfuses the straight tubules of the medullary rays mixes afterwards with the blood that perfuses the convoluted tubules (*vide supra*).

Medulla

The three regions of the medulla contain different populations of nephron segments. The outer stripe contains straight parts of the proximal tubule (S_3 segments), straight parts of the distal tubule (thick ascending limbs), and collecting ducts. The inner stripe is composed of descending thin limbs, ascending thick limbs (distal straight tubules), and collecting ducts. The inner medulla contains thin descending and ascending limbs, and collecting ducts.

The architectural organization of the medulla can best be described by considering the vascular bundles as central axes and studying how the tubules are arranged around them.[33,112] A "simple" and a "complex" type of renal medulla are distinguished (Figure 20.22); the differences between both are mainly found in the inner stripe.

The vascular bundles develop in the outer stripe (Figures 20.20 and 20.23). At the very beginning of the bundles the straight proximal and distal tubules of juxtamedullary nephrons are grouped immediately around the bundles. In the continuation of the medullary rays, the tubules of superficial and midcortical nephrons, together with the collecting ducts, fill the spaces between the bundles and their adjacent juxtamedullary tubules. In the outer stripe straight proximal tubules and straight distal tubules (thick ascending limbs) should theoretically be present in equal numbers; however, a cross-section through the outer stripe shows that proximal tubular profiles are much more numerous than distal tubules. In the rat, proximal tubules occupy roughly 68% of the space in the outer stripe, in contrast to approximately 13% by the thick ascending limbs, and 5% by the collecting ducts.[41] The dominance of the proximal tubules is rooted in the fact that the straight proximal tubules of juxtamedullary nephrons are not straight (as their name indicates), but rather take a tortuous course when descending through the outer stripe; this holds true for the mouse kidney.[113] In addition, straight proximal tubules are much thicker in diameter than the straight distal tubules, and proximal tubules of juxtamedullary nephrons are even thicker than those of the midcortical and superficial nephrons.[5]

The tubules of the outer stripe are perfused by a specific "capillary" plexus. "True" capillaries, derived from direct branches of efferent arterioles, are few; the dominating "capillary" vessels in the outer stripe are the ascending vasa recta (Figures 20.3 and 20.4b). They traverse the outer stripe as wide tortuous channels closely contacting the tubules like proper capillaries. Because these vessels carry the entire venous blood from the medulla, the outer stripe tubules are mainly supplied by venous blood from deeper parts of the medulla.

The outer stripe varies considerably in thickness among species; in the rat[33] and mouse,[34] it is very well-developed and constitutes approximately one-third of the outer medulla. In contrast, in *Psammomys*,[32] cat,[37] dog,[114] and humans,[37] the outer stripe is very thin.

The inner stripe (Figures 20.20 and 20.24) of the outer medulla is the most constant part of the renal medulla, consisting of the regularly distributed vascular bundles (VB) leaving between them the interbundle region (IBR). Two types of vascular bundles can be distinguished, which form the basis for the discrimination of a "simple" and a "complex" type of medulla.

In most species[5,115] vascular bundles of the simple type are present, which exclusively contain descending and ascending vasa recta. The tubules are found in the IBR and are arranged around the bundles in a pattern similar to that found in the outer stripe. The loops of

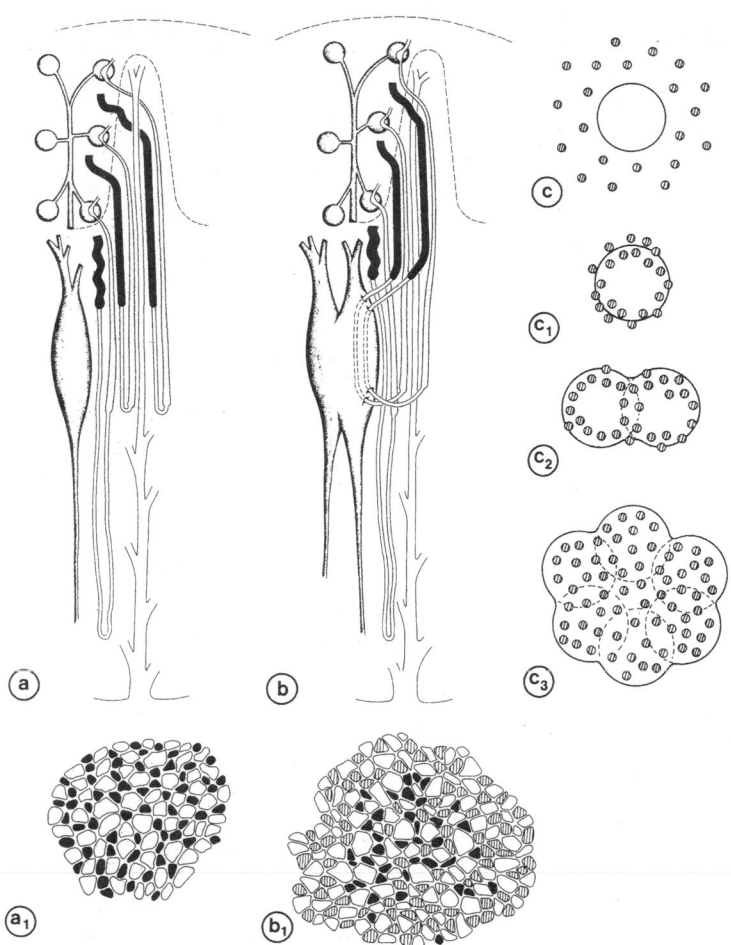

FIGURE 20.22 **Schematic to demonstrate the difference between the simple (a and a₁) and complex (b and b₁) types of medulla.** In the simple medulla (a), loops of Henle surround the vascular bundle according to the pattern established in the cortex. The long loops lie nearest to the bundle, the short loops of superficial nephrons farthest away. The collecting ducts are situated at a distance from the bundle. The bundle itself (a₁) contains only descending (black) and ascending (white) vasa recta. In the complex medulla (b), the descending thin limbs of short loops descend within the vascular bundles. The complex bundle (b₁) contains, in addition to descending (black) and ascending (white) vasa recta, the descending thin limbs of short loops (hatched). *(From ref. [133], with permission.)* (c–c₃): Schematics of cross-sections through vascular bundles to show different degrees of bundle fusing and loop integration in the complex type of renal medulla (c1–c3) compared with the simple type (c) (Large circle: Vascular bundle; Small hatched circles: Descending thin limbs of short loops). In the simple type of medulla (c), the descending thin limbs of short loops are all located outside the bundle. Complex bundles (c₁–c₃) may be established in different degrees. In rat (c₁), descending thin limbs of short loops are arranged in the periphery of the bundles; bundles generally do not fuse. In mouse (c₂), bundles frequently fuse; descending thin limbs of short loops have penetrated deeper into the bundle. In *Psammomys* or *Meriones* (c₃), bundle fusing has produced giant bundles; descending thin limbs of short loops are distributed over the entire bundle area. *(From ref. [115], with permission.)*

Henle, originating from juxtamedullary nephrons (generally the longest long loops), lie nearest to the bundles, whereas the loops derived from superficial and midcortical nephrons (in most species, short loops) lie distant from the bundles. The collecting ducts are generally arranged in distant rings around the bundles, and are intermingled with loops derived from superficial and midcortical nephrons. Altogether, they are perfused by the dense capillary plexus of the IBR.

The complex type of vascular bundle (Figure 20.25) is present in several rodent species with a high urine concentrating ability, including rat,[33] mouse,[16,34] *Meriones*,[116] and *Psammomys*.[32] It differs from the simple type in that the descending thin limbs of short loops (only of short loops!) descend within the vascular bundle (Figure 20.26). Consequently, the bundles within the inner stripe change from the classic countercurrent arrangement of a rete mirabile, consisting of DVRs and AVRs, to a system in which one ascending tube (AVRs) is closely packed together with two descending tubes (DVRs and SDTLs). In addition, the vascular bundles in the complex type of medulla tend to fuse and to form larger bundles, up to giant bundles (*Psammomys*). These complex bundles are developed at the transition from the outer stripe to the inner stripe, and are maintained only throughout the inner stripe.

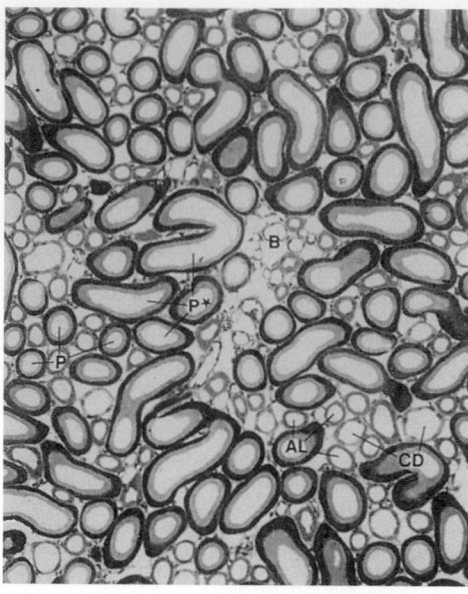

FIGURE 20.23   Outer stripe of rat kidney; 1 μm cross-section. The vascular bundle (VB) is surrounded by the straight proximal tubules of juxtamedullary nephrons (asterisk), which are larger in diameter than those of superficial and midcortical nephrons (P), which lie distant from the bundles (Asterisks: thick ascending limb; C: collecting duct). Interstitial spaces are sparsely developed (×~220).

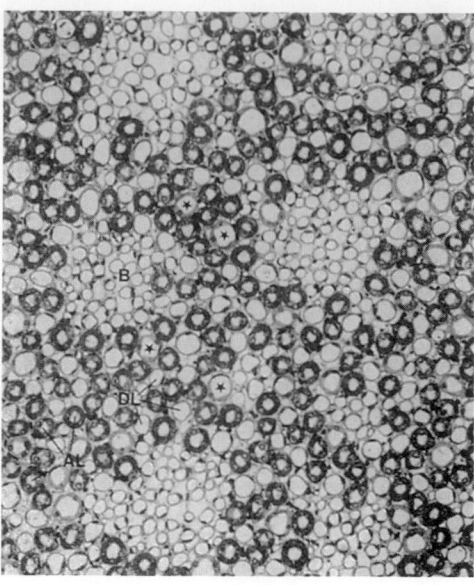

FIGURE 20.24   Inner stripe of rabbit kidney (simple medulla); 1 μm cross-section. The vascular bundles (VB) are regularly distributed. The collecting ducts (C) lie distant from the bundles. Descending thin limbs (asterisks) and thick ascending limbs (stars) are situated within the interbundle regions (×~200).

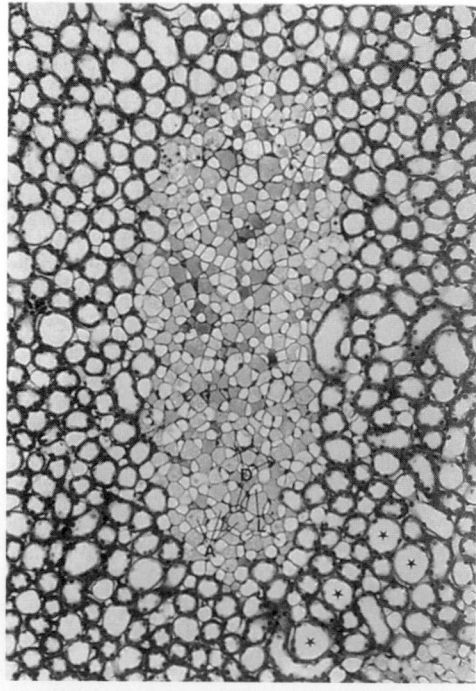

FIGURE 20.25   Inner stripe of *Meriones shawii* kidney (complex medulla); paraffin cross-section. The large vascular bundle originates by fusing of primary bundles. In addition to descending (D) and ascending (A) vasa recta, complex vascular bundles contain descending thin limbs of short loops (L). Collecting ducts (some are marked by asterisks) are situated distant from the bundles (×~190).

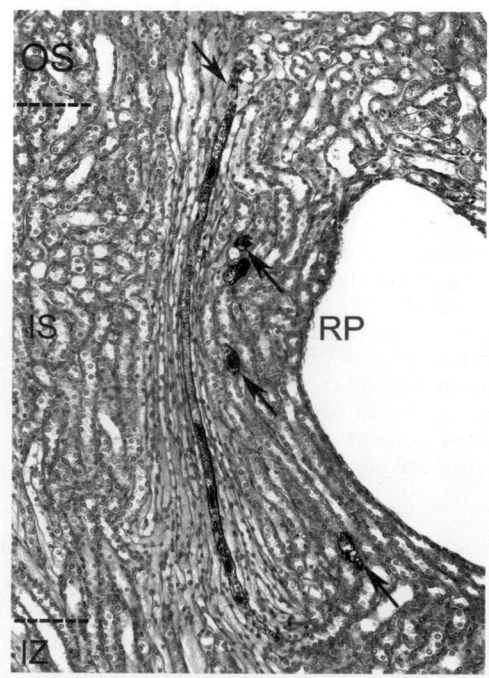

FIGURE 20.26   Longitudinal section through a vascular bundle in the inner stripe of a gerbil kidney (complex medulla); paraffin section. One superficial nephron has been injected with microfill; at the transition from the outer (OS) to the inner stripe (IS) the proximal tubule transforms to the intermediate tubule (thin descending limb; left arrow) which descends within the vascular bundle; the tubule leaves the bundle at the border between the inner stripe and the inner zone (IZ), and ascends as thick ascending limb (right arrows) within the interbundle region (RP: Extension of the renal pelvis; ×~200).

At the border to the inner medulla, the SDTLs leave the bundles, and the fused bundles split into the original number of bundles. The characteristics of the complex type are developed to different degrees in the species so far investigated. A somewhat "gradual" transition from the rat, via the mouse, to *Meriones* and *Psammomys* is observed.

The tubular pattern around these complex bundles is different from that of the simple type. At the border between the outer stripe and inner stripe, the SDTLs leave their position distant from the bundles, then turn toward a bundle and descend within the bundle. Their TALs maintain a position distant from the bundles and near to a collecting duct throughout the outer medulla. As observed in the simple type, the tubules of the interbundle regions are embedded in the dense capillary plexus of the IBR. In contrast to what is observed in the simple type, it is worthwhile to stress the fact that in the complex type only the LDTLs, scattered among the TALs of short and long loops, traverse IBR. Specific variations of this pattern in mice[117] and *Psammomys*[17,32] are described elsewhere.

To understand the possible functional implications of the inner stripe architecture, as well as the differences between the simple type and the complex type, we have to consider precisely the composition of the vascular bundles. The vascular bundles of the simple type contain all descending and all ascending vasa recta servicing the inner medulla. Furthermore, they contain most of the descending vasa recta, which service the inner stripe, but only few of the ascending vasa recta, which drain the inner stripe. The numerical relationship between descending and ascending vasa recta is about 1 to 1 (at the level of the inner stripe). Thus, in the simple type of vascular bundle, the venous blood from the inner medulla contacts the arterial blood that supplies both the inner medulla and the inner stripe of the outer medulla in a countercurrent arrangement. Therefore, inner medullary venous blood may exchange not only with the arterial blood that is predetermined for the inner medulla, but also with blood predetermined for the inner stripe. Substances originating from the inner medulla could be trapped by countercurrent exchange to the inner medulla, but could also be shifted to the inner stripe capillary plexus, and thereby be offered to inner stripe tubules (see below).

In the complex type of medulla, the vascular bundles incorporate the descending thin limbs of short loops. In *Psammomys*, at the level of the inner stripe, the bundles consist of approximately 10% descending vasa recta, 45% ascending vasa recta, and 45% descending thin limbs,[32] with the descending thin limbs being completely surrounded by ascending vasa recta. The difference between the simple and the complex types of bundles is even more pronounced when it is realized that the bundles in *Psammomys* no longer contain any vasa recta servicing the inner stripe. All vasa recta present in the giant bundles of *Psammomys* either descend to the inner medulla or ascend from the inner medulla. The vasa recta servicing the inner stripe in *Psammomys* descend or ascend, respectively, independent of the bundles. Thus, the giant bundles of the inner stripe in *Psammomys* appear to form a countercurrent trap for the inner medullary blood that is located in the inner stripe. In other species with complex bundles (rat, mouse), vasa recta servicing the inner stripe are not as strictly excluded from the bundles as in *Psammomys*; even in these species the vascular bundles appear to be a countercurrent trap for mainly the inner medullary circulation.

The inner medulla develops very differently among species. Species with only short loops of Henle[6] do not have an inner medulla; their urine concentrating ability is poor. All species with high urine concentrating ability have a well-developed inner medulla.[3,118] It is characteristic for the inner medulla to taper from a broad basis to a papilla (or crest). The mass of the inner medulla is therefore unevenly distributed along the longitudinal axis. A study in the rat[2,119] has shown that the decrease in the mass of the inner medulla along the longitudinal axis follows an exponential function. The upper half of the inner medulla accounts for roughly 80% of the total inner medullary volume, and consequently only 20% are left for the papillary half.

With regard to the ratio between Henle's loops and collecting ducts along the inner medulla, considerable differences are found when comparing the base with the tip of the inner medulla, as well as notable interspecies differences.[42] In the rat, the ratio is about 2.5 (2.5 loops per one collecting duct) at the beginning of the inner medulla; this ratio rapidly decreases to about 1 toward the papilla. In the rabbit, the ratio increases from 3 at the beginning of the inner medulla to 9 within the papilla, then later decreases to 5 in the papillary tip. These data all await functional interpretation, thus indicating the limitation of our knowledge concerning structure–function correlations in the inner medulla.

An architectural pattern within the inner medulla is less apparent than in the outer medulla.[5,34,120] Constant histotopographical relationships between certain structures or spatial separations of others do not seem to be as important to the function of the inner medulla compared to the outer medulla. When entering the inner medulla, the vascular bundles already contain a drastically decreased number of vasa recta. Towards the papilla, this number continues to decrease; finally single descending vasa recta enter the tip of the papilla. Ascending vasa recta in the inner medulla generally ascend independent of the bundles, which they finally

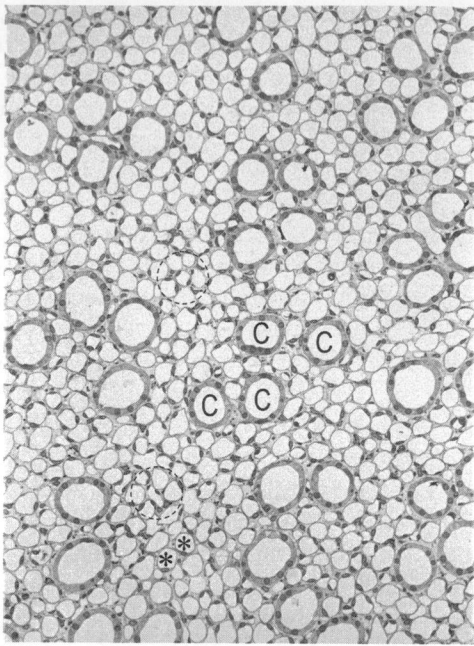

FIGURE 20.27 **Inner medulla of the rabbit kidney; 1 μm cross-section through the upper part.** The collecting ducts are still arranged in groups, reflecting the pattern in the medullary rays of the cortex. Vascular bundles (dashed circles) are poorly delineated. Thin loop limbs (asterisks) lie near collecting ducts (C), as well as near vasa recta of the vascular bundles (× ~240).

join at the border of the inner stripe. Thus, in the inner medulla, the vasa recta are never as closely packed to bundles as they are in the inner stripe.

As far as vascular bundles are discernible, the collecting ducts are generally distanced from them. At the very beginning of the inner medulla, collecting ducts are still arranged in groups that reflect their grouping within the medullary rays of the cortex (Figure 20.27). Joining of collecting ducts first occurs among the ducts of one group. Descending and ascending thin loop limbs, together with individually running vasa recta and capillaries, fill the spaces between the bundle centers and the collecting ducts. DTLs in general tend to be more distant from CDs, whereas ATLs tend to be positioned more closely to CDs[120,121]; a thin limb of Henle, regardless of whether descending or ascending, may be associated with both collecting ducts and/or vasa recta. Obviously, the interactions of the structures in the inner medulla are mediated through the wide interstitial spaces.

With regard to the functional connections of the inner medulla with the outer medulla, it is notable that all descending vasa recta servicing the inner medulla have already been established as individual vessels in the outer stripe and traverse the inner stripe within the bundles. All ascending vasa recta from the inner medulla traverse the inner stripe within the bundles

without joining with ascending vasa recta from the inner stripe. The blood flow of the inner stripe and that of the inner medulla are apparently distinct from each other. In the outer stripe, however, venous vasa recta coming up from the inner medulla and those from the inner stripe finally take a similar route. Both traverse the outer stripe as wide capillary channels representing the major capillary supply of the outer stripe tubules.

GLOMERULUS (RENAL CORPUSCLE)

The renal corpuscle consists of a tuft of specialized capillaries that protrudes into Bowman's space (urinary space) surrounded by Bowman's capsule (BC). The tuft consists of specialized capillaries held together by the mesangium and covered — as a whole — by the glomerular basement membrane (GBM), followed by a layer of unique epithelial cells, the podocytes. Traditionally, this layer is called the visceral epithelium of BC, which — at the vascular pole of the glomerular tuft — reflects into the parietal epithelium of BC. Nowadays, the term Bowman's capsule is generally used only for this parietal cell layer which — together with its basement membrane (parietal, BM, PBM) — forms the outer wall of a glomerulus. At the urinary pole, BC transforms into the proximal tubule epithelium, Bowman's space opens into the tubular lumen (Figures 20.28 and 20.29).

The diameters of the — more or less — spherical renal corpuscles in different species range from approximately 100 μm (mouse) up to 300 μm (elephant), in humans they are approximately 200 μm, in rat 120 μm, and in rabbit 150 μm.[29,36,37] In many species (rodents) the diameter of juxtamedullary renal corpuscles may exceed that of midcortical and superficial nephrons by up to 50[22,29,34,37]; this does not hold true for the human kidney.[122]

Architecture of the Glomerulus

The reflection of the parietal epithelium of Bowman's capsule into the visceral epithelium creates an oval opening in the glomerulus, which is called the glomerular hilum. Actually, it is the reflection of the GBM into the PBM (i.e., the basement membrane of the parietal epithelium of Bowman's capsule) that borders the opening. Through it the glomerular arterioles, together with the glomerular mesangium, enter the inner space of the GBM, which forms a complex folded sack. Inside this sack the glomerular capillaries pursue a tortuous course around centrally located mesangial axes. Together, capillaries and mesangium totally fill the labyrinthine spaces inside the GBM. The outer

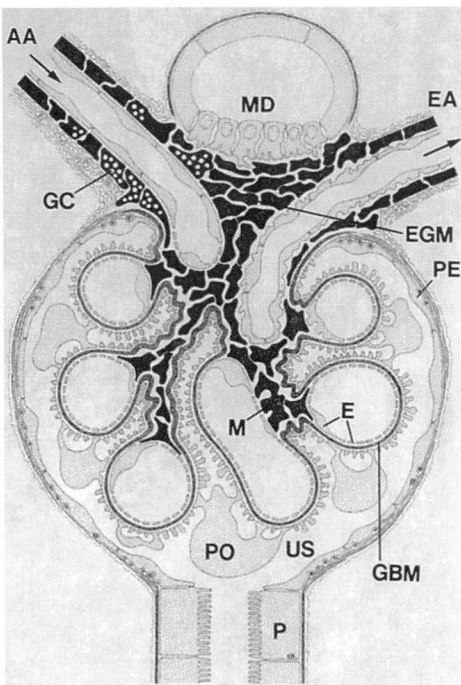

FIGURE 20.28 **Diagram of a longitudinal section through a glomerulus and its juxtaglomerular apparatus (JGA).** The capillary tuft consists of a network of specialized capillaries, which are outlined by a fenestrated endothelium. *(From Cunningham, R. et al. (2005). Am. J. Physiol. Renal Physiol. 289(4), F933–938.)* Defective PTH regulation of sodium-dependent phosphate transport in NHERF1$^{-/-}$ renal proximal tubule cells and wild-type cells adapted to low-phosphate media. At the vascular pole, the afferent arteriole (AA) branches into capillaries immediately after its entrance; the efferent arteriole (EA) is established inside the tuft and passes through the glomerular stalk before leaving at the vascular pole. The capillary network, together with the mesangium, is enclosed in a common compartment bounded by the glomerular basement membrane (GBM). Note that there is no basement membrane at the interface between the capillary endothelium and the mesangium. The glomerular visceral epithelium consists of highly-branched podocytes (PO) which, in a typical interdigitating pattern, cover the outer aspect of the GBM. At the vascular pole, the visceral epithelium and the GBM are reflected into the parietal epithelium (PE) of Bowman's capsule, which passes over into the epithelium of the proximal tubule (PT) at the urinary pole. At the vascular pole, the glomerular mesangium is continuous with the extraglomerular mesangium (EGM) consisting of extraglomerular mesangial cells and an extraglomerular mesangial matrix. The extraglomerular mesangium, together with the granular cells (G) of the afferent arteriole and the macula densa (MD), establish the JGA. All cells which are suggested to be of smooth muscle origin are shown in black (F: foot processes; N: sympathetic nerve terminals; US: urinary space). *(Adapted from Kriz, W., and Sakai, T. et al. (1988). Morphological aspects of glomerular function. In "Nephrology," A. M. Davison, Vol. 1, Proceedings of the X International Congress of Nephrology," 3–23. Bailliere Tindall, London.)*

aspect of the GBM is covered by the visceral epithelium, i.e., by the podocytes. The glomerular tuft therefore consists of the glomerular capillaries and the mesangium inside the sack of the GBM (frequently called the "endocapillary compartment"), and the

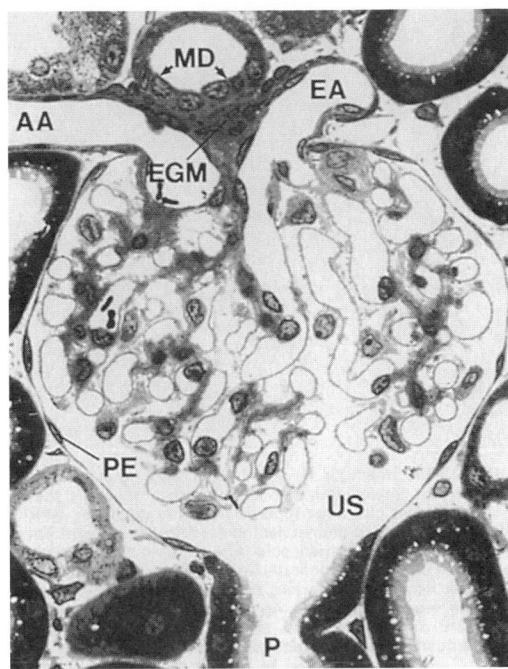

FIGURE 20.29 **Longitudinal section through a glomerulus (rat).** At the vascular pole the afferent arteriole (AA), the efferent arteriole (EA), the extraglomerular mesangium (EGM), and the macula densa (MD) are seen. At the urinary pole the beginning of the proximal tubule is seen (P) (PE: Parietal epithelial of Bowman's capsule; US: Urinary space; LM $\times\sim$490).

podocytes covering this sack from outside ("exocapillary compartment").

The glomerular capillaries are derived from the afferent arteriole which — strictly at the entrance level — divides into several (two to five) primary capillary branches.[20,123] Each of these branches gives rise to an anastomosing capillary network which runs toward the urinary pole and then turns back, running toward the vascular pole. Thereby, the glomerular tuft is subdivided into several (2–5) lobules, each of which contains an afferent and efferent capillary portion. The lobules are not strictly separated from each other; some anastomoses between lobules occur. The efferent portions of all lobules together establish the efferent domain of the capillary network out of which the efferent arteriole develops.

In contrast to the afferent arteriole, the efferent arteriole is already established inside the glomerular tuft; thus, the efferent arteriole has a significant intraglomerular segment which runs through the glomerular stalk (Figures 20.30, 20.31 and 20.32).[20] At this site, the efferent arteriole has close spatial relationships to the first branching of the afferent arteriole. After leaving the tuft, the efferent arteriole has a segment which is narrowly associated with the extraglomerular mesangium (see below). The intraglomerular segment is

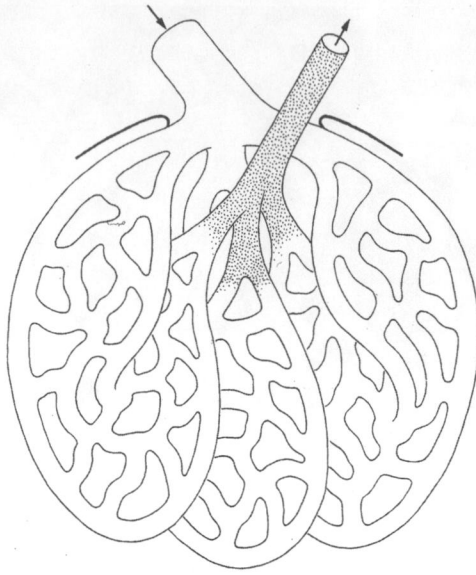

FIGURE 20.30   Schematic to show the branching pattern of the glomerular tuft. Immediately after its entrance into the tuft, the afferent arteriole splits into large superficially located capillaries which are the supplying vessels of glomerular lobules (three are shown). The capillaries run toward the urinary pole. After turning back they unite to establish the efferent arteriole still inside the glomerular tuft. Thus, in contrast to the afferent arteriole, the efferent arteriole has an intraglomerular segment (stippled). An afferent and an efferent capillary domain are distinguished. The efferent capillary domain occupies roughly a quarter sector of the tuft; it is partly covered by the afferent domain. *(From Winkler, D., and Elger, M. et al. (1991). Branching and confluence pattern of glomerular arterioles in the rat. Kidney Int. Suppl 32, S2—8, with permission.)*

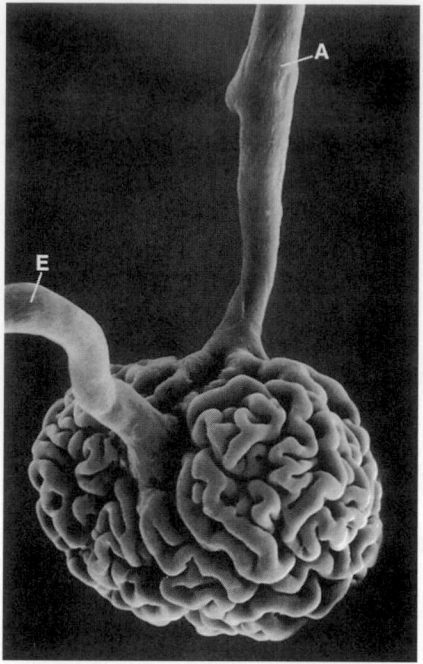

FIGURE 20.31   Scanning electron micrograph of a vascular cast of a dog glomerulus with afferent (A) and efferent (E) arterioles. Note the superficially located branching pattern of the afferent arteriole, out of which the afferent capillary domain is supplied. The efferent arteriole emerges from inside of the glomerular tuft.

made up by a continuous endothelium which is fully separated from the GBM by a "mesangial layer" consisting of mesangial cell processes and matrix. Thus, this initial segment of the EA is fully embedded into the mesangium. Along the course through the extraglomerular mesangium, the mesangial and/or extraglomerular mesangial cells in its wall are gradually replaced by smooth muscle cells.[20] Thereafter, the efferent vessel is established as a proper arteriole.

Glomerular capillaries are a specific type of blood vessel whose wall is made up of an endothelial tube only. A small strip of the outer circumference of this tube is in contact with the mesangium, the major part bulges toward the urinary space and is covered by the GBM, followed by the layer of podocyte foot processes. Taken together, these peripheral portions of the capillary wall represent the filtration area. The small juxtamesangial portion of the capillary wall is not underlain by a basement membrane, but directly abuts the mesangium.[124] The glomerular mesangium constitutes the axis of a glomerular lobule, to which the glomerular capillaries are attached by their juxtamesangial portion. Apart from this attachment site, the mesangium is

bounded by the perimesangial part of the GBM. Like the peripheral GBM, it is covered at its outer aspect by podocyte processes. At the turning points of the GBM the opposing parts of the GBM are interconnected by podocyte processes that are strongly armed with actin filaments.

The Glomerular Basement Membrane (GBM)

The glomerular basement membrane represents the skeletal backbone of the glomerular tuft. Topographically, the GBM consists of a peripheral (pericapillary) and a perimesangial part. At the border between both parts, the GBM changes from a convex pericapillary into a concave perimesangial course; the turning points are called mesangial angles.[124]

During development, the GBM originates from the fusion of an endothelial and a podocytic basement membrane. In the adult, the collagen component of the GBM is solely derived from podocytes, whereas the laminin component originates from both podocytes and endothelial cells.[125] The GBM is a remarkably stable structure; the *in vivo* loss of protein radioactivity suggests a half-life of more than 100 days.[126] Nevertheless, a continuous turnover occurs,[127,128] but few details are known about where and how new

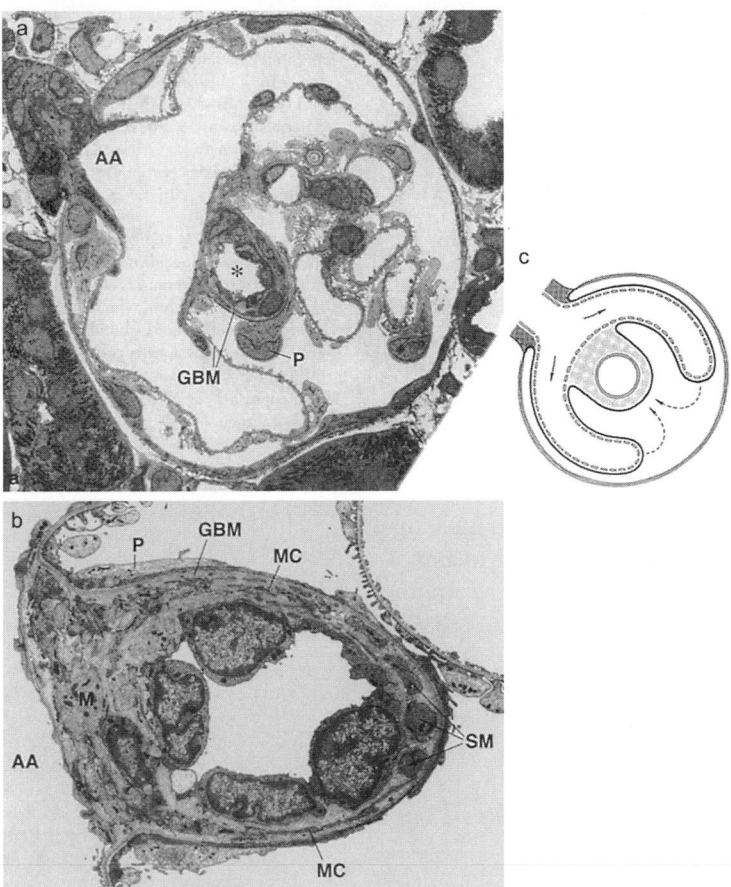

FIGURE 20.32 (a) Narrow association between the afferent arteriole (AA) and the intraglomerular segment of the efferent arteriole (*, EA) as seen in a section approximately 15 μm inside a glomerulus. The afferent arteriole (AA) splits into primary branches. The branching point of the AA has a narrow spatial relationship to the inraglomerular segment of the EA (asterisk), which is located in the center of the tuft. The intraglomerular segment of the EA is enclosed — together with the AA — in a common compartment bordered by the GBM. (b) Higher magnification of the intraglomerular segment in a subsequent section with several conspicuous features: the lumen is narrow; the continuous endothelium consists of four cell bodies that bulge into the lumen; the endothelium is surrounded by a mesangial envelope made up of mesangial cells (MC) and matrix; a few smooth muscle cell processes (*SM*) are interspersed. AA and EA are separated only by mesangial tissue (*M*); there is no basement membrane separating the AA and EA. *P*, cell body of a podocyte attached to the GBM surrounding the EA. (c) Schematic of a cross-section through the glomerular vascular pole, showing the spatial relationships of the AA and EA within the glomerular stalk corresponding to the situation in (a). Immediately after its entry into the glomerulus, the AA splits into wide capillary branches with open endothelial pores. The branching point of the AA has a narrow spatial association with the outflow segment of the EA. The outflow segment is enclosed, together with the AA, in a common compartment bordered by the GBM. The EA is completely surrounded by a layer of mesangial tissue (shown in gray), and is separated from the AA only by this layer; there is no basement membrane between AA and EA. Broken arrows represent blood flow from afferent branches through the capillary network to the outflow segment (TEMs: (a) ×~1500; (b) ×~4300). (*From ref. [20], with permission.*)

components are added, and others removed and degraded. Several extracellular matrix degrading enzymes have been found to be produced by podocytes and mesangial cells[129–131]; however, the relevance of these enzymes to the turnover of the GBM remains to be established.

The GBM varies in width among species. In humans the thickness ranges between 240 and 370 nm, in rat and other experimental animals it is between 110 and 190 nm. In electron micrographs of traditionally fixed tissue the GBM appears as a trilaminar structure made up of a lamina densa bounded by two less dense layers — the lamina rara interna and externa. Recent studies using freeze techniques reveal only one dense layer directly attached to the bases of the epithelium and endothelium.[132]

The major components of the mature GBM include type IV collagen, type II laminin (= laminin 521), heparan sulphate proteoglycans (agrin, perlecan), and the glycoproteins entactin/nidogen[133,134]; type V and VI collagen have also been demonstrated.[135]

The mature GBM is established during the development of a glomerulus from the S-shaped body to the capillary loop stage. During this transition, the collagen

IV α_1 and α_2 chains are replaced by α_3, α_4, and α_5 chains, and the laminin α_1 and β_1 chains are replaced by α_5 and β_2 chains, the γ_1 chain remains preserved, together forming laminin 521.[136,137] The components of the mature GBM are all synthesized by the podocytes. The functional importance of this specific composition of the GBM compared to basement membranes elsewhere in the body becomes evident when looking at their involvement in glomerular diseases: the various forms of Alport syndrome are caused by mutations in the genes encoding the α_3, α_4, and α_5 chains of collagen type IV; Goodpasture syndrome is mediated by antibodies against the α_3 collagen IV chain.[138]

Current models depict the basic structure of the basement membrane as a three-dimensional network of collagen type IV.[139] Monomers of type IV collagen consist of a triple helix of α_3, α_4, and α_5 chains measuring 400 nm in length which, at its carboxy-terminal end, has a large non-collagenous globular domain, called NC1. At the amino-terminus the helix possesses a triple helical rod 60 nm in length, the 7S domain. Interactions between the 7S domains of two triple helices or the NC1 domains of four triple helices allow collagen type IV monomers to form dimers and tetramers. In addition, triple helical strands interconnect by lateral associations via binding of NC1 domains to sites along the collagenous region.

Fibronectin, laminin, and entactin are the glycoproteins of the GBM[140]; the major one is laminin 521. Laminin forms a second network that is superimposed onto the collagenous network. Laminin is a noncollagenous glycoprotein consisting of three polypeptide chains, two of which are glycolylated and cross-linked by disulfide bridges.[137] Laminin, via entactin, binds to specific sites on the polymerized network of type IV collagen, as well as to integrin and dystroglycan surface receptors of the podocytes and endothelial cells (see later). This combined network of type IV collagen and laminin is considered to provide mechanical strength to the basement membrane, and to serve as a scaffold for alignment of other matrix components.

The proteoglycans of the GBM consist of core proteins and covalently bound glycosaminoclycans which are concentrated in the laminae rarae internae and externae. The electronegative charge of the GBM is mainly due to these polyanionic proteoglycans.[141] The major proteoglycans of the GBM are heparan sulfate proteoglycans; most prominent is agrin but perlecan is also present.[142,143] Proteoglycan molecules aggregate to form a meshwork that is kept highly hydrated by water molecules trapped in the interstices of the matrix. Within the GBM heparan sulfate proteoglycans may act as an anticlogging agent to prevent hydrogen bonding and adsorption of anionic plasma proteins and maintain an efficient flow of water through the membrane.

The Cells of the Glomerular Tuft

Within the glomerular tuft three cell types (Figure 20.33) are found which all contact the GBM: (1) mesangial cells; (2) endothelial cells; and (3) podocytes (visceral epithelial cells).

Mesangial cells, together with the mesangial matrix, establish the glomerular mesangium (Figure 20.34). Mesangial cells are quite irregular in shape, with many processes extending from the cell body towards the GBM.[144,145] In these processes (to a lesser extent also in cell bodies) dense assemblies of microfilaments are found which have been shown to contain actin, myosin, and α-actinin.[146]

The processes of mesangial cells run towards the GBM, to which they are attached either directly or mediated by the interposition of microfibrils (see below). The GBM represents the effector structure of mesangial contractility.[124,147] Mesangial-cell-GBM connections are

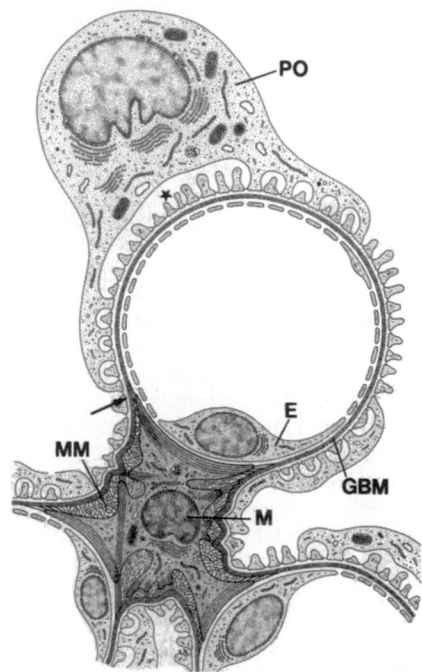

FIGURE 20.33   Schematic to show the arrangement of the structures in the glomerular tuft. Part of a glomerular lobule is shown with three glomerular capillaries (two are only partly shown) attached to a mesangial center. The glomerular capillary is made up of a fenestrated endothelium. The peripheral part of the endothelial tube is surrounded by the GBM which, at the mesangial angles (arrow), deviates from a pericapillary course and covers the mesangium. The interdigitated pattern of the podocyte (PO) foot processes form the external layer of the filtration barrier. Note the subcell body space (star). Podocyte foot processes are also found covering the paramesangial GBM. In the center a mesangial cell (M) is shown. Its many processes contain microfilament bundles and run towards the GBM, to which they are connected. The mesangial matrix (MM) contains an interwoven network of microfilaments. *(From Venkatachalam, M. A., and Kriz, W. (1992). In "Anatomy of the Kidney. Pathology of the Kidney," 1–92, Heptinstall, R. Little, Brown and Company, Boston, with permission.)*

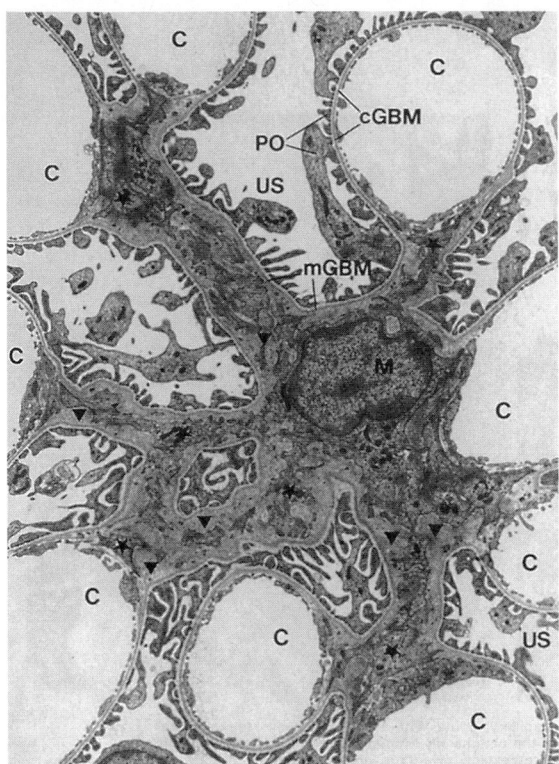

FIGURE 20.34 Section through a glomerular lobule (rat). The relationships of glomerular capillaries to the mesangium in the lobule center are seen. Glomerular capillaries (C) and the glomerular mesangium occupy a common compartment enclosed by the glomerular basement membrane (GBM). The mesangial cell body (M) gives rise to several processes (some are marked by stars) which extend toward the peripherally located capillaries. Note the abundant mesangial matrix (triangles). The layer of podocytes (PO) covers the outer aspect of the GBM. Thus, neither the GBM, nor the podocyte layer encircle the capillaries completely; both together form a common surface cover around the entire lobule. Therefore, two subdomains of the GBM (as well as of the podocyte layer) can be delineated: the pericapillary (peripheral) GBM (cGBM; faced by podocytes and the endothelium); and the perimesangial GBM (mGBM) bordered by podocytes and the mesangium. The peripheral part of the capillary wall establishes the filtration barrier. Note the mesangial cell body (M) giving rise to many cell processes (some are marked by stars) which are embedded in the mesangial matrix (triangles) (US: Urinary space; TEM: $\times \sim 5500$).

especially prominent alongside the capillaries. At these sites mesangial cell processes (densely stuffed with microfilament bundles) extend underneath the capillary endothelium towards the mesangial angles of the GBM where they are anchored. Generally, these processes interconnect the GBM from two opposing mesangial angles (Figure 20.35b). Functionally, the microfilament bundles bridge the entire distance between both mesangial angles. In the axial mesangial region as well, numerous microfilament bundles extending through mesangial cell bodies and processes bridge opposing parts of the GBM. The connection of mesangial cell processes to the GBM is mediated by the integrin $\alpha3\beta1$ and the Lutheran glycoprotein, which both adhere to the laminin $\alpha5$ chain.[148]

The mesangial matrix fills the highly irregular spaces between the mesangial cells and the perimesangial GBM (for review see [147,149]). A large number of common extracellular matrix proteins have been demonstrated within the mesangial matrix, including several types of collagen (III, IV, V, and VI), heparin sulfate proteoglycans (including the small proteoglycans biglycan and decorin),[150] fibronectin, laminin, and entactin, as well as fibrillin 1 and other specific elastic fiber proteins.[140,151–153] Among these components, fibronectin is the most abundant, and has been shown to be associated with microfibrils.[151,154]

The basic ultrastructural organization of the matrix is a network of microfibrils. In specimens prepared for TEM by routine methods a fine filamentous network is seen, which possibly corresponds to collagenous filaments. In specimens prepared by a technique that avoids osmium tetroxide and uses tannic acid for staining, the mesangial matrix is seen to contain abundant elastic microfibrils.[124,155] Microfibrils are unbranched, noncollagenous tubular structures that have an indefinite length and are about 15 nm in diameter. They form a dense three-dimensional network establishing a functionally continuous medium anchoring the mesangial cells to the GBM.[147,153] Distinct bundles of microfibrils may be regarded as "microtendons" that allow the transmission of contractile force of mesangial cells to specific sites of the GBM, predominantly to the mesangial angles.[124,155] α-8 integrin serves as a specific matrix receptor in the mesangium.[156]

Glomerular endothelial cells (Figures 20.33, 20.34 and 20.35) are large flat cells consisting of a cell body (which contains all the usual cell organelles) and densely perforated peripheral parts. These regions are extremely attenuated and characterized by round to oval pores varying in diameter between 50 and 100 nm. Unlike fenestrae (unfortunately, these pores are frequently also called "fenestrae"), the pores of glomerular endothelial cells lack a diaphragm, they are virtually open[26]; (Figures 20.36b and 20.37b). Fenestrae bridged by diaphragms in glomerular capillaries are only found along the intraglomerular segment of the efferent arteriole and its tributaries.[20] In rat, about 60% of the capillary surface is covered by the porous regions; the total area of pores occupies about 13% of the capillary surface.[157] Micropinocytotic vesicles are very rare in glomerular endothelial cells, corroborating the fact that the open pores make transcytotic processes unnecessary.

Glomerular endothelial cells contain the usual inventory of cytoplasmic organelles, generally located within the cell body cytoplasm. The endothelial skeleton comprises intermediate filaments and microtubules; individual pores are lined by clusters of microfilaments.[158]

The luminal membrane of endothelial cells is highly negatively charged, due to a cell coat that also fills the

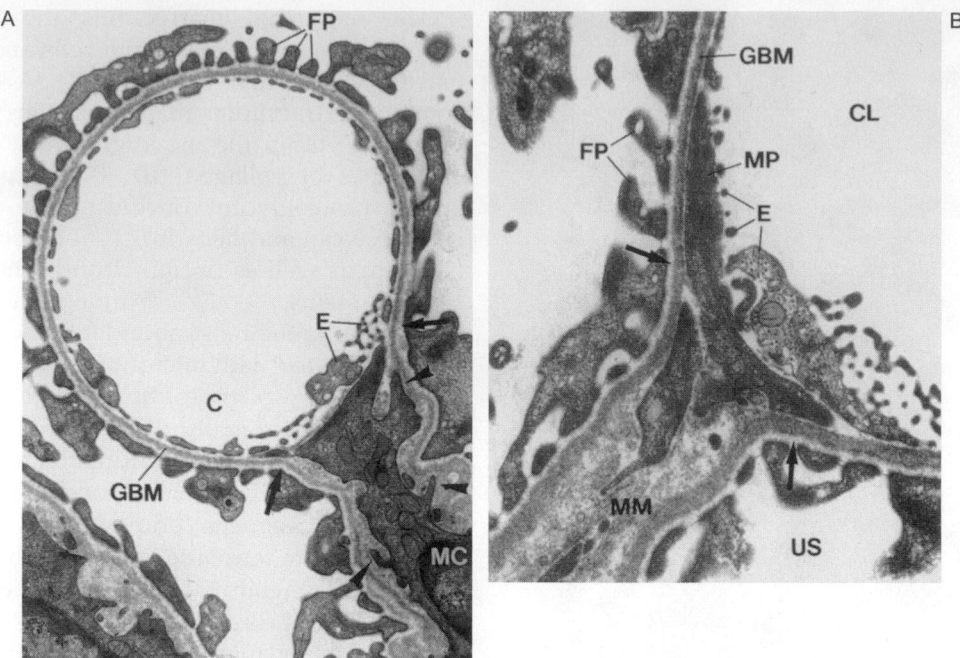

FIGURE 20.35 **(a) Overview of a glomerular capillary (mouse).** Within the mesangium, a mesangial cell (MC) is seen whose processes extend toward the peripherally located capillary (C). Microprojections (arrowheads) originating from the primary process extend toward the GBM. Note that the GBM (as well as the podocyte layer) deviates from its pericapillary course at the two mesangial angles (marked by arrows), continuing as a cover of the mesangium. Thus, the juxtamesangial part of the glomerular capillary lacks a basement membrane; at this site the endothelium is directly exposed to the mesangium. The capillary endothelium is thin and fenestrated. The podocyte layer consists of interdigitating foot processes (FP) which abut the GBM on its outside surface (TEM: × ∼13,500). **(b) Capillary–mesangium interface (rat).** At this site a basement membrane is not developed. Beneath the endothelium, tongue-like mesangial cell processes (MP) are found which run toward both opposing mesangial angles. They contain microfilament bundles, which obviously interconnect the GBM of both mesangial angles (marked by arrows) (CL: capillary lumen; US: urinary space; MM: mesangial matrix; FP: foot processes; TEM: × ∼23,000).

pores like "sieve plugs".[159] It consists of several polyanionic glycoproteins including a sialoprotein called podocalyxin, which is considered as the major surface polyanion of glomerular endothelial as well as epithelial cells.[160] Endothelial cells are active participants in the processes controlling coagulation, inflammation and immune processes. Glomerular endothelial cells synthesize and release endothelin-1, endothelium-derived relaxing factor (EDRF),[161] and PDGF B.[162] Glomerular endothelial cells have receptors for VEGF A and angiopoetin that are produced by podocytes.[163,164] The continuous stimulation of glomerular endothelial cells by podocyte-derived VEGF A has major relevance for the maintenance of glomerular capillaries and the formation of pores instead of fenestrae.[165]

Within the conspicuously narrow portion of the efferent arteriole (outflow segment) the endothelial cells are arranged in an eye-catching pattern: their cell bodies bulge into the lumen being longitudinally stretched, suggesting a specific shear stress receptor of glomerular capillaries.[20,166]

Mature podocytes are highly-differentiated cells. In the developing glomerulus at the S-shaped body stage, podocytes are a simple polygonal shape connected by

apical tight junctions. At the transition to the capillary loop stage the mitotic activity of the cells is completed, the interdigitating foot process pattern with basally located slit membranes instead of apical tight junctions is established, and the final number of podocytes is determined. In rat this point is reached soon after birth, in man it is established during prenatal life. Differentiated podocytes are unavailable for regenerative cell replication[167]; thus in the adult, lost podocytes cannot be replaced by division of the remaining cells. The only way to replace the function of lost podocytes is the hypertrophy of the remaining podocytes.

Podocytes have a voluminous smooth surfaced cell body (Figures 20.36a and 20.37a), which floats within the urinary space; it appears to adapt in shape to the surrounding flow conditions created by the filtrate. The cells give rise to long primary processes (frequently branching another time) that extend towards the capillaries, finally splitting apart into terminal processes, called foot processes, which affix to the GBM (Figures 20.36 and 20.37a). The foot processes of neighbouring podocytes regularly interdigitate with each other, leaving meandering slits (filtration slits) between them, which are bridged by an extracellular structure,

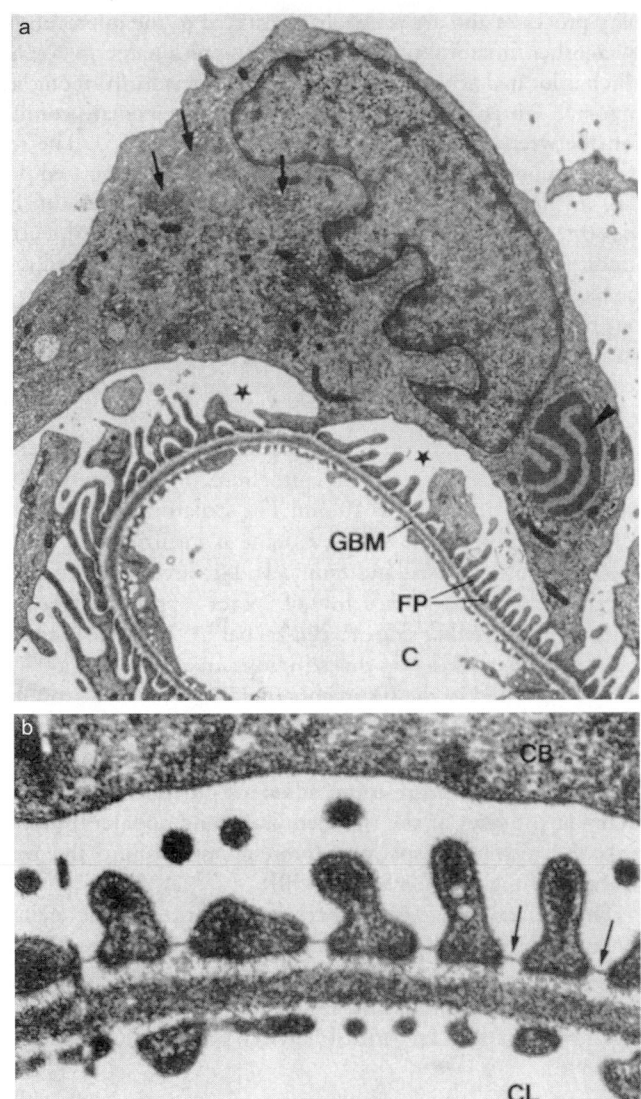

FIGURE 20.36 **(a) Podocyte (rat)**. The cell body contains a large nucleus with indentations. The cytoplasm contains a well-developed Golgi apparatus (arrows), and a conspicuous lamellated inclusion body (arrowhead). The cell processes run toward the GBM forming the inter-digitating pattern of foot processes (FP) there. Note the subcellbody space (stars) (C: capillary; TEM: × ~7600). **(b) Filtration barrier (rat)**. The peripheral part of the glomerular capillary wall comprises three layers: the endothelium with large open pores; the basement membrane (GBM); and the layer of interdigitating podocyte foot processes. The GBM consists of a lamina densa, a lamina rara interna toward the endothelium, and a lamina rara externa toward the epithelium. Note the slit diaphrams bridging the floor of the filtrations slits (arrows) (CL: capillary lumen; CB: cell body of a podocyte; TEM: × ~57,000).

the so-called slit diaphragm. Podocytes are polarized epithelial cells with a luminal and a basal cell membrane domain; the latter corresponds to the sole plates of the foot processes which are embedded into the GBM to a depth of 40 to 60 nm. The border between basal and luminal membrane is represented by the insertion of the slit diaphragm.[167]

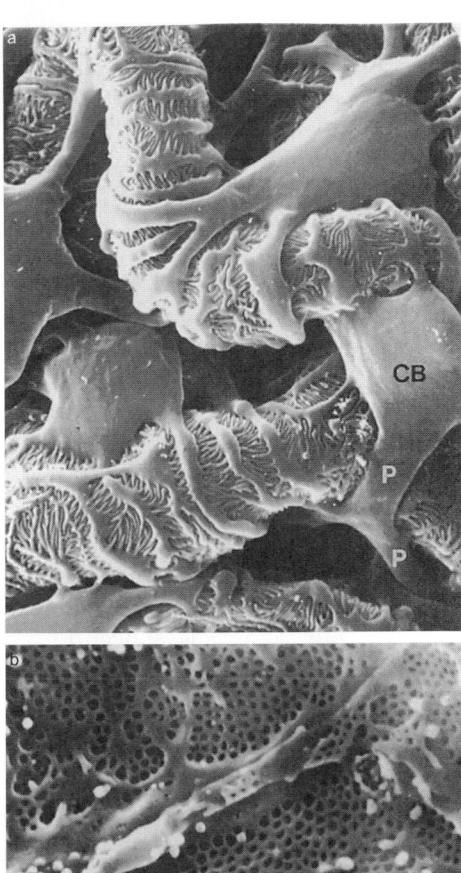

FIGURE 20.37 **(a) Outer surface of glomerular capillaries (rat)**. Processes (P) of podocytes run from the cellbody (CB) toward the capillaries where they ultimately split into foot processes. By inter-digitation, foot processes from neighbouring cells create the filtration slits (SEM: × ~3400). **(b) Inner surface of a glomerular capillary (rat)**. The open fenestrations (not bridged by a diaphragm) are shown (SEM: × ~16,000).

The cell body contains a prominent nucleus, a well-developed Golgi system (Figure 20.36a), abundant rough and smooth endoplasmic reticulum, prominent lysosomes (including abundant multivesicular bodies), and many mitochondria. In contrast to the cell body, the cell processes contain only a few organelles (except from multivesicular bodies). The density of organelles in the cell body indicates a high level of anabolic, as well as catabolic, activity. In addition to the work necessary to sustain the structural integrity of these specialized cells, all components of the GBM are synthesized by podocytes.[133,143]

A well-developed cytoskeleton accounts for the complex shape of the cells. In the cell body and the primary processes, microtubules and intermediate filaments (vimentin, desmin) dominate, whereas microfilaments are densely accumulated in the foot processes. In addition, in the cell body and the primary processes, microfilaments are seen as a thin layer underlying the cell membrane.[168,169]

The prominent bundles of microtubules in the large processes are associated with microtubule-associated proteins, including MAP3/MAP4 and tau.[170] Moreover, like in neuronal dendrites, the microtubules of the podocyte foot processes are non-uniformly arranged with peripheral plus- and minus-end microtubules associated with the specific protein CHO1/MKLP1.[171] In addition, the large processes contain the intermediate type filament protein vimentin.[168]

In the foot processes a complete microfilament-based contractile apparatus is present. The microfilaments form loop-shaped bundles, with their limbs running in the longitudinal axis of the foot processes. The bends of these loops are located centrally at the transition to the primary processes, and are probably connected to the microtubules by "tau" which is concentrated at those sites.[172] Tau is known from other places to mediate connections between microtubules and microfilaments.[173] The microfilament bundles contain actin, myosin II,

α-actinin, and synaptopodin[168,174,175]; synaptopodin, a novel podocyte-specific actin-associated protein interacts with α-actinin inducing the formation of long unbranched parallel bundles of microfilaments.[176] Peripherally, the actin bundles anchor in the dense cytoplasm associated with the basal cell membrane of podocytes, i.e., the sole plates of foot processes.[167]

Anchoring of the sole plates to the GBM is achieved by specific transmembrane receptors; two systems are so far known (Figure 20.38). First, a specific integrin heterodimer, consisting of $\alpha_3\beta_1$ integrins, which bind within the GBM to collagen type IV, fibronectin, and laminin 521.[177–179] Second, a dystroglycan complex connects the intracellular molecule utrophin to laminin 521, agrin, and perlecan in the GBM.[180,181] Both integrins and dystroglycans are coupled via adapter molecules (paxillin, vinculin, α-actinin) to the podocyte cytoskeleton, allowing outside-in and inside-out signaling, as well as transmission of mechanical force in both directions. A major role in this issue is played by the integrin-linked kinase.[182]

A huge body of data has been accumulated in recent years concerning the inventory of receptors and signaling processes starting from podocytes. cGMP signaling

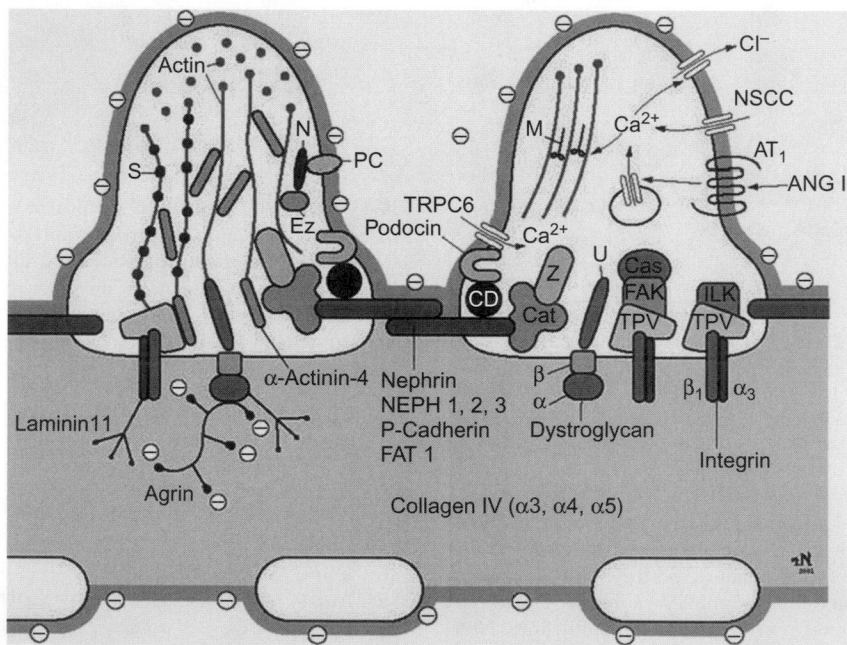

FIGURE 20.38 Glomerular filtration barrier. (*Modified from Endlich, K. H., Kriz, W., and Witzgall, R. (2001). Update in podocyte biology. Curr. Opin. Nephrol. Hypertens. 10, 331–340.*) Two podocyte foot processes bridged by the slit membrane, the GBM, and the porous capillary endothelium are shown. The surfaces of podocytes and of the endothelium are covered by a negatively-charged glycocalyx containing the sialoprotein podocalyxin (PC). The GBM is mainly composed of collagen IV (α_3, α_4, and α_5), of laminin 11 (α_5, β_2, and γ_1 chains) and the heparan sulphate proteoglycan agrin. The slit membrane represents a porous proteinaceous membrane composed of (as far as is known) Nephrin, Neph1, 2, and 3, P-cadherin, and FAT1. The actin-based cytoskeleton of the foot processes connects to both the GBM and the slit membrane. With regard to the GBM, β_1/α_3 integrin dimers specifically interconnect the TVP complex (talin, paxillin, vinculin) to laminin 11; the β and α dystroglycans interconnect utrophin to agrin. The slit membrane proteins are joined to the cytoskeleton via various adaptor proteins, including Podocin, Zonula occludens protein 1 (ZO-1; Z), CD2-associated protein (CD), and catenins (Cat). TRPC6 associates with podocin (and nephrin; not shown) at the slit membrane. Among the many surface receptors only the angiotensin II (ANG II) type 1 receptor (AT1) is shown (Additional abbreviations: Cas: P130Cas; Ez: ezrin; FAK: focal adhesion kinase; ILK: integrin-linked kinase; M: myosin; N: NHERF2 (Na$^+$-H$^+$ exchanger regulatory factor); NSCC: Non-selelctive cation channel; S: Synaptopodin).

(stimulated by ANP, BNP, and CNP, as well as by NO), cAMP signaling (stimulated by prostaglandin E_2, dopamine, isoproterenol, PTH/PTHrP), and Ca^{2+} signaling (stimulated by a huge number of ligands including angiotensin II, acetylcholine, PGF_2, AVP, ATP, endothelin, histamine) have been identified. Among the cation channels, TRPC6, a nonselective Ca^{2+} channel, has recently received attention, since mutations in the respective gene lead to hereditary FSGS.[183,184] The major target of this signaling orchestra is the cytoskeleton, the concrete effects, however, are poorly-understood. Other receptors, such as for C3b,[185] TGFß,[186,187] FGF2,[188] and various other cytokines and chemokines have been shown to be involved in the development of podocyte diseases (for details see [189]). Megalin, a multi-ligand endocytotic receptor, is associated with coated bits[190–192]; it represents the major antigen of rat Heymann nephritis.[193]

The filtration slits are the site of convective fluid flow through the visceral epithelium. They have a width of 30 to 40 nm and are bridged by the slit membrane. The structure and molecular composition of this proteinaceous membrane is insufficiently understood. Chemically fixed and tannic acid treated tissue reveals a zipper-like structure with a row of "pores" approximately 4×14 nm on either side of a central bar.[194] According to its dimension and its components (as far as is known) the slit diaphragm may be considered as a specific adherens-like intercellular junction. Intensive research in recent years has uncovered several transmembrane proteins that participate in the formation of the slit membrane, including nephrin,[195] Neph1,[196] P-cadherin,[197] and FAT[198] (Figure 20.38). Other molecules, such as ZO1,[199] Podocin,[200] CD2AP,[201] and catenins mediate the connection to the actin cytoskeleton (see below). Nephrin is a member of the immunoglobin superfamily (IgCAM); its gene NPHS1 has been identified as the gene whose mutations cause congenital nephritic syndrome of the Finnish type.[195] In addition to its role as a structural component, nephrin acts as a signaling molecule that can activate MAP kinase cascades.[202] Neph1 is considered as a ligand for nephrin. Podocin belongs to the raft associated stomatin family, whose gene NPHS2 is mutated in a subgroup of patients with autosomol-recessive stereoid-resistent nephrotic syndrome.[200] These patients show disease onset in early childhood and rapid progression to end-stage renal failure. Podocin interacts with nephrin and CD2AP.[203] FAT is a novel member of the cadherin superfamily, with 34 tandem cadherin-like extracellular repeats and a molecular weight of 516 kDa.[204] Because FAT has a huge extracellular domain, it is speculated that it dominates the molecular structure of the slit membrane[198]; the FAT mutant mouse fails to develop a slit membrane.[205] P-cadherin[197] is thought to mediate the linkage to ß- and γ-catenin with its intracellular domain, a complex which then connects to the actin cytoskeleton via α-catenin and α-actinin. Taken together, many components of the slit membrane are known, but an integrative model of its substructure including all components is so far lacking.

The luminal membrane and the slit diaphragm are covered by a thick surface coat which is rich in sialoglycoproteins (including podocalyxin, podoendin, and others) that are responsible for the high negative surface charge of the podocytes.[206,207] Podocalyxin is anchored to the actin cytoskeleton beneath the cell membrane via the linker protein NHERF 2 (Na^+/H^+ exchanger regulatory factor 2) and ezrin.[208,209] The surface charge of podocytes contributes to the maintenance of the interdigitating pattern of the foot processes. In response to neutralization of the surface charge by cationic substances (e.g., protamine sulfate), the foot processes retract, resulting in what is called "foot process effacement".[210]

Filtration Barrier

The walls of glomerular capillaries represent a specific barrier which is very permeable to water, and yet able to prevent all but very minute losses of serum albumin and other major plasma proteins from the circulation. The glomerular capillary wall consists of three distinct layers (Figures 20.36b and 20.37). Starting at the capillary lumen, there is the porous endothelium, followed by the GBM, and the layer of interdigitating foot processes with the filtration slits in between.

The high hydraulic permeability of this barrier suggests that the filtrate pathway is entirely extracellular, passing through the endothelial fenestrae, across the GBM, and through the slit diaphragms of the filtration slits. According to a calculation by Drumond and Deen,[211] the hydraulic resistance of the endothelium is negligible. The GBM and the filtration slits each make up roughly one half of the total hydraulic resistance of the filtration barrier.

Charge, size, and shape determine the specific permeability of a macromolecule. It is now generally accepted that the charge barrier plays an important part in preventing polyanionic macromolecules such as albumin from passing through the glomerular filter. All components of the glomerular filter are heavily laden with negative charges.[212] Recent investigation[213,214] suggests that the negative residues of the endothelium play the major role in establishing a negative charge field which considerably decreases the entry of polyanionic macromolecules, i.e., albumin, into the filter.

With regard to the size selectivity, direct experimental findings,[211,215,216] as well as recent findings about the molecular composition of the slit membrane (see above) and the consequences of genetic mutations in these components, suggest that it is for the major part the slit membrane which is responsible for the size selectivity; it appears to be the main barrier for uncharged large molecules.

There is another major unresolved problem in glomerular physiology, namely the regulation of the ultrafiltration coefficient Kf. Kf is the product of the local hydraulic permeability and the filtration area. There has been a widespread belief that Kf is regulated through changes in the filtration area due to an action of the mesangium.[217] However, the structural arrangement of the mesangium,[124] as well as several morphometric studies,[218,219] do not support such an assumption. Dimensional changes in just the slit membrane area have also been regarded as a reasonable and, theoretically, very effective site to change Kf.[220] In pathological conditions, e.g., in membranous nephropathy,[221] the decrease in Kf correlates perfectly with the decrease in total slit length. With respect to acute regulatory mechanisms under physiological conditions, however, no convincing morphometric data have been published showing that changes in Kf are correlated with corresponding dimensional changes in the slit membrane. Thus, the question of where and how Kf is regulated remains an open problem.

Stability of the Glomerular Tuft

The glomerular tuft is constantly exposed to comparably high intraglomerular pressures within glomerular capillaries and mesangium. The high intraglomerular pressures challenge not only the glomerular capillaries themselves, but also the folding pattern of the glomerular tuft. Increased pressures lead to loss of the folding pattern, and to dilation of the glomerular capillaries. Therefore, we have to ask what are the specific structures and mechanisms that counteract the expansile forces in the glomerular tuft. To answer this question we have to distinguish between the structures and mechanisms maintaining: (1) the folding pattern of the glomerular tuft; and those maintaining (2) the width of glomerular capillaries (Figure 20.39).

The folding pattern of the glomerular tuft is primarily sustained by the mesangium.[124,147,222] Mesangial cells are connected to the GBM by their contractile processes (see above); by centripetal contractions they maintain the infoldings of the GBM, thereby allowing the capillaries to arrange in the peripheral expansion of the GBM. This supporting role of mesangial cells is best illustrated under circumstances with loss of mesangial cells, such as Thy-1 nephritis.[223] Under those circumstances the folding pattern of the GBM is progressively lost, finally resulting in mesangial aneurysms. Podocytes clearly contribute to the maintenance of the folding pattern by specific cell processes that interconnect opposing parts of the GBM from outside within the niches of the infoldings. This function is again clearly illustrated in Thy-1 nephritis under circumstances with loss of mesangial support: podocytes are capable of maintaining a high degree of the GBM folding pattern for 2—4 days, after which they fail and mesangial aneurysms become prominent.[223]

The width of glomerular capillaries, in the long run, is probably controlled by growth processes accounting for different-sized capillaries. The width of a given capillary, in an acute situation being exposed to changes in blood pressure, appears to be stabilized by the GBM which is a strong elastic structure[224] and, together with the mesangial cell bridges (see above), is capable of developing wall tension.[147,225] In addition, the tensile strength of the GBM is reinforced by podocytes. Podocytes are a kind of pericyte; their foot processes represent a unique type of pericyte process which, like elsewhere in the body, counteract the dilation of the vessel. Podocyte processes are firmly attached to the underlying GBM (see above); their cytoskeletal tonus counteracts the elastic extension of the GBM. Podocytes cannot be replaced by any other cell; failure in this function will lead to capillary dilation.

Parietal Epithelium of Bowman's Capsule

The parietal layer of Bowman's capsule consists of squamous epithelial cells resting on a basement

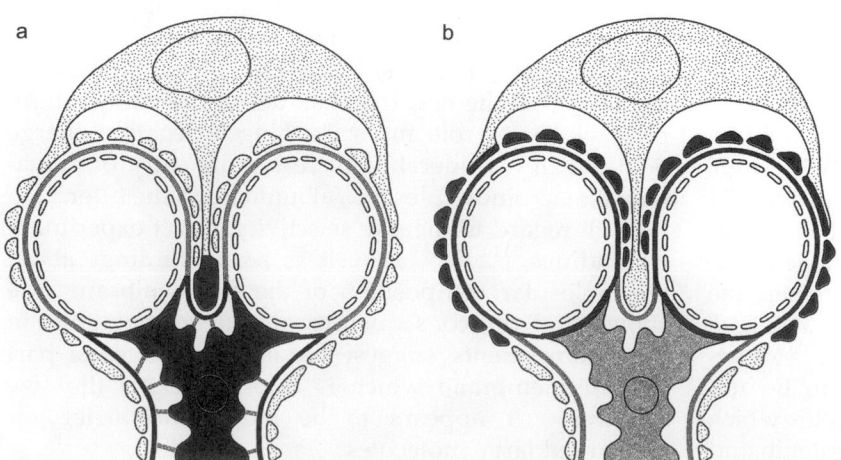

FIGURE 20.39 Schematic to show the mechanisms that stabilize the glomerular tuft against expansion (relevant structures are highlighted in dark gray). The folding pattern of the GBM is thus stained by mesangial cells from inside, and by specific podocyte processes located in the depth between two capillaries from outside. The width of capillaries against transmural pressure gradients is maintained by wall tension, which is generated by the rigidity of the GBM, by the mesangial cell processes that interconnect opposing turning points of the GBM, and by the tonus of podocyte foot processes.

membrane (Figure 20.29). The cells are of polygonal shape and contain prominent bundles of actin filaments running in all directions. Microfilament bundles are especially prominent in the parietal cells surrounding the vascular pole, where they are located within cytoplasmic ridges that run in a circular fashion around the glomerular entrance.[20]

The basement membrane of the parietal epithelium (PBM) is, at variance with the GBM, composed of several dense layers which are separated by translucent layers and contain bundles of fibrils.[226] Recent studies suggest a role of type XIV collagen in the organization of the multilayered PBM.[227] In contrast to the GBM, the predominant proteoglycan of the PBM is a chondroitin sulfate proteoglycan.[149] The transition from the GBM to the PBM borders the glomerular entrance. This transitional region is mechanically connected to the smooth muscle cells of the afferent and efferent arterioles as well as to extraglomerular mesangial cells.

At the urinary pole, the flat parietal cells transform into proximal tubule cells. In some cases the flat cells may continue for a certain distance as a so-called neck segment of the tubule (rabbit)[228] or the typical proximal tubule epithelium generally starts within the glomerular capsule. This is the case in the mouse,[824] most pronounced in males.

In rare cases, parietal epithelial cells may be replaced by podocytes ("parietal podocytes") which display a process pattern identical to that of podocyte proper of the tuft.[229] At such sites, the PBM is similar to the GBM and capillaries may attach from outside. As shown recently, parietal podocytes are regularly found when ß-catenin is deleted in renal epithelial cells during development at the S-shaped body stage.[230] Recent observations suggest that a niche of glomerular epithelial stem cells resides within the parietal epithelium at the transition to the proximal tubule.[231,232]

It is an intriguing hypothesis that proliferating stem cells from this locus may transform into podocytes and may reach the tuft via the transitions of the epithelia at the glomerular vascular pole. Migration of parietal cells via the vascular pole and subsequent transition into podocytes has been shown to occur in the new-born mouse.[233] However, evidence that such a process may be of any relevance in the adult has so far not been presented.[233]

STRUCTURAL ORGANIZATION OF RENAL ELECTROLYTE TRANSPORTING EPITHELIA

General Overview of Renal Epithelial Organization

The renal tubular epithelia function as selective barriers between the tubular fluid in the luminal compartment and the interstitial compartment that communicates with the blood compartment. The epithelium consists of a single layer of cells, resting on a basement membrane composed of extracellular matrix. The cells are interconnected by *junctional complexes* that encircle each individual cell like a belt. The *tight junction* (zonula occludens) separates the luminal compartment from the lateral intercellular space and is the boundary between the apical plasma membrane domain, facing the tubular fluid, and the basolateral membrane domain, which lines the intercellular compartments and is in contact with the basement membrane. The *intermediate junctions* (zonula adherens), and the patches of *desmosomes* (maculae adherentes) provide mechanical adherence. Gap junctions that provide intercellular communication exist exclusively in the proximal tubule.

This basic organization of the epithelium (Figure 20.40) implies two *transepithelial transport pathways* for solutes and macromolecules: (1) the paracellular pathway across the tight junctions and the lateral intercellular spaces (the passage of solutes through the paracellular pathway is driven by the transepithelial electrochemical and oncotic gradients); (2) the transcellular pathway across the luminal membrane domain, the cellular cytoplasm and the basolateral membrane domain, and *vice versa* (the passage of solutes via the transcellular pathway occurs mostly against electrochemical gradients and is energy-dependent).

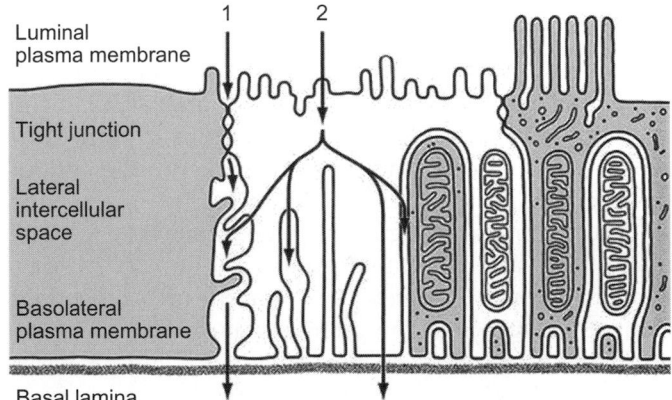

Luminal plasma membrane

Tight junction

Lateral intercellular space

Basolateral plasma membrane

Basal lamina

FIGURE 20.40 **Schematic drawing, demonstrating the essential structural features of renal transporting epithelia.** (1) Paracellular route through the tight junction and the lateral intercellular spaces; (2) Transcellular route, across the apical plasma membrane, which may be augmented by short microvilli, microfolds (not shown) or long microvilli of uniform length, called " brush border," across the cytoplasm, and across the basolateral plasma membrane; the latter may be augmented by infoldings of the basal plasma membrane or by basolateral processes of the cells, which narrowly interdigitate with each other. The lateral interdigitating processes contain large mitochondria.

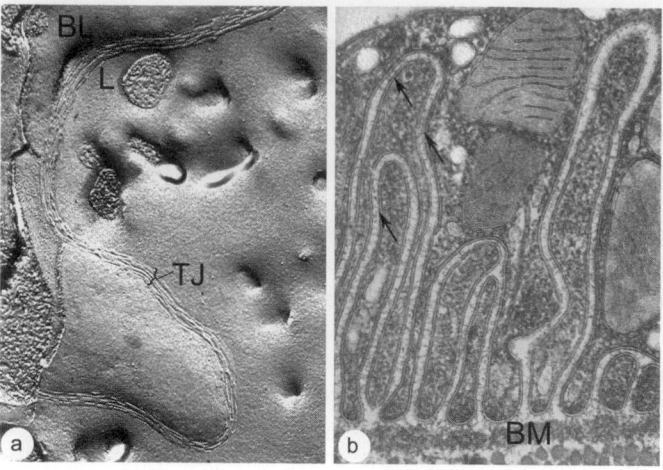

FIGURE 20.41 Tight junction and intercellular space. (a) Freeze-fracture electron micrograph of thick ascending limb cells. (b) The tight junction (TJ) consists of several densely arranged parallel strands (BL: basolateral membrane; L: luminal membrane; Rabbit: ×~45,000). (Cooperation with A.Schiller and R.Taugner).

Paracellular Pathway

As seen in freeze-fracture replicas, tight junctions are composed of globular particles, arranged in one or several roughly parallel strands or in a net-like pattern[234] (Figure 20.41a). The more-or-less densely packed particles in the strands presumably represent the transmembrane proteins that participate in the junction's formation.

The tight junctions function as barriers between the luminal compartment and the lateral intercellular spaces. At the same time they allow a selective, regulated paracellular flow of small inorganic cations,[235,236] and the passage of some large organic cations and of some uncharged molecules.[234,237] The selectivity of tight junctions for different solutes varies among the different tubular epithelia.[238,239] Claudins, a large family of integral membrane proteins, make up the bulk of tight junctional strands,[240–243] and play a key role in determining and regulating the paracellular permeability for small inorganic cations.[244] They act as size-, charge-, ion concentration- and pH-dependent channels or pores in the intercellular space,[245–247] and seem to be targets of the serine-threonine kinases WNK1 and WNK4.[248–251] The dynamic regulation of paracellular flux does not seem to involve structural changes of the tight junctional complexes. Mutations in claudin members[252,253] or defects in the WNK-signaling cascades may have major implications on volume homeostasis.[250,251,254–257] Occludin, another integral membrane protein, is interspersed with claudins in the tight junctional strands. The cytoplasmic domain of occludin is associated with ZO1, thereby providing a linkage for the membrane to its scaffolding actin cytoskeleton.[234,244] The interaction of occludins with the actin skeleton may be important in regulating the paracellular passage for larger molecules, and for "macropermeation" across the epithelium, as well as in the transduction of signals from apoptotic cells.[258] Further, ZO1 seems to be associated with the "fence" function of tight junctions,[258] i.e., the ability of the tight junction to prevent diffusion of lipids from the apical to the basolateral membrane domain. Via transcription factor zonula occludens 1 (ZO-1)-associated nucleic acid binding protein (ZONAB), it can also be involved in controlling cell proliferation.[259]

Cell adhesion proteins at the extracellular face of the basolateral surface of renal tubular cells maintain a basal level of cell–cell adhesion, in addition to strong cellular adhesion provided by the junctional complexes and/or desmosomes. The cell adhesion proteins in the intercellular spaces can be made visible by electron-microscopy with specific fixation procedures.[260] The "classical" cell adhesion proteins N- and E-cadherin,[261–264] as well as the "atypical" kidney-specific (ksp) cadherin 16[265,266] have been located by immunostainings on the basolateral membranes all along the tubular system. The classical cell adhesion molecules are linked to the scaffolding actin skeleton, as well as to β-catenin, at the cytoplasmic face of the basolateral cell membranes.[267] This connection provides a pathway for coupling extracellular signals (among others, binding of a hormone to its receptor, mechanical stresses) to intracellular signaling cascades that control various cellular responses, such as endocytosis, ubiquitination of proteins, transcription, proliferation or apotosis.[267]

Transcellular Pathway

The prerequisite for transcellular vectorial transport of solutes across epithelia is the asymmetric or polarized allocation of co-transporters, exchangers, channels, and enzymes, to the luminal and basolateral plasma membrane

LUMINAL MEMBRANE DOMAIN

The uptake of most solutes into the cell is coupled to passage of sodium via solute-specific co-transporters, via channels or via exchange against protons (H^+) in the luminal plasma membrane. The given assembly of transport proteins in the luminal membrane of the cells of a segment determines the segment-specific solute transport pattern. Enzymes (e.g., phosphatases, peptidases) in the luminal membrane hydrolyze poorly permeable organic compounds to readily permeable ones, and various receptor proteins (e.g., megalin, cubilin etc.[268]) mediate the uptake of their ligands into the cell.

Many of the apical transport proteins are linked to the actin-based cytoskeleton under the plasma

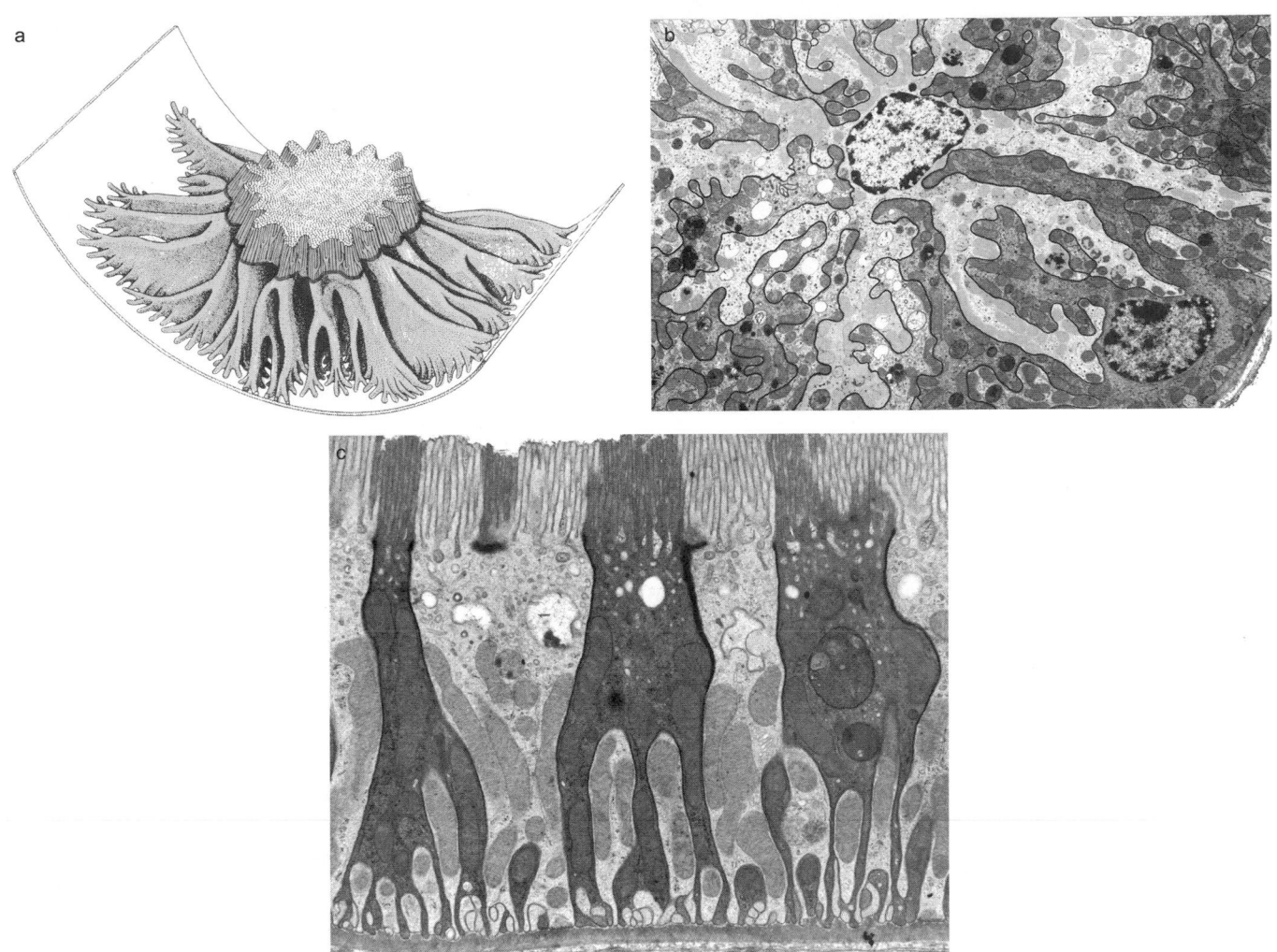

FIGURE 20.42 Augmentation of apical and basolateral plasma membrane surfaces by microvilli and interdigitating lateral cell processes. (a) Three-dimensional model of a rabbit proximal tubule cell. *(From Welling, L. W., and Welling, D. J. (1975). Surface areas of brush border and lateral cell walls in the rabbit proximal nephron. Kidney Int. 8(6), 343–348 ,with permission.)* The dark line indicates the position of the tight junctional belt between the apical and basolateral membrane domains; the apical membrane domain is amplified by microvilli, which form a brush border; the basolateral membrane domain is augmented by interdigitating lateral cell processes that split in an apico–basal direction to primary and secondary processes and basal plicae; the latter are anchored in the basement membrane. (b) and (c): Sections through S1 proximal tubule (*Psammomys obesus*); the dark contrast of the intercellular spaces (black lines), and the differential contrast of adjacent cells result from fixation with reduced osmium; (b) the section, cut approximately in parallel to the basement membrane through the center of the cell reveals the complex interdigitation of the lateral cell processes; (c) in the section in an apico–basal direction apical interdigitation by lateral processes is revealed by the different contrast in the brush border; the lateral interdigitating processes increasingly split up towards the cell base; the larger ones are filled out with mitochondria (TEM: × ~9000).

membrane via adaptor proteins containing PDZ interactive domains,[269–273] namely NHERF1, 2, 3, and are thereby maintained in the specific cell membrane areas.[274]

The given assembly of transport proteins in the apical plasma membrane of a segment confers the *specificity* for transported solutes. The *rate* of solute permeation across the membrane critically depends on type (co-transporter, exchanger, channels) and *quantity of active transport systems* in the apical cell membrane domain. The latter is ultimately related to the available *surface area*. Thus, in many epithelia with high transport rates the apical membrane area is much larger than the area of a virtual plane at the level of the tight junctional belt.

Three modes of amplification of apical plasma membrane surface are distinguished (Figure 20.40): (1) densely arranged finger-like microvilli, all of similar dimensions, evenly distributed over the entire cell surface, forming the so-called "brush border" (Figures 20.42 and 20.44). The microvilli have an axial cytoskeleton of actin filaments, arranged in a 6 + 1 pattern, associated with villin and fimbrin in the micro-villar core.[275] The actin filaments extend into the terminal web, located in the subapical cytoplasm immediately beneath the base of the microvilli. Brush border formation characterizes the proximal tubule: (2) short microvilli, found on all other tubular cells; their density and distribution on the cell surface varies considerably; (3) microfolds, found on cells in which regulation of the permeation rates for given solutes is associated with rapid transient modulation of the luminal cell surface area (subtypes of intercalated cells and occasionally also in collecting duct cells; see below).

BASOLATERAL MEMBRANE DOMAIN

The entry of sodium-coupled solutes across the luminal membrane is driven by the enzymatic splitting of ATP by the Na-K-ATPase, the so-called sodium pump.[276] In renal epithelia ATP is mainly made available by mitochondria. The Na-K-ATPase is inserted in the basolateral membrane domain of all tubular cells, and is firmly linked to the actin cytoskeleton by interacting proteins, such as ankyrin, spectrin/fodrin, and NHERF.[277]

Segment-specific differences in Na-K-ATPase activity/protein[278,279] per unit tubular length rely on cell type-specific differences in the density of the enzyme molecules per area basolateral membrane, and on the available surface area of basolateral membrane per unit tubular length.[280,281] Basically two modes of increases of the basolateral membrane surface per unit tubular length are distinguished in renal epithelia:

1. *Lateral folding and interdigitation (basolateral interdigitations)*: this mode increases the lateral membrane area[282] and implies an increase of the lateral intercellular space, the common compartment of para- and transcellular transport routes.[40] The width of the lateral intercellular spaces (about 20–50 nm) varies little with function.
In interdigitated epithelia the tight junctions are composed of one or several parallel strands with more-or-less high particle density. The tall lateral plasma membrane folds, equipped with Na-K-ATPase, narrowly enclose large mitochondria. The folds split into complex basal ridges with densely packed actin filaments (but no Na-K-ATPase[283,284]), arranged in a circular manner,[285–287] which provide attachment to the underlying basememt membrane. This arrangement prevails in proximal (Figures 20.42, 20.43 and 20.44) and distal tubules (Figures 20.52, 20.53, 20.54, 20.56 and 20.57), and causes the characteristic basal striation of these segments in histological sections.
2. *Infoldings of the basal plasma membrane* into the cell body; the spaces between the infolded (Na-K-

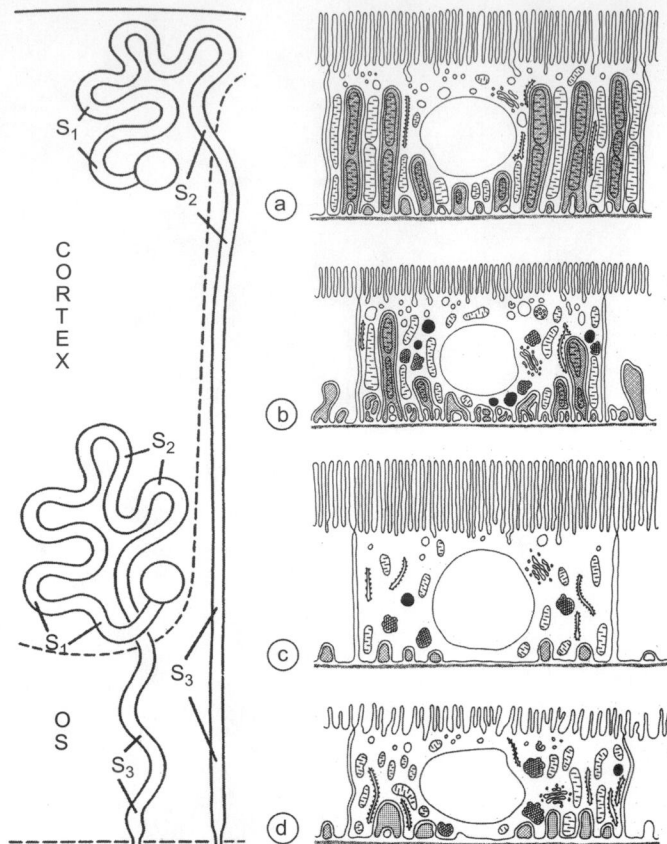

FIGURE 20.43 Survey on location and ultrastructure of proximal tubule segments. (a) S1 segments start at the urinary pole of the renal corpuscle in the cortex, and transform gradually to S2 segments within the labyrinth, S2 segments give way to S3 at different levels (depending on the nephron generation) within the medullary rays; S3 terminates at the border (dashed line) of the outer stripe (OS) and the inner stripe. (b) Salient features of S1, S2, and S3 proximal tubule cells; neighbouring cells are shaded in order to reveal the interdigitation by lateral cell processes; the vacuolar apparatus in the subapical cytoplasm, mitochondria, ER, Golgi apparatus, lysosomes (black spots), and peroxisomes (cross-hatched) are indicated; in rat S3 segments (c) the brush border micovilli are the highest, in rabbit (d) and most other species they are the shortest. (*Adapted from ref. [5], with permission*).

ATPase carrying) membranes open via so-called basal slits directly towards the underlying basement membrane, and have no continuity with the lateral intercellular spaces. Consequently, trans- and paracellular solute transport pathways are largely separated. The tight junctional belt consists of networks of anastomosing strands with high particle density. The width of the intercellular spaces can be narrow or dilated, depending on the functional conditions. The lateral membranes carry small finger-like villi or folds, and are often interconnected by small desmosomes, These might help to maintain mechanical cohesion under

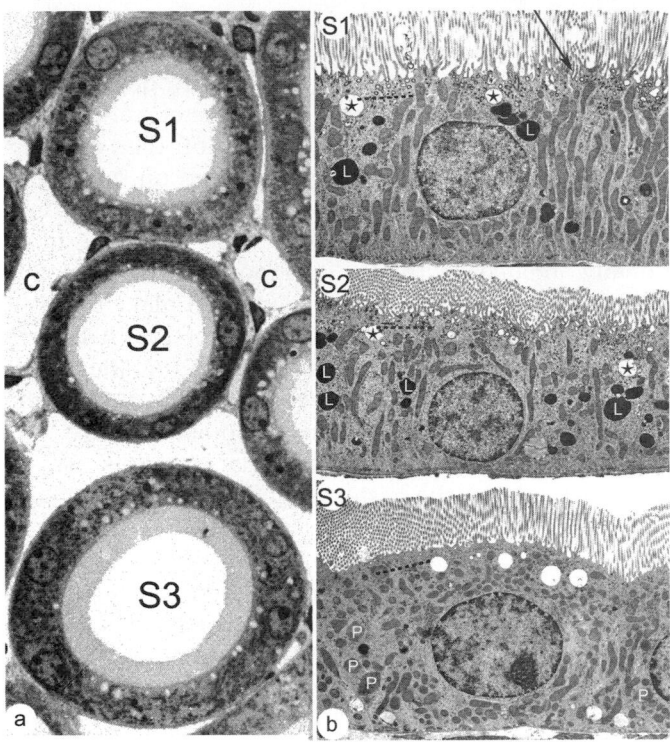

FIGURE 20.44 Proximal tubule (rat). (a) Profiles of S1, S2, and S3 segments of juxtamedullary proximal tubules; note the differences in brush border length, in cell height, cytoplasmic density, and outer diameter (c: Peritubular capillaries; Rat: 1 mm Epon section; × ~1000). (b) Ultrastructure of S1, S2, and S3 proximal tubule cells (Rat). The mitochondria in S1 and S2 are located in lateral cell processes, in S3 they are mainly scattered throughout the cytoplasm; the endocytotic apparatus in the subapical cytoplasm (roughly delimited by broken lines) is most prominent in S1 and early S2; endosomes (stars) and lysosomes (L) are located deeper in the cytoplasm; in S3 the vacuolar apparatus and lysosomes are virtually absent, whereas peroxisomes (P) are more frequent than in S1 and S2; interdigitation by lateral folds is almost lacking (TEM: × ~5400).

availability of active transport systems in the cell, and can be effected by several mechanisms, e.g., by gating of transport channels (e.g., ENaC in collecting duct cells), that are present in the luminal plasma membrane,[277] by redistribution of the given protein between microdomains in the apical membrane (e.g., NHE3 in the brush border of proximal tubuli,[297,298] by cycling of luminal and vesicular membrane domains containing the respective transport proteins (e.g., AQP2 in collecting duct cells; H[+]ATPase in intercalated cells) between the cell surface and intracellular vesicles[299] or by exocytotic insertion and endocytotic retraction of specific transport proteins into and from, respectively, the luminal membrane (e.g., ENaC[300]; NaPiIIa[301,302]).

Prolonged duration of increased transcellular flow rates stimulates, in addition to the acute responses, the transcription rates for the given transport proteins,[303] and finally results in cellular and epithelial hypertrophy, including cell proliferation.[304,305] Inversely, chronic decreases in Na-transport rates may result in epithelial hypotrophy, including a reduction of cell mass by apoptosis.[293,305–307] On this background it is tempting to interpret the internephron heterogeneity as a reflection of their different filtration and transport rates. In rats the juxtamedullary nephrons with the largest glomeruli and highest filtration rates[308] display the largest tubular diameter, the largest basolateral membrane area, Na-K-ATPase activity, and mitochondrial volume density.[41] The superficial nephrons have the smallest glomeruli, filtration rates, and tubular dimensions.

Primary Single Cilia

All renal cell types, except the intercalated cells, carry a central single primary cilium on their luminal surface. Primary cilia are regarded as mechanosensors that sense changes in luminal flow rate and circumferential stretch.[309–312] The extracellular mechanical stimulus caused by the urinary flow is transduced via the transmembrane proteins Polycystin 1 (PC-1) and Polycystin 2 (PC-2),[313] located in the membrane of the cilium.[314,315] Both together form a complex required for flow-mediated calcium entry in response to the deflection of the axoneme.[316] This subsequently results in release of calcium stores from the endoplasmic reticulum, possibly mediated by Polycystin 2.[309,311] On the one hand, this might induce local purinergic signaling and modulate renal tubular transport[317]; on the other hand, the primary cilia may be involved in the functional differentiation of polarized cells,[318] in the maintenance of normal tubular architecture,[309] in regulation of tissue morphogenesis,[319] and in gene transcription.[320] Cilia seem also to help to regulate and control mTOR and temper the response of this pathway to growth factors.[321] Loss-of-

functionally-induced dilation of the intercellular space. This epithelial organization characterizes the collecting duct system. Increases in membrane area by lateral interdigitating folds and basal infoldings may well be found in the same cell (e.g., connecting tubule cells; Figures 20.56 and 20.58).

Correlation Between Structure and Transport

In defined nephron segments rather constant ratios have been found between Na-transport rates, Na-K-ATPase activity, basolateral plasma membrane surface area, and mitochondrial density.[276,279–281,288–294]

Acute changes in flow rates for a given solute across the luminal cell membrane may be sensed by local purinergic signaling and responded to by rapid adjustment in transport rates.[295,296] They depend on the function mutations in the genes for PC-1 or PC-2 cause ciliary abnormalities[322] and the autosomal dominant form of polycystic kidney disease (ADPKD).[315,323]

PROXIMAL TUBULE

The proximal tubule takes up the glomerular filtrate and recovers the major fraction of water, sodium, and solutes by reabsorption from the tubular lumen back to the blood compartment, and it clears the blood of various organic compounds by uptake from the blood compartment and secretion into the tubular lumen.[324,325] Furthermore, the epithelium removes almost completely filtered proteins from the tubular fluid by endocytosis.

The proximal tubule begins at the urinary pole of the renal corpuscle, and ends at the transition to the descending thin limb of Henle's loop which defines the border between the outer and the inner stripes. It has a convoluted part, situated in the cortical labyrinth, and a straight part (pars recta: the thick descending limb of Henle's loop), located in the cortical medullary rays and in the outer stripe (Figure 20.43). The volume fraction of proximal tubules is about 48% in the rat cortex and about 54% in the outer stripe.[41] From the collected tubular volume in the cortical labyrinth of an adult rat the convoluted proximal tubule takes a fraction of 80 to 85%.[38]

Morphology of Proximal Tubular Epithelium

The proximal tubule is lined by cells with complex, interdigitating folding of the basolateral plasma membrane and characteristic formation of a brush border at the apical pole. The largely amplified apical and basolateral plama membrane surfaces correspond to the high transcellular solute transport rates (see "Organization of Electrolyte Transporting Epithelia"). The lateral foldings narrowly ensheath large mitochondria. At the base the foldings are split into numerous basal ridges, which are densely filled with circular running f-actin filaments, and provide the anchoring of the cell to the underlying extracellular basement membrane. The tight junctions are shallow, mostly consisting of a single strand with low particle density,[275] in agreement with the low-resistance shunt pathway in parallel with a high-resistance pathway across the limiting cell membranes.[326,327] The proximal tubule cells are electrically coupled by gap junctions.

The subapical cytoplasm immediately under the base of the brush border microvilli is a membrane-rich region, called the "vacuolar apparatus".[268] It is the structural correlate of the early endocytotic apparatus

(Figure 20.45a) and contains intermicrovillar more or less deep infoldings ("clefts") into the cytoplasm, small clathrin-coated vesicles, uncoated "dense apical tubules" (DAT) 70–90 nm in diameter, and large uncoated vesicles. The dimensions of the vacuolar apparatus are very variable, and depend on the rate of endocytosis (see below). The more or less abundant lysosomes, present in the center of the cells, are functionally related with the degradation of proteins. The nucleus is encircled in its equatorial plane by well-developed Golgi apparatus. Cisterns of rough ER are preferentially extended in parallel with the lateral cell membranes; ribosomes are abundant throughout the cytoplasm. Fenestrated cisterns of smooth ER are particularly abundant. In the terminal portions of the proximal tubule the cisterns of smooth ER contain xenobiotc-metabolizing enzymes[328] which contribute to detoxification processes. The cisterns of the smooth ER often extend along the lateral membranes and narrowly enwrap mitochondria and peroxisomes.[329] The latter are generally situated in the basal portions of the cells.[330] The amount of lysosomes, peroxisomes, and lipid droplets in proximal tubule cells strongly varies with the functional stage of the animal, food intake, and sex hormones.[331–333]

The proximal tubule is subdivided into three segments, S1, S2 and S3.[334,335] The subdivision is based on more-or-less gradually occurring quantitative changes along the proximal tubule. S1 cells line the initial half of the convoluted portion, and have the largest basolateral plasma membrane surface, Na-K-ATPase activity per unit membrane area, and mitochondrial density. They transform to S2 cells within the second half of the convoluted portion. All proximal tubule segments touching the renal capsule are S2 cella,[336] and S2 cells also form the beginning of the straight part in the medullary rays. In rats and rabbits the microvilli in S2 are markedly shorter than in S1 (in rat S1: ~4.5 to 4.0 μm; S2: ~4.0 to 1.5 μm). S2 cells usually have very prominent lysosomes. The basolateral surface area, Na-K-ATPase activity per unit membrane area, and mitochondrial density decrease from S1 to S3. S3 cells supersede S2 cells at various levels (depending on the nephron generation) in the medullary rays[34,113,268,336] and line the terminal portion of the proximal tubule. In rabbits, dog, and human the height of microvilli further decreases along S3.[5,114,334,335] In mice differences in the length of the brushborder microvilli among the three segments are little apparent,[113] whereas in rats the brush border microvilli of S3 are the longest from the three proximal tubule subsegments (Figure 20.44a). Lateral folding of the plasma membrane is lacking, and the S3 cells usually have a polygonal outline and a comparably small basolateral plasma membrane surface and

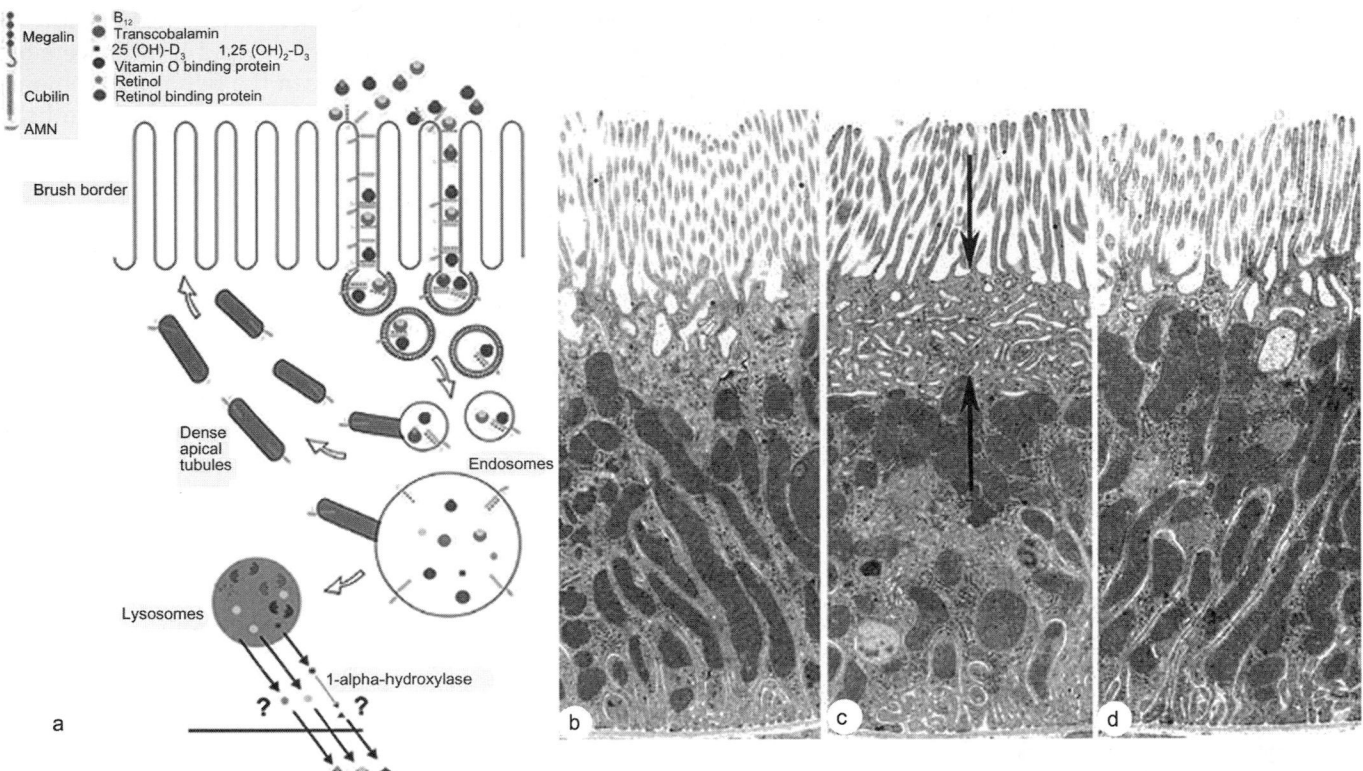

FIGURE 20.45 (a) Schematic representation of receptor-mediated endocytosis in the proximal tubule, exemplified for the megalin- and cubilin-mediated uptake of three vitamin carrier protein complexes: DBP-vitamin D3, TC-vitamin B12, and RBP-retinol in renal proximal tubule. Likewise, the cubilin chaperone protein amnionless, AMN, is indicated. Following receptor-mediated endocytosis via apical coated pits, the complexes accumulate in lysosomes for degradation of the proteins, while the receptors recycle to the apical plasma membrane via dense apical tubules. Megalin mediates the uptake of cubilin and its ligands. The mechanisms for the cellular release of the vitamins remain to be clarified. *(From ref. [346].)* (b)—(d) Transmission electron micrographs of S1 cells of the proximal tubule of rats; (b) control; (c) 15 min and (d) 60 min after a single PTH-injection; PTH induces rapid downregulation of the sodium phosphate co-transporter NaPi-IIa in the brush border membrane by endocytotic mechanisms, associated with a transient expansion of the vacuolar apparatus (between arrows) in the subapical vesicular compartment (TEM ~10,000). *(Modified from ref. [356].)*

Na-K-ATPase activity. Yet, the volume density of mitochondria in S3 of rat and mice is rather high. The mitochondria are scattered throughout the cytoplasm. Structural correlates for endocytosis and lysosomes are almost absent in S3, whereas amount and size of peroxisomes increases from S2 towards S3.

Functional Aspects

Structural Correlate for Receptor-Mediated Endocytosis

Receptor-mediated endocytosis (Figure 20.45a) is the most efficient mechanism for cellular uptake of filtered proteins[268,337,338] and plays an important role in the acute downregulation of transport rates by selective retraction of transport proteins from the microvillous membrane rapid (e.g., NaPiIIa, Figures 20.45b,c,d; see below). By multiphoton microscopy the passage of proteins across the different endocytotic compartments has been directly observed *in vivo*.[339,340]

The first requirement for cellular uptake of a protein by endocytosis is binding of a ligand to a receptor protein on the surface of the tubular cell. The multireceptors megalin, cubilin, and amnionless[341,342] have all been located in the proximal tubule, mainly on the base of the microvillous plasma membrane, in the intermicrovillar membrane invaginations ("clefts"), and in subapical clathrin-coated pits. Megalin belongs to the LDL-receptor family, and is bound with its cytoplasmic tail to cytoplasmic adaptor proteins.[343,344] It forms a tandem with the peripheral protein cubilin which is associated with the membrane by amnionless.[345,346] Megalin is responsible for the internalization of its own ligands and of cubilin with its ligands.[338] The receptor—ligand complexes are gathered in the clathrin-coated membrane pits, and are directed by clathrin-coated vesicles to larger, uncoated early and late endosomes, located slightly deeper in the cytoplasm. In the endosomes the receptors are cleaved from the ligands and travel back to the luminal membrane via uncoated "dense apical tubules" (DAT).[347-350] The DAT form an elaborate, moving dynamic network of anastomosing tubules,[348,351] which are transiently connected to the larger endosomes, and which display at their other end small clathrin-coated domains.[352-354] From the endosomes the ligands are sorted either for degradation to lysosomes or for ubiquitination via the proteasome pathway.

The trafficking of internalized material from the vacuolar apparatus to lysosomes critically depends on the microtubular system.[355] Microtubules normally form a loose network across the proximal tubule cells, and become highly oriented in the apico–basal direction during vesicular transport of endocytosed cargo to lysosomes.[356] The dimensions of the vacuolar apparatus and the abundance of megalin in proximal tubule cells are correlated with the rate of endocytosis. If endocytosis does not take place, either due to paucity of ligands in the tubular fluid (e.g., normally in S3) or due to lack or low levels of the endocytosis receptor,[338,357,358] the vacuolar apparatus is barely developed.

The processing of material in the vesicular compartments of the endocytotic pathway relies on acidification. NHE3, the proton-ATPase, and the chloride channel ClC-5 (for a review see [359]), are all highly expressed and co-localized in the intermicrovillous clefts and in the vesicular membranes of the early endocytotic pathway.[360-362] Dysfunction of one or several of these acidifying proteins may cause primary defects in endocytosis. Knockout of the ClC-5 channel, for instance, impairs the clearance of PTH from the tubular fluid, bringing about hyperphosphaturia and hypercalciuria.[361,362] This mechanism can explain the high incidence of kidney stones in Dent's disease, with functionally impaired ClC-5 channels.[363-367]

The role of basolateral endocytosis is interesting, since the basolateral cell membrane is the site of different hormone receptors,[368] e.g., the insulin receptor. After binding to the receptors peptide hormones seem to be, at least in part, taken up by the cells and are transported to the lysosomes.[369]

Sodium Proton Exchange

Apical Na^+-H^+ exchange in the proximal tubule and the reabsorption of the bulk of filtered sodium is mediated by the sodium/hydrogen exchanger NHE3 in the microvillous plasma membrane[361,370-372] and in the plasma membrane of the intermicrovillous invaginations.[297] The sodium/hydrogen exchanger is enriched in the intermicrovillar microdomain,[370] where it interacts with the scavenger receptor megalin (see above, [298]). Changes in Na/H exchange activity

correlate with changes in cell surface expression of NHE-3, mediated by sgk2.[373] Rapid and reversible redistribution of NHE3 between the two microdomains in the microvillous plasma membrane domain and the intervillous plasma membrane invaginations ("clefts") may also alter the surface expression of NHE3 and activity of Na/H exchange.[298,374-377]

Reabsorption of Water and Solutes

The plasma membrane of the microvilli is covered by a glycocalyx containing hydrolases (phosphatases, peptidases, nucleotidases) which cleave their substrates in the tubular fluid (ecto-enzymes). The microvillous membrane holds a large variety of transport proteins for uptake of water and solutes from the tubular fluid. The density of a given transport protein in the microvillous membrane can be dissimilar along the segments of the proximal tubule and among nephron generations. Many of the transport proteins are anchored by adaptor proteins, such as PDZ-proteins and NHERF1/2, to the underlying apical scaffold.[372,373,378,379]

Transcellular water reabsorption in the proximal tubule is mediated by the constitutive water channel, aquaporin 1 (AQP1) located in the microvillous- and basolateral plasma membrane domains.[380-384] Orthogonal arrays of intramembrane particles in the basolateral membranes of S3 of mice[385] are associated with another water channel, AQP4, AQP7, which is probably involved in the reabsorption of glycerol (see review in [386]) and is expressed in the brush border, especially of S3 in rats and mice, as shown by immunocytochemistry.[387,388]

Sodium-coupled solute uptake from the lumen into the cells is mediated by co-transport proteins located in the plasma membrane of the microvilli. The proximal tubule usually recovers all filtered glucose. The sodium–glucose co-transporter SGLT2 is found primarily in S1, and is responsible for 90% of glucose reabsorption. SLGT1 is located in S3, and is responsible for only 10% of reabsorption (reviewed by Hediger and Rhoads[389,390]). SGLT1 is more highly expressed in females than in males.[391] The exit of glucose across the basolateral plasma membrane occurs by the glucose transporters GLUT2 (low affinity in S1) and GLUT1 (high affinity in S3).[392]

Inorganic phosphate (Pi) transport is mediated by at least three different brush border $Na^+/P(i)$ co-transporter proteins, the electrogenic transporter NaPi IIa, Pit-2, and the electroneutral transporter NaPi Iic.[393,394] Their expressions and activities appear to be tightly regulated.

Low dietary intake of Pi increases mRNA and brush border expression of NaPi IIa.[395] High dietary Pi intake, parathyroid hormone (PTH) and activation of dopamine receptors[358] rapidly downregulate NaPiIIa-mRNA[395] and NaPiIIa in the brush border,[396-398] and induce phosphaturia. Downregulation of NaPiIIa in the brush border involves receptor-mediated endocytosis (see above) and subsequent lysosomal degradation.[355,356,358,399,400]

The passage of NaPi-IIa across the successive endocytotic compartments namely, the megalin-containing clefts, the clathrin-coated-vesicle compartment,[401] through the early and late endosomal compartment, and finally its disposal in lysosomes, where NaPi-IIa is degraded, has been tracked by immunofluorescence.[301] The shifting of the protein through the early endocytotic compartments goes along with a dramatic, rapidly transient expansion and remodeling of the vacuolar apparatus in the subapical compartment[356] (Figure 20.45). PTH also reduces Pit-2 expression and activity, whereas NaPi-IIc is inhibited and internalized with a delay of several hours after PTH application.[394]

Recently Klotho has been recognized as a phosphatonin, and an important regulator of phosphate homeostasis. In partnership with the FGF-R, Klotho functions as an obligate co-receptor for FGF23.[402] Secreted soluble Klotho inhibits Pi transport by altering the trafficking of the proximal tubule Na-coupled phosphate transporter.[402]

Neutral amino acids, which represent about 80% of circulating amino acids, are transported by the low affinity Na^+-co-transporter B(0)AT1, located in the early proximal tubule. The high affinity transporter B(0)AT3 is located in the late proximal tubule, at least in mice. In addition, there are several other apical and basolateral amino acid transporters (for a recent review see [403]). Similarly the short-chain peptide, di-, and tripeptide carriers PEPT1, high capacity, low affinity, and PEPT2 low capacity, high affinity are located in mainly S1 and S3, respectively.[404,405]

Secretion of organic amphiphilic electrolytes from the blood into the tubular fluid is a pathway for clearance and detoxification of xenobiotics and drugs, including diuretics.[325,406−410] The uptake into the proximal tubule epithelium proceeds via multispecific organic anion transporters (OAT) and organic cation transporters (OCT) in the basolateral membrane domain. The majority of members of the OAT- and OCT-family have been immunolocalized to the basolateral cell membrane of S3 proximal tubule,[411−413] yet OAT 1 has been detected mainly in S2,[414] a few also in S1. The expression of the OATs and OCTs is strongly regulated by sex hormones.[415−420]

The export into the tubular lumen of both conjugated and unconjugated lipophilic anionic substrates involves various OATs and primarily active transporters with ATP-binding casette motifs, belonging to the MRP-family,[421] and located in the brush border membrane of S1, S2, and S3 proximal tubule segments.[421,422]

The role of basolateral endocytosis is interesting, since the basolateral cell membrane is the site of different hormone receptors,[368] e.g., the insulin receptor. After binding to the receptors peptide hormones seem to be, at least in part, taken up by the cells and are transported to the lysosomes.[369]

THIN LIMBS OF HENLE'S LOOP (INTERMEDIATE TUBULE)

The intermediate tubule comprises the thin tubular portions, interposed between the proximal and the distal tubules (Figure 20.46). Ultrastructurally, the intermediate tubule has four structurally different segments: (1) the descending thin limbs of short loops (SDTL); (2) the upper part; (3) the lower part of descending thin limbs of long loops (LDTLup and LDTL lp); and (4) the ascending thin limbs (ATL). This pattern has been observed in various species, including rat,[423,424] mouse,[34,425] golden hamster,[426] rabbit,[5,427] *Perognathus*,[428] *Octodon degus*,[429] *Meriones shawii*,[116] and *Psammomys obesus*.[430−432] An additional subsegment of thin limbs has been identified in Chinchilla.[433] The thin limbs in human have so far not been studied in comparable completeness.[434−436]

Surprisingly, by lightmicroscopy these simple-looking epithelia are strikingly different from each other with respect to ultrastructure and function, not only the ascending from the descending limbs but, most remarkably, the descending limbs of short from those of long loops. Furthermore, within the descending segments (SDTL, LDTLup, LDTLlp) the proximal portion, although structurally no different from the distal portion, displays considerable functional differences. In the IM a high percentage of thin limbs was found that consisted of a patchwork of descending and ascending type epithelia.[437,438] Beyond all these heterogeneities, there are prominent differences among species. This complex situation appears to account for the persistent discussion about the integrated function of thin limbs in the urine concentrating process.

The type I epithelium (Figure 20.47), which is characteristic for descending thin limbs of short loops (SDTL), has a simple and uniform organization. It is composed of flat, non-interdigitating cells reposing on a thin basement membrane. The luminal cell membrane bears only a few short microvilli that are mainly found along the cell borders. The tight junction consists of several anastomosing junctional strands; desmosomes are frequently encountered. The SDTLs in the rat have, among all other thin limb segments, a particularly prominent cytoskeleton with a high content of cytokeratins and desmoplakins.[439] Cell organelles, such as mitochondria, profiles of rough and smooth

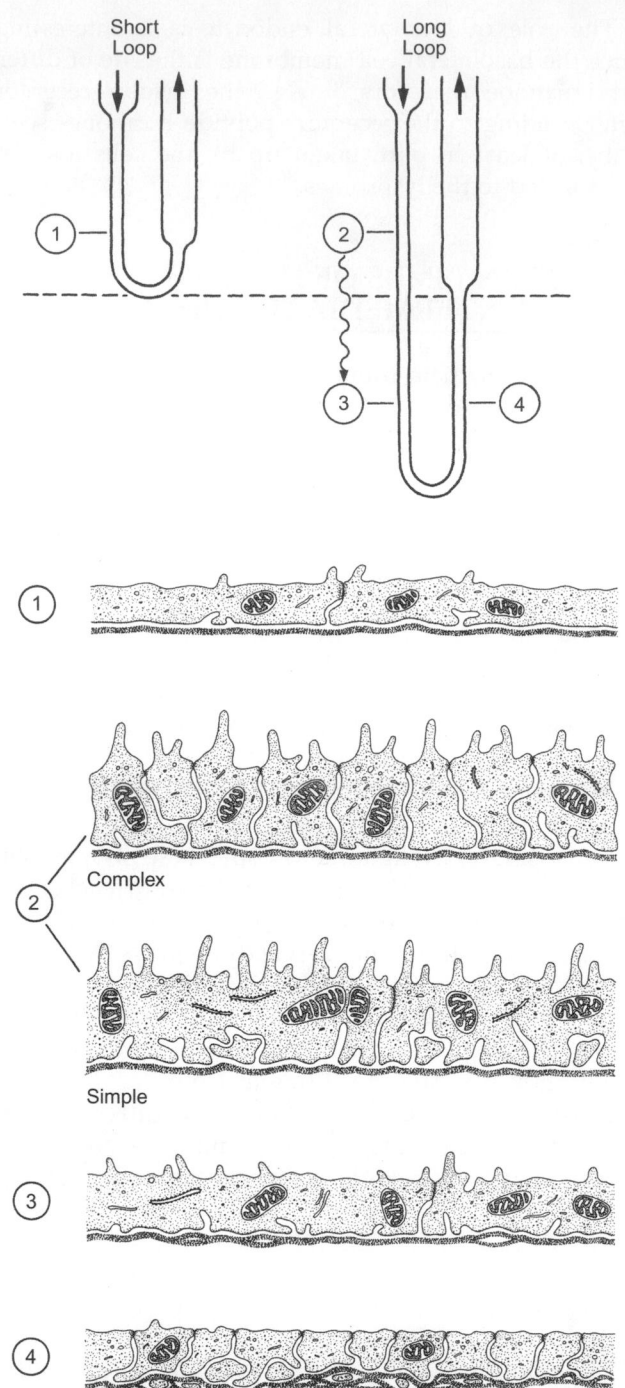

FIGURE 20.46 Survey of thin limb ultrastructure. Four thin limb segments are discernible: (1) Descending thin limb of short loops. (2) Descending thin limbs of long loops, upper part. This segment is differently developed among species: a complex type (upper panel) found e.g., in rat, mouse, and *Psammomys* is distinguished from a simple type (lower panel) found e.g., in rabbit and guinea pig. (3) Descending thin limb of long loops, lower part. The transition between upper and lower parts is gradual. (4) Ascending thin limb. (*Adapted from Kriz, W., and Schiller, A. et al. (1980). In "Comparative and Functional Aspects of Thin Loop Limb Ultrastructure. Functional Ultrastructure of the Kidney," 239–250, Maunsbach, A. B. Academic Press, London, and Kaissling, B., and Kriz, W. (1992). In "Morphology of the Loop of Henle, Distal Tubule and Collecting Duct. Handbook of Physiology: Section on Renal Physiology," 109–167, Windhager, E. E. Oxford University Press, New York, with permission).*

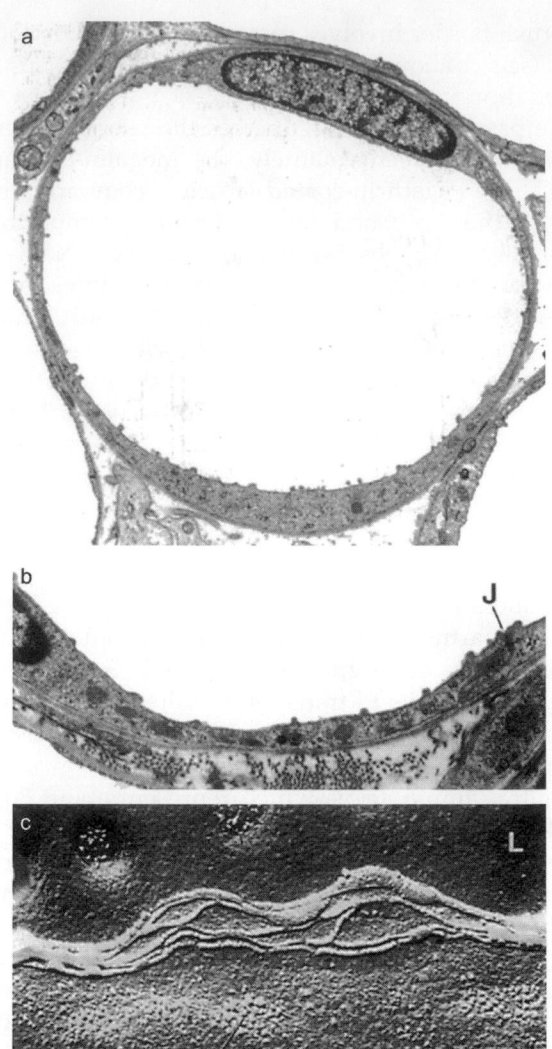

FIGURE 20.47 Thin descending limbs of short loops. (a) Cross-sectional profile (rat; TEM: ×~4100). (b) The simplicity of the epithelium is demonstrated (J: Junctional complex; Rat: TEM: × ~11,000). (c) Freeze-fracture electron micrograph. The tight junction consists of several anastomosing strands (L: luminal membrane; BL: basolateral membrane; D: desmosome; Rabbit: ×~71,000).

endoplasmic reticulum, etc., are exceedingly sparse in type I epithelium.

Apart from an initial stretch of maximally 400 μm in about 10% of SDTLs in mouse, these nephron segments do not show any labeling for aquaporin 1 (AQP1), thus they are rather impermeable to water.[440] The lower parts of SDTLs contain the urea transporter UT-A2 in its cell membranes.[382,441,442] In species with complex vascular bundles (e.g., rat, mouse), the short descending limbs lie within the vascular bundles[115]; in these surroundings, the thin limbs are in an ideal position to recycle urea from the ascending vasa recta into the short loop nephrons (see below).

This simple type I epithelium is also found in many descending loop profiles in the inner stripe of feline and canine kidneys which, by microanatomical definition, possess only "long" loops. Consequently, it may be assumed that these simple profiles belong to those long loops that descend into the inner medulla for only very short distances, frequently less than 500 μm.[443] The epithelial characteristics of these loops may be more important than their short descent into the inner zone for determining their functional role. From this point of view, "short loops" are also present in the cat kidney. The short descending thin limbs of cortical loops — studied in the minipig[444] and guinea pig (unpublished results from our laboratory) — are also established by the simple type 1 epithelium.

The descending thin limbs of long loops are generally much larger in diameter, and have a thicker epithelium than those of short loops. Moreover, the LDTLs are heterogeneous; obviously, those of the "longest" long loops begin in the inner stripe as a much thicker tubule than those of "shorter" long loops. The character of the epithelium gradually changes as the limbs descend toward and into the inner medulla. The subdivision of these thin limbs into an upper part (type 2 epithelium) (Figure 20.48a) and a lower part (type 3 epithelium) (Figure 20.48b) is an approximation, and reflects the gradual change to a more and more structurally simplified epithelium. Moreover, this process of epithelial simplification appears to be individually related to the length of each loop. It occurs earlier and more quickly in "short" long loops and is delayed in the longest of the long loops.[34,260,424,432,445] This explains the heterogeneity among descending thin

limb profiles in a given cross-section through the medulla: profiles lined with the lower-part epithelium (type 3) may already be found at the end of the inner stripe. Even deep in the inner medulla, profiles with the upper part epithelium (type 2; in reduced elaboration) are still present.

Furthermore, considerable interspecies differences, concerning in particular the upper parts of LDTLs, complicate understanding of the long descending thin limbs. Two patterns may be distinguished[260]; in one group of species (mouse, rat, golden hamster, *Perognathus, Psammomys, O. degus*, cat), the epithelium (type 2) of the LDTLup is characterized by an extremely high degree of cellular interdigitation. In a single cross-section, more than 100 cell processes may be encountered (Figures 20.48a and 20.49a,b). The tight junctions are extremely shallow, usually consisting of one junctional strand. Thus, the most characteristic features of this epithelium are the prominent paracellular pathways. The junctions are "leaky," and the amount of junctional area available per unit area of epithelial surface is increased several-fold by the tortuosity of the junction due to cellular interdigitation. The lateral cellular spaces form an elaborate "labyrinth," bordered by correspondingly amplified basolateral membranes. Additional structural characteristics of the epithelium are numerous apical microvilli, considerable numbers of mitochondria, and a strikingly high density of uniform intramembranous particles in the luminal and basolateral membrane. In addition, cytochemical and immunohistochemical studies have revealed that the LDTLup exhibits a sodium–potassium ATPase in both membranes,[446,447] suggesting active salt secretion. In addition, salt transport may occur through the tight

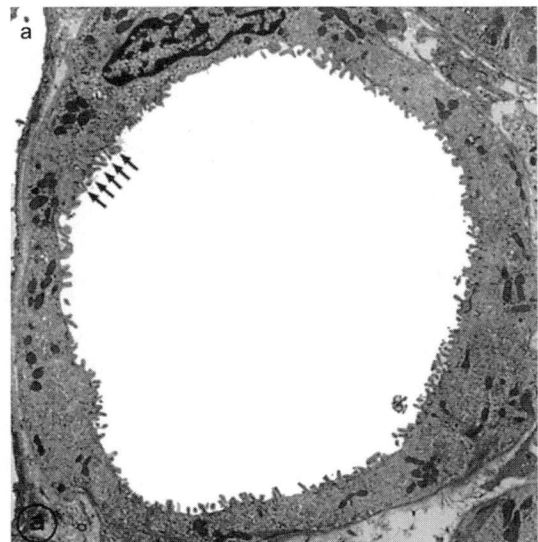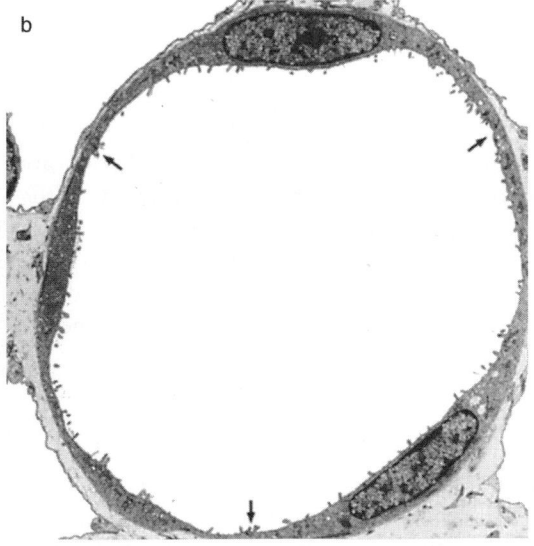

FIGURE 20.48 Descending thin limbs of long loops, upper part. (a) Complex type; note the many tight junctions (arrows) (*Psammomys*: TEM: ×~3000). (b) Simple type; only three junctions are encountered (arrows) (rabbit: TEM: × ~3000).

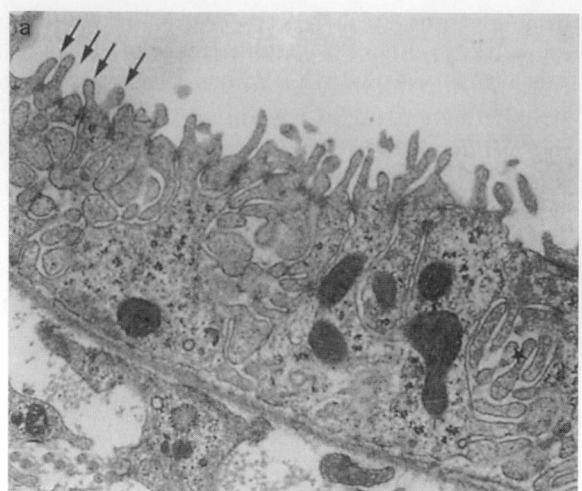
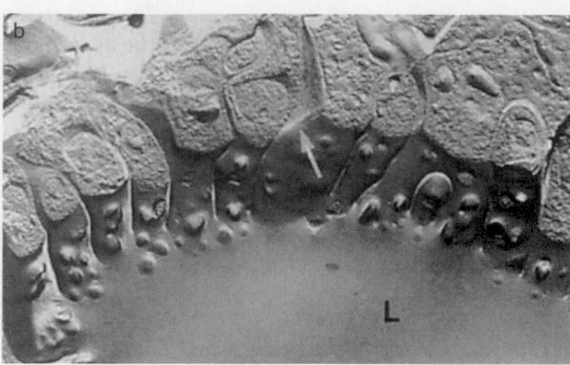
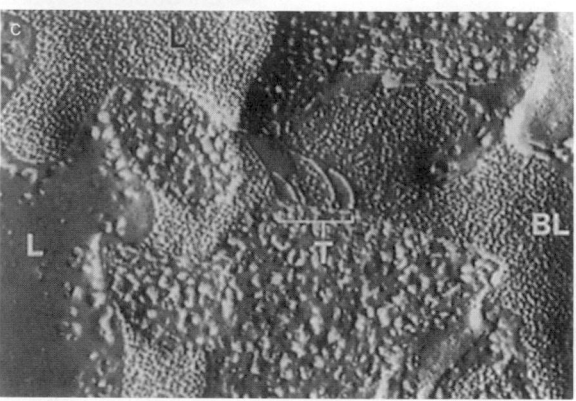

FIGURE 20.49   Descending thin limbs of long loops, upper part. (a) The complex epithelium is characterized by numerous tight junctions (arrows) indicating the extensive intercellular digitation. The interdigitation of the basolateral membrane forms a "labyrinth" of extracellular spaces within the cell body (*) (rat: TEM: ×∼11,000). (b) Freeze-fracture electron micrograph exhibiting the luminal aspect of the complex epithelium demonstrating the extensive cellular interdigitation. The tight junction consists of one strand only (arrow) (L: lumen of the tubule; Rat: TEM: × ∼13,000). *(From Kriz, W., and Schiller, A. et al. (1980). In "Comparative and Functional Aspects of Thin Loop Limb Ultrastructure. Functional Ultrastructure of the Kidney," 239−250, Maunsbach, A. B. Academic Press, London, with permission.)* (c) Freeze-fracture electron micrograph of the simple type epithelium. The tight junction (T) consists of several junctional strands. Note the dense pattern of intramembrane particles on the P face of luminal (L) and basolateral (BL) membranes (an equally dense particle pattern is also found in the complex type) (L: Tubular lumen; Rabbit: × ∼66,000). *(From Schiller, A., and Taugner, R. et al. (1980). The thin limbs of Henle's loop in the rabbit. A freeze fracture study. Cell Tissue Res.* **207**(2), 249−265, with permission.)

junctions, which contain claudin 2.[261,448] LDTLups are highly permeable to water due to the abundancy of the constitutive water channel aquaporin 1 (AQD1) in both membranes,[449] probably correlating with the high density of intramembrane particles. Carbonic anhydrase activity was found in both short and long descending thin limbs.[450]

In a second group of species that includes rabbit,[427,451] minipig[444] and guinea pig (unpublished data from our laboratory), the upper parts of LDTLs are more simply organized. The prominent paracellular pathway typical of the first group is lacking. The epithelial cells in this group do not interdigitate, and are joined by much deeper tight junctions consisting of several anastomosing junctional strands

(Figures 20.48b and 20.49c). In other respects, however, the epithelia are similar in the two groups. Numerous luminal microvilli, many mitochondria, and the dense assembly of intramembrane particles in luminal and basolateral membranes are present in type 2 epithelium also in this group. The high density of intramembrane particles may be partially due to the high density of aquaporin 1 (AQP1) channels in both membranes; corresponding to the decrease of particle density along its descending course the density of AQP1 channels decreases.[452−454]

The epithelium of the lower part of LDTL (type 3 epithelium) is comparably simple (Figure 20.50); interspecies differences are no longer prominent. The epithelium consists of relatively flat, noninterdigitating

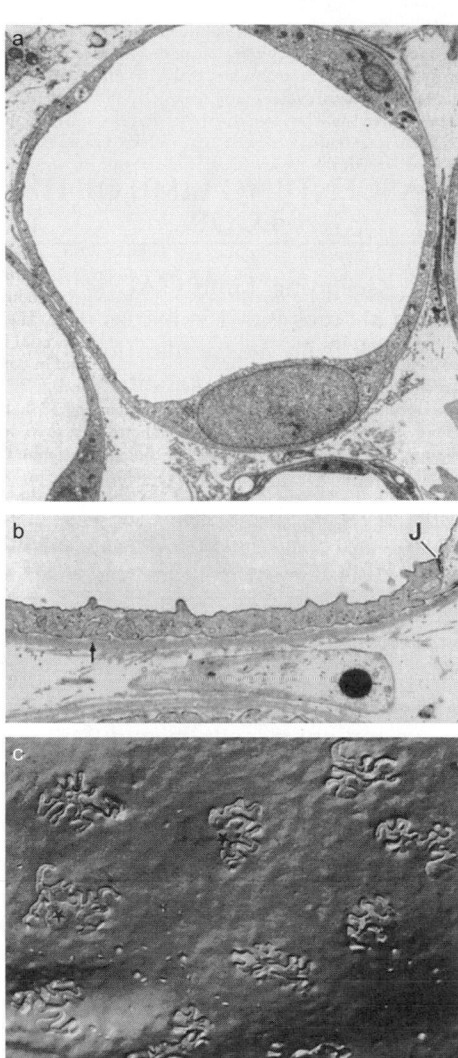

FIGURE 20.50 Descending thin limbs of long loops, lower part. (a) Cross-sectional profile (rat: TEM: ×~3800). (b) The epithelium is simply organized; basal infoldings (arrow) are regularly encountered (J: Junctional complex; Rabbit: TEM: ×~10,200). (c) Freeze-fracture electron micrograph demonstrating the regular pattern of basal infoldings within the basal cell membrane (*) (*Psammomys*: ×~12,800). (*In cooperation with A. Schiller and R. Taugner.*)

typical for the upper parts, has disappeared. This appears to correlate with the decrease in density of AQP1 channels that, in the terminal portions of this segment, may completely disappear. Thus, the water permeability probably decreases toward the loop bend[452,453]; the terminal segment may accordingly be thought to have a very low water permeability. Regarding the permeability to urea and the distribution of the urea transporter UT-A, conflicting data are published, especially when comparing data from different species.[438,442,452,455−457] In the mouse in antidiuretic conditions, the UTA2 urea transporter is upregulated in LDTLep.[458] Also, claudin 8 has been found in this segment.[240]

With respect to the descending thin limbs of the human kidney, the published data do not allow a final conclusion. In an older TEM investigation[459] a thin limb profile is shown with a heavily interdigitated epithelium corresponding to the thin limb epithelium described above as the complex type in other species. However, in the text the descending thin limbs in the human kidney are described as being outlined by a simply structured epithelium. In 1967, when this paper was published, it was not yet known that there were four different thin limb epithelia.

The axial, the internephron, as well as the interspecies differences in descending thin limb epithelia, is surprisingly prominent compared to all other nephron segments. Differences among thin limb segments were also found with respect to the cholesterol content of their cell membranes.[460] Binding studies with various lectins have revealed distinct labeling patterns in the descending, as well as the ascending, thin limbs in rat and rabbit.[461−463]

The ascending thin limb is present only in long loop nephrons, and is uniformly organized among mammals (Figure 20.51). Generally, the transition from the type 3 epithelium of the descending limb to the type 4 epithelium of the ascending limb occurs a short, but fairly constant, distance before the bend ("pre-bend segment[34,120,121,431]"). Therefore, functionally, the entire bend should be regarded as part of the ascending thin limb. The type 4 epithelium is characterized by very flat but heavily interdigitating cells joined by shallow tight junctions, consisting of only one prominent junctional strand. This leaky organization of the paracellular pathways corresponds with functional studies,[464,465] which all demonstrate that the ascending thin limbs are highly permeable for ions.

The change from the type 3 epithelium to the type 4 epithelium coincides with the disappearance of the urea transporter UT-A 2, and the abrupt beginning of the expression of the chloride channel ClC-K1[437,452,466]; aquaporins are completely lacking. Thus, the ascending thin limb is water- and urea-impermeable, but highly

cells bearing some sparse microvilli; in the rat it is covered by an unusually thick surface coat.[424] The tight junctions are of an intermediate apicobasal depth, composed of several junctional strand (in rabbit: 138 ± 37 nm and 3.5 ± 0.7 strands; in *Psammomys*, 51 ± 28 nm).[260] The basolateral membrane regularly forms basal infoldings, similar to those found in the simple type of LDTLup.[260] The fluid spaces between the infoldings are not continuous with the lateral intercellular spaces, and thus they are not part of a paracellular pathway route. The pattern and density of intramembrane particles in the luminal and basolateral membranes are inconspicuous; the dense packing,

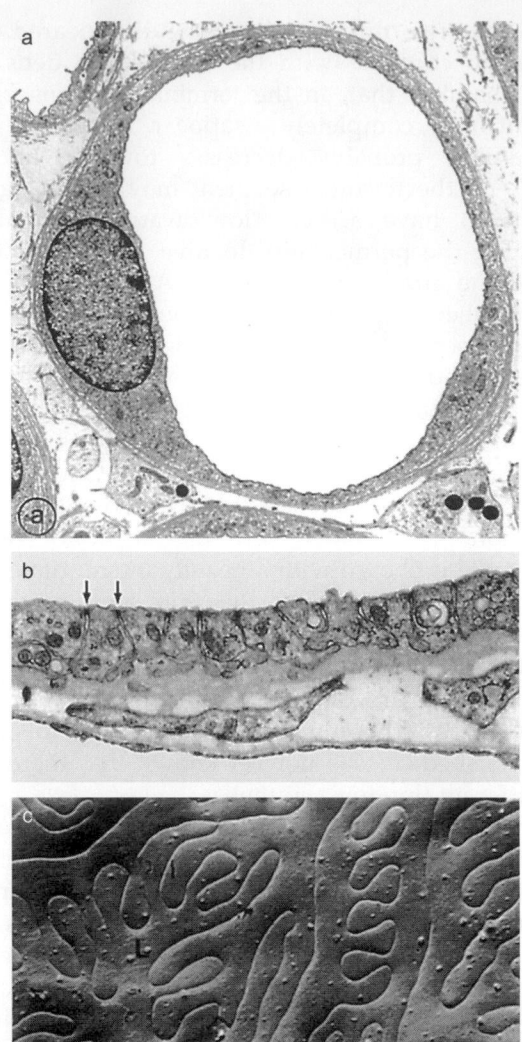

FIGURE 20.51   Ascending thin limbs. (a) Cross-sectional profile; note the many junctions (arrows) (*Psammomys*: TEM: ×∼3500). (b) Epithelium exhibiting extensive intercellular interdigitation; numerous tight junctions are encountered (arrows) (C: Capillary; Golden hamster: TEM: ×∼13,500). (c) Freeze-fracture electron micrograph. Luminal aspect of the tubule demonstrating the mode of cellular interdigitation and the shallow tight junction (arrow) (L: luminal membrane; BL: basolateral membrane; *Psammomys*: ×∼4800). *(From Kriz, W., and Schiller, A. et al. (1981). Freeze-fracture studies on the thin limbs of Henle's loop in Psammomys obesus. Am. J. Anat. **162**(1), 23–33, with permission.)*

permeable for Cl^- and also Na^+. The relevance of the expression of claudin 4[261] is poorly-understood. Surprisingly, in mouse, rat, and rabbit a high fraction of "mixed" thin limbs was found consisting of alternating stretches of descending and ascending type epithelia.

In most species the transition from the ascending thin limb to the thick ascending limb (distal straight tubule) is abrupt over the length of one cell. The level of this transition defines the border between the inner medulla and the inner stripe of the outer medulla. In the canine[467] and human kidney,[459] a gradual transition between the thin and thick ascending parts of the limb has been observed.

THICK ASCENDING LIMB OF HENLE'S LOOP

The Thick Ascending Limb (TAL = distal straight tubule − DST) absorbs NaCl in excess of water.[468] The subtraction of salt from the tubular fluid contributes to rendering the surrounding interstitium hypertonic, a crucial prerequisite for the urinary concentration process. The tubular fluid delivered by the segment into the cortex becomes progressively diluted. In addition, the TAL plays a prominent role in acid–base homeostasis, and recovers important fractions of filtered Mg^{2+} and Ca^{2+} via the paracellular transport route.

The beginning and end of the TAL epithelium are sharply demarcated from the preceding thin limb epithelium, and the successive DCT epithelium. The TAL of nephrons with long loops begins at the border between inner and outer medulla, and that of nephrons with short loops at various levels within the inner stripe of the outer medulla (in cortical loops even in the medullary rays in the cortex). It ascends through the outer medulla and the cortical medullary rays, enters the cortical labyrinth for a short distance, and contacts with the "macula densa," the vascular pole of its parent glomerulus (Figure 20.52). After a short "post-macula" segment the TAL transforms to the distal convoluted tubule (DCT). The length of the post-macula segment varies not only among species (< 500 μm in rabbits), but also among nephrons within the same kidney.[5,37,260] An association of its length with nephron types has not been established.

Long-looped nephrons have a thinner epithelium than nephrons with short loops.[5,308,469] The thickness of the epithelium decreases gradually, although considerably in the flow direction along the segment (Figures 20.52 and 20.53).[308]

The organization of the TAL-epithelium is exemplary for electrolyte transporting epithelia (see above: "Organization of Electrolyte Transporting Epithelia") (Figure 20.52). The cells display prominent lateral membrane foldings (Figure 20.22a)[5,470] which narrowly interdigitate with adjacent cells and enclose plate-like large mitochondria, and occasionally a few cisterns of rough endoplasmic reticulum (rER)[470] (Figure 20.53). Except in the deep inner stripe the lateral folding extends over the entire cell height. Hence, the luminal outline and tight junctional belt are much longer in upstream portions than in the deep inner stripe,[471] evident by the very frequent hits of the tortuous tight junctional belt in sections of cortical TAL

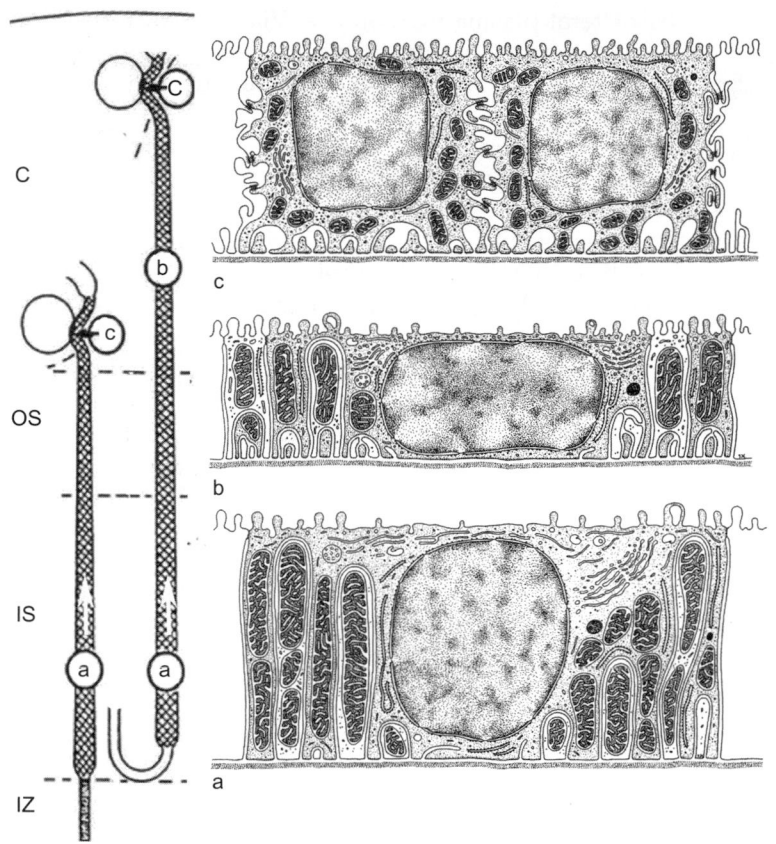

FIGURE 20.52 Survey on location and ultrastructure of the thick ascending limb of Henle's loop. (TAL: distal straight tubule, including macula densa; C: cortex; IS: inner stripe; OS: outer stripe; IZ: inner zone.) The direction of the urinary flow is indicated by white arrows, interdigitated cells with large mitochondria, enclosed in the lateral processes; (a) medullary part; (b) cortical part; (c) macula densa; note the difference in the organization of the lateral intercellular spaces between macula densa cells and other TAL cells. *(Adapted from Kaissling, B., and Kriz, W. (1979). Structural analysis of the rabbit kidney. Adv. Anat. Embryol. Cell Biol. 56, 1–123, and Kaissling, B., and Kriz, W. (1992). In "Morphology of the Loop of Henle, Distal Tubule and Collecting Duct. Handbook of Physiology: Section on Renal Physiology," 109–167, Windhager, E. E. Oxford University Press, New York, with permission).*

epithelium (Figure 20.53b). The tight junction is organized by a few strands, arranged in parallel, and with a high particle density (Figure 20.41a).

The large nucleus usually (except in the deep inner stripe) spans the entire cell height. The cytoplasm in the nuclear region displays small, round mitochondrial profiles, a particularly extensive Golgi apparatus,[308] polyribosomes, and some short cisterns of rER. The varying amounts of narrow tubular profiles and smooth vesicles in the subapical cytoplasm might be related with trafficking of apical transport proteins (see below). The apical membrane of the cells carries short stubby microvilli,[114,472] which usually border the tight junctional belt[471] and are less abundant in the center of the cell and in the vicinity of the single cilium. Scanning electron microscopy revealed that "rough" cells with numerous microvilli may be present side-by-side with rather smooth cells with only a few microvilli.[469] The latter cells display strong immunoreactivity for EGF, which seems to play a role in the regulation of growth and differentiation of cells in the loop of Henle.[473]

Role of the TAL in NaCl Reabsorption

The major fraction of salt reabsorption by the TAL (including the macula densa cells) proceeds via the $Na^+,K^+,2Cl^-$ (NKCC2) symporter[468] in the luminal membrane[474–476] which is specifically inhibited by loop diuretics, such as bumetanide and furosemide.[477] The apical entry of Na^+,K^+ and $2Cl^-$ is driven by the Na-K-ATPase in the basolateral plasma membrane. The density of Na-K-ATPase in the TAL exceeds by far that of more proximal tubular sites.[278,279]

The inwardly rectifying renal outer medullary K channel, ROMK, which recycles the K^+ ions entering the cell via NKCC2 over the apical membrane, is particularly abundant in the apical plasma membrane of TAL cells.[365,478–483] The basolateral extrusion of Cl^- occurs passively through ClC-K and ClC-Kb channels.[479,484]

Role in Bicarbonate Reabsorption

In addition to its role in salt reabsorption, the TAL has also an important function in maintaining acid—base homeostasis. It reabsorbs about 15–20% of the filtered bicarbonate[485–488] via the sodium/hydrogen exchangers NHE3 and NHE2 in the luminal plasma membrane of the TAL cells[370,489–491] and the NEM-sensitive vacuolar H^+-ATPase.[492] The apical Na/H exchange is tightly coupled with the basolateral Cl^-/HCO_3^- exchange that proceeds by the Cl^-/HCO_3^-

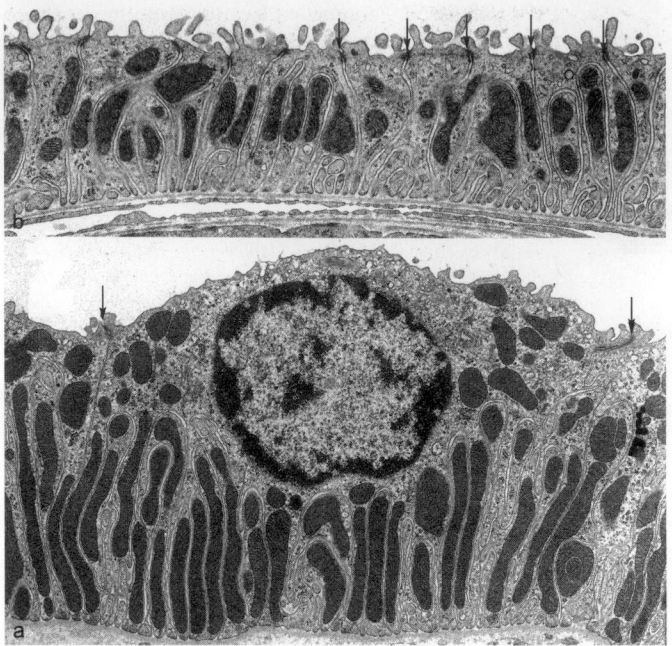

FIGURE 20.53 **Thick ascending limb cells.** (a) Deep level of the inner stripe; the lateral interdigitated foldings contain large mitochondria and do not reach up to the lumen; (b) Cortical part; in the much lower cells the lateral interdigitated foldings reach up to the lumen, causing a folded course of the tight junctions (arrows) (rat: TEM: × ~14,500). (*Adapted from and Kaissling, B., and Kriz, W. (1992). In "Morphology of the Loop of Henle, Distal Tubule and Collecting Duct. Handbook of Physiology: Section on Renal Physiology," 109–167, Windhager, E. E. Oxford University Press, New York, with permission*).

exchanger AE2.[493,494] The abundance of the NHE3 protein in the apical plasma membrane of the TAL has been shown to increase with functional adaptation to reduced renal mass,[487] under metabolic acidosis,[495] and with high levels of glucocorticoids.[496]

Role in Mg^{2+} and Ca^{2+} Recovery

Although virtually impermeable to water, the junctions in the TAL display a selective permeability for Mg^{2+} and Ca^{2+}. 40–70% of the filtered Mg^{2+} is recovered by the TAL in a passive paracellular manner facilitated by tight junction proteins claudin-16 and claudin-19 protein.[252,497] The much greater length of the tight junctional belt in the CTAL than in the MTAL might explain the higher paracellular movement of Mg^{2+} and Ca^{2+} in the CTAL than in the MTAL.[497,498] Impaired function of paracellin 1 (claudin 16) leads to urinary losses, specifically of magnesium and calcium.[499–506]

Regulation of salt transport rates in the TAL involves peptide hormones, among them vasopressin and glucagons, which bind to receptors on the basolateral plasma membranes. Via the cAMP messenger system they increase the abundance of the NKCC2 co-transporter and the K-channel in the luminal membrane.[106,117,474,468,507–512]

The acute response to decreases or increases of cAMP seem to involve endocytotic and exocytotic, respectively, membrane translocation.[513] The various amounts of NKCC2-displaying vesicular and tubular structures in the apical cytoplasm of TAL cells[270,510,514] might well be part of the membrane pool, available for translocation. Similar to the proximal tubule, endocytosis requires NHE3-mediated acidification, and needs the chloride channel CLC5. NHE3 and ClC5 are both located in the apical cytoplasm of TAL cells.[480,515] The basolateral extrusion of Cl occurs passively through ClC-K and ClC-Kb channels.[479] The trafficking of ClC-K to the basolateral membrane depends on the protein barttin.[479]

Cyclooxygenase 2 (COX2) has been located in the TAL cells, including the macula densa cells, and contributes through local production of prostaglandins[479,516–518] to the handling of ions by the TAL.

All maneuvers that chronically affect the salt transport rates by the TAL finally result in structural hyper- or hypotrophy of the TAL epithelium. The plasticity of the TAL epithelium in response to variations in plasma levels of vasopressin (ADH) or cAMP had been revealed by studies on Brattleboro rats, which genetically lack ADH and suffer from diabetes insipidus (DI).[519] In these rats the medullary and cortical portion of the TAL are equally thin.[520] In healthy rats with chronic low plasma levels of ADH due to chronic high water intake the structural appearance of the TAL resembles that seen in DI-rats.[521] Several weeks of substitution of ADH in DI rats or of endogenously increased ADH-levels, associated with chronic water restriction, restore the normal axial heterogeneity.[522,523]

The transport rates by the TAL epithelium are correlated with the DNA synthesis rate of TAL cells. Specific inhibition of NaCl reabsorption in the TAL of rats by furosemide transiently reduces the incidence of TAL cells showing DNA synthesis (assessed by nuclear detection of the proliferating cell nuclear antigen, PCNA, and incorporation of the thymidine analog bromodesoxyuridine) from about 1%, the basal rate in the rat TAL epithelium, to zero.[305]

With the given background it is likely that the structural heterogeneity regarding cell height, mitochondrial density, and basolateral plasma membrane surface along the TAL represents the physiologically lower tubular salt load, and ensuing lower transport rates in the cortical than in the medullary portions.[468] In rabbits the overall reduction of the cell height, membrane area and mitochondrial volume (per unit tubular length) along the TAL is much more pronounced than in rats and mice.

Disruption of genes coding for NKCC2 (SLC12A1) or for one or several proteins and/or channels associated with the NaCl-transport via NKCC2 (e.g., chloride channels ClCKA, ClCkB or the Barttin subunit, CLC5, NHE3), involved in regulation of its surface expression, or of the respective signaling cascades causes more or less severe renal salt-wasting, characteristic of "Bartter" syndrome. Symptoms of the Bartter syndrome are, e.g., lowered blood pressure, hypokalemic metabolic alkalosis, and hypercalciuria, with variable risk of kidney stones.[479,483–484,524–527]

The Tamm-Horsfall glycoprotein (THP), the most abundant urinary protein in mammals, is synthesized exclusively by the renal TAL epithelium. It is located in high density on the apical plasma membrane, in low density also on the basolateral plasma membrane.[528,529] Uromodulin has been linked to water–electrolyte balance and to kidney innate immunity.[530] THP is thought to be relevant in the pathogenesis of cast nephropathy and urolithiasis. By its property to compete efficiently with urothelial cell receptors, such as uroplakins, in adhering to type I fimbriated *Escherichia coli*, it may play a role in defense against urinary tract infection.[531] Mutations in the gene encoding uromodulin lead to rare autosomal dominant diseases, collectively referred to as uromodulin-associated kidney diseases.[532] Recently, it has been shown that THP-deficient (THP$^{-/-}$) mice showed moderately impaired urinary concentrating abilityuromodulin plays a permissive role in TAL reabsorptive fu/uromodulin plays a permissive role in TAL reabsorptive function.[533]

SEGMENTS DOWNSTREAM OF THE TAL: DISTAL CONVOLUTED TUBULE, CONNECTING TUBULE, AND COLLECTING DUCT

Electrolyte transports by the tubular epithelia distal of the loop of Henle provide the fine tuning of urinary electrolyte- and water-excretion. Located downstream of the macula densa, their transepithelial solute transport rates are no more directly submitted to tubuloglomerular feedback control but, rather, they are regulated by systemic hormones and a multitude of local factors.[296,317]

The structural subdivision of these portions in the cortex into the distal convoluted tubule (DCT), the connecting tubule (CNT), and the cortical collecting duct (CCD) goes back to light microscopic observations made in sections and microdissected tubules from kidneys of rabbits, human, mouse, sheep, cat, pig, beef,

and dolphin by Karl Peter early in the 20th century.[37] More than half-a-century later, microdissection studies of nephrons from rabbits and mice by the group of Morel[534] revealed that the distribution of sensitivities for several peptide hormones was bound to the morphological segmentation. Detailed electron microscopic investigations of the distal tubular portions in rabbits,[5] rats,[291,535,536] *Psammomys obesus*,[35] and mice[537,538] further confirmed and extended the earlier findings. The few studies on the human nephron[459,539–541] agree with the data obtained from experimental animals.

In contrast to the preceding tubular portions, the epithelial lining of each of the segments following the TAL display at least two distinct cell types: one cell type is segment-specific and called accordingly DCT cell, CNT cell, and CD cell; the other one, the intercalated cell (IC cell), is interspersed in differing amounts among the specific cells of each segment.[542] The transition from one segment to the next may be sharp and unequivocally definable, e.g., as in rabbits[5,268] or they may develop gradually, involving more-or-less long transitional portions with a mixture of cells from the successive segments or with cells showing features intermediate between the segment-specific cell types of the given segments.[535] The presence of a rather long transitional portion between the definite DCT and CNT in rats,[543,544] in mice,[537,538] and in humans[539] claimed a subdivision of the DCT in these species into the "early" DCT and the "transitional portion"[538,545] or the DCT 1 and the DCT 2,[537] respectively. Taken the morphological data of the various species (except rabbits!) together it is obvious that the segmentation of the cortical tubular portion distal of Henle's loop is a matter of definition.[544] The nowadays conventionally-used segment definitions for the DCT, the CNT and the CCD (Figure 20.55) take into account the structural data and the distribution of the major apical salt and water transport proteins (Figure 20.55). The uptake by the cell type-specific transport proteins in the luminal plasma membrane into the cell and the movement across and out of the cell is facilitated by a bunch of "auxiliary" cytoplasmic and/or basolateral membrane proteins (e.g., Na-K-ATPase, Ca-binding proteins, K-channels, hormone receptors, etc.). These "auxiliary" proteins are not restricted to the given cell type and thus, are not segment-specific. The inventory of gene expressions (*in situ* hybridization of mouse kidney sections with annotations) in given segments can be looked up in the "Euregene Expression Database." "The Kidney Atlas" (http://www.euregene.org/portal/pages/index.html).

The segmentation of the CD into cortical (CCD), outer medullary (OMCD), and inner medullary CD (IMCD) is based mainly on the location in the given zones. The structural differences between the CCD and

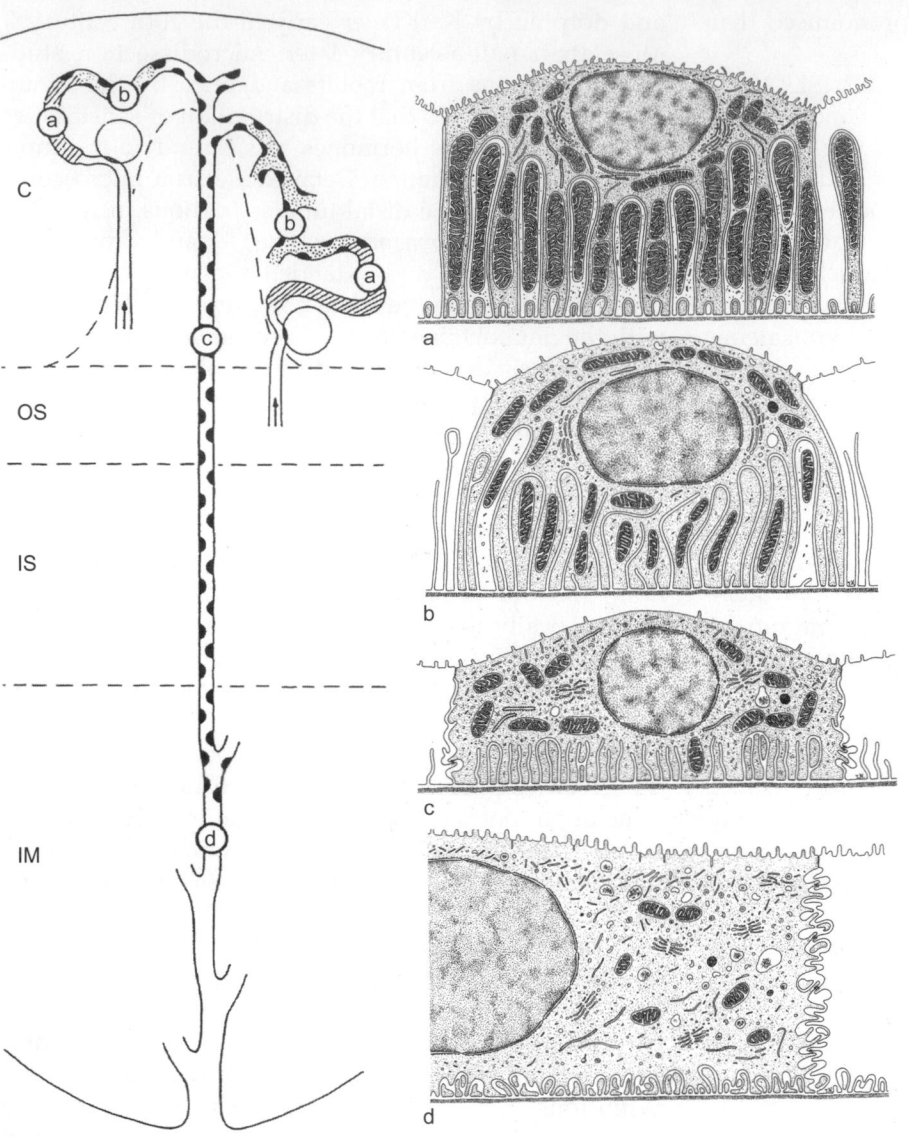

FIGURE 20.54 Survey on organization of the cortical distal segments and collecting ducts (left panel) and on ultrastructure of the segment-specific cells (right panel). (C: cortex; OS: outer stripe; IS: inner stripe of the outer medulla; IM: inner medulla; Dashed line: delimits the medullary ray; (a): distal convoluted tubule (DCT) and DCT-cell; (b): connecting tubule (CNT) and CNT-cell; (c): CCD and CCD cell; (d): inner medulla (IM) and IMCD cell; Black semicircles indicate the occurrence of intercalated (IC) cells.) Each DCT opens into one CNT. In superficial nephrons the CNT opens directly into a CCD; connecting tubules of deeper nephrons join to form an arcades which ascend in the cortical labyrinth, before they open into a CCD. The collecting ducts descend in the medullary rays and through the outer and inner stripes of the outer medulla; the lower two-thirds of the collecting duct are lined by IMCD cells exclusively; the IMCD open as papillary ducts on the renal papilla. *(Adapted from and Kaissling, B., and Kriz, W. (1992). In "Morphology of the Loop of Henle, Distal Tubule and Collecting Duct. Handbook of Physiology: Section on Renal Physiology," 109–167, Windhager, E. E. Oxford University Press, New York, with permission).*

OMCD cells are quantitative rather than qualitative. Usually, the IMCD does not display any more IC cells in its two lower thirds and the lining cells (IMCD cells) are regarded as a separate cell type[546] (Figure 20.54).

Distal Convoluted Tubule (DCT)

The DCT reabsorbs 5–10% of the filtered Na-load[547] and determines the final urinary Mg^{2+} concentration through active transcellular transport.[548] In addition, the transitional portion (DCT2) participates (together with the subsequent CNT; see below) in regulation of calcium excretion by transcellular calcium reabsorption.[538,549] The DCT epithelium is water-impermeable, similar as the preceding TAL.

The abrupt increase in epithelial height (Figure 20.56)[550,544] marks the beginning of the DCT. This prominent feature in the tubular epithelium has been observed in all mammalian species investigated so far, and it coincides exactly with the replacement in the luminal membrane of the NKCC2, characterizing the TAL cells, by the thiazide-inhibitable sodium chloride co-transporter, NCC, characterizing the DCT cells.[547] The NCC characterizes all DCT cells (DCT1 and DCT2). The breaking off of NCC expression defines the end of the DCT.[537] It is sharp in rabbits,[551] but it drops off over a more or less long distance in mice and rat.[538]

The DCT epithelium is organized by laterally interdigitating cells (Figures 20.57 and 20.58a) similar to the TAL, yet the lateral folding excludes the apical cell portion in DCT cells. The amount of Na-K-ATPase,[279] the

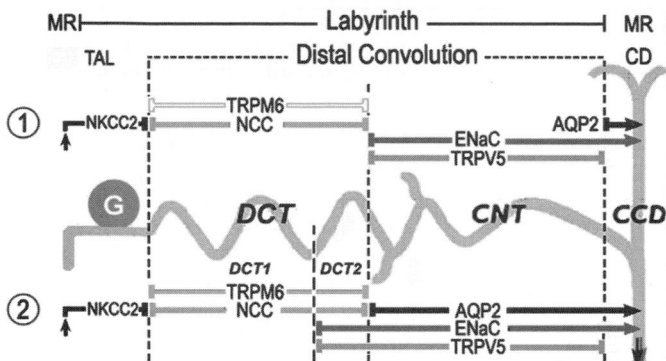

FIGURE 20.55 **Schematic distribution of the major apical transport proteins (NKCC2, NCC, TRPM6, TRPV5, ENaC, and AQP2) along the cortical distal segments.** (1) In rabbit; and (2) in rat, mouse, and human (MR: medullary ray; TAL: thick ascending limb; G: renal corpuscle; DCT: distal convoluted tubule; CNT: connecting tubule; CCD: cortical collecting duct). Sharp beginning and stop of a transporter along the cortical nephron is indicated by vertical bars, the continuation along the CD by arrows.

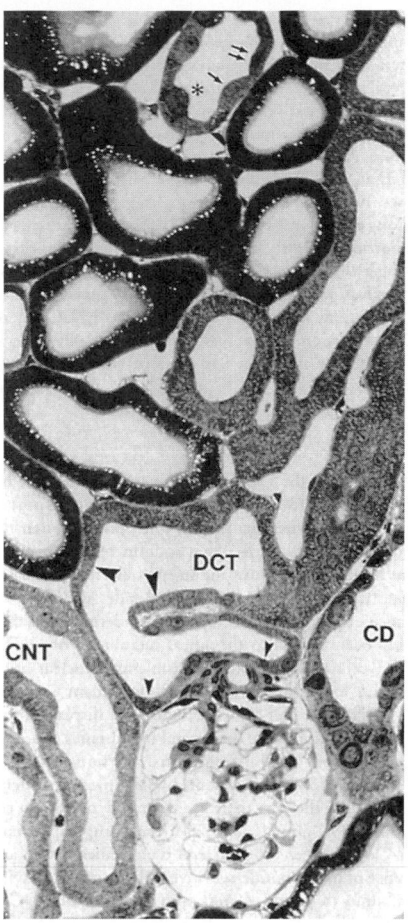

FIGURE 20.56 **Distal tubular segments beyond the macula densa.** Small arrowheads delimit the macula densa, large arrowheads point to the transition from the epithelium of the thick ascending limb to the distal convoluted tubule (DCT) (CNT: connecting tubule; CD: cortical collecting duct). The tubule profile in the upper portion of the micrograph has a mixed cell population, composed of CNT cells (arrow), CD cells (double arrow), and IC cells (asterisk) and represents the transition from a CNT to a cortical CD (rat: TEM: ×~500).

surface area of basolateral membranes and the volume density of mitochondria[280] are the highest of all tubular cells[41] (Figure 20.26). The large lamella-like mitochondria are narrowly enveloped by the lateral interdigitating plasma membrane foldings, all other cell organelles are situated in the apical cytoplasm: the nucleus; the distinct Golgi apparatus; numerous small mitochondrial profiles; short cisterns of rough endoplasmic reticulum; and abundant smooth small, invaginated vesicles closely beneath the apical plasma membrane.[260,552] Lysosomes are less frequently observed in DCT cells. The microtubular system in DCT cells is much more prominent than in proximal tubule cells. The tight junctional belt has a similar organization as in the TAL, but is shorter since the apical portions of the DCT cells have a polygonal outline. The intercellular space has a regular width of about 50 nm and is bridged by an intercellular skeleton.[553] The apical plasma membrane carries numerous stubby microvilli. Single cilia are present on the center of all DCT cells.

In the transitional portion (DCT-2) the lateral folding is progressively superseded by infoldings of the basal plasmalemma which may extend into the apical cell pole. The infolded membranes carry a few caveolae on their cytoplasmic face.[260] This structural observation is confirmed by the finding of caveolin in late DCT cells.[554,555] Size and volume density of mitochondria slightly decrease along the DCT2.

In rats, mice, and humans the appearance of basal plasmalemma infoldings of the DCT cells coincides with the most upstream appearance of intercalated cells. In rabbits, a species that lacks a transitional segment (DCT2), infoldings of the basal plasmalemma and

the most upstream appearance of IC cells mark the beginning of the CNT.

Functional Data

Sodium chloride reabsorption by the DCT proceeds via the electro-neutral Na^+-Cl^- co-transporter (NCC) in the apical plasma membrane of DCT cells. NCC is specifically inhibitable by thiazide diuretics,[547,556] which are frequently used in the treatment of hypertension.[547] The driving force for influx of NaCl via NCC is generated by the Na-K-ATPase activity in the basolateral membrane of DCT cells. The basolateral chloride channel, subunit b (ClC-Kb),[479,556,557] extrudes Cl^- ions at the basolateral side of DCT cells. Potassium handling, associated with NCC-mediated transport,

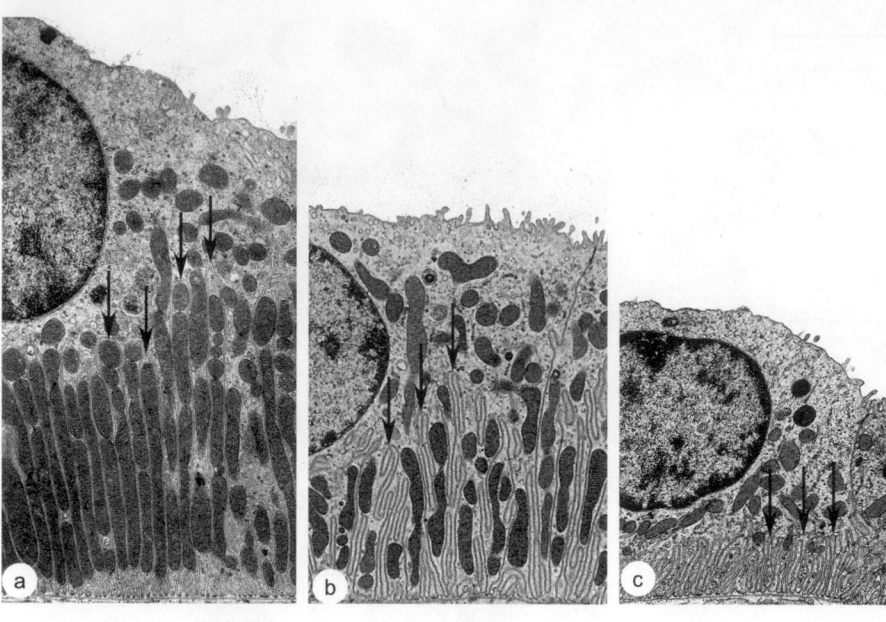

FIGURE 20.57 Organization of distal and collecting duct cells in the renal cortex; (a) and (b) *Psammomys obesus*; (c) rat; fixation by reduced osmium. (a) DCT cell, interdigitating, lateral cell processes (arrows) narrowly enclose large mitochondria; (b) CNT cell, displaying a few interdigitating lateral cell processes and abundant infoldings of the basal plasma membrane (arrows), extending up into the apical cell half; most mitochondria are aligned between the infolded membranes; (c) non-interdigitating CCD cell; all infoldings of the basal plasma membrane are restricted to the basal cell portion; the location of mitochondria above the basal rim of infolded membranes is characteristic for CD cells (TEM: ×~10 000).

involves ROMK, detectable by immunomethods in the cytoplasm of DCT1,[481,558] and in the apical membrane of DCT2 cells, and BK channels.[558,559]

The NaCl transport rates by the DCT epithelium are linked with NCC surface expression. It is regulated (among others) by the luminal NaCl-load,[560] dietary salt,[561] by angiotensin II,[562–564] and by sex hormones.[565] Although mineralocorticoid receptors have been detected in the DCT,[547] aldosterone has no effect on NCC-mediated transport since beta hydroxysteroid-dehydrogenase, which confers mineralocorticoid specificity to the receptor, is lacking in DCT1.[562]

Changes in NCC surface expression are effected by trafficking of the co-transporter from the subapical vesicular compartment into[564] and removal by endocytosis[566] from, respectively, the apical plasmalemma, and by altering the NCC degradation rate through the lysosomal pathway.[567,568]

Kinases, such as the serum- and glucocorticoid-inducible kinase, SGK1, with-no-lysine kinases WNK1 and WNK4, both themselves controlled by NaCl intake, play an important role in this regulation.[559,561,569–571] WNKs promote NCC-targeting to the lysosome for degradation.[572] WNK signaling is implicated in the coordination of transcellular and paracellular flux to achieve NaCl and K$^+$ homeostasis.[250]

Recent data obtained in genetically vasopressin-deficient Brattleboro rats suggest that vasopressin and the vasopressin-V2 receptor-NCC signaling cascade might play a role in the short-term regulation of NCC in the apical plasmalemma of DCT cells.[573,574] Vasopressin-dependent increases in cAMP had not been recorded in the DCT of rats and other species.[534,575]

Chronic increases in the NaCl-transport rates in the DCT, induced in rabbits by high dietary Na-intake combined with low K-intake[280,281] or in rats by rises in NaCl-delivery due to impaired NaCl-reabsorption in the preceding TAL, provoke extensive structural compensatory hypertrophy in the DCT,[290,292,304,576,577] including substantial increases in the DNA synthesis rate in DCT cells.[305,578] These changes occur in the presence, but also in the absence, of increased plasma levels of mineralocorticoids,[578] and are mediated most probably by angiotensin II.[562]

In line with these earlier structural observations are recent studies in a ROMK-deficient mice model for Bartter's syndrome with loss of TAL function. The ROMK-deficient mice reveal hypertrophy of the DCT epithelium, with compensatory upregulation of NaCl reabsorption via the thiazide-sensitive NCC co-transporter.[579,580]

The renal abundance and the NCC-labeling in DCT were found to be profoundly and selectively decreased in aldosterone-escape rats, suggesting that the thiazide-sensitive NaCl co-transporter may be the chief molecular target for regulatory processes responsible for mineralocorticoid escape via a post-transcriptional mechanism.[581]

The DCT determines the final urinary Mg^{2+} concentration through active transcellular transport.[504,548,582,583] The transient receptor potential channel melastatin subtype 6 (TRPM6),[548,584] co-localizes with NCC, at least in the early DCT (DCT1), and is regarded as a likely candidate for influx of Mg^{2+} across the luminal membrane. This influx apparently requires the presence of the gamma subunit of the renal Na-K-APTase in the basolateral membrane of the

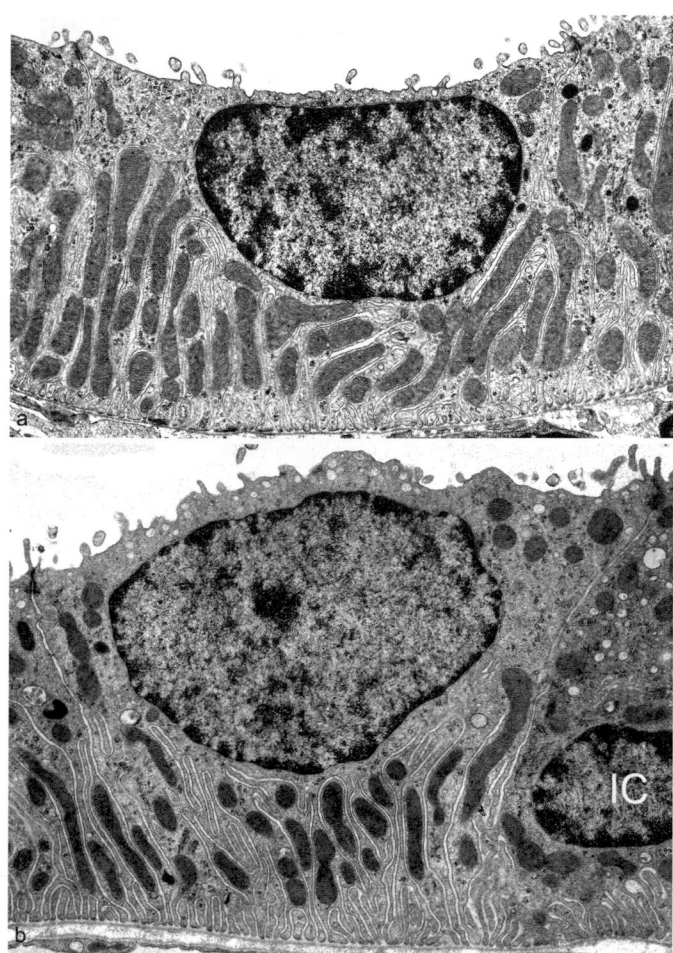

FIGURE 20.58 Ultrastructure of distal convoluted tubule cells (rat kidney). (a) Cell in the early and (b) late portion of the DCT; in (a) characteristic apical position of the nucleus and location of the mitochondria in basolateral interdigitating cell processes; the volume density of mitochondria is high; in (b) the amount of basal plasma membrane infoldings is higher than in (a), the amount of mitochondria is lower; the most upstream appearance of intercalated cells (IC) is in the late DCT (TEM: ×~5400).

calbindinD28k, and is prominent in the early part of the DCT of mice.[537,538] PV seems also to play a role in the endogenous NCC expression in DCT cells by modulating intracellular Ca^{2+} signaling in response to ATP.[590]

The key players for paracellular Mg^{2+}-transport, Claudin 16 (paracellin1) and Claudin 19, are both detected in the DCT tight junction,[497] and may enable paracellular Mg^{2+}-movement across the DCT epithelium in addition to the transcellular Mg^{2+}-transport. The tight junction protein Claudin 7 has been found to be highly expressed in the distal convoluted tubules (and collecting ducts) of the mature kidney, suggesting that it may play a role in paracellular NaCl and K handling.[240,591,592]

DCT 2

This transitional segment expresses, in addition to NCC, the amiloride-sensitive epithelial sodium channel, ENaC. The onset of ENaC in the apical plasma membrane coincides with the most upstream appearance of intercalated cells (see below), apical immunoexpression of ROMK. The eyecatching beginning of prominent cytoplasmic immunostaining for Vitamin D-dependent calbindin-D28k, and the marked increase in immunostaining for PMCA and NCX in the basolateral plasma membrane go along with the onset in the luminal membrane of the epithelial calcium channel, TRPV5,[538] the gatekeeper for renal epithelial Ca^{2+} transport.[593] ENaC and TRPV5 are coexpressed in the CNT and will be discussed there.

Rabbits have no DCT2; in this species the transition from the DCT to the CNT is sharp and marked by an abrupt change in cell structure,[280] coinciding with the abrupt onset of ENaC[538] in the apical membrane, as well as the onset of the TRPV5[594] (Figure 20.55), and also the appearance of IC cells.

Dysfunctions of NaCl Reabsorption in the DCT

Inhibition of NCC in rats treated for three to four days with thiazide diuretics induces massive rates of apoptotic cell death of DCT cells in the early part of the DCT, while the late part of the segment with the additional sodium entry pathway ENaC remains intact.[307] If the transport activity of the early DCT cells is inhibited for only a few days, the epithelium rapidly and fully recovers within a few days after removal of the drug.

In loss-of-function mutations of the NCC gene in mice,[595] permanent, dramatic atrophy of the early DCT portion is seen.[545] These data highlight the eminent importance of the transport activity in maintaining and modeling the tubular epithelium. Loss-of-function mutations in the NCC-gene in humans cause "Gitelman's syndrome." This syndrome is characterized by mild

DCT cells.[276,585] Transcription factor HNF1B (hepatocyte nuclear factor 1 homeobox B) is proposed to regulate the expression of the g-subunit of the Na^+/K^+-ATPase.[586] In addition to the Na-K-ATPase, the DCT cells weakly display the plasma membrane $Ca^{2+}(Mg^{2+})$-ATPase (PMCA)[307,587] and the sodium—calcium exchanger (NCX).[544]

The epidermal growth factor (EGF) expressed by the DCT epithelium[473,588,589] seems to be involved in TRPM6-mediated regulation of active Mg^{2+} reabsorption. Transcellular magnesium reabsorption via TRPM6 seems to critically depend on low levels of free intracellular magnesium, putatively kept low by the cytoplasmic calcium-binding protein parvalbumin (PV). PV has a several-fold higher binding capacity for magnesium than the calcium-binding protein renal sodium-wasting, hypocalciuria, hypomagnesaemia, hypokaliemic alkalosis, and reduced blood pressure in humans.[596-599]

Mutations in the NCC-regulating WNK1 and WNK4 increase NCC activity, and cause Gordon's Syndrome (Pseudohypoaldosteronism type II - PAH II). The symptoms of this disease comprise arterial hypertension, hyperkaliaemia, hypercalciuria and hypermagnesaemia, and mirror Gitelman's disease.[251,567,600] Loss-of-function mutations of one or several of the genes involved in Mg^{2+} reabsorption are associated with hypomagnesemia,[601] characteristic for Gordon's syndrome.[602]

Connecting Tubule (CNT)

In all species the epithelium of the CNT is lined by two distinct cell types (Figure 20.59): the segment-specific CNT cells; and the intercalated cells (IC cells) (see below). The segment-specific CNT cells display the calcium channel TRPV5 and the amiloride-sensitive epithelial sodium channel (ENaC) in their apical plasma membrane. In rats, mice, and humans they display, in addition, the vasopressin-regulated water channel, aquaporin-2 (AQP2) (Figure 20.55). In these species the emergence of AQP2 in the apical plasmalemma in the epithelial lining defines the beginning of the CNT, since TRPV5 and ENaC already appear in the transitional region (DCT2) (see Figure 20.55). Contrastingly, in rabbits vasopressin-regulated water channels are lacking in the CNT. In rabbits the beginning of the CNT is defined by a distinct change in epithelial structure, expression of TRPV5 and ENaC, and the first incidence of intercalated cells[544] (Figure 20.55). Evidently, the CNT shares cytological and functional features ascribed to both the nephron (derived from the metanephrogenic blastema) and the collecting duct (derived from the ureteric bud). The assignment of the CNT to either the nephron or the collecting ducts is disputed.[36,37,603,604]

CNT Cell Organization

The organization of CNT cells (Figures 20.54b, 20.57b, and 20.59b) is similar to that of DCT2 cells, i.e., intermediate between the DCT cells with basolateral membrane surface augmentation by interdigitating lateral folds and the non-interdigitating epithelia (CD cells) with basal plasma membrane infoldings.

The apical and the basal outlines of CNT cells approach a polygonal shape, and the cells are smoothly apposed to each other. The basolateral plasma membrane area is increased predominantly by folding of the basal plasma membrane into the cell. The infolded plasma membranes may extend into the most apical

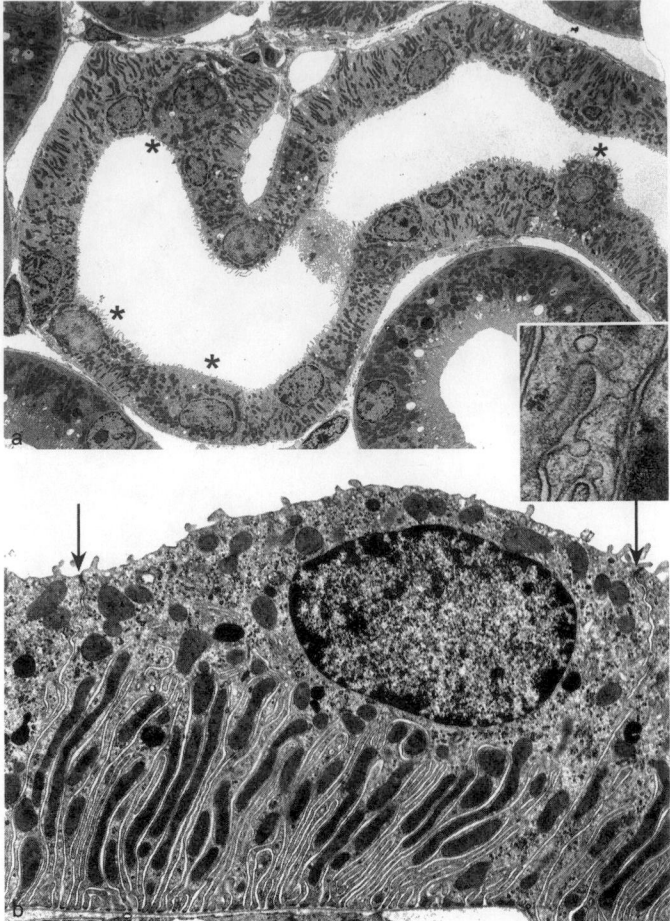

FIGURE 20.59　Connecting tubule (rat kidney). (a) The epithelium is composed of CNT cells and IC cells, (asterisks). (b) Characteristic CNT cell with abundant infoldings of the basal cell membrane; the arrows point to the tight junction. Insert: The infolded plasma membranes reveal numerous caveolae (TEM (a): ×~1400; (b): ×~6100).

cell portion, and are endowed with abundant caveolae on their cytoplasmic face[260,554] (Figure 20.59). The extracellular spaces between the basal plasma membrane foldings and the lateral intercellular spaces have no direct continuity and are usually narrow.[260] The apical plasma membrane with short slender microvilli is delimited from the lateral plasma membrane by rather deep tight junctions, composed of several anastomosing strands.[427] The nucleus, the Golgi apparatus, polyribosomes, very short profiles of rER, and elongated and small round mitochondrial profiles are located in the cytoplasm between or above the infolded membranes. Smooth vesicles are particularly abundant in the apical half of CNT cells. In contrast to DCT cells, small lysosomes are frequent in CNT cells.

From the beginning to the end of the segment, the height of the CNT cells, the extent of basal plasma membrane, and their volume density of mitochondria decrease. The steepness of the axial changes is more pronounced in rabbits[280] and mice than in rats, and varies with the functional conditions.[605,606]

Functional Aspects

Calcium Reabsorption

Microperfusion[607] and micropuncture studies had located active Ca^{2+} reabsorption to the distal convolution, including the DCT and CNT (for review see [608]) a long time before the specific Ca^{2+}-channel in the distal segments, TRPV5, was known.. The localization of TRPV5[609] in the apical plasmalemma of the late distal tubule (DCT2 cells and CNT cells[538]) (Figure 20.55) unequivocally identified these segments as sites for active transcellular Ca^{2+} reabsorption in the kidney. The paracellular pathway in these segments is impermeable for Ca^{2+}.

The cytoplasmic calcium-binding protein, calbindin D28k, the sodium calcium exchanger, NCX, and the plasma membrane calcium-Mg ATPase, PMCA, located in the basolateral plasma membrane, are auxiliary proteins necessary for TRPV5-mediated transcellular calcium movement. All three reveal very heavy immunostaining in DCT2 and CNT cells.[537,538] Upon its entry into the cell via TRPV5, calbindinD28k buffers Ca^{2+} and the basolateral Ca^{2+} transporters NCX and PMCA extrude Ca^{2+} into the interstitial compartment.[593] Interestingly, in tubular flow direction immunostaining for TRPV5 progressively shifts from the apical plasma membrane into the cytoplasm,[538] associated with parallel decreases of immuno-traceability for cytoplasmic calbindinD28k, for basolateral PMCA and for NCX. These changes most probably indicate respective changes of transcellular calcium transport rates.

Regulation of transcellular Ca^{2+} transport rates involves changes in the apical channel abundance and direct TRPV5 channel activation.[610] Via binding to its receptor (PTH/PTHrP) in the basolateral plasma membrane of CNT cells,[611–613] parathyroid hormone (PTH) increases the protein expression of TRPV5[593,614] and via a cAMP-PKA signaling pathway PTH increases the channel opening probability.[615] Transcription of the Ca^{2+} channel is regulated by the active form of vitamin D_3, 1,25-dihydroxyvitamin D_3 (1,25$(OH)_2D_3$).[594,616] The male and female sex hormones, estrogens and androgens, also play a role in renal Ca^{2+} handling.[617] Urinary klotho stimulates TRPV5 channel activity at the apical membrane, whereas intracellular klotho enhances basolateral Na-K-ATPase surface expression

that activates NCX-mediated Ca^{2+} efflux.[593] Urinary tissue kallikrein (TK) activates a bradykinin receptor (BK2) in the apical membrane of segment-specific CNT cells,[618] and thereby stimulates TRPV5-mediated Ca^{2+} influx.[615,619–621] The sites of TK synthesis in the kidney are approximately congruent with the sites of calcium reabsorption, i.e, the late DCT and CNT.[618] These findings suggest that TK may be a physiologic regulator of renal tubular calcium transport.[622,623] Kallikrein synthesis in the CNT and its subsequent release into the urine are stimulated by aldosterone,[624] dietary Na^+ restriction,[618] and in particular by dietary K^+ loading.[625,626] TK knockout mice display a somewhat delayed kaliuretic response to potassium loading.[623,627]

Sodium Reabsorption

The amiloride-sensitive sodium channel, ENaC, is the key player in the final sodium recovery by the kidney.[628,629] ENaC is a heteromultimeric channel composed of three homologous subunits (α, β, γ).[630] Full activity of ENaC requires the co-expression of all three subunits in the luminal membrane.

The activity of amiloride-sensitive transport is under the tight control of aldosterone.[631] Therefore, all segments with ENaC-mediated sodium reabsorption — DCT2, CNT, and CD — are collectively designated as "aldosterone-sensitive distal nephron" (ASDN[632]). While the mineralocorticoid receptor (MR) is expressed in all distal segments,[633] only the renal ENaC-expressing portions display the enzyme 11-β-hydroxysteroid dehydrogenase type 2 (11βHSD2),[605,606,634–639] which confers mineralocorticoid specificity to the MR. The rate-limiting factor for transepithelial Na^+ transport in the ASDN is the activity and abundance of ENaC in the luminal membrane of the ENaC-expressing cells.

Under control conditions[605,606] all three EnaC subunits are well detectable by immunostainings in the apical plasma membrane of the DCT2- and CNT-cells.[605,606] Along the course of the CNT and CD-segments all three subunits become undetectable in the apical plasmalemma, but heavily accumulate in the cytoplasm.[605,606,639] The decline in available channels in the luminal membrane is paralleled by reduction of basal infoldings and of mitochondria, most evident along the CNT epithelium and by a respective progressive decline of Na^+ transport activity along the axis of the ASDN (CNT > CCD).[604,640] The physiological relevance of ENaC-mediated Na^+ transport in the CNT is highlighted by the observation that the collecting duct-specific deletion of the alpha ENaC gene in mice[604] is fully compensated by the residual activity of ENaC in the upstream located CNT (and in the DCT2).[604]

In fact, recent data on the three-dimensional reconstruction of the mouse nephron show that five to seven nephrons are connected via a CNT to a single CCD.[34] Thus, the collected luminal surface for ENaC-mediated sodium reabsorption in the late DCTs and the CNT,[37,641] is several-fold greater than that available in the CCD itself.

All factors involved in regulation of sodium transport rates in the ASDN (hormones, proteases, intra-, and extracellular ion concentrations, tubular flow rate, as well as kinases and interacting proteins (for review see [562,642–644]), ultimately target the ENaC channel activity or abundance in the apical plasma membrane. Changes in ENaC abundance in the luminal plasma membrane involve channel synthesis, exocytotic delivery of subunits to the cell surface, and endocytotic retrieval of channels from the luminal membrane and their degradation.[300,562,628,644,645]

Endogeneous increases in plasma aldosterone levels rapidly induce (within hours) activation and redistribution of ENaC subunits from intracellular compartments to the apical plasma membrane[605,631,639,646] and a decrease of internalization of ENaC through the synthesis of SGK1.[647–649] Prolonged changes in EnaC-mediated sodium transport promote respective changes in cell height, abundance of basolateral plasma membrane infoldings, and the density of mitochondria,[280,290,292,293] which all together reflect the changes in Na^+ transport rates.

ENaC channel activity and abundance in the apical plasma membrane of the ASDN is also target of other hormones. The co-expression of ENaC with vasopressin receptors (V1 and V2) and vasopressin-sensitive water channels AQP2 in rat-, mice-, and human-segment-specific CNT (not in rabbit CNT cells) suggests the mutual interaction of sodium and water transport.[650,651] Indeed, vasopressin facilitates the translocation of ENaC to the apical membrane[652] and on removal of a V2R agonist ENaC is endocytosed from the membrane surface and reorganized into recycling vesicles, with a mechanism similar to that described for AQP2 regulation.[653] The delivery of somewhat water-depleted tubular fluid from the CNTs to the cortical collecting duct might enhance the urinary concentration process in the CD. Interestingly, in rabbits, in which the CNT lacks vasopressin-sensitive water channels, the arcades open at a much higher cortical level into the cortical collecting duct than in rats, mice or humans.[37]

Insulin and insulin-like growth factor,[610] angiotensin II[654–656] kinases, interacting proteins, intra-, and extracellular ion concentrations, osmolarity (for review see [645]), locally released nucleotides, and tubular flow rate (for review see [657]) have also been shown to modulate ENaC-mediated Na-transport activity.

Potassium Transport

In all ENaC-displaying cells renal outer medulla potassium channel ROMK is strongly expressed in the luminal membrane, where it co-localizes with PDZ proteins (NHERF2).[272] ENaC-mediated sodium reabsorption is coupled in a fixed ratio with K secretion via the ROMK. K^+ enters the cell by the activity of the Na-K-ATPase in the basolateral membrane, and exits into the tubular fluid via ROMK. The ratio of sodium-reabsorption and K-secretion by the segment-specific (CNT; CD cells)[658] can be modulated by intercalated cells which are bound to ENaC-displaying epithelia. The proton secretion by IC cells via a H-K-ATPase can apparently be coupled with K reabsorption.[659] Therefore, the ASDN is also the tubular site for net renal potassium (K^+) excretion.[482,660] The main factors regulating K^+ secretion are dietary K^+ intake and aldosterone (for review see [562]).

Mutations in the genes coding for ENaC subunits,[628,629] and for proteins involved in ENaC-associated K-secretion (ROMK),[661] as well as the correct targeting into or removal from the membrane (e.g., SGK1, Nedd4-2; for review see [645]) are associated with severe disturbances of blood pressure regulation.[662]

Transition From CNT tO CCD

In rodents and humans no marked structural change indicates the transition from the CNT to the CCD. Morphologically, the CCD can be defined by its location in the medullary ray. In difference, in rabbits the clear-cut onset of vasopressin-regulated water permeability marks the beginning of the CCD. It is associated with the appearance of dilated intercellular spaces in the epithelium[5,280] and the change of segment-specific cells, i.e., from CNT- to CD-cells.

By immunostaining, the beginning of the CCD is defined in rodents and rabbits by the break-off of TRPV5 (Figure 20.55) and related proteins (NCX, calbindin D28k[538,544]). In humans, NCX and calbindin D28k have also been detected in the CCD.[539]

Collecting Ducts

The CCD, the OMCD, and the upper part of the IMCD are composed of segment-specific cells (CD cells) and intercalated cells (IC cells; see subsequent sections) (Figure 20.54). The CD cells (Figures 20.54, 20.57, 20.60 and 20.61) have simple polygonal basal and apical outlines. Their most characteristic feature is the narrowly arranged basal plasmalemma infoldings of uniform height (Figures 20.54, 20.57, and 20.60) at the base of the cells, easily recognizable in light- and electron-microscopy as a basal light rim. All major cell organelles — the nucleus, small mitochondria, numerous small Golgi-fields, abundant profiles of smooth ER, and a few of rough ER, lysosomes, multivesicular bodies, and occasional glycogen accumulations — are located in the zone above the infolded membranes. The subapical zone often reveals small round or elongated vesicles, oriented either perpendicularly or at an oblique angle to the luminal membrane (Figure 20.61c). These vesicles contain aggregates of AQP2, and are called aggrephores. Many of the aggrephores carry spherical clathrin-coated heads. The tight junctional belt is deep and consists of anastomosing strands with high particle density.[663] The apical plasma membrane generally bears only a few short slender microvilli or microfolds. The prominent central single cilia on the collecting duct-specific cells (Figure 20.62a) have been proposed as the key structural element in the Ca^{2+} response to fluid shear stress.[312,664] Short microvilli or folds of the lateral plasma membrane project into

the intercellular space, and are connected by small desmosomes with those of adjacent cells (Figure 20.62b). In marked contrast to the water-impermeable epithelia of the TAL and the DCT, the width of the intercellular spaces between CD cells as well as the space between the infolded basal plasma membranes may be largely dilated or narrow, correlating with bulk water flow across the epithelium (see below).

The cytoskeleton is particularly prominent in CD cells. Actin filaments and microtubules form a dense meshwork along the apical and lateral plasma membrane. The cytoskeleton is essential for the shuttling of AQP2 to and from the plasmalemma (see below). Furthermore, the prominent cytoskeleton may be one mean, among others, to withstand the varying osmotic pressure in the collecting duct.

The CD cell undergoes gradual, although considerable, changes from the deep cortex (CCD) downstream to the upper third of the inner zone (IMCD) (Figure 20.61). The extent of basal plasma membrane foldings and the volume density of mitochondria decrease from the cortex towards the inner zone, whereas the volume density of lysosomes and the density of cytoskeletal proteins increase. The degree of changes along the CD differs among species.[5,260,540]

The CD cells in the lower two-thirds of the inner medulla are distinguished as inner medullary collecting duct cells (IMCD cells).[552] In rabbit[5] and guinea pig, IMCD cells increase in height toward the papilla up to 20-fold. A substantial, albeit less dramatic, increase occurs in rhesus monkey[665] and in human kidney.[540] In other species (e.g., rat, mouse, *Psammomys*, and dog[260]) the epithelium near the tip of the papilla is cuboidal or low columnar. The luminal membrane of IMCD cells is covered by numerous stubby microvilli, and generally lacks the central cilium.[546] The lateral intercellular spaces are conspicuous by their dense assembly of microvilli and microfolds, projecting from the lateral cell membranes. In the beginning of the inner medullary collecting duct (IMCD) the tight junctions are complex and consist of several anastomosing strands.[260] Toward the papillary tip in rat and rabbit, there is a considerable decrease in the number of strands, and in the apico—basal depth of the junction.[260]

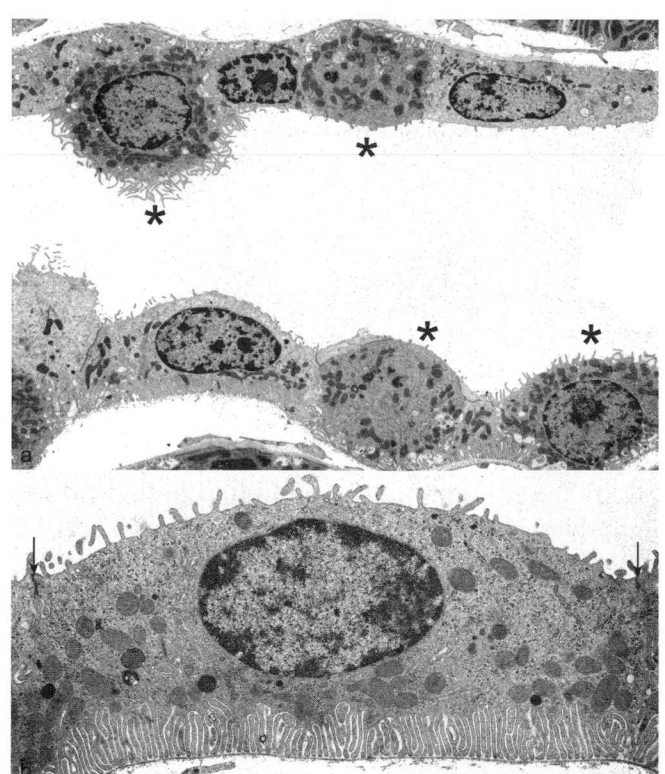

FIGURE 20.60 Cortical collecting duct (rat kidney). (a) The epithelium is composed of CD cells and IC cells. (b) CCD cell — infoldings of the basal plasma membrane are restricted to the basal cell portion; all mitochondria and cell organelles are located above the infolded membranes (Arrows: Tight junctions; TEM (a): $\times \sim 2700$; (b): $\times \sim 8500$). *(Adapted from and Kaissling, B., and Kriz, W. (1992). In "Morphology of the Loop of Henle, Distal Tubule and Collecting Duct. Handbook of Physiology: Section on Renal Physiology," 109—167, Windhager, E. E. Oxford University Press, New York, with permission).*

Sodium Reabsorption in the Collecting Duct

Together with the vasopressin-regulated water-channel AQP2, the CD cells consistently express the amiloride-sensitive Na-channel ENaC (see CNT)[666] (Figure 20.55) and ROMK. The coexistence of the differentially regulated pathways for water- and Na-reabsorption in the same cell suggest the possibility for mutual interactions.[650,666,667]

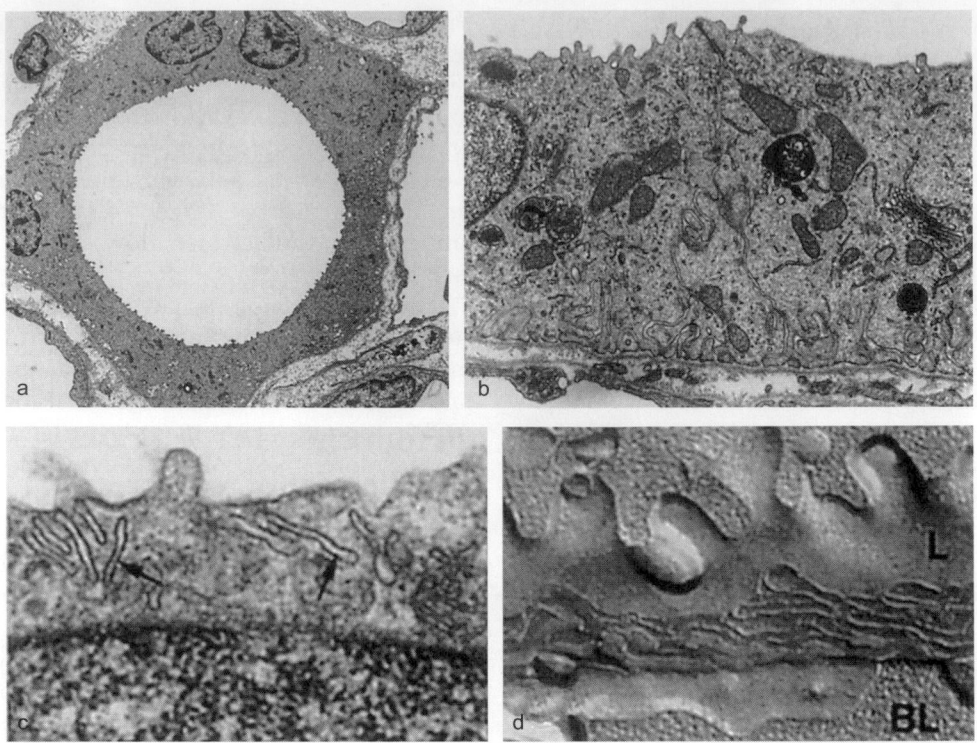

FIGURE 20.61 Inner medullary collecting duct. (a) Tubular profile showing the homogenous epithelium (rat: TEM: ×~3400). (b) Epithelium of the middle portion of an IMCD. Within the epithelium three zones are seen: a basal zone with basal infoldings, a middle zone containing Golgi fields, mitochondria and lysosomal elements, and a thin apical zone with tubular and vesicular profiles. Note the deep tight junction (rat: TEM: ×~17,000). (c) Apical zone of a CD cell with many elongated tubular profiles (arrows) which are believed to represent agrophores (rat: TEM: ×~38,000). (d) Freeze-fracture electron micrograph to show the multistranded tight junction of the collecting duct epithelium (L: luminal membrane; BL: basolateral membrane; Rabbit: ×~34,000).

Recently, a second pathway for electroneutral NaCl absorption has been revealed in the collecting duct epithelium, This pathway is located in the intercalated cells (see below) and is insensitive to amiloride but inhibited by thiazides, and couples 2 anion exchangers, pendrin and Na-driven chloride/bicarbonate exchanger (NDCBE)[668,669] (see "Intercalated Cells").

Paracrine and autocrine regulation by the purinergic system[296,657,670,671] mediates flow-and metabolic rate-dependent changes of Na^+ and water transport in the collecting duct.

Vasopressin-Regulated Water and Urea Reabsorption in the Collecting Duct

Collecting ducts are the canonical targets for vasopressin-sensitive water and urea reabsorption.[672] They display receptors for vasopressin (V_1 and V_2) in the basolateral plasma membrane of the segment-specific cells, the CD cells,[519] and vasopressin-sensitive water channels AQP2. Water permeability of the luminal membrane is achieved by exocytotic insertion of the vasopressin-regulated water-channel AQP2 from subapical vesicles (aggrephores) into the apical cell membrane. The exocytosis is triggered by binding of vasopressin (ADH) to the V2-receptor at the basolateral membrane of CD cells and the subsequent signal transduction cascade. The aggregates of AQP2 in the aggrephores are colocalized with dynein and dynactin.[673] Many of the aggrephores carry spherical clathrin-coated heads. With low levels of vasopressin, the AQP2-containing membrane portions recycle back into the subapical cytoplasm.[299,674−676] The movement of aggrephores critically depends on microtubules and actin filaments in the apical cytoplasm.

High levels of vasopressin-independent AQP2 surface expression have been observed under long-term[677] and acute[678] exposure of rats and mice to statins. Applied chronically, statins decrease membrane cholesterol[679] and clathrin-mediated endocytosis of AQP2. Acutely, the statins seem to decrease endocytosis of AQP2 and vesicle trafficking by modulating Rho-GTPase,[678] which is involved in regulation of the cytoskeleton, endocytosis, and vesicle trafficking.[680,681] The water channels AQP3 and AQP4 are both located in the basolateral membrane of CD cells.[682] AQP3 is permeable to glycerol, urea, and water; AQP4 is associated with orthogonal arrays of intramembrane particles, as

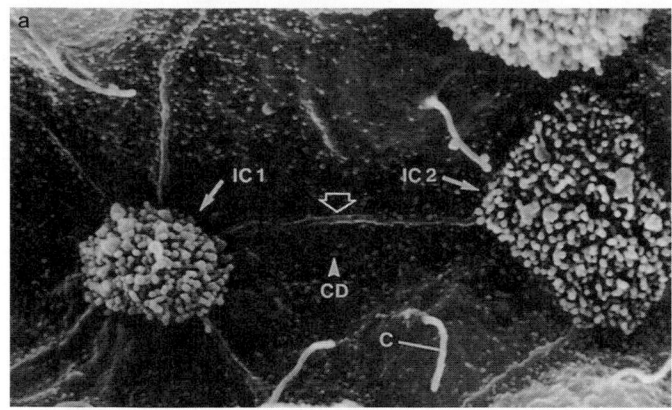

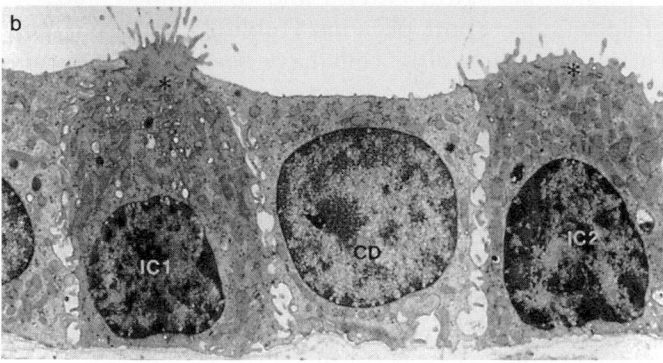

FIGURE 20.62 **Intercalated cells from the rabbit.** (a) Scanning electron micrograph of a cortical collecting duct with collecting duct-specific CD cells (CD) and intercalated cells (IC). The CD cells carry single cilia (C) and short microvilli (arrowhead). The straight ridges (open arrow) represent the cell borders between CD cells. From the IC cells one (IC 1) has a narrow, constricted apical cell pole, the other one (IC 2) a large apical cell pole, both adorned with numerous long microvilli (TEM: ×~13,000). (b) Section across corresponding cells. Note the position and accumulation of flat vesicles (asterisk) in the apical cell pole of the IC cells (TEM: ×~7500).

revealed by freeze-fracture studies in the outer medullary collecting duct.[683,684]

The IMCD cells co-express, in addition to vasopressin-regulated AQP2, the vasopressin-regulated urea transporters UT-A1/3 and possibly UT-A4 (for review see [148]). The abundance of UT-A1/3 in the apical membrane is rate-limiting for transepithelial, vasopressin-dependent urea reabsorption.[571,685] The basolateral membranes of the IMCD cells display the water channel AQP3. The abundance of UT-A1/3 in the apical membrane is rate-limiting for transepithelial, vasopressin-dependent urea reabsorption.[571,685] In the basolateral membranes of the IMCD cells the water channels AQP3,[682] permeability to glycerol, urea and water,[686] and AQP4[683,687] with an apparently low urea permeability have been demonstrated.

The genes coding for proteins, which are involved in cellular accumulation of organic osmolytes, such as the vasopressin-regulated urea transporter UT-A and

heat shock protein 70,[688] are target genes of the tonicity-response enhancer binding protein (TonEBP), a transcriptional activator of the REL-family. During kidney development, expression of TonEBP precedes that of the urea transporter. It is first detected in the renal medulla of mice at the fetal age of 16 days and increases up to postnatal day 21, when the medulla is fully developed and the urinary concentrating ability is achieved.[689]

Intercalated Cells (IC Cells)

Intercalated cells (IC cells) are interspersed as single cells among the epithelium of the ASDN (i.e., among ENaC-displaying epithelia, the late DCT (DCT2), the CNT (Figure 20.59a), and the CD (Figure 20.60a). IC cells play a decisive role in the final regulation by the collecting system of acid–base excretion, in potassium reabsorption and secretion, in ammonia excretion and, as discovered recently, intercalated cells participate together with the segment-specific cells in electro-neutral sodium reabsorption.

Consistent Structural Features of Intercalated Cells

Intercalated cells reveal conspicuous structural heterogeneity (Figure 20.61). IC cells usually do not form a continous epithelial layer, but at least their luminal poles are entirely surrounded by the segment-specific cells. The luminal outline of IC cells is in most cases rather circular (Figure 20.62a),[291,540,690–692] IC cells generally reveal a specific surface pattern of microprojections (Figure 20.62a) and lack, at least in the cortex, the central cilium which is apparent on other cells (Figure 20.62b). Among the most consistent distinguishing intracellular features is the distribution pattern of mitochondria: the often rounded mitochondrial profiles lack the systematic association to basolateral cell membranes[35,693,694] evident in other tubular cells. The generally small, more or less round vesicles often reveal an invagination bordered by a thin smooth membrane ("invaginated vesicles"[5]); they participate in endocytosis[695–697]; the elongated slender profiles — "tubules" — probably represent sections through flat saccules or collapsed large spherical vesicles ("flat vesicles").[5] Occasionally they are found to be continuous with the luminal membrane, and are often in close juxtaposition with mitochondria.[5] Transitional forms between the two vesicle types can be seen; the presence of specific particles in one or several membrane domains (luminal, basolateral, and/or tubulo-vesicular) have been observed. In TEM preparations the membranes reveal a coat of densely arranged, approximately rectangular large particles, so-called "studs," on their cytoplasmic face. The "studs" are 10 nm spherical structures (Figure 20.65a,c,d), which represent the H^+-ATPase.[698,699] In freeze-fracture preparations dense arrays of intramembrane particles, so-called "rod-shaped" particles appear on the P-face of the membranes (Figure 20.65b).[543,700] The presence of "studs" and of "rod-shaped" particles on the cytoplasmic membrane faces often coincides. Clathrin-coated pits on either the luminal or the basal cell membrane and clathrin heads on the "studded" vesicles are regularly found. The nucleus generally reveals more heterochromatin condensations and looks darker than that of the adjacent CNT or CD cells.

Proteins Related to Intercalated Cell Functions

All intercalated cells display high levels of cabonic anhydrase II in the cytoplasm.[450,472,701−704] All IC cells express the electrogenic V-type proton-ATPase, the proton pump[698] in at least one of their membrane domains, and all express an anion exchanger, either anion exchanger 1 (AE1, gene Slc4A1; band 3[705]) or Pendrin (Slc 26A4[706]) in one membrane domain. Pendrin is an aldosterone-sensitive Na^+-independent Cl^-/HCO_3^- exchanger that mediates Cl^- absorption and HCO_3^- secretion in the cortical collecting duct (CCD).[669] Furthermore, studies on isolated CCDs suggested that the parallel action of the Na^+-driven Cl^-/HCO_3^- exchanger (NDCBE/SLC4A8) and the Na^+-independent Cl^-/HCO_3^- exchanger (pendrin/SLC26A4) account for the electroneutral thiazide-sensitive sodium transport in the CCD (where the thiazide sensitive electroneutral NaCl co-transporter NCC is not expressed), a finding that challenges the current concept of a functional separation between principal cells for the regulation of sodium and potassium balance, and intercalated cells for acid−base regulation.[668]

All IC cells express the Rhesus glycoproteins, Rh B Glycoprotein (Rhbg[707]) and Rh C Glycoprotein (Rhcg[708]). These proteins are recently recognized ammonia transporters in the distal tubule and collecting duct. Rhcg is present in both the apical and basolateral plasma membrane, is expressed in parallel with renal ammonia excretion, and mediates a critical role in renal ammonia excretion and collecting duct ammonia transport. Rhbg is expressed specifically in the basolateral plasma membrane.[709]

Subtypes of Intercalated Cells

By morphological criteria and distribution patterns of specific transport proteins (Table 20.1) three different manifestation of IC cells have been described, type A cells, type B cells,[694] and type nonA-nonB cells.[710]

TYPE A IC CELLS

Morphologically, the type A IC cells usually have a broad protruding apical cell pole, which is adorned with numerous slender microfolds and/or finger-like microvilli giving rise to a very complex surface pattern[5,691,694](Figures 20.63a and 20.64a). The cytoplasmic membrane face of the microprojections and of the esicles in the apical cell pole are "studded"[594] (Figure 20.65a). "Rod-shaped" particles (Figure 20.64b) have also been demonstrated.[700] The mitochondria are particularly numerous, and are accumulated in the apical cell pole above the large round nucleus (Figure 20.64a). They are often found very closely adjacent to the luminal cell membrane. They possess narrower cristae, and their matrix appears more electron-dense than in other cell types. The Golgi apparatus and other cell organelles are only slightly apparent among the numerous mitochondria. Polyribosomes may be exceedingly frequent. Some profiles of RER are

TABLE 20.1   Proteins with Defined Functional Relevance (see text) in Renal Intercalated Cell (IC) Subtypes

Intercalated Cells Protein	Type A	Type B	Type nonA-nonB	References
Carbonic anhydrase II	yes; a	yes; c	yes; c	450,812−819
H^+-ATPase	**yes; a**	**yes; b**	yes; **diff**	698,699,714−719
AE1 (Slc4A1; Band 3)	**yes; a**	absent	absent	705,709,721,740,820
Pendrin(Slc 26A4)	absent	**yes; a**	**yes; a**	740,820
RhBG	yes; b	absent	yes; b	494,709,730
RhCG	yes; a	absent	yes; a	709,730,732,821,822
H + -K-ATPase (gastric and non-gastric)	yes; a	?	?	823−830
5′NT	yes; a	yes; a (b)	?	57,753

Localization in: a: apical membrane domain; b: basolateral membrane domain; (b): occasionally; diff: diffuse vesicular; c: cytoplasmic; ?: not determined. bold: marker combination for IC subtype diagnosis.

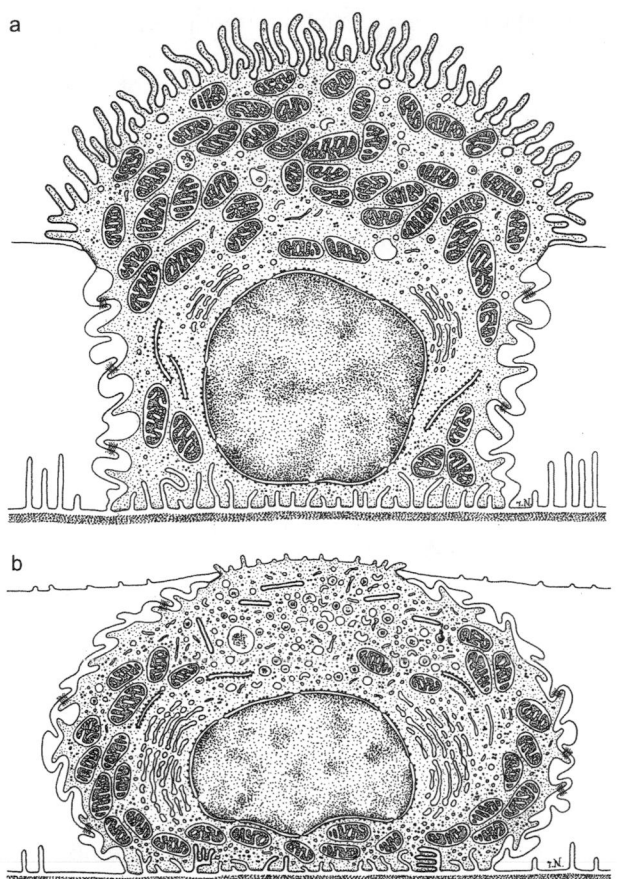

FIGURE 20.63 **Survey of ultrastructure of intercalated cells.** (a) A-type IC cell; (b) B-type IC cell. . *(Adapted from and Kaissling, B., and Kriz, W. (1992). In "Morphology of the Loop of Henle, Distal Tubule and Collecting Duct. Handbook of Physiology: Section on Renal Physiology," 109–167, Windhager, E. E. Oxford University Press, New York, with permission)*

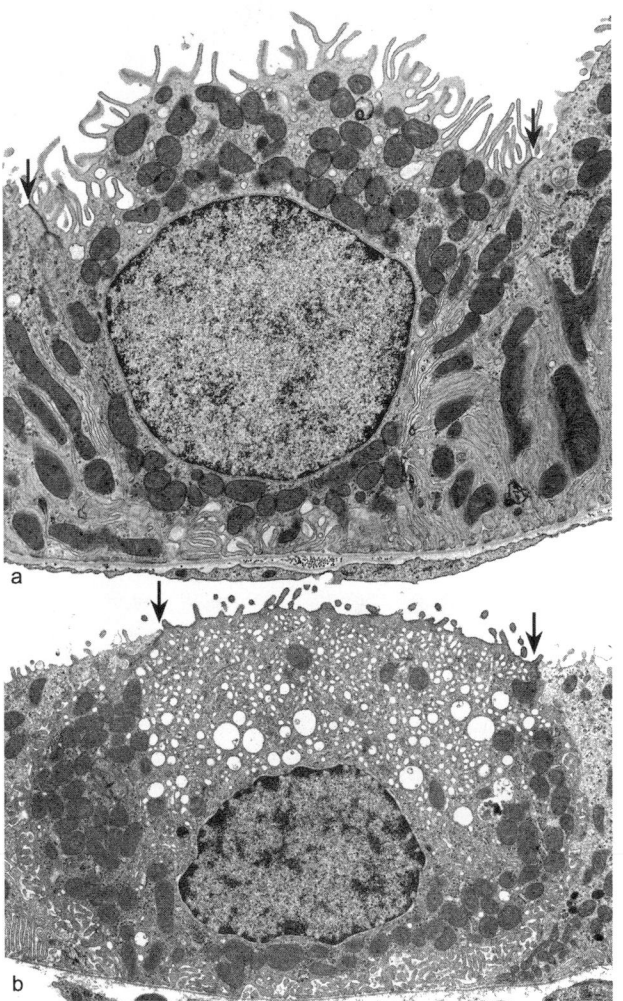

FIGURE 20.64 **Intercalated cells (rat).** (a) Type A cell with many luminal microfolds and abundant mitochondria in the apical cell pole. (b) Type B cell with a rather narrow apical cell pole, a narrow rim of dense cytoplasm with no vesicles under the apical plasma membrane, abundant smooth-surfaced vesicles in the apical cytoplasm, and a huge Golgi complex (G), with abundant mitochondria along the basolateral plasma membrane (Arrows: Tight junction; TEM: $\times \sim 7000$).

generally found in basal cell portions. Basal infoldings can be extensive in the rat,[694,711] yet in the rabbit they are virtually absent.[712]

Some structural variation within type A cells exist among and even within individuals. They concern essentially the extent of studded membrane projections on the luminal cell surface, and the abundance of studded tubulo-vesicular profiles in the apical cell pole. The membrane surface area of the microfolds seems to be inversely related that of the tubular-vesicular profiles; both vary with functional conditions. For instance, under acute metabolic and respiratory acidosis[711] and/or potassium depletion the vesicular pool decreases and the apical membrane increases. Mitochondria with rather short profiles and narrowly arranged cristae are amassed in the apical cell pole, in particularly close vicinity to the apical cell membrane. Many microtubules and clathrin-coated vesicles are apparent between the tubulo-vesicular profiles and

the mitochondria. The nucleus is shifted to the basal cell portion (Figures 20.63a and 20.64a) (for review see [492,698,713]).

IC cells in the outer medulla and the initial part of the inner medullary CD (rats) appear slightly different from the cortical type A cells. In rats, the apical cell pole is often narrower than the basal cell pole.[268] The mitochondrial profiles are fewer and smaller than in cortical type A, the Golgi apparatus and the SER are less apparent than in cortical type A cells, the basal infoldings are less extensive compared to cortical type A cells and the nucleus has a characteristic elongated flattened profile. Among the "studded" vesicles in the apical cell pole very large round profiles and

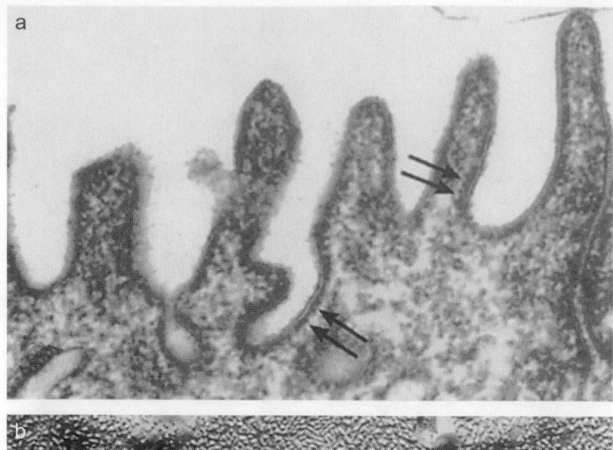

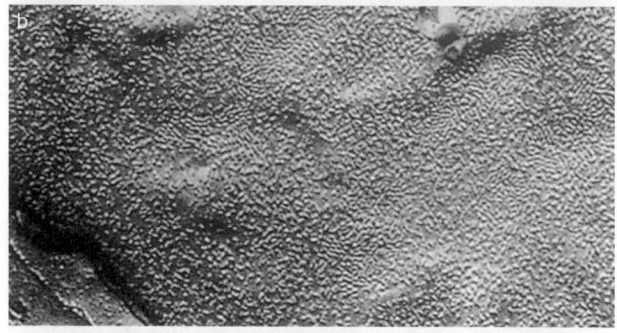

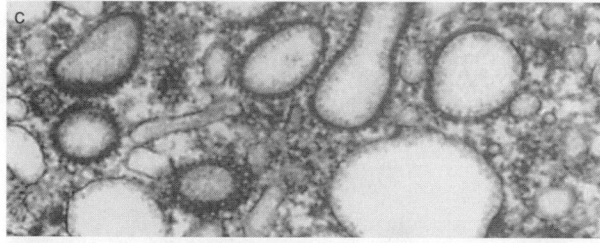

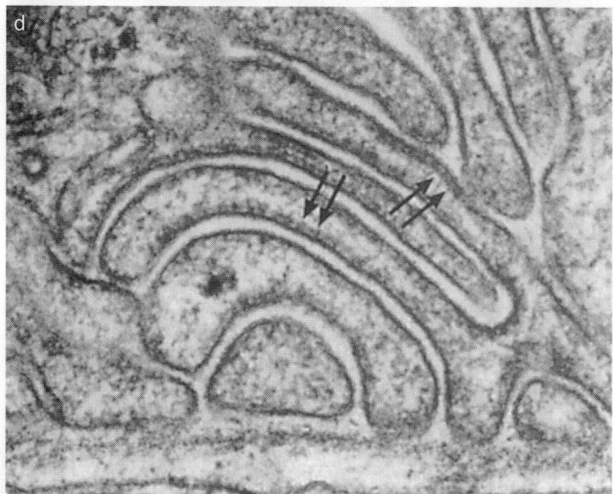

FIGURE 20.65 Intercalated cells (rat). (a) Luminal membrane; its cytoplasmic face is coated with studs (arrows) (TEM: ×~61,000). **(b)** Freeze-fracture electron micrograph showing the rod-shaped intramembrane particles (stars) of a luminal membrane (TEM: ×~32,000). **(c)** Apical cytoplasm of a type A cell. The specific vesicles are coated with studs (TEM: ×~64,000). **(d)** Membrane of basal infoldings of type B cell; its cytoplasmic face is covered with studs (arrows) (TEM: ×~61,000).

particularly long flat vesicles often predominate over other cell organelles.

Type A IC cells are considered as the proton-secreting cells. Their apical membrane domain possesses various subunits of H^+-ATPase, among them the B1- and d-subunits which possess a high selectivity for intercalated cells.[698,699,715–719] The proton-ATPase functions in series with a bicarbonate/Cl (HCO_3^-/Cl^-) exchanger located in the basolateral membrane domain (for review see [492]). In type A IC cells the HCO_3^-/Cl^- exchanger is the anion exchanger AE1 (SLC4A1, band 3), a splice variant product of the erythrocyte band 3 gene.[705,720] The presence of AE1 in the basolateral membrane is decisive for diagnosis of type A IC cells.[705,721]

In addition to the V-type proton-ATPase type A IC cells — at least in the outer stripe — also display a P-type (gastric-type) K-H-ATPase, shown so far in rat and rabbit.[578,659,722–726] This K-reabsorbing ATPase seems to be associated with clusters of rod-shaped particles, revealed by freeze-fracture studies on the P-face of cell membranes in rabbit IC cells.[700] Thus, the type A IC cells could be involved in recovering potassium, secreted via ROMK, in association with EnaC-mediated Na-reabsorption by the segment-specific cells. Type A cells also express the chloride channel ClC 5.[727] The secretory isoform of the Na-K-Cl-co-transporter, NKCC 1, has been detected in the basolateral membrane of type A cells in the outer stripe.[728]

The type A IC cells express apically and basolaterally non-erythroid Rh-associated glycoproteins Rhcg and basolaterally Rhbg,[492,494,709,729–731] which mediate transport of ammonia/ammonium (NH_4^+/NH_3)[494,732] when expressed in *Xenopus laevis* oocytes.[733]

In chronic metabolic acidosis and prolonged high proton secretion the type A IC cells hypertrophy (for review see [492]), and IC cells in the OMCD and IMCD show increased RhCG expression.[734] However, genetic ablation of the RhBG gene is not a critical determinant of NH_4^+ excretion by the kidney under acidic or under control conditions.[729] Under chronic acidosis the type A IC cells proliferate, as evidenced by upregulation of cell cycle proteins, by incorporation of the thymidine analog bromo-deoxyuridine (BrdU) and mitotic figures.[735]

TYPE B IC CELLS

Morphologically, Type B IC cells reveal a relatively small, occasionally slightly polygonal luminal outline and protrude only slightly into the lumen (Figures 20.60a, 20.63b, and 20.64b[711]). The cells seem to be partly covered by the adjacent CD cells, and their sectional profiles often appear almost elliptical (Figures 20.63b and 20.64b). The luminal membrane, with only a few short microprojections, lacks "studs".[736] In contrast, "studs" may be apparent on fragments or even along the entire lateral and often extensive formation of infoldings of the basal plasma membrane (Figure 20.65d). The small short mitochondria are accumulated in the basal cell portion and along the lateral cell faces (Figures 20.63b and 20.64b), but they are never found immediately beneath the luminal membrane. The cytoplasm above the plane of the tight junctional belt may be completely devoid of any cell organelles. The nucleus often reveals some basal indentations,[711] and is often situated eccentrically. The center of the cell is occupied by a conspicuously developed Golgi apparatus, a few short profiles of RER, polyribosomes, and microtubules, as well as lysosomes of varying dimensions, and autophagosomes containing frequently recognizable remnants of mitochondria or membranes. A striking feature of these cells is the high abundance of narrow-meshed profiles of smooth ER, often with clathrin-coated heads.[329] The SER is intermingled with a great amount of small, generally "unstudded" invaginated vesicles, which are preferentially found in the apical cell portion, but may be accumulated also in the direct vicinity of the basal cell membrane. "Studded" vesicles are sparse or lacking.

The type B cells also display different manifestations. Between cells which are densely stuffed with SER and display very few mitochondria and very few "studded" membrane domains, and cells which contain large amounts of mitochondria, of "studded" vesicles, and which may be even densely covered with short microvilli, all intermediates can be found. Another configuration of possibly type B cells is found in the cortex of rabbits. These cells appear "constricted" at the level of the tight junctional belt where a prominent web of microfilaments is evident. Some elongated profiles of "studded" vesicles are found within and beneath this web. The narrow, apical cell pole is adorned with a tuft of long microvilli.[260]

Type B IC cells mediate secretion of HCO_3^- through apical Cl^- / HCO_3^- exchange, which functions in series with H^+-ATPase-mediated H^+ efflux across the basolateral plasma membrane.[737] They are characterized by apical pendrin (Slc4A1)[738–740] and basolateral H^+-ATPase. Type B cells reveal less carbonic anhydric activity than type A cells,[702] and they express the chloride channel ClC 3[727] in the apical cell pole.

Metabolic alkalosis is compensated in the kidney by reducing bicarbonate reabsorption and increased bicarbonate secretion by type B IC cells. Type B IC cells adapt under chronic metabolic alkalosis with cellular hypertrophy.[741] DNA synthesis and mitoses of type B cells have been recorded under this situation.[742] Adaptive downregulation of pendrin in metabolic acidosis indicates the important role of this exchanger in acid−base regulation in the CCD.[741] The type B

intercalated cell does not express either Rhbg or Rhcg detectable by immunohistochemistry.

NON A-NON B CELLS

A third type of IC cells without evident polarity with respect to proton-APTase, and so far with undefined function, are called "non A-non B" cells.[738] These cells are often much larger and protrude much more into the lumen than type A or B.[709] In contrast to type A and B IC cells, neither the luminal nor the basolatreal plasma membranes reveal "studs," at best "studs" are found on membranes of vesicular profiles in the cytoplasm. In mice this latter population of intercalated cells is more frequent than in rats.[743] It decreases in either pronounced chronic metabolic acidosis or pronounced chronic metabolic alkalosis.[492,711,744]

On their apical plasma membrane they display, similar to type B IC cells, the anion exchanger pendrin (Slc4A1) and diffusely distributed H^+-ATPase, occasionally also in the apical membrane. They express apical, but not basolatreal, Rhcg and basolateral Rhbg.[709]

The observations on non A-non B cells, the striking structural diversity[713,745] and the apparent plasticity of IC cells raised the question whether one, two or more distinct cell types are subsumed in the IC cell population or whether the different appearances are manifestations of different functional stages of the same cell type. Based on studies in collecting ducts *in vitro* from adult rabbits and IC cells cultured *in vitro*,[746−749] (IC cells with the morphology of type B were identified by apical binding to peanut lectin),[750] it was speculated that the IC cells might reverse their polarity in response to specific functional environmental conditions. Type A would present the terminal differentiation of IC cells. This hypothesis received support from studies *in vitro* showing that the matrix protein hensin could reverse the functional phenotype of cultured intercalated cells (for review see [492]), and induce the type A IC cells. The non A-non B cells might represent intermediate stages. The diminution of this latter population under chronic acidotic or alkalotic conditions would agree with this hypothesis.

Another view was that the non A-non B cells could be precursors for either A or B cells or only of B cells (for review see [492]). This hypothesis would also be supported by the finding of a diminution of non A-non-B cells under chronic acidosis or alkalosis. The observations on mitosis in fully-differentiated type A,[735,751] as well as in type B IC cells[742] do not agree with the hypothesis on reversal of polarity, nor with the hypothesis claiming a common precursor cell of type A and B.

Most IC cells also display on at least one membrane domain (more often on the luminal and vesicular than on the basolateral) the AMP-degrading phosphatidyl-inositol-anchored ecto-enzyme 5'nucleotidase

(5′NT)[57,60,740,752,753] and the protein Connexin 30, that might function as plasma membrane ATP channel.[754] It has been shown that increased flow in the distal nephron induces K secretion through the large-conductance, calcium-activated K channel (BK), which is primarily expressed in intercalated cells (IC). High distal flows and shear stress induce BK-dependent K efflux and ATP release from IC cells.[295] These mechanisms might play a role in the purinergic autocrine and/or paracrine regulation of salt and water reabsorption.[317]

The intergral membrane proteins syntaxin 3[755] and synaptotagmin VIII demonstrated in the basolateral membrane of IC cells,[756] are possibly involved in the targeting of acid—base transporters and may participate in the basolateral membrane remodeling of IC cells in response to systemic acid—base perturbations.

Interestingly, it had been reported that IC cells lack significant levels of Na-K-ATPase in the basolateral membranes.[283] However, more recently, weak to moderate Na-K-ATPase was revealed in cortical and outer medullary IC cells, whereas IC cells in the upper part of the inner medullary collecting duct showed a staining intensity that was similar or even stronger to that in adjacent IMCD cells.[757]

Distribution of IC Cells

The ratio of intercalated cells to other tubular cell types varies among and within species, and along the distal segments (DCT, CNT, upper and lower half of cortical collecting duct, outer and inner stripe collecting duct). Possibly, it may be altered by some functional conditions.[744] Discrepancies in reported data for a given species may be rooted in poor definition of the investigated kidney region, and also in the criteria used for the recognition of cells. The relative number of intercalated cells (all forms) in the various segments is roughly ~25–30% in the CNT, ~40% in the CCD and OMCD, and ~10% in the initial IMCD.[699,718,743,758] IC cells are absent in deeper levels of the inner medulla in most species.

In the rat, taking the morphological, cyto-, and immunochemical data together, it can be deduced that among the IC cells in the CNT the type A cells prevail. Type B cells are in the minority among the IC cells in the CNT in rat, but not in mouse. Type B IC cells constitute the majority of IC cells in the CCD, of which a varying proportion may present proton-ATPase in the basolateral cell membrane. Based on the different distribution of the proton-ATPase in non-type A intercalated cells, it has been suggested type B IC cells with only basolateral proton-ATPase staining and non-A/non-B IC cells with bipolar or luminal proton-ATPase staining should be distinguished.[743] However, both subpopulations carry pendrin staining, and may represent different states of activity.

In the CCD type A cells are in the minority, and often appear in their apparently functionally less active form, with less microprojections, but more intracellular "studded" vesicles than type A cells in the CNT.[759] Accordingly, they display a slightly weaker luminal, but often a diffuse cytoplasmic, staining for the proton-ATPase. Apparently only one type of IC cells exists in the OMCD of rats, mice, and humans. It resembles the type A cells in the cortex.

Disruption of IC Cell Characteristic Genes

Inheritable forms of distal renal tubular acidosis (dRTA) most often affect the physiology of type A IC cells.[760] Disruption of one of the IC cell characteristic genes leads to profound structural alterations of IC cell types. In mice with functional deletion of carbonic anhydrase II, the frequency of IC cells is drastically reduced.[701]

The genetic disruption of pendrin (Slc26a4) leads to marked reduction of type B cell size, with reduced H^+/OH^- transporter expressions.[506,738] In mice with disruption of the Foxi1 gene, upstream of several anion transporters, proton pumps, and anion exchange proteins expressed by intercalated cells, and of the collecting ducts cells, the normal collecting duct epithelium with its two major cell populations — collecting ducts cells (principal) and intercalated cells — has been replaced by a single cell type positive for both principal and intercalated cell markers.[761]

ARCHITECTURAL—FUNCTIONAL RELATIONSHIPS

So far we have always emphasized the relationships between structure and function. However, we have neglected the important relationships between architecture and function — i.e., arrangements through which the close relationships between certain nephron and vascular portions permit the carrying out and coordination of complex regulatory functions. The two most obvious examples in this respect are the juxtaglomerular apparatus (JGA), regulating glomerular perfusion and renin secretion, and the renal medulla permitting the production of urine, varying in dilution and concentration.

Juxtaglomerular Apparatus

The juxtaglomerular apparatus (JGA) is a composite assembly of specialized structures at the vascular pole of the glomerulus (Figures 20.28 and 20.29). The thick ascending limb of Henle's loop (TAL) returns to its parent glomerulus and extends through the angle

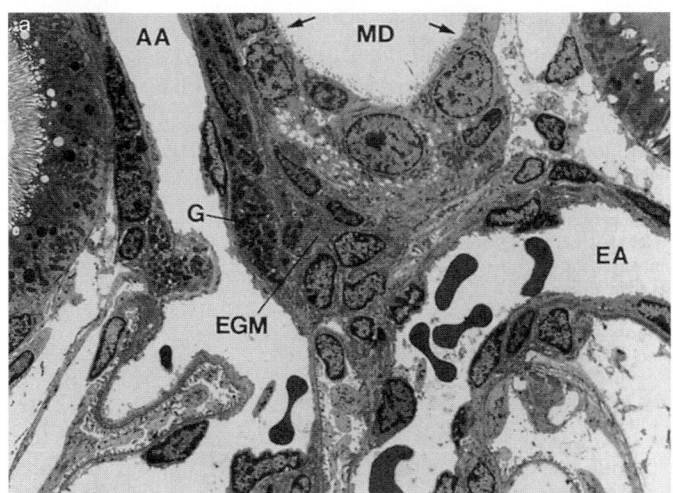

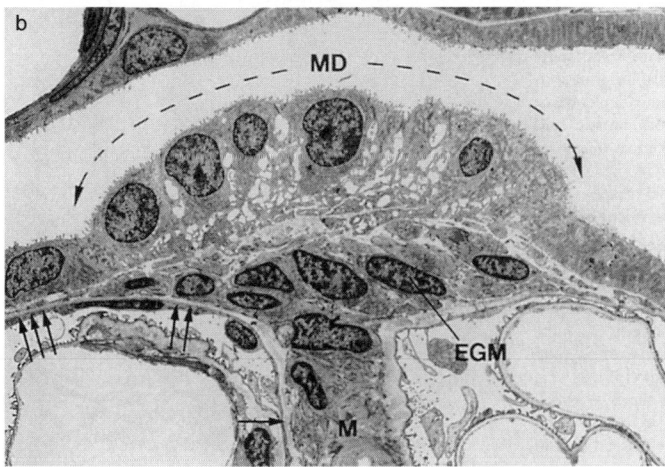

FIGURE 20.66 Juxtaglomerular apparatus. (a) Meridional section through a glomerulus which runs through both glomerular arterioles (rat). The macula densa (MD) is attached to the extraglomerular mesangium (EGM), which fills the angle between the afferent (AA) and efferent (EA) arteriole. Within the wall of the afferent arteriole granular cells (G) are seen. Note the intraglomerular segment of the efferent arteriole (TEM: ×~1850). (b) Meridional section through a glomerulus running in between both arterioles (rabbit). The macula densa (MD) is a prominent cell plaque within the thick ascending limb. It covers the extraglomerular mesangium (EGM). Within the glomerular stalk the EGM continues into the mesangium (M). The EGM interconnects opposing parts of the GBM (one arrow) to the basement membrane of Bowman's capsule (BCBM) (two arrows), as well as the first parts of the BCBM (three arrows). Note the dilated intercellular spaces between macula densa cells (TEM: ×~8100).

between afferent and efferent arterioles, where it is firmly attached to the extraglomerular mesangium (Figure 20.66a). At the attachment point, the TAL changes its character: a plaque of specialized cells, known as the macula densa (MD), represents the contact site of the tubule. Around this attachment, other specialized structures are developed which, together with the macula densa, comprise the JGA. These are:

the terminal portion of the afferent arteriole housing the renin producing granular cells; the initial portion of the efferent arteriole; and the extraglomerular mesangium (EGM). The latter is in continuity with the intraglomerular mesangium, and has intimate relationships with the parietal epithelium of Bowman's capsule.[20] The JGA, more precisely the granular cells and the smooth muscle cells of afferent and efferent arterioles, are richly innervated by sympathetic nerves.

Macula Densa

Shortly before its end, the TAL passes between the afferent and efferent arterioles of its original glomerulus. At this site the basal face of the tubule is affixed to the extracellular matrix, enveloping the cells of the extraglomerular mesangium (EGM), tying together both arterioles. The TAL cells in contact with the EGM are transformed into the "macula densa" (MD). The MD is a cell plaque comprising some 20 to 30 specialized epithelial cells (in juxtamedullary nephrons more than in superficial nephrons). The MD completely and consistently overlaps the EGM, and may extend over variable portions of the afferent and efferent arterioles.[429,762] The specific histo-topographical relationship of the epithelial tubular cells and the other components of the JGA at the glomerular vascular pole are established already during nephron formation. The prospective MD cells are affixed to the mesenchymal cells accompanying the capillary loops that invade the distal cleft of the S-shaped body of the nephron-anlage to form the glomerular tuft.[763] This occurs before the epithelial cells of the prospective loop of Henle have elongated into a tubule.

The cells of the MD (Figure 20.66) differ from the surrounding cells of the thick ascending limb in several aspects. The most eye-catching feature of the MD are the closely packed nuclei, usually located in the apical cell pole.[5,764] This feature, well recognizable even in light microscopic preparations at low magnification, conferred the name "macula densa" to the cell plaque.

Most importantly, and in marked contrast to the cells of the thick ascending limb, MD cells do not interdigitate with each other by large lateral folding; rather, the lateral cell membranes of MD cells run in a fairly straight fashion from the tight junction toward the base of the epithelium.[5,764] They possess slender microplicae or microvilli that protrude into the lateral intercellular spaces, and contact (frequently by desmosomes) corresponding protrusions from opposite cells. At the very base the cells ramify into slender processes. They are fixed to the basement membrane of the MD cells which is fused with the basement membrane-like material surrounding the extraglomerular mesangial cells. The tight junctions are morphologically similar as in the TAL, but they may be slightly deeper (e.g., in rabbit). Like all other TAL cells, MD cells do not display gap junctions.

The cytoplasm of MD cells is relatively sparse and displays the usual organelles comprising some small mitochondria. The Golgi apparatus is large, smooth endoplasmic reticulum and free ribosomes are abundant, but rough endoplasmic reticulum is infrequent.

The luminal cell membrane is densely studded by short stubby microvilli and displays, like the other tubular cells, single cilia. In some species (e.g., rabbit[5]) the MD cells are distinctly taller than the surrounding TAL cells, so that the entire plaque of the MD protrudes into the tubule lumen.

The inventory of transport proteins in MD cells is essentially the same as in the other TAL cells, i.e., they display the bumetanide-sensitive NKCC2 co-transporter,[537,765,766] ROMK,[767,768] and NHE3[769] in the apical plasma membrane, and express cyclooxygenase-1.[516] They specifically express cyclooxygenase-2[516] and nitric oxide synthetase 1.[770,771] In contrast to the TAL, MD cells lack the Tamm-Horsfall protein.[528]

Recent findings[772] detected by RT-PCR and by immunohistochemistry demonstrated olfactory-related adenylate cyclase 3 (AC3) and the olfactory G-protein limited to the distal convoluted tubule and especially the MD.[772] These findings suggest a role of the olfactory machinery in the regulation of renin secretion and glomerular filtration rate.[772]

In contrast to all other TAL cells, the lateral intercellular spaces in the MD epithelium have been found to be dilated under most physiological conditions, usually regarded as "normal" conditions.[754,764,773-776] In agreement with the suggestion that water flow through the MD-epithelium is secondary to active sodium reabsorption, compounds that block sodium transport by MD cells (e.g., furosemide), as well as high osmolalities of impermeable solutes in the tubular fluid (e.g., mannitol), are associated with narrow intercellular spaces.[764,773] These observations suggested that the MD epithelium might be a water-permeable cell plaque within the water-impermeable TAL epithelium,[764] but so far direct evidence for this suggestion is missing. The lack of immunoreactivity for TRPV4, a nonselective cation channel of the transient receptor potential (TRP) family, gated by hypotonicity, had been interpreted as indirect support for this assumption.[777]

The granular cells (often termed juxtaglomerular cells) (Figure 20.67)[778] are assembled in clusters (up to 15 cells, but generally not more than 4 or 5) within the wall of the terminal portion of the afferent arteriole, replacing ordinary smooth muscle cells. Occasionally, they are also found within the wall of the efferent arteriole, again occupying the space where one would otherwise expect to find an ordinary smooth muscle cell. In rare cases, extraglomerular mesangial cells may also be replaced by granular cells. The name "granular" cell points to the specific cytoplasmic granules which may densely fill the cell body cytoplasm. They are electrondense, membrane-bound, and irregular in size and

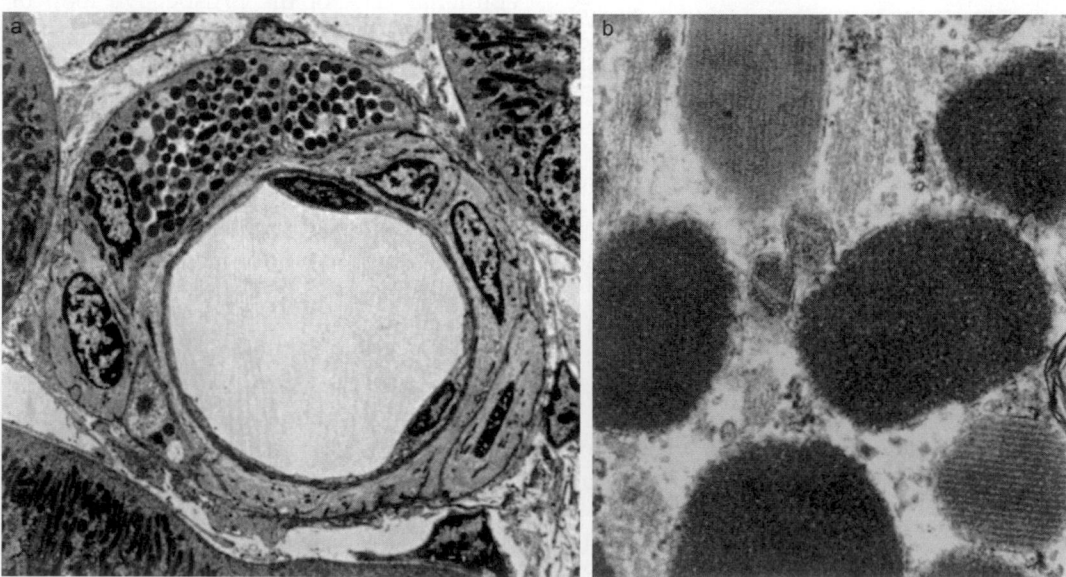

FIGURE 20.67   (a) Juxtaglomerular portion of an afferent arteriole. Smooth muscle cells are replaced by two granular cells (rabbit: TEM: ×~2700). (b) Granular cell. Renin granules are membrane-bound. Granules with a crystalline substructure are considered as "protogranules" which will develop into mature amorphous granules (rat: TEM: ×~48,000).

shape. Small granules with crystalline substructure represent protogranules, which are developed within the prominent Golgi apparatus and are then transformed into the major amorphous granules. Immunocytochemical studies with two antibodies against the renin prosegment and against mature renin have shown that only protogranules are prosegment-positive, whereas a signal of mature renin was found in mature as well as protogranules. These findings show that the cleavage of the prosegment, i.e., the maturation of renin, takes place in the juvenile granules; mature renin is then stored in the electron-dense granules. However, it is suggested that a major fraction of pro-renin never matures to renin, but is constitutively secreted as pro-renin — together with an unknown fraction of renin. Mature renin is segregated into storage granules for regulated release. The release mode of renin is not fully-understood. In addition to classic exocytosis, other mechanisms may also be involved.[18] It is important to know that renin release occurs into the surrounding interstitium, not into the lumen of the afferent arteriole, as has been frequently suggested.

Granular cells are modified smooth muscle cells. Within the peripheral parts of the cytoplasm, especially within the many cell processes, granular cells contain myofibrils. In situations that require enhanced renin synthesis (e.g., volume depletion or stenosis of the renal artery) additional smooth muscle cells located upstream in the wall of the afferent arteriole transform into granular cells.[19]

Granular cells have processes of manifold shapes.[99] Because of them, granular cells have extensive membrane contacts to all surrounding cells, e.g., other granular cells, smooth muscle cells, and extraglomerular mesangial cells. At these contacts, gap junctions are frequently encountered.[19] Like ordinary smooth muscle cells, granular cells also have membrane contacts to endothelial cells, in the manner that foot-like processes of endothelial cells penetrate the basement membrane and come into contact with granular cells; gap junctions are found at these contact sites.[99]

Peripolar cells have first been described in sheep, where they are regularly found[779]; in most other species, including man, they are rare.[780] Peripolar cells are parietal cells of Bowman's capsule which are located around the glomerular hilum (i.e., at the vascular pole, therefore: peripolar), and which contain numerous cytoplasmic membrane-bound granules filled homogeneously with electron-dense fibrillogranular material.[779] Subsequent studies have shown that these granules contain a neuron-specific enolase-like protein[781] and transthyretin[782]; their function is unknown. The number of cells and the number of granules per cell vary greatly among species and, furthermore, are dependent on age.[780] In the rat kidney, granulated peripolar cells have only rarely been found.[780]

Extraglomerular mesangial cells (EGM-cells, Goormaghtigh cells, lacis cells) together with the surrounding matrix establish the extraglomerular mesangium (polar cushion). The EGM represents a solid cell complex that is not penetrated by blood vessels or lymphatic capillaries. Nerves pass on both sides of it from the afferent to the efferent arteriole, but do not enter the cell complex.[99]

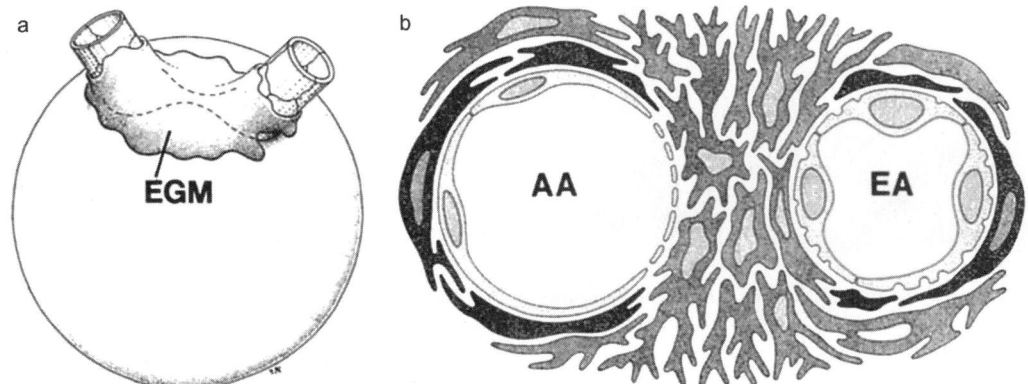

FIGURE 20.68 (a) Schematic of the extraglomerular mesangium (*EGM*). The glomerulus is shown as a globe. Its outer aspect is represented by the parietal basement membrane of Bowman's capsule (*PBM*). The EGM lies between the two arterioles above the opening of Bowman's capsule (broken line). It is attached to the PBM and has extensive contacts with the two arterioles. The macula densa and the smooth muscle layers of the arterioles are not shown. (b) Schematic cross-section through the vascular pole just above Bowman's capsule. Afferent and efferent arterioles (*AA, EA*) are cut transversely. Extraglomerular mesangial cells (*EGM*) are shown in moderate gray, smooth muscle cells in dark gray, and endothelial cells in light gray. Note differences in the walls of AA and EA; the AA already displays endothelial fenestration on the side facing the EGM. Conversely, the EA has a continuous endothelium with many cell bodies. In both AA and EA the smooth muscle layer (*SM*) is not complete; towards the center of the EGM the SM cells are replaced by EGM cells. *(Elger, M., and Sakai, T. et al. (1998). The vascular pole of the renal glomerulus of rat. Adv. Anat. Embryol. Cell Biol.**139**, 1–98, with permission).*

The EGM is located within the triangular space bordered by the two glomerular arterioles and the macula densa (Figures 20.66 and 20.68).[778] Reconstruction studies have shown that EGM-cells are flat and elongated, separating into two bunches of long cell processes at their poles.[783] They are arranged in several layers parallel to the base of the macula densa. The cells nearest to the glomerular stalk, thus filling the deepest portion of the triangle, lose this parallel grouping, but extend into the stalk of the glomerular tuft mixing with mesangial cells proper. The cells are separated by a conspicuous matrix which appears to be different from the intraglomerular mesangial matrix by the fact that microfibrils are rarely found in the EGM[20]; details are largely unknown.

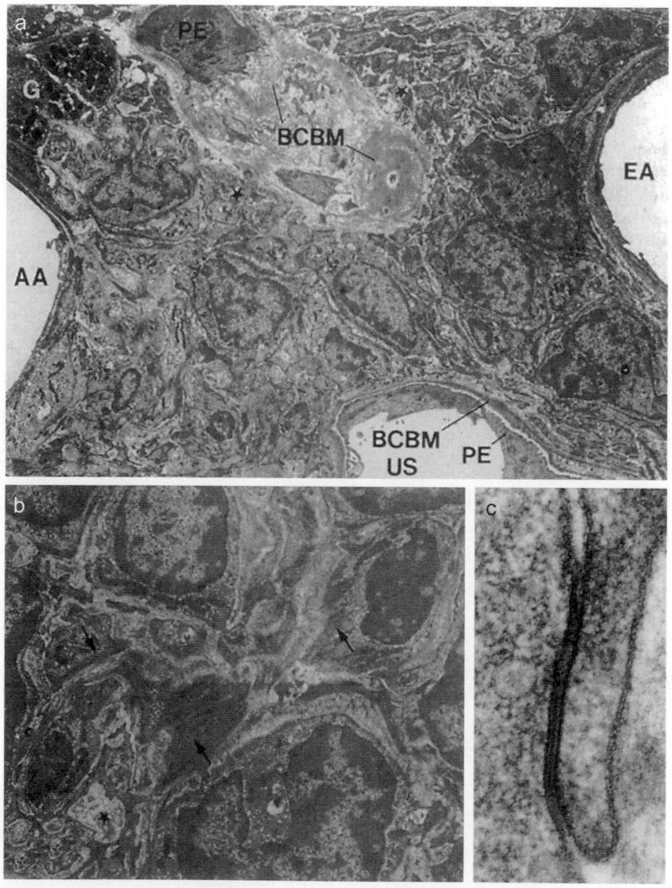

EGM cells are characterized by the scantness of their cytoplasm and their extensive ramifications (Figure 20.69).[778,784] A Golgi apparatus and some profiles of granulated endoplasmic reticulum are regularly encountered. Although direct evidence is lacking, EGM-cells can be expected to be contractile for several reasons. First, they contain a good amount of microfilaments, mainly in their processes and peripherally within cell bodies. Second, intimate structural similarities are found among arteriolar smooth muscle cells, granular cells, and intra- and EGM cells, suggesting that they have the same origin. Third, they are extensively coupled by gap junctions. Gap junctions not only bridge different cells, but also regularly bridge individual processes of the same cell.[785] Moreover, gap junction contacts consistently occur to all other cells of the JGA (except the macula densa!), i.e., to granular cells, to ordinary smooth muscle cells of both arterioles, and to the mesangial cells proper.[19]

From a biomechanical point of view, the contractile apparatus of EGM cells is conspicuous. Microfilament bundles are contained within the periphery of cell bodies and within the cell processes, which are connected to the walls of both glomerular arterioles and to the basement membrane of the parietal layer of Bowman's capsule (PBM) surrounding the glomerular hilum (Figures 20.68 and 20.69). As a whole, the EGM can be considered as a spider-like contractile clamp sitting above the glomerular entrance interconnecting all structures at this site.[20] The EGM probably represents some sort of closure device of the glomerular entrance, maintaining the structural integrity of the entrance against the distending forces exerted on it by the high intraglomerular pressure. Moreover, from the viewpoint that the glomerular mesangium represents a high pressure compartment (mesangial interstitial pressures are expected to range in the same magnitude as glomerular capillary pressures[147]), the EGM would seem to be the structure which mediates a gradual pressure drop toward the cortical interstitium and toward the base of the macula densa.[20]

The function of the EGM cells is obscure. Because of their central position within the JGA, their constant relationships to the macula densa and their gap junction coupling to all smooth muscle-derived cells of the JGA, the EGM cells have repeatedly been considered as the necessary functional link between the macula densa and any possible effector cell within the regulatory mechanisms of the JGA.[20,99] Thus, they are widely considered as an integrating system of signals derived

FIGURE 20.69 Flat section through the extraglomerular mesangium (rat). (a) The section crosses the afferent (AA) and the efferent (EA) arteriole; it grazes the top of Bowman's capsule, showing the basement membrane of Bowman's capsule (BCBM), and the parietal epithelium (PE), as well as the urinary space (US). The extraglomerular mesangium forms a complicated texture by which the structures of the vascular pole are interconnected. Note that toward their insertion in the BCBM the extraglomerular mesangial cells fall apart into many processes (stars) (G: Granular cells; TEM: $\times \sim 2650$). (b) Higher magnification of extraglomerular mesangial cells. Note the microfilament bundles within the periphery of cell bodies, as well as within cell processes (arrows). Note the irregular extracellular spaces filled with a matrix of varying appearance (star) (TEM: $\times \sim 6000$). (c) Gap junction between two mesangial cells (rat: TEM: $\times \sim 147,000$).

from the reabsorptive function of the MD and the function of the EGM as a pressure sentinel mirroring the blood pressure in the afferent–efferent arteriolar system, but details are unknown.

The intimate and systematic juxtaposition of tubular and vascular cells within the JGA has given rise to early speculations about a feedback system between tubular and glomerular function.[786] It has now become clear that the JGA serves two different functions: it regulates the flow resistance of afferent arterioles in the so-called tubuloglomerular feedback mechanism; and it participates in the control of renin synthesis and release from granular cells in the afferent arteriole.[787] Researchers originally assumed that the two responses might be related to each other, in that renin released from the granular cells not only has systematic relevance, but locally triggers the formation of angiotensin II, and thus is responsible for afferent vasoconstriction as well; however, it now appears that the final activation of smooth muscle and granular effector cells occurs through largely independent pathways. Renin release from granular cells is the major source of systemic angiotensin II, and thus plays an essential role in controlling extracellular volume and blood pressure, whereas the vasoconstriction of the afferent arteriole locally serves to modulate the filtration of this nephron.

For both mechanisms, it is well-established that a change in NaCl concentration in the tubular fluid at the MD initiates the appropriate signal. Thus, the MD, situated at the very end of the TAL, controls the work of the TAL; the short postmacula segment of the TAL may be interpreted to guarantee that the composition of the tubular fluid at the MD might not be influenced by the function of the subsequent DCT. Expressed in general terms, the MD translates changes in the tubular fluid Na-Cl concentration into a graded release of mediators that reach their target by diffusion, thus acting in a paracrine fashion. Note that the extraglomerular mesangium that mediates the contact between the MD and the effector cells is not vascularized, so that the build-up of any paracrine agent would not be perturbed by blood flow.

With respect to renin release, the most likely paracrine mediators of this process are prostaglandin E 2 and nitric oxide.[18,788–790] With respect to the vasoconstrictor response purinergic mediators, either ATP or adenosine, as first suggested by Oswald and colleagues[791] appear to play the major role.[62,787,792] For an up to-date discussion of the function of the JGA see the reviews by Schnermann and Levine,[787,793] Persson and colleagues,[794] and Komlosi and colleagues.[795,796]

THE RENAL MEDULLA

During phylogeny the renal medulla has developed in response to the necessity to conserve water by excreting concentrated urine.[29] Loops of Henle, collecting ducts, and a specific blood supply through vascular bundles have developed into a complex structural system that accounts for this function. However, the details are insufficiently understood.

The overall mechanism (Figure 20.70) is clear: reabsorption of NaCl from the MTALs in the outer medulla represents the driving force to produce an interstitial cortico-medullary osmotic gradient that provokes osmotic water withdrawal from the collecting duct when the latter descend toward the papillary tip. The reabsorbed water is brought back into the systemic circulation by venous vasa.[2,797]

The unresolved problem is the generation of a cortico-papillary solute gradient, notably in the inner medulla. In discussions concerning the formation of a medullary solute gradient "countercurrent multiplication" has occupied a center-stage as the decisive mechanism. This mechanism has been experimentally established in artificial tubes,[798] and has been imposed on the renal medulla, conceding immense deviations from the original conditions. From a structural point of view, the preconditions for countercurrent multiplication in the renal medulla would appear to be quite incompletely developed: at no site are the limbs of Henle's loop juxtaposed to each other. Even when allowing a mediating interstitial space between both loop limbs, the DTLs do not case behave homogenously in an adequate way, but they change their function gradually on their descent, and even change their transport characteristics to the ascending limb type a considerable distance before the bend; most relevant in the present context is that the terminal third of the SDTLs in the mouse kidney is equipped with TAL epithelium.[16,34] Without going into more details, everyone who has been engaged in this problem knows that the principle of countercurrent multiplication has been extensively bent to make it fit with the structural organization of the renal medulla — in our view, with little benefit in facilitating the understanding of the function of the renal medulla. If at all, this principle can only be applied to describe the mechanism in the outer medulla. In the inner medulla, a process that could be regarded as a "single concentrating effect" is not apparent. Several "passive models"[452,799–802] attempting to explain the concentrating mechanism in the inner medulla have greatly refined our understanding of the problem, but have never reached the level of a convincing theory.

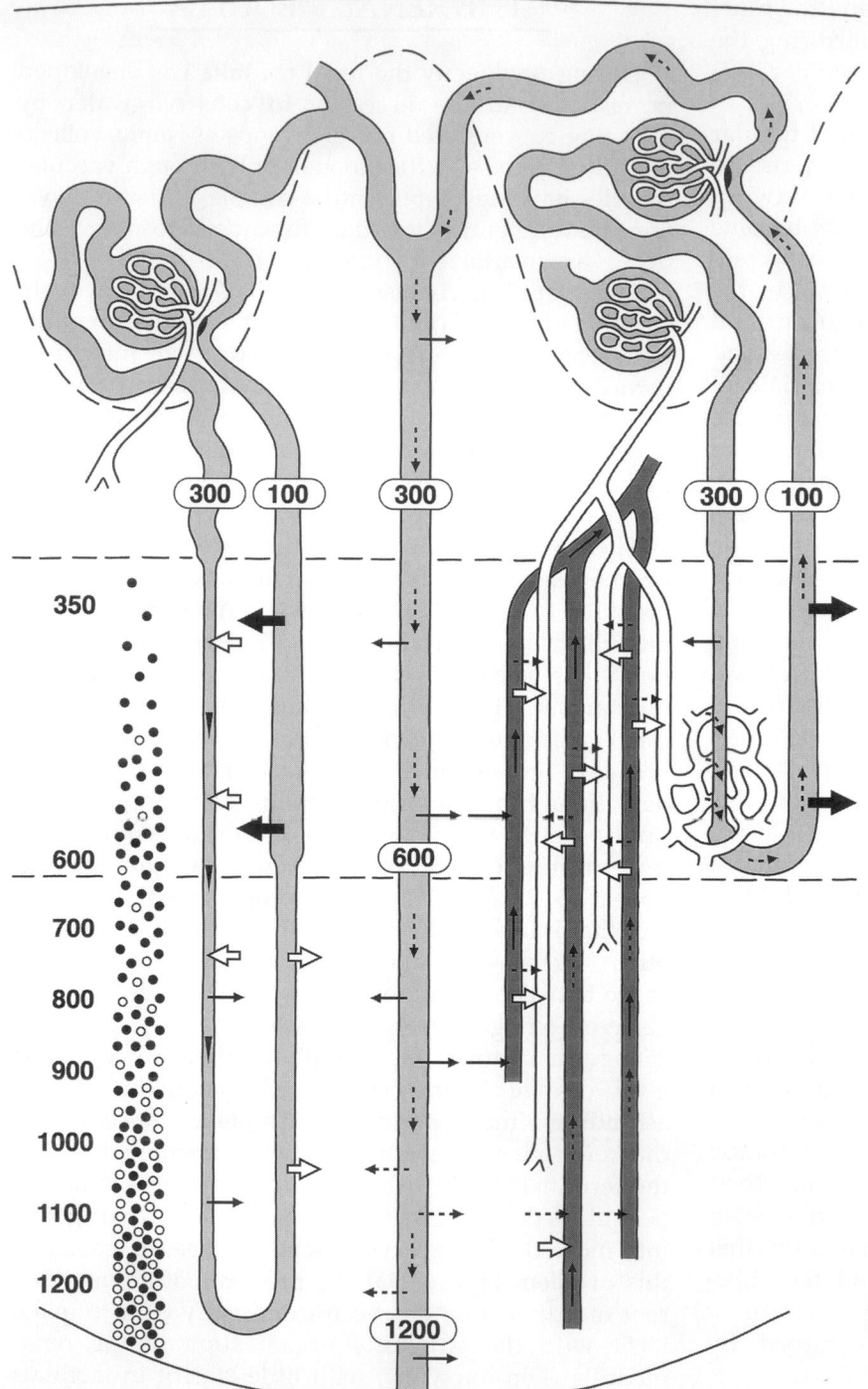

FIGURE 20.70 Schematic to show the functional interactions in the medulla as they are derived from the histotopography of the structures, the distribution of channels and transporters and direct measurements of transport characteristics in the various tubular and vessel segments. A long looped nephron, a short looped nephron, and a collecting duct are shown in light gray. Descending vasa recta (DVRs) derived from the efferent arteriole of a juxtamedullary glomerulus are shown in white (including the capillaries), ascending vasa recta (AVRs) in dark gray: both together establish a vascular bundle. The osmolar concentration in the medulla rises from the cortico-medullary border to the papillary tip from 300 to 12,000 mosmol/l, mainly established by the increase in the concentration of salt (indicated by dark dots) and urea (indicated by open circles). The driving force of the concentrating mechanism is the dumping of salt into the medullary interstitium from TALs (thick black arrows), leaving behind a diluted fluid (indicated by an osmolar concentration of 100 mosmol/l at the re-entry into the cortex). Osmotic water withdrawal from CCDs (slim arrows) into the cortical circulation again elevates the tubular urine to 300 mosmol/l upon re-entry into the medulla. Continuous water reabsorption along the MCDs (slim arrows) will produce a final urine concentration of about 12,000 mosmol/l (in humans). The source for the inner medullary solute gradient is shown to consist of: (1) dragging of salt from the IS into the IM by LDTLs (arrow heads); and (2) re-entry of urea from the CDs into the terminal portion of the IM (hatched arrows). The gain in osmotic energy by urea re-entry originates from urea recycling, which starts with a shift of urea from the AVRs into the SDTLs in the IS (follow the hatched arrows), and concentration of this urea by water reabsorption in the CCDs, OMCDs, and starting portions of IMCDs (see text for further explanation). The removal of the water from the medulla regained from the CDs (thus the final step in urine concentration) is effected by AVRs (follow the slim arrows). These vessels are the core structures in the complex countercurrent exchange system of the medulla equilibrating at any level with the local concentrations of salt and urea. Open thick arrows show passive movements of salt (see text).

In this situation it might be worth an attempt, opposite to the usual, to start with the available functional data – including the recent data on the distribution of transporters – confronting them with the structure, i.e., the architecture of the renal medulla, as well as the cellular organization of the individual components, in order to arrive at a novel view of "function–structure–correlation."

Let us first regard the three regions of the medulla with such an approach. The most constant region is the IS; there is no renal medulla known without an IS. In contrast, an OS is frequently quite incompletely developed, and an IM may be fully absent.

The Inner Stripe of the Outer Medulla

The IS (Figures 20.20 and 20.24) is made up of two portions: the vascular bundles (VBs) and the interbundle region (IBR). The IBR contains the tubules (DTLs, TALs, CDs) supplied by a dense capillary plexus which is drained upwards by the gradual transition of capillaries into AVRs that directly ascend into the OS. Since all the salt reabsorbed by MTALs accumulates in this area, the interstitium of the IBR is rich in salt.[803]

The VBs, structurally, are part of the IS but, functionally, they belong to the IM. They represent a quite perfectly developed countercurrent exchange system primarily handling the blood descending to and ascending from the IM by respective DVRs and AVRs. However, since the DVRs also supplying the capillary plexus of the IBR of the IS are contained within the VBs (not the respective AVRs), the VBs provide the possibility of shifting solutes coming up from the IM into the IBR of the IS. Since the dominating solute of the IM is urea, the VBs are rich in urea. The handling of urea as a main function of the VBs becomes most obvious in the complex bundles (see below).

The Inner Medulla

The IM (Figures 20.20 and 20.27) including the papilla, at the transverse level, is homogenously organized; a separation into VBs and an IBR is no longer possible. Even if there may be a certain prevalence that the ATLs are more frequently gathered around CDs than DTLs,[34,804] it appears quite doubtful that this is of any functional relevance. The AVRs (including the capillaries) are homogenously distributed among all other components and, most importantly, a wide homogenous interstitial space permits the interaction of every descending tube with every ascending tube. The IM provides strict countercurrent arrangements of all involved structures, but without giving prevalence to any specific lateral interaction. Thus, the IM as a whole may be considered as a countercurrent system that allows countercurrent exchange – mediated by the interstitium – between all descending (DVRs, DTLs, CDs) and all ascending tubes (AVRs, ATLs), according to the transport characteristics of the individual tubes.

A most important feature of the IM is its particular shape reflecting its longitudinal organization. The inner medulla tapers from a broad basis to a tiny papilla[2] (see also above). This shape perfectly reflects what happens with the structures within the inner medulla: loops of Henle, vasa recta, and collecting ducts (by fusing together) all decrease rapidly in number from the base to the tip of the papilla.[119,805] For the rat, it has been calculated that, of an estimated 10,000 long loops entering the inner medulla at its base, only about 1500 reach the papillary half of the inner medulla, and only a few of these the papillary tip.[2] The majority of long loops, the "short" long loops, turn back shortly after entering the inner medulla, a smaller but still substantial number of long loops reach the middle part of the inner medulla, and only a small population of "long" long loops really reach the papilla.

The Outer Stripe of the Outer Medulla

The OS (Figures 20.20 and 20.23) is a transitional region which separates the medulla from the cortex, mediating the transition between an hyperosmotic and an isoosmotic environment. The OS does not seem to make any particular contribution to the creation of the cortico-medullary solute gradient, but it greatly helps to maintain it. The OS contains the nascent (or dissolving) VBs (performing the same function as in the IS but quantitatively of minor importance) and the AVRs which are directly coming up form the IBR of the IS (Figure 20.71). Together with the AVRs spreading out from the dissolving VBs, the AVRs as a whole traverse the OS as individual vessels intimately associated with the tubules of this region; actually they represent the major "capillary" supply of the OS (see above). In addition, among all regions of the kidney, the OS exhibits the smallest fraction of interstitial space, thus the vessels are most closely juxtaposed to the tubules (note: lymphatics are absent from the entire medulla[25]). Since the PSTs of juxtamedullary nephrons, in contrast to their name, take a tortuous course when descending through the OS, the majority of tubular profiles in the OS consists of PSTs (S3 segments). This arrangement – AVRs closely associated with descending PTs (and, to some extent, also CDs) represent an ultimate countercurrent trap to prevent the loss of osmotic energy into the systemic circulation (Figure 20.71 right panel). Since reabsorption from PTs is isoosmotic, the hypertonic environment created by AVRs will allow water withdrawal not only from CDs (starting the concentrating process), but also from the PTs, increasing their osmolarity already at the level of the OS – with a clear prevalence of the PTs of juxtamedullary nephrons (tortuous course!) that give rise to the "long long loops." The TALs of the OS are already of the cortical type (equipped with a comparably flat epithelium; see above) capable of maintaining and even increasing a large salt gradient, but incapable of transporting large quantities.[308]

So far, we have a summary of the essential architectural features of the three medullary regions; let us now talk about the functional connections between them. This needs, first, to talk about the overall mechanism

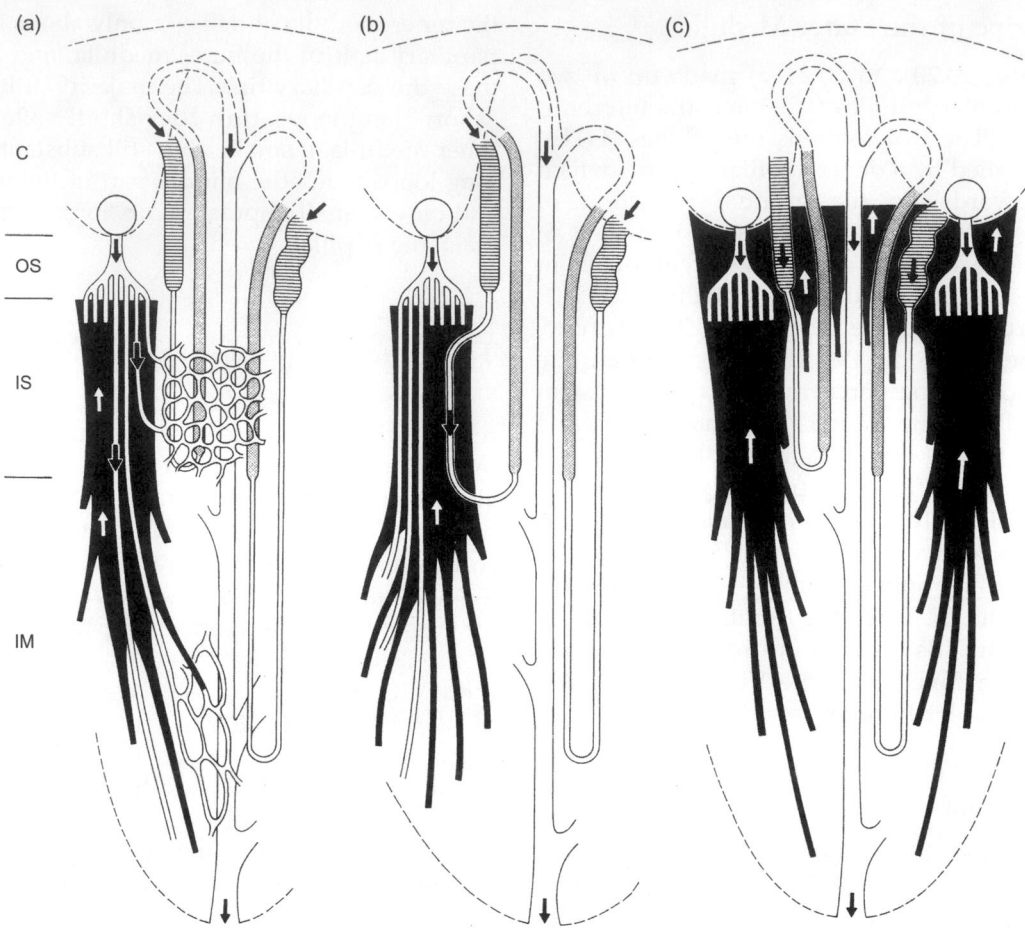

FIGURE 20.71   Schematics to demonstrate the possible recycling routes within the medulla. A short loop and a long loop of Henle and a collecting duct are shown. The straight proximal tubules are hatched; the thin limbs, collecting ducts, and capillaries are white; the thick ascending limbs are gray. Ascending vasa recta are drawn black en bloc (C: cortex; OS: outer stripe; IS: inner stripe; IM: inner medulla). (a) Simple type of medulla: recycling route from the ascending vasa recta in the inner stripe, via descending vasa recta, to inner stripe tubules. (b) Complex type of medulla: recycling route from ascending vasa recta in the inner stripe to descending thin limbs of short loops. (c) Recycling route from the ascending vasa recta in the outer stripe to descending tubules (proximal tubules and collecting ducts); valid for both the simple type and the complex type of medulla. *(Adapted from Kaissling, B., and Kriz, W. (1979). Structural analysis of the rabbit kidney. Adv. Anat. Embryol. Cell Biol. 56, 1–123, and Kriz, W., and Barrett, J. M. et al. (1976). The renal vasculature. In "Anatomical–Functional Aspects. Kidney and Urinary Tract Physiology II, 1–21, Thruau, K. Tokyo University Park Press, Baltimore, London.)*

underlying urine concentration in some more detail, and afterwards to talk about the individual mechanisms.

The Basic Mechanism in Some Detail

The renal medulla contains the phylogenetically ancient "diluting segments" of the nephron, i.e., the TALs which separate salt from water (Figure 20.70). The salt is dumped into the medullary interstitium, the water is carried up into the cortex and — in the case that ADH is available — is recovered by the systemic circulation through osmotic withdrawl from the CCDs. Thus, the tubular urine that re-enters the renal medulla in the collecting duct is isoosmotic with respect to plasma concentration, and considerably reduced in quantity compared to the amount that originally entered the renal medulla in descending limbs after filtration.

Thus, the salt that is available to drive the concentrating mechanism has emerged from a much larger quantity of isoosmotic fluid than the quantity of isoosmotic fluid that is subject to concentration. Moreover, along with the increasing concentration of the CD urine, less and less water has to be reclaimed to achieve the same increment in concentration; the work that is necessary to account for a progressively increasing urine concentration decreases steeply toward the tip of the papilla.

In the IM, in addition to salt, urea is a major solute accounting for the solute gradient toward the tip of the papilla. Since in the IM neither any up-hill transport of salt nor of urea is known, the crucial problem consists of explaining the increasing concentration of salt (flat increase) and of urea (steep increase) in the IM toward the papillary tip. If both depend on the work of the TALs in the OM, how can part of the osmotic energy be carried down from the OM into the IM and piled up there to a steep solute gradient toward the tip of the papilla?

In our view, three major mechanisms have become apparent that are responsible for the distribution of salt and urea into a cortico-papillary gradient in the IM (Figure 20.70). They all depend on salt reabsorption by TALs in the OM; they all fit with the morphology, even more: specific structural elaborations in highly concentrating species support their relevance. These are: (1) salt dragging by flow to deeper medullary levels; (2) countercurrent exchange of solutes and water to maintain the cortico-papillary gradient; and (3) urea recycling by short loops of Henle as a major mechanism to create the solute gradient toward the papilla.

Dragging of Solutes by Flow to Deeper Medullary Levels

In all descending tubes of the renal medulla (DVRs, DTLs, CDs) solutes are dragged by flow to deeper medullary levels. This appears to be relevant for salt in the DTLs and for urea in the CDs (see urea recycling).

Continuous uptake and dragging of salt by SDTLs down to their bends at the end of the IS has been considered as an essential mechanism in the original countercurrent multiplication concept. In the light of current knowledge such a mechanism in short DTLs may not be of crucial importance. In contrast to previous reports, SDTLs (apart from some of them; see above) do not express aquaporin, and thus must be considered as fairly water-impermeable. Also, the Na^+ and Cl^- permeability was found to be low.[806] Thus, the increasing concentration towards the bend of SDTLs seems to be predominantly accounted for by urea entry into the lower part (see below: urea recycling). However, in any case the salt left from filtration at the end of the proximal tubule that enters the SDTLs in the OS will be dragged down by flow until the loop bends and will return in the TALs to be reabsorbed there. In case that, despite low salt permeability, a small part of the reabsorbed salt may − via the interstitium − re-enter the descending limb, thus being trapped within the SDTLs, this salt transfer from the TALs to the SDTLs represents the only esssential step that would be left from the countercurrent multiplication principle.

In contrast, continuous uptake of salt by LDTLs in the OM and dragging it by flow down into the IM appears to be the essential mechanism for salt accumulation in the IM; no other source of salt (apart from a small quantity reabsorbed by IMCDs) for the IM is obvious. Available models of the inner medullary concentrating process do not put so much emphasis on this mechanism, but the structural data strongly do suggest it. Layton and colleagues[452] were the first to include this idea into a model. The structural arguments are the following:

1. The upper portions of the LDTLs, most obvious in the IS, have an epithelial organization that suggests ion transport through extensively developed (Figure 20.48a) claudin 2 (cation pore) and claudin 10 (anion and cation pore) containing tight junctions.[261,807] Since the salt concentration is certainly higher outside the LDTLs (see below), salt can readily be expected to diffuse into the lumen. This process may become reinforced by active salt-secretion into the lumen, based on the abundant occurrence of Na^+-K^+-ATPase in the upper portions of LDTLs.[446,447] Moreover, the LDTLups are the only thin limb segments with abundant expression of aquaporin 1 channels (see below). No question, the salt concentrations within LDTLs at the transition from the OM to the IM may be expected to be quite high. Measured data are not available, but it seems reasonable to suggest considerably higher salt concentrations inside than outside.

2. The LDTLs on their descent through the inner stripe always pass through the sodium richest area, i.e., distant from the vascular bundles among the TALs of short loops[803] (Figure 20.22). In the mouse kidney, two specific modifications in this system appear to reinforce the ability of LDTLs for salt uptake. First, the LDTLs take a tortuous course when descending through the IS (increasing their length by 27%[34]) and, second, at the end of the IS before entering the IM, they traverse the so-called "innermost stripe," which has a thickness of about half of the IS proper and in which the SDTLs are already equipped with the TAL epithelium.[16,34] Thus, the density of TALs dumping salt into the interstitium at this level is dramatically higher (5 versus 3 per unit area) than at any other level of the OM. Consequently, the interstitial salt concentration should be very high. The LDTLs traverse this region and may readily be expected to take up some of the accumulated salt.

3. After challenging urine concentration in rats by water deprivation (or treatment with ADH) the TALs hypertrophy, with the most prominent increase in epithelial salt transport capacity of the initial portions in the deep IS.[520,808] Thus again, a prominent "surplus" in salt accumulation occurs just at the border to the inner medulla.

4. As described above, the LDTLs are quite heterogeneous with respect to their actual length,

and with respect to the epithelial differentiation of their upper parts.[435,803] Most important, the actual length of an LDTL strictly correlates with the degree of epithelial elaboration of its upper part in the IS. The small fraction of longest long loops extending down into the papilla clearly have the most prominent upper parts in the IS: they are thicker, with larger lumina and with more elaborate epithelia composed of heavily interdigitating cells; also their abundance in Na-K-ATPase is spectacular.[446] Comparing these longest long loops with those extending down into the IM for only short or intermediate distances, there is a continuous spectrum also with respect to the epithelial elaboration in the IS. Thus, the idea is plausible that salt is taken up by the upper portions of LDTLs, and subsequently carried down through the salt impermeable lower portions to the bend region. Beginning abruptly with a prebend segment, the loop becomes ion-permeable, allowing the salt to be dumped into the interstitium. In the mouse, the prebend segments are quite prominent comprising a length up to 700 μm.[34] Thus, the entire loop bend appears to represent a loop segment that delivers salt into the interstitium.

Since the lower portions of LDTLS are also water-permeable (to what extent is not clear[452,453]), water withdrawal may further increase the salt concentration in these segments. The problem consists of the driving force for such a process. A possibility offered from a structural view is that the heterogeneous longitudinal distribution of loops within the inner medulla (as describe above) might account for a cascade-like transport of salt toward the papilla. The large fraction of "short" long loops carries salt into the first third of the IM. Together with some urea (emerging from reabsorption by papillary CDs and subsequent recycling; see later) the total interstitial osmolality will be elevated above DTL fluid osmolality at the respective level allowing reclaimation of water from DTLs, elevating the total osmolality and salt concentration in all the DTLs underway to deeper medullary levels. A major fraction of those will reach an intermediate level of the IM before bending, dumping a major fraction of its salt at this level into the interstitium. Again, together with some urea a driving force will be established accounting for some water withdrawal from the small fraction of "long" long loops that will carry their salt into the papillary tip. No question, this is quite a hypothetical idea, but from a structural point of view would be worth modeling. Ideas in this direction have been published previously,[435] and also mathematical models for some features of such a mechanism have been presented.[452]

Countercurrent Exchange of Solutes and Water

Countercurrent exchange in a U-type countercurrent exchanger may have two functions: (1) trapping of solutes within the system by transfer of solutes from the ascending to the descending limb; and (2) preventing water from entering the system by short circuiting from the descending to the ascending limb. Both mechanisms *per se* do not build up any solute gradient; they are only capable of maintaining a gradient (with little loss). However, incorporated into the complex countercurrent arrangement of the renal medulla they decisively participate in the creation of the cortico-papillary gradient. In agreement with others,[797] in our view, the relevance of countercurrent exchange has always been underestimated compared to countercurrent multiplication in the urine concentrating mechanism. Actually, from a structural point of view, the renal medulla should best be considered as an extremely complex countercurrent exchange system that is fuelled by two mechanisms at two sites: by salt reabsorption through TALs in the OS; and by urea addition through terminal CDs in the IM. These solutes are distributed by countercurrent exchange into a cortico-medullary gradient that — due to continuous fueling — allows water withdrawal from CDs and the transport of this water into the systemic circulation in the cortex.

As already discussed above, a more-or-less direct countercurrent exchange between juxtaposed countercurrent tubes may only occur within the VBs of the IS. In contrast, in the IBR of the IS, and within the entire IM, the countercurrent tubes are consistently separated from each other by comparably wide interstitial spaces, thus any exchange at a transverse level is mediated by the interstitium. No doubt, this decreases the effectiveness of the exchanges, but allows countercurrent exchanges between more than two structures. Any solute dumped into the inner medullary interstitium, i.e., predominantly salt from LDTLs (at their bends) and urea from CDs (at their terminal portion) or left in ATL and AVRs at their beginning in the IM, will be subject to countercurrent trapping (or used to drive countercurrent short-circuiting of water; see below), between AVRs and ATLs on the one site and DVRs and DTLs on the other.

In addition to solute trapping, countercurrent exchange of water preventing the flow of water to deeper levels by short circuiting seems of major relevance. The recent elucidation of the distribution of aquaporins in medullary structures has shed considerable light on the handling of water in the urine concentrating process. Among the thin limbs only the LDTLups have regularly been found to be equipped with aquaporin 1 channels; in rat, also, the LDTLlps have been reported to express AQP1[453]; DVRs are abundantly equipped with AQP1 channels[453]; the water permeability of CDs is ADH-dependent (see above). The only ascending structures that are water-permeable are the AVRs (based on the hydrophilic fenestrae providing a direct route of water flow through the endothelium). Thus, any water withdrawn from any descending structure finally enters an AVR, by which it is brought back to the cortex. This cardinal function of AVRs has recently been analyzed in detail by Pallone and colleagues.[797]

The ability of AVRs to take up water appears to be based on an elevated oncotic pressure (resulting from short circuiting of water between DVRs and AVRs within the VBs), and on the reasonable assumption that the blood in capillaries at any level of the medulla is in osmotic equilibrium with the interstitial fluid (due to the hydrophilic fenestrae in capillary and AVR endothelia). Thus, when capillary blood at any level of the medulla starts to assemble in AVRs and to ascend, it will − after any small ascent − become hyperosmotic compared to the surrounding interstitium. Due to the abundant hydrophilic fenestrae of the AVR endothelium osmotic equilibrium will most easily be achieved by water uptake.

The water to be taken up originates mainly from the CDs, but water may also originate from DTLs. In LTDLs, the upper parts have abundant aquaporins (type 1) in both membranes surprisingly contained in an epithelium that exhibits the features of an ion-permeable epithelium, i.e., an extremely lengthened leaky tight junction due to extensive cellular interdigitation. Thus, this epithelium, in addition to being water-permeable, obviously allows the transport of large amounts of ions. From what we have argued above, that salt dragging by flow in LDTLs appears to be the only mechanism to bring down the salt into the IM, large volumes of salt-enriched urine would be the best precondition for this goal. It appears to us that the actual transport capabilities of the upper portions of LDTLs have not been completely elucidated. Along the lower portions of LDTLs in the IM, the water permeability progressively decreases and fully ceases at the transition to the prebend segment.[437,438] This offers the possibility (described already above) that water withdrawal from the LDTLs by an osmotic driving force established at each medullary level by salt and urea might lead to a "cascade-like" transport of salt toward the tip of the papilla.

Urea Recycling

Solute recycling is a different mechanism compared to solute trapping by countercurrent exchange; this difference is rarely appreciated. Urea appears to be the only solute, recycling of which plays an essential role in the urine concentrating process. Recycling of urea defines a process that starts with a molecule of urea in the inner medullary interstitium and brings this molecule back into the IM via the normal tubular route, finally re-entering the inner medullary interstitium via exit from the terminal IMCD (Figure 20.70). As described above, the terminal portion of the IMCDs contains the urea transporters UTA$_1$ and UTA$_3$ which allow the facilitated diffusion of urea from the CD into the surrounding interstitium.[809] A precondition for this reuptake of urea is that the concentration of urea in the tubular urine of IMCDs has reached a higher level than in the medullary interstitium at the same level. This is achieved by water removal through urea-impermeable tubular segments, i.e., CNTs and CCDs in the cortex, OMCDs and upper IMCDs in the medulla. The reabsorption of urea through IMCDs compromises the reclaiming of water through IMCDs, decreasing urine concentration instead of increasing it. Thus, urea does both: on the one hand, reabsorption of urea increases the inner medullary solute gradient, thereby decreasing urine osmolality; on the other hand, the increased solute gradient increases the driving force for water reabsorption, thereby increasing urine osmolality. This sounds like a story from Baron Münchhausen, who was able to help himself getting out of a swamp by pulling on his own hairs.

However, the two opposing functions of urea have a solid base: a given molecule of urea may become active a second (or a third) time, this is what urea recycling means. After entering the inner medullary interstitium from an IMCD, a given molecule of urea will travel towards the cortex within an AVR, thereby balancing (together with other molecules and other solutes) a certain amount of water that enters the AVR along its ascent, and that finally has to be delivered into the systemic circulation at the cortico-medullary border. However, this specific molecule of urea participates in water balancing on its way from a hyperosmotic to an isoosmotic environment only up to an intermediate level, i.e., up to the IS. Here it re-enters the nephron; its relevance in balancing water that continuously enters the AVR and needs to be transported further up into the cortex is taken over by salt which, due to the active Na$^+$ reabsorption by TALs, is available in abundance at this level. Thus, the urea molecule has spent only part of its osmotic energy for the transport of water before it re-enters the nephron, precisely the SDTL, and becomes again subject of a concentrating process in subsequent urea-impermeable, but water-permeable, tubular segments. This urea molecule started the intratubular concentrating process at a higher energy level than a urea molecule that entered the tubule by filtration. In our view, this difference in osmotic energy between a recycling and a freshly filtered urea molecule, entering the nephron in the IS versus in the cortex, and becoming subject to a concentrating process by water removal along the DCT, CNT, CCD, OMCD, and upper IMCD represents a real gain in osmotic energy that is finally available for water reabsorption in the inner medulla. Entry of urea to the LTDLs somewhere in the IM (i.e., recycling of urea via long loops) would not have a similar effect, simply because at this site there is no surplus salt available to replace urea in its role of water balancing.

At the present stage of knowledge, urea recycling via short loops appears as an essential process in urine concentration, and represents the most obvious evidence for the numerical dominance of short loops of Henle in every highly concentrating species. Note that also species which by definition are commonly reported to have 100% long loops (e.g., *Psammomys obesus*) in reality have a majority of short loops.

Moreover, as described above, the SDTLs in such highly concentrating rodent species are directly incorporated into the vascular bundles, and thus provide a more direct route for urea recycling than the simple bundles (Figures 20.22, 20.25, 20.26, and 20.71).[16,32,115,435] Within the VBs of such species, AVRs coming up from the IM are arranged in a countercurrent fashion not only with DVRs but, most prominently, also with the SDTLs. Thus urea, by countercurrent exchange, may directly enter the SDTLs through the urea transporter UT-A2[441,809] (the hydrophilic fenestrae of the endothelium of the AVRs may readily be expected to be highly permeable for urea). In a renal medulla with "simple" vascular bundles (as they are found in most species) countercurrent exchange of urea first occurs from AVRs to DVRs (which contain the urea transporter UT-B1[810,811]), which afterwards will deliver their blood to the capillary plexus of the IBR in the IS, which perfuses the SDTLs on their descending way. Thus, even if probably much less effective, urea from the inner medulla has access to the SDTLs[435,803,809] and may start its recycling route to the terminal CD in the papilla.[435,809,811]

The locus of urea redelivery, i.e., in the papilla, thus at the "ultimate bend" of the complex countercurrent exchange system in the papilla, is optimal, since by countercurrent exchange in vasa recta and thin limbs, urea is largely trapped and distributed in a longitudinal gradient within the inner medulla. The fraction of urea that escapes this process in the inner medulla is subject to recycling via short loops (starting in the IS) back into the inner medulla, and is thus available another time within the papillary interstitium ready to withdraw and/or to balance water reabsorption from the collecting duct.

CONCLUSION

The urine concentrating mechanism certainly does not belong to the most urgent of problems in medicine, but it represents a highly challenging biological enigma. We are aware that several aspects of our view are hypothetical, but they are based on particular structural features (the ultrastructural organization and particular histotopographical relationships of LDTLs, the incorporation of SDTLs into the VBs in highly concentrating rodent species) for which no better functional relevance is available. Whether the proposed mechanisms are sufficient to build up an effective solute gradient in the IM (in rodents up to several osmoles) or whether there are additional sources complementing the solute gradients (continuous production of osmotic active substances) is presently unknown.

References

[1] Hodson J. The lobar structure of the kidney. Br J Urol 1972;44:246.

[2] Jamison R, Kriz W. Urinary concentrating mechanism. Structure and function. New York: Oxford University Press; 1982.

[3] Sperber J. Studies of the mammalian kidney. Zool Bidrag 1944;22:249–431.

[4] Inke G. The protolobar structure of the human kidney. New York: Alan R. Liss, Inc; 1988.

[5] Kaissling B, Kriz W. Structural analysis of the rabbit kidney. Adv Anat Embryol Cell Biol 1979;56:1–123.

[6] Schmidt-Nielsen B, Pfeiffer E. Urea and urinary concentrating ability in the mountain beaver, *Aplodontia rufa*. Am J Physiol 1970;218:1370–5.

[7] Lacy E. The mammalian renal pelvis: physiological implications from morphometric analyses. Anat Embryol 1980; 160:131–44.

[8] Fourman J, Moffat D. The blood vessels of the kidney. Oxford: Blackwell Scientific; 1971.

[9] Lemley K, Kriz W. Structure and function of the renal vasculature. In: Tisher C, Brenner B, editors. Renal pathology. Philadelphia: Lippincott,J.B.; 1989. p. 926–64.

[10] Moffat D, Fourman J. The vascular pattern of the rat kidney. J Anat 1963;97:543–53.

[11] Rollhäuser H, Kriz W, Heinke W. Das Gefässsystem der Rattenniere. Z Zellforsch Mikrosk Anat 1964;64:381–403.

[12] Beeuwkes R. Efferent vascular patterns and early vascular-tubular relations in the dog kidney. Am J Physiol 1971;221:1361–74.

[13] Casellas D, Mimran A. Shunting in renal microvasculature of the rat: a scanning electron microscopic study of corosion casts. Anat Rec 1981;201:237–48.

[14] Moffat D. The Mammalian Kidney. London: Cambridge University; 1975.

[15] Beeuwkes R, Bonventre J. Tubular organization and vascular–tubular relations in the dog kidney. Am J Physiol 1975;229:695–713.

[16] Kriz W, Koepsell H. The structural organization of the mouse kidney. Z Anat Entwicklungsgesch 1974;144:137–63.

[17] Bankir L, Kaissling B, de Rouffignac C, Kriz W. The vascular organization of the kidney of *Psammomys obesus*. Anat Embryol 1979;155:149–60.

[18] Kurtz A. Renin release: sites, mechanisms, and control. Annu Rev Physiol 2011;73:377—99.

[19] Taugner R, Hackenthal E. In: Springer-Verlag, editor. The juxtaglomerular apparatus. Berlin,Heidelberg: Springer-Verlag; 1989.

[20] Elger M, Sakai T, Kriz W. The vascular pole of the renal glomerulus of rat. Adv Anat Embryol Cell Biol 1998;139:1—98.

[21] Schnabel E, Kriz W, Steinhausen M. Outflow segment of the efferent arteriole of the rat glomerulus investigated by *in vivo* and electron microscopy. Ren Physiol 1987;10:318—26.

[22] Bankir L, Farman N. Hétérogénéité des glomérules chez le lapin. Arch Anat Microsc Morphol Exp 1973;62:281—91.

[23] Dieterich H. Die Struktur der Blutgefäbe in der Rattenniere. In: Bargmann W, Doerr W, editors. Normale und pathologische anatomie. Bd.35. Stuttgart: Thieme; 1978. p. 1—127.

[24] Edwards J. Efferent arterioles of glomeruli in the juxtamedullary zone of the human kidney. Anat Rec 1956;125:521—9.

[25] Kriz W, Dieterich H. The supplying and draining vessels of the renal medulla in mammals. Proceedings of the 4th international congress of nephrology. Basel: Karger; 1970138—144

[26] Bearer E, Orci L. Endothelial fenestral diaphragms: a quick-freeze, deep-etch study. J Cell Biol 1985;100:418—28.

[27] Stan R, Kubitza M, Palade G. PV-1 is a component of the fenestral and stomatal diaphragms in fenestrated endothelia. Proc Natl Acad Sci USA 1999;96:13203—7.

[28] Baines A, de Rouffignac C. Functional heterogeneity of nephrons. II. Filtration rates, intraluminal flow velocities and fractional water reasorption. Pflugers Arch 1969;308:260—76.

[29] Smith H. The kidney: structure and function in health and disease. New York: Oxford University Press; 1951.

[30] Amann K, Plank C, Dotsch J. Low nephron number — a new cardiovascular risk factor in children? Pediatr Nephrol 2004; 19:1319—23.

[31] Bertram J, Douglas-Denton R, Diouf B, Hughson M, Hoy W. Human nephron number: implications for health and disease. Pediatr Nephrol 2011;26:1529—33.

[32] Kaissling B, de Rouffignac C, Barrett J, Kriz W. The structural organization of the kidney of the desert rodent *Psammomys obesus*. Anat Embryol 1975;148:121—43.

[33] Kriz W. Der architektonische und funktionelle Aufbau der Rattenniere. Z Zellforsch Mikrosk Anat 1967;82:495—535.

[34] Zhai X, Thomsen J, Birn H, Kristoffersen I, Andreasen A, Christensen E. Three-dimensional reconstruction of the mouse nephron. J Am Soc Nephrol 2006;17:77—88.

[35] Kaissling B. Ultrastructural organization of the transition from the distal nephron to the collecting duct in the desert rodent *Psammomys obesus*. Cell Tissue Res 1980;212:475—95.

[36] Oliver J. Nephrons and kidneys. New York/Evanston/London: Harper & Row, Hoeber Medical; 1968.

[37] Peter K. Untersuchungen über bau und entwicklung der niere. Jena: Gustav Fischer; 1909.

[38] Kaissling B, Spiess S, Rinne B, Le Hir M. Effects of anemia on the morphology of the renal cortex of rats. Am J Physiol 1993;264:F608—17.

[39] Kriz W, Napiwotzky P. Structural and functional aspects of the renal interstitium. In: Berlyne G, editor. Contr Nephrol. Basel: Karger; 1979. p. 104—8.

[40] Pedersen J, Persson A, Maunsbach A. Ultrastructure and quantitative characterization of the cortical interstitium in the rat kidney. In: Maunsbach A, Olsen T, Christensen E, editors. Functional ultrastructure of the kidney. London: Academic Press; 1980. p. 443—57.

[41] Pfaller W. Structure function correlation in rat kidney. Quantitative correlation of structure and function in the normal and injured rat kidney. Adv Anat Embryol Cell Biol 1982; 70:1—106.

[42] Knepper M, Danielson R, Saidel G, Post R. Quantitative analysis of renal medullary anatomy in rats and rabbits. Kidney Int 1977;12:313—23.

[43] Wolgast M, Larson M, Nygren K. Functional characteristics of the renal interstitium. Am J Physiol 1981;241:F105—11.

[44] Lemley K, Kriz W. Anatomy of the renal interstitium. Kidney Int 1991;39:370—81.

[45] Kaissling B, Le Hir M. Characterization and distribution of interstitial cell types in the renal cortex of rat. Kidney Int 1994;45:709—20.

[46] Eddy A, McCulloch L, Adams J, Liu E. Interstitial nephritis induced by protein-overload proteinuria. Am J Pathol 1989; 135:718—9.

[47] Kaissling B, Hegyi I, Loffing J, Le Hir M. Morphology of interstitial cells in the healthy kidney. Anat Embryol 1996;193:303—18.

[48] Kaissling B, Le Hir M. The renal cortical interstitium: morphological and functional aspects. Histochem Cell Biol 2008;130:247—62.

[49] Schiller A, Taugner R. Junctions between interstitial cells of the renal medulla: a freeze-fracture study. Cell Tissue Res 1979; 203:231—40.

[50] Takahashi-Iwanaga H. The three-dimensional spaces of the kidney. Cell Tissue Res 1991;264:269—81.

[51] Fletcher D, Mullins R. Cell mechanics and the cytoskeleton. Nature 2010;463:485—92.

[52] Fujigaki Y, Muranaka Y, Sun D, Goto T, Zhou H, Sakakima M, et al. Transient myofibroblast differentiation of interstitial fibroblastic cells relevant to tubular dilatation in uranyl acetate-induced acute renal failure in rats. Virchows Arch 2005;446:164—76.

[53] van Kooten C, Daha M. Cytokine cross-talk between tubular epithelial cells and interstitial immunocompetent cells. Curr Opin Nephrol Hypertens 2001;10:55—9.

[54] Postlethwaite A, Kang A. Fibroblasts and matrix proteins. In: Gallin J, Goldstein I, Snyderman R, editors. Inflammation: basic principles and clinical correlates. New York: Raven Press; 1992. p. 747—73.

[55] Karkavelas G, Kefalides N. Comparative ultrastructural localization of collagen types III, IV, VI and laminin in rat uterus and kidney. J Ultrastruct Mol Struct Res 1988;100:137—55.

[56] Pitcock J, Lyons H, Brown P, Rightsel W, Muirhead E. Glycosaminoglycans of the rat renomedullary interstitium: ultrastructural and biochemical observations. Exp Mol Pathol 1988;49:373—87.

[57] Le Hir M, Kaissling B. Distribution and regulation of renal ecto-5'-nucleotidase: implications for physiological functions of adenosine. Am J Physiol 1993;264:F377—87.

[58] Eltzschig H, Ibla J, Furuta G, Leonard M, Jacobson K, Enjyoji K, et al. Coordinated adenine nucleotide phosphohydrolysis and nucleoside signaling in posthypoxic endothelium: role of ectonucleotidases and adenosine A2B receptors. J Exp Med 2003; 198:783—96.

[59] Vallon V. Tubuloglomerular feedback and the control of glomerular filtration rate. News Physiol Sci 2003;18:169—74.

[60] Gandhi R, Le Hir M, Kaissling B. Immunolocalization of ecto-5'nucleotidase in the kidney by a monoclonal antibody. Histochemie 1990;95:165—74.

[61] Franco M, Bautista R, Tapia E, Soto V, Santamaria J, Osorio H, et al. Contribution of renal purinergic receptors to renal vasoconstriction in angiotensin II-induced hypertensive rats. Am J Physiol Renal Physiol 2011;300:F1301—9.

[62] Castrop H, Huang Y, Hashimoto S, Mizel D, Hansen P, Theilig F, et al. Impairment of tubuloglomerular feedback regulation

of GFR in ecto-5′-nucleotidase/CD73-deficient mice. J Clin Invest 2004;114:634–42.

[63] Theilig F, Bostanjoglo M, Pavenstadt H, Grupp C, Holland G, Slosarek I, et al. Cellular distribution and function of soluble guanylyl cyclase in rat kidney and liver. J Am Soc Nephrol 2001;12:2209–20.

[64] Bachmann S, Ramasubbu K. Immunohistochemical colocalization of the alpha-subunit of neutrophil NADPH oxidase and ecto-5′-nucleotidase in kidney and liver. Kidney Int 1997;51:479–82.

[65] Bachmann S, Le Hir M, Eckardt K. Co-localization of erythropoietin mRNA and ecto-5′-nucleotidase immunoreactivity in peritubular cells of rat renal cortex indicates that fibroblasts produce erythropoietin. J Histochem Cytochem 1993;41: 335–41.

[66] Fisher J, Koury S, Ducey T, Mendel S. Erythropoietin production by interstitial cells of hypoxic monkey kidneys. Br J Haematol 1996;95:27–32.

[67] Maxwell P, Osmond M, Pugh C, Heryet A, Nicholls L, Tan C, et al. Identification of the renal erythropoietin-producing cells using transgenic mice. Kidney Int 1993;44:1149–62.

[68] Rosenberger C, Griethe W, Gruber G, Wiesener M, Frei U, Bachmann S, et al. Cellular responses to hypoxia after renal segmental infarction. Kidney Int 2003;64:874–86.

[69] Rosenberger C, Rosen S, Heyman S. Current understanding of HIF in renal disease. Kidney Blood Press Res 2005;28: 325–40.

[70] Maxwell P. HIF-1: an oxygen response system with special relevance to the kidney. J Am Soc Nephrol 2003;14: 2712–22.

[71] Eckardt K, Koury S, Tan C, Schuster S, Kaissling B, Ratcliffe P, et al. Distribution of erythropoietin producing cells in rat kidneys during hypoxic hypoxia. Kidney Int 1993;43: 815–23.

[72] Alpers C, Hudkins K, Floege J, Johnson R. Human renal cortical interstitial cells with some features of smooth muscle cells participate in tubulointerstitial and crescentic glomerular injury. J Am Soc Nephrol 1994;5:201–10.

[73] Desmouliere A, Gabbiani G. Myofibroblast differentiation during fibrosis. Exp Nephrol 1995;3:134–9.

[74] Diamond J, van Goor H, Ding G, Engelmyer E. Myofibroblasts in experimental hydronephrosis. Am J Pathol 1995;146:121–9.

[75] Picard N, Baum O, Vogetseder A, Kaissling B, Le Hir M. Origin of renal myofibroblasts in the model of unilateral ureter obstruction in the rat. Histochem Cell Biol 2008;130: 141–55.

[76] Sappino A, Schurch W, Gabbiani G. Different repertoire of fibroblastic cells: expression of cytoskeletal proteins as markers of phenotypic modulations. Lab Invest 1990;63: 144–61.

[77] Grupp C, Lottermoser J, Cohen D, Begher M, Franz H, Mueller G. Transformation of rat inner medullary fibroblasts to myofibroblasts in vitro. Kidney Int 1997;52:1279–90.

[78] Lüllmann-Rauch R. Lysosomal storage of sulfated glycosaminoglycans in renal interstitial cells of rats treated with tilorone. Cell Tissue Res 1987;250:641–8.

[79] Muirhead E. Discovery of the renomedullary system of blood pressure control and its hormones. Hypertension 1990; 15:114–6.

[80] Vernace M, Mento P, Maita M, Girardi E, Chang M, Nord E, et al. Osmolar regulation of endothelin signaling in rat medullary interstitial cells. J Clin Invest 1995;96:183–91.

[81] Breyer M, Harris R. Cyclooxygenase 2 and the kidney. Curr Opin Nephrol Hypertens 2001;10:89–98.

[82] Jensen B, Kurtz A. Differential regulation of renal cyclooxygenase mRNA by dietary salt intake. Kidney Int 2004;52: 1242–9.

[83] Yang T, Singh I, Pham H, Sun D, Smart A, Schnermann J, et al. Regulation of cyclooxygenase expression in the kidney by dietary salt intake. Am J Physiol 1998;274:F481–9.

[84] Ye W, Zhang H, Hillas E, Kohan D, Miller R, Nelson R, et al. Expression and function of COX isoforms in renal medulla: evidence for regulation of salt sensitivity and blood pressure. Am J Physiol Renal Physiol 2006;290:F542–9.

[85] Austyn J, Hankins D, Larsen C, Morris P, Rao A, Roake J. Isolation and characterization of dendritic cells from mouse heart and kidney. J Histochem Cytochem 1994;41:335–41.

[86] Dong X, Swaminathan S, Bachman L, Croatt A, Nath K, Griffin M. Antigen presentation by dendritic cells in renal lymph nodes is linked to systemic and local injury to the kidney. Kidney Int 2005;68:1096–108.

[87] John R, Nelson P. Dendritic cells in the kidney. J Am Soc Nephrol 2011;18:2628–35.

[88] Soos T, Sims T, Barisoni L, Link K, Littman D, Dustin M, et al. CX3CR1 + interstitial dendritic cells form a contiguous network throughout the entire kidney. Kidney Int 2006; 70:591–6.

[89] Kruger T, Benke D. Identification and functional characterization of dendritic cells in the healthy murine kidney and in experimental glomerulonephritis. J Am Soc Nephrol 2004;15:613–21.

[90] McDermott R, Ziylan U, Spehner D, Bausinger H, Lipsker D, Mommaas M, et al. Birbeck granules are subdomains of endosomal recycling compartment in human epidermal Langerhans cells, which form where Langerin accumulates. Mol Biol Cell 2002;13:317–35.

[91] Le Hir M, Hegyi I, Loffing-Cueni D, Loffing J, Kaissling B. Characterization of renal interstitial fibroblast-specific protein 1/S100A4-positive cells in healthy and inflamed rodent kidneys. Histochem Cell Biol 2005;123:335–46.

[92] Kriz W. A periarterial pathway for intrarenal distribution of renin. Kidney Int 1987;31:S-51–6.

[93] Matusi K, Nagy-Bojarsky K, Laakkonen P, Krieger S, Mechtler K, Uchida S, et al. Lymphatic microvessels in the rat remnant kidney model of renal fibrosis: aminopeptidase p and podoplanin are discriminatory markers for endothelial cells of blood and lymphatic vessels 4432. J Am Soc Nephrol 2003;14:1981–9.

[94] Gardiner B, Smith D, O'Connor P, Evans R. A mathematical model of diffusional shunting of oxygen from arteries to veins in the kidney. Am J Physiol Renal Physiol 2011;300: F1339–52.

[95] Schurek H, Jost U, Baumgärtl H, Bertram H, Heckmann U. Evidence for a preglomerular oxygen diffusion shunt in rat renal cortex. Am J Physiol 1990;259:F910–5.

[96] Barajas L, Wang P. Myelinated nerves of the rat kidney. A light and electron microscopic study. J Ultrastruct Res 1978; 65:148–62.

[97] Barajas L, Wang P. Demonstration of acetylcholinesterase in the adrenergic nerves of the renal glomerular arterioles. J Ultrastruct Res 1975;53:244–53.

[98] Dolezel S, Edvinsson L, Owman C, Owman T. Fluorescence histochemistry and autoradiography of adrenergic nerves in the renal juxtaglomerular complex of mammals and man, with special regard to the efferent arteriole. Cell Tissue Res 1976;169:211–20.

[99] Gorgas K. Structure and innervation of the juxtaglomerular apparatus of the rat. Adv Anat Embryol Cell Biol 1978;54:5–84.

[100] Dinerstein R, Vannice J, Henderson R, Roth L, Goldberg L, Hoffmann P. Histofluorescence techniques provide evidence for dopamine-containing neuronal elements in canine kidney. Science 1979;205:497—9.

[101] Unwin R, Ganz M, Sterzel R. Brain-gut peptides, renal function and cell growth. Kidney Int 1990;37:1031—47.

[102] Dieterich H. Electron microscopic studies of the innervation of the rat kidney. Z Anat Entwicklungsgesch 1974;145:169—86.

[103] Fourman J. The adrenergic innervation of the efferent arterioles and the vasa recta in the mammalian kidney. Experientia 1970;26:293—4.

[104] Barajas L, Powers K. Innervation of the renal proximal convoluted tubule of the rat. Am J Anat 1989;186:378—88.

[105] DiBona G, Kopp U. Neural control of renal function. Physiol Rev 1997;77:75—197.

[106] Morel F, Chabardes D, Imbert-Teboul M. Heterogeneity of hormonal control in the distal nephron. In: Barcelo R, editor. Proceedings of the VII international congress of nephrology. Basel: Karger; 1978. p. 209—16.

[107] Ciriello J, de Oliveira C. Renal afferents and hypertension. Curr Hypertens Rep 2002;4:136—42.

[108] DiBona G. Differentiation of vasoactive renal sympathetic nerve fibers. Acta Physiol Scand 2000;168:195—200.

[109] Eppel G, Luff S, Denton K, Evans R, Neuropeptide Y. (Y1) receptors and {alpha}1-adrenoceptors in the neural control of regional renal perfusion. Am J Physiol Regul Integr Comp Physiol 2006;290(2):R331—40.

[110] Ferguson M, Bell C. Ultrastructural localization and characterization of sensory nerves in the rat kidney. J Comp Neurol 1988;274:9—16.

[112] von Mollendorff W. Der Exkretionsapparat. Berlin: Springer-Verlag; 1930.

[113] Zhai X, Birn H, Jensen K, Thomsen J, Andreasen A, Christensen E. Digital three-dimensional reconstruction und ultrastructure of the mouse proximal tubule. J Am Soc Nephrol 2003;14:611—9.

[114] Bulger R, Cronin R, Dobyan D. Survey of the morphology of the dog kidney. Anat Rec 1979;194:41—66.

[115] Kriz W. Structural organization of the renal medulla: comparative and functional aspects. Am J Physiol 1981;241:R3—16.

[116] Kriz W, Dieterich H, Hoffmann S. Aufbau der Gefässbündel im Nierenmark von Wüstenmäusen. Naturwissenschaften 1968;55:40.

[117] Morel F, Imbert-Teboul M, Chabardes D. Receptors to vasopressin and other hormones in the mammalian kidney. Kidney Int 1987;31:512—20.

[118] Schmidt-Nielsen B, O'Dell R. Structure and concentrating mechanism in the mammalian kidney. Am J Physiol 1961;200:1119—24.

[119] Han J, Thompson K, Chou C, Knepper M. Experimental tests of three-dimensional model of urinary concentrating mechanism. J Am Soc Nephrol 1992;2:1677—88.

[120] Kriz W, Schnermann J, Koepsell H. The position of short and long loops of Henle in the rat kidney. Z Anat Entwicklungsgesch 1972;138:301—19.

[121] Pannabecker T, Dantzler W. Three-dimensional lateral and vertical relationships of inner medullary loops of Henle and collecting ducts. Am J Physiol Renal Physiol 2004;287:F767—74.

[122] Samuel T, Hoy W, Douglas-Denton R, Hughson M, Bertram J. Determinants of glomerular volume in different cortical zones of the human kidney. J Am Soc Nephrol 2005;16:3102—9.

[123] Murakami T, Miyoshi M, Fujita T. Glomerular vessels of the rat kidney with special reference to double efferent arterioles. A scanning electron microscope study of corrosion casts. Arch Histol Jpn 1971;3:179—98.

[124] Sakai T, Kriz W. The structural relationship between mesangial cells and basement membrane of the renal glomerulus. Anat Embryol 1987;176:373—86.

[125] Abrahamson D, Hudson B, Stroganova L, Borza D, St John P. Cellular origins of type IV collagen networks in developing glomeruli. J Am Soc Nephrol 2009;20:1471—9.

[126] Price R, Spiro R. Studies on the metabolism of the renal glomerular basement membrane. Turnover measurements in the rat with the use of radiolabeled amino acids. J Biol Chem 1977;252:8597—602.

[127] Abrahamson D. Origin of the glomerular basement membrane visualized after in vivo labeling of laminin in newborn rat kidneys. J Cell Biol 1985;100:1988—2000.

[128] Reddi A. Metabolism of glomerular basement membrane in normal, hypophysectomized, and growth-hormone-treated diabetic rats. Exp Mol Pathol 1985;43:196—208.

[129] Davies M, Thomas G, Shrewing L, Mason R. Mesangial cell proteoglycans: synthesis and metabolism. J Am Soc Nephrol 1992;2(10 Suppl):S88—94.

[130] Martin J, Eynstone L, Davies M, Steadman R. Induction of metalloproteinases by glomerular mesangial cells stimulated by proteins of the extracellular matrix. J Am Soc Nephrol 2001;12:88—96.

[131] Martin J, Steadman R, Knowlden J, Williams J, Davies M. Differential regulation of matrix melalloproteinases and their inhibitors in human glomerular epithelial cells in vitro. J Am Soc Nephrol 1998;9:1629—37.

[132] Inoue S. Ultrastructural architecture of basement membranes. Contrib Nephrol 1994;107:21—8.

[133] Abrahamson D. Structure and development of the glomerular capillary wall and basement membrane. Am J Physiol 1987;253:F783—94.

[134] Yurchenco P. Assembly of laminin and type IV collagen into basement membrane networks. In: Yurchenco P, Birk D, Mecham R, editors. Extracellular matrix assembly and structure. San Diego: Academic Press; 1994. p. 351—88.

[135] Martinez-Hernandez A, Gay S, Miller E. Ultrastructural localization of type V collagen in rat kidney. J Cell Biol 1982;92:343.

[136] Miner J. Building the glomerulus: a matricentric view. J Am Soc Nephrol 2005;16:857—61.

[137] Miner J, Yurchenco P. Laminin functions in tissue morphogenesis. Annu Rev Cell Dev Biol 2004;20:255—84.

[138] Hudson B, Reeders S, Tryggvason K. Type IV collagen: structure, gene organization and role in human diseases. J Biol Chem 1993;268:26033—6.

[139] Timpl R, Brown J. Supramolecular assembly of basement membranes. BioEssays 1996;18(2):123—32.

[140] Martinez-Hernandez A, Chung A. The ultrastructural localization of two basement membrane components entactin and laminin — in rat tissue. J Histochem Cytochem 1984;32:289.

[141] Stow J, Sawada H, Farquhar M. Basement membrane heparan sulfate proteoglycans are concentrated in the laminae rarae and in the podocytes of the rat renal glomerulus. Proc Natl Acad Sci USA 1985;82:3296.

[142] Groffen A, Buskens C, van Kuppevelt T, Veerkamp J, Monnens L, van den Heuvel L. Primary structure and high expression of human agrin in basement membranes of adult lung and kidney. Eur J Biochem 1998;254:123—8.

[143] Miner J. Renal basement membrane components. Kidney Int 1999;56:2016—24.

[144] Farquhar M, Palade G. Functional evidence for the existence of a third cell type in the renal glomerulus. Phagocytosis of filtration residues by a distinctive "third" cell. J Cell Biol 1962;13:55—87.

[145] Zimmermann K. Ueber den Bau des Glomerulus der Saeugerniere. Z Mikrosk Anat Forsch 1933;32:176–278.

[146] Elger M, Drenckhahn D, Nobiling R, Mundel P, Kriz W. Cultured rat mesangial cells contain smooth muscle a-actin not found in vivo. Am J Pathol 1993;142:497–509.

[147] Kriz W, Elger M, Mundel P, Lemley K. Structure-stabilizing forces in the glomerular tuft. J Am Soc Nephrol 1995;5:1731–9.

[148] Kikkawa Y, Virtanen I, Miner J. Mesangial cells organize the glomerular capillaries by adhering to the G domain of laminin a5 in the glomerular basement membrane. J Cell Biol 2003; 161:187–96.

[149] Couchman J, Beavan L, McCarthy K. Glomerular matrix: synthesis, turnover and role in mesangial expansion. Kidney Int 1994;45:328–35.

[150] Schaefer L, Gröne H, Raslik I, Robenek H, Ugorcakova J, Budny S, et al. Small proteoglycans of normal adult human kidney: distinct expression patterns of decorin, biglycan, fibromodulin, and lumican. Kidney Int 2000;58:1557–68.

[151] Courtoy P, Timpl R, Farquhar M. Comparative distribution of laminin, type IV collagen and fibronectin in the rat glomerulus. J Histochem Cytochem 1982;30:874.

[152] Madri J, Roll F, Furthmayr H, Foidart J. Ultrastructural localization of fibronectin and laminin in the basement membranes of the murine kidney. J Cell Biol 1980;86:G82–7.

[153] Sterzel R, Hartner A, Schlotzer-Schrehard U, Voit S, Hausknecht B, Doliana R, et al. Elastic fiber proteins in the glomerular mesangium in vivo and in cell culture. Kidney Int 2000;58:1588–602.

[154] Schwartz E, Goldfischer S, Coltoff-Schiller B, Blumenfeld O. Extracellular matrix microfibrils are composed of core proteins coated with fibronectin. J Histochem Cytochem 1985;33: 268–74.

[155] Mundel P, Elger M, Sakai T, Kriz W. Microfibrils are a major component of the mesangial matrix in the glomerulus of the rat kidney. Cell Tissue Res 1988;254:183–7.

[156] Bieritz B, Spessotto P, Colombatti A, Jahn A, Prols F, Hartner A. Role of alpha8 integrin in mesangial cell adhesion, migration, and proliferation. Kidney Int 2003;64:119–27.

[157] Bulger R, Eknoyan G, Purcell D, Dobyan D. Endothelial characteristics of glomerular capillaries in normal, mercuric chloride-induced, and gentamicin-induced acute renal failure in the rat. J Clin Invest 1983;72:128–41.

[158] Vasmant D, Maurice M, Feldmann G. Cytoskeleton ultrastructure of podocytes and glomerular endothelial cells in man and in the rat. Anat Rec 1984;210:17–24.

[159] Rostgaard J, Qvortrup K. Sieve plugs in fenestrae of glomerular capillaries – site of the filtration barrier? Cells Tissues Organs 2002;170:132–8.

[160] Horvat R, Hovorka A, Dekan G, Poczewski H, Kerjaschki D. Endothelial cell membranes contain podocalyxin: the major sialoprotein of visceral glomerular epithelial cells. J Cell Biol 1986;102:484–91.

[161] Savage C. The biology of the glomerulus: endothelial cells. Kidney Int 1994;45:314–9.

[162] Betsholtz C, Lindblom P, Bjarnegard M, Enge M, Gerhardt H, Lindahl P. Role of platelet-derived growth factor in mesangium development and vasculopathies: lessons from platelet-derived growth factor and platelet-derived growth factor receptor mutations in mice. Curr Opin Nephrol Hypertens 2005;13:45–52.

[163] Eremina V, Quaggin S. The role of VEGF-A in glomerular development and function. Curr Opin Nephrol Hypertens 2004; 13:9–15.

[164] Satchell S, Anderson K, Mathieson P. Angiopoietin 1 and vascular endothelial growth factor modulate human glomerular cell barrier properties. Am Soc Nephrol 2004;15: 566–74.

[165] Ballermann B. Glomerular endothelial cell differentiation. Kidney Int 2005;67:1668–71.

[166] Fretschner M, Endlich K, Fester C, Parekh N, Steinhausen M. A narrow segment of the efferent arteriole controls efferent resistance in the hydronephrotic rat kidney. Kidney Int 1990; 37:1227–39.

[167] Mundel P, Kriz W. Structure and function of podocytes: an update. Anat Embryol 1995;192:385–97.

[168] Drenckhahn D, Franke R. Ultrastructural organization of contractile and cytoskeletal proteins in glomerular podocytes of chicken, rat, and man. Lab Invest 1988;59:673–82.

[169] Ichimura K, Kurihara H, Sakai T. Actin filament organization of foot-processes in rat podocytes. J Histochem Cytochem 2003;51:1589–600.

[170] Huber G, Matus A. Microtubule-associated protein 3 (MAP3) expression in non-neuronal tissues. J Cell Sci 1990;95: 237–46.

[171] Kobayashi N, Reiser J, Kuriyama R, Kriz W, Mundel P. Nonuniform microtubular polarity established by CHO1/MKLP1 motor protein is necessary for process formation of podocytes. J Cell Biol 1998;143:1961–70.

[172] Sanden W, Elger M, Mundel P, Kriz W. The architecture of podocyte cytoskeleton suggests a role in glomerular filtration dynamics. Ann Anat 1995;177:44–5.

[173] Cross D, Vial C, Maccioni R. A tau-like protein interacts with stress fibers and microtubules in human and rodent cultured cell lines. J Cell Sci 1993;105:51–60.

[174] Lloyd C, Minto A, Dorf M, Proudfoot A, Wells T, Salant D, et al. RANTES and monocyte chemoattractant protein-1 (MCP-1) play an important role in the inflammatory phase of crescentic nephritis, but only MCP-1 is involved in crescent formation and interstitial fibrosis. J Exp Med 1997;185:1371–80.

[175] Volk K, Sigmund R, Snyder P, McDonald F, Welsh M, Stokes J. rENaC is the predominant Na^+ channel in the apical membrane of the rat renal inner medullary collecting duct. J Clin Invest 1995;96:2748–57.

[176] Asanuma K, Kim K, Oh J, Giardino L, Chabanis S, Faul C, et al. Synaptopodin regulates the actin-bundling activity of alpha-actinin in an isoform-specific manner. J Clin Invest 2005;1:1.

[177] Adler S. Characterization of glomerular epithelial cell matrix receptors. Am J Pathol 1992;141:571–8.

[178] Cybulsky A, Carbonetto S, Huang Q, McTavish A, Cyr M. Adhesion of rat glomerular epithelial cells to extracellular matrices: role of b1 integrins. Kidney Int 1992;42:1099–106.

[179] Kreidberg J, Symons J. Integrins in kidney development, function, and disease. Am J Physiol Renal Physiol 2000;279(2): F233–42.

[180] Raats C, van den Born J, Bakker M, Oppers-Walgreen B, Pisa B, Dijkman H, et al. Expression of agrin, dystroglycan, and utrophin in normal renal tissue and in experimental glomerulopathies. Am J Pathol 2000;156(5):1749–65.

[181] Regele H, Fillipovic E, Langer B, Poczewski H, Kraxberger I, Bittner R, et al. Glomerular expression of dystroglycans is reduced in minimal change nephrosis but not in focal segmental glomerulosclerosis. J Am Soc Nephrol 2000;11(3): 403–12.

[182] Blattner S, Kretzler M. Integrin-linked kinase in renal disease: connecting cell–matrix interaction to the cytoskeleton. Curr Opin Nephrol Hypertens 2005;14:404–10.

[183] Reiser J, Polu K, Moller C, Kenlan P, Altintas M, Wei C, et al. TRPC6 is a glomerular slit diaphragm-associated channel required for normal renal function. Nat Genet 2005;37: 739–44.

[184] Winn M, Conlon P, Lynn K, Farrington M, Creazzo T, Hawkins A, et al. A mutation in the TRPC6 cation channel causes familial focal segmental glomerulosclerosis. Science 2005;308:1801–4.

[185] Kazatchkine M, Fearon D, Appay M, Mandet C, Bariety J. Immunohistochemical study of the human glomerular C3b receptor in normal kidney and in seventy-five cases of renal diseases. J Clin Invest 1982;69:900—12.

[186] Schiffer M, Schiffer L, Gupta A, Shaw A, Roberts I, Mundel P, et al. Inhibitory smads and TGF-ß signaling in glomerular cells. J Am Soc Nephrol 2002;13:2657—66.

[187] Wogensen L, Nielsen C, Hjorth P. Under control of the Ren-1c promoter, locally produced transforming growth factor-beta1 induced accumulation of glomerular extracellular matrix in transgenic mice. Diabetes 1999;48:182—92.

[188] Kriz W, Haehnel B, Rosener S, Elger M. Long-term treatment of rats with FGF-2 results in focal segmental glomerulosclerosis. Kidney Int 1995;48:1435—50.

[189] Pavenstadt H, Kriz W, Kretzler M. Cell biology of the glomerular podocyte. Physiol Rev 2003;83:253—307.

[190] Kerjaschki D, Exner M, Ullrich R, Susani M, Curtiss L, Witztum J, et al. Pathogenic antibodies inhibit the binding of apolipoproteins to megalin/gp330 in passive Heymann nephritis. J Clin Invest 1997;100:2303—9.

[191] Kerjaschki D, Farquhar M. Immunocytochemical localization of the Heymann antigen (gp 330) in glomerular epithelial cells of normal Lewis rats. J Exp Med 1983;157:667—86.

[192] Orlando R, Rader K, Authier F, Yamazaki H, Posner B, Farquhar M. Megalin is an endocytic receptor for insulin. J Am Soc Nephrol 1998;9:1759—66.

[193] Saito A, Pietromonaco S, Loo A, Farquhar M. Complete cloning and sequencing of rat gp330/"megalin," a distinctive member of the low density lipoprotein receptor gene family. Proc Natl Acad Sci USA 1994;91:9725—9.

[194] Rodewald R, Karnovsky M. Porous substructure of the glomerular slit diaphragm in the rat and mouse. J Cell Biol 1974;60:423—33.

[195] Ruotsalainen V, Ljungberg P, Wartiovaara J, Lenkkeri U, Kestila M, Jalanko H, et al. Nephrin is specifically located at the slit diaphragm of glomerular podocytes. Proc Natl Acad Sci USA 1999;96(14):7962—7.

[196] Donoviel D, Freed D, Vogel H, Potter D, Hawkins E, Barrish J, et al. Proteinuria and perinatal lethality in mice lacking NEPH1, a novel protein with homology to nephrin. Mol Cell Biol 2001;21:4829—36.

[197] Reiser J, Kriz W, Kretzler M, Mundel P. The glomerular slit diaphragm is a modified adherens junction. J Am Soc Nephrol 2000;11:1—8.

[198] Inoue T, Yaoita E, Kurihara H, Shimizu F, Sakai T, Kobayashi T, et al. Fat is a component of glomerular slit diaphragms. Kidney Int 2001;59:1003—12.

[199] Schnabel E, Anderson J, Farquhar M. The tight junction protein ZO-1 is concentrated along slit diaphragms of the glomerular epithelium. J Cell Biol 1990;111:1255—63.

[200] Boute N, Gribouval O, Roselli S, Benessy F, Lee H, Fuchshuber A, et al. NPHS2, encoding the glomerular protein podocin, is mutated in autosomal recessive steroid-resistant nephrotic syndrome. Nat Genet 2000;24:349—54.

[201] Li C, Ruotsalainen V, Tryggvason K, Shaw A, Miner J. CD2AP is expressed with nephrin in developing podocytes and is found widely in mature kidney and elsewhere. Am J Physiol Renal Physiol 2000;279(4):F785—92.

[202] Huber T, Kottgen M, Schilling B, Walz G, Benzing T. Interaction with podocin facilitates nephrin signaling. J Biol Chem 2001; 276:41543—6.

[203] Schwarz K, Simons M, Reiser J, Saleem M, Faul C, Kriz W, et al. Podocin, a raft-associated component of the glomerular slit diaphragm, interacts with CD2AP and nephrin. J Clin Invest 2001;108:1621—9.

[204] Dunne J, Hanby A, Poulsom R, Jones T, Sheer D, Chin W, et al. Molecular cloning and tissue expression of FAT, the human homologue of the Drosophila fat gene that is located on chromosome 4q34-q35 and encodes a putative adhesion molecule. Genomics 1995;30:207—23.

[205] Ciani L, Patel A, Allen N, ffrench-Constant C. Mice lacking the giant protocadherin mFAT1 exhibit renal slit junction abnormalities and a partially penetrant cyclopia and anophthalmia phenotype. Mol Cell Biol 2003;23:3575—82.

[206] Huang T, Langlois J. Podoendin. A new cell surface protein of the podocyte and endothelium. J Exp Med 1985;162:245—67.

[207] Sawada H, Stukenbrok H, Kerjaschki D, Farquhar M. Epithelial polyanion (podocalyxin) is found on the sides but not the soles of the foot processes of the glomerular epithelium. Am J Pathol 1986;125:309—18.

[208] Hugo C, Nangaku M, Shankland S, Pichler R, Gordon K, Amieva M, et al. The plasma membrane-actin linking protein, ezrin, is a glomerular epithelial cell marker in glomerulogenesis, in the adult kidney and in glomerular injury. Kidney Int 1998;54:1934—44.

[209] Takeda T, McQuistan T, Orlando R, Farquhar M. Loss of glomerular foot processes is associated with uncoupling of podocalyxin from the actin cytoskeleton. J Clin Invest 2001;108:289—301.

[210] Seiler M, Rennke H, Venkatachalam M, Cotran R. Pathogenesis of polycation-induced alteration (fusion) of glomerular epithelium. Lab Invest 1977;36:48—61.

[211] Drumond M, Deen W. Structural determinants of glomerular hydraulic permeability. Am J Physiol 1994;266:F1—12.

[212] Kanwar Y, Venkatachalam M. Renal Physiology. In: Windhager E, editor. Handbook of physiology. New York: Oup; 1992. p. 3—40.

[213] Bolton G, Deen W, Daniels B. Assessment of the charge selectivity of glomerular basement membrane using Ficoll sulfate. Am J Physiol 1998;274:F889—96.

[214] Daniels B. Increased albumin permeability in vitro following alterations of glomerular charge is mediated by the cells of the filtration barrier. J Lab Clin Med 1994;124(2):224—30.

[215] Drumond M, Deen W. Hindered transport of macromolecules through a single row of cylinders: application to glomerular filtration. J Biomech Eng 1995;117:414—22.

[216] Edwards A, Daniels B, Deen W. Hindered transport of macromolecules in isolated glomeruli. II. Convection and pressure effects in basement membrane. Biophys J 1997;72:214—22.

[217] Dworkin L, Brenner B. Biophysical basis of glomerular filtration. In: Seldin D, Giebisch G, editors. The kidney: physiology and pathophysiology. New York: Raven Press; 1992. p. 979—1016.

[218] Anderson W, Alcorn D, Gilchrist A, Whiting J, Ryan G. Glomerular actions of ANG II during reduction of renal artery pressure: a morphometric analysis. Am J Physiol 1989;256:F1021—6.

[219] Denton K, Fennessy P, Alcorn D, Anderson W. Morphometric analysis of the actions of angiotensin II on renal arterioles and glomeruli. Am J Physiol 1992;262:F367—72.

[220] Andrews P. Morphological alterations of the glomerular (visceral) epithelium in response to pathological and experimental situations. J Electron Microsc Tech 1988;9:115—44.

[221] Drumond M, Kristal B, Myers B, Deen W. Structural basis for reduced glomerular filtration capacity in nephrotic humans. J Clin Invest 1994;94:1187—95.

[222] Kriz W, Elger M, Lemley K, Sakai T. Structure of the glomerular mesangium: a biomechanical interpretation. Kidney Int 1990;38:S2—9.

[223] Kriz W, Haehnel B, Hosser H, Ostendorf T, Kränzlin B, Gretz N, et al. Pathways to recovery and loss of nephrons in anti-Thy-1 nephritis. J Am Soc Nephrol 2003;14:1904–26.

[224] Welling L, Zupka M, Welling D. Mechanical properties of basement membrane. News Physiol Sci 1995;10(1):30–5.

[225] Kriz W, Mundel P, Elger M. The contractile apparatus of podocytes is arranged to counteract GBM expansion. Contrib Nephrol 1994;107:1–9.

[226] Mbassa G, Elger M, Kriz W. The ultrastructural organization of the basement membrane of Bowman's capsule in the rat renal corpuscle. Cell Tissue Res 1988;253:151–63.

[227] Lethias C, Aubert-Foucher E, Dublet B, Eichenberger D, Font B, Goldschmidt D, et al. Structure, molecular assembly and tissue distribution of facit collagen molecules. Contrib Nephrol 1994; 107:57–63.

[228] Schonheyder H, Maunsbach A. Ultrastructure of a specialized neck region in the rabbit nephron. Kidney Int 1975;7:145–53.

[229] Gibson I, Downie I, Downie T, Han S, More I, Lindop G. The parietal podocyte: a study of the vascular pole of the human glomerulus. Kidney Int 1992;41:211–4.

[230] Grouls S, Iglesias D, Wentzensen N, Moeller M, Bouchard M, Kemler R, et al. ß-catenin/wnt-signaling is required for lineage specification of parietal epithelial cells of the glomerulus. J Am Soc Nephrol 2011;: in press:nn.

[231] Ronconi E, Sagrinati C, Angelotti M, Lazzeri E, Mazzinghi B, Ballerini L, et al. Regeneration of glomerular podocytes by human renal progenitors. J Am Soc Nephrol 2009;20:322–32.

[232] Sagrinati C, Netti G, Mazzinghi B, Lazzeri E, Liotta F, Frosali F, et al. Isolation and characterization of multipotent progenitor cells from the Bowman's capsule of adult human kidneys. J Am Soc Nephrol 2006;17:2443–56.

[233] Appel D, Kershaw D, Smeets B, Yuan G, Fuss A, Freye B, et al. Recruitment of podocytes from glomerular parietal epithelial cells. J Am Soc Nephrol 2008;20:333–43.

[234] Schneeberger E, Lynch R. Sodium transport deficiency and sodium balance in gene-targeted mice. Am J Physiol Cell Physiol 2004;286:C1213–28.

[235] Mitic L, Anderson J. Molecular architecture of tight junctions. Annu Rev Physiol 1998;60:121–42.

[236] Tsukita S, Furuse M. Multifunctional strands in tight junctions 4437. Nat Rev Mol Cell Biol 2001;2:285–93.

[237] Matlin K. Clues to occludin. Focus on "Knockdown of occludin expression leads to diverse phenotypic alterations in epithelial cells.". Am J Physiol Cell Physiol 2011;288:C1191–2.

[238] Denker B, Sabath E. The biology of epithelial cell tight junctions in the kidney. J Am Soc Nephrol 2011;22:622–5.

[239] Madara J. Regulation of the movement of solutes across tight junctions. Annu Rev Physiol 1998;60:143–59.

[240] Li W, Huey C, Yu A. Expression of claudin-7 and -8 along the mouse nephron. Am J Physiol Renal Physiol 2004;286:F1063–71.

[241] Peter Y, Goodenough D. Claudins. Curr Opin Cell Biol 2004;14:R293–4.

[242] Yu A. Claudins and epithelial paracellular transport: the end of the beginning 4441. Curr Opin Nephrol Hypertens 2003;12:503–9.

[243] Yu A, Enck A. Claudin-8 expression in Madin–Darby canine kidney cells augments the paracellular barrier to cation permeation. J Biol Chem 2003;278:17350–9.

[244] Tsukita S, Furuse M. Claudin-based barrier in simple and stratified cellular sheets. Curr Opin Cell Biol 2002;14:531–6.

[245] Colegio O, Van Itallie C. Claudins create charge-selective channels in the paracellular pathway between epithelial cells. Am J Physiol Cell Physiol 2002;283:C142–7.

[246] Colegio O, Van Itallie C. Claudin extracellular domains determine paracellular charge selectivity and resistance but not tight junction fibril architecture. Am J Physiol Cell Physiol 2003;284:C1346–54.

[247] Tang V, Goodenough D. Paracellular ion channel at the tight junction. Biophys J 2003;84:1660–73.

[248] Clarke H, Marano C. Modification of tight junction function by protein kinase C isoforms. Adv Drug Delivery Rev 2000;41:283–301.

[249] Hopkins A, Li D. Modulation of tight junction function by G protein-coupled events. Adv Drug Delivery Rev 2000; 41:329–40.

[250] Kahle K, Gimenez I. WNK4 regulates apical and basolateral Cl⁻ flux in extrarenal epithelia. Proc Natl Acad Sci USA 2004;101:2064–9.

[251] Yang C, Angell J. WNK kinases regulate thiazide-sensitive Na-Cl co-transport. J Clin Invest 2003;111:1039–45.

[252] Simon D, Lu Y. Paracellin-1 a renal tight junction protein required for paracellular Mg^{2+} resorption. Science 1999; 285:103–6.

[253] Wilcox E, Burton Q. Mutations in the gene encoding tight junction claudin-14 cause autosomal recessive deafness. Cell 2001;104:165–72.

[254] Choate K, K. Kahle. WNK1 a kinase mutated in inherited hypertension with hyperkalemia, localizes to diverse Cl⁻-transporting epithelia. Proc Natl Acad Sci USA 2003;100:663–8.

[255] Kahle K, Wilson F. WNK4 regulates the balance between renal NaCl reabsorption and K^+ secretion. Nat Genet 2003;35:372–6.

[256] Wilson F, Disse-Nicodeme S. Human hypertension caused by mutations in WNK kinases. Science 2001;293:1107–12.

[257] Wilson F, Kahle K. Molecular pathogenesis of inherited hypertension with hyperkalemia: the Na-Cl co-transporter is inhibited by wild-type but not mutant WNK4. Proc Natl Acad Sci USA 2003;100:680–4.

[258] Yu A, McCarthy K. Knockdown of occludin expression leads to diverse phenotypic alterations in epithelial cells. Am J Physiol Cell Physiol 2005;288:C1231–41.

[259] Lima WR, Parreira K, Devuyst O, Caplanusi A, N'kuli F, Marien B, et al. ZONAB promotes proliferation and represses differentiation of proximal tubule epithelial cells. J Am Soc Nephrol 2010;21:478–88.

[260] Kaissling B, Kriz W. Morphology of the loop of Henle, distal tubule and collecting duct. In: Windhager E, editor. Handbook of physiology: section on renal physiology. New York, N.Y.: Oxford University Press; 1992. p. 109–67.

[261] Kiuchi-Saishin Y, Gotoh S, Furuse M, Takasuga A, Tano Y, Tsukita S. Differential expression patterns of claudins, tight junction membrane proteins, in mouse nephron segments. J Am Soc Nephrol 2002;13:875–86.

[262] Piepenhagen P, Nelson W. Differential expression of cell–cell and cell–substratum adhesion proteins along the kidney nephron 4461. Am J Physiol 1995;269:C1433–49.

[263] Piepenhagen P, Peters L, Lux S, Nelson W. Differential expression of Na(+)-K(+)-ATPase, ankyrin, fodrin, and E-cadherin along the kidney nephron. Am J Physiol 1995;269: C1417–32.

[264] Prozialeck W, Lamar P, Appelt D. Differential expression of E-cadherin, N-cadherin and beta-cadherin in proximal and distal segments of the rat nephron. BMC Physiol 2004;4:10.

[265] Rybak J, Ettorre A, Kaissling B, Giavazzi R, Neri D, Elia G. In vivo protein biotinylation for identification of organ-specific antigens accessible from the vasculature. Nat Methods 2005; 2:291–8.

[266] Thomson R, Aronson P. Immunolocalization of Ksp-cadherin in the adult and developing rabbit kidney. Am J Physiol Renal Physiol 1999;277:F146–56.

[267] Nelson W, Nusse R. Convergence of Wnt, beta-catenin, and cadherin pathways. Science 2004;303:1483–7.

[268] Christensen E, Wagner C, Kaissling B. The uriniferous tubule: structural and functional organization. In: American Physiological Society, editor. Compr physiol. Wiley Blackwell; 2012. p. 1–57.

[269] Donowitz M, Cha B, Zachos N, Brett C, Sharma A, Tse C, et al. Family and NHE3 regulation 4469. J Physiol 2005;567:3–11.

[270] Ecelbarger C, Kim G, Wade J, Knepper M. Regulation of the abundance of renal sodium transporters and channels by vasopressin 4467. Exp Neurol 2001;171:227–34.

[271] Wade J, Stanton B, Brown D. Structural correlates of transport in distal tubule and collecting duct segments. In: Windhager E, editor. Handbook of physiology: renal. New York: Oxford Univerity Press; 1992. p. 1–10.

[272] Wade J, Welling P, Donowitz M, Shenolikar S, Weinman E. Differential renal distribution of NHERF isoforms and their colocalization with NHE3, ezrin, and ROMK. Am J Physiol Cell Physiol 2001;280:C192–8.

[273] Weinman E, Cunningham R, Wade J, Shenolikar S. The role of NHERF-1 in the regulation of renal proximal tubule sodium-hydrogen exchanger 3 and sodium-dependent phosphate co-transporter 2a 4470. J Physiol 2005;567:27–32.

[274] Cha B, Kenworthy A, Murtazina R, Donowitz M. The lateral mobility of NHE3 on the apical membrane of renal epithelial OK cells is limited by the PDZ domain proteins NHERF1/2, but is dependent on an intact actin cytoskeleton as determined by FRA. J Cell Sci 2004;117:3353–65.

[275] Rodman J, Mooseker M, Farquhar M. Cytoskeletal proteins of the rat kidney proximal tubule brush border. Eur J Cell Biol 1986;42:313.

[276] Geering K. FXYD proteins: new regulators of Na-K-ATPase. J Physiol Renal Physiol 2006;290:F241–50.

[277] Brown D. Targeting of membrane transporters in renal epithelia: when cell biology meets physiology. Am J Physiol Renal Physiol 2000;278:F192–201.

[278] Doucet A, Katz A, Morel F. Determination of Na-K-ATPase activity in single segments of the mammalian nephron 4474. Am J Physiol 1979;237:F105–13.

[279] Katz A, Doucet A, Morel F. Na-K-ATPase activity along the rabbit, rat and mouse nephron. Am J Physiol 1979;237: F114–20.

[280] Kaissling B, Le Hir M. Distal tubular segments in the rabbit kidney after adaptation to altered Na- and K-intake. I. Structural changes. Cell Tissue Res 1982;224:469–92.

[281] Le Hir M, Kaissling B, Dubach U. Distal tubular segments of the rabbit kidney after adaption to altered Na- and K-intake. II. Changes in Na-K-ATPase activity. Cell Tissue Res 1982; 224:493–504.

[282] Welling D, Urani J, Welling L, Wagner E. Fractal analysis and imaging of the proximal nephron cell. Am J Physiol 1996;270: C953–63.

[283] Kashgarian M, Biemesderfer D, Caplan M, Forbush B. Monocloal antibody to Na,K-ATPase: immunocytochemical localization along nephron segments. Kidney Int 1985; 28:899–913.

[284] Koob R, Zimmermann M, Schoner W, Drenckhahn D. Colocalization and coprecipitation of ankyrin and Na$^+$,K$^+$-ATPase in kidney epithelial cells. Eur J Cell Biol 1988; 45:230–7.

[285] Rostgaard J, Kristensen B, Nielsen L. Electron microscopy of filaments in the basal part of rat kidney tubule cells, and their *in situ* interaction with heavy meromyosin. Z Zellforsch Mikrosk Anat 1972;132:497–521.

[286] Rostgaard J, Thuneberg L. Electron microscopic evidence suggesting a contractile system in the base of tubular cells of rat kidney. J Ultrastruct Res 1969;29:570–7.

[287] Trenchev P, Dorling J, Webb J, Holborrow E. Localization of smooth muscle-like contractile proteins in kidney by immunoelectron microscopy. J Anat 1976;121:85–95.

[288] Guder W, Wagner S, Wirthensohn G. Metabolic fuels along the nephron: pathways and intracellular mechanisms of interaction. Kidney Int 1986;29:41–5.

[289] Kaissling B. Structural aspects of adaptive changes in renal electrolyte excretion. Am J Physiol 1982;243:F211–26.

[290] Kaissling B, Stanton B. Adaptation of distal tubule and collecting duct to increased sodium delivery. I. Ultrastructure. Am J Physiol 1988;255:F1256–68.

[291] Madsen K, Verlander J, Tisher C. Relationship between structure and function in distal tubule and collecting duct. J Electron Microsc Tech 1988;9:187–208.

[292] Stanton B, Kaissling B. Adaptation of distal tubule and and collecting duct to increased Na delivery. II. Na$^+$ and K$^+$ transport. Am J Physiol 1988;255:F1269–75.

[293] Stanton B, Kaissling B. Regulation of renal ion transport and cell growth by sodium. Am J Physiol 1989;257:F1–10.

[294] Wade J, O'Neil R, Pryor J, Boulpaep E. Modulation of cell membrane area in renal collecting tubules by corticosteroid hormones. J Cell Biol 1979;81:439–45.

[295] Holtzclaw J, Cornelius R, Hatcher L, Sansom S. Coupled ATP and potassium efflux from intercalated cells. Am J Physiol Renal Physiol 2011;300:F1319–26.

[296] Praetorius H, Leipziger J. Intrarenal purinergic signaling in the control of renal tubular transport. Annu Rev Physiol 2010; 72:377–93.

[297] Biemesderfer D, DeGray D. Active (9.6 s) and inactive (21 s) oligomers of NHE3 in microdomains of the renal brush border 4478. J Biol Chem 2001;276:10161–7.

[298] McDonough A, Biemesderfer D. Does membrane trafficking play a role in regulating the sodium/hydrogen exchanger isoform 3 in the proximal tubule? Curr Opin Nephrol Hypertens 2003;12:533–41.

[299] Brown D. The ins and outs of aquaporin-2 trafficking. Am J Physiol Renal Physiol 2003;284:F893–901.

[300] Butterworth M. Regulation of the epithelial sodium channel (ENaC) by membrane trafficking. Biochim Biopyhs Acta 2010;1802:1166–77.

[301] Bacic D, Le Hir M, Biber J, Kaissling B, Murer H, Wagner C. The renal Na$^+$/phosphate co-transporter NaPi-IIa is internalized via the receptor-mediated endocytic route in response to parathyroid hormone. Kidney Int 2006;69:495–503.

[302] Thomas C, Itani O. New insights into epithelial sodium channel function in the kidney: site of action, regulation by ubiquitin ligases, serum- and glucocorticoid-inducible kinase and proteolysis 4482. Curr Opin Nephrol Hypertens 2004; 13:541–8.

[303] Ecelbarger C, Knepper M. Increased abundance of distal sodium transporters in rat kidney during vasopressin escape. J Am Soc Nephrol 2001;12:207–17.

[304] Kaissling B, Bachmann S, Kriz W. Structural adaptation of the distal convoluted tubule to prolonged furosemide treatment. Am J Physiol Renal Fluid Electrolyte Physiol 1985;248:F374–81.

[305] Loffing J, Le Hir M, Kaissling B. Modulation of salt transport rate affects DNA sythesis *in vivo* in rat renal tubules. Kidney Int 1995;47:1615–23.

[306] Kaissling B, Loffing J. Cell growth and cell death in renal distal tubules, associated with diuretic treatment. Nephrol Dial Transplant 1998;13:1341–3.

[307] Loffing J, Loffing-Cueni D, Hegyi I, Kaplan M, Hebert S, Le Hir M, et al. Thiazide treatment of rats provokes apoptosis in distal tubule cells. Kidney Int 1996;50:1180–90.

[308] Bankir L, Bouby N, Trinh-Trang-Tan M, Kaissling B. The thick ascending limb of Henle's loop. Anatomical and functional

characteristics and role in the urine concentration mechanism. In: Crosnier J, Funck-Brentano J, Bach J, Grünfeld J, editors. Actualités nephrologiques de l'Hopital Necker. Paris: Flammarion Medicine-Sciences; 1987.

[309] Calvert J. New insights into ciliary function: kidney cysts and photoreceptors 4484. Proc Natl Acad Sci USA 2003;100: 5583–5.

[310] Liu W, Xu S, Woda C, Kim P, Weinbaum S, Satlin L. Effect of flow and stretch on the $[Ca^{2+}]i$ response of principal and intercalated cells in cortical collecting duct. Am J Physiol Renal Physiol 2003;285:F998–1012.

[311] Luo Y, Vassilev P, Li X, Kawanabe Y, Zhou J. Native polycystin 2 functions as a plasma membrane Ca^{2+}-permeable cation channel in renal epithelia. Mol Biol Cell 2003;23:2600–7.

[312] Weinbaum S, Duan Y, Satlin L, Wang T, Weinstein A. Mechanotransduction in the renal tubule 4491. Am J Physiol Renal Physiol 2010;299:F1220–36.

[313] Yoder B, Hou X, Guay-Woodford L. The polycystic kidney disease proteins, polycystin-1, polycystin-2, polaris, and cystin, are co-localized in renal cilia. J Am Soc Nephrol 2002;13: 2508–16.

[314] Li Q, Montalbetti N, Shen P, Dai X, Cheeseman C, Karpinski E, et al. Alpha-actinin associates with polycystin-2 and regulates its channel activity. Hum Mol Genet 2005;14:1587–603.

[315] Zhang Q, Taulman P, Yoder B. Cystic kidney diseases: all roads lead to the cilium 4489. Physiology 2004;19:225–30.

[316] Davenport J, Yoder B. An incredible decade for the primary cilium: a look at a once-forgotten organelle 4486. Am J Physiol Renal Physiol 2005;289:F1159–69.

[317] Leipziger J. Luminal nucleotides are tonic inhibitors of renal tubular transport. Curr Opin Nephrol Hypertens 2011; 20:518–22.

[318] Hou X, Mrug M, Yoder B, Lefkowitz E, Kremmidiotis G, D'Eustachio P, et al. Cystin, a novel cilia-associated protein, is disrupted in the cpk mouse model of polycystic kidney disease. J Clin Invest 2002;109:533–40.

[319] Nauli S, Alenghat F, Luo Y, Williams E, Vassilev P, Li X, et al. Polycystins 1 and 2 mediate mechanosensation in the primary cilium of kidney cells 4494. Nat Genet 2003;33:129–37.

[320] Zhou J. Polycystins and primary cilia: primers for cell cycle progression. Annu Rev Physiol 2009;71:83–113.

[321] Bell P, Fitzgibbon W, Sas K, Stenbit A, Amria M, Houston A, et al. Loss of primary cilia upregulates renal hypertrophic signaling and promotes cystogenesis 4496. J Am Soc Nephrol 2011; 22:839–48.

[322] Igarashi P, Somlo S. Genetics and pathogenesis of polycystic kidney disease. J Am Soc Nephrol 2002;13:2384–98.

[323] Nishio S, Hatano M, Nagata M, Horie S, Koike T, Tokuhisa T, et al. Pkd1 regulates immortalized proliferation of renal tubular epithelial cells through p53 induction and JNK activation. J Clin Invest 2005;115:910–8.

[324] Orlando R, Takeda T, Zak B, Schmieder S, Benoit V, McQuistan T, et al. The glomerular epithelial cell anti-adhesion podocalyxin associates with the actin cytoskeleton through interactions with ezrin. J Am Soc Nephrol 2001;12:1589–98.

[325] Wright S, Dantzler W. Molecular and cellular physiology of renal organic cation and anion transport. Physiol Rev 2004;84:987–1049.

[326] Grandchamp A, Boulpaep E. Pressure control of sodium reabsorption and intercellular backflux across proximal kidney tubule. J Clin Invest 1974;54:69.

[327] Lutz M, Cardinal J, Burg B. Electrical resistance of renal proximal tubule perfused in vitro. Am J Physiol 1973;225:729.

[328] Lock E, Reed C. Xenobiotic metabolizing enzymes of the kidney. Toxicol Pathol 1998;26:18–25.

[329] Bergeron M, Gaffiero P, Thiery G. Segmental variations in the organization of the endoplasmic reticulum of the rat nephron. A stereomicroscopic study. Cell Tissue Res 1987;247: 215–25.

[330] Zaar K. Structure and function of peroxisomes in the mammalian kidney. Eur J Cell Biol 1992;59:233–54.

[331] Daigeler R. Sex-dependent changes in the rat kidney after hypophysectomy. Cell Tissue Res 1981;216:423–43.

[332] Schiebler T, Danner K. The effect of sex hormones on the proximal tubules in the rat kidney. Cell Tissue Res 1978; 192:527–49.

[333] Zabel M, Schiebler T. Histochemical, autoradiographic and electron microscopic investigations of the renal proximal tubule of male and female rats after castration. Histochemie 1980;69:255–76.

[334] Maunsbach A. The influence of different fixatives and fixation methods on the ultrastructure of rat kidney proximal tubule cells: I. Comparison of different perfusion fixation methods and of glutaraldehyde, formaldehyde and osmium tetroxide fixatives. J Ultrastruct Res 1966;15:242–82.

[335] Maunsbach A. The influence of different fixatives and fixation methods on the ultrastructure of rat kidney proximal tubule cells: II. Effects of varying osmolality, ionic strength, buffer system and fixative concentration of glutaraldehyde solutions. J Ultrastruct Res 1966;15:283.

[336] Dorup J, Maunsbach A. Three-dimensional organization and segmental ultrastructure of rat proximal tubules. Exp Nephrol 1997;5:305–17.

[337] Birn H, Willnow T, Nielsen R, Norden A, Bönsch C, Moestrup S, et al. Megalin is essential for renal proximal tubule reabsorption and accumulation of transcobalamin-B(12). Am J Physiol Renal Physiol 2002;282:F408–16.

[338] Christensen E, Gburek J. Protein reabsorption in renal proximal tubule – function and dysfunction in kidney pathophysiology. Pediatr Nephrol 2004;19:714–21.

[339] Hall A, Crawford C, Unwin R, Duchen M, Peppipiatt-Wildman C. Multiphoton imaging of the functioning kidney. J Am Soc Nephrol 2011;22:1297–304.

[340] Molitoris B, Sandoval R. Intravital multiphoton mircroscopy of dynamic renal processes. Am J Physiol Renal Physiol 2005;288: F1084–9.

[341] He Q, Madsen M. Amnionless function is required for cubilin brush-border expression and intrinsic factor-cobalamin (vitamin B12) absorption in vivo. Blood 2005;106:1447–53.

[342] Moestrup S, Nielsen L. The role of the kidney in lipid metabolism. Curr Opin Lipidol 2005;16:301–6.

[343] Nagai J, Christensen E. Mutually dependent localization of megalin and Dab2 in the renal proximal tubule. Am J Physiol Renal Physiol 2005;289:F569–76.

[344] Takeda T, Yamazaki H, Farquhar M. Identification of an apical sorting determinant in the cytoplasmic tail of megalin. Am J Physiol Cell Physiol 2003;284:C1105–13.

[345] Verroust P, Birn H, Nielsen R, Kozyraki R, Christensen E. The tandem endocytic receptors megalin and cubilin are important proteins in renal pathology. Kidney Int 2002;62:745–56.

[346] Verroust P, Christensen E. Megalin and cubilin – the story of two multipurpose receptors unfolds. Nephrol Dial Transplant 2002;17:1867–71.

[347] Christensen E, Nielsen S, Moestrup S, Borre C, Maunsbach A, de Heer E, et al. Segmental distribution of the endocytosis receptor gp330 in renal proximal tubules. Eur J Cell Biol 1995;66:349–64.

[348] Hatae T, Ichimura T, Ishida T, Sakurai T. Apical tubular network in the rat kidney proximal tubule cells studied by thick-section and scanning electron microscopy. Cell Tissue Res 1997;288:317–25.

[349] Maunsbach A. Observations on the segmentation of the proximal tubule in the rat kidney. J Ultrastruct Res 1966; 16:239–58.

[350] Maunsbach A. Functional ultrastructure of the proximal tubule. In: Windhager E, editor. Handbook of physiology: section on renal physiology. New York, N.Y.: Oxford University Press; 1992. p. 41–108.

[351] Cui S, Mata L, Maunsbach A, Christensen E. Ultrastructure of the vacuolar apparatus in the renal proximal tubule microinfused in vivo with the cytological stain light green. Exp Nephrol 1998;6:359–67.

[352] Cui S, Christensen E. Three-dimensional organization of the vacuolar apparatus involved in endocytosis and membrane recycling of rat kidney proximal tubule cells. An electronmicroscopic study of serial sections. Exp Nephrol 1993;1: 175–84.

[353] Cui S, Verroust P, Moestrup S, Christensen E. Megalin/gp 330 mediates uptake of albumin in renal proximal tubule. Am J Physiol 1996;271:F900–7.

[354] Farquhar M, Saito A, Kerjaschki D, Orlando R. The Heymann nephritis antigenic complex: megalin (gp330) and RAP. J Am Soc Nephrol 1995;6:35–47.

[355] Lotscher M, Kaissling B, Biber J, Murer H, Levi M. Role of microtubules in the rapid regulation of renal phosphate transport in response to acute alterations in dietary phosphate content. J Clin Invest 1997;99:1302–12.

[356] Lotscher M, Scarpetta Y, Levi M, Halaihel N, Wang H, Zajicek H, et al. Rapid downregulation of rat renal Na/P(i) co-transporter in response to parathyroid hormone involves microtubule rearrangement. J Clin Invest 1999;104:483–94.

[357] Bachmann S, Schlichting U, Geist B, Mutig K, Petsch T, Bacic D, et al. Kidney-specific inactivation of the megalin gene impairs trafficking of renal inorganic sodium phosphate co-transporter (NaPi-IIa). J Am Soc Nephrol 2004; 15:892–900.

[358] Bacic D, Capuano P, Gisler S, Pribanic S, Christensen E, Biber J, et al. Impaired PTH-induced endocytotic down-regulation of the renal type IIa Na$^+$/Pi-co-transporter in RAP-deficient mice with reduced megalin expression. Pflugers Arch 2003; 446:475–84.

[359] Marshansky V, Ausiello D, Brown D. Physiological importance of endosomal acidification: potential role in proximal tubulopathies. Curr Opin Nephrol Hypertens 2002;11: 527–37.

[360] Gekle M, Völker K, Mildenberger S, Freudinger R, Shull G, Wiemann M. NHE3 Na$^+$/H + exchanger supports proximal tubular protein reabsorption in vivo. Am J Physiol Renal Physiol 2004;287:F469–73.

[361] Honegger K, Capuano P, Winter C, Bacic D, Stange G, Wagner C, et al. Regulation of sodium-proton exchanger isoform 3 (NHE3) by PKA and exchange protein directly activated by cAMP (EPAC). Proc Natl Acad Sci USA 2006;103:803–8.

[362] Wang Y, Cai H, Cebotaru L, Hryciw D, Weinman E, Donowitz M, et al. ClC-5: role in endocytosis in the proximal tubule. Am J Physiol Renal Physiol 2005;289:F850–62.

[363] Devuyst O. Chloride channels and endocytosis: new insights from Dent's disease and CLC-5 knockout mice. Bull Mem Acad R Med Belg 2004;159:212–7.

[364] Jentsch T. Chloride transport in the kidney: lessons from human disease and knockout mice. J Am Soc Nephrol 2005;16:1549–61.

[365] Jentsch T, Hübner C, Fuhrmann J. Ion channels: function unravelled by dysfunction. Nat Cell Biol 2004;6:1039–47.

[366] Marshanky V, Ausiello D, Brown D. Physiological importance of endosomal acidification: potential role in proximal tubulopathies. Curr Opin Nephrol Hypertens 2002;11:527–37.

[367] Novarino G, Weinert S, Rickheit G, Jentsch T. Endosomal chloride-proton exchange rather than chloride conductance is crucial for renal endocytosis. Science 2010;328:1398–401.

[368] Rabkin R, Mahoney C. Hormones and the kidney. In: Schrier R, Gottschalk C, editors. Diseases of the kidney. Boston: Little Brown; 1988. p. 309.

[369] Nielsen S, Nielsen J, Christensen E. Luminal and basolateral uptake of insulin in isolated, perfused proximal tubules. Am J Physiol Renal Fluid Electrolyte Physiol 1987;253: F857–67.

[370] Amemiya M, Loffing J, Lötscher M, Kaissling B, Alpern R, Moe O. Expression of NHE-3 in the apical membrane of rat renal proximal tubule and thick ascending limb. Kidney Int 1995;48:1206–15.

[371] Aronson P. Ion exchangers mediating NaCl transport in the renal proximal tubule. Cell Biochem Biophys 2002; 36:147–53.

[372] Bobulescu I, Moe O. Luminal Na(+)/H (+) exchange in the proximal tubule. Pflugers Arch 2009;458:5–21.

[373] Pao A, Bhargava A, Di Sole F, Quigley R, Saho X, Wang J, et al. Expression and role of serum and glucocorticoid-regulated kinase 2 in the regulation of Na$^+$/H$^+$ exchanger 3 in the mammalian kidney. Am J Physiol Renal Physiol 2010;299: F1496–506.

[374] Besse-Eschmann V, Klisic J, Nief V, Le Hir M, Kaissling B, Ambühl P. Regulation of the proximal tubular sodium/proton exchanger NHE3 in rats with puromycin aminonucleoside (PAN)-induced nephrotic syndrome. J Am Soc Nephrol 2002;13:2199–206.

[375] Kobayashi K, Monkawa T, Hayashi M, Saruta T. Expression of the Na$^+$/H$^+$ exchanger regulatory protein family in genetically hypertensive rats. J Hypertens 2004;22:1723–30.

[376] McDonough A, Leong P, Yang L. Mechanisms of pressure natriuresis: how blood pressure regulates renal sodium transport. Ann NY Acad Sci 2003;986:669–77.

[377] Yang L, Maunsbach A, Leong P, McDonough A. Differential traffic of proximal tubule Na$^+$ transporters during hypertension or PTH: NHE3 to base of microvilli vs. NaPi2 to endosomes. Am J Physiol Renal Physiol 2004;287:F896–906.

[378] Biber J, Gisler S, Hernando N, Wagner C, Murer H. PDZ interactions and proximal tubular phosphate reabsorption. Am J Physiol Renal Physiol 2004;287:F871–5.

[379] Gisler S, Pribanic S, Bacic D, Forrer P, Gantenbein A, Sabourin L, et al. PDZK1: I. A major scaffolder in brush borders of proximal tubular cells. Kidney Int 2003;64:1733–45.

[380] Maunsbach A, Marples D, Chin E, Ning G, Bondy C, Agre P, et al. Aquaporin-1 water channel expression in human kidney. J Am Soc Nephrol 1997;8:1–14.

[381] Nielsen S. Renal aquaporins: an overview. BJU Int 2002;90:1–6.

[382] Nielsen S, Frokiaer J. Aquaporins in the kidney: from molecules to medicine. Physiol Rev 2002;82:205–44.

[383] Sabolic I, Valenti G, Verbavatz J, van Hoek A, Verkman A. Localization of the CHIP28 water channel in rat kidney. Am J Physiol 1992;263:C1225–33.

[384] Schnermann J, Chou C, Ma T, Traynor T, Knepper M, Verkman A. Defective proximal tubular fluid reabsorption in transgenic aquaporin-1 null mice. Proc Natl Acad Sci USA 1998;95:9660–4.

[385] van Hoek A, Ma T, Yang B, Verkman A, Brown D. Aquaporin-4 is expressed in basolateral membranes of proximal tubule S3 segments in mouse kidney. Am J Physiol Renal Physiol 2000;278:F310–6.

[386] Sohara E, Uchida S, Sasaki S. Function of aquaporin-7 in the kidney and the male reproductive system. Handb Exp Pharmacol 2009;190:219–31.

II. STRUCTURAL ORGANIZATION OF THE MAMMALIAN KIDNEY

[387] Ishibashi K, Imai M, Sasaki S. Cellular localization of aquaporin 7 in the rat kidney. Exp Nephrol 2000;8:252—7.

[388] Nesjum L, Elkjaer M, Hager H, Frokiaer J, Kwon T, Nielsen S. Localization of aquaporin-7 in rat and mouse kidney using RT-PCR, immunoblotting, and immunocytochemistry. Biochem Biophys Res Commun 2000;277:164—70.

[389] Bakris G, Fonseca V, Sharma K, Wright E. Renal sodium-glucose transport: role in diabetes mellitus and potential clinical implications. Kidney Int 2009;75:1272—7.

[390] Hediger M, Rhoads D. Molecular physiology of sodium-glucose co-transporters. Physiol Rev 1994;74:993—1026.

[391] Sabolic I, Skarica M, Gorboulev V, Ljubojevic M, Balen D, Herak-Kramberger C, et al. Rat renal glucose transporter SGLT1 exhibits zonal distribution and androgen-dependent gender differences. Am J Physiol Renal Physiol 2006;290:F913—26.

[392] Rahmoune H, Thompson P, Ward J, Smith C, Hong G, Brown J. Glucose transporters in human renal proximal tubular cells isolated from the urine of patients with non-insulin-dependent diabetes. Diabetes 2005;54:3427—34.

[393] Forster I, Hernando N, Biber J, Murer H. Proximal tubular handling of phosphate: a molecular perspective. Kidney Int 2006;70:1548—59.

[394] Villa-Bellosta R, Ravera S, Sorribas V, Stange G, Levi M, Murer H, et al. The Na$^+$-Pi co-transporter PiT-2 (SLC20A2) is expressed in the apical membrane of rat renal proximal tubules and regulated by dietary Pi. Am J Physiol Renal Physiol 2009;296:F691—9.

[395] Ritthaler T, Traebert M, Lötscher M, Biber J, Murer H, Kaissling B. Effects of phosphate intake on distribution of type ll Na/P-co-transporter mRNA in rat kidney. Kidney Int 1998;:.

[396] Levi M, Lötscher M, Sorribas V, Custer M, Arar M, Kaissling B, et al. Cellular mechanisms of acute and chronic adaptation of rat renal Pi-transporter to alterations in dietary Pi. Am J Physiol 1994;267:F900—8.

[397] Lötscher M, Kaissling B, Biber J, Murer H, Levi M. Role of microtubules in the rapid regulation of renal phosphate transport in response to acute alterations in dietary phosphate content. J Clin Invest 1997;99:1302—12.

[398] Murer H, Forster I, Hernando N, Biber J. Proximal tubular handling of phosphate: Na/Pi-co-transporters and their regulation. In: Alpern R, Hebert S, editors. Seldin and Giebisch's the kidney. New York: Academic Press; 2008. p. 1979—88.

[399] Kempson S, Lötscher M, Kaissling B, Biber J, Murer H, Levi M. Parathyroid hormone action on phosphate transporter mRNA and protein in rat renal proximal tubules. Am J Physiol 1995;268:F784—91.

[400] Keusch I, Traebert M, Lotscher M, Kaissling B, Murer H, Biber J. Parathyroid hormone and dietary phosphate provoke a lysosomal routing of the proximal tubular Na/Pi cotransporter type II. Kidney Int 1998;54:1224—32.

[401] Traebert M, Roth J, Biber J, Murer H, Kaissling B. Internalization of proximal tubular type II Na-P(i) co-transporter by PTH: Immunogold electron microscopy. Am J Physiol Renal Physiol 2000;278:F148—54.

[402] Huang C, Moe O. Klotho: a novel regulator of calcium and phosphorus homeostasis. Pflugers Arch 2011;462:185—93.

[403] Verrey F, Singer D, Ramadan T, Vuille-dit-Bille R, Mariotta L, Camargo S. Kidney amino acid transport. Pflugers Arch 2009;458:53—60.

[404] Daniel H, Rubio-Aliaga I. An update on renal peptide transporters. Am J Physiol Renal Physiol 2003;284:F885—92.

[405] Shen H, Smith D, Yang T, Huang Y, Schnermann J, Brosius F3. Localization of PEPT1 and PEPT2 proton-coupled oligopeptide transporter mRNA and protein in rat kidney. Am J Physiol 1999;276:F658—65.

[406] Koepsell H. Polyspecific organic cation transporters: their functions and interactions with drugs. Trends Pharmacol Sci 2004;25:375—81.

[407] Lee W, Kim R. Transporters and renal drug elimination. Annu Rev Pharmacol Toxicol 2004;44:137—66.

[408] Rafey M, Lipkowitz M, Leal-Pinto E, Abramson R. Uric acid transport. Curr Opin Nephrol Hypertens 2003;12:511—6.

[409] Wright S. Role of organic cation transporters in the renal handling of therapeutic agents and xenobiotics. Toxicol Appl Pharmacol 2005;204:309—19.

[410] You G. Structure, function, and regulation of renal organic anion transporters. Med Res Rev 2011;22:602—16.

[411] Karbach U, Kricke J, Meyer-Wentrup F, Gorboulev V, Volk C, Loffing-Cueni D, et al. Localization of organic cation transporters OCT1 and OCT2 in rat kidney. Am J Physiol Renal Physiol 2000;279:F679—87.

[412] Urakami Y, Okuda M, Masuda S, Akazawa M, Saito H, Inui K. Distinct characteristics of organic cation transporters, OCT1 and OCT2, in the basolateral membrane of renal tubules. Pharm Res 2001;18:1528—34.

[413] Urakami Y, Okuda M, Masuda S, Saito H, Inui K. Functional characteristics and membrane localization of rat multispecific organic cation transporters, OCT1 and OCT2, mediating tubular secretion of cationic drugs. J Pharmacol Exp Ther 1998;287:800—5.

[414] Tojo A, Sekine T, Nakajima N, Hosoyamada M, Kanai Y, Kimura K, et al. Immunohistochemical localization of multispecific renal organic anion transporter 1 in rat kidney. J Am Soc Nephrol 1999;10:464—71.

[415] Burckhardt B, Burckhardt G. Transport of organic anions across the basolateral membrane of proximal tubule cells. Rev Physiol Biochem Pharmacol 2003;146:95—158.

[416] Kato Y, Kuge K, Kusuhara H, Meier P, Sugiyama Y. Gender difference in the urinary excretion of organic anions in rats. J Pharmacol Exp Ther 2002;302:483—9.

[417] Kato Y, Sai Y, Yoshida K, Watanabe C, Hirata T, Tsuji A. PDZK1 directly regulates the function of organic cation/carnitine transporter OCTN2. Mol Pharmacol 2005;67:734—43.

[418] Ljubojevic M, Herak-Kramberger C, Hagos S, Bahn A, Endou H, Burckhardt G, et al. Rat renal cortical OAT1 and OAT3 exhibit gender differences determined by both androgen stimulation and estrogen inhibition. Am J Physiol Renal Physiol 2004;287:F124—38.

[419] Urakami Y, Nakamura N, Takahashi K, Okuda M, Saito H, Hashimoto Y, et al. Gender differences in expression of organic cation transporter OCT2 in rat kidney. FEBS Lett 1999;461:339—42.

[420] Urakami Y, Okuda M, Saito H, Inui K. Hormonal regulation of organic cation transporter OCT2 expression in rat kidney. FEBS Lett 2000;473:173—6.

[421] Sekine T, Miyazaki H, Endou H. Molecular physiology of renal organic anion transporters. Am J Physiol Renal Physiol 2006;290:F251—61.

[422] Schaub T, Kartenbeck J, König J, Vogel O, Witzgall R, Kriz W, et al. Expression of the conjugate export pump encoded by the mrp2 gene in the apical membrane of kidney proximal tubules. J Am Soc Nephrol 1997;8:1213—21.

[423] Kriz W, Schnermann J, Dieterich H. Differences in the morphology of descending limbs of short and long loops of Henle in the rat kidney. In: Wirz H, Spinelli F, editors. Recent advances in renal physiology. Basel: Karger; 1972. p. 140—4.

[424] Schwartz M, Venkatachalam M. Structural differences in thin limbs of Henle: physiological implications. Kidney Int 1974;6:193—208.

[425] Dieterich H, Barrett J, Kriz W, Bülhoff J. The ultrastructure of the thin loop limbs of the mouse kidney. Anat Embryol 1975;147:1—18.

[426] Bachmann S, Kriz W. Histotopography an ultrastructure of the thin limbs of the loop of Henle in the hamster. Cell Tissue Res 1982;225:111—27.

[427] Schiller A, Forssmann W, Taugner R. The tight junctions of the renal tubules in the cortex and outer medulla. A quantitative study of the kidney of six species. Cell Tissue Res 1980; 212:395—413.

[428] Nagle R, Altschuler E, Dobyan D, Dong S, Bulger R. The ultrastructure of the thin limbs of Henle in kidneys of the desert heteromyid (Perognathus penicillatus). Am J Anat 1981; 161:33—47.

[429] Barajas L. The ultrastructure of the juxtaglomerular apparatus as disclosed by three-dimensional reconstruction from serial sections: the anatomical relationship between the tubular and vascular components. J Ultrastruct Res 1970;33: 116—47.

[430] Barrett J, Kriz W, Kaissling B, de Rouffignac C. The ultrastructure of the nephrons of the desert rodent (Psammomys obesus) kidney. I. Thin limbs of Henle of short looped nephrons. Am J Anat 1978;151:487—98.

[431] Barrett J, Kriz W, Kaissling B, de Rouffignac C. The ultrastructure of the nephrons of the desert rodent (Psammomys obesus) kidney. II. Thin limbs of Henle of long-looped nephrons. Am J Anat 1978;151:499—514.

[432] Kriz W, Schiller A, Taugner R. Freeze-fracture studies on the thin limbs of Henle's loop in Psammomys obesus. Am J Anat 1981;162:23—34.

[433] Chou C, Nielsen S, Knepper M. Structural—functional correlation in chinchilla long loop of Henle thin limbs: a novel papillary subsegment. Am J Physiol 1993;265:F863—74.

[434] Dobyan D, Jamison R. Structure and function of the renal papilla. Semin Nephrol 1984;4:5.

[435] Kriz W. Structural organization of the renal medullary counterflow system. Fed Proc 1983;42:2379—85.

[436] Kriz W, Kaissling B. Structural organization of the mammalian kidney. In: Seldin D, Giebisch G, editors. The kidney. Philadelphia: Lippincott Williams and Wilkens; 2000. p. 587—654.

[437] Pannabecker T, Abbott D, Dantzler W. Three-dimensional functional reconstruction of inner medullary thin limbs of Henle's loop. Am J Physiol Renal Physiol 2004;286: F38—45.

[438] Pannabecker T, Dahmann A, Brokl O, Dantzler W. Mixed descending- and ascending-type thin limbs of Henle's loop in mammalian renal inner medulla. Am J Physiol Renal Physiol 2000;278:F202—8.

[439] Bachmann S, Kriz W, Kuhn C, Franke W. Differentiation of cell types of the mammalian kidney by immunofluorescence microscopy using antibodies to intermediate filament proteins and desmoplakins. Histochemistry 1983;77:365—94.

[440] Zhai X, Fenton R, Andreasen A, Thomsen J, Christensen E. Aquaporin-1 is not expressed in descending thin limbs of short-loop nephrons. J Am Soc Nephrol 2007;18:2937—44.

[441] Bankir L, Trinh-Trang-Tan M. Renal urea transporters. Direct and indirect regulation by vasopressin. Exp Physiol 2000;85:243S—52S.

[442] Kim Y, Kim D, Han K, Jung J, Sands J, Knepper M, et al. Expression of urea transporters in the developing rat kidney. Am J Physiol Renal Physiol 2002;282:F530—40.

[443] Küttler T. Verlauf und histotopographische beziehungen oberflächlich gelegener nephrone der katzenniere. Heidelberg: Dissertation; 1980.

[444] Dobyan D, Bulger R. Morphology of the minipig kidney. J Electron Microsc Tech 1988;9:213—34.

[445] Schwartz M, Karnovsky M, Venkatachalam M. Ultrastructural differences between rat inner medullary descending and ascending vasa recta. Lab Invest 1976;35:161—70.

[446] Ernst S, Schreiber J. Ultrastructural localization of Na+, K+-ATPase in rat and rabbit kidney medulla. J Cell Biol 1981;91:803—13.

[447] Majack R, Paull W, Barrett J. The ultrastructural localization of membrane ATPase in rat thin limbs of the loop of Henle. Histochemie 1979;63:23—33.

[448] Van Itallie C, Anderson J. Claudins and epithelial paracellular transport. Annu Rev Physiol 2006;68:403—29.

[449] Nielsen S, Digiovanni S, Christensen E, Knepper M, Harris H. Cellular and subcellular immunolocalization of vasopressin-regulated water channel in rat kidney. Proc Natl Acad Sci USA 1993;90:11663—7.

[450] Dobyan D, Magill L, Friedman P, Herbert S, Bulger R. Carbonic anhydrase histochemistry in rabbit and mouse kidneys. Anat Rec 1982;204:185—97.

[451] Schiller A, Taugner R, Kriz W. The thin limbs of Henle's loop in the rabbit: a freeze-fracture study. Cell Tissue Res 1980; 207:249—65.

[452] Layton A, Pannabecker T, Dantzler W, Layton H. Two modes for concentrating urine in rat inner medulla. Am J Physiol Renal Physiol 2004;287:F816—39.

[453] Nielsen S, Pallone T, Smith B, Christensen E, Agre P, Maunsbach A. Aquaporin-1 water channels in short and long loop descending thin limbs and in descending vasa recta in rat kidney. Am J Physiol Renal Physiol 1995; 268:1023—37.

[454] Verbavatz J, Brown D, Sabolic I, Valenti G, Ausiello D, van Hoek A, et al. Tetrameric assembly of CHIP28 water channels in liposomes and cell membranes: a freeze-fracture study. J Cell Biol 1993;123:605—18.

[455] Hediger M, Knepper M. Introduction: recent insights into the urinary concentrating mechanism: from cDNA cloning to dodelin renal function. Am J Physiol 1998;275:F317.

[456] Shayakul C, Knepper M, Smith C, Digiovanni S, Hediger M. Segmental localization of urea transporter mRNAa in rat kidney. Am J Physiol 1997;272:F654—60.

[457] Trinh-Trang-Tan M, Bankir L. Integrated function of urea transporters in the mammalian kidney. Exp Nephrol 1998; 6:471—9.

[458] Wade J, Lee A, Liu C, Ecelbarger C, Mitchell C, Bradford A, et al. UT-A2: A 55-kDa urea transporter in thin descending limb whose abundance is regulated by vasopressin. Am J Physiol Renal Physiol 2000;278:F52—62.

[459] Bulger R, Tisher C, Myers C, Trump B. Human renal ultrastructure. II. The thin limb of Henle's loop and the interstitium in healthy individuals. Lab Invest 1967;16:124—41.

[460] Orci L, Brown D. Distribution of filipin-sterol complexes in plasma membranes of the kidney. II. The thin limbs of Henle's loop. Lab Invest 1983;48:80—9.

[461] Le Hir M, Dubach U. The cellular specificity of lectin binding in the kidney. I. A light microscopical study in the rat. Histochemie 1982;74:521—30.

[462] Le Hir M, Dubach U. The cellular specificity of lectin binding in the kidney. II. A light microscopical study in the rabbit. Histochemie 1982;74:531—40.

[463] Roth J, Taatjes D. Glycocalix heterogeneity of rat kidney urinary tubule: demonstration with lectin-gold technique specific for sialic acid. Eur J Cell Biol 1985;39:449—57.

[464] Imai M. Function of the thin ascending limb of Henle of rats and hamsters perfused in vitro. Am J Physiol 1977;232:F201—9.

[465] Jamison R. Micropuncture study of segments of thin loops of Henle in the rat. Am J Physiol 1968;215:236—42.

[466] Uchida S, Sasaki S, Nitta K, Uchida K, Horita S, Nihei H, et al. Localization and functional characterization of rat kidney-specific chloride channel, CIC-K1. J Clin Invest 1995;95: 104—13.

[467] Bulger R. The shape of rat kidney tubular cells. Am J Anat 1965;116:237—56.

[468] Hebert S, Culpepper R, Andreoli T. NaCl transport in mouse medullary thick ascending limbs. I. Functional nephron heterogeneity and ADH-stimulated NaCl co-transport. Am J Physiol 1981;241:F412—31.

[469] Allen F, Tisher C. Morphology of the ascending thick limb of Henle. Kidney Int 1976;9:8—22.

[470] Welling L, Welling D, Hill J. Shape of cells and intercellular channals in rabbit thick ascending limb of Henle. Kidney Int 1978;13:144—51.

[471] Kone B, Madsen K, Tisher C. Ultrastructure of the thick ascending limb of Henle in the rat kidney. Am J Anat 1984;171:217—26.

[472] Bulger R, Dobyan D. Recent structure—function relationships in normal and injured mammalian kidneys. Anat Rec 1983; 205:1—11.

[473] Jung J, Song J, Li C, Yang C, Kang T, Won M, et al. Expression of epidermal growth factor in the developing rat kidney. Am J Physiol Renal Physiol 2005;288:F227—35.

[474] Ecelbarger C, Terris J, Hoyer J, Nielsen S, Wade J, Knepper M. Localization and regulation of the rat renal Na$^+$-K$^+$-2Cl$^-$ co-transporter,BSC-1. Am J Physiol 1996;271:F619—28.

[475] Nielsen S, Maunsbach A, Ecelbarger C, Knepper M. Ultrastructural localization of Na-K-2Cl co-transporter in thick ascending limb and macula densa of rat kidney. Am J Physiol Renal Physiol 1998;275:F885—93.

[476] Obermüller N, Kunchaparty S, Ellison D, Bachmann S. Expression of the Na-K-2Cl co-transporter by macula densa and thick ascending limb cells of rat and rabbit nephron. J Clin Invest 1996;98:635—40.

[477] Greger R, Schlatter E, Lang F. Evidence for electroneutral sodium chloride co-transport in the cortical thick ascending limb of Henle's loop of rabbit kidney. Pflugers Arch 1983;396:308—14.

[478] Giebisch G. Renal potassium channels: function, regulation, and structure. Kidney Int 2001;60:436—45.

[479] Hebert S. Bartter syndrome. Curr Opin Nephrol Hypertens 2003;12:527—32.

[480] Lin D, Sterling H, Wang W. The protein tyrosine kinase-dependent pathway mediates the effect of K intake on renal K secretion. Physiology 2005;20:140—6.

[481] Wade J, Fang L, Coleman R, Liu J, Grimm P, Wang T, et al. Differential regulation of ROMK (Kir1.1) in distal nephron segments by dietary potassium. Am J Physiol Renal Physiol 2011;300:F1385—93.

[482] Wang W. Renal potassium channels: recent developments. Curr Opin Nephrol Hypertens 2004;13:549—55.

[483] Wang W. Regulation of ROMK (Kir1.1) channels: new mechanisms and aspects. Am J Physiol Renal Physiol 2006;290: F14—9.

[484] Krämer B, Bergler T, Stoelcker B, Waldegger S. Mechanisms of disease: the kidney-specific chloride channels CICKA and CICKB, the Barttin subunit and their clinical relevance. Nat Clin Pract Nephrol 2008;4:38—46.

[485] Burckhardt G, Di Sole F, Helmle-Kolb C. The Na$^+$/H$^+$ exchanger gene family. J Nephrol 2002;(Suppl. 5):S3—21.

[486] Burckhardt G, Wolff N, Bahn A. Molecular characterization of the renal organic anion transporter 1. Cell Biochem Biophys 2002;36:169—74.

[487] Capasso G, Rizzo M, Pica A, Di Maio F, Moe O, Alpern R, et al. Bicarbonate reabsorption and NHE-3 expression: abundance and activity are increased in Henle's loop of remnant rats. Kidney Int 2002;62:2126—35.

[488] Capasso G, Unwin R. Bicarbonate transport along the loop of Henle: molecular mechanisms and regulation. J Nephrol 2002; (Suppl. 5):S88—96.

[489] Biemesderfer D, Rutherford P, Nagy T, Pizzonnia J, Abu-Alfa A, Aronson P. Monoclonal antibodies for high-resolution localization of NHE-3 in adult and neonatal rat kidney. Am J Physiol 1997;273:F289—99.

[490] Sun A, Liu Y, Dworkin L, Tse C, Donowitz M, Yip K. Na$^+$/H$^+$ exchanger isoform 2 (NHE2) is expressed in the apical membrane of the medullary thick ascending limb. J Membr Biol 1997;160:85—90.

[491] Wright F, Giebisch G. Regulation of potassium excretion. In: Seldin D, Giebisch G, editors. The kidney: physiology and pathophysiology. New York: Raven Press; 1985. p. 1223—49.

[492] Wagner C, Finberg K, Breton S, Marshansky V, Brown D, Geibel J. Renal vacuolar H$^+$-ATPase. Physiol Rev 2004; 84:1263—314.

[493] Pushkin A, Kurtz I. SLC4 base (HCO$_3^-$, CO$_3^{2-}$) transporters: classification, function, structure, genetic diseases, and knockout models. Am J Physiol Renal Physiol 2006;290: F580—99.

[494] Quentin F, Eladari D, Cheval L, Lopez C, Goossens D, Colin Y, et al. RhBG and RhCG, the putative ammonia transporters, are expressed in the same cells in the distal nephron. J Am Soc Nephrol 2003;14:545—54.

[495] Ambühl P, Amemiya M, Danzkay M, Lötscher M, Kaissling B, Moe O, et al. Chronic metabolic acidosis inicreases NHE-3 protein abundance in rat kidney. Am J Physiol 1996;271:F917—25.

[496] Loffing J, Lötscher M, Kaissling B, Biber J, Murer H, Seikaly M, et al. Renal Na/H exchanger NHE-3 and Na-PO$_4$ co-transporter NaPi-2 protein expression in glucocorticoid excess and deficient states. J Am Soc Nephrol 1998;9:1560—7.

[497] Konrad M, Schlingmann K, Gudermann T. Insights into the molecular nature of magnesium homeostasis. Am J Physiol Renal Physiol 2004;286:F599—605.

[498] Konrad M, Weber S. Recent advances in molecular genetics of hereditary magnesium-losing disorders. J Am Soc Nephrol 2003;14:249—60.

[499] Ellison D. Divalent cation transport by the distal nephron: insights from Bartter's and Gitelman's syndromes. Am J Physiol Renal Physiol 2000;279:F616—25.

[500] Gunzel D, Yu A. Function and regulation of claudins in the thick ascending limb of Henle. Pflugers Arch 2009;458:77—88.

[501] Hou J, Renigunta A, Gomes A, Hou M, Paul D, Waldegger S, et al. Claudin-16 and claudin-19 interaction is required for their assembly into tight junctions and for renal reabsorption of magnesium. Proc Natl Acad Sci USA 2009;106:15350—5.

[502] Knohl S, Scheinman S. Inherited hypercalciuric syndromes: dent's disease (CLC-5) and familial hypomagnesemia with hypercalciuria (paracellin-1). Semin Nephrol 2004;24: 55—60.

[503] Konrad M, Schaller A, Seelow D, Pandey A, Waldegger S, Lesslauer A, et al. Mutations in the tight-junction gene claudin 19 (CLDN19) are associated with renal magnesium wasting, renal failure, and severe ocular involvement. Am J Hum Genet 2006;79:949—57.

[504] Quamme G, de Rouffignac C. Epithelial magnesium transport and regulation by the kidney. Front Biosci 2000;5:D694—711.

[505] Unwin R, Capasso G, Shirley D. An overview of divalent cation and citrate handling by the kidney. Nephron Physiol 2004;98:15—20.

[506] Wagner C. Metabolic acidosis: new insights from mouse models. Curr Opin Nephrol Hypertens 2007;16:471–6.

[507] Chabardes D, Gagnan-Brunette M, Imbert-Teboul M, Gontcharevskaia O, Montegut M, Clique A, et al. Adenylate cyclase responsiveness to hormones in various portions of the human nephron. J Clin Invest 1980;65:439–48.

[508] de Rouffignac C, Di Stefano A, Wittner M, Roinel N, Elalouf J. Consequences of differential effects of ADH and other peptide hormones on thick ascending limb of mammalian kidney. Am J Physiol 1991;260:R1023–35.

[509] Hebert S, Andreoli T. Control of Nal transport in the thick ascending limb. Am J Physiol 1984;246:F745–56.

[510] Knepper M, Kim G, Fernandez-Llama P, Ecelbarger C. Regulation of thick ascending limb transport by vasopressin. J Am Soc Nephrol 1999;10:628–34.

[511] Molony D, Reeves W, Hebert S, Andreoli T. ADH increases apical Na^+, K^+, $2Cl^-$ entry in mouse medullary thick ascending limbs of Henle. Am J Physiol 1987;252:F177–87.

[512] Wittner M, Di Stefano A, Mandon B, Roinel N, de Rouffignac C. Stimulation of NaCl reabsorption by antidiuretic hormone in the cortical thick ascending limb of Henle's loop of the mouse. Pflugers Arch 1991;419:212–4.

[513] Meade P, Hoover R, Plata C, Vázquez N, bobadilla N, Gamba G, et al. cAMP-dependent activation of the renal-specific Na^+-K^+-$2Cl^-$ co-transporter is mediated by regulation of co-transporter trafficking. Am J Physiol Renal Physiol 2003;284: F1145–54.

[514] Kim G, Ecelbarger C, Mitchell C, Packer R, Wade J, Knepper M. Vasopressin increases Na-K-2Cl co-transporter expression in thick ascending limb of Henle's loop. Am J Physiol 1999;276: F96–103.

[515] Pham P, Devuyst O, Phamt P, Matsumoto N, Shih R, Jo O, et al. Hypertonicity increases CLC-5 expression in mouse medullary thick ascending limb cells. Am J Physiol Renal Physiol 2004;287:F747–52.

[516] Harris R, McKanna J, Akai Y, Jacobson H, Dubois R, Breyer M. Cyclooxygenase-2 is associated with the macula densa of rat kidney and increases with salt restriction. J Clin Invest 1994;94:2504–10.

[517] Jeck N, Schlingmann K, Reinalter S, Kömhoff M, Peters M, Waldegger S, et al. Salt handling in the distal nephron: lessons learned from inherited human disorders. Am J Physiol Regul Integr Comp Physiol 2005;288:R782–95.

[518] Vio C, Cespedes C, Gallardo P, Masferrer J. Renal identification of cyclooxygenase-2 in a subset of thick ascending limb cells. Hypertension 1997;30:687–92.

[519] Valtin H. Physiological effects of vasopressin on the kidney. In: Gash D, Boer G, editors. Vasopressin. New York: Plenum; 1987. p. 369–87.

[520] Trinh-Trang-Tan M, Bouby N, Kriz W, Bankir L. Functional adaptation of the thick ascending limb and internephron heterogeneity to urine concentration. Kidney Int 1987;31:549–55.

[521] Bankir L, Fischer C, Fischer S, Jukkala K, Specht H, Kriz W. Adaptation of the rat kidney to altered water intake and urine concentration. Pflugers Arch 1988;412:42–53.

[522] Bouby N, Bankir L. Effect of high protein intake on sodium, potassium-dependent adenosine triphosphatase activity in the thick ascending limb of Henle's loop in the rat. Clin Sci 1988;74:319–29.

[523] Bouby N, Trinh-Trang-Tan M, Coutaud C, Bankir L. Vasopressin is involved in renal effects of high-protein diet: study in homozygous Brattleboro rats. Am J Physiol 1991;260: F96–100.

[524] Lu M, Wang T, Yan Q, Wang W, Giebisch G, Hebert S. ROMK is required for expression of the 70-pS K channel in the thick ascending limb. Am J Physiol Renal Physiol 2004;286:F490–5.

[525] Nomura N, Tajima M, Sugawara N, Morimoto T, Kondo Y, Ohno M, et al. Generation and analyses of R8L barttin knockin mouse. Am J Physiol Renal Physiol 2011;301:F297–307.

[526] Schnermann J. Sodium transport deficiency and sodium balance in gene-targeted mice. Acta Physiol Scand 2001; 173:59–66.

[527] Teulon J, Eladari D. A new mouse model for Bartter's syndrome. Am J Physiol Renal Physiol 2011;301:F295–6.

[528] Bachmann S, Koeppen-Hagemann I, Kriz W. Ultrastructural localization of Tamm-Horsfall glycoprotein (THP) in rat kidney as revealed by protein A-gold immunocytochemistry. Histochemistry 1985;83:531–8.

[529] Bachmann S, Metzger R, Bunnemann B. Tamm-Horsfall protein-mRNA synthesis is localized to the thick ascending limb of Henle's loop in rat kidney. Histochemistry 1990;94:517–23.

[530] Rampoldi L, Scolari F, Amoroso A, Ghiggeri G, Devuyst O. The rediscovery of uromodulin (Tamm-Horsfall protein): from tubulointerstitial nephropathy to chronic kidney disease. Kidney Int 2011;80:338–47.

[531] Serafini-Cessi F, Malagolini N, Cavallone D. Tamm-Horsfall glycoprotein: biology and clinical relevance. Am J Kidney Dis 2003;42:658–76.

[532] Bernascone J, Janas S, Ikehata M, Trudu M, Corbelli A, Schaeffer C, et al. A transgenic mouse model for uromodulin-associated kidney diseases shows specific tubulo-interstitial damage, urinary concentrating defect and renal failure. Hum Mol Genet 2010;19:2898–3010.

[533] Mutig K, Kahl T, Godes M, Persson P, Bates J, Raffi H, et al. Activation of the bumetanide-sensitive Na^+,K^+,$2Cl^-$ co-transporter (NKCC2) is facilitated by Tamm-Horsfall protein in a chloride-sensitive manner. J Biol Chem 2011;286:30200–10.

[534] Morel F, Chabardes D, Imbert-Teboul M. Functional segmentation of the rabbit distal tubule by microdetermination of hormone-dependent adenylate cyclase activity. Kidney Int 1976; 9:264–77.

[535] Crayen M, Thoenes W. Architecture and cell structures in the distal nephron of the rat kidney. Cytobiol 1978;17:197–211.

[536] Schmitt R, Ellison D, Farman N, Rossier B, Reilly R, Reeves W, et al. Developmental expression of sodium entry pathways in rat nephron. Am J Physiol 1999;276:F367–81.

[537] Campean V, Kricke J, Ellison D, Luft F, Bachmann S. Localization of thiazide-sensitive Na(+)-Cl(−) co-transport and associated gene products in mouse DCT. Am J Physiol Renal Physiol 2001;281:F1028–35.

[538] Loffing J, Loffing-Cueni D, Valderrabano V, Klausli L, Hebert S, Rossier B, et al. Distribution of transcellular calcium and sodium transport pathways along mouse distal nephron. Am J Physiol Renal Physiol 2001;281:F1019–20.

[539] Biner H, Arpin-Bott M, Loffing J, Wang X, Kneper M, Hebert S, et al. Human cortical distal nephron: distribution of electrolyte and water transport pathways. J Am Soc Nephrol 2002; 13:836–47.

[540] Myers C, Bulger R, Tisher C, Trump B. Human renal ultrastructure. IV. Collecting duct of healthy individuals. Lab Invest 1966;15:1921–50.

[541] Tisher C, Bulger R, Trump B. Human renal ultrastructure. III. The distal tubule in healthy individuals. Lab Invest 1968; 18:655–68.

[542] Kriz W, Bankir L. A standard nomenclature for structure of the kidney. The Renal Commission of the International Union of Physiological Sciences (IUPS). Kidney Int 1988;33:1–7.

[543] Dorup J. Ultrastructure of distal nephron cells in rat renal cortex. J Ultrastruct Res 1985;92:101–18.

[544] Loffing J, Kaissling B. Sodium and calcium transport pathways along the mammalian distal nephron from rabbit to human. Am J Physiol Renal Physiol 2003;284:F628–43.

[545] Loffing J, Vallon V, Loffing-Cueni D, Aregger F, Richter K, Pietri L, et al. Altered renal distal tubule structure and renal Na($^+$) and Ca($^{2+}$) handling in a mouse model for Gitelman's syndrome. J Am Soc Nephrol 2004;15:2276–88.

[546] Clapp W, Madsen K, Verlander J, Tisher C. Intercalated cells of the rat inner medullary collecting duct. Kidney Int 1987;31:1080–7.

[547] Reilly R, Ellison D. Mammalian distal tubule: physiology, pathophysiology, and molecular anatomy. Physiol Rev 2000;80:277–313.

[548] Voets T, Nilius B, Hoefs S, van der Kemp A, Droogmans G, Bindels R, et al. TRPM6 forms the Mg^{2+} influx channel involved in interstitial and renal Mg^{2+} absorption. J Biol Chem 2004;279:19–25.

[549] Nijenhuis T, Hoenderop J, Loffing J, van der Kemp A, van Os C, Bindels R. Thiazide-induced hypocalciuria is accompanied by a decreased expression of Ca^{2+} transport proteins in kidney. Kidney Int 2003;64:555–64.

[550] Kaissling B, Peter S, Kriz W. The transition of the thick ascending limb of Henle's loop into the distal convoluted tubule in the nephron of the rat kidney. Cell Tissue Res 1977;182:111–8.

[551] Loffing J, Loffing-Cueni D, Macher A, Hebert S, Olson B, Knepper M, et al. Localization of epithelial sodium channel and aquaporin-2 in rabbit cortex. Am J Physiol Renal Physiol 2000;272:530.

[552] Madsen K, Clapp W, Verlander J. Structure and function of the inner medullary-collecting duct. Kidney Int 1988;34:441–54.

[553] Stoessel A, Himmerkus N, Bleich M, Bachmann S, Theilig F. Connexin 37 is localized in renal epithelia and responds to changes in dietary salt intake. Am J Physiol Renal Physiol 2010;298:F216–23.

[554] Breton S, Lisanti M, Tyszkowski R, McLaughlin M, Brown D. Basolateral distribution of caveolin-1 in the kidney: absence from H^+-ATPase-coated endocytic vesicles in intercalated cells. J Histochem Cytochem 1998;46:205–14.

[555] Voldstedlund M, Thuneberg L, Tranum-Jensen J, Vinten J, Christensen E. Caveolae, caveolin and cav-p60 in smooth muscle and renin-producing cells in the rat kidney. Acta Physiol Scand 2003;179:179–88.

[556] Gamba G. The thiazide-sensitive Na^+-Cl-co-transporter: molecular biology, functional properties, and regulation by WNKs. Am J Physiol Renal Physiol 2009;297:F838–48.

[557] Estevez R, Boettger T, Stein V, Birkenhager R, Otto E, Hildebrandt F, et al. Barttin is a Cl^- channel beta-subunit crucial for renal Cl-reabsorption and inner ear K^+ secretion. Nature 2001;414:558–61.

[558] Rieg T, Vallon V, Sausbier M, Kaissling B, Ruth P, Osswald H. The role of the BK channel in potassium homeostasis and flow-induced renal potassium excretion. Kidney Int 2007; 72:566–73.

[559] Rodan A, Cheng C, Huang C. Recent advances in distal tubular potassium handling. Am J Physiol Renal Physiol 2011;300: F821–7.

[560] Yang L, Sandberg M, Can A, Pihakaski-Maunsbach K, McDonough A. Effects of dietary salt on renal Na^+ transporter subcellular distribution, abundance, and phosphorylation status. Am J Physiol Renal Physiol 2008;295: F1003–16.

[561] Vallon V, Schroth J, Lang F, Kuhl D, Uchida S. Expression and phosphorylation of the Na^+-Cl^- co-transporter NCC *in vivo* is regulated by dietary salt, potassium, and SGK1. Am J Physiol Renal Physiol 2009;297:F704–12.

[562] Arroyo P, Ronzaud C, Lagnaz D, Staub O, Gamba G. Aldosterone paradox: differential regulation of ion transport in distal nephron. Physiology 2011;26:115–23.

[563] Lee D, Riquier A, Yang L, Leong P, Maunsbach A, McDonough A. Acute hypertension provokes acute trafficking of distal tubule Na-Cl-co-transporter (NCC) to subapical cytoplasmic vesicles. Am J Physiol Renal Physiol 2009;296: F810–8.

[564] Sandberg M, Riquier A, Pihakaski-Maunsbach K, McDonough A, Maunsbach A. ANG II provokes acute trafficking of distal tubule Na^+-Cl^-($^-$) co-transporter to apical membrane. Am J Physiol Renal Physiol 2007;293:F662–9.

[565] Verlander J, Tran T, Zhang L, Kaplan M, Hebert S. Estradiol enhances thiazide-sensitive NaCl co-transporter density in the apical plasma membrane of the distal convoluted tubule in ovariectomized rats. J Clin Invest 1998;101:1661–9.

[566] Ko B, Kamsteeg E, Cooke L, Moddes L, Deen P, Hoover R. RasGRP1 stimulation enhances ubiquitation and endocytosis. Am J Physiol Renal Physiol 2010;299:F300–9.

[567] Golbang A, Cope G, Hamad A, Murthy M, Liu C, Cuthbert A, et al. Regulation of the expression of the Na/Cl co-transporter by WNK4 and WNK1: evidence that accelerated dynamin-dependent endocytosis is not involved. Am J Physiol Renal Physiol 2006;291:F1369–76.

[568] Subramanya A, Ellison D. Sorting out lysosomal trafficking of the thiazide-sensitive Na-Cl co-transporter. J Am Soc Nephrol 2010;21:7–9.

[569] Gamba G. Role of WNK kinases in regulating tubular salt and potassium transport and in the development of hypertension. Am J Physiol Renal Physiol 2005;288:F245–52.

[570] Hadouchel J, Soukaseum C, Büsst C, Zhou X, Baudrie V, Zürrer T, et al. Decreased ENaC expression compensates the increased NCC activity following inactivation of the kidney specific isoform of WNK1 and prevents hypertension. Proc Natl Acad Sci USA 2010;107:18109–14.

[571] Yang B, Bankir L. Urea and urine concentrating ability: new insights from studies in mice. Am J Physiol Renal Physiol 2005;288:F881–96.

[572] Zhou B, Zhuang J, Gu D, Wang H, Cebotaru L, Guggino W, et al. WNK4 enhances the degradation of NCC through a sortilin-mediated lysosomal pathway. J Am Soc Nephrol 2010;21:82–92.

[573] Mutig K, Saritas T, Uchida S, Kahl T, Borowski T, Paliege A, et al. Short-term stimulation of the thiazide-sensitive Na^+-Cl^- co-transporter by vasopressin involves phosphorylation and membrane translocation. Am J Physiol Renal Physiol 2010;298: F502–9.

[574] Pedersen N, Hofmeister M, Rosenbaek L, Nielsen J, Fenton R. Vasopressin induces phosphorylation of the thiazide-sensitive chloride co-transporter in the distal convoluted tubule. Kidney Int 2010;78:160–9.

[575] Imbert-Teboul M, Chabardes D, Morel F. Vasopressin and catecholamine sites of action along rabbit, mouse and rat nephron. In: Bahlman J, Brod J, editors. Contributions to nephrology: disturbance of water and electrolyte metabolism. Basel: Karger; 1980. p. 41–7.

[576] Ellison D, Velazquez H, Wright F. Thiazide-sensitive sodium chloride co-transport in early distal tubule. Am J Physiol 1987; 253:F546–54.

[577] Koechlin N, Elalouf J, Kaissling B, Roinel N, de Rouffignac C. A structural study of the rat proximal and distal nephron:

effect of peptide and thyroid hormones. Am J Physiol 1989;256:F814—22.

[578] Stanton B. Renal potassium transport: morphological and functional adaptations. Am J Physiol 1989;257:R989—97.

[579] Cantone A, Yang X, Yan Q, Giebisch G, Hebert S, Wang T. Mouse model of type II Bartter's syndrome. I. Upregulation of thiazide-sensitive Na-Cl co-transporter activity. Am J Physiol Renal Physiol 2008;294:F1366—72.

[580] Wagner C, Loffing-Cueni D, Yan Q, Schulz N, Fakitsas P, Carrel M, et al. Mouse model of type II Bartter's syndrome. II. Altered expression of renal soldium- and water-transporting proteins. Am J Physiol Renal Physiol 2008;294:F1373—80.

[581] Wang X, Masilamani S, Nielsen S, Kwon T, Brooks H, Nielsen S, et al. The renal thiazide-sensitive Na-Cl co-transporter as mediator of the aldosterone-escape phenomenon. J Clin Invest 2001;108:215—22.

[582] Glaudermans B, Knoers N, Hoenderop J, Bindels R. New molecular players facilitating Mg^{2+} reabsorption in the distal convoluted tubule. Kidney Int 2010;77:17—22.

[583] Satoh J, Romero M. Mg^{2+} transport in the kidney. Biometals 2002;15:285—95.

[584] Schlingmann K, Gudermann T. A critical role of TRPM channel-kinase for human magnesium transport. J Physiol 2005;566:301—8.

[585] Meij I, Koenderink J, de Jong J, De Pont J, Monnens L, van den Heuvel L, et al. Dominant isolated renal magnesium loss is caused by misrouting of the Na^+,K^+-ATPase gamma-subunit. Ann NY Acad Sci 2003;986:437—43.

[586] Adalat S, Woolf A, Johnstone K, Wirsing A, Harries L, Long D, et al. HNF1B mutations associate with hypomagnesemia and renal magnesium wasting. J Am Soc Nephrol 2009;20:1123—31.

[587] Borke J, Caride A, Verma A, Penniston J, Kumari R. Plasma membrane calcium pump and 28-KDa calcium binding protein in cells of rat kidney distal tubules. Am J Physiol 1989;257:F842—9.

[588] Salido E, Fisher D, Barajas L. Immunoelectron microscopy of epidermal growth factor in mouse kidney. J Ultrastruct Mol Struct Res 1986;96:105—13.

[589] Salido E, Lakshmanan J, Fisher D, Shapiro L, Barajas L. Expression of epidermal growth factor in the rat kidney. An immunocytochemical and in situ hybridization study. Histochemie 1991;96:65—72.

[590] Belge H, Gailly P, Schwaller B, Loffing J, Debaix H, Riveira-Munoz E, et al. Renal expression of parvalbumin is critical for NaCl handling and response to diuretics. Proc Natl Acad Sci USA 2007;104:14849—54.

[591] Tatum R, Zhang Y, Salleng K, Lu Z, Lin J, Lu Q, et al. Renal salt wasting and chronic dehydration in claudin-7-deficient mice. Am J Physiol Renal Physiol 2010;298:F24—34.

[592] Turksen K. Wasted salts and wasted bodies: new insight into the role of claudin-7 in the kidney. Am J Physiol Renal Physiol 2010;298:F22—3.

[593] Boros S, Bindels R, Hoenderop J. Active Ca^{2+} reabsorption in the connecting tubule. Pflugers Arch 2009;458:99—109.

[594] van Abel M, Hoenderop J, van der Kemp A, Friedlaender M, van Leeuwen J, Bindels R. Coordinated control of renal Ca^{2+} transport proteins by parathyroid hormone. Kidney Int 2005;68:1708—21.

[595] Schultheis P, Lorenz J, Meneton P, Nieman M, Riddle T, Flagella M, et al. Phenotype resembling Gitelman's syndrome in mice lacking the apical Na^+-Cl^- co-transporter of the distal convoluted tubule. J Biol Chem 1998;273:29150—5.

[596] Cruz D, Shaer A, Bia M, Lifton R, Simon D. Gitelman's syndrome revisited: an evaluation of symptoms and health-related quality of life. Kidney Int 2001;59:710—7.

[597] De Jong J, Van der Vliet W, van den Heuvel L, Willems P, Knoers N, Bindels R. Functional expression of mutations in the human NaCl co-transporter: evidence for impaired routing mechanisms in Gitelman's syndrome. J Am Soc Nephrol 2002;13:1442—8.

[598] Melander O, Orho-Melander M, Bengtsson K, Lindblad U, Rastam L, Groop L, et al. Genetic variants of thiazide-sensitive NaCl-co-transporter in Gitelman's syndrome and primary hypertension. Hypertension 2000;36:389—94.

[599] Reissinger A, Ludwig M, Utsch B, Prömse A, Baulmann J, Weisser B, et al. Novel NCCT gene mutations as a cause of Gitelman's syndrome and a systematic review of mutant and polymorphic NCCT alleles. Kidney Blood Press Res 2002;25:354—62.

[600] Kahle K, Macgregor G, Wilson F, van Hoek A, Brown D, Ardito T, et al. Paracellular Cl^- permeability is regulated by WNK4 kinase: insight into normal physiology and hypertension. Proc Natl Acad Sci USA 2004;101:14877—82.

[601] San-Cristobal P, Dimke H, Hoenderop J, Bindels R. Novel molecular pathways in renal Mg^{2+} transport: a guided tour along the nephron. Curr Opin Nephrol Hypertens 2010;19:456—62.

[602] Lang F, Capasso G, Schwab M, Waldegger S. Renal tubular transport and the genetic basis of hypertensive disease. Clin Exp Nephrol 2005;9:91—9.

[603] Osathanondh V, Potter E. Development of human kidney as shown by microdissection. III. Formation and interrelationship of collecting tubules and nephrons. Arch Pathol 1963;76:290—302.

[604] Rubera I, Loffing J, Palmer L, Frindt G, Fowler-Jaeger N, Sauter D, et al. Collecting duct-specific gene inactivation of alphaENacC in the mouse kidney does not impair sodium and potassium balance. J Clin Invest 2003;112:554—65.

[605] Loffing J, Pietri L, Aregger F, Bloch-Faure M, Ziegler U, Meneton P, et al. Differential subcellular localization of ENaC subunits in mouse kidney in response to high- and low-Na diets. Am J Physiol Renal Physiol 2000;279:F252—8.

[606] Loffing J, Zecevic M, Feraille S, Kaissling B, Asher C, Rossier B, et al. Aldosterone induces rapid apical translocation of ENaC in early portion of renal collecting system: possible role of SGK. Am J Physiol Renal Physiol 2001;280:F675—82.

[607] Costanzo L, Windhager E. Calcium and sodium transport by the distal convoluted tubule of the rat. Am J Physiol 1978;235:F492—506.

[608] Friedman P. Mechanism of renal calcium transport. Exp Nephrol 2000;8:343—50.

[609] Hoenderop J, van der Kemp A, Hartog A, van de Graaf S, van Os C, Willems P, et al. Molecular identification of the apical Ca^{2+} channel in 1, 25-dihydroxyvitamin D3-responsive epithelia. J Biol Chem 1999;274:8375—8.

[610] Markadieu N, Bindels R, Hoenderop J. The renal connecting tubule: resolved and unresolved issues in Ca^{2+} transport. Int J Biochem Cell Biol 2011;43:1—4.

[611] Riccardi D, Hall A, Chattopadhyay N, Yu J, Brown E, Hebert S. Localization of the extracellular Ca^{2+}/polyvalent cation-sensing protein in rat kidney. Am J Physiol 1998;274:F611—22.

[612] Riccardi D, Lee W, Lee K, Segre G, Brown E, Hebert S. Localization of the extracellular Ca^{2+}-sensing receptor and PPTH/PTHrP receptor in rat kidney. Am J Physiol 1996;271:F951—6.

[613] Yang T, Hassan S, Huang Y, Smart A, Briggs J, Schnermann J. Expression of PTHrP, PTH/PTHrP receptor, and Ca^{2+}-sensing

receptor mRNAs along the rat nephron. Am J Physiol 1997; 272:F751–8.

[614] Riccardi D, Brown E. Physiology and pathophysiology of the calcium-sensing receptor in the kidney. Am J Physiol Renal Physiol 2010;298:F485–99.

[615] de Groot T, Bindels R, Hoenderop J. TRPV5: an ingeniously controlled calcium channel. Kidney Int 2008;74:1241–6.

[616] Hoenderop J, Nilius B, Bindels R. ECaC: the gatekeeper of transepithelial Ca^{2+} transport. Biochim Biopyhs Acta 2002; 1600:6–11.

[617] Hsu Y, Dimke H, Schoeber J, Hsu S, Lin S, Chu P, et al. Testosterone increases urinary calcium excretion and inhibits expression of renal calcium transport proteins. Kidney Int 2010;77:601–8.

[618] Omata K, Carretero O, Itoh S, Scicli A. Active and inactive kallikrein in rabbit connecting tubules and urine during low and normal sodium intake. Kidney Int 1983;24:714–8.

[619] Cha S, Huang C. WNK4 kinase stimulates caveola-mediated endocytosis of TRPV5 amplifying the dynamic range of regulation of the channel by protein kinase C. J Biol Chem 2010;285:6604–11.

[620] Gkika D, Topala C, Chang Q, Picard N, Thebault S, Houillier P, et al. Tissue kallikrein stimulates $Ca^{(2+)}$ reabsorption via PKC-dependent plasma membrane accumulation of TRPV5. EMBO J 2006;25:4707–16.

[621] Topala C, Bindels R, Hoenderop J. Regulation of the epithelial calcium channel TRPV5 by extracellular factors. Curr Opin Nephrol Hypertens 2007;16:319–24.

[622] Ardiles L, Loyola F, Ehrenfeld P, Burgos M, Flores C, Valderrama G, et al. Modulation of renal kallikrein by a high potassium diet in rats with intense proteinuria. Kidney Int 2006;69:53–9.

[623] Picard N, Van A, Campone C, Seiler M, Bloch-Faure M, Hoenderop J, et al. Tissue kallikrein-deficient mice display a defect in renal tubular calcium absorption. J Am Soc Nephrol 2005;16:3602–10.

[624] Marchetti J, Imbert-Teboul M, Alhenc-Gelas F, Allegrini J, Menard J, Morel F. Kallikrein along the rabbit microdissected nephron: a micromethod for its measurement. Effect of adrenalectomy and DOCA treatment. Pflugers Arch 1984; 401:27–33.

[625] Guder W, Hallbach J, Fink E, Kaissling B, Wirthensohn G. Kallikrein (kininogenese) in the mouse nephron: effect of dietary potassium. Biol Chem Hoppe Seyler 1987;368:637–45.

[626] Vio C, Figueroa C. Evidence for a stimulatory effect of high potassium diet on renal kallikrein. Kidney Int 1987;31: 1327–34.

[627] El Moghrabi S, Houillier P, Picard N, Sohet F, Wootla B, Bloch-Faure M, et al. Tissue kallikrein permits early renal adaptation of potassium load. Proc Natl Acad Sci USA 2010;107:13526–31.

[628] Rossier B, Pradervand S, Schild L, Hummler E. Epithelial sodium channel and the control of sodium balance: interaction between genetic and enviromental factors. Annu Rev Physiol 2002;64:877–97.

[629] Warnock D, Rossier B. Renal sodium handling: the role of the epithelial sodium channel. J Am Soc Nephrol 2005;322:302–7.

[630] Duc C, Farman N, Canessa C, Bonvalet J, Rossier B. Cell-specific expression of epithelial sodium channel a,b,and G subunits in aldosterone-responsive epithelia from the rat: localization by in situ hybridization and immunocytochemistry. J Cell Biol 1994;127:1907–21.

[631] Masilamani S, Kim G, Mitchell C, Wade J, Knepper M. Aldosterone-mediated regulation of ENaC alpha, beta and gama subunit proteins in the rat kidney. J Clin Invest 1999;104: R19–23.

[632] Verrey F, Loffing J, Zecevic M, Heitzmann D, Staub O. SGK1: aldosterone-induced relay of Na^+ transport regulation in distal kidney nephron cells. Cell Physiol Biochem 2003; 13:21–8.

[633] Ellison D. The thiazide-sensitive Na-CL co-transporter and human disease: reemergence of an old player. J Am Soc Nephrol 2003;14:538–40.

[634] Ackermann D, Gresko N, Carrel M, Loffing-Cueni D, Habermehl D, Gomez-Sanchez C, et al. In vivo nuclear translocation of mineralocorticoid and glucocorticoid receptors in rat kidney: differential effect of corticosteroids along the distaltubule. Am J Physiol Renal Physiol 2011;299: F1473–85.

[635] Bostanjoglo M, Reeves W, Reilly R, Velazquez H, Robertson N, Litwack G, et al. Molecular segmentation of the rat distal tubule: Co-expression of the thiazide-sensitive Na-Cl co-transporter with 11b-hydroxysteroid dehydrogenase. J Am Soc Nephrol 1998;9:1347–58.

[636] Brown R, Diaz R, Robson A, Kotelevtsev Y, Mullins J, Kaufman M, et al. The ontogeny of 11b-hydroxysteroid dehydrogenase type 2 and mineralocorticoid receptor gene expression reveal intricate control of glucocorticoid action in development. Endocrinology 1996;137:794–7.

[637] Farman N, Rafestin-Oblin M. Multiple aspects of mineralocorticoid selectivity. Am J Physiol Renal Physiol 2001;280: F181–92.

[638] Kyossev Z, Walker P, Reeves W. Immunolocalization of NAD-dependent 11b-hydroxysteroid dehydrogenase in human kidney and colon. Kidney Int 1996;49:271–81.

[639] Loffing J, Summa V, Zecevic M, Verrey F. Mediators of aldosterone action in the renal tubule. Curr Opin Nephrol Hypertens 2001;10:667–75.

[640] Frindt G, Palmer L. Surface expression of sodium channels and transporters in rat kidney: effects of dietary sodium. Am J Physiol Renal Physiol 2009;297:F1249–55.

[641] Coleman R, Wu D, Liu J, Wade J. Expression of aquaporin in the renal connecting tubule. Am J Physiol Renal Physiol 2000;279:F874–83.

[642] Kleyman T, Myerburg M, Hughey R. Regulation of ENaC by protease: an increasingly complex story. Kidney Int 2006; 70:1391–2.

[643] Planes C, Caughey G. Regulation of the epithelial Na^+ channel by peptidase. Curr Top Dev Biol 2007;78:23–46.

[644] Rossier B, Stutts M. Activation of the epithelial sodium channel (ENaC) by serine protease. Annu Rev Physiol 2009; 71:361–79.

[645] Loffing J, Korbmacher C. Regulated sodium transport in the renal connecting tubule (CNT) via the epithelial sodium channel (ENaC). Pflugers Arch 2009;458:111–35.

[646] Dijkink L, Hartog A, Deen P, van Os C, Bindels R. Time-dependent regulation by aldosterone of the amiloride-sensitive Na^+ channel in rabbit kidney. Pflugers Arch 1999;438:354–60.

[647] Debonneville C, Flores S, Kamynina E, Plant P, Tauxe C, Thomas M, et al. Phosphorylation of Nedd4-2 by Sgk1 regulates epithelial $Na^{(+)}$ channel cell surface expression. EMBO J 2001;20:7052–9.

[648] Flores S, Loffing-Cueni D, Kamynina E, Daidié D, Gerbex C, Chabanel S, et al. Aldosterone-induced serum and glucocorticoid-induced kinase 1 expression is accompanied by Nedd4-2 phosphorylation and increased Na^+ transport in cortical collecting duct cells. J Am Soc Nephrol 2005;16:2279–87.

[649] Snyder P, Olson D, Thomas B. Serum and glocotorticoid-regulated kinase modulates Nedd4-2-mediated inhibition of the epithelial Na channel. J Biol Chem 2002;277:5–8.

[650] Bankir L, Bichet D, Bouby N. Vasopressin V2 receptors. ENaC, and sodium reabsorption: a risk factor for hypertension? Am J Physiol Renal Physiol 2010;299:F917—28.

[651] Bugaj V, Pochynyuk O, Stockand J. Activation of the epithelial Na^+ chanel in the collecting duct by vasopressin contributes to water reabsorption. Am J Physiol Renal Physiol 2009;297: F1411—8.

[652] Boulkroun S, Ruffieux-Daidiè D, Vitagliano J, Poirot O, Charles R, Lagnaz D, et al. Vasopressin-inducible ubiquitin-specific protease 10 increases ENaC cell surface expression by deubiquitylating and stabilizing sorting nexin 3. Am J Physiol Renal Physiol 2008;295:F889—900.

[653] Butterworth M, Edinger R, Johnson J, Frizzell R. Acute ENaC stimulation by cAMP in a kidney cell line is mediated by exocytic insertion from a recycling channel pool. J Gen Physiol 2005;125:81—101.

[654] Cruz D, Simon D, Nelson-Williams C, Farhi A, Finberg K, Burleson L, et al. Mutations in the Na-Cl co-transporter reduce blood pressure in humans. Hypertension 2001;37:1458—64.

[655] Harrison-Bernard L, Navar L, Ho H, Vinson G, El-Dahr S. Immunohistochemical localization of ANG II AT1 receptor in adult rat kidney using a monoclonal antibody. Am J Physiol 1997;273:F170—7.

[656] Mujais S, Kauffman S, Katz A. Aingiotensin II binding sites in individual segments of the rat nephron. J Clin Invest 1986; 77:315—8.

[657] Vallon V, Rieg T. Regulation of renal NaCl and water transport by the ATP/UTP/P2Y2 receptor system. Am J Physiol Renal Physiol 2011;301:F463—75.

[658] Wang T, Giebisch G. Effects of angiotensin II on electrolyte transport in the early and late distal tubule in rat kidney. Am J Physiol 1996;271:F143—9.

[659] Wingo C, Smolka A. Function and structure of H-K-ATPase immunoreactivity in cortical and outer medullary collecting duct. Am J Physiol Renal Physiol 1995;269:F1—16.

[660] Kovacikova J, Winter D, Loffing-Cueni D, Loffing J, Finberg K, Lifton R, et al. The connecting tubule is the main site of the furosemide-induced urinary acidification by the vacuolar H^+-ATPase. Kidney Int 2006;70:1706—16.

[661] Simon D, Karet F, Rodriguez-Soriano J, Hamdan J, DiPietro A, Trachtman H, et al. Genetic heterogeneity of Bartter's syndrome revealed by mutations in the K^+ channel, ROMK. Nat Genet 1996;14:152—6.

[662] Palmer B, Alpern R. Liddle's syndrome. Am J Med 1998; 104:301—9.

[663] Schiller A, Taugner R. Heterogeneity of tight junctions along the collecting duct in the renal medulla. A freeze-fracture study in rat and rabbit. Cell Tissue Res 1982;223:603—14.

[664] Liu W, Morimoto T, Woda C, Kleyman T, Satlin L. Ca^{2+} dependence of flow-stimulated K secretion in the mammalian cortical collecting duct. Am J Physiol Renal Physiol 2007;293:F227—35.

[665] Andrews P. Scanning electron microscopy of human and rhesus monkey kidneys. Lab Invest 1975;32:610—8.

[666] Nielsen J, Kwon T, Praetorius J, Frokiaer J, Knepper M, Nielsen S. Aldosterone increases urine production and decreases apical AQP2 expression in rats with diabetes insipitus. Am J Physiol Renal Physiol 2006;290:F438—49.

[667] Nicco C, Wittner M, DiStefano A, Jounier S, Bankir L, Bouby N. Chronic exposure to vasopressin upregulates ENaC and sodium transport in the rat renal collecting duct and lung. Hypertension 2001;38:1143—9.

[668] Leviel F, Hübner C, Houillier P, Morla L, El Moghrabi S, Brideau G, et al. The Na^+-dependent chloride-bicarbonate exchanger SLC4A8 mediates an electroneural Na^+ reabsorption process in the renal cortical collecting duct of mice. J Clin Invest 2010;120:1627—35.

[669] Pech V, Pham T, Hong S, Weinstein A, Spencer K, Duke B, et al. Pendrin modulates ENaC function by changing luminal HCO_3. J Am Soc Nephrol 2010;21:1928—41.

[670] Kishore B, Nelson R, Miller R, Carlson N, Kohan D. P2Y2 receptors and water transport in the kidney. Purinergic Signal 2009;5:491—9.

[671] Shirley D, Vekaria R, Sévigny J. Ectonucleotidases in the kidney. Purinergic Signal 2009;5:501—11.

[672] Moeller H, Olesen E, Fenton R. Regulation of the water channel aquaporin-2 by posttranslational modifications. Am J Physiol Renal Physiol 2011;300:F1062—73.

[673] Marples D, Schroer T, Ahrens N, Taylor A, Knepper M, Nielsen S. Dynein and dynactin colocalize with AQP2 water channels in intracellular vesicles from kidney collecting duct. Am J Physiol 1998;274:F384—94.

[674] Nielsen S, Chou C, Marples D, Christensen E, Kishore B, Knepper M. Vasopressin increases water permeability of kidney collecting duct by inducing translocation of aquaporin-CD water channels to plasma membrane. Proc Natl Acad Sci USA 1995;92:1013—7.

[675] Sabolic I, Brown D. Water channels in renal and nonrenal tissues. News Physiol Sci 1995;10:12—7.

[676] Verkman A, Shi L, Frigeri A, Hasegawa H, Farinas J, Mitra A, et al. Structure and function of kidney water channels. Kidney Int 1995;48:1081—96.

[677] Lu H, Sun T, Bouley R, Blackburn K, McLaughlin M, Brown D. Inhibition of endocytosis causes phosphorylation (S256)-independent plasma membrane accumulation of AQP2. Am J Physiol Renal Physiol 2004;286:F233—43.

[678] Li W, Zhang Y, Bouley R, Chen Y, Matsuzaki T, Nunes P, et al. Simvastatin enhances aquaporin-2 surface expression and urinary concentration in vasopressin-deficient Brattleboro rats through modulation of Rho GTPase. Am J Physiol Renal Physiol 2011;301:F309—18.

[679] Procino G, Barbieri C, Carmosino M, Rizzo F, Valenti G, Svelto M. Lovastatin-induced cholesterol depletion affects both apical sorting and endocytosis of aquaporin-2 in renal cells. Am J Physiol Renal Physiol 2010;298:F266—78.

[680] Ridley A. Rho GTPase and actin dynamics in membrane protrusions and vesicle trafficking. Trends Cell Biol 2011; 16:522—9.

[681] Rikitake Y, Liao J. Rho GTPase, statins, and nitric oxide. Circ Res 2005;97:1232—5.

[682] Knepper M, Wade J, Terris J, Ecelbarger C, Marples D, Mandon B, et al. Renal aquaporins. Kidney Int 1996;49:1712—7.

[683] Terris J, Ecelbarger C, Marples D, Knepper M, Nielsen S. Distribution of aquaporin-4 water channel expression within rat kidney. Am J Physiol 1995;269:F775—85.

[684] Verkman A. Lessons on renal physiology from transgenic mice lacking aquaporin wter channels. J Am Soc Nephrol 1999; 10:1126—35.

[685] Nielsen S, Knepper M. Vasopressin activates collecting duct urea transporters and water channels by distinct physical processes. Am J Physiol 1993;265:F204—13.

[686] Ishibashi K, Sasaki S, Fushimi K, Yamamoto T, Kuwahara M, Marumo F. Immunolocalization and effect of dehydration on AQP3, a basolateral water channel of kidney collecting ducts. Am J Physiol 1997;272:F235—41.

[687] Frigeri A, Gropper M, Truck C, Verkman A. Immunolocalization of the mercurial-insensitive water channel and glycerol intrinsic protein in epithelial cell plasma membranes. Proc Natl Acad Sci USA 1995;92:4328—31.

[688] Han K, Woo S, Kim W, Park S, Cha J, Kim J, et al. Maturation of TonEBP expression in developing rat kidney. Am J Physiol Renal Physiol 2004;287:F878—85.

[689] Kultz D. Hypertonicity and TonEBP promote development of the renal concentrating system. Am J Physiol Renal Physiol 2004;287:F876—7.

[690] Dorup J. Structural adaptation of intercalated cells in rat renal cortex to acute metabolic acidosis and lakalosis. J Ultrastruct Res 1985;92:119—31.

[691] LeFurgey A, Tisher C. Morphology of rabbit collecting duct. Am J Anat 1979;155:111—24.

[692] Tisher C, Madsen K. Anatomy of the kidney. In: Brenner B, editor. The kidney. Philadelphia: Saunders; 1996. p. 3—71.

[693] Kaissling B. Cellular heterogeneity of the distal nephron and its relation to function. Klin Wochenschr 1985;63:868—76.

[694] Madsen K, Tisher C. Structural—functional relationships along the distal nephron. Am J Physiol 1986;250:F1—15.

[695] Brown D, Weyer P, Orci L. Nonclathrin-coated vesicles are involved in endocytosis in kidney collecting duct intercalated cells. Anat Rec 1987;218:237—42.

[696] Gluck S, Cannon C, Al-Awqati Q. Exocytosis regulates urinary acidification in turtle bladder by rapid insertion of H^+ pumps into the luminal membrane. Proc Natl Acad Sci USA 1982; 79:4327—31.

[697] Schwartz G, Barasch J, Al-Awqati Q. Plasticity of functional epithelial polarity. Nature 1985;318:368—71.

[698] Brown D, Gluck S, Hartwig J. Structure of the novel membrane-coating material in proton-secreting epithelial cells and identification as an H^+-ATPase. J Cell Biol 1987;105: 1637—48.

[699] Brown D, Hirsch S, Gluck S. Localization of a proton-pumping ATPase in rat kidney. J Clin Invest 1988;82:2114—26.

[700] Stetson D, Wade J, Giebisch G. Morphologic alterations in the rat medullary collecting duct following potassium depletion. Kidney Int 1980;17:45—56.

[701] Breton S, Alper S, Gluck S, Sly W, Barker J, Brown D. Depletion of intercalated cells from collecting ducts of carbonic anhydrase ll-deficient (CAR null) mice. Am J Physiol 1995;269:F761—74.

[702] Kim J, Tisher C, Linser P, Madsen K. Ultrastructural localization of carbonic anhydrase ll in subpopulations of intercalated cells of the rat kidney. J Am Soc Nephrol 1990;1:245—56.

[703] Ridderstrale Y, Wistrand P, Tashian R. Membrane-associated carbonic anhydrase activity in the kidney of CA ll-deficient mice. J Histochem Cytochem 1992;40:1665—73.

[704] Schwartz G, Winkler C, Zavilowitz B, Bargiello T. Carbonic anhydrase ll mRNA is induced in rabbit kidney cortex during chronic metabolic acidosis. Am J Physiol 1993;265: F764—72.

[705] Drenckhahn D, Schluter K, Allen D, Bennett V. Colocalization of band 3 with ankyrin and spectrin at the basal membrane of intercalated cells in the rat kidney. Science 1985;230:1287—9.

[706] Verlander J, Kim Y, Shin W, Pham T. Dietary $Cl^{(-)}$ restriction upregulates pendrin expression within the apical plasma membrane of type B intercalated cells. Am J Physiol Renal Physiol 2006;291:F833—9.

[707] Bishop J, Verlander J, Lee H, Nelson R, Weiner A, Handlogten M, et al. Role of the Rhesus glycoprotein, RhB glycoprotein, in renal ammonia excretion. Am J Physiol Renal Physiol 2010;299: F1065—77.

[708] Lee H, Verlander J, Bishop J, Nelson R, Handlogten M, Weiner I. Effect of intercalated cell-specific Rh C glycoprotein deletion on basal and metabolic acidosis-stimulated renal ammonia excretion. Am J Physiol Renal Physiol 2010; 299:F369—79.

[709] Weiner I, Verlander J. Role of NH3 and NH4 transporters in renal acid—base transport. Am J Physiol Renal Physiol 2011; 300:F11—23.

[710] Kim J, Kim Y, Cha J, Tisher C, Madsen K. Intercalated cells subtypes in connecting tubule and cortical collecting duct of rat and mouse. J Am Soc Nephrol 1999;10:1—12.

[711] Verlander J, Madsen K, Tisher C. Effect of acute respiratory acidosis on two populations of intercalated cells in rat cortical collecting duct. Am J Physiol Renal Fluid Electrolyte Physiol 1987;253:F1142—56.

[712] Kaissling B, Koeppen B, Wade J. Effect of mineralocorticoids on the structure of intercalated cells. Acta Anat 1981;111:72.

[713] Bastani B. Immunocytochemical localization of the vacuolar H^+-ATPase pump in the kidney. Histopathology 1997; 12:769—79.

[714] Brown D, Hirsch S, Gluck S, An H. ATPase in opposite plasma membrane domains in kidney epithelial cell subpopulations. Nature 1988;331:622—4.

[715] Nelson R, Guo X, Masood K, Kalkbrenner M, Gluck S. Selectively amplified expression of an isoform of the vacuolar H(+)-ATPase 56-kilodaltons subunit in renal intercalated cells. Proc Natl Acad Sci USA 1992;89:3541—5.

[716] Oka T, Murata Y, Namba M, Yoshimizu T, Toyumura T, Yamamoto A, et al. A4, a unique kidney-specific isoform of mouse vacuolar H^+-ATPase subunit a. J Biol Chem 2001;276:40050—4.

[717] Smith A, Jouret F, Bord S, Brothwick K, Al-Lamki R, Wagner C, et al. Vacuolar H^+-ATPase d2 subunit: molecular characterization, developmental regulation, and localization to specialized proton pumps in kidney and bone. J Am Soc Nephrol 2005;16:1245—56.

[718] Stehberger P, Schulz N, Finberg K, Karet F, Giebisch G, Lifton R, et al. Localization and regulation of the ATP6V0A4 (a4) vacuolar H^+-ATPase subunit defective in an inherited form of distal renal tubular acidosis. J Am Soc Nephrol 2003;14: 3027—38.

[719] Sun-Wada G, Murata Y, Namba M, Yamamoto A, Wada Y, Futai M. Mouse proton pump ATPase C subunit isoforms (C2-a and C2-b9) specifically expressed in kidney and lung. J Biol Chem 2003;278:44843—51.

[720] Alper S. The band 3-related anion exchanger (AE) gene family. Annu Rev Physiol 1991;53:549—64.

[721] Alper S, Natale J, Gluck S, Lodish H, Brown D. Subtypes of intercalated cells in rat kidney collecting duct defined by antibodies against erythroid band 3 and renal vascular H^+-ATPase. Proc Natl Acad Sci USA 1989;80:5429—33.

[722] Emmons C, Kurtz I. H^+/base transport pathways in the cortical collecting duct. Exp Nephrol 1993;1:325—33.

[723] Greenlee M, Lynch I, Gumz M, Cain B, Wingo C. Mineralocorticoids stimulate the activity and expression of renal H^+,K^+-ATPases. J Am Soc Nephrol 2011;22:49—58.

[724] Gunz M, Lynch I, Greenlee M, Cain B, Wingo C. The renal H-K-ATPases: physiology, regulation, and structure. Am J Physiol Renal Physiol 2010;298:F12—21.

[725] Silver R, Frindt G, Mennitt P, Satlin L. Characterization and regulation of H-K-ATPase in intercalated cells of rabbit cortical collecting duct. J Exp Zool 1997;279:443—55.

[726] Wingo C, Cain B. The renal H-K-ATPase: physiological significance and role in potassium homeostasis. Annu Rev Physiol 1993;55:323.

[727] Obermüller N, Gretz N, Kriz W, Reilly R, Witzgall R. The swelling-activated chloride channel CIC-2, the chloride channel CIC-3, and CIC-5, a chloride channel mutated in kidney stone disease, are expressed in distinct subpopulations of renal epithelial cells. J Clin Invest 1998;101:635—42.

[728] Ginns S, Knepper M, Ecelbarger C, Terris J, Coleman R, He X, et al. Immunolocalization of the secretory isoform of Na-K-Cl co-transporter in rat renal intercalated cells. J Am Soc Nephrol 1996;7:2533–42.

[729] Chambrey R, Goossens D, Bourgeois S, Picard N, Bloch-Faure M, Leviel F, et al. Genetic ablation of Rhbg in the mouse does not impair renal ammonium excretion. Am J Physiol Renal Physiol 2005;289:F1281–90.

[730] Verlander J, Miller R, Frank A, Royaux I, Kim Y, Weiner I. Localization of the ammonium transporter proteins RhBG and RhCG in mouse kidney. Am J Physiol 2003;284:F323–37.

[731] Weiner I, Miller R, Verlander J. Localization of the ammonium transporters, Rh B glycoprotein and Rc C glycoprotein, in the mouse liver. Gastroenterology 2011;5:1432–40.

[732] Eladari D, Cheval L, Quentin F, Bertrand O, Mouro I, Cherif-Zahar B, et al. Expression of RhCG, a new putative NH(3)/NH (4)(+) transporter, along the rat nephron. J Am Soc Nephrol 2002;13:1999–2008.

[733] Mak D, Dang B, Weiner I, Foskett J, Westhoff C. Characterization of ammonia transport by the kidney Rh glycoproteins RhBG and RhCG. Am J Physiol Renal Physiol 2006;290:F297–305.

[734] Seshadri R, Klein J, Kozlowski S, Sands J, Kim Y, Han K, et al. Renal expression of the ammonia transporters, Rhbg and Rhcg, in response to chronic metabolic acidosis. Am J Physiol Renal Physiol 2006;290:397–408.

[735] Welsh-Bacic D, Nowik M, Kaissling B, Wagner C. Proliferation of acid-secretory 1 cells in the kidney during adaptive remodelling of the collecting duct. PLOS one 2011;6 (10):e25240.

[736] Munkacsi I. Distribution of the intrarenal moonoaminergic nerves in the kidney of the desert rat (*Dipodomys merriami*) and the white rat (*Rattus norvegicus*). Acta Anat 1969;73: 56–68.

[737] Milton A, Weiner I. Regulation of B-type intercalated cell apical anion exchange activity by CO2/HCO3. Am J Physiol 1998;275:F1086–94.

[738] Kim Y, Verlander J, Matthews S, Kurtz I, Shin W, Weiner I, et al. Intercalated cell H^+/OH^- transporter expression is reduced in Slc26a4 null mice. Am J Physiol Renal Physiol 2005;289: F262–72.

[739] Quentin F, Eladari D, Frische S, Cambillau M, Nielsen S, Alper S, et al. Regulation of the Cl^-/HCO_3^- exchanger AE2 in rat thick ascending limb of Henle's loop in response to changes in acid–base and sodium balance. J Am Soc Nephrol 2004;15:2988–97.

[740] Royaux I, Wall S, Karniski L, Everett L, Suzuki K, Knepper M, et al. Pendrin, encoded by the Pendred syndrome gene, resides in the apical region of renal intercalated cells and mediates bicarbonate secretion. Proc Natl Acad Sci USA 2001; 98:4221–6.

[741] Petrovic S, Wang Z, Ma L, Soleimani M. Regulation of the apical $Cl^-/IICO-3$ exchanger pendrin in rat cortical collecting duct in metabolic acidosis. Am J Physiol Renal Physiol 2003; 284:F103–12.

[742] Wehrli P, Loffing-Cueni D, Kaissling B, Loffing J. Replication of segment-specific and intercalated cells in the mouse renal collecting system. Histochem Cell Biol 2007;127: 389–98.

[743] Teng-Umnuay P, Verlander J, Yuan W, Tisher C, Madsen K. Identification of distinct subpopulations of intercalated cells in the mouse collecting duct. J Am Soc Nephrol 1996;7: 260–74.

[744] Wagner C, Devuyst O, Bourgeois S, Mohebbi N. Regulated acid–base transport in the collecting duct. Pflugers Arch 2009;458:137–56.

[745] Bastani B, Haragsim L. Immunocytochemistry of renal H-ATPase. Miner Electrolyte Metab 1996;22:382–95.

[746] Matsumoto T, Fejes-Toth G, Schwartz G. Postnatal differentiation of rabbit collecting duct intercalated cells. Pediatr Res 1996;39:1–12.

[747] Matsumoto T, Feyes-Toth G, Schwartz G. Developmental expression of acid–base-related proteins in the rabbit kidney. Pediatr Nephrol 1993;7:792–7.

[748] Schwaderer A, Vijayakumar S, Al-Awqati Q, Schwartz G. Glectin-3 expression is induced in renal beta-intercalated cells during metabolic acidosis. Am J Physiol Renal Physiol 2006;290:F148–58.

[749] Schwartz G, Satlin L. Fluorescent characterization of intercalated cells in the rabbit renal cortical collecting duct. Semin Nephrol 1989;9:79–82.

[750] Le Hir M, Kaissling B, Koeppen B, Wade J. Binding of peanut lectin to specific epithelial cell types in the kidney. Am J Physiol 1982;242:C117–20.

[751] van Huyen D, Cheval L, Bloch-Faure M, Belair M, Heudes D, Bruneval P, et al. GDF15 triggers homeostatic proliferation of acid-secreting collecting duct cells. J Am Soc Nephrol 2008; 19:1965–74.

[752] Brown D, Waneck G. Glycosyl-phosphatidylinositol-anchored membrane proteins. J Am Soc Nephrol 1992;3:895–906.

[753] Dawson T, Gandhi R, Le Hir M, Kaissling B. Ecto-5'-nucleotidase: localization in rat kidney by light microscopic histochemical methods. J Histochem Cytochem 1989;37:39–47.

[754] McCulloch F, Chambrey R, Eladari D, Peti-Peterdi J. Localization of connexin 30 in the luminal membrane of cells in the distal nephron. Am J Physiol Renal Physiol 2005;289: F1304–12.

[755] Mandon B, Nielsen S, Kishore B, Knepper M. Expression of syntaxins in rat kidney. Am J Physiol 1997;273:F718–30.

[756] Kishore B, Wade J, Schorr K, Inoue T, Mandon B, Knepper M. Expression of synaptotagmin Vlll in rat kidney. Am J Physiol 1998;275:F131–42.

[757] Sabolic I, Herak-Kramberger C, Breton S, Brown D. Na/KATPase in intercalated cells along the rat nephron revealed by antigen. J Am Soc Nephrol 1999;10:913–22.

[758] Kim J, Kim Y, Cha J, Tisher C, Madsen K. Intercalated cell subtypes in connecting tubule and cortical collecting duct of rat and mouse. J Am Soc Nephrol 1999;10:1–12.

[759] Schon D, Backman K, Hayslett J. Role of the medullary collecting duct in potassium excretion in potassium-adapted animals. Kidney Int 1981;20:655–62.

[760] Nicoletta J, Schwartz G. Distal renal tubular acidosis. Curr Opin Pediatr 2004;16:194–8.

[761] Blomqvist S, Vidarsson H, Fitzgerald S, Johansson B, Ollerstam A, Brown R, et al. Distal renal tubular acidosis in mice that lack the forkhead transcription factor Foxi1. J Clin Invest 2004;113:1560–70.

[762] Christensen J, Bjaerke H, Meyer D, Bohle A. The normal juxtaglomerular apparatus in the human kidney. A morphological study. Acta Anat 1979;103:374–83.

[763] Kriz W. Ontogenetic development of the filtration barrier. Nephron Exp Nephrol 2007;106:e44–50.

[764] Kaissling B, Kriz W. Variability of intercellular spaces between macula densa cells: a transmission electron microscopic study in rabbits and rats. Kidney Int 1982;22:9–17.

[765] Bachmann S, Velazquez H, Obermüller N, Reilly R, Moser D, Ellison D. Expression of the thiazide-sensitive Na-Cl co-transporter in rat and human kidney. Am J Physiol 1995;96: 2510–4.

[766] Haas M, Forbush Bl. The Na-K-Cl contransporters. J Bioenerg Biomembr 1998;30:161–72.

[767] Boim M, Ho K, Shuck M, Bienkowski M, Block J, Slighton J, et al. ROMK inwardly rectifying ATP-sensitive K$^+$ channel. II. Cloning and distribution of alternative forms. Am J Physiol 1995;268:F1132–40.

[768] Mennitt P, Wade J, Ecelbarger C, Palmer L, Frindt G. Localization of ROMK channels in the rat kidney. J Am Soc Nephrol 1997;8:1823–30.

[769] Kim G, Ecelbarger C, Knepper M, Packer R. Regulation of thick ascendig limb ion transporter abundance in response to altered acid/base intake. J Am Soc Nephrol 1999;10:935–42.

[770] Mundel P, Bachmann S, Bader M, Fischer A, Kummer W, Mayer B, et al. Expression of nitric oxide synthase in kidney macula densa cells. Kidney Int 1992;42:1017–9.

[771] Wilcox C, Welch W. Macula densa nitric oxide synthase: expression, regulation, and function. Kidney Int 1998;67:7–53.

[772] Pluznick J, Zou D, Zhang X, Yan Q, Rodriguez-Gil D, Eisner C, et al. Functional expression of the olfactory signaling system in the kidney. Proc Natl Acad Sci USA 2009;106:2059–64.

[773] Alcorn D, Anderson W, Ryan G. Morphological changes in the renal macula densa during natriuresis and diuresis. Ren Physiol 1986;9:335–47.

[774] Bell P, Komlosi P, Zhang Z. ATP as a mediator of macula densa cell signaling. Purinergic Sigal 2009;5:461–71.

[775] Kirk K, Bell P, Barfuss D, Ribadeneira M. Direct visualization of the isolated and perfused macula densa. Am J Physiol 1985;248:F890–4.

[776] Rosivall L, Mirzahosseini S, Toma I, Sipos A, Peti-Peterdi J. Fluid flow in the juxtaglomerular interstitium visualized in vivo. Am J Physiol Renal Physiol 2006;291:F1241–7.

[777] Tian W, Salanova M, Xuk H, Lindsley J, Oyama T, Anderson S, et al. Renal expression of osmotically responsive cation channel TRPV4 is restricted to water-impermeant nephron segments. Am J Physiol Renal Physiol 2004;287:F17–24.

[778] Barajas L. The JGA: anatomical considerations in feedback control of glomerular filtration rate. Fed Proc 1981;40:78–86.

[779] Ryan G, Coghlan J, Scoggins B. The granulated peripolar epithelial cell: a potential secretory component of the renal juxtaglomerular complex. Nature 1979;277:655–6.

[780] Gall J, Alcorn D, Butkus A, Coghlan J, Ryan G. Distribution of glomerular peripolar cells in different mammalian species. Cell Tissue Res 1986;244:203–4.

[781] Trahair J, Ryan G. Co-localization of neuron-specific enolase-like and kallikrein-like immunoreactivity in ductal and tubular epithelium of sheep salivary gland and kidney. J Histochem Cytochem 1989;37:309–14.

[782] Hollywell C, Jaworowski A, Thumwood C, Alcorn D, Ryan G. Immunohistochemical localization of transthyretin in glomerular peripolar cells of newborn sheep. Cell Tissue Res 1992;267:193–7.

[783] Spanidis A, Wunsch H, Kaissling B, Kriz W. Three-dimensional shape of a Goormaghtigh cell and its contact with a granular cell in the rabbit kidney. Anat Embryol 1982;165:239–52.

[784] Satlin G, Schwartz J. Cellular remodeling of HCO$_3$-secreting cells in rabbit renal collecting duct in response to an acidic environment. J Cell Biol 1989;109:1279–88.

[785] Spanidis A, Wunsch H. Rekonstruktion einer goormaghtigh'schen und einer epitheloiden zelle der kaninchenniere. Heidelberg: Dissertation University of Heidelberg; 1979.

[786] Goormaghtigh N. Facts in favour of an endocrine function of the renal arterioles. J Pathol Bacteriol 1945;57:392.

[787] Schnermann J, Levine D. Paracrine factors in tubuloglomerular feedback: adenosine, ATP, and nitric oxide. Annu Rev Physiol 2003;65:501–29.

[788] Peti-Peterdi J, Komlosi P, Fuson A, Guan Y, Schneider A, Qi Z, et al. Luminal NaCl delivery regulates basolateral PGE$_2$ release from macla densa cells. J Clin Invest 2003;112:76–82.

[789] Schweda F, Kurtz A. Cellular mechanism of renin release. Acta Physiol Scand 2004;181:383–90.

[790] Wilcox C, Welch W, Murad F, Gross S, Taylor G, Levi R, et al. Nitric oxide synthase in macula densa regulates glomerular capillary pressure. Proc Natl Acad Sci USA 1992;89:11993–7.

[791] Osswald H, Nabakowski G, Hermes H. Adenosine as a possible mediator of metabolic control of glomerular filtration rate. Int J Biochem 1980;12:263–7.

[792] Thomson S, Bao D, Deng A, Vallon V. Adenosine formed by 5'-nucleotidase mediates tubuloglomerular feedback. J Clin Invest 2000;106:289–98.

[793] Schnermann J, Briggs J. Tubuloglomerular feedback: mechanistic insights from gene-manipulated mice. Kidney Int 2008;74:418–26.

[794] Persson A, Ollerstam A, Liu R, Brown R. Mechanism for macula densa cell release of renin. Acta Physiol Scand 2004;181:471–4.

[795] Komlosi P, Fintha A, Bell P. Current mechanisms of macula densa cell signaling. Acta Physiol Scand 2004;181:463–9.

[796] Vallon V, Mühlbauer B, Osswald H. Adenosine and kidney function. Physiol Rev 2006;86:901–40.

[797] Pallone T, Turner M, Edwards A, Jamison R. Countercurrent exchange in the renal medulla. Am J Physiol Regul Integr Comp Physiol 2003;284:R1153–75.

[798] Wirz H. Countercurrent principle. Protoplasma 1967;63:322–7.

[799] Kokko J, Rector Jr F. Countercurrent multiplication system without active transport in inner medulla. Kidney Int 1972;2:214–23.

[800] Stephenson J. Concentration of urine in a central core model of the renal counterflow system. Kidney Int 1972;2:85–94.

[801] Thomas S. Cycles and separations in a model of the renal medulla. Am J Physiol 1998;275:F671–90.

[802] Wexler A, Kalaba R, Marsh D. Three-dimensional anatomy and renal concentrating mechanism. I. Modeling results. Am J Physiol 1991;260:F368–83.

[803] Lemley K, Kriz W. Cycles and separations: the histotopography of the urinary concentrating process. Kidney Int 1987;31:538–48.

[804] Koepsell H, Kriz W, Schnermann J. Pattern of luminal diameter changes along the descending and ascending thin limbs of the loop of Henle in the inner medullary zone of the rat kidney. Z Anat Entwicklungsgesch 1972;138: 321–8.

[805] Becker B. Quantitative beschreibung der innenzone der rattenniere. Muenster: Inaugural Dissertation; 1978.

[806] Imai M, Hayashi M, Araki M. Functional heterogeneity of the descending limbs of Henle's loop. I. Internephron heterogeneity in the hamster kidney. Pflugers Arch 1984;402:385–92.

[807] Van Itallie C, Anderson J. The molecular physiology of tight junction pores. Physiology 2004;19:331–8.

[808] Bankir L, Kriz W. Adaptation of the kidney to protein intake and to urine concentrating activity: similar consequences in health and CFR. Kidney Int 1995;47:7–24.

[809] Bankir L, Trinh-Trang-Tan M. Urea and the kidney. In: Brenner B, editor. The kidney. Philadelphia: Saunders; 2000. p. 637–79.

[810] Bankir L, Chen K, Yang B. Lack of UT-B in vasa recta and red blood cells prevents urea-induced improvement of urinary concentrating ability. Am J Physiol Renal Physiol 2004;286:F144–51.

[811] Trinh-Trang-Tan M, Lasbennes F, Gane P, Roudier N, Ripoche P, Cartron J, et al. UT-B1 proteins in rat: tissue distribution and regulation by antidiuretic hormone in kidney. Am J Physiol Renal Physiol 2002;283:F912—22.

[812] Brown D, Kumpulainen J, Roth J, Orci L. Immunohistochemical localization of carbonic anhydrase in postnatal and adult rat kidney. Am J Physiol 1983;245:F110—8.

[813] Brown D, Kumpulainen T. Immunocytochemical localization of carbonic anhydrase on ultrathin frozen sections with protein A-gold. Histochemistry 1985;83:153—8.

[814] Brown D, Roth J, Kumpulainen T, Orci L. Ultrastructural immunocytochemical localization of carbonic anhydrase. Presence in intercalated cells of the rat collecting tubule. Histochemistry 1982;75:209—13.

[815] Dobyan D, Bulger R. Renal carbonic anhydrase. Am J Physiol 1982;243:F311—24.

[816] Holthofer H, Schulte B, Pasternack G, Siegel G, Spicer S. Immunocytochemical characterization of carbonic anhydrase-rich cells in the rat kidney collecting duct. Lab Invest 1987; 57:150—6.

[817] Holthofer H, Schulte B, Pasternack G, Siegel G, Spicer S. Three distinct cell populations in rat kidney collecting duct. Am J Physiol 1987;253:C323—8.

[818] Lönnerholm G, Ridderstrale Y. Intracellular distribution of carbonic anhydrase in the rat kidney. Kidney Int 1980;17:162—74.

[819] Lönnerholm G, Wistrand P. Carbonic anhydrase in the human kidney: a histochemical and immunocytochemical study. Kidney Int 1984;25:86—898.

[820] Kim Y, Kwon T, Frische S, Kim J, Tisher C, Madsen K, et al. Immunocytochemical localization of pendrin in intercalated cell subtypes in rat and mouse kidney. Am J Physiol Renal Physiol 2002;283:F744—54.

[821] Brown A, Hallouane D, Mawby W, Karet F, Saleem M, Howie A, et al. RhCG is the mahor putative ammonia transporter expressed in the human kidney, and RhBG is not expressed at detectable levels. Am J Physiol Renal Physiol 2009;296: F1279—90.

[822] Kim H, Verlander J, Bishop J, Cain B, Han K, Igarashi P, et al. Basolateral expression of the ammonia transporter family member Rh C glycoprotein in the mouse kidney. Am J Physiol Renal Physiol 2009;296:F543—55.

[823] Ahn K, Park K, Kim K, Kone B. Chronic hypokalemia enhances expression of the H(+)-K(+)-ATPase alpha 2-subunit gene in renal medulla. Am J Physiol 1996;271:F314—21.

[824] Codina J, Delmas-Mata J, DuBose TJ. Expression of HKalpha2 protein is increased selectively in renal medulla by chronic hypokalemia. Am J Physiol 1998;275:F433—40.

[825] DuBose TJ, Codina J, Burges A, Pressley T. Regulation of H (+)-K(+)-ATPase expression in kidney. Am J Physiol 1995;269: F500—7.

[826] Jaisser F, Escoubet B, Coutry N, Eugene E, Bonvalet J, Farman N. Differential regulation of putative K($^+$)-ATPase by low K^+ diet and corticocosteroids in rat distal colon and kidney. Am J Physiol 1996;270:C679—87.

[827] Kraut J, Helander K, Helander H, Iroezi N, Marcus E, Sachs G. Detection and localization of H^+-K^+-ATPase isoforms in human kidney. Am J Physiol Renal Physiol 2001;281:F763—8.

[828] Ryan G, Karnovsky M. Distribution of endogenous albumin in the rat glomerulus. Role of hemodynamic factors in glomerular barrier function. Kidney Int 1976;9:36—45.

[829] Sangan P, Rajendran V, Mann A, Kashgarian M, Binder H. Regulation of colonic H-K-ATPase in large intestine and kidney by dietary Na depletion and dietary K depletion. Am J Physiol 1987;272:C685—96.

[830] Verlander J, Moudy R, Campbell W, Cain B, Wingo C. Immunohistochemical localization of H-K-ATPase alpha(2c)-subunit in rabbit kidney. Am J Physiol Renal Physiol 2001;281: F357—65.

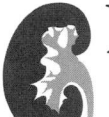

Biophysical Basis of Glomerular Filtration

Scott C. Thomson and Roland C. Blantz

University of California and VA San Diego Healthcare System, San Diego, CA, USA

INTRODUCTION

Marcello Malpighi (1628—1694) discovered the renal corpuscle and proposed that each glomerular body embraces the ampullar extremity of a tubule to form a "glandular follicle".[81] Thereafter, progress toward understanding the structure and function of the nephron stalled for two centuries, until William Bowman finally established the proper anatomic relationship between the glomerular arterioles, capillary tuft, and uriniferous tubule in 1842.[1,16] In that same year, Carl Ludwig, in his *Habilitations* thesis, addressed the driving force that separates the watery and crystalloid constituents of the plasma from its "proteid" constituents. He dismissed both the "nonexistent" vital force and chemical theories for converting blood to urine, and deduced from geometric considerations that local hydraulic forces drive filtration of blood plasma through porous glomerular capillary walls[78] (Figure 21.1). Ludwig's theory was not universally accepted at the time and other influential figures, such as Heidenhain, continued to advocate the secretory formation of urine.[54] Ludwig also had the foresight to envision that the hyperproteinemia resulting from glomerular filtration causes concentration of the urine by endosmosis into the peritubular capillaries.[79] Several decades later, vant Hoff and others began to describe osmosis in terms of pressure using thermodynamic principles,[143] which inspired Ernest Henry Starling to contemplate a role for the osmotic pressure of the plasma colloids in glomerular filtration. Starling wondered whether the minimum blood pressure below which formation of urine ceases might equal the osmotic pressure of the plasma colloids that oppose filtration. In 1897, he tested this hypothesis using a colloid osmometer of his own design[131] with which he estimated the osmotic pressure of the blood plasma protein to be 25—30 mmHg or about 0.4 mmHg-gram^{-1}/liter^{-1}. Then

he observed that raising the ureteral pressure to within 30—45 mmHg of the arterial blood pressure would stop the flow of urine in a dog undergoing diuresis. Thus, the hydraulic pressure across the glomerular epithelium must exceed the plasma colloid osmotic pressure by some small amount in order for urine to form. On this basis, Ludwig's filtration hypothesis was deemed credible. Further evidence for glomerular filtration was published in 1924 by Wearn and Richards, who directly visualized the passage of indigo carmine into Bowman's space from the blood in the course of performing the first-ever micropuncture experiments. Wearn and Richards interpreted their own findings as "indirect evidence that the process in the glomerulus is physical".[148]

Glomerular filtration eventually received theoretical consideration as a case of coupled transport, subject to the basic rules of non-equilibrium thermodynamics, which were articulated by Onsager in 1931[95] and adapted to describe the permeability of biological membranes by several investigators in the 1950s. Prior to the 1950s, the conventional description of transport through membranes simply combined Fick's diffusion equation for solute flux with Darcy's equation for water flux, such that the function of a membrane which is to "prescribe the road along which the system strives toward equilibrium",[132] was defined by two permeability coefficients, one for diffusion of solute and one for bulk flow of water. By the 1950s it had become clear that these "conventional" permeability equations for solute and volume flow could not fully describe the physical behavior of membranes, so attempts were made to supplement them. The most cited contribution in this area came from Kedem and Katchalsky,[69] who pointed out that the prior approach was incomplete due to the fact that it included only two coefficients, whereas Onsager's theory calls for exactly three coefficients to characterize permeability for a solute—solvent system. Qualitatively, the

Seldin and Giebisch's The Kidney, Fifth Edition.
DOI: http://dx.doi.org/10.1016/B978-0-12-381462-3.00021-5

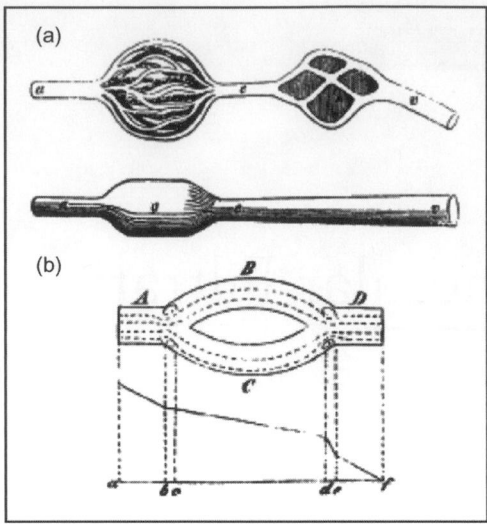

FIGURE 21.1 Ludwig's representation of renal microvasculature (a) and (b) pressure profiles along the glomerular capillary *(from ref. [56]).*

hydrodynamic resistance to free diffusion is due to friction between solute and solvent alone, and is determined by a single diffusion coefficient. But passage through a membrane involves two additional factors, namely, the friction between solute and membrane, and the friction between solvent and membrane. Hence, three processes are at play, and three coefficients are required to account for them all. Kedem and Katchalsky then proceeded with a formal argument, starting from the rate of entropy production and invoking Onsager's theory for a solute–solvent system which is paraphrased as follows:

For present purposes, we are interested in the transmembrane flux of a two-component system consisting of a water (w) and a non-electrolyte solute (s). Each of these components is driven by a conjugate force equivalent to its difference in free energy across the membrane. The conjugate forces for water and non-electrolyte solute are:

$$\Delta\mu_w = V_w\Delta P + RT\Delta\ln\gamma_w X_w \qquad (21.1a)$$

$$\Delta\mu_s = V_s\Delta P + RT\Delta\ln\gamma_s X_s \qquad (21.1b)$$

where V is a partial molar volume, ΔP is the pressure difference, X is the mole fraction, and γ is an activity function, empirically derived as a function of X. Since water flux affects X_s and solute flux affects X_w, the two conjugate forces and fluxes are coupled. For a small deviation from equilibrium this coupling can be taken into account by the following linear flux equations:

$$J_w = L_{11}\Delta\mu_w + L_{12}\Delta\mu_s \qquad (21.2a)$$

$$J_s = L_{21}\Delta\mu_w + L_{22}\Delta\mu_s \qquad (21.2b)$$

where Lxy are the so-called phenomenological constants. Onsager's theory says that $L_{21} = L_{12}$. Therefore,

if the three coefficients, L_{11}, L_{22}, and $L_{21} = L_{12}$ are known, along with baseline values of J_w and J_s, then one can predict the changes in J_w and J_s that will arise from any alteration in $\Delta\mu_w$ or $\Delta\mu_s$. However, the physical meanings of the phenomenological constants are difficult to appreciate, and a more familiar form of the Onsager equations was provided in 1958 by Kedem and Katchalsky to describe transport across biological membranes[69]:

$$J_v = L_P\cdot(\Delta P - \sigma_s\Delta\Pi) \qquad (21.3a)$$

$$J_s = P_s\cdot\Delta C_s + J_V(1 - \sigma_s)\cdot\overline{C_s} \qquad (21.3b)$$

When applied to movement across a capillary wall, J_v and J_s denote respectively the flux of volume (substituting volume for water is allowable for dilute solutions) and solute; ΔP, $\Delta\Pi$, and ΔC are differences in hydrostatic pressure, osmotic pressure, and concentration integrated across the membrane; σ_s is the reflection coefficient of the membrane for s; L_p is the hydraulic permeability per unit area of membrane; and P_s is the diffusive permeability of the membrane to s; $\overline{C_s}$ is the mean concentration of s within the membrane. Π is a function of C. σ_s assumes a value between zero and one. Three of these parameters, L_p, P_s, and σ_s, are characteristics of the membrane, in keeping with the Onsager theory which requires exactly three coefficients to describe the coupled transport of the two entities, v and s. Equation (21.3a) is often referred to as the "Starling equation." Equation (21.3b) expresses J_s as the sum of diffusive and convective components. Equations (21.3a) and (21.3b) are coupled. J_s explicitly depends on J_v. J_v depends on J_s because J_s affects $\Delta\Pi$.

There are limitations to irreversible thermodynamics and to the simplified equations, beginning with the assumption of a linear relationship between fluxes and forces. For example, one can imagine how increasing ΔP might cause a capillary wall to stretch, thereby changing the geometry of its pores and altering L_p. Also, $\overline{C_s}$ can take a variety of forms, depending on whether σ is taken to be active throughout the membrane or to be a membrane entrance phenomenon, and this will affect how J_s is parsed into its diffusive and convective components.[67] Finally, protein accumulates near the capillary wall during filtration, which could raise the local colloid osmotic pressure at the wall and cause L_p to be underestimated when calculated based on Π for the bulk plasma. Nonetheless, these equations remain the basis for all current understanding of the physical factors that determine transport of water and solutes between the glomerular capillary plasma and the urinary space.

Depending on the context, different simplifying assumptions are made that streamline the description of capillary flux in the glomerulus. For example, when considering J_v (i.e., glomerular filtration), the solutes are divided into two groups, large and small. Large solutes are the colloids, and it is assumed that P_s for these is zero and σ_s is unity. All other solutes are assumed to be small, and it is assumed that σ_s (and ΔC) for these is zero. Solutes with intermediate permeability are ignored. Therefore, $\Delta\Pi$ can be substituted by the colloid osmotic pressure of the glomerular plasma, and a full description of J_v is provided by Eq. (21.3a). This obviates the need to consider coupled transport. Although the contribution of filtered macromolecules to the transcapillary oncotic pressure may be negligible, there are times when it is critical to understand the sieving properties of the glomerulus for large molecules. In such cases, simplifying assumptions are made regarding the geometry of the filtration barrier and the shape of the solute molecules, so that the process can be conveniently described using hydrodynamic theory.

THE MAGNITUDE OF RENAL BLOOD FLOW AND GLOMERULAR FILTRATION

In humans, the kidneys constitute 0.5% of the body weight, but receive 20% of the cardiac output. The low resistance to renal blood flow is owing to the large number of parallel conductances, with each human kidney containing about 1 million glomeruli.[124] Approximately 8000 liters per day of blood plasma transits the extrarenal organs, of which about 20 liters is filtered into interstitial spaces and returned to the blood as lymph.[71] In contrast, the kidneys form 180 liters per day of glomerular filtrate from 900 liters of blood plasma. The high rate of filtration by the kidney relative to other organs is due to a greater ultrafiltration coefficient, not to greater Starling force.[44,99,149] The surface area available for filtration in the human kidney is in the order of 1.2 m^2 overall or 0.6 mm^2 per glomerulus. A meaningful number is difficult to assign to the capillary surface area in other major organs where the number of capillaries perfused at any given moment is highly variable. The hydraulic permeability L_p of fenestrated glomerular capillaries has been estimated from 2.5−4.0 μl/min/mmHg/cm^2 in rats and humans,[33,114,115] which is 50-fold higher than L_p for non-fenestrated skeletal muscle.[123]

GLOMERULAR HEMODYNAMICS BY INFERENCE

Having first identified inulin and PAH as a markers of GFR renal plasma flow (RPF),[121,126] Homer Smith and colleagues used clearance of these markers to make logical judgments about the regulation of GFR. Smith observed a reciprocal relationship between RPF and

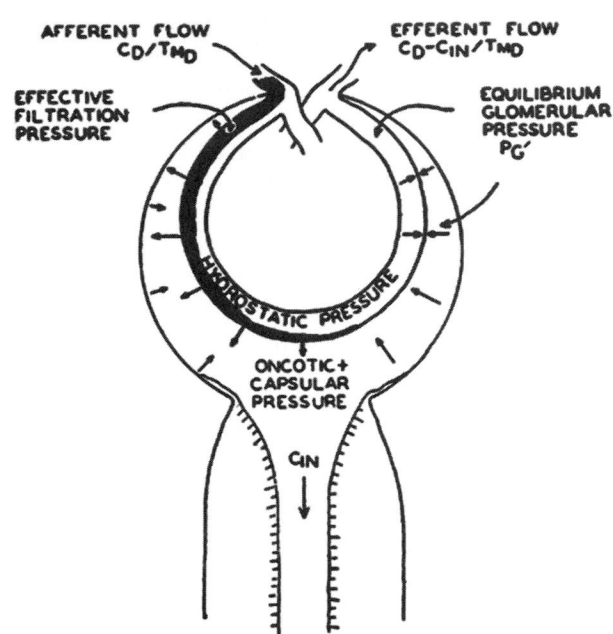

FIGURE 21.2 Filtration equilibrium illustrated in the glomerulus (*from ref. [29]*).

filtration fraction in human subjects injected with pyrogens,[23] and recognized that this is contrary to what should occur if the changes in RPF were mediated by a preglomerular resistance. He used equations to argue that the renal resistance changed in these experiments due to dilation and constriction of the efferent arteriole. His formulation required a strong inverse effect of efferent resistance on filtration fraction, which could be achieved by assuming that the net ultrafiltration pressure vanishes at some point along the capillary, as hydrostatic pressure declines and plasma oncotic pressure increases. Based on knowledge that this occurs in the mesenteric circulation, Smith was willing to assume that this also happens in the kidney, and coined the term "filtration pressure equilibrium" in reference to the phenomenon[125] (see Figure 21.2). Smith later recanted his notion of filtration pressure equilibrium in the glomerular capillary, arguing on teleologic grounds that the hydrostatic null point should occur in the proximal portion of the efferent arteriole in order to promote maximal GFR and maximal reabsorption in the peritubular capillary.[124] His revised thinking was likely influenced by the contemplations of Gomez.[47]

GLOMERULAR HEMODYNAMICS AND MICROPUNCTURE

A full and direct assessment of the filtration forces and hydraulic permeability in a mammalian glomerulus was first published by Brenner et al. in 1971.[19] Three developments made this possible. First, a mutant rat strain (Munich Wistar) was discovered with glomeruli on the kidney surface making them accessible for glomerular micropuncture. Second, a servo-null device was invented that enabled accurate and rapid pressure measurements in capillaries and tubules.[41] Third, a microadaptation of the Lowry method[77] was developed for measuring the protein concentration in a few nanoliters of plasma which could be obtained by micropuncture from a postglomerular arteriole.[17]

Given values for the pressure in the glomerular capillary P_{GC} and Bowman's space P_{BS}, pre- and postglomerular plasma protein concentrations c_0 and c_1, single nephron ^{3}H-inulin clearance $SNGFR$, and a simple mathematical model for computing changes in the ultrafiltration pressure P_{UF} along the glomerular capillary, it is possible to obtain values for the glomerular plasma flow Q_0 and ultrafiltration coefficient LpA. LpA is the product of the hydraulic permeability Lp (see Eq. (21.3a)) and the filtration surface area A.

The mathematical model for computing the physical determinants of $SNGFR$ from micropuncture data was developed by Deen, Robertson, and Brenner in 1972.[31] This model treats the glomerular capillary as a circular cylinder of unit length and surface area, uniform permeability to water and small solutes, and zero permeability to protein (see Figure 21.3). As in Eq. (21.3a), the filtration flux at any point along the capillary is equal to the product of the Starling force, $\Delta P - \Delta\Pi$, and the hydraulic permeability, Lp. $SNGFR$ is obtained by integrating the flux along the capillary length:

$$
\begin{aligned}
SNGFR &= \int_0^1 Jv \cdot dx \\
&= LpA \int_0^1 (\Delta P - \Delta\Pi) dx \\
&= LpA \langle P_{UF} \rangle
\end{aligned}
\tag{21.4}
$$

where $\Delta P = P_{GC} - P_{BS}$, $\Delta\Pi + \Pi_{GC} - \Pi_{BS}$ and $\langle P_{UF} \rangle$ is the mean ultrafiltration pressure. The term LpA represents the product of the hydraulic permeability Lp and filtration surface area A. For the non-dimensionalized capillary, A equals unity. For the real capillary, micropuncture data do not distinguish between changes in Lp and changes in A.

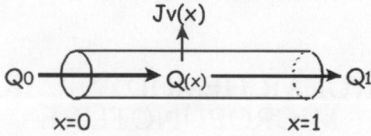

FIGURE 21.3　Glomerular capillary represented by a homogerous circular circular cylinder with unit length and surface area (Q: Plasma flow; Jv: Filtration water flux; X: Axial position along the capillary).

To perform the integration in Eq. (21. 4) it is necessary to know how the integrand varies along the capillary. In theory, both ΔP and $\Delta\Pi$ should change along the capillary, since P_{GC} must decline due to axial flow resistance and Π_{GC} must rise as water moves from the plasma into Bowman's space. It has always been assumed that the decline in P_{GC} along the capillary is small relative to the increase in Π_{GC}. This assumption was eventually justified by a three-dimensional reconstruction of the rat glomerulus submitted to computational analysis.[104] It is our custom to ignore the small axial pressure drop and represent ΔP as a constant, since including a 1–2 mmHg axial pressure drop in the model has a minimal effect on $\langle P_{UF} \rangle$. However, to better illustrate certain principles in this chapter, we have incorporated a 1 mmHg decline in P_{GC} from the beginning to the end of the glomerular capillary.

For the purposes of determining $\Delta\Pi$ it is assumed that all solutes in the system are either completely impermeant plasma proteins that exert their full osmotic potential ($\sigma = 1$, $Ps = 0$) and reside solely in the plasma or small molecules that are freely filtered ($\sigma = 0$) and contribute nothing to $\Delta\Pi$. Thus, $\Delta\Pi$ is reduced to the plasma oncotic pressure, Π_{GC}. The oncotic pressure in a plasma sample is determined from the protein concentration c, according to an empiric relationship developed by Landis and Pappenheimer:

$$
\Pi = \alpha_1 c + \alpha_2 c^2
\tag{21.5}
$$

The values of α_1 and α_2 in Eq. (21.5) vary according to the ratio of albumin to globulin in the plasma. When Π is expressed in mmHg and c in grams per 100 ml, for rat plasma, α_1 and α_2 are 1.73 and 0.28, respectively.[71] According to Eq. (21.5), Π_{GC} will increase from 18 to 35 mmHg along the length of a glomerular capillary if the systemic plasma contains 6 g/dl of protein and the nephron filtration fraction is 0.29. Such values are typical of the rat.

LpA is computed from $SNGFR$ and $\langle P_{UF} \rangle$, according to Eq. (21.4). To obtain $\langle P_{UF} \rangle$ it is necessary to know the profile for Π_{GC} along the capillary. This profile is computed from the following mass balance considerations for protein and water. First are three conservation of mass equations:

$$
Q_0 = SNGFR \left(\frac{c_1}{c_1 - c_0} \right)
\tag{21.6a}
$$

$$
cQ = c_0 Q_0
\tag{21.6b}
$$

$$
J_v = -\frac{dQ}{dx}
\tag{21.6c}
$$

where Q_0 is the nephron plasma flow and c_0 and c_1 are the pre- and post-capillary plasma protein concentrations. Differentiating Eq. (21.6b) and substituting Eqs. (21.6c), (21.5), and (21.3a):

$$\frac{dc}{dx} = \frac{c^2}{c_0 Q_0} J_v \tag{21.7a}$$

$$= \frac{Lp \cdot c^2}{c_0 Q_0}(\Delta P - (\alpha_1 c + \alpha_2 c^2)) \tag{21.7b}$$

A standard root-finding algorithm is used to obtain a value for LpA by numerical integration of Eq. (21.7) along the entire capillary to obtain an estimate for the plasma protein concentration at the end of the capillary (c_1^*) and adjust the value of LpA until c_1^* is arbitrarily close to the measured value of c_1.

$$c_1^* = c_0 + \frac{LPA}{c_0 Q_0}\int_0^1 c^2(\Delta P - (\alpha_1 c + \alpha_2 c^2)) \cdot dx \tag{21.8}$$

In a typical experiment, $SNGFR$, ΔP, and c_1 are measured in several nephrons. Most often, these parameters are not obtained from the same nephrons. The mean values for an experiment are inserted into the model to calculate the determinants of SNGFR for an idealized nephron.

From the foregoing description, we see that $SNGFR$ is fully determined by ΔP, Q_0, c_0, and LpA. Typical values for these parameters are shown in Table 21.1 for Munich Wistar rats from two different breeding colonies under different volume states. Conceptually, $SNGFR$ can be made to increase by raising ΔP, Q_0 or LpA or by reducing c_0. But the magnitude of the dependence on each of the four determinants depends on the values of the other three. Some of these interactions are shown in Figures 21.4–21.7 and discussed below.

Ultrafiltration Coefficient, *LpA*, and Filtration Pressure Equilibrium

If the ratio of LpA to Q_0 is great enough, then Π_{GC} will rise to become arbitrarily near to ΔP at some point along the glomerular capillary, resulting in filtration pressure equilibrium. The remaining capillary surface downstream from the equilibration point will not contribute to the flux. It is possible to infer the presence of filtration equilibrium from micropuncture data, but it is not possible to know at what point along the length of the capillary equilibrium occurs. Therefore, it is not possible to compute actual values for $\langle P_{UF}\rangle$ or LpA for nephrons in filtration equilibrium. When Eqs. (21.4)–(21.8) are applied to data from a nephron in filtration pressure equilibrium, the values generated for LpA and $\langle P_{UF}\rangle$ are respective

TABLE 21.1 Representative Micropuncture Data in Munich Wistar Rats from the Blantz Lab in San Diego and Brenner Lab in Boston.

Laboratory	State of Hydration	SNGFR (nl/min)	ΔP (mmHg)	Π_0 (mmHg)	Q_0 (nl/min)	LpA (nl/s/mmHg)	Filtration Pressure Equilibrium	Reference
Blantz	Hydropenia	30	30.5	18.3	86	0.08*	Yes	9
	Euvolemia	31	37.2	19.7	121	0.06	No	137
	Acute 2.5% plasma volume expansion	45	42.2	18.2	177	0.05	No	137
Brenner	Hydropenia	21	35.3	19.4	65	0.08*	Yes	19
	Euvolemia	32	33.4	19.4	114	0.08*	Yes	59
	Acute 5% plasma volume expansion	50	41.2	22.9	201	0.08	No	33

*Minimum estimate due to filtration pressure equilibrium. LpA values that show differently from the original papers were originally calculated based on a linear estimate of the oncotic pressure profile and are recalculated here using the non-linear model.

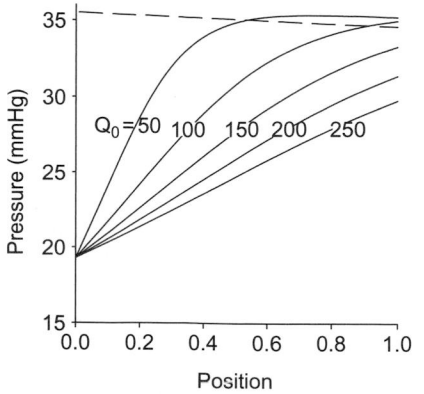
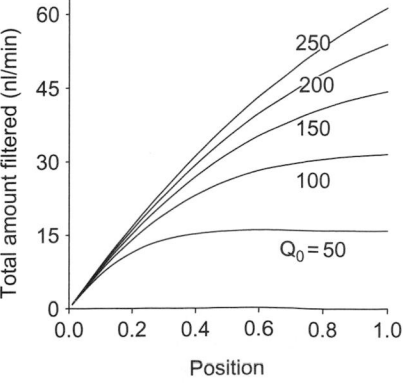

FIGURE 21.4 **Pressure (left) and total flux (right) along the length of the glomerular capillary.** In left panel solid curves represent plasma oncotic pressure which rises due to removal of water, while dashed line represents ΔP, which declines by 1 mmHg along the capillary due to flow resistance. $SNGFR$ is the total amount filtered at position 1. Other inputs include systemic plasma protein concentration 5.8 mg/dl, and LpA 0.08 nl/s/mmHg. Filtration ceases where oncotic pressure rises to equal ΔP, which occurs when incoming plasma flow, Q_0, is low.

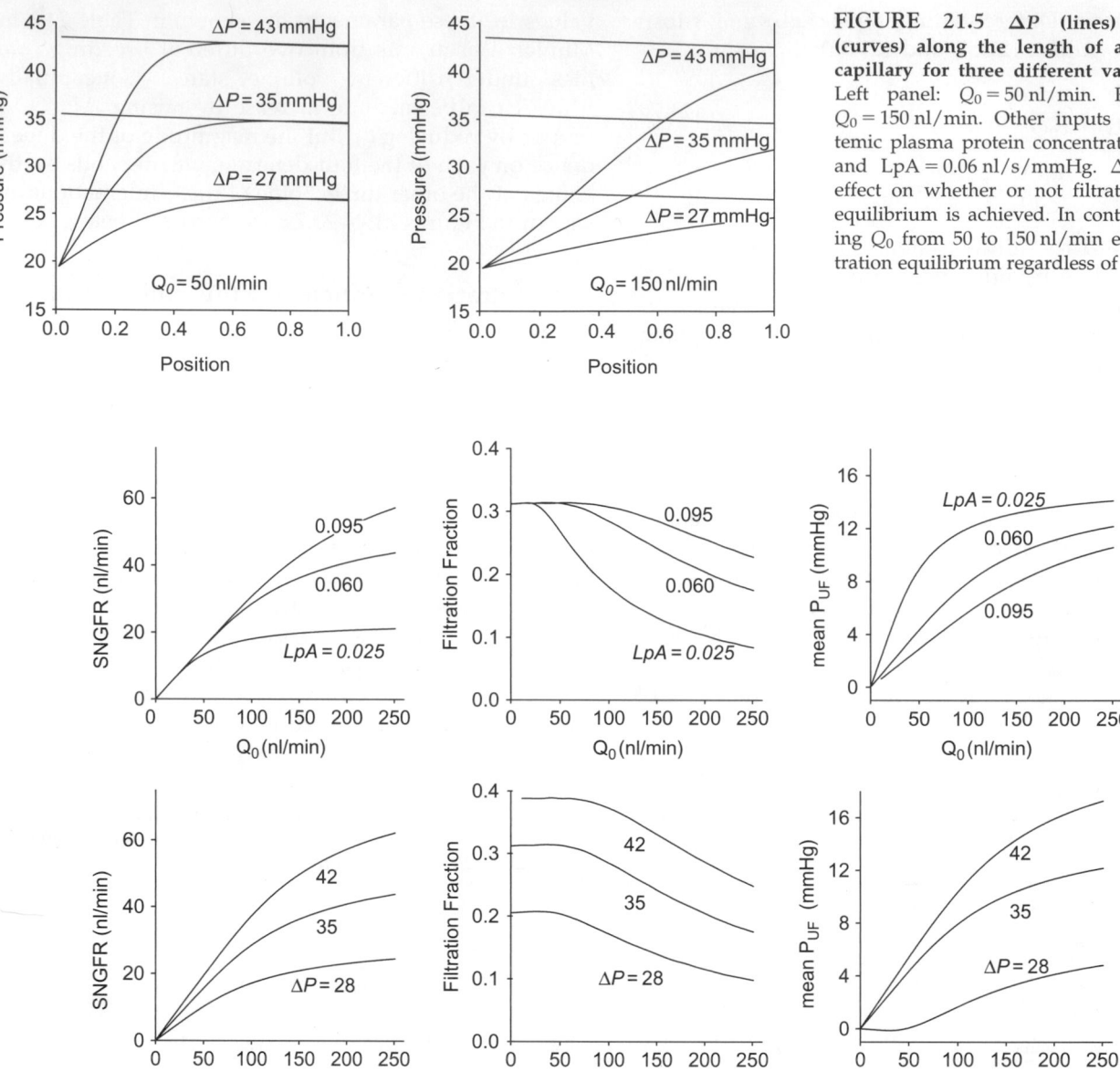

FIGURE 21.5 ΔP **(lines) and** Π_{GC} **(curves) along the length of a glomerular capillary for three different values of** ΔP. Left panel: $Q_0 = 50$ nl/min. Right panel: $Q_0 = 150$ nl/min. Other inputs include systemic plasma protein concentration 5.8 g/dl, and LpA = 0.06 nl/s/mmHg. ΔP has little effect on whether or not filtration pressure equilibrium is achieved. In contrast, increasing Q_0 from 50 to 150 nl/min eliminates filtration equilibrium regardless of ΔP.

FIGURE 21.6 *SNGFR, filtration fraction or mean ultra-filtration pressure (P_{UF}) as a function of nephron plasma flow, Q_0.* Curves in top panels were generated for three different values of LpA. Curves in the bottom panel were generated for three values of ΔP. Unless otherwise stated, LpA = 0.06 nl/s/mmHg; $\Delta P = 35$ mmHg; Systemic plasma oncotic pressure = 19.5 mmHg. Values over this range occur in the rat under varying levels of volume expansion.

minimum and maximum estimates for actual *LpA* and $\langle P_{UF} \rangle$. If a change in *LpA* occurs while a nephron remains in filtration pressure equilibrium, the equilibrium point will shift along the capillary, but *SNGFR* will not be affected. In order for *SNGFR* to be affected by a change in *LpA*, the nephron must not be in filtration equilibrium.

A debate over whether filtration pressure equilibrium occurs dates back to Homer Smith, who used conjecture and teleology to argue both sides of the issue at different points in his career (*vide supra*). Brenner and colleagues found filtration equilibrium in each of 12 consecutive

published series, suggesting that filtration equilibrium is universal for hydropenic or euvolemic Munich Wistar rats. However, contrary data were generated by other micropuncture laboratories. At one point, this led to consternation.[92] The issue was resolved after experiments done with rats exchanged between different laboratories led to the conclusion that filtration equilibrium prevails in some rat strains or breeding colonies but not in others, and that the difference is attributable to differences in *LpA*.[4] This finding detracts somewhat from teleologic arguments for or against filtration pressure equilibrium.

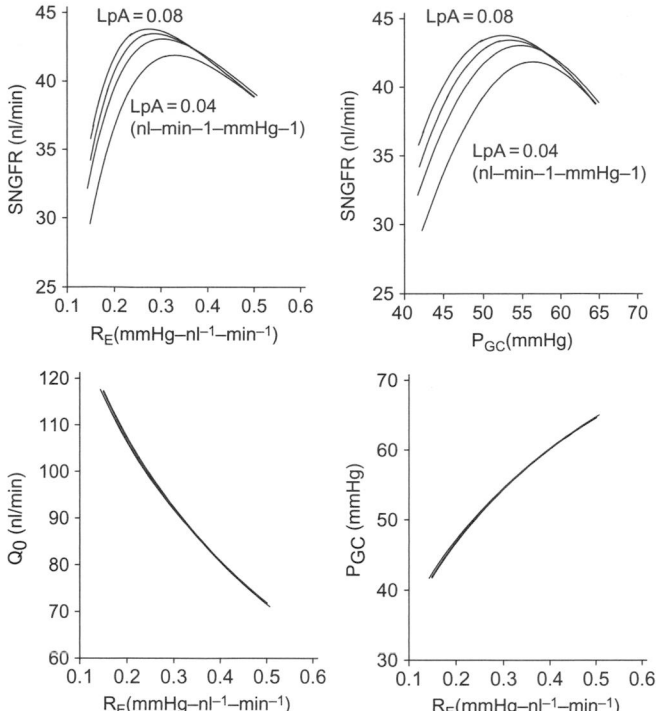

FIGURE 21.7 **Effects of efferent arteriolar resistance (R_E) on SNGFR, nephron plasma flow (Q_0), and glomerular capillary pressure (P_{GC}).** In top right panel, P_{GC} is made an independent variable by manipulating R_E. Effects on Q_0 and P_{GC} are nonlinear, because the filtration fraction rises along with R_E such that a lesser fraction of the blood flow transits the efferent arteriole. The Q_0 and P_{GC} curves (bottom) are insensitive to LpA. The apex of the SNGFR curve occurs within the physiological range of P_{GC} (48–52 mmHg). Medical treatments for glomerular capillary hypertension that reduce R_E until P_{GC} is normal will not reduce SNGFR. However, for P_{GC} <48 mmHg, reducing R_E will cause SNGFR to decline.

Nephron Plasma Flow, Q_0

Q_0 does not appear in the Starling equation for water flux (Eq. (21.3a)) or in the flux integral that defines SNGFR (Eq. (21.4)). Nonetheless, Q_0 is an important determinant of SNGFR. In fact, increased renal plasma flow underlies many of the physiologic increases in GFR that occur in the normal course of life, such as during pregnancy[6] or after protein feeding.[57,103,120] SNGFR is the simple product of LpA and $\langle P_{UF} \rangle$ (Eq. (21.4)). $\langle P_{UF} \rangle$ becomes greater if the average plasma oncotic pressure along the capillary is less. Removing a given amount of water from the plasma will cause a lesser increase in the plasma oncotic pressure if that water is subtracted from a larger initial plasma volume. Hence, increasing Q_0 will cause oncotic pressure to rise more slowly along the capillary. Therefore, increasing Q_0 causes $\langle P_{UF} \rangle$ to increase. The precise effect of Q_0 on the rate of rise in plasma protein concentration along the nephron is described mathematically in Eq. (21.7). SNGFR will be most sensitive to

changes in Q_0 under conditions of filtration pressure equilibrium where the filtration fraction remains constant as Q_0 increases. In filtration disequilibrium, c_1, ergo filtration fraction, will decline with increasing Q_0 to reduce the impact of Q_0 on SNGFR. Homer Smith recognized that renal plasma flow should affect GFR by this mechanism, and that his experiments (vide supra) failed to confirm a plasma flow dependence of GFR only because the particular tools that he employed to manipulate the renal blood flow were confounded by offsetting effects on P_{GC}.[125]

Systemic Plasma Protein Concentration, c_0

In the idealized glomerulus, an isolated change in c_0 will cause opposite changes in $\langle P_{UF} \rangle$ and, therefore, SNGFR. However, it is difficult to demonstrate this experimentally because it is nearly impossible to manipulate oncotic pressure of the arterial plasma without affecting the neurohumoral milieu of the entire body, thereby altering other determinants of SNGFR. In fact, the circumstances associated with low oncotic pressure in real life (e.g., generalized capillary leak, sepsis, malnutrition or nephrosis) are generally associated with a low GFR. When c_0 is manipulated by whatever means, changes in other determinants occur to offset the impact on SNGFR. These changes are discussed below under "Interactions Among the Determinants of SNGFR."

Hydrostatic Pressure, P_{GC}, and ΔP

Whereas SNGFR is insensitive to LpA when Q_0 is low and insensitive to Q_0 when LpA is low, SNGFR will always be sensitive to an isolated change in ΔP unless ΔP is so low as to be exceeded by the incoming plasma oncotic pressure, in which case SNGFR will be zero. This is true because the proportional increase in $\langle P_{UF} \rangle$ brought about by any increment in $\Delta P - \Pi_0$ is relatively insensitive to the other determinants of SNGFR. This is illustrated in Figure 21.5 and in the lower half of Figure 21.6.

The interposition of the efferent arteriole between the glomerulus and peritubular capillary provides a simple mechanism for regulating ΔP independently of Q_0. Furthermore, this arrangement provides an opportunity to elicit reciprocal changes in P_{GC} and pressure in the downstream peritubular capillary P_{PTC}. Tying an increase in P_{GC} to a decrease in P_{PTC} has teleologic appeal, as this will facilitate homeostasis of the effective circulating blood volume while stabilizing GFR. If the efferent arteriole reacts to sustain P_{GC} and reduce P_{PTC} during a decline in renal perfusion pressure or effective circulating blood volume, then GFR will be relatively spared from declining while filtration fraction will increase, thus affecting both the hydraulic and oncotic components of the Starling force that drives reabsorption by the peritubular capillary.

Regulating the efferent arteriole in this way is largely the purview of the renin—angiotensin system, which figures prominently among the myriad neurohumoral mechanisms contained in models of blood pressure and salt homeostasis. Angiotensin II is antinatriuretic and constricts arterioles throughout the body but, on balance, its effect on the glomerulus is always to elevate ΔP.[52,55,119,142] Thus, in spite of being a renal vasoconstrictor, angiotensin II protects GFR from total decline when the arterial blood pressure is low or when the preglomerular resistance is high.

While unduly low P_{GC} must impair glomerular filtration, P_{GC} and SNGFR are poorly correlated under normal circumstances, as are P_{GC} and arterial blood pressure. This implies that the kidney generally protects P_{GC} against the influence of arterial blood pressure and employs determinants other than ΔP to effect physiologically those changes in SNGFR that normally occur throughout life. Furthermore, it has recently been demonstrated that the preglomerular myogenic elements, long associated with static renal blood flow autoregulation, efficiently buffer the glomerular capillary against systolic pressure pulses delivered at the heart-rate frequency.[76] Teleologic reasoning behind sheltering the glomerular capillary from high pressure is that high P_{GC} augments wall stress in the glomerular capillary, which elicits a trophic response. If unchecked, this response will ultimately sclerose and destroy the glomerulus. Therefore, high P_{GC} is always pathologic, and treating glomerular capillary hypertension has been a cornerstone of nephrology practice for more than two decades. Some examples of glomerular capillary hypertension include angiotensin II-mediated hypertension,[46] experimental glomerulonephritis,[10,45] and residual nephrons after subtotal nephrectomy.[3] It has been asserted, and commonly accepted, that glomerular capillary hypertension also underlies glomerular hyperfiltration in early diabetes mellitus.[58,151] However, there are more than 10 published micropuncture studies in which diabetic hyperfiltration occurred in the absence of glomerular capillary hypertension or in which glomerular capillary hypertension was treated with no mitigating effect on diabetic hyperfiltration.[27,62,79,83,84,89,90,106,118,122,141,152] This does not detract from the salutary effect of therapy to reduce P_{GC}, which applies to all glomerular diseases.[5,73,82,136]

Interactions Among the Determinants of SNGFR

According to the standard model of Deen and Brenner, SNGFR is completely determined by a set of four parameters, which include P, Q_0, LpA, and c_0 (or Π_0). To state that SNGFR can be calculated from these four determinants is a mathematical truism which requires no consideration of how the four determinants might correlate in actual physiology. In fact, the individual components of the glomerular microvasculature that influence determinants of SNGFR generally affect more than one of them at a time. For example, an isolated increase in resistance of the preglomerular arteriole will directly reduce both ΔP and Q_0 and will reliably reduce SNGFR. In contrast, an isolated increase in resistance of the efferent arteriole will directly augment ΔP and reduce Q_0. Since these two effects exert opposing influences on SNGFR, increasing efferent arteriolar resistance might cause SNGFR to increase, decrease or remain the same, depending on other circumstances. For example if P_{GC} is low enough to be at or below Π_{GC}, then raising the efferent resistance can only cause SNGFR to increase whereas, if efferent resistance increases toward infinity, Q_0 must tend toward zero while P_{GC} cannot exceed the arterial blood pressure and, therefore, SNGFR must decline. The point where the impact of increasing the efferent resistance switches from positive to negative is within the domain of values that occur *in vivo*. Much of the acute renal failure encountered in contemporary medical practice occurs when drugs that reduce the ratio of efferent:afferent resistance are taken by patients who operate to the left of that point (see Figure 21.7).

There are other correlations between determinants of SNGFR that are more difficult to explain. For example, since LpA is computed as the ratio of SNGFR to $\langle P_{UF} \rangle$, random uncorrelated errors in ΔP and SNGFR will cause an inverse correlation to appear between ΔP and LpA. Also, an isolated reduction in LpA, if sufficient to reduce SNGFR, will remove a shunt pathway for fluid to bypass the efferent arteriole, thereby increasing ΔP. Furthermore, the physical orientation of the glomerular mesangium relative to the intraglomerular portion of the efferent arteriole allows activation of the same contractile elements to simultaneously reduce LpA and constrict the efferent arteriole.[40] This appears to explain why angiotensin II, the prototype effector of glomerular hemodynamics, simultaneously increases ΔP and reduces LpA,[12] and why lyzing mesangial cells with an antibody negates the effects of angiotensin II on both ΔP and LpA.[11]

Another interesting interaction among two determinants of SNGFR involves ΔP and the systemic plasma oncotic pressure Π_0. As mentioned above, experiments targeted at confirming the role of Π_0 as a determinant of SNGFR are encumbered by the difficulty in manipulating the plasma protein concentration independent of the neurohumoral environment. To get around this, Brenner[7] and Blantz[9,13,140] drew upon a wide variety of infusion and exchange protocols to alter the systemic plasma protein concentration in multiple ways that were likely to yield contrary effects on the effective circulating volume and hematocrit. These differences were roughly intended to cancel each other out and reveal the underlying impact of Π_0 on $SNGFR$, ΔP, Q_0, and LpA. Both groups of investigators confirmed that the four determinants of $SNGFR$ are not independent of one another. In particular, they discovered that, regardless of the experimental means for invoking a change in Π_0, a change in Π_0 causes a parallel change in ΔP, and reciprocal change in LpA. In contrast, neither $SNGFR$ nor Q_0 are predictably tied to Π_0. Most remarkably, ΔP is so strongly dependent on Π_0 that the afferent effective filtration pressure, $\Delta P - \Pi_0$, is independent of Π_0. A biophysical or anatomic explanation for this interaction between Π_0 and ΔP has not been forthcoming. It seems, instead, that a physiological mechanism is involved in autoregulating the afferent effective filtration pressure (see Table 21.2).

Brenner and Blantz also both observed an inverse correlation between Π_0 and LpA. It is possible that this is an artifact of concentration polarization which causes plasma proteins to accumulate near the capillary wall. Concentration polarization will lead to an overestimate of P_{UF}, because the calculation of P_{UF} will be based on a lower value of Π than is present at the plasma interface with the capillary wall. Using an overestimate of $\langle P_{UF} \rangle$ in Eq. (21.4) will lead to an underestimate for LpA. If concentration polarization occurs in the glomerular capillary, the effect will be greatest when c_0 is least. Hence, the appearance could arise of an inverse dependence of LpA on c_0, even though c_0 has no actual effect on the capillary wall. However, there is likely to be enough scrubbing by red blood cells to prevent concentration polarization. Furthermore, concentration polarization cannot explain the correlation between Π_0 and ΔP. Finally, we have already discussed a mechanism for the inverse relationship between ΔP and LpA.

TABLE 21.2 Multivariate Regression Applied to Combined Micropuncture Data from Brenner[7] and Blantz[126] to Test for Interactions between ΔP and the other Determinants of SNGFR*

Dependent Variable	Independent Terms in Multivariate Regression		
P (mmHg)	Π_0 (mmHg)	LpA (nl/sec/mmHg)	Q_0 (nl/min)
Regression coefficient	0.84 ± 0.09	-72 ± 10	~ 0
P-Value associated with regression coefficient	2×10^{-10}	1×10^{-10}	0.750

*The original regression model included the protocol for manipulating the systemic plasma protein and the lab where the work was performed, neither of which influenced the result.

Therefore, the inverse correlation of between LpA and Π_0 might arise because LpA is affected, as an innocent bystander, by a mechanism that is postulated to autoregulate afferent P_{UF}.

THE FILTRATION BARRIER AND FILTRATION OF MACROMOLECULES

A striking feature of glomerular filtration is the ability of the capillary wall to discriminate among molecules of varying size. Solutes up to the size of inulin pass freely from the plasma to Bowman's space, while passage becomes progressively difficult for substances that are larger such that all but the smallest plasma proteins are screened almost entirely. Hence, when describing the determinants of SNGFR, the concentration of macromolecules in the filtrate is low enough that these contribute negligibly to the Starling forces. However, the filtration of small amounts of macromolecules is important for other reasons. For example, the plasma transiting a normal pair of human kidneys in one day contains 50,000 grams of protein, while the appearance of one gram per day of protein in the urine is sufficient to establish the presence of glomerular disease. Discerning how this small amount of protein winds up in Bowman's space is key to explaining how the filtration barrier operates normally, and to understanding the physical aspects of glomerular disease.

The filtration of a macromolecule is most often quantified in terms of its sieving coefficient, Θ, which is the ratio of solute concentration in the filtrate relative to filtrand. The earliest direct test for protein in mammalian glomerular filtrate was performed by Walker in 1941, who reported that micropuncture fluid obtained from Bowman's space in rat, guinea pig or opossum contained "either no protein or, at most, very small amounts." The assay in use at the time would have detected an overall sieving coefficient for protein of 0.4%, which made it insensitive by later standards.[146] Several subsequent micropuncture studies during the 1970s yielded widely varying amounts of albumin in proximal tubular fluid, even within an experiment. This variability was reasonably ascribed to contamination of samples by extratubular proteins, since only 1% contamination of a tubular fluid sample with plasma from the peritubular capillary would markedly alter the apparent result.[93] Performing micropuncture with a system of concentric pipettes to reduce contamination, Tojo succeeded in confirming a strong inverse relationship between TF/P inulin and albumin concentration in fluid collected from rat proximal tubules due to removal of filtered albumin along the proximal tubule. By linear extrapolation to TF/P inulin of unity,

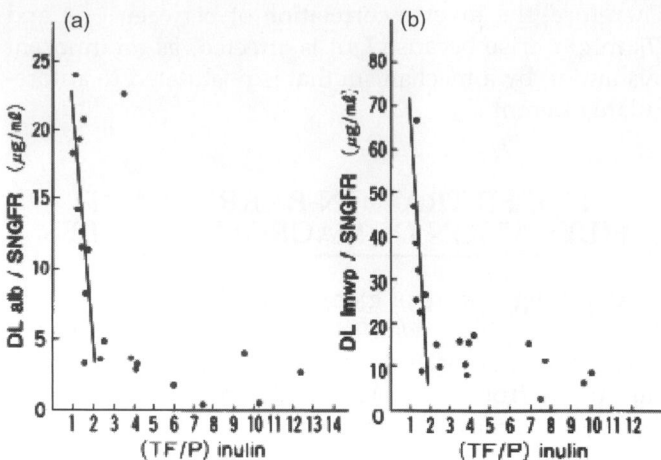

FIGURE 21.8 Albumin (a) and low molecular weight protein (LMWP) delivery (b) along the nephron. Linear regression over the domain of TF/Pinulin from 1 to 2 was used to calculate the protein concentration in Bowman's space *(from ref. [80])*.

which represents Bowman's space, the sieving coefficient for albumin was estimated at 0.062%. Meanwhile, the sieving coefficient of low molecular weight proteins was almost 99%, confirming the size-selective nature of protein sieving[138] (see Figure 21.8). However, micropuncture remains an unwieldy technique for studying glomerular sieving of macromolecules, and most of what is known about glomerular sieving has been learned by other means (*vide infra*).

Pore Theory

The glomerular capillary wall clearly screens solutes according to size, and it is usually taught that the glomerulus also screens macromolecules according to charge. The physical basis of molecular sieving is often modeled using pore theory. In pore theory, the coupled flux equations (Eq. (21.3a,b)) are modified to fit an idealized model of the glomerular capillary wall. The usual model consists of a solid barrier perforated by cylindrical pores. In some models, the pores form a homogenous population, while other models employ a mixture of pores of different sizes. This paradigm for describing the flow of material through porous membranes was applied to diffusion and filtration of solutes by capillaries, and an early review of the subject was published by Pappenheimer in 1953.[98] Mathematical descriptions were developed for pores shaped like circular cylinders or rectangular slits. At about the same time, theories were developed by others to explain the migration of large solutes through fibrous gels.[91] Given what is now known about the physical structure of the

glomerular capillary wall, pores, slits, and fibrous gels are all relevant to glomerular sieving. Hence, descriptions based solely on cylindrical pores have become more obviously phenomenological. Nonetheless, pore theory remains the most popular paradigm for describing nuances of glomerular sieving in humans.[13,29,72,86]

Pore theory builds on the Kedem–Katchalsky flux equations (Eq. (21.3a,b)) by associating the three membrane parameters, Lp, P_s, and σ_s with an idealized physical structure. This structure incorporates the membrane geometry, the Stokes–Einstein radius of the solute molecules, temperature, viscosity, and the Boltzman constant. The solutes are represented by rigid spheres that interact with the solvent medium and with the pores, but not with each other. This makes the problem mathematically tractable. The filtration properties of a membrane with circular pores turn out to depend on two things: (1) the ratio of pore diameter to membrane thickness; and (2) the overall fraction of the membrane area covered by pores.

An explanation begins with Fick's first law of diffusion for a solute s:

$$J_s^{diffusion} = -D_s \frac{dC_s}{dx} \qquad (21.9)$$

where:

$$D_s = \frac{RT}{fN} \qquad (21.10)$$

is the diffusion coefficient, N is Avogadro's number, and f is the frictional force that opposes diffusion of s.

According to Stokes' law, a sphere of radius a falling at unit velocity in a medium of viscosity:

$$J_s^{diffusion} = D_0 \frac{A_p}{\delta} \Delta C_s$$

η faces a frictional force given by:

$$f = 6\pi\eta a \qquad (21.11)$$

Einstein[39] combined Fick's law of diffusion and Stokes law to derive the diffusion coefficient for a spherical molecule in free solution, D_0, in terms of its molecular radius a:

$$D_0 = \frac{RT}{6\pi\eta aN} \qquad (21.12)$$

Since actual molecules are not spherical, the Stokes–Einstein radius, a, of a molecule is a virtual quantity represented by a sphere of equivalent radius. Using the Stokes–Einstein radius of a marker solute to estimate the size of pores in a membrane will overestimate the actual pore radius if the marker solute is flexible and can squeeze through a smaller pore than a rigid sphere with the same Stokes-Einstein radius.

For the diffusion of small molecules through a membrane that contains large pores, Fick's first law is rewritten:

$$J_s^{diffusion} = D_0 \frac{A_p}{\delta} \Delta C_s \qquad (21.13)$$

where A_p is the fraction of the membrane surface covered by pores and δ is the membrane thickness. Therefore, the diffusion through a membrane of a small solute with known D_0 is a convenient method to determine the ratio of pore area to thickness for the membrane.

However, when the molecular radius of the solute molecule is on the same scale as the pore size, diffusion through the membrane is less than predictable from Eq. (21.13). In other words, mobility of the solute is restricted. There are two factors that contribute to restricted mobility. First, there is steric hindrance to the solute entering or residing within the pore. Second, solute molecules within the pore experience greater friction than predicted by Stokes' law for solute molecules in free solution. While it makes sense to us to represent the steric hindrance by a reduced effective pore area and the increased friction as a reduced effective diffusion coefficient, most of the literature combines both effects into an expression for the effective pore area. This is described below.

Diffusion through a Porous Membrane: Steric Hindrance and Altered Friction

Restricted passage of solutes of increasing molecular radius is a basic property of membrane structures made of impermeable matrix with pores or fibrous gels. The basis for molecular sieving in all cases is the exclusion of large solute molecules from a portion of the membrane that is otherwise available to be occupied by water and other small molecules. The formulae for describing steric hindrance are different for pores than for gels. Here we will describe the phenomenon for cylindrical pores.

The center of a spherical molecule cannot approach any closer than its own radius to the edge of any pore. Hence, the fraction of a cylindrical pore, area Vp and radius r, that is available to be occupied by a solute with molecular radius a, is:

$$\frac{V}{V_p} = \frac{\pi(r-a)^2}{\pi r^2} = \left(1 - \frac{a}{r}\right)^2 \qquad (21.14)$$

Introducing solvent flow makes the steric hindrance more complex. This was first addressed by Ferry who added a term to account for laminar flow within the pore[43]:

$$\frac{V}{Vp} = \left(1 - \frac{a}{r}\right)^2 \cdot \left(2 - \left(1 - \frac{a}{r}\right)^2\right) \qquad (21.15)$$

The frictional drag on a solute molecule moving through a pore is also different from that described by Stokes' law for a solute in an unbounded free solution. The drag according to Stokes' law for the unbounded condition and the drag encountered in a pore are given by Eq. (21.16a,b) for a solute moving with velocity u in a fluid with velocity v. k_1 and k_2 are component drag coefficients that weight the contributions of the particle and fluid velocities. k_1 and k_2 are functions of a/r.

Theoretical treatments have provided approximate solutions for k_1 and k_2 for particles in cylindrical tubes.[51] Determining values for k_1 and k_2 is computationally intense. For this reason, k_1 and k_2 were originally provided for only a few values of a/r and a polynomial equation was fit to these points to allow interpolation. This approximation expression was inaccurate for $a/r > 0.6$, but this was the only method available until better computers were built in the 1970s.[97]

$$f_{unbounded} = 6\pi\eta a(u - v) \qquad (21.16a)$$

$$f_{pore} = 6\pi\eta a(u \cdot k_1 - v \cdot k_2) \qquad (21.16b)$$

Accounting for steric hindrance and dividing Eq. (21.16b) by Eq. (21.16a) to correct for the departure from Stokes' law, the diffusive flux is rewritten from Eq. (13) to become:

$$\begin{aligned} J_s^{diffusion} &= D_0 \frac{A_p}{\delta} \left(\left(1 - \frac{a}{r}\right)^2 \left(2 - \left(1 - \frac{a}{r}\right)^2\right) \right) \\ &\quad \cdot \left(\frac{u - v}{uk_1 - vk_2} \right) \Delta C_s \qquad (21.17) \\ &= D_0 \frac{A_{eff}}{\delta} \Delta C_s \end{aligned}$$

where A_{eff} represents the "effective" pore area and depends on a/r as well as the solute and bulk flow velocities. The combined effects of steric hindrance and friction on A_{eff} are illustrated in Figure 21.9 using published values for k_1 and k_2.[97] The approximation equation used by Landis and Pappenheimer in 1963 is also shown[71] where:

$$\frac{f_{unbounded}}{f_{pore}} = 1 - 2.104 \cdot \left(\frac{a}{r}\right) + 2.09 \left(\frac{a}{r}\right)^3 - 0.95 \left(\frac{a}{r}\right)^5 + \cdots$$

$$(21.18)$$

From Figure 21.9 it is clear that restricted diffusion will cause a membrane to discriminate between two solute molecules of different radii, even when the radii of both are considerably less than the radius of the pore. Also, note that Eq. (21.17) reduces to Eq. (21.13) in the absence of bulk flow and as a/r approaches zero.

Pore Theory and Hydrodynamic Flow

It is allowable to describe bulk flow within a cylindrical pore using Poiseulle's law as long as the pore

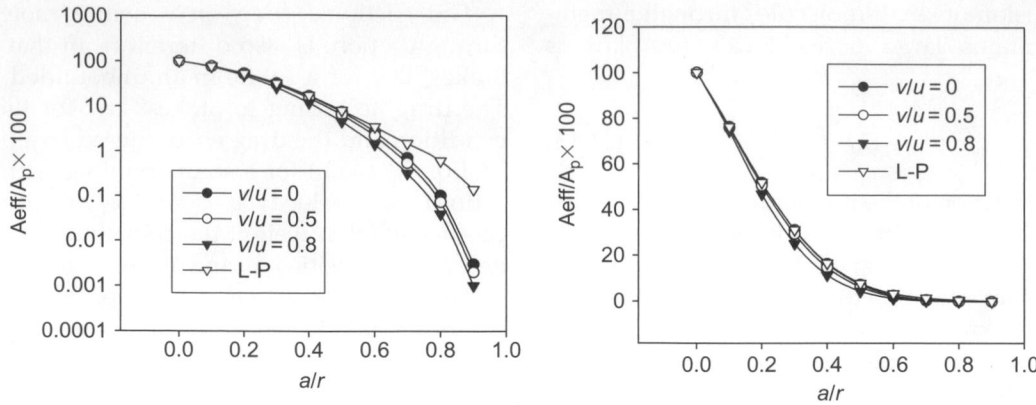

FIGURE 21.9 **Ratio of effective pore area A_{eff} to physical pore area A_P that applies to diffusion of solute with radius a through circular pore with radius r.** The model accounts for steric hindrance and for friction; u and v are respective solute and bulk flow velocities. Friction is calculated based on published coefficients.[97] L−P refers to result generated by older method of Landis and Pappenheimer, which works well for $a/r < 0.6$. Results shown in semi-log (left) and linear (right) formats.

radius is several-fold the radius of a water molecule. Accordingly:

$$q = \frac{-\pi r^4}{8\eta} \frac{dP}{dy} \tag{21.19}$$

where q represents bulk flow within a single pore and dP/dy is the axial pressure gradient along the pore. For flow per unit area across a membrane, pressure is replaced by the Starling forces[113,117] such that:

$$Jv = \frac{n\pi r^4}{8\eta\delta}(\Delta P - \Delta \Pi) = \frac{A_w r^2}{8\eta\delta}(\Delta P - \Delta \Pi) \tag{21.20}$$

where n is the number of pores per unit area and A_w is the restricted pore area available to water. Comparing Eq. (20) to Eq. (3a), the hydraulic permeability L_p for an isoporous membrane is given in terms of the pore radius r and the ratio of total pore area to membrane thickness A_w/δ.

$$L_p = \frac{A_w r^2}{8\eta\delta} \tag{21.21}$$

Combining Bulk Flow and Restricted Diffusion

The solute flux equation (Eq. (21.3b)) includes terms for diffusion and advection. Advective transport and restricted diffusion occur simultaneously in the glomerulus, and each contributes to the presence of large molecules in the filtrate. Furthermore, convection and diffusion are coupled, and this coupling must be unraveled for a full understanding of glomerular sieving. We shall present two approaches to this that are both based on pore theory and rely on the sieving coefficient, Θ, to draw inferences regarding the filtration barrier. The first approach is the early work of Pappenheimer, and the second approach is that of

Chang and Deen who based their method on the prior work of Patlak. It is the latter approach to interpreting sieving data that is used by most authors who publish in the physiology or clinical literature nowadays.

There are some intuitive features of glomerular sieving, and some that are not so intuitive. First, it is intuitive that Θ cannot be a negative number, nor can it exceed unity. If Θ exceeds unity, a model other than pore theory is required to explain the flux. It is also intuitive that Θ will approach unity for small solutes, and that Θ will equal zero for any solute that is larger than the largest pore. A feature that is not so intuitive is how intermediate Θ can arise from an isoporous membrane, although we have shown intermediate A_{eff} for an isoporous membrane in Figure 21.9. Intermediate Θ also owes to the effect of filtration rate on molecular sieving, which appears as the second term in Eq. (21.3b). If the passage of a solute is restricted relative to the passage of water, then the filtrate will become diluted during filtration. This will give rise to a concentration gradient for diffusion. Thus, the overall sieving coefficient is determined by competition between the filtration rate, which tends to dilute the filtrate, and the restricted diffusion, which fights to reduce the concentration difference that arises from molecular sieving.

It is intuitive that, if A_{eff} is non-zero and J_v is low enough, then solute will eventually equilibrate between the plasma and Bowman's space ($\Theta = 1$). It is also intuitive that, at high rates of J_v, Θ will approach the ratio of restricted pore area for solute relative to water. Pappenheimer provided a quantitative expression for Θ that satisfies these two conditions.[71] This derivation begins with a bulk-flow sieving step to create an initial filtrate to plasma concentration ratio:

$$\frac{C_{filtrate}}{C_{plasma}} = (1 - \sigma_s) = \frac{A_s}{A_w} \tag{21.22}$$

where C is the concentration of the solute in question, A_w and A_s are the effective pore areas for water and solute, and σ_s is the sieving coefficient from Eq. (21.3). Next, diffusion is superimposed according to Fick's law. Assuming that the concentration gradient is constant within the membrane:

$$J_s^{diffusion} = D_0 \frac{A_s}{\delta}(C_{plasma} - C_{filtrate}) \tag{21.23}$$

where D_0 is the free solute diffusion coefficient and δ is the membrane thickness. Summing the effects of bulk-flow sieving and diffusion:

$$C_{filtrate} = \left(\frac{A_s}{A_w}\right)C_{plasma} + \frac{J_s^{diffusion}}{J_v} \tag{21.24}$$

Inserting Eq. (21.23) into Eq. (21.24) and rearranging yields:

$$\Theta = \frac{C_{filtrate}}{C_{plasma}} = \frac{\left(1 + \frac{D_0 A_w}{J_v \delta}\right)}{\left(\frac{A_w}{A_s} + \frac{D_0 A_w}{J_v \delta}\right)} \tag{21.25}$$

The assumption of a constant solute gradient within the membrane is a shortcoming of Pappenheimer's approach. This shortcoming was later overcome, based on the work of Patlak[100] who developed a more rigorous approach for quantifying filtration–diffusion interactions in isoporous membranes. Variations on the Patlak approach form the basis for the pore models that are applied to animal and clinical investigations of glomerular sieving nowadays.[2] A modified Patlak equation for solute flux begins again with the Kedem–Katchalsky solute flux equation (Eq. (21.3b)). Diffusion-advection coupling in Eq. (21.3b) is contained in the parameter $\overline{C_s}$, which is the average value of C_s within the membrane. However, $\overline{C_s}$ can't be measured or derived without prior knowledge of the coupled flux that we are trying to determine. Therefore, the challenge is to come up with a form of Eq. (21.3b) that doesn't contain $\overline{C_s}$. The first step toward accomplishing this is to divide the capillary wall of thickness δ into a series of infinitesimally thin laminae. The Kedem–Katchalsky equation for a thin lamina is:

$$J_s = -D_s \frac{dC_s}{dy} + J_v(1 - \sigma_s)C_s \tag{21.26}$$

where y is the position along the length of the pore, which runs perpendicular to the membrane surface. Next, separating variables and integrating across the membrane yields:

$$\int_{plasma}^{filtrate} \frac{dy}{-D_s} = \int_{plasma}^{filtrate} \frac{dC_s}{J_s - J_v(1 - \sigma_s)C_s} \tag{21.27a}$$

$$\frac{\delta}{-D_s} = \frac{1}{-P_s} = \frac{1}{-J_v(1 - \sigma_s)}[\ln(J_s - J_v(1 - \sigma_s)C_s)]_{plasma}^{filtrate} \tag{21.27b}$$

$$\exp\left(\frac{J_v(1 - \sigma_s)}{P_s}\right) = \left[\frac{J_s - J_v(1 - \sigma_s)C_{filtrate}}{J_s - J_v(1 - \sigma_s)C_{plasma}}\right] \tag{21.27c}$$

Making the substitutions:

$$P_e = \frac{J_v(1 - \sigma_s)}{P_s} \quad \text{and} \quad C_{filtrate} = \frac{J_s}{J_v} \tag{21.28}$$

and rearranging Eq. (21.24c) to solve for J_s yields:

$$J_s = \frac{C_{plasma}J_v(1 - \sigma_s)}{1 - \sigma_s\exp(-P_e)} \tag{21.29}$$

Equation (21.29) expresses the solute flux as a function of plasma solute concentration, filtration rate, and the membrane characteristics σ_s and P_s, without referring to C_s anywhere inside the membrane. P_e is the Peclet number, which represents the ratio of advective to diffusive solute flux.

The remaining steps involve relating P_s and σ_s to the idealized membrane geometry using the equations for the hydrodynamics of cylindrical pores developed above.

$$P_s = \frac{D_0 A_s}{\delta A_p} \quad \text{and} \quad \sigma_s = 1 - \frac{A_s}{A_w} \tag{21.30}$$

PORE THEORY AND EXPERIMENTS IN THE GLOMERULUS

To characterize the filtration properties of a particular membrane by applying pore theory as described above, one begins with tracer solute(s) of known concentration (s) and Stokes–Einstein radii and a membrane of unknown microscopic dimensions. The water flux and sieving coefficient of the tracer solute(s) are measured along with the filtrand tracer concentration(s) and transmembrane pressure. A best fit of these data is made to the theoretical model, in order to determine the size and density of idealized pore(s). A better fit can always be achieved by allowing subpopulations of pores with various sizes. This is often justifiable on grounds of common sense. For example, in glomerular disease there is increased permeability to macromolecules, but not to water. This is easily explained by the appearance of a small population of large pores (sometimes called "shunts") that allow for the passage of macromolecules that are excluded from the main population of small pores. A scant population of shunt pores could account for most of the macromolecular sieving, but contribute negligibly to the ultrafiltration coefficient, LpA, because the pore area available to water is much larger.

To convert solute flux to overall sieving for the glomerulus, flux must be integrated over the entire capillary surface. Using C_{plasma} to represent the plasma concentration of s and x as the position along the capillary:

$$\Theta_s = \frac{1}{C_{plasma}(0)} \cdot \frac{\int_0^1 J_s dx}{\int_0^x J_v dx} \tag{21.31}$$

But the forces driving J_v and J_s change along the length of the capillary, since C_{plasma} rises as filtration occurs and J_v declines as oncotic pressure in the capillary pressure rises. For the idealized cylindrical capillary of unit length:

$$C_{plasma}(x) = \frac{C_{plasma}(0)Q_0 - \int_0^x J_s(z)dz}{Q_0 - \int_0^x J_v(z)dz} \tag{21.32a}$$

$$J_v(x) = Lp(\Delta P - \Pi(x)) \tag{21.32b}$$

where Q_0 is the incident plasma flow, and the oncotic pressure Π is given by Eq. (21.5).

To solve for the total sieving of solute by a glomerular capillary, Eq. (21.32) is iterated to provide the inputs for Eq. (21.29), which is then integrated along the capillary according to Eq. (21.31). Although the actual glomerular capillary bed is a complex and heterogeneous network of branching blood vessels, the sieving coefficients predicted for the idealized homogeneous circular cylinder differ negligibly from those predicted from a reconstruction that incorporates the complex anatomy.[105]

SIEVING CURVES

In order to compute the size-selective properties of the glomerular barrier it is necessary to know the sieving coefficient Θ for multiple tracer solutes with different radii. Therefore, tracer solutes are required whose concentration in Bowman's space can be measured or inferred. Direct sampling from Bowman's space is inconvenient or impossible in most circumstances, so it is usually necessary to infer sieving coefficient(s) from urinary clearance(s). The sieving coefficient of a tracer solute is equal to its urinary clearance divided by the GFR, as long as the test solute is not secreted, reabsorbed or metabolized by the tubule. Polysaccharides fulfill this criterion of being impervious to processing by the tubule. Also, it is possible to generate mixtures of polysaccharides with a range of Stokes–Einstein radii. These mixtures can be used to plot Θ as a function of Stokes–Einstein radius with many data points in a single experiment. These sieving curves can be used to determine pore size and relative abundance of different pores in heteroporous models.

The most commonly used tracer polysaccharide is dextran, an inert polymer of glucopyranose. There are over 50 published human and animal studies in which the size selective characteristics of the glomerular barrier have been analyzed from dextran sieving curves. As a rule, dextran sieving data are consistent with a two pore model[109] of the glomerular capillary wall where the vast majority are small pores with radius of 4.8–6.0 nm and the remainder are shunt pores with radius exceeding 10 nm (reviewed in [144]). However,

this use of dextran is seriously encumbered because the equations of pore theory were developed for rigid spheres, whereas dextran exists as a flexible random coil.[48] Due to its flexibility, a dextran molecule is far less hindered at crossing the filtration barrier than a rigid spherical molecule of equivalent Stokes–Einstein radius.[108] Based on pore sizes computed from dextran sieving data, Θ for albumin (Stokes–Einstein radius 3.6 nm) should exceed the experimental value by roughly 500-fold. The realization that this discrepancy in Θ between albumin and 3.6 nm neutral dextran owes mainly to the flexibility of the dextran molecule has reduced the need explain the low sieving coefficient for albumin based on something other than size. Hence, there is a lesser emphasis placed on the charge selectivity of the glomerular capillary wall these days than there was during the 1970s. Clearly, one must be cautious when using dextran sieving data to predict the sieving of non-dextrans. Nonetheless, dextran sieving is reproducible and precise, and predicts the structural changes that befall diseased glomeruli, even though they give a biased estimate of pore size.

Ficoll is an inert spherical sucrose polymer with internal cross-linking that confers some rigidity.[14] Ficoll has been tested against dextran in rats and found to have a sieving coefficient substantially less than size-matched dextran for Stokes–Einstein radii greater than 3 nm.[15,94] Lower sieving coefficients for Ficoll relative to size-matched dextran have also been confirmed in healthy and nephrotic humans.[1,13] However, Ficoll is less convenient to use than dextran in humans, because potential toxicity limits the amount that can be given. Also, Ficoll molecules are more compressible than globular proteins, such that pore sizes estimated from Ficoll sieving data will overestimate the sieving coefficients of like-sized globular proteins, albeit to a lesser degree than dextran.[144]

The glomerular sieving of polysaccharides is useful to the extent that it helps explain the permselectivity for endogenous proteins. Ultimately, however, the predictions based on polysaccharide sieving must be verified for proteins. As already discussed, the direct approach of measuring protein sieving by micropuncture is difficult. There are other strategies that have been employed to estimate sieving coefficients for proteins without requiring micropuncture. We will mention two of these. One alternative to micropuncture is to reduce the tubular processing of proteins by cooling the isolated perfused rat kidney to 8°C (cold IPK) to stop the tubule from degrading or transporting filtered proteins, then assuming that the filtered protein equals the protein excretion. Adding furosemide and nitroprusside to the cold IPK eliminates water reabsorption almost completely, and reportedly yields stable values for albumin fractional clearance. However, GFR is low in the cold IPK and perfusate flow is high, which means that the determinants of glomerular filtration are quite different than *in vivo*. This should pose a problem for the cold IPK, since fractional solute clearance must depend on the determinants of glomerular filtration rate given that convection and diffusion both contribute to solute transport.[22] Nonetheless, cooling seems to have minimal effect on the urine to plasma ratio for Ficoll, and the cold IPK has been used to address a variety of issues related to glomerular protein sieving.[53,64−66,74,75,128]

More recently, Tenstad et al. have made direct estimates of glomerular sieving coeffients for proteins based on tracer radioactivity retained in the kidney six minutes after administering radiolabeled proteins to rats. The rationale behind this approach is that there exists a several-minute window of opportunity when a tracer protein will remain in the kidney after being filtered and taken up by the proximal tubule, and before being degraded or reabsorbed back into the body. An estimate of this time window was first made using cystatin C, which is a freely filtered protein that is completely degraded by the tubule. As such, the rate at which cystatin C enters the urinary space is equal to its plasma concentration × GFR. Administering a bolus of labeled cystatin C along with a GFR marker, then stopping the experiment at various time points and counting tracer activity in the kidney, revealed that cystatin C remains in the kidney for at least six minutes after undergoing filtration.[135] In tracer uptake experiments using neutral horseradish peroxidase, myoglobin, and charge-neutralized albumin, the sieving coefficients for each of these proteins was significantly less than for Ficoll or dextran of equal hydrodynamic radius.[80] The principle pore radius computed by pore theory is 3.75, 4.6, and 5.5 nm for protein, Ficoll, and dextran, respectively[144] (see Figure 21.10).

COMBINING FIBER MATRIX THEORY WITH THE PORE MODEL

Using a wider range of dextran radii than previously employed by others, Katz generated dextran sieving curves that were not uniformly convex upward, but flattened out slightly above 4 nm.[68] This nuance could be explained by a two-pore model in which the pores were filled with a fiber matrix, but it could not be explained by any open-pore model of equal complexity. Citing the location of albumin molecules found in glomerular sections[112] and confocal tracking of dextran in isolated glomeruli,[25] it was hypothesized that the albumin barrier does not reside in the GBM anyway, and that the endothelial fenestrae, filled with fibrous glycocalyx, justify the mathematical model. The pore-matrix model has features corresponding to the pore theory model described above. For example, there is steric

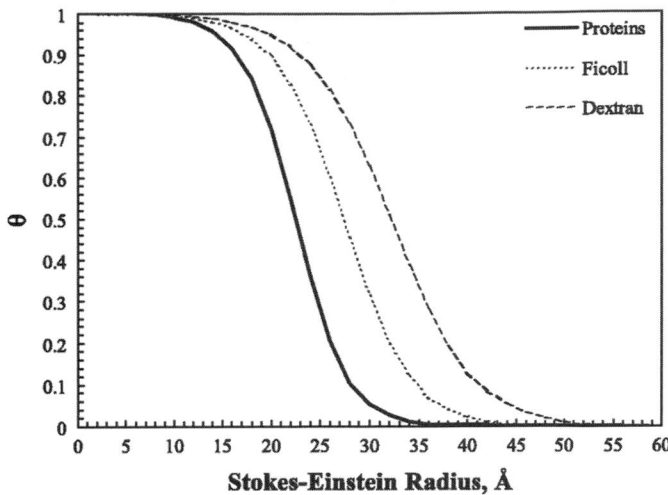

FIGURE 21.10 Sieving curves for dextran, Ficoll, and neutral proteins constructed from the literature *(taken from ref. [98]).*

hindrance due to the presence of the gel fibers. There is also reduced solute mobility due to the gel fibers. The specific formulae for these were developed from the theoretical groundwork for gel permeation by solutes provided by Ogston,[91] and combined with pore theory by Katz.[68]

Intravital Microscopy and Albumin Sieving

Glomerular permeability to albumin has also been examined using intravital dual-photon microscopy. The first measurements of glomerular albumin sieving by the dual-photon method were reported in 2007 by Russo et al. who administered fluorophore-labeled albumin to rats, compared fluorescence intensity in Bowman's space to plasma, and concluded that the albumin sieving coefficient is approximately 0.03, which is 50-fold higher than previously reported by any other method dating from the 1940s.[113] Subsequent application of the dual-photon technique by Tanner, who used the same facility but a different brand of microscope, failed to reproduce the finding, instead corroborating the traditional view of an albumin sieving coefficient less than 0.004, which was his lower limit of detection.[133] Peti-Peterdi also examined the filtration barrier using dual-photon microscopy and came to the same conclusion as Tanner, namely that the Russo finding was in error.[101] Peti-Peterdi has also argued that fluorescence imaging is poorly suited to measuring glomerular sieving coefficients, because light absorption and scattering by RBCs suppresses the apparent fluorescence of plasma proteins, which will lead to an overestimate of Θ.[102] So, after initial excitement over the Russo finding, the prevailing opinion among investigators in this field remains that the glomerular sieving coefficient of albumin is approximately 0.0006.

Charge Selectivity of the Filtration Barrier

Since the 1970s it has been generally accepted that the glomerular capillary wall is less permeable to proteins that are negatively charged. In addition to the low Θ for albumin compared to neutral dextran for equivalent Stokes—Einstein radius, the impression of charge selectivity was supported by experiments that compared sieving of anionic, neutral, and cationic dextrans.[18,21] It has since been learned that anionic dextran sulfate can be taken up by glomerular cells, desulfated, then secreted to appear in the urine as neutral dextran.[134,145] In addition, sieving of dextran sulfate is reduced through binding to plasma proteins.[49] These effects could create the appearance of charge selectivity of the filtration barrier where none exists. Furthermore, other experiments using Ficoll or hydroxyethyl starch failed to show a charge-selective barrier to either of these alternative polysaccharide molecules.[50,116]

Although the notion of charge selectivity for polysaccharides has lost some of its currency, the bulk of evidence still favors the notion that charge selectivity applies to the filtration of globular proteins. Rennke showed a lesser sieving coefficient for anionic horseradish peroxidase (HRP) than neutral HRP in rats,[107] allowing that part of the effect may have been due to degradation of anionic HRP during filtration.[96] Lindström showed charge selectivity for the somewhat larger protein, lactate dehydrogenase.[75] Making use of the tissue tracer uptake technique described above, Lund calculated sieving coefficients and reflection coefficients for several proteins, including charge-neutralized and native anionic human serum albumin. Θ for anionic albumin was remarkably similar to the micropuncture result of Tojo (*vide supra*) while Θ for neutral albumin was 10-fold higher[80] (Table 21.3).

TABLE 21.3 Charge Permselectivity of the Glomerulus in Rats Confirmed by the Tracer Uptake Method Using Neutralized or Native Anionic Human Serum Albumin

	Stokes—Einstein Radius (Å)	Isoelectric pH	Θ	σ
neutral albumin	35.0	7.4	0.0055	0.996
anionic albumin	35.5	4.9	0.0006	0.9997

Adapted from data in Lund et al. (2003). Am. J. Physiol.[80]
Θ: glomerular sieving coefficient; σ: Staverman reflection coefficient. Since these experiments were performed *in vivo*, they reflect the normal contributions of diffusion and convection to albumin flux.

Theory of Charge Selective Sieving

Deen presented a theory for glomerular filtration of charged solutes based on a homogeneous distribution of fixed negative charges within the glomerular capillary wall[32] as idealized in Figure 21.11. The mathematical description of this model begins with an equation for flux through an imaginary thin surface within a membrane. This is the same as Eq. (21.26), except that the full electrochemical potential is included in the diffusion force to yield:

$$J_s = -D_s \left(\frac{dC_s}{dx} + z_s C_s \frac{d\psi}{dx} \right) + J_v (1 - \sigma_s) C_s \qquad (21.33)$$

where $D_s = D_0 \cdot A_{eff}$, z_s is the valence of s and ψ is a dimensionless electrical potential.

Next, it is assumed that there is electrochemical equilibrium at both membrane-solution interfaces. This allows the step change in C_s at each interface to be calculated from the Nernst equation and the steric hindrance:

$$C_s'(0) = C_{plasma}(1 - \sigma_s)\exp(z_s(\psi_{plasma} - \psi'(0)))$$
$$C_s'(\delta) = C_{filtrate}(1 - \sigma_s)\exp(z_s(\psi_{B.S.} - \psi'(\delta))) \qquad (21.34)$$

where (') refers to values within the membrane just inside its interface with the plasma or Bowman's space, and *B.S.* refers to Bowman's space. Within the membrane, $d\psi/dx$ is small so that the same integration can be done as was done to Eq. (21.27). Integrating from 0 to δ within the membrane and substituting and rearranging yields the following charged-solute flux equation which is analogous to Eq. (21.29):

$$J_s = \frac{C_{plasma}J_v(1 - \sigma)\exp(z_s(\psi_{plasma} - \psi'(0)))}{1 - \exp(-P_e)(1 - (1 - \sigma)\exp(z_s(\psi_{B.S.} - \psi'(\delta))))} \qquad (21.35)$$

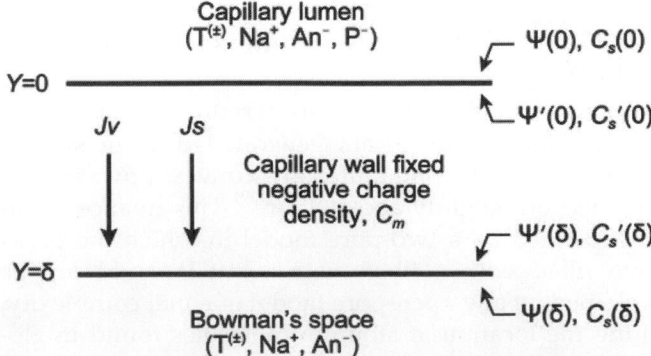

FIGURE 21.11 Idealized capillary wall with fixed negative charge density C_m, which causes Donnan potentials ($\Psi - \Psi'$) to form at interfaces of the membrane with the capillary lumen and Bowman's space. These Donnan potentials retard the flux of anionic tracer T^- and accelerate the flux of cationic tracer T^+ according to formulae developed in the text (A_n: mobile anions; P^-: anionic proteins) (adapted from ref. [125]).

The two electrical potential differences in Eq. (21.35) are next to be determined. These cannot be measured, but are given by the Donnan potentials for Na^+:

$$\psi - \psi' = \ln\left(\frac{C'_{Na^+}}{C_{Na^+}}\right) \quad (21.36)$$

Since there must be zero net charge in each compartment:

$$C_{Na} = C_{An} \quad \text{and} \quad C'_{Na} = C'_{An} + C_m \quad (21.37)$$

where An refers to mobile anions and Cm is the density of negative charges in the membrane. At Donnan equilibrium:

$$\frac{C'_{An}}{C_{An}} = \frac{C_{Na}}{C'_{Na}} \quad (21.38)$$

Combining Eqs. (21.37) and (21.38) yields a quadratic equation for C'_{Na} with the positive root:

$$C'_{Na^+} = \frac{C_m + \sqrt{C_m^2 + 4C_{Na^+}C_{An^-}}}{2} \quad (21.39)$$

Inserting Eq. (21.39) into the numerator of Eq. (21.36) gives the Donnan potentials. Inserting these into Eq. (21.35) gives an expression for solute flux that incorporates the effect of C_m. If C_m or z_s is zero, this reduces to Eq. (21.29), as it should. Θ_s for the glomerulus is obtained by integrating J_s along the capillary surface as per Eq. (21.31).

Deen's model predicts that a single parameter, C_m, can account for charge selective sieving. This is shown in Figure 21.12, where the theory was applied to anionic dextran sulfate based on other model inputs from the normal rat in which neutral dextran was used to determine a pore radius.

This theory of charge-selective filtration has been criticized, because isolated GBM was found to have too low a density of anionic charge to satisfy model predictions for what is required of the GBM to operate as barrier to albumin.[24] However, the inflated 5 nm pore radius calculated from neutral dextran sieving may account for the discrepancy. It should also be noted that this model explains charge-related sieving entirely on the basis of Donnan potentials at the two membrane interfaces. It makes no allowance for any effect that the fixed membrane charges might have on the steric hindrance or friction within the pore. Such effects are likely, and would further reduce the amount of fixed negative membrane charge required to account for any degree of charge selectivity. To date, there is no theory for quantifying this, although it has been argued that the phenomenon of "charge screening" can be used to show reduced partitioning of anionic proteins in the glomerular capillary wall (vide infra). Furthermore, the relevant Donnan potential may arise at the plasma

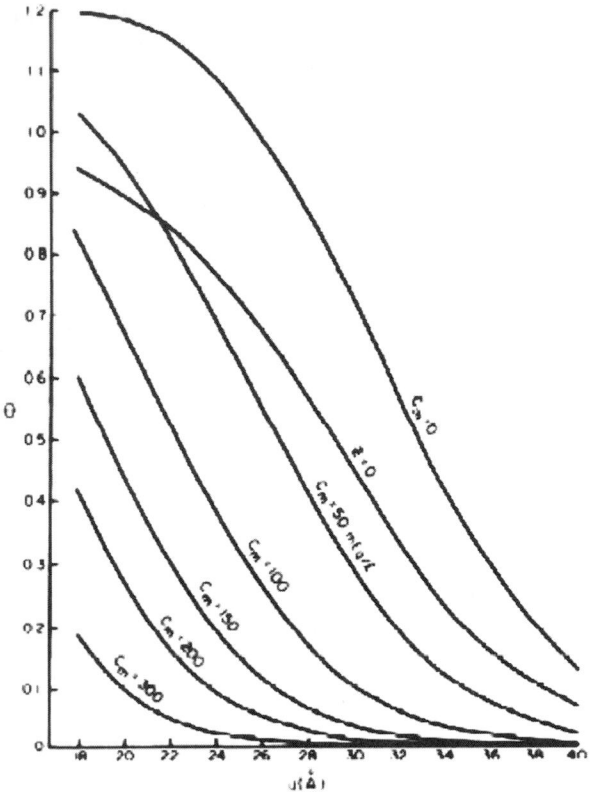

FIGURE 21.12 Sieving coefficent (Θ) for dextran sulfate as function of Stokes–Einstein radius, a. Cm-membrane fixed negative charge density in mEq/liter. Valence, z, of dextran = 0.245 × a. z = 0 is curve for neutral dextran (from ref. [126]).

interface with the negatively charged endothelial glycocalyx rather than the basement membrane, in which case the charge density of the GBM is not the appropriate straw man for arguments against charge-based sieving (vide infra).

Endothelial Glycocalyx as the Barrier to Macromolecules

It has been a challenge to determine which individual layer of the glomerular filtration barrier contributes most to macromolecular sieving. Various investigators at various times and with various methods have argued for the GBM,[20,42,60] filtration slit diaphragm,[139] and endothelium.[112] Overall, the glomerular endothelium has received less attention than GBM and slit diaphragm with respect to permselectivity. Nonetheless, it is arguably unwise to ignore the possibility of a proximal barrier, since the filter should clog if albumin is allowed to permeate downstream and wedge against the slit diaphragm.[127]

The glomerular endothelium is perforated with fenestrae 20 times the diameter of albumin. So if the endothelium serves as a selective barrier to filtration of macromolecules this property owes to the glycocalyx that fills these fenestrae. Information about the molecular dimensions and electrical properties of the endothelial glycocalyx has accrued slowly, and lack of such information has forestalled a definitive analysis. Nonetheless, both experimental data and logical arguments have emerged for the glycocalyx as an important size and charge-selective barrier. The endothelial glycocalyx forms a hydrated gel within the fenestrae, and contains fixed negative charges on its gel fibers. The effective permeability of a solute in a gel relative to free solution (D_{eff}) can be expressed as the product of its diffusion coefficient in the gel relative to free solution (D_{gel}/D_0) and the fraction of the gel volume available to be occupied by the protein (e.g., its partition coefficient, Φ).

$$D_{eff} = \frac{D_{gel}}{D_0}\Phi \qquad (21.40)$$

Considering charge selectivity, it is conceivable that electrostatic interactions with a negatively charged gel might impede the transit of like-charged molecules by reducing D_{gel} or Φ.

One way to study the role of electrostatic interactions between proteins and gels is to inhibit these interactions by increasing the ionic strength of the solvent, which is the standard method for separating proteins by size and charge on agarose gels in the laboratory. Ions in the solvent have the effect of screening the charged solute protein from the coulomb forces that would otherwise be exerted on it by the fixed charges on the gel fibers.

The following brief digression into the physical theory of colloids (also known as Debye—Hückel theory) explains how this phenomenon works. Adding a point charge at a fixed position in any medium generates an electric field that attracts mobile ions of opposite charge. An electric field formed by those charges will offset the field associated with the fixed charge so that at some distance from the fixed charge, one can no longer "sense" its presence. If a fixed charge is added, mobile charges will reposition in response, and it can be shown from the density of repositioned charges that the influence of the fixed charge decays exponentially with distance. The reciprocal of the decay constant is known as the Debye length. The Debye length can be deduced by rearranging the equation for electrochemical potential into a Boltzman distribution for the concentration of redistributed charges, using a linear approximation for the Boltzmann distribution to obtain charge concentration as a function of voltage, then inserting the result into the Poisson equation from classical electrical theory, which expresses the second derivative of voltage as a function of charge density. This yields:

$$C(r) = \frac{l}{d}\exp\left(\frac{-r}{d}\right) \text{ where } d = \sqrt{\frac{k_B T \varepsilon}{q^2 C_0}} \qquad (21.41)$$

$C(r)$ is the probability density of relocated charges at distance r from the fixed charge, d is the Debye length, k_B is Boltzmann's constant, ε is the permittivity, q is the elementary charge, and C_0 is the baseline concentration of mobile charges, e.g., the ionic strength of the buffer. Accordingly, increasing the salinity of the buffer will shorten the Debye length and the influence of the fixed charge wanes almost completely beyond two or three Debye lengths. For a material with a typical dielectric constant and 0.15 molar mobile charges, the Debye length is about 0.2 nm, which is similar to the difference between the main pore radius estimated from sieving of neutral proteins (3.75 nm, *vide supra*) and the molecular radius of albumin (3.6 nm).

Johnson et al. made use of charge screening to examine the role of electrostatic interactions on diffusion and partitioning of bovine serum albumin in 6% sulfated agarose gels by varying the ionic strength of the buffer from 0.01 to 1.0 molar. Increasing the ionic strength to shorten the Debye length and reduce the distance over which repulsive coulomb forces from gel anions can be "felt" had minimal effect on the diffusion coefficient for albumin, but caused a major increase in its partitioning coefficient, Φ. Therefore, the anionic gel poses a selective barrier to sieving of anionic proteins not because it restricts the diffusive mobility of albumin within the gel, but because electrostatic forces reduce the amount of space available within the gel to be occupied by albumin.[63]

The notion of altering buffer strength to manipulate the Debye length has also been applied to study the filtration of charged proteins in the cold isolated perfused kidney.[129] Perfusion with physiologic concentration of buffer salts (152 mM) yielded respective sieving coefficients of 0.11 and 0.045 for neutral and anionic horseradish peroxidase (HRP). Reducing the total salts in the buffer from 152 to 34 mM did not affect the sieving of neutral HRP, but reduced the sieving coefficient for anionic HRP by about half. Thus, there appears to be selective screening-out of anionic HRP by the glomerulus that increases along with the distance over which coulomb forces between the barrier and albumin are able to act. A note of caution is warranted when ascribing the effect of buffer salinity to charge screening within the membrane, since increasing the buffer salinity will also reduce the Donnan potential at the membrane—solution interface, according to Eqs. (21.35)–(21.39).

Glomerular sieving properties have also been examined in the cold isolated perfused kidney of mice treated with glycosaminoglycan-degrading enzymes intended to disrupt the endothelial glycocalyx. This treatment was estimated to reduce the fiber charge density by 10% and increased the sieving coefficient for albumin by five-fold, but only increased sieving of Ficoll by 1.5-fold, thus demonstrating that hyaluronic acid, chondroitin sulfate, and heparan sulfate are important for glomerular charge selectivity.[61] If the endothelial glycocalyx contributes to the screening of albumin, this removes some of the burden of showing how the GBM can do this when it appears that the GBM contains too few fixed charges. Screening by the glycocalyx at the interface with the well-stirred plasma also reduces the burden on the epithelial slit diaphragm which might otherwise clog.

Recent inroads to understanding the filtration properties of the endothelial glycocalyx have also been made with mathematics. Using computed autocorrelation functions of electron micrographs, Squire et al. found quasi-periodic 20 nm spacing of 10 nm fibers in the endothelial glycocalyx of frog mesentery, and suggested that the glycocalyx in fenestrated glomerular capillaries could be similarly organized.[131] Inspired by Squire et al., Zhang developed a formula for reflection coefficients in a periodic array of parallel fibers. The Zhang model predicts a reflection coefficient for albumin of approximately 0.6, but it does not account for electrical charge, and requires that flow occurs parallel to the fiber axis.[150] Bhalla and Deen also developed a model based on Squire's version of glycocalyx geometry in which they applied Debye–Hückel theory to incorporate the effects of charge on osmotic reflection coefficients of macromolecules in a membrane of parallel fibers bearing like surface charge with flow parallel to the fiber axis.[8] This involved computing the electrostatic free energy for a charged sphere interacting with a hexagonal array of charged fibers. The sphere was assigned a size and surface charge resembling albumin (-0.2 coulomb-m^{-2}). Charge densities were ascribed to the fiber array up to the predicted charge density on chondroitin sulfate. At zero fiber charge, the reflection coefficient matched the prediction of the Zhang model. The reflection coefficient was steeply dependent on fiber charge, rising almost to unity within the tested range. So the current idealized models suggest that the endothelium is a major barrier to albumin, whereas the GBM is probably not.

Serial Membrane Models

The glomerular filtration barrier is built of multiple layers arranged in series. The sieving coefficient for the whole assembly differs from what is predicted by deriving individual sieving coefficients for each layer based on its own physical properties, then multiplying these coefficients together. Conversely, the physical characteristics of a given layer cannot be inferred from its sieving coefficient as measured *in situ*. This is because the sieving coefficient of a given layer is determined by its own physical characteristics, and by the physical characteristics of all downstream layers. In other words, for a filtration barrier consisting of two layers arranged in series with upstream and downstream layers denoted by respective subscripts 1 and 2 and overall sieving coefficient $\Theta = \Theta_1\Theta_2$, it can be shown that Θ_1 depends on Θ_2. There are several consequences of this. The most striking is that placing a less selective layer upstream of a more selective layer actually causes the upstream sieving coefficient to exceed unity, and causes the overall barrier function to deteriorate. This counterintuitive result can be deduced from the solute flux equation, as follows.

We wish to describe the sieving of a solute that exists in low concentration in the plasma. Solute concentration at the boundary interface between the two layers is C_B. By conservation of mass, J_s and J_v are constant throughout the barrier and solute concentration in the terminal filtrate is J_s/J_v. $\Theta_2 = C_{filtrate}/C_B$ rearranges to $C_B = J_s/(J_v\Theta_2)$. Starting with the solute flux equation for the downstream layer, separating variables, integrating, defining the Peclet number, and rearranging to solve for Θ_2 gives:

$$\exp(-Pe_2) = \frac{J_s - J_v(1-\sigma_2)C_B}{J_s - J_v(1-\sigma_2)C_{filtrate}}$$

$$\Theta_2 \equiv \frac{C_{filtrate}}{C_B} = \frac{1-\sigma_2}{1-\exp(-Pe_2)+(1-\sigma_2)\exp(-Pe_2)}$$

(21.42)

Next, we take the same approach to the upstream layer and substitute $J_s/(J_v\Theta_2)$ for C_B to yield

$$\exp(-Pe_1) = \frac{J_s - J_v(1-\sigma_1)C_{plasma}}{J_s - J_v(1-\sigma_1)\left(\frac{J_s}{J_v\cdot\Theta_2}\right)}$$

$$\Theta_1 \equiv \frac{C_B}{C_{plasma}} = \frac{1-\sigma_1}{\Theta_2(1-\exp(-Pe_1))+(1-\sigma_1)\exp(-Pe_1)}$$

(21.43)

Note that the expression for Θ_2 (Eq. (21.42)) contains no reference to upstream events, whereas Θ_1 is affected by Θ_2 (Eq. (21.43)) such that reducing the sieving coefficient of the downstream membrane increases the sieving coefficient of the upstream membrane without altering any of its physical properties Extending this approach to the *i*th component of a membrane with *n* series components gives:

$$\Theta_i = \frac{1-\sigma_i}{\Theta_{i+1}\Theta_{i+2}\ldots\Theta_n(1-\exp(-Pe_i))+(1-\sigma_i)\exp(-Pe_i)}$$

(21.44)

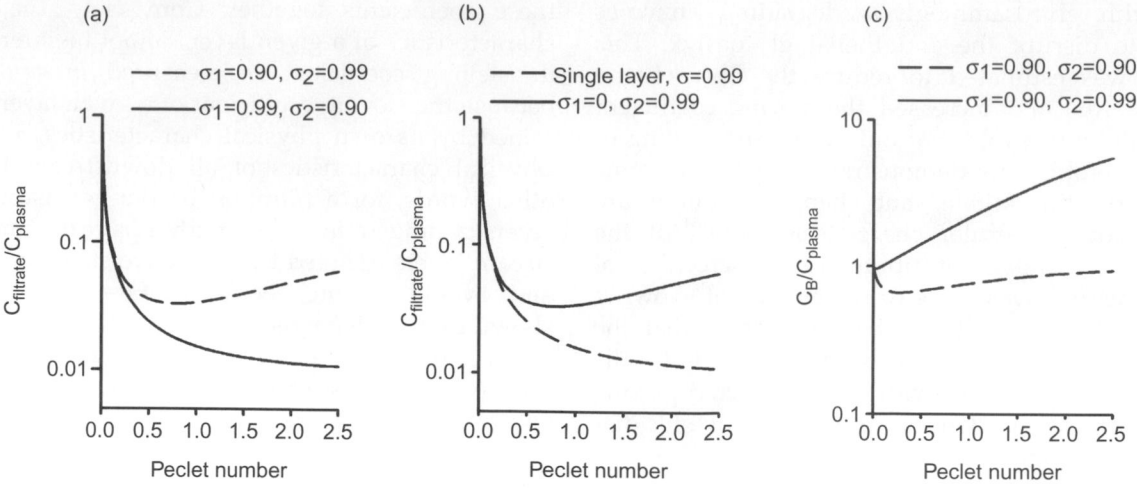

FIGURE 21.13 Sieving coefficients for a filtration barrier consisting of two layers shown over a range of Peclet numbers. The upstream and downstream layers are designated *1* and *2*, respectively. Each layer has its own inherent reflection coefficient, σ. C_{plasma}, $C_{filtrate}$, and C_B are the respective solute concentrations in plasma, filtrate, and at the boundary between the two layers. When the Peclet number is zero, there is no bulk flow and the system comes to diffusion equilibrium with equal solute concentrations everywhere (all sieving coefficients = unity). (a) One layer has $\sigma = 0.99$ and the other has $\sigma = 0.90$. The overall efficiency as a filtration barrier is markedly diminished when the less restrictive layer is placed upstream of the more restrictive layer. (b) Placing a permeable layer ($\sigma = 0$) upstream of a restrictive layer yields a barrier that is less efficient than the restrictive layer alone. (c) The sieving coefficient of the upstream layer (C_B/C_{plasma}) is strongly influenced by the reflection coefficient of the downstream layer. Remarkably, when the downstream layer is only 10% more restrictive than the upstream layer, the upstream sieving coefficient can exceed unity by several-fold. In other words, there is concentration polarization in the upstream layer. This acts like a force for diffusion through the downstream layer, and explains the separation of the two curves in panel (a).

Some implications of the double layer filtration barrier are shown graphically in Figure 21.13. Note that all components of Θ approach unity as the Peclet number approaches zero. This corresponds to zero *SNGFR*, where the solute comes to diffusion equilibrium across the membrane. For a single layer membrane at high Peclet number (corresponding to high *SNGFR*) diffusion becomes irrelevant, and Θ approaches $1 - \sigma$. Placing a more selective layer downstream of a less selective layer actually causes the upstream sieving coefficient, Θ_1, to exceed unity, and the overall barrier function deteriorates. Adding an upstream layer of equivalent selectivity to the downstream layer is equivalent to doubling the thickness of a homogeneous membrane. As expected, this halves the diffusion permeability, as manifest by $\Theta_1 \approx 0.5$ at low Peclet number. Peclet numbers haven't been measured for cell layers of the glomerular filtration barrier, but Deen has presented a logical argument against small Pe for albumin in the endothelial or epithelial layers.[28]

Structure-Based Models of the Glomerular Capillary

Since the 1990s there has been progress toward relating the filtration properties of the glomerulus to its actual physical structure. This is mainly the work of Deen and colleagues, who apply modern numerical

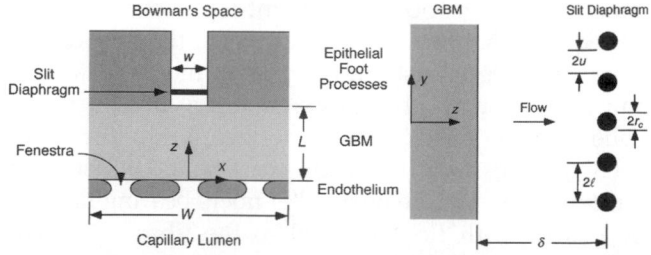

FIGURE 21.14 Left: Idealized structural unit of glomerular capillary wall corresponding to one filtration slit. Right: Idealized structure of slit diaphragm in relation to GBM. Dimensions in nm: W 360, L 200, w 39, rf 30, rc 2, 2u 20 ± 15, Δ 500, fractional area of fenestrae 0.2, fractional area of filtration slits 0.11 *(from ref. [145])*.

methods in fluid mechanics to a specific structural model that is based on morphometry.[30,35] The defined structural elements of the model include the endothelial cells and fenestrae, the GBM represented as homogeneous porous material, and the epithelial cell foot processes with filtration slits bridged by slit diaphragms. These elements form a filtering subunit that is repeated many times to comprise the glomerular capillary. Each filtration subunit consists of one filtration slit, several fenestrae, and the GBM in between (see Figure 21.14). Water movement is assumed to be paracellular. In some instances consideration is given to the endothelial glycocalyx, although untestable assumptions are required for this, since the permeability characteristics of the glycocalyx are not known.

The hydraulic conductances of the endothelium, GBM and filtration slits are treated as separate conductances arranged in series such that the overall conductance is given by a reciprocal of summed resistance:

$$\frac{P_{UF}}{Jv} = \frac{1}{k} = \frac{1}{k_{endo}} + \frac{1}{k_{GBM}} + \frac{1}{k_{epi}} \tag{21.45}$$

where P_{UF} is the ultrafiltration pressure and k is the hydraulic permeability.

By analogy to the first term in Eq. (21.3a), the hydraulic permeability for a single endothelial fenestra is equal to:

$$k_{endo} = \frac{\varepsilon_F \overline{v}_Z}{(P_G - \overline{P_0})} \tag{21.46}$$

where z is the direction perpendicular to the membrane, v_Z is the average z-component of the flow velocity within the fenestra, P_0 is the average pressure at the outflow, P_G is the capillary pressure, and ε_F is the fraction of the endothelial surface covered by fenestrae. P_0 and v_Z are determined from pressure and velocity fields calculated by finite element analysis applied to a simplified Navier–Stokes'equation, which relates fluid flow to pressure and external forces acting on a fluid.

Hydraulic permeability of the basement membrane is estimated from Darcy's law, which describes the flow of water through porous media when the structural details of the media are unknown:

$$v = -\nabla P \frac{k_D}{\mu} \tag{21.47}$$

where v is the velocity vector, μ is the viscosity and k_D is the so-called Darcy permeability of the medium. The Darcy permeability is related to Lp in Eq. (21.3a), and must be determined empirically. Values for k_D/μ are available from measurements made on isolated glomerular basement membrane.[26,37,110] It is a complicated problem to solve for the pressures and flows within the GBM due to streaming and bulging of the velocity and pressure fields that arise, because fluid must enter only through fenestrae and leave only through epithelial slits that cover only part of the basement membrane. These pressure and flow fields are determined numerically after setting the appropriate conditions for zero flow in the z-direction at boundary areas covered by cells, and setting the divergence of flow equal to zero to satisfy conservation of mass for a noncompressible fluid. Calculating k_{GBM} in this way is somewhat artificial, inasmuch as the apparent conductance of the GBM will increase along with the fraction of its surface

that is covered by fenestrae and filtration slits. Therefore, as the number of fenestrae and filtration slits declines, the apparent hydraulic resistance of the GBM will increase even though there has been no actual change to the GBM.

Hydraulic permeability of the epithelial layer is calculated, again by applying the simplified Navier–Stokes' equation, this time to an ultrastructural model of the filtration slit as a rectangular channel bridged by fibers.[34] This particular geometry for the slit diaphragm is based on microscopy of Rodewald and Karnovsky, who suggested that the filtration slit consists of a central fiber connected by bridging fibers to the cell membranes on either side (see Figure 21.15).[111] Solving the model reveals that the slit diaphragm is the main site of resistance to flow through the filtration slit, and that there is little resistance to flow along the remainder of the filtration slit, which is a channel whose walls are formed by two adjacent foot processes. One caveat to these predictions has arisen from molecular sieving data, which suggest that the true pore dimensions provided by the Rodewald–Karnovsky model are too small, and are better explained if the slit diaphragm is represented by a single row of parallel cylindrical fibers rather than two rows of pores separated by a central fiber.[38] However, a more detailed image of the slit diaphragm has now been obtained by electron tomography which validates the basic zipper-like configuration with pores on each side that approximate the dimension of

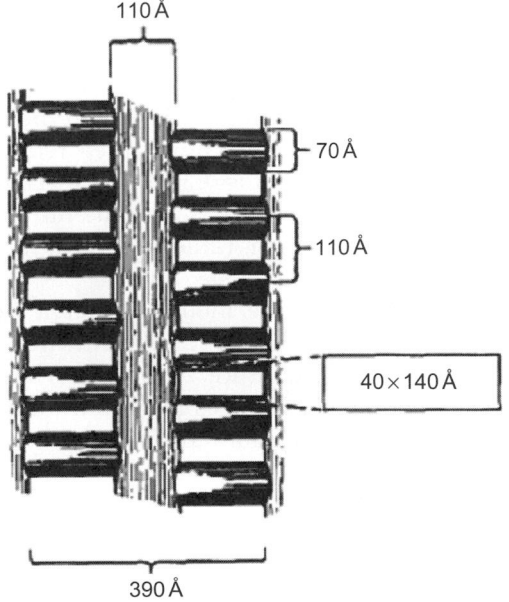

FIGURE 21.15 Schematic drawing of the epithelial slit diaphragm. Typical cross-sectional dimensions of pores between crossbridges are 40 × 140 D *(from ref. [144]).*

TABLE 21.4 Microstructural Parameters and Ultrafiltration Coefficient in the Rat used by Drumond et al.*

Width of filtration unit	360 nm
Thickness of GBM	200 nm
Width of filtration slit	39 nm
Fractional area of fenestrae	0.2
Number of fenestrae per unit	3
Fractional area of slits	0.11
Darcy permeability of GBM	2.7 nm^2
k_{endo}	$2.0 \times 10^{-7} \text{ m-s}^{-1}\text{-Pa}^{-1}$
k_{GBM}	$8.3 \times 10^{-9} \text{ m-s}^{-1}\text{-Pa}^{-1}$
k_{epi}	$8.6 \times 10^{-9} \text{ m-s}^{-1}\text{-Pa}^{-1}$
k	$4.1 \times 10^{-9} \text{ m-s}^{-1}\text{-Pa}^{-1}$
k estimated from micropuncture and morphometry	$3 \times 10^{-9} - 5 \times 10^{-9} \text{ m-s}^{-1}\text{-Pa}^{-1}$

*Drumond et al. (1994). Am. J. Physiol. Renal Fluid Electrolyte Physiol. 266, F1–F12.[35] See also Figure 21.14.

albumin. As depicted by electron tomography, these pores appear more irregular and tortuous than previously imagined.[147]

The morphometric parameters and hydraulic permeabilities calculated from the ultrastructural model of Deen et al. are shown in Table 21.4, which also shows that the hydraulic permeability predicted by the model is consistent with values obtained by micropuncture in normal rats. Some other predictions of the model cannot be tested by micropuncture. For example, a main prediction of the model is that the GBM and epithelial layers contribute equally and, together, account for most of the resistance to glomerular filtration. The endothelial fenestrae pose little resistance to bulk flow, except that reducing their fractional area reduces the apparent permeability of the GBM. Furthermore, as already mentioned, most resistance of the filtration slit is due to the slit diaphragm, rather than to drag along the length of the slit.

An important test of the model is that it predicts changes in the ultrafiltration coefficient that occur when the glomerular structure is altered. The model has successfully forecast changes in ultrafiltration coefficient brought about by manipulating dietary protein and/or renal mass to alter glomerular morphology in rats with adriamycin nephrosis.[85]

Computation based on morphometry has also been employed to estimate glomerular ultrafiltration coefficient from renal biopsies in patients with reduced GFR due to membranous or minimal change nephropthies[36] and pre-eclampsia.[70] In each of these conditions, GFR was reduced in spite of normal PAH clearance. In order for GFR to decline while nephron plasma flow remains constant, there must be a decrease in either glomerular ultrafiltration pressure or ultrafiltration coefficient. While it is not possible to measure ultrafiltration pressure in humans, the determinants of SNGFR have been extensively evaluated in a wide range of animal models of glomerular disease. With the single exception of cyclosporine toxicity,[137] low pressure in the glomerular capillary does not provide the basis for low SNGFR in any of these models. Therefore, it is reasonable to assume that ultrafiltration pressure is not reduced in humans with idiopathic nephrotic syndrome or pre-eclampsia, and that the low filtration fraction in these patients is likely to be the consequence of a decline in ultrafiltration coefficient. Once this premise is accepted, there are several potential explanations for an apparent decline in ultrafiltration coefficient in a glomerulus. First, this could be due to a loss of capillary surface area. Second, it could result from mismatched blood flow among capillary loops within the glomerulus, such that those loops with low flow manifest filtration equilibrium early in their course, which eliminates their latter portions from contributing to the working area. A third mechanism for reducing ultrafiltration coefficient could be to alter the chemical composition of the GBM or slit diaphragm to make them less permeable to water. Finally, ultrafiltration coefficient could decline due to changes in geometry of the individual filtration unit. The latter of these possibilities is amenable to testing by applying computational fluid dynamics to morphometry. Based on this approach, changes in geometry of the filtration unit predict that the ultrafiltration coefficient will be different between normal subjects and those with minimal change disease, membranous nephropthy, and pre-eclampsia. Although each disease has its own morphology, reduced frequency of filtration slits, increased basement membrane thickness, loss of fenestral area or loss of capillary surface area predicted changes in the ultrafiltration coefficient consistent with what would be necessary to explain the associated declines in GFR, given the reasonable assumption that glomerular capillary pressure was not profoundly reduced, and a less certain assumption that the Darcy permeability for the GBM is unaffected. One interesting prediction of the model is that, while the GBM is thickened in membranous nephropathy, this has little importance to the GFR because an even greater augmentation of the average distance traveled from fenestra to slit diaphragm results from the lower filtration slit density, which requires much of the filtrate to stream obliquely through the GBM rather than crossing it directly.

In 2005 it was recognized that the visceral epithelial cell body attaches to the GBM in such a way as to create a semi-confined space downstream of the filtration

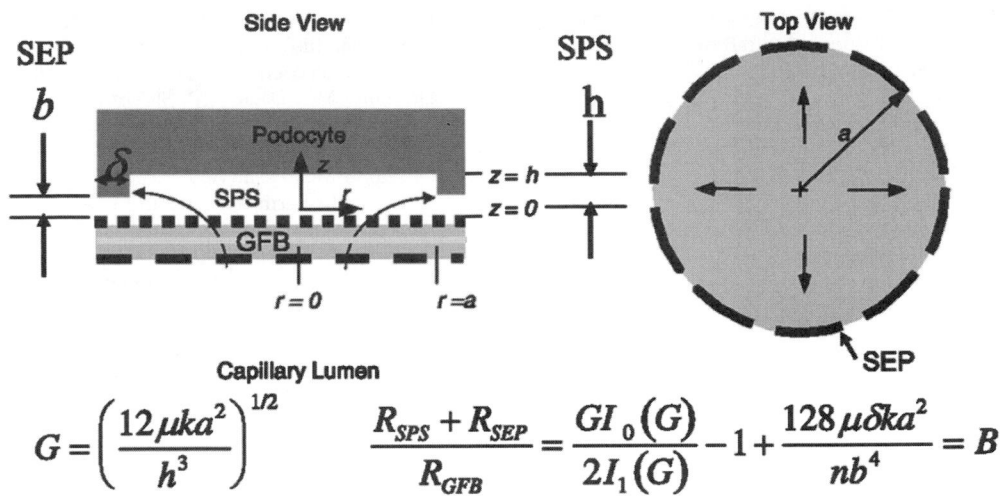

FIGURE 21.16 **Flow across the glomerular filtration barrier and through the subpodocyte space (SPS).** Resistance depends on height of subpodocyte space (h), the path length (a), and the area draining into SPS (πa^2) *(reprinted from ref. [88]).*

slit and upstream of the rest of Bowman's space[87] (see Figure 21.16). It was further estimated that 60% of the filtration surface is covered by this subpodocyte space, and that the space between attachments constitute pores through which filtrate must pass en route to Bowman's space. When analyzed in greater detail and subject to mathematical modeling, it was estimated that the resistance encountered by filtrate in exiting the subepithelial space is likely to exceed that of the traditional 3-layer filtration barrier, and that pressure in this space could, therefore, be three-fold greater than in Bowman's space.[88] This poses a problem for prior structure-based models, which accurately predict the hydraulic permeability without this contribution to the barrier.

SUMMARY

Details about the physics of glomerular filtration have become known over the past century. Different approaches to describing glomerular filtration employ different admixtures of phenomenology and structural detail. The spectrum of useful models extends from the glomerular capillary as an idealized circular cylinder with homogenous permeability to water and small solutes and zero permeability to macromolecules, to a tube perforated by discreet cylindrical pores with differential permeability to solutes based on size and electrical charge, to fiber matrix models based on the physical theory of colloids, to representations that incorporate actual physical dimensions to determine the contributions of endothelial, basement membrane, and epithelial layers to the filtration barrier.

Acknowledgment

This work was performed with grant support from NIH, RO1 DK28602 and RO1 DK56248 and the Department of Veterans Affairs Research Service.

References

[1] Andersen S, Blouch K, Bialek J, Deckert M, Parving HH, Myers BD. Glomerular permselectivity in early stages of overt diabetic nephropathy. Kidney Int 2000;58:2129—37.

[2] Anderson JL, Quinn JA. Restricted transport in small pores. A model for steric exclusion and hindered particle motion. Biophys J 1974;14:130—50.

[3] Anderson S, Meyer TW, Rennke HG, Brenner BM. Control of glomerular hypertension limits glomerular injury in rats with reduced renal mass. J Clin Invest 1985;76(2):612—9.

[4] Arendshorst WJ, Gottschalk CW. Glomerular ultrafiltration dynamics: historical perspective. Am J Physiol 1985;248(2 Pt 2): F163—74.

[5] Bakris GL, Weir MR. Angiotensin-converting enzyme inhibitor-associated elevations in serum creatinine: is this a cause for concern? Arch Intern Med 2000;160(5):685—93.

[6] Baylis C. The mechanism of the increase in glomerular filtration rate in the twelve-day pregnant rat. J Physiol 1980;305:405—14.

[7] Baylis C, Ichikawa I, Willis WT, Wilson CB, Brenner BM. Dynamics of glomerular ultrafiltration. IX. Effects of plasma protein concentration. Am J Physiol 1977;232(1):F58—71.

[8] Bhalla G, Deen WM. Effects of charge on osmotic reflection coefficients of macromolecules in fibrous membranes. Biophys J 2009;97(6):1595—605.

[9] Blantz RC. Effect of mannitol on glomerular ultrafiltration in the hydropenic rat. J Clin Invest 1974;54(5):1135—43.

[10] Blantz RC, Gabbai F, Gushwa LC, Wilson CB. The influence of concomitant experimental hypertension and glomerulonephritis. Kidney Int 1987;32(5):652—63.

[11] Blantz RC, Gabbai FB, Tucker BJ, Yamamoto T, Wilson CB. Role of mesangial cell in glomerular response to volume and angiotensin II. Am J Physiol 1993;264(1 Pt 2):F158—65.

[12] Blantz RC, Konnen KS, Tucker BJ. Angiotensin II effects upon the glomerular microcirculation and ultrafiltration coefficient of the rat. J Clin Invest 1976;57(2):419–34.

[13] Blantz RC, Rector Jr FC, Seldin DW. Effect of hyperoncotic albumin expansion upon glomerular ultrafiltration in the rat. Kidney Int 1974;6(4):209–21.

[14] Blouch K, Deen WM, Fauvel JP, Bialek J, Derby G, Myers BD. Molecular configuration and glomerular size selectivity in healthy and nephrotic humans. Am J Physiol 1997;273:F430–7.

[15] Bohrer MP, Deen WM, Robertson CR, Troy JL, Brenner BM. Influence of molecular configuration on the passage of macromolecules across the glomerular capillary wall. J Gen Physiol 1979;74(5):583–93.

[16] Bowman W. On the Structure and Use of the Malpighian Bodies of the Kidney, with Observations on the Circulation. London: Printed by R. and J. E. Taylor, 1842. Offprint from *Philosophical Transactions of the Royal Society, Part I for 1842.*

[17] Brenner BM, Falchuk KH, Keimowitz RI, Berliner RW. The relationship between peritubular capillary protein concentration and fluid reabsorption by the renal proximal tubule. J Clin Invest 1969;48(8):1519–31.

[18] Brenner BM, Hostetter TH, Humes HD. Glomerular permselectivity: barrier function based on discrimination of molecular size and charge. Am J Physiol Renal Fluid Electrolyte Physiol 1978;234:F455–60.

[19] Brenner BM, Troy JL, Daugharty TM. The dynamics of glomerular ultrafiltration in the rat. J Clin Invest 1971;50(8):1776–80.

[20] Caulfield JP, Farquhar MG. The permeability of glomerular capillaries to graded dextrans. Identification of the basement membrane as the primary filtration barrier. J Cell Biol 1974; 63(3):883–903.

[21] Chang RL, Deen WM, Robertson CR, Brenner BM. Permselectivity of the glomerular capillary wall. III. Restricted transport of polyanions. Kidney Int 1975;8:212–8.

[22] Chang RL, Robertson CR, Deen WM, Brenner BM. Permselectivity of the glomerular capillary wall to macromolecules. I. Theoretical considerations. Biophys J 1975;15(9):861–86.

[23] Chasis H, Ranges HA, Goldring W, Smith HW. The control of renal blood flow and glomerular filtration in normal man. J Clin Invest 1938;17:683–97.

[24] Comper WD, Lee AS, Tay M, Adal Y. Anionic charge concentration of rat kidney glomeruli and glomerular basement membrane. Biochem J. 1993;289:647–52.

[25] Daniels BS, Deen WM, Mayer G, Meyer T, Hostetter TH. Glomerular permeability barrier in the rat. Functional assessment by *in vitro* methods. J Clin Invest 1993;92(2):929–36.

[26] Daniels BS, Hauser EH, Deen WM, Hostetter TH. Glomerular basement membrane: *in vitro* studies of water and protein permeability. Am J Physiol Renal Fluid Electrolyte Physiol 1992;262:F919–26.

[27] De Nicola L, Blantz RC, Gabbai FB. Renal functional reserve in the early stage of experimental diabetes. Diabetes 1992;41 (3):267–73.

[28] Deen WM. Cellular contributions to glomerular size selectivity. Kidney Int 2006;69(8):1295–7.

[29] Deen WM, Bridges CR, Brenner BM, Myers BD. Heteroporous model of glomerular size selectivity: application to normal and nephrotic humans. Am J Physiol 1985;249:F374 –F389.

[30] Deen WM, Lazzara MJ, Myers BD. Structurual determinants of glomerular permeability. Am J Physiol Renal Physiol 2001;281: F579–96.

[31] Deen WM, Robertson CR, Brenner BM. A model of glomerular ultrafiltration in the rat. Am J Physiol 1971;223:1178–83.

[32] Deen WM, Satvat B, Jamieson JM. Theoretical model for glomerular filtration of charged solutes. Am J Physiol 1980;238(2):F126–39.

[33] Deen WM, Troy JL, Robertson CR, Brenner BM. Dynamics of glomerular ultrafiltration in the rat. IV. Determination of the ultrafiltration coefficient. J Clin Invest 1973;52(6):1500–8.

[34] Drumond MC, Deen WM. Stokes flow through a row of cylinders between parallel walls: model for the glomerular slit diaphragm. J Biomech Eng 1994;116(2):184–9.

[35] Drumond MC, Deen WH. Structural determinants of glomerular hydraulic permeability. Am J Physiol Renal Fluid Electrolyte Physiol 1994;266:F1–12.

[36] Drumond MC, Kristal B, Myers BD, Deen WM. Structural basis for reduced glomerular filtration capacity in nephrotic humans. J Clin Invest 1994;94(3):1187–95.

[37] Edwards A, Daniels BS, Deen WM. Hindered transport of macromolecules in isolated glomeruli II. Convection and pressure effects in basememt membrane. Biophys J 1997;72: 214–22.

[38] Edwards A, Daniels BS, Deen WM. Ultrastructural model for size selectivity in glomerular filtration. Am J Physiol 1999;276(6 Pt 2):F892–902.

[39] Einstein A. Uber die von der molekularkinetistchen Theorie der Waerme geforderte Bewegung von in ruhenden Fluessigkeiten suspendierten Teilchen. Ann Physik 1905;17:549–60.

[40] Elger M, Sakai T, Kriz W. The vascular pole of the renal glomerulus of rat. Adv Anat Embryol Cell Biol 1998;139:1–98.

[41] Falchuk HK, Berliner RW. Hydrostatic pressures in peritubular capillaries and tubules in the rat kidney. Am J Physiol 1971;220:1422–6.

[42] Farquhar MG, Palade GE. Glomerular permeability. II. Ferritin transfer across the glomerular capillary wall in nephrotic rats. J Exp Med 1961;114:699–716.

[43] Ferry JD. Ultrafilter membranes and ultrafiltration. Chem Rev 1936;18:373.

[44] Fronek K, Zweifach BW. Microvascular pressure distribution in skeletal muscle and the effect of vasodilation. Am J Physiol 1975;228(3):791–6.

[45] Gabbai FB, Gushwa LC, Wilson CB, Blantz RC. An evaluation of the development of experimental membranous nephropathy. Kidney Int 1987;31(6):1267–78.

[46] Gabbai FB, Gushwa LC, Peterson OW, Wilson CB, Blantz RC. Analysis of renal function in the two-kidney Goldblatt model. Am J Physiol 1987;252(1 Pt 2):F131–7.

[47] Gomez DM. Evaluation of renal resistances, with special reference to changes in essential hypertension. J Clin Invest 1951;30:1143–55.

[48] Granath KA. Solution properties of branched dextrans. J Colloid Sci 1958;13:308–28.

[49] Guasch A, Deen WM, Myers BD. Charge selectivity of the glomerular filtration barrier in healthy and nephrotic humans. J Clin Invest 1993;92:2274–82.

[50] Guimarães MA, Nikolovski J, Pratt LM, Greive K, Comper WD. Anomalous fractional clearance of negatively charged Ficoll relative to uncharged Ficoll. Am J Physiol Renal Physiol 2003;285:F1118–24.

[51] Haberman WL, Sayre RM. David Taylor Model Basin. Report No. 1143 Motion of rigid and fluid spheres in stationary and moving liquids inside cylindrical tubes. Washington DC: U.S. Navy; 1958

[52] Hall JE, Guyton AC, Smith Jr MJ, Coleman TG. Blood pressure and renal function during chronic changes in sodium intake: role of angiotensin. Am J Physiol 1980;239(3):F271–80.

[53] Haraldsson BS, Johnsson EK, Rippe B. Glomerular permselectivity is dependent on adequate serum concentrations of orosomucoid. Kidney Int 1992;41(2):310–6.

[54] Heidenhain RP. Absonderungsvorgaenge. Sechster Abschnitt. Die Harnabsonderung (Viertes Capitel. Die Absonderung der

festen Harnbestandteile). In: Leipzig HL, editor. Handbuch d Physiol Fuenfter Teil. Germany: Vogel; 1883. p. 341—3.

[55] Heller J, Horacek V. Angiotensin II: preferential efferent constriction? Ren Physiol 1986;9(6):357—65.

[56] Hierholzer K, Ullrich KJ. History of renal physiology in Germany during the 19th century. Am J Nephrol 1999; 19(2):243—56.

[57] Hostetter TH. Human renal response to a meat meal. Am J Physiol 1986;250(4 Pt 2):F613—8.

[58] Hostetter TH, Troy JL, Brenner BM. Glomerular hemodynamics in experimental diabetes mellitus. Kidney Int 1981;19(3):410—5.

[59] Ichikawa I, Brenner BM. Local intrarenal vasoconstrictor—vasodilator interactions in mild partial ureteral obstruction. Am J Physiol 1979;236(2):F131—40.

[60] Jarad G, Cunningham J, Shaw AS, Miner JH. Proteinuria precedes podocyte abnormalities inLamb2$^{-/-}$ mice, implicating the glomerular basement membrane as an albumin barrier. J Clin Invest 2006;116(8):2272—9.

[61] Jeansson M, Haraldsson B. Glomerular size and charge selectivity in the mouse after exposure to glucosaminoglycan-degrading enzymes. J Am Soc Nephrol 2003;14(7):1756—65.

[62] Jensen PK, Christiansen JS, Steven K, Parving HH. Renal function in streptozotocin-diabetic rats. Diabetologia 1981; 21(4):409—14.

[63] Johnson EM, Berk DA, Jain RK, Deen WM. Diffusion and partitioning of proteins in charged agarose gels. Biophys J 1995; 68(4):1561—8.

[64] Johnsson E, Haraldsson B. An isolated perfused rat kidney preparation designed for assessment of glomerular permeability characteristics. Acta Physiol Scand 1992;144(1): 65—73.

[65] Johnsson E, Rippe B, Haraldsson B. Analysis of the pressure-flow characteristics of isolated perfused rat kidneys with inhibited tubular reabsorption. Acta Physiol Scand 1994; 150(2):189—99.

[66] Johnsson E, Rippe B, Haraldsson B. Reduced permselectivity in isolated perfused rat kidneys following small elevations of glomerular capillary pressure. Acta Physiol Scand 1994; 150(2):201—9.

[67] Katz MA, Bressler EH. Osmosis. In: Staub N, Taylor A, editors. Edema: Basic science and clinical manifestations. NY: Raven Press; 1984. p. 39—60.

[68] Katz MA, Schaeffer Jr RC, Gratrix M, Mucha D, Carbajal J. The glomerular barrier fits a two-pore-and-fiber-matrix model: derivation and physiologic test. Microvasc Res 1999;57(3): 227—43.

[69] Kedem O, Katchalsky A. Thermodynamic analysis of the permeability of biological membranes to non-electrolytes. Biochim Biophys Acta 1958;27:229—46.

[70] Lafayette RA, Druzin M, Sibley R, Derby G, Malik T, Huie P, et al. Nature of glomerular dysfunction in pre-eclampsia. Kidney Int 1998;54(4):1240—9.

[71] Landis EM, Pappenheimer JR. Exchange of substances through the capillary walls. In: Hamilton WF, Dow P, editors. *Handbook of Physiology. Circulation.* Washington DC: Am Physiol Soc; 1963. p. p961—1034. Section 2. Vol II. Chapter 29

[72] Lemley KV, Blouch K, Abdullah I, Boothroyd DB, Bennett PH, Myers BD, et al. Glomerular permselectivity at the onset of nephropathy in type 2 diabetes mellitus. J Am Soc Nephrol 2000;11:2095—105.

[73] Lewis EJ, Hunsicker LG, Bain RP, Rohde RD, for the Collaborative Study Group. The effect of angiotensin-converting-enzyme inhibition on diabetic nephropathy. N Engl J Med 1993;329:1456—62.

[74] Lindströöm KE, Blom A, Johnsson E, Haraldsson B, Fries E. High glomerular permeability of bikunin despite similarity in charge and hydrodynamic size to serum albumin. Kidney Int 1997;51(4):1053—8.

[75] Lindströöm KE, Johnsson E, Haraldsson B. Glomerular charge selectivity for proteins larger than serum albumin as revealed by lactate dehydrogenase isoforms. Acta Physiol Scand 1998;162 (4):481—8.

[76] Loutzenhiser R, Bidani A, Chilton L. Renal myogenic response: kinetic attributes and physiological role. Circ Res 2002;90 (12):1316—24.

[77] Lowry OH, Rosebrough NJ, Farr AL, Randall RJ. Protein measurement with the Folin phenol reagent. J Biol Chem 1951;193:265—75.

[78] Ludwig CFW. Beitraege zur lehre vom mechanismus der harnsekretion. Marburg: N.G. Elwert; 1843.

[79] Ludwig C. De viribus physicis secretionem urinae adjuvantibus Thesis, Marburg. 1842. Reprinted with a translation into English in Kidney Int 1994;(Suppl 46):1—23.

[80] Lund U, Rippe A, Venturoli D, Tenstad O, Grubb A, Rippe B. Glomerular filtration rate dependence of sieving of albumin and some neutral proteins in rat kidneys. Am J Physiol Renal Physiol 2003;284:F1226—34.

[81] Malpighi M. De viscerum structura exercitatio anatomica Bononias Iacoi Montiz, 1666. For English translation see: JM Hayman Jr. Maipighi's "Concerning the structure of the kidney." Ann Med Hist 1925;7:242—63.

[82] Maschio G, Alberti D, Janin G, Locatelli F, Mann JF, Motolese M, et al. Effect of the angiotensin-converting-enzyme inhibitor benazepril on the progression of chronic renal insufficiency: The Angiotensin-Converting-Enzyme Inhibition in Progressive Renal Disease trial. N Engl J Med 1996;334: 939—45.

[83] Michels LD, Davidman M, Keane WF. Determinants of glomerular filtration and plasma flow in experimental diabetic rats. J *Lab Clin Med* 1981;8(6):869—85.

[84] Michels LD, O'Donnell MP, Keane WF. Glomerular hemodynamic and structural correlations in long-term experimental diabetic rats. J Lab Clin Med 1984;103(6):840—7.

[85] Miller PL, Scholey JW, Rennke HG, Meyer TW. Glomerular hypertrophy aggravates epithelial cell injury in nephrotic rats. J Clin Invest 1990;85(4):1119—26.

[86] Myers BD, Nelson RG, Williams GW, Bennett PH, Hardy SA, Berg RL, et al. Glomerular function in Pima Indians with noninsulin-dependent diabetes mellitus of recent onset. J Clin Invest 1991;88(2):524—30.

[87] Neal CR, Crook H, Bell E, Harper SJ, Bates DO. Three-dimensional reconstruction of glomeruli by elecron microscopy reveals a distinct restrictive urinary subpodocyte space. J Am Soc Nephrol 2005;16:1223—35.

[88] Neal CR, Muston PR, Njegovan D, Verrill R, Harper SJ, Deen WM, et al. Glomerular filtration into the subpodicyte space is highly restricted under physiological perfusion conditions. Am J Physiol 2007;293(6):F1787—98.

[89] O'Donnell MP, Kasiske BL, Daniels FX, Keane WF. Effects of nephron loss on glomerular hemodynamics and morphology in diabetic rats. Diabetes 1986;35(9):1011—5.

[90] O'Donnell MP, Kasiske BL, Keane WF. Glomerular hemodynamic and structural alterations in experimental diabetes mellitus. FASEB J 1988;8:2339—47.

[91] Ogston AG. The spaces in a uniform random suspension of fibres. Trans Faraday Soc 1958;54:1754—7.

[92] Oken DE, Choi SC. Filtration pressure equilibrium: a statistical analysis. Am J Physiol 1981;241(2):F196—200.

[93] Oken DE, Flamenbaum W. Micropuncture studies of proximal tubule albumin concentrations in normal and nephrotic rats. J Clin Invest 1971;50(7):1498—505.

II. STRUCTURAL AND FUNCTIONAL ORGANIZATION OF THE KIDNEY

[94] Oliver JD, Anderson S, Troy JL, Brenner BM, Deen WH. Determination of glomerular size-selectivity in the normal rat with Ficoll. J Am Soc Nephrol 1992;3:214–8.

[95] Onsager L. Reciprocal relations in irreversible processes. I. I *Phys Rev* 1931;37:405–91.

[96] Osicka TM, Comper WD. Glomerular charge selectivity for anionic and neutral horseradish peroxidase. Kidney Int 1995;47:1630–7.

[97] Paine PL, Scherr P. Drag coefficients for the movement of rigid spheres through liquid-filled cylindrical pores. Biophysical Journal 1975;15:1087–91.

[98] Pappenheimer JR. Passage of molecules through capillary walls. Physiol Rev 1953;33:387–423.

[99] Parazynski SE, Tucker BJ, Aratow M, Crenshaw A, Hargens AR. Direct measurement of capillary blood pressure in the human lip. J Appl Physiol 1993;74(2):946–50.

[100] Patlak CS, Goldstein DA, Hoffman JF. The flow of solute and solvent across a two-membrane system. J. Theoretical Biology 1963;5:426–42.

[101] Peti-Peterdi J. Independent two-photon measurements of albumin GSC give low values. Am J Physiol Renal Physiol 2009;296(6):F1255–7.

[102] Peti-Peterdi J, Sipos A. A high-powered view of the filtration barrier. J Am Soc Nephrol 2010;21(11):1835–41.

[103] Pullman TN, Alving AS, Dern RJ, Landowne M. The influence of dietary protein intake on specific renal functions in normal man. J Lab Clin Med 1954;44:320–32.

[104] Remuzzi A, Brenner BM, Pata V, Tebaldi G, Mariano R, Belloro A, et al. Three-dimensional reconstructed glomerular capillary network: Blood flow distribution and local filtration. Am J Physiol 1992;263(3 Pt 2):F562–72.

[105] Remuzzi A, Ene-Iordache B. Capillary network structure does not affect theoretical analysis of glomerular size selectivity. Am J Physiol 1995;268(5 Pt 2):F972–9.

[106] Remuzzi A, Fassi A, Sangalli F, Malanchini B, Mohamed EI, Bertani T, et al. Prevention of renal injury in diabetic MWF rats by angiotensin II antagonism. Exp Nephrol 1998;6(1):28–38.

[107] Rennke HG, Patel Y, Venkatachalam MA. Glomerular filtration of proteins: clearance of anionic, neutral, and cationic horseradish peroxidase in the rat. Kidney Int 1978;13:278–88.

[108] Rennke HG, Venkatachalam MA. Glomerular permeability of macromolecules. Effect of molecular configuration on the fractional clearance of uncharged dextran and neutral horseradish peroxidase in the rat. J Clin Invest 1979;63(4):713–7.

[109] Rippe B, Haraldsson B. Transport of macromolecules across microvascular walls: the two-pore theory. Physiol Rev 1994;74:163–219.

[110] Robinson GB, Walton HA. Glomerular basement membrane as a compressible ultrafilter. Microvasc Res 1989;38:36–48.

[111] Rodewald R, Karnovsky MJ. Porous substructure of the glomerular slit diaphragm in the rat and mouse. J Cell Biol 1974;60(2):423–33.

[112] Russo PA, Bendayan M. Distribution of endogenous albumin in the glomerular wall of proteinuric patients. Am J Pathol 1990;137(6):1481–90.

[113] Russo LM, Sandoval RM, McKee M, Osicka TM, Collins AB, Brown D, et al. The normal kidney filters nephrotic levels of albumin retrieved by proximal tubule cells: retrieval is disrupted in nephrotic states. Kidney Int 2007;71(6):504–13.

[114] Savin VJ. Ultrafiltration in single isolated human glomeruli. Kidney Int 1983;24(6):748–53.

[115] Savin VJ, Terreros DA. Filtration in single isolated mammalian glomeruli. Kidney Int 1981;20(2):188–97.

[116] Schaeffer Jr RC, Gratrix ML, Mucha DR, Carbajal JM. The rat glomerular filtration barrier does not show negative charge selectivity. Microcirculation 2002;9:329–42.

[117] Schlogl R. Zurtheorie der anomalen Osmose. Z *Physik Chem* 1955;3:73–102.

[118] Scholey JW, Meyer TW. Control of glomerular hypertension by insulin administration in diabetic rats. J Clin Invest 1989; 83(4):1384–9.

[119] Schor N, Ichikawa I, Brenner BM. Glomerular adaptations to chronic dietary salt restriction or excess. Am J Physiol 1980; 238(5):F428–36.

[120] Shannon JA, Jolliffe N, Smith HW. The excretion of urine in the dog IV. The effect of maintenance diet, feeding, etc., upon the quantity of the glomerular filtrate. Am J Physiol 1932;101:625–38.

[121] Shannon JA, Smith HW. The excretion of inulin, xylose and urea by normal and phlorinized man. J Clin Invest 1935;112:405–13.

[122] Slomowitz LA, Peterson OW, Thomson SC. Converting enzyme inhibition and the glomerular hemodynamic response to glycine in diabetic rats. J Am Soc Nephrol 1999;10(7): 1447–54.

[123] Smaje L, Zweifach BW, Intaglietta M. Micropressures and capillary filtration coefficients in single vessels of the cremaster muscle of the rat. Microvasc Res 1970;2(1):96–110.

[124] Smith HW. The kidney: Structure and function in health and disease. New York: Oxford Univ. Press; 1951.

[125] Smith HW, Chasis H, Goldring W, Ranges HA. Glomerular dynamics in the normal human kidney. J Clin Invest 1940;19:751–64.

[126] Smith HW, Finkelstein N, Aliminosa L, Crawford B, Graber M. The renal clearance of substituted hippuric acid derivatives and other aromatic acids in dog and man. J Clin Invest 1945;24:388–404.

[127] Smithies O. Why the kidney glomerulus does not clog: a gel permeation/diffusion hypothesis of renal function. Proc Natl Acad Sci USA 2003;100(7):4108–13.

[128] Sorensson J, Ohlson M, Lindströom K, Haraldsson B. Glomerular charge selectivity for horseradish peroxidase and albumin at low and normal ionic strengths. Acta Physiol Scand 1998;163(1):83–91.

[129] Sorensson J, Ohlson M, Lindströom K, Haraldsson B. Glomerular charge selectivity for horseradish peroxidase and albumin at low and normal ionic strengths. Acta Physiol Scand 1998;163(1):83–91.

[130] Squire JM, Chew M, Nneji G, Neal C, Barry J, Michel C. Quasi-periodic substructure in the microvessel endothelial glycocalyx: a possible explanation for molecular filtering? J Struct Biol 2001;136(3):239–55.

[131] Starling EH. The glomerular functions of the kidney. J Physiol London 1899;24:317–30.

[132] Staverman AJ. Non-equilibrium thermodynamics of membrane processes. Trans Faraday Soc 1952;48:176–85.

[133] Tanner GA. Glomerular sieving coefficient of serum albumin in the rat: a two-photon microscopy study. Am J Physiol Renal Physiol 2009;296(6):F1258–65.

[134] Tay M, Comper WD, Singh AK. Charge selectivity in kidney ultrafiltration is associated with glomerular uptake of transport probes. Am J Physiol Renal Fluid Electrolyte Physiol 1991;260: F549–54.

[135] Tenstad O, Roald AB, Grubb A, Aukland K. Renal handling of radiolabelled human cystatin C in the rat. Scand J Clin Lab Invest 1996;56:409–14.

[136] The Sixth Report of the Joint National Committee on Prevention, Detection, Evaluation and Treatment of High Blood Pressure. Arch Intern Med. 1997;157:2413-2446

[137] Thomson SC, Tucker BJ, Gabbai FB, Blantz RC. Functional effects on glomerular hemodynamics of short-term chronic cyclosporine in male rats. J Clin Invest 1989;83:960—9.

[138] Tojo A, Endou H. Intrarenal handling of proteins in rats using fractional micropuncture technique. Am J Physiol 1992;263(4 Pt 2):F601—6.

[139] Tryggvason K, Wartiovaara J. Molecular basis of glomerular permselectivity. Curr Opin Nephrol Hypertens 2001;10:543—9.

[140] Tucker BJ, Blantz RC. Effects of glomerular filtration dynamics on the glomerular permeability coefficient. Am J Physiol 1981;240(3):F245—54.

[141] Tucker BJ, Anderson CM, Thies RS, Collins RC, Blantz RC. Glomerular hemodynamic alterations during acute hyperinsulinemia in normal and diabetic rats. Kidney Int 1992;42(5): 1160—8.

[142] Tucker BJ, Mundy CA, Blantz RC. Adrenergic and angiotensin II influences on renal vascular tone in chronic sodium depletion. Am J Physiol 1987;252(5 Pt 2):F811—7.

[143] van't Hoff J. Chemical equilibria in gaseous systems or strongly diluted solutions), 1885. From *Nobel Lectures, Chemistry 1901-1921* L'Équilibre chimique dans les Systè mes gazeux ou dissous à I'État dilué. Amsterdam: Elsevier Publishing Company; 1966

[144] Venturoli D, Rippe B. Ficoll and dextran vs. globular proteins as probes for testing glomerular permselectivity: effects of molecular size, shape, charge, and deformability. Am J Physiol Renal Physiol 2005;288(4):F605—13.

[145] Vyas SV, Comper WD. Dextran sulfate binding to isolated rat glomeruli and glomerular basement membrane. Biochim Biophys Acta 1994;1201:367—72.

[146] Walker AM, Bott PA, Oliver J, MacDowell M. The collection and analysis of fluid from single nephrons of the mammalian kidney. Am J Physiol 1941;134:580—5.

[147] Wartiovaara J, Ofverstedt LG, Khoshnoodi J, Zhang J, Makela E, Sandin S, et al. Nephrin strands contribute to a porous slit diaphragm scaffold as revealed by electron tomography. J Clin Invest 2004;114(10):1475—83.

[148] Wearn JT, Richards AN. From: Observations on the composition of glomerular urine, with particular reference to the problem of reabsorption in the renal tubules. Am J Physiol 1924;71:209 —227.

[149] Wiederhielm CA, Weston BV. Microvascular, lymphatic, and tissue pressures in the unanesthetized mammal. Am J Physiol 1973;225(4):992—6.

[150] Zhang X, Curry FR, Weinbaum S. Mechanism of osmotic flow in a periodic fiber array. Am J Physiol Heart Circ Physiol 2006;290(2):H844—52.

[151] Zatz R, Dunn BR, Meyer TW, Anderson S, Rennke HG, Brenner BM. Prevention of diabetic glomerulopathy by pharmacological amelioration of glomerular capillary hypertension. J Clin Invest 1986;77(6):1925—30.

[152] Zatz R, Meyer TW, Rennke HG, Brenner BM. Predominance of hemodynamic rather than metabolic factors in the pathogenesis of diabetic glomerulopathy. Proc Natl Acad Sci USA 1985;82(17):5963—7.

Glomerular Cell Biology

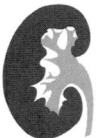

Yoshiro Maezawa[1], Davide Cina[1,2] and Susan E. Quaggin[1,2,3]

[1]Samuel Lunenfeld Research Institute, Mount Sinai Hospital
[2]Institute of Medical Science
[3]Division of Nephrology, St. Michael's Hospital University of Toronto, Toronto, Ontario, Canada

CELL BIOLOGY OF THE GLOMERULUS

Structure and Function of the Glomerulus (Renal Corpuscle)

The glomerulus or renal corpuscle is comprised of the glomerular tuft surrounded by Bowman's capsule and space. The tuft is a specialized microvascular bed which contains three cell types including the fenestrated or sinusoidal glomerular endothelial cells, the visceral epithelial cells known as podocytes, and mesangial cells. The glomerular filtration barrier is made up of the endothelial cells and podocytes together with an intervening glomerular basement membrane, and is the site of formation of the primary urinary filtrate. In the average adult human with normal renal function, 180 L of primary urinary filtrate is formed each day. The filtration barrier must permit free passage of water and small solutes into the urine, while retaining larger macromolecules in the blood. The demands of such "high flux" filtration require that the cell types of the glomerulus exhibit many specialized features, which will be discussed in this chapter.

In all mammals, the renal corpuscle appears as a spherical structure, although its diameter varies to some degree with the size of the organism. In humans, glomeruli are approximately 200 μm in diameter, in elephants 300 μm, in rats 120 μm, and in rabbits 150 μm.[209,215,271] A normal human kidney contains approximately one million individual glomeruli.

The central component of the renal corpuscle is composed of a plexus of sinusoidal or fenestrated capillaries that extend into Bowman's space where the primary urinary filtrate accumulates. The capillary loops are held together by the mesangial cells, and they are covered by a continuous layer of podocytes (Figure 22.1). At the vascular pole, the podocyte layer is continuous with the parietal epithelium of Bowman's capsule. Cells with intermediate phenotypes (between podocyte and parietal epithelium) can be observed at the transition zone. At the urinary pole of the renal corpuscle, the parietal epithelium is continuous with the epithelium of the proximal tubule (Figure 22.2c).

At the site of transition between parietal and visceral epithelium, the afferent and efferent arterioles enter and exit the glomerulus respectively, this is known as the glomerular hilum. After entering, the afferent arteriole branches to form a complex plexus of fenestrated capillaries with loops at the urinary pole.[64,197] The mesangium is required for proper structure and formation of this plexus, and in its absence only a single ballooned capillary loop forms.[64] The capillary loops come into direct contact with the mesangium at discrete points in a small region known as the juxtamesangial portion. However, the majority of the loops are found within Bowman's space and are covered entirely by the glomerular basement membrane and podocyte foot processes.[246] This is the surface area across which filtration occurs. The branches of the afferent arteriole give rise to individual vascular lobules within the glomerular tuft; each of these lobules contains its own afferent and efferent capillary with some connections between lobules. After looping at the urinary pole, the efferent capillaries join to form the larger efferent arteriole, which exits the tuft at the glomerular hilum. Along the length of the efferent arteriole, the

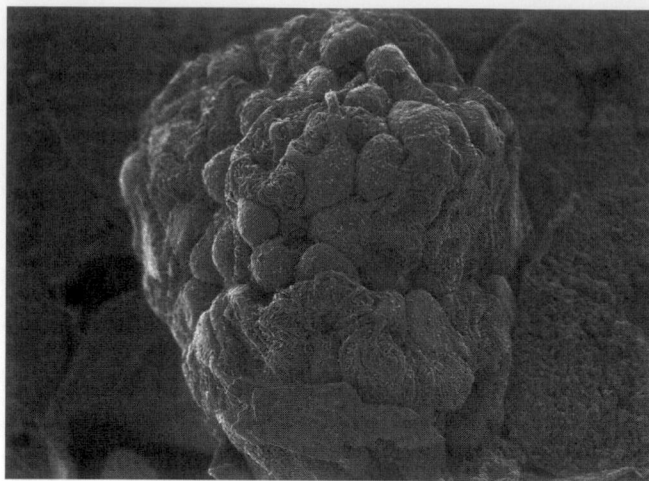

FIGURE 22.1   **Scanning electron micrograph of a normal mouse glomerulus.** Glomeruli are spherical bundles of capillary loops, covered by structurally unique podocytes and their foot processes (SEM × 1900). *(Courtesy of Dr. Marie Jeansson, Mount Sinai Hospital, Toronto, ON.)*

extraglomerular mesangium is gradually replaced by typical smooth muscle cells[64] (Figures 22.3 and 22.4).

GLOMERULAR ENDOTHELIAL CELLS

General Description

Glomerular endothelial cells are large, highly flattened cells that form the innermost layer of the glomerular capillary. Peripherally these cells are extremely thin, and the cell body contains the nucleus and all the cell organelles. The peripheral portions of the endothelial cells contain numerous fenestrae, which are 50−100 nm pores that penetrate the cytoplasm[158,241] (Figure 22.5). The luminal side of endothelial cells is covered by a thick layer consisting of glycoproteins that form "sieve plugs" in the fenestrae and the glycocalyx.[241]

Formation of Glomerular Capillaries

Several transplantation studies have demonstrated that the glomerular capillaries are formed largely by vasculogenesis: endothelial cells are derived from angioblasts believed to be intrinsic to the metanephric mesenchyme.[120,234,235] At E12.5, in mice before the formation of immature vasculature, kinase insert domain receptor (Kdr, also known as vascular endothelial growth factor receptor 2 (Vegfr-2) or Flk-1) positive angioblasts are present in the metanephric mesenchyme.[235] In the S-shaped stage of the developing nephron, immature podocytes start expressing vascular endothelial growth factor-A (Vegfa), thereby attracting Kdr-expressing endothelial cells to migrate to the vascular cleft.[65,68,225] Transforming growth factor-β1 (Tgfb1) induces apoptosis of the endothelial cells and opens the capillary lumens.[73]

Fenestrae and Diaphragms

Ultrastructural analysis demonstrates that diaphragms are often observed in fenestrae of glomerular endothelial cells in rodent embryos. Diaphragmed fenestrae are formed in the S-shaped stage, and then the diaphragms disappear from the capillary loop stage onwards.[121] The main component of the fenestration diaphragm is type II transmembrane glycoprotein plasmalemmal vesicle-associated protein-1 (Pv-1), but its precise function is still unknown.[249] Fenestrae in adult glomerular endothelial cells do not have diaphragms[121] (Figure 22.5); however, fenestrae bridged by diaphragms can be found along the intraglomerular segment of the efferent arteriole and its derivatives.[64] Diaphragms can also be observed in a drug-induced nephritis model, suggesting that diaphragms are required in the development and remodeling of fenestrations, thereby compensating for the immaturity of the barrier function in these settings.[121]

Glycocalyx/Sieve Plugs

The luminal membrane of endothelial cells is covered by a highly negatively-charged layer called the endothelial surface layer (ESL). The relatively dense, membrane-associated part of this layer is called the glycocalyx, and the larger, less compact component is known as the endothelial cell coat (Figure 22.6). The main components of the ESL are glycoproteins, glycoaminoglycans (GAGs), and membrane-associated and secreted proteoglycans.[104] Ultrastructural examinations with sophisticated specialized fixation techniques have revealed that this layer also fills the fenestrae with slit diaphragm-like "sieve plugs".[241] The thickness of the glycocalyx is estimated to be 50−100 nm, and that of the loose endothelial cell coat is considered to be 200−400 nm.[115,129,165,242] The relative importance of the ESL and sieve plug in the glomerular filtration barrier is still controversial.

Functional Maintenance of Glomerular Endothelial Cells: Insights from Studies of Angiogenic Factors

A number of factors are involved in the maintenance of glomerular endothelial structure and function, and coordinate an elaborate cross-talk between endothelial

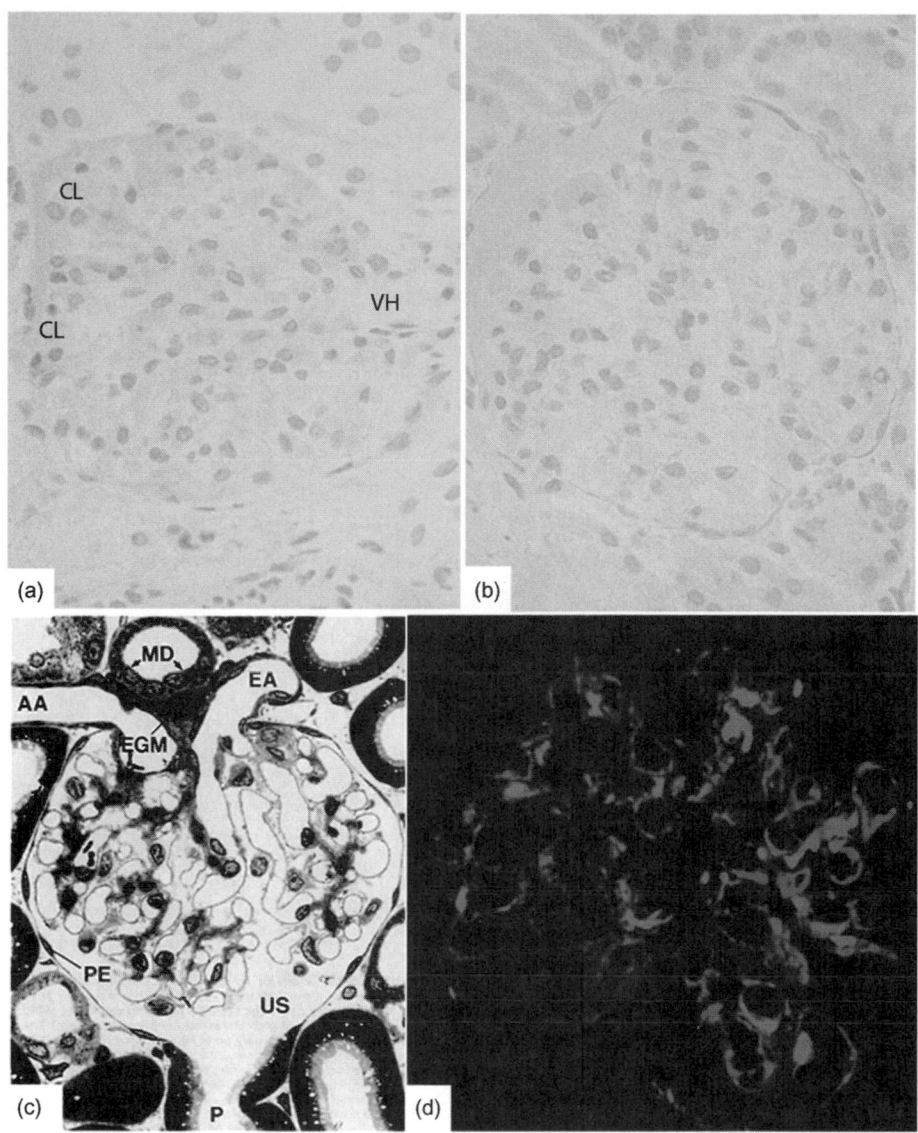

FIGURE 22.2 (a): Histology of normal human glomerulus. Hematoxylin-eosin (HE) staining showing patent capillary loops (CL) and vascular hilum (VH) (LM × 600). (b): Histology of normal human glomerulus. Periodic acid Schiff (PAS) staining (LM × 600). (c): Rat glomerulus sectioned through the vascular pole and the urinary pole. The afferent arteriole (AA), the efferent arteriole (EA), the extraglomerular mesangium (EGM), and the macula densa (MD) can be observed in this section. The orifice of proximal tubule (P) can be seen at the urinary pole (PE: parietal epithelial cells of Bowman's capsule; US: urinary space; LM × 490). (d): Immunostaining shows the three cell types found within the glomerular tuft (mouse glomerulus is shown) (Green: Zo-1 = podocytes; red: CD31 = endothelial cells; yellow: desmin = mesangial cells). The capillary loops are outlined by podocytes. Mesangial cells are located within the capillary tuft and connect capillary loops with each other (× 400). *(a and b: Courtesy of Dr. Paul S. Thorner, The Hospital for Sick Children, Toronto, ON.)* See color section at the back of the book.

cells and other cell types of the glomerulus (Figure 22.7).

Pdgfb/Pdgfrb

Platelet-derived growth factor B (Pdgfb) is secreted from endothelial cells and binds its receptor (Pdgfrb) on mesangial cells.[161,165,272] Pdgfb or Pdgfrb knockout mice have a defect in mesangial migration and a single, dilated glomerular capillary loop[14,161,272] (Figure 22.8). Endothelial specific deletion of Pdgfb results in the same phenotype as that seen in mice with a systemic knockout.[14,166] Also, this paracrine system requires retention of the ligands in the pericellular space, because mutants with deletion of the Pdgfb retention motif demonstrate delayed mesangial migration and, later on, proteinuria and glomerulosclerosis.[69,166]

Vegfa

Vegfa facilitates the formation of fenestrae in cultured glomerular endothelial cells.[67,69] Podocytes produce large amounts of Vegfa that can bind to Kdr on endothelial cells.[67,68] Cell-selective deletion of Vegfa from podocytes demonstrates that Vegfa signaling is required for formation and maintenance of the glomerular vasculature, its fenestrated phenotype and the filtration barrier. Mice treated with soluble fms-related tyrosine kinase-1 (sFlt-1, discussed below), a decoy receptor of Vegfa, show striking attenuation of endothelial fenestration, highlighting the necessity for Vegfa in the maintenance of fenestration[132] (Figure 22.5). In mutant mice that carry a podocyte-specific gene deletion of *Vegfa*, a few endothelial cells migrate into the developing glomeruli but they fail

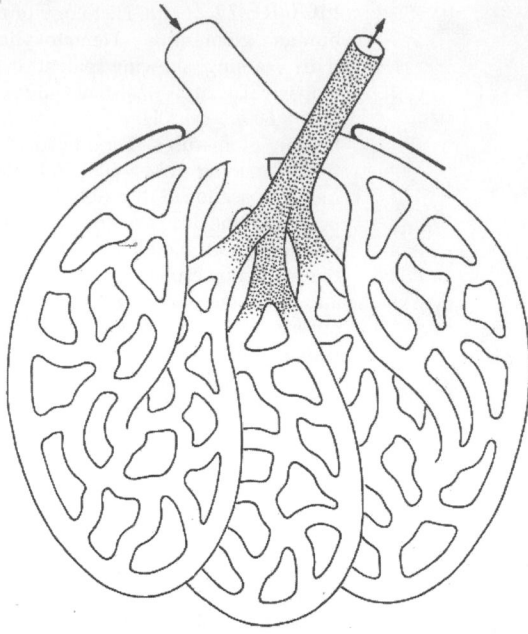

FIGURE 22.3 **Schematic diagram shows the branching pattern of glomerular capillaries.** As soon as the afferent arteriole enters the glomerulus, it divides into two to five branches to form the glomerular capillaries. The capillaries run toward the urinary pole, continuing to branch, and then loop back to the vascular pole to unify and form the efferent arteriole within the glomerular tuft. The efferent arteriole possesses a significant intraglomerular portion (*stippled*), whereas the afferent arteriole does not. *(From Winkler, D., Elger, M., et al. (1991). Branching and confluence pattern of glomerular arterioles in the rat. Kidney Int. Suppl. 32: S2—8, with permission.)*

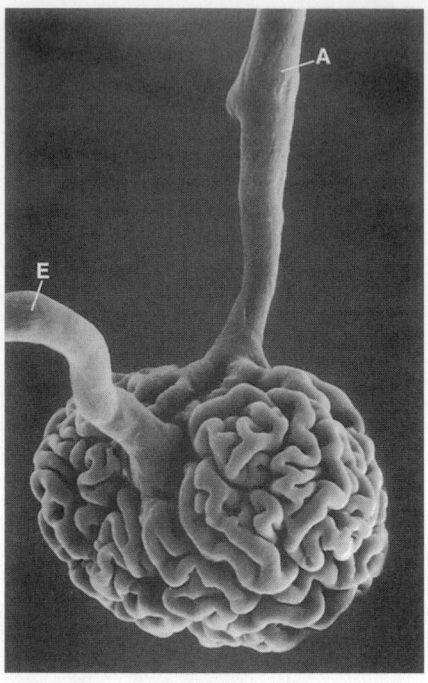

FIGURE 22.4 **Scanning electron micrograph of a glomerular vascular cast.** Afferent (A) and efferent (E) arterioles can be seen.

to develop fenestrations and rapidly disappear, causing renal failure and neonatal death.[67,68] The deletion of one allele of the *Vegfa* gene from podocytes leads to a glomerular defect known as endotheliosis, characterized by endothelial swelling and loss of fenestrations — a universal feature found in thrombotic microangiopathies. Overexpression of the major angiogenic Vegfa 164 isoform in podocytes results in collapse of the glomerular tuft.[67,98] Additionally, patients receiving anti-VEGF therapy may develop proteinuria due to thrombotic microangiopathy (TMA) of the glomerulus with prominent endotheliosis[66,98] (Figure 22.9). Indeed, deletion of *Vegfa* in mature podocytes of adult mice leads to TMA.[66,162] Taken together, these results indicate an indispensable role for Vegfa in the development, maintenance, and function of the glomerular vasculature and filtration barrier. They also highlight the importance of Vegfa paracrine signaling from the podocyte to Kdr on glomerular endothelial cells.

sFlt-1 is an alternatively spliced soluble form of VEGF receptor 1 (VEGFR-1)/Flt-1, and binds to VEGF as a decoy, thereby acting as a potent inhibitor of VEGF activity. Treatment of mice with adenoviral-induced sFlt-1 leads to a massive reduction of endothelial fenestrae[133] (Figure 22.5b). sFlt-1 blood levels are elevated in patients with pre-eclampsia[162,179] and administration of sFlt-1 to pregnant rats causes hypertension and proteinuria with histological glomerular endotheliosis. The endothelium is the most common glomerular region affected in pre-eclampsia,[157,179] suggesting a functional role for sFlt-1 in the function of the glomerular endothelium. A recent study also implicated sFlt-1 in the pathogenesis of PR3-ANCA-associated vasculitis affecting the glomeruli.[157,167]

Tgfb1

Infusion of a neutralizing antibody against transforming growth factor β1 (Tgfb1) to neonatal rats causes a delay in glomerular capillary formation, including the development of fenestrations.[167,173] In the choroid plexus, neutralization of both Tgfb1 and Vegfa leads to decreased cerebral perfusion, vascular thorombi, and a defect of fenestration, which does not occur when either of these treatments are administered individually.[173,279] Thus, Tgfb1 also plays a crucial role in the development and maintenance of glomerular endothelial cells, and may work in concert with Vegfa. Additionally, blood levels of soluble endoglin, an antagonist of Tgfb1 are elevated in patients with preeclampsia, and correlate with disease severity. Administration of soluble endoglin in combination with sFlt-1 to pregnant rats results in severe pre-

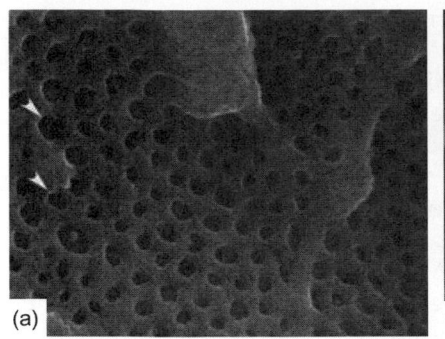
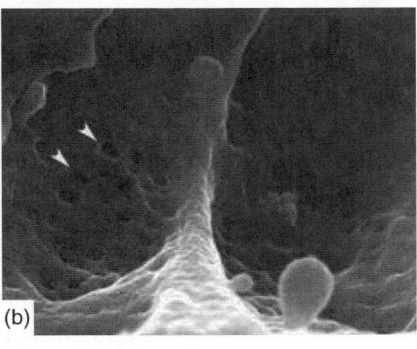

FIGURE 22.5 (a): Scanning electron micrograph shows the inner surface of a healthy glomerular capillary and its beautifully fenestrated endothelium. (B): Endothelial fenestrae are largely reduced after 14 days treatment of mice with soluble Flt-1 (SEM × 18,000). *(From Kamba, T., and McDonald, D. M. (2007). Mechanisms of adverse effects of anti-VEGF therapy for cancer. British Journal of Cancer **96**: 1788–1795, with permission.)*

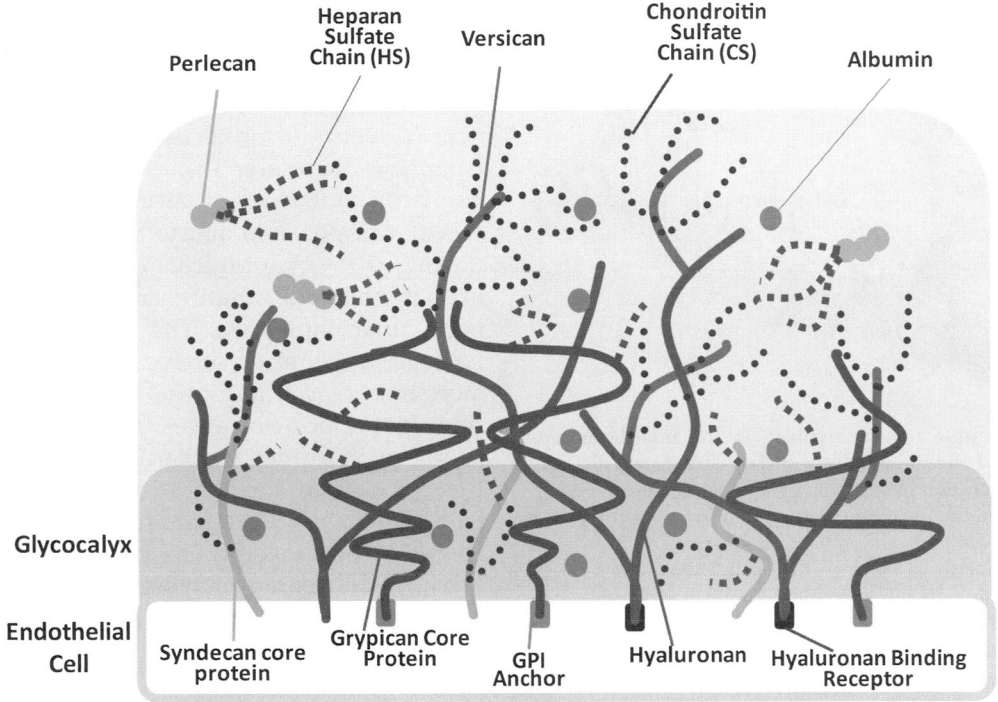

FIGURE 22.6 **Schematic diagram showing the endothelial surface layer (ESL).** The relatively dense part of the layer close to the endothelial cells form the glycocalyx, which consists of membrane-bound proteoglycans (PG), including syndecan and glypican. Syndecan carries both chondroitin sulfate (CS) and heparan sulfate (HS) side chains, and glypican carries HS side chains. The ESL is comprised of secreted proteoglycans such as perlecan (mainly HS) and versican (mainly CS), as well as secreted glycosaminoglycans (GAG) including hyaluronan. It also traps some plasma proteins such as albumin. *(Modified from Haraldsson, B., Nystrom, J., and Deen, W. M. (2008). Properties of the glomerular barrier and mechanisms of proteinuria. Physiol. Rev. **88**: 451–487, with permission.)*

eclampsia, including HELLP syndrome (hemolysis, elevated liver enzymes, and low platelets).[292]

Angiopoietins

Another family of angiogenic factors required for the development and homeostasis of glomerular endothelial cells is the Angiopoetin–Tek signaling system. Angiopoietin 1 (Angpt1) and Angiopoietin 2 (Angpt2) are ligands for Tek tyrosine kinase (Tek/Tie-2). Angpt1 binds to the Tek receptor expressed on endothelial cells, and causes its phosphorylation. This signal leads to enhanced survival of endothelial cells, stabilization of the endothelial cell-to-cell connection, and reduced permeability.[174,253,279] Angpt2 is considered to be a competitive antagonist of Angpt1 by binding Tek but not activating any intracellular signaling.[174,253,320] There is some data, however, that suggests that Angpt2 can activate Tek signaling under certain conditions.[319,320] Angpt1, Angpt2 and Tek are all expressed in developing kidneys.[319] Angpt1 is expressed widely in the condensing mesenchyme in the developing kidney and its derivatives,[250,319] and in mature podocytes.[250,318] Angpt2 shows a more restricted expression pattern, localizing to endothelial cells, pericytes, smooth muscle cells of cortical and large blood vessels, and immature mesangial cells.[318,319] Tek is expressed both in mature and immature glomerular endothelial cells.[279,319] Angpt1 conventional knockout mice die at embryonic day 12.5, thus precluding any analysis of its role in the glomerular vasculature.[146,279] In mouse metanephric organ culture, recombinant Angpt1 enhances the growth of interstitial capillaries.[146,247] A recent report demonstrated that Angpt1 treatment of

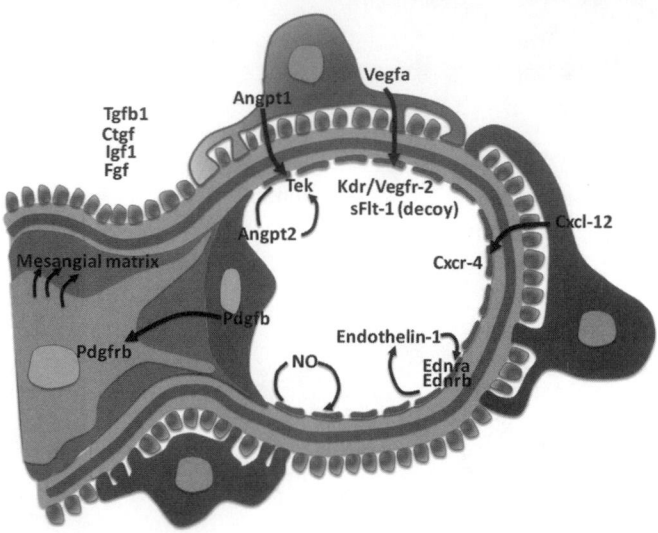

FIGURE 22.7 Soluble factors involved in the maintenance of endothelial cells and the glomerular capillary structure. Schematic diagram shows the location of secretion of soluble factors, and where the associated receptors are expressed. Vegfa from podocytes is required for the recruitment, survival, and maintenance of the endothelial cells, and binds to its receptor Kdr. sFlt-1 works as a decoy, but its precise function is still unknown. Angpt-1 is expressed in podocytes and binds to the endothelial Tie-2/Tek receptor in a paracrine fashion, whereas its antagonist, Angpt-2 is secreted from endothelial cells and binds to the Tie-2/Tek receptor in an autocrine fashion. Cxcl12 is secreted from podocytes and interstitial cells, and acts on Cxcr4 in endothelial cells to regulate vascular development and function. Pdgfb secreted by endothelial cells signals to the Pdgfrb receptor expressed by mesangial cells, and is a critical factor for their migration and maintenance. Endothelial cells also express some vasoactive factors including NO and endothelins. Expression of growth factors such as Tgfb, Ctgf, Igf, and Fgf are increased in disease conditions such as diabetic nephropathy, but their precise functions under normal conditions are still unclear.

isolated rat glomeruli reduced vascular permeability and increased the depth of the glycocalyx layer.[159,247] Cell type-specific/inducible knockout approaches, however, have revealed a crucial role for Angpt1 in glomeruli. Deletion of Angpt1 at E10.5 leads to a single, dilated glomerular capillary loop without mesangial migration in a portion (~10%) of glomeruli that is reminiscent of the Pdgfb/Pdgfrb mouse mutant phenotype (Figure 22.10a,b). Although deletion of Angpt1 after E13.5 doesn't cause any immediate vascular phenotype, streptozotocin-induced diabetic mice with global or glomerular-specific Angpt1 deletion develop increased urinary albumin excretion, severe mesangial expansion, glomerular sclerosis, and early mortality (Figure 22.10c,d). Another report also demonstrated that treatment of diabetic mice with Angpt1 recombinant protein is protective for renal function.[127,159] Angpt1 is therefore dispensable in quiescent, mature glomeruli, but is essential in development and in the vascular response to injury.[80,127,217]

Angpt2 knockout mice are briefly viable in the postnatal period, and exhibit increased pericyte coverage of peritubular capillaries. The mice die soon after birth however, precluding analysis of the role of Angpt2 in more mature capillary beds.[52,80,217] Angpt2 overexpression in podocytes causes proteinuria and podocyte apoptosis in formed glomeruli.[52,308]

Angiopoietin ligands seem to function in concert with Vegfa. In Vegfa-rich conditions, Vegfa and Angpt2 work together to promote sprouting.[84,299,308] The precise degree of cross-talk between these pathways is still under investigation.

Ephrin-Eph Family

Ephrin-Eph molecules are another family of tyrosine kinase signaling factors that are widely expressed in the developing kidney. In other organs, they are involved in the specification of arteries and veins, as well as in neural development.[84,282,299] In the developing kidney, the Ephrin B2 ligand is expressed in podocyte precursors, but later it is expressed by endothelial

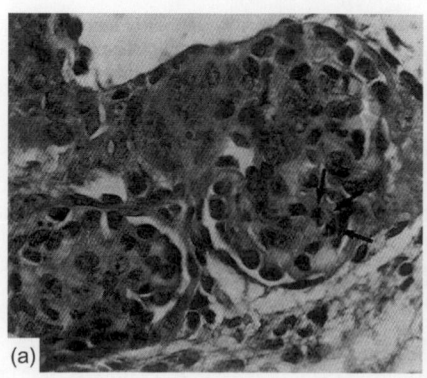 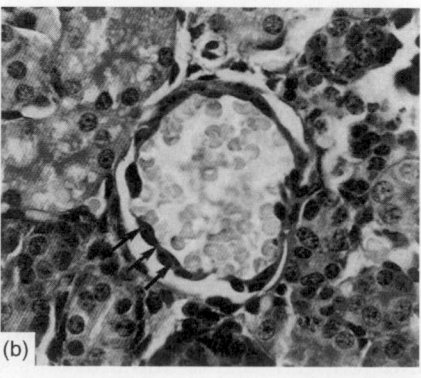

FIGURE 22.8 PAS stain of glomeruli from E17.5 mouse embryos. (a): Normal mouse glomerulus. Arrows show normal fold of the basement membrane. (b): Pdgfb−/− glomerulus shows a single open aneurysm-like capillary loop without any mesangium (failure of mesangial migration). There is no fold of basement membrane (arrows). (*From Betsholtz, C. (1995). Role of platelet-derived growth factor in mouse development. Int. J. Dev. Biol. 39: 817–825 with permission.*) See color plate section at the back of the book.

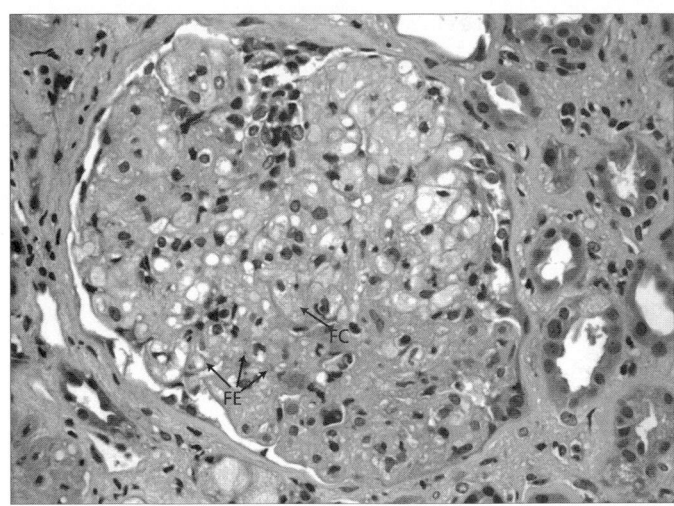

FIGURE 22.9 A glomerulus showing thrombotic microangiopathy from a patient who received anti-VEGF therapy, showing fragmentation of erythrocytes (FE: arrows) and foamy change (FC: arrow) of endothelium. *(Courtesy of Dr. Laura Barisoni, New York University School of Medicine, New York, NY.)* See color plate section at the back of the book.

and mesangial cells.[282,307] In adults, the EphB4 receptor is mainly expressed in podocytes.[5,307] Overexpression of the EphB4 receptor causes defects of glomerular arteriolar formation.[5,307] Deletion of Ephrin B2 from Pdgfrb-expressing pericytes and the mesangial cell population results in abnormal glomerular tuft formation.[7,76] Pharmacologic inhibition of EphB4 leads to delayed recovery and extended injury of endothelial cells and podocytes in a rat mesangial injury model.[280,307] Therefore, it seems this family is involved in glomerular tuft formation and maintenance, but the precise mechanism is still unclear.

CXCR4/CXCR7/CXCL12 Axis

Chemokine CXC motif receptor type 4 (CXCR4), CXCR7, and Chemokine CXC motif ligand 12 (CXCL12) are also critical factors in the development and maintenance of glomerular vasculature. Cxcr4 and Cxcr7 are seven-transmembrane G-protein coupled receptors, and Sdf-1/Cxcl12 is their cognate chemokine ligand.[7,281] A deficiency of Cxcr4 or Cxcl12 leads to a

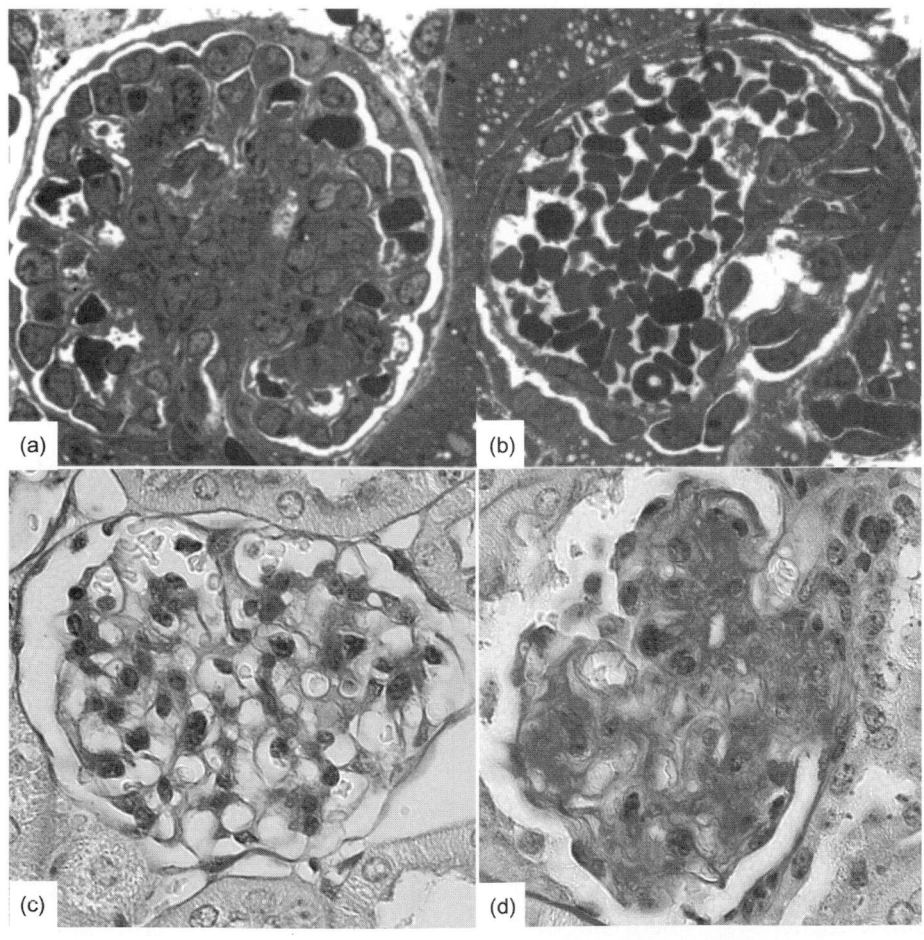

FIGURE 22.10 **Conditional deletion of Angpt1 results in glomerular developmental defects and enhanced diabetic glomerular injury.** (a): A normal glomerulus at embryonic day 17.5 (E17.5). (b): Early conditional deletion of Angpt1 gene at embryonic day 10.5 (midgestation) results in some abnormal glomeruli with single open capillary loops similar to that of Pdgfb-null mouse at E17.5. (c) and (d): Late deletion of Angpt1 at E16.5 doesn't lead to any immediate phenotype. However, after 20 weeks of streptozotocin-induced diabetes, the diabetic mutant mice that carry Angpt1 deletion show an increase in mesangial matrix expansion and sclerosis (d) compared with that of diabetic controls (c) (LM × 1000). *(Courtesy of Dr. Marie Jeansson, Mount Sinai Hospital, Toronto, ON.)* See color plate section at the back of the book.

failure of vasculogenesis and embryonic lethality.[55,280] During renal development, Cxcr4[−/−] or Cxcl12[−/−] knockout mice show a ballooning of the glomerular capillary loops which is reminiscent of Pdgfb/Pdgfrb knockout mice.[51,251,281] On the other hand, activation of the CXCR4/CXCR7/CXCL12 axis appears to underlie some glomerular diseases, such as rapidly progressive glomerulonephritis (RPGN),[55,216] diabetic nephropathy,[51,251,281] and hemolytic uremic syndrome (HUS).[116,212,216] It appears that Cxcl12 is secreted from podocytes or interstitial cells, and acts on Cxcr4 expressed by the endothelial cells to regulate vascular development and function.[212,281]

Glomerular Endothelial Cells as a Source of Vasoregulators

Glomerular endothelial cells produce both nitric oxide, a vasodilator, and endothelin-1, a vasoconstrictor. Nitric oxide is produced by NO synthases. Both endothelial and inducible NO synthases are expressed by glomerular endothelial cells *in vitro* and *in vivo*.[116,212,288,310] eNOS expression and activation is at least partially influenced by Vegfa.[212,288] In many rodent disease models and human patients with kidney diseases, overproduction of NO and its derivatives has been observed.[116,288,310] It is considered that excessive NO production generated by inducible NO synthase (iNOS) results in glomerular injury, whereas NO generated from endothelial NO synthase (eNOS) is protective by preserving endothelial survival and function.[200,288,324] In diabetic patients, eNOS expression is increased in renal endothelial cells, whereas iNOS expression is preferentially upregulated in inflammatory cells. The degree of eNOS expression is related to the severity of the glomerular lesion and proteinuria.[116,286] Diabetic eNOS knockout mice develop more severe glomerular lesions and greater albuminuria.[114,200,324] In addition, excretion of NO-related products is often reduced in diabetic patients with nephropathy.[286,305]

Endothelin-1 is a potent vasoconstrictor which binds to one of two receptors: endothelin receptor type A (Ednra); and endothelin receptor type B (Ednrb). Binding of endothelin-1 to Ednra results in vasconstriction, while binding to Ednrb causes vasodilation.[114,315] In glomerular endothelial cells, Ednrb is dominant, whereas Ednra is expressed by mesangial cells.[71,305]

Glomerular endothelial cells are also involved in the renin−angiotensin−aldosterone system (RAAS). They express angiotensin-converting enzyme (ACE) and produce angiotensin II.[63,315] The relative contribution of the glomerular endothelium compared to the systemic endothelium with regard to angiotensin II production, however, is still unknown. Furthermore, the potential role of angiotensin receptors in endothelial cells is also unknown.

Summary

Glomerular endothelial cells form the first permselective barrier in the glomerulus. The relationship between their elaborate, fenestrated cell shape and function is maintained by a network of various angiogenic factors. Glomerular endothelial cells also contribute to the charge-selective barrier through the negatively-charged glycocalyx.

MESANGIAL CELLS

Description

Mesangial cells are irregularly shaped cells which extend processes from their cell body towards the glomerular basement membrane (GBM). The "mesangium" refers to the mesangial cells together with the mesangial matrix they produce[71,141] (Figures 22.11 and 22.12). Mesangial cells provide structural support to the glomerular tuft, produce and maintain mesangial matrix, communicate with other glomerular cells by secreting soluble factors, and may contribute to the glomerular capillary flow via their contractile properties.

Mesangial Cells Provide Structural Support to the Glomerular Tuft

The mesangium forms the central core of the glomerular tuft. The processes which they extend towards the GBM are densely populated by bundles of actin, myosin, and β-actinin microfilaments.[63,152] These processes attach directly or by interposition of microfibrils to the GBM. They also extend underneath glomerular endothelial cells toward the mesangial angles of the GBM, anchoring two opposing mesangial angles together through their microfilament bundles (Figure 22.12b). These microfilament bundles cross the mesangial cells to tether opposing parts of the GBM through α3β1 integrin and the basal cell adhesion molecule (BCAM) glycoprotein, which bind laminin α5 in the GBM.[141] These structures are believed to supply protection from hydraulic pressure by providing inward-directed tension.[152]

Mesangial Cells Produce and Maintain Mesangial Matrix

The *mesangial matrix* fills the remaining spaces between the mesangial cells and the perimesangial glomerular basement membrane (GBM, for review

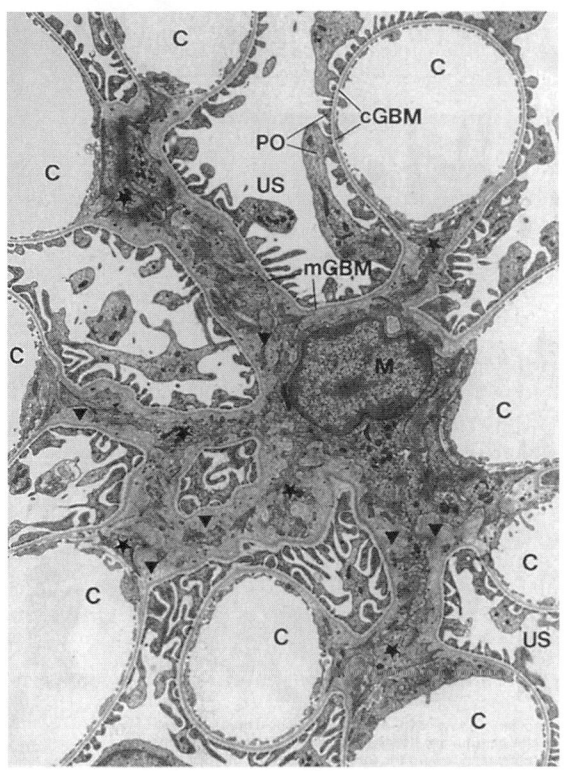

FIGURE 22.11 **Transmission electron micrograph showing all components of the glomerular tuft.** The glomerular tuft is marked by the GBM, which includes the pericapillary GBM (cGBM; between podocytes and the endothelium) and the perimesangial GBM (mGBM; between podocytes and mesangium). Glomerular capillaries (C) are covered by podocytes at the periphery, and connected to the mesangium, proximally. The mesangial cell body (M) possesses several processes (some are marked by *stars*) which extend toward the peripherally located capillaries. In the mesangial area, abundant mesangial matrix (*triangles*) can be seen (US: urinary space; TEM × 5500).

see [152]). This matrix is composed of a diverse array of common matrix proteins including collagens type III, IV, V, and VI; heparan sulfate proteoglycans including biglycan and decorin[252]; and the elastic fiber proteins fibronectin, laminin, entactin, and fibrillin-1, among others.[42,87,172,177,276] Fibronectin is the most abundant of these, and is associated with microfibrils which network to form the basic ultrastructure of the matrix.[42,260] These microfibrils are unbranched and non-collagenous with a diameter of 15 nm, and form a dense three-dimensional network that contributes to the anchoring of mesangial cells to the GBM.[152] It is thought that these microfibrils allow for the transmission of mesangial cell contractile forces to the GBM.

Mesangial phenotypic changes are a hallmark of certain glomerular diseases such as diabetic nephropathy. This condition is characterized by glomerular sclerosis due to an accumulation of mesangial matrix and thickening of the GBM. The sclerotic lesion contains an abundance of type IV collagen normally present in the glomerulus, but also contains types I and III collagen which are usually absent but are produced by injured mesangial cells.[175]

Signaling Molecules Involved in Mesangial Cell Biology

Integrins

In addition to α3β1 integrin observed in connections between the GBM and mesangial processes, α1β1, α2β1, and fibronectin receptors α5β1 and α8β1 integrins are expressed in the mesangial cells,[13,142] and are able to activate integrin-linked cell signaling. In the

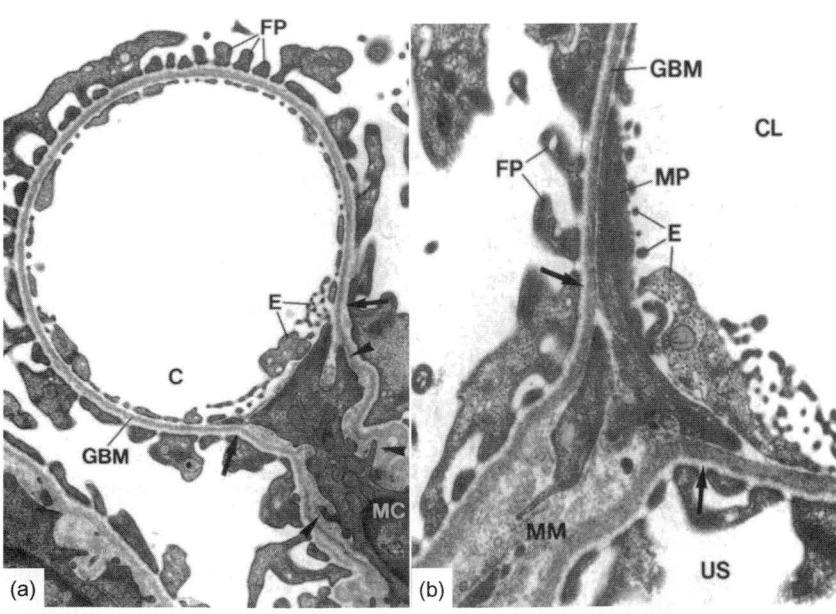

FIGURE 22.12 (a): Transmission electron micrograph showing a mouse glomerular capillary. A mesangial cell (MC) extends its processes to a capillary loop (C). Microprojections (*arrowheads*) from the primary process run toward the glomerular basement membrane (GBM). As shown by arrows, the endothelial cells are directly connected to the mesangium. Podocyte foot processes (FP) and fenestrated endothelium (E) are shown (TEM × 13,500). (b): High magnification of the juxtamesangial part of the capillary loop showing direct contact of mesangium to endothelium. Endothelial cells are attached to the mesangial cell processes (MP) that connect opposing mesangial angles. (arrows) (CL: capillary lumen; US: urinary space; MM: mesangial matrix; FP: foot processes; TEM × 23,000).

absence of α1 integrin, cultured mesangial cells show decreased proliferation, increased matrix production, and altered intracellular signaling. Mice lacking α1 integrin exhibit more severe Adriamycin and diabetes-induced glomerular injury,[34,323] highlighting the importance of matrix-related signaling. On the other hand, removal of α2 integrin in mice leads to amelioration of glomerular damage in an Adriamycin and partial renal ablation model.[18] α8 integrin seems to promote adhesion, but inhibits migration and proliferation of mesangial cells *in vitro*.[13]

Pdgfrb

Pdgfb is secreted from endothelial cells and binds to Pdgfrb expressed in mesangial cells, where it exerts a crucial role in mesangial migration and glomerular tuft formation. Without mesangial cell migration, the looping of glomerular capillaries does not occur. This interaction is discussed further in the endothelial section.

Ephrin B2

As mentioned in the section on the glomerular endothelium, deletion of Ephrin B2 from mesangial cells and pericytes leads to abnormal glomerular tuft formation and reduced numbers of capillary loops.[76] It's receptor, EphB4 is expressed in podocytes, suggesting an interaction between the mesangium and podocytes.

Other Secretary Molecules and Receptors

Mesangial cells produce, and are also influenced by, many growth factors including Tgfb1,[257] connective tissue growth factor (Ctgf),[44,297] insulin like growth factor (Igf),[220,221] fibroblast growth factor (Fgf),[75,221] and hepatocyte growth factor (Hgf).[46,48] Among these factors, Hgf antagonizes the pro-fibrotic actions of Tgfb1, whereas the other factors are upregulated by mesangial cells in disease conditions including diabetes or Thy1.1 nephritis, and facilitate glomerular matrix accumulation.[75,297] Vasoactive factors such as angiotensin II and endothelins promote mesangial proliferation, and this effect may be mediated by transactivation of the Egf receptor.[54,118] However, because of the lack of effective tools for deleting genes specifically from mesangial cells, the precise functions of these factors in normal physiology remain to be determined.

Contractile Ability of Mesangial Cells

Because of the microfibrils and the contractile ability of cultured mesangial cells, it has been assumed that the mesangial cells regulate glomerular filtration by controlling the capillary surface area, but concrete *in vivo* evidence is lacking.[85]

THE GLOMERULAR BASEMENT MEMBRANE

Description

The glomerular basement membrane (GBM) is a specialized extracellular matrix that sits between the podocytes and vascular side of the filtration barrier. During glomerulogenesis, components of the GBM are synthesized by both the glomerular endothelial cells and podocytes, forming a bilayered structure that later fuses.[189] Compared to basement membranes in other tissues the GBM is unusually thick, measuring 240−370 nm in adults.[189,210,274] Ultrastructural analysis of the mature GBM shows a trilaminar structure made up of a lamina densa surrounded by the lamina rara interna and externa, which appear less dense.

Similar to other basement membranes, the GBM is primarily made up of laminin, collagen type IV, nidogen, and heparan sulfate proteoglycans. However, the GBM contains different members of some of these families compared to other basement membranes, including laminin-521, collagen a3a4a5(IV), and agrin.[2] Laminin and collagen type IV appear to be particularly important for function of the GBM, as mutations in these factors are associated with glomerular filtration defects and renal disease.[189] Components of the GBM are continuously "turned over",[1] but it is not yet clear how new components are added and old ones removed.

Given the location of the GBM between the relatively "open pores" of the endothelium and the podocyte foot processes and filtration slits bridged by the slit diaphragms, a major role for the GBM is to restrict the passage of plasma proteins into Bowman's space. From the time of classic electron micrographic studies of the GBM in the 1950s attempting to define the specific characteristics of the GBM that impart its permselective properties, to the current molecular era, it is still hotly debated which component represents the major barrier. Current models suggest that all three layers of the filtration barrier are likely important (including the glycocalyx of the endothelial layer), but relative contributions remain unknown. However, it is clear that mutations in genes encoding specific GBM proteins are sufficient to cause proteinuria and renal failure, underscoring the importance of this layer to the barrier.[189]

Laminin

Laminins are secreted as heterotrimers, which are stabilized by disulfide interchain bonding. Each laminin heterotrimer is composed of α, β, and γ chains that combine with each other in nonrandom combinations to form at least 15 different heterotrimers. The laminins are named by their composition; for example: α5β2γ1 is named laminin-521 or LM-521.[40,192] The heterotrimer structure appears as a "cross" with one longer and three shorter arms. At the COOH end of all α chains is a laminin globular chain (LG) that extends beyond the long arm. This LG domain interacts with cell surface receptors such as integrins and dystroglycans that are expressed by the podocytes.

Interactions between the laminin heterotrimers themselves are mediated by subdomains found in the shorter arms of the "cross." Laminin also binds to the network of type IV collagen via nidogen, and to agrin, a heparan sulfate proteoglycan of the GBM.[189] The combined network of type IV collagen (see below) and laminin provides mechanical properties to the basement membrane, serving as a scaffold for the placement of other matrix components.

During glomerular formation, laminin trimer compostion changes from LM-111 to LM-511, and finally to LM-521.[150,187,192] In the adult, laminins continue to be produced by both endothelial cells and podocytes, as the protein can be identified in the endoplasmic reticula of both cell types.[273]

A series of reports confirm an important role for laminins in GBM function. A mutation of laminin β2 results in Pierson syndrome in humans that is characterized by ocular and neurological symptoms, and congenital nephrotic syndrome.[204] This observation was confirmed using knockout mice of laminin β2 that develop proteinuria even before the onset of visible ultrastructural changes to the podocytes.[125] Recently, the phenotype of the laminin β2 knockout mouse was rescued by overexpression of laminin β1, suggesting redundancy between laminin β1 and β2.[117] Also, deletion of laminin α5 in mice prevents the transition from LM-111 to the mature LM-521 that leads to breakdown of the GBM and failure of glomerular vascularization.[185] A mouse carrying a hypomorphic mutation of laminin α5 also shows glomerular proteinuria, hematuria, and cystic kidneys, suggesting the gene dosage of the laminin α5 chain is crucial for the maintenance of the GBM.[119]

Type IV Collagen

Collagen IV is another major component of the GBM. Similar to other collagens, collagen IV is a trimeric extracelluluar matrix component made up of α chains that are rich in Gly-X-Y amino acid repeats.[119,154] The type IV collagen family includes six genetically distinct α chains that trimerize with each other in specific combinations to make three types of trimers with each other: (α1)₂α2; α3α4α5; and (α5)₂α6. Each of these trimers is referred to as a protomer. Protomers are secreted into the extracellular matrix, where they self-polymerize and are subsequently cross-linked by specific enzymes.[188]

Similar to laminin, the composition of type IV collagen trimers undergoes a developmental switch in the GBM. Early in glomerulogenesis (S-shaped stage), the GBM is composed of α2/α1 chains, which are replaced at the capillary loop stage by α3α4α5.[3] Although a basement membrane can form in the absence of type IV collagen its structure is compromised, resulting in variable defects in the filtration barrier depending on the specific genetic mutation.[188] In the adult kidney, the type IV collagen α3α4α5 network is produced only by podocytes.[3]

Mutations in any of the α3, α4 or α5 genes are associated with glomerular disease in patients, emphasizing the key role that type IV collagen plays in glomerular barrier function. The defects can be minimal, as observed in patients with thin basement membrane disease (also known as benign familial hematuria). This disease is inherited in an autosomal dominant fashion, and patients present with isolated microscopic hematuria. As suggested by its name, the GBMs show thinning. Thirty to forty per cent of the patients exhibit mutations in COL4A3 or COL4A4. Although originally assumed to be benign, FSGS has been reported in Cypriot families with this disease.[295]

The same mutations in COL4A3 and COL4A4 inherited in a homozygous fashion as an autosomal recessive disease result in a more severe disease known as Alport's syndrome, a hereditary basement membrane disease associated with progressive glomerulopathy that leads to renal failure, and is associated with deafness and ocular abnormalities. The commonest form of Alport syndrome is X-linked, caused by mutations in the α5 chain (Figure 22.13). Goodpasture syndrome, an autoimmune disease characterized by glomerulonephritis and lung hemorrhage, is mediated by antibodies against the type IV collagen α3 chain.[119]

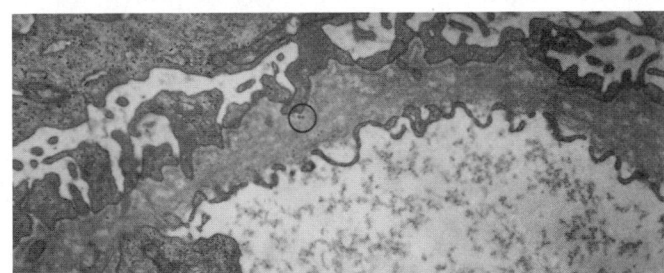

FIGURE 22.13 Transmission electron micrograph of the GBM in a patient with Alport syndrome. Thickening, splitting and lamination of the GBM can be seen (TEM × 14,900). *(From Rumpelt, H. J. (1987). Alport's syndrome: Specificity and pathogenesis of glomerular basement membrane alterations. Pediatr. Nephrol. **1**: 422–427, with permission.)*

Intriguingly, recent studies have shown that a mutation of the type IV collagen α1 chain causes hereditary angiopathy with nephropathy, aneurysms, and muscle cramps (HANAC syndrome); the renal manifestations are characterized by hematuria and large bilateral cysts.[107] A rodent model of this mutation leads to defects of the GBM,[89] suggesting a functional role for the α1 chain in the GBM, despite the prominence of a3a4a5 trimers in mature type IV collagen.

Nidogen

Nidogen-1 and -2 (previously known as entactin-1 and entactin-2) are virtually ubiquitous basement membrane glycoproteins. Nidogen-1 binds both laminin and type IV collagen,[77] suggesting that it is involved in forming the GBM. However, it was demonstrated that a single knockout of either nidogen-1 or nidogen-2 in mice results in no GBM phenotype.[199,262] Although deletion of both nidogen genes results in perinatal lethality, suggesting some overlapping roles of the two genes,[11] the glomerular basement membrane still forms apparently normally. The exact role and requirement of nidogen in the GBM is not yet known.

Proteoglycans

Heparan sulfate proteoglycans of the GBM are concentrated in the laminae rarae internae and externae, and provide an electronegative charge to the GBM.[136,277] The major proteoglycans of the GBM are heparan sulfate proteoglycans; most prominent is agrin, but perlecan is also present.[92,205] Although classical studies suggested that the negative charge of the GBM was essential to retard passage of neutral and negatively-charged macromolecules across the barrier, this model has been challenged due to results obtained from genetically modified mice. Podocyte-specific knockout mice for agrin and/or perlecan, either in isolation or together, does not result in proteinuria or overt filtration defects.[88,108] Current thoughts on the glomerular charge barrier are discussed later in the chapter.

PODOCYTES

Podocyte Morphology

Mature podocytes are highly-differentiated, polarized epithelial cells that sit on the glomerular basement membrane in Bowman's space. They function as vascular support cells, wrapping around the underlying glomerular capillaries, providing growth factors necessary for endothelial health and survival. Podocytes are characterized by a highly arborized and unique cytoskeleton. They have a large cell body (Figure 22.14a) that gives rise to a complex network of processes including primary, major processes, which then continue to branch as they extend around the glomerular capillary loops until they form terminal foot processes. The foot processes are the only point of contact between the podocyte and the GBM (Figure 22.15a). The foot processes of neighbouring podocytes interdigitate (Figure 22.14b), and are connected to one another through a specialized intercellular junction known as the slit diaphragm (SD). The SD bridges the porous filtration slits; these structures have been recently visualized at high magnification[79,236] (Figures 22.14b, and 22.15b). In disease, these structures can be dysregulated, causing a disorganization of foot processes and breakdown of the GFB (Figure 22.15c,d).

While the podocyte is terminally differentiated and largely post-mitotic, the podocyte cell body contains a number of organelles that are crucial to maintain its high metabolic activity and secretory function, including a large nucleus, abundant lysosomes, and many mitochondria.[196] In addition to producing factors necessary for maintaining their own specialized architectural cytoskeleton and protecting adjacent endothelial cells, podocytes must synthesize many of the components of the GBM in the mature glomerulus (reviewed in [189]).

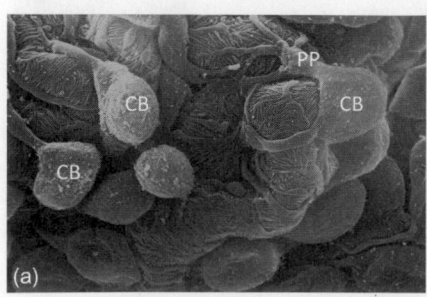
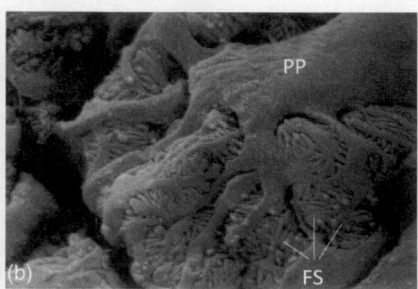

FIGURE 22.14 Scanning electron micrograph shows podocytes wrapping around glomerular capillary loops. (a): Mouse podocytes have a large, smooth-surfaced cell body (CB) which branches into primary processes (PP), which continue to branch as they wrap around the capillary loop forming the actin-based foot processes (SEM × 5600). (b): Scanning electron micrograph of rat podocytes. The filtration slits are created between the interdigitating foot processes, the terminal ends of the branching processes (FS) (SEM × 5670). (Courtesy of Dr. Monika Wnuk, Mount Sinai Hospital, Toronto, ON.)

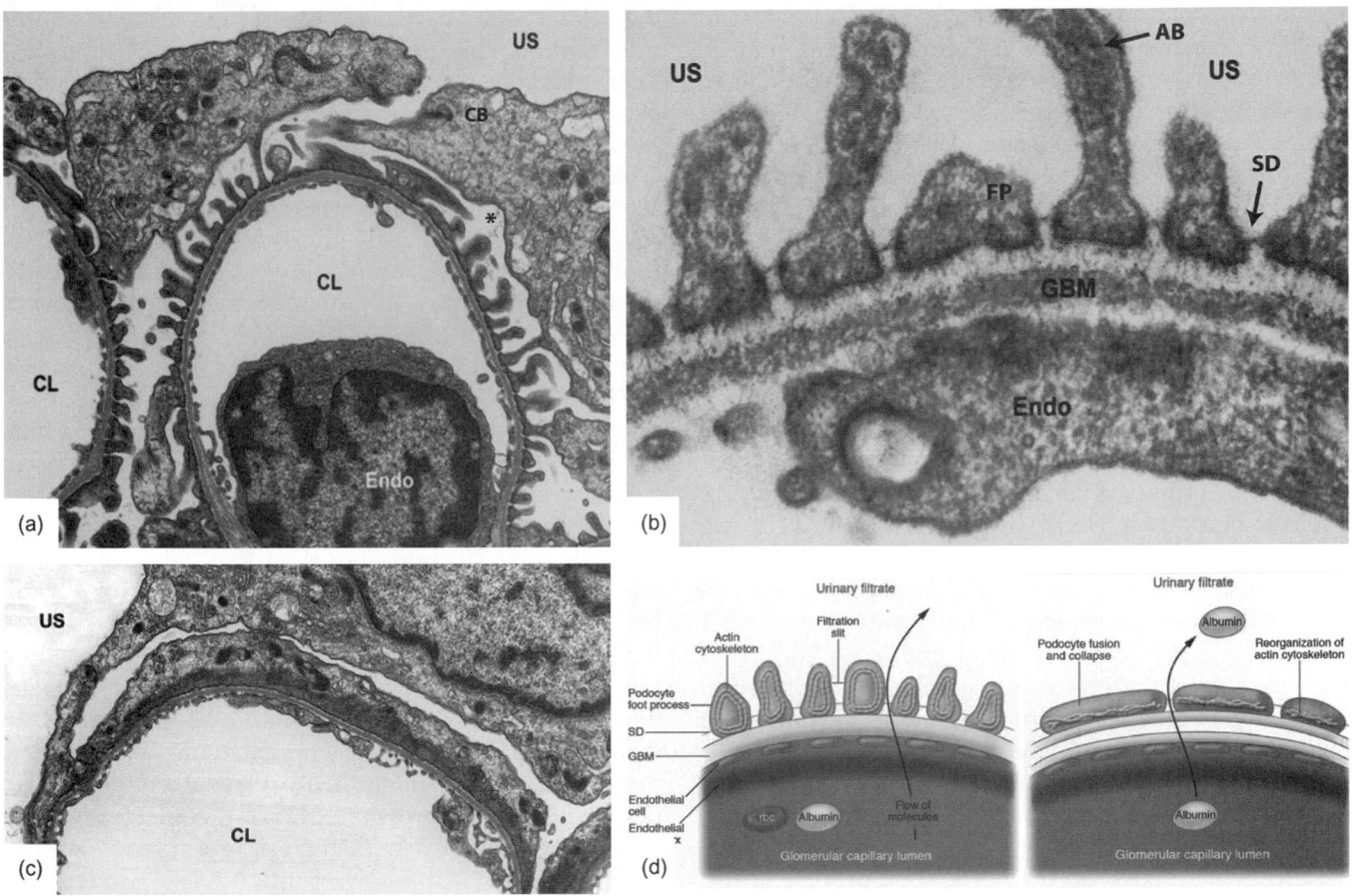

FIGURE 22.15 Transmission electron micrograph of a normal and abnormal human podocytes. (a): Coronal section of a podocyte intimately associated and lining a glomerular capillary loop (CL) cell body (CB) can be seen. Note the space (*) between the cell body and the basement membrane as the foot processes are the only point of contact between the podocyte and the GBM. (b): High power transmission EM shows podocyte foot processes (FP) attached to the glomerular basement membrane (GBM). Foot processes contain actin bundles (AB), and adjacent foot processes are attached by their slit diaphragms (SDs). (c): Transmission electron micrograph of podocyte foot process effacement in human focal segmental glomerulosclerosis (FSGS). (d): Scheme of podocyte foot process flattening. Left panel shows normal podocyte foot processes, actin cytoskeleton supports its elaborated shape. Once the actin cytoskeleton is disorganized, podocytes are no longer able to keep the foot process assembly, which results in fusion and flattening of foot processes (right panel). *((a)–(c): Courtesy of Dr. Dontscho Kerjaschki, Medical University Vienna, Vienna, Austria; (b): From Ronco, P. (2007). Proteinuria: Is it all in the foot? J. Clin. Invest. 117: 2079–2082, with permission.)* See color plate section at the back of the book.

The structure of the cell body and the primary major processes is determined by microtubules and intermediate filaments (vimentin, desmin, and nestin), while the shape (width and length) of the foot processes is largely determined by actin microfilament bundles. The actin bundles form continuous loops that run longitudinally in the foot processes and end at the sole plates, connecting adjacent foot processes associated with a single, primary, major process (Figure 22.15b). The loops of actin bundles are tethered to the microtubules and intermediate filaments of the major processes.[196] This connection is thought to be mediated by Tau, which is known to form connections between microtubules and microfilaments and is concentrated at these areas.[145] In the foot processes, a complex system links the slit diaphragm proteins, GBM receptors on the basolateral side, and the actin cytoskeleton to regulate the functional morphology of podocytes; this will be discussed at greater length later.

Podocyte Development, Transcription Factors, and Notch

Podocyte precursors first appear in the "S-shaped body" phase of glomerular development as a columnar epithelium attached along their lateral membrane by a cadherin junction containing P-cadherin.[36] This nascent glomerulus is also populated by a thin epithelial layer called the Bowman's capsule, and a capillary loop that begins to enter the glomerular cleft. As glomerular development progresses, the primitive podocytes extend themselves around the capillary loop by an unknown mechanism and differentiate into mature podocytes. A number of transcription factors have been identified that are expressed in the immature and mature podocytes, including Wt-1, Pod1 (Tcf21), Lmx1b, Kreisler (Maf1), and Foxc2.

Wt-1

The transcription factor Wt-1 is first expressed in the metanephric mesenchyme, which contains progenitors of the tubular and glomerular epithelium. As renal development continues, its expression becomes restricted to the renal vesicle, comma, and the S-shaped body. Later on, its expression is observed in immature and mature podocytes, which persists throughout life.

Wt-1 is a transcription factor with four zinc fingers that can bind both DNA and RNA.[24,25,61] There are four major splice variants of Wt-1 mRNA, which may be responsible for its variety of functions in development and normal physiology.[99] Embryonic loss of Wt-1 in mice leads to complete renal and gonadal agenesis,[149] defects in the epicardium, lack of sub-epicardial mesenchymal cells, and adrenal agenesis,[194] suggesting its important role in multiple organs.

Several mouse models underscore the importance of Wt-1 function during nephrogenesis and in podocytes. Postnatal deletion of the Wt-1 gene results in glomerulosclerosis with loss of podocyte foot processes and molecular markers of differentiation such as nephrin, atrophy of the exocrine pancreas and spleen, severe reduction in bone and fat mass, and failure of erythropoiesis.[30] In Wt-1 knockout mice, restitution of Wt-1 expression using a human derived Wt-1-YAC transgene leads to a rescue of cardiac defects, but incomplete glomerular development.[194] Furthermore, Wt-1 haploinsufficient mice develop adult onset mesangiosclerosis and glomerulonephritis.[96,184]

In humans, Wt-1 mutations are associated with two glomerulopathies: Denys–Drash syndrome (DDS) and Frasier syndrome (FS), which can both present early in life and cause abnormal glomerular development. DDS is caused by heterozygous mutations of the Wt-1 gene that predominantly affect the zinc finger regions in exons 8 (zinc finger II) and 9 (zinc finger III), and directly interfere with the DNA-binding capacity of Wt-1.[214] The characteristic clinical picture of DDS is a triad of congenital nephrotic syndrome, XY pseudohermaphroditism, and Wilm's tumor.[53,59] The characteristic renal lesion in these patients is diffuse mesangiosclerosis due to increased matrix deposition on the vascular side of the glomerular basement membrane. Expression of the DDS mutation in mice, either in podocytes or systemically, leads to various glomerular lesions similar to those of humans. Wt-1 is expressed in podocytes, which are found on the opposite side of

the glomerular basement membrane (GBM) to the mesangium. The glomerular lesion in DDS therefore highlights the importance of interactions that occur between podocytes on one side of the GBM and endothelial cells or mesangial cells on the other side of the GBM. Frasier syndrome (FS) is characterized by focal segmental glomerular sclerosis, male-to-female sex reversal, but no tumors. It results from a dominant mutation that causes an inability to include an alternatively spliced lysine-threonine-serine (KTS) sequence after the third zinc finger[102] of Wt-1. Interestingly, mice engineered to exclusively express the variant that is +KTS or −KTS display normal induction of the metanephric mesenchyme by the ureteric bud, but have malformed glomeruli. These findings suggest different roles for the alternatively spliced variants of Wt-1 in glomerular development and maintenance.

While the contribution of Wt-1 to renal development and maintenance is undeniable, its precise role is still being elucidated. Human and animal models seem to indicate it plays a role in regulating the expression of a number of developmental genes. During early renal development the regulatory gene Pax-2 is expressed in the induced metanephric mesenchyme and ureteric bud, but is absent in the mature renal epithelium. In podocytes, the expression of Wt-1 coincides with a downregulation of Pax-2, suggesting a role for Wt-1 in transcriptional repression of this gene.[244] Indeed, in patients with DDS, downregulation of Wt-1 was associated with increased Pax-2 expression[311]; however, it is unclear if this increased Pax-2 expression is pathogenic. Recent advances in high-throughput technology for assessing transcription factor activity have elucidated a number of other Wt-1 regulated genes that are known to play a role in renal development, including Six2, Bmp7, Sall1, and HeyL.[107]

Wt-1 also plays a role in maintaining podocyte homeostasis beyond development. The essential podocyte slit diaphragm protein nephrin has been identified as a transcriptional target of Wt-1, and is downregulated in the glomeruli of mice lacking the Wt-1(−KTS) splice variant.[95,298] Furthermore, Wt-1 modulates the podocyte glycocalyx through transcriptional regulation of Podocalyxin[213] and 6-O-endosulfatases Sulf1 and Sulf2,[259] which play a role in maintaining the charge of the glomerular filtration barrier, podocyte foot process separation, and bioavailability of essential growth factors such as vascular endothelial growth factor-α (Vegfa) and fibroblast growth factor (Fgf)-2. In addition to post-translational regulation of Vegfa bioavailability, Wt-1 can also directly regulate expression of Vegfa, which is essential to the maintenenance of the glomerular vasculature.[103,107] Given this wide range of regulatory functions, it is still unclear what is responsible for the pathology observed in DDS and FS patients, but it is likely a convergence of a number of these signaling networks.

Lmx1b

Lmx1b encodes a Lim-domain protein that is mutated in Nail–Patella syndrome.[31,60] In mice lacking Lmx1b, podocytes retain their immature cuboidal phenotype, fail to form foot processes or endothelial fenestrations, and have a split glomerular basement membrane.[237] These findings are associated with a concomitant downregulation of Vegfa, Synaptopodin, Nphs2, type III collagen α4 (Col3a4), and type IV collagen α4 (Col4a4). Lmx1b-binding elements in the Nphs2 and Col4a4 promoter regions suggest that this occurs through direct transcriptional regulation.[191,237]

Tcf21

Tcf21 (also known as Pod1/Capsulin/Epicardin) encodes a basic helix-loop-helix transcription factor that is highly-expressed in the developing kidney, lung, intestine, and pancreas at sites of mesenchymal–epithelial interaction.[224] In the developing mouse kidney, it is expressed in the condensing mesenchyme, and knockdown of Tcf21 expression in renal explants causes decreased mesenchymal condensation and ureteric bud branching.[224] Subsequently, *Tcf21* expression is restricted to the primitive podocytes of the S-shaped bodies, and genetic deletion of Tcf21 in mice leads to failure of podocyte terminal differentiation[223] (Figure 22.16). Tcf21[−/−] knockout mice have a marked reduction in glomerular number, and the remaining glomeruli are developmentally arrested between S-shaped body and capillary loop stages.

Kreisler

Kreisler (Mafb) encodes a basic domain leucine zipper transcription factor that is expressed in podocytes at the capillary loop stage of glomerular development.[245] Mice with a homozygous enu mutation of Kreisler show a similar but milder phenotype to those with a Tcf21 deletion. They are born with glomeruli arrested at the capillary loop stage, and podocytes that adhere to the GBM but fail to form foot processes.[245]

Kreisler mutants, however, express Tcf21, suggesting that Tcf21 is either upstream of Kreisler in podocyte development or acts by a different mechanism.

Foxc2

Foxc2 is a winged helix transcription factor that was identified during a screen of enriched genes in mRNA isolated from glomeruli at different stages of development.[284] Foxc2 is first expressed in putative podocytes during the comma shaped body stage of glomerular development, and as such is the earliest known podocyte marker. Glomeruli from Foxc2[−/−] mice display aberrant podocyte foot process formation, mesangial cell clustering at the base of the glomerular tuft, and swollen endothelial cells lacking fenestrae,[284] similar to Tcf21[−/−] mutant mice. In these mice, the endothelial and mesangial defects are thought to be secondary to the podocyte defects. Gene array of Foxc2[−/−] glomeruli identified over 700 differentially regulated genes. Notably, however, there was a strong downregulation of Nphs2, Col4α3, and Col4α4, which are fundamental to slit diaphragm assembly and GBM formation.

Notch

The Notch family includes four well-conserved genes that encode transmembrane receptors involved in cell fate specification and development from invertebrates to mammals. Notch is fundamental in the segmentation of the metanephric mesenchyme into 20 functionally-distinct cell types segregated into different compartments along the nephron.

During normal development, Notch2 is expressed in condensing structures of the metanephric mesenchyme, such as the metanephric vesicles, comma-shaped bodies, and S-shaped bodies, but is eventually restricted to differentiating podocytes in more mature glomeruli.[181] Jag1 is the Notch2 ligand thought to be important for glomerular differentiation. During development, it is expressed in renal vesicles, comma-shaped bodies, and S-shaped bodies.[32] In more mature glomeruli it then localizes to the inner region of the glomerular tuft to endothelial and/or mesangial cells.[181] Mice homozygous for a hypomorphic mutation

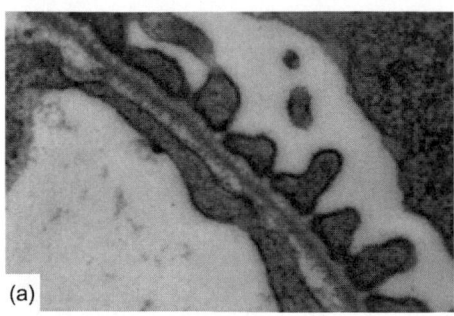 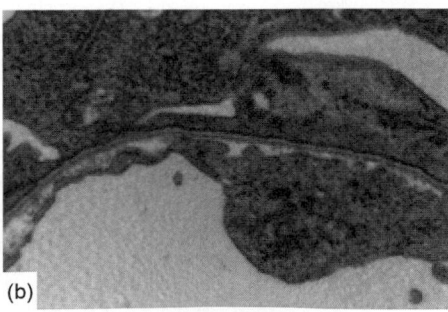

FIGURE 22.16 Transmission electron micrograph of podocyte foot processes at E18.5. Normal mouse podocytes show organized foot processes assembly (a), whereas Tcf21 null mouse podocytes demonstrate defects of foot process development (b).

(a)   (b)

in the *Notch2* gene exhibit hypoplastic kidneys, and an arrest of glomerular development prior to the capillary loop stage.[181] A conditional inactivation of Notch2 from nephron progenitor cells results in a more severe "distal tubule only" phenotype, with a complete failure of glomerulogenesis and proximal tubule formation.[35]

In humans, mutations in Jag1 or Notch2 cause Alagille syndrome, an autosomal dominant disorder characterized by the presence of cholestatic liver disease, cardiac disease, ocular abnormalities, skeletal abnormalities, and characteristic facial features.[164,182,206] A large proportion of Alagille patients also develop renal disease characterized by glomerular lesions, cystic kidneys, and ultimately renal failure.[182] Taken together these studies suggest an important role for Notch signaling in establishing the proximal–distal orientation of the nephron, and segmentation of the proximal structures.

Recent evidence also reports a crucial role for the Notch pathway in the maintenance of mature podocytes. In patients with a variety of proteinuric nephropathies, including diabetic nephropathy and FSGS, activation of the Notch pathway was observed in podocytes.[198,202] Furthermore, upregulation of Notch expression in podocytes of transgenic mice results in severe proteinuria and glomerulosclerosis with dedifferentiation of podocytes.[300]

Podocyte Slit Diaphragm Assembly

The attachments between foot processes are comprised of the "slit diaphragm" (SD). SD assembly is an important part of glomerular development, as it is integral to the correct interdigitation of podocyte foot processes. The SD, which is visible by high power electron microscopy, is a structure that connects adjacent foot processes. It consists of a complex of transmembrane proteins and cytoskeletal adaptor proteins that link adjacent foot processes to the complex actin cytoskeleton of the podocyte and make up a component of the protein barrier (reviewed in [101,115,129,242,289]). While the relative importance of the endothelial layer versus the glomerular basement membrane versus the podocyte SD in maintaining the perm-selectivity of the glomerular filtration barrier is debatable, studies in humans and mice have shown that SD components are essential to this function.

In 1974 Rodewald and Karnovsky described the slit diaphragm as rod-like units connected in the center to a linear bar forming a zipper-like pattern with pores.[76,236] They hypothesized that because of the size of these pores (40 Å × 140 Å), the slit-diaphragm was the principal filtration barrier to plasma proteins in the kidney.

Nephrin

While this first description of the SD shed light on the filtration function of podocytes, the molecular composition of the SD remained poorly-defined. However, the discovery that a mutation in the *NPHS1* gene causes Congenital Nephrotic syndrome of the Finnish variety[143,160] suggested that dysregulation of SD structure can cause glomerular disease. This disease is characterized by massive proteinuria *in utero*, lack of a slit diaphragm, and abnormal foot process formation. The *NPHS1* gene encodes a 180 kDa transmembrane protein of the immunoglobulin superfamily called nephrin that is expressed in the glomerular podocyte, and localizes specifically to the SD.[117,243] These findings defined the importance of nephrin to the formation and maintenance of a normal SD, and led to the postulation of a "zipper-like model" of nephrin assembly in the SD. Accordingly, it is considered that the SD is the principle structure of the glomerular filtaration barrier and nephrin is its main component. Subsequent work, however, has also elucidated an important role for nephrin as a mediator of actin cytoskeletal organization by binding Src homology domain SH2/SH3 containing Nck adaptor proteins.[131] The cytoplasmic tail of nephrin contains three tyrosine-aspartic acid-x-valine (YDxV) residues which, when phosphrylated by Src family kinases, recruit the SH2 Nck adaptor proteins and induce local actin polymerization[15] (Figure 22.17). Following the identification of nephrin, intensive research has led to the discovery of several other transmembrane proteins that participate in the formation of the slit diaphragm (Figure 22.18).

Podocin

NPHS2 is a gene that is mutated in some forms of steroid-resistant nephrotic syndrome[19] that cause early onset proteinuria, and focal and segmental glomerulosclerosis. This gene encodes a protein called podocin, which associates in podocyte lipid rafts with nephrin and another SD component, CD2AP, via its C-terminal domain.[163,261,268] Nephrin is thought to contribute directly to the formation of the SD, while podocin and CD2AP are thought to mediate its connection to the podocyte actin cytoskeleton. Mouse models in which any of these three components are disrupted lead to a congenital nephrotic syndrome.[222,239,269]

Neph Proteins

The C-terminal domain of podocin also interacts with another group of three immunoglobulin superfamily transmembrane proteins called Neph1, 2, and 3 that bear significant homology to nephrin. This family is defined by their well-conserved cytoplasmic tail with a centrally located tyrosine residue required for

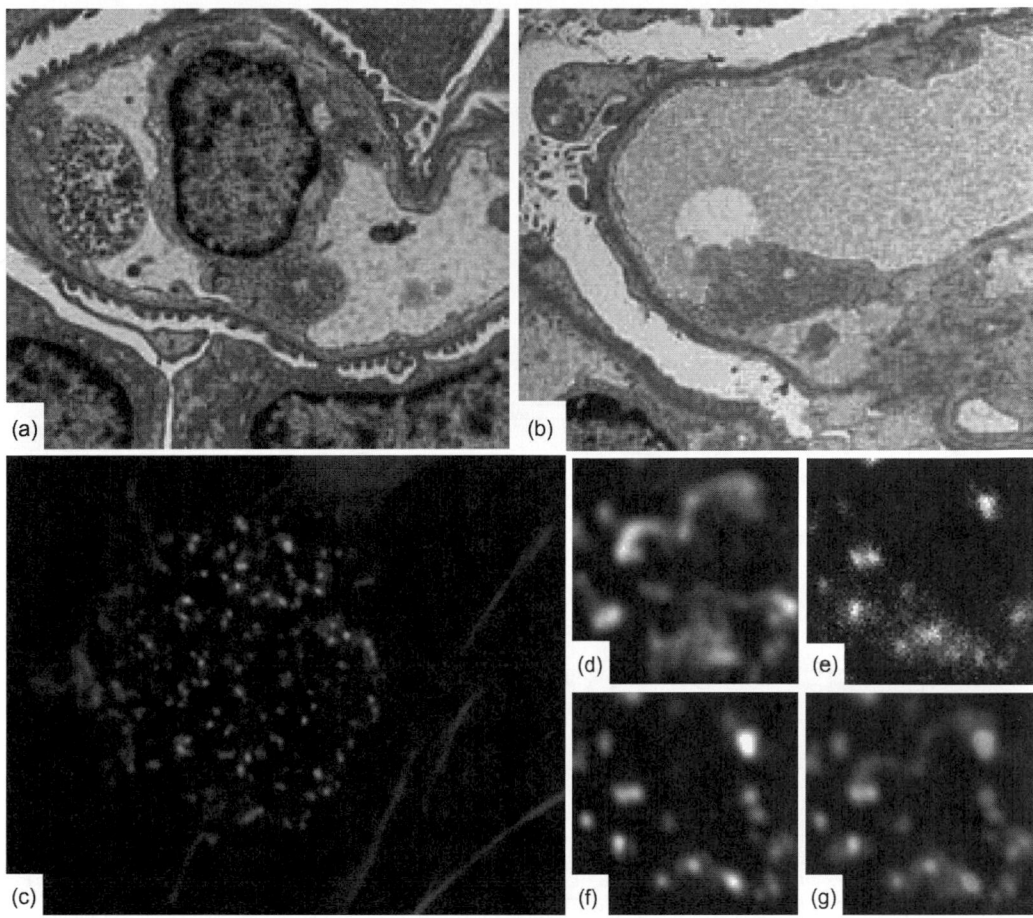

FIGURE 22.17 Transmission electron micrograph of distinct mouse podocyte foot-processes present at 4 days of birth (a), but absent in Nck knockout mice (b). (c)−(g): Cellular immunostaining showing co-localization of Nck2, nephrin at the actin tail. Nck-nephrin interaction is required for nephrin-dependent actin reorganization (Green: nephrin; purple: Nck2; red: palloidin = actin). (d), (e), and (f) show actin, nck2, and nephrin staining, respectively. *((a) and (b): From Jones, N., et al. (2006). Nck adaptor proteins link nephrin to the actin cytoskeleton of kidney podocytes. Nature **440**: 818−823, with permission; (c)−(g): Courtesy of Drs. Tony Pawson and Nina Jones.)* See color section at the back of the book.

interacting with podocin.[265] The extracellular domain of Neph1 interacts with nephrin in the SD, and is essential for the regulation of glomerular perm-selectivity.[168] In addition to podocin, the C-terminal (intracellular) domain binds the tight junction protein-1 (Tjp-1/ZO-1), which in turn tethers it to the podocyte actin cytoskeleton.[168] Like nephrin, Neph1 plays a role in intracellular signaling, and is tyrosine phosphorylated at the SD, particularly in certain disease models.[105] Mutations in Neph1 result in proteinuria and perinatal lethality in mice, but the phenotype is less dramatic than that observed in nephrin knockout mice, suggesting that nephrin may be more crucial to maintain the SD.[57] This Nephrin-centric view of the slit diaphragm was called into question by a recent study showing that chickens and developing chicks lack nephrin, but express all three Neph proteins.[296] Ultrastructurally, however, chickens are still able to

assemble a SD in the glomerular filtration barrier. These SDs lacking nephrin still express P-cadherin and the large protocadherin Fat-1, suggesting that heterophilic interactions between Neph proteins and these other cadherins may be sufficient to allow SD assembly.[190]

Cadherin and Catenins

In addition to these atypical junctions, the slit diaphragm contains adherens junction proteins P-cadherin, and α, β, γ catenins.[230] P-cadherin is a transmembrane protein, and the extracellular domain is thought to contribute to slit diaphragm formation, while its cytoplasmic tail connects to β or γ catenin. Linkage of this complex to the actin cytoskeleton is believed to occur through an interaction between α catenin and Tjp-1/ZO-1 or α-actinin-4, both of which can directly bind actin.

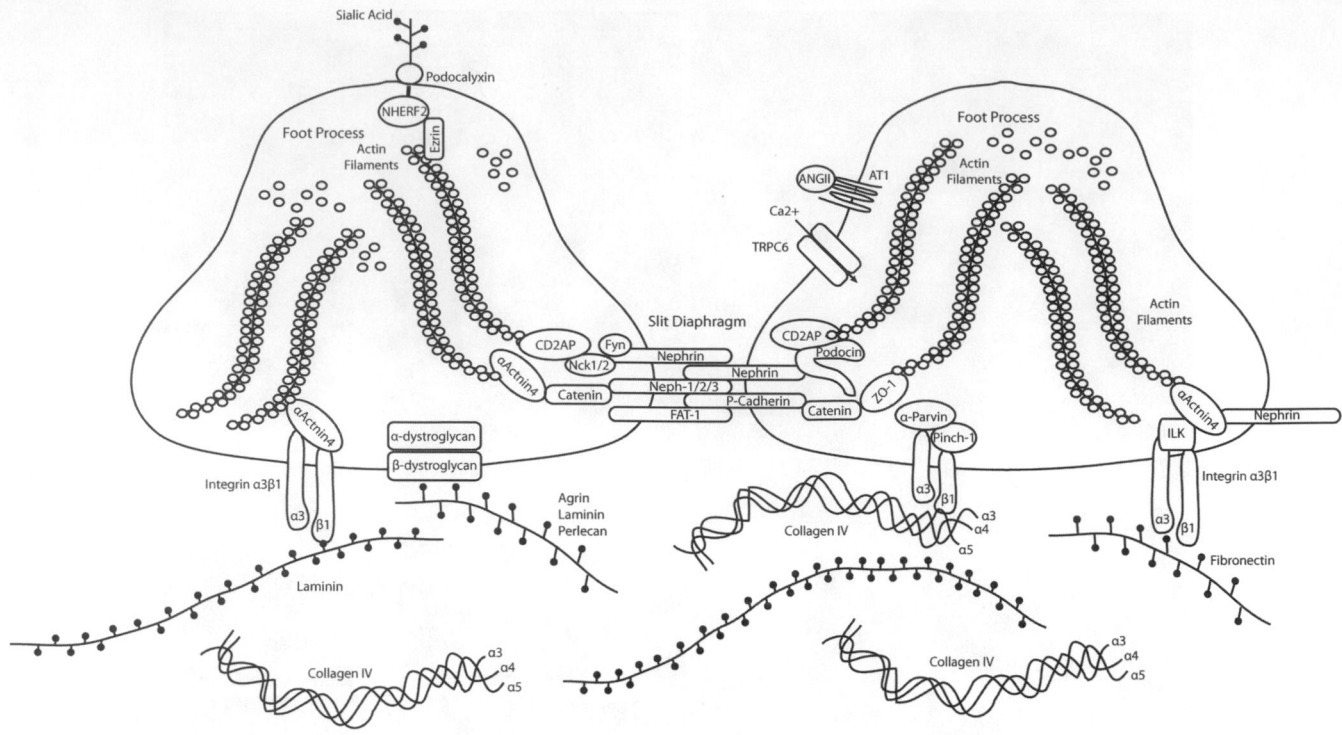

FIGURE 22.18   Schematic diagram of the podocyte foot process and slit diaphragm with associated molecules.

The occludens protein Tjp-1/ZO-1 is expressed specifically at the points of insertion of the slit diaphragms in mature glomeruli.[256] Tjp-1/ZO-1 appears early on in podocyte development when the apical junctional complexes between podocytes are composed of typical tight and adherens junctions, and persists as these junctional complexes migrate to the basolateral side and ultimately form the SDs. These findings suggest that tight junction proteins play a role in podocyte SD development and function, independent of their ability to form tight junctions.

α-Actinin-4

In humans, mutations in α-actinin-4 result in an autosomal dominant familial FSGS.[111,137] *In vitro* the mutant form of α-actinin-4 binds F-actin more strongly than wild-type. This is thought to reduce the podocytes' ability to respond dynamically to the hydrostatic pressure required for normal glomerular filtration, and ultimately leads to podocyte injury.[303] In addition, α-actinin-4 is thought to mediate the interaction between the actin cytoskeleton and integrins to regulate podocyte adhesion to the glomerular basement membrane.[50]

FAT1

FAT1 is another member of the cadherin superfamily expressed in the podocyte at the SD, and has 34 tandem cadherin-like extracellular repeats. With its large extracellular domain, FAT1 is a major molecular component of the SD, and is required for normal foot process formation as FAT1 knockout mice lack SDs.[37,123] Because of its localization to the cell–cell contact sites and tips of cellular processes, FAT1 may be involved in the initial steps of cell–cell interaction between podocytes.[313]

Rho GTPases

Given the actin rich nature of the podocyte cytoskeleton, it is not surprising that Rho GTPases — master regulators of cytoskeletal dynamics — are important in podocyte biology. At the leading edge, Rac1 and Cdc42 promote lamellipodia and fillipodia formation, thus enhancing cell motility. In contrast, RhoA promotes a contractile phenotype by inducing formation of actin-myosin stress fibers.[70,227] In this sense, it is believed that a balance between the opposing activities of RhoA and Cdc42/Rac1 regulates podocyte cytoskeletal dynamics. Both overexpression and inhibition of these small Rho GTPases in podocytes causes glomerular injury in mouse models. Podocyte-specific deletion of Cdc42 leads to a congenital nephropathy in transgenic mice by impairing actin polymerization at sites of nephrin clustering[263] (Figure 22.19), while RhoA deletion does not result in proteinuria. By contrast, overexpression of RhoA in podocytes results in an FSGS phenotype in mice.[325]

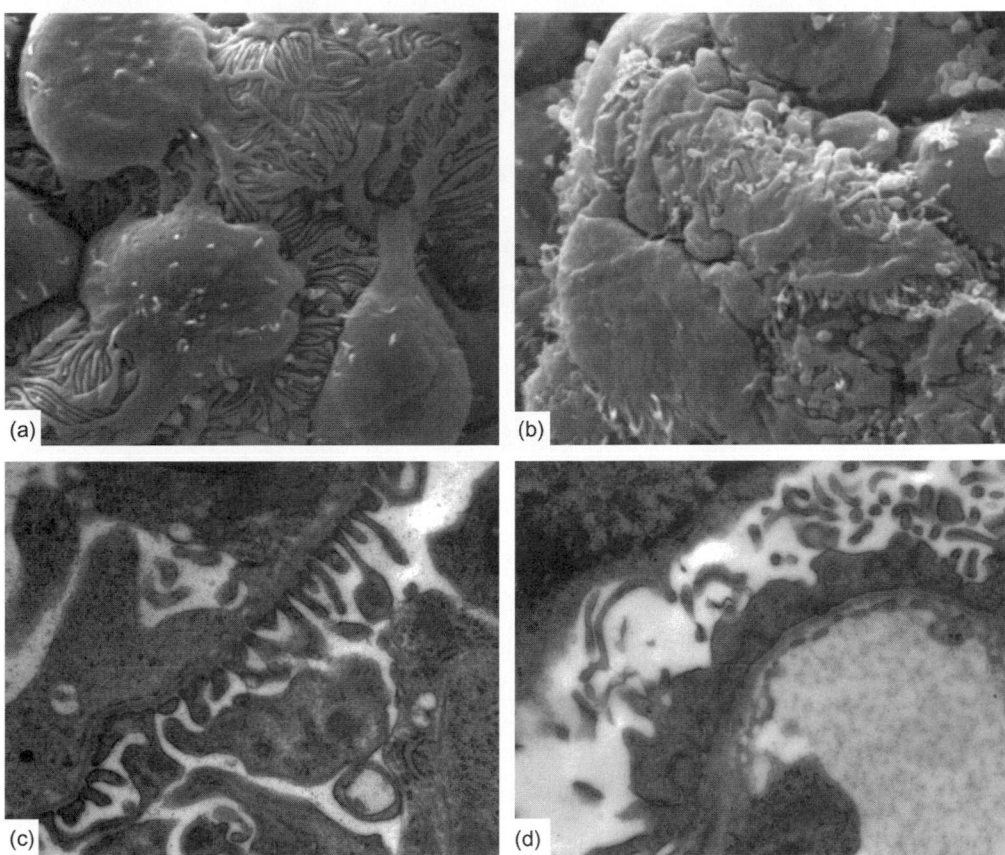

FIGURE 22.19 Scanning ((a) and (b)) and transmission ((c) and (d)) electron micrograph of murine podocytes. (a) and (c): Normal appearance of podocytes. (b) and (d): Podocytes lacking Cdc42 show extensive effacement of foot process at postnatal day 5 ((a), (b) × 11, 000; (c), (d) × 27,000). *(From Scott, R. P., et al. (2012) Podocyte-specific loss of Cdc42 leads to congenital nephropathy. J. Am. Soc. Nephrol.* **23***(7): 1149–1154 with permission.)*

Recently, dysregulation of Rho-GTPase signaling has also been linked to human glomerular disease. *ARHGAP24* is a RhoA-activated Rac1 GTPase-activating protein (Rac1-GAP); a mutation that impairs Rac1-GAP activity results in FSGS in humans.[4] Two recent reports also showed that mutations in the Inverted Formin 2 (*IFN2*) gene result in autosomal dominant FSGS.[20,82] INF2 interacts with other diaphanous related formins such as Cdc42; disease causing mutations in *INF2* result in decreased CDC42 targeting to the plasma membrane, and impaired actin polymerization and depolymerization in podocytes.[20]

Podocyte–GBM Interaction

The podocyte actin cytoskeleton is not only required for formation of podocyte foot processes and the slit diaphragm, but is also involved in a dynamic and bidirectional cross-talk with the glomerular basement membrane (GBM). In addition to production of GBM components, podocytes also express transmembrane molecules on their basolateral surface which interact with the GBM to regulate intracellular signaling. These include α3β1 integrin, αvβ3 integrin, and α- and β-dystroglycans.

α3β1 Integrin

α3β1 integrin is a heterodimeric cell adhesion receptor with specificity for collagen types I and VI, laminins, fibronectin, and nidogen.[147] α3β1 integrin is highly-expressed on the basolateral surface of mature and developing podocytes, and plays an important role in the development and maintenance of podocyte foot processes.[147,228] Mice with a targeted mutation of the α3 integrin gene lack podocyte foot processes, and have a reduced number of capillary loops.[148] Furthermore, the podocyte-derived basement membrane fails to fuse with the endothelium-derived basement membrane and becomes fragmented and disorganized. A recent paper reported three paediatric patients who have mutations in *ITGA3*, which encodes α3 integrin; they presented with congenital nephrotic syndrome and severe basement membrane abnormalities.[109] Taken together, these findings indicate that α3β1 integrin is not only a receptor for GBM components, but is also required for its development and maintenance. Similarly, podocyte specific ablation of the β1 integrin gene in mice results in massive proteinuria, abnormal capillary morphogenesis, podocyte foot process effacement, and podocyte apoptosis.[134,219]

αvβ3 Integrin

While α3β1 integrin is the primary integrin expressed in podocytes, more recent work has identified a role for αvβ3 integrin in podocyte homeostasis. αvβ3 integrin is a vitronectin receptor that localizes to podocyte foot processes, and is predominantly associated with non-lipid raft fractions of the cell membrane. Genetic deletion of β3 integrin does not result in an overt renal phenotype, but these mice are protected from LPS-induced proteinuria,[302] suggesting that αvβ3 integrin activation may play a role in the pathogenesis of proteinuria in the setting of glomerular injury. Further work by Wei et al. showed that activation of β3 integrin by soluble urokinase receptor (suPAR) may occur in primary focal segmental glomerular sclerosis; the authors suggest that suPAR may be the circulating factor responsible for recurrence of FSGS after transplant.[301] While these data suggest that αvβ3 integrin activation may injure the podocyte, other work shows that αv integrins act as receptors for osteopontin, which is a protective factor in stretch-induced podocyte injury.[258]

Dystroglycan

Integrins are not the only adhesion proteins to be expressed in podocyte foot processes. The dystrophin—glycoprotein complex (DGC) is a group of proteins that includes α- and β-dystroglycan, utrophin, and dystrophin, and plays a central role in stabilizing skeletal muscle cell membranes by tethering the cytoskeleton to the basement membrane components laminin, perlecan, and agrin. α- and β-dystroglycan have also been localized to podocyte foot processes, and their expression is diminished in several mouse models of glomerular disease and human minimal change disease.[226,229] However, recent studies have shown that genetic deletion of dystroglycan from podocytes in mice does not result in a glomerular phenotype or increased susceptibility to injury, suggesting that integrins may be the primary functional extracellular matrix receptors in the podocyte.[126]

Integrin-Linked Kinase

Given the central, non-redundant role of α3β1 integrin in the development and maintenance of the glomerular filtration barrier, it is of interest to identify its interacting proteins in podocytes. Integrin-linked kinase (ILK) is a serine/threonine kinase with kinase-dependent and -independent functions that interact with the cytoplasmic domains of β1 and β3 integrins.[309] Detailed molecular studies have elucidated a role for ILK in podocyte morphology and health. ILK forms a complex with Pinch1 and α-Parvin to regulate matrix adhesion, foot process formation, and inhibit podocyte apoptosis.[312] ILK also forms a ternary complex with α-actinin-4 and α3β1 integrin, providing a link between the GBM, the actin cytoskeleton, and nephrin in the SD.[47] ILK was first identified as a potential mediator of glomerular disease by two groups showing that it is upregulated in glomeruli of patients with diabetic nephropathy,[97] congenital nephrotic syndrome of the Finnish type, and two proteinuric mouse models.[151] Indeed, activation of ILK in vivo using a rodent model of puromycin-associated nephropathy, and in vitro by overexpression of a kinase-active ILK transgene, caused activation of β-catenin, podocyte detachment and apoptosis, and transcriptional repression of the SD components P-cadherin and Cd2ap.[285] However, while ILK activation may contribute to podocyte injury in disease, it also plays a fundamentally important role in normal podocyte physiology. Mice with a podocyte-specific deletion of the ILK gene appear normal at birth, but develop focal segmental glomerular sclerosis with GBM thickening, and podocyte foot process effacement characterized by an aberrant distribution of α-actinin-4 and nephrin.[47,62,134] The deletion of ILK causes an upregulation of focal adhesion kinase (FAK),[134] a non-receptor tyrosine kinase which is involved in focal adhesion turnover, cell spreading, and motility. This result is supported by recent work showing that FAK is activated in LPS and anti-GBM models of podocyte injury, and genetic deletion of FAK protects mice from proteinuria.[171]

Tetraspanin CD151

CD151 is a tetraspanin family protein with affinity for α3β1 integrin[314] that is expressed abundantly in the glomerulus.[275] While CD151 is not absolutely required for α3β1 integrin binding to the extracellular matrix, it stabilizes the active conformation of α3β1 integrin and strengthens this interaction.[203] A nonsense mutation in CD151 causes hereditary nephropathy in patients characterized by a splitting and thickening of the GBM, along with pretibial epidermis bullosa, sensorineural deafness, and thalassemia.[138] A podocyte specific knockout mouse model recapitulates this renal phenotype. Mechanistically, CD151 causes a redistribution of α3β1 integrin at the interface between the podocyte and GBM, increasing its binding affinity for laminin-511/521. These findings suggest that CD151 may strengthen the adhesion of podocytes to the GBM, protecting them from higher glomerular pressures.

Negative Charge on the Surface of Podocytes

Although heparan sulfate proteoglycans are key components of the GBM and endothelial cell layer (as discussed above), they are also expressed by podocytes. The two major families of heparan sulfates expressed by the podocyte are Podocalyxin and Syndecans (primarily Syndecan I and Syndecan IV). Podocalyxin and Syndecans are transmembrane proteins involved in regulation of the podocyte actin cytoskeleton through regulation of signaling pathways (see below). While heparan sulfates provide a negative charge to the surface of the podocyte, sialyation of glycoproteins (including podocalyxin) and gangliosides also imparts a negative charge. Both are important components of glomerular barrier function.[33]

Podocalyxin

Podocalyxin is a CD34-related sialomucin protein that is highly-expressed by podocytes and also by mesothelia, vascular endothelial cells, hematopoietic stem cells, and platelets. Mice with a conventional knockout of the podocalyxin gene die within the first 24 hours of life from renal failure. Importantly, podocyte foot processes do not form, and intercellular junctions between adjacent foot processes are abnormal and appear immature. These data provide functional evidence that podocalyxin is a key molecule in podocyte development.[58] Cell biologic experiments have shown that podocalyxin interacts with the Na^+/H^+ exchanger regulatory factor 2 (NHERF2) and phosphorylated ezrin in a complex, connecting it to the actin cytoskeleton of the podocyte foot process. Disruption of this interaction results in nephrotic syndrome.[178,255,283] Podocalyxin appears to regulate foot process architecture through activation of the small Rho-GTPase, RhoA, mediated by its interaction with the NHERF/Ezrin complex.[255]

Sialyation Defects and the Podocyte

Podocytes express a number of sialyated proteins including podocalyxin (as described above), other proteoglycans, and gangliosides. Loss of sialyation of podocalyxin has been identified in various nephrotic syndrome experimental models, such as in rodents injected with sialidase, puromycin aminonucleoside or protaimine sulfate, which neutralizes negative charges.[140,153,264] All of these compounds cause an abrupt onset of proteinuria, together with foot process effacement. Simultaneous infusion of sialic acid prevents the proteinuria and podocyte foot process fusion observed with puromycin injection, presumably due to resialylation of critical glomerular proteins.[195] More recently, loss of sialyation of podocalyxin was observed

in a transgenic rat model of minimal change disease due to overexpression of Anptl4.[39]

Although many studies have focused on sialylation defects of podocalyxin, the podocyte expresses other sialylated glycoproteins and gangliosides. Mutations in sialylating enzymes have also been associated with glomerular defects and proteinuria. For example, a point mutation in a gene encoding one of the key enzymes needed for sialic acid biosynthesis (uridine disphospho-N-acetylglucosamine (UDP-GlcNAc) 2-epimerase/N-acetyl-mannosamine (ManNAc) kinase (GNE/MNK)) results in severe perinatal glomerular disease in mice, characterized by splitting of the glomerular basement membrane, hematuria, and proteinuria.[81] The phenotype was partially rescued by dietary supplementation with ManNAc. Intriguingly, ManNAc supplementation also appeared to rescue the Anptl4-induced sialyation defect in rats, suggesting it might represent a new therapy for certain forms of glomerular disease.

Podocytes and Metabolism

Although the majority of podocyte studies to date have focused on its unique cytoskeletal architecture and its role as a structural component of the filtration barrier, recent studies have highlighted the importance of metabolic regulatory pathways in podocyte function.

mTOR

The mechanistic target of rapamycin (mTOR) is an evolutionarily-conserved serine-threonine kinase that interacts with regulatory associated protein of mTOR (Rptor) or Rptor-independent companion of MTOR (Rictor) to form mTORC1 and mTORC2 complexes, respectively. mTORC1 is a key regulator of cellular metabolism, including protein translation, ribosomal biogenesis, cell growth and proliferation, and suppression of autophagy in response to amino acids, growth factors, and elevated cellular ATP levels.[326] mTORC2 is regulated primarily by growth factors to promote actin cytoskeletal rearrangement, cell survival, and cell cycle progression.[124] Rapamycin is an mTOR inhibitor that is used clinically and is thought to specifically inhibit mTORC1 function.[94] In certain cell types including the podocyte, however, chronic inhibition of mTORC1 by rapamycin also results in downregulation of mTORC2 functions.[248,294,321] The importance of mTOR in podocyte biology was first suggested by the clinical observation that rapamycin causes proteinuria.[23,266]

Deletion of mTOR itself or Rptor in podocytes of mice results in proteinuria.[38,90] Conversely, ectopic mTORC1 activation in mouse podocytes, accomplished by deletion of its suppressor Tsc1, results in kidney disease with many of the features of diabetic nephropathy (DN), including podocyte hypertrophy and loss and proteinuria, and is attributed to endoplasmic reticulum stress.[122] Although mTORC1 appears to be crucial for podocyte function, loss of Rictor from podocytes of mice does not result in a phentoype.[90]

Given its central role in cellular metabolism, mTOR is likely to play multiple roles in podocyte biology. Regulation of autophagy is one pathway regulated by mTOR that appears to be crucial for podocyte function. Autophagy is a lysosomal-dependent cellular survival response to starvation or lack of growth factors in which cells degrade cellular constituents from proteins to entire organelles, such as mitochondria, in order to provide a supply of nutrients under conditions of stress. A basal level of autophagy is, however, necessary to remove damaged organelles, excessive lipids, and long-lived or misfolded proteins. The basal level of autophagy

appears to be increased in podocytes,[106,201] and it has been suggested that autophagy may be required to protect this long-living cell from injury. In keeping with this model, deletion of Atg5, a key component of the autophagic pathway, results in late onset of glomerular disease in mice at 20 to 24 months of age due to the accumulation of damaged organelles and ubiquitinated protein complexes.[106] In contrast, deletion of mTOR from podocytes results in disruption of autophagic flux, with subsequent accumulation of autophagolysomes in the podocyte[38] (Figure 22.20). Clinically, dysregulation of autophagy is observed in patients with lysosomal storage diseases such as Fabry's disease, Aspartilglucoseaminuria or Scheie's disease, where the inability to acidify lysosomes causes a failure of lysosomal reformation[317]; these patients are prone to developing proteinuria,[74] providing additional support that the autophagic pathway is clinically relevant.

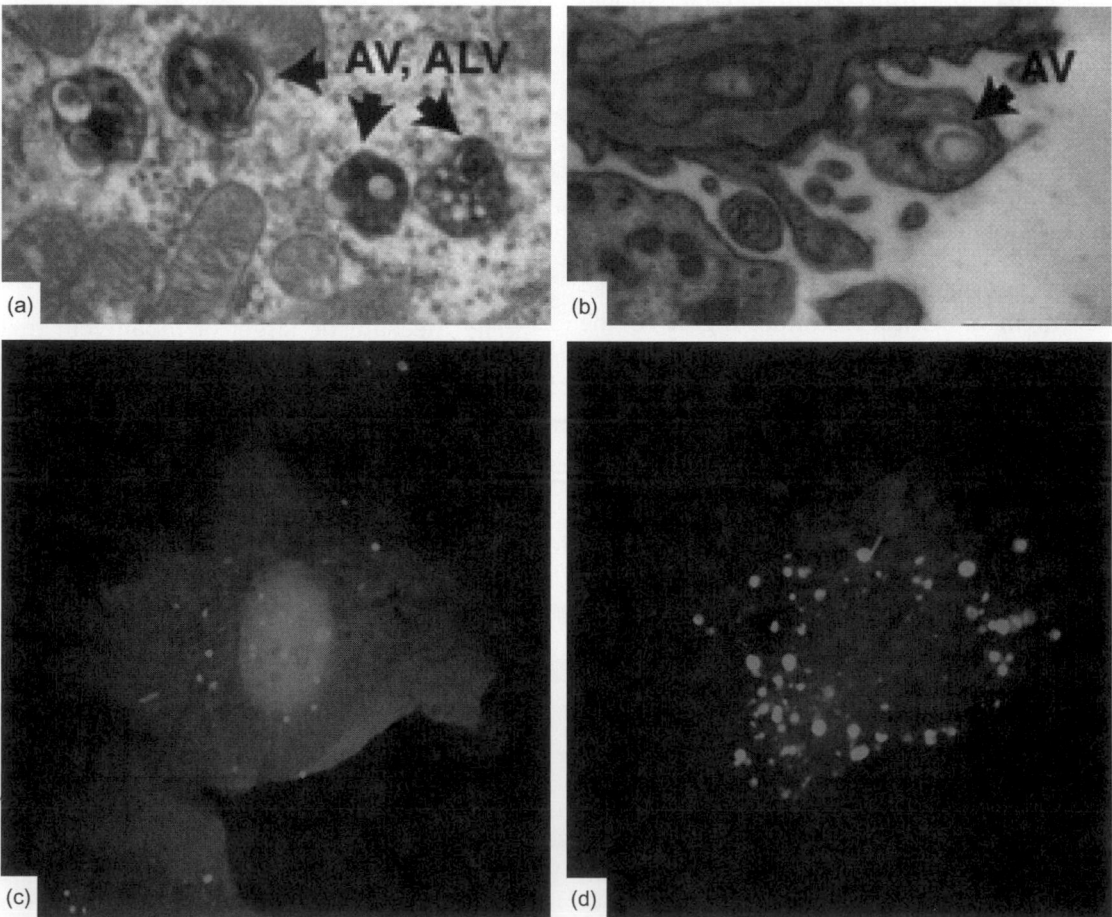

FIGURE 22.20 (a) and (b): Transmission electron micrographs of podocytes from 3 week old podocyte-specific mTor knockout mice showing an accumulation of autophagosomal vesicles (AV) and autophagolysosomal vesicles (ALV). *(From Cina, D. et al. (2012). Inhibition of MTOR disrupts autophagic flux in podocytes. J. Am. Soc. Nephrol. 23: 412–420, with permission.)* (c): LC3 positive autophagosomes are visualized by green fluorescent protein in cultured human podocyte. (d): Treatment of the podocytes with rapamycin induces massive activation of autophagy. See color section at the end of the book.

Insulin Signaling

mTORC1 hyperactivation is associated with a phosphorylation of IRS1/2 and decreased insulin sensitivity, suggesting that podocytes might be a direct cellular target for insulin.[155] A recent study confirmed this hypothesis; genetic deletion of the insulin receptor from podocytes recapitulates many of the features of diabetic nephropathy (DN).[304] *In vitro*, insulin binds the insulin receptor on podocytes and acts through the mitogen-activated protein kinase and phosphor-inositol-3-kinase pathways to induce cytoskeletal rearrangement.[43,304] Taken together, these findings suggest that strategies aimed at increasing insulin sensitivity in podocytes may be a therapeutic option in DN.

Calcium Signaling

TRPC6

The identification of mutations in the Transient Receptor Potential Cation Channel 6 (TRPC6) in patients with autosomal dominant familial FSGS[231,306] emphasizes the key role that calcium signaling plays in glomerular function. Atlhough a variety of different mutations were identified, a number of them result in enhanced calcium signaling within the podocyte. These human genetic findings helped explain results why other factors (such as complement 5b-9,[45] protamine sulfate,[264] bradykinin,[8] and angiotensin (ANG) II[112]), which are associated with increased cytosolic Ca^{2+} concentrations in cultured podocytes, also cause injury. Furthermore, ANG II was shown to signal to the nonselective cation channels TRPC5 and TRPC6 through the AT1 receptor,[287] suggesting that these channels may play a role in podocyte injury beyond the familial FSGS described by Winn et al.[306]

Calcineurin and Synaptopodin

Calcineurin-mediated, NFAT-independent[72] and -dependent[254] signaling pathways in podocytes have also been associated with activating mutations of TRPC6. The link between Ca^{2+}, calcineurin, and synaptopodin provided a clue that TRPC channels may be involved in regulating the actin cytoskeleton, as synaptopodin is known to regulate small Rho GTPases — master regulators of actin cytoskeletal dynamics. The opposing action of RhoGTPases — RhoA which promotes F-actin stabilization, and Cdc42 or Rac1 that promote F-actin turnover — are thought to maintain the podocyte FP dynamic.[91] Podocyte-specific overexpression of TRPC6 led to a Ca^{2+}-mediated increase in RhoA activity,[130] while genetic deletion of TRPC6 led to increased Rac1 activity and podocyte motility.[287] This cumulative body of work outlines an important role for intracellular Ca^{2+} in regulating the actin cytoskeleton of podocytes, and more work in the area will yield interesting insights into the intersection of metabolism, Ca^{2+} signaling, and cytoskeleton in podocytes.

GLOMERULAR PARIETAL EPITHELIUM

Description

The parietal layer of Bowman's capsule consists of a heterogenous population of squamous and cuboidal epithelial cells resting on a basement membrane.[100] The heterogeneity of this population is rendered more complex by the identification of a peripolar cell population, which by morphology[86] and molecular markers[12] resemble visceral podocytes, and extend up to 100 μm along Bowman's capsule. The glomerular parietal epithelial cells (PECs) are rich in actin microfilament bundles which are particularly prominent in the cells surrounding the vascular pole.[64] In this cell population, the actin bundles are located in cytoplasmic grooves that run circularly around the vascular stalk.[64]

As the visceral and parietal layers of the glomerulus are continuous, so are the basement membranes. The transition region occurs around the vascular stalk, and is connected to the smooth muscle cells of the afferent and efferent arterioles and the extraglomerular mesangial cells. Despite this continuity, however, the parietal basement membrane layer is considerably different. Ultrastructurally, the parietal basement membrane is multilayered, with translucent laminae on the extracellular matrix.[180] Further immunohistochemical studies have identified type I, III, IV, and V collagens, heparin sulfate proteoglycans, laminin, enactin, fibronectin, and nidogen.[180] Of these, however, only type IV and V collagen[238] and heparin sulfated proteoglycans[277] have been confirmed by electron microscopy. Compared to the tubular and glomerular basement membrane, the parietal basement membrane is particularly enriched in collagen type IV as opposed to laminin.[238]

Podocyte Progenitors

It has been long assumed that because of podocytes' limited replicative ability, podocyte loss is a largely irreversible event, ultimately leading to end-stage kidney disease. However, under physiologic conditions and in the event of reversible glomerular disease in humans and animals, podocytes are reportedly shed into the urine at a rate that is not compatible with recovery.[78,176,293,316] This would suggest that there is another mechanism allowing for the replenishment of podocytes. Indeed, seminal experiments involving irreversible triple labeling of parietal epithelial cells in the Bowman's capsule of mice show the existence of a population of cells near the glomerular vascular stalk that can migrate into the glomerulus and differentiate into podocytes.[6]

Parietal Epithelial Cell-Fate Specification and Wnt Signaling

Given the presence of podocyte progenitors in the parietal epithelium and the podocyte-like cells that seem to populate the transition zone between visceral and parietal epithelium, it is important to understand the developmental cues that push their common progenitors in the S-shaped body stage of glomerular development towards either phenotype. To elucidate this, a conditional deletion of *β-catenin* from the renal epithelium and developing collecting ducts showed that in the absence of β-catenin/Wnt signaling, well-differentiated podocytes replace the parietal epithelium of Bowman's capsule.[93] These "parietal podocytes" were not a result of podocytes migrating from the glomerular tuft, but rather were derived from parietal precursors in the S-shaped body phase by direct lineage switch.

PECs in Glomerular Injury

Glomerulosclerosis

While PECs can promote recovery from physiologic podocyte loss or milder forms of injury, they can also contribute to sclerotic lesions in certain mouse models of glomerulosclerosis.[270] Lineage tracing of podocytes in a mouse model of podocyte depletion showed that PECs, but not podocytes, avidly proliferated and migrated into the visceral side, developing a lesion that is similar to idiopathic FSGS.[10]

Crescent Formation

A role for PECs has also been demonstrated in crescentic formation in inflammatory models of murine glomerular injury. Unlike in the sclerotic lesions, anti-GBM glomerular nephritis induced the proliferation of both podocytes and PECs.[193] In this model, podocytes undergo a profound phenotypic change, losing all their typical markers, and form a bridge between the tuft and Bowman's capsule.[156,193] This bridging event then induces the proliferation of PECs, and both cell types can be found in the cellular crescents that are the hallmark of severe inflammatory glomerular injury.[270]

Glomerular Permeability

In the setting of inflammatory injury, the tight junctions between PECs are also disturbed and become permeable to texas-red labeled dextran and ovalbumin.[207] These findings suggest that, along with their basement membrane, PECs also form a second barrier to protein, and the perturbation of this cell layer may be responsible for the periglomerular inflammation typical of anti-GBM glomerulonephritis.

THE GLOMERULAR FILTRATION BARRIER

As discussed above, the glomerular filtration barrier has multiple components that contribute to its size and charge perm-selectivity.[104] It begins at the glomerular capillary loop with its fenestrated endothelium, endothelial surface layer, and glycocalyx, then progresses to the glomerular basement membrane, and finally to the podocyte foot processes with their filtration slits bridged by the slit diaphragms.

Size Barrier

Many classical experiments using dextrans,[29] ficolls,[16] and proteins[170] have incontrovertibly established the existence of a size barrier to permeability. Some reports support the idea that the GBM is the principle filtration barrier. Infusion of dextrans with different molecular weights in rats shows that the particles can reach the subendothelial part of the GBM, but cannot go further.[26] Knockout mice for laminin β2, a major component of the GBM, develop massive proteinuria, even before the onset of visible ultrastructural changes to the podocytes.[125] Mutations in this gene cause Pierson syndrome in patients, an autosomal recessive condition characterized by nephrotic syndrome and ocular abnormalities.[322] Mutations in the gene encoding type IV collagen α5 chain (*COL4A5*) cause X-linked Alport syndrome, characterized by hereditary nephrotic syndrome, hearing loss, and lens defects. Furthermore, homozygous mutations in *COL4A3* or *COL4A4* also affect the collagen network of the GBM structure, and result in an autosomal recessive form of Alport syndrome.[139]

On the other hand, the sieve-like structure of the slit diaphragm[290] also seems to be of paramount importance to the size-selective glomerular filtration barrier. Evidence from human mutations and genetic mouse models which affect slit diaphragm components (discussed above), leads to massive proteinuria, providing evidence that the slit membrane plays a major role in size selectivity. Therefore, current literature supports a role for both the GBM and the podocyte slit diaphragm in size perm-selectivity.

TABLE 22.1 Genetic Mutations that Result in Glomerular Disease (Humans)

Gene	Protein	Disease	Inheritance	Clinical Features	Reference
NPHS1	Nephrin	Congenital nephrotic syndrome of the Finnish type	AR	Massive proteinuria *in utero* and treatment resistant nephrotic syndrome	143
NPHS2	Podocin	Steroid-resistant nephrotic syndrome	AR	Variable onset nephropathy that is steroid resistant	19
CD2AP	CD2AP	Sporadic FSGS	n/a	FSGS	144
ACTN4	α-Actinin-4	FSGS	AD	Progressive proteinuria starting in adolescence with adult onset FSGS (variable penetrance)	137
COQ2	Coenzyme Q10 biosynthesis mono-oxigenase 2	Steroid-resistant nephrotic syndrome	AR	Steroid resistant nephrotic syndrome, epileptic encephalopathy	56
COQ6	Coenzyme Q10 biosynthesis mono-oxigenase 6	Steroid-resistant nephrotic syndrome	AR	Nephrotic syndrome with sensorineural deafness	110
PLCE1	PLCε1	Inherited nephrotic syndrome	AR	Nephrosis and diffuse mesangial sclerosis leading to renal failure	113
LAMB2	Laminin β2	Pierson's syndrome	AR	Congenital nephrosis, mesangial sclerosis, and microcoria	322
ITGA3	Integrin α3	Congenital nephrotic syndrome	AR	Congenital nephrotic syndrome, interstitial lung disease, and skin fragility	109
TRPC6	TRPC6	FSGS	AD	High grade proteinuria with adult onset, and progression to renal failure	306
MYH9	MYH9	Epstein syndrome Fechtner's syndrome	AD	Proteinuria, microhematuria, thrombocytopenia, and sensorineural deafness	9
LMX1B	LMX1B	Nail−Patella syndrome	AD	Nephrotic syndrome with nail and skeletal abnormalities in children	60
WT1	WT1	Denis−Drash syndrome (DDS) Frasier syndrome (FS)	AD	Pseudohermaphroditism, diffuse mesangial sclerosis and renal failure with varying onset depending on the mutation	214
SYNPO	Synaptopodin	Sporadic FSGS	n/a	FSGS risk in Chinese patients	49
MYOE1	Myosin 1E	Childhood FSGS	n/a	Childhood onset FSGS	183
APOL1	Apolipoprotein L-1	Sporadic FSGS	n/a	Risk of FSGS in African-American patients	83
GPC5	Glypican 5	Acquired nephrotic syndrome	n/a	Increased risk of nephrotic syndrome	208
INF2	Formin	Charcot−Marie Tooth	AD	Adolescent onset proteinuria with progression to FSGS and renal failure	20,82
PTPRO/ GLEPP1	Protein-tyrosine phosphatase receptor type O [PTPRO or GLEPP1]	FSGS	AR	Childhood nephrotic syndrome with FSGS and progression to renal failure	211
COL4A1	Collagen IV α1	Alport's syndrome	X-linked	Nephrotic syndrome with hematuria and sensorineural hearing loss (α1,3,4,5)	41,169,186,218,233
COL4A3	Collagen IV α3		AR		
COL4A4	Collagen IV α4		AR		
COL4A5	Collagen IV α5			Intracerebral hemorrhage and strokes (α1)	
ARHGAP24	Arhgap24	FSGS	AD	Early onset FSGS	4

AR: autosomal recessive; AD: autosomal dominant.

II. STRUCTURAL AND FUNCTIONAL ORGANIZATION OF THE KIDNEY

Charge Barrier

The presence of a charge barrier was demonstrated by sequential classical analyses that show retardation of anionic macromolecules from passing through the glomerular filtration barrier as compared to neutral molecules with a similar size.[21,22,28]

GBM as a Charge Barrier

Electron microscopy with perfusion of cationic lysozyme demonstrated the presence of anionic sites in all three layers of the GBM.[27] Studies using ferritins with different isometric points showed that cationic ferritin could distribute widely into the GBM, whereas filtration of its neutral counterpart was restricted at the level of the endothelium and subendothelial layer of the GBM.[232] Treatment of rats with heparinase reduced the restriction of neutral ferritin and allowed the ferritin particles[135] and bovine albumin[240] into the GBM. These results were considered to be conclusive evidence that the negative charges of heparan sulfate proteoglycans in the GBM play a major role in maintaining the charge barrier. Recently, however, podocyte-specific genetic deletion of agrin, both agrin and the heparan sulfated side chains of perlecan, and a systemic deletion of COLXVIII[88,108,291] were reported. Although they are the main components of heparan sulfate proteoglycans in the GBM, none of the mutant mice developed significant proteinuria, as discussed above in the section on GBM. Moreover, a study using isolated GBM showed the sieving coefficients of negatively-charged ficoll sulfate were not different from those of neutral ficoll at physiological ionic strength.[17] Given these recent results, it is unlikely that the GBM is the main charge selective barrier in the glomerulus.

Endothelial Surface Layer as a Charge Barrier

Several experiments have been performed to reduce the endothelial charge barrier by enzymatic digestion of glycosaminoglycans (GAGs). GAGs are major contributors to the GBM negative charge, but they are also expressed on the endothelial surface layer. Perfusion of mice with heparanase, chondroitinase, and hyaluronidase reduces the charge density and thickness of the endothelial surface layer and increases the fractional clearance of albumin.[128,129] In these studies the authors assume that it is most unlikely that the enzymes affect the GBM or podocytes, because they are large molecules and are therefore restricted largely to the vascular lumen. Indeed, the ultrastructure of the endothelium, GBM, and podocytes were not affected by this enzymatic digestion. Since the GBM is no longer considered as the principal charge barrier, these data support the notion of an endothelial charge barrier.

References

[1] Abrahamson DR. Origin of the glomerular basement membrane visualized after in vivo labeling of laminin in newborn rat kidneys. J Cell Biol 1985;100(6):1988–2000.
[2] Abrahamson DR. Structure and development of the glomerular capillary wall and basement membrane. Am J Physiol 1987;253 (5 Pt 2):F783–94.
[3] Abrahamson DR, Hudson BG, Stroganova L, Borza D-B St, John PL. Cellular origins of type IV collagen networks in developing glomeruli. J Am Soc Nephrol 2009;20(7):1471–9.
[4] Akilesh S, Suleiman H, Yu H, Stander MC, Lavin P, Gbadegesin R, et al. Arhgap24 inactivates Rac1 in mouse podocytes, and a mutant form is associated with familial focal segmental glomerulosclerosis. J Clin Invest 2011;121(10):4127–37.
[5] Andres A-C, Munarini N, Djonov V, Bruneau S, Zuercher G, Loercher S, et al. EphB4 receptor tyrosine kinase transgenic mice develop glomerulopathies reminiscent of aglomerular vascular shunts. Mech Dev 2003;120(4):511–6.
[6] Appel D, Kershaw DB, Smeets B, Yuan G, Fuss A, Frye B, et al. Recruitment of podocytes from glomerular parietal epithelial cells. J Am Soc Nephrol 2009;20(2):333–43.
[7] Ara T, Tokoyoda K, Okamoto R, Koni PA, Nagasawa T. The role of CXCL12 in the organ-specific process of artery formation. Blood 2005;105(8):3155–61.
[8] Ardaillou N, Blaise V, Costenbader K, Vassitch Y, Ardaillou R. Characterization of a B2-bradykinin receptor in human glomerular podocytes. Am J Physiol 1996;271(3 Pt 2):F754–61.
[9] Arrondel C, Vodovar N, Knebelmann B, Grünfeld J-P, Gubler M-C, Antignac C, et al. Expression of the nonmuscle myosin heavy chain IIA in the human kidney and screening for MYH9 mutations in Epstein and Fechtner syndromes. J Am Soc Nephrol 2002;13(1):65–74.
[10] Asano T, Niimura F, Pastan I, Fogo AB, Ichikawa I, Matsusaka T. Permanent genetic tagging of podocytes: fate of injured podocytes in a mouse model of glomerular sclerosis. J Am Soc Nephrol 2005;16(8):2257–62.
[11] Bader BL, Smyth N, Nedbal S, Miosge N, Baranowsky A, Mokkapati S, et al. Compound genetic ablation of nidogen 1 and 2 causes basement membrane defects and perinatal lethality in mice. Mol Cell Biol 2005;25(15):6846–56.
[12] Bariety J, Mandet C, Hill GS, Bruneval P. Parietal podocytes in normal human glomeruli. J Am Soc Nephrol 2006;17 (10):2770–80.
[13] Bieritz B, Spessotto P, Colombatti A, Jahn A, Prols F, Hartner A. Role of alpha8 integrin in mesangial cell adhesion, migration, and proliferation. Kidney Int 2003;64(1):119–27.
[14] Bjarnegård M, Enge M, Norlin J, Gustafsdottir S, Fredriksson S, Abramsson A, et al. Endothelium-specific ablation of PDGFB leads to pericyte loss and glomerular, cardiac and placental abnormalities. Development 2004;131(8):1847–57.
[15] Blasutig IM, New LA, Thanabalasuriar A, Dayarathna TK, Goudreault M, Quaggin SE, et al. Phosphorylated YDXV motifs and Nck SH2/SH3 adaptors act cooperatively to induce actin reorganization. Mol Cell Biol 2008;28(6):2035–46.
[16] Blouch K, Deen WM, Fauvel JP, Bialek J, Derby G, Myers BD. Molecular configuration and glomerular size selectivity in healthy and nephrotic humans. Am J Physiol 1997;273(3 Pt 2):F430–7.
[17] Bolton GR, Deen WM, Daniels BS. Assessment of the charge selectivity of glomerular basement membrane using Ficoll sulfate. Am J Physiol 1998;274(5 Pt 2):F889–96.
[18] Borza CM, Su Y, Chen X, Yu L, Mont S, Chetyrkin S, et al. Inhibition of integrin α2β1 ameliorates glomerular injury. J Am Soc Nephrol 2012;23(6):1027–38.

[19] Boute N, Gribouval O, Roselli S, Benessy F, Lee H, Fuchshuber A, et al. NPHS2, encoding the glomerular protein podocin, is mutated in autosomal recessive steroid-resistant nephrotic syndrome. Nat Genet 2000;24(4):349—54.

[20] Boyer O, Nevo F, Plaisier E, Funalot B, Gribouval O, Benoit G, et al. INF2 mutations in Charcot-Marie-Tooth disease with glomerulopathy. N Engl J Med 2011;365(25):2377—88.

[21] Brenner BM, Baylis C, Deen WM. Transport of molecules across renal glomerular capillaries. Physiol Rev 1976;56(3):502—34.

[22] Brenner BM, Bohrer MP, Baylis C, Deen WM. Determinants of glomerular permselectivity: insights derived from observations *in vivo*. Kidney Int 1977;12(4):229—37.

[23] Budde K, Becker T, Arns W, Sommerer C, Reinke P, Eisenberger U, et al. Everolimus-based, calcineurin-inhibitor-free regimen in recipients of *de novo* kidney transplants: an open-label, randomised, controlled trial. Lancet 2011;377 (9768):837—47.

[24] Call KM, Glaser T, Ito CY, Buckler AJ, Pelletier J, Haber DA, et al. Isolation and characterization of a zinc finger polypeptide gene at the human chromosome 11 Wilms' tumor locus. Cell 1990;60(3):509—20.

[25] Caricasole A, Duarte A, Larsson SH, Hastie ND, Little M, Holmes G, et al. RNA binding by the Wilms tumor suppressor zinc finger proteins. Proc Natl Acad Sci USA 1996;93 (15):7562 6.

[26] Caulfield JP, Farquhar MG. The permeability of glomerular capillaries to graded dextrans. Identification of the basement membrane as the primary filtration barrier. J Cell Biol 1974;63 (3):883—903.

[27] Caulfield JP, Farquhar MG. Distribution of annionic sites in glomerular basement membranes: their possible role in filtration and attachment. Proc Natl Acad Sci USA 1976;73(5): 1646—50.

[28] Chang RL, Deen WM, Robertson CR, Brenner BM. Permselectivity of the glomerular capillary wall: III. Restricted transport of polyanions. Kidney Int 1975;8(4):212—8.

[29] Chang RL, Ueki IF, Troy JL, Deen WM, Robertson CR, Brenner BM. Permselectivity of the glomerular capillary wall to macromolecules. II. Experimental studies in rats using neutral dextran. Biophys J 1975;15(9):887—906.

[30] Chau Y-Y, Brownstein D, Mjoseng H, Lee W-C, Buza-Vidas N, Nerlov C, et al. Acute multiple organ failure in adult mice deleted for the developmental regulator Wt1. PLoS Genet 2011;7 (12):e1002404.

[31] Chen H, Lun Y, Ovchinnikov D, Kokubo H, Oberg KC, Pepicelli CV, et al. Limb and kidney defects in Lmx1b mutant mice suggest an involvement of LMX1B in human Nail Patella syndrome. Nat Genet 1998;19(1):51—5.

[32] Chen L, Al-Awqati Q. Segmental expression of Notch and Hairy genes in nephrogenesis. Am J Physiol Renal Physiol 2005;288(5):F939—52.

[33] Chen S, Wassenhove-McCarthy DJ, Yamaguchi Y, Holzman LB, van Kuppevelt TH, Jenniskens GJ, et al. Loss of heparan sulfate glycosaminoglycan assembly in podocytes does not lead to proteinuria. Kidney Int 2008;74(3):289—99.

[34] Chen X, Moeckel G, Morrow JD, Cosgrove D, Harris RC, Fogo AB, et al. Lack of integrin alpha1beta1 leads to severe glomerulosclerosis after glomerular injury. Am J Pathol 2004;165 (2):617—30.

[35] Cheng H-T, Kim M, Valerius MT, Surendran K, Schuster-Gossler K, Gossler A, et al. Notch2, but not Notch1, is required for proximal fate acquisition in the mammalian nephron. Development 2007;134(4):801—11.

[36] Cho EA, Patterson LT, Brookhiser WT, Mah S, Kintner C, Dressler GR. Differential expression and function of cadherin-6

during renal epithelium development. Development 1998;125 (5):803—12.

[37] Ciani L, Patel A, Allen ND, ffrench-Constant C. Mice lacking the giant protocadherin mFAT1 exhibit renal slit junction abnormalities and a partially penetrant cyclopia and anophthalmia phenotype. Mol Cell Biol 2003;23(10):3575—82.

[38] Cinà DP, Onay T, Paltoo A, Li C, Maezawa Y, De Arteaga J, et al. Inhibition of MTOR disrupts autophagic flux in podocytes. J Am Soc Nephrol 2011;23(3):412—20.

[39] Clement LC, Avila-Casado C, Macé C, Soria E, Bakker WW, Kersten S, et al. Podocyte-secreted angiopoietin-like-4 mediates proteinuria in glucocorticoid-sensitive nephrotic syndrome. Nat Med 2011;17(1):117—22.

[40] Colognato H, Yurchenco PD. Form and function: the laminin family of heterotrimers. Dev Dyn 2000;218(2):213—34.

[41] Cosgrove D, Meehan DT, Grunkemeyer JA, Kornak JM, Sayers R, Hunter WJ, et al. Collagen COL4A3 knockout: a mouse model for autosomal Alport syndrome. Genes Dev 1996;10 (23):2981—92.

[42] Courtoy PJ, Timpl R, Farquhar MG. Comparative distribution of laminin, type IV collagen, and fibronectin in the rat glomerulus. J Histochem Cytochem 1982;30(9):874—86.

[43] Coward RJM, Welsh GI, Yang J, Tasman C, Lennon R, Koziell A, et al. The human glomerular podocyte is a novel target for insulin action. Diabetes 2005;54(11):3095—102.

[44] Crean JKG, Finlay D, Murphy M, Moss C, Godson C, Martin F, et al. The role of p42/44 MAPK and protein kinase B in connective tissue growth factor induced extracellular matrix protein production, cell migration, and actin cytoskeletal rearrangement in human mesangial cells. J Biol Chem 2002;277 (46):44187—94.

[45] Cybulsky AV, Bonventre JV, Quigg RJ, Lieberthal W, Salant DJ. Cytosolic calcium and protein kinase C reduce complement-mediated glomerular epithelial injury. Kidney Int 1990;38 (5):803—11.

[46] Dai C, Liu Y. Hepatocyte growth factor antagonizes the profibrotic action of TGF-beta1 in mesangial cells by stabilizing Smad transcriptional corepressor TGIF. J Am Soc Nephrol 2004;15(6):1402—12.

[47] Dai C, Stolz DB, Bastacky SI, St-Arnaud R, Wu C, Dedhar S, et al. Essential role of integrin-linked kinase in podocyte biology: Bridging the integrin and slit diaphragm signaling. J Am Soc Nephrol 2006;17(8):2164—75.

[48] Dai C, Yang J, Bastacky S, Xia J, Li Y, Liu Y. Intravenous administration of hepatocyte growth factor gene ameliorates diabetic nephropathy in mice. J Am Soc Nephrol 2004;15(10):2637—47.

[49] Dai S, Wang Z, Pan X, Wang W, Chen X, Ren H, et al. Functional analysis of promoter mutations in the ACTN4 and SYNPO genes in focal segmental glomerulosclerosis. Nephrol Dial Transplant 2010;25(3):824—35.

[50] Dandapani SV, Sugimoto H, Matthews BD, Kolb RJ, Sinha S, Gerszten RE, et al. Alpha-actinin-4 is required for normal podocyte adhesion. J Biol Chem 2007;282(1):467—77.

[51] Darisipudi MN, Kulkarni OP, Sayyed SG, Ryu M, Migliorini A, Sagrinati C, et al. Dual blockade of the homeostatic chemokine CXCL12 and the proinflammatory chemokine CCL2 has additive protective effects on diabetic kidney disease. Am J Pathol 2011;179(1):116—24.

[52] Davis B, Dei Cas A, Long DA, White KE, Hayward A, Ku C-H, et al. Podocyte-specific expression of angiopoietin-2 causes proteinuria and apoptosis of glomerular endothelia. J Am Soc Nephrol 2007;18(8):2320—9.

[53] Denys P, Malvaux P, Van Den Berghe H, Tanghe W, Proesmans W. Association of an anatomo-pathological syndrome of male pseudohermaphroditism, Wilms' tumor, parenchymatous

nephropathy and XX/XY mosaicism. Arch Fr Pediatr 1967;24 (7):729—39.

[54] Ding G, Zhang A, Huang S, Pan X, Zhen G, Chen R, et al. ANG II induces c-Jun NH2-terminal kinase activation and proliferation of human mesangial cells via redox-sensitive transactivation of the EGFR. Am J Physiol Renal Physiol 2007;293(6): F1889—97.

[55] Ding M, Cui S, Li C, Jothy S, Haase V, Steer BM, et al. Loss of the tumor suppressor Vhlh leads to upregulation of Cxcr4 and rapidly progressive glomerulonephritis in mice. Nat Med 2006;12(9):1081—7.

[56] Diomedi-Camassei F, Di Giandomenico S, Santorelli FM, Caridi G, Piemonte F, Montini G, et al. COQ2 nephropathy: A newly described inherited mitochondriopathy with primary renal involvement. J Am Soc Nephrol 2007;18(10): 2773—80.

[57] Donoviel DB, Freed DD, Vogel H, Potter DG, Hawkins E, Barrish JP, et al. Proteinuria and perinatal lethality in mice lacking NEPH1, a novel protein with homology to nephrin. Mol Cell Biol 2001;21(14):4829—36.

[58] Doyonnas R, Kershaw DB, Duhme C, Merkens H, Chelliah S, Graf T, et al. Anuria, omphalocele, and perinatal lethality in mice lacking the CD34-related protein podocalyxin. J Exp Med 2001;194(1):13—27.

[59] Drash A, Sherman F, Hartmann WH, Blizzard RM. A syndrome of pseudohermaphroditism, Wilms' tumor, hypertension, and degenerative renal disease. J Pediatr 1970;76(4):585—93.

[60] Dreyer SD, Zhou G, Baldini A, Winterpacht A, Zabel B, Cole W, et al. Mutations in LMX1B cause abnormal skeletal patterning and renal dysplasia in nail patella syndrome. Nat Genet 1998;19 (1):47—50.

[61] Drummond IA, Rupprecht HD, Rohwer-Nutter P, Lopez-Guisa JM, Madden SL, Rauscher FJ, et al. DNA recognition by splicing variants of the Wilms' tumor suppressor, WT1. Mol Cell Biol 1994;14(6):3800—9.

[62] El-Aouni C, Herbach N, Blattner SM, Henger A, Rastaldi MP, Jarad G, et al. Podocyte-specific deletion of integrin-linked kinase results in severe glomerular basement membrane alterations and progressive glomerulosclerosis. J Am Soc Nephrol 2006;17(5):1334—44.

[63] Elger M, Drenckhahn D, Nobiling R, Mundel P, Kriz W. Cultured rat mesangial cells contain smooth muscle alpha-actin not found in vivo. Am J Pathol 1993;142(2):497—509.

[64] Elger M, Sakai T, Kriz W. The vascular pole of the renal glomerulus of rat. Adv Anat Embryol Cell Biol 1998;139:1—98.

[65] Eremina V, Cui S, Gerber H, Ferrara N, Haigh J, Nagy A, et al. Vascular endothelial growth factor a signaling in the podocyte-endothelial compartment is required for mesangial cell migration and survival. J Am Soc Nephrol 2006;17 (3):724—35.

[66] Eremina V, Jefferson JA, Kowalewska J, Hochster H, Haas M, Weisstuch J, et al. VEGF inhibition and renal thrombotic microangiopathy. N Engl J Med 2008;358(11):1129—36.

[67] Eremina V, Quaggin SE. The role of VEGF-A in glomerular development and function. Curr Opin Nephrol Hypertens 2004;13(1):9—15.

[68] Eremina V, Sood M, Haigh J, Nagy A, Lajoie G, Ferrara N, et al. Glomerular-specific alterations of VEGF-A expression lead to distinct congenital and acquired renal diseases. J Clin Invest 2003;111(5):707—16.

[69] Esser S, Wolburg K, Wolburg H, Breier G, Kurzchalia T, Risau W. Vascular endothelial growth factor induces endothelial fenestrations in vitro. J Cell Biol 1998;140(4):947—59.

[70] Etienne-Manneville S, Hall A. Rho GTPases in cell biology. Nature 2002;420(6916):629—35.

[71] Farquhar MG, Palade GE. Functional evidence for the existence of a third cell type in the renal glomerulus: phagocytosis of filtration residues by a distinctive "third" cell. J Cell Biol 1962;13 (1):55—87.

[72] Faul C, Donnelly M, Merscher-Gomez S, Chang YH, Franz S, Delfgaauw J, et al. The actin cytoskeleton of kidney podocytes is a direct target of the antiproteinuric effect of cyclosporine A. Nat Med 2008;14(9):931—8.

[73] Fierlbeck W, Liu A, Coyle R, Ballermann BJ. Endothelial cell apoptosis during glomerular capillary lumen formation in vivo. J Am Soc Nephrol 2003;14(5):1349—54.

[74] Fischer EG, Moore MJ, Lager DJ. Fabry disease: a morphologic study of 11 cases. Mod Pathol 2006;19(10):1295—301.

[75] Floege J, Burg M, Hugo C, Gordon KL, Van Goor H, Reidy M, et al. Endogenous fibroblast growth factor-2 mediates cytotoxicity in experimental mesangioproliferative glomerulonephritis. J Am Soc Nephrol 1998;9(5):792—801.

[76] Foo SS, Turner CJ, Adams S, Compagni A, Aubyn D, Kogata N, et al. Ephrin-B2 controls cell motility and adhesion during blood-vessel-wall assembly. Cell 2006;124(1):161—73.

[77] Fox JW, Mayer U, Nischt R, Aumailley M, Reinhardt D, Wiedemann H, et al. Recombinant nidogen consists of three globular domains and mediates binding of laminin to collagen type IV. EMBO J 1991;10(11):3137—46.

[78] Fries JW, Sandstrom DJ, Meyer TW, Rennke HG. Glomerular hypertrophy and epithelial cell injury modulate progressive glomerulosclerosis in the rat. Lab Invest 1989;60(2):205—18.

[79] Gagliardini E, Conti S, Benigni A, Remuzzi G, Remuzzi A. Imaging of the porous ultrastructure of the glomerular epithelial filtration slit. J Am Soc Nephrol 2010;21(12):2081—9.

[80] Gale NW, Thurston G, Hackett SF, Renard R, Wang Q, McClain J, et al. Angiopoietin-2 is required for postnatal angiogenesis and lymphatic patterning, and only the latter role is rescued by Angiopoietin-1. Dev Cell 2002;3(3):411—23.

[81] Galeano B, Klootwijk R, Manoli I, Sun M, Ciccone C, Darvish D, et al. Mutation in the key enzyme of sialic acid biosynthesis causes severe glomerular proteinuria and is rescued by N-acetylmannosamine. J Clin Invest 2007;117(6):1585—94.

[82] Gbadegesin RA, Lavin PJ, Hall G, Bartkowiak B, Homstad A, Jiang R, et al. Inverted formin 2 mutations with variable expression in patients with sporadic and hereditary focal and segmental glomerulosclerosis. Kidney Int 2012;81(1):94—9.

[83] Genovese G, Friedman DJ, Ross MD, Lecordier L, Uzureau P, Freedman BI, et al. Association of trypanolytic ApoL1 variants with kidney disease in African Americans. Science 2010;329 (5993):841—5.

[84] Gerety SS, Anderson DJ. Cardiovascular ephrinB2 function is essential for embryonic angiogenesis. Development 2002;129 (6):1397—410.

[85] Ghayur MN, Krepinsky JC, Janssen LJ. Contractility of the renal glomerulus and mesangial cells: lingering doubts and strategies for the future. Med Hypotheses Res 2008;4(1):1—9.

[86] Gibson IW, Downie I, Downie TT, Han SW, More IA, Lindop GB. The parietal podocyte: a study of the vascular pole of the human glomerulus. Kidney Int 1992;41(1):211—4.

[87] Gibson MA, Kumaratilake JS, Cleary EG. The protein components of the 12-nanometer microfibrils of elastic and nonelastic tissues. J Biol Chem 1989;264(8):4590—8.

[88] Goldberg S, Harvey SJ, Cunningham J, Tryggvason K, Miner JH. Glomerular filtration is normal in the absence of both agrin and perlecan-heparan sulfate from the glomerular basement membrane. Nephrol Dial Transplant 2009;24(7):2044—51.

[89] Gould DB, Phalan FC, van Mil SE, Sundberg JP, Vahedi K, Massin P, et al. Role of COL4A1 in small-vessel disease and hemorrhagic stroke. N Engl J Med 2006;354(14):1489—96.

[90] Gödel M, Hartleben B, Herbach N, Liu S, Zschiedrich S, Lu S, et al. Role of mTOR in podocyte function and diabetic nephropathy in humans and mice. J Clin Invest 2011;121(6):2197–209.

[91] Greka A, Mundel P. Cell biology and pathology of podocytes. Annu Rev Physiol 2012;74:299–323.

[92] Groffen AJ, Ruegg MA, Dijkman H, van de Velden TJ, Buskens CA, van den Born J, et al. Agrin is a major heparan sulfate proteoglycan in the human glomerular basement membrane. J Histochem Cytochem 1998;46(1):19–27.

[93] Grouls S, Iglesias DM, Wentzensen N, Moeller MJ, Bouchard M, Kemler R, et al. Lineage specification of parietal epithelial cells requires β-catenin/Wnt signaling. J Am Soc Nephrol 2012;23(1):63–72.

[94] Guertin DA, Sabatini DM. The pharmacology of mTOR inhibition. Sci Signal 2009;2(67):pe24.

[95] Guo G, Morrison DJ, Licht JD, Quaggin SE. WT1 activates a glomerular-specific enhancer identified from the human nephrin gene. J Am Soc Nephrol 2004;15(11):2851–6.

[96] Guo J-K, Menke AL, Gubler M-C, Clarke AR, Harrison D, Hammes A, et al. WT1 is a key regulator of podocyte function: reduced expression levels cause crescentic glomerulonephritis and mesangial sclerosis. Hum Mol Genet 2002;11(6): 651–9.

[97] Guo L, Sanders PW, Woods A, Wu C. The distribution and regulation of integrin-linked kinase in normal and diabetic kidneys. Am J Pathol 2001;159(5):1735–42.

[98] Gurevich F, Perazella MA. Renal effects of anti-angiogenesis therapy: update for the internist. Am J Med 2009;122(4):322–8.

[99] Haber DA, Sohn RL, Buckler AJ, Pelletier J, Call KM, Housman DE. Alternative splicing and genomic structure of the Wilms tumor gene WT1. Proc Natl Acad Sci USA 1991;88 (21):9618–22.

[100] Haensly WE, Lee JC. Metaplasia of the parietal layer of Bowman's capsule: a histopathological survey of the human kidney. Histol Histopathol 1986;1(4):363–7.

[101] Hamano Y, Grunkemeyer JA, Sudhakar A, Zeisberg M, Cosgrove D, Morello R, et al. Determinants of vascular permeability in the kidney glomerulus. J Biol Chem 2002;277(34): 31154–62.

[102] Hammes A, Guo JK, Lutsch G, Leheste JR, Landrock D, Ziegler U, et al. Two splice variants of the Wilms' tumor 1 gene have distinct functions during sex determination and nephron formation. Cell 2001;106(3):319–29.

[103] Hanson J, Gorman J, Reese J, Fraizer G. Regulation of vascular endothelial growth factor, VEGF, gene promoter by the tumor suppressor, WT1. Front Biosci 2007;12:2279–90.

[104] Haraldsson B, Nyström J, Deen WM. Properties of the glomerular barrier and mechanisms of proteinuria. Physiol Rev 2008;88(2):451–87.

[105] Harita Y, Kurihara H, Kosako H, Tezuka T, Sekine T, Igarashi T, et al. Neph1, a component of the kidney slit diaphragm, is tyrosine-phosphorylated by the Src family tyrosine kinase and modulates intracellular signaling by binding to Grb2. J Biol Chem 2008;283(14):9177–86.

[106] Hartleben B, Gödel M, Meyer-Schwesinger C, Liu S, Ulrich T, Köbler S, et al. Autophagy influences glomerular disease susceptibility and maintains podocyte homeostasis in aging mice. J Clin Invest 2010;120(4):1084–96.

[107] Hartwig S, Ho J, Pandey P, Macisaac K, Taglienti M, Xiang M, et al. Genomic characterization of Wilms' tumor suppressor 1 targets in nephron progenitor cells during kidney development. Development 2010;137(7):1189–203.

[108] Harvey SJ, Jarad G, Cunningham J, Rops AL, van der Vlag J, Berden JH, et al. Disruption of glomerular basement membrane charge through podocyte-specific mutation of agrin does not alter glomerular permselectivity. Am J Pathol 2007;171 (1):139–52.

[109] Has C, Spartà G, Kiritsi D, Weibel L, Moeller A, Vega-Warner V, et al. Integrin α3 mutations with kidney, lung, and skin disease. N Engl J Med 2012;366(16):1508–14.

[110] Heeringa SF, Chernin G, Chaki M, Zhou W, Sloan AJ, Ji Z, et al. COQ6 mutations in human patients produce nephrotic syndrome with sensorineural deafness. J Clin Invest 2011;121 (5):2013–24.

[111] Henderson JM, Alexander MP, Pollak MR. Patients with ACTN4 mutations demonstrate distinctive features of glomerular injury. J Am Soc Nephrol 2009;20(5):961–8.

[112] Henger A, Huber T, Fischer KG, Nitschke R, Mundel P, Schollmeyer P, et al. Angiotensin II increases the cytosolic calcium activity in rat podocytes in culture. Kidney Int 1997;52 (3):687–93.

[113] Hinkes B, Wiggins RC, Gbadegesin R, Vlangos CN, Seelow D, Nürnberg G, et al. Positional cloning uncovers mutations in PLCE1 responsible for a nephrotic syndrome variant that may be reversible. Nat Genet 2006;38(12):1397–405.

[114] Hirata Y, Emori T, Eguchi S, Kanno K, Imai T, Ohta K, et al. Endothelin receptor subtype B mediates synthesis of nitric oxide by cultured bovine endothelial cells. J Clin Invest 1993;91(4):1367–73.

[115] Hjalmarsson C, Johansson BR, Haraldsson B. Electron microscopic evaluation of the endothelial surface layer of glomerular capillaries. Microvasc Res 2004;67(1):9–17.

[116] Hohenstein B, Hugo CPM, Hausknecht B, Boehmer KP, Riess RH, Schmieder RE. Analysis of NO-synthase expression and clinical risk factors in human diabetic nephropathy. Nephrol Dial Transplant 2008;23(4):1346–54.

[117] Holthöfer H, Ahola H, Solin ML, Wang S, Palmen T, Luimula P, et al. Nephrin localizes at the podocyte filtration slit area and is characteristically spliced in the human kidney. Am J Pathol 1999;155(5):1681–7.

[118] Hua H, Munk S, Whiteside CI. Endothelin-1 activates mesangial cell ERK1/2 via EGF-receptor transactivation and caveolin-1 interaction. Am J Physiol Renal Physiol 2003;284(2): F303–12.

[119] Hudson BG, Tryggvason K, Sundaramoorthy M, Neilson EG. Alport's syndrome, Goodpasture's syndrome, and type IV collagen. N Engl J Med 2003;348(25):2543–56.

[120] Hyink DP, Tucker DC St, John PL, Leardkamolkarn V, Accavitti MA, Abrass CK, et al. Endogenous origin of glomerular endothelial and mesangial cells in grafts of embryonic kidneys. Am J Physiol 1996;270(5 Pt 2):F886–99.

[121] Ichimura K, Stan RV, Kurihara H, Sakai T. Glomerular endothelial cells form diaphragms during development and pathologic conditions. J Am Soc Nephrol 2008;19(8):1463–71.

[122] Inoki K, Mori H, Wang J, Suzuki T, Hong S, Yoshida S, et al. mTORC1 activation in podocytes is a critical step in the development of diabetic nephropathy in mice. J Clin Invest 2011;121 (6):2181–96.

[123] Inoue T, Yaoita E, Kurihara H, Shimizu F, Sakai T, Kobayashi T, et al. FAT is a component of glomerular slit diaphragms. Kidney Int 2001;59(3):1003–12.

[124] Jacinto E, Loewith R, Schmidt A, Lin S, Rüegg MA, Hall A, et al. Mammalian TOR complex 2 controls the actin cytoskeleton and is rapamycin insensitive. Nat Cell Biol 2004;6(11):1122–8.

[125] Jarad G, Cunningham J, Shaw AS, Miner JH. Proteinuria precedes podocyte abnormalities inLamb2$^{-/-}$ mice, implicating the glomerular basement membrane as an albumin barrier. J Clin Invest 2006;116(8):2272–9.

[126] Jarad G, Pippin JW, Shankland SJ, Kreidberg JA, Miner JH. Dystroglycan does not contribute significantly to kidney

development or function, in health or after injury. Am J Physiol Renal Physiol 2011;300(3):F811—20.

[127] Jeansson M, Gawlik A, Anderson G, Li C, Kerjaschki D, Henkelman M, et al. Angiopoietin-1 is essential in mouse vasculature during development and in response to injury. J Clin Invest 2011;121(6):2278—89.

[128] Jeansson M, Haraldsson B. Glomerular size and charge selectivity in the mouse after exposure to glucosaminoglycan-degrading enzymes. J Am Soc Nephrol 2003;14(7):1756—65.

[129] Jeansson M, Haraldsson B. Morphological and functional evidence for an important role of the endothelial cell glycocalyx in the glomerular barrier. Am J Physiol Renal Physiol 2006;290 (1):F111—6.

[130] Jiang L, Ding J, Tsai H, Li L, Feng Q, Miao J, et al. Over-expressing transient receptor potential cation channel 6 in podocytes induces cytoskeleton rearrangement through increases of intracellular Ca^{2+} and RhoA activation. Exp Biol Med (Maywood) 2011;236(2):184—93.

[131] Jones N, Blasutig IM, Eremina V, Ruston JM, Bladt F, Li H, et al. Nck adaptor proteins link nephrin to the actin cytoskeleton of kidney podocytes. Nature 2006;440(7085):818—23.

[132] Kamba T, McDonald DM. Mechanisms of adverse effects of anti-VEGF therapy for cancer. Br J Cancer 2007;96(12):1788—95.

[133] Kamba T, Tam BYY, Hashizume H, Haskell A, Sennino B, Mancuso MR, et al. VEGF-dependent plasticity of fenestrated capillaries in the normal adult microvasculature. Am J Physiol Heart Circ Physiol 2006;290(2):H560—76.

[134] Kanasaki K, Kanda Y, Palmsten K, Tanjore H, Lee SB, Lebleu VS, et al. Integrin beta1-mediated matrix assembly and signaling are critical for the normal development and function of the kidney glomerulus. Dev Biol 2008;313(2):584—93.

[135] Kanwar YS, Linker A, Farquhar MG. Increased permeability of the glomerular basement membrane to ferritin after removal of glycosaminoglycans (heparan sulfate) by enzyme digestion. J Cell Biol 1980;86(2):688—93.

[136] Kanwar YS, Danesh FR, Chugh SS. Contribution of proteoglycans towards the integrated functions of renal glomerular capillaries: a historical perspective. Am J Pathol 2007;171 (1):9—13.

[137] Kaplan JM, Kim SH, North KN, Rennke H, Correia LA, Tong HQ, et al. Mutations in ACTN4, encoding alpha-actinin-4, cause familial focal segmental glomerulosclerosis. Nat Genet 2000;24(3):251—6.

[138] Karamatic Crew V, Burton N, Kagan A, Green CA, Levene C, Flinter F, et al. CD151, the first member of the tetraspanin (TM4) superfamily detected on erythrocytes, is essential for the correct assembly of human basement membranes in kidney and skin. Blood 2004;104(8):2217—23.

[139] Kashtan CE. Alport syndromes: phenotypic heterogeneity of progressive hereditary nephritis. Pediatr Nephrol 2000;14 (6):502—12.

[140] Kerjaschki D. Polycation-induced dislocation of slit diaphragms and formation of cell junctions in rat kidney glomeruli: the effects of low temperature, divalent cations, colchicine, and cytochalasin B. Lab Invest 1978;39(5):430—40.

[141] Kerjaschki D, Farquhar MG. Immunocytochemical localization of the Heymann nephritis antigen (GP330) in glomerular epithelial cells of normal Lewis rats. J Exp Med 1983;157 (2):667—86.

[142] Kerjaschki D, Ojha PP, Susani M, Horvat R, Binder S, Hovorka A, et al. A beta 1-integrin receptor for fibronectin in human kidney glomeruli. Am J Pathol 1989;134(2):481—9.

[143] Kestilä M, Lenkkeri U, Männikkö M, Lamerdin J, McCready P, Putaala H, et al. Positionally cloned gene for a novel glomerular protein — nephrin — is mutated in congenital nephrotic syndrome. Mol Cell 1998;1(4):575—82.

[144] Kim JM, Wu H, Green G, Winkler CA, Kopp JB, Miner JH, et al. CD2-associated protein haploinsufficiency is linked to glomerular disease susceptibility. Science 2003;300(5623): 1298—300.

[145] Kobayashi N, Mundel P. A role of microtubules during the formation of cell processes in neuronal and non-neuronal cells. Cell Tissue Res 1998;291(2):163—74.

[146] Kolatsi-Joannou M, Li XZ, Suda T, Yuan HT, Woolf AS. Expression and potential role of angiopoietins and Tie-2 in early development of the mouse metanephros. Dev Dyn 2001;222(1):120—6.

[147] Kreidberg JA. Functions of alpha3beta1 integrin. Curr Opin Cell Biol 2000;12(5):548—53.

[148] Kreidberg JA, Donovan MJ, Goldstein SL, Rennke H, Shepherd K, Jones RC, et al. Alpha 3 beta 1 integrin has a crucial role in kidney and lung organogenesis. Development 1996;122 (11):3537—47.

[149] Kreidberg JA, Sariola H, Loring JM, Maeda M, Pelletier J, Housman D, et al. WT-1 is required for early kidney development. Cell 1993;74(4):679—91.

[150] Kreidberg JA, Symons JM. Integrins in kidney development, function, and disease. Am J Physiol Renal Physiol 2000;279(2): F233—42.

[151] Kretzler M, Teixeira VP, Unschuld PG, Cohen CD, Wanke R, Edenhofer I, et al. Integrin-linked kinase as a candidate downstream effector in proteinuria. FASEB J 2001;15(10):1843—5.

[152] Kriz W, Elger M, Mundel P, Lemley KV. Structure-stabilizing forces in the glomerular tuft. J Am Soc Nephrol 1995;5 (10):1731—9.

[153] Kurihara H, Anderson JM, Kerjaschki D, Farquhar MG. The altered glomerular filtration slits seen in puromycin aminonucleoside nephrosis and protamine sulfate-treated rats contain the tight junction protein ZO-1. Am J Pathol 1992;141 (4):805—16.

[154] Kühn K. Basement membrane (type IV) collagen. Matrix Biol 1995;14(6):439—45.

[155] Laplante M, Sabatini DM. mTOR signaling in growth control and disease. Cell 2012;149(2):274—93.

[156] Le Hir M, Keller C, Eschmann V, Hähnel B, Hosser H, Kriz W. Podocyte bridges between the tuft and Bowman's capsule: an early event in experimental crescentic glomerulonephritis. J Am Soc Nephrol 2001;12(10):2060—71.

[157] Le Roux S, Pepper RJ, Dufay A, Néel M, Meffray E, Lamandé N, et al. Elevated soluble Flt1 inhibits endothelial repair in PR3-ANCA-associated vasculitis. J Am Soc Nephrol 2012;23 (1):155—64.

[158] Lea PJ, Silverman M, Hegele R, Hollenberg MJ. Tridimensional ultrastructure of glomerular capillary endothelium revealed by high-resolution scanning electron microscopy. Microvasc Res 1989;38(3):296—308.

[159] Lee S, Kim W, Kim DH, Moon S-O, Jung YJ, Lee AS, et al. Protective effect of COMP-angiopoietin-1 on cyclosporine-induced renal injury in mice. Nephrol Dial Transplant 2008;23 (9):2784—94.

[160] Lenkkeri U, Männikkö M, McCready P, Lamerdin J, Gribouval O, Niaudet PM, et al. Structure of the gene for congenital nephrotic syndrome of the Finnish type (NPHS1) and characterization of mutations. Am J Hum Genet 1999;64(1):51—61.

[161] Levéen P, Pekny M, Gebre-Medhin S, Swolin B, Larsson E, Betsholtz C. Mice deficient for PDGF B show renal, cardiovascular, and hematological abnormalities. Genes Dev 1994;8 (16):1875—87.

[162] Levine RJ, Maynard SE, Qian C, Lim K-H, England LJ, Yu KF, et al. Circulating angiogenic factors and the risk of preeclampsia. N Engl J Med 2004;350(7):672—83.

[163] Li C, Ruotsalainen V, Tryggvason K, Shaw AS, Miner JH. CD2AP is expressed with nephrin in developing podocytes and is found widely in mature kidney and elsewhere. Am J Physiol Renal Physiol 2000;279(4):F785—92.

[164] Li L, Krantz ID, Deng Y, Genin A, Banta AB, Collins CC, et al. Alagille syndrome is caused by mutations in human Jagged1, which encodes a ligand for Notch1. Nat Genet 1997;16 (3):243—51.

[165] Lindahl P, Hellström M, Kalén M, Karlsson L, Pekny M, Pekna M, et al. Paracrine PDGF-B/PDGF-Rbeta signaling controls mesangial cell development in kidney glomeruli. Development 1998;125(17):3313—22.

[166] Lindblom P, Gerhardt H, Liebner S, Abramsson A, Enge M, Hellstrom M, et al. Endothelial PDGF-B retention is required for proper investment of pericytes in the microvessel wall. Genes Dev 2003;17(15):1835—40.

[167] Liu A, Dardik A, Ballermann BJ. Neutralizing TGF-beta1 antibody infusion in neonatal rat delays in vivo glomerular capillary formation 1. Kidney Int 1999;56(4):1334—48.

[168] Liu G, Kaw B, Kurfis J, Rahmanuddin S, Kanwar YS, Chugh SS. Neph1 and nephrin interaction in the slit diaphragm is an important determinant of glomerular permeability. J Clin Invest 2003;112(2):209—21.

[169] Lu W, Phillips CL, Killen PD, Hlaing T, Harrison WR, Elder FF, et al. Insertional mutation of the collagen genes Col4a3 and Col4a4 in a mouse model of Alport syndrome. Genomics 1999;61(2):113—24.

[170] Lund U, Rippe A, Venturoli D, Tenstad O, Grubb A, Rippe B. Glomerular filtration rate dependence of sieving of albumin and some neutral proteins in rat kidneys. Am J Physiol Renal Physiol 2003;284(6):F1226—34.

[171] Ma H, Togawa A, Soda K, Zhang J, Lee S, Ma M, et al. Inhibition of podocyte FAK protects against proteinuria and foot process effacement. J Am Soc Nephrol 2010;21(7):1145—56.

[172] Madri JA, Roll FJ, Furthmayr H, Foidart JM. Ultrastructural localization of fibronectin and laminin in the basement membranes of the murine kidney. J Cell Biol 1980;86(2):682—7.

[173] Maharaj ASR, Walshe TE, Saint-Geniez M, Venkatesha S, Maldonado AE, Himes NC, et al. VEGF and TGF-beta are required for the maintenance of the choroid plexus and ependyma. J Exp Med 2008;205(2):491—501.

[174] Maisonpierre PC, Suri C, Jones PF, Bartunkova S, Wiegand SJ, Radziejewski C, et al. Angiopoietin-2, a natural antagonist for Tie2 that disrupts in vivo angiogenesis. Science 1997;277 (5322):55—60.

[175] Makino H, Kashihara N, Sugiyama H, Kanao K, Sekikawa T, Shikata K, et al. Phenotypic changes of the mesangium in diabetic nephropathy. J Diabetes Complicat 1995;9(4):282—4.

[176] Marshall CB, Shankland SJ. Cell cycle and glomerular disease: a minireview. Nephron Exp Nephrol 2006;102(2):e39—48.

[177] Martinez-Hernandez A, Chung AE. The ultrastructural localization of two basement membrane components: entactin and laminin in rat tissues. J Histochem Cytochem 1984;32 (3):289—98.

[178] Matsui T, Maeda M, Doi Y, Yonemura S, Amano M, Kaibuchi K, et al. Rho-kinase phosphorylates COOH-terminal threonines of ezrin/radixin/moesin (ERM) proteins and regulates their head-to-tail association. J Cell Biol 1998;140(3):647—57.

[179] Maynard SE, Min J-Y, Merchan J, Lim K-H, Li J, Mondal S, et al. Excess placental soluble fms-like tyrosine kinase 1 (sFlt1) may contribute to endothelial dysfunction, hypertension, and proteinuria in preeclampsia. J Clin Invest 2003;111(5):649—58.

[180] Mbassa G, Elger M, Kriz W. The ultrastructural organization of the basement membrane of Bowman's capsule in the rat renal corpuscle. Cell Tissue Res 1988;253(1):151—63.

[181] McCright B, Gao X, Shen L, Lozier J, Lan Y, Maguire M, et al. Defects in development of the kidney, heart and eye vasculature in mice homozygous for a hypomorphic Notch2 mutation. Development 2001;128(4):491—502.

[182] McDaniell R, Warthen DM, Sanchez-Lara PA, Pai A, Krantz ID, Piccoli DA, et al. NOTCH2 mutations cause Alagille syndrome, a heterogeneous disorder of the notch signaling pathway. Am J Hum Genet 2006;79(1):169—73.

[183] Mele C, Iatropoulos P, Donadelli R, Calabria A, Maranta R, Cassis P, et al. MYO1E mutations and childhood familial focal segmental glomerulosclerosis. N Engl J Med 2011;365 (4):295—306.

[184] Menke AL, IJpenberg A, Fleming S, Ross A, Medine CN, Patek CE, et al. The wt1-heterozygous mouse; a model to study the development of glomerular sclerosis. J Pathol 2003;200 (5):667—74.

[185] Miner JH, Li C. Defective glomerulogenesis in the absence of laminin alpha5 demonstrates a developmental role for the kidney glomerular basement membrane. Dev Biol 2000;217 (2):278—89.

[186] Miner JH, Sanes JR. Molecular and functional defects in kidneys of mice lacking collagen alpha 3(IV): implications for Alport syndrome. J Cell Biol 1996;135(5):1403—13.

[187] Miner JH. Building the glomerulus: a matricentric view. J Am Soc Nephrol 2005;16(4):857—61.

[188] Miner JH. Organogenesis of the kidney glomerulus: focus on the glomerular basement membrane. Organogenesis 2011;7 (2):75—82.

[189] Miner JH. The glomerular basement membrane. Exp Cell Res 2012;318(9):973—8.

[190] Miner JH. Life without nephrin: it's for the birds. J Am Soc Nephrol 2012;23(3):369—71.

[191] Miner JH, Morello R, Andrews KL, Li C, Antignac C, Shaw AS, et al. Transcriptional induction of slit diaphragm genes by Lmx1b is required in podocyte differentiation. J Clin Invest 2002;109(8):1065—72.

[192] Miner JH, Yurchenco PD. Laminin functions in tissue morphogenesis. Annu Rev Cell Dev Biol 2004;20:255—84.

[193] Moeller MJ, Soofi A, Hartmann I, Le Hir M, Wiggins R, Kriz W, et al. Podocytes populate cellular crescents in a murine model of inflammatory glomerulonephritis. J Am Soc Nephrol 2004;15(1):61—7.

[194] Moore AW, McInnes L, Kreidberg J, Hastie ND, Schedl A. YAC complementation shows a requirement for Wt1 in the development of epicardium, adrenal gland and throughout nephrogenesis. Development 1999;126(9):1845—57.

[195] Muchitsch E, Pichler L, Schwarz HP, Ulrich W. Effects of human alpha-1-acid glycoprotein on aminonucleoside-induced minimal change nephrosis in rats. Nephron 1999;81(2):194—9.

[196] Mundel P, Kriz W. Structure and function of podocytes: an update. Anat Embryol 1995;192(5):385—97.

[197] Murakami T, Miyoshi M, Fujita T. Glomerular vessels of the rat kidney with special reference to double efferent arterioles. A scanning electron microscope study of corrosion casts. Arch Histol Jpn 1971;33(3):179—98.

[198] Murea M, Park J-K, Sharma S, Kato H, Gruenwald A, Niranjan T, et al. Expression of Notch pathway proteins correlates with albuminuria, glomerulosclerosis, and renal function. Kidney Int 2010;78(5):514—22.

[199] Murshed M, Smyth N, Miosge N, Karolat J, Krieg T, Paulsson M, et al. The absence of nidogen 1 does not affect murine basement membrane formation. Mol Cell Biol 2000;20 (18):7007−12.

[200] Nakagawa T, Sato W, Glushakova O, Heinig M, Clarke T, Campbell-Thompson M, et al. Diabetic endothelial nitric oxide synthase knockout mice develop advanced diabetic nephropathy. J Am Soc Nephrol 2007;18(2):539−50.

[201] Narita M, Young ARJ, Arakawa S, Samarajiwa SA, Nakashima T, Yoshida S, et al. Spatial coupling of mTOR and autophagy augments secretory phenotypes. Science 2011;332(6032):966−70.

[202] Niranjan T, Bielesz B, Gruenwald A, Ponda MP, Kopp JB, Thomas DB, et al. The Notch pathway in podocytes plays a role in the development of glomerular disease. Nat Med 2008;14(3):290−8.

[203] Nishiuchi R, Sanzen N, Nada S, Sumida Y, Wada Y, Okada M, et al. Potentiation of the ligand-binding activity of integrin alpha3beta1 via association with tetraspanin CD151. Proc Natl Acad Sci USA 2005;102(6):1939−44.

[204] Noakes PG, Miner JH, Gautam M, Cunningham JM, Sanes JR, Merlie JP. The renal glomerulus of mice lacking s-laminin/laminin beta 2: nephrosis despite molecular compensation by laminin beta 1. Nat Genet 1995;10(4):400−6.

[205] Noonan DM, Fulle A, Valente P, Cai S, Horigan E, Sasaki M, et al. The complete sequence of perlecan, a basement membrane heparan sulfate proteoglycan, reveals extensive similarity with laminin A chain, low density lipoprotein-receptor, and the neural cell adhesion molecule. J Biol Chem 1991;266 (34):22939−47.

[206] Oda T, Elkahloun AG, Pike BL, Okajima K, Krantz ID, Genin A, et al. Mutations in the human Jagged1 gene are responsible for Alagille syndrome. Nat Genet 1997;16(3):235−42.

[207] Ohse T, Chang AM, Pippin JW, Jarad G, Hudkins KL, Alpers CE, et al. A new function for parietal epithelial cells: A second glomerular barrier. Am J Physiol Renal Physiol 2009;297(6): F1566−74.

[208] Okamoto K, Tokunaga K, Doi K, Fujita T, Suzuki H, Katoh T, et al. Common variation in GPC5 is associated with acquired nephrotic syndrome. Nat Genet 2011;43(5):459−63.

[209] Oliver J, MacDowell M. Nephrons and kidneys: a quantitative study of developmental and evolutionary mammalian renal architectonics. New York: Hoeber Medical Division, Harper & Row; 1968.

[210] Osterby R. Morphometric studies of the peripheral glomerular basement membrane in early juvenile diabetes. I. Development of initial basement membrane thickening. Diabetologia 1972;8 (2):84−92.

[211] Ozaltin F, Ibsirlioglu T, Taskiran EZ, Baydar DE, Kaymaz F, Buyukcelik M, et al. Disruption of PTPRO causes childhood-onset nephrotic syndrome. Am J Hum Genet 2011;89(1): 139−47.

[212] Pala L, Cresci B, Manuelli C, Maggi E, Yamaguchi YF, Cappugi P, et al. Vascular endothelial growth factor receptor-2 and low affinity VEGF binding sites on human glomerular endothelial cells: biological effects and advanced glycosilation end products modulation. Microvasc Res 2005;70(3):179−88.

[213] Palmer RE, Kotsianti A, Cadman B, Boyd T, Gerald W, Haber DA. WT1 regulates the expression of the major glomerular podocyte membrane protein Podocalyxin. Curr Biol 2001;11 (22):1805−9.

[214] Pelletier J, Bruening W, Kashtan CE, Mauer SM, Manivel JC, Striegel JE, et al. Germline mutations in the Wilms' tumor suppressor gene are associated with abnormal urogenital development in Denys−Drash syndrome. Cell 1991;67(2):437−47.

[215] Peter K. Untersuchungen über bau und entwickelung der niere. Jena: Gustav Fischer; 1909.

[216] Petruzziello-Pellegrini TN, Yuen DA, Page AV, Patel S, Soltyk AM, Matouk CC, et al. The CXCR4/CXCR7/SDF-1 pathway contributes to the pathogenesis of Shiga toxin-associated hemolytic uremic syndrome in humans and mice. J Clin Invest 2012;122(2):759−76.

[217] Pitera JE, Woolf AS, Gale NW, Yancopoulos GD, Yuan HT. Dysmorphogenesis of kidney cortical peritubular capillaries in angiopoietin-2-deficient mice. Am J Pathol 2004;165 (6):1895−906.

[218] Plaisier E, Gribouval O, Alamowitch S, Mougenot B, Prost C, Verpont MC, et al. COL4A1 mutations and hereditary angiopathy, nephropathy, aneurysms, and muscle cramps. N Engl J Med 2007;357(26):2687−95.

[219] Pozzi A, Jarad G, Moeckel GW, Coffa S, Zhang X, Gewin L, et al. Beta1 integrin expression by podocytes is required to maintain glomerular structural integrity. Dev Biol 2008;316(2):288−301.

[220] Pricci F, Pugliese G, Romano G, Romeo G, Locuratolo N, Pugliese F, et al. Insulin-like growth factors I and II stimulate extracellular matrix production in human glomerular mesangial cells. Comparison with transforming growth factor-beta. Endocrinology 1996;137(3):879−85.

[221] Pugliese G, Pricci F, Locuratolo N, Romeo G, Romano G, Giannini S, et al. Increased activity of the insulin-like growth factor system in mesangial cells cultured in high glucose conditions. Relation to glucose-enhanced extracellular matrix production. Diabetologia 1996;39(7):775−84.

[222] Putaala H, Soininen R, Kilpeläinen P, Wartiovaara J, Tryggvason K. The murine nephrin gene is specifically expressed in kidney, brain and pancreas: inactivation of the gene leads to massive proteinuria and neonatal death. Hum Mol Genet 2001;10(1):1−8.

[223] Quaggin SE, Schwartz L, Cui S, Igarashi P, Deimling J, Post M, et al. The basic-helix-loop-helix protein pod1 is critically important for kidney and lung organogenesis. Development 1999;126(24):5771−83.

[224] Quaggin SE, Vanden Heuvel GB, Igarashi P. Pod-1, a mesoderm-specific basic-helix-loop-helix protein expressed in mesenchymal and glomerular epithelial cells in the developing kidney. Mech Dev 1998;71(1−2):37−48.

[225] Quaggin SE, Kreidberg JA. Development of the renal glomerulus: good neighbors and good fences. Development 2008;135 (4):609−20.

[226] Raats CJ, van den Born J, Bakker MA, Oppers-Walgreen B, Pisa BJ, Dijkman HB, et al. Expression of agrin, dystroglycan, and utrophin in normal renal tissue and in experimental glomerulopathies. Am J Pathol 2000;156(5):1749−65.

[227] Raftopoulou M, Hall A. Cell migration: rho GTPases lead the way. Dev Biol 2004;265(1):23−32.

[228] Rahilly MA, Fleming S. Differential expression of integrin alpha chains by renal epithelial cells. J Pathol 1992;167 (3):327−34.

[229] Regele HM, Fillipovic E, Langer B, Poczewki H, Kraxberger I, Bittner RE, et al. Glomerular expression of dystroglycans is reduced in minimal change nephrosis but not in focal segmental glomerulosclerosis. J Am Soc Nephrol 2000;11 (3):403−12.

[230] Reiser J, Kriz W, Kretzler M, Mundel P. The glomerular slit diaphragm is a modified adherens junction. J Am Soc Nephrol 2000;11(1):1−8.

[231] Reiser J, Polu KR, Möller CC, Kenlan P, Altintas MM, Wei C. TRPC6 is a glomerular slit diaphragm-associated channel required for normal renal function. Nat Genet 2005;37 (7):739−44.

[232] Rennke HG, Venkatachalam MA. Glomerular permeability: *in vivo* tracer studies with polyanionic and polycationic ferritins. Kidney Int 1977;11(1):44–53.

[233] Rheault MN, Kren SM, Thielen BK, Mesa HA, Crosson JT, Thomas W, et al. Mouse model of X-linked Alport syndrome. J Am Soc Nephrol 2004;15(6):1466–74.

[234] Robert B St, John PL, Abrahamson DR. Direct visualization of renal vascular morphogenesis in Flk1 heterozygous mutant mice. Am J Physiol 1998;275(1 Pt 2):F164–72.

[235] Robert B St, John PL, Hyink DP, Abrahamson DR. Evidence that embryonic kidney cells expressing flk-1 are intrinsic, vasculogenic angioblasts. Am J Physiol 1996;271(3 Pt 2): F744–53.

[236] Rodewald R, Karnovsky MJ. Porous substructure of the glomerular slit diaphragm in the rat and mouse. J Cell Biol 1974;60(2):423–33.

[237] Rohr C, Prestel J, Heidet L, Hosser H, Kriz W, Johnson RL, et al. The LIM-homeodomain transcription factor Lmx1b plays a crucial role in podocytes. J Clin Invest 2002;109(8):1073–82.

[238] Roll FJ, Madri JA, Albert J, Furthmayr H. Codistribution of collagen types IV and AB2 in basement membranes and mesangium of the kidney. An immunoferritin study of ultrathin frozen sections. J Cell Biol 1980;85(3):597–616.

[239] Roselli S, Heidet L, Sich M, Henger A, Kretzler M, Gubler M-C, et al. Early glomerular filtration defect and severe renal disease in podocin-deficient mice. Mol Cell Biol 2004;24 (2):550–60.

[240] Rosenzweig LJ, Kanwar YS. Removal of sulfated (heparan sulfate) or nonsulfated (hyaluronic acid) glycosaminoglycans results in increased permeability of the glomerular basement membrane to 125I-bovine serum albumin. Lab Invest 1982;47 (2):177–84.

[241] Rostgaard J, Qvortrup K. Electron microscopic demonstrations of filamentous molecular sieve plugs in capillary fenestrae. Microvasc Res 1997;53(1):1–13.

[242] Rostgaard J, Qvortrup K. Sieve plugs in fenestrae of glomerular capillaries — site of the filtration barrier? Cells Tissues Organs (Print) 2002;170(2–3):132–8.

[243] Ruotsalainen V, Ljungberg P, Wartiovaara J, Lenkkeri U, Kestilä M, Jalanko H, et al. Nephrin is specifically located at the slit diaphragm of glomerular podocytes. Proc Natl Acad Sci USA 1999;96(14):7962–7.

[244] Ryan G, Steele-Perkins V, Morris JF, Rauscher FJ, Dressler GR. Repression of Pax-2 by WT1 during normal kidney development. Development 1995;121(3):867–75.

[245] Sadl V, Jin F, Yu J, Cui S, Holmyard D, Quaggin S, et al. The mouse Kreisler (Krml1/MafB) segmentation gene is required for differentiation of glomerular visceral epithelial cells. Dev Biol 2002;249(1):16–29.

[246] Sakai T, Kriz W. The structural relationship between mesangial cells and basement membrane of the renal glomerulus. Anat Embryol 1987;176(3):373–86.

[247] Salmon AHJ, Neal CR, Sage LM, Glass CA, Harper SJ, Bates DO. Angiopoietin-1 alters microvascular permeability coefficients *in vivo* via modification of endothelial glycocalyx. Cardiovasc Res 2009;83(1):24–33.

[248] Sarbassov DD, Ali SM, Sengupta S, Sheen J-H, Hsu PP, Bagley AF, et al. Prolonged rapamycin treatment inhibits mTORC2 assembly and Akt/PKB. Mol Cell 2006;22(2): 159–68.

[249] Satchell SC, Braet F. Glomerular endothelial cell fenestrations: an integral component of the glomerular filtration barrier. Am J Physiol Renal Physiol 2009;296(5):F947–56.

[250] Satchell SC, Harper SJ, Tooke JE, Kerjaschki D, Saleem MA, Mathieson PW. Human podocytes express angiopoietin 1, a

[251] Sayyed SG, Hägele H, Kulkarni OP, Endlich K, Segerer S, Eulberg D, et al. Podocytes produce homeostatic chemokine stromal cell-derived factor-1/CXCL12, which contributes to glomerulosclerosis, podocyte loss and albuminuria in a mouse model of type 2 diabetes. Diabetologia 2009;52 (11):2445–54.

[252] Schaefer L, Grone HJ, Raslik I, Robenek H, Ugorcakova J, Budny S, et al. Small proteoglycans of normal adult human kidney: distinct expression patterns of decorin, biglycan, fibromodulin, and lumican. Kidney Int 2000;58(4):1557–68.

[253] Scharpfenecker M, Fiedler U, Reiss Y, Augustin HG. The Tie-2 ligand angiopoietin-2 destabilizes quiescent endothelium through an internal autocrine loop mechanism. J Cell Sci 2005;118(Pt 4):771–80.

[254] Schlondorff J, Del Camino D, Carrasquillo R, Lacey V, Pollak MR. TRPC6 mutations associated with focal segmental glomerulosclerosis cause constitutive activation of NFAT-dependent transcription. Am J Physiol, Cell Physiol 2009;296(3): C558–69.

[255] Schmieder S, Nagai M, Orlando RA, Takeda T, Farquhar MG. Podocalyxin activates RhoA and induces actin reorganization through NHERF1 and Ezrin in MDCK cells. J Am Soc Nephrol 2004;15(9):2289–98.

[256] Schnabel E, Anderson JM, Farquhar MG. The tight junction protein ZO-1 is concentrated along slit diaphragms of the glomerular epithelium. J Cell Biol 1990;111(3):1255–63.

[257] Schnaper HW, Hayashida T, Hubchak SC, Poncelet A-C. TGF-beta signal transduction and mesangial cell fibrogenesis. Am J Physiol Renal Physiol 2003;284(2):F243–52.

[258] Schordan S, Schordan E, Endlich K, Endlich N. AlphaV-integrins mediate the mechanoprotective action of osteopontin in podocytes. Am J Physiol Renal Physiol 2011;300(1):F119–32.

[259] Schumacher VA, Schlötzer-Schrehardt U, Karumanchi SA, Shi X, Zaia J, Jeruschke S. WT1-dependent sulfatase expression maintains the normal glomerular filtration barrier. J Am Soc Nephrol 2011;22(7):1286–96.

[260] Schwartz E, Goldfischer S, Coltoff-Schiller B, Blumenfeld OO. Extracellular matrix microfibrils are composed of core proteins coated with fibronectin. J Histochem Cytochem 1985;33 (4):268–74.

[261] Schwarz K, Simons M, Reiser J, Saleem MA, Faul C, Kriz W, et al. Podocin, a raft-associated component of the glomerular slit diaphragm, interacts with CD2AP and nephrin. J Clin Invest 2001;108(11):1621–9.

[262] Schymeinsky J, Nedbal S, Miosge N, Pöschl E, Rao C, Beier DR, et al. Gene structure and functional analysis of the mouse nidogen-2 gene: nidogen-2 is not essential for basement membrane formation in mice. Mol Cell Biol 2002;22(19):6820–30.

[263] Scott RP, Hawley SP, Ruston J, Du J, Brakebusch C, Jones N, et al. Podocyte-specific loss of Cdc42 leads to congenital nephropathy. J Am Soc Nephrol 2012;: [epub ahead of print]

[264] Seiler MW, Rennke HG, Venkatachalam MA, Cotran RS. Pathogenesis of polycation-induced alterations ("fusion") of glomerular epithelium. Lab Invest 1977;36(1):48–61.

[265] Sellin L, Huber TB, Gerke P, Quack I, Pavenstädt H, Walz G. NEPH1 defines a novel family of podocin interacting proteins. FASEB J 2003;17(1):115–7.

[266] Serra AL, Poster D, Kistler AD, Krauer F, Raina S, Young J, et al. Sirolimus and kidney growth in autosomal dominant polycystic kidney disease. N Engl J Med 2010;363(9):820–9.

[267] Shannon MB, Patton BL, Harvey SJ, Miner JH. A hypomorphic mutation in the mouse laminin alpha5 gene causes polycystic kidney disease. J Am Soc Nephrol 2006;17(7):1913–22.

[268] Shih NY, Li J, Cotran R, Mundel P, Miner JH, Shaw AS. CD2AP localizes to the slit diaphragm and binds to nephrin via a novel C-terminal domain. Am J Pathol 2001;159 (6):2303–8.

[269] Shih NY, Li J, Karpitskii V, Nguyen A, Dustin ML, Kanagawa O, et al. Congenital nephrotic syndrome in mice lacking CD2-associated protein. Science 1999;286(5438):312–5.

[270] Smeets B, Kuppe C, Sicking E-M, Fuss A, Jirak P, van Kuppevelt TH, et al. Parietal epithelial cells participate in the formation of sclerotic lesions in focal segmental glomerulosclerosis. J Am Soc Nephrol 2011;22(7):1262–74.

[271] Smith HW. The kidney. USA: Oxford University Press; 1951.

[272] Soriano P. Abnormal kidney development and hematological disorders in PDGF beta-receptor mutant mice. Genes Dev 1994;8(16):1888–96.

[273] St John PL, Abrahamson DR. Glomerular endothelial cells and podocytes jointly synthesize laminin-1 and -11 chains. Kidney Int 2001;60(3):1037–46.

[274] Steffes MW, Barbosa J, Basgen JM, Sutherland DE, Najarian JS, Mauer SM. Quantitative glomerular morphology of the normal human kidney. Lab Invest 1983;49(1):82–6.

[275] Sterk LMT, Geuijen CAW, van den Berg JG, Claessen N, Weening JJ, Sonnenberg A. Association of the tetraspanin CD151 with the laminin-binding integrins alpha3beta1, alpha6-beta1, alpha6beta4 and alpha7beta1 in cells in culture and in vivo. J Cell Sci 2002;115(Pt 6):1161–73.

[276] Sterzel RB, Hartner A, Schlotzer-Schrehardt U, Voit S, Hausknecht B, Doliana R, et al. Elastic fiber proteins in the glomerular mesangium in vivo and in cell culture. Kidney Int 2000;58(4):1588–602.

[277] Stow JL, Sawada H, Farquhar MG. Basement membrane heparan sulfate proteoglycans are concentrated in the laminae rarae and in podocytes of the rat renal glomerulus. Proc Natl Acad Sci USA 1985;82(10):3296–300.

[278] Suh JH, Jarad G, VanDeVoorde RG, Miner JH. Forced expression of laminin beta1 in podocytes prevents nephrotic syndrome in mice lacking laminin beta2, a model for Pierson syndrome. Proc Natl Acad Sci USA 2011;108(37):15348–53.

[279] Suri C, Jones PF, Patan S, Bartunkova S, Maisonpierre PC, Davis S, et al. Requisite role of angiopoietin-1, a ligand for the TIE2 receptor, during embryonic angiogenesis. Cell 1996;87 (7):1171–80.

[280] Tachibana K, Hirota S, Iizasa H, Yoshida H, Kawabata K, Kataoka Y, et al. The chemokine receptor CXCR4 is essential for vascularization of the gastrointestinal tract. Nature 1998;393(6685):591–4.

[281] Takabatake Y, Sugiyama T, Kohara H, Matsusaka T, Kurihara H, Koni PA, et al. The CXCL12 (SDF-1)/CXCR4 axis is essential for the development of renal vasculature. J Am Soc Nephrol 2009;20(8):1714–23.

[282] Takahashi T, Takahashi K, Gerety S, Wang H, Anderson DJ, Daniel TO. Temporally compartmentalized expression of ephrin-B2 during renal glomerular development. J Am Soc Nephrol 2001;12(12):2673–82.

[283] Takeda T, McQuistan T, Orlando RA, Farquhar MG. Loss of glomerular foot processes is associated with uncoupling of podocalyxin from the actin cytoskeleton. J Clin Invest 2001;108 (2):289–301.

[284] Takemoto M, He L, Norlin J, Patrakka J, Xiao Z, Petrova T, et al. Large-scale identification of genes implicated in kidney glomerulus development and function. EMBO J 2006;25(5): 1160–74.

[285] Teixeira V de PC, Blattner SM, Li M, Anders H-J, Cohen CD, Edenhofer I, et al. Functional consequences of integrin-linked kinase activation in podocyte damage. Kidney Int 2005;67(2):514–23.

[286] Tessari P, Cecchet D, Cosma A, Vettore M, Coracina A, Millioni R, et al. Nitric oxide synthesis is reduced in subjects with type 2 diabetes and nephropathy. Diabetes 2010;59(9): 2152–9.

[287] Tian D, Jacobo SMP, Billing D, Rozkalne A, Gage SD, Anagnostou T, et al. Antagonistic regulation of actin dynamics and cell motility by TRPC5 and TRPC6 channels. Sci Signal 2010;3(145):ra77.

[288] Trachtman H. Nitric oxide and glomerulonephritis. Semin Nephrol 2004;24(4):324–32.

[289] Tryggvason K, Wartiovaara J. Molecular basis of glomerular permselectivity. Curr Opin Nephrol Hypertens 2001;10 (4):543–9.

[290] Tryggvason K, Patrakka J, Wartiovaara J. Hereditary proteinuria syndromes and mechanisms of proteinuria. N Engl J Med 2006;354(13):1387–401.

[291] Utriainen A, Sormunen R, Kettunen M, Carvalhaes LS, Sajanti E, Eklund L, et al. Structurally altered basement membranes and hydrocephalus in a type XVIII collagen deficient mouse line. Hum Mol Genet 2004;13(18):2089–99.

[292] Venkatesha S, Toporsian M, Lam C, Hanai J-I, Mammoto T, Kim YM, et al. Soluble endoglin contributes to the pathogenesis of preeclampsia. Nat Med 2006;12(6):642–9.

[293] Vogelmann SU, Nelson WJ, Myers BD, Lemley KV. Urinary excretion of viable podocytes in health and renal disease. Am J Physiol Renal Physiol 2003;285(1):F40–8.

[294] Vollenbröker B, George B, Wolfgart M, Saleem MA, Pavenstädt H, Weide T. mTOR regulates expression of slit diaphragm proteins and cytoskeleton structure in podocytes. Am J Physiol Renal Physiol 2009;296(2):F418–26.

[295] Voskarides K, Damianou L, Neocleous V, Zouvani I, Christodoulidou S, Hadjiconstantinou V, et al. COL4A3/COL4A4 mutations producing focal segmental glomerulosclerosis and renal failure in thin basement membrane nephropathy. J Am Soc Nephrol 2007;18(11):3004–16.

[296] Völker LA, Petry M, Abdelsabour-Khalaf M, Schweizer H, Yusuf F, Busch T, et al. Comparative analysis of Neph gene expression in mouse and chicken development. Histochem Cell Biol 2012;137(3):355–66.

[297] Wada J, Makino H, Kanwar YS. Gene expression and identification of gene therapy targets in diabetic nephropathy. Kidney Int 2002;61(1 Suppl):S73–8.

[298] Wagner N, Wagner K-D, Xing Y, Scholz H, Schedl A. The major podocyte protein nephrin is transcriptionally activated by the Wilms' tumor suppressor WT1. J Am Soc Nephrol 2004;15(12):3044–51.

[299] Wang HU, Anderson DJ. Eph family transmembrane ligands can mediate repulsive guidance of trunk neural crest migration and motor axon outgrowth. Neuron 1997;18(3): 383–96.

[300] Waters AM, Wu MYJ, Onay T, Scutaru J, Liu J, Lobe CG, et al. Ectopic notch activation in developing podocytes causes glomerulosclerosis. J Am Soc Nephrol 2008;19(6):1139–57.

[301] Wei C, Hindi El S, Li J, Fornoni A, Goes N, Sageshima J, et al. Circulating urokinase receptor as a cause of focal segmental glomerulosclerosis. Nat Med 2011;17(8):952–60.

[302] Wei C, Möller CC, Altintas MM, Li J, Schwarz K, Zacchigna S, et al. Modification of kidney barrier function by the urokinase receptor. Nat Med 2008;14(1):55–63.

[303] Weins A, Schlondorff JS, Nakamura F, Denker BM, Hartwig JH, Stossel TP, et al. Disease-associated mutant alpha-actinin-4 reveals a mechanism for regulating its F-actin-binding affinity. Proc Natl Acad Sci USA 2007;104(41):16080–5.

[304] Welsh GI, Hale LJ, Eremina V, Jeansson M, Maezawa Y, Lennon R, et al. Insulin signaling to the glomerular podocyte is

critical for normal kidney function. Cell Metab 2010;12 (4):329—40.

[305] Wendel M, Knels L, Kummer W, Koch T. Distribution of endothelin receptor subtypes ETA and ETB in the rat kidney. J Histochem Cytochem 2006;54(11):1193—203.

[306] Winn MP, Conlon PJ, Lynn KL, Farrington MK, Creazzo T, Hawkins AF, et al. A mutation in the TRPC6 cation channel causes familial focal segmental glomerulosclerosis. Science 2005;308(5729):1801—4.

[307] Wnuk M, Hlushchuk R, Janot M, Tuffin G, Martiny-Baron G, Holzer P, et al. Podocyte EphB4 signaling helps recovery from glomerular injury. Kidney Int 2012;81(12):1212—25.

[308] Woolf AS. Angiopoietins: Vascular growth factors looking for roles in glomeruli. Curr Opin Nephrol Hypertens 2010;19 (1):20—5.

[309] Wu C, Dedhar S. Integrin-linked kinase (ILK) and its interactors: A new paradigm for the coupling of extracellular matrix to actin cytoskeleton and signaling complexes. J Cell Biol 2001;155(4):505—10.

[310] Yamagishi S-I, Matsui T. Nitric oxide, a janus-faced therapeutic target for diabetic microangiopathy: friend or foe? Pharmacol Res 2011;64(3):187—94.

[311] Yang Y, Jeanpierre C, Dressler GR, Lacoste M, Niaudet P, Gubler MC. WT1 and PAX-2 podocyte expression in Denys—Drash syndrome and isolated diffuse mesangial sclerosis. Am J Pathol 1999;154(1):181—92.

[312] Yang Y, Guo L, Blattner SM, Mundel P, Kretzler M, Wu C. Formation and phosphorylation of the PINCH-1-integrin linked kinase-alpha-parvin complex are important for regulation of renal glomerular podocyte adhesion, architecture, and survival. J Am Soc Nephrol 2005;16(7):1966—76.

[313] Yaoita E, Kurihara H, Yoshida Y, Inoue T, Matsuki A, Sakai T, et al. Role of Fat1 in cell—cell contact formation of podocytes in puromycin aminonucleoside nephrosis and neonatal kidney. Kidney Int 2005;68(2):542—51.

[314] Yauch RL, Kazarov AR, Desai B, Lee RT, Hemler ME. Direct extracellular contact between integrin alpha(3)beta(1) and TM4SF protein CD151. J Biol Chem 2000;275(13):9230—8.

[315] Ye M, Wysocki J, William J, Soler MJ, Cokic I, Batlle D. Glomerular localization and expression of Angiotensin-converting enzyme 2 and Angiotensin-converting enzyme:

[316] Yu D, Petermann A, Kunter U, Rong S, Shankland SJ, Floege J. Urinary podocyte loss is a more specific marker of ongoing glomerular damage than proteinuria. J Am Soc Nephrol 2005;16(6):1733—41.

[317] Yu L, McPhee CK, Zheng L, Mardones GA, Rong Y, Peng J, et al. Termination of autophagy and reformation of lysosomes regulated by mTOR. Nature 2010;465(7300):942—6.

[318] Yuan HT, Suri C, Landon DN, Yancopoulos GD, Woolf AS. Angiopoietin-2 is a site-specific factor in differentiation of mouse renal vasculature. J Am Soc Nephrol 2000;11 (6):1055—66.

[319] Yuan HT, Suri C, Yancopoulos GD, Woolf AS. Expression of angiopoietin-1, angiopoietin-2, and the Tie-2 receptor tyrosine kinase during mouse kidney maturation. J Am Soc Nephrol 1999;10(8):1722—36.

[320] Yuan HT, Khankin EV, Karumanchi SA, Parikh SM. Angiopoietin 2 is a partial agonist/antagonist of Tie2 signaling in the endothelium. Mol Cell Biol 2009;29(8):2011—22.

[321] Zeng Z, Sarbassov DD, Samudio IJ, Yee KWL, Munsell MF, Ellen Jackson C, et al. Rapamycin derivatives reduce mTORC2 signaling and inhibit AKT activation in AML. Blood 2007;109 (8):3509—12.

[322] Zenker M, Aigner T, Wendler O, Tralau T, Müntefering H, Fenski R, et al. Human laminin beta2 deficiency causes congenital nephrosis with mesangial sclerosis and distinct eye abnormalities. Hum Mol Genet 2004;13(21):2625—32.

[323] Zent R, Yan X, Su Y, Hudson BG, Borza D-B, Moeckel GW. Glomerular injury is exacerbated in diabetic integrin alpha1-null mice. Kidney Int 2006;70(3):460—70.

[324] Zhao HJ, Wang S, Cheng H, Zhang M-Z, Takahashi T, Fogo AB, et al. Endothelial nitric oxide synthase deficiency produces accelerated nephropathy in diabetic mice. J Am Soc Nephrol 2006;17(10):2664—9.

[325] Zhu L, Jiang R, Aoudjit L, Jones N, Takano T. Activation of RhoA in podocytes induces focal segmental glomerulosclerosis. J Am Soc Nephrol 2011;22(9):1621—30.

[326] Zoncu R, Efeyan A, Sabatini DM. mTOR: from growth signal integration to cancer, diabetes and ageing. Nat Rev Mol Cell Biol 2011;12(1):21—35.

Implications for albuminuria in diabetes. J Am Soc Nephrol 2006;17(11):3067—75.

23

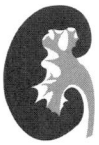

Function of the Juxtaglomerular Apparatus: Control of Glomerular Hemodynamics and Renin Secretion

Jürgen B. Schnermann[1] and Hayo Castrop[2]

[1]National Institute of Diabetes, and Digestive and Kidney Diseases, National Institutes of Health, Bethesda, MD, USA

[2]Institute of Physiology, University of Regensburg, Germany

CELLULAR ELEMENTS OF THE JUXTAGLOMERULAR APPARATUS (JGA)

More than a century ago, Golgi observed that "the ascending limb of the loop of Henle returns with invariable constancy to its capsule of origin".[1] At this point of contact at the glomerular hilum, the afferent and efferent arterioles together with the adherent distal tubule form a wedge-shaped compartment which contains the three defining cell types of the juxtaglomerular apparatus (JGA) (Figure 23.1). The *macula densa* (MD) cells in the wall of the tubule abut on a cushion of closely packed interstitial cells called *Goormaghtigh* or lacis cells. These cells are indistinguishable in their fine structure from mesangial cells[2] and are also referred to as extraglomerular mesangial (EGM) cells. The third specialized cell type of the JGA is the *juxtaglomerular granular* (JG) cell, a modified smooth muscle cell in the media of the arteriolar wall.

The anatomical relationships in the vicinity of the JGA have been extensively studied, since they may reveal pathways for functional connections. The most extensive and regular contact of the MD cells is with the underlying extraglomerular mesangium.[3] Regions of adherence between the afferent arteriole and the thick ascending limb outside the MD, and between afferent arterioles and the distal and connecting tubule, have also been observed.[4–7] Less extensive and consistent contacts exist between the MD and efferent arterioles, although the efferent arteriole can be adjacent to the distal tubule and to the thick ascending limb, either immediately before or immediately after the MD.[2,8]

Macula Densa Cells

Morphology

The MD cells form an elliptical plaque of epithelial cells located at the distal end of the thick ascending limb, approximately 100 to 200 µm upstream from the transition to the distal convoluted tubule.[2,9] An MD plaque has been reported to consist of 14 cells in rat and about 25 cells in rabbit.[10,11] Cellular plasticity is suggested by the finding that this number increased by about 30% following chronic angiotensin II receptor blockade, probably by transdifferentiation of adjacent TAL cells.[11] MD cells are morphologically characterized by a high nucleus-to-cytoplasm ratio, absence of basal infoldings, and numerous mitochondria that are typically not in contact with the basal membrane.[2,12] The basement membrane is thinner than that found in other areas of the tubule, and shows discontinuities in scanning electron micrographs.[13] The difference in basement membrane appearance is paralleled by a macromolecular composition that differs from that of adjacent TAL cells.[14]

NaCl and Water Movement

Although morphologically distinct, MD cells and neighboring thick ascending limb (TAL) cells share similar NaCl transport mechanisms (Figure 23.2). As in TAL cells, NaCl uptake is mostly through the apical Na,K,2Cl co-transporter (NKCC2/BSC1). Conventional electrophysiology and patch-clamp evidence has established its presence functionally.[15–17] Presence of the NKCC2 co-transporter has also been shown at mRNA

Seldin and Giebisch's The Kidney, Fifth Edition.
DOI: http://dx.doi.org/10.1016/B978-0-12-381462-3.00023-9

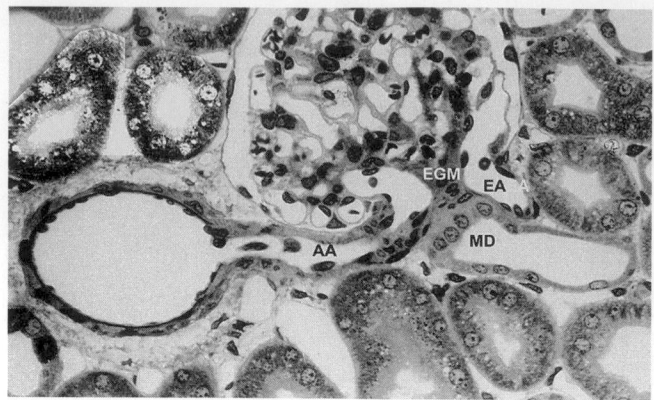

FIGURE 23.1   Low power electron micrograph of the juxtaglomerular apparatus and surrounding cortical tissue (mag. ×320) (AA: afferent arteriole; EA: efferent arteriole; MD: macula densa; EGM: extraglomerular mesangium). *(Courtesy of Brigitte Kaissling and Wilhelm Kriz.)*

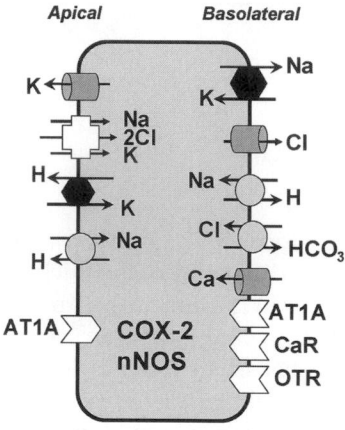

FIGURE 23.2   Representation of transport proteins and receptors in apical and basolateral membranes of macula densa cells. Experimental evidence comes from work in both rats and rabbits.

and protein expression levels.[18–20] Of the three full length isoforms of the co-transporter, both the A and the B types are expressed in the MD.[20–23] In contrast to TAL cells, in which NKCC2 phosphorylation is strongly enhanced by vasopressin, MD cells have a constitutively high presence of phospho-NKCC2 even in the complete absence of vasopressin.[24] From the rates of MD cell acidification by luminal ammonium it has been concluded that apical NKCC2-mediated flux rates are not markedly different from those in TAL cells.[25] Apical membranes of MD cells are rich in low conductance K channels of the ROMK type that are required for K recycling.[16,17,26–28] Na/H exchange through NHE2 provides a second pathway for a smaller fraction of Na uptake by MD cells.[29–32] In the rabbit, the apical membrane may also be a site of active Na extrusion, since the luminal presence of ouabain has been found to elevate intracellular Na concentration in both MD

and TAL cells; in addition, luminal ouabain prevented the recovery of intracellular Na from the elevated levels resulting from increased luminal NaCl.[33] Apical Na efflux in MD cells may be mediated by a luminal H,K-ATPase, as colonic H,K-ATPase has been shown previously to mediate active Na efflux.[34] Its presence in MD cells is supported by immunocytochemical and functional evidence.[33,35]

Na,K-ATPase abundance and activity in the basolateral membrane of MD cells in rabbit kidneys appears to be low compared to neighboring TAL cells, a finding that is probably mainly due to the absence of basolateral membrane infoldings.[33,36,37] In the rat, basolateral membranes of MD cells identified by nNOS counterstaining clearly express α1 Na,K-ATPase, together with β1- and γ-subunits.[38–43] Cl exit across the basolateral membrane occurs through abundant Cl channels.[17,44] Immunocytochemical evidence indicates the presence of the AE2 anion exchanger in basolateral membranes of MD cells in both the rat and the mouse, and Cl/HCO$_3$ exchange activity has been observed in isolated rabbit JGA preparations.[45,46] Together with the apical Na/H exchanger, basolateral AE2 may play a role in the absorption of HCO$_3$ or it may act as a pHi-controlling housekeeping gene.

The effect of changes in luminal fluid composition on the volume of macula densa cells has remained a controversial issue. At constant luminal osmolarity of around 300 mOsm, changes in luminal NaCl concentration caused parallel changes in the volume of MD cells.[47–49] Changes in volume were to some extent transient, indicating some ability of MD cells for volume regulation.[49] Both increases and decreases in MD cell volume have been observed with concomitant increments in Na (25 to 135 mM) and osmolarity (210 to 300 mOsm).[10,47] When NaCl concentration was kept constant, MD cells behaved like osmometers, swelling with a reduction and shrinking with an increase in osmolarity.[49] Transcellular osmotic water permeability of MD cells, assessed from the initial cell volume change in response to an osmotic step change, was estimated to be similar to that of cortical collecting tubules in the absence of ADH.[50,51] The main restriction to water movement resides in the apical membrane.[50] Transmembrane channels for water movement have not been identified; apical membranes of MD cells lack aquaporin 1,[52] and the presence of other aquaporins has not been established. Vasopressin receptors of both the V1a and V2 varieties have been found in MD cells, but there is no evidence that MD water permeability is regulated.[24,53]

Other Cellular Characteristics

Nitric oxide synthase type I (NOS I or nNOS), a constitutive and Ca-dependent NOS isoform, is highly and selectively expressed in MD cells, and has become a useful marker of this cell type.[54,55] Alternative splicing leads to the generation of several nNOS variants with NO synthase activity.[56] The presence of three of these variants, nNOSα, β, and γ in MD cells and their regulation by salt intake has recently been demonstrated.[57] Catalysis of the conversion of L-arginine to NO and L-citrulline by NOS requires the participation of a number of co-factors. One of these co-factors is NADPH, and it is possible that the relatively high activity of glucose-6-phosphate dehydrogenase (G6PDH) in MD cells is related to the NADPH requirement of NOS.[58] A functional connection between nNOS and G6PDH is suggested by the parallel upregulation of the expression of both enzymes during NaCl restriction.[58-60] Alternatively, the high pentose shunt activity suggested by the abundance of G6PDH may serve to provide ribose-5-phosphate for nucleic acid synthesis. Avid uptake of labeled uridine has been shown to occur in MD cells, a process inhibited by actinomycin D, and therefore indicative of incorporation of the pyrimidine precursor into the RNA pool.[61]

Cyclooxygenase-2 (COX-2), typically induced by LPS and cytokines in the inflammatory process, is constitutively expressed both in the renal medulla and to a lesser extent in the cortex.[62,63] Cortical expression of COX-2 in the mature rat and rabbit kidney is restricted to a subgroup of MD and perimacular cells of the TAL.[62,64-66] MD expression of COX-2 has also been observed in humans older than 60 years, and in patients with Bartter syndrome.[67,68] Condensation of COX-2 expression is the remnant of a more intense expression in early postnatal kidneys, where the enzyme can be found in a more contiguous pattern in TAL cells proximal and distal of the MD. At this early stage, COX-2 appears to be specifically excluded from MD cells.[69] Conversion of PGH$_2$ into the bioactive PGE$_2$ is catalyzed by prostaglandin E2 synthases, of which both a microsomal and cytosolic isoform have been described.[70] Immunocytochemical evidence has demonstrated the presence of a membrane-associated PGE$_2$ synthase in MD cells of both rats and rabbits.[71,72] Co-localization of COX-2 with phospholipase A2 has been described in the MD at the level of single cells.[66] Table 23.1 lists a number of other differences in the expression pattern of MD compared to surrounding TAL cells where the function has remained unclear.

Extraglomerular Mesangial (EGM) Cells

Morphology

The EGM cells (Goormaghtigh or lacis cells are synonyms) are the cells of the JGA which have the most intimate and regular contact with the MD.[3] MD

TABLE 23.1 List of Proteins with an Expression Pattern that Differs between Macula Densa and Surrounding Tubular Cells

Macula Densa	Comments	Reference
Tamm-Horsfall protein	Neg, ideal negative selection marker	596
Epidermal growth factor	Neg, present in TAL and DCT	597
Hepcidin	Neg, present in TAL, apical	598
PKD2	Neg, present in TAL, mostly basolateral	599
TRPV4	Neg, present in TAL and DCT	600
Oxytocin receptors	Pos, not in TAL, mostly basolateral	601
Angiotensin II receptors	Pos, apical and basolateral	602
Benzodiazepine receptors	Pos, peripheral type receptors	603
Ca-sensing receptor	Pos, basolateral	604
PTHrP	Pos, microvessels, PCT and DCT	605
Stanniocalcin	Pos, also in TAL, DCT, and CD	606
Integrin-β6	Pos, fibronectin receptor	607
P2Y receptors	Pos, basolateral	608
WNK4	Pos also in TAL and DCT	609
P38 MAP Kinase	Pos more than other tubular segments	610
SGLT1	Pos also in cTAL	611
IQGAP1	Pos apical, also in DCT, less inTAL	612

cells and EGM cells are separated by an interstitial cleft of variable width that does not appear to be bridged by gap junctional connections. In three-dimensional reconstructions EGM cells are elongated cells with long cytoplasmic processes, which in general run parallel to the base of the MD cells.[73] Commensurate with extensive gap junctional coupling of EGM cells with each other as well as with mesangial cells and granular cells,[74,75] connexins 40, 37, and perhaps 43 or 45 are expressed to various degrees in extra- and intraglomerular mesangium.[76,77] The presence of myofilaments in EM cells suggests that EGM cells, like mesangial cells, have contractile potential.[78]

The extraglomerular mesangial cell field is free of capillaries, lymph terminals or nerve fibers. The absence of blood capillaries may cause a retardation of fluid entry and fluid removal from this compartment. In fact, the interstitial volume density of the EGM cell field increased from 17% during volume depletion to 29% during volume expansion, while no changes were noted in the peritubular interstitium.[79] Nevertheless, recent studies of the flow dynamics across the JGA interstitium using lucifer yellow as a fluorescent marker indicate rapid exchange between afferent arterioles and tubular lumen, presumably mediated by bulk fluid flow.[80]

Biochemical and Functional Aspects

Localization studies using histochemical, autoradiographic or immunological methods usually do not distinguish between intra- and extraglomerular mesangial expression patterns. Nevertheless, in some cases it seems justified to assume parallel expression in both cell types. For example, autoradiographic localization of angiotensin II and atrial natriuretic factor binding suggests the presence of receptors on both intra- and extraglomerular mesangial cells.[81,82] Relative predominance of AT1 receptor mRNA in EGM cells has been observed by *in situ* hybridization.[83] While EGM cells normally do not synthesize renin, they can be recruited to form renin with long-standing stimulation such as chronic diuretic abuse.[7,84]

Differential expression patterns in intra- and extraglomerular mesangium are relatively discrete. EGM cells do not stain with antibodies against Thy-1, while the glomerular mesangium does.[85] Conversely, decay accelerating factor (DAF), a glycoprotein that limits complement activation on cell surfaces, is restricted to the EGM cells, at least in the human kidney.[86] HSP 25 expression has also been reported in extraglomerular, but not intraglomerular, mesangium.[87] Of unknown significance is the observation that two Na,K-ATPase-associated proteins, the FXYD protein phospholemman (FXYD1) and the β2-subunit, are expressed in the extraglomerular mesangium, while being excluded from both MD cells and intraglomerular mesangial cells.[43] Conventional mesangial cell cultures have been used as a model to study JGA-specific issues such as NO and PGE$_2$ production, but whether or not this approach permits inferences about the JGA signaling mechanisms *in vivo* has remained unclear.[88–90]

Granular Cells

Morphology

The granular cells in the arteriolar walls are the main renin-producing cells of the kidney. With a rough endoplasmic reticulum, a well-developed Golgi apparatus, and numerous cytoplasmic granules, they have the fine structure of protein-secreting cells.[2,78] The renin-containing granules are membrane-bound. Some granules, believed to be the more newly formed, have a crystalline lattice appearance and may mainly contain pro-renin; others, with an amorphous electron-dense content, are believed to represent the mature form.[7,91] Myofibrils and smooth muscle myosin are sparse, and may be even absent in granular cells at the vascular pole.[92] In the mature rat kidney under control conditions, granular cells are clustered at the vascular pole over a length of about 30 μm or about 20% of the afferent arteriole, but single ring-like renin-positive regions in more proximal locations are sometimes seen.[93] In the developing kidney, as well as during stimulation of renin synthesis, for example with converting enzyme blockade, renin-positive cells can be found all along the afferent arteriole and also in larger vessels.[94,95]

Coexistence of renin and angiotensin II in granules of rat and human epithelioid cells has been shown by light and electron microscopy.[96,97] Granular angiotensin II appears to increase in parallel to renin following adrenalectomy and renal artery stenosis.[97,98] Granular angiotensin II may reflect uptake through either nonspecific endocytosis, receptor internalization or intracellular *de novo* generation.[99,100] Not unexpectedly, granular cells contain AT1 receptor mRNA, with rats expressing both AT1A and AT1B receptor mRNA and mice expressing only AT1A receptor mRNA.[101,102] Granular cells express the mRNA for both D1-like and D2-like dopamine receptors mediating stimulation and inhibition of renin secretion.[103,104] The gap junctional connexins 40 and 37 have been shown to co-localize with renin, indicating functional connections among granular cells.[105–107] Other proteins found in JG cells include cyclic guanylate kinase II,[108] the ubiquitous basolateral form of the Na,2Cl,K co-transporter NKCC1/BSC2,[109] and GLUT4.[110]

Functional Aspects

Renin release has been found to be episodic or quantal, an observation most consistent with granule exocytosis.[111] Nevertheless, EM images rarely document the classic omega configuration with an open pore to the cell exterior,[7] and no evidence in support of the presence of vesicle or target membrane SNARE proteins in JG cells has been published. On the other hand, isoproterenol and cAMP caused an increase in membrane capacitance in isolated JG cells, an observation usually interpreted to be the result of an exocytotic membrane fusion event.[112] An attempt to observe exocytosis has been made in dissected glomerulus/vessel preparations using optical labeling of renin granules with quinacrine and LysoTracker-Red, fluorophores that are taken up into acidic organelles. When stimulated by isoproterenol or a low arteriolar pressure, labeled granules disappeared at a rate of about 5–10 granules per minute.[113] In renin-releasing As4.1 cells, the extinction of individual granules was followed by the appearance of an extracellular quinacrine cloud, presumably representing the released granule contents.[113]

Studies of the membrane characteristics of JG cells in the hydronephrotic mouse kidney by the whole cell patch-clamp technique have identified an inward rectifying K current whose inhibition was shown to be partly responsible for the depolarizing effect of angiotensin II.[114] In addition, JG cells expressed Ca-activated Cl channels in high density.[114] In contrast, inwardly rectifying K channels were not detected in isolated JG cells from rat kidneys.[115] Instead, Ca-dependent and voltage-gated large conductance K channels (BK_{Ca}) were identified that largely determined the resting potential of -32 mV.[115] Presence of BK_{Ca} channels was verified at the mRNA level by RT-PCR, and at the protein level by immunocytochemistry. The increased outward current caused by cAMP was also due to activation of BK_{Ca} channels, suggesting that they were of the cAMP-stimulated ZERO splice variant.[115] There is also evidence for the presence of K-ATP channels in JG cells, but their functional role is not clear.[116] While earlier studies failed to obtain functional evidence for the presence of voltage-dependent Ca channels,[117] the presence of L-type Ca channels and their activation by strong depolarizations has been established in isolated JG cells.[118] JG cells express NKCC1, the ubiquitous isoform of the Na,K,2Cl co-transporter, and its inhibition by furosemide stimulates renin exocytosis, as evidenced by increased membrane capacitance.[119]

MACULA DENSA CONTROL OF VASCULAR TONE

The Tubuloglomerular Feedback Loop

Effect of Distal Tubule Flow Perturbations on SNGFR

The tubuloglomerular feedback (TGF) response is defined as the change of *SNGFR* resulting from a change in tubular fluid flow exiting the proximal convoluted tubule, a practical experimental variable to predictably alter tubular fluid composition in the MD segment of the tubule.[120] The average reduction of *SNGFR* in superficial nephrons of rats caused by a saturating flow increase in 15 independent studies was 13 $\pm$ 1 nl/min or 40 $\pm$ 3%.[52] In addition to the rat, TGF responses were found in all mammalian species tested thus far (dog, hamster, mouse, humans), as well as in two non-mammalian species (*Amphiuma means* and *Necturus maculosus*).[52] Fitting *SNGFR* measurements at eight different loop perfusion rates to a four parameter logistic equation (Figures 23.3 and 23.4) revealed that TGF responses occur over a defined flow range and show nonlinear saturation kinetics.[121] $V_{1/2}$, the flow resulting in the half-maximum response, was 17.5 nl/min, a value close to the ambient end-proximal flow

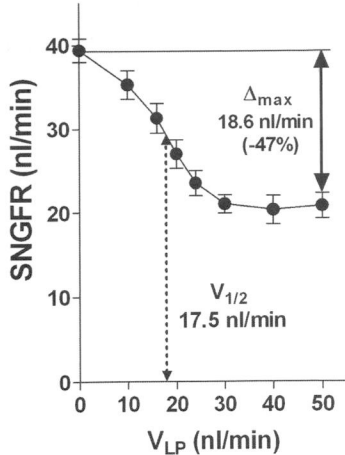

FIGURE 23.3 Relationship between *SNGFR* and loop of Henle perfusion rate (V_{LP}). The diagram shows mean values from 9 tubules in which *SNGFR* was determined at 8 different flow rates[121] (Δ_{max}: maximum reduction of *SNGFR*; $V_{1/2}$: perfusion rate causing half-maximal reduction of *SNGFR*).

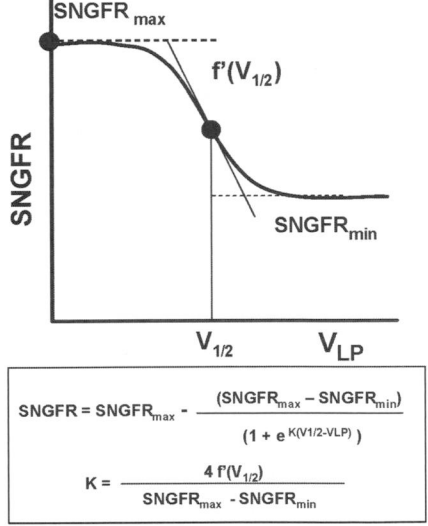

FIGURE 23.4 Four parameter equation (logistic equation) used to describe the sigmoidal relationship between *SNGFR* and lat proximal flow rate (V_{LP}). Parameters are $SNGFR_{max}$, $SNGFR_{min}$, $V_{1/2}$, the flow rate at which the response is half-maximum, and f' $V_{1/2}$, the slope at the midpoint.[594]

rate in the rat (Figure 23.3). The precise location of the TGF operating point has been determined by adding or withdrawing small volumes of fluid from the proximal tubule and determining the resulting changes in proximal flow rate.[122] In these studies, small increases and decreases in loop flow rate were equally and maximally effective in altering *SNGFR*, an observation that directly demonstrates the position of the operating point at the midpoint of the feedback function curve.[122,123] Consistent with the conclusion of tonic suppression of GFR by TGF are observations showing that *SNGFR* based on fluid collections in the proximal tubule where the TGF signal is eliminated is usually higher than *SNGFR* based on distal collections where the TGF signal is intact (Figure 23.5[52]). Systematically higher values of *SNGFR* of superficial nephrons determined in proximal compared to distal tubule segments have also been demonstrated in the dog and mouse.[124,125] TGF responses were also observed in juxtamedullary nephrons of both rats and hamsters, where increased flow past the MD by perfusion of thin ascending limbs produced a reduction in *SNGFR* by about 25 nl/min or approximately 50%.[126,127]

The vasoconstriction elicited by TGF at the level of the JGA may be partially offset by a tubular vasodilator effect that appears to be mediated by a tubulovascular contact area at the level of the connecting tubule.[128] This dilator mechanism, called cTGF, is activated by high Na concentrations and inhibited by amiloride or benzamil, suggesting that it is initiated by activation of ENaC-dependent Na transport.[128] Activation of cTGF seems to require relatively high flow rates, and may therefore play an important role only under special circumstances.[129] Nevertheless, the implications of these observations are potentially far-reaching for the interpretation of previous microperfusion studies, and for the understanding of the physiology of TGF regulation of GFR.

TGF Oscillations

In both rats and mice the operation of the TGF system in the closed-loop mode can result in stable oscillations of filtration pressure and filtration rate with a periodicity of 2–3 cycles/min (30–50 mHz).[125,134,135] Synchronous pressure oscillations were seen in efferent arteriolar blood flow, with blood flow leading tubular pressure by about a 1 second lag. This phase shift suggests that oscillations in blood flow were the cause of changes in tubular pressure.[130] Oscillations were principally of single nephron origin, since oscillations in random nephrons were not in phase.[131] However, synchronized pressures were

observed in adjacent nephrons whose afferent arterioles originate from the same interlobular artery.[132,133] The simultaneous assessment of the oscillatory pattern of many nephrons on the surface of the kidney using the novel approach of laser speckle contrast imaging has shown that synchronized TGF oscillations can sometimes be observed among nephrons that are not located in the immediate vicinity of each other.[134] Pressure oscillations were abolished by loop diuretics, and they were absent in mice that lack TGF responses, suggesting that they were generated by the TGF system.[125,135] This contention was further supported by the finding that distal flow rate and Cl concentrations oscillate with the same frequency, but with a fixed phase shift.[136] Mathematical modeling of the TGF system indicates that oscillations are the result of a relatively high feedback gain, in combination with delays in the transmission of the signal across the JGA and along the nephron.[137,138]

In addition to the slow TGF-dependent oscillations, laser-Doppler velocimetry identified oscillations in star vessel blood flow with a frequency of about 100–200 mHz, probably reflecting myogenic vessel activity.[130] Since TGF and myogenic mechanisms are targeted to identical arteriolar smooth muscle cells, they are expected to interact and become synchronized. As an expression of the interaction, the power of the myogenic oscillations increased during inhibition of TGF, and decreased during TGF saturation.[130,139] In contrast to the synchronized oscillations of normal animals, irregular fluctuations of proximal tubular pressure have been observed in spontaneously hypertensive as well as Goldblatt hypertensive rats, but not in salt-sensitive Dahl rats with hypertension.[140–142] Mathematical modeling has shown that desynchronizations like those seen in the hypertensive models can result from parameter variations of the TGF system or from increases in interaction strength, particularly when nephrons are electrotonically coupled.[143,144] Oxygen tension on the renal surface has also been found to oscillate at the 30 mHz TGF frequency,

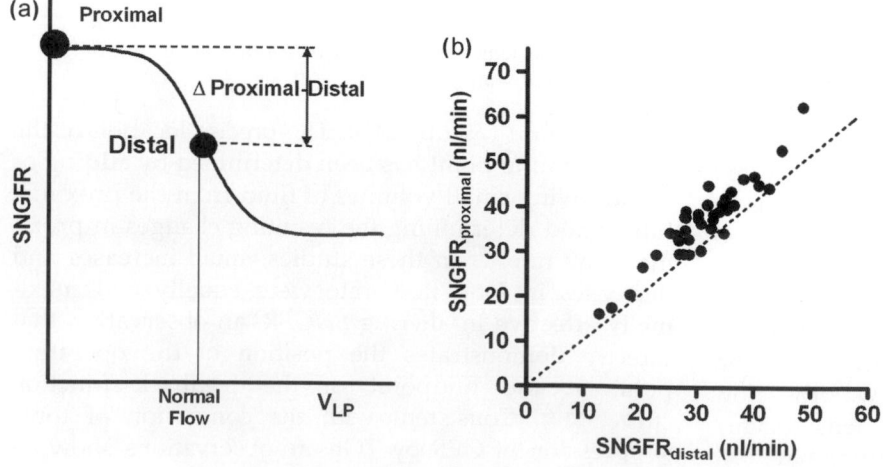

FIGURE 23.5 (a) Difference between *SNGFR* measured in the distal and in the proximal tubule (Δ proximal–distal); its magnitude is an index of the *SNGFR*-reducing effect of ambient flow rates past the macula densa. (b) Relationship between measurements of *SNGFR* in proximal and distal segments of the same nephron. Each point is the mean of an experimental series taken from the literature (for references see [52]). Proximal *SNGFR* exceeded distal *SNGFR* by an average of 6.0 ± 0.54 nl/min, suggesting TGF-dependent suppression of the GFR of superficial nephrons by about 16%

and it has been speculated that a switch of TAL cell energy production from aerobic to anaerobic metabolism may cause the instability in MD NaCl concentration that activates TGF oscillations.[145]

The Tubular Signal and the Sensing Mechanism

Effect of Loop of Henle Flow on MD NaCl Concentration

Although flow rate changes are frequently used to activate TGF, their mechanical consequences *per se* do not appear to be sufficient cause for vasomotor responses *in vivo*. Flow rate changes do not elicit TGF responses as long as they are not accompanied by changes in NaCl, and conversely, full TGF responses can be induced by low flows, as long as NaCl is supplied at sufficiently high concentrations.[120,146–148] Furthermore, widely varying TGF responses can be observed at identical flow rates.[148,149] However, in a recent study using the isolated perfused JGA preparation, changes in flow even in the absence of NaCl were observed to elicit vasoconstriction and increases of cytosolic calcium in vascular cells at the glomerular pole, an effect attributed to the consequences of mechanical deflection of the central cilium of MD cells.[150,151] The reasons for this major discrepancy between the *in vivo* and *in vitro* effects of flow are not known.

Nevertheless, extensive experimental evidence *in vivo* favors the notion that the MD cells respond to changes in luminal NaCl concentration, and that the flow dependency of TGF responses reflects flow dependence of luminal [NaCl] in the MD region of the nephron.[152] *In situ* microperfusion of loops of Henle has revealed a biphasic relationship between flow rate and distal [NaCl] measured 300–600 µm downstream from the MD, the earliest accessible site along the distal convoluted tubule.[120,153,154] The increase of distal solute concentrations at subnormal flow rates is the result of modifications of tubular fluid between the MD region and the distal tubule. NaCl influx along the early post-MD epithelium causes [NaCl] to increase over the levels existing at the MD, and the effect of this addition of NaCl is particularly evident at low flow rates.[153,155]

Effect of MD NaCl Concentration on SNGFR

The precise relationship between MD NaCl concentration and *SNGFR* was established by perfusing loops of Henle from their distal ends in a retrograde direction.[148] In this approach, the distance between perfusion and sensing sites is greatly shortened, the changes in perfusate composition by tubular transport activities are minimized, and the effects of perfusate composition on *SNGFR* can be studied at constant flow rate and pressure. At a flow rate of 20 nl/min, *SNGFR* varied inversely with changes in perfusate NaCl concentration between 15 and 60 mM (or 30 and 120 mOsm), values which extend over the hypotonic range normally occurring at the end of the thick ascending limb.[146,148,156] Increments in NaCl concentration above 60 mM did not further suppress filtration rate. Maximum changes of *SNGFR* caused by saturating flow rates during orthograde perfusion and by saturating NaCl concentrations during retrograde perfusion were identical. Fitting the equation of a hyperbolic tangent to these results (Figure 23.6) indicates that the half-maximum decrease in *SNGFR* is caused by a NaCl concentration of 33.5 mM, and that the maximum slope is about 0.5 nl/min mM.

Studies designed to discriminate between ionic or osmotic effects of the perfusion fluid indicate that total solute concentration at the MD does not seem to measurably participate in TGF-mediated reductions of *SNGFR*. Orthograde perfusion with isotonic mannitol solutions in the rat is usually not associated with sustained reductions in *SNGFR*, even though distal tubular fluid osmolality is greatly increased.[120,147,157] TGF responses correlating with alterations in osmolality have been observed during orthograde perfusion with various perfusion solutions, but the variations in distal osmolality were outside the critical osmolality range of 30 to 120 mOsm observed in retrograde perfusion studies.[158] In retrograde perfusion experiments in which fluid osmolality and NaCl concentration were varied independently, TGF responses were exclusively determined by NaCl concentration, and not by osmolality in a range between 130 and 400 mOsm.[149] Finally, the pattern of *SNGFR* responses during retrograde perfusion with isotonic solutions in which either Na or Cl was replaced, but in which osmolality was kept constant, indicates dependence on the ionic composition and independence of osmolality.[148,156]

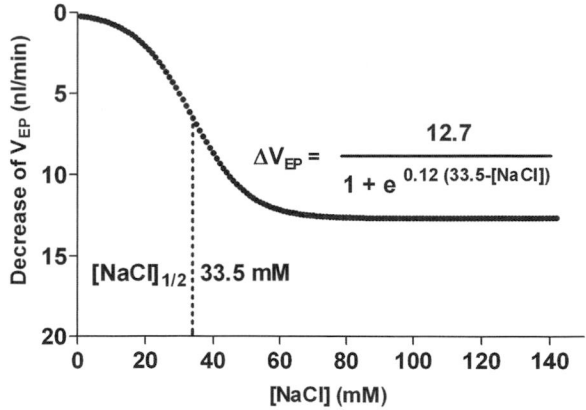

FIGURE 23.6 Logistic equation describing the relationship between NaCl at the macula densa and early proximal flow rate (V_{EP}), a close correlate of *SNGFR*. Changes in NaCl concentration at the macula densa were produced by retrograde microperfusion.[148] $[NaCl]_{1/2}$, NaCl concentration causing half-maximum reduction of V_{EP}.

TGF Response and NaCl Transport

EFFECTS OF LOOP DIURETICS

The observation that inhibition of NaCl transport along the loop of Henle is associated with blockade of the TGF mechanism has been of fundamental importance in understanding the initiation of the TGF signaling pathway.[159] TGF inhibition has been rather uniformly observed in the presence of loop diuretics such as furosemide, bumetanide, piretanide, ethacrynic acid, triflocin or l-ozolinone.[52] Concentrations causing half-maximal inhibition of transport and feedback appear to be similar, about 5×10^{-5} M for furosemide and about 10^{-6} M for bumetanide[160] (own unpublished data). Furosemide also blocked TGF responses during retrograde perfusion, suggesting that metabolic consequences of TAL inhibition are not transmitted by convective transport to the MD cells.[161,162] Since distal Na and Cl concentrations are greatly elevated during loop NaCl transport inhibition, TGF responses do not appear to be caused by luminal NaCl concentration changes *per se*, but by changes in cellular NaCl uptake mediated by the furosemide-inhibitable Na,K,2Cl co-transporter NKCC2. The concentration dependence of feedback responses is probably the result of concentration dependence of NaCl uptake. Studies in mice with selective deletions of the A or B isoform of NKCC2 indicate that NKCC2B mediates TGF in the low NaCl concentration range, while NKCC2A is required for responsiveness to higher NaCl concentrations.[22,163] Thus, the presence of two isoforms of NKCC2 in the macula densa extends the NaCl range over which TGF operates (Figure 23.7). The concept that TGF responses are generated by the successive activation of NKCC2B and NKCC2A is supported by expression studies in *Xenopus* oocytes that have shown a higher Cl

affinity of NKCC2B than NKCC2A, 9 mM versus 45 mM.[21] Other aspects, such as the dependence of the inhibitory potency of furosemide on Cl concentration, have also been found to hold true for the TGF response.[162,164] Diuretic agents with primary actions outside the loop of Henle such as acetazolamide, chlorothiazide, and amiloride do not possess TGF-inhibitory properties.[159,165]

EFFECT OF K CHANNEL BLOCKADE

Retrograde application of the K channel blocker U37883A caused an almost complete inhibition of TGF responses.[166] This effect is mediated by inhibition of ROMK type K channels, since TGF responses were largely absent in mice with targeted ROMK deletion,[167] a finding that has been confirmed in mice in which selective breeding of surviving animals has generated ROMK-deficient mice with less compromised kidney function and well-maintained blood pressure.[168,169] The observation that inhibition of NKCC2 and ROMK has similar effects on TGF responses argues against a specific "sensor" function of these transport proteins, and for a critical role of some consequence of MD NaCl transport. Since ambient distal K concentrations near the MD are close to the K affinity of the co-transporter, it is possible that variations in luminal K may in part regulate TGF response magnitude.[166] Nevertheless, the increase in distal K concentration accompanying acute hyperkalemia was associated with attenuation, not enhancement, of TGF responses.[170]

ION SUBSTITUTION STUDIES

That NaCl uptake by NKCC2 is the initial step in the feedback transmission pathway is further supported by parallels in the ionic requirements for both TGF- and NKCC2-mediated NaCl transport across TALH. During retrograde perfusion of the MD segment (Figure 23.8a), TGF responses were not seen during perfusion with isotonic or hypotonic solutions of Na salts such as $NaHCO_3$, $NaNO_3$, NaI, NaSCN, Na acetate, Na gluconate or Na isethionate.[148,156] In contrast, isotonic solutions of Cl salts (Figure 23.8b) accompanied by small monovalent cations such as K, Rb, Cs or NH_4 elicited full TGF responses, as did the bromide salts of Na and K[148]. It is to be noted that some of these small cations have been found to be substrates for either the Na or the K site on the NKCC2 co-transporter.[164,171]

The requirement for sizable Cl or Br concentrations, and the apparent lack of dependence on Na concentration, are consistent with an involvement of Na,K,2Cl co-transport, since the apparent overall affinity of NKCC2 for Cl in both TAL and MD cells is much lower than that for Na or K.[172,173] Thus, the relatively low Cl affinity would predictably create an apparent Cl dependency of transport, while the small amounts of Na or K entering

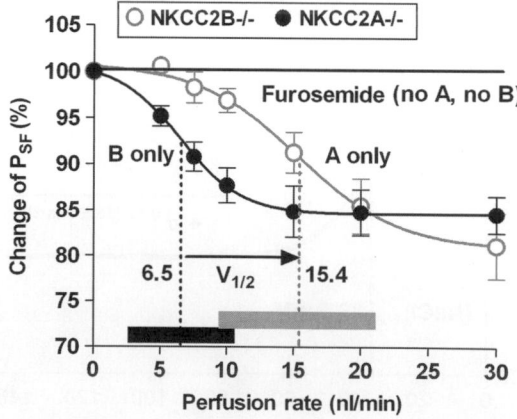

FIGURE 23.7 Relationship between loop of Henle perfusion rate and the relative reduction of P_{SF} ($\pm$ SEM) in mice lacking NKCC2B (circles: (A) only) or NKCC2A (dots: (B) only). Dashed lines indicate the positions of $V_{1/2}$, the flow rates causing half-maximum reduction of P_{SF}; bars indicate the flow ranges over which 90% of the total responses occur. (*Data from .[22,163]*)

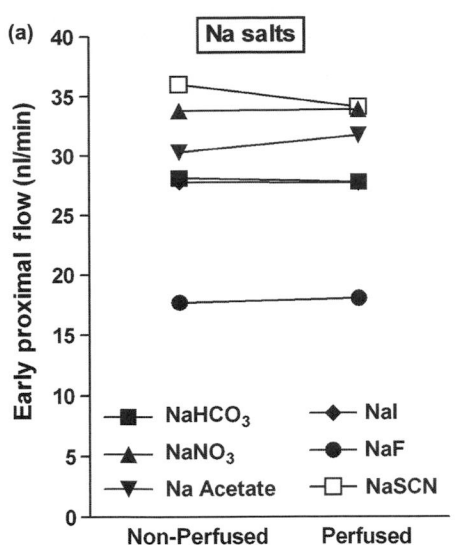

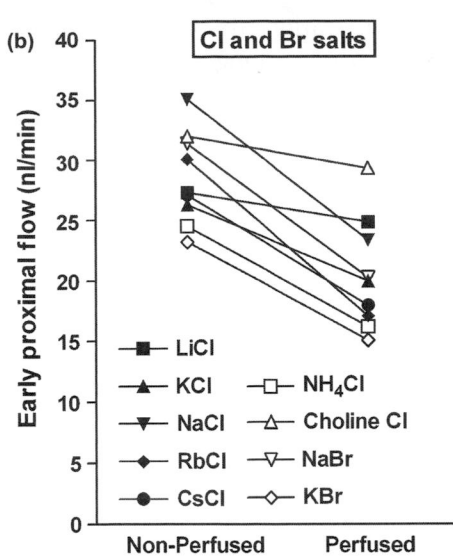

FIGURE 23.8 (a) Effect of Na salts with various anionic substitutions on the response of V_{EP} to retrograde perfusion of the macula densa segment. (b) Effect of Cl and Br salts with various cationic substitutions on the response of V_{EP} to retrograde perfusion of the macula densa segment. *(Data from ref. [148]).*

initially Na- or K-free solutions are sufficient to sustain near normal NKCC2 activity. When Na was replaced with large cations such as choline or TMA, TGF responses of normal magnitude were not seen, even though Cl was present in sufficiently high concentrations.[148,156] Considering the cationic selectivity of the paracellular shunt, replacing luminal Na for choline will result in a sizable lumen positive Na diffusion potential[172] that is predicted to reduce NaCl absorption by increasing Cl backflux. This explanation is consistent with the observation that NaCl transport rates of isolated TAL were found unaltered when studied under symmetric conditions with high choline Cl on both sides of the epithelium.[172] In this case, Na backdiffusion and voltage-dependent inhibition of NaCl absorption is not to be expected as long as low concentrations of Na and K are present.

ACTIVE NaCl TRANSPORT

Transport inhibition caused by metabolic inhibitors such as cyanide, antimycin A or uncouplers of oxidative phosphorylation has also been found to reduce TGF responsiveness.[159,174] TGF responses are not affected by peritubular application of ouabain, and this is probably related to the fact that the $\alpha 1$ Na,K-ATPase in rodents is rather insensitive to cardiac glycoside inhibition.[175] In fact, when $\alpha 1$ Na,K-ATPase was genetically engineered to become ouabain-sensitive, intravenous or luminal administration of the glycoside caused marked reductions of TGF responses.[176] The effect of luminal ouabain may not be related to H,K-ATPase inhibition, since TGF responses were unaltered in H,K-ATPase-deficient mice.[176] The striking effect of loop transport blockade suggests that NaCl uptake through the furosemide sensitive Na,K,2Cl co-transporter, and Na extrusion through an energy-dependent pathway are critical steps in generating feedback responses.

The Vascular Effector Mechanism

The vascular response to a change in perfusion of single loops of Henle occurs without alterations in systemic arterial pressure, renal sympathetic tone or in the resistance of larger renal vessels such as the cortical radial arteries (interlobular arteries). Therefore, the alteration in the hemodynamic determinants of filtration must be caused by a change in the contractile state of glomerular vascular elements. To determine the effect of TGF on glomerular arteriolar resistance, both the pressure fall and the rate of arteriolar blood flow have to be assessed while the perfusion in the loop of Henle of the same nephron is altered.

Pressure Gradients

GLOMERULAR CAPILLARY PRESSURE (P_{GC})

Direct measurements in superficial glomeruli of Munich-Wistar rats have shown that saturating flow increments cause a significant fall in P_{GC}, with fractional decreases ranging between 15 and 22%.[123,177−180] The slope of the P_{GC} change in the most sensitive flow range was 1.3 mmHg min/nl.[123] P_{GC} measured directly in an *in vitro* preparation of juxtamedullary nephrons also fell during TGF activation.[181] P_{GC} in nephrons without superficial glomeruli can be estimated from measurements of stop flow pressure (P_{SF}).[182] In response to a saturating increase in loop flow, mean P_{SF} of 23 studies fell by 22%, from 39.0 ± 0.8 to 30.3 ± 0.8 mmHg.[52] A reduction in P_{SF} was also observed in the dog when loop flow was increased from zero to normal and supranormal values.[183,184] In the mouse, TGF responses of P_{SF} are similar in magnitude as those seen in rats, but the sensitivity range is shifted to lower flows.[185] Since multiple determinations of P_{SF} can be made in the same nephron with small perfusion flow increments, the nonlinear relationship between loop of Henle flow and P_{SF} was apparent long before a similar feedback function for *SNGFR* was defined.[186] In 15 experimental series, the maximum P_{SF} decrease averaged 7.9 ± 0.6 mmHg, with a mean $V_{1/2}$ of 20.1 ± 1.1 nl/min. The maximum sensitivity varied substantially between different studies, but in general was between 1 and 2 mmHg min/nl.[52] Two laboratories have reported that the TGF-induced change in P_{SF} was identical to the TGF-induced change in P_{GC}.[178,179]

The main uncertainty in the determination of feedback-induced changes in the glomerular arteriolar pressure drop results from the evidence that, at least in the rat, a portion of the preglomerular resistance resides in the cortical radial arteries rather than in the afferent arterioles.[187,188] As a consequence, afferent arteriolar resistance, calculated from the artery-to-glomerulus pressure difference, overestimates true afferent resistance, while the relative change caused by the TGF mechanism is underestimated. If preglomerular resistance is equally apportioned between interlobular artery and afferent arteriole, the TGF-induced resistance change along the afferent arteriole would be about 15% greater.

Glomerular Plasma Flow

Estimation of glomerular plasma flow (GPF) by micropuncture requires measurements of *SNGFR* and single nephron filtration fraction (SNFF), with SNFF being derived from the increase in protein concentration or hematocrit in collected samples of early postglomerular blood. Increasing loop perfusion rate reduced plasma flow entering the glomerulus by about 20%, a change accompanied by a fall in SNFF.[189,190] Laser-Doppler shift analysis showed that saturation of the TGF mechanism caused about a 40% reduction in efferent arteriolar blood flow, while TGF inhibition with furosemide increased blood flow by about 25%.[130] Supportive evidence for TGF-induced reductions in GPF came from the observation that glomerular blood flow, estimated from the change in the arrival of fluorescent particles in a single glomerular capillary,[191] fell by about 25–30% when loop flow was increased (M. Steinhausen and J. Schnermann, unpublished). A 30% reduction in afferent arteriolar blood flow was also seen in *Amphiuma* and *Necturus* kidneys when distal flow rate was increased.[192,193]

Effector Site

PREGLOMERULAR RESISTANCE

The micropuncture studies agree that increasing loop of Henle flow produces a 30–40% increase in preglomerular resistance.[189,190] TGF-induced reductions in afferent arteriolar diameter have been directly observed in the blood-perfused juxtamedullary nephron preparation, and in an isolated perfused tubule/vessel preparation.[181,194,195] TGF-induced resistance changes estimated from such diameter observations are consistently much larger than those measured with the micropuncture approach. As suggested above, the location of a sizable resistance along large intrarenal arteries would lead to an underestimation of the TGF-induced resistance change. It is also possible that in the small preglomerular arterioles resistance estimates may deviate from Poiseuille's law. Finally, cTGF, the vasodilator effect at the level of the connecting tubule, may blunt TGF *in vivo*, but would be absent in the perfused tubule.[128,196]

The ultimate cause for TGF-induced vasoconstriction is a rise in intracellular calcium that, at least to a large extent, is mediated by activation of voltage-dependent calcium channels. Depolarization of afferent arteriolar smooth muscle cells during TGF activation has recently been demonstrated using voltage-sensitive dyes.[197] A role for the resulting activation of L-type Ca channels in TGF is supported by the TGF inhibitory effects of intravenous or peritubular application of Ca channel blockers.[198–200] A decrease in protein kinase A activation may be an additional component of TGF-mediated vasoconstriction of the afferent arteriole, since Db-cAMP in the presence of 50 μM IBMX or the luminal application of forskolin, a stimulator of adenyl cyclase, significantly reduced the TGF response magnitude.[201,202]

Observation of the TGF response indicates that the afferent arteriole immediately adjacent to the glomerulum is the main direct target of the TGF mediator.[181] The glomerular entrance segment of the vessel is the part of the afferent arteriole in which agents affecting TGF response magnitude, such as adenosine and angiotensin II, exert their largest constrictor action.[203,204] TGF-induced local constriction may elicit a vascular conducted response that spreads to proximal portions of the arteriole by electrotonic coupling or myogenic excitation.[205,206] Spreading of contractile responses during local application of KCl has been observed in juxtamedullary nephrons, indicating electrotonic coupling of afferent arteriolar smooth muscle cells.[207] Upstream propagation of TGF-induced vasoconstriction is also responsible for the functional coupling of nephrons that are supplied by a common interlobular artery.[132,208,209] It is probable that conducted vasoconstriction relies on the presence of various connexins in endothelial and smooth muscle cells.[76,210] In view of the functional connection between afferent arteriolar smooth muscle cells, one may conclude that the total vasoconstrictor response to a NaCl step-change is composed of a local MD-generated effect and an upstream myogenic constrictor component.

POSTGLOMERULAR RESISTANCE

Evidence for a concomitant constriction of efferent arterioles during TGF activation has been obtained by micropuncture studies showing a reduction of GFR with unaltered glomerular capillary pressure, therefore suggesting proportional increases in the tone of afferent and efferent vessels.[179,190,211] Furthermore, an increase of flow within the low-to-ambient flow range is associated with a greater change of *SNGFR* than of P_{SF}, suggesting that either there was balanced afferent and efferent vasoconstriction, with the *SNGFR* fall being a consequence of the reduced plasma flow or that total resistance did not change and the *SNGFR* change was a consequence of a reduced K_f.[123,212] Direct observations of juxtamedullary efferent arterioles during TGF activation did not reveal any vasoactivity.[181] In contrast to these observations, luminal NaCl has been observed to dilate efferent vessels in the double-perfused nephron preparation of the rabbit, an effect that was prevented by antagonists of A2 adenosine receptors.[213] There is some experimental evidence in support of the possibility that a reduction in the filtration coefficient may contribute to TGF-induced reduction of GFR.[190]

Purinergic Mediation of the Vascular Response

As discussed in the previous sections, an increase in loop of Henle flow rate produces increases in NaCl concentration and NaCl transport at the MD, and this functional alteration elicits a vasoconstrictor response of the glomerular microvasculature, as well as a reduction in the rate of renin secretion. Propagation of the signal across the JGA interstitium and subsequent changes in vasomotor tone occurs through the transport-dependent generation and action of purinergic mediators (Figure 23.9).

ADENOSINE

Adenosine was originally proposed as a mediator of the TGF response, since it provided a conceptual link between the energy expended for NaCl transport and the generation of a vasoactive ATP metabolite.[214,215] Stimulation of Na transport in the proximal tubule is in fact associated with a decrease in cellular ATP, and increased NaCl secretion in the shark rectal gland causes a decrease in ATP, as well as an increase in adenosine release.[216,217]

The vasomotor action of adenosine in most organs and vascular beds consists of vasorelaxation that reflects the wide distribution of the two types of A2 adenosine receptors, A2aAR and A2bAR. Although the kidney is usually considered an exception to this rule,[218] several studies have shown that the steady-state response to an intravenous administration of adenosine is a clear reduction of renal vascular resistance, whereas

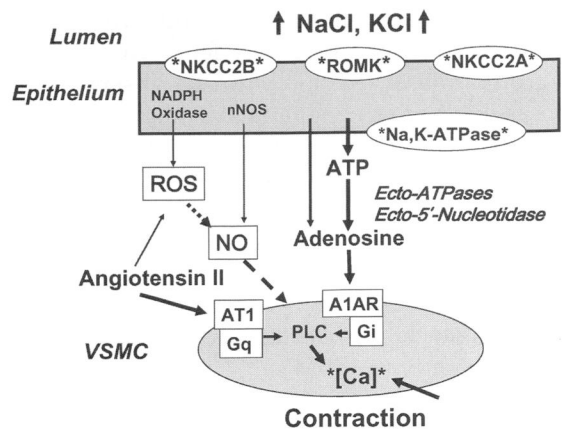

FIGURE 23.9 Schematic summary of our current understanding of the pathway by which an increase in luminal NaCl at the macula densa causes activation of vascular smooth muscle cells (VSMC) in the afferent arteriole. Some consequence of NaCl uptake is linked to the release of ATP, subsequent generation of adenosine, interaction with adenosine 1 receptors (A1AR), Gi-dependent activation of PLC, and increases in Ca by release from stores and opening of Ca channels. Angiotensin II is an important co-factor that augments the impact of A1AR activation. NO is a response-attenuating factor whose levels are to some extent modulated by reactive oxygen species (ROS).

the initial constrictor response is only short-lasting.[219] In contrast, persistent vasoconstriction of afferent arterioles by adenosine and A1 adenosine (A_1) analogs was observed in the hydronephrotic kidney and in isolated perfused afferent arterioles when adenosine receptors were activated from the interstitial aspect of the vessel.[203,220–222] The constrictor effect was absent in arterioles from A1 adenosine receptor (A1AR)-deficient mice.[203,223] Thus, adenosine causes a lasting vasoconstriction only when the nucleoside is generated in a restricted interstitial region so that A1AR can be accessed without general activation of the more dominant A2 receptors. Expression data, as well as functional observations, indicate that the terminal afferent arteriole is a vessel with high representation of A1AR.[222,224] A1AR-mediated vasoconstriction of afferent arterioles is initiated by Gi-dependent activation of phospholipase C, release of Ca from intracellular stores, and subsequent Ca entry through L-type Ca channels.[203,225,226] The A1AR-mediated vasoconstrictor effect of adenosine in afferent arterioles was stable for extended periods of time, indicating absence of rapid receptor desensitization.[203,225] Tubular administration of A1AR agonists augments the vasoconstrictor response to increased loop flow rates.[161,227] This effect does not appear to be mediated through apical A1AR, but rather to reflect a direct interaction with A1AR on afferent arterioles, and it thereby demonstrates the vasoconstrictor potency of A1AR activation and its effect on glomerular capillary pressure *in vivo*.[28]

Two laboratories have independently generated mouse strains with targeted deletion of A1AR, and both groups observed a complete absence of TGF responses in A1AR$^{-/-}$ animals using micropuncture measurements of stop flow pressure or single nephron GFR (Figure 23.10).[229,230] Furthermore, specific A1AR antagonists such as 8-cyclopentyl-1,3-dipropylxanthine (DPCPX) or PSB-36 inhibit TGF responses when added to either the tubular lumen or the peritubular blood.[228,231] A similar effect has been seen earlier with non-specific blockers such as theophylline or 3-isobutyl-1-methylxanthine, IBMX.[161,201,214,232] Addition of the nonxanthine A$_1$ receptor antagonist FK838 to the perfusate or bath also eliminated TGF responses in an isolated tubule preparation.[233] There is evidence that adenosine generated during TGF activation may also interact with A2 adenosine receptors, but the site of action is unclear. Enhanced TGF responses have been observed during A2AR blockade, suggesting that activation of A2AR tonically diminishes A1AR-mediated vasoconstriction of afferent arterioles, perhaps through the release of nitric oxide.[231,234] On the other hand, adenosine is able to vasodilate preconstricted efferent arterioles through A2AR, and A2AR inhibition has been found to block TGF-mediated vasodilatation of efferent arterioles in the isolated perfused JGA preparation.[213,235] The latter findings are difficult to reconcile with the absence of *in vivo* evidence for a reduction of efferent arteriolar resistance during TGF activation.

ATP

The preponderance of current evidence indicates that extracellular ATP serves as the major source for the generation of adenosine in the JG interstitium.

Strong support for this notion is furnished by the demonstration that basolateral membranes of MD cells appear to have an ATP release pathway that is modulated by changes in luminal NaCl. Release of ATP by MD cells is suggested by the observation that PC12 or mesangial cells placed near the basolateral MD cell membrane responded to changes in luminal NaCl over the 20−60 mM range with an increase in cytosolic calcium.[236,237] This Ca response of the biosensor cells reflects P2 receptor activation, since it was inhibited by suramin.[236,237] Patch-clamp studies in cell-attached and excised patches of the basolateral membrane of MD cells showed the presence of an anion channel of 380 pS whose activity was dependent on the presence of extracellular NaCl, and that was active in the presence of ATP as the only anion.[236,237] Channel activity was blocked by gadolinium, but not by the Cl channel inhibitors DPC or NPPB.[236] The molecular nature of this large conductance anion channel has not been identified, but it may be identical to a functionally described maxi-anion channel that is widely expressed throughout the body.[238] Release of ATP across connexin hemichannels would be another possibility, but the evidence for the presence of connexins in the basolateral membrane of MD cells is weak.[76,239]

It is likely that ATP released into the JGA interstitium serves as substrate for membrane-bound ecto-ATPases and nucleotidases, ultimately resulting in the formation of the vascular mediator adenosine. In fact, TGF responses have been found to be greatly reduced in mice with deletion of NTPDase1/CD39, the major renal ecto-ATPase that dephosphorylates both ATP and ADP to AMP.[240] Furthermore, evidence has been obtained suggesting that adenosine formation by

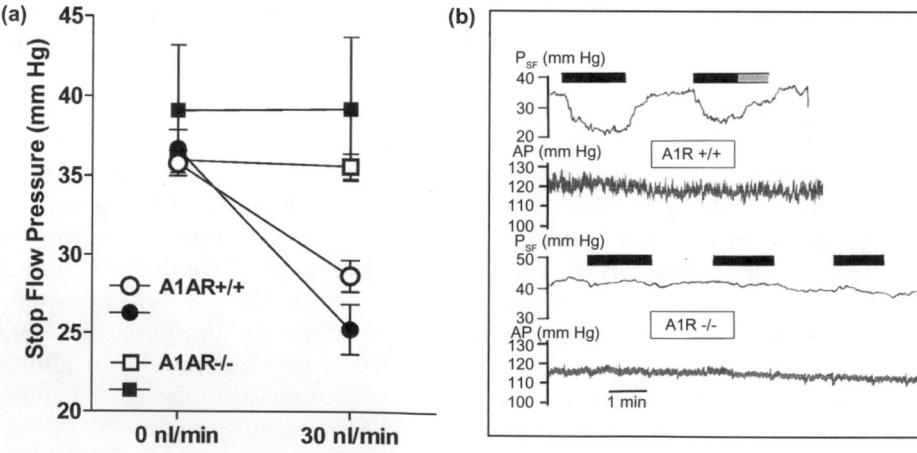

FIGURE 23.10   (a) Mean responses of stop flow pressure to an increase in loop of Henle perfusion rate from 0 to 30 nl/min in wild-type (A1AR$^{+/+}$) and in adenosine 1 receptor-deficient mice (A1AR$^{-/-}$). Gene targeting and phenotypic studies were performed by two independent groups of investigators (Closed symbols: data from [229]; Open symbols: data from [230]). (b) Recordings of stop-flow pressure (P$_{SF}$) and arterial blood pressure (AP) in a wild-type mouse (A1R$^{+/+}$) and in an adenosine 1 receptor-deficient mouse (A1R$^{-/-}$). During periods indicated by black bars, loop of Henle perfusion rate was increased to activate the TGF mechanism. Note absence of perfusion-related changes of P$_{SF}$ in the nephron of the A1 receptor-deficient animal.

e-5'NT/CD73 may be critical in the generation of adenosine during the TGF response. Blocking adenosine formation with the e-5'NT-inhibitor α,β-methylene adenosine 5'-diphosphate (MADP) significantly reduced the compensatory TGF efficiency and the slope of the TGF relationship.[241] When the level of TGF activation was fixed by saturating concentrations of CHA, TGF efficiency was further reduced, and retrograde administration of MADP in combination with CHA caused vasoconstriction and abolition of TGF response.[241] Consistent with these data are observations in mice with targeted deletion of e-5'NT/CD73 in which TGF responses were found to be markedly compromised.[242,243] Finally, in the double-perfused JGA preparation, bath addition of the ecto-ATPase apyrase enhanced, and MADP abolished, TGF responses, suggesting that extracellular generation of adenosine from ATP is critical for JGA signaling.[244] Exogenous e-5'NT was also found to improve the defective TGF component of renal autoregulation in Thy-1 nephritic rats.[245] Dephosphorylation of ATP and AMP is likely to occur through enzymes anchored to the surface of mesangial cells.[246,247] Whether adenosine levels in the JG interstitium are regulated by adenosine release across equilibrative nucleoside transporters (ENT) is unclear, since evidence based on the effect of ENT inhibitors such as dipyridamole or dilazep on TGF responses is inconclusive.[214,248,249]

As an alternative to a role of ATP as precursor for adenosine, it has been proposed that ATP may directly elicit TGF responses, most likely through activation of P2 receptors on extraglomerular mesangial cells and gap junctional transmission of the resulting increase of cytosolic Ca to the afferent arteriole.[150,236,250,251] ATP may also directly activate arteriolar P2 receptors, with P2X1 receptors being the most likely receptor subtype since its presence in afferent arterioles has been well-documented.[252] In fact, ATP causes rapid and reversible constriction of afferent arterioles, an effect that may be more pronounced in juxtamedullary than superficial nephrons.[222,250] A similar effect is seen with the P2X receptor-specific ligand α,ß-methylene ATP, suggesting mediation of vasoconstriction by P2X purinoceptors.[250] Nevertheless, unequivocal evidence in support of a P2 receptor-mediated action of ATP in TGF *in vivo* is not available. TGF responses in superficial nephrons of P2X1 knockout mice were not statistically distinguishable from wild-type animals.[169] Likewise, TGF responses were not significantly affected by the infusion of the broad-spectrum inhibitors of P2 receptors PPADS or suramin, although these agents clearly diminished the blood pressure response to the P2 agonist α,ß-methylene ATP.[253] Results from the double-perfused JGA preparation are controversial. In an earlier study on rabbit tissue, suramin had been without effect on the response of afferent arteriolar diameter to an increase of luminal NaCl.[244] Since acceleration of ATP breakdown enhanced, and inhibition of 5'-ecto nucleotidase and of A1 adenosine receptors blocked, the arteriolar diameter response, these results were consistent with the ATP dephosphorylation/adenosine paradigm.[233,244] However, in similar preparations from rabbit or mouse, suramin was recently found to abolish afferent arteriolar Ca and constrictor responses, while the A1AR antagonist DPCPX was without effect.[150,151] The reasons for this divergence are presently unclear, but it is to be noted that a novel approach was used in at least part of the latter study, in that only the macula densa cells of the perfused nephron were maintained, while all thick ascending limb cells were removed by microdissection.[151] While it is conceivable that the presence of thick ascending limb cells is required for the "conventional" TGF response that is flow-independent, NaCl-dependent, and affects vascular tone through A1AR activation, the possibility of technical reasons for the obvious discrepancies cannot be excluded.

LINK BETWEEN NaCl TRANSPORT AND TGF

Exactly how an increase of NaCl transport by MD cells is coupled to the release of ATP or the subsequent activation of the purinergic signaling pathway is one of the major open questions in TGF physiology. Cell swelling is a very common cause for eliciting ATP release, and this mechanism may be the critical factor for linking NaCl transport to ATP egress in MD cells. Nevertheless, as discussed above, the relationship between the compositional changes associated with elevated loop flow rates and MD cell volume is not entirely clear. ATP release could also be related to any of the changes caused by stimulation of NaCl transport acrosss apical or basal membranes of MD cells. NKCC2 activation is followed by increases in cytosolic Na and Cl concentrations, increases in cytosolic pH, and membrane depolarization.[16,30,33,173,254] MD depolarization by about 30 mV following an increase of luminal [NaCl] to 150 mM occurs over the 20—60 mM range, and it therefore parallels the TGF response curve.[255] Depolarization may be directly involved in TGF responses, since the cation ionophore nystatin elicited afferent arteriolar vasoconstriction in the presence of low luminal NaCl and furosemide.[256] TGF responses were also seen when MD cells were depolarized by luminal application of the K ionophore valinomycin, together with 50 mM KCl. The valinomycin-induced vascular response was not affected by the Cl channel inhibitor NPPB (5-nitro-2-(3-phenylpropylamino) benzoic acid), whereas the normal NaCl-induced response was fully blocked by NPPB.[256] Thus, it appears that TGF responses depend upon MD cell depolarization independent of the specific mechanism underlying the PD change, but evidence is needed to establish that the depolarization by valinomycin or nystatin is restricted to MD cells, and does not affect arteriolar smooth muscle cells.

MD cell depolarization may be linked to TGF responsiveness through its effect on MD cytosolic calcium $[Ca]_i$. Transport-induced changes in MD $[Ca]_i$ have been suggested to play a specific role in coupling the luminal electrolyte signal to the vascular response.[257] The Ca ionophore A 23187 in the presence of luminal Ca enhanced TGF responsiveness, whereas blocking Ca release from intracellular stores with 8-(N,N-diethyl-amino)-octyl-3,4,5-trimethoxybenzoate (TMB 8) and chelation of Ca with BAPTA-AM diminished it.[257–259] Ca entry may occur through a voltage-activated and nifedipine-sensitive Ca channel in the basolateral membrane,[260] but increased flux across a 20 pS non-selective cation channel with finite Ca permeability reduced Ca extrusion by Na/Ca exchange, and utilization of a conductive Ca entry pathway across the apical cell membrane is an alternative possibility.[259,261,262] Despite the evidence supporting an important role of $[Ca]_i$ it is far from certain that the $[Ca]_i$ changes occurring in response to fluctuations of luminal NaCl between 20 and 60 mM *in vivo* are large and consistent enough to establish a systematic and causal association between MD $[Ca]_i$ and the TGF response. In fact, the relationship between luminal NaCl and MD cytosolic calcium has been described as positive,[260] negative[49] or entirely absent,[150] perhaps indicating that the changes of $[Ca]^i$ in MD cells may be too small to be safely distinguishable from experimental noise in this technically demanding experimental approach.

A novel role for MD cell depolarization may be activation of NADPH oxidase and generation of superoxide that may directly or by scavenging NO enhance TGF.[263] An increase in NaCl delivery to the MD in the isolated perfused JGA preparation caused about a three-fold increase in superoxide production that was largely inhibited by tempol or apocynin.[264,265] Activation of NADPH oxidase appears to be the direct result of depolarization, since depolarization with valinomycin increased superoxide production and the hyperpolarization following furosemide-induced inhibition of NaCl uptake reduced it.[265] The enhanced activity of the NOX2 isoform of NADPHase oxidase following membrane depolarization may be associated with translocation of the small GTP-binding protein Rac to the plasma membrane.[266–268]

Integrated Function of the TGF Mechanism

The JGA control system is constructed as a negative, homeostatic feedback loop. The physiological purpose of this regulatory loop has been the subject of a substantial body of investigation using both experimental approaches and mathematical modeling. One potential effect of the operation of the TGF feedback loop is to reduce fluctuations of NaCl concentration at the MD, thus reducing the variability in the delivery of NaCl into the relatively low-capacity transport system of the distal nephron. Another role hypothesized for the TGF loop is in the autoregulatory adjustments in vascular resistance that promote constancy of GFR when arterial pressure changes.

The two hypothesized roles, regulation of distal salt delivery and control of GFR, are functionally interrelated; the feedback loop may contribute to stabilization of NaCl excretion, rendering it relatively independent of fast and irregular fluctuations in perturbing forces that are not the expression of an adaptation to a change in body Na balance. Such variations are represented, for example, by the marked fluctuations in blood pressure that have been observed to occur throughout the day and with changing body activities.[269] In the absence of tight control of vascular resistance, glomerular capillary pressure, and hence GFR, would be expected to fluctuate in parallel with blood pressure, causing changes in Na excretion unrelated to the NaCl status of the organism. Since, however, changes in GFR will in general be followed by parallel changes in distal NaCl concentration, the TGF system can dampen the amplitude of the predicted GFR changes. Similar rapid hemodynamic adjustments will occur with other acute perturbations of MD NaCl concentration resulting from variations in cardiac output, renal blood flow or proximal tubular transport. As discussed below, the TGF mechanism changes its response characteristics when perturbations of MD NaCl concentration are sustained for extended periods of time.[270] The homeostatic efficiency of TGF in the regulation of distal salt delivery and *SNGFR* is greatest in the vicinity of the operating point where fractional compensations of small input perturbations may be between 0.6 and 0.75, corresponding to an open loop gain of around 3.[122,271]

Participation of TGF in autoregulation

Acute changes in mean arterial pressure induce adjustments in renal vascular resistance which stabilize renal blood flow and glomerular filtration rate over a wide range of pressures. Pressure-induced resistance changes in the kidney have been proposed to be TGF-mediated.[272,273] A role of TGF in steady-state autoregulation was first supported by the observation in both dogs and rats that interruption of the TGF loop in single nephrons causes *SNGFR* and P_{SF} to vary directly with arterial pressure.[124,184,274–279] Pressure dependency of *SNGFR* was noted regardless of whether the TGF loop was physically disrupted by injecting an oil block, blocked acutely by adding furosemide to the perfusate[274] or inhibited by chronic treatment with DOCA and a high salt diet.[274] In contrast, arterial pressure had little effect on GFR when the TGF loop was intact.[124,274–278] In the *in vitro* perfused juxtamedullary nephron preparation, interference with the TGF mechanism by furosemide or physical interruption of the feedback loop markedly diminished autoregulatory diameter alterations of afferent arterioles,[195,280,281] and constancy of afferent arteriolar blood flow was no longer maintained.[281]

There is equally solid evidence for the existence of TGF-independent autoregulatory resistance changes. Glomerular arterioles in kidney tissue transplanted to the cheek pouch of the hamster showed marked autoregulation of vessel diameters.[282] In the hydronephrotic kidney model which does not possess an operating TGF system, a decrease in arterial pressure increased vessel diameters along the entire preglomerular vasculature, except for the portion of the afferent arteriole near the glomerulus.[283] Isolated afferent arterioles and interlobular arteries of the rabbit maintained their diameter when luminal pressure increased,[284,285] while perfused afferent arterioles from the mouse showed an 11% diameter reduction with a doubling of perfusion pressure from 40–80 mmHg accompanied by a linear increase in wall tension.[286] The nature of the TGF-independent regulator is unclear, but an intrinsic myogenic mechanism responding to wall tension or mechanical stress is the most likely possibility.

Existence of at least two regulators is further supported by studies in which the dynamic response of renal blood flow to random fluctuations of blood pressure has been analyzed. Frequency domain analysis of renal blood flow using linear techniques revealed the presence of a regulator with a frequency response compatible with the TGF mechanism, about 0.01 Hz, and a faster mechanism with a frequency characteristic consistent with myogenic vasomotion, about 0.1 Hz.[287–289] Since the TGF system is nonlinear, it is important that a similar conclusion has been reached from the more recent application of nonlinear system analysis.[290–292] The existence of two regulators with similar frequencies has also been established in spontaneously hypertensive and Dahl rats.[293–295] There is evidence for the operation of two regulating mechanisms in conscious dogs and mice.[296,297] Interference with the slow component was observed in a number of experimental models of TGF interruption, including A1AR-deficient mice, ureteral obstruction, converting enzyme inhibition, and the perfused hydronephrotic kidney.[294,298–300] Temporal resolution of the adjustment of renal vascular resistance to step-changes in renal arterial pressure is consistent with the sequential operation of several mechanisms with different

response times.[301–303] Various approaches and analyses have concluded that the quantitative contribution of TGF to autoregulation may be between 30 and 60%.[181,274,275,278,281,302] In addition to the TGF and myogenic components, evidence for the presence of a third mechanism with a slow response time has been obtained that may be of particular importance at low perfusion pressures.[302,303] Furthermore, an afferent arteriolar constrictor mechanism has been identified that responds to the systolic pressure peaks rather than to mean arterial pressure, and therefore must possess a response time in the frequency of the heart rate.[304,305] This mechanism is thought to protect the glomerular vasculature against the high pressures exerted during systole.

Interaction between the two autoregulatory mechanisms may lead to amplification of vascular responses. Models of autoregulation suggest that a TGF-dependent vasoconstriction can induce a myogenic response in upstream vascular regions and amplify the resistance increase.[206,306,307] In fact, mathematical modeling suggests that a myogenic contribution from proximal vascular segments is necessary for distal mechanisms such as TGF to contribute to resistance regulation.[308] Spatial separation between the two regulatory mechanisms along the afferent arteriole has been noted, with TGF being most effective in the region of the afferent arteriole close to the glomerulus, and the myogenic component being more pronounced in more proximal portions of the afferent arteriole.[195] Interactions between the myogenic response and TGF have been demonstrated at both the single nephron and the whole kidney level,[290,309] and they have been the subject of extensive mathematical modeling.[292,310,311] One of the conclusions is that elimination of a variable TGF signal enhances myogenic responsiveness.[301,309,310,312] Recent evidence indicates that the restraining effect of TGF on the myogenic mechanism is mediated by nitric oxide.[313,314] Functional coupling of small ensembles of nephrons by ascending myogenic or conducted vascular responses adds to the complexity of regulation of preglomerular vascular tone.[132,209] Enhanced nephron-to-nephron coupling has been suggested to be responsible for the more efficient dynamic autoregulation in spontaneously hypertensive rats.[133,207,293]

Role of TGF in Response to Transport Alterations

HYPERTONIC NaCl

Administration of hypertonic NaCl causes vasodilatation in most vascular beds, but in the kidney it results in an anomalous vasoconstriction.[315] This response may be a whole kidney equivalent of the response of *SNGFR* to increased loop flow rate. Both TGF- and NaCl-induced vasoconstriction are enhanced by salt depletion[316,317] and inhibited by furosemide, theophylline or DOCA-salt treatment.[159,232,318–320] Furthermore, hypertonic non-chloride containing solutions usually do not produce vasoconstriction.[317] A micropuncture study in the rat revealed that an infusion of hypertonic NaCl reduced proximal tubular fluid absorption and increased loop flow rate, and that *SNGFR* fell as a result of these changes.[321]

PROTEIN FEEDING

The vasodilatation caused by acute and chronic protein feeding may include a TGF-dependent component. In conscious dogs, furosemide and ethacrynic acid blocked the acute rise in GFR following a meat meal, suggesting that the postprandial vasodilatation may be TGF-dependent.[322] It has been proposed that the rise in filtered amino acids causes an increase in proximal Na and fluid absorption, and a decrease in MD Na delivery.[322]

Chronic consumption of a high-protein diet induced a rightward resetting in the feedback curve of normal and Goldblatt hypertensive rats, so that higher flows were necessary to suppress GFR than in control or low-protein fed animals.[323,324] In normotensive animals the response amplitude and the slope of the feedback function were unaltered.[324] These effects appear to be due to alterations in transport along the loop of Henle, since NaCl concentrations in distal tubular fluid during loop perfusion were 30% lower in rats on a high-protein diet than in rats on a low-protein diet.[325] Consistent with this notion is the observation that TGF responses were the same in the two groups of rats when loops of Henle were perfused in a retrograde fashion, indicating that functional changes in the loop of Henle rather than at the level of the JGA were responsible for the protein-induced changes in TGF characteristics. The increased rate of NaCl transport along the loop of Henle caused by high-protein feeding may result from structural adaptations.[326]

INHIBITION OF PROXIMAL TRANSPORT

Diuretics that inhibit predominantly proximal tubular fluid absorption may cause a TGF-dependent decrease in GFR as a result of increased distal NaCl delivery. In support of this hypothesis, several studies using carbonic anhydrase inhibitors, as well as chlorothiazide, suggest that these agents cause *SNGFR* to fall more with the TGF loop intact than with the TGF loop interrupted.[165,211,327] In view of the Cl dependency of TGF, however, the acute TGF activation by carbonic anhydrase inhibition is unexpected since these drugs, while causing an increase of early distal [Na], do not elevate distal Cl concentrations.[165,327] There is no evidence to show that HCO_3 can substitute for Cl in initiating TGF responses. In fact, recent studies have

shown that the effect of benzolamide to reduce GFR and RBF was maintained in A1AR[−/−] mice which are unable to generate a TGF response.[328] Thus, the mechanism of the renal vasoconstriction caused by CA inhibitors is not entirely clear, but a rise in tubular pressure may be an important contributor.[329,330] In addition, studies in rats and mice indicate that major increases in urine flow, including those caused by furosemide, may lead to increases in total renal vascular resistance even when participation of TGF is *a priori* unlikely.[331,332]

SNGFR of mice with targeted deletion of AQP1 was found to be significantly reduced compared to wild-type when it was determined in distal nephron segments with the TGF pathway intact.[333] The fall in GFR was dependent upon distal fluid delivery, since it was not observed when *SNGFR* was measured in the proximal tubule with the TGF loop interrupted.[333] Mice deficient in both AQP1 and A1AR which combine a proximal transport defect with absent TGF responsiveness, have been found to have a normal distal *SNGFR*, supporting the notion that the fall of GFR in AQP1[−/−] mice is TGF-mediated.[334]

Very similar results were obtained in mice with a knockout mutation in the apical Na/H exchanger NHE3, another model of established proximal tubular NaCl and fluid malabsorption.[335] Considering that distal flow rates were not different between wild-type and AQP1 or NHE3 knockout mice, it seems unlikely that TGF activation is due to an increased NaCl concentration at the MD. Resetting of the TGF function curve (discussed below) subsequent to extracellular volume depletion seems to be more likely as causation for enhanced TGF engagement.

Adaptation of TGF Response Characteristics
EXTRACELLULAR FLUID VOLUME

Adaptations in the TGF function occur whenever MD NaCl concentrations deviate from normal for an extended period of time. Typically, such deviations result from alterations in body Na content, with volume expansion associated with persistently increased, and volume depletion associated with decreased, MD NaCl concentrations. Formally, two types of adaptation in the TGF relationship can be distinguished. TGF *resetting* refers to a shift in the range over which the system is operating, either a shift to the right, to higher flows or concentrations or a shift to the left, to lower flows or concentrations. A change in TGF response *sensitivity* refers to an altered response, either altered slope and/or maximum response magnitude. By and large, volume depletion is associated with a left shift and an increase in response magnitude, and volume expansion with the opposite, but the actual adaptation observed has varied with the protocol used.

A number of studies have established that acute expansion of the extracellular space by infusion of isotonic saline or plasma reduces the TGF response magnitude and slope, and increases $V_{1/2}$ in both superficial and juxtamedullary nephrons.[127,336-341] Impaired TGF responses have been observed during chronic volume expansion caused by the administration of DOCA together with isotonic saline as drinking fluid.[274,320,342] The combination of a right shift and a reduced response magnitude is not invariant. Short-term volume expansion by a bolus injection of dilute rat plasma shifted the responsive range to higher flows, although this protocol produced an increase rather than a decrease in the maximum response magnitude[343]; *SNGFR* at zero loop flow rose 60%, whereas kidney GFR and free flow *SNGFR* rose only moderately with the position of the operating point and a large proximal–distal *SNGFR* difference indicating that the suppressing effect of the TGF mechanism was greater than normal. Thus, in these studies, the TGF mechanism appeared to counteract TGF-independent vasodilator influences on the renal vasculature. These data are consistent with closed-loop studies in which acute volume expansion with plasma did not reduce the maximum homeostatic efficiency, but shifted it away from ambient flows to lower flows, enhancing its dilatory and reducing its constrictor potency.[122]

The effects of an acute decrease of ECV have been studied in rats after acute hypotensive hemorrhage,[344,345] and in dehydrated rats.[346] In general, these interventions are accompanied by an increase in TGF response magnitude. Hypotensive hemorrhage induced a shift of the feedback curve to the left.[344,345,347] Since proximal absorption increased at the same time, the operating point tended to move toward the shoulder of the reset feedback function.[344] Thus, in this circumstance, the resetting results in reduced dilatory and enhanced constrictor capacity.

Studies have been performed to determine the time course of TGF adaptation. When single nephrons were perfused for extended periods of time, resetting developed over the initial 30–40 minutes of hyperperfusion, whereas changes in response magnitude were slower, requiring 40–60 minutes.[270] Similarly, acute volume depletion by furosemide restored TGF responses in chronically volume-expanded rats within 60–120 minutes.[342]

Other Conditions Associated with TGF Adaptation

URETERAL AND NEPHRON OBSTRUCTION

In the first few hours following complete unilateral ureteral obstruction (UUO), TGF reactivity appears to be completely abolished.[348-350] Elimination of the restraining effect of TGF is reflected by increased renal

and glomerular plasma flows and elevated glomerular capillary pressures.[351] After persistence of ureteral obstruction for 24 hours, TGF activity is restored and possibly slightly enhanced, as indicated by a reduced $V_{1/2}$.[350,352] Augmentation of TGF responses in hydronephrotic kidneys appears to be caused by increased superoxide formation and NO deficiency, since nNOS blockade was without effect and tempol administration normalized TGF responsiveness in hydronephrotic animals.[353,354] The dominant effect of prolonged ureteral obstruction is a marked reduction of glomerular capillary pressure and glomerular plasma flow, changes which result in a dramatic reduction of GFR.[349,355] The apparent absence of a luminal signal suggests that vasoconstriction is not equivalent to the standard TGF response discussed so far. On the other hand, obstruction of a single nephron for 4 hours also causes marked vasoconstriction, indicating that persistent interruption of distal delivery produces a local constrictor signal of unknown nature.[356-358]

Following release of short-lasting ureteral obstruction TGF reactivity is increased,[349] and it is maintained in its somewhat activated state after release of an obstruction of 24 hours duration.[350,352] It is possible that the activated TGF mechanism is in part responsible for the continued vasoconstriction following release of both ureteral and single nephron obstruction.[352] However, additional mechanisms appear to contribute to the reduction in filtration after release of obstruction, since *SNGFR* at zero flow increased only slightly above distal values.[352] Furthermore, nephron and kidney filtration rates were also markedly suppressed after release of bilateral ureteral obstruction, even though in this experimental condition TGF responses were blunted rather than enhanced.[350,352]

During partial unilateral ureteral obstruction for 3–6 weeks, TGF reactivity appears to be in the normal range.[359,360] During volume expansion, on the other hand, TGF reactivity increased in the hydronephrotic kidney whereas it was strongly inhibited in the non-obstructed contralateral kidney.[359] The enhanced TGF reactivity seen in hydronephrotic kidneys during volume expansion could be prevented by thromboxane synthase inhibition.[360] A similar paradoxical enhancement of TGF reactivity by volume expansion was less pronounced during chronic bilateral ureteral obstruction.[361]

LOSS OF RENAL MASS

In the first hours following unilateral nephrectomy, TGF responses in the residual kidney may be enhanced and ambient distal flows may exert a GFR-depressing effect as judged from an increase in the proximal–distal *SNGFR* difference, without a change in the proximal value.[362] However, at later time points uninephrectomy or 5/6 ablation has been shown to shift the TGF function to the right, with[363] or without increasing the maximum response.[364,365] A similar response to nephrectomy was noted in transplanted kidneys.[364] On the other hand, a striking variability in SNGFR responses to loop of Henle perfusion was noted in rats with subtotal nephrectomy, in which the average TGF response was zero. Unexpectedly, AT1 blockade restored TGF responses for reasons that are not clear.[366] To the extent that the most striking change is a TGF-independent increase in GFR (Y-intercept of the TGF function or proximal SNGFR) these results are reminiscent of the findings during growth-related increases in renal weight, and suggest an adaptation of the TGF function curve to a primary increase in GFR.[121,367]

HYPERGLYCEMIA

Moderate hyperglycemia produced by either acute glucose infusion[368] or streptozotocin-induced diabetes mellitus[369] reduced the amplitude of the TGF response and shifted $V_{1/2}$ to higher flow rates.[368] Type 2 diabetic rats of the OLETF strain have significantly diminished TGF responses accompanied by reduced autoregulatory efficiency even in the pre-diabetic stage.[370] Reduced TGF responses have also been observed in the Akita mouse model of type 1 diabetes mellitus, as well as in hydrated db/db mice, a model of type 2 diabetes.[371,372] This reduced capacity to compensate for experimentally-induced perturbations was also demonstrable under closed-loop conditions.[373] The reduction in the TGF response magnitude may in part be caused by a reduction in NaCl concentration, and the presence of glucose in tubular perfusion fluid.[368,374,375]

It has been suggested that the hyperfiltration of early diabetes is caused by TGF, as a result of excessive salt reabsorption in nephron segments upstream from the MD and the resulting reduction in MD NaCl concentration.[376,377] This hypothesis is supported by the demonstration that tubular transport proximal to the macula densa is in fact enhanced in diabetic animals.[378,375] Structural adaptations participate in tubular hyper-reabsorption; inhibition of the enzyme ornithine decarboxylase blocked the renal hypertrophy in a rat model of diabetes mellitus,[379] and attenuated both the enhanced proximal reabsorption and the increase in GFR.[378] On the other hand, it has been argued that TGF may actually prevent excessive hyperfiltration in diabetes.[380] A protective action of TGF is supported by the finding that diabetic mice of the Akita strain display an exaggerated hyperfiltration when TGF is rendered inoperative by A1AR deletion.[371] Hyperfiltration in alloxan-diabetic mice deficient in A1AR also suggests that TGF is not the primary cause of hyperfiltration in this diabetic model.[381]

Both in streptozotocin-treated rats and in diabetic humans, a paradoxical relationship between salt intake and GFR or renal plasma flow has been observed, with high salt intake producing a decrease instead of the expected rise of GFR,[375,382] an effect which was absent when kidney growth was suppressed by inhibition of ornithine decarboxylase.[383] These observations are consistent with the notion that the TGF adaptation during changes in extracellular fluid volume may be defective in diabetic animals. Whereas TGF desensitization normally prevents a non-homeostatic reduction of GFR during volume expansion, absent or incomplete resetting of TGF in diabetes appears to permit persistent GFR deviations. Altered resetting in diabetic animals could be a consequence of abnormal RAS activation or dysregulation of NO generation, factors thought to be involved in TGF adaptation.[372,384,385] Nevertheless, the paradoxical low salt-induced increase and high salt-induced decrease of GFR has not been found in all studies of diabetic patients and animals.[386–388] Differences in the dietary background, aside from NaCl content, may be an important modifying factor.[389]

RENAL SYMPATHETIC NERVE ACTIVITY

Whereas some experiments did not detect an effect of acute denervation or renal nerve stimulation on the TGF function curve in normotensive animals,[390,391] other studies have reported that denervation causes a time-dependent resetting of TGF to higher values of $V_{1/2}$ without changes in the maximum response.[392] Changes in TGF function persisted for at least one week, and were associated with increased GFR and Na excretion.[393]

Mechanisms of TGF Adaptation
RENIN—ANGIOTENSIN SYSTEM

The local activity of the renin—angiotensin system appears to be the most consistent determinant of TGF sensitivity. Converting enzyme inhibitors or angiotensin-receptor blockers in relatively high doses cause a reduction of the TGF response magnitude by about 50—60%.[394–398] An essentially complete inhibition of TGF responsiveness was seen in mice with a null mutation in the AT1A receptor, the major renal receptor for angiotensin I[185]. Similarly, TGF responses were essentially absent in ACE knockout mice, an effect that was in part reversible with infusion of subpressor doses of angiotensin II.[399] Studies in mice with deletion of tissue ACE or with selective expression of ACE in either blood vessels or proximal tubules suggest that the angiotensin II that is required for full TGF responsiveness is derived both from the action of membrane-associated ACE in endothelial cells, and from systemic

ACE,[400] while exclusive expression of ACE in proximal tubules is unable to sustain normal TGF responses.[401] This conclusion is consistent with earlier observations that angiotensin infusion partly restored feedback responsiveness during captopril-induced TGF inhibition.[402,403] Intravenous or peritubular infusion of angiotensin II enhanced TGF responses in untreated control rats, a property not shared by other vasoconstrictors such as vasopressin and norepinephrine.[404,212] Conversely, the arteriolar constrictor response to angiotensin II was greater during simultaneous TGF activation in both the isolated afferent arteriole/MD double-perfusion approach, and in the blood-perfused juxtamedullary nephron preparation.[405,406] Since local adenosine levels are thought to increase during TGF activation, this augmentation is possibly due to the effect of adenosine in preventing angiotensin II desensitization.[407] In accordance with the role of TGF in autoregulation, angiotensin II has been noted to enhance the TGF component of dynamic autoregulation.[408–410] The suppression of TGF responsiveness caused by acute volume expansion could be fully overcome by the infusion of angiotensin II at doses that restored normal plasma angiotensin II levels.[341] Taken together, these results indicate that an AT1A receptor-mediated effect of angiotensin II is a required constituent of the TGF pathway. The requirement for angiotensin II may result from the well-described synergistic interaction between the vascular effects of angiotensin II and of the TGF mediator adenosine.[223,226,411–413] The mechanism of this interaction has been suggested to result from an intracellular action of adenosine that enhances the calcium sensitivity of myosin light chain phosphorylation or prevents desensitization of angiotensin II receptors.[407,414] Contributing factors may be upregulation of MD NaCl transport by angiotensin II or enhanced production of feedback-enhancing superoxide radicals.[266,415]

The TGF-modifying effect of angiotensin II gains special importance in view of the fact that changes in NaCl in the tubular fluid in the MD region not only affect vascular tone, but also regulate renin secretion (see below). This dual effect of MD NaCl has the potential to automatically adjust TGF sensitivity to the NaCl status of the organism. When the combined external forces determining GFR and proximal and loop of Henle absorption cause deflections in MD NaCl concentration which exceed the range over which TGF operates effectively, persistent changes in MD NaCl occur which will cause an inverse change in renin secretion. The change in angiotensin II concentration resulting from the altered rate of renin secretion, in turn, is predicted to alter TGF sensitivity. For example, an increase in MD NaCl resulting from extracellular volume expansion will decrease renin secretion, and the decrease of angiotensin II concentration expected to gradually develop is then predicted to uncouple GFR from MD control.

EICOSANOIDS

The presence of both isoforms of cyclooxygenase (COX) in the juxtaglomerular region raises the possibility of a participation of prostaglandins in JGA cell-to-cell signaling. COX-1 is expressed in mesangial cells and in endothelial cells of afferent arterioles,[416] whereas COX-2 activity has been demonstrated in epithelial cells of thick ascending limb and MD.[417] Maximum TGF responses have been found to be inhibited by the intravenous or luminal application of high concentrations of non-specific COX inhibitors, as well as specific inhibitors of both COX-2 and COX-1.[418–422] The conclusion that the net effect of PGs on TGF is enhanced vasoconstriction is supported by the finding that arachidonic acid elicits a constrictor rather than a dilator response when administered by retrograde luminal infusion.[423] Thromboxane (TP) is a vasoconstrictor prostaglandin that has been implicated in TGF on the basis of the finding that the intravenous administration of inhibitors of TP receptors or of TP synthesis reduced the magnitude of the TGF-induced vasoconstrictor response.[360,398,422] TP receptor blockade also interfered with the TGF reducing effects of COX-2 and COX-1 inhibitors, indicating that these effects were TP-dependent.[418] Conversely, activation of TP receptors by U-46,619 or by the isoprostane 8-isoprostaglandin F2α enhanced TGF responses,[424] and COX-1 generated prostaglandins, presumably TP, may contribute to the TGF-enhancing effects of angiotensin II.[425] Low levels of glomerular thromboxane synthase may limit thromboxane formation under basal and low-salt conditions[426,427]; in fact, attenuation of TGF responses by systemic or luminal application of blockers of TP receptors or of TP synthesis has not been found in all laboratories,[360,398,422,423] and normal TGF responses have been observed in TP receptor knockout mice.[428] Administration of a high-salt diet, on the other hand, caused a 20-fold increase of thromboxane synthase expression, as well as a stimulation of TP receptor levels.[426,429] These observations provide an explanation for the finding that the TGF response in the presence of the TP mimetic U-46,619 is augmented in high-salt fed animals.[426] TP receptor activation may also contribute to the exaggerated TGF responses observed in young spontaneously hypertensive rats (SHR).[430] In contrast to these conclusions, studies in the blood-perfused juxtamedullary nephron preparation indicate that TGF activation is accompanied by nNOS-dependent enhancement of COX-2 activity and subsequent generation of vasodilatory PG metabolites which counteract TGF-mediated vasoconstriction.[431]

There is some evidence that 20-hydroxyeicosatetrae-noic acid (20-HETE), an arachidonic acid metabolite endogenously generated in afferent arterioles by the 4A family of cytochrome P450 enzymes, may be involved in the TGF response.[432] Two inhibitors of cytochrome P450 enzymes, 17-octadecynoic acid (ODYA) and clotrimazole, caused a marked attenuation of the TGF response when added to the luminal perfusate for an extended period of time, and this inhibition could be overcome by the administration of exogenous 20-HETE.[433] The presence of the mRNAs for cytochrome P450 4A2, 4A3, and 4A8 has recently been demonstrated by RT-PCR in glomeruli and most segments of the tubule, while preglomerular arterioles appear to express only the 4A2 isoform.[434] Immunocytochemistry with a polyclonal non-specific P450 4A antibody showed cortical presence of P450 4A protein in proximal tubules, thick ascending limbs, glomeruli, and preglomerular arterioles.[434] Exactly how locally formed 20-HETE affects the TGF pathway is unclear. In addition to its vasoconstrictor properties, 20-HETE has been shown to inhibit TAL NaCl transport by blocking Na,K,2Cl co-transport, Na,K-ATPase, and by closing K channels.[435] This combination of effects should result in a powerful inhibition of NaCl transport in thick ascending limb and presumably MD cells, so that increments in 20-HETE production would be expected to attenuate, not enhance, TGF responses. It is conceivable, therefore, that ODYA and clotrimazole inhibit the TGF response in a non-specific way by causing a reduction in baseline afferent arteriolar tone.[436] It is also possible that 20-HETE acts as an intracellular second messenger for the TGF-mediating agent.[432,437]

NITRIC OXIDE

Luminal application of non-specific and nNOS-selective inhibitors of NO synthases has been shown to enhance MD-mediated vasoconstrictor responses both *in vivo* and *in vitro*.[55,438–441] These findings demonstrate tonic attenuation of TGF responsiveness by NO generated by nNOS in MD cells, an effect that is cGMP-dependent.[442] TGF responses of stop flow pressure *in situ* and afferent arteriolar diameter reductions *in vitro* in response to elevated MD [NaCl] were similar in nNOS-deficient and wild-type mice,[443,444] but the specific mutation in these mice does not exclude the possibility of maintained expression of β and γ splice variants of nNOS.[57] Nevertheless, the proximal–distal *SNGFR* difference was significantly higher in the nNOS$^{-/-}$ animals, and luminal administration of a non-specific NOS inhibitor (NLA 10^{-3} M) caused an augmentation of TGF responses only in wild-type, but not in nNOS knockout, mice.[444] Luminal and systemic administration of NOS inhibitors reversed the

attenuation of TGF responses caused by an acute saline infusion, suggesting that NO contributes to the TGF resetting caused by volume expansion.[445]

NO may affect TGF by altering the function of MD cells. In the isolated double-perfused JGA preparation, inhibition of soluble guanylate cyclase or cGMP-dependent protein kinase mimicked the TGF-potentiating effect of a nNOS inhibitor when administered from the tubular side, whereas there was no effect when inhibitors were added to the vascular perfusate.[446] The cGMP-dependent mechanism may be inhibition of NaCl uptake, since inhibition of Cl fluxes by NO is mediated by soluble guanylate cyclase in TAL cells.[447] Formation of NO may occur in MD cells, but a contribution of NO produced by eNOS in TAL cells appears to also affect MD cell function.[448]

The relationship between luminal NaCl concentration and NO formation in MD cells has been addressed by using the NO-binding agents DAF-AM DA and DAF-AM. Two independent studies agree that an increase in luminal NaCl causes an increase in fluorescence in MD cells, as well as in their surroundings, and that this increase was prevented by an inhibitor of nNOS.[48,449,450] Since the concentration steps causing increased NO formation were between 35 and 135 mM in one study and between 60 and 150 mM in the other, it has been concluded that supraphysiological NaCl changes are necessary to stimulate NOS.[449] That the stimulation of nNOS activity by high luminal NaCl is Ca-dependent is unlikely, since NaCl does not consistently elevate [Ca]$_i$, and since an activation of NOS was seen in Ca-free medium.[48] Another explanation for the increased formation of NO is based on the fact that the pH optimum of NOS is in the slightly alkaline range.[451] Since an increase in luminal NaCl caused cell alkanization, it is conceivable that pH-dependent disinhibition of nNOS is responsible for the enhanced NO generation.[30] This notion is supported by the observation that dimethyl amiloride increased TGF responses, and that an nNOS-specific inhibitor in the presence of the NHE blocker did not further enhance the TGF reaction.[450,452] Furthermore, amiloride as well as 7-nitroindazole blunted the increase in NO formation caused by elevated luminal NaCl.[450] Stimulation of NO formation by high-luminal NaCl is consistent with the earlier observations that the effect of NOS blockade on TGF-dependent vasoconstriction is greater at high than at low flows.[453] Increases in luminal flow rate also stimulate NO formation by TAL cells, but in contrast to MD cells stimulation is strictly shear stress-dependent, and independent of NaCl transport.[454,455] NaCl independence is difficult to reconcile with direct NO measurements performed with carbon fiber electrodes in the distal tubule which have shown an increase in the amount of NO and in NO concentration during perfusion of loops of

Henle with furosemide, suggesting that transport inhibition along the entire loop of Henle stimulates emission and downstream convection of NO.[456] These results seem consistent with observations in an MD cell line showing increased NO generation during exposure to low chloride or furosemide.[457]

In the absence of hemoglobin, the biological half-life of NO in relation to the diffusion distance across the JGA would seem long enough to permit a direct interaction of NO released by MD cells with smooth muscle cells of the afferent arterioles. Nevertheless, NO inactivation may be an important modulator of the effect of NO on TGF. Reactive oxygen species have been identified as a factor that can markedly reduce bioactive NO levels. MD cells express NADPH oxidase isoforms NOX2 and NOX4, together with the required constituents of the active enzyme complex p47phox, p67phox, p22phox, and Rac.[268,458] A high-luminal NaCl appears to activate NADPH oxidase, and this activation is pH-dependent since blocking Na/H exchange with dimethyl amiloride or acidification of the luminal perfusate diminished superoxide production.[459] Production of the NO scavenger may limit the impact of NO that is stimulated in MD cells at the same time by the same mechanism. The membrane-permeant superoxide dismutase mimetic tempol can diminish TGF responses *in vivo* and in the perfused JGA preparation, but this effect is usually not very pronounced under control conditions.[263,354,460,461] Since tempol had no effect in the presence of a NOS inhibitor, it appears that any effect is due to an increase in NO bioavailability.[263,460] In spontaneously hypertensive rats (SHR) the expression of NADPH oxidase subunits is elevated, and the TGF-inhibiting effect of tempol is enhanced compared to normotensive controls, suggesting increased oxidative stress in SHR and reduced bioavailability of NO.[458,461] This observation is in accordance with the earlier finding that inhibition of nNOS did not enhance TGF responses in SHR.[462] Angiotensin II may be in part responsible for the activation of NADPH oxidase in SHR, since candesartan restored normal TGF responses to NOS inhibition.[463] A high salt intake may be another situation in which the generation of superoxide is increased as indicated by increased expression of NADPH oxidase subunits, and increased excretion of isoprostanes.[464] However, the TGF-enhancing effect of NOS inhibition was augmented rather than reduced in rats on a high-salt diet.[465,466] NO availability may also be regulated by ADMA (asymmetric dimethylarginine), an endogenous NOS inhibitor that also inhibits cellular uptake of the NOS substrate arginine. In fact, ADMA in the luminal perfusate enhanced TGF responses, and this effect appears to be the result of both inhibition of arginine uptake and of NOS activity.[467,468] Finally, NO may reduce TGF responses by inhibition of ecto-5′-nucleotidase, an intervention that would be predicted to reduce extracellular adenosine levels.[469,470]

OTHER VASOACTIVE FACTORS

A reduction in TGF reactivity has been observed subsequent to the systemic administration of renal vasodilators such as atrial natriuretic factor,[471,472] histamine,[436] dopamine,[473] high concentrations of PGI_2,[474] bradykinin,[348] uroguanylin,[475] and a number of vasodilating drugs.[199,200,436,476] Inhibition of heme oxygenase with stannous mesoporphyrin enhanced TGF-induced vasoconstriction in the isolated tubule/vessel preparation, and the administration of the CO-releasing agent CORM-3 (tricarbonylchloro[glycinato]rutheniumII) inhibited it, suggesting that carbon monoxide reduces TGF.[477] Since the presence of heme oxygenases in the MD has not been established, it is likely that carbon monoxide affects TGF by its vasodilatory properties.[478,479] Furthermore, TGF reactivity is decreased by an acute reduction of arterial blood pressure,[309] probably as a consequence of non-TGF-mediated autoregulatory vasodilatation. It seems unlikely that all these agents specifically interact with the TGF mechanism at the JGA level to cause a reduction of renal vascular resistance. Rather, the adjustment of TGF responsiveness may be the non-specific consequence of vasodilatation, reflecting a dependency of vascular resistance changes on the initial wall thickness—radius ratio.[480] Since the predominant effector of the TGF response is the afferent arteriole, a resistance change at this site would appear to be most likely to modulate TGF sensitivity.

INTERSTITIAL PRESSURE

TGF reactivity has been shown to increase during peritubular capillary perfusion with a hyperoncotic solution, whereas perfusion with protein-free solutions reduced TGF responses.[481] Changes in response were seen after a time delay of about 20 minutes.[481] Based on these observations, the concept was developed that net interstitial pressure (the difference between interstitial hydrostatic pressure and interstitial oncotic pressure) may be an important determinant of TGF reactivity in general. It was subsequently shown that TGF reactivity correlated inversely with net interstitial pressure during acute NaCl infusion,[336,337,339,482] during short-lasting ureteral obstruction,[349] and after contralateral nephrectomy.[363,483] In all these conditions, $V_{1/2}$ increased and the TGF response amplitude decreased. Conversely, net interstitial pressure was found to be reduced by 24 hours of dehydration,[346,482] and before and after release of 24 hour unilateral ureteral occlusion.[350] TGF reactivity was increased in these experimental situations. Exactly how net interstitial pressure affects TGF reactivity is unclear.

RESETTING BY LUMINAL FACTORS

There are a number of circumstances in which unidentified factors in tubular fluid have been shown to modify responses. During chronic dietary salt-loading, TGF control was inhibited when native tubular fluid was used as perfusate, whereas responses were only slightly blunted during perfusion with an artificial fluid.[484] A luminal factor has also been reported to modify TGF during the infusion of atrial natriuretic peptide,[485] but this factor appears to enhance TGF responses compared to the blunting observed with artificial solutions. Loop of Henle perfusion with electrolyte-free plasma dialysates from patients with acute renal failure and liver dysfunction produced exaggerated TGF responses which could not be blocked by furosemide,[486] suggesting that the plasma in certain disease states contains a factor which can elicit NaCl-independent vasoconstriction when present in the tubular lumen.

MACULA DENSA CONTROL OF RENIN SECRETION

Following Goormaghtigh's early speculation,[487] Vander suggested that renin release might be influenced by tubular fluid composition at the macula densa.[488] During a variety of experimental conditions, plasma renin activity and sodium excretion appeared to be inversely correlated, whereas there was no correlation between renin and mean arterial pressure or renal blood flow.[489,490] The overall conclusion from these studies was that an increased delivery of NaCl to the MD cells inhibits renin secretion. These early observations have now been corroborated by additional evidence from whole animal studies and from isolated *in vitro* systems which have established the concept that a high NaCl concentration at the macula densa inhibits renin secretion.[488,491]

Evidence for Macula Densa Control of Renin Secretion

Studies in Intact Animals

Vander's proposal that renin secretion depends upon MD NaCl concentration was studied more directly by comparing renin secretion from normal or nonfiltering kidneys. In dogs in which basal levels of renin were elevated by thoracic caval constriction, intrarenal infusion of NaCl or KCl inhibited renin secretion, but such a response was not seen in similarly treated animals in which the infused kidney had been rendered nonfiltering by ureteral occlusion.[492] In conscious mice, acute infusion of isotonic saline, a maneuver that has been shown to result in increased distal tubular NaCl concentrations, leads to a suppression of renin secretion.[493,494]

Attempts have been made to evaluate the effect of changes in MD NaCl concentration at the single nephron level *in vivo*. In these studies in rats, renin concentration in proximal tubular fluid and in postglomerular blood collected by micropuncture was found to vary inversely with changes in distal NaCl.[495]

Studies in the Isolated Perfused TAL/Glomerulus Preparation

With the isolated perfused tubule technique it has been possible to study MD-dependent renin secretion in the absence of baroreceptor and regulated adrenergic inputs, and during precise control of tubular fluid composition.[491] Another important aspect of the isolated JGA preparation is that it limits the possible sites of tubulovascular information transfer to MD cells and possibly a small number of surrounding TAL cells as the only cells present in the area of contact. In this preparation (Figure 23.11) there is unequivocal

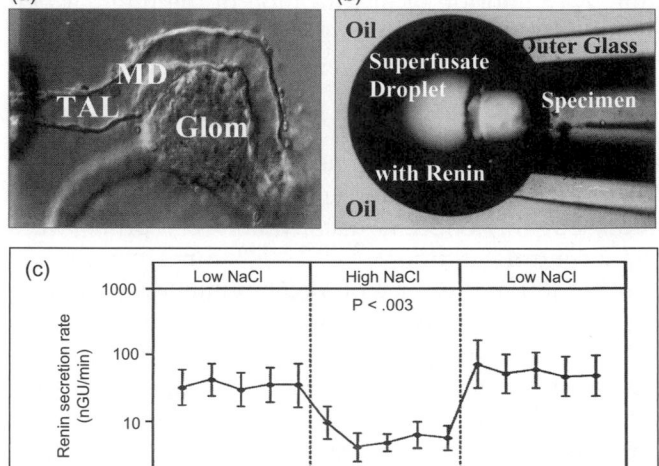

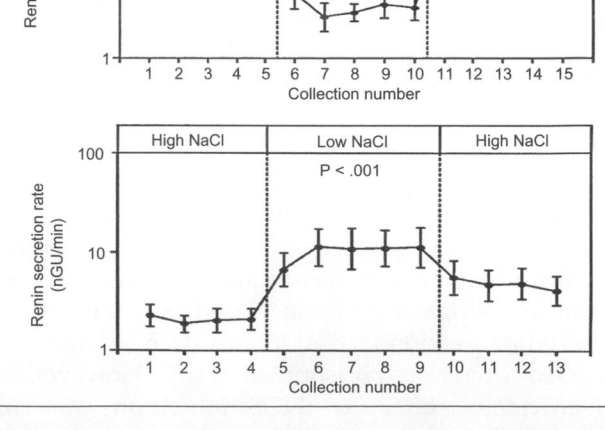

FIGURE 23.11   (a) Isolated perfused thick ascending limb (TAL) with attached glomerulus (glom); macula densa (MD) cells can be seen to protrude into the luminal space. (b) The perfused specimen is superfused through an outer glass pipette; emerging superfusate containing the secreted renin is collected under oil in defined time intervals.[595] (c) Macula densa-mediated changes in renin secretion showing the time course of changes in renin release to an increase (top) and decrease (bottom) in perfusate NaCl concentration.[497,498] See color plate section at the back of the book.

evidence that increasing NaCl concentration in the tubular perfusate suppresses renin secretion and reducing NaCl concentration stimulates it.[496−499] MD-dependent renin secretion is characterized by a rapid onset and offset following step-changes in NaCl concentration, and by reversibility of the induced changes.[497,499] Renin responses were independent of whether the tubule was perfused in an orthograde fashion from the TALH or in a retrograde fashion from the distal convoluted tubule.[497] Similar to the TGF response, MD-dependent renin secretion was not altered when NaCl concentration was reduced from isotonicity to about 80 mM, but the full renin response was seen when NaCl concentrations were varied between 7 and 61 mM of Cl and between 26 and 80 mM of Na, i.e., within the range that is physiologically relevant.[500] In the most sensitive concentration range between 7 and 47 mM of Cl, renin secretion increased by about 2 nGU/min per mM, whereas it fell by 0.4 nGU/min per mM when NaCl concentration was raised from 47 to 87 mM.[500] The NaCl concentration causing a half-maximum renin response is between 25 and 30 mM, values close to the estimated ambient NaCl concentration and close to the NaCl concentration causing a half-maximum TGF response. Although both decreases and increases of NaCl concentration are predicted to affect renin secretion, MD-dependent renin secretion is asymmetric around the operating point, with most of the responses occurring in the subnormal concentration range. Quantitative extrapolation from this *in vitro* system to the *in vivo* response must be made with caution, mainly because renin secretory responses *in vitro* are assessed in the absence of stabilizing feedback loops that may dampen MD-dependent changes in renin secretion *in vivo*.

Sensing Mechanism for Macula Densa-Mediated Renin Secretion

Renin Secretory Response and NaCl Transport

Early studies in intact animals suggested that, in certain conditions, renin secretion correlates more closely with distal tubular NaCl load than NaCl concentration, for example, during the infusion of hypertonic mannitol.[490,501,502] However, a reinvestigation of early distal NaCl concentration during mannitol diuresis showed a clear concentration decrease, in agreement with the stimulation of renin release typically seen in this condition.[503] In the isolated JGA preparation, an 80% reduction in luminal NaCl load by decreasing perfusate flow at constant NaCl concentration caused only a small, approximately two-fold increase in the rate of renin secretion. In contrast, when NaCl load was reduced to a similar degree by decreasing perfusate NaCl concentration, renin secretion increased nearly eight-fold, indicating that NaCl concentration is a more important determinant of renin release than NaCl delivery.[497]

Based on the stimulatory effect of loop diuretics in intact animals, it was concluded that MD NaCl transport plays a critical role as an early step in NaCl-dependent control of renin secretion.[488,490,504−507] Recent studies in mice deficient in the NKCC2A isoform of the co-transporter have shown that the inhibitory effect of an acute volume load on renin release is absent, supporting the notion that intact salt transport is required for salt-sensing by MD cells.[163] Direct evidence for an MD-mediated effect of transport inhibition on renin secretion was obtained in non-perfused afferent arterioles in which furosemide stimulated renin release only when the MD segment was included in the dissected specimen, but not in its absence.[508] In the isolated perfused JGA preparation, luminal application of bumetanide at $10^{−6}$ M increased renin secretion during perfusion with high NaCl solutions.[498] Furthermore, the presence of furosemide at $5 \times 10^{−5}$ M essentially abolished the dependence of renin secretion on luminal NaCl concentration.[500]

Although NKCC2 mediates the bulk of MD Na reabsorption, apical expression of the Na^+/H^+ exchanger 2 (NHE2) may contribute to Na^+ transport, as well as to the regulation of intracellular pH.[30,32] In NHE2-deficient mice, renal renin content and plasma renin concentration were elevated compared to wild-type controls, and the stimulation of the renin system by a salt-depleted diet was blunted.[509] Increased baseline renin secretion in NHE2$^{−/−}$ mice was paralleled by enhanced MD COX-2 and mPGES expression. Recent studies have shown that plasma renin concentration is significantly elevated in NKCC1-deficient compared to wild-type mice.[510] Studies in isolated JG cells indicate that NKCC1 exerts a direct inhibitory effect on basal renin release.[119] This effect appears to be independent of the NKCC2-dependent inhibitory pathway through the macula densa, since the stimulatory effect of furosemide on renin release was essentially normal in NKCC1$^{−/−}$ mice.

Ion Specificity of Renin Secretion

MD control of renin secretion shows an apparent Cl dependency that is reminiscent of that described for TGF responses. Whereas the acute or chronic administration of various Cl or Br salts without Na inhibited renin secretion, Na salts without Cl as the accompanying anion had no effect.[493,511] Furthermore, changes in renin secretion under these conditions correlated with loop of Henle Cl absorption.[512] Conversely, an acute selective depletion of Cl by peritoneal dialysis increased plasma renin activity,[513] and substitution of

Cl by nitrate or thiocyanate in the perfusate of isolated kidneys stimulated renin secretion.[514] In the isolated perfused JGA, ion selectivity has been examined by measuring the inhibitory effect of adding various Na and Cl salts to a low NaCl perfusate. The inhibitory response was unchanged when most luminal Na was replaced by choline or rubidium.[498] On the other hand, substituting Cl by isethionate or acetate virtually eliminated the response to increased Na concentration.[498] Cl dependency is supported by studies in conscious mice showing that suppression of renin secretion following acute intravenous salt-loading is observed with infusion of NaCl, but not $NaHCO_3$.[515] These results support the hypothesis that the initiating signal for MD control of renin secretion is a change in the rate of NaCl uptake predominantly via a luminal Na,K,2Cl cotransporter whose physiological activity is determined by a change in luminal Cl concentration.

Organic Compounds and Renin Secretion

In addition to their function as sensors of TAL Cl concentration, MD cells are equipped with receptors for organic compounds, like the citric acid intermediate succinate. The succinate receptor GPR91 (succinate receptor 1, SUCNR1) has been shown to be localized in the apical membrane of cells of the cortical TAL, including the MD.[516] Increases in tubular succinate concentration result in the induction of the same intracellular signaling pathways that are activated by a low NaCl concentration. Incubation of cultured MD cells with succinate induced phosphorylation of p38 and Erk1/2 MAP kinases, and subsequent stimulation of COX-2 activity and expression in MD cells and enhanced PGE_2 release.[517] During streptozotocin-induced diabetes mellitus, renocortical COX-2 and renin content were upregulated in wild-type mice, and this stimulation of the renin system was markedly reduced in GPR91-deficient mice.[517] GPR91 expression in the vicinity of the JG cells, however, is not restricted to MD cells. GPR91 is also present in endothelial cells of the afferent arteriole, and may mediate renin release by stimulating endothelial prostanoid and NO formation.[518,519]

Furthermore, components of the olfactory system are present in MD cells.[520] MD cells rather specifically express the olfactory adenylate cyclase isoform 3 (AC3), as well as the olfactory trimeric G-protein G_{olf}. The olfactory receptor Olfr90 was detected in a MD cell line, and was also present in the native kidney.[520] Plasma renin concentration in AC3-deficient mice was reduced by about 50% compared to wild-types, despite increased MD COX-2 expression and augmented nNOS activity. The reason for these alterations of the MD–JG axis is unclear, and the ligands that may activate olfactory receptors on MD cells *in vivo* remain to be determined.

The Stimulus—Response Coupling Mechanism

Nitric Oxide

The presence of NOS I in MD cells raises the possibility that NO may act as an epithelium-derived factor that participates in MD control of renin secretion. This notion is supported by observations showing that the expression of MD nNOS changes in parallel with renin expression in a number of circumstances. MD cells of rats on a low-salt diet have increased levels of nNOS mRNA and protein expression.[59,60,521−523] Furthermore, the administration of furosemide also causes a marked increase in MD nNOS expression,[59,521] as does renal artery constriction.[59,521] The mechanism responsible for the upregulation of nNOS expression in these states is unclear, but a reduced NaCl transport at the MD is a common feature. Since the expression and secretion of renin is known to be elevated in these conditions, it is possible that NO generation is an upstream signal in the control of the RAS. The suggestion that a chronically reduced NaCl transport may stimulate MD nNOS expression is not immediately reconcilable with the evidence discussed earlier that acute increases in NaCl concentration appear to increase nNOS activity and NO formation. The expression of nNOS in MD cells is stabilized by negative feedback influences exerted by angiotensin II and PGE_2, since nNOS expression was markedly upregulated in mice with AT1 receptor or angiotensinogen deficiencies, as well as in COX-2$^{-/-}$ mice.[524−526]

Understanding the role of NO in renin secretion is complicated by the fact that NO can elicit both stimulatory and inhibitory effects. The inhibitory effect appears to result from activation of cGMP-dependent protein kinases (cGK), while the stimulatory effects are related to changes in intracellular cAMP levels. Two isoforms of cGK have been identified, cGK I and cGK II, and both isoforms have been found in granular cells.[108] A direct activator of cGK, 8-para-chlorophenylthio-cGMP, has been shown to inhibit isoproterenol- or forskolin-stimulated renin secretion in isolated perfused rat kidneys and microdissected afferent arterioles, and this stimulation could be reversed by an inhibitor of cGK.[527] A role for cGKII is suggested by the finding that 8-bromo-cGMP reduced basal and forskolin stimulated renin secretion in JG cells isolated from wild-type and cGK I$^{-/-}$ mice, but that it had no effect in cultures from cGK II$^{-/-}$ mice.[528]

The mechanism of the stimulatory effect of NO on renin secretion is related to an activation of the cAMP/protein kinase A pathway, and this activation results from an inhibition of PDEIII, a cAMP degrading phosphodiesterase that is inhibited by cGMP.[529] An early report showing that the PDEIII inhibitor milrinone increased basal and isoproterenol stimulated renin release in conscious rabbits has now been corroborated by substantial additional evidence.[530] In the isolated perfused rat kidney, Na nitroprusside increased renin secretion, and this increase was attenuated by the protein kinase A inhibitor Rp-8-CPT-cAMPS. Since membrane-permeable cGMP analogs also reduced the stimulatory effect of SNP, stimulation of renin secretion by NO was clearly related to the A kinase, not G kinase pathway.[531] Inhibition of PDE IV, a phosphodiesterase with predominant effects on cGMP degradation, also increased renin secretion,[532] and this effect was blunted by nNOS inhibition suggesting that nNOS contributed to cGMP formation.

NO IN MD-DEPENDENT RENIN RELEASE

In view of the dual effects of NO on renin secretion and the ambiguity about the directional changes of juxtaglomerular NO with changes in loop of Henle flow rates, it is not surprising that the precise role of NO in MD control of renin release has remained equivocal. In the isolated perfused JGA preparation during perfusion with a low NaCl concentration, the luminal addition of l-arginine stimulated renin secretion and this stimulation was abolished by NOS blockade, suggesting that in this setting NO is renin-stimulatory.[533] Consistent with this conclusion is the observation that the NaCl dependency of renin secretion was essentially abolished in the presence of an NOS blocker in the tubular lumen, a change that was due entirely to prevention of the rise of renin secretion caused by a low luminal NaCl.[533] The conclusion that a low NaCl concentration at the MD stimulates renin secretion in an NO-dependent fashion is also supported by findings showing that the increased renin secretion caused by a reduction in arterial or perfusion pressure in kidneys of conscious dogs and in isolated rat kidneys was markedly and consistently blunted by NOS inhibition.[534,535] In other studies, the administration of a loop diuretic has been used to simulate a reduction in MD NaCl concentration. In dissected rat renal microvessels, NOS inhibition abolished the increase in renin release caused by furosemide pretreatment.[536] Similarly, the stimulation of renin secretion by furosemide *in vivo* was inhibited by the administration of NOS inhibitors.[504,537,538] Plasma renin activity in nNOS knockout mice and basal renin secretion in isolated perfused kidneys from nNOS[−/−] or eNOS[−/−] mice were found to be consistently lower than in wild-type animals, suggesting that tonic release of NO enhances renin release in mice.[505,526] The relative increases of renin secretion by furosemide were essentially normal in nNOS[−/−] or eNOS[−/−] mice, but were markedly reduced by general NOS inhibition.[505] Furthermore, the administration of the NO donor SNAP in kidneys in which endogenous NO production was blocked by L-NAME completely

restored the stimulatory effect of loop diuretics. According to this recent evidence, it would appear that exposition of JG cells to NO regardless of its exact cellular source is necessary for the MD pathway to operate normally. The nature of this permissive effect of NO may be to inhibit PDEIII, and thereby to sensitize the renin secretory mechanism to the renin mediator that we assume to act through activation of the cAMP/PKA pathway (Figure 23.12).

Prostaglandins

Starting with the early observations by Larsson et al. that arachidonic acid increases and indomethacin reduces plasma renin activity,[539] various metabolites of arachidonic acid, most notably prostaglandins, have been established as potent regulators of renin secretion in a variety of experimental conditions.[506] Stimulation of renin secretion is most consistently seen with administration of prostaglandins of the E and I series.[540] The effect of prostaglandins on renin secretion are mediated by G_s-protein-coupled receptors, IP receptors in the case of PGI2, and EP2/EP4 receptors in the case of PGE2.[541] Selective deletion of floxed $G_{s\alpha}$ in JG cells by cre recombinase driven by the endogenous renin promoter was associated with marked reductions of plasma renin concentration.[542]

RELATIONSHIP BETWEEN MD COX-2 AND RENIN

Cyclooxygenases catalyze the hydroxylation and oxygenation of arachidonic acid that lead to the generation of endoperoxides (or PGH2). Subsequent processing by a number of enzymes converts PGH2 into the biologically active spectrum of prostaglandins. The potential of prostaglandins to regulate renin secretion became highly relevant for the MD-dependent pathway by the demonstration that one of the cyclooxygenases, the inducible isoform COX-2, was constitutively expressed in MD

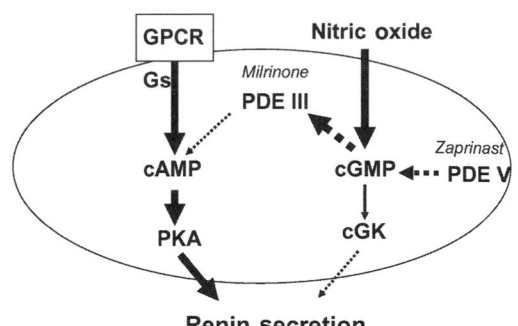

FIGURE 23.12 Schematic representation of the pathways by which nitric oxide can inhibit or stimulate renin secretion. Inhibition of PDEIII by cGMP and subsequent reduced degradation of cAMP appears to be the dominant pathway under many conditions. Milrinone, an inhibitor of PDEIII, consistently stimulates renin secretion.

cells.[62] The abundance of COX-2 in the MD and adjacent TAL cells is highly regulated, and the pattern of COX-2 regulation parallels that of nNOS in the macula densa and of renin in JG cells. Parallel increases in COX-2 and renin have been observed in rats treated chronically with furosemide, and in patients with Bartter syndrome, suggesting that COX-2 expression, like nNOS, may be in some way linked to NaCl uptake by MD cells.[543–547] An increase of MD COX-2 expression and of JG cell renin is induced by administration of a low NaCl diet or by renal artery stenosis.[62,63,548–550] Stimulation of COX-2 expression has also been found following partial renal ablation and in active lupus nephritis.[551,552] A low NaCl diet also caused a two- to three-fold increase in the expression of PGE_2 synthase in MD cells.[71] Conversely, mice with genetic COX-2 deficiency have a marked reduction of renin expression and of plasma renin concentration.[553,554] On the other hand, angiotensin II appears to play the role of a negative feedback regulator of COX-2 synthesis: a strong and consistent stimulation of COX-2 expression is induced by ACE inhibition or AT1 receptor blockade, and COX-2 expression is increased in AT1 receptor knockout mice,[543,555,556] as well as in other states of low angiotensin action.[542]

REGULATION OF PGE_2 PRODUCTION

The application of a biosensor technique has provided a missing piece of evidence linking MD NaCl delivery to local PGE_2 release.[557] In this approach, HEK293 cells were stably transfected with the mouse PGE_2 receptor EP1, a receptor subtype that is coupled to the IP3 pathway, and whose activation therefore causes an increase in cytosolic Ca. In perfused TAL/MD preparations dissected from kidneys of salt-restricted rabbits, a transfected and fura-2 loaded sensor cell was positioned at the basolateral aspect of MD cells, and changes in $[Ca]_i$ were used as an index of PGE_2 release. In this preparation, removal of luminal NaCl caused a significant increase in sensor cell $[Ca]_i$, while no effect was seen when NaCl was reduced to zero in the presence of luminal furosemide (Figure 23.13b). This effect appeared to be cell-specific, since the positioning of the sensor cell close to a TAL cell had no effect on $[Ca]_i$. Of major importance is the observation that most of the change in $[Ca]_i$ occurred in a NaCl concentration range of between 20 and 40 mM, exactly the concentration range in which NaCl concentration affects renin secretion in a similar preparation (Figure 23.13a).

Studies in the isolated rabbit JGA have shown that acute, non-specific COX inhibition with flufenamic acid or flurbiprofen virtually completely abolished the increase in renin secretion caused by a decrease in MD NaCl concentration.[496] Since the concentration change from minimal to maximal was done in a single step, it is not clear whether the effect of these agents was symmetrical around the midpoint or whether it mainly affected the stimulation in the subnormal concentration range. Direct evidence for a role of COX-2 has been obtained in an extension of these studies in which the specific COX-2 inhibitor NS-398 was also found to prevent the stimulation of renin secretion by low NaCl, while the putative COX-1 blocker valerylsalicylate did not have this effect (Figure 23.13c).[558] The significance of these findings is substantial since as pointed out earlier, the isolated perfused rabbit JGA preparation is the only currently available technique capable of assessing MD-dependent renin release unencumbered by simultaneous sympathetic and baroreceptor input.

The mechanisms by which a reduction in luminal NaCl may cause stimulation of PGE_2 release and COX-2 expression have been studied in cell lines derived from the MD and from TAL cells.[559,560] In both lines of cells a reduction in medium NaCl caused a prompt and dose-dependent increase in PGE_2 release that was essentially completely inhibited by NS-398, and was therefore largely mediated by COX-2. The onset of this response preceded any increase in COX-2 expression, suggesting that it was the result of an increase in COX-2 activity and/or of an activation of PLA2 followed by increased availability of arachidonic acid. Presence of PLA2 in macula densa cells and regulation of PLA2 in parallel to that of COX-2 has recently been demonstrated.[66] In both TAL and MD cells in culture, a reduction in medium NaCl also augmented the expression of the mRNA and protein expression of COX-2.[559,560] Ion substitution studies indicate that the extracellular signal for COX-2 stimulation appears to be a reduction in Cl rather than in Na concentration, a finding that is remarkably concordant with the Cl-dependency of renin secretion shown earlier in an entirely different preparation. The intracellular signaling events leading to the stimulation of COX-2 activity and expression are initiated by rapid phosphorylation of p38 and Erk1/2 kinases (Figure 23.14).[560] Participation of MAP kinases in COX-2 expression is supported by the inhibitory effects of SB 203580 and PD 98059, inhibitors of p38- and Erk1/2-mediated signaling events.[559,560] The role of the MAP kinase pathway in Cl-dependent COX-2 expression that appears to reflect both a transcriptional activation and an increased stability of the mRNA[561] is similar to the involvement of MAP kinases in mediating the effects of cytokines, growth factors, and hypertonicity on COX-2 expression in other cell types.[562–564]

Chronic interference with COX-2 signaling is associated with a reduction of renin expression that has secondary consequences for acute renin secretory responses. Thus, COX-2-deficient mice have been shown to have a markedly reduced renin mRNA expression and plasma renin, and this effect was greater on 129J or C57Bl/6 than on mixed genetic

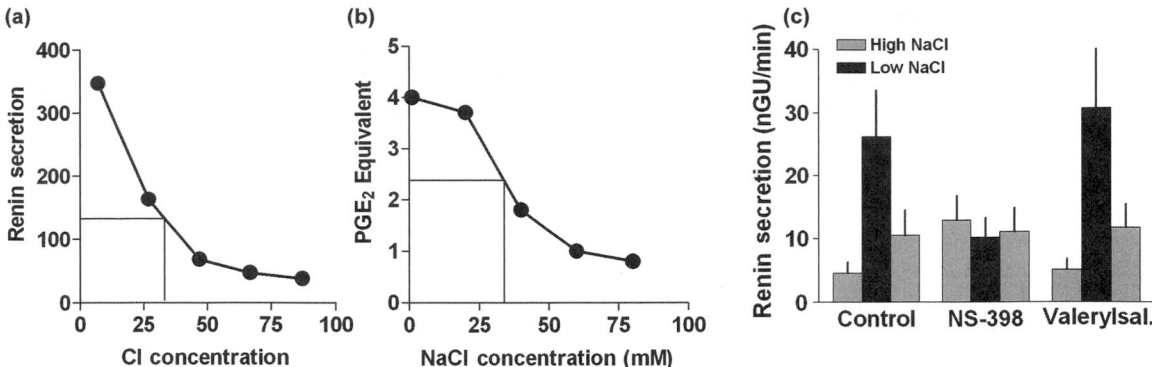

FIGURE 23.13 (a) Relationship between perfusate Cl concentration and renin release in the isolated perfused JGA preparation; data from [500]. (b) Relationship between perfusate NaCl concentration and PGE₂ release by macula densa cells.[557] The PGE2 equivalent corresponds to the EP1-mediated increase in cytosolic Ca in HEK cells transfected with EP1 receptor cDNA, and placed at the basolateral aspect of macula densa cells.[557] (c) Renin secretion in the perfused thick ascending limb/glomerulus preparation of the rabbit in response to perfusion with solutions containing high and low NaCl concentrations during control conditions, during inhibition of COX-2 with NS-398, and during inhibition of COX-1 with valerylsalicylate.[558]

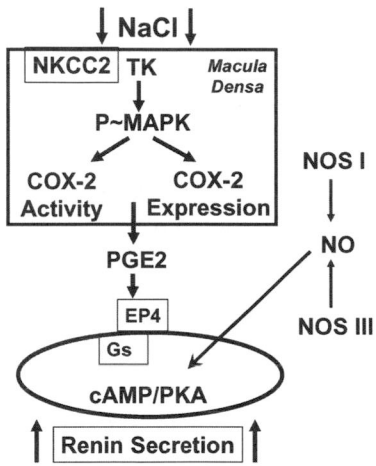

FIGURE 23.14 **Schematic summary of the pathway by which a decrease in luminal NaCl concentration causes stimulation of renin secretion.** Activation of several MAP kinases causes activation of COX-2, as well as transcriptional upregulation of COX-2 synthesis, augmented release of PGE2, and stimulation of the cAMP/PKA pathway through EP4 receptors. Nitric oxide, derived from both NOS I and NOC III, supports renin secretion by stabilizing cAMP.

background.[553,554,565] Chronic administration of COX-2 blockers, on the other hand, did not consistently reduce renin expression.[566–568] Acute stimulation of renin release by furosemide, hydralazine or isoproterenol was markedly reduced in COX-2-deficient compared to wild-type mice, suggesting that the acute release response was dependent upon basal renin expression levels.[553] Thus, when low renin release in COX-2-deficient mice was overcome by chronic prestimulation of their renin system, *acute* renin secretory responses to various stimuli were reconstituted to levels observed in wild-type animals. Furthermore, stimulation of renin release by angiotensin converting enzyme or AT1 blockers was also markedly reduced in animals with

genetic or pharmacologic COX-2-deficiency.[553,555,565] Overall these studies reveal that the level of renin expression is an important and non-specific determinant of the acute secretory response, independent of whether the stimulus acts through the MD, baroreceptor, sympathetic or any other pathway. The strong relationship between basal levels of renin release or its surrogate, plasma renin, and the acute release response suggests the existence of an acutely releasable renin pool in JG cells whose magnitude depends on renin synthesis.[553,569]

In addition to the MD, the renal vasculature including the afferent arteriole appears to be a significant source of prostanoids in the vicinity of the JGA in some species. In humans, expression levels of COX-2 in the MD are low and are exceeded by vascular COX-2 expression, in particular in close vicinity to the JG cells.[570] In patients with renal artery stenosis this vascular expression of COX-2 was enhanced, and therefore prostaglandins from non-MD sources may contribute to enhanced renin secretion in this condition. In addition, stimulation of the renin system *in vivo* after loop diuretics may not be exclusively mediated by the MD pathway, but may be at least partly related to enhanced vascular prostanoid formation.[571] Furthermore, the reduced stimulatory capacity of loop diuretics on renin secretion in the presence of COX inhibitors appears to be to some extent related to blockade of vascular prostanoid formation.[572,573]

Adenosine

In general, exogenous adenosine inhibits renin release in intact rats or dogs,[574–576] an effect that is produced by activation of A1AR.[575] Nevertheless, it is unclear to what extent adenosine participates in the renin inhibition caused by high luminal NaCl concentrations. In the isolated perfused JGA, the selective A1AR blocker 8-cyclopentyl-1,3-dipropylxanthine (CPX) blunted the fall in renin secretion caused by an elevation in luminal NaCl, but did not abolish it.[499] Adenosine itself was found to be only a weak inhibitor of MD-stimulated renin secretion when added to the bathing fluid.[577] This may reflect effective degradation of exogenous adenosine, since the addition of the adenosine deaminase inhibitor pentostatin (deoxycoformycin) augmented the renin-inhibitory effect of adenosine somewhat.[577] Additional studies may have clarified the role of adenosine in MD-dependent renin release. In isolated perfused kidneys, it was found that the stimulation of renin release by bumetanide was not measurably different between wild-type and A1AR-deficient mice.[578] This observation argues against a role of A1AR and adenosine in the stimulation of renin secretion during inhibition of NaCl transport below ambient levels. On the other hand, renin secretion fell when NaCl at the MD was acutely increased by a bolus injection of NaCl, and this effect was not seen in A1AR-deficient mice, suggesting that the renin-inhibitory effect of increased NaCl concentrations is mediated by adenosine, whereas the renin-stimulatory effect is not (Figure 23.15).

The cellular mechanisms of inhibition of renin release by adenosine are not clear, but it is likely that an increase in $[Ca]_i$ may play a role. Considerable progress has been made in understanding the paradoxical inhibition of renin release by elevated $[Ca]_i$. In primary cultures of JG cells it has been observed that an increase of $[Ca]_i$ by thapsigargin, angiotensin II or endothelin was associated with a marked decrease in isoproterenol- or forskolin-stimulated cellular cAMP and a decrease of renin release.[579] Conversely, a decrease of $[Ca]_i$ by the Ca chelator BAPTA-AM caused an increase in cellular cAMP, accompanied by an increase in renin release.[580] The inverse relation between $[Ca]_i$ and cAMP was suggested to reflect regulation of adenylyl cyclase (AC) by $[Ca]_i$. In fact, the Ca-inhibitable AC5 and AC6 isoforms were shown to be expressed in JG cells,[579,580] and siRNAs directed against AC5 and AC6 were able to prevent cAMP stimulation by forskolin or isoproterenol, as well as renin secretion in As4.1 cells (Figure 23.16).[579]

Ionic and Osmotic Effects

Changes in external juxtaglomerular osmolarity may mediate the renin secretory response to a change of luminal NaCl. In a number of different preparations hypoosmolarity stimulates and hyperosmolarity inhibits renin secretion, and such changes would seem to be directionally plausible in mediating MD-dependent renin release.[581–584] Hypotonicity-stimulated renin secretion appears to be initiated by AQP1-mediated water flux leading to COX-2-dependent PGE_2 production and cAMP formation.[585] However, a recent study in isolated perfused rat or mouse kidneys established a direct rather than an inverse relationship between renin release and external osmolarity,[569] a finding that confirms an earlier *in vivo* observation.[586] Osmotic stimulation of renin release was not prevented by L-NAME, indomethacin or bumetanide, and was therefore

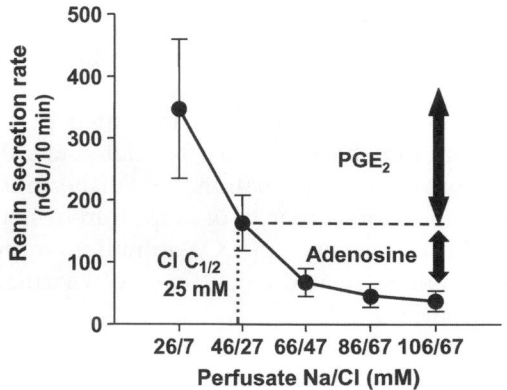

FIGURE 23.15 Control of macula densa-dependent renin secretion by PGE2 and adenosine, with PGE2 being responsible for the larger stimulatory effect during reduced luminal NaCl, and adenosine causing a smaller inhibitory effect during increases in macula densa NaCl.

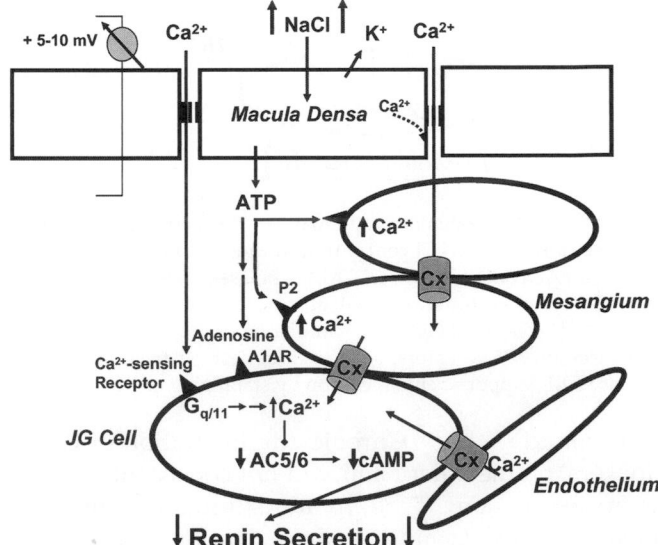

FIGURE 23.16 Schematic summary of the pathways by which an increase in TAL/macula densa NaCl reabsorption mediates Ca-dependent suppression of renin secretion. TAL/macula densa transepithelial NaCl transport and concomitant K recycling generate a lumen-positive potential which drives paracellular Ca absorption. Ca-sensing receptors on JG cells translate changes in interstitial Ca into a modulation of Ca_i. Cell coupling by calcium-permeable connexins (Cx), activation of Ca_i-mobilizing P2 receptors by ATP, and A1AR activation in JG cells are additional pathways for raising JG cell calcium. Ca-inhibited adenylyl cyclases (AC5 and AC6) link the increase of Ca_i to a reduction of cAMP formation in JG cells.

suggested to reflect a direct effect on JG cells.[569] In addition to changes in interstitial osmolarity, direct ionic effect may influence renin secretion. Thus, JG cells express the calcium receptor CaR which renders renin-producing cells capable of translating changes in extracellular calcium into changes in intracellular calcium.[587] In fact, the calcimimetic R-568 partially blunted the stimulation of renin secretion in response to isoproterenol, furosemide, and enalapril, while having little effect on basal renin release.[588] It remains to be determined under which conditions changes in interstitial Ca concentrations may occur *in vivo*. In theory, increased TAL/MD NaCl reabsorption would be expected to augment the tubular lumen-positive potential, and would enhance the driving force for paracellular Ca uptake; this would result in an increased interstitial Ca concentration. In line with this concept, interstitial renal cortical Ca concentration as determined by *in situ* microdialysis techniques in Wistar rats was shown to rise by 25% during chronic oral salt loading.[589] A role of Ca in the MD-JG signal transmission is further supported by the finding that an increased tubular flow rate triggers a Ca wave that originates around the MD, spreads throughout the JGA, and eventually increases Ca_i of the JG cells. Both cell–cell coupling in the JGA via connexins and ATP-dependent mechanisms appear to participate in the propagation of this Ca wave.[150,590]

Gap junction uncoupling by α-glycyrrhetinic acid and ATP degradation by apyrase markedly diminished changes in Ca_i in the most distal portion of the afferent arteriole.[150] Connexin 45 expression was detected in vascular smooth muscle cells of the afferent and efferent arteriole, the mesangium, and JG cells. In cultured vascular smooth muscle cells from mice with local deletion of connexin 45 the speed of a cell-to-cell Ca wave was reduced by 60% compared to wild-type controls.[590] Furthermore, mice with deletion of connexin 45 in the JGA showed increased PRC accompanied by elevated blood pressure suggesting an inadequate inhibitory input on renin secretion.[590] However, connexin 45 probably is not the only connexin involved in a Ca-dependent signal transmission from MD cells to renin granular cells. In particular, connexin 40 was shown to mediate Ca transmission from endothelial to JG cells,[591] a finding consistent with major derangements in JG cell renin secretion and topology in connexin 40-deficient mice.[592,593]

Acknowledgment

Research from the laboratory of the authors was supported by intramural funds of the National Institute of Diabetes, and Digestive and Kidney Diseases, National Institutes of Health, and by funding from the Deutsche Forschungsgemeinschaft.

References

[1] Golgi C. Annotazioni intorno all'istologia dei reni dell'uomo e di altri mammiferi e sull'istogenesi dei canalicoli oriniferi. Atti della Reale Accademia dei Lincei 1889;5:334–42.

[2] Kaissling B, Kriz W. Structural analysis of the rabbit kidney. Adv Anat Embryol Cell Biol 1979;56:1–123.

[3] Christensen JA, Meyer DS, Bohle A. The structure of the human juxtaglomerular apparatus. A morphometric, lightmicroscopic study on serial sections. Virchows Arch A Pathol Anat Histol 1975;367:83–92.

[4] Christensen JA, Bohle A. The juxtaglomerular apparatus in the normal rat kidney. Virchows Arch A Pathol Anat Histol 1978;379:143–50.

[5] Dorup J, Morsing P, Rasch R. Tubule–tubule and tubule–arteriole contacts in rat kidney distal nephrons. A morphologic study based on computer-assisted three-dimensional reconstructions. Lab Invest 1992;67:761–9.

[6] Komlosi P, Banizs B, Fintha A, Steele S, Zhang ZR, Bell PD. Oscillating cortical thick ascending limb cells at the juxtaglomerular apparatus. J Am Soc Nephrol 2008;19:1940–6.

[7] Taugner R, Hackenthal E. The juxtaglomerular apparatus. Berlin Heidelberg: Springer-Verlag; 1989.

[8] Barajas L. Anatomy of the juxtaglomerular apparatus. Am J Physiol 1979;237:F333–343.

[9] Kaissling B, Peter S, Kriz W. The transition of the thick ascending limb of Henle's loop into the distal convoluted tubule in the nephron of the rat kidney. Cell Tissue Res 1977;182:111–8.

[10] Peti-Peterdi J, Morishima S, Bell PD, Okada Y. Two-photon excitation fluorescence imaging of the living juxtaglomerular apparatus. Am J Physiol Renal Physiol 2002;283:F197–201.

[11] Razga Z, Nyengaard JR. The effect of angiotensin II on the number of macula densa cells through the AT1 receptor. Nephron Physiol 2009;112:37–43.

[12] Zimmermann KW. Ueber den Bau des Glomerulus der Saeugerniere. Z Mikr Anat Forsch 1933;32:176–278.

[13] Bonsib SM. The macula densa tubular basement membrane: a unique plaque of basement membrane specialization. J Ultrastruct Mol Struct Res 1986;97:103–8.

[14] Ojeda JL, Piedra S. Lectin-binding sites and silver affinity of the macula densa basement membranes in the rabbit kidney. J Anat 1994;185:529–35.

[15] Lapointe JY, Bell PD, Cardinal J. Direct evidence for apical Na^+:$2Cl^-$:K^+ co-transport in macula densa cells. Am J Physiol Renal Physiol 1990;258:F1466–1469.

[16] Schlatter E, Salomonsson M, Persson AE, Greger R. Macula densa cells sense luminal NaCl concentration via furosemide sensitive $Na^+2Cl^-K^+$ co-transport. Pflugers Arch 1989;414:286–90.

[17] Schlatter E. Effect of various diuretics on membrane voltage of macula densa cells. Whole-cell patch-clamp experiments. Pflugers Arch 1993;423:74–7.

[18] Nielsen S, Maunsbach AB, Ecelbarger CA, Knepper MA. Ultrastructural localization of Na-K-2Cl co-transporter in thick ascending limb and macula densa of rat kidney. Am J Physiol Renal Physiol 1998;275:F885–893.

[19] Obermuller N, Kunchaparty S, Ellison DH, Bachmann S. Expression of the Na-K-2Cl co-transporter by macula densa and thick ascending limb cells of rat and rabbit nephron. J Clin Invest 1996;98:635–40.

[20] Yang T, Huang YG, Singh I, Schnermann J, Briggs JP. Localization of bumetanide- and thiazide-sensitive Na-K-Cl co-transporters along the rat nephron. Am J Physiol 1996;271: F931–939.

[21] Gimenez I, Isenring P, Forbush B. Spatially distributed alternative splice variants of the renal Na-K-Cl co-transporter exhibit

dramatically different affinities for the transported ions. J Biol Chem 2002;277:8767–70.

[22] Oppermann M, Mizel D, Huang G, et al. Macula densa control of renin secretion and preglomerular resistance in mice with selective deletion of the B isoform of the Na,K,2Cl co-transporter. J Am Soc Nephrol 2006;17:2143–52.

[23] Payne JA, Forbush B. Alternatively spliced isoforms of the putative renal Na-K-Cl co-transporter are differently distributed within the rabbit kidney. Proc Nat Acad Sci USA 1994; 91:4544–8.

[24] Mutig K, Paliege A, Kahl T, Jons T, Muller-Esterl W, Bachmann S. Vasopressin V2 receptor expression along rat, mouse, and human renal epithelia with focus on TAL. Am J Physiol Renal Physiol 2007;293:F1166–1177.

[25] Laamarti MA, Lapointe JY. Determination of NH_4^+/NH_3 fluxes across apical membrane of macula densa cells: A quantitative analysis. Am J Physiol Renal Physiol 1997;273:F817–824.

[26] Hurst AM, Lapointe JY, Laamarti A, Bell PD. Basic properties and potential regulators of the apical K^+ channel in macula densa cells. J Gen Physiol 1994;103:1055–70.

[27] Nusing RM, Pantalone F, Grone HJ, Seyberth HW, Wegmann M. Expression of the potassium channel ROMK in adult and fetal human kidney. Histochem Cell Biol 2005;123:553–9.

[28] Xu JZ, Hall AE, Peterson LN, Bienkowski MJ, Eessalu TE, Hebert SC. Localization of the ROMK protein on apical membranes of rat kidney nephron segments. Am J Physiol Renal Physiol 1997;273:F739–48.

[29] Amemiya M, Loffing J, Lotscher M, Kaissling B, Alpern RJ, Moe OW. Expression of NHE-3 in the apical membrane of rat renal proximal tubule and thick ascending limb. Kidney Int 1995;48:1206–15.

[30] Fowler BC, Chang YS, Laamarti A, Higdon M, Lapointe JY, Bell PD. Evidence for apical sodium proton exchange in macula densa cells. Kidney Int 1995;47:746–51.

[31] Kwon TH, Nielsen J, Kim YH, Knepper MA, Frokiaer J, Nielsen S. Regulation of sodium transporters in the thick ascending limb of rat kidney: response to angiotensin II. Am J Physiol Renal Physiol 2003;285:F152–165.

[32] Peti-Peterdi J, Chambrey R, Bebok Z, Biemesderfer St D, John PL, Abrahamson DR, et al. Macula densa $Na^{(+)}/H^{(+)}$ exchange activities mediated by apical NHE2 and basolateral NHE4 isoforms. Am J Physiol Renal Physiol 2000;278:F452–463.

[33] Peti-Peterdi J, Bebok Z, Lapointe JY, Bell PD. Novel regulation of cell $[Na^{(+)}]$ in macula densa cells: apical $Na^{(+)}$ recycling by H-K-ATPase. Am J Physiol Renal Physiol 2002;282:F324–329.

[34] Rajendran VM, Sangan P, Geibel J, Binder HJ, Ouabain-sensitive H. K-ATPase functions as Na,K-ATPase in apical membranes of rat distal colon. J Biol Chem 2000;275:13035–40.

[35] Verlander JW, Moudy RM, Campbell WG, Cain BD, Wingo CS. Immunohistochemical localization of H-K-ATPase alpha(2c)-subunit in rabbit kidney. Am J Physiol Renal Physiol 2001;281: F357–365.

[36] Kashgarian M, Biemesderfer D, Caplan M, Forbush III B. Monoclonal antibody to Na,K-ATPase: immunocytochemical localization along nephron segments. Kidney Int 1985; 28:899–913.

[37] Schnermann J, Marver D. ATPase activity in macula densa cells of the rabbit kidney. Pflugers Arch 1986;407:82–6.

[38] Arystarkhova E, Wetzel RK, Sweadner KJ. Distribution and oligomeric association of splice forms of $Na^{(+)}-K^{(+)}$-ATPase regulatory gamma-subunit in rat kidney. Am J Physiol Renal Physiol 2002;282:F393–407.

[39] Farman N, Fay M, Cluzeaud F. Cell-specific expression of three members of the FXYD family along the renal tubule. Ann NY Acad Sci 2003;986:428–36.

[40] Pu HX, Cluzeaud F, Goldshleger R, Karlish SJ, Farman N, Blostein R. Functional role and immunocytochemical localization of the gamma a and gamma b forms of the Na,K-ATPase gamma subunit. J Biol Chem 2001;276:20370–8.

[41] Sweadner KJ, Arystarkhova E, Donnet C, Wetzel RK. FXYD proteins as regulators of the Na,K-ATPase in the kidney. Ann NY Acad Sci 2003;986:382–7.

[42] Wetzel RK, Sweadner KJ. Immunocytochemical localization of Na-K-ATPase alpha- and gamma-subunits in rat kidney. Am J Physiol Renal Physiol 2001;281:F531–545.

[43] Wetzel RK, Sweadner KJ. Phospholemman expression in extraglomerular mesangium and afferent arteriole of the juxtaglomerular apparatus. Am J Physiol Renal Physiol 2003;285: F121–129.

[44] Lapointe JY, Bell PD, Hurst AM, Cardinal J. Basolateral ionic permeabilities of macula densa cells. Am J Physiol Renal Physiol 1991;260:F856–860.

[45] Alper SL, Stuart-Tilley AK, Biemesderfer D, Shmukler BE, Brown D. Immunolocalization of AE2 anion exchanger in rat kidney. Am J Physiol Renal Physiol 1997;273:F601–614.

[46] Komlosi P, Frische S, Fuson AL, Fintha A, Zsmbery A, Peti-Peterdi J, et al. Characterization of basolateral chloride/bicarbonate exchange in macula densa cells. Am J Physiol Renal Physiol 2005;288:F380–386.

[47] Komlosi P, Fintha A, Bell PD. Unraveling the relationship between macula densa cell volume and luminal solute concentration/osmolality. Kidney Int 2006;70:865–71.

[48] Liu R, Pittner J, Persson AE. Changes of cell volume and nitric oxide concentration in macula densa cells caused by changes in luminal NaCl concentration. J Am Soc Nephrol 2002;13:2688–96.

[49] Liu R, Persson AE. Simultaneous changes of cell volume and cytosolic calcium concentration in macula densa cells caused by alterations of luminal NaCl concentration. J Physiol 2005;205:895–901.

[50] Gonzalez E, Salomonsson M, Muller-Suur C, Persson AE. Measurements of macula densa cell volume changes in isolated and perfused rabbit cortical thick ascending limb. II. Apical and basolateral cell osmotic water permeabilities. Acta Physiol Scand 1988;133:159–66.

[51] Gonzalez E, Salomonsson M, Muller-Suur C, Persson AE. Measurements of macula densa cell volume changes in isolated and perfused rabbit cortical thick ascending limb. I. Isosmotic and anisosmotic cell volume changes. Acta Physiol Scand 1988;133:149–57.

[52] Schnermann J, Briggs JP. Function of the juxtaglomerular apparatus: control of glomerular hemodynamics and renin secretion. In: Seldin DW, Giebisch G, editors. The kidney physiology and pathophysiology, vol. 1. Philadelphia: Lippincott Williams &Wilkins; 2000. p. 945–80.

[53] Aoyagi T, Izumi Y, Hiroyama M, Matsuzaki T, Yasuoka Y, Sanbe A, et al. Vasopressin regulates the renin–angiotensin–aldosterone system via V1a receptors in macula densa cells. Am J Physiol Renal Physiol 2008;295:F100–107.

[54] Mundel P, Bachmann S, Bader M, Fischer A, Kummer W, Mayer B, et al. Expression of nitric oxide synthase in kidney macula densa cells. Kidney Int 1992;42:1017–9.

[55] Wilcox CS, Welch WJ, Murad F, Gross SS, Taylor G, Levi R, et al. Nitric oxide synthase in macula densa regulates glomerular capillary pressure. Proc Natl Acad Sci USA 1992;89:11993–7.

[56] Brenman JE, Chao DS, Gee SH, McGee AW, Craven SE, Santillano DR, et al. Interaction of nitric oxide synthase with the postsynaptic density protein PSD-95 and alpha1-syntrophin mediated by PDZ domains. Cell 1996;84:757–67.

[57] Lu D, Fu Y, Lopez-Ruiz A, Juncos R, Liu H, Manning Jr RD, et al., Salt-sensitive splice variant of nNOS expressed in the macula densa cells. Am J Physiol Renal Physiol 298: F1465–71.

[58] Norgaard T. Quantitation of glucose-6-phosphate dehydrogenase activity in cortical fractions of the nephron in sodium-depleted and sodium-loaded rabbits. Histochemistry 1980;69:49–59.

[59] Schricker K, Potzl B, Hamann M, Kurtz A. Coordinate changes of renin and brain-type nitric-oxide-synthase (b-NOS) mRNA levels in rat kidneys. Pflugers Arch 1996;432:394–400.

[60] Singh I, Grams M, Wang WH, Yang T, Killen P, Smart A, et al. Coordinate regulation of renal expression of nitric oxide synthase, renin, and angiotensinogen mRNA by dietary salt. Am J Physiol Renal Physiol 1996;270:F1027–1037.

[61] Vandewalle A, Farman N, Cluzeaud F, Bonvalet JP. Heterogeneity of uridine incorporation along the rabbit nephron. I. Autoradiographic study. Am J Physiol 1984;246:F417–426.

[62] Harris RC, McKanna JA, Akai Y, Jacobson HR, Dubois RN, Breyer MD. Cyclooxygenase-2 is associated with the macula densa of rat kidney and increases with salt restriction. J. Clin. Invest 1994;94:2504–10.

[63] Yang T, Singh I, Pham H, Sun D, Smart A, Schnermann JB, et al. Regulation of cyclooxygenase expression in the kidney by dietary salt intake. Am J Physiol Renal Physiol 1998;274: F481–9.

[64] Guan Y, Chang M, Cho W, Zhang Y, Redha R, Davis L, et al. Cloning, expression, and regulation of rabbit cyclooxygenase-2 in renal medullary interstitial cells. Am J Physiol Renal Physiol 1997;273:F18–26.

[65] Hartner A, Goppelt-Struebe M, Hilgers KF. Coordinate expression of cyclooxygenase-2 and renin in the rat kidney in renovascular hypertension. Hypertension 1998;31:201–5.

[66] Mangat H, Peterson LN, Burns KD. Hypercalcemia stimulates expression of intrarenal phospholipase A_2 and prostaglandin H synthase-2 in rats. J Clin Invest 1997;100:1941–50.

[67] Komhoff M, Seyberth HW, Nusing RM, Breyer MD. Cyclooxygenase-2 expression is associated with the macula densa in kidneys from patients with Bartter like syndrome. J Am Soc Nephrol 1999;10:437A (abstract)

[68] Nantel F, Meadows E, Denis D, Connolly B, Metters KM, Giaid A. Immunolocalization of cyclooxygenase-2 in the macula densa of human elderly. FEBS Lett 1999;457:475–7.

[69] Zhang MZ, Wang JL, Cheng HF, Harris RC, McKanna JA. Cyclooxygenase-2 in rat nephron development. Am J Physiol Renal Physiol 1997;273:F994–1002.

[70] Murakami M, Nakatani Y, Tanioka T, Kudo I. Prostaglandin E synthase. Prostaglandins Other Lipid Mediat 2002;68-69:383–99.

[71] Campean V, Theilig F, Paliege A, Breyer M, Bachmann S. Key enzymes for renal prostaglandin synthesis: site-specific expression in rodent kidney (rat, mouse). Am J Physiol Renal Physiol 2003;285:F19–32.

[72] Fuson AL, Komlosi P, Unlap TM, Bell PD, Peti-Peterdi J. Immunolocalization of a microsomal prostaglandin E synthase in rabbit kidney. Am J Physiol Renal Physiol 2003;285:F558–564.

[73] Spanidis A, Wunsch H, Kaissling B, Kriz W. Three-dimensional shape of a Goormaghtig cell and its contact with a granular cell in the rabbit kidney. Anat Embryol (Berl) 1982;165:239–52.

[74] Pricam C, Humbert F, Perrelet A, Orci L. Gap junctions in mesangial and lacis cells. J Cell Biol 1974;63:349–54.

[75] Taugner R, Schiller A, Kaissling B, Kriz W. Gap junctional coupling between the JGA and the glomerular tuft. Cell Tissue Res 1978;186:279–85.

[76] Hanner F, Sorensen CM, Holstein-Rathlou NH, Peti-Peterdi J. Connexins and the kidney. Am J Physiol Regul Integr Comp Physiol 2010;298:R1143–1155.

[77] Kurtz L, Madsen K, Kurt B, Jensen BL, Walter S, Banas B, et al. High-level connexin expression in the human juxtaglomerular apparatus. Nephron Physiol 2010;116:p1–8.

[78] Latta H, Maunsbach AB. The juxtaglomerular apparatus as studied electron microscopically. J Ultrastruct Res 1962;6:547–61.

[79] Schnabel E, Kriz W. Morphometric studies of the extraglomerular mesangial cell field in volume expanded and volume depleted rats. Anat Embryol (Berl) 1984;170:217–22.

[80] Rosivall L, Mirzahosseini S, Toma I, Sipos A, Peti-Peterdi J. Fluid flow in the juxtaglomerular interstitium visualized in vivo. Am J Physiol Renal Physiol 2006;291:F1241–1247.

[81] Bacay AC, Mantyh CR, Cohen AH, Mantyh PW, Fine LG. Glomerular atrial natriuretic factor receptors in primary glomerulopathies: studies on human renal biopsies. Am J Kidney Dis 1989;14:386–95.

[82] Osborne MJ, Droz B, Meyer P, Morel F, Angiotensin II. Renal localization in glomerular mesangial cells by autoradiography. Kidney Int 1975;8:245–54.

[83] Kakinuma Y, Fogo A, Inagami T, Ichikawa I. Intrarenal localization of angiotensin II type 1 receptor mRNA in the rat. Kidney Int 1993;43:1229–35.

[84] Christensen JA, Bohle A, Mikeler E, Taugner R. Renin-positive granulated Goormaghtig cells. Immunohistochemical and electron-microscopic studies on biopsies from patients with pseudo-Bartter syndrome. Cell Tissue Res 1989;255:149–53.

[85] Paul LC, Rennke HG, Milford EL, Carpenter CB. Thy-1.1 in glomeruli of rat kidneys. Kidney Int 1984;25:771–7.

[86] Cosio FG, Sedmak DD, Mahan JD, Nahman Jr. NS. Localization of decay accelerating factor in normal and diseased kidneys. Kidney Int 1989;36:100–7.

[87] Muller E, Neuhofer W, Ohno A, Rucker S, Thurau K, Beck FX. Heat shock proteins HSP25, HSP60, HSP72, HSP73 in isoosmotic cortex and hyperosmotic medulla of rat kidney. Pflugers Arch 1996;431:608–17.

[88] Kremer SG, Breuer WV, Skorecki KL. Vasoconstrictor hormones depolarize renal glomerular mesangial cells by activating chloride channels. J Cell Physiol 1989;138:97–105.

[89] Okuda T, Yamashita N, Kurokawa K. Angiotensin II and vasopressin stimulate calcium-activated chloride conductance in rat mesangial cells. J Clin Invest 1986;78:1443–8.

[90] Tsukahara H, Krivenko Y, Moore LC, Goligorsky MS. Decrease in ambient [Cl$^-$] stimulates nitric oxide release from cultured rat mesangial cells. Am J Physiol Renal Physiol 1994;267: F190–195.

[91] Barajas L. The development and ultrastructure of the juxtaglomerular cell granule. J Ultrastruct Res 1966;15:400–13.

[92] Taugner R, Rosivall L, Buhrle CP, Groschel-Stewart U. Myosin content and vasoconstrictive ability of the proximal and distal (renin-positive) segments of the preglomerular arteriole. Cell Tissue Res 1987;248:579–88.

[93] Casellas D, Dupont M, Kaskel FJ, Inagami T, Moore LC. Direct visualization of renin–cell distribution in preglomerular vascular trees dissected from rat kidney. Am J Physiol Renal Physiol 1993;265:F151–156.

[94] Gomez RA, Chevalier RL, Everett AD, Elwood JP, Peach MJ, Lynch KR, et al. Recruitment of renin gene-expressing cells in adult rat kidneys. Am J Physiol 1990;259:F660–665.

[95] Sauter A, Machura K, Neubauer B, Kurtz A, Wagner C. Development of renin expression in the mouse kidney. Kidney Int 2008;73:43–51.

[96] Celio MR, Inagami T. Angiotensin II immunoreactivity coexists with renin in the juxtaglomerular granular cells of the kidney. Proc Natl Acad Sci USA 1981;78:3897–900.

[97] Taugner R, Mannek E, Nobiling R, Buhrle CP, Hackenthal E, Ganten D, et al. Coexistence of renin and angiotensin II in

epitheloid cell secretory granules of rat kidney. Histochemistry 1984;81:39−45.

[98] Cantin M, Gutkowska J, Lacasse J, Ballack M, Ledoux S, Inagami T, et al. Ultrastructural immunocytochemical localization of renin and angiotensin II in the juxtaglomerular cells of the ischemic kidney in experimental renal hypertension. Am J Pathol 1984;115:212−24.

[99] Mercure C, Ramla D, Garcia R, Thibault G, Deschepper CF, Reudelhuber TL. Evidence for intracellular generation of angiotensin II in rat juxtaglomerular cells. FEBS Lett 1998;422:395−9.

[100] Naruse K, Inagami T, Celio MR, Workman RJ, Takii Y. Immunohistochemical evidence that angiotensins I and II are formed by intracellular mechanism in juxtaglomerular cells. Hypertension 1982;4:70−4.

[101] Burson JM, Aguilera G, Gross KW, Sigmund CD. Differential expression of angiotensin receptor 1A and 1B in mouse. Am J Physiol 1994;267:E260−267.

[102] Gasc JM, Shanmugam S, Sibony M, Corvol P. Tissue-specific expression of type 1 angiotensin II receptor subtypes. An *in situ* hybridization study. Hypertension 1994;24:531−7.

[103] Sanada H, Yao L, Jose PA, Carey RM, Felder RA. Dopamine D3 receptors in rat juxtaglomerular cells. Clin Exp Hypertens 1997;19:93−105.

[104] Yamaguchi I, Yao L, Sanada H, Ozono R, Mouradian MM, Jose PA, et al. Dopamine D1A receptors and renin release in rat juxtaglomerular cells. Hypertension 1997;29:962−8.

[105] Haefliger JA, Demotz S, Braissant O, Suter E, Waeber B, Nicod P, et al. Connexins 40 and 43 are differentially regulated within the kidneys of rats with renovascular hypertension. Kidney Int 2001;60:190−201.

[106] Kurtz L, Janssen-Bienhold U, Kurtz A, Wagner C. Connexin expression in renin-producing cells. J Am Soc Nephrol 2009;20:506−12.

[107] Wagner C, de Wit C, Kurtz L, Grunberger C, Kurtz A, Schweda F. Connexin40 is essential for the pressure control of renin synthesis and secretion. Circ Res 2007;100:556−63.

[108] Gambaryan S, Hausler C, Markert T, Pohler D, Jarchau T, Walter U, et al. Expression of type II cGMP-dependent protein kinase in rat kidney is regulated by dehydration and correlated with renin gene expression. J Clin Invest 1996;98:662−70.

[109] Kaplan MR, Plotkin MD, Brown D, Hebert SC, Delpire E. Expression of the mouse Na-K-2Cl co-transporter, mBSC2, in the terminal inner medullary collecting duct, the glomerular and extraglomerular mesangium, and the glomerular afferent arteriole. J Clin Invest 1996;98:723−30.

[110] Anderson TJ, Martin S, Berka JL, James DE, Slot JW, Stow JL. Distinct localization of renin and GLUT-4 in juxtaglomerular cells of mouse kidney. Am J Physiol 1998;274:F26−33.

[111] Skott O. Episodic release of renin from single isolated superfused rat afferent arterioles. Pflugers Arch 1986;407:41−5.

[112] Friis UG, Jensen BL, Hansen PB, Andreasen D, Skott O. Exocytosis and endocytosis in juxtaglomerular cells. Acta Physiol Scand 2000;168:95−9.

[113] Peti-Peterdi J, Fintha A, Fuson AL, Tousson A, Chow RH. Real-time imaging of renin release *in vitro*. Am J Physiol Renal Physiol 2004;287:F329−335.

[114] Kurtz A, Penner R. Angiotensin II induces oscillations of intracellular calcium and blocks anomalous inward rectifying potassium current in mouse renal juxtaglomerular cells. Proc Natl Acad Sci USA 1989;86:3423−7.

[115] Friis UG, Jorgensen F, Andreasen D, Jensen BL, Skott O. Molecular and functional identification of cyclic AMP-sensitive BKCa potassium channels (ZERO variant) and L-type voltage-dependent calcium channels in single rat juxtaglomerular cells. Circ Res 2003;93:213−20.

[116] Russ U, Rauch U, Quast U. Pharmacological evidence for a KATP channel in renin-secreting cells from rat kidney. J Physiol 1999;517(Pt 3):781−90.

[117] Kurtz A, Skott O, Chegini S, Penner R. Lack of direct evidence for a functional role of voltage-operated calcium channels in juxtaglomerular cells. Pflugers Arch 1990;416:281−7.

[118] Friis UG, Jorgensen F, Andreasen D, Jensen BL, Skott O. Membrane potential and cation channels in rat juxtaglomerular cells. Acta Physiol Scand 2004;181:391−6.

[119] Castrop H, Lorenz JN, Hansen PB, Friis U, Mizel D, Oppermann M, et al. Contribution of the basolateral isoform of the Na-K-2Cl⁻ co-transporter (NKCC1/BSC2) to renin secretion. Am J Physiol Renal Physiol 2005;289:F1185−1192.

[120] Schnermann J, Wright FS, Davis JM, Stackelberg WV, Grill G. Regulation of superficial nephron filtration rate by tubuloglomerular feedback. Pflugers Arch 1970;318:147−75.

[121] Briggs JP, Schubert G, Schnermann J. Quantitative characterization of the tubuloglomerular feedback response: effect of growth. Am J Physiol Renal Physiol 1984;247:F808−15.

[122] Thomson SC, Blantz RC. Homeostatic efficiency of tubuloglomerular feedback in hydropenia, euvolemia, and acute volume expansion. Am J Physiol Renal Physiol 1993;264: F930−936.

[123] Thomson S, Vallon V, Blantz RC. Asymmetry of tubuloglomerular feedback effector mechanism with respect to ambient tubular flow. Am J Physiol Renal Physiol 1996;271:F1123−30.

[124] Navar LG, Burke TJ, Robinson RR, Clapp JR. Distal tubular feedback in the autoregulation of single nephron glomerular filtration rate. J Clin Invest 1974;53:516−25.

[125] Vallon V, Richter K, Huang DY, Rieg T, Schnermann J. Functional consequences at the single-nephron level of the lack of adenosine A1 receptors and tubuloglomerular feedback in mice. Pflugers Arch 2004;448:214−21.

[126] Muller-Suur R, Ulfendahl HR, Persson AE. Evidence for tubuloglomerular feedback in juxtamedullary nephrons of young rats. Am J Physiol Renal Physiol 1983;244:F425−431.

[127] Muller-Suur R, Persson AE. Influence of water-diuresis or saline volume expansion on deep nephron tubuloglomerular feedback. Acta Physiol Scand 1986;126:139−46.

[128] Ren Y, Garvin JL, Liu R, Carretero OA. Crosstalk between the connecting tubule and the afferent arteriole regulates renal microcirculation. Kidney Int 2007;71:1116−21.

[129] Wang H, Garvin JL, D'Ambrosio MA, Ren Y, Carretero OA. Connecting tubule glomerular feedback (CTGF) antagonizes tubuloglomerular feedback (TGF) *in vivo*. Am J Physiol Renal Physiol 2010;299:F1374−8.

[130] Yip KP, Holstein-Rathlou NH, Marsh DJ. Mechanisms of temporal variation in single-nephron blood flow in rats. Am J Physiol Renal Physiol 1993;264:F427−434.

[131] Leyssac PP, Baumbach L. An oscillating intratubular pressure response to alterations in Henle loop flow in the rat kidney. Acta Physiol Scand 1983;117:415−9.

[132] Holstein-Rathlou NH. Synchronization of proximal intratubular pressure oscillations: evidence for interaction between nephrons. Pflugers Arch 1987;408:438−43.

[133] Yip KP, Holstein-Rathlou NH, Marsh DJ. Dynamics of TGF-initiated nephron−nephron interactions in normotensive rats and SHR. Am J Physiol Renal Physiol 1992;262:F980−988.

[134] Holstein-Rathlou NH, Sosnovtseva OV, Pavlov AN, Cupples WA, Sorensen CM, Marsh DJ. Nephron blood flow dynamics measured by laser speckle contrast imaging. Am J Physiol Renal Physiol 2011;300:F319−29.

[135] Leyssac PP, Holstein-Rathlou NH. Effects of various transport inhibitors on oscillating TGF pressure responses in the rat. Pflugers Arch 1986;407:285−91.

[136] Holstein-Rathlou NH, Marsh DJ. Oscillations of tubular pressure, flow, and distal chloride concentration in rats. Am J Physiol Renal Physiol 1989;256:F1007—1014.

[137] Holstein-Rathlou NH, Marsh DJ. A dynamic model of the tubuloglomerular feedback mechanism. Am J Physiol Renal Physiol 1990;258:F1448—1459.

[138] Layton HE, Pitman EB, Moore LC. Bifurcation analysis of TGF-mediated oscillations in SNGFR. Am J Physiol Renal Physiol 1991;261:F904—919.

[139] Marsh DJ, Sosnovtseva OV, Pavlov AN, Yip KP, Holstein-Rathlou NH. Frequency encoding in renal blood flow regulation. Am J Physiol Regul Integr Comp Physiol 2005;288:R1160—1167.

[140] Holstein-Rathlou NH, Leyssac PP. TGF-mediated oscillations in the proximal intratubular pressure: differences between spontaneously hypertensive rats and Wistar-Kyoto rats. Acta Physiol Scand 1986;126:333—9.

[141] Karlsen FM, Leyssac PP, Holstein-Rathlou NH. Tubuloglomerular feedback in Dahl rats. Am J Physiol Renal Physiol 1998;274:R1561—1569.

[142] Yip KP, Holstein-Rathlou NH, Marsh DJ. Chaos in blood flow control in genetic and renovascular hypertensive rats. Am J Physiol Renal Physiol 1991;261:F400—408.

[143] Laugesen JL, Sosnovtseva OV, Mosekilde E, Holstein-Rathlou NH, Marsh DJ. Coupling-induced complexity in nephron models of renal blood flow regulation. Am J Physiol Regul Integr Comp Physiol 298:R997—1006.

[144] Layton AT, Moore LC, Layton HE. Multistability in tubuloglomerular feedback and spectral complexity in spontaneously hypertensive rats. Am J Physiol Renal Physiol 2006;291:F79—97.

[145] Schurek HJ, Johns O. Is tubuloglomerular feedback a tool to prevent nephron oxygen deficiency? Kidney Int 1997;51:386—92.

[146] Bell PD, Navar LG. Relationship between tubulo-glomerular feedback responses and perfusate hypotonicity. Kidney Int 1982;22:234—9.

[147] Briggs J, Schubert G, Schnermann J. Further evidence for an inverse relationship between macula densa NaCl concentration and filtration rate. Pflugers Arch 1982;392:372—8.

[148] Schnermann J, Ploth DW, Hermle M. Activation of tubuloglomerular feedback by chloride transport. Pfluegers Arch 1976;362:229—40.

[149] Briggs JP, Schnermann J, Wright FS. Failure of tubule fluid osmolarity to affect feedback regulation of glomerular filtration. Am J Physiol Renal Physiol 1980;239:F427—432.

[150] Peti-Peterdi J. Calcium wave of tubuloglomerular feedback. Am J Physiol Renal Physiol 2006;291:F473—480.

[151] Sipos A, Vargas SL, Peti-Peterdi J. Direct demonstration of tubular fluid flow sensing by macula densa cells. Am J Physiol Renal Physiol 2010;299:F1087—93.

[152] Thurau K, Schnermann J. The Na concentration at the macula densa cells as a factor regulating glomerular filtration rate (micropuncture studies). 1965 [classical article]. J Am Soc Nephrol 1998;9:925—34.

[153] Gutsche HU, Muller-Suur R, Hegel U, Hierholzer K. Electrical conductivity of tubular fluid of the rat nephron. Micropuncture study of the diluting segment in situ. Pflugers Arch 1980;383:113—21.

[154] Morgan T, Berliner RW. A study by continuous microperfusion of water and electrolyte movements in the loop of Henle and distal tubule of the rat. Nephron 1969;6:388—405.

[155] Schnermann J, Briggs J, Schubert G. In situ studies of the distal convoluted tubule in the rat. I. Evidence for NaCl secretion. Am J Physiol 1982;243:F160—166.

[156] Seney FD, Wright FS. Signal for tubuloglomerular feedback control of GFR: separate changes of sodium and chloride at constant osmolality. Kidney Int 1986;29:388.

[157] Wright FS, Mandin H, Persson AE. Studies of the sensing mechanism in the tubuloglomerular feedback pathway. Kidney Int Suppl 1982;12:S90—96.

[158] Bell PD, McLean CB, Navar LG. Dissociation of tubuloglomerular feedback responses from distal tubular chloride concentration in the rat. Am J Physiol Renal Physiol 1981;240:F111—119.

[159] Wright FS, Schnermann J. Interference with feedback control of glomerular filtration rate by furosemide, triflocin, and cyanide. J Clin Invest 1974;53:1695—708.

[160] Mason J, Takabatake T, Olbricht C, Thurau K. The early phase of experimental acute renal failure. III. Tubuloglomerular feedback. Pflugers Arch 1978;373:69—76.

[161] Franco M, Bell PD, Navar LG. Effect of adenosine A1 analogue on tubuloglomerular feedback mechanism. Am J Physiol Renal Physiol 1989;257:F231—236.

[162] Schnermann J, Briggs JP. Concentration-dependent sodium chloride transport as the signal in feedback control of glomerular filtration rate. Kidney Int 1982;22(Suppl. 12):S82—9.

[163] Oppermann M, Mizel D, Kim SM, Chen L, Faulhaber-Walter R, Huang Y, et al. Renal function in mice with targeted disruption of the A isoform of the Na-K-2Cl co-transporter. J Am Soc Nephrol 2007;18:440—8.

[164] Kinne R, Koenig B, Hannafin J, Kinne-Saffran E, Scott DM, Zierold K. The use of membrane vesicles to study the NaCl/KCl co-transporter involved in active transepithelial chloride transport. Pflugers Arch 1985;405(Suppl. 1):S101—105.

[165] Okusa MD, Persson AE, Wright FS. Chlorothiazide effect on feedback-mediated control of glomerular filtration rate. Am J Physiol Renal Physiol 1989;257:F137—144.

[166] Vallon V, Osswald H, Blantz RC, Thomson S. Potential role of luminal potassium in tubuloglomerular feedback. J Am Soc Nephrol 1997;8:1831—7.

[167] Lorenz JN, Baird NR, Judd LM, Noonan WT, Andringa A, Doetschman T, et al. Impaired renal NaCl absorption in mice lacking the ROMK potassium channel, a model for type II Bartter's syndrome. J Biol Chem 2002;277:37871—80.

[168] Lu M, Wang T, Yan Q, Yang X, Dong K, Knepper MA, et al. Absence of small conductance K⁺ channel (SK) activity in apical membranes of thick ascending limb and cortical collecting duct in ROMK (Bartter's) knockout mice. J Biol Chem 2002;277:37881—7.

[169] Schnermann J, Briggs JP. Tubuloglomerular feedback: mechanistic insights from gene-manipulated mice. Kidney Int 2008;74:418—26.

[170] Braam B, Boer P, Koomans HA. Tubuloglomerular feedback and tubular reabsorption during acute potassium loading in rats. Am J Physiol Renal Physiol 1994;267:F223—230.

[171] Kinne R, Kinne-Saffran E, Schutz H, Scholermann B. Ammonium transport of medullary thick ascending limb of rabbit kidney: involvement of the Na⁺,K⁺,Cl-co-transporter. J Membr Biol 1986;94:279—84.

[172] Greger R. Ion transport mechanism in thick ascending limb of Henle's loop of mammalian nephron. Physiol Rev 1985;65:760—97.

[173] Lapointe JY, Laamarti A, Hurst AM, Fowler BC, Bell PD. Activation of Na:2Cl:K co-transport by luminal chloride in macula densa cells. Kidney Int 1995;47:752—7.

[174] Briggs JP, Schnermann J. The effect of metabolic inhibitors on feedback response of nephron filtration rate. Pflugers Arch 1981;389(Suppl):R40.

[175] Price EM, Lingrel JB. Structure—function relationships in the Na,K-ATPase alpha subunit: Site-directed mutagenesis of

glutamine-111 to arginine and asparagine-122 to aspartic acid generates a ouabain-resistant enzyme. Biochemistry 1988;27:8400–8.

[176] Lorenz JN, Dostanic-Larson I, Shull GE, Lingrel JB. Ouabain inhibits tubuloglomerular feedback in mutant mice with ouabain-sensitive alpha1 Na,K-ATPase. J Am Soc Nephrol 2006;17:2457–63.

[177] Bell PD, Reddington M, Ploth D, Navar LG. Tubuloglomerular feedback-mediated decreases in glomerular pressure in Munich-Wistar rats. Am J Physiol Renal Physiol 1984;247:F877–880.

[178] Briggs JP. Effect of loop of Henle flow rate on glomerular capillary pressure. Ren Physiol 1984;7:311–20.

[179] Persson AE, Gushwa LC, Blantz RC. Feedback pressure-flow responses in normal and angiotensin-prostaglandin-blocked rats. Am J Physiol Renal Physiol 1984;247:F925–931.

[180] Peterson OW, Gushwa LC, Wilson CB, Blantz RC. Tubuloglomerular feedback activity after glomerular immune injury. Am J Physiol Renal Physiol 1989;257:F67–71.

[181] Casellas D, Moore LC. Autoregulation and tubuloglomerular feedback in juxtamedullary glomerular arterioles. Am J Physiol Renal Physiol 1990;258:F660–669.

[182] Gertz KH, Mangos JA, Braun G, Pagel HD. Pressure in the glomerular capillaries of the rat kidney and its relation to arterial blood pressure. Pflugers Arch Gesamte Physiol Menschen Tiere 1966;288:369–74.

[183] Bell PD, Thomas C, Williams RH, Navar LG. Filtration rate and stop-flow pressure feedback responses to nephron perfusion in the dog. Am J Physiol 1978;234:F154–165.

[184] Navar LG, Chomdej B, Bell PD. Absence of estimated glomerular pressure autoregulation during interrupted distal delivery. Am J Physiol 1975;229:1596–603.

[185] Schnermann J, Traynor T, Yang T, Huang YG, Oliverio MI, Coffman T, et al. Absence of tubuloglomerular feedback responses in AT1A receptor-deficient mice. Am J Physiol Renal Physiol 1997;273:F315–320.

[186] Schnermann J, Persson AE, Agerup B. Tubuloglomerular feedback. Nonlinear relation between glomerular hydrostatic pressure and loop of Henle perfusion rate. J Clin Invest 1973;52:862–9.

[187] Boknam L, Ericson AC, Aberg B, Ulfendahl HR. Flow resistance of the interlobular artery in the rat kidney. Acta Physiol Scand 1981;111:159–63.

[188] Heyeraas Tonder KJ, Aukland K. Interlobular arterial pressure in the rat kidney. Renal Physiol 1979/80;2:214–21.

[189] Briggs JP, Wright FS. Feedback control of glomerular filtration rate: site of the effector mechanism. Am J Physiol 1979;236:F40–47.

[190] Ichikawa I. Direct analysis of the effector mechanism of the tubuloglomerular feedback system. Am J Physiol Renal Physiol 1982;243:F447–455.

[191] Steinhausen M, Zimmerhackl B, Thederan H, Dussel R, Parekh N, Esslinger HU, et al. Intraglomerular microcirculation: measurements of single glomerular loop flow in rats. Kidney Int 1981;20:230–9.

[192] Persson BE, Sakai T, Marsh DJ. Juxtaglomerular interstitial hypertonicity in *Amphiuma*: tubular origin-TGF signal. Am J Physiol 1988;254:F445–449.

[193] Persson BE, Sakai T, Ekblom M, Marsh DJ. Effect of bumetanide on tubuloglomerular feedback in *Necturus maculosus*. Acta Physiol Scand 1989;137:93–9.

[194] Ito S, Carretero OA. An *in vitro* approach to the study of macula densa-mediated glomerular hemodynamics. Kidney Int 1990;38:1206–10.

[195] Moore LC, Casellas D. Tubuloglomerular feedback dependence of autoregulation in rat juxtamedullary afferent arterioles. Kidney Int 1990;37:1402–8.

[196] Morsing P, Velazquez H, Ellison D, Wright FS. Resetting of tubuloglomerular feedback by interrupting early distal flow. Acta Physiol Scand 1993;148:63–8.

[197] Marsh DJ, Toma I, Sosnovtseva OV, Peti-Peterdi J, Holstein-Rathlou NH. Electrotonic vascular signal conduction and nephron synchronization. Am J Physiol Renal Physiol 2009;296:F751–761.

[198] Haberle DA, Kawata T, Davis JM. The site of action of nitrendipine in the rat kidney. J Cardiovasc Pharmacol 1987;9(Suppl. 1):S17–23.

[199] Mitchell KD, Navar LG. Tubuloglomerular feedback responses during peritubular infusions of calcium channel blockers. Am J Physiol Renal Physiol 1990;258:F537–544.

[200] Muller-Suur R, Gutsche HU, Schurek HJ. Acute and reversible inhibition of tubuloglomerular feedback mediated afferent vasoconstriction by the calcium-antagonist verapamil. Curr Probl Clin Biochem 1976;6:291–8.

[201] Bell PD. Cyclic AMP-calcium interaction in the transmission of tubuloglomerular feedback signals. Kidney Int 1985;28:728–32.

[202] Schnermann J. Juxtaglomerular cell complex in the regulation of renal salt excretion. Am J Physiol Renal Physiol 1998;274: R263–279.

[203] Hansen PB, Castrop H, Briggs J, Schnermann J. Adenosine induces vasoconstriction through GI-dependent activation of phospholipase C in isolated perfused afferent arterioles of mice. J Am Soc Nephrol 2003;14:2457–65.

[204] Weihprecht H, Lorenz JN, Briggs JP, Schnermann J. Vasoconstrictor effect of angiotensin and vasopressin in isolated rabbit afferent arterioles. Am J Physiol Renal Physiol 1991;261:F273–282.

[205] Gustafsson F, Holstein-Rathlou N. Conducted vasomotor responses in arterioles: characteristics, mechanisms and physiological significance. Acta Physiol Scand 1999;167:11–21.

[206] Moore LC, Rich A, Casellas D. Ascending myogenic autoregulation: interactions between tubuloglomerular feedback and myogenic mechanisms. Bull Math Biol 1994;56:391–410.

[207] Wagner AJ, Holstein-Rathlou NH, Marsh DJ. Internephron coupling by conducted vasomotor responses in normotensive and spontaneously hypertensive rats. Am J Physiol 1997;272: F372–379.

[208] Chen YM, Yip KP, Marsh DJ, Holstein-Rathlou NH. Magnitude of TGF-initiated nephron–nephron interactions is increased in SHR. Am J Physiol Renal Physiol 1995;269:F198–204.

[209] Kallskog O, Marsh DJ. TGF-initiated vascular interactions between adjacent nephrons in the rat kidney. Am J Physiol Renal Physiol 1990;259:F60–64.

[210] Wagner C. Function of connexins in the renal circulation. Kidney Int 2008;73:547–55.

[211] Tucker BJ, Steiner RW, Gushwa LC, Blantz RC. Studies on the tubulo-glomerular feedback system in the rat. The mechanism of reduction in filtration rate with benzolamide. J Clin Invest 1978;62:993–1004.

[212] Schnermann J, Briggs JP. Single nephron comparison of the effect of loop of Henle flow on filtration rate and pressure in control and angiotensin II-infused rats. Miner Electrolyte Metab 1989;15:103–7.

[213] Ren Y, Garvin JL, Carretero OA. Efferent arteriole tubuloglomerular feedback in the renal nephron. Kidney Int 2001;59:222–9.

[214] Osswald H, Nabakowski G, Hermes H. Adenosine as a possible mediator of metabolic control of glomerular filtration rate. Int J Biochem 1980;12:263–7.

[215] Spielman WS, Thompson CI. A proposed role for adenosine in the regulation of renal hemodynamics and renin release. Am J Physiol 1982;242:F423–435.

[216] Beck JS, Breton S, Mairbaurl H, Laprade R, Giebisch G. Relationship between sodium transport and intracellular ATP in isolated perfused rabbit proximal convoluted tubule. Am J Physiol 1991;261:F634—639.

[217] Kelley GG, Aassar OS, Forrest Jr. JN. Endogenous adenosine is an autacoid feedback inhibitor of chloride transport in the shark rectal gland. J Clin Invest 1991;88:1933—9.

[218] Vallon V, Muhlbauer B, Osswald H. Adenosine and kidney function. Physiol Rev 2006;86:901—40.

[219] Hansen PB, Hashimoto S, Oppermann M, Huang Y, Briggs JP, Schnermann J. Vasoconstrictor and vasodilator effects of adenosine in the mouse kidney due to preferential activation of A1 or A2 adenosine receptors. J Pharmacol Exp Ther 2005;315:1150—7.

[220] Holz FG, Steinhausen M. Renovascular effects of adenosine receptor agonists. Renal Physiol 1987;10:272—82.

[221] Nishiyama A, Inscho EW, Navar LG. Interactions of adenosine A_1 and A_{2a} receptors on renal microvascular reactivity. Am J Physiol Renal Physiol 2001;280:F406—14.

[222] Weihprecht H, Lorenz JN, Briggs JP, Schnermann J. Vasomotor effects of purinergic agonists in isolated rabbit afferent arterioles. Am J Physiol Renal Physiol 1992;263:F1026—1033.

[223] Lai EY, Patzak A, Steege A, Mrowka R, Brown R, Spielmann N, et al. Contribution of adenosine receptors in the control of arteriolar tone and adenosine—angiotensin II interaction. Kidney Int 2006;70:690—8.

[224] Weaver DR, Reppert SM. Adenosine receptor gene expression in rat kidney. Am J Physiol Renal Physiol 1992;263:F991—995.

[225] Hansen PB, Schnermann J. Vasoconstrictor and vasodilator effects of adenosine in the kidney. Am J Physiol Renal Physiol 2003;285:F590—599.

[226] Lai EY, Patzak A, Persson AE, Carlstrom M. Angiotensin II enhances the afferent arteriolar response to adenosine through increases in cytosolic calcium. Acta Physiol (Oxf) 2009;196:435—45.

[227] Schnermann J. Effect of adenosine analogues on tubuloglomerular feedback responses. Am J Physiol Renal Physiol 1988;255:F33—42.

[228] Schnermann J, Weihprecht H, Briggs JP. Inhibition of tubuloglomerular feedback during adenosine1 receptor blockade. Am J Physiol Renal Physiol 1990;258:F553—561.

[229] Brown R, Ollerstam A, Johansson B, Skøtt O, Gebre-Medhin S, Fredholm B, et al. Abolished tubuloglomerular feedback and increased plasma renin in adenosine A1 receptor-deficient mice. Am J Physiol Regul Integr Comp Physiol 2001;281:R1362—1367.

[230] Sun D, Samuelson LC, Yang T, Huang Y, Paliege A, Saunders T, et al. Mediation of tubuloglomerular feedback by adenosine: evidence from mice lacking adenosine 1 receptors. Proc Natl Acad Sci USA 2001;98:9983—8.

[231] Carlstrom M, Wilcox CS, Welch WJ. Adenosine A(2) receptors modulate tubuloglomerular feedback. Am J Physiol Renal Physiol 2010;299:F412—417.

[232] Schnermann J, Osswald H, Hermle M. Inhibitory effect of methylxanthines on feedback control of glomerular filtration rate in the rat. Pflugers Arch 1977;369:39—48.

[233] Ren Y, Arima S, Carretero OA, Ito S. Possible role of adenosine in macula densa control of glomerular hemodynamics. Kidney Int 2002;61:169—76.

[234] Carlstrom M, Wilcox CS, Welch WJ. Adenosine A2A receptor activation attenuates tubuloglomerular feedback responses by stimulation of endothelial nitric oxide synthase. Am J Physiol Renal Physiol 2011;300:F457—64.

[235] Al-Mashhadi RH, Skott O, Vanhoutte PM, Hansen PB. Activation of A(2) adenosine receptors dilates cortical efferent arterioles in mouse. Kidney Int 2009;75:793—9.

[236] Bell PD, Lapointe JY, Sabirov R, Hayashi S, Peti-Peterdi J, Manabe K, et al. Macula densa cell signaling involves ATP release through a maxi anion channel. Proc Natl Acad Sci USA 2003;100:4322—7.

[237] Komlosi P, Peti-Peterdi J, Fuson AL, Fintha A, Rosivall L, Bell PD. Macula densa basolateral ATP release is regulated by luminal [NaCl] and dietary salt intake. Am J Physiol Renal Physiol 2004;286:F1054—1058.

[238] Sabirov RZ, Okada Y. The maxi-anion channel: a classical channel playing novel roles through an unidentified molecular entity. J Physiol Sci 2009;59:3—21.

[239] Stoessel A, Himmerkus N, Bleich M, Bachmann S, Theilig F. Connexin 37 is localized in renal epithelia and responds to changes in dietary salt intake. Am J Physiol Renal Physiol 2010;298:F216—223.

[240] Oppermann M, Friedman DJ, Faulhaber-Walter R, Mizel D, Castrop H, Enmjyoji K, et al. Tubuloglomerular feedback and renin secretion in NTPDase1/CD39-deficient mice. Am J Physiol Renal Physiol 2008;294:F965—970.

[241] Thomson S, Bao D, Deng A, Vallon V. Adenosine formed by 5'-nucleotidase mediates tubuloglomerular feedback. J Clin Invest 2000;106:289—98.

[242] Castrop H, Huang Y, Hashimoto S, Mizel D, Hansen P, Theilig F, et al. Impairment of tubuloglomerular feedback regulation of GFR in ecto-5'-nucleotidase/CD73-deficient mice. J Clin Invest 2004;114:634—42.

[243] Huang DY, Vallon V, Zimmermann H, Koszalka P, Schrader J, Osswald H. Ecto-5'-nucleotidase (cd73)-dependent and -independent generation of adenosine participates in the mediation of tubuloglomerular feedback in vivo. Am J Physiol Renal Physiol 2006;291:F282—288.

[244] Ren Y, Garvin JL, Liu R, Carretero OA. Role of macula densa adenosine triphosphate (ATP) in tubuloglomerular feedback. Kidney Int 2004;66:1479—85.

[245] Takenaka T, Okada H, Kanno Y, Inoue T, Ryuzaki M, Nakamoto H, et al. Exogenous 5'-nucleotidase improves glomerular autoregulation in Thy-1 nephritic rats. Am J Physiol Renal Physiol 2006;290:F844—853.

[246] Le Hir M, Kaissling B. Distribution and regulation of renal ecto-5'-nucleotidase: implications for physiological functions of adenosine. Am J Physiol 1993;264:F377—387.

[247] Stefanovic V, Savic V, Vlahovic P, Ardaillou N, Ardaillou R. Ecto-5'-nucleotidase of cultured rat mesangial cells. Ren Physiol Biochem 1988;11:89—102.

[248] Kawabata M, Haneda M, Wang T, Imai M, Takabatake T. Effects of a nucleoside transporter inhibitor, dilazep, on renal microcirculation in rats. Hypertens Res 2002;25:615—21.

[249] Vallon V, Osswald H. Dipyridamole prevents diabetes-induced alterations of kidney function in rats. Naunyn Schmiedebergs Arch Pharmacol 1994;349:217—22.

[250] Inscho EW. P2 receptors in regulation of renal microvascular function. Am J Physiol Renal Physiol 2001;280:F927—944.

[251] Navar LG, Inscho EW, Majid SA, Imig JD, Harrison-Bernard LM, Mitchell KD. Paracrine regulation of the renal microcirculation. Physiol Rev 1996;76:425—536.

[252] Chan CM, Unwin RJ, Bardini M, Oglesby IB, Ford AP, Townsend-Nicholson A, et al. Localization of P2X1 purinoceptors by autoradiography and immunohistochemistry in rat kidneys. Am J Physiol 1998;274:F799—804.

[253] Schnermann J. Maintained tubuloglomerular feedback responses during acute inhibition of P2 purinergic receptors in mice. Am J Physiol Renal Physiol 2011;300:F339—44.

[254] Salomonsson M, Gonzalez E, Westerlund P, Persson AE. Chloride concentration in macula densa and cortical thick ascending limb cells. Kidney Int Suppl 1991;32:S51—54.

[255] Bell PD, Lapointe JY, Cardinal J. Direct measurement of baso-lateral membrane potentials from cells of the macula densa. Am J Physiol Renal Physiol 1989;257:F463−468.

[256] Ren Y, Yu H, Wang H, Carretero OA, Garvin JL. Nystatin and valinomycin induce tubuloglomerular feedback. Am J Physiol Renal Physiol 2001;281:F1102−1108.

[257] Bell PD, Navar LG. Cytoplasmic calcium in the mediation of macula densa tubulo-glomerular feedback responses. Science 1982;215:670−3.

[258] Bell PD, Reddington M. Intracellular calcium in the transmission of tubuloglomerular feedback signals. Am J Physiol Renal Physiol 1983;245:F295−302.

[259] Ren Y, Liu R, Carretero OA, Garvin JL. Increased intracellular Ca^{++} in the macula densa regulates tubuloglomerular feedback. Kidney Int 2003;64:1348−55.

[260] Peti-Peterdi J, Bell PD. Cytosolic $[Ca^{2+}]$ signaling pathway in macula densa cells. Am J Physiol Renal Physiol 1999;277:F472−476.

[261] Lapointe JY, Bell PD, Sabirov RZ, Okada Y. Calcium-activated nonselective cationic channel in macula densa cells. Am J Physiol Renal Physiol 2003;285:F275−280.

[262] Naruse M, Inoue T, Nakayama M, Sato T, Kurokawa K. Effect of luminal Cl^- and Ca^{2+} on tubuloglomerular feedback mechanism. Jpn J Physiol 1994;44:S269−272.

[263] Liu R, Ren Y, Garvin JL, Carretero OA. Superoxide enhances tubuloglomerular feedback by constricting the afferent arteriole. Kidney Int 2004;66:268−74.

[264] Hong NJ, Garvin JL. Flow increases superoxide production by NADPH oxidase via activation of Na-K-2Cl co-transport and mechanical stress in thick ascending limbs. Am J Physiol Renal Physiol 2007;292:F993−998.

[265] Liu R, Garvin JL, Ren Y, Pagano PJ, Carretero OA. Depolarization of the macula densa induces superoxide production via NAD(P)H oxidase. Am J Physiol Renal Physiol 2007;292:F1867−1872.

[266] Fu Y, Zhang R, Lu D, Liu H, Chandrashekar K, Juncos LA, Liu R. NOX2 is the primary source of angiotensin II-induced superoxide in the macula densa. Am J Physiol Regul Integr Comp Physiol 2010;298:R707−712.

[267] Liu R, Juncos LA. GTPase-Rac enhances depolarization-induced superoxide production by the macula densa during tubuloglomerular feedback. Am J Physiol Regul Integr Comp Physiol 2010;298:R453−458.

[268] Zhang R, Harding P, Garvin JL, Juncos R, Peterson E, Juncos LA, et al. Isoforms and functions of NAD(P)H oxidase at the macula densa. Hypertension 2009;53:556−63.

[269] Marsh DJ, Osborn JL, Cowley Jr. AW. 1/f fluctuations in arterial pressure and regulation of renal blood flow in dogs. Am J Physiol 1990;258:F1394−1400.

[270] Thomson SC, Blantz RC, Vallon V. Increased tubular flow induces resetting of tubuloglomerular feedback in euvolemic rats. Am J Physiol Renal Physiol 1996;270:F461−468.

[271] Holstein-Rathlou NH. A closed-loop analysis of the tubuloglomerular feedback mechanism. Am J Physiol Renal Physiol 1991;261:F880−889.

[272] Guyton AC, Langston JB, Navar G. Theory for renal autoregulation by feedback at the juxtaglomerular apparatus. Circ Res. 1964;15(Suppl):187−97.

[273] Thurau K. Renal hemodynamics. Am J Med 1964;36:850−60.

[274] Moore LC, Schnermann J, Yarimizu S. Feedback mediation of SNGFR autoregulation in hydropenic and DOCA- and salt-loaded rats. Am J Physiol Renal Physiol 1979;237:F63−74.

[275] Moore LC. Tubuloglomerular feedback and SNGFR autoregulation in the rat. Am J Physiol Renal Physiol 1984;247:F267−276.

[276] Ploth DW, Schnermann J, Dahlheim H, Hermle M, Schmidmeier E. Autoregulation and tubuloglomerular feedback in normotensive and hypertensive rats. Kidney Int 1977;12:253−67.

[277] Ploth DW, Dahlheim H, Schmidmeier E, Hermle M, Schnermann J. Tubuloglomerular feedback and autoregulation of glomerular filtration rate in Wistar-Kyoto spontaneously hypertensive rats. Pflugers Arch 1978;375:261−7.

[278] Schnermann J, Briggs JP, Weber PC. Tubuloglomerular feedback, prostaglandins, and angiotensin in the autoregulation of glomerular filtration rate. Kidney Int 1984;25:53−64.

[279] Sjoquist M, Goransson A, Kallskog O, Ulfendahl HR. The influence of tubulo-glomerular feedback on the autoregulation of filtration rate in superficial and deep glomeruli. Acta Physiol Scand 1984;122:235−42.

[280] Sanchez-Ferrer CF, Roman RJ, Harder DR. Pressure-dependent contraction of rat juxtamedullary afferent arterioles. Circ Res 1989;64:790−8.

[281] Takenaka T, Harrison-Bernard LM, Inscho EW, Carmines PK, Navar LG. Autoregulation of afferent arteriolar blood flow in juxtamedullary nephrons. Am J Physiol Renal Physiol 1994;267:F879−887.

[282] Gilmore JP, Cornish KG, Rogers SD, Joyner WL. Direct evidence for myogenic autoregulation of the renal microcirculation in the hamster. Circ Res 1980;47:226−30.

[283] Steinhausen M, Blum M, Fleming JT, Holz FG, Parekh N, Wiegman DL. Visualization of renal autoregulation in the split hydronephrotic kidney of rats. Kidney Int 1989;35:1151−60.

[284] Edwards RM. Segmental effects of norepinephrine and angiotensin II on isolated renal microvessels. Am J Physiol 1983;244:F526−534.

[285] Harder DR, Gilbert R, Lombard JH. Vascular muscle cell depolarization and activation in renal arteries on elevation of transmural pressure. Am J Physiol 1987;253:F778−781.

[286] Lai EY, Onozato ML, Solis G, Aslam S, Welch WJ, Wilcox CS. Myogenic responses of mouse isolated perfused renal afferent arterioles: effects of salt intake and reduced renal mass. Hypertension 2010;55:983−9.

[287] Daniels FH, Arendshorst WJ. Tubuloglomerular feedback kinetics in spontaneously hypertensive and Wistar-Kyoto rats. Am J Physiol Renal Physiol 1990;259:F529−534.

[288] Holstein-Rathlou NH, Wagner AJ, Marsh DJ. Tubuloglomerular feedback dynamics and renal blood flow autoregulation in rats. Am J Physiol Renal Physiol 1991;260:F53−68.

[289] Young DK, Marsh DJ. Pulse wave propagation in rat renal tubules: implications for GFR autoregulation. Am J Physiol 1981;240:F446−458.

[290] Chon KH, Chen YM, Marmarelis VZ, Marsh DJ, Holstein-Rathlou NH. Detection of interactions between myogenic and TGF mechanisms using nonlinear analysis [published erratum appears in Am J Physiol Renal Physiol 1994 Dec;267(6 Pt 3): section F following table of contents] Am J Physiol Renal Physiol 1994;267:F160−173.

[291] Chon KH, Chen YM, Holstein-Rathlou NH, Marmarelis VZ. Nonlinear system analysis of renal autoregulation in normotensive and hypertensive rats. IEEE Trans Biomed Eng 1998;45:342−53.

[292] Holstein-Rathlou NH, Marsh DJ. Renal blood flow regulation and arterial pressure fluctuations: a case study in nonlinear dynamics. Physiol Rev 1994;74:637−81.

[293] Chen YM, Holstein-Rathlou NH. Differences in dynamic autoregulation of renal blood flow between SHR and WKY rats. Am J Physiol Renal Physiol 1993;264:F166−174.

[294] Daniels FH, Arendshorst WJ, Roberds RG. Tubuloglomerular feedback and autoregulation in spontaneously hypertensive rats. Am J Physiol Renal Physiol 1990;258:F1479–1489.

[295] Karlsen FM, Andersen CB, Leyssac PP, Holstein-Rathlou NH. Dynamic autoregulation and renal injury in Dahl rats. Hypertension 1997;30:975–83.

[296] Iliescu R, Cazan R, McLemore Jr. GR, Venegas-Pont M, Ryan MJ. Renal blood flow and dynamic autoregulation in conscious mice. Am J Physiol Renal Physiol 2008;295:F734–740.

[297] Wittmann U, Nafz B, Ehmke H, Kirchheim HR, Persson PB. Frequency domain of renal autoregulation in the conscious dog. Am J Physiol 1995;269:F317–322.

[298] Cupples WA, Loutzenhiser RD. Dynamic autoregulation in the in vitro perfused hydronephrotic rat kidney. Am J Physiol Renal Physiol 1998;275:F126–130.

[299] He J, Marsh DJ. Effect of captopril on fluctuations of blood pressure and renal blood flow in rats. Am J Physiol Renal Physiol 1993;264:F37–44.

[300] Just A, Arendshorst WJ. A novel mechanism of renal blood flow autoregulation and the autoregulatory role of A1 adenosine receptors in mice. Am J Physiol Renal Physiol 2007;293:F1489–1500.

[301] Just A, Ehmke H, Toktomambetova L, Kirchheim HR. Dynamic characteristics and underlying mechanisms of renal blood flow autoregulation in the conscious dog. Am J Physiol Renal Physiol 2001;280:F1062–1071.

[302] Just A, Arendshorst WJ. Dynamics and contribution of mechanisms mediating renal blood flow autoregulation. Am J Physiol Regul Integr Comp Physiol 2003;285:R619–631.

[303] Wronski T, Seeliger E, Persson PB, Forner C, Fichtner C, Scheller J, et al. The step response: a method to characterize mechanisms of renal blood flow autoregulation. Am J Physiol Renal Physiol 2003;285:F758–764.

[304] Loutzenhiser R, Bidani A, Chilton L. Renal myogenic response: kinetic attributes and physiological role. Circ Res 2002;90:1316–24.

[305] Loutzenhiser R, Bidani AK, Wang X. Systolic pressure and the myogenic response of the renal afferent arteriole. Acta Physiol Scand 2004;181:407–13.

[306] Davis JM, Haberle DA, Kawata T. The control of glomerular filtration rate and renal blood flow in chronically volume-expanded rats. J Physiol (Lond) 1988;402:473–95.

[307] Haberle DA. Hemodynamic interactions between intrinsic blood flow control mechanisms in the rat kidney. Ren Physiol Biochem 1988;11:289–315.

[308] Feldberg R, Colding-Jorgensen M, Holstein-Rathlou NH. Analysis of interaction between TGF and the myogenic response in renal blood flow autoregulation. Am J Physiol Renal Physiol 1995;269:F581–593.

[309] Schnermann J, Briggs JP. Interaction between loop of Henle flow and arterial pressure as determinants of glomerular pressure. Am J Physiol Renal Physiol 1989;256:F421–9.

[310] Chon KH, Raghavan R, Chen YM, Marsh DJ, Yip KP. Interactions of TGF-dependent and myogenic oscillations in tubular pressure. Am J Physiol Renal Physiol 2005;288:F298–307.

[311] Marsh DJ, Sosnovtseva OV, Chon KH, Holstein-Rathlou NH. Nonlinear interactions in renal blood flow regulation. Am J Physiol Regul Integr Comp Physiol 2005;288:R1143–1159.

[312] Walker III M, Harrison-Bernard LM, Cook AK, Navar LG. Dynamic interaction between myogenic and TGF mechanisms in afferent arteriolar blood flow autoregulation. Am J Physiol Renal Physiol 2000;279:F858–865.

[313] Just A, Arendshorst WJ. Nitric oxide blunts myogenic autoregulation in rat renal but not skeletal muscle circulation via tubuloglomerular feedback. J Physiol 2005;569:959–74.

[314] Shi Y, Wang X, Chon KH, Cupples WA. Tubuloglomerular feedback-dependent modulation of renal myogenic autoregulation by nitric oxide. Am J Physiol Regul Integr Comp Physiol 2006;290:R982–991.

[315] Nashat FS, Tappin JW, Wilcox CS. The renal blood flow and the glomerular filtration rate of anaesthetized dogs during acute changes in plasma sodium concentration. J Physiol 1976;256:731–45.

[316] Dev B, Drescher C, Schnermann J. Resetting of tubulo-glomerular feedback sensitivity by dietary salt intake. Pflugers Arch 1974;346:263–77.

[317] Wilcox CS. Regulation of renal blood flow by plasma chloride. J Clin Invest 1983;71:726–35.

[318] Gerber JG, Branch RA, Nies AS, Hollifield JW, Gerkens JF. Influence of hypertonic saline on canine renal blood flow and renin release. Am J Physiol 1979;237:F441–446.

[319] Gerkens JF, Heidemann HT, Jackson EK, Branch RA. Aminophylline inhibits renal vasoconstriction produced by intrarenal hypertonic saline. J Pharmacol Exp Ther 1983;225:611–5.

[320] Schnermann J, Hermle M, Schmidmeier E, Dahlheim H. Impaired potency for feedback regulation of glomerular filtration rate in DOCA escaped rats. Pflugers Arch 1975;358:325–38.

[321] Schnermann J, Briggs J, Wright FS. Feedback-mediated reduction of glomerular filtration rate during infusion of hypertonic saline. Kidney Int 1981;20:462–8.

[322] Woods LL, DeYoung DR, Smith BE. Regulation of renal hemodynamics after protein feeding: effects of loop diuretics. Am J Physiol Renal Physiol 1991;261:F815–823.

[323] Schnermann J, Gokel M, Weber PC, Schubert G, Briggs JP. Tubuloglomerular feedback and glomerular morphology in Goldblatt hypertensive rats on varying protein diets. Kidney Int 1986;29:520–9.

[324] Seney Jr. FD, Wright FS. Dietary protein suppresses feedback control of glomerular filtration in rats. J Clin Invest 1985;75:558–68.

[325] Seney Jr. FD, Persson EG, Wright FS. Modification of tubulo-glomerular feedback signal by dietary protein. Am J Physiol Renal Physiol 1987;252:F83–90.

[326] Bouby N, Trinh-Trang-Tan MM, Kriz W, Bankir L. Possible role of the thick ascending limb and of the urine concentrating mechanism in the protein-induced increase in GFR and kidney mass. Kidney Int Suppl 1987;22:S57–61.

[327] Persson AEG, Wright FS. Evidence for feedback mediated reduction of glomerular filtration rate during infusion of acetazolamide. Acta Physiol Scand 1982;114:1–7.

[328] Hashimoto S, Huang YG, Castrop H, Hansen PB, Mizel D, Briggs J, et al. Effect of carbonic anhydrase inhibition on GFR and renal hemodynamics in adenosine-1 receptor-deficient mice. Pflugers Arch 2004;448:621–8.

[329] Leyssac PP, Karlsen FM, Skott O. Dynamics of intrarenal pressures and glomerular filtration rate after acetazolamide. Am J Physiol Renal Physiol 1991;261:F169–178.

[330] Leyssac PP, Karlsen FM, Holstein-Rathlou NH, Skott O. On determinants of glomerular filtration rate after inhibition of proximal tubular reabsorption. Am J Physiol Renal Physiol 1994;266:R1544–1550.

[331] Janssen BJ, Eerdmans PH, Smits JF. Mechanisms of renal vasoconstriction following furosemide in conscious rats. Naunyn Schmiedebergs Arch Pharmacol 1994;349:528–37.

[332] Oppermann M, Hansen PB, Castrop H, Schnermann J. Vasodilatation of afferent arterioles and paradoxical increase

of renal vascular resistance by furosemide in mice. Am J Physiol Renal Physiol 2007;293:F279−287.

[333] Schnermann J, Chou C-L, Ma T, Traynor T, Knepper MA, Verkman AS. Defective proximal tubular fluid reabsorption in transgenic aquaporin-1 null mice. Proc Natl Acad Sci 1998;95:9660−4.

[334] Hashimoto S, Huang Y, Mizel D, Briggs J, Schnermann J. Compensation of proximal tubule malabsorption in AQP1-deficient mice without TGF-mediated reduction of GFR. Acta Physiol Scand 2004;181:455−62.

[335] Lorenz JN, Schultheis PJ, Traynor T, Shull GE, Schnermann J. Micropuncture analysis of single-nephron function in NHE3-deficient mice. Am J Physiol Renal Physiol 1999;277:F447−53.

[336] Boberg U, Persson AE. Tubuloglomerular feedback during elevated renal venous pressure. Am J Physiol Renal Physiol 1985;249:F524−531.

[337] Boberg U, Persson AE. Increased tubuloglomerular feedback activity in Milan hypertensive rats. Am J Physiol Renal Physiol 1986;250:F967−974.

[338] Persson AE, Schnermann J, Wright FS. Modification of feedback influence on glomerular filtration rate by acute isotonic extracellular volume expansion. Pflugers Arch 1979;381:99−105.

[339] Persson AE, Bianchi G, Boberg U. Tubuloglomerular feedback in hypertensive rats of the Milan strain. Acta Physiol Scand 1985;123:139−46.

[340] Ploth DW, Rudulph J, Thomas C, Navar LG. Renal and tubuloglomerular feedback responses to plasma expansion in the rat. Am J Physiol Renal Physiol 1978;235:F156−162.

[341] Schnermann J, Briggs JP. Restoration of tubuloglomerular feedback in volume-expanded rats by angiotensin II. Am J Physiol Renal Physiol 1990;259:F565−572.

[342] Moore LC, Yarimizu S, Schubert G, Weber PC, Schnermann J. Dynamics of tubuloglomerular feedback adaptation to acute and chronic changes in body fluid volume. Pflugers Arch 1980;387:39−45.

[343] Davis JM, Takabatake T, Kawata T, Haberle DA. Resetting of tubuloglomerular feedback in acute volume expansion in rats. Pflugers Arch 1988;411:322−7.

[344] Moore LC, Mason J. Perturbation analysis of tubuloglomerular feedback in hydropenic and hemorrhaged rats. Am J Physiol Renal Physiol 1983;245:F554−563.

[345] Moore LC, Mason J. Tubuloglomerular feedback control of distal fluid delivery: effect of extracellular volume. Am J Physiol Renal Physiol 1986;250:F1024−1032.

[346] Selen G, Muller-Suur R, Persson AE. Activation of the tubuloglomerular feedback mechanism in dehydrated rats. Acta Physiol Scand 1983;117:83−9.

[347] Kaufman JS, Hamburger RJ, Flamenbaum W. Tubuloglomerular feedback response after hypotensive hemorrhage. Ren Physiol 1982;5:173−81.

[348] Morsing P, Persson AE. Kinin and tubuloglomerular feedback in normal and hydronephrotic rats. Am J Physiol Renal Physiol 1991;260:F868−873.

[349] Persson AE, Wahlberg J, Safirstein R, Wright FS. The effect of 2 hours of complete unilateral ureteral obstruction on tubuloglomerular feedback control. Acta Physiol Scand 1984;122:35−43.

[350] Wahlberg J, Stenberg A, Wilson DR, Persson AE. Tubuloglomerular feedback and interstitial pressure in obstructive nephropathy. Kidney Int 1984;26:294−301.

[351] Dal Canton A, Stanziale R, Corradi A, Andreucci VE, Migone L. Effects of acute ureteral obstruction on glomerular hemodynamics in rat kidney. Kidney Int 1977;12:403−11.

[352] Tanner GA. Tubuloglomerular feedback after nephron or ureteral obstruction. Am J Physiol Renal Physiol 1985;248: F688−697.

[353] Carlstrom M, Brown RD, Edlund J, Sällström J, Larsson E, Teerlink T, et al. Role of nitric oxide deficiency in the development of hypertension in hydronephrotic animals. Am J Physiol Renal Physiol 2008;294:F362−370.

[354] Carlstrom M, Brown RD, Sallstrom J, Larsson E, Zilmer M, Zabihi S, et al. SOD1 deficiency causes salt sensitivity and aggravates hypertension in hydronephrosis. Am J Physiol Regul Integr Comp Physiol 2009;297:R82−92.

[355] Dal Canton A, Corradi A, Stanziale R, Maruccio G, Migone L. Effects of 24-hour ureteral obstruction on glomerular hemodynamics in rat kidney. Kidney Int 1979;15:457−62.

[356] Arendshorst WJ, Finn WF, Gottschalk CW. Nephron stop-flow pressure response to obstruction for 24 hours in the rat kidney. J Clin Invest 1974;53:1497−500.

[357] Tanner GA. Effects of kidney tubule obstruction on glomerular function in rats. Am J Physiol 1979;237:F379−385.

[358] Tanner GA. Nephron obstruction and tubuloglomerular feedback. Kidney Int Suppl 1982;12:S213−218.

[359] Morsing P, Stenberg A, Muller-Suur C, Persson AE. Tubuloglomerular feedback in animals with unilateral, partial ureteral occlusion. Kidney Int 1987;32:212−8.

[360] Morsing P, Stenberg A, Persson AE. Effect of thromboxane inhibition on tubuloglomerular feedback in hydronephrotic kidneys. Kidney Int 1989;36:447−52.

[361] Morsing P, Stenberg A, Wahlin N, Persson AE. Tubuloglomerular feedback in rats with chronic partial bilateral ureteral obstruction. Ren Physiol Biochem 1995;18:27−34.

[362] Blantz RC, Peterson OW, Thomson SC. Tubuloglomerular feedback responses to acute contralateral nephrectomy. Am J Physiol Renal Physiol 1991;260:F749−756.

[363] Muller-Suur R, Norlen BJ, Persson AE. Resetting of tubuloglomerular feedback in rat kidneys after unilateral nephrectomy. Kidney Int 1980;18:48−57.

[364] Norlen BJ, Muller-Suur R, Persson AE. Tubulo-glomerular feedback response and excretory characteristics of the transplanted rat kidney. Scand J Urol Nephrol 1978;12:27−33.

[365] Salmond R, Seney FJ. Reset tubuloglomerular feedback permits and sustains glomerular hyperfunction after extensive renal ablation. Am J Physiol Renal Physiol 1991;260:F395−401.

[366] Singh P, Deng A, Blantz RC, Thomson SC. Unexpected effect of angiotensin AT1 receptor blockade on tubuloglomerular feedback in early subtotal nephrectomy. Am J Physiol Renal Physiol 2009;296:F1158−1165.

[367] Pollock CA, Bostrom TE, Dyne M, Gyory AZ, Field MJ. Tubular sodium handling and tubuloglomerular feedback in compensatory renal hypertrophy. Pflugers Arch 1992;420:159−66.

[368] Blantz RC, Peterson OW, Gushwa L, Tucker BJ. Effect of modest hyperglycemia on tubuloglomerular feedback activity. Kidney Int Suppl 1982;12:S206−212.

[369] Jensen PK, Kristensen KS, Rasch R, Persson AEG. Decreased sensitivity of the tubuloglomerular feedback mechanism in experimental diabetic rats. In: Persson AEG, Boberg U, editors. The Juxtaglomerular Apparatus. Amsterdam: Elsevier; 1988. p. 333−8.

[370] Hashimoto S, Yamada K, Kawata T, Mochizuki T, Schnermann J, Koike T. Abnormal autoregulation and tubuloglomerular feedback in prediabetic and diabetic OLETF rats. Am J Physiol Renal Physiol 2009;296:F598−604.

[371] Faulhaber-Walter R, Chen L, Oppermann M, Kim SMK, Huang Y, Hiramatsu MJ, et al. Lack of A1 adenosine receptors augments diabetic hyperfiltration and glomerular injury. J Am Soc Nephrol 2008;19:722−30.

[372] Levine DZ, Iacovitti M, Robertson SJ, Mokhtar GA. Modulation of single-nephron GFR in the db/db mouse model

of type 2 diabetes mellitus. Am J Physiol Regul Integr Comp Physiol 2006;290:R975—981.

[373] Vallon V, Blantz RC, Thomson S. Homeostatic efficiency of tubuloglomerular feedback is reduced in established diabetes mellitus in rats. Am J Physiol Renal Physiol 1995;269:F876—883.

[374] Blantz RC, Konnen KS. Relation of distal tubular delivery and reabsorptive rate to nephron filtration. Am J Physiol Renal Physiol 1977;233:F315—324.

[375] Vallon V, Huang DY, Deng A, Richter K, Blantz RC, Thomson S. Salt-sensitivity of proximal reabsorption alters macula densa salt and explains the paradoxical effect of dietary salt on glomerular filtration rate in diabetes mellitus. J Am Soc Nephrol 2002;13:1865—71.

[376] Thomson SC, Vallon V, Blantz RC. Kidney function in early diabetes: the tubular hypothesis of glomerular filtration. Am J Physiol Renal Physiol 2004;286:F8—15.

[377] Vallon V, Blantz RC, Thomson S. Glomerular hyperfiltration and the salt paradox in early [corrected] type 1 diabetes mellitus: a tubulo-centric view. J Am Soc Nephrol 2003;14:530—7.

[378] Thomson SC, Deng A, Bao D, Satriano J, Blantz RC, Vallon V. Ornithine decarboxylase, kidney size, and the tubular hypothesis of glomerular hyperfiltration in experimental diabetes. J Clin Invest 2001;107:217—24.

[379] Pedersen SB, Flyvbjerg A, Richelsen B. Inhibition of renal ornithine decarboxylase activity prevents kidney hypertrophy in experimental diabetes. Am J Physiol 1993;264:C453—456.

[380] Pollock CA, Lawrence JR, Field MJ. Tubular sodium handling and tubuloglomerular feedback in experimental diabetes mellitus. Am J Physiol Renal Physiol 1991;260:F946—952.

[381] Sallstrom J, Carlsson PO, Fredholm BB, Larsson E, Persson AE, Palm F. Diabetes-induced hyperfiltration in adenosine A(1)-receptor deficient mice lacking the tubuloglomerular feedback mechanism. Acta Physiol (Oxf) 2007;190:253—9.

[382] Vallon V, Kirschenmann D, Wead LM, Lortie MJ, Satriano J, Blantz RC, et al. Effect of chronic salt loading on kidney function in early and established diabetes mellitus in rats. J Lab Clin Med 1997;130:76—82.

[383] Miracle CM, Rieg T, Mansoury H, Vallon V, Thomson SC. Ornithine decarboxylase inhibitor eliminates hyperresponsiveness of the early diabetic proximal tubule to dietary salt. Am J Physiol Renal Physiol 2008;295:F995—1002.

[384] Bell TD, DiBona GF, Biemiller R, Brands MW. Continuously measured renal blood flow does not increase in diabetes if nitric oxide synthesis is blocked. Am J Physiol Renal Physiol 2008;295:F1449—1456.

[385] Thomson SC, Deng A, Komine N, Hammes JS, Blantz RC, Gabbai FB. Early diabetes as a model for testing the regulation of juxtaglomerular NOS I. Am J Physiol Renal Physiol 2004;287:F732—738.

[386] Allen TJ, Waldron MJ, Casley D, Jerums G, Cooper ME. Salt restriction reduces hyperfiltration, renal enlargement, and albuminuria in experimental diabetes. Diabetes 1997;46:19—24.

[387] Bank N, Lahorra G, Aynedjian HS, Wilkes BM. Sodium restriction corrects hyperfiltration of diabetes. Am J Physiol 1988;254: F668—676.

[388] Campese VM, Wurgaft A, Safa M, Bianchi S. Dietary salt intake, blood pressure and the kidney in hypertensive patients with non-insulin dependent diabetes mellitus. J Nephrol 1998;11:289—95.

[389] O'Neill H, Kwon TH, Ring T, et al. Restriction of dietary NaCl decreases urinary output in diabetic rats: absence of the salt paradox in uncontrolled type 1 diabetes mellitus. J Am Soc Nephrol 2008;19:849A (abstract).

[390] Hermansson K, Kallskog O, Wolgast M. Effect of renal nerve stimulation on the activity of the tubuloglomerular feedback mechanism. Acta Physiol Scand 1984;120:381—5.

[391] Takabatake T, Ushiogi Y, Ohta K, Hattori N. Attenuation of enhanced tubuloglomerular feedback activity in SHR by renal denervation. Am J Physiol Renal Physiol 1990;258:F980—985.

[392] Thorup C, Kurkus J, Morsing P, Persson AE. Acute renal denervation causes time-dependent resetting of the tubuloglomerular feedback mechanism. Acta Physiol Scand 1995;153:43—9.

[393] Thorup C, Kurkus J, Ollerstam A, Persson AE. Effects of acute and chronic unilateral renal denervation on the tubuloglomerular feedback mechanism. Acta Physiol Scand 1996;156:139—45.

[394] Ploth DW, Rudulph J, LaGrange R, Navar LG. Tubuloglomerular feedback and single nephron function after converting enzyme inhibition in the rat. J Clin Invest 1979;64:1325—35.

[395] Ploth DW, Roy RN. Renal and tubuloglomerular feedback effects of [Sar1,Ala8]angiotensin II in the rat. Am J Physiol Renal Physiol 1982;242:F149—157.

[396] Schnermann J, Briggs JP, Schubert G, Marin-Grez M. Opposing effects of captopril and aprotinin on tubuloglomerular feedback responses. Am J Physiol Renal Physiol 1984;247: F912—918.

[397] Stowe N, Schnermann J, Hermle M. Feedback regulation of nephron filtration rate during pharmacologic interference with the renin—angiotensin and adrenergic systems in rats. Kidney Int 1979;15:473—86.

[398] Welch WJ, Wilcox CS. Feedback responses during sequential inhibition of angiotensin and thromboxane. Am J Physiol Renal Physiol 1990;258:F457—466.

[399] Traynor T, Yang T, Huang YG, Krege JH, Briggs JP, Smithies O, et al. Tubuloglomerular feedback in ACE-deficient mice. Am J Physiol Renal Physiol 1999;276:F751—757.

[400] Hashimoto S, Adams JW, Bernstein KE, Schnermann J. Micropuncture determination of nephron function in mice without tissue angiotensin converting enzyme. Am J Physiol Renal Physiol 2005;288:F445—52.

[401] Kessler SP, Hashimoto S, Senanayake PS, Gaughan C, Sen GC, Schnermann J. Nephron function in transgenic mice with selective vascular or tubular expression of Angiotensin-converting enzyme. J Am Soc Nephrol 2005;16:3535—42.

[402] Huang WC, Bell PD, Harvey D, Mitchell KD, Navar LG. Angiotensin influences on tubuloglomerular feedback mechanism in hypertensive rats. Kidney Int 1988;34:631—7.

[403] Ploth DW, Roy RN. Renin—angiotensin influences on tubuloglomerular feedback activity in the rat. Kidney Int Suppl 1982;12:S114—121.

[404] Mitchell KD, Navar LG. Enhanced tubuloglomerular feedback during peritubular infusions of angiotensins I and II. Am J Physiol Renal Physiol 1988;255:F383—390.

[405] Ikenaga H, Fallet RW, Carmines PK. Contribution of tubuloglomerular feedback to renal arteriolar angiotensin II responsiveness. Kidney Int 1996;49:34—9.

[406] Ren YL, Carretero OA, Ito S. Influence of NaCl concentration at the macula densa on angiotensin II-induced constriction of the afferent arteriole. Hypertension 1996;27:649—52.

[407] Lai EY, Martinka P, Fahling M, Mrowka R, Steege A, Gericke A, et al. Adenosine restores angiotensin II-induced contractions by receptor-independent enhancement of calcium sensitivity in renal arterioles. Circ Res 2006;99:1117—24.

[408] DiBona GF, Sawin LL. Effect of endogenous angiotensin II on the frequency response of the renal vasculature. Am J Physiol Renal Physiol 2004;287:F1171—1178.

[409] Guan Z, Willgoss DA, Matthias A, Manley SW, Crozier S, Gobe G, et al. Facilitation of renal autoregulation by angiotensin II is mediated through modulation of nitric oxide. Acta Physiol Scand 2003;179:189—201.

II. STRUCTURAL AND FUNCTIONAL ORGANIZATION OF THE KIDNEY

[410] Just A, Ehmke H, Wittmann U, Kirchheim HR. Role of angiotensin II in dynamic renal blood flow autoregulation of the conscious dog. J Physiol 2002;538:167—77.

[411] Schnermann J, Levine DZ. Paracrine factors in tubuloglomerular feedback: adenosine, ATP, and nitric oxide. Annu Rev Physiol 2003;65:501—29.

[412] Traynor T, Yang T, Huang YG, Arend L, Oliverio MI, Coffman T, et al. Inhibition of adenosine-1 receptor-mediated preglomerular vasoconstriction in AT1A receptor-deficient mice. Am J Physiol Renal Physiol 1998;275:F922—927.

[413] Weihprecht H, Lorenz JN, Briggs JP, Schnermann J. Synergistic effects of angiotensin and adenosine in the renal microvasculature. Am J Physiol Renal Physiol 1994;266:F227—239.

[414] Patzak A, Lai EY, Fahling M, Sendeski M, Martinka P, Persson PB, et al. Adenosine enhances long term the contractile response to angiotensin II in afferent arterioles. Am J Physiol Regul Integr Comp Physiol 2007;293:R2232—2242.

[415] Kovacs G, Peti-Peterdi J, Rosivall L, Bell PD. Angiotensin II directly stimulates macula densa Na-2Cl-K co-transport via apical AT(1) receptors. Am J Physiol Renal Physiol 2002;282: F301—306.

[416] Smith WL, Bell TG. Immunohistochemical localization of the prostaglandin-forming cyclooxygenase in renal cortex. Am J Physiol Renal Physiol 1978;235:F451—7.

[417] Harris RC, Breyer MD. Physiological regulation of cyclooxygenase-2 in the kidney. Am J Physiol Renal Physiol 2001;281: F1—11.

[418] Araujo M, Welch WJ. Cyclooxygenase 2 inhibition suppresses tubuloglomerular feedback: Roles of thromboxane receptors and nitric oxide. Am J Physiol Renal Physiol 2009;296:F790—794.

[419] Morsing P, Persson AE. Effect of prostaglandin synthesis inhibition on the tubuloglomerular feedback control in the rat kidney. Ren Physiol Biochem 1992;15:66—72.

[420] Schnermann J, Schubert G, Hermle M, Herbst R, Stowe NT, Yarimizu S, et al. The effect of inhibition of prostaglandin synthesis on tubuloglomerular feedback in the rat kidney. Pflugers Arch 1979;379:269—79.

[421] Schnermann J, Weber PC. Reversal of indomethacin-induced inhibition of tubuloglomerular feedback by prostaglandin infusion. Prostaglandins 1982;24:351—61.

[422] Welch WJ, Wilcox CS. Modulating role for thromboxane in the tubuloglomerular feedback response in the rat. J Clin Invest 1988;81:1843—9.

[423] Franco M, Bell PD, Navar LG. Evaluation of prostaglandins as mediators of tubuloglomerular feedback. Am J Physiol Renal Physiol 1988;254:F642—649.

[424] Welch WJ. Effects of isoprostane on tubuloglomerular feedback: roles of TP receptors, NOS, and salt intake. Am J Physiol Renal Physiol 2005;288:F757—762.

[425] Araujo M, Welch WJ. Tubuloglomerular feedback is decreased in COX-1 knockout mice after chronic angiotensin II infusion. Am J Physiol Renal Physiol 2010;298:F1059—1063.

[426] Welch WJ, Peng B, Takeuchi K, Abe K, Wilcox CS. Salt loading enhances rat renal TxA2/PGH2 receptor expression and TGF response to U-46,619. Am J Physiol Renal Physiol 1997;273: F976—983.

[427] Yanagisawa H, Jin Z, Kurihara N, Klahr S, Morrissey J, Wada O. Increases in glomerular eicosanoid production in rats with bilateral ureteral obstruction are mediated by enhanced enzyme activities of both the cyclooxygenase and 5-lipoxygenase pathways. Proc Soc Exp Biol Med 1993;203:291—6.

[428] Schnermann J, Traynor T, Pohl H, Thomas DW, Coffman TM, Briggs JP. Vasoconstrictor responses in thromboxane receptor knockout mice: tubuloglomerular feedback and ureteral obstruction. Acta Physiol Scand 2000;168:201—7.

[429] Wilcox CS, Welch WJ. Thromboxane synthase and TP receptor mRNA in rat kidney and brain: effects of salt intake and ANG II. Am J Physiol Renal Physiol 2003;284:F525—531.

[430] Brannstrom K, Arendshorst WJ. Thromboxane A_2 contributes to the enhanced tubuloglomerular feedback activity in young SHR. Am J Physiol Renal Physiol 1999;276:F758—66.

[431] Ichihara A, Imig JD, Inscho EW, Navar LG. Cyclooxygenase-2 participates in tubular flow-dependent afferent arteriolar tone: interaction with neuronal NOS. Am J Physiol Renal Physiol 1998;275:F605—612.

[432] Zhao X, Imig JD. Kidney CYP450 enzymes: biological actions beyond drug metabolism. Curr Drug Metab 2003;4:73—84.

[433] Zou AP, Imig JD, Ortiz de Montellano PR, Sui Z, Falck JR, Roman RJ. Effect of P-450 omega-hydroxylase metabolites of arachidonic acid on tubuloglomerular feedback. Am J Physiol Renal Physiol 1994;266:F934—941.

[434] Ito O, Alonso-Galicia M, Hopp KA, Roman RJ. Localization of cytochrome P-450 4A isoforms along the rat nephron. Am J Physiol 1998;274:F395—404.

[435] Sarkis A, Roman RJ. Role of cytochrome P450 metabolites of arachidonic acid in hypertension. Curr Drug Metab 2004;5:245—56.

[436] Schnermann J. Vascular tone as a determinant of tubuloglomerular feedback responsiveness. In: Persson AEG, Boberg U, editors. The juxtaglomerular apparatus. Amsterdam: Elsevier; 1988. p. 167—76.

[437] Harder DR, Lange AR, Gebremedhin D, Birks EK, Roman RJ. Cytochrome P450 metabolites of arachidonic acid as intracellular signaling molecules in vascular tissue. J Vasc Res 1997;34:237—43.

[438] Braam B, Koomans HA. Reabsorption of nitro-L-arginine infused into the late proximal tubule participates in modulation of TGF responsiveness. Kidney Int 1995;47:1252—7.

[439] Ito S, Ren YL. Evidence for the role of nitric oxide in macula densa control of glomerular hemodynamics. J Clin Invest 1993;92:1093—8.

[440] Thorup C, Persson AE. Macula densa derived nitric oxide in regulation of glomerular capillary pressure. Kidney Int 1996;49:430—6.

[441] Vallon V, Thomson S. Inhibition of local nitric oxide synthase increases homeostatic efficiency of tubuloglomerular feedback. Am J Physiol Renal Physiol 1995;269:F892—9.

[442] Thomson SC, Deng A. Cyclic GMP mediates influence of macula densa nitric oxide over tubuloglomerular feedback. Kidney Blood Press Res 2003;26:10—8.

[443] Ren YL, Garvin JL, Ito S, Carretero OA. Role of neuronal nitric oxide synthase in the macula densa. Kidney Int 2001;60:1676—83.

[444] Vallon V, Traynor T, Barajas L, Huang YG, Briggs JP, Schnermann J. Feedback control of glomerular vascular tone in neuronal nitric oxide synthase knockout mice. J Am Soc Nephrol 2001;12:1599—606.

[445] Brown R, Ollerstam A, Persson AE. Neuronal nitric oxide synthase inhibition sensitizes the tubuloglomerular feedback mechanism after volume expansion. Kidney Int 2004; 65:1349—56.

[446] Ren YL, Garvin JL, Carretero OA. Role of macula densa nitric oxide and cGMP in the regulation of tubuloglomerular feedback. Kidney Int 2000;58:2053—60.

[447] Ortiz PA, Garvin JL. NO Inhibits NaCl absorption by rat thick ascending limb through activation of cGMP-stimulated phosphodiesterase. Hypertension 2001;37:467—71.

[448] Wang H, Carretero OA, Garvin JL. Nitric oxide produced by THAL nitric oxide synthase inhibits TGF. Hypertension 2002;39:662—6.

[449] Kovacs G, Komlosi P, Fuson A, Peti-Peterdi J, Rosivall L, Bell PD. Neuronal nitric oxide synthase: its role and regulation in macula densa cells. J Am Soc Nephrol 2003;14:2475–83.

[450] Liu R, Carretero OA, Ren Y, Garvin JL. Increased intracellular pH at the macula densa activates nNOS during tubuloglomerular feedback. Kidney Int 2005;67:1837–43.

[451] Yaqoob M, Edelstein CL, Wieder ED, Alkhunaizi AM, Gengaro PA, Nemenoff RA, et al. Nitric oxide kinetics during hypoxia in proximal tubules: effects of acidosis and glycine. Kidney Int 1996;49:1314–9.

[452] Wang H, Carretero OA, Garvin JL. Inhibition of apical Na^+/H^+ exchangers on the macula densa cells augments tubuloglomerular feedback. Hypertension 2003;41:688–91.

[453] Welch WJ, Wilcox CS. Tubuloglomerular feedback and macula densa-derived NO. In: Goligorsky MS, Gross SS, editors. Nitric oxide and the kidney. New York: Chapman & Hall; 1997. p. 216–32.

[454] Cabral PD, Hong NJ, Garvin JL. Shear stress increases nitric oxide production in thick ascending limbs. Am J Physiol Renal Physiol 2010;299:F1185–1192.

[455] Ortiz PA, Hong NJ, Garvin JL. Luminal flow induces eNOS activation and translocation in the rat thick ascending limb. Am J Physiol Renal Physiol 2004;287:F274–280.

[456] Levine DZ, Burns KD, Jaffey J, Iacovitti M. Short-term modulation of distal tubule fluid nitric oxide in vivo by loop NaCl reabsorption. Kidney Int 2004;65:184–9.

[457] Kawada H, Yasuoka Y, Fukuda H, Kawahara K. Low [NaCl]-induced neuronal nitric oxide synthase (nNOS) expression and NO generation are regulated by intracellular pH in a mouse macula densa cell line (NE-MD). J Physiol Sci 2009;59:165–73.

[458] Chabrashvili T, Tojo A, Onozato ML, Kitiyakara C, Quinn MT, Fujita T, et al. Expression and cellular localization of classic NADPH oxidase subunits in the spontaneously hypertensive rat kidney. Hypertension 2002;39:269–74.

[459] Liu R, Carretero OA, Ren Y, Wang H, Garvin JL. Intracellular pH regulates superoxide production by the macula densa. Am J Physiol Renal Physiol 2008;295:F851–856.

[460] Ren Y, Carretero OA, Garvin JL. Mechanism by which superoxide potentiates tubuloglomerular feedback. Hypertension 2002;39:624–8.

[461] Welch WJ, Tojo A, Wilcox CS. Roles of NO and oxygen radicals in tubuloglomerular feedback in SHR. Am J Physiol Renal Physiol 2000;278:F769–776.

[462] Welch WJ, Tojo A, Lee JU, Kang DG, Schnackenberg CG, Wilcox CS. Nitric oxide synthase in the JGA of the SHR: expression and role in tubuloglomerular feedback. Am J Physiol Renal Physiol 1999;277:F130–138.

[463] Welch WJ, Wilcox CS. AT1 receptor antagonist combats oxidative stress and restores nitric oxide signaling in the SHR. Kidney Int 2001;59:1257–63.

[464] Kitiyakara C, Chabrashvili T, Chen Y, Blau J, Karber A, Aslam S, et al. Salt intake, oxidative stress, and renal expression of NADPH oxidase and superoxide dismutase. J Am Soc Nephrol 2003;14:2775–82.

[465] Welch WJ, Wilcox CS. Role of nitric oxide in tubuloglomerular feedback: effects of dietary salt. Clin Exp Pharmacol Physiol 1997;24:582–6.

[466] Wilcox CS, Deng X, Welch WJ. NO generation and action during changes in salt intake: roles of nNOS and macula densa. Am J Physiol 1998;274:R1588–1593.

[467] Tojo A, Welch WJ, Bremer V, Kimoto M, Kimura K, Omata M, et al. Colocalization of demethylating enzymes and NOS and functional effects of methylarginines in rat kidney. Kidney Int 1997;52:1593–601.

[468] Welch WJ, Wilcox CS. Macula densa arginine delivery and uptake in the rat regulates glomerular capillary pressure. Effects of salt intake. J Clin Invest 1997;100:2235–42.

[469] Satriano J, Wead L, Cardus A, Deng A, Boss GR, Thomson SC, et al. Regulation of ecto-5'-nucleotidase by NaCl and nitric oxide: potential roles in tubuloglomerular feedback and adaptation. Am J Physiol Renal Physiol 2006;291:F1078–1082.

[470] Siegfried G, Amiel C, Friedlander G. Inhibition of ecto-5'-nucleotidase by nitric oxide donors. Implications in renal epithelial cells. J Biol Chem 1996;271:4659–64.

[471] Briggs JP, Steipe B, Schubert G, Schnermann J. Micropuncture studies of the renal effects of atrial natriuretic substance. Pflugers Arch 1982;395:271–6.

[472] Huang CL, Cogan MG. Atrial natriuretic factor inhibits maximal tubuloglomerular feedback response. Am J Physiol Renal Physiol 1987;252:F825–828.

[473] Schnermann J, Todd KM, Briggs JP. Effect of dopamine on the tubuloglomerular feedback mechanism. Am J Physiol Renal Physiol 1990;258:F790–798.

[474] Boberg U, Hahne B, Persson AE. The effect of intraarterial infusion of prostacyclin on the tubuloglomerular feedback control in the rat. Acta Physiol Scand 1984;121:65–72.

[475] Wang T, Kawabata M, Haneda M, Takabatake T. Effects of uroguanylin, an intestinal natriuretic peptide, on tubuloglomerular feedback. Hypertens Res 2003;26:577–82.

[476] Wang T, Takabatake T. Effects of vasopeptidase inhibition on renal function and tubuloglomerular feedback in spontaneously hypertensive rats. Hypertens Res 2005;28:611–8.

[477] Ren Y, D'Ambrosio MA, Wang H, Liu R, Garvin JL, Carretero OA. Heme oxygenase metabolites inhibit tubuloglomerular feedback (TGF). Am J Physiol Renal Physiol 2008;295:F1207–1212.

[478] Kozma F, Johnson RA, Zhang F, Yu C, Tong X, Nasjletti A. Contribution of endogenous carbon monoxide to regulation of diameter in resistance vessels. Am J Physiol 1999;276:R1087–1094.

[479] Thorup C, Jones CL, Gross SS, Moore LC, Goligorsky MS. Carbon monoxide induces vasodilation and nitric oxide release but suppresses endothelial NOS. Am J Physiol 1999;277:F882–889.

[480] Folkow B. Physiological aspects of primary hypertension. Physiol Rev 1982;62:347–504.

[481] Persson AE, Muller-Suur R, Selen G. Capillary oncotic pressure as a modifier for tubuloglomerular feedback. Am J Physiol Renal Physiol 1979;236:F97–102.

[482] Selen G, Persson AE. Hydrostatic and oncotic pressures in the interstitium of dehydrated and volume expanded rats. Acta Physiol Scand 1983;117:75–81.

[483] Hahne B, Persson AEG. Prevention of interstitial pressure change at unilateral nephrectomy by prostaglandin synthesis inhibition. Kidney Int 1984;25:42–6.

[484] Haberle DA, Davis JM. Resetting of tubuloglomerular feedback: evidence for a humoral factor in tubular fluid. Am J Physiol Renal Physiol 1984;246:F495–500.

[485] Pollock DM, Arendshorst WJ. Native tubular fluid attenuates ANF-induced inhibition of tubuloglomerular feedback. Am J Physiol Renal Physiol 1990;258:F189–198.

[486] Wunderlich PF, Brunner FP, Davis JM, Haberle DA, Tholen H, Thiel G. Feedback activation in rat nephrons by sera from patients with acute renal failure. Kidney Int 1980;17:497–506.

[487] Goormaghtigh N. Une glande endocrine dans la paroi des arterioles renales. Bruxelles Med 1939;19:1541–9.

[488] Vander AJ. Control of renin release. Physiol Rev 1967;47:359–82.

[489] Vander AJ, Miller R. Control of renin secretion in the anesthetized dog. Am J Physiol 1964;207:537–46.

II. STRUCTURAL AND FUNCTIONAL ORGANIZATION OF THE KIDNEY

[490] Vander AJ. Renin secretion during mannitol diuresis and ureteral occlusion. Proc Soc Exp Biol Med 1968;128:518—20.

[491] Skott O, Briggs JP. Direct demonstration of macula densa-mediated renin secretion. Science 1987;237:1618—20.

[492] Shade RE, Davis JO, Johnson JA, Witty RT. Effects of renal arterial infusion of sodium and potassium on renin secretion in the dog. Circ Res 1972;31:719—27.

[493] Kirchner KA, Kotchen TA, Galla JH, Luke RG. Importance of chloride for acute inhibition of renin by sodium chloride. Am J Physiol 1978;235:F444—450.

[494] Kotchen TA, Galla JH, Luke RG. Contribution of chloride to the inhibition of plasma renin by sodium chloride in the rat. Kidney Int 1978;13:201—7.

[495] Leyssac PP. Changes in single nephron renin release are mediated by tubular fluid flow rate. Kidney Int 1986;30:332—9.

[496] Greenberg SG, Lorenz JN, He XR, Schnermann JB, Briggs JP. Effect of prostaglandin synthesis inhibition on macula densa-stimulated renin secretion. Am J Physiol Renal Physiol 1993;265:F578—583.

[497] Lorenz JN, Weihprecht H, Schnermann J, Skott O, Briggs JP. Characterization of the macula densa stimulus for renin secretion. Am J Physiol Renal Physiol 1990;259:F186—193.

[498] Lorenz JN, Weihprecht H, Schnermann J, Skott O, Briggs JP. Renin release from isolated juxtaglomerular apparatus depends on macula densa chloride transport. Am J Physiol Renal Physiol 1991;260:F486—493.

[499] Weihprecht H, Lorenz JN, Schnermann J, Skott O, Briggs JP. Effect of adenosine1-receptor blockade on renin release from rabbit isolated perfused juxtaglomerular apparatus. J Clin Invest 1990;85:1622—8.

[500] He XR, Greenberg SG, Briggs JP, Schnermann J. Effects of furosemide and verapamil on the NaCl dependency of macula densa-mediated renin secretion. Hypertension 1995;26:137—42.

[501] Churchill PC, Churchill MC, McDonald FD. Effects of saline and mannitol on renin and distal tubule Na in rats. Circ Res 1979;45:786—92.

[502] DiBona GF. Effect of mannitol diuresis and ureteral occlusion on distal tubular reabsorption. Am J Physiol 1971;221:511—4.

[503] Leyssac PP, Holstein-Rathlou NH, Skott O. Renal blood flow, early distal sodium, and plasma renin concentrations during osmotic diuresis. Am J Physiol Regul Integr Comp Physiol 2000;279:R1268—1276.

[504] Beierwaltes WH. Selective neuronal nitric oxide synthase inhibition blocks furosemide- stimulated renin secretion in vivo. Am J Physiol Renal Physiol 1995;269:F134—139.

[505] Castrop H, Schweda F, Mizel D, Huang Y, Briggs J, Kurtz A, et al. Permissive role of nitric oxide in macula densa control of renin secretion. Am J Physiol Renal Physiol 2004;286(5):F848—857 .

[506] Keeton TK, Campbell WB. The pharmacologic alteration of renin release. Pharmacol Rev 1980;32:81—227.

[507] Vander AJ, Carlson J. Mechanism of the effects of furosemide on renin secretion in anesthetized dogs. Circ Res 1969;25:145—52.

[508] Itoh S, Carretero OA. Role of the macula densa in renin release. Hypertension 1985;7:I49—54.

[509] Hanner F, Chambrey R, Bourgeois S, Meer E, Mucsi I, Rosivall L, et al. Increased renal renin content in mice lacking the Na$^+$/H$^+$ exchanger NHE2. Am J Physiol Renal Physiol 2008;294:F937—944.

[510] Castrop HW, Hansen PB, Huang YG, et al. Direct effects of furosemide on renin secretion and preglomerular resistance. J Am Soc Nephrol 2004;15:199A (abstract)

[511] Kotchen TA, Luke RG, Ott CE, Galla JH, Whitescarver S. Effect of chloride on renin and blood pressure responses to sodium chloride. Ann Intern Med 1983;98:817—22.

[512] Welch WJ, Ott CE, Lorenz JN, Kotchen TA. Effects of chlorpropamide on loop of Henle function and plasma renin. Kidney Int 1986;30:712—6.

[513] Abboud HE, Luke RG, Galla JH, Kotchen TA. Stimulation of renin by acute selective chloride depletion in the rat. Circ Res 1979;44:815—21.

[514] Rostand SG, Work J, Luke RG. Effect of reduced chloride reabsorption on renin release in the isolated rat kidney. Pflugers Arch 1985;405:46—51.

[515] Kim SM, Mizel D, Huang YG, Briggs JP, Schnermann J. Adenosine as a mediator of macula densa-dependent inhibition of renin secretion. Am J Physiol Renal Physiol 2006;290:F1016—1023.

[516] Robben JH, Fenton RA, Vargas SL, Schweer H, Peti-Peterdi J, Deen PM, et al. Localization of the succinate receptor in the distal nephron and its signaling in polarized MDCK cells. Kidney Int 2009;76:1258—67.

[517] Vargas SL, Toma I, Kang JJ, Meer EJ, Peti-Peterdi J. Activation of the succinate receptor GPR91 in macula densa cells causes renin release. J Am Soc Nephrol 2009;20:1002—11.

[518] Baumbach L, Leyssac PP, Skinner SL. Studies on renin release from isolated superfused glomeruli: effects of temperature, urea, ouabain and ethacrynic acid. J Physiol 1976;258:243—56.

[519] Toma I, Kang JJ, Sipos A, Vargas S, Bansal E, Hanner F, et al. Succinate receptor GPR91 provides a direct link between high glucose levels and renin release in murine and rabbit kidney. J Clin Invest 2008;118:2526—34.

[520] Pluznick JL, Zou DJ, Zhang X, Yan Q, Rodriguez-Gil DJ, Eisner C, et al. Functional expression of the olfactory signaling system in the kidney. Proc Natl Acad Sci USA 2009;106:2059—64.

[521] Bosse HM, Bohm R, Resch S, Bachmann S. Parallel regulation of constitutive NO synthase and renin at JGA of rat kidney under various stimuli. Am J Physiol Renal Physiol 1995;269:F793—805.

[522] Murakami K, Tsuchiya K, Naruse M, Naruse K, Demura H, Arai J, et al. Nitric oxide synthase I immunoreactivity in the macula densa of the kidney is angiotensin II dependent. Kidney Int Suppl 1997;63:S208—210.

[523] Tojo A, Madsen KM, Wilcox CS. Expression of immunoreactive nitric oxide synthase isoforms in rat kidney. Effects of dietary salt and losartan. Jpn Heart J 1995;36:389—98.

[524] Kihara M, Umemura S, Kadota T, Yabana M, Tamura K, Nyuui N, et al. The neuronal isoform of constitutive nitric oxide synthase is up-regulated in the macula densa of angiotensinogen gene-knockout mice. Lab Invest 1997;76:285—94.

[525] Kihara M, Umemura S, Sugaya T, Toya Y, Yabana M, Kobayashi S, et al. Expression of neuronal type nitric oxide synthase and renin in the juxtaglomerular apparatus of angiotensin type-1a receptor gene-knockout mice. Kidney Int 1998;53:1585—93.

[526] Paliege A, Mizel D, Medina C, Pasumarthy A, Huang YG, Bachmann S, et al. Inhibition of nNOS expression in the macula densa by COX-2-derived prostaglandin E(2). Am J Physiol Renal Physiol 2004;287:F152—159.

[527] Gambaryan S, Wagner C, Smolenski A, Walter U, Poller W, Haase W, et al. Endogenous or overexpressed cGMP-dependent protein kinases inhibit cAMP-dependent renin release from rat isolated perfused kidney, microdissected glomeruli, and isolated juxtaglomerular cells. Proc Natl Acad Sci USA 1998;95:9003—8.

[528] Wagner C, Pfeifer A, Ruth P, Hofmann F, Kurtz A. Role of cGMP-kinase II in the control of renin secretion and renin expression. J Clin Invest 1998;102:1576—82.

[529] Harrison SA, Reifsnyder DH, Gallis B, Cadd GG, Beavo JA. Isolation and characterization of bovine cardiac muscle cGMP-inhibited phosphodiesterase: a receptor for new cardiotonic drugs. Mol Pharmacol 1986;29:506—14.

[530] Chiu T, Reid IA. Role of cyclic GMP-inhibitable phosphodiesterase and nitric oxide in the beta adrenoceptor control of renin secretion. J Pharmacol Exp Ther 1996;278:793—9.

[531] Kurtz A, Gotz KH, Hamann M, Kieninger M, Wagner C. Stimulation of renin secretion by NO donors is related to the cAMP pathway. Am J Physiol Renal Physiol 1998;274:F709—717.

[532] Sayago CM, Beierwaltes WH. Nitric oxide synthase and cGMP-mediated stimulation of renin secretion. Am J Physiol Regul Integr Comp Physiol 2001;281:R1146—1151.

[533] He XR, Greenberg SG, Briggs JP, Schnermann JB. Effect of nitric oxide on renin secretion. II. Studies in the perfused juxtaglomerular apparatus. Am J Physiol Renal Physiol 1995;268:F953—959.

[534] Persson PB, Baumann JE, Ehmke H, Hackenthal E, Kirchheim HR, Nafz B, et al. Endothelium-derived NO stimulates pressure-dependent renin release in conscious dogs. Am J Physiol 1993;264:F943—947.

[535] Scholz H, Kurtz A. Involvement of endothelium-derived relaxing factor in the pressure control of renin secretion from isolated perfused kidney. J Clin Invest 1993;91:1088—94.

[536] Chatziantoniou C, Pauti MD, Pinet F, Promeneur D, Dussaule JC, Ardaillou R. Regulation of renin release is impaired after nitric oxide inhibition. Kidney Int 1996;49:626—33.

[537] Reid IA, Chou L. Effect of blockade of nitric oxide synthesis on the renin secretory response to frusemide in conscious rabbits. Clin Sci (Colch) 1995;88:657—63.

[538] Schricker K, Hamann M, Kurtz A. Nitric oxide and prostaglandins are involved in the macula densa control of the renin system. Am J Physiol Renal Physiol 1995;269:F825—830.

[539] Larsson C, Weber P, Anggard E. Arachidonic acid increases and indomethacin decreases plasma renin activity in the rabbit. Eur J Pharmacol 1974;28:391—4.

[540] Jensen BL, Schmid C, Kurtz A. Prostaglandins stimulate renin secretion and renin mRNA in mouse renal juxtaglomerular cells. Am J Physiol Renal Physiol 1996;271:F659—69.

[541] Jensen BL, Mann B, Skott O, Kurtz A. Differential regulation of renal prostaglandin receptor mRNAs by dietary salt intake in the rat. Kidney Int 1999;56:528—37.

[542] Chen L, Kim SM, Oppermann M, Faulhaber-Walter R, Huang Y, Mizel D, et al. Regulation of renin in mice with Cre recombinase-mediated deletion of G protein Gsalpha in juxtaglomerular cells. Am J Physiol Renal Physiol 2007;292:F27—37.

[543] Castrop H, Schweda F, Schumacher K, Wolf K, Kurtz A. Role of renocortical cyclooxygenase-2 for renal vascular resistance and macula densa control of renin secretion. J Am Soc Nephrol 2001;12:867—74.

[544] Kammerl MC, Nusing RM, Richthammer W, Kramer BK, Kurtz A. Inhibition of COX-2 counteracts the effects of diuretics in rats. Kidney Int 2001;60:1684—91.

[545] Komhoff M, Jeck ND, Seyberth HW, Grone HJ, Nusing RM, Breyer MD. Cyclooxygenase-2 expression is associated with the renal macula densa of patients with Bartter-like syndrome. Kidney Int 2000;58:2420—4.

[546] Mann B, Hartner A, Jensen BL, Kammerl M, Kramer BK, Kurtz A. Furosemide stimulates macula densa cyclooxygenase-2 expression in rats. Kidney Int 2001;59:62—8.

[547] Reinalter SC, Jeck N, Brochhausen C, Watzer B, Nüsing RM, Seyberth HW, et al. Role of cyclooxygenase-2 in hyperprostaglandin E syndrome/antenatal Bartter syndrome. Kidney Int 2002;62:253—60.

[548] Hartner A, Cordasic N, Goppelt-Struebe M, Veelken R, Hilgers KF. Role of macula densa cyclooxygenase-2 in renovascular hypertension. Am J Physiol Renal Physiol 2003;284:F498—502.

[549] Jensen BL, Kurtz A. Differential regulation of renal cyclooxygenase mRNA by dietary salt intake. Kidney Int 1997;52:1242—9.

[550] Wang JL, Cheng HF, Harris RC. Cyclooxygenase-2 inhibition decreases renin content and lowers blood pressure in a model of renovascular hypertension. Hypertension 1999;34:96—101.

[551] Tomasoni S, Noris M, Zappella S, Gotti E, Casiraghi F, Bonazzola S, et al. Upregulation of renal and systemic cyclooxygenase-2 in patients with active lupus nephritis. J Am Soc Nephrol 1998;9:1202—12.

[552] Wang JL, Cheng HF, Zhang MZ, McKanna JA, Harris RC. Selective increase of cyclooxygenase-2 expression in a model of renal ablation. Am J Physiol Renal Physiol 1998;275:F613—622.

[553] Kim SM, Chen L, Mizel D, Huang YG, Briggs JP, Schnermann J. Low plasma renin and reduced renin secretory responses to acute stimuli in conscious COX-2-deficient mice. Am J Physiol Renal Physiol 2007;292:F415—22.

[554] Yang T, Endo Y, Huang YG, Smart A, Briggs JP, Schnermann J. Renin expression in COX-2-knockout mice on normal or low-salt diets. Am J Physiol Renal Physiol 2000;279:F819—825.

[555] Cheng HF, Wang JL, Zhang MZ, Miyazaki Y, Ichikawa I, McKanna JA, et al. Angiotensin II attenuates renal cortical cyclooxygenase-2 expression. J Clin Invest 1999;103:953—61.

[556] Wolf K, Castrop H, Hartner A, Goppelt-Strube M, Hilgers KF, Kurtz A. Inhibition of the renin-angiotensin system upregulates cyclooxygenase-2 expression in the macula densa. Hypertension 1999;34:503—7.

[557] Peti-Peterdi J, Komlosi P, Fuson AL, Guan Y, Schneider A, Qi Z, et al. Luminal NaCl delivery regulates basolateral PGE2 release from macula densa cells. J Clin Invest 2003;112:76—82.

[558] Traynor TR, Smart A, Briggs JP, Schnermann J. Inhibition of macula densa-stimulated renin secretion by pharmacological blockade of cyclooxygenase-2. Am J Physiol Renal Physiol 1999;277:F706—10.

[559] Cheng HF, Wang JL, Zhang MZ, McKanna JA, Harris RC. Role of p38 in the regulation of renal cortical cyclooxygenase-2 expression by extracellular chloride. J Clin Invest 2000;106:681—8.

[560] Yang T, Park JM, Arend L, Huang Y, Topaloglu R, Pasumarthy A, et al. Low chloride stimulation of prostaglandin E2 release and cyclooxygenase-2 expression in a mouse macula densa cell line. J Biol Chem 2000;275:37922—9.

[561] Cheng HF, Harris RC. Cyclooxygenase-2 expression in cultured cortical thick ascending limb of Henle increases in response to decreased extracellular ionic content by both transcriptional and post-transcriptional mechanisms. Role of p38-mediated pathways. J Biol Chem 2002;277:45638—43.

[562] Guan Z, Buckman SY, Miller BW, Springer LD, Morrison AR. Interleukin-1beta-induced cyclooxygenase-2 expression requires activation of both c-Jun NH2-terminal kinase and p38 MAPK signal pathways in rat renal mesangial cells. J Biol Chem 1998;273:28670—6.

[563] Xie W, Herschman HR. Transcriptional regulation of prostaglandin synthase 2 gene expression by platelet-derived growth factor and serum. J Biol Chem 1996;271:31742—8.

[564] Yang T, Huang Y, Heasley LE, Berl T, Schnermann JB, Briggs JP. MAPK mediation of hypertonicity-stimulated cyclooxygenase-2 expression in renal medullary collecting duct cells. J Biol Chem 2000;275:23281—6.

[565] Cheng HF, Wang JL, Zhang MZ, Wang SW, McKanna JA, Harris RC. Genetic deletion of COX-2 prevents increased renin expression in response to ACE inhibition. Am J Physiol Renal Physiol 2001;280:F449—456.

[566] Fujino T, Nakagawa N, Yuhki K, Hara A, Yamada T, Takayama K, et al. Decreased susceptibility to renovascular hypertension in mice lacking the prostaglandin I2 receptor IP. J Clin Invest 2004;114:805—12.

[567] Hocherl K, Kammerl MC, Schumacher K, Endemann D, Grobecker HF, Kurtz A. Role of prostanoids in regulation of the renin—angiotensin—aldosterone system by salt intake. Am J Physiol Renal Physiol 2002;283:F294—301.

[568] Kammerl MC, Nusing RM, Seyberth HW, Riegger GA, Kurtz A, Kramer BK. Inhibition of cyclooxygenase-2 attenuates urinary prostanoid excretion without affecting renal renin expression. Pflugers Arch 2001;442:842—7.

[569] Kurtz A, Schweda F. Osmolarity-induced renin secretion from kidneys: evidence for readily releasable renin pools. Am J Physiol Renal Physiol 2006;290:F797—805.

[570] Therland KL, Stubbe J, Thiesson HC, Ottosen PD, Walter S, Sørensen GL, et al. Cycloxygenase-2 is expressed in vasculature of normal and ischemic adult human kidney and is colocalized with vascular prostaglandin E2 EP4 receptors. J Am Soc Nephrol 2004;15:1189—98.

[571] Liguori A, Casini A, Di Loreto M, Andreini I, Napoli C. Loop diuretics enhance the secretion of prostacyclin in vitro, in healthy persons, and in patients with chronic heart failure. Eur J Clin Pharmacol 1999;55:117—24.

[572] Hocherl K, Kees F, Kramer BK, Kurtz A. Cyclosporine A attenuates the natriuretic action of loop diuretics by inhibition of renal COX-2 expression. Kidney Int 2004;65:2071—80.

[573] Stichtenoth DO, Marhauer V, Tsikas D, Gutzki FM, Frolich JC. Effects of specific COX-2-inhibition on renin release and renal and systemic prostanoid synthesis in healthy volunteers. Kidney Int 2005;68:2197—207.

[574] Arend LJ, Haramati A, Thompson CI, Spielman WS. Adenosine-induced decrease in renin release: dissociation from hemodynamic effects. Am J Physiol Renal Physiol 1984;247:F447—452.

[575] Churchill PC, Churchill MC. A1 and A2 adenosine receptor activation inhibits and stimulates renin secretion of rat renal cortical slices. J Pharmacol Exp Ther 1985;232:589—94.

[576] Tagawa H, Vander AJ. Effects of adenosine compounds on renal function and renin secretion in dogs. Circ Res 1970;26:327—38.

[577] Lorenz JN, Weihprecht H, He XR, Skott O, Briggs JP, Schnermann J. Effects of adenosine and angiotensin on macula densa-stimulated renin secretion. Am J Physiol Renal Physiol 1993;265:F187—194.

[578] Schweda F, Wagner C, Kramer BK, Schnermann J, Kurtz A. Preserved macula densa-dependent renin secretion in A1 adenosine receptor knockout mice. Am J Physiol Renal Physiol 2003;284:F770—777.

[579] Grunberger C, Obermayer B, Klar J, Kurtz A, Schweda F. The calcium paradoxon of renin release: Calcium suppresses renin exocytosis by inhibition of calcium-dependent adenylate cyclases AC5 and AC6. Circ Res 2006;99:1197—206.

[580] Ortiz-Capisano MC, Ortiz PA, Harding P, Garvin JL, Beierwaltes WH. Decreased intracellular calcium stimulates renin release via calcium-inhibitable adenylyl cyclase. Hypertension 2007;49:162—9.

[581] Frederiksen O, Leyssac PP, Skinner SL. Sensitive osmometer function of juxtaglomerular cells in vitro. J Physiol 1975;252:669—79.

[582] Jensen BL, Skott O. Osmotically sensitive renin release from permeabilized juxtaglomerular cells. Am J Physiol 1993;265: F87—95.

[583] Schricker K, Kurtz A. Role of membrane-permeable ions in renin secretion by renal juxtaglomerular cells. Am J Physiol 1995;269:F64—69.

[584] Skott O. Do osmotic forces play a role in renin secretion? Am J Physiol 1988;255:F1—10.

[585] Friis UG, Madsen K, Svenningsen P, Hansen PB, Gulaveerasingam A, Jorgensen F, et al. Hypotonicity-induced Renin exocytosis from juxtaglomerular cells requires aquaporin-1 and cyclooxygenase-2. J Am Soc Nephrol 2009;20:2154—61.

[586] Young DB, Rostorfer HH. Renin release responses to acute alterations in renal arterial osmolarity. Am J Physiol 1973;225:1009—14.

[587] Ortiz-Capisano MC, Ortiz PA, Garvin JL, Harding P, Beierwaltes WH. Expression and function of the calcium-sensing receptor in juxtaglomerular cells. Hypertension 2007;50:737—43.

[588] Maillard MP, Tedjani A, Perregaux C, Burnier M. Calcium-sensing receptors modulate renin release in vivo and in vitro in the rat. J Hypertens 2009;27:1980—7.

[589] Palmer CE, Rudd MA, Bukoski RD. Renal interstitial Ca^{2+} during sodium loading of normotensive and Dahl-salt hypertensive rats. Am J Hypertens 2003;16:771—6.

[590] Hanner F, von Maltzahn J, Maxeiner S, Toma I, Sipos A, Kruger O, et al. Connexin45 is expressed in the juxtaglomerular apparatus and is involved in the regulation of renin secretion and blood pressure. Am J Physiol Regul Integr Comp Physiol 2008;295:R371—380.

[591] Toma I, Bansal E, Meer EJ, Kang JJ, Vargas SL, Peti-Peterdi J. Connexin 40 and ATP-dependent intercellular calcium wave in renal glomerular endothelial cells. Am J Physiol Regul Integr Comp Physiol 2008;294:R1769—1776.

[592] Krattinger N, Capponi A, Mazzolai L, Aubert JF, Caille D, Nicod P, et al. Connexin40 regulates renin production and blood pressure. Kidney Int 2007;72:814—22.

[593] Kurtz L, Schweda F, de Wit C, Kriz W, Witzgall R, Warth R, et al. Lack of connexin 40 causes displacement of renin-producing cells from afferent arterioles to the extraglomerular mesangium. J Am Soc Nephrol 2007;18:1103—11.

[594] Briggs J. A simple steady-state model for feedback control of glomerular filtration rate. Kidney International 1982;22(Suppl. 12):S143—50.

[595] Skott O, Briggs JP. A method for superfusion of the isolated perfused tubule. Kidney Int 1988;33:1009—12.

[596] Hoyer JR, Sisson SP, Vernier RL. Tamm-Horsfall glycoprotein: Ultrastructural immunoperoxidase localization in rat kidney. Lab Invest 1979;41:168—73.

[597] Salido EC, Yen PH, Shapiro LJ, Fisher DA, Barajas L. In situ hybridization of prepro-epidermal growth factor mRNA in the mouse kidney. Am J Physiol 1989;256:F632—638.

[598] Kulaksiz H, Theilig F, Bachmann S, Gehrke SG, Rost D, Janetzko A, et al. The iron-regulatory peptide hormone hepcidin: expression and cellular localization in the mammalian kidney. J Endocrinol 2005;184:361—70.

[599] Obermuller N, Gallagher AR, Cai Y, Gassler N, Gretz N, Somlo S, et al. The rat pkd2 protein assumes distinct subcellular distributions in different organs. Am J Physiol 1999;277: F914—925.

[600] Tian W, Salanova M, Xu H, Lindsley JN, Oyama TT, Anderson S, et al. Renal expression of osmotically responsive cation channel TRPV4 is restricted to water-impermeant nephron segments. Am J Physiol Renal Physiol 2004;287:F17—24.

[601] Stoeckel ME, Freund-Mercier MJ. Autoradiographic demonstration of oxytocin-binding sites in the macula densa [published erratum appears in Am J Physiol Renal Physiol 1990 Jan;258(1 Pt 2):preceding F1] Am J Physiol Renal Physiol. 1989;257:F310−314.

[602] Harrison-Bernard LM, Navar LG, Ho MM, Vinson GP, el-Dahr SS. Immunohistochemical localization of ANG II AT1 receptor in adult rat kidney using a monoclonal antibody. Am J Physiol 1997;273:F170−177.

[603] Beaumont K, Healy DP, Fanestil DD. Autoradiographic localization of benzodiazepine receptors in the rat kidney. Am J Physiol 1984;247:F718−724.

[604] Riccardi D, Hall AE, Chattopadhyay N, Xu JZ, Brown EM, Hebert SC. Localization of the extracellular Ca^{2+}/polyvalent cation-sensing protein in rat kidney. Am J Physiol 1998;274: F611−622.

[605] Massfelder T, Stewart AF, Endlich K, Soifer N, Judes C, Helwig JJ. Parathyroid hormone-related protein detection and interaction with NO and cyclic AMP in the renovascular system. Kidney Int 1996;50:1591−603.

[606] Haddad M, Roder S, Olsen HS, Wagner GF. Immunocytochemical localization of stanniocalcin cells in the rat kidney. Endocrinology 1996;137:2113−7.

[607] Breuss JM, Gillett N, Lu L, Sheppard D, Pytela R. Restricted distribution of integrin beta 6 mRNA in primate epithelial tissues. J Histochem Cytochem 1993;41:1521−7.

[608] Liu R, Bell PD, Peti-Peterdi J, Kovacs G, Johansson A, Persson AE. Purinergic receptor signaling at the basolateral membrane of macula densa cells. J Am Soc Nephrol 2002;13:1145−51.

[609] O'Reilly M, Marshall E, Macgillivray T, Mittel M, Xue W, Kenyon CJ, et al. Dietary electrolyte-driven responses in the renal WNK kinase pathway *in vivo*. J Am Soc Nephrol 2006;17:2402−13.

[610] Komers R, Lindsley JN, Oyama TT, Cohen DM, Anderson S. Renal p38 MAP kinase activity in experimental diabetes. Lab Invest 2007;87:548−58.

[611] Balen D, Ljubojevic M, Breljak D, Brzica H, Zlender V, Koepsell H, et al. Revised immunolocalization of the Na^{+}-D-glucose co-transporter SGLT1 in rat organs with an improved antibody. Am J Physiol Cell Physiol 2008;295: C475−489.

[612] Lai LW, Yong KC, Lien YH. Site-specific expression of IQGAP1, a key mediator of cytoskeleton, in mouse renal tubules. J Histochem Cytochem 2008;56:659−66.

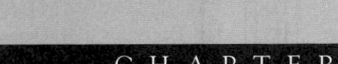

Renal Cortical and Medullary Microcirculations: Structure and Function

Thomas L. Pallone and Chunhua Cao

Division of Nephrology, Department of Medicine, University of Maryland at Baltimore, Baltimore, MD, USA

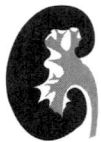

ANATOMY OF THE RENAL CIRCULATION

Cortical Microcirculation

The basic vascular pattern of the kidney is preserved across mammalian species[1,3–9] (Figure 24.1). The renal artery branches into interlobar arteries that ascend within the renal pelvis to enter the parenchyma. In multipapillate organisms, the interlobar arteries travel toward the cortex along the columns of Bertin. These vessels change direction and follow an arc-like course near the corticomedullary border to become arcuate arteries. The arcuate artery gives rise to the interlobular arteries that ascend, in radial fashion, toward the cortical surface. Afferent arterioles arise from interlobular arteries at angles that vary with their cortical depth. Afferents that supply deep glomeruli near the corticomedullary junction (juxtamedullary glomeruli) leave the interlobular artery at a recurrent angle. In contrast, superficial afferent arterioles that supply glomeruli near the surface of the kidney line up with the interlobular artery at its termination.

In some species (rat, cat, dog, and *Meriones*) a pair of intra-arterial "cushions" exist as parallel ridges that project from the origin of the juxtamedullary afferent arteriole into the lumen of the parent intralobular artery (Figure 24.2a).[10,11] The cushions are 18–30 μm in length, composed of a ground substance in which smooth muscle cells are embedded and covered by a layer of continuous endothelium (Figure 24.2b).[12] The cushions are ideally placed to regulate blood flow

distribution within the cortex. Given that blood flow to the renal medulla arises largely from the efferent flow of juxtamedullary glomeruli, it is also plausible that the cushions play a role in the regulation of blood flow to the medulla. The cushions have been hypothesized to separate plasma and red blood cells, and alter medullary hematocrit by "skimming" plasma from a red cell-free layer near the vessel wall.[10,13]

The structure of afferent and efferent arterioles varies with cortical location. Afferent arterioles are composed of one to three layers of smooth muscle cells. Muscle and elastic tissue diminish near the glomerulus and the media is replaced by granular cells of the juxtaglomerular apparatus. The diameters of efferent arterioles vary from as small as 12 μm in the superficial cortex to 28 μm for juxtamedullary glomeruli. Efferent arterioles in the superficial cortex branch to form a dense peritubular capillary plexus. Ten different branching patterns have been described.[14] In contrast to the efferent arterioles of superficial glomeruli, those of juxtamedullary glomeruli most frequently cross the corticomedullary junction to enter the outer stripe of the outer medulla, where they give rise to descending vasa recta (DVR). DVR are transitional vessels along which smooth muscle is replaced by contractile pericytes.[8,15] A small fraction of blood flow to the renal medulla may bypass juxtamedullary glomeruli in "shunt" vessels (dashed line, Figure 24.1). Casellas and Mimran have described variations of those shunts as: (1) branches of afferent arterioles; (2) continuous vessels from which afferent arterioles arise as side branches; (3) short vascular connections between

Seldin and Giebisch's The Kidney, Fifth Edition.
DOI: http://dx.doi.org/10.1016/B978-0-12-381462-3.00024-0

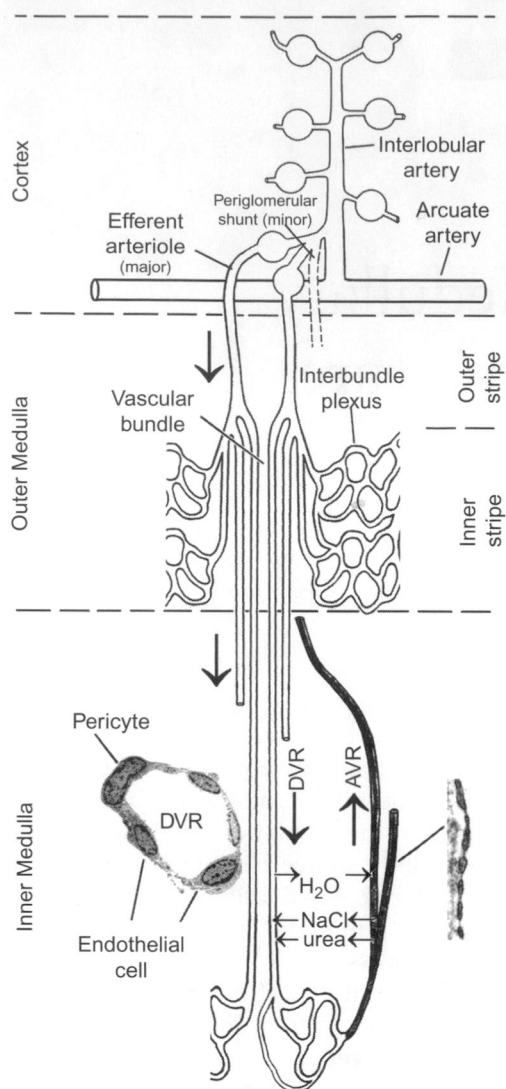

FIGURE 24.1   Microcirculation of the renal cortex and medulla. Within the renal cortex, interlobular arteries, derived from the arcuate artery, ascend toward the cortical surface. Superficial and midcortical glomeruli arise at obtuse and right angles, while juxtamedullary glomeruli arise at an acute, recurrent angle from the interlobular artery. The majority of blood flow to the medulla arises from juxtamedullary efferent arterioles. A minor fraction might also be derived from periglomerular shunt pathways (dashed lines). In the outer stripe of the outer medulla, juxtamedullary efferent arterioles give rise to DVR that combine with AVR, and sometimes thin descending limbs of Henle, to form vascular bundles. Vascular bundles are the prominent feature of the inner stripe of the outer medulla. DVR on the periphery of vascular bundles perfuse the interbundle capillary plexus that supplies nephrons (thick ascending limb, collecting duct, long looped thin descending limbs, not shown). DVR in the center of the bundles continue across the inner–outer medullary junction to perfuse the inner medulla. In some species, thin descending limbs of short looped nephrons migrate toward or become associated with vascular bundles. In the inner medulla, vascular bundles disappear and vasa recta become dispersed with thin loops of Henle and collecting ducts. Blood from the interbundle capillary plexus is returned without rejoining vascular bundles. DVR have a continuous endothelium (inset) and are surrounded by contractile pericytes. Like cortical peritubular capillaries, the AVR endothelium is highly fenestrated. As blood flows toward the papillary tip, NaCl and urea diffuse into DVR and out of AVR. Transmural gradients of NaCl and urea drive water efflux across the DVR wall via aquaporin-1 water channels. The increasing size of the circled "P" is to represent the rise in DVR plasma protein concentration with medullary depth. *(Reproduced with permission from ref. [31].)*

afferent and efferent arterioles; and (4) pelvic arterioles derived from afferent arterioles near the renal hilus (Figure 24.3).[16] Several reviews of arteriolar patterns in the renal cortex have been written.[4,11,17]

The bulk of glomerular filtrate is reabsorbed by the proximal convoluted tubule. That reabsorbate is conducted through the cortical interstitium and taken up by peritubular capillaries. The peritubular interstitium of the cortex has been divided into "narrow" and "wide" portions comprising 0.6 and 3.4% of tissue volume.[18,19] The narrow interstitium is flanked by a highly fenestrated capillary wall on one side and the basolateral membrane of the PCT on the other (Figure 24.4).[9,20] Since only 26% of the tubular surface faces the narrow interstitium it follows that substantial quantities of fluid must flow from the wide to the narrow portion, implying that hydrostatic pressure gradients exist within the cortical interstitium.[18,21]

Medullary Microcirculation

Blood flow to the renal medulla is supplied by DVR. Descending vasa recta (DVR) arise largely from efferent arterioles of juxtamedullary glomeruli and supply all blood flow to the renal medulla (Figure 24.1). The afferent arterioles that supply juxtamedullary glomeruli arise from interlobular arterioles (cortical penetrating arterioles) at recurrent angles. Muscular intra-arterial cushions exist at the origins of afferent arterioles (Figure 24.2), particularly near the corticomedullary junction, and have been proposed to participate in reduction of medullary hematocrit by "plasma skimming" (see below).[10,11] Juxtamedullary efferent arterioles are larger, longer, and have a more robust smooth muscle layer than those derived from superficial or midcortical glomeruli (Figure 24.5).[15,17] They often divide into branches that either remain in the cortex to supply cortical peritubular

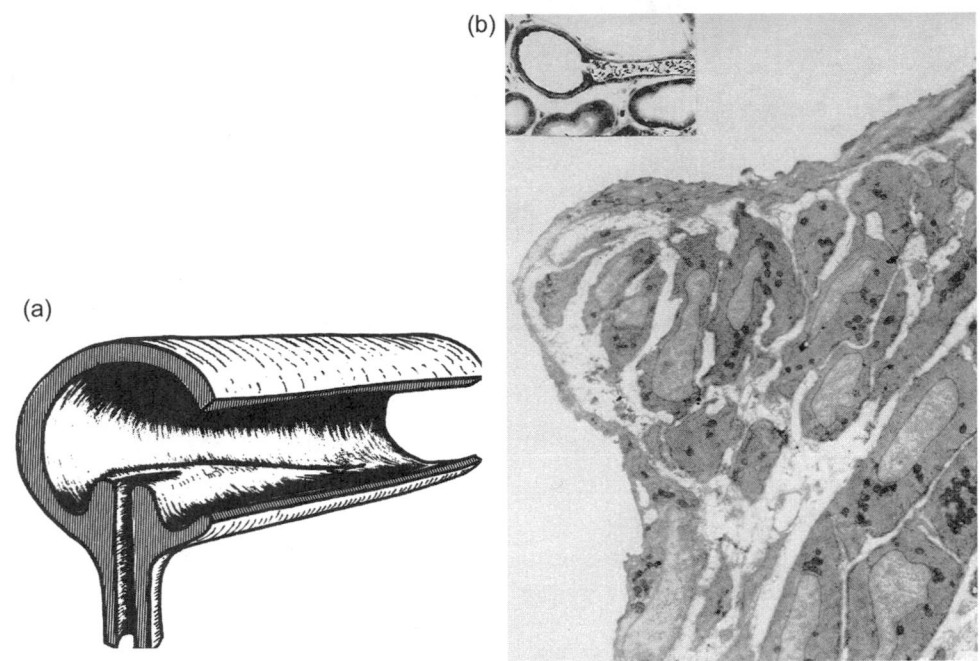

FIGURE 24.2 **The intra-arterial cushion.** (a) In some species intra-arterial cushions are present where juxtamedullary afferent arterioles arise from interlobular arterioles. (b) A longitudinal section through an afferent arteriole shows an intra-arterial cushion at its origin from the interlobular artery (inset: ×160). The cushion protrudes into the lumen of the parent vessel. Smooth muscle cells of the cushion are embedded in a copious matrix (×4000). Intra-arterial cushions might affect the relative volume fraction of RBCs versus plasma (hematocrit) that is directed from intralobular arterioles to juxtamedullary glomeruli and renal medulla. It is also conceivable that they regulate the relative distribution of blood flow between the superficial and juxtamedullary cortex (see text). *(Reproduced with permission from ref. [11,12]).*

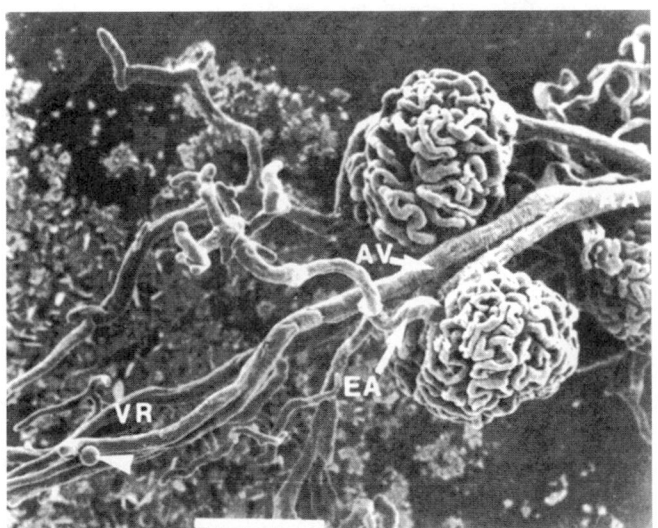

FIGURE 24.3 **Corrosion cast showing a periglomerular shunt vessel at the corticomedullary junction.** The afferent arteriole (AA) of a juxtamedullary glomerulus gives rise to a side branch (AV) which forms descending vasa recta (VR). The efferent arteriole (EA) of the juxtamedullary glomerulus is visible (Arrowhead: 16 μm sphere; Bar: 100 μm). It is probable that some blood flow that reaches the renal medulla bypasses juxtamedullary glomeruli by shunts such as the one illustrated, but the overall fraction of medullary blood flow derived from shunts is probably small (i.e., <10%). *(Reproduced with permission from ref. [16]).*

capillaries or, alternatively, descend into the medulla to form DVR.[14,22,23] DVR are about one half of the diameter of parent juxtamedullary efferent arterioles, in the range of 12 to 18 μm; some may be as large as 20 μm. DVR branch from their parent efferent arteriole in the outer stripe of the outer medulla and then coalesce within vascular bundles in the inner stripe of the outer medulla[4,5,8,24,25] (Figure 24.1). Larger diameter DVR lie in the center of vascular bundles and penetrate to the deepest regions of the inner medulla.[15,17,26] DVR are transitional vessels, wherein smooth muscle is replaced by contractile pericytes.[27] Pericytes become increasingly scarce with medullary depth, but are retained well into the inner medulla[28] (Figure 24.6). DVR have a continuous endothelium with tight junctions. In contrast, ascending vasa recta (AVR) that arise from DVR are highly fenestrated[25,29,30] (Figure 24.7). DVR peel off from the periphery of the vascular bundles as they pass through the inner stripe to supply the interbundle capillary plexus (Figure 24.8a,b,c). AVR within vascular bundles are only those that originate from the inner medulla.[24] Blood flow from the outer medullary interbundle capillary plexus returns to the cortex without rejoining vascular bundles. Thus, countercurrent exchange in the vascular bundles of the inner stripe of the outer medulla involves all DVR, but only those AVR that return from the inner medulla.

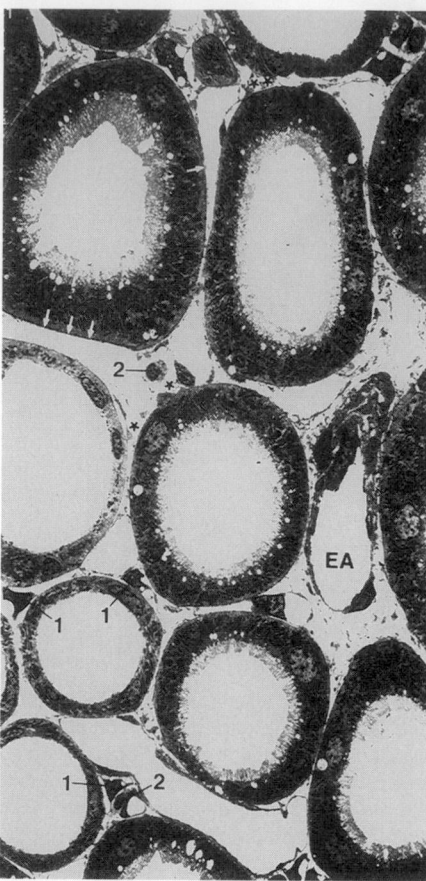

FIGURE 24.4 Peritubular interstitium of the renal cortex. The narrow portion of the cortical interstitium (arrows) lies immediately adjacent to the basement membrane of the proximal tubule. The wide portion (stars) lies between peritubular capillaries and cortical nephrons. Interstitial cells are fibroblast-like[780] or rounded[746] (EA: efferent arteriole ($\times 1000$). *(Reproduced with permission from ref. [20]).*

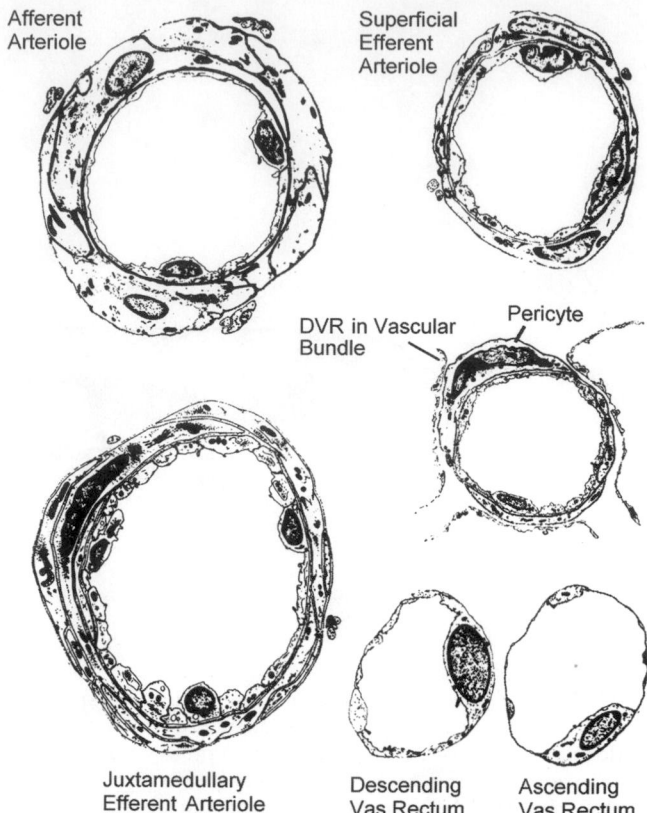

FIGURE 24.5 Structure and transition of cortical and medullary vessels. The proximal afferent arteriole is composed of at least two layers of smooth muscle cells. The muscularity and size of cortical efferent arterioles differ with location. Note the difference between the superficial and juxtamedullary efferent arterioles. The juxtamedullary efferent arteriole is larger, has a thicker, multilayered media, and its endothelium is composed of more numerous endothelial cells. In the illustration, a descending vas rectum (DVR) in a vascular bundle is adjacent to three fenestrated ascending vasa recta (AVR). The DVR wall is surrounded by a contractile pericyte. At the bottom right, DVR and AVR from the inner medulla are shown. Inner medullary DVR have a continuous endothelium through most of their length as pericytes become scarcer with medullary depth. Terminal DVR and the entire AVR wall is fenestrated. *(Reproduced with permission from ref. [15]).*

The most striking characteristic of the outer medullary circulation is its separation into vascular bundles and the dense capillary plexus that supplies the interbundle region of the inner stripe[4,5,15,17,24–26,31] (Figures 24.1, and 24.8). Species variation exists with respect to the association of nephrons with vascular bundles. The "simple" vascular bundle of the rabbit, guinea pig, dog, cat, monkey, and man is comprised only of DVR and AVR, excluding nephrons.[4,17,26] The "complex" vascular bundle of some rodents incorporates the descending thin limbs of short looped nephrons (nephrons that return from the inner–outer medullary junction). The degree to which thin descending limbs of Henle are incorporated into vascular bundles varies with species, and is highly developed in the mouse[4,17,26,32] (Figure 24.9). *Psammomys obesus* is a desert-dwelling rodent in which vascular bundles combine in the outer stripe of the outer medulla to form "giant" vascular bundles (Figure 24.8a).[5] By anatomical inference, the parallel arrangement of DVR within vascular bundles of all species contributes to the

regulation of regional blood flow distribution in the kidney. Constriction of DVR on the vascular bundle periphery should favor perfusion of the inner medulla. Conversely, constriction of DVR in the bundle center should preferentially favor flow to the capillary plexus of the interbundle region. Experimental evidence that supports such differential regulation of perfusion of the outer and inner medulla is sparse, because few studies have simultaneously measured outer and inner medullary blood flow.[33]

The vascular bundles that are characteristic of the inner stripe of the outer medulla disappear below the inner–outer medullary junction. Throughout the medulla, AVR are larger and more numerous than DVR. As a consequence, during passage of blood from the

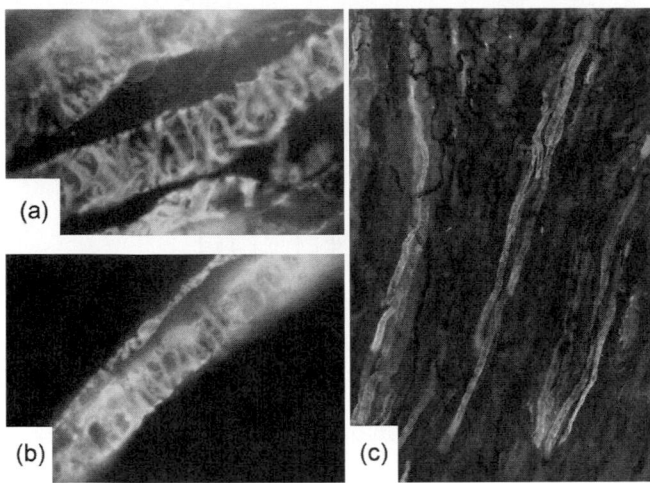

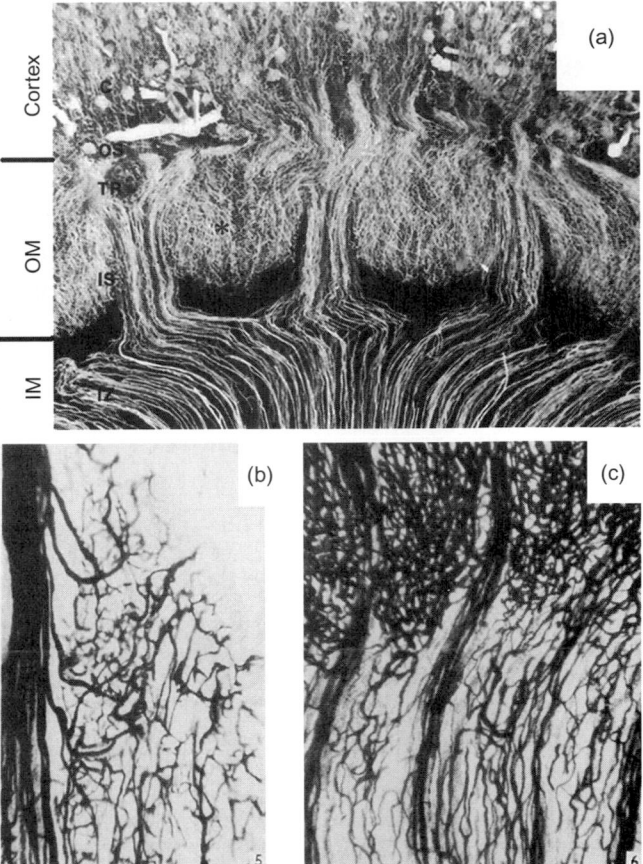

FIGURE 24.6 Distribution of descending vasa recta pericytes. (a) (b) Immunofluorescent staining of DVR pericytes using anti α-smooth muscle actin as primary antibody. The pericytes are present on DVR from outer medullary vascular bundles (Panel a), and those from the inner medulla (Panel b) (×1000). (c) Low power image of immunofluorescent staining of DVR pericytes using anti α-smooth muscle actin antibody. Some vessels show pericytes throughout their length to the papillary tip. Black vessels are filled with Indian ink (×100). *(Reproduced with permission from ref. [28]).*

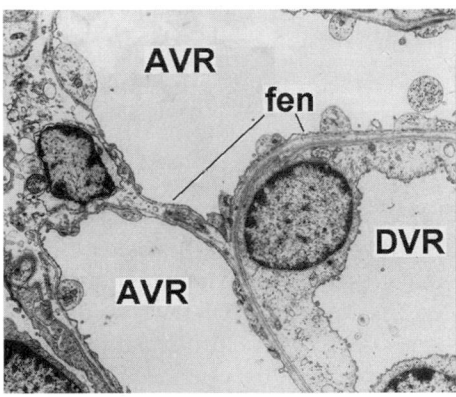

FIGURE 24.7 Electron micrograph of DVR and AVR. Electron micrograph of DVR and AVR in rat vascular bundles. DVR have a continuous endothelium and AVR are fenestrated. Note the minimal interstitium that exists between vessels in this region (×12,400). *(Reproduced with permission from ref. [111]).*

FIGURE 24.8 Arterial injection of *Psammomys obesus*. (a) Photograph of the microvasculature of the desert rodent *Psammomys obesus* obtained by injecting the arteries of the kidney with Microfil and digesting the tissue. The distinct arteriolar patterns of the cortex, outer, and inner medulla are apparent. In *Psammomys*, the separation of the outer medulla into vascular bundles and the dense capillary plexus of the interbundle region (*) is striking, because vasa recta coalesce into giant vascular bundles (OM: outer medulla; IM: inner medulla). Designations on the original figure are: c: cortex; TR: transitional region (outer stripe of the outer medulla); IS: inner stripe of the outer medulla; IZ: inner zone (inner medulla). *(Reproduced with permission from ref. [5]).* (b),(c) Indian ink injection study of vascular bundles in the outer medulla of the rat. In contrast to *Psammomys*, individual vascular bundles do not coalesce into giant bundles. The bundles are more evenly dispersed throughout the inner stripe of the outer medulla. This pattern is typical of many mammalian species including the rat, mouse and human. *(Reproduced with permission from ref. [790]).*

juxtamedullary efferent arteriole to DVR and then AVR, single vessel flow rate falls as overall microvessel cross-sectional area increases.[17,31,34−36] The latter increases transit time, presumably to favor greater equilibration of solute concentrations between AVR blood and interstitium. Outer medullary vascular bundles have little interstitial space. In contrast, the fraction of medullary cross-section attributable to interstitium rises substantially toward the deepest regions of the inner medulla, particularly near the papillary tip.[17,20,37] In some species, renal medullary interstitial cells (RMIC) of the inner medulla appear to be tethered between thin limbs of

Henle and vasa recta[20,25,36] (Figure 24.10). It is likely that the horizontal arrangement of RMIC helps to preserve corticomedullary solute gradients by limiting axial diffusion along the medulla.[20,38] RMIC have receptors for vasoactive peptides such as angiotensin II, bradykinin, and endothelin. In addition, they release vasoactive agents such as PGE_2 and medullipin. RMIC are contractile and respond to various paracrine factors.[39−42]

Three-dimensional computer reconstructions of images derived from immunostained serial sections have yielded insight into relationships between tubules,

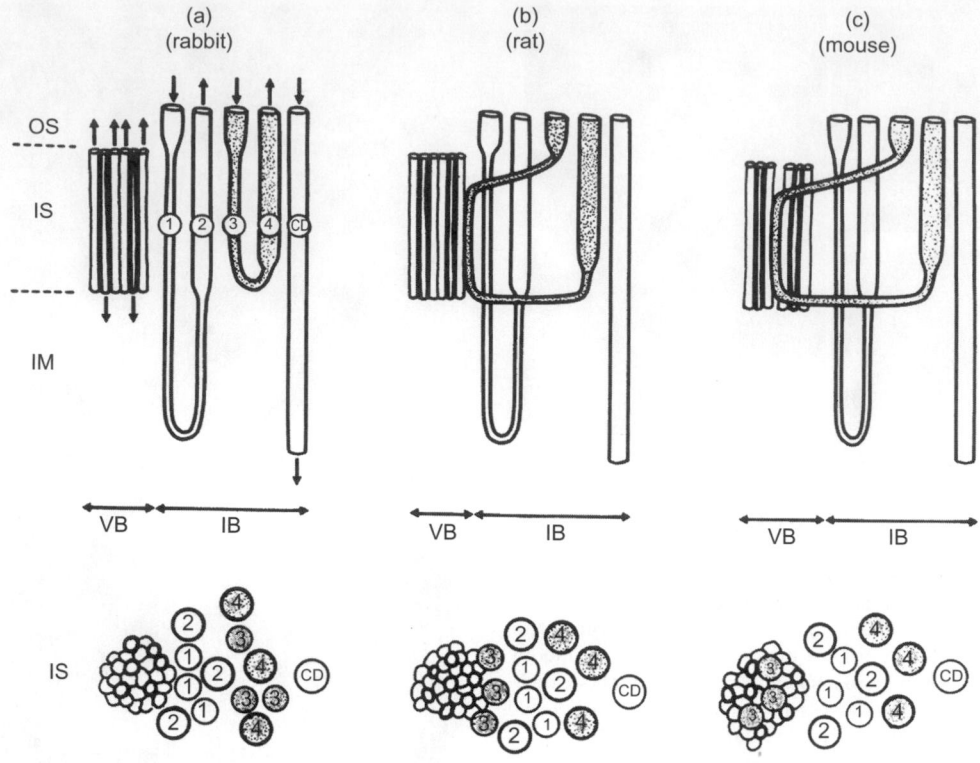

FIGURE 24.9   Tubular-vascular relationships in the outer medulla. Organization of the inner stripe of the outer medulla. Top and bottom panels show longitudinal and cross-sectional views, respectively. The extent to which the thin descending limbs (tDLH) of short looped nephrons associate with vascular bundles varies between species. In the rabbit (a) no association exists, whereas in the rat (b) and mouse (c), the tDLH migrates to the periphery or becomes incorporated within vascular bundles, respectively (Abbreviations: VB: vascular bundle; IB: interbundle region; 1 and 2: thin descending and thick ascending limbs of long looped nephrons; 3 and 4: thin descending and thick ascending limbs of short looped nephrons.) *(Reproduced with permission from ref. [4]).*

collecting ducts, and the vasculature in rats and mice.[25,32,43–46] Specifically, collecting ducts (CD), descending thin limbs of Henle (DLH), ascending thin limbs of Henle (ALH), descending vasa recta (DVR), and ascending vasa recta (AVR) are identified by their respective expression of aquaporin 2 (AQP2), aquaporin 1 (AQP1), chloride channel (ClCK1), urea transporter type B (UTB), and the fenestral protein, PV-1. Thin DLH frequently lack AQP1 expression, and are identified as thin limbs lacking ClCK1 but expressing α,β-crystallin, an antigen that is present along the entire loop of Henle.[47,48] Thin DLH include an entirely AQP1-null group that turns early in the inner medulla, and longer limbs that are AQP1-positive for the first ~40% of their length; the latter turn to form thin ALH within deeper regions of the inner medulla. More than 50% of the AQP1-positive DLH also express ClC-K1. AQP1-positive segments have semilunar cell bodies that regularly jut into the lumen.[49] Murine tubulovascular relationships in the outer medulla may exhibit an important characteristic, in that some thick ascending limbs of long looped nephrons may lie within vascular bundles. In that species, short looped thin DLH are known to be incorporated into the more peripheral parts of vascular bundles.[4,20,26,32]

Pannabecker and colleagues have described clustering of collecting ducts that eventually coalesce to form single large collecting ducts in the deep medulla (Figure 24.11). The tubules and vessels that surround the collecting duct clusters occupy structured patterns.[43,46–48] DVR and DLH occupy regions outside the clusters, while AVR and ALH are diffusely distributed both within the central regions of the CD clusters and throughout the surrounding inner medulla. Within clusters, four AVR abut individual CDs.[25] AVR closely approach the CD wall and appear to be tethered to it. That arrangement may be critical to vascular reabsorption in the medulla, allowing interstitial pressure to exceed AVR luminal pressure without inducing collapse.[38,50,51] The implications of those tubulovascular relationships have been examined in mathematical simulations.[52–55] The organization of the outer medulla into vascular bundles and the peribundle region enhances the delivery of high osmolality fluid to the inner medulla by long looped DLH and CD. Reduction of the number of DVR that reach the inner–outer medullary junction is predicted to favor enhancement of urinary concentration, as is a high AVR solute permeability. The striking observation of thick ascending limbs of Henle within vascular bundles

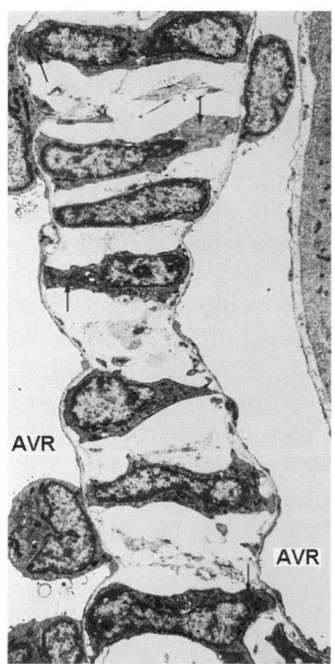

FIGURE 24.10   Renal medullary interstitial cells (RMIC). RMIC from the rat kidney appear to be tethered between thin limbs and vasa recta in the inner medulla. Interstitial spaces lie between the cells, and the cells are stacked like rungs of a ladder. RMIC are contractile and secrete vasoactive paracrine agents (see text). The stacked arrangement or RMICs in some species has been suggested to help retard axial diffusion that would otherwise tend to dissipate cortico-medullary gradients of NaCl and urea (V: venous or ascending vasa recta; Arrows point to lipid droplets within RMIC). *(Reproduced with permission from ref. [20]).*

of the mouse[32] may have important implications for urinary concentration, because sodium chloride reabsorption from those structures might raise vicinal osmolality to favor water uptake from AQP1-expressing DVR, thereby concentrating their contents en route to the inner medulla.

TRANSPORT FUNCTIONS AND PROPERTIES

The Renal Cortex and Capillary Uptake of Tubular Reabsorbate

Cortical peritubular capillaries are fenestrated, have a large surface area and high hydraulic conductivity. It is generally accepted that fluid is driven into the cortical interstitium from the PCT due to the generation of a locally hypertonic fluid within the lateral intercellular space between PCT epithelial cells. The local hypertonicity results from the secretion of small hydrophilic solutes by proximal tubular cells. Dilution of the interstitium in the vicinity of the capillary wall with protein-free fluid both lowers interstitial oncotic pressure and

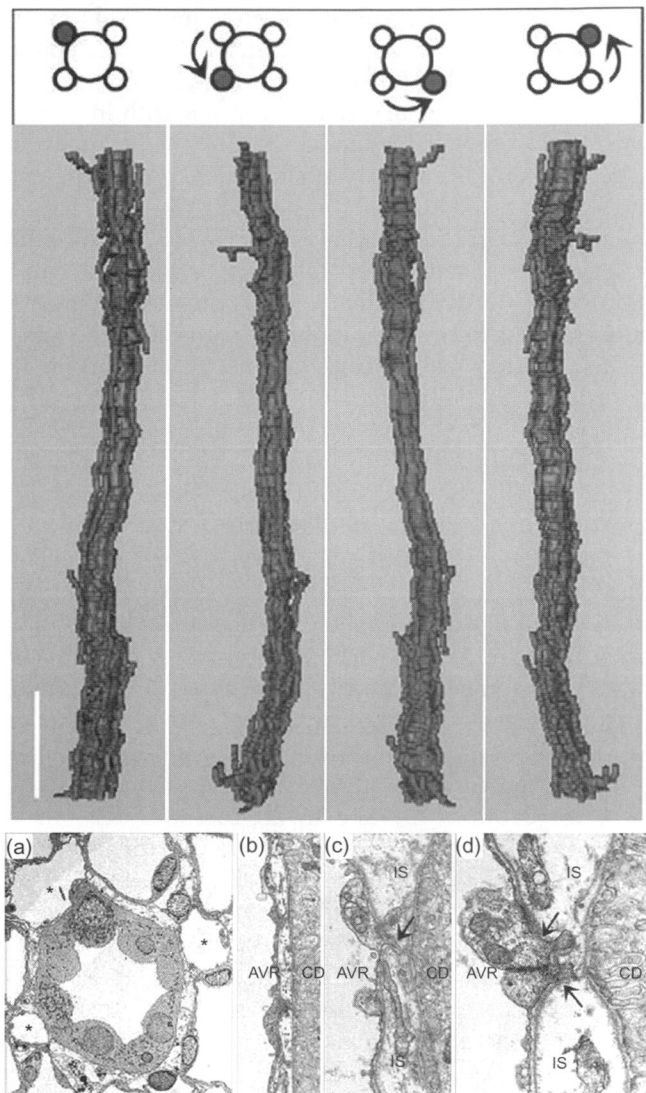

FIGURE 24.11   Relationship between vasa recta and collecting duct clusters. Upper panel: A single collecting duct (blue) with adjacent AVR (red) is shown in four 90° rotated views (Bar = 100 microns). Lower panel: (a–c) Electron micrographs of sections through a collecting duct (CD) and adjacent AVR, demonstrating the close apposition and interstitial space (IS). (d) Close approximation of AVR and CD where the two appear to be tethered with microvilli (arrows). *(Reproduced with permission from ref. [25]).* See color plate section at the back of the book.

raises interstitial hydraulic pressure. These effects generate Starling forces that favor capillary reabsorption.

A substantial body of evidence has demonstrated that modulation of cortical peritubular capillary oncotic pressure alters PCT reabsorption. Intra-aortic injection or peritubular perfusion of colloid free or hyperoncotic fluid leads to decreases or increases proximal reabsorption, respectively.[56-58] While it seems inviting to surmise that protein oncotic pressure acts directly to enhance fluid movement out of the PCT, several lines of evidence suggest otherwise. Oncotic pressure changes fail to modulate reabsorption when active transport by PCT epithelia is inhibited,[59] PCT reabsorption rates correlate with GFR (glomerulotubular balance) but not with interstitial Starling forces,[60] hydropenia blunts the capacity of hyperoncotic albumin to enhance PCT reabsorption,[61] and elevation of luminal pressure in the PCT fails to enhance reabsorption.[62] The osmotic water permeability of the proximal convoluted tubule ($P_f = 0.1 - 0.4$ cm/s) is probably too low for small oncotic pressure changes to substantially affect transmembrane water flux.[63,64] It has been suggested that peritubular oncotic pressure might modulate PCT volume reabsorption by affecting solute reabsorption rate[65,66] or by enhancing paracellular backleak into the PCT lumen.[67] More recently, attention has turned to mechanosensation of luminal shear forces as a transducer of glomerulotubular balance.[68–70]

Whatever mechanisms converge to influence PCT reabsorption it is immense, and its removal from the interstitium is the task of the cortical microcirculation. Since lymphatics remove less than 1% of the reabsorbate,[71] the route for return to the systemic circulation must be via peritubular capillaries. As reviewed by Aukland et al., the high oncotic pressure of postglomerular plasma cannot be invoked as the primary driving force for capillary uptake in all cases. Older rats in which renal lymphatic (and therefore presumably interstitial) protein concentration is equal to that of plasma continue to reabsorb tubular fluid.[18,71] Furthermore, PCT reabsorption occurs even in kidneys perfused with colloid free solutions.[72] Particularly in the latter case, it is apparent that interstitial pressure must exceed intracapillary luminal pressure to provide the driving force for transcapillary volume flux. It also follows that the peritubular capillaries must be tethered to the interstitium in a way that prevents an inwardly directed transmural pressure from collapsing the lumen.

The Renal Medulla and Countercurrent Exchange

Like the capillary bed of other organs, the renal medullary microcirculation supplies oxygen and nutrients to the surrounding tissue. Additionally, however, corticomedullary gradients of NaCl and urea must be preserved to enable urinary concentration. This task is accommodated by countercurrent exchange between DVR and AVR.[17,31,73,74] Countercurrent exchange is an adaptation found throughout nature. The maintenance of high gas tensions in swim bladders of deep sea fish, and the minimization of heat loss from the extremities of aquatic and arctic animals relies upon this strategy.[31,75]

The microcirculation of the renal medulla traps NaCl and urea deposited to the interstitium by the loops of Henle and collecting ducts. Countercurrent exchange provides the means by which blood flow through the medulla is concentrated and then diluted to preserve corticomedullary solute gradients established by countercurrent multiplication. The hypothesis that vasa recta are a purely "U-tube" diffusive countercurrent exchanger implies the following function. NaCl and urea diffuse from interstitium into DVR plasma en route from the corticomedullary junction toward the papillary tip. The solutes diffuse out from AVR plasma to be returned to the interstitium as blood returns to the cortex. That theory predicts that countercurrent exchanger efficiency will be enhanced if permeability to solute is high.

In fact, vasa recta probably do not function as a purely diffusive countercurrent exchanger. Several features point to greater complexity. Tubulovascular relationships in the outer and inner medulla differ markedly (Figures 24.1, 24.9, 24.11), and the endothelium of DVR and AVR are continuous and fenestrated, respectively (Figure 24.7). The discoveries of aquaporin-1 (AQP1) water channels and the facilitated urea carrier, UTB, in DVR endothelia (see below) shows that transcellular as well as paracellular pathways involving water and urea are involved in equilibration of DVR plasma with the interstitium. Efflux of water across the DVR wall to the medullary interstitium occurs across AQP1 water channels, and AQP1 excludes NaCl and urea implying that both water removal and diffusive influx of solute contribute to transmural equilibration.[31,76–78] Expression of AQP1 within the vasculature has been found to vary with axial location, greater in those DVR that turn in the outer portion of the inner medulla.[45,46]

Transport of Small Solutes and Water by Vasa Recta and Red Blood Cells

Transport of Water across the DVR Wall: Small Solutes, Osmotic Pressure, and Starling Forces

Mass balance dictates that water, NaCl, and urea must be removed from the medullary interstitium at a rate that equals deposition by the loops of Henle and collecting tubules.[17,79] Papillary micropuncture studies in the hydropenic rat[80] and hamster[81,82] have shown that DVR and AVR plasma osmolality rises in parallel with tubular fluid from the loops of Henle and collecting ducts. DVR plasma protein also becomes concentrated along the direction of flow, implying that water is lost from DVR lumen to the interstitium (Table 24.1, Figure 24.1).[83,84] Uptake of fluid into AVR exceeds that lost from DVR, accounting for mass balance in the medulla.[15,85–88] Volume efflux from the DVR occurs despite an intracapillary oncotic pressure that exceeds hydraulic pressure, so that "Starling forces" cannot fully explain transmural volume efflux. According to Starling, volume flux (J_v) across a

TABLE 24.1 Vasa Recta Plasma Protein Concentration, Hydraulic and Oncotic Pressures Measured in Rats and Hamsters

Location	VR/P	Cp (g/dl)	Oncotic Pressure (mmHg)	Hydraulic Pressure (mmHg)	Osmolality (mOsm)	Condition (Reference)
DVR-base	1.76	7.1	26.0	9.2		Hydropenia
DVR-tip	—	—	—	—		83
AVR-base	1.38	5.6	18.1	7.8		
DVR-base	1.43	7.1	26.0	6.6	688	Hydropenia
DVR-tip	1.66	6.4	21.8	7.4	759	84
AVR-base	—	—	—	—		
DVR-base	1.0 to 1.8[a]					Hydropenia
DVR-tip	2.1 to 2.9					87
DVR-base	1.42	5.1	16.0	—		Hydropenia
DVR-tip	—	—	—	—		88
AVR-base	1.11	4.0	11.2	—		
DVR-base				15.7		Hydropenia
DVR-tip				11.4		429
AVR-base				10.2		
DVR-base	1.08	5.2	16.7	9.5	573	Hydropenia
DVR-tip	1.42	6.8	18.2	9.1	1011	86
AVR-base	—	—	—	—	—	
DVR-base	1.10	5.4	17.6	12.2	356	Furosemide
DVR-tip	1.12	5.5	18.2	11.2	377	86
AVR-base	—	—	—	—	—	
DVR-base	1.19	5.7	18.6	11.7	380	Furosemide
DVR-tip	—	—	—	11.2	386	187
AVR-base	1.17	5.6	18.4	9.6	—	
AVR-mid		5.2	16.7	8.0		Hydropenia
AVR-mid		5.2	16.7	16.0		Furosemide
						143
DVR-mid				9.1 to 15.5[b]		Plasma/ANP[c]
AVR-mid				7.8 to 14.3		Plasma/ANP
DVR-mid				8.4 to 10.8		Plasma/Furosemide
AVR-mid				7.8 to 10.0		Plasma/Furosemide
						792

[a]Ratio measured from ^{131}I-albumin activity.
[b]Values refer to changes before and after administration of either ANP or furosemide.
[b]Measured after replacement of surgical fluid losses with plasma.
Abbreviations: VR/P: vasa recta to plasma ratio; Cp: plasma protein concentration; DVR: descending vasa recta; AVR: ascending vasa recta; base, mid, tip, micropuncture site along exposed papilla (inner 1/3 of the inner medulla, blood flows from base to tip in DVR and tip to base in AVR); ANP: atrial natriuretic peptide.

capillary wall is a function of capillary (P_c) and interstitial hydraulic pressure (P_i), and luminal (π_c) and interstitial (π_i) oncotic pressure.[89]

$$J_V = L_P[(P_c - P_i) - (\pi_c - \pi_i)] \tag{24.1}$$

where L_p is the hydraulic conductivity. In order to explain volume efflux from the DVR in a manner compatible with Eq. (24.1), a negative interstitial hydraulic pressure or very high interstitial oncotic pressure has to be postulated. In either of those cases, however, interstitial driving forces would prevent volume uptake by AVR violating mass balance. Neither possibility can be the explanation.[17,84,90]

Due to the lag in equilibration of DVR plasma with the interstitium, NaCl and urea concentrations in the interstitium exceed those in DVR so that a transendothelial osmotic gradient favors water efflux across the DVR wall. That driving force could account for water efflux only if there is a transendothelial pathway across which small solutes are effective to drive water movement.[84] Volume flux across a membrane can be simulated by Eq. (24.2) that accounts for osmotic reflection coefficients (σ) to individual solutes. In the current context, small solutes (σ_{ss}) and proteins (σ_{pr}) are of importance, leading to[91]:

$$J_V = L_P[\Delta P - \sigma_{pr}\Delta\pi_{pr} - \sigma_{ss}\Delta\pi_{ss}] \tag{24.2}$$

where ΔP is transmembrane hydraulic pressure, and $\Delta\pi_{pr}$ and $\Delta\pi_{ss}$ are the transmembrane osmotic pressure due to protein and small solutes, respectively.[84] The hypothesis that small solutes act to promote volume movement across the DVR is equivalent to postulating that $\sigma_{ss} > 0$. Support for this was readily obtained. Volume efflux from DVR was prevented by elimination of corticomedullary (and therefore transendothelial) NaCl and urea gradients by furosemide,[86] and *in vivo* microperfusion of DVR with buffers made hypertonic or hypotonic to the papillary interstitium generated volume uptake or efflux, respectively ($\sigma_{NaCl} > 0$).[92]

DVR Hydraulic Conductivity and Osmotic Water Permeability

The predominant pathway that conducts water efflux across the DVR is the AQP1 water channel. AQP1 but not other aquaporins are expressed by DVR endothelia.[36,45,93,94] *Diffusional* water permeability (P_D) of isolated, microperfused DVR, measured by efflux of ^3H_2O, was reduced by the AQP1 blocking mercurial agent p-chloromercuribenzene sulfonate (pCMBS). Dramatic confirmation was provided by the demonstration that *osmotic* water permeability (P_f) of microperfused DVR, measured by driving water flux with transmural gradients of NaCl, was driven from $\sim 1100\ \mu m/s$ to nearly zero by pCMBS (Figure 24.12a).

In contrast, when albumin rather than NaCl was used to drive water flux, P_f was much higher, $\sim 16,700\ \mu m/s$ and insensitive to pCMBS, implying that a different pathway conducts transmural volume flux driven by oncotic pressure.[77,78] The results support the notion that NaCl and urea drive water flux across the DVR wall exclusively through AQP1 (contribution to total transmural water conductivity is $P_f \sim 1100\ \mu m/s$), while hydraulic pressure and oncotic pressure drive most water flux through a high conductivity parallel pathway (paracellular or other). Mathematically, the AQP1 and parallel pathways are best stimulated as[85,95]:

$$J_{V,P} = L_{P,P}[\Delta P - \sigma_{pr}\Delta\pi_{pr}] \text{ and, } J_{V,C} = L_{P,C}[\Delta P - \textstyle\sum_i \Delta\pi_i] \tag{24.3a, b}$$

where the additional subscript "P" (probably pericellular) refers to the high conductivity pathway for which $\sigma_{NaCl} = \sigma_{urea} = 0$,[96] and the subscript "C" refers to the transcellular AQP1 pathway for which $\sigma_{NaCl} = \sigma_{urea} = 1$. Hydraulic conductivity (Lp) and osmotic water permeability (P_f) are related according to Lp = ($P_f \times V_w$)/(RT), where V_W is the partial molar volume of water. Existing measurements of DVR osmotic water permeability are summarized in Table 24.2. A rigorous discussion of the measurement of, and relationships between, these transport parameters has been provided.[78,96]

The AQP1 knockout mouse provided additional confirmation of the role of AQP1 in DVR water transport. P_f of DVR in AQP1 knockout mice, driven by NaCl, was indeed very low (Figure 24.12b). An intriguing finding was that urea and larger solutes (raffinose, MW 594, glucose, MW[97]) drive significant water flux despite AQP1 deletion, a finding that implies the existence of a non-AQP1 route across which those solutes are osmotically active. A potential candidate for the non-AQP1, pCMBS insensitive pathway is the UTB urea transporter (see below) which is expressed by the DVR endothelium and can function as a water channel.[98–102]

Insights from Modeling: AQP1 and the Enhancement of Exchanger Efficiency

Mathematical models of urinary concentration have played an important role in the evolution of our understanding. Simulation of both nephrons and the microcirculation is difficult, so that investigators prefer to account for one while neglecting the other. Vasa recta models typically assume specified corticomedullary solute concentrations, and simulate transport properties of the vessel wall. Wang and Michel revised this approach by specifying the rate of deposition of NaCl, urea, and water to the medullary interstitium as though they are generated within the interstitium. In agreement with electron probe measurements, they predicted an exponential increase in corticomedullary solute

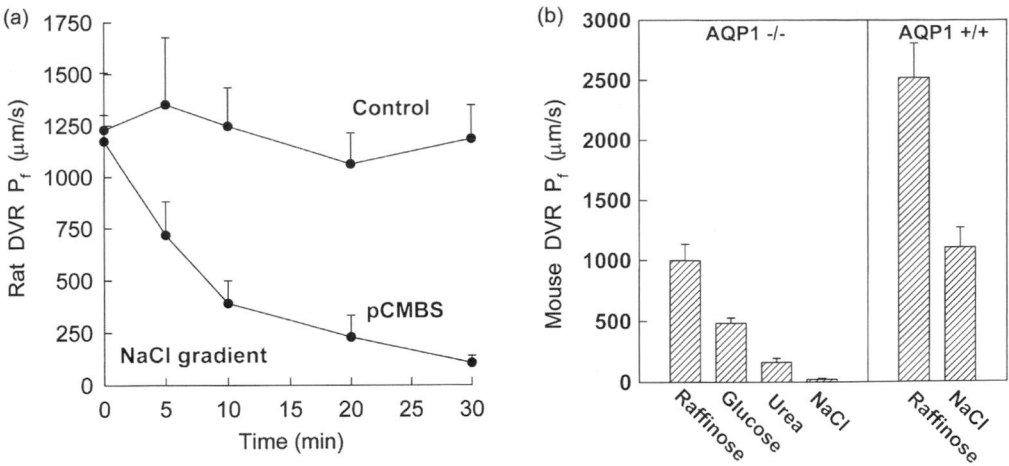

FIGURE 24.12   Osmotic water permeability (P_f) of outer medullary DVR. (a) Pf was measured in glutaraldehyde-fixed rat DVR by measuring the rate of transmural water flux generated by a bath > lumen NaCl gradient. Sequential measurements in controls were stable. In contrast, exposure to p-chloromercuribenzene sulfonate (pCMBS, 2 mM), an agent that covalently binds to cysteine residues on aquaporin-1, reduced Pf to nearly zero. In these experiments, glutaraldehyde fixation was necessary to prevent deterioration of the vessel caused by pCMBS and other harsh conditions of the experiment. (b) Pf was measured in AQP1-null($^{-/-}$) or replete($^{+/+}$) murine DVR by transmural gradients of NaCl, urea, glucose or raffinose. When NaCl was the solute used to drive water flux, deletion of AQP1 reduced Pf from $\sim$1100 μm/s to nearly zero. Water flux driven by raffinose (MW 564) was markedly reduced by AQP1deletion (compare AQP1$^{-/-}$ to $^{+/+}$), but remained unexpectedly high. Similarly, glucose (MW 180) and urea (MW 60) gradients drove measurable water flux across AQP1($^{-/-}$) DVR. *(Reproduced with permission from ref. [76,77]).*

TABLE 24.2   Hydraulic Conductivity, Osmotic Water Permeability and Solute Reflection Coefficients of Vasa Recta

Parameter	Driving Force	OMDVR	IMDVR	IMAVR	Reference
$L_p \times 10^{-613}$ (cm•s^{-780}•mmHg^{-780})	Albumin Gradient		1.4[a]		187
$L_p \times 10^{-613}$ (cm•s^{-780}•mmHg^{-780})	Albumin Gradient	1.6			96
$L_p \times 10^{-613}$ (cm•s^{-780}•mmHg^{-780})	NaCl Gradient	0.12[b]			76,77
$L_p \times 10^{-613}$ (cm•s^{-780}•mmHg^{-780})	Hydraulic Pressure			12.5	50,92

Parameter	Method	OMDVR	IMDVR	IMAVR	Reference
$\sigma_{albumin}$	Sieving	0.89[c]			96
$\sigma_{albumin}$	Sieving			0.78	128
$\sigma_{albumin}$	Osmotic			0.70	50
σ_{Na}	Osmotic		<0.05[d]	0.00[d]	92,129
σ_{Na}	Osmotic	$\sim$0.03[d]			78
σ_{Na}	Sieving	$\sim$1.0[e]			78
$\sigma_{Raffinose}$	Sieving	$\sim$1.0[e]			78

[a]*Assumes a reflection coefficient to albumin of 1.0.*
[b]*Evidence shows that transmural NaCl gradients drive water flux exclusively through water channels, whereas albumin drives water flux predominantly through water channels along with a small component via other pathway(s), see text and references.[77,78,96]*
[c]*Not significantly different from 1.0.*
[d]*Measurement of σ_{Na} for the vessel wall as a whole.*
[e]*σ_{Na}, $\sigma_{Raffinose}$ for the putative aquaporin 1 water channel pathway through which NaCl gradients drive water flux, see text and references [77,78].*

concentration in the medulla.[103–105] A weakness of models that neglect simulation of loops of Henle and collecting ducts is that solute generation rates in the interstitium are assigned as inputs and interstitial solute concentrations calculated as predictions. Variations of blood flow and transport properties cannot affect the interstitial appearance of NaCl, urea, and water from nephrons as would occur *in vivo*. Convincing evidence has been provided that structure and properties of nephrons can abruptly vary with medullary depth.[28,40,49,106,107]

Many key parameters needed to simulate microvascular exchange in the renal medulla (solute permeabilities, reflection coefficients, hydraulic conductivities) have been measured. That data has been combined with more complete simulations of transcellular pathways for urea and water transport to perform additional simulations. The models predict that AQP1 might play an important role to raise medullary interstitial osmolality by driving water efflux from DVR to the medullary interstitium across AQP1 water channels (see above); that water movement effectively shunts DVR plasma volume to the AVR reducing blood flow to the deep medulla; and that favors high diffusive exchanger efficiency in the deep inner medulla where urea is added to the interstitium from the collecting duct. Stated another way, it reduces the lag in equilibration that leads to solute "washout" from the deep medulla.[76,108,109] The net effect is to enhance interstitial osmolality (Figure 24.13). Interest in this intriguing prediction is heightened by the observation that transmural water flux can be driven across the wall of AQP1-null mice by solutes other than NaCl (Figure 24.12b). If the non-AQP1 pathway is important *in vivo*, it might also enhance shunting of water from DVR to AVR.[31,76,108]

Transport of Small Hydrophilic Solutes across the DVR Wall

It is likely that the majority of NaCl and urea equilibration across the DVR wall occurs by diffusive influx. AQP1 contributes to the process of equilibration through molecular sieving. Evidence supports the notion that small hydrophilic solutes (NaCl, urea) diffuse through the same "shared" pathway that conducts the component of water flux driven by Starling forces, because DVR permeability to tracers (^{22}Na, ^{36}Cl, ^{3}Hraffinose, ^{14}Cinulin) correlate with each other and hydraulic conductivity.[31,96,110,111] Urea transport across the DVR wall is more complicated, because it diffuses both via paracellular and transcellular routes. A summary of available solute diffusive permeability measurements is provided in Table 24.3.

Facilitated Transport of Urea across DVR and RBCs

Transmural flux of urea across the DVR wall is complicated, because DVR endothelia express a facilitated

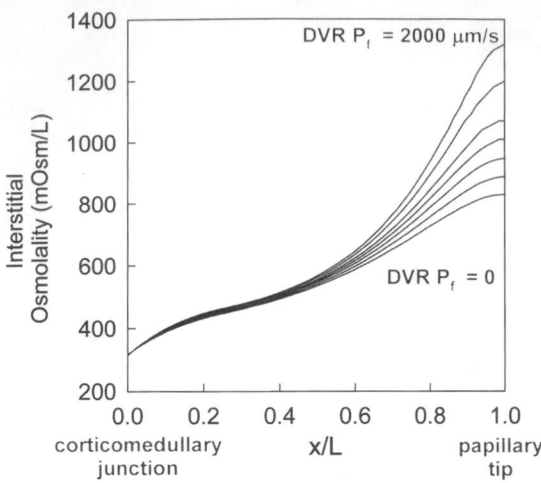

FIGURE 24.13   Effect of AQP1 deletion on predictions of renal medullary interstitial osmolality. A mathematical simulation of the renal medulla was solved to predict interstitial osmolality. Interstitial osmolality is shown as a function of corticomedullary axis ($x/L = 0$ is the corticomedullary junction; $x/L = 1$ is the papillary tip). Various curves denote predictions for different values of Pf (DVR osmotic water permeability). Pf was varied between 0 (equivalent to AQP1 deletion) and 2000 μm/s. AQP1 expression in DVR is predicted to enhance concentrating ability by conducting water flux from DVR to interstitium where after it is taken up by AVR. The net result is a secondary reduction of blood flow in the deepest regions of the inner medulla (papillary tip). *(Reproduced with permission from ref. [76]).*

urea carrier.[112,113] Sodium and urea have similar free water diffusivity, and are therefore expected to have the same transvessel permeability if they diffuse, sterically unrestricted, through a large pore. In contrast to this, some outer medullary DVR have low or moderate P_{Na} but high P_U (Figure 24.14). DVR permeability to ^{14}C urea can be partially inhibited by phloretin, pCMBS, and structural analogs of urea, verifying the presence of an endothelial carrier.[111,112] Histochemical evidence and *in situ* hybridization studies have shown that the DVR urea carrier is the same as that in the RBC (urea transporter type B, UTB), and is distinct from the urea carrier in the thin limbs of Henle (UTA2) and collecting duct (UTA1, UTA3, UTA4).[100,114–118]

Rat UTB carries the Kidd blood group antigen, has 62% identity to UTA2, and is expressed in RBCs, DVR endothelium, papillary surface, and pelvic epithelium of the kidney.[100,119] The presence of UTB in the DVR endothelium and RBCs facilitates medullary urea recycling. Urea tends to exit the renal medulla in AVR plasma and RBCs. To prevent associated dissipation of corticomedullary urea gradients, urea recycles from AVR into DVR plasma and RBCs via UTB, and into thin limbs of Henle via UTA2 (Figure 24.15). Those processes are highly evolved in the outer medullary inner stripe where DVR and AVR are closely

TABLE 24.3 Diffusional Permeability of Vasa Recta to Hydrophilic Solutes

Permeability $\times 10^{-590}$ cm/s	Species	OMDVR[a]	IMDVR[b]	IMAVR[b]	Reference
P_{Na}	Hamster		28	51	35
P_{Na}	Rat	76	75	115	111
P_{Na}	Rat		67	116	92,129
P_{Na}	Mouse	207–314			76
P_{Urea}	Rat		47		130
P_{Urea}	Rat	360	76	121	111
P_{Urea}	Rat	$343 \rightarrow 191$[c]			112
P_{Urea}	Mouse	661[d]			76
P_D	Rat	476[e]			93,110
$P_{raffinose}$	Rat	40			110,96
$P_{raffinose}$	Mouse	80, 111[d]			76

Permeability Ratio	Species	OMDVR[a]	IMDVR[b]	IMAVR[b]	Reference
P_{Urea}/P_{Na}	Rat	4.7	1.1	0.98	76,110,111
	Mouse[d]	3.2			
P_{Cl}/P_{Na}	Rat	1.3			
$P_{raffinose}/P_{Na}$	Rat	0.35			
	Mouse	0.35, 0.39[d]			
P_{Inulin}/P_{Na}	Rat	0.22			
	Mouse	0.31[d]			

[a]*Values obtained with* in vitro *microperfusion are highly dependent upon perfusion rate, see text and references* [77,110,96].
[b]*Values obtained with* in vivo *microperfusion in the exposed papilla, probably underestimated due to boundary layer effects, see text.*
[c]*Values are before and after inhibition with 50 mM thiourea.*
[d]*Value from DVR of AQP1 null mice.*[76]
[e]*Diffusional water permeability measured with* ^3H_2O *efflux.*
Abbreviations: OMDVR: outer medullary descending vasa recta; IMDVR: inner medullary descending vasa recta; IMAVR: inner medullary ascending vasa recta.

positioned in vascular bundles. Many water-conserving species also incorporate UTA2 expressing thin limbs of Henle within or on the periphery of vascular bundles[5,6,15,24,26] (Figure 24.9). Interesting insights into function have been obtained from the study of UTB-null mice. UTB deficiency results in reduced urinary concentrating ability, reduced urea clearance, and an increased plasma urea concentration.[100,114,118] In contrast to wild-type mice, infusion of urea into UTB-null animals fails to enhance urinary concentrating ability.[114] Acute regulation of UTB by vasopressin or other factors has not been demonstrated. In contrast to upregulation of UTA transporters,[119] chronic vasopressin treatment may reduce UTB expression.[99,120] UTB expression in the renal medulla increases during osmotic diuresis induced by urea, but not NaCl or glucose infusion.[121] In contrast, UTB expression is depressed by ureteral obstruction, lithium treatment, potassium deficiency, and cyclosporine toxicity.[122–125]

UTB expression in RBCs should limit AQP1-mediated water transport and the associated osmotic shrinking and swelling that would otherwise accompany RBC transit through the medulla. Macey and Yousef proposed that this might prevent osmotic lysis.[126] Against this hypothesis is the finding that humans devoid of Kidd antigen have mildly depressed urinary concentrating ability, but no hemolytic anemia. It seems most likely that RBC expression of UTB serves to increase the overall mass of urea that is efficiently recycled from the AVR and DVR lumens in the renal inner medulla.[98,100,102]

Transport of Solutes and Water across the AVR Wall

Transport of solutes and water in AVR has not been as thoroughly evaluated as that in DVR, because AVR cannot be isolated for *in vitro* microperfusion. Measurements of AVR transport properties have been performed by *in vivo* micropuncture and microperfusion of vessels on the surface of the exposed papilla (inner

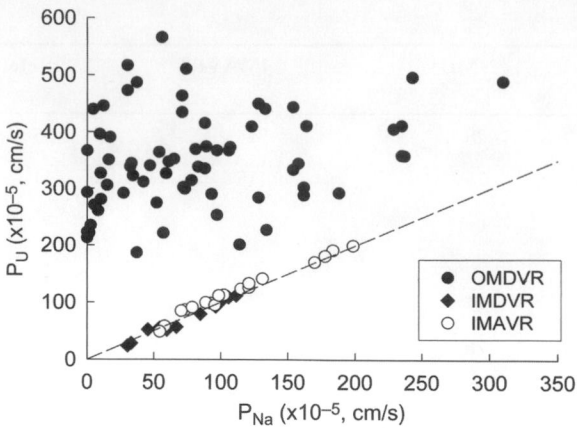

FIGURE 24.14 Vasa recta solute permeabilities. [^{14}C]urea permeability (P_U, ordinate) versus ^{22}Na permeability (P_{Na}: abscissa) is shown for outer medullary DVR (OMDVR) isolated from Sprague-Dawley rats and perfused *in vitro*. Results are also shown for inner medullary DVR and AVR (IMDVR, IMAVR) perfused on the surface of the exposed papilla of Munich-Wistar rats *in vivo*. The dashed line is identity. P_U and P_{Na} are highly correlated and nearly equal in inner medullary vasa recta. In contrast, P_U of outer medullary DVR is always very high and is not correlated with P_{Na}. The dissociation of P_{Na} and P_U in OMDVR results (at least in part) from the expression of the UTB facilitated urea carrier. In separate experiments (not shown), P_U of OMDVR was inhibited by exposure to urea analogs or phloretin. *(Data reproduced with permission from ref. [111]).*

third of the inner medulla) of rats. Some reliable measurements of AVR hydraulic conductivity (Lp) have been obtained. Consistent with the highly fenestrated endothelium, Lp is high, about 12.5×10^{-613} cm/(s•mmHg) ($P_f = 13.4$ cm/s).[50,127] The reflection coefficient of the AVR wall to albumin has been measured by molecular sieving[128] and by osmosis.[50] Mean values of 0.78 and 0.70 were obtained, respectively. A summary of AVR hydraulic conductivity and reflection coefficient measurements is provided in Table 24.2.

When blood ascends toward the cortex in AVR it encounters decreasing NaCl and urea concentrations, so that luminal osmolality exceeds that of the adjacent interstitium. Perfusing AVR *in vivo* with buffers made hypertonic or hypotonic to the papillary interstitium with NaCl generated no measurable water flux, suggesting that, for the AVR wall, $\sigma_{SS} = 0$ (Eq. (24.2)).[129] Transmural AVR NaCl and urea gradients *in vivo* are likely to be smaller than those in DVR, because AVR blood flow rates are lower. AVR are larger in diameter and more numerous than DVR.[34,35,88] Consequently, high permeability, high surface area, and an increased transit time of blood all favor a high degree of equilibration between AVR plasma and interstitium.[90,95]

Vasa recta diffusional solute permeabilities, measured in the rat[129,130] and hamster,[35] are higher than those in DVR (Table 24.3). Even so, AVR permeabilities

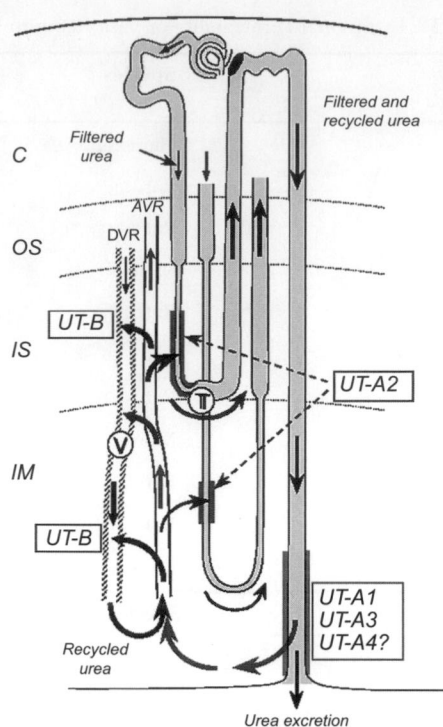

FIGURE 24.15 UTB and urea recycling in the medulla. Schematic of vascular and tubular urea recycling in the kidney. Short and long loops of Henle and vasa recta are shown. The UTA2 urea transporter is expressed in the thin descending limbs of Henle. The UTB urea transporter is expressed in DVR endothelium and red blood cells (not shown). Thin descending limbs of short looped nephrons become associated with vascular bundles (see Figure 24.9) so that urea recycling from thin limbs to DVR via UTA2 and UTB is accommodated. UTB is not expressed by the AVR endothelium, but AVR are fenestrated and urea permeability is high. Thus, urea in AVR plasma and RBCs can readily recycle back to DVR in vascular bundles using UTB in the RBC membrane and DVR endothelium. The UTA1, A3, and A4 collecting duct urea transporters conduct urea from the lumen to the inner medullary interstitium (C: cortex; OS: outer stripe of outer medulla; IS: inner stripe of outer medulla; IM: inner medulla). *(Reproduced with permission from ref. [100]).*

have probably been underestimated, because all measurements relied upon ^{22}Na and ^{14}Curea efflux during microperfusion *in vivo*. That method probably underestimates permeability, because accumulation of tracers near the abluminal surface during microperfusion violates the assumption that abluminal tracer concentrations are zero.[92,129]

Transport of Macromolecules in the Cortex and Medulla

It is generally accepted that lymphatics are sparse in the outer medulla, and absent from the inner medulla.[79,131] It has long been recognized that proteins permeate the walls of capillaries[89,132,133] to be drained by lymphatics and returned to the systemic circulation. Given the absence of lymphatics in the inner medulla, the mechanisms that regulate interstitial oncotic pressure and protein trafficking through the interstitium have been enigmatic. Early studies led to the conclusion that a large extravascular pool of albumin is present within the medulla.[134–136] Leakage of fluorescent albumin[137,138] and Evans blue dye-labeled albumin[139,140] into the medullary interstitium were observed. Ultrastructural studies with horseradish peroxidase (molecular radius 50 Å), catalase (elliptical molecule, 240,000 Da, major axis 240 Å), and ferritin (spherical molecule, 500,000 D, 110 Å) demonstrated that these markers can cross the fenestrations of cortical peritubular cortical capillaries[141] and medullary AVR.[142]

Measurements of albumin transport rates across the DVR and AVR walls have been technically limited. Using molecular sieving of Texas red-labeled albumin, Turner estimated the reflection coefficient of the DVR wall to albumin to be 0.89 (not significantly different from unity).[96] In separate studies with different methods, the reflection coefficient of the AVR wall to albumin was estimated to be 0.7 and 0.78.[50,128] No reliable measurements of the diffusional permeability of either the DVR or AVR wall to albumin exist. Attempts have been made to determine Starling forces within the medullary interstitium through direct measurement of interstitial protein concentration. Using a differential centrifugation technique, MacPhee and Michel obtained a mean value of 0.9 g/dl.[50] By an alternative approach, interstitial protein concentrations of 4 to 6 g/dl were predicted and interstitial hydraulic pressures in the range of 5 to 10 mmHg were found.[143]

Whatever the concentration of albumin in the medullary interstitium, the fundamental question remains, in the absence of lymphatics, how is medullary interstitial protein deposited and cleared by the microcirculation? Protein transport into the AVR lumen by convective influx is the most likely answer.[50,74,143] Michel pointed out that molecular sieving at the AVR wall would indicate convective movement of protein into the AVR lumen, were it not for continuous deposition of protein-free fluid by medullary nephrons.[74] The plausibility of convective protein uptake is also supported by the finding that papillary AVR withstand an inwardly-directed hydraulic pressure without collapsing.[51] Pinter and colleagues have suggested that the combined effects of negative charge exclusion resulting from compartmentation of hyaluron and albumin, Donnan equilibrium, and hydrostatic pressure variation from ureteral contractions provide key driving forces for fluid movements and urinary concentration.[144,145]

INTRARENAL HEMATOCRIT

When the volumes of distribution of plasma and red blood cells within the kidney were examined by injecting labeled albumin and red blood cells (RBCs), intrarenal hematocrit was found to be less than systemic hematocrit. Given the observation of Fahraeus that red cells migrate to the center of small vessels, Pappenheimer and Kinter proposed that cell free blood is "skimmed" from the periphery of the interlobular arteries to enter the afferent arterioles of deep glomeruli,[13,146] an effect which might be facilitated by intra-arterial cushions[10–12] (Figure 24.2). This possibility was tested by Lilienfield et al. who found that RBC transit time was shorter than plasma transit time, and that tissue hematocrit varies with medullary axis.[147] Rasmussen performed a technically superior examination using ^{131}I-IgM, a larger and therefore more reliable plasma marker. Simultaneous injection with ^{51}Cr-RBCs, led to the estimates of tissue hematocrit shown in Figure 24.16.[148] Using videomicroscopic techniques, Zimmerhackl estimated the "dynamic" or "tube" hematocrit of the papillary DVR and AVR to be 26 and 25%, respectively.[149] Direct measurements with micropuncture gave similar results. A low microvessel hematocrit in the renal medulla has been consistently found.

In addition to plasma skimming,[10,13] other mechanisms could reduce medullary hematocrit. Fahraeus demonstrated that the hematocrit of a microvessel is reduced by migration of RBCs to the centerline where the velocity of flow is highest.[146] Based on this alone,

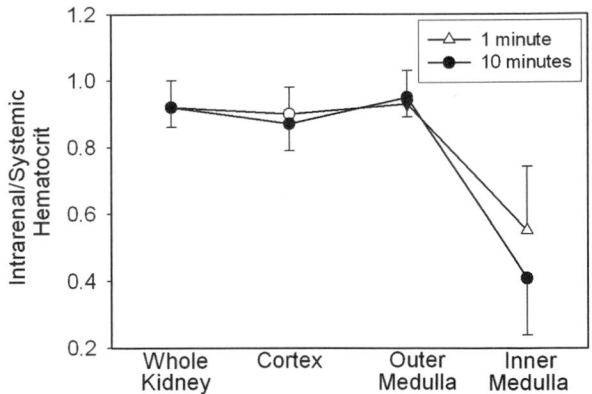

FIGURE 24.16 **Distribution of hematocrit in the kidney.** ^{51}Cr-RBC's and ^{131}I-IgM (plasma volume marker) were simultaneously infused into the kidney. An equilibration period of either 1 or 10 minutes followed before ligation of the renal artery and vein. The distribution of RBCs and plasma were inferred by measuring activity of the isotopes in tissue and dividing their ratio by the systemic ratio. Results show that the hematocrit of inner medullary blood is lower than that whole kidney, cortex or outer medulla. (*Data redrawn with permission from ref. [148]*).

vasa recta (10–20 μm diameter) are expected to have hematocrits reduced by 40 to 50% of that in a large vessel.[150] Pries et al. have shown that a "network" Fahraeus effect can further reduce microvessel hematocrit by as much as 20%. When a vessel bifurcates, the higher flow branch receives blood of higher hematocrit. Conservation of RBC and plasma dictates that the increase of hematocrit in one branch must be less than the reduction in the other branch, tending to reduce average capillary hematocrit.[151] Shrinkage of RBCs in the hypertonic medulla must also tend to lower medullary microvessel hematocrit.[17]

METHODS FOR MEASUREMENT OF REGIONAL BLOOD FLOW TO THE CORTEX AND MEDULLA

The relative contribution of various renal microvessels to renal vascular resistance can be inferred from the luminal hydrostatic pressure profile. As shown in Figure 24.17, the largest pressure drop, and therefore the dominant resistance, is the afferent arteriole. Glomerular capillaries, due to their large combined cross-sectional area, are thought to offer little resistance to flow. Efferent arterioles and DVR contribute significantly to renal vascular resistance, but less than that

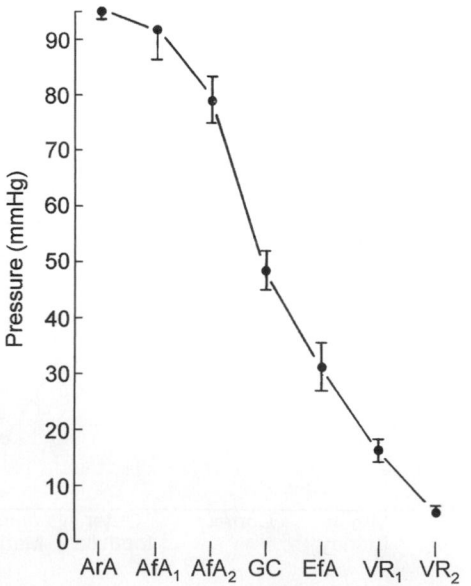

FIGURE 24.17 Microvessel pressure distribution within the kidney. The values on the ordinate were obtained by micropuncture and servo-nulling pressure measurements using the juxtamedullary nephron preparation. Pressure falls successively from the arcuate artery to vasa recta (ArA: arcuate artery; AfA$_1$ and AfA$_2$: early and late afferent arteriole; GC: glomerular capillaries; EfA: efferent arterioles; VR$_1$: descending vasa recta; VR$_2$: ascending vasa recta). *(Reproduced with permission from ref. [202]).*

attributed to afferent arterioles. Vasoactivity of the afferent arteriole is governed by myogenic autoregulation and tubuloglomerular feedback via the macula densa, important topics that are covered by other chapters of this text. The afferent and efferent arterioles may also be influenced by other nephron to vascular cross-talk mechanisms.[152,153] Measurement of regional blood flows in the kidney that result from the actions and distributions of resistance arterioles has been the frequently pursued. Early approaches to the measurement of regional blood flow within the kidney relied upon tracers, gave widely varying estimates of tissue blood flow, and have fallen into disfavor. Results from those methods are summarized in Table 24.4 from which one can conclude that inner medullary tissue blood flow rate is much lower than that of the cortex.[34,148,154–173] The associated details have been reviewed in prior versions of this text and other sources.[1,17,174] Videomicroscopic measurement of RBC velocity is a more reliable means for calculating single vessel blood flow rates, but it is limited to surface microvessels in the cortex or exposed papilla.[149,175] Use of a pencil lens camera for measurement of glomerular and cortical peritubular RBC velocities has been described by Goligorsky and colleagues.[176] It has been used to examine effects of pharmaceutical calcium channel blockers on glomerular arteriolar tone *in situ*.[177] Laser-Doppler flowmetry is the dominant method for examining regional blood flow, due to the ease of applying optical fibers to the kidney surface or inserting them into otherwise inaccessible regions within the parenchyma[167]; laser speckle[178,179] and ultrasound imaging of microbubbles[180,181] may offer future improvements.

Videomicroscopy

Measurement of microvessel diameter and RBC velocity (V$_{RBC}$) can be combined to calculate single vessel blood flow rates.[35] Gussis and colleagues measured V$_{RBC}$ in vasa recta on the surface of the exposed renal papilla, following which Holliger and co-workers coupled V$_{RBC}$ with diameter measurement to calculate single vessel blood flow rates.[34,182] In later refinements, contrast between red cells, plasma, and the capillary wall was enhanced by injection of fluorescein isothiocyanate-labeled gamma globulin, and V$_{RBC}$ was determined from the video images captured with a silicon intensified target camera. Additionally, the Fahraeus effect[146] was accounted for by calibrating RBC streaming effects in quartz capillaries.[175] Application of videomicroscopy to measurement of renal blood flow is limited by regional accessibility. Observation of the medulla for videomicroscopy is limited to the papilla (distal third of the inner medulla) because only that

TABLE 24.4 Regional Tissue Plasma Inflow Rates Measured in the Kidney

| Method | Species | Inflow Rate, ml • min • g^{-780} | | | Reference |
		Cortex	Outer Medulla	Inner Medulla	
Dye Transit	Dog		1.3	0.2–0.7	171
	Dog	5.35	3.22	0.38	165
^{32}P Transit	Dog		1.8	0.5–0.7	172
^{85}Kr Washout	Dog	4.72	1.32	0.17	170
H$_2$ Washout	Dog	2.6–5.0			154
^{86}Rb Uptake	Dog	4.4–7.4	1.2–2.3	1.1	169
	Dog	4.84	2.81	0.8	155
	Rat	4.76	1.35	0.66	163
	Rat		0.60–0.88[a]	0.2–0.3[a]	159
	Rat	5.2	1.5–2.2	0.69	164
	Rat	4.7–7.3	2.4	2.4	173
Albumin Accumulation	Dog			0.25	166
	Dog			0.22	160
	Dog			0.23	157
	Rat			0.38–0.42	161,162
	Rat			0.32	168
	Rat			0.27	156
	Rat			0.36	158
	Rat			0.38–0.64	148
	Rat			0.06–0.08[b]	148
	Rat			0.18[c,d]	167
	Rat			0.31[c,e]	167
RBC velocity	Rat			1.3–5.9[c,f]	34

[a]*Probably underestimated.*
[b]*RBC inflow rate.*
[c]*Total blood (RBC and plasma) inflow rate.*
[d]*Young rats.*
[e]*Old rats.*
[f]*Probably overestimated.*
Abbreviations: RBC: red blood cell.

part of the medulla can be exposed for visualization by excising the ureter of young rodents.

Laser-Doppler

The laser-Doppler method for measuring tissue blood flow rates relies upon the frequency shift of light emitted from a laser due to scattering by flowing RBCs.[183] Among other advantages, sequential measurements in the same region are possible, and signals can be obtained on the renal surface or from optical fibers implanted into the parenchyma. The counterflow arrangement of vasa recta within the medulla would appear to violate the requirement that the laser-Doppler receive random backscattered light. Despite this concern, agreement between laser-Doppler and videomicroscopy[184] or ^{51}Cr-RBC accumulation[167] has been demonstrated. The laser-Doppler device provides a voltage proportional to tissue perfusion in the immediate vicinity of the fiber-optic probe. Calibration to convert the signal to absolute units that quantitatively describe local perfusion is generally not possible. This limits absolute comparisons of measurements between regions of the kidney of the same or different animals.

METHODS FOR DIRECT MEASUREMENTS OF MICROVESSEL REACTIVITY

Other important methods for investigation of the regulation of regional blood flow examine the effects of vasoactive agents on pressurized microvessels. Important information on the sites of action, the concentrations at which specific hormones modulate reactivity, and receptor subtypes responsible for mediating vasoactivity can be obtained. Extrapolation of results to arrive at conclusions concerning the effects of hormones and autocoids on regional blood flow within the kidney is fraught with uncertainty. This topic has been frequently reviewed.[1,2,15,185–188]

In Vitro Microperfusion

The *in vitro* microperfusion method commonly used for study of transport processes in renal tubules has also been applied to microvessels[189,190] (Figure 24.18). The first applications of this method were in canine glomeruli.[191] Subsequent adaptations in rabbits permitted examination of vasomotor tone in afferent and efferent arterioles.[192–196] Using this approach, it has been possible to measure effects of vasoactive agents on afferent arterioles (Figure 24.19a) and vasa recta[111,197,198] (Figure 24.19b,c). As with all methods, limitations exist. Hormones that cause vasoconstriction often activate compensatory mechanisms that inhibit their actions. Endothelium-dependent vasodilators such as nitric oxide, prostacyclin, and hyperpolarizing factors[199] might be blunted, substrate-limited[200] or simply diluted into the bathing buffer. The actions of nitric oxide (NO) might be enhanced *in vitro* due to the absence of hemoglobin, a NO scavenger[201] or reduced by endothelial damage during vessel isolation.

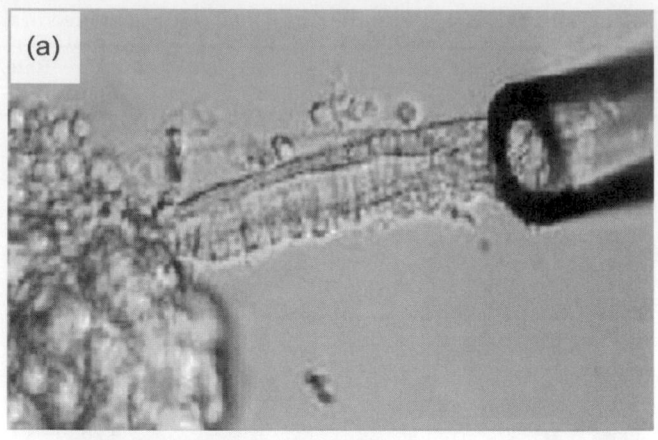

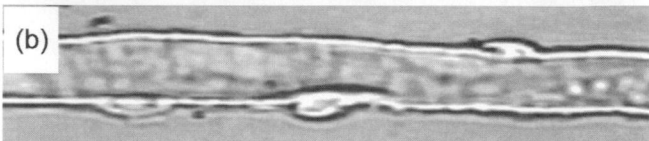

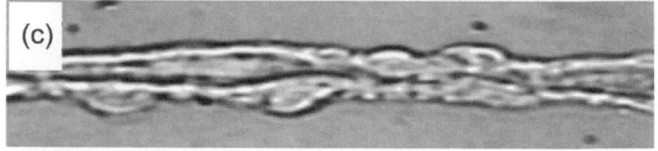

FIGURE 24.19 *In vitro* **microperfusion.** (a) An afferent arteriole is cannulated with concentric pipettes and perfused toward the glomerulus. *(Reproduced with permission from ref. [197]).* (b), (c) Perfusion of an isolated DVR. Images obtained before (b) and after (c) exposure to angiotensin II. Compare the thick smooth muscle layer of the afferent arteriole to the sporadically distributed pericyte cell bodies of DVR.

Juxtamedullary Nephron Preparation

The ingenious blood-perfused juxtamedullary nephron preparation was devised by Casellas and Navar (Figure 24.20, top panel). The surgically isolated kidney, perfused with artificial buffers or blood, is hemisected. Dissection of perihilar fat and reflection of the papilla exposes the juxtamedullary circulation to enable observation of RBC flow and microvessel diameters. Advantages of the method are many, including relative preservation of tubulovascular relationships, continuous oxygenation of the tissue under study, the ability to measure pressures by servo-nulling, and the ability to control hormone concentrations in the perfusate and superfusate.[202]

The Split Hydronephrotic Kidney

Steinhausen et al. developed a method for reducing the kidney to a transparent layer of tissue within which transilluminated microvessels are readily visualized. After transient ischemia to the kidney, ureteral ligation is performed, inducing hydronephrosis. Weeks later,

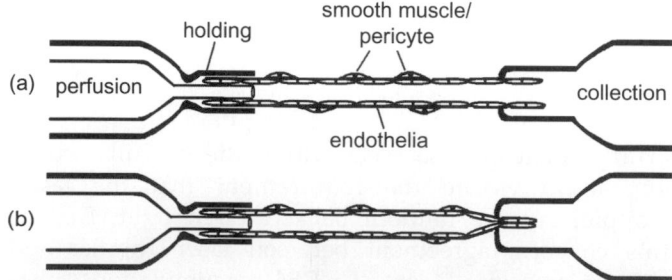

FIGURE 24.18 *In vitro* **microperfusion.** (a) An isolated microvessel is cannulated on concentric pipettes by drawing the vessel into an outer holding pipette and cannulating its orifice with a perfusion pipette. By pressurizing the perfusion pipette, fluid is forced to flow through the vessel lumen into a collection pipette. (b) The collection end can be crimped to create a "stop-flow" condition in which the lumen is pressurized to that of the holding pipette in the absence of flow. *(Reproduced with permission from ref. [393]).*

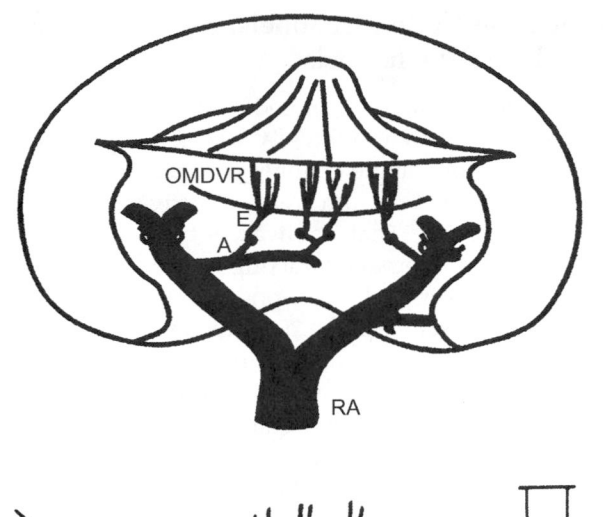

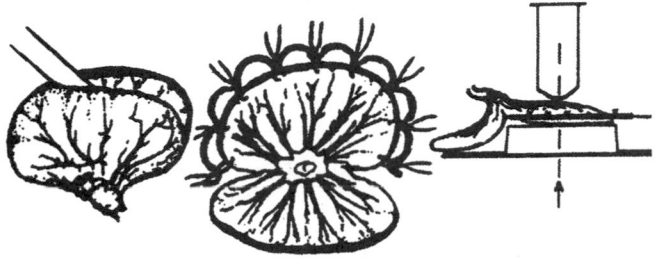

FIGURE 24.20 Juxtamedullary nephron and split hydronephrotic kidney preparations. Top panel: The juxtamedullary nephron preparation is created by perfusing the kidney, sectioning it longitudinally and reflecting the papilla to expose the underlying microvasculature (RA: renal artery; A and E: afferent and efferent arterioles; OMDVR: outer medullary descending vasa recta). Bottom panel: The split hydronephrotic kidney preparation is created by ligating the ureter for 3 to 10 weeks prior to isolation of the kidney. Ureteral ligation eventually reduces the kidney to a thin sheet of tissue in which tubules have atrophied but the vasculature remains. The kidney is exposed, split along the greater curvature, and sutured onto a chamber for observation and experimentation. *(Reproduced with permission from ref. [2]).*

the hydronephrotic kidney, reduced to a thin layer, can be split along its curvature and suspended on a microscope stage for study[203,204] (Figure 24.20, bottom panel). The actions of vasoactive agents can be studied by infusing them into the rat or by applying them directly onto the preparation. Changes in blood flow rate can be measured by videomicroscopy, and the reactivity of microvessels quantitated as changes in luminal diameter. The possibility of phenotypic drift in the altered tissue has to be considered.

VASOACTIVITY OF THE RENAL MICROCIRCULATION: ION CHANNEL ARCHITECTURE

Voltage-Gated Ca^{2+} Channels

Contraction of microvessels is generally tied to elevation of cytoplasmic calcium ($[Ca^{2+}]_{CYT}$) of smooth muscle cells (SMC). The increase of $[Ca^{2+}]_{CYT}$ is often mediated by influx through voltage-gated channels that are activated by membrane depolarization. This is observed experimentally, exposing SMC to high extracellular KCl induces depolarization by raising the K^+ equilibrium potential (Keq), activating voltage-gated Ca^{2+} entry and inducing vasoconstriction. Studies have shown that KCl depolarization constricts afferent arterioles more than efferent arterioles.[205-207] A role for high voltage-gated, L-type channels to mediate afferent SMC contraction is supported by the observation that both $[Ca^{2+}]_{CYT}$ elevation and vasoconstriction are blocked by diltiazem.[208,209] In the split hydronephrotic kidney preparation, angiotensi II constricts both afferent and efferent arterioles, but depolarizes only the former.[210] Application of agonists such as angiotensin II, endothelin, and ATP to preglomerular smooth muscle preparations consistently elicits $[Ca^{2+}]_{CYT}$ and current responses that are sensitive to L-type antagonists.[211-215] Taken together, sensitivity of the preglomerular microcirculation to L-type calcium channel blockade has been a very consistent finding.[216-221] Reduction of afferent vasoconstriction due to impairment of L-channel function could conceivably lead to transmission of elevated pressures to the glomerulus, resulting in injury. Such a mechanism has been invoked in rodent models of diabetes and hypertension.[222-224]

Voltage-gated Ca^{2+} channels (CaV) exist as a variety of subtypes and splice variants thereof. The nomenclature has evolved. Modern CaV classification follows the identity of the pore forming α-subunit (Table 24.5). Isoforms of classic high voltage-activated (HVA), L-channels are CaV 1.1– 1.3, and those of low voltage-activated (LVA) T-type channels are CaV 3.1–3.3. Other HVA types, originally identified in neurons, are the P/Q, R, and N which are CaV 2.1–2.3. Recently, RT-PCR and immunochemistry have been used to examine the distribution of voltage-gated Ca^{2+} channel α-subunits in the kidney. In addition to the anticipated expression of L-type (CaV 1.x) in the afferent circulation, T-type as well as unexpected P/Q-type Ca^{2+} channels were found.[206,225-229] Consistent with the earlier literature (see above), superficial efferent arterioles were not found to express L-type channels.[206]

Functional confirmation of CaV expression in the afferent and efferent circulation has been obtained in various studies. The CaV 1.x, L-type blocker diltiazem, partially reversed angiotensin II vasoconstriction and $[Ca^{2+}]_{CYT}$ elevation in DVR pericytes.[230,231] Similarly, the L-type blocker calciseptine and nonselective T-type blockers nilvadipine, mibefradil, pimozide, and Ni^{2+} reversed KCl and angiotensin II-induced constriction of afferent and efferent arterioles.[206,227,228,232,233] Elegant patch-clamp recordings by Gordienko et al. demonstrated signature currents consistent with both

TABLE 24.5 Expression of Voltage Activated Ca^{2+} Cannels (CaV) in the Renal Microcirculation[225,206,226,227,228,355,320,236]

		CaV	α-subunit	Renal SMC[a]	Locations Found
HVA	L	1.1	1S	−	Preglomerular SMC
	L	1.2	1C	+	Afferent arteriole
	L	1.3	1D	−	Mesangial cells
	L	1.4	1F	−	JM efferent arteriole
					DVR
HVA	P/Q	2.1	1A	+	Afferent arteriole
	N	2.2	1B	−	Mesangial cells
	R	2.3	1E	−	DVR
LVA	T	3.1	1G	+	Afferent arteriole
	T	3.2	1H	+	Efferent arteriole
	T	3.3	1I	−	DVR

[a]*Detection by immunochemistry, polymerase chain reaction.*
Abbreviations: SMC: smooth muscle cell; HVA: high voltage activated by depolarization to > -40 mV; LVA: low voltage activated by depolarization to > -55 mV.

high (L-type) and low (T-type) voltage-gated Ca^{2+} entry into isolated preglomerular smooth muscle.[234] Glomerular mesangial cells have a smooth muscle phenotype and express L-type dihydropyridine-sensitive voltage-gated Ca^{2+} channels.[235]

It is now clear that CaV are not just confined to the preglomerular circulation; juxtamedullary efferent arterioles and DVR express them. Despite positive immunostaining for T-type and P/Q-type channels in DVR pericytes,[206,225] a rigorous search for signature currents found only L-type activity.[236] Feng and colleagues examined the roles of arteriolar CaV with the juxtamedullary nephron preparation. Pimozide and mibefradil (T-type blockers) reduced basal tone of both afferent and efferent arterioles. In contrast, successful blockade with diltiazem (L-type blocker) occurred only in afferent arteriole, except when generation of NO was prevented by NO synthase inhibition. In their hands, T-type channel blockade with pimozide reversed both afferent and efferent contraction by angiotensin II.[232,237,238] Elegant studies in the renal cortex, performed *in vivo* using a pencil lens camera, have also documented that efferent arterioles are dilated by nonselective CCB, such as efonidipine and mibefradil.[239] Taken together, a role for CaV, particularly T-type channels, to participate in myogenic tone and agonist-induced contraction of juxtamedullary efferent arterioles is well-supported, and the ability of combined T- and L-type blockade to provide renoprotection through efferent dilation has thus become the subject of clinical investigation.[240-242]

Nonselective Cation Channels, Store Operated Channels, TRP Channels

Early study of store operated Ca^{2+} entry (SOC) in mast cells pointed to a highly Ca^{2+} selective pathway of immeasurably low single channel conductance that was referred to as a "calcium release activated current" (CRAC or I_{CRAC}).[243] That pathway is been attributed to the ER anchored stromal interacting molecule (STIM1) as the putative sensor and Orai, possibly interacting with TRPC1 as the selective pore.[244-247] Other pathways may participate in cellular Ca^{2+} entry in response to receptor activation and intracellular Ca^{2+} store depletion.[248] The routes involved are not always highly selective for Ca^{2+}, but instead also conduct other cations including Na^+. Their promiscuous transport of cations led to the designation "nonselective cation channels" (NSCC). Both receptor operated and store operated Ca^{2+} entry into cells can occur via NSCC, and channels of the transient receptor potential (TRP) families are now recognized as the major participants.[249] Fellner and Arendshorst showed that store operated Ca^{2+} entry into renal SMCs occurs and may be increased in the spontaneously hypertensive rat,[223,250] and that using SKF-96365 as an NSCC blocker, it has been shown that angiotensin II induced Ca^{2+} responses[215] and vasoconstriction[251] of the efferent arteriole involves NSCC. Assigning subtype-specific functional roles to the ubiquitously expressed TRP channel family members has proven generally difficult.[249] Takenaka and colleagues demonstrated that TRPC1 is expressed in glomerular arterioles and might conduct store or receptor operated Ca^{2+} entry.[249,251] The presence and activation of SOC has been most thoroughly examined in glomerular mesangial cells. Sansom and colleagues identified a small, 2.1 pS cation channel that is activated by thapsigargin-induced store depletion.[249,252] In whole cell patch-clamp experiments, identical currents were elicited by either thapsigargin or epidermal growth factor activation.[253,254] Activation of the pathway requires signaling through PKCα.[255,256] TRPC1 and TRPC4 are expressed in the murine mesangium, where antisense-induced suppression of TRPC4 was accompanied by inhibition of store operated currents.[257] TRPC4 has also been identified in DVR pericytes and endothelium, where it is in physical association with isoform 2 of the Na^+/H^+ exchange regulatory factor (NHERF-2), a scaffolding protein that facilitates protein−protein interactions.[258] The function of the NHERF-TRPC4 association is unknown.

Chloride Channels

For CaV to mediate Ca^{2+} entry into smooth muscle, they must depolarize the cell membrane to potentials greater than the CaV activation threshold. The equilibrium potential for K^+ ion is about -90 mV and SMC membrane potential is held at negative values because overall conductance of the cell membrane is dominated by permeability to K^+. In many SMCs, depolarization that presages CaV-mediated Ca^{2+} entry is achieved by increasing the conductance to Cl^- ion, the equilibrium potential of which is generally -35 to -20 mV. This is accomplished through activation of Ca^{2+}-dependent Cl^- channels (CaCC).[259,260] The identity of CaCC had been confusing and enigmatic, but has recently been traced to TMEM16A and the family of proteins dubbed "anoctamins".[261,262] It seems likely that anoctamins are SMC CaCC, but confirmatory evidence in the renal vasculature is currently lacking. In the kidney, activation of CaCC channels has been described to participate in angiotnsin II-, endothelin-, and adenosine-induced constriction of afferent but not efferent arterioles.[263−267] Presumably, based on the juxtamedullary efferent expression of CaV,[206] CaCC plays a similar role in that location, but this has not been demonstrated. DVR pericyte depolarization and constriction is dependent upon CaCC activation.[268−270] In pericytes, cyclic CaCC stimulation participates in angiotensin II-induced oscillations of membrane potential,[271,272] and CaCC activity can be regulated by kinase blockade.[273] It has also been shown that high concentrations of angiotensin II also depolarize DVR pericytes by inhibiting K^+ channels.[274] The extent to which Cl^- channel activity regulates overall renal vascular resistance is uncertain.[229,248,275]

Potassium Channels

Most smooth muscle cells (SMC) express an array of K^+ channels. These include inward rectifier (K_{IR}), calcium-dependent (K_{Ca}), voltage-dependent (K_V), and ATP-dependent (K_{ATP}) varieties.[276] SMC of renal vessels are no exception, and many studies have been dedicated to the determination of their distribution and function (Table 24.6).

K_{Ca} channels are activated by depolarization and elevation of $[Ca^{2+}]_{CYT}$. They can be further subdivided into larger conductance (maxiK_{Ca} or BK_{Ca}) channels sensitive to charybdotoxin and iberotoxin, and medium and low conductance channels blocked by apamin. K_{Ca} channels are ubiquitous in smooth muscle. When stimulated by Ca^{2+} entry, they may provide a "breaking" function that opposes depolarization and deactivates CaV.

K_V channels, also refered to as delayed rectifiers, activate with depolarization, are insensitive to $[Ca^{2+}]_{CYT}$, and are specifically blocked by 4-aminopyridine. K_V can contribute to resting potential, and their voltage-dependent activation probably limits membrane depolarization.

K_{IR} are named for their avid permeation of K^+ at membrane potentials that lie below Keq. Above Keq, where the physiological function of K_{IR} occurs, K_{IR}

TABLE 24.6 Potassium Channel Expression in the Renal Microcirculation

Site	K_{Ca}	Kv	K_{IR}	K_{ATP}	Reference
Main renal artery	+	+	N.D.	N.D.	281,284,285
Preglomerular SMCs	+	+	+	+	283,291,292,299,301,302,307
Interlobular artery	+	+	N.D.	N.D.	234,282,296,300
Arcuate artery	+	+	+	N.D.	234,282,286,289,290
Interlobular arteriole	+	+	N.D.	N.D.	287,288,293,294
Afferent arteriole	+	+	+	+	298,303−306,308−310−316
Mesangial cells	+	+	N.D.	+	320−328,330−334,793
Efferent arteriole	+	N.D.	+	+	311,317
DVR	+	N.D.	+	+	231,274,318,319,467

Table entries are + for existence of functional evidence based on electrophysiology, vasoactivity and use of specific channel blockers. Abbreviations: K_{Ca}: small, medium or large/maxi calcium dependent potassium channel; Kv: voltage-gated (delayed rectifier) potassium channel; K_{IR}: inward rectifier potassium channel; K_{ATP}: ATP-dependent potassium channel; N.D.: no data; DVR: descending vasa recta.

conduct K^+ efflux from cells in a complex manner. Conductance, at membrane potentials greater than Keq, declines as the difference between membrane potential and Keq increases. The latter property imparts a very important characteristic. Small elevations of extracellular K^+ (e.g., 5−20 mM) raise Keq to a level that enhances K_{IR} conductance, but still lies below the resting membrane potential. The result is hyperpolarization of the membrane that favors inhibition of Ca^{2+} entry and vasodilation.[277] That mechanism may enable extracellular K^+ ion to function as an endothelium-dependent hyperpolarizing factor (EDHF). The increase in extracellular K^+ needed for the EDHF process to occur is thought to arise from endothelial K^+ secretion. Vasodilators, such as bradykinin and acetylcholine, increase $[Ca^{2+}]_{CYT}$ and stimulate endothelial K_{Ca} channels so that they secrete K^+ ion into the extracellular space of adjacent SMCs.[97,278−280] Stated another way, K^+ may be an EDHF, the function of which depends upon endothelial K^+ secretion and SMC K_{IR} expression. Extracellular K^+ can also activate electrogenic Na^+K^+-ATPase activity in SMC which, by exchanging $3Na^+$ for $2K^+$, favors hyperpolarization. Participation of Na^+ pumps versus K_{IR} in SMC hyperpolarization must be experimentally distinguished, generally by examining the component that is sensitive to ouabain.

SMC K_{ATP} channels are generally comprised of four K_{IR} 6.1 α-subunits combined with four type 2B sulfonurea receptors (SUR2B). Despite the participation of K_{IR} 6.1, K_{ATP} channels lack the strongly inward rectifying characteristics of other K_{IR} isoforms. K_{ATP} channels are widely expressed in SMC and, with high specificity, are inhibited by antagonists such as glybenclamide that bind to the SUR-subunits. K_{ATP} channels are named for their inhibition by intracellular ATP. In addition to ATP, nucleotide diphosphates (NDPs) regulate most K_{ATP} channels. It was historically thought that reduction of cellular ATP related to metabolic stress activates K_{ATP} channels favoring hyperpolarization, microvessel dilation, and enhancement of perfusion. It is now recognized that this is an oversimplification, because K_{ATP} channels can contribute to resting potential and are sensitive to a variety of regulatory influences.[277]

SMC of the main renal artery, interlobular, and arcuate arteries have been shown to express both BK_{Ca} and K_V channels that exhibit slow inactivation after depolarization.[234,281–286] Preglomerular renal microvessels of varying caliber obtained by hand dissection or by filling them with iron oxide particles and isolating them from collagenase-digested tissue with a magnet have provided preparations for study. SK_{Ca}, BK_{Ca}, and K_V channels have been observed in afferent SMCs.[287–289] The P450 cyclooxygenase constrictor, 20-hydroxyeicosatetraenoic acid (20-HETE), inhibits preglomerular K_{Ca} channel activity,[290–292] probably through activation of MAP kinase.[293] Preglomerular K_{Ca} channels can be activated by NO,[294] 11,12-epoxyeicosatrienoic acid (11, 12-EET),[295] and CO generated by hemoxygenase.[296] The cytochrome P450 synthesis of epoxyeicosatrienoic acids (EETs) has been shown to activate BK_{Ca}, and may participate in the function of EETs as an EDHF.[297–299] NO-mediated inhibition of 20-HETE synthesis may be the primary mechanism (versus cyclic GMP generation) that favors BK_{Ca} activation in preglomerular SMC.[291,300] Preglomerular expression of K_{ATP} component subunits has been variably observed.[301,302]

Afferent arterioles are the dominant resistance of the renal microcirculation, and play vital roles in autoregulation through myogenic constriction and tubuloglomerular feedback. The K^+ channel architecture of afferent arterioles has been intensely studied, and evidence for expression of K_{Ca}, K_{IR}, K_V, and K_{ATP} channels has been obtained. Afferent dilation by acetylcholine during inhibition of NO and prostaglandin synthesis has been traced to the participation of K_{IR} and K_{Ca} channels, because it is blocked by the combined K_{Ca} inhibitors, charybdotoxin and apamin.[298,303] As described above, the EDHF response may be related to local elevations of K^+ outside the SMC membrane. Direct participation of K_{IR} has been demonstrated by Chilton and Loutzenhiser, who found that small elevations of K^+ dilate afferent arterioles. The dilation is sensitive to low concentrations of Ba^{2+} ($<100\ \mu M$) that selectively blocks K_{IR} channels.[304–306] Juxtaglomerular cells express the strong inward rectifier, K_{IR} 2.1, where it plays a role in setting membrane potential.[307] Vasodilation of afferent arterioles by the K^+ channel activator, NS-1619, supports a role for K_{Ca} channels in that structure.[307,308] Myogenic constriction appears to be modulated through PKC that acts, at least in part, by inhibiting 4-aminopyridine sensitive K_V channels.[309] A role for K_{ATP} channel activity to affect afferent arterioles has been repeatedly verified. K_{ATP} channels activated by hypoxia, pinacidil, calcitonin gene related peptide (CGRP) or adenosine modulate constriction[310–313] and levakromlin hyperpolarizes renin-secreting cells of the afferent arteriole.[314] K_{ATP} expression in afferent arterioles is supported by the observation of $[^3H]P$-1075 binding to membranes.[315] Multiple classes of K^+ channels contribute to resting tone of afferent arterioles, and enhancement of K_{IR} and K_{ATP} activity may contribute to vasodilation and glomerular hypertension in diabetes.[316]

The role of K^+ channels in the activity of the efferent circulation has not been as thoroughly explored as that of afferent smooth muscle. The K_{ATP} opener, pinacidil, dilates the efferent arteriole.[311] Pinacidil both dilates DVR and hyperpolarizes DVR smooth muscle/pericytes.[231] High concentrations of angiotensin II inhibit DVR K^+ channel activity.[274] A modulatory role for K_{IR} and K_{Ca} channels to affect $[Ca^{2+}]_{CYT}$ signaling by angiotensin II in efferent arteriolar smooth muscle has been described.[317] Roles for strong K_{IR} isoforms to modulate contraction and membrane potential of glomerular arterioles and vasa recta pericytes have been verified.[304,318,319]

Mesangial cells are smooth muscle pericytes that contract to modulate filtration by glomerular capillaries.[320] The ability to study mesangial cells in culture has permitted study of their channel architecture. Molecular evidence exists for expression of K_V, K_{ATP}, and K_{Ca} channels in rat primary and immortalized murine mesangial cells.[321,322] Both medium and large conductance K_{Ca} channels are present.[289,323–328] The BK_{Ca} channel in mesangial cells is activated by arachidonic acid[329] and Ca^{2+}-calmodulin-dependent protein kinase.[330] Atrial natriuretic peptide[331] or nitric oxide, acting through cGMP-dependent protein kinase, also activates K_{Ca} channels through phosphorylation of the β1-subunit.[332] Mesangial BK_{Ca} activation is favored by protein phosphatase 2A inhibition,[333] and enhancement of activity and expression by insulin-induced MAPK activation.[334]

Connexins

In addition to permitting exchange of ions with the extracellular space, specialized channel proteins, the connexins, electrically couple smooth muscle and endothelia in the vascular wall. Of more than 20 connexins, Cx37, Cx40, Cx43, and Cx45 have been found in the vasculature where they form endothelial and myoendothelial gap junctions. Connexins are four transmembrane spanning proteins with two extracellular loops that combine as homomeric or heteromeric hexamers. Docking of the extracellular loops combines two hexameric hemichannels from adjacent cells into the transcellular "connexon" conduit that mediates cell—cell communication. Mimetic peptides have been designed that interfere with binding of the extracellular loops.[335] Connexons are true channels that generally have high conductivity (15—300 pS), high open probability, and can occupy multiple subconductance states. They are regulated by pH, Ca^{2+}, signaling molecules, and phosphorylation events. Their pores are sufficiently large to pass signaling molecules, anions, and cations. Communication between cells is often documented by cell-to-cell spreading of fluorescent molecules (e.g., Lucifer yellow 457 Da).[336—338] The physiological roles of vascular gap junctions are under study. A role for endothelial to smooth muscle transfer of vasodilators has been postulated.[97,278] This has received support from the observation that Cx40 deficient mice are hypertensive, have abnormal vasomotion, and deficient spreading of vasodilation.[336,339,340] Endothelial deficiency of Cx43 also leads to abnormal spreading of vasodilation,[341,342] and targeting of Cx43 and Cx37 with the extracellular peptide mimetic, Gap27, inhibits myogenic responses.[343]

The renal microcirculation expresses gap junctions Cx37, Cx40, Cx43, and Cx45.[29,344—352] NO- and COX-independent (EDHF-mediated) dilation of the main renal artery with carbachol was shown to be sensitive to Gap27.[353] Similarly, arachidonic acid- and bradykinin-mediated, NO- and COX-independent dilation of arcuate and interlobar arterioles was inhibited by the gap junction blocker, 18-α glycyrrhetinic acid.[354] Salmonsson and colleagues have documented Ca^{2+} spreading along interlobular arterioles that is likely to be mediated by gap junctions.[355] Cx40 is highly expressed in endothelial cells of renal vessels and glomeruli,[347,356] and may play an important role in tubuloglomerular feedback and autoregulation.[348] Endothelial cells of preglomerular arteries and arterioles also express Cx37 and Cx43. Cx37 is found in arcuate and interlobular arteries, and afferent arterioles.[352] Cx40 bridging endothelial cells are most abundantly localized in large intrarenal arteries, including interlobular artery and the proximal portion of the afferent arteriole, but then markedly decreases as the arteriole approaches a glomerulus.[347] Deficiency of Cx40 leads to ectopic renin production.[357—359] Afferent arterioles have considerably more connexin expression than efferent

arterioles where Cx43 is largely present in the endothelium. Cx37 and Cx40 are expressed in juxtaglomerular cells and extraglomerular mesangial cells.[352] Cx43 is localized to extraglomerular mesangium and is found in isolated glomeruli.[360,361,362] Intraglomerular mesangial cells have primarily Cx40.[352,363] In the renal medullary microcirculation, DVR pericytes express Cx37 while the endothelia express Cx40 and Cx43 (Figure 24.21). DVR endothelia, but not pericytes, are highly connected as an electrical syncytium. DVR conduct Ca^{2+} responses to mechanical stimulation that can be inhibited by gap junction blockade.[364]

REGULATION OF BLOOD FLOW AND MICROVESSEL CONTRACTION

The most effective locations at which regional perfusion of cortex and medulla can be controlled are readily inferred from renal microanatomy (Figure 24.1). For example, constriction of intralobular arterioles should favor redistribution of blood flow toward the medulla via the juxtamedullary glomeruli. Similarly, closure of juxtamedullary intra-arterial cushions (Figure 24.2) or constriction of juxtamedullary afferent or efferent arterioles should favor perfusion of the superficial cortex. DVR are the final resistance vessels involved in the

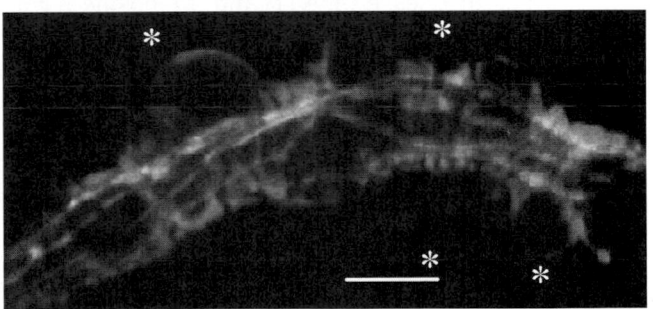
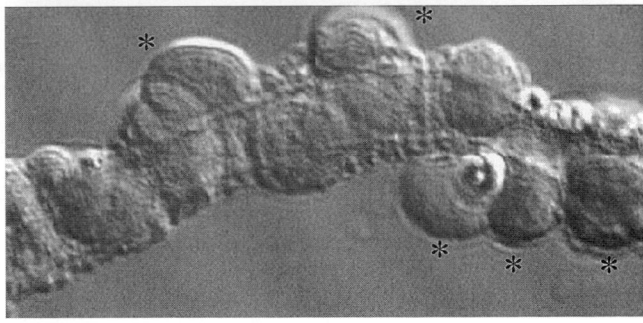

FIGURE 24.21 **Connexin staining in DVR.** Immunostaining with antibody directed against α-smooth muscle actin (SMA red, pericyte marker) or Cx40 (green) along with corresponding white light micrograph. Cx40 is linear and confined to the endothelium with very little SMA colocalization. Abluminal pericyte cell bodies (*) protrude from the outer rim of the vessel (Bar = 10 microns). *(Reproduced with permission from ref. [364]).* See color plate section at the back of the book.

control of medullary perfusion. The fraction of the total resistance to blood flow into the renal medulla accounted for by DVR, versus juxtamedullary afferent and efferent arterioles, is uncertain. The parallel arrangement of DVR within vascular bundles does, however, imply a probable role for them to modulate regional perfusion to the outer versus inner medulla. For example, contraction of DVR that are destined to perfuse the inner medulla should favor redirection of blood flow toward the outer medullary interbundle capillary plexus. Factors that control regional perfusion within the kidney are the subject of intense investigation.

Autoregulation and Pressure Natriuresis

Blood flow to the kidney remains relatively constant despite physiological variation of renal perfusion pressure (RPP), a phenomenon called autoregulation. Two major mechanisms account for renal autoregulation. The first is "myogenic," whereby stretch of the afferent arteriole leads to reflex vasoconstriction.[365] The second component, that reacts more slowly than the myogenic reflex, is tubuloglomerular feedback (TGF). TGF occurs when an increase in renal perfusion pressure, transiently transmitted to glomerular capillaries, results in a rise in glomerular filtration rate. After a delay traversing the nephron, the increased tubular fluid delivery is sensed at the macula densa, where a signaling cascade leads to release of ATP and adenosine formation via 5'-ecto-nucleotidase. The adenosine so formed constricts the afferent arteriole, thereby reducing filtration pressure and returning glomerular filtration rate to its set point.[366–371]

The phenomenon of "pressure natriuresis" may be tied to variation of medullary autoregulation. Pressure natriuresis refers to the observation that elevation of renal perfusion pressure (RPP) causes natriuresis even in isolated, denervated kidneys.[372,373] Increased RPP leads to increased sodium delivery to papillary thin descending limbs of Henle, implying that a mechanism exists to inhibit reabsorption by the proximal tubule of deep nephrons.[374,375] Internalization of proximal Na^+/H^+ exchanger from the apical membrane might participate. Pressure natriuresis has been traced to alteration of renal interstitial hydrostatic pressure (RIHP). An increase in RIHP occurs when RPP is elevated,[376] and both the increase in RIHP and natriuresis can be blunted through renal decapsulation.[377] Garcia-Estan and Roman have suggested that residual effects after decapsulation might be traced to the inability of decapsulation to modulate interstitial pressure in the renal medulla.[378] A role for RIHP in the phenomenon of pressure natriuresis is supported by experiments in which it has been altered without changing RPP. Infusion of 2.5% albumin into the

renal interstitium increases RIHP and causes natriuresis through inhibition of sodium reabsorption by superficial and deep nephrons.[379,380]

It is accepted that renal cortical blood flow is autoregulated over a physiological range of renal perfusion pressure. In contrast, the extent to which medullary blood flow is autoregulated is controversial. It has been proposed that lack of medullary autoregulation is essential to pressure natriuresis, and the control of salt and water excretion.[76,184,381–385] The renal medulla is largely perfused by postglomerular blood. Flow through a small population of shunt vessels that bypass glomeruli has been invoked to explain the escape of the medulla from tubuloglomerular feedback-mediated autoregulation (Figures 24.1 and 24.3).[16,381] Nearly 50 years of investigation have failed to completely support or refute the hypothesis that blood flow to the renal medulla lacks autoregulation. Work with microvascular transit time indicators favored lack of autoregulation,[171] but several early studies favored its presence.[183,386,387] Studies performed in the rat suggest that the efficiency of medullary autoregulation is a function of volume status. Measurement of blood flow to the cortex and medulla using videomicroscopy or laser-Doppler probes placed on the renal surface[388] or within the parenchyma[389] showed that medullary blood flow of volume-expanded rats does not autoregulate, but instead increases with perfusion pressure (Figure 24.22). Both an increase in single vessel blood flow rate and recruitment of flow through

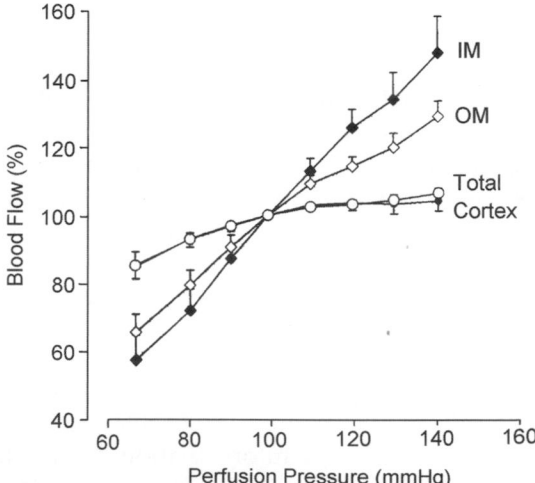

FIGURE 24.22 Autoregulation in different regions of the kidney. An electromagnetic flow device on the renal artery was used to measure total renal blood flow. Laser-Doppler flow probes were inserted into the renal parenchyma at various depths to measure regional blood flow in the outer and inner medulla. Total renal blood flow and cortical tissue blood flow shows intact autoregulation (stability of blood flow over a range of perfusion pressure). In contrast, in these volume-expanded rats (see text) the small fraction of blood flow that reaches the outer or inner medulla is not autoregulated. *(Reproduced with permission from ref. [389]).*

previously unperfused vasa recta may contribute to the process.[388] In contrast to volume-expanded animals, hydropenic rats autoregulate medullary blood flow and minimal pressure natriuresis[381,382,384,390] (Figure 24.23). Studies of regional blood flow in sodium-replete dogs by Majid, and in rabbits by Eppel et al. support intact medullary autoregulation.[391,392] Zhang and colleagues recently demonstrated that pressurizing the DVR lumen leads to endothelial $[Ca^{2+}]_{CYT}$ elevation and generation of NO.[393] If transmission of pressure to the medulla is a key event in pressure natriuresis, release of NO could conceivably inhibit salt reabsorption by adjacent nephrons generating pressure natriuresis. Such a paracrine role for NO to signal between the vasculature and nephrons is frequently postulated.[382,394–397]

Blood flow to the renal medulla is dependent on generation of NO.[382,384] This is particularly true in the spontaneously hypertensive rat (SHR).[398] Roald and colleagues observed poor autoregulation of juxtamedullary blood flow in the SHR. They proposed that the tendency toward early tissue damage in the juxtaglomerular cortex is due to poor autoregulation.[399] The superoxide dismutase mimetic, tempol, enhances tissue NO levels by eliminating its reaction with superoxide.[400] Feng and colleagues found that tempol reduced blood pressure and enhanced medullary blood flow in the SHR.[401]

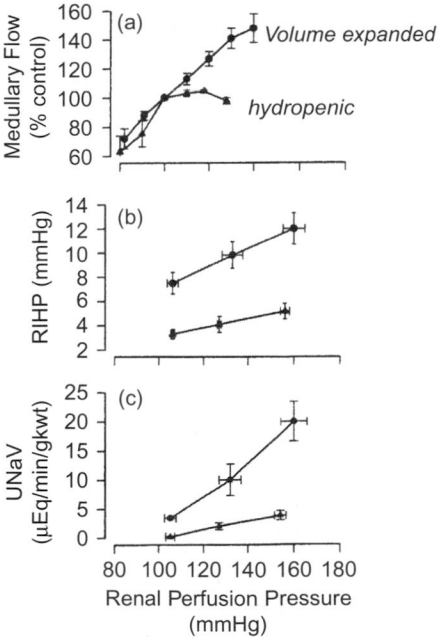

FIGURE 24.23 **Pressure natriuresis.** Panel a: Medullary blood flow is autoregulated in hydropenic but not volume-expanded rats. Panel b: Renal interstitial hydrostatic pressure (RIHP) is higher and increases to a greater degree with renal perfusion pressure in volume-expanded animals. Panel c: When renal perfusion pressure is increased, urinary sodium excretion (UNaV) increases much more markedly in volume-expanded than in hydropenic animals. *(Reproduced with permission from ref. [381]).*

Vasopressin and Excretion of Water

Changes in medullary blood flow might have a diuretic effect by reducing the efficiency of countercurrent exchange, leading to "solute washout" and loss of corticomedullary axial gradients of NaCl and urea.[17] The role of vasopressin to modulate medullary blood flow during antidiuresis has been the focus of much investigation.[2,381,390,402] Early studies, based on indicator transit times, showed that vasopressin reduces medullary blood flow.[171] Homozygous Brattleboro rats that lack vasopressin secretion have elevated papillary plasma flow.[156] The effect of vasopressin and specific V_1 (vasoconstrictor) and V_2 (antidiuretic) receptor subtype inhibitors on vasa recta blood flow was studied with videomicroscopy. Vasopressin reduces vasa recta blood flow in a manner that was partially blocked with either vasopressin V1 or V2 receptor subtype inhibitors.[403–405]

Studies with laser-Doppler and implantable probes confirmed that intrarenal infusion of a selective V_1 receptor agonist reduces inner medullary blood flow more than outer medullary blood flow.[406] Similarly, elevation of circulating vasopressin, stimulated by depriving conscious rats of water, led to selective reduction of only inner medullary blood flow, sparing perfusion of the cortex and outer medulla. Infusion of a V_1-antagonist into the medullary parenchyma blocked the decline in inner medullary perfusion and interfered with urinary concentration.[33] When vasopressin was infused into decerebrate rats to maintain plasma levels within a physiological range of 2.9 to 11.2 pg/ml (about 1 to 10 pM), inner medullary blood flow fell to an extent that correlated with urinary osmolality[33] (Figure 24.24). Those studies support the V_1-mediated vascular effect of vasopressin as a modulator of inner medullary blood flow favoring antidiuresis. The renal cortex might be spared from V_1

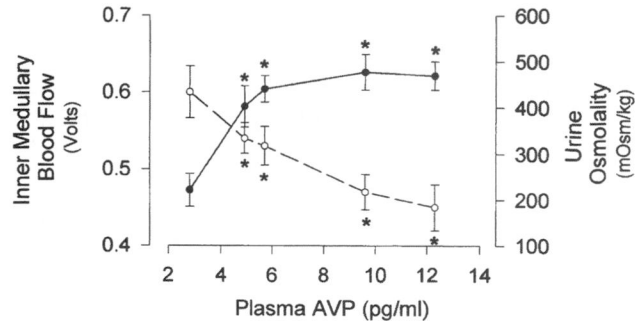

FIGURE 24.24 **Effect of arginine vasopressin (AVP) on inner medullary blood flow and urine osmolality.** To control plasma vasopressin concentrations, decerebrate rats were infused with AVP. Increasing AVP concentration within the physiological range caused a reduction of inner medullary blood flow and an improvement in urinary concentration. *(Reproduced with permission from ref. [33]).*

receptor-mediated vasoconstriction by reflex generation of vasodilator epoxyeicosatrienoic acids.[407]

Vasopressin reduces inner medullary perfusion by acting at various sites. It constricts juxtamedullary afferent (1 pM–1 nM) and efferent (1 nM) arterioles in isolated, perfused rat kidneys.[408] Afferent AVP constriction is dependent upon voltage-gated Ca^{2+} entry, whereas efferent constriction may be related to Ca^{2+} mobilization from stores.[409] Vasopressin also constricts rabbit afferent arterioles,[410] efferent arterioles (0.1 pM–100 nM), and rat outer medullary DVR (100 pM–1 microM) *in vitro*.[411,412] Correia and colleagues showed that vasopressin V_1-agonist reduced medullary blood flow in rabbits, but did not constrict either juxtamedullary afferent or efferent arterioles. They concluded that DVR might be the primary site at which vasopressin acts to regulate inner medullary blood flow.[413]

In addition to the constrictor effects of vasopressin, mediated by the V1 receptor, it has been demonstrated that vasodilation of some vessels can be mediated through vascular V2 receptors, leading to elevation of nitric oxide.[414–417] Selective V2 agonists have been shown to dilate preconstricted afferent arterioles[418] and outer medullary DVR[412] *in vitro*. In contrast, however, efforts to date have failed to show V2 receptor mRNA in dissected renal microvessels by RT-PCR.[419] Chronic infusion of the V2 agonist dDAVP was shown to elevate renal medullary nitric oxide and increase medullary blood flow,[420] an effect that may be related to release of NO by collecting duct.[421,422] Blockade of NO production during vasopressin elevation leads to hypertension. That finding suggests that V2-mediated NO production in the medulla serves as a buffer to protect the outer medulla from ischemia, as well as to prevent salt retention and hypertension.[423,424] The probable source of V2-mediated NO production is the inner medullary collecting duct.[421]

Angiotensins

Studies that employ isolated microvessel perfusion,[193,194,198,396,410,421,425,426] the juxtamedullary nephron preparation[205,263,427] or the split hydronephrotic kidney,[204,210] have all shown that angiotensin II constricts afferent arterioles, efferent arterioles, and DVR. Cultured mesangial cells also contract in response to angiotensin II.[320] Angiotensin II tonically constricts the juxtamedullary microcirculation *in vivo*[160,428–430] in a manner that is modulated by vasodilators and renal nerves.[431–435] Several vasodilators modulate angiotensin II-induced vasoconstriction. Blockade of NOS induces basal constriction of afferent arterioles and DVR, and intensifies constriction by angiotensin II stimulation.[193,194,436–438] Paracrine agents such as prostaglandin E_2 (PGE$_2$) and

adenosine counteract angiotensin II constriction of glomerular arterioles and DVR.[198,439–441] Blockade of prostaglandin production may have a greater effect in augmenting constriction of juxtamedullary than superficial glomerular arterioles.[439]

Angiotensin II exerts its effects through type 1 (AT1$_A$ and AT1$_B$) and type 2 (AT2) receptors. AT1 stimulation activates phospholipase C (PLC) to generate inositol trisphosphate (IP$_3$) and elevate $[Ca^{2+}]_{CYT}$.[211,215] AT1$_A$ receptor-null mice have blunted afferent and absent efferent arteriolar responses to angiotensin II.[442] Study of the distribution of receptors on juxtamedullary efferent arterioles revealed expression of AT1$_A$, AT1$_B$, and AT2 on muscular efferents destined to perfuse the medulla. In contrast, the AT1$_B$ subtype was absent in efferent arterioles that give rise to juxtamedullary capillary plexus in the cortex.[443] AT2 receptor activation has been reported to favor vasodilation via generation of nitric oxide.[444,445] In the afferent arteriole, however, AT2 stimulation favors synthesis of vasodilatory CYP450 epoxygenase products (EETs)[436,437,446] rather than NO. The evidence favors compensatory NO generation due to AT1 stimulation.[447,448] AT2 activation also vasodilates efferent arterioles[449] and DVR, where it both inhibits reactive oxygen species formation and facilitates endothelium-dependent $[Ca^{2+}]_{CYT}$ signaling in response to vasodilators.[395,450,451] The vasodilatory response to AT2 receptors may be impaired in forms of hypertension.[452,453] Both AT1 and AT2 receptors are widely expressed in vascular and tubular elements of the kidney.[454]

The role of angiotensin II AT1 and AT2 receptors to modulate regional perfusion in the kidney has been investigated. Angiotensin II constricts DVR that supply the medulla,[198,395] but angiotensin II infusion largely reduces blood flow to the renal cortex, sparing the medulla.[432,434,435] Moreover, there are reports that angiotensin II enhances medullary perfusion in rats and rabbits.[431,455,456] The resistance of the renal medulla to angiotensin II-induced vasoconstriction has been traced to reflex generation of compensatory vasodilators, particularly NO.[394,395,455,457–459] Recent studies favor the role of endothelial nitric oxide synthase (eNOS, NOS3) to maintain basal perfusion and stimulation of neuronal nitric oxide synthase (nNOS, NOS1) to blunt vasoconstriction by angiotensin II.[460] Pressure natriuresis has been tied to renal medullary perfusion (see above). Possibly related to this, AT2 receptor-null mice are hypertensive and lack the pressure natriuretic response.[461]

Angiotensin II constricts renal microvessels over a broad range of concentrations, with efferent arterioles and DVR showing the greatest sensitivity (EC$_{50}$ ~0.5 nM). Although circulating plasma angiotensin II concentrations are in the range of 100 pM, renal interstitial and intratubular concentrations approach 1 to 10 nM, implying that there is an intrarenal mechanism for generation and sequestration (Figure 24.25). Interstitial concentrations are greatest in the renal medulla, where angiotensin II receptor density is high.[462-466] At very high concentrations of 1 to 10 nM, angiotensin II acting via the AT1 receptor blunts DVR endothelial $[Ca^{2+}]_{CYT}$ responses to bradykinin and acetylcholine, an effect that is partially counteracted by concomitant AT2 receptor activation.[395,450] At high concentrations, angiotensin II inhibits K^+ channel activity of DVR pericytes[274,467,468] while stimulating Ca^{2+}-dependent Cl^- channel-mediated depolarization[268,270,273] to favor voltage-gated Ca^{2+} entry.[231,236] In DVR pericytes, angiotensin II often induces oscillations of $[Ca^{2+}]_{CYT}$ and Cl^- ion conductance.[271,272] Taken together, the results favor the interpretation that high levels of angiotensin II prevent vasodilatory compensation within vasa recta by blocking NO generation and K^+ channel activation, while stimulating NO generation by adjacent nephrons. Hypothetically, DVR on the vascular bundle periphery dilate in response to NO from adjacent epithelia to preferentially maintain outer medullary perfusion.[394,459,469-471]

Angiotensin II is derived from angiotensin I through the actions of angiotensin-converting enzyme (ACE).

Angiotensin II has a short half-life, and is itself degraded by angiotensinases to form several fragments, including angiotensin [1-7] and angiotensin [3-8]. Angiotensin-converting enzyme type 2 (ACE2) is a metalloprotease that hydrolyzes angiotensin I and angiotensin II to form the heptapeptide, angiotensin [1-7]. ACE2 is not blocked by conventional converting enzyme inhibitors. ACE2 reduces formation of angiotensin II by degrading angiotensin I to other fragments.[444,464,472] Angiotensin [1-7] is a dilator of the renal and other capillary beds,[473] and accumulates during ACE inhibition, potentially contributing to antihypertensive actions of those pharmaceuticals.[474] In the kidney, angiotensin [1-7] specifically binds to the Mas receptor. Mas-null mice lack binding, aortic relaxation, and antidiuretic response to angiotensin [1-7].[475] Renoprotective roles for angiotensin [1-7] are emerging.[476-478]

Aldosterone

Aldosterone increases transcription of molecular machinery dedicated to salt reabsorption in the distal nephron. It has been shown to increase mRNA for renin in juxtaglomerular cells in a manner that is blocked by the mineralocorticoid receptor antagonist, spironoloactone.[479] Recently, it has also been shown that aldosterone acts as a paracrine agent in the vasculature to have acute "nongenomic" effects on vasoactivity.[480] This was uncovered by Schmidt and colleagues, who showed that aldosterone increased human forearm blood flow. With NOS inhibition, aldosterone enhanced blood flow reduction mediated by phenyephrine. The data were interpreted to show that aldosterone causes vasoconstriction via smooth muscle activation and compensatory vasodilation via release of NO.[481] Similarly, Arima et al. showed that aldosterone caused concentration-dependent constriction of both afferent and efferent arterioles, an effect that was insensitive to spironoloactone. The constriction was prevented by PLC inhibition, involved voltage-gated Ca^{2+} entry mediated principally by L-type and T-type channels in the afferent and efferent arterioles, respectively, and is partially offset by NO generation.[482-485]

Adrenomedullin

Adrenomedullin and adrenomedullin-2/intermedin are peptide hormones with homology to calcitonin gene related peptide (CGRP). It circulates in picomolar concentrations and is widely synthesized by tissues including vascular smooth muscle and endothelium. It has potent vasodilatory and hypotensive effects, at least partially mediated by NO.[486-488] Deletion of the gene for adrenomedullin is lethal *in utero*.

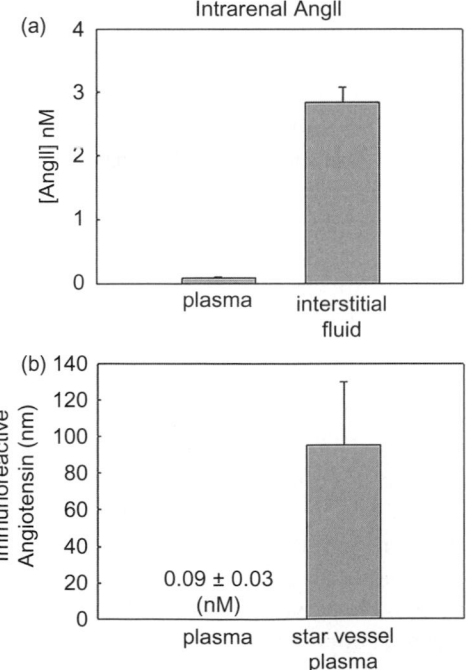

FIGURE 24.25 Intrarenal angiotensin II concentrations. (a) Graph shows a comparison of angiotensin II concentration in plasma and renal interstitial fluid obtained by microdialysis. Cortical interstitial angiotensin II concentrations are markedly higher than plasma values. (b) Comparison of immunoreactive angiotensins in systemic plasma and star vessel plasma (efferent arteriolar, precapillary blood) by micropuncture of the rat kidney. Angiotensin II concentration is estimated to be ~10-25% of the immunoreactive angiotensins in various compartments. (*Results redrawn from published data [465,466]*).

Heterozygotes live to adulthood but are hypertensive, have defective synthesis of NO, and are vulnerable to renal ischemia.[489,490] Renal synthesis of adrenomedullin is enhanced by hypoxia.[491] Intrarenal infusion induces vasodilation that is attenuated by NO synthase inhibition[492–494] and was found to increase canine cortical and medullary blood flow.[493] Adrenomedullin has been shown to dilate both afferent and efferent arterioles of the hydronephrotic kidney preparation.[495] Chronic infusion of adrenomedullin was found to limit hypertensive injury in deoxycorticosterone (DOCA) salt hypertensive rats[496,497] and limits injury during ureteral obstruction.[498] It may partially act by limiting generation of reactive oxygen species.[499]

Intermedin, also known as adrenomedullin-2, shares many of the properties of adrenomedullin. Its receptor profile overlaps that of CGRP and adrenomedullin, and its adult expression is largely in the hypothalamus, pituitary, and kidney.[500,501] Intra-arterial infusion enhances renal blood flow and induces diuresis.[502] Like adrenomedullin, intermedin has been found to ameliorate renal tissue damage in pathological models,[503] and its expression is reduced in forms of renal injury.[504]

Nitric Oxide

Endothelia and transporting epthelia secrete paracrine modulators of vascular tone, including nitric oxide (NO), prostacyclin (prostaglandin I_2, PGI_2), and endothelium-derived hyperpolarizing factors (EDHF). Nitric oxide regulates vessel tone, regional distribution of blood flow, autoregulation, pressure natriuresis, tubuloglomerular feedback, and salt reabsorption. Its effects on the microcirulation of the kidney are protean and have been frequently reviewed.[382–385,457,505–517] Nitric oxide synthase (NOS) isoforms are expressed by nephrons and vessels throughout the kidney,[384,385,510,513] but expression is greatest in the inner medullary collecting duct and vasa recta.[518] It has also been shown that NO generation by collecting duct is regulated by uptake of L-arginine via the CAT1 cationic amino acid transporter.[519–522] Infusion of competing cationic amino acids reduced medullary NO, reduced medullary blood flow, and induced hypertension.[519] Asymmetric dimethyl arginine (ADMA) is an endogenous NOS inhibitor that is metabolized by dimethylaminohydrolase (DDAH).[523–525] ADMA equilibrates with the cytoplasm via cationic amino acid transporters (CATs), competes with their ability to transport L-arginine, and inhibits NOS.[524] The DDAH2 isoform predominates to remove ADMA in the vasculature. The role of ADMA and DDAH in endothelial function and dysfunction is the subject of much current investigation.[526,527]

Infusion of the NO synthase inhibitor Nw-nitro-L-arginine methyl ester (L-NAME) into the renal artery of rats and dogs increases renal vascular resistance and blunts pressure natriuresis.[528,529] NOS inhibition constricts the preglomerular microcirculation of the juxtamedullary nephron preparation, an effect that is enhanced when RBCs, that consume NO, are included in the perfusate.[530,531] The ability of NO to modulate afferent arteriolar tone results both from its synthesis by the endothelium[193–195,532] and signaling in the macula densa.[196] Similar to cortical microvessels, NOS inhibition constricts isolated DVR, largely by preventing the consumption of superoxide by NO.[425,438]

NOS inhibition interferes with pressure natriuresis.[531,533] Infusion of an NO synthase inhibitor into rats was found to restore medullary autoregulation and blunt the pressure natriuretic response.[383] Similarly, infusion of L-arginine both altered medullary autoregulation and normalized pressure natriuresis in the spontaneously hypertensive rat (SHR).[534] Exogenous L-arginine increases NO production in cultured cells and the isolated perfused kidney.[535] Moreover, it can abrogate hypertension and renal damage in hypertension induced by chronic angiotensin II infusion.[536,537]

Chronic, global NOS inhibition causes a selective reduction of renal medullary blood flow.[538,539] Nitric oxide (NO) production in the renal medulla exceeds that in the cortex.[385,540–543] L-arginine supplementation enhances NO levels in the renal medullary interstitium,[543] and abrogates hypertension in the Dahl rat and SHR.[534,544,545] In contrast to global NOS inhibition, reduction of nNOS activity induces hypertension without affecting medullary perfusion, suggesting that the saliuretic effects of NO generated by those isoforms is of predominant importance.[546–549] Thus, NO generated by eNOS may primarily affect basal vascular resistance, while NO derived from other NOS isoforms, particularly nNOS, affects renal epithelial Na^+ reabsorption and adaptation to a high-salt diet.[550–552]

NO is released in response to administration of the vasoconstrictor agents norepinephrine, angiotensin II, and vasopressin.[420,424,458,459,553,554] Evidence also favors an important role for NO to abrogate tissue hypoxia that would otherwise arise from the action of vasoconstrictors. Low dose, subpressor infusion of L-NAME into the renal interstitium does not affect MBF or pO_2, but enables otherwise ineffective doses of angiotensin II,[459] norepinephrine[553,554] or vasopressin[424,555] to reduce those parameters. Reduced expression of NOS isoforms and NO generation in the Dahl rat may contribute to its sensitivity to angiotensin II and hypertension.[458] In the absence of NOS blockade, constrictors enhance medullary NO levels, implying that a reflex increase in medullary NO probably serves to protect the hypoxic medulla from ischemia. NO generation has also been found to protect the medulla from the blood flow redistribution induced by endotoxemic hypotension[556,557] and radiocontrast agents.[558]

Given that NO has both vasodilatory and saliuretic effects and is widely synthesized by nephrons and endothelium, attention has been drawn to possible tubulovascular interactions. NO generated by the medullary thick ascending limb has been proposed to influence DVR tone to mitigate medullary hypoperfusion and hypoxia.[269,382,394,395,450,559,560] NO generation by DVR is highly perfusion-dependent,[393] and NOS inhibition constricts *in vitro* perfused DVR, implying a substantial tonic role for intrinsic endothelial NO generation to modify DVR function.[425] The bioavailability and actions of NO are predicted to be under the influence of opposing generation of reactive oxygen species.[471,561] Mathematical simulations of NO and superoxide trafficking in the medulla favor a role for DVR endothelial NO generation to influence tissue NO levels,[469,470] leading to the consideration that DVR might influence salt reabsorption by adjacent nephrons. The latter might mechanistically link medullary perfusion and pressure natriuresis.[393] Stated another way, hemoglobin in outer medullary vascular bundles degrades NO so that NO from transporting epithelia and DVR endothelium must generate gradients directed toward the vascular bundle centers. Accordingly, elevation of NO outside vascular bundles in the vicinity of nephrons is likely to arise from both epithelial and endothelial NO generation.

Reactive Oxygen Species

Oxygen free radicals are generated by one and two electron reductions of O_2 that generate superoxide (O_2^-) and hydrogen peroxide (H_2O_2). In turn, reactions of those species yield hypochlorous acid and hydroxyl radical (OH). Reaction of NO with O_2^- forms peroxynitrite ($ONOO^-$), reducing the availability of NO to act as a vasodilator. Oxygen-derived radicals are collectively referred to as "reactive oxygen species" (ROS). ROS can be generated through many pathways. Autooxidation of cysteine can generate O_2^- and H_2O_2. Oxygen utilizing enzymes such as cyclooxygenase, lipoxygenase, epoxygenase, and xanthine oxidase can generate ROS. When oxidative stress reduces the ratio of the NOS co-factor tetrahydrobiopterin (BH_4) relative to dihydrobiopterin (BH_2), NOS produces O_2^- rather than NO. It is generally accepted that the dominant source of ROS for bacterocidal activity in leukocytes and signaling in other cells is NADPH oxidase. NADPH oxidase consists of cytosolic components ($p47^{phox}$, $p67^{phox}$), a G-protein (Rac1 or Rac2), and membrane-associated cytochrome b_{558} comprised of

$p22^{phox}$ and $gp91^{phox}$. In nonphagocytic cells, the $gp91^{phox}$-subunit may be substituted by another isoform, such as RENOX/NOX4.[400] Antioxidant systems exist within all cells. Superoxide dismutase (SOD) catalyzes the conversion of O_2^- to H_2O_2 which is then converted to water by catalase. Extracellular, cytoplasmic (Cu/ZnSOD), and mitochondrial (MnSOD) forms of SOD participate in the control of oxidative stress. Endogenous free radical scavengers also serve to limit the potential for oxidative damage to cellular macromolecules.[562]

Tissue NO levels are modulated through reaction with ROS. Generation of oxygen free radicals is known to affect agonist-induced constriction of renal microvessels in cortex and medulla,[563–565] and play a prominent role in hypertension.[516,566] The cell permeant superoxide dismutase (SOD) mimetic, tempol, prevents afferent arteriolar constriction by the TxA_2/prostaglandin H_2 (TP) receptor agonist U-46,619.[567] Similarly, tempol increased detection of NO in bradykinin stimulated DVR and vasodilated DVR preconstricted with angiotensin II.[560] Zhang et al. found that ROS are generated upon stimulation of DVR with angiotensin II and protein kinase C agonists, and angiotensin II-stimulated ROS generation was enhanced when AT2 receptors were blocked with PD123,319.[451] The role of ROS in the mediation of vasoconstriction probably varies with the vasoactive stimulus.[568] Studies of ROS generation by the medullary thick ascending limb show that reactions with superoxide from the mTAL might limit NO delivery and vasodilation of vascular bundle DVR.[394,569,570]

Intrarenal generation of ROS plays a role in vasoactivity and generation of hypertension.[506,515,566,571,572] Blood pressure elevation in the SHR is associated with enhanced urinary excretion of the ROS marker, 8-iso prostaglandin F2α. Both hypertension and 8-Iso PGF2α excretion are blunted by the superoxide dismutase (SOD) mimetic, tempol. Infusion of L-NAME eliminates the antihypertensive effect of tempol, implying that reduction of NO availability through reaction with O_2^- partially underlies the genesis of SHR hypertension.[573,574] Slow pressor hypertension due to chronic infusion of angiotensin II is also associated with an increase in cortical ROS generation,[575] but the medulla may be spared in that model.[576] Intrarenal oxygen tension and the efficiency of renal oxygen utilization are low in rodent models of hypertension, suggesting a shunt of oxygen toward formation of ROS.[577–579]

Enhancement of renal medullary ROS generation occurs in hypertensive models and intramedullary infusion of the SOD inhibitor, diethylthiocarbamate, reduces medullary blood flow and raises arterial blood pressure.[580–582] Conversely, infusion of the SOD mimetic, tempol, increases medullary blood flow and sodium excretion, an effect that is enhanced when H_2O_2 is eliminated with catalase.[580,581,583] A role for renal medullary generation of ROS was reinforced by Meng et al. who showed that hypertension of Dahl salt-sensitive rats is accompanied by reduced expression of Cu/Zn SOD and Mn SOD in the medulla.[584] In contrast to those findings, slow pressor hypertension generated by chronic angiotensin II infusion failed to increase ROS generation by isolated DVR.[576] Instead, angiotensin II hypertension was accompanied by increased DVR generation of NO, a finding that agrees with earlier reports by Zou and Cowley.[382,459] It is possible that ROS production by medullary nephrons contributes to angiotensin II, slow pressor hypertension. NO is an endogenous diuretic, and its consumption by ROS could favor hypertension.[550,551] Enhanced generation of ROS may also play a role in enhancing arteriolar constriction in diabetes.[316,585-589]

Carbon Monoxide and Hemoxygenase

Hemoxygenases-1 and -2 (HO-1, HO-2) are microsomal enzymes that degrade heme to form carbon monoxide (CO) and biliverdin. CO, like NO, induces vasodilation via cGMP generation, while biliverdin is converted to bilirubin by biliverdin reductase. Bilirubin is a highly effective free radical scavenger and inhibits ROS generation via NADPH oxidase and protein kinase C.[590] Constitutive expression of HO isoforms in the kidney predominate in the medulla[591] under transcriptional control of oxygen and superoxide anion. Hypoxia inducible factor $\alpha 1$,[592,593] urea concentration, and medullary hypertonicity[594] all influence HO expression. HO inhibition with zinc deuteroporphyrin 2,4-bis glycol via the renal interstitium reduces medullary blood flow and cGMP content.[591] Treatment with cobalt protoporphyrin upregulates HO-1, reduces intrarenal levels of 20-HETE, and ameliorates SHR hypertension.[595] Exacerbation and protection of the kidney from ischemic injury can be accomplished by inhibiting or upregulating HO-1.[596] Acute HO inhibition blunts pressure natriuresis, and chronic inhibition raises blood pressure.[597-599] HO pre-induction blocks slow-pressor angiotensin II-induced hypertension.[600,601] Inducing HO also minimizes radiocontrast injury.[602,603] The protean and beneficial effects of HO upregulation have attracted considerable attention, pointing to a potential target for therapeutic intervention.[590,604]

Adenosine and P1 Purinoceptors

Adenosine acts via A1, A2$_A$, A2$_B$, and A3 receptors (P$_1$ purinoceptors). In the kidney, A1 and A2 receptors predominate, A2$_A$ are primarily vascular, and A3 may

be absent.[605,606] Through its action, adenosine modulates vasoactivity and epithelial transport.[605,607-610] Acting via the P2X1 receptor, adenosine may be a primary mediator of renal autoregulation.[611] The microvascular effects of adenosine vary with intrarenal location.[612] Adenosine A1 receptor activation transiently reduces cortical and medullary blood flow, and constricts afferent arterioles.[613-615] When afferent A1 receptors are blocked, however, A2 mediated vasodilation can be elicited.[616] The effects of adenosine in the efferent arteriole may be primarily vasodilatory.[153,617,618] Afferent constriction by adenosine is of particular importance, because evidence supports it as a key mediator of tubuloglomerular feedback (TGF).[619-624] ATP release from macula densa cells via maxi-anion channels followed by ecto-5'-nucleotidase-mediated hydrolysis are the likely steps in its formation.[366-368,370,625] A role for adenosine to act on both afferent and efferent arterioles has been proposed as integral to the TGF response.[153,626] Adenosine constriction of the afferent arteriole is complex, because proximal portions away from the glomerulus may be regulated by both A2-mediated dilatory and A1-mediated contractile interactions. In contrast, the afferent arteriole near the glomerlar hilus may lack A2 receptors, so that it constricts as adenosine concentration is increased.[264,607]

Adenosine A2 receptor stimulation leads to preferential vasodilation, saliuresis, and enhanced perfusion of the medulla[612,613,627] (Figure 24.26). Both A1 and A2 receptors are expressed by DVR,[628] and their respective stimulation induces constriction or dilation.[396] Interstitial adenosine concentrations are near the affinity for the A2 receptor, so that changes should modulate vasodilatory and saliuretic effects.[629] In preglomerular vessels, A1-induced constriction is mediated by pertussis toxin sensitive G$_i$-protein and phospholipase C activation.[630] A2-mediated dilation has been traced to activation of K$_{ATP}$ channels,[313] probably activated through 11,12-epoxyeicosatrienoic acid.[631]

Evidence for and against synergism between angiotensin II and adenosine exists.[197,625] Several studies have favored the interdependence of adenosine A1 receptor- and angiotensin II AT1 receptor-mediated constriction,[632-636] while others have not.[614,637,638] The availability of adenosine A1 and angiotensin II AT1$_A$ receptor-deficient mice have permitted re-examination of the issue. Infusion of angiotensin II led to less reduction of renal blood flow and less constriction of afferent arterioles in A1 knockout mice.[197] Similarly, favoring synergism, intranephron infusion of an adenosine A1 agonist induced greater reduction of stop-flow pressure (reflecting afferent constriction) in wild-type than in angiotensin II AT1$_A$ receptor-deficient mice.[639]

A consequence of countercurrent exchange is that renal medullary oxygen tensions (pO$_2$) are low[640]

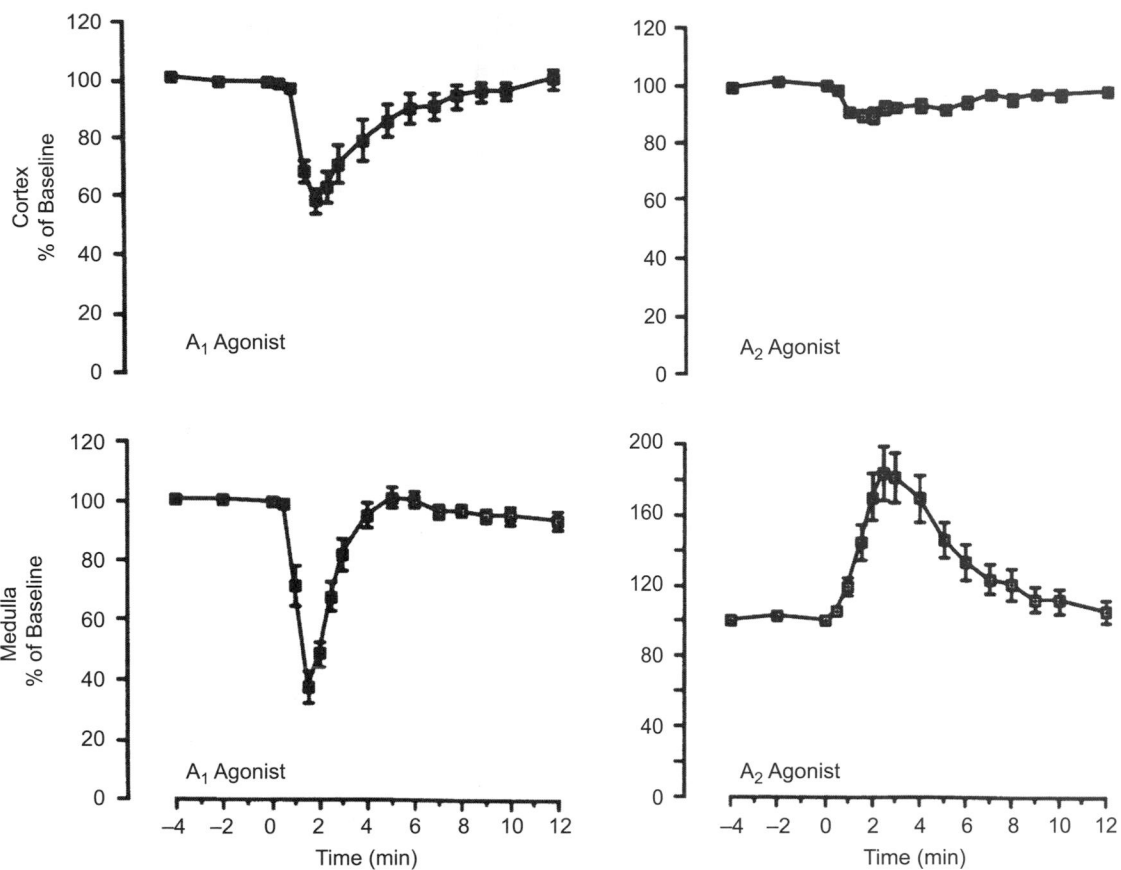

FIGURE 24.26 **Effect of intrarenal infusion of adenosine receptor A1 or A2 subtype agonists.** Top and bottom panels show the effect of adenosine agonist infusions on intrarenal blood flow. Cortical and medullary measurements were obtained using laser-Doppler flowmetry with optical fibers placed on the kidney surface or inserted into the renal parenchyma, respectively. Left and right panels show the respective effects of either A1 or A2 receptor stimulation with subtype specific agonists. At time = 0, the A1 agonist N^6-cyclopentyladenosine (left panels) or the A2 agonist CGS-21680C (right panels) were transiently infused (1 minute) into the renal parenchyma. The A1 agonist transiently reduced both cortical and medullary blood flow, while the A2 agonist caused a preferential increase in blood flow to the medulla. (*Reproduced with permission from ref. [613,465]*).

(Figure 24.27). During hypoxia, the medullary thick ascending limb of Henle (mTAL) synthesizes adenosine.[641] That finding, coupled with the close proximity of the mTAL to outer medullary vascular bundles, led to the hypothesis that adenosine, like NO and prostaglandins (see above), acts as a paracrine vasodilator to preserve medullary perfusion, raising medullary pO_2.[642] Inhibition of mTAL transport by adenosine A2 receptor activation, like the effects of furosemide, probably raises medullary pO_2 by reducing O_2 consumption.[642,643] Rats fed a high-salt diet increase tissue adenosine levels and downregulate A1 receptor expression, the activation of which encourages sodium reabsorption.[644]

Extracellular ATP and Renal P_2 Purinoceptors

In addition to the actions of adenosine mediated by P1 purinoceptors (A1, A2 adenosine receptors),

micromolar concentrations of ATP modulate vasoactivity through P2 purinoceptors.[611,625,638,645−647] P2 receptors are subdivided into P2X and P2Y families, encoded by separate genes, that yield either ligand-gated nonselective cation channels or seven transmembrane spanning G-protein coupled receptors, respectively. Unlike adenosine receptors, P2 receptors seem confined to the preglomerular microcirculation.[648−650] P2 antagonists such as suramin are somewhat nonselective, however α,β-methylene-ATP and β,γ-methylene-ATP are relatively selective agonists for P2X receptors. UTP largely stimulates P2Y.[638,648,651,652] The experimental effects of ATP on the vasculature are variable, depending upon luminal versus abluminal application, the preparation, and species.[651] Both constrictor and dilator effects can be observed. Intrarenal infusion of α,β-methylene-ATP leads to constriction, but ATP (mixed P2X, P2Y agonist) and UTP (selective P2Y agonist) yield NO dependent dilation at low concentrations or constriction at high

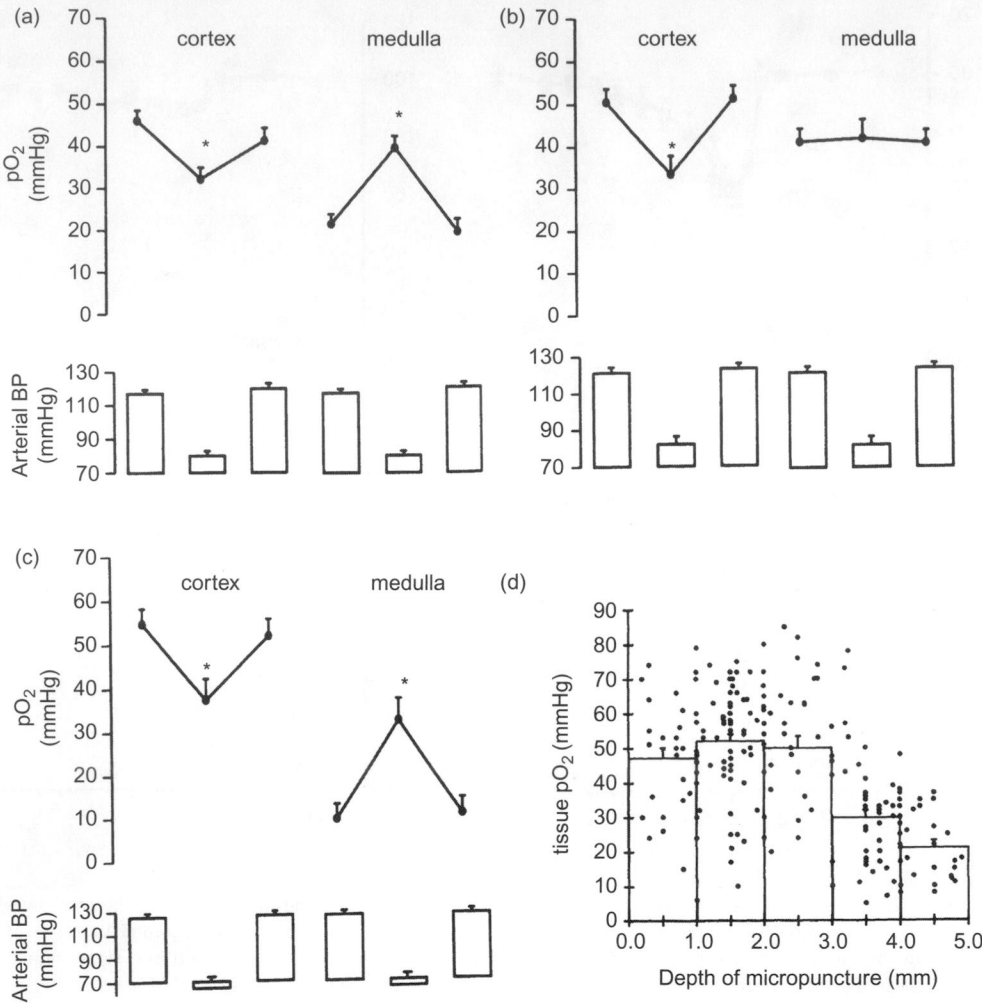

FIGURE 24.27   **Hemodynamic effects on intrarenal oxygenation.** Intrarenal oxygen tension (pO_2) was measured in the cortex and medulla with a microelectrode. Cortical pO_2 falls and medullary pO_2 increases during an episode of hypotension induced by hemorrhage, aortic ligation or nitroprusside infusion (Panel a). Inhibition of transport in the thick ascending limb of Henle with a loop diuretic (Panel b) increases basal pO_2 in the medulla (compare to Panel a), and eliminates the effect of hypotension to raise medullary pO_2. Inhibition of vasodilatory prostaglandins and nitric oxide or blockade of adenosine receptors reduces basal pO_2 in the medulla and accentuates the increase in pO_2 caused by hypotension (Panel c). Intrarenal tissue pO_2 decreases with medullary depth (Panel d). *(Reproduced with permission from ref. [643,791]).*

concentrations.[653] Exposure of preconstricted afferent arterioles of rabbit and human kidneys to ATP leads to dilation via NO generation.[647,651,654] In the juxtamedullary nephron preparation of the rat, activation of P2X leads to afferent but not efferent constriction that is dependent upon generation of 20-HETE and Ca^{2+} influx involving L-type Ca^{2+} channel blockade.[655−658] Stimulation of P2Y receptors yields sustained constriction that is independent of 20-HETE, and dependent upon Ca^{2+} release from cellular stores.[213,659,660]

Of great importance, myogenic autoregulatory constriction of afferent arterioles has been traced to activation of P2 receptors (Figure 24.28). In the juxtamedullary nephron preparation, prior desensitization or nonspecific blockade of P2 receptors attenuated pressure-induced afferent constriction.[661] Similarly,

infusion of excess ATP into the dog kidney during NO sythase blockade eliminated autoregulatory constriction.[662,663] Finally, P2X1 receptor-deficient mice were shown to retain tubuloglomerular feedback responses, but to lack autoregulatory adjustments to changes in perfusion pressure.[611,645,664] Pharmacological blockade of P2X1 receptors eliminates renal whole-organ autoregulation in the rat.[611]

Arachidonic Acid Metabolites

Once liberated from the membrane by phospholipases, arachidonic acid undergoes metabolism to a very large array of metabolites that function as paracrine, autocrine, and intracellular signaling molecules (Figure 24.29). These metabolites have profound effects

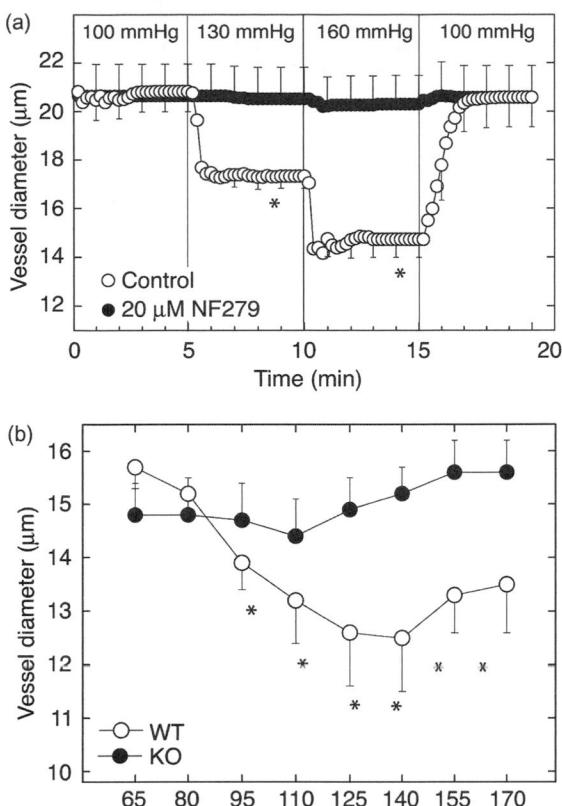

FIGURE 24.28 Autoregulation and purinoceptors. (a) Panel shows the effect of a P2X receptor blocker (NF279) on autoregulatory afferent arteriolar constriction resulting from step-changes in perfusion pressure from 100 to 120 and 160 mmHg. P2X blockade eliminates the afferent myogenic response associated with autoregulation. (b) Summary of the changes in murine afferent arteriolar diameter elicited by graded change of perfusion pressure. Autoregulatory vasoconstriction occurs in wild-type (WT) but not P2X$_1$ receptor-null mice. Data obtained using the juxtamedullary nephron preparation. *(Reproduced with permission from ref. [664]).*

on vascular tone, as well as on solute and water excretion. Three generalized pathways are recognized, cyclo-oxygenases (COX) that generate prostaglandins (PG) and thromboxanes (TBX), lipoxygenases that generate leukotrienes (LT) and hydroxyeicosatetraenoic acids (HETE), and cytochrome P450 pathways that synthesize HETEs and epoxyeicosatrienoic acids (EET).

Prostaglandins

Prostaglandins (PGs) are generated from arachidonic acid by cyclooxygenase (COX) (Figure 24.29a) and exert wide effects on solute reabsorption, tubuloglomerular feedback, and intrarenal hemodynamics. When injected into the renal artery, PGE$_2$ and PGI$_2$ enhance renal blood flow.[665] Early efforts showed that stimulation of PG synthesis redistributes blood flow toward the juxtamedullary cortex.[666,667] A consistent finding has been that renal medullary perfusion is

protected from vasoconstrictors by NO (see above) and PGs.[668,669] Nonselective COX blockade decreased vasa recta blood flow,[670] and augmented the ability of angiotensin II infusion to decrease single vessel blood flow in the exposed papilla.[428] Laser-Doppler studies indicate that COX blockade reduces medullary blood flow with relative sparing of cortical perfusion.[671–674] Radiocontrast agents can lower cortical and medullary oxygen content, predisposing to hypoxic insult. Indomethacin potentiates medullary hypoxia and the parenchymal damage induced by either radiocontrast agents or ureteral excision.[675–677]

COX-1 and COX-2 isoforms contribute to renal PG synthesis. Of the two, COX-1 is expressed to a greater extent, while COX-2 is more highly regulated.[678–682] In a manner that predicts the effects of its inhibition, COX-2 expression is pronounced in macula densa.[678] Release of renin by juxtaglomerular cells and release of PGE$_2$ by the macula densa is COX-2-dependent.[683–685] In the macula densa, COX-2 is co-expressed with NOS1. Simultaneous inhibition of COX-2 and NOS in the dog markedly enhances sensitivity to vasoconstriction. Norepinephrine infusion, which otherwise has minor effects, induces a remarkable rise in renal vascular resistance and sharp reduction of GFR.[686] COX-2 blockade blunts adaptation of tubuloglomerular feedback[687] and augments afferent constriction associated with benzolamide inhibition of proximal transport.[688] Renomedullary interstitial cells express receptors for vasoconstrictors, release paracrine substances such as PGE$_2$ and medullipin, and express both COX-1 and COX-2.[41,678] Zhang et al. showed that COX-2 expression is stimulated by medullary tonicity.[689] Genetic deficiency of COX-2 or its inhibition leads to reduction of medullary perfusion, salt-sensitive hypertension, and enhanced response to infusion of angiotensin II.[690–694]

In isolated vessels, Edwards first showed that prostaglandins dilate *in vitro* perfused rabbit afferent (PGE$_2$ and PGI$_2$) and efferent (PGI$_2$) arterioles.[695] In contrast, Inscho et al. found that PGE$_2$ enhanced angiotensin II and norepinephrine constriction of the afferent arteriole, while PGI$_2$ counteracted their effects.[696] In rabbit afferent arterioles, indomethacin enhanced vasoconstriction when perfusate passed through the glomerulus, but not during retrograde perfusion, implying that glomerular PGs influence efferent vasoactivity.[697] Abluminal PGE$_2$ blunts angiotensin II-induced constriction of DVR.[198,397] Few studies of the effects of selective COX-2 inhibition in isolated vessel preparations are available. Wang et al. determined that augmented constriction of afferent arterioles during slow pressor angiotensin II hypertension is partially mediated by a COX-2 product from the endothelium.[698] PGE$_2$ is very abundant in the kidney, and its local actions are governed by the receptor subtype activated.

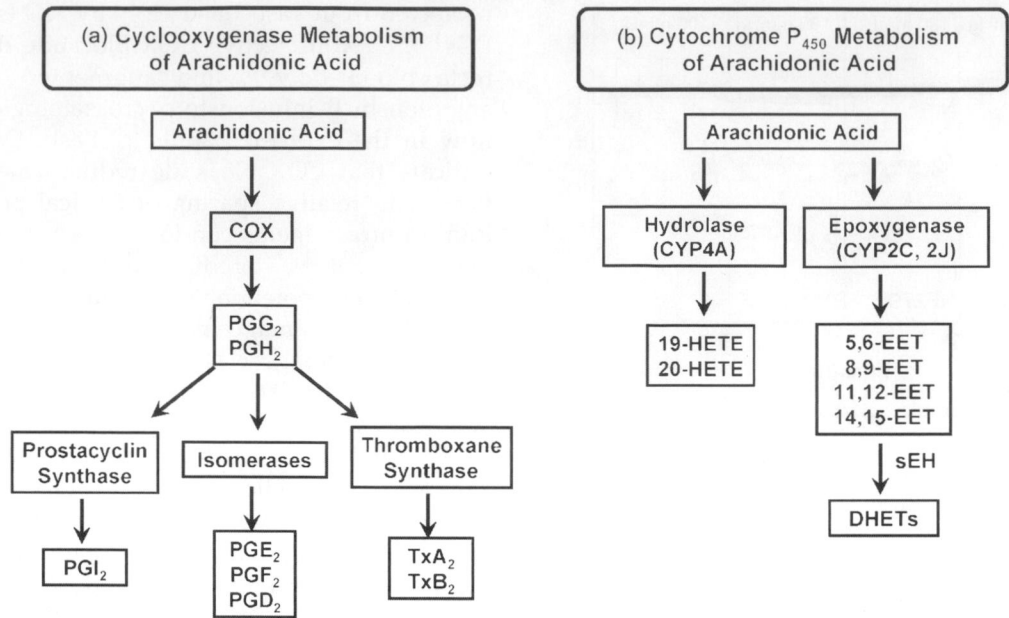

FIGURE 24.29 **Arachidonic acid metabolites.** (a) Abbreviated schematic showing signaling molecules generated from arachadonic acid by cyclo-oxygenase (COX). Prostaglandins (PG) and thromboxanes (Tx) are vasoactive end products. (b) Abbreviated schematic showing signaling molecules generated cytochrome P450 metabolism of arachidonic acid (COX). Hydrolases generate the potent constrictor 20-hydroxyeicosatetraenoic acid (20-HETE), and epoxygenases generate the epoxyeicosatrienoic acids (EETs) that most often function as vasodilators. The lipoxygenase pathway of arachidonic acid metabolism is not shown.

For example, stimulation of the EP3 receptor inhibits cAMP formation, favoring vasoconstriction, while stimulation of EP2 and EP4 receptors increases cAMP, favoring vasodilation.[297] The ability of PGE_2 to act as a vasoconstrictor has also been observed,[696] and EP3 receptor deficiency leads to reduction of renal vascular resistance.[297,699]

COX products can be metabolized by thromboxane synthase to stimulate the thromboxane/PGH_2 receptor and induce vasoconstriction. In the afferent arteriole and DVR, angiotensin II-induced constriction is reduced by TP receptor blockade, inhibition of COX with indomethacin or inhibition of thromboxane synthesis.[440,700−702] Thromboxane-mediated constriction may be exaggerated during angiotensin II slow pressor hypertension, due to enhanced sythesis of reactive oxygen species.[698,703]

Cytochrome P450 Metabolites of Arachadonic Acid

Vasoactive products of arachidonic acid are generated by cytochrome P450 (CYP) isoforms (Figure 24.29B) in the form of epoxyeicosatrienoic acids (EETs), the hydroxyeicosatetraenoic acids (HETEs) and their products, dihydroxyeicosatetraneoic acids (DHETs).[704] More than 400 CYP isoforms are recognized in various species. Those that have >40% homology are classified by an Arabic numeral and those with >55% homology by a capital letter. CYP monooxygenases metabolize arachadonic acid to 19- and 20-HETE (ω/ω-1 hyroxylase) and

to 5,6-, 8,9-, 11,12-, and 14,15-EETs (epoxygenases). For the purposes of focusing on the microvasculature of the kidney, it is important to recognize that CYP2C and CYC2J isoforms are largely responsible for synthesis of EETs, and CYP4A isoforms for synthesis of the HETEs. This topic has been frequently reviewed.[280,291,704−714]

The 20 ω-hydroxylation product, 20-HETE, is a potent vasoconstrictor the synthesis of which is rate-limited by O_2.[715,716] 20-HETE depolarizes and increases $[Ca^{2+}]_{CYT}$ in smooth muscle[290] and mediates constriction by angiotensin II,[436,717] endothelin-1,[708,718] and ATP via P2X stimulation.[658] 20-HETE plays an important role in blood flow autoregulation of the cerebral and renal microcirculations.[704,719] 20-HETE inhibits K_{Ca} channel activity[292−294,299,713,716] through the actions of tyrosine and MAP kinases.[293] It is generally recognized that NO inhibits vascular smooth muscle contraction through cGMP formation. Roman and colleagues have shown that the majority of NO effects in the kidney involve inhibition of CYP4A and reduction of 20-HETE synthesis.[300,720] 20 ω-Hydroxylation products play a role in blood pressure regulation, and blockade of 20-HETE synthesis interferes with pressure natriuresis.[721] Chronic inhibition of 20-HETE synthesis induces salt-sensitive hypertension in the rat,[722,723] and exacerbates ischemia reperfusion injury.[711] Similarly, disruption of murine CYP4A14 leads to hypertension, and a variant of the CYP4A11 homolog in humans has been associated with essential hypertension.[724−726]

The EET epoxygenase metabolite arachidonic acid has several important roles in the renal microcirculation. In addition, EETs have been broadly identified as endothelium-dependent hyperpolarizing factors (EDHF).[97,278] The EETs are largely vasodilatory, but some of their metabolites can induce COX-dependent vasoconstriction.[297,727,728] Stimulation of preglomerular arteriolar $A2_A$ adenosine receptors leads to enhanced synthesis of EETs and vasodilation.[631] Similarly, angiotensin II dilation via AT2 receptor stimulation has been traced to these epoxygenase products.[436,446] Afferent vasodilation by 11,12-EET is partially mediated by PKA.[729] In contrast to inhibition by 20-HETE, 11,12-EET and 5,6-EET are associated with K_{Ca} channel activation.[292,295,713,730−732]

The ability to activate large conductance K_{Ca} channels may be tied to the role of 11,12-EET as an EDHF. Putative EDHFs are agents that elevate endothelial $[Ca^{2+}]_{CYT}$, hyperpolarize endothelium and smooth muscle and vasodilate, independent of NO and COX. Work in this area has failed to identify a single EDHF, but much evidence points to a role for EET formation and K_{Ca} channel activation in the endothelium. Adjacent smooth muscle hyperpolarization may be tied to diffusion of secondary signaling molecules or electrogenic spread of current from the endothelium via myoendothelial gap junctions.[279,280] It might also be tied to release of K^+ ion into the myoendothelial intercellular space via EET-stimulated endothelial K_{Ca} channels, resulting in hyperpolarization via activation of smooth muscle K_{IR} or Na^+,K^+-ATPase.[97,278] In the kidney, evidence points to a role for afferent arteriolar EET formation in the EDHF related actions of bradykinin[733] and acetylcholine.[298] Evidence for K_{IR} expression in afferent smooth muscle has been provided.[304,305] Reduction of vasodilatory EET formation may accompany hypertension. Imig et al. showed that enhanced afferent constriction during slow pressor angiotensin II hypertension is reversed by an 11,12-EET analog, and that reduction of EET degradation through soluble epoxide hydrolase inhibition reverses angiotensin II hypertension.[734,735] Lack of ability to upregulate CYP2C and CYP2J isoforms of P450 might underlie the abnormality.[736] Similarly, it has been found that enhancement of EET through inhibition of soluble epoxide hydrolase reverses hypertension, and protects the kidney from damage.[694,706,707,737,738]

Endothelins

Endothelins are 21 amino acid vasoactive peptides synthesized by a variety of cell types in the kidney. Three ETs have been identified (ET1, ET2, ET3). These agents are autocrine/paracrine hormones derived from ~200 amino acid preproendothelins that undergo successive proteolytic cleavage to form large (Big ET) intermediates that are processed by endothelin-converting enzymes. ETs stimulate ETA and ETB receptors on smooth muscle to induce potent vasoconstriction. Endothelia express ETB receptors, stimulation of which leads to synthesis of NO. In addition to their vascular actions, ETs have an important role to inhibit sodium reabsorption through inhibition of transport by NO and downregulation of the epithelial Na^+ of the collecting duct.[739−742] Renal ET receptors have been identified on collecting ducts, vascular bundles, and RMIC.[743−745]

The highest concentrations of ET1 occur in the renal medulla where it is synthesized by collecting duct and other cells.[746,747] ET1 is a potent vasoconstrictor and reduces overall renal blood flow via combined ETA and ETB stimulation. Isolated ETB receptor stimulation, however, can have net vasodilatory effects.[748] In the renal cortex, ET1 constricts afferent and efferent arterioles, arcuate and interlobular arteries.[2,749−754] Afferent constriction by ET1 partially depends upon voltage-gated Ca^{2+} entry, is modulated by endothelial generation of NO,[195,755] and is mediated by 20-HETE and COX products.[708,718] Preglomerular smooth muscle cells show biphasic $[Ca^{2+}]_{CYT}$ responses to ETA agonists, but small or absent responses to ETB agonists.[756−758] Isolated DVR from the outer medulla are intensely constricted by low concentrations of endothelins.[27,269,397]

The actions of ETB stimulation in the medulla favor natriuresis and vasodilation, at least partially by activating NO generation through NOS1.[743,759,760] Bolus injection of ET1 (a mixed ETA and ETB receptor agonist) selectively reduced cortical blood flow while transiently increasing medullary blood flow. Medullary vasodilation and saliuresis is abrogated by blocking ETB receptors or synthesis of NO.[423,752,753,761,762] The effects on medullary blood flow may vary with dietary salt intake.[763] ETB receptor deficient "spotted lethal" rats have been identified that have been rescued from lethal abnormalities by selective ETB gene replacement into ganglionic cells of the intestine. Those rats have salt-sensitive hypertension.[764,765] Injection of Big ET1 into ETB receptor-deficient rats or wild-type rats in which ETB receptor has been blocked fails to elicit saliuresis.[753,766] Chronic angiotensin II infusion, combined with salt-loading, increases cortical and medullary immunoreactive ET.[767,768] Reduction of endothelin-induced saliuresis may play a role in human and rodent models of hypertension.[740,767,769−771] ETs might play a significant roles in other pathological states.[743,747,772]

Natriuretic Peptides

The diuretic effect of injection of extracts of atrial tissue extracts into rats led to the discovery of atrial

(ANP), brain (BNP), and C natriuretic peptides (CNP). Each is derived by proteolytic cleavage of different gene products. They act through stimulation of guanylyl cyclase A (GC-A) (ANP, BNP ligands), GC-B type (CNP ligand), and GC-C receptors. GC-C may play a role in peptide clearance and inhibition. Deletion of ANP or its receptor leads to hypertension, while over-expression results in hypotension.[773] In the kidney, expression and alternate processing of ANP prohormone yields urodilatin.[774,775] Studies showed that that ANP infusions increased renal blood flow, glomerular filtration rate, papillary plasma flow, and sodium excretion. Diuresis and natriuresis, however, begin before the increase in medullary blood flow, so that medullary dilation is not required for the natriuretic effect.[776–779] Examination of the vasoactive effects of natriuretic peptides generally uncovered dilation of preglomerular vasculature.[780–783] Edwards and Weidley found no effect of ANP on *in vitro* perfused rabbit afferent or efferent arterioles.[784] In the efferent arteriole, either a lack of effect[783,784] or constriction[785] was reported, while urodilatin mediated vasodilation.[786] Vasodilatory effects of ANP may be mediated through cGMP formation, activation of smooth muscle K_{Ca} channels, hyperpolarization and inhibition of Ca^{2+} signaling.[320,332] Natriuresis from an oral salt load is more brisk than that from an intravenous route, a finding that may be related to intestinal release of guanylin and uroguanylin, peptide hormones that activate ANP receptors. Like ANP, these agents inhibit tubuloglomerular feedback, but their specific effects on renal arterioles have not been reported.[787,788] Trials of ANP as a renoprotective agent have yielded inconclusive results.[789]

Acknowledgments

Efforts have been supported by NIH R37 DK42495, R01 DK67621, and P01 HL078870.

References

[1] Navar LG, Arendshorst WJ, Pallone TL, Inscho EW, Imig JD, Bell PD. The Renal Microcirculation. In: Tuma RF, Duran WN, Ley K, editors. Handbook of physiology: microcirculation. San Diego: Elsevier; 2008. p. 550–683.

[2] Navar LG, Inscho EW, Majid SA, Imig JD, Harrison-Bernard LM, Mitchell KD. Paracrine regulation of the renal microcirculation. Physiol Rev 1996;76:425–536.

[3] Bankir L, Bouby N, Trinh-Trang-Tan MM. Heterogeneity of nephron anatomy. Kidney Int Suppl 1987;20:S25–39.

[4] Bankir L, de Rouffignac C. Urinary concentrating ability: insights from comparative anatomy. Am J Physiol 1985;249: R643–66.

[5] Bankir L, Kaissling B, de Rouffignac C, Kriz W. The vascular organization of the kidney of *Psammomys obesus*. Anat Embryol (Berl) 1979;155:149–60.

[6] Kaissling B, de Rouffignac C, Barrett JM, Kriz W. The structural organization of the kidney of the desert rodent *Psammomys obesus*. Anat Embryol (Berl) 1975;148:121–43.

[7] Kaissling B, Kriz W. Structural analysis of the rabbit kidney. Adv Anat Embryol Cell Biol 1979;56:1–123.

[8] Kriz W. Structural organization of the renal medulla: comparative and functional aspects. Am J Physiol-Regul, Integr Comp Physiol 1981;241:R3–16.

[9] Kriz W, Napiwotzky P. Structural and functional aspects of the renal interstitium. Contrib Nephrol 1979;16:104–8.

[10] Fourman J, Moffat DB. The effect of intra-arterial cushions on plasma skimming in small arteries. J Physiol 1961;158:374–80.

[11] Fourman J, Moffat DB. The blood vessels of the kidney. Blackwell Scientific, Oxford, UK. 1971.

[12] Moffat DB, Creasey M. The fine structure of the intra-arterial cushions at the origins of the juxtamedullary afferent arterioles in the rat kidney. J Anat 1971;110:409–19.

[13] Pappenheimer JR, Kinter WB. Hematocrit ratio of blood within mammalian kidney and its significance for renal hemodynamics. Am J Physiol 1956;185:377–90.

[14] Beeuwkes III R. The vascular organization of the kidney. Ann Rev Physiol 1980;42:531–42.

[15] Jamison RL, Kriz W. Urinary concentrating mechanism: structure and function. New York-Oxford, Oxford University Press, 1982.

[16] Casellas D, Mimran A. Shunting in renal microvasculature of the rat: a scanning electron microscopic study of corrosion casts. Anat Rec 1981;201:237–48.

[17] Pallone TL, Robertson CR, Jamison RL. Renal medullary microcirculation. Physiol Rev 1990;70:885–920.

[18] Aukland K, Bogusky RT, Renkin EM. Renal cortical interstitium and fluid absorption by peritubular capillaries. Am J Physiol 1994;266:F175–84.

[19] Pedersen JC, Persson AEG, Maunsbach AB. Ultrastructure and quantitative characterization of the cortical interstitium in the rat kidney. Functional ultrastructure of the kidney. London: Academic Press; 1980443–457

[20] Lemley KV, Kriz W. Anatomy of the renal interstitium. Kidney Int 1991;39:370–81.

[21] Wolgast M, Larson M, Nygren K. Functional characteristics of the renal interstitium. Am J Physiol 1981;241:F105–11.

[22] Beeuwkes III R, Bonventre JV. Tubular organization and vascular–tubular relations in the dog kidney. Am J Physiol 1975;229:695–713.

[23] Evan AP, Dail Jr WG. Efferent arterioles in the cortex of the rat kidney. Anat Rec 1977;187:135–45.

[24] Lemley KV, Kriz W. Cycles and separations: the histotopography of the urinary concentrating process. Kidney Int 1987;31:538–48.

[25] Pannabecker TL, Dantzler WH. Three-dimensional architecture of inner medullary vasa recta. Am J Physiol Renal Physiol 2006;290:F1355–66.

[26] Kriz W. Structural organization of the renal medulla: comparative and functional aspects. Am J Physiol 1981;241:R3–16.

[27] Pallone TL, Silldorff EP. Pericyte regulation of renal medullary blood flow. Exp Nephrol 2001;9:165–70.

[28] Park F, Mattson DL, Roberts LA, Cowley Jr AW. Evidence for the presence of smooth muscle alpha-actin within pericytes of the renal medulla. Am J Physiol 1997;273:R1742–8.

[29] Mink D, Schiller A, Kriz W, Taugner R. Interendothelial junctions in kidney vessels. Cell Tissue Res 1984;236:567–76.

[30] Schwartz MM, Karnovsky MJ, Vehkatachalam MA. Ultrastructural differences between rat inner medullary descending and ascending vasa recta. Lab Invest 1976;35:161–70.

[31] Pallone TL, Turner MR, Edwards A, Jamison RL. Countercurrent exchange in the renal medulla. Am J Physiol Regul Integr Comp Physiol 2003;284:R1153–75.

[32] Zhai XY, Thomsen JS, Birn H, Kristoffersen IB, Andreasen A, Christensen EI. Three-dimensional reconstruction of the mouse nephron. J Am Soc Nephrol 2006;17:77—88.

[33] Franchini KG, Cowley Jr AW. Renal cortical and medullary blood flow responses during water restriction: role of vasopressin. Am J Physiol 1996;270:R1257—64.

[34] Holliger C, Lemley KV, Schmitt SL, Thomas FC, Robertson CR, Jamison RL. Direct determination of vasa recta blood flow in the rat renal papilla. Circ Res 1983;53:401—13.

[35] Marsh DJ, Segel LA. Analysis of countercurrent diffusion exchange in blood vessels of the renal medulla. Am J Physiol 1971;221:817—28.

[36] Pannabecker TL, Dantzler WH. Three-dimensional architecture of collecting ducts, loops of Henle, and blood vessels in the renal papilla. Am J Physiol Renal Physiol 2007;293:F696—704.

[37] Knepper MA, Danielson RA, Saidel GM, Post RS. Quantitative analysis of renal medullary anatomy in rats and rabbits. Kidney Int 1977;12:313—23.

[38] Takahashi-Iwanaga H. The three-dimensional cytoarchitecture of the interstitial tissue in the rat kidney. Cell Tissue Res 1991;264:269—81.

[39] Hughes AK, Barry WH, Kohan DE. Identification of a contractile function for renal medullary interstitial cells. J Clin Invest 1995;96:411—6.

[40] Thomas CJ, Woods RL, Evans RG, Alcorn D, Christy IJ, Anderson WP. Evidence for a renomedullary vasodepressor hormone. Clin Exp Pharmacol Physiol 1996;23:777—85.

[41] Zhuo JL. Renomedullary interstitial cells: a target for endocrine and paracrine actions of vasoactive peptides in the renal medulla. Clin Exp Pharmacol Physiol 2000;27:465—73.

[42] Zusman RM, Keiser HR. Prostaglandin biosynthesis by rabbit renomedullary interstitial cells in tissue culture. Stimulation by angiotensin II, bradykinin, and arginine vasopressin. J Clin Invest 1977;60:215—23.

[43] Kim J, Pannabecker TL. Two-compartment model of inner medullary vasculature supports dual modes of vasopressin-regulated inner medullary blood flow. Am J Physiol Renal Physiol 2010;299:F273—9.

[44] Pannabecker TL. Loop of Henle interaction with interstitial nodal spaces in the renal inner medulla. Am J Physiol Renal Physiol 2008;295:F1744—51.

[45] Pannabecker TL, Henderson CS, Dantzler WH. Quantitative analysis of functional reconstructions reveals lateral and axial zonation in the renal inner medulla. Am J Physiol Renal Physiol 2008;294:F1306—14.

[46] Yuan J, Pannabecker TL. Architecture of inner medullary descending and ascending vasa recta: pathways for countercurrent exchange. Am J Physiol Renal Physiol 2010; 299:F265—72.

[47] Pannabecker TL, Abbott DE, Dantzler WH. Three-dimensional functional reconstruction of inner medullary thin limbs of Henle's loop. Am J Physiol Renal Physiol 2004;286:F38—45.

[48] Pannabecker TL, Dantzler WH. Three-dimensional lateral and vertical relationships of inner medullary loops of Henle and collecting ducts. Am J Physiol Renal Physiol 2004;287:F767—74.

[49] Pannabecker TL, Dahlmann A, Brokl OH, Dantzler WH. Mixed descending- and ascending-type thin limbs of Henle's loop in mammalian renal inner medulla. Am J Physiol Renal Physiol 2000;278:F202—8.

[50] MacPhee PJ, Michel CC. Fluid uptake from the renal medulla into the ascending vasa recta in anaesthetized rats. J Physiol 1995;487(Pt 1):169—83.

[51] MacPhee PJ, Michel CC. Subatmospheric closing pressures in individual microvessels of rats and frogs. J Physiol 1995; 484(Pt 1):183—7.

[52] Layton AT, Layton HE. A region-based mathematical model of the urine concentrating mechanism in the rat outer medulla. I. Formulation and base-case results. Am J Physiol Renal Physiol 2005;289:F1346—66.

[53] Layton AT, Layton HE. A region-based mathematical model of the urine concentrating mechanism in the rat outer medulla. II. Parameter sensitivity and tubular inhomogeneity. Am J Physiol Renal Physiol 2005;289:F1367—81.

[54] Layton AT, Pannabecker TL, Dantzler WH, Layton HE. Two modes for concentrating urine in rat inner medulla. Am J Physiol Renal Physiol 2004;287:F816—39.

[55] Layton AT, Pannabecker TL, Dantzler WH, Layton HE. Functional implications of the three-dimensional architecture of the rat renal inner medulla. Am J Physiol Renal Physiol 2010;298:F973—87.

[56] Brenner BM, Falchuk KH, Keimowitz RI, Berliner RW. The relationship between peritubular capillary protein concentration and fluid reabsorption by the renal proximal tubule. J Clin Invest 1969;48:1519—31.

[57] Brenner BM, Troy JL. Postglomerular vascular protein concentration: evidence for a causal role in governing fluid reabsorption and glomerulotublar balance by the renal proximal tubule. J Clin Invest 1971;50:336—49.

[58] Spitzer A, Windhager EE. Effect of peritubular oncotic pressure changes on proximal tubular fluid reabsorption. Am J Physiol 1970;218:1188—93.

[59] Sapirstein LA. Regional blood flow by fractional distribution of indicators. Am J Physiol 1958;193:161—8.

[60] Tucker BJ, Blantz RC. Determinants of proximal tubular reabsorption as mechanisms of glomerulotubular balance. Am J Physiol 1978;235:F142—50.

[61] Ott CE, Haas JA, Cuche JL, Knox FG. Effect of increased peritubule protein concentration on proximal tubule reabsorption in the presence and absence of extracellular volume expansion. J Clin Invest 1975;55:612—20.

[62] Grantham JJ, Qualizza PB, Welling LW. Influence of serum proteins on net fluid reabsorption of isolated proximal tubules. Kidney Int 1972;2:66—75.

[63] Andreoli TE, Schafer JA, Troutman SL. Perfusion rate-dependence of transepithelial osmosis in isolated proximal convoluted tubules: estimation of the hydraulic conductance. Kidney Int 1978;14:263—9.

[64] Green R, Giebisch G. Luminal hypotonicity: a driving force for fluid absorption from the proximal tubule. Am J Physiol 1984;246:F167—74.

[65] Baum M, Berry CA. Peritubular protein modulates neutral active NaCl absorption in rabbit proximal convoluted tubule. Am J Physiol 1985;248:F790—5.

[66] Green R, Giebisch G, Unwin R, Weinstein AM. Coupled water transport by rat proximal tubule. Am J Physiol 1991;261:F1046—54.

[67] Imai M, Kokko JP. Effect of peritubular protein concentration on reabsorption of sodium and water in isolated perfused proxmal tubules. J Clin Invest 1972;51:314—25.

[68] Du Z, Yan Q, Duan Y, Weinbaum S, Weinstein AM, Wang T. Axial flow modulates proximal tubule NHE3 and H-ATPase activities by changing microvillus bending moments. Am J Physiol Renal Physiol 2006;290:F289—96.

[69] Wang T. Flow-activated transport events along the nephron. Curr Opin Nephrol Hypertens 2006;15:530—6.

[70] Weinstein AM, Weinbaum S, Duan Y, Du Z, Yan Q, Wang T. Flow-dependent transport in a mathematical model of rat proximal tubule. Am J Physiol Renal Physiol 2007;292:F1164—81.

[71] Pinter GG, Gartner K. Peritubular capillary, interstitium, and lymph of the renal cortex. Rev Physiol Biochem Pharmacol 1984;99:184—202.

[72] Schurek HJ, Alt JM. Effect of albumin on the function of perfused rat kidney. Am J Physiol 1981;240:F569—76.

[73] Kuhn W, Ryffel R. Herstellung konzentrierter Losungen aus verdunnten durch blosse Membranwirkung. (Ein Modellversuch zur Function der Niere). Hoppe-Seylers Z Physiol Chem 1942;276:145—78.

[74] Michel CC. Renal medullary microcirculation: architecture and exchange. Microcirculation 1995;2:125—39.

[75] Scholander PF. The wonderful net. Scient Am 1957;196:96—107.

[76] Pallone TL, Edwards A, Ma T, Silldorff EP, Verkman AS. Requirement of aquaporin-1 for NaCl-driven water transport across descending vasa recta. J Clin Invest 2000;105:215—22.

[77] Pallone TL, Kishore BK, Nielsen S, Agre P, Knepper MA. Evidence that aquaporin-1 mediates NaCl-induced water flux across descending vasa recta. Am J Physiol 1997;272:F587—96.

[78] Pallone TL, Turner MR. Molecular sieving of small solutes by outer medullary descending vasa recta. Am J Physiol 1997;272: F579—86.

[79] Kriz W, Dieterich HJ. [The lymphatic system of the kidney in some mammals. Light and electron microscopic investigations]. Z Anat Entwicklungsgesch 1970;131:111—47.

[80] Johnston PA, Battilana CA, Lacy FB, Jamison RL. Evidence for a concentration gradient favoring outward movement of sodium from the thin loop of Henle. J Clin Invest 1977;59:234—40.

[81] Gottschalk CW, Mylle M. Micropuncture study of the mammalian urinary concentrating mechanism: evidence for the countercurrent hypothesis. Am J Physiol 1959;196:927—36.

[82] Marsh DJ, Azen SP. Mechanism of NaCl reabsorption by hamster thin ascending limbs of Henle's loop. Am J Physiol 1975;228:71—9.

[83] Sanjana VM, Johnston PA, Deen WM, Robertson CR, Brenner BM, Jamison RL. Hydraulic and oncotic pressure measurements in inner medulla of mammalian kidney. Am J Physiol 1975;228:1921—6.

[84] Sanjana VM, Johnston PA, Robertson CR, Jamison RL. An examination of transcapillary water flux in renal inner medulla. Am J Physiol 1976;231:313—8.

[85] Edwards A, Pallone TL. A multiunit model of solute and water removal by inner medullary vasa recta. Am J Physiol 1998;274: H1202—10.

[86] Pallone TL, Yagil Y, Jamison RL. Effect of small-solute gradients on transcapillary fluid movement in renal inner medulla. Am J Physiol 1989;257:F547—53.

[87] Thurau K, Sugiura T, Lilienfield LS. Micropuncture of renal vasa recta in hydropenic hamsters. Circ Res 1960;8:383.

[88] Zimmerhackl B, Robertson CR, Jamison RL. Fluid uptake in the renal papilla by vasa recta estimated by two methods simultaneously. Am J Physiol 1985;248:F347—53.

[89] Landis EM, Pappenheimer JR. Exchange of substances through the capillary wall. Handbook of physiology. Circulation. Washington: Am. Physiol. Soc; 1963962—1034.

[90] Pallone TL, Morgenthaler TI, Deen WM. Analysis of microvascular water and solute exchanges in the renal medulla. Am J Physiol 1984;247:F303—15.

[91] Kedem O, Katchalsky A. Thermodynamic analysis of the permeability of biological membranes to non-electrolytes. Biochim Biophys Acta 1958;27:229—46.

[92] Pallone TL. Effect of sodium chloride gradients on water flux in rat descending vasa recta. J Clin Invest 1991;87:12—9.

[93] Nielsen S, Pallone T, Smith BL, Christensen EI, Agre P, Maunsbach AB. Aquaporin-1 water channels in short and long loop descending thin limbs and in descending vasa recta in rat kidney. Am J Physiol 1995;268:F1023—37.

[94] Nielsen S, Smith BL, Christensen EI, Agre P. Distribution of the aquaporin CHIP in secretory and resorptive epithelia and capillary endothelia. Proc Natl Acad Sci U S A 1993;90:7275—9.

[95] Edwards A, Pallone TL. Facilitated transport in vasa recta: theoretical effects on solute exchange in the medullary microcirculation. Am J Physiol 1997;272:F505—14.

[96] Turner MR, Pallone TL. Hydraulic and diffusional permeabilities of isolated outer medullary descending vasa recta from the rat. Am J Physiol 1997;272:H392—400.

[97] Fleming I. Cytochrome P450 epoxygenases as EDHF synthase (s). Pharmacol Res 2004;49:525—33.

[98] Layton AT. Role of UTB urea transporters in the urine concentrating mechanism of the rat kidney. Bull Math Biol 2007;69:887—929.

[99] Promeneur D, Bankir L, Hu MC, Trinh-Trang-Tan MM. Renal tubular and vascular urea transporters: influence of antidiuretic hormone on messenger RNA expression in Brattleboro rats. J Am Soc Nephrol 1998;9:1359—66.

[100] Yang B, Bankir L. Urea and urine concentrating ability: new insights from studies in mice. Am J Physiol Renal Physiol 2005;288:F881—96.

[101] Yang B, Verkman AS. Urea transporter UT3 functions as an efficient water channel. Direct evidence for a common water/urea pathway. J Biol Chem 1998;273:9369—72.

[102] Zhang W, Edwards A. Theoretical effects of UTB urea transporters in the renal medullary microcirculation. Am J Physiol Renal Physiol 2003;285:F731—47.

[103] Koepsell H, Nicholson WA, Kriz W, Hohling HJ. Measurements of exponential gradients of sodium and chlorine in the rat kidney medulla using the electron microprobe. Pflugers Arch 1974;350:167—84.

[104] Wang W, Michel CC. Effects of anastomoses on solute transcapillary exchange in countercurrent systems. Microcirculation 1997;4:381—90.

[105] Wang W, Parker KH, Michel CC. Theoretical studies of steady-state transcapillary exchange in countercurrent systems. Microcirculation 1996;3:301—11.

[106] Chou CL, Knepper MA. In vitro perfusion of chinchilla thin limb segments: segmentation and osmotic water permeability. Am J Physiol 1992;263:F417—26.

[107] Chou CL, Nielsen S, Knepper MA. Structural—functional correlation in chinchilla long loop of Henle thin limbs: a novel papillary subsegment. Am J Physiol 1993;265:F863—74.

[108] Edwards A, Delong MJ, Pallone TL. Interstitial water and solute recovery by inner medullary vasa recta. Am J Physiol Renal Physiol 2000;278:F257—69.

[109] Thomas SR. Cycles and separations in a model of the renal medulla. Am J Physiol 1998;275:F671—90.

[110] Pallone TL, Nielsen S, Silldorff EP, Yang S. Diffusive transport of solute in the rat medullary microcirculation. Am J Physiol 1995;269:F55—63.

[111] Pallone TL, Work J, Myers RL, Jamison RL. Transport of sodium and urea in outer medullary descending vasa recta. J Clin Invest 1994;93:212—22.

[112] Pallone TL. Characterization of the urea transporter in outer medullary descending vasa recta. Am J Physiol 1994;267: R260—7.

[113] Promeneur D, Rousselet G, Bankir L, Bailly P, Cartron JP, Ripoche P, et al. Evidence for distinct vascular and tubular urea transporters in the rat kidney. J Am Soc Nephrol 1996;7:852—60.

[114] Bankir L, Chen K, Yang B. Lack of UT-B in vasa recta and red blood cells prevents urea-induced improvement of urinary concentrating ability. Am J Physiol Renal Physiol 2004;286:F144—51.

[115] Shayakul C, Knepper MA, Smith CP, DiGiovanni SR, Hediger MA. Segmental localization of urea transporter mRNAs in rat kidney. Am J Physiol 1997;272:F654—60.

[116] Shayakul C, Steel A, Hediger MA. Molecular cloning and characterization of the vasopressin-regulated urea transporter of rat kidney collecting ducts. J Clin Invest 1996;98:2580–7.

[117] Xu Y, Olives B, Bailly P, Fischer E, Ripoche P, Ronco P, et al. Endothelial cells of the kidney vasa recta express the urea transporter HUT11. Kidney Int 1997;51:138–46.

[118] Yang B, Bankir L, Gillespie A, Epstein CJ, Verkman AS. Urea-selective concentrating defect in transgenic mice lacking urea transporter UT-B. J Biol Chem 2002;277:10633–7.

[119] Sands JM. Renal urea transporters. Curr Opin Nephrol Hypertens 2004;13:525–32.

[120] Trinh-Trang-Tan MM, Lasbennes F, Gane P, Roudier N, Ripoche P, Cartron JP, et al. UT-B1 proteins in rat: tissue distribution and regulation by antidiuretic hormone in kidney. Am J Physiol Renal Physiol 2002;283:F912–22.

[121] Kim D, Klein JD, Racine S, Murrell BP, Sands JM. Urea may regulate urea transporter protein abundance during osmotic diuresis. Am J Physiol Renal Physiol 2005;288:F188–97.

[122] Jung JY, Madsen KM, Han KH, Yang CW, Knepper MA, Sands JM, et al. Expression of urea transporters in potassium-depleted mouse kidney. Am J Physiol Renal Physiol 2003;285: F1210–24.

[123] Klein JD, Gunn RB, Roberts BR, Sands JM. Down-regulation of urea transporters in the renal inner medulla of lithium-fed rats. Kidney Int 2002;61:995–1002.

[124] Li C, Klein JD, Wang W, Knepper MA, Nielsen S, Sands JM, et al. Altered expression of urea transporters in response to ureteral obstruction. Am J Physiol Renal Physiol 2004;286:F1154–62.

[125] Lim SW, Li C, Sun BK, Han KH, Kim WY, Oh YW, et al. Long-term treatment with cyclosporine decreases aquaporins and urea transporters in the rat kidney. Am J Physiol Renal Physiol 2004;287:F139–51.

[126] Macey RI, Yousef LW. Osmotic stability of red cells in renal circulation requires rapid urea transport. Am J Physiol 1988;254:C669–74.

[127] Pallone TL. Resistance of ascending vasa recta to transport of water. Am J Physiol 1991;260:F303–10.

[128] Pallone TL. Molecular sieving of albumin by the ascending vasa recta wall. J Clin Invest 1992;90:30–4.

[129] Pallone TL. Transport of sodium chloride and water in rat ascending vasa recta. Am J Physiol 1991;261:F519–25.

[130] Morgan T, Berliner RW. Permeability of the loop of Henle, vasa recta, and collecting duct to water, urea, and sodium. Am J Physiol 1968;215:108–15.

[131] Bell RD, Keyl MJ, Shrader FR, Jones EW, Henry LP. Renal lymphatics: the internal distribution. Nephron 1968;5:454–63.

[132] LeBrie SJ. Renal peritubular capillary permeability to macromolecules. Am J Physiol 1967;213:1225–32.

[133] Renkin EM. Capillary transport of macromolecules: pores and other endothelial pathways. J Appl Physiol 1985;58:315–25.

[134] Lassen NA, Longley JB, Lilienfield LS. Concentration of albumin in renal papilla. Science 1958;128:720–1.

[135] Lilienfield LS, Maganzini HC, Bauer MH. Blood flow in the renal medulla. Circ Res 1961;9:614–7.

[136] Slotkoff LM, Lilienfield LS. Extravascular renal albumin. Am J Physiol 1967;212:400–6.

[137] Carone FA, Everett BA, Blondeel NJ, Stolarczyk J. Renal localization of albumin and its function in the concentrating mechanism. Am J Physiol 1967;212:387–93.

[138] Pomerantz RM, Slotkoff LM, Lilienfield LS. Histochemical and microanatomical differences between renal cortical and medullary interstitium. In: Kass EH, editor. Progress in pyelonephritis. Philadelphia: F.A. Davis Co.; 1965. p. 434–525.

[139] Moffat DB. Extravascular protein in the renal medulla. Q J Exp Physiol Cogn Med Sci 1969;54:60–7.

[140] Wilde WS, Vorburger C. Albumin multiplier in kidney vasa recta analyzed by microspectrophotometry of T-1824. Am J Physiol 1967;213:1233–43.

[141] Venkatachalam MA, Karnovsky MJ. Extravascular protein in the kidney. An ultrastructural study of its relation to renal peritubular capillary permeability using protein tracers. Lab Invest 1972;27:435–44.

[142] Shimamura T, Morrison AB. Vascular permeability of the renal medullary vessels in the mouse and rat. Am J Pathol 1973;71:155–63.

[143] Pallone TL. Extravascular protein in the renal medulla: analysis by two methods. Am J Physiol 1994;266:R1429–36.

[144] Pinter GG, Shohet JL. Two fluid compartments in the renal inner medulla: a view through the keyhole of the concentrating process. Philos Transact A Math Phys Eng Sci 2006;364:1551–61.

[145] Pinter GG, Shohet JL. An inner medullary concentrating process actuated by renal pelvic/calyceal muscle contractions: assessment and hypothesis. Nephron Physiol 2009;113:1–6.

[146] Fahraeus R. The suspension stability of blood. Physiol Rev 1929;9:241–74.

[147] Lilienfield LS, Rose JC, Lassen NA. Diverse distribution of red cells and albumin in the dog kidney. Circ Res 1958;6:810–5.

[148] Rasmussen SN. Red cell and plasma volume flows to the inner medulla of the rat kidney: determinations by means of a step function input indicator technique. Pflugers Arch 1978;373:153–9.

[149] Zimmerhackl B, Dussel R, Steinhausen M. Erythrocyte flow and dynamic hematocrit in the renal papilla of the rat. Am J Physiol 1985;249:F898–902.

[150] Gaehtgens P. Flow of blood through narrow capillaries: Rheological mechanisms determining capillary hematocrit and apparent viscosity. Biorheology 1980;17:183–9.

[151] Pries AR, Ley K, Gaehtgens P. Generalization of the Fahraeus principle for microvessel networks. Am J Physiol 1986;251: H1324–32.

[152] Ren Y, Garvin JL, Liu R, Carretero OA. Crosstalk between the connecting tubule and the afferent arteriole regulates renal microcirculation. Kidney Int 2007;71:1116–21.

[153] Ren Y, Garvin JL, Liu R, Carretero OA. Possible mechanism of efferent arteriole (Ef-Art) tubuloglomerular feedback. Kidney Int 2007;71:861–6.

[154] Aukland K, Bower BF, Berliner RW. Measurement of local blood flow with hydrogen gas. Circ Res 1964;14:164–87.

[155] Balint P, Bartha J, Fekete A. Intrarenal distribution of blood flow in the dog. Acta Physiol Acad Sci Hung 1969;36:1–11.

[156] Bayle F, Eloy L, Trinh-Trang-Tan MM, Grunfeld JP, Bankir L. Papillary plasma flow in rats. I. Relation to urine osmolality in normal and Brattleboro rats with hereditary diabetes insipidus. Pflugers Arch 1982;394:211–6.

[157] Chou SY, Spitalewitz S, Faubert PF, Park IY, Porush JG. Inner medullary hemodynamics in chronic salt-depleted dogs. Am J Physiol 1984;246:F146–54.

[158] Chuang EL, Reineck HJ, Osgood RW, Kunau Jr RT, Stein JH. Studies on the mechanism of reduced urinary osmolality after exposure of renal papilla. J Clin Invest 1978;61:633–9.

[159] Coelho JB. Heterogeneity of intracortical peritubular plasma flow in the rat kidney. Am J Physiol 1977;233:F333–41.

[160] Faubert PF, Chou SY, Porush JG. Regulation of papillary plasma flow by angiotensin II. Kidney Int 1987;32:472–8.

[161] Ganguli M, Tobian L, Azar S, O'Donnell M. Evidence that prostaglandin synthesis inhibitors increase the concentration of sodium and chloride in rat renal medulla. Circ Res 1977;40: I135–9.

[162] Ganguli M, Tobian L, Dahl L. Low renal papillary plasma flow in both Dahl and Kyoto rats with spontaneous hypertension. Circ Res 1976;39:337–41.

[163] Harsing L, Pelley K. [The determination of renal medullary blood flow based on Rb-86 deposit and distribution]. Pflugers Arch Gesamte Physiol Menschen Tiere 1965;285:302—12.

[164] Karlberg L, Kallskog O, Ojteg G, Wolgast M. Renal medullary blood flow studied with the 86-Rb extraction method. Methodological considerations. Acta Physiol Scand 1982;115:11—8.

[165] Kramer K, Thurau K, Deetjen P. [Hemodynamics of kidney medullary substance. Part I. Capillary passage time, blood volume, circulation, tissue hematocrit and oxygen consumption of kidney medullary substance in situ.]. Pflugers Arch Gesamte Physiol Menschen Tiere 1960;270:251—69.

[166] Lilienfield LS, Maganzini HC, Bauer MH. Renal medullary blood flow. Fed Proc 1960;19:363—5.

[167] Roman RJ, Smits C. Laser-Doppler determination of papillary blood flow in young and adult rats. Am J Physiol 1986;251: F115—24.

[168] Solez K, Kramer EC, Fox JA, Heptinstall RH. Medullary plasma flow and intravascular leukocyte accumulation in acute renal failure. Kidney Int 1974;6:24—37.

[169] Steiner SH, King RD. Nutrient renal blood flow and its distribution in the unanesthetized dog. J Surg Res 1970;10:133—46.

[170] Thorburn GD, Kopald HH, Herd JA, Hollenberg M, O'Morchoe CC, Barger AC. Intrarenal distribution of nutrient blood flow determined with krypton 85 in the unanesthetized dog. Circ Res 1963;13:290—307.

[171] Thurau K. Renal hemodynamics. Am J Med 1964;36:698—719.

[172] Wolgast M. Studies on the regional renal blood flow with p32-labelled red cells and small beta-sensitive semiconductor detectors. Acta Physiol Scand Suppl 1968;313:1—109.

[173] Yarger WE, Boyd MA, Schrader NW. Evaluation of methods of measuring glomerular and nutrient blood flow in rat kidneys. Am J Physiol 1978;235:H592—600.

[174] Pallone TL. The extraglomerular circulation of the kidney. In: Seldin DW, Giebisch G, editors. The kidney: physiology and pathophysiology. Philadelphia, PA: Lippincott Williams and Wilkins; 2000. p. 791—822.

[175] Zimmerhackl B, Tinsman J, Jamison RL, Robertson CR. Use of digital cross-correlation for on-line determination of single-vessel blood flow in the mammalian kidney. Microvasc Res 1985;30:63—74.

[176] Yamamoto T, Tada T, Brodsky SV, Tanaka H, Noiri E, Kajiya F, et al. Intravital videomicroscopy of peritubular capillaries in renal ischemia. Am J Physiol Renal Physiol 2002;282:F1150—5.

[177] Hayashi K, Wakino S, Sugano N, Ozawa Y, Homma K, Saruta T. Ca^{2+} channel subtypes and pharmacology in the kidney. Circ Res 2007;100:342—53.

[178] Draijer M, Hondebrink E, van LT, Steenbergen W. Review of laser speckle contrast techniques for visualizing tissue perfusion. Lasers Med Sci 2009;24:639—51.

[179] Humeau A, Steenbergen W, Nilsson H, Stromberg T. Laser-Doppler perfusion monitoring and imaging: novel approaches. Med Biol Eng Comput 2007;45:421—35.

[180] Correas JM, Claudon M, Tranquart F, Helenon AO. The kidney: imaging with microbubble contrast agents. Ultrasound Q 2006;22:53—66.

[181] Sullivan JC, Wang B, Boesen EI, D'Angelo G, Pollock JS, Pollock DM. Novel use of ultrasound to examine regional blood flow in the mouse kidney. Am J Physiol Renal Physiol 2009;297:F228—35.

[182] Gussis GL, Jamison RL, Robertson CR. Determination of erythrocyte velocities in the mammalian inner renal medulla by a video velocity-tracking system. Microvasc Res 1979;18:370—83.

[183] Stern MD, Bowen PD, Parma R, Osgood RW, Bowman RL, Stein JH. Measurement of renal cortical and medullary blood

flow by laser-Doppler spectroscopy in the rat. Am J Physiol 1979;236:F80—7.

[184] Fenoy FJ, Roman RJ. Effect of volume expansion on papillary blood flow and sodium excretion. Am J Physiol 1991;260: F813—22.

[185] Aukland K. Methods for measuring renal blood flow: total flow and regional distribution. Annu Rev Physiol 1980;42:543—55.

[186] Carmines PK, Fleming JT. Control of the renal microvasculature by vasoactive peptides. FASEB J 1990;4:3300—9.

[187] Pallone TL, Work J, Jamison RL. Resistance of descending vasa recta to the transport of water. Am J Physiol 1990;259:F688—97.

[188] Roman RJ, Carmines PK, Loutzenhiser R, Conger JD. Direct studies on the control of the renal microcirculation. J Am Soc Nephrol 1991;2:136—49.

[189] Burg M, Grantham J, Abramow M, Orloff J. Preparation and study of fragments of single rabbit nephrons. Am J Physiol 1966;210:1293—8.

[190] Pallone TL. Microdissected perfused vessels. Methods Mol Med 2003;86:443—56.

[191] Osgood RW, Patton M, Hanley MJ, Venkatachalam M, Reineck HJ, Stein JH. In vitro perfusion of the isolated dog glomerulus. Am J Physiol 1983;244:F349—54.

[192] Edwards RM. Segmental effects of norepinephrine and angiotensin II on isolated renal microvessels. Am J Physiol 1983;244: F526—34.

[193] Ito S, Arima S, Ren YL, Juncos LA, Carretero OA. Endothelium-derived relaxing factor/nitric oxide modulates angiotensin II action in the isolated microperfused rabbit afferent but not efferent arteriole. J Clin Invest 1993;91:2012—9.

[194] Ito S, Johnson CS, Carretero OA. Modulation of angiotensin II-induced vasoconstriction by endothelium-derived relaxing factor in the isolated microperfused rabbit afferent arteriole. J Clin Invest 1991;87:1656—63.

[195] Ito S, Juncos LA, Nushiro N, Johnson CS, Carretero OA. Endothelium-derived relaxing factor modulates endothelin action in afferent arterioles. Hypertension 1991;17:1052—6.

[196] Ito S, Ren Y. Evidence for the role of nitric oxide in macula densa control of glomerular hemodynamics. J Clin Invest 1993;92:1093—8.

[197] Hansen PB, Hashimoto S, Briggs J, Schnermann J. Attenuated renovascular constrictor responses to angiotensin II in adenosine 1 receptor knockout mice. Am J Physiol Regul Integr Comp Physiol 2003;285:R44—9.

[198] Pallone TL. Vasoconstriction of outer medullary vasa recta by angiotensin II is modulated by prostaglandin E2. Am J Physiol 1994;266:F850—7.

[199] Newby AC, Henderson AH. Stimulus-secretion coupling in vascular endothelial cells. Annu Rev Physiol 1990;52:661—74.

[200] Buckley BJ, Mirza Z, Whorton AR. Regulation of Ca($^{2+}$)-dependent nitric oxide synthase in bovine aortic endothelial cells. Am J Physiol 1995;269:C757—65.

[201] Martin W, Villani GM, Jothianandan D, Furchgott RF. Selective blockade of endothelium-dependent and glyceryl trinitrate-induced relaxation by hemoglobin and by methylene blue in the rabbit aorta. J Pharmacol Exp Ther 1985;232:708—16.

[202] Casellas D, Navar LG. In vitro perfusion of juxtamedullary nephrons in rats. Am J Physiol 1984;246:F349—58.

[203] Steinhausen M, Ballantyne D, Fretschner M, Parekh N. Sex differences in autoregulation of juxtamedullary glomerular blood flow in hydronephrotic rats. Am J Physiol 1990;258:F863—9.

[204] Steinhausen M, Kucherer H, Parekh N, Weis S, Wiegman DL, Wilhelm KR. Angiotensin II control of the renal microcirculation: effect of blockade by saralasin. Kidney Int 1986;30:56—61.

[205] Carmines PK, Morrison TK, Navar LG. Angiotensin II effects on microvascular diameters of *in vitro* blood-perfused juxtamedullary nephrons. Am J Physiol 1986;251:F610−8.

[206] Hansen PB, Jensen BL, Andreasen D, Skott O. Differential expression of T- and L-type voltage-dependent calcium channels in renal resistance vessels. Circ Res 2001;89:630−8.

[207] Loutzenhiser R, Hayashi K, Epstein M. Divergent effects of KCl-induced depolarization on afferent and efferent arterioles. Am J Physiol 1989;257:F561−4.

[208] Conger JD, Falk SA. KCl and angiotensin responses in isolated rat renal arterioles: effects of diltiazem and low-calcium medium. Am J Physiol 1993;264:F134−40.

[209] Inscho EW, Mason MJ, Schroeder AC, Deichmann PC, Stiegler KD, Imig JD. Agonist-induced calcium regulation in freshly isolated renal microvascular smooth muscle cells. J Am Soc Nephrol 1997;8:569−79.

[210] Loutzenhiser R, Chilton L, Trottier G. Membrane potential measurements in renal afferent and efferent arterioles: actions of angiotensin II. Am J Physiol 1997;273:F307−14.

[211] Arendshorst WJ, Brannstrom K, Ruan X. Actions of angiotensin II on the renal microvasculature. J Am Soc Nephrol 1999;10 (Suppl. 11):S149−61.

[212] Helou CM, Marchetti J. Morphological heterogeneity of renal glomerular arterioles and distinct [Ca^{2+}]*i* responses to ANG II. Am J Physiol 1997;273:F84−96.

[213] Inscho EW, Schroeder AC, Deichmann PC, Imig JD. ATP-mediated Ca^{2+} signaling in preglomerular smooth muscle cells. Am J Physiol 1999;276:F450−6.

[214] Iversen BM, Arendshorst WJ. ANG II and vasopressin stimulate calcium entry in dispersed smooth muscle cells of preglomerular arterioles. Am J Physiol 1998;274:F498−508.

[215] Loutzenhiser K, Loutzenhiser R. Angiotensin II-induced $Ca^{(2+)}$ influx in renal afferent and efferent arterioles: differing roles of voltage-gated and store-operated $Ca^{(2+)}$ entry. Circ Res 2000;87:551−7.

[216] Carmines PK, Navar LG. Disparate effects of Ca channel blockade on afferent and efferent arteriolar responses to ANG II. Am J Physiol 1989;256:F1015−20.

[217] Fleming JT, Parekh N, Steinhausen M. Calcium antagonists preferentially dilate preglomerular vessels of hydronephrotic kidney. Am J Physiol 1987;253:F1157−63.

[218] Loutzenhiser R, Epstein M, Horton C. Inhibition by diltiazem of pressure-induced afferent vasoconstriction in the isolated perfused rat kidney. Am J Cardiol 1987;59:72A−5A.

[219] Loutzenhiser RD, Epstein M, Fischetti F, Horton C. Effects of amlodipine on renal hemodynamics. Am J Cardiol 1989;64:122I−7I.

[220] Navar LG, Inscho EW, Imig JD, Mitchell KD. Heterogeneous activation mechanisms in the renal microvasculature. Kidney Int Suppl 1998;67:S17−21.

[221] Takenaka T, Ohno Y, Hayashi K, Saruta T, Suzuki H. Governance of arteriolar oscillation by ryanodine receptors. Am J Physiol Regul Integr Comp Physiol 2003;285:R125−31.

[222] Carmines PK, Ohishi K, Ikenaga H. Functional impairment of renal afferent arteriolar voltage-gated calcium channels in rats with diabetes mellitus. J Clin Invest 1996;98:2564−71.

[223] Fellner SK, Arendshorst WJ. Store-operated Ca^{2+} entry is exaggerated in fresh preglomerular vascular smooth muscle cells of SHR. Kidney Int 2002;61:2132−41.

[224] Iversen BM, Arendshorst WJ. Exaggerated Ca^{2+} signaling in preglomerular arteriolar smooth muscle cells of genetically hypertensive rats. Am J Physiol 1999;276:F260−70.

[225] Hansen PB, Jensen BL, Andreasen D, Friis UG, Skott O. Vascular smooth muscle cells express the alpha(1A) subunit of a P-/Q-type voltage-dependent $Ca^{(2+)}$ channel, and it is functionally important in renal afferent arterioles. Circ Res 2000;87:896−902.

[226] Jensen BL, Friis UG, Hansen PB, Andreasen D, Uhrenholt T, Schjerning J, et al. Voltage-dependent calcium channels in the renal microcirculation. Nephrol Dial Transplant 2004;19:1368−73.

[227] Ozawa Y, Hayashi K, Nagahama T, Fujiwara K, Saruta T. Effect of T-type selective calcium antagonist on renal microcirculation: studies in the isolated perfused hydronephrotic kidney. Hypertension 2001;38:343−7.

[228] Ozawa Y, Hayashi K, Nagahama T, Fujiwara K, Wakino S, Saruta T. Renal afferent and efferent arteriolar dilation by nilvadipine: studies in the isolated perfused hydronephrotic kidney. J Cardiovasc Pharmacol 1999;33:243−7.

[229] Salomonsson M, Sorensen CM, Arendshorst WJ, Steendahl J, Holstein-Rathlou NH. Calcium handling in afferent arterioles. Acta Physiol Scand 2004;181:421−9.

[230] Rhinehart K, Zhang Z, Pallone TL. $Ca^{(2+)}$ signaling and membrane potential in descending vasa recta pericytes and endothelia. Am J Physiol Renal Physiol 2002;283:F852−60.

[231] Zhang Z, Rhinehart K, Pallone TL. Membrane potential controls calcium entry into descending vasa recta pericytes. Am J Physiol Regul Integr Comp Physiol 2002;283:R949−57.

[232] Feng MG, Navar LG. Angiotensin II-mediated constriction of afferent and efferent arterioles involves T-type Ca channel activation. Am J Nephrol 2004;24:641−8.

[233] Hayashi K, Ozawa Y, Wakino S, Kanda T, Homma K, Takamatsu I, et al. Cellular mechanism for mibefradil-induced vasodilation of renal microcirculation: studies in the isolated perfused hydronephrotic kidney. J Cardiovasc Pharmacol 2003;42:697−702.

[234] Gordienko DV, Clausen C, Goligorsky MS. Ionic currents and endothelin signaling in smooth muscle cells from rat renal resistance arteries. Am J Physiol 1994;266:F325−41.

[235] Hall DA, Carmines PK, Sansom SC. Dihydropyridine-sensitive $Ca^{(2+)}$ channels in human glomerular mesangial cells. Am J Physiol Renal Physiol 2000;278:F97−103.

[236] Zhang Z, Lin H, Cao C, Khurana S, Pallone TL. Voltage gated divalent currents in descending vasa recta pericytes. Am J Physiol Renal Physiol 2010.

[237] Feng MG, Li M, Navar LG. T-type calcium channels in the regulation of afferent and efferent arterioles in rats. Am J Physiol Renal Physiol 2004;286:F331−7.

[238] Feng MG, Navar LG. Nitric oxide synthase inhibition activates L- and T-type Ca^{2+} channels in afferent and efferent arterioles. Am J Physiol Renal Physiol 2006;290:F873−9.

[239] Honda M, Hayashi K, Matsuda H, Kubota E, Tokuyama H, Okubo K, et al. Divergent renal vasodilator action of L- and T-type calcium antagonists *in vivo*. J Hypertens 2001;19:2031−7.

[240] Hart P, Bakris GL. Calcium antagonists: do they equally protect against kidney injury? Kidney Int 2008;73:795−6.

[241] Saruta T, Kanno Y, Hayashi K, Konishi K. Antihypertensive agents and renal protection: calcium channel blockers. Kidney Int Suppl 1996;55:S52−6.

[242] Sasaki H, Saiki A, Endo K, Ban N, Yamaguchi T, Kawana H, et al. Protective effects of efonidipine, a T- and L-type calcium channel blocker, on renal function and arterial stiffness in type 2 diabetic patients with hypertension and nephropathy. J Atheroscler Thromb 2009;16:568−75.

[243] Parekh AB. Store-operated Ca^{2+} entry: dynamic interplay between endoplasmic reticulum, mitochondria and plasma membrane. J Physiol 2003;547:333−48.

[244] Cioffi DL, Barry C, Stevens T. Store-operated calcium entry channels in pulmonary endothelium: the emerging story of TRPCS and Orai1. Adv Exp Med Biol 2010;661:137−54.

[245] Putney Jr JW. Capacitative calcium entry: sensing the calcium stores. J Cell Biol 2005;169:381–2.

[246] Putney JW. Capacitative calcium entry: from concept to molecules. Immunol Rev 2009;231:10–22.

[247] Vaca L. SOCIC: the store-operated calcium influx complex. Cell Calcium 2010;47:199–209.

[248] Fellner SK, Arendshorst WJ. Angiotensin II-stimulated Ca^{2+} entry mechanisms in afferent arterioles: role of transient receptor potential canonical channels and reverse Na^+/Ca^{2+} exchange. Am J Physiol Renal Physiol 2008;294:F212–9.

[249] Clapham DE. TRP channels as cellular sensors. Nature 2003;426:517–24.

[250] Fellner SK, Arendshorst WJ. Capacitative calcium entry in smooth muscle cells from preglomerular vessels. Am J Physiol 1999;277:F533–42.

[251] Takenaka T, Suzuki H, Okada H, Inoue T, Kanno Y, Ozawa Y, et al. Transient receptor potential channels in rat renal microcirculation: actions of angiotensin II. Kidney Int 2002;62:558–65.

[252] Ma R, Smith S, Child A, Carmines PK, Sansom SC. Store-operated $Ca^{(2+)}$ channels in human glomerular mesangial cells. Am J Physiol Renal Physiol 2000;278:F954–61.

[253] Li WP, Tsiokas L, Sansom SC, Ma R. Epidermal growth factor activates store-operated Ca^{2+} channels through an inositol 1,4,5-trisphosphate-independent pathway in human glomerular mesangial cells. J Biol Chem 2004;279:4570–7.

[254] Ma R, Sansom SC. Epidermal growth factor activates store-operated calcium channels in human glomerular mesangial cells. J Am Soc Nephrol 2001;12:47–53.

[255] Ma R, Kudlacek PE, Sansom SC. Protein kinase C-alpha participates in activation of store-operated Ca^{2+} channels in human glomerular mesangial cells. Am J Physiol Cell Physiol 2002;283:C1390–8.

[256] Ma R, Pluznick J, Kudlacek P, Sansom SC. Protein kinase C activates store-operated $Ca^{(2+)}$ channels in human glomerular mesangial cells. J Biol Chem 2001;276:25759–65.

[257] Wang X, Pluznick JL, Wei P, Padanilam BJ, Sansom SC. TRPC4 forms store-operated Ca^{2+} channels in mouse mesangial cells. Am J Physiol Cell Physiol 2004;287:C357–64.

[258] Lee-Kwon W, Wade JB, Zhang Z, Pallone TL, Weinman EJ. Expression of TRPC4 channel protein that interacts with NHERF-2 in rat descending vasa recta. Am J Physiol Cell Physiol 2005;288:C942–9.

[259] Kitamura K, Yamazaki J. Chloride channels and their functional roles in smooth muscle tone in the vasculature. Jpn J Pharmacol 2001;85:351–7.

[260] Large WA, Wang Q. Characteristics and physiological role of the $Ca^{(2+)}$-activated Cl^- conductance in smooth muscle. Am J Physiol 1996;271:C435–54.

[261] Duran C, Thompson CH, Xiao Q, Hartzell HC. Chloride channels: often enigmatic, rarely predictable. Annu Rev Physiol 2010;72:95–121.

[262] Hartzell HC, Yu K, Xiao Q, Chien LT, Qu Z. Anoctamin/TMEM16 family members are Ca^{2+}-activated Cl^- channels. J Physiol 2009;587:2127–39.

[263] Carmines PK. Segment-specific effect of chloride channel blockade on rat renal arteriolar contractile responses to angiotensin II. Am J Hypertens 1995;8:90–4.

[264] Hansen PB, Friis UG, Uhrenholt TR, Briggs J, Schnermann J. Intracellular signalling pathways in the vasoconstrictor response of mouse afferent arterioles to adenosine. Acta Physiol (Oxf) 2007;191:89–97.

[265] Hansen PB, Jensen BL, Skott O. Chloride regulates afferent arteriolar contraction in response to depolarization. Hypertension 1998;32:1066–70.

[266] Jensen BL, Ellekvist P, Skott O. Chloride is essential for contraction of afferent arterioles after agonists and potassium. Am J Physiol 1997;272:F389–96.

[267] Takenaka T, Kanno Y, Kitamura Y, Hayashi K, Suzuki H, Saruta T. Role of chloride channels in afferent arteriolar constriction. Kidney Int 1996;50:864–72.

[268] Pallone TL, Huang JM. Control of descending vasa recta pericyte membrane potential by angiotensin II. Am J Physiol Renal Physiol 2002;282:F1064–74.

[269] Pallone TL, Zhang Z, Rhinehart K. Physiology of the renal medullary microcirculation. Am J Physiol Renal Physiol 2003;284:F253–66.

[270] Zhang Z, Huang JM, Turner MR, Rhinehart KL, Pallone TL. Role of chloride in constriction of descending vasa recta by angiotensin II. Am J Physiol Regul Integr Comp Physiol 2001;280:R1878–86.

[271] Edwards A, Pallone TL. Mechanisms underlying angiotensin II-induced calcium oscillations. Am J Physiol Renal Physiol 2008;295:F568–84.

[272] Zhang Q, Cao C, Zhang Z, Wier WG, Edwards A, Pallone TL. Membrane current oscillations in descending vasa recta pericytes. Am J Physiol Renal Physiol 2008;294:F656–66.

[273] Lin H, Pallone TL, Cao C. Murine vasa recta pericyte chloride conductance is controlled by calcium, depolarization andkinase activity. Am J Physiol Regul Integr Comp Physiol 2010 .

[274] Pallone TL, Cao C, Zhang Z. Inhibition of K^+ conductance in descending vasa recta pericytes by ANG II. Am J Physiol Renal Physiol 2004;287:F1213–22.

[275] Steendahl J, Holstein-Rathlou NH, Sorensen CM, Salomonsson M. Effects of chloride channel blockers on rat renal vascular responses to angiotensin II and norepinephrine. Am J Physiol Renal Physiol 2004;286:F323–30.

[276] Nelson MT, Quayle JM. Physiological roles and properties of potassium channels in arterial smooth muscle. Am J Physiol 1995;268:C799–822.

[277] Quayle JM, Nelson MT, Standen NB. ATP-sensitive and inwardly rectifying potassium channels in smooth muscle. Physiol Rev 1997;77:1165–232.

[278] Busse R, Edwards G, Feletou M, Fleming I, Vanhoutte PM, Weston AH. EDHF: bringing the concepts together. Trends Pharmacol Sci 2002;23:374–80.

[279] Popp R, Brandes RP, Ott G, Busse R, Fleming I. Dynamic modulation of interendothelial gap junctional communication by 11,12-epoxyeicosatrienoic acid. Circ Res 2002;90:800–6.

[280] Quilley J, Fulton D, McGiff JC. Hyperpolarizing factors. Biochem Pharmacol 1997;54:1059–70.

[281] Betts LC, Kozlowski RZ. Electrophysiological effects of endothelin-1 and their relationship to contraction in rat renal arterial smooth muscle. Br J Pharmacol 2000;130:787–96.

[282] Fergus DJ, Martens JR, England SK. Kv channel subunits that contribute to voltage-gated K^+ current in renal vascular smooth muscle. Pflugers Arch 2003;445:697–704.

[283] Gebremedhin D, Kaldunski M, Jacobs ER, Harder DR, Roman RJ. Coexistence of two types of $Ca^{(2+)}$-activated K^+ channels in rat renal arterioles. Am J Physiol 1996;270:F69–81.

[284] Gelband CH, Hume JR. Ionic currents in single smooth muscle cells of the canine renal artery. Circ Res 1992;71:745–58.

[285] Gelband CH, Ishikawa T, Post JM, Keef KD, Hume JR. Intracellular divalent cations block smooth muscle K^+ channels. Circ Res 1993;73:24–34.

[286] Prior HM, Yates MS, Beech DJ. Functions of large conductance Ca^{2+}-activated (BKCa), delayed rectifier (KV) and background K^+ channels in the control of membrane potential in rabbit renal arcuate artery. J Physiol 1998;511(Pt 1):159–69.

[287] Martens JR, Gelband CH. Alterations in rat interlobar artery membrane potential and K$^+$ channels in genetic and nongenetic hypertension. Circ Res 1996;79:295–301.

[288] Martens JR, Gelband CH. Ion channels in vascular smooth muscle: alterations in essential hypertension. Proc Soc Exp Biol Med 1998;218:192–203.

[289] Prior HM, Yates MS, Beech DJ. Role of K$^+$ channels in A2A adenosine receptor-mediated dilation of the pressurized renal arcuate artery. Br J Pharmacol 1999;126:494–500.

[290] Ma YH, Gebremedhin D, Schwartzman ML, Falck JR, Clark JE, Masters BS, et al. 20-Hydroxyeicosatetraenoic acid is an endogenous vasoconstrictor of canine renal arcuate arteries. Circ Res 1993;72:126–36.

[291] Maier KG, Roman RJ. Cytochrome P450 metabolites of arachidonic acid in the control of renal function. Curr Opin Nephrol Hypertens 2001;10:81–7.

[292] Zou AP, Fleming JT, Falck JR, Jacobs ER, Gebremedhin D, Harder DR, et al. 20-HETE is an endogenous inhibitor of the large-conductance Ca^{2+}-activated K$^+$ channel in renal arterioles. Am J Physiol 1996;270:R228–37.

[293] Sun CW, Falck JR, Harder DR, Roman RJ. Role of tyrosine kinase and PKC in the vasoconstrictor response to 20-HETE in renal arterioles. Hypertension 1999;33:414–8.

[294] Sun CW, Alonso-Galicia M, Taheri MR, Falck JR, Harder DR, Roman RJ. Nitric oxide-20-hydroxyeicosatetraenoic acid interaction in the regulation of K$^+$ channel activity and vascular tone in renal arterioles. Circ Res 1998;83:1069–79.

[295] Imig JD, Dimitropoulou C, Reddy DS, White RE, Falck JR. Afferent arteriolar dilation to 11,12-EET analogs involves PP2A activity and Ca^{2+}-activated K$^+$ channels. Microcirculation 2008;15:137–50.

[296] Kaide JI, Zhang F, Wei Y, Jiang H, Yu C, Wang WH, et al. Carbon monoxide of vascular origin attenuates the sensitivity of renal arterial vessels to vasoconstrictors. J Clin Invest 2001;107:1163–71.

[297] Imig JD. Eicosanoid regulation of the renal vasculature. Am J Physiol Renal Physiol 2000;279:F965–81.

[298] Wang D, Borrego-Conde LJ, Falck JR, Sharma KK, Wilcox CS, Umans JG. Contributions of nitric oxide, EDHF, and EETs to endothelium-dependent relaxation in renal afferent arterioles. Kidney Int 2003;63:2187–93.

[299] Zou AP, Fleming JT, Falck JR, Jacobs ER, Gebremedhin D, Harder DR, et al. Stereospecific effects of epoxyeicosatrienoic acids on renal vascular tone and K$^+$-channel activity. Am J Physiol 1996;270:F822–32.

[300] Alonso-Galicia M, Sun CW, Falck JR, Harder DR, Roman RJ. Contribution of 20-HETE to the vasodilator actions of nitric oxide in renal arteries. Am J Physiol 1998;275:F370–8.

[301] Li L, Wu J, Jiang C. Differential expression of Kir6.1 and SUR2B mRNAs in the vasculature of various tissues in rats. J Membr Biol 2003;196:61–9.

[302] Sun X, Cao K, Yang G, Huang Y, Hanna ST, Wang R. Selective expression of Kir6.1 protein in different vascular and non-vascular tissues. Biochem Pharmacol 2004;67:147–56.

[303] Wang X, Trottier G, Loutzenhiser R. Determinants of renal afferent arteriolar actions of bradykinin: evidence that multiple pathways mediate responses attributed to EDHF. Am J Physiol Renal Physiol 2003;285:F540–9.

[304] Chilton L, Loutzenhiser K, Morales E, Breaks J, Kargacin GJ, Loutzenhiser R. Inward rectifier K$^+$ currents and Kir2.1 expression in renal afferent and efferent arterioles. J Am Soc Nephrol 2008;19:69–76.

[305] Chilton L, Loutzenhiser R. Functional evidence for an inward rectifier potassium current in rat renal afferent arterioles. Circ Res 2001;88:152–8.

[306] Eckman DM, Nelson MT. Potassium ions as vasodilators: role of inward rectifier potassium channels. Circ Res 2001;88:132–3.

[307] Leichtle A, Rauch U, Albinus M, Benohr P, Kalbacher H, Mack AF, et al. Electrophysiological and molecular characterization of the inward rectifier in juxtaglomerular cells from rat kidney. J Physiol 2004;560:365–76.

[308] Fallet RW, Bast JP, Fujiwara K, Ishii N, Sansom SC, Carmines PK. Influence of Ca^{2+}-activated K$^+$ channels on rat renal arteriolar responses to depolarizing agonists. Am J Physiol Renal Physiol 2001;280:F583–91.

[309] Kirton CA, Loutzenhiser R. Alterations in basal protein kinase C activity modulate renal afferent arteriolar myogenic reactivity. Am J Physiol 1998;275:H467–75.

[310] Loutzenhiser RD, Parker MJ. Hypoxia inhibits myogenic reactivity of renal afferent arterioles by activating ATP-sensitive K$^+$ channels. Circ Res 1994;74:861–9.

[311] Reslerova M, Loutzenhiser R. Divergent mechanisms of ATP-sensitive K$^+$ channel-induced vasodilation in renal afferent and efferent arterioles. Evidence of L-type Ca^{2+} channel-dependent and -independent actions of pinacidil. Circ Res 1995;77:1114–20.

[312] Reslerova M, Loutzenhiser R. Renal microvascular actions of calcitonin gene-related peptide. Am J Physiol 1998;274:F1078–85.

[313] Tang L, Parker M, Fei Q, Loutzenhiser R. Afferent arteriolar adenosine A2a receptors are coupled to KATP in in vitro perfused hydronephrotic rat kidney. Am J Physiol 1999;277:F926–33.

[314] Russ U, Rauch U, Quast U. Pharmacological evidence for a KATP channel in renin-secreting cells from rat kidney. J Physiol 1999;517(Pt 3):781–90.

[315] Metzger F, Quast U. Binding of [^{3}H]-P1075, an opener of ATP-sensitive K$^+$ channels, to rat glomerular preparations. Naunyn Schmiedebergs Arch Pharmacol 1996;354:452–9.

[316] Troncoso Brindeiro CM, Fallet RW, Lane PH, Carmines PK. Potassium channel contributions to afferent arteriolar tone in normal and diabetic rat kidney. Am J Physiol Renal Physiol 2008;295:F171–8.

[317] Marchetti J, Praddaude F, Rajerison R, Ader JL, Alhenc-Gelas F. Bradykinin attenuates the [Ca^{2+}]$_{(i)}$ response to angiotensin II of renal juxtamedullary efferent arterioles via an EDHF. Br J Pharmacol 2001;132:749–59.

[318] Cao C, Goo JH, Lee-Kwon W, Pallone TL. Vasa recta pericytes express a strong inward rectifier K$^+$ conductance. Am J Physiol Regul Integr Comp Physiol 2006;290:R1601–7.

[319] Cao C, Lee-Kwon W, Payne K, Edwards A, Pallone TL. Descending vasa recta endothelia express inward rectifier potassium channels. Am J Physiol Renal Physiol 2007;293:F1248–55.

[320] Stockand JD, Sansom SC. Glomerular mesangial cells: electrophysiology and regulation of contraction. Physiol Rev 1998;78:723–44.

[321] Barber RD, Woolf AS, Henderson RM. Potassium conductances and proliferation in conditionally immortalized renal glomerular mesangial cells from the H-2Kb-tsA58 transgenic mouse. Biochim Biophys Acta 1997;1355:191–203.

[322] Szamosfalvi B, Cortes P, Alviani R, Asano K, Riser BL, Zasuwa G, et al. Putative subunits of the rat mesangial KATP: a type 2B sulfonylurea receptor and an inwardly rectifying K$^+$ channel. Kidney Int 2002;61:1739–49.

[323] Grimm PR, Sansom SC. BK channels in the kidney. Curr Opin Nephrol Hypertens 2007;16:430–6.

[324] Matsunaga H, Yamashita N, Miyajima Y, Okuda T, Chang H, Ogata E, et al. Ion channel activities of cultured rat mesangial cells. Am J Physiol 1991;261:F808–14.

[325] Sansom SC, Stockand JD. Physiological role of large, Ca^{2+}-activated K^+ channels in human glomerular mesangial cells. Clin Exp Pharmacol Physiol 1996;23:76–82.

[326] Stockand JD, Sansom SC. Large $Ca^{(2+)}$-activated K^+ channels responsive to angiotensin II in cultured human mesangial cells. Am J Physiol 1994;267:C1080–6.

[327] Stockand JD, Sansom SC. Activation by methylene blue of large $Ca^{(2+)}$-activated K^+ channels. Biochim Biophys Acta 1996;1285:123–6.

[328] Stockand JD, Sansom SC. Role of large $Ca^{(2+)}$-activated K^+ channels in regulation of mesangial contraction by nitroprusside and ANP. Am J Physiol 1996;270:C1773–9.

[329] Stockand JD, Silverman M, Hall D, Derr T, Kubacak B, Sansom SC. Arachidonic acid potentiates the feedback response of mesangial BKCa channels to angiotensin II. Am J Physiol 1998;274:F658–64.

[330] Sansom SC, Ma R, Carmines PK, Hall DA. Regulation of $Ca^{(2+)}$-activated $K^{(+)}$ channels by multifunctional $Ca^{(2+)}$/calmodulin-dependent protein kinase. Am J Physiol Renal Physiol 2000;279:F283–8.

[331] Cermak R, Kleta R, Forssmann WG, Schlatter E. Natriuretic peptides increase a K^+ conductance in rat mesangial cells. Pflugers Arch 1996;431:571–7.

[332] Kudlacek PE, Pluznick JL, Ma R, Padanilam B, Sansom SC. Role of hbeta1 in activation of human mesangial BK channels by cGMP kinase. Am J Physiol Renal Physiol 2003;285:F289–94.

[333] Sansom SC, Stockand JD, Hall D, Williams B. Regulation of large calcium-activated potassium channels by protein phosphatase 2A. J Biol Chem 1997;272:9902–6.

[334] Foutz RM, Grimm PR, Sansom SC. Insulin increases the activity of mesangial BK channels through MAPK signaling. Am J Physiol Renal Physiol 2008;294:F1465–72.

[335] Dhein S. Peptides acting at gap junctions. Peptides 2002;23:1701–9.

[336] De Wit C. Connexins pave the way for vascular communication. News Physiol Sci 2004;19:148–53.

[337] Evans WH, Martin PE. Gap junctions: structure and function (Review). Mol Membr Biol 2002;19:121–36.

[338] Figueroa XF, Isakson BE, Duling BR. Connexins: gaps in our knowledge of vascular function. Physiology (Bethesda) 2004;19:277–84.

[339] De Wit C, Roos F, Bolz SS, Kirchhoff S, Kruger O, Willecke K, et al. Impaired conduction of vasodilation along arterioles in connexin40-deficient mice. Circ Res 2000;86:649–55.

[340] De Wit C, Roos F, Bolz SS, Pohl U. Lack of vascular connexin 40 is associated with hypertension and irregular arteriolar vasomotion. Physiol Genomics 2003;13:169–77.

[341] Figueroa XF, Paul DL, Simon AM, Goodenough DA, Day KH, Damon DN, et al. Central role of connexin40 in the propagation of electrically activated vasodilation in mouse cremasteric arterioles in vivo. Circ Res 2003;92:793–800.

[342] Liao Y, Day KH, Damon DN, Duling BR. Endothelial cell-specific knockout of connexin 43 causes hypotension and bradycardia in mice. Proc Natl Acad Sci USA 2001;98:9989–94.

[343] Earley S, Resta TC, Walker BR. Disruption of smooth muscle gap junctions attenuates myogenic vasoconstriction of mesenteric resistance arteries. Am J Physiol Heart Circ Physiol 2004;287:H2677–86.

[344] Arensbak B, Mikkelsen HB, Gustafsson F, Christensen T, Holstein-Rathlou NH. Expression of connexin 37, 40, and 43 mRNA and protein in renal preglomerular arterioles. Histochem Cell Biol 2001;115:479–87.

[345] Braunstein TH, Sorensen CM, Holstein-Rathlou NH. Connexin abundance in resistance vessels from the renal microcirculation in normo- and hypertensive rats. APMIS 2009;117:268–76.

[346] Gustafsson F, Mikkelsen HB, Arensbak B, Thuneberg L, Neve S, Jensen LJ, et al. Expression of connexin 37, 40 and 43 in rat mesenteric arterioles and resistance arteries. Histochem Cell Biol 2003;119:139–48.

[347] Hwan SK, Beyer EC. Heterogeneous localization of connexin40 in the renal vasculature. Microvasc Res 2000;59:140–8.

[348] Just A, Kurtz L, de WC, Wagner C, Kurtz A, Arendshorst WJ. Connexin 40 mediates the tubuloglomerular feedback contribution to renal blood flow autoregulation. J Am Soc Nephrol 2009;20:1577–85.

[349] Silverstein DM, Thornhill BA, Leung JC, Vehaskari VM, Craver RD, Trachtman HA, et al. Expression of connexins in the normal and obstructed developing kidney. Pediatr Nephrol 2003;18:216–24.

[350] Takenaka T, Inoue T, Kanno Y, Okada H, Hill CE, Suzuki H. Connexins 37 and 40 transduce purinergic signals mediating renal autoregulation. Am J Physiol Regul Integr Comp Physiol 2008;294:R1–11.

[351] Takenaka T, Inoue T, Kanno Y, Okada H, Meaney KR, Hill CE, et al. Expression and role of connexins in the rat renal vasculature. Kidney Int 2008;73:415–22.

[352] Zhang J, Hill CE. Differential connexin expression in preglomerular and postglomerular vasculature: accentuation during diabetes. Kidney Int 2005;68:1171–85.

[353] Karagiannis J, Rand M, Li CG. Role of gap junctions in endothelium-derived hyperpolarizing factor-mediated vasodilatation in rat renal artery. Acta Pharmacol Sin 2004;25:1031–7.

[354] Udosen IT, Jiang H, Hercule HC, Oyekan AO. Nitric oxide–epoxygenase interactions and arachidonate-induced dilation of rat renal microvessels. Am J Physiol Heart Circ Physiol 2003;285:H2054–63.

[355] Salomonsson M, Gustafsson F, Andreasen D, Jensen BL, Holstein-Rathlou NH. Local electric stimulation causes conducted calcium response in rat interlobular arteries. Am J Physiol Renal Physiol 2002;283:F473–80.

[356] Haefliger JA, Krattinger N, Martin D, Pedrazzini T, Capponi A, Doring B, et al. Connexin43-dependent mechanism modulates renin secretion and hypertension. J Clin Inves 2006;116:405–13.

[357] Kurtz L, Gerl M, Kriz W, Wagner C, Kurtz A. Replacement of connexin 40 by connexin 45 causes ectopic localization of renin-producing cells in the kidney but maintains in vivo control of renin gene expression. Am J Physiol Renal Physiol 2009;297:F403–9.

[358] Kurtz L, Madsen K, Kurt B, Jensen BL, Walter S, Banas B, et al. High-level connexin expression in the human juxtaglomerular apparatus. Nephron Physiol 2010;116:1–8.

[359] Kurtz L, Schweda F, De Wit C, Kriz W, Witzgall R, Warth R, et al. Lack of connexin 40 causes displacement of renin-producing cells from afferent arterioles to the extraglomerular mesangium. J Am Soc Nephrol 2007;18:1103–11.

[360] Barajas L, Liu L, Tucker M. Localization of connexin43 in rat kidney. Kidney Int 1994;46:621–6.

[361] Guo R, Liu L, Barajas L. RT-PCR study of the distribution of connexin 43 mRNA in the glomerulus and renal tubular segments. Am J Physiol 1998;275:R439–47.

[362] Hillis GS, Duthie LA, Mlynski R, McKay NG, Mistry S, MacLeod AM, et al. The expression of connexin 43 in human kidney and cultured renal cells. Nephron 1997;75:458–63.

[363] Haefliger J-A, Demotz S, Braissant O, Suter E, Waeber B, Nicod P, et al. Connexins 40 and 43 are differentially regulated within the kdineys of rats with renovascular hypertension. Kidney Int 2001;60:190–201.

[364] Zhang Q, Cao C, Mangano M, Zhang Z, Silldorff EP, Lee-Kwon W, et al. Descending vasa recta endothelium is an

electrical syncytium. Am J Physiol Regul Integr Comp Physiol 2006;291:R1688−99.

[365] Loutzenhiser R, Bidani AK, Wang X. Systolic pressure and the myogenic response of the renal afferent arteriole. Acta Physiol Scand 2004;181:407−13.

[366] Bell PD, Lapointe JY, Peti-Peterdi J. Macula densa cell signaling. Annu Rev Physiol 2003;65:481−500.

[367] Bell PD, Lapointe JY, Sabirov R, Hayashi S, Peti-Peterdi J, Manabe K, et al. Macula densa cell signaling involves ATP release through a maxi anion channel. Proc Natl Acad Sci USA 2003;100:4322−7.

[368] Castrop H, Huang Y, Hashimoto S, Mizel D, Hansen P, Theilig F, et al. Impairment of tubuloglomerular feedback regulation of GFR in ecto-5′-nucleotidase/CD73-deficient mice. J Clin Invest 2004;114:634−42.

[369] Komlosi P, Fintha A, Bell PD. Current mechanisms of macula densa cell signalling. Acta Physiol Scand 2004;181:463−9.

[370] Ren Y, Garvin JL, Liu R, Carretero OA. Role of macula densa adenosine triphosphate (ATP) in tubuloglomerular feedback. Kidney Int 2004;66:1479−85.

[371] Schnermann J, Homer W. Smith Award lecture. The juxtaglomerular apparatus: from anatomical peculiarity to physiological relevance. J Am Soc Nephrol 2003;14:1681−94.

[372] Granger JP, Alexander BT, Llinas M. Mechanisms of pressure natriuresis. Curr Hypertens Rep 2002;4:152−9.

[373] Kaloyanides GJ, DiBona GF, Raskin P. Pressure natriuresis in the isolated kidney. Am J Physiol 1971;220:1660−6.

[374] Haas JA, Granger JP, Knox FG. Effect of renal perfusion pressure on sodium reabsorption from proximal tubules of superficial and deep nephrons. Am J Physiol 1986;250:F425−9.

[375] Roman RJ. Pressure-diuresis in volume-expanded rats. Tubular reabsorption in superficial and deep nephrons. Hypertension 1988;12:177−83.

[376] Khraibi AA, Haas JA, Knox FG. Effect of renal perfusion pressure on renal interstitial hydrostatic pressure in rats. Am J Physiol 1989;256:F165−70.

[377] Khraibi AA, Knox FG. Effect of renal decapsulation on renal interstitial hydrostatic pressure and natriuresis. Am J Physiol 1989;257:R44−8.

[378] Garcia-Estan J, Roman RJ. Role of renal interstitial hydrostatic pressure in the pressure diuresis response. Am J Physiol 1989;256:F63−70.

[379] Granger JP, Haas JA, Pawlowska D, Knox FG. Effect of direct increases in renal interstitial hydrostatic pressure on sodium excretion. Am J Physiol 1988;254:F527−32.

[380] Haas JA, Granger JP, Knox FG. Effect of intrarenal volume expansion on proximal sodium reabsorption. Am J Physiol 1988;255:F1178−82.

[381] Cowley Jr AW. Role of the renal medulla in volume and arterial pressure regulation. Am J Physiol 1997;273:R1−15.

[382] Cowley Jr AW, Mori T, Mattson D, Zou AP. Role of renal NO production in the regulation of medullary blood flow. Am J Physiol Regul Integr Comp Physiol 2003;284:R1355−69.

[383] Fenoy FJ, Ferrer P, Carbonell L, Garcia-Salom M. Role of nitric oxide on papillary blood flow and pressure natriuresis. Hypertension 1995;25:408−14.

[384] Mattson DL. Importance of the renal medullary circulation in the control of sodium excretion and blood pressure. Am J Physiol Regul Integr Comp Physiol 2003;284:R13−27.

[385] Mattson DL, Wu F. Control of arterial blood pressure and renal sodium excretion by nitric oxide synthase in the renal medulla. Acta Physiol Scand 2000;168:149−54.

[386] Cohen HJ, Marsh DJ, Kayser B. Autoregulation in vasa recta of the rat kidney. Am J Physiol 1983;245:F32−40.

[387] Galskov A, Nissen OI. Autoregulation of directly measured blood flows in the superficial and deep venous drainage areas of the cat kidney. Circ Res 1972;30:97−103.

[388] Roman RJ, Cowley Jr AW, Garcia-Estan J, Lombard JH. Pressure-diuresis in volume-expanded rats. Cortical and medullary hemodynamics. Hypertension 1988;12:168−76.

[389] Mattson DL, Lu S, Roman RJ, Cowley Jr AW. Relationship between renal perfusion pressure and blood flow in different regions of the kidney. Am J Physiol 1993;264:R578−83.

[390] Cowley Jr AW. Control of the renal medullary circulation by vasopressin V1 and V2 receptors in the rat. Exp Physiol 2000;85: Spec No:223S-231S

[391] Eppel GA, Bergstrom G, Anderson WP, Evans RG. Autoregulation of renal medullary blood flow in rabbits. Am J Physiol Regul Integr Comp Physiol 2003;284:R233−44.

[392] Majid DS, Godfrey M, Omoro SA. Pressure natriuresis and autoregulation of inner medullary blood flow in canine kidney. Hypertension 1997;29:210−5.

[393] Zhang Z, Pallone TL. Response of descending vasa recta to luminal pressure. Am J Physiol Renal Physiol 2004;287:F535−42.

[394] Dickhout JG, Mori T, Cowley Jr AW. Tubulovascular nitric oxide crosstalk: buffering of angiotensin II-induced medullary vasoconstriction. Circ Res 2002;91:487−93.

[395] Pallone TL, Silldorff EP, Zhang Z. Inhibition of calcium signaling in descending vasa recta endothelia by ANG II. Am J Physiol Heart Circ Physiol 2000;278:H1248−55.

[396] Silldorff EP, Kreisberg MS, Pallone TL. Adenosine modulates vasomotor tone in outer medullary descending vasa recta of the rat. J Clin Invest 1996;98:18−23.

[397] Silldorff EP, Yang S, Pallone TL. Prostaglandin E2 abrogates endothelin-induced vasoconstriction in renal outer medullary descending vasa recta of the rat. J Clin Invest 1995;95:2734−40.

[398] Racasan S, Joles JA, Boer P, Koomans HA, Braam B. NO dependency of RBF and autoregulation in the spontaneously hypertensive rat. Am J Physiol Renal Physiol 2003;285:F105−12.

[399] Roald AB, Ofstad J, Iversen BM. Attenuated buffering of renal perfusion pressure variation in juxtamedullary cortex in SHR. Am J Physiol Renal Physiol 2002;282:F506−11.

[400] Taniyama Y, Griendling KK. Reactive oxygen species in the vasculature: molecular and cellular mechanisms. Hypertension 2003;42:1075−81.

[401] Feng MG, Dukacz SA, Kline RL. Selective effect of tempol on renal medullary hemodynamics in spontaneously hypertensive rats. Am J Physiol Regul Integr Comp Physiol 2001;281:R1420−5.

[402] Bankir L. Antidiuretic action of vasopressin: quantitative aspects and interaction between V1a and V2 receptor-mediated effects. Cardiovasc Res 2001;51:372−90.

[403] Gussis GL, Robertson CR, Jamison RL. Erythrocyte velocity in vasa recta: effect of antidiuretic hormone and saline loading. Am J Physiol 1979;237:F326−32.

[404] Kiberd B, Robertson CR, Larson T, Jamison RL. Effect of V2-receptor-mediated changes on inner medullary blood flow induced by AVP. Am J Physiol 1987;253:F576−81.

[405] Zimmerhackl B, Robertson CR, Jamison RL. Effect of arginine vasopressin on renal medullary blood flow. A videomicroscopic study in the rat. J Clin Invest 1985;76:770−8.

[406] Nakanishi K, Mattson DL, Gross V, Roman RJ, Cowley Jr AW. Control of renal medullary blood flow by vasopressin V1 and V2 receptors. Am J Physiol 1995;269:R193−200.

[407] Rajapakse NW, Roman RJ, Falck JR, Oliver JJ, Evans RG. Modulation of V1-receptor-mediated renal vasoconstriction by epoxyeicosatrienoic acids. Am J Physiol Regul Integr Comp Physiol 2004;287:R181−7.

II. STRUCTURAL AND FUNCTIONAL ORGANIZATION OF THE KIDNEY

[408] Harrison-Bernard LM, Carmines PK. Juxtamedullary microvascular responses to arginine vasopressin in rat kidney. Am J Physiol 1994;267:F249–56.

[409] Fallet RW, Ikenaga H, Bast JP, Carmines PK. Relative contributions of Ca^{2+} mobilization and influx in renal arteriolar contractile responses to arginine vasopressin. AJP - Renal Physiology 2005;288:F545–51.

[410] Weihprecht H, Lorenz JN, Briggs JP, Schnermann J. Vasoconstrictor effect of angiotensin and vasopressin in isolated rabbit afferent arterioles. Am J Physiol 1991;261:F273–82.

[411] Edwards RM, Trizna W, Kinter LB. Renal microvascular effects of vasopressin and vasopressin antagonists. Am J Physiol 1989;256:F274–8.

[412] Turner MR, Pallone TL. Vasopressin constricts outer medullary descending vasa recta isolated from rat kidneys. Am J Physiol 1997;272:F147–51.

[413] Correia AG, Denton KM, Evans RG. Effects of activation of vasopressin-V1-receptors on regional kidney blood flow and glomerular arteriole diameters. J Hypertens 2001;19:649–57.

[414] Aki Y, Tamaki T, Kiyomoto H, He H, Yoshida H, Iwao H, et al. Nitric oxide may participate in V2 vasopressin-receptor-mediated renal vasodilation. J Cardiovasc Pharmacol 1994;23:331–6.

[415] Liard JF. L-NAME antagonizes vasopressin V2-induced vasodilatation in dogs. Am J Physiol 1994;266:H99–106.

[416] Naitoh M, Suzuki H, Murakami M, Matsumoto A, Ichihara A, Nakamoto H, et al. Arginine vasopressin produces renal vasodilation via V2 receptors in conscious dogs. Am J Physiol 1993;265:R934–42.

[417] Rudichenko VM, Beierwaltes WH. Arginine vasopressin-induced renal vasodilation mediated by nitric oxide. J Vasc Res 1995;32:100–5.

[418] Tamaki T, Kiyomoto K, He H, Tomohiro A, Nishiyama A, Aki Y, et al. Vasodilation induced by vasopressin V2 receptor stimulation in afferent arterioles. Kidney Int 1996;49:722–9.

[419] Park F, Mattson DL, Skelton MM, Cowley Jr AW. Localization of the vasopressin V1a and V2 receptors within the renal cortical and medullary circulation. Am J Physiol 1997;273:R243–51.

[420] Park F, Zou AP, Cowley Jr AW. Arginine vasopressin-mediated stimulation of nitric oxide within the rat renal medulla. Hypertension 1998;32:896–901.

[421] Mori T, Dickhout JG, Cowley Jr AW. Vasopressin increases intracellular NO concentration via $Ca^{(2+)}$ signaling in inner medullary collecting duct. Hypertension 2002;39:465–9.

[422] O'Connor PM, Cowley Jr AW. Vasopressin-induced nitric oxide production in rat inner medullary collecting duct is dependent on V2 receptor activation of the phosphoinositide pathway. Am J Physiol Renal Physiol 2007;293:F526–32.

[423] Evans RG, Madden AC, Denton KM. Diversity of responses of renal cortical and medullary blood flow to vasoconstrictors in conscious rabbits. Acta Physiol Scand 2000;169:297–308.

[424] Szentivanyi Jr M, Park F, Maeda CY, Cowley Jr AW. Nitric oxide in the renal medulla protects from vasopressin-induced hypertension. Hypertension 2000;35:740–5.

[425] Cao C, Edwards A, Sendeski M, Lee-Kwon W, Cui L, Cai CY, et al. Intrinsic nitric oxide and superoxide production regulates descending vasa recta contraction. Am J Physiol Renal Physiol 2010.

[426] Yuan BH, Robinette JB, Conger JD. Effect of angiotensin II and norepinephrine on isolated rat afferent and efferent arterioles. Am J Physiol 1990;258:F741–50.

[427] Harrison-Bernard LM, Carmines PK. Impact of cyclo-oxygenase blockade on juxtamedullary microvascular responses to angiotensin II in rat kidney. Clin Exp Pharmacol Physiol 1995;22:732–8.

[428] Cupples WA, Sakai T, Marsh DJ. Angiotensin II and prostaglandins in control of vasa recta blood flow. Am J Physiol 1988;254:F417–24.

[429] Goransson A, Sjoquist M, Ulfendahl HR. Superficial and juxtamedullary nephron function during converting enzyme inhibition. Am J Physiol 1986;251:F25–33.

[430] Roman RJ, Kaldunski ML, Scicli AG, Carretero OA. Influence of kinins and angiotensin II on the regulation of papillary blood flow. Am J Physiol 1988;255:F690–8.

[431] Evans RG, Head GA, Eppel GA, Burke SL, Rajapakse NW. Angiotensin II and neurohumoral control of the renal medullary circulation. Clin Exp Pharmacol Physiol 2010;37:e58–69.

[432] Mori T, Cowley Jr AW, Ito S. Molecular mechanisms and therapeutic strategies of chronic renal injury: physiological role of angiotensin II-induced oxidative stress in renal medulla. J Pharmacol Sci 2006;100:2–8.

[433] Navar LG, Prieto-Carrasquero MC, Kobori H. Molecular aspects of the renal renin–angiotensin system. In: Re R, DiPette DJ, Schiffrin EL, Sowers JR, editors. *Molecular mechanisms in hypertension*. Taylor & Francis group. 2006. p. 3–14.

[434] Patzak A, Persson AE. Angiotensin II–nitric oxide interaction in the kidney. Curr Opin Nephrol Hypertens 2007;16:46–51.

[435] Sadowski J, Badzynska B. Specific features and roles of renal circulation: angiotensin II revisited. J Physiol Pharmacol 2006;57(Suppl. 11):169–78.

[436] Kohagura K, Arima S, Endo Y, Chiba Y, Ito O, Abe M, et al. Involvement of cytochrome P450 metabolites in the vascular action of angiotensin II on the afferent arterioles. Hypertens Res 2001;24:551–7.

[437] Kohagura K, Endo Y, Ito O, Arima S, Omata K, Ito S. Endogenous nitric oxide and epoxyeicosatrienoic acids modulate angiotensin II-induced constriction in the rabbit afferent arteriole. Acta Physiol Scand 2000;168:107–12.

[438] Yang S, Silldorff EP, Pallone TL. Effect of norepinephrine and acetylcholine on outer medullary descending vasa recta. Am J Physiol 1995;269:H710–6.

[439] Matsuda H, Hayashi K, Arakawa K, Kubota E, Honda M, Tokuyama H, et al. Distinct modulation of superficial and juxtamedullary arterioles by prostaglandin in vivo. Hypertens Res 2002;25:901–10.

[440] Silldorff EP, Pallone TL. Adenosine signaling in outer medullary descending vasa recta. Am J Physiol Regul Integr Comp Physiol 2001;280:R854–61.

[441] Tang L, Loutzenhiser K, Loutzenhiser R. Biphasic actions of prostaglandin E(2) on the renal afferent arteriole: role of EP(3) and EP(4) receptors. Circ Res 2000;86:663–70.

[442] Harrison-Bernard LM, Cook AK, Oliverio MI, Coffman TM. Renal segmental microvascular responses to ANG II in AT1A receptor null mice. Am J Physiol Renal Physiol 2003;284:F538–45.

[443] Helou CM, Imbert-Teboul M, Doucet A, Rajerison R, Chollet C, Alhenc-Gelas F, et al. Angiotensin receptor subtypes in thin and muscular juxtamedullary efferent arterioles of rat kidney. Am J Physiol Renal Physiol 2003;285:F507–14.

[444] Carey RM. Update on the role of the AT2 receptor. Curr Opin Nephrol Hypertens 2005;14:67–71.

[445] Carey RM, Jin X, Wang Z, Siragy HM. Nitric oxide: a physiological mediator of the type 2 (AT2) angiotensin receptor. Acta Physiol Scand 2000;168:65–71.

[446] Arima S, Endo Y, Yaoita H, Omata K, Ogawa S, Tsunoda K, et al. Possible role of P-450 metabolite of arachidonic acid in vasodilator mechanism of angiotensin II type 2 receptor in the isolated microperfused rabbit afferent arteriole. J Clin Invest 1997;100:2816–23.

[447] Patzak A, Kleinmann F, Lai EY, Kupsch E, Skelweit A, Mrowka R. Nitric oxide counteracts angiotensin II induced contraction in efferent arterioles in mice. Acta Physiol Scand 2004;181:439—44.

[448] Patzak A, Lai EY, Mrowka R, Steege A, Persson PB, Persson AE. AT1 receptors mediate angiotensin II-induced release of nitric oxide in afferent arterioles. Kidney Int 2004;66:1949—58.

[449] Endo Y, Arima S, Yaoita H, Omata K, Tsunoda K, Takeuchi K, et al. Function of angiotensin II type 2 receptor in the postglomerular efferent arteriole. Kidney Int Suppl 1997;63:S205—7.

[450] Rhinehart K, Handelsman CA, Silldorff EP, Pallone TL. ANG II AT2 receptor modulates AT1 receptor-mediated descending vasa recta endothelial Ca^{2+} signaling. Am J Physiol Heart Circ Physiol 2003;284:H779—89.

[451] Zhang Z, Rhinehart K, Kwon W, Weinman E, Pallone TL. ANG II signaling in vasa recta pericytes by PKC and reactive oxygen species. Am J Physiol Heart Circ Physiol 2004;287:H773—81.

[452] Endo Y, Arima S, Yaoita H, Tsunoda K, Omata K, Ito S. Vasodilation mediated by angiotensin II type 2 receptor is impaired in afferent arterioles of young spontaneously hypertensive rats. J Vasc Res 1998;35:421—7.

[453] Goto M, Mukoyama M, Sugawara A, Suganami T, Kasahara M, Yahata K, et al. Expression and role of angiotensin II type 2 receptor in the kidney and mesangial cells of spontaneously hypertensive rats. Hypertens Res 2002;25:125—33.

[454] Miyata N, Park F, Li XF, Cowley Jr AW. Distribution of angiotensin AT1 and AT2 receptor subtypes in the rat kidney. Am J Physiol 1999;277:F437—46.

[455] Badzynska B, Grzelec-Mojzesowicz M, Dobrowolski L, Sadowski J. Differential effect of angiotensin II on blood circulation in the renal medulla and cortex of anaesthetised rats. J Physiol 2002;538:159—66.

[456] Duke LM, Eppel GA, Widdop RE, Evans RG. Disparate roles of AT2 receptors in the renal cortical and medullary circulations of anesthetized rabbits. Hypertension 2003;42:200—5.

[457] Navar LG, Ichihara A, Chin SY, Imig JD. Nitric oxide-angiotensin II interactions in angiotensin II-dependent hypertension. Acta Physiol Scand 2000;168:139—47.

[458] Szentivanyi Jr M, Zou AP, Mattson DL, Soares P, Moreno C, Roman RJ, et al. Renal medullary nitric oxide deficit of Dahl S rats enhances hypertensive actions of angiotensin II. Am J Physiol Regul Integr Comp Physiol 2002;283:R266—72.

[459] Zou AP, Wu F, Cowley Jr AW. Protective effect of angiotensin II-induced increase in nitric oxide in the renal medullary circulation. Hypertension 1998;31:271—6.

[460] Mattson DL, Meister CJ. Renal cortical and medullary blood flow responses to L-NAME and ANG II in wild-type, nNOS null mutant, and eNOS null mutant mice. Am J Physiol Regul Integr Comp Physiol 2005;289:R991—7.

[461] Gross V, Schunck WH, Honeck H, Milia AF, Kargel E, Walther T, et al. Inhibition of pressure natriuresis in mice lacking the AT2 receptor. Kidney Int 2000;57:191—202.

[462] Navar LG. The intrarenal renin—angiotensin system in hypertension. Kidney Int 2004;65:1522—32.

[463] Navar LG, Nishiyama A. Why are angiotensin concentrations so high in the kidney? Curr Opin Nephrol Hypertens 2004;13:107—15.

[464] Nishiyama A, Seth DM, Navar LG. Renal interstitial fluid angiotensin I and angiotensin II concentrations during local angiotensin-converting enzyme inhibition. J Am Soc Nephrol 2002;13:2207—12.

[465] Nishiyama A, Seth DM, Navar LG. Angiotensin II type 1 receptor-mediated augmentation of renal interstitial fluid angiotensin II in angiotensin II-induced hypertension. J Hypertens 2003;21:1897—903.

[466] Seikaly MG, Arant Jr BS, Seney Jr FD. Endogenous angiotensin concentrations in specific intrarenal fluid compartments of the rat. J Clin Invest 1990;86:1352—7.

[467] Cao C, Lee-Kwon W, Silldorff EP, Pallone TL. KATP channel conductance of descending vasa recta pericytes. Am J Physiol Renal Physiol 2005;289:F1235—45.

[468] Pallone TL, Turner MR. Ion channel architecture of the renal microcirculation. Current Hypertension Reviews 2006;2:69—81.

[469] Edwards A, Layton AT. Nitric oxide and superoxide transport in a cross-section of the rat outer medulla. I. Effects of low medullary oxygen tension. Am J Physiol Renal Physiol 2010.

[470] Edwards A, Layton AT. Nitric oxide and superoxide transport in a cross-section of the rat outer medulla. II. Reciprocal interactions and tubulo-vascular cross-talk. Am J Physiol Renal Physiol 2010.

[471] Zhang W, Edwards A. A model of nitric oxide tubulovascular cross talk in a renal outer medullary cross section. Am J Physiol Renal Physiol 2007;292:F711—22.

[472] Ferrario CM, Chappell MC. Novel angiotensin peptides. Cell Mol Life Sci 2004;61:2720—7.

[473] Sampaio WO, Nascimento AA, Santos RA. Systemic and regional hemodynamic effects of angiotensin-(1—7) in rats. Am J Physiol Heart Circ Physiol 2003;284:H1985—94.

[474] Stegbauer J, Oberhauser V, Vonend O, Rump LC. Angiotensin-(1—7) modulates vascular resistance and sympathetic neurotransmission in kidneys of spontaneously hypertensive rats. Cardiovasc Res 2004;61:352—9.

[475] Santos RA, Simoes e Silva AC, Maric C, Silva DM, Machado RP, de BI, et al. Angiotensin-(1—7) is an endogenous ligand for the G protein-coupled receptor Mas. Proc Natl Acad Sci USA 2003;100:8258—63.

[476] Batlle D, Soler MJ, Wysocki J. New aspects of the renin—angiotensin system: angiotensin-converting enzyme 2 — a potential target for treatment of hypertension and diabetic nephropathy. Curr Opin Nephrol Hypertens 2008;17:250—7.

[477] Chappell MC. Emerging evidence for a functional angiotensin-converting enzyme 2-angiotensin-(1—7)-MAS receptor axis: more than regulation of blood pressure? Hypertension 2007;50:596—9.

[478] Dilauro M, Burns KD. Angiotensin-(1—7) and its effects in the kidney. Scientific World Journal 2009;9:522—35.

[479] Klar J, Vitzthum H, Kurtz A. Aldosterone enhances renin gene expression in juxtaglomerular cells. Am J Physiol Renal Physiol 2004;286:F349—55.

[480] Uhrenholt TR, Jensen BL, Skott O. Rapid nongenomic effect of aldosterone on vasoconstriction. Hypertension 2004;43:e30.

[481] Schmidt BM, Oehmer S, Delles C, Bratke R, Schneider MP, Klingbeil A, et al. Rapid nongenomic effects of aldosterone on human forearm vasculature. Hypertension 2003;42:156—60.

[482] Arima S. Aldosterone and the kidney: rapid regulation of renal microcirculation. Steroids 2006;71:281—5.

[483] Arima S. Rapid non-genomic vasoconstrictor actions of aldosterone in the renal microcirculation. J Steroid Biochem Mol Biol 2006;102:170—4.

[484] Arima S, Kohagura K, Xu HL, Sugawara A, Abe T, Satoh F, et al. Nongenomic vascular action of aldosterone in the glomerular microcirculation. J Am Soc Nephrol 2003;14:2255—63.

[485] Arima S, Kohagura K, Xu HL, Sugawara A, Uruno A, Satoh F, et al. Endothelium-derived nitric oxide modulates vascular action of aldosterone in renal arteriole. Hypertension 2004;43:352—7.

[486] Brain SD, Grant AD. Vascular actions of calcitonin gene-related peptide and adrenomedullin. Physiol Rev 2004;84:903—34.

[487] Bunton DC, Petrie MC, Hillier C, Johnston F, McMurray JJ. The clinical relevance of adrenomedullin: a promising profile? Pharmacol Ther 2004;103:179—201.

[488] Hinson JP, Kapas S, Smith DM. Adrenomedullin, a multifunctional regulatory peptide. Endocr Rev 2000;21:138—67.

[489] Nishimatsu H, Hirata Y, Shindo T, Kurihara H, Kakoki M, Nagata D, et al. Role of endogenous adrenomedullin in the regulation of vascular tone and ischemic renal injury: studies on transgenic/knockout mice of adrenomedullin gene. Circ Res 2002;90:657—63.

[490] Shindo T, Kurihara Y, Nishimatsu H, Moriyama N, Kakoki M, Wang Y, et al. Vascular abnormalities and elevated blood pressure in mice lacking adrenomedullin gene. Circulation 2001;104:1964—71.

[491] Nagata D, Hirata Y, Suzuki E, Kakoki M, Hayakawa H, Goto A, et al. Hypoxia-induced adrenomedullin production in the kidney. Kidney Int 1999;55:1259—67.

[492] Gardiner SM, Kemp PA, March JE, Bennett T. Regional haemodynamic effects of human and rat adrenomedullin in conscious rats. Br J Pharmacol 1995;114:584—91.

[493] Majid DS, Kadowitz PJ, Coy DH, Navar LG. Renal responses to intra-arterial administration of adrenomedullin in dogs. Am J Physiol 1996;270:F200—5.

[494] Minami K, Segawa K, Uezono Y, Shiga Y, Shiraishi M, Ogata J, et al. Adrenomedullin inhibits the pressor effects and decrease in renal blood flow induced by norepinephrine or angiotensin II in anesthetized rats. Jpn J Pharmacol 2001;86:159—64.

[495] Hirata Y, Hayakawa H, Suzuki Y, Suzuki E, Ikenouchi H, Kohmoto O, et al. Mechanisms of adrenomedullin-induced vasodilation in the rat kidney. Hypertension 1995;25:790—5.

[496] Mori Y, Nishikimi T, Kobayashi N, Ono H, Kangawa K, Matsuoka H. Long-term adrenomedullin infusion improves survival in malignant hypertensive rats. Hypertension 2002;40:107—13.

[497] Nishikimi T, Mori Y, Kobayashi N, Tadokoro K, Wang X, Akimoto K, et al. Renoprotective effect of chronic adrenomedullin infusion in Dahl salt-sensitive rats. Hypertension 2002;39:1077—82.

[498] Ito K, Yoshii H, Asano T, Seta K, Mizuguchi Y, Yamanaka M, et al. Adrenomedullin increases renal nitric oxide production and ameliorates renal injury in mice with unilateral ureteral obstruction. J Urol 2010;183:1630—5.

[499] Oba S, Hino M, Fujita T. Adrenomedullin protects against oxidative stress-induced podocyte injury as an endogenous antioxidant. Nephrol Dial Transplant 2008;23:510—7.

[500] Bell D, McDermott BJ. Intermedin (adrenomedullin-2): a novel counter-regulatory peptide in the cardiovascular and renal systems. Br J Pharmacol 2008;153(Suppl. 1):S247—62.

[501] Fujisawa Y, Nagai Y, Miyatake A, Miura K, Shokoji T, Nishiyama A, et al. Roles of adrenomedullin 2 in regulating the cardiovascular and sympathetic nervous systems in conscious rats. Am J Physiol-Heart Circ Physiol 2006;290:H1120—7.

[502] Fujisawa Y, Nagai Y, Miyatake A, Takei Y, Miura K, Shoukouji T, et al. Renal effects of a new member of adrenomedullin family, adrenomedullin2, in rats. Eur J Pharmacol 2004;497:75—80.

[503] Hagiwara M, Bledsoe G, Yang ZR, Smith Jr RS, Chao L, Chao J. Intermedin ameliorates vascular and renal injury by inhibition of oxidative stress. Am J Physiol Renal Physiol 2008;295:F1735—43.

[504] Hirose T, Totsune K, Mori N, Mori T, Morimoto R, Metoki H, et al. Expression of adrenomedullin 2/intermedin, a possible reno-protective peptide, is decreased in the kidneys of rats with hypertension or renal failure. Am J Physiol Renal Physiol 2010;299:F128—34.

[505] Baylis C. Nitric oxide deficiency in chronic kidney disease. Am J Physiol Renal Physiol 2008;294:F1—9.

[506] Cowley Jr AW. Renal medullary oxidative stress, pressure-natriuresis, and hypertension. Hypertension 2008;52:777—86.

[507] Goligorsky MS, Brodsky SV, Noiri E. NO bioavailability, endothelial dysfunction, and acute renal failure: new insights into pathophysiology. Semin Nephrol 2004;24:316—23.

[508] Goligorsky MS, Li H, Brodsky S, Chen J. Relationships between caveolae and eNOS: everything in proximity and the proximity of everything. Am J Physiol Renal Physiol 2002;283:F1—10.

[509] Kone BC. Nitric oxide synthesis in the kidney: isoforms, biosynthesis, and functions in health. Semin Nephrol 2004;24:299—315.

[510] Kone BC, Baylis C. Biosynthesis and homeostatic roles of nitric oxide in the normal kidney. Am J Physiol 1997;272:F561—78.

[511] Kone BC, Kuncewicz T, Zhang W, Yu ZY. Protein interactions with nitric oxide synthases: controlling the right time, the right place, and the right amount of nitric oxide. Am J Physiol Renal Physiol 2003;285:F178—90.

[512] Majid DS, Navar LG. Nitric oxide in the control of renal hemodynamics and excretory function. Am J Hypertens 2001;14:74S—82S.

[513] Mattson DL, Lu S, Cowley Jr AW. Role of nitric oxide in the control of the renal medullary circulation. Clin Exp Pharmacol Physiol 1997;24:587—90.

[514] Pallone TL, Mattson DL. Role of nitric oxide in regulation of the renal medulla in normal and hypertensive kidneys. Curr Opin Nephrol Hypertens 2002;11:93—8.

[515] Wilcox CS. Effects of tempol and redox-cycling nitroxides in models of oxidative stress. Pharmacol Ther 2010;126:119—45.

[516] Wilcox CS, Pearlman A. Chemistry and antihypertensive effects of tempol and other nitroxides. Pharmacol Rev 2008;60:418—69.

[517] Zou AP, Cowley Jr AW. Reactive oxygen species and molecular regulation of renal oxygenation. Acta Physiol Scand 2003;179:233—41.

[518] Mattson DL, Wu F. Nitric oxide synthase activity and isoforms in rat renal vasculature. Hypertension 2000;35:337—41.

[519] Kakoki M, Kim HS, Arendshorst WJ, Mattson DL. L-Arginine uptake affects nitric oxide production and blood flow in the renal medulla. Am J Physiol Regul Integr Comp Physiol 2004;287:R1478—85.

[520] Kakoki M, Wang W, Mattson DL. Cationic amino acid transport in the renal medulla and blood pressure regulation. Hypertension 2002;39:287—92.

[521] Wu F, Cholewa B, Mattson DL. Characterization of L-arginine transporters in rat renal inner medullary collecting duct. Am J Physiol Regul Integr Comp Physiol 2000;278:R1506—12.

[522] Zewde T, Wu F, Mattson DL. Influence of dietary NaCl on L-arginine transport in the renal medulla. Am J Physiol Regul Integr Comp Physiol 2004;286:R89—93.

[523] Palm F, Onozato ML, Luo Z, Wilcox CS. Dimethylarginine dimethylaminohydrolase (DDAH): expression, regulation, and function in the cardiovascular and renal systems. Am J Physiol Heart Circ Physiol 2007;293:H3227—45.

[524] Teerlink T, Luo Z, Palm F, Wilcox CS. Cellular ADMA: regulation and action. Pharmacol Res 2009;60:448—60.

[525] Tojo A, Welch WJ, Bremer V, Kimoto M, Kimura K, Omata M, et al. Colocalization of demethylating enzymes and NOS and functional effects of methylarginines in rat kidney. Kidney Int 1997;52:1593—601.

[526] Wang D, Gill PS, Chabrashvili T, Onozato ML, Raggio J, Mendonca M, et al. Isoform-specific regulation by N^G,N^G-dimethylarginine dimethylaminohydrolase of rat serum asymmetric dimethylarginine and vascular endothelium-derived relaxing factor/NO. Circ Res 2007;101:627—35.

[527] Wang D, Strandgaard S, Iversen J, Wilcox CS. Asymmetric dimethylarginine, oxidative stress, and vascular nitric oxide

synthase in essential hypertension. Am J Physiol Regul Integr Comp Physiol 2009;296:R195−200.

[528] Beierwaltes WH, Sigmon DH, Carretero OA. Endothelium modulates renal blood flow but not autoregulation. Am J Physiol 1992;262:F943−9.

[529] Majid DS, Williams A, Navar LG. Inhibition of nitric oxide synthesis attenuates pressure-induced natriuretic responses in anesthetized dogs. Am J Physiol 1993;264:F79−87.

[530] Imig JD, Gebremedhin D, Harder DR, Roman RJ. Modulation of vascular tone in renal microcirculation by erythrocytes: role of EDRF. Am J Physiol 1993;264:H190−5.

[531] Imig JD, Roman RJ. Nitric oxide modulates vascular tone in preglomerular arterioles. Hypertension 1992;19:770−4.

[532] Juncos LA, Ito S, Carretero OA, Garvin JL. Removal of endo-thelium-dependent relaxation by antibody and complement in afferent arterioles. Hypertension 1994;23:I54−9.

[533] Hoffend J, Cavarape A, Endlich K, Steinhausen M. Influence of endothelium-derived relaxing factor on renal microvessels and pressure-dependent vasodilation. Am J Physiol 1993;265:F285−92.

[534] Larson TS, Lockhart JC. Restoration of vasa recta hemodynam-ics and pressure natriuresis in SHR by L-arginine. Am J Physiol 1995;268:F907−12.

[535] Kakoki M, Kim HS, Edgell CJ, Maeda N, Smithies O, Mattson DL. Amino acids as modulators of endothelium-derived nitric oxide. Am J Physiol Renal Physiol 2006;291:F297−304.

[536] Rajapakse NW, De MC, Das S, Mattson DL. Exogenous L-arginine ameliorates angiotensin II-induced hypertension and renal damage in rats. Hypertension 2008;52:1084−90.

[537] Rajapakse NW, Mattson DL. Role of L-arginine in nitric oxide production in health and hypertension. Clin Exp Pharmacol Physiol 2009;36:249−55.

[538] Mattson DL, Lu S, Nakanishi K, Papanek PE, Cowley Jr AW. Effect of chronic renal medullary nitric oxide inhibition on blood pressure. Am J Physiol 1994;266:H1918−26.

[539] Nakanishi K, Mattson DL, Cowley Jr AW. Role of renal medul-lary blood flow in the development of L-NAME hypertension in rats. Am J Physiol 1995;268:R317−23.

[540] Biondi ML, Dousa T, Vanhoutte P, Romero JC. Evidence for the existence of endothelium-derived relaxing factor in the renal medulla. Am J Hypertens 1990;3:876−8.

[541] McKee M, Scavone C, Nathanson JA. Nitric oxide, cGMP, and hormone regulation of active sodium transport. Proc Natl Acad Sci USA 1994;91:12056−60.

[542] Moridani BA, Kline RL. Effect of endogenous L-arginine on the measurement of nitric oxide synthase activity in the rat kidney. Can J Physiol Pharmacol 1996;74:1210−4.

[543] Zou AP, Cowley Jr AW. Nitric oxide in renal cortex and medulla. An in vivo microdialysis study. Hypertension 1997;29:194−8.

[544] Miyata N, Cowley Jr AW. Renal intramedullary infusion of L-arginine prevents reduction of medullary blood flow and hyper-tension in Dahl salt-sensitive rats. Hypertension 1999;33:446−50.

[545] Miyata N, Zou AP, Mattson DL, Cowley Jr AW. Renal medul-lary interstitial infusion of L-arginine prevents hypertension in Dahl salt-sensitive rats. Am J Physiol 1998;275:R1667−73.

[546] Kakoki M, Zou AP, Mattson DL. The influence of nitric oxide synthase 1 on blood flow and interstitial nitric oxide in the kid-ney. Am J Physiol Regul Integr Comp Physiol 2001;281:R91−7.

[547] Mattson DL, Bellehumeur TG. Neural nitric oxide synthase in the renal medulla and blood pressure regulation. Hypertension 1996;28:297−303.

[548] Mattson DL, Maeda CY, Bachman TD, Cowley Jr AW. Inducible nitric oxide synthase and blood pressure. Hypertension 1998;31:15−20.

[549] Mattson DL, Meister CJ. Sodium sensitivity of arterial blood pressure in L-NAME hypertensive but not eNOS knockout mice. Am J Hypertens 2006;19:327−9.

[550] Garvin JL, Ortiz PA. The role of reactive oxygen species in the regulation of tubular function. Acta Physiol Scand 2003;179:225−32.

[551] Ortiz PA, Garvin JL. Role of nitric oxide in the regulation of nephron transport. Am J Physiol Renal Physiol 2002;282:F777−84.

[552] Ortiz PA, Garvin JL. Superoxide stimulates NaCl absorption by the thick ascending limb. Am J Physiol Renal Physiol 2002;283:F957−62.

[553] Szentivanyi Jr M, Zou AP, Maeda CY, Mattson DL, Cowley Jr AW. Increase in renal medullary nitric oxide synthase activity protects from norepinephrine-induced hypertension. Hypertension 2000;35:418−23.

[554] Zou AP, Cowley Jr AW. Alpha²-adrenergic receptor-mediated increase in NO production buffers renal medullary vasocon-striction. Am J Physiol Regul Integr Comp Physiol 2000;279:R769−77.

[555] Yuan B, Cowley Jr AW. Evidence that reduced renal medullary nitric oxide synthase activity of Dahl S rats enables small ele-vations of arginine vasopressin to produce sustained hyperten-sion. Hypertension 2001;37:524−8.

[556] Heyman SN, Rosen S, Darmon D, Goldfarb M, Bitz H, Shina A, et al. Endotoxin-induced renal failure. II. A role for tubular hypoxic damage. Exp Nephrol 2000;8:275−82.

[557] James PE, Bacic G, Grinberg OY, Goda F, Dunn JF, Jackson SK, et al. Endotoxin-induced changes in intrarenal PO_2, measured by in vivo electron paramagnetic resonance oximetry and mag-netic resonance imaging. Free Radic Biol Med 1996;21:25−34.

[558] Sendeski M, Patzak A, Pallone TL, Cao C, Persson AE, Persson PB. Iodixanol, constriction of medullary descending vasa recta, and risk for contrast medium-induced nephropathy. Radiology 2009;251:697−704.

[559] Mori T, Cowley Jr AW. Angiotensin II-NAD(P)H oxidase-stimulated superoxide modifies tubulovascular nitric oxide cross-talk in renal outer medulla. Hypertension 2003;42:588−93.

[560] Rhinehart KL, Pallone TL. Nitric oxide generation by isolated descending vasa recta. Am J Physiol Heart Circ Physiol 2001;281:H316−24.

[561] Zhang W, Pibulsonggram T, Edwards A. Determinants of basal nitric oxide concentration in the renal medullary microcircula-tion. Am J Physiol Renal Physiol 2004;287:F1189−203.

[562] Droge W. Free radicals in the physiological control of cell func-tion. Physiol Rev 2002;82:47−95.

[563] Araujo M, Welch WJ. Oxidative stress and nitric oxide in kid-ney function. Curr Opin Nephrol Hypertens 2006;15:72−7.

[564] Schnackenberg CG. Physiological and pathophysiological roles of oxygen radicals in the renal microvasculature. Am J Physiol Regul Integr Comp Physiol 2002;282:R335−42.

[565] Welch WJ. Angiotensin II-dependent superoxide: effects on hypertension and vascular dysfunction. Hypertension 2008;52:51−6.

[566] Wilcox CS. Oxidative stress and nitric oxide deficiency in the kidney: a critical link to hypertension? Am J Physiol Regul Integr Comp Physiol 2005;289:R913−35.

[567] Schnackenberg CG, Welch WJ, Wilcox CS. TP receptor-mediated vasoconstriction in microperfused afferent arterioles: roles of O$(_2)(^-)$ and NO. Am J Physiol Renal Physiol 2000;279:F302−8.

[568] Ozawa Y, Hayashi K, Wakino S, Kanda T, Homma K, Takamatsu I, et al. Free radical activity depends on underlying vasoconstrictors in renal microcirculation. Clin Exp Hypertens 2004;26:219−29.

[569] Abe M, O'Connor P, Kaldunski M, Liang M, Roman RJ, Cowley Jr AW. Effect of sodium delivery on superoxide and nitric oxide in the medullary thick ascending limb. Am J Physiol Renal Physiol 2006;291:F350−7.

[570] Mori T, O'Connor PM, Abe M, Cowley Jr AW. Enhanced superoxide production in renal outer medulla of Dahl salt-sensitive rats reduces nitric oxide tubular-vascular cross-talk. Hypertension 2007;49:1336−41.

[571] Palm F, Onozato M, Welch WJ, Wilcox CS. Blood pressure, blood flow, and oxygenation in the clipped kidney of chronic 2-kidney, 1-clip rats: effects of tempol and angiotensin block-ade. Hypertension 2010;55:298−304.

[572] Sedeek M, Hebert RL, Kennedy CR, Burns KD, Touyz RM. Molecular mechanisms of hypertension: role of Nox family NADPH oxidases. Curr Opin Nephrol Hypertens 2009;18:122−7.

[573] Schnackenberg CG, Welch WJ, Wilcox CS. Normalization of blood pressure and renal vascular resistance in SHR with a membrane-permeable superoxide dismutase mimetic: role of nitric oxide. Hypertension 1998;32:59−64.

[574] Schnackenberg CG, Wilcox CS. Two-week administration of tempol attenuates both hypertension and renal excretion of 8-Iso prostaglandin f2alpha. Hypertension 1999;33:424−8.

[575] Chabrashvili T, Kitiyakara C, Blau J, Karber A, Aslam S, Welch WJ, et al. Effects of ANG II type 1 and 2 receptors on oxidative stress, renal NADPH oxidase, and SOD expression. Am J Physiol Regul Integr Comp Physiol 2003;285:R117−24.

[576] Zhang Z, Rhinehart K, Solis G, Pittner J, Lee-Kwon W, Welch WJ, et al. Chronic ANG II infusion increases NO generation by rat descending vasa recta. Am J Physiol Heart Circ Physiol 2005;288:H29−36.

[577] Welch WJ. Intrarenal oxygen and hypertension. Clin Exp Pharmacol Physiol 2006;33:1002−5.

[578] Welch WJ, Baumgartl H, Lubbers D, Wilcox CS. Renal oxygen-ation defects in the spontaneously hypertensive rat: role of AT1 receptors. Kidney Int 2003;63:202−8.

[579] Welch WJ, Blau J, Xie H, Chabrashvili T, Wilcox CS. Angiotensin-induced defects in renal oxygenation: role of oxidative stress. Am J Physiol Heart Circ Physiol 2005;288: H22−8.

[580] Chen YF, Cowley Jr AW, Zou AP. Increased $H_{(2)}O_{(2)}$ counter-acts the vasodilator and natriuretic effects of superoxide dis-mutation by tempol in renal medulla. Am J Physiol Regul Integr Comp Physiol 2003;285:R827−33.

[581] Makino A, Skelton MM, Zou AP, Cowley Jr AW. Increased renal medullary H_2O_2 leads to hypertension. Hypertension 2003;42:25−30.

[582] Makino A, Skelton MM, Zou AP, Roman RJ, Cowley Jr AW. Increased renal medullary oxidative stress produces hyperten-sion. Hypertension 2002;39:667−72.

[583] Zou AP, Li N, Cowley Jr AW. Production and actions of super-oxide in the renal medulla. Hypertension 2001;37:547−53.

[584] Meng S, Roberts LJ, Cason GW, Curry TS, Manning Jr RD. Superoxide dismutase and oxidative stress in Dahl salt-sensitive and -resistant rats. Am J Physiol Regul Integr Comp Physiol 2002;283:R732−8.

[585] Carmines PK. The renal vascular response to diabetes. Curr Opin Nephrol Hypertens 2010;19:85−90.

[586] Ishii N, Patel KP, Lane PH, Taylor T, Bian K, Murad F, et al. Carmines PK. Nitric oxide synthesis and oxidative stress in the renal cortex of rats with diabetes mellitus. J Am Soc Nephrol 2001;12:1630−9.

[587] Kanwar YS, Wada J, Sun L, Xie P, Wallner EI, Chen S, et al. Diabetic nephropathy: mechanisms of renal disease progres-sion. Exp Biol Med (Maywood) 2008;233:4−11.

[588] Pollock JS, Carmines PK. Diabetic nephropathy: nitric oxide and renal medullary hypoxia. Am J Physiol Renal Physiol 2008;294:F28−9.

[589] Schoonmaker GC, Fallet RW, Carmines PK. Superoxide anion curbs nitric oxide modulation of afferent arteriolar ANG II responsiveness in diabetes mellitus. Am J Physiol Renal Physiol 2000;278:F302−9.

[590] Abraham NG, Kappas A. Heme oxygenase and the cardiovas-cular−renal system. Free Radic Biol Med 2005;39:1−25.

[591] Zou AP, Billington H, Su N, Cowley Jr AW. Expression and actions of heme oxygenase in the renal medulla of rats. Hypertension 2000;35:342−7.

[592] Yang ZZ, Zhang AY, Yi FX, Li PL, Zou AP. Redox regulation of HIF-1alpha levels and HO-1 expression in renal medullary interstitial cells. Am J Physiol Renal Physiol 2003;284: F1207−15.

[593] Yang ZZ, Zou AP. Transcriptional regulation of heme oxyge-nases by HIF-1alpha in renal medullary interstitial cells. Am J Physiol Renal Physiol 2001;281:F900−8.

[594] Tian W, Bonkovsky HL, Shibahara S, Cohen DM. Urea and hypertonicity increase expression of heme oxygenase-1 in murine renal medullary cells. Am J Physiol Renal Physiol 2001;281:F983−91.

[595] Abraham NG, Botros FT, Rezzani R, Rodella L, Bianchi R, Goodman AI. Differential effect of cobalt protoporphyrin on distributions of heme oxygenase in renal structure and on blood pressure in SHR. Cell Mol Biol (Noisy-le-grand) 2002;48:895−902.

[596] Akagi R, Takahashi T, Sassa S. Cytoprotective effects of heme oxygenase in acute renal failure. Contrib Nephrol 2005;148:70−85.

[597] Li N, Chen L, Yi F, Xia M, Li PL. Salt-sensitive hypertension induced by decoy of transcription factor hypoxia-inducible fac-tor-1alpha in the renal medulla. Circ Res 2008;102:1101−8.

[598] Li N, Yi F, dos Santos EA, Donley DK, Li PL. Role of renal medullary heme oxygenase in the regulation of pressure natriuresis and arterial blood pressure. Hypertension 2007;49:148−54.

[599] Li N, Yi F, Sundy CM, Chen L, Hilliker ML, Donley DK, et al. Expression and actions of HIF prolyl-4-hydroxylase in the rat kidney. Am J Physiol Renal Physiol 2007;292:F207−16.

[600] Vera T, Kelsen S, Stec DE. Kidney-specific induction of heme oxygenase-1 prevents angiotensin II hypertension. Hypertension 2008;52:660−5.

[601] Vera T, Kelsen S, Yanes LL, Reckelhoff JF, Stec DE. HO-1 induction lowers blood pressure and superoxide production in the renal medulla of angiotensin II hypertensive mice. Am J Physiol Regul Integr Comp Physiol 2007;292:R1472−8.

[602] Curtis LM, Agarwal A. Hope for contrast-induced acute kid-ney injury. Kidney Int 2007;72:907−9.

[603] Goodman AI, Olszanecki R, Yang LM, Quan S, Li M, Omura S, et al. Heme oxygenase-1 protects against radiocontrast-induced acute kidney injury by regulating anti-apoptotic pro-teins. Kidney Int 2007;72:945−53.

[604] Jarmi T, Agarwal A. Heme oxygenase and renal disease. Curr Hypertens Rep 2009;11:56−62.

[605] Jackson EK, Zhu C, Tofovic SP. Expression of adenosine recep-tors in the preglomerular microcirculation. Am J Physiol Renal Physiol 2002;283:F41−51.

[606] Vitzthum H, Weiss B, Bachleitner W, Kramer BK, Kurtz A. Gene expression of adenosine receptors along the nephron. Kidney Int 2004;65:1180−90.

[607] Hansen PB, Schnermann J. Vasoconstrictor and vasodilator effects of adenosine in the kidney. Am J Physiol Renal Physiol 2003;285:F590−9.

[608] Jackson EK, Dubey RK. Role of the extracellular cAMP-adenosine pathway in renal physiology. Am J Physiol Renal Physiol 2001;281:F597−612.

[609] Vallon V, Muhlbauer B, Osswald H. Adenosine and kidney function. Physiol Rev 2006;86:901−40.

[610] Vallon V., Osswald H. Adenosine receptors and the kidney. Handb Exp Pharmacol 2009;(193):443−70.

[611] Osmond DA, Inscho EW. P2X(1) receptor blockade inhibits whole kidney autoregulation of renal blood flow *in vivo*. Am J Physiol Renal Physiol 2010;298:F1360−8.

[612] McCoy DE, Bhattacharya S, Olson BA, Levier DG, Arend LJ, Spielman WS. The renal adenosine system: structure, function, and regulation. Semin Nephrol 1993;13:31−40.

[613] Agmon Y, Dinour D, Brezis M. Disparate effects of adenosine A1- and A2-receptor agonists on intrarenal blood flow. Am J Physiol 1993;265:F802−6.

[614] Carmines PK, Inscho EW. Renal arteriolar angiotensin responses during varied adenosine receptor activation. Hypertension 1994;23:I114−9.

[615] Weihprecht H, Lorenz JN, Briggs JP, Schnermann J. Vasomotor effects of purinergic agonists in isolated rabbit afferent arterioles. Am J Physiol 1992;263:F1026−33.

[616] Nishiyama A, Inscho EW, Navar LG. Interactions of adenosine A1 and A2a receptors on renal microvascular reactivity. Am J Physiol Renal Physiol 2001;280:F406−14.

[617] Al-Mashhadi RH, Skott O, Vanhoutte PM, Hansen PB. Activation of A^2 adenosine receptors dilates cortical efferent arterioles in mouse. Kidney Int 2009;75:793−9.

[618] Blantz RC, Vallon V. Tubuloglomerular feedback responses of the downstream efferent resistance: unmasking a role for adenosine? Kidney Int 2007;71:837−9.

[619] Brown R, Ollerstam A, Johansson B, Skott O, Gebre-Medhin S, Fredholm B, et al. Abolished tubuloglomerular feedback and increased plasma renin in adenosine A1 receptor-deficient mice. Am J Physiol Regul Integr Comp Physiol 2001;281:R1362−7.

[620] Castrop H. Mediators of tubuloglomerular feedback regulation of glomerular filtration: ATP and adenosine. Acta Physiol (Oxf) 2007;189:3−14.

[621] Oppermann M, Mizel D, Kim SM, Chen L, Faulhaber-Walter R, Huang Y, et al. Renal function in mice with targeted disruption of the A isoform of the Na-K-2Cl co-transporter. J Am Soc Nephrol 2007;18:440−8.

[622] Oppermann M, Qin Y, Lai EY, Eisner C, Li L, Huang Y, et al. Enhanced tubuloglomerular feedback in mice with vascular overexpression of A1 adenosine receptors. Am J Physiol Renal Physiol 2009;297:F1256−64.

[623] Schnermann J. Adenosine mediates tubuloglomerular feedback. Am J Physiol Regul Integr Comp Physiol 2002;283: R276−7.

[624] Thomson S, Bao D, Deng A, Vallon V. Adenosine formed by 5'-nucleotidase mediates tubuloglomerular feedback. J Clin Invest 2000;106:289−98.

[625] Inscho EW, Cook AK, Imig JD, Vial C, Evans RJ. Renal autoregulation in P2X1 knockout mice. Acta Physiol Scand 2004;181:445−53.

[626] Blantz RC, Deng A. Coordination of kidney filtration and tubular reabsorption: considerations on the regulation of metabolic demand for tubular reabsorption. Acta Physiol Hung 2007;94:83−94.

[627] Miyamoto M, Yagil Y, Larson T, Robertson C, Jamison RL. Effects of intrarenal adenosine on renal function and medullary blood flow in the rat. Am J Physiol 1988;255:F1230−4.

[628] Kreisberg MS, Silldorff EP, Pallone TL. Localization of adenosine-receptor subtype mRNA in rat outer medullary descending vasa recta by RT-PCR. Am J Physiol 1997;272:H1231−8.

[629] Baranowski RL, Westenfelder C. Estimation of renal interstitial adenosine and purine metabolites by microdialysis. Am J Physiol 1994;267:F174−82.

[630] Hansen PB, Castrop H, Briggs J, Schnermann J. Adenosine induces vasoconstriction through Gi-dependent activation of phospholipase C in isolated perfused afferent arterioles of mice. J Am Soc Nephrol 2003;14:2457−65.

[631] Cheng MK, Doumad AB, Jiang H, Falck JR, McGiff JC, Carroll MA. Epoxyeicosatrienoic acids mediate adenosine-induced vasodilation in rat preglomerular microvessels (PGMV) via A2A receptors. Br J Pharmacol 2004;141:441−8.

[632] Dietrich MS, Endlich K, Parekh N, Steinhausen M. Interaction between adenosine and angiotensin II in renal microcirculation. Microvasc Res 1991;41:275−88.

[633] Hall JE, Granger JP. Adenosine alters glomerular filtration control by angiotensin II. Am J Physiol 1986;250:F917−23.

[634] Osswald H, Schmitz HJ, Heidenreich O. Adenosine response of the rat kidney after saline loading, sodium restriction and hemorrhagia. Pflugers Arch 1975;357:323−33.

[635] Spielman WS, Osswald H. Blockade of postocclusive renal vasoconstriction by an angiotensin II antagonists: evidence for an angiotensin−adenosine interaction. Am J Physiol 1979;237: F463−7.

[636] Weihprecht H, Lorenz JN, Briggs JP, Schnermann J. Synergistic effects of angiotensin and adenosine in the renal microvasculature. Am J Physiol 1994;266:F227−39.

[637] Barrett RJ, Droppleman DA. Interactions of adenosine A1 receptor-mediated renal vasoconstriction with endogenous nitric oxide and ANG II. Am J Physiol 1993;265:F651−9.

[638] Inscho EW. Modulation of renal microvascular function by adenosine. Am J Physiol Regul Integr Comp Physiol 2003;285: R23−5.

[639] Traynor T, Yang T, Huang YG, Arend L, Oliverio MI, Coffman T, et al. Inhibition of adenosine-1 receptor-mediated preglomerular vasoconstriction in AT1A receptor-deficient mice. Am J Physiol 1998;275:F922−7.

[640] Dinour D, Brezis M. Effects of adenosine on intrarenal oxygenation. Am J Physiol 1991;261:F787−91.

[641] Beach RE, Watts III BA, Good DW, Benedict CR, DuBose Jr TD. Effects of graded oxygen tension on adenosine release by renal medullary and thick ascending limb suspensions. Kidney Int 1991;39:836−42.

[642] Beach RE, Good DW. Effects of adenosine on ion transport in rat medullary thick ascending limb. Am J Physiol 1992;263: F482−7.

[643] Brezis M, Agmon Y, Epstein FH. Determinants of intrarenal oxygenation. I. Effects of diuretics. Am J Physiol 1994;267: F1059−62.

[644] Zou AP, Wu F, Li PL, Cowley Jr AW. Effect of chronic salt loading on adenosine metabolism and receptor expression in renal cortex and medulla in rats. Hypertension 1999; 33:511−6.

[645] Guan Z, Osmond DA, Inscho EW. P2X receptors as regulators of the renal microvasculature. Trends Pharmacol Sci 2007;28: 646−52.

[646] Guan Z, Osmond DA, Inscho EW. Purinoceptors in the kidney. Exp Biol Med (Maywood) 2007;232:715−26.

[647] Inscho EW. Renal microvascular effects of P2 receptor stimulation. Clin Exp Pharmacol Physiol 2001;28:332−9.

[648] Bailey MA, Hillman KA, Unwin RJ. P2 receptors in the kidney. J Auton Nerv Syst 2000;81:264−70.

[649] Chan CM, Unwin RJ, Bardini M, Oglesby IB, Ford AP, Townsend-Nicholson A, et al. Localization of P2X1 purinoceptors by autoradiography and immunohistochemistry in rat kidneys. Am J Physiol 1998;274:F799−804.

[650] Lewis CJ, Evans RJ. P2X receptor immunoreactivity in different arteries from the femoral, pulmonary, cerebral, coronary and renal circulations. J Vasc Res 2001;38:332—40.

[651] Inscho EW. P2 receptors in regulation of renal microvascular function. Am J Physiol Renal Physiol 2001;280:F927—44.

[652] Ralevic V, Burnstock G. Receptors for purines and pyrimidines. Pharmacol Rev 1998;50:413—92.

[653] Churchill PC, Ellis VR. Pharmacological characterization of the renovascular P2 purinergic receptors. J Pharmacol Exp Ther 1993;265:334—8.

[654] Rump LC, Oberhauser V, von KI. Purinoceptors mediate renal vasodilation by nitric oxide dependent and independent mechanisms. Kidney Int 1998;54:473—81.

[655] Inscho EW, Ohishi K, Cook AK, Belott TP, Navar LG. Calcium activation mechanisms in the renal microvascular response to extracellular ATP. Am J Physiol 1995;268:F876—84.

[656] Inscho EW, Ohishi K, Navar LG. Effects of ATP on pre- and postglomerular juxtamedullary microvasculature. Am J Physiol 1992;263:F886—93.

[657] Zhao X, Falck JR, Gopal VR, Inscho EW, Imig JD. P2X receptor-stimulated calcium responses in preglomerular vascular smooth muscle cells involves 20-hydroxyeicosatetraenoic acid. J Pharmacol Exp Ther 2004;311:1211—7.

[658] Zhao X, Inscho EW, Bondlela M, Falck JR, Imig JD. The CYP450 hydroxylase pathway contributes to P2X receptor-mediated afferent arteriolar vasoconstriction. Am J Physiol Heart Circ Physiol 2001;281:H2089—96.

[659] Inscho EW, LeBlanc EA, Pham BT, White SM, Imig JD. Purinoceptor-mediated calcium signaling in preglomerular smooth muscle cells. Hypertension 1999;33:195—200.

[660] White SM, Imig JD, Kim TT, Hauschild BC, Inscho EW. Calcium signaling pathways utilized by P2X receptors in freshly isolated preglomerular MVSMC. Am J Physiol Renal Physiol 2001;280:F1054—61.

[661] Inscho EW, Cook AK, Navar LG. Pressure-mediated vasoconstriction of juxtamedullary afferent arterioles involves P2-purinoceptor activation. Am J Physiol 1996;271:F1077—85.

[662] Majid DS, Inscho EW, Navar LG. P2 purinoceptor saturation by adenosine triphosphate impairs renal autoregulation in dogs. J Am Soc Nephrol 1999;10:492—8.

[663] Majid DS, Navar LG. Suppression of blood flow autoregulation plateau during nitric oxide blockade in canine kidney. Am J Physiol 1992;262:F40—6.

[664] Inscho EW, Cook AK, Imig JD, Vial C, Evans RJ. Physiological role for P2X1 receptors in renal microvascular autoregulatory behavior. J Clin Invest 2003;112:1895—905.

[665] Chatziantoniou C, Arendshorst WJ. Prostaglandin interactions with angiotensin, norepinephrine, and thromboxane in rat renal vasculature. Am J Physiol 1992;262:F68—76.

[666] Itskovitz HD, Stemper J, Pacholczyk D, McGiff JC. Renal prostaglandins: determinants of intrarenal distribution of blood flow in the dog. Clin Sci Mol Med Suppl 1973;45(Suppl. 1):321s—4s.

[667] Larsson C, Anggard E. Increased juxtamedullary blood flow on stimulation of intrarenal prostaglandin biosynthesis. Eur J Pharmacol 1974;25:326—34.

[668] Gomez SI, Strick DM, Romero JC. Role of nitric oxide and prostaglandin in the maintenance of cortical and renal medullary blood flow. Braz J Med Biol Res 2008;41:170—5.

[669] Sadowski J, Badzynska B. Intrarenal vasodilator systems: NO, prostaglandins and bradykinin. An integrative approach. J Physiol Pharmacol 2008;59(Suppl. 9):105—19.

[670] Lemley KV, Schmitt SL, Holliger C, Dunn MJ, Robertson CR, Jamison RL. Prostaglandin synthesis inhibitors and vasa recta erythrocyte velocities in the rat. Am J Physiol 1984;247:F562—7.

[671] Badzynska B, Grzelec-Mojzesowicz M, Sadowski J. Prostaglandins but not nitric oxide protect renal medullary perfusion in anaesthetised rats receiving angiotensin II. J Physiol 2003;548:875—80.

[672] Oliver JJ, Eppel GA, Rajapakse NW, Evans RG. Lipoxygenase and cyclo-oxygenase products in the control of regional kidney blood flow in rabbits. Clin Exp Pharmacol Physiol 2003;30:812—9.

[673] Parekh N, Zou AP. Role of prostaglandins in renal medullary circulation: response to different vasoconstrictors. Am J Physiol 1996;271:F653—8.

[674] Roman RJ, Lianos E. Influence of prostaglandins on papillary blood flow and pressure-natriuretic response. Hypertension 1990;15:29—35.

[675] Agmon Y, Peleg H, Greenfeld Z, Rosen S, Brezis M. Nitric oxide and prostanoids protect the renal outer medulla from radiocontrast toxicity in the rat. J Clin Invest 1994;94:1069—75.

[676] Heyman SN, Brezis M, Epstein FH, Spokes K, Silva P, Rosen S. Early renal medullary hypoxic injury from radiocontrast and indomethacin. Kidney Int 1991;40:632—42.

[677] Heyman SN, Fuchs S, Jaffe R, Shina A, Ellezian L, Brezis M, et al. Renal microcirculation and tissue damage during acute ureteral obstruction in the rat: effect of saline infusion, indomethacin and radiocontrast. Kidney Int 1997;51:653—63.

[678] Campean V, Theilig F, Paliege A, Breyer M, Bachmann S. Key enzymes for renal prostaglandin synthesis: site-specific expression in rodent kidney (rat, mouse). Am J Physiol Renal Physiol 2003;285:F19—32.

[679] Cheng HF, Harris RC. Cyclooxygenases, the kidney, and hypertension. Hypertension 2004;43:525—30.

[680] Harris RC, Breyer MD. Physiological regulation of cyclooxygenase-2 in the kidney. Am J Physiol Renal Physiol 2001;281: F1—11.

[681] Harris RC, Zhang MZ, Cheng HF. Cyclooxygenase-2 and the renal renin—angiotensin system. Acta Physiol Scand 2004;181:543—7.

[682] Yang T. Regulation of cyclooxygenase-2 in renal medulla. Acta Physiol Scand 2003;177:417—21.

[683] Fujino T, Nakagawa N, Yuhki K, Hara A, Yamada T, Takayama K, et al. Decreased susceptibility to renovascular hypertension in mice lacking the prostaglandin I2 receptor IP. J Clin Invest 2004;114:805—12.

[684] Paliege A, Mizel D, Medina C, Pasumarthy A, Huang YG, Bachmann S, et al. Inhibition of nNOS expression in the macula densa by COX-2-derived prostaglandin E(2). Am J Physiol Renal Physiol 2004;287:F152—9.

[685] Peti-Peterdi J, Komlosi P, Fuson AL, Guan Y, Schneider A, Qi Z, et al. Luminal NaCl delivery regulates basolateral PGE2 release from macula densa cells. J Clin Invest 2003;112:76—82.

[686] Lopez R, Llinas MT, Roig F, Salazar FJ. Role of nitric oxide and cyclooxygenase-2 in regulating the renal hemodynamic response to norepinephrine. Am J Physiol Regul Integr Comp Physiol 2003;284:R488—93.

[687] Deng A, Wead LM, Blantz RC. Temporal adaptation of tubuloglomerular feedback: effects of COX-2. Kidney Int 2004;66:2348—53.

[688] Ichihara A, Imig JD, Inscho EW, Navar LG. Cyclooxygenase-2 participates in tubular flow-dependent afferent arteriolar tone: interaction with neuronal NOS. Am J Physiol 1998;275: F605—12.

[689] Zhang MZ, Sanchez LP, McKanna JA, Harris RC. Regulation of cyclooxygenase expression by vasopressin in rat renal medulla. Endocrinology 2004;145:1402—9.

[690] Birck R, Krzossok S, Knoll T, Braun C, Der Woude FJ, Rohmeiss P. Preferential COX-2 inhibitor, meloxicam,

compromises renal perfusion in euvolemic and hypovolemic rats. Exp Nephrol 2000;8:173–80.

[691] Green T, Rodriguez J, Navar LG. Augmented cyclooxygenase-2 effects on renal function during varying states of angiotensin II activity. Am J Physiol Renal Physiol 2010;299(5):F954–962.

[692] Qi Z, Hao CM, Langenbach RI, Breyer RM, Redha R, Morrow JD, et al. Opposite effects of cyclooxygenase-1 and -2 activity on the pressor response to angiotensin II. J Clin Invest 2002;110:61–9.

[693] Zewde T, Mattson DL. Inhibition of cyclooxygenase-2 in the rat renal medulla leads to sodium-sensitive hypertension. Hypertension 2004;44:424–8.

[694] Zhao X, Yamamoto T, Newman JW, Kim IH, Watanabe T, Hammock BD, et al. Soluble epoxide hydrolase inhibition protects the kidney from hypertension-induced damage. J Am Soc Nephrol 2004;15:1244–53.

[695] Edwards RM. Effects of prostaglandins on vasoconstrictor action in isolated renal arterioles. Am J Physiol 1985;248:F779–84.

[696] Inscho EW, Carmines PK, Navar LG. Prostaglandin influences on afferent arteriolar responses to vasoconstrictor agonists. Am J Physiol 1990;259:F157–63.

[697] Arima S, Ren Y, Juncos LA, Carretero OA, Ito S. Glomerular prostaglandins modulate vascular reactivity of the downstream efferent arterioles. Kidney Int 1994;45:650–8.

[698] Wang D, Chabrashvili T, Wilcox CS. Enhanced contractility of renal afferent arterioles from angiotensin-infused rabbits: roles of oxidative stress, thromboxane prostanoid receptors, and endothelium. Circ Res 2004;94:1436–42.

[699] Audoly LP, Ruan X, Wagner VA, Goulet JL, Tilley SL, Koller BH, et al. Role of EP(2) and EP(3) PGE(2) receptors in control of murine renal hemodynamics. Am J Physiol Heart Circ Physiol 2001;280:H327–33.

[700] Hayashi K, Loutzenhiser R, Epstein M. Direct evidence that thromboxane mimetic U44069 preferentially constricts the afferent arteriole. J Am Soc Nephrol 1997;8:25–31.

[701] Silldorff EP, Hilbun LR, Pallone TL. Angiotensin II constriction of rat vasa recta is partially thromboxane dependent. Hypertension 2002;40:541–6.

[702] Wilcox CS, Welch WJ, Snellen H. Thromboxane mediates renal hemodynamic response to infused angiotensin II. Kidney Int 1991;40:1090–7.

[703] Kawada N, Dennehy K, Solis G, Modlinger P, Hamel R, Kawada JT, et al. TP receptors regulate renal hemodynamics during angiotensin II slow pressor response. Am J Physiol Renal Physiol 2004;287:F753–9.

[704] Harder DR, Campbell WB, Roman RJ. Role of cytochrome P-450 enzymes and metabolites of arachidonic acid in the control of vascular tone. J Vasc Res 1995;32:79–92.

[705] Fleming I. Cytochrome p450 and vascular homeostasis. Circ Res 2001;89:753–62.

[706] Imig JD. Eicosanoids and renal vascular function in diseases. Clin Sci (Lond) 2006;111:21–34.

[707] Imig JD. Targeting epoxides for organ damage in hypertension. J Cardiovasc Pharmacol 2010;56(4):329–35.

[708] Imig JD, Pham BT, LeBlanc EA, Reddy KM, Falck JR, Inscho EW. Cytochrome P450 and cyclooxygenase metabolites contribute to the endothelin-1 afferent arteriolar vasoconstrictor and calcium responses. Hypertension 2000;35:307–12.

[709] McGiff JC, Quilley J. 20-HETE and the kidney: resolution of old problems and new beginnings. Am J Physiol 1999;277:R607–23.

[710] Ortiz PA, Garvin JL. Intrarenal transport and vasoactive substances in hypertension. Hypertension 2001;38:621–4.

[711] Regner KR, Zuk A, Van Why SK, Shames BD, Ryan RP, Falck JR, et al. Protective effect of 20-HETE analogues in experimental renal ischemia reperfusion injury. Kidney Int 2009;75:511–7.

[712] Roman RJ. P-450 metabolites of arachidonic acid in the control of cardiovascular function. Physiol Rev 2002;82:131–85.

[713] Roman RJ, Maier KG, Sun CW, Harder DR, Alonso-Galicia M. Renal and cardiovascular actions of 20-hydroxyeicosatetraenoic acid and epoxyeicosatrienoic acids. Clin Exp Pharmacol Physiol 2000;27:855–65.

[714] Sarkis A, Lopez B, Roman RJ. Role of 20-hydroxyeicosatetraenoic acid and epoxyeicosatrienoic acids in hypertension. Curr Opin Nephrol Hypertens 2004;13:205–14.

[715] Harder DR, Narayanan J, Birks EK, Liard JF, Imig JD, Lombard JH, et al. Identification of a putative microvascular oxygen sensor. Circ Res 1996;79:54–61.

[716] Imig JD, Zou AP, Stec DE, Harder DR, Falck JR, Roman RJ. Formation and actions of 20-hydroxyeicosatetraenoic acid in rat renal arterioles. Am J Physiol 1996;270:R217–27.

[717] Alonso-Galicia M, Maier KG, Greene AS, Cowley Jr AW, Roman RJ. Role of 20-hydroxyeicosatetraenoic acid in the renal and vasoconstrictor actions of angiotensin II. Am J Physiol Regul Integr Comp Physiol 2002;283:R60–8.

[718] Hercule HC, Oyekan AO. Cytochrome P450 omega/omega-1 hydroxylase-derived eicosanoids contribute to endothelin(A) and endothelin(B) receptor-mediated vasoconstriction to endothelin-1 in the rat preglomerular arteriole. J Pharmacol Exp Ther 2000;292:1153–60.

[719] Zou AP, Imig JD, Kaldunski M, Ortiz de Montellano PR, Sui Z, Roman RJ. Inhibition of renal vascular 20-HETE production impairs autoregulation of renal blood flow. Am J Physiol 1994;266:F275–82.

[720] Alonso-Galicia M, Drummond HA, Reddy KK, Falck JR, Roman RJ. Inhibition of 20-HETE production contributes to the vascular responses to nitric oxide. Hypertension 1997;29:320–5.

[721] Williams JM, Sarkis A, Lopez B, Ryan RP, Flasch AK, Roman RJ. Elevations in renal interstitial hydrostatic pressure and 20-hydroxyeicosatetraenoic acid contribute to pressure natriuresis. Hypertension 2007;49:687–94.

[722] Hoagland KM, Flasch AK, Roman RJ. Inhibitors of 20-HETE formation promote salt-sensitive hypertension in rats. Hypertension 2003;42:669–73.

[723] Stec DE, Mattson DL, Roman RJ. Inhibition of renal outer medullary 20-HETE production produces hypertension in Lewis rats. Hypertension 1997;29:315–9.

[724] Capdevila JH, Falck JR. The CYP P450 arachidonic acid monooxygenases: from cell signaling to blood pressure regulation. Biochem Biophys Res Commun 2001;285:571–6.

[725] Capdevila JH, Nakagawa K, Holla V. The CYP P450 arachidonate monooxygenases: enzymatic relays for the control of kidney function and blood pressure. Adv Exp Med Biol 2003;525:39–46.

[726] Gainer JV, Bellamine A, Dawson EP, Womble KE, Grant SW, Wang Y, et al. Functional variant of CYP4A11 20-hydroxyeicosatetraenoic acid synthase is associated with essential hypertension. Circulation 2005;111:63–9.

[727] Imig JD, Navar LG, Roman RJ, Reddy KK, Falck JR. Actions of epoxygenase metabolites on the preglomerular vasculature. J Am Soc Nephrol 1996;7:2364–70.

[728] Spiecker M, Liao JK. Vascular protective effects of cytochrome p450 epoxygenase-derived eicosanoids. Arch Biochem Biophys 2005;433:413–20.

[729] Imig JD, Inscho EW, Deichmann PC, Reddy KM, Falck JR. Afferent arteriolar vasodilation to the sulfonimide analog of 11,12-epoxyeicosatrienoic acid involves protein kinase A. Hypertension 1999;33:408–13.

[730] Fukao M, Mason HS, Kenyon JL, Horowitz B, Keef KD. Regulation of BK(Ca) channels expressed in human embryonic

kidney 293 cells by epoxyeicosatrienoic acid. Mol Pharmacol 2001;59:16—23.

[731] Pomposiello SI, Quilley J, Carroll MA, Falck JR, McGiff JC. 5,6-Epoxyeicosatrienoic acid mediates the enhanced renal vasodilation to arachidonic acid in the SHR. Hypertension 2003;42:548—54.

[732] Regner KR, Zuk A, Van Why SK, Shames BD, Ryan RP, Falck JR, et al. Protective effect of 20-HETE analogues in experimental renal ischemia reperfusion injury. Kidney Int 2009;75:511—7.

[733] Imig JD, Falck JR, Wei S, Capdevila JH. Epoxygenase metabolites contribute to nitric oxide-independent afferent arteriolar vasodilation in response to bradykinin. J Vasc Res 2001;38:247—55.

[734] Imig JD, Zhao X, Capdevila JH, Morisseau C, Hammock BD. Soluble epoxide hydrolase inhibition lowers arterial blood pressure in angiotensin II hypertension. Hypertension 2002;39:690—4.

[735] Imig JD, Zhao X, Falck JR, Wei S, Capdevila JH. Enhanced renal microvascular reactivity to angiotensin II in hypertension is ameliorated by the sulfonimide analog of 11,12-epoxyeicosatrienoic acid. J Hypertens 2001;19:983—92.

[736] Zhao X, Pollock DM, Inscho EW, Zeldin DC, Imig JD. Decreased renal cytochrome P450 2C enzymes and impaired vasodilation are associated with angiotensin salt-sensitive hypertension. Hypertension 2003;41:709—14.

[737] Yu Z, Huse LM, Adler P, Graham L, Ma J, Zeldin DC, et al. Increased CYP2J expression and epoxyeicosatrienoic acid formation in spontaneously hypertensive rat kidney. Mol Pharmacol 2000;57:1011—20.

[738] Yu Z, Xu F, Huse LM, Morisseau C, Draper AJ, Newman JW, et al. Soluble epoxide hydrolase regulates hydrolysis of vasoactive epoxyeicosatrienoic acids. Circ Res 2000;87:992—8.

[739] Kotelevtsev Y, Webb DJ. Endothelin as a natriuretic hormone: the case for a paracrine action mediated by nitric oxide. Cardiovasc Res 2001;51:481—8.

[740] Krum H, Viskoper RJ, Lacourciere Y, Budde M, Charlon V. The effect of an endothelin-receptor antagonist, bosentan, on blood pressure in patients with essential hypertension. Bosentan Hypertension Investigators. N Engl J Med 1998;338:784—90.

[741] Naicker S, Bhoola KD. Endothelins: vasoactive modulators of renal function in health and disease. Pharmacol Ther 2001;90:61—88.

[742] Plato CF, Garvin JL. Nitric oxide, endothelin and nephron transport: potential interactions. Clin Exp Pharmacol Physiol 1999;26:262—8.

[743] Kohan DE. The renal medullary endothelin system in control of sodium and water excretion and systemic blood pressure. Curr Opin Nephrol Hypertens 2006;15:34—40.

[744] Terada Y, Tomita K, Nonoguchi H, Marumo F. Different localization of two types of endothelin receptor mRNA in microdissected rat nephron segments using reverse transcription and polymerase chain reaction assay. J Clin Invest 1992;90:107—12.

[745] Zhuo J, Dean R, Maric C, Aldred PG, Harris P, Alcorn D, et al. Localization and interactions of vasoactive peptide receptors in renomedullary interstitial cells of the kidney. Kidney Int Suppl 1998;67:S22—8.

[746] Abassi ZA, Ellahham S, Winaver J, Hoffman A. The intrarenal endothelin system and hypertension. News Physiol Sci 2001;16:152—6.

[747] Kohan DE. Endothelins in the normal and diseased kidney. Am J Kidney Dis 1997;29:2—26.

[748] Just A, Olson AJ, Arendshorst WJ. Dual constrictor and dilator actions of ET(B) receptors in the rat renal microcirculation: interactions with ET(A) receptors. Am J Physiol Renal Physiol 2004;286:F660—8.

[749] Bloom IT, Bentley FR, Wilson MA, Garrison RN. In vivo effects of endothelin on the renal microcirculation. J Surg Res 1993;54:274—80.

[750] Cavarape A, Bartoli E. Effects of BQ-123 on systemic and renal hemodynamic responses to endothelin-1 in the rat split hydronephrotic kidney. J Hypertens 1998;16:1449—58.

[751] Endlich K, Hoffend J, Steinhausen M. Localization of endothelin ETA and ETB receptor-mediated constriction in the renal microcirculation of rats. J Physiol 1996;497(Pt 1): 211—8.

[752] Kitamura K, Tanaka T, Kato J, Eto T, Tanaka K. Regional distribution of immunoreactive endothelin in porcine tissue: abundance in inner medulla of kidney. Biochem Biophys Res Commun 1989;161:348—52.

[753] Konishi F, Okada Y, Takaoka M, Gariepy CE, Yanagisawa M, Matsumura Y. Role of endothelin ET(B) receptors in the renal hemodynamic and excretory responses to big endothelin-1. Eur J Pharmacol 2002;451:177—84.

[754] Loutzenhiser R, Epstein M, Hayashi K, Horton C. Direct visualization of effects of endothelin on the renal microvasculature. Am J Physiol 1990;258:F61—8.

[755] Edwards RM, Trizna W, Ohlstein EH. Renal microvascular effects of endothelin. Am J Physiol 1990;259:F217—21.

[756] Fellner SK, Arendshorst WJ. Endothelin A and B receptors of preglomerular vascular smooth muscle cells. Kidney Int 2004;65:1810—7.

[757] Pollock DM, Jenkins JM, Cook AK, Imig JD, Inscho EW. L-type calcium channels in the renal microcirculatory response to endothelin. Am J Physiol Renal Physiol 2004.

[758] Schroeder AC, Imig JD, LeBlanc EA, Pham BT, Pollock DM, Inscho EW. Endothelin-mediated calcium signaling in preglomerular smooth muscle cells. Hypertension 2000;35:280—6.

[759] Nakano D, Pollock DM. Contribution of endothelin A receptors in endothelin 1-dependent natriuresis in female rats. Hypertension 2009;53:324—30.

[760] Nakano D, Pollock JS, Pollock DM. Renal medullary ETB receptors produce diuresis and natriuresis via NOS1. Am J Physiol Renal Physiol 2008;294:F1205—11.

[761] Gurbanov K, Rubinstein I, Hoffman A, Abassi Z, Better OS, Winaver J. Differential regulation of renal regional blood flow by endothelin-1. Am J Physiol 1996;271:F1166—72.

[762] Hoffman A, Abassi ZA, Brodsky S, Ramadan R, Winaver J. Mechanisms of big endothelin-1-induced diuresis and natriuresis: role of ET(B) receptors. Hypertension 2000;35:732—9.

[763] Vassileva I, Mountain C, Pollock DM. Functional role of ETB receptors in the renal medulla. Hypertension 2003;41:1359—63.

[764] Gariepy CE, Ohuchi T, Williams SC, Richardson JA, Yanagisawa M. Salt-sensitive hypertension in endothelin-B receptor-deficient rats. J Clin Invest 2000;105:925—33.

[765] Gariepy CE, Williams SC, Richardson JA, Hammer RE, Yanagisawa M. Transgenic expression of the endothelin-B receptor prevents congenital intestinal aganglionosis in a rat model of Hirschsprung disease. J Clin Invest 1998;102:1092—101.

[766] Pollock DM. Contrasting pharmacological ETB receptor blockade with genetic ETB deficiency in renal responses to big ET-1. Physiol Genomics 2001;6:39—43.

[767] Pollock DM. Renal endothelin in hypertension. Curr Opin Nephrol Hypertens 2000;9:157—64.

[768] Sasser JM, Pollock JS, Pollock DM. Renal endothelin in chronic angiotensin II hypertension. Am J Physiol Regul Integr Comp Physiol 2002;283:R243—8.

[769] Dhaun N, Goddard J, Kohan DE, Pollock DM, Schiffrin EL, Webb DJ. Role of endothelin-1 in clinical hypertension: 20 years on. Hypertension 2008;52:452—9.

[770] Dhaun N, Goddard J, Webb DJ. The endothelin system and its antagonism in chronic kidney disease. J Am Soc Nephrol 2006;17:943—55.

[771] Molero MM, Giulumian AD, Reddy VB, Ludwig LM, Pollock JS, Pollock DM, et al. Decreased endothelin binding and $[Ca^{2+}]_i$ signaling in microvessels of DOCA-salt hypertensive rats. J Hypertens 2002;20:1799—805.

[772] Kohan DE. Biology of endothelin receptors in the collecting duct. Kidney Int 2009.

[773] Kuhn M. Molecular physiology of natriuretic peptide signalling. Basic Res Cardiol 2004;99:76—82.

[774] Levin ER, Gardner DG, Samson WK. Natriuretic peptides. N Engl J Med 1998;339:321—8.

[775] Vesely DL. Atrial natriuretic peptides in pathophysiological diseases. Cardiovasc Res 2001;51:647—58.

[776] Janssen WM, Beekhuis H, de Bruin R, de Jong PE, de Zeeuw D. Noninvasive measurement of intrarenal blood flow distribution: kinetic model of renal 123I-hippuran handling. Am J Physiol 1995;269:F571—80.

[777] Kiberd BA, Larson TS, Robertson CR, Jamison RL. Effect of atrial natriuretic peptide on vasa recta blood flow in the rat. Am J Physiol 1987;252:F1112—7.

[778] Takezawa K, Cowley Jr AW, Skelton M, Roman RJ. Atriopeptin III alters renal medullary hemodynamics and the pressure diuresis response in rats. Am J Physiol 1987;252: F992—1002.

[779] Tsuchiya K, Sanaka T, Nitta K, Ando A, Sugino N. Effects of atrial natriuretic peptide on regional renal blood flow measured by a thermal diffusion technique. Jpn J Exp Med 1989;59:27—35.

[780] Aalkjaer C, Mulvany MJ, Nyborg NC. Atrial natriuretic factor causes specific relaxation of rat renal arcuate arteries. Br J Pharmacol 1985;86:447—53.

[781] Hayashi K, Epstein M, Loutzenhiser R. Determinants of renal actions of atrial natriuretic peptide. Lack of effect of atrial natriuretic peptide on pressure-induced vasoconstriction. Circ Res 1990;67:1—10.

[782] Marin-Grez M, Fleming JT, Steinhausen M. Atrial natriuretic peptide causes pre-glomerular vasodilatation and post-glomerular vasoconstriction in rat kidney. Nature 1986;324:473—6.

[783] Veldkamp PJ, Carmines PK, Inscho EW, Navar LG. Direct evaluation of the microvascular actions of ANP in juxtamedullary nephrons. Am J Physiol 1988;254:F440—4.

[784] Edwards RM, Weidley EF. Lack of effect of atriopeptin II on rabbit glomerular arterioles *in vitro*. Am J Physiol 1987;252: F317—21.

[785] Endlich K, Steinhausen M. Natriuretic peptide receptors mediate different responses in rat renal microvessels. Kidney Int 1997;52:202—7.

[786] Endlich K, Forssmann WG, Steinhausen M. Effects of urodilatin in the rat kidney: comparison with ANF and interaction with vasoactive substances. Kidney Int 1995;47:1558—68.

[787] Lorenz JN, Nieman M, Sabo J, Sanford LP, Hawkins JA, Elitsur N, et al. Uroguanylin knockout mice have increased blood pressure and impaired natriuretic response to enteral NaCl load. J Clin Invest 2003;112:1244—54.

[788] Wang T, Kawabata M, Haneda M, Takabatake T. Effects of uroguanylin, an intestinal natriuretic peptide, on tubuloglomerular feedback. Hypertens Res 2003;26:577—82.

[789] Ejaz AA, Heinig ME, Kazory A, Bihorac A, Hobson CE, Beaver TM. The rise and fall of natriuretic peptides in acute kidney injury: a misunderstood relationship? Rev Cardiovasc Med 2007;8(Suppl 5):S32—7.

[790] Moffat DB, Fourman J. The vascular pattern of the rat kidney. J Anat 1963;97:543—53.

[791] Brezis M, Heyman SN, Dinour D, Epstein FH, Rosen S. Role of nitric oxide in renal medullary oxygenation. Studies in isolated and intact rat kidneys. J Clin Invest 1991;88:390—5.

[792] Mendez RE, Dunn BR, Troy JL, Brenner BM. Atrial natriuretic peptide and furosemide effects on hydraulic pressure in the renal papilla. Kidney Int 1988;34:36—42.

[793] Ma R, Pluznick JL, Sansom SC. Ion channels in mesangial cells: function, malfunction, or fiction. Physiology (Bethesda) 2005;20:102—11.

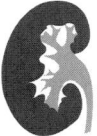

Molecular and Cellular Mechanisms of Kidney Development

Kevin T. Bush[1], Hiroyuki Sakurai[2] and Sanjay K. Nigam[1,3,4,5]

[1]Departments of Pediatrics, University of California San Diego, La Jolla, CA, USA

[2]Kyorin University School of Medicine, Mitaka, Tokyo, Japan

[3]Cellular and Molecular Medicine, University of California San Diego, La Jolla, CA, USA

[4]Medicine (Division of Nephrology and Hypertension), University of California San Diego, La Jolla, CA, USA

[5]Bioengineering, University of California San Diego, La Jolla, CA, USA

OVERVIEW

In the course of its development, the mammalian kidney goes through three distinct forms: the pronephros; the mesonephros; and the metanephros, ultimately leading to the formation of the mature kidney (Figure 25.1). At day 22 of gestation in humans or at day 8 in mice, an epithelial streak called the pronephric duct arises in the cervical region of the developing embryo from intermediate mesodermal cells induced to undergo the transition to epithelial cells in response to signals arising from the somite and surface ectoderm.[1–3] The pronephric duct then extends caudally to form the nephric duct or Wolffian duct. The most primitive kidney, the pronephros, is formed as the pronephric duct induces surrounding mesenchyme to form the pronephric tubules. Glomerulus-like structures (glomera) are also seen, but are not physically connected to the tubules forming a non-integrated nephron.[4] The pronephros is functional only in fish and amphibians; it is thought to be rudimentary and non-functional in higher vertebrates.

Next, a more complex "protokidney," the mesonephros, arises just caudal to the pronephros at day 24 in humans or day 9.5 in mice. As with the pronephros, mesonephric development starts with induction of the surrounding mesenchyme by the Wolffian duct. Unlike the pronephros, however, the mesonephros glomeruli are linked to the Wolffian duct via mesonephric tubules. In humans, about 30 nephrons are observed in

the mesonephros; their function is unclear. The mesonephric duct and some tubules persist, and are ultimately integrated into the male genital system forming, in part, the vas deferens and tubules of the epididymis.[5] In females, the mesonephros degenerates and disappears.

The permanent kidney of amniotes, the metanephros, starts to form at day 28 in humans or day 11 in mice. Unlike the pronephros and mesonephros, which are induced by the Wolffian duct, metanephric tubules are induced by an epithelial structure derived from the Wolffian duct: the ureteric bud. The ureteric bud is induced to evaginate from the Wolffian duct in response to signals arising from the metanephric mesenchyme, a loose aggregation of intermediate mesodermal cells.[6,7] The emergence of this epithelial progenitor tissue of the metanephric kidney is a key initiating event, and depends upon differentiation of the metanephric mesenchyme from the intermediate mesodermal cells.[8,9] As the ureteric bud invades the surrounding mesenchyme, it induces the mesenchymal cells to form epithelial metanephric tubules that eventually differentiate into the proximal through distal portions of the nephron. The ureteric bud, reciprocally induced by the metanephric mesenchyme, undergoes branching morphogenesis, eventually giving rise to the collecting system. Morphologically, nephron formation is completed by birth in humans, although only after birth does the nephron become fully functional.[7]

Seldin and Giebisch's The Kidney, Fifth Edition.
DOI: http://dx.doi.org/10.1016/B978-0-12-381462-3.00025-2

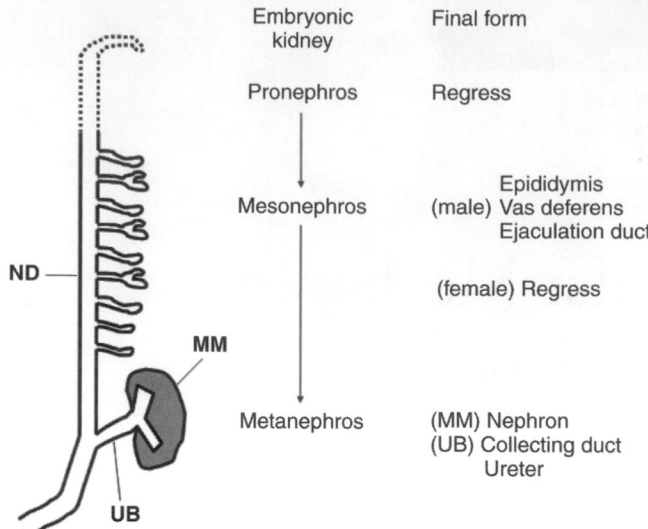

FIGURE 25.1 Schematic illustration of mammalian kidney development. The pronephros appears at a relatively higher position in the embryo. Then the mesonephros forms caudally around the nephric duct (ND) or Wolffian duct. In the male, the mesonephric tubules become a part of the genital system. The permanent kidney, the metanephros, forms caudally to the mesonephros. The ureteric bud (UB) derives from the Wolffian duct, ultimately becoming the collecting system. The metanephric mesenchyme, induced by the ureteric bud, forms nephron tubules and glomeruli.

DEVELOPMENT OF THE METANEPHROS

Here, the development of the metanephros is described in more detail (Figure 25.2), since it becomes the final kidney in mammals. As discussed in the previous section, the ureteric bud, the inducer of metanephric development, is formed from the Wolffian duct. This structure invades the metanephric mesenchyme, whereupon mesenchymal cells condense at the tip of the ureteric bud. The condensed mesenchymal cells then differentiate into epithelial cells: the so-called mesenchymal-to-epithelial transformation (MET). The newly formed epithelial cells gradually develop into distinct structures called "comma-shaped bodies," which subsequently become "S-shaped bodies." The S-shaped bodies, which begin to exhibit tubular morphology, continue to elongate; the end closest to the ureteric bud connects to it, while the opposite end forms podocytes and Bowman's capsule. The middle part ultimately differentiates into the proximal through distal tubules of the nephron. At the same time, the tips of the ureteric bud, induced by the metanephric mesenchyme, continue to branch to ultimately form the collecting ducts, renal pelvis, calyces, and papillae.

The process of collecting system development has been studied in detail by microdissection of the human kidney.[10,11] Initial ureteric bud branching is dichotomous and symmetric; the ureteric bud takes on a T-shape in this early stage of metanephrogenesis. Subsequently, the ureteric bud elongates and bifurcates at the tips, and eventually branches again dichotomously. At later branching events, the angle between branches lessens and branching may not be completely symmetrical, so that somehow the ureteric tree structure "fits" into the final shape of the kidney.[8] The initial branches become dilated to form the renal pelvis, while terminal branches become collecting

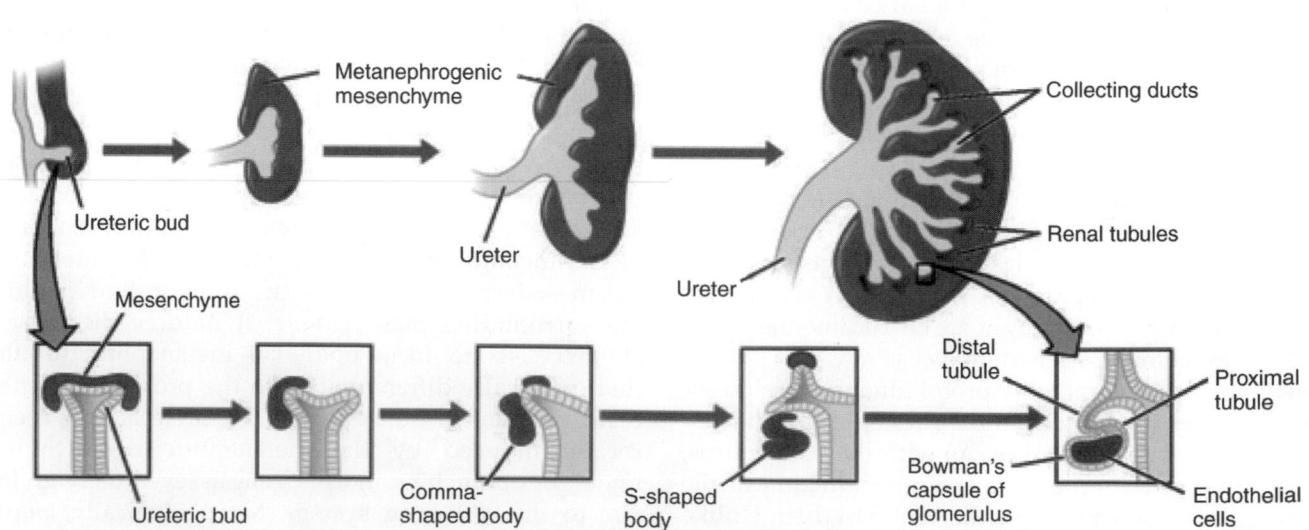

FIGURE 25.2 Schematic illustration of metanephros development. Top panels show a macroscopic view of kidney collecting system development through ureteric bud branching morphogenesis. Bottom panels show nephron development from metanephric mesenchyme. *adapted from ref. [82]).*

ducts. As the ureteric bud undergoes branching morphogenesis, its tips continue to induce more nephrons from the metanephric mesenchyme.

Vascular development occurs along with nephron development. Dissection of the developing kidney reveals that large vessels branch off from the dorsal aorta invading into the kidneys.[12] As will be discussed later, the extent to which the microvasculature of the kidney is derived from cells of the metanephric mesenchyme versus cells from outside the kidney is still unclear (reviewed in [13]). The origin of the mesangial cells, which closely associate with the endothelial cells in the glomerulus, also remains uncertain.

Thus, the reciprocal mutual induction and feedback between the ureteric bud and the metanephric mesenchyme represent key events in metanephric epithelial tissue development leading to a functional kidney. These reciprocal interactions induce branching morphogenesis of the ureteric bud, together with epithelialization and tubulogenesis of the metanephric mesenchyme (Figure 25.3). To better understand the mechanisms underlying induction, it is necessary to identify and analyze the key molecules that mediate signals between the metanephric mesenchyme and the ureteric bud.

EXPERIMENTAL APPROACHES TO KIDNEY DEVELOPMENT

Over the years, a variety of experimental approaches have been used for evaluation of the mechanistic details of the induction process between the ureteric bud and metanephric mesenchyme. For example, the

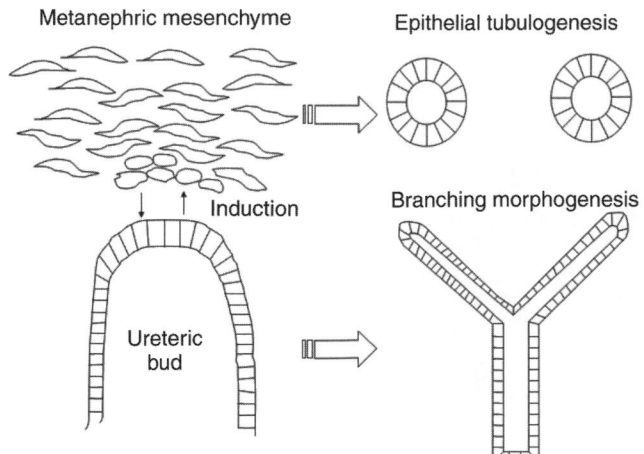

FIGURE 25.3 Schematic illustrations of mutual induction. The metanephric mesenchyme cells become epithelial nephron tubules (induced by the ureteric bud), while the ureteric bud undergoes branching morphogenesis to form the collecting system (induced by the metanephric mesenchyme).

developing kidney has been found to be amenable to extensive *in vitro* analysis. In addition to this "whole embryonic kidney organ culture," it has been demonstrated that progenitor tissues (i.e., Wolffian duct, ureteric bud, and metanephric mesenchyme) can be isolated and cultured individually. Advances in genetic manipulation have allowed the analysis of kidney development *in vivo* in genetically-engineered mice. As *in vitro* culture techniques and *in vivo* genetic manipulation become increasingly sophisticated, it is becoming clear that these approaches should be viewed as complementary.

Organ Culture

Whole Embryonic Kidney Organ Culture

The transfilter culture system, used by Grobstein and co-workers in the 1950s,[14−16] has been the mainstay of *in vitro* organ culture work in the developing kidney. In this system, microdissected kidneys, from as early as the beginning of metanephrogenesis (gestational day 11.5 in mice or day 13.5 in rats), are cultured on top of filters for several days. In the presence of appropriately defined serum-free medium, kidney rudiments grow and differentiate.[17] It is possible to observe branching morphogenesis of the ureteric bud, induction of the metanephric mesenchyme, and formation of nephrons by microscopy as the cultured embryonic kidneys develop (Figure 25.4a). Only vascular development does not occur to an appreciable extent. Thus, not only does the whole embryonic kidney culture resemble *in vivo* developmental processes, but it also appears to retain the inherent spatiotemporal complexity.

In this whole embryonic kidney culture, it is possible to manipulate humoral factors that play a role in nephrogenesis. The effects of growth factors or their inhibitors on kidney development can be evaluated *in vitro* by analysis of total kidney size, ureteric bud branching events, and metanephric mesenchyme tubulogenesis. For example, ureteric bud branching can be assayed by staining with a fluorescently-labeled lectin from *Dolichos biflorus*, which has been shown to bind specifically to the cells derived from the ureteric bud[18] (Figure 25.4b). However, the organ culture method is not without its limitations. For example, when antibodies and antisense oligonucleotides are used to perturb *in vitro* nephrogenesis, care must be taken to ensure that the agent is delivered to the sites of interest, since antisense oligonucleotides do not seem to penetrate the ureteric bud as well as the metanephric mesenchyme.[19] In addition, oligonucleotide toxicity may, in some instances, nonspecifically inhibit kidney growth.[19] However, recent development of RNAi technology to perturb specific gene function may prove useful in this setting.[20,21]

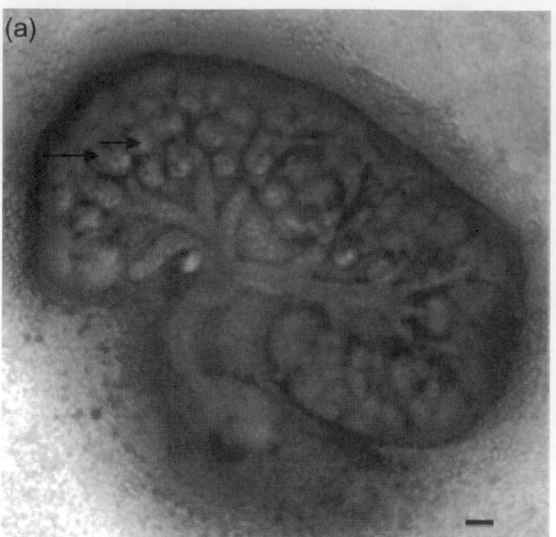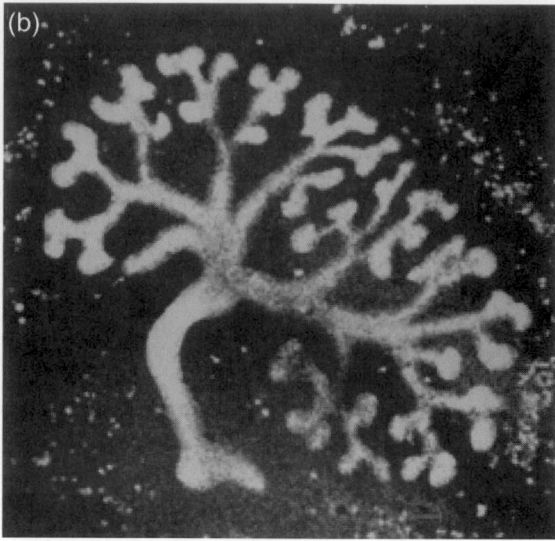

FIGURE 25.4   **(a) Embryonic rat kidney isolated at embryonic day 13 and cultured for 3 days on Transwell filter. Ureteric bud branches and epithelial nephron formation (arrows) are visible. (b) Cultured kidney stained with fluorescent-labeled lectin from Dolichos biflorus to visualize ureteric bud-derived structures** (Bars: 100 μm). See color plate section at the end of the book.

Isolated Wolffian Duct Culture

It is possible to culture the entire mesonephros —metanephros area on top of transfilters. Addition of humoral factors can induce outgrowth of ureteric bud-like structures from the Wolffian duct.[22–26] For example, the addition of glial cell-derived neurotrophic factor (GDNF) induces numerous budding events at multiple foci along the length of the cultured Wolffian duct (Figure 25.5). The epithelial Wolffian ducts can also be dissected away from most of the non-epithelial mesoderm and cultured in the presence of soluble growth factors to induce the outgrowth of ureteric bud-like structures.[23–25,27–30] However, in this culture system GDNF alone is insufficient to induce the outgrowth of ureteric bud-like structures, and supplementation with other growth factors is required[23,24] (Figure 25.6). The Wolffian duct can also be cultured as a "naked" epithelial tube cleared of all surrounding mesodermal cells, although these isolated ducts must be cultured within a three-dimensional extracellular matrix.[25] The ureteric bud-like structures can be excised from the Wolffian duct and induced to branch in culture (Figure 25.7), indicating that the *in vitro* ureteric bud possesses the ability to branch and grow in a manner similar to that seen with the *in vivo* ureteric bud (see below). These *ex vivo* culture systems have proven useful in the elucidation of the mechanism of ureteric bud budding, and have allowed for the identification of multiple modulators/regulators (e.g., growth factors, signal transduction pathways, etc.) of this process.[23–25,27–30]

Isolated Ureteric Bud Culture

Since the 1950s, *in vitro* culture of the two individual components of metanephros, the ureteric bud and the metanephric mesenchyme, has been attempted. Of the two progenitor tissues, *in vitro* growth of the isolated ureteric bud proved to be more difficult, and it was argued that cell—cell contact between the ureteric bud

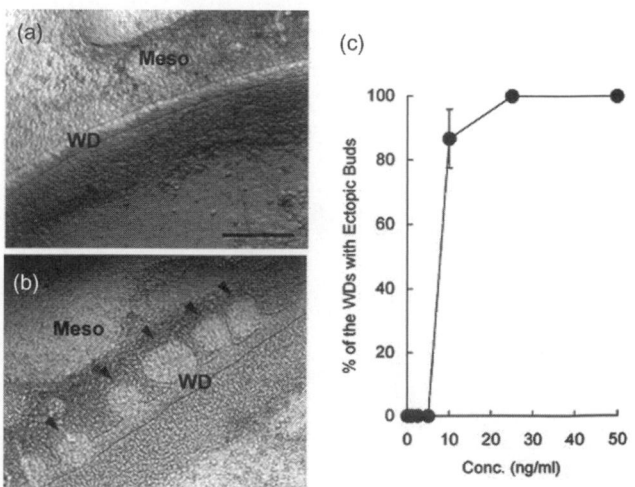

FIGURE 25.5   (a), (b) Photomicrographs of whole mesonephros (Meso) with attached Wolffian duct (WD) cultured for 4 days in the absence (a) or presence (b) of GDNF. (c) Graph depicting quantitative analysis of ureteric bud emergence (Scale bar: 200 μm; Arrowheads: ectopic ureteric buds). *(from ref. [24]).*

Day 0 Day 3

WD +
Mesonephros

WD +
Mesoderm

Isolated WD

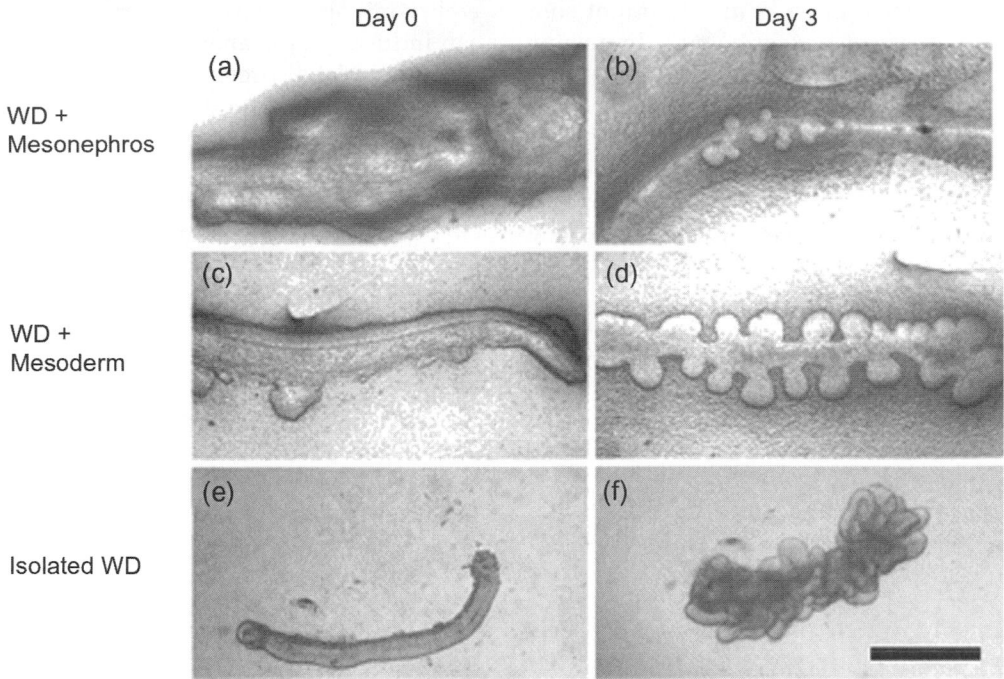

FIGURE 25.6 (a–f) Photomicrographs of isolated mesonephric tissues at Day 0 (a, c, e) or after 3 days of culture in the presence of GDNF (b, d, f). (a), (b) Entire mesonephros with attached Wolffian duct (WD). (c), (d) Wolffian duct (WD) dissected free from most of surrounding mesonephros. (e), (f) Wolffian duct (isolated WD) isolated free of surrounding mesonephros and mesodermal cells which must be cultured within an extracellular matrix gel (Scale bar: 500 μm). *(from ref. [25]).*

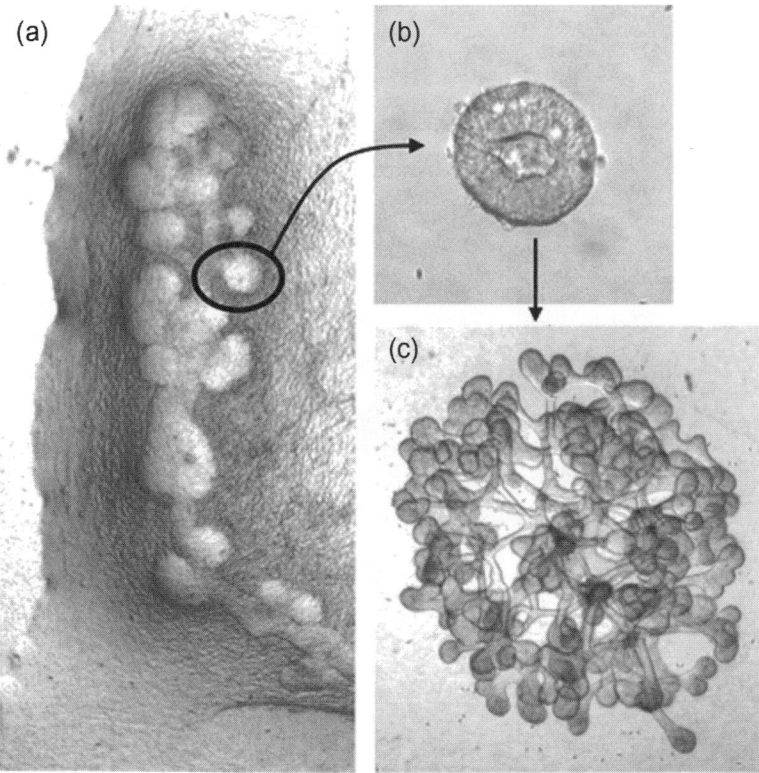

FIGURE 25.7 (a) Wolffian duct dissected free from most of mesonephros cultured for 4 days in the presence of GDNF. (b) High magnification view of a single ureteric bud-like structure isolated from cultured Wolffian duct in (a). (c) Single ureteric bud-like structure in (b) cultured within a three-dimensional extracellular matrix gel in the presence of branch-inducing growth factors. *(from ref. [25]).*

and metanephric mesenchyme was an important component in the process of ureteric bud branching. However, the isolated ureteric bud has since been shown to grow and branch extensively in the presence of appropriate extracellular matrix and soluble factors in the absence of direct contact with the metanephric mesenchyme[31] (Figure 25.8). The epithelial cells of the ureteric bud in this culture system appear to retain similar morphological characteristics to those of the ureteric bud in the whole embryonic kidney culture.[32] This system has allowed for the isolation and identification of numerous molecules, including soluble factors that modulate ureteric bud branching morphogenesis.[31–47]

Isolated Metanephric Mesenchyme Culture: Recombination with Heterologous Inductive Tissues

Another setting in which organ culture has been used focuses on metanephric mesenchyme induction and transformation to an epithelial phenotype. In this system, the isolated mesenchyme is cultured on one side of a filter while, on the other side of the filter, heterologous inducing tissues are placed. Various stages of metanephric mesenchyme induction (i.e., condensation, epithelialization, and tubulogenesis) can be observed, depending on the inductive capacity of the tissue. Using this method, it has been shown that embryonic spinal cord, salivary gland, and other tissues can induce the metanephric mesenchyme.[48,49] As is the case for isolated ureteric bud branching described previously, a key question here is the relative contribution of humoral factor(s) or cell–cell contact in this process. Electron microscopic examination revealed that the inducing tissue can contact the metanephric mesenchyme via cellular processes extending through the filter.[50] In fact, filters with pore sizes greater than 0.1 μm are unable to block cell-to-cell contact completely,[7] indicating the importance of cell–cell contact. However, complete mesenchymal induction has been demonstrated in the presence of soluble factors without cell–cell contact with inductive tissue.[51,52]

Isolated Metanephric Mesenchyme Culture: Recombination with Isolated Ureteric Bud

It has been shown that when co-cultured with freshly isolated metanephric mesenchyme, the isolated ureteric bud in culture (as described previously) is capable of inducing nephron tubules from the metanephric mesenchyme.[31] At the same time, the pattern of ureteric bud growth is altered by the presence of the metanephric mesenchyme; it is only through contact with metanephric mesenchyme that the ureteric bud undergoes vectorial branching with elongation and tapering of newly induced branches, similar to those seen in cultured whole embryonic kidneys[44] (Figure 25.9). Although this

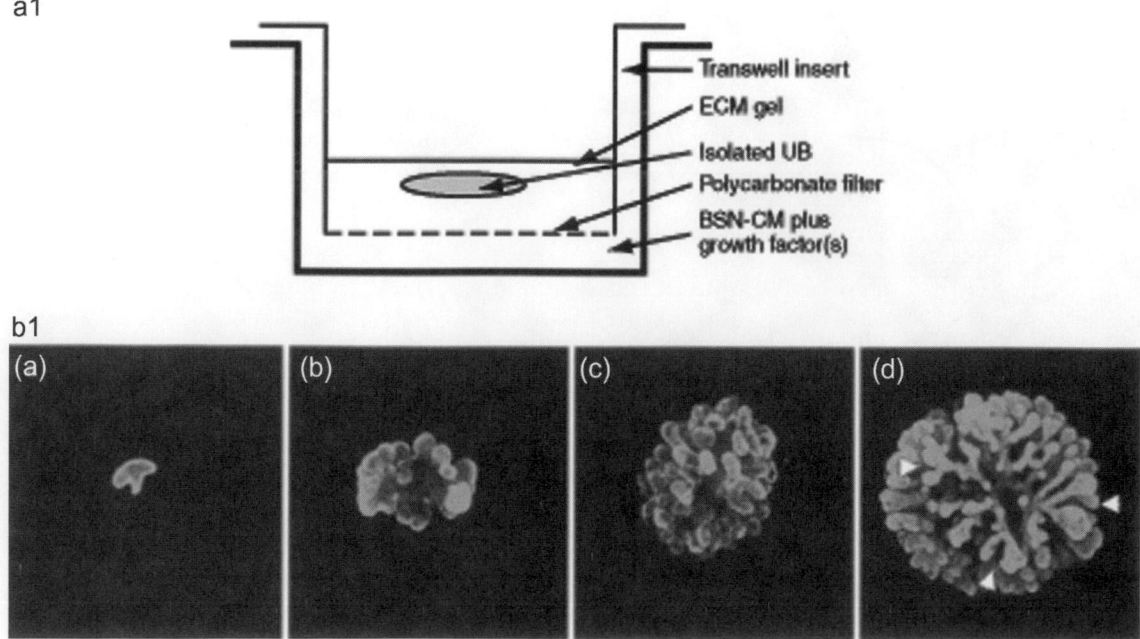

FIGURE 25.8   (a1) Illustration of isolated ureteric bud culture system. (b1) Cultured ureteric buds stained with fluorescein-conjugated lectin from Dolichos biflorus at (a) 0 days; (b) 3 days; (c) 6 days; and (d) 12 days. Arrows indicate branch points. *(adapted from ref. [31]).* See color plate section at the end of the book.

patterning effect on the ureteric bud appears to be modulated, in part, by soluble factors, cell contact with the metanephric mesenchyme and/or short-acting factors produced by the interaction of these two progenitor tissues plays a key role in determining the arborization pattern.[44] Another potential application of this "recombination" system is to pinpoint the defective tissue in knockout mice with a kidney phenotype. Through recombination of wild-type and gene knockout tissues (e.g., wild-type ureteric bud with knockout metanephric mesenchyme), it may be possible to determine the source of the kidney defect. For example, kidneys lacking heparan sulfate 2-O sulfotransferase (Hs2st$^{-/-}$) display renal agenesis, presumably due to defects in the inductive responsiveness of the ureteric bud to undergo branching morphogenesis.[53] However, examination of cultures of recombined wild-type and Hs2st$^{-/-}$ ureteric buds and metanephric mesenchyme (Figure 25.10) provided evidence that the key defect in the knockout kidney is the inability of the metanephric mesenchyme to undergo induction.[46]

The aforementioned tissue culture systems allow one to observe certain key phenomenon in metanephric kidney development *in vitro/ex vivo*. The analysis of genetically-engineered kidneys (and/or their component tissues) in these *in vitro* systems, in combination with an advanced method of gene perturbation (e.g., RNAi), will undoubtedly provide a more mechanistic picture of kidney development.

Genetically-Engineered Mice

Genetically-engineered mice allow one to manipulate the process of kidney development *in vivo*. Introducing null mutations of the gene of interest into mouse embryonic stem cells can be used to generate gene knockout mice.[54–56] Generally speaking, knockout mice grow from conception without normal expression of the gene product. If the mice develop beyond the stage of kidney development, the effect of the gene disruption on nephrogenesis can be observed *in vivo* by direct examination of the tissue histology. In such cases, the abnormal kidney phenotype can be directly or indirectly ascribed to disruption of the gene. In fact, many important molecules involved in kidney development have been identified by gene knockout technology.[57,58] In particular, the contribution of many transcription factors, molecules acting in the nucleus to regulate gene expression in the cell, have been demonstrated by this technique. However, knockout technology has its limitations. For example, although gene knockout mice can demonstrate the indispensability of a particular gene, how the gene product acts in the complex process of kidney development often remains unclear, owing to the spatiotemporal complexity of the

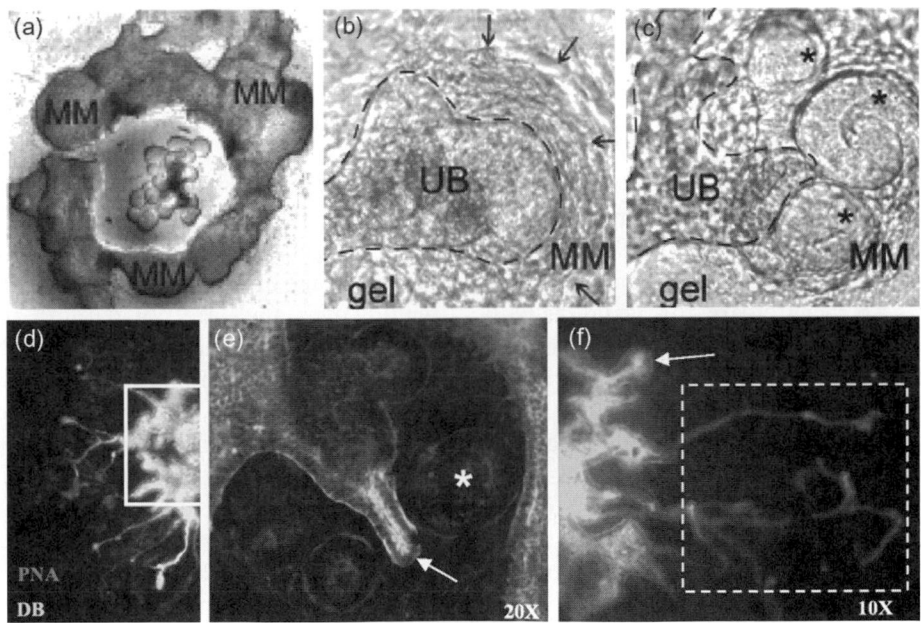

FIGURE 25.9 (a–c) Photomicrogrpahs of uninduced metanephric mesenchyme (MM) placed around the cultured UB (a); and co-cultured for 7 days (b–c). (d–f) UB and MM recombinations after 8 days of co-culture visualized with UB-specific lectin (*Dolichos biflorus*) and antibody against E-cadherin. Structures derived from mesenchymal-to-epithelial transformation, including cap-condensate (b: arrows) and coronas (indicated by asterisks) are observed. (f) Boxed area indicates elongation of UB branches and vectorial growth toward the MM; arrow indicates an area of the UB that has not undergone recombination with the MM and maintains its original architecture. *(adapted from ref. [44]).*

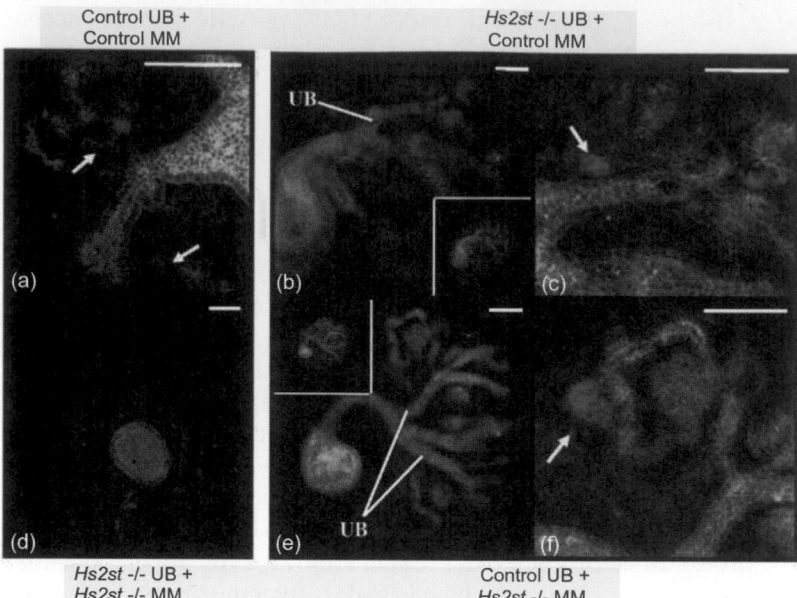

Control UB + Control MM

Hs2st -/- UB + Control MM

Hs2st -/- UB + *Hs2st -/-* MM

Control UB + *Hs2st -/-* MM

FIGURE 25.10 (a–f) Confocal photomicrographs of mix-and-match recombination cultures between heparan sulfate 2-O-sulfotransferase (Hs2st) knockout and control tissues. E-cadherin staining reveals epithelial structures derived from either ureteric bud (UB) or metanpehric mesenchyme (arrows). Mutual induction can be seen in co-cultures of control tissues recombined with control (a) or Hs2st$^{-/-}$ tissues (b), (c), (e), (f). Recombination of UB and MM from Hs2st$^{-/-}$ kidneys results in no mutual induction (d) (Scale bars: 100 μm). *(from ref. [46]).*

developing organ. Thus, if one observes defective ureteric bud branching in knockout mice, the deleted/disrupted gene product could be affecting the ureteric bud directly or it could be affecting the metanephric mesenchyme, resulting in incompetent induction of the ureteric bud. To resolve this problem, some have used organ culture type approaches ("recombination").[46,59] Another limitation of gene knockouts is that the mice may not have an apparent phenotype due to redundancy. In other words, the expression of other molecules with features or functions that overlap with the targeted gene could compensate for the defect from the gene knockout.

Perhaps the major drawback of conventional knockouts for studying genes involved in development of the kidney is the possibility that the targeted gene is critical for early embryonic survival, rendering the analysis of kidney development impossible as the embryo dies before organogenesis. In recent years, this issue (as well as some of the others listed above) has been overcome by the use of tissue-specific knockout technologies which provides the means for gene disruption in a time- and organ-specific manner.[60] This gene targeting system utilizes site-specific recombinases to excise out genes or portions of genes from the genomic DNA, resulting in the inactivation of the gene of interest.[61] Cre-loxP is the most commonly employed site-specific recombinase for these "conditional" deletions, although other site-specifc recombinases are available, including Flp-FRT and Dre-Rox. In the case of the Cre-loxP system (although the general principles are shared), conditional deletion of a gene of interest is performed by crossing two transgenic mouse lines: (1) "floxed" mice that carry the gene of interest with flanking loxP sites

which can be cleaved by the enzyme; and (2) Cre-recombinase transgenic mice under the control of a tissue-specific promoter.[62] For example, deletion of β1 integrin from the epithelial cells destined to become the ureteric bud using Cre recombinase under the control of the HoxB7 promoter disrupts ureteric bud branching morphogenesis, and variably retards kidney growth, leading in a few instances to renal agenesis.[45,63] While such approaches have proven useful, the main drawback of these conditional deletions in the study of the kidney is the availability of cell-specific promoters.[61] The use of tet-operon and tamoxifen to induce recombinase activity and the modulation of gene activity have also proven to be useful.[61] In these systems, animals are exposed to tetracycline or tamoxifen which activates the site-specific recombinase under its control, resulting in the modulation of gene activity. These systems have the advantage of being under the control of the investigator; however, they are not without problems, including the toxicity of the inducing agent.[61] Nevertheless, these spatiotemporal conditional deletions have rapidly established themselves as an invaluable tool for investigating the development of the kidney.

Cell Culture

Cell culture models have the advantage of simplicity. Since they use homogenous cell populations grown under controlled conditions, it is possible to perform biochemical analysis in great detail. Moreover, gene introduction by plasmid transfection and gene knockdown by RNAi is simpler in comparison to the organ culture system. Here, the most relevant system for branching morphogenesis of the ureteric bud, the three-dimensional cell culture system, is discussed.

When certain kidney-derived epithelial cells are suspended in an extracellular matrix gel (type I collagen or a collagen—Matrigel mixture) in the presence of morphogenetic humoral factors, they form tubules and undergo branching morphogenesis *in vitro*. The tubules in the three-dimensional culture have lumens and retain apical—basolateral polarity.[64] The effect of humoral factors in epithelial tube and/or branch formation can be studied here. In addition to the humoral factors, the effect of extracellular matrix composition on morphogenesis and the cellular details of morphogenesis can be examined in this system. MDCK cells and murine inner medullary collecting duct (mIMCD3) cells have been used in the past,[65–68] but these have the limitation of being derived from mature renal epithelial cells. To address this issue, an *in vitro* cell culture system using ureteric bud (UB) cells directly derived from embryonic day (E) 11.5 mouse ureteric bud has also been established.[69] Although there is some difference in the responsiveness of the different cell lines to growth factors, all three cell lines respond to soluble factors produced by the metanephric mesenchyme by forming branching tubules.

A detailed mechanism of hepatocyte growth factor (HGF)-induced MDCK cell tubulogenesis model has been described.[70] There appear to be two steps involved in this process of invasion: epithelial—mesenchymal transition; and the re-establishment of epithelial intercellular junctions. However, it has also been shown that ureteric buds in *in vitro* culture undergo branching morphogenesis through budding, a process in which epithelial cells never lose their junctions.[32] It remains to be seen where and when these two morphogenetic processes, branching through invasion ("invadopodia") and branching through budding, are utilized *in vivo*.[71]

MOLECULAR APPROACHES TO KIDNEY DEVELOPMENT

The development of high-density DNA microarray technology and global gene profiling has made it possible to analyze patterns of gene expression throughout embryonic and postnatal development and into adulthood in the whole developing rodent kidney.[72,73] It has also been possible to analyze gene expression changes in *in vitro* culture systems such as the isolated UB and MM.[39,42,74] For example, initial microarray analysis of a global time series of gene expression in the developing rat kidney revealed five discrete patterns or groups of gene expression[72] (Figure 25.11). mRNA encoding transcription factors and growth factors were found to be upregulated early in organogenesis (group 1). Among the genes

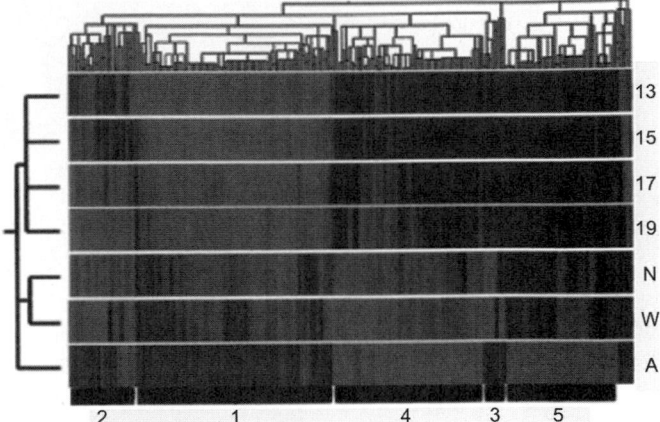

FIGURE 25.11   Hierarchical clustering of 873 genes identified as changing significantly at some point in kidney development (out of 8740 genes examined). Numbers at the bottom indicate group numbers derived from k-means clustering. Group 1 genes are upregulated (red) in the early embryonic period and decrease thereafter. Group 2 genes rise to a mid-late embryonic peak. Group 3 genes peak in the neonatal period. Group 4 genes rise somewhat linearly throughout development. Group 5 genes display a distinct peak in the adult versus all earlier times (13, 15, 17, 19: embryonic days; N: newborn; W: 1 week old; A: adult). *(from ref. [72]).* See color plate section at the end of the book.

whose expression level peaked in the middle of kidney organogenesis (group 2), many extracellular matrix related genes were found.[72] Further representing the global time series gene expression data as self-organizing maps (SOMs) made it possible to define roughly six stages of gene expression during pre- and postnatal kidney development in the rat.[73] Computational analysis suggested points of stability and transition based solely on gene expression and correlations where classically described anatomical changes were not intuitively obvious[73] (Figure 25.12). The most profound changes appear to occur at birth, when there is a sudden burst in the expression of many genes involved in redox metabolism and transport, including multispecific drug transporters such as Oat1 and Oct1.[75]

There has also been a massive effort to create an atlas of gene expression in the developing kidney, the genitourinary developmental molecular anatomy project or GUDMAP.[76–80] This multi-group international project is still continuing and has not only provided an atlas of localization information (e.g., ureteric bud, comma-shaped bodies, S-shaped bodies, renal vesicle), but has also yielded specific gene signatures for developing structures like branching ureteric bud tips. Although the function of many of these genes remains unknown, at a minimum they represent useful markers.

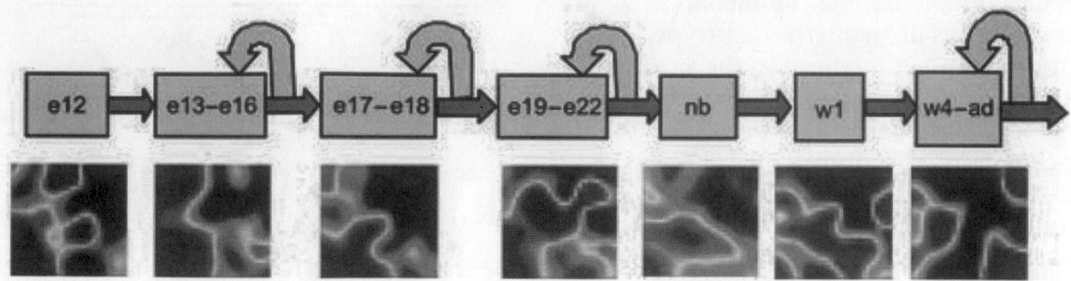

FIGURE 25.12 **Representative SOMs from each stage (Stage 1: e12; stage 2: e13 to e16; stage 3: e17 to e18; stage 4: e19 to e22; stage 5: nb (P0 to P1); stage 6: w1; stage 7: w4 to ad).** Curved arrows represent putative negative feedback loops that potentially stabilize the previous stage. *(from ref. [73]).*

One of the key tasks in the future will be to place this localization information in the context of global gene expression time series data, to obtain a more accurate picture of the dynamics of kidney organogenesis and suggest new points of regulation. Growth factor-selective heparan sulfation interactions have been proposed as important regulators of the switching between stages.[46,47] Moreover, based on current knockout and *in vitro* data, it has been suggested that key "hubs" in the network of genes regulating kidney development include the process of GDNF-dependent budding early on, and late tubulogenesis involving cilia-associated genes such as those implicated in various types of cystic kidney disease.[81,82] It is becoming increasingly clear that an abundance of knockouts reported to have "renal phenotypes" cluster around these processes. *In vivo* branching morphogenesis, especially in the middle phases, appears largely protected from disruption in many knockouts of gene products known to be involved in *in vitro* branching. When branching phenotypes are reported, it is usually in the form of a small reduction in nephron number. One interpretation, supported by a wealth of *in vitro* data, is that there are many growth factor—heparan sulfate-dependent pathways regulating branching, and deletion of any single one is likely to be compensated by another. Double knockouts, for example of the EGF receptor and the HGF receptor (c-met), are beginning to provide support for this view.[83]

In addition to these high-throughput gene profiling approaches, epigenetic transcriptional controls are becoming rapidly appreciated. These dynamic cell-inheritable processes alter transcriptional activity without affecting DNA sequence, and include covalent modifications of DNA and histones, DNA packaging, chromatin folding, and regulatory noncoding microRNAs (miRNAs).[84,85] For example, conditional deletion of Dicer, the RNase involved in the production of miRNAs (which control gene expression at the post-transcriptional level), from cells of the nephron lineage lead to elevated apoptosis and premature termination of nephrogenesis.[86] In addition, deletion of Dicer from ureteric bud epithelium disrupts branching morphogenesis, and leads to the development of renal cysts.[86] Together with other studies on Dicer and miRNAs, the data clearly indicate a role for Dicer and Dicer-dependent miRNA activity in the development of the kidney, as well as in the development and progression of kidney disease.[84,86–93]

Ultimately, high-throughput gene profiling, together with a thorough epigenetic analysis, may provide mechanistic insight into the very complex system of gene expression regulating kidney development. This may enable the development of a systems perspective on nephrogenesis. Attempts at creation of "coarse grained" models of kidney development have clearly begun.[40,82,94,95] In the following section, a number of molecules which have been shown to be involved in kidney development are discussed. Over the past two decades, a large number of developing kidney phenotypes has been reported in gene knockout studies. Together with *in vitro* studies, they provide a great deal of functional information. We will highlight some of the results below. Several recent reviews describe them in much more detail.[96–98] Moreover, we do not discuss in great detail the impressive amount of work that has been done in relation to the formation of the glomerular filtration barrier (reviewed in [99]), polycystic kidney disease (reviewed in [100]) or late nephron differentiation and acquisition of mature transport function (reviewed in [96–98,101]). We focus largely on the WD, UB, and early MM-derived structures.

TRANSCRIPTION FACTORS IN METANEPHROGENESIS

Transcription factors bind to DNA and regulate the expression of other genes that are involved in, among other things, morphogenesis and differentiation. As a result of many gene disruption studies, several important transcription factors in kidney development have been demonstrated. With careful molecular marker analysis, it will soon be possible to draw a whole network of these molecules in this process.

Transcription Factors Regulating Glial Cell Line-Derived Neurotrophic Growth Factor

As will be described later, a key molecule in the process of the initial stage of metanephros development (i.e., ureteric bud formation and outgrowth from the Wolffian duct) is glial cell line-derived neurotrophic growth factor (GDNF). Many transcription factors regulating expression of this growth factor affect ureteric bud development, and thus kidney development.

Hox Genes

Hox genes, mammalian homologs of *Drosophilia* homeotic genes, have been shown to be critically important for early nephrogenesis. While null mutants for *Hoxa11* or *Hoxd11* mice do not have a kidney phenotype, double knockouts of *Hoxa11* and *Hoxd11* show kidney agenesis or hypogenesis.[102] Moreover, complete elimination of *Hox11* paralogs (*Hoxa11*, *Hoxc11*, and *Hoxd11*) result in a lack of ureteric bud outgrowth from the Wolffian duct.[103] In this mutant, expression of another transcription factor, *Six2* as well as *Gdnf* is lacking, suggesting that *Hox11* paralogs regulate *Gdnf* expression.

Pax Genes

Additional members of the homeotic gene family, the *Pax* genes, have been implicated in nephrogenesis. Compared with *Hox* genes, *Pax* genes appear to be restricted to certain tissues or organs. *Pax2* and *Pax8* have been shown to be expressed in the kidney. These *Pax* genes can be considered as early nephric lineage specification genes, as they are first expressed in the pronephric duct, and their simultaneous disruption causes failure in the formation of the epithelial pronephric duct from the intermediate mesoderm.[1] After the pronephric duct, *Pax2* expression is sequentially found in its extension, the Wolffian duct, the ureteric bud, as well as the condensed metanephric mesenchyme and the newly formed nephron tubules. As the kidney tubules mature, *Pax2* expression decreases.[104,105] The expression pattern suggests a role for *Pax2* in mesenchymal–epithelial transformation. Homozygous null mutant mice lacking *Pax2* show only a partially developed Wolffian duct, leading to kidney agenesis.[106] It has also been shown that the mutant Wolffian duct does not respond to GDNF to form the ureteric bud. Furthermore, the mutant metanephric mesenchyme not only lacks *Gdnf* expression, it is not competent to form nephron tubules in response to wild-type spinal cord.[22] Heterozygous *Pax2* mutant mice have hypoplastic kidneys.[106] In fact, there are Pax2-binding sites in the promoter region of *Gdnf*, and Pax2 can promote *Gdnf* expression *in vitro*.[22] Pax2 has also been shown to promote the assembly of an H3K4 methyltransferase complex, which is involved in epigenetic transcriptional regulation.[85]

Pax8 has a similar tissue expression pattern to *Pax2*; however, *Pax8* expression peaks later than *Pax2*.[107] Although kidney development is apparently normal in *Pax8* knockout mice,[108] double knockouts of *Pax2* and *Pax8* show a complete absence of a urogenital system, due to failure in the formation of the pronephric duct from the intermediate mesoderm,[1] suggesting some overlap in the roles of these two *Pax* genes in pronephric duct induction. Analysis of kidney development in mice heterozygous for *Pax2* and for *Pax8*, which form kidneys (albeit hypodysplastic with fewer ureteric bud tips and a reduced nephron number), indicates a dramatic reduction in the expression levels of *Lim1*.[109] Although normal levels of *Ret* and *Gdnf* were seen, *Wnt11* (an important downstream target of Gdnf signaling, see below) was reduced. Thus, it has been postulated that *Pax2* and *Pax8* play a key cooperative role in nephron differentiation and branching of the ureteric bud.[109]

Eya1, Six1, and Six2 Genes

These genes have been implicated in *Drosophila* eye development together with *Pax6*,[110] and are expressed in the metanephric mesenchyme in the kidney. Homozygous null mutants for *Eya1* show kidney agenesis with loss of *Gdnf* and *Six* expression,[111] suggesting that EYA1 acts upstream of SIX, and together they regulate *Gdnf* expression. In fact, EYA1 is shown to act as a co-activator[111] of the genes regulated by SIX.[112] In *Six1* knockouts, which show various kidney phenotypes ranging from hypogenesis to agenesis, *Gdnf* expression is reduced, but *Eya1* expression is preserved.[112,113] Interestingly, metanephric mesenchyme derived from *Six1* knockout mice is not competent in nephron tubule formation when it is cultured with spinal cord, a potent inducer of nephron tubulogenesis, suggesting that these factors not only control *Gdnf* expression, but also have a role in maintaining certain characteristics of metanephric mesenchyme.[113] As described previously, another member of the *Six* family, *Six2* appears to regulate *Gdnf* expression downstream of *Hox11* paralogs.[103] Although *Six1* and *Six2* show overlapping areas of expression, the fact that *Six2* expression is reduced in *Six1* knockouts[112,113] suggests a close relationship between these two molecules. *Six2* expression *in vivo* has been found to be directly activated by a novel protein complex composed of the Hox11 paralogous proteins, Pax2 and Eya1, which clearly demonstrates that *Six2* and *Gdnf* are downstream targets of the Hox11 paralogs.[114] Moreover, *Six2* defines nephron progenitor populations in the metanephric mesenchyme and it cell-autonomously maintains progenitor populations.[6]

Sall1

Sall1 is a transcription-related protein expressed in the metanephric mesenchyme of the developing kidney.[115] It is also expressed in extrarenal tissues such as the limb buds and central nervous systems. Knockout of this gene results in failure of the ureteric bud to undergo branching after invading the metanephric mesenchyme.[116] Although *Gdnf* expression just before ureteric bud formation is reported to be normal, its expression in the metanephric mesenchyme subsequently decreases.[115] It is unclear whether this reduction of *Gdnf* expression is due to a direct effect of the *Sall1* mutation or if it is secondary to a loss of a ureteric bud-derived signal. Interestingly, exogenous Gdnf was unable to rescue branching in cultures of *Sall1* knockout kidneys despite expression of *Ret*, suggesting that the ureteric buds are unable to respond to Gdnf.[116] *In situ* hybridization demonstrates the expression of the stalk-specific marker, *Wnt9b*, as well as the β-catenin target gene *Axin2*, in the ureteric bud tips of *Sall1* knockout kidneys.[116] Since reduction of β-catenin levels in *Sall1* mutants rescued ureteric bud branching and overexpression of *Wnt9b*-inhibited branching in normal ureteric buds, the data indicate that *Sall1*-dependent signals regulate the initiation of ureteric bud branching by modulating the expression of ureteric bud tip-specific genes.[116] In addition, among metanephric mesenchyme cells, only those cells which express high levels of *Sall1* are capable of nephron formation, suggesting the possibility that activation of this gene is key for nephron-forming capacity in the metanephric mesenchyme.[117] Given the fact that *Six2* maintains nephron progenitor cells, *Sall1* may act together with *Six2* to ensure multipotency of nephron progenitors.

Foxc1

Although some of the aforementioned genes affect a number of other genes, they all normally stimulate *Gdnf* expression. However, it is also important to restrict the area of *Gdnf* expression, to avoid multiple kidneys arising from a single Wolffian duct. In this regard, a member of the forkhead transcription factor superfamily, *Foxc1*, appears to restrict *Gdnf* expression to the intermediate mesoderm around the Wolffian duct (i.e., metanephric mesenchyme). *Foxc1* homozygous null mutants display ectopic ureteric bud

outgrowth resulting in duplex kidneys.[118] In this mutant, the restrictive expression pattern of *Gdnf* as well as *Eya1* is perturbed, and is abnormally extended along the Wolffian duct.

Transcription Factors Regulating Ureteric Bud Formation (or Early Kidney Development)

Lim1

Lim1 is a homeotic gene expressed in both the central nervous system and kidneys. By whole-mount *in situ* hybridization, its transcript is detected from the pronephric stage to the metanephros.[119] In the metanephros, its expression is detected in the renal vesicles, S-shaped bodies, and ureteric bud branches.[119] Knockout of *Lim1* leads to kidney agenesis, suggesting its distinct role in early nephrogenesis.[120] Since *Pax2* expression in the mesonephros is detected in *Lim1* knockouts,[121] and the ectopic expression of *Pax2* was found to induce *Lim1* in the intermediate mesoderm,[1] it is likely that *Lim1* acts downstream of *Pax2* in pronephros development. However, the exact role of *Lim1* in metanephrogenesis remains to be determined.

Wt1

One of the Wilms tumor suppressor genes, *Wt1*, a zinc-finger transcription factor, is required for kidney development. *Wt1* generally acts as a transcriptional repressor, and has been shown to repress *Igf2*,[122] *Igf1* receptor,[123] *Pax2*,[124] *Myc*,[125] and *Bcl2*[125] expression. Most of these genes are related to cell proliferation, supporting the notion that loss of *Wt1*-mediated repression could lead to disregulated proliferation (i.e., cancer). It seems paradoxical that the *Wt1* knockout suffers from kidney agenesis, not tumors.[126] In the homozygous deletion mutant of *Wt1*, the ureteric bud fails to form, despite relatively normal development of the mesonephros and in the presence of *Gdnf* expression,[127] suggesting that factor(s) other than GDNF might be required for ureteric bud initiation. In normal embryonic kidneys, *Wt1* is expressed in uninduced mesenchyme, renal vesicles, and glomerular podocytes.[128] *Wt1* mutant mesenchyme is not responsive to the inductive signal from wild-type spinal cord, while the mutant Wolffian duct can induce wild-type metanephric mesenchyme, suggesting that the primary defect is in the mesenchyme.[127] Interestingly, the mechanism(s) of WT1 remain to be fully elucidated. Genome-wide expression profiling analysis in cells expressing inducible WT1 identified some direct WT1-target genes, including EGF receptor ligands, chemokines, and transcription factors.[129]

Limb Deformity Gene/*Fmn1*

Kidney agenesis is observed in mice homozygous for the *limb deformity* (*ld*) gene, *Fmn1*, mutation. The initial outgrowth of the ureteric bud is not observed in mutant mice. The metanephric mesenchyme from *Fmn1* mutant mice is induced by embryonic spinal cord, suggesting that the defect is in the ureteric bud.[130] The *Fmn* gene encodes formin, a gene product, which is present in both the ureteric bud and the metanephric mesenchyme.[131,132] Although knockouts of certain formin isoforms display limb deformity and kidney defects, specific elimination of isoform 4 results in a pure kidney phenotype.[133]

Myc Genes

The *Myc* family members were first recognized as proto-oncogenes that function as transcription factors. While *Myc* is expressed in the uninduced metanephric mesenchyme and newly formed epithelium, *Nmyc1* is transiently expressed in the area of mesenchymal–epithelial transformation.[134] Another *Myc* family member, *Lmyc1*, is expressed in ureteric bud-derived structures, and its expression increases as these structures mature.[134] Both *Myc* and *Nmyc1* gene knockouts are lethal at E9.5–10.5 and E10.5–12.5, respectively.[135–137] *Myc* mutants apparently have no specific kidney phenotype. In *Nmyc1* mutants, mesonephric development is affected. In both cases, mice die before metanephric development, which therefore cannot be assessed. The distinct pattern of expression of the various *Myc* genes makes them useful as markers: mesenchymal stromal cells are negative for *Myc*; *Nmyc1* is a marker for induced mesenchyme or early mesenchymal epithelialization; *Lmyc1* is a marker for the collecting duct.

Transcription Factors Regulating Ureteric Bud Survival/Branching

Emx2

Disruption of a homeotic gene, *Emx2* results in urogenital defects in mice.[59] In mutant mice, the initial formation of the Wolffian duct and ureteric bud is normal, as is the initial induction of the metanephric mesenchyme. Normal *Pax2* expression is observed in these structures. However, the ureteric bud starts to degenerate around E12.5. At the same time, the expression of *Pax2* and *Ret*, a receptor tyrosine kinase normally expressed at the tip of growing ureteric bud, is greatly reduced. Recombinant organ culture between wild-type and mutant ureteric bud and metanephric mesenchyme indicates a defect in the ureteric bud. *Emx2* expression is observed at a later stage of epithelialization than *Pax2* in normal mice. The expression pattern suggests that *Emx2* regulates maturation and/or survival of epithelial cells, rather than formation of epithelial cells.

Timeless

By differential gene expression screening in the epithelial cell three-dimensional culture system for branching tubulogenesis, the mammalian ortholog of *Timeless* gene was identified as a candidate for regulation of epithelial branching morphogenesis. Its expression is detected in the active region of ureteric bud branching in the developing kidney. Selective inhibition of this gene in various *in vitro* culture models resulted in inhibition of ureteric bud branching.[33] Deletion of this gene is embryonic lethal prior to the onset of kidney development.[138] The kidney (or ureteric bud)-specific knockout data are needed to provide a definitive role of this molecule in kidney development.

ETS Transcription Factor Genes

Etv4 and *Etv5*, two members of the Pea3 family of E-twenty six (ETS) domain transcription factors, which are believed to function as transcriptional activator proteins,[139] were identified in an analysis of gene expression in ureteric buds cultured in the absence or presence of Gdnf.[140,141] *Etv4* and *Etv5* were found to have overlapping expression in ureteric bud tips which was positively enhanced by Gdnf.[140,141] Gene dosage reductions and/or deletions of these transcription factors indicated a role in the formation of the ureteric bud tip domain.[140,141]

Sox Genes

Sox genes are developmental regulators containing a DNA-binding domain with high homology with the HMG box of the sex-determining gene *Sry*. Mice with double deletions of *Sox9* and *Sox8* have kidney defects, including renal agenesis.[142] *In situ* hybridization demonstrates reduced expression of a number of downstream targets of Gdnf-Ret signaling, including *Etv4*, *Etv5*, *Met*, and *Spry1* in the ureteric bud tips. Together, the data indicate that *Sox8* and *Sox9* have key roles in Gdnf-Ret signaling regulating/modulating ureteric bud branching morphogenesis.[142]

Transcription Factors Regulating Stroma Development

Foxd1

Study of one of the forkhead box transcription factor superfamily members, *Foxd1* (*Bf2*), shed light on the role of the third cellular component of the developing kidney, the stroma. In developing kidneys, *Foxd1* is expressed by the cortical stromal mesenchyme. Homozygous null mutants for *Foxd1* die soon after birth due to renal failure. Mutant kidneys are small, fused, and located in the pelvis.[143] Both ureteric bud branching morphogenesis and kidney tubulogenesis in the metanephric mesenchyme-derived segments are perturbed. Further analysis of this knockout mouse reveals that the mutant kidney capsule abnormally contains cells expressing bone morphogenetic protein (BMP) 4 or PECAM (endothelial marker). Abnormal signals from these cells are likely to cause disruption of normal ureteric bud branching and nephrogenesis.[144] One of the target genes for this transcription factor is placental growth factor, a family member of vascular endothelial growth factor.[145]

Pod1

The *Pod1* gene, a transcription factor expressed in mesenchymal cells surrounding the ureteric bud and visceral glomerular podocytes in the developing kidney,[146] also plays a role in regulating ureteric bud branching and nephron formation. Null mutants for this gene exhibit a phenotype similar to that seen in *Foxd1* knockouts; initial ureteric budding and mesenchymal condensation occurs, but the process appears to slow down beyond this point.[147] By chimeric mouse analysis, *Pod1* expression was shown to be critical for the medullary stroma.[148]

Pbx1

Pbx1 gene encodes a homeodomain containing transcription factor expressed in metanephric mesenchyme, and both cortical and medullary stroma in the developing kidney. The kidney phenotype of *Pbx1* knockouts is similar to that of *Pod1/Foxd1* knockouts.[149] It appears that expression of these genes is not dependent upon the others, and all three genes are required for the functioning stroma to be capable of supporting ureteric bud branching and nephron differentiation. Identifying the molecular nature of this "stromal effect" will provide considerable insight into kidney development.

Retinoic Acid Receptor Genes

One possible mechanism for control of ureteric bud branching morphogenesis by the stromal cells is through the vitamin A/retinoic acid pathway. Vitamin A deficiency has been known to result in small kidneys.[150] Dietary vitamin A is converted to its active form, retinoic acid, and its signal is mediated through the retinoic acid receptor, which acts as a transcription factor. Retinoic acid synthesizing enzyme localizes to the cortical stromal cells,[151] and double knockout of retinoic acid receptor *Rara* and *Rarb2* results in *Ret* downregulation and impaired ureteric branching.[152]

Transcription Factors Regulating Functional Maturation of Nephron Tubules

Hnf1

Hepatocyte nuclear factor (Hnf)-1 is a homeotic gene mainly expressed in liver and kidney. *Hnf1* knockout mice have an enlarged liver and Fanconi syndrome, resulting in urinary wasting of sugars, amino acids, and electrolytes that normally are reabsorbed in the renal proximal tubules,[153] suggesting an important role for *Hnf1* in regulating the expression of proximal tubule transporters.

Brn1

Maturation of Henle's loop and distal tubule is controlled by *Brn1*, a POU transcription factor. *Brn1* is expressed only in part of the mesenchymal condensate, then the prospective Henle's loop and distal tubule in the maturing kidney. There is no expression in the glomerulus, proximal tubule or collecting duct. Knockout of this transcription factor results in an elongation and maturation defect of the Henle's loop, macula densa, and distal tubule.[154]

URETERIC BUD OUTGROWTH FROM THE WOLFFIAN DUCT

Outgrowth of the ureteric bud from the Wolffian duct in response to signals arising from the metanephric mesenchyme is the initiating event in the development of the mammalian kidney.[7] The major growth factor involved in this process is Glial-derived neurotrophic factor (Gdnf) (see below). There are several levels of regulation surrounding the GDNF pathway.

Restriction of GDNF Expressed Region by *Slit-Robo*

The secreted protein *Slit2* and its receptor *Robo2*, previously reported as a chemo-repellant factor for axon guidance,[155] also functions to restrict *Gdnf* expression. Null mutations of either *Slit2* or *Robo2* result in supernumerary ureteric buds, caused by an abnormally extended *Gdnf* expression area.[156]

Regulators for GDNF Signaling Pathway

Sprouty

Sprouty (Spry) is an intercellular protein that acts as a negative feedback regulator for FGF and other receptor tyrosine kinase-mediated signaling.[157] Knockouts of Spry1 display multiple ureters and multiplex kidneys.[158] It appears that mutant Wolffian ducts are abnormally more sensitive to GDNF, as reduction of Gdnf expression rescues the phenotype.[158] Double knockouts of Spry and Gdnf (Spry[−/−]; Gdnf[−/−]) rescue normal ureteric bud outgrowth and kidney development.[159] When Fgf10 was also deleted from these mice ureteric bud outgrowth failed to occur, suggesting that Fgf10 is likely to function as the receptor tyrosine kinase responsible for ureteric bud outgrowth in the absence of Spry and Gdnf.[159]

Activin and FGF

One of the puzzles in early nephrogenesis has been that a substantial fraction of Ret knockouts develop very rudimentary kidneys, suggesting the existence of a "bypass" pathway for ureteric bud formation. A GDNF-independent pathway for in vitro budding has been described that appears to involve a FGF,[22] but it is possible that inhibition of activin signaling also enables a "bypass" of the GDNF-ret pathway.[23,24] The FGF-dependent bypass pathway has been recently supported by in vivo evidence.[159]

NPY and BMP through PKA

Utilizing ex vivo cultured Wolffian ducts, microarray analysis of ducts maintained in the absence or presence of Gdnf identified neuropeptide Y (Npy) as a novel modulator of ureteric bud outgrowth.[28] Npy also rescues budding in Bmp4-treated Wolffian ducts, suggesting that this neuropeptide is reciprocally regulated by Gdnf and Bmps.[28] Comparison of budded and non-budded portions of Gdnf-induced cultured Wolffian ducts also reveals an almost 15-fold increase in protein kinase A (PKA) activity in non-budded Wolffian ducts.[30] Microarray analysis reveals a marked decrease in the expression of Ret following activation of the PKA pathway in cultured Wolffian duct. Bmp2 expression is also increased in unbudded Wolffian ducts, and exogenous Bmp2 inhibits ex vivo budding from the Wolffian duct with a three-fold increase in PKA activity.[30] Taken together, the data suggest a role for PKA in regulating the site of ureteric bud outgrowth, potentially via a Bmp-dependent downregulation of Ret/Gfrα1 co-receptor expression.[30]

GDF11

Another member of this family, growth/differentiation factor (Gdf)11 is expressed in the Wolffian duct and the metanephric mesenchyme. Knockouts of this gene result in kidney hypoplasia to agenesis, thought to be caused by downregulation of Gdnf in the mesenchyme.[160,161] In these mice, molecules known to regulate Gdnf expression such as Eya1, Six2, Pax2, and Wt1 are expressed in the metanephric mesenchyme region, and the metanephric mesenchyme from this mutant undergoes nephron tubule formation when it is cultured with embryonic spinal cord. Molecular markers for the Wolffian duct such as Ret, Pax2, Emx2, and Lim1 were expressed in the right place, and mutant Wolffian duct responds to exogenous GDNF.[160] Thus, GDF11 is likely to be indispensable for Gdnf expression.

Outside the kidney, this mutant mouse shows deranged anterior/posterior patterning, with alteration of Hox gene expression pattern.[161] Given the fact that Hox11 paralogs control Gdnf expression,[103] downregulation of Gdnf in Gdf11 mutants may be mediated through Hox11 expression. GDF11 acts through the activin receptor (ACVR) IIA and IIB,[162] and knockouts of Acvr2b result in a similar though milder phenotype than that of Gdf11 knockouts.[163]

Unidentified Signal(s) from Metanephric Mesenchyme

Another pathway involved in the regulation of ureteric bud outgrowth is revealed by single deletions of Fgfr2 (but not Fgfr1, which appeared to be normal) from the metanephric mesenchyme, which leads to the outgrowth of duplicated ureteric buds from the Wolffian duct.[164] Although it is not clear which factors are secreted from metanephric mesenchyme, this result suggests that certain FGF signaling plays a role in the metanephric mesenchyme to suppress ectopic ureteric bud formation.

URETERIC BUD BRANCHING MORPHOGENESIS

As discussed previously, ureteric bud branching morphogenesis is induced by signals from the metanephric mesenchyme. Soluble growth factors, direct cell-to-cell contact, and cell−matrix contact play key roles in the process. The molecules likely to be involved in ureteric bud branching morphogenesis are summarized in Table 25.1.

TABLE 25.1 Molecules Likely to be Involved in Ureteric Bud Outgrowth and Branching Morphogenesis

Process	Soluble Factors	Transcription Factors	ECM/ Protease/ Integrin
Initiation	GDNF	*Pax2*	
	WNT2b	*Lim1*	
	Slit/Robo	*Six1, 2*	
	Activin (inhibitory)	*Eya1*	
	BMP2/4 (inhibitory)	*Wt1*	
	Sprouty (intracellular molecule)	*Hox11 paralogs*	
		Formin	
		Foxc1	
		Sox9	
		Sall1	
Branching morphogenesis	GDNF	*Sall1*	Proteoglycans
	Pleiotrophin	*Timeless*	MMP9
	Wnt11	*Sox9*	Integrin $\alpha_3\beta_1$
	Gremlin	*Etv4*	Integrin β1
	TGFβ superfamily	*Etv5*	
	HGF		
	IGF		
	FGFs		
	FGFR2		
Maintenance/ maturation of collecting system	EGFR ligands	*Emx2*	
	Wnt9b, Wnt7b	*Foxd1*	
		Pbx1	
		Pod1	

ECM: extracellular matrix; EGFR: epidermal growth factor receptor; GDNF: glial cell line-derived neurotrophic growth factor; HGF: hepatocyte growth factor; IGF: insulin-like growth factor; TGF: transforming growth factor.

Growth Factors

The embryonic kidney or isolated metanephric mesenchyme can induce branching morphogenesis of MDCK, mIMCD3 or UB cells grown in type I collagen gels in the absence of apparent cell contact.[65,69,165] Moreover, isolated ureteric buds from E13 rats have been shown to undergo branching morphogenesis in the presence of soluble factors.[31] This suggests that the metanephric mesenchyme elaborates soluble growth factors capable of inducing branching morphogenesis

in the ureteric bud. A number of key growth factors have been identified.

Glial Cell Line-Derived Neurotrophic Factor

The importance of GDNF and its receptors GFRa1 and RET in kidney development is strongly supported by gene knockout data. Kidney agenesis or severe kidney hypogenesis is found in *Gdnf*,[166–168] *Gfra1*[169] or *Ret* knockout mice.[170,171] GDNF is expressed in the prospective metanephric mesenchyme area, while GFRa1 and RET are expressed in the Wolffian duct at the time of ureteric bud induction. As discussed previously, a wide variety of genetic manipulations affecting the transcription of the GDNF/GFRα1/Ret axis lead to disruption of kidney development. Moreover, *in vitro* application of GDNF-soaked beads to the whole genitourinary tract culture induces ectopic budding of the Wolffian duct.[172] GDNF is also important in subsequent branching morphogenesis of the ureteric bud, as inhibition of this factor perturbs further branching of the isolated ureteric bud *in vitro*.[31] Gene dosage of *Gdnf* is important, as heterozygous null mutants of this gene have smaller kidneys.[173] However, unlike ureteric budding from the Wolffian duct, where GDNF appears necessary and sufficient, GDNF is necessary but not sufficient to support ureteric bud branching morphogenesis, at least in the isolated ureteric bud culture system.[31]

Fibroblast Growth Factors and Receptors

Many fibroblast growth factors (FGFs) and their receptors are expressed in the developing kidney.[174] Initial demonstration of the importance of this signaling pathway came from an analysis of transgenic mice that overexpress a soluble chimera of FGFR 2IIIb and human IgG Fc. In these animals, where FGF signaling is broadly inhibited, kidney agenesis or severe hypogenesis ensues.[175] In addition, minor kidney defects are reported in *Fgf7*,[176] *Fgf10*,[177] and *Fgfr2IIIb*[178] knockout mice. In the isolated ureteric bud culture system, FGF2 and FGF7 induce a less branched globular ureteric bud growth, while FGF1 and FGF10 support branching growth,[36] suggesting that FGFs may play a role in ureteric bud morphogenesis. Consistent with this, a ureteric bud-specific knockout of *Fgfr2*, (but not *Fgfr1*) was found to result in abnormal ureteric bud growth, as well as abnormally thickened cortical stroma.[164] Three-dimensional reconstructive imaging reveals decreases in ureteric bud tip number and increases in the length of the ureteric bud segments.[179,180]

Pleiotrophin

This heparin-binding growth factor has been implicated in neurite outgrowth[181] and mesenchymal–epithelial interaction during organogenesis.[182] In the context of kidney development, pleiotrophin (isolated from the conditioned medium made by metanephric mesenchyme-derived cells) was found to induce ureteric bud branching morphogenesis in the presence of GDNF in the *in vitro* culture system.[37] It is present in the developing kidney at the basement membrane of the ureteric bud. Although pleiotrophin may act as a mitogen for the ureteric bud after its budding through GDNF action, knockout of this gene does not appear to have a major affect in kidney development.[183]

Wnts and Related Molecules (Frizzled-Related Proteins)

A member of the WNT family of secreted glycoprotein, WNT2b is expressed in the stroma, and its presence promotes ureteric bud branching *in vitro*.[184] Null mutants of the gene encoding another member of WNT family, *Wnt11*, result in decreased ureteric bud branching with reduced *Gdnf* expression in the mesenchyme.[185] *Ret* knockout mice also show reduced expression of *Wnt11*.[185] In the trunk or stalk region of the ureteric bud, *Wnt9b* is expressed, and genetic deletion of this molecule results in cystic kidneys, presumably due to the disruption of the planar cell polarity (non-canonical beta catenin-independent) pathway of Wnt signaling.[186] Later in collecting duct development, collecting duct-specific inactivation of *Wnt7b* displays a similar phenotype.[187]

Secreted frizzled-related proteins (sFRPs) are secreted proteins that function as WNT modulators. sFRP1 is expressed in the stroma and periureter area; sFRP2 is expressed in early mesenchymal condensates and also in the periureter area in the developing kidney.[188,189] Exogenous administration of sFRP1 to embryonic kidney organ culture leads to decreased ureteric bud branching and nephron induction. While exogenous sFRP2 alone does not have a major effect, its administration to the organ culture treated with sFRP1 partially reverses the inhibitory effect of sFRP1.[189]

Transforming Growth Factor β Superfamily

Most of the soluble factors discussed thus far facilitate ureteric bud branching and growth. However, unopposed proliferation and branching is not desirable for normal kidney development. Potential candidates for these "negative regulators" include members of the transforming growth factor (TGF) β superfamily. Generally, TGFβ inhibits epithelial cell growth. In organ culture, exogenous TGFβ1 or another member of the TGFβ superfamily, activin, inhibits ureteric bud development and/or disrupts the branching pattern,[190] suggesting their role not only in regulating proliferation, but also in correct patterning. In this regard, it is interesting that TGFβ selectively inhibits HGF-induced mIMCD3 branching events with little effect on tubule formation[67]; HGF plus TGFβ induces long, straight tubules, whereas HGF alone induces branching tubules. Furthermore, detailed image analysis reveals alteration in the ureteric bud branching pattern in embryonic kidneys treated with TGFβ superfamily members.[40] In isolated ureteric bud culture, administration of TGFβ superfamily members causes growth inhibition, as well as morphological changes similar (although not so striking) to that observed in mIMCD cell culture.[40]

Heterozygous mutation of another family member, bone morphogenetic protein (*Bmp*) 4 reveals loss of ureteric bud elongation, together with ectopic budding from the Wolffian duct.[191] Its expression is detected at the intermediate mesoderm surrounding the Wolffian duct and metanephric mesenchyme surrounding the stalk of the ureteric bud.[191,192] Taken together, these data suggest that TGFβ superfamily members inhibit branching events, but have somewhat less effect on ureteric bud elongation (and may even facilitate it in the presence of stimulatory growth factors), and play a role in regulating the pattern of ureteric bud branching.

Gremlin

Gremlin is a secreted BMP antagonist[193] expressed initially in the Wolffian duct, followed by induced mesenchyme in metanephros development.[194] Knockout of this gene results in kidney agenesis. The ureteric bud forms but fails to invade the metanephric mesenchyme.[194] Subsequently, the metanephric mesenchyme undergoes apoptosis. Although the kidney phenotype of *Gremlin1* knockouts resembles that of *Sall1* knockouts, *Sall1* expression is unchanged in *Gremlin1* knockouts.[194] However, inactivation of one copy of the *Bmp4* gene or the complete absence of *Bmp7* in gremlin knockout animals rescues ureteric bud invasion and branching.[191,192] Thus, it possible that gremlin antagonization of BMP activity at ureteric bud tips acts to restrict and guide ureteric bud outgrowth and branching, although the mechanism remains unclear.[195,196] Furthermore, treatment of embryonic kidneys from *Six1* knockout animals with gremlin restores ureteric bud branching morphogenesis, while heterozygous inactivation of *Bmp4* (*Bmp4*$^{+/-}$) also rescues ureteric bud branching morphogenesis and kidney development in Six1 knockout animals.[197] Taken together, the data indicate that interplay between Bmps, gremlin, and Six1 likely plays a key role in the regulation/modulation of ureteric bud growth and branching.[197]

Hepatocyte Growth Factor

Embryonic kidneys express HGF and its receptor Met.[165] Neutralizing anti-HGF antibodies inhibit the growth of the embryonic kidney and disrupt ureteric bud branching morphogenesis in serum-free organ culture.[165] These results support the notion that HGF is an important morphogen for the ureteric bud that is secreted from metanephric mesenchyme. However, kidney development appears to be unaffected up to embryonic day 14 in *Hgf* or *Met* knockout mice, which die around this time from liver failure.[198,199] Although HGF may act at later stages of ureteric bud branching morphogenesis, it is probably not critically important in the initial stages.

Epidermal Growth Factor Receptor Ligands

Epidermal growth factor (EGF), transforming growth factor α (TGFα), heparin-binding epidermal growth factor-like growth factor (HBEGF), amphiregulin, and betacellulin all bind and activate the EGF receptor.[200] TGFα is present in the embryonic kidney, and disruption of TGFα signaling by neutralizing antibodies results in a small, less well-developed kidney in organ culture.[201] As mentioned above, when mIMCD3 cells grown in collagen gels are co-cultured with embryonic kidney, the cells undergo branching morphogenesis. Unlike MDCK cells, which only undergo branching morphogenesis in the presence of HGF,[165,202] mIMCD3 cells respond to EGF receptor ligands as well.[65,68] Similar results are obtained with the UB cell three-dimensional culture system.[69] Moreover, *Met* (HGF receptor) knockout kidney epithelial cells grown in three-dimensional extracellular matrix (ECM) gels undergo *in vitro* tubulogenesis in response to EGF or TGFα.[203] A conditional deletion of *Met* from the ueteric bud results in kidneys with a reduced number of nephrons and increased epidermal growth factor (EGF) receptor expression.[83] Mice which lack both normal *Egfr* and *Met* signaling have decreased ureteric bud branching and small kidneys with a reduced number of glomeruli, suggesting that *Met* and *Egfr* can act cooperatively to regulate ureteric bud branching.[83] Although *Tgfα* knockout mice do not have a kidney phenotype,[204,205] knockout of the *EGF* receptor in mice with a certain genetic background leads to dilated collecting ducts and renal dysfunction.[206] These results suggest an important role for EGF receptor ligands in later collecting duct development.

Insulin-Like Growth Factors

In serum-free organ culture, the embryonic kidney produces insulin-like growth factors (IGFs) 1 and 2.[207] When neutralizing antibodies against IGFs are added to the culture, kidney growth is suppressed.[207] The ureteric bud expresses IGF1 receptor.[208] Addition of antisense oligonucleotides against IGF1 receptor to the embryonic kidney in organ culture leads to a small kidney with disrupted ureteric bud branching morphogenesis.[208] However, knockout mice for either *Igf1* or *Igf2* do not display a kidney phenotype.[209,210] Molecular redundancy may be part of the explanation; however, as with HGF, the apparent discrepancies between the *in vitro* and *in vivo* data need to be addressed experimentally.

Extracellular Matrix

Soluble growth factors are not the only molecules involved in ureteric bud branching morphogenesis. Cells of the ureteric bud are surrounded by ECM proteins, and to form branching tubules the cells must digest the ECM. Cells have receptors for ECM proteins, such as integrins, as well as other specific receptors. Integrins can transmit signals to cytosolic and intranuclear proteins in a fashion similar to growth factor receptors. The cell modifies its behavior in response to the combined signals from growth factors and ECM proteins.[211]

The importance of the specific composition of the ECM in kidney epithelial cell branching morphogenesis has been shown using the three-dimensional cell culture model. When MDCK cells are cultured in type I collagen gels in the presence of HGF, the cells undergo branching morphogenesis. When MDCK cells are suspended in growth factor-reduced Matrigel, a basement membrane protein mixture secreted by EHS sarcoma cells, HGF-induced tubulogenesis is inhibited.[212] By mixing individual Matrigel component proteins into type I collagen gels, it was found that collagen I, laminin, fibronectin, and entactin facilitate MDCK cell tubulogenesis, whereas collagen IV, vitronectin, and heparan sulfate proteoglycan inhibit it.[212] However, a mixture of type I collagen and Matrigel, not pure type I collagen, is the optimum ECM for UB cell (a cell line derived from embryonic kidney tissue) tubulogenesis. Interestingly, when these cells are cultured in growth factor-reduced Matrigel alone, UB cells develop into cystic structures (Figure 25.13).[69] Together with the fact that isolated ureteric buds can be cultured in an ECM containing Matrigel but not in pure type 1 collagen gels,[31] this indicates that ECM composition modulates tubulogenesis and branching morphogenesis.

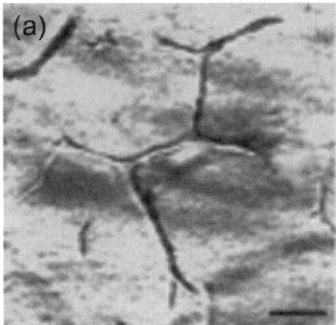 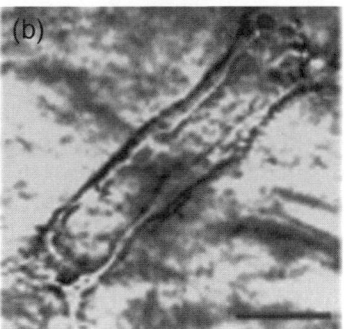 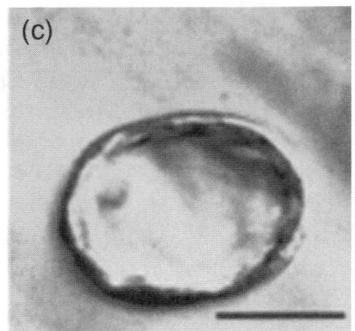

FIGURE 25.13 **Photomicrograph of ureteric bud (UB) cells cultured in three-dimensional extracellular matrix (ECM) gels.** In the presence of conditioned medium from metanephric mesenchyme cells, UB cells form branching cordlike structures in 3 to 5 days (a). In 10 to 15 days tubules with clear lumens can be observed (b). UB cells form multicellular cysts when cultured in pure Matrigel (c) instead of collagen I/Matrigel mixture (A and B) (Bars: 50 μm). *(from ref. [69]).*

Laminin

Laminins are the major component of the mature basement membrane. The role of laminin in epithelial branching morphogenesis has been shown in lung organ culture *in vitro*. Antilaminin antibodies perturb branching morphogenesis of embryonic lung in culture.[213] In the kidney, studies have shown a role for laminin in epithelial cell formation from the induced metanephric mesenchyme. It is known that antibodies against nidogen, a basement membrane protein secreted by mesenchymal cells, perturb epithelial morphogenesis in lung and kidney.[214] Nidogen binds to the γ1 chain of laminin. Thus, it is conceivable that the mesenchyme regulates epithelial branching morphogenesis through nidogen–laminin interaction. Moreover, knockouts of one of the laminin receptors, α3β1 integrin, result in decreased ureteric bud branching morphogenesis.[215] In *in vitro* whole organ culture and isolated ureteric bud culture, branching is inhibited in the presence of blocking antibodies against integrins α3, α6, β1 or β4. Interestingly, a common ligand for α3β1 and α6β4, laminin-5, is present in the developing ureteric bud, and its inhibition results in decreased branching in both whole embryonic kidney culture and isolated ureteric bud culture.[38]

Proteoglycans

Proteoglycans are protein molecules containing many bound glycosaminoglycan (GAG) chains.[216] The common GAG chains include chondroitin sulfate, dermatan sulfate, heparan sulfate, heparin, and keratan sulfate. Proteoglycans are mostly found at the cell surface or in the extracellular matrix. In embryonic kidneys, sulfated proteoglycans are concentrated around the tip of the ureteric bud, and perturbation of their synthesis by β-D-xyloside results in the inhibition of ureteric bud branching morphogenesis.[217,218] This perturbation also abolishes the expression of *Wnt11* at the tip of the ureteric bud.[219] As described previously, loss of *Wnt11* expression at the tip of the ureteric bud can lead to loss of *Gdnf* expression in the metanephric mesenchyme. However, the linking mechanism between inhibition of sulfated proteoglycan and the loss of *Wnt11* expression is unclear. Along the same lines, genetic inactivation of an enzyme, heparan sulfate 2-O-sulfotransferase, involved in heparan sulfate proteoglycan synthesis results in kidney agenesis.[53] In this case, the ureteric bud forms from the Wolffian duct, but subsequent invasion of the metanephric mesenchyme is perturbed. As for the mesenchyme, initial specification of the metanephric mesenchyme appears intact, but subsequent mesenchymal condensation is affected. Consistent with the *in vitro* result described above, heparan sulfate biosynthesis perturbation results in loss of *Wnt11* expression and reduced *Gdnf* expression. Given the fact that many growth factors that regulate branching morphogenesis of the ureteric bud are heparin (a heavily sulfated form of GAG chain)-binding, it is likely that global inhibition of GAG chain synthesis or its sulfation could compromise actions of these heparin-binding growth factors.

In contrast, inhibition of specific heparan sulfate proteoglycans results in less clear effects. One exception is *glypican* (*Gpc*) 3, a gene encoding a heparan sulfate proteoglycan linked to the cell surface via a glycosyl-phosphatidylinositol anchor. *Gpc3* knockout mice display enhanced ureteric branching and dysplastic kidneys.[220] *Gpc3* is expressed in the ureteric bud cells and modulates BMP and FGF action on the ureteric bud.[220] A potent angiogenesis inhibitor, endostatin, a breakdown product of extracellular proteoglycan, collagen XVIII, inhibits ureteric bud branching morphogenesis.[35] Interestingly, this action is likely to be mediated through its binding to glypicans.[35]

Although it is not a proteoglycan in the strict sense, because it lacks a protein core, hyaluronic acid (HA) also plays a role in branching morphogenesis. Synthetic enzymes for this GAG are expressed in the developing kidney, and the addition of HA to three-dimensional culture of UB cells promotes tubulogenesis and survival of cells. Blocking antibodies against its receptor CD44 abolishes this effect.[221] In addition, supplementation of cultures of isolated ureteric bud or whole kidneys with hyaluronidase inhibited branching morphogenesis.[222] Specific sizes and concentrations of HA were also found to act independently in regulating UB branching, and in tubular maturation.[222]

While the protein core of proteoglycans, particularly the heparan sufate proteoglycans, play important roles in many developmental and physiologic processes, most of the function of these proteoglycans are mediated by the variably sulfated heparan sulfate GAG chain. For example, mice deficient in heparan sufate 2-O sulfotransferase, a heparan sulfate biosynthetic enzyme, display renal agenesis.[53] As described above, this is likely due to a defect in the induction of the metanephric mesenchyme.[46] On the other hand, ureteric bud branching morphogenesis appears to be more dependent upon 6-O sulfated heparan sulfate.[47]

Fibrillin1

Fibrillin1 is made in the metanephric mesenchyme and binds to integrin $\alpha3\beta1$, which is expressed in the ureteric bud. Antisense oligonucleotides directed against this extracellular matrix molecule induce dysmorphogenesis of cultured metanephros,[223] suggesting a role for this protein in kidney development.

Extracellular Proteinases and their Inhibitors

The idea that ECM-degrading proteases are involved in branching morphogenesis is supported by work from *in vitro* three-dimensional culture and organ culture. Two classes of proteases appear to be involved: metalloproteases (MMPs) and serine proteases. In HGF-induced MDCK cell tubulogenesis, inhibitors of collagenase (MMP1) perturb the morphogenetic events when the cells are suspended in type I collagen gels.[224] The broadly active MMP inhibitor, 1,10-phenanthroline, inhibits TGFα- or HGF-induced mIMCD3 cell tubulogenesis in collagen gels.[68] Furthermore, tubulogenic growth factors, such as HGF or EGF receptor ligands, upregulate the expression of MMPs and urokinase in the epithelial cells as they undergo tubulogenesis.[68,71] Interestingly, in the case of long, non-

branching mIMCD3 cell tubules induced by HGF plus TGFβ, the balance between proteases (MMP1 and urokinase) and their inhibitors (TIMP1 and PAI1) expressed by mIMCD3 cells changes in parallel with tubular morphology.[67] In embryonic ureteric bud-derived UB cells, expression of MMPs and TIMPs changes in response to surrounding ECM and soluble factors.[34] These results suggest that tubulogenic growth factors act, at least in part, through changing the expression patterns of extracellular proteases and their inhibitors in *in vitro* tubulogenesis. It has also been shown that "tubulogenic ECM" and highly tubulogenic conditioned medium secreted by metanephric mesenchyme-derived cells contain MMP activity, and that the expression level of regulators for these MMPs in UB cells alters as branching morphogenesis progresses,[34] suggesting local control of proteolytic activity is important in the morphogenetic process. In the embryonic kidney in organ culture, antibodies against MMP9, but not MMP2, inhibit the branching morphogenesis of the ureteric bud.[225] Although *Mmp9* knockout mice do not show a kidney phenotype in some genetic backgrounds,[226] in the C57BL/6 background deletion of Mmp9 results in a ~30% reduction in nephron number.[227] This is most likely through its anti-apoptotic effect in the mesenchyme, and its ability to stimulate ureteric bud branching morphogenesis.[227] Both of these enzymes act as a gelatinase, which is required to digest ECMs in basement membranes. In another study, however, antisense oligonucleotides against mesenchymal MMP2 or epithelial cell surface-expressed membrane type (MT)1-MMP inhibit metanephrogenesis in organ culture.[228]

In summary, ureteric bud branching outgrowth and morphogenesis is modulated in large part by a combination of positive and negative soluble growth factors secreted by the metanephric mesenchyme that act synergistically. In many cases, these pathways are more parallel than interdependent. These growth factors subsequently regulate downstream effector molecules such as ECM or ECM-degrading proteinases (Figure 25.14).

TUBULOGENESIS AFTER INDUCTION OF THE METANEPHRIC MESENCHYME

Early mesenchymally-derived nephrons, which will go on to form Bowman's capsule, as well as the proximal and distal tubules, are induced in the metanephric mesenchyme by the ureteric bud. In the process, mesenchymal cells transform into epithelial cells. The induced epithelial cells differentiate into kidney tubules. This transformation can be induced by a number of inducer tissues other than the ureteric bud, including embryonic spinal cord, embryonic salivary

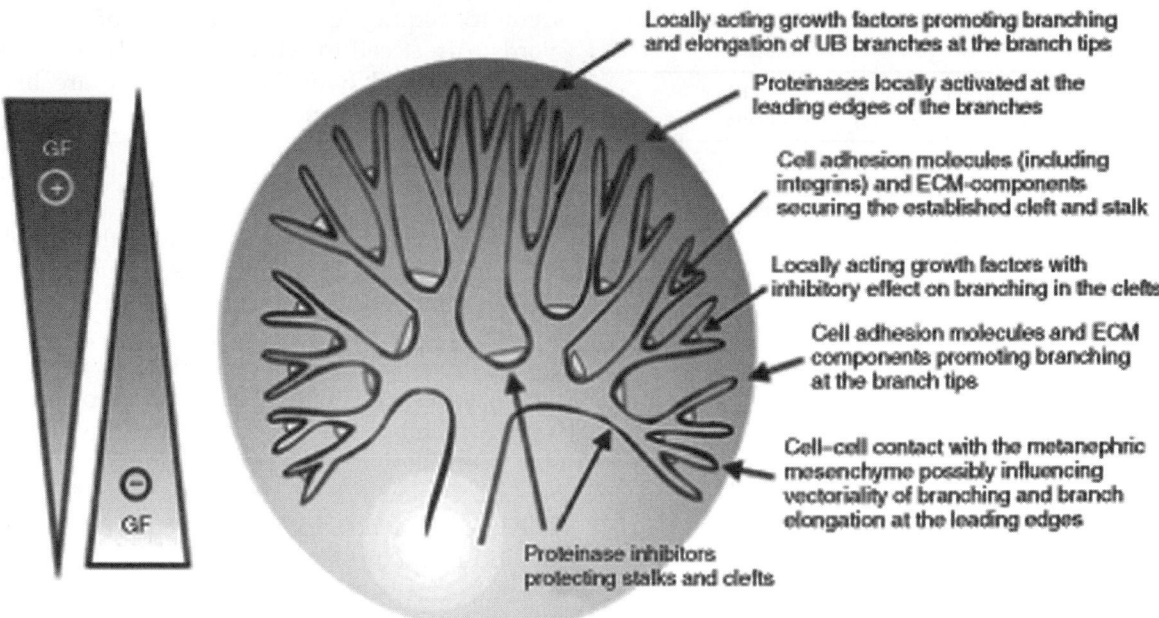

Locally acting growth factors promoting branching and elongation of UB branches at the branch tips

Proteinases locally activated at the leading edges of the branches

Cell adhesion molecules (including integrins) and ECM-components securing the established cleft and stalk

Locally acting growth factors with inhibitory effect on branching in the clefts

Cell adhesion molecules and ECM components promoting branching at the branch tips

Cell-cell contact with the metanephric mesenchyme possibly influencing vectoriality of branching and branch elongation at the leading edges

Proteinase inhibitors protecting stalks and clefts

FIGURE 25.14 Model for ureteric bud branching morphogenesis. After induction of the ureteric bud (UB), in which GDNF appears to play a critical role, branching may be guided by gradients of promoting (GF +) and inhibiting growth factors (GF −). Distal effector molecules probably include facilitating and inhibiting extracellular matrix (ECM) components, together with signal transducing–cell adhesion molecules such as integrins, CD44, membrane-bound proteinase activators such as MT1-MMP, and active proteinases (e.g., MMP9), as well as proteinase inhibitors such as TIMP3, which binds to the ECM and could protect the matrix around the stalks from degradation. *(Reprinted with permission from the* Annual Review of Physiology, *Volume 62* © *2000 by Annual Reviews www.annualreviews.org.)*

mesenchyme, and embryonic bone.[48,49,229] Many embryonic epithelial, neural or mesenchymal tissues can thus induce the metanephric mesenchyme, although various tissues have different potency. For example, brain can only induce metanephric mesenchyme to the condensation stage, while spinal cord can induce tubule formation.[230] Thus, it is conceivable that there are several steps in the induction process: (1) rescue of metanephric mesenchyme and/or later tubular structures from apoptosis; (2) mesenchymal cell condensation; (3) epithelial polarization and junction formation; and (4) tubule formation. The molecules likely involved in the process are summarized in Table 25.2.

Prevention of Apoptosis

During kidney tubule development, apoptosis is observed among cells surrounding newly formed epithelial tubules.[231] In fact, significant levels of apoptosis appear to be occurring in many parts of the kidney during development.[232] When the metanephric mesenchyme is cultured with inducer tissues or EGF, apoptosis becomes less prominent.[231,232] These results suggest that an important early signal from the inducer tissue prevents metanephric mesenchyme cell apoptosis. In *in vitro* culture of metanephric mesenchyme,

conditioned medium from UB cells also exhibits an anti-apoptotic effect.[233] One of the anti-apoptotic molecules in UB-conditioned medium is FGF2.[234] Consistent with these findings, RUB cell (derived from rat ureteric bud)-conditioned medium requires supplementation of FGF2 and TGFα to induce kidney tubule formation in the absence of inductive tissues.[235]

In addition, analysis of bone morphogenetic protein (*Bmp*)7-deficient mice suggests that BMP7 may act as an anti-apoptotic factor.[236,237] BMP7 belongs to the TGFβ superfamily and is expressed in the Wolffian duct, ureteric bud, and nephron structures after induction.[236] *Bmp7* knockout mice exhibit defects in eye and kidney development. Although there is a difference in the early kidney phenotype between knockout mice created by different groups, ureteric bud formation and initial induction appears unaffected; at least a few comma- and S-shaped bodies are observed at E12.5.[236,237] However, soon after this, both the ureteric bud and the metanephric mesenchyme start to degenerate, ultimately resulting in nonfunctioning disorganized kidneys. This raises the possibility that BMP7 maintains induced tubules, inhibiting them from apoptosis rather than directly inducing the metanephric mesenchyme.[236] On the other hand, *in vitro* application of BMP7 has been reported to induce E11.5 mouse metanephric mesenchyme to form epithelial glomeruli

TABLE 25.2 Molecules Likely to be Involved in Metanephric Mesenchyme Induction

Process	Transcription Factors	Soluble Factors	ECM/Other Molecules
Define	Wt1		
nephrogenic	Pax2		
mesenchyme	Six1 Six2 Sall1 high		
	Myc (uninduced MM)		
Rescue from apoptosis		FGF2, FGF8	
		EGFR ligands	
		BMP7	
Condensation/ epithelialization	Pax2	Wnt9b	Laminin
	Pax8	LIF	(γ1chain)/laminin receptor
	Nmyc	TGFβ2	(α6β1 integrin, nonmuscle dystroglycan)
	Foxd1	Lipocalin	
	Pod1	Wnt4	
	Pbx1		α8β1 integrin
Tubule formation	Hnf1 (proximal tubule)		Laminin (γ1chain)/laminin
	Brn1 (Henle, distal)		receptor

ECM: extracellular matrix; LIF: leukemia-inhibiting factor; TGF: transforming growth factor.

without inductive tissues.[238] Whether BMP7 directly induces the metanephric mesenchyme remains to be determined.

Molecules Involved in Metanephric Mesenchyme Induction and Nephron Tubule Formation

As discussed in the transcription factor section, certain transcription factors such as *Pax2*, *Wt1*, *Six1*, *Six2* or *Sall1* are necessary to retain competency of the metanephric mesenchyme to respond to the signals from the ureteric bud. Early experiments using transfilter co-culture of the metanephric mesenchyme with various inductive tissues defined several expected characteristics of "inductive molecules".[7] Experiments using different pore-size filters and multiple filters to separate the metanephric mesenchyme and inducer suggest that inductive molecules do not simply diffuse, rather, they

seem to require close association of cells. In other words, direct cell-to-cell contact and/or soluble molecules associated with the cell surface are likely to be required for induction. In fact, direct interaction between the inductive tissue and the metanephric mesenchyme cells have been observed through the filter pores by electron microscopy.[239]

However, *in vitro* work indicates that combinations of soluble factors are sufficient to induce tubulogenesis of the metanephric mesenchyme. Leukemia inhibitory factor (LIF), FGF2, and TGFβ[51] or this combination plus TGFβ2[52] can induce nephron tubules in metanephric mesenchyme cultured in the absence of inductive tissues. A member of the lipocalin superfamily, 24p3, has also been shown to induce epithelialization of metanephric mesenchyme in the presence of FGFs,[240] and to deliver iron to the cell (iron is required for mesenchymal induction by this molecule[240]).

Cell surface glycoproteins of the Wnt family are candidate molecules for coordinating morphogenesis at the interface of metanephric mesenchyme and inductive tissues, as WNT1-expressing fibroblasts induce the metanephric mesenchyme to form glomeruli.[241] Although the *Wnt1* gene is not expressed in embryonic kidneys,[242] this result raises the possibility of an important role for other Wnt family members in nephrogenesis. Another Wnt family member, *Wnt4*, is expressed in the embryonic kidneys; it first appears in condensed metanephric mesenchyme, and its expression continues in comma- and S-shaped bodies, finally becoming restricted to the area where newly formed epithelial tubules are connected to collecting ducts.[243] WNT9b, secreted from the ureteric bud, triggers mesenchymal epithelial transformation, as metanephric mesenchyme induction is not observed in *Wnt9b*$^{-/-}$ mice.[244] Six2, a transcription factor important for nephron progenitor maintenance, counteracts WNT9b signaling.[6] Downstream of WNT9b, WNT4 plays an important role in metanephric mesenchyme induction as an autocrine factor for metanephric mesenchymal cells.[244] The metanephric mesenchyme of mutant mice lacking the *Wnt4* gene is able to condense around the branching ureteric bud, but fails to form peritubular aggregates.[243] There is no apparent kidney tubule development in these knockout animals. The expression of markers for early mesenchymal induction, *Pax2* and *Nmyc*, does not seem to be affected in *Wnt4* mutant mice, suggesting that *Wnt4* acts at a later stage than *Pax2* or *Nmyc*. However, *Pax8* expression by metanephric mesenchyme-derived structures cannot be detected in the mutant mice.

Another autocrine factor for metanephric mesenchyme induction is FGF8. Site specific, conditional deletion of Fgf8, either in the metanephric mesenchyme[245] or in all mesodermal tissues,[179,246] results in hypolastic, dysmorphic kidneys displaying disruptions in nephron formation. Conditional deletion of both *Fgfr1* and *Fgfr2* from the metanephric mesenchyme results in renal dysgenesis, due to defects in the formation of the metanephric mesenchyme and early ureteric bud.[247]

The cell-surface-signaling molecule Notch has also been implicated in tubulogenesis. Binding of Notch by its ligands (Jagged1 (Jag1), Jag2, Delta-like (Dll) 1, Dll3 or Dll4)) results in the shedding of its extracellular domain, cleavage of its transmembrane domain by γ-secretase, and translocation of its intracellular domain to the nucleus where it promotes transcription of target genes (reviewed in [248–250]). *Notch 1, 2,* and *3* have been shown to be expressed in the developing kidney.[58,251–255] *Notch2* mutation leads to hypoplastic kidneys with glomerular defects,[256] while conditional deletion of *Notch2*, but not *Notch1*, causes the loss of glomeruli and proximal tubules.[248] However, proteolytic cleavage of Notch1 by γ-secretase is required for Notch activation, and this inhibition in kidney organ culture results in decreased S-shaped bodies despite having normal condensation.[257] Knockout and partial rescue of *Presenilin1* and *2* that are required for γ-secretase activity lead to a similar phenotype.[258] In addition, augmenting Notch1 signaling by inactivating Mint (an inhibitor of Notch-mediated transcription[250,259–262]) has the ability to partially rescue nephron development in Notch2 knockout kidneys.[250] Taken together, the data suggest that Notch1 and Notch2 likely act in concert to regulate proximal tubule and glomerular development.[250]

Extracellular matrix proteins are important for maintaining epithelial tubular structures. Much work has been done on the basement membrane glycoprotein laminin and the integrins that bind laminin. Laminin1 is composed of three chains: α1; β1; and γ1. Of these, β1- and γ1-expression increases early (day 1) when the metanephric mesenchyme is induced, while the α1 chain is expressed after epithelial cell polarization begins.[263,264] The laminin α1 chain is exclusively expressed by the epithelial cells,[263] and perturbation of this chain by antibodies inhibits kidney tubulogenesis *in vitro*.[265] The kidney epithelial cell has at least two laminin receptors: $\alpha_6\beta_1$ integrin and nonmuscle dystroglycan. Perturbation of these receptors inhibits kidney tubulogenesis *in vitro*.[38,266] Moreover, in *in vitro* culture of embryonic lung, it has been demonstrated that heterotypic cell-to-cell contact between epithelial cells and mesenchymal cells is required to synthesize the laminin α_1 chain.[267] If this result is applicable to embryonic kidney, further differentiation after cell-to-cell contact may be a function of expression of the laminin α_1 chain.

In addition to laminin-binding integrins, knockouts of integrin α8 have been shown to produce severe defects in kidney development.[268] The ureteric bud initiation and initial mesenchymal induction appear unaffected; the metanephric mesenchyme cells condense around the ureteric bud and start to express *Pax2* and p75 NGFR. However, further steps toward epithelialization and tubule formation are not observed. In normal mice, α8β1 integrin is transiently expressed in the condensing mesenchymal cells. Both spatiotemporal localization and knockout phenotype suggest that $\alpha_8\beta_1$ integrin plays an important role after the initial induction step of mesenchymal–epithelial transformation.

Evidence is beginning to accumulate on the functional maturation of the kidney tubules. Kidney tubules further differentiate into several segments. In each segment the tubular cells express different sets of transporters. For example, Northern blot analysis shows that the organic anion transporter Oat1 begins to be expressed at around E16 kidney.[269] It is likely that expression of many transporters, characteristic of mature tubules, is tightly regulated. In this regard, elucidation of the roles of transcription factors *Hnf1* (proximal tubules) and *Brn1* (Henle's loop and distal tubule) is important, and other unknown factors may be involved in this process.

VASCULAR AND GLOMERULAR DEVELOPMENT

The origin of glomerular endothelial cells and mesangial cells, and how the vascular system is integrated in the developing kidney, has been an area of controversy for years (reviewed in[13]). Vascular development occurs by: (1) angiogenesis, in which new vessels arise from existing vasculature; and/or (2) vasculogenesis, in which *de novo* endothelial cells are formed. As mentioned previously, *in vitro* kidney organ culture gives rise to epithelial glomerular structures, not mesangial cells nor endothelial cells, suggesting that either the culture conditions are not suitable for endothelial cell growth or there are no angioblasts in the metanephric mesenchyme. To study kidney vascular development, interspecies grafting techniques have been used in which E11 murine embryonic kidneys are transplanted into chick chorioallantoic-membranes (CAM).[270] When E11 mouse kidneys, which have no apparent vascular development, are grown in chick CAM, the kidneys form glomeruli containing blood vessels from the chick, as determined by staining with species-specific antibodies against basement membranes.[271,272] However, when E11 mouse kidneys are grafted into the rat anterior eye chamber, newly formed glomerular endothelial cells appear to be derived from the graft.[273] Moreover, the same group has demonstrated that vascular endothelial cell growth factor (Vegf) receptor FLK1-positive cells are found in the E12 mouse kidney, and these cells are likely to be angioblasts, which differentiate into blood vessels in the glomeruli.[274] Thus, depending on the culture and grafting conditions, glomerular capillaries can be derived by an angiogenic process (i.e., outside of the metanephric mesenchyme or a vasculogenic process; inside of the metanephric mesenchyme). Which of these processes is more important *in vivo* remains uncertain, and it is of course possible that both are important.

The origin of mesangial cells also remains uncertain, although it has been recently proposed that they are derived from cap mesenchymal cells.[6,275] In the aforementioned different kidney graft systems, mesangial cells appear to behave similarly to glomerular endothelial cells: in CAM grafts, the mesangial cells are derived from the hosts[276,277]; while in the anterior eye chamber grafts, they are derived from the grafts.[273] Platelet-derived growth factor (*Pdgf*)-B receptor knockout mice do not have mesangial cells, and exhibited dilated capillary loops resulting in defective glomeruli.[278,279]

Recently, genetic fate tracing of *Six2*-positive nephron progenitor cells revealed that neither vasucular endothelial cells nor mesangial cells are derived from nephron progenitors.[280] This does not mean that blood vessel and mesangial cells are extrarenal in origin, because metanephric mesenchyme contains non-nephron progenitor cells. Nevertheless, it should be noted that endothelial and mesangial cells and nephron epithelial cells are derived from distinct sources.

In addition, deletion of *Crim1*, a transmembrane protein expressed in mesangial cells and podocytes, was found to induce abnormal glomerular development, characterized by simplified glomerular capillary networks with dilated capillaries.[281–283] Together with the observed mislocalization of Vegf-A, as well as increased activation of Flk1, *Crim1* appears to regulate the spatial distribution of Vegf-A during glomerular development.[282] Knockout of Semaphorin3a (*Sema3a*) also disrupts kidney vascular patterning.[101,284,285] Decreased apoptosis of endothelial cells is observed in kidneys from *Sema3a* knockout animals, while whole organ culture also indicates that Sema3a is a chemorepellant and inhibits endothelial cell migration.[101,284,285] Together with the fact that Vegf-A promotes endothelial cell survival and acts as a chemoattractant for endothelial cells,[286,287] the data suggest that endothelial cell number and vascular patterning is regulated by a balance of Vegf-A and Sema3a signaling.[284,285]

TERMINATION OF KIDNEY DEVELOPMENT

Despite the wealth of literature describing the molecules and mechanisms regulating the various morphogenetic processes involved in the development of the metanephric kidney, how the overall process is brought to an end has received little attention. In humans, kidney organogenesis is complete before birth; however, in other mammals, including rats and mice, kidney development continues into the postnatal period. Examination of this postnatal period in mice reveals the loss of nephrogenic mesenchyme by day three after birth.[288] This was not due to an increase in apoptosis, but rather appeared to result from the synchronous conversion of the remaining nephrogenic mesenchyme into new nephrons.[288] Since, during this time, the ureteric bud tips retain the capacity to induce nephrogenesis *in vitro*, this indicates that this loss of nephrogeneic mesenchyme demarcates the beginning of the end of kidney development.[288] This time period also correlates with the observed sudden burst in the expression of many genes involved in redox metabolism and transport, including multispecific drug transporters such as Oat1 and Oct1.[75] Together, the data suggest that parturition and the end of kidney development is characterized by rapid changes in: (1) the remaining metanephric mesenchyme, leading to the formation of new nephrons (which completes metanephrogenesis and sets the final nephron number); and (2) the differentiation state of existing nephrons.[75,288]

Acknowledgments

The authors thank Dr. Wei Wu for providing valuable comments on this manuscript. S. K. Nigam is funded by the National Institutes of Health.

References

[1] Bouchard M, Souabni A, Mandler M, Neubuser A, Busslinger M. Nephric lineage specification by Pax2 and Pax8. Genes Dev 2002;16(22):2958–70.

[2] Mauch TJ, Yang G, Wright M, Smith D, Schoenwolf GC. Signals from trunk paraxial mesoderm induce pronephros formation in chick intermediate mesoderm. Dev Biol 2000;220(1):62–75.

[3] Obara-Ishihara T, Kuhlman J, Niswander L, Herzlinger D. The surface ectoderm is essential for nephric duct formation in intermediate mesoderm. Development 1999;126(6):1103–8.

[4] Vize PD, Seufert DW, Carroll TJ, Wallingford JB. Model systems for the study of kidney development: use of the pronephros in the analysis of organ induction and patterning. Dev Biol 1997;188(2):189–204.

[5] Smith C, Mackay S. Morphological development and fate of the mouse mesonephros. J Anat 1991;174:171–84.

[6] Kobayashi A, Valerius MT, Mugford JW, Carroll TJ, Self M, Oliver G, et al. Six2 defines and regulates a multipotent self-renewing nephron progenitor population throughout mammalian kidney development. Cell Stem Cell 2008;3(2):169–81.

[7] Saxen L, Organogenesis of the Kidney. In: Barlow P, Green P, White C, editors. Cambridge, U.K.: Cambridge University Press; 1987; 184.

[8] Costantini F. GDNF/Ret signaling and renal branching morphogenesis: from mesenchymal signals to epithelial cell behaviors. Organogenesis 2010;6(4):252—62.

[9] Sajithlal G, Zou D, Silvius D, Xu PX. Eya 1 acts as a critical regulator for specifying the metanephric mesenchyme. Dev Biol 2005;284(2):323—36.

[10] Osathanondh V, Potter EL. Development of human kidney as shown by microdissection. III. Formation and interrelationship of collecting tubules and nephrons. Arch Pathol 1963; 76:290—302.

[11] Osathanondh V, Potter EL. Development of human kidney as shown by microdissection. II. Renal pelvis, calyces, and papillae. Arch Pathol 1963;76:277—89.

[12] Osathanondh V, Potter EL. Development of human kidney as shown by microdissection. V. Development of vascular pattern of glomerulus. Arch Pathol 1966;82(5):403—11.

[13] Sequeira Lopez ML, Gomez RA. Development of the renal arterioles. J Am Soc Nephrol 2011;22(12):2156—65.

[14] Grobstein C. Morphogenetic interaction between embryonic mouse tissues separated by a membrane filter. Nature 1953;172 (4384):869—70.

[15] Grobstein C. Inductive epitheliomesenchymal interaction in cultured organ rudiments of the mouse. Science 1953;118(3054): 52—5.

[16] Grobstein C. Inductive tissue interaction in development. Adv Cancer Res 1956;4:187—236.

[17] Ekblom P, Thesleff I, Miettinen A, Saxen L. Organogenesis in a defined medium supplemented with transferrin. Cell Differ 1981;10(5):281—8.

[18] Laitinen L, Virtanen I, Saxen L. Changes in the glycosylation pattern during embryonic development of mouse kidney as revealed with lectin conjugates. J Histochem Cytochem 1987;35 (1):55—65.

[19] Durbeej M, Soderstrom S, Ebendal T, Birchmeier C, Ekblom P. Differential expression of neurotrophin receptors during renal development. Development 1993;119(4):977—89.

[20] Davies JA, Ladomery M, Hohenstein P, Michael L, Shafe A, Spraggon L, et al. Development of an siRNA-based method for repressing specific genes in renal organ culture and its use to show that the Wt1 tumour suppressor is required for nephron differentiation. Hum Mol Genet 2004;13(2):235—46.

[21] Sakai T, Larsen M, Yamada KM. Fibronectin requirement in branching morphogenesis. Nature 2003;423(6942):876—81.

[22] Brophy PD, Ostrom L, Lang KM, Dressler GR. Regulation of ureteric bud outgrowth by Pax2-dependent activation of the glial derived neurotrophic factor gene. Development 2001;128 (23):4747—56.

[23] Maeshima A, Sakurai H, Choi Y, Kitamura S, Vaughn DA, Tee JB, et al. Glial cell-derived neurotrophic factor independent ureteric bud outgrowth from the Wolffian duct. J Am Soc Nephrol 2007;18(12):3147—55.

[24] Maeshima A, Vaughn DA, Choi Y, Nigam SK. Activin A is an endogenous inhibitor of ureteric bud outgrowth from the Wolffian duct. Dev Biol 2006;295(2):473—85.

[25] Rosines E, Sampogna RV, Johkura K, Vaughn DA, Choi Y, Sakurai H, et al. Staged in vitro reconstitution and implantation of engineered rat kidney tissue. Proc Natl Acad Sci USA 2007;104(52):20938—43.

[26] Tang MJ, Cai Y, Tsai SJ, Wang YK, Dressler GR. Ureteric bud outgrowth in response to RET activation is mediated by phosphatidylinositol 3-kinase. Dev Biol 2002;243(1):128—36.

[27] Bush KT, Vaughn DA, Li X, Rosenfeld MG, Rose DW, Mendoza SA, et al. Development and differentiation of the ureteric bud into the ureter in the absence of a kidney collecting system. Dev Biol 2006;298(2):571—84.

[28] Choi Y, Tee JB, Gallegos TF, Shah MM, Oishi H, Sakurai H, et al. Neuropeptide Y functions as a facilitator of GDNF-induced budding of the Wolffian duct. Development 2009;136(24): 4213—24.

[29] Rosines E, Johkura K, Zhang X, Schmidt HJ, Decambre M, Bush KT, et al. Constructing kidney-like tissues from cells based on programs for organ development: toward a method of in vitro tissue engineering of the kidney. Tissue Eng Part A 2010;6 (18):2441—55.

[30] Tee JB, Choi Y, Shah MM, Dnyanmote A, Sweeney DE, Gallegos TF, et al. Protein kinase A regulates GDNF/RET-dependent but not GDNF/Ret-independent ureteric bud outgrowth from the Wolffian duct. Dev Biol 2010;347(2):337—47.

[31] Qiao J, Sakurai H, Nigam SK. Branching morphogenesis independent of mesenchymal-epithelial contact in the developing kidney. Proc Natl Acad Sci USA 1999;96(13):7330—5.

[32] Meyer TN, Schwesinger C, Bush KT, Stuart RO, Rose DW, Shah MM, et al. Spatiotemporal regulation of morphogenetic molecules during in vitro branching of the isolated ureteric bud: toward a model of branching through budding in the developing kidney. Dev Biol 2004;275(1):44—67.

[33] Li Z, Stuart RO, Qiao J, Pavlova A, Bush KT, Pohl M, et al. A role for Timeless in epithelial morphogenesis during kidney development. Proc Natl Acad Sci USA 2000;97(18):10038—43.

[34] Pohl M, Sakurai H, Bush KT, Nigam SK. Matrix metalloproteinases and their inhibitors regulate in vitro ureteric bud branching morphogenesis. Am J Physiol Renal Physiol 2000;279(5): F891—900.

[35] Karihaloo A, Karumanchi SA, Barasch J, Jha V, Nickel CH, Yang J, et al. Endostatin regulates branching morphogenesis of renal epithelial cells and ureteric bud. Proc Natl Acad Sci USA 2001;98(22):12509—14.

[36] Qiao J, Bush KT, Steer DL, Stuart RO, Sakurai H, Wachsman W, et al. Multiple fibroblast growth factors support growth of the ureteric bud but have different effects on branching morphogenesis. Mech Dev 2001;109(2):123—35.

[37] Sakurai H, Bush KT, Nigam SK. Identification of pleiotrophin as a mesenchymal factor involved in ureteric bud branching morphogenesis. Development 2001;128(17):3283—93.

[38] Zent R, Bush KT, Pohl ML, Quaranta V, Koshikawa N, Wang Z, et al. Involvement of laminin binding integrins and laminin-5 in branching morphogenesis of the ureteric bud during kidney development. Dev Biol 2001;238(2):289—302.

[39] Stuart RO, Bush KT, Nigam SK. Changes in gene expression patterns in the ureteric bud and metanephric mesenchyme in models of kidney development. Kidney Int 2003;64(6): 1997—2008.

[40] Bush KT, Sakurai H, Steer DL, Leonard MO, Sampogna RV, Meyer TN, et al. TGF-beta superfamily members modulate growth, branching, shaping, and patterning of the ureteric bud. Dev Biol 2004;266(2):285—98.

[41] Steer DL, Shah MM, Bush KT, Stuart RO, Sampogna RV, Meyer TN, et al. Regulation of ureteric bud branching morphogenesis by sulfated proteoglycans in the developing kidney. Dev Biol 2004;272(2):310—27.

[42] Sakurai H, Bush KT, Nigam SK. Heregulin induces glial cell line-derived neurotrophic growth factor-independent, non-branching growth and differentiation of ureteric bud epithelia. J Biol Chem 2005;280(51):42181—7.

[43] Meyer TN, Schwesinger C, Sampogna RV, Vaughn DA, Stuart RO, Steer DL, et al. Rho kinase acts at separate steps in ureteric bud and metanephric mesenchyme morphogenesis during kidney development. Differentiation 2006;74(9-10):638—47.

[44] Shah MM, Tee JB, Meyer T, Meyer-Schwesinger C, Choi Y, Sweeney DE, et al. The instructive role of metanephric

mesenchyme in ureteric bud patterning, sculpting, and maturation and its potential ability to buffer ureteric bud branching defects. Am J Physiol Renal Physiol 2009;297(5):F1330—41.

[45] Wu W, Kitamura S, Truong DM, Rieg T, Vallon V, Sakurai H, et al. Beta1-integrin is required for kidney collecting duct morphogenesis and maintenance of renal function. Am J Physiol Renal Physiol 2009;297(1):F210—7.

[46] Shah MM, Sakurai H, Sweeney DE, Gallegos TF, Bush KT, Esko JD, et al. Hs2st mediated kidney mesenchyme induction regulates early ureteric bud branching. Dev Biol 2010;339(2):354—65.

[47] Shah MM, Sakurai H, Gallegos TF, Sweeney DE, Bush KT, Esko JD, et al. Growth factor-dependent branching of the ureteric bud is modulated by selective 6-O sulfation of heparan sulfate. Dev Biol 2011;356(1):19—27.

[48] Grobstein C. Trans-filter induction of tubules in mouse metanephrogenic mesenchyme. Exp Cell Res 1956;10(2):424—40.

[49] Saxen L, Lehtonen E. Embryonic kidney in organ culture. Differentiation 1987;36(1):2—11.

[50] Lehtonen E, Wartiovaara J, Nordling S, Saxen L. Demonstration of cytoplasmic processes in Millipore filters permitting kidney tubule induction. J Embryol Exp Morphol 1975; 33(1):187—203.

[51] Barasch J, Yang J, Ware CB, Taga T, Yoshida K, Erdjument-Bromage H, et al. Mesenchymal to epithelial conversion in rat metanephros is induced by LIF. Cell 1999;99(4):377—86.

[52] Plisov SY, Yoshino K, Dove LF, Higinbotham KG, Rubin JS, Perantoni AO. TGF beta 2, LIF and FGF2 cooperate to induce nephrogenesis. Development 2001;128(7):1045—57.

[53] Bullock SL, Fletcher JM, Beddington RS, Wilson VA. Renal agenesis in mice homozygous for a gene trap mutation in the gene encoding heparan sulfate 2-sulfotransferase. Genes Dev 1998;12(12):1894—906.

[54] Capecchi MR. Altering the genome by homologous recombination. Science 1989;244(4910):1288—92.

[55] Capecchi MR. Targeted gene replacement. Sci Am 1994;270 (3):52—9.

[56] Galli-Taliadoros LA, Sedgwick JD, Wood SA, Korner H. Gene knock-out technology: a methodological overview for the interested novice. J Immunol Methods 1995;181(1):1—15.

[57] Lechner MS, Dressler GR. The molecular basis of embryonic kidney development. Mech Dev 1997;62(2):105—20.

[58] Yu J, McMahon AP, Valerius MT. Recent genetic studies of mouse kidney development. Curr Opin Genet Dev 2004;14 (5):550—7.

[59] Miyamoto N, Yoshida M, Kuratani S, Matsuo I, Aizawa S. Defects of urogenital development in mice lacking Emx2. Development 1997;124(9):1653—64.

[60] Ly JP, Onay T, Quaggin SE. Mouse models to study kidney development, function and disease. Curr Opin Nephrol Hypertens 2011;20(4):382—90.

[61] Birling MC, Gofflot F, Warot X. Site-specific recombinases for manipulation of the mouse genome. Methods Mol Biol 2009;561:245—63.

[62] Gawlik A, Quaggin SE. Deciphering the renal code: advances in conditional gene targeting. Physiology (Bethesda) 2004;19: 245—52.

[63] Zhang X, Mernaugh G, Yang DH, Gewin L, Srichai MB, Harris RC, et al. beta1 integrin is necessary for ureteric bud branching morphogenesis and maintenance of collecting duct structural integrity. Development 2009;136(19):3357—66.

[64] Santos OF, Moura LA, Rosen EM, Nigam SK. Modulation of HGF-induced tubulogenesis and branching by multiple phosphorylation mechanisms. Dev Biol 1993;159(2):535—48.

[65] Barros EJ, Santos OF, Matsumoto K, Nakamura T, Nigam SK. Differential tubulogenic and branching morphogenetic activities

of growth factors: implications for epithelial tissue development. Proc Natl Acad Sci USA 1995;92(10):4412—6.

[66] Cantley LG, Barros EJ, Gandhi M, Rauchman M, Nigam SK. Regulation of mitogenesis, motogenesis, and tubulogenesis by hepatocyte growth factor in renal collecting duct cells. Am J Physiol 1994;267(2 Pt 2):F271—80.

[67] Sakurai H, Nigam SK. Transforming growth factor-beta selectively inhibits branching morphogenesis but not tubulogenesis. Am J Physiol 1997;272(1 Pt 2):F139—46.

[68] Sakurai H, Tsukamoto T, Kjelsberg CA, Cantley LG, Nigam SK. EGF receptor ligands are a large fraction of in vitro branching morphogens secreted by embryonic kidney. Am J Physiol 1997; 273(3 Pt 2):F463—72.

[69] Sakurai H, Barros EJ, Tsukamoto T, Barasch J, Nigam SK. An in vitro tubulogenesis system using cell lines derived from the embryonic kidney shows dependence on multiple soluble growth factors. Proc Natl Acad Sci USA 1997;94(12):6279—84.

[70] Zegers MM, O'Brien LE, Yu W, Datta A, Mostov KE. Epithelial polarity and tubulogenesis in vitro. Trends Cell Biol 2003;13 (4):169—76.

[71] Stuart RO, Barros EJ, Ribeiro E, Nigam SK. Epithelial tubulogenesis through branching morphogenesis: relevance to collecting system development. J Am Soc Nephrol 1995;6(4):1151—9.

[72] Stuart RO, Bush KT, Nigam SK. Changes in global gene expression patterns during development and maturation of the rat kidney. Proc Natl Acad Sci USA 2001;98(10):5649—54.

[73] Tsigelny IF, Kouznetsova VL, Sweeney DE, Wu W, Bush KT, Nigam SK. Analysis of metagene portraits reveals distinct transitions during kidney organogenesis. Sci Signal 2008;1 (49):ra16.

[74] Schmidt-Ott KM, Masckauchan TN, Chen X, Hirsh BJ, Sarkar A, Yang J, et al. Beta-catenin/TCF/Lef controls a differentiation-associated transcriptional program in renal epithelial progenitors. Development 2007;134(17):3177—90.

[75] Sweeney DE, Vallon V, Rieg T, Wu W, Gallegos TF, Nigam SK. Functional maturation of drug transporters in the developing, neonatal, and postnatal kidney. Mol Pharmacol 2011;80 (1):147—54.

[76] Brunskill EW, Aronow BJ, Georgas K, Rumballe B, Valerius MT, Aronow J, et al. Atlas of gene expression in the developing kidney at microanatomic resolution. Dev Cell 2008;15(5): 781—91.

[77] Georgas KM, Chiu HS, Lesieur E, Rumballe BA, Little MH. Expression of metanephric nephron-patterning genes in differentiating mesonephric tubules. Dev Dyn 2011;240(6):1600—12.

[78] Harding SD, Armit C, Armstrong J, Brennan J, Cheng Y, Haggarty B, et al. The GUDMAP database—an online resource for genitourinary research. Development 2011;138(13):2845—53.

[79] Little MH, Brennan J, Georgas K, Davies JA, Davidson DR, Baldock RA, et al. A high-resolution anatomical ontology of the developing murine genitourinary tract. Gene Expr Patterns 2007;7(6):680—99.

[80] McMahon AP, Aronow BJ, Davidson DR, Davies JA, Gaido KW, Grimmond S, et al. GUDMAP: the genitourinary developmental molecular anatomy project. J Am Soc Nephrol 2008;19(4): 667—71.

[81] Nigam SK, Shah MM. How does the ureteric bud branch? J Am Soc Nephrol 2009;20(7):1465—9.

[82] Sampogna RV, Nigam SK. Implications of gene networks for understanding resilience and vulnerability in the kidney branching program. Physiology (Bethesda) 2004;19:339—47.

[83] Ishibe S, Karihaloo A, Ma H, Zhang J, Marlier A, Mitobe M, et al. Met and the epidermal growth factor receptor act cooperatively to regulate final nephron number and maintain collecting duct morphology. Development 2009;136(2):337—45.

[84] Pastorelli LM, Wells S, Fray M, Smith A, Hough T, Harfe BD, et al. Genetic analyses reveal a requirement for Dicer1 in the mouse urogenital tract. Mamm Genome 2009;20(3): 140−51.

[85] Patel SR, Kim D, Levitan I, Dressler GR. The BRCT-domain containing protein PTIP links PAX2 to a histone H3, lysine 4 methyltransferase complex. Dev Cell 2007;13(4): 580−92.

[86] Nagalakshmi VK, Ren Q, Pugh MM, Valerius MT, McMahon AP, Yu J. Dicer regulates the development of nephrogenic and ureteric compartments in the mammalian kidney. Kidney Int 2011;79(3):317−30.

[87] Harvey SJ, Jarad G, Cunningham J, Goldberg S, Schermer B, Harfe BD, et al. Podocyte-specific deletion of dicer alters cytoskeletal dynamics and causes glomerular disease. J Am Soc Nephrol 2008;19(11):2150−8.

[88] Ho J, Ng KH, Rosen S, Dostal A, Gregory RI, Kreidberg JA. Podocyte-specific loss of functional microRNAs leads to rapid glomerular and tubular injury. J Am Soc Nephrol 2008;19(11): 2069−75.

[89] Ho JJ, Marsden PA. Dicer cuts the kidney. J Am Soc Nephrol 2008;19(11):2043−6.

[90] Saal S, Harvey SJ. MicroRNAs and the kidney: coming of age. Curr Opin Nephrol Hypertens 2009;18(4):317−23.

[91] Shi S, Yu L, Chiu C, Sun Y, Chen J, Khitrov G, et al. Podocyte-selective deletion of dicer induces proteinuria and glomerulosclerosis. J Am Soc Nephrol 2008;19(11):2159−69.

[92] Tang KF, Song GB, Shi YS, Yuan L, Li YH. Dicer knockdown induces fibronectin-1 expression in HEK293T cells via induction of Egr1. Biochim Biophys Acta 2010;1800(3):380−4.

[93] Wei Q, Bhatt K, He HZ, Mi QS, Haase VH, Dong Z. Targeted deletion of Dicer from proximal tubules protects against renal ischemia-reperfusion injury. J Am Soc Nephrol 2010;21(5): 756−61.

[94] Monte JC, Sakurai H, Bush KT, Nigam SK. The developmental nephrome: systems biology in the developing kidney. Curr Opin Nephrol Hypertens 2007;16(1):3−9.

[95] Nigam SK. From the ureteric bud to the penome. Kidney Int 2003;64(6):2320−2.

[96] Costantini F, Kopan R. Patterning a complex organ: branching morphogenesis and nephron segmentation in kidney development. Dev Cell 2010;18(5):698−712.

[97] Dressler GR. Patterning and early cell lineage decisions in the developing kidney: the role of Pax genes. Pediatr Nephrol 2011;26(9):1387−94.

[98] Little M, Georgas K, Pennisi D, Wilkinson L. Kidney development: two tales of tubulogenesis. Curr Top Dev Biol 2010; 90:193−229.

[99] Miner JH. Organogenesis of the kidney glomerulus: focus on the glomerular basement membrane. Organogenesis 2011;7 (2):75−82.

[100] Chapin HC, Caplan MJ. The cell biology of polycystic kidney disease. J Cell Biol 2010;191(4):701−10.

[101] Reidy KJ, Rosenblum ND. Cell and molecular biology of kidney development. Semin Nephrol 2009;29(4):321−37.

[102] Davis AP, Witte DP, Hsieh-Li HM, Potter SS, Capecchi MR. Absence of radius and ulna in mice lacking hoxa-11 and hoxd-11. Nature 1995;375(6534):791−5.

[103] Wellik DM, Hawkes PJ, Capecchi MR. Hox11 paralogous genes are essential for metanephric kidney induction. Genes Dev 2002;16(11):1423−32.

[104] Dressler GR, Deutsch U, Chowdhury K, Nornes HO, Gruss P. Pax2, a new murine paired-box-containing gene and its expression in the developing excretory system. Development 1990; 109(4):787−95.

[105] Dressler GR, Douglass EC. Pax-2 is a DNA-binding protein expressed in embryonic kidney and Wilms tumor. Proc Natl Acad Sci USA 1992;89(4):1179−83.

[106] Torres M, Gomez-Pardo E, Dressler GR, Gruss P. Pax-2 controls multiple steps of urogenital development. Development 1995;121(12):4057−65.

[107] Plachov D, Chowdhury K, Walther C, Simon D, Guenet JL, Gruss P. Pax8, a murine paired box gene expressed in the developing excretory system and thyroid gland. Development 1990;110(2):643−51.

[108] Mansouri A, Chowdhury K, Gruss P. Follicular cells of the thyroid gland require Pax8 gene function. Nat Genet 1998;19 (1):87−90.

[109] Narlis M, Grote D, Gaitan Y, Boualia SK, Bouchard M. Pax2 and pax8 regulate branching morphogenesis and nephron differentiation in the developing kidney. J Am Soc Nephrol 2007;18(4):1121−9.

[110] Wawersik S, Purcell P, Maas RL. Pax6 and the genetic control of early eye development. Results Probl Cell Differ 2000; 31:15−36.

[111] Xu PX, Adams J, Peters H, Brown MC, Heaney S, Maas R. Eya1-deficient mice lack ears and kidneys and show abnormal apoptosis of organ primordia. Nat Genet 1999;23(1):113−7.

[112] Li X, Oghi KA, Zhang J, Krones A, Bush KT, Glass CK, et al. Eya protein phosphatase activity regulates Six1-Dach-Eya transcriptional effects in mammalian organogenesis. Nature 2003;426(6964):247−54.

[113] Xu PX, Zheng W, Huang L, Maire P, Laclef C, Silvius D. Six1 is required for the early organogenesis of mammalian kidney. Development 2003;130(14):3085−94.

[114] Gong KQ, Yallowitz AR, Sun H, Dressler GR, Wellik DM. A Hox-Eya-Pax complex regulates early kidney developmental gene expression. Mol Cell Biol 2007;27(21):7661−8.

[115] Nishinakamura R, Matsumoto Y, Nakao K, Nakamura K, Sato A, Copeland NG, et al. Murine homolog of SALL1 is essential for ureteric bud invasion in kidney development. Development 2001;128(16):3105−15.

[116] Kiefer SM, Robbins L, Stumpff KM, Lin C, Ma L, Rauchman M. Sall1-dependent signals affect Wnt signaling and ureter tip fate to initiate kidney development. Development 2010;137 (18):3099−106.

[117] Nishinakamura R, Osafune K. Essential roles of Sall family genes in kidney development. J Physiol Sci 2006;56(2):131−6.

[118] Kume T, Deng K, Hogan BL. Murine forkhead/winged helix genes Foxc1 (Mf1) and Foxc2 (Mfh1) are required for the early organogenesis of the kidney and urinary tract. Development 2000;127(7):1387−95.

[119] Fujii T, Pichel JG, Taira M, Toyama R, Dawid IB, Westphal H. Expression patterns of the murine LIM class homeobox gene lim1 in the developing brain and excretory system. Dev Dyn 1994;199(1):73−83.

[120] Shawlot W, Behringer RR. Requirement for Lim1 in head-organizer function. Nature 1995;374(6521):425−30.

[121] Tsang TE, Shawlot W, Kinder SJ, Kobayashi A, Kwan KM, Schughart K, et al. Lim1 activity is required for intermediate mesoderm differentiation in the mouse embryo. Dev Biol 2000;223(1):77−90.

[122] Drummond IA, Madden SL, Rohwer-Nutter P, Bell GI, Sukhatme VP, Rauscher III FJ. Repression of the insulin-like growth factor II gene by the Wilms tumor suppressor WT1. Science 1992;257(5070):674−8.

[123] Werner H, Re GG, Drummond IA, Sukhatme VP, Rauscher III FJ, Sens DA, et al. Increased expression of the insulin-like growth factor I receptor gene, IGF1R, in Wilms tumor is correlated with modulation of IGF1R promoter activity by the WT1

Wilms tumor gene product. Proc Natl Acad Sci USA 1993;90 (12):5828–32.

[124] Ryan G, Steele-Perkins V, Morris JF, Rauscher III FJ, Dressler GR. Repression of Pax-2 by WT1 during normal kidney development. Development 1995;121(3):867–75.

[125] Hewitt SM, Hamada S, McDonnell TJ, Rauscher III FJ, Saunders GF. Regulation of the proto-oncogenes bcl-2 and c-myc by the Wilms' tumor suppressor gene WT1. Cancer Res 1995;55(22):5386–9.

[126] Kreidberg JA, Sariola H, Loring JM, Maeda M, Pelletier J, Housman D, et al. WT-1 is required for early kidney development. Cell 1993;74(4):679–91.

[127] Donovan MJ, Natoli TA, Sainio K, Amstutz A, Jaenisch R, Sariola H, et al. Initial differentiation of the metanephric mesenchyme is independent of WT1 and the ureteric bud. Dev Genet 1999;24(3-4):252–62.

[128] Mundlos S, Pelletier J, Darveau A, Bachmann M, Winterpacht A, Zabel B. Nuclear localization of the protein encoded by the Wilms' tumor gene WT1 in embryonic and adult tissues. Development 1993;119(4):1329–41.

[129] Kim HS, Kim MS, Hancock AL, Harper JC, Park JY, Poy G, et al. Identification of novel Wilms' tumor suppressor gene target genes implicated in kidney development. J Biol Chem 2007;282 (22):16278–87.

[130] Maas R, Elfering S, Glaser T, Jepeal L. Deficient outgrowth of the ureteric bud underlies the renal agenesis phenotype in mice manifesting the limb deformity (ld) mutation. Dev Dyn 1994;199(3):214–28.

[131] Chan DC, Wynshaw-Boris A, Leder P. Formin isoforms are differentially expressed in the mouse embryo and are required for normal expression of fgf-4 and shh in the limb bud. Development 1995;121(10):3151–62.

[132] Mass RL, Zeller R, Woychik RP, Vogt TF, Leder P. Disruption of formin-encoding transcripts in two mutant limb deformity alleles. Nature 1990;346(6287):853–5.

[133] Wynshaw-Boris A, Ryan G, Deng CX, Chan DC, Jackson-Grusby L, Larson D, et al. The role of a single formin isoform in the limb and renal phenotypes of limb deformity. Mol Med 1997;3(6):372–84.

[134] Mugrauer G, Ekblom P. Contrasting expression patterns of three members of the myc family of protooncogenes in the developing and adult mouse kidney. J Cell Biol 1991;112(1):13–25.

[135] Charron J, Malynn BA, Fisher P, Stewart V, Jeannotte L, Goff SP, et al. Embryonic lethality in mice homozygous for a targeted disruption of the N-myc gene. Genes Dev 1992;6 (12A):2248–57.

[136] Davis AC, Wims M, Spotts GD, Hann SR, Bradley A. A null c-myc mutation causes lethality before 10.5 days of gestation in homozygotes and reduced fertility in heterozygous female mice. Genes Dev 1993;7(4):671–82.

[137] Stanton BR, Perkins AS, Tessarollo L, Sassoon DA, Parada LF. Loss of N-myc function results in embryonic lethality and failure of the epithelial component of the embryo to develop. Genes Dev 1992;6(12A):2235–47.

[138] Gotter AL, Manganaro T, Weaver DR, Kolakowski Jr. LF, Possidente B, Sriram S, et al. A time-less function for mouse timeless. Nat Neurosci 2000;3(8):755–6.

[139] Guo B, Panagiotaki N, Warwood S, Sharrocks AD. Dynamic modification of the ETS transcription factor PEA3 by sumoylation and p300-mediated acetylation. Nucleic Acids Res 2011;39 (15):6403–13.

[140] Kuure S, Chi X, Lu B, Costantini F. The transcription factors Etv4 and Etv5 mediate formation of the ureteric bud tip domain during kidney development. Development 2010;137 (12):1975–9.

[141] Lu BC, Cebrian C, Chi X, Kuure S, Kuo R, Bates CM, et al. Etv4 and Etv5 are required downstream of GDNF and Ret for kidney branching morphogenesis. Nat Genet 2009;41(12): 1295–302.

[142] Reginensi A, Clarkson M, Neirijnck Y, Lu B, Ohyama T, Groves AK, et al. SOX9 controls epithelial branching by activating RET effector genes during kidney development. Hum Mol Genet 2011;20(6):1143–53.

[143] Hatini V, Huh SO, Herzlinger D, Soares VC, Lai E. Essential role of stromal mesenchyme in kidney morphogenesis revealed by targeted disruption of Winged Helix transcription factor BF-2. Genes Dev 1996;10(12):1467–78.

[144] Levinson RS, Batourina E, Choi C, Vorontchikhina M, Kitajewski J, Mendelsohn CL. Foxd1-dependent signals control cellularity in the renal capsule, a structure required for normal renal development. Development 2005;132(3):529–39.

[145] Zhang H, Palmer R, Gao X, Kreidberg J, Gerald W, Hsiao L, et al. Transcriptional activation of placental growth factor by the forkhead/winged helix transcription factor FoxD1. Curr Biol 2003;13(18):1625–9.

[146] Quaggin SE, Vanden Heuvel GB, Igarashi P. Pod-1, a mesoderm-specific basic-helix-loop-helix protein expressed in mesenchymal and glomerular epithelial cells in the developing kidney. Mech Dev 1998;71(1-2):37–48.

[147] Quaggin SE, Schwartz L, Cui S, Igarashi P, Deimling J, Post M, et al. The basic-helix-loop-helix protein pod1 is critically important for kidney and lung organogenesis. Development 1999;126(24):5771–83.

[148] Cui S, Schwartz L, Quaggin SE. Pod1 is required in stromal cells for glomerulogenesis. Dev Dyn 2003;226(3):512–22.

[149] Schnabel CA, Godin RE, Cleary ML. Pbx1 regulates nephrogenesis and ureteric branching in the developing kidney. Dev Biol 2003;254(2):262–76.

[150] Wilson JG, Roth CB, Warkany J. An analysis of the syndrome of malformations induced by maternal vitamin A deficiency. Effects of restoration of vitamin A at various times during gestation. Am J Anat 1953;92(2):189–217.

[151] Batourina E, Gim S, Bello N, Shy M, Clagett-Dame M, Srinivas S, et al. Vitamin A controls epithelial/mesenchymal interactions through Ret expression. Nat Genet 2001;27(1):74–8.

[152] Mendelsohn C, Batourina E, Fung S, Gilbert T, Dodd J. Stromal cells mediate retinoid-dependent functions essential for renal development. Development 1999;126(6):1139–48.

[153] Pontoglio M, Barra J, Hadchouel M, Doyen A, Kress C, Bach JP, et al. Hepatocyte nuclear factor 1 inactivation results in hepatic dysfunction, phenylketonuria, and renal Fanconi syndrome. Cell 1996;84(4):575–85.

[154] Nakai S, Sugitani Y, Sato H, Ito S, Miura Y, Ogawa M, et al. Crucial roles of Brn1 in distal tubule formation and function in mouse kidney. Development 2003;130(19):4751–9.

[155] Wong K, Park HT, Wu JY, Rao Y. Slit proteins: molecular guidance cues for cells ranging from neurons to leukocytes. Curr Opin Genet Dev 2002;12(5):583–91.

[156] Grieshammer U, Le M, Plump AS, Wang F, Tessier-Lavigne M, Martin GR. SLIT2-mediated ROBO2 signaling restricts kidney induction to a single site. Dev Cell 2004;6(5):709–17.

[157] Kramer S, Okabe M, Hacohen N, Krasnow MA, Hiromi Y. Sprouty: a common antagonist of FGF and EGF signaling pathways in Drosophila. Development 1999;126(11):2515–25.

[158] Basson MA, Akbulut S, Watson-Johnson J, Simon R, Carroll TJ, Shakya R, et al. Sprouty1 is a critical regulator of GDNF/RET-mediated kidney induction. Dev Cell 2005;8(2):229–39.

[159] Michos O, Cebrian C, Hyink D, Grieshammer U, Williams L, D'Agati V, et al. Kidney development in the absence of Gdnf and Spry1 requires Fgf10. PLoS Genet 2010;6(1):e1000809.

[160] Esquela AF, Lee SJ. Regulation of metanephric kidney development by growth/differentiation factor 11. Dev Biol 2003;257 (2):356—70.

[161] McPherron AC, Lawler AM, Lee SJ. Regulation of anterior/posterior patterning of the axial skeleton by growth/differentiation factor 11. Nat Genet 1999;22(3):260—4.

[162] Oh SP, Yeo CY, Lee Y, Schrewe H, Whitman M, Li E. Activin type IIA and IIB receptors mediate Gdf11 signaling in axial vertebral patterning. Genes Dev 2002;16(21):2749—54.

[163] Oh SP, Li E. The signaling pathway mediated by the type IIB activin receptor controls axial patterning and lateral asymmetry in the mouse. Genes Dev 1997;11(14):1812—26.

[164] Zhao H, Kegg H, Grady S, Truong HT, Robinson ML, Baum M, et al. Role of fibroblast growth factor receptors 1 and 2 in the ureteric bud. Dev Biol 2004;276(2):403—15.

[165] Santos OF, Barros EJ, Yang XM, Matsumoto K, Nakamura T, Park M, et al. Involvement of hepatocyte growth factor in kidney development. Dev Biol 1994;163(2):525—9.

[166] Moore MW, Klein RD, Farinas I, Sauer H, Armanini M, Phillips H, et al. Renal and neuronal abnormalities in mice lacking GDN. Nature 1996;382(6586):76—9.

[167] Pichel JG, Shen L, Sheng HZ, Granholm AC, Drago J, Grinberg A, et al. Defects in enteric innervation and kidney development in mice lacking GDN. Nature 1996;382(6586):73—6.

[168] Sanchez MP, Silos-Santiago I, Frisen J, He B, Lira SA, Barbacid M. Renal agenesis and the absence of enteric neurons in mice lacking GDN. Nature 1996;382(6586):70—3.

[169] Enomoto H, Araki T, Jackman A, Heuckeroth RO, Snider WD, Johnson Jr. EM, et al. GFR alpha1-deficient mice have deficits in the enteric nervous system and kidneys. Neuron 1998;21 (2):317—24.

[170] Durbec P, Marcos-Gutierrez CV, Kilkenny C, Grigoriou M, Wartiowaara K, Suvanto P, et al. GDNF signalling through the Ret receptor tyrosine kinase. Nature 1996;381(6585):789—93.

[171] Schuchardt A, D'Agati V, Pachnis V, Costantini F. Renal agenesis and hypodysplasia in ret-k-mutant mice result from defects in ureteric bud development. Development 1996;122 (6):1919—29.

[172] Sainio K, Suvanto P, Davies J, Wartiovaara J, Wartiovaara K, Saarma M, et al. Glial-cell-line-derived neurotrophic factor is required for bud initiation from ureteric epithelium. Development 1997;124(20):4077—87.

[173] Cullen-McEwen LA, Drago J, Bertram JF. Nephron endowment in glial cell line-derived neurotrophic factor (GDNF) heterozygous mice. Kidney Int 2001;60(1):31—6.

[174] Cancilla B, Davies A, Cauchi JA, Risbridger GP, Bertram JF. Fibroblast growth factor receptors and their ligands in the adult rat kidney. Kidney Int 2001;60(1):147—55.

[175] Celli G, LaRochelle WJ, Mackem S, Sharp R, Merlino G. Soluble dominant-negative receptor uncovers essential roles for fibroblast growth factors in multi-organ induction and patterning. Embo J 1998;17(6):1642—55.

[176] Qiao J, Uzzo R, Obara-Ishihara T, Degenstein L, Fuchs E, Herzlinger D. FGF-7 modulates ureteric bud growth and nephron number in the developing kidney. Development 1999;126 (3):547—54.

[177] Ohuchi H, Hori Y, Yamasaki M, Harada H, Sekine K, Kato S, et al. FGF10 acts as a major ligand for FGF receptor 2 IIIb in mouse multi-organ development. Biochem Biophys Res Commun 2000;277(3):643—9.

[178] Revest JM, Spencer-Dene B, Kerr K, De Moerlooze L, Rosewell I, Dickson C. Fibroblast growth factor receptor 2-IIIb acts upstream of Shh and Fgf4 and is required for limb bud maintenance but not for the induction of Fgf8, Fgf10, Msx1, or Bmp4. Dev Biol 2001;231(1):47—62.

[179] Bates CM. Role of fibroblast growth factor receptor signaling in kidney development. Am J Physiol Renal Physiol 2011;301 (2):F245—51.

[180] Sims-Lucas S, Argyropoulos C, Kish K, McHugh K, Bertram JF, Quigley R, et al. Three-dimensional imaging reveals ureteric and mesenchymal defects in Fgfr2-mutant kidneys. J Am Soc Nephrol 2009;20(12):2525—33.

[181] Li YS, Milner PG, Chauhan AK, Watson MA, Hoffman RM, Kodner CM, et al. Cloning and expression of a developmentally regulated protein that induces mitogenic and neurite outgrowth activity. Science 1990;250(4988):1690—4.

[182] Mitsiadis TA, Salmivirta M, Muramatsu T, Muramatsu H, Rauvala H, Lehtonen E, et al. Expression of the heparin-binding cytokines, midkine (MK) and HB-GAM (pleiotrophin) is associated with epithelial-mesenchymal interactions during fetal development and organogenesis. Development 1995;121 (1):37—51.

[183] Amet LE, Lauri SE, Hienola A, Croll SD, Lu Y, Levorse JM, et al. Enhanced hippocampal long-term potentiation in mice lacking heparin-binding growth-associated molecule. Mol Cell Neurosci 2001;17(6):1014—24.

[184] Lin Y, Liu A, Zhang S, Ruusunen T, Kreidberg JA, Peltoketo H, et al. Induction of ureter branching as a response to Wnt-2b signaling during early kidney organogenesis. Dev Dyn 2001;222(1):26—39.

[185] Majumdar A, Vainio S, Kispert A, McMahon J, McMahon AP. Wnt11 and Ret/Gdnf pathways cooperate in regulating ureteric branching during metanephric kidney development. Development 2003;130(14):3175—85.

[186] Karner CM, Chirumamilla R, Aoki S, Igarashi P, Wallingford JB, Carroll TJ. Wnt9b signaling regulates planar cell polarity and kidney tubule morphogenesis. Nat Genet 2009;41 (7):793—9.

[187] Yu J, Carroll TJ, Rajagopal J, Kobayashi A, Ren Q, McMahon APA. Wnt7b-dependent pathway regulates the orientation of epithelial cell division and establishes the cortico-medullary axis of the mammalian kidney. Development 2009;136(1): 161—71.

[188] Lescher B, Haenig B, Kispert A. sFRP-2 is a target of the Wnt-4 signaling pathway in the developing metanephric kidney. Dev Dyn 1998;213(4):440—51.

[189] Yoshino K, Rubin JS, Higinbotham KG, Uren A, Anest V, Plisov SY, et al. Secreted Frizzled-related proteins can regulate metanephric development. Mech Dev 2001;102(1-2):45—55.

[190] Ritvos O, Tuuri T, Eramaa M, Sainio K, Hilden K, Saxen L, et al. Activin disrupts epithelial branching morphogenesis in developing glandular organs of the mouse. Mech Dev 1995;50 (2-3):229—45.

[191] Miyazaki Y, Oshima K, Fogo A, Hogan BL, Ichikawa I. Bone morphogenetic protein 4 regulates the budding site and elongation of the mouse ureter. J Clin Invest 2000;105(7): 863—73.

[192] Raatikainen-Ahokas A, Hytonen M, Tenhunen A, Sainio K, Sariola H. BMP-4 affects the differentiation of metanephric mesenchyme and reveals an early anterior—posterior axis of the embryonic kidney. Dev Dyn 2000;217(2):146—58.

[193] Hsu DR, Economides AN, Wang X, Eimon PM, Harland RM. The Xenopus dorsalizing factor Gremlin identifies a novel family of secreted proteins that antagonize BMP activities. Mol Cell 1998;1(5):673—83.

[194] Michos O, Panman L, Vintersten K, Beier K, Zeller R, Zuniga A. Gremlin-mediated BMP antagonism induces the epithelial—mesenchymal feedback signaling controlling metanephric kidney and limb organogenesis. Development 2004;131 (14):3401—10.

II. STRUCTURAL AND FUNCTIONAL ORGANIZATION OF THE KIDNEY

[195] Goncalves A, Zeller R. Genetic analysis reveals an unexpected role of BMP7 in initiation of ureteric bud outgrowth in mouse embryos. PLoS One 2011;6(4):e19370.

[196] Michos O, Goncalves A, Lopez-Rios J, Tiecke E, Naillat F, Beier K, et al. Reduction of BMP4 activity by gremlin 1 enables ureteric bud outgrowth and GDNF/WNT11 feedback signalling during kidney branching morphogenesis. Development 2007;134(13):2397—405.

[197] Nie X, Xu J, El-Hashash A, Xu PX. Six1 regulates Grem1 expression in the metanephric mesenchyme to initiate branching morphogenesis. Dev Biol 2011;352(1):141—51.

[198] Bladt F, Riethmacher D, Isenmann S, Aguzzi A, Birchmeier C. Essential role for the c-met receptor in the migration of myogenic precursor cells into the limb bud. Nature 1995;376 (6543):768—71.

[199] Schmidt C, Bladt F, Goedecke S, Brinkmann V, Zschiesche W, Sharpe M, et al. Scatter factor/hepatocyte growth factor is essential for liver development. Nature 1995;373(6516): 699—702.

[200] Massague J, Pandiella A. Membrane-anchored growth factors. Annu Rev Biochem 1993;62:515—41.

[201] Rogers SA, Ryan G, Hammerman MR. Metanephric transforming growth factor-alpha is required for renal organogenesis in vitro. Am J Physiol 1992;262(4 Pt 2):F533—9.

[202] Montesano R, Matsumoto K, Nakamura T, Orci L. Identification of a fibroblast-derived epithelial morphogen as hepatocyte growth factor. Cell 1991;67(5):901—8.

[203] Kjelsberg C, Sakurai H, Spokes K, Birchmeier C, Drummond I, Nigam S, et al. Met$^{-/-}$ kidneys express epithelial cells that chemotax and form tubules in response to EGF receptor ligands. Am J Physiol 1997;272(2 Pt 2):F222—8.

[204] Luetteke NC, Qiu TH, Peiffer RL, Oliver P, Smithies O, Lee DC. TGF alpha deficiency results in hair follicle and eye abnormalities in targeted and waved-1 mice. Cell 1993;73(2): 263—78.

[205] Mann GB, Fowler KJ, Gabriel A, Nice EC, Williams RL, Dunn AR. Mice with a null mutation of the TGF alpha gene have abnormal skin architecture, wavy hair, and curly whiskers and often develop corneal inflammation. Cell 1993;73(2):249—61.

[206] Threadgill DW, Dlugosz AA, Hansen LA, Tennenbaum T, Lichti U, Yee D, et al. Targeted disruption of mouse EGF receptor: effect of genetic background on mutant phenotype. Science 1995;269(5221):230—4.

[207] Rogers SA, Ryan G, Hammerman MR. Insulin-like growth factors I and II are produced in the metanephros and are required for growth and development in vitro. J Cell Biol 1991;113 (6):1447—53.

[208] Wada J, Liu ZZ, Alvares K, Kumar A, Wallner E, Makino H, et al. Cloning of cDNA for the alpha subunit of mouse insulin-like growth factor I receptor and the role of the receptor in metanephric development. Proc Natl Acad Sci USA 1993;90 (21):10360—4.

[209] Baker J, Liu JP, Robertson EJ, Efstratiadis A. Role of insulin-like growth factors in embryonic and postnatal growth. Cell 1993;75(1):73—82.

[210] Powell-Braxton L, Hollingshead P, Warburton C, Dowd M, Pitts-Meek S, Dalton D, et al. IGF-I is required for normal embryonic growth in mice. Genes Dev 1993;7(12B):2609—17.

[211] Kanwar YS, Wada J, Lin S, Danesh FR, Chugh SS, Yang Q, et al. Update of extracellular matrix, its receptors, and cell adhesion molecules in mammalian nephrogenesis. Am J Physiol Renal Physiol 2004;286(2):F202—15.

[212] Santos OF, Nigam SK. HGF-induced tubulogenesis and branching of epithelial cells is modulated by extracellular matrix and TGF-beta. Dev Biol 1993;160(2):293—302.

[213] Schuger L, O'Shea S, Rheinheimer J, Varani J. Laminin in lung development: effects of anti-laminin antibody in murine lung morphogenesis. Dev Biol 1990;137(1):26—32.

[214] Ekblom P, Ekblom M, Fecker L, Klein G, Zhang HY, Kadoya Y, et al. Role of mesenchymal nidogen for epithelial morphogenesis in vitro. Development 1994;120(7):2003—14.

[215] Kreidberg JA, Donovan MJ, Goldstein SL, Rennke H, Shepherd K, Jones RC, et al. Alpha 3 beta 1 integrin has a crucial role in kidney and lung organogenesis. Development 1996;122(11): 3537—47.

[216] Kjellen L, Lindahl U. Proteoglycans: structures and interactions. Annu Rev Biochem 1991;60:443—75.

[217] Klein DJ, Brown DM, Moran A, Oegema Jr. TR, Platt JL. Chondroitin sulfate proteoglycan synthesis and reutilization of beta-D-xyloside-initiated chondroitin/dermatan sulfate glycosaminoglycans in fetal kidney branching morphogenesis. Dev Biol 1989;133(2):515—28.

[218] Lelongt B, Makino H, Dalecki TM, Kanwar YS. Role of proteoglycans in renal development. Dev Biol 1988;128(2):256—76.

[219] Kispert A, Vainio S, Shen L, Rowitch DH, McMahon AP. Proteoglycans are required for maintenance of Wnt-11 expression in the ureter tips. Development 1996;122(11):3627—37.

[220] Grisaru S, Cano-Gauci D, Tee J, Filmus J, Rosenblum ND. Glypican-3 modulates BMP- and FGF-mediated effects during renal branching morphogenesis. Dev Biol 2001;231(1): 31—46.

[221] Pohl M, Sakurai H, Stuart RO, Nigam SK. Role of hyaluronan and CD44 in in vitro branching morphogenesis of ureteric bud cells. Dev Biol 2000;224(2):312—25.

[222] Rosines E, Schmidt HJ, Nigam SK. The effect of hyaluronic acid size and concentration on branching morphogenesis and tubule differentiation in developing kidney culture systems: potential applications to engineering of renal tissues. Biomaterials 2007;28(32):4806—17.

[223] Kanwar YS, Ota K, Yang Q, Kumar A, Wada J, Kashihara N, et al. Isolation of rat fibrillin-1 cDNA and its relevance in metanephric development. Am J Physiol 1998;275(5 Pt 2):F710—23.

[224] Montesano R, Soriano JV, Pepper MS, Orci L. Induction of epithelial branching tubulogenesis in vitro. J Cell Physiol 1997;173 (2):152—61.

[225] Lelongt B, Trugnan G, Murphy G, Ronco PM. Matrix metalloproteinases MMP2 and MMP9 are produced in early stages of kidney morphogenesis but only MMP9 is required for renal organogenesis in vitro. J Cell Biol 1997;136(6):1363—73.

[226] Andrews KL, Betsuyaku T, Rogers S, Shipley JM, Senior RM, Miner JH, et al. (MMP-9) is not essential in the normal kidney and does not influence progression of renal disease in a mouse model of Alport syndrome. Am J Pathol 2000;157(1): 303—11.

[227] Arnould C, Lelievre-Pegorier M, Ronco P, Lelongt B. MMP9 limits apoptosis and stimulates branching morphogenesis during kidney development. J Am Soc Nephrol 2009;20(10): 2171—80.

[228] Kanwar YS, Ota K, Yang Q, Wada J, Kashihara N, Tian Y, et al. Role of membrane-type matrix metalloproteinase 1 (MT-1-MMP), MMP-2, and its inhibitor in nephrogenesis. Am J Physiol 1999;277(6 Pt 2):F934—47.

[229] Unsworth B, Grobstein C. Induction of kidney tubules in mouse metanephrogenic mesenchyme by various embryonic mesenchymal tissues. Dev Biol 1970;21(4):547—56.

[230] Lombard MN, Grobstein C. Activity in various embryonic and postembryonic sources for induction of kidney tubules. Dev Biol 1969;19(1):41—51.

[231] Koseki C, Herzlinger D, al-Awqati Q. Apoptosis in metanephric development. J Cell Biol 1992;119(5):1327—33.

[232] Coles HS, Burne JF, Raff MC. Large-scale normal cell death in the developing rat kidney and its reduction by epidermal growth factor. Development 1993;118(3):777–84.

[233] Barasch J, Pressler L, Connor J, Malik A. A ureteric bud cell line induces nephrogenesis in two steps by two distinct signals. Am J Physiol 1996;271(1 Pt 2):F50–61.

[234] Barasch J, Qiao J, McWilliams G, Chen D, Oliver JA, Herzlinger D. Ureteric bud cells secrete multiple factors, including bFGF, which rescue renal progenitors from apoptosis. Am J Physiol 1997;273(5 Pt 2):F757–67.

[235] Karavanova ID, Dove LF, Resau JH, Perantoni AO. Conditioned medium from a rat ureteric bud cell line in combination with bFGF induces complete differentiation of isolated metanephric mesenchyme. Development 1996;122(12):4159–67.

[236] Dudley AT, Lyons KM, Robertson EJ. A requirement for bone morphogenetic protein-7 during development of the mammalian kidney and eye. Genes Dev 1995;9(22):2795–807.

[237] Luo G, Hofmann C, Bronckers AL, Sohocki M, Bradley A, Karsenty G. BMP-7 is an inducer of nephrogenesis, and is also required for eye development and skeletal patterning. Genes Dev 1995;9(22):2808–20.

[238] Vukicevic S, Kopp JB, Luyten FP, Sampath TK. Induction of nephrogenic mesenchyme by osteogenic protein 1 (bone morphogenetic protein 7). Proc Natl Acad Sci USA 1996;93(17):9021–6.

[239] Lehtonen E. Epithelio–mesenchymal interface during mouse kidney tubule induction in vivo. J Embryol Exp Morphol 1975;34(3):695–705.

[240] Yang J, Blum A, Novak T, Levinson R, Lai E, Barasch J. An epithelial precursor is regulated by the ureteric bud and by the renal stroma. Dev Biol 2002;246(2):296–310.

[241] Herzlinger D, Qiao J, Cohen D, Ramakrishna N, Brown AM. Induction of kidney epithelial morphogenesis by cells expressing Wnt-1. Dev Biol 1994;166(2):815–8.

[242] Wilkinson DG, Bailes JA, McMahon AP. Expression of the proto-oncogene int-1 is restricted to specific neural cells in the developing mouse embryo. Cell 1987;50(1):79–88.

[243] Stark K, Vainio S, Vassileva G, McMahon AP. Epithelial transformation of metanephric mesenchyme in the developing kidney regulated by Wnt-4. Nature 1994;372(6507):679–83.

[244] Carroll TJ, Park JS, Hayashi S, Majumdar A, McMahon AP. Wnt9b plays a central role in the regulation of mesenchymal to epithelial transitions underlying organogenesis of the mammalian urogenital system. Dev Cell 2005;9(2):283–92.

[245] Grieshammer U, Cebrian C, Ilagan R, Meyers E, Herzlinger D, Martin GR. FGF8 is required for cell survival at distinct stages of nephrogenesis and for regulation of gene expression in nascent nephrons. Development 2005;132(17):3847–57.

[246] Perantoni AO, Timofeeva O, Naillat F, Richman C, Pajni-Underwood S, Wilson C, et al. Inactivation of FGF8 in early mesoderm reveals an essential role in kidney development. Development 2005;132(17):3859–71.

[247] Poladia DP, Kish K, Kutay B, Hains D, Kegg H, Zhao H, et al. Role of fibroblast growth factor receptors 1 and 2 in the metanephric mesenchyme. Dev Biol 2006;291(2):325–39.

[248] Cheng HT, Kim M, Valerius MT, Surendran K, Schuster-Gossler K, Gossler A, et al. Notch2 but not Notch1, is required for proximal fate acquisition in the mammalian nephron. Development 2007;134(4):801–11.

[249] Kopan R, Cheng HT, Surendran K. Molecular insights into segmentation along the proximal–distal axis of the nephron. J Am Soc Nephrol 2007;18(7):2014–20.

[250] Surendran K, Boyle S, Barak H, Kim M, Stomberski C, McCright B, et al. The contribution of Notch1 to nephron segmentation in the developing kidney is revealed in a sensitized Notch2 background and can be augmented by reducing Mint dosage. Dev Biol 2010;337(2):386–95.

[251] Mitsiadis TA, Lardelli M, Lendahl U, Thesleff I. Expression of Notch 1, 2 and 3 is regulated by epithelial–mesenchymal interactions and retinoic acid in the developing mouse tooth and associated with determination of ameloblast cell fate. J Cell Biol 1995;130(2):407–18.

[252] Mitsiadis TA, Gayet O, Zhang N, Carroll P. Expression of Deltex1 during mouse embryogenesis: comparison with Notch1, 2 and 3 expression. Mech Dev 2001;109(2):399–403.

[253] McCright B. Notch signaling in kidney development. Curr Opin Nephrol Hypertens 2003;12(1):5–10.

[254] Chen L, Al-Awqati Q. Segmental expression of Notch and Hairy genes in nephrogenesis. Am J Physiol Renal Physiol 2005;288(5):F939–52.

[255] Cheng HT, Kopan R. The role of Notch signaling in specification of podocyte and proximal tubules within the developing mouse kidney. Kidney Int 2005;68(5):1951–2.

[256] McCright B, Gao X, Shen L, Lozier J, Lan Y, Maguire M, et al. Defects in development of the kidney, heart and eye vasculature in mice homozygous for a hypomorphic Notch2 mutation. Development 2001;128(4):491–502.

[257] Cheng HT, Miner JH, Lin M, Tansey MG, Roth K, Kopan R. Gamma-secretase activity is dispensable for mesenchyme-to-epithelium transition but required for podocyte and proximal tubule formation in developing mouse kidney. Development 2003;130(20):5031–42.

[258] Wang P, Pereira FA, Beasley D, Zheng H. Presenilins are required for the formation of comma- and S-shaped bodies during nephrogenesis. Development 2003;130(20):5019–29.

[259] Oswald F, Kostezka U, Astrahantseff K, Bourteele S, Dillinger K, Zechner U, et al. SHARP is a novel component of the Notch/RBP-Jkappa signalling pathway. Embo J 2002;21(20):5417–26.

[260] Oswald F, Winkler M, Cao Y, Astrahantseff K, Bourteele S, Knochel W, et al. RBP-Jkappa/SHARP recruits CtIP/CtBP corepressors to silence Notch target genes. Mol Cell Biol 2005;25(23):10379–90.

[261] Tsuji M, Shinkura R, Kuroda K, Yabe D, Honjo T. Msx2-interacting nuclear target protein (Mint) deficiency reveals negative regulation of early thymocyte differentiation by Notch/RBP-J signaling. Proc Natl Acad Sci USA 2007;104(5):1610–5.

[262] Yabe D, Fukuda H, Aoki M, Yamada S, Takebayashi S, Shinkura R, et al. Generation of a conditional knockout allele for mammalian Spen protein Mint/SHARP. Genesis 2007;45(5):300–6.

[263] Ekblom M, Klein G, Mugrauer G, Fecker L, Deutzmann R, Timpl R, et al. Transient and locally restricted expression of laminin A chain mRNA by developing epithelial cells during kidney organogenesis. Cell 1990;60(2):337–46.

[264] Klein G, Ekblom M, Fecker L, Timpl R, Ekblom P. Differential expression of laminin A and B chains during development of embryonic mouse organs. Development 1990;110(3):823–37.

[265] Klein G, Langegger M, Timpl R, Ekblom P. Role of laminin A chain in the development of epithelial cell polarity. Cell 1988;55(2):331–41.

[266] Falk M, Salmivirta K, Durbeej M, Larsson E, Ekblom M, Vestweber D, et al. Integrin alpha 6B beta 1 is involved in kidney tubulogenesis in vitro. J Cell Sci 1996;109(Pt 12):2801–10.

[267] Schuger L, Skubitz AP, Zhang J, Sorokin L, He L. Laminin alpha1 chain synthesis in the mouse developing lung: requirement for epithelial–mesenchymal contact and possible role in bronchial smooth muscle development. J Cell Biol 1997;139(2):553–62.

II. STRUCTURAL AND FUNCTIONAL ORGANIZATION OF THE KIDNEY

[268] Muller U, Bossy B, Venstrom K, Reichardt LF. Integrin alpha 8 beta 1 promotes attachment, cell spreading, and neurite outgrowth on fibronectin. Mol Biol Cell 1995;6(4):433–48.

[269] Lopez-Nieto CE, You G, Bush KT, Barros EJ, Beier DR, Nigam SK. Molecular cloning and characterization of NKT, a gene product related to the organic cation transporter family that is almost exclusively expressed in the kidney. J Biol Chem 1997;272(10):6471–8.

[270] Preminger GM, Koch WE, Fried FA, Mandell J. Utilization of the chick chorioallantoic membrane for in vitro growth of the embryonic murine kidney. Am J Anat 1980;159(1):17–24.

[271] Ekblom P, Sariola H, Karkinen-Jaaskelainen M, Saxen L. The origin of the glomerular endothelium. Cell Differ 1982;11 (1):35–9.

[272] Sariola H, Ekblom P, Lehtonen E, Saxen L. Differentiation and vascularization of the metanephric kidney grafted on the chorioallantoic membrane. Dev Biol 1983;96(2):427–35.

[273] Hyink DP, Abrahamson DR. Origin of the glomerular vasculature in the developing kidney. Semin Nephrol 1995;15(4):300–14.

[274] Robert St B, John PL, Hyink DP, Abrahamson DR. Evidence that embryonic kidney cells expressing flk-1 are intrinsic, vasculogenic angioblasts. Am J Physiol 1996;271(3 Pt 2):F744–53.

[275] Faa G, Gerosa C, Fanni D, Monga G, Zaffanello M, Van Eyken P, et al. Morphogenesis and molecular mechanisms involved in human kidney development. J Cell Physiol 2012;227 (3):1257–68.

[276] Sariola H, Kuusela P, Ekblom P. Cellular origin of fibronectin in interspecies hybrid kidneys. J Cell Biol 1984;99(6):2099–107.

[277] Sariola H, Timpl R, von der Mark K, Mayne R, Fitch JM, Linsenmayer TF, et al. Dual origin of glomerular basement membrane. Dev Biol 1984;101(1):86–96.

[278] Leveen P, Pekny M, Gebre-Medhin S, Swolin B, Larsson E, Betsholtz C. Mice deficient for PDGF B show renal, cardiovascular, and hematological abnormalities. Genes Dev 1994;8 (16):1875–87.

[279] Soriano P. Abnormal kidney development and hematological disorders in PDGF beta-receptor mutant mice. Genes Dev 1994;8(16):1888–96.

[280] Humphreys BD, Valerius MT, Kobayashi A, Mugford JW, Soeung S, Duffield JS, et al. Intrinsic epithelial cells repair the kidney after injury. Cell Stem Cell 2008;2(3):284–91.

[281] Wilkinson L, Gilbert T, Sipos A, Toma I, Pennisi DJ, Peti-Peterdi J, et al. Loss of renal microvascular integrity in postnatal Crim1 hypomorphic transgenic mice. Kidney Int 2009;76 (11):1161–71.

[282] Wilkinson L, Gilbert T, Kinna G, Ruta LA, Pennisi D, Kett M, et al. Crim1KST264/KST264 mice implicate Crim1 in the regulation of vascular endothelial growth factor-A activity during glomerular vascular development. J Am Soc Nephrol 2007;18 (6):1697–708.

[283] Pennisi DJ, Wilkinson L, Kolle G, Sohaskey ML, Gillinder K, Piper MJ, et al. Crim1KST264/KST264 mice display a disruption of the Crim1 gene resulting in perinatal lethality with defects in multiple organ systems. Dev Dyn 2007;236(2): 502–11.

[284] Reidy K, Tufro A. Semaphorins in kidney development and disease: modulators of ureteric bud branching, vascular morphogenesis, and podocyte-endothelial crosstalk. Pediatr Nephrol 2011;26(9):1407–12.

[285] Reidy KJ, Villegas G, Teichman J, Veron D, Shen W, Jimenez J, et al. Semaphorin3a regulates endothelial cell number and podocyte differentiation during glomerular development. Development 2009;136(23):3979–89.

[286] Tufro A, Norwood VF, Carey RM, Gomez RA. Vascular endothelial growth factor induces nephrogenesis and vasculogenesis. J Am Soc Nephrol 1999;10(10):2125–34.

[287] Tufro A. VEGF spatially directs angiogenesis during metanephric development in vitro. Dev Biol 2000;227(2):558–66.

[288] Hartman HA, Lai HL, Patterson LT. Cessation of renal morphogenesis in mice. Dev Biol 2007;310(2):379–87.

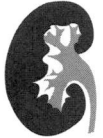

Molecular and Cellular Mechanisms of Glomerular Capillary Development

Jeffrey H. Miner[1] *and Dale R. Abrahamson*[2]

[1]Department of Medicine, Renal Division, Washington University School of Medicine, St. Louis, MO, USA

[2]Department of Anatomy and Cell Biology, University of Kansas Medical Center, Kansas City, KS, USA

Among all of the capillaries in the body, the glomerulus is arguably the most unusual and important, if not the most aesthetically interesting. In this chapter, we review the morphogenesis of this unique capillary, discuss the origins of its cells and extracellular matrices, and describe some of the primary regulatory events that occur during glomerular development.

GLOMERULAR MORPHOGENESIS

Formation of the permanent, metanephric kidney begins at embryonic day 11 in mice, day 12 in rats, and during the 4th-5th week of gestation in humans. As the ureteric bud projects from the mesonephric duct and enters the metanephric anlage, mesenchymal cells condense around the bud's advancing tip. Soon thereafter, the condensed mesenchyme converts to an epithelial phenotype and proceeds through a developmental sequence of nephric structures, which are termed vesicle, comma-, and S-shaped, developing capillary loop, and maturing glomerulus stages.[1,2] Bud tip stimulation of mesenchymal cell induction and aggregation, conversion to epithelium, and glomerular and tubule differentiation occur repeatedly until the full complement of nephrons has developed. Nephrogenesis concludes ~1 week after birth in rodents,[2] and during the 34th gestational week in humans.[3]

Vesicle Stage

At the inception of the vesicle stage of nephron development, the aggregated mesenchymal cells near the ureteric bud tips convert to a cluster of epithelial cells (vesicle), and begin assembling a basement membrane matrix containing collagen type IV, laminin, and basement membrane proteoglycans around the basal surface of the vesicle.[4-6] As development progresses through the comma- and then S-shaped stages, a groove (vascular cleft) forms in the lower aspect of the vesicle, into which endothelial precursor cells (angioblasts) migrate (Figure 26.1). Two epithelial layers can be distinguished beneath the vascular cleft: visceral epithelial cells (which ultimately differentiate into podocytes); and parietal epithelial cells (which will become the thin epithelium lining Bowman's capsule of the mature nephron). Epithelial cells above the vascular cleft ultimately develop into proximal, Henle's loop, and distal tubule epithelium. During the S-shaped phase of nephron development, the distal segment fuses with the same ureteric bud branch tip that initially induced the nephric structure, so that the lumen of the forming nephron is now continuous with that of the developing collecting system. Continued growth and branching of the ureteric bud leads to the induction of new mesenchymal aggregates, and glomerulo- and tubulogenesis continues until the full complement of nephrons is achieved.[2]

Vascular Clefts of Comma- and S-Shaped Stage

With the progressive invasion and differentiation of endothelial cells, the developing capillary endothelium assembles a subendothelial basement membrane matrix.

Seldin and Giebisch's The Kidney, Fifth Edition.
DOI: http://dx.doi.org/10.1016/B978-0-12-381462-3.00026-4

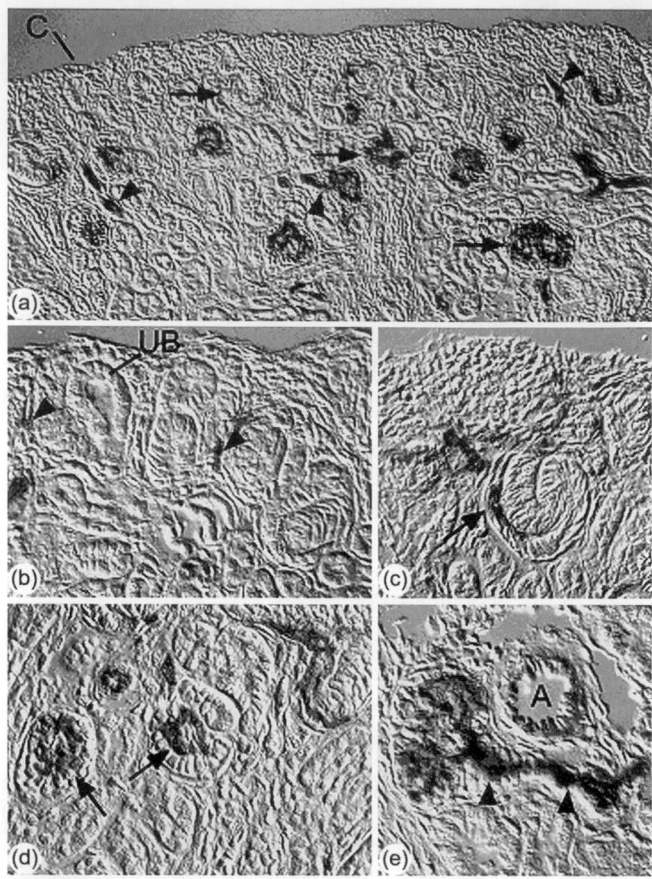

FIGURE 26.1   Sections of developing kidney from a heterozygous Flk1/LacZ transgenic mouse. Blue reaction product reflects cellular sites of Flk1 (VEGFR2) gene transcription. (a) Kidney cortex contains a range of glomeruli at different stages of development (arrows) that are lined by endothelial cells expressing Flk1. Vascular endothelium throughout the cortex also express Flk1 (arrowheads) (C: capsule). (b) Higher magnification view of outer cortex. Note blue cells scattered in mesenchyme (arrowheads) (UB: branch of ureteric bud). (c) Nephric figure at S-shaped stage. Endothelial cells expressing Flk1 can be seen migrating into the vascular cleft (arrow), which is the initial site of glomerular formation. (d) Two capillary loop stage glomeruli can be seen (arrows). (e) Maturing stage glomerulus with attached arteriole (arrowheads) (A: small artery). *(Reprinted from ref. [26], with permission).*

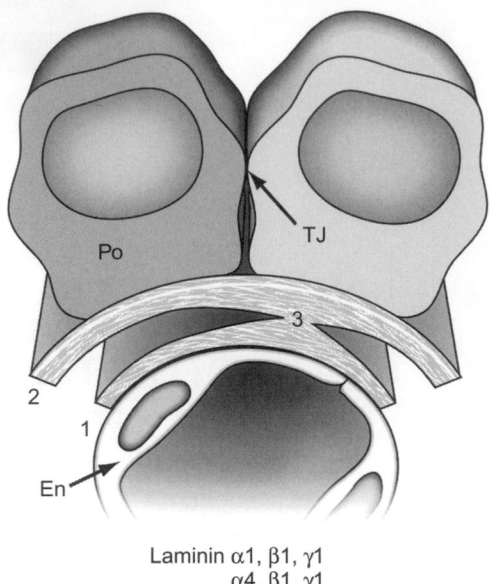

Laminin α1, β1, γ1
α4, β1, γ1
Collagen α1, α2(IV)

FIGURE 26.2   Diagram showing spatial relationships during development of glomerular capillary wall. During initial glomerular development, endothelial cells (En) migrate into vascular clefts of comma- and S-shaped nephrons. Dual sheets of subendothelial (1) and subepithelial (2) basement membranes separate the endothelium from the developing podocyte (Po) cell layers. Areas of basement membrane fusion can be seen (3). The immature GBM contains laminin α1,β1,γ1, laminin α4,β1,γ1 and collagen α1,α2(IV) at this time point. Apical tight junctional complexes (TJ) exist between immature podocytes.

Similarly, the developing podocyte cell layer assembles a subepithelial basement membrane, so that two distinct basal laminae can be seen between the endothelial and epithelial cells (Figure 26.2). As nephrons develop further, these two basement membranes layers merge to form the glomerular basement membrane (GBM), with endothelial cells lining its inner surface, and podocytes adherent to its outer surface.[7]

Capillary Loop

As glomerular capillary loops begin to form, the endothelial cells gradually flatten and become extensively fenestrated (Figures 26.3 and 26.4). Initially, the fenestrations are spanned by diaphragms, but these structures soon disappear. The epithelial podocytes, which originally were columnar with apical junctional complexes, also begin to flatten and begin sending out basolateral cytoplasmic projections that interdigitate with similar projections from neighboring cells (Figure 26.3). As glomeruli mature, these projections go on to develop into the podocyte pedicels or foot processes (Figures 26.3 and 26.4). The apical junctional complexes migrate basolaterally between these cellular projections and, although the mechanism is not fully-understood (see below), convert into the slit diaphragm complex between foot processes[8] (Figure 26.4). Metabolic labeling studies, histochemical and immunohistochemical techniques, and inter-species transplantation experiments[6,9–12] have all shown that both the endothelium and epithelium are actively synthesizing glomerular basement membrane (GBM) proteins at this time.[4]

Maturing Glomeruli

Here, capillary loop diameters expand, and endothelial and podocyte cell layers differentiate further until the

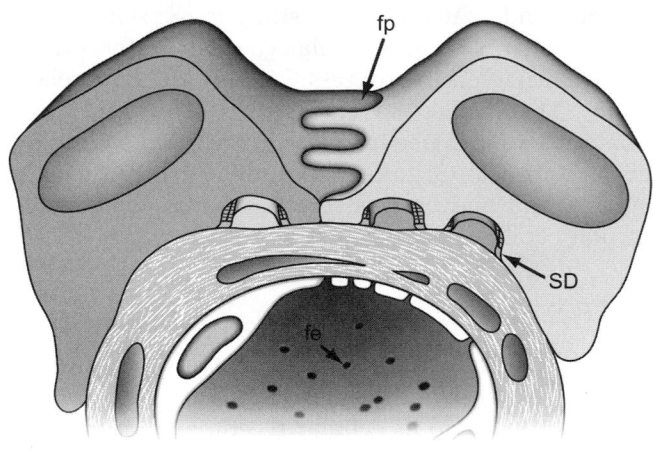

Laminin α5, β1, γ1
α5, β2, γ1
Collagen α1, α2(IV)
α3, α4, α5 (IV)

FIGURE 26.3 **During intermediate, capillary loop and maturing stages of glomerular development, fenestrae form in the endothelial cells.** Foot process (fp) extension occurs between podocytes and epithelial slit diaphragms (SD) first appear. Remodeling and splicing of newly synthesized GBM into existing, fused, GBM takes place, and new isoforms of GBM laminin and type IV collagen are seen.

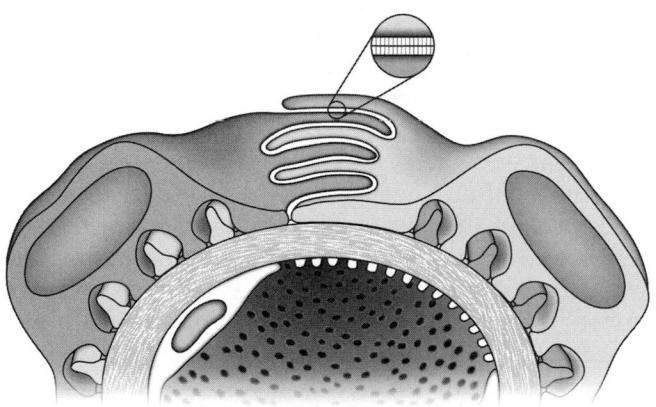

Laminin α5, β2, γ1
Collagen α3, α4, α5 (IV)

FIGURE 26.4 **As glomeruli approach full maturation, the endothelium becomes extensively fenestrated, and the mature GBM laminin and collagen type IV isoforms are now in place.** In the podocyte layer, foot process extension and interdigitation finalizes, and epithelial slit diaphragms completely span the filtration slits. Inset shows structure of SD viewed *en face*.

fully mature glomerular morphology is achieved. Unfused basement membranes are rarely seen in maturing glomeruli. On the other hand, complex, irregular projections of basement membrane are commonly found beneath podocytes at this stage, particularly in areas where foot processes are broad and their formation into relatively narrow pedicels is still incomplete. *In vivo*

labeling studies have shown that these subepithelial basement membrane segments are somehow spliced or inserted into the existing fused GBM, possibly to provide the additional GBM material necessary for the inflating capillaries.[13,14] Shortly after the initial, vascular cleft stage, and continuing into maturing glomeruli, modification and remodeling of the GBM occurs, with the appearance of new basement membrane protein isoforms and the disappearance of earlier species. As discussed later, however, we do not understand how these events are regulated at either the gene or protein level. Additionally, once the glomerulus is fully mature (Figure 26.4), matrix synthesis and cell morphogenesis virtually halt (except for some poorly-understood activities responsible for GBM "maintenance" or "turnover"), and how these processes are downregulated is also not known.

ORIGIN OF THE GLOMERULAR ENDOTHELIUM

Extrarenal Origins

Although compelling evidence has accumulated showing that nephron epithelial cells, including the visceral and parietal epithelium of Bowman's capsule, all derive originally from the metanephric mesenchyme, the origin of vascular endothelial cells during kidney organogenesis has been more difficult to understand.[15] Studies conducted nearly 30 years ago convincingly showed that cells of extrarenal origin grew into the metanephros and established the microvasculature, including the glomerular capillary tufts. These studies involved the grafting of embryonic, avascular mouse or quail kidney rudiments onto avian chorioallantoic membranes. After culturing *in ovo*, the kidney grafts contained glomerular endothelial and mesangial cells stemming from host chorioallantoic tissues, therefore signifying the ingress of vessel progenitors from sites outside the kidney.[12,16]

Intrarenal Origins

Contrary to the results discussed above, several lines of evidence from a number of more recent experiments have shown that the metanephros contains its own pool of endothelial progenitors (angioblasts) capable of vascularizing nephrons *in vivo*.[17] The first clues about the existence of these intrinsic metanephric angioblasts came from transplantation studies between mice and rats. For example, when E12 mouse kidneys are grafted into anterior eye chambers of rats, the vascular and glomerular basement membranes that develop within the grafts after transplantation are almost entirely of mouse (graft) origin.[18] Similarly, when E12 kidneys are transplanted under kidney capsules of adult ROSA26 mice (which bear a ubiquitously expressed LacZ reporter gene useful as a cell lineage marker), all of the microvascular and glomerular endothelial *cells* within grafts are derived from the engrafted kidney, not from the host.[19] Furthermore, when kidneys from E12 ROSA26 mice are grafted into the nephrogenic renal cortices of newborn wild-type hosts, endothelial cells stemming from the grafts can be seen integrating into host vasculature.[19] In additional experiments, when embryonic kidneys from Flk1 (VEGF receptor-2)–LacZ heterozygous mice are grown under routine organ culture conditions, Flk1-LacZ-positive microvessels do not develop *in vitro*, despite the extensive formation of metanephric tubules and avascular glomerular epithelial tufts.[20] When these same cultured kidneys are then transplanted into anterior eye chambers of wild-type host mice, the grafts develop microvessels and vascularized glomeruli lined by Flk1-LacZ-expressing cells, indicating again that the endothelium originates from the engrafted kidney itself, and not from the host.[20] Several other research groups have reached similar conclusions independently. For example, when avascular metanephroi from E11 Tie1/LacZ transgenic mice are transplanted into newborn wild–type hosts, widespread expression of Tie1/LacZ is found within glomeruli developing within grafts.[21] Others have immunolocalized putative angioblasts in the metanephric mesenchyme of prevascular embryonic rat kidney.[22]

Although current evidence shows that the embryonic kidney contains a pool of angioblasts capable of establishing the glomerular endothelium, whether these progenitors originate initially from outside the metanephric blastema or instead stem directly from metanephric mesenchyme is not yet clear. Nevertheless, immunolabeling experiments in developing rat kidney shows that endothelial, as well as mesangial, cell precursors share common markers during glomerulogenesis (RECA-1 and Thy1.1, respectively), suggesting that they may indeed derive from metanephric mesenchyme.[23] Other immunolocalization and transplantation experiments have shown that juxtaglomerular cells in developing kidney also originate from metanephric mesenchyme, although they appear to stem from a different lineage than endothelial and mesangial cells.[24]

ENDOTHELIAL CELL RECRUITMENT AND DIFFERENTIATION

Mechanisms controlling vascular development are highly complex and involve several different transcription factors, cell-cell and cell-matrix interactions, and many membrane receptor–ligand signaling cascades. Although our knowledge of these systems in a variety of vascular beds has improved dramatically during the past several years, many key questions regarding

temporal and spatial controls still persist. With respect to the formation of glomerular capillaries, the process can be considered to progress through four interrelated events: (1) angioblast survival, proliferation and differentiation into endothelium; (2) glomerular endothelial cell recruitment; (3) initial assembly of the glomerular capillary tuft and associated mesangium; and (4) glomerular capillary stabilization and maturation.[25,26]

VEGF Signaling

Among all of the mechanisms involved with development of the systemic vasculature, signals evoked by binding of VEGF to its cellular receptors, VEGFR-1 and VEGFR-2, are singularly critical. Mice with homozygous *Vegfa* gene deletions die by E9.5 with severe vascular deficits. Remarkably, *Vegfa* heterozygote mutants also succumb by E12 with vascular phenotypes, indicating that a single *Vegfa* allele is insufficient to direct normal vascular development.[27,28] Homozygous (but not heterozygous) *Vegfr1* and *Vegfr2* mutants die at midgestation, due to failure of endothelial differentiation[29] and vessel integrity,[30] respectively.

Developing podocytes are key sources of VEGF,[31] and its secretion and binding to angioblasts bearing VEGF receptors may initiate their recruitment into the vascular cleft of comma- and S-shaped nephrons,[32] which is the initial site of glomerulogenesis. Because *Vegfa* and *Vegfr2* knockout mice die with vascular phenotypes before glomerulogenesis commences, the precise role of this ligand-receptor pair in mediating glomerular endothelial development has been difficult to analyze fully. Nevertheless, and underscoring the importance of the VEGF signaling system, injection of VEGF-blocking antibodies into developing mouse kidney cortex inhibits glomerular capillary formation *in vivo*.[33] With the advent of cell selective and/or inducible gene deletion technologies, additional evidence for the importance of podocyte-derived VEGF has been obtained. For example, homozygous deletion of *Vegfa* selectively in podocytes (obtained in bi-transgenic mice carrying nephrin-cre recombinase and floxed *Vegfa* alleles) results in animals which die perinatally with non-vascularized glomeruli.[34] Heterozygous deletion of *Vegfa* causes no evident phenotype initially. By 2.5 weeks of age, however, mice become proteinuric, and glomeruli contain swollen endothelial cells and hyaline deposits similar to those seen in patients with pre-eclampsia. By contrast, overexpression of the VEGF$_{164}$ isoform specifically in podocytes leads to collapsing glomerulopathy and death at ~5 days of age.[35] When *Vegfa* is selectively deleted in podocytes of adult mice (using a Tet-On conditional expression model), mice become severely proteinuric and hypertensive, and glomeruli resemble those of humans with thrombotic microangiopathy (mesangiolysis, endothelial swelling, red cell fragmentation, and fibrin deposition).[196] Clearly, the cellular controls for maintaining VEGF protein expression within an optimal range are critically important for the appropriate establishment and maintenance of the glomerular capillary.

Regulation of Endothelial Development

Hypoxia-Inducible Transcription Factors (HIFs)

Transcription of VEGF and VEGFR genes is activated by hypoxia-inducible transcription factors (HIFs), which consist of heterodimers of HIF α- and β-subunits.[36] Under normal oxygen concentrations, the HIF α-subunit undergoes prolyl hydroxylation, binding to von Hippel Lindau protein (VHL), polyubiquitination, and proteasomal degradation. In hypoxia, the prolyl hydroxylase enzyme is inhibited, and HIF α chain degradation is avoided. Hypoxia-stabilized HIF α/β heterodimers bind to hypoxia-responsive elements (HREs) located in promoter/enhancer regions of inducible genes,[37] many of which are proteins expressed in response to hypoxic stress. For example, erythropoietin, transferrin, VEGF, VEGFR1, and VEGFR2 are among the more than 70 distinct genes known to be transcriptionally activated by HIFs.[36]

There are at least three distinct HIF α- and two β-subunits known at present, making a variety of different HIF isoforms possible. Because HIF stabilization is enhanced in cells experiencing subnormal oxygen tensions, such as those in rapidly growing tissues, robust VEGF and VEGFR synthesis commonly occurs during organogenesis. Increased VEGF/VEGFR signaling stimulates mitosis in endothelial progenitor cells, phosphorylation of the antiapoptotic kinases Akt/PKB[38] and focal adhesion kinase (FAK),[39] and upregulation of the survival factors Bcl2 and A1.[38] In time, these events can lead to the creation of new blood vessels, which can then provide appropriate levels of oxygen specifically to the formerly hypoxic tissue sites.

Renal HIF Expression

The expression patterns for several of the different HIF α- and β-subunits have been documented in developing human, rat, and mouse kidney using in situ hybridization and immunohistochemistry. In general, both HIF-1 and HIF-2α are found in glomeruli, with specific immunolocalization of HIF-2α protein to immature podocytes (which are rich sources of VEGF).[40,41] HIF-2α is also expressed by developing vascular endothelial cells in the kidney (most of which express VEGFR-2), whereas HIF-1α is found in cortical and medullary collecting duct epithelium. HIF-1α and HIF-2α protein are undetectable in fully mature glomeruli. Mice with a global deletion of Hif2α show no defects in glomerular development or function, and no deficits in VEGF or Flk1 expression.[197] Interestingly, HIF-1β is apparently ubiquitously expressed by all cells in the kidney, but HIF-2β distribution is greatly restricted during development and, in mice, becomes confined to nuclei in cells of the thick ascending limb of Henle's loop.[42]

The selective expression of certain HIF isoforms in different tissue compartments of developing kidney may reflect the coordinated regulation of different sets of HIF target genes.[43] Importantly, individuals with mutations in VHL, a key protein in mediating HIF α chain degradation, and thereby reducing expression of HIF target genes, are prone to developing hemangioblastomas and clear cell-renal cell carcinomas.[44–46] Some studies have shown that HIF-1α and HIF-2α had differential and sometimes antagonistic effects on the growth of clear cell-renal cell carcinomas, with HIF-1α retarding and HIF-2α promoting tumor growth.[47] These findings provide further evidence for differential effects of different HIF isoforms, and call for more studies examining the expression of HIF and HIF gene targets in the developing kidney. Surprisingly, when Vhl is selectively deleted in podocytes, glomerular vascularization patterns are not affected, and kidneys develop normally.[198] On the other hand, mice become proteinuric by 4 weeks of age, and there is ectopic deposition of collagen $(\alpha 1)_2 \alpha 2(IV)$ in peripheral loop GBMs, and upregulation of an ancient oxygen-binding protein, neuroglobin, specifically in podocytes.[198]

Once glomeruli are vascularized and fully mature, podocytes still continue VEGF synthesis. Likewise, expression of Flk1 is also maintained by glomerular endothelial cells of mature kidneys. VEGF-Flk1 signaling in glomeruli therefore probably exerts functions extending well beyond those needed for mobilization of angioblasts and initial formation of the capillary tuft. For example, in co-cultures of epithelial cells with endothelium, epithelial-derived VEGF has been shown to induce fenestrae formation in the endothelium.[48] When Vegfr2 is inducibly deleted in adult mice, podocytes appear normal, but there is loss of viable glomerular endothelial cells.[199] Perhaps the continued expression of VEGF by podocytes and Flk1 by glomerular endothelial cells in vivo is necessary for maintenance of the highly-differentiated state seen in the endothelium.

Other Growth Factor/Receptors

Beyond VEGF and VEGFR, several other growth factor-receptor signaling systems important for vessel development systemically are also crucial for glomerular capillary formation, including the Tie/angiopoietin and PDGFR/PDGF families.[25,26] Developing glomerular endothelial cells express Tie-2, and and one of its ligands, angiopoietin-1, is important for vascular organization and remodeling. Another Tie-2 ligand, angiopoietin-2, may mediate vascular integrity and permeability. The coordinated expression of these two angiopoietins may therefore regulate the maturation and stabilization phases of glomerular development (reviewed in [49]). Additionally, Tie-2 and at least some members of the angiopoietins contain defined HREs in their promoters, making their transcriptional regulation by hypoxia/HIFs seem likely.[36] Similarly, an HRE is found in the PDGFB gene promoter, although this may not necessarily be responsive to hypoxia.[50] During early glomerular development, PDGFB protein is expressed by podocytes. This may be important for the glomerular recruitment of immature mesangial cells, which express the PDGFB receptor, PDGFRβ.[51] In later developmental stages, both PDGF and PDGFRβ expression becomes confined to the mesangium, which may provide autocrine signals required for mesangial cell proliferation and/or maturation[51] (see below).

Like other developing vessels, at least some neuronal axon guidance receptors and ligands are also found in developing glomeruli.[52–54] For example, neuropilin-1 (Np1), which is a co-receptor with VEGFR2 for VEGF$_{164}$ (but lacks a cytoplasmic signaling domain), immunolocalizes to glomerular endothelial cells. Semaphorins-3A and -3F, which are ligands for Np1, have been found on podocytes, suggesting that semaphorin-Np1 signaling between podocytes and endothelium may help pattern glomerular morphogenesis.[55] One study, however, has also reported that Np1 is expressed by podocytes in vivo.[56] Recent experiments also showed that podocyte-derived VEGF may act as an autocrine survival factor for cultured podocytes in vitro.[57] Additionally, these same studies found an upregulation of VEGFR2 in cultured podocytes, suggesting that VEGF/VEGFR2 signaling is important not only for glomerular capillary formation and maintenance, but also for podocyte differentiation.[57]

Other receptor-ligand signaling systems probably crucial for glomerular capillary formation include members of the Eph/ephrin receptor/counter-receptor families.[20,25] Specifically, the receptor tyrosine kinase EphB1 and its ligand, ephrin-B1, which itself is also a transmembrane protein receptor, are both expressed in similar distribution patterns in developing kidney microvasculature.[58] Although the precise roles for Eph/ephrin signaling in the glomerulus are still uncertain, knockout mice display lethal vascular phenotypes, including defects in vessel patterning, sprouting, and remodeling (reviewed in [25]). Reciprocal gradients of Eph and ephrin protein concentrations have been identified in the developing brain, where they appear to direct accurate neuronal patterning in the visual system. Perhaps analogous events take place in the developing glomerulus, where spatial signals conveyed between endothelial cells help target them to correct microanatomical domains.[25]

DEVELOPMENT OF THE MESANGIUM

Fundamentals regarding the development of the intercapillary mesangium, as well as the origin and recruitment of mesangial cell progenitors, are still largely unresolved issues in glomerular biology. Nevertheless, we have known for some time that PDGFB and its receptor, PDGFRβ, are both expressed by mesangial cells of mature glomeruli.[51] Additionally, studies in developing kidney have shown that immature podocytes produce PDGFB which may help recruit mesangial cell progenitors expressing PDGFRβ into glomeruli. Later, podocyte expression of PDGF declines, and the synthesis of both PDGF and PDGFRβ becomes confined to the mesangial cells, perhaps to promote their proliferation or maturation.[51] Gene deletion studies in mice have conclusively shown an absolute requirement for PDGFB/PDGFRβ signaling. Null mutants for either genes die perinatally, with massive hemorrhaging systemically.[59,60] Importantly, glomeruli in these mutants entirely lack mesangial cells and consist of one or only a few large, swollen capillary loops.[59,60]

Interestingly, once the glomerulus has fully matured, there appears to be a small population of extraglomerular mesangial cells capable of completely repopulating the glomerulus if the intraglomerular mesangium becomes severely injured. These mesangial reserve cells reside in the juxtaglomerular apparatus, and are distinct from renin-secreting cells, macrophages, vascular smooth muscle cells, and endothelial cells.[61] In an anti-Thy-1 model of proliferative glomerulonephritis in rats, these extraglomerular mesangial reserve cells migrate into the glomerulus and entirely restore the depleted intraglomerular mesangium.[61] Alternatively, some studies suggest that bone marrow hematopoitic stem cells can be a source of mesangial cells.[62] Perhaps additional studies based on these fascinating observations can shed more light on the origin and development of mesangial cells during glomerulogenesis. Similarly, much more work needs to be done on the assembly and maintenance of the mesangial matrix. Although this matrix undergoes morphologic and compositional changes throughout glomerulogenesis, it has not yet been the topic of thorough study. Whether the mesangial matrix is produced exclusively by mesangial cells or whether glomerular endothelial cells and podocytes also contribute components, are also not understood. On the other hand, and as discussed later, considerable progress has been made in understanding the assembly of the GBM (see below).

FACTORS REGULATING PODOCYTE DIFFERENTIATION

Determination of podocyte identity and regulation of podocyte differentiation are fundamental aspects of glomerulogenesis about which much remains to be learned. Although the podocyte transcription factors described below have been shown to be crucial for proper differentiation, exactly how these regulators interact to orchestrate the complex acquisition of the podocyte phenotype remains a mystery. Studies aimed at defining the entire glomerular transcriptome[63,64] have been very useful for defining what genes may play important roles in podocyte determination, differentiation, and function; however, we have only just begun to gain an understanding of how the podocyte achieves its unique and important properties through interacting pathways.[65]

WT1

The protein that likely has one of the earliest roles in podocyte differentiation is Wilms tumor 1 (WT1), a zinc-finger protein that is involved in both transcription and RNA processing.[66] WT1 is expressed at the initial stages of nephrogenesis, when it has been shown to regulate such developmentally important genes as *Bmp7*, *Six2*, and *Sall1*.[67] But once glomerulogenesis begins, there is a dramatic increase in the level of WT1 in podocyte precursors, and podocytes continue to express WT1 throughout life (reviewed in [68]). One potentially important function of WT1 is to downregulate expression of Pax2 in the immature podocytes of S-shape stage nephrons,[69] as artificial overexpression of Pax2 widely, including in podocytes, causes severe nephrotic syndrome.[70] In addition, WT1 has been shown to regulate a number of genes, including NPHS1,[71,72] the gene encoding nephrin (discussed below). This provides a clear mechanism whereby alteration in WT1 function directly affects glomerular function.

Several lines of investigation reveal important roles for WT1 in promoting proper podocyte differentiation (reviewed in [66,68,73]). Most notable is that heterozygous mutations that affect the zinc-finger structure of WT1 cause Denys—Drash syndrome in humans. This rare disease is characterized by proteinuria, nephrotic syndrome, diffuse mesangial sclerosis, and ESRD. Expression of mutant WT1 forms associated with Denys—Drash syndrome in transgenic mice, either globally or specifically in podocytes, causes various glomerular and podocyte defects that are consistent with the human pathology.[66,74] Moreover, heterozygous mutations in WT1 that affect the normal pattern of WT1 RNA alternative splicing to generate the so-called +KTS and −KTS isoforms of WT1, cause Frasier syndrome.[75] The renal component of this disease includes proteinuria that begins in early childhood and progresses to FSGS, but the course to ESRD is slower than observed in Denys—Drash syndrome. Mice engineered to express only the +KTS or the −KTS isoforms develop severe podocyte and glomerular defects, further emphasizing the important role that WT1 and these specific splice variants play in glomerular development and function.[76]

Lmx1b

Lmx1b, a LIM-homeodomain protein, is another transcription factor expressed in podocytes that is affected in human disease. Heterozygous mutations in LMX1B cause Nail—Patella syndrome,[77] an autosomal dominant disease with skeletal abnormalities, nail hypoplasia, and variably penetrant nephropathy associated with accumulation of fibrillar material in the GBM that appears to be collagen type III.[78] Although Lmx1b$^{+/-}$ mice do not exhibit a phenotype, Lmx1b$^{-/-}$ mice die shortly after birth with abnormalities in dorsal limb structures, including absence of nails and patellae, abnormal glomeruli, attenuated podocyte maturation with lack of normal slit diaphragms, and tubular protein casts.[79] Analysis of gene expression in Lmx1b$^{-/-}$ podocytes has revealed decreases in collagen α3 and α4(IV), podocin, and CD2AP,[80–82] which are all known to be important for proper glomerular filtration. The reduced expression in Lmx1b$^{-/-}$ mice suggests a basis for the partially penetrant nephropathy in LMX1B$^{+/-}$ humans, but gene expression studies in affected individuals do not support this hypothesis.[78] Thus, exactly how LMX1B haploinsufficiency causes nephropathy in humans remains a mystery. If there really is no reduction in the expression of relevant podocyte genes, then perhaps there is a lack of repression, either direct or indirect, of genes injurious to glomerular function, as previously proposed.[83]

Pod1/Tcf21

Pod1, a basic helix-loop-helix transcription factor also known as epicardin, capsulin, and Tcf21, is highly expressed early during kidney development in condensing metanephric mesenchyme and in stromal cells. In the developing nephron, Pod1 is expressed in podocyte precursors at the S-shaped stage, and persists in adult podocytes.[73,84] The kidney phenotype in Pod1[−/−] mice, which die at birth due to heart and lung defects, is complex, but it is clear that there are fewer glomeruli associated with defects in ureteric bud branching. In addition, there is a striking arrest of glomerular development at the capillary loop stage, and podocytes fail to mature properly, elaborating only rudimentary foot processes.[85] Gene expression profiling studies of Pod1[−/−] glomeruli revealed 3986 genes expressed differently than in wild-type glomeruli, demonstrating that Pod1 has profound effects on gene expression.[86]

Kreisler/Mafb

Kreisler/Mafb is a basic domain leucine zipper transcription factor expressed in podocytes from the capillary loop stage onwards.[87] Mice that are homozygous for a point mutation affecting the kreisler DNA-binding domain die within 24 hours of birth. The podocytes of these mice fail to extend foot processes or establish slit diaphragms, and there is a significant reduction in expression of nephrin, podocin, and CD2AP.[88] Interestingly, whereas Pod1 is expressed in kreisler[−/−] podocytes, kreisler is not expressed in Pod1[−/−] podocytes. This suggests the existence of a transcriptional hierarchy in which Pod1 may activate expression of kreisler.[87]

Foxc2

Foxc2 is a member of the forkhead/winged-helix family of transcription factors. During nephrogenesis, Foxc2 is first expressed in a subset of cells in the comma-shaped body and then is expressed in developing podocytes at the S-shaped and capillary loop stages, and more weakly at maturity.[89] Foxc2[−/−] mice exhibit small kidneys and reduced numbers of glomeruli with ballooned capillaries, suggesting a defect in adhesion of mesangial cells (which are present) to the glomerular basement membrane (GBM). Ultrastructural analyses revealed that podocytes fail to extend processes or assemble slit diaphragms, and endothelial cells fail to become fenestrated, suggesting an arrest of differentiation of these two cell types. Gene expression profiling studies of Foxc2[−/−] glomeruli showed reductions in a number of known podocyte genes, such as kreisler/Mafb, Nphs2 (podocin), and Podxl1 (podocalyxin), although others, such as Nphs1, Wt1, and Cd2ap, were not affected.[89] Interestingly, in the Xenopus pronephros, the combined knockdown of WT1 and Foxc2 resulted in the loss of all podocyte marker gene expression.[65]

Notch2

Notch2 is expressed in developing podocytes from as early as the comma-shaped stage.[90] Although the total absence of Notch2 in mice results in embryonic lethality at E11.5 before glomerulogenesis begins, homozygosity for a hypomorphic Notch2 allele allows survival until 24 hours after birth. These latter Notch2[−/−] mice exhibit small kidneys with cortical vascular lesions. Some glomeruli arrested before the capillary loop stage and were not vascularized, whereas others became vascularized but had ballooned capillaries due to an absence of mesangial cells. In addition, genetic interaction studies demonstrated that Jagged1, a Notch ligand, is required for proper Notch2 signaling during glomerulogenesis.[90] Additional studies using a conditional Notch2 allele showed that Notch2 (but not Notch1) is required for acquisition of podocyte and proximal tubule cell fates.[91,92]

FORMATION OF THE SLIT DIAPHRAGM COMPLEX

In mature glomeruli, the slit diaphragm (SD) represents the only known connection between adjacent podocytes and podocyte foot processes. The SD spans the space between the interdigitated foot processes (Figure 26.4), and has been proposed to play a crucial role in glomerular filtration by serving as the major barrier to albumin,[93] although some data do not support this view.[94,95] The SD has also been shown to mediate important signaling events that are responsible for maintaining podocyte survival and differentiation,[96,97] suggesting that it plays dual roles in ensuring proper glomerular function. But interestingly, mutant mice without slit diaphragms due to lack of nephrin have dramatic leakage of albumin into the urine, but they do not have major alterations in podocyte survival or gene expression.[98]

Slit Diaphragm Components

Nephrin and the Neph Family

The explosion of research into SD composition and function began with the identification of the nephrin gene (NPHS1), as mutated in congenital nephrotic syndrome of the Finnish type,[99] and the nephrin protein as an integral component of the SD[100,101] (Figure 26.5). Nephrin is an immunoglobulin superfamily member containing eight extracellular Ig-like domains, a

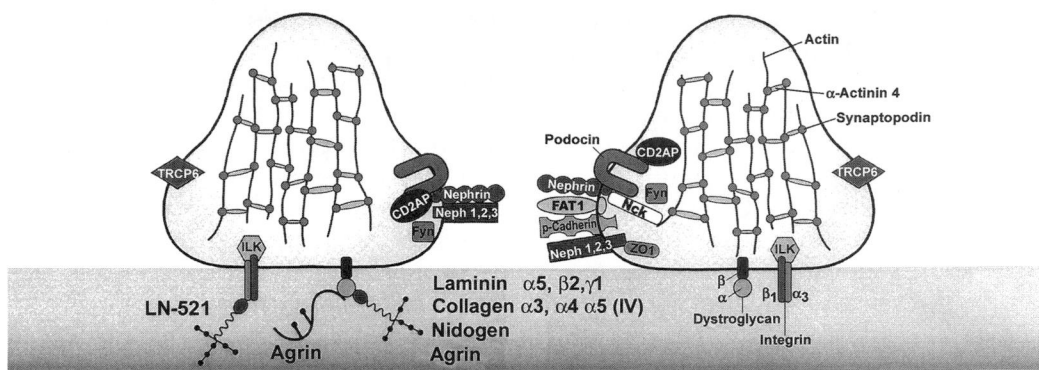

FIGURE 26.5 Diagram showing clustering of the slit diaphragm complex proteins at the basolateral surfaces of podocyte foot processes, which are attached to the underlying GBM (shown in blue). Molecules are not drawn to scale, but many known extracellular and intracellular protein:protein interactions are represented. Exactly how the several protein ectodomains interact to form the characteristic SD ultrastructure is not yet fully defined. See text for details. See color section at the end of the book.

fibronectin type III domain, a single-pass transmembrane domain, and a cytoplasmic tail of ~155 amino acids, including several tyrosines that have been predicted to be important for its function, perhaps by interacting with actin-binding Nck adapter proteins.[102−106] Humans and mice lacking nephrin never establish SDs, demonstrating the importance of nephrin for SD formation. A group of three related Ig superfamily molecules that interact with nephrin, Neph1-3, are also found at the SD, as well as in other tissues, and it is clear that at least Neph1 is required for maintenance of the filtration barrier.[107] Interestingly, nephrin interacts directly with the Neph proteins[108−110] (Figure 26.5), and disturbing their association *in vivo* causes proteinuria.[111]

Further evidence for the importance of nephrin-Neph interactions come from the model organisms *Drosophila* (fruitflies) and *C. elegans* (nematodes), which have conserved homologs of nephrin and Neph proteins. In both these invertebrates, a nephrin homolog on one cell interacts with a Neph homolog on another cell to promote a developmental event.[112−114] Amazingly, all three mouse Neph proteins can partially compensate for the nematode Neph-like protein SYG-1.[115] Together with data from mouse, these results suggest that nephrin-Neph interactions are conserved across phyla.

ZO-1 and Podocin

Before the identification of nephrin, zonula occludens-1 (ZO-1), an epithelial tight junction protein, was shown to be localized to the cytoplasmic face of the SD.[116] ZO-1 has recently been shown to interact with Neph1−3, which may serve to anchor it to the SD. In turn, podocin, whose encoding gene (*NPHS2*) is mutated in familial steroid resistant nephrotic syndrome, appears important for anchoring nephrin and the Neph family to the SD (Figure 26.5). Podocin is a hairpin-shaped integral membrane protein that interacts with the cytoplasmic tails of nephrin and Neph family members,[117] and is required to target nephrin to lipid raft microdomains, which have been proposed to be crucial for SD organization and function.[118]

Cadherins

Consistent with the notion that the SD is a modified adherens junction,[119] two cadherins, P-cadherin and the FAT1 protocadherin, have been localized to the SD. P-cadherin was found to associate with ZO-1 and the catenins at the SD, but the functional importance of P-cadherin at the SD has yet to be demonstrated, and humans with mutations in the P-cadherin gene (*CDH3*) are not reported to have kidney disease. FAT1, an extremely large member of the cadherin family, is involved in regulating actin cytoskeleton dynamics and cell polarization.[120] Mice lacking FAT1 die within two days of birth, and their podocytes lack SDs and significant foot process formation. This underscores the importance of FAT1 in the establishment or maintenance of SDs. A model of the SD that can accommodate the very large extracellular domain of FAT1 has not yet been presented, but FAT1 may somehow contribute to the central density of the SD that is apparent in ultrastructural analyses.[93,121]

CD2AP

CD2-associated protein (CD2AP) is a modular cytoplasmic docking protein that interacts with multiple slit diaphragm components, including nephrin and podocin, as well as with the actin cytoskeleton[122,123] (Figure 26.5). Mice lacking CD2AP exhibit congenital nephrotic syndrome with progressive loss of SDs and foot processes, and they die at 6−7 weeks of age.[124] In addition, CD2AP haploinsufficiency has been associated with renal disease in both mice and humans,[125,126] and a patient homozygous for a premature stop codon mutation (R612X) lacking the final 28 amino acids of 639 total exhibited proteinuria, FSGS, and kidney failure by 3 years of age.[127] CD2AP is thought to be an adaptor that forms a bridge between the SD and the cytoskeleton,[128] but it also appears to play a role in the trafficking of endocytic vesicles.[122,126] Although CD2AP is very widely expressed, it seems to be required only in the podocyte[129]; this could be due to compensation by a paralog of CD2AP, CIN85, although CIN85 activity in podocytes appears to be detrimental.[130]

Nck

That mice lacking CD2AP are able to form normal foot processes and SDs initially suggests the existence of other adaptor proteins in podocytes that might play an earlier role in organizing SDs and linking them to the cytoskeleton. Indeed, the Nck adaptor proteins (Nck1 and Nck2), which contain three Src homology 3 (SH3) domains and one SH2 domain, bind to phosphotyrosine-containing motifs in the cytoplasmic tail of nephrin via their SH2 domains. In addition, clustering of nephrin-Nck complexes reorganized the actin cytoskeleton in transfected cells.[102,105] Importantly, genetically-engineered mice lacking Nck1 and Nck2 in podocytes failed to elaborate foot processes or assemble SDs,[102] and inducible deletion of Nck1 and Nck2 in adult podocytes rapidly leads to proteinuria and glomerulosclerosis.[131] These exciting findings establish a potentially pivotal role for the Nck adaptor proteins in organizing and maintaining SDs, and suggest one mechanism whereby the Fin minor mutation in NPHS1, which results in a nephrin protein lacking most of its cytoplasmic tail and all of the intracellular tyrosines,[99] causes congenital nephrotic syndrome.

TRPC6

TRPC6 is a member of the transient receptor potential family of cation channel proteins, and is associated with the SD. Mutations in TRPC6 have been shown to cause autosomal dominant FSGS in several different families, and this was associated with increased calcium current amplitude in some cases.[132,133] Calcium flux mediated by TRPC6 could have an important role in regulating podocyte and SD homeostasis, perhaps by regulating actin dynamics and motility[134] and calcium-sensitive transcription factors such as those in the NFAT family.[135]

Slit Diaphragm Assembly Mechanisms

As mentioned earlier, the slit diaphragm bears some relationship to adherens junctions, and ZO-1 immunolocalizes to the cytoplasmic domains on the lateral surfaces of podocytes adjacent to the extracellular diaphragm spanning the slit pore. The synthetic patterns of all of the SD components during glomerular development have not yet been studied in detail. However, nephrin and podocin first appear during the late S-shaped and early capillary loop stages of nephron development, which is when foot process interdigitation first occurs, simultaneous with the first ultrastructural appearance of SDs.[100,136] Also occurring at this stage of development is the apical-to-basal translocation of protein complexes involved in cell polarity, an event crucial for proper slit diaphragm and foot process formation.[137,138] The precise sequence of SD assembly, including how the linkages between the ectodomains of SD proteins are made, as well as connections with the internal cytoskeleton and associated elements, are not known. Similarly, the extent to which the SD may be dynamic and undergo modification with age is poorly-understood. Nevertheless, an increasing number of studies have shown that the SD does not merely represent a static component of the glomerular filtration barrier, but it also functions to influence podocyte behavior.[97]

Signaling at the Slit Diaphragm

The first evidence that the SD complex may have a signaling role came from studies of nephrin activity in cultured cells. Transfection of cells with nephrin increased activator protein-1 (AP1)-mediated transcriptional activation, and this effect on intracellular signaling was augmented by cotransfection with podocin, to which nephrin binds.[139] These authors later showed that podocin recruits nephrin to lipid rafts,[118] which are cholesterol-enriched plasma membrane microdomains associated with high concentrations of signaling proteins and high levels of signaling activity. Furthermore, as alluded to above, nephrin contains multiple tyrosines in its cytoplasmic tail. Some of these can be phosphorylated by the Src-family tyrosine kinase, Fyn,[106] and clustering of nephrin by Fyn increases phosphorylation.[103] Phosphorylation of nephrin both augments its interaction with podocin[104] and allows Nck adaptor proteins to bind its tail and influence the organization of the adjacent actin cytoskeleton.[102,105] Consistent with this, $Fyn^{-/-}$ mice have variably coarsened or effaced foot processes.[106] In addition, trans-heterozgyous $Fyn^{+/-}$; $Cd2ap^{+/-}$ mice exhibit marked proteinuria and FSGS, and CD2AP can be immunoprecipitated with Fyn from glomerular lysates. These findings demonstrate that Fyn-mediated signaling likely depends upon interactions with CD2AP.[125]

Nephrin-mediated signaling has also been shown to involve stimulation of phosphoinositide 3-OH kinase (PI3K). Nephrin and CD2AP interact with the p85 regulatory subunit of PI3K, recruit PI3K to the plasma membrane and, in conjunction with podocin, stimulate PI3K activation of AKT signaling in podocytes.[140] This is proposed to regulate the behavior of podocytes and protect them from detachment—induced apoptosis (anoikis), which suggests that proper signaling at the SD is important for maintaining podocyte health.

Neph family proteins, like nephrin, have cytoplasmic tails containing tyrosines that can be phosphorylated. Also like nephrin, Neph1 can induce AP-1-mediated transcriptional activation.[117] ZO-1, which binds to the cytoplasmic tail of Neph proteins, enhances tyrosine phosphorylation of Neph1 and augments AP-1 activation.[141] As ZO-1 can also interact with the actin cytoskeleton, one can envisage how the podocin-CD2AP-nephrin-Neph-ZO-1 complex can activate signaling in podocytes and provide stability to the SD via linkage to actin (Figure 26.5). Interfering with any of these interactions likely leads to abnormal podocyte behavior and proteinuria; in this regard, the actin cytoskeleton in podocyte foot processes also has specialized components. These include α-actinin-4, which is mutated in autosomal dominant FSGS,[142] and synaptopodin, which regulates α-actinin's actin bundling activity[143] and binds to CD2AP.[125] That trans-heterozygous $Synpo^{+/-}$; $Cd2ap^{+/-}$ mice develop proteinuria and FSGS-like lesions[125] underscores the importance of the SD-actin cytoskeleton linkage in maintaining podocyte health, structure, and function. Further support comes from a study showing that the action of cyclosporine A in reducing proteinuria has to do with a protective effect on synaptopodin and on the podocyte's actin cytoskeleton.[144]

DEVELOPMENTAL-ORGANIZATIONAL ROLE OF THE GLOMERULAR BASEMENT MEMBRANE

An important extracellular matrix component of developing and mature glomeruli is the glomerular basement membrane (GBM). Basement membranes are the thin sheets of specialized extracellular matrix that underlie all epithelial cells, including the vascular endothelium. The GBM is somewhat unique in that it is an unusually thick basement membrane that forms by fusion of two independent basement membranes, one secreted by podocytes and one by endothelial cells. Thus, both cell types contribute components to the GBM. Like all basement membranes, the GBM contains laminin, type IV collagen, nidogen/entactin, and sulfated proteoglycans.[145] These are all relatively large glycoproteins of which there are multiple isoforms, but only specific ones are found in the GBM.[146] These isoforms are thought to impart properties to the GBM that

are important for maintaining glomerular structure and function.

Laminin

Most laminins are cruciform heterotrimers consisting of evolutionarily related α, β, and γ chains.[147] There are five α, four β, and three γ chains that associate nonrandomly and become disulfide bonded to each other to form at least 15 different heterotrimers, most of which are $\sim$800 kDa.[148] Assembly of trimers occurs intracellularly within the endoplasmic reticulum, and then trimers are secreted into the extracellular space where they interact with cellular receptors, such as integrins and dystroglycan, and polymerize with each other to form laminin networks.[149] This network provides the foundation of the basement membrane; as shown in knockout mice, basement membranes do not form without laminin.[148]

Only a subset of the known laminin heterotrimers are expressed in glomeruli, and only a single heterotrimer, laminin $\alpha5\beta2\gamma1$ (designated LM-521),[147] is found in the mature GBM[146] (Figure 26.4). The mesangial matrix, on the other hand, which is structurally and compositionally similar but distinct from basement membranes, contains an assortment of laminins, including LM-111, LM-211, LM-411, and LM-511.[146] Whether these mesangial laminins have any specific functions in glomerular biology is not yet clear, but they could certainly influence the behavior of mesangial cells and interact with laminins or other components of the GBM to strengthen the adhesion of the mesangium to GBM segments at the bases of the glomerular capillary loops. In contrast, as discussed below, the laminin content of the GBM is well-known to be extremely important for both glomerular development and function.

Developmental Transitions in GBM Laminin Composition

During glomerulogenesis there are well-characterized developmental transitions in the deposition of laminin isoforms in the GBM and its precursor.[150] From the comma-shape through the S-shape stage, LM-111 and LM-411 are present, but they are eliminated from the GBM during the transition to the capillary loop stage (Figures 26.2 and 26.3). At the S-shape stage, LM-511 is first deposited in the nascent GBM by the presumptive podocytes and the invading endothelial cells. At the capillary loop stage, both LM-511 and LM-521 are present in the maturing GBM, but LM-511 is gradually eliminated as the glomerulus begins functioning as a filter. LM-521 is from then on the major GBM laminin.[150] While little is known about the transcriptional control of these isoform transitions during glomerular development, it is clear that the *in vivo* setting is important, as metanephroi grown *ex vivo* do not deposit LM-521. This deficiency is rescued upon reimplantation and subsequent glomerular vascularization *in vivo*, suggesting that glomerular endothelial cells are required for proper laminin isoform substitution.[151]

LAMININ A CHAIN TRANSITIONS

Experiments primarily in knockout mice have revealed the importance of some of these developmental transitions for successful glomerulogenesis and proper glomerular function. A targeted mutation in Lama5, the gene encoding laminin α5, results in breakdown of the GBM at the stage when LM-511 should begin to replace LM-111 (late S-shape stage).[152] In the absence of LM-511, LM-111 is still eliminated from the nascent GBM, and without a full-size laminin trimer, GBM architecture cannot be maintained. The loss of the GBM at this critical stage of glomerulogenesis has severe consequences, as podocytes lose their cup-shaped arrangement and instead contract into a ball of cells, leaving no place for the endothelial and mesangial cells to form capillaries. Thus, glomerular vascularization completely fails.[152] Additional studies aimed at defining the function of the laminin α5 COOH-terminal globular (α5LG) domain in glomerulogenesis showed that this domain is not important for maintenance of GBM integrity, but rather serves as a ligand for mesangial cells to adhere to the GBM at the bases of the glomerular capillary loops so that they can maintain and perhaps modulate capillary loop structure and diameter, as previously proposed.[153] When this ligand is missing, the capillaries balloon in a fashion similar to that observed in the absence of mesangial cells (discussed above), yet here mesangial cells are clearly present but apparently unable to adhere to the GBM under the stress of capillary blood flow.[154] These studies show that the GBM and the laminin that it contains serve important organizational roles, both during and after glomerulogenesis.

LAMININ β CHAIN TRANSITIONS

In contrast to the requirement for laminin α5 for successful glomerulogenesis, laminin β2 is dispensable. This is best demonstrated by the structurally normal glomeruli that form in Lamb2[−/−] mice, which correlates with maintenance of GBM integrity during glomerulogenesis.[155] The GBM is able to remain intact without LM-521, the only isoform normally found in mature GBM, because of the persistence or continued expression of laminin β1, resulting in a GBM containing LM-511 instead of LM-521. However, despite normal glomerulogenesis, Lamb2[−/−] mice exhibit

congenital nephrotic syndrome and are proteinuric.[155] Similarly, humans with mutations in LAMB2 exhibit congenital nephrotic syndrome and diffuse mesangial sclerosis that is sometimes associated with distinct ocular and other abnormalities, a disease entity called Pierson syndrome.[156−158] Together these results show that laminin β2 in the GBM (as part of LM-521) is uniquely qualified to ensure that the glomerular barrier to protein is intact. This could be due to either direct effects on GBM porosity or indirect effects on behavior of the attached endothelium and overlying podocytes, as well as assembly and function of the slit diaphragm complex.

Post-fixation immunoelectron microscopy of wild-type mouse kidney has shown that the laminin α1, α5, β1, and β2 chains all originate in both glomerular endothelial cells and podocytes during glomerular development.[151] Similarly, in transgenic mice that overexpress human *LAMA5*, endothelial cells and podocytes were both positive for human laminin α5 protein.[200]

Collagen Type IV

There are six genetically distinct collagen IV chains, called α chains, that assemble in a defined fashion to form three different triple helical protomers.[159,160] These are designated $(\alpha1)_2\alpha2$, $\alpha3\alpha4\alpha5$, and $(\alpha5)_2\alpha6$. Like all collagen chains, collagen IV chains contain long stretches of Gly-X-Y amino acid triplet repeats that favor formation of a triple helix. However, unlike most other collagens, type IV contains interspersed interruptions of the triplet repeats that provide flexibility both to the protomers and to the collagen IV network. This is in turn thought to impart needed flexibility to basement membranes.[161]

Collagen IV protomers interact with each other via both covalent and non-covalent interactions to form a chicken wire-like network, and a substantial amount of cross-linking stabilizes the network. Surprisingly, knockout mice demonstrate that collagen IV is not absolutely required for basement membrane formation, but it is crucial for basement membrane maintenance and stability.[162]

Most basement membranes in the body contain the $\alpha(1)_2\alpha2$ protomer, and this is also true of the early nephrogenic epithelial structures (Figure 26.2). As is the case for the laminins, α1α2α1 collagen(IV) originates in both endothelial cells and podocytes.[163] However, at the capillary loop stage, the α3, α4, and α5 chains become detectable in the GBM[150] (Figure 26.3), and have been shown to be made exclusively by podocytes.[163] At maturity, the α3α4α5 protomer represents the major collagen IV component of the

GBM (Figure 26.4), although apparently small amounts of presumably residual $(\alpha1)_2\alpha2$ can also be detected, more so in human than in mouse GBM. On the other hand, the $\alpha1$ and $\alpha2$(IV) chains are abundant in the mesangial matrix, whereas the $\alpha3$, $\alpha4$, and $\alpha5$ chains are absent.[146] Interestingly, the basement membrane of Bowman's capsule contains $(\alpha1)_2\alpha2$ and $(\alpha5)_2\alpha6$ protomers.[164]

As implied by the existence of only three different collagen IV protomers *in vivo*, the $\alpha3$ and $\alpha4$(IV) chains exist exclusively in combination with $\alpha5$(IV) to make the $\alpha3\alpha4\alpha5$ protomer.[159,160] Thus, if any one of the three genes encoding these chains is altered by genetic mutation, this protomer is affected. Mutations that prevent proper assembly of this protomer cause Alport syndrome or hereditary glomerulonephritis, in humans, dogs, and mice,[159,160] as discussed in detail in Chapter 90. In the absence of the $\alpha3\alpha4\alpha5$ protomer, there are no defects in glomerulogenesis, primarily due to compensation by the collagen IV network containing the $(\alpha1)_2\alpha2$ protomer. However, as affected individuals age, the abnormal GBM develops characteristic lesions, including thickening and splitting, that eventually lead to renal failure in most cases.[165] Heterozygous mutations in human and mouse Col4a1 have also been shown to cause disease that includes defects in kidney function.[166–169]

Nidogen—Entactin

Nidogens are dumbbell-shaped molecules.[145] There are two isoforms of nidogen, nidogen-1 and -2, and both have been reported to be present in the GBM.[170] Nidogen-1 was previously considered to be an obligatory link between the laminin and collagen IV networks, because it binds well to each of them.[145] However, mutant mice lacking both nidogens-1 and -2 survive to birth with most basement membranes intact, demonstrating that nidogen is not required for the integrity of all basement membranes.[171] Although the double knockouts died on the day of birth, urine removed from their bladders showed only a marginal increase in low molecular weight proteins,[171] suggesting that the glomerular barrier to albumin was intact and therefore not dependent on the presence of nidogen in the GBM.

Nidogen-1 binds to laminin trimers via a high-affinity interaction with a specific domain of the laminin $\gamma1$ chain.[172] To determine the biological importance of this interaction, 56 amino acids encompassing this domain of $\gamma1$ were deleted in mice such that nidogen-1 could no longer bind laminin.[173] Interestingly, the result was a phenotype that is in many ways more severe than the total absence of both nidogen-1 and -2. For example,

homozygotes died immediately after birth rather than surviving for many hours. Renal agenesis was very common, and glomerular capillary aneurisms and hydronephrosis occurred in those few kidneys that did form.[173] Together, the results of these two studies[171,173] suggest that the alteration to laminin $\gamma1$ affects more than just its ability to bind nidogens, but the phenotype of this Lamc1 mutant also underscores the importance of laminin for proper glomerulogenesis.

Sulfated Proteoglycans

Proteoglycans consist of a core protein with covalently attached glycosaminoglycan side chains (GAGs). Those proteoglycans present in basement membranes are usually modified further on their GAGs by addition of heparan sulfate and/or chondroitin sulfate. The anionic character of these sulfate-containing adducts provides much of the basement membrane's net negative charge. A large number of experiments performed in animals suggest that the glomerular filtration barrier possesses charge selectivity, and the sulfated proteoglycans that are present in the GBM are attractive candidates to provide the basis for at least part of this selectivity against the passage of negatively charged molecules into the urine. However, recent studies suggest that anionic charges within the GBM may not be involved in establishment of the glomerular filtration barrier under normal circumstances.[174,175]

Perlecan

There are four major sulfated proteoglycans with relevance to the glomerulus, and the best-studied biochemically is perlecan. Perlecan consists of a 400 kDa core protein with three heparan sulfate chains linked to residues near the NH2-terminus. It is widely found in basement membranes, and is abundant in the mesangial matrix, but perlecan is only weakly detected in the GBM.[176] Cleavage of the COOH-terminus of perlecan produces a fragment with antiangiogenic activity called endorepellin.[177]

Knockout mice lacking perlecan die during embryogenesis or in the neonatal period with multiple developmental defects. Most basement membranes form normally, but mechanical stress causes disruptions in meningeal and cardiomyocyte basement membranes. Perlecan is also normally found in cartilage extracellular matrix, and this matrix is severely disrupted in perlecan mutants.[178,179] No defects in kidneys were noted in these mice.

To investigate further the function of perlecan as a heparan sulfate proteoglycan, a deletion was made that affects only the small part of the protein to which the GAGs are normally attached. Mice carrying this mutation are viable, but they have defects in the lens capsule.[180] Neither functional nor structural defects were noted in kidney glomeruli under normal circumstances, but these mice exhibit elevated levels of urinary protein after bovine serum albumin overload.[181] Because little perlecan is detectable in the GBM, it is somewhat surprising that removal of its GAGs can have an effect on the filtration barrier.

Agrin

Agrin is a widely expressed modular proteoglycan that consists of a core protein of ∼220 kDa with two glycosaminoglycan side chains that carry heparan sulfate and/or chondroitin sulfate. These increase the molecular weight of agrin to greater than 400 kDa. Agrin exhibits robust binding to the coiled-coil domain of the laminin γ1 chain *in vitro*,[182] and this might indicate that agrin is involved in organization of basement membrane architecture.

Agrin has been intensively studied by the neuroscience community because a specific splice form of agrin is deposited by motor neurons on developing skeletal muscle fibers, where it serves as a signal that is in part responsible for maintaining the aggregation of acetylcholine receptors to ensure the proper assembly of the neuromuscular junction.[183,184] In kidney, agrin is highly concentrated in the GBM,[185] significantly more so than perlecan, but there is as yet no evidence that it serves any signaling functions. Agrin has, however, been proposed to be responsible for the anionic charge that is present in the GBM, and that is presumed to be involved in establishing the charge-selective aspect of the glomerular barrier to protein.

Several different mutations have been made in the mouse agrin gene. Whereas all but the most subtle of these have dramatic effects on the differentiation of the neuromuscular junction, no defects in the kidney have been found. Because agrin mutant mice die at birth due to an inability to breathe, agrin-null kidneys beyond the neonatal period have not been studied. Nevertheless, no defects in glomerulogenesis were noted in agrin-deficient kidneys at perinatal stages.[175] In addition, a conditional knockout of agrin in podocytes using the Cre/loxP system was successful at removing both agrin and fixed anionic sites from the GBM, yet there were no detectable defects in glomerular filtration.[175] These results show that agrin likely plays no role either in glomerulogenesis or in establishment of the glomerular barrier to protein. Further, these findings suggest that glomerular charge selectivity may be contributed by podocyte and endothelial cell surface molecules, rather than by GBM proteoglycans.

Other Proteoglycans

Although perlecan and agrin are the best-studied GBM proteoglycans, two others have been shown to be present. Collagen XVIII, the COOH-terminus of which is cleaved to form the antiangiogenic molecule endostatin,[177] is unique in that it is a basement membrane collagen with heparan sulfate glycosaminoglycan side chains.[186] It is present in the GBM, but its function there, if any, is unknown. Mutant mice lacking collagen XVIII have no reported glomerular defects, but do exhibit abnormal blood vessel formation in the eye and retinal defects.[187] Consistent with this, Knobloch syndrome in humans is caused by mutations in COL18A1.[188]

A basement membrane chondroitin sulfate proteoglycan that exhibits transient deposition in postnatal rat GBM has been described.[189] Although nothing is known about the function of this protein, of potential interest is the fact that increased levels of this proteoglycan were detected in the GBM of diabetic rats, compared to the normal situation where it is not detected in mature GBM.[190]

RECEPTORS AND RECEPTOR-ASSOCIATED PROTEINS MEDIATING GLOMERULAR CELL INTERACTIONS WITH THE GBM

In order for glomerular cells to interact appropriately with the GBM, they must express the required matrix receptors and the associated cytoplasmic proteins that mediate responses to the engagement of ligand. While there is a plethora of these molecules, only a limited set have been studied in the context of glomerulogenesis and glomerular function.

The best characterized matrix receptors are the integrins. Integrins are a large family of transmembrane αβ heterodimers that bind to extracellular matrix proteins, mediate adhesion, and transduce signals that govern cell proliferation, survival, and migration. The most studied integrin in the glomerulus is α3β1. This is primarily a laminin-binding integrin, although it has also been shown to bind collagen IV. Biochemical studies suggest that α3β1 preferentially binds laminins containing the α3 and α5 chains. This would include the LM-511 and LM-521 heterotrimers that, as discussed above, are so important for glomerular development and function.

The first indication that integrin α3β1 is important for glomerulogenesis came from studies of Itga3 mutant mice, which lack integrin α3.[191] These mice die in the neonatal period due to defects in both kidney and lung. Glomerulogenesis occurs in a mostly normal fashion, but ultrastructural analysis reveals that formation of podocyte foot processes is defective, and the GBM appears highly disorganized.[191] These data are consistent with the fact that podocytes express integrin α3β1 at a high level, and suggest that α3β1 is involved in organizing GBM architecture, perhaps by modulating polymerization of secreted laminins, and in regulating foot process extension. Integrin α3β1 also serves as a mesangial cell receptor for the COOH-terminal LG domain of laminin α5 in the GBM. Their interaction at the base of the glomerular capillary loops allows mesangial cells to maintain loop structure. If this interaction is impaired, either by alteration of the composition of the LG domain or by deletion of integrin α3, then capillary ballooning occurs.[154,191] Ballooning is more severe in the former case, indicating that there is likely a receptor on mesangial cells besides integrin α3β1 that mediates binding to the GBM. One possibility is integrin α8β1, as older Itga8$^{-/-}$ mice exhibit widening of the glomerular capillaries, although the effect is mild.[192]

Integrin α3β1 is one of many integrins that use the integrin-linked kinase (ILK) as an intermediate in signal transduction. ILK binds to integrins and to various actin-binding proteins, and therefore serves to bridge the actin cytoskeleton with the cell's major linkage to the extracellular matrix. Whereas mice lacking ILK die as very early peri-implantation embryos, mice with a podocyte-specific deletion of ILK survive for a few months, but they eventually succumb to an end-stage renal disease that begins with thickening and broadening of the GBM, followed by focal segmental glomerulosclerosis.[193] Mutation of CD151, a tetraspanin family protein expressed by podocytes that interacts with and modulates integrin function, can also cause GBM defects and glomerular disease.[194,195] These data further underscore the importance of the podocyte in organizing GBM architecture.

CONCLUDING REMARKS

Although much progress has been made in understanding certain aspects of glomerular development, many important questions remain. First and foremost, the fundamental morphogenic events that initiate, propel, and conclude glomerulogenesis are still poorly-defined. In this chapter, we discussed a series of different transcription factors, intracellular and transmembrane proteins, growth factors, and various signaling mechanisms associated with glomerular endothelial cell and podocyte biology. With only a few exceptions, however, most of these individual proteins and processes are expressed by many other cells and tissues throughout the body, and therefore are not likely to be solely or directly responsible for development of the glomerulus. On the other hand, there are a few features of the glomerulus that are both compositionally and structurally distinct, and these include the GBM and epithelial slit diaphragm. Similarly, the intercapillary mesangial cell and its matrix are also unusual structures not found in other vascular beds. We believe that more research aimed at investigating the regulation of the synthesis, assembly, and maintenance of the GBM, SD, and mesangium specifically may yield detailed new insights into how the glomerulus develops and is maintained normally. Perhaps new therapies that retrace parts of the normal developmental pathway could then be designed and used successfully to repair injured glomeruli.

Acknowledgments

We thank Erin Cambron and the late Eileen Roach for help with the illustrations. Our supporting funds came from the National Institutes of Health.

References

[1] Abrahamson DR. Glomerulogenesis in the developing kidney. Sem Nephrol 1991;11:375—89.

[2] Saxen L. Organogenesis of the kidney. Cambridge, UK: Cambridge University Press; 1987.

[3] Woolf AS. The life of the human kidney before birth: its secrets unfold. Pediatr Res 2001;49:8—10.

[4] Abrahamson DR. Structure and development of the glomerular capillary wall and basement membrane. Am J Physiol 1987;253: F783—794.

[5] Ekblom P. Formation of basement membranes in the embryonic kidney: an immunohistological study. J Cell Biol 1981;91:1—10.

[6] Lelongt B, Makino H, Kanwar YS. Maturation of the developing renal glomerulus with respect to basement membrane proteoglycans. Kidney Int 1987;32:498—506.

[7] Abrahamson DR, Wang R. Development of the glomerular capillary and its basement membrane. In: Vize PD, Woolf AS, Bard JBL, editors. The Kidney. From normal development to congenital disease. London: Academic Press; 2003. p. 221—49.

[8] Reeves W, Caulfield JP, Farquhar MG. Differentiation of epithelial foot processes and filtration slits: sequential appearance of occluding junctions, epithelial polyanion, and slit membranes in developing glomeruli. Lab Invest 1978;39:90—100.

[9] Abrahamson DR. Origin of the glomerular basement membrane visualized after in vivo labeling of laminin in newborn rat kidneys. J Cell Biol 1985;100:1988—2000.

[10] Kanwar YS, Jakubowski ML, Rosenzweig LJ, Gibbons JT. De novo cellular synthesis of sulfated proteoglycans of the developing renal glomerulus in vivo. Proc Natl Acad Sci USA 1984;81:7108—11.

[11] Reeves WH, Kanwar YS, Farquhar MG. Assembly of the glomerular filtration surface. differentiation of anionic sites in glomerular capillaries of newborn rat kidney. J Cell Biol 1980;85:735—53.

[12] Sariola H, Peault B, LeDouarin N, Buck C, Dieterlen-Lievre F, Saxen L. Extracellular matrix and capillary ingrowth in interspecies chimeric kidneys. Cell Diff 1984;15:43 51.

[13] Abrahamson DR, Perry EW. Evidence for splicing new basement membrane into old during glomerular development in newborn rat kidneys. J Cell Biol 1986;103:2489—98.

[14] Desjardins M, Bendayan M. Ontogenesis of glomerular basement membrane: structural and functional properties. J Cell Biol 1991;113:689—700.

[15] Hyink DP, Abrahamson DR. Origin of the glomerular vasculature in the developing kidney. Semin Nephrol 1995;15:300—14.

[16] Sariola H, Ekblom P, Lehtonen E, Saxen L. Differentiation and vascularization of the metanephric kidney grafted on the chorioallantoic membrane. Dev Biol 1983;96:427—35.

[17] Abrahamson DR. Development of kidney glomerular endothelial cells and their role in basement membrane assembly. Organogenesis 2009;5:275—87.

[18] Hyink DP, Tucker DC, St John PL, Leardkamolkarn V, Accavitti MA, Abrass CK, et al. Endogenous origin of glomerular endothelial and mesangial cells in grafts of embryonic kidneys. Am J Physiol 1996;270:F886—899.

[19] Robert St. B, John PL, Hyink DP, Abrahamson DR. Evidence that embryonic kidney cells expressing flk-1 are intrinsic, vasculogenic angioblasts. Am J Physiol 1996;271:F744—753.

[20] Robert B, St John PL, Abrahamson DR. Direct visualization of renal vascular morphogenesis in Flk1 heterozygous mutant mice. Am J Physiol 1998;275:F164—172.

[21] Loughna S, Hardman P, Landels E, Jussila L, Alitalo K, Woolf AS. A molecular and genetic analysis of renalglomerular capillary development. Angiogenesis 1997;1:84—101.

[22] Tufro A, Norwood VF, Carey RM, Gomez RA. Vascular endothelial growth factor induces nephrogenesis and vasculogenesis. J Amer Soc Nephrol 1999;10:2125—34.

[23] Ricono JM, Xu YC, Arar M, Jin DC, Barnes JL, Abboud HE. Morphological insights into the origin of glomerular endothelial and mesangial cells and their precursors. J Histochem Cytochem 2003;51:141—50.

[24] Sequeira Lopez ML, Pentz ES, Robert B, Abrahamson DR, Gomez RA. Embryonic origin and lineage of juxtaglomerular cells. Am J Physiol Renal Physiol 2001;281:F345—356.

[25] Daniel TO, Abrahamson D. Endothelial signal integration in vascular assembly. Annu Rev Physiol 2000;62:649—71.

[26] Robert B, Abrahamson DR. Control of glomerular capillary development by growth factor/receptor kinases. Pediatr Nephrol 2001;16:294—301.

[27] Carmeliet P, Ferreira V, Breier G, Pollefeyt S, Kieckens L, Gertsenstein M, et al. Abnormal blood vessel development and lethality in embryos lacking a single VEGF allele. Nature 1996;380:435—9.

[28] Ferrara N, Carver-Moore K, Chen H, Dowd M, Lu L, O'Shea KS, et al. Heterozygous embryonic lethality induced by targeted inactivation of the VEGF gene. Nature 1996;380:439—42.

[29] Shalaby F, Rossant J, Yamaguchi TP, Gertsenstein M, Wu XF, Breitman ML, et al. Failure of blood-island formation and vasculogenesis in Flk-1-deficient mice. Nature 1995;376:62—6.

[30] Fong GH, Rossant J, Gertsenstein M, Breitman ML. Role of the Flt-1 receptor tyrosine kinase in regulating the assembly of vascular endothelium. Nature 1995;376:66—70.

[31] Simon M, Grone HJ, Johren O, Kullmer J, Plate KH, Risau W, et al. Expression of vascular endothelial growth factor and its receptors in human renal ontogenesis and in adult kidney. Am J Physiol 1995;268:F240—250.

[32] Tufro A. VEGF spatially directs angiogenesis during metanephric development in vitro. Dev Biol 2000;227:558—66.

[33] Kitamoto Y, Tokunaga H, Tomita K. Vascular endothelial growth factor is an essential molecule for mouse kidney development: Glomerulogenesis and nephrogenesis. J Clin Invest 1997;99:2351—7.

[34] Eremina V, Cui S, Gerber H, Ferrara N, Haigh J, Nagy A, et al. Vascular endothelial growth factor-A signaling in the podocyte-endothelial compartment is required for mesangial cell migration and survival. J Am Soc Nephrol 2006;17:724—35.

[35] Eremina V, Sood M, Haigh J, Nagy A, Lajoie G, Ferrara N, et al. Glomerular-specific alterations of VEGF-A expression lead to distinct congenital and acquired renal diseases. J Clin Invest 2003;111:707—16.

[36] Wenger RH, Stiehl DP, Camenisch G. Integration of oxygen signaling at the consensus HRE. Sci STKE 2005;306:re12.

[37] Maxwell PH, Ratcliffe PJ. Oxygen sensors and angiogenesis. Semin Cell Dev Biol 2002;13:29—37.

[38] Gerber HP, Dixit V, Ferrara N. Vascular endothelial growth factor induces expression of the antiapoptotic proteins Bcl-2 and A1 in vascular endothelial cells. J Biol Chem 1998;273:13313—6.

[39] Abedi H, Zachary I. Vascular endothelial growth factor stimulates tyrosine phosphorylation and recruitment to new focal adhesions of focal adhesion kinase and paxillin in endothelial cells. J Biol Chem 1997;272:15442—51.

[40] Bernhardt WM, Schmitt R, Rosenberger C, Munchenhagen PM, Grone HJ, Frei U, et al. Expression of hypoxia-inducible transcription factors in developing human and rat kidneys. Kidney Int 2006;69:114—22.

[41] Freeburg PB, Robert St B, John PL, Abrahamson DR. Podocyte expression of hypoxia-inducible factor (HIF)-1 and HIF-2 during glomerular development. J Am Soc Nephrol 2003;14:927—38.

[42] Freeburg PB, Abrahamson DR. Divergent expression patterns for hypoxia-inducible factor-1beta and aryl hydrocarbon receptor nuclear transporter-2 in developing kidney. J Am Soc Nephrol 2004;15:2569—78.

[43] Freeburg PB, Abrahamson DR. Hypoxia-inducible factors and kidney vascular development. J Amer Soc Nephrol 2003;14:2723—30.

[44] Haase VH. Hypoxia-inducible factors in the kidney. Am J Physiol Renal Physiol 2006;291:F271—281.

[45] Haase VH. The VHL/HIF oxygen-sensing pathway and its relevance to kidney disease. Kidney Int 2006;69:1302—7.

[46] Kaelin Jr WG. The von Hippel-Lindau tumor suppressor gene and kidney cancer. Clin Cancer Res 2004;10:6290S—5S.

[47] Raval RR, Lau KW, Tran MG, Sowter HM, Mandriota SJ, Li JL, et al. Contrasting properties of hypoxia-inducible factor 1 (HIF-1) and HIF-2 in von Hippel-Lindau-associated renal cell carcinoma. Mol Cell Biol 2005;25:5675—86.

[48] Esser S, Wolburg K, Wolburg H, Breier G, Kurzchalia T, Risau W. Vascular endothelial growth factor induces endothelial fenestrations in vitro. J Cell Biol 1998;140:947—59.

[49] Woolf AS, Yuan HT. Angiopoietin growth factors and Tie receptor tyrosine kinases in renal vascular development. Pediatr Nephrol 2001;16:177—84.

[50] Ulleras E, Wilcock A, Miller SJ, Franklin GC. The sequential activation and repression of the human PDGF-B gene during chronic hypoxia reveals antagonistic roles for the depletion of oxygen and glucose. Growth Factors 2001;19:233—45.

[51] Alpers CE, Seifert RA, Hudkins KL, Johnson RJ, Bowen-Pope DF. Developmental patterns of PDGF B-chain, PDGF-receptor, and alpha-actin expression in human glomerulogenesis. Kidney Int 1992;42:390—9.

[52] Eichmann A, Makinen T, Alitalo K. Neural guidance molecules regulate vascular remodeling and vessel navigation. Genes Dev 2005;19:1013—21.

[53] Klagsbrun M, Eichmann A. A role for axon guidance receptors and ligands in blood vessel development and tumor angiogenesis. Cytokine Growth Factor Rev 2005;16:535—48.

[54] Robert B, Zhao X, Abrahamson DR. Coexpression of neuropilin-1, Flk1, and VEGF(164) in developing and mature mouse kidney glomeruli. Am J Physiol Renal Physiol 2000;279:F275—282.

[55] Villegas G, Tufro A. Ontogeny of semaphorins 3A and 3F and their receptors neuropilins 1 and 2 in the kidney. Mech Dev 2002;119(Suppl. 1):S149—153.

[56] Harper SJ, Xing CY, Whittle C, Parry R, Gillatt D, Peat D, et al. Expression of neuropilin-1 by human glomerular epithelial cells *in vitro* and *in vivo*. Clin Sci 2001;101:439—46.

[57] Guan F, Villegas G, Teichman J, Mundel P, Tufro A. Autocrine VEGF-A system in podocytes regulates podocin and its interaction with CD2AP. Am J Physiol Renal Physiol 2006;291:F422—428.

[58] Daniel TO, Stein E, Cerretti DP, St John PL, Robert B, Abrahamson DR. ELK and LERK-2 in developing kidney and microvascular endothelial assembly. Kidney Int Supp 1996;57: S73—81.

[59] Leveen P, Pekny M, Gebre-Medhin S, Swolin B, Larsson E, Betsholtz C. Mice deficient for PDGF B show renal, cardiovascular, and hematological abnormalities. Genes Dev 1994;8:1875—87.

[60] Soriano P. Abnormal kidney development and hematological disorders in PDGF beta- receptor mutant mice. Genes Dev 1994;8:1888—96.

[61] Hugo C, Shankland SJ, Bowen-Pope DF, Couser WG, Johnson RJ. Extraglomerular origin of the mesangial cell after injury. A new role of the juxtaglomerular apparatus. J Clin Invest 1997;100:786—94.

[62] Masuya M, Drake CJ, Fleming PA, Reilly CM, Zeng H, Hill WD, et al. Hematopoietic origin of glomerular mesangial cells. Blood 2003;101:2215—8.

[63] Lindenmeyer MT, Eichinger F, Sen K, Anders HJ, Edenhofer I, Mattinzoli D, et al. Systematic analysis of a novel human renal glomerulus-enriched gene expression dataset. PLoS ONE 2010;5:e11545.

[64] Takemoto M, He L, Norlin J, Patrakka J, Xiao Z, Petrova T, et al. Large-scale identification of genes implicated in kidney glomerulus development and function. EMBO J 2006;25:1160—74.

[65] White JT, Zhang B, Cerqueira DM, Tran U, Wessely O. Notch signaling, wt1 and foxc2 are key regulators of the podocyte gene regulatory network in *Xenopus*. Development 2010;137: 1863—73.

[66] Hastie ND. Life, sex, and WT1 isoforms—three amino acids can make all the difference. Cell 2001;106:391—4.

[67] Hartwig S, Ho J, Pandey P, Macisaac K, Taglienti M, Xiang M, et al. Genomic characterization of Wilms' tumor suppressor 1 targets in nephron progenitor cells during kidney development. Development 2010;137:1189—203.

[68] Kreidberg JA. Podocyte differentiation and glomerulogenesis. J Am Soc Nephrol 2003;14:806—14.

[69] Ryan G, Steele-Perkins V, Morris JF, Rauscher 3rd FJ, Dressler GR. Repression of Pax-2 by WT1 during normal kidney development. Development 1995;121:867—75.

[70] Dressler GR, Wilkinson JE, Rothenpieler UW, Patterson LT, Williams-Simons L, Westphal H. Deregulation of Pax-2 expression in transgenic mice generates severe kidney abnormalities. Nature 1993;362:65—7.

[71] Guo G, Morrison DJ, Licht JD, Quaggin SE. WT1 activates a glomerular-specific enhancer identified from the human nephrin gene. J Am Soc Nephrol 2004;15:2851—6.

[72] Wagner N, Wagner KD, Xing Y, Scholz H, Schedl A. The major podocyte protein nephrin is transcriptionally activated by the Wilms' tumor suppressor WT1. J Am Soc Nephrol 2004;15: 3044—51.

[73] Quaggin SE. Transcriptional regulation of podocyte specification and differentiation. Microsc Res Tech 2002;57:208—11.

[74] Natoli TA, Liu J, Eremina V, Hodgens K, Li C, Hamano Y, et al. A mutant form of the Wilms' tumor suppressor gene WT1 observed in Denys-Drash syndrome interferes with glomerular capillary development. J Am Soc Nephrol 2002;13:2058—67.

[75] Salomon R, Gubler MC, Niaudet P. Genetics of the nephrotic syndrome. Curr Opin Pediatr 2000;12:129—34.

[76] Hammes A, Guo JK, Lutsch G, Leheste JR, Landrock D, Ziegler U, et al. Two splice variants of the Wilms' tumor 1 gene have distinct functions during sex determination and nephron formation. Cell 2001;106:319—29.

[77] Dreyer SD, Zhou G, Baldini A, Winterpacht A, Zabel B, Cole W, et al. Mutations in LMX1B cause abnormal skeletal patterning and renal dysplasia in nail patella syndrome. Nat Genet 1998;19:47—50.

[78] Heidet L, Bongers EM, Sich M, Zhang SY, Loirat C, Meyrier A, et al. *In vivo* expression of putative LMX1B targets in nail-patella syndrome kidneys. Am J Pathol 2003;163:145—55.

[79] Chen H, Lun Y, Ovchinnikov D, Kokubo H, Oberg KC, Pepicelli CV, et al. Limb and kidney defects in Lmx1b mutant mice suggest an involvement of LMX1B in human nail patella syndrome. Nat Genet 1998;19:51—5.

[80] Miner JH, Morello R, Andrews KL, Li C, Antignac C, Shaw AS, et al. Transcriptional induction of slit diaphragm genes by Lmx1b is required in podocyte differentiation. J Clin Invest 2002;109:1065—72.

[81] Morello R, Zhou G, Dreyer SD, Harvey SJ, Ninomiya Y, Thorner PS, et al. Regulation of glomerular basement membrane collagen expression by LMX1B contributes to renal disease in nail patella syndrome. Nat Genet 2001;27:205—8.

[82] Rohr C, Prestel J, Heidet L, Hosser H, Kriz W, Johnson RL, et al. The LIM-homeodomain transcription factor Lmx1b plays a crucial role in podocytes. J Clin Invest 2002;109:1073—82.

[83] Mutter WP, Peng H, Goldring MB, Knebelmann B, Karumanchi A. Role of LMX1B in proteinuria. J Am Soc Nephrol 2005;16:670A.

[84] Quaggin SE, Vanden Heuvel GB, Igarashi P. Pod-1, a mesoderm-specific basic-helix-loop-helix protein expressed in mesenchymal and glomerular epithelial cells in the developing kidney. Mech Dev 1998;71:37—48.

[85] Quaggin SE, Schwartz L, Cui S, Igarashi P, Deimling J, Post M, et al. The basic-helix-loop-helix protein pod1 is critically important for kidney and lung organogenesis. Development 1999;126: 5771—83.

[86] Cui S, Li C, Ema M, Weinstein J, Quaggin SE. Rapid isolation of glomeruli coupled with gene expression profiling identifies downstream targets in Pod1 knockout mice. J Am Soc Nephrol 2005;16:3247—55.

[87] Sadl V, Jin F, Yu J, Cui S, Holmyard D, Quaggin S, et al. The mouse Kreisler (Krml1/MafB) segmentation gene is required for differentiation of glomerular visceral epithelial cells. Dev Biol 2002;249:16—29.

[88] Moriguchi T, Hamada M, Morito N, Terunuma T, Hasegawa K, Zhang C, et al. MafB is essential for renal development and F4/80 expression in macrophages. Mol Cell Biol 2006;26:5715—27.

[89] Takemoto M, Asker N, Gerhardt H, Lundqvist A, Johansson BR, Saito Y, et al. A new method for large scale isolation of kidney glomeruli from mice. Am J Pathol 2002;161:799—805.

[90] McCright B, Gao X, Shen L, Lozier J, Lan Y, Maguire M, et al. Defects in development of the kidney, heart and eye vasculature in mice homozygous for a hypomorphic Notch2 mutation. Development 2001;128:491—502.

[91] Cheng HT, Kim M, Valerius MT, Surendran K, Schuster-Gossler K, Gossler A, et al. Notch2, but not Notch1, is required for proximal fate acquisition in the mammalian nephron. Development 2007;134:801—11.

[92] Cheng HT, Miner JH, Lin M, Tansey MG, Roth K, Kopan R. Gamma-secretase activity is dispensable for mesenchyme-to-epithelium transition but required for podocyte and proximal tubule formation in developing mouse kidney. Development 2003;130:5031—42.

[93] Wartiovaara J, Ofverstedt LG, Khoshnoodi J, Zhang J, Makela E, Sandin S, et al. Nephrin strands contribute to a porous slit diaphragm scaffold as revealed by electron tomography. J Clin Invest 2004;114:1475–83.

[94] Gagliardini E, Conti S, Benigni A, Remuzzi G, Remuzzi A. Imaging of the porous ultrastructure of the glomerular epithelial filtration slit. J Amer Soc Nephrol 2010;21:2081–9.

[95] Jarad G, Cunningham J, Shaw AS, Miner JH. Proteinuria precedes podocyte abnormalities in Lamb2$^{-/-}$ mice, implicating the glomerular basement membrane as an albumin barrier. J Clin Invest 2006;116:2272–9.

[96] Aaltonen P, Holthofer H. The nephrin-based slit diaphragm: new insight into the signalling platform identifies targets for therapy. Nephrol Dial Transplant 2007;22:3408–10.

[97] Huber TB, Benzing T. The slit diaphragm: a signaling platform to regulate podocyte function. Curr Opin Nephrol Hypertens 2005;14:211–6.

[98] Done SC, Takemoto M, He L, Sun Y, Hultenby K, Betsholtz C, et al. Nephrin is involved in podocyte maturation but not survival during glomerular development. Kidney Int 2008;73:697–704.

[99] Kestila M, Lenkkeri U, Mannikko M, Lamerdin J, McCready P, Putaala H, et al. Positionally cloned gene for a novel glomerular protein— nephrin— is mutated in congenital nephrotic syndrome. Mol Cell 1998;1:575–82.

[100] Holzman LB, John PL, Kovari IA, Verma R, Holthofer H, Abrahamson DR. Nephrin localizes to the slit pore of the glomerular epithelial cell. Kidney Int 1999;56:1481–91.

[101] Ruotsalainen V, Ljungberg P, Wartiovaara J, Lenkkeri U, Kestila M, Jalanko H, et al. Nephrin is specifically located at the slit diaphragm of glomerular podocytes. Proc Natl Acad Sci USA 1999;96:7962–7.

[102] Jones N, Blasutig IM, Eremina V, Ruston JM, Bladt F, Li H, et al. Nck adaptor proteins link nephrin to the actin cytoskeleton of kidney podocytes. Nature 2006.

[103] Lahdenpera J, Kilpelainen P, Liu XL, Pikkarainen T, Repenon P, Ruotsalainen V, et al. Clustering-induced tyrosine phosphorylation of nephrin by Src family kinases. Kidney Int 2003;64:404–13.

[104] Li H, Lemay S, Aoudjit L, Kawachi H, Takano T. SRC-family kinase Fyn phosphorylates the cytoplasmic domain of nephrin and modulates its interaction with podocin. J Am Soc Nephrol 2004;15:3006–15.

[105] Verma R, Kovari I, Soofi A, Nihalani D, Patrie K, Holzman LB. Nephrin ectodomain engagement results in Src kinase activation, nephrin phosphorylation, Nck recruitment, and actin polymerization. J Clin Invest 2006;116:1346–59.

[106] Verma R, Wharram B, Kovari I, Kunkel R, Nihalani D, Wary KK, et al. Fyn binds to and phosphorylates the kidney slit diaphragm component Nephrin. J Biol Chem 2003;278:20716–23.

[107] Donoviel DB, Freed DD, Vogel H, Potter DG, Hawkins E, Barrish JP, et al. Proteinuria and perinatal lethality in mice lacking neph1, a novel protein with homology to nephrin. Mol Cell Biol 2001;21:4829–36.

[108] Barletta GM, Kovari IA, Verma RK, Kerjaschki D, Holzman LB. Nephrin and Neph1 co-localize at the podocyte foot process intercellular junction and form cis hetero-oligomers. J Biol Chem 2003;278:19266–71.

[109] Gerke P, Huber TB, Sellin L, Benzing T, Walz G. Homodimerization and heterodimerization of the glomerular podocyte proteins nephrin and NEPH1. J Am Soc Nephrol 2003;14:918–26.

[110] Gerke P, Sellin L, Kretz O, Petraschka D, Zentgraf H, Benzing T, et al. NEPH2 is located at the glomerular slit diaphragm, interacts with nephrin and is cleaved from podocytes by metalloproteinases. J Am Soc Nephrol 2005;16:1693–702.

[111] Liu G, Kaw B, Kurfis J, Rahmanuddin S, Kanwar YS, Chugh SS. Neph1 and nephrin interaction in the slit diaphragm is an important determinant of glomerular permeability. J Clin Invest 2003;112:209–21.

[112] Shelton C, Kocherlakota KS, Zhuang S, Abmayr SM. The immunoglobulin superfamily member Hbs functions redundantly with Sns in interactions between founder and fusion-competent myoblasts. Development 2009;136:1159–68.

[113] Shen K, Fetter RD, Bargmann CI. Synaptic specificity is generated by the synaptic guidepost protein SYG-2 and its receptor, SYG-1. Cell 2004;116:869–81.

[114] Zhuang S, Shao H, Guo F, Trimble R, Pearce E, Abmayr SM. Sns and Kirre, the *Drosophila* orthologs of Nephrin and Neph1, direct adhesion, fusion and formation of a slit diaphragm-like structure in insect nephrocytes. Development 2009;136:2335–44.

[115] Neumann-Haefelin E, Kramer-Zucker A, Slanchev K, Hartleben B, Noutsou F, Martin K, et al. A model organism approach: defining the role of Neph proteins as regulators of neuron and kidney morphogenesis. Hum Mol Genet 2010;19:2347–59.

[116] Schnabel E, Anderson JM, Farquhar MG. The tight junction protein ZO-1 is concentrated along slit diaphragms of the glomerular epithelium. J Cell Biol 1990;111:1255–63.

[117] Sellin L, Huber TB, Gerke P, Quack I, Pavenstadt H, Walz G. NEPH1 defines a novel family of podocin interacting proteins. FASEB J 2003;17:115–7.

[118] Huber TB, Simons M, Hartleben B, Sernetz L, Schmidts M, Gundlach E, et al. Molecular basis of the functional podocin-nephrin complex: mutations in the NPHS2 gene disrupt nephrin targeting to lipid raft microdomains. Hum Mol Genet 2003;12:3397–405.

[119] Reiser J, Kriz W, Kretzler M, Mundel P. The glomerular slit diaphragm is a modified adherens junction. J Am Soc Nephrol 2000;11:1–8.

[120] Moeller MJ, Soofi A, Braun GS, Li X, Watzl C, Kriz W, et al. Protocadherin FAT1 binds Ena/VASP proteins and is necessary for actin dynamics and cell polarization. EMBO J 2004;23:3769–79.

[121] Rodewald R, Karnovsky MJ. Porous substructure of the glomerular slit diaphragm in the rat and mouse. J Cell Biol 1974;60:423–33.

[122] Welsch T, Endlich N, Gokce G, Doroshenko E, Simpson JC, Kriz W, et al. Association of CD2AP with dynamic actin on vesicles in podocytes. Am J Physiol Renal Physiol 2005;289:F1134–1143.

[123] Yuan H, Takeuchi E, Salant DJ. Podocyte slit-diaphragm protein nephrin is linked to the actin cytoskeleton. Am J Physiol Renal Physiol 2002;282:F585–591.

[124] Shih N-Y, Li J, Karpitskii V, Nguyen A, Dustin ML, Kanagawa O, et al. Congenital nephrotic syndrome in mice lacking CD2-associated protein. Science 1999;286:312–5.

[125] Huber TB, Kwoh C, Wu H, et al. A bigenic mouse model of focal segmental glomerulosclerosis involving pairwise interaction of CD2AP, Fyn and synaptopodin. J Clin Invest 2006;116:1337–45.

[126] Kim JM, Wu H, Green G, Winkler CA, Kopp JB, Miner JH, et al. CD2-associated protein haploinsufficiency is linked to glomerular disease susceptibility. Science 2003;300:1298–300.

[127] Lowik MM, Groenen PJ, Pronk I, Lilien MR, Goldschmeding R, Dijkman HB, et al. Focal segmental glomerulosclerosis in a patient homozygous for a CD2AP mutation. Kidney Int 2007;72:1198–203.

[128] Shih N-Y, Li J, Cotran R, Mundel P, Miner JH, Shaw AS. CD2AP localizes to the slit diaphragm and binds to nephrin via a novel C-terminal domain. Am J Pathol 2001;159:2303–8.

[129] Grunkemeyer JA, Kwoh C, Huber TB, Shaw AS. CD2-associated protein (CD2AP) expression in podocytes rescues lethality of CD2AP deficiency. J Biol Chem 2005;280:29677—81.

[130] Tossidou I, Teng B, Drobot L, Meyer-Schwesinger C, Worthmann K, Haller H, et al. CIN85/RukL is a novel binding partner of nephrin and podocin and mediates slit diaphragm turnover in podocytes. J Biol Chem 2010;285:25285—95.

[131] Jones N, New LA, Fortino MA, Eremina V, Ruston J, Blasutig IM, et al. Nck proteins maintain the adult glomerular filtration barrier. J Amer Soc Nephrol 2009;20:1533—43.

[132] Reiser J, Polu KR, Moller CC, Kenlan P, Altintas MM, Wei C, et al. TRPC6 is a glomerular slit diaphragm-associated channel required for normal renal function. Nat Genet 2005;37:739—44.

[133] Winn MP, Conlon PJ, Lynn KL, Farrington MK, Creazzo T, Hawkins AF, et al. A mutation in the TRPC6 cation channel causes familial focal segmental glomerulosclerosis. Science 2005;308:1801—4.

[134] Tian D, Jacobo SM, Billing D, Rozkalne A, Gage SD, Anagnostou T, et al. Antagonistic regulation of actin dynamics and cell motility by TRPC5 and TRPC6 channels. Sci Signal 2010;3:ra77.

[135] Wang Y, Jarad G, Tripathi P, Pan M, Cunningham J, Martin DR, et al. Activation of NFAT signaling in podocytes causes glomerulosclerosis. J Amer Soc Nephrol 2010;21:1657—66.

[136] Moeller MJ, Sanden SK, Soofi A, Wiggins RC, Holzman LB. Podocyte-specific expression of cre recombinase in transgenic mice. Genesis 2003;35:39—42.

[137] Hartleben B, Schweizer H, Lubben P, Bartram MP, Moller CC, Herr R, et al. Neph-Nephrin proteins bind the Par3-Par6-atypical protein kinase C (aPKC) complex to regulate podocyte cell polarity. J Biol Chem 2008;283:23033—8.

[138] Huber TB, Hartleben B, Winkelmann K, Schneider L, Becker JU, Leitges M, et al. Loss of podocyte aPKClambda/iota causes polarity defects and nephrotic syndrome. J Amer Soc Nephrol 2009;20:798—806.

[139] Huber TB, Kottgen M, Schilling B, Walz G, Benzing T. Interaction with podocin facilitates nephrin signaling. J Biol Chem 2001;276:41543—6.

[140] Huber TB, Hartleben B, Kim J, Schmidts M, Schermer B, Keil A, et al. Nephrin and CD2AP associate with phosphoinositide 3-OH kinase and stimulate AKT-dependent signaling. Mol Cell Biol 2003;23:4917—28.

[141] Huber TB, Schmidts M, Gerke P, Schermer B, Zahn A, Hartleben B, et al. The carboxy terminus of Neph family members binds to the PDZ domain protein Zonula occludens-1. J Biol Chem 2003;278:13417—21.

[142] Kaplan JM, Kim SH, North KN, Rennke H, Correia LA, Tong HQ, et al. Mutations in ACTN4, encoding alpha-actinin-4, cause familial focal segmental glomerulosclerosis. Nat Genet 2000;24:251—6.

[143] Asanuma K, Kim K, Oh J, Giardino L, Chabanis S, Faul C, et al. Synaptopodin regulates the actin-bundling activity of alpha-actinin in an isoform-specific manner. J Clin Invest 2005;115:1188—98.

[144] Faul C, Donnelly M, Merscher-Gomez S, Chang YH, Franz S, Delfgaauw J, et al. The actin cytoskeleton of kidney podocytes is a direct target of the antiproteinuric effect of cyclosporine A. Nat Med 2008;14:931—8.

[145] Timpl R. Structure and biological activity of basement membrane proteins. Eur J Biochem 1989;180:487—502.

[146] Miner JH. Renal basement membrane components. Kidney Int 1999;56:2016—24.

[147] Aumailley M, Bruckner-Tuderman L, Carter WG, et al. A simplified laminin nomenclature. Matrix Biol 2005;24:326—32.

[148] Miner JH, Yurchenco PD. Laminin functions in tissue morphogenesis. Annu Rev Cell Dev Biol 2004;20:255—84.

[149] Colognato H, Yurchenco PD. Form and function: the laminin family of heterotrimers. Dev Dyn 2000;218:213—34.

[150] Miner JH. Developmental biology of glomerular basement membrane components. Curr Opin Nephrol Hypertens 1998;7:13—9.

[151] St. John PL, Wang R, Yin Y, Miner JH, Robert B, Abrahamson DR. Glomerular laminin isoform transitions: errors in metanephric culture are corrected by grafting. Am J Physiol Renal Physiol 2001;280:F695—705.

[152] Miner JH, Li C. Defective glomerulogenesis in the absence of laminin α5 demonstrates a developmental role for the kidney glomerular basement membrane. Dev Biol 2000;217:278—89.

[153] Kriz W, Elger M, Mundel P, Lemley KV. Structure-stabilizing forces in the glomerular tuft. J Am Soc Nephrol 1995;5:1731—9.

[154] Kikkawa Y, Virtanen I, Miner JH. Mesangial cells organize the glomerular capillaries by adhering to the G domain of laminin alpha5 in the glomerular basement membrane. J Cell Biol 2003;161:187—96.

[155] Noakes PG, Miner JH, Gautam M, Cunningham JM, Sanes JR, Merlie JP. The renal glomerulus of mice lacking s-laminin/laminin beta2: nephrosis despite molecular compensation by laminin beta1. Nat Genet 1995;10:400—6.

[156] Zenker M, Aigner T, Wendler O, Tralau T, Müntefering H, Fenski R, et al. Human laminin beta2 deficiency causes congenital nephrosis with mesangial sclerosis and distinct eye abnormalities. Hum Mol Genet 2004;13:2625—32.

[157] Zenker M, Pierson M, Jonveaux P, Reis A. Demonstration of two novel LAMB2 mutations in the original Pierson syndrome family reported 42 years ago. Am J Med Genet A 2005;138:73—4.

[158] Zenker M, Tralau T, Lennert T, Pitz S, Mark K, Madlon H, et al. Congenital nephrosis, mesangial sclerosis, and distinct eye abnormalities with microcoria: an autosomal recessive syndrome. Am J Med Genet A 2004;130:138—45.

[159] Hudson BG. The molecular basis of Goodpasture and Alport syndromes: beacons for the discovery of the collagen IV family. J Am Soc Nephrol 2004;15:2514—27.

[160] Hudson BG, Tryggvason K, Sundaramoorthy M, Neilson EG. Alport's syndrome, Goodpasture's syndrome, and type IV collagen. N Engl J Med 2003;348:2543—56.

[161] Hudson BG, Reeders ST, Tryggvason K. Type IV collagen: structure, gene organization, and role in human diseases. J Biol Chem 1993;268:26033—6.

[162] Poschl E, Schlotzer-Schrehardt U, Brachvogel B, Saito K, Ninomiya Y, Mayer U. Collagen IV is essential for basement membrane stability but dispensable for initiation of its assembly during early development. Development 2004;131:1619—28.

[163] Abrahamson DR, Hudson BG, Stroganova L, Borza DB, St John PL. Cellular origins of type IV collagen networks in developing glomeruli. J Am Soc Nephrol 2009;20:1471—9.

[164] Ninomiya Y, Kagawa M, Iyama K, Naito I, Kishiro Y, Seyer JM, et al. Differential expression of two basement membrane collagen genes, COL4A6 and COL4A5, demonstrated by immunofluorescence staining using peptide-specific monoclonal antibodies. J Cell Biol 1995;130:1219—29.

[165] Kashtan CE. Alport syndrome. Kidney Int 1997;51(Suppl. 58): S-69—71.

[166] Gould DB, Phalan FC, Breedveld GJ, van Mil SE, Smith RS, Schimenti JC, et al. Mutations in Col4a1 cause perinatal cerebral hemorrhage and porencephaly. Science 2005;308:1167—71.

[167] Gould DB, Phalan FC, van Mil SE, Sundberg JP, Vahedi K, Massin P, et al. Role of COL4A1 in small-vessel disease and hemorrhagic stroke. N Engl J Med 2006;354:1489—96.

II. STRUCTURAL AND FUNCTIONAL ORGANIZATION OF THE KIDNEY

[168] Plaisier E, Chen Z, Gekeler F, Benhassine S, Dahan K, Marro B, et al. Novel COL4A1 mutations associated with HANAC syndrome: a role for the triple helical CB3[IV] domain. Am J Med Genet A 2010;152A:2550—5.

[169] Plaisier E, Gribouval O, Alamowitch S, Mougenot B, Prost C, Verpont MC, et al. COL4A1 mutations and hereditary angiopathy, nephropathy, aneurysms, and muscle cramps. N Engl J Med 2007;357:2687—95.

[170] Miosge N, Kother F, Heinemann S, Kohfeldt E, Herken R, Timpl R. Ultrastructural colocalization of nidogen-1 and nidogen-2 with laminin-1 in murine kidney basement membranes. Histochem Cell Biol 2000;113:115—24.

[171] Bader BL, Smyth N, Nedbal S, Miosge N, Baranowsky A, Mokkapati S, et al. Compound genetic ablation of nidogen 1 and 2 causes basement membrane defects and perinatal lethality in mice. Mol Cell Biol 2005;25:6846—56.

[172] Mayer U, Nischt R, Poschl E, Mann K, Fukuda K, Gerl M, et al. A single EGF-like motif of laminin is responsible for high affinity nidogen binding. EMBO J 1993;12:1879—85.

[173] Willem M, Miosge N, Halfter W, Smyth N, Jannetti I, Burghart E, et al. Specific ablation of the nidogen-binding site in the laminin gamma1 chain interferes with kidney and lung development. Development 2002;129:2711—22.

[174] Goldberg S, Harvey SJ, Cunningham J, Tryggvason K, Miner JH. Glomerular filtration is normal in the absence of both agrin and perlecan-heparan sulfate from the glomerular basement membrane. Nephrol Dial Transplant 2009;24:2044—51.

[175] Harvey SJ, Jarad G, Cunningham J, Rops AL, van der Vlag J, Berden JH, et al. Disruption of glomerular basement membrane charge through podocyte-specific mutation of agrin does not alter glomerular permselectivity. Am J Pathol 2007;171:139—52.

[176] Groffen AJA, Hop FWH, Tryggvason K, Dijkman H, Assmann KJ, Veerkamp JH, et al. Evidence for the existence of multiple heparan sulfate proteoglycans in the human glomerular basement membrane and mesangial matrix. Eur J Biochem 1997;247:175—82.

[177] Bix G, Iozzo RV. Matrix revolutions: "Tails" of basement-membrane components with angiostatic functions. Trends Cell Biol 2005;15:52—60.

[178] Arikawa-Hirasawa E, Watanabe H, Takami H, Hassell JR, Yamada Y. Perlecan is essential for cartilage and cephalic development. Nat Genet 1999;23:354—8.

[179] Costell M, Gustafsson E, Aszodi A, Morgelin M, Bloch W, Hunziker E, et al. Perlecan maintains the integrity of cartilage and some basement membranes. J Cell Biol 1999;147:1109—22.

[180] Rossi M, Morita H, Sormunen R, Airenne S, Kreivi M, Wang L, et al. Heparan sulfate chains of perlecan are indispensable in the lens capsule but not in the kidney. EMBO J 2003;22: 236—45.

[181] Morita H, Yoshimura A, Inui K, Ideura T, Watanabe H, Wang L, et al. Heparan sulfate of perlecan is involved in glomerular filtration. J Am Soc Nephrol 2005;16:1703—10.

[182] Kammerer RA, Schulthess T, Landwehr R, Schumacher B, Lustig A, Yurchenco PD, et al. Interaction of agrin with laminin requires a coiled-coil conformation of the agrin-binding site within the laminin gamma1 chain. EMBO J 1999;18: 6762—70.

[183] Gautam M, Noakes PG, Moscoso L, Rupp F, Scheller RH, Merlie JP, et al. Defective neuromuscular synaptogenesis in agrin-deficient mutant mice. Cell 1996;85:525—35.

[184] Misgeld T, Kummer TT, Lichtman JW, Sanes JR. Agrin promotes synaptic differentiation by counteracting an inhibitory effect of neurotransmitter. Proc Natl Acad Sci USA 2005;102: 11088—93.

[185] Groffen AJ, Ruegg MA, Dijkman H, van de Velden TJ, Buskens CA, van den Born J, et al. Agrin is a major heparan sulfate proteoglycan in the human glomerular basement membrane. J Histochem Cytochem 1998;46:19—27.

[186] Halfter W, Dong S, Schurer B, Cole GJ. Collagen XVIII is a basement membrane heparan sulfate proteoglycan. J Biol Chem 1998;273:25404—12.

[187] Fukai N, Eklund L, Marneros AG, Oh SP, Keene DR, Tamarkin L, et al. Lack of collagen XVIII/endostatin results in eye abnormalities. EMBO J 2002;21:1535—44.

[188] Suzuki OT, Sertie AL, Der Kaloustian VM, Kok F, Carpenter M, Murray J, et al. Molecular analysis of collagen XVIII reveals novel mutations, presence of a third isoform, and possible genetic heterogeneity in Knobloch syndrome. Am J Hum Genet 2002;71:1320—9.

[189] McCarthy KJ, Bynum St. K, John PL, Abrahamson DR, Couchman JR. Basement membrane proteoglycans in glomerular morphogenesis: chondroitin sulfate proteoglycan is temporally and spatially restricted during development. J Histochem Cytochem 1993;41:401—14.

[190] McCarthy KJ, Abrahamson DR, Bynum St KR, John PL, Couchman JR. Basement membrane-specific chondroitin sulfate proteoglycan is abnormally associated with the glomerular capillary basement membrane of diabetic rats. J Histochem Cytochem 1994;42:473—84.

[191] Kreidberg JA, Donovan MJ, Goldstein SL, Rennke H, Shepherd K, Jones RC, et al. Alpha3 beta1 integrin has a crucial role in kidney and lung organogenesis. Development 1996;122:3537—47.

[192] Haas CS, Amann K, Schittny J, Blaser B, Muller U, Hartner A. Glomerular and renal vascular structural changes in alpha8 integrin-deficient mice. J Am Soc Nephrol 2003;14:2288—96.

[193] El-Aouni C, Herbach N, Blattner SM, Henger A, Rastadi MP, Jarad G, et al. Podocyte specific deletion of integrin-linked kinase results in severe glomerular basement membrane alterations and progressive glomerulosclerosis. J Am Soc Nephrol 2006;17:1334—44.

[194] Baleato RM, Guthrie PL, Gubler MC, Ashman LK, Roselli S. Deletion of CD151 results in a strain-dependent glomerular disease due to severe alterations of the glomerular basement membrane. Am J Pathol 2008;173:927—37.

[195] Sachs N, Kreft M, van den Bergh WMA, Beynon AJ, Peters TA, et al. Kidney failure in mice lacking the tetraspanin CD151. J Cell Biol 2006;175:33—9.

[196] Eremina V, Jefferson JA, Kowalewska J, Hochster H, Haas M, Weisstuch J, et al. VEGF inhibition and renal thrombotic microangiopathy. N England J Med 2008;358:1129—36.

[197] Steenhard BM, Freeburg PB, Isom K, Stroganova L, Borza DB, Hudson BG, et al. Kidney development and gene expression in the HIF2α knockout mouse. Dev Dyn 2007;236:1115—25.

[198] Steenhard BM, Isom K, Stroganova L, St John PL, Zelenchuk A, Freeburg PB, et al. Deletion of von Hippel-Lindau in gomerular podocytes results in glomerular basement membrane thickening, extopic subepithelial deposition of collagen α1, α2, α1(IV), expression of neuroglobin, and proteinuria. Am J Pathol 2010;177:84—96.

[199] Sison K, Eremina V, Baelde H, Min W, Hirashima M, Fantus IG, et al. Glomerular structure and function require paracrine, not autocrine, VEGFVEGFR-2 signaling. J Am Soc Nephrol 2010;21:1691—701.

[200] Steenhard BM, Zelenchuk A, Stroganova L, Isom K, St John PL, Andrews GK, et al. TRansgenic expression of human LAMA5 suppresses murine LAma5 mRNA and laminin α5 protein deposition. PLoS ONE 2011;6(9):e23926.

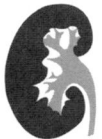

Postnatal Renal Development

Michel Baum[1,2], Jyothsna Gattineni[1] and Lisa M. Satlin[3]

[1]Departments of Pediatrics and University of Texas Southwestern Medical Center, Dallas, TX, USA
[2]Internal Medicine, University of Texas Southwestern Medical Center, Dallas, TX, USA
[3]Departments of Pediatrics and Medicine, Mount Sinai School of Medicine, New York, NY, USA

RENAL BLOOD FLOW AND GLOMERULAR FILTRATION RATE

Renal Blood Flow

The renal blood flow in the adult human is 660 ml/min which is 20–25% of the cardiac output. In contrast, the fetal kidney receives only 2% of the cardiac output from mid-gestation to term.[178] The developmental increase in renal blood flow is due in part to an increase in cardiac output, but predominantly to a decrease in renal vascular resistance.[92,117,220] When corrected for a body surface area of 1.73 m[2], the human neonate has a renal blood flow of only 15–20% of that measured in adults.[51,177] Renal blood flow doubles in the first month of life, and is comparable to adults by one to two years of age when corrected for body surface area.[177] The maturational changes in renal vascular resistance are due to anatomical changes in the renal vasculature, as well as changes in the balance between vasoconstrictors, such as catecholamines and angiotensin II, and vasodilators, such as nitric oxide.[169] The kidney develops in a centrifugal fashion. Juxtamedullary nephrons are formed before those in the superficial cortex. The renal blood flow distribution, measured by both xenon washout and injection of microspheres, shows a paucity of blood flow to the outer cortex compared to the deep cortex in neonates.[18,117,155] During postnatal maturation there is a redistribution of blood flow, with enhanced perfusion of the outer cortex due to a decrease in renal vascular resistance.[18,117,155]

Autoregulation

Renal blood flow (RBF) and glomerular filtration rate (GFR) remain stable over a wide range of perfusion pressures.[251] As perfusion pressure falls there is vasodilatation of the afferent arteriole and vasoconstriction of the efferent arteriole which maintains RBF and GFR. As blood pressure increases during development, the range in pressure where autoregulation of renal blood flow and GFR occurs shifts accordingly.[118] While neonates can autoregulate GFR in response to changes in blood pressure, this protective mechanism is far less developed than the autoregulatory capability of adults due, at least in part, to an attenuated release and efferent arteriolar response to angiotensin II.[251]

Glomerular Filtration Rate

Initiation of glomerular filtration, as evidenced by the flow of urine, begins between nine and twelve weeks gestation in the human.[85] The glomerular filtration rate (GFR) is lower in neonates than adults, even when corrected for body surface area.[15,177] In premature human infants creatinine clearance increases as a function of postconceptual age (the sum of gestational age and postnatal age).[15] GFR is constant at ~0.5 ml/min in infants with a postconceptional age of 28–34 weeks, despite the increase in renal size.[14] GFR increases to 1.0 ml/min at 34–37 weeks and to 2 ml/min at a postconceptional age of 40 weeks.[14] In absolute terms, the GFR increases 25-fold from birth to adulthood. Corrected for a surface area of 1.73 m[2], the GFR in the human term neonate is 30 ml/min/1.73 m[2] in the first week of life.[15,67] GFR continues to increase during the first ~1–2 years of life to reach adult levels when factored for body surface area[177] (Figure 27.1).

At birth, juxtamedullary glomeruli have a larger volume and greater single nephron GFR than superficial

Seldin and Giebisch's The Kidney, Fifth Edition.
DOI: http://dx.doi.org/10.1016/B978-0-12-381462-3.00027-6

911

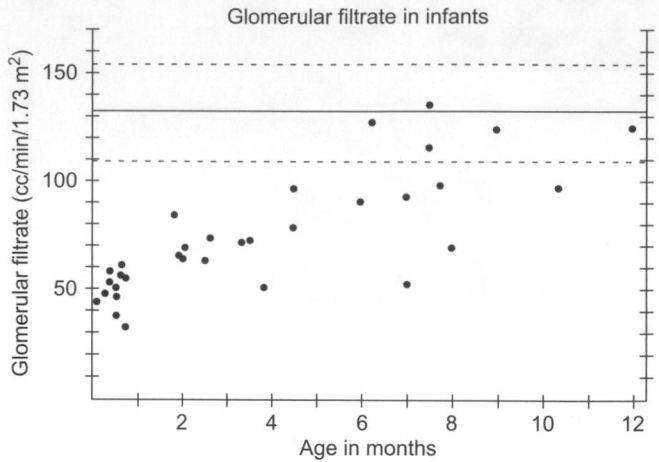

FIGURE 27.1 **Glomerular filtration rate (GFR) in infants in the first year of life (values are corrected for a surface area of 1.73 m^2).** The horizontal line is the mean adult value, and the broken line represents one standard deviation. *(from ref. [177] with permission.)*

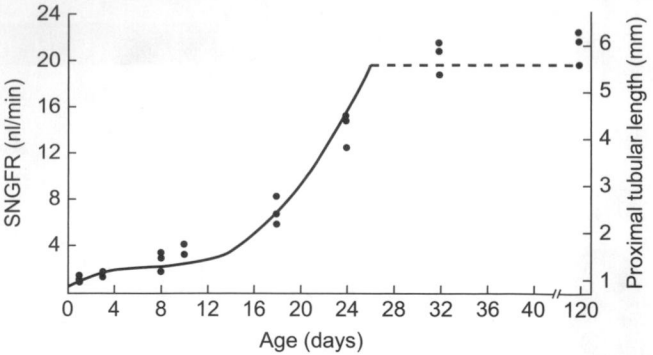

FIGURE 27.2 **Single nephron GFR (SNGFR) in guinea pigs with age.** Each point represents two to six determinations of SNGFR in an animal *(from ref. [219]).*

nephrons.[219] In the guinea pig there is a 7-fold increase in GFR in the first month of life.[219] The increase in total kidney GFR during the first week of life, a time when superficial nephron GFR is relatively constant, is predominantly due to an increase in juxtamedullary nephron GFR.[219] After two weeks of age, however, the rise in total kidney GFR is predominantly due to an increase in GFR in superficial nephrons[219] (Figure 27.2).

The increase in single nephron GFR with postnatal maturation is due to a number of factors. Single nephron GFR is the product of the net ultrafiltration pressure and the glomerular ultrafiltration coefficient, K_f. The effective ultrafiltration pressure is the difference between the hydrostatic and oncotic pressures across the glomerular capillary bed. Studies comparing newborn rats and guinea pigs to adults have shown a maturational increase in effective ultrafiltration pressure.[3,220] However, these changes contribute at most 10% to the 20-fold increase in single nephron GFR.[113,220,232] The maturational increase in GFR is predominantly the result of the increase in K_f, which is the product of the hydraulic permeability of the glomerular capillary and the glomerular capillary surface area.[88,115,129,232] Studies using neutral dextrans have found that the permeability characteristics change only slightly with maturation.[88] The increase in K_f, and thus single nephron GFR, is predominately due to the 7.5-fold increase in glomerular capillary surface area during renal maturation.[115,129]

SODIUM CHLORIDE TRANSPORT

The transition from fetal to neonatal life is characterized by a dramatic decrease in urinary sodium excretion, despite an increase in GFR. The early fetus excretes ~20% of the filtered sodium, while the late gestation fetus excretes only ~0.2%.[173,211] Term neonates are able to maintain a positive sodium balance over a wide range of sodium intake which is essential for growth.[9,218] Compared to adults, neonates have a limited capacity to excrete an acute sodium load, and will develop volume expansion and hypernatremia with a sodium load.[9,65] This phenomenon is exemplified in a study where adult and neonatal dogs were given an isotonic saline infusion equal in volume to 10% of the animal's weight.[87] The results of the cumulative excretion of sodium with time are shown in Figure 27.3. Adult dogs had a brisk natriuresis and diuresis, excreting 50% of the sodium within two hours of the infusion. Dogs less than one week of age excreted less than 10% of the sodium infused by two hours. The limited ability to excrete a sodium load in neonates was not explained by a low GFR, since there was a comparable change with volume expansion in neonates and adults. Premature neonates have high urinary sodium losses and fractional excretion of sodium compared to term neonates.[2,7,9,75] The following section discusses the maturation of tubular transport, which maintains the positive sodium balance in growing neonates.

Glomerulotubular Balance

Glomerulotubular balance remains fairly constant under a number of conditions which alter the GFR in the adult. During postnatal development, the maturational increase in the GFR is paralleled by a concomitant increase in the rate of tubule solute absorption.[109,219] If this did not occur, there would be loss of essential solutes which would jeopardize the life of the neonate as GFR increases during development.[109,219]

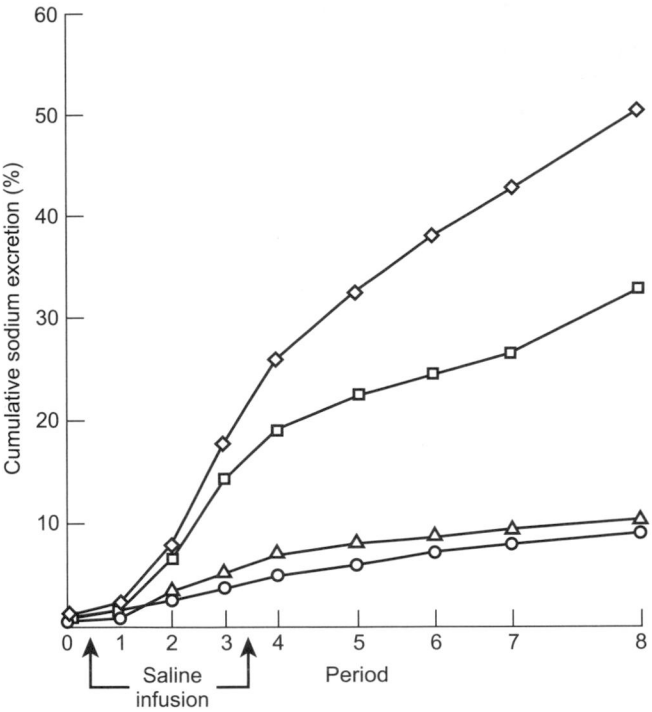

FIGURE 27.3 Cumulative sodium excretion in dogs of various ages after infusion of isotonic saline equal to 10% of body weight over 30 minutes. Period 8 is approximately 120 minutes after initiation of saline infusion. *(from ref. [87]).*

In the fetus, however, the GFR and delivery of solutes and water to the tubules can surpass the reabsorptive capacity of the tubules. In a clearance study examining the fractional reabsorption of volume and sodium after salt-loading in fetal, young, and adult guinea pigs, the fractional reabsorption of volume and sodium were lower in the fetus and in one-day-old animals. By 2–5 days of age, the fractional reabsorption of sodium and water were at the adult level.[149] The glomerular–tubular imbalance is not only present in the fetus, but can also be manifest in the premature neonate. This is exemplified by the fact that glucosuria is frequently present in premature human neonates born before 30 weeks of gestation.[14,235] In human neonates born before 34 weeks gestation, 93% of the filtered glucose is reabsorbed,[14] which is comparable to the fractional reabsorption in the guinea pig fetus.[149] By 34 weeks of gestation, the human neonate can reabsorb over 99% of the filtered glucose load.[14]

Maturation of Proximal Tubule Volume Reabsorption

The developing kidney exhibits a centrifugal pattern of nephron maturation, with juxtamedullary nephrons being formed before superficial nephrons.[76] The glomerular and tubular morphology of juxtamedullary nephrons are more mature than those in the superficial cortex.[76] In many species, including the mouse, rat, and rabbit, nephrogenesis continues after birth in the superficial cortex. Nephrogenesis also continues postnatally in humans born prior to 34 weeks gestation.

The reabsorptive capacity of the neonatal superficial and juxtamedullary proximal tubule is less than that of adults. The rate of volume absorption in superficial proximal convoluted tubules increases two-fold between a 22–24-day-old weanling and a 40–45-day-old adult rat.[11] In rabbit superficial proximal tubules the rate of volume absorption increased four-fold between one week and one month of age,[130] while the rate of volume absorption in rabbit juxtamedullary proximal convoluted tubules did not change appreciably during that time.[190] However, there is a two-fold increase in volume absorption in juxtamedullary nephrons between 4 and 6 weeks of age in the rabbit.[190] Proximal tubule transport for each solute is the sum of transport mediated by passive diffusion, solvent drag, and active transport, which are discussed below.

Na$^+$/K$^+$-ATPase Activity

The basolateral Na$^+$/K$^+$-ATPase provides the driving force for all sodium-dependent transport along the nephron by generating and maintaining a low intracellular sodium concentration. Inhibition of Na$^+$/K$^+$-ATPase with ouabain reduces the rate of volume absorption to zero in neonatal and adult isolated rabbit proximal convoluted tubules.[190] Thus, maturation of Na$^+$/K$^+$-ATPase activity plays a key role in the maturation of solute transport along the nephron.

The Na$^+$/K$^+$-ATPase is made up of an α-subunit and a regulatory ß-subunit. There are four α isoforms and three ß isoforms.[41] The α-subunit is the catalytic subunit, and has an ATP-binding site as well as the binding site for cardiac glycosides. The adult kidney predominantly expresses the α1 and ß1 isoforms. There is a postnatal increase in renal Na$^+$/K$^+$-ATPase activity.[12,13,188,191] In dissected rabbit tubules, the neonatal Na$^+$/K$^+$-ATPase activity is lower than the adult in each nephron segment examined[188] (Figure 27.4). The V$_{max}$ Na$^+$/K$^+$-ATPase activity increases five-fold during renal maturation, with no change in the K$_m$ for sodium, potassium or ATP.

The increase in Na$^+$/K$^+$-ATPase activity in the rabbit juxtamedullary proximal convoluted tubule lags behind the maturational increase in bicarbonate and volume absorption by one week,[188] consistent with the maturational increase in apical membrane transport being the driving force for the increase in basolateral

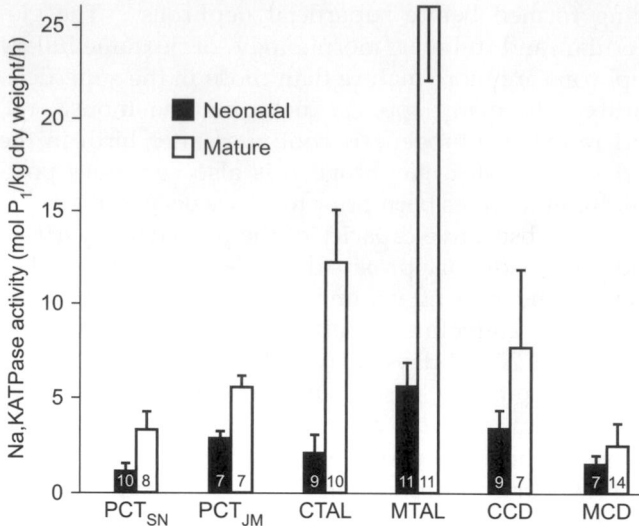

FIGURE 27.4 **Na⁺/K⁺-ATPase activity in neonatal and adult rabbit nephron segments** (PCT$_{SN}$: superficial proximal convoluted tubule; PCT$_{JM}$: juxtamedullaryproximal convoluted tubule; CTAL and MTAL: cortical and medullary thick ascending limbs; CCD and MCD: cortical and medullary collecting ducts) *(from ref. [188]).*

Na⁺/K⁺-ATPase. Several studies have supported this hypothesis. In rat proximal tubule cells in culture, stimulation of the Na⁺/H⁺ exchanger increases intracellular sodium and leads to an increase in Na⁺/K⁺-ATPase activity.[101] An increase in intracellular sodium not only increases pump activity, but also increases α and ß Na⁺/K⁺-ATPase subunit mRNA and protein abundance.[61] Chronic increases in Na⁺/H⁺ exchanger activity in rats induced by metabolic acidosis result in an increase in Na⁺/K⁺-ATPase activity in growing but not adult rats, an effect not seen when the rats were administered amiloride, an inhibitor of the Na⁺/H⁺ exchanger.[81] Thus, the maturational increase in Na⁺/H⁺ exchanger activity may be responsible for the increase in Na⁺/K⁺-ATPase activity.

Maturation of Proximal Tubule NaCl Transport

In the early proximal tubule there is preferential reabsorption of bicarbonate over chloride ions. This leaves the proximal tubule luminal fluid with a higher chloride concentration and a lower bicarbonate concentration than the peritubular fluid. Chloride transport is the sum of active transcellular reabsorption and chloride diffusion across the paracellular pathway down its concentration gradient. In the adult rabbit proximal convoluted tubule, two-thirds of NaCl transport is active and transcellular and one-third is passive and paracellular.[23] In the adult rat proximal convoluted

tubule one-third of NaCl transport is active, and two-thirds is mediated by passive diffusion.[4]

Active chloride transport by the proximal convoluted tubule is mediated by the parallel operation of the Na⁺/H⁺ and Cl⁻/base exchangers.[17,204,208] Cl⁻/OH⁻, Cl⁻/oxalate, and Cl⁻/formate exchange have all been found to mediate chloride uptake into the proximal tubule[17]; however, the relative importance of these transporters remains controversial. In the rabbit superficial convoluted tubule there is evidence for both Cl⁻/OH⁻ and Cl⁻/formate exchangers.[208] However, in juxtamedullary proximal convoluted tubules only Cl⁻/OH⁻ exchange is present.[208] In the guinea pig there is a large increase in Na⁺/H⁺ exchanger activity and Cl⁻/formate exchange in brush border membrane vesicles during the transition from fetus to newborn.[93] In isolated perfused rabbit proximal straight tubules the rate of active NaCl transport was two-fold greater in adult proximal straight tubules compared to neonatal tubules.[203] Both Cl⁻/OH⁻ and Na⁺/H⁺ exchange activities were five-fold less in neonatal tubules compared to that in adult tubules.[203]

The relative contribution of passive chloride transport to total NaCl transport may be species-specific. In the adult rat the late proximal tubular chloride concentration is significantly higher than that in the glomerular ultrafiltrate.[133] However, in the neonatal rat, the proximal tubule luminal chloride concentration remains the same as that in the glomerular ultrafiltrate. The constant luminal chloride concentration could be due to equal rates of chloride and bicarbonate reabsorption by the immature segment or to a higher chloride permeability in the neonate mediating higher rates of passive chloride transport than in adults.[133] Direct measurements of chloride permeability and the relative contributions of passive chloride transport have not been examined *in vivo*. Thus, the reason for the lack of the chloride gradient in neonatal rat proximal tubules is unknown.

Developmental Changes in the Paracellular Transport

Direct measurements of rabbit proximal convoluted tubule chloride and bicarbonate permeabilities demonstrate that neonatal segments have a lower permeability to both solutes than in the adult.[162,165,206] In addition, the resistance of the proximal tubule is higher in the neonatal rabbit proximal tubule than the adult, providing further evidence that there are developmental changes in the paracellular pathway.[165] Finally, studies have demonstrated that solvent drag does not contribute significantly to volume absorption in the neonatal tubule, as the reflection coefficients for both

NaCl and NaHCO$_3$ were not different from one.[164] Passive chloride transport has been characterized in the rabbit using *in vitro* microperfusion.[165,203,206] In both neonates and adults chloride permeability is extremely low, indicating that passive chloride transport does not contribute significantly to chloride absorption in this nephron segment.[206] The permeability of chloride in neonatal juxtamedullary proximal convoluted tubules is more than 10-fold lower than that of the adult segment.[206] In adult rabbit proximal straight tubules there is a substantive rate of passive chloride transport[165,203]; however, the neonatal rabbit proximal straight tubule is impermeable to chloride. Thus, there is no passive NaCl transport in the neonatal proximal straight tubule.[165,203]

The maturational changes in passive paracellular transport indicate there must be a developmental change in the composition of tight junction proteins. The tight junction creates a barrier and mediates the paracellular properties of the paracellular pathway.[236] Occludin, a protein with a ubiquitous distribution, and claudins, a family of tight junction proteins that number over 20, have four membrane spanning domains forming two extracellular loops that adjoin with their partner on the neighboring cell.[236] The permeability properties, including the ion permeability and resistance of epithelia, are determined predominantly by the isoforms of the claudins in the tight junction. Using semiquantitative real-time PCR of individually dissected tubules, there was no difference in the mRNA expression of claudins 1, 2, 10a, 12, and occludin in neonates compared to adult proximal tubules. However, claudins 6 and 9 were present in neonatal proximal tubules, but were absent in the adult segment.[1] Expression of claudins 6 and 9 in Madin−Darby canine kidney II (MDCK II) cells, which have a low resistance and do not express these claudin isoforms, resulted in an increase in the paracellular resistance and increased sodium-to-chloride and bicarbonate-to-chloride permeability ratios.[179] In addition, expression of claudin 6 and claudin 9 in MDCK II cells resulted in a decrease in the transepithelial chloride permeability.[179] Thus, the expression of claudin 6 and 9 in neonatal proximal tubule is likely the cause for the higher resistance and the lower chloride permeability than in the adult tubule.

Distal Tubule NaCl Transport

The thick ascending limb and distal convoluted tubule reabsorb NaCl, and are impermeable to water. The osmolality of the luminal fluid collected by micropuncture of rat early distal tubules is 40% lower in adults compared to neonates,[253] and the fraction of filtered sodium remaining in the early distal tubule is higher in neonatal than adult rats,[10] consistent with a maturational increase in the rate of sodium transport in the thick ascending limb. *In vivo* micropuncture of 13- to 39-day-old rats showed an increase in loop NaCl reabsorption during postnatal maturation,[133] and *in vitro* microperfusion of the rabbit cortical thick ascending limb demonstrated that the rate of sodium transport in the adult segment is five-fold greater than that of the neonate.[107] Both rat and rabbit cortical and medullary thick ascending limb Na$^+$/K$^+$-ATPase activity increase approximately four-fold during postnatal maturation, consistent with a large developmental increase in sodium reabsorption by both segments.[167,188] A direct comparison of NaCl transport in neonatal and adult medullary thick ascending limb has not been performed; however, there is a maturational increase in Na$^+$/K$^+$-ATPase activity in this segment.[69,167,188]

Compared to adults, neonates have a limited capacity to excrete a sodium load which is not due solely to a lower GFR.[9,65,87] None of the nephron segments discussed thus far is responsible for this phenomenon, as this requires a segment where the relative transport rates are higher in neonates than in adults. The adult distal convoluted tubule reabsorbs only 5% of the filtered sodium, but sodium transport rates are higher in neonates.[10] In an *in vivo* micropuncture study, distal tubule transport was assayed during hydropenia and during volume expansion in 24- and 40-day-old rats. While 24-day-old hydropenic rats had a higher fraction of filtered sodium remaining in the early distal tubule than 40-day-old animals, this difference had disappeared by the late distal tubule puncture site. With volume expansion there was a comparable fraction of filtered sodium remaining in the early distal tubule in the two age groups, but there was enhanced late distal tubule sodium reabsorption in the younger rats.[10] Thus this segment is, at least in part, responsible for the blunted natriuresis with salt-loading in neonates.

The cortical collecting duct is the nephron segment responsible for the final modulation of sodium transport under the control of aldosterone. In the isolated perfused cortical collecting tubule, there is a three- to five-fold increase in sodium transport between one-week-old and adult rabbits.[180,237] Most of the maturational increase occurs between the first and second weeks of life. Sodium entry in the neonatal and adult cortical collecting tubule is via an apical sodium channel termed ENaC. ENaC is the rate-limiting step in collecting tubule sodium transport, and neonatal cortical collecting ducts have fewer apical conducting sodium channels than adult segments[112,184](Figure 27.5). ENaC is composed of α-, ß-, and γ- subunits, and the mRNA and protein abundance of each increases during postnatal life.[112,238,241,254] The driving force for conductive sodium entry across the apical conductance is the

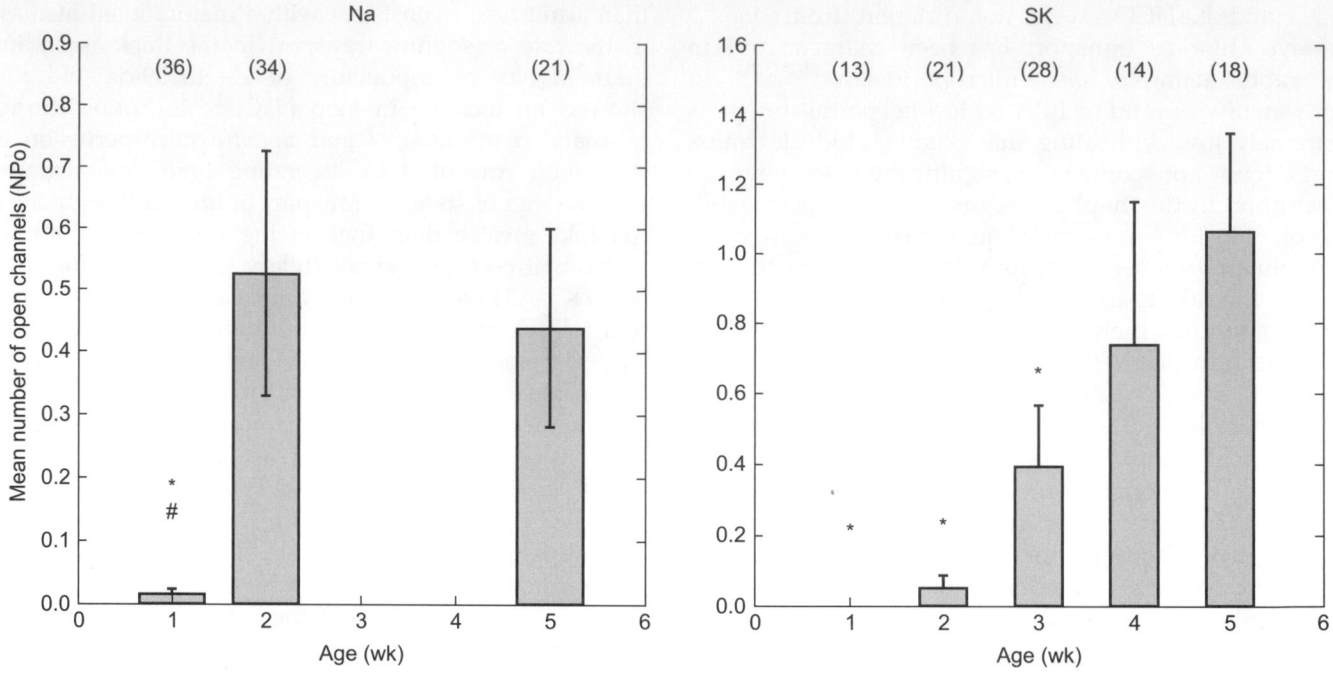

FIGURE 27.5 **Postnatal changes in number of conducting Na (ENaC) and secretory potassium (SK) channels per cell-attached patch of apical membrane of rabbit principal cells.** The number of functional Na channels increased ~30-fold between the first and second weeks of life, whereas the number of SK channels increased gradually after the second postnatal week *(from ref. [184] with permission)*.

basolateral Na^+/K^+-ATPase, which increases in activity two-fold during maturation in this segment.[188] Interestingly, the fetal collecting duct expresses the Na^+/K^+-ATPase on the apical membrane; the significance of this is unknown.[50,108]

REGULATION OF SODIUM TRANSPORT

Renin–Angiotensin–Aldosterone

Plasma renin activity is higher in the neonate than the adult, and increases appropriately to a reduction in extracellular fluid volume in the fetus, premature infant, and neonate.[71,86,141,225] Plasma aldosterone levels are also significantly higher in preterm and term neonates than in adults.[8,34,141,210,225] Cord blood from term infants born to mothers who ingested a normal salt diet had significantly lower plasma aldosterone levels than those whose mothers ingested a low-salt diet or who were taking diuretics.[34] These data imply that the human fetus can also respond to volume contraction with an increase in serum aldosterone. The plasma aldosterone level has also been shown to vary inversely with sodium intake in preterm infants with respiratory distress syndrome.[210] Although the

newborn can increase aldosterone secretion, the effect of aldosterone to increase distal tubule sodium reabsorption and potassium secretion is blunted compared to adults.[8,141,225] For example, in adult rats, adrenalectomy produces a 40-fold increase in urinary Na/K ratio, but in neonatal rats adrenalectomy has no effect on urinary electrolyte excretion.[222] Administration of exogenous aldosterone to adult adrenalectomized rats decreases the urinary Na/K ratio profoundly, but administration of aldosterone has no effect on urinary electrolytes in adrenalectomized neonatal rats.[222] Isolated perfused cortical collecting tubules from adult rabbits treated with mineralocorticoid had a significant increase in sodium absorption compared to control rabbits, but neonatal cortical collecting tubules were unaffected by prior mineralocorticoid treatment.[237] This resistance to aldosterone in neonatal rats is not due to a paucity of mineralocorticoid receptors, but is a postreceptor phenomenon.[222] However, in the mouse the blunted effect of aldosterone may also be due to fewer mineralocorticoid receptors compared to adults.[141]

Angiotensin II augments proximal and distal tubule sodium reabsorption by binding to both basolateral and luminal receptors. While neonatal rats have a blunted diuresis and natriuresis in response to volume expansion, this was not the case in neonates which received Losartan, an AT_I receptor blocker, consistent with angiotensin II playing an important role in the regulation of sodium absorption in the neonate.[56]

Renal Nerves and Catecholamines

Renal nerve stimulation produces an increase in renal vascular resistance and reduction in renal blood flow in the fetus and newborn, although the effect is less in immature animals compared to adults.[174] Renal denervation of the fetal and neonatal lamb does not significantly alter renal blood flow, GFR or renal sodium handling, indicating that basal renal function is not significantly affected by renal nerves.[172,214,215] However, in the transition from fetal to neonatal life, renal nerves play a role in the decrease in sodium excretion that occurs during this period.[216] Sheep with denervated kidneys had a greater urine volume and sodium excretion in the first 24 hours after birth, as well as lower plasma atrial natriuretic peptide and renin levels.[216] There is no difference in urinary sodium or volume excretion after the first day of life, indicating that other unknown variables play an important role in mediating the profound decrease in urinary sodium and volume excretion after birth.[216]

Dopamine is a natriuretic hormone whose plasma levels are increased with volume expansion. Dopamine increases renal blood flow and GFR, and inhibits sodium transport in the proximal tubule, thick ascending limb, and collecting duct.[6] The concentration of dopamine is higher in fetal rat plasma and amniotic fluid than in the maternal blood.[39] Administration of exogenous dopamine to human premature neonates with respiratory distress syndrome increases GFR, and produces a natriuresis and diuresis.[234] However, comparative studies demonstrate that the effect of dopamine on the Na^+/H^+ exchanger and Na^+/K^+-ATPase is less in neonatal than adult tubules.[6,82,119,136]

RENAL ACIDIFICATION

The serum bicarbonate concentration in human infants in the first year of life averages 22 mEq/l, a value significantly less than that of adults.[74] Premature human neonates can have serum bicarbonate levels as low as 14.5 mEq/l.[193] The lower serum bicarbonate concentration in neonates and infants is due to a lower threshold for bicarbonate by the immature kidney.[74] This section will discuss the salient differences between the neonatal and adult kidney with regard to renal acidification.

Proximal Tubules

The adult proximal tubule reabsorbs 80% of the filtered bicarbonate. The lower bicarbonate threshold in neonates is, in large part, due to a lower bicarbonate reabsorptive capacity of the neonatal proximal tubule. In rabbit juxtamedullary proximal convoluted tubules perfused in vitro, the rate of bicarbonate reabsorption in proximal tubules from one-week-old rabbits is one-third that of the adult proximal tubule.[190] The rate of bicarbonate absorption does not change significantly until the time of weaning at four weeks of age. At six weeks of age, the rate of bicarbonate absorption is comparable to the adult. The maturational pattern of glucose and total volume reabsorption is quite similar to that for bicarbonate absorption.[190] The rate of bicarbonate absorption has not been directly measured in superficial nephrons. However, micropuncture studies in rats and in vitro microperfusion studies in rabbits have demonstrated a similar maturational increase in the rate of volume absorption in these segments.[11,130,133] Since a substantial fraction of volume absorption reflects bicarbonate absorption, a similar maturational pattern for bicarbonate is likely.

There are several potential explanations for the lower rate of bicarbonate transport in neonatal proximal tubules. In the adult proximal tubule there is a preferential reabsorption of bicarbonate over chloride ions. This leaves the luminal fluid with a higher chloride concentration and a lower bicarbonate concentration than that in the peritubular capillaries. This bicarbonate concentration difference could potentially allow bicarbonate to diffuse from the peritubular capillaries back to the luminal fluid. The amount of bicarbonate passive backflux is dependent upon the permeability of the paracellular pathway of the neonatal proximal tubule to bicarbonate.[123,162,165,203,205,206] However, bicarbonate permeability in juxtamedullary rabbit proximal convoluted tubules is less in neonatal juxtamedullary proximal tubules perfused in vitro than that of the adult segment.[162] Thus, the lower rate of bicarbonate transport in neonatal juxtamedullary proximal tubules is not explained by enhanced back diffusion, but is entirely due to a lower rate of active transcellular bicarbonate transport.

In the adult proximal tubule, two-thirds of apical proton secretion is mediated by the Na^+/H^+ exchanger and one-third is via an H^+-ATPase.[21,160] The driving force for the Na^+/H^+ exchanger is the low intracellular sodium concentration generated by the Na^+/K^+-ATPase. In the adult proximal tubule bicarbonate, exit is via the $Na(HCO_3)_3$ co-transporter. A lower rate of bicarbonate reabsorption by the neonatal proximal tubule could be due to a lower activity of any of these transport processes.

Studies using a variety of different techniques have demonstrated a maturational increase in proximal tubule apical membrane Na$^+$/H$^+$ exchanger activity.[20,21,31,202] In isolated perfused rabbit juxtamedullary proximal convoluted tubules the rate of Na$^+$/H$^+$ exchanger activity is approximately one-third that of the adult rate, and adult values are reached at six weeks of age.[20] These results compare well to the maturational changes in bicarbonate absorption measured in isolated perfused rabbit convoluted tubules.[190] While this study solely examined juxtamedullary proximal tubules, similar findings have been demonstrated in brush border membrane vesicles from the renal cortex.[31] Na$^+$/H$^+$ exchanger activity in late rabbit fetal kidney cortex is 25% that of the adult cortex. This difference is entirely due to a lower V$_{max}$, and not to a difference in the K$_M$ for sodium.[31]

The H$^+$-ATPase, present on the apical membrane of the adult proximal tubules, does not contribute significantly to bicarbonate absorption in the neonatal proximal tubule. To study the relative contribution of the Na$^+$/H$^+$ exchanger and the H$^+$-ATPase to proximal tubule acidification, the rates of these two transporters were assayed by measuring proton secretory rates in adult and neonatal proximal convoluted tubules in response to an intracellular acid load.[21] As has previously been demonstrated, the rate of neonatal Na$^+$/H$^+$ exchanger activity is less than that in the adult. In the adult rabbit proximal tubule two-thirds of the pH recovery from an acid load is due to the Na$^+$/H$^+$ exchanger, and one-third is due to the the H$^+$-ATPase. In the neonate, 95% of pH recovery is due to the Na$^+$/H$^+$ exchanger, and only 5% is due to a sodium-independent mechanism. Thus, both the Na$^+$/H$^+$ exchanger and the H$^+$-ATPase undergo a significant increase in activity during maturation, and presumably limit bicarbonate absorption by the neonatal proximal tubule.

Three isoforms of the Na$^+$/H$^+$ exchanger, NHE1, NHE3, and NHE8 have been localized to the proximal tubule.[39,40,91,255] NHE1 has a ubiquitous distribution in tissues, and is found on the basolateral membrane of the proximal tubule.[40] NHE1 protein abundance does not vary significantly with postnatal maturation.[24] NHE3 is the apical membrane Na$^+$/H$^+$ exchanger mediating most luminal proton secretion by the adult proximal tubule.[39,249] There is a substantive postnatal maturational increase in NHE3 mRNA and protein abundance.[24] Interestingly, neonates have Na$^+$/H$^+$ exchanger activity at a time when NHE3 protein abundance is barely detectable.[202] The disparity between the presence of Na$^+$/H$^+$ exchanger activity and the paucity of NHE3 in the proximal tubule of neonates is due to the presence of NHE8.[33] NHE8 is predominantly an intracellular sodium–hydrogen exchanger that is also abundantly expressed on the apical membrane in neonates. Brush border membrane NHE8 decreases in abundance during postnatal maturation[33] (Figure 27.6). The factors responsible for this isoform switch will be discussed below.

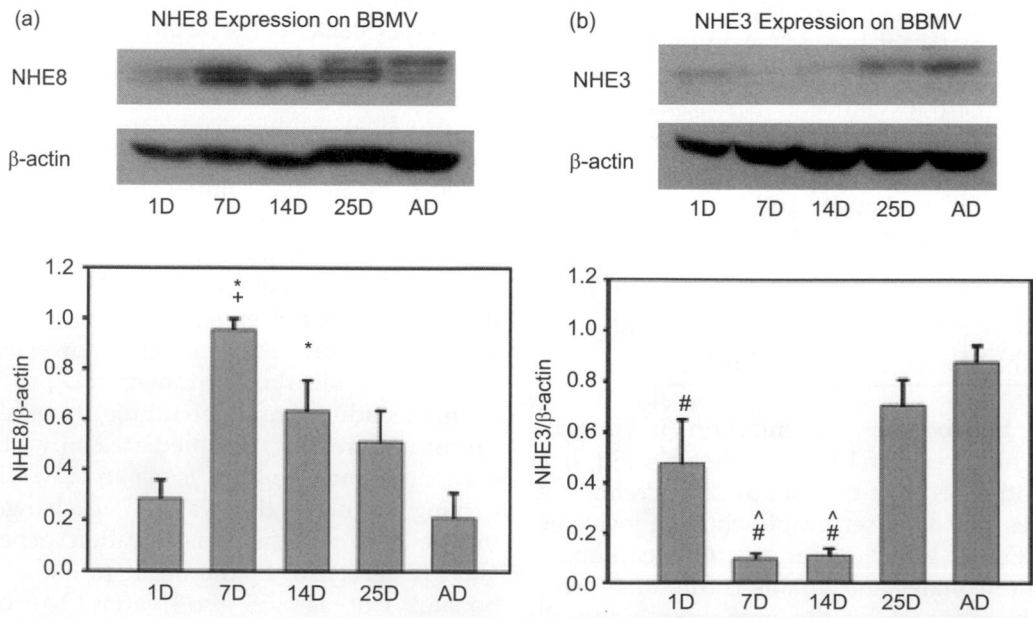

FIGURE 27.6   **Developmental change in brush border membra 33 ne NHE8 (a) and NHE3 (b) compared to β-actin.** NHE8 increased during postnatal development with a reciprocal increase in NHE3. *$P < 0.05$ vs. 1D and AD; $+ P < 0.05$ vs. 26D; #$P < 0.05$ vs. 26D and AD; ^$P < 0.05$ vs. 1D. (*from ref. [33] with permission*).

The basolateral membrane $Na(HCO_3)_3$ co-transporter facilitates bicarbonate exit from the proximal tubule. $Na(HCO_3)_3$ symporter activity in neonates is only slightly less than that of adults.[20] This transporter not only plays a role in bicarbonate exit, but is also the predominate mechanism for the defense against changes in intracellular pH by the proximal tubule.[20]

Distal Tubule Acidification

The adult cortical collecting duct can absorb or secrete bicarbonate depending on the acid–base status of the animal.[146] Proton and bicarbonate secretion are mediated by α- and β-intercalated cells, respectively, which are far fewer in number than principal cells, the predominant cell in the cortical collecting duct. The number of α- and β-intercalated cells per millimeter of tubular length increases several-fold during maturation of the rabbit cortical collecting duct.[77,183] β-intercalated cells start to appear in the mouse cortical collecting tubule in the first week of life.[217] While β-intercalated cells are present in the outer medullary collecting duct of the neonate, they disappear by apoptosis and are no longer present in this segment by 2–3 weeks of age.[48,217]

Net bicarbonate transport in the cortical collecting tubule is dependent on the relative rates of bicarbonate absorption and secretion. In isolated perfused cortical collecting tubules from neonatal rabbits there is no net bicarbonate transport, whereas adult cortical collecting ducts secrete bicarbonate.[147] Bicarbonate secretion by the β-intercalated cell is via an apical chloride-bicarbonate exchanger that functions at a reduced rate in the neonatal segment.[183] Removal of bath chloride inhibits basolateral membrane chloride-base exchange on α-intercalated cells and inhibits luminal proton secretion. Removal of bath chloride had no effect on the rate of bicarbonate transport in cortical collecting tubules from neonatal rabbits, but increased net bicarbonate secretion in adult segments, indicating that there is a maturational increase in the cortical collecting tubule to secrete bicarbonate.[147] The bicarbonate absorptive capacity of the α-intercalated cell in the cortical collecting duct also increases during postnatal maturation.[183,186] The outer medullary collecting duct is an important segment for urinary acidification. Unlike the cortical collecting tubule, the number of intercalated cells per millimeter of tubular length does not change significantly with postnatal development.[77,186] The rate of bicarbonate absorption is only slightly less in the neonatal outer medullary collecting ducts compared to the adult rabbit segment.[147] Thus, there is a significant difference in the relative maturity of the cortical and medullary segments in neonates.

Titratable Acid and Ammonia Excretion

In addition to reclaiming the filtered load of bicarbonate, the kidney must excrete an amount of acid equivalent to the acid generated from metabolism. The growing animal must also excrete protons liberated during the formation of bone.[125,126] This is in part compensated for by the gastrointestinal absorption of alkali in the neonate,[125,126,240] but as in the adult, the neonatal kidney plays a major role in acid excretion. Thus, the kidney of the growing neonate must excrete 50–100% more acid per kg than the adult.

To excrete the quantity of acid generated from metabolism of proteins and growing bones, there must be urinary buffers to accept the secreted protons. If there were no titratable acids and ammonia in our urine, the secretion of a few protons would decrease the urine pH to levels that would inhibit further proton secretion. Net acid excretion, the sum of ammonium and titratable acid excretion per kg body weight, is significantly less in neonates than adults.[144] However, by seven days of age cows milk formula-fed infants have comparable rates of ammonium and titratable acid excretion as that of adults when normalized per kg of body weight.[142,144] Breast milk-fed infants, however, have significantly less phosphate intake and lower rates of titratable acid excretion than infants fed cows milk formula.[66,80,102,144] Thus, the rate of renal maturation of net acid excretion is quite brisk. However, unlike adults, human neonates function at near maximal capacity of net acid excretion to eliminate metabolically generated acid,[142] and have a limited ability to respond to an exogenous acid-load by increasing titratable acid and ammonia excretion.[142] In comparison to adults, neonates given an acid-load have a smaller increase in both titratable acid and ammonium excretion, making them more prone to develop acidosis when so challenged.[60,102] By one month of age the rate of net acid excretion in response to an acid-load is comparable to that of adults.[74,90,152,158,228] However, young infants respond to an acid-load with higher rates of titratable acid excretion to compensate for the lower rates of ammonium excretion.[74,152] In vitro studies have shown that the rate of renal ammonia production in kidney slices is lower in neonates compared to adults.[105] The low rate of ammonia production is in part due to lower glutamine synthetase activity limiting glutamine availability, but predominantly due to lower glutaminase activity.[89,239] As in adults, glutaminase activity increases substantively in response to an acid-load.[36] Premature neonates have significantly lower rates of titratable acid and ammonia excretion than term infants.[124,226,229] Preterm infants are thus less tolerant of a high protein formula than term infants, because sulfur containing amino acids generate an acid-load which cannot be eliminated due to the low rates of net acid excretion.[63,228] Administration of NH_4Cl to premature infants resulted in an increase in net acid excretion, but premature infants had lower rates of ammonium and titratable acid excretion, and a higher urine pH, than term neonates.[90,124,226,227,229] As with term infants, there is a rapid maturation of the ability of premature infants to excrete an exogenous acid-load.[124,226,229]

Carbonic Anhydrase Activity

Carbonic anhydrase facilitates the reversible hydration of CO_2 to H_2CO_3.[161,192] Carbonic anhydrase is localized to all acidifying nephron segments, where it plays an important role in acidification. For example, carbonic anhydrase inhibition results in a 90% decrease in the rate of proximal tubule bicarbonate reabsorption.[139] There are 15 carbonic acid isoforms, with both species- and nephron segment-specificity.[161]

Carbonic anhydrase II is located in the cytosol of all acidifying renal tubules, and comprises 95% of carbonic anhydrase activity in the kidney.[120] Carbonic anhydrase IV comprises approximately 5% of total renal carbonic anhydrase activity, and is located on the apical and basolateral membrane of the proximal tubule and on the apical membrane of acid-secreting cells in the distal nephron.[192,194,195,245] Carbonic anhydrase XII is present on the basolateral membrane of acidifying segments.[156] In rodents, carbonic anhydrase XIV is also expressed on the apical membrane of the proximal tubule and thick ascending limb.[161] Carbonic anhydrase II protein abundance, normalized per millimeter of tubular length, increases approximately 10-fold in rat proximal convoluted tubules, cortical collecting tubules, and outer medullary collecting tubules between one and twelve weeks of age.[120] In the rabbit, carbonic anhydrase II increases only two-fold during postnatal maturation compared to carbonic anhydrase IV, which undergoes a ten-fold increase in mRNA and protein abundance with cortical maturation.[195,245] Thus, the developmental increase in carbonic anhydrase may be a factor in the postnatal increase in renal acidification.

INDUCTION OF NEPHRON MATURATION

As noted above, there are a number of quantitative and qualitative changes that occur in all nephron segments during postnatal development. Most of the studies examining the factors responsible for the postnatal changes during development come from studies of the proximal tubule, which will be the focus here. There are a number of potential factors which may be responsible for the postnatal maturational changes in proximal tubule transport. The maturational increase in GFR may induce the maturation of transporters on the apical membrane by increasing solute delivery. As previously discussed, an increase in apical membrane sodium transport could increase intracellular sodium and play a potential role in the maturational increase in Na^+/K^+-ATPase activity.[61,101,131] There are also significant postnatal maturational changes in several hormones which affect proximal tubular transport, including thyroid hormone and glucocorticoids, which increase 3-fold and 20-fold, respectively, in the postnatal period.[104]

Glucocorticoids increase renal cortical Na^+/H^+ exchanger activity. This effect can, in part, be mediated by an increase in GFR which will increase sodium delivery to the proximal tubule. However, glucocorticoids and thyroid hormone have a direct epithelial action on the proximal tubule to increase the rate of bicarbonate absorption and Na^+/H^+ exchanger activity.[22,25] This effect of glucocorticoids and thyroid hormone on NHE3 is due to an increase in NHE3 transcription.[22,52] However, glucocorticoids also increase apical membrane NHE3 by increasing the rate of exocytosis.[42] Administration of glucocorticoids to pregnant rabbits two days prior to the delivery increases the V_{max} of the Na^+/H^+ exchanger in neonates to levels the same as those seen in adults.[31] The K_m for sodium is comparable in neonates and adults. Similarly, proximal convoluted tubules from neonatal rabbits whose mothers received dexamethasone before delivery had infants with an almost two-fold increase in the rate of bicarbonate absorption to levels comparable to that measured in adult animals.[27] In addition, the rate of Na^+/H^+ exchanger and $Na(HCO_3)_3$ activity in proximal tubules increased two-fold in dexamethasone treated neonates.[27] The effect of dexamethasone is specific for the NHE3 isoform, the isoform present on the apical membrane of the proximal tubule and responsible for the majority of Na^+/H^+ exchanger activity in adults.[24] Prevention of the maturational increase of either glucocorticoids or thyroid hormone prevents the maturational increase in Na^+/H^+ exchanger activity and NHE3 protein abundance.[26,95] While glucocorticoids are the most important factor causing the maturational increase in NHE3, adrenalectomy in the neonatal period does not totally prevent an increase in both Na^+/H^+ exchanger activity and NHE3 protein and mRNA abundance, suggesting that thyroid hormone can compensate, to some extent, in the absence of glucocorticoids.[95] This was definitively demonstrated in studies using hypothyroid-glucocorticoid-deficient rats, where the maturational increase in both hormones was prevented, and where Na^+/H^+ exchanger activity, NHE3 protein, and mRNA abundance remained at neonatal levels into adulthood.[94] As noted, there is an isoform switch from NHE8 to NHE3 during postnatal development.[33] The maturational decrease in NHE8 on the apical membrane of the proximal tubule is due the postnatal increase in thyroid hormone.[84] Administration of thyroid hormone to neonates resulted in a premature decrease in NHE8 and increase in NHE3 on brush border membranes, while prevention of developmental increase in thyroid hormone prevented the decrease in brush border membrane NHE8 abundance.[84] The regulation of NHE8 by thyroid hormone is due to a direct epithelial effect to decrease NHE8 surface expression, likely by post-transcriptional regulation.[84]

As will be discussed, there is a maturational decrease in the rate of phosphate transport during postnatal maturation.[57,66,106] This is observed at a time when there is an increase in serum glucocorticoid levels.[104] Administration of glucocorticoids to neonatal rats produced a significant inhibition in the rate of sodium-dependent phosphate uptake. This is due to a reduction in the V_{max} with no change in the K_M for phosphate.[16] This glucocorticoid-induced decrease in phosphate uptake was not accompanied by a change in NaPi-2a mRNA abundance; however, there was a three-fold decrease in NaP_i transporter protein abundance.[16] Thus, glucocorticoids play a role in the maturational decrease in phosphate transport.

Thyroid hormone appears to play an important role in postnatal development of mitochondrial enzymes in the rat proximal convoluted tubule. The normal maturational increase in the proximal tubule mitochondrial enzymes 3-keto acid-CoA transferase, an enzyme involved in ketone body oxidation, and citrate synthase and carnitine acetyltransferase were impaired in hypothyroid rats.[243] The enzyme activities were restored with thyroid replacement. Acetoacetyl-CoA thiolase, however, is not decreased in 21-day-old hypothyroid rats.[243] Finally, thyroid hormone plays a role in the maturational changes that occur in the permeability properties of the paracellular pathway.[28,205] As noted above, the adult rabbit proximal straight tubule has a high chloride permeability which results in high rates of passive chloride transport.[205] The neonatal rabbit proximal straight tubule is impermeable to chloride.[165] Neonatal proximal straight tubules have higher P_{Na}/P_{Cl} (sodium to chloride permeability ratio) and P_{HCO3}/P_{Cl} ratios than adult segments. Many, but not all, of the maturational changes in paracellular permeability properties of the proximal tubule can be accelerated by administration of thyroid hormone to neonates[205] or prevented if the neonates are made hypothyroid.[205]

PHOSPHATE TRANSPORT

Phosphate is essential for growth, and unlike adults growing animals are in positive phosphate balance. Human neonates and infants have a higher serum phosphate concentration than that of adults. While the high serum phosphate in neonates could be due to the lower GFR compared to adults, this is not the case. Studies have demonstrated that increasing the GFR by arginine infusion in young rats does not increase phosphate excretion, and lowering the GFR in adult rats by constricting the abdominal aorta does not increase the rate of phosphate absorption to that seen in the neonate.[99] The tubular reabsorptive capacity for phosphate is higher in neonates and infants than in adults.[57,66,106,171] Approximately 90—95% of the filtered phosphate is reabsorbed in human neonates during the first week of life, and growing children continue to maintain a higher maximal tubular reabsorption of phosphate than adults.[57,106]

A number of variables, such as intrinsic properties of phosphate transport in the proximal tubule, dietary phosphate content, parathyroid hormone, and growth factors can modulate phosphate transport, and could potentially explain the higher rate of phosphate transport by the neonatal kidney. The role of these factors has been extensively studied and will be reviewed in this section. A higher intrinsic rate of renal phosphate transport has been demonstrated in the isolated perfused guinea pig kidney where other in vivo factors were eliminated.[116] The maximal tubular reabsorption of phosphate per volume of glomerular filtrate in 3—7-day-old neonatal guinea pig kidneys is 40% greater than that measured in adult animals.[107] A higher intrinsic rate of proximal tubular phosphate reabsorption was also directly demonstrated in micropuncture studies, where 5—14 day neonatal guinea pigs reabsorbed a higher fraction of filtered phosphate than adults.[122] The maximal rate of phosphate uptake in brush border membrane vesicles (V_{max}) is five-fold higher in neonates than in adults, in the absence of a maturational change in the K_M for phosphate in growing animals.[154]

In addition to the difference in the rate of sodium-dependent phosphate co-transport with maturation, other intrinsic proximal tubular factors may play a role in the higher rates of phosphate transport in growing animals. The intracellular phosphate concentration (P_i) measured in isolated perfused kidneys using NMR was 40% lower in growing animals than in adults.[19] This provides a greater driving force for phosphate transport in growing animals. The lower intracellular phosphate concentration in the presence of a higher rate of apical phosphate transport implies that the rate of basolateral phosphate exit is also higher in growing animals, although this has not been directly examined.

Membrane fluidity also has been shown to affect phosphate transport.[134,135,151] The brush border membrane content of cholesterol, sphingomyelin, and phosphatidylinositol increases with age.[135] This change in lipid composition decreases membrane fluidity,[135,151] which directly decreases the rate of phosphate transport.[134,151] Thus, the lipid composition and high membrane fluidity of the neonate and growing animal provides an environment which increases the V_{max} of the NaPi co-transporter. Glucocorticoids, which increase during the time of weaning, decrease membrane fluidity, and likely play a role in the postnatal decrease in phosphate transport.[16]

There are two sodium-dependent phosphate co-transporters, designated as NaPi-2a and NaPi-2c, present on the apical membrane of the proximal tubule that are primarily responsible for phosphate reabsorption.[140,197] In mice, NaPi-2a has been identified as the most important phosphate transporter in the kidney, responsible for $\sim 70\%$ of phosphate reabsorption.[32] NaPi-2a mRNA is first detected in early proximal convolutions in the post S-shaped body segment of the developing nephron.[189] However, NaPi-2a protein is not detected until the proximal tubules have a distinct brush border membrane.[231] Brush border membrane NaPi-2a expression is two-fold higher in 4-week-old juvenile rats than in adult rats, consistent with the higher rate of phosphate transport in growing animals.[246] A growth-specific NaPi co-transporter was postulated to be responsible for the increased phosphate transport in the weaning animals,[213] which was later identified as NaPi-2c.[197] NaPi-2c mRNA and protein expression is highest in the brush border of the convoluted proximal tubules of weanling rodents,[197] whereas it plays a negligible role in renal phosphate absorption in adults.[150,199,200] In contrast to rodents, NaPi-2c plays an important role in phosphate transport in humans. Mutations in NaPi-2c result in an autosomal recessive disorder termed hereditary hypophosphatemic rickets with hypercalciuria that is characterized by hypophosphatemia, due to renal phosphate-wasting, rickets, hypervitaminosis D, hypercalcemia, and hypercalciuria.[37,114]

Dietary phosphate content regulates renal phosphate transport in adult and in growing animals.[54,121,153,246] Thyroparathyroidectomized growing rats had a greater increase in their maximal tubular capacity for phosphate reabsorption in response to a low-phosphate diet and a blunted decrease in phosphate reabsorption on a high-phosphate diet compared to adult thyroparathyroidectomized rats.[54,153] In addition, the adaptive increase in maximal tubular capacity of phosphate reabsorption in response to phosphate deprivation took longer to occur in adult animals than in growing animals.[54] A low phosphate diet increases the rate of sodium-dependent phosphate uptake by brush border membrane vesicles in growing rats.[55] In addition, ingestion of a low-phosphate diet increases the abundance of Na-Pi transporters on the apical membrane of the proximal tubule, whereas a high-phosphate diet produces the opposite effect.[246] The dietary changes in phosphorus affect both brush border membrane NaPi-2a and NaPi-2c expression.[197,198]

The plasma concentration of PTH is lower in human neonates than in adults.[64] Fetal and neonatal rats can respond to changes in serum calcium with appropriate changes in PTH levels,[230] although there is a blunted response to PTH secretion.[242] Infusion of PTH in one-day-old human neonates produces no increase in urinary phosphate excretion.[57,137] By three days of age, infusion of parathyroid hormone results in an increase in phosphate excretion and increase in urinary cAMP.[57,137,145] However, the phosphaturic response to PTH is markedly lower in neonates than adults.[137] Furthermore, in micropuncture studies, the proximal tubule response to infusion of pharmacologic doses of PTH is attenuated in young rats compared to adults.[246] Despite the fact that PTH did not significantly increase phosphate excretion in young animals, the urinary cAMP corrected for GFR in response to PTH infusion was similar in all ages.[242] Thus, there is clearly a disassociation between the PTH-induced increase in cAMP production in neonates and the effect on phosphate excretion. The blunted response to PTH in the neonate compared to the adult is due to lower levels of phospholipase A2 activity in response to PTH and cAMP.[207]

Growth hormone administration can result in an increase in serum phosphate.[103] Brush border membrane vesicle phosphate transport is increased in dogs that received growth hormone compared to controls.[97] The effect of growth hormone on phosphate transport is mediated by IGF-1.[163] While growth hormone is not a significant regulator of phosphate transport in the adult, this may not be the case in the growing animal. Administration of growth hormone-releasing factor antagonist, which suppresses growth hormone secretion, has no effect on the maximal rate of phosphate absorption in adult rats, but significantly reduces phosphate absorption in growing rats.[100]

In addition to PTH, there are a number of hormones, known as phosphatonins, that regulate phosphate transport, including fibroblast growth factor-23 (FGF23),[29,209] secreted frizzled-related protein 4 (sFRP-4),[38] matrix extracellular phosphoglycoprotein,[49] fibroblast growth factor 7 (FGF7),[53] and dentin matrix protein-1(DMP1).[78] These hormones are dysregulated in a number of diseases with aberrant phosphate regulation, incuding X-linked hypophosphatemia and tumor-induced osteomalacia.[83] The role of these phosphatonins in the developmental changes in phosphate transport remains to be elucidated.

POTASSIUM TRANSPORT

Potassium is transported actively across the placenta from mother to fetus,[201] ensuring that the fetal plasma potassium concentration is maintained at levels exceeding 5 mEq/L, even in the face of maternal potassium deficiency.[62,201] Both premature and term neonates have very low rates of renal potassium excretion, which maintains a positive potassium balance necessary for growth.[68,225] The low rate of renal potassium excretion is also responsible, at least in part, for the higher serum potassium concentration in neonates than in adults.[225] Renal potassium clearance in infants less than one year of age is less than that of older children, even if corrected for GFR.[181,225] Neonates can respond to potassium-loading with net tubular secretion, but this response is less than that of adults.[138,233]

The proximal tubule of neonatal and adult rats reabsorbs approximately 50% of the filtered potassium.[133] There is a maturational increase in potassium reabsorption by the loop of Henle.[70,133] The loop of Henle of adult rats has been shown to reabsorb 79% of the delivered load, while only 56% was reabsorbed by 13−15-day-old neonates.[133] The limited capability of the thick ascending limb of the neonate to reabsorb potassium will increase distal delivery of potassium. Thus, neither the proximal tubule nor the loop of Henle is responsible for the limited capability of the neonate to excrete potassium.

The distal convoluted and connecting tubules and cortical collecting duct ultimately regulate potassium excretion in adults and neonates. Clearance studies in dogs have demonstrated that the amiloride-sensitive (i.e., EnaC-dependent) component of potassium secretion is substantially less in neonates than adults, providing indirect evidence for a limited distal nephron potassium secretory capacity.[138] The developmental maturation of potassium transport in the distal nephron has been directly examined in the rabbit cortical collecting duct by in vitro microperfusion.[180] Baseline potassium secretory rates are not different than zero during the first three weeks of life, and did not reach mature rates until six weeks of age.[180]

The limited capacity of the distal nephron for net potassium secretion could be due to either an unfavorable electrochemical gradient across the apical membrane and/or a limited apical potassium permeability. The rate of net sodium absorption in the cortical collecting duct of the two-week-old animal is approximately 60% of that measured in the adult,[81] reflecting the rapid appearance of conducting ENaC channels in the apical membrane of this segment between the first and second weeks of life.[184] Thus, the electrochemical gradient is not considered to be limiting for potassium secretion at this age. While low rates of luminal flow and distal sodium delivery can limit potassium secretion in adults, these are unlikely to be significant variables in neonates, which have high rates of distal nephron flow and sodium delivery.[10,133]

In support of the notion that a paucity of plasma membrane potassium channels limits potassium secretion early in life is the observation that the intracellular potassium concentration in the distal nephron at birth is comparable to that measured in the adult,[182] despite Na^+/K^+-ATPase activity that is only 50% of that measured in adult.[59,188] Direct analysis of the apical potassium conductance of CCDs isolated from maturing rabbits showed that the mean number of open channels per patch (NPo) increased progressively after birth[185] (Figure 27.5).

Two populations of apical potassium channels have been identified by patch-clamp analysis in the collecting duct. The secretory K (SK) channel, encoded by ROMK and restricted to principal cells, is a small conductance channel with a high open probability. The SK/ROMK channel is considered to mediate baseline potassium secretion.[185] High conductance BK channels, present in both principal and intercalated cells, are activated by increases in intracellular calcium concentration and stretch, but are rarely open at physiological membrane potentials. BK channels mediate flow-induced potassium secretion, which does not appear until the fifth week of postnatal life.[247,248] The temporal delay between the postnatal increases in SK/ROMK and BK channel activity accounts for the sequential appearance of basal- and then flow-induced net potassium secretion at 3 and 5 weeks, respectively, of postnatal life in the rabbit. Specifically, SK/ROMK channel activity increases progressively after the second week of postnatal life,[185] whereas functional BK channel activity does not appear until 5 weeks of age in the cortical collecting duct.[248] Both developmental processes closely parallel increases in channel-specific mRNA levels and immunodetectable protein at the apical membrane of the CCD.[35,248,254]

The H^+/K^+-ATPase is a third potassium transporter, present in the apical membrane of intercalated cells in the distal nephron. The H^+/K^+-ATPase has little functional role except under conditions of potassium deficiency and metabolic acidosis, when it mediates potassium absorption and proton secretion. The activity of this transporter is comparable in neonates and adult collecting tubules.[58]

URINARY CONCENTRATING AND DILUTING ABILITY

Deprived of water for sufficient time, an adult human can concentrate urine to 1200 mOsm/Kg water, while the term and premature neonatal kidney can achieve urine osmolalities of only 400–600 mOsm/Kg water.[79,98,157,159] By six months of age, the human infant can increase the urine osmolality to 600 mOsm/Kg water[159] and by 1 to 1.5 years the human infant can concentrate the urine to levels comparable to that of an adult.[159,244] The neonate also has a limited capacity to excrete free water compared to that of adults.[132,143] However, both term and premature infants can excrete dilute urine with an osmolality approaching 50 mOsm/Kg water.[176] Thus, the primary limiting factor in the ability of the neonate to excrete free water is the low GFR that limits the distal delivery of fluid.

The ability to maximally concentrate urine requires vasopressin secretion from the neurohypophysis, a hypertonic renal medulla and a renal collecting duct that responds to vasopressin by increasing water permeability. In the developing human, there are a number of factors in the concentrating mechanism that limit the ability to maximally concentrate urine. The neonate and late gestation fetus respond to changes in plasma osmolality and volume with appropriate changes in plasma vasopressin.[96,168] These changes in plasma vasopressin are of comparable magnitude to that measured under similar conditions in the adult.[168] Perinatal stress also results in the secretion of vasopressin.[96,170] However, infusion of vasopressin in the late gestation fetal sheep resulted in a smaller increase in urinary osmolality than that measured in adult animals.[175] Thus, while the fetus and neonate can secrete vasopressin at concentrations comparable to the adult, there is a hyporesponsiveness to the renal effect of vasopressin to increase urinary osmolality.

The osmotic gradient in the renal medulla is composed of urea and sodium chloride. The urea concentration in the neonatal renal medulla is limited in part by the low dietary protein intake and the high volume of fluid ingested.[72,73] Augmentation of protein or addition of urea to the diet of neonates increases their maximal concentrating ability, albeit not to the levels measured in adults.[72,73] Urea must get into the interstitium, which is facilitated by the urea transporter (UTA) located in the inner medulla. The abundance of UTA-1, which is also regulated by vasopressin, increases during postnatal maturation.[128] The capacity of the thick ascending limb to reabsorb sodium chloride, necessary to generate a hypertonic medulla, is less in the neonate compared to that of an adult.[10,107,110,167,188,253] The developmental changes that occur in transport with age in the thick

ascending limb are paralleled by an increase in the concentration of sodium and urea in the medulla and papilla.[168,221] In addition, the sorbitol concentration in the inner medulla, a major intracellular osmolyte formed by aldose reductase, is significantly less than that in the adult.[196] Fluid restriction increases aldose reductase activity in the adult medulla, but not in the neonate.[196]

The urinary concentrating ability of neonatal rats can be induced prematurely by the administration of glucocorticoids,[168,224] likely due to the premature induction of the NKCC2 in the medullary thick limb.[224,252] Adrenalectomy in rats on day 16 of life prevents the maturational increase in papillary sodium and urea concentration, but not the growth of the papilla, consistent with a role of glucocorticoids in the maturation of the tubular transport processes responsible for development of maximally concentrated urine.[168] However, adrenalectomy at 10 days of life in rats results in a poorly-developed papilla and an increase in medullary cyclooxygenase-2 protein abundance and PGE_2 levels. Administration of glucocorticoids alone to adrenalectomized neonatal rats increased, but did not normalize, urine osmolality,[223] which required both glucocorticoid and mineralocorticoid replacement.[223] The requirement for mineralocorticoids may be due to their effect of decreasing medullary cyclooxygenase-2 levels, since prostaglandins cause a natriuresis and diuresis.[223]

The osmotic water permeability of the adult and neonatal inner medullary collecting duct are very low in the absence of vasopressin.[212] Vasopressin causes an increase in cAMP that increases protein kinase A activity. Protein kinase A phosphorylates aquaporin 2, resulting in trafficking of the protein to the apical membrane and an increase in apical membrane water permeability.[43] In both the outer and inner medullary collecting collecting duct, vasopressin results in an increase in osmotic permeability, yet the response is far less than that measured in the adult segment.[111,212]

The limited response to vasopressin by the neonatal collecting tubule is due to several factors. There are fewer vasopressin-binding sites in the medullary and cortical collecting duct in the neonatal rat compared to the adult,[5,43] but is not likely to be a significant factor limiting renal concentrating ability.[30,166] Aquaporin-2 is less abundant in the renal medulla of neonatal rats than in adult animals.[45,250,252] Both aquaporin-2 mRNA and protein abundance increase with neonatal betamethasone administration,[252] providing further evidence that glucocorticoids are important in the maturation of the urinary concentrating mechanism. In the neonatal rat kidney aquaporin-2 expression and trafficking increase appropriately in response to both water deprivation and vasopressin administration.[45] The basolateral water channels, aquaporin-3 and -4 do not change significantly with postnatal development.[30,127,250]

The basal cAMP level is comparable in immature and adult cortical collecting ducts. However, there is a diminished stimulation of cAMP production in response to vasopressin in neonates compared to that of adults.[46] Forskolin, which directly activates adenylate cyclase, does not stimulate cAMP levels in the cortical collecting duct to the same extent as the adult tubule,[46] due to elevated phosphodiesterase activity which degrades cAMP in neonatal tubules compared to adult tubules.[166] In the presence of inhibitor of phosphodiesterase IV, the neonatal collecting duct water permeability was comparable to the adult in response to vasopressin.[166] Thus, developmental change in phosphodiesterase plays an important role in the development of the concentrating ability by degrading the generated cAMP. The limited vasopressin-mediated increase in cAMP levels in the neonatal collecting tubule due to increased degradation is the predominant factor impairing the action of vasopressin to increase water permeability.[46]

Prostaglandins could also play a role in the limited response of the neonatal collecting duct to vasopressin, since prostaglandins impair cAMP production.[46] While one study showed decreased PGE_2 production in neonatal cortical collecting tubules,[187] others have demonstrated both higher rates of production and greater abundance of G_i-coupled EP_3 (prostaglandin) receptors.[44,148] cAMP production in response to forskolin and vasopressin in neonatal and adult tubules are comparable when incubated with indomethacin to inhibit prostaglandin production.[44] However, when neonatal collecting ducts were perfused *in vitro*, there was no difference in water permeability in the response to vasopressin in presence or absence of indomethacin.[47] Thus, the role of prostaglandins in the limited response to vasopressin in the neonatal collecting duct remains unclear.

References

[1] Abuazza G, Becker A, Williams SS, Chakravarty S, Truong HT, Lin F, Baum M. Claudins 6, 9, and 13 are developmentally expressed renal tight junction proteins. Am J Physiol Renal Physiol 2006;291(6):F1132–41.

[2] Al-Dahhan J, Haycock GB, Chantler C, Stimmler L. Sodium homeostasis in term and preterm neonates. Arch Dis Child 1983;58:335–42.

[3] Allison ME, Lipham EM, Gottschalk CW. Hydrostatic pressure in the rat kidney. Am J Physiol 1972;223(4):975–83.

[4] Alpern RJ, Howlin KJ, Preisig PA. Active and passive components of chloride transport in the rat proximal convoluted tubule. J Clin Invest 1985;76(4):1360–6.

[5] Ammar A, Roseau S, Butlen D. Postnatal ontogenesis of vasopressin receptors in the rat collecting duct. Mol Cell Endocrinol 1992;86(3):193–203.

[6] Aperia A. Intrarenal dopamine: a key signal in the interactive regulation of sodium metabolism. Annu Rev Physiol 2000;62:621–47.

[7] Aperia A, Broberger O, Elinder G, Herin P, Zetterstrom R. Postnatal development of renal function in pre-term and full-term infants. Acta Paediatr Scand 1981;70(2):183–7.

[8] Aperia A, Broberger O, Herin P, Zetterstrom R. Sodium excretion in relation to sodium intake and aldosterone excretion in newborn preterm and fullterm infants. Acta Paediatr Scand 1979;68:813–7.

[9] Aperia A, Broberger O, Thodenius K, Zetterstrom R. Renal response to an oral sodium load in newborn full-term infants. Acta Paediatr Scand 1972;61:670–6.

[10] Aperia A, Elinder G. Distal tubular sodium reabsorption in the developing rat kidney. Am J Physiol 1981;240(6):F487–91.

[11] Aperia A, Larrson L. Corrrelation between fluid reabsorption and proimal tubule ultrastructure during development of the rat kidney. Acta Physiol Scand 1979;105:11–22.

[12] Aperia A, Larrson L. Induced development of proximal tublar Na,K-ATPase, basolateral cell membranes and fluid reabsorption. Acta Physiol Scand 1984;121:133–41.

[13] Aperia A, Larrson L, Zetterstrom R. Hormonal induction of Na-K-ATPase in developing proximal tubular cells. Am J Physiol 1981;241:F356–60.

[14] Arant Jr BS. Developmental patterns of renal functional maturation compared in the human neonate. J Pediatr 1978;92:705–12.

[15] Arant Jr BS, Edelmann Jr CM, Nash MA. The renal reabsorption of glucose in the developing canine kidney: a study of glomerulotubular balance. Pediatr Res 1974;8:638–46.

[16] Arar M, Levi M, Baum M. Maturational effects of glucocorticoids on neonatal brush-border membrane phosphate transport. Pediatr Res 1994;35:474–8.

[17] Aronson PS. Role of ion exchangers in mediating NaCl transport in the proximal tubule. Kidney Int 1996;49(6):1665–70.

[18] Aschinberg LC, Goldsmith DI, Olbing H, Spitzer A, Edelmann Jr CM, Blaufox MD. Neonatal changes in renal blood flow distribution in puppies. Am J Physiol 1975;228(5):1453–61.

[19] Barac-Nieto M, Dowd TL, Gupta RK, Spitzer A. Changes in NMR-visible kidney cell phosphate with age and diet: relationship to phosphate transport. Am J Physiol 1991;261(1 Pt 2): F153–62.

[20] Baum M. Neonatal rabbit juxtamedullary proximal convoluted tubule acidification. J Clin Invest 1990;85:499–506.

[21] Baum M. Developmental changes in rabbit juxtamedullary proximal convoluted tubule acidification. Pediatr Res 1992;31(4 Pt 1):411–4.

[22] Baum M, Amemiya M, Dwarakanath V, Alpern RJ, Moe OW. Glucocorticoids regulate NHE-3 transcription in OKP cells. Am J Physiol 1996;270(1 Pt 2):F164–9.

[23] Baum M, Berry CA. Evidence for neutral transcellular NaCl transport and neutral basolateral chloride exit in the rabbit convoluted tubule. J Clin Invest 1984;74:205–11.

[24] Baum M, Biemesderfer D, Gentry D, Aronson PS. Ontogeny of rabbit renal cortical NHE3 and NHE1: effect of glucocorticoids. Am J Physiol 1995;268(5 Pt 2):F815–20.

[25] Baum M, Cano A, Alpern RJ. Glucocorticoids stimulate Na^+/H^+ antiporter in OKP cells. Am J Physiol 1993;264(6 Pt 2): F1027–31.

[26] Baum M, Dwarakanath V, Alpern RJ, Moe OW. Effects of thyroid hormone on the neonatal renal cortical Na^+/H^+ antiporter. Kidney Int 1998;53(5):1254–8.

[27] Baum M, Quigley R. Prenatal glucocorticoids stimulate neonatal juxtamedullary proximal convoluted tubule acidification. Am J Physiol 1991;261(5 Pt 2):F746–52.

[28] Baum M, Quigley R. Thyroid hormone modulates rabbit proximal straight tubule paracellular permeability. Am J Physiol-Renal Physiol 2004;286(3):F477−82.

[29] Baum M, Schiavi S, Dwarakanath V, Quigley R. Effect of fibroblast growth factor-23 on phosphate transport in proximal tubules. Kidney Int 2005;68(3):1148−53.

[30] Baum MA, Ruddy MK, Hosselet CA, Harris HW. The perinatal expression of aquaporin-2 and aquaporin-3 in developing kidney. Pediatr Res 1998;43(6):783−90.

[31] Beck JC, Lipkowitz MS, Abramson RG. Ontogeny of Na/H antiporter activity in rabbit renal brush border membrane vesicles. J Clin Invest 1991;87(6):2067−76.

[32] Beck L, Karaplis AC, Amizuka N, Hewson AS, Ozawa H, et al. Targeted inactivation of Npt2 in mice leads to severe renal phosphate wasting, hypercalciuria, and skeletal abnormalities. Proc Natl Acad Sci USA 1998;95(9):5372−7.

[33] Becker AM, Zhang J, Goyal S, Dwarakanath V, Aronson PS, Moe OW, et al. Ontogeny of NHE8 in the rat proximal tubule. Am J Physiol Renal Physiol 2007;293:F255−61.

[34] Beitins IZ, Bayard F, Levitsky L, Ances IG, Kowarski A, Migeon CJ. Plasma aldosterone concentration at delivery and during the newborn period. J Clin Invest 1972;51(2):386−94.

[35] Benchimol C, Zavilowitz B, Satlin LM. Developmental expression of ROMK mRNA in rabbit cortical collecting duct. Pediatr Res 2000;47(1):46−52.

[36] Benyajati S, Goldstein L. Renal glutaminase adaptation and ammonia excretion in infant rats. Am J Physiol 1975;228 (3):693−8.

[37] Bergwitz C, Roslin NM, Tieder M, Loredo-Osti JC, Bastepe M, Abu-Zahra H, et al. SLC34A3 mutations in patients with hereditary hypophosphatemic rickets with hypercalciuria predict a key role for the sodium-phosphate co-transporter NaPi-IIc in maintaining phosphate homeostasis. Am J Hum Genet 2006;78 (2):179−92.

[38] Berndt T, Craig TA, Bowe AE, Vassiliadis J, Reczek D, Finnegan R, et al. Secreted frizzled-related protein 4 is a potent tumor-derived phosphaturic agent. J Clin Invest 2003;112(5):785−94.

[39] Biemesderfer D, Pizzonia J, Abu-Alfa A, Exner M, Reilly R, Igarashi P, et al. NHE3: a Na$^+$/H$^+$ exchanger isoform of renal brush border. Am J Physiol 1993;265(5 Pt 2):F736−42.

[40] Biemesderfer D, Reilly RF, Exner M, Igarashi P, Aronson PS. Immunocytochemical characterization of Na$^{(+)}$-H$^+$ exchanger isoform NHE-1 in rabbit kidney. Am J Physiol 1992;263(5 Pt 2): F833−40.

[41] Blanco G, Mercer RW. Isozymes of the Na-K-ATPase: heterogeneity in structure, diversity in function. Am J Physiol 1998;275(5 Pt 2):F633−50.

[42] Bobulescu IA, Dwarakanath V, Zou L, Zhang J, Baum M, Moe OW. Glucocorticoids acutely increase cell surface Na$^+$/H$^+$ exchanger-3 (NHE3) by activation of NHE3 exocytosis. Am J Physiol Renal Physiol 2005;289(4):F685−91.

[43] Bonilla-Felix M. Development of water transport in the collecting duct. Am J Physiol Renal Physiol 2004;287(6):F1093−101.

[44] Bonilla-Felix M, Jiang W. Expression and localization of prostaglandin EP3 receptor mRNA in the immature rabbit kidney. Am J Physiol 1996;271(1 Pt 2):F30−6.

[45] Bonilla-Felix M, Jiang W. Aquaporin-2 in the immature rat: expression, regulation, and trafficking. J Am Soc Nephrol 1997;8 (10):1502−9.

[46] Bonilla-Felix M, John-Phillip C. Prostaglandins mediate the defect in AVP-stimulated cAMP generation in immature collecting duct. Am J Physiol 1994;267(1 Pt 2):F44−8.

[47] Bonilla-Felix M, Vehaskari VM, Hamm LL. Water transport in the immature rabbit collecting duct. Pediatr Nephrol 1999;13 (2):103−7.

[48] Bonnici B, Wagner CA. Postnatal expression of transport proteins involved in acid−base transport in mouse kidney. Pflugers Arch 2004;448(1):16−28.

[49] Bresler D, Bruder J, Mohnike K, Fraser WD, Rowe PS. Serum MEPE-ASARM-peptides are elevated in X-linked rickets (HYP): implications for phosphaturia and rickets. J Endocrinol 2004;183 (3):R1−9.

[50] Burrow CR, Devuyst O, Li X, Gatti L, Wilson PD. Expression of the beta2-subunit and apical localization of Na$^+$-K$^+$-ATPase in metanephric kidney. Am J Physiol 1999;277(3 Pt 2):F391−403.

[51] Calcagno PL, Rubin MI. Renal extraction of para-aminohippurate in infants and children. J Clin Invest 1963;42:1632−9.

[52] Cano A, Baum M, Moe OW. Thyroid hormone stimulates the renal Na/H exchanger NHE3 by transcriptional activation. Am J Physiol 1999;276(1 Pt 1):C102−8.

[53] Carpenter TO, Ellis BK, Insogna KL, Philbrick WM, Sterpka J, Shimkets R. Fibroblast growth factor 7: an inhibitor of phosphate transport derived from oncogenic osteomalacia-causing tumors. J Clin Endo Med 2005;90(2):1012−20.

[54] Caverzasio J, Bonjour JP, Fleisch H. Tubular handling of Pi in young growing and adult rats. Am J Physiol 1982;242(6): F705−10.

[55] Caverzasio J, Murer H, Fleisch H, Bonjour JP. Phosphate transport in brush border membrane vesicles isolated from renal cortex of young growing and adult rats. Comparison with whole kidney data. Pflugers Arch 1982;394(3):217−21.

[56] Chevalier RL, Thornhill BA, Belmonte DC, Baertschi AJ. Endogenous angiotensin II inhibits natriuresis after acute volume expansion in the neonatal rat. Am J Physiol 1996;270(2 Pt 2):R393−7.

[57] Connelly JP, Crawford JD, Watson J. Studies of neonatal hyperphosphatemia. Pediatrics 1962;30:425−32.

[58] Constantinescu A, Silver RB, Satlin LM. H-K-ATPase activity in PNA-binding intercalated cells of newborn rabbit cortical collecting duct. Am J Physiol 1997;272(2 Pt 2):F167−77.

[59] Constantinescu AR, Lane JC, Mak J, Zavilowitz B, Satlin LM. Na$^{(+)}$-K$^{(+)}$-ATPase-mediated basolateral rubidium uptake in the maturing rabbit cortical collecting duct. Am J Physiol Renal Physiol 2000;279(6):F1161−8.

[60] Cort JP, McCrane RA. The renal response of puppies to an acidosis. J Physiol (London) 1954;124:358−69.

[61] Cramb G, Cutler CP, Lamb JF, McDevitt T, Ogden PH, Owler D, et al. The effects of monensin on the abundance of mRNA (alpha) and of sodium pumps in human cultured cells. Q J Exp Physiol 1989;74(1):53−63.

[62] Dancis J, Springer D. Fetal homeostasis in maternal malnutrition: potassium and sodium deficiency in rats. Pediatr Res 1970;4(4):345−51.

[63] Darrow DC, DaSilva MM, Stevenson SS. Production of acidosis in premature infants by protein milk. J Pediatr 1945;27:43−58.

[64] David L, Anast CS. Calcium metabolism in newborn infants. The interrelationship of parathyroid function and calcium, magnesium, and phosphorus metabolism in normal, "sick," and hypocalcemic newborns. J Clin Invest 1974;54(2):287−96.

[65] Dean RF, McCance RA. The renal response of infants and adults to the administration of hypertonic solutions of sodium chloride and urea. J Physiol (London) 1949;109:81−7.

[66] Dean RF, McCance RA. Phosphate clearance in infants and adults. J Physiol (London) 1948;107:182−6.

[67] Dean RFA, McCance RA. Inulin, diodone, creatinine and urea clearance in newborn infants. J Physiol (London) 1947;106:431−9.

[68] Delgado MM, Rohatgi R, Khan S, Holzman IR, Satlin LM. Sodium and potassium clearances by the maturing kidney: clinical–molecular correlates. Pediatr Nephrol 2003;18 (8):759–67.

[69] Djouadi F, Wijkhuisen A, Bastin J. Coordinate development of oxidative enzymes and Na-K-ATPase in thick ascending limb: role of corticosteroids. Am J Physiol 1992;263(2 Pt 2):F237–42.

[70] Dlouha H. A micropuncture study of the development of renal function in the young rat. Biol Neonate 1976;29(1–2):117–28.

[71] Drukker A, Goldsmith DI, Spitzer A, Edelmann Jr. CM, Blaufox MD. The renin angiotensin system in newborn dogs: developmental patterns and response to acute saline loading. Pediatr Res 1980;14(4 Pt 1):304–7.

[72] Edelmann Jr CM, Barnett HL, Stark H. Effect of urea on concentration of urinary nonurea solute in premature infants. J Appl Physiol 1966;21(3):1021–5.

[73] Edelmann Jr CM, Barnett HL, Troupkou V. Renal concentrating mechanisms in newborn infants. Effect of dietary protein and water content, role of urea, and responsiveness to antidiuretic hormone. J Anat 1960;1062–9.

[74] Edelmann CMJ, Soriano JR, Boichis H, Gruskin AB, Acosta M. Renal bicarbonate reabsorption and hydrogen ion excretion in normal infants. J Clin Invest 1967;46:1309–17.

[75] Engelke SC, Shah GL, Vasan J, Raye JR. Sodium blance in very low-birth-weight infants. J Pediatr 1978;93:837–41.

[76] Evan AP, Gattone II, Schwartz GJ. Development of solute transport in rabbit proximal tubule. II. Morphologic segmentation. Am J Physiol 1983;245:F391–407 Renal Fluid Electrolyte Physiol 14

[77] Evan AP, Satlin LM, Gattone VH, Connors B, Schwartz GJ. Postnatal maturation of rabbit renal collecting duct. II. Morphological observations. Am J Physiol 1991;261(1 Pt 2): F91–107.

[78] Feng JQ, Ward LM, Liu SG, Lu YB, Xie YX, Yuan BZ, et al. Loss of DMP1 causes rickets and osteomalacia and identifies a role for osteocytes in mineral metabolism. Nat Genet 2006;38 (11):1310–5.

[79] Fisher DA, Pyle Jr HR, Porter JC, Beard AG, Panos TC. Control of water balance in the newborn. Am J Dis Child 1963;106:137–46.

[80] Fomon SJ, Harris DM, Jensen RL. Acidification of the urine by infants fed human milk and whole cow's milk. Pediatrics 1959;23:113–20.

[81] Fukuda Y, Aperia A. Differentiation of Na$^+$-K$^+$ pump in rat proximal tubule is modulated by Na$^+$-H$^+$ exchanger. Am J Physiol 1988;255(3 Pt 2):F552–7.

[82] Fukuda Y, Bertorello A, Aperia A. Ontogeny of the regulation of Na$^+$,K($^+$)-ATPase activity in the renal proximal tubule cell. Pediatr Res 1991;30(2):131–4.

[83] Gattineni J, Baum M. Regulation of phosphate transport by fibroblast growth factor 23 (FGF23): implications for disorders of phosphate metabolism. Pediatr Nephrol 2010;25(4):591–601.

[84] Gattineni J, Sas D, Dagan A, Dwarakanath V, Baum M. Effect of thyroid hormone on the postnatal renal expression of NHE8. Am J Physiol Renal Physiol 2008;294(1):F198–204.

[85] Gersh I. The correlation of structure and function in the developing mesonephros and metanephros. Contrib Embryol 1937;153:35–58.

[86] Godard C, Geering JM, Geering K, Vallotton MB. Plasma renin activity related to sodium balance, renal function and urinary vasopressin in the newborn infant. Pediatr Res 1979;13 (6):742–5.

[87] Goldsmith DI, Drukker A, Blaufox MD, Edelmann Jr CM, Spitzer A. Hemodynamic and excretory response of the neonatal canine kidney to acute volume expansion. Am J Physiol 1979;237(5):F392–7.

[88] Goldsmith DI, Jodorkovsky RA, Sherwinter J, Kleeman SR, Spitzer A. Glomerular capillary permeability in developing canines. Am J Physiol 1986;251(3 Pt 2):F528–31.

[89] Goldstein L. Ammonia metabolism in kidneys of suckling rats. Am J Physiol 1971;220(1):213–7.

[90] Gordon HH, McNamara H, Benjamin HR. The response of young infants to ingestion of ammonium chloride. Pediatrics 1948;2:290–302.

[91] Goyal S, Vanden Heuvel G, Aronson PS. Renal expression of novel Na$^+$/H$^+$ exchanger isoform NHE8. Am J Physiol Renal Physiol 2003;284(3):F467–73.

[92] Gruskin AB, Edelmann Jr CM, Yuan S. Maturational changes in renal blood flow in piglets. Pediatr Res 1970;4 (1):7–13.

[93] Guillery EN, Huss DJ. Developmental regulation of chloride/formate exchange in guinea pig proximal tubules. Am J Physiol 1995;269(5 Pt 2):F686–95.

[94] Gupta N, Dwarakanath V, Baum M. Maturation of the Na/H antiporter (NHE3) in the proximal tubule of the hypothroid adrenalectomized rat. Am J Physiol Renal Physiol 2004;287: F521–7.

[95] Gupta N, Tarif SR, Seikaly M, Baum M. Role of glucocorticoids in the maturation of the rat renal Na$^+$/H$^+$ antiporter (NHE3). Kidney Int 2001;60(1):173–81.

[96] Hadeed AJ, Leake RD, Weitzman RE, Fisher DA. Possible mechanisms of high blood levels of vasopressin during the neonatal period. J Pediatr 1979;94:805–8.

[97] Hammerman MR, Karl IE, Hruska KA. Regulation of canine renal vesicle Pi transport by growth hormone and parathyroid hormone. Biochim Biophys Acta 1980;603(2):322–35.

[98] Hansen JOL, SmithC. A. Effects of withholding fluid in the immediate post-natal period. Pediatrics 1953;12:99–113.

[99] Haramati A, Mulroney SE. Enhanced tubular capacity for phosphate reabsorption in immature rats: role of glomerular–filtration rate (Gfr). Fed Proc 1987;46(4):1288.

[100] Haramati A, Mulroney SE, Lumpkin MD. Regulation of renal phosphate reabsorption during development: implications from a new model of growth hormone deficiency. Pediatr Nephrol 1990;4(4):387–91.

[101] Harris RC, Seifter JL, Lechene C. Coupling of Na-H exchange and Na-K pump activity in cultured rat proximal tubule cells. Am J Physiol 1986;251(5 Pt 1):C815–24.

[102] Hatemi N, McCance RA. Response to acidifying drugs. Acta Paediatr Scand 1961;50:603–16.

[103] Henneman PH, Forbes AP, Moldawer M, Dempsey EF, Carroll EL. Effects of human growth hormone in man. J Clin Invest 1960;39:1223–38.

[104] Henning SJ. Plasma concentrations of total and free corticosterone during development in the rat. Am J Physiol 1978;235(5): E451–6.

[105] Hines HE, McCance RA. Ammonia formation from glutamine by kidney slices from adult and newborn animals. J Physiol (London) 1954;124:8–16.

[106] Hohenauer L, Rosenberg TF, Oh W. Calcium and phosphorus homeostasis on the first day of life. Biol Neonate 1970;15 (12):49–56.

[107] Horster M. Loop of Henle functional differentiation: in vitro perfusion of the isolated thick ascending segment. Pflugers Arch 1978;378(1):15–24.

[108] Horster M, Huber S, Tschop J, Dittrich G, Braun G. Epithelial nephrogenesis. Pflugers Arch 1997;434(6):647–60.

[109] Horster M, Valtin H. Postnatal development of renal function: micropuncture and clearance studies in the dog. J Clin Invest 1971;50(4):779–95.

[110] Horster MF, Gilg A, Lory P. Determinants of axial osmotic gradients in the differentiating countercurrent system. Am J Physiol 1984;246(2 Pt 2):F124−32.

[111] Horster MF, Zink H. Functional differentiation of the medullary collecting tubule: influence of vasopressin. Kidney Int 1982;22(4):360−5.

[112] Huber SM, Braun GS, Horster MF. Expression of the epithelial sodium channel (ENaC) during ontogenic differentiation of the renal cortical collecting duct epithelium. Pflugers Arch 1999;437(3):491−7.

[113] Ichikawa I, Maddox DA, Brenner BM. Maturational development of glomerular ultrafiltration in the rat. Am J Physiol 1979;236(5):F465−71.

[114] Ichikawa S, Sorenson AH, Imel EA, Friedman NE, Gertner JM, Econs MJ. Intronic deletions in the SLC34A3 gene cause hereditary hypophosphatemic rickets with hypercalciuria. J Clin Endocrinol Metab 2006;91(10):4022−7.

[115] John E, Goldsmith DI, Spitzer A. Quantitative changes in the canine glomerular vasculature during development: physiologic implications. Kidney Int 1981;20(2):223−9.

[116] Johnson V, Spitzer A. Renal reabsorption of phosphate during development: whole-kidney events. Am J Physiol 1986;251(2 Pt 2):F251−6.

[117] Jose PA, Slotkoff LM, Lilienfield LS, Calcagno PL, Eisner GM. Sensitivity of neonatal renal vasculature to epinephrine. Am J Physiol 1974;226(4):796−9.

[118] Jose PA, Slotkoff LM, Montgomery S, Calcagno PL, Eisner G. Autoregulation of renal blood flow in the puppy. Am J Physiol 1975;229(4):983−8.

[119] Kaneko S, Albrecht F, Asico LD, Eisner GM, Robillard JE, Jose PA. Ontogeny of DA1 receptor-mediated natriuresis in the rat: in vivo and in vitro correlations. Am J Physiol 1992;263(3 Pt 2): R631−8.

[120] Karashima S, Hattori S, Ushijima T, Furuse A, Nakazato H, Matsuda I. Developmental changes in carbonic anhydrase II in the rat kidney. Pediatr Nephrol 1998;12(4):263−8.

[121] Karlen J. Renal response to low and high phosphate intake in weanling, adolescent and adult rats. Acta Physiol Scand 1989;135(3):317−22.

[122] Kaskel FJ, Kumar AM, Feld LG, Spitzer A. Renal reabsorption of phosphate during development: tubular events. Pediatr Nephrol 1988;2(1):129−34.

[123] Kaskel FJ, Kumar AM, Lockhart EA, Evan A, Spitzer A. Factors affecting proximal tubular reabsorption during development. Am J Physiol 1987;252:F188−97 Renal Fluid Electrolyte Physiol. 21

[124] Kerpel-Fronius E, Heim T, Sulyok E. The development of the renal acidifying processes and their relation to acidosis in low-birth-weight infants. Biol Neonate 1979;15:156−68.

[125] Kildeberg P, Engel K, Winters RW. Balance of net acid in growing infants. Endogenous and transintestinal aspects. Acta Paediatr Scand 1969;58(4):321−9.

[126] Kildeberg P, Winters R. Infant feeding and blood acid−base status. Pediatrics 1972;49(6):801−2.

[127] Kim YH, Earm JH, Ma T, Verkman AS, Knepper MA, Madsen KM, et al. Aquaporin-4 expression in adult and developing mouse and rat kidney. J Am Soc Nephrol 2001;12 (9):1795−804.

[128] Kim YH, Kim DU, Han KH, Jung JY, Sands JM, Knepper MA, et al. Expression of urea transporters in the developing rat kidney. Am J Physiol Renal Physiol 2002;282(3): F530−40.

[129] Knutson DW, Chieu F, Bennett CM, Glassock RJ. Estimation of relative glomerular capillary surface area in normal and hypertrophic rat kidneys. Kidney Int 1978;14(5):437−43.

[130] Larsson L, Horster M. Ultrastructure and net fluid transport in isolated perfused developing proximal tubules. J Ultrastruct Res 1976;54:276−85.

[131] Larsson SH, Rane S, Fukuda Y, Aperia A, Lechene C. Changes in Na influx precede post-natal increase in Na, K-ATPase activity in rat renal proximal tubular cells. Acta Physiol Scand 1990;138(1):99−100.

[132] Leake RD, Zakauddin S, Trygstad CW, Fu P, Oh W. The effects of large volume intravenous fluid infusion on neonatal renal function. J Pediatr 1976;89(6):968−72.

[133] Lelievre-Pegorier M, Merlet-Benichou D, Roinel N, DeRouffignac C. Developmental pattern of water and electrolyte transport in rat superficial nephrons. Am J Physiol 1983;245:F15−21.

[134] Levi M, Baird BM, Wilson PV. Cholesterol modulates rat renal brush border membrane phosphate transport. J Clin Invest 1990;85:231−7.

[135] Levi M, Jameson DM, van der Meer BW. Role of BBM lipid composition and fluidity in impaired renal pi transport in aged rat. Am J Physiol 1989;256(1 Pt 2):F85−94.

[136] Li XX, Albrecht FE, Robillard JE, Eisner GM, Jose PA. Gbeta regulation of Na/H exchanger-3 activity in rat renal proximal tubules during development. Am J Physiol Regul Integr Comp Physiol 2000;278(4):R931−6.

[137] Linarelli LG. Nephron urinary cyclic AMP and developmental renal responsiveness to parathyroid hormone. Pediatrics 1972;50:14−23.

[138] Lorenz JM, Kleinman LI, Disney TA. Renal response of newborn dog to potassium loading. Am J Physiol 1986;251(3 Pt 2): F513−9.

[139] Lucci MS, Pucacco LR, DuBose Jr. TD, Kokko JP, Carter NW. Direct evaluation of acidification by rat proximal tubule: role of carbonic anhydrase. Am J Physiol 1980;238(5):F372−9.

[140] Magagnin S, Werner A, Markovich D, Sorribas V, Stange G, Biber J, et al. Expression cloning of human and rat renal cortex Na/Pi co-transport. Proc Natl Acad Sci USA 1993;90 (13):5979−83.

[141] Martinerie L, Pussard E, Foix-L'Helias L, Petit F, Cosson C, Boileau P, et al. Physiological partial aldosterone resistance in human newborns. Pediatr Res 2009;66(3):323−8.

[142] McCance RA, Hatemi N. Control of acid−base stability in the newly born. Lancet 1961;1:293−7.

[143] McCance RA, Naylor NJ, Widdowson EM. The response of infants to a large dose of water. Arch Dis Child 1954;29 (144):104−9.

[144] McCance RA, Widdowson EM. Renal aspects of acid−base control in the newly born. Acta Paediatr Scand 1960;49:409−14.

[145] McCrory WW, Forman CW, McNamara H, Barnett HL. Renal excretion of inorganic phosphate in newborn infants. J Clin Invest 1952;31(4):357−66.

[146] McKinney TD, Burg MB. Bicarbonate transport by rabbit cortical collecting tubules. Effect of acid and alkali loads in vivo on transport in vitro. J Clin Invest 1977;60(3):766−8.

[147] Mehrgut FM, Satlin LM, Schwartz GJ. Maturation of HCO_3^- transport in rabbit collecting duct. Am J Physiol 1990;259(5 Pt 2):F801−8.

[148] Melendez E, Reyes JL, Escalante BA, Melendez MA. Development of the receptors to prostaglandin E2 in the rat kidney and neonatal renal functions. Dev Pharmacol Ther 1989;14(2):125−34.

[149] Merlet-Benichou C, Pegorier M, Muffat-Joly M, Augeron D. Functional and morphologic patterns of renal maturation in the developing guinea pig. Am J Physiol 1981;36:H1467−75.

[150] Miyamoto K, Ito M, Tatsumi S, Kuwahata M, Segawa H. New aspect of renal phosphate reabsorption: the type IIc sodium-

dependent phosphate transporter. Am J Nephrol 2007;27(5):503−15.

[151] Molitoris BA, Simon FR. Renal cortical brush-border and basolateral membranes: cholesterol and phospholipid composition and relative turnover. J Membr Biol 1985;83(3):207−15.

[152] Monnens L, Schretlen E, van Munster P. The renal excretion of hydrogen ions in infants and children. Nephron 1973;12:29−43.

[153] Mulroney SE, Haramati A. Renal adaptation to changes in dietary phosphate during development. Am J Physiol 1990;258(6 Pt 2):F1650−6.

[154] Neiberger RE, Barac-Nieto M, Spitzer A. Renal reabsorption of phosphate during development: transport kinetics in BBMV. Am J Physiol 1989;257(2 Pt 2):F268−74.

[155] Olbing H, Blaufox MD, Aschinberg LC, Silkalns GI, Bernstein J, Spitzer A, et al. Postnatal changes in renal glomerular blood flow distribution in puppies. J Clin Invest 1973;52(11):2885−95.

[156] Parkkila S, Parkkila AK, Saarnio J, Kivela J, Karttunen TJ, Kaunisto K, et al. Expression of the membrane-associated carbonic anhydrase isozyme XII in the human kidney and renal tumors. J Histochem Cytochem 2000;48(12):1601−8.

[157] Pellegrini L, Burke DF, von Delft F, Mulloy B, Blundell TL. Crystal structure of fibroblast growth factor receptor ectodomain bound to ligand and heparin. Nature 2000;407(6807):1029−34.

[158] Peonides A, Levin B, Young WF. The renal excretion of hydrogen ions in infants and children. Arch Dis Child 1965;40:33−9.

[159] Polacek E, Vocel J, Neugebaurova L, Sebkova M, Vechetova E. The osmotic concentrating ability in healthy infants and children. Arch Dis Child 1965;40:291−5.

[160] Preisig PA, Ives HE, Cragoe Jr. EJ, Alpern RJ, Rector Jr. FC. Role of the Na$^+$/H$^+$ antiporter in rat proximal tubule bicarbonate absorption. J Clin Invest 1987;80(4):970−8.

[161] Purkerson JM, Schwartz GJ. The role of carbonic anhydrases in renal physiology. Kidney Int 2007;71(2):103−15.

[162] Quigley R, Baum M. Developmental changes in rabbit juxtamedullary proximal convoluted tubule bicarbonate permeability. Pediatr Res 1990;28(6):663−6.

[163] Quigley R, Baum M. Effects of growth hormone and insulin-like growth factor I on rabbit proximal convoluted tubule transport. J Clin Invest 1991;88(2):368−74.

[164] Quigley R, Baum M. Developmental changes in rabbit juxtamedullary proximal convoluted tubule water permeability. Am J Physiol 1996;271(4 Pt 2):F871−6.

[165] Quigley R, Baum M. Developmental changes in rabbit proximal straight tubule paracellular permeability. Am J Physiol Renal Physiol 2002;283(3):F525−31.

[166] Quigley R, Chakravarty S, Baum M. Antidiuretic hormone resistance in the neonatal cortical collecting tubule is mediated in part by elevated phosphodiesterase activity. Am J Physiol Renal Physiol 2004;286(2):F317−22.

[167] Rane S, Aperia A. Ontogeny of Na-K-ATPase activity in thick ascending limb and of concentrating capacity. Am J Physiol 1985;249(5 Pt 2):F723−8.

[168] Rane S, Aperia A, Eneroth P, Lundin S. Development of urinary concentrating capacity in weaning rats. Pediatr Res 1985;19(5):472−5.

[169] Ratliff B, Rodebaugh J, Sekulic M, Dong KW, Solhaug M. Nitric oxide synthase and renin−angiotensin gene expression and NOS function in the postnatal renal resistance vasculature. Pediatr Nephrol 2009;24(2):355−65.

[170] Rees L, Forsling ML, Brook CG. Vasopressin concentrations in the neonatal period. Clin Endocrinol (Oxf) 1980;12(4):357−62.

[171] Richmond JB, Kravitz H, Segar W, Kravitz H. Renal clearance of endogenous phosphate in infants and children. Proc Soc Exp Biol Med 1951;77:83−7.

[172] Robillard JE, Nakamura KT, DiBona GF. Effects of renal denervation on renal responses to hypoxemia in fetal lambs. Am J Physiol 1986;250(2 Pt 2):F294−301.

[173] Robillard JE, Sessions C, Kennedey RL, Hamel-Robillard L, Smith Jr FG. Interrelationship between glomerular filtration rate and renal transport of sodium and chloride during fetal life. Am J Obstet Gynecol 1977;128(7):727−34.

[174] Robillard JE, Smith FG, Nakamura KT, Sato T, Segar J, Jose PA. Neural control of renal hemodynamics and function during development. Pediatr Nephrol 1990;4(4):436−41.

[175] Robillard JE, Weitzman RE. Developmental aspects of the fetal renal response to exogenous arginine vasopressin. Am J Physiol 1980;238(5):F407−14.

[176] Rodriguez-Soriano J, Vallo A, Oliveros R, Castillo G. Renal handling of sodium in premature and full-term neonates: a study using clearance methods during water diuresis. Pediatr Res 1983;17(12):1013−6.

[177] Rubin MI, Bruck E, Rapoport M. Maturation of renal function in childhood: clearance studies. J Clin Invest 1949;28:1144−62.

[178] Rudolph AM, Heymann MA. Circulatory changes during growth in the fetal lamb. Circ Res 1970;26(3):289−99.

[179] Sas D, Hu MC, Moe OW, Baum M. Effect of claudins 6 and 9 on paracellular permeability in MDCK II cells. Am J Physiol-Regul Integr and Comp Physiol 2008;295(5):R1713−9.

[180] Satlin LM. Postnatal maturation of potassium transport in rabbit cortical collecting duct. Am J Physiol 1994;266(1 Pt 2):F57−65.

[181] Satlin LM. Regulation of potassium transport in the maturing kidney. Semin Nephrol 1999;19(2):155−65.

[182] Satlin LM, Evan AP, Gattone III VH, Schwartz GJ. Postnatal maturation of the rabbit cortical collecting duct. Pediatr Nephrol 1988;2(1):135−45.

[183] Satlin LM, Matsumoto T, Schwartz GJ. Postnatal maturation of rabbit renal collecting duct. III. Peanut lectin-binding intercalated cells. Am J Physiol 1992;262(2 Pt 2):F199−208.

[184] Satlin LM, Palmer LG. Apical Na$^+$ conductance in maturing rabbit principal cell. Am J Physiol 1996;270(3 Pt 2):F391−7.

[185] Satlin LM, Palmer LG. Apical K$^+$ conductance in maturing rabbit principal cell. Am J Physiol 1997;272(3 Pt 2):F397−404.

[186] Satlin LM, Schwartz GJ. Postnatal maturation of rabbit renal collecting duct: Intercalated cell function. Am J Physiol 1987;253(4 Pt 2):F622−35.

[187] Schlondorff D, Satriano JA, Schwartz GJ. Synthesis of prostaglandin E2 in different segments of isolated collecting tubules from adult and neonatal rabbits. Am J Physiol 1985;248(1 Pt 2):F134−44.

[188] Schmidt U, Horster M. Na-K-activated ATPase: activity maturation in rabbit nephron segments dissected in vitro. Am J Physiol 1977;233(1):F55−60.

[189] Schmitt R, Ellison DH, Farman N, Rossier BC, Reilly RF, Reeves WB, et al. Developmental expression of sodium entry pathways in rat nephron. Am J Physiol 1999;276(3 Pt 2):F367−81.

[190] Schwartz GH, Evan AP. Development of solute transport in rabbit proximal tubule. I. HCO3 and glucose absorption. Am J Physiol 1983;245:F382−90 Renal Fluid Electrolyte Physiol. 14

[191] Schwartz GH, Evan AP. Development of solute transport in rabbit proximal tubule. III. Na-K-ATPase activity. Am J Physiol 1984;246:F845−52 Renal Fluid Electrolyte Physiol. 15

[192] Schwartz GJ. Physiology and molecular biology of renal carbonic anhydrase. J Nephrol 2002;15(Suppl 5):S61−74.

II. STRUCTURAL AND FUNCTIONAL ORGANIZATION OF THE KIDNEY

[193] Schwartz GJ, Haycock GB, Edelmann Jr. CM, Spitzer A. Late metabolic acidosis: a reassessment of the definition. J Pediatr 1979;95(1):102−7.

[194] Schwartz GJ, Kittelberger AM, Barnhart DA, Vijayakumar S. Carbonic anhydrase IV is expressed in H($^+$)-secreting cells of rabbit kidney. Am J Physiol Renal Physiol 2000;278(6): F894−904.

[195] Schwartz GJ, Olson J, Kittelberger AM, Matsumoto T, Waheed A, Sly WS. Postnatal development of carbonic anhydrase IV expression in rabbit kidney. Am J Physiol 1999;276(4 Pt 2): F510−20.

[196] Schwartz GJ, Zavilowitz BJ, Radice AD, Garcia-Perez A, Sands JM. Maturation of aldose reductase expression in the neonatal rat inner medulla. J Clin Invest 1992;90(4):1275−83.

[197] Segawa H, Kaneko I, Takahashi A, Kuwahata M, Ito M, Ohkido I, et al. Growth-related renal type II Na/Pi co-transporter. J Biol Chem 2002;277(22):19665−72.

[198] Segawa H, Kawakami E, Kaneko I, Kuwahata M, Ito M, Kusano K, et al. Effect of hydrolysis-resistant FGF23-R179Q on dietary phosphate regulation of the renal type-II Na/Pi transporter. Pflugers Arch 2003;446(5):585−92.

[199] Segawa H, Onitsuka A, Furutani J, Kaneko I, Aranami F, Matsumoto N, et al. Npt2a and Npt2c in mice play distinct and synergistic roles in inorganic phosphate metabolism and skeletal development. Am J Physiol Renal Physiol 2009;297(3): F671−8.

[200] Segawa H, Onitsuka A, Kuwahata M, Hanabusa E, Furutani J, Kaneko I, et al. Type IIc sodium-dependent phosphate transporter regulates calcium metabolism. J Am Soc Nephrol 2009;20(1):104−13.

[201] Serrano CV, Talbert LM, Welt LG. Potassium deficiency in the pregnant dog. J Clin Invest 1964;43:27−31.

[202] Shah M, Gupta N, Dwarakanath V, Moe OW, Baum M. Ontogeny of Na$^+$/H$^+$ antiporter activity in rat proximal convoluted tubules. Pediatr Res 2000;48(2):206−10.

[203] Shah M, Quigley R, Baum M. Maturation of rabbit proximal straight tubule chloride/base exchange. Am J Physiol 1998;274 (5 Pt 2):F883−8.

[204] Shah M, Quigley R, Baum M. Neonatal rabbit proximal tubule basolateral membrane Na$^+$/H$^+$ antiporter and Cl$^-$/base exchange. Am J Physiol 1999;276(6 Pt 2):R1792−7.

[205] Shah M, Quigley R, Baum M. Maturation of proximal straight tubule NaCl transport: role of thyroid hormone. Am J Physiol Renal Physiol 2000;278(4):F596−602.

[206] Sheu JN, Baum M, Bajaj G, Quigley R. Maturation of rabbit proximal convoluted tubule chloride permeability. Pediatr Res 1996;39(2):308−12.

[207] Sheu JN, Baum M, Harkins EW, Quigley R. Maturational changes in rabbit renal cortical phospholipase A2 activity. Kidney Int 1997;52(1):71−8.

[208] Sheu JN, Quigley R, Baum M. Heterogeneity of chloride/base exchange in rabbit superficial and juxtamedullary proximal convoluted tubules. Am J Physiol 1995;268(5 Pt 2):F847−53.

[209] Shimada T, Kakitani M, Hasegawa H, Yamazaki Y, Ohguma A, Takeuchi Y, et al. Targeted ablation of FGF-23 causes hyperphosphatemia, increased 1,25-dihydroxyvitamin D level and severe growth retardation. J Bone Miner Res 2002;17:S168.

[210] Siegel SR, Fisher DA, Oh W. Serum aldosterone concentrations related to sodium balance in the newborn infant. Pediatrics 1974;53(3):410−3.

[211] Siegel SR, Oh W. Renal function as a marker of human fetal maturation. Acta Paediatr Scand 1976;65:481−5.

[212] Siga E, Horster MF. Regulation of osmotic water permeability during differentiation of inner medullary collecting duct. Am J Physiol 1991;260(5 Pt 2):F710−6.

[213] Silverstein DM, Barac-Nieto M, Murer H, Spitzer A. A putative growth-related renal Na($^+$)-Pi co-transporter. Am J Physiol 1997;273(3 Pt 2):R928−33.

[214] Smith FG, Sato T, McWeeny OJ, Klinkefus JM, Robillard JE. Role of renal sympathetic nerves in response of the ovine fetus to volume expansion. Am J Physiol 1990;259(5 Pt 2):R1050−5.

[215] Smith FG, Sato T, McWeeny OJ, Torres L, Robillard JE. Role of renal nerves in response to volume expansion in conscious newborn lambs. Am J Physiol 1989;257(6 Pt 2):R1519−25.

[216] Smith FG, Smith BA, Guillery EN, Robillard JE. Role of renal sympathetic nerves in lambs during the transition from fetal to newborn life. J Clin Invest 1991;88(6):1988−94.

[217] Song HK, Kim WY, Lee HW, Park EY, Han KH, Nielsen S, et al. Origin and fate of pendrin-positive intercalated cells in developing mouse kidney. J Am Soc Nephrol 2007;18 (10):2672−82.

[218] Spitzer A. The role of the kidney in sodium homeostasis during maturation. Kidney Int 1982;21(4):539−45.

[219] Spitzer A, Brandis M. Functional and morphologic maturation of the superficial nephrons. Relationship to total kidney function. J Clin Invest 1974;53(1):279−87.

[220] Spitzer A, Edelmann Jr CM. Maturational changes in pressure gradients for glomerular filtration. Am J Physiol 1971;221 (5):1431−5.

[221] Stanier MW. Development of intra-renal solute gradients in foetal and post-natal life. Pflugers Arch 1972;336(3):263−70.

[222] Stephenson G, Hammet M, Hadaway G, Funder JW. Ontogeny of renal mineralocorticoid receptors and urinary electrolyte responses in the rat. Am J Physiol 1984;247(4 Pt 2):F665−71.

[223] Stubbe J, Madsen K, Nielsen FT, Bonde RK, Skott O, Jensen BL. Postnatal adrenalectomy impairs urinary concentrating ability by increased COX-2 and leads to renal medullary injury. Am J Physiol Renal Physiol 2007;293(3):F780−9.

[224] Stubbe J, Madsen K, Nielsen FT, Skott O, Jensen BL. Glucocorticoid impairs growth of kidney outer medulla and accelerates loop of Henle differentiation and urinary concentrating capacity in rat kidney development. Am J Physiol Renal Physiol 2006;291(4):F812−22.

[225] Sulyok E, Nemeth M, Tenyi I, Csaba IF, Varga F, Gyory E, et al. Relationship between maturity, electrolyte balance and the function of the renin−angiotensin−aldosterone system in newborn infants. Biol Neonate 1979;35(1−2):60−5.

[226] Sulyok EHT. Assessment of maximal urinary acidification in prematuare infants. Biol Neonate 1971;19:200−10.

[227] Sulyok EHT. The influence of matauarity on renal control of acidosis in newborn infants. Biol Neonate 1972;21:418−35.

[228] Svenningsen NW. Renal acid−base titration studies in infants with and without metabolic acidosis in the postneonatal period. Pediatr Res 1973;8:659−72.

[229] Svenningsen NW, Lindquist B. Postnatal development of renal hydrogen ion excretion capacity in relation to age and protein intake. Acta Paediatr Scand 1974;63:721−31.

[230] Thomas ML, Anast CS, Forte LR. Regulation of calcium homeostasis in the fetal and neonatal rat. Am J Physiol 1981;240(4):E367−72.

[231] Traebert M, Lotscher M, Aschwanden R, Ritthaler T, Biber J, Murer H, et al. Distribution of the sodium/phosphate transporter during postnatal ontogeny of the rat kidney. J Am Soc Nephrol 1999;10(7):1407−15.

[232] Tucker BJ, Blantz RC. Factors determining superficial nephron filtration in the mature, growing rat. Am J Physiol 1977;232(2): F97−104.

[233] Tudvad F, McNamara H, Barnett HL. Renal response of premature infants to administration of bicarbonate and potassium. Pediatrics 1954;13(1):4−16.

[234] Tulassay T, Rascher W, Hajdu J, Lang RE, Toth M, Seri I. Influence of dopamine on atrial natriuretic peptide level in premature infants. Acta Paediatr Scand 1987;76(1):42–6.

[235] Tuvad F, Vesterdal J. The maximal tubular transfer of glucose and para-aminohippurate in premature infants. Acta Paediatr Scand 1953;42:337–45.

[236] Van Itallie CM, Anderson JM. Claudins and epithelial paracellular transport. Annu Rev Physiol 2006;68:403–29.

[237] Vehaskari VM. Ontogeny of cortical collecting duct sodium transport. Am J Physiol 1994;267(1 Pt 2):F49–54.

[238] Vehaskari VM, Hempe JM, Manning J, Aviles DH, Carmichael MC. Developmental regulation of ENaC subunit mRNA levels in rat kidney. Am J Physiol 1998;274(6 Pt 1):C1661–6.

[239] Wacker GR, Zarkowsky HS, Bruch HB. Changes in kidney enzymes of rats after birth. Am J Physiol 1961;200:367–9.

[240] Wamberg S, Kildeberg P, Engel K. Balance of net base in the rat. II. Reference values in relation to growth rate. Biol Neonate 1976;28:171–90.

[241] Watanabe S, Matsushita K, McCray Jr. PB, Stokes JB. Developmental expression of the epithelial Na^+ channel in kidney and uroepithelia. Am J Physiol 1999;276(2 Pt 2):F304–14.

[242] Webster SK, Haramati A. Developmental changes in the phosphaturic response to parathyroid hormone in the rat. Am J Physiol 1985;249(2 Pt 2):F251–5.

[243] Wijkhuisen A, Djouadi F, Vilar J, Merlet-Benichou C, Bastin J. Thyroid hormones regulate development of energy metabolism enzymes in rat proximal convoluted tubule. Am J Physiol 1995;268(4 Pt 2):F634–42.

[244] Winberg J. Determination of renal concentrating capacity in infants and children without renal disease. Acta Paediatrica Scandinavia 1959;48:318–28.

[245] Winkler CA, Kittelberger AM, Watkins RH, Maniscalco WM, Schwartz GJ. Maturation of carbonic anhydrase IV expression in rabbit kidney. Am J Physiol Renal Physiol 2001;280(5): F895–903.

[246] Woda C, Mulroney SE, Halaihel N, Sun L, Wilson PV, Levi M, et al. Renal tubular sites of increased phosphate transport and NaPi-2 expression in the juvenile rat. Am J Physiol Regul Integr Comp Physiol 2001;280(5):R1524–33.

[247] Woda CB, Bragin A, Kleyman TR, Satlin LM. Flow-dependent K^+ secretion in the cortical collecting duct is mediated by a maxi-K channel. Am J Physiol Renal Physiol 2001;280(5): F786–93.

[248] Woda CB, Miyawaki N, Ramalakshmi S, Ramkumar M, Rojas R, Zavilowitz B, et al. Ontogeny of flow-stimulated potassium secretion in rabbit cortical collecting duct: Functional and molecular aspects. Am J Physiol Renal Physiol 2003;285(4): F629–39.

[249] Wu MS, Biemesderfer D, Giebisch G, Aronson PS. Role of NHE3 in mediating renal brush border Na^+-H^+ exchange. Adaptation to metabolic acidosis. J Biol Chem 1996;271 (51):32749–52.

[250] Yamamoto T, Sasaki S, Fushimi K, Ishibashi K, Yaoita E, Kawasaki K, et al. Expression of AQP family in rat kidneys during development and maturation. Am J Physiol 1997;272(2 Pt 2):F198–204.

[251] Yared A, Yoshioka T. Autoregulation of glomerular filtration in the young. Semin Nephrol 1989;9(1):94–7.

[252] Yasui M, Marples D, Belusa R, Eklof AC, Celsi G, Nielsen S, et al. Development of urinary concentrating capacity: role of aquaporin-2. Am J Physiol 1996;271(2 Pt 2):F461–8.

[253] Zink H, Horster M. Maturation of diluting capacity in loop of Henle of rat superficial nephrons. Am J Physiol 1977;233(6): F519–24.

[254] Zolotnitskaya A, Satlin LM. Developmental expression of ROMK in rat kidney. Am J Physiol 1999;276(6 Pt 2):F825–36.

[255] Zweifach A, Desir GV, Aronson PS, Giebisch G. Inhibition of Ca-activated K^+ channels from renal microvillus membrane vesicles by amiloride analogs. J Membr Biol 1992;128 (2):115–22.

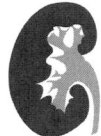

Renal Hyperplasia and Hypertrophy

Paul T. Brinkkoetter[1], Sian V. Griffin[2] and Stuart J. Shankland[3]

[1]University Hospital Cologne, Cologne, Germany
[2]University Hospital Wales, Health Park, Cardiff, Wales
[3]University of Washington, Seattle, Washington, USA

INTRODUCTION

The tight regulation of cell growth and division within an organ is essential for the development and maintenance of correct structure and function. Perturbations of renal growth occurring either developmentally or following injury to mature renal cells contribute to the abnormalities observed in a wide range of diseases. The changes in growth are increasingly recognized as an influence on the progression of the initial disease process, and the ultimate clinical outcome. Abnormal cell growth is classified according to the presence of an increase in cell number or cell size. Hyperplasia refers to abnormal growth resulting in an increased absolute number of cells, whereas hypertrophy refers to an increase in individual cell size. Both processes may be present in a given cell population and contribute to the increase in overall kidney size.

Of particular interest to clinical nephrologists and renal pathologists is the fact that the kidney has several different resident cell types. Within the glomerulus, the growth responses of the mesangial cell, podocyte, parietal epithelial cell, and endothelial cell differ. The tubulointerstitial cells and vascular smooth muscle cells also vary in their growth responses following injury. Thus, characterizing the mechanisms that regulate each cell's growth response enables the potential development of specific therapies that will modify the response to injury. We recognize that renal cell hyperplasia and hypertrophy are regulated by numerous pathways, involving growth factors, signaling pathways, and transcription factors. However, the focus of this review is to update the reader on recent advances in the regulation of these growth processes at the level of the cell

cycle. We will first describe cell cycle regulation by specific cell cycle proteins, and then discuss hyperplasia and hypertrophy for individual glomerular and tubular cell types.

Although highly metabolically active, under normal conditions the cells of the mature kidney are relatively quiescent with respect to cell cycle entry. Following injury to either the glomerulus or the tubules, cell cycle progression with proliferation is often an essential part of the reparative process. However, if unchecked, proliferation can lead to compromise of renal function. Similarly, renal hypertrophy may occur as a compensatory physiological response, but unregulated hypertrophy is maladaptive, and is one of the hallmarks of diabetic nephropathy.

Cell proliferation is ultimately regulated at the level of the cell cycle, which occurs within the nucleus. Within the kidney, the control of the cell cycle is particularly intriguing, given the contrasting responses of the various resident cell types to injury. For example, the mesangial cell is capable of marked proliferation, often accompanied by the deposition of extracellular matrix. In contrast, the podocyte has been considered a relatively inert cell, although this view has recently been challenged, and the reparative proliferation of glomerular endothelial cells following injury has also been described. Renal tubular cells readily undergo both proliferative and hypertrophic responses following injury. The last decade has seen a rapid expansion in our understanding of the molecular mechanisms underlying the cell cycle, and therapeutic options for its manipulation are becoming available. There is currently increasing awareness of the need to reduce the progression of renal diseases. Knowledge of the cell cycle and an understanding of how this can be

Seldin and Giebisch's The Kidney, Fifth Edition.
DOI: http://dx.doi.org/10.1016/B978-0-12-381462-3.00028-8

influenced may be crucial to the prevention, control, and amelioration of a wide range of renal diseases.

MEASUREMENT OF CELL GROWTH

Hyperplasia

During a hyperplastic response, the number of proliferating cells is increased. A number of methods are available for measuring this increase, both *in vivo* and in cell culture. The majority of these have as their basis the detection of increased DNA synthesis. This may be done by determining the presence of proteins known to be associated with DNA synthesis, such as proliferating cell nuclear antigen (PCNA) or Ki-67, or by exogenously labeling cells with a compound known to be incorporated into newly synthesized DNA, such as ^{3}H thymidine or bromodeoxyuridine (BrdU). In cell culture, a convenient and high-throughput method for determining cell number is the MTT assay, in which the yellow tetrazolium salt is reduced in metabolically active cells to form insoluble formazan crystals, which are solubilized by the addition of detergent. The color intensity may then be quantified spectrophotometrically, allowing quantification of changes in proliferation. A caveat for this method is that a decrease in cell viability will mimic a decrease in proliferation, and concomitant apoptosis should be excluded. Analysis by fluorescent activated cell sorting (FACS) is a valuable tool for the assessment of hyperplasia, because it also allows quantification of the number of cells in each phase of the cell cycle.

Hypertrophy

Cellular hypertrophy may be defined as an increase in cell size due to an increase in protein and RNA content without DNA replication,[1,2] and this forms the basis for the majority of methods for detection of hypertrophy. Upon entry into G1, cells undergo a physiologic increase in protein synthesis prior to the DNA synthesis of S-phase. Thus, one mechanism underlying hypertrophy is cell cycle arrest at the G1/S checkpoint, so that while protein synthesis and hence content, increase, there is no subsequent increase in DNA. Hypertrophy may also occur independently of the cell cycle, due to an inhibition of protein synthesis, and this mechanism is considered to contribute to tubular cell hypertrophy.[3,4] Measurement of leucine or proline incorporation and comparison to ^{3}H thymidine incorporation allow determination of cell protein/DNA content, and hence assessment of hypertrophy. FACS analysis is also useful and enables direct measurement of cell size. Defining the growth response to a given stimulus as either hyperplastic or hypertrophic is important, as each will result from different alterations in cell signaling pathways, with implications for possible interventions.

CELL CYCLE AND CELL CYCLE REGULATORY PROTEINS

Cell Cycle

The cell cycle is divided into distinct phases, each representing a different function, and each being regulated by specific proteins[5] (Figure 28.1). Quiescent cells are termed as in G0, and upon mitogenic stimuli enter the cell cycle at early G1. Cells pass through the restriction point in late G1, beyond which they are typically unresponsive to extracellular cues, and are committed to complete the cell cycle despite the withdrawal of mitogenic stimuli. DNA synthesis occurs in S-phase. Cells then progress through G2, in preparation for mitosis (M-phase). Ultimately, cell division follows during cytokinesis. Our current understanding suggests there are at least two checkpoints to ensure fidelity of DNA duplication, at G1/S and G2/M, where cell cycle progression may be arrested. The length of the cell cycle is cell-type-specific, but this variability is largely due to differences in the duration of G1. For mammalian cells, the typical duration of G1 is approximately 12 hours, S- and G2-phases 6 hours, and mitosis 30 minutes.

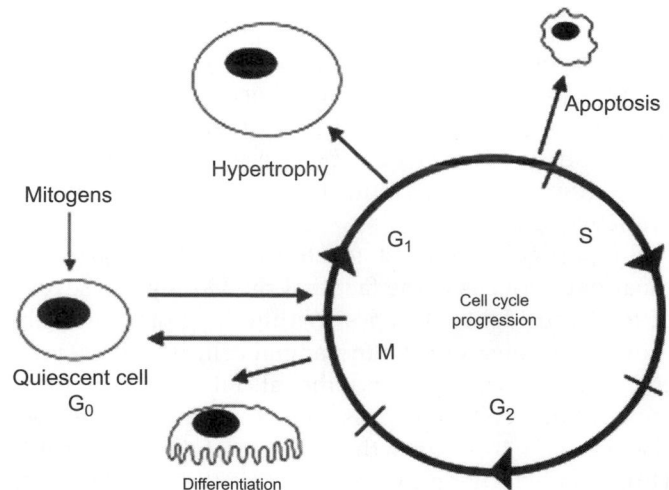

FIGURE 28.1 The cell cycle and possible consequences of cell cycle exit. Mitogens stimulate quiescent cells to engage the cell cycle at G1-phase. Hyperplasia then requires a coordinated and sequential series of events, including DNA synthesis at S-phase, followed by a resting G2-phase and mitosis in M-phase. This is followed by cell division. Cells that then exit the cell cycle and are quiescent again are in many cases differentiated. Of note is that if cells arrest at the G1/S-phase, they can develop a hypertrophic phenotype. Cell cycle exit with apoptosis may also occur.

Cyclins and Cyclin-Dependent Kinases: Positive Regulators of the Cell Cycle

Overview

The progress of a somatic cell through the cell cycle is dependent on the sequential and coordinated activation of the cyclin-dependent kinases (Cdks) by their specific partners, called cyclins (Figure 28.2). Cdks belong to the family of proline-directed serine/threonine kinases with a specific (K/R) (S*/T*) PX (K/H/R)-phosphorylation motif. Once active, Cdks phosphorylate downstream targets, ultimately to induce DNA synthesis.[6] While the levels of the Cdk catalytic subunits remain constant throughout the cell cycle, they are only functional following the binding of their specific cyclin partners. In contrast, cyclins are unstable proteins that are sequentially expressed and subsequently degraded by ubiquitination throughout the cell cycle,[7] which activate their partner Cdks by inducing conformational changes. Originally described for their fluctuation during the cell cycle,[8] members of the cyclin family are now defined by the presence of a conserved 100 amino acid cyclin box, which binds their complementary Cdk. In addition, the binding of inhibitors and accessory proteins, subcellular localization, and both inhibitory and activating phosphorylations influence the functional activity of the Cdk—cyclin complex.[9]

Jumpstarting the Cycle

The cell cycle is initiated by the mitogen-driven induction of cyclin D.[10–12] Depending on the cell type, three forms of cyclin D have been described (D1, D2, and D3), which interact allosterically with Cdk4 and Cdk6. Receptor-activated Ras signaling pathways lead to accumulation of cyclin D by three mechanisms: gene transcription; assembly; and stabilization of the cyclin D—Cdk complex.[13] The Ras-Raf-1-mitogen-activated, protein kinase kinase (MEK), extracellular signal-related protein kinase (ERK) pathway both induces cyclin D transcription and promotes assembly of cyclin D—Cdk.[14,15] The rate of degradation of cyclin D is controlled by a separate Ras signaling pathway involving phosphatidylinositol 3-kinase (PI3K) and protein kinase B (PKB/Akt), which inhibits the phosphorylation of cyclin D on threonine-286 (Thr-286) by glycogen synthase kinase 3β (GSKβ).[16] Thr-286 phosphorylated cyclin D would otherwise be exported to the cytoplasm for ubiquitination and degradation.[17] This requirement for mitogen signaling prevents the cell from autonomous cycling. Although ectopic expression of cyclin D is insufficient to drive cell cycle progression, constitutive activation of the cyclin D pathway can reduce the reliance of the cell on mitogenic stimulation, and lower the threshold for oncogenic transformation.[18] The cyclin D—Cdk4/6 complex enters the cell nucleus and is phosphorylated by Cdk-activating kinase (CAK).[19]

Once DNA replication begins, active cyclin D-dependent kinase activity is not required until mitosis is complete, and the cell re-enters the next G1 phase.[20] In continuously dividing cells, cyclin D1 is exported to the cytoplasm during S-phase, and its turnover is accelerated.[16,21] However, cyclin D1 synthesis stimulated by Ras is stabilized in G2 as described above, allowing reaccumulation before cells divide.[22] Hence, in the presence of continuous mitogen stimulation, the second and subsequent cell cycles are shorter than the first. Withdrawal of mitogens results in a rapid decline in cyclin D kinase activity, and cell cycle exit.

Active cyclin D-dependent kinases phosphorylate the retinoblastoma protein (pRb), which in quiescent cells has a growth-inhibitory effect.[23,24] In its hypophosphorylated state, pRb suppresses the transcription of several genes whose proteins are required for DNA synthesis, including the E2F transcription factors. Upon phosphorylation of pRb, the E2Fs are released from inhibition, leading to the transcription of cyclins E and A, and many genes whose products are required for DNA replication.[25] Furthermore, cyclin D—Cdk4 complexes also phosphorylate Smad3, negatively regulating the functions of transcriptional proteins responsible for mediating the growth inhibitory effects of transforming growth factor β (TGFβ).[26] Cyclin D-dependent kinases therefore affect the activity of at least two pathways that

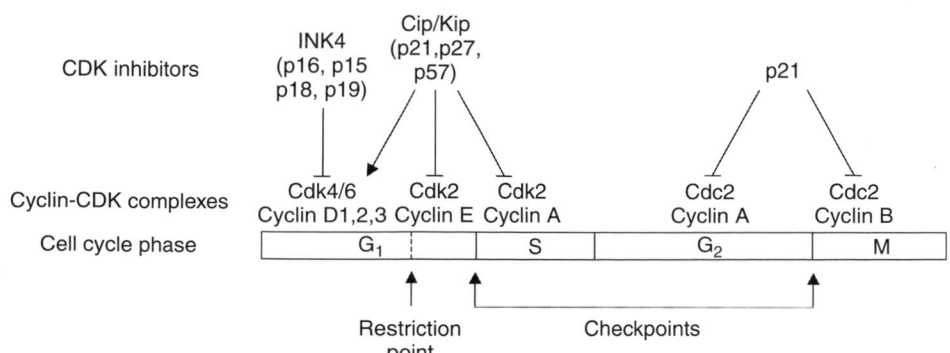

FIGURE 28.2 Cell cycle progression: timing of activation of cyclins and Cdks, and site of action of Cdk inhibitors. Each Cdk is activated by a partner cyclin in each phase of the cell cycle, and the resulting cyclin—Cdk complex can be inhibited by specific Cdk inhibitors.

independently inhibit the expression of cell cycle promoting genes.

The activity of cyclin E–Cdk2 is maximal at the G1- to S-phase transition,[27,28] when its function to further phosphorylate pRb releases the cell from mitogen dependency.[29,30] In addition to preferentially phosphorylating pRb on different sites to the cyclin D-dependent kinases, which may modify the interaction with E2Fs,[31] cyclin E–Cdk2 phosphorylates a second set of substrates involved in cell replication, thus affecting histone gene expression, and centrosome duplication.[32] The timing of expression and wider range of substrates suggest a role for cyclin E–Cdk2 in coordinating G1 regulation and the core cell cycle machinery.

The abrupt decline in cyclin E–Cdk2 activity in early S-phase results from cyclin E degradation. Phosphorylation by GSK-3β and Cdk2 itself target cyclin E for ubiquitination by the SCF^{Fbw7} E3 ligase, leading to proteasomal destruction.[33−35]

Low levels of cyclin A–Cdk2 activity are first detected in late G1-phase, increase as cells begin to replicate their DNA, and decline as cyclin A is degraded in early mitosis. The substrate specificity of cyclin A–Cdk2 is different from that of cyclin E–Cdk2. In S-phase, cyclin A–Cdk2 is thought to phosphorylate substrates that control the start of DNA replication from preassembled replication initiation complexes,[36−38] and control the integration of the end of S-phase with the activation of the mitotic Cdks.[39] The apparently central role of Cdk2 in coordinating cell cycle progression through S-phase and entry into mitosis has been challenged by the surprising observation that Cdk2 null mice are viable.[40,41] The possibility that other Cdks compensate for the loss of Cdk2 is currently a focus of intense research.

The entry to mitosis is controlled by cyclin B–Cdc2.[42,43] Cell cycle-regulated transcription of cyclin B begins at the end of S-phase. Phosphorylation on Thr161 by CAK parallels cyclin B binding to Cdc2.[44] During G2, cyclin B–Cdc2 complexes are maintained in an inactive state by phosphorylation on two inhibitory sites, Thr14 and tyrosine 15 (Tyr15) (Figure 28.3). Phosphorylation on Tyr15 is mediated by the nuclear Wee1 kinases,[166] and that on Thr14 by the membrane-bound Myt1.[45] In late G2 phase, both Thr14 and Tyr15

are dephosphorylated by Cdc25, thus activating cyclin B–Cdc2, and initiating mitosis.[46] Inappropriate triggering of mitosis is also prevented by the translocation of cyclin B to the cytoplasm by the nuclear export factor CRM1 (exportin 1) during S- and G2-phases.[47] Phosphorylation of cyclin B is thought to promote nuclear import at the G2/M transition.[48] Cyclin B–Cdc2 phosphorylates numerous downstream targets responsible for the structural reorganization of the cell to enable mitosis.

Although what is described above represents the basic paradigm of the control of cell cycle progression in mammalian cells, recent studies of knockout mice have demonstrated that much fetal development can occur normally despite the absence of cyclins and Cdks formerly considered to be vital.[49] Clearly, individual cyclins and Cdks are able to act more promiscuously than previously appreciated to enable compensation for the lack of a specific cell cycle protein.

Stopping the Cell Cycle: Cdk Inhibitors Act as Negative Regulators

In essence, Cdk inhibitors bind and inhibit target cyclin–Cdk complexes. Two classes of Cdk inhibitors have been described, the *INK4 proteins* and the *Cip/Kip family*.[50,51] Within each family, individual proteins are named according to their molecular weight. INK4 proteins were originally named for their ability to *in*hibit Cd*k4*. This family comprises four proteins, namely p16^{INK4a}, p15^{INK4b}, p18^{INK4c}, and p19^{INK4d}. Structurally these proteins are made up of multiple ankyrin repeats, and bind only to the catalytic subunits Cdk4 and Cdk6, thus inhibiting G1 progression. An alternate reading frame of the genetic locus encoding p16^{INK4a} also encodes a second structurally and functionally unrelated protein named p19^{ARF} in the mouse (p14^{ARF} in the human).[52] Whereas p16^{INK4a} acts to stabilize Rb by inhibition of Cdk4/6, p19^{ARF} stabilizes p53 by binding its negative regulator, Mdm2.[53] Data from knockout mice suggest that p19^{ARF}, rather than p16^{INK4a}, is responsible for the tumor suppressor function of this locus.[54]

The second class of Cdk inhibitors is the Cip/Kip family, which includes p21^{Cip1}, p27^{Kip1}, and p57^{Kip2},

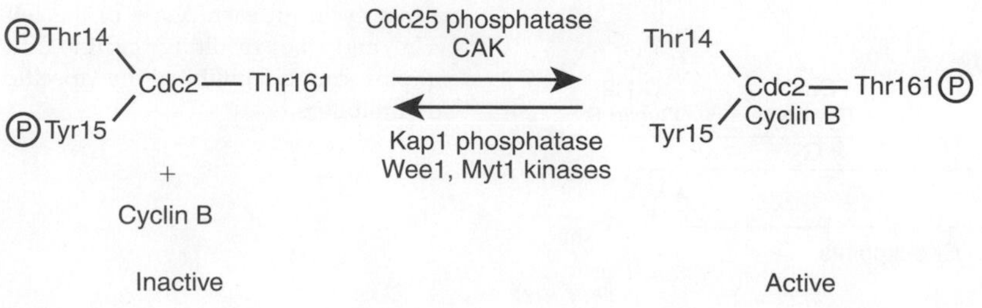

FIGURE 28.3 **Regulation of the phosphorylation status of Cdc2.** Wee1 and Myt1 kinases phosphorylate Cdc2 on Thr14 and Tyr15, inhibiting activity. Phosphorylation by CAK on Thr161 results in a 200-fold increase in kinase activity. Cdk2 is similarly phosphorylated on Thr160.

which share a conserved N-terminal Cdk-binding domain.[50] They are capable of binding a wider range of targets, and can variably affect the activities of cyclin D-, E-, A-, and B-dependent kinases.[43,51,55,56] Although potent inhibitors of cyclin E- and A-dependent CDK2, and to a lesser extent Cdc2, the Cip/Kip proteins have recently also been characterized, paradoxically, as positive regulators of the cyclin D-dependent kinases.[57]

The first member of the family to be identified was p21[Cip1],[58–60] and it is usually present at a low level in quiescent cells. As the cell enters the replicative cycle, p21[Cip1] levels rise, displace INK4 proteins from binding to Cdk 4/6, and promote the assembly of cyclin D-Cdk complexes.[61,62] This stabilizes the active complex and additionally provides a nuclear localization signal (NLS). The transcription of p21[Cip1] is increased by both p53-dependent[27] and -independent[63] pathways, such as those mediated by TGFβ.[64] The inhibitory role of p21[Cip1] becomes dominant later in the cell cycle, and levels are also increased in senescent cells.[65]

In contrast to p21[Cip1], the level of p27[Kip1] is usually high in quiescent cells, where its primary role is as an inhibitor of cell division.[66,67] Whereas p21[Cip1] is a principal mediator of the p53-dependent G1 arrest that occurs following DNA damage,[37] p27[Kip1] appears to be primarily responsible for mediating extracellular antiproliferative signals.[66,67] The levels and activity of p27[Kip1] are post-transcriptionally regulated by changes in the rates of translation, ubiquitination, and phosphorylation.[68,69] As cyclin D levels rise in response to mitogens, both p21[Cip1] and p27[Kip1] are sequestered by cyclin D–Cdk complexes, and therefore are unable to inhibit Cdk2.[51] Cyclin E–Cdk2 phosphorylates p27[Kip1] on Thr 187,[70,71] proving a recognition motif for an E3 ligase that targets p27[Kip1] for ubiquitination and proteasomal degradation.[72,73]

The most recently identified member of the family, p57[Kip2], was cloned in 1995.[74,75] While tissue expression of p21[Cip1] and p27[Kip1] is widespread, that of p57[Kip2] is restricted to placenta, muscle, heart, brain, lung, and kidney. In addition to the Cdk inhibitory domain and putative C terminal NLS, p57[Kip2] also has a proline-rich domain containing a consensus ERK phosphorylation site, and an acidic domain, the functions of which are not known.[74,75] A role for p57[Kip2] in the cell cycle exit that accompanies terminal differentiation has been suggested.

Despite their structural similarities, knockout studies have demonstrated divergent roles for the three Cip/Kip Cdk inhibitors. While p21[Cip1] and p27[Kip1] are not essential for normal embryogenesis,[50,76,77] lack of p57[Kip2] results in profound developmental abnormalities.[78–80] Most p57[Kip2] null mice die shortly after birth and have severe cleft palates, abdominal wall and gastrointestinal tract defects, and abnormal skeletal ossification. Unlike adult p21[Cip1−/−] mice,[81,82] p27[Kip1−/−] mice are larger than wild-type animals, and have hyperplasia of organs that usually express high levels of p27[Kip1], such as the thymus, spleen, adrenal and pituitary glands, testes, and ovaries.[50,76] In contrast, only 10% of p57[Kip2−/−] mice survive the weaning period and are much smaller than wild-type.[78] The kidneys of p57[Kip2−/−] mice have medullary dysplasia, although glomerular development appears normal.

HYPERPLASIA: AN INCREASE IN CELL NUMBER DUE TO PROLIFERATION

Glomerular Hyperplasia

Mesangial Cell Proliferation

Mesangial cell proliferation characterizes many forms of both experimental and human glomerular disease, including IgA nephropathy, lupus nephritis, diabetic nephropathy, and other forms of membranoproliferative glomerulonephritis (Figure 28.4). It is frequently associated with, and likely underlies, matrix expansion and subsequent glomerulosclerosis, the significance of which has been shown in a range of experimental models.[83–89] This simple observation provides the impetus for understanding what switches mesangial proliferation on and what switches it off. Several growth factors and cytokines are mitogens for mesangial cells, including platelet-derived growth factor (PDGF),[90,91] basic fibroblast growth factor (bFGF),[92] interleukin 6,[93,94] and the product of growth arrest-specific gene 6 (Gas6).[95] Intervention to reduce mesangial proliferation also reduces matrix

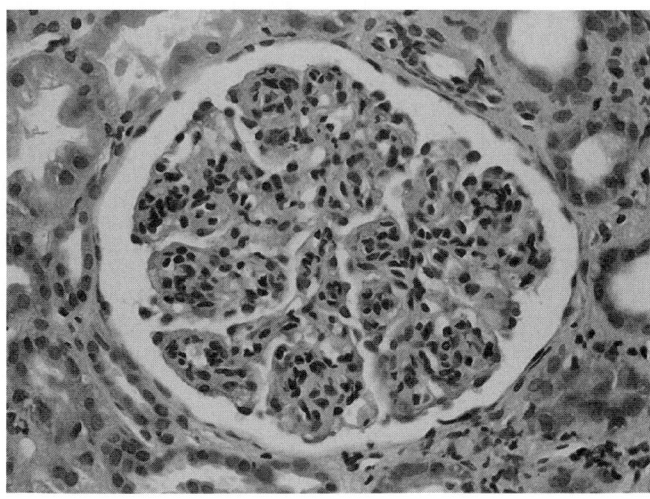

FIGURE 28.4 Global mesangial cell proliferation occurring in the context of membranoproliferative glomerulonephritis (haematoxylin and eosin × 400). *(Histology courtesy of Dr Meryl Griffiths, Addenbrooke's Hospital, Cambridge.)*

expansion, confirming the tight link between these two processes. This has been achieved in experimental models using complement depletion,[96,97] heparin infusion,[91] blocking the action PDGF[92,98] and bFGF,[83] and inhibiting their specific intracellular signaling pathways with phosphodiesterase inhibitors.[86] Warfarin has been used with mixed results in the treatment of glomerular diseases since the 1970s, and was originally hypothesized to reduce fibrin deposition. However, low-dose warfarin may also be effective, suggesting a mechanism of action not directly related to anticoagulation. Gas6 is a vitamin K-dependent growth factor for mesangial cells, and its inhibition by warfarin is likely to underlie the reported benefits of this treatment in human disease.[95] Careful research since the mid-1990s has delineated the role of individual cell cycle proteins in mesangial cell proliferation, and also its resolution by apoptosis (Figure 28.5).

ROLE OF CDK2 IN MESANGIAL CELL PROLIFERATION

Cdk2 protein and kinase activity increase in cultured mesangial cells in response to mitogenic growth

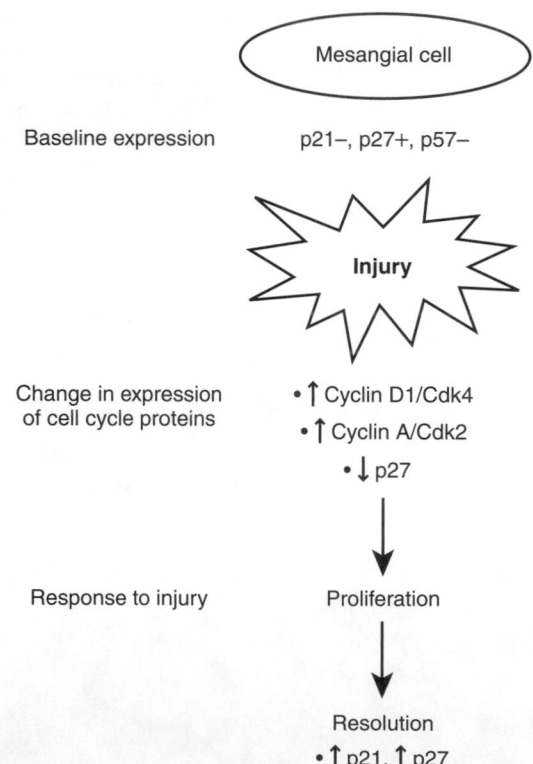

FIGURE 28.5 **Changes in cell cycle protein activity following injury to glomerular mesangial cells.** At baseline, quiescent mesangial cells express p27[Kip1], but not p21[Cip1] or p57[Kip2]. Following injury, there is an increase in the positive cell cycle regulators cyclin D1/Cdk4 and cyclin A/Cdk2, with a decline in p27[Kip1], resulting in promotion of cell cycle progression and proliferation. During the resolution phase, there is an increase in the Cdk-inhibitors p21[Cip1] and p27[Kip1], with cessation of proliferation.

factors.[99,100] The Thy1 model of experimental mesangial proliferative glomerulonephritis, induced in rats by an antibody directed against the mesangial Thy1 antigen, has provided an opportunity to study the regulation and consequences of mesangial cell proliferation *in vivo*.[101,102] The initial complement-dependent mesangiolysis is followed by a phase of marked mesangial proliferation, paralleled by an increase in extracellular matrix accumulation and a decline in renal function. This model is useful as not only may the fluctuations of cell cycle proteins during proliferation be defined, but also the effect of their manipulation. Mesangial cell proliferation is associated with an increase in cyclin D1 and A, and their partners Cdk4 and Cdk2.[103] Cdk2 expression is absent in the normal rat glomerulus. Proliferation is associated with increased Cdk2 activity, measured by the histone H1 kinase assay on protein extracted from isolated glomeruli. Bokemeyer et al. identified activation of the map kinase ERK as an upstream regulator of Cdk2 activity in the Thy1 model.[104] Inhibition of ERK was associated with decreased cell proliferation by 67%.[105] Cdk2 protein levels are also increased in the remnant kidney model, a nonimmune glomerular disease associated with mesangial proliferation.[106] Taken together, these studies show that in contrast to most nonrenal cells,[103] Cdk2 protein is at low levels in quiescent mesangial cells, and its levels and activity increase following injury.

Cdk Inhibitors and Mesangial Cell Proliferation

The Cdk inhibitor p27[Kip1] is constitutively expressed in quiescent mesangial cells both *in vitro*[107] and *in vivo*,[103] whereas p21[Cip1] and p57[Kip2] are essentially absent.[103,108] In cultured mesangial cells, proliferation induced by mitogenic growth factors reduces p27[Kip1] levels.[107] Mesangial cells derived from p27[Kip1−/−] mice have augmented proliferation in response to mitogens,[109] and lowering p27[Kip1] levels with antisense oligonucleotides has a similar effect in rat mesangial cells.[107]

Complement-induced injury in the Thy1 model is associated with a marked decrease in p27[Kip1] levels.[103] However, there is *de novo* synthesis of p21[Cip1] in the resolution phase of the disease, coincident with a decrease in proliferation. To further explore the role of p27[Kip1] in inflammatory disease, we induced experimental glomerulonephritis in p27[Kip1−/−] mice.[110] Our results showed a marked increase in the onset and magnitude of glomerular cell proliferation and cellularity in nephritic p27[Kip1−/−] mice compared to control nephritic p27[Kip1+/+] mice. Moreover, this was associated with increased extracellular matrix proteins and a decline in renal function. To demonstrate that this result was not specific to glomerular cells or immune-mediated injury, we also obstructed a ureter by ligation to induce nonimmune injury to tubuloepithelial cells.[110] Our results showed that tubuloepithelial proliferation was increased in obstructed $p27^{Kip1-/-}$ mice compared to obstructed $p27^{Kip1+/+}$ mice. Taken together, these studies were the first to show that in inflammatory diseases, renal cell proliferation is regulated by the CKI $p27^{Kip1}$, supporting a role for $p27^{Kip1}$ in controlling the threshold at which proliferation occurs.

Little is known about the role of the Cdk inhibtiors $p21^{Cip1}$ and $p57^{Kip2}$. In an immune-mediated model of MC disease, the absence $p21^{Cip1}$ was associated with increased focal segmental tuft necrosis, mesangiolysis, and mesangial hypercellularity.[111]

Role of Cell Cycle Proteins in Resolution of Mesangial Hyperplasia: Apoptosis

Although a characteristic response to mesangial cell injury is proliferation, apoptosis is often simultaneously increased.[85] Studies have shown that apoptosis is a vital mechanism required to normalize cell number in the reparative phase of injury.[112] However, the cellular pathways linking these opposing responses remain unclear. Many cells undergoing apoptosis have entered the cell cycle, but rather than completing their replication, they are destined to leave by programmed cell death. This suggests a role for the cell cycle proteins in directing these alternative outcomes.

Evidence to support this hypothesis was the observation that the resolution phase of Thy1 mesangial proliferation in the rat is characterized by mesangial cell apoptosis, a process that peaks when the levels of $p27^{Kip1}$ are at their lowest.[103] Considering glomerulonephritis or unilateral ureteric obstruction in $p27^{Kip1-/-}$ mice as described above, in addition to the increase in either glomerular or tubuloepithelial cell proliferation following injury, there was a marked increase in apoptosis in the $p27^{Kip1-/-}$ mice compared to wild-type disease controls.[110] Moreover, apoptosis was also increased in $p27^{Kip1-/-}$ mesangial cells in culture following growth factor deprivation or cycloheximide, and reconstituting $p27^{Kip1}$ levels by transfection-rescued cells from apoptosis.[109] In wild-type rat mesangial cells, apoptosis was increased following treatment with anti-$p27^{Kip1}$ antisense oligonucleotides.[109] These results showed for the first time that $p27^{Kip1}$ has a role beyond the regulation of proliferation, in that it also protects cells from apoptosis. This dual role of regulating the proliferative threshold and governing apoptosis makes $p27^{Kip1}$ a potent regulator of overall mesangial cell numbers. In contrast, $p21^{Cip1}$ showed no effect on MC apoptosis.[111]

HOW DOES $P27^{KIP1}$ PROTECT CELLS FROM APOPTOSIS?

A clue to a possible mechanism was the increase in Cdk2 activity in $p27^{Kip1-/-}$ mesangial cells when deprived of growth factors.[109] The increase was due specifically to cyclin A—Cdk2, and not cyclin E—Cdk2. Moreover, inhibition of cyclin A—Cdk2 activity by roscovitine or a dominant negative mutant reduced apoptosis in mesangial cells and fibroblasts. In apoptotic $p27^{Kip1-/-}$ mesangial cells, Cdk2 was bound to cyclin A, without a preceding increase in cyclin E—Cdk2 activity. We suggest that, in the absence of $p27^{Kip1}$, uncoupling of Cdk2 activity from the scheduled sequence of cell cycle protein expression may lead to an inappropriate and premature initiation of G_1/S-phase transition, causing the cell to respond by undergoing apoptosis, rather than inappropriately progressing through an unscheduled cell cycle.

HOW MIGHT Cdk2 CONTROL GROWTH AND APOPTOTIC FATE OF CELLS?

Apoptosis typically begins in the cytoplasm, whereas DNA synthesis and mitosis are nuclear events. Accordingly, we tested the hypothesis that the subcellular localization of Cdk2 determines if cells undergo apoptosis or proliferation.[113] As expected, Cdk2 protein was cytoplasmic in quiescent, and nuclear in proliferating, mesangial cells. However, in proliferating cells injured by an apoptotic stimulus, Cdk2 localized to the cytoplasm, was no longer nuclear, and importantly, remained active. Our results also showed that cyclin A, and not cyclin E, co-localized to the cytoplasm with Cdk2 in apoptotic cells, to form an active cytoplasmic cyclin A—Cdk2 complex. The translocation of Cdk2 is not p53-dependent, and inhibiting the nuclear localization signal has no effect. That inhibiting Cdk2 decreased apoptosis provides further support for a critical role for cytoplasmic Cdk2 in triggering programmed cell death. Thus, the subcellular localization of active Cdk2 determines the fate of a cell: when nuclear, cells proliferate; when cytoplasmic, cells die by apoptosis. The mechanism by which nuclear Cdk2 is translocated to the cytoplasm remains to be elucidated. These studies provide the novel paradigm that specific cell cycle regulatory proteins have a role in glomerular disease beyond the regulation of proliferation.

Therapeutic Inhibition of Mesangial Proliferation at Cell Cycle Level

In vitro and animal studies have recently revealed the potential of several novel therapies to modulate glomerular cell proliferation: the purine analog roscovitine, which inhibits Cdk2 activity; retinoids, derived from vitamin A; and lipoxins, endogenously produced eicosanoids. Roscovitine and retinoids have also been used to beneficial effect in the treatment of podocyte diseases, discussed in the next sections.

ROSCOVITINE

The significance of increased Cdk2 activity in mesangial proliferation was demonstrated by Pippin et al.,[114] using roscovitine to inhibit Cdk2 in rats with Thy1 mesangioproliferative gomerulonephritis. Given immediately after disease induction, roscovitine significantly reduced mesangial cell proliferation. Moreover, administering roscovitine to rats once mesangial proliferation was already established also reduced proliferation. This inhibition of Cdk2 activity was accompanied by a marked reduction in the accumulation of glomerular extracellular matrix proteins (collagen IV, laminin, and fibronectin), and an improvement in renal function compared to controls. These results suggest that inhibiting Cdk2 may be a potential therapeutic target in glomerular diseases characterized by proliferation.

RETINOIDS

Retinoic acid (RA) has an established role in kidney development.[115,116] RA binds to specific nuclear receptors, and the RA receptor complex then binds to DNA–RA response elements to cause the transcription of target genes.[117] RA is used therapeutically in acute promyelocytic leukemia to slow proliferation and promote differentiation. RA-induced cell cycle arrest in nonrenal cells has been reported to involve reduction in c-Myc, cyclin D1, and cyclin E levels, with upregulation of p21^{Cip1} and p27^{Kip1}.[118–120] The treatment of rats with experimental Thy1 glomerulonephritis with RA reduced mesangial cell proliferation, glomerular lesions, and albuminuria.[121] In addition to a direct antiproliferative action, RA has also been reported to modulate both the renin–angiotensin system[122] and TGFβ signaling,[123] in addition to anti-inflammatory and immune modulatory effects.[116] The efficacy of RA in the treatment of glomerulonephritis is likely due to its pleiotropic effects on these numerous pathways.

LIPOXINS

Lipoxins are endogenously produced eicosanoids with potent anti-inflammatory actions,[124] and are generated during the resolution phase of an acute inflammatory insult.[125] Lipoxin A_4 biosynthesis has been demonstrated in glomerulonephritis,[126] and its effects include modulation of leukocyte trafficking and phagocytic clearance of apoptotic cells.[124,125] In vitro, lipoxin A4 inhibits PDGF-induced activation of Akt/PKB in human mesangial cells, and modulates PDGF-induced decrements of p21^{Cip1} and p27^{Kip1}.[127] PDGF-induced increases in Cdk2–cyclin E complex formation are also inhibited by lipoxin A_4. Prolonged exposure

of mesangial cells to PDGF is associated with autocrine TGFβ production, and this is ameliorated by lipoxin A_4.

In vivo, lipoxins are rapidly metabolized. To enable study of these compounds in disease models, stable synthetic analogs have been developed that are modified at C-15, C-16, and/or C20.[128] These compounds retain the biological activity and receptor-binding affinity of the native lipoxin. The effect of a lipoxin A_4 analog, 15-epi-16-(FPho)-LXA-Me, has been studied in the immediate phase of experimental anti-GBM nephritis in mice, and found to inhibit neutrophil infiltration and glomerular nitrotyrosine staining.[129] Although animal studies with lipoxins are at an earlier stage than those with roscovitine or retinoids, their potential to augment the resolution phase of glomerulonephritis suggests that they may in the future have an important therapeutic role.

The Podocyte and Cell Cycle: Why Is Lack of Podocyte Proliferation Important?

The podocyte, or visceral glomerular epithelial cell, is a highly specialized, terminally differentiated cell overlying the outer aspect of the glomerular basement membrane. In contrast to the mesangial cell, numerous studies of both animal models and human disease have shown that aside from a few specific conditions, podocytes do not typically proliferate in vivo (Figure 28.6). Indeed, following injury, podocyte numbers may become depleted, because following cell loss by detachment or apoptosis, the lack of proliferation prevents normalization of podocyte number. Although initially the remaining podocytes may undergo a degree of compensatory hypertrophy, the decrease in podocyte number will eventually result in areas of "denuded" basement membrane, which is thought to predispose to the formation of synechiae between the GBM and Bowman's capsule, leading to the development of secondary focal glomerulosclerosis and subsequent decline in renal function.[130–134] Podocytes provide a size- and charge-dependent barrier to protein leakage into the urine, and are therefore a critical component of the glomerular filtration apparatus. Several studies in diverse renal diseases have shown a close correlation between the onset and progression of proteinuria and reduced podocyte number.[135–141] These events provide a compelling rationale to define the mechanisms underlying the lack of podocyte proliferation.

MATURE PODOCYTE HAS EXITED CELL CYCLE AND IS POSTMITOTIC

During glomerulogenesis, immature podocytes are capable of proliferation.[108,142] However, during the critical S-shaped body stage of glomerular development,

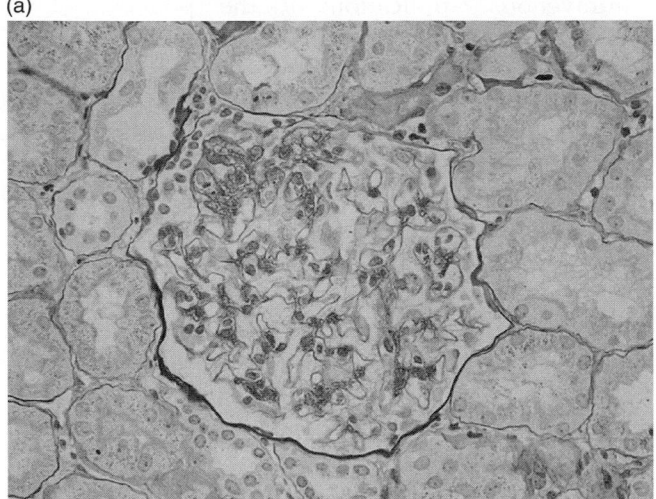

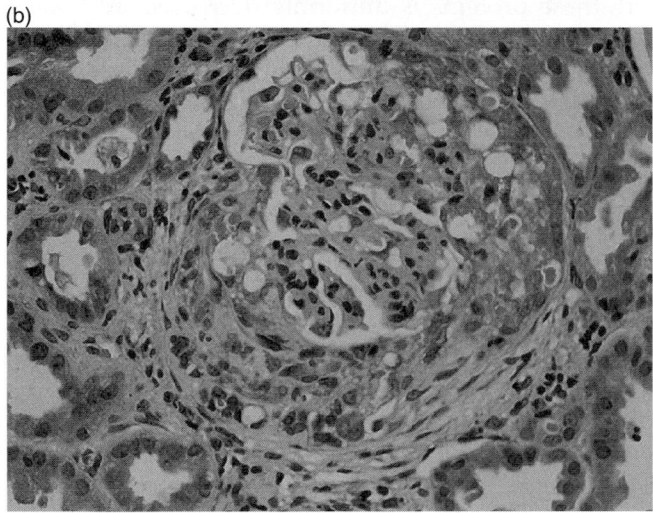

FIGURE 28.6 **The podocyte response to injury in human glomerulonephritis – to proliferate or not to proliferate?** (a) No proliferation, with development of segmental sclerosis, as occurs in idiopathic focal and segmental. (b) Proliferation, with the glomerulosclerosis (Periodic Acid Schiff, development of a cellular crescent in a patient with vasculitis (haematoxylin and eosin $\times 400$). (*Histology courtesy of Dr Meryl Griffiths, Addenbrooke's Hospital, Cambridge.*)

podocytes exit the cell cycle in order to become terminally differentiated and quiescent, which are necessary requirements for normal function. Thus, in podocytes, proliferation and differentiation are closely linked, akin to neurons and cardiac myocytes. In both mouse and human glomerulogenesis, immunostaining for p27^{Kip1} and p57^{Kip2} is absent in proliferating podocytes during the S-shaped body stage.[108,142] On cessation of proliferation, there is strong expression of both Cdk inhibitors, so that p27^{Kip1} and p57^{Kip2} are constitutively expressed in mature podocytes. The Cdk inhibitors p21^{Cip1}, p27^{Kip1}, and p57^{Kip2} alone are not required for normal glomerular development because, as described previously, the glomeruli from null mice are histologically

normal. However, functional redundancy of p27^{Kip1} and p57^{Kip2}, at least within the podocyte, has been suggested by studies of E13.5 embryonic metanephroi from double p27^{Kip1}/p57$^{Kip2-/-}$ mice. Glomeruli from these mice have been reported to be significantly larger than those from wild-type or single mutants, due to an increase in podocyte number. Differentiation of podocytes was judged to be normal by electron microscopy and immunostaining for WT-1, suggesting a synergistic role for p27^{Kip1} and p57^{Kip2} in determining the final complement of podocytes.

RESISTANCE OF PODOCYTES TO PROLIFERATION: ROLE OF CELL CYCLE REGULATORY PROTEINS

Studies have shown that the frequently observed lack of podocyte proliferation may be due to abnormalities in DNA synthesis or mitosis and cytokinesis (Figure 28.7).

The passive Heymann nephritis (PHN) model, induced by the administration of an antibody reactive against the Fx1A antigen on the rat podocyte, has many similarities to human membranous nephropathy.[143,144] In common with the Thy1 model of mesangial proliferative glomerulonephritis, PHN is complement (C5b-9)-dependent. However, in contrast to the observed mesangial cell proliferation in response

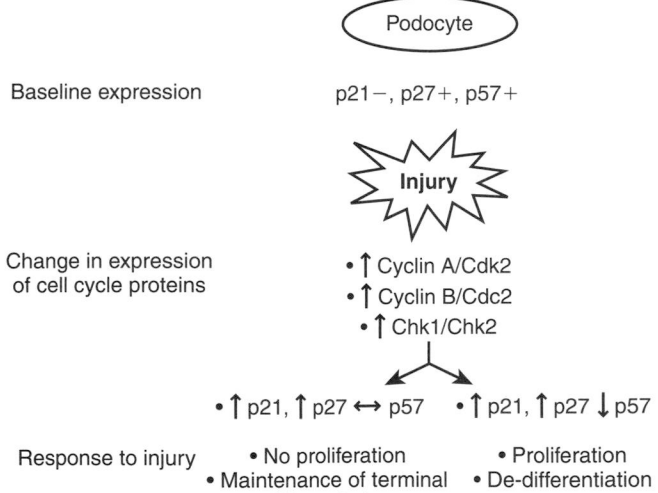

FIGURE 28.7 **Changes in cell cycle protein activity following injury to glomerular podocytes: the critical role of Cdk inhibitors in determining podocyte fate.** In contrast to mesangial cells, at baseline quiescent podocytes express both p27^{Kip1} and p57^{Kip2}. Following injury, there is an increase in the positive cell cycle regulators cyclin A/Cdk2 and cyclin B/Cdc2; however, this is accompanied by an increase in checkpoint kinases 1 and 2. The subsequent podocyte response depends on changes in the Cdk inhibitors. If p21^{Cip1} and p27^{Kip1} increase, cell cycle entry remains inhibited, there is no proliferation, and terminal differentiation is maintained. However, if there is a decline in the levels of p21^{Cip1}, p27^{Kip1}, and p57^{Kip2}, then the cell cycle is engaged and proliferation and de-differentiation occur.

to complement-mediated injury, there is no increase in podocyte number. Mitotic figures and an increase in ploidy are seen in the acute phase of disease, but over time the number of podocytes decreases. The comparison of patterns of expression of cell cycle proteins between the PHN and Thy-1 disease models has provided an opportunity to elucidate the role of cell cycle proteins in experimental podocyte disease.

Following C5b-9-induced injury in PHN rats, protein levels for cyclin A and Cdk2 rise,[145] indicating engagement of the cell cycle. However, only a limited increase in DNA synthesis occurs, suggesting the presence of an inhibitor to cell cycle progression. Indeed, the levels of the Cdk inhibitors p21^{Cip1} and p27^{Kip1} increase specifically in podocytes following the induction of PHN.[145] The increase in p21^{Cip1} is attenuated by administering the mitogen bFGF to PHN rats, and this augments the increase in podocyte DNA synthesis and ploidy. Furthermore, upregulation of M-phase cell cycle proteins Cdc2 and cyclin B is also observed in PHN podocytes, suggesting that a disturbance in cytokinesis is ultimately responsible for the development of polynucleated cells and lack of podocyte proliferation in this experimental glomerular disease.[146]

Cell culture studies have further explored the inability of podocytes to proliferate following C5b-9-induced injury, and support the hypothesis of a defect in completing mitosis. When cultured podocytes are exposed to sublytic C5b-9 attack, the cells engage the cell cycle. However, there is a delay or inhibition in entering mitosis, suggesting a block in the G_2/M transition, and involvement of mechanisms that regulate this checkpoint. This response is typical of that following DNA damage, to which podocytes appear to be particularly susceptible. The occurrence of DNA damage following exposure to sublytic C5b-9 has subsequently been confirmed,[147] together with increased checkpoint kinase-1 and -2 protein levels, thus arresting cells at G_2/M. The mechanism by which DNA damage occurs in podocytes is not currently well-understood, but is thought to involve the generation of reactive oxygen radicals.

A key role for p21^{Cip1} in limiting the proliferative response of podocytes has been demonstrated in studies using p21^{Cip1} knockout mice.[148,149] The administration of an antiglomerular antibody to induce experimental podocyte injury caused podocyte dedifferentiation and proliferation in p21$^{Cip1-/-}$ mice compared to control mice receiving the same antibody. Glomerular extracellular matrix accumulation was also increased in p21$^{Cip1-/-}$ mice, and was associated with a significant decrease in renal function. Additional *in vitro* data could link the pro-apoptotic effect of TGF-beta1 in podocytes to p21^{Cip1}.[150] Podocyte apoptosis induced by TGF-beta1 required sufficient p21^{Cip1} levels.

Intravenous application of the podocyte toxin Adriamycin resembles the histological findings of focal segmental glomerulosclerosis (FSGS) in mice. Diseased p21$^{Cip1-/-}$ mice presented with increased podocyte apotosis and decreased podocyte number, leading to aggravated glomerular disease including worse albuminuria, glomerulosclerosis, and increased BUN compared to control animals.[151]

The resistance of podocytes to proliferation in the majority of animal models has been confirmed in human diseases, and similar underlying mechanisms have been observed. Normal quiescent podocytes express p27^{Kip1} and p57^{Kip2}, and immunostaining for these proteins is maintained in conditions without proliferation, namely minimal change diseases and membranous glomerulopathy.[152] In contrast, expression of both these proteins is uniformly decreased in diseases characterized by podocyte proliferation, that is, cellular FSGS, collapsing glomerulopathy, and HIV-associated nephropathy. This is accompanied by the *de novo* expression of p21^{Cip1}. The mechanisms by which the podocyte eludes the usual constraints on proliferation are discussed below.

RESISTANCE OF PODOCYTES TO PROLIFERATION: ROLE OF MECHANICAL STRETCH

An additional factor reported to influence the proliferative capacity of the podocyte is the presence of mechanical stress.[153] Independent of the site of initial injury, a common pathway to progressive glomerulosclerosis is an increase in intraglomerular pressure, also known as glomerular hypertension.[130,132,154] Lowering intraglomerular pressure reduces progression in a number of glomerular diseases, including diabetic nephropathy.[155] Glomerular hypertension is associated with glomerular hypertrophy (see below), and the resultant mechanical stretch causes injury to all three glomerular cell types. Whereas applying mechanical stretch to cultured mesangial cells increases proliferation,[156] the opposite response is seen in cultured podocytes.[157,171] Stretching mouse podocytes in culture decreased the levels of cyclins D1, A, B1, and Cdc2, in association with an increase in the Cdk inhibitors. Stretch caused an early increase in p21^{Cip1}, followed by an increase in p27^{Kip1} at 24 hours and p57^{Kip2} at 72 hours. In contrast to the growth arrest seen in wild-type cells exposed to stretch, p21$^{Cip1-/-}$ podocytes exposed to stretch continued to proliferate, suggesting a role for p21^{Cip1} in the inability of the podocyte to progress through the cell cycle in response to stretch. These studies show that in addition to being injurious to mesangial cells, mechanical stretch affects podocytes and reduces their proliferative potential by altering specific cell cycle proteins.

PODOCYTE PROLIFERATION

Although the majority of both experimental animal models of podocyte injury and human podocyte diseases are not associated with proliferation, this has been reported to occur in a limited number of settings. The true ability of the mature podocyte to proliferate remains controversial, principally because glomerular cells believed to be proliferating podocytes frequently lack defining cell-type-specific markers.[158] However, the use of transgenic animals has been invaluable in resolving the debate. A well-studied animal model of podocyte proliferation is crescentic glomerulonephritis in the mouse, which has been examined in detail by several groups. In this model, predictable proliferation of glomerular cells occurs, and early in the course of the disease this is not associated with rupture of Bowman's capsule, nor with the presence of infiltrating cells.[159] It is therefore a useful model for studying the contribution of intrinsic glomerular cells to crescent formation. Moeller et al. generated a mouse with constitutive expression of β galactosidase specifically in podocytes in vivo.[160] Experimental crescentic nephritis was induced by injecting rabbit IgG ip, followed six days later by an intravenous injection of rabbit anti-mouse GBM antibody. The crescents contained numerous β-galactosidase-expressing cells, confirming their podocyte origin. Furthermore, expression of the nuclear proliferation marker Ki-67 by these cells demonstrated the capability of these podocyte-derived cells to undergo proliferation. Matsusaka et al. generated a transgenic mouse with podocyte-specific expression of human CD25.[161] Injury was then induced using an immunotoxin, resulting in a proliferative glomerular lesion. However, immunohistochemistry indicated that the proliferating cells were of parietal epithelial origin, not podocytes. The disparity between these two results likely results from the different initiating injuries used, but illustrates the ongoing debate which was further fueled by recent data.[162] Smeets et al. could show, by lineage tracing of either podocytes or parietal epithelial cells (PECs), that the majority of cells within extracapillary proliferative leasions were PECs, and only a minority were of podocyte origin. This held true in the nephrotoxic nephritis model of inflammatory crescentic glomerulonephritis, and in the Thy-1.1 transgenic mouse model of collapsing glomerulopathy. As described above, once podocytes proliferate they lose several of their defining characteristic proteins, such as WT-1, making identification difficult. However, there is broad agreement that the proliferating resident glomerular cells making up crescents are of epithelial origin, although the relative contributions of parietal cells and podocytes remains disputed.

In human disease, podocyte proliferation is considered to occur in collapsing glomerulopathy, cellular focal segmental glomerulosclerosis, and HIV-associated nephropathy.[163,164] In these diseases, there is increased expression of cyclin A and the proliferation marker Ki-67, with a marked reduction in p27^{Kip1} and p57^{Kip2}.[152,164] In contrast, all other diseases of podocytes in humans, including membranous nephropathy, minimal change disease, and focal segmental glomerulosclerosis, are not associated with a decrease in Cdk inhibitor levels, and typical markers of proliferation are absent. Interestingly, the rate of progression to end-stage renal failure is increased in glomerular diseases characterized by podocyte proliferation.[165,166] The pathogenesis of HIV-associated nephropathy has been further detailed using transgenic mice expressing HIV-1 genes.[167–169] The Tg26 mouse model develops murine HIVAN secondary o renal expression of HIV-1 mRNAs from the HIV-1 NL4-3 gag-pol proviral transgene.[169] This model has enabled characterization of the cellular effects of HIV-1 using both the intact animal and conditionally immortalized podocytes in culture. HIV-1 induces loss of contact inhibition in podocytes,[170] and expression of cyclin D1 and phosphorylation of pRb.[171] The cells become dedifferentiated, with loss of specific podocyte-expressed proteins.[167,172] Interestingly, there have been reports of reversibility of HIV nephropathy in both mice (discussed below) and human disease[173] following treatment with highly active antiretroviral therapy, suggesting that once the virus is cleared the podocyte is capable of exiting the cell cycle and redifferentiating to its mature phenotype.

ATYPICAL EFFECTS OF CELL CYCLE PROTEINS ON PODOCYTES

The traditional view of cell cycle proteins focuses on the regulation of cellular proliferation. The view on cell cycle proteins has since been broadened by the discovery of atypical cyclin proteins and dependent kinases. These include cyclin C-Cdk8, cyclin H-cdk7, cyclin K-Cdk9, cyclin T-Cdk9 or cyclin I-Cdk5.[174] We could show that cyclin I null mice are normal consistent with the notion that cyclin I is not required for cell differentation. Cyclin I is predominantly expressed in terminally differentiated cells, including neurons and podocytes. Lack of cyclin I rendered podocytes more susceptible to apoptosis.[175] A potential mechanism included a decreased expression and protein stability of p21.

The Cdk partner of cyclin I remained elusive since its discovery. We could identify Cdk5 as the Cdk partner of cyclin I.[176] Cdk5 itself is essential for normal development, as Cdk5 null mice die from developmental deficits, but little is known about its function in the kidney. Cdk5 is mainly activated by the non-cyclin proteins p35 and p39. The latter is not expressed in podocytes, but p35–Cdk5 has been shown to be present in podocytes.[177] In 2004, Griffin et al. demonstrated an essential role for p35–Cdk5 in podocyte differentiation, proliferation, and maintenance. Cdk5 levels decline in experimental disease associated with podocyte dedifferentiation and proliferation, including anti-glomerular antibody disease and HIV-associated nephropathy. More recent *in vivo* and *in vitro* data support the model that Cdk5 is central to podocyte survival, and is dually regulated by cyclin I and p35. Downstream targets of Cdk5 were the pro-survival proteins Bcl-2 and Bcl-XL.[174,176,178]

Therapeutic Inhibition of Podocyte Proliferation at Cell Cycle Level

As with glomerular diseases principally affecting the mesangial cell, both roscovitine and retinoids have shown promise as therapeutic agents in modulating the podocyte response to injury. In addition, recent data suggest a direct effect of glucocorticoids on podocytes at the cell cycle level.

ROSCOVITINE

We hypothesized that inhibition of podocyte proliferation with the Cdk2 inhibitor roscovitine in a mouse model of crescentic glomerulonephritis would improve renal outcome,[179] similar to that observed following inhibition of mesangial cell proliferation in Thy 1 nephritis described previously.[114] Inhibition of Cdk2 activity was confirmed by a histone kinase assay, and podocyte DNA synthesis measured by incorporation of BrdU. Compared to control nephritic animals receiving the vehicle, in mice treated with roscovitine there was a significant decrease in BrdU at day 5 of nephritis. This was accompanied by less accumulation of laminin at day 14, and significantly improved renal function, suggesting a similar intervention may be beneficial in human diseases. Roscovitine has also been demonstrated to be beneficial in the treatment of Tg26 mice at doses that did not decrease HIV-1 transgene expression, suggesting an effect mediated by inhibition of cell cycle progression.[180]

RETINOIDS

Retinoids are particularly attractive agents for the treatment of podocyte disease, as it has been demonstrated that following podocyte injury, both decrease podocyte proliferation and maintain the expression of markers of differentiation.[181,182] The promoter region of the human nephrin gene (NPHS1) contains three putative retinoic acid-response elements, and shows enhancer activity in response to all-trans-retinoic acid

(ATRA) in a dose-dependent manner. We have recently demonstrated that ATRA *in vitro* significantly retards podocyte proliferation, as measured by the MTT assay, while inducing process formation and increasing the expression of both nephrin and podocin.[182] Similarly, in mice with antiglomerular antibody nephritis, treatment with ATRA both reduces podocyte proliferation and prevents the decreases in nephrin, podocin, and synaptopodin in experimental animals. This was accompanied by a reduction in proteinuria. The dual roles of retinoids to both inhibit proliferation while promoting differentiation underscore their potential value as therapeutic agents for human podocyte diseases.

GLUCOCORTICOIDS

Glucocorticods are the clinical backbone to treat patients with glomerular diseases. Their mode of action is poorly-understood, particularly in patients with steroid-sensitive nephritic syndrome which lacks any signs of inflammation in the glomerulus. *In vitro* data in human podocytes revealed direct effects of dexamethasone on human podocytes.[183] Incubation with steroids led to decreased expression of p21 and suppression of inflammatory chemokines (IL-6/IL-8), but did not induce apoptosis.

Parietal Epithelial Cell Proliferation

As outlined above, there is an ongoing debate on the cellular origin of extracapillary proliferative lesions in glomerular disease. The parietal epithelial cell (PEC) has long been neglected, but recently moved into the center of glomerular research.[184] PECs share a common lineage with podocytes until the S-shaped stage of glomerulogenesis. Between the S-shaped body and capillary loop stages, each cell begins to express distinct genes, used as "cell-specific markers." For example, Wilm's tumor suppressor protein 1 (WT-1) expression is no longer detected in PECs, whereas podocytes maintain WT-1 and gain vimentin expression. In mice, PECs express CD10 in the capillary loop stage of development.[158] Potential mechanisms underlying PEC proliferation result from studies of cell cycle proteins. In contrast to podocytes, expression of the Cdk inhibitors p21^{Cip1} and p57^{Kip2} were not detected in healthy PECs, whereas p27^{Kip1} was expressed at low levels. In experimental and human forms of FSGS, PECs showed increased DNA-synthesis. The increased expression of Ki-67 and cyclin A were accompanied by decreased p27^{Kip1} expression in the absence of p21^{Cip1} and p57^{Kip2}.[185] Suzuki et al. recently showed in a mouse model of FSGS, that PEC proliferation was in part regulated by p21^{Cip1}.[186]

Glomerular Endothelial Cell Proliferation

The endothelial cells of mature glomeruli are quiescent, but retain the capacity to proliferate and form new capillaries following injury.[187] The degree of proliferation appears to be dependent on the local balance of proangiogenic factors, such as vascular endothelial growth factor (VEGF), and antiangiogenic factors, such as thrombospondin-1. An inadequate proliferative response may lead to loss of the glomerular microvasculature, and contribute to glomerulosclerosis and progressive renal impairment. The beneficial effects of VEGF administration have been demonstrated in animal models of acute glomerulonephritis,[188–190] suggesting that amelioration of human diseases may be achieved by augmenting the reparative potential of the glomerular endothelial cells. However, the underlying role of individual cyclins, Cdk, and Cdk inhibitors in these cells remains unknown.

Tubular Cell Hyperplasia

Renal tubular hyperplasia is most frequently encountered during the reparative phase following an acute injury, such as ischemia or toxin exposure.[191] Tubular injury results in cell loss by either necrosis or apoptosis, and therefore there is a requirement for the remaining cells to spread and migrate to cover the exposed basement membrane. These cells then dedifferentiate and proliferate to restore cell number, and finally differentiate again to restore the functional integrity of the nephron. Interestingly, the tubular repair recapitulates organogenesis in patterns of gene expression, including vimentin, neural cell adhesion molecule, growth factors such as IGF-1, fibroblast growth factor, and hepatocyte growth factor; and matrix molecules such as osteopontin.[191] This dedifferentiated phenotype is likely to be important for the spreading and proliferative properties of the viable tubular epithelial cells as they cover the denuded basement membrane to replace lost cells. However, the factors controlling the reversion to a less-differentiated phenotype, and the subsequent re-establishment of the mature phenotype, remain poorly-understood.

As might be expected, the proliferation observed following a transient ischemic injury is associated with an increase in the mRNA and protein expression of cyclins D1, D3, and B, mRNA expression of cyclin A, and protein expression of Cdks 2 and 4.[192] Both cyclin-D and -E kinase activities are increased.[192] Thus, the proliferative response is due to increased expression of both the regulatory and catalytic subunits of the G1 kinases, and an increase in their activity.

The Cdk inhibitors appear to have a critical role in limiting the proliferative response. Following acute renal injury induced by ischemia, ureteral obstruction or cisplatin, $p21^{Cip1}$ protein expression is increased in the thick ascending limb of the loop of Henle, and in the distal convoluted tubule.[193] Induction of the same injury in $p21^{Cip1-/-}$ mice was associated with increased proliferation, as assessed by BrdU incorporation and PCNA staining.[194] The $p21^{Cip-/-}$ mice had a more rapid onset of acute renal failure, developed more severe morphological damage, and had a higher mortality, emphasizing the requirement for proliferation following injury to be at a controlled and appropriate level.

HYPERTROPHY

Hypertrophy has been described in most segments of the nephron, but proximal tubular hypertrophy is observed most frequently. Hypertrophy of the proximal tubule has been described in compensatory renal growth, chronic metabolic acidosis and chronic hypokalemia, diabetes mellitus, and during protein-loading.[195] In compensatory renal growth, there is also hypertrophy of the glomerulus and collecting tubules; in diabetes, hypertrophy of glomerular cells is well-described, and with prolonged protein-loading hypertrophy of the initial segments of the thick ascending limb occurs.

As mentioned previously, cellular hypertrophy may result from either cell cycle-dependent or -independent mechanisms. Within the glomerulus, an increase in cell size is predominantly due to cell cycle re-entry without progression, whereas in the tubules there appears to be a more significant contribution from the inhibition of protein synthesis.

Glomerular Hypertrophy

Glomerular cell hypertrophy occurs during many forms of chronic renal disease, and may herald the development of glomerulosclerosis.[130,196,197] Glomerular diseases associated with glomerular hypertrophy include diabetic nephropathy,[198] minimal change nephropathy,[199] focal segmental glomerulosclerosis,[200,201] and a reduction in renal mass.[202] However, there are clear differences in the prognosis of glomerular hypertrophy, depending on the underlying disease. Following uninephrectomy, the hypertrophy is compensatory, and is not typically associated with the development of glomerulosclerosis. In contrast, the hypertrophy of diabetic nephropathy antecedes and probably underlies the development of glomerulosclerosis.[169] Diabetic nephropathy is the leading cause of end-stage renal disease in Western countries, and is discussed further below. Pathological glomerular hypertrophy leads to progressive glomerulosclerosis and scarring by a number of different mechanisms.[196] The increased metabolic rate of cells undergoing hypertrophy results in enhanced mitochondrial oxygen consumption, which may lead to tissue injury due to the generation of reactive oxygen radicals and the subsequent peroxidation of proteins and lipids. The hypertrophy is often initiated by growth factors that also stimulate the cells to increase production of extracellular matrix components, such as type IV collagen.

Diabetic Nephropathy

Diabetes mellitus is now the most frequent cause of end-stage renal failure in Western countries, and the pathogenesis of diabetic nephropathy is discussed in detail elsewhere in this book. The focus of this chapter is on the disordered cell growth seen in association with diabetic renal involvement. The hallmarks of human diabetic nephropathy are similar in both type I and type II diabetes, and consist of mesangial cell hypertrophy and podocyte loss, with accumulation of extracellular matrix in the mesangium and tubulointerstitium, resulting in glomerulosclerosis and tubulointerstitial fibrosis.[203−205] Research has concentrated principally on the ability of hyperglycemia and TGF-β to induce mesangial cell hypertrophy, and more recently the roles of RAGE[206] and hyperinsulinemia[207] have also been studied.

DIABETES AND MESANGIAL CELLS

HYPERGLYCEMIA *In vitro* culture of mesangial cells in high glucose media causes cell cycle entry and a biphasic growth response.[208] Following initial proliferation, the cells arrest in G1-phase, and there is progressive hypertrophy. Both kidney and glomerular hypertrophy induced by hyperglycemia are associated with an early and sustained increase in expression of cyclin D1 and activation of Cdk4.[209] An arrested cell cycle suggests a role for the Cdk inhibitors in mediating hypertrophy, and indeed high glucose increases the levels of both p21^{Cip1} [210] and p27^{Kip1} [211] in cultured mesangial cells. This is mediated by a number of factors, including glucose itself, TGF-β, which then acts in an autocrine fashion,[212,213] and CTGF.[214] High glucose directly stimulates the transcription of p21^{Cip1},[215] and activates MAP kinases, which prolong the half-life of p27^{Kip1} by phosphorylation on serine residues.[216] Lowering p21^{Cip1} [217] or p27^{Kip1} [211] levels with antisense oligonucleotides reduces the hypertrophic effects of high glucose. Moreover, hypertrophy is not induced by high glucose in p21$^{Cip1-/-}$ (unpublished observations) and p27$^{Kip1-/-}$[218] mesangial cells *in vitro*. Indeed, high glucose increases proliferation in p27$^{Kip1-/-}$ mesangial cells, whereas it arrests cell cycle progression in p27$^{Kip1+/+}$ mesangial cells.[218] Reconstituting p27^{Kip1} levels in p27$^{Kip1-/-}$ mesangial cells by transfection restores the hypertrophic phenotype.[218] These studies show a compelling role for the Cdk inhibitors p21^{Cip1} and p27^{Kip1} in mediating the hypertrophy induced by high glucose.

These *in vitro* findings have been confirmed in experimental models of both type I and type II diabetic nephropathy. Considering type I diabetes, the glomerular protein levels of p21^{Cip1} are increased in the streptozotocin (STZ)-induced model in the mouse,[210] and both p21^{Cip1} and p27^{Kip1} levels are increased in the glomeruli of diabetic BBdp rats.[64] A similar increase was noted in glomeruli of *db/db* mice[215] and the Zucker diabetic fatty rat,[219] models of type II diabetic nephropathy. Diabetic p21$^{Cip1-/-}$ mice are protected from glomerular hypertrophy.[220] Diabetic p27$^{Kip1-/-}$ mice have only mild mesangial expansion and no glomerular or renal hypertrophy compared to control diabetic p27$^{Kip1+/+}$ mice, despite upregulation of glomerular TGF-β.[221] These results support a critical role for the Cdk inhibitors p21^{Cip1} and p27^{Kip1} in mediating the glomerular hypertrophy seen not only in association with diabetes, but also as described in the following, a reduction in nephron number.

TRANSFORMING GROWTH FACTOR β The cytokine TGF-β has been shown in numerous settings to be a key mediator of progressive fibrosis in renal disease.[222−224] TGF-β also decreases proliferation in mesangial cells, an effect that appears to be independent of p21^{Cip1} and p27^{Kip1}, and induces cell hypertrophy.[225−227] To determine the role of Cdk inhibitors in mediating the hypertrophic effects of TGF-β, mesangial cells derived from single and double null mice were studied.[226] Compared to wild-type mice, hypertrophy was significantly reduced in double p21^{Cip1}/p27$^{Kip1-/-}$ mesangial cells. A less marked reduction in hypertrophy was seen in the single p21$^{Cip1-/-}$ and p27$^{Kip1-/-}$ cells. These results show that although p21^{Cip1} and p27^{Kip1} each contribute to the hypertrophic action of TGF-β, the presence of both is required for maximal effect.

The expression of Cdk inhibitors has also been explored in response to CTGF, considered to be a principle mediator of the downstream effects of TGF-β. Abdel Wahab et al.[214] demonstrated that CTGF is a hypertrophic factor for human mesangial cells, and that this hypertrophy is associated with the induction of p15^{INK4b}, p21^{Cip1}, and p27^{Kip1}, with the maintenance of pRb in a hypophosphorylated state.

Diabetes and Podocytes

Morphometric analyses have demonstrated that the podocyte undergoes hypertrophy early in the course of both animal models of diabetic nephropathy[219,228-230] and in human disease.[140,231] This hypertrophy may be in direct response to the metabolic changes associated with diabetes or compensatory, consequent to the loss of podocytes that is known to occur.[232,233]

At the level of the cell cycle, mRNA and protein expression of p27[Kip1] is increased in both cultured podocytes exposed to high glucose, and in glomeruli isolated from streptozotocin-induced diabetic rats.[230] The p27[Kip1] gene appears to be haplo-insufficient, as diabetic p27[Kip1+/−] mice exhibited an intermediate degree of functional and structural renal injury.[234] High glucose also significantly increased angiotensin II levels both in cell lysates and media compared with normal glucose, and exogenous angiotensin II increased p27[Kip1] mRNA and protein expression. Exposure of cultured cells and treatment of diabetic rats with an angiotensin II receptor antagonist (ARB) inhibited the increase in p27[Kip1]. Glomerular hypertrophy was also significantly prevented by ARB treatment. It appears likely that similar cell cycle mechanisms drive both mesangial cell and podocyte hypertrophy in diabetic nephropathy, suggesting that podocytes in this setting are also capable of engaging the cell cycle.

Compensatory Glomerular Hypertrophy

A reduction in nephron number results in compensatory hypertrophy in the remaining viable nephron.[235] Uninephrectomy does not alter the protein expression of cyclins D1 or D2, nor of Cdk2 or Cdk4, when total renal lysates are studied at day 7.[236] However, there may be a differential effect in specific renal compartments,[187] and an increase in tubular cyclin E–Cdk2 activity was demonstrated during compensatory hypertrophy following uninephrectomy. Prior to hypertrophy, severe renal ablation produced by 5/6 nephrectomy resulted in an early proliferative glomerular response, associated with an increase in cyclin E expression and phosphorylation of pRb.[106]

A role for the Cdk inhibitors is now emerging in the pathogenesis of glomerular hypertrophy. Following partial renal ablation, p21[Cip1−/−] mice develop glomerular hyperplasia rather than hypertrophy and increased intraglomerular pressure, with protection from the development of progressive renal failure.[237] Increased intraglomerular pressure is a final pathway toward glomerulosclerosis in systemic hypertension, diabetes, and focal segmental glomerulosclerosis (FSGS). This glomerular hypertension causes stress-tension, or stretch, on resident glomerular cells, with differing consequences for the different cell types. Exposure of mesangial cells to cyclical mechanical stretch results in cell cycle entry and proliferation.[238] In contrast, mechanical stretch reduces cell cycle

progression and induces podocyte hypertrophy *in vitro*.[157] This is unchanged in p27[Kip1−/−] cells, but hypertrophy was not induced in p21[Cip1] and double p21[Cip1]/p27[Kip1−/−] podocytes, indicating a requirement for p21[Cip1]. Stretch-induced hypertrophy required cell cycle entry, and was prevented by specifically blocking Erk1/2 or Akt. However, it is not clear whether podocyte hypertrophy represents a beneficial adaptive response to raised intraglomerular pressure or whether this change in podocyte phenotype is accompanied by a disturbance in function that is detrimental to the glomerulus.

TUBULAR HYPERTROPHY

The compensatory growth capacity of the kidney was known to the ancient Greeks: Aristotle (384−322 BC) described that animals born with a single kidney have a larger organ compared to those born with two. More contemporary studies have documented that the increase in renal size following nephron reduction by disease or surgical resection is due primarily to proximal tubular epithelial hypertrophy.[183,239] The initial hypertrophic response is considered adaptive;[77,235,240] however, with time persistent hypertrophy is associated with the infiltration of macrophages, T-cells, and fibroblasts into the tubulointerstitial space.[87,196] This hypertrophy is no longer beneficial to organ function, and the cellular infiltrate results in tubular atrophy and tubulointerstitial fibrosis, the final convergent pathway of many renal diseases of diverse etiologies.

Cell Cycle-Dependent Tubular Cell Hypertrophy
TRANSFORMING GROWTH FACTOR β

As in the glomerulus, TGF-β is an important mediator of tubular cell hypertrophy. The hypertrophy induced by both angiotensin II and high glucose[241] is also dependent on TGF-β. TGF-β converts a mitogen-induced proliferative response to cellular hypertrophy, and this has been studied in detail in cultures of proximal tubule cells by examining the effects of epidermal growth factor (EGF) plus TGF-β. TGF-β alone has an antiproliferative effect on tubular cell growth, but does not induce hypertrophy.[242] EGF-induced hyperplasia is associated with cell cycle entry, hyperphosphorylation of pRb, and an increase in thymidine incorporation, but no change in cell size or protein/DNA ratio.[242] In the presence of additional TGF-β, cell cycle entry is not impaired and cyclin-E protein levels increase, but there is no increase in DNA synthesis and pRb remains hypophosphorylated, with arrest of the cells in mid- to late-G1. Inactivation of pRb by expression of either SV40 large-T antigen (inactivates both pRb and p53) or

HPV E7 (inactivates pRb alone) prevents TGF-β from converting EGF-induced hyperplasia to hypertrophy. In contrast, inactivation of p53 alone with HPV E6 has no effect on the induction of hypertrophy, confirming the importance of pRb in the cell cycle arrest of tubular cells resulting from TGF-β.

The maintenance of pRb in its hypophosphorylated state suggests TGF-β modifies the activity of G1 kinases. Consistent with the observation that cell cycle entry is not impaired in the presence of TGF-β, TGF-β has no effect on EGF-induced increase in Cdk4/6−cyclin D kinase activity.[243,244] However, there is no increase in cyclin E kinase activity, with a decreased number of Cdk2−cyclin E complexes and retention of p57, but not p27 or p21, in those complexes that do form.

In summary, the proposed paradigm for the development of hypertrophy in response to TGF-β in renal tubular cells is as follows. After a proliferative stimulus, there is cell cycle entry and activation of cyclin D kinase. This is associated with an increase in protein synthesis, and hence cell size. As the cell reaches mid- to late-G1, if cyclin E kinase is sufficiently activated, pRb is further phosphorylated and becomes inactivated, allowing the cell to progress to S-phase and hyperplasia to occur. However, in the presence of TGF-β, cyclin E kinase is not sufficiently activated, pRb remains hypophosphorylated, the cell is arrested, and hypertrophy results.

ANGIOTENSIN II

Angiotensin II has an established role in stimulating hypertrophy of proximal tubular cells, mediated by the high-affinity AT_1 receptor.[245] Both angiotensin II and EGF induce the expression of early immediate genes in tubule cells, suggesting that angiotensin II-mediated hypertrophy is also dependent on cell cycle entry.[246] Indeed, angiotensin II-treated cells are arrested in G1, and do not progress to S-phase,[245,247] reminiscent of cells exposed to TGF-β. It has subsequently been shown that angiotensin II stimulates the transcription and protein synthesis of TGF-β in proximal tubule cells.[248] Exposure of cells to a neutralizing antibody to TGF-β abrogated the ability of angiotensin II to induce hypertrophy, demonstrating its dependency on the induction and autocrine activity of TGF-β.[248] In contrast to proximal tubules cells exposed to EGF and TGF-β, angiotensin II increases protein (but not mRNA) levels for $p27^{Kip1}$.[249] To characterize the functional role of $p27^{Kip1}$ in angiotensin II-mediated hypertrophy, proximal tubule cells were cultured from $p27^{Kip1}$ null mice,[250] which responded to angiotensin II with cell cycle progression but no hypertrophy. Cdk4/6−cyclin D kinase activity was stimulated in both wild-type and null cells, but Cdk2−cyclin E kinase activity only increased in the null cells, indicating that $p27^{Kip1}$ inhibits this

complex, and is required for angiotensin II-mediated hypertrophy of proximal tubular cells.

The mechanism by which angiotensin II increases $p27^{Kip1}$ expression has been studied in detail.[251] Angiotensin II upregulates p22phox, a subunit of membrane-bound NADPH oxidase, and hence increases the concentration of intracellular reactive oxygen species. This results in phosphorylation and activation of the mitogen-activated protein kinases Erk 1,2, that in turn leads to serine phosphorylation of $p27^{Kip1}$.[216,252] Serine phosphorylated $p27^{Kip1}$ has increased stability and decreased degradation by the ubiquitin pathway.[216] Atrial natriuretic peptide attenuates angiotensin II-mediated $p27^{Kip1}$ expression and proximal tubule cell hypertrophy, by a mechanism that appears to involve activation of the phosphatase MKP-1, which dephosphorylates Erk1,2.[253] The importance of this pathway has also been shown in vivo.[254] Infusion of angiotensin II into normal rats for 7 days increased the formation of reactive oxygen species in tubular cells and augmented $p27^{Kip1}$ expression. Immunostaining for PCNA decreased, indicating G1 cell cycle arrest, although hypertrophy was not observed.

As occurs with mesangial cells, a role for CTGF has been described in mediating tubular cell hypertrophy in response to angiotensin II. Systemic infusion of angiotensin II into normal rats induced overexpression of CTGF in glomeruli, tubules, and renal arteries, with associated tubular injury and increase in fibronectin expression.[255] A similar effect was demonstrated in cultured tubular cells, with angiotensin II acting through the AT_1 receptor. The importance of CTGF in angiotensin II-mediated hypertrophy was explored in detail by another group using HK2 cells.[256] Angiotensin II induced CTGF expression, G1 cell cycle arrest, and cell hypertrophy, which were reversed by treatment with an anti-CTGF antibody. In addition to the well-described roles in apoptosis and fibrosis, further detrimental renal effects of angiotensin II are likely to be secondary to its recently described effects of cell cycle arrest and hypertrophy.

A summary of the changes in cell cycle proteins occurring in glomerular and tubular hyperplasia, and in cell cycle-dependent hypertrophy, is shown in Table 28.1. Data from knockout mice are shown in Table 28.2.

Cell Cycle-Independent Tubular Cell Hypertrophy

In addition to increased new protein synthesis, a decrease in the rate of protein breakdown may contribute to cell hypertrophy.[3] Within the kidney, this is best characterized for tubular cells. Although diabetes and acidosis are catabolic states, both are associated with decreases in renal proteolysis, which makes a significant contribution to the associated growth of the kidney.[257−259]

TABLE 28.1 Summary of Cell Cycle Proteins in Hyperplasia and Hypertrophy of Renal Cells

	Experiment	Cyclin CDK			CDK Inhibitor			Reference
		Increased	Decreased	No Change	Increased	Decreased	No Change	
MESANGIAL CELL								
Proliferation	*In vitro* exposure to mitogens (PDGF, bFGF)	D1, E, A			p21	p27	p57	176,193,99
	Animal models		Cdk4,2					
	Thy1	D1, E Cdk4, 2			p15, p21	p27		200
	Remnant kidney	E, Cdk2		Cdk4				199
Suppression of proliferation hypertrophy	*In vitro* exposure to antimitogens (TGFβ, SPARC, heparin)		D1, E, A Cdk4, 2		p15, p21, p27			193,203,246
	In vitro exposure Glucose			Cdk2	p21, p27			112,245
	TGFβ				p16, p21, p27			201,248
	CTGF				p15, p21, p27			1
	Animal models							
	Type I diabetes (STZ mouse, BBdp rat)			E, A	p21, p27			112,248
	Type II diabetes (*db/db* mouse, Zucker rat)			Cdk2	p27			88,243
Apoptosis	Cytoplasmic location of Cdk2							85
PODOCYTE								
Immune injury	*In vitro* exposure to C5b9				p21			43
	Animals models							
	PHN	A, Cdk2			p21	p57		176,98
	Antiglomerular antibody	A, Cdk2			p21, p27	p57		203
Proliferation	*In vitro* exposure to HIV-1	D₁						151
	Human disease							
	Collapsing GN	A				p27, p57		10,202
Response to stretch	*In vitro*		D, A, B		D, A p21, p27, p57			171
TUBULAR EPITHELIAL CELL								
Proliferation	Animal models							
	Uninephroctomy	E, Cdk2						122
	Ischemic injury	D1, D3, A, B Cdk2, 4						137,164
	UUO, cisplatin				p21			164
Hypertrophy	In vitro exposure EGF + TGFβ	D, Cdk4	E					62,120

TABLE 28.2 Data from Knockout Mice

	Experiment	Outcome	Reference
p21$^{-/-}$	Mesangial cells exposed to high glucose *in vitro*	Resistant to hypertrophy	—[a]
	Animal models STZ diabetes Antiglomerular antibody Remnant kidney Acute tubular injury (ischemia, UUO, cisplatin)	Reduced glomerular hypertrophy	3
		Increased podocyte proliferation	100
		Glomerular hyperplasia, not hypertrophy	135
		Increased proliferation, worse renal function, increased mortality	136
p27$^{-/-}$	Mesangial cells exposed to high glucose *in vitro*	Resistant to hypertrophy	244
	Mesangial cells deprived of growth factors	Increased apoptosis	84
	Animal models STZ diabetes Antiglomerular antibody	Reduced glomerular hypertrophy	5
		Increased mesangial cell proliferation and apoptosis	158
	UUO	Increased tubular apoptosis	158
p57$^{-/-}$	Unmanipulated animal	Normal glomerulogenesis in embryonic mice	217,257,263

[a]*Unpublished.*
UUO: Unilateral ureteral obstruction.

An estimated 60% of total intracellular proteolysis in renal tubular cells occurs by the ubiquitin—proteasome pathway;[260] however, this does not appear to be a major factor in the regulation of proteolysis during the hypertrophic response of renal tubular cells. Two lines of evidence support an alteration in lysosomal function as underlying the reduced proteolysis observed in certain cases of tubular hypertrophy, and a possible mechanism by which this occurs has recently begun to be clarified.[261] First, in addition to stimulating cell cycle entry, EGF increases protein half-life by approximately 30% in cultured primary proximal tubular cells, primarily by affecting lysosomal proteolysis.[260] Second, exposure of tubular cells to ammonia leads to alkalinization of acidic intracellular compartments, including lysosomes, thus modifying their function, and stimulates hypertrophy that is independent of cell cycle entry.[262]

Several studies have demonstrated proximal tubule cell hypertrophy in response to ammonia *in vitro*,[262−264] and renal ammonia synthesis is increased in several apparently diverse clinical conditions associated with hypertrophy.[195,265] In chronic metabolic acidosis and chronic hypokalemia, mitochondrial ammoniagenesis is directly stimulated. In contrast, the increase in ammonia in diabetes mellitus, following uninephrectomy and during protein-loading, is thought to be stimulated by an increase in single-nephron glomerular filtration rate (SNGFR). Cell culture studies involving either reducing the media pH[182] or lowering potassium concentration[266] do not induce hypertrophy, indicating that it is not changes in the extracellular milieu *per se* that initiate the hypertrophic growth response. The results from direct application of ammonium chloride suggest that the accumulation of this molecule, in response to acidosis or hypokalemia, drives the development of hypertrophy. This hypothesis is supported by studies of hypertrophy in the setting of chronic hypokalemia in the rat.[267] In this model, renal ammonia production is significantly increased. Administration of bicarbonate both decreases the rate of ammonia synthesis and the hypertrophy. Renal generation of ammonia has recently been studied in patients with metabolic acidosis and normal renal function.[263] Compared to individuals with normal acid— base balance, kidney protein degradation was significantly lower and urinary ammonia excretion significantly higher. As with cell and animal studies, it was suggested that in human metabolic acidosis the increased ammonia synthesis drives the decrease in protein degradation, and is potentially responsible for kidney hypertrophy.

What is the mechanism by which altered lysosomal function affects protein degradation? Chaperone-mediated autophagy allows lysosomal import of proteins containing a specific consensus sequence, KFERQ, by the binding of heat-shock cognate protein 73 (Hsc73) to lysosomal membrane protein 2a (LAMP2a). In cultured

NRK-52E cells (a rat kidney epithelial cell line) exposed to EGF or ammonia (but not TGF-β alone), there was an increase in the half-life of KFERQ-containing proteins[261] associated with a decrease in total cellular and lysosomal LAMP2a. Furthermore, declines in LAMP2a and Hsc73 have also been demonstrated in lysosomes isolated from the hypertrophied cortex of acutely diabetic rats, and was accompanied by an increase in KFERQ-containing proteins.[268] Other lysosomal pathways may also be affected during renal hypertrophy.[3] EGF-induced suppression of proteolysis in NRK-52E cells was prevented by inhibitors of Ras and PI-3 kinase, but not by inhibitors of MAP kinase or Src.[269] PI-3 kinase and Akt activities are increased in the renal cortex of diabetic *db/db* mice and correlate with hypertrophy.[270] Products of the PI-3 kinase pathway control membrane and protein trafficking, and the suppression of chaperone-mediated autophagy may be part of a generalized abnormality in trafficking to and from lysosomes.

CONCLUSIONS

The last two decades have seen an explosion in our understanding of the underlying mechanisms governing renal hyperplasia and hypertrophy which has literally burgeoned since 1991. The goal for the next 15 years will be to identify specific modifiable targets to alter or even reverse these pathological processes. Numerous agents have been demonstrated to be beneficial in ameliorating the course of animal models of disease, and the hope is that certain of these will transfer to be of use in human disease. Indeed, Cdk2 inhibitors are now in human trials for treatment of proliferative glomerulonephritis. With the discovery of drugs that target either the network of mitogens responsible for stimulating abnormal cell growth or specific cell cycle-regulatory proteins, potential therapies may be on the horizon for patients with renal diseases in which hyperplasia or hypertrophy is a dominant feature. Much has been learned, but in addition to characterizing the role of conventional cyclins, Cdks, and Cdk inhibitors, the challenge remains to identify novel cell cycle proteins, determine their role in renal disease, and the consequences of their manipulation.

References

[1] Fine L. The biology of renal hypertrophy. Kidney Int 1986;29 (3):619—34.

[2] Fine LG, Norman J. Cellular events in renal hypertrophy. Annu Rev Physiol 1989;51:19—32.

[3] Franch HA. Pathways of proteolysis affecting renal cell growth. Curr Opin Nephrol Hypertens 2002;11(4):445—50.

[4] Preisig P. A cell cycle-dependent mechanism of renal tubule epithelial cell hypertrophy. Kidney Int 1999;56(4):1193—8.

[5] Nurse P. A long twentieth century of the cell cycle and beyond. Cell 2000;100(1):71—8.

[6] Harper JW, Adams PD. Cyclin-dependent kinases. Chem Rev 2001;101(8):2511—26.

[7] Koepp DM, Harper JW, Elledge SJ. How the cyclin became a cyclin: regulated proteolysis in the cell cycle. Cell 1999;97(4):431—4.

[8] Evans T, Rosenthal ET, Youngblom J, Distel D, Hunt T. Cyclin: a protein specified by maternal mRNA in sea urchin eggs that is destroyed at each cleavage division. Cell 1983;33(2):389—96.

[9] Pines J. Cyclins and cyclin-dependent kinases: a biochemical view. Biochem J 1995;308(Pt 3):697—711.

[10] Aktas H, Cai H, Cooper GM. Ras links growth factor signaling to the cell cycle machinery via regulation of cyclin D1 and the Cdk inhibitor p27KIP1. Mol Cell Biol 1997;17(7):3850—7.

[11] Filmus J, Robles AI, Shi W, Wong MJ, Colombo LL, Conti CJ. Induction of cyclin D1 overexpression by activated ras. Oncogene 1994;9(12):3627—33.

[12] Winston JT, Coats SR, Wang YZ, Pledger WJ. Regulation of the cell cycle machinery by oncogenic ras. Oncogene 1996;12(1):127—34.

[13] Gille H, Downward J. Multiple ras effector pathways contribute to G(1) cell cycle progression. J Biol Chem 1999;274 (31):22033—40.

[14] Cheng M, Sexl V, Sherr CJ, Roussel MF. Assembly of cyclin D-dependent kinase and titration of p27Kip1 regulated by mitogen-activated protein kinase kinase (MEK1). Proc Natl Acad Sci USA 1998;95(3):1091—6.

[15] Peeper DS, Upton TM, Ladha MH, Neuman E, Zalvide J, Bernards R, et al. Ras signalling linked to the cell-cycle machinery by the retinoblastoma protein. Nature 1997;386 (6621):177—81.

[16] Diehl JA, Cheng M, Roussel MF, Sherr CJ. Glycogen synthase kinase-3beta regulates cyclin D1 proteolysis and subcellular localization. Genes Dev 1998;12(22):3499—511.

[17] Diehl JA, Zindy F, Sherr CJ. Inhibition of cyclin D1 phosphorylation on threonine-286 prevents its rapid degradation via the ubiquitin-proteasome pathway. Genes Dev 1997;11(8):957—72.

[18] Sherr CJ. Mammalian G1 cyclins. Cell 1993;73(6):1059—65.

[19] Kaldis P, Sutton A, Solomon MJ. The Cdk-activating kinase (CAK) from budding yeast. Cell 1996;86(4):553—64.

[20] Matsushime H, Roussel MF, Ashmun RA, Sherr CJ. Colony-stimulating factor 1 regulates novel cyclins during the G1 phase of the cell cycle. Cell 1991;65(4):701—13.

[21] Baldin V, Lukas J, Marcote MJ, Pagano M, Draetta G. Cyclin D1 is a nuclear protein required for cell cycle progression in G1. Genes Dev 1993;7(5):812—21.

[22] Guo Y, Stacey DW, Hitomi M. Post-transcriptional regulation of cyclin D1 expression during G2 phase. Oncogene 2002;21 (49):7545—56.

[23] Matsushime H, Quelle DE, Shurtleff SA, Shibuya M, Sherr CJ, Kato JY. D-type cyclin-dependent kinase activity in mammalian cells. Mol Cell Biol 1994;14(3):2066—76.

[24] Weinberg RA. The retinoblastoma protein and cell cycle control. Cell 1995;81(3):323—30.

[25] Trimarchi JM, Lees JA. Sibling rivalry in the E2F family. Nat Rev Mol Cell Biol 2002;3(1):11—20.

[26] Matsuura I, Denissova NG, Wang G, He D, Long J, Liu F. Cyclin-dependent kinases regulate the antiproliferative function of Smads. Nature 2004;430(6996):226—31.

[27] Dulic V, Lees E, Reed SI. Association of human cyclin E with a periodic G1-S phase protein kinase. Science 1992;257 (5078):1958—61.

[28] Koff A, Giordano A, Desai D, Yamashita K, Harper JW, Elledge S, et al. Formation and activation of a cyclin E-cdk2 complex during the G1 phase of the human cell cycle. Science 1992;257(5077):1689—94.

[29] Kitagawa M, Higashi H, Jung HK, Suzuki-Takahashi I, Ikeda M, Tamai K, et al. The consensus motif for phosphorylation by cyclin D1-Cdk4 is different from that for phosphorylation by cyclin A/E-Cdk2. EMBO J 1996;15(24):7060—9.

[30] Lundberg AS, Weinberg RA. Functional inactivation of the retinoblastoma protein requires sequential modification by at least two distinct cyclin-cdk complexes. Mol Cell Biol 1998;18(2):753—61.

[31] Harbour JW, Dean DC. The Rb/E2F pathway: expanding roles and emerging paradigms. Genes Dev 2000;14(19):2393—409.

[32] Yu Q, Sicinski P. Mammalian cell cycles without cyclin E-CDK2. Cell Cycle 2004;3(3):292—5.

[33] Clurman BE, Sheaff RJ, Thress K, Groudine M, Roberts JM. Turnover of cyclin E by the ubiquitin-proteasome pathway is regulated by cdk2 binding and cyclin phosphorylation. Genes Dev 1996;10(16):1979—90.

[34] Welcker M, Singer J, Loeb KR, Grim J, Bloecher A, Gurien-West M, et al. Multisite phosphorylation by Cdk2 and GSK3 controls cyclin E degradation. Mol Cell 2003;12(2):381—92.

[35] Won KA, Reed SI. Activation of cyclin E/CDK2 is coupled to site-specific autophosphorylation and ubiquitin-dependent degradation of cyclin E. EMBO J 1996;15(16):4182—93.

[36] Coverley D, Laman H, Laskey RA. Distinct roles for cyclins E and A during DNA replication complex assembly and activation. Nat Cell Biol 2002;4(7):523—8.

[37] Hua XH, Newport J. Identification of a preinitiation step in DNA replication that is independent of origin recognition complex and cdc6, but dependent on cdk2. J Cell Biol 1998;140(2):271—81.

[38] Krude T, Jackman M, Pines J, Laskey RA. Cyclin/Cdk-dependent initiation of DNA replication in a human cell-free system. Cell 1997;88(1):109—19.

[39] Mitra J, Enders GH. Cyclin A/Cdk2 complexes regulate activation of Cdk1 and Cdc25 phosphatases in human cells. Oncogene 2004;23(19):3361—7.

[40] Berthet C, Aleem E, Coppola V, Tessarollo L, Kaldis P. Cdk2 knockout mice are viable. Curr Biol 2003;13(20):1775—85.

[41] Ortega S, Prieto I, Odajima J, Martin A, Dubus P, Sotillo R, et al. Cyclin-dependent kinase 2 is essential for meiosis but not for mitotic cell division in mice. Nat Genet 2003;35(1):25—31.

[42] Atherton-Fessler S, Parker LL, Geahlen RL, Piwnica-Worms H. Mechanisms of p34cdc2 regulation. Mol Cell Biol 1993;13(3):1675—85.

[43] Smits VA, Medema RH. Checking out the G(2)/M transition. Biochim Biophys Acta 2001;1519(1—2):1—12.

[44] Krek W, Nigg EA. Differential phosphorylation of vertebrate p34cdc2 kinase at the G1/S and G2/M transitions of the cell cycle: identification of major phosphorylation sites. EMBO J 1991;10(2):305—16.

[45] Li J, Meyer AN, Donoghue DJ. Requirement for phosphorylation of cyclin B1 for *Xenopus* oocyte maturation. Mol Biol Cell 1995;6(9):1111—24.

[46] Nilsson I, Hoffmann I. Cell cycle regulation by the Cdc25 phosphatase family. Prog Cell Cycle Res 2000;4:107—14.

[47] Yang J, Bardes ES, Moore JD, Brennan J, Powers MA, Kornbluth S. Control of cyclin B1 localization through regulated binding of the nuclear export factor CRM1. Genes Dev 1998;12(14):2131—43.

[48] Hagting A, Jackman M, Simpson K, Pines J. Translocation of cyclin B1 to the nucleus at prophase requires a phosphorylation-dependent nuclear import signal. Curr Biol 1999;9(13):680—9.

[49] Sherr CJ, Roberts JM. Living with or without cyclins and cyclin-dependent kinases. Genes Dev 2004;18(22):2699—711.

[50] Nakayama K, Ishida N, Shirane M, Inomata A, Inoue T, Shishido N, et al. Mice lacking p27(Kip1) display increased body size, multiple organ hyperplasia, retinal dysplasia, and pituitary tumors. Cell 1996;85(5):707—20.

[51] Sherr CJ, Roberts JM. CDK inhibitors: positive and negative regulators of G1-phase progression. Genes Dev 1999;13(12):1501—12.

[52] Quelle DE, Zindy F, Ashmun RA, Sherr CJ. Alternative reading frames of the INK4a tumor suppressor gene encode two unrelated proteins capable of inducing cell cycle arrest. Cell 1995;83(6):993—1000.

[53] Sherr CJ. The INK4a/ARF network in tumour suppression. Nat Rev Mol Cell Biol 2001;2(10):731—7.

[54] Sherr CJ. Parsing Ink4a/Arf: "pure" p16-null mice. Cell 2001;106(5):531—4.

[55] Bunz F, Dutriaux A, Lengauer C, Waldman T, Zhou S, Brown JP, et al. Requirement for p53 and p21 to sustain G2 arrest after DNA damage. Science 1998;282(5393):1497—501.

[56] Smits VA, Klompmaker R, Vallenius T, Rijksen G, Makela TP, Medema RH. p21 inhibits Thr161 phosphorylation of Cdc2 to enforce the G2 DNA damage checkpoint. J Biol Chem 2000;275(39):30638—43.

[57] Cheng M, Olivier P, Diehl JA, Fero M, Roussel MF, Roberts JM, et al. The p21(Cip1) and p27(Kip1) CDK "inhibitors" are essential activators of cyclin D-dependent kinases in murine fibroblasts. EMBO J 1999;18(6):1571—83.

[58] el-Deiry WS, Tokino T, Velculescu VE, Levy DB, Parsons R, Trent JM, et al. WAF1, a potential mediator of p53 tumor suppression. Cell 1993;75(4):817—25.

[59] Harper JW, Adami GR, Wei N, Keyomarsi K, Elledge SJ. The p21 Cdk-interacting protein Cip1 is a potent inhibitor of G1 cyclin-dependent kinases. Cell 1993;75(4):805—16.

[60] Xiong Y, Hannon GJ, Zhang H, Casso D, Kobayashi R, Beach D. p21 is a universal inhibitor of cyclin kinases. Nature 1993;366(6456):701—4.

[61] LaBaer J, Garrett MD, Stevenson LF, Slingerland JM, Sandhu C, Chou HS, et al. New functional activities for the p21 family of CDK inhibitors. Genes Dev 1997;11(7):847—62.

[62] Parry D, Mahony D, Wills K, Lees E. Cyclin D-CDK subunit arrangement is dependent on the availability of competing INK4 and p21 class inhibitors. Mol Cell Biol 1999;19(3):1775—83.

[63] Parker SB, Eichele G, Zhang P, Rawls A, Sands AT, Bradley A, et al. p53-independent expression of p21Cip1 in muscle and other terminally differentiating cells. Science 1995;267(5200):1024—7.

[64] Wolf G, Wenzel U, Ziyadeh FN, Stahl RA. Angiotensin converting-enzyme inhibitor treatment reduces glomerular p16INK4 and p27Kip1 expression in diabetic BBdp rats. Diabetologia 1999;42(12):1425—32.

[65] Noda A, Ning Y, Venable SF, Pereira-Smith OM, Smith JR. Cloning of senescent cell-derived inhibitors of DNA synthesis using an expression screen. Exp Cell Res 1994;211(1):90—8.

[66] Polyak K, Lee MH, Erdjument-Bromage H, Koff A, Roberts JM, Tempst P, et al. Cloning of p27Kip1, a cyclin-dependent kinase inhibitor and a potential mediator of extracellular antimitogenic signals. Cell 1994;78(1):59—66.

[67] Toyoshima H, Hunter T. p27, a novel inhibitor of G1 cyclin-Cdk protein kinase activity, is related to p21. Cell 1994;78(1):67—74.

[68] Hengst L, Reed SI. Translational control of p27Kip1 accumulation during the cell cycle. Science 1996;271(5257):1861–4.

[69] Pagano M, Tam SW, Theodoras AM, Beer-Romero P, Del Sal G, Chau V, et al. Role of the ubiquitin-proteasome pathway in regulating abundance of the cyclin-dependent kinase inhibitor p27. Science 1995;269(5224):682–5.

[70] Sheaff RJ, Groudine M, Gordon M, Roberts JM, Clurman BE. Cyclin E-CDK2 is a regulator of p27Kip1. Genes Dev 1997;11(11):1464–78.

[71] Vlach J, Hennecke S, Amati B. Phosphorylation-dependent degradation of the cyclin-dependent kinase inhibitor p27. EMBO J 1997;16(17):5334–44.

[72] Bloom J, Pagano M. Deregulated degradation of the cdk inhibitor p27 and malignant transformation. Semin Cancer Biol 2003;13(1):41–7.

[73] Elledge SJ, Harper JW. The role of protein stability in the cell cycle and cancer. Biochim Biophys Acta 1998;1377(2):M61–70.

[74] Lee MH, Reynisdottir I, Massague J. Cloning of p57KIP2, a cyclin-dependent kinase inhibitor with unique domain structure and tissue distribution. Genes Dev 1995;9(6):639–49.

[75] Matsuoka S, Edwards MC, Bai C, Parker S, Zhang P, Baldini A, et al. p57KIP2, a structurally distinct member of the p21CIP1 Cdk inhibitor family, is a candidate tumor suppressor gene. Genes Dev 1995;9(6):650–62.

[76] Fero ML, Rivkin M, Tasch M, Porter P, Carow CE, Firpo E, et al. A syndrome of multiorgan hyperplasia with features of gigantism, tumorigenesis, and female sterility in p27(Kip1)-deficient mice. Cell 1996;85(5):733–44.

[77] Wolf G, Neilson EG. Molecular mechanisms of tubulointerstitial hypertrophy and hyperplasia. Kidney Int 1991;39(3):401–20.

[78] Takahashi K, Nakayama K. Mice lacking a CDK inhibitor, p57Kip2, exhibit skeletal abnormalities and growth retardation. J Biochem 2000;127(1):73–83.

[79] Yan Y, Frisen J, Lee MH, Massague J, Barbacid M. Ablation of the CDK inhibitor p57Kip2 results in increased apoptosis and delayed differentiation during mouse development. Genes Dev 1997;11(8):973–83.

[80] Zhang P, Liegeois NJ, Wong C, Finegold M, Hou H, Thompson JC, et al. Altered cell differentiation and proliferation in mice lacking p57KIP2 indicates a role in Beckwith-Wiedemann syndrome. Nature 1997;387(6629):151–8.

[81] Deng C, Zhang P, Harper JW, Elledge SJ, Leder P. Mice lacking p21CIP1/WAF1 undergo normal development, but are defective in G1 checkpoint control. Cell 1995;82(4):675–84.

[82] Wolf G, Ziyadeh FN. Molecular mechanisms of diabetic renal hypertrophy. Kidney Int 1999;56(2):393–405.

[83] Couser WG, Johnson RJ. Mechanisms of progressive renal disease in glomerulonephritis. Am J Kidney Dis 1994;23(2):193–8.

[84] Fogo A, Ichikawa I. Evidence for the central role of glomerular growth promoters in the development of sclerosis. Semin Nephrol 1989;9(4):329–42.

[85] Baker AJ, Mooney A, Hughes J, Lombardi D, Johnson RJ, Savill J. Mesangial cell apoptosis: the major mechanism for resolution of glomerular hypercellularity in experimental mesangial proliferative nephritis. J Clin Invest 1994;94(5):2105–16.

[86] Tsuboi Y, Shankland SJ, Grande JP, Walker HJ, Johnson RJ, Dousa TP. Suppression of mesangial proliferative glomerulonephritis development in rats by inhibitors of cAMP phosphodiesterase isozymes types III and IV. J Clin Invest 1996;98(2):262–70.

[87] Klahr S, Schreiner G, Ichikawa I. The progression of renal disease. N Engl J Med 1988;318(25):1657–66.

[88] Pesce CM, Striker LJ, Peten E, Elliot SJ, Striker GE. Glomerulosclerosis at both early and late stages is associated with increased cell turnover in mice transgenic for growth hormone. Lab Invest 1991;65(5):601–5.

[89] Striker LJ, Doi T, Elliot S, Striker GE. The contribution of glomerular mesangial cells to progressive glomerulosclerosis. Semin Nephrol 1989;9(4):318–28.

[90] Hudkins KL, Gilbertson DG, Carling M, Taneda S, Hughes SD, Holdren MS, et al. Exogenous PDGF-D is a potent mesangial cell mitogen and causes a severe mesangial proliferative glomerulopathy. J Am Soc Nephrol 2004;15(2):286–98.

[91] Floege J, Eng E, Young BA, Couser WG, Johnson RJ. Heparin suppresses mesangial cell proliferation and matrix expansion in experimental mesangioproliferative glomerulonephritis. Kidney Int 1993;43(2):369–80.

[92] Floege J, Eng E, Lindner V, Alpers CE, Young BA, Reidy JM, et al. Rat glomerular mesangial cells synthesize basic fibroblast growth factor. Release, upregulated synthesis, and mitogenicity in mesangial proliferative glomerulonephritis. J Clin Invest 1992;90(6):2362–9.

[93] Ruef C, Budde K, Lacy J, Northemann W, Baumann M, Sterzel RB, et al. Interleukin 6 is an autocrine growth factor for mesangial cells. Kidney Int 1990;38(2):249–57.

[94] Ryffel B, Car BD, Gunn H, Roman D, Mihatsch MJ. Interleukin-6 exacerbates glomerulonephritis in (NZB × NZW)F1 mice. Am J Pathol 1994;144(5):927–37.

[95] Yanagita M. The role of the vitamin K-dependent growth factor Gas6 in glomerular pathophysiology. Curr Opin Nephrol Hypertens 2004;13(4):465–70.

[96] Brandt J, Pippin J, Schulze M, Hansch GM, Alpers CE, Johnson RJ, et al. Role of the complement membrane attack complex (C5b-9) in mediating experimental mesangioproliferative glomerulonephritis. Kidney Int 1996;49(2):335–43.

[97] Floege J, Johnson RJ, Gordon K, Iida H, Pritzl P, Yoshimura A, et al. Increased synthesis of extracellular matrix in mesangial proliferative nephritis. Kidney Int 1991;40(3):477–88.

[98] Gesualdo L, Di Paolo S, Ranieri E, Schena FP. Trapidil inhibits human mesangial cell proliferation: effect on PDGF beta-receptor binding and expression. Kidney Int 1994;46(4):1002–9.

[99] Caspary T, Cleary MA, Perlman EJ, Zhang P, Elledge SJ, Tilghman SM. Oppositely imprinted genes p57(Kip2) and igf2 interact in a mouse model for Beckwith-Wiedemann syndrome. Genes Dev 1999;13(23):3115–24.

[100] Schoecklmann HO, Rupprecht HD, Zauner I, Sterzel RB. TGF-beta1-induced cell cycle arrest in renal mesangial cells involves inhibition of cyclin E-cdk 2 activation and retinoblastoma protein phosphorylation. Kidney Int 1997;51(4):1228–36.

[101] Yamamoto T, Wilson CB. Complement dependence of antibody-induced mesangial cell injury in the rat. J Immunol 1987;138(11):3758–65.

[102] Yamamoto T, Wilson CB. Quantitative and qualitative studies of antibody-induced mesangial cell damage in the rat. Kidney Int 1987;32(4):514–25.

[103] Shankland SJ, Hugo C, Coats SR, Nangaku M, Pichler RH, Gordon KL, et al. Changes in cell-cycle protein expression during experimental mesangial proliferative glomerulonephritis. Kidney Int 1996;50(4):1230–9.

[104] Bokemeyer D, Panek D, Kitahara M, et al. The map kinase ERK regulates renal activity of cyclin-dependent kinase 2 in experimental glomerulonephritis. Nephrol Dial Transplant 2007;22(12):3431–41.

[105] Bokemeyer D, Panek D, Kramer HJ, Lindemann M, Kitahara M, Boor P, et al. In vivo identification of the mitogen-activated protein kinase cascade as a central pathogenic pathway in experimental mesangioproliferative glomerulonephritis. J Am Soc Nephrol 2002;13(6):1473–80.

[106] Shankland SJ, Hamel P, Scholey JW. Cyclin and cyclin-dependent kinase expression in the remnant glomerulus. J Am Soc Nephrol 1997;8(3):368–75.

[107] Shankland SJ, Pippin J, Flanagan M, Coats SR, Nangaku M, Gordon KL, et al. Mesangial cell proliferation mediated by PDGF and bFGF is determined by levels of the cyclin kinase inhibitor p27Kip1. Kidney Int 1997;51(4):1088–99.

[108] Hiromura K, Haseley LA, Zhang P, Monkawa T, Durvasula A, Petermann AT, et al. Podocyte expression of the CDK-inhibitor p57 during development and disease. Kidney Int 2001;60 (6):2235–46.

[109] Hiromura K, Pippin JW, Fero ML, Roberts JM, Shankland SJ. Modulation of apoptosis by the cyclin-dependent kinase inhibitor p27(Kip1). J Clin Invest 1999;103(5):597–604.

[110] Ophascharoensuk V, Fero ML, Hughes J, Roberts JM, Shankland SJ. The cyclin-dependent kinase inhibitor p27Kip1 safeguards against inflammatory injury. Nat Med 1998;4 (5):575–80.

[111] Monkawa T, Pippin J, Yo Y, Kopp JB, Alpers CE, Shankland SJ. The cyclin-dependent kinase inhibitor p21 limits murine mesangial proliferative glomerulonephritis. Nephron Exp Nephrol 2006;102(1):e8–18.

[112] Savill J. Regulation of glomerular cell number by apoptosis. Kidney Int 1999;56(4):1216–22.

[113] Hiromura K, Pippin JW, Blonski MJ, Roberts JM, Shankland SJ. The subcellular localization of cyclin dependent kinase 2 determines the fate of mesangial cells: role in apoptosis and proliferation. Oncogene 2002;21(11):1750–8.

[114] Pippin JW, Qu Q, Meijer L, Shankland SJ. Direct *in vivo* inhibition of the nuclear cell cycle cascade in experimental mesangial proliferative glomerulonephritis with Roscovitine, a novel cyclin-dependent kinase antagonist. J Clin Invest 1997;100 (10):2512–20.

[115] Gilbert T, Merlet-Benichou C. Retinoids and nephron mass control. Pediatr Nephrol 2000;14(12):1137–44.

[116] Xu Q, Lucio-Cazana J, Kitamura M, Ruan X, Fine LG, Norman JT. Retinoids in nephrology: promises and pitfalls. Kidney Int. 2004;66(6):2119–31.

[117] Marill J, Idres N, Capron CC, Nguyen E, Chabot GG. Retinoic acid metabolism and mechanism of action: a review. Curr Drug Metab 2003;4(1):1–10.

[118] Dimberg A, Bahram F, Karlberg I, Larsson LG, Nilsson K, Oberg F. Retinoic acid-induced cell cycle arrest of human myeloid cell lines is associated with sequential down-regulation of c-Myc and cyclin E and posttranscriptional up-regulation of p27(Kip1). Blood 2002;99(6):2199–206.

[119] Hsu SL, Hsu JW, Liu MC, Chen LY, Chang CD. Retinoic acid-mediated G1 arrest is associated with induction of p27(Kip1) and inhibition of cyclin-dependent kinase 3 in human lung squamous carcinoma CH27 cells. Exp Cell Res 2000;258 (2):322–31.

[120] Seewaldt VL, Dietze EC, Johnson BS, Collins SJ, Parker MB. Retinoic acid-mediated G1-S-phase arrest of normal human mammary epithelial cells is independent of the level of p53 protein expression. Cell Growth Differ 1999;10(1):49–59.

[121] Dechow C, Morath C, Peters J, Lehrke I, Waldherr R, Haxsen V, et al. Effects of all-trans retinoic acid on renin–angiotensin system in rats with experimental nephritis. Am J Physiol Renal Physiol 2001;281(5):F909–19.

[122] Wagner J, Dechow C, Morath C, Lehrke I, Amann K, Waldherr R, et al. Retinoic acid reduces glomerular injury in a rat model of glomerular damage. J Am Soc Nephrol 2000; 11(8):1479–87.

[123] Morath C, Dechow C, Lehrke I, Haxsen V, Waldherr R, Floege J, et al. Effects of retinoids on the TGF-beta system and extracellular matrix in experimental glomerulonephritis. J Am Soc Nephrol 2001;12(11):2300–9.

[124] McMahon B, Mitchell S, Brady HR, Godson C. Lipoxins: revelations on resolution. Trends Pharmacol Sci. 2001;22(8):391–5.

[125] Levy BD, Clish CB, Schmidt B, Gronert K, Serhan CN. Lipid mediator class switching during acute inflammation: signals in resolution. Nat Immunol 2001;2(7):612–9.

[126] Papayianni A, Serhan CN, Phillips ML, Rennke HG, Brady HR. Transcellular biosynthesis of lipoxin A4 during adhesion of platelets and neutrophils in experimental immune complex glomerulonephritis. Kidney Int 1995;47(5):1295–302.

[127] Mitchell D, Rodgers K, Hanly J, McMahon B, Brady HR, Martin F, et al. Lipoxins inhibit Akt/PKB activation and cell cycle progression in human mesangial cells. Am J Pathol 2004;164(3):937–46.

[128] Clish CB, Gronert K, Serhan CN. Local and systemic delivery of an aspirin-triggered lipoxin stable analog inhibits neutrophil trafficking. Ann NY Acad Sci 2000;905:274–8.

[129] Ohse T, Ota T, Kieran N, Godson C, Yamada K, Tanaka T, et al. Modulation of interferon-induced genes by lipoxin analogue in anti-glomerular basement membrane nephritis. J Am Soc Nephrol 2004;15(4):919–27.

[130] Fries JW, Sandstrom DJ, Meyer TW, Rennke HG. Glomerular hypertrophy and epithelial cell injury modulate progressive glomerulosclerosis in the rat. Lab Invest 1989;60(2):205–18.

[131] Kriz W. Podocyte is the major culprit accounting for the progression of chronic renal disease. Microsc Res Tech 2002;57 (4):189–95.

[132] Kriz W, Gretz N, Lemley KV. Progression of glomerular diseases: is the podocyte the culprit? Kidney Int 1998;54 (3):687–97.

[133] Kriz W, Lemley KV. The role of the podocyte in glomerulosclerosis. Curr Opin Nephrol Hypertens 1999;8(4):489–97.

[134] Rennke HG. How does glomerular epithelial cell injury contribute to progressive glomerular damage? Kidney Int Suppl 1994;45:S58–63.

[135] Dalla Vestra M, Masiero A, Roiter AM, Saller A, Crepaldi G, Fioretto P. Is podocyte injury relevant in diabetic nephropathy? Studies in patients with type 2 diabetes. Diabetes 2003;52 (4):1031–5.

[136] Hishiki T, Shirato I, Takahashi Y, Funabiki K, Horikoshi S, Tomino Y. Podocyte injury predicts prognosis in patients with IgA nephropathy using a small amount of renal biopsy tissue. Kidney Blood Press Res 2001;24(2):99–104.

[137] Lemley KV, Lafayette RA, Safai M, Derby G, Blouch K, Squarer A, et al. Podocytopenia and disease severity in IgA nephropathy. Kidney Int 2002;61(4):1475–85.

[138] Meyer TW, Bennett PH, Nelson RG. Podocyte number predicts long-term urinary albumin excretion in Pima Indians with Type II diabetes and microalbuminuria. Diabetologia 1999;42 (11):1341–4.

[139] Nakamura T, Ushiyama C, Hara M, Osada S, Ugai K, Shimada N, et al. Comparative effects of plasmapheresis and intravenous cyclophosphamide on urinary podocyte excretion in patients with proliferative Lupus nephritis. Clin Nephrol 2002;57(2):108–13.

[140] White KE, Bilous RW. Structural alterations to the podocyte are related to proteinuria in type 2 diabetic patients. Nephrol Dial Transplant 2004;19(6):1437–40.

[141] White KE, Bilous RW, Marshall SM, El Nahas M, Remuzzi G, Piras G, et al. Podocyte number in normotensive type 1 diabetic patients with albuminuria. Diabetes 2002;51(10):3083–9.

[142] Nagata M, Nakayama K, Terada Y, Hoshi S, Watanabe T. Cell cycle regulation and differentiation in the human podocyte lineage. Am J Pathol 1998;153(5):1511–20.

[143] Cybulsky AV, Rennke HG, Feintzeig ID, Salant DJ. Complement-induced glomerular epithelial cell injury. Role of the membrane attack complex in rat membranous nephropathy. J Clin Invest 1986;77(4):1096−107.

[144] Salant DJ, Darby C, Couser WG. Experimental membranous glomerulonephritis in rats. Quantitative studies of glomerular immune deposit formation in isolated glomeruli and whole animals. J Clin Invest 1980;66(1):71−81.

[145] Shankland SJ, Floege J, Thomas SE, Nangaku M, Hugo C, Pippin J, et al. Cyclin kinase inhibitors are increased during experimental membranous nephropathy: potential role in limiting glomerular epithelial cell proliferation in vivo. Kidney Int 1997;52(2):404−13.

[146] Petermann AT, Pippin J, Hiromura K, Monkawa T, Durvasula R, Couser WG, et al. Mitotic cell cycle proteins increase in podocytes despite lack of proliferation. Kidney Int 2003;63(1):113−22.

[147] Pippin JW, Durvasula R, Petermann A, Hiromura K, Couser WG, Shankland SJ. DNA damage is a novel response to sublytic complement C5b-9-induced injury in podocytes. J Clin Invest 2003;111(6):877−85.

[148] Kim YG, Alpers CE, Brugarolas J, Johnson RJ, Couser WG, Shankland SJ. The cyclin kinase inhibitor p21CIP1/WAF1 limits glomerular epithelial cell proliferation in experimental glomerulonephritis. Kidney Int 1999;55(6):2349−61.

[149] Shankland SJ, Wolf G. Cell cycle regulatory proteins in renal disease: role in hypertrophy, proliferation, and apoptosis. Am J Physiol Renal Physiol 2000;278(4):F515−29.

[150] Wada T, Pippin JW, Terada Y, Shankland SJ. The cyclin-dependent kinase inhibitor p21 is required for TGF-beta1-induced podocyte apoptosis. Kidney Int 2005;68(4):1618−29.

[151] Marshall CB, Krofft RD, Pippin JW, Shankland SJ. The CDK-inhibitor p21 is pro-survival in adriamycin(R)-induced podocyte injury, in vitro and in vivo. Am J Physiol Renal Physiol 2010.

[152] Shankland SJ, Eitner F, Hudkins KL, Goodpaster T, D'Agati V, Alpers CE. Differential expression of cyclin-dependent kinase inhibitors in human glomerular disease: role in podocyte proliferation and maturation. Kidney Int 2000;58(2):674−83.

[153] Petermann AT, Hiromura K, Blonski M, Pippin J, Monkawa T, Durvasula R, et al. Mechanical stress reduces podocyte proliferation in vitro. Kidney Int 2002;61(1):40−50.

[154] Brenner BM. Nephron adaptation to renal injury or ablation. Am J Physiol 1985;249(3 Pt 2):F324−37.

[155] Weir MR. Diabetes and hypertension: blood pressure control and consequences. Am J Hypertens 1999;12(12 Pt 1−2):170S−8S.

[156] Harris RC, Haralson MA, Badr KF. Continuous stretch-relaxation in culture alters rat mesangial cell morphology, growth characteristics, and metabolic activity. Lab Invest 1992;66(5):548−54.

[157] Petermann AT, Pippin J, Durvasula R, Pichler R, Hiromura K, Monkawa T, et al. Mechanical stretch induces podocyte hypertrophy in vitro. Kidney Int 2005;67(1):157−66.

[158] Nagata M, Tomari S, Kanemoto K, Usui J, Lemley KV. Podocytes, parietal cells, and glomerular pathology: the role of cell cycle proteins. Pediatr Nephrol 2003;18(1):3−8.

[159] Ophascharoensuk V, Pippin JW, Gordon KL, Shankland SJ, Couser WG, Johnson RJ. Role of intrinsic renal cells versus infiltrating cells in glomerular crescent formation. Kidney Int 1998;54(2):416−25.

[160] Moeller MJ, Soofi A, Hartmann I, Le Hir M, Wiggins R, Kriz W, et al. Podocytes populate cellular crescents in a murine model of inflammatory glomerulonephritis. J Am Soc Nephrol 2004;15(1):61−7.

[161] Matsusaka T, Xin J, Niwa S, Kobayashi K, Akatsuka A, Hashizume H, et al. Genetic engineering of glomerular sclerosis in the mouse via control of onset and severity of podocyte-specific injury. J Am Soc Nephrol 2005;16(4):1013−23.

[162] Smeets B, Uhlig S, Fuss A, Mooren F, Wetzels JF, Floege J, et al. Tracing the origin of glomerular extracapillary lesions from parietal epithelial cells. J Am Soc Nephrol 2009;20(12):2604−15.

[163] Barisoni L, Kriz W, Mundel P, D'Agati V. The dysregulated podocyte phenotype: a novel concept in the pathogenesis of collapsing idiopathic focal segmental glomerulosclerosis and HIV-associated nephropathy. J Am Soc Nephrol 1999;10(1):51−61.

[164] Barisoni L, Mokrzycki M, Sablay L, Nagata M, Yamase H, Mundel P. Podocyte cell cycle regulation and proliferation in collapsing glomerulopathies. Kidney Int 2000;58(1):137−43.

[165] Detwiler RK, Falk RJ, Hogan SL, Jennette JC. Collapsing glomerulopathy: a clinically and pathologically distinct variant of focal segmental glomerulosclerosis. Kidney Int 1994;45(5):1416−24.

[166] Schwartz MM, Evans J, Bain R, Korbet SM. Focal segmental glomerulosclerosis: prognostic implications of the cellular lesion. J Am Soc Nephrol 1999;10(9):1900−7.

[167] Barisoni L, Bruggeman LA, Mundel P, D'Agati VD, Klotman PE. HIV-1 induces renal epithelial dedifferentiation in a transgenic model of HIV-associated nephropathy. Kidney Int 2000;58(1):173−81.

[168] Bruggeman LA, Dikman S, Meng C, Quaggin SE, Coffman TM, Klotman PE. Nephropathy in human immunodeficiency virus-1 transgenic mice is due to renal transgene expression. J Clin Invest 1997;100(1):84−92.

[169] Dickie P, Felser J, Eckhaus M, Bryant J, Silver J, Marinos N, et al. HIV-associated nephropathy in transgenic mice expressing HIV-1 genes. Virology 1991;185(1):109−19.

[170] Schwartz EJ, Cara A, Snoeck H, Ross MD, Sunamoto M, Reiser J, et al. Human immunodeficiency virus-1 induces loss of contact inhibition in podocytes. J Am Soc Nephrol 2001;12(8):1677−84.

[171] Nelson PJ, Sunamoto M, Husain M, Gelman IH. HIV-1 expression induces cyclin D1 expression and pRb phosphorylation in infected podocytes: cell-cycle mechanisms contributing to the proliferative phenotype in HIV-associated nephropathy. BMC Microbiol 2002;2:26.

[172] Conaldi PG, Bottelli A, Baj A, Serra C, Fiore L, Federico G, et al. Human immunodeficiency virus-1 that induces hyperproliferation and dysregulation of renal glomerular epithelial cells. Am J Pathol 2002;161(1):53−61.

[173] Scheurer D. Rapid reversal of renal failure after initiation of HAART: a case report. AIDS Read 2004;14(8):443−7.

[174] Brinkkoetter PT, Pippin JW, Shankland SJ. Cyclin I-Cdk5 governs survival in post-mitotic cells. Cell Cycle 2010;9(9):1729−31.

[175] Griffin SV, Olivier JP, Pippin JW, Roberts JM, Shankland SJ. Cyclin I protects podocytes from apoptosis. J Biol Chem 2006;281(38):28048−57.

[176] Brinkkoetter PT, Olivier P, Wu JS, Henderson S, Krofft RD, Pippin JW, et al. Cyclin I activates Cdk5 and regulates expression of Bcl-2 and Bcl-XL in postmitotic mouse cells. J Clin Invest 2009.

[177] Griffin SV, Hiromura K, Pippin J, Petermann AT, Blonski MJ, Krofft R, et al. Cyclin-dependent kinase 5 is a regulator of podocyte differentiation, proliferation, and morphology. Am J Pathol 2004;165(4):1175−85.

[178] Brinkkoetter PT, Wu JS, Ohse T, Krofft RD, Schermer B, Benzing T, et al. p35, the non-cyclin activator of Cdk5, protects

podocytes against apoptosis *in vitro* and *in vivo*. Kidney Int 2010;77(8):690—9.

[179] Griffin SV, Krofft RD, Pippin JW, Shankland SJ. Limitation of podocyte proliferation improves renal function in experimental crescentic glomerulonephritis. Kidney Int 2005;67(3):977—86.

[180] Gherardi D, D'Agati V, Chu TH, Barnett A, Gianella-Borradori A, Gelman IH, et al. Reversal of collapsing glomerulopathy in mice with the cyclin-dependent kinase inhibitor CYC202. J Am Soc Nephrol 2004;15(5):1212—22.

[181] Suzuki A, Ito T, Imai E, Yamato M, Iwatani H, Kawachi H, et al. Retinoids regulate the repairing process of the podocytes in puromycin aminonucleoside-induced nephrotic rats. J Am Soc Nephrol 2003;14(4):981—91.

[182] Tovbin D, Franch HA, Alpern RJ, Preisig PA. Media acidification inhibits TGF beta-mediated growth suppression in cultured rabbit proximal tubule cells. Proc Assoc Am Physicians 1997;109(6):572—9.

[183] Xing CY, Saleem MA, Coward RJ, Ni L, Witherden IR, Mathieson PW. Direct effects of dexamethasone on human podocytes. Kidney Int 2006;70(6):1038—45.

[184] Ohse T, Pippin JW, Chang AM, Krofft RD, Miner JH, Vaughan MR, et al. The enigmatic parietal epithelial cell is finally getting noticed: a review. Kidney Int 2009;76 (12):1225—38.

[185] Nitta K, Horita S, Honda K, Uchida K, Watanabe T, Nihei H, et al. Glomerular expression of cell-cycle-regulatory proteins in human crescentic glomerulonephritis. Virchows Arch 1999;435 (4):422—7.

[186] Suzuki T, Matsusaka T, Nakayama M, Asano T, Watanabe T, Ichikawa I, et al. Genetic podocyte lineage reveals progressive podocytopenia with parietal cell hyperplasia in a murine model of cellular/collapsing focal segmental glomerulosclerosis. Am J Pathol 2009;174(5):1675—82.

[187] Kang DH, Kanellis J, Hugo C, Truong L, Anderson S, Kerjaschki D, et al. Role of the microvascular endothelium in progressive renal disease. J Am Soc Nephrol 2002;13 (3):806—16.

[188] Kang DH, Hughes J, Mazzali M, Schreiner GF, Johnson RJ. Impaired angiogenesis in the remnant kidney model: II. Vascular endothelial growth factor administration reduces renal fibrosis and stabilizes renal function. J Am Soc Nephrol 2001;12(7):1448—57.

[189] Kim YG, Suga SI, Kang DH, et al. Vascular endothelial growth factor accelerates renal recovery in experimental thrombotic microangiopathy. Kidney Int 2000;58(6):2390—9.

[190] Masuda Y, Shimizu A, Mori T, Ishiwata T, Kitamura H, Ohashi R, et al. Vascular endothelial growth factor enhances glomerular capillary repair and accelerates resolution of experimentally induced glomerulonephritis. Am J Pathol 2001;159 (2):599—608.

[191] Bonventre JV. Dedifferentiation and proliferation of surviving epithelial cells in acute renal failure. J Am Soc Nephrol 2003;14 (Suppl. 1):S55—61.

[192] Park SK, Kang MJ, Kim W, Koh GY. Renal tubule regeneration after ischemic injury is coupled to the up-regulation and activation of cyclins and cyclin dependent kinases. Kidney Int 1997;52(3):706—14.

[193] Megyesi J, Udvarhelyi N, Safirstein RL, Price PM. The p53-independent activation of transcription of p21 WAF1/CIP1/ SDI1 after acute renal failure. Am J Physiol 1996;271(6 Pt 2): F1211—6.

[194] Megyesi J, Safirstein RL, Price PM. Induction of p21WAF1/ CIP1/SDI1 in kidney tubule cells affects the course of cis-platin-induced acute renal failure. J Clin Invest 1998;101 (4):777—82.

[195] Kurtz I. Role of ammonia in the induction of renal hypertrophy. Am J Kidney Dis 1991;17(6):650—3.

[196] Hostetter TH. Progression of renal disease and renal hypertrophy. Annu Rev Physiol 1995;57:263—78.

[197] Zatz R, Fujihara CK. Glomerular hypertrophy and progressive glomerulopathy. Is there a definite pathogenetic correlation? Kidney Int Suppl. 1994;45:S27—29; discussion S30-21.

[198] Ziyadeh FN, Sharma K. Role of transforming growth factor-beta in diabetic glomerulosclerosis and renal hypertrophy. Kidney Int Suppl 1995;51:S34—6.

[199] Toth T, Takebayashi S. Glomerular hypertrophy in relapsing minimal change nephropathy. Nephron 1996;74(1):64—71.

[200] Fogo A, Hawkins EP, Berry PL, Glick AD, Chiang ML, MacDonell Jr RC, et al. Glomerular hypertrophy in minimal change disease predicts subsequent progression to focal glomerular sclerosis. Kidney Int 1990;38(1):115—23.

[201] Muda AO, Feriozzi S, Cinotti GA, Faraggiana T. Glomerular hypertrophy and chronic renal failure in focal segmental glomerulosclerosis. Am J Kidney Dis 1994;23(2):237—41.

[202] Tenschert S, Elger M, Lemley KV. Glomerular hypertrophy after subtotal nephrectomy: relationship to early glomerular injury. Virchows Arch 1995;426(5):509—17.

[203] McGowan T, McCue P, Sharma K. Diabetic nephropathy. Clin Lab Med 2001;21(1):111—46.

[204] Pagtalunan ME, Miller PL, Jumping-Eagle S, Nelson RG, Myers BD, Rennke HG, et al. Podocyte loss and progressive glomerular injury in type II diabetes. J Clin Invest 1997;99(2):342—8.

[205] Ritz E, Keller C, Bergis K, Strojek K. Pathogenesis and course of renal disease in IDDM/NIDDM: differences and similarities. Am J Hypertens 1997;10(9 Pt 2):202S—7S.

[206] Brizzi MF, Dentelli P, Rosso A, et al. RAGE- and TGF-beta receptor-mediated signals converge on STAT5 and p21waf to control cell-cycle progression of mesangial cells: a possible role in the development and progression of diabetic nephropathy. FASEB J 2004;18(11):1249—51.

[207] Cusumano AM, Bodkin NL, Hansen BC, Iotti R, Owens J, Klotmant PE, et al. Glomerular hypertrophy is associated with hyperinsulinemia and precedes overt diabetes in aging rhesus monkeys. Am J Kidney Dis 2002;40(5):1075—85.

[208] Young BA, Johnson RJ, Alpers CE, Eng E, Gordon K, Floege J, et al. Cellular events in the evolution of experimental diabetic nephropathy. Kidney Int 1995;47(3):935—44.

[209] Feliers D, Frank MA, Riley DJ. Activation of cyclin D1-Cdk4 and Cdk4-directed phosphorylation of RB protein in diabetic mesangial hypertrophy. Diabetes 2002;51(11):3290—1.

[210] Kuan CJ, al-Douahji M, Shankland SJ. The cyclin kinase inhibitor p21WAF1, CIP1 is increased in experimental diabetic nephropathy: potential role in glomerular hypertrophy. J Am Soc Nephrol 1998;9(6):986—93.

[211] Wolf G, Schroeder R, Ziyadeh FN, Thaiss F, Zahner G, Stahl RA. High glucose stimulates expression of p27Kip1 in cultured mouse mesangial cells: relationship to hypertrophy. Am J Physiol 1997;273(3 Pt 2):F348—56.

[212] Wolf G, Sharma K, Chen Y, Ericksen M, Ziyadeh FN. High glucose-induced proliferation in mesangial cells is reversed by autocrine TGF-beta. Kidney Int 1992;42(3):647—56.

[213] Ziyadeh FN, Sharma K, Ericksen M, Wolf G. Stimulation of collagen gene expression and protein synthesis in murine mesangial cells by high glucose is mediated by autocrine activation of transforming growth factor-beta. J Clin Invest 1994;93 (2):536—42.

[214] Abdel-Wahab N, Weston BS, Roberts T, Mason RM. Connective tissue growth factor and regulation of the mesangial cell cycle: role in cellular hypertrophy. J Am Soc Nephrol 2002;13(10):2437—45.

[215] Wolf G, Schroeder R, Thaiss F, Ziyadeh FN, Helmchen U, Stahl RA. Glomerular expression of p27Kip1 in diabetic db/db mouse: role of hyperglycemia. Kidney Int 1998;53(4):869—79.

[216] Wolf G, Reinking R, Zahner G, Stahl RA, Shankland SJ. Erk 1,2 phosphorylates p27(Kip1): functional evidence for a role in high glucose-induced hypertrophy of mesangial cells. Diabetologia 2003;46(8):1090—9.

[217] Fan YP, Weiss RH. Exogenous attenuation of p21(Waf1/Cip1) decreases mesangial cell hypertrophy as a result of hyperglycemia and IGF-1. J Am Soc Nephrol 2004;15(3):575—84.

[218] Wolf G, Schroeder R, Zahner G, Stahl RA, Shankland SJ. High glucose-induced hypertrophy of mesangial cells requires p27 (Kip1), an inhibitor of cyclin-dependent kinases. Am J Pathol 2001;158(3):1091—100.

[219] Hoshi S, Shu Y, Yoshida F, Inagaki T, Sonoda J, Watanabe T, et al. Podocyte injury promotes progressive nephropathy in zucker diabetic fatty rats. Lab Invest 2002;82(1):25—35.

[220] Al-Douahji M, Brugarolas J, Brown PA, Stehman-Breen CO, Alpers CE, Shankland SJ. The cyclin kinase inhibitor p21WAF1/CIP1 is required for glomerular hypertrophy in experimental diabetic nephropathy. Kidney Int 1999;56 (5):1691—9.

[221] Awazu M, Omori S, Ishikura K, Hida M, Fujita H. The lack of cyclin kinase inhibitor p27(Kip1) ameliorates progression of diabetic nephropathy. J Am Soc Nephrol 2003;14(3):699—708.

[222] Kopp JB, Factor VM, Mozes M, Nagy P, Sanderson N, Böttinger EP, et al. Transgenic mice with increased plasma levels of TGF-beta 1 develop progressive renal disease. Lab Invest 1996;74(6):991—1003.

[223] Roberts AB, McCune BK, Sporn MB. TGF-beta: regulation of extracellular matrix. Kidney Int 1992;41(3):557—9.

[224] Shankland SJ, Johnson RJ. TGF-beta in glomerular disease. Miner Electrolyte Metab 1998;24(2—3):168—73.

[225] MacKay K, Striker LJ, Stauffer JW, Doi T, Agodoa LY, Striker GE. Transforming growth factor-beta. Murine glomerular receptors and responses of isolated glomerular cells. J Clin Invest 1989;83(4):1160—7.

[226] Monkawa T, Hiromura K, Wolf G, Shankland SJ. The hypertrophic effect of transforming growth factor-beta is reduced in the absence of cyclin-dependent kinase-inhibitors p21 and p27. J Am Soc Nephrol 2002;13(5):1172—8.

[227] Wolf G. Molecular mechanisms of renal hypertrophy: role of p27Kip1. Kidney Int 1999;56(4):1262—5.

[228] Gross ML, El-Shakmak A, Szabo A, Koch A, Kuhlmann A, Munter K, et al. ACE-inhibitors but not endothelin receptor blockers prevent podocyte loss in early diabetic nephropathy. Diabetologia 2003;46(6):856—68.

[229] Gross ML, Ritz E, Schoof A, Adamczak M, Koch A, Tulp O, et al. Comparison of renal morphology in the Streptozotocin and the SHR/N-cp models of diabetes. Lab Invest 2004;84 (4):452—64.

[230] Xu ZG, Yoo TH, Ryu DR, Cheon Park H, Ha SK, Han DS, et al. Angiotensin II receptor blocker inhibits p27Kip1 expression in glucose-stimulated podocytes and in diabetic glomeruli. Kidney Int 2005;67(3):944—52.

[231] White KE, Bilous RW. Estimation of podocyte number: a comparison of methods. Kidney Int 2004;66(2):663—7.

[232] Bhathena DB. Glomerular basement membrane length to podocyte ratio in human nephronopenia: implications for focal segmental glomerulosclerosis. Am J Kidney Dis 2003;41 (6):1179—88.

[233] Petermann AT, Pippin J, Krofft R, Blonski M, Griffin S, Durvasula R, et al. Viable podocytes detach in experimental diabetic nephropathy: potential mechanism underlying glomerulosclerosis. Nephron Exp Nephrol 2004;98(4):e114—23.

[234] Wolf G, Schanze A, Stahl RA, Shankland SJ, Amann K. p27 (Kip1) Knockout mice are protected from diabetic nephropathy: evidence for p27(Kip1) haplotype insufficiency. Kidney Int 2005;68(4):1583—9.

[235] Wolf G. Changing concepts of compensatory renal growth: from humoral pathology to molecular biology. Am J Nephrol 1992;12(5):369—73.

[236] Park SK, Kang SK, Lee DY, Kang MJ, Kim SH, Koh GY. Temporal expressions of cyclins and cyclin dependent kinases during renal development and compensatory growth. Kidney Int 1997;51(3):762—9.

[237] Megyesi J, Price PM, Tamayo E, Safirstein RL. The lack of a functional p21(WAF1/CIP1) gene ameliorates progression to chronic renal failure. Proc Natl Acad Sci USA 1999;96 (19):10830—5.

[238] Ingram AJ, Ly H, Thai K, Kang M, Scholey JW. Activation of mesangial cell signaling cascades in response to mechanical strain. Kidney Int 1999;55(2):476—85.

[239] Rabkin R, Fervenza FC. Renal hypertrophy and kidney disease in diabetes. Diabetes Metab Rev 1996;12(3):217—41.

[240] Wolf G. Cellular mechanisms of tubule hypertrophy and hyperplasia in renal injury. Miner Electrolyte Metab 1995;21 (4—5):303—16.

[241] Chen S, Hoffman BB, Lee JS, Kasama Y, Jim B, Kopp JB, et al. Cultured tubule cells from TGF-beta1 null mice exhibit impaired hypertrophy and fibronectin expression in high glucose. Kidney Int 2004;65(4):1191—204.

[242] Franch HA, Shay JW, Alpern RJ, Preisig PA. Involvement of pRB family in TGF beta-dependent epithelial cell hypertrophy. J Cell Biol 1995;129(1):245—54.

[243] Liu B, Preisig P. TGF-beta1-mediated hypertrophy involves inhibiting pRB phosphorylation by blocking activation of cyclin E kinase. Am J Physiol 1999;277(2 Pt 2):F186—94.

[244] Preisig P. What makes cells grow larger and how do they do it? Renal hypertrophy revisited. Exp Nephrol 1999;7(4):273—83.

[245] Wolf G, Neilson EG. Angiotensin II induces cellular hypertrophy in cultured murine proximal tubular cells. Am J Physiol 1990;259(5 Pt 2):F768—77.

[246] Wolf G, Kuncio GS, Sun MJ, Neilson EG. Expression of homeobox genes in a proximal tubular cell line derived from adult mice. Kidney Int 1991;39(5):1027—33.

[247] Burns KD, Harris RC. Signaling and growth responses of LLC-PK1/Cl4 cells transfected with the rabbit AT1 ANG II receptor. Am J Physiol 1995;268(4 Pt 1):C925—35.

[248] Wolf G, Mueller E, Stahl RA, Ziyadeh FN. Angiotensin II-induced hypertrophy of cultured murine proximal tubular cells is mediated by endogenous transforming growth factor-beta. J Clin Invest 1993;92(3):1366—72.

[249] Wolf G, Stahl RA. Angiotensin II-stimulated hypertrophy of LLC-PK1 cells depends on the induction of the cyclin-dependent kinase inhibitor p27Kip1. Kidney Int 1996;50(6): 2112—9.

[250] Wolf G, Jablonski K, Schroeder R, Reinking R, Shankland SJ, Stahl RA. Angiotensin II-induced hypertrophy of proximal tubular cells requires p27Kip1. Kidney Int 2003;64(1): 71—81.

[251] Hannken T, Schroeder R, Stahl RA, Wolf G. Angiotensin II-mediated expression of p27Kip1 and induction of cellular hypertrophy in renal tubular cells depend on the generation of oxygen radicals. Kidney Int 1998;54(6):1923—33.

[252] Hannken T, Schroeder R, Zahner G, Stahl RA, Wolf G. Reactive oxygen species stimulate p44/42 mitogen-activated protein kinase and induce p27(Kip1): role in angiotensin II-mediated hypertrophy of proximal tubular cells. J Am Soc Nephrol 2000;11(8):1387—97.

[253] Hannken T, Schroeder R, Stahl RA, Wolf G. Atrial natriuretic peptide attenuates ANG II-induced hypertrophy of renal tubular cells. Am J Physiol Renal Physiol 2001;281(1): F81−90.

[254] Wolf G, Wenzel U, Hannken T, Stahl RA. Angiotensin II induces p27(Kip1) expression in renal tubules *in vivo*: role of reactive oxygen species. J Mol Med 2001;79(7):382−9.

[255] Ruperez M, Ruiz-Ortega M, Esteban V, Lorenzo O, Mezzano S, Plaza JJ, et al. Angiotensin II increases connective tissue growth factor in the kidney. Am J Pathol 2003;163(5): 1937−47.

[256] Liu BC, Sun J, Chen Q, Ma KL, Ruan XZ, Phillips AO. Role of connective tissue growth factor in mediating hypertrophy of human proximal tubular cells induced by angiotensin II. Am J Nephrol 2003;23(6):429−37.

[257] Olbricht CJ, Geissinger B. Renal hypertrophy in streptozotocin diabetic rats: role of proteolytic lysosomal enzymes. Kidney Int 1992;41(4):966−72.

[258] Shechter P, Boner G, Rabkin R. Tubular cell protein degradation in early diabetic renal hypertrophy. J Am Soc Nephrol 1994;4(8):1582−7.

[259] Shechter P, Shi JD, Rabkin R. Renal tubular cell protein breakdown in uninephrectomized and ammonium chloride-loaded rats. J Am Soc Nephrol 1994;5(5):1201−7.

[260] Franch HA, Curtis PV, Mitch WE. Mechanisms of renal tubular cell hypertrophy: mitogen-induced suppression of proteolysis. Am J Physiol 1997;273(3 Pt 1):C843−51.

[261] Franch HA, Sooparb S, Du J, Brown NS. A mechanism regulating proteolysis of specific proteins during renal tubular cell growth. J Biol Chem 2001;276(22):19126−31.

[262] Franch HA, Preisig PA. NH4Cl-induced hypertrophy is mediated by weak base effects and is independent of cell cycle processes. Am J Physiol 1996;270(3 Pt 1):C932−8.

[263] Garibotto G, Sofia A, Robaudo C, Saffioti S, Sala MR, Verzola D, et al. Kidney protein dynamics and ammoniagenesis in humans with chronic metabolic acidosis. J Am Soc Nephrol 2004;15(6):1606−15.

[264] Ling H, Vamvakas S, Gekle M, Schaefer L, Teschner M, Schaefer RM, et al. Role of lysosomal cathepsin activities in cell hypertrophy induced by NH4Cl in cultured renal proximal tubule cells. J Am Soc Nephrol 1996;7(1):73−80.

[265] Nath KA, Hostetter MK, Hostetter TH. Increased ammoniagenesis as a determinant of progressive renal injury. Am J Kidney Dis 1991;17(6):654−7.

[266] Walsh-Reitz MM, Toback FG. Kidney epithelial cell growth is stimulated by lowering extracellular potassium concentration. Am J Physiol 1983;244(5):C429−32.

[267] Tolins JP, Hostetter MK, Hostetter TH. Hypokalemic nephropathy in the rat. Role of ammonia in chronic tubular injury. J Clin Invest 1987;79(5):1447−58.

[268] Sooparb S, Price SR, Shaoguang J, Franch HA. Suppression of chaperone-mediated autophagy in the renal cortex during acute diabetes mellitus. Kidney Int 2004;65(6):2135−44.

[269] Franch HA, Wang X, Sooparb S, Brown NS, Du J. Phosphatidylinositol 3-kinase activity is required for epidermal growth factor to suppress proteolysis. J Am Soc Nephrol 2002;13(4):903−9.

[270] Feliers D, Duraisamy S, Faulkner JL, Duch J, Lee AV, Abboud HE, et al. Activation of renal signaling pathways in *db/db* mice with type 2 diabetes. Kidney Int 2001;60(2):495−504.

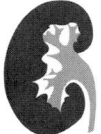

Stem Cells and Generation of New Cells in the Adult Kidney

Juan A. Oliver[1] and Qais Al-Awqati[2]

[1]Department of Medicine, Columbia University, New York, NY, USA
[2]Departments of Medicine and Physiology, Columbia University, New York, NY, USA

EMBRYONIC ORIGIN OF RENAL CELLS

The idea that the kidney is an organ needs to be tempered by the realization that it is the nephron that is the organ. Each nephron, as far as we know, is independent from other nephrons, and the kidney is to a first approximation a collection of these mini-organs put together in a complex three-dimensional assembly. The nephrons of all mammals are remarkably similar in size, function, and origin (as far as we know), and the differences among species are largely if not entirely due to the number of these units in the assembly, with mice having 10,000 and whales having 250 million in each kidney. But while the epithelial character of the nephron garners most of the attention, one needs to be reminded that the kidney has a very extensive vascular network with multiple distinct morphological and functional domains, as well as an abundant interstitial cell population that unfortunately is still poorly understood (see Kaissiling and Le Hir[1] for a review). While the taxonomy of the renal epithelial cells is nearly complete, that of the cells of the vascular and interstitial compartments awaits detailed characterization. Hence, analysis of renal regeneration after injury, as well as search for putative renal stem cells in the adult kidney, has essentially been restricted to the epithelial compartment. However, as epithelial cells are likely instructed by mesenchymal signals and epithelia-mesenchymal cross-talk is critical for renal epithelial differentiation and function,[2] there is a need for deeper understanding of the cell types that comprise the renal vascular and interstitial compartments, and their roles in kidney homeostasis and repair from injury. For example, in many organs including the kidney, mesenchymal cells with characteristics of precursor/stem cells have been found to reside near or in the vascular wall,[3–5] but the exact origin and normal function of these cells is unknown.

The different cellular compartments of the adult kidney have been traditionally recognized by their morphological characteristics or by their embryonic origin, since it was long ago recognized that the adult (metanephric) kidney derives from two distinct elements of the intermediate mesoderm: the metanephric mesenchyme and the ureteric bud. Within the kidney, the ureteric bud gives rise to the collecting duct cells, while some metanephric mesenchyme cells give rise to the rest of the nephron.[6] However, over the last few decades, the discovery of several genes that are expressed in the restricted group of cells of the renal anlage has allowed a different taxonomic approach that has greatly illuminated our understanding of the distinct cell populations in the adult kidney. Moreover, it has allowed development of research tools with which it is possible to probe in the adult kidney the function of specific cells, of specific genes in specific cells, and importantly for the present discussion, to identify the daughter cells of different cell types by *in vivo* genetic cell lineage methods. Thus, we briefly review the embryonic origin of the distinct cells in the adult kidney, emphasizing those aspects that might clarify the origin of new cells in the adult organ.

Epithelial Cells

All epithelial cells of the adult kidney are believed to derive from the intermediate mesoderm, from which both the ureteric bud (a branch of the Wolffian duct) and the metanephric mesenchyme originate. Renal

Seldin and Giebisch's The Kidney, Fifth Edition.
DOI: http://dx.doi.org/10.1016/B978-0-12-381462-3.00029-X

morphogenesis starts when the ureteric bud invades the metanephric mesenchyme and starts branching. The cells in the tip of each ureteric bud branch give rise to the collecting duct cells and the metanephric mesenchyme cells in contact with each ureteric bud tip give rise, after a series of morphogenic steps, to the cells of the remaining nephron segments spanning from the connecting tubule to the glomerulus. The ureteric bud, like the Wolffian duct, expresses the homeobox gene *HoxB7*,[7] and transgenic mice expressing *HoxB7*-GFP or *HoxB7*-Cre recombinase have been used to label most, if not all, of the cells in the ureteric bud branches of the embryonic collecting duct,[8] and their progeny in the adult kidney.

The metanephric mesenchymal cells undergo simultaneous differentiation (to generate a nephron for each ureteric bud tip) and growth, so that the appropriate number of nephrons will be generated for the branches of the ureteric bud. It was recently found that the metanephric mesenchymal cells that are in contact with the tips of the ureteric bud, referred to as the cap mesenchyme, are the progenitor cells of all nephron epithelia (except the collecting duct). These cells were found to express the transcription factors *Cited1*[9] and *Six2*,[10] thereby allowing generation of transgenic mice that label all nephron epithelial cells except those of the collecting ducts. More relevant to the present discussion is that these mice can be used to permanently identify the progeny of adult nephron epithelial cells,[9,10] thus providing an invaluable tool for analysis of epithelial cell regeneration after kidney injury and/or disease,[11] as discussed below.

Mesenchymal/Stromal Cells

Like renal epithelial cells, the vast majority of the stroma cells in the adult kidney derive from the intermediate mesoderm[12] that in the kidney gives rise to a cell population that expresses the forkhead transcription factor *Foxd1*.[2,13,14] These cells generate many renal interstitial cells, as well as mesangial cells, vascular smooth muscle, pericytes, and renal capsule, and likely mesenchymal stem cells.[5] *Foxd1*-expressing cells are absolutely required for normal kidney development,[2,13,14] and their adult progeny is of extreme interest because it likely contains pluripotent MSC[5] and pericytes,[4] although a clear-cut distinction between these two cell types is not yet possible. In addition, identification of *Foxd1* as marker of these cells has made it possible to develop transgenic mice that can be used to label the stroma cell progeny in the adult kidney.[15]

Another population of renal stromal cells derives from the paraxial mesoderm,[16] but the precise contribution of these cells to the interstitial and mesenchymal cell populations of the adult kidney remains to be defined. Finally, an area of the intermediate mesoderm located ventro—lateral to the dorsal aorta generates renal interstitial cells that express the stem cell factor receptor (*c-kit*).[17] During embryogenesis, these cells appear to be involved in the maintenance of the metanephric mesenchyme-derived cells, but identification of their progeny in the adult kidney remains to be established.

Endothelial Cells

The renal circulation is both anatomically and functionally complex, and likely contains many types of endothelial cells. Their exact origin is still poorly-understood. It is clear that once kidney development starts, the renal anlage contains angioblats[18,19] that give rise to endothelial cells. It is currently unknown whether these endothelial precursors migrate into the developing kidney or differentiated from cells that reside in the metanephric mesenchyme. The latter appears more likely, as we found that many cells in the renal anlage express tyrosine kinases that are characteristic of adult endothelial cells.[20] Interestingly, in addition to being endothelial precursors, angioblasts in the renal anlage appear to provide signals important for development and differentiation of the metanephric mesenchyme.[21] It is currently unknown if there exists interaction in the adult kidney between endothelial cells and either interstitial or epithelial cells that might be involved in maintaining kidney homeostasis or repair from injury. Recent work by Lin et al.[22] suggests that endothelial-to-pericyte cross-talk is involved in the generation of kidney myofibroblats, as detailed below.

NEW CELLS IN THE ADULT KIDNEY

Normal Conditions

As assayed by a variety of methods, the normal adult kidney has a low rate of cellular proliferation.[23–26] Using antibodies to Ki67, a nuclear protein expressed in cycling cells during G0 and G1, between 0.4—1% of all cells were cycling in the adult rat kidney.[24,25] Interestingly, age has a profound effect in the abundance of proliferating cells found in the kidney. Vogesterder et al.[25] found that while only ~0.4% of all renal cells were positive for Ki67 in the kidneys of 16- to 20-week-old rats, in animals that were only 4 weeks old the number of cycling cells was ~5%. This suggests that in the kidney there is an age-dependent progressive decline in the number of cycling cells, and that workers examining renal cell proliferation should take into account the age of the animal as an important variable.

Proliferating cells in the renal cortex of 4-week-old rats were found preferentially located to the S3 segment of the proximal tubule, when compared to the S1 and S2 segments.[25] This interesting result might have important implications in designing strategies to identify renal stem cells, a subject to which we will return below. In contrast, in 1-year-old rats, we found that most of the kidney parenchyma had a homogeneous fraction of ~1% of Ki67 positive cells Figure 29.1. There were two exceptions to this, however, the body of the papilla where there were extremely low numbers of cycling cells (<0.1% of the cells were positive for Ki67), and the upper part of the papilla (at the papilla—medullary junction), where we found the highest frequency of cycling cells (~2.5%),[24] indicating that it is an area of privileged cellular proliferation in the adult rat. Detailed morphological observations indicate that terminally differentiated tubular epithelia cells can generate new cells,[27,28] but these observations don't exclude the possibility that there are epithelial stem cells.

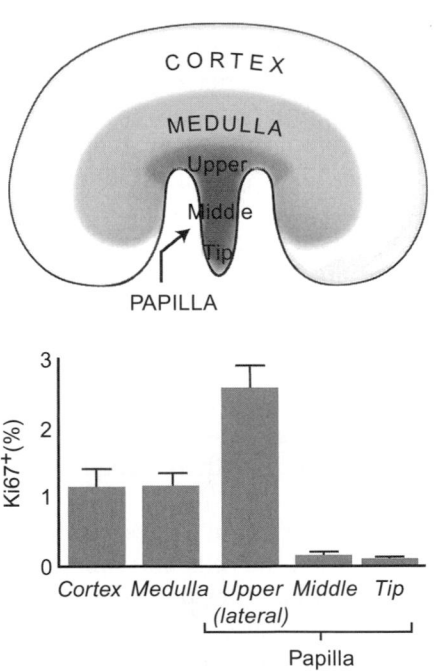

FIGURE 29.1 Cellular proliferation in adult kidney. Top: Kidney regions were examined for cellular proliferation. Bottom: Fraction of Ki67-positive cells in different kidney regions. Cortex and medulla had a similar number of Ki67-positive cells, but the lateral side of the papilla had significantly more Ki67-positive cells than the cortex and medulla, as well as the other regions of the papilla. The middle and tip of the papilla had significantly fewer Ki67 positive cells than other regions of the kidney. *(From ref. [27].)*

Organ Repair from Injury

In contrast to normal conditions, the kidney displays a remarkable proliferation capacity shortly after transient injury. For example, injury induced by 30—45 minutes of complete renal artery occlusion in rodents causes functional failure, and widespread cellular apoptosis and necrosis that are followed by diffuse cellular proliferation and functional recovery. What is the origin of these new cells? While the kidney has multiple cell types, studies on the generation of new cells after injury have fundamentally focused on the epithelial cells, likely because of their better-understood functional importance and easier identification. It is now established that the new epithelial cells after kidney injury develop from within the parenchyma, rather than being derived from extrarenal sources such as the bone marrow,[29,30] and thus three possibilities appear likely: (1) any surviving terminally differentiated epithelial cell can generate identical cells; (2) there exist kidney epithelial stem cells capable of generating any epithelial cell type, similar to what was found in the interfollicular epidermis;[31,32] and (3) pluripotent renal stem cells generate epithelial as well as other cell types, as in the case of the stem cells in the bulge of the skin.[33—36]

Morphological observations[35,37] and functional studies with nucleotide analogs[27,38] have provided strong evidence that terminally-differentiated epithelial cells generate new epithelial cells after injury. More recent elegant genetic cell fate-mapping studies have confirmed this suspicion; Humpreys et al.[11] used reporter mice in which the renal epithelial cell compartment was labeled by a Cre recombinase driven by the promoter of *Six2*, a gene that is specifically expressed in embryonic epithelial precursors (see above), and examined their response to acute kidney injury. They found that injury induced massive cellular proliferation, and that all new epithelial cells expressed the reporter gene (Figure 29.2). Since RT-PCR of adult kidney tissue could neither detect *Six2* nor *Cre*, it is apparent that the labeled cells originated from epithelial cells labeled previously during kidney development, thus excluding the interstitial/stroma cell compartment as the origin of new epithelial cells. Needless to say, this experiment does not address whether there exists a group of restricted epithelial cells that are responsible for all the new epithelia generated after injury; these cells could function as adult renal epithelial stem cells. In a recent study, Humphreys et al.[39] examined this possibility by labeling cycling cells after transient kidney injury with two different thymidine analogs administered sequentially. Since the number of epithelial cells that were positive for both nucleotides was very low, these workers concluded that surviving epithelial cells repopulate the nephron epithelium in a stochastic manner,

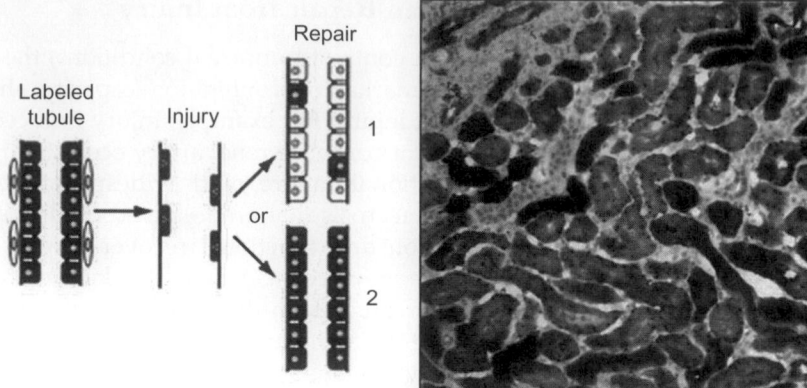

FIGURE 29.2   Surviving epithelial cells after injury generate new epithelial cells. (Left) New cells after acute kidney injury in mice with genetically labeled epithelial tubules will not carry the label if they derive from cells outside the epithelial cell compartment (#1), but will carry the label if they derive from terminally differentiated epithelial cells (#2). (Right) Fifteen days after transient ischemic injury and repair, there was no dilution on the number of labeled cells (dark) despite marked cellular proliferation, indicating that they derived from epithelial cells. *(From ref. [14].)* See color plate section at the back of the book.

suggesting that the nephron epithelia has no stem cells.[39] However, while control experiments clearly showed appropriate specificity of both antibodies, detection of closely related thymidine analogs during conditions that, unlike in the control experiments, probably result in incorporation of very different amounts of the two analogs in a given cell are fraught with potential problems. More importantly, their conclusion is based on the implicit assumption that a putative population of epithelial stem cells would be a small fraction of the total number of cells. Under these conditions, to repopulate the damaged epithelia the stem cell progeny would need to divide rapidly, and would thus incorporate both nucleotide analogs. However, as detailed below, stem cells in *Drosophila* Malpighian tubules are a very large fraction of the total cells, and there is no reason why this may not also be the case in mammalian kidneys. Similarly, in organs other than the kidney such as the adult airway epithelia, stem cells account for about one-third of the total number of cells.[40,41]

Identification of the site where cellular proliferation first starts after transient injury could potentially facilitate identification of precursor/stem cells. Unfortunately, for most insults that cause acute kidney injury with functional failure, cellular proliferation has most often been examined one or a few days afterwards, at which time cell proliferation, while very prominent in the S3 segment of the proximal tubule, is also widespread in other parts of the kidney parenchyma, particularly the medulla.[38,42–44]

Following acute kidney injury by renal artery occlusion we could not detect proliferating cells until ~24 hours later when we examined kidney sections of ~5 μm thickness, as is done routinely. However, with 100 μm vibrotome sections, one hour after injury we found that the upper part of the papilla had more proliferative cells than other parts of the kidney[24] (see Figure 29.3), suggesting that this is the site of initial cellular proliferation after kidney injury, which we previously found to be the site of enhanced cell cycling under normal conditions (see above). Interestingly, Vinsonneau et al.[45] reported that the first cells that they found cycling after ischemia reperfusion injury to the kidney were uro-epithelial cells in the upper part of the urinary (intrarenal) space and neighboring interstitial cells; detailed analysis with Ki67 and BrdU incorporation showed that these cells were proliferating ~16 hours after ischemic injury and ~4 hours before proliferation could be detected elsewhere in the kidney. The site identified by Vinsonneau et al.[45] is where the base of the papilla attaches to the medulla, it is in close proximity to the cortex, and appears to be the same proliferating site we identified in the upper papilla. Needless to say, identification of these "early" proliferating cells and of their progeny would be of extreme interest.

An additional observation merits mention. In the few studies that identified the cells that first started proliferating after injury, either after transient ischemic injury[44] or aminoglycoside toxicity,[46,47] it is remarkable that in all instances they were interstitial cells, perhaps suggesting that some interstitial cell plays a critical role in initiating epithelial regeneration. Indeed, the likelihood of renal functional recovery after injury was found to correlate with increases in the number of interstitial cells, many of which were likely myofibroblasts.[43,48,49] Although these results raise the possibility that myofibroblasts might be involved in epithelial regeneration, other interstitial cells such as macrophages are known

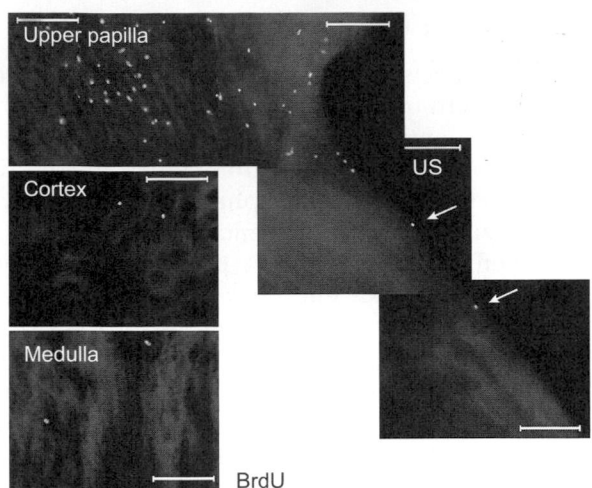

BrdU

FIGURE 29.3 Cellular proliferation was first detected in the upper papilla following kidney injury. There was a selective increase of cells in S-phase in the upper papilla during the first hour after transient ischemic injury. Note abundant BrdU-labeled cells in the upper papilla, whereas the cortex and medulla revealed very rare BrdU-labeled cells (US: urinary space). Photomicrographs were done in 100 μm tissue sections obtained with a vibratome.*(From ref. [27].)* See color plate section at the back of the book.

to be involved in kidney repair,[50] and a detailed characterization of the interstitial cell compartment following transient kidney injury is lacking.

Effect of Age

For many organs, including the kidney,[51] the capacity to recover from injury decreases with age, an observation familiar to most practicing nephrologists. In most organs, it remains to be determined whether this is due to a decrease in the number of organ-specific stem cells or to the inability of the stem cells to be activated, but recent work suggest that the latter is more likely (reviewed by Liu and Rando[52]). For example, it was recently found that aging muscle had a normal number of satellite cells, but the cells failed to activate in response to exercise.[53] Interestingly, progenitor/stem cells in advanced age can display a "young" response by exposure to a young systemic environment,[54] indicating that the changes responsible for the functional decrease of precursor/stem cells are potentially reversible.

While the effect of age on the renal proliferative capacity after injury has not been studied in detail, it appears that cell proliferation after acute kidney injury decreases with age,[55] in agreement with the poor prognosis of recovery from acute kidney injury in elderly patients.[51] Mechanisms that could account for these observations include telomere shortening[56] and increased expression by renal epithelial cells of

zinc-α^2-glycoprotein (Zag), an adipokine associated with cachexia.[58] To examine whether the poor regenerative capacity of the aging kidney is due to a decrease in the numbers or in the functionality of putative renal stem/progenitor cells awaits definitive identification of these cells.

In sum, both during normal conditions and particularly after transient kidney injury, the S3 segment of the proximal tubule is a site of intense cell proliferation, suggesting the presence of progenitor cells in this part of the nephron. In addition, the upper part of the papilla and close to the urinary space is also a site of robust cell cycling, both under normal conditions[24] and after transient kidney injury.[24,45]

IDENTIFICATION OF POTENTIAL PRECURSOR/STEM CELLS IN THE ADULT KIDNEY

Studies from several laboratories have presented evidence characterizing renal precursor cells in the adult kidney, but none of these cells meet strict criteria for traditional adult, organ-specific stem cells; i.e., asymmetric cell division and multipotency. Nonetheless, since our ultimate aim is to understand the origin of new cells in the adult kidney so that the responsible mechanisms might be manipulated, these studies are worth reviewing. In addition, the results of these studies are likely to be useful for future work to identify adult renal stem cells. Several strategies have been used to identify and characterize adult kidney precursor/stem cells, and the robustness of the obtained results varies widely. In our view, the methodological approach used for cell identification and/or isolation of the cells best separates these studies.

Cellular Markers

Several workers have isolated cells from the adult kidney using a candidate gene approach. For example, Busolatti et al.[59] used the transmembrane glycoprotein Cd133, which is expressed in hematopoietic stem cells, endothelial progenitor cells, neuronal, glial, and glioblastoma stem cells, as well as some other cell types (see Mizrak et al.[60] for a review), to select cells from the adult human kidney. The isolated cells showed strong clonogenic capacity, and when subcutaneously transplanted to SCID mice formed tubules which expressed some renal epithelial markers. Finally, when the cells were injected intravenously into mice with glycerol-mediated acute kidney injury, they integrated into tubules. However, the functional significance of the integration was not explored.

Using a somewhat similar approach, Dekel et al.[61] used Sca-1, a protein identified in several progenitor cells, to isolate a cell population from mouse kidneys. However, because Sca-1 is also expressed in renal epithelia, these workers used a collagenase digestion approach that appeared to yield interstitial cells. The *in vitro* differentiation of these cells suggested that they were mesenchymal-like stem cells, since they differentiated into myogenic, osteogenic, adipogenic, and neural lineages. When injected into kidneys with acute kidney injury, they also incorporated into tubules.

In Vitro Growth Behavior

Several laboratories have isolated cells from adult kidneys based on their characteristics when cultured *in vitro*. For example, cells were selected because of their high clonogenic potential, ability to outlast all other cultured cells or their ability to change their phenotype. For example, Gupta et al.,[62] cultured cells from collagenase digested rat kidneys, and after ~5 weeks in culture they obtained a cell population with substantial proliferative potential (which in fact was the characteristic that lead to isolation of the cells) and expressing transcription factors such as *Pax-2* and *Oct4* that are either involved in renal development or in determining cell fate. When the cells were injected into the subcapsular space of normal kidneys, some of them incorporated into tubules.

Kitamura et al.[63] used a slightly different strategy by isolating single nephrons from adult rat kidneys and culturing them *in vitro*. Cells growing out from these nephrons were harvested and individually cultured; and the clone with the fastest proliferation capacity was characterized. These clonal cells expressed several proteins important in kidney development and proteins characteristic of mature nephrons. When the cells were injected in the subcapsular region of a kidney with acute kidney injury, the cells engrafted into renal tubules.

More recently, Lee et al.[64] used a mouse with a targeted mutation in which GFP is expressed under the control of *Myh9*, a gene expressed in interstitial cells (among others). After isolation of the GFP⁺ cells from the kidney and subsequent culture for eight weeks, they isolated a cell line that expressed renal embryonic or stem cell markers such as *Oct-4*, *Pax-2*, *Wnt-4*, and *WT-1*. Immunolocation of the endogenous Oct-4⁺ and GFP⁺ cells in the kidney found them in the interstitial space of the medulla and papilla. Finally, when the cells were injected directly into kidneys after acute kidney injury, they incorporated into tubules and partially decreased the functional consequences of the injury.

In Vivo Growth Behavior

The hypothesis that adult, organ-specific stem cells divide infrequently has been a powerful tool in locating and identifying several stem/precursor cells. According to this hypothesis, due to their low cycling behavior, stem cells retain S-phase labels (traditionally ³H-Thymidine or a thymidine analog such as BrdU) when given as a short pulse followed by a long time of chase. Recent work has, however, demonstrated that there is more complexity than originally thought[65–67] (see Fuchs[68] for an informed discussion), as not all stem cells are low cycling and "label retention" experiments identify a heterogeneous group of cells. Nonetheless, populations of "label-retaining cells" from several organs are enriched for stem cells,[66,69–72] and identification of a "label-retaining" group of cells is of great interest. To detect low cycling cells, an S-phase label is only administered during a short period of intense growth (e.g., embryonic life or shortly after birth), so that all cells are cycling and incorporate the label; during the subsequent period of chase the label is diluted and lost by the progeny of dividing cells and selectively retained by low- or non-cycling cells. Cells cycling infrequently were thus named "label-retaining cells" (LRC). Several investigators have used this approach in the kidney.

Maeshima et al.[38] administered BrdU for one week to adult rats that were then "chased" for two weeks, and found that there were many BrdU-retaining cells the kidney parenchyma, particularly in the proximal tubules. Following transient ischemic injury, most of the tubular cells that were proliferating (expressing proliferating nuclear antigen; PCNA) were also BrdU-labeled cells. These results led Maeshima et al.[38] to conclude that a "label-retaining" cell population was the precursor of new cells during kidney repair from injury. However, the long pulse and short period of chase complicate the interpretation of these results. In addition, the increased number of BrdU-labeled cells after injury was likely due to detection of the cells loaded with BrdU during the "pulse" plus their immediate progeny after injury. Nonetheless, because a relatively small population of cells were labeled during the one-week "pulse" and many of these cells were also PCNA positive after injury, this experiment suggests that both during normal conditions and during repair from injury a group of renal epithelial cells cycles at a much higher frequency that most other epithelial cells. This raises the possibility that these cells could be adult, renal epithelial precursors.

We exploited the low cycling frequency of adult stem cells by giving BrdU to newborn rats or mice during a short pulse, and "chased" the animals to adulthood.[73] In addition, to circumvent the use of BrdU, we[24] also followed the suggestion of Tumbar et al.[74] and used transgenic mice that expressed a fusion protein of histone 2B and GFP (referred as H2B-GFP mice) under the control of a tetracycline-responsive element. Pregnant females given doxycycline give birth to pups where all cells are GFP+ cells, but when these pups are chased to adulthood, only low-cycling cells remain GFP+. As shown in the Figure 29.4, after 2−3 months of chase, label-retaining cells were only found in the kidney papilla. When isolated, the cells showed pluripotency and, like other stem cells, formed spheres.[24,73]

Under normal conditions, most of these papillary label-retaining cells (LRC) in the adult kidney are, unsurprisingly, in growth arrest, but we found in the upper papilla a small population of them that were cycling[24] (see Figure 29.5), indicating that they generate new cells and explaining that the number of papillary LRC slowly decreased with age. In marked contrast to the normally low-cycling frequency of the papillary LRC, many of these cells proliferated shortly after acute kidney injury, likely generating many daughter cells, since after a few weeks the S-phase label disappeared from the papilla (see Figure 29.6). Hence, the cells we identified in the kidney papilla showed two cycling characteristics: first, during normal homeostasis, the cells are low-cycling (and thus they are LRC) except for a small population of them that are cycling in the upper papilla; second, and in marked contrast to normal conditions, may of the papillary LRC start cycling shortly after injury. These results strongly suggest that the population of LRC of the kidney papilla is involved in kidney repair, and that within the LRC cells are renal stem/precursor cells.

Because the renal capsule contains a population of nestin-expressing cells,[75] and this intermediate filament protein has been found in a variety of precursor cells,[76] Park and co-workers[77] searched for low-cycling cells in this part of the kidney. They administered a short pulse of BrdU to 4-week-old mice, and followed the pulse by a chase period of two months. They found that the kidney capsule had a sparse population of BrdU-retaining cells which further characterization showed them to be CD29+, Sca-1+, vimentin+, and nestin+, but that did not express hematopoietic or endothelial markers. These cells showed marked proliferative and clonogenic capacities, and could differentiate towards adipogenic, chondrogenic, and osteogenic lineages, suggesting that they were MSC or MSC-like. The function of these cells *in vivo* remains unknown, and it would be of great interests to determine whether kidney injury induces their proliferation.

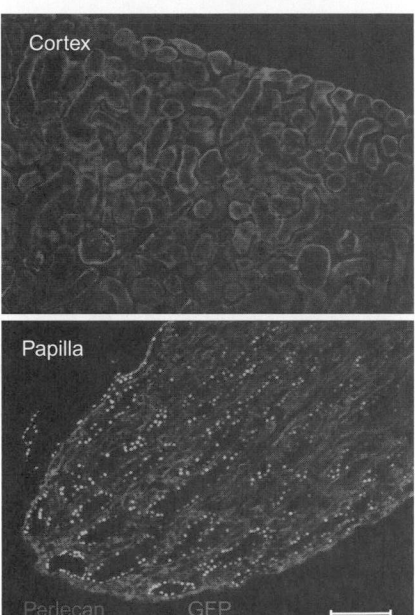

FIGURE 29.4 Papillary LRCs in mice expressing histone 2B-GFP. The kidney of an 11-week-old mouse pulsed with doxycycline during embryonic life showed low cycling cells (i.e., GFP- retaining) in the papilla but not the cortex or medulla. *(From ref. [27].) See color section at the end of the book.*

Cellular Function

Since first used to enrich for hematopoietic stem cells,[78−80] the *Side Population* discrimination assay has been used to identify stem cells and progenitor cells in a variety of organs and tumors.[81] The assay can be useful when stem cell-specific markers are not available, and it is based on the differential ability of cells to efflux a lipophilic fluorescent dye via the ATP-binding cassette transporter protein ABCG2. Many stem/precursor cells rapidly efflux the Hoechst 33342 dye, a process that can be blocked with ABC transporter inhibitors. By flow cytometry, such cells are recognized as being "Hoechst low" (versus "Hoechst high") and as they are a very small fraction of the total cells, they were termed side population (SP) cells. Because the assay is dependent on normal cellular metabolic function in freshly isolated cells, it is extremely challenging (for a detailed discussion see Golebiewska et al.[81]), and uncertainty exists about the significance of some of the results. Nonetheless several workers have isolated SP cells from the adult kidney.[82−85] The frequency of these cells has been reported to vary from ~5%[84] to ~0.1%.[83,85] In one study, exogenous administration of the isolated cells to mice with cisplatin-induced acute kidney injury improved the kidney's functional response.[84] These provocative results need further analysis, particularly because the SP of the kidney

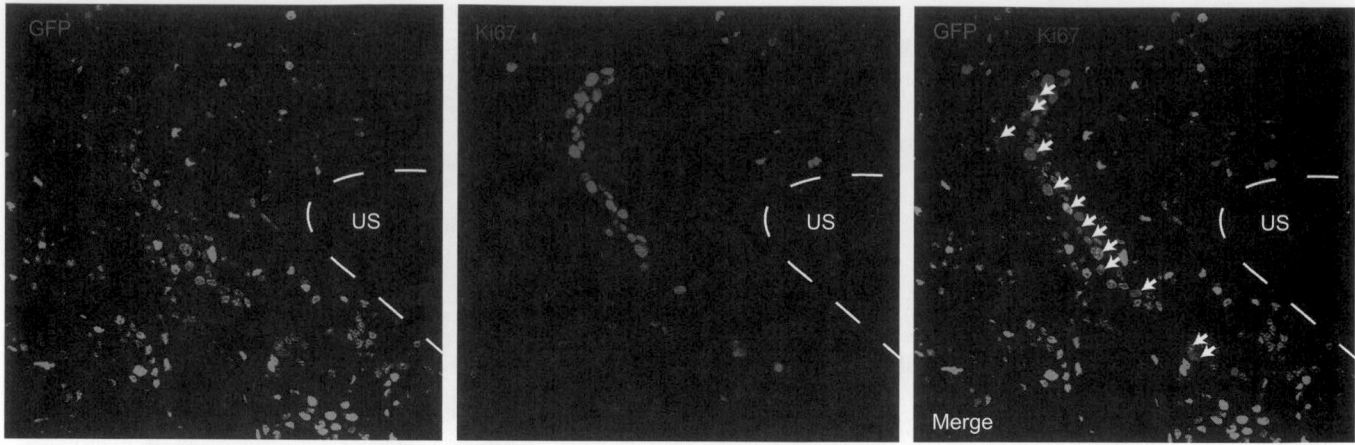

FIGURE 29.5 **LRC in the upper papilla from chains of proliferating cells.** LRCs (GFP+: top) and proliferating cells (Ki67-positive: middle) in the upper papilla. The merged image shows that several cells are positive for both Ki67 and GFP (arrows). Broken white line depicts papillary edge (US: urinary space). *(From ref. [27].)* See color section at the end of the book.

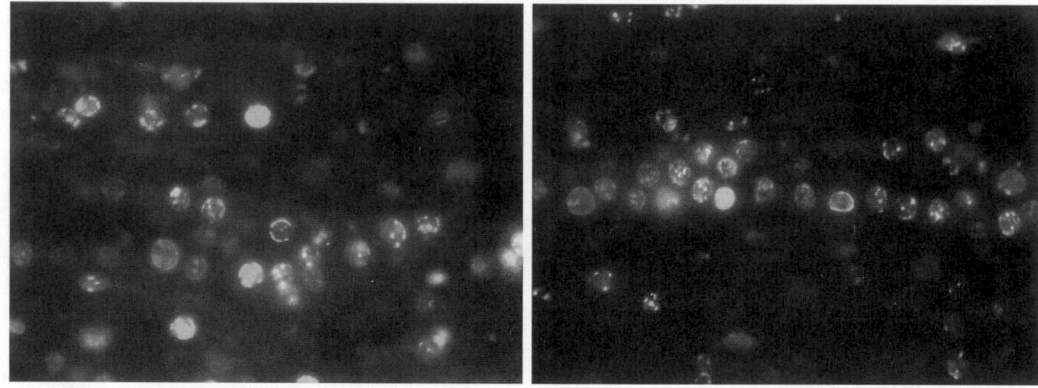

FIGURE 29.6 **Proliferation of papillary LRC after transient ischemic injury.** Cellular proliferation of papillary LRC after transient renal ischemia. Thirty-six hours after ischemic injury, many LRC of the papilla (FITC fluorescin) were cycling and labeled by a Ki67 antibody (rhodamine) (Scale bars: 50 μm). *(From ref. [76].)* See color section at the end of the book.

appears to show considerable heterogeneity.[83] However, the kidney is a transporting organ with a large number of ABC-type transporters expressed in several of its segments including ABCG2, the putative transporter of the Hoechst33342 dye. Hence, the presence of cells that pump the dye out may not be the best marker for progenitor cells.

Another cellular function that has been exploited to isolate putative renal stem/precursor cells is the *aldehyde dehydrogenase activity* (ALDH). This enzyme oxidizes intracellular aldehydes (for a review see Sophos and Vasiliou[86]), and it is believed to have a role in cellular differentiation by its ability to oxidize retinol to retinoic acid.[87] Hematopoietic, neural, and some cancer stem/precuror cells were found to have high ALDH enzymatic activity.[88] Similarly, Lindgren et al.[89] recently isolated from the human kidneys cells with progenitor characteristics. Using an ALDH enzymatic

assay in suspensions of renal cortical cells deprived of glomeruli, they separated the cells into ALDH^low and ALDH^high populations. Interestingly, transcription analysis of the populations showed that one of the most upregulated genes in the ALDH^high cells was Cd133, a membrane protein found in some progenitor/stem cells and used to isolate other renal progenitors (see above and the section on podocyte precursors next). *In vitro*, the cells showed some stem/precursor cell characteristics, but of particular interest is their finding by immunohistochemistry that there is a population of Cd133-positive cells scattered through the proximal tubule, clearly showing that there is some heterogeneity in the proximal tubular cells. Analyses of kidney biopsies of patients with acute tubular necrosis showed that in areas of regeneration tubular cells positive for Cd133 in their luminal membrane were frequently found to be also positive for vimentin in their basolateral membrane. Since tubular epithelial cells expressing vimentin have been observed during the recovery phase of acute kidney injury,[90,91] it is possible that these Cd133- and vimentin-expressing cells might be specialized epithelial precursors.

Podocyte Precursors

It had long been assumed that in adult kidneys podocytes, the specialized epithelial cells that surround the glomerular capillary loops, have extremely low or no cycling activity. Yet, these cells are clearly renewed because they can be captured in the urine of normal subjects.[92] Interest in the origin of podocytes and their life cycle has been spurred by observations that their numbers can decrease during diseases caused by several mutations that disrupt their proteins, leading to glomerular sclerosis (reviewed by D'Agati[93]). In addition, it was recently found that a variable fraction of the cells in the glomerular "crescents" (layers of abnormal cells attached to the Bowman's capsule) often present in glomerulonephritis were found to express nestin.[94] Since normal podocytes express nestin, these results raised the possibility that cells in crescents might derive from podocytes or that podocytes and cells in crescents share a common lineage. Regardless, these interesting observations suggested that both podocyte loss and/or their uncontrolled proliferation might be involved in renal diseases.

Analyzing human kidney sections, Sagrinati et al.[95] found that a subpopulation of the parietal epithelial cells of Bowman's capsule expressed Cd24 and Cd133, two cell surface proteins found in a variety of adult stem cells. Isolation of these cells from glomerular cultures showed them to possess high cloning efficiency and some differentiation potential. In addition, when the cells were intravenously administered to mice with acute kidney injury, there was improvement in the morphological and functional renal response.[95,96] The observation that some epithelial cells in the parietal side of the Bowman's capsule had progenitor characteristics led to the hypothesis that these cells could be podocyte precursors.[97,98] With this in mind, Ronconi et al.[98] analyzed human kidneys sections, and confirmed that a group of cells in the parietal epithelia of the Bowman's capsule expressed Cd133 and Cd24 and that, in contrast, fully differentiated podocytes only expressed proteins used to identify them such as nestin, complement receptor-1, and podocalyxin. Interestingly, they also identified a third cell population that expressed Cd133, Cd24, and podocyte markers, suggesting that it could be a podocyte precursor. Isolation of these three different cell populations by FACS using Cd133, Cd24, and podocalyxin and their culture *in vitro* showed that a cell clone derived from a cell only positive for Cd133 and Cd24 contained cells that expressed both tubular epithelial markers and podocyte markers. In contrast, clones of cells derived from cells positive for Cd133, Cd24 plus podocalyxin only expressed podocyte markers. When these two different types of cells were intravenously administered to mice that had received the podocyte toxin adriamycin, they found that cells only positive for Cd133 and Cd24, but not cells positive for Cd133, Cd24, and podocalyxin, were capable of reducing urinary protein excretion and morphologic damage. Finally, labeling the cells with vital dyes showed that the former, but not the latter, localized to glomeruli. These results were interpreted as indicating that in adult kidney, podocytes derive from a precursor cell population that resides in the parietal epithelium of Bowman's capsule. One might conclude that the study shows heterogeneity in the parietal epithelial cells of Bowman's capsule, and that *in vitro* these cell types express different genes. The mechanism responsible for the functional recovery after cell injection and its significance is harder to define, since the large majority of epithelial cells administered intravenously are likely to lodge into the lung vascular bed.

The hypothesis that parietal epithelial cells might migrate into the glomerular capillaries and differentiate into podocytes was also examined by Appel et al.[97] in a detailed and elegant study. These authors reported that in adult rats, cells that had morphological characteristics of both glomerular parietal epithelial cells and podocytes could be detected by electron microscopy in the glomerular vascular stacks. That these cells could be transitional cells between parietal epithelial cells and podocytes was examined in 10-day-old mice with a variety of approaches. By immune-detection they found that some cells had markers of both parietal epithelial cells and podocytes. Administration of BrdU to young rats for two weeks showed that, while a substantial number of parietal epithelial cells were labeled with BrdU, only ~0.5% of podocytes were labeled. However, as the animals aged, the number of BrdU$^+$ parietal epithelial cells decreased, while that of BrdU$^+$ podocytes increased, suggesting that the latter derived from the former. In a final genetic fate-mapping experiment, these workers generated triple-transgenic mice in which labeling of the parietal epithelial cells and their progeny could be temporarily controlled by doxycycline administration. In 5-day-old and 10-day-old mice they found that the number of podocytes that derived from parietal epithelial cells increased as the animals aged. This elegant study provides strong evidence that podocytes derive from parietal epithelial cells, at least in the young. This is a very exciting result, because even if this process only occurs at very young ages, understanding of its controlling mechanisms might allow its modulation. An additional conclusion appears also important; it is clear that as our understanding of the homeostasis of the renal cell populations advances, the distinction between embryonic and adult lives is becoming less clear-cut than previously believed (i.e., "development" appears to be a life-long process), a subject to which we return below.

Because a variety of glomerulonephritis types are associated with hyperplasia of Bowman's capsule (a histological finding long ago termed "crescents"), the possibility that unregulated proliferation of a precursor cell could be responsible for their generation was examined. In a study of human kidney biopsies, the hypercellular lesions of crescentic glomerulonephritis were analyzed with antibodies and RT-PCR after laser capture of the lesions.[99] The authors found that these lesions contained three kinds of cells: Cd133[+], Cd24[+], podocalyxin[−] and nestin[−] (presumed podocyte precursors), Cd133[+], Cd24[+], podocalyxin[+] and nestin[+] (named intermediate cells), and finally, Cd133[−], Cd24[−] but podocalyxin[+] and nestin[+] (same profile as that of differentiated podocytes). When the lesions were examined for the presence of proliferating cells with a Ki67 antibody, most of the cells that were cycling were only positive for Cd133[+], Cd24[+]. Further, in vitro, Cd133[+], Cd24[+], podocalyxin[−] and nestin[−] cells responded robustly to TGFβ induction of extracellular proteins. These results were taken as evidence that generation of glomerular crescents is likely due to proliferation of "podocyte progenitors." In a related experimental study, Smeets et al.[100] induced crescentic glomerulonephritis in triple-transgenic mice in which parietal epithelial cells and their progeny could be labeled by the administration of doxycycline. In these mice, "crescents" could be detected to be positive by enzymatic X-gal staining, strongly suggesting that these cells derived from epithelial cells of the Bowman's capsule. In contrast, podocyte genetic labeling experiments did not show that the cells in the crescents derived from podocytes. These interesting results strongly suggest that some cells in the parietal epithelium of the Bowman's capsule, and not the podocytes, proliferate in response to injury.

However, in a fascinating study, Ding et al.[101] found that deletion of the product of the von Hippel-Lindau gene (Vhlh, encoding VHL) specifically in podocytes caused glomerulonephritis with crescent formation. Loss of VHL stabilizes the hypoxia-inducible factor (HIF) α-subunit and activates hypoxia-response genes. Of great interest is their finding that the cells in the crescents were derived from podocytes; this was elegantly shown by laser-capture of the crescents and PCR demonstrating the rearrangement of the genomic DNA induced in the podocytes (a tour de force control experiment which unfortunately is rarely done). In addition, because the gene expression profile revealed induction of Cxcr4 expression in glomeruli, Ding and co-workers overexpressed this receptor in podocytes; this resulted in podocyte proliferation and glomerulonephritis. This extremely interesting study therefore indicates that under some conditions, podocytes can proliferate, likely by the effect of Cxcl12 (SDF-1) the ligand of Cxcr4, and that their proliferation can lead to "crescent" formation.

Renal Mesenchymal Stem Cells and/or Pericytes

Mesenchymal stem cells (MSC) from the bone marrow were originally characterized by their ability to adhere to culture surfaces and when cultured with appropriate differentiation media, by their differentiation potential into adipocytes, osteoblasts, chondrocytes, and, sometimes, myoblasts. In other organs including the kidneys, MSC identification and characterization remains to be formalized, since they might be a heterogeneous population that expresses a variety of cell surface markers.[5] Nonetheless, there is widespread interest in MSC because, in addition to their differentiation potential, they appear to be present in most if not all organs[4,5] including the kidney,[5,102] and their precise function remains to be defined. They preferentially locate in the perivascular space[4,5] of even large blood vessels such as the aorta and vena cava,[5] and have pericyte-like characteristics.[3] In the kidney, mesangial cells also have MSC-like characteristics,[5] and might be the glomerular cells that express Cd146[+] and Cd133[−] found by Bruno et al.[103] in glomeruli. Because of their perivascular location and mesenchymal origin, pericytes are difficult to distinguish from MSCs, and how these two cells differ and relate is still poorly-understood. Although true renal pericytes can only be unambiguously identified by their anatomical location surrounding capillary endothelial cells, these cells have been implicated in myofibroblast generation during renal fibrogenesis,[15] and are discussed in detail below. In organs other than the kidney, pericytes have been found to have MSC-like characteristics,[104] and in the most detailed study to date, perivascular cells from skeletal muscle, bone marrow, and adipose tissue were found to express several pericyte markers, as well as MSC markers and MSC differentiation potential,[4] suggesting that MSC and pericytes might be the same cells in different locations. It has been shown that during tooth growth and in response to injury, pericytes can give rise to MSC, although in the same organ MSC have an additional, pericyte-independent origin,[105] so that lineage analysis between MSC and pericytes is likely to be complex. In the kidney, mesangial cells, vascular smooth muscle, pericytes, and likely, MSC derive from the *Foxd1* embryonic cellular compartment described above but as stated, the exact relationship among these different cells remains to be defined.

It is currently unknown whether renal pericytes/ MSCs generate daughter cells important for normal kidney homeostasis or for repair from injury. However, recent studies showing that pericytes characterized as Cd73[+], platelet-derived growth factor receptor[+] and smooth muscle actin negative, give rise to myofibroblasts during renal fibrosis[15] have generated a great deal of interest, a finding that we discuss below. However, morphological observations indicating the transient presence of myofibroblasts after transient kidney injury[43,106] suggest that these cells, long studied from a pathogenic perspective, might also be involved in organ repair, a possibility that we believe deserves attention. Regardless, since like other organs, the kidney contains perivascular cells that are pericytes, MSC or their immediate progenitors,[15] their full characterization and role in normal renal homeostasis and if any, in organ repair from injury, would be of great interest.

POTENTIAL SITES HARBORING RENAL STEM CELLS

Given the kidney's anatomical complexity, identification of stem cells within it might be facilitated by focusing on sites that might harbor them. Several strategies are possible to locate candidate sites, but we believe that current evidence already suggests the presence of sites likely to contain stem cells.

Highly Proliferative Regions

Because many adult stem cells are low-cycling (see [37] and [107] for recent reviews), to generate needed new cells they frequently give rise to an immediate progeny that experience several "transit amplifying" (TA) divisions prior to their differentiation. In this way, many new cells can be regenerated from infrequent stem cell cycling. Hence, adult stem cells can be located close to sites of increased cell cycling. Indeed a seminal discovery in this field showed that there was postnatal neurogenesis in the granular zone of the dentate gyrus in the hippocampus,[57] and led to the discovery that the subgranular zone harbored neural stem cells (reviewed in Zhao et al.[108]). Hence, proliferative regions during normal homeostasis or after kidney injury are good candidates to harbor renal stem cells.

After nephrogenesis is completed in young rats and during normal homeostasis, it was found that the S3 segment of the proximal tubule displayed high cycling activity[25,28]: over a two-week period in 4-week-old rats, 90% of the cells of the S3 segment had cycled, a remarkable rate of proliferation. While this may reflect morphogenetic requirements of a growing kidney, the high proliferative capacity of these cells raises the possibility that they could be "transit amplifying" daughter cells of a proximal tubule stem cell. Other findings support that the S3 segment of the proximal tubule might contain stem cells. Shortly after several types of kidney injury, high proliferation activity was particularly prominent in cells from the S3 segment.[25,42,43] Moreover, Gupta et al.[62] found cells in the cortico—medullary junction which expressed Oct-4 and had progenitor characteristics, and Kitamura et al.[63] isolated a highly proliferative cell type from the S3 segment of rat kidneys that, at least *in vitro*, also expressed precursor cell markers. Whether these putative stem cells relate to the recently described podocyte precursor (see above) or renal proximal tubule progenitors[95] remains to be determined.

The S3 segment of the proximal tubule is of additional interest as a potential site to harbor renal stem cells, because indirect determinations of oxygen tension have shown that this part of the nephron surprisingly exists in a hypoxic environment quite different from other parts of the kidney cortex.[109] A low oxygen tension is characteristic of sites where stem cells in other organs reside, a subject that we discuss below.

To determine whether the adult kidney contained regions of increased cell proliferation, we used kidneys of one-year-old rats, because we reasoned that fully grown older animals would not have proliferating cells needed for organ growth. We found cycling cells by staining for Ki67, a marker of cellular proliferation.[24] As shown in Figure 29.1, Ki67-positive cells were rare in the cortex and medulla, and were solitary and of a similar frequency (~1 % of the total cells). In contrast, the papilla showed marked heterogeneity in its abundance of Ki67-positive cells; they were extremely rare in its tip and middle part (~0.1 %), but were readily apparent in the upper part of the peripheral papilla, adjacent to the urinary space (US) where the kidney parenchyma forms a narrow angle which provides an easily identifiable landmark and the papilla meets the medulla; it is also very close to the kidney cortex. In this region, and unlike other areas of the kidney, Ki67-positive cells frequently formed chain-like structures and accounted for ~2.5 % of the total cells, a significant difference from other parts of the kidney. When cellular proliferation was assayed 24 hours after labeling cells in S-phase by administration of a single dose of BrdU, proliferating cells were very rarely detected in the cortex and medulla but again, the lateral part of the upper papilla consistently contained cycling cells; i.e.,

BrdU-labeled (not shown). We also obtained similar results in kidney of six-month-old rats.

Interestingly, after acute kidney injury, the lateral part of the upper papilla is also the site in which we first detected the increased cell cycling that follows injury; rats were subjected to 45 minutes of unilateral kidney ischemia, following which were given a single dose of BrdU and sacrificed one hour later. Thus, only cells that were in S-phase during this hour could be labeled, and using 5 μm kidney sections, we saw only equally rare labeled cells in normal kidneys or in the kidneys subjected to ischemia. However, examination of 100 μm vibratome sections showed abundant cells in S-phase in the upper papilla (Figure 29.3), next to the urinary space (US) only in the kidneys subjected to ischemia. In the aggregate, these results indicate that the lateral upper part of the kidney papilla contains more proliferating cells than other parts of the kidney under normal conditions, and that it contains the first cells that start cycling in response to transient injury. As reviewed above, Vinsonneau et al.[45] found that the first intrarenal area that contains Ki67 positive cells after ischemia reperfusion injury was the uro-epithelium and adjacent interstitial space in the upper part of the urinary space at the papilla—medullary junction.

In sum, because of their proliferative behavior, both under homeostatic conditions and during repair from several types of kidney injury, the S3 segment of the proximal tubule and the lateral part of the upper papilla are domains of the kidney where stem cells appear likely to reside.

Stem Cell "Niches"

Adult stem cells receive critical signaling from their immediate microenvironment, a domain that is distinct from the rest of the organ (see Morrison and Spradling[110] for a review). In these locations (referred to as "niches"), stem cells interact with other cells and the extracellular matrix, a process that is best understood in the *Drosophila* germline stem cells (see Fuller and Spradling for a review[111]). The stem cell "niche" provides positional information that regulates both proliferation activity and cell fate identity, and in fact it can even redirect cell fate similar to what often happens during embryogenesis.[112] While characterization of mammalian stem cell niches is still very limited, some common motifs are emerging that might be useful to identify the location of renal stem cells. Among those, a hypoxic environment is a prominent characteristic. Several organ-specific stem cells such as hematopoietic stem cells[113–115] and neural stem cells[116] reside in hypoxic regions, and a large body of *in vitro* work has shown the critical role of oxygen on stem cell

regulation (see Mohyeldin et al.[117] for a review). Moreover, in both hematopoietic stem cells and neural stem cells, it was recently found that regulation of the oxygen-sensitive gene *HIF-1α* is critical for the cells' maintenance and fate decisions.[114–116,118]

The kidney parenchyma possesses steep oxygen gradients,[119] and variations in renal oxygenation are undoubtedly sensed as they regulate erythropoietin synthesis. While direct determinations of oxygen tension in the kidney papilla have not been reported, it is likely that papillary pO_2 ranges are ~4–10 mmHg.[119] The presence of low-cycling cells in this very hypoxic environment[24,39,73,120] and that many of these cells express nestin,[24] an intermediate filament protein identified in a variety of progenitor/stem cells,[76] suggests that the papilla harbors renal stem cells. Interestingly, using a nestin-GFP-expressing mouse,[75] nestin$^+$ cells were detected in large clusters within the papilla, along the *vasa rectae* and, at least *in vitro*, these papillary nesting-expressing cells were found to migrate upwards in the papilla towards the cortex, an observation compatible with our *in vivo* experiments with vital dyes in which we found upward migration of papillary cells, some of which were "label-retaining cells".[24]

Several other findings also suggest that the kidney papilla is a niche for renal stem/precursor cells. Dekel and co-workers[61] isolated a population of purportedly renal stem cells from the renal interstitium that expressed the stem cell antigen-1 (Sca-1) and were enriched for β1-integrin; when the cells were located *in vivo*, they were found to be particularly abundant in the renal papilla. Using a different approach, Lee et al.[64] identified a renal interstitial cell that expressed several potential renal progenitor cell markers, such as *Oct-4*, *Pax-2*, *Wnt-4*, and *WT-1*. *In vivo*, Oct-4$^+$ cells were located in the medulla as well as in the papilla, leading these authors to suggest that the interstitium in these regions of the kidney is a "niche" for renal stem cells. Finally, and with a very different approach, Curtis et al.[121] examined whether cells from different regions of the kidneys were equally capable of contributing to cell regeneration after acute kidney injury. These workers isolated from mice constitutively expressing β-galactosidase in certain cells from the kidney cortex, medulla or papilla, and implanted them under the capsule of kidneys subjected to ischemia-reperfusion injury. Seven days later, implanted cells deriving from the three different regions of the kidney could be detected in the tubules of the renal medulla, but cells obtained from the papilla exhibited the most robust engraftment. These results suggest that cells deriving from all regions of the kidney might contribute to the reparative response of the organ after injury, and that some cells in the papilla are particularly capable of contributing to repair and might be stem cells.

RENAL STEM CELLS IN NON-MAMMALS

Renal Progenitors in Fish

Unlike mammals, fish appear to be capable of generating new nephrons during adult life, and their kidneys possess a clearly identifiable "nephrogenic zone".[122] This zone decreases in volume as the animal ages, likely because the nephron number increases with age.[123] In addition and of great interest, the nephrogenic zone can be stimulated in adult fish. For example, in the little skate the cellular proliferation and morphological complexity of the zone increased after partial nephrectomy,[122] a process that resembled embryonic nephrogenesis in mammals. While this morphological response strongly suggests *de novo* generation of nephrons, confirmation that new and functional nephrons developed remains to be established. Following acute kidney injury due to gentamicin, zebrafish can regenerate their nephrons, a process that starts shortly after injury with expression of *wt1b* (the zebrafish homolog of *Wilm's Tumor 1*) in individually dispersed cells of the mesonephric interstitium.[123]

These studies suggest that the fish could be a useful model to explore mechanisms of kidney repair where one can derive information that might facilitate identification of mammalian adult renal stem cells. Indeed, in a recent elegant study, Diep et al.[124] used zebrafish to search for potential nephron precursor cells. They reasoned that if adult kidney contains nephron progenitors these cells could be transplanted. They induced acute kidney injury by gentamicin administration, and performed a series of transplant experiments using cells from transgenic fish expressing reporters such as EGFP or Cherry with *cdh17*, thereby locating the fluorescent reporters in the distal nephron. When they injected unpurified whole kidney marrow cells (5×10^2 cells), mostly comprised of non-tubular interstitial cells, they found that the donor cells generated new nephrons in the host in 100% of the cases (Figure 29.7). Nephron number increased with time after injection and at later times, donor-derived nephrons were found at sites distal from the injection site, indicating that the cells migrated. Importantly, they found that these donor-generated nephrons connected to the host renal tubules and to the host's circulation, as shown by the fact that they could filter fluorescent dextran. Because in cell transplantation experiments it is frequently impossible to be certain that fusion of donor and recipient cells did not occur, to exclude this possibility Diep et al.[124] injected Cherry labeled cells into EGFP recipients and found that all engrafted nephrons were Cherry+ and EGFP negative, indicating that cell-to-cell fusion did not take place. To identify the cells responsible for the genesis of new nephrons, the authors examined the zebrafish homologs of transcription factors know to be expressed in the mammalian renal vesicles (the precursors of the nephron). They found that kidneys from adult zebrafish transgenics expressing *lhx1:EFGP* (the homolog of Lh1/Lim 1[125,126]) contained ~100 aggregates of ~30 EGFP+ cells per kidney. Examination of the evolution of these aggregates showed that they emerged from the assembly of ~3-4*lhx1:EFGP*+ cells that expanded to form a renal vesicle (expressing *wt1b*, the homolog of mammalian *WT1*), which in turn elongated into a nephron. Interestingly, laser ablation of a single aggregate of *lhx1:EFGP*+ cells prevented nephron formation without affecting neighboring nephrons, indicating that *lhx1:EFGP*+ cells are required for nephrogenesis. However, transplantation of single *lhx1:EGFP*+ cells to conditioned hosts failed to engraft, but transplantation of aggregates of *lhx1:EFGP*+ cells generated nephrons. Thus, *lhx1:EFGP*+ aggregates contain nephron progenitors and several cells are needed to generate a nephron. Whether the cell aggregates are clonal or contain several nephron progenitors with more restrictive differentiation potential is unclear. Nonetheless, demonstration in adult zebrafish of nephron progenitors capable of kidney regeneration and identification of their "genetic signature" is likely to facilitate design of new studies searching for renal stem cells in adult mammalian kidney.

Renal Progenitors in Invertebrates

The nephron is the basic structure of the vertebrate kidney, but many insects have tubular excretory systems with "nephron-like" features, suggesting that at least some components of the vertebrate kidneys derive from invertebrate ancestors. In addition, to regulate the composition of hemolymph, *Drosophila* has filtration cells that possess fly orthologs of the major components of the slit diaphragm, indicating that these cells are podocyte-like.[127] The similarity of the fly's excretory system to that of the nephron in vertebrates suggests that analysis of renal stem cells in *Drosophila* might be of considerable interest. Indeed, Singh et al.[128] used lineage tracing, molecular marking analysis, and BrdU incorporation to follow the fate of the different cells in the Malpigian tubules of adult flies. These tubules contain four types of cells, and Singh et al.[128] found that one type of cell was multipotent and could generate all the cell types of the Malpigian tubules of adult flies, indicating that they are renal stem cells. Singh et al. additionally found that autocrine JAK-STAT signaling in the renal stem cells regulated their renewal, and absence of signaling promoted their differentiation with loss of the stem cell

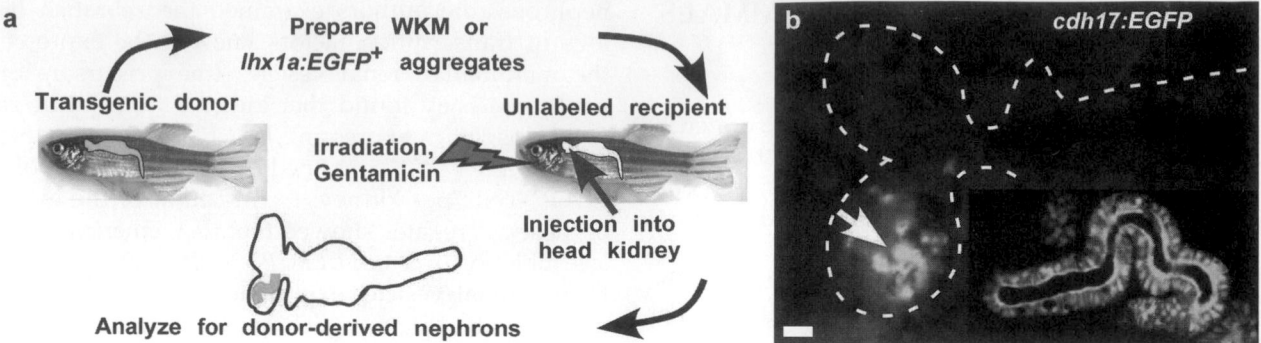

FIGURE 29.7 **The kidney of the adult zebrafish contains progenitor cells that generate new nephrons.** (a) Transplantation assay. Whole kidney marrow cells mostly comprising interstitial cells were isolated from genetically labeled donors. (b) Injection of the cells into recipients with damaged nephrons due to genatmicin injection resulted in donor-derived nephrons. *(From ref. [127].)* See color plate section at the back of the book.

population. Of great interest was their additional finding that these stem cells are present in the lower tubules and ureters, very much resembling the initial location of the nephron precursors recently identified in zebrafish,[124] and raising the possibility that the sharp distinction currently being made in mammalian adult kidneys between collecting ducts and the rest of the nephron might require re-evaluation. Also remarkable is that these stem cells are a large fraction of the total number of cells of the Malpighian tubules, rather than the anticipated small minority, another characteristic worth noting for workers on the renal stem field.

NEW CELLS IN DISEASED KIDNEYS

Renal Fibroblast and Myofibroblasts

In addition to dendritic cells, the normal adult kidney contains a network of interstitial fibroblasts and other cells that remain poorly-characterized, as they are technically difficult to detect and there is no general agreement on markers that identify them.[1] However, during many kidney diseases the renal interstitial compartment changes dramatically, with a marked increase in the number of renal fibroblasts and the invasion of the interstitium by a new type of cell called a myofibroblast. Myofibroblasts have fibroblast-like characteristics, but also express α smooth muscle actin (αSMA), and are believed to have great migratory capacity. It is currently thought that the marked proliferation of fibroblasts and myofibroblasts plus the expansion of their secreted extracellular matrix, i.e., renal fibrogenesis, is itself pathogenic as it disrupts the normal renal architecture and is the final common pathway of many kidney diseases. Indeed, expansion of the fibroblast and myofibroblast populations and the extracellular matrix are tightly correlated with the slow and

inexorable progressive loss-of-function that characterizes many kidney diseases. There is thus great interest in the mechanisms responsible for appearance of these cells during diseases.

Several possibilities have attracted attention. First, the cells might derive from resident renal interstitial "fibroblasts." In this view, the disease process induces fibroblast proliferation and in some of them, a change in their phenotype that results in expression of αSMA. Detailed morphological studies suggest that at least in some forms of renal fibrosis, such as that due to unilateral ureteral obstruction (UUO), this is likely the case.[129] More recent genetic cell fate tracing studies by Humphreys et al.[15] have suggested that myofibroblasts after unilateral ureteral obstruction (UUO) or after acute ischemic kidney injury derive from interstitial cells that are likely pericytes, since they were positive for Cd73 and platelet-derived growth factor receptor β (PGDFR β). Interestingly, pericyte differentiation and proliferation appears to be dependent on endothelial cell action, since blockade of their VEGF receptor 2 attenuates the fibrogenic process.[22] However, while Cd73 and PGDFR β appear to be present in most pericytes, there is no definitive marker profile for these cells, as they can only be unambiguously identified by their location around capillary endothelium. Moreover, new studies have shown that most, if not all, organs possess a population of perivascular mesenchymal stem cells,[4,5] and the distinction between these cells and pericytes is poorly-understood (see Corselli et al.[130] for a review). Hence, whether myofibroblasts solely derive from resident interstitial fibroblasts, pericytes, mesenchymal stem cells or from a combination of these cells remains to be clarified, and must await a detailed characterization of these three interstitial cell types.

Another possibility is that myofibroblasts could derive from bone marrow mesenchymal stem cells

(MSC); i.e., cells characterized by their ability to differentiate into adipocytes, osteoblasts, chondrocytes, and, sometimes, myoblasts. While Iwano et al.[131] found a small number of bone marrow-derived fibroblasts in the renal interstitium, little additional evidence has been obtained to support that bone marrow precursor cells could be the origin of the myofibroblasts.

Another possible origin of the renal fibroblasts and myofibroblasts found in kidney diseases is that they derive from renal epithelial cells by epithelial-mesenchymal transition (EMT), a process in which epithelial cells lose the ability to maintain close contacts with their neighbors as well as apico—basal polarity, and instead develop a mesenchymal phenotype that includes migratory capacity. The process of EMT is of course widely used during embryogenesis and in some disease processes, particularly cancer (for a recent review see Thiery et al.[132]). It is of great interest that in nonrenal cells, it has been found that EMT might generate cells with the properties of stem cells,[133] but this possibility appears not to have been examined in the kidney.

There is little doubt, at least *in vitro*, that epithelial cells from both embryonic[134] and adult kidneys[15,135] can undergo EMT. However, there is currently a debate whether this process might generate fibroblasts and myofibroblasts *in vivo* (see Kapus and Quaggin[136] and Kriz et al.[137] for informed discussions). Morphological and cell marker studies during renal fibrosis have provided some evidence supporting EMT *in vivo*, both in experimental models[90,138—142] and in human diseases,[90,91,143,144] but other studies have failed to support this.[129,145] The most robust method currently to determine whether myofibroblasts might derive from renal epithelial cells is based on studies using genetic cell fate analysis. In these studies epithelial cells are genetically labeled so that their progeny (e.g., fibroblasts or myofibroblasts) can be easily identified. Using the UUO model of renal fibrogenesis, Iwano et al.[131] found that a substantial number of renal fibroblasts derived from renal epithelial cells. However, three subsequent studies with UUO plus other models of renal fibrogenesis and using different epithelial genes to drive Cre recombinase and label epithelial cells in reporter mice found no evidence that renal fibroblasts and myofibroblasts derived from epithelial cells.[15,146,147] There is currently no clear explanation for these conflicting results, and it is apparent that additional studies are needed.

Finally, another potential origin of renal fibroblasts and myofibroblasts are endothelial cells. Genetic cell fate experiments have shown that Cre recombinase driven by Tie2 (a tyrosine kinase receptor believed to be endothelial-specific in the adult) identified a reporter gene in renal fibroblasts in UUO and streptozotocin-induced renal fibrogenesis.[148,149] This unexpected result is of particular interest, because adult endothelial cells have been shown to have the capacity to transform into mesenchymal stem-like cells by activation of activin-like kinase-2,[153] and two ligands well-known to be involved in renal fibrogenesis, TGFβ and BMP4, phosphorylated activin-like kinase-2 and induced a mesenchymal phenotype in cultured endothelial cells.[150]

This brief survey shows that the precise origin of the renal fibroblasts and myofibroblasts during renal diseases remains undefined, and given the medical importance of this issue additional studies are needed. Needless to say, it is also likely that these cells might have more than one origin. While studies based on morphology and/or cell identification by cell-specific markers offer at best indirect evidence, genetic-based cell lineage tracing experiments have their own potential pitfalls (see the review by Matthaei[151]). In particular, two potential problems might complicate their interpretation. The first is that it is assumed that the reporter gene is expressed in all cells and for the duration of the animal's life, as well as during the disease process. Definitive proof of this is lacking and, for example, in the adult kidney, the robustness of the reporter expression in the *Rosa26* locus (frequently used to introduce the reporter gene) was found to be less than anticipated ([152] and our unpublished results). In addition, cell fate-mapping studies can give markedly different results depending on the genetic construct of the reporter.[153] The second, and potentially more confounding, problem in the interpretation of genetic cell-fate analyses is that the gene used to activate the reporter gene is chosen because of its restricted expression to a specific cell type during embryogenesis, and lack of expression during adult life and after injury, when the analysis is done. However, the possibility that the gene is activated later in life or by the disease process in a small number of cells might be very difficult to detect.

KIDNEY REPAIR BY EXOGENOUS STEM/PRECURSOR CELLS

While analysis of the kidney's ability to repair from injury has naturally focused on the intrinsic renal cell population, reports that cells derived from the bone marrow could generate new renal cells and perhaps contribute to organ repair generated a great deal of interest.[154—157] However, subsequent studies have firmly established that most if not all the new cells generated after kidney injury derived from other renal cells.[29,30] Nonetheless, and stimulated from work in other organs, the possibility that exogenous cells might either facilitate kidney repair or diminish the consequences of injury has been examined in multiple studies. Indeed, clinical trials with bone marrow-derived MSC are already underway or in planned stages in a variety of diseases, particularly for myocardial infarction, but also including the kidney (http://www3. niddk.nih.gov/fund/other/akiworkshop/). In experimental animals, the potential therapeutic effect of several cell types in acute kidney injury has been examined under a variety of protocols.

Mesenchymal Stem Cells (MSC)

When HSC and bone marrow-derived MSC were administered to mice it was found that the latter, but not the former, protected the animals from the functional consequences of acute kidney injury due to cisplatin.[156] Multiple studies have confirmed that extrarenal MSC can either diminish the functional consequences of acute kidney injury or accelerate recovery of kidney function after injury. In addition to MSC derived from the bone marrow,[23,158−161] MSC from human cord blood[162] or even the kidney[163] have been shown to be effective. In these studies, acute kidney injury was induced by several methods and the cells were administered through a variety of routes: intravenously, intra-arterially and by direct intrarenal injection.

What are the potential mechanisms by which exogenous MSC might protect the kidney from injury or facilitate its repair? Although initial observations suggested incorporation of the cells into the renal parenchyma,[156] more recent studies have shown that their mechanism of action is likely to be that the cells provide endocrine/paracrine factors, perhaps growth factors[23,161,164] or chemokines such as IL10.[161] In this view, the mechanism of action of the MSC would be similar to that of directly delivering growth factors in transient kidney injury (reviewed by Hammerman and Miller[165]). Unfortunately, very little information is available on the identity of these beneficial factors, and whether MSC are more or less effective than isolated growth factors alone.

Another possible mechanism is that the transplanted MSC might modulate the host immune response by effects on macrophages,[166,167] dendritic cells,[168,169] T-cells[168] or B-cells.[170] Given the complexity of the kidney's response to the insults used to induce functional acute renal failure, it is apparent that there might be multiple mechanisms whereby exogenous cells could protect this organ from injury or facilitate its repair. An additional problem complicating analysis of these studies is that because MSC are identified *a posteriori* (based on a variety of characteristics such as high proliferation capacity and ability to differentiate into several mesenchymal lineages) there are no strict identification criteria for the administered cells, making comparison across studies extremely difficult.

Regardless, given the clinical severity and epidemiological importance of acute kidney failure, the finding that MSC can improve its evolution is of extreme interest, and studies that illuminate their mechanisms of action are urgently needed. Work in other organs has begun to provide answers. In an elegant study in myocardial repair from ischemic myocardial infarction, Lee et al.[171] found that human MSC (hMSC) administered intravenously acutely embolized into the lungs where they upregulated multiple genes, including the anti-inflamatory protein TSG-6 (the product of tumor necrosis factor-stimulated gene 6). Similar to the observations in kidney injury, the injected hMSC reduced the myocardial inflammatory response to ischemia, decreased infarct size, and improved myocardial function. Administration of recombinant TSG-6 had similar effects as hMSC, but hMSC that were transduced with TSG-6 siRNA did not. This interesting study provides a detailed mechanistic explanation of why hMSC facilitate myocardial repair without engraftment into the organ, and opens new therapeutic avenues for research.

Other Bone Marrow-Derived Cells

Earlier experiments with bone marrow-derived stem cells (other than MSC) suggested that they could ameliorate the functional consequences of transient acute kidney injury.[154] While the possibility that these cells exerted this effect by generating significant numbers of renal epithelia cells has been ruled out,[29,30] their mechanism of action remains unexplained and little explored. Lie et al.[172] used human $Cd34^+$ hematopoietic stem/progenitor cells isolated from peripheral blood after granulocyte colony stimulating factor mobilization, and injected them into mice. They found that, whereas the cells did not localize to normal kidneys, they did so in injured kidneys. Moreover, administration of the cells increased cellular proliferation in the injured kidneys, accelerated kidney functional recovery, and increased animal survival. The exact mechanism(s) whereby these cells exerted these effects remain to be determined, and many possibilities exist. For example, in the heart where bone marrow-derived cells also had significant regenerative effects, their action appears to be mediated by resident cardiac stem cells. In a model of myocardial infarction by coronary ligation, Loffredo et al.[173] administered a population of purified $c-kit^+$ bone marrow-derived cells and found that they stimulated endogenous cardiomyocite progenitors. These progenitors are capable of differentiating into several cell types, including cardiac muscle cells, and their stimulation resulted in improved cardiac repair and enhanced function. In contrast, MSC were unable to stimulate endogenous myocardial progenitors.

Kidney Cells

A variety of studies have examined whether administration of cells derived from the kidney might facilitate this organ's repair from injury. All the cells used in these studies possess some "precursor/stem" characteristics, but were poorly-characterized and even their exact *in vivo* location is somewhat uncertain. Administration of cells derived from the S3 segment of the proximal tubule had no effect on the functional response to acute kidney injury due to ischemia-reperfusion.[62,63] However, when the kidney was injured by cisplatin, subcapsular transplantation of the cells facilitated kidney functional recovery.[174]

Several studies have used cells from the kidney that were captured by their expression of Cd24 and Cd133, either from embryonic kidney[175] or adult kidneys.[95,96] In these studies, intravenous administration of the cells facilitated kidney functional recovery from rhabdomyolysis induced by glycerol administration. Lee et al.[64] used a renal interstitial cell population expressing *Oct4*, *Pax2*, *Wnt 4*, and *WT1* (discussed above), and found that intrarenal injection of the cells markedly blunted the functional consequences of kidney injury from transient ischemia.

What is to be concluded form these experiments with exogenous cells? That the administration of MSC might improve the kidney's functional response to injury appears well-established; however, that of other bone marrow cells or renal-derived cells appears to be less robust. Significant problems in many of these studies include: (1) poor characterization of the cell population used; (2) less than ideal monitoring of the kidney functional response, notoriously difficult to do in mice; and (3) lack of analysis of where the majority of the injected cells locate. Most cells injected into the renal artery are retained by glomeruli[176] and the vast majority of intravenously injected cells remain in the lungs.[171] The recent discovery that under specific culture conditions, MSC reduce their size such that when they are injected intravenously they can cross the pulmonary circulation[166] is a finding that may allow the systemic delivery of MSC to the kidney. It is of course possible that injected cells that locate at sites other than the kidney might be responsible for the observed beneficial effects on renal function. Regardless of the location and potential mechanism of action of the injected cells, these initial results suggesting that exogenous cell therapy might be beneficial in acute kidney injury need confirmation and further analysis.

CONCLUDING REMARKS

Whether the adult mammalian kidney contains stem cells that self-renew and are pluripotent is currently unknown. However, given its multiple cell types and by analogy with other organs, it is very likely that renal stem cells might indeed be present. In contrast to the mammalian kidney, it is established that the Malpighian tubule of *Drosophila* contains true stem cells, and that the zebrafish kidney can be regenerated from a small number of specialized epithelial precursor cells, strongly suggesting that it also contains stem cells. Most work searching for a renal stem cell has focused on the epithelial cellular compartment, likely because of its understood important functional role and the relative ease with which it can be identified. However, the adult kidney also contains an abundant population of interstitial cells that are just now beginning to be understood; the discovery that the transcription factor *Foxd1* (*Bcl2*) is expressed during embryonic development in many of these cells has provided an important new research tool that should illuminate their role.

While *bona fide* adult stem cells in the mammalian kidney remain to be identified, several observations suggest that some stem/precursor cells exist in several locations. Perhaps the best evidence that a specialized precursor exists is in the glomerular podocytes, although it also appears likely that, at least under pathological conditions, podocytes themselves can generate other cell types. Perhaps podocytes are not solely terminally-differentiated cells, but can give rise to other cell progeny. A surprisingly variable cell identity was recently discovered in some of the progeny of hair follicle stem cells; these daughter cells were found to return to the stem cell niche and serve as future stem cells.[177]

Confirming classical morphological observations, new genetic cell lineage tracing experiments have provided strong evidence that after acute kidney injury epithelial cells give rise to new epithelia cells, but it remains unclear whether there exist distinct epithelial stem/precursor cells. In fact, multiple observations are compatible with the presence of specialized epithelial progenitors/stem cells in the S3 segment of the proximal tubule. Is it possible that some of the conflicting results could be explained by the presence of two types of stem/precursor cells: one that normally divides to provide new cells during homeostatic conditions and a low-cycling stem cell that is activated during organ repair, as appears to be the case in other organs (see Fuchs[68] and Li and Clevers[107] for reviews)?

Finally, several lines of evidence strongly suggest that the kidney papilla is a "niche" for renal stem cells. This very hypoxic part of the kidney contains many low-cycling cells (identified as "label-retaining cells") that slowly disappear as the animal ages, and that after acute kidney injury quickly start cycling and markedly decrease in number after repair. While *in vitro* characterization of these cells has shown them to have many properties of stem/precursor cells, no array of specific cell markers can yet identify them, so that their identity and the identity of their progeny remains to be defined. It is our hope that genetic cell lineage analysis will allow us to answer these questions.

References

[1] Kaissling B, Le Hir M. The renal cortical interstitium: morphological and functional aspects. Hematol Cell Biol 2008;130:247–62.

[2] Hatini V, Huh SO, Herzlinger D, Soares VC, Lai E. Essential role of stromal mesenchyme in kidney morphogenesis revealed by targeted disruption of Winged Helix transcription factor BF-2. Genes Dev 1996;10:1467–78.

[3] Covas DT, Panepucci RA, Fontes AM, Silva Jr WA, Orellana MD, Freitas MC, et al. Multipotent mesenchymal stromal cells obtained from diverse human tissues share functional properties and gene-expression profile with CD146+ perivascular cells and fibroblasts. Exp Hematol 2008;36:642–54.

[4] Crisan M, Yap S, Casteilla L, Chen CW, Corselli M, Park TS, et al. A perivascular origin for mesenchymal stem cells in multiple human organs. Cell Stem Cell 2008;3:301–13.

[5] da Silva Meirelles L, Chagastelles PC, Nardi NB. Mesenchymal stem cells reside in virtually all post-natal organs and tissues. J Cell Sci 2006;119:2204–13.

[6] Herzlinger D, Koseki C, Mikawa T, al-Awqati Q. Metanephric mesenchyme contains multipotent stem cells whose fate is restricted after induction. Development 1992;114:565–72.

[7] Kress C, Vogels R, De Graaff W, Bonnerot C, Meijlink F, Nicolas JF, et al. Hox-2.3 upstream sequences mediate lacZ expression in intermediate mesoderm derivatives of transgenic mice. Development 1990;109:775–86.

[8] Srinivas S, Goldberg MR, Watanabe T, D'Agati V, al-Awqati Q, Costantini F. Expression of green fluorescent protein in the ureteric bud of transgenic mice: a new tool for the analysis of ureteric bud morphogenesis. Dev Genet 1999;24:241–51.

[9] Boyle S, Misfeldt A, Chandler KJ, Deal KK, Southard-Smith EM, Mortlock DP, et al. Fate mapping using Cited1-CreERT2 mice demonstrates that the cap mesenchyme contains self-renewing progenitor cells and gives rise exclusively to nephronic epithelia. Dev Biol 2008;313:234–45.

[10] Kobayashi A, Valerius MT, Mugford JW, Carroll TJ, Self M, Oliver G, et al. Six2 defines and regulates a multipotent self-renewing nephron progenitor population throughout mammalian kidney development. Cell Stem Cell 2008;3:169–81.

[11] Humphreys BD, Valerius MT, Kobayashi A, Mugford JW, Soeung S, Duffield JS, et al. Intrinsic epithelial cells repair the kidney after injury. Cell Stem Cell 2008;2:284–91.

[12] Mugford JW, Sipila P, McMahon JA, McMahon AP. Osr1 expression demarcates a multi-potent population of intermediate mesoderm that undergoes progressive restriction to an Osr1-dependent nephron progenitor compartment within the mammalian kidney. Dev Biol 2008;324:88–98.

[13] Levinson RS, Batourina E, Choi C, Vorontchikhina M, Kitajewski J, Mendelsohn CL. Foxd1-dependent signals control cellularity in the renal capsule, a structure required for normal renal development. Development 2005;132:529–39.

[14] Mendelsohn C, Batourina E, Fung S, Gilbert T, Dodd J. Stromal cells mediate retinoid-dependent functions essential for renal development. Development 1999;126:1139–48.

[15] Humphreys BD, Lin SL, Kobayashi A, Hudson TE, Nowlin BT, Bonventre JV, et al. Fate tracing reveals the pericyte and not epithelial origin of myofibroblasts in kidney fibrosis. Am J Pathol 2010;176:85–97.

[16] Guillaume R, Bressan M, Herzlinger D. Paraxial mesoderm contributes stromal cells to the developing kidney. Dev Biol 2009;329:169–75.

[17] Schmidt-Ott KM, Chen X, Paragas N, Levinson RS, Mendelsohn CL, Barasch J. c-kit delineates a distinct domain of progenitors in the developing kidney. Dev Biol 2006;299:238–49.

[18] Robert B St, John PL, Abrahamson DR. Direct visualization of renal vascular morphogenesis in Flk1 heterozygous mutant mice. Am J Physiol 1998;275:F164–72.

[19] Robert B St, John PL, Hyink DP, Abrahamson DR. Evidence that embryonic kidney cells expressing flk-1 are intrinsic, vasculogenic angioblasts. Am J Physiol 1996;271:F744–53.

[20] Oliver JA, Barasch J, Yang J, Herzlinger D, Al-Awqati Q. Metanephric mesenchyme contains embryonic renal stem cells. Am J Physiol Renal Physiol 2002;283:F799–809.

[21] Gao X, Chen X, Taglienti M, Rumballe B, Little MH, Kreidberg JA. Angioblast-mesenchyme induction of early kidney development is mediated by Wt1 and Vegfa. Development 2005;132:5437–49.

[22] Lin SL, Chang FC, Schrimpf C, Chen YT, Wu CF, Wu VC, et al. Targeting endothelium-pericyte cross talk by inhibiting VEGF receptor signaling attenuates kidney microvascular rarefaction and fibrosis. Am J Pathol 2011;178:911–23.

[23] Bi B, Schmitt R, Israilova M, Nishio H, Cantley LG. Stromal cells protect against acute tubular injury via an endocrine effect. J Am Soc Nephrol 2007;18:2486–96.

[24] Oliver JA, Klinakis A, Cheema FH, Friedlander J, Sampogna RV, Martens TP, et al. Proliferation and migration of label-retaining cells of the kidney papilla. J Am Soc Nephrol 2009;20:2315–27.

[25] Vogetseder A, Picard N, Gaspert A, Walch M, Kaissling B, Le Hir M. Proliferation capacity of the renal proximal tubule involves the bulk of differentiated epithelial cells. Am J Physiol Cell Physiol 2008;294:C22–28.

[26] Witzgall R, Brown D, Schwarz C, Bonventre JV. Localization of proliferating cell nuclear antigen, vimentin, c-Fos, and clusterin in the postischemic kidney. Evidence for a heterogenous genetic response among nephron segments, and a large pool of mitotically active and dedifferentiated cells. J Clin Invest 1994;93:2175–88.

[27] Vogetseder A, Karadeniz A, Kaissling B, Le Hir M. Tubular cell proliferation in the healthy rat kidney. Histochem Cell Biol 2005;124:97–104.

[28] Vogetseder A, Palan T, Bacic D, Kaissling B, Le Hir M. Proximal tubular epithelial cells are generated by division of differentiated cells in the healthy kidney. Am J Physiol Cell Physiol 2007;292:C807–13.

[29] Duffield JS, Park KM, Hsiao LL, Kelley VR, Scadden DT, Ichimura T, et al. Restoration of tubular epithelial cells during repair of the postischemic kidney occurs independently of bone marrow-derived stem cells. J Clin Invest 2005;115:1743–55.

[30] Lin F, Moran A, Igarashi P. Intrarenal cells, not bone marrow-derived cells, are the major source for regeneration in postischemic kidney. J Clin Invest 2005;115:1756–64.

[31] Ghazizadeh S, Taichman LB. Multiple classes of stem cells in cutaneous epithelium: a lineage analysis of adult mouse skin. Embo J 2001;20:1215–22.

[32] Ro S, Rannala B. A stop-EGFP transgenic mouse to detect clonal cell lineages generated by mutation. EMBO Rep 2004;5:914–20.

[33] Blanpain C, Lowry WE, Geoghegan A, Polak L, Fuchs E. Self-renewal, multipotency, and the existence of two cell populations within an epithelial stem cell niche. Cell 2004;118:635–48.

[34] Morris RJ, Liu Y, Marles L, Yang Z, Trempus C, Li S, et al. Capturing and profiling adult hair follicle stem cells. Nat Biotechnol 2004;22:411–7.

[35] Oliver J, Mac DM, Tracy A. The pathogenesis of acute renal failure associated with traumatic and toxic injury; renal ischemia, nephrotoxic damage and the ischemic episode. J Clin Invest 1951;30:1307–439.

[36] Oshima H, Rochat A, Kedzia C, Kobayashi K, Barrandon Y. Morphogenesis and renewal of hair follicles from adult multipotent stem cells. Cell 2001;104:233–45.

[37] Haagsma BH, Pound AW. Mercuric chloride-induced tubulonecrosis in the rat kidney: the recovery phase. Br J Exp Pathol 1980;61:229–41.

[38] Maeshima A, Yamashita S, Nojima Y. Identification of renal progenitor-like tubular cells that participate in the regeneration processes of the kidney. J Am Soc Nephrol 2003;14:3138–46.

[39] Humphreys BD, Czerniak S, Dirocco DP, Hasnain W, Cheema R, Bonventre JV. Repair of injured proximal tubule does not involve specialized progenitors. Proc Natl Acad Sci USA 2011;108:9226–31.

[40] Rock JR, Gao X, Xue Y, Randell SH, Kong YY, Hogan BL. Notch-dependent differentiation of adult airway basal stem cells. Cell Stem Cell 2011;8:639–48.

[41] Rock JR, Onaitis MW, Rawlins EL, Lu Y, Clark CP, Xue Y, et al. Basal cells as stem cells of the mouse trachea and human airway epithelium. Proc Natl Acad Sci U S A 2009;106:12771–5.

[42] Fujigaki Y, Goto T, Sakakima M, Fukasawa H, Miyaji T, Yamamoto T, et al. Kinetics and characterization of initially regenerating proximal tubules in S3 segment in response to various degrees of acute tubular injury. Nephrol Dial Transplant 2006;21:41–50.

[43] Sun DF, Fujigaki Y, Fujimoto T, Yonemura K, Hishida A. Possible involvement of myofibroblasts in cellular recovery of uranyl acetate-induced acute renal failure in rats. Am J Pathol 2000;157:1321–35.

[44] Vanthertem D, Caron N, Decleves AE, Cludts S, Gossiaux A, Nonclercq D, et al. Label-retaining cells and tubular regeneration in postischaemic kidney. Nephrol Dial Transplant 2008;23:3786–97.

[45] Vinsonneau C, Girshovich A, M'Rad MB, Perez J, Mesnard L, Vandermersch S, et al. Intrarenal urothelium proliferation: an unexpected early event following ischemic injury. Am J Physiol Renal Physiol 2010;299:F479–86.

[46] Nonclercq D, Wrona S, Toubeau G, Zanen J, Heuson-Stiennon JA, Schaudies RP, et al. Tubular injury and regeneration in the rat kidney following acute exposure to gentamicin: a time-course study. Ren Fail 1992;14:507–21.

[47] Nouwen EJ, Verstrepen WA, Buyssens N, Zhu MQ, De Broe ME. Hyperplasia, hypertrophy, and phenotypic alterations in the distal nephron after acute proximal tubular injury in the rat. Lab Invest 1994;70:479–93.

[48] Kwon O, Hong SM, Sutton TA, Temm CJ. Preservation of peritubular capillary endothelial integrity and increasing pericytes may be critical to recovery from postischemic acute kidney injury. Am J Physiol Renal Physiol 2008;295:F351–9.

[49] Sun DF, Fujigaki Y, Fujimoto T, Goto T, Yonemura K, Hishida A. Mycophenolate mofetil inhibits regenerative repair in uranyl acetate-induced acute renal failure by reduced interstitial cellular response. Am J Pathol 2002;161:217–27.

[50] Lin SL, Li B, Rao S, Yeo EJ, Hudson TE, Nowlin BT, et al. Macrophage Wnt7b is critical for kidney repair and regeneration. Proc Natl Acad Sci U S A 2010;107:4194–9.

[51] Schmitt R, Coca S, Kanbay M, Tinetti ME, Cantley LG, Parikh CR. Recovery of kidney function after acute kidney injury in the elderly: a systematic review and meta-analysis. Am J Kidney Dis 2008;52:262–71.

[52] Liu L, Rando TA. Manifestations and mechanisms of stem cell aging. J Cell Biol 2011;193:257–66.

[53] Carlson ME, Suetta C, Conboy MJ, Aagaard P, Mackey A, Kjaer M, et al. Molecular aging and rejuvenation of human muscle stem cells. EMBO Mol Med 2009;1:381–91.

[54] Conboy IM, Conboy MJ, Wagers AJ, Girma ER, Weissman IL, Rando TA. Rejuvenation of aged progenitor cells by exposure to a young systemic environment. Nature 2005;433:760–4.

[55] Schmitt R, Cantley LG. The impact of aging on kidney repair. Am J Physiol Ren Physiol 2008;294:F1265–1272.

[56] Westhoff JH, Schildhorn C, Jacobi C, Homme M, Hartner A, Braun H, et al. Telomere shortening reduces regenerative capacity after acute kidney injury. J Am Soc Nephrol 2010;21:327–36.

[57] Altman J, Das GD. Postnatal neurogenesis in the guinea-pig. Nature 1967;214:1098–101.

[58] Schmitt R, Marlier A, Cantley LG. Zag expression during aging suppresses proliferation after kidney injury. J Am Soc Nephrol 2008;19:2375–83.

[59] Bussolati B, Bruno S, Grange C, Buttiglieri S, Deregibus MC, Cantino D, et al. Isolation of renal progenitor cells from adult human kidney. Am J Pathol 2005;166:545–55.

[60] Mizrak D, Brittan M, Alison MR. CD133: molecule of the moment. J Pathol 2008;214:3–9.

[61] Dekel B, Zangi L, Shezen E, Reich-Zeliger S, Eventov-Friedman S, Katchman H, et al. Isolation and characterization of nontubular sca-1 + lin − multipotent stem/progenitor cells from adult mouse kidney. J Am Soc Nephrol 2006;17:3300–14.

[62] Gupta S, Verfaillie C, Chmielewski D, Kren S, Eidman K, Connaire J, et al. Isolation and characterization of kidney-derived stem cells. J Am Soc Nephrol 2006;17:3028–40.

[63] Kitamura S, Yamasaki Y, Kinomura M, Sugaya T, Sugiyama H, Maeshima Y, et al. Establishment and characterization of renal progenitor like cells from S3 segment of nephron in rat adult kidney. Faseb J 2005;19:1789–97.

[64] Lee PT, Lin HH, Jiang ST, Lu PJ, Chou KJ, Fang HC, et al. Mouse kidney progenitor cells accelerate renal regeneration and prolong survival after ischemic injury. Stem Cells 2010;28:573–84.

[65] Barker N, van Es JH, Kuipers J, Kujala P, van den Born M, Cozijnsen M, et al. Identification of stem cells in small intestine and colon by marker gene Lgr5. Nature 2007;449:1003–7.

[66] Foudi A, Hochedlinger K, Van Buren D, Schindler JW, Jaenisch R, Carey V, et al. Analysis of histone 2B-GFP retention reveals slowly cycling hematopoietic stem cells. Nat Biotechnol 2009;27:84–90.

[67] Kiel MJ, He S, Ashkenazi R, Gentry SN, Teta M, Kushner JA, et al. Haematopoietic stem cells do not asymmetrically segregate chromosomes or retain BrdU. Nature 2007;449:238–42.

[68] Fuchs E. The tortoise and the hair: slow-cycling cells in the stem cell race. Cell 2009;137:811–9.

[69] Cotsarelis G, Cheng SZ, Dong G, Sun TT, Lavker RM. Existence of slow-cycling limbal epithelial basal cells that can be preferentially stimulated to proliferate: implications on epithelial stem cells. Cell 1989;57:201–9.

[70] Marshman E, Booth C, Potten CS. The intestinal epithelial stem cell. Bioessays 2002;24:91–8.

[71] Wilson A, Laurenti E, Oser G, van der Wath RC, Blanco-Bose W, Jaworski M, et al. Hematopoietic stem cells reversibly switch from dormancy to self-renewal during homeostasis and repair. Cell 2008;135:1118–29.

II. STRUCTURAL AND FUNCTIONAL ORGANIZATION OF THE KIDNEY

[72] Zhang YV, Cheong J, Ciapurin N, McDermitt DJ, Tumbar T. Distinct self-renewal and differentiation phases in the niche of infrequently dividing hair follicle stem cells. Cell Stem Cell 2009;5:267–78.

[73] Oliver JA, Maarouf O, Cheema FH, Martens TP, Al-Awqati Q. The renal papilla is a niche for adult kidney stem cells. J Clin Invest 2004;114:795–804.

[74] Tumbar T, Guasch G, Greco V, Blanpain C, Lowry WE, Rendl M, et al. Defining the epithelial stem cell niche in skin. Science 2004;303:359–63.

[75] Patschan D, Michurina T, Shi HK, Dolff S, Brodsky SV, Vasilieva T, et al. Normal distribution and medullary-to-cortical shift of Nestin-expressing cells in acute renal ischemia. Kidney Int 2007;71:744–54.

[76] Wiese C, Rolletschek A, Kania G, Blyszczuk P, Tarasov KV, Tarasova Y, et al. Nestin expression: a property of multi-lineage progenitor cells? Cell Mol Life Sci 2004;61:2510–22.

[77] Park HC, Yasuda K, Kuo MC, Ni J, Ratliff BB, Chander PN, et al. Renal capsule as a stem cell niche. Am J Physiol Renal Physiol 2010;298:F1254–62.

[78] Goodell MA, Brose K, Paradis G, Conner AS, Mulligan RC. Isolation and functional properties of murine hematopoietic stem cells that are replicating *in vivo*. J Exp Med 1996;183:1797–806.

[79] Matsuzaki Y, Kinjo K, Mulligan RC, Okano H. Unexpectedly efficient homing capacity of purified murine hematopoietic stem cells. Immunity 2004;20:87–93.

[80] Zhou S, Schuetz JD, Bunting KD, Colapietro AM, Sampath J, Morris JJ, et al. The ABC transporter Bcrp1/ABCG2 is expressed in a wide variety of stem cells and is a molecular determinant of the side-population phenotype. Nat Med 2001;7:1028–34.

[81] Golebiewska A, Brons NH, Bjerkvig R, Niclou SP. Critical appraisal of the side population assay in stem cell and cancer stem cell research. Cell Stem Cell 2011;8:136–47.

[82] Asakura A, Rudnicki MA. Side population cells from diverse adult tissues are capable of *in vitro* hematopoietic differentiation. Exp Hematol 2002;30:1339–45.

[83] Challen GA, Bertoncello I, Deane JA, Ricardo SD, Little MH. Kidney side population reveals multilineage potential and renal functional capacity but also cellular heterogeneity. J Am Soc Nephrol 2006;17:1896–912.

[84] Hishikawa K, Marumo T, Miura S, Nakanishi A, Matsuzaki Y, Shibata K, et al. Musculin/MyoR is expressed in kidney side population cells and can regulate their function. J Cell Biol 2005;169:921–8.

[85] Iwatani H, Ito T, Imai E, Matsuzaki Y, Suzuki A, Yamato M, et al. Hematopoietic and nonhematopoietic potentials of Hoechst (low)/side population cells isolated from adult rat kidney. Kidney Int 2004;65:1604–14.

[86] Sophos NA, Vasiliou V. Aldehyde dehydrogenase gene superfamily: the 2002 update. Chem Biol Interact 2003;143–144:5–22.

[87] Chute JP, Muramoto GG, Whitesides J, Colvin M, Safi R, Chao NJ, et al. Inhibition of aldehyde dehydrogenase and retinoid signaling induces the expansion of human hematopoietic stem cells. Proc Nat Acad Sci USA 2006;103:11707–12.

[88] Ginestier C, Hur MH, Charafe-Jauffret E, Monville F, Dutcher J, Brown M, et al. ALDH1 is a marker of normal and malignant human mammary stem cells and a predictor of poor clinical outcome. Cell Stem Cell 2007;1:555–67.

[89] Lindgren D, Bostrom AK, Nilsson K, Hansson J, Sjolund J, Moller C, et al. Isolation and characterization of progenitor-like cells from human renal proximal tubules. Am J Pathol 2011;178:828–37.

[90] Grone HJ, Weber K, Grone E, Helmchen U, Osborn M. Coexpression of keratin and vimentin in damaged and regenerating tubular epithelia of the kidney. Am J Pathol 1987;129:1–8.

[91] Moll R, Hage C, Thoenes W. Expression of intermediate filament proteins in fetal and adult human kidney: modulations of intermediate filament patterns during development and in damaged tissue. Lab Invest 1991;65:74–86.

[92] Vogelmann SU, Nelson WJ, Myers BD, Lemley KV. Urinary excretion of viable podocytes in health and renal disease. Am J Physiol Renal Physiol 2003;285:F40–8.

[93] D'Agati VD. Podocyte injury in focal segmental glomerulosclerosis: lessons from animal models (a play in five acts). Kidney Int 2008;73:399–406.

[94] Thorner PS, Ho M, Eremina V, Sado Y, Quaggin S. Podocytes contribute to the formation of glomerular crescents. J Am Soc Nephrol: J Am Soc Nephrol 2008;19:495–502.

[95] Sagrinati C, Netti GS, Mazzinghi B, Lazzeri E, Liotta F, Frosali F, et al. Isolation and characterization of multipotent progenitor cells from the Bowman's capsule of adult human kidneys. J Am Soc Nephrol: J Am Soc Nephrol 2006;17:2443–56.

[96] Mazzinghi B, Ronconi E, Lazzeri E, Sagrinati C, Ballerini L, Angelotti ML, et al. Essential but differential role for CXCR4 and CXCR7 in the therapeutic homing of human renal progenitor cells. J Exp Med 2008;205:479–90.

[97] Appel D, Kershaw DB, Smeets B, Yuan G, Fuss A, Frye B, et al. Recruitment of podocytes from glomerular parietal epithelial cells. J Am Soc Nephrol 2009;20:333–43.

[98] Ronconi E, Sagrinati C, Angelotti ML, Lazzeri E, Mazzinghi B, Ballerini L, et al. Regeneration of glomerular podocytes by human renal progenitors. J Am Soc Nephrol 2009;20:322–32.

[99] Smeets B, Angelotti ML, Rizzo P, Dijkman H, Lazzeri E, Mooren F, et al. Renal progenitor cells contribute to hyperplastic lesions of podocytopathies and crescentic glomerulonephritis. J Am Soc Nephrol 2009;20:2593–603.

[100] Smeets B, Uhlig S, Fuss A, Mooren F, Wetzels JF, Floege J, et al. Tracing the origin of glomerular extracapillary lesions from parietal epithelial cells. J Am Soc Nephrol 2009;20:2604–15.

[101] Ding M, Cui S, Li C, Jothy S, Haase V, Steer BM, et al. Loss of the tumor suppressor Vhlh leads to upregulation of Cxcr4 and rapidly progressive glomerulonephritis in mice. Nat Med 2006;12:1081–7.

[102] Plotkin MD, Goligorsky MS. Mesenchymal cells from adult kidney support angiogenesis and differentiate into multiple interstitial cell types including erythropoietin-producing fibroblasts. Am J Physiol Renal Physiol 2006;291:F902–12.

[103] Bruno S, Bussolati B, Grange C, Collino F, di Cantogno LV, Herrera MB, et al. Isolation and characterization of resident mesenchymal stem cells in human glomeruli. Stem Cells Dev 2009;18:867–80.

[104] Farrington-Rock C, Crofts NJ, Doherty MJ, Ashton BA, Griffin-Jones C, Canfield AE. Chondrogenic and adipogenic potential of microvascular pericytes. Circulation 2004;110:2226–32.

[105] Feng J, Mantesso A, De Bari C, Nishiyama A, Sharpe PT. Dual origin of mesenchymal stem cells contributing to organ growth and repair. Proc Natl Acad Sci U S A 2011;108:6503–8.

[106] Fujigaki Y, Muranaka Y, Sun D, Goto T, Zhou H, Sakakima M, et al. Transient myofibroblast differentiation of interstitial fibroblastic cells relevant to tubular dilatation in uranyl acetate-induced acute renal failure in rats. Virchows Arch 2005;446:164–76.

[107] Li L, Clevers H. Coexistence of quiescent and active adult stem cells in mammals. Science 2010;327:542–5.

[108] Zhao C, Deng W, Gage FH. Mechanisms and functional implications of adult neurogenesis. Cell 2008;132:645–60.

[109] Rosenberger C, Rosen S, Paliege A, Heyman SN. Pimonidazole adduct immunohistochemistry in the rat kidney: detection of tissue hypoxia. Methods Mol Biol 2009;466:161—74.

[110] Morrison SJ, Spradling AC. Stem cells and niches: mechanisms that promote stem cell maintenance throughout life. Cell 2008;132:598—611.

[111] Fuller MT, Spradling AC. Male and female *drosophila* germline stem cells: two versions of immortality. Science 2007;316:402—4.

[112] Bonfanti P, Claudinot S, Amici AW, Farley A, Blackburn CC, Barrandon Y. Microenvironmental reprogramming of thymic epithelial cells to skin multipotent stem cells. Nature 2010;466:978—82.

[113] Parmar K, Mauch P, Vergilio JA, Sackstein R, Down JD. Distribution of hematopoietic stem cells in the bone marrow according to regional hypoxia. Proc Natl Acad Sci U S A 2007;104:5431—6.

[114] Simsek T, Kocabas F, Zheng J, Deberardinis RJ, Mahmoud AI, Olson EN, et al. The distinct metabolic profile of hematopoietic stem cells reflects their location in a hypoxic niche. Cell Stem Cell 2010;7:380—90.

[115] Takubo K, Goda N, Yamada W, Iriuchishima H, Ikeda E, Kubota Y, et al. Regulation of the HIF-1alpha level is essential for hematopoietic stem cells. Cell Stem Cell 2010;7:391—402.

[116] Mazumdar J, O'Brien WT, Johnson RS, LaManna JC, Chavez JC, Klein PS, et al. O_2 regulates stem cells through Wnt/beta-catenin signalling. Nat Cell Biol 2010;12:1007—13.

[117] Mohyeldin A, Garzon-Muvdi T, Quinones-Hinojosa A. Oxygen in stem cell biology: a critical component of the stem cell niche. Cell Stem Cell 2010;7:150—61.

[118] Kranc KR, Schepers H, Rodrigues NP, Bamforth S, Villadsen E, Ferry H, et al. Cited2 is an essential regulator of adult hematopoietic stem cells. Cell Stem Cell 2009;5:659—65.

[119] Zhang W, Edwards A. Oxygen transport across vasa recta in the renal medulla. Am J Physiol Heart Circ Physiol 2002;283:H1042—55.

[120] Adams DC, Oxburgh L. The long-term label retaining population of the renal papilla arises through divergent regional growth of the kidney. Am J Physiol Renal Physiol 2009;297:F809—15.

[121] Curtis LM, Chen S, Chen B, Agarwal A, Klug CA, Sanders PW. Contribution of intrarenal cells to cellular repair after acute kidney injury: subcapsular implantation technique. Am J Physiol Renal Physiol 2008;295:F310—4.

[122] Elger M, Hentschel H, Litteral J, Wellner M, Kirsch T, Luft FC, et al. Nephrogenesis is induced by partial nephrectomy in the elasmobranch *Leucoraja erinacea*. J Am Soc Nephrol 2003;14:1506—18.

[123] Zhou W, Boucher RC, Bollig F, Englert C, Hildebrandt F. Characterization of mesonephric development and regeneration using transgenic zebrafish. Am J Physiol Renal Physiol 2010;299:F1040—7.

[124] Diep CQ, Ma D, Deo RC, Holm TM, Naylor RW, Arora N, et al. Identification of adult nephron progenitors capable of kidney regeneration in zebrafish. Nature 2011;470:95—100.

[125] Georgas K, Rumballe B, Valerius MT, Chiu HS, Thiagarajan RD, Lesieur E, et al. Analysis of early nephron patterning reveals a role for distal RV proliferation in fusion to the ureteric tip via a cap mesenchyme-derived connecting segment. Dev Biol 2009;332:273—86.

[126] Kobayashi A, Kwan KM, Carroll TJ, McMahon AP, Mendelsohn CL, Behringer RR. Distinct and sequential tissue-specific activities of the LIM-class homeobox gene Lim1 for tubular morphogenesis during kidney development. Development 2005;132:2809—23.

[127] Weavers H, Prieto-Sanchez S, Grawe F, Garcia-Lopez A, Artero R, Wilsch-Brauninger M, et al. The insect nephrocyte is a podocyte-like cell with a filtration slit diaphragm. Nature 2009;457:322—6.

[128] Singh SR, Liu W, Hou SX. The adult *Drosophila* malpighian tubules are maintained by multipotent stem cells. Cell Stem Cell 2007;1:191—203.

[129] Picard N, Baum O, Vogetseder A, Kaissling B, Le Hir M. Origin of renal myofibroblasts in the model of unilateral ureter obstruction in the rat. Histochem Cell Biol 2008;130:141—55.

[130] Corselli M, Chen CW, Crisan M, Lazzari L, Peault B. Perivascular ancestors of adult multipotent stem cells. Arterioscler Thromb Vasc Biol 2010;30:1104—9.

[131] Iwano M, Plieth D, Danoff TM, Xue C, Okada H, Neilson EG. Evidence that fibroblasts derive from epithelium during tissue fibrosis. J Clin Invest 2002;110:341—50.

[132] Thiery JP, Acloque H, Huang RY, Nieto MA. Epithelial-mesenchymal transitions in development and disease. Cell 2009;139:871—90.

[133] Mani SA, Guo W, Liao MJ, Eaton EN, Ayyanan A, Zhou AY, et al. The epithelial—mesenchymal transition generates cells with properties of stem cells. Cell 2008;133:704—15.

[134] Oliver JA, Barasch J, Yang J, Herzlinger D, Al-Awqati Q. Metanephric mesenchyme contains embryonic renal stem cells. Am J Physiol Renal Physiol 2002;283:F799—809.

[135] Okada H, Danoff TM, Kalluri R, Neilson EG. Early role of Fsp1 in epithelial-mesenchymal transformation. Am J Physiol 1997;273:F563—74.

[136] Quaggin SE, Kapus A. Scar wars: mapping the fate of epithelial—mesenchymal—myofibroblast transition. Kidney Int 2011;80:41—50.

[137] Kriz W, Kaissling B, Le Hir M. Epithelial—mesenchymal transition (EMT) in kidney fibrosis: fact or fantasy? J Clin Invest 2011;121:468—74.

[138] Burns WC, Twigg SM, Forbes JM, Pete J, Tikellis C, Thallas-Bonke V, et al. Connective tissue growth factor plays an important role in advanced glycation end product-induced tubular epithelial-to-mesenchymal transition: implications for diabetic renal disease. J Am Soc Nephrol 2006;17:2484—94.

[139] Cheng S, Lovett DH. Gelatinase A (MMP-2) is necessary and sufficient for renal tubular cell epithelial—mesenchymal transformation. Am J Pathol 2003;162:1937—49.

[140] Li Y, Yang J, Dai C, Wu C, Liu Y. Role for integrin-linked kinase in mediating tubular epithelial to mesenchymal transition and renal interstitial fibrogenesis. J Clin Invest 2003;112:503—16.

[141] Strutz F, Okada H, Lo CW, Danoff T, Carone RL, Tomaszewski JE, et al. Identification and characterization of a fibroblast marker: FSP1. J Cell Biol 1995;130:393—405.

[142] Zhang G, Kernan KA, Collins SJ, Cai X, Lopez-Guisa JM, Degen JL, et al. Plasmin(ogen) promotes renal interstitial fibrosis by promoting epithelial-to-mesenchymal transition: role of plasmin-activated signals. J Am Soc Nephrol 2007;18:846—59.

[143] Nishitani Y, Iwano M, Yamaguchi Y, Harada K, Nakatani K, Akai Y, et al. Fibroblast-specific protein 1 is a specific prognostic marker for renal survival in patients with IgAN. Kidney Int 2005;68:1078—85.

[144] Rossini M, Cheunsuchon B, Donnert E, Ma LJ, Thomas JW, Neilson EG, et al. Immunolocalization of fibroblast growth factor-1 (FGF-1), its receptor (FGFR-1), and fibroblast-specific protein-1 (FSP-1) in inflammatory renal disease. Kidney Int 2005;68:2621—8.

[145] Faulkner JL, Szcykalski LM, Springer F, Barnes JL. Origin of interstitial fibroblasts in an accelerated model of angiotensin II-induced renal fibrosis. Am J Pathol 2005;167:1193—205.

[146] Koesters R, Kaissling B, Lehir M, Picard N, Theilig F, Gebhardt R, et al. Tubular overexpression of transforming growth factor-beta1 induces autophagy and fibrosis but not mesenchymal transition of renal epithelial cells. Am J Pathol 2010;177:632—43.

[147] Li L, Zepeda-Orozco D, Black R, Lin F. Autophagy is a component of epithelial cell fate in obstructive uropathy. Am J Pathol 2010;176:1767—78.

[148] Li J, Qu X, Bertram JF. Endothelial—myofibroblast transition contributes to the early development of diabetic renal interstitial fibrosis in streptozotocin-induced diabetic mice. Am J Pathol 2009;175:1380—8.

[149] Zeisberg EM, Potenta SE, Sugimoto H, Zeisberg M, Kalluri R. Fibroblasts in kidney fibrosis emerge via endothelial-to-mesenchymal transition. J Am Soc Nephrol 2008;19:2282—7.

[150] Medici D, Shore EM, Lounev VY, Kaplan FS, Kalluri R, Olsen BR. Conversion of vascular endothelial cells into multipotent stem-like cells. Nat Med 2010;16:1400—6.

[151] Matthaei KI. Genetically manipulated mice: a powerful tool with unsuspected caveats. J Physiol 2007;582:481—8.

[152] Duffield JS, Humphreys BD. Origin of new cells in the adult kidney: results from genetic labeling techniques. Kidney Int 2011;79:494—501.

[153] Madisen L, Zwingman TA, Sunkin SM, Oh SW, Zariwala HA, Gu H, et al. A robust and high-throughput Cre reporting and characterization system for the whole mouse brain. Nat Neurosci 2010;13:133—40.

[154] Kale S, Karihaloo A, Clark PR, Kashgarian M, Krause DS, Cantley LG. Bone marrow stem cells contribute to repair of the ischemically injured renal tubule. J Clin Invest 2003;112:42—9.

[155] Lin F, Cordes K, Li L, Hood L, Couser WG, Shankland SJ, et al. Hematopoietic stem cells contribute to the regeneration of renal tubules after renal ischemia-reperfusion injury in mice.. J Am Soc Nephrol 2003;14:1188—99.

[156] Morigi M, Imberti B, Zoja C, Corna D, Tomasoni S, Abbate M, et al. Mesenchymal stem cells are renotropic, helping to repair the kidney and improve function in acute renal failure. J Am Soc Nephrol 2004;15:1794—804.

[157] Poulsom R, Forbes SJ, Hodivala-Dilke K, Ryan E, Wyles S, Navaratnarasah S, et al. Bone marrow contributes to renal parenchymal turnover and regeneration. J Pathol 2001;195:229—35.

[158] Hauser PV, De Fazio R, Bruno S, Sdei S, Grange C, Bussolati B, et al. Stem cells derived from human amniotic fluid contribute to acute kidney injury recovery. Am J Pathol 2010;177:2011—21.

[159] Herrera MB, Bussolati B, Bruno S, Morando L, Mauriello-Romanazzi G, Sanavio F, et al. Exogenous mesenchymal stem cells localize to the kidney by means of CD44 following acute tubular injury. Kidney Int 2007;72:430—41.

[160] Lange C, Togel F, Ittrich H, Clayton F, Nolte-Ernsting C, Zander AR, et al. Administered mesenchymal stem cells enhance recovery from ischemia/reperfusion-induced acute renal failure in rats. Kidney Int 2005;68:1613—7.

[161] Togel F, Hu Z, Weiss K, Isaac J, Lange C, Westenfelder C. Administered mesenchymal stem cells protect against ischemic acute renal failure through differentiation-independent mechanisms. Am J Physiol Renal Physiol 2005;289:F31—42.

[162] Morigi M, Rota C, Montemurro T, Montelatici E, Lo Cicero V, Imberti B, et al. Life-sparing effect of human cord blood-mesenchymal stem cells in experimental acute kidney injury. Stem Cells 2010;28:513—22.

[163] Chen J, Park HC, Addabbo F, Ni J, Pelger E, Li H, et al. Kidney-derived mesenchymal stem cells contribute to vasculogenesis, angiogenesis and endothelial repair. Kidney Int 2008;74:879—89.

[164] Togel F, Weiss K, Yang Y, Hu Z, Zhang P, Westenfelder C. Vasculotropic, paracrine actions of infused mesenchymal stem cells are important to the recovery from acute kidney injury. Am J Physiol Renal Physiol 2007;292:F1626—35.

[165] Hammerman MR, Miller SB. Therapeutic use of growth factors in renal failure. J Am Soc Nephrol 1994;5:1—11.

[166] Bartosh TJ, Ylostalo JH, Mohammadipoor A, Bazhanov N, Coble K, Claypool K, et al. Aggregation of human mesenchymal stromal cells (MSCs) into 3D spheroids enhances their antiinflammatory properties. Proc Natl Acad Sci U S A 2010;107:13724—9.

[167] Nemeth K, Leelahavanichkul A, Yuen PS, Mayer B, Parmelee A, Doi K, et al. Bone marrow stromal cells attenuate sepsis via prostaglandin E(2)-dependent reprogramming of host macrophages to increase their interleukin-10 production. Nat Med 2009;15:42—9.

[168] Huang Y, Johnston P, Zhang B, Zakari A, Chowdhry T, Smith RR, et al. Kidney-derived stromal cells modulate dendritic and T cell responses. J Am Soc Nephrol 2009;20:831—41.

[169] Zhang B, Liu R, Shi D, Liu X, Chen Y, Dou X, et al. Mesenchymal stem cells induce mature dendritic cells into a novel Jagged-2-dependent regulatory dendritic cell population. Blood 2009;113:46—57.

[170] Corcione A, Benvenuto F, Ferretti E, Giunti D, Cappiello V, Cazzanti F, et al. Human mesenchymal stem cells modulate B-cell functions. Blood 2006;107:367—72.

[171] Lee RH, Pulin AA, Seo MJ, Kota DJ, Ylostalo J, Larson BL, et al. Intravenous hMSCs improve myocardial infarction in mice because cells embolized in lung are activated to secrete the anti-inflammatory protein TSG-6. Cell Stem Cell 2009;5:54—63.

[172] Li B, Cohen A, Hudson TE, Motlagh D, Amrani DL, Duffield JS. Mobilized human hematopoietic stem/progenitor cells promote kidney repair after ischemia/reperfusion injury. Circulation 2010;121:2211—20.

[173] Loffredo FS, Steinhauser ML, Gannon J, Lee RT. Bone marrow-derived cell therapy stimulates endogenous cardiomyocyte progenitors and promotes cardiac repair. Cell Stem Cell 2011;8:389—98.

[174] Kinomura M, Kitamura S, Tanabe K, Ichinose K, Hirokoshi K, Takazawa Y, et al. Amelioration of cisplatin-induced acute renal injury by renal progenitor-like cells derived from the adult rat kidney. Cell Transplant 2008;17:143—58.

[175] Lazzeri E, Crescioli C, Ronconi E, Mazzinghi B, Sagrinati C, Netti GS, et al. Regenerative potential of embryonic renal multipotent progenitors in acute renal failure. J Am Soc Nephrol 2007;18:3128—38.

[176] Kunter U, Rong S, Boor P, Eitner F, Muller-Newen G, Djuric Z, et al. Mesenchymal stem cells prevent progressive experimental renal failure but maldifferentiate into glomerular adipocytes. J Am Soc Nephrol 2007;18:1754—64.

[177] Hsu YC, Pasolli HA, Fuchs E. Dynamics between stem cells, niche, and progeny in the hair follicle. Cell 2011;144:92—105.

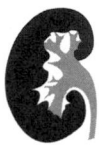

FLUID AND ELECTROLYTE REGULATION AND DYSREGULATION

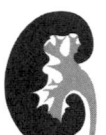

Epithelial Na$^+$ Channels

Shaohu Sheng[1], Kenneth R. Hallows[1,2] and Thomas R. Kleyman[1,2]

[1]Renal-Electrolyte Division, Department of Medicine, University of Pittsburgh, Pittsburgh, PA, USA
[2]Department of Cell Biology and Physiology, University of Pittsburgh, Pittsburgh, PA, USA

INTRODUCTION

From the late distal convoluted tubule, connecting tubule, and throughout the collecting duct, Na$^+$ exits the urinary space by passive diffusion through an apical membrane epithelial Na$^+$ channel, referred to as ENaC. Na$^+$ exits cells across basolateral membranes via the Na$^+$,K$^+$-ATPase. Koefoed-Johnson and Ussing initially proposed this model of electrogenic transepithelial Na$^+$ transport, with diffusion of Na$^+$ across an apical membrane conductance pathway, in 1958.[1] Studies using both noise analysis and single channel recordings demonstrated the presence of apical membrane Na$^+$ selective ion channels.[2–4] Subsequent to the cloning of ENaC, knockout studies have confirmed the role of ENaC in the reabsorption of filtered Na$^+$ in the distal nephron, as well as its role in facilitating renal K$^+$ secretion.[5–7]

Electrophysiologic Characteristics

The basic electrophysiologic characteristics of epithelial Na$^+$ channels have been defined using both macroscopic and single channel studies, and are presented in Figure 30.1. ENaCs are Na$^+$- and Li$^+$-permeable channels that exhibit negligible K$^+$ conductance, with a single channel conductance of 4 to 5 pS at room temperature with Na$^+$ as the charge carrier.[3,8,9] These channels exhibit a slight increase in open probability under hyperpolarizing membrane potentials.[10,11] ENaCs characteristically exhibit long open and closed times, in the order of seconds to tens of seconds, although a population of ENaCs has been described that has brief open times and long closed times that likely represent channels that have not been processed by proteases.[11–13] Channels are blocked by

submicromolar concentrations of amiloride, a pyrazinoylguanidine derivative.[14,15] Amiloride is a weak base and has a pK$_a$ of 8.8 in water. It is the charged, or protonated, form of amiloride that blocks ENaC.[15] Other organic weak bases, including triamterene, trimethoprim, and pentamidine also inhibit ENaC.[16–19]

Biochemical and Molecular Characteristics of ENaC

Amiloride was first demonstrated to inhibit electrogenic transepithelial Na$^+$ transport in 1968.[14] With an IC$_{50}$ of ∼100 nM, amiloride and several related compounds proved to be highly selective Na$^+$ channel inhibitors.[15] Prior to the cloning of ENaC subunits, several different approaches were used to isolate a Na$^+$ channel complex.[20–22] The relationship of this channel complex to ENaC is still unclear, although antibodies raised against a subunit of the cloned Na$^+$ channel have been observed to recognize a polypeptide within the purified channel complex.[23]

The molecular characteristics of this channel were elucidated in studies from Canessa and co-workers and Lingueglia and co-workers in 1993 and 1994.[9,24–26] An expression cloning technique led to the identification of a cDNA, termed α ENaC, whose cRNA induced expression of amiloride-sensitive Na$^+$ currents when injected into *Xenopus* oocytes.[24,25] However, Na$^+$ currents were lower than expected. Two subsequent cDNA clones were isolated based on their ability to complement α ENaC cRNA in the expression of amiloride-sensitive Na$^+$ currents in *Xenopus* oocytes, and were termed β and γ ENaC.[9] *Xenopus* oocytes coinjected with the three cRNA species expressed amiloride-sensitive Na$^+$ channels with characteristics nearly identical to that of Na$^+$ channels expressed in renal

Seldin and Giebisch's The Kidney, Fifth Edition.
DOI: http://dx.doi.org/10.1016/B978-0-12-381462-3.00030-6

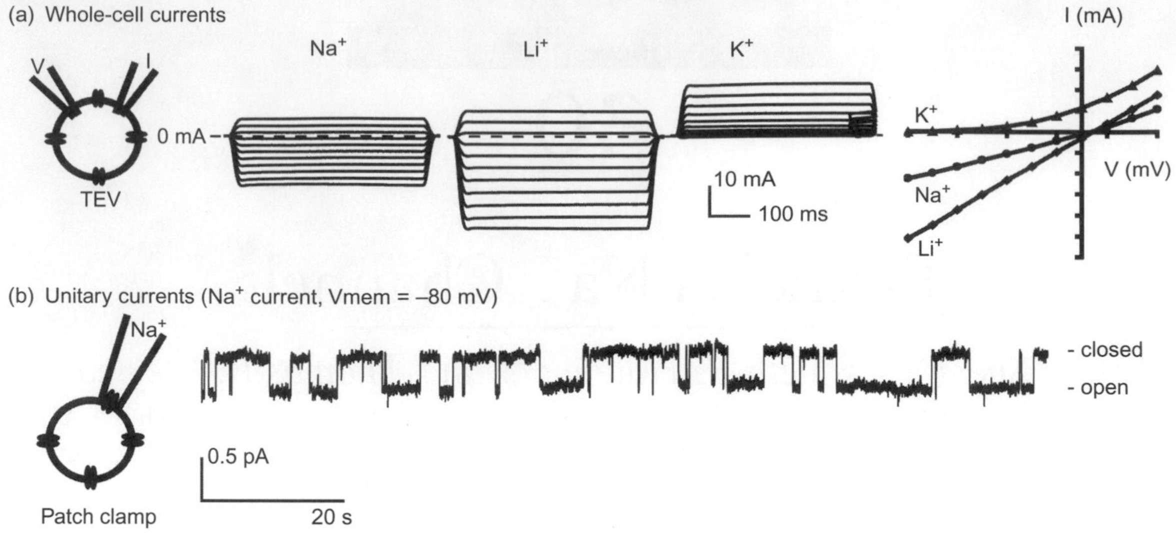

(a) Whole-cell currents

Na⁺   Li⁺   K⁺

0 mA –

TEV

10 mA

100 ms

I (mA)

K⁺

V (mV)

Na⁺

Li⁺

(b) Unitary currents (Na⁺ current, Vmem = –80 mV)

Na⁺

- closed

- open

0.5 pA

Patch clamp

20 s

FIGURE 30.1   Biophysical properties of epithelial Na⁺ channels. (a) Whole-cell currents were recorded in *Xenopus* oocytes expressing αβγ ENaC that were bathed with NaCl, LiCl or KCl solutions. Current-voltage curves are shown on the right. (b) Single channel recording was performed with cell-attached patch and NaCl in the pipette *(Recordings in part (a) are reprinted with permission from ref. [170]).*

cortical collecting tubules and in cultured cell lines derived from the distal nephron. Na⁺ currents were not observed when either the β- or γ-subunits were expressed alone.

The three ENaC subunits are likely derived from a common ancestral gene, given their limited (~30 to 40%) sequence identity. ENaC subunits have been cloned from a variety of species, including rat, human, mouse, rabbit, guinea pig, chicken, cattle, sheep, salamander, clawed African frog (*Xenopus laevis*), and bullfrog.[9,24–34] The human α-subunit gene *Scnn1a* spans 17 kb on human chromosome 12p13. The β- and γ-subunit genes *Scnn1b* and *Scnn1g* are closely linked on human chromosome 16p12-p13.[35,36] The genes encoding the three ENaC subunits have a conserved exon–intron architecture, with 13 exons.[37,38] Splice variants have been described that alter the cytoplasmic N-termini or alter the extracellular domains.[39–41] Variants that result in a termination codon in the region coding the extracellular domain of the α-subunit have also been reported.[41–43] Some of these variants are associated with a reduction or loss of channel activity when expressed in heterologous systems, and with an autosomal recessive loss of function phenotype (pseudohypoaldosteronism) in humans.[42]

ENaC/Degenerin Gene Family

Canessa and co-workers noted that ENaC subunits were related to genes identified in *Caenorhabditis elegans* that participate in mechanosensation specific mutations of which result in degeneration of selected neurons.[44–46] ENaCs belong to the ENaC/Degenerin gene

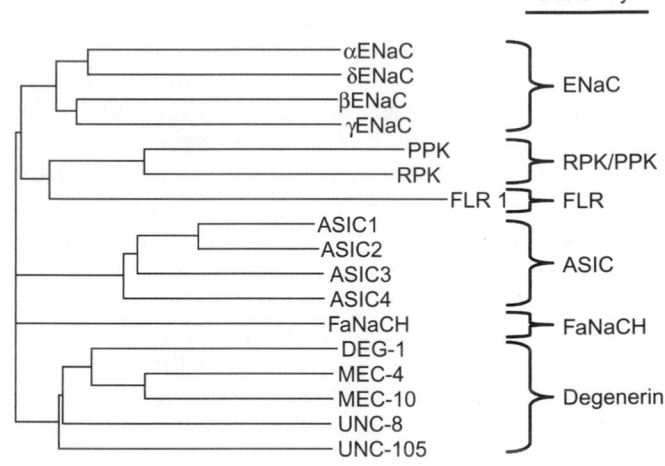

Subfamily

αENaC
δENaC   ENaC
βENaC
γENaC
PPK   RPK/PPK
RPK
FLR 1   FLR
ASIC1
ASIC2
ASIC3   ASIC
ASIC4
FaNaCH   FaNaCH
DEG-1
MEC-4
MEC-10   Degenerin
UNC-8
UNC-105

FIGURE 30.2   Phylogenetic tree of the ENaC/DEG superfamily. Family members are grouped into six subfamilies: ENaCs: RPK (ripped pocket)/PPK (pickpocket), expressed in *Drosophila*; FLR: expressed in *C. elegans*; ASICs or acid-sensing ion channels; FaNaCh: a peptide-gated channel expressed in marine snails; and degenerins: expressed in *C. elegans*.

family (Figure 30.2). There are two additional ENaC subunits, referred to as δ and ε, that appear to be functionally related to the α-subunit. δ ENaC is a proton-activated channel expressed in primates, although its physiologic role is still unclear.[47,48] The ε-subunit was identified in *Xenopus*, and has an altered Na⁺ self-inhibition response suggesting altered gating properties.[49] Members of this family also include genes identified in *C. elegans* that are involved in mechanosensation (*mecs* and *degs*) or control of defecation rhythm (*flrs*);

H$^+$-gated channels (referred to as acid-sensing ion channels (or ASICs)) that are expressed in mammalian central and peripheral nervous systems and have a role in nociception, mechanosensation, fear-related behavior, and seizure termination;[50−55] a family of 16 genes expressed in *Drosophila*, referred to as pickpocket, that may have roles in airway fluid clearance, mechanosensation, salt sensation, and detection of pheromones;[56−61] and peptide-gated channels expressed in marine snails.[62−64]

Structure and Function of ENaC

Each ENaC subunit has only two predicted membrane spanning domains, similar to the topology of members of the Kir family of K$^+$ channels, and members of the P2X family of purinergic receptors that are ligand-gated ion channels[65,66] (Figure 30.3). Three independent groups published topologic analyses of ENaC subunits.[67,68] Each subunit has intracellular amino and carboxyl termini and two α helical membrane spanning domains connected by a large extracellular domain. The cytoplasmic domains have kinase phosphorylation sites, as well as protein−protein and protein−lipid interaction motifs that affect channel gating or trafficking.

Jasti and colleagues resolved the crystal structure of ASIC1, a member of the ENaC/Degenerin family.[69,70] Although initially lacking the N- and C-terminal cytoplasmic regions, this structure provided important insights into the structural organization of ASIC and related family members, including ENaC. ASIC1 is a trimer, suggesting that ENaC has a subunit stoichiometry of α1β1γ1, in contrast to the higher ordered stoichiometry that had been proposed based on biophysical and biochemical studies.[71−74] The extracellular region is a highly ordered structure that resembles an outstretched hand containing a ball, and has clearly defined domains termed wrist, finger, thumb, palm, knuckle, and β-ball[69] (see Figure 30.3). Jasti et al. suggested that ASIC1 proton-dependent gating occurs in conjunction with conformational changes within the thumb and finger domains, which are transmitted to the transmembrane domains.[69] The three ENaC subunits contribute residues that line the channel's pore. The resolved ASIC1 structure suggests that the channel's gate resides in the outer part of the pore,[70,75] in the vicinity of the "degenerin" site where the introduction of bulky residues in: (1) ENaC subunits; (2) mec4 or mec10 (a component of the mechanosensitive channel in *C. elegans*); and (3) ASIC subunits result in a dramatic increase in channel open probability.[46,76−79]

ASIC1 is the only member of the ENaC/Degenerin gene family whose structure has been resolved.[69] This

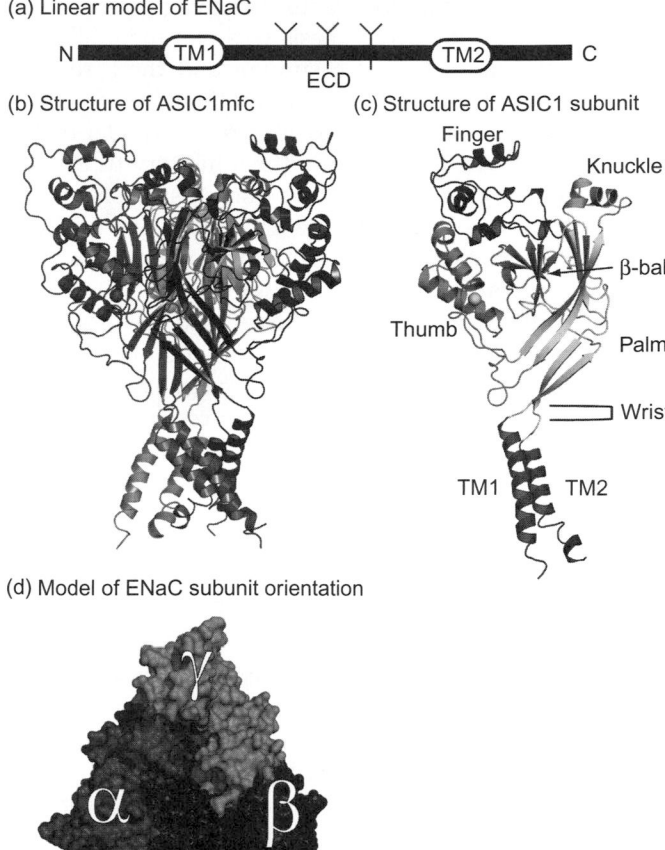

(a) Linear model of ENaC

(b) Structure of ASIC1mfc

(c) Structure of ASIC1 subunit

(d) Model of ENaC subunit orientation

FIGURE 30.3   Structural features of ENaC subunits. (a) Linear model of an ENaC subunit (TM1, TM2: the first and second transmembrane domains; ECD: extracellular domain connecting TM1 and TM2; N: amino terminus; C: carboxyl terminus). Several glycosylation sites are shown as branched lines. (b) Structure of the minimally functional chicken ASIC1.[70] Three identical ASIC1 subunits are shown as ribbons with colors of red, green, and blue for the three subunits. (c) Defined subdomains within the large extracellular domain. (d) Proposed subunit orientation of ENaC, viewed from above.[187,191] Surface rendering of the relative locations of the α- (red), β- (blue), and γ- (green) subunits are shown. The structural models in this figure were generated from coordinates of ASIC1.[70] See color section at the back of the book.

structure provides a starting point to generate models of ENaC subunits. Kashlan and co-workers have built models of the extracellular region of the α-subunit of ENaC based, in part, on homology to ASIC1.[80−82] The extracellular regions of ENaC subunits and ASIC1 are reasonably homologous, except in the finger domain. For example, the α-subunit of ENaC has 73 additional residues when compared to ASIC (see [81,82]). The α-subunit is proteolytically processed at specific sites within its finger domain, releasing an inhibitory tract.[83−85] To determine the molecular architecture of the α-subunit finger domain, sites within α ENaC that interact with an 8 residue inhibitory peptide derived from the portion of the α-subunit that is removed by furin cleavage were determined.[86] The working hypothesis was that the inhibitory tract within a non-cleaved α-subunit and the 8 residue inhibitory peptide share common binding sites. Distance constraints were introduced to construct a model of the α-subunit.[81,82] The model places the inhibitory tract at an interface of the finger and thumb domains. Kashlan and co-workers suggested that the inhibitory tract blocks channel activity by stabilizing the movement of the finger domain relative to the thumb domain.[81,82]

Stockand and co-workers have also generated a model of an ENaC trimer, based on the structure of ASIC1.[87] To generate the model areas that lacked sequence similarity within the finger regions of ENaC subunits were removed. Although this limits the utility of the model, the model provides important insights regarding sites of intersubunit interactions.

ENaC Biogenesis

Na⁺ channel subunits likely undergo assembly in the endoplasmic reticulum (ER), where core, high mannose Asn- (or N)-linked glycans are added at specific sites.[88-97] Each subunit is modified by N-linked glycosylation at multiple sites. For example, rat α-, β-, and γ-subunits have six, twelve, and five consensus sites (Asn-X-Ser/Thr) for N-linked oligosaccharide addition, respectively. Exit of assembled channels from the ER appears to be inefficient.[96,98] A motif that facilitates the exit of ENaC from the ER was found in the proximal cytoplasmic carboxyl terminus of the α-subunit.[98]

Channel subunits that do not exit the ER are likely degraded via proteasome-mediated ER associated degradation (ERAD).[99-102] Integral membrane proteins such as ENaC are co-translationally inserted into the ER. The proper folding and assembly of polypeptides synthesized in the ER involves interactions with a variety of chaperone proteins.[103-105] Specific chaperones that participate in ENaC folding and assembly or targeting misfolded subunits for degradation are starting to be defined. These include members of the luminal Hsp40s, the small heat shock protein alpha A-crystallin, and calreticulin.[100-102,106,107] Cytoplasmic Hsp70s also have roles in channel trafficking, although at present it is unclear whether their roles are related to facilitating ER exit or post-ER trafficking events.[106]

The half-life of newly synthesized subunits, determined by metabolic labeling/pulse-chase experiments, is approximately an hour,[89,91-93,96,99,108] consistent with the notion that the majority of ENaC subunits synthesized within the ER are targeted for degradation via ERAD. A longer-lived pool of channels is apparent in pulse-chase studies, which likely reflects properly assembled channels that have exited the ER.[99] Several

groups have determined the half-life of channels that have reached the surface. The rate of degradation of channels that have reached the surface may be in the order of many hours to days,[92,109-111] although some investigators have reported a shorter half-life for channels that have reached the cell surface of A6 cells and MDCK cells expressing exogenous ENaCs.[91,93] These differences in the half-life of channels that have reached the cell surface could result from differences in cell type, and whether ENaCs are expressed endogenously or exogenously.

ENaC Processing in the Biosynthetic Pathway

As assembled ENaCs exit the ER, it has been thought that channels follow the route used by other proteins in the secretory pathway. This involves trafficking through the Golgi where most N-glycans are processed, and the trans-Golgi network where channels are sorted into endosomes that are delivered to the apical membrane. N-glycan processing is often monitored by the enzyme endoglycosidase H, an enzyme that removes high mannose N-linked glycans prior to processing events that occur in the medial Golgi complex.

N-glycans on all three subunits of assembled channels are modified to complex-type Endo H-resistant forms.[93,97] Surprisingly, subunits with endoglycosidase H sensitive N-glycans have also been described.[97] Hughey and co-workers reported that two distinct pools of ENaC subunits were expressed at the plasma membrane: subunits with processed N-glycans and cleaved α- and γ-subunits; and full-length subunits that have non-processed N-glycans.[97] Processing of subunits within a channel complex appears to be an all-or-nothing event.[112] These findings suggest that a population of channel complexes exiting the ER transits through Golgi and post-Golgi compartments where subunits are processed (Figure 30.4). These processed channels likely represent the pool of active, functional channels. A distinct population of channels exiting the ER appears to bypass Golgi and post-Golgi processing events. This distinct pool of non-processed channels is likely a functionally inactive pool, as proteolysis of ENaC subunits appears to have a dramatic effect on increasing channel open probability.[13,83,113-115] Proteolytic cleavage of these inactive channels provides a potential mechanism to increase rates of Na⁺ transport in the distal nephron. The role of proteolysis of ENaC subunits in regulating channel gating is discussed in detail later in this chapter.

Intracellular Trafficking of ENaC

Functional channels are delivered to the apical plasma membrane via the traditional secretory

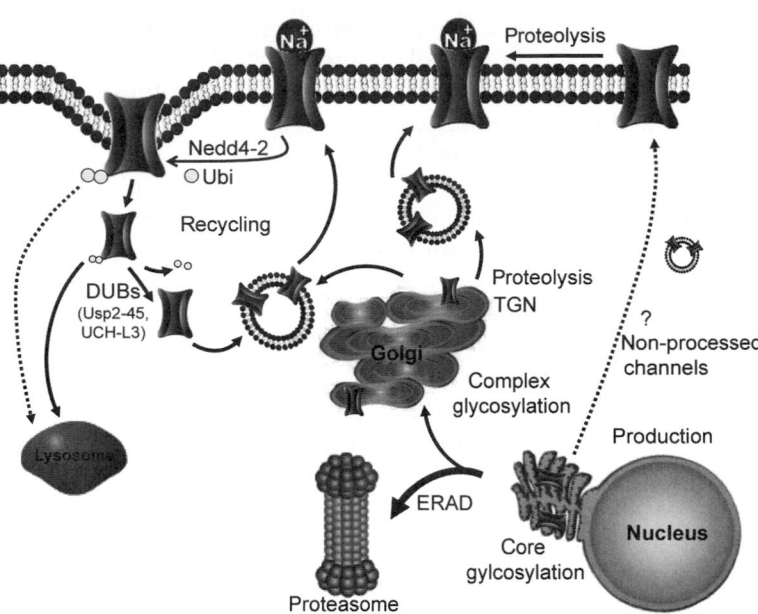

FIGURE 30.4 Model of ENaC biogenesis and intracellular trafficking. ENaC subunits are assembled and undergo addition of high mannose asparagine (N)-linked glycans within the endoplasmic reticulum (ER). The majority of newly synthesized subunits are targeted for ER associated degradation (ERAD) that occurs within proteasomes. Assembled ENaCs that exit the ER transit to the apical plasma membrane via distinct routes. ENaCs traffic through the Golgi, where most N-glycans are processed, and through the trans-Golgi network (TGN), where channels are processed by the protease furin prior to delivery to the apical membrane. Alternatively, ENaCs exiting the ER may be delivered directly to the apical plasma membrane, bypassing processing steps that occur in the Golgi and TGN. These non-processed channels are functionally inactive, but are potentially activated by proteases present at the plasma membrane or within the urinary space. ENaCs at the plasma membrane are targeted for internalization following Nedd4-2-dependent ubiquitination (Ubi). Internalized channels are degraded within lysosomes or proteasomes. Alternatively, internalized channels are likely deubiquitinated by specific deubiquitinating enzymes (DUBs), and recycled to the plasma membrane in a regulated manner.

pathway[112] (Figure 30.4). The exocytic insertion of channels into the apical plasma membrane occurs as a regulated process that is increased in response to a variety of hormones, including vasopressin, aldosterone, and insulin. Vesicle and target SNAREs (soluble N-ethylmaleimide sensitive factor attachment protein receptors) participate in this process, and overexpression of specific SNARE proteins disrupts the intracellular trafficking of ENaC subunits.[116–119] Channels at the plasma membrane appear to reside within specific compartments. Several groups have reported that a population of channels resides within lipid-rich microdomains, referred to as lipid rafts,[120,121] although other groups have not confirmed this finding.[91] While lipid rafts have been reported to facilitate the co-localization of membrane proteins and signaling molecules, the functional consequences of ENaCs within lipid rafts are still unclear. ENaCs interact with cytoskeletal elements, including actin and α-spectrin, which may have a role in localizing the channel to the plasma membrane and in modulating ENaC activity.[122–125]

The residency time of channels at the plasma membrane has been examined by several groups, with reported half-lives in the order of minutes to hours.[91,93,110,111,126,127] Mutations within a carboxyl-terminal PY motif within the β- and γ-subunits are associated with increases in the half-life of the channel at the plasma membrane via mechanisms that are discussed later in this chapter.[126,128] Internalization of channels from the plasma membrane has been proposed to occur via a dynamin-dependent process.[126] Dynamin is required for clathrin-dependent endocytosis, as well as for caveolae-dependent endocytosis.[129–131] Ubiquitin conjugation of defined lysine residues within ENaC subunits at the plasma membrane targets the channels for endocytosis,[132] presumably via a clathrin-dependent mechanism (Figure 30.4).[133] Once internalized, some channels are targeted for degradation via proteasomes or possibly lysosomes.[93,108,132] A significant fraction of the pool of endocytosed channels may undergo recycling to the plasma membrane in a regulated manner[111] (Figure 30.4). Specific deubiquitination enzymes have a role in removing ubiquitin from internalized channels, facilitating the recycling of channels to the plasma membrane.[134–136]

Localization within the Kidney and Other Organs

The aldosterone-sensitive distal nephron is the final site of Na$^+$ reabsorption within the nephron. ENaCs are expressed in principal cells in the late distal convoluted tubule, connecting tubule, and through the collecting duct, and are the major pathway for Na⁺ entry across the apical plasma membrane. In the more proximal segments of the aldosterone-sensitive distal nephron, Na⁺ reabsorption via ENaC is coupled to K⁺ secretion mediated by apical membrane K⁺ channels, including Kir1.1 (or ROMK) and the large conductance Ca²⁺-activated K⁺ channel (maxi-K).[137-139] ENaC-dependent reabsorption of Na⁺ in the distal nephron has a major role in the control of extracellular fluid volume, blood pressure, and renal K⁺ secretion.

The cellular localization of individual ENaC subunits may differ within the nephron. When maintained on normal laboratory diet, β- and γ-subunits were localized within an intracellular compartment in principal cells within the cortical and outer medullary segments of the rat aldosterone-sensitive distal nephron.[140] One group reported that the α-subunit was localized primarily to apical part of principal cells,[140] whereas other groups have observed either modest cytoplasmic localization or have failed to detect the α-subunit.[141,142] Within the inner medullary collecting duct, all three ENaC subunits were localized primarily within an intracellular compartment.[140] When placed on a low-Na⁺ diet or following administration of aldosterone, all three subunits were expressed at the apical membrane of principal cells.[141,143]

Mice lacking expression of the β- or γ-subunits or that have reduced expression of the α-subunit exhibit renal Na⁺-wasting.[5-7,144] Mice that lack expression of the α-subunit are unable to clear airway fluids at birth, leading to death in the early postnatal period.[145] Recent work suggests that the density of ENaC expression may be greatest in the connecting tubule, an early segment within the aldosterone-sensitive distal nephron that connects the distal convoluted tubule to the collecting tubule.[146] Mice that lack expression of α ENaC beyond the connecting tubule are able to maintain Na⁺ and K⁺ balance, even in the setting of dietary Na⁺ restriction or K⁺-loading.[147]

In addition to its expression in the nephron, ENaCs are expressed within numerous other organs. They are expressed throughout the airways, as well as in both type I and type II alveolar cells.[148-152] ENaC has a key role in the reabsorption of airway fluids.[145,153] Maintaining an appropriate volume of airway surface liquids has an important role in facilitating mucociliary clearance.[153,154] ENaCs are also expressed in the distal colon, sweat ducts, salivary ducts, inner ear, lingular epithelium, keratinocytes, lymphocytes, and vascular smooth muscle. ENaC expression has also been reported in endothelia and in various sites within the eye, including epithelia within the retina, lens, and pigmented ciliary body and iris.[9,155-162] The functional roles of ENaCs within many of these tissues are unclear.

ENaC STRUCTURE AND FUNCTION

Specific structural features within channel subunits have key roles in defining the biophysical properties of ENaC. All three ENaC subunits contribute to the formation of the conduction pore, as pore properties are altered by mutations within each of the three subunits.[163] The published structures of ASIC1 reveal a homomeric trimer[69,70] (Figure 30.3). The structures of the extracellular domain (ECD) and transmembrane domain (TM) are well-defined, while the cytoplasmic amino- and carboxyl-terminal domains are not resolved in the crystal structures. The cASIC1 structures confirm a longstanding notion that the channel pore is formed largely by the second transmembrane domain (TM2s) that determines the basic biophysical properties of ENaC. Both the extracellular and cytoplasmic domains have roles in modulating channel-gating and trafficking. The functional roles of individual domains within ENaC subunits, and potential mechanisms of ion permeation, ion selectivity, channel-gating, and amiloride block are reviewed below with insights from the ASIC1 structures.

Functional Domains within ENaC Subunits

Amino-Terminus

The cytoplasmic amino-termini have regions that affect channel-gating, trafficking, and regulation by intracellular factors. Chalfant and co-workers identified a Lys-Gly-Asp-Lys tract within the rat α-subunit corresponding to residues 47–50, that may function as an endocytic signal that regulates the number of channels in the plasma membrane.[164] A domain that affects channel-gating has been characterized within the distal portion of the amino-terminus of the α-subunit, which includes a highly-conserved His-Gly tract.[165,166] A mutation in the corresponding Gly in the β-subunit was described in a patient with pseudohypoaldosteronism. Reduced channel activity attributed to a decreased open probability was observed with a mutation of the conserved Gly in each subunit, suggesting that the His-Gly tract within the amino termini of all three subunits influences channel-gating.[42,165,166] A recent study showed that mutations of this Gly in the α and γ ENaC subunits induced a strong inward rectification in the whole cell currents, reflecting voltage-dependent gating.[167] Mutations at other sites have also been found to reduce channel activity and induce voltage-dependent gating.[168–171]

Phosphatidylinositol 4,5-bisphosphate (PIP2) activates ENaCs,[172,173] an effect that reflects an increase in channel open probability as a result of direct interactions between PIP2 and ENaC. Several groups have proposed that the amino-termini of the β- and γ-subunits of ENaC harbor putative PIP2-binding domains containing basic amino acid residues.[172,174,175] In addition, Helms and co-workers suggest that PIP3 mediates aldosterone-induced ENaC activity and trafficking, and interacts with γ ENaC.[176] The ENaC amino-termini also contain Cys residues that may interact with intracellular metals (Cd^{2+} and Zn^{2+}) and thiol-reactive chemicals, leading to a reduction in channel open probability.[177] Palmitoylation of amino-terminal Cys-43 and carboxyl-terminal Cys-557 of mouse β ENaC enhances channel open probability (see below).[98]

First Transmembrane Domain (TM1)

The ASIC1 structures were apparently resolved in a desensitized state. In these structures, the channel pore is primarily lined by TM2 helices from three identical subunits, with the three TM1 helices packed tangentially behind the TM2 helices and contacting the lipid bilayer. The TM1 helix from an individual subunit also makes extensive interactions with the TM2 helix of the same subunit, as well as specific contacts with helices from an adjacent subunit.[70] The closed-pore conformation of ENaC may be similar to that of ASIC1. A Trp scanning of the TM1 of α ENaC showed that mutations within the amino-terminal portion of αTM1 alter channel activity, selectivity, and gating,[178] consistent with the extensive intrasubunit interaction between TM1 and TM2 helices revealed in the ASIC1 structures.[69,70] A recent Cys scanning of ASIC1 TM domains is also consistent with the relative locations of TM1 and TM2 helices in the resolved structures.[75]

Extracellular Domain (ECD)

Each ENaC subunit has a large, ~450 residue extracellular region with 16 conserved Cys residues clustered within two Cys-rich domains.[179] Other members of the ENaC/DEG family also possess extracellular Cys-rich domains.[180] The size and the apparently conserved structural organization of the extracellular domain suggest that this region has important functional roles. Recent studies have examined the role of the ECD in modulating channel-gating in response to proteases, sheer stress, external Na^+, metals, H^+, and Cl^-.[49,80,97,179,181–193] These functional studies and insights from the ASIC1 structure suggest that the ECD of ENaC functions as a sensor or receptor for a variety of extracellular signals. The extracellular domains also facilitate the assembly of the heteroligomeric channel complex within the endoplasmic reticulum, and influence intracellular trafficking.[179,193,194]

Several proteases, including prostasin and related channel-activating proteases, furin, trypsin, chymotrypsin, and elastase have been shown to activate ENaC.[83,113,114,195–199] Activation of ENaC by proteases is a result of proteolytic cleavage of ENaC subunits within their extracellular domains at defined sites, releasing intrinsic inhibitory tracts.[81,84,85,200] Mechanisms by which proteases activate ENaCs are discussed below.

ENaCs are inhibited by extracellular Na^+, which presumably binds to sites within the ECD. This response, referred to as self-inhibition, reflects a reduction in channel open probability.[2,115,182,185,201,202] The structural basis of Na^+ self-inhibition has begun to emerge from mutagenesis studies.[80,182,185,186,188,190–193] At present, the sites of Na^+-binding, as well as the subsequent allosteric changes that lead to a reduction in channel open probability, have not been defined. In addition to Na^+, other external cations such as Ni^{2+}, Zn^{2+}, Cu^{2+}, Cd^{2+}, and Hg^{2+} affect ENaC activity, presumably by binding to sites within the ECDs and altering channel open probability.[181,184,187,203–206] The effects of these metals on ENaC are both metal- and species-specific.

Extracellular anions also interact at sites within the extracellular domains of ENaC subunits and alter ENaC gating. Collier and Snyder found that external Cl^- regulates ENaC activity in part through enhancing Na^+ self-inhibition. Their findings provide a mechanism by which changes in extracellular Cl^- modulates epithelial Na^+ absorption.[190] They identified two Cl^- inhibitory sites in ENaC, one formed by residues in the thumb domain of the α-subunit and the palm domain of the β-subunit, and the other formed by residues at the interface of the thumb domain of the β-subunit and the palm domain of the γ-subunit. Based on the effects of mutagenesis on Cl^- inhibition, the additive nature of mutations, and on differences in the mechanisms of Cl^- inhibition, the authors propose a model in which ENaC subunits assemble in an αγβ-orientation when viewed from above[191] (Figure 30.3). This subunit arrangement is also suggested by Chen et al., based on the identification of a putative Cu^{2+}-binding site at the α- and β-subunit interface within the ECD of human ENaC.[187] However, the model is based on the assumption that the functional ENaC complex is a heterotrimer. The possibility that multiple arrangements co-exist needs to be tested.

Within the ENaC extracellular domains are 16 Cys residues, which are largely conserved among other members of the ENaC/degenerin family. Firsov and colleagues proposed that specific Cys residues (the first and sixth Cys in all three subunits, as well as the eleventh and twelfth Cys in the α- and β-subunits) have an essential role in the efficient transport of assembled channels to the plasma membrane.[179] A mutation of the first cysteine residue in the human α-subunit (αC133Y) is associated with PHA-1.[207] Sheng et al. proposed that there are several intrasubunit disulfide bonds, based on analyses of additivity of double Cys mutations and responses to sulfhydryl reagent of single and double mutants.[183] These predicted disulfide bonds (Cys1-Cys6, Cys4-Cys5, Cys7-Cys16, Cys11-Cys12, Cys10-Cys13, and Cys8-Cys15 (conserved Cys numbered sequentially)) were present in the resolved ASIC1 structure.[69] ASIC subunits have 14 conserved Cys residues within the ECD that form seven intrasubunit disulfide bonds, one in β-ball, one in palm, and five in thumb domain.[69] The locations of the disulfide bonds are consistent with their roles in stabilizing the conformations of these domains.

Second Transmembrane Domain (TM2)

The TM2 region is thought to be the segment that lines the conduction pore and contains important functional sites, including the degenerin (DEG) site, amiloride-binding site, and selectivity filter site[169,208,209] (Figure 30.5). The structure of the ENaC pore is expected to be similar to that of ASIC1, given the high degree of sequence homology and similar biophysical properties. For example, three ENaC TM2s likely line the channel pore, while TM1s contact the lipid bilayer. As the resolved ASIC1 structures likely represent non-conducting states, they provide limited information regarding the roles of TM2 residues in ion permeation and selectivity. Two distinct TM domain structures of ASIC1 have been described,[69,70] adding an additional layer of complexity in interpreting structure and function relationships of the TM2 domains from the resolved ASIC1 structures. Here we discuss mutagenesis results, mainly in reference to the most recent ASIC1 structure.[70]

AMILORIDE BINDING

Schild and co-workers identified a ring of residues at homologous positions within each of the three subunits (αS583, βG525, and γG537 in rat ENaC) as a putative amiloride-binding site[163] (Figure 30.5). The substitution of βG525 or γG537 weakened amiloride IC$_{50}$ by about three orders of magnitude. In contrast, the substitution of αS583 with amino acids bearing side chains with different functional groups (e.g., Gly, Leu, Asn, Gln) had only a slight effect on amiloride block, suggesting that the side chain of αS583 does not participate in amiloride binding.[171] However, amino acids with aromatic side chains introduced at αS583 led to a large reduction in amiloride affinity, suggesting that large side chains at position α583

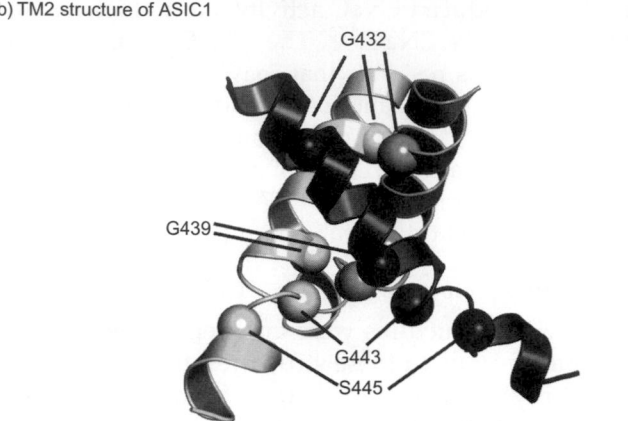

(a) TM2 sequence alignments

FIGURE 30.5   ENaC/ASIC pore structures. (a) Sequence alignments of the second transmembrane domains (TM2) of mouse α-, β- and γ-subunits and chicken ASIC1. Identical residues are shown as boxed and bold letters and the similar residues are shaded. Key functional sites are labeled. Selected ASIC1 residues are identified below by residue numbers. Location of the proposed desensitization gate of ASIC1[70] is indicated by a square bracket. (b) Model of the TM2 bundles of ASIC1.[70] The three TM2 helices are shown. Spheres represent α-carbons of ASIC1 residues identified in panel (a).

protrude into the pore, and limit access of amiloride to this site.[171] The effects of Cys substitutions at the amiloride-binding ring on the inhibitory constant largely reflected an increase in the microscopic k_{off} rate, consistent with an effect on the bound complex.[210] An adjacent three residue Gly/Ser-X-Ser tract that forms the primary selectivity filter may also have an important role in amiloride binding. Mutations introduced in the first position of this tract in the α- or β-subunit were associated with a large reduction in amiloride affinity,[211–213] suggesting that amiloride also interacts with this site.

The introduction of Cys residues at the amiloride-binding ring rendered channels sensitive to block by external Zn^{2+}-, Cd^{2+}-, and sulfhydryl-reactive methanthiosulfonate (MTS) derivatives.[72,76,163,209,212] Moreover, mutations of these residues reduced single channel conductance.[163,171] This site was also shown to be located within the membrane electrical field.[76,163,171] These observations suggest that this ring of residues line the conducting pore, as was observed in the homologous residue in the resolved ASIC1 structure.[70]

SELECTIVITY FILTER

A three residue tract (Gly/Ser-X-Ser) starting four residues distal to the amiloride-binding site has a key role in conferring cation selectivity (Figure 30.5). Systematic examination of the ENaC TM2 domains by several groups found that mutations of either the first and/or third residue within the Gly/Ser-X-Ser tract of the α-, β-, and γ-subunits resulted in significant K[+] permeation.[169,208,209,211,212,214] Certain substitutions of the third residue within this tract in the α-subunit allow for permeation of divalent cations.[208]

It is unclear whether backbone carbonyl oxygens or side chains within this three residue Gly/Ser-X-Ser tract face the lumen.[213–215] Kellenberger et al. initially proposed that carbonyl oxygen atoms from third position Ser residues provide a Na[+]-binding site, based on a positive correlation between increases in K[+] permeability and the volumes of several substituted residues at αSer589.[214] Alternatively, Sheng et al. proposed that the side chains of the selectivity filter residues faced the pore lumen, based on the sensitivity of channels with an introduced Cys at the first or third residue in the selectivity filter to externally applied Cd[2+].[213] This proposed side chain orientation is also consistent with the need for a hydroxyl group at position α589 to prevent K[+] permeation.[169] The dispute regarding the orientation of residue side chains within the selectivity filter will likely remain until a high-resolution structure of ENaC or ASIC in an open state is available.

The distal (C-terminal) portions of the TM2 domains have three well-conserved negatively charged residues that likely line one face of an α helix. The introduction of mutations at specific sites containing acidic residues has been reported to reduce channel activity without altering surface expression[216] and result in K[+] permeation, suggesting that some of these residues may also have a direct or indirect role in conferring cation selectivity.[170]

CHANNEL GATE

A five residue motif (G[432]DIGG[436]) in the outer part of the ASIC1 TM2 domain has been proposed to function as the desensitization gate[70] (Figure 30.5). Gly432 is conserved among ASICs and is homologous to Ala442 in MEC4, the degenerin site where substitutions with a bulky residue result in degeneration of specific neurons in *Caenorhabditis elegans*.[217,218] The three ENaC subunits bear a Ser at this site. Mutations at the degeneration site in MECs, ASICs, and ENaCs have the common phenotype of an increase in channel open probability,[76,78,79,219] suggesting similar gating

machinery. ENaCs with a Cys substitution at the degenerin site are activated by externally applied sulfhydryl reagents.[76,79,219] Modification of Cys residues at the degenerin site is dependent on channels being in an open state, suggesting that either: (1) there is an extracellular gate controlling access to the degenerin site or (2) that this site undergoes a conformational change in association with channel-gating that alters the accessibility of the cysteine side chain to chemical reagents.[79] The desensitization gate of ASIC1 is formed by a helical bundle crossing, which favors the second possibility.[70]

In addition to the degenerin site, external sulfhydryl reagents activate channels with Cys substitutions at nearby sites with a periodicity suggestive of an α-helical structure,[76] suggesting that an extended helical region functions as a gating domain.[76] Consistent with the hypothesis, the sulfhydryl reactive agent MTSET transitions channels with an introduced Cys distal to the α-subunit degenerin site to a high open probability state. Furthermore, these modified channels lose their response to external Na[+] and to laminar shear stress.[182,220] Carattino and co-workers reported that mutations at multiple sites within the TM2 of the α-subunit altered the magnitude and time course of ENaC activation by laminar shear stress, suggesting that this region has a role in the channel's response to external mechanical forces.[221] While ENaCs do not undergo desensitization, these results suggest that the primary gate within ENaCs is located in the same region as the ASIC1 desensitization gate.

Previous studies also suggest that there are additional sites within the TM1 and TM2 domains that affect rates of ion permeation or channel-gating. Several amiloride-binding site mutants (see above) exhibited an altered single channel conductance, although cation selectivity was preserved.[72,163,171] Moreover, channels with a cysteine residue at the γ-subunit amiloride-binding site (γG537) had a high open probability, failed to respond to shear stress stimulus, and lacked a Na[+] self-inhibition response.[222] These results suggest that the αS583-βG525-γG537 ring participates, either directly or indirectly, in ion permeation and channel-gating, in addition to its role in amiloride-binding. The carboxyl-terminal portion of TM2 may also have a role in the regulation of gating.[223,224]

STRUCTURE OF THE PORE

Analogous to the ASIC1 pore structure, the ENaC pore is likely lined primarily by the TM2 helices. The TM1 helices may insulate the TM2 helices from the lipid bilayer. However, uncertainties regarding the ENaC pore structure remain, due in part to the distinct pore structures of the two ASIC1 structures that apparently were resolved from channels in the desensitized state.[69,70] It is not clear which structure represents the native pore conformation and the extent to which structural distortion was generated by crystal lattice contacts. It remains possible that these two structures represent two native conformations that are captured at different stages of desensitization. The TM domains in the original structure[69] are asymmetric with the TM2 helices of two of the subunits showing a $\sim 30-33°$ kink at Gly 435, with the third subunit being nearly straight. The kinks bring the TM2 helices close together, allowing Leu 440 side chains to occlude the pore and separate the outer and inner vestibules. In contrast, the second structure has a symmetric pore design with all TM helices tilted at $\sim 50°$ relative to the membrane normal, with the TM2 helices crossing at the proposed desensitization gate ($G^{432}DIGG^{436}$) that separates the extracellular and intracellular vestibules.[70] The defined degenerin site is located at the top of the gate. Assuming that the ENaC pore has a similar structure, the amiloride-binding and selectivity filter sites would be located within the intracellular vestibule. Mutagenesis studies of the ENaC pore are consistent with an asymmetric open state pore structure.[76,163,169,171,208,210–213,219]

Cytoplasmic Carboxyl-Terminus

The region immediately following TM2 contains clusters of basic residues that effect channel-gating through interactions with acidic phospholipids, such as PIP3, as well as cation selectivity.[175,225–228] A major function of the carboxyl-termini appears to be related to the internalization of the channel complex, through a well-characterized Pro-Tyr (PY) motif (PPPXYXXL) that interacts with the ubiquitin ligase Nedd4-2.[128,132,229,230] ENaC subunit ubiquitination serves as a signal for channel internalization from the plasma membrane.[132] It is unclear whether the YXXL sequence within this motif serves as an independent signal for channel internalization. Other sites within the carboxyl termini may influence rates of channel endocytosis. For example, an A663T polymorphism in the α-subunit of the human ENaC affects rates of channel internalization from the plasma membrane.[231,232] ER exit of ENaC is regulated by a signal within the α-subunit carboxyl cytoplasmic tail.[99]

The carboxyl-termini have sites that are targeted by specific protein kinases that modulate ENaC activity via phosphorylation. These kinases include an extracellular regulated kinase (ERK), casein kinase 2 (CK2), a serum and glucocorticoid regulated kinase (SGK1), and a G-protein-coupled receptor kinase (Grk2).[233–237] ERK1/2-dependent phosphorylation of the carboxyl-termini of the β- and γ-subunits enhances ENaC's interactions with Nedd4.[233] Both forskolin and phorbol 12-myristate 13-acetate (PMA) have been reported to enhance phosphorylation of the β- and γ-subunits, although the target residues that are phosphorylated have not been identified.[238] A region in the proximal part of the carboxyl-terminus of the α-subunit has a role in conferring sensitivity to a staurosporine-sensitive kinase that has not been identified.[239] The carboxyl termini also bind α spectrin and possibly actin, linking the channel to the cytoskeleton.[122,124] Grk2 activates ENaC by phosphorylating the carboxyl terminus of the β-subunit, and prevents Nedd4-2-dependent inhibition of ENaC.[236] Cysteine residues in the amino and carboxyl termini of ENaC subunits may participate in the inhibition of ENaC that is observed with intracellular thiol reactive reagents.[177] Selected cytoplasmic cysteine residues in the β- and γ-subunits are targets of modified palmitoylation.[98] β-Subunit palmitoylation modulates channel-gating, possibly by facilitating interactions between cytoplasmic domains and the plasma membrane.[98]

Cation Permeation and Selectivity

While a detailed understanding of the molecular mechanisms underlying permeation and selectivity awaits a high-resolution structure of ENaC in the open state, there is a growing body of information regarding ion permeation and selectivity.[81,240,241] Organic or inorganic cations larger than Na⁺ are unable to pass through the channel, in contrast to voltage-gated Na⁺ channels, suggesting that permeant cations must dehydrate to cross the narrowest part of the channel pore (i.e., the selectivity filter).[242,243] Within the Gly/Ser-X-Ser tract that comprises ENaCs selectivity filter,[169,211,214] backbone carbonyl oxygens or hydroxyl oxygens present on the side chains of Ser residues may coordinate permeating Na⁺ or Li⁺ ions.[213,214]

The selectivity sequence of ENaC (Li⁺ > Na⁺ >>> K⁺, organic cations) suggests that the relative permeability of an ion is inversely related to its ionic size, a relationship consistent with a mechanism in which ENaC discriminates cations through molecular sieving.[208,214] Alternatively, cation selectivity could be achieved by placing a negatively (or partially negatively) charged site with strong field strength that preferentially binds small cations within the channel pore.[242,243] In this regard, the selectivity sequence for ENaC corresponds to sequence XI of Eisenman. This sequence was determined based on the presence of strong electrostatic interactions between ions and the selectivity site that override differences in dehydration energies for ions.[244] Interestingly, the selectivity filter of a voltage-gated Na⁺ channel has a high-field-strength anionic coordination site.[245]

Selectivity filters appear to be flexible, not static, structures.[246–250] A dynamic selectivity filter of ENaC has been suggested,[76] and appears to be likely in the light of the resolved ASIC1 structures. Both ASIC1 structures likely represent a desensitized state, and the selectivity filter residues are not in close proximity.[81] We speculate that these residues are brought sufficiently close in the open state to interact with permeating cations. A recent study of ASIC1 is consistent with this notion.[75]

Mechanisms of ENaC-Gating

ENaC-gating is characterized by unusually long open and closed times (up to seconds or even tens of seconds) compared to other channels such as voltage-gated channels (Figure 30.1). This gating pattern seems appropriate for this channel, given its major physiological role of mediating bulk Na^+ transport across the apical membrane of epithelial cells, for which slow transitions between open and closed states may be beneficial for transport efficiency. Transitions between open and closed states appear to occur spontaneously. Another feature of ENaC-gating is the high variability in open probability observed in patch-clamp recordings.[11,251,252] Subunit composition and regulatory factors that affect gating may account for this variability.[252,253] As discussed in detail below, proteolytic cleavage of ENaC subunits converts channels that have a low open probability to channels that exhibit either an intermediate or high open probability.[13,83,97,113] Mechanical forces, external metals, and temperature have also been shown to affect channel-gating.[181,182,184,202,220,221] Studies on Na^+ self-inhibition and effects of metals on ENaC-gating have raised the question of whether ENaCs should be considered a ligand-gated channel, similar to FaNaCh and ASIC.[81,184,254]

A detailed understanding of ENaC-gating mechanisms is lacking, despite the identification of several sites within ENaC where the introduction of mutations affects ENaC-gating kinetics. These sites are present within the amino-terminal domain,[165,166] the extracellular domain,[13,83,113,181,182,184,255] TM2,[76,79,219,221,224] and the intracellular carboxyl-terminal domain.[226,227,256] However, it is unclear whether these different regions control channel-gating in an independent or coordinated manner, nor is it known whether there is a single gate or multiple gates. The location of the ENaC gate is another open question, although the region corresponding to the desensitization gate of ASIC1 is an attractive candidate.

Several recent studies have suggested that the pore helix of cation channels may be a central gating structure.[221,257–260] Yeh and co-workers suggested that the regulation of TRPV5 (a member of the transient receptor potential channel subfamily)-gating by extracellular and intracellular protons is mediated by a rotational movement of the pore helix, and the subsequent closing of a gate within the selectivity filter gate.[260] As the amino-terminal helical portion of the TM2 helices of ENaC participates in channel-gating,[76,79,219] it is possible that rotation of the TM2 helix that is initiated by conformational changes at other sites of the channels alters ENaC-gating kinetics, as suggested for ASIC1.[261] Li and co-workers proposed a gating motion for ASIC1 involving a straightening of the tilt of TM2 without significant rotation.[75]

Permeation and gating of ion channels were proposed to be two independent processes 60 years ago.[262] While previous studies have supported this concept, recent studies suggest that connections exist between permeation and gating.[263,264] For example, channel gating is often modulated by permeant or blocking ions.[265,266] Mutations within selectivity filters are associated with changes in gating kinetics in K^+ channels, voltage-gated Na^+ channels, and ENaC.[168,211,221] Lu and co-workers provided evidence suggesting conformational changes of the selectivity filter contribute directly to the spontaneous gating of an inward rectifier K^+ channel (Kir2.1).[267] Significant differences in the selectivity filter structure of KcsA K^+ channel were observed when the crystals were soaked in low-K^+ and high-K^+ solutions,[268] suggesting that the selectivity filter of this channel is flexible. Molecular simulations using the high resolution structures of bacterial K^+ channels support this idea of a flexible selectivity filter.[269,270] Conformational changes in the selectivity filter have been proposed to occur in the ligand-initiated gating of cyclic nucleotide-gated ion channels.[271] A similar notion has been proposed for inward rectifier K^+ channels.[272,273] We anticipate that future studies will examine whether ENaC's selectivity filter also serves as a gate.

ENaC REGULATION

ENaC is subject to a wide variety of regulatory influences that alter channel activity over long or short time periods in order to respond to the physiologic needs of the organism. In the kidney, these regulatory influences determine the final Na^+ concentration of urine, which may vary from virtually Na^+ free to >100 mM. Abnormalities in these regulatory mechanisms in the cortical collecting duct have been convincingly linked to excess Na^+ reabsorption and hypertension, when disordered regulation leads to gain-of-function; and salt-wasting, hypotension and hyperkalemia when abnormal regulation leads to loss-of-function.[207] Altered or abnormal regulation of ENaC in the lung has been linked to abnormal alveolar fluid clearance in disease states such as cystic fibrosis, high altitude pulmonary edema, and acute lung injury.[153,154,274–276] In many cases, studies of abnormal ENaC function in disease states have complemented basic observations concerning channel function made in experimental settings, and led to remarkable insights concerning molecular mechanisms of regulation of channel activity.

Channel activity is subject to regulation through alteration of one of its intrinsic kinetic properties, either its number, open probability or single channel conductance. Since significant changes in single channel conductance are not found under physiologic conditions, channel regulation may be considered primarily as a matter of alterations in channel number and/or open probability. Thinking about channel regulation from this perspective would seem to simplify the subject, and certainly provides a framework within which regulation may be considered. However, the subject remains enormously complex given the number of regulatory influences that may modify either channel number or open probability.

There has been a significant paradigm shift, in that we now recognize that "near silent" channels are present in the membrane, in addition to constitutively active channels.[11–13] These "near silent" channels are capable of activation and may be viewed as the extreme case of open probability regulation, where channels move from very low to a measurable open probability, giving the appearance of increased numbers of channels.[13] The levels of "near silent" channel expression in the distal nephron under various physiological and pathological conditions are currently unclear. Channel regulation serves to either enhance or diminish Na⁺ reabsorption from luminal fluids of the distal nephron, lung or colon, in accord with the needs of the organism. Given the wide variations in rates of Na⁺ reabsorption and luminal Na⁺ gradients that this involves, other intrinsic regulatory influences are required to maintain constant cell volume and ion gradients. To respond to these needs under normal physiologic conditions, channel activity is regulated by a number of hormones, including steroids, vasopressin, and insulin; by a variety of accessory proteins; by kinases, proteases, methyltransferases, and other signaling mediators; by other channels such as CFTR; and by ion concentrations and pH.

Cellular Regulation

Ubiquitination and Deubiquitination

Liddle syndrome is a hereditary form of salt-sensitive hypertension associated with increased ENaC activity.[207,277,278] The most common defects in ENaC primary structure leading to this disorder involve the proline-rich regions in carboxyl-termini of the β- or γ-subunit.[277,279–281] Rotin and colleagues used this region of the β-subunit as bait in a yeast two-hybrid screen to identify proteins that interact with ENaC and might regulate ENaC expression. They isolated the protein Nedd4 (Neuronal precursor cells Expressed Developmentally Downregulated) using this technique. In a series of elegant studies they examined the role of this protein in the regulation of ENaC expression.[132,282,283] Nedd4 is an E3 ubiquitin ligase composed of a C2 domain, three or four WW domains that are protein interaction modules, and a ubiquitin ligase Hect domain. The WW domains of Nedd4 bind ENaC, with the strongest interaction being between the carboxyl-terminus of the β-subunit and the third WW domain.[284] The Hect domain is an E3 ligase that receives ubiquitin from an E2 protein and transfers ubiquitin to lysines on target proteins. The C2 region is a Ca²⁺- and phospholipid-binding domain. It is not present on all Nedd4 isoforms and, based on oocyte studies, does not appear to be essential for inhibition of ENaC expression.[230,285,286] This domain does, however, serve to localize Nedd4 to plasma membrane in response to an increase in cytosolic [Ca²⁺],[287] and mediates association with annexin XIIIb, which may be involved in apical membrane targeting in epithelia.[288]

Nedd4-2, the isoform most active in binding ENaC, is detected in tissues that express ENaC. The Nedd4-2 WW domains interact *in vitro* with the proline-rich region of carboxyl terminus of the β- and γ- (and possibly α-) subunits of ENaC.[289–291] Considerable evidence indicates that the interaction between Nedd4-2 and ENaC results in ubiquitination of the channel (Figure 30.6). ENaC has been shown to be ubiquitinated in endogenously expressing A6 cells, and when overexpressed along with Nedd4-2 in HEK-293 cells.[108,132] Co-expression studies with Nedd4-2 and ENaC in oocytes demonstrated that Nedd4-2 decreases ENaC surface expression, and that this is dependent both on the E3 ligase domain of Nedd4-2 and on the presence of Lys residues on the amino-termini of the target subunits.[132] Taken together, these studies strongly support the model that surface expression of ENaC is regulated by ubiquitination, which serves as a signal for retrieval from the plasma membrane. It is likely that ENaC is ubiquitinated at other cellular sites, including the endoplasmic reticulum. Unassembled subunits are likely degraded by the proteasome by a process involving polyubiquitination, while fully assembled trimeric channels are degraded by either the proteasome or lysosomal–endosomal pathway following ubiquitination at the cell surface.[93,95,108,132] At present, it is unclear whether monoubiquitination of

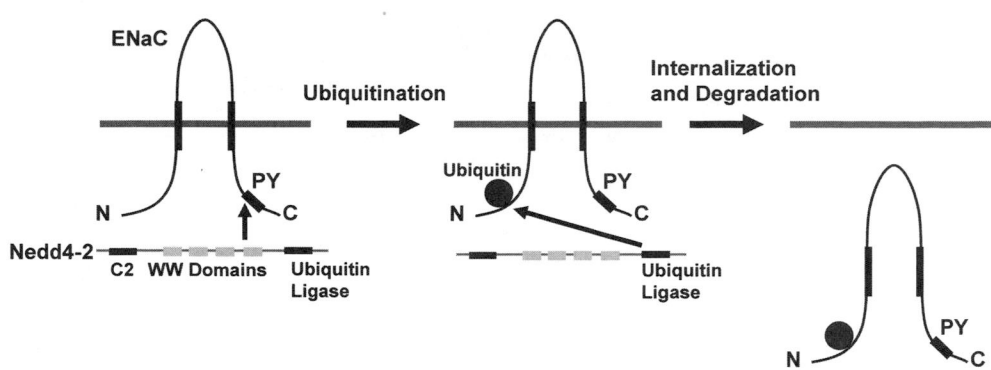

FIGURE 30.6   Nedd4-2-dependent regulation of ENaC surface expression. Nedd4-2 binding to ENaC subunits is facilitated through interactions between WW domains on Nedd4-2 and the PY motifs on the β- and γ-subunits. Nedd4-2-dependent ubiquitination of ENaC subunits targets the channel for internalization and degradation. *(adapted from ref. [295]).*

ENaC occurs at the cell surface. However, there is considerable evidence suggesting that ubiquitination is a signal for channel internalization from the plasma membrane,[292] and that channel internalization is a dynamin-dependent,[126] clathrin-dependent,[133] as well as caveolin-dependent process.[293]

The interaction between Nedd4-2 and ENaC is itself subject to regulation by specific hormones and kinases.[233,236,294–300] The regulation of ENaC by Nedd4-2 represents a final common pathway of several regulatory influences affecting ENaC surface expression, providing further evidence for the importance of this interaction in ENaC regulation (see below).

Recent work has elucidated an important role for deubiquitinating enzymes (DUBs) in the regulation of ENaC expression and trafficking in cells.[134,135] Specifically, the DUB Usp2-45 was found to be upregulated by aldosterone in mouse polarized collecting duct (mpkCCD$_{c14}$) cells, which causes deubiquitination of ENaC, and an increase in ENaC surface expression and activity.[134] The subcellular site(s) of action of Usp2-45 on ENaC and its precise physiological role are currently unclear. Butterworth and colleagues identified another DUB, UCH-L3, in the early endosomal compartment of these cells, which also deubiquitinates ENaC, and enhances the recycling of ENaC to the apical membrane.[135] UCH-L3 may play an important role in reversing Nedd4-2-mediated ubiquitination of ENaC upon retrieval from the plasma membrane, thereby rescuing ENaC from degradation and promoting apical recycling of the channel (Figure 30.4). Finally, Usp10 was recently identified as a vasopressin-stimulated DUB, leading to enhanced ENaC abundance and activity at the plasma membrane.[301] In summary, DUBs may respond to hormonal inputs and appear to antagonize Nedd4-2-dependent ubiquitination and inhibition of ENaC, promoting ENaC stabilization and function at the plasma membrane.[302]

Kinases

Protein phosphatase inhibitors, such as okadaic acid, activate ENaC,[303] while nonspecific kinase inhibitors, such as staurosporine, inhibit basal channel activity,[239,304] suggesting that kinases play an important role in regulating the channel. In many cases, the regulation of ENaC by a protein kinase is indirect, with kinase activation occurring within a pathway of hormonal regulation or cellular stress. Examples of this are: (1) SGK1 activation by steroid hormones induces SGK1-dependent phosphorylation of Nedd4-2 (the subsequent binding of 14-3-3 proteins to phosphorylated Nedd4-2 prevents the interaction of Nedd4-2 with ENaC subunits, and reduces ubiquitin-based retrieval of channels from the plasma membrane[305–309]) (Figure 30.7); (2) insulin-dependent activation of phosphatidyl-inositol 3 kinase and 3-phosphoinositide-dependent kinase 1 results in the phosphorylation and activation of SGK1 and ENaC;[307,310] (3) activation of protein kinase A by adenylate cyclase and cAMP in response to vasopressin or beta-adrenergic agonists leads to phosphorylation of Nedd4-2 at sites that overlap the SGK1 phosphorylation sites, and a reduction in ENaC endocytosis,[297] as well as exocytotic insertion of Na$^+$ channels into the plasma membrane;[111,311,312] (4) activated IKKβ, the kinase-regulating NF-κB, interacts with the cytoplasmic carboxyl terminus of β ENaC[313] and phosphorylates Nedd4-2 at a residue that is also targeted by SGK1 and PKA, reducing channel endocytosis[300] (IKKβ provides a mechanism of integrating inflammatory cascades and ENaC activation); (5) endothelin-dependent activation of Src kinase results in a decrease in channel open probability without directly phosphorylating channel subunits[314]; (6) selected protein kinase C isoforms also reduce channel open probability in a Ca^{2+}-dependent manner, protein kinase C also decreases expression of the β- and γ-subunits, which is dependent on activated

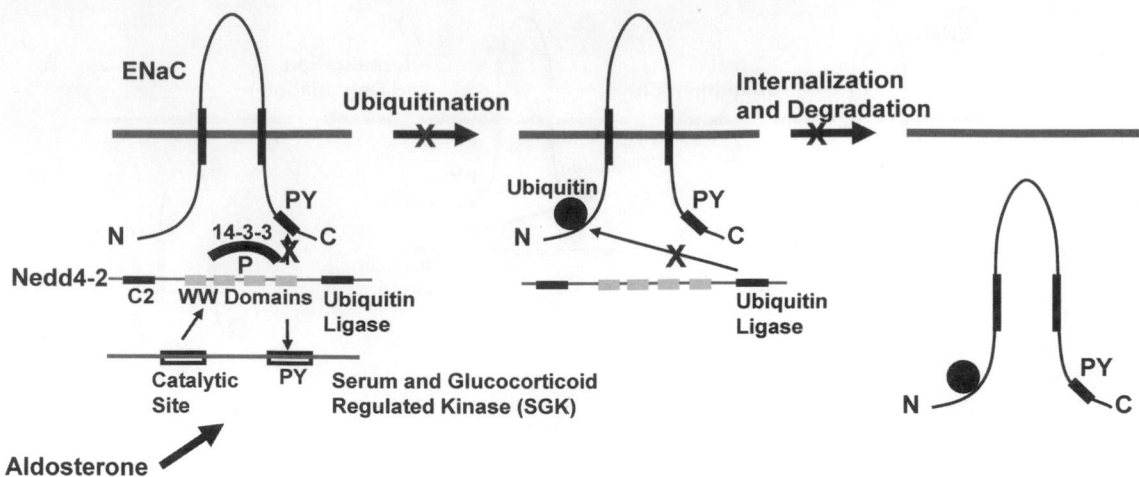

FIGURE 30.7 Aldosterone modulates the interaction between Nedd4-2 and ENaC. Sgk1 is targeted to Nedd4-2 through interactions between a PY motif on Sgk1 and WW domains on Nedd4-2. Sgk1-dependent phosphorylation of Nedd4-2 results in the recruitment of a 14-3-3 protein that prevents Nedd4-2 binding to ENaC. *(adapted from ref. [295]).*

ERK kinase[315–317]; (7) AMP-activated protein kinase (AMPK) is a ubiquitous metabolic sensor that phosphorylates Nedd4-2, enhances Nedd4-2 binding to β ENaC, and inhibits ENaC activity and surface expression.[77,299,318]

ENaC is also a substrate for kinases that are involved in its regulation. Studies of ENaC expressed in MDCK cells have demonstrated increased phosphorylation of the β- and γ-subunits in response to stimulation by aldosterone and insulin.[238] Phosphopeptide mapping indicated that the phosphorylated sites were carboxyl terminal Ser and Thr residues.[238] Shi and colleagues described phosphorylation of Ser631 in the β-subunit and Thr599 in the γ-subunit by the pleiotropic but essential kinase CK2.[234] Kunzelmann and colleagues found that a specific CK2 inhibitor blocked ENaC activity, and expression of a trimeric channel lacking both CK2 sites inhibited ENaC conductance and rendered ENaC insensitive to CK2.[237] They concluded that phosphorylation by CK2 is essential for ENaC activation and partly regulates ENaC surface expression. Garty and colleagues also described phosphorylation of βThr613 and γThr623 by the extracellular regulated kinase (ERK).[233] ERK-dependent phosphorylation of ENaC facilitates interactions between the channel and Nedd4-2, thereby inhibiting ENaC activity. SGK1 increases channel open probability by directly phosphorylating the carboxyl-terminus of the α-subunit at Ser-621.[235] Finally, insulin has been described to increase phosphorylation of a fully mature 65 kDa form of α ENaC in cultured epithelial cells, which correlated with an increase in channel activity.[319] The kinase-mediating of this effect was not directly identified, but the protein kinase C inhibitor

chelerythrine blocked the insulin stimulation of transport and subunit phosphorylation.

It has also been reported that the G-protein-coupled receptor kinase, Grk2, phosphorylates Ser-633 in the carboxyl-terminus of the β-subunit.[236] Phosphorylation at this site renders the channel insensitive to regulation by Nedd4-2, resulting in increased surface expression and channel activity. This finding is intriguing, as: (1) it is the first report of a G-protein receptor kinase directly regulating an ion channel; and (2) increased Grk2 activity has been associated with hypertension.[320] Grk2 may also phosphorylate Nedd4-2, although the relevant site(s) and functional significance of this phosphorylation are unclear.[321] A recent study suggests that Grk2 may also stimulate ENaC via a kinase-independent mechanism that requires its interaction with α-subunits of the Gq/11 family.[322]

Another family of kinases linked to human hypertension is the WNK (with no lysine) family of serine-threonine kinases.[323] These kinases are prominently expressed in the distal convoluted tubule, connecting segment, and cortical collecting duct of the kidney (i.e., the aldosterone-sensitive distal nephron), where they coordinate with angiotensin II and aldosterone signaling pathways.[324] WNK mutations lead to hypertension and hyperkalemia typical of pseudohypoaldosteronism type II (PHA II).[325] WNK4 inhibits the renal Na,Cl cotransporter (NCC) and ROMK, and mutations associated with hypertension relieve the inhibition of NCC, but enhance inhibition of ROMK.[323] These observations suggested that under normal physiologic conditions, WNK4 regulates the balance between renal Na⁺ reabsorption and K⁺ excretion, but mutations would lead to exaggerated Na⁺ reabsorption and hypertension with hyperkalemia, due to impaired K^+ excretion. In addition to NCC and ROMK, one group found that WNK4 also inhibits ENaC *in vitro*, and this inhibition by WNK4 is relieved by SGK1 phosphorylation near the WNK4 C-terminus.[326] In contrast, another group suggested that WNK4 activates ENaC.[327] Another member of this family, WNK1, has also been implicated in activating ENaC.[327] Interestingly, intronic deletions that could lead to hypertension and hyperkalemia result in overexpression of WNK1.[328] Aldosterone has also been shown to stimulate expression of a kidney-specific isoform of WNK1, and overexpression of this kinase stimulates Na^+ reabsorption in cultured collecting duct cells, and in overexpression systems.[329] WNK1 expression activates SGK1 in a PI-3 kinase-dependent manner, indicating that the kinase activates ENaC by increasing its expression at the apical membrane of collecting duct cells, contributing to the human hypertension seen in association with PHA II.[327,330]

As suggested above, the E3 ubiquitin ligase Nedd4-2 has emerged as a central convergence point for the regulation of ENaC and other transport proteins in cells. A growing number of kinases have been shown to phosphorylate Nedd4-2, modulate Nedd4-2 function, and thereby regulate ENaC.[331] These include the aldosterone-induced kinase SGK1,[306] vasopressin-stimulated PKA,[297] the metabolic sensor AMPK,[299] the NF-κB inflammatory mediator IKKβ,[300] Grk2,[321] and the insulin-stimulated kinase Akt1.[332] In general, these kinases modulate the apparent binding affinity of Nedd4-2 for ENaC and/or 14-3-3 scaffolding proteins. Of note, additional putative Nedd4-2 phosphorylation sites have been recently identified by mass spectrometry that may be targets of the c-Jun N-terminal kinase (JNK1), and possibly other kinases.[333] Unlike the above paradigm, where kinases regulate protein–protein interactions involving Nedd4-2, these novel target phosphorylation sites appear to play an important role in regulating Nedd4-2 catalytic function.[333]

Proteases

Proteolysis of ENaC subunits has an important role in regulating ENaC activity. The first hint that proteases modulated ENaC activity was that serine protease inhibitors reduced transepithelial Na^+ transport across toad urinary bladder.[334] Subsequent studies identified a channel-activating protease, or CAP,[195] and demonstrated that extracellular trypsin activated ENaC by increasing channel open probability.[114] Following these initial observations, other proteases have been identified that activate ENaC when either co-expressed with the channel in heterologous expression systems or when added to a solution bathing cells expressing ENaCs. These channel activating proteases

include prostasin (also referred to as CAP1), TMPRSS4 (transmembrane protease serine 4 or CAP2), and matriptase (or CAP3), elastase, chymotrypsin, kallikrein, and plasmin.[113,114,195,199,335–339]

Proteolytic processing of ENaC subunits occurs within the biosynthetic pathway. This is likely mediated by furin, a member of the proprotein convertase family of serine proteases that is expressed primarily in the trans-Golgi network.[83,340] There are two furin cleavage sites within the extracellular domain of the α-subunit, and a single site within the extracellular domain of the γ-subunit.[83,85] Furin-dependent cleavage of the α-subunit excises a 26 residue inhibitory fragment. Simply deleting this 26 residue tract from the α-subunit in the absence of subunit cleavage was sufficient to activate the channel.[84] Furthermore, a synthetic peptide corresponding to the released fragment is a reversible channel inhibitor.[84] An 8 residue tract, embedded within the 26 residue fragment, is responsible for the inhibitory properties of this fragment.[86]

While the α-subunit is cleaved by furin twice, releasing an inhibitory fragment, the γ-subunit is cleaved only once by furin. As was observed with α-subunit processing by furin, cleavage at two sites spanning an inhibitory tract within the γ-subunit increases channel activity. While furin cleaves the γ-subunit at a site preceding an embedded inhibitory tract,[200] multiple proteases have been shown to cleave the γ-subunit at sites distal to the inhibitory tract. Among the proteases that cleave the γ-subunit distal to the inhibitory tract are prostasin, TMPRSS4 (CAP2), elastase, and plasmin.[199,200,338,339,341] Deleting the γ-subunit inhibitory tract dramatically increases channel activity, even in the absence of γ-subunit cleavage.[200,342] An 11 residue tract is responsible for the inhibitory properties of the released fragment.[342] With regard to channel activation, release of the γ-subunit inhibitory tract has a more profound effect than release of the α-subunit inhibitory tract.[343]

At the single channel level, ENaCs exhibit a highly variable open probability. While ENaCs often exhibit open and closed times in the order of seconds to tens of seconds, a distinct population of ENaCs have very brief open times and long closed times.[11–13] Caldwell and co-workers have shown that this latter population of channels responds to external trypsin, with a dramatic increase in channel open probability.[13] These inactive channels likely represent a population of channels whose subunits have not been processed by proteases. Channels with α-subunit furin site mutations that have retained α- and γ-subunit inhibitory tracts have a very low open probability that reflects a dramatically enhanced reduction in ENaC activity in response to external Na^+ (referred to as Na^+ self-inhibition). When these channels are examined in the presence of a low external [Na$^+$], their activity dramatically increases.[115]

Both processed (i.e., cleaved) and unprocessed subunits are expressed at the cell surface.[93,112] These nonprocessed channels provide a pool of ENaCs that could be activated by proteases in a regulated manner. In this regard, rats placed on a low-Na$^+$ diet or receiving exogenous aldosterone have increased levels of whole kidney expression of the processed form of the γ-subunit.[142,344–347]

The sites of protease cleavage in the α- and γ-subunits are located with the finger domain. A model of the α-subunit generated by Kashlan and co-workers suggests that the α-subunit inhibitory tract binds to sites at an interface of the finger and thumb domains. They proposed that the inhibitory tract reduces channel activity by stabilizing the movement of the finger domain relative to the thumb domain.[81,82]

Syntaxins

The factors regulating ENaC delivery to the apical membrane in epithelial cells have not been fully-defined. The SNARE proteins (soluble N-ethylmaleimide sensitive factor attachment protein receptors) have been linked to directed exocytosis and intracellular trafficking in a number of tissues.[348] A typical interaction involves binding of vesicle-associated v-SNARES to target membrane-associated t-SNARES. These interactions may be regulated by accessory proteins such as Munc 18.[349] The t-SNARE syntaxin 1A has been demonstrated to interact directly with ENaC in co-immunoprecipitation experiments, and overexpression of this protein inhibited ENaC expression in oocytes.[116,350] This effect was blocked by co-expression of Munc 18. These findings implicate the SNARE proteins in the process of exocytosis of ENaC, but are somewhat counterintuitive in that overexpression of the trafficking partners results in downregulation of the channel. The results suggest that the balance of t- and v-SNAREs may regulate this process, and that overexpression alters this interaction in a negative fashion.

The direct interaction of syntaxin 1A and ENaC suggests that there are cargo-specific interactions between SNARE proteins and apical membrane resident proteins such as ENaC. In a series of studies, Condliffe and colleagues identified domain-specific interactions between the carboxyl-termini of ENaC subunits and the H3 domain of syntaxin 1A. Interestingly, there was an effect of the H3 domain to decrease ENaC open probability, suggesting that SNARE proteins may regulate both channel exocytosis and gating.[118,119] A more recent study suggests that syntaxin 1A regulates ENaC function by multiple mechanisms that include PKA, phospholipase C, PI-3 kinase, and MAP kinase

signaling systems.[351] Distinct inhibitory and stimulatory domains of syntaxin 1A interact with ENaC subunits, and the overall effect of syntaxin 1A on ENaC function depends on distinct physiological conditions.

Cystic Fibrosis Transmembrane Conductance Regulator (CFTR)

Patients with cystic fibrosis (CF) have increased amiloride-sensitive transport in airway epithelia.[352] Indeed, increased ENaC activity in airway epithelia has been proposed as one mechanism for the drying of airway fluids, which promotes progression of airway disease. Lung specific overexpression of β ENaC or knockout of Nedd4-2 in mice results in a phenotype similar to CF airway disease in humans.[153,353] CF is caused by function impairing mutations in the cystic fibrosis transmembrane conductance regulator (CFTR), an ATP-gated Cl$^-$ channel.[354] On the basis of studies comparing ENaC activity in the presence and absence of CFTR expressed in MDCK cells, Stutts and colleagues proposed that CFTR functions as a cAMP-dependent regulator of ENaC, and the absence of this function in CF airways explained the increased ENaC activity in CF patients.[355,356] Ling and co-workers demonstrated that inhibiting CFTR expression in a renal distal nephron cell line (A6) led to an increase in ENaC open probability.[357] Studies in *Xenopus* oocytes or other overexpression systems have demonstrated that CFTR inhibits ENaC activity,[355,358,359] although this has been disputed.[360,361] However, several recent studies have questioned the role of CFTR in modulating ENaC activity.[362,363] There is also evidence that ENaC enhances the activity of CFTR, due to an increase in the number of channels expressed at the plasma membrane, as well as an increase in CFTR open probability.[364]

It is unclear if the interaction between CFTR and ENaC is indirect or results from a direct physical interaction. Changes in the intracellular [Cl$^-$], as well as electrochemical coupling, have been proposed as potential mechanisms by which CFTR regulates ENaC.[360,365] One group has proposed that there are interactions between the regulatory domain of CFTR and ENaC,[366] although the manner in which this interaction results in ENaC regulation is not clear. Moreover, ENaC–CFTR interactions appear to vary depending on the tissue of expression. For example, in sweat ducts, CFTR enhances ENaC activity.[367] Although both CFTR and ENaC are expressed in collecting duct principal cells, no significant abnormalities of renal Na$^+$ handling have been described in CF patients. In airway epithelial cells, CFTR and ENaC co-immunoprecipitate, and interestingly expression of the most common CF-causing ΔF508 CFTR mutation was recently found to increase the proportion of cleaved to uncleaved α ENaC that was bound to CFTR.[368] These findings suggest that wild-type CFTR may normally impede the proteolytic stimulation of ENaC in airway cells, although mechanistic details of how this may occur are unclear. Elastase is one of perhaps several proteases that are present in inflamed CF airways and could contribute to an increase in the extent of γ ENaC subunit proteolysis.[113,199,337] Another recent study suggested that CFTR regulates the whole cell and surface expression of ENaC in airway epithelial cells, and that absence of this regulation may foster ENaC hyperactivity in CF airway epithelia.[369] In summary, with current data it is difficult to explain the regulatory interactions between CFTR and ENaC solely on the basis of physical interactions or alterations in electrochemical driving forces or the intracellular Cl⁻ concentration. The regulatory interactions may reflect changes in ENaC open probability (cleavage status) and surface expression, and vary among differing tissues, suggesting that other proteins or factors not yet recognized may be critical for functional CFTR–ENaC interactions.[370]

Methyltransferases

Methylation reactions have long been implicated in the activation of ENaC by aldosterone.[371,372] Aldosterone stimulates carboxylmethylation of proteins and phospholipids, and inhibition of these reactions blunts the ENaC response to steroid stimulation.[373] A few potential targets of methyltransferases have been identified: k-ras, β ENaC, and more recently, histones involved in the aldosterone-dependent control of transcription. Aldosterone induces k-ras in a *Xenopus* distal nephron cell line (A6) cells, and this small G-protein is methylated by isoprenylcysteine carboxylmethyltransferase (PCMTase). PCMTase is not induced by aldosterone, but is regulated by the enzyme S-adenosyl-homocysteine hydrolase that is stimulated by aldosterone and results in increased activity of PCMTase.[374] The enzyme (PCMTase) itself does not appear to stimulate ENaC, so it is unlikely to directly methylate the channel. Induction and processing of k-ras appears to be important for regulation of ENaC in A6 cells, but it is not clear that this occurs in mammalian tissues.[375] Direct methylation of β ENaC has been demonstrated using a partially purified membrane preparation as a source of enzyme, but the enzyme itself has not been identified. Methylation of ENaC in planar lipid bilayers has been shown to lead to an increase in open probability of the channel.[376] Edinger and co-workers identified a methyltransferase that activates ENaC when co-expressed with the channel in oocytes.[377] Methylation does not appear to play a role in basal channel activity.

Several recent studies have explored the role of Dot1a, which has histone H3K79 methyltransferase activity and is widely expressed in the kidney,[378] in the transcriptional control of α ENaC in response to aldosterone.[379] Aldosterone releases repression of α ENaC by reducing expression of Dot1a and its partner AF9,[380] and by impairing Dot1a–AF9 interaction via SGK1-mediated AF9 phosphorylation.[381] This network also appears to regulate transcription of several other aldosterone target genes, including SGK1.[382]

Calcium

Increases in intracellular calcium have been shown to inhibit ENaC activity by several groups.[252,383–385] This appears to happen as a biphasic process with a very quick early response and a slower downregulation after 5 minutes.[385] This is likely an indirect effect on the channel, as the activity of channels from cortical collecting ducts in excised patches exposed to increased cytosolic $[Ca^{2+}]$ was not altered.[383] Activation of protein kinase C has been suggested to mediate the Ca^{2+}-dependent inhibition of ENaC, since this is known to decrease channel activity.[315] A second intriguing possibility, related to the delayed effect of Ca^{2+} on ENaC activity, is Ca^{2+}-dependent recruitment of Nedd4-2 isoforms that possess the Ca^{2+}-binding C2 domain to the plasma membrane,[285,286] with a subsequent increase in channel retrieval from the apical membrane.

pH and Oxidative Stress

Acidic intracellular pH, below 7.2, has been shown to decrease amiloride-sensitive Na^+ transport in isolated epithelial tissues, suggesting that intracellular pH may act as an intrinsic regulator of ENaC activity.[383,386,387] In conditions of ischemia or hypoxia where intracellular pH might fall, activation of AMPK might act to decrease channel activity, as noted above.[77] Hypoxia is known to decrease activity of ENaC through a decrease in channel expression in cultured type II alveolar cells, but the mechanism of this response is unknown. The effect of pH on channel activity appears to be direct. In excised, inside-out patches from apical membranes of rat cortical collecting tubule, a fall in pH from 7.4 to 6.4 resulted in a progressive and dramatic fall in open probability of the channel. The mechanism of this regulation is unknown. However, ENaC activity is clearly downregulated under cellular conditions where ATP is limiting.[388] It has been proposed that ENaC may be sensitive to changes in intracellular redox potential through oxidation of intracellular cysteine residues.[177] It has also been shown that transcription and expression of α ENaC subunit variants are suppressed by oxidative stress in lung epithelial cells.[389] Conversely, oxidative stress induced by hydrogen peroxide exposure appears to stimulate ENaC activity through a PI 3-kinase-dependent pathway in cultured kidney collecting duct cells.[390] Such oxidative stress-induced stimulation of

ENaC has been proposed to contribute to the pathogenesis of salt-sensitive hypertension. Similarly, superoxide formation and release by NADPH oxidase (NOX2) downstream of epidermal growth factor and Rac1 has been reported to stimulate ENaC open probability in the lung.[391]

Nitric Oxide

Several studies have shown that nitric oxide (NO) inhibits ENaC activity in both alveolar type II (AT II) cells and in cultured renal epithelial cells.[392–394] This effect may be important in inflammatory conditions such as acute respiratory distress syndrome, where NO levels may be elevated due to increased expression of inducible nitric oxide synthase (iNOS).[393] NO appears to inhibit the open probability of the channel in a cGMP-dependent manner.[392] Interestingly, aldosterone has also been shown to inhibit NO production from ATII cells, and this appears to be related to an effect of SGK1.[395] These results suggest a second, novel mechanism by which SGK1 could enhance ENaC activity through downregulation of iNOS activity, and a decrease in NO inhibition of ENaC open probability. In addition, the superoxide generation that occurs with oxidative stress appears to antagonize the NO-mediated inhibition of ENaC in lung slice patch-clamp experiments.[396]

Lipids

A number of membrane lipids and lipid intermediates have been shown to modify ENaC activity, often in complex ways. Inhibition of phospholipase A2 (PLA2) by aristolochic acid reduced arachidonic acid (AA) levels and increased ENaC activity in both *Xenopus* oocytes and A6 cells in culture.[127,397] Direct application of AA to rat cortical collecting ducts markedly reduced ENaC activity in a dose-dependent manner. While this effect was not reproduced by application of a non-metabolized analog of AA, 5,8,11,14-eicosatetraynoic acid (ETYA), it was reproduced by the CYP-epoxygenase metabolite 11,12-epoxyeicosatrienoic acid (EET).[398] A recent study found that, along with 11,12-EET, 8,9-EET, and 14,15-EET are additional eicosanoids that inhibit ENaC activity downstream of CYP2C8.[399] These results suggest that arachidonic acid effects are mediated by CYP epoxygenase metabolites. In contrast, in A6 cells current stimulation by PLA2 inhibition was blocked by ETYA, suggesting a direct effect of arachidonic acid on the channel, rather than the effect of a metabolite. The effect of ETYA on ENaC was to reduce open probability.[397] In oocytes, however, both arachidonic acid and ETYA inhibited ENaC, and this was due to an alteration in the number of surface channels. Analysis of ENaC surface expression showed a downregulation of channels consistent with a trafficking effect mediated by both increased endocytosis and decreased exocytosis.[127] Taken together, these experimental observations indicate that PLA2 activity leads to increased arachidonic acid levels that inhibit ENaC activity, but the precise molecular mechanisms remain in dispute.

Cellular phosphoinositides also affect ENaC function. Phosphatidylinositol-4,5-bisphosphate (PIP2) is a signaling molecule related to a number of intracellular processes, including endocytosis[400] and exocytosis.[401] It has also been implicated in the activation of several ion channels.[401] Patch-clamp studies have shown that anionic phospholipids, including PIP2 and PI-3,4,5-P3, can directly alter channel activity presumably by binding to cationic sequences within β and γ ENaC.[172,173] A distinct PIP3-binding site has been identified in the initial part of the carboxyl-terminus of the γ-subunit.[227] PIP2 also directly interacts with ENaC at a site distinct from the PIP3 binding site, and may be permissive for channel gating.[228] Interestingly, increases in cellular PIP2 levels have also been shown to increase surface expression of ENaC, presumably by stimulating exocytosis.[402] Kunzelmann and colleagues demonstrated that purinergic inhibition of ENaC by extracellular ATP in tracheal epithelia resulted in depletion of PIP2 from cells, and appeared to require a PIP2-binding region of the amino-terminus of the β-subunit.[174]

There are three isoforms of phosphoinositide-5-kinase, which produces PI-4,5-P2 from PI4P. These kinases have differing effects on cellular processes such as endocytosis.[400,403] PIP2 may thus induce varying effects on ENaC function, depending on the isoform of PI5K that is activated or the spatial localization of kinases and phosphatases that regulate PIP2 activity within the cellular microenvironment.[404] In summary, phosphoinositides functioning either as signaling agents or directly binding to ENaC affect channel activity.

Intracellular cytoplasmic Cys residues in β- and γ-subunits are modified by palmitoylation. Two Cys residues (Cys43 and Cys557) in the mouse β-subunit were shown to be modified by palmitoylation. Mutation of these Cys to Ala to prevent palmitoylation at these sites was associated with a reduction in channel open probability.[98] Secondary structural predictions suggest that Cys557 is within an amphipathic α helix near the second transmembrane domain, while Cys43 is in proximity to the first transmembrane α helix. Mueller and co-workers suggested that β-subunit palmitoylation modulates channel-gating by enhancing interactions between cytoplasmic domains and the plasma membrane.[98]

Intracellular Na⁺

Since ENaC is present in epithelia that generate a steep lumen-to-bath Na⁺ gradient, it is potentially exposed to significant variations in both internal and external [Na$^+$]. ENaC is modulated by both intracellular and extracellular [Na$^+$]. Low levels of extracellular [Na$^+$] increase ENaC activity while elevated levels decrease activity, a process known as Na$^+$ self-inhibition.[405] Cytoplasmic [Na$^+$] is usually maintained quite low through the action of the Na$^+$,K$^+$-ATPase on the basolateral surface of epithelial cells. Since the pump is normally functioning well below its maximum capacity, Na$^+$ entry into cells is the rate-limiting step for Na$^+$ reabsorption. Under conditions of rapid increases in ENaC activity, regulation may also be achieved through increases in the intracellular [Na$^+$], a process referred to as feedback inhibition. This phenomenon has been observed in epithelial cells and *Xenopus* oocytes.[385,406] Feedback inhibition in response to an increase in the intracellular [Na$^+$] is a slow process that occurs over a period of minutes, in contrast to Na$^+$ self-inhibition, which occurs over seconds.[252] Studies in rat cortical collecting ducts suggested that PKC activation plays an important role in ENaC feedback inhibition.[407] Studies in oocytes indicated that this feedback inhibition was not readily seen in cells expressing ENaC with Liddle mutations that inhibit Nedd4-2-binding and ubiquitin-dependent internalization.[408] This finding focused attention on Nedd4-2 as the potential mediator of Na$^+$ feedback inhibition. In a series of studies in mouse mandibular duct cells, it was demonstrated that Na$^+$ feedback inhibition was dependent on Nedd4-2, and required binding of the second and third WW domains to carboxyl termini of β and γ ENaC.[409,410] More recent studies have suggested that the A-kinase anchoring protein 15 (AKAP-15) may bind to PKC and act in concert with PKC to regulate Na$^+$ feedback inhibition[411] or that intracellular [Na$^+$] may directly modulate the proteolytic activation of ENaC.[412] In summary, a few potential signaling pathways/mechanisms have been implicated in ENaC feedback inhibition by intracellular [Na$^+$], although the relative contributions for each and how they may integrate with one another in different cell types are still unclear.

Extracellular Na$^+$

Increases in extracellular [Na$^+$] inhibit ENaC activity, a process referred to as Na$^+$ self-inhibition. This phenomenon was originally observed in studies of native epithelial tissues in the setting of a rapid increase in extracellular Na$^+$ concentration.[413] This process reflects a decrease in channel open probability, and is not dependent on Na$^+$ influx.[2,182,201,202] Chraibi and Horisberger demonstrated that Na$^+$ self-inhibition is an intrinsic property of EnaC, and can be abolished by treatment with extracellular proteases.[202] Na$^+$ self-inhibition is a temperature-dependent phenomenon

and has a large activation energy, suggesting that a conformational change occurs in association with the inhibition of channel activity by extracellular Na$^+$ that is presumably initiated by Na$^+$-binding to an extracellular site.[202,414] Numerous sites within the extracellular domains of the α- and γ-subunits have been identified where mutations alter Na$^+$ self-inhibition.[80,182,185,186,188,191,192] A number of important questions remain to be addressed regarding the Na$^+$ self-inhibition response, including: (1) where are the external Na$^+$-binding site(s); (2) what are the conformational changes that occur in response to Na$^+$-binding that result in a reduction in channel open probability; and (3) how do external proteases, presumably by cleaving ENaC subunits, diminish the Na$^+$ self-inhibition response?

Peroxisome Proliferators-Activated Receptors (PPARs)

The peroxisome proliferators-activated receptors (PPAR) have been implicated in the regulation of a wide variety of cellular processes. PPARγ is the pharmacological target of thiazolidinediones (TZDs) that have been used in the management of hyperglycemia associated with type II diabetes mellitus.[415] PPARγ is localized along the collecting duct in kidney,[416] and it is known that a side-effect of PPAR stimulation by TZDs is fluid retention.[417] It has been shown that TZD-induced weight gain was prevented in mice by amiloride or by deletion of the gene encoding PPARγ from collecting duct.[417] These studies suggested that TZDs increase ENaC activity in collecting duct cells, and increased mRNA for γ ENaC. These interesting results implicate PPARs in the regulation of transcription of at least one ENaC subunit that apparently leads to increased ENaC activity. More recent studies have suggested that the PPARγ-induced Na$^+$ reabsorption via ENaC in the kidney may be mediated through increased SGK1 expression.[418,419] In contrast, work from other groups suggest that PPARγ agonists do not activate ENaC[420] in cultured principal cells or decrease ENaC expression in the kidney.[421]

ATP

Luminal ATP signals through P2Y2 receptors and inhibits ENaC activity through activation of phospholipase C, activation of protein kinase C, and reducing cellular levels of PIP2 and channel open probability.[228,422,423] Recent studies suggest that this signaling pathway may have an important role in aldosterone escape, and the enhanced rates of Na$^+$ excretion in animals on a high-Na$^+$ diet.[424–426] Cellular release of ATP may be occurring through connexin 30 hemi-channels.[426]

Hormonal Regulation

Aldosterone

The major hormones regulating ENaC activity in a broad variety of tissues are corticosteroids. ENaC regulation by steroids is the subject of a separate chapter in this volume, and will not be discussed in detail here. Although non-genomic actions of aldosterone have been described in vascular and non-absorptive tissues,[427] the bulk of the available evidence supports the notion that steroid regulation of ENaC in Na^+-absorptive epithelia is mediated by processes dependent on transcription and translation. This transcriptional activity is driven by translocation of the steroid receptor to the nucleus following binding to its cognate ligand, and binding to specific domains within the genome. Interestingly, ENaC regulation varies somewhat by tissue. Steroid regulation of ENaC activity is largely due to an increase in the number of active channels in the apical membrane, although there is evidence for effects on open probability as well.[12,428,429] The increase in the number of active channels is not apparently a simple one-step procedure. An early increase in channels appears to be a trafficking event, with altered insertion or retrieval of already synthesized subunits.[142,143] A large part, but not all, of this effect is regulated by the aldosterone-induced proteins SGK1 and GILZ1 altering Nedd4-2-ENaC interactions and leading to increased membrane expression of the channel[305–307,430–433] (Figure 30.7). Synthesis and delivery of new channel subunits can be detected somewhat later in the course of steroid action in responsive tissues and, interestingly, also varies somewhat by tissue. In kidney, the predominant induced subunit is α, while in colon, the β- and γ-subunits are primarily induced.[434] This is true both at the mRNA and protein level. This phenomenon has been referred to as non-coordinate regulation, and suggests a degree of complexity of ENaC trafficking that is still not fully-understood.[92,435]

Vasopressin

Vasopressin has been shown to stimulate ENaC activity in the kidney and a number of epithelial cell lines derived from kidney.[252,312,436] The response is relatively rapid, with a time course of minutes, and does not appear to depend on transcription or translation of new proteins, at least in its initial phase.[252] Vasopressin binds to V_2 receptors on the basolateral surface of responsive epithelia, and activates adenylate cyclase. In almost all tissues studied, the action of vasopressin on Na^+ transport is fully reproduced by exogenous cAMP, and is felt to be secondary to activation of protein kinase A (PKA).[252,437,438] PKA has not been shown to phosphorylate any subunit of the channel, so its actions are felt to be indirect.[437] There has been no consistent demonstration of an effect of PKA on ENaC open probability, so it is likely that the primary effect of PKA on ENaC is to increase the number of channels at the plasma membrane. Indeed, there are now numerous demonstrations that PKA stimulation leads to an increase in surface expression of ENaC by biochemical, immunohistochemical, and electrophysiologic techniques.[111,312,439–441] By analogy to its well-described effects on insertion of aquaporins in kidney cortex and medulla, it seems reasonable to expect that the primary event in PKA stimulation of ENaC is the exocytosis of channels into the apical membrane from some pre-existing cytoplasmic pool. Strong evidence supports this likelihood. Studies by patch-clamp indicate a rapid increase in the number of surface channels in response to cAMP stimulation.[442] Stimulation of adenylate cyclase by forskolin or by addition of cAMP analogs leads to an increase in biochemical and immunohistochemically measured apical channel number,[312,439] and this increase is temporally associated with an increase in apical membrane capacitance typical of exocytic events.[111,441] Butterworth and colleagues have recently proposed that cAMP stimulation leads to exocytic insertion of channels from a subapical recycling pool of channels that is distinct from constitutive turnover of the channel, analogous to vasopressin regulation of water channels[111] (Figure 30.4).

It is also likely that vasopressin, acting through cAMP and Nedd4-2, alters channel retrieval. Snyder and colleagues reported that Nedd4-2 is a substrate for PKA phosphorylation, and they related cAMP regulation of ENaC to inhibition of Nedd4-ENaC interactions.[297] Indeed, PKA appears to phosphorylate Nedd4-2 at sites that overlap the SGK1 target phosphorylation sites, suggesting a similar mechanism of action in promoting the sequestration of Nedd4-2 through binding to 14-3-3 proteins.[308,309] There is an obvious interplay between the hormonal regulation of ENaC by aldosterone and vasopressin, and it is possible that it occurs at the point of kinase regulation. However, the fact that aldosterone and vasopressin are synergistic, and that ENaCs with Liddle's mutations which should be unresponsive to Nedd4-2 inhibition are still responsive to vasopressin stimulation,[436] suggests that, at a minimum, some distinct pathways are involved in the regulation of ENaC by these two hormones. It is also interesting to note that a long-term (days) effect of vasopressin to stimulate transcription of ENaC subunits would clearly complement and be synergistic with aldosterone effects in situations of significant Na^+ avidity.[443]

Insulin

Insulin stimulates ENaC activity in renal epithelia.[252,444] The exact mechanism(s) of this effect are a subject of considerable controversy. This would seem odd, as it is clear that insulin stimulates phosphoinositide 3-kinase (PI3K), which in turn regulates the activity of 3-phosphoinositide-dependent kinase 1. The latter kinase phosphorylates SGK1 and converts it to an active form.[445] This represents an obvious convergence point for the effects of aldosterone and insulin, which have been shown to be synergistic, on the stimulation of ENaC activity.[445−447] Indeed, noise analysis indicates that the primary effect of insulin is to increase the number of active apical membrane channels, with little effect on open probability.[446] All of these observations are consistent with insulin increasing ENaC activity via decreasing Nedd4-2-dependent retrieval.

It is possible, however, that the action of insulin is more complex. Stimulation of ENaC activity by insulin is quite rapid (minutes), and has been associated with exocytosis and delivery of preformed channels to the apical membrane in a PI3K-dependent manner.[310] Additionally it has been proposed that insulin may directly activate channels by phosphorylation that is dependent on protein kinase C[319] or by interaction with active metabolites of PI3K, phosphoinositol 3,4 phosphate, and phosphoinositol 3,4,5 phosphate, both of which activate ENaC in excised patches.[448] As with aldosterone and vasopressin, although a great deal has been learned about the regulation and trafficking of ENaC, the final control mechanisms by which hormones regulate the channel are complex and only partially-understood.

Angiotensin II

Angiotensin II activates ENaC by signaling through angiotensin II type 1 receptors.[449−451] The signaling mechanism appears to involve activation of a Ca^{2+}-independent protein kinase C isoform and activation of NADPH oxidase, leading to an increase in channels at the plasma membrane, as well as an increase in channel open probability.[450,451]

Endothelin

Endothelin-1 signaling through ETB receptors results in a decrease in ENaC open probability. The intracellular signaling pathways subsequent to ETB receptor activation involve Src kinase and MAP kinase 1/2 signaling pathways.[314,452,453]

Regulation by Mechanical Forces

Members of the ENaC/DEG family expressed in *C. elegans* are mechanosensitive ion channels. Early studies directed at examining the mechanosensitivity of ENaC produced conflicting results that have led to lively debates.[454] Different responses of ENaC

expressed in *Xenopus* oocytes to cell swelling or shrinking have been reported.[455,456] Application of a negative hydrostatic pressure to rat CCD cells by patch pipettes led to a variable increase in the open probability of Na^+ channels.[11]

The distal nephron is subject to varying flow rates and volumes, dependent in part on extracellular volume status and the use of pharmacologic agents, such as loop and thiazide diuretics. Changes in flow rates within the distal nephron affect ENaC activity. Micropuncture and microperfusion studies of distal nephron segments have demonstrated that increases in flow rates within the physiologic range led to increases in the rates of net transepithelial Na^+ flux.[457−459] Increases in tubular flow rates expose channels to a variety of mechanical forces, including hydrostatic pressure and shear stress. Carattino and co-workers demonstrated that ENaCs expressed in oocytes are activated when exposed to laminar shear stress at levels that are likely to be present at the surface of principal cells within collecting ducts exposed to flow rates within a physiologic range.[220,221] The increase in ENaC activity is due to an increase in channel open probability.[204,220,221,460] While mutations introduced at sites within the channel pore alter the channel's response to shear stress, evidence suggest that the large extracellular regions function as flow sensors.[188,221,461,462] ENaC subunits are also expressed in vascular smooth muscle, where they are also exposed to mechanical forces. ENaC subunits, possibly in conjunction with ASIC subunits, form mechanosensitive channels that function as arterial baroreceptors and participate in the myogenic response in vascular beds.[160,463−470]

ENaC AND HUMAN DISORDERS

Liddle syndrome is a rare, autosomal dominant disorder characterized by extracellular fluid volume expansion, hypertension, and hypokalemia. Mutations have been described in patients with this disorder in genes encoding the β- or γ-subunits of ENaC that result in either a truncation or frameshift within the intracellular carboxyl termini or amino acid substitutions within the PY motifs.[277,279−281] These mutations disrupt the binding of Nedd4-2 to ENaC, prevent Nedd4-2-dependent ubiquitination of ENaC subunits, and significantly retard rates of channel internalization from the plasma membrane and degradation.[126,128,282,471,472] Liddle's mutations are also associated with an increase in channel open probability that may reflect an increase in the proteolytic processing of subunits, in association with an increased residency time at the plasma membrane.[473]

It is likely that rare mutations that result in a Liddle syndrome phenotype that are not associated with the

PY motif will be identified. These mutations would result in either an increase in channel open probability or an increase in surface expression. For example, a γ-subunit N530K mutation has been described in a patient with diabetic nephropathy.[474] This mutation is within a region where mutations or chemical modification of substituted cysteine residues lead to an increase in channel open probability.[76,79,219] Common human epithelial Na⁺ channel polymorphisms segregate with blood pressure, including βT594M and αA663T,[475,476] and are associated with altered channel activity.[231,477,478] A homozygous missense mutation in the gene encoding SCNN1A (α-subunit) resulting in a Ser243Pro mutation was noted in an infant with severe renal Na⁺-wasting.[479] This mutation was associated with enhanced Na⁺ self-inhibition, as well as enhanced Na⁺ feedback inhibition (an inhibition of channel activity due to an increase in intracellular [Na⁺]). Another report described an individual with atypical cystic fibrosis who was heterozygous for the ΔF508 CFTR mutation.[192] This individual also had a mutation in the α-subunit (αW493R) that resulted in a profound loss in Na⁺ self-inhibition. While it is unclear whether the αW493R mutation contributed to the pulmonary symptoms, individuals who are heterozygous for the ΔF508 mutation in the cystic fibrosis transmembrane conductance regulator (CFTR) generally lack overt pulmonary symptoms. Specific disorders of mineralocorticoid and glucocorticoid metabolism are also associated with increases in ENaC activity and hypertension.

A decrease in airway fluid volume has been observed in patients with cystic fibrosis. As discussed above, it has been suggested the CFTR, a cAMP-regulated Cl⁻ channel, inhibits ENaC activity in airway epithelia. In the absence of functional CFTR, the activity of ENaC in airways appears to be increased,[352,355,357] although conflicting observations have been reported.[362,363]

Renal Na⁺ retention occurs in nephrotic syndrome, even in the absence of activation of known volume regulatory hormones. Recent studies suggest that plasminogen is filtered by damaged glomeruli, and is converted to plasmin by urokinase that lines kidney tubules.[338,339,480] Plasmin cleaves the γ-subunit and activates ENaC, raising the possibility that aberrant activation of ENaC by plasmin may have an important role in the activation of renal Na⁺ retaining mechanisms in nephrotic syndrome.[338,339,480]

ENaC loss-of-function mutations have been described in the autosomal recessive variant of type I pseudohypoaldosteronism. This disorder is characterized by volume depletion, hypotension, and hyperkalemia. Many of the mutations described to date are due to a frameshift or premature stop codon.[42] A missense mutation within the β-subunit G37S led to the identification of an N-terminal domain that affects channel-gating.[165,166]

References

[1] Koefoed-Johnson V, Ussing HH. The nature of frog skin potential. Acta Physiol Scand 1958;42:298—308.

[2] Van Driessche W, Lindemann B. Concentration dependence of currents through single sodium-selective pores in frog skin. Nature 1979;282(5738):519—20.

[3] Palmer LG, Frindt G. Epithelial sodium channels: characterization by using the patch-clamp technique. Fed Proc 1986;45 (12):2708—12.

[4] Hamilton KL, Eaton DC. Single-channel recordings from amiloride-sensitive epithelial sodium channel. Am J Physiol 1985;249(3 Pt 1):C200—7.

[5] Hummler E, Barker P, Talbot C, Wang Q, Verdumo C, Grubb B, et al. A mouse model for the renal salt-wasting syndrome pseudohypoaldosteronism. Proc Natl Acad Sci USA 1997;94 (21):11710—5.

[6] McDonald FJ, Yang B, Hrstka RF, Drummond HA, Tarr DE, McCray Jr PB, et al. Disruption of the beta subunit of the epithelial Na⁺ channel in mice: Hyperkalemia and neonatal death associated with a pseudohypoaldosteronism phenotype. Proc Natl Acad Sci USA 1999;96(4):1727—31.

[7] Pradervand S, Barker PM, Wang Q, Ernst SA, Beermann F, Grubb BR, et al. Salt restriction induces pseudohypoaldosteronism type 1 in mice expressing low levels of the beta-subunit of the amiloride-sensitive epithelial sodium channel. Proc Natl Acad Sci USA 1999;96(4):1732—7.

[8] Hamilton KL, Eaton DC. Single-channel recordings from two types of amiloride-sensitive epithelial Na⁺ channels. Membr Biochem 1986;6(2):149—71.

[9] Canessa CM, Schild L, Buell G, Thorens B, Gautschi I, Horisberger JD, et al. Amiloride-sensitive epithelial Na⁺ channel is made of three homologous subunits. Nature 1994;367 (6462):463—7.

[10] Palmer LG, Frindt G. Conductance and gating of epithelial Na channels from rat cortical collecting tubule. Effects of luminal Na and Li. J Gen Physiol 1988;92(1):121—38.

[11] Palmer LG, Frindt G. Gating of Na channels in the rat cortical collecting tubule: effects of voltage and membrane stretch. J Gen Physiol 1996;107(1):35—45.

[12] Kemendy AE, Kleyman TR, Eaton DC. Aldosterone alters the open probability of amiloride-blockable sodium channels in A6 epithelia. Am J Physiol 1992;263(4 Pt 1):C825—37.

[13] Caldwell RA, Boucher RC, Stutts MJ. Serine protease activation of near-silent epithelial Na⁺ channels. Am J Physiol Cell Physiol 2004;286(1):C190—4.

[14] Bentley PJ. Amiloride: a potent inhibitor of sodium transport across the toad bladder. J Physiol 1968;195(2):317—30.

[15] Kleyman TR, Cragoe Jr EJ. Cation transport probes: the amiloride series. Methods Enzymol 1990;191:739—55.

[16] Salako LA, Smith AJ. Effects of the diuretics, triamterene and mersalyl on active sodium transport mechanisms in isolated frog skin. Br J Pharmacol 1971;41(3):552—7.

[17] Choi MJ, Fernandez PC, Patnaik A, Coupaye-Gerard B, D'Andrea D, Szerlip H, et al. Brief report: trimethoprim-induced hyperkalemia in a patient with AIDS. N Engl J Med 1993;328(10):703—6.

[18] Schlanger LE, Kleyman TR, Ling BN. K(⁺)-sparing diuretic actions of trimethoprim: inhibition of Na⁺ channels in A6 distal nephron cells. Kidney Int 1994;45(4):1070—6.

[19] Kleyman TR, Roberts C, Ling BN. A mechanism for pentamidine-induced hyperkalemia: inhibition of distal nephron sodium transport. Ann Intern Med 1995;122(2):103–6.

[20] Benos DJ, Saccomani G, Brenner BM, Sariban-Sohraby S. Purification and characterization of the amiloride-sensitive sodium channel from A6 cultured cells and bovine renal papilla. Proc Natl Acad Sci USA 1986;83(22):8525–9.

[21] Benos DJ, Saccomani G, Sariban-Sohraby S. The epithelial sodium channel. Subunit number and location of the amiloride binding site. J Biol Chem 1987;262(22):10613–8.

[22] Kleyman TR, Kraehenbuhl JP, Ernst SA. Characterization and cellular localization of the epithelial Na$^+$ channel. Studies using an anti-Na$^+$ channel antibody raised by an antiidiotypic route. J Biol Chem 1991;266(6):3907–15.

[23] Ismailov II, Berdiev BK, Bradford AL, Awayda MS, Fuller CM, Benos DJ. Associated proteins and renal epithelial Na$^+$ channel function. J Membr Biol 1996;149(2):123–32.

[24] Canessa CM, Horisberger JD, Rossier BC. Epithelial sodium channel related to proteins involved in neurodegeneration. Nature 1993;361(6411):467–70.

[25] Lingueglia E, Voilley N, Waldmann R, Lazdunski M, Barbry P. Expression cloning of an epithelial amiloride-sensitive Na$^+$ channel. A new channel type with homologies to *Caenorhabditis elegans* degenerins. FEBS Lett 1993;318(1):95–9.

[26] Lingueglia E, Renard S, Waldmann R, Voilley N, Champigny G, Plass H, et al. Different homologous subunits of the amiloride-sensitive Na$^+$ channel are differently regulated by aldosterone. J Biol Chem 1994;269(19):13736–9.

[27] Ahn YJ, Brooker DR, Kosari F, Harte BJ, Li J, Mackler SA, et al. Cloning and functional expression of the mouse epithelial sodium channel. Am J Physiol 1999;277(1 Pt 2):F121–9.

[28] McDonald FJ, Price MP, Snyder PM, Welsh MJ. Cloning and expression of the beta- and gamma-subunits of the human epithelial sodium channel. Am J Physiol 1995;268(5 Pt 1):C1157–63.

[29] McDonald FJ, Snyder PM, McCray Jr PB, Welsh MJ. Cloning, expression, and tissue distribution of a human amiloride-sensitive Na$^+$ channel. Am J Physiol 1994;266(6 Pt 1):L728–34.

[30] Fuller CM, Awayda MS, Arrate MP, Bradford AL, Morris RG, Canessa CM, et al. Cloning of a bovine renal epithelial Na$^+$ channel subunit. Am J Physiol 1995;269(3 Pt 1):C641–54.

[31] Puoti A, May A, Canessa CM, Horisberger JD, Schild L, Rossier BC. The highly selective low-conductance epithelial Na channel of *Xenopus laevis* A6 kidney cells. Am J Physiol 1995;269(1 Pt 1):C188–97.

[32] Jensik P, Holbird D, Cox T. Cloned bullfrog skin sodium (fENaC) and xENaC subunits hybridize to form functional sodium channels. J Comp Physiol [B] 2002;172(7):569–76.

[33] Goldstein O, Asher C, Garty H. Cloning and induction by low NaCl intake of avian intestine Na$^+$ channel subunits. Am J Physiol 1997;272(1 Pt 1):C270–7.

[34] Schnizler M, Mastroberardino L, Reifarth F, Weber WM, Verrey F, Clauss W. cAMP sensitivity conferred to the epithelial Na$^+$ channel by alpha-subunit cloned from guinea-pig colon. Pflugers Arch 2000;439(5):579–87.

[35] Voilley N, Bassilana F, Mignon C, Merscher S, Mattei MG, Carle GF, et al. Cloning, chromosomal localization, and physical linkage of the beta and gamma subunits (SCNN1B and SCNN1G) of the human epithelial amiloride-sensitive sodium channel. Genomics 1995;28(3):560–5.

[36] Brooker DR, Kozak CA, Kleyman TR. Epithelial sodium channel genes Scnn1b and Scnn1g are closely linked on distal mouse chromosome 7. Genomics 1995;29(3):784–6.

[37] Ludwig M, Bolkenius U, Wickert L, Marynen P, Bidlingmaier F. Structural organisation of the gene encoding the alpha-subunit of the human amiloride-sensitive epithelial sodium channel. Hum Genet 1998;102(5):576–81.

[38] Thomas CP, Auerbach SD, Zhang C, Stokes JB. The structure of the rat amiloride-sensitive epithelial sodium channel gamma subunit gene and functional analysis of its promoter. Gene 1999;228(1–2):111–22.

[39] Thomas CP, Auerbach S, Stokes JB, Volk KA. 5′ heterogeneity in epithelial sodium channel alpha-subunit mRNA leads to distinct NH2-terminal variant proteins. Am J Physiol 1998;274(5 Pt 1):C1312–23.

[40] Chraibi A, Verdumo C, Merillat AM, Rossier BC, Horisberger JD, Hummler E. Functional analyses of a N-terminal splice variant of the alpha subunit of the epithelial sodium channel. Cell Physiol Biochem 2001;11(3):115–22.

[41] Tucker JK, Tamba K, Lee YJ, Shen LL, Warnock DG, Oh Y. Cloning and functional studies of splice variants of the alpha-subunit of the amiloride-sensitive Na$^+$ channel. Am J Physiol 1998;274(4 Pt 1):C1081–9.

[42] Chang SS, Grunder S, Hanukoglu A, Rosler A, Mathew PM, Hanukoglu I, et al. Mutations in subunits of the epithelial sodium channel cause salt wasting with hyperkalaemic acidosis, pseudohypoaldosteronism type 1. Nat Genet 1996;12(3):248–53.

[43] Bonny O, Chraibi A, Loffing J, Jaeger NF, Grunder S, Horisberger JD, et al. Functional expression of a pseudohypoaldosteronism type I mutated epithelial Na$^+$ channel lacking the pore-forming region of its alpha subunit. J Clin Invest 1999;104(7):967–74.

[44] Huang M, Chalfie M. Gene interactions affecting mechanosensory transduction in *Caenorhabditis elegans*. Nature 1994;367(6462):467–70.

[45] Corey DP, Garcia-Anoveros J. Mechanosensation and the DEG/ENaC ion channels. Science 1996;273(5273):323–4.

[46] Goodman MB, Ernstrom GG, Chelur DS, O'Hagan R, Yao CA, Chalfie M. MEC-2 regulates *C. elegans* DEG/ENaC channels needed for mechanosensation. Nature 2002;415(6875):1039–42.

[47] Waldmann R, Champigny G, Bassilana F, Voilley N, Lazdunski M. Molecular cloning and functional expression of a novel amiloride-sensitive Na$^+$ channel. J Biol Chem 1995;270(46):27411–4.

[48] Yamamura H, Ugawa S, Ueda T, Nagao M, Shimada S. Protons activate the delta-subunit of the epithelial Na$^+$ channel in humans. J Biol Chem 2004;279(13):12529–34.

[49] Babini E, Geisler HS, Siba M, Grunder S. A new subunit of the epithelial Na$^+$ channel identifies regions involved in Na$^+$ self-inhibition. J Biol Chem 2003;278(31):28418–26.

[50] Waldmann R, Champigny G, Bassilana F, Heurteaux C, Lazdunski M. A proton-gated cation channel involved in acid-sensing. Nature 1997;386(6621):173–7.

[51] Price MP, Snyder PM, Welsh MJ. Cloning and expression of a novel human brain Na$^+$ channel. J Biol Chem 1996;271(14):7879–82.

[52] Wemmie JA, Askwith CC, Lamani E, Cassell MD, Freeman Jr JH, Welsh MJ. Acid-sensing ion channel 1 is localized in brain regions with high synaptic density and contributes to fear conditioning. J Neurosci 2003;23(13):5496–502.

[53] Wemmie JA, Coryell MW, Askwith CC, Lamani E, Leonard AS, Sigmund CD, et al. Overexpression of acid-sensing ion channel 1a in transgenic mice increases acquired fear-related behavior. Proc Natl Acad Sci USA 2004;101(10):3621–6.

[54] Ziemann AE, Allen JE, Dahdaleh NS, Drebot II, Coryell MW, Wunsch AM, et al. The amygdala is a chemosensor that detects carbon dioxide and acidosis to elicit fear behavior. Cell 2009;139(5):1012–21.

[55] Ziemann AE, Schnizler MK, Albert GW, Severson MA, Howard III MA, Welsh MJ, et al. Seizure termination by acidosis depends on ASIC1a. Nat Neurosci 2008;11(7):816—22.

[56] Adams CM, Anderson MG, Motto DG, Price MP, Johnson WA, Welsh MJ. Ripped pocket and pickpocket, novel *Drosophila* DEG/ENaC subunits expressed in early development and in mechanosensory neurons. J Cell Biol 1998;140(1):143—52.

[57] Darboux I, Lingueglia E, Pauron D, Barbry P, Lazdunski M. A new member of the amiloride-sensitive sodium channel family in *Drosophila melanogaster* peripheral nervous system. Biochem Biophys Res Commun 1998;246(1):210—6.

[58] Take-Uchi M, Kawakami M, Ishihara T, Amano T, Kondo K, Katsura I. An ion channel of the degenerin/epithelial sodium channel superfamily controls the defecation rhythm in *Caenorhabditis elegans*. Proc Natl Acad Sci USA 1998;95(20):11775—80.

[59] Liu L, Johnson WA, Welsh MJ. *Drosophila* DEG/ENaC pickpocket genes are expressed in the tracheal system, where they may be involved in liquid clearance. Proc Natl Acad Sci USA 2003;100(4):2128—33.

[60] Liu L, Leonard AS, Motto DG, Feller MA, Price MP, Johnson WA, et al. Contribution of *Drosophila* DEG/ENaC genes to salt taste. Neuron 2003;39(1):133—46.

[61] Lin H, Mann KJ, Starostina E, Kinser RD, Pikielny CWA. *Drosophila* DEG/ENaC channel subunit is required for male response to female pheromones. Proc Natl Acad Sci USA 2005;102(36):12831—6.

[62] Lingueglia E, Champigny G, Lazdunski M, Barbry P. Cloning of the amiloride-sensitive FMRFamide peptide-gated sodium channel. Nature 1995;378(6558):730—3.

[63] Cottrell GA. The first peptide-gated ion channel. J Exp Biol 1997;200(Pt 18):2377—86.

[64] Jeziorski MC, Green KA, Sommerville J, Cottrell GA. Cloning and expression of a FMRFamide-gated Na(⁺) channel from *Helisoma trivolvis* and comparison with the native neuronal channel. J Physiol 2000;526(Pt 1):13—25.

[65] Ho K, Nichols CG, Lederer WJ, Lytton J, Vassilev PM, Kanazirska MV, et al. Cloning and expression of an inwardly rectifying ATP-regulated potassium channel. Nature 1993;362(6415):31—8.

[66] Valera S, Hussy N, Evans RJ, Adami N, North RA, Surprenant A, et al. A new class of ligand-gated ion channel defined by P2x receptor for extracellular ATP. Nature 1994;371(6497):516—9.

[67] Renard S, Lingueglia E, Voilley N, Lazdunski M, Barbry P. Biochemical analysis of the membrane topology of the amiloride-sensitive Na⁺ channel. J Biol Chem 1994;269(17):12981—6.

[68] Canessa CM, Merillat AM, Rossier BC. Membrane topology of the epithelial sodium channel in intact cells. Am J Physiol 1994;267(6 Pt 1):C1682—90.

[69] Jasti J, Furukawa H, Gonzales EB, Gouaux E. Structure of acid-sensing ion channel 1 at 1.9 A resolution and low pH. Nature 2007;449(7160):316—23.

[70] Gonzales EB, Kawate T, Gouaux E. Pore architecture and ion sites in acid-sensing ion channels and P2X receptors. Nature 2009;460(7255):599—604.

[71] Firsov D, Gautschi I, Merillat AM, Rossier BC, Schild L. The heterotetrameric architecture of the epithelial sodium channel (ENaC). Embo J 1998;17(2):344—52.

[72] Kosari F, Sheng S, Li J, Mak DO, Foskett JK, Kleyman TR. Subunit stoichiometry of the epithelial sodium channel. J Biol Chem 1998;273(22):13469—74.

[73] Snyder PM, Cheng C, Prince LS, Rogers JC, Welsh MJ. Electrophysiological and biochemical evidence that DEG/ENaC cation channels are composed of nine subunits. J Biol Chem 1998;273(2):681—4.

[74] Anantharam A, Palmer LG. Determination of epithelial Na⁺ channel subunit stoichiometry from single-channel conductances. J Gen Physiol 2007;130(1):55—70.

[75] Li T, Yang Y, Canessa CM. Outlines of the pore in open and closed conformations describe the gating mechanism of ASIC1. Nat Commun 2011;2:399.

[76] Sheng S, Li J, McNulty KA, Kieber-Emmons T, Kleyman TR. Epithelial sodium channel pore region. Structure and role in gating. J Biol Chem 2001;276(2):1326—34.

[77] Carattino MD, Edinger RS, Grieser HJ, Wise R, Neumann D, Schlattner U, et al. Hallows KR. Epithelial sodium channel inhibition by AMP-activated protein kinase in oocytes and polarized renal epithelial cells. J Biol Chem 2005;280(18):17608—16.

[78] Adams CM, Snyder PM, Price MP, Welsh MJ. Protons activate brain Na⁺ channel 1 by inducing a conformational change that exposes a residue associated with neurodegeneration. J Biol Chem 1998;273(46):30204—7.

[79] Snyder PM, Bucher DB, Olson DR. Gating induces a conformational change in the outer vestibule of ENaC. J Gen Physiol 2000;116(6):781—90.

[80] Kashlan OB, Boyd CR, Argyropoulos C, Okumura S, Hughey RP, Grabe M, et al. Allosteric inhibition of the epithelial Na⁺ channel through peptide binding at peripheral finger and thumb domains. J Biol Chem 2010;285(45):35216—23.

[81] Kashlan OB, Kleyman TR. ENaC structure and function in the wake of a resolved structure of a family member. Am J Physiol Renal Physiol 2011;301(4):F684—96.

[82] Kashlan OB, Adelman JL, Okumura S, Blobner BM, Zuzek Z, Hughey RP, et al. Constraint-based, homology model of the extracellular domain of the epithelial Na⁺ channel alpha subunit reveals a mechanism of channel activation by proteases. J Biol Chem 2011;286(1):649—60.

[83] Hughey RP, Bruns JB, Kinlough CL, Harkleroad KL, Tong Q, Carattino MD, et al. Epithelial sodium channels are activated by furin-dependent proteolysis. J Biol Chem 2004;279(18):18111—4.

[84] Carattino MD, Sheng S, Bruns JB, Pilewski JM, Hughey RP, Kleyman TR. The epithelial Na⁺ channel is inhibited by a peptide derived from proteolytic processing of its alpha subunit. J Biol Chem 2006;281(27):18901—7.

[85] Kleyman TR, Carattino MD, Hughey RP. ENaC at the cutting edge: regulation of epithelial sodium channels by proteases. J Biol Chem 2009;284(31):20447—51.

[86] Carattino MD, Passero CJ, Steren CA, Maarouf AB, Pilewski JM, Myerburg MM, et al. Defining an inhibitory domain in the alpha-subunit of the epithelial sodium channel. Am J Physiol Renal Physiol 2008;294(1):F47—52.

[87] Stockand JD, Staruschenko A, Pochynyuk O, Booth RE, Silverthorn DU. Insight toward epithelial Na⁺ channel mechanism revealed by the acid-sensing ion channel 1 structure. IUBMB Life 2008;60(9):620—8.

[88] Adams CM, Snyder PM, Welsh MJ. Interactions between subunits of the human epithelial sodium channel. J Biol Chem 1997;272(43):27295—300.

[89] May A, Puoti A, Gaeggeler HP, Horisberger JD, Rossier BC. Early effect of aldosterone on the rate of synthesis of the epithelial sodium channel alpha subunit in A6 renal cells. J Am Soc Nephrol 1997;8(12):1813—22.

[90] Prince LS, Welsh MJ. Cell surface expression and biosynthesis of epithelial Na⁺ channels. Biochem J 1998;336(Pt 3):705—10.

[91] Hanwell D, Ishikawa T, Saleki R, Rotin D. Trafficking and cell surface stability of the epithelial Na⁺ channel expressed in epithelial Madin—Darby canine kidney cells. J Biol Chem 2002;277(12):9772—9.

[92] Weisz OA, Wang JM, Edinger RS, Johnson JP. Non-coordinate regulation of endogenous epithelial sodium channel (ENaC) subunit expression at the apical membrane of A6 cells in response to various transporting conditions. J Biol Chem 2000;275(51):39886−93.

[93] De La Rosa DA, Li H, Canessa CM. Effects of aldosterone on biosynthesis, traffic, and functional expression of epithelial sodium channels in A6 cells. J Gen Physiol 2002;119(5): 427−42.

[94] Cheng C, Prince LS, Snyder PM, Welsh MJ. Assembly of the epithelial Na$^+$ channel evaluated using sucrose gradient sedimentation analysis. J Biol Chem 1998;273(35):22693−700.

[95] Rotin D, Kanelis V, Schild L. Trafficking and cell surface stability of ENaC. Am J Physiol Renal Physiol 2001;281(3):F391−9.

[96] Valentijn JA, Fyfe GK, Canessa CM. Biosynthesis and processing of epithelial sodium channels in *Xenopus* oocytes. J Biol Chem 1998;273(46):30344−51.

[97] Hughey RP, Mueller GM, Bruns JB, Kinlough CL, Poland PA, Harkleroad KL, et al. Maturation of the epithelial Na$^+$ channel involves proteolytic processing of the alpha- and gamma-subunits. J Biol Chem 2003;278(39):37073−82.

[98] Mueller GM, Maarouf AB, Kinlough CL, Sheng N, Kashlan OB, Okumura S, et al. Cys palmitoylation of the beta subunit modulates gating of the epithelial sodium channel. J Biol Chem 2010;285(40):30453−62.

[99] Mueller GM, Kashlan OB, Bruns JB, Maarouf AB, Aridor M, Kleyman TR, et al. Epithelial sodium channel exit from the endoplasmic reticulum is regulated by a signal within the carboxyl cytoplasmic domain of the alpha subunit. J Biol Chem 2007;282(46):33475−83.

[100] Kashlan OB, Mueller GM, Qamar MZ, Poland PA, Ahner A, Rubenstein RC, et al. Small heat shock protein alphaA-crystallin regulates epithelial sodium channel expression. J Biol Chem 2007;282(38):28149−56.

[101] Buck TM, Kolb AR, Boyd CR, Kleyman TR, Brodsky JL. The endoplasmic reticulum-associated degradation of the epithelial sodium channel requires a unique complement of molecular chaperones. Mol Biol Cell 2010;21(6):1047−58.

[102] Kolb AR, Buck TM, Brodsky JL. *Saccharomyces cerivisiae* as a model system for kidney disease: what can yeast tell us about renal function? Am J Physiol Renal Physiol 2011;301(1):F1−11.

[103] Kopito RR. ER quality control: the cytoplasmic connection. Cell 1997;88(4):427−30.

[104] Ellgaard L, Molinari M, Helenius A. Setting the standards: quality control in the secretory pathway. Science 1999;286 (5446):1882−8.

[105] Fewell SW, Travers KJ, Weissman JS, Brodsky JL. The action of molecular chaperones in the early secretory pathway. Annu Rev Genet 2001;35:149−91.

[106] Goldfarb SB, Kashlan OB, Watkins JN, Suaud L, Yan W, Kleyman TR, et al. Differential effects of Hsc70 and Hsp70 on the intracellular trafficking and functional expression of epithelial sodium channels. Proc Natl Acad Sci USA 2006;103 (15):5817−22.

[107] Sugahara T, Koga T, Ueno-Shuto K, Shuto T, Watanabe E, Maekawa A, et al. Calreticulin positively regulates the expression and function of epithelial sodium channel. Exp Cell Res 2009;315(19):3294−300.

[108] Malik B, Schlanger L, Al-Khalili O, Bao HF, Yue G, Price SR, et al. ENaC degradation in A6 cells by the ubiquitin-proteosome proteolytic pathway. J Biol Chem 2001;276(16):12903−10.

[109] Kleyman TR, Zuckerman JB, Middleton P, McNulty KA, Hu B, Su X, et al. Cell surface expression and turnover of the alpha-subunit of the epithelial sodium channel. Am J Physiol Renal Physiol 2001;281(2):F213−21.

[110] Mohan S, Bruns JR, Weixel KM, Edinger RS, Bruns JB, Kleyman TR, et al. Differential current decay profiles of epithelial sodium channel subunit combinations in polarized renal epithelial cells. J Biol Chem 2004;279(31):32071−8.

[111] Butterworth MB, Edinger RS, Johnson JP, Frizzell RA. Acute ENaC stimulation by cAMP in a kidney cell line is mediated by exocytic insertion from a recycling channel pool. J Gen Physiol 2005;125(1):81−101.

[112] Hughey RP, Bruns JB, Kinlough CL, Kleyman TR. Distinct pools of epithelial sodium channels are expressed at the plasma membrane. J Biol Chem 2004;279(47):48491−4.

[113] Caldwell RA, Boucher RC, Stutts MJ. Neutrophil elastase activates near-silent epithelial Na$^+$-channels and increases airway epithelial Na$^+$-transport. Am J Physiol Lung Cell Mol Physiol 2005;288(5):L813−9.

[114] Chraibi A, Vallet V, Firsov D, Hess SK, Horisberger JD. Protease modulation of the activity of the epithelial sodium channel expressed in *Xenopus* oocytes. J Gen Physiol 1998;111 (1):127−38.

[115] Sheng S, Carattino MD, Bruns JB, Hughey RP, Kleyman TR. Furin cleavage activates the epithelial Na$^+$ channel by relieving Na$^+$ self-inhibition. Am J Physiol Renal Physiol 2006;290(6): F1488−96.

[116] Saxena S, Quick MW, Tousson A, Oh Y, Warnock DG. Interaction of syntaxins with the amiloride-sensitive epithelial sodium channel. J Biol Chem 1999;274(30):20812−7.

[117] Berdiev BK, Jovov B, Tucker WC, Naren AP, Fuller CM, Chapman ER, et al. ENaC subunit-subunit interactions and inhibition by syntaxin 1A. Am J Physiol Renal Physiol 2004;286 (6):F1100−6.

[118] Condliffe SB, Zhang H, Frizzell RA. Syntaxin 1A regulates ENaC channel activity. J Biol Chem 2004;279(11):10085−92.

[119] Condliffe SB, Carattino MD, Frizzell RA, Zhang H. Syntaxin 1A regulates ENaC via domain-specific interactions. J Biol Chem 2003;278(15):12796−804.

[120] Hill WG, An B, Johnson JP. Endogenously expressed epithelial sodium channel is present in lipid rafts in A6 cells. J Biol Chem 2002;277(37):33541−4.

[121] Shlyonsky VG, Mies F, Sariban-Sohraby S. Epithelial sodium channel activity in detergent-resistant membrane microdomains. Am J Physiol Renal Physiol 2003;284(1):F182−8.

[122] Rotin D, Bar-Sagi D, O'Brodovich H, Merilainen J, Lehto VP, Canessa CM, et al. An SH3 binding region in the epithelial Na$^+$ channel (alpha rENaC) mediates its localization at the apical membrane. Embo J 1994;13(19):4440−50.

[123] Zuckerman JB, Chen X, Jacobs JD, Hu B, Kleyman TR, Smith PR. Association of the epithelial sodium channel with Apx and alpha-spectrin in A6 renal epithelial cells. J Biol Chem 1999;274 (33):23286−95.

[124] Copeland SJ, Berdiev BK, Ji HL, Lockhart J, Parker S, Fuller CM, et al. Regions in the carboxy terminus of alpha-bENaC involved in gating and functional effects of actin. Am J Physiol Cell Physiol 2001;281(1):C231−40.

[125] Berdiev BK, Latorre R, Benos DJ, Ismailov II. Actin modifies Ca^{2+} block of epithelial Na$^+$ channels in planar lipid bilayers. Biophys J 2001;80(5):2176−86.

[126] Shimkets RA, Lifton RP, Canessa CM. The activity of the epithelial sodium channel is regulated by clathrin-mediated endocytosis. J Biol Chem 1997;272(41):25537−41.

[127] Carattino MD, Hill WG, Kleyman TR. Arachidonic acid regulates surface expression of epithelial sodium channels. J Biol Chem 2003;278(38):36202−13.

[128] Schild L, Lu Y, Gautschi I, Schneeberger E, Lifton RP, Rossier BC. Identification of a PY motif in the epithelial Na channel subunits as a target sequence for mutations causing channel

activation found in Liddle syndrome. Embo J 1996;15 (10):2381–7.

[129] Takei K, McPherson PS, Schmid SL, De Camilli P. Tubular membrane invaginations coated by dynamin rings are induced by GTP-gamma S in nerve terminals. Nature 1995;374 (6518):186–90.

[130] Henley JR, Krueger EW, Oswald BJ, McNiven MA. Dynamin-mediated internalization of caveolae. J Cell Biol 1998;141 (1):85–99.

[131] Oh P, McIntosh DP, Schnitzer JE. Dynamin at the neck of caveolae mediates their budding to form transport vesicles by GTP-driven fission from the plasma membrane of endothelium. J Cell Biol 1998;141(1):101–14.

[132] Staub O, Gautschi I, Ishikawa T, Breitschopf K, Ciechanover A, Schild L, et al. Regulation of stability and function of the epithelial Na$^+$ channel (ENaC) by ubiquitination. Embo J 1997;16 (21):6325–36.

[133] Wang H, Traub LM, Weixel KM, Hawryluk MJ, Shah N, Edinger RS, et al. Clathrin-mediated endocytosis of the epithelial sodium channel. Role of epsin J Biol Chem 2006;281 (20):14129–35.

[134] Fakitsas P, Adam G, Daidie D, van Bemmelen MX, Fouladkou F, Patrignani A, et al. Early aldosterone-induced gene product regulates the epithelial sodium channel by deubiquitylation. J Am Soc Nephrol 2007;18(4):1084–92.

[135] Butterworth MB, Edinger RS, Ovaa H, Burg D, Johnson JP, Frizzell RA. The deubiquitinating enzyme UCH-L3 regulates the apical membrane recycling of the epithelial sodium channel. J Biol Chem 2007;282(52):37885–93.

[136] Oberfeld B, Ruffieux-Daidie D, Vitagliano JJ, Pos KM, Verrey F, Staub O. Ubiquitin-specific protease 2-45 (Usp2-45) binds to epithelial Na$^+$ channel (ENaC)-ubiquitylating enzyme Nedd4-2. Am J Physiol Renal Physiol 2011;301(1):F189–96.

[137] Xu JZ, Hall AE, Peterson LN, Bienkowski MJ, Eessalu TE, Hebert SC. Localization of the ROMK protein on apical membranes of rat kidney nephron segments. Am J Physiol 1997;273 (5 Pt 2):F739–48.

[138] Woda CB, Miyawaki N, Ramalakshmi S, Ramkumar M, Rojas R, Zavilowitz B, et al. Ontogeny of flow-stimulated potassium secretion in rabbit cortical collecting duct: functional and molecular aspects. Am J Physiol Renal Physiol 2003;285(4): F629–39.

[139] Woda CB, Bragin A, Kleyman TR, Satlin LM. Flow-dependent K$^+$ secretion in the cortical collecting duct is mediated by a maxi-K channel. Am J Physiol Renal Physiol 2001;280(5): F786–93.

[140] Hager H, Kwon TH, Vinnikova AK, Masilamani S, Brooks HL, Frokiaer J, et al. Immunocytochemical and immunoelectron microscopic localization of alpha-, beta-, and gamma-ENaC in rat kidney. Am J Physiol Renal Physiol 2001;280(6):F1093–106.

[141] Loffing J, Pietri L, Aregger F, Bloch-Faure M, Ziegler U, Meneton P, et al. Differential subcellular localization of ENaC subunits in mouse kidney in response to high- and low-Na diets. Am J Physiol Renal Physiol 2000;279(2):F252–8.

[142] Masilamani S, Kim GH, Mitchell C, Wade JB, Knepper MA. Aldosterone-mediated regulation of ENaC alpha, beta, and gamma subunit proteins in rat kidney. J Clin Invest 1999;104 (7):R19–23.

[143] Loffing J, Zecevic M, Feraille E, Kaissling B, Asher C, Rossier BC, et al. Aldosterone induces rapid apical translocation of ENaC in early portion of renal collecting system: possible role of SGK. Am J Physiol Renal Physiol 2001;280(4): F675–82.

[144] Barker PM, Nguyen MS, Gatzy JT, Grubb B, Norman H, Hummler E, et al. Role of gammaENaC subunit in lung liquid clearance and electrolyte balance in newborn mice. Insights into perinatal adaptation and pseudohypoaldosteronism. J Clin Invest 1998;102(8):1634–40.

[145] Hummler E, Barker P, Gatzy J, Beermann F, Verdumo C, Schmidt A, et al. Early death due to defective neonatal lung liquid clearance in alpha-ENaC-deficient mice. Nat Genet 1996;12(3):325–8.

[146] Frindt G, Palmer LG. Na channels in the rat connecting tubule. Am J Physiol Renal Physiol 2004;286(4):F669–74.

[147] Rubera I, Loffing J, Palmer LG, Frindt G, Fowler-Jaeger N, Sauter D, et al. Collecting duct-specific gene inactivation of alphaENaC in the mouse kidney does not impair sodium and potassium balance. J Clin Invest 2003;112(4):554–65.

[148] Burch LH, Talbot CR, Knowles MR, Canessa CM, Rossier BC, Boucher RC. Relative expression of the human epithelial Na$^+$ channel subunits in normal and cystic fibrosis airways. Am J Physiol 1995;269(2 Pt 1):C511–8.

[149] Talbot CL, Bosworth DG, Briley EL, Fenstermacher DA, Boucher RC, Gabriel SE, et al. Quantitation and localization of ENaC subunit expression in fetal, newborn, and adult mouse lung. Am J Respir Cell Mol Biol 1999;20(3):398–406.

[150] Matsushita K, McCray Jr PB, Sigmund RD, Welsh MJ, Stokes JB. Localization of epithelial sodium channel subunit mRNAs in adult rat lung by in situ hybridization. Am J Physiol 1996;271(2 Pt 1):L332–9.

[151] Jain L, Chen XJ, Malik B, Al-Khalili O, Eaton DC. Antisense oligonucleotides against the alpha-subunit of ENaC decrease lung epithelial cation-channel activity. Am J Physiol 1999;276(6 Pt 1):L1046–51.

[152] Borok Z, Liebler JM, Lubman RL, Foster MJ, Zhou B, Li X, et al. Na transport proteins are expressed by rat alveolar epithelial type I cells. Am J Physiol Lung Cell Mol Physiol 2002;282 (4):L599–608.

[153] Mall M, Grubb BR, Harkema JR, O'Neal WK, Boucher RC. Increased airway epithelial Na$^+$ absorption produces cystic fibrosis-like lung disease in mice. Nat Med 2004;10 (5):487–93.

[154] Boucher RC. Regulation of airway surface liquid volume by human airway epithelia. Pflugers Arch 2003;445 (4):495–8.

[155] Duc C, Farman N, Canessa CM, Bonvalet JP, Rossier BC. Cell-specific expression of epithelial sodium channel alpha, beta, and gamma subunits in aldosterone-responsive epithelia from the rat: localization by in situ hybridization and immunocytochemistry. J Cell Biol 1994;127(6 Pt 2):1907–21.

[156] Kretz O, Barbry P, Bock R, Lindemann B. Differential expression of RNA and protein of the three pore-forming subunits of the amiloride-sensitive epithelial sodium channel in taste buds of the rat. J Histochem Cytochem 1999;47(1): 51–64.

[157] Brouard M, Casado M, Djelidi S, Barrandon Y, Farman N. Epithelial sodium channel in human epidermal keratinocytes: expression of its subunits and relation to sodium transport and differentiation. J Cell Sci 1999;112(Pt 19):3343–52.

[158] Grunder S, Muller A, Ruppersberg JP. Developmental and cellular expression pattern of epithelial sodium channel alpha, beta and gamma subunits in the inner ear of the rat. Eur J Neurosci 2001;13(4):641–8.

[159] Couloigner V, Fay M, Djelidi S, Farman N, Escoubet B, Runembert I, et al. Location and function of the epithelial Na channel in the cochlea. Am J Physiol Renal Physiol 2001;280(2): F214–22.

[160] Drummond HA, Gebremedhin D, Harder DR. Degenerin/epithelial Na$^+$ channel proteins: components of a vascular mechanosensor. Hypertension 2004;44(5):643–8.

[161] Mirshahi M, Nicolas C, Mirshahi S, Golestaneh N, d'Hermies F, Agarwal MK. Immunochemical analysis of the sodium channel in rodent and human eye. Exp Eye Res 1999;69(1):21–32.

[162] Bubien JK, Watson B, Khan MA, Langloh AL, Fuller CM, Berdiev B, et al. Expression and regulation of normal and polymorphic epithelial sodium channel by human lymphocytes. J Biol Chem 2001;276(11):8557–66.

[163] Schild L, Schneeberger E, Gautschi I, Firsov D. Identification of amino acid residues in the alpha, beta, and gamma subunits of the epithelial sodium channel (ENaC) involved in amiloride block and ion permeation. J Gen Physiol 1997;109(1):15–26.

[164] Chalfant ML, Denton JS, Langloh AL, Karlson KH, Loffing J, Benos DJ, et al. The NH_2 terminus of the epithelial sodium channel contains an endocytic motif. J Biol Chem 1999;274 (46):32889–96.

[165] Grunder S, Firsov D, Chang SS, Jaeger NF, Gautschi I, Schild L, et al. A mutation causing pseudohypoaldosteronism type 1 identifies a conserved glycine that is involved in the gating of the epithelial sodium channel. Embo J 1997;16(5):899–907.

[166] Grunder S, Jaeger NF, Gautschi I, Schild L, Rossier BC. Identification of a highly conserved sequence at the N-terminus of the epithelial Na^+ channel alpha subunit involved in gating. Pflugers Arch 1999;438(5):709–15.

[167] Kucher V, Boiko N, Pochynyuk O, Stockand JD. Voltage-dependent gating underlies loss of ENaC function in Pseudohypoaldosteronism type 1. Biophys J 2011;100 (8):1930–9.

[168] Waldmann R, Champigny G, Lazdunski M. Functional degenerin-containing chimeras identify residues essential for amiloride-sensitive Na^+ channel function. J Biol Chem 1995;270 (20):11735–7.

[169] Sheng S, Li J, McNulty KA, Avery D, Kleyman TR. Characterization of the selectivity filter of the epithelial sodium channel. J Biol Chem 2000;275(12):8572–81.

[170] Sheng S, McNulty KA, Harvey JM, Kleyman TR. Second transmembrane domains of ENaC subunits contribute to ion permeation and selectivity. J Biol Chem 2001;276(47):44091–8.

[171] Kashlan OB, Sheng S, Kleyman TR. On the interaction between amiloride and its putative alpha-subunit epithelial Na^+ channel binding site. J Biol Chem 2005;280(28):26206–15.

[172] Yue G, Malik B, Yue G, Eaton DC. Phosphatidylinositol 4,5-bisphosphate (PIP2) stimulates epithelial sodium channel activity in A6 cells. J Biol Chem 2002;277(14):11965–9.

[173] Ma HP, Saxena S, Warnock DG. Anionic phospholipids regulate native and expressed epithelial sodium channel (ENaC). J Biol Chem 2002;277(10):7641–4.

[174] Kunzelmann K, Bachhuber T, Regeer R, Markovich D, Sun J, Schreiber R. Purinergic inhibition of the epithelial Na^+ transport via hydrolysis of PIP2. Faseb J 2005;19(1):142–3.

[175] Pochynyuk O, Tong Q, Medina J, Vandewalle A, Staruschenko A, Bugaj V, et al. Molecular determinants of PI(4,5)P2 and PI (3,4,5)P3 regulation of the epithelial Na^+ channel. J Gen Physiol 2007;130(4):399–413.

[176] Helms MN, Liu L, Liang YY, Al-Khalili O, Vandewalle A, Saxena S, et al. Phosphatidylinositol 3,4,5-trisphosphate mediates aldosterone stimulation of epithelial sodium channel (ENaC) and interacts with gamma-ENaC. J Biol Chem 2005;280 (49):40885–91.

[177] Kellenberger S, Gautschi I, Pfister Y, Schild L. Intracellular thiol-mediated modulation of epithelial sodium channel activity. J Biol Chem 2005;280(9):7739–47.

[178] Kashlan OB, Maarouf AB, Kussius C, Denshaw RM, Blumenthal KM, Kleyman TR. Distinct structural elements in the first membrane-spanning segment of the epithelial sodium channel. J Biol Chem 2006;281(41):30455–62.

[179] Firsov D, Robert-Nicoud M, Gruender S, Schild L, Rossier BC. Mutational analysis of cysteine-rich domains of the epithelium sodium channel (ENaC). Identification of cysteines essential for channel expression at the cell surface. J Biol Chem 1999;274 (5):2743–9.

[180] Mano I, Driscoll M. DEG/ENaC channels: a touchy superfamily that watches its salt. Bioessays 1999;21(7):568–78.

[181] Sheng S, Perry CJ, Kleyman TR. External nickel inhibits epithelial sodium channel by binding to histidine residues within the extracellular domains of alpha and gamma subunits and reducing channel open probability. J Biol Chem 2002;277 (51):50098–111.

[182] Sheng S, Bruns JB, Kleyman TR. Extracellular histidine residues crucial for Na^+ self-inhibition of epithelial Na^+ channels. J Biol Chem 2004;279(11):9743–9.

[183] Sheng S, Maarouf AB, Bruns JB, Hughey RP, Kleyman TR. Functional role of extracellular loop cysteine residues of the epithelial Na^+ channel in Na^+ self-inhibition. J Biol Chem 2007;282(28):20180–90.

[184] Sheng S, Perry CJ, Kleyman TR. Extracellular Zn^{2+} activates epithelial Na^+ channels by eliminating Na^+ self-inhibition. J Biol Chem 2004;279(30):31687–96.

[185] Maarouf AB, Sheng N, Chen J, Winarski KL, Okumura S, Carattino MD, et al. Novel determinants of epithelial sodium channel gating within extracellular thumb domains. J Biol Chem 2009;284(12):7756–65.

[186] Winarski KL, Sheng N, Chen J, Kleyman TR, Sheng S. Extracellular allosteric regulatory subdomain within the gamma subunit of the epithelial Na^+ channel. J Biol Chem 2010;285(34):26088–96.

[187] Chen J, Myerburg MM, Passero CJ, Winarski KL, Sheng S. External Cu^{2+} inhibits human epithelial Na^+ channels by binding at a subunit interface of extracellular domains. J Biol Chem 2011;286(31):27436–46.

[188] Shi S, Ghosh DD, Okumura S, Carattino MD, Kashlan OB, Sheng S, et al. Base of the thumb domain modulates epithelial sodium channel gating. J Biol Chem 2011;286(17):14753–61.

[189] Collier DM, Snyder PM. Extracellular protons regulate human ENaC by modulating Na^+ self-inhibition. J Biol Chem 2009;284 (2):792–8.

[190] Collier DM, Snyder PM. Extracellular chloride regulates the epithelial sodium channel. J Biol Chem 2009;284(43):29320–5.

[191] Collier DM, Snyder PM. Identification of epithelial Na^+ channel (ENaC) intersubunit Cl^- inhibitory residues suggests a trimeric alpha gamma beta channel architecture. J Biol Chem 2011;286(8):6027–32.

[192] Rauh R, Diakov A, Tzschoppe A, Korbmacher J, Azad AK, Cuppens H, et al. A mutation of the epithelial sodium channel associated with atypical cystic fibrosis increases channel open probability and reduces Na^+ self inhibition. J Physiol 2010;588 (Pt 8):1211–25.

[193] Edelheit O, Hanukoglu I, Dascal N, Hanukoglu A. Identification of the roles of conserved charged residues in the extracellular domain of an epithelial sodium channel (ENaC) subunit by alanine mutagenesis. Am J Physiol Renal Physiol 2011;300(4):F887–97.

[194] Bruns JB, Hu B, Ahn YJ, Sheng S, Hughey RP, Kleyman TR. Multiple epithelial Na^+ channel domains participate in subunit assembly. Am J Physiol Renal Physiol 2003;285(4):F600–9.

[195] Vallet V, Chraibi A, Gaeggeler HP, Horisberger JD, Rossier BC. An epithelial serine protease activates the amiloride-sensitive sodium channel. Nature 1997;389(6651):607–10.

[196] Vuagniaux G, Vallet V, Jaeger NF, Pfister C, Bens M, Farman N, et al. Activation of the amiloride-sensitive epithelial sodium channel by the serine protease mCAP1 expressed in a mouse

[196] cortical collecting duct cell line. J Am Soc Nephrol 2000;11 (5):828—34.

[197] Adachi M, Kitamura K, Miyoshi T, Narikiyo T, Iwashita K, Shiraishi N, et al. Activation of epithelial sodium channels by prostasin in Xenopus oocytes. J Am Soc Nephrol 2001;12 (6):1114—21.

[198] Guipponi M, Vuagniaux G, Wattenhofer M, Shibuya K, Vazquez M, Dougherty L, et al. The transmembrane serine protease (TMPRSS3) mutated in deafness DFNB8/10 activates the epithelial sodium channel (ENaC) in vitro. Hum Mol Genet 2002;11(23):2829—36.

[199] Adebamiro A, Cheng Y, Rao US, Danahay H, Bridges RJ. A segment of gamma ENaC mediates elastase activation of Na+ transport. J Gen Physiol 2007;130(6):611—29.

[200] Bruns JB, Carattino MD, Sheng S, Maarouf AB, Weisz OA, Pilewski JM, et al. Epithelial Na+ channels are fully activated by furin- and prostasin-dependent release of an inhibitory peptide from the gamma-subunit. J Biol Chem 2007;282 (9):6153—60.

[201] Garty H, Benos DJ. Characteristics and regulatory mechanisms of the amiloride-blockable Na+ channel. Physiol Rev 1988;68 (2):309—73.

[202] Chraibi A, Horisberger JD. Na self inhibition of human epithelial Na channel: temperature dependence and effect of extracellular proteases. J Gen Physiol 2002;120(2):133—45.

[203] Segal A, Cucu D, Van Driessche W, Weber WM. Rat ENaC expressed in Xenopus laevis oocytes is activated by cAMP and blocked by Ni$^{(2+)}$. FEBS Lett 2002;515(1—3):177—83.

[204] Althaus M, Bogdan R, Clauss WG, Fronius M. Mechano-sensitivity of epithelial sodium channels (ENaCs): laminar shear stress increases ion channel open probability. FASEB J 2007;21 (10):2389—99.

[205] Chen J, Winarski KL, Sheng S. Mutations in extracellular domains reverse Zn^{2+}. Activation of human epithelial Na+ channels. Biophys J 2010;98(3, Suppl. 1):532a.

[206] Yu L, Eaton DC, Helms MN. Effect of divalent heavy metals on epithelial Na+ channels in A6 cells. Am J Physiol Renal Physiol 2007;293(1):F236—44.

[207] Rossier BC, Pradervand S, Schild L, Hummler E. Epithelial sodium channel and the control of sodium balance: interaction between genetic and environmental factors. Annu Rev Physiol 2002;64:877—97.

[208] Kellenberger S, Gautschi I, Schild L. A single point mutation in the pore region of the epithelial Na+ channel changes ion selectivity by modifying molecular sieving. Proc Natl Acad Sci USA 1999;96(7):4170—5.

[209] Snyder PM, Olson DR, Bucher DB. A pore segment in DEG/ENaC Na$^{(+)}$ channels. J Biol Chem 1999;274(40): 28484—90.

[210] Kellenberger S, Gautschi I, Schild L. Mutations in the epithelial Na+ channel ENaC outer pore disrupt amiloride block by increasing its dissociation rate. Mol Pharmacol 2003;64 (4):848—56.

[211] Kellenberger S, Hoffmann-Pochon N, Gautschi I, Schneeberger E, Schild L. On the molecular basis of ion permeation in the epithelial Na+ channel. J Gen Physiol 1999;114(1):13—30.

[212] Li J, Sheng S, Perry CJ, Kleyman TR. Asymmetric organization of the pore region of the epithelial sodium channel. J Biol Chem 2003;278(16):13867—74.

[213] Sheng S, Perry CJ, Kashlan OB, Kleyman TR. Side chain orientation of residues lining the selectivity filter of epithelial Na+ channels. J Biol Chem 2005;280(9):8513—22.

[214] Kellenberger S, Auberson M, Gautschi I, Schneeberger E, Schild L. Permeability properties of ENaC selectivity filter mutants. J Gen Physiol 2001;118(6):679—92.

[215] Takeda AN, Gautschi I, van Bemmelen MX, Schild L. Cadmium trapping in an epithelial sodium channel pore mutant. J Biol Chem 2007;282(44):31928—36.

[216] Langloh AL, Berdiev B, Ji HL, Keyser K, Stanton BA, Benos DJ. Charged residues in the M2 region of alpha-hENaC play a role in channel conductance. Am J Physiol Cell Physiol 2000;278(2): C277—91.

[217] Driscoll M, Chalfie M. The mec-4 gene is a member of a family of Caenorhabditis elegans genes that can mutate to induce neuronal degeneration. Nature 1991;349(6310):588—93.

[218] Hong K, Driscoll M. A transmembrane domain of the putative channel subunit MEC-4 influences mechanotransduction and neurodegeneration in C. elegans. Nature 1994;367 (6462):470—3.

[219] Kellenberger S, Gautschi I, Schild L. An external site controls closing of the epithelial Na+ channel ENaC. J Physiol 2002;543 (Pt 2):413—24.

[220] Carattino MD, Sheng S, Kleyman TR. Epithelial Na+ channels are activated by laminar shear stress. J Biol Chem 2004;279 (6):4120—6.

[221] Carattino MD, Sheng S, Kleyman TR. Mutations in the pore region modify epithelial sodium channel gating by shear stress. J Biol Chem 2005;280(6):4393—401.

[222] Carattino MD, Sheng S, Kleyman TR. Mutations in the pore region modify epithelial sodium channel gating by shear stress. J Biol Chem 2005;280(6):4393—401.

[223] Zhang P, Fyfe GK, Grichtchenko II, Canessa CM. Inhibition of alphabeta epithelial sodium channels by external protons indicates that the second hydrophobic domain contains structural elements for closing the pore. Biophys J 1999;77(6):3043—51.

[224] Fyfe GK, Zhang P, Canessa CM. The second hydrophobic domain contributes to the kinetic properties of epithelial sodium channels. J Biol Chem 1999;274(51):36415—21.

[225] Ji HL, Parker S, Langloh AL, Fuller CM, Benos DJ. Point mutations in the post-M2 region of human alpha-ENaC regulate cation selectivity. Am J Physiol Cell Physiol 2001;281(1):C64—74.

[226] Booth RE, Tong Q, Medina J, Snyder PM, Patel P, Stockand JD. A region directly following the second transmembrane domain in gamma ENaC is required for normal channel gating. J Biol Chem 2003;278(42):41367—79.

[227] Pochynyuk O, Staruschenko A, Tong Q, Medina J, Stockand JD. Identification of a functional phosphatidylinositol 3,4,5-trisphosphate binding site in the epithelial Na+ channel. J Biol Chem 2005;280(45):37565—71.

[228] Pochynyuk O, Bugaj V, Stockand JD. Physiologic regulation of the epithelial sodium channel by phosphatidylinositides. Curr Opin Nephrol Hypertens 2008;17(5):533—40.

[229] Snyder PM, Price MP, McDonald FJ, Adams CM, Volk KA, Zeiher BG, et al. Mechanism by which Liddle's syndrome mutations increase activity of a human epithelial Na+ channel. Cell 1995;83(6):969—78.

[230] Kamynina E, Debonneville C, Bens M, Vandewalle A, Staub O. A novel mouse Nedd4 protein suppresses the activity of the epithelial Na+ channel. Faseb J 2001;15(1):204—14.

[231] Samaha FF, Rubenstein RC, Yan W, Ramkumar M, Levy DI, Ahn YJ, et al. Functional polymorphism in the carboxyl terminus of the alpha-subunit of the human epithelial sodium channel. J Biol Chem 2004;279(23):23900—7.

[232] Yan W, Suaud L, Kleyman TR, Rubenstein RC. Differential modulation of a polymorphism in the carboxyl terminus of the alpha subunit of the human epithelial sodium channel by protein kinase C {delta}. Am J Physiol Renal Physiol 2005;290(2): F279—88.

[233] Shi H, Asher C, Chigaev A, Yung Y, Reuveny E, Seger R, et al. Interactions of beta and gamma ENaC with Nedd4 can be

facilitated by an ERK-mediated phosphorylation. J Biol Chem 2002;277(16):13539—47.

[234] Shi H, Asher C, Yung Y, Kligman L, Reuveny E, Seger R, et al. Casein kinase 2 specifically binds to and phosphorylates the carboxy termini of ENaC subunits. Eur J Biochem 2002;269 (18):4551—8.

[235] Diakov A, Korbmacher C. A novel pathway of epithelial sodium channel activation involves a serum- and glucocorticoid-inducible kinase consensus motif in the C terminus of the channel's alpha-subunit. J Biol Chem 2004;279(37):38134—42.

[236] Dinudom A, Fotia AB, Lefkowitz RJ, Young JA, Kumar S, Cook DI. The kinase Grk2 regulates Nedd4/Nedd4-2-dependent control of epithelial Na$^+$ channels. Proc Natl Acad Sci USA 2004;101(32):11886—90.

[237] Bachhuber T, Almaca J, Aldehni F, Mehta A, Amaral MD, Schreiber R, et al. Regulation of the epithelial Na$^+$ channel by the protein kinase CK2. J Biol Chem 2008;283(19):13225—32.

[238] Shimkets RA, Lifton R, Canessa CM. *In vivo* phosphorylation of the epithelial sodium channel. Proc Natl Acad Sci USA 1998;95(6):3301—5.

[239] Volk KA, Snyder PM, Stokes JB. Regulation of epithelial sodium channel activity through a region of the carboxyl terminus of the alpha-subunit. Evidence for intracellular kinase-mediated reactions. J Biol Chem 2001;276(47):43887—93.

[240] Palmer LG. Epithelial Na channels: the nature of the conducting pore. Ren Physiol Biochem 1990;13(1—2):51—8.

[241] Kellenberger S, Schild L. Epithelial sodium channel/degenerin family of ion channels: a variety of functions for a shared structure. Physiol Rev 2002;82(3):735—67.

[242] Benos DJ, Mandel LJ, Simon SA. Cationic selectivity and competition at the sodium entry site in frog skin. J Gen Physiol 1980;76(2):233—47.

[243] Palmer LG. Ion selectivity of the apical membrane Na channel in the toad urinary bladder. J Membr Biol 1982;67(2):91—8.

[244] Eisenman G. Cation selective glass electrodes and their mode of operation. Biophys J 1962;2((2)Pt 2):259—323.

[245] Payandeh J, Scheuer T, Zheng N, Catterall WA. The crystal structure of a voltage-gated sodium channel. Nature 2011;475 (7356):353—8.

[246] Khakh BS, Lester HA. Dynamic selectivity filters in ion channels. Neuron 1999;23(4):653—8.

[247] Roux B. Ion conduction and selectivity in K$^{(+)}$ channels. Annu Rev Biophys Biomol Struct 2005;34:153—71.

[248] Berneche S, Roux B. A gate in the selectivity filter of potassium channels. Structure (Camb) 2005;13(4):591—600.

[249] Cuello LG, Jogini V, Cortes DM, Pan AC, Gagnon DG, Dalmas O, et al. Structural basis for the coupling between activation and inactivation gates in K$^{(+)}$ channels. Nature 2010;466 (7303):272—5.

[250] Cuello LG, Jogini V, Cortes DM, Perozo E. Structural mechanism of C-type inactivation in K$^{(+)}$ channels. Nature 2010;466 (7303):203—8.

[251] Chalfant ML, Peterson-Yantorno K, O'Brien TG, Civan MM. Regulation of epithelial Na$^+$ channels from M-1 cortical collecting duct cells. Am J Physiol 1996;271(4 Pt 2):F861—70.

[252] Garty H, Palmer LG. Epithelial sodium channels: function, structure, and regulation. Physiol Rev 1997;77(2):359—96.

[253] Fyfe GK, Canessa CM. Subunit composition determines the single channel kinetics of the epithelial sodium channel. J Gen Physiol 1998;112(4):423—32.

[254] Horisberger JD, Chraibi A. Epithelial sodium channel: a ligand-gated channel? Nephron Physiol 2004;96(2):p37—41.

[255] Kelly O, Lin C, Ramkumar M, Saxena NC, Kleyman TR, Eaton DC. Characterization of an amiloride binding region in the alpha-subunit of ENaC. Am J Physiol Renal Physiol 2003;285 (6):F1279—90.

[256] Ji HL, Fuller CM, Benos DJ. Intrinsic gating mechanisms of epithelial sodium channels. Am J Physiol Cell Physiol 2002;283(2): C646—50.

[257] Liu J, Siegelbaum SA. Change of pore helix conformational state upon opening of cyclic nucleotide-gated channels. Neuron 2000;28(3):899—909.

[258] Alagem N, Yesylevskyy S, Reuveny E. The pore helix is involved in stabilizing the open state of inwardly rectifying K$^+$ channels. Biophys J 2003;85(1):300—12.

[259] Seebohm G, Westenskow P, Lang F, Sanguinetti MC. Mutation of colocalized residues of the pore helix and transmembrane segments S5 and S6 disrupt deactivation and modify inactivation of KCNQ1 K$^+$ channels. J Physiol 2005; 563(Pt 2):359—68.

[260] Yeh BI, Kim YK, Jabbar W, Huang CL. Conformational changes of pore helix coupled to gating of TRPV5 by protons. Embo J 2005;24(18):3224—34.

[261] Tolino LA, Okumura S, Kashlan OB, Carattino MD. Insights into the mechanism of pore opening of acid-sensing ion channel 1a. J Biol Chem 2011;286(18):16297—307.

[262] Hodgkin AL, Huxley AF. A quantitative description of membrane current and its application to conduction and excitability in nerve. Journal of Physiology 1952;117:500—44.

[263] Zheng J, Sigworth FJ. Selectivity changes during activation of mutant Shaker potassium channels. J Gen Physiol 1997;110 (2):101—17.

[264] Zhang ZR, McDonough SI, McCarty NA. Interaction between permeation and gating in a putative pore domain mutant in the cystic fibrosis transmembrane conductance regulator. Biophys J 2000;79(1):298—313.

[265] Swenson Jr. RP, Armstrong CM. K.$^+$ channels close more slowly in the presence of external K$^+$ and Rb$^+$. Nature 1981;291(5814):427—9.

[266] Demo SD, Yellen G. Ion effects on gating of the Ca$^{(2+)}$-activated K$^+$ channel correlate with occupancy of the pore. Biophys J 1992;61(3):639—48.

[267] Lu T, Ting AY, Mainland J, Jan LY, Schultz PG, Yang J. Probing ion permeation and gating in a K$^+$ channel with backbone mutations in the selectivity filter. Nat Neurosci 2001;4 (3):239—46.

[268] Zhou Y, Morais-Cabral JH, Kaufman A, MacKinnon R. Chemistry of ion coordination and hydration revealed by a K$^+$ channel-Fab complex at 2.0 Å resolution. Nature 2001;414 (6859):43—8.

[269] Domene C, Grottesi A, Sansom MS. Filter flexibility and distortion in a bacterial inward rectifier K$^+$ channel: simulation studies of KirBac1.1. Biophys J 2004;87(1):256—67.

[270] Domene C, Sansom MS. Potassium channel, ions, and water: simulation studies based on the high resolution X-ray structure of KcsA. Biophys J 2003;85(5):2787—800.

[271] Matulef K, Zagotta WN. Cyclic nucleotide-gated ion channels. Annu Rev Cell Dev Biol 2003;19:23—44.

[272] Xiao J, Zhen XG, Yang J. Localization of PIP2 activation gate in inward rectifier K$^+$ channels. Nat Neurosci 2003;6(8):811—8.

[273] Proks P, Antcliff JF, Ashcroft FM. The ligand-sensitive gate of a potassium channel lies close to the selectivity filter. EMBO Rep 2003;4(1):70—5.

[274] Matalon S, Lazrak A, Jain L, Eaton DC. Invited review: Biophysical properties of sodium channels in lung alveolar epithelial cells. J Appl Physiol 2002;93(5):1852—9.

[275] Donaldson SH, Boucher RC. Sodium channels and cystic fibrosis. Chest 2007;132(5):1631—6.

[276] Eaton DC, Helms MN, Koval M, Bao HF, Jain L. The contribution of epithelial sodium channels to alveolar function in health and disease. Annu Rev Physiol 2009;71:403—23.

[277] Shimkets RA, Warnock DG, Bositis CM, Nelson-Williams C, Hansson JH, Schambelan M, et al. Liddle's syndrome: heritable human hypertension caused by mutations in the beta subunit of the epithelial sodium channel. Cell 1994;79 (3):407—14.

[278] Warnock DG. Liddle syndrome: genetics and mechanisms of Na⁺ channel defects. Am J Med Sci 2001;322(6):302—7.

[279] Tamura H, Schild L, Enomoto N, Matsui N, Marumo F, Rossier BC. Liddle disease caused by a missense mutation of beta subunit of the epithelial sodium channel gene. J Clin Invest 1996;97(7):1780—4.

[280] Hansson JH, Schild L, Lu Y, Wilson TA, Gautschi I, Shimkets R, et al. A de novo missense mutation of the beta subunit of the epithelial sodium channel causes hypertension and Liddle syndrome, identifying a proline-rich segment critical for regulation of channel activity. Proc Natl Acad Sci USA 1995;92 (25):11495—9.

[281] Hansson JH, Nelson-Williams C, Suzuki H, Schild L, Shimkets R, Lu Y, et al. Hypertension caused by a truncated epithelial sodium channel gamma subunit: Genetic heterogeneity of Liddle syndrome. Nat Genet 1995;11(1):76—82.

[282] Staub O, Dho S, Henry P, Correa J, Ishikawa T, McGlade J, et al. WW domains of Nedd4 bind to the proline-rich PY motifs in the epithelial Na⁺ channel deleted in Liddle's syndrome. Embo J 1996;15(10):2371—80.

[283] Staub O, Abriel H, Plant P, Ishikawa T, Kanelis V, Saleki R, et al. Regulation of the epithelial Na⁺ channel by Nedd4 and ubiquitination. Kidney Int 2000;57(3):809—15.

[284] Snyder PM, Olson DR, McDonald FJ, Bucher DB. Multiple WW domains, but not the C2 domain, are required for inhibition of the epithelial Na⁺ channel by human Nedd4. J Biol Chem 2001;276(30):28321—6.

[285] Itani OA, Campbell JR, Herrero J, Snyder PM, Thomas CP. Alternate promoters and variable splicing lead to hNedd4-2 isoforms with a C2 domain and varying number of WW domains. Am J Physiol Renal Physiol 2003;285(5):F916—29.

[286] Itani OA, Stokes JB, Thomas CP. Nedd4-2 isoforms differentially associate with ENaC and regulate its activity. Am J Physiol Renal Physiol 2005;289(2):F334—46.

[287] Plant PJ, Yeger H, Staub O, Howard P, Rotin D. The C2 domain of the ubiquitin protein ligase Nedd4 mediates Ca²⁺-dependent plasma membrane localization. J Biol Chem 1997;272(51):32329—36.

[288] Plant PJ, Lafont F, Lecat S, Verkade P, Simons K, Rotin D. Apical membrane targeting of Nedd4 is mediated by an association of its C2 domain with annexin XIIIb. J Cell Biol 2000;149 (7):1473—84.

[289] Fotia AB, Dinudom A, Shearwin KE, Koch JP, Korbmacher C, Cook DI, et al. The role of individual Nedd4-2 (KIAA0439) WW domains in binding and regulating epithelial sodium channels. Faseb J 2003;17(1):70—2.

[290] Lott JS, Coddington-Lawson SJ, Teesdale-Spittle PH, McDonald FJ. A single WW domain is the predominant mediator of the interaction between the human ubiquitin-protein ligase Nedd4 and the human epithelial sodium channel. Biochem J 2002;361(Pt 3):481—8.

[291] Kamynina E, Staub O. Concerted action of ENaC, Nedd4-2, and Sgk1 in transepithelial Na⁺ transport. Am J Physiol Renal Physiol 2002;283(3):F377—87.

[292] Lu C, Pribanic S, Debonneville A, Jiang C, Rotin D. The PY motif of ENaC, mutated in Liddle syndrome, regulates channel internalization, sorting and mobilization from subapical pool. Traffic 2007;8(9):1246—64.

[293] Lee IH, Campbell CR, Song SH, Day ML, Kumar S, Cook DI, et al. The activity of the epithelial sodium channels is regulated by caveolin-1 via a Nedd4-2-dependent mechanism. J Biol Chem 2009;284(19):12663—9.

[294] McCormick JA, Bhalla V, Pao AC, Pearce D. SGK1: a rapid aldosterone-induced regulator of renal sodium reabsorption. Physiology (Bethesda) 2005;20:134—9.

[295] Snyder PM. The epithelial Na⁺ channel: cell surface insertion and retrieval in Na⁺ homeostasis and hypertension. Endocr Rev 2002;23(2):258—75.

[296] Snyder PM. Regulation of epithelial Na⁺ channel trafficking. Endocrinology 2005;146(12):5079—85.

[297] Snyder PM, Olson DR, Kabra R, Zhou R, Steines JC. cAMP and serum and glucocorticoid-inducible kinase (SGK) regulate the epithelial Na(⁺) channel through convergent phosphorylation of Nedd4-2. J Biol Chem 2004;279(44):45753—8.

[298] Bhalla V, Daidie D, Li H, Pao AC, LaGrange LP, Wang J, et al. Serum- and glucocorticoid-regulated kinase 1 regulates ubiquitin ligase neural precursor cell-expressed, developmentally downregulated protein 4-2 by inducing interaction with 14-3-3. Mol Endocrinol 2005;19(12):3073—84.

[299] Bhalla V, Oyster NM, Fitch AC, Wijngaarden MA, Neumann D, Schlattner U, et al. AMP-activated kinase inhibits the epithelial Na⁺ channel through functional regulation of the ubiquitin ligase Nedd4-2. J Biol Chem 2006;281(36):26159—69.

[300] Edinger RS, Lebowitz J, Li H, Alzamora R, Wang H, Johnson JP, et al. Functional regulation of the epithelial Na⁺ channel by IkappaB kinase-beta occurs via phosphorylation of the ubiquitin ligase Nedd4-2. J Biol Chem 2009;284(1):150—7.

[301] Boulkroun S, Ruffieux-Daidie D, Vitagliano JJ, Poirot O, Charles RP, Lagnaz D, et al. Vasopressin-inducible ubiquitin-specific protease 10 increases ENaC cell surface expression by deubiquitylating and stabilizing sorting nexin 3. Am J Physiol Renal Physiol 2008;295(4):F889—900.

[302] Rotin D, Staub O. Role of the ubiquitin system in regulating ion transport. Pflugers Arch 2011;461(1):1—21.

[303] Becchetti A, Malik B, Yue G, Duchatelle P, Al-Khalili O, Kleyman TR, et al. Phosphatase inhibitors increase the open probability of ENaC in A6 cells. Am J Physiol Renal Physiol 2002;283(5):F1030—45.

[304] Volk KA, Husted RF, Snyder PM, Stokes JB. Kinase regulation of hENaC mediated through a region in the COOH-terminal portion of the alpha-subunit. Am J Physiol Cell Physiol 2000;278(5):C1047—54.

[305] Snyder PM, Olson DR, Thomas BC. Serum and glucocorticoid-regulated kinase modulates Nedd4-2-mediated inhibition of the epithelial Na⁺ channel. J Biol Chem 2002;277(1):5—8.

[306] Debonneville C, Flores SY, Kamynina E, Plant PJ, Tauxe C, Thomas MA, et al. Phosphorylation of Nedd4-2 by Sgk1 regulates epithelial Na(⁺) channel cell surface expression. Embo J 2001;20(24):7052—9.

[307] Flores SY, Loffing-Cueni D, Kamynina E, Daidie D, Gerbex C, Chabanel S, et al. Aldosterone-induced serum and glucocorticoid-induced kinase 1 expression is accompanied by Nedd4-2 phosphorylation and increased Na + transport in cortical collecting duct cells. J Am Soc Nephrol 2005;16(8):2279—87.

[308] Bhalla V, Daidie D, Li H, Pao AC, Lagrange LP, Wang J, et al. SGK1 regulates ubiquitin ligase Nedd4-2 by inducing interaction with 14-3-3. Mol Endocrinol 2005;19(12):3073—84.

[309] Ichimura T, Yamamura H, Sasamoto K, Tominaga Y, Taoka M, Kakiuchi K, et al. 14-3-3 proteins modulate the expression of epithelial Na⁺ channels by phosphorylation-dependent

interaction with Nedd4-2 ubiquitin ligase. J Biol Chem 2005;280(13):13187–94.

[310] Blazer-Yost BL, Esterman MA, Vlahos CJ. Insulin-stimulated trafficking of ENaC in renal cells requires PI 3-kinase activity. Am J Physiol Cell Physiol 2003;284(6):C1645–53.

[311] Snyder PM. Liddle's syndrome mutations disrupt cAMP-mediated translocation of the epithelial Na$^{(+)}$ channel to the cell surface. J Clin Invest 2000;105(1):45–53.

[312] Morris RG, Schafer JA. cAMP increases density of ENaC subunits in the apical membrane of MDCK cells in direct proportion to amiloride-sensitive Na$^{(+)}$ transport. J Gen Physiol 2002;120(1):71–85.

[313] Lebowitz J, Edinger RS, An B, Perry CJ, Onate S, Kleyman TR, et al. Ikappab kinase-beta (ikkbeta) modulation of epithelial sodium channel activity. J Biol Chem 2004;279(40):41985–90.

[314] Gilmore ES, Stutts MJ, Milgram SL. SRC family kinases mediate epithelial Na^{+} channel inhibition by endothelin. J Biol Chem 2001;276(45):42610–7.

[315] Ling BN, Eaton DC. Effects of luminal Na^{+} on single Na^{+} channels in A6 cells, a regulatory role for protein kinase C. Am J Physiol 1989;256(6 Pt 2):F1094–103.

[316] Yue G, Edinger RS, Bao HF, Johnson JP, Eaton DC. The effect of rapamycin on single ENaC channel activity and phosphorylation in A6 cells. Am J Physiol Cell Physiol 2000;279(1):C81–8.

[317] Booth RE, Stockand JD. Targeted degradation of ENaC in response to PKC activation of the ERK1/2 cascade. Am J Physiol Renal Physiol 2003;284(5):F938–47.

[318] Woollhead AM, Scott JW, Hardie DG, Baines DL. Phenformin and 5-aminoimidazole-4-carboxamide-1-beta-D-ribofuranoside (AICAR) activation of AMP-activated protein kinase inhibits transepithelial Na^{+} transport across H441 lung cells. J Physiol 2005;566(Pt 3):781–92.

[319] Zhang YH, Alvarez de la Rosa D, Canessa CM, Hayslett JP. Insulin-induced phosphorylation of ENaC correlates with increased sodium channel function in A6 cells. Am J Physiol Cell Physiol 2005;288(1):C141–7.

[320] Feldman RD. Deactivation of vasodilator responses by GRK2 overexpression: a mechanism or the mechanism for hypertension? Mol Pharmacol 2002;61(4):707–9.

[321] Sanchez-Perez A, Kumar S, Cook DI. GRK2 interacts with and phosphorylates Nedd4 and Nedd4-2. Biochem Biophys Res Commun 2007;359(3):611–5.

[322] Lee IH, Song SH, Campbell CR, Kumar S, Cook DI, Dinudom A. Regulation of the epithelial Na^{+} channel by the RH domain of G protein-coupled receptor kinase, GRK2, and Galphaq/11. J Biol Chem 2011;286(22):19259–69.

[323] Kahle KT, Wilson FH, Leng Q, Lalioti MD, O'Connell AD, Dong K, et al. WNK4 regulates the balance between renal NaCl reabsorption and K^{+} secretion. Nat Genet 2003;35(4):372–6.

[324] Furgeson SB, Linas S. Mechanisms of type I and type II pseudohypoaldosteronism. J Am Soc Nephrol 2010;21(11):1842–5.

[325] Wilson FH, Disse-Nicodeme S, Choate KA, Ishikawa K, Nelson-Williams C, Desitter I, et al. Human hypertension caused by mutations in WNK kinases. Science 2001;293 (5532):1107–12.

[326] Ring AM, Leng Q, Rinehart J, Wilson FH, Kahle KT, Hebert SC, et al. An SGK1 site in WNK4 regulates Na^{+} channel and K^{+} channel activity and has implications for aldosterone signaling and K^{+} homeostasis. Proc Natl Acad Sci USA 2007;104 (10):4025–9.

[327] Heise CJ, Xu BE, Deaton SL, Cha SK, Cheng CJ, Earnest S, et al. Serum and glucocorticoid-induced kinase (SGK) 1 and the epithelial sodium channel are regulated by multiple with

no lysine (WNK) family members. J Biol Chem 2010;285(33): 25161–7.

[328] Xu BE, Stippec S, Chu PY, Lazrak A, Li XJ, Lee BH, et al. WNK1 activates SGK1 to regulate the epithelial sodium channel. Proc Natl Acad Sci USA 2005;102(29):10315–20.

[329] Naray-Fejes-Toth A, Snyder PM, Fejes-Toth G. The kidney-specific WNK1 isoform is induced by aldosterone and stimulates epithelial sodium channel-mediated Na^{+} transport. Proc Natl Acad Sci USA 2004;101(50):17434–9.

[330] Xu BE, Stippec S, Lazrak A, Huang CL, Cobb MH. WNK1 activates SGK1 by a PI-3 kinase-dependent and non-catalytic mechanism. J Biol Chem 2005;280(40):34218–23.

[331] Snyder PM. Downregulating destruction: Phosphorylation regulates the E3 ubiquitin ligase Nedd4-2. Sci Signal 2009;2(79): pe41.

[332] Lee IH, Dinudom A, Sanchez-Perez A, Kumar S, Cook DI. Akt mediates the effect of insulin on epithelial sodium channels by inhibiting Nedd4-2. J Biol Chem 2007;282(41):29866–73.

[333] Hallows KR, Bhalla V, Oyster NM, Wijngaarden MA, Lee JK, Li H, et al. Phosphopeptide screen uncovers novel phosphorylation sites of Nedd4-2 that potentiate its inhibition of the epithelial Na^{+} channel. J Biol Chem 2010;285(28):21671–8.

[334] Orce GG, Castillo GA, Margolius HS. Inhibition of short-circuit current in toad urinary bladder by inhibitors of glandular kallikrein. Am J Physiol 1980;239(5):F459–65.

[335] Vuagniaux G, Vallet V, Jaeger NF, Hummler E, Rossier BC. Synergistic activation of ENaC by three membrane-bound channel-activating serine proteases (mCAP1, mCAP2, and mCAP3) and serum- and glucocorticoid-regulated kinase (Sgk1) in Xenopus oocytes. J Gen Physiol 2002;120(2):191–201.

[336] Picard N, Eladari D, El Moghrabi S, Planes C, Bourgeois S, Houillier P, et al. Defective ENaC processing and function in tissue kallikrein-deficient mice. J Biol Chem 2008;283(8): 4602–11.

[337] Harris M, Firsov D, Vuagniaux G, Stutts MJ, Rossier BC. A novel neutrophil elastase inhibitor prevents elastase activation and surface cleavage of the epithelial sodium channel expressed in Xenopus laevis oocytes. J Biol Chem 2007;282(1): 58–64.

[338] Svenningsen P, Bistrup C, Friis UG, Bertog M, Haerteis S, Krueger B, et al. Plasmin in nephrotic urine activates the epithelial sodium channel. J Am Soc Nephrol 2009;20(2):299–310.

[339] Passero CJ, Mueller GM, Rondon-Berrios H, Tofovic SP, Hughey RP, Kleyman TR. Plasmin activates epithelial Na^{+} channels by cleaving the gamma subunit. J Biol Chem 2008;283 (52):36586–91.

[340] Thomas G. Furin at the cutting edge: from protein traffic to embryogenesis and disease. Nat Rev Mol Cell Biol 2002;3 (10):753–66.

[341] Passero CJ, Mueller GM, Myerburg MM, Carattino MD, Hughey RP, Kleyman TR. TMPRSS4-dependent activation of the epithelial sodium channel requires cleavage of the gamma subunit distal to the furin cleavage site. Am J Physiol Renal Physiol 2011;302(1):F1–8.

[342] Passero CJ, Carattino MD, Kashlan OB, Myerburg MM, Hughey RP, Kleyman TR. Defining an inhibitory domain in the gamma subunit of the epithelial sodium channel. Am J Physiol Renal Physiol 2010;299(4):F854–61.

[343] Carattino MD, Hughey RP, Kleyman TR. Proteolytic processing of the epithelial sodium channel gamma subunit has a dominant role in channel activation. J Biol Chem 2008;283 (37):25290–5.

[344] Nielsen J, Kwon TH, Masilamani S, Beutler K, Hager H, Nielsen S, et al. Sodium transporter abundance profiling in

III. FLUID AND ELECTROLYTE REGULATION AND DYSREGULATION

kidney: effect of spironolactone. Am J Physiol Renal Physiol 2002;283(5):F923–33.

[345] Frindt G, Masilamani S, Knepper MA, Palmer LG. Activation of epithelial Na channels during short-term Na deprivation. Am J Physiol Renal Physiol 2001;280(1):F112–8.

[346] Frindt G, Ergonul Z, Palmer LG. Surface expression of epithelial Na channel protein in rat kidney. J Gen Physiol 2008;131 (6):617–27.

[347] Frindt G, Palmer LG. Surface expression of sodium channels and transporters in rat kidney: effects of dietary sodium. Am J Physiol Renal Physiol 2009;297(5):F1249–55.

[348] Gerst JE. SNAREs and SNARE regulators in membrane fusion and exocytosis. Cell Mol Life Sci 1999;55(5):707–34.

[349] Sollner TH. Regulated exocytosis and SNARE function (Review). Mol Membr Biol 2003;20(3):209–20.

[350] Qi J, Peters KW, Liu C, Wang JM, Edinger RS, Johnson JP, et al. Regulation of the amiloride-sensitive epithelial sodium channel by syntaxin 1A. J Biol Chem 1999;274(43):30345–8.

[351] Saxena SK, Singh M, Kaur S, George C. Distinct domain-dependent effect of syntaxin1A on amiloride-sensitive sodium channel (ENaC) currents in HT-29 colonic epithelial cells. Int J Biol Sci 2007;3(1):47–56.

[352] Mall M, Bleich M, Greger R, Schreiber R, Kunzelmann K. The amiloride-inhibitable Na$^+$ conductance is reduced by the cystic fibrosis transmembrane conductance regulator in normal but not in cystic fibrosis airways. J Clin Invest 1998;102(1):15–21.

[353] Kimura T, Kawabe H, Jiang C, Zhang W, Xiang YY, Lu C, et al. Deletion of the ubiquitin ligase Nedd4L in lung epithelia causes cystic fibrosis-like disease. Proc Natl Acad Sci USA 2011;108(8):3216–21.

[354] Dalemans W, Barbry P, Champigny G, Jallat S, Dott K, Dreyer D, et al. Altered chloride ion channel kinetics associated with the delta F508 cystic fibrosis mutation. Nature 1991;354(6354):526–8.

[355] Stutts MJ, Canessa CM, Olsen JC, Hamrick M, Cohn JA, Rossier BC, et al. CFTR as a cAMP-dependent regulator of sodium channels. Science 1995;269(5225):847–50.

[356] Stutts MJ, Rossier BC, Boucher RC. Cystic fibrosis transmembrane conductance regulator inverts protein kinase A-mediated regulation of epithelial sodium channel single channel kinetics. J Biol Chem 1997;272(22):14037–40.

[357] Ling BN, Zuckerman JB, Lin C, Harte BJ, McNulty KA, Smith PR, et al. Expression of the cystic fibrosis phenotype in a renal amphibian epithelial cell line. J Biol Chem 1997;272(1): 594–600.

[358] Chabot H, Vives MF, Dagenais A, Grygorczyk C, Berthiaume Y, Grygorczyk R. Downregulation of epithelial sodium channel (ENaC) by CFTR co-expressed in Xenopus oocytes is independent of Cl$^-$ conductance. J Membr Biol 1999;169(3):175–88.

[359] Konstas AA, Koch JP, Korbmacher C. cAMP-dependent activation of CFTR inhibits the epithelial sodium channel (ENaC) without affecting its surface expression. Pflugers Arch 2003; 445(4):513–21.

[360] Horisberger JD. ENaC-CFTR interactions: the role of electrical coupling of ion fluxes explored in an epithelial cell model. Pflugers Arch 2003;445(4):522–8.

[361] Nagel G, Barbry P, Chabot H, Brochiero E, Hartung K, Grygorczyk R. CFTR fails to inhibit the epithelial sodium channel ENaC, when expressed in Xenopus laevis oocytes. J Physiol 2005;564(Pt 3):671–82.

[362] Itani OA, Chen JH, Karp PH, Ernst S, Keshavjee S, Parekh K, et al. Human cystic fibrosis airway epithelia have reduced Cl$^-$ conductance but not increased Na$^+$ conductance. Proc Nat Acad Sci USA 2011;108(25):10260–5.

[363] Chen JH, Stoltz DA, Karp PH, Ernst SE, Pezzulo AA, Moninger TO, et al. Loss of anion transport without increased sodium absorption characterizes newborn porcine cystic fibrosis airway epithelia. Cell 2010;143(6):911–23.

[364] Jiang Q, Li J, Dubroff R, Ahn YJ, Foskett JK, Engelhardt J, et al. Epithelial sodium channels regulate cystic fibrosis transmembrane conductance regulator chloride channels in Xenopus oocytes. J Biol Chem 2000;275(18):13266–74.

[365] Bachhuber T, Konig J, Voelcker T, Murle B, Schreiber R, Kunzelmann K. Cl$^-$ interference with the epithelial Na$^+$ channel ENaC. J Biol Chem 2005;280(36):31587–94.

[366] Schreiber R, Hopf A, Mall M, Greger R, Kunzelmann K. The first-nucleotide binding domain of the cystic-fibrosis transmembrane conductance regulator is important for inhibition of the epithelial Na$^+$ channel. Proc Natl Acad Sci USA 1999;96 (9):5310–5.

[367] Reddy MM, Quinton PM. Functional interaction of CFTR and ENaC in sweat glands. Pflugers Arch 2003;445(4):499–503.

[368] Gentzsch M, Dang H, Dang Y, Garcia-Caballero A, Suchindran H, Boucher RC, et al. The cystic fibrosis transmembrane conductance regulator impedes proteolytic stimulation of the epithelial Na$^+$ channel. J Biol Chem 2010;285(42):32227–32.

[369] Rubenstein RC, Lockwood SR, Lide E, Bauer R, Suaud L, Grumbach Y. Regulation of endogenous ENaC functional expression by CFTR and DeltaF508-CFTR in airway epithelial cells. Am J Physiol Lung Cell Mol Physiol 2011;300(1): L88–101.

[370] Huang P, Gilmore E, Kultgen P, Barnes P, Milgram S, Stutts MJ. Local regulation of cystic fibrosis transmembrane regulator and epithelial sodium channel in airway epithelium. Proc Am Thorac Soc 2004;1(1):33–7.

[371] Sariban-Sohraby S, Burg M, Wiesmann WP, Chiang PK, Johnson JP. Methylation increases sodium transport into A6 apical membrane vesicles: possible mode of aldosterone action. Science 1984;225(4663):745–6.

[372] Stockand JD, Edinger RS, Eaton DC, Johnson JP. Toward understanding the role of methylation in aldosterone-sensitive Na$^{(+)}$ transport. News Physiol Sci 2000;15:161–5.

[373] Wiesmann WP, Johnson JP, Miura GA, Chaing PK. Aldosterone-stimulated transmethylations are linked to sodium transport. Am J Physiol 1985;248(1 Pt 2):F43–7.

[374] Stockand JD, Edinger RS, Al-Baldawi N, Sariban-Sohraby S, Al-Khalili O, Eaton DC, et al. Isoprenylcysteine-O-carboxyl methyltransferase regulates aldosterone-sensitive Na$^{(+)}$ reabsorption. J Biol Chem 1999;274(38):26912–6.

[375] Stockand JD, Spier BJ, Worrell RT, Yue G, Al-Baldawi N, Eaton DC. Regulation of Na$^{(+)}$ reabsorption by the aldosterone-induced small G protein K-Ras2A. J Biol Chem 1999;274(50): 35449–54.

[376] Rokaw MD, Wang JM, Edinger RS, Weisz OA, Hui D, Middleton P, et al. Carboxylmethylation of the beta subunit of xENaC regulates channel activity. J Biol Chem 1998;273 (44):28746–51.

[377] Edinger RS, Yospin J, Perry C, Kleyman TR, Johnson JP. Regulation of epithelial Na$^+$ channels (ENaC) by methylation: a novel methyltransferase stimulates ENaC activity. J Biol Chem 2006;281(14):9110–7.

[378] Zhang W, Hayashizaki Y, Kone BC. Structure and regulation of the mDot1 gene, a mouse histone H3 methyltransferase. Biochem J 2004;377(Pt 3):641–51.

[379] Zhang W, Xia X, Jalal DI, Kuncewicz T, Xu W, Lesage GD, et al. Aldosterone-sensitive repression of ENaCalpha transcription by a histone H3 lysine-79 methyltransferase. Am J Physiol Cell Physiol 2006;290(3):C936–46.

[380] Zhang W, Xia X, Reisenauer MR, Hemenway CS, Kone BC. Dot1a-AF9 complex mediates histone H3 Lys-79 hypermethylation and repression of ENaCalpha in an aldosterone-sensitive manner. J Biol Chem 2006;281(26):18059−68.

[381] Zhang W, Xia X, Reisenauer MR, Rieg T, Lang F, Kuhl D, et al. Aldosterone-induced Sgk1 relieves Dot1a-Af9-mediated transcriptional repression of epithelial Na$^+$ channel alpha. J Clin Invest 2007;117(3):773−83.

[382] Reisenauer MR, Wang SW, Xia Y, Zhang W. Dot1a contains three nuclear localization signals and regulates the epithelial Na$^+$ channel (ENaC) at multiple levels. Am J Physiol Renal Physiol 2010;299(1):F63−76.

[383] Palmer LG, Frindt G. Effects of cell Ca and pH on Na channels from rat cortical collecting tubule. Am J Physiol 1987;253(2 Pt 2):F333−9.

[384] Garty H, Asher C, Yeger O. Direct inhibition of epithelial Na$^+$ channels by a pH-dependent interaction with calcium, and by other divalent ions. J Membr Biol 1987;95(2):151−62.

[385] Ishikawa T, Marunaka Y, Rotin D. Electrophysiological characterization of the rat epithelial Na$^+$ channel (rENaC) expressed in MDCK cells. Effects of Na$^+$ and Ca^{2+}. J Gen Physiol 1998;111(6):825−46.

[386] Harvey BJ, Thomas SR, Ehrenfeld J. Intracellular pH controls cell membrane Na$^+$ and K$^+$ conductances and transport in frog skin epithelium. J Gen Physiol 1988;92(6):767−91.

[387] Chalfant ML, Denton JS, Berdiev BK, Ismailov II, Benos DJ, Stanton BA. Intracellular H$^+$ regulates the alpha-subunit of ENaC, the epithelial Na$^+$ channel. Am J Physiol 1999;276(2 Pt 1):C477−86.

[388] Ishikawa T, Jiang C, Stutts MJ, Marunaka Y, Rotin D. Regulation of the epithelial Na$^+$ channel by cytosolic ATP. J Biol Chem 2003;278(40):38276−86.

[389] Xu H, Chu S. ENaC alpha-subunit variants are expressed in lung epithelial cells and are suppressed by oxidative stress. Am J Physiol Lung Cell Mol Physiol 2007;293(6):L1454−62.

[390] Ma HP. Hydrogen peroxide stimulates the epithelial sodium channel through a phosphatidylinositide 3-kinase-dependent pathway. J Biol Chem 2011;286(37):32444−53.

[391] Takemura Y, Goodson P, Bao HF, Jain L, Helms MN. Rac1-mediated NADPH oxidase release of O$_2^-$ regulates epithelial sodium channel activity in the alveolar epithelium. Am J Physiol Lung Cell Mol Physiol 2010;298(4):L509−20.

[392] Jain L, Chen XJ, Brown LA, Eaton DC. Nitric oxide inhibits lung sodium transport through a cGMP-mediated inhibition of epithelial cation channels. Am J Physiol 1998;274(4 Pt 1):L475−84.

[393] Ding JW, Dickie J, O'Brodovich H, Shintani Y, Rafii B, Hackam D, et al. Inhibition of amiloride-sensitive sodium-channel activity in distal lung epithelial cells by nitric oxide. Am J Physiol 1998;274(3 Pt 1):L378−87.

[394] Hardiman KM, McNicholas-Bevensee CM, Fortenberry J, Myles CT, Malik B, Eaton DC, et al. Regulation of amiloride-sensitive Na$^+$ transport by basal nitric oxide. Am J Respir Cell Mol Biol 2004;30(5):720−8.

[395] Helms MN, Yu L, Malik B, Kleinhenz DJ, Hart CM, Eaton DC. Role of SGK1 in nitric oxide inhibition of ENaC in Na$^+$-transporting epithelia. Am J Physiol Cell Physiol 2005;289(3):C717−26.

[396] Helms MN, Jain L, Self JL, Eaton DC. Redox regulation of epithelial sodium channels examined in alveolar type 1 and 2 cells patch-clamped in lung slice tissue. J Biol Chem 2008;283(33):22875−83.

[397] Worrell RT, Bao HF, Denson DD, Eaton DC. Contrasting effects of cPLA2 on epithelial Na$^+$ transport. Am J Physiol Cell Physiol 2001;281(1):C147−56.

[398] Wei Y, Lin DH, Kemp R, Yaddanapudi GS, Nasjletti A, Falck JR, et al. Arachidonic acid inhibits epithelial Na channel via cytochrome P450 (CYP) epoxygenase-dependent metabolic pathways. J Gen Physiol 2004;124(6):719−27.

[399] Pavlov TS, Ilatovskaya DV, Levchenko V, Mattson DL, Roman RJ, Staruschenko A. Effects of cytochrome P-450 metabolites of arachidonic acid on the epithelial sodium channel (ENaC). Am J Physiol Renal Physiol 2011;301(3):F672−81.

[400] Padron D, Wang YJ, Yamamoto M, Yin H, Roth MG. Phosphatidylinositol phosphate 5-kinase Ibeta recruits AP-2 to the plasma membrane and regulates rates of constitutive endocytosis. J Cell Biol 2003;162(4):693−701.

[401] Hilgemann DW, Feng S, Nasuhoglu C. The complex and intriguing lives of PIP2 with ion channels and transporters. Sci STKE 2001;2001(111):RE19.

[402] Staruschenko A, Nichols A, Medina JL, Camacho P, Zheleznova NN, Stockand JD. Rho small GTPases activate the epithelial Na$^{(+)}$ channel. J Biol Chem 2004;279(48):49989−94.

[403] Weixel KM, Edinger RS, Kester L, Guerriero CJ, Wang H, Fang L, et al. Phosphatidylinositol 4-phosphate 5-kinase reduces cell surface expression of the epithelial sodium channel (ENaC) in cultured collecting duct cells. J Biol Chem 2007;282(50):36534−42.

[404] Butterworth MB, Edinger RS, Frizzell RA, Johnson JP. Regulation of the epithelial sodium channel by membrane trafficking. Am J Physiol Renal Physiol 2009;296(1):F10−24.

[405] Van Driessche W, Zeiske W. Ionic channels in epithelial cell membranes. Physiol Rev 1985;65(4):833−903.

[406] Awayda MS. Regulation of the epithelial Na$^{(+)}$ channel by intracellular Na$^{(+)}$. Am J Physiol 1999;277(2 Pt 1):C216−24.

[407] Frindt G, Palmer LG, Windhager EE. Feedback regulation of Na channels in rat CCT. IV. Mediation by activation of protein kinase C. Am J Physiol 1996;270(2 Pt 2):F371−6.

[408] Kellenberger S, Gautschi I, Rossier BC, Schild L. Mutations causing Liddle syndrome reduce sodium-dependent downregulation of the epithelial sodium channel in the *Xenopus* oocyte expression system. J Clin Invest 1998;101(12):2741−50.

[409] Harvey KF, Dinudom A, Cook DI, Kumar S. The Nedd4-like protein KIAA0439 is a potential regulator of the epithelial sodium channel. J Biol Chem 2001;276(11):8597−601.

[410] Harvey KF, Dinudom A, Komwatana P, Jolliffe CN, Day ML, Parasivam G, et al. All three WW domains of murine Nedd4 are involved in the regulation of epithelial sodium channels by intracellular Na. J Biol Chem 1999;274(18):12525−30.

[411] Bengrine A, Li J, Awayda MS. The A-kinase anchoring protein 15 regulates feedback inhibition of the epithelial Na$^+$ channel. FASEB J 2007;21(4):1189−201.

[412] Knight KK, Wentzlaff DM, Snyder PM. Intracellular sodium regulates proteolytic activation of the epithelial sodium channel. J Biol Chem 2008;283(41):27477−82.

[413] Fuchs W, Larsen EH, Lindemann B. Current−voltage curve of sodium channels and concentration dependence of sodium permeability in frog skin. J Physiol 1977;267(1):137−66.

[414] Chraibi A, Horisberger JD. Dual effect of temperature on the human epithelial Na$^+$ channel. Pflugers Arch 2003;447(3):316−20.

[415] Yki-Jarvinen H. Thiazolidinediones. N Engl J Med 2004;351(11):1106−18.

[416] Guan Y, Zhang Y, Davis L, Breyer MD. Expression of peroxisome proliferator-activated receptors in urinary tract of rabbits and humans. Am J Physiol 1997;273(6 Pt 2):F1013−22.

[417] Guan Y, Hao C, Cha DR, Rao R, Lu W, Kohan DE, et al. Thiazolidinediones expand body fluid volume through PPARgamma stimulation of ENaC-mediated renal salt absorption. Nat Med 2005;11(8):861−6.

III. FLUID AND ELECTROLYTE REGULATION AND DYSREGULATION

[418] Artunc F, Sandulache D, Nasir O, Boini KM, Friedrich B, Beier N, et al. Lack of the serum and glucocorticoid-inducible kinase SGK1 attenuates the volume retention after treatment with the PPARgamma agonist pioglitazone. Pflugers Arch 2008;456 (2):425–36.

[419] Renauld S, Tremblay K, Ait-Benichou S, Simoneau-Roy M, Garneau H, Staub O, et al. Stimulation of ENaC activity by rosiglitazone is PPARgamma-dependent and correlates with SGK1 expression increase. J Membr Biol 2010;236(3):259–70.

[420] Nofziger C, Chen L, Shane MA, Smith CD, Brown KK, Blazer-Yost BL. PPARgamma agonists do not directly enhance basal or insulin-stimulated Na$^{(+)}$ transport via the epithelial Na$^{(+)}$ channel. Pflugers Arch 2005;451(3):445–53.

[421] Borsting E, Cheng VP, Glass CK, Vallon V, Cunard R. Peroxisome proliferator-activated receptor gamma agonists repress epithelial sodium channel expression in the kidney. Am J Physiol Renal Physiol 2012;302(5):F540–51.

[422] Pochynyuk O, Bugaj V, Vandewalle A, Stockand JD. Purinergic control of apical plasma membrane PI(4,5)P2 levels sets ENaC activity in principal cells. Am J Physiol Renal Physiol 2008;294(1):F38–46.

[423] Ma HP, Chou CF, Wei SP, Eaton DC. Regulation of the epithelial sodium channel by phosphatidylinositides: experiments, implications, and speculations. Pflugers Arch 2007;455(1): 169–80.

[424] Pochynyuk O, Rieg T, Bugaj V, Schroth J, Fridman A, Boss GR, et al. Dietary Na$^+$ inhibits the open probability of the epithelial sodium channel in the kidney by enhancing apical P2Y2-receptor tone. FASEB J 2010;24(6):2056–65.

[425] Stockand JD, Mironova E, Bugaj V, Rieg T, Insel PA, Vallon V, et al. Purinergic inhibition of ENaC produces aldosterone escape. J Am Soc Nephrol 2010;21(11):1903–11.

[426] Mironova E, Peti-Peterdi J, Bugaj V, Stockand JD. Diminished paracrine regulation of the epithelial Na$^+$ channel by purinergic signaling in mice lacking connexin 30. J Biol Chem 2011;286 (2):1054–60.

[427] Zhou ZH, Bubien JK. Nongenomic regulation of ENaC by aldosterone. Am J Physiol Cell Physiol 2001;281(4):C1118–30.

[428] Stockand JD, Zeltwanger S, Bao HF, Becchetti A, Worrell RT, Eaton DC. S-adenosyl-L-homocysteine hydrolase is necessary for aldosterone-induced activity of epithelial Na$^{(+)}$ channels. Am J Physiol Cell Physiol 2001;281(3):C773–85.

[429] Thomas SV, Kathpalia PP, Rajagopal M, Charlton C, Zhang J, Eaton DC, et al. Epithelial sodium channel regulation by cell surface-associated serum- and glucocorticoid-regulated kinase 1. J Biol Chem 2011;286(37):32074–85.

[430] Soundararajan R, Melters D, Shih IC, Wang J, Pearce D. Epithelial sodium channel regulated by differential composition of a signaling complex. Proc Natl Acad Sci USA 2009;106 (19):7804–9.

[431] Soundararajan R, Wang J, Melters D, Pearce D. Glucocorticoid-induced Leucine zipper 1 stimulates the epithelial sodium channel by regulating serum- and glucocorticoid-induced kinase 1 stability and subcellular localization. J Biol Chem 2010;285(51):39905–13.

[432] Soundararajan R, Zhang TT, Wang J, Vandewalle A, Pearce D. A novel role for glucocorticoid-induced leucine zipper protein in epithelial sodium channel-mediated sodium transport. J Biol Chem 2005;280(48):39970–81.

[433] Soundararajan R, Pearce D, Hughey RP, Kleyman TR. Role of epithelial sodium channels and their regulators in hypertension. J Biol Chem 2010;285(40):30363–9.

[434] Asher C, Wald H, Rossier BC, Garty H. Aldosterone-induced increase in the abundance of Na$^+$ channel subunits. Am J Physiol 1996;271(2 Pt 1):C605–11.

[435] Weisz OA, Johnson JP. Noncoordinate regulation of ENaC: Paradigm lost? Am J Physiol Renal Physiol 2003;285(5): F833–42.

[436] Auberson M, Hoffmann-Pochon N, Vandewalle A, Kellenberger S, Schild L. Epithelial Na$^+$ channel mutants causing Liddle's syndrome retain ability to respond to aldosterone and vasopressin. Am J Physiol Renal Physiol 2003;285(3): F459–71.

[437] Benos DJ, Awayda MS, Ismailov II, Johnson JP. Structure and function of amiloride-sensitive Na$^+$ channels. J Membr Biol 1995;143(1):1–18.

[438] Ecelbarger CA, Kim GH, Wade JB, Knepper MA. Regulation of the abundance of renal sodium transporters and channels by vasopressin. Exp Neurol 2001;171(2):227–34.

[439] Kleyman TR, Ernst SA, Coupaye-Gerard B. Arginine vasopressin and forskolin regulate apical cell surface expression of epithelial Na$^+$ channels in A6 cells. Am J Physiol 1994;266(3 Pt 2): F506–11.

[440] Erlij D, De Smet P, Mesotten D, Van Driessche W. Forskolin increases apical sodium conductance in cultured toad kidney cells (A6) by stimulating membrane insertion. Pflugers Arch 1999;438(2):195–204.

[441] Butterworth MB, Helman SI, Els WJ. cAMP-sensitive endocytic trafficking in A6 epithelia. Am J Physiol Cell Physiol 2001;280 (4):C752–62.

[442] Marunaka Y, Eaton DC. Effects of vasopressin and cAMP on single amiloride-blockable Na channels. Am J Physiol 1991;260 (5 Pt 1):C1071–84.

[443] Ecelbarger CA, Kim GH, Terris J, Masilamani S, Mitchell C, Reyes I, et al. Vasopressin-mediated regulation of epithelial sodium channel abundance in rat kidney. Am J Physiol Renal Physiol 2000;279(1):F46–53.

[444] Wiesmann WP, Sinha S, Klahr S. Insulin stimulates active sodium transport in toad bladder by two mechanisms. Nature 1976;260(5551):546–7.

[445] Pearce D. The role of SGK1 in hormone-regulated sodium transport. Trends Endocrinol Metab 2001;12(8):341–7.

[446] Blazer-Yost BL, Liu X, Helman SI. Hormonal regulation of ENaCs: Insulin and aldosterone. Am J Physiol 1998;274(5 Pt 1): C1373–9.

[447] Faletti CJ, Perrotti N, Taylor SI, Blazer-Yost BL. sgk: an essential convergence point for peptide and steroid hormone regulation of ENaC-mediated Na$^+$ transport. Am J Physiol Cell Physiol 2002;282(3):C494–500.

[448] Tong Q, Gamper N, Medina JL, Shapiro MS, Stockand JD. Direct activation of the epithelial Na$^{(+)}$ channel by phosphatidylinositol 3,4,5-trisphosphate and phosphatidylinositol 3,4-bisphosphate produced by phosphoinositide 3-OH kinase. J Biol Chem 2004;279(21):22654–63.

[449] Peti-Peterdi J, Warnock DG, Bell PD. Angiotensin II directly stimulates ENaC activity in the cortical collecting duct via AT (1) receptors. J Am Soc Nephrol 2002;13(5):1131–5.

[450] Sun P, Yue P, Wang WH. Angiotensin II stimulates epithelial sodium channels (ENaC) in the cortical collecting duct of the rat kidney. Am J Physiol Renal Physiol 2012;302(6): F679–87.

[451] Mamenko M, Zaika O, Ilatovskaya DV, Staruschenko A, Pochynyuk O. Angiotensin II increases activity of the epithelial Na$^+$ channel (ENaC) in distal nephron additively to aldosterone. J Biol Chem 2012;287(1):660–71.

[452] Bugaj V, Pochynyuk O, Mironova E, Vandewalle A, Medina JL, Stockand JD. Regulation of the epithelial Na$^+$ channel by endothelin-1 in rat collecting duct. Am J Physiol Renal Physiol 2008;295(4):F1063–70.

[453] Bugaj V, Mironova E, Kohan DE, Stockand JD. Collecting duct-specific endothelin B receptor knockout increases ENaC activity. Am J Physiol Cell Physiol 2012;302(1):C188−94.

[454] Rossier BC. Mechanosensitivity of the epithelial sodium channel (ENaC): Controversy or pseudocontroversy? J Gen Physiol 1998;112(2):95−6.

[455] Awayda MS, Subramanyam M. Regulation of the epithelial Na$^+$ channel by membrane tension. J Gen Physiol 1998;112(2):97−111.

[456] Ji HL, Fuller CM, Benos DJ. Osmotic pressure regulates alpha beta gamma-rENaC expressed in *Xenopus* oocytes. Am J Physiol 1998;275(5 Pt 1):C1182−90.

[457] Engbretson BG, Stoner LC. Flow-dependent potassium secretion by rabbit cortical collecting tubule *in vitro*. Am J Physiol 1987;253(5 Pt 2):F896−903.

[458] Malnic G, Berliner RW, Giebisch G. Flow dependence of K$^+$ secretion in cortical distal tubules of the rat. Am J Physiol 1989;256(5 Pt 2):F932−41.

[459] Satlin LM, Sheng S, Woda CB, Kleyman TR. Epithelial Na($^+$) channels are regulated by flow. Am J Physiol Renal Physiol 2001;280(6):F1010−8.

[460] Morimoto T, Liu W, Woda C, Carattino MD, Wei Y, Hughey RP, et al. Mechanism underlying flow stimulation of sodium absorption in the mammalian collecting duct. Am J Physiol Renal Physiol 2006;291(3):F663−9.

[461] Carattino MD, Liu W, Hill WG, Satlin LM, Kleyman TR. Lack of a role of membrane-protein interactions in flow-dependent activation of ENaC. Am J Physiol Renal Physiol 2007;293(1):F316−24.

[462] Abi-Antoun T, Shi S, Tolino LA, Kleyman TR, Carattino MD. Second transmembrane domain modulates epithelial sodium channel gating in response to shear stress. Am J Physiol Renal Physiol 2011;300(5):F1089−95.

[463] Drummond HA, Price MP, Welsh MJ, Abboud FM. A molecular component of the arterial baroreceptor mechanotransducer. Neuron 1998;21(6):1435−41.

[464] Drummond HA, Welsh MJ, Abboud FM. ENaC subunits are molecular components of the arterial baroreceptor complex. Ann NY Acad Sci 2001;940:42−7.

[465] Drummond HA, Grifoni SC, Jernigan NL. A new trick for an old dogma: ENaC proteins as mechanotransducers in vascular smooth muscle. Physiology (Bethesda) 2008;23:23−31.

[466] Jernigan NL, Drummond HA. Vascular ENaC proteins are required for renal myogenic constriction. Am J Physiol Renal Physiol 2005;289(4):F891−901.

[467] Jernigan NL, Drummond HA. Myogenic vasoconstriction in mouse renal interlobar arteries: role of endogenous beta and gammaENaC. Am J Physiol Renal Physiol 2006;291(6):F1184−91.

[468] Jernigan NL, LaMarca B, Speed J, Galmiche L, Granger JP, Drummond HA. Dietary salt enhances benzamil-sensitive component of myogenic constriction in mesenteric arteries. Am J Physiol Heart Circ Physiol 2008;294(1):H409−20.

[469] Guan Z, Pollock JS, Cook AK, Hobbs JL, Inscho EW. Effect of epithelial sodium channel blockade on the myogenic response of rat juxtamedullary afferent arterioles. Hypertension 2009;54(5):1062−9.

[470] Grifoni SC, Chiposi R, McKey SE, Ryan MJ, Drummond HA. Altered whole kidney blood flow autoregulation in a mouse model of reduced beta-ENaC. Am J Physiol Renal Physiol 2010;298(2):F285−92.

[471] Kamynina E, Tauxe C, Staub O. Distinct characteristics of two human Nedd4 proteins with respect to epithelial Na($^+$) channel regulation. Am J Physiol Renal Physiol 2001;281(3):F469−77.

[472] Goulet CC, Volk KA, Adams CM, Prince LS, Stokes JB, Snyder PM. Inhibition of the epithelial Na$^+$ channel by interaction of Nedd4 with a PY motif deleted in Liddle's syndrome. J Biol Chem 1998;273(45):30012−7.

[473] Knight KK, Olson DR, Zhou R, Snyder PM. Liddle's syndrome mutations increase Na$^+$ transport through dual effects on epithelial Na$^+$ channel surface expression and proteolytic cleavage. Proc Natl Acad Sci USA 2006;103(8):2805−8.

[474] Melander O, Orho M, Fagerudd J, Bengtsson K, Groop PH, Mattiasson I, et al. Mutations and variants of the epithelial sodium channel gene in Liddle's syndrome and primary hypertension. Hypertension 1998;31(5):1118−24.

[475] Baker EH, Dong YB, Sagnella GA, Rothwell M, Onipinla AK, Markandu ND, et al. Association of hypertension with T594M mutation in beta subunit of epithelial sodium channels in black people resident in London. Lancet 1998;351(9113):1388−92.

[476] Ambrosius WT, Bloem LJ, Zhou L, Rebhun JF, Snyder PM, Wagner MA, et al. Genetic variants in the epithelial sodium channel in relation to aldosterone and potassium excretion and risk for hypertension. Hypertension 1999;34(4 Pt 1):631−7.

[477] Baker EH, Duggal A, Dong Y, Ireson NJ, Wood M, Markandu ND, et al. Amiloride, a specific drug for hypertension in black people with T594M variant? Hypertension 2002;40(1):13−7.

[478] Cui Y, Su YR, Rutkowski M, Reif M, Menon AG, Pun RY. Loss of protein kinase C inhibition in the beta-T594M variant of the amiloride-sensitive Na$^+$ channel. Proc Natl Acad Sci USA 1997;94(18):9962−6.

[479] Dirlewanger M, Huser D, Zennaro MC, Girardin E, Schild L, Schwitzgebel VM. A homozygous missense mutation in SCNN1A is responsible for a transient neonatal form of pseudohypoaldosteronism type 1. Am J Physiol Endoc M 2011;301(3):E467−73.

[480] Passero CJ, Hughey RP, Kleyman TR. New role for plasmin in sodium homeostasis. Curr Opin Nephrol Hypertens 2010;19(1):13−9.

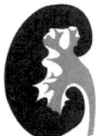

Anion Channels

Owen M. Woodward and William B. Guggino

Department of Physiology, The Johns Hopkins University School of Medicine, Baltimore, MD, USA

INTRODUCTION

The mammalian kidney evolved to allow for the efficient secretion of metabolic waste without excess loss of water in terrestrial environments, for the maintenance of the ionic balance in the extracellular milieu, for the regulation of blood pressure, and for the recapture of essential solutes like proteins and sugars. These functions all deferentially depended on the conductance/transport of Cl^- and other anions across individual cell membranes. A classic example is NaCl reabsorption in the distal nephron, where Na^+, Cl^-, and K^+ enter the cell across the apical membrane via the NKCC2 co-transporter, driven by the Na^+ gradient established by the Na^+/K^+-ATPase, and the Cl^- gradient maintained by basolateral ClC-Kb Cl^- channels. Mutations in these basolateral Cl^- channels result in the severe salt-wasting characteristic of Type III Bartter's syndrome. As more of the major Cl^- channel family molecular identities are resolved, our understanding of the role of Cl^- channels in kidney disease will increase proportionally, and hopefully shed light on some of the long-standing mysteries of kidney function.

Although anions and negatively charged organic solutes were appreciated as necessary to balance the charges accumulated by the cations, Na^+, K^+, and Ca^{2+}, they were believed to be passive players. Cl^-, by far the most abundant physiological anion, was believed to be balanced across the membrane, a belief supported by early studies of skeletal muscle, where the resting Cl^- permeability was found to be very high,[27] and thus Cl^- was mostly known for its contribution to the "leak" current.[131] Even as later studies demonstrated that Cl^- was being actively transported in squid axons or secreted as HCl in the stomach,[27] less interest was given to anion conductances. Initial patch-

clamp studies of Cl^- channels discovered that Cl^- channels are not really even Cl^- channels; their general promiscuity toward all anions makes them more accurately described as anion channels. The tide first began to change as neuroscientists found, and later cloned, the GABA- and glycine-gated Cl^- channels that worked to inhibit synaptic transmission, proving that Cl^- was not in equilibrium at rest and could be harnessed by cells to do work. But it was the cloning of two major classes of Cl^- channels, the CLCs and CFTR, which lead to an explosion of interest in Cl^- channels, and exponentially increased our understanding of their ubiquity, importance in human disease, and function in the mammalian kidney.

Anion channels are usually grouped into five major classes, based on how they are activated or regulated. There are the voltage-dependent Cl^- channels (the CLCs); ligand-gated Cl^- channels (the GABA and glycine receptor channels); cAMP-activated channels (CFTR); Ca^{2+}-activated Cl^- channels (the TMEM16 channels); and the volume-regulated anion channels (the VRAC channels). This chapter will examine the expression and function of these major classes of Cl^- channels in the kidney, but will also discuss at length Cl^- channels that are expressed ubiquitously or for which expression and functional information does not yet exist. The chapter dives right in to survey the major anion channel families and their relevance in the kidney, focusing on the CLC, CFTR, TMEM16, VRAC, and SLC26A7/9 Cl^- channels. However, the chapter will also look at a number of less well-understood anion channel genes that have currently unclear physiological relevance. Lastly, we will delve deeply into Cl^- channelopathies that affect the kidney both directly and indirectly, seeking insight into how Cl^- channels contribute to normal kidney physiology.

What's "New"?

Recent work on Cl^- channels has paid disproportionate dividends for Cl^- channel researchers, including advances in our understanding of Cl^- channel structure, molecular identity, and discovery of new Cl^- channels in familiar but surprising places. The most important advance in Cl^- channel knowledge came in 2008, when three independent groups using three novel approaches all identified the TMEM16A gene as the molecular identity of the classic Ca^{2+}-activated Cl^- channel (CaCC). The TMEM16 family of genes has 10 human homologs that are expressed widely, including in the kidney. As more and more work is done describing their function, biophysical characteristics, and expression patterns, the more certain it becomes that TMEM16a is the classic CaCC. Second, crystal structures solved for bacterial orthologs of the voltage-dependent CLC Cl^- channel family revealed via homology that a number of the human CLCs (ClC-3, 4, 5, 6, and 7) are not in fact channels, but H^+/Cl^- exchangers, a finding with ramifications in the kidney. And third, two members of a well-known anion transporter family, SLC26A7 and A9, appear to behave almost exclusively as anion channels, with no appreciable transport of bicarbonate. Which, taken in conjunction with the recent reclassification of a number of the CLC channels as exchangers, suggests a fine line between anion transporter and anion channel. Each of the recent advances mentioned above will be discussed in depth in the following chapter.

MAJOR CLASSES OF IDENTIFIED ANION CHANNELS

Similar to the study of other ion channels, extensive research into the biophysical and physiological characteristics and functions of Cl^- channels preceded the identification of their molecular identity or their corresponding human genes. One reason that the molecular identification of Cl^- channels lagged far behind that of cation channels is that there were no highly specific inhibitors that could be used for cloning Cl^- channels in a manner similar to that done for many cation channels. However, with a considerable amount of effort, more and more of the Cl^- channels recognized for their biophysical characteristics now have mammalian gene candidates, identifications of which have quickly expanded our knowledge of the roles of Cl^- channels in cellular functions and in human disease. The molecular identification has also shown just how difficult identification of all the Cl^- channels is. There is no homology between any of the identified gene families containing Cl^- channels, and very little commonality in structure.[27] Their demonstrated convergence of function, so different from the common homology of many of the families of cation channels, presents no easy bioinformatic road map to the discovery of Cl^- channel identities. Instead, a narrowly focused approach has been used on each of the functional classes of Cl^- channels to identify the known Cl^- channel families (Figure 31.1), a growing list that now includes the CLC voltage-dependent channels, CFTR, TMEM16/Anoctamins Ca^{2+}-activated Cl^- channels,

Anion Channel	Regulation	Channel Properties	Kidney Localization	Physiological Role	Human Disease
CFTR	Activated by cAMP-dependent phosphorylation	Linear I/V; $Cl^->I^-$	Proximal and distal tubule, collecting duct	Cl^- secretion from epithelium	Cystic fibrosis; Polycystic kidney disease
ClC-2	Activated by hyperpolarization and cell swelling	Inward rectifying I/V; $Cl^->I^-$	Proximal tubule	Unknown	Unknown
ClC-Ka and Kb	Weak voltage activation and requires barttin subunit	Moderate outward rectifying I/V; $Cl^->I^-$	ClC-Ka: tAL; ClC-Ka: TAL, distal tubule, collecting duct	Basolateral Cl^- secretion	Bartter's syndrome type III and IV
TMEM16 (A)	Activated by cytosolic Ca^{2+}	Outward rectifying I/V; $I^->Cl^-$	Unknown	Ca^+ dependent Cl^- secretion from epithelium	Unknown
SLC26A7	Constitutively active and pH sensitive	Linear I/V; $Cl^->I^-$	Collecting duct	pH sensor or Cl^- shunt in acid secreting cells	Unknown
VRAC/Maxi-anion	Activated by cell swelling	Outward rectifying, depolarization induced inactivation; $I^->Cl^-$	Ubiquitous; maxi-anion; macula densa cells	Regulatory volume decrease; salt-sensing and ATP secretion	Unknown

FIGURE 31.1   Anion Channels of the human kidney.

SLC26A7/9, GABA and glycine receptor channels, VDAC, and a myriad of less well-studied groups including the bestrophins, intracellular CLICs, CLCA, and twety (hTTYH3). The long search for molecular identities of the Cl⁻ channels has lead to many ambiguous discoveries, dead ends, and great success stories. Below we review the Cl⁻ channels with known molecular identities, and known physiological and kidney specific functions, but we will also discuss those genes that code for proteins that can conduct Cl⁻, but do not yet have known physiological functions.

CLC Cl⁻ Channels

Our discussion about the specific families of Cl⁻ channels begins with CLC Cl⁻ channels (Figure 31.2). Unlike CFTR, which was not immediately recognized as a Cl⁻ channel and appeared to be a very divergent type of ABC transporter,[27] the canonical ClC-0 shared close homology with proteins from a large gene family with members expressed across all phyla, including nine members expressed in humans. Two decades of subsequent work have revealed much about the CLC family, their biophysical properties, and their importance in human disease, yet many of the mammalian orthologs still only have vaguely defined physiological functions. However, the relevance of the CLCs in the human kidney is clear. Eight of nine human CLC orthologs are expressed in the kidney, and their dysfunction leads directly to Dent's disease and Type III Bartter's syndrome.[25]

For years the mammalian CLCs were divided into two classes, based on cellular localization with ClC-1, 2, and ClC-Ka, b channels being expressed in the plasma membranes, and the remaining ClC-3, 4, 5, 6, and 7 all being expressed on intracellular membranes. Recent evidence has substantially shifted this paradigm of understanding, with the plasma membrane CLCs now simply classified as the voltage-dependent Cl⁻ channel CLCs with the rest now classified as Cl⁻/H⁺ exchangers. It turns out that the vast majority of all CLC family members across all phyla are Cl⁻/H⁺ exchangers and not Cl⁻ channels. For the mammalian CLC proteins this has meant a revision of functions and physiological roles for the previously designated intracellular CLCs. Intrinsically, the difference between a CLC Cl⁻ channel and a CLC Cl⁻/H⁺ exchanger is little more than a few strategically placed glutamate residues; extrinsically, their thermodynamic properties are completely different.[79] These newly classified exchangers will be covered briefly below, but this section will mostly focus on the remaining CLC Cl⁻ channels and their functions in the kidney.

The early work investigating CLC Cl⁻ channels found they have very distinct biophysical properties, which immediately set them apart from the known cation channels and would later set them apart from all other known Cl⁻ channels. ClC-0 can be described as voltage-dependent, pH-dependent, and dependent on the Cl⁻ gradient across the pore, as can most of the CLC Cl⁻ channels.[19] The "kidney" Cl⁻ channels, ClC-Ka and ClC-Kb, are additionally dependent on a smaller beta-subunit, barttin (BSND); a dependence with ramifications for NaCl reuptake in the thick ascending loop and Bartter's syndrome. The halide selectivity sequence for ClC-0 is Cl⁻ > Br⁻ > I⁻, and in most physiological circumstances it forms functional homodimers, although heterodimers from ClC-0, 1, and 2 can be formed heterologously.[19,54] ClC-0 single channel currents appeared at first glance to be two separate channels, albeit with identical conductances; however, even though the two conductances or protopores appeared to open and close independently, sporadically they both closed simultaneously and remained closed for prolonged periods before opening again.[19,70a,78] The coexpression of ClC-0 and ClC-2 heterodimers resulted in the same strange phenomenon, but this time the two protopore conductances were different. The difference in protopore conductances correlated with the varying protopore size between ClC-0, 1, and 2, being 10 pS, 1.5 pS, and 3 pS respectively.[27] This prompted the conclusion that ClC Cl⁻ channels function as dimers, with two separate protopores, each independently gated by a separate "fast" gate, but both gated simultaneously by a "slow" gate.[55]

This hypothesis was proven correct after the crystallization of the prokaryotic CLC proteins from *E. coli* and *Salmonella typhimurium*.[28] These prokaryotic CLCs formed dimers, with each subunit forming its own protopore. Each subunit consists of 18 membrane "embedded" domains, where many of the helices do not project completely through the bilayer.[28] Interestingly, each subunit has structurally similar halves that "twist" in an antiparallel structure that forms an hourglass shaped protopore toward the center.[28] Further work on the *E. coli* CLC, EcClC-1, crystal revealed that there are three Cl⁻-binding sites within the hourglass shaped pore, and in the outermost site the Cl⁻ appears to compete with the carboxyl group of a negatively-charged glutamate.[29] When this glutamate is replaced with a non-charged amino acid in the ClC-0 channel, the voltage-dependent gating properties are altered.[29] This suggests that the central "gating" glutamate is key in the voltage- and Cl⁻-dependence of CLC gating,[55] and represents the fast gate regulating each protopore. The possible protonation of the gating glutamate, thereby allowing Cl⁻ to enter the pore, may also help explain the pH-dependence observed for many CLCs.[27]

The reconstitution of EcClC-1 in lipid bilayers revealed that it is not a Cl⁻ channel, but a Cl⁻/H⁺

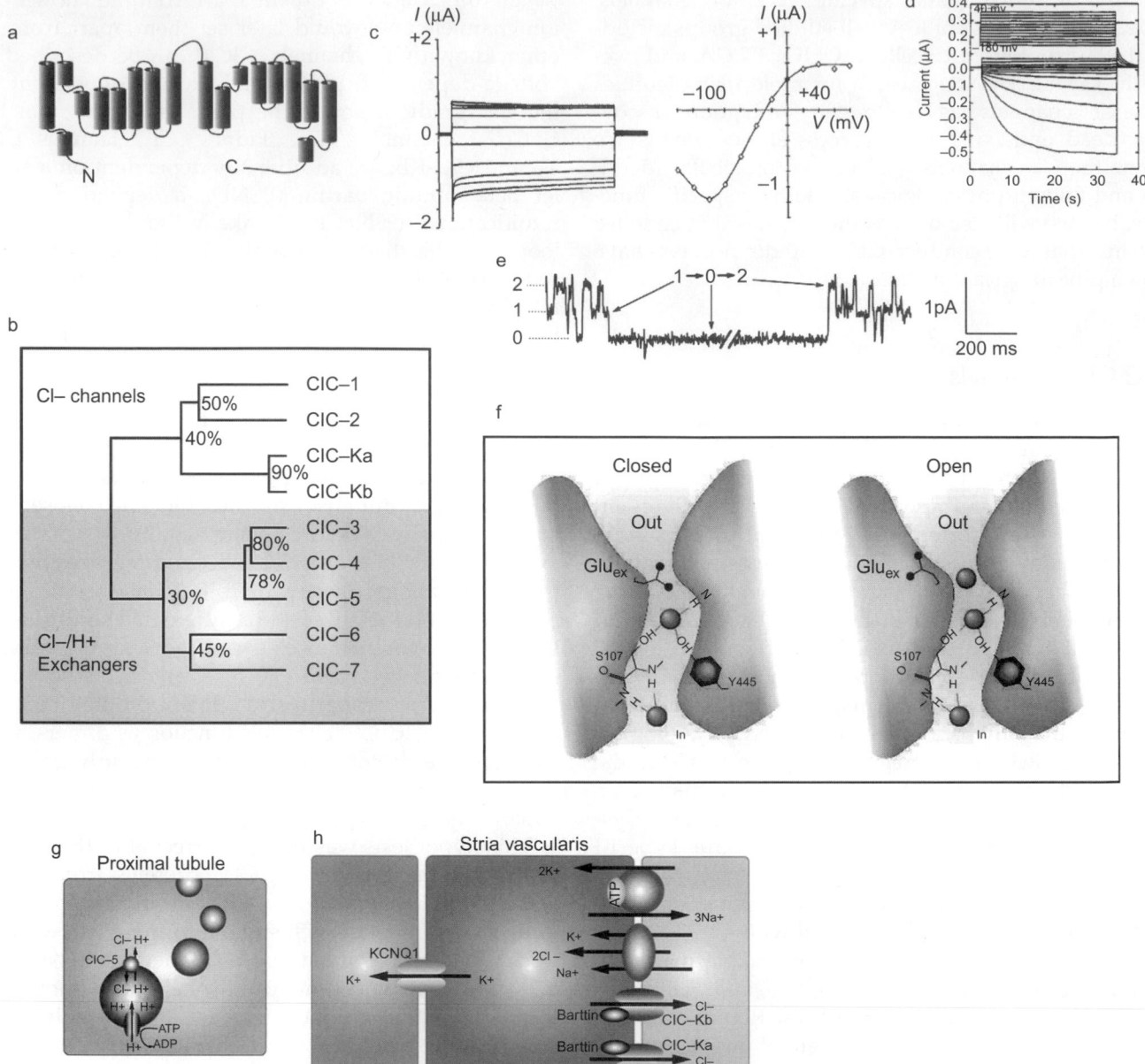

FIGURE 31.2   CLC Gene family. (a) Topography of representative CLC protein. (b) Dendrogram of mammalian CLC proteins. (c) Whole cell currents and I/V relationship of ClC-1 expressed in *Xenopus* oocytes. (d) Whole cell currents from ClC-2 expressing *Xenopus* oocytes. (e) Single channel ClC-0 openings with two clear substates or protopores. (f) Drawing of the closed and opened states of ClC channels and exchangers. In the closed state the "gating" glutamate side chain is bound to the uppermost Cl⁻ binding site, to open the channel the side chain must be moved or bind an H⁺. (g) ClC-5 acts to balance the positive charge build-up resulting from the acidification of endosomes. (h) In the inner ear the two ClC proteins Ka and Kb secret Cl⁻ across the basolateral membrane, allowing high concentrations of K⁺ to be conducted across the apical membrane into the stria media facilitating the function of the hair cells. ((c), (d), (e), (f): *Reprinted by permission from Macmillan Publishers Ltd. (c) Steinmeyer, K., Ortland, C., Jentsch, T. J. (1991). Primary structure and functional expression of a developmentally regulated skeletal muscle chloride channel. Nature 354, 301–304.*[118] *(d) Thiemann, A., Grunder, S., Pusch, M., Jentsch, T. J. (1992). A chloride channel widely expressed in epithelial and non-epithelial cells. Nature 356, 57–60.* [125]*(e) Lisal, J., and Maduke, M. (2008). The ClC-0 chloride channel is a broken Cl⁻/H⁺ antiporter. Nat. Struct. Mol. Bio. 15, 805–810.*[71a] *(f) Miller, C. (2006). ClC chloride channels viewed through a transporter lens. Nature 440, 484–489.*[79])

exchanger, where two Cl⁻ ions are substituted for one H⁺.[55] Further mutational studies discovered the H⁺ exchange depended on both the gating glutamate, and a second glutamate near the cytosolic surface, but not in the protopore.[79] These characteristics suggest that both protons and Cl⁻ are gated by the "gating" glutamate, after which they travel separate permeation paths to the cytoplasm. This theory is supported by experiments where this second glutamate was mutated in the EcClC-1, making the protein exclusively a Cl^- channel, not an exchanger.[1] The human CLCs ClC-3, 4, 5, 6, and 7 all have this second glutamate marking them as exchangers, and mutating both glutamates in ClC-4 and 5 converted them into Cl^- channels,[96,109] demonstrating just how fine the line is between Cl^- channel and exchanger.

The pharmacology of CLC Cl^- channels, like many of the other anion channels, has been plagued by the lack of specific high affinity inhibitors. Although the mammalian CLCs are highly conserved, they do differ somewhat in their susceptibility to the classic Cl^- channel inhibitors. ClC-0, ClC-1, and ClC-2 all differ in their affinity for 9-anthracene carboxylic acid (9-AC), with ClC-1 effectively blocked by 100 μM, whereas ClC-0 and ClC-2 require mM levels.[118,125] The CLCs are also affectively inhibited by the clofibric acid derivatives 2-(-p-chlorophenoxy) propionic acid (CPP) and 2-(-p-chlorophenoxy) acetic acid (CPA).[19,131] Stilibenes can also be weakly inhibitory and can block ClC-2, as can DPC and NPPB at 0.5 to >1 mM concentrations.[131] ClC-2 is also inhibited by divalent cations like zinc and cadmium with IC_{50} in the μM range[131] as the other CLC Cl^- channels can be. Because of their human disease relevance the kidney CLCs, Ka and Kb have been scrutinized more than the others. Specifically, inhibitors could regulate dieresis and possibly blood pressure, and therapeutic activators could aid patients with Bartter's Syndrome.[70] The close shared homology of the ClC-Ks obviously suggested similar sensitivities to inhibitors, but both CPP and DIDS are more affective at blocking CLC-Ka than Kb.[28,131] Niflumic acid (NFA), another classic Cl^- channel inhibitor, was actually shown to activate the CLC-Ks at low concentrations (50−100 μM),[70] but inhibit them at higher concentrations,[131] a finding that prompted Liantonio et al.[70] to manipulate the CPP structure to recapitulate characteristics of the NFA molecule, in order to create a better inhibitor. They found that their rationally designed benzofuran carboxyl acid derivatives could inhibit both ClC-Ka and Kb with low μM IC_{50}s.[70] Their work, and the insight provided by the EcClC-1 crystal structure, make finding potential therapeutic activators and inhibitors of the CLC-Ks a real likelihood, therapies that could impact millions of patients.

Physiological Function of Mammalian CLC Cl⁻ Channels

With the recent identification of the intracellular CLCs as exchangers, only four human CLCs remain for further in-depth discussion: ClC-1, ClC-2, and the CLC-Ks. ClC-1 (the human gene is *CLCN1*), is the only CLC that is not expressed in the kidney.[25] It is a plasma membrane localized Cl^- channel found almost exclusively in skeletal muscle. There it represents about 80% of the resting conductance of the muscle.[55] When the muscle depolarizes along the T-tubule, and Ca^{2+} is released from the sarcoplasmic reticulum, ClC-1 is further activated. The ClC-1 activation repolarizes the muscle cell and brings it back to its negative resting potential. Cl^- and not K^+, as in most other excitable cells, is used for repolarization because it is thought that in the microdomains of T-tubules extracellular K^+ would quickly build up, causing unsolicited depolarizations.[55] The physiological importance of ClC-1 became clear after causal ClC-1 mutations were found first in myotonic mice and later in humans.[55] The human form of the disease, myotonia or "muscle stiffness" is characterized by muscles that suffer prolonged contractions, exactly the phenotype expected if repolarization cannot occur after the initial depolarizing stimulus. Humans can have either the recessive form of the disease (Becker type) with complete ClC-1 functionality loss or the dominant form (Thomsen's) with the retention of some ClC-1 function and less severe debilitation.[55,131]

ClC-2

ClC-2 is broadly expressed in many different tissues, but is prominent in epithelium (including kidney), neurons, glia, and heart muscle.[125] Unlike ClC-1, ClC-2 is inwardly rectifying and hyperpolarization activated.[108,131] It can also be activated by cell swelling, but is clearly not the ubiquitous VRAC current, which differs in selectivity, voltage-dependence, rectification, and single channel conductance.[55] Unfortunately, little is yet known about its function. Even the development of $Clnc2^{-/-}$ knockout mice has provided only minimal hints at its broad functions. $Clcn2^{-/-}$ mice did display some disease phenotypes; however, knockout mice displayed degeneration of photo receptors and seminiferous tubules in testicles.[131] There is also some evidence that ClC-2 is involved in Cl^- secretion in lung epithelium, and that it could provide an alternative source of Cl^- secretion in patients with aberrant CFTR function.[112] To that end, the FDA approved lubiprostone, the only CLC-targeted drug yet approved, for treatment in cystic fibrosis (CF).[23,131] More recent work suggests that ClC-2 may be localized more on the basolateral membrane and not apical, at least in gut epithelium,[55] and that lubiprostome may also activate CFTR or other apical Cl^- channels, not necessarily just ClC-2.[6,131] Unfortunately, $Clcn2^{-/-}$ mice have no kidney phenotype, even though ClC-2 is believed to be expressed in the proximal tubule.[128] It is possible that, like in the gut, they may be expressed on the basolateral membrane and involved in the reabsorption of Cl^- along the nephron, but to what extent is unclear.

CLC Exchangers

Before progressing to the in-depth analysis of the remaining kidney CLC Cl⁻ channels, it is necessary to briefly touch on the CLC intracellular exchangers, in particular ClC-5 because of its relevance in kidney function. Like most other CLCs, ClC-5 is a Cl⁻/H⁺ exchanger that exchanges two Cl⁻ for every H⁺. ClC-5 is localized to the proximal tubule and to the α-intercalated cells of the cortical collecting duct.[25] ClC-5 is specifically localized to the endosomes in these cell types, alongside the v-type H⁺-ATPase.[25,43,98] The human ClC-5 gene CLCN5 was identified independently, first through positional cloning in families with Dent's disease,[25] and confirmed through homology cloning.[55] Dent's disease is an X-linked renal tubular disorder characterized by low molecular weight proteinuria (LMWP), hypercalciuria, nephrocalcinosis, kidney stones, and renal failure.[25] More than 40 mutations have been identified in human CLCN5 that cause Dent's disease, with a wide range of severity.[55] Recapitulating some of the disease-causing mutations in ClC-5 expressed in heterologous systems showed they almost universally resulted in reduction or loss of Cl⁻ conductance (ClC-5 when overexpressed reaches the plasma membrane).[25] This, along with its known localization to subapical endosomes alongside H⁺-ATPases, prompted the hypothesis that ClC-5 was functioning to provide Cl⁻ influx to offset the positive charge build-up from the acidification of the endosomes.[25,98] A Cl⁻ shunt would prevent a slowdown of H⁺ pumping into the endosomes from positive charge build-up. Importantly, the then presumed channel characteristics of ClC-5 didn't match this function well, ClC-5 is outwardly rectifying, and most importantly is inhibited by acidic pH.[25] The creation of a Clcn5⁻/⁻ knockout mouse allowed the testing of the role ClC-5 plays in endosomal acidification. The two models[97,135] both reproduced the LWMP and defective apical endocytosis, seemingly supporting the hypothesis that ClC-5 aids in acidification.[25,55,128] In addition, in vitro disruption of ClC-5 function caused reduced acidification of the endosomes.[87] But with the discovery that ClC-5 is not in fact a Cl⁻ channel, but a Cl⁻/H⁺ exchanger it became far less clear how it could provide the shunt current for acidification, and how it could be influencing the endocytosis of low molecular weight proteins. Recent work by Noarino et al.[87] addressed this question directly by comparing mouse models with either Clcn5⁻/⁻ knockout or the knockin of a mutated Clcn5 (Clcn5unc) that removed the "gating" glutamate, uncoupling the Cl⁻/H⁺ exchange and thereby creating a ClC-5 Cl⁻ channel, not exchanger. They found, as reported previously, endosomes from the Clcn5 knockout showed reduced acidification and defective endocytosis; however, the Clcn5unc knockin mice showed normal acidification, but still had defective endocytosis.[87] These data strongly suggest that ClC-5 plays a role in acidification by acting as a charge shunt; however, as a Cl⁻/H⁺ exchanger it plays a further yet to be explained role in endocytosis unrelated to its role as a shunt. Novarino et al.[87] suggest the intra-endosome absolute Cl⁻ concentration may be key in regulating endocytosis, not just the negative charge.

CLC-Ks

There are two mammalian CLC-K channels, named because of their localization to kidney tissues, although they are now also known to be expressed in the inner ear. Mammals possess two CLC-Ks, ClC-K1 and K2, and the human orthologs are termed ClC-Ka and -Kb, respectively. The CLC-Ks are highly conserved with the rodent homologs, ClC-K1 and K2, sharing 80% homology and the human pair being over 90% homologous.[61] After the homology cloning of rodent ClC-K1 and -K2, they were heterologously expressed in Xenopus oocytes, but only ClC-K1 expression resulted in Cl⁻ currents.[127] These ClC-K1 currents displayed a linear I/V relationship, with little voltage-dependence.[133] Like the rodent ClC-K2 that failed to produce currents, the heterologous expression of the human ClC-Ka and -Kb failed to yield any Cl⁻ currents,[61] prompting the supposition that a β-subunit may be necessary for function. The discovery of the subunit came tangentially from the successful positional cloning of a gene mutated in human type IV Bartter's syndrome, BSND, which codes for the protein barttin.[14] Barttin has two transmembrane domains, and both N- and C-termini located in the cytoplasm.[32] The expression of barttin along with either of the human CLC-Ks resulted in robust Cl⁻ currents with ion selectivity similar to that of other CLC Cl⁻ channels, inhibited by low extracellular pH, and stimulated by extracellular Ca²⁺.[62] The main function of barttin appears to be to increase dramatically the amount of CLC-Ks that make it to the plasma membrane, although it also appears to subtly alter gating.[134] Interestingly, the voltage-dependence described for other CLCs is absent in the CLC-Ks,[128] a phenomenon that appears connected to the "gating" glutamate described in the EcClC-1 exchanger; the two ClC-K channels in humans lack the gating glutamate and instead have a valine at the same position. However, if the valine is mutated to a glutamate, strong voltage dependence is recapitulated.[133]

Although human CLC-Ks share close homology and do have overlapping kidney expression patterns, there does appear to be some divergence in localization that is supported by a divergence in function as well. ClC-

K1 (and presumably ClC-Ka) is expressed in the cortex, inner, and outer medulla, specifically localized in the thin ascending limb (tAL) of the loop of Henle; ClC-K2 is expressed in the cortex, inner, and outer medulla, specifically localizing to the thick ascending limb (TAL), distal convoluted tubule, and the α-intercalated cells of the collecting duct. Barttin expression is co-localized with the two CLC-Ks.[25,55,61,130] All three proteins, ClC-Ka, b, and barttin, are also expressed together in the stria vascularis of the inner ear.[61]

Function of the CLC-Ks

The discussion on function will concentrate on three areas, the tAL, the TAL, and the inner ear. These are not the only areas of the nephron where the CLC-Ks have significant function, but they are the areas most directly attributed to their roles in human disease. An additional discussion of Bartter's syndrome and CLC-Kb will come at the end of the chapter.

Currently there are no described human diseases with an isolated defect in the ClC-Ka gene, *CLCNKA*.[61] Although there has been one report of an association between salt-sensitive hypertension and single nucleotide polymorphisms in humans *CLCNKA*,[7] it is not clear how the SNPs or resulting haplotypes would alter ClC-Ka function. This lack of recognized human diseases from mutant ClC-Ka may be due to functional redundancies or poor sampling, because evidence has accumulated suggesting that ClC-Ka plays an important role in the urine concentrating mechanism of the loop of Henle. As mentioned above, ClC-K1 (Ka) is localized to the tAL, the area of the nephron with the highest Cl^- permeability,[25] and early studies comparing the characteristics of heterologously expressed ClC-K1/barttin currents versus those described from *in vitro* perfusion studies found striking similarities.[128] Subsequent work demonstrated that ClC-K1 was expressed in both the basolateral and apical membranes of tAL epithelium,[25] and interestingly, dehydration appears to increase the tAL expression of ClC-K1 in rats.[61] This loose connection between volume sensing and ClC-K1 expression in the tAL may be through the skg1 protein kinase. The SKG1 gene and protein expression increases when the cell volume diminishes and, in turn, can upregulate ClC-K1/barttin currents.[31] Barttin has a PY site on its C-terminus which facilitates the binding of WW domain-containing ubiquitin ligases like Nedd4-2; sgk1 can phosphorylate Nedd4-2, preventing the ubiquitination of barttin and increasing the half-life of ClC-K1/barttin at the plasma membrane.[31] Upregulation of Cl^- vectorial transport in the tAL in times of dehydration would work to increase the concentrating mechanism of the inner medulla, and allow for increased water reabsorption via Aquaporin-2 in the collecting duct principle cells. However, it

wasn't until the creation of the $Clcnk1^{-/-}$ knockout mouse that the physiological significance of ClC-K1 was clearly demonstrated.

$Clcnk1^{-/-}$ mice display no physical phenotypes, no renal organ phenotype or changes in plasma creatinine, Na^+, K^+ or HCO_3^-. However, they do display a four- to five-fold increase in the volume of excreted urine and other symptoms similar to the human condition nephrogenic diabetes insipidus (NDI).[77,128] The concentrating of urine depends on the reuptake of water in the collecting duct, a process which in turn depends on the osmolarity gradient across the inner medulla.[25] The high interstitial osmolarity of the inner medulla depends on the reabsorption of $NaCl^-$ and the recycling of urea in the tAL. The dysfunction of any part of the complicated concentrating mechanism will lead to diabetes insipidus, qualified as "nephrogenic" if the application of vasopressin (AVP) has no effect on the water lost in urine.[25] The $Clcnk1^{-/-}$ mice demonstrated an increase in urinary AVP secretion, no tAL Cl^- transport, and reduction in papillary osmolarity due to decreased accumulation of NaCl and urea in the inner medulla.[77] These results clearly and unambiguously demonstrated that ClC-K1 (Ka) is solely responsible for the vectorial Cl^- transport of the tAL, and that it constitutes an important part of the urine concentrating mechanism.

The function of ClC-K2 (Kb) became clear after the mapping of human mutations in the *CLCNKB* in patients with Bartter's syndrome, a condition that includes renal salt-wasting.[61] This discovery, coupled with the localization of ClC-Kb to the TAL, prompted a model of NaCl reapportion in the TAL, where the ClC-K2 (Kb) is responsible for the basolateral Cl^- conductance out of the cell. More specifically, in TAL cells, the apical membrane contains the NKCC2 co-transporter (SLC12A1) and ROMK K^+ channels; Na^+, Cl^-, and K^+ all enter the cell via the NKCC2, K^+ exits again apically via the ROMK channel, Na^+ is pumped into the interstitium via the Na^+/K^+-ATPase, and the Cl^- moves down its gradient through basolateral ClC-Kb channels into the interstitium.[61] This model is well-supported by the human genetics underlying Bartter's syndrome, and will be discussed further at the end of the chapter. In contrast, gain-of-function mutations have also been identified in the human *CLCNKB*, most notably the T481S polymorphism prevalent in both African and Caucasian populations, with minor allele frequencies of 0.22 and 0.12 respectively.[53] The T481S mutation in ClC-Kb increases currents 20-fold, possibly by alterations to the channels open probability,[53] and was thought therefore to lead to increased salt reabsorption and thus hypertension; however, studies have mostly shown that there is no association between the T481S mutation and hypertension.[55]

More recently, ClC-Ka, ClC-Kb, and barttin have all been shown to be expressed outside the kidney, in the stria vascularis of the inner ear. This was discovered only after a connection between deafness in some patients suffering from Bartter's syndrome was made to a mutation in the barttin protein. Barttin and the CLC-Ks are expressed on the basolateral membrane of the stria vascularis epithelium, where they function to reduce the Cl^- concentration in the stria vascularis. The fluid of the stria media has a very high concentration of K^+, and an unusually low concentration of Na^+. The excess K^+ is necessary to depolarize the hair cells via mechanosensory apical K^+ channels. The high K^+ is established by the movement of K^+ out of the stria vascularis epithelium via apical KCNQ1/KCNE1 K^+ channels. The K^+ enters the stria vascularis cells via basolateral Na^+/K^+-ATPases and the NKCC1 transporter, which imports two Cl^- for every K^+. Excess Na^+ is pumped out via the Na^+/K^+-ATPase and the Cl^- is extruded through basolateral CLC-K channels.[55,61] Human mutations in either one or the other CLC-K does not result in deafness, only in the dysfunction of their common barttin subunit or in very rare cases an individual has a mutation in both CLC-K genes.[55] This suggests redundancy in function that may also occur in the kidney and help explain why human disease does not result from *CLCNKA* mutations. Intriguingly, individuals carrying at least one copy of the T481S ClC-Kb gain-of-function mutation mentioned above display a lower hearing threshold than wild-type individuals.[35]

CFTR

Cystic fibrosis (CF) is the most common autosomal recessive genetic disease in Caucasians, and is debilitating and fatal; thus, long before the cloning of the Cystic Fibrosis Transmembrane Conductance Regulator (CFTR) gene, CF had been the focus of extensive physiological study. It was apparent that lung epithelium from patients with CF was lacking cAMP-activated Cl^- conductance, as well as dramatically increased apical Na^+ conductance.[25] These seemingly irreconcilable phenotypes resulted in the naming of the "CF" gene as a regulator of conductances, not as a Cl^- channel.[103] In fact, even after the successful cloning of the CFTR gene in 1989,[57,103,104] it wasn't until the creation of a $CFTR^{-/-}$ knockout mouse in 1993 that CFTR was definitively described as a Cl^- channel.[38] The $CFTR^{-/-}$ knockout demonstrated that there are actually two Cl^- conductances that are dysfunctional in CF patients and in the $CFTR^{-/-}$ mouse, and that the CFTR biophysical characteristics did not match the large outwardly rectifying currents (ORCC) that were for years believed to be the dominant Cl^- conductance.[38] Instead, CFTR regulated these ORCC currents.[25] Later work demonstrated that CFTR could regulate other channels like the epithelial sodium channel ENaC and the ATP sensitive K^+ channel ROMK2.[113]

CFTR (Figure 31.3) is now known to be a member of the ABC (ATP-binding cassette) superfamily of transporters; a vast gene family found in all phyla, responsible for transporting everything from metabolic products, lipids, and sterols, to drugs[3] and uric acid.[140] CFTR is a member of the C branch of the ABC family (ABCC7), characterized by having two large multi-helix transmembrane domains (TMD) and two intracellular nucleotide-binding domains (NBD).[3] CFTR, uniquely among the ABC proteins, also possesses an extra, highly-charged cytoplasmic domain, termed the regulatory or "R" domain.[103] Perhaps not coincidentally, CFTR is also the only ABC transporter, among 48 expressed in humans,[3] shown to conduct Cl^-. Both the N- and C-terminus of the protein are cytosolic, and the C-terminus contains the amino acid sequence DTRL, a sequence that is known to interact with the "PDZ" domains often found on scaffolding and linker proteins upon which regulatory protein complexes can be built.[41,82] CFTR is therefore a single channel among a large family of anion transporters, much like the CLC and SLC26A gene families, further demonstrating the relative uniqueness of proteins that are Cl^- channels and how many appear to be derivatives of exchangers or transporters.

CFTR can most aptly be characterized as activated by cAMP-dependent phosphorylation, although the activation of the channel is actually a complicated and slow process. First, the R domain needs to be phosphorylated by the catalytic subunit of protein kinase A (PKA) (activated directly by cAMP-binding)[38]; second, ATP needs to be bound (and hydrolyzed) within the conserved walker A- and B-binding sites of the NBD domains.[39] Once activated, the Cl^- currents show little or no voltage-dependence, display a linear I/V relation, show no Ca^{2+}-dependence, and have an anion selectivity sequence of $Br^- > Cl^- > I^- > F^-$.[3,131] Single channel properties are reflective of the whole cell current characteristics: linear I/V relationship under symmetrical Cl^- concentrations; 10−11 pS single channel conductance; activation by catalytic subunit of PKA; and channel-gating coupled to ATP hydrolysis.[145]

In a recurring theme that may be the single common characteristic among the various identified Cl^- channels, for many years there was no identified high affinity or specific CFTR inhibitors. Common Cl^- channel inhibitors like glibenclamide, DPC, NPPB, and niflumic acid provided low affinity pore blocking, but DIDS and other stilbene derivatives have little effect. In the CF lung there would be little use for CFTR

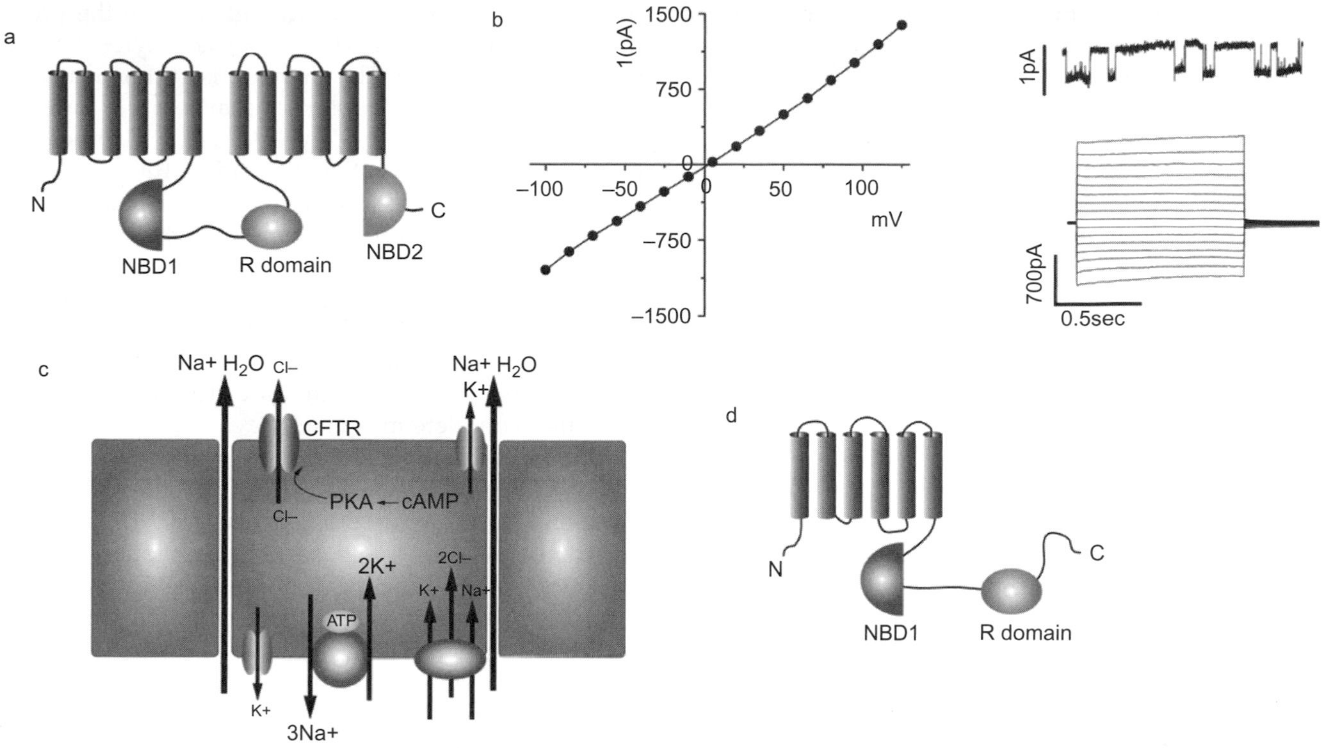

FIGURE 31.3 **Cystic fibrosis transmembrane conductance regulator (CFTR).** (a) Topography of CFTR. (b) I/V relationship, single channel recordings, and whole cell current records of CFTR heterologously expressed in CHO cells (Woodward and Guggino, unpublished data). (c) CFTR mediated Cl^- conductance drives fluid secretion in secretory airway epithelium cells. (d) Topography of kidney localized CFTR splice variant TNR-CFTR.

inhibitors therapeutically; however, CFTR expression has also been linked to fluid secretion in the kidney (see discussion of polycystic kidney disease below) and in the human gut. Specifically, toxin from *Cholera* increases cAMP levels and induces secretory diarrhea, a loss of fluids and salts that can be lethal.[74,131] The severity and pervasiveness of cholera has led to a substantial commitment of time and money to finding specific inhibitors of the cAMP-dependent Cl^- secretion of the gut epithelium. High-throughput screens of small drug-like molecules, using a fluorescent halide-based assay has yielded two classes of specific CFTR inhibitors.[74,131] The first class includes members of the 2-thioxo-4-thiazolidinone chemical class, in particular a compound named CFTRinh-172 with an IC_{50} of 300 nM.[74] CFTRinh-172 inhibits by blocking the intracellular pore in a voltage-independent fashion and prolongs the channels closed time, is non-toxic at high concentrations, is excreted with little metabolism,[131] and has been shown to effectively reduce *Cholera*-induced fluid loss by 90% in mouse models.[74] The second class of inhibitors includes the glycine hydrazides, and specifically GlyH-101.[83] It appears to block the CFTR pore from the extracellular side, is voltage- and Cl^- concentration-dependent, and in a closed loop model of cholera, GlyH-101 reduced fluid secretion by

80%.[83,131] Both classes and their lead compounds, CFTRinh-172 and GlyH-101, appear to represent therapeutic avenues for cholera and polycystic kidney disease; however, the assays used to find them also present the possibility of finding CFTR activators. The past decade has seen the discovery of a number of correctors and potentiators, small molecules targeted to bind directly to the CFTR molecule and aid in folding or in changing the gating characteristics. A number of these compounds have begun clinical trials for treating CF patients, and represent a valid avenue for chronic CF therapy.

Before progressing to a discussion of CFTRs specific role in the kidney, it is appropriate to introduce CFTR function first in the context of the human lung. CFTR was originally cloned as the gene responsible for cystic fibrosis, a disease characterized by chronic lung infection, deteriorating lung function, pancreatic exocrine insufficiency, male infertility, meconium ileus, and gastrointestinal complications.[131] In each phenotype the dysfunction stems from the reduction in fluid secretion at each relevant epithelium. CFTR is normally apically localized, and when activated Cl^- leaves the cells and enters the lumen or airway this drives paracellular Na^+, leading to water movement into the lumen.[68] In the lung, the loss of the CFTR Cl^- conductance lowers the airway surface liquid volume (ASL), reduces the activity of the epithelial cilia, and reduces or abolishes the mucus clearance, leading to chronic infection.[124]

Currently, over 1500 CFTR mutations have been found in CF patients, representing a spectrum of disease severity directly proportional to the level of residual CFTR function. Null mutations result in no protein being produced, whereas other mutations can result in minor changes to channel-gating or cell surface expression. By far the most common CFTR mutation is the deletion of phenylalanine residue at position 508 (Δ508), carried by 90% of CF patients,[131] a mutation that causes misprocessing and trafficking, and results in no CFTR being expressed at the cell surface. Human CFTR mutations have been classified based on their severity into five classes. Class I mutants produce no CFTR, Class II includes the folding and processing mutants like Δ508, and Class III mutants produce CFTR that is trafficked to the membrane but have dysfunctional Cl⁻ conductance; all three classes result in severe lung disease and pancreatic insufficiency. Class IV mutants display less pronounced conductance abnormalities and often have no lung phenotypes, and Class V mutants are often asymptomatic and diagnosed only after they are found to be infertile or present with idiopathic pancreatitis.[20,21]

CFTR in the Kidney

CFTR expression is abundant in the human kidney. Early studies looking at CFTR mRNA or using RT-PCR found evidence for CFTR expression generally in the cortex and outer medulla. More specifically, CFTR was found all along the nephron, including proximal and distal tubules, thin and thick ascending limbs, and the collecting duct.[80,81] Immunostaining of CFTR protein showed CFTR expression again in the proximal and distal tubules, the tAL, and the cortical and inner medullary collecting ducts.[81] Functional studies using patch-clamp have identified CFTR-like currents in the proximal and distal tubules and the collecting ducts.[81] CFTR is also known to be expressed in the embryonic kidney, with upregulation in the ureteric bud during the later stages of branching morphogenesis.[25] Intriguingly, a large proportion of the overall CFTR expression in the kidney consists of a CFTR splice variant termed TNR-CFTR.[80] The TNR-CFTR mRNA is missing the final 145 bp including exons 13 and 14, creating an early stop codon. The splicing may be regulated by snRNAs U11 and U12, which co-localize to the same areas of the kidney as the TNR-CFTR isoform.[117] This truncation corresponds to a loss of the second TMD and NBD, as well as 7% of the R domain in the final protein. The TNR-CFTR is therefore a "half" transporter, similar to many other members of the ABC family, and like those other ABC transporters, the remaining half molecule is enough to give the protein function. When expressed in *Xenopus* oocytes the TNR-CFTR is a functional Cl⁻ channel, is still activated my cAMP and PKA, and possesses many of the same biophysical traits as the wild-type CFTR.[80] Its processing, however, seems less efficient,[80] and little makes it to the plasma membrane, but instead it localizes to intracellular vesicles.[81] More generally, TNR-CFTR is found mostly in the renal medulla, and has an interesting developmental expression pattern. In mice, the expression of TNR-CFTR increases throughout embryonic kidney development, reaching its highest level at birth.[81] The functional significance of TNR-CFTR remains a complete mystery.

CFTR as a Kidney Cl⁻ Channel

Although the expression levels of CFTR in kidney are comparable to those of the lung, there is no clear CF kidney phenotype, with the exception of increased risk of hyperoxaluria or insufficient citrate-induced kidney stones; a fact that many have taken as evidence that CFTR is not very important in salt handling in the kidney, and yet CFTR is known to play important roles in renal diseases like ADPKD. Many have attributed the lack of phenotypes to a redundancy in Cl⁻ channels present in the kidney. Mouse CFTR⁻/⁻ knockout models often show little or no lung CF phenotype, a discrepancy explained by the upregulation of Ca²⁺-activated Cl⁻ channels (TMEM16s;[62]) to compensate for the loss of CFTR Cl⁻ conductances. Likewise in the kidney, other types of Cl⁻ channels could be compensating for the missing functional CFTR in CF patients. However, CFTRs functional role in the kidney could be more regulatory, thus CF renal phenotypes more subtle. Recent work looking at CFTR in the apical membrane of mouse cortical collecting duct principal cells demonstrates the difficulty in establishing CFTRs function as a Cl⁻ channel and not as a regulator of other channels. Lu et al.[72] definitively demonstrated CFTR Cl⁻ channel activity on the apical membrane of mouse principal cells, and plausibly suggest that it could represent a short-circuit current meant to regulate Na⁺ absorption and K⁺ secretion. However, they concede that it is just as likely that phosphorylation of CFTR could act as a modulatory switch on ROMK activity, and thus exert an influence on K⁺ secretion.[72] To complicate matters further, the prevailing model of ion movement in principal cells has Cl⁻ being reabsorbed mainly through a paracellular pathway, suggesting that for CFTR to have an effect it would need to represent a very large conductance, much larger than that measured by Lu et al. in mouse principal cells.[72] In fact, there is ample evidence that in the kidney and elsewhere CFTRs main function may be to regulate other ion channels.

CFTR as a Regulator of ENaC

From before its initial molecular identification, CFTR has been shown to regulate an ORCC Cl⁻ conductance and a Na⁺ conductance.[113] In the airway of CF patients (but not in the sweat ducts), increased Na⁺ absorption via the epithelial sodium channel, ENaC, is observed due to loss of the normal CFTR-mediated inhibition; however, the mechanism of regulation remains unclear. Currently, there are multiple hypotheses to explain how CFTR regulates ENaC. One possibility is that intracellular Cl⁻ regulates ENaC activity. This is supported by data showing that CFTR Cl⁻ conductance is necessary for ENaC regulation, and in some but not all cell types replacing CFTR Cl⁻ current with CLC-mediated Cl⁻ currents can also inhibit ENaC currents.[12] These data are conflicted by the lack of identified Cl⁻-binding sites on ENaCs intracellular domains, and by studies showing that alternative Cl⁻ channels like CaCCs cannot inhibit ENaC.[12]

A second theory proposes CFTR exerts its regulatory effects through intermediary proteins as part of a large protein complex. CFTR contains a PDZ-binding domain that enables it to interact with linking proteins like ezrin-binding phosphoprotein 50 (EB50) and NHERF1. NHERF1, through its PZD2 region, can bind YAP65 which recognizes the PY motif on the C-terminus of ENaC, creating a complex with both CFTR and ENaC. C-Yes, a c-Src kinase, is a known inhibitor of ENaC and can bind to YAP65. Thus, CFTR, in aiding the assembly of the protein complex, inhibits the activity of ENaC and the dissolution of the complex, e.g., from CFTR dysfunction or mutation, liberates ENaC from C-Yes inhibition.[42] However, this possibility has not been demonstrated in heterologous expression systems.[12]

A third possibility involves CFTR interacting directly with ENaC to cause inhibition. Patch-clamp studies of ENaC subunits and CFTR in proteoliposomes, presumably free of contaminating complex proteins, showed that CFTR directly affects the gating of ENaC single channels. FRET studies have demonstrated an association of less than 10 nM of the two proteins in vitro, and co-immunoprecipitation experiments show the two physically interact.[12] However, with the exception of the single channel results, the evidence does not strictly rule out the possibility of CFTR and ENaC interacting indirectly as part of a protein complex.

The relationship between CFTR and ENaC in the kidney appears as conflicting as that found for the airways and seat ducts. Some work has shown that CFTR inhibits ENaC in the kidney, similar to the relationship found in airways. Experiments in M-1 cortical collecting duct cells showed that activation of PKA reduced the amiloride-sensitive apical Na⁺ current.[66] However, other studies have found CCD cells from mice carrying a mutation in ENaC, known to cause Liddles's syndrome (deletion of the PY motif in the c-terminus as the β-subunit ENaC), display increased Na⁺ absorption as compared to wild-type when treated with dD-arginine vasopressin. A similar increase is seen in the CFTR-mediated apical current, implying vasopressin causes increases in both conductances,[130] an idea consistent with the cAMP-induced increases in both CFTR and ENaC seen in sweat ducts.[101] Simply put, the evidence for CFTR regulating ENaC in the kidney is sparse, and it remains unknown whether or not it acts as an inhibitor, activator or neither. It may require a final determination of how CFTR regulates ENaC in airway tissue before a renewed focus can be brought on CFTR and ENaC in the kidney.

CFTR as a Regulator of ROMK

The inward rectifier potassium channel ROMK (Kir1.1) and its isoforms are expressed highly in the distal nephron, where it plays a major role in ATP sensitive K⁺ secretion.[72] Some of their defining traits are lack of sensitivity to the common K⁺ channel blocker tetraethylammonium (TEA), and inhibition by ATP and sulfonylureas like glibenclamide.[113] But when the ROMK2 isoform was expressed in the Xenopus oocytes, it was no longer sensitive to glibenclamide. Other ATP-sensitive K⁺ channels require ABC transporter subunits, SUR1 and SUR2 (ABCC8 and ABCC9), for glibenclamide sensitivity, but neither SUR1 nor SUR2 is known to be expressed in the kidney. However, CFTR is expressed in the same distal nephron cells as ROMK channels, and when CFTR and ROMK2 are co-expressed in Xenopus oocytes, the glibenclamide sensitivity is restored.[113] Subsequent work has demonstrated that CFTR is also necessary for ROMK's sensitivity to Mg-ATP in CCD mouse cells. Lu et al.[72] hypothesize that water diuresis and the resulting low cAMP-PKA would promote the CFTR–ROMK interaction, and so cytoplasmic ATP would inhibit excessive K⁺ secretion. However, during antidiuresis when PKA levels are high, the phosphorylation of CFTR will free ROMK from ATP sensitivity and promote K⁺ secretion.[72] The specifics of the ROMK–CFTR interaction are unknown, but it is probably similar to the better-understood Kir6.x/SUR complex of pancreatic β-cells. Kir6.x-subunits form tetramers, with each subunit associated with a SURx subunit to create an eight unit complex.[2] Although the CFTR regulation of ROMK appears functionally very important, there is no reported K⁺ secretion phenotype in the distal nephron in CF patients.

CFTR as a Regulator of SLC26As

CFTR is also a demonstrated regulator of transporters from the SLC family of anion transporters. Earlier research showed that CFTR could interact with and activate SLC26A3 and A6, conferring cAMP sensitivity on these two transporters.[116] In the pancreatic ducts, HCO_3 secretion is a critical component of the function of the secretory epithelium, a function disrupted in patients with severe CF. Wang et al.[136] showed specifically that the SLC26A6 HCO_3^-/Cl^- exchanger was critical for HCO_3^- secretion, and that its function was regulated by co-localized CFTR expression in the luminal membrane. Further work demonstrated that a conserved region of the SLC26A transporters, the STAS domain, interacted directly with the R domain of CFTR.[59] The binding of the STAS and R domains activates SLC26A6, but also dramatically increase the Cl^- conductance of CFTR by increasing the channels open probability six-fold.[59] Interestingly, SLC26A6 is expressed throughout the kidney, but appears most prominently in the apical–luminal membrane of the proximal tubule where it is responsible for Cl^-, HCO_3^-, oxalate, and formate exchange.[59] CFTR expression is also reported in the proximal tubule, and although there is no current evidence of their interaction in the kidney it seems plausible.

CFTR more recently has also been demonstrated to be a regulator of one of the two true Cl^- channel members of the SLC26A family, SLC26A9. Both SLC26A9 and CFTR co-localize to the apical membrane of human bronchial epithelial (HBE) cells, where cAMP leads to the co-activation of SLC26A9 and CFTR Cl^- channels.[13] The nature of the CFTR–SLC26A9 interaction is similar to the other CFTR–SLC interactions, the conserved STAS domain of SLC26A9 binds directly to the R domain of CFTR.[17] However, there are conflicting reports as to the exact regulatory nature of the CFTR–SLC26A9 relationship. Bertrand et al.[13] report that endogenous SLC26 currents in HBE cells are activated by functional CFTR; whereas Chang et al.[17] report heterologous co-expression of an NBD + R domain CFTR construct with SLC26A9 in *Xenopus* oocytes results in the inhibition of SLC26A9 currents. What is clear is that the conserved STAS domain of the SLC26A channels and transporters strongly interacts with CFTR, an interaction that may extend to many of the SLC26A members. SLC26A9 is expressed mainly in the lung, but the other described SLC26A pure Cl^- channel, SLC26A7, is expressed throughout the kidney, and in particular cells of the cortical collecting ducts, an area also high in CFTR expression. The role of a possible interaction between SLC26A7 and CFTR in the cortical collecting duct is an important area for future investigation.

CFTR and Endocytosis

A new area of CFTR research has begun investigating CFTRs role in acidification of endosomes of the proximal tubule. Generally, CF patients have shown increased renal clearance of some drugs including aminoglycosides, and more specifically a cohort of patients with at least one copy of the Δ508 CFTR mutation showed significantly higher levels of albuminuria and LMW proteinuria.[56] $CFTR^{-/-}$ knockout mice have significantly increased excretion of LMW Clara Cell protein (CC16), and decreased uptake of radio-labeled ^{124}I-β2microglobulin and aminoglycosides, similar to human CF patients. Significantly, the $CFTR^{-/-}$ mice also demonstrated decreased cubilin expression in the S3 segment of the proximal tubule, a finding correlating with the observed increase of cubilin excretion.[56] Cubilin is a lipoprotein receptor and, along with megalin, is critical for the uptake of LMW proteins. In the $CFTR^{-/-}$ mouse, however, megalin is not affected, thus it appears CFTR is specifically reducing cubilin expression. Cubilin recycling to the apical membrane via endosomes is critical to maintain apical cubilin expression and for LWM protein uptake. The sorting and recycling of endosomes is pH-dependent.[56] CFTR has been localized to the apical region in proximal tubule cells and specifically it co-distributes with ClC-5 and Rab5a in endosomes,[56] where it is proposed to aid in providing a negative current shunt for the interior of the endosomes. CFTR would offset the build-up of positively-charged H^+ during acidification, a role similar to that proposed for the Cl^-/H^+ exchanger ClC-5.[56] The evidence of CFTRs involvement in receptor-mediated endocytosis from CF patient studies and $CFTR^{-/-}$ mice is compelling, but the mechanism remains unconfirmed, although it seems likely CFTR, along with ClC-5 and possibly other Cl^- channels, all contribute to the pH regulation of the proximal tubule endosomes.

Ca^{2+}-Activated Cl^- Channels (CaCC): TMEM16/Anoctamin

For 30 years Ca^{2+}-activated Cl^- channels (CaCC) with similar biophysical characteristics have been studied in a wide range of tissue and cell types, including secretory epithelia, egg cells, cardiac, smooth, and skeletal muscles, neurons, olfactory and photoreceptors, hepatocytes, and beta cells.[45,47] The classic CaCC characteristics are best described by the endogenous CaCCs of *Xenopus* oocytes or the CaCCs of acinar cells in the salivary gland (Figure 31.4). These classic CaCC channels are activated by small amounts of cytosolic Ca^{2+} (0.2–5 μM)[45] either from extracellular influx or store release. Activation appears to occur through direct binding of Ca^{2+} to the channel. When cytosolic Ca^{2+} is

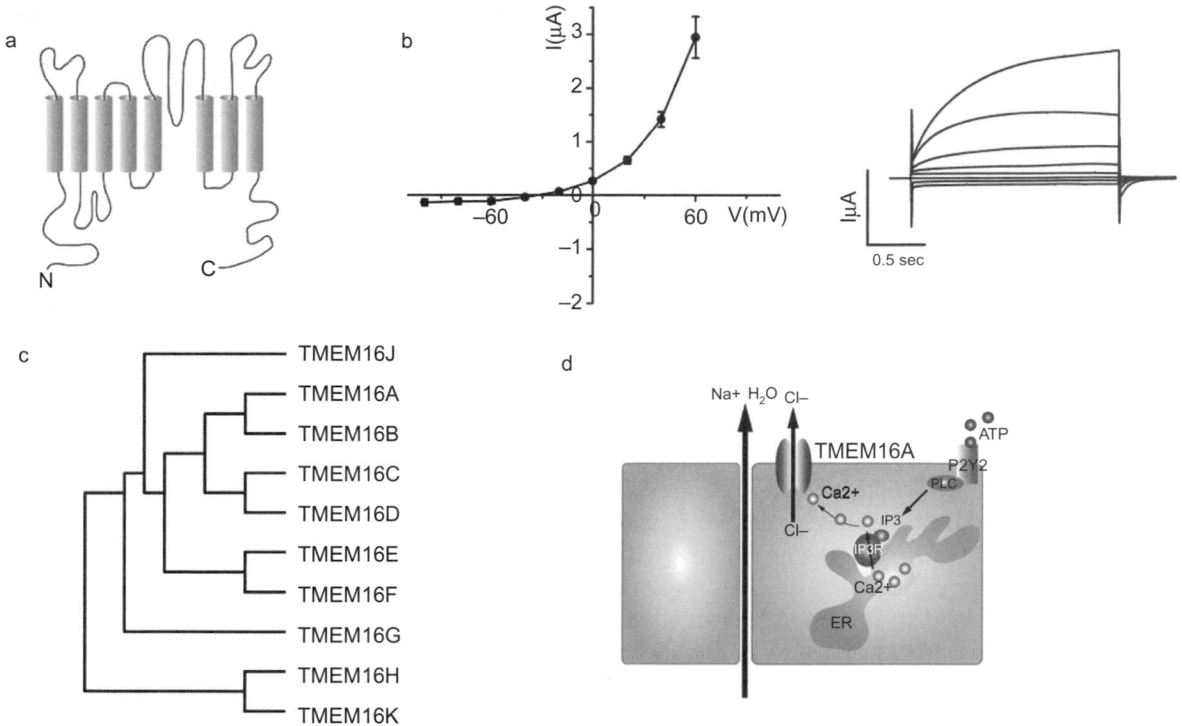

FIGURE 31.4 **Ca²⁺ activated Cl⁻ channels (CaCC), the TMEM16s.** (a) Topography of TMEM16A. (b) I/V relationship and whole cell classical endogenous CaCC currents of *Xenopus* oocytes mediated by TMEM16A (Woodward and Guggino, unpublished data). (c) Phylogenetic tree of human TMEM16 members. (*Reprinted from Schroeder, B. C., Cheng, T., Jan, Y. N., and Jan, L. Y. (2008). Expression cloning of TMEM16A as a calcium-activated chloride channel subunit. Cell* **134**, *1019−1029, with permission from Elsevier.[111]*) (d) Typical ATP/Ca²⁺-activated Cl⁻ and fluid secretion in secretory epithelium mediated by TMEM16A.

limiting, CaCC shows an outward rectifying I/V relationship, but as cytosolic Ca²⁺ increases the rectification diminishes.[45,85,138,139] The open probability appears to be voltage-dependent and the single channel conductance is small 1−3 pS, although a variety of conductance sizes has been reported.[45] Classic CaCCs, like other anion channels, are relatively non-selective, with Na⁺ permeability being roughly 10% that of Cl⁻. Among anions the selectivity sequence is $SCN^- > NO_3^- > I^- > Br^- > Cl^- > F^-$.[45]

The ubiquitous nature of CaCC channels makes describing their physiological function difficult; it plays different roles in each cell type. In *Xenopus* oocytes CaCC plays a major role in blocking polyspermy fertilization of the egg. Fertilization generates a Ca²⁺ wave across the membrane, activating the CaCC channels and depolarizing the egg.[45] In secretory epithelia Cl⁻ secretion is critical to draw Na⁺ and water across the apical membrane, and CaCCs appear to contribute to the Cl⁻ conductance across the apical membrane, often in an ATP-dependent manner.[45]

Similar to many other epithelial cell types, kidney epithelia have demonstrated CaCC currents and channels, including rabbit distal convoluted tubules, proximal convoluted tubules, and cortical collecting duct.

However, most of the work has been done on a mouse medullary collecting duct cell line, IMCD-K2.[15,99] Using the IMCD-K2 line, Qu et al.[99] described CaCC currents that they suggested were the same as those found endogenously in *Xenopus* oocytes. These currents can be activated by ATP and rely on intracellular Ca²⁺ store release for activation.[15] They are co-expressed in IMCD-K2 cells with CFTR, and while their specific function in the collecting duct is not known, it may be similar to the Cl⁻ secretory role they play in airway epithelium. Because CaCC currents may be controlled by hormones, the CaCC-mediated Cl⁻ secretion in the distal kidney may help fine-tune urine composition.[45]

The molecular identity of the CaCC channels was for decades an elusive dream, with a stream of potential candidates including the CLCAs and the bestrophins, whose biophysical characteristics matched some of the classic CaCC characteristics, but not all. Recently, a new family of genes has been proposed to represent the CaCCs, the TMEM16 or Anoctamin gene family which, unlike previous candidates, shares all of the biophysical characteristics of the classic CaCC channels. The confidence in this new family of proteins as CaCC comes from a number of factors, not the least of which was the methods used to discover their identities. Three different research groups, using three totally different methodologies, each independently arrived at the conclusion that TMEM16A/Aco 1 was the classic CaCC. Schroeder et al.[111] took advantage of the unique property of Axolotl (*Ambystoma mexicanum*) salamander oocytes of not having any CaCC currents. They used these oocytes to screen a cDNA library from size fractionated RNA isolated from *Xenopus* oocytes resulting in the identification and cloning of a gene that coded for a 979 amino acid protein, the *Xenopus* ortholog to the human TMEM16A gene. Expression of TMEM16A in the Axolotl oocytes produced Cl⁻ currents identical in most of the biophysical properties that define the classic CaCCs. Schroeder et al.[111] also showed that TMEM16s are expressed in salivary glands, as expected if they are the CaCCs. A second group, Yang et al.[146] used a bioinformatic search targeting putative channel or transporter-like genes with more than two transmembrane domains. Their search turned up TMEM16A, which met their criteria but became their focus because it had no described function, and the TMEM16 family has 10 human homologs. They renamed the TMEM16s anoctamins because the channels appeared to be anion selective with eight (OCT) transmembrane domains.[47] Yang et al.[146] tested the biophysical properties of TMEM16A when expressed in HEK cells, and like Schroeder et al.[111] found their properties to be very similar to those described above for the classic CaCCs, although the pharmacological sensitivities of the overexpressed TMEM16A channels in HEK cells were far more sensitive to the classic anion channel blockers DIDS, NPPB, and NFA than their endogenous counterparts.[47] Yang et al.[146] went further, and showed that mutating the putative poor region, between TM5 and TM6, disrupted anion permeability markedly. Importantly, like Schroeder et al. they showed that TMEM16s were expressed in tissues where classic CaCCs have been described, and demonstrated that knocking-down TMEM16A in acinar cells of the salivary gland reduced the endogenous CaCC currents, and reduced saliva production upon pilocarpine application. And finally, a third group, Caputo et al.,[16] identified TMEM16s through a microarray screen of airway epithelial cells treated with IL-4, a treatment known to increase CaCC currents in these cells. They isolated a group of membrane proteins with no known function, including TMEM16A, then generated RNAi against each of the most likely candidates and attempted to knock-down the endogenous CaCC activity inCFPAC-1 and CFBE410 cells. Activity was assayed using a halide sensitive YFP protein and short-circuit currents, and siRNA TMEM16A was found to very effectively reduce the endogenous CaCC currents. Caputo et al.[16] went on to express TMEM16A in FRT cells, and again

described their biophysical properties as being almost identical as those known for the classic CaCC currents.

The TMEM16 family of genes is well-conserved, with members found throughout eukaryotic phyla; however, there appears to be an increased representation in mammals.[47] Humans have 10 members of the TMEM16 family (A—H, J—K) or Ano 1—10, and their predicted topology has both N- and C-termini intracellular, eight transmembrane domains, and the pore region located between TM5 and TM6.[146] Interestingly, no clear Ca^{2+}-binding domain has yet been discovered in the TMEM16s. In TMEM16A there is no EF hand region or CaM-binding sites.[47] However, there does appear to be a Ca^{2+} bowl structure, similar to that found in BK Ca^{2+}-activated K^+ channels. This same structure was predicted by Hartzell et al.[45] for classical CaCCs before the identification of the TMEM16 genes based on the demonstrated μmolar range Ca^{2+} affinity.[45] The molecular diversity of the TMEM16 family could help explain the differences in described biophysical properties of endogenous CaCCs in different cell and tissue types. Members of the TMEM16 family may have different channel properties or they may heterodimerize to create chimera channels. The TMEM16s also exhibit multiple splice variants, TMEM16A has at least four,[16] and these variants were found to have different channel properties.[16] The likelihood that members of the TMEM16 family other than TMEM16A are anion channels is high, because of the close sequence homology among the members. And although most of the descriptive work has focused on TMEM16A, Cl⁻ currents have also been described for TMEM16B (Ano2) which is found in olfactory receptors,[27] and for TMEM16F and TMEM16K (Ano 6 and 10).[110] In each case, like TMEM16A they share many similarities with the classic CaCC, but each has some differences as well, supporting the idea that the diversity of the TMEM16 family corresponds to the diversity of CaCCs.

The TMEM16s are only now getting the in-depth attention necessary to discern how TMEM16s function as CaCCs, which ones are expressed in which cell and tissue type, and what role if any they may play in human disease. Even before TMEM16A was known to be a Cl⁻ channel it had been observed to be upregulated in tumors, but why is unknown.[27,47] Initial reports on the Cl⁻ channel functions of TMEM16A have focused on tissues and cells historically known to have large CaCC currents, including airway epithelial cells. In these cells CaCC currents have long been seen as a potential target in treating cystic fibrosis; by upregulating CaCC currents the lost anion conductance from dysfunctional CFTR could be replaced, and disease severity lessened. Mouse models of CF, strangely devoid of the debilitating lung systems found in

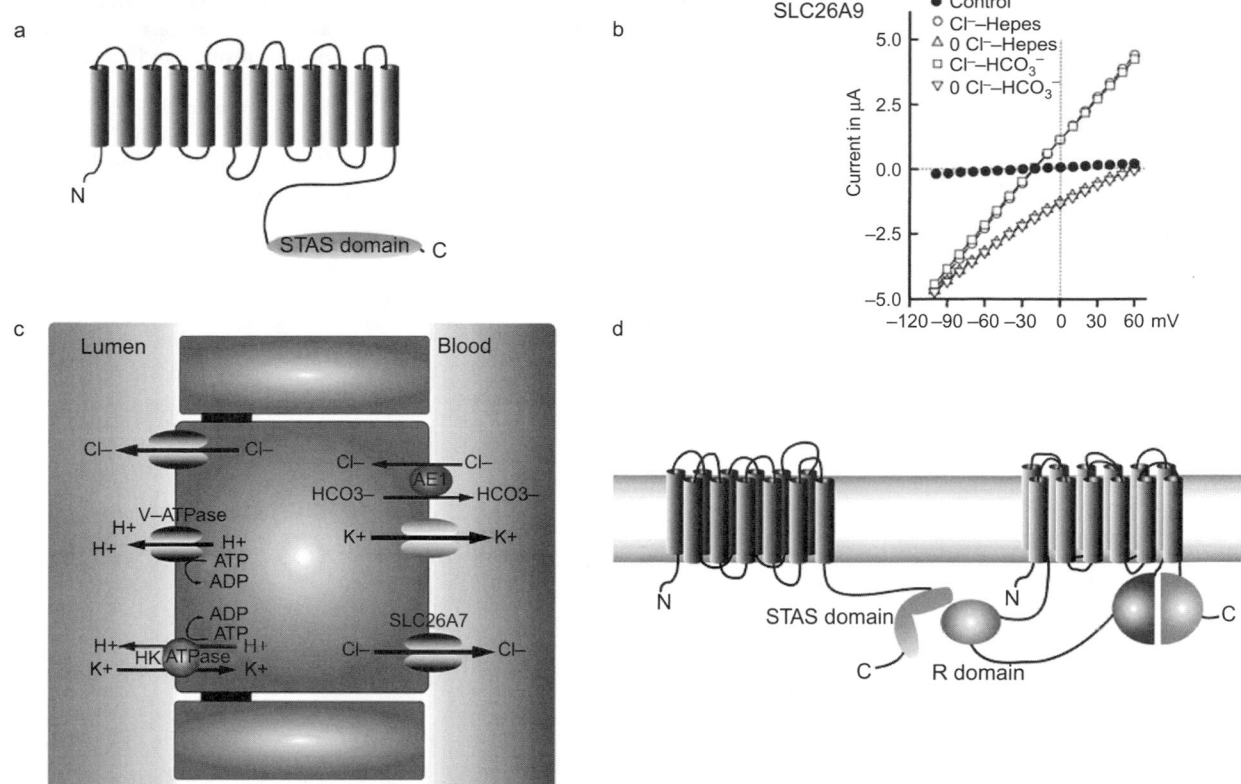

FIGURE 31.5   Solute carrier (SLC) 26A7 and A9. (a) Proposed, although not experimentally verified, topography of the SLC26 proteins. (b) I/V relationship from whole cell currents in *Xenopus* oocytes cells expressing SLC26A9. *(Reprinted with permission from Dorwart, M. R., Shcheynikov, N., Wang, Y., Stippec, S., and Muallem, S. (2007). SLC26A9 is a Cl⁻ channel regulated by the WNK kinases. J. Physiol. 584(1), 333–345.[26a])* (c) SLC26A7 provides a pH sensitive basolateral Cl⁻ conductance in α-intercalated cells of the collecting duct. (d) SLC26A9 is regulated through direct interactions between the SLC26A9s STAS domain and the R domain of CFTR.

humans, have been shown to express TMEM16A at much higher levels than in wild-type airway epithelia, strongly supporting the targeting of TMEM16A in humans as a CF treatment.[62] It is not clear what functional role the TMEM16s play in the kidney. Presumably they underlie the known CaCC currents identified in the kidney, but which ones and how remains unknown. Yang et al.[146] showed specifically that TMEM16A is expressed in the epithelia of proximal tubules and the distal renal tubules. In mice TMEM16F mRNA was found in the kidney at high levels, as were slightly lower levels of TMEM16K and H. Going forward it will be exciting to learn more about the TMEM16 family, and specifically their role in anion regulation in the kidney and the role they play in diseases such as ADPKD.

Solute Carrier 26 Transporters

As discussed earlier, the distinction between Cl⁻ transporter and Cl⁻ channel can be the position of one or two amino acids, and just as recently resolved crystal structures revealed members of the CLC Cl⁻ channel

family to be transporters, recent studies of the large SLC26 transporter family revealed at least two of its members bear the hallmarks of Cl⁻ channels, not transporters. Specifically, SLC26A9 and SLC26A7 appear to operate solely as Cl⁻ channels, and have little or no bicarbonate permeability.[89] The SLC26 family is large and very diverse, much like the CLC gene family, and many of its members still lack identified physiological function, including SLC26A7 and SLC26A9 (Figure 31.5). However, present work does suggest both may play important roles in secretory epithelia in areas of the lung and kidney. As discussed earlier, SLC26A9 is expressed highly in lung epithelia, and may be regulated by CFTR[13] via the highly-conserved SLC26 STAS domain.[17] When expressed in HEK cells or *Xenopus* oocytes, the SLC26A9 channel is constitutively active, with a linear to slight inward rectification I/V relation,[13,17,26,26a,89] is only slightly permeable to bicarbonate, and is not pH sensitive.[26,26a,89] And while SLC26A9 is most highly expressed in ciliated bronchial airway epithelial and alveolar cells, its expression is widespread.[26]

SLC26A7, on the other hand, is very highly expressed in the human kidney, including in the renal

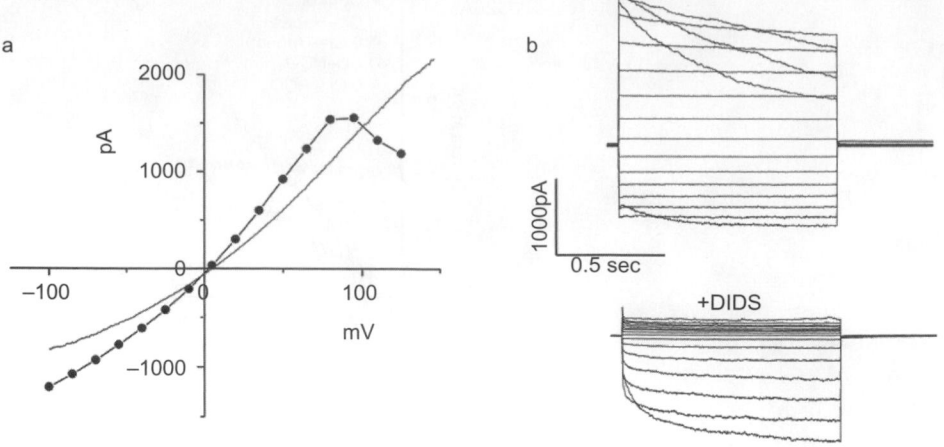

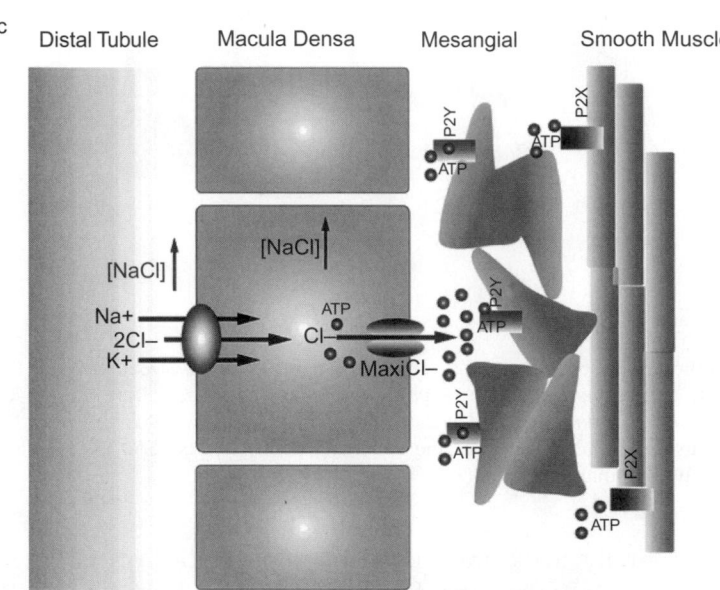

outer medullary collecting duct, the thick ascending limb, and the apical membrane of proximal tubule.[26] Like SLC26A9, SLC26A7 is constitutively active, has a linear I/V relation, is not permeable to bicarbonate,[58] but unlike SLC26A9, SLC26A7 is very sensitive to pH.[26,89] Acidic pHi increases the selectivity of SLC26A7 to Cl^-,[58] apparently through intracellular H^+ regulation of the channel. SLC26A7s pHi sensitivity has prompted the hypothesis that it may function as a pHi sensor[89] or function in Cl^--loading in parietal cells. The physiological function of SLC26A7 in the kidney remains unknown, although it is expressed on the basolateral membrane of the alpha-intercalated cells of the outer medullary collecting duct, cells that secrete acid[116,120] as part of the kidney's role in regulating the blood's acid–base balance (Figure 31.5). It would seem that the pHi sensitivity of SLC26A7 would make it an affective pHi sensor in alpha-intercalating cells just as in parietal cells, and it could again function as a Cl^--loading mechanism and therefore would be important

in the apical secretion of H^+ from the cells. Currently no human diseases are associated with SLC26A7 or SLC27A9 dysfunction; however, it seems likely that further work will reveal their importance in human and kidney physiology.

Volume-Regulated Anion Channels

The recent success in discovering the molecular identity of the CaCC only highlights the need to identify the last remaining functional group of Cl^- channels, the volume-regulated anion channels (VRAC) (Figure 31.6). VRACs are found in every cell type as part of the normal housekeeping functions possessed by all cells. In mammalian cells when an osmotic imbalance occurs and water moves into the cell, threatening the integrity of the membrane, the cell initiates the regulatory volume decrease (RVD) response consisting of the efflux of K^+ and Cl^- ions, as well as bicarbonate and amino acids; through the loss of these osmolites the osmotic balance can be regained and the cell shrinks. In the dynamic osmotic conditions along the mammalian nephron the VRAC channels may play a dominant role in the RVD response, protecting the cells from osmotic harm. In addition to cell volume regulation, VRAC channels are known to play roles in maintaining resting potentials, aiding in vectorial Cl⁻ transport, salt and fluid secretion, cell proliferation and differentiation,[85] cell migration,[92] apoptosis,[91] and ATP secretion.[85,92] In addition to VRACs role in RVD in kidney cells, another role has been described for the large conductance maxi-anion type of VRAC channels which appear concentrated in the macula densa cells of the thick ascending limb (TAL). Macular densa cells function to sense changes in the luminal NaCl concentration, and signal the regulator mechanism necessary to bring salt levels back to normal via tubuloglomerular feedback (TGF).[10] Bell et al.[10] found that maxi-anion channels in the macula densa cells could conduct ATP, and did so under conditions of experimentally high luminal NaCl. It is not yet clear how the maxi-anion channels are activated by the high luminal NaCl concentrations, nor is it clear exactly what role ATP plays in signaling as compared to NO and PGE2.[11] But it is clear that ATP is important, and that the maxi-anion channels are the only described mechanism for its secretion from the macula densa cells, implying a very important role for the VRAC channels in the TAL. Ultimately only the molecular identity of the VRAC channels will further our understanding of their function in the kidney.

The general biophysical characteristics of the VRAC channels are similar to other known anion channels, including its relative non-selectivity, and its outward rectification. The most unique characteristics of VRAC channels are their voltage-dependence: depolarization above $+60$ mV causes time and voltage inactivation, with negative potentials removing inactivation.[84,85] Intracellular Mg^{2+} and extracellular protons appear to accelerate this inactivation. The anion selectivity sequence is $SNC^- > I^- > NO_3^- > Br^- > Cl^- > F^-$, but VRAC channels are also permeable to amino acids like glutamate and aspartate, polyols, and ATP.[84,85] This promiscuity is in part due to the large calculated pore size of ~ 11 Å.[85] Pharmacologically, the usual nonspecific anion channel blockers also work on VRAC channels, $NPPB > DIDS > NFA$,[84] some, like DIDS, show a strong voltage-dependence to its block, demonstrating it can only block from one direction. The single channel properties suggest VRAC channels are a heterogeneous group consisting of mini-anion channels (0.1–8 pS), volume-sensitive outwardly rectifying channels (VSOR: 20–80 pS), and maxi-anion channels (100–400 pS), although most fall into either the VSOR or maxi-anion groups.

Because of their extremely important physiological role in TGF, a further look at the maxi-anion channel subclass of VRAC channels is deserved. As mentioned above, maxi-anion channels have very large single channel conductances that increase with saturating concentrations of Cl⁻ in excess of 640 pS.[107] In contrast to the characteristics described above for the classic VSOR type of VRAC channels, the maxi-anion channels have a much larger pore size of 1.16–1.42 nm, which again helps to explain its ability to conduct ATP. Like other VRAC channels, maxi-anion channels are voltage-dependent with inactivation at depolarizing potentials, but unlike other VRAC channels it also inactivates at hyperpolarizing potentials, resulting in a bell shaped voltage-dependence of open channel probability.[107] At potentials with little or no inactivation, the I/V relationship is linear. Further questions about maxi-anion channel structure and function in both the kidney and beyond will, as for the entire VRAC group, depend on resolving its molecular identity. This is perhaps the most pressing issue in all of anion channel research currently, and remains a gaping hole in our fundamental understanding of how anion conductances shape cellular function and life.

Other Cl⁻ Channels

GABA and Glycine Receptor Channels

The GABA (GABAA, GABAC) and glycine receptor (GlyR) Cl⁻ channels represent the only examples of anion channels within the cation channel gene families. Both GABA- and glycine-gated channels are members of the ligand-gated ion channel (LGIC) superfamily,[18] and share a large amount of structure homology with cation members of the same LGIC family, including the nicotinic acetylcholine (nACh) receptor channels and the 5HT3 receptors.[18] Like nACh channels, both the GABA and glycine receptor channels have a 5 subunit structure, with two alpha-, two beta-, and one gamma-subunit.[88] There are two GABA receptor channel groups that conduct anions, GABAA and GABAC, both are important for inhibitory synaptic transmission in the nervous system, and both have a $I^- > Cl^-$ permeability.[131] GABA receptors may play key roles in human disorders including epilepsy, multiple sleep disorders, and Alzheimer's.[18] GlyR channels are also important in synaptic inhibition in the nervous system, and have been linked to hyperekplexia[73,131] or human startle disease. GlyR channels have an ion selectivity sequence, $I^- > Br^- > Cl^- > F^-$, similar to the GABA channels, with a pore size around 5–6 Å,[88] slightly smaller than the other cation members of the LGIC family. The GlyR single channel conductance is variable depending on the arrangement and type of subunits, but most frequently is around 90 ps.[88] Though the GABA and GlyR channels play significant roles in human disease and are very important in the function of the human nervous system, they have not been shown to express in the human kidney and therefore their discussion will remain superficial.

Voltage-Dependent Anion-Selective Channel (VDAC)

Often in a discussion of anion channels the voltage-dependent anion selective channels (VDAC) are omitted, because of their believed confinement to the outer membranes of the mitochondria (hence their alternative name of mitochondria porins),[24] loose anion selectivity, and giant poor size. Thus, the logic goes, the VDAC channels are not comparable to the Cl^- channels that inhabit the other cellular membranes. However, their recent localization to the plasma membrane has elevated them to Cl^- channel status, if just barely. VDACs were first discovered on the membrane in human B-lymphocytes, and the subsequent development of an antibody lead to the description of VDAC surface localization in numerous cell types including epithelium. Subsequent work confirmed VDAC1 to be located within caveolins, or plasma membrane subcompartments, and found VDAC in proteomic surveys of the plasma membrane of human cells.[24] Perhaps most convincingly, VDAC proteins have been purified from both the plasma membrane (using a NH-SS-biotin label) and from the mitochondria, and compared via electrophoretic mobility, antibodies, and electrophysiological recordings in reconstructed lipid bilayers.[8,9,52] The question remained, however, what were they doing there? In the mitochondria, the VDAC family of proteins resident in the outer mitochondrial membrane is responsible for a number of functions, but probably not the regulation of Cl^- conductance. The VDAC proteins are 30–35 kDa proteins that contain a single alpha helix and 13, 16 or 19 transmembrane beta sheets.[24,114] When reconstituted in a lipid bilayer VDAC forms a very large 2–3 nm pore,[114] and is loosely voltage-dependent (40% of the initial conductance persists in the "closed" state).[107] Its Cl^-/K^+ permeability ratio is an astoundingly low 1.7–1.9,[107] but its single channel conductance of Cl^- is linear up to 10 nS with no saturation.[107] However, its primary function in mitochondria is probably more related to metabolite flux (including ATP, cytochrome c, and superoxide anions),[105] membrane composition, and an important role in apoptosis.[40]

There are a number of hypotheses as to the nature of the VDAC function on the plasma membrane. The voltage-dependence of VDAC means that at most resting potentials the channel should be closed,[24] alleviating the obvious lethal potential of a large, relatively nonselective pore in the plasma membrane. There is some evidence that VDAC may be an ATP release channel,[90,114] although there is also evidence that VDAC may inhibit ATP release.[24] Other proposed functions include plasma membrane VDAC1 as a redox enzyme which reduces extracellular ferricyanide in the presence of NADH.[5] Its role as a redox enzyme is supported by evidence that transfection of COS-7 cells with a VDAC1 construct increased the plasma membrane NADH:ferricyanide reductase activity 40-fold.[5] This VDAC1 function may play a role in the reductive activation of the anticancer drug 2-methyl-furanonaphthoquinone.[115] Finally, plasma membrane VDAC has been long hypothesized to be the maxi-anion channel found in many tissue types including the kidney. There exist many superficial similarities in the biophysical properties of each, which has lead for years to the acceptance that VDAC was the molecular identity of maxi-anion channels, even though there appear to be some vast differences in characteristics and localization. For instance, surface VDAC has been shown in epithelium,[24] but not specifically in kidney. Recently this hypothesis was tested directly by Sabirov et al.,[106] where they either knocked-out or knocked-down expression of the three VDAC isoforms, and found the endogenous maxi-anion channel of mouse embryonic fibroblasts (MEFs) unaltered, strongly arguing against VDACs being the molecular identity of maxi-anion channels. However, it is worth noting that expression of surface VDAC channels is not universal and could be very cell type-specific, thus in cell types other than MEFs VDAC could still be the previously identified maxi-anion channels that are critical for renal salt balance in the human kidney (see discussion above).

Tweety (Human Homolog hTTYH3)

The VDAC proteins are not the only recent entrant in the race to win the title "identity of maxi-anion channel." Using a rather novel bioinformatic methodology Susuki[122] screened for *Drosophila* genes that coded for proteins with four or more predicted transmembrane domains and a described behavioral abnormality. Suzuki found a gene, *tweety*, within the *flightless* locus, which matched his criteria, and its knockout resulted in loss of normal flight. Suzuki further found that *tweety* has a human homology, hTTYH3, a gene encoding a 523 amino acid protein. mRNA expression of mouse TTYH3 is found in most excitable tissues as well as kidney, fat cells, thymus, and uterus, and also a number of cell lines including kidney epithelial cells (OK, HEK, and MDCK lines).[122] Using a c-terminal antibody, TTYH3 was positively localized in the glomerulus of the kidney.[122] Other *tweety* genes may also be important in the human kidney, hTTYH2 mRNA has been shown to be upregulated in renal cell carcinoma.[48]

The electrophysiological characteristics of hTTYH3 do certainly show similarities to maxi-anion channels, but also to large conductance Ca^{2+}-activated Cl^- channels. Expression of hTTYH3 in CHO cells in the presence of ionomycin results in large linear Cl^- currents.[122] The ion selectivity for the hTTYH channel is $I^- > Br^- > Cl^-$, and the mutations of positively-charged amino acids in the pore region result in an appropriate reduction in the gluconate/Cl^- permeability ratio.[122] The large linear Cl^- currents of hTTYH3-expressing cells were not blocked by niflumic acid, DTT, ZnCl or SITS; however, the hTTYH3 currents were blocked by DIDS (10 µm).[122] Suzuki[122] also reports the single channels characteristic of the human *tweety* channel: large single channel conductance (250 pS) in the presence of high cytosolic Ca^{2+}; and a linear I−V relationship.

Although, like the VDAC channels, *tweety* channels share characteristics with the well-defined maxi-anion channels, but like the VDAC channels, recent experiments suggest they probably do not represent the molecular indentity of the maxi-anion channels.[107] They could, however, represent a novel class of large conductance CaCC channels or a prototype Cl^- channel based on its 6TMD topology and homology to other *Drosophila* cation channels.[122] Their localization to kidney epithelium and upregulation in renal cell carcinoma demands further exploration for this very interesting, newly discovered group of Cl^- channels.

CLCAs

Despite early promise, the possibility that the family of proteins called the Ca^{2+}-activated Cl^- channels (CLCAs) function as anion channels has become very remote. The CLCAs were the first cloned proteins to demonstrate CaCC characteristics under experimental conditions.[37] Specifically, expression of the bovine homolog, bCLCA1, in *Xenopus* oocytes resulted in an increase in CaCC current.[37] Single channel characteristics also seemed to fit with those previously described for CaCC channels: a single channel conductance of 25−30 pS; a mostly linear I−V relationship; and a selectivity profile of $I^- > Br^- > Cl^-$.[22,123] CLACs possible CaCC activity, its expression in airway epithelia, and its connection to airway inflammation in cystic fibrosis attracted a lot of research attention to the new family of proteins.[36] Unfortunately, the increased scrutiny brought with it increased evidence that the structure of the CLCA proteins made them unlikely candidates as integral channel proteins.[93] Newly performed structure and sequence analysis now predicts that CLCA are soluble proteins that may be secreted from the cell as signaling molecules.[93] More recent work has focused on

the very real connection between the CLCAs and chronic obstructive disease (COPD), and CLCAs revised localization to the airway mucal cells, not epithelium. Specifically, mouse Clca3 expression was sufficient to drive mucin production *in vitro*, and in multiple animal models CLCAs were found to play an important role in mucal cell metaplasia and airway hyperactivity.[93] Thus, now yoked with an unfortunate name, it seems a consensus exists concluding that CLCAs do not function physiologically as anion channels.

Bestrophin

Until the discovery of the TMEM16/Anoctamin gene, the four mammalian bestrophin genes, Best 1−4, were the most obvious candidate for the CaCC channel. There is overwhelming evidence that bestrophins are Cl^- channels, and recent clear evidence that they are critical in a number of channnelopathies. However, slight discrepancies in their characteristics and localization always created questions as to their identity[27] as the classic CaCC. The identification of this new family of Cl^- channels came from a study of the disease Best Vitelliform Macular Dystrophy (BVMD) within a large Swedish family.[86] Linkage analysis identified a region of chromosome 11 (11q13) as the locus for BVMD, which lead to the cloning of the VMD2 gene.[34,76,95,119] Subsequent syntax revision has renamed VMD2 as Best 1, and the other mammalian members of the gene family as Best 2, 3, and 4.

All the members of the Best gene family code for Cl^- channels. Early recordings done in HEK cells demonstrated novel Cl^- conductances in cells expressing the Best genes; however, the biophysical characteristics varied for each, strongly supporting the idea that each is a Cl^- channel and not a regulatory or support protein.[46] In HEK cells, Best 1 proved to be Ca^{2+}-dependent; removal and chelation of Ca^{2+} in the pipette substantially reduced current amplitudes. The currents showed some outward rectification, but were not time-dependent.[46] However, other Best channels display linear I−V (Best 2), strong inward rectification and time-dependence (Best 3), and linear I−V but with time-dependent inactivation.[46] The Best channels are weakly inhibited by niflumic acid and stilbenes[131] including DIDS (at 500 µM). The selectivity sequence is $I^- > Br^- > Cl^-$. Mutagenesis of the Best proteins provides further evidence that the Best proteins are Cl^- channels. A mutation W93H in mbest2 changes the channel gating, the I−V relation from linear to inwardly rectifying, and activates slowly upon hyperpolarization[100,126]; whereas an S79C mutation in mbest2 increases the IC_{50} of DIDS blockage by a factor of 5.[100] Regulation of the Best channels by calcium has also received recent attention. Extensive work has demonstrated that Ca^{2+} can activate bestrophins with a KD of 200 nM without the need for any diffusible intermediate,[27] suggesting that Ca^{2+} can bind bestrophins directly. Structural analysis revealed an EF-hand region in the C-terminus of the bestrophin proteins, and mutation of the region reduces the channels Ca^{2+} affinity 20-fold.[27]

Clearly, bestrophins are Cl^- channels, but where they function and their role in human disease has become increasingly controversial. Best gene mutations were known from the beginning to cause the human disease BVMD, and were known to be expressed highly in the retinal pigment epithelium (RPE). BVMD results in increased fluid in the subretinal and sub-RPE spaces, and an abnormal electro-oculogram[46]; phenotypes that appeared to be related to the function of basolateral CaCC channels in the RPE cells. hBest1 seemed a logical candidate channel to mediate these important Cl^- currents. However, recent studies using mouse knockout models of mBest1 do not phenocopy the human disease, and the mice have no retinal dysfunction.[75] Further, it appears that the newly discovered TMEM16/Anoctamin CaCC channels are also expressed in the basolateral membrane of RPE cells, and are now thought more likely to mediate the CaCC currents of these cells.[27] So although hBest1 is a Cl^- channel, in this case it does not appear to be essential for the conductance of Cl^-. Subsequent work suggests that hBest1 may regulate other channels (voltage-gated Ca^{2+} channels) or be a HCO_3^- channel, and therefore be important in cellular pH regulation.[27]

The characteristics of the four hBest channels are similar to a number of Cl^- currents identified in the kidney, and mRNA expression of all four hBest genes has been demonstrated in large mRNA expression surveys. However, there is currently no specific evidence that hBest proteins are expressed in the kidney or have any involvement in kidney function.

Chloride Intracellular Channel (CLIC)

Chloride intracellular channels (CLICs) were initially discovered in an attempt to identify the elusive Cl^- channel responsible for cystic fibrosis. Landry et al.[64] affinity purified a 64 kDa protein from bovine kidney cortex membrane vesicles using a weak Cl^- channel inhibitor, IAA-94 (indanyloxyacetic acid), and found when reconstituted into a lipid bilayer it produced a novel Cl^- conductance. Using an antibody against the 64 kDa protein, they localized it to the apical membrane and to intracellular vesicles in CFPAC-1 cells.[102] Using the same antibody, the 64 kDa protein was cloned[63] from a kidney cDNA library, and subsequent work showed it to be a member of a large family of proteins that became known as the CLICs, with the original 64 kDa protein becoming CLIC5B. In humans,

six homologs exist, each representative of a highly-conserved paralog; however, the most extensive research has been done on CLIC1 and CLIC4.

The early work on CLICB showed that it could insert into the membrane and can act as a Cl^- channel, but only in a reconstituted bilayer system, presumably because the protein was exclusively in intracellular membranes. Experiments overexpressing human CLIC1 in CHO-K1 cells managed to record a novel Cl^- current, and were able to measure some single channel characteristics.[4] The overexpressed CLIC1 localized to both the nuclear and plasma membrane, and patch recordings were done from both. CLIC1 demonstrated a slight inward rectification and voltage-dependent inactivation,[71] a selectivity sequence of $F^- > Cl^- > I^-$ (unfortunately from a single experiment), a single channel conductance of approximately 30 pS,[4,71] and was reversibly inhibited by 10 μM IAA-94.[4] Further work demonstrated that CLIC1 actually forms tetramers, each with a pore conductance of approximately 8 pS.[71] Importantly, a single point mutation in CLIC1 (C24A) changes the channel characteristics, demonstrating that CLIC1 is unambiguously a Cl^- channel when inserted into a membrane.[71] In contrast, overexpression of CLIC4 in HEK cells produces channels with a significantly smaller single channel conductance, 1 pS, but a similar selectivity sequence, $I^- > Cl^-$,[4] although CLIC4 appears to be poorly selective generally with K^+ and Cl^- having similar permeability.[71]

The most interesting recent CLIC protein discovery concerns their switch hitting life-style. It is clear that CLIC1 can be both a stable globular soluble protein, and an integral membrane protein. The solved crystal structure of CLIC1 demonstrated its nature as a soluble protein, and more importantly marked it as a member of the superfamily of glutathione s-transferase (GST) genes.[71] This revelation dramatically altered the hypothesized function of the CLICs; they may not act as Cl^- channels, but instead as soluble enzymes like the rest of the GST family. It appears their putative function depends on whether the CLIC proteins insert into the membrane or not, and recent work has concentrated on environmental factors that can manipulate CLIC tertiary structure. It turns out that, like other GST proteins, oxidation can drastically alter the structure of CLIC1, creating a second stable tertiary structure, marking it as a metamorphic protein.[71] This second oxidized stable state appears likely to insert into membranes, thus oxidation may control the function of CLIC1, channel or enzyme. Separate unfolding experiments on soluble CLIC1 suggest that low pH "primes" the protein for insertion into membranes.[33] These two environmental modulators of CLIC1 may point to its possible *in vivo* physiological function. The localization of CLIC1 and CLIC4 to acidified intracellular vesicles and endosomes may imply a coupling of CLIC Cl^- channel activity to the acidification by a proton pump reminiscent of CLC5 or CFTR. A link between CFTR and CLIC1 is supported by work done by Edwards,[30] who demonstrated in *Xenopus* oocytes that the co-expression of CFTR and CLIC1 lead to a synergistic increase in cAMP-activated current, part of which was IAA-94 sensitive. A similar regulator relationship between CLIC1 and CFTR could be even further enhanced in the acidic environment of endosomes, where more of the CLIC1 protein would form Cl^- channels. As genetic tools continue to evolve, a number of mouse knockout models have been developed to test the physiological role of CLIC *in vivo*. Both the $CLIC1^{-/-}$ and $CLIC4^{-/-}$ showed very slight phenotypes; however, a study of the intracellular vesicles of the $CLC4^{-/-}$ mice revealed that the large intracellular vesicles were less acidic than wild-type, although the endosomes demonstrated no change in acidification.[129] The potential redundancy of the CLICs may have masked many phenotypic changes from single CLIC knockouts. To further grasp the role of the CLICs specifically in the intracellular vesicles, multiple knockout models are needed.

ANION CHANNELOPATHIES OF THE KIDNEY

Thus far, only a single anion channelopathy has been described in human kidney, dysfunction of ClC-Kb which causes type III and IV Bartter's syndrome. Recent evidence has shown that ClC-5 is a Cl^-/H^+ exchanger, and thus has removed Dent's disease from the ranks of anion channelopathies, so it will be discussed elsewhere. In fact, the dearth of anion channelopathies in the kidney does not suggest that Cl^- conductances are not important in the nephron, but perhaps instead is illustrative of our limited knowledge of Cl^- channels' functional roles. The physiological functions of the newly identified TMEM16 Cl^- channel family are only beginning to be understood, and the missing molecular identities of the vast collection of volume-sensitive Cl^- channels still represent a significant hole in our understanding. Learning more about Cl^- channels in the kidney will undoubtedly teach us more about the cause of human diseases and how to treat them.

Bartter's Syndrome

Bartter's syndrome is a collection of kidney diseases that result in mishandling of salts in the thick ascending limb (TAL), and result in renal salt-wasting, hypokalemic metabolic alkalosis, elevated rennin and aldosterone levels, normal or low blood pressure, and hypercalciuria.[50] Traditionally, Bartter's was divided into two classes based on the age of the onset of symptoms: either neonatal or classic Bartter's. More recent genetic analysis of Bartter's patients revealed that mutations in five separate genes could cause the symptoms associated with Bartter's, prompting a further division into five classes, each demonstrating a separate dysfunction in the NaCl absorption pathway of the TAL[55] (Figure 31.7). Na^+, K^+, and Cl^- anions are imported across the apical membrane from the tubule lumen in the cells of the TAL via the NKCC2 co-transporter; mutations causing dysfunction in the NKCC2 co-transporter result in type I Bartter's syndrome. The K^+ leaves the cell via apical ROMK K^+ channels to return to the lumen; mutations in the ROMK K^+ channels result in type II Bartter's. The Cl^- exits the cell across the basolateral membrane through the ClC-Kb/Barttin channel complex; mutations in the ClC-Kb channel cause type III Bartter's, and mutations in the ClC-Kb channel subunit Barttin cause type IV.[55] Type V Bartter's syndrome results from gain-of-function mutations in the calcium sensing receptor protein, CaSR, a member of the G-protein receptor superfamily.[50] CaSR is activated by high extracellular Ca^{2+}, and in turn inhibits salt transport, thus overactive CaSR inappropriately inhibits salt absorption, resulting in symptoms typical in Bartter's syndrome.[49]

Interestingly, type III and type IV Bartter's does not result in the same phenotype, which would be expected if only the ClC-Kb—Barttin complex was being affected. Patients with mutations in the Barttin subunit have more severe salt-wasting than those with type III, in addition to sensorineural deafness. The deafness is now known to be caused by dysfunction of both ClC-Ka and ClC-Kb channels in the inner ear (see previous CLC section), demonstrating that Barttin is a required subunit for both ClC-Ks. In humans, the increased severity of type IV Bartter's therefore suggests a role of ClC-Ka in salt absorption in the TAL, although dysfunction in ClC-Ka alone is not associated with any renal disease phenotype.[61]

Polycystic Kidney Disease

Unlike type III and IV Bartter's syndrome, autosomal dominant polycystic kidney disease (ADPKD) is not a Cl^- channelopathy; however, the progress of ADPKD depends directly on an inappropriate increase in Cl^- channel function. ADPKD is the most common genetic disorder found in humans, effecting 1 out of 800 births.[137] It results in the slow and progressive accumulation of fluid filled cysts in the kidney and the liver, which by adulthood can result in renal failure and necessitate kidney transplantation or result in patient death.[137] Two genes have been causally associated with ADPKD, the two polycystin genes, PKD1

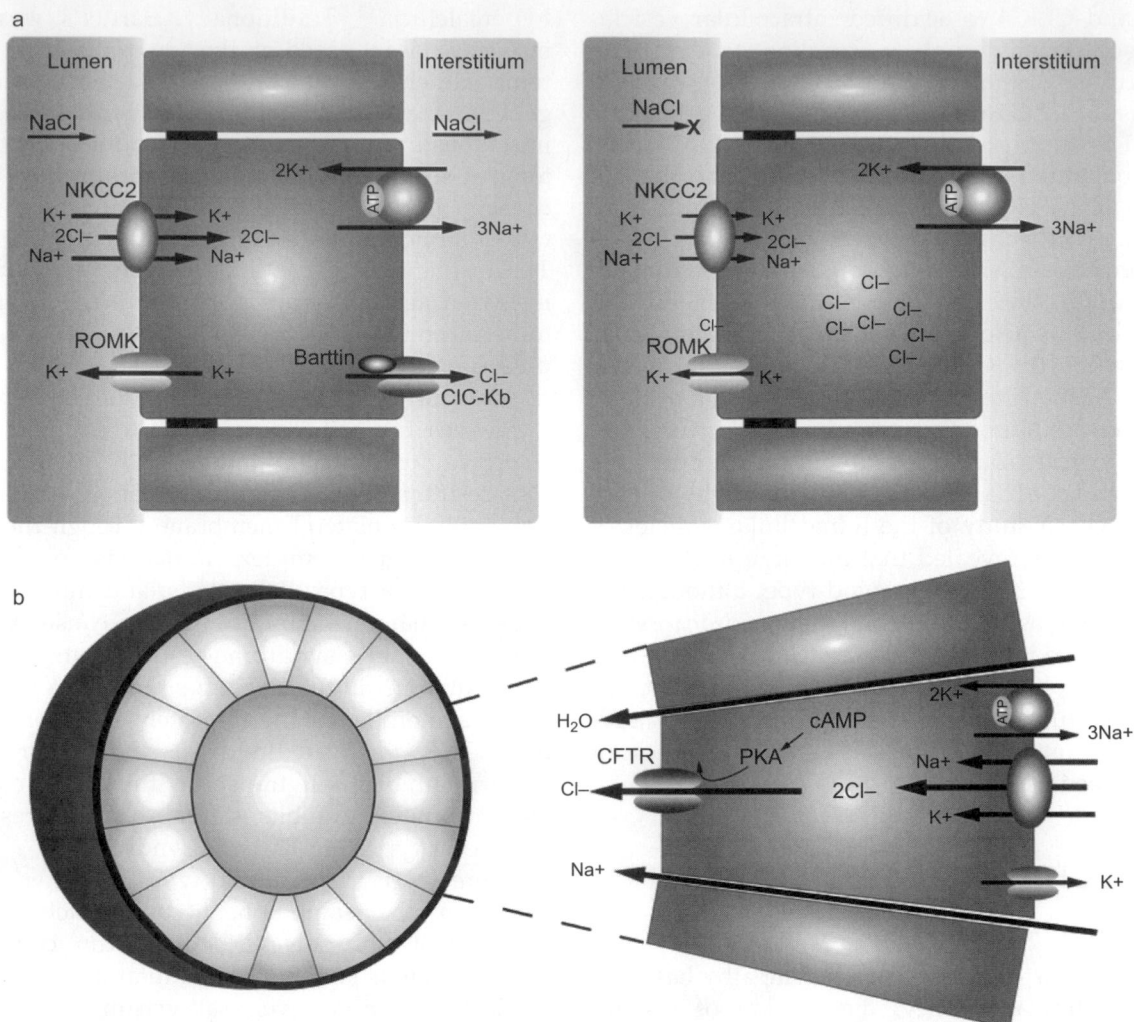

FIGURE 31.7 Anion channelopathies of the kidney. (a) Bartter's syndrome type III and IV. In normal cells of the thick ascending loop (TAL), NaCl is absorbed from the lumen and moved into the interstitium, a process that requires the transport of K^+, $2Cl^-$, and Na^+ across the apical membrane (NKCC2), and the subsequent efflux of Na^+ (Na^+/K^+-ATPase) and Cl^- (ClC-Kb) across the basolateral membrane. When either the ClC-Kb or its barttin subunit is dysfunctional, Cl^- builds within the cell, slowing apical transport of Na^+, Cl^-, and K^+. Without NaCl absorption in the TAL potentially severe salt-wasting will occur. (b) Mutations of either PKD1 or PKD2 genes causes tubule epithelial cells to form cysts and not tubules. Cyst growth and expansion, however, relies on fluid secretion into the cyst lumen driven by an apical CFTR Cl^- conductance that pulls paracellular Na^+ and H_2O along with it.

and PKD2[137]; how mutations in these genes and their gene products, PC1 and PC2/TRPP2 respectively, lead to cyst development remains unclear. PC1 is a large membrane protein that includes an extensive extracellular domain and may be part of focal adhesion complexes at the plasma membrane,[60] but it has also been shown to cleave into numerous functional products including P100, which has been shown to inhibit the ER Ca^{2+} sensor protein STIM1.[141] PC1 may also regulate the function of PC2. PC2 is a calcium channel that may reside on either the ER or plasma membranes. PC2 has been shown to be a key regulator of ER Ca^{2+} stores and ATP-mediated Ca^{2+} release.[60,69] A PC1–PC2 complex on an extended non-motile cilium has

been proposed to detect intertubule flow, a key developmental signal during tubulogenesis. Under this hypothesis, a dysfunction in flow directionality may lead to abnormal tubule growth and the creation of cysts.[148] Alternative hypotheses have PC1 and PC2 playing key roles in regulating proliferation and apoptosis, both key elements in normal tubulogenesis, and being co-opted for cyst development.[121]

Although the mechanism that begins cytogenesis is not yet understood, the mechanisms contributing to cyst growth and enlargement are better understood. The development of ADPKD cysts requires the proliferation of epithelial cells and fluid accumulation within the cyst cavity.[67] Both of these are accelerated by the cAMP signal transduction pathway.[68] In studies of primary cultures of ADPKD cells, apical cAMP-activated Cl^- conductances were identified using the patch-clamp technique. These currents were sensitive to glibenclamide and DPC, but not DIDS, and had a selectivity sequence of $Br^- > Cl^- > I^-$; these are all hallmark characteristics of the CFTR Cl^- channel.[44] Immunohistochemistry showed CFTR to be in the apical membranes of ADPKD cells and in cyst linings of ADPKD kidneys.[44] The movement of fluid, therefore, is believed to be facilitated by Cl^- secretion into the lumen of the cysts by apical CFTR channels, pulling both Na^+ and water along with it via paracellular pathways (Figure 31.7). This model of CFTR-mediated secretion is very similar to the role of CFTR in the airway, where it maintains the airway surface liquid (ASL). The apical Cl^- secretion in cyst epithelia is made possible by the accumulation of cytosolic Cl^- via the basolateral NKCC1 co-transporter, which transports in two Cl^- for every Na^+ and K^+ ion.[65] More recent work has also confirmed a more direct connection between CFTR and the polycystin proteins. Ikeda et al.[51] demonstrated in a MDCK model system that the expression of PC1 downregulated the amount of apical CFTR expression, concluding that mutant PC1 would promote increased CFTR plasma membrane expression, and increased Cl^- and fluid secretion into the cyst lumen. Thus, the increased function of CFTR may lead to fluid accumulation in the cysts; perhaps demonstrating better than any of the numerous experiments mentioned earlier in the CFTR section that CFTR is in the kidney and it functions there just as it does elsewhere: facilitating salt and fluid secretion.

To test the role CFTR plays in cyst growth in humans, researchers looked specifically at families with members who suffered from both ADPKD and CF. Although very few of these individuals have been studied, it does appear that ADPKD patients who also suffer from CF have fewer and smaller renal and hepatic cysts than do their age-matched siblings with ADPKD but not CF.[143] However, in another study where a single CF ($\Delta508CFTR$) patient with ADPKD was compared to non-siblings with ADPKD but no CF, there appeared to be no difference in kidney volume or renal function.[94] Obviously, in humans it will require further accumulation of the very rare occurrence of families with both ADPKD and CF before we can really know whether CF patients receive some renal protection. Surprisingly, $CFTR^{-/-}$ knockout mice have not been crossed with any ADPKD mouse models to see if cytogenesis or cyst growth is diminished; this type of experiment could increase our understanding of CFTRs role in ADPKD.

Recent work has focused on CFTR as a target for a therapeutic approach to control ADPKD-mediated cyst growth and expansion using specific, high-affinity CFTR inhibitors. MDCK cells with endogenous CFTR and low levels of PC1 will form cysts when grown in a collagen matrix and given the cAMP agonist forskolin, but cyst growth is inhibited with the application of the specific CFTR inhibitor CFTRinh-172.[67] Similarly, when CFTR inhibitor compounds CFTRinh-172 and Ph-GlyH-101 were used to treat embryonic cystic mouse kidneys in a 4 day culture model system, they reduced cyst number and growth by more than 80%. Further, direct treatment of PKD1 knockout mice with the CFTR inhibitor slowed the normally fast development of kidney cysts and preserved kidney function.[144,131] These studies strongly support targeting CFTR as a therapy for ADPKD patients that may prove efficacious in decreasing cyst size and preserving kidney function.

SUMMARY

Recent years have marked an exciting time in the field of Cl^- channel research. More and more of the molecular identities of the functional Cl^- channel groups have been discovered, and this new knowledge has given us an expanded view of the importance of Cl^- channels in both kidney physiology and human physiology. So, too, we must acknowledge the shifting landscape that has redefined many anion channels as exchangers, and accept that perhaps that the characteristics that separate the two groups are far less significant than previously believed. But what hasn't changed is the importance of anion channels in kidney function. Each year increases our understanding of their role in secretion of waste, water retention, ionic balance, blood pressure regulation, and the recapture of essential solutes. We now add the TMEM16 and SLC26a gene families to those expressed in the kidney that conduct anions, and look forward to what these newly discovered Cl^- channels can tell us. But not all recent discoveries have been on the large-scale, many incremental but significant discoveries have also been made that slowly progress our understanding of human diseases like Bartter's Syndrome and PKD, and bring us one step closer to developing more effective therapies. The same questions persist: how do anion channels work in the context of the human kidney? How does their dysfunction lead to human disease? Can we develop new or more effective pharmacologic therapies for human kidney disease? But we now have even greater tools, knockout animals, siRNA, vast drug libraries, and the ability for large-scale molecular screens with which to answer these fundamental questions.

References

[1] Accardi A, Miller C. Secondary active transport mediated by a prokaryotic homologue of ClC Cl⁻ channels. Nature 2004;427:803−7.

[2] Akrouh A, Halcomb SE, Nichols CG, Sala-Rabanal M. Molecular biology of K(ATP) channels and implications for health and disease. IUBMB Life 2009;61:971−8.

[3] Anderson MP, Gregory RJ, Thompson S, Souza DW, Paul S, Mulligan RC, et al. Demonstration that CFTR is a chloride channel by alteration of its anion selectivity. Science 1991;253:202−5.

[4] Ashley RH. Challenging accepted ion channel biology: p64 and the CLIC family of putative intracellular anion channel proteins (Review). Mol Membr Biol 2003;20:1−11.

[5] Baker MA, Lane DJ, Ly JD, De Pinto V, Lawen A. VDAC1 is a transplasma membrane NADH-ferricyanide reductase. J Biol Chem 2004;279:4811−9.

[6] Bao HF, Liu L, Self J, Duke BJ, Ueno R, Eaton DC. A synthetic prostone activates apical chloride channels in A6 epithelial cells. Am J Physiol Gastrointest Liver Physiol 2008;295:G234−51.

[7] Barlassina C, Dal FC, Lanzani C, Manunta P, Guffanti G, Ruello A, et al. Common genetic variants and haplotypes in renal CLCNKA gene are associated to salt-sensitive hypertension. Hum Mol Genet 2007;16:1630−8.

[8] Bathori G, Parolini I, Tombola F, Szabo I, Messina A, Oliva M, et al. Porin is present in the plasma membrane where it is concentrated in caveolae and caveolae-related domains. J Biol Chem 1999;274:29607−12.

[9] Bathori G, Parolini I, Szabo I, Tombola F, Messina A, Oliva M, et al. Extramitochondrial porin: facts and hypotheses. J Bioenerg Biomembr 2000;32:79−89.

[10] Bell PD, Lapointe JY, Sabirov R, Hayashi S, Peti-Peterdi J, Manabe K, et al. Macula densa cell signaling involves ATP release through a maxi anion channel. Proc Natl Acad Sci USA 2003;100:4322−7.

[11] Bell PD, Komlosi P, Zhang ZR. ATP as a mediator of macula densa cell signalling. Purinergic Signal 2009;5:461−71.

[12] Berdiev BK, Qadri YJ, Benos DJ. Assessment of the CFTR and ENaC association. Mol Biosyst 2009;5:123−7.

[13] Bertrand CA, Zhang R, Pilewski JM, Frizzell RA. SLC26A9 is a constitutively active, CFTR-regulated anion conductance in human bronchial epithelia. J Gen Physiol 2009;133:421−38.

[14] Birkenhager R, Otto E, Schurmann MJ, Vollmer M, Ruf EM, Maier-Lutz I, et al. Mutation of BSND causes Bartter syndrome with sensorineural deafness and kidney failure. Nat Genet 2001;29:310−4.

[15] Boese SH, Aziz O, Simmons NL, Gray MA. Kinetics and regulation of a Ca²⁺-activated Cl⁻ conductance in mouse renal inner medullary collecting duct cells. Am J Physiol Renal Physiol 2004;286:F682−92.

[16] Caputo A, Caci E, Ferrera L, Pedemonte N, Barsanti C, Sondo E, et al. TMEM16A, a membrane protein associated with calcium-dependent chloride channel activity. Science 2008;322:590−4.

[17] Chang MH, Plata C, Sindic A, Ranatunga WK, Chen AP, Zandi-Nejad K, et al. Slc26a9 is inhibited by the R-region of the cystic fibrosis transmembrane conductance regulator via the STAS domain. J Biol Chem 2009;284:28306−18.

[18] Chebib M. GABAC receptor ion channels. Clin Exp Pharmacol Physiol 2004;31:800−4.

[19] Chen TY. Structure and function of clc channels. Annu Rev Physiol 2005;67:809−39.

[20] Chillon M, Casals T, Mercier B, Bassas L, Lissens W, Silber S, et al. Mutations in the cystic fibrosis gene in patients with congenital absence of the vas deferens. N Engl J Med 1995;332:1475−80.

[21] Choudari CP, Lehman GA, Sherman S. Pancreatitis and cystic fibrosis gene mutations. Gastroenterol Clin North Am 1999;28:543−9 [vii-viii]

[22] Cunningham SA, Awayda MS, Bubien JK, Ismailov II, Arrate MP, Berdiev BK, et al. Cloning of an epithelial chloride channel from bovine trachea. J Biol Chem 1995;270:31016−26.

[23] Cuppoletti J, Malinowska DH, Tewari KP, Li QJ, Sherry AM, Patchen ML, et al. SPI-0211 activates T84 cell chloride transport and recombinant human ClC-2 chloride currents. Am J Physiol Cell Physiol 2004;287:C1173−83.

[24] De Pinto V, Messina A, Lane DJ, Lawen A. Voltage-dependent anion-selective channel (VDAC) in the plasma membrane. FEBS Lett 2010;584:1793−9.

[25] Devuyst O, Guggino WB. Chloride channels in the kidney: lessons learned from knockout animals. Am J Physiol Renal Physiol 2002;283:F1176−91.

[26] Dorwart MR, Shcheynikov N, Yang D, Muallem S. The solute carrier 26 family of proteins in epithelial ion transport. *Physiology* (Bethesda) 2008;23:104−14.

[26a] Dorwart MR, Shcheynikon N, Wang Y, Stippec S, Muallem S. SLC26A9 is a Cl − channel regulated by the WNK kinases. J Physiol 2007;584(1):333−45.

[27] Duran C, Thompson CH, Xiao Q, Hartzell HC. Chloride channels: often enigmatic, rarely predictable. Annu Rev Physiol 2010;72:95−121.

[28] Dutzler R, Campbell EB, Cadene M, Chait BT, MacKinnon R. X-ray structure of a ClC chloride channel at 3.0 Å reveals the molecular basis of anion selectivity. Nature 2002;415:287−94.

[29] Dutzler R, Campbell EB, MacKinnon R. Gating the selectivity filter in ClC chloride channels. Science 2003;300:108−12.

[30] Edwards JC. The CLIC1 chloride channel is regulated by the cystic fibrosis transmembrane conductance regulator when expressed in *Xenopus* oocytes. J Membr Biol 2006;213:39−46.

[31] Embark HM, Bohmer C, Palmada M, Rajamanickam J, Wyatt AW, Wallisch S, et al. Regulation of CLC-Ka/barttin by the ubiquitin ligase Nedd4-2 and the serum- and glucocorticoid-dependent kinases. Kidney Int 2004;66:1918−25.

[32] Estevez R, Boettger T, Stein V, Birkenhager R, Otto E, Hildebrandt F, et al. Barttin is a Cl⁻ channel beta-subunit crucial for renal Cl⁻ reabsorption and inner ear K⁺ secretion. Nature 2001;414:558−61.

[33] Fanucchi S, Adamson RJ, Dirr HW. Formation of an unfolding intermediate state of soluble chloride intracellular channel protein CLIC1 at acidic pH. Biochemistry 2008;47:11674−81.

[34] Forsman K, Graff C, Nordstrom S, Johansson K, Westermark E, Lundgren E, et al. The gene for Best's macular dystrophy is located at 11q13 in a Swedish family. Clin Genet 1992;42:156−9.

[35] Frey A, Lampert A, Waldegger S, Jeck N, Waldegger P, Artunc F, et al. Influence of gain of function epithelial chloride channel ClC-Kb mutation on hearing thresholds. Hear Res 2006;214:68−75.

[36] Fuller CM, Benos DJ. Ca²⁺-activated Cl⁻ channels: a newly emerging anion transport family. News Physiol Sci 2000;15:165−71.

[37] Fuller CM, Ji HL, Tousson A, Elble RC, Pauli BU, Benos DJ. Ca²⁺-activated Cl⁻ channels: a newly emerging anion transport family. Pflugers Arch 2001;443(Suppl. 1):S107−10.

[38] Gabriel SE, Clarke LL, Boucher RC, Stutts MJ. CFTR and outward rectifying chloride channels are distinct proteins with a regulatory relationship. Nature 1993;363:263−8.

[39] Gadsby DC, Vergani P, Csanady L. The ABC protein turned chloride channel whose failure causes cystic fibrosis. Nature 2006;440:477−83.

[40] Goncalves RP, Buzhysnskyy N, Scheuring S. Mini review on the structure and supramolecular assembly of VDAC. J Bioenerg Biomembr 2008;40:133−8.

[41] Guggino WB. The cystic fibrosis transmembrane regulator forms macromolecular complexes with PDZ domain scaffold proteins. Proc Am Thorac Soc 2004;1:28—32.

[42] Guggino WB, Stanton BA. New insights into cystic fibrosis: molecular switches that regulate CFTR. Nat Rev Mol Cell Biol 2006;7:426—36.

[43] Gunther W, Luchow A, Cluzeaud F, Vandewalle A, Jentsch TJ. ClC-5, the chloride channel mutated in Dent's disease, colocalizes with the proton pump in endocytotically active kidney cells. Proc Natl Acad Sci USA 1998;95:8075—80.

[44] Hanaoka K, Devuyst O, Schwiebert EM, Wilson PD, Guggino WB. A role for CFTR in human autosomal dominant polycystic kidney disease. Am J Physiol 1996;270:C389—99.

[45] Hartzell C, Putzier I, Arreola J. Calcium-activated chloride channels. Annu Rev Physiol 2005;67:719—58.

[46] Hartzell HC, Qu Z, Yu K, Xiao Q, Chien LT. Molecular physiology of bestrophins: multifunctional membrane proteins linked to Best disease and other retinopathies. Physiol Rev 2008;88:639—72.

[47] Hartzell HC, Yu K, Xiao Q, Chien LT, Qu Z. Anoctamin/TMEM16 family members are Ca^{2+}-activated Cl^- channels. J Physiol 2009;587:2127—39.

[48] He Y, Ramsay AJ, Hunt ML, Whitbread AK, Myers SA, Hooper JD. N-glycosylation analysis of the human Tweety family of putative chloride ion channels supports a penta-spanning membrane arrangement: impact of N-glycosylation on cellular processing of Tweety homologue 2 (TTYH2). Biochem J 2008;412:45—55.

[49] Hebert SC. Extracellular calcium-sensing receptor: implications for calcium and magnesium handling in the kidney. Kidney Int 1996;50:2129—39.

[50] Hebert SC. Bartter syndrome. Curr Opin Nephrol Hypertens 2003;12:527—32.

[51] Ikeda M, Fong P, Cheng J, Boletta A, Qian F, Zhang XM, et al. A regulatory role of polycystin-1 on cystic fibrosis transmembrane conductance regulator plasma membrane expression. Cell Physiol Biochem 2006;18:9—20.

[52] Jakob C, Gotz H, Hellmann T, Hellmann KP, Reymann S, Florke H, et al. Studies on human porin: XIII. The type-1 VDAC "porin 31HL" biotinylated at the plasmalemma of trypan blue excluding human B lymphocytes. FEBS Lett 1995;368:5—9.

[53] Jeck N, Waldegger S, Lampert A, Boehmer C, Waldegger P, Lang PA, et al. Activating mutation of the renal epithelial chloride channel ClC-Kb predisposing to hypertension. Hypertension 2004;43:1175—81.

[54] Jentsch TJ, Poet M, Fuhrmann JC, Zdebik AA. Physiological functions of CLC Cl^- channels gleaned from human genetic disease and mouse models. Annu Rev Physiol 2005;67:779—807.

[55] Jentsch TJ. CLC chloride channels and transporters: from genes to protein structure, pathology and physiology. Crit Rev Biochem Mol Biol 2008;43:3—36.

[56] Jouret F, Devuyst O. CFTR and defective endocytosis: new insights in the renal phenotype of cystic fibrosis. Pflugers Arch 2009;457:1227—36.

[57] Kerem B, Rommens JM, Buchanan JA, Markiewicz D, Cox TK, Chakravarti A, et al. Identification of the cystic fibrosis gene: Genetic analysis. Science 1989;245:1073—80.

[58] Kim KH, Shcheynikov N, Wang Y, Muallem S. SLC26A7 is a Cl^- channel regulated by intracellular pH. J Biol Chem 2005;280:6463—70.

[59] Ko SB, Zeng W, Dorwart MR, Luo X, Kim KH, Millen L, et al. Gating of CFTR by the STAS domain of SLC26 transporters. Nat Cell Biol 2004;6:343—50.

[60] Kottgen M. TRPP2 and autosomal dominant polycystic kidney disease. Biochim Biophys Acta 2007;1772:836—50.

[61] Kramer BK, Bergler T, Stoelcker B, Waldegger S. Mechanisms of disease: the kidney-specific chloride channels ClCKA and ClCKB, the Barttin subunit, and their clinical relevance. Nat Clin Pract Nephrol 2008;4:38—46.

[62] Kunzelmann K, Kongsuphol P, Aldehni F, Tian Y, Ousingsawat J, Warth R, et al. Bestrophin and TMEM16-Ca^{2+} activated Cl $(^-)$ channels with different functions. Cell Calcium 2009;46:233—41.

[63] Landry D, Sullivan S, Nicolaides M, Redhead C, Edelman A, Field M, et al. Molecular cloning and characterization of p64, a chloride channel protein from kidney microsomes. J Biol Chem 1993;268:14948—55.

[64] Landry DW, Akabas MH, Redhead C, Edelman A, Cragoe Jr EJ, al-Awqati Q. Purification and reconstitution of chloride channels from kidney and trachea. Science 1989;244:1469—72.

[65] Lebeau C, Hanaoka K, Moore-Hoon ML, Guggino WB, Beauwens R, Devuyst O. Basolateral chloride transporters in autosomal dominant polycystic kidney disease. Pflugers Arch 2002;444:722—31.

[66] Letz B, Korbmacher C. cAMP stimulates CFTR-like Cl^- channels and inhibits amiloride-sensitive Na^+ channels in mouse CCD cells. Am J Physiol 1997;272:C657—66.

[67] Li H, Findlay IA, Sheppard DN. The relationship between cell proliferation, Cl^- secretion, and renal cyst growth: a study using CFTR inhibitors. Kidney Int 2004;66:1926—38.

[68] Li H, Sheppard DN. Therapeutic potential of cystic fibrosis transmembrane conductance regulator (CFTR) inhibitors in polycystic kidney disease. BioDrugs 2009;23:203—16.

[69] Li Y, Santoso NG, Yu S, Woodward OM, Qian F, Guggino WB. Polycystin-1 interacts with inositol 1,4,5-trisphosphate receptor to modulate intracellular Ca^{2+} signaling with implications for polycystic kidney disease. J Biol Chem 2009;284:36431—41.

[70] Liantonio A, Picollo A, Carbonara G, Fracchiolla G, Tortorella P, Loiodice F, et al. Molecular switch for CLC-K Cl^- channel block/activation: Optimal pharmacophoric requirements towards high-affinity ligands. Proc Natl Acad Sci USA 2008;105:1369—73.

[71] Littler DR, Harrop SJ, Goodchild SC, Phang JM, Mynott AV, Jiang L, et al. The enigma of the CLIC proteins: Ion channels, redox proteins, enzymes, scaffolding proteins? FEBS Lett 2010;584:2093—101.

[71a] Lisal J, Maduke M. The ClC-0 chloride channel is a broken Cl^-/H^+ antiporter. Nat Struct Mol Bio 2008;15:805—10.

[72] Lu M, Dong K, Egan ME, Giebisch GH, Boulpaep EL, Hebert SC. Mouse cystic fibrosis transmembrane conductance regulator forms cAMP-PKA-regulated apical chloride channels in cortical collecting duct. Proc Natl Acad Sci USA 2010;107:6082—7.

[73] Lynch JW. Molecular structure and function of the glycine receptor chloride channel. Physiol Rev 2004;84:1051—95.

[74] Ma T, Thiagarajah JR, Yang H, Sonawane ND, Folli C, Galietta LJ, et al. Thiazolidinone CFTR inhibitor identified by high-throughput screening blocks cholera toxin-induced intestinal fluid secretion. J Clin Invest 2002;110:1651—8.

[75] Marmorstein LY, Wu J, McLaughlin P, Yocom J, Karl MO, Neussert R, et al. The light peak of the electroretinogram is dependent on voltage-gated calcium channels and antagonized by bestrophin (best-1). J Gen Physiol 2006;127:577—89.

[76] Marquardt A, Stohr H, Passmore LA, Kramer F, Rivera A, Weber BH. Mutations in a novel gene, VMD2, encoding a protein of unknown properties cause juvenile-onset vitelliform macular dystrophy (Best's disease). Hum Mol Genet 1998;7:1517—25.

III. FLUID AND ELECTROLYTE REGULATION AND DYSREGULATION

[77] Matsumura Y, Uchida S, Kondo Y, Miyazaki H, Ko SB, Hayama A, et al. Overt nephrogenic diabetes insipidus in mice lacking the CLC-K1 chloride channel. Nat Genet 1999;21:95–8.

[78] Matulef K, Maduke M. The CLC "chloride channel" family: revelations from prokaryotes. Mol Membr Biol 2007;24:342–50.

[79] Miller C. ClC chloride channels viewed through a transporter lens. Nature 2006;440:484–9.

[80] Morales MM, Carroll TP, Morita T, Schwiebert EM, Devuyst O, Wilson PD, et al. Both the wild-type and a functional isoform of CFTR are expressed in kidney. Am J Physiol 1996;270:F1038–48.

[81] Morales MM, Falkenstein D, Lopes AG. The cystic fibrosis transmembrane regulator (CFTR) in the kidney. An Acad Bras Cienc 2000;72:399–406.

[82] Moyer BD, Denton J, Karlson KH, Reynolds D, Wang S, Mickle JE, et al. A PDZ-interacting domain in CFTR is an apical membrane polarization signal. J Clin Invest 1999;104:1353–61.

[83] Muanprasat C, Sonawane ND, Salinas D, Taddei A, Galietta LJ, Verkman AS. Discovery of glycine hydrazide pore-occluding CFTR inhibitors: Mechanism, structure–activity analysis, and in vivo efficacy. J Gen Physiol 2004;124:125–37.

[84] Nilius B, Eggermont J, Voets T, Buyse G, Manolopoulos V, Droogmans G. Properties of volume-regulated anion channels in mammalian cells. Prog Biophys Mol Biol 1997;68:69–119.

[85] Nilius B, Droogmans G. Amazing chloride channels: an overview. Acta Physiol Scand 2003;177:119–47.

[86] Nordstrom S, Barkman Y. Hereditary macular degeneration (HMD) in 246 cases traced to one gene-source in central Sweden. Hereditas 1977;84:163–76.

[87] Novarino G, Weinert S, Rickheit G, Jentsch TJ. Endosomal chloride–proton exchange rather than chloride conductance is crucial for renal endocytosis. Science 2010;328:1398–401.

[88] Nutt D. GABAA receptors: subtypes, regional distribution, and function. J Clin Sleep Med 2006;2:S7–11.

[89] Ohana E, Yang D, Shcheynikov N, Muallem S. Diverse transport modes by the solute carrier 26 family of anion transporters. J Physiol 2009;587:2179–85.

[90] Okada SF, O'Neal WK, Huang P, Nicholas RA, Ostrowski LE, Craigen WJ, et al. Voltage-dependent anion channel-1 (VDAC-1) contributes to ATP release and cell volume regulation in murine cells. J Gen Physiol 2004;124:513–26.

[91] Okada Y, Shimizu T, Maeno E, Tanabe S, Wang X, Takahashi N. Volume-sensitive chloride channels involved in apoptotic volume decrease and cell death. J Membr Biol 2006;209:21–9.

[92] Okada Y, Sato K, Numata T. Pathophysiology and puzzles of the volume-sensitive outwardly rectifying anion channel. J Physiol 2009;587:2141–9.

[93] Patel AC, Brett TJ, Holtzman MJ. The role of CLCA proteins in inflammatory airway disease. Annu Rev Physiol 2009;71:425–49.

[94] Persu A, Devuyst O, Lannoy N, Materne R, Brosnahan G, Gabow PA, et al. CF gene and cystic fibrosis transmembrane conductance regulator expression in autosomal dominant polycystic kidney disease. J Am Soc Nephrol 2000;11:2285–96.

[95] Petrukhin K, Koisti MJ, Bakall B, Li W, Xie G, Marknell T, et al. Identification of the gene responsible for Best macular dystrophy. Nat Genet 1998;19:241–7.

[96] Picollo A, Pusch M. Chloride/proton antiporter activity of mammalian CLC proteins ClC-4 and ClC-5. Nature 2005;436:420–3.

[97] Piwon N, Gunther W, Schwake M, Bosl MR, Jentsch TJ. ClC-5 Cl−-channel disruption impairs endocytosis in a mouse model for Dent's disease. Nature 2000;408:369–73.

[98] Plans V, Rickheit G, Jentsch TJ. Physiological roles of CLC Cl(−)/H(+) exchangers in renal proximal tubules. Pflugers Arch 2009;458:23–37.

[99] Qu Z, Wei RW, Hartzell HC. Characterization of Ca2+-activated Cl− currents in mouse kidney inner medullary collecting duct cells. Am J Physiol Renal Physiol 2003;285:F326–35.

[100] Qu Z, Fischmeister R, Hartzell C. Mouse bestrophin-2 is a bona fide Cl(−) channel: identification of a residue important in anion binding and conduction. J Gen Physiol 2004;123:327–40.

[101] Reddy MM, Quinton PM. Functional interaction of CFTR and ENaC in sweat glands. Pflugers Arch 2003;445:499–503.

[102] Redhead CR, Edelman AE, Brown D, Landry DW, al-Awqati Q. A ubiquitous 64-kDa protein is a component of a chloride channel of plasma and intracellular membranes. Proc Natl Acad Sci USA 1992;89:3716–20.

[103] Riordan JR, Rommens JM, Kerem B, Alon N, Rozmahel R, Grzelczak Z, et al. Identification of the cystic fibrosis gene: cloning and characterization of complementary DNA. Science 1989;245:1066–73.

[104] Rommens JM, Iannuzzi MC, Kerem B, Drumm ML, Melmer G, Dean M, et al. Identification of the cystic fibrosis gene: Chromosome walking and jumping. Science 1989;245:1059–65.

[105] Roy SS, Ehrlich AM, Craigen WJ, Hajnoczky G. VDAC2 is required for truncated BID-induced mitochondrial apoptosis by recruiting BAK to the mitochondria. EMBO Rep 2009;10:1341–7.

[106] Sabirov RZ, Sheiko T, Liu H, Deng D, Okada Y, Craigen WJ. Genetic demonstration that the plasma membrane maxianion channel and voltage-dependent anion channels are unrelated proteins. J Biol Chem 2006;281:1897–904.

[107] Sabirov RZ, Okada Y. The maxi-anion channel: a classical channel playing novel roles through an unidentified molecular entity. J Physiol Sci 2009;59:3–21.

[108] Sanchez-Rodriguez JE, De Santiago-Castillo JA, Arreola J. Permeant anions contribute to voltage dependence of ClC-2 chloride channel by interacting with the protopore gate. J Physiol 2010;588:2545–56.

[109] Scheel O, Zdebik AA, Lourdel S, Jentsch TJ. Voltage-dependent electrogenic chloride/proton exchange by endosomal CLC proteins. Nature 2005;436:424–7.

[110] Schreiber R, Uliyakina I, Kongsuphol P, Warth R, Mirza M, Martins JR, et al. Expression and function of epithelial anoctamins. J Biol Chem 2010;285:7838–45.

[111] Schroeder BC, Cheng T, Jan YN, Jan LY. Expression cloning of TMEM16A as a calcium-activated chloride channel subunit. Cell 2008;134:1019–29.

[112] Schwiebert EM, Cid-Soto LP, Stafford D, Carter M, Blaisdell CJ, Zeitlin PL, et al. Analysis of ClC-2 channels as an alternative pathway for chloride conduction in cystic fibrosis airway cells. Proc Natl Acad Sci USA 1998;95:3879–84.

[113] Schwiebert EM, Benos DJ, Egan ME, Stutts MJ, Guggino WB. CFTR is a conductance regulator as well as a chloride channel. Physiol Rev 1999;79:S145–66.

[114] Shoshan-Barmatz V, Israelson A. The voltage-dependent anion channel in endoplasmic/sarcoplasmic reticulum: characterization, modulation and possible function. J Membr Biol 2005;204:57–66.

[115] Simamura E, Shimada H, Ishigaki Y, Hatta T, Higashi N, Hirai K. Bioreductive activation of quinone antitumor drugs by mitochondrial voltage-dependent anion channel 1. Anat Sci Int 2008;83:261–6.

[116] Sindic A, Chang MH, Mount DB, Romero MF. Renal physiology of SLC26 anion exchangers. Curr Opin Nephrol Hypertens 2007;16:484–90.

[117] Souza-Menezes J, Tukaye DN, Novaira HJ, Guggino WB, Morales MM. Small nuclear RNAs U11 and U12 modulate expression of TNR-CFTR mRNA in mammalian kidneys. Cell Physiol Biochem 2008;22:93–100.

[118] Steinmeyer K, Ortland C, Jentsch TJ. Primary structure and functional expression of a developmentally regulated skeletal muscle chloride channel. Nature 1991;354:301−4.

[119] Stone EM, Nichols BE, Streb LM, Kimura AE, Sheffield VC. Genetic linkage of vitelliform macular degeneration (Best's disease) to chromosome 11q13. Nat Genet 1992;1:246−50.

[120] Sun X, Petrovic S. Increased acid load and deletion of AE1 increase Slc26a7 expression. Nephron Physiol 2008;109:29−35.

[121] Sutters M, Germino GG. Autosomal dominant polycystic kidney disease: molecular genetics and pathophysiology. J Lab Clin Med 2003;141:91−101.

[122] Suzuki M. The *Drosophila* tweety family: molecular candidates for large-conductance Ca^{2+}-activated Cl^- channels. Exp Physiol 2006;91:141−7.

[123] Suzuki M, Morita T, Iwamoto T. Diversity of $Cl(^-)$ channels. Cell Mol Life Sci 2006;63:12−24.

[124] Tarran R, Button B, Boucher RC. Regulation of normal and cystic fibrosis airway surface liquid volume by phasic shear stress. Annu Rev Physiol 2006;68:543−61.

[125] Thiemann A, Grunder S, Pusch M, Jentsch TJ. A chloride channel widely expressed in epithelial and non-epithelial cells. Nature 1992;356:57−60.

[126] Tsunenari T, Sun H, Williams J, Cahill H, Smallwood P, Yau KW, et al. Structure−function analysis of the bestrophin family of anion channels. J Biol Chem 2003;278:41114−25.

[127] Uchida S, Sasaki S, Furukawa T, Hiraoka M, Imai T, Hirata Y, et al. Molecular cloning of a chloride channel that is regulated by dehydration and expressed predominantly in kidney medulla. J Biol Chem 1993;268:3821−4.

[128] Uchida S, Sasaki S. Function of chloride channels in the kidney. Annu Rev Physiol 2005;67:759−78.

[129] Ulmasov B, Bruno J, Gordon N, Hartnett ME, Edwards JC. Chloride intracellular channel protein-4 functions in angiogenesis by supporting acidification of vacuoles along the intracellular tubulogenic pathway. Am J Pathol 2009;174:1084−96.

[130] Vandewalle A. Expression and function of CLC and cystic fibrosis transmembrane conductance regulator chloride channels in renal epithelial tubule cells: pathophysiological implications. Chang Gung Med J 2007;30:17−25.

[131] Verkman AS, Galietta LJ. Chloride channels as drug targets. Nat Rev Drug Discov 2009;8:153−71.

[132] Waldegger S, Jentsch TJ. Functional and structural analysis of ClC-K chloride channels involved in renal disease. J Biol Chem 2000;275:24527−33.

[133] Waldegger S, Jeck N, Barth P, Peters M, Vitzthum H, Wolf K, et al. Barttin increases surface expression and changes current properties of ClC-K channels. Pflugers Arch 2002;444: 411−8.

[134] Wang SS, Devuyst O, Courtoy PJ, Wang XT, Wang H, Wang Y, et al. Mice lacking renal chloride channel, CLC-5, are a model for Dent's disease, a nephrolithiasis disorder associated with defective receptor-mediated endocytosis. Hum Mol Genet 2000;9:2937−45.

[135] Wang Y, Soyombo AA, Shcheynikov N, Zeng W, Dorwart M, Marino CR, et al. Slc26a6 regulates CFTR activity *in vivo* to determine pancreatic duct HCO_3^- secretion: relevance to cystic fibrosis. EMBO J 2006;25:5049−57.

[136] Wilson PD. Polycystic kidney disease. N Engl J Med 2004;350:151−64.

[137] Woodward OM, Willows AO. Dopamine modulation of $Ca(^{2+})$ dependent $Cl(^-)$ current regulates ciliary beat frequency controlling locomotion in *Tritonia diomedea*. J Exp Biol 2006;209:2749−64.

[138] Woodward OM, Willows AO. Nervous control of ciliary beating by $Cl(^-)$, $Ca(^{2+})$ and calmodulin in *Tritonia diomedea*. J Exp Biol 2006;209:2765−73.

[139] Woodward OM, Kottgen A, Coresh J, Boerwinkle E, Guggino WB, Kottgen M. Identification of a urate transporter, ABCG2, with a common functional polymorphism causing gout. Proc Natl Acad Sci USA 2009;106:10338−42.

[140] Woodward OM, Li Y, Yu S, Greenwell P, Wodarczyk C, Boletta A, et al. Identification of a polycystin-1 cleavage product, P100, that regulates store operated Ca entry through interactions with STIM1. PLoS One 2010;5(8):e12305.

[141] Xu J, Song P, Nakamura S, Miller M, Barone S, Alper SL, et al. Deletion of the chloride transporter slc26a7 causes distal renal tubular acidosis and impairs gastric acid secretion. J Biol Chem 2009;284:29470−9.

[142] Xu N, Glockner JF, Rossetti S, Babovich-Vuksanovic D, Harris PC, Torres VE. Autosomal dominant polycystic kidney disease coexisting with cystic fibrosis. J Nephrol 2006;19:529−34.

[143] Yang B, Sonawane ND, Zhao D, Somlo S, Verkman AS. Small-molecule CFTR inhibitors slow cyst growth in polycystic kidney disease. J Am Soc Nephrol 2008;19:1300−10.

[144] Yang IC, Cheng TH, Wang F, Price EM, Hwang TC. Modulation of CFTR chloride channels by calyculin A and genistein. Am J Physiol 1997;272:C142−55.

[145] Yang YD, Cho H, Koo JY, Tak MH, Cho Y, Shim WS, et al. TMEM16A confers receptor-activated calcium-dependent chloride conductance. Nature 2008;455:1210−5.

[146] Zhou J. Polycystins and primary cilia: primers for cell cycle progression. Annu Rev Physiol 2009;71:83−113.

III. FLUID AND ELECTROLYTE REGULATION AND DYSREGULATION

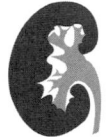

Physiology and Pathophysiology of the NaCl Co-Transporters in the Kidney

Gerardo Gamba

Molecular Physiology Unit, Department of Nephrology and Mineral Metabolism, Instituto Nacional de Ciencias Médicas y Nutrición Salvador Zubirán, and Instituto de Investigaciones Biomédicas, Universidad Nacional Autónoma de México, Mexico City, Mexico

INTRODUCTION

There are four types of electroneutral co-transporter systems that have been identified: (1) the sulfamoylbenzoic (or bumetanide)-sensitive Na^+-K^+-$2Cl^-$ co-transporter; (2) the sulfamoylbenzoic (or bumetanide)-sensitive Na^+-Cl^- co-transporter; (3) the benzothiadiazine (or thiazide)-sensitive Na^+-Cl^- co-transporter; and (4) the dihydroindenyloxy-alkanoic acid (DIOA)-sensitive K^+-Cl^- co-transporter. All these possibilities are encoded by members of the family of solute carriers SLC12, according to the classification of the Human Genome Organization.[1] Two genes of this family, SLC12A1 encoding the apical Na^+:K^+:$2Cl^-$ co-transporter, NKCC2 (also known as BSC1), and SLC12A3, encoding the Na^+:Cl^- co-transporter, NCC (also known as TSC1), are particularly relevant to kidney physiology, pharmacology, and pathophysiology. NKCC2 and NCC play a key role in salt reabsorption of the thick ascending limb of Henle's loop and distal convoluted tubule, respectively, with consequent effects in potassium, calcium, and acid–base homeostasis. They also serve as receptors for the loop diuretics (furosemide, bumetanide, ethacrinic acid) and thiazide-type diuretics (chlortalidone, hydrochlorothiazide, metolazone), respectively, that are heavily used in the management of patients with arterial hypertension or edematous states, such a cardiac failure, chronic liver disease, chronic renal disease or nephrotic syndrome. Inactivating mutations of NKCC2 cause Bartter syndrome type I, and of NCC cause Gitelman's syndrome. Additionally, dysregulation of NCC is implicated in the genesis of pseudohypoaldosteronism type II, and it is proposed that both co-transporters belong to the hypertension susceptibility genes. In this chapter we will discuss the cation-coupled chloride co-transporters, with particular emphasis on NKCC2 and NCC.

The SLC12A family was identified in the early 1990s with the cloning of the thiazide-sensitive Na^+-Cl^- co-transporter,[2,3] followed by two genes encoding the Na^+-K^+-$2Cl^-$ co-transporters,[3–6] and is composed of nine related genes.[7,8] Later, the four genes encoding K^+:Cl^- co-tranporters that were named KCC1,[9] KCC2,[10] KCC3,[11,12] and KCC4[12] were identified.

Figure 32.1 depicts a phylogenetic tree of all members of the SLC12 family for which functional properties are known, as well as the chromosome to which each gene has been mapped in humans, the inherited disease that results from inactivating mutations of the gene, and the consequence of knocking-out each gene in the mouse. Two branches within the family are clearly identified. The Na^+-driven branch encompasses three genes: SLC12A1 and SLC12A2 encode the Na^+:K^+:$2Cl^-$ co-transporters, NKCC2 and NKCC1, respectively. NKCC2 is a kidney-specific gene, with expression restricted to the apical membrane of the thick ascending limb of Henle's loop (TAL).[3,5,13,14] In contrast, NKCC1 is a ubiquitously expressed protein that is located at the basolateral membrane of secretory epithelial cells, as well as in many non-epithelial cells (neurons, fibroblasts, erythrocytes, etc.).[15,16] SCL12A3 is the third gene of the Na^+-driven branch, and encodes the thiazide-sensitive Na^+:Cl^- co-transporter,

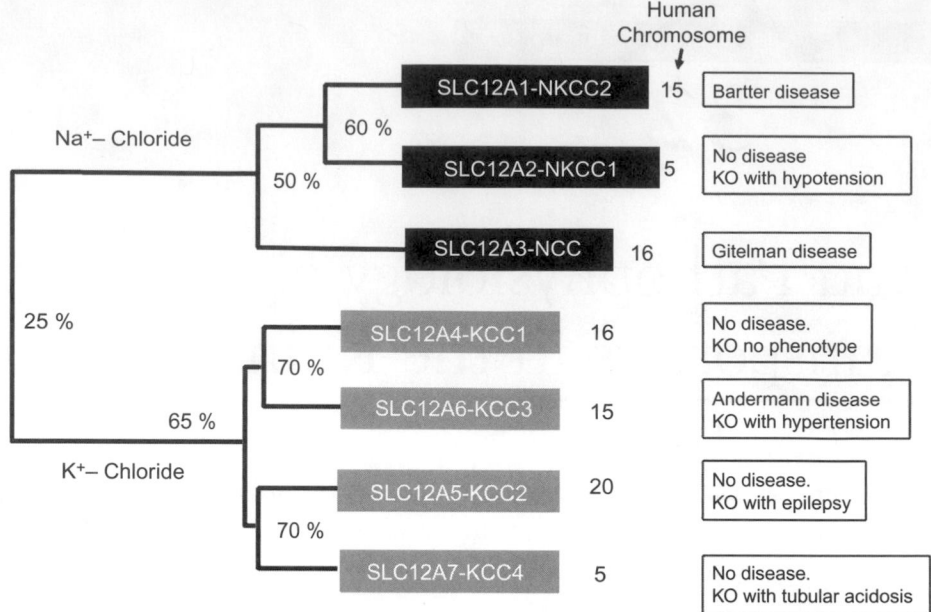

FIGURE 32.1 SLC12 phylogenetic tree. The family is divided in two branches: the Na-coupled and the K-coupled co-transporters. The degree of identity between members is shown in percentages. Chromosome location, inherited diseases, consequences in corresponding knockout mice, and the tissue specific expression is shown.

NCC.[2,3,17] It is mainly expressed in the apical membrane of the distal convoluted tubule (DCT). Initially it was thought that NCC is a gene with restrictive expression in the kidney; however, later it was demonstrated to be expressed at the protein level along the gut,[18] in bone,[19] and in the lens.[20] Although a thiazide-sensitive Na$^+$-Cl$^-$ co-transporter has been postulated to exist in other tissues,[21] blood vessels,[22] pancreas,[23] peripheral blood mononuclear cells,[24] gallbladder[25] and heart,[26] its presence at the molecular level has not been demonstrated. In bone, NCC activity is associated with the rate of bone formation. Many clinical studies have shown that thiazide diuretics in elderly subjects promote an increase in bone mineral density and help to prevent pathological fractures.[27,28] Consistent with this beneficial effect of thiazides, NCC is expressed in osteoblasts of rat and human bones, and addition of thiazides to osteoblasts in culture increases the formation of mineralized nodules. This effect of thiazides was not present after NCC expression was reduced by transfecting cells with an NCC antisense plasmid.[19]

The degree of identity at the protein level between NKCC1 and NKCC2 is ~60%, and between NCC and the NKCCs is ~50%. The degree varies, however, within specific domains of the co-transporters. It is >80% in some of the central hydrophobic membrane spanning domains, ~50% in the carboxyl terminal domain, and <10% in the amino terminal domain and most of the interconnecting loops that are oriented toward the extracellular side.

The K$^+$-driven branch is composed of four genes, SLC12A4 to SLC12A7, encoding the K$^+$:Cl$^-$ co-transporters KCC1 to KCC4, respectively. KCC1 is ubiquitously expressed, while KCC2 is only present in neurons. KCC3 and KCC4 are expressed in several tissues, including the kidney.[7,8,29] Along the nephron KCC3 has been shown to be present only in the proximal tubule, while KCC4 is also expressed in the basolateral membrane of TAL and the intercalated cells of collecting duct (CD).[30–32] The degree of identity is about 60% between KCCs and about 25% with the members of the Na$^+$-driven branch.

Two additional genes are classified within the SLC12A family (not shown in Figure 32.1) due to a degree of identity of ~20% with either the Na$^+$-driven or the K$^+$-driven branches. SLC12A8 gene (human chromosome 3) encodes a protein of 714 amino acid residues that has been identified as a psoriasis susceptibility gene by two independent groups.[33,34] One report suggests that this protein may translocate polyamines and amino acids across the plasma membrane.[35] SLC12A9 (human chromosome 7) encodes a 918 residue protein originally named as co-transporter interacting protein (CIP) for its ability to modulate the activity of NKCC1.[36] Its topological similarity and the 25% identity with other members of the family suggest that it is likely that CIP transports substrates that have not been identified.

THE PHYSIOLOGY OF NaCl CO-TRANSPORTERS IN THE KIDNEY

The electroneutral cation—chloride co-transporters translocate Cl$^-$ ions together with a cation, which can be Na$^+$, K$^+$ or both, maintaining the requirement of electroneutrality: $1Na^+$-$1Cl^-$, or $1K^+$-$1Cl^-$ or $1Na^+$-$1K^+$-$2Cl^-$ stoichiometry. The direction of the transport process is defined by the cation gradient. Therefore, NKCC1, NKCC2, and NCC move ions inward across the plasma membrane, while KCCs move ions outward. Because Na^+ and K^+ are returned to the steady-state by the Na^+:K^+-ATPase, the activity of the SLC12A co-transporters is considered to be primarily regulation of the intracellular chloride concentration $[Cl^-]_i$, a role that is critical to some physiological processes. One of these is cell volume regulation. During cell shrinking, due to increased osmolarity of the extracellular medium, the regulatory volume increase response stimulates transport mechanisms to enhance the intracellular osmolarity, including activation of NKCC1 > NKCC2 > NCC. In contrast, during cell swelling, the regulatory volume decrease promotes the activation of KCCs to reduce intracellular osmolarity. Because basically every cell expresses NKCC1 and KCC1, this cell volume regulatory mechanism is universal.[37]

Another major function of electroneutral cation–chloride co-transporters is the setting of the intraneuronal chloride concentration, either above or below its electrochemical equilibrium potential. For this reason, the activity of these co-transporters is critical in determining the polarity and magnitude of the effect of neurotransmitters that gate Cl^- channels in postsynaptic membranes, such as GABA.[16,38] It is known that before birth GABA behaves mostly as an excitatory neurotransmitter, in neurons in which intracellular chloride is above the electrochemical equilibrium due to more prominent expression of NKCC1 than KCC2. After birth, however, GABA becomes predominantly an inhibitor transmitter, due to the inversion of NKCC1/KCC2 ratio of expression that lowers intracellular chloride below equilibrium.[39]

A third major role of the SLC12A co-transporters that will occupy our interest for the rest of this chapter is the transepithelial movement of ions. NCC and NKCC2 are polarized to the apical membrane of DCT and TAL, respectively, where they participate in renal salt reabsorption. NKCC1 is expressed in the basolateral membrane of several chloride-secreting epithelia, where its activity is critical to provide the cell with chloride ions to be secreted in the apical membrane. The K^+:Cl^- co-transporters are also involved in epithelial movement of ions. One example is KCC4 that is expressed in the intercalated cells of the CD, where it plays a role in the chloride efflux required to maintain hydrogen secretion and thus, acid–base homeostasis.[31]

The Thiazide-Sensitive Na^--Cl^- Co-Transporter

NCC is the major salt transport pathway in the apical membrane of mammalian DCT cells[40–44] which mediates reabsorption of 5–10% of glomerular filtrate. In the early DCT (DCT1) NCC is fully in charge of salt reabsorption, while in the late DCT (DCT2) it shares the responsibility with the sodium channel ENaC.[45–49] This is an important difference, since DCT1 is not considered to be part of the aldosterone-sensitive distal nephron, due to the lack of 11β-hydroxysteroid dehydrogenase type 2 (11β-HSD2), which prevents illicit occupation of the mineralocorticoid receptor by cortisol.[46,49–52] Thus, NCC is susceptible to aldosterone regulation only in DCT2 cells. The molecular mechanism of salt reabsorption in DCT is illustrated in Figure 32.2. The Na^+ gradient that drives transport from the lumen to the interstitium is generated and maintained by the intense activity of Na^+/K^+-ATPase that is polarized to the basolateral membrane.[53] Potassium entering the cell through the Na^+/K^+ pump is secreted by the luminal membrane via K^+ channels[54] and by an apical K^+-Cl^- co-transporter.[55] Thus, potassium secretion rate is determined, at least in part, by the rate of Na^+-Cl^- reabsorption. In addition, NCC modulates magnesium and calcium reabsorption, the latter in an inverse relationship with sodium reabsorption. The lower the sodium reabsorption, the higher the calcium reabsorption, and vice versa.[42] As shown in Figure 32.2, NCC is the target for thiazide-type diuretics (metolazone, hydrochlorothiazide, chlortalidone, bendroflumethiazide).[3,43,56] Because thiazides are recommended for the treatment of arterial hypertension, some edematous states, and renal stone disease,[57,58] this group of drugs are among the most commonly prescribed medicines in the world.

The Loop-Diuretic-Sensitive Na^+-K^+-$2Cl^-$ Co-Transporter 2 (NKCC2)

NKCC2 is the major salt transport pathway in the apical membrane of the mammalian TAL, a nephron segment where 15–20% of glomerular filtrate is reabsorbed.[59–64] In addition to its role in salt reabsorption, NKCC2 activity also serves to keep the countercurrent multiplication mechanism by promoting salt concentration in the renal medulla and thus, the renal ability to concentrate urine. Divalent cation (Ca^{2+} and Mg^{2+}) and ammonium (NH_4^+) reabsorption in the TAL also requires the activity of NKCC2 (for reviews see [64–66]). As shown in Figure 32.2, in the case of Ca^{2+} and Mg^{2+} this is due to the fact that simultaneous

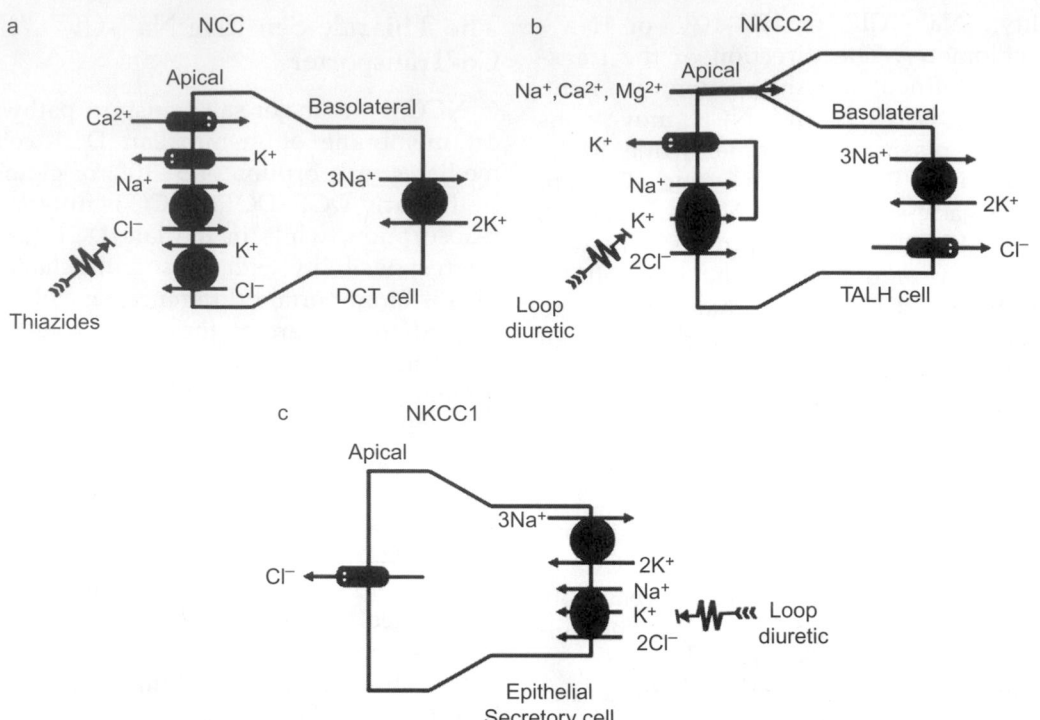

FIGURE 32.2   Transepithelial ion transport by NCC, NKCC2, and NKCC1. (a) Distal convoluted tubule. Expression of NCC is polarized towards the apical membrane. (b) Thick ascending limb of Henle's loop. NKCC2 expression is located to the apical membrane. (c) An example of secretory epithelial cell that could be from trachea, gills, intestine, salivary gland, etc. NKCC1 present in the basolateral membrane provides the cell with the chloride to be secreted through the apical membrane.

operation of NKCC2 with the basolateral chloride channels CLC-KB, the Na^+/K^+-ATPase, and the apical inwardly rectifying K^+ channel known as ROMK, promotes the generation of positive voltage within the TAL lumen, which in turn drives the reabsorption of a second cation via a paracellular pathway, which could be Na^+, Ca^{2+} or Mg^{2+}. Thus, in contrast to what occurs in DCT, in the TAL reducing salt reabsorption is associated with reducing calcium reabsorption. Because of this, loop diuretics are often used in the clinical setting for the management of life-threatening hypercalcemia. In the case of ammonium, this is due to the fact that NH_4 can use potassium transport pathways for its translocation through the plasma membrane. Thus, NKCC2 can also operate as the Na^+:NH_4^+:$2Cl^-$ co-transporter.[67,68]

NKCC2 is an important target in cardiovascular and renal pharmacology, because inhibition of this co-transporter is the base of the loop diuretic actions that are the most potent natriuretic agents available for clinical use (furosemide, ethacrinic acid, bumetanide). Loop diuretics decrease the salt reabsorption in TAL, producing significant natriuresis and diuresis. Because loop diuretics reduce interstitial osmolarity of the renal medulla, another mechanism of action is to reduce the concentration capacity of the kidney. Any increase in salt delivery to the macula densa is expected to be compensated by reducing the glomerular filtration rate due to the tubuloglomerular balance.[69] This compensation is absent, however, in the presence of loop diuretics, because the salt-sensing protein in macula densa is also NKCC2.[70] Since the B variant of NKCC2 is the most abundant variant in macula densa cells,[71] and it is not expressed in shark kidney, which also lacks a macula densa,[72] it has been proposed that NKCC2B is the Cl^- sensor in TAL cells. It has been difficult to prove this hypothesis because the variant-specific knockout mice lacking NKCC2B developed a compensatory increase in NKCC2A expression in the TAL cells, and only exhibited a very slight shift to the right of the tubuloglomerular feedback curve.[73] Similarly, the isoform-specific null mice for NKCC2A variant also showed slight changes in tubuloglomerular feedback.[74] These observations suggest that both isoforms working together compose the Cl^- sensor in the macula densa.

Increasing net NaCl reabsorption in TAL by hormones generating cAMP via Gs-coupled receptors such as vasopressin, glucagon, parathyroid hormone, β-adrenergic, and calcitonin is a fundamental mechanism for regulating salt transport in this nephron segment.[75,76] Of these hormones, the most important is the antidiuretic hormone vasopressin, which increases NaCl absorption by TAL through a mechanism that appears to involve trafficking of NKCC2 to the apical plasma membrane.[77–79] Supporting this proposal it has been observed in medullary TAL that most NKCC2 protein is located in intracellular vesicles, and that addition of cAMP increases the expression of NKCC2 in the apical membrane by activating the exocytosis, rather than by inhibiting the endocytosis of NKCC2-containing vesicles.[80,81] Additionally, long-term increases in vasopressin are associated with increased expression of NKCC2 and maximal urinary concentration ability.[82,83]

The Loop-Diuretic Sensitive Na$^+$-K$^+$-2Cl$^-$ Co-Transporter 1 (NKCC1)

NKCC1 is the Na$^+$-K$^+$-2Cl$^-$ co-transporter that is present in secretory epithelium, as well as in many non-epithelial cells. At the cellular physiology level, NKCC1 is very important for cell volume and [Cl$^-$]$_i$ regulation.[7,15,37,84] The diverse phenotypes of NKCC1 knockout mice illustrate the role of this transporter in numerous physiological processes.[85-87] NKCC1 knockout mice feature deafness due to both disrupted epithelial secretion in the labyrinth and a sensorineural defect, infertility due to a deficiency in spermatocyte production, cecum bleeding and blockade of the colon due to impaired intestinal secretion, salivation impairment, and low blood pressure due to vascular and renal effects.[88] Blood pressure in NKCC1 null mice is decreased due to reduced vascular tone.[86,88–90] In this regard, the loop diuretic bumetanide decreased blood pressure in normal mice by inhibiting the activity of NKCC1 in vascular beds, and reduced the vascular smooth muscle cells' myogenic tone. Both effects are not present in the NKCC1 null mice, strongly suggesting that are the results of inhibiting NKCC1 in blood vessels.[91,92] Of note, however, one study using telemetry to monitor blood pressure day and night for several days failed to confirm hypotension in the NKCC1 knockout mice, and suggested a salt-sensitive component because a significant increase in blood pressure was produced by a high-salt diet.[93] Finally, NKCC1 is expressed in the basolateral membrane of the macula densa cells,[94] where it has been suggested that it modulates renin secretion.[95]

MOLECULAR BIOLOGY OF THE SODIUM-DEPENDENT CHLORIDE CO-TRANSPORTERS

The Thiazide-Sensitive Na$^+$-Cl$^-$ Co-Transporter

Following an expression cloning strategy using the functional expression system of *Xenopus laevis* oocytes, NCC cDNA was first identified at the molecular level from the winter flounder (*Pseudopleuronectes americanus*) urinary bladder.[2] This clone was named as TSC (for thiazide-sensitive co-transporter), and later changed to NCC. The flounder's transcript produced a 3.7 kb cDNA clone containing a 3609 bp open reading frame that predicted a 1023 amino acid residues protein with a core molecular mass of 112 kDa. The computer-based analysis hydrophobicity/hydrophylicity[96] suggested the putative basic topology of the Na$^+$-coupled-Cl$^-$ co-transporters shown in Figure 32.3a. The short amino terminal domain is followed by a central hydrophobic domain containing what appear to be 12 α-helices compatible with transmembrane-spanning segments. A long carboxyl terminal domain follows this. The amino and carboxyl terminal domains are predicted to be located within the cell. The long loop between transmembrane segments 7 and 8 is glycosylated in NCC[97,98] and NKCC2,[99] and thus presumably in all members of the SLC12A family. In flounder, a shorter 3.0 kb transcript due to alternative splicing is expressed in several tissues including the brain, eye, heart, intestine, gonads, and skeletal muscle.[2] The functional consequence of this variant remains elusive.[100] After the cloning of NCC from the flounder urinary bladder, cDNAs encoding NCC from a variety of mammalian sources were isolated, including rat (*Rattus norvegicus*),[3] mouse (*Mus musculus*),[177] rabbit (*Oryctolagus cuniculus*),[101] and human (*Homo sapiens*).[102,103] Additionally, the NCC cDNA sequence has been deposited in gene databases for at least another 10 species, mostly mammalians and one birth.[104] The degree of identity between mammalian NCCs is ~90%, and of any mammalian with flounder is ~60%. Molecular identification of putative NCC sequences in eel suggests the existence of two different NCC genes.[105] NCCα is expressed only in eel kidney, while NCCβ was observed in many tissues, but more abundantly in intestine. The amino acid residues of NCCα and NCCβ are 1027 and 1043, respectively. No functional expression was analyzed, but the extend of identity of NCCα or NCCβ with any NCC, NKCC1 or NKCC2 supports the proposition that these eel sequences probably correspond to NCC, since degree of identity of NCCα or NCCβ with any NCC sequence is higher than with any NKCC1 or NKCC2. In mammals, rabbit and human NCC is longer than other species due to the presence of 17–26 amino acid residues in the carboxyl terminal domain. These extra residues were shown to be encoded in humans by a separate exon (exon 20) which is not present in rodents.[7,104] It is noteworthy that in humans, there is a putative protein kinase A (PKA) site (RPS) within the extra fragment. No functional significance for this extra exon in humans has been reported, but an extensive proteomic analysis of human urinary

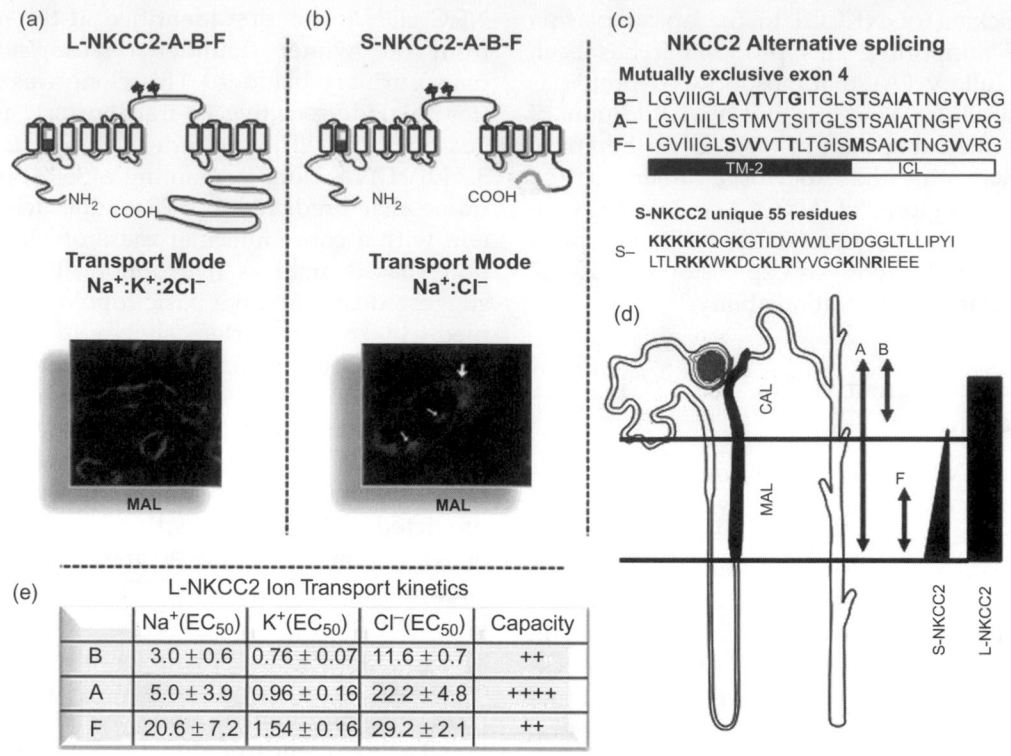

FIGURE 32.3   **Molecular physiology of the Na$^+$-K$^+$-2Cl$^-$ co-transporter, NKCC2.** (a) Proposed topology (similar to NCC and NKCC1), transport mode, and immunolocalization of the long isoform of NKCC2 (L-NKCC2). The intracellular short amino-terminal domain is followed by 12 transmembrane segments and a long carboxyl terminal domain. The long hydrophilic loop between TM segments 7 and 8 is gylcosylated.[97,99] Several threonines/serine residues in the amino-terminal domain are known to be critical for the regulation of the co-transporters. The mutually exclusive cassette exons A, B, and F are shown in red. (b) Proposed topology, transport mode, and immunolocalization of the short isoform of NKCC2 (L-NKCC2). Location of the mutually exclusive cassette exons is shown in red, and the unique 55 piece at the end is shown in orange. In the picture the white arrows points to positive cells. (c) Sequence and alignment of the exon cassettes A, B, and F. Swapping the red or green residues between B and F isoforms switches their ion transport kinetics between each other (TM-2: transmembrane domain 2; ICL: interconnecting segment between TM2 and TM3). The 55 unique fragment of the short NKCC2 is shown. Positively charged residues are shown in blue. (d) Distribution of L-NKCC2 and S-NKCC2, as well as exons A, B, and F along the limb of Henle, as stated. (e) Ion transport kinetics and capacity of transport for L-NKCC2 A, B, and F variants, as informed by Plata et al.[77] *(Modified from ref. [64].)* See color section at the back of the book.

exosomes revealed, among may proteins found, the presence of several fragments of NCC, some of which have the serine 811 phosphorylated, that correspond to the putative protein kinase A site RPS contained by the human exon 20.[106] The expression of NCC protein has been confirmed using specific antibodies in intestine,[18] bone cells,[19] and lens.[20] Additionally, *in silico* analysis of NCC expression revealed that NCC transcripts are abundantly present in sensory ganglia, such as trigeminal and dorsal root ganglion.[104] No report has confirmed the presence of NCC protein in this tissue, and its functional significance is unknown.

The Loop-Diuretic-Sensitive Na$^+$-K$^+$-2Cl$^-$ Co-Transporter 2 (NKCC2)

The product of SLC12A1 is the Na$^+$-K$^+$-2Cl$^-$ co-transporter known as NKCC2, and it has been located

exclusively in the apical membrane of the TAL. Two groups simultaneously identified the cDNA encoding both Na$^+$:K$^+$:2Cl$^-$ co-transporter isoforms. Hebert and co-workers cloned the cDNA encoding NKCC2/BSC1 from rat renal outer medulla, and then NKCC1/BSC2 from a mouse inner medullary collecting cells cDNA library,[6] while Forbush and co-workers first identified NKCC1/BSC2 cDNA from a shark rectal gland cDNA library,[4] and later NKCC2/BSC1 from rabbit renal outer medulla.[5] Later, human and mouse NKCC2 sequences were reported.[14,107] Isolated cDNA clones were about 4.5 kb in size, with an open reading frame of 3285 bp encoding a 1095 residue protein. The predicted NKCC2 topology (Figure 32.3A) is highly similar to NCC, featuring the central hydrophobic domain with 12 putative membrane-spanning segments that is flanked by the predominantly hydrophilic amino terminal domain (~165 amino acids) and carboxyl terminal domain (~450 residues). Functional expression analysis in *Xenopus laevis* oocytes demonstrated that NKCC2 encodes a bumetanide-sensitive Na$^+$-K$^+$-2Cl$^-$ co-transporter.[3] It was observed, in a tissue distribution analysis using Northern blot, that NKCC2 transcripts are exclusively present in the renal outer medulla. All other tissues were negative and, until today, no study has confirmed the presence of NKCC2 protein in any other tissue or culture cell. It was proposed that this is due to the presence of a tissue-specific promoter.[108] Interestingly, however, as shown for NCC, *in silico* distribution analysis suggests the existence of NKCC2 transcripts in the sensory ganglia, such as trigeminal and dorsal root ganglion.[104]

SLC12A1 gives rise to a number of alternative splicing variants. At least six isoforms have been suggested to be present in the mouse kidney. Two independent alternatively splicing mechanisms are responsible[7,13,109] (Figure 32.3a,b). One splicing event was first observed in rabbit,[5] and later also in mouse,[14] rat,[110] and human[107] kidney. Three isoforms or variants arise from this splicing mechanism that involve the existence of three mutually-exclusive cassette exons nominated as A, B, and F (Figure 32.3a). These cassettes are composed of 96 bp encoding a 32 amino acid that is part of the second part of the transmembrane segment 2 and the first part of the intracellularly-located interconnecting segment between TM2 and 3 (Figure 32.3c). Thus, three NKCC2 proteins are produced differing only in the 32 amino acid residues, and all three are present in the mammalian NKCC2s known to date.[104] Only variants A and F have been identified from *Squalus acanthias* (shark) kidney.[72]

Another splicing of *SLC12A1* gene that was observed in the mouse kidney is due to the presence of a poly-adenylation site located in the intron between exons 16 and 17, resulting in a shorter C-terminal domain with an extra 55 amino acid residues, not present in the long isoform (Figure 32.3b).[13] Thus, two NKCC2 proteins are produced. These are identical from the first residue in the amino terminal domain to residue 74 of the carboxyl terminal domain. After this point, the longer isoform contains 383 residues not present in the shorter isoform, while the shorter contains 55 residues not present in the longer variant (Figure 32.3c). The existence of the shorter isoform in mouse kidney was demonstrated by a specific polyclonal antibody directed against the 55 unique piece of the shorter isoform.[13] By means of RT-PCR, it was shown that mouse kidney exhibits transcripts of the three isoforms A, B, and F, combined with both possibilities for the carboxyl terminal domain, suggesting that both splicing mechanisms are independent of each other and thus, that a total of six isoforms are predicted to be produced in mouse kidney: three long NKCC2 isoforms (A, B, and F), and three short NKCC2 isoforms (A, B and F).[13] The possible functional significance of spliced isoforms is discussed below.

The Ubiquitous Bumetanide-Sensitive Na$^+$-K$^+$-2Cl$^-$ Co-Transporter (NKCC1)

The SLC12A2 gene encodes the ubiquitously expressed Na$^+$-K$^+$-2Cl$^-$ co-transporter. NKCC1 is expressed in the plasma membrane of both epithelial and non-epithelial cells. In the first case, it is limited to the basolateral membrane in which the activity NKCC1 serves to provide the cell with the potassium or chloride ions to be secreted through the apical membrane. The only exception is the choroid plexus, in which both the Na$^+$-K$^+$-ATPase and NKCC1 are expressed in the apical membrane.[111] NKCC1 has been identified at the molecular level in several species, including mouse,[6] rat,[112] human,[113] *Bos taurus* (bovine),[114] shark,[4] *Anguilla anguilla* (eel),[115] and *Dicentrarchus labrax* (sea bass),[116] and even from the plant *Arabidopsis thaliana*.[117] The existence of one alternatively-spliced isoform of NKCC1 has been suggested.[118] This is a slightly shorter splice variant present in mouse brain total RNA due to the lack of 48 bp corresponding to the entire exon 21. This exon contains a potential PKA phosphorylation site. The existence of a splice transcript was supported by an RNAse protection assay. Distribution analysis within the brain showed that an NKCC1 transcript lacking exon 21 is present in all areas examined except in the choroid plexus, where only the full-length isoform containing exon 21 is expressed. Functional expression in heterologous systems revealed that the shorter variant behaves as a Na$^+$-K$^+$-2Cl$^-$ co-transporter.[119] Interestingly, it was recently shown that exon 21 of NKCC1 is implicated in differential sorting in polarized epithelial cells.[120]

Genes, Promoters, and Phylogenetic Analysis

The location of *SLC12A1*, the gene encoding NKCC2 in humans is within chromosome 15,[107] in rat within chromosome 3,[121] and in mouse within chromosome 2.[122] *SLC12A1* is composed of more than 80 kb and 26 exons have been clearly described to encode for the full length 1095 amino acid residue protein.[104] Mouse is the only species from which the *SLC12A1* promoter region has been cloned.[108] The NKCC2 transcript starts with the first exon of 34 bp that is non-coding, followed by a first intron of 1101 bp and a second exon containing the translation start codon. The promoter is composed of 2255 bp. There is a TATA box located at position -29 and consensus recognition sites for several transcription factors, of which the most interesting could be a binding site for HNF-1 at -211 bp. In developing mouse kidney, the expression of HNF-1 precedes the expression of NKCC2.[123] HNF-1 has been implicated in the regulation of tissue-specific expression of genes in liver, pancreas, kidney, and intestine. Deletion of −2255 to −1529 bp of the promoter resulted in a ~three-fold increase in gene transcription rate, suggesting the presence of negative regulatory elements in this segment. No further effect was observed by deleting −1529 to −469 bp, but a significant reduction in gene expression was obtained by elimination from −469 to −190, suggesting that this region contains positive regulatory elements. An HFN-1-binding site is located in this region. A cAMP response element-binding protein is located at nucleotide −1111, and this could be of major importance because it is known that NKCC2 expression is stimulated by vasopressin.[75,82,124]

The gene *SLC12A2* encodes NKCC1 and is located to chromosome 5q23 in humans,[113] and to chromosome 18 in mouse.[6] The complete gene encompasses a region of 75 kb[118] and is made up of 28 exons. Significant luciferase activity was produced by transfection of mouse IMDC3 cells with a 2063 bp promoter region, together with a luciferase reporter gene. Deletions of >1 kb that reduced the promoter region to 702 or 516 bp resulted in a significant increase in luciferase activity, suggesting the existence of silencer sequences in the deleted bases. Additional deletions resulted in progressive reduction of luciferase activity, suggesting the presence of enhancer elements. Expression of NKCC1 in vascular smooth muscle cells has been suggested to be associated with the development of hypertension in rat models of hypertension. In this regard, a recent report showed that SLC2A2 gene promoter hypomethylation upregulates NKCC1 expression in aorta and heart of spontaneously hypertensive rats.[125,126]

SLC12A3, the gene encoding the thiazide sensitive Na$^+$-Cl$^-$ co-transporter, is located in humans to chromosome 16q13,[102,103] in rat to chromosome 19p12-14,[127] and in mouse to chromosome 8.[128] Human *SLC12A3* is 55 kb long and contains 26 exons.[102] Transcription initiation is confined to an area from -18 to -6 bp upstream of the translation start codon. The promoter activity observed in the mouse distal convoluted cell line (MDCT),[129] with a construct containing 1019 bp of the 5′ flanking region was reduced only 25% by eliminating the first 885 bp. Sequence analysis of the promoter revealed the presence of a TATA element, two Sp-binding sites, and potential binding sites for NF-1/CTF or NY-I/CP-I. Interestingly, the promoter activity of the rat NCC gene is inhibited by acidosis. This is consistent with a marked fall in renal cortical abundance of NCC protein assessed by Western blot,[130] and by [^{3}H] Metolazone-binding to plasma membranes from the renal cortex[131] of rats exposed to chronic NH$_4$Cl-loading.

FUNCTIONAL PROPERTIES

The member of the family that has been more extensively characterized is NKCC1. This is because it is expressed in many different cell types that, on one hand, made it accessible for functional characterization, even before the cDNA was identified, and on the other hand, it attracted the interest of many groups of researchers in a variety of fields such as neuroscience, cell volume regulation, red blood cell, and epithelial transport mechanism (for an in-depth review see [15]). In contrast, before identification of the corresponding genes, functional characterization of NKCC2 and NCC was relatively scarce,[57,132,133] and most of the knowledge came from analysis of renal outer medulla or cortical plasma membrane-binding of tracer [^{3}H] Bumetanide or [^{3}H]Metolazone, respectively.[134−136] With the cloning of cDNAs encoding the SLC12A co-transporter proteins and several variants, in-depth characterization of their major functional, pharmacologic, and some regulatory properties has been made possible.

The Thiazide-Sensitive-Na$^+$-Cl$^-$ Co-Transporter

Heterologous expression of teleost, rat, mouse, and human NCC has been achieved in *Xenopus laevis* oocytes.[2,3,137−140] Oocytes are not epithelial cells; however, this expression system is a useful tool for robust and reproducible NCC expression. Unfortunately, expression of NCC in mammalian cells transfected with NCC cDNAs has been almost impossible to achieve, and so far has been reported only by two independent groups in MDCK[141] and HEK-293.[142] However, in both cases, the level of NCC expression was low, and not sufficient for that required to define the functional properties of the co-transporter. Thus, *Xenopus laevis* continued to be the best cells to assess NCC activity, and basically all of what is known today regarding the functional properties and regulation of NCC activity comes from studies performed in oocytes. Recent reports from Hoover and co-workers[143,144] showed that a subcloned version of the immortal mouse DCT cell line originally produced by Gesek, Friedman and co-workers[145] exhibit what appears to be a robust expression of endogenous NCC, promising an excellent tool for NCC functional analysis in a mammalian cell system.

As shown in Table 32.1, a number of interesting differences have been observed between fish (flounder) and mammalian (rat and mouse) NCC. The affinity for Na$^+$ and Cl$^-$ in rat[137] or mouse NCC proteins[139] is significantly higher than the affinity observed in the flounder NCC.[146] In addition, the Km values for Na[+] and Cl[−] in mammalian NCCs are similar, whereas in flounder the Km value for extracellular Cl[−] is lower than the value for Na[+]. NCC activity is inhibited by thiazide-type diuretics with the following profile: polythiazide > metolazone > bendroflumethiazide > trichloromethiazide > chlorthalidone. However, for all thiazides, flounder's NCC exhibited lower affinity. At a concentration of 100 μM, the thiazides with lower potency, trichloromethiazide and chlorthalidone, reduced flounder NCC activity by only 68 and 46%, respectively,[146] whereas the same concentration of all thiazides inhibited rat NCC by >95% .[137]

Two proposals for the order of ion-binding to NCC have been suggested. By assessing the [3H]metolazone-binding to membranes extracted from rat renal cortex, Tran and collaborators[147] observed that Na[+] increased tracer-binding to the putative thiazide-sensitive transport protein. In contrast, Cl[−] decreased the affinity for metolazone. Thus, the model that was proposed included two binding sites within the thiazide receptor: one selective for Na[+]; and the other that recognizes either Cl[−] or metolazone in a competitive fashion. In this model, occupation of the Na[+] site increases the affinity of the second site for either Cl[−] and/or metolazone.[148]

The second model was based on observations of functional properties of NCC as expressed in *Xenopus laevis* oocytes. Monroy et al.[137] observed that affinity for Na[+] or Cl[−] changed as a function of counterion concentration. The lower the extracellular Na[+] concentration, the lower the Cl[−] affinity, a relationship that supports the initial conclusions of Tran et al.[147] However, it was also observed that lower extracellular Cl[−] concentrations coincided with lower Na[+] affinity. In addition, it was observed that the IC$_{50}$ for metolazone inhibition increased when the thiazide dose−response curves were measured in lower Na[+] or Cl[−] conditions, suggesting that both ions compete with metolazone for binding to the co-transporter. Thus, the proposed model included a random order of binding, with both ions affecting affinity for the counterion and

competing with thiazide diuretics.[137] Supporting this model, data produced later that is discussed below suggest that affinity-defining domains or residues for Cl[−] and thiazide-binding are located in different parts of the protein.[98]

The Loop-Diuretic-Sensitive Na[+]-K[+]-2Cl[−] Co-Transporter 2 (NKCC2)

Several NKCC2 splice variants in different species have been analyzed at tissue-specific expression and functional level, including shark,[72] rat,[3] mouse,[78] rabbit,[5] and human.[149] As previously discussed, there are three variants of NKCC2 named A, B, and F (Figure 32.3c). The three variants from mouse perform as Na[+]-K[+]-2Cl[−], suggesting that the difference between variants could be in the kinetic properties for ion transport and/or bumetanide affinity.[78] This hypothesis was supported by intrarenal localization studies that demonstrated axial distribution of these variants along TAL.[5,14,110] As shown in Figure 32.3d, the A isoform is present in both cortical and medullary TAL. In contrast, the B isoform is present only in cortical TAL, and the F variant is expressed only in the inner stripe of the outer medulla. Early studies[150−152] demonstrated that the NaCl transport rate in mTAL is significantly more rapid than in the cTAL, but with greater diluting power in the later segment. Thus, the possibility for heterogeneity of the transport process was suggested. Evidence supporting this hypothesis was obtained simultaneously by Plata et al.[153] and Gimenez et al.[71] using mouse and rabbit NKCC2 variants, respectively (Figure 32.3e). NKCC2F exhibits the lowest affinity for co-transported ions, and is more sensitive to changes in extracellular osmolarity. As shown in Figure 32.3d, NKCC2F is predominantly expressed in the inner stripe of the outer medulla, where the salt concentration is very high, and where greater changes in extracellular osmolarity occur. NKCC2A exhibits the highest transport capacity and is expressed along all TAL. Finally, NKCC2B, the variant that is expressed only the cTAL where ion concentration of the tubular fluid has decreased to values even below those in plasma, is the variant with the highest affinity for the co-transported ions. Thus, the dilution power along TAL is explained by the presence of three alternatively-spliced variants of NKCC2 with distinct functional characteristics. The NKCC2 influx data from Plata et al.[153] were later used to construct a mathematical model for the NKCC2 co-transporter isoforms.[154]

As discussed above, a shorter variant containing 55 amino acid residues at the end that are not present in the longer NKCC2 isoform has been described

TABLE 32.1 Ion Transport and Thiazide-Sensitive Kinetics of Mammalian and Flounder NCC Expressed in *Xenopus laevis* Oocytes

	Rat NCC[98,137]	Mouse NCC[139]	Flounder NCC[98,137]
Na[+] Km (mM)	5.5 ± 1.0	7.2 ± 0.4	30.0 ± 6.0
Cl[−] Km (mM)	2.6 ± 0.6	5.6 ± 0.6	15.2 ± 2.0
Metolazone IC$_{50}$ μM	0.3 ± 0.001	0.4 ± 0.001	4.0 ± 0.08

Modified from references [98,137,139].

(Figure 32.3b,c). This variant is only present in mTAL, not in cTAL[13] and performs as a K$^+$-independent, but nevertheless, loop diuretic-sensitive Na$^+$-Cl$^-$ co-transporter that is activated by hypotonicity and inhibited by cAMP.[155] Therefore, the shorter NKCC2 variant may provide a molecular explanation for previous physiological studies that suggested a switch from Na$^+$-Cl$^-$ to Na$^+$-K$^+$-Cl$^-$ co-transporter mode in TAL by extracellular osmolarity or by the presence of vasopressin. Eveloff and co-workers[156,157] observed, in rabbit TAL cells, the existence of a K$^+$-independent, furosemide-sensitive Na$^+$-Cl$^-$ co-transporter in hypotonic conditions that became K$^+$-dependent, constituting the Na$^+$-K$^+$-2Cl$^-$ co-transporter, when cells were changed to isotonic medium. In addition, Sun et al.[158] found that in mouse TAL cells, vasopressin (i.e., cAMP) shifts the mode of apical co-transport from Na$^+$-Cl$^-$ (in its absence) to Na$^+$-K$^+$-2Cl$^-$ (in its presence). Consistent with these studies, the large NKCC2 is a Na$^+$-K$^+$-2Cl$^-$ co-transporter that is activated by increased tonicity or the presence of vasopressin, while the shorter NKCC2 is a Na$^+$-Cl$^-$ co-transporter that is activated in hypotonicity or by inhibition of protein kinase A activity.

The shorter variant also exerts a dominant-negative effect upon the activity of the longer NKCC2 that can be abrogated by cAMP.[78] Using confocal microcopy, in oocytes injected with both the long (NKCC2F) and the short variant of mouse NKCC2, Meade et al.[79] observed that the short NKCC2 reduced the activity and surface expression of the long NKCC2. This effect could be prevented by cAMP, and correlated with the observation that the short NKCC2 variant prevented co-transporter trafficking and surface membrane expression of the long NKCC2. These studies thus suggested that in mouse medullary TAL, activation of Na$^+$-K$^+$-2Cl$^-$ co-transporter by hormones that increase intracellular cAMP (e.g., vasopressin, PTH) requires the presence of the short NKCC2 protein. The absence of cAMP allows the short form of NKCC2 to reduce co-transporter activity, whereas in the presence of cAMP, the negative effect of the short isoform on NKCC2 is inhibited. In this regard, Mount and collaborators[13] observed that expression of the short NKCC2 is axially distributed along TAL, as cortical TAL appears to lack this isoform. This heterogeneity may explain the observation that in mouse the vasopressin effect is present only in the medullary TAL.[63] Interestingly, the short isoform is also expressed in the thin ascending limb (Figure 32.3d), but its significance in this region is not known.

STRUCTURE–FUNCTION RELATIONSHIPS

The proposed topology for the Na-coupled chloride co-transporters NKCC1, NKCC2, and NCC is shown in Figure 32.3. There is only one study that has addressed the topology at the biochemical level. Gerelsaikhan and Turner[159] used an *in vitro* translation experiment with a variety of human NKCC1 constructs with the carboxyl-terminal reporter sequence containing multiple N-linked glycosylation sites located after each of the putative transmembrane domain. The authors concluded that the amino- and carboxyl-terminal domains are located intracellulary and flank the central hydrophobic domain in which the first eight TM segments are easily identifiable, exhibiting the classical ~20 residue α-helices. It was impossible to differentiate between TMs 9 and 10, and between TMs 11 and 12, and thus it was proposed that probably there are only two large TMs of ~36 residues in length that form tight hairpin-like structures in the membrane or take up either a non-helical or a partial-helical structure.

Ion or Diuretic Affinity Modifier Domains or Residues

Several attempts to begin to understand structure–function relationship issues in the Na$^+$-coupled Cl$^-$-co-transporters have been made on NKCC1 (for review see [160]), NKCC2,[71,153,161–163] and NCC.[98] In most cases, functional differences in NKCC1 or NCC between fish and mammalian orthologs have been exploited to design chimeric proteins to begin to define domains, regions or individual residues that are defining the ion transport or diuretic-binding affinities and/or specificity. In the case of NKCC2, most of the structure–function information available comes from the functional analysis of alternatively spliced variants.

The identity degree between shark and human NKCC1 is 74%, and interesting functional differences occurs between these orthologs (Table 32.2). Several chimeric constructs were studied by interchanging fragments of NKCC1 between human and shark cDNAs. First, the amino- and carboxyl-terminal domains between both species were swapped, providing evidence that residues located within the central hydrophobic core define ion affinity.[164] Then, a variety of chimeras were constructed and analyzed by in-depth kinetic analysis.[164–166] The chimeric design took into account the transmembrane segments that are identical in NKCC1 of both species. According to the results,[160] the three TM segments playing an important

TABLE 32.2 Ion Transport Kinetics and Bumetanide Affinity of the Na^+-K^+-$2Cl^-$ Co-Transporter NKCC1 from Human and Shark

	Sodium Km (mM)	Rubidium Km (mM)	Chloride Km (mM)	Bumetanide Ki (μM)	Reference
hNKCC1	19.6 ± 4.9	2.68 ± 0.72	26.5 ± 1.3	0.16	113
hNKCC1	15.2 ± 1.5	1.6–2.5	31 ± 1.0	0.044–0.079	164
HEK-293	22	12	110	0.054	4
sNKCC1	42	12	110	0.54	4
sNKCC1	165 ± 34	14 ± 8.0	101 ± 24	0.57	113
sNKCC1	113 ± 11	9.6–11.6	102 ± 7	0.22–0.30	164

hNKCC1: human NKCC1; sNKCC1: shark NKCC1.

role in ion transport kinetics in NKCC1 are TM2, TM4, and TM7. TM2 is involved in Na^+ and Rb^+ kinetics, TM 4 in Rb^+ and Cl^- kinetics, and TM7 in Na^+, Rb^+, and Cl^- kinetics. Interestingly, the behavior of several chimeric proteins with respect to bumetanide inhibition was completely different from that observed in ion transport kinetics. In the case of bumetanide, data suggested that TM segments 2—6 and 10—12 play a role in defining affinity for loop diuretics. Thus, results from studies using shark and human NKCC1 chimeric co-transporters argued against a previous hypothesis that loop diuretics and Cl^- compete for the same binding site.[167]

Analysis of the spliced variants A, B, and F of NKCC2 revealed a clear role of the segments encoded by these exons (TM2) in transport kinetics properties, not only for Na^+ and Rb^+, but also for Cl^- and bumetanide[71,153] (Figure 32.3). Further studies[72] showed that NKCC2 variants A and F, but not B, are present in the shark kidney, and that also in shark, the affinity for transported ions of the NKCC2A variant is higher than the NKCC2F variant. Additional chimeric proteins were constructed: chimera A/F contained the TM2 sequence of variant A followed by an interconnecting sequence of variant F, and *vice versa*.[168] The results suggested that Cl^- transport affinity-defining domains between isoforms A and F were located within the predicted interconnecting segment between TM2 and TM3, rather than within the TM2 segment. The chimeras' behavior with respect to bumetanide affinity was opposite to that of Cl^- affinity, suggesting that residues located within TM2, and not within the TM2—TM3 interconnecting segment, play a role in defining bumetanide affinity. The most recent study regarding structure—function relationship on the NKCC2 variants included a series of single or multiple point mutations of rabbit NKCC2 variants B and F or A and B, in order to switch one or few residues between variants.[162] The results demonstrated that replacement of six residues in NKCC2B resulted in a variant with Na^+ and Cl^- affinities identical to those of NKCC2F. Interestingly, three of these residues are located within the TM2 segment (ATG in B isoform were switched to TAY), and the other three within the interconnecting segment between TM2 and TM3 (SVT in B isoform were changed to MCV). The six mutations (ATG-TAY/SVT-MCV) turned NKCC2B into the F variant (Figure 32.3c), suggesting that the interconnecting loop between TM2 and TM3 might actually be part of a membrane-embedded domain.

The domains or residues defining the affinity for co-transporter ions or inhibitors may not be the same as the residues critical for the specificity for certain ions or inhibitors. All studies discussed above were performed in native, chimeric, and/or mutant NKCC1 or NKCC2 that were expected to behave as Na^+-K^+-$2Cl^-$ co-transporters. Thus, no information was obtained concerning structural requirements to define specificity for ions or diuretics. In this regard, the short isoform of NKCC2 in mouse perform as a K^+-independent, but loop diuretic-sensitive, Na^+-Cl^- co-transporter,[155] suggesting that sequences within the carboxyl-terminal domain could be critical to endow NKCC2 with K^+ transport ability. However, a study in which chimeras were constructed by swapping the amino- and carboxyl-terminal domains between NCC and NKCC2F[161] showed that chimera with the central hydrophobic domain of NKCC2, flanked by amino- and carboxyl-terminal domains of rat NCC, exhibit NKCC2 behavior. That is, as a bumetanide-sensitive Na^+-K^+-$2Cl^-$ co-transporter, indicating that the residues that endow rat NKCC2F with its functional properties should be located within the central hydrophobic domain. Thus, the explanation on how the short NKCC2 variant performs as a bumetanide-sensitive Na^+-Cl^- co-transporter remains elusive. The unique 55 amino acid segment at the end of this isoform contains several negatively-charged residues, suggesting that this fragment could interact with the co-transporter core to prevent K^+ translocation, like the ball and chain mechanism proposed for some membrane channels.[169]

Similar chimera construction and directed point mutation approaches have been used to gain insight into the structure—function relationships of NCC. It was first observed that rat[137] and mouse[139] NCCs exhibit similar functional properties that are, however, significantly different from those shown for flounder NCC.[146] Differences in functional properties and primary sequences between rat and flounder NCCs were

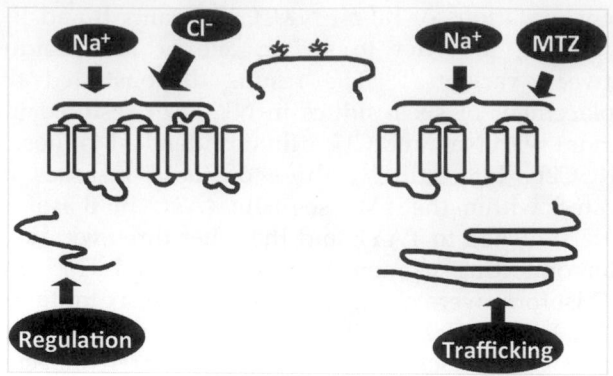

FIGURE 32.4   Affinity modifying domains in the thiazide-sensitive Na$^+$-Cl$^-$ co-transporter, NCC. *(Modified from ref. [98].)*

exploited to define affinity-modifying domains and residues.[98,170] Figure 32.4 depicts what is known regarding the structure–function relationship of NCC. By means of silent restriction sites, NCC cDNAs from rat and flounder were divided into five fragments: amino terminal domain; TM segments 1–7; extracellular glycosylated loop; TM segments 8–12; and the entire carboxyl-terminal domain, and then fragments were swapped between them to obtain a variety of combinations. The results first indicated that the central hydrophobic domains define functional characteristics of NCC. Chimeras in which the TM segments 1–7 were interchanged between flounder and rat NCCs demonstrated that affinity-defining residues for Cl$^-$ are located within these segments. Similarly, affinity-defining residues for thiazide inhibition are located within TM segments 8–12. The observation that Cl$^-$ affinity is defined by residues located within TM segments 1–7 is supported by another study, in which functional consequences of single nucleotide polymorphisms (SNP) located within the exons of the human *SLC12A3* gene changed the primary structure of NCC.[171] The results revealed that a highly-conserved glycine within the fourth transmembrane domain plays a critical role in defining the level of co-transporter activity and the affinity for Cl$^-$. Accordingly, it was observed that a glycine-to-alanine SNP at position 264 resulted in decreased activity of the co-transporter by 50%, with increased affinity for Cl$^-$ by one order of magnitude. Based on these observations, it was later observed that this SNP on NCC increases the response of humans to loop diuretics, probably because of the reduced capacity of DCT to compensate for the effect of inhibiting salt reabsorption in TAL.[172] The information that thiazide affinity-defining residues were located within TM8 to TM12 was further explored by site directed mutagenesis, revealing that a single residue in rNCC and flNCC is responsible for the differences in affinity for thiazides between mammalian and fish co-transporters. The serine 575 in rat NCC corresponds to the cysteine 576 in flounder NCC. By changing this residue, the affinity for thiazides can be transformed from mammalian to fish affinity, and *vice versa*.[170] It is worth noticing that the NCC mutants that changed the affinity for thiazides had no effect upon the co-transporter affinity for Cl$^-$, arguing against the proposal that thiazide diuretics and Cl$^-$ compete for the same binding site.[147]

Analysis of the putative glycosylation sites in rat NCC by means of mutagenesis revealed that glycosylation itself is another component of the co-transporter that affects thiazide affinity. In one study, eliminating the glycosylation sites located within the extracellular loop between TM segments 7 and 8 has remarkable consequences in NCC transport activity and properties.[97] Elimination of one site (either N204 or N242) resulted in a 50% reduction of NCC activity, and elimination of both sites was associated with a 95% reduction. Interestingly, prevention of glycosylation was associated with increased affinity for extracellular Cl$^-$ and metolazone. This effect of glycosylation on thiazide affinity seems to be unique to rat NCC, since it was not observed after preventing glycosylation of flounder NCC[98] or rat NKCC2F.[99] In this last co-transporter, elimination of glycosylation by means of site directed mutagenesis was associated with increased affinity for extracellular chloride, but no effect was observed on the affinity for the loop diuretic bumetanide.

The carboxyl terminal domain appears to have an important role in maturation and trafficking of the co-transporters. A region of 77 amino acid residues of NKCC2 (amino acid 708–884), that is not present in NKCC1, seems to be required for driving NKCC2 to the apical membrane in polarized cells,[120] while there is a dileucine motif NKCC1, not present in NKCC2, that directs this co-transporter to the basolateral membrane.[173] A LLV motif in NKCC2 was identified as an ER retaining signal.[174] A protein known as SCMP2 influences NKCC2 expression through recycling endosomes and interfering with its exocytotic trafficking.[175]

The Na-Coupled Chloride Co-Transporters Form Homodimers

Moore-Hoon and Turner[176] used rat parotid plasma membrane to analyze NKCC1 using the reversible chemical cross-linker DTSSP (3,3'-dithiobis-[sulfosuccinimidyl propionate]). They observed that NKCC1 migrates at ~335 kDa. After protein denaturation, single monomers of approximately ~170 kDa were obtained, in which the investigators were unable to detect the presence of any additional protein. Similar results were later observed on human NKCC2 by Starremans et al.,[177] and on NCC by De Jong et al.[178] These studies were performed in *Xenopus laevis* oocytes injected with *in vitro*-transcribed cRNA from FLAG- and/or HA-tagged wild-type co-transporters and concatamer constructions. These experiments revealed that FLAG-NKCC2 and HA-NKCC2 are physically linked.[177] Similar observations were obtained for FLAG-NCC and HA-NCC constructs.[178] Thus, NKCC1, NKCC2, and NCC are able to form homodimers, and might be functional in this conformation. Because dimers are sensitive to reducing agents such as β-mercaptoethanol, it is likely that disulfide bonds between cysteines are involved.[170] Additionally, some data suggest that members of the *SLC12A* family can build heterocomplexes comprised of different members of the family. For example, an orphan gene of the family known as CIP appears to inhibit transport activity of NKCC1[36] or activate KCC2.[179] However, it does not affect the activity of other family members, raising the possibility that CIP may form an activating heterocomplex specifically with NKCC1.[36] A recent study has shown, by means of yeast two-hybrid and pull down assays, that K$^+$-Cl$^-$ co-transporter isoforms can interact among themselves, and even with NKCC1.[180]

REGULATION OF SODIUM CATION-COUPLED CO-TRANSPORTERS

The activity of the sodium—cation coupled chloride co-transporters, as occurs with many other ion transport proteins, can be modulated at multiple levels. One is the level of expression of the protein, which in turn can be due to increase in the rate of gene transcription, in the stability of the messenger RNA or post-translationally by affecting the turnover rate of the protein. This level of regulation requires activation/deactivation of synthesis/degradation mechanisms that usually take time to install, and thus are preferred with increased or decreased activity of the co-transporters required for longer periods of time. Another level of regulation is the balance between endocytosis and exocytosis of the co-transporter containing vesicles into the plasma membrane, as only the fraction of co-transporters inserted in the membrane are able to translocate ions. Finally, a co-transporter that is already in the membrane can be regulated to increase or decrease its turnover rate due to conformational changes that affect their activity. The presence of a co-transporter in the cell surface and its intrinsic level of activity are often modulated by phosphorylation/dephosphorylation processes and thus, are subjected to a rapid regulation through cascades of second messengers induced by a variety of hormonal signals.

With the availability of cDNA probes, primers, and high-quality polyclonal antibodies against NCC or NKCC2, several strategies have been implemented to study patterns of these co-transporters abundance, and changes under several physiological and pathophysiological circumstances.[7,181] Discussion of each model is beyond the scope of this chapter, but Tables 32.3 and 32.4 summarize the several experimental, physiological or pathophysiological conditions in which the level of NCC or NKCC2 protein and/or mRNA expression has been analyzed. In general, increased expression of either NCC or NKCC2 is observed in models in which salt retention is induced, while decreased expression is observed by salt-wasting stimuli.

The knowledge of the cation-coupled chloride co-transporters regulation by phosphorylation/dephosphorylation processes has expanded enormously in the last few years, thanks to the discovery of a kinase network that works in conjunction to modulate the ion transport mechanisms. It is well-known that activity of NKCC1/2 and NCC is tightly regulated by means of phosphorylation/dephosphorylation processes, and several lines of evidence suggest that intracellular chloride concentration $[Cl^-]_i$ is a common pathway of NKCCs regulation. When $[Cl^-]_i$ falls, the co-transporters become phosphorylated and activated, whereas when $[Cl^-]_i$ rises, the co-transporters are dephosphorylated and inhibited.[182,183] These effects of $[Cl^-]_i$ on co-transporter activity have been demonstrated for NKCC1,[182,184,185] NKCC2,[186] and NCC.[142,187] In all cases, it was observed that activation of the co-transporter by intracellular Cl$^-$ depletion is associated with increased phosphorylation of the co-transporter in several conserved threonine residues located within the amino-terminal domain.

A great tool to advance in our understanding of NKCC1, NKCC2, and NCC regulation came from the discovery that certain threonine/serine residues in the amino-terminal domain become phosphorylated in association with activation of the co-transporters. The first evidence was obtained for activation of the NKCC1 with phosphorylation of a threonine residue by Lytle and Forbush,[188] in suspensions of shark rectal gland tubules. The peptide FGHNTIDAVP, which became phosphorylated, was isolated and corresponds to amino acid residues 184—194, which are located within the amino-terminal domain of NKCC1.[4] It was later demonstrated by mass spectrophotometry that in phospho-acceptor amino acid sites within the co-transporter amino-terminal domain threonines located at positions 184, 189, and 202 of NKCC1 become phosphorylated in associated with the co-transporter's activation.[184] Of these, threonine 189 is absolutely required for NKCC1 to be functional. Then, analysis *in vivo* was performed using a specific antiphospho-NKCC1

TABLE 32.3   Analysis of NCC Expression in Different Experimental, Physiological or Pathophysiological Conditions

	mRNA	Protein	References
Low Na$^+$ diet	$\leftrightarrow^{****}\uparrow^{**}$	$\uparrow$	289–296
Loop diuretics	$\leftrightarrow^*\uparrow^{****}$	$\uparrow$	294,295,297
Spironolactone[&]	$\leftrightarrow^*$	$\uparrow$	297
Thiazide diuretics	—	$\uparrow$	298
Low-protein diet	—	$\uparrow^+$	299
L-NAME therapy	—	$\uparrow$	300
Aldosterone	—	$\uparrow$	293
Aldosterone + high-salt diet (4%)	$\uparrow$	$\uparrow$	296
Fludrocortisone		$\uparrow$	293
dDAVP	—	$\uparrow^b\leftrightarrow^c$	b:301; c:194
Vasopressin escape	—	$\uparrow^\#$	302
dDAVP + candesartan	—	$\uparrow^d\leftrightarrow^c$	d:303; c:194
Obesity	—	$\uparrow$	304
Angiotensin II	—	$\uparrow$	197
Metabolic acidosis	—	$\uparrow$	130,305
Estradiol	—	$\uparrow$	306
Prenatally programmed hypertension[a]	$\uparrow^{**}$	$\uparrow$	307
Chronic renal failure + dDAVP (surgical reduction of renal mass)	—	$\uparrow$	308
KS-WNK1 KO model	—	$\uparrow$	221
Dexamethasone	—	$\uparrow$	309
Tacroliums	—	$\uparrow$	310
Isoproterenol	—	$\uparrow$	311
WNK4 BAC transgenic mice. Two wild-type and two PHAII WNK4 alleles	—	$\uparrow$	214
PHAII WNK4 knockin mice (WNK4$^{+/D561A}$)	—	$\uparrow$	215
Conditional kidney-specific Nedd4-2 knockout mice	—	$\uparrow$	279
WNK1 knockout	—	$\uparrow$	312
Kidney specific OSR1 knockout	—	$\uparrow$	235
Gentamicin	—	$\leftrightarrow$	313
Water restriction	—	$\leftrightarrow$	301
Insulin	—	$\leftrightarrow$	314
Chronic noradrenaline infusion	—	$\leftrightarrow$	315
Lithium (low dose or high dose) 40 versus 60 mmol lithium/kg dry food	—	$\leftrightarrow$	316
Chronic renal failure (surgical reduction of renal mass)	—	$\leftrightarrow$	308
High-K$^+$ diet	—	$\downarrow$	290,317
High-K$^+$ diet and HS diet after unilateral nephrectomy	—	$\downarrow$	318
Low-K$^+$ diet	$\downarrow^*$	$\downarrow$	319,320
DOCA	—	$\downarrow$	321

(Continued)

III. FLUID AND ELECTROLYTE REGULATION AND DYSREGULATION

TABLE 32.3 (*Continued*)

	mRNA	Protein	References
Candesartan	−	$\downarrow^e \leftrightarrow^c$	e:322; c:194
Chronic renal failure + candesartan	−	$\downarrow$	323
Aldosterone escape	$\leftrightarrow^{****}$	$\downarrow$	324
L-NAME + aldosterone escape	−	$\downarrow$	325
Bilateral ureteral obstruction	−	$\downarrow$	326
Bilateral ureteral obstruction and release of obstruction (Day 14)	−	$\downarrow$	327
Puromycin-induced nephrotic syndrome	−	$\downarrow$	328
Spironolactone infusion in low-salt (0.7%) diet	$\downarrow$	$\downarrow$	296
SGK1 inducible knockout mouse model	$\leftrightarrow$	$\downarrow$	329
Cyclosporine	−	$\downarrow$	330
WNK4 BAC transgenic mice. Four wild-type WNK4 alleles	$\downarrow$	$\downarrow$	214
SPAK knockin mice (SPAK$^{T243A/T243A}$)	$\downarrow$	$\downarrow$	192
SPAK knockout mice	−	$\downarrow$	234
Overexpression of WNK1	−	$\downarrow$	312
Dehydration	$\uparrow^{****}$	−	294
High-Na$^+$ diet	$\leftrightarrow^{***} \downarrow^{**}$	$\downarrow$	294−296
Saline-loading	$\leftrightarrow^{***}$	−	294
Water-loading	$\leftrightarrow^{***}$	−	294

*Northern Blot.
**Real-time PCR.
***Semi-quantitative PCR.
****mRNA Protection Assay.
&in loop- diuretic treated animals.
+ Associated with high plasma aldosterone levels.
#Increased NCC protein during days 1 and 2, no difference in days 3 or 7.
aPrenatal hypertension induced by low-protein diets in pregnant rats.

antibody named R5, which was raised against a synthetic peptide of the amino-terminal domain containing threonines 212 and 217 of human NKCC1 (corresponding to threonines 184 and 189 of shark NKCC1).[185,189] The results demonstrated that activation of NKCC1 by intracellular Cl$^-$ depletion is associated with phosphorylation of these threonines.

The same R5 phospho-antibody was used to demonstrate that activation of NKCC2 or NCC by cell volume changes or intracellular Cl$^-$ depletion is associated with phosphorylation of the conserved threonines 96−101 in rat NKCC2 and 53−58 in rat NCC.[186,187,190] Later, specific phospho-antibodies for these and other threonine/serines in the amino-terminal domain were raised against each rat or human co-transporter, confirming the role of the residues detected by R5 antibody and suggesting other sites within the amino-terminal domain as potential residues to be involved.[142,191] Similar to NKCC1, threonine 60 of

human NCC (corresponding to 189 from shark NKCC1) is required for NCC to be functional,[187] and when activated by phosphorylation it appears that T60 is the first to be phosphorylated; this opens the possibility to phosphorylate nearby threonine/serine residues.[191] None of these phospho-acceptor sites are individually required for NKCC2 to be functional, because elimination of each one at a time reduces, but does not prevent, the activity of the co-transporter.[186]

Figure 32.5 shows an alignment analysis of a region of the amino-terminal domain of NCC, NKCC2, and NKCC1 highlighting the conserved threonine/serine phosphorylation sites among species that have been implicated in activation of the co-transporters in different studies. Tables 32.5 and 32.6 contain detailed information on all the works in which phosphorylation of specific site or sites on NCC or NKCC2 have been studied. Several works *in vitro* and *in vivo* have shown that some of the amino-terminal domain phosphorylation

TABLE 32.4 Analysis of NKCC2 Expression in Different Experimental, Physiological or Pathophysiological Conditions

	mRNA	Protein	References
Low-Na$^+$ diet	↔*	↔,↑	289,292,294,295
Loop diuretics	↔*	↑	294,295,298
Low-protein diet	−	↑ +	299
Dexamethasone	↑****	↑	331,309
High-fat diet	−	↑	332
Lipopolysacharide injections	−	↑ + +	333
Candesartan	−	↑	322
Chronic renal failure + candesartan	−	↑	323
L-NAME therapy	−	↑	334
Diclofenac/indomethacin	−	↑	335
Growth hormone	−	↑$	201
Obesity	−	↓↑	336,304
Rosiglitazone	−	↑	336
Hyperosmolarity	−	↑	337
Bilateral ureteral obstruction and release of obstruction (Day 14)	−	↑	327
Angiotensin II	−	↑	338
dDAVP	−	↑	82,301,303
Water restriction	−	↑	82,301
Lithium	−	↑	339
Chronic noradrenaline infusion	−	↑	315
Prenatally programmed hypertensiona	↑**	↑	307
Lithium (high dose) 60 mmol lithium/kg dry food	−	↑	340
Sildenafil in the presence of lithium-induced DI	−	↑	341
Vasopressin escape	−	↑↓#	302
Chronic renal failure + dDAVP	−	↑	308
(Surgical reduction of renal mass.)			
Hypothyroid rat model	−	↑	342
Dahl salt-sensitive rats	−	↑##	343
SPAK knockout mice	−	↑	234,236
WNK1 knockout	−	↑	312,221
P2Y2 receptor KO mice with high-salt diet	−	↑	344
Aldosterone	−	↔	197
Candesartan	−	↔	345
Aldosterone escape	−	↔	324
dDAVP + candesartan	−	↔	303
Chronic metabolic acidosis	↑****	↔,↑	130,346−348
Lithium (low dose) 40 mmol lithium/kg dry food	−	↔	340

(Continued)

III. FLUID AND ELECTROLYTE REGULATION AND DYSREGULATION

TABLE 32.4 *(Continued)*

	mRNA	Protein	References
Chronic renal failure (surgical reduction of renal mass)	−	↔	308
Low-K⁺ diet	↓*	↓	319,320
DOCA	−	↓	321
Cyclosporine	−	↓	349
Parecoxib	↓***	↓	350
Gentamicin	−	↓	313
Bilateral ureteral obstruction	−	↓	326,351
17-Beta-estradiol	−	↓	352
L-NAME + aldosterone escape	↔**	↓	325
Puromycin-induced nephrotic syndrome	−	↓	328
SGK1 inducible knockout mouse model	−	↓	329
High-K⁺ diet and high-salt diet after unilateral nephrectomy	−	↓#$	318
Dahl salt-resistant rats	−	↓###	343
P2Y2 receptor knockout mice with high-salt diet	−	↓	344
SPAK knockin mice (SPAK^T243A/T243A)	−	↓	192
Overexpression WNK1	−	↓	312
Kidney-specific OSR1 knockout	−	↓	235
High-Na⁺ diet	↔*	−	294,295
Saline-loading	↔*	−	294
Dehydration	↔*	−	294
Water-loading	↔*	−	294

*Northern Blot.
**Real time PCR.
***Semi-quantitative PCR.
****RT PCR.
⁺ Associated with high plasma aldosterone levels.
⁺⁺Increased in inner stripe of outer medulla.
$Increased total protein in outer stripe of outer medulla, increased phosphorylation with no change in NKCC2 total protein in inner stripe.
#Increased during day 2 of dDAVP and decreased by day 7. No change in days 1 or 3.
##Increase in surface NKCC2 with no change in total/G6PD.
###Decrease in surface NKCC2 with no change in total/G6PD.
ªPrenatal hypertension induced by low protein diets in pregnant rats.
#$Change in NKCC2 after 3 wks, no change after 1 wk with HS + KCl diet. L-NAME - N-nitro-L-arginine-methyl esterase.

residues are involved in activation of NCC by intracellular chloride depletion,[142,187] low-salt diet,[192,193] vasopressin,[194,195] angiotensin II[196,197] or aldosterone[193,198]; and NKCC2 by hypertonicity,[199] intracellular chloride depletion,[186,200] vasopressin,[77] and growth hormone.[201] Thus, NKCC1, NKCC2 or NCC are activated by phosphorylation of particular amino-terminal domain threonine/serine residues by different stimuli and intracellular cascades such as Gαs receptor-cAMP-PKA (vasopressin), Gαq receptor-IP3-PKC (angiotensin II), tyrosine kinase-associated receptor (growth hormone) or activation of an intracellular soluble kinase by [Cl⁻]ᵢ or changes in cell volume (see below). These data suggest that different cascades probably combine in

activation of a particular kinase pathway that is responsible for the phosphorylation of these particular sites.

The kinase cascade that has been shown to be involved in the phosphorylation of the amino terminal threonine or serine residues of NKCC1, NKCC2 or NCC is the WNK-SPAK pathway. The WNK family of serine/threonine kinases is closely related to MAP kinases. Members of this family lack the conserved catalytic lysine (K) present in subdomain II of all the other serine/threonine kinases, hence the name WNK for "with no lysine (K)".[202] The crystal structure of the WNK1 catalytic domain later revealed that the catalytic lysine is present in subdomain I.[203] The family is

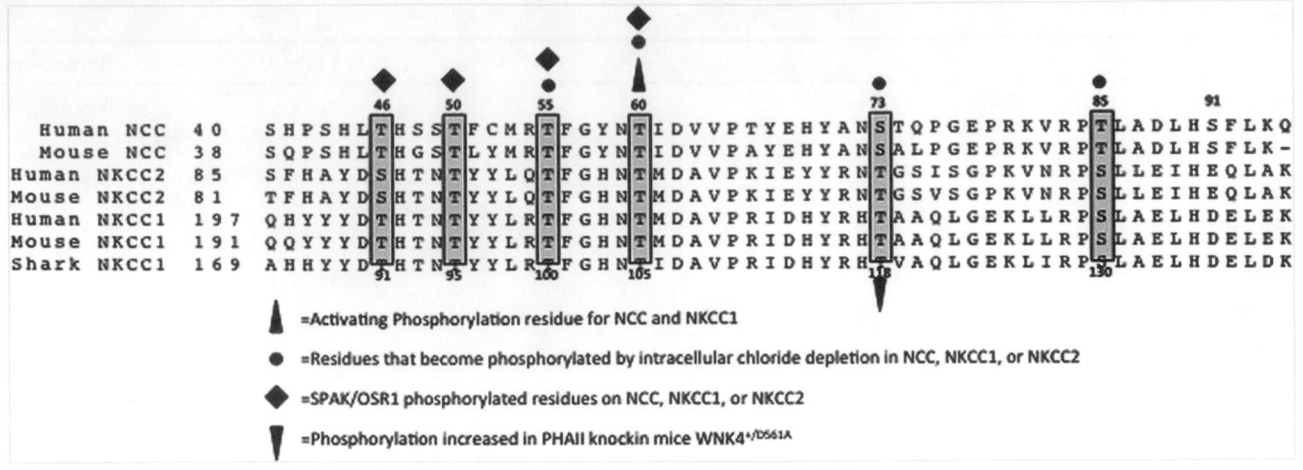

FIGURE 32.5   Sequence alignment of a region of the amino-terminal domain containing the conserved residues (highlighted in gray) that have been associated with phosphorylation/activation of the co-transporters. Numbering above alignment indicates residues in NCC. Numbering below alignment indicates numbering in NKCC2.

composed of four members, known as WNK1 to WNK4,[204] each containing a serine/threonine kinase domain of 294 residues flanked by a short amino-terminal domain (146 to 220 amino acid residues) and a long carboxyl terminal domain (796 to 1888 residues) exhibiting two coiled-coil domains for protein interaction, and a conserved auto-inhibitory motif shown to inhibit autophosphorylation in WNK1.[202,205] The degree of conservation among the four isoforms is high within the kinase domain (>80%), but low within the amino- or carboxyl-terminal domains (<15%).

The importance of WNKs to renal physiology and pathophysiology was highlighted by the demonstration that intronic deletions of WNK1 or missense mutations in an acidic conserved region of WNK4 are the cause of a human form of an inherited syndrome featuring arterial hypertension, hyperkalemia, and metabolic acidosis known as pseudohypoaldosteronism type II (PHAII), Familiar Hyperkalemic Hypertension (FHH) or Gordon's disease.[206–208] Because PHAII is a mirror image of Gitelman's disease and it is treatable with low doses of thiazides (see below), it was suspected that activity of NCC was implicated in the pathophysiology of the disease. This was first demonstrated using the heterologous expression system of *Xenopus laevis* oocytes.[209,210] WNK4 inhibits the activity of NCC, and this effect is prevented by either eliminating the catalytic activity of WNK4[209,211–213] or by the introduction of one of the PHAII-type mutations in WNK4,[209,213] thus suggesting that the activity of NCC in PHAII patients is increased due to elimination of the WNK4-induced inhibition of NCC. The activation/ phosphorylation of NCC as the major mechanism for hypertension and hyperkalemia was confirmed in two animal models of PHAII[214,215] (Table 32.5). The

mechanism for PHAII in families with intronic deletion of WNK1 is less-understood. WNK1 does not seem to have a direct effect upon NCC. Instead, it has been observed that WNK1 prevents the WNK4-induced inhibition of NCC.[210] Thus, if WNK1 expression is increased, as is suggested to occur as a consequence of WNK1 intronic 1 deletion,[206] the WNK4 inhibitory effect upon NCC will be prevented and thus, NCC activity will increase. Interestingly, there is a shorter variant of WNK1, lacking the entire amino and kinase domain that is exclusively expressed in the kidney, specifically in DCT.[216–218] The short WNK1 prevents the WNK1 effect on WNK4.[219] Thus, it is postulated that under physiological conditions the expression of the short WNK1 in DCT modulates the interaction between WNK1 and WNK4, regulating NCC activity. In PHAII, however, increased expression of the long WNK1 surpasses the regulatory capacity of short-WNK1, thus inhibiting WNK4 with the consequent activation of NCC. This model, however, awaits definitive confirmation by *in vivo* models.[220–222]

Two kinases related to the yeast Ste-20p family known as SPAK (Ste20p-related proline-alanine rich kinase) and OSR1 (oxidative stress response 1) have been shown to be located downstream of WNKs, at least for their effects on the cation-coupled chloride co-transporters.[223,224] The first evidence of the WNK-SPAK/OSR1 interaction was obtained in a study in which the K-Cl co-transporter, KCC3, was shown to interact with SPAK/OSR1 in a two-hybrid yeast system. The co-transporter interacting with SPAK/OSR1 using a specific binding domain was determined to be RFx(V/I).[225] One such binding site is located in the amino-terminal domain of NCC and NKCC2, two are present in NKCC1, and two or three sites in each

TABLE 32.5 Phosphorylation of NCC in Different Sites and Conditions

Experimental System/Model	Phospho-site*	Effect	Stimuli	Kinase Involved	Reference
In tube	T^{55}, T^{60}, S^{73}	−	SPAK	WNK1/SPAK	190
Xenopus oocytes	T^{55}, T^{60}, S^{73}	↑↑	Intracellular Cl^- depletion	¿?	187
Mouse	S^{73}	↑↑	WNK4 knockin	WNK4	215
HEK-293 cells	$T^{46}, T^{55}, T^{60}, S^{91}$	↑↑	Intracellular Cl^- depletion	SPAK	142
Rat	T^{55}, T^{60}, S^{73}	↑↑	Low-salt diet	¿?	193
Human urine	S^{811}	↑	None	¿?	106
Xenopus oocytes/mpkDCT cells	T^{55}, T^{60}	↑↑	Angiotensin II	WNK4-SPAK	196
Mouse	T^{55}, T^{60}, S^{73}	↑	Low-K^+ diet	SGK1	290
Mouse	T^{55}, T^{60}, S^{73}	↓	WNK4 hypomorphic	WNK4	280
Brattleboro rats	T^{55}, S^{73}	↑↑	dDAVP	¿?	195
Brattleboro rats/wistar rats	T^{55}, T^{60}	↑↑	dDAVP	SPAK	194
Mouse	T^{55}, T^{60}, S^{91}	↓↓	SPAK knockin	SPAK	192
mpkDCT cells/mouse	T^{55}, T^{60}, S^{73}	↑↑	Angiotensin II/aldosterone	SPAK	198
Adrenalectomized rats	T^{55}, T^{60}	↑↑	Angiotensin II/aldosterone	WNK4-SPAK	197
Mouse	$T^{45}, T^{55}, T^{60}, S^{73}$	↑↑	KS-WNK1 knockout	WNK1/WNK4	221
In tube	$T^{46}, T^{55}, T^{60}, S^{91}$	↑	Incubation with MO25	SPAK/OSR1	353
Mouse	T^{55}, T^{60}, S^{73}	↓↓	SPAK knockout	SPAK	234
Mouse	T^{55}, S^{73}	↓↓	SPAK knockout	SPAK	236
mDCT cells/Rats	T^{55}, T^{60}, S^{73}	↑	Cyclosporine	¿?	354
Mouse	T^{55}	↑	Tacrolimus	WNK3/WNK4	310
Mouse	T^{55}	↔	NCC transgenic	¿?	355
Mouse	T^{60}	↓↓	WNK4 knockout	WNK4/SPAK	356
mpkDCT cells/mouse	T^{55}, T^{60}, S^{73}	↑	Insulin	WNK4/SPAK	357
Xenopus oocytes *Ex vivo* kidney	T^{60}	↑	Insulin	WNK4/SPAK	358
Mouse	T^{55}	↑	KS-OSR1 knockout	OSR1/SPAK	235
Mouse	T^{55}, S^{73}	↑	Isoproterenol salt-sensitive hypertension	WNK4	311
Xenopus oocytes	T^{60}	↑↑	WNK3	WNK3/SPAK	226

Numbers correspond to human NCC sequence.

WNKs support the interaction between WNKs and co-transporters with SPAK.[142,225,226] In fact, among all proteins in the human proteome, WNK1 and NKCC1 are the ones with higher numbers of SPAK-binding domains.[227] Functional and biochemical studies using NKCC1 demonstrated that both WNK1 or WNK4, as well as SPAK or OSR1, must be present to induce amino-terminal domain phosphorylation and activation of the co-transporter.[190,223,228] It was shown that WNKs lie upstream of SPAK/OSR1, and that WNK phosphorylates SPAK/OSR1 on two specific threonine and serine residues (T243 and S383 in SPAK), inducing activation of the kinase.[192,223] Thus, it is believed that SPAK/OSR1 are the kinases that actually phosphorylate the amino-terminal threonine residues of NKCC1, NKCC2 or NCC, and that WNKs modulate this effect by activating SPAK/OSR1.[191,229–232]

The interaction between SPAK and NCC has been confirmed, and also the requirement for the amino-terminal domain SPAK-binding site of NCC.[142,191,226] To find out the importance of the interaction and phosphorylation between SPAK and NCC *in vivo*, Rafiqui et al.[192] generated a mice knockin model by eliminating the threonine residue of the T-loop in SPAK (T243A) or OSR1 (T185A) that is phosphorylated by WNK1 or WNK4. The OSR1[185A/185A] mice died on embryonic

TABLE 32.6　Phosphorylation of NKCC2 in Different Sites and Conditions

Experimental System/Model	Phospho-site*	Effect	Stimuli	Kinase Involved	Reference
Mice	T^{100}, T^{105}	↑↑	Vasopressin	¿?	77
Xenopus oocytes	T^{100}, T^{105}	↑↑	Hypertonicity	¿?	199
In tube	Amino terminal fragment 1–181	−	SPAK/OSR1	WNK1/SPAK	190
Xenopus oocytes	T^{100}, T^{105}	↑↑	WNK3	WNK3	239
Rat	T^{100}, T^{105}	↑↑	Growth hormone	¿?	201
Xenopus oocytes/MMDD1 cells	S^{130}	↑	Hypertonicity	AMPK	359
Xenopus oocytes	T^{100}, T^{105}	↑↑	Intracellular Cl⁻ depletion/WNK3	WNK3/SPAK	186
Mouse	T^{55}, T^{60}, S^{91}	↓↓	SPAK knockin	SPAK	192
Dahl TAL cells	T^{100}, T^{105}	↔	High-salt diet	¿?	343
HEK-293 cells	$T^{95}, T^{100}, T^{105}, S^{130}$	↑↑	Intracellular Cl⁻ depletion	SPAK	200
In tube	T^{95}, T^{100}, T^{105}	↑	Incubation with MO25	SPAK/OSR1	353
HEK-293 cells	T^{100}, T^{105}	↑↑	Ouabain Calyculin A	SPAK	360
Milan rats	T^{100}, T^{105}	↑	−	SPAK	361
Mice/culture TAL	T^{118}	↑↑	dDAVP	¿?	362
THP knockout mice/culture TAL	T^{118}	↓	dDAVP	¿?	362
Mouse	T^{100}, T^{105}	↑↑	SPAK knockout	SPAK	234
Mouse	T^{100}, T^{105}	↓	KS-OSR1 knockout	OSR1/SPAK	235

*Numbers correspond to human NKCC2 sequence.

day 17.5, while the SPAK[234A/234A] mice were viable, grew normally and thus were further analyzed. Along the nephron, SPAK is specifically expressed in TAL and DCT. The blood pressure of SPAK[234A/234A] mice is reduced and consistent with reduction in salt reabsorption as the mechanism of hypotension; blood pressure was normalized after feeding the SPAK[234A/234A] mice with a high-salt diet for several days. In fact, SPAK[234A/234A] mice developed a Gitelman-like syndrome, with hypomagnesemia and hypocalciuria. Hypokalemia was not observed in a normal-sodium diet, but became apparent with a low-sodium diet. Using specific phosphoantibodies for NCC amino-terminal threonine residues, it was shown that in SPAK[234A/234A] mice expression of NCC in the kidney was reduced by 30% and phosphorylation at residues T53, T58, and S89 were reduced by about 80% (Tables 32.3 and 32.5). Similar observations were obtained using specific antibodies against NKCC2 (Tables 32.4 and 32.6). All these observations together indicate that absence of SPAK activity resulted in decreased activity of NKCC2 and/or NCC. Because the phenotype resembles Gitelman's rather than Bartter's disease, it was suggested that the effect of SPAK inactivation upon NCC was stronger. Crossing the PHAII

knockin mice generated by Yang et al.[215] with the SPAK[234A/234A] mice[192] demonstrated that hypertension and the whole PHAII syndrome were prevented, indicating the major role of SPAK-induced regulation of NCC in this syndrome.[233] Thus, the SPAK knockin mice model provided compelling evidence of the key role of SPAK in modulation of NKCC2 and NCC activity.

Interestingly, the complete elimination of SPAK in a SPAK knockout model also resulted in decreased expression and phosphorylation of NCC, but in contrast to the SPAK[234A/234A] mice, resulted in increased phosphorylation of NKCC2[234] (Tables 32.4 and 32.6). In contrast, a recent study in which a kidney tissue-specific elimination of OSR1 was achieved (KS-OSR1[−/−] mice) resulted in an incomplete form of Bartter's syndrome, with decreased expression and phosphorylation of NKCC2, together with increased expression of SPAK and NCC phosphorylation[235] (Tables 32.4 and 32.6). Thus, it is possible that NKCC2 is preferentially under the control of OSR1, while NCC is under the control of SPAK. Several SPAK splicing isoforms are expressed in the kidney that could serve to explain the different regulation of NKCC2 and NCC under different circumstances.[236]

WNK2 and WNK3 also exert effects on the cation-coupled chloride co-transporters that are of interest. WNK3 is expressed along the entire nephron, as well as in several epithelial and non-epithelial cells outside the kidney,[232,237] and strongly activates NKCC1, NKCC2, and NCC, while it inhibits all four KCCs.[238–240] Thus, WNK3 activates chloride influx pathways and inactivates chloride efflux pathways. Activation of NKCC1, NKCC2, and NCC by WNK3 is associated with phosphorylation of the same amino-terminal domain threonines in the several models discussed above[226,238,239] (Tables 32.5 and 32.6). WNK3 activation of NCC is associated with increased expression of NCC on the cell surface, suggesting that it promotes the trafficking of NCC vesicles into the plasma membrane.[239] One study suggests that the effect of WNK3 and WNK4 on NCC can be achieved by the carboxyl-terminal domain of the kinase alone, that is, in the complete absence of the kinase domain.[241] Other studies, however, have shown that the effect of WNK3 and WNK4 on NCC are kinase-dependent,[209,212,213,239,241] and unlike what occurs with WNK1 variants[216,217] there is no evidence that such truncated variants of WNK3 or WNK4 are expressed in the DCT. One study in which chimeric proteins between WNK3 and WNK4 domains were constructed suggested that the type of effect of WNK3 or WNK4 upon NCC resides within the amino-terminal domain.[211]

The WNK3-induced activation of NKCCs or inhibition of KCCs occurs even during cell swelling, which is a well-known inhibitor of NKCCs and activator of KCCs.[3,137,199] WNK3 catalytic activity can be prevented by the substitution of D294A. By doing this, the effect on the co-transporters is not only prevented, indicating the requirement for catalytic activity, but additionally, catalytically inactive WNK3 becomes an inhibitor of NKCC1, NKCC2, and NCC, and an activator of KCCs, even in isotonic conditions in which KCCs are non-functional. Because activation of KCCs by WNK3-D294A can be prevented with calyculin A and/or cyclosporine A, it is likely due to a catalytically inactive WNK3-induced activation of protein phosphatases.[240] Because the effect of WNK3 upon the sodium-coupled chloride co-transporters is associated with phosphorylation of the SPAK phospho-acceptor sites in the co-transporter's amino-terminal domain, it is likely that WNK3 also lies upstream of SPAK/OSR1 for its effect on the SLC12A co-transporters. Supporting this possibility, the positive effect of WNK3 on NKCC2 or NCC can be prevented by elimination of SPAK-binding sites located in WNK3.[186,226] Thus, WNK3 modulates the activity of all members of the SLC12 family and, in

doing so, bypasses the changes in cell volume and/or intracellular chloride concentration that are usually required for their activation or inhibition. It is believed that WNK3/SPAK is the intracellular kinase pathway sensitive to cell volume and/or intracellular chloride concentration.[184,232,242] WNK2 is preferentially expressed in the central nervous system, and is apparently absent in kidney. Its effects on NKCC1 and KCCs are similar to those of WNK3.[243]

THE ROLE OF THE SODIUM-COUPLED CATION CHLORIDE CO-TRANSPORTERS IN INHERITED DISEASE

Given the major roles that NCC and NKCC2 play in renal physiology, it is of no surprise that inactivating mutations of these co-transporter genes are associated with monogenic disease, such as Gitelman's and type I Bartter's diseases, respectively. In addition, by affecting the modulation of NCC by certain kinases, increased activity of this co-transporter (and other ion transport protein in the distal nephron) is the mechanism behind another monogenic disease known as PHAII.

Gitelman's Disease

Gitelman's disease is an autosomal recessive monogenic disease featuring hypokalemic metabolic alkalosis, arterial hypotension, hypocalciuria, and hypomagenesemia. The clinical presentation usually becomes evident by the second decade of life. All these manifestations are due to a lack of salt transport capacity of the DCT, and resemble the clinical consequences of thiazide diuretic intoxication. Because of this, NCC became a strong candidate for the cause of the disease, and links between Gitelman's disease and the locus for *SLC12A3* in human chromosome 16 was found by several groups.[102,244–246] At present, nearly 350 different mutations of NCC have been reported to be associated with Gitelman's disease or with low blood pressure in an open population (see the human gene mutation data base at www.hgmd.or). Supporting the studies on genomic associations, phenotypes resembling Gitelman's disease have been obtained in mice by targeted disruption of NCC.[247,248] Interestingly, total knockout of NCC produces an incomplete Gitelman syndrome, while substituting the serine residue at the position 707 by a stop codon completely expunges the disease. Functional analysis of human or rat NCC containing some of the reported point mutations revealed that mutant NCC proteins are non-functional.[138–140]

Although Gitelman's disease is an autosomal recessive disorder, surprisingly, not all patients have shown mutations in both SLC12A3 alleles. About 30% of the Gitelman patients have been diagnosed with mutations in only one allele, another 45% are compound heterozygous; that is, they exhibit mutations in both alleles, but the mutation is different for each one, and near 20% are homozygous.[7,102,249−254] Because inheritance of Gitelman's disease is clearly recessive, and heterozygous relatives of patients with Gitelman's disease are clinically and metabolically asymptomatic, it is likely that undetected mutations in the other allele also exist. Most of the studies usually search for mutation within exons, but it is possible that mutations within the promoter or even in some introns or in the 3' untranslated region affect expression of the protein. Most of the Gitelman's mutations are single point mutations in residues that are highly-conserved from fish to humans, and the mechanisms by which mutations reduce or abolish transporter activity are several, including impairment of protein synthesis, impairment of protein processing, impairment of insertion of an otherwise functional protein into the plasma membrane, impairment of functional properties of the co-transporter, and acceleration of protein removal from the membrane or degradation. Initial reports of missense mutations reported along the NCC protein revealed that the co-transporter is not glycosylated and thus, is not present at the plasma membrane.[138] It is known that preventing NCC glycosylation remarkably reduces the activity of the co-transporter due to deficient insertion into the plasma membrane.[97] Later studies of more mutants of NCC[139,140] showed that some missense mutations in NCC causing partially functional proteins are explained by a defect in the trafficking of the co-transporter to the plasma membrane which possesses normal functional and kinetic properties, but in which insertion into plasma membrane is seriously impaired.

Bartter's Disease

The characteristic clinical picture of Bartter's syndrome includes a salt-wasting state with low blood pressure due to dehydration, metabolic alkalosis with hypokalemia, hypercalciuira, hypereninemia, and secondary aldosteronism.[255] This picture is clearly due to a reduction in the salt transporting capacity of the TAL. The disease is usually apparent at birth or even earlier, due to excessive accumulation of amniotic fluid (polyhydramnios). A striking difference with Gitelman's disease is that Bartter's patients exhibit hypercalciuria and some develop nephrocalcinosis (Table 32.7), while in Gitelman's syndrome the expected presentation is hypocalciuria. Although Bartter's disease is monogenic, it is heterogeneous, because mutations in five different genes expressed in TAL can produce a very similar disease. Of these, three are directly involved in salt reabsorption in TAL and two other genes modulate the activity and/or trafficking of salt transporters. Thus, Bartter's disease is classified into five types. Types I to IV (Table 32.7) are the consequence of inactivating mutations of NKCC2 (type I), the potassium channel ROMK (type II), the basolateral Cl⁻ channel CLC-KB (type III), and the CLC-KB chaperon protein Barttin (type IV).[66,107,256−258] The absence of ROMK prevents NKCC2 activity, because recycling of potassium to the TAL lumen is prevented. Reduction of CLC-KB activity, due to mutations on the channel or because of the absence of barttin, probably decreases the activity of NKCC2, because the co-transporter is sensitive to intracellular chloride concentration.[186] Bartter's disease type V is the result of activating mutations in the calcium sensing receptor located in the basolateral membrane.[64,259−261] The

TABLE 32.7   Clinical Presentation of Patients with Bartter's Disease According To Genomic Classification in Types I to IV

	Type I	Type II	Type III	Type IV
Affected gene	SLC12A1	KCNJ1/ROMK	ClCNKB	BSND
Age of onset	Neonatal	Neonatal	First decade	Neonatal
Polyhydramnios	Yes	Yes	No	Yes
Sensorineural deafness	Rare	Rare	No	Yes
Poliuria	Yes	Yes	Uncommon	Yes
End-stage renal disease	No	No	No	Yes
Hypokalemia	Severe	Severe	Moderate	Severe
Metabolic alkalosis	Moderate	Moderate	Mild	Moderate
Nephrocalcinosis	Yes	Yes	No	Yes

stimulation of the calcium sensing receptor by extracellular calcium activates a second messenger cascade within the TAL that inhibits NKCC2 and ROMK. This way, an increase in extracellular calcium reduces salt reabsorption in the TAL that is followed by a reduction in calcium reabsorption, thus increasing calciuria. In patients with active mutations of the calcium sensing receptor, the receptor is activated with normal extracellular calcium concentration inducing a permanent reduction in NKCC2/ROMK activity. Bartter's disease in this case is usually a mild syndrome.

At present, nearly 75 different mutations of NKCC2 have been reported to be associated with Bartter's disease or with low blood pressure in an open population (see the human gene mutation data base at www. hgmd.or). It is possible to suggest the molecular nature of Bartter's syndrome just by analyzing the clinical picture, although a confirmation by specific gene sequencing is desirable (Table 32.7). For instance, all patients present hypokalemia and metabolic alkalosis, which are less severe in type III patients. Antenatal presentation and polyhydroamnios are much more often seen in Bartter's type I, II, and IV than in type III disease. Patients with type III disease do not develop nephrocalcinosis. Type IV is associated with deafness and development of chronic renal failure.[66,262] Therefore, age of clinical presentation and certain features such as nephrocalcinosis, deafness, and chronic renal failure help the clinician to identify of the appropriate molecular target.

Pseudohypoaldosteronism Type II/Familial Hypekalemia Hypertension

PHAII/FHH is the mirror image of Gitelman's disease. It is an autosomal dominant inherited disease featuring arterial hypertension with hyperkalemia, despite a normal glomerular filtration rate, and hyperchloremic metabolic acidosis as a consequence of decreased urinary H^+ excretion.[207,208] In addition, while Gitelman's patient's develop hypocalciuria, PHAII patients develop hypercalciuria.[263] This is translated into bone, because the first exhibit is increased bone mineral density,[264,265] whereas later a significant decrease in bone density develops.[266] As shown above, Gitelman's disease is the consequence of inactivating mutations of NCC. In contrast, all clinical features in PHAII patients are corrected by treatment with low dose, thiazide-type diuretics,[208,266] suggesting that increased activity of NCC is required for PHAII. No significant linkage was found between PHAII and the SLC12A3 locus on chromosome 16,[267] eliminating the possibility that activating mutations of NCC are behind the development of this syndrome. Instead, four

different genes have been shown to be the cause of PHAII. As discussed above, the gene responsible in families linked to chromosomes 12 and 17 have been observed to be WNK1 and WNK4, respectively.[206,268-274] Two other genes can be the cause of the disease: Kelch-like 3 (KLHL3) and cullin 3 (CUL3).[275] While KLHL3 mutations can be dominant or recessive, CUL3 are dominant and most of them are *de novo* mutations.

Extensive work has been done with WNKs regarding NCC modulation. Nothing is known yet regarding KLHK3 and CUL3 modulation of NCC activity. However, because most of the pathophysiology of PHAII seems to be explained by increased activity of NCC,[17,191,276,277] it is highly likely that these proteins modulate the activity of NCC. KLHL3 and CUL3 together form a protein complex that provides a RING-type of E3-ubiquitin ligase.[278] It has been demonstrated that the HECT-type of E3-ubiquitin ligase known as Nedd4-2 modulates NCC activity.[279] Thus, it is possible that the KLHL3–CUL3 complex regulates either NCC, some of the WNKs, or SPAK by ubiquitination or another known or unknown associated protein that in turn affects the activity of NCC.

WNK4 has been proposed to be a negative regulator of NCC activity that becomes a positive regulator when it harbors PHAII-type mutations.[209,210,212,213] A PHAII syndrome develops in BAC transgenic mice containing two wild-type WNK4 alleles and two PHAII-type mutant alleles,[214] indicating that haploinsufficiency does not explain the disease, because this model contains two wild-type WNK4 alleles. The disease is also present in a knockin mouse harboring WNK4 with a PHAII type mutation.[215] In these models, PHAII clinical features were rescued by treatment of mice with a thiazide-type diuretic, by crossing the mouse with the NCC null mice or with the SPAK knockin mice,[214,215,233] highlighting the importance of SPAK-NCC in producing the disease. Thus, it is possible that under certain conditions WNK4 inhibits NCC activity and in patients with PHAII mutations this inhibition is not present, leading to a chronic increase in the activity of NCC that produces arterial hypertension and hyperkalemia. One study proposed that PHAII mutations in WNK4 reconstitute the effect of angiotensin II upon the WNK4-SPAK-NCC cascade, suggesting that PHAII is a gain-of-function disease producing a state of hyperactivity of angiotensin II in the DCT.[17,196] There are, however, other proposals. One is that NCC activation is the result of altered interactions between the NCC activating WNK3 and the inhibitory WNK4.[241] The other, based on observations on hypomorphic WNK4 mice, is that WNK4 could be an activator of NCC that increases its potency by PHAII mutations.[280]

POTENTIAL ROLE IN POLYGENIC DISEASES

The physiological roles of sodium—chloride co-transporters and the diseases that are produced by their inactivating mutations or misregulation by WNKs support that they are implicated in the development of complex polygenic diseases, such as arterial hypertension. This is a highly prevalent disease (>20% of the adult population) with an important genetic component. NCC and NKCC2 are genes that clearly play a role in defining blood pressure levels, since inactivation of these transport proteins is associated with hypotension. Inhibition of NCC with thiazides is the base of the most recommended first line therapy for arterial hypertension.[281] Supporting the role of NCC or NKCC2 in defining blood pressure levels in an open population, a work based on genetic analysis of the Framingham Population Study sequenced the NCC, NKCC2, and ROMK genes in 3125 subjects. It was observed that 49 out of the 3125 exhibited a rare mutation in one allele of one these genes. This is 1.5% of the studied population. Subjects harboring such mutations have lower blood pressure, a reduced risk for developing hypertension, and a reduced risk of death due to cardiovascular disease.[282] Although several of the mutations detected in this study were not reported previously as causing Gitelman's or Bartter's disease, it was later shown that they indeed reduced the activity of NCC[283] or NKCC2.[283,284] A genome-wide association study in an Amish population revealed that SPAK or STK39 is a hypertension risk gene.[285] Thus, genome studies are beginning to reveal the role of SLC12A co-transporter genes in essential hypertension.

Osteoporosis is a polygenic disease of the skeleton that is secondary to a decrease in bone mineral density, with a disruption of the normal bone architecture and a consequent increase in the risk of fractures. Due to the functional interaction of NCC with calcium-transport mechanisms, this co-transporter is involved in renal calcium absorption. Inactivating mutations of NCC in Gitelman's disease are associated with high bone mineral density,[264,265] whereas activation of NCC in PHAII subjects is accompanied by decreased bone mineral density.[266] In addition, there is strong epidemiological evidence that hypertensive patients treated with thiazides are at a lower risk for osteoporosis.[27,28,286–288] In this regard, it has been shown that the NCC protein is expressed in osteoblasts in rat and human bones, and that addition of thiazides to osteoblast cells in culture increases the formation of mineralized nodules by a mechanism that may involve NCC.[19] Therefore, it is likely that osteoporosis is another polygenic disease in which this co-transporter could be implicated.

Acknowledgments

This chapter is dedicated with endless gratitude to the memory of my mentor Steven C. Hebert MD for his invaluable help and collaboration of over 20 years. Experimental work performed in the author's laboratory has been supported by The Mexican Council of Science and Technology (CONACYT), NIH grants DK36803 and DK064635, the Wellcome Trust, The Foundation Leducq for the Transatlantic Network on Hypertension—Renal Salt Handling in the Control of Blood Pressure.

References

[1] Hediger MA, Romero MF, Peng JB, Rolfs A, Takanaga H, Bruford EA. The ABCs of solute carriers: physiological, pathological and therapeutic implications of human membrane transport proteins. Introduction. Pflugers Arch 2004;447:465—8.

[2] Gamba G, Saltzberg SN, Lombardi M, Miyanoshita A, Lytton J, Hediger MA, et al. Primary structure and functional expression of a cDNA encoding the thiazide-sensitive, electroneutral sodium-chloride co-transporter. Proc Natl Acad Sci USA 1993;90:2749—53.

[3] Gamba G, Miyanoshita A, Lombardi M, Lytton J, Lee WS, Hediger MA, et al. Molecular cloning, primary structure and characterization of two members of the mammalian electroneutral sodium-(potassium)-chloride co-transporter family expressed in kidney. J Biol Chem 1994;269:17713—22.

[4] Xu J-C, Lytle C, Zhu TT, Payne JA, Benz Jr E, Forbush III B. Molecular cloning and functional expression of the bumetanide-sensitive Na-K-Cl co-transporter. Proc Natl Acad Sci USA 1994;91:2201—5.

[5] Payne JA, Forbush III B. Alternatively spliced isoforms of the putative renal Na-K-Cl co-transporter are differentially distributed within the rabbit kidney. Proc Natl Acad Sci USA 1994;91:4544—8.

[6] Delpire E, Rauchman MI, Beier DR, Hebert SC, Gullans SR. Molecular cloning and chromosome localization of a putative basolateral Na$^+$-K$^+$-2Cl$^-$ co-transporter from mouse inner medullary collecting duct (mIMCD-3) cells. J Biol Chem 1994;269:25677—83.

[7] Gamba G. Molecular physiology and pathophysiology of the electroneutral cation-chloride co-transporters. Physiol Rev 2005;85:423—93.

[8] Hebert SC, Mount DB, Gamba G. Molecular physiology of cation-coupled Cl($^-$) co-transport: the SLC12 family. Pflugers Arch 2004;447:580—93.

[9] Gillen CM, Brill S, Payne JA, Forbush III B. Molecular cloning and functional expression of the K-Cl co-transporter from rabbit, rat and human. A new member of the cation-chloride co-transporter family. J Biol Chem 1996;271:16237—44.

[10] Payne JA, Stevenson TJ, Donaldson LF. Molecular characterization of a putative K-Cl co-transporter in rat brain. A neuronal-specific isoform. J Biol Chem 1996;271:16245—52.

[11] Hiki K, D'Andrea RJ, Furze J, Crawford J, Woollatt E, Sutherland GR, et al. Cloning, characterization, and chromosomal location of a novel human K$^+$-Cl$^-$ co-transporter. J Biol Chem 1999;274:10661—7.

[12] Mount DB, Mercado A, Song L, Xu J, George Jr AL, Delpire E, et al. Cloning and characterization of KCC3 and KCC4, new members of the cation-chloride co-transporter gene family. J Biol Chem 1999;274:16355—62.

[13] Mount DB, Baekgard A, Hall AE, Plata C, Xu J, Beier DR, et al. Isoforms of the Na-K-2Cl transporter in murine TAL I.

Molecular characterization and intrarenal localization. Am J Physiol (Renal Physiol) 1999;276:F347–58.

[14] Igarashi P, Vanden Heuver GB, Payne JA, Forbush III B. Cloning, embryonic expression, and alternative splicing of a murine kidney-specific Na-K-Cl co-transporter. Am J Physiol (Renal Fluid Electrolyte Physiol) 1995;269:F406–18.

[15] Russell JM. Sodium-potassium-chloride co-transport. Physiol Rev 2000;80:211–76.

[16] Kahle KT, Staley KJ, Nahed BV, Gamba G, Hebert SC, Lifton RP, et al. Roles of the cation-chloride co-transporters in neurological disease. Nat Clin Pract Neurol 2008;4:490–503.

[17] Gamba G. The thiazide-sensitive Na⁺-Cl⁻ co-transporter: molecular biology, functional properties, and regulation by WNKs. Am J Physiol Renal Physiol 2009;297:F838–48.

[18] Bazzini C, Vezzoli V, Sironi C, Dossena S, Ravasio A, Debiasi S, et al. Thiazide-sensitive NaCl co-transporter in the intestine: possible role of HCTZ in the intestinal Ca²⁺ uptake. J Biol Chem 2005;280:19902–10.

[19] Dvorak MM, De Joussineau C, Carter DH, Pisitkun T, Knepper MA, Gamba G, et al. Thiazide diuretics directly induce osteoblast differentiation and mineralized nodule formation by interacting with a sodium chloride co-transporter in bone. J Am Soc Nephrol 2007;18:2509–16.

[20] Chee KN, Vorontsova I, Lim JC, Kistler J, Donaldson PJ. Expression of the sodium potassium chloride co-transporter (NKCC1) and sodium chloride co-transporter (NCC) and their effects on rat lens transparency. Mol Vis 2010;16:800–12.

[21] Deng L, Chen G. Cyclothiazide potently inhibits gamma-aminobutyric acid type a receptors in addition to enhancing glutamate responses. Proc Natl Acad Sci USA 2003;100:13025–9.

[22] Clader JA, Schacheter M, Sever PS. Direct vascular actions of hydrochlorothaizide and indapamide in isolated small vessels. Eur J Pharmacol 1992;220:19–26.

[23] Bernstein PL, Zawalach W, Bartiss A, Reilly R, Palcso M, Ellison DH. The thiazide-sensitive Na-Cl co-transporter is expressed in rat endocrine pancreas. J Am Soc Nephrol 1995;6:732.

[24] Abuladze N, Yanagawa N, Lee I, Jo OD, Newman D, Hwang J, et al. Peripheral blood mononuclear cells express mutated NCCT mRNA in Gitelman's syndrome: evidence for abnormal thiazide-sensitive NaCl co-transport. J Am Soc Nephrol 1998;9:819–26.

[25] Cremaschi D, Porta C, Botta G, Bazzini C, Baroni MD, Garavaglia M. Apical Na(⁺)-Cl(⁻) symport in rabbit gallbladder epithelium: a thiazide- sensitive co-transporter (TSC). J Membr Biol 2000;176:53–65.

[26] Drewnowska K, Baumgarten CM. Regulation of cellular volume in rabbit ventricular myocytes: Bumetanide, chlorthiazide, and ouabain. *Am J Physiol* (*Cell Physiol*) 1991;260:C122–31.

[27] Jones G, Nguyen T, Sambrook PN, Eisman JA. Thiazide diuretics and fractures: can meta-analysis help? J Bone Miner Res 1995;10:106–11.

[28] Schoofs MW, van der KM, Hofman A, de Laet CE, Herings RM, Stijnen T, et al. Thiazide diuretics and the risk for hip fracture. Ann Intern Med 2003;139:476–82.

[29] Mount DB, Gamba G. Renal potassium-chloride co-transporters. Curr Opin Nephrol Hypertens 2001;10:685–91.

[30] Mercado A, Vazquez N, Song L, Cortes R, Enck AH, Welch R, et al. Amino-terminal heterogeneity in the KCC3 K⁺-Cl⁻ co-transporter. Am J Physiol Renal Physiol 2005;289:F1246–61.

[31] Boettger T, Hubner CA, Maier H, Rust MB, Beck FX, Jentsch TJ. Deafness and renal tubular acidosis in mice lacking the K-Cl co-transporter Kcc4. Nature 2002;416:874–8.

[32] Jentsch TJ. Chloride transport in the kidney: lessons from human disease and knockout mice. J Am Soc Nephrol 2005;16:1549–61.

[33] Hewett D, Samuelsson L, Polding J, Enlund F, Smart D, Cantone K, et al. Identification of a psoriasis susceptibility candidate gene by linkage disequilibrium mapping with a localized single nucleotide polymorphism map. Genomics 2002;79:305–14.

[34] Huffmeier U, Lascorz J, Traupe H, Bohm B, Schurmeier-Horst F, Stander M, et al. Systematic linkage disequilibrium analysis of SLC12A8 at PSORS5 confirms a role in susceptibility to psoriasis vulgaris. J Invest Dermatol 2005;125:906–12.

[35] Daigle ND, Carpentier GA, Frenette-Cotton R, Simard MG, Lefoll MH, Noel M, et al. Molecular characterization of a human cation-Cl⁻ co-transporter (SLC12A8A, CCC9A) that promotes polyamine and amino acid transport. J Cell Physiol 2009;220:680–9.

[36] Caron L, Rousseau F, Gagnon E, Isenring P. Cloning and functional characterization of a cation C1-co-transporter interacting protein. J Biol Chem 2000;275:32027–36.

[37] Lang F, Busch GL, Ritter M, Volkl H, Waldegger S, Gulbins E, et al. Functional significance of cell volume regulatory mechanisms. Physiol Rev 1998;78:247–306.

[38] Mercado A, Mount DB, Gamba G. Electroneutral cation-chloride co-transporters in the central nervous system. Neurochem Res 2004;29:17–25.

[39] Blaesse P, Airaksinen MS, Rivera C, Kaila K. Cation-chloride co-transporters and neuronal function. Neuron 2009;61:820–38.

[40] Kunau RT, Weller DR, Webb HL. Clarification of the site of action of chlorothiazide in the rat nephron. J Clin invest 1975;56:401–7.

[41] Velazquez H, Good DW, Wright FS. Mutual dependence of sodium and chloride absorption by renal distal tubule. Am J Physiol (Renal Fluid Electrolyte Physiol) 1984;247:F904–11.

[42] Costanzo LS. Localization of diuretic action in microperfused rat distal tubules: Ca and Na transport. Am J Physiol (Renal Fluid Electrolyte Physiol) 1985;248:F527–35.

[43] Ellison DH, Velazquez H, Wright FS. Thiazide-sensitive sodium chloride co-transport in early distal tubule. Am J Physiol (Renal Fluid Electrolyte Physiol) 1987;253:F546–54.

[44] Plotkin MD, Kaplan MR, Verlander JM, Lee W-S, Brown D, Poch E, et al. Localization of the thiazide sensitive Na-Cl co-transporter, rTSC1, in the rat kidney. Kidney Int 1996;50:174–83.

[45] Loffing J, Kaissling B. Sodium and calcium transport pathways along the mammalian distal nephron: from rabbit to human. Am J Physiol Renal Physiol 2003;284:F628–43.

[46] Loffing J, Loffing-Cueni D, Valderrabano V, Klausli L, Hebert SC, Rossier BC, et al. Distribution of transcellular calcium and sodium transport pathways along mouse distal nephron. Am J Physiol Renal Physiol 2001;281:F1021–7.

[47] Obermuller N, Bernstein P, Velázquez H, Reilly R, Moser D, Ellison DH, et al. Expression of the thiazide-sensitive Na-Cl co-transporter in rat and human kidney. Am J Physiol (Renal Fluid Electrolyte Physiol) 1995;269:F900–10.

[48] Campean V, Kricke J, Ellison D, Luft FC, Bachmann S. Localization of thiazide-sensitive Na(⁺)-Cl(⁻) co-transport and associated gene products in mouse DCT. Am J Physiol Renal Physiol 2001;281:F1028–35.

[49] Reilly RF, Ellison DH. Mammalian distal tubule: physiology, pathophysiology, and molecular anatomy. Physiol Rev 2000;80:277–313.

[50] Bostanjoglo M, Reeves WB, Reilly RF, Velazquez H, Robertson N, Litwack G, et al. 11 Beta-hydroxysteroid dehydrogenase, mineralocorticoid receptor, and thiazide-sensitive Na-Cl co-transporter expression by distal tubules. J Am Soc Nephrol 1998;9:1347–58.

[51] Bonvalet JP, Doignon I, Blot-Chabaud M, Pradelles P, Farman N. Distribution of 11 beta-hydroxysteroid dehydrogenase along the rabbit nephron. J Clin Invest 1990;86:832–7.

[52] Rusvai E, Naray-Fejes-Toth A. A new isoform of 11 beta-hydroxysteroid dehydrogenase in aldosterone target cells. J Biol Chem 1993;268:10717–20.

[53] Doucet A. Function and control of Na-K-ATPase in single nephron segments of the mammalian kidney. Kidney Int 1988;34:749–60.

[54] Xu JZ, Hall AE, Peterson LN, Bienkowski MJ, Eessalu TE, Hebert SC. Localization of the ROMK protein on apical membranes of rat kidney nephron segments. Am J Physiol Renal Physiol 1997;273:F739–49.

[55] Amorim JB, Bailey MA, Musa-Aziz R, Giebisch G, Malnic G. Role of luminal anion and pH in distal tubule potassium secretion. Am J Physiol Renal Physiol 2003;284:F381–8.

[56] Stokes JB, Lee I, D'Amico M. Sodium chloride absorption by the urinary bladder of the winter flounder. A thiazide-sensitive, electrically neutral transport system. J Clin invest 1984;74:7–16.

[57] Rose BD. Diuretics. Kidney Int 1991;39:336–52.

[58] Gamba G. Molecular biology of distal nephron sodium transport mechanisms. Kidney Int 1999;56:1606–22.

[59] Greger R. Chloride reabsorption in the rabbit cortical thick ascending limb of the loop of Henle. A sodium dependent process. Pflugers Arch 1981;390:38–43.

[60] Greger R, Schlatter E. Presence of luminal K$^+$, a prerequisite for active NaCl transport in the cortical thick ascending limb of Henle's loop of rabbit kidney. Pflugers Arch 1981;392:92–4.

[61] Greger R, Schlatter E, Lang F. Evidence for electroneutral sodium chloride co-transport in the cortical thick ascending limb of Henle's loop of rabbit kidney. Pflugers Arch 1983;396:308–14.

[62] Greger R, Schlatter E. Properties of the lumen membrane of the cortical thick ascending limb of Henle's loop of rabbit kidney. Pflugers Arch 1983;396:315–24.

[63] Hebert SC, Culpepper RM, Andreoli TE. NaCl transport in mouse medullary thick ascending limbs. I. Functional nephron heterogeneity and ADH-stimulated NaCl co-transport. Am J Physiol (Renal Fluid Electrolyte Physiol) 1981;241:F412–31.

[64] Gamba G, Friedman PA. Thick ascending limb: the Na($^+$):K($^+$):2Cl($^-$) co-transporter, NKCC2, and the calcium-sensing receptor, CaSR. Pflugers Arch 2009;458:61–76.

[65] Greger R. Ion transport mechanisms in thick ascending limb of Henle's loop of mammalian nephron. Physiol Rev 1985;65:760–97.

[66] Hebert SC. Bartter syndrome. Curr Opin Nephrol Hypertens 2003;12:527–32.

[67] Amlal H, Paillard M, Bichara M. Cl($^-$)-dependent NH$_4^+$ transport mechanisms in medullary thick ascending limb cells. Am J Physiol 1994;267:C1607–15.

[68] Attmane-Elakeb A, Amlal H, Bichara M. Ammonium carriers in medullary thick ascending limb. Am J Physiol Renal Physiol 2001;280:F1–9.

[69] Schnermann J. Juxtaglomerular cell complex in the regulation of renal salt excretion. Am J Physiol (Regulatory Integrative Comp Physiol) 1998;274:R263–79.

[70] Nielsen S, Maunsbach AB, Ecelbarger CA, Knepper MA. Ultrastructural localization of Na-K-2Cl co-transporter in thick ascending limb and macula densa of rat kidney. Am J Physiol 1998;275:F885–93.

[71] Gimenez I, Isenring P, Forbush III B. Spatially distributed alternative splice variants of the renal Na-K-Cl co-transporter exhibit dramatically different affinities for the transported ions. J Biol Chem 2002;277:8767–70.

[72] Gagnon E, Forbush B, Flemmer AW, Gimenez I, Caron L, Isenring P. Functional and molecular characterization of the shark renal Na-K-Cl co-transporter: novel aspects. Am J Physiol Renal Physiol 2002;283:F1046–55.

[73] Oppermann M, Mizel D, Huang G, Li C, Deng C, Theilig F, et al. Macula densa control of renin secretion and preglomerular resistance in mice with selective deletion of the B isoform of the Na,K,2Cl co-transporter. J Am Soc Nephrol 2006;17:2143–52.

[74] Oppermann M, Mizel D, Kim SM, Chen L, Faulhaber-Walter R, Huang Y, et al. Renal function in mice with targeted disruption of the a isoform of the Na-K-2Cl co-transporter. J Am Soc Nephrol 2007;18:440–8.

[75] Hebert SC, Culpepper RM, Andreoli TE. NaCl transport in mouse medullary thick ascending limbs. II. ADH enhancement of transcellular NaCl cotransport; origin of transepithelial voltage. Am J Physiol (Renal Fluid Electrolyte Physiol) 1981;241:F432–42.

[76] Hebert SC, Culpepper RM, Andreoli TE. NaCl transport in mouse medullary thick ascending limbs. III. Modulation of ADH efect by peritubular osmolality. Am J Physiol (Renal Fluid Electrolyte Physiol) 1981;241:F443–51.

[77] Gimenez I, Forbush B. Short-term stimulation of the renal Na-K-Cl co-transporter (NKCC2) by vasopressin involves phosphorylation and membrane translocation of the protein. J Biol Chem 2003;278:26946–51.

[78] Plata C, Mount DB, Rubio V, Hebert SC, Gamba G. Isoforms of the Na-K-2Cl co-transporter in murine TAL. II. Functional characterization and activation by cAMP. Am J Physiol (Renal Physiol) 1999;276:F359–66.

[79] Meade P, Hoover RS, Plata C, Vazquez N, Bobadilla NA, Gamba G, et al. cAMP-dependent activation of the renal-specific Na$^+$-K$^+$-2Cl$^-$ co-transporter is mediated by regulation of co-transporter trafficking. Am J Physiol Renal Physiol 2003;284:F1145–54.

[80] Ortiz PA. cAMP increases surface expression of NKCC2 in rat thick ascending limbs: role of VAMP. Am J Physiol Renal Physiol 2006;290:F608–16.

[81] Caceres PS, Ares GR, Ortiz PA. cAMP stimulates apical exocytosis of the renal Na-K-2Cl co-transporter NKCC2 in the thick ascending limb: Role of protein kinase A (PKA). J Biol Chem 2009;284:24965–71.

[82] Kim G-H, Ecelbarger CA, Mitchell C, Packer RK, Wade JB, Knepper MA. Vasopressin increases Na-K-2Cl co-transporter expression in thick ascending limb of Henle's loop. Am J Physiol (Renal Physiol) 1999;276:F96–103.

[83] Knepper MA, Kim GH, Fernandez-Llama P, Ecelbarger CA. Regulation of thick ascending limb transport by vasopressin. J Am Soc Nephrol 1999;10:628–34.

[84] Alvarez-Leefmans FJ. Intracellular chloride regulation. 3rd ed. 2001:301-318.

[85] Delpire E, Mount DB. Human and murine phenotypes associated with defects in cation-chloride co-transport. Annu Rev Physiol 2002;64:803–43.

[86] Flagella M, Clarke LL, Miller ML, Erway LC, Giannella RA, Andringa A, et al. Mice lacking the basolateral Na-K-2Cl co-transporter have impaired epithelial chloride secretion and are profoundly deaf. J Biol Chem 1999;274:26946–55.

[87] Delpire E, Lu J, England R, Dull C, Thorne T. Deafness and imbalance associated with inactivation of the secretory Na-K-2Cl co-transporter. Nat Genet 1999;22:192–5.

[88] Orlov SN, Tremblay J, Hamet P. NKCC1 and hypertension: a novel therapeutic target involved in the regulation of vascular tone and renal function. Curr Opin Nephrol Hypertens 2010;19:163–8.

[89] Meyer JW, Flagella M, Sutliff RL, Lorenz JN, Nieman ML, Weber CS, et al. Decreased blood pressure and vascular smooth muscle tone in mice lacking basolateral Na$^{(+)}$-K$^{(+)}$-2Cl$^{(-)}$ co-transporter. Am J Physiol Heart Circ Physiol 2002;283: H1846−55.

[90] Wall SM, Knepper MA, Hassell KA, Fischer MP, Shodeinde A, Shin W, et al. Hypotension in NKCC1 null mice: role of the kidneys. Am J Physiol Renal Physiol 2006;290:F409−16.

[91] Garg P, Martin CF, Elms SC, Gordon FJ, Wall SM, Garland CJ, et al. Effect of the Na-K-2Cl co-transporter NKCC1 on systemic blood pressure and smooth muscle tone. Am J Physiol Heart Circ Physiol 2007;292:H2100−5.

[92] Koltsova SV, Kotelevtsev SV, Tremblay J, Hamet P, Orlov SN. Excitation-contraction coupling in resistance mesenteric arteries: evidence for NKCC1-mediated pathway. Biochem Biophys Res Commun 2009;379:1080−3.

[93] Kim SM, Eisner C, Faulhaber-Walter R, Mizel D, Wall SM, Briggs JP, et al. Salt sensitivity of blood pressure in NKCC1-deficient mice. Am J Physiol Renal Physiol 2008;295:F1230−8.

[94] Kaplan MR, Plotkin MD, Brown D, Hebert SC, Delpire E. Expression of the mouse Na-K-2Cl co-transporter, mBSC2, in the terminal inner medullary collecting duct, the glomerular and extraglomerular masangium, and the glomerular afferent arteriole. J Clin invest 1996;98:723−30.

[95] Castrop H, Lorenz JN, Hansen P, Friis U, Mizel D, Oppermann M, et al. Contribution of the basolateral isoform of the Na, K,2Cl-co-transporter (NKCC1/BSC2) to renin secretion. Am J Physiol Renal Physiol 2005;289:F1185−92.

[96] Kyte J, Doolittle RF. A simple method for displaying the hydropathic character of a protein. J Mol Biol 1982;157:105−32.

[97] Hoover RS, Poch E, Monroy A, Vazquez N, Nishio T, Gamba G, et al. N-Glycosylation at two sites critically alters thiazide binding and activity of the rat thiazide-sensitive Na$^{(+)}$:Cl$^{(-)}$ co-transporter. J Am Soc Nephrol 2003;14:271−82.

[98] Moreno E, San Cristobal P, Rivera M, Vazquez N, Bobadilla NA, Gamba G. Affinity defining domains in the Na-Cl co-transporter: different location for Cl$^-$ and thiazide binding. J Biol Chem 2006;281:17266−75.

[99] Paredes A, Plata C, Rivera M, Moreno E, Vazquez N, Munoz-Clares R, et al. Activity of the renal Na$^+$:K$^+$:2Cl$^-$ co-transporter is reduced by mutagenesis of N-glycosylation sites: role for protein surface charge in Cl$^-$ transport. Am J Physiol Renal Physiol 2006;290:F1094−102.

[100] Merino A, Hebert SC, Gamba G. Correlation between water salinity and tissue expression of the thiazide-sensitive co-transporter (TSC) in teleost. J Am Soc Nephrol 1999;10:39A.

[101] Velazquez H, Naray-Fejes-Toth A, Silva T, Andujar E, Reilly RF, Desir GV, et al. Rabbit distal convoluted tubule coexpresses NaCl co-transporter and 11 beta-hydroxysteroid dehydrogenase II mRNA. Kidney Int 1998;54:464−72.

[102] Simon DB, Nelson-Williams C, Johnson-Bia M, Ellison D, Karet FE, Morey-Molina A, et al. Gitelman's variant of Bartter's syndrome, inherited hypokalaemic alkalosis, is caused by mutations in the thiazide-sensitive Na-Cl co-transporter. Nature Genetics 1996;12:24−30.

[103] Mastroianni N, DeFusco M, Zollo M, Arrigo G, Zuffardi O, Bettinelli A, et al. Molecular cloning, expression pattern, and chromosomal localization of the human Na-Cl thiazide-sensitive co-transporter (SLC12A3). Genomics 1996;35:486−93.

[104] Di Fulvio M, Alvarez-Leefmans FJ. The NKCC and NCC genes: an *in silico* view. In: Alvarez-Leefmans FJ, Delpire E, editors. Physiology and pathology of chloride transporters and channels in the nervous system. New York: Elsevier; 2009. p. 169−208.

[105] Cutler CP, Cramb G. Differential expression of absorptive cation-chloride-co-transporters in the intestinal and renal tissues of the European eel (*Anguilla anguilla*). Comp Biochem Physiol B Biochem Mol Biol 2008;149:63−73.

[106] Gonzales PA, Pisitkun T, Hoffert JD, Tchapyjnikov D, Star RA, Kleta R, et al. Large-scale proteomics and phosphoproteomics of urinary exosomes. J Am Soc Nephrol 2009;20:363−79.

[107] Simon DB, Karet FE, Hamdan JM, Di Pietro A, Sanjad SA, Lifton RP. Bartter's syndrome, hypokalaemic alkalosis with hypercalciuria, is caused by mutations in the Na-K-2Cl co-transporter NKCC2. Nature Genetics 1996;13:183−8.

[108] Igarashi P, Whyte DA, Kui L, Nagami GT. Cloning and kidney cell-specific activity of the promoter of the murine renal Na-K-Cl co-transporter gene. J Biol Chem 1996;271:9666−74.

[109] Gamba G. Alternative splicing and diversity of renal transporters. Am J Physiol Renal Physiol 2001;281:F781−94.

[110] Yang T, Huang YG, Singh I, Schnermann J, Briggs JP. Localization of bumetanide- and thiazide-sensitive Na-K-Cl co-transporters along the rat nephron. Am J Physiol (Renal Fluid Electrolyte Physiol) 1996;271:F931−9.

[111] Plotkin MD, Kaplan MR, Peterson LN, Gullans SR, Hebert SC, Delpire E. Expression of the Na$^+$-K$^+$-2Cl$^-$ co-transporter BSC2 in the nervous system. Am J Physiol (Cell Physiol) 1997;272: C173−83.

[112] Moore-Hoon ML, Turner RJ. Molecular and topological characterization of the rat parotid Na$^+$-K$^+$-2Cl$^-$ co-transporter1. Biochim Biophys Acta 1998;1373:261−9.

[113] Payne JA, Xu J-C, Haas M, Lytle CY, Ward D, Forbush III B. Primary structure, functional expression, and chromosomal localization of the bumetanide-sensitive Na-K-Cl co-transporter in human colon. J Biol Chem 1995;270:17977−85.

[114] Yerby TR, Vibat CRT, Sun D, Payne JA, O'Donnell ME. Molecular characterization of the Na-K-Cl co-transporter of bovine aortic endothelial cells. Am J Physiol (Cell Physiol) 1997;273:C188−97.

[115] Cutler CP, Cramb G. Two isoforms of the Na$^+$/K$^+$/2Cl$^-$ co-transporter are expressed in the European eel (*Anguilla anguilla*). Biochim Biophys Acta 2002;1566:92−103.

[116] Lorin-Nebel C, Boulo V, Bodinier C, Charmantier G. The Na$^+$/K$^+$/2Cl$^-$ co-transporter in the sea bass *dicentrarchus labrax* during ontogeny: involvement in osmoregulation. J Exp Biol 2006;209:4908−22.

[117] Colmenero-Flores JM, Martinez G, Gamba G, Vazquez N, Iglesias DJ, Brumos J, et al. Identification and functional characterization of cation-chloride co-transporters in plants. Plant J 2007;50:278−92.

[118] Randall J, Thorne T, Delpire E. Partial cloning and characterization of Slc12a2: the gene encoding the secretory Na$^+$-K$^+$-2Cl$^-$ co-transporter. Am J Physiol (Cell Physiol) 1997;273: C1267−77.

[119] Vibat CR, Holland MJ, Kang JJ, Putney LK, O'Donnell ME. Quantitation of Na$^+$-K$^+$-2Cl$^-$ co-transport splice variants in human tissues using kinetic polymerase chain reaction. Anal Biochem 2001;298:218−30.

[120] Carmosino M, Gimenez I, Caplan M, Forbush B. Exon loss accounts for differential sorting of Na-K-Cl co-transporters in polarized epithelial cells. Mol Biol Cell 2008;19:4341−51.

[121] Wang J, Pravenec M, Kren V, Kurtz TW. Linkage mapping of the Na-K-2Cl co-transporter gene (Slc12a1) to rat chromosome 3. Mamm Genome 1997;8:379.

[122] Quaggin SE, Payne JA, Forbush III B, Igarashi P. Localization of the renal Na-K-Cl co-transporter gene (Slc12a1) on mouse chromosome 2. Mamm Genome 1995;6:557−8.

III. FLUID AND ELECTROLYTE REGULATION AND DYSREGULATION

[123] Lazzaro D, De S V, De Magistris L, Lehtonen E, Cortese R. LFB1 and LFB3 homeoproteins are sequentially expressed during kidney development. Development 1992;114:469–79.

[124] Molony DA, Reeves WB, Hebert SC, Andreoli TE. ADH increases apical Na$^+$,K$^+$,2Cl$^-$ entry in mouse medullary thick ascending limbs of Henle. Am J Physiol (Renal Fluid Electrolyte Physiol) 1987;252:F177–87.

[125] Lee HA, Baek I, Seok YM, Yang E, Cho HM, Lee DY, et al. Promoter hypomethylation upregulates Na$^+$-K$^+$-2Cl$^-$ co-transporter 1 in spontaneously hypertensive rats. Biochem Biophys Res Commun 2010;396:252–7.

[126] Cho HM, Lee HA, Kim HY, Han HS, Kim IK. Expression of Na$^+$-K$^+$-2Cl$^-$ co-transporter 1 is epigenetically regulated during postnatal development of hypertension. Am J Hypertens 2011;24:1286–93.

[127] Taniyama Y, Sato K, Sugawara A, Uruno A, Ikeda Y, Kudo M, et al. Renal tubule-specific transcription and chromosomal localization of rat thiazide-sensitive Na-Cl co-transporter gene. J Biol Chem 2001;276:26260–8.

[128] Pathak BG, Shaughnessy Jr JD, Meneton P, Greeb J, Shull GE, Jenkins NA, et al. Mouse chromosomal location of three epithelial sodium channel subunit genes and an apical sodium chloride co-transporter gene. Genomics 1996;33:124–7.

[129] MacKenzie S, Vaitkevicius H, Lockette W. Sequencing and characterization of the human thiazide-sensitive Na-Cl co-transporter (SLC12A3) gene promoter. Biochem Biophys Res Commun 2001;282:991–1000.

[130] Kim GH, Martin SW, Fernandez-Llama P, Masilamani S, Packer RK, Knepper MA. Long-term regulation of renal Na-dependent co-transporters and ENaC: response to altered acid–base intake. Am J Physiol Renal Physiol 2000;279:F459–67.

[131] Fanestil DD, Vaughan DA, Blakely P. Metabolic acid–base influences on renal thiazide receptor density. Am J Physiol (Regulatory Integrative Comp Physiol) 1997;272:R2004–8.

[132] O'Grady SM, Palfrey HC, Field M. Characteristics and function of Na-K-Cl co-transport in epithelial tissues. Am J Physiol (Cell Physiol) 1987;253:C177–92.

[133] Bachmann S, Bostanjoglo M, Schmitt R, Ellison DH. Sodium transport-related proteins in the mammalian distal nephron — distribution, ontogeny and functional aspects. Anat Embryol (Berl) 1999;200:447–68.

[134] Haas M. Properties and diversity of (Na-K-Cl) co-transporters. Annu Rev Physiol 1989;51:443–57.

[135] Haas M, Dunham PB, Forbush III B. [^{3}H]Bumetanide binding to mouse kidney membranes: identification of corresponding membrane proteins. Am J Physiol (Cell Physiol) 1991;260:C791–804.

[136] Fanestil DD, Tran JM, Vaughn DA, Maciejewski AR, Beaumont K. Investigation of the metolazone receptor 1990:195–204.

[137] Monroy A, Plata C, Hebert SC, Gamba G. Characterization of the thiazide-sensitive Na$^{(+)}$-Cl$^{(-)}$ co-transporter: a new model for ions and diuretics interaction. Am J Physiol Renal Physiol 2000;279:F161–9.

[138] Kunchaparty S, Palcso M, Berkman J, Velazquez H, Desir GV, Bernstein P, et al. Defective processing and expression of thiazide-sensitive Na-Cl co-transporter as a cause of Gitelman's syndrome. Am J Physiol 1999;277:F643–9.

[139] Sabath E, Meade P, Berkman J, De Los Heros P, Moreno E, Bobadilla NA, et al. Pathophysiology of functional mutations of the thiazide-sensitive Na-Cl co-transporter in Gitelman disease. Am J Physiol Renal Physiol 2004;287:F195–203.

[140] De Jong JC, Van Der Vliet WA, van den Heuvel LP, Willems PH, Knoers NV, Bindels RJ. Functional expression of mutations in the human NaCl co-transporter: evidence for impaired

[141] routing mechanisms in Gitelman's syndrome. J Am Soc Nephrol 2002;13:1442–8.

De Jong JC, Willems PH, van den Heuvel LP, Knoers NV, Bindels RJ. Functional expression of the human thiazide-sensitive NaCl co-transporter in Madin–Darby canine kidney cells. J Am Soc Nephrol 2003;14:2428–35.

[142] Richardson C, Rafiqi FH, Karlsson HK, Moleleki N, Vandewalle A, Campbell DG, et al. Activation of the thiazide-sensitive Na$^+$-Cl$^-$ co-transporter by the WNK-regulated kinases SPAK and OSR1. J Cell Sci 2008;121:675–84.

[143] Ko B, Joshi LM, Cooke LL, Vazquez N, Musch MW, Hebert SC, et al. Phorbol ester stimulation of RasGRP1 regulates the sodium-chloride co-transporter by a PKC-independent pathway. Proc Natl Acad Sci USA 2007;104:20120–5.

[144] Ko B, Kamsteeg EJ, Cooke LL, Moddes LN, Deen PM, Hoover RS. RasGRP1 stimulation enhances ubiquitination and endocytosis of the sodium-chloride co-transporter. Am J Physiol Renal Physiol 2010;299:F300–9.

[145] Gesek FA, Friedman PA. Mechanism of calcium transport stimulated by chlorothiazide in mouse distal convoluted tubule cells. J Clin Invest 1992;90:429–38.

[146] Vazquez N, Monroy A, Dorantes E, Munoz-Clares RA, Gamba G. Functional differences between flounder and rat thiazide-sensitive Na-Cl co-transporter. Am J Physiol Renal Physiol 2002;282:F599–607.

[147] Tran JM, Farrell MA, Fanestil DD. Effect of ions on binding of the thiazide-type diuretic metolazone to kidney membrane. Am J Physiol (Renal Fluid Electrolyte Physiol) 1990;258:F908–15.

[148] Chang H, Fujita T. A kinetic model of the thaizide-sensitive Na-Cl co-transporter. Am J Physiol (Renal Physiol) 1999;276:F952–9.

[149] Starremans PG, Kersten FF, Knoers NV, van den Heuvel LP, Bindels RJ. Mutations in the human Na-K-2Cl Co-transporter (NKCC2) identified in Bartter syndrome Type I consistently result in nonfunctional transporters. J Am Soc Nephrol 2003;14:1419–26.

[150] Burg MB. Thick ascending limb of Henle's loop. Kidney Int 1982;22:454–64.

[151] Rocha AS, Kokko JP. Sodium chloride and water transport in the medullary thick ascending limb of Henle. Evidence for active chloride transport. J Clin Invest 1973;52:612–23.

[152] Reeves WB, Molony DA, Andreoli TE. Diluting power of thick limbs of Henle. III. Modulation of in vitro diluting power. Am J Physiol 1988;255:F1145–54.

[153] Plata C, Meade P, Vazquez N, Hebert SC, Gamba G. Functional properties of the apical Na$^+$-K$^+$-2Cl$^-$ co-transporter isoforms. J Biol Chem 2002;277:11004–12.

[154] Marcano M, Yang HM, Nieves-Gonzalez A, Clausen C, Moore LC. Parameter estimation for mathematical models of NKCC2 co-transporter isoforms. Am J Physiol Renal Physiol 2009;296:F369–81.

[155] Plata C, Meade P, Hall AE, Welch RC, Vazquez N, Hebert SC, et al. Alternatively spliced isoform of the apical Na-K-Cl co-transporter gene encodes a furosemide sensitive Na-Cl co-transporter. Am J Physiol Renal Physiol 2001;280:F574–82.

[156] Eveloff J, Calamia J. Effect of osmolarity on cation fluxes in medullary thick ascending limb cells. Am J Physiol (Renal Fluid Electrolyte Physiol) 1986;250:F176–80.

[157] Alvo M, Calamia J, Eveloff J. Lack of potassium effect on Na-Cl co-transport in the medullary thick ascending limb. Am J Physiol (Renal Fluid Electrolyte Physiol) 1985;249:F34–9.

[158] Sun A, Grossman EB, Lombardi M, Hebert SC. Vasopressin alters the mechanism of apical Cl$^-$ entry from Na$^+$:Cl$^-$ to Na$^+$:K$^+$:2Cl$^-$ co-transport in mouse medullary thick ascending limb. J Membrane Biol 1991;120:83–94.

[159] Gerelsaikhan T, Turner RJ. Transmembrane topology of the secretory Na$^+$-K$^+$-2Cl$^-$ co-transporter (NKCC1) studied by *in vitro* translation. J Biol Chem 2000;275:40471–7.

[160] Isenring P, Forbush B. Ion transport and ligand binding by the Na-K-Cl co-transporter, structure–function studies. Comp Biochem Physiol A Mol Integr Physiol 2001;130:487–97.

[161] Tovar-Palacio C, Bobadilla NA, Cortes P, Plata C, De Los Heros P, Vazquez N, et al. Ion and diuretic specificity of chimeric proteins between apical Na$^+$:K + :2Cl$^-$ and Na$^+$:Cl$^-$ co-transporters. Am J Physiol Renal Physiol 2004;287:F570–7.

[162] Gimenez I, Forbush B. The residues determining differences in ion affinities among the alternative splice variants F, A, and B of the mammalian renal Na-K-Cl co-transporter (NKCC2). J Biol Chem 2007;282:6540–7.

[163] Gagnon E, Bergeron MJ, Daigle ND, Lefoll MH, Isenring P. Molecular mechanisms of cation transport by the renal Na$^+$-K$^+$-Cl$^-$ co-transporter: structural insight into the operating characteristics of the ion transport sites. J Biol Chem 2005;280:32555–63.

[164] Isenring P, Forbush III B. Ion and bumetanide binding by the Na-K-Cl co-transporter. Importance of transmembrane domains. J Biol Chem 1997;272:24556–62.

[165] Isenring P, Jacoby SC, Forbush III B. The role of transmembrane domain 2 in cation transport by the Na-K-Cl co-transporter. Proc Natl Acad Sci USA 1998;95:7179–84.

[166] Isenring P, Jacoby SC, Chang J, Forbush III B. Mutagenic mapping of the Na-K-Cl co-transporter for domains involved in ion transport and bumetanide binding. J Gen Physiol 1998;112:549–58.

[167] Forbush III B, Palfrey HC. [^{3}H]Bumetanide binding to membranes isolated from dog kidney outer medulla. Relationship to the Na,K,Cl co-transport system. J Biol Chem 1983;258:11787–92.

[168] Gagnon E, Bergeron MJ, Brunet GM, Daigle ND, Simard CF, Isenring P. Molecular mechanisms of Cl transport by the renal Na-K-Cl co-transporter: identification of an intracellular locus that may form part of a high affinity Cl-binding site. J Biol Chem 2003;279:5648–54.

[169] Malysiak K, Grzywna ZJ. On the possible methods for the mathematical description of the ball and chain model of ion channel inactivation. Cell Mol Biol Lett 2008;13:535–52.

[170] Castaneda-Bueno M, Vazquez N, Bustos-Jaimes I, Hernandez D, Rodriguez-Lobato E, Pacheco-Alvarez D, et al. A single residue in transmembrane domain 11 defines the different affinity for thiazides between mammalian and flounder NaCl transporter. Am J Physiol Renal Physiol 2010;299:F1111–9.

[171] Moreno E, Tovar-Palacio C, De Los Heros P, Guzman B, Bobadilla NA, Vazquez N, et al. A single nucleotide polymorphism alters the activity of the renal Na$^+$:Cl$^-$ co-transporter and reveals a role for transmembrane segment 4 in chloride and thiazide affinity. J Biol Chem 2004;279:16553–60.

[172] Vormfelde SV, Sehrt D, Toliat MR, Schirmer M, Meineke I, Tzvetkov M, et al. Genetic variation in the renal sodium transporters NKCC2, NCC, and ENaC in relation to the effects of loop diuretic drugs. Clin Pharmacol Ther 2007;82:300–9.

[173] Nezu A, Parvin MN, Turner RJ. A conserved hydrophobic tetrad near the C terminus of the secretory Na$^+$-K$^+$-2Cl$^-$ co-transporter (NKCC1) is required for its correct intracellular processing. J Biol Chem 2009;284:6869–76.

[174] Zaarour N, Demaretz S, Defontaine N, Mordasini D, Laghmani K. A highly conserved motif at the C-terminus dictates ER exit and cell-surface expression of NKCC2. J Biol Chem 2009;284:21752–64.

[175] Zaarour N, Defontaine N, Demaretz S, Azroyan A, Cheval L, Laghmani K. Secretory carrier membrane protein 2 regulates exocytic insertion of NKCC2 into the cell membrane. J Biol Chem 2011;286:9489–502.

[176] Moore-Hoon ML, Turner RJ. The structural unit of the secretory Na$^+$-K$^+$-2Cl$^-$ co-transporter (NKCC1) is a homodimer. Biochemistry 2000;39:3718–24.

[177] Starremans PG, Kersten FF, van den Heuvel LP, Knoers NV, Bindels RJ. Dimeric architecture of the human bumetanide-sensitive Na-K-Cl Co-transporter. J Am Soc Nephrol 2003;14:3039–46.

[178] De Jong JC, Willems PH, Mooren FJ, van den Heuvel LP, Knoers NV, Bindels RJ. The structural unit of the thiazide-sensitive NaCl co-transporter is a homodimer. J Biol Chem 2003;278:24302–7.

[179] Wenz M, Hartmann AM, Friauf E, Nothwang HG. CIP1 is an activator of the K$^{(+)}$-Cl$^{(-)}$ co-transporter KCC2. Biochem Biophys Res Commun 2009;381(3):388–92.

[180] Simard CF, Bergeron MJ, Frenette-Cotton R, Carpentier GA, Pelchat ME, Caron L, et al. Homooligomeric and heterooligomeric associations between K$^+$-Cl$^-$ co-transporter isoforms and between K$^+$-Cl$^-$ and Na$^+$-K$^+$-Cl$^-$ co-transporters. J Biol Chem 2007;282:18083–93.

[181] Knepper MA, Brooks HL. Regulation of the sodium transporters NHE3, NKCC2 and NCC in the kidney. Curr Opin Nephrol Hypertens 2001;10:655–9.

[182] Lytle C, McManus T. Coordinate modulation of Na-K-2Cl cotransport and K-Cl co-transport by cell volume and chloride. Am J Physiol Cell Physiol 2002;283:C1422–31.

[183] McManus ML, Churchwell KB, Strange K. Regulation of cell volume in health and disease. N Engl J Med 1995;333:1260–6.

[184] Dowd BF, Forbush B. PASK (proline-alanine-rich STE20-related kinase), a regulatory kinase of the Na-K-Cl co-transporter (NKCC1). J Biol Chem 2003;278:27347–53.

[185] Flemmer AW, Gimenez I, Dowd BF, Darman RB, Forbush B. Activation of the Na-K-Cl cotransporter NKCC1 detected with a phospho-specific antibody. J Biol Chem 2002;277:37551–8.

[186] Ponce-Coria J, San Cristobal P, Kahle KT, Vazquez N, Pacheco-Alvarez D, De Los Heros P, et al. Regulation of NKCC2 by a chloride-sensing mechanism involving the WNK3 and SPAK kinases. Proc Natl Acad Sci USA 2008;105:8458–63.

[187] Pacheco-Alvarez D, San Cristobal P, Meade P, Moreno E, Vazquez N, Munoz E, et al. The Na-Cl co-transporter is activated and phosphorylated at the amino terminal domain upon intracellular chloride depletion. J Biol Chem 2006;281:28755–63.

[188] Lytle C, Forbush III B. The Na-K-Cl co-transport protein of shark rectal gland. II Regulation by direct phosphorylation. J Biol Chem 1992;267:25438–43.

[189] Darman RB, Forbush B. A regulatory locus of phosphorylation in the N terminus of the Na-K-Cl co-transporter, NKCC1. J Biol Chem 2002;277:37542–50.

[190] Moriguchi T, Urushiyama S, Hisamoto N, Iemura S, Uchida S, Natsume T, et al. WNK1 regulates phosphorylation of cation-chloride-coupled co-transporters via the STE20-related kinases, SPAK and OSR1. J Biol Chem 2005;280:42685–93.

[191] Richardson C, Alessi DR. The regulation of salt transport and blood pressure by the WNK-SPAK/OSR1 signalling pathway. J Cell Sci 2008;121:3293–304.

[192] Rafiqi FH, Zuber AM, Glover M, Richardson C, Fleming S, Jovanovic S, et al. Role of the WNK-activated SPAK kinase in regulating blood pressure. EMBO Mol Med 2010;2:63–75.

[193] Chiga M, Rai T, Yang SS, Ohta A, Takizawa T, Sasaki S, et al. Dietary salt regulates the phosphorylation of OSR1/SPAK kinases and the sodium chloride co-transporter through aldosterone. Kidney Int 2008;74:1403–9.

[194] Pedersen NB, Hofmeister MV, Rosenbaek LL, Nielsen J, Fenton RA. Vasopressin induces phosphorylation of the thiazide-sensitive sodium chloride co-transporter in the distal convoluted tubule. Kidney Int 2010;78:160—9.

[195] Mutig K, Saritas T, Uchida S, Kahl T, Borowski T, Paliege A, et al. Short-term stimulation of the thiazide-sensitive Na$^+$,Cl$^-$-co-transporter by vasopressin involves phosphorylation and membrane translocation. Am J Physiol Renal Physiol 2010;298:F502—9.

[196] San Cristobal P, Pacheco-Alvarez D, Richardson C, Ring AM, Vazquez N, Rafiqi FH, et al. Angiotensin II signaling increases activity of the renal Na-Cl co-transporter through a WNK4-SPAK-dependent pathway. Proc Natl Acad Sci USA 2009;106:4384—9.

[197] van der LN, Lim CH, Fenton RA, Meima ME, Jan Danser AH, Zietse R, et al. Angiotensin II induces phosphorylation of the thiazide-sensitive sodium chloride co-transporter independent of aldosterone. Kidney Int 2011;79:66—76.

[198] Talati G, Ohta A, Rai T, Sohara E, Naito S, Vandewalle A, et al. Effect of angiotensin II on the WNK-OSR1/SPAK-NCC phosphorylation cascade in cultured mpkDCT cells and *in vivo* mouse kidney. Biochem Biophys Res Commun 2010;393:844—8.

[199] Gimenez I, Forbush B. Regulatory phosphorylation sites in the N-terminus of the renal Na-K-Cl co-transporter (NKCC2). Am J Physiol Renal Physiol 2005;289:F1341—5.

[200] Richardson C, Sakamoto K, De Los Heros P, Deak M, Campbell DG, Prescott AR, et al. Regulation of the NKCC2 ion co-transporter by SPAK-OSR1-dependent and -independent pathways. J Cell Sci 2011;124:789—800.

[201] Dimke H, Flyvbjerg A, Bourgeois S, Thomsen K, Frokiaer J, Houillier P, et al. Acute growth hormone administration induces antidiuretic and antinatriuretic effects and increases phosphorylation of NKCC2. Am J Physiol Renal Physiol 2007;292:F723—35.

[202] Xu B, English JM, Wilsbacher JL, Stippec S, Goldsmith EJ, Cobb MH. WNK1, a novel mammalian serine/threonine protein kinase lacking the catalytic lysine in subdomain II. J Biol Chem 2000;275:16795—801.

[203] Min X, Lee BH, Cobb MH, Goldsmith EJ. Crystal structure of the kinase domain of WNK1, a kinase that causes a hereditary form of hypertension. *Structure (Camb)* 2004;12:1303—11.

[204] Verissimo F, Jordan P. WNK kinases, a novel protein kinase subfamily in multi-cellular organisms. Oncogene 2001;20:5562—9.

[205] Lenertz LY, Lee BH, Min X, Xu BE, Wedin K, Earnest S, et al. Properties of WNK1 and implications for other family members. J Biol Chem 2005;280:26653—8.

[206] Wilson FH, Disse-Nicodeme S, Choate KA, Ishikawa K, Nelson-Williams C, Desitter I, et al. Human hypertension caused by mutations in WNK kinases. Science 2001;293:1107—12.

[207] Gordon RD. Syndrome of hypertension and hyperkalemia with normal glomerular filtration rate. Hypertension 1986;8:93—102.

[208] Gordon RD, Hodsman GP. The syndrome of hypertension and hyperkalaemia without renal failure: long term correction by thiazide diuretic. Scott Med J 1986;31:43—4.

[209] Wilson FH, Kahle KT, Sabath E, Lalioti MD, Rapson AK, Hoover RS, et al. Molecular pathogenesis of inherited hypertension with hyperkalemia: the Na-Cl co-transporter is inhibited by wild-type but not mutant WNK4. Proc Natl Acad Sci USA 2003;100:680—4.

[210] Yang CL, Angell J, Mitchell R, Ellison DH. WNK kinases regulate thiazide-sensitive Na-Cl co-transport. J Clin Invest 2003;111:1039—45.

[211] San Cristobal P, Ponce-Coria J, Vazquez N, Bobadilla NA, Gamba G. WNK3 and WNK4 amino terminal domain defines their effect on the renal Na$^+$:Cl$^-$ co-transporter. Am J Physiol Renal Physiol 2008;295:F1199—206.

[212] Golbang AP, Cope G, Hamad A, Murthy M, Liu CH, Cuthbert AW, et al. Regulation of the expression of the Na/Cl co-transporter (NCCT) by WNK4 and WNK1: evidence that accelerated dynamin-dependent endocytosis is not involved. Am J Physiol Renal Physiol 2006;291:F1369—76.

[213] Cai H, Cebotaru V, Wang YH, Zhang XM, Cebotaru L, Guggino SE, et al. WNK4 kinase regulates surface expression of the human sodium chloride co-transporter in mammalian cells. Kidney Int 2006;69:2162—70.

[214] Lalioti MD, Zhang J, Volkman HM, Kahle KT, Hoffmann KE, Toka HR, et al. Wnk4 controls blood pressure and potassium homeostasis via regulation of mass and activity of the distal convoluted tubule. Nat Genet 2006;38:1124—32.

[215] Yang SS, Morimoto T, Rai T, Chiga M, Sohara E, Ohno M, et al. Molecular pathogenesis of pseudohypoaldosteronism type II: generation and analysis of a Wnk4(D561A/ +) knockin mouse model. Cell Metab 2007;5:331—44.

[216] Delaloy C, Lu J, Houot AM, Disse-Nicodeme S, Gasc JM, Corvol P, et al. Multiple promoters in the WNK1 gene: one controls expression of a kidney-specific kinase-defective isoform. Mol Cell Biol 2003;23:9208—21.

[217] Faure S, Delaloy C, Leprivey V, Hadchouel J, Warnock DG, Jeunemaitre X, et al. WNK kinases, distal tubular ion handling and hypertension. Nephrol Dial Transplant 2003;18:2463—7.

[218] O'Reilly M, Marshall E, Speirs HJ, Brown RW. WNK1, a gene within a novel blood pressure control pathway, tissue-specifically generates radically different isoforms with and without a kinase domain. J Am Soc Nephrol 2003;14:2447—56.

[219] Subramanya AR, Yang CL, Zhu X, Ellison DH. Dominant-negative regulation of WNK1 by its kidney-specific kinase-defective isoform. Am J Physiol Renal Physiol 2006;290:F619—24.

[220] Huang CL, Kuo E. Mechanisms of disease: WNK-ing at the mechanism of salt-sensitive hypertension. Nat Clin Pract Nephrol 2007;3:623—30.

[221] Hadchouel J, Soukaseum C, Busst C, Zhou XO, Baudrie V, Zurrer T, et al. Decreased ENaC expression compensates the increased NCC activity following inactivation of the kidney-specific isoform of WNK1 and prevents hypertension. Proc Natl Acad Sci USA 2010;107:18109—14.

[222] Delaloy C, Elvira-Matelot E, Clemessy M, Zhou XO, Imbert-Teboul M, Houot AM, et al. Deletion of WNK1 first intron results in misregulation of both isoforms in renal and extrarenal tissues. Hypertension 2008;52:1149—59.

[223] Vitari AC, Deak M, Morrice NA, Alessi DR. The WNK1 and WNK4 protein kinases that are mutated in Gordon's hypertension syndrome, phosphorylate and activate SPAK and OSR1 protein kinases. Biochem J 2005;391:17—24.

[224] Gamba G. WNK lies upstream of kinases involved in regulation of ion transporters. Biochem J 2005;391:e1—3.

[225] Piechotta K, Lu J, Delpire E. Cation chloride co-transporters interact with the stress-related kinases Ste20-related proline-alanine-rich kinase (SPAK) and oxidative stress response 1 (OSR1). J Biol Chem 2002;277:50812—9.

[226] Pacheco-Alvarez D, Vazquez N, Castaneda-Bueno M, de los Heros P, Cortes-Gonzalez C, Moreno E, et al. WNK3-SPAK interaction is required for the modulation of NCC and other members of the SLC12 family. Cell Physiol Biochem 2012;29:291—302.

[227] Delpire E, Gagnon KB. Genome-wide analysis of SPAK/OSR1 binding motifs. Physiol Genomics 2007;28:223—31.

[228] Gagnon KB, England R, Delpire E. Volume sensitivity of cation-Cl- co-transporters is modulated by the interaction of two kinases: Ste20-related proline-alanine-rich kinase and WNK4. Am J Physiol Cell Physiol 2006;290:C134—42.

[229] Delpire E. The mammalian family of sterile 20p-like protein kinases. Pflugers Arch 2009;458:953—67.

[230] Delpire E, Gagnon KB. SPAK and OSR1, key kinases involved in the regulation of chloride transport. Acta Physiol (Oxf) 2006;187:103—13.

[231] Delpire E, Gagnon KB. SPAK and OSR1: STE20 kinases involved in the regulation of ion homoeostasis and volume control in mammalian cells. Biochem J 2008;409:321—31.

[232] Kahle KT, Rinehart J, Ring A, Gimenez I, Gamba G, Hebert SC, et al. WNK protein kinases modulate cellular Cl$^-$ flux by altering the phosphorylation state of the Na-K-Cl and K-Cl co-transporters. Physiology (Bethesda) 2006;21:326—35.

[233] Chiga M, Rafiqi FH, Alessi DR, Sohara E, Ohta A, Rai T, et al. Phenotypes of pseudohypoaldosteronism type II caused by the WNK4 D561A missense mutation are dependent on the WNK-OSR1/SPAK kinase cascade. J Cell Sci 2011;124:1391—5.

[234] Yang SS, Lo YF, Wu CC, Lin SW, Yeh CJ, Chu P, et al. SPAK-knockout mice manifest Gitelman syndrome and impaired vasoconstriction. J Am Soc Nephrol 2010;21:1868—77.

[235] Lin SH, Yu IS, Jiang ST, Lin SW, Chu P, Chen A, et al. Impaired phosphorylation of Na$^+$-K$^+$-2Cl$^-$ co-transporter by oxidative stress-responsive kinase-1 deficiency manifests hypotension and Bartter-like syndrome. Proc Natl Acad Sci USA 2011;108:17538—43.

[236] McCormick JA, Mutig K, Nelson JH, Saritas T, Hoorn EJ, Yang CL, et al. A SPAK isoform switch modulates renal salt transport and blood pressure. Cell Metab 2011;14:352—64.

[237] San Cristobal P, De Los Heros P, Ponce-Coria J, Moreno E, Gamba G. WNK kinases, renal ion transport and hypertension. Am J Nephrol 2008;28:860—70.

[238] Kahle KT, Rinehart J, De Los Heros P, Louvi A, Meade P, Vazquez N, et al. WNK3 modulates transport of Cl$^-$ in and out of cells: implications for control of cell volume and neuronal excitability. Proc Natl Acad Sci USA 2005;102:16783—8.

[239] Rinehart J, Kahle KT, De Los Heros P, Vazquez N, Meade P, Wilson FH, et al. WNK3 kinase is a positive regulator of NKCC2 and NCC, renal cation-Cl$^-$ co-transporters required for normal blood pressure homeostasis. Proc Natl Acad Sci USA 2005;102:16777—82.

[240] De Los Heros P, Kahle KT, Rinehart J, Bobadilla NA, Vazquez N, San Cristobal P, et al. WNK3 bypasses the tonicity requirement for K-Cl co-transporter activation via a phosphatase-dependent pathway. Proc Natl Acad Sci USA 2006;103:1976—81.

[241] Yang CL, Zhu X, Ellison DH. The thiazide-sensitive Na-Cl co-transporter is regulated by a WNK kinase signaling complex. J Clin Invest 2007;117:3403—11.

[242] Kahle KT, Ring AM, Lifton RP. Molecular physiology of the WNK kinases. Annu Rev Physiol 2008;70:329—55.

[243] Rinehart J, Vazquez N, Kahle KT, Hodson CA, Ring AM, Gulcicek EE, et al. WNK2 is a novel regulator of essential neuronal cation-chloride co-transporters. J Biol Chem 2011;286:30171—80.

[244] Pollak MR, Delaney VB, Graham RM, Hebert SC. Gitelman's syndrome (Bartter's variant) maps to the thiazide-sensitive co-transporter gene locus on chromosome 16q13 in a large kindred. J Am Soc Nephrol 1996;7:2244—8.

[245] Mastroianni N, Bettinelli A, Bianchetti M, Colussi G, de Fusco M, Sereni F, et al. Novel molecular variants of the Na-Cl co-transporter gene are responsible for Gitelman syndrome. Am J Hum Genet 1996;59:1019—26.

[246] Lemmink HH, van den Heuvel LP, van Dijk HA, Merkx GF, Smilde TJ, Taschner PE, et al. Linkage of Gitelman syndrome to the thiazide-sensitive sodium-chloride co-transporter gene with identification of mutations in Dutch families. Pediatr Nephrol 1996;10:403—7.

[247] Schultheis PJ, Lorenz JN, Meneton P, Nieman ML, Riddle TM, Flagella M, et al. Phenotype resembling Gitelman's syndrome in mice lacking the apical Na$^+$-Cl$^-$ co-transporter of the distal convoluted tubule. J Biol Chem 1998;273:29150—5.

[248] Yang SS, Lo YF, Yu IS, Lin SW, Chang TH, Hsu YJ, et al. Generation and analysis of the thiazide-sensitive Na$^+$-Cl$^-$ co-transporter (Ncc/Slc12a3) Ser707X knockin mouse as a model of Gitelman syndrome. Hum Mutat 2010;31:1304—15.

[249] Cruz DN, Shaer AJ, Bia MJ, Lifton RP, Simon DB. Gitelman's syndrome revisited: an evaluation of symptoms and health-related quality of life. Kidney Int 2001;59:710—7.

[250] Maki N, Komatsuda A, Wakui H, Ohtani H, Kigawa A, Aiba N, et al. Four novel mutations in the thiazide-sensitive Na-Cl co-transporter gene in Japanese patients with Gitelman's syndrome. Nephrol Dial Transplant 2004;19(7):1761—6.

[251] Lemmink HH, Knoers NV, Karolyi L, van Dijk H, Niaudet P, Antignac C, et al. Novel mutations in the thiazide-sensitive NaCl co-transporter gene in patients with Gitelman syndrome with predominant localization to the C-terminal domain. Kidney Int 1998;54:720—30.

[252] Lin SH, Cheng NL, Hsu YJ, Halperin ML. Intrafamilial phenotype variability in patients with Gitelman syndrome having the same mutations in their thiazide-sensitive sodium/chloride co-transporter. Am J Kidney Dis 2004;43:304—12.

[253] Syren ML, Tedeschi S, Cesareo L, Bellantuono R, Colussi G, Procaccio M, et al. Identification of fifteen novel mutations in the SLC12A3 gene encoding the Na-Cl Co-transporter in Italian patients with Gitelman syndrome. Hum Mutat 2002;20:78.

[254] Vargas-Poussou R, Dahan K, Kahila D, Venisse A, Riveira-Munoz E, Debaix H, et al. Spectrum of mutations in Gitelman syndrome. J Am Soc Nephrol 2011;22:693—703.

[255] Shaer AJ. Inherited primary renal tubular hypokalemic alkalosis: a review of Gitelman and Bartter syndromes. Am J Med Sci 2001;322:316—32.

[256] Simon DB, Karet FE, Rodriguez-Soriano J, Hamdan JH, DiPietro A, Trachtman H, et al. Genetic heterogeneity of Bartter's syndrome revealed by mutations in the K$^+$ channel, ROM. Nature Genetics 1996;14:152—6.

[257] Simon DB, Bindra RS, Mansfield TA, Nelson-Williamns C, Mendonca E, Stone R, et al. Mutations in the chloride channel gene, CLCNKB, cause Bartter's syndrome type III. Nature Genetics 1997;17:171—8.

[258] Estevez R, Boettger T, Stein V, Birkenhager R, Otto E, Hildebrandt F, et al. Barttin is a Cl$^-$ channel beta-subunit crucial for renal Cl$^-$ reabsorption and inner ear K$^+$ secretion. Nature 2001;414:558—61.

[259] Watanabe S, Fukumoto S, Chang H, Takeuchi Y, Hasegawa Y, Okazaki R, et al. Association between activating mutations of calcium-sensing receptor and Bartter's syndrome. Lancet 2002;360:692—4.

[260] Vargas-Poussou R, Huang C, Hulin P, Houillier P, Jeunemaitre X, Paillard M, et al. Functional characterization of a calcium-sensing receptor mutation in severe autosomal dominant hypocalcemia with a Bartter-like syndrome. J Am Soc Nephrol 2002;13:2259—66.

[261] Vezzoli G, Arcidiacono T, Paloschi V, Terranegra A, Biasion R, Weber G, et al. Autosomal dominant hypocalcemia with mild type 5 Bartter syndrome. J Nephrol 2006;19:525—8.

III. FLUID AND ELECTROLYTE REGULATION AND DYSREGULATION

[262] Meade P, Sabath E, Gamba G. Fisiopatología molecular del síndrome de Bartter. Rev Invest Clin 2003;55:74—83.

[263] Mayan H, Munter G, Shaharabany M, Mouallem M, Pauzner R, Holtzman EJ, et al. Hypercalciuria in familial hyperkalemia and hypertension accompanies hyperkalemia and precedes hypertension: description of a large family with the Q565E WNK4 mutation. J Clin Endocrinol Metab 2004;89:4025—30.

[264] Cruz DN. The renal tubular Na-Cl co-transporter (NCCT): a potential genetic link between blood pressure and bone density? Nephrol Dial Transplant 2001;16:691—4.

[265] Nicolet-Barousse L, Blanchard A, Roux C, Pietri L, Bloch-Faure M, Kolta S, et al. Inactivation of the Na-Cl co-transporter (NCC) gene is associated with high BMD through both renal and bone mechanisms: analysis of patients with Gitelman syndrome and Ncc null mice. J Bone Miner Res 2005;20:799—808.

[266] Mayan H, Vered I, Mouallem M, Tzadok-Witkon M, Pauzner R, Farfel Z. Pseudohypoaldosteronism type II: marked sensitivity to thiazides, hypercalciuria, normomagnesemia, and low bone mineral density. J Clin Endocrinol Metab 2002;87:3248—54.

[267] Simon DB, Farfel Z, Ellison D, Bia M, Tucci J, Lifton RP. Examination of the thiazide-sensitive Na-Cl co-transporter as a candidate gene in Gordon's syndrome. J Am Soc Nephrol 1995;6:632.

[268] Brooks AM, Owens M, Sayer JA, Salzmann M, Ellard S, Vaidya B. Pseudohypoaldosteronism type 2 presenting with hypertension and hyperkalaemia due to a novel mutation in the WNK4 gene. QJM 2011;: e-pub ahead of print

[269] Zhang C, Wang Z, Xie J, Yan F, Wang W, Feng X, et al. Identification of a novel WNK4 mutation in Chinese patients with pseudohypoaldosteronism type II. Nephron Physiol 2011;118:53—61.

[270] Gong H, Tang Z, Yang Y, Sun L, Zhang W, Wang W, et al. A patient with pseudohypoaldosteronism type II caused by a novel mutation in WNK4 gene. Endocrine 2008;33:230—4.

[271] Golbang AP, Murthy M, Hamad A, Liu CH, Cope G, Hoff WV, et al. A new kindred with pseudohypoaldosteronism type II and a novel mutation (564D > H) in the acidic motif of the WNK4 gene. Hypertension 2005;46(2):295—300.

[272] Kamide K, Takiuchi S, Tanaka C, Miwa Y, Yoshii M, Horio T, et al. Three novel missense mutations of WNK4, a kinase mutated in inherited hypertension, in Japanese hypertensives: implication of clinical phenotypes. Am J Hypertens 2004;17:446—9.

[273] Achard JM, Warnock DG, Disse-Nicodeme S, Fiquet-Kempf B, Corvol P, Fournier A, et al. Familial hyperkalemic hypertension: phenotypic analysis in a large family with the WNK1 deletion mutation. Am J Med 2003;114:495—8.

[274] Bergaya S, Vidal-Petiot E, Jeunemaitre X, Hadchouel J. Pathogenesis of pseudohypoaldosteronism type 2 by WNK1 mutations. Curr Opin Nephrol Hypertens 2012;21:39—45.

[275] Boyden LM, Choi M, Choate KA, Nelson-Williams CJ, Farhi A, Toka HR, et al. Mutations in kelch-like 3 and cullin 3 cause hypertension and electrolyte abnormalities. Nature 2012;482(7383):98—102.

[276] Welling PA, Chang YP, Delpire E, Wade JB. Multigene kinase network, kidney transport, and salt in essential hypertension. Kidney Int 2010;77:1063—9.

[277] Huang CL, Yang SS, Lin SH. Mechanism of regulation of renal ion transport by WNK kinases. Curr Opin Nephrol Hypertens 2008;17:519—25.

[278] Zimmerman ES, Schulman BA, Zheng N. Structural assembly of cullin-RING ubiquitin ligase complexes. Curr Opin Struct Biol 2010;20:714—21.

[279] Arroyo JP, Lagnaz D, Ronzaud C, Vazquez N, Ko BS, Moddes L, et al. Nedd4-2 modulates renal Na^+-Cl^- co-transporter via the aldosterone-SGK1-Nedd4-2 pathway. J Am Soc Nephrol 2011;22:1707—19.

[280] Ohta A, Rai T, Yui N, Chiga M, Yang SS, Lin SH, et al. Targeted disruption of the Wnk4 gene decreases phosphorylation of Na-Cl co-transporter, increases Na excretion, and lowers blood pressure. Hum Mol Genet 2009;18:3978—86.

[281] Chobanian AV, Bakris GL, Black HR, Cushman WC, Green LA, Izzo Jr. JL, et al. The seventh report of the joint national committee on prevention, detection, evaluation, and treatment of high blood pressure: the JNC 7 Report. JAMA 2003;289:2560—71.

[282] Ji W, Foo JN, O'Roak BJ, Zhao H, Larson MG, Simon DB, et al. Rare independent mutations in renal salt handling genes contribute to blood pressure variation. Nat Genet 2008;40:592—9.

[283] Acuna R, Martinez-de-la-Maza L, Ponce-Coria J, Vazquez N, Ortal-Vite P, Pacheco-Alvarez D, et al. Rare mutations in SLC12A1 and SLC12A3 protect against hypertension by reducing the activity of renal salt co-transporters. J Hypertens 2011;29:475—83.

[284] Monette MY, Rinehart J, Lifton RP, Forbush B. Rare mutations in the human Na-K-Cl co-transporter (NKCC2) associated with lower blood pressure exhibit impaired processing and transport function. Am J Physiol Renal Physiol 2011;300:F840—7.

[285] Wang Y, O'Connell JR, McArdle PF, Wade JB, Dorff SE, Shah SJ, et al. Whole-genome association study identifies STK39 as a hypertension susceptibility gene. Proc Natl Acad Sci USA 2009;106:226—31.

[286] Ray WA, Griffin MR, Downey W, Melton III LJ. Long-term use of thiazide diuretics and risk of hip fracture. The Lancet 1989; I:687—90.

[287] Sebastian A. Thiazides and bone. Am J Med 2000;109:429—30.

[288] Reid IR, Ames RW, Orr-Walker BJ, Clearwater JM, Horne AM, Evans MC, et al. Hydrochlorothiazide reduces loss of cortical bone in normal postmenopausal women: a randomized controlled trial. Am J Med 2000;109:362—70.

[289] Frindt G, Palmer LG. Surface expression of sodium channels and transporters in rat kidney: effects of dietary sodium. Am J Physiol Renal Physiol 2009;297:F1249—55.

[290] Vallon V, Schroth J, Lang F, Kuhl D, Uchida S. Expression and phosphorylation of the Na-Cl-co-transporter NCC in vivo is regulated by dietary salt, potassium and SGK1. Am J Physiol Renal Physiol 2009;297:F704—12.

[291] Masilamani S, Kim GH, Mitchell C, Wade JB, Knepper MA. Aldosterone-mediated regulation of ENaC alpha, beta, and gamma subunit proteins in rat kidney. J Clin Invest 1999;104: R19—23.

[292] Masilamani S, Wang X, Kim GH, Brooks H, Nielsen J, Nielsen S, et al. Time course of renal Na-K-ATPase, NHE3, NKCC2, NCC, and ENaC abundance changes with dietary NaCl restriction. Am J Physiol Renal Physiol 2002;283:F648—57.

[293] Kim G-H, Masilamani S, Turner R, Mitchell C, Wade JB, Knepper MA. The thiazide-sensitive Na-Cl co-transporter is an aldosterone-induced protein. Proc Natl Acad Sci USA 1998;95:14552—7.

[294] Moreno G, Merino A, Mercado A, Herrera JP, González-Salazar J, Correa-Rotter R, et al. Electronuetral Na-coupled co-transporter expression in the kidney during variations of NaCl and water metabolism. Hypertension 1998;31:1002—6.

[295] Wolf K, Castrop H, Riegger GA, Kurtz A, Kramer BK. Differential gene regulation of renal salt entry pathways by salt load in the distal nephron of the rat. Pflugers Arch 2001;442:498—504.

[296] Lai L, Feng X, Liu D, Chen J, Zhang Y, Niu B, et al. Dietary salt modulates the sodium chloride co-transporter expression likely through an aldosterone-mediated WNK4-ERK1/2 signaling pathway. Pflugers Arch 2012;463:477–85.

[297] Abdallah JG, Schrier RW, Edelstein C, Jennings SD, Wyse B, Ellison DH. Loop diuretic infusion increases thiazide-sensitive Na$^+$/Cl$^-$ co-transporter abundance: role of aldosterone. J Am Soc Nephrol 2001;12:1335–41.

[298] Na KY, Oh YK, Han JS, Joo KW, Lee JS, Earm JH, et al. Upregulation of Na$^+$ transporter abundance in response to chronic thiazide or loop diuretic treatment in rats. Am J Physiol Renal Physiol 2003;284:F133–43.

[299] Ruete MC, Carrizo LC, Bocanegra MV, Valles PG. Altered renal expression of Na($^+$) transporters and ROMK in protein-deprived rats. Nephron Physiol 2009;111:17–29.

[300] Kim JS, Choi KC, Jeong MH, Kim SW, Oh YW, Lee JU. Increased expression of sodium transporters in rats chronically inhibited of nitric oxide synthesis. J Korean Med Sci 2006;21:1–4.

[301] Ecelbarger CA, Kim GH, Wade JB, Knepper MA. Regulation of the abundance of renal sodium transporters and channels by vasopressin. Exp Neurol 2001;171:227–34.

[302] Ecelbarger CA, Knepper MA, Verbalis JG. Increased abundance of distal sodium transporters in rat kidney during vasopressin escape. J Am Soc Nephrol 2001;12:207–17.

[303] Kwon TH, Nielsen J, Knepper MA, Frokiaer J, Nielsen S. Angiotensin II AT1 receptor blockade decreases vasopressin-induced water reabsorption and AQP2 levels in NaCl-restricted rats. Am J Physiol Renal Physiol 2005;288:F673–84.

[304] Bickel CA, Verbalis JG, Knepper MA, Ecelbarger CA. Increased renal Na-K-ATPase, NCC, and beta-ENaC abundance in obese Zucker rats. Am J Physiol Renal Physiol 2001;281:F639–48.

[305] Faroqui S, Sheriff S, Amlal H. Metabolic acidosis has dual effects on sodium handling by rat kidney. Am J Physiol Renal Physiol 2006;291:F322–31.

[306] Verlander JM, Tran TM, Zhang L, Kaplan MR, Hebert SC. Estradiol enhances thiazide-sensitive NaCl co-transporter density in the apical plasma membrane of the distal convoluted tubule in ovariectomized rats. J Clin Invest 1998;101:1661–9.

[307] Manning J, Beutler K, Knepper MA, Vehaskari VM. Upregulation of renal BSC1 and TSC in prenatally programmed hypertension. Am J Physiol Renal Physiol 2002;283:F202–6.

[308] Kwon TH, kiaer J, ndez-Llama P, Maunsbach AB, Knepper MA, Nielsen S. Altered expression of Na transporters NHE-3, NaPi-II, Na-K-ATPase, BSC-1, and TSC in CRF rat kidneys. Am J Physiol 1999;277:F257–70.

[309] Frindt G, Palmer LG. Regulation of epithelial Na$^+$ channels by adrenal steroids: Mineralocorticoid and glucocorticoid effects. Am J Physiol Renal Physiol 2012;302:F20–6.

[310] Hoorn EJ, Walsh SB, McCormick JA, Furstenberg A, Yang CL, Roeschel T, et al. The calcineurin inhibitor tacrolimus activates the renal sodium chloride co-transporter to cause hypertension. Nat Med 2011;17:1304–9.

[311] Mu S, Shimosawa T, Ogura S, Wang H, Uetake Y, Kawakami-Mori F, et al. Epigenetic modulation of the renal beta-adrenergic-WNK4 pathway in salt-sensitive hypertension. Nat Med 2011;17:573–81.

[312] Liu Z, Xie J, Wu T, Truong T, Auchus RJ, Huang CL. Downregulation of NCC and NKCC2 co-transporters by kidney-specific WNK1 revealed by gene disruption and transgenic mouse models. Hum Mol Genet 2011;20:855–66.

[313] Sassen MC, Kim SW, Kwon TH, Knepper MA, Miller RT, Frokiaer J, et al. Dysregulation of renal sodium transporters in gentamicin-treated rats. Kidney Int 2006;70:1026–37.

[314] Song J, Hu X, Riazi S, Tiwari S, Wade JB, Ecelbarger CA. Regulation of blood pressure, the epithelial sodium channel (ENaC), and other key renal sodium transporters by chronic insulin infusion in rats. Am J Physiol Renal Physiol 2006;290:F1055–64.

[315] Sonalker PA, Tofovic SP, Bastacky SI, Jackson EK. Chronic noradrenaline increases renal expression of NHE-3, NBC-1, BSC-1 and aquaporin-2. Clin Exp Pharmacol Physiol 2008;35:594–600.

[316] Kwon TH, Laursen UH, Marples D, Maunsbach AB, Knepper MA, Frokiaer J, et al. Altered expression of renal AQPs and Na($^+$) transporters in rats with lithium-induced NDI. Am J Physiol Renal Physiol 2000;279:F552–64.

[317] Frindt G, Palmer LG. Effects of dietary K on cell-surface expression of renal ion channels and transporters. Am J Physiol Renal Physiol 2010;299:F890–7.

[318] Jung JY, Kim S, Lee JW, Jung ES, Heo NJ, Son MJ, et al. Effects of potassium on expression of renal sodium transporters in salt-sensitive hypertensive rats induced by uninephrectomy. Am J Physiol Renal Physiol 2011;300:F1422–30.

[319] Amlal H, Wang Z, Soleimani M. Potassium depletion downregulates chloride-absorbing transporters in rat kidney. J Clin Invest 1998;101:1045–54.

[320] Elkjaer ML, Kwon TH, Wang W, Nielsen J, Knepper MA, Frokiaer J, et al. Altered expression of renal NHE3, TSC, BSC-1, and ENaC subunits in potassium-depleted rats. Am J Physiol Renal Physiol 2002;283:F1376–88.

[321] Bae EH, Kim IJ, Ma SK, Kim SW. Altered regulation of renal sodium transporters and natriuretic peptide system in DOCA-salt hypertensive rats. Regul Pept 2009;157:76–83.

[322] Madala H V, Tiwari S, Riazi S, Hu X, Ecelbarger CM. Chronic candesartan alters expression and activity of NKCC2, NCC, and ENaC in the obese Zucker rat. Am J Physiol Renal Physiol 2008;294:F1222–31.

[323] Kim EJ, Jung YW, Kwon TH. Angiotensin II AT1 receptor blockade changes expression of renal sodium transporters in rats with chronic renal failure. J Korean Med Sci 2005;20:248 55.

[324] Wang XY, Masilamani S, Nielsen J, Kwon TH, Brooks HL, Nielsen S, et al. The renal thiazide-sensitive Na-Cl co-transporter as mediator of the aldosterone-escape phenomenon. J Clin Invest 2001;108:215–22.

[325] Turban S, Wang XY, Knepper MA. Regulation of NHE3, NKCC2 and NCC abundance in kidney during aldosterone-escape phenomenon: role of NO. Am J Physiol Renal Physiol 2003;285:F841–3.

[326] Kim SW, Lee J, Jung K, Ma SK, Oh Y, Kim WY, et al. Diminished expression of sodium transporters in the ureteral obstructed kidney in rats. Nephron Exp Nephrol 2004;96:e67–76.

[327] Li C, Wang W, Kwon TH, Knepper MA, Nielsen S, Frokiaer J. Altered expression of major renal Na transporters in rats with bilateral ureteral obstruction and release of obstruction. Am J Physiol Renal Physiol 2003;285:F889–901.

[328] Kim SW, Wang W, Nielsen J, Praetorius J, Kwon TH, Knepper MA, et al. Increased expression and apical targeting of renal ENaC subunits in puromycin aminonucleoside-induced nephrotic syndrome in rats. Am J Physiol Renal Physiol 2004;286:F922–35.

[329] Faresse N, Lagnaz D, Debonneville A, Ismailji A, Maillard M, Fejes-Toth G, et al. Inducible kidney specific Sgk1 knock-out mice show a salt losing phenotype. Am J Physiol Renal Physiol 2012;302(8):F977–85.

[330] Ledeganck KJ, Boulet GA, Horvath CA, Vinckx M, Bogers JJ, Van Den BR, et al. Expression of renal distal tubule transporters TRPM6 and NCC in a rat model of cyclosporine nephrotoxicity and effect of EGF treatment. Am J Physiol Renal Physiol 2011;301:F486–93.

[331] Attmane-Elakeb A, Sibella V, Vernimmen C, Belenfant X, Hebert SC, Bichara M. Regulation by glucocorticoids of expression and activity of rBSC1, the Na$^+$-K$^+$(NH$_4^+$)-2Cl$^-$ co-transporter of medullary thick ascending limb. J Biol Chem 2000;275:33548−53.

[332] Riazi S, Tiwari S, Sharma N, Rash A, Ecelbarger CM. Abundance of the Na-K-2Cl co-transporter NKCC2 is increased by high-fat feeding in Fischer 344 X Brown Norway (F1) rats. Am J Physiol Renal Physiol 2009;296:F762−70.

[333] Olesen ET, de Seigneux S, Wang G, Lutken SC, Frokiaer J, Kwon TH, et al. Rapid and segmental specific dysregulation of AQP2, S256-pAQP2 and renal sodium transporters in rats with LPS-induced endotoxaemia. Nephrol Dial Transplant 2009;24:2338−49.

[334] Wangensteen R, Rodriguez-Gomez I, Moreno JM, Vargas F, Alvarez-Guerra M. Chronic nitric oxide blockade modulates renal Na-K-2Cl co-transporters. J Hypertens 2006;24:2451−8.

[335] Fernandez-Llama P, Ecelbarger CA, Ware JA, Andrews P, Lee AJ, Turner R, et al. Cyclooxygenase inhibitors increase Na-K-2Cl co-transporter abundance in thick ascending limb of Henle's loop. Am J Physiol 1999;277:F219−26.

[336] Riazi S, Khan O, Tiwari S, Hu X, Ecelbarger CA. Rosiglitazone regulates ENaC and Na-K-2Cl co-transporter (NKCC2) abundance in the obese Zucker rat. Am J Nephrol 2006;26:245−57.

[337] Li C, Wang W, Summer SN, Cadnapaphornchai MA, Falk S, Umenishi F, et al. Hyperosmolality in vivo upregulates aquaporin 2 water channel and Na-K-2Cl co-transporter in Brattleboro rats. J Am Soc Nephrol 2006;17:1657−64.

[338] Kwon TH, Nielsen J, Kim YH, Knepper MA, Frokiaer J, Nielsen S. Regulation of sodium transporters in the thick ascending limb of rat kidney: response to angiotensin II. Am J Physiol Renal Physiol 2003;285:F152−65.

[339] Blount MA, Sim JH, Zhou R, Martin CF, Lu W, Sands JM, et al. Expression of transporters involved in urine concentration recovers differently after cessation of lithium treatment. Am J Physiol Renal Physiol 2010;298:F601−8.

[340] Kwon TH, Laursen UH, Marples D, Maunsbach AB, Knepper MA, Frokiaer J, et al. Altered expression of renal AQPs and Na($^+$) transporters in rats with lithium-induced NDI. Am J Physiol Renal Physiol 2000;279:F552−64.

[341] Sanches TR, Volpini RA, Massola Shimizu MH, Braganca AC, Oshiro-Monreal F, Seguro AC, et al. Sildenafil reduces polyuria in rats with lithium-induced NDI. Am J Physiol Renal Physiol 2012;302:F216−25.

[342] Moreno JM, Perez-Abud R, Wangensteen R, Rodriguez G I, Lopez M I, Osuna A, et al. Function and expression of renal epithelial sodium transporters in rats with thyroid dysfunction. J Endocrinol Invest 2011;: e-pub ahead of print

[343] Haque MZ, Ares GR, Caceres PS, Ortiz PA. High salt differentially regulates surface NKCC2 expression in thick ascending limbs of Dahl salt-sensitive and salt-resistant rats. Am J Physiol Renal Physiol 2011;300:F1096−104.

[344] Zhang Y, Listhrop R, Ecelbarger CM, Kishore BK. Renal sodium transporter/channel expression and sodium excretion in P2Y2 receptor knockout mice fed a high-NaCl diet with/without aldosterone infusion. Am J Physiol Renal Physiol 2011;300:F657−68.

[345] Beutler KT, Masilamani S, Turban S, Nielsen J, Brooks HL, Ageloff S, et al. Long-term regulation of ENaC expression in kidney by angiotensin II. Hypertension 2003;41:1143−50.

[346] Attmane-Elakeb A, Mount DB, Sibella V, Vernimmen C, Micheli L, Hebert SC, et al. Chronic metabolic acidosis upregulates expression of mRNA and protein of the MTAL Na$^+$-K$^+$(NH$_4^+$)-2Cl$^-$ co-transporter BSC1 (NKCC2). J Am Soc Nephrol 1998;9:2A.

[347] Attmane-Elakeb A, Mount DB, Sibella V, Vernimmen C, Hebert SC, Bichara M. Stimulation by in vivo and in vitro metabolic acidosis of expression of rBSC-1, the Na$^+$-K$^+$(NH$_4^+$)-2Cl$^-$ co-transporter of the rat medullary thick ascending limb. J Biol Chem 1998;273:33681−91.

[348] Karim Z, Attmane-Elakeb A, Sibella V, Bichara M. Acid pH increases the stability of BSC1/NKCC2 mRNA in the medullary thick ascending limb. J Am Soc Nephrol 2003;14:2229−36.

[349] Lim SW, Ahn KO, Sheen MR, Jeon US, Kim J, Yang CW, et al. Downregulation of renal sodium transporters and tonicity-responsive enhancer binding protein by long-term treatment with cyclosporin A. J Am Soc Nephrol 2007;18:421−9.

[350] Norregaard R, Jensen BL, Topcu SO, Diget M, Schweer H, Knepper MA, et al. COX-2 activity transiently contributes to increased water and NaCl excretion in the polyuric phase after release of ureteral obstruction. Am J Physiol Renal Physiol 2007;292:F1322−33.

[351] Jensen AM, Li C, Praetorius HA, Norregaard R, Frische S, Knepper MA, et al. Angiotensin II mediates downregulation of aquaporin water channels and key renal sodium transporters in response to urinary tract obstruction. Am J Physiol Renal Physiol 2006;291:F1021−32.

[352] Riazi S, Maric C, Ecelbarger CA. 17-beta Estradiol attenuates streptozotocin-induced diabetes and regulates the expression of renal sodium transporters. Kidney Int 2006;69:471−80.

[353] Filippi BM, De Los Heros P, Mehellou Y, Navratilova I, Gourlay R, Deak M, et al. MO25 is a master regulator of SPAK/OSR1 and MST3/MST4/YSK1 protein kinases. EMBO J 2011;30:1730−41.

[354] Melnikov S, Mayan H, Uchida S, Holtzman EJ, Farfel Z. Cyclosporine metabolic side effects: association with the WNK4 system. Eur J Clin Invest 2011;41(10):1113−20.

[355] McCormick JA, Nelson JH, Yang CL, Curry JN, Ellison DH. Overexpression of the sodium chloride co-transporter is not sufficient to cause familial hyperkalemic hypertension. Hypertension 2011;58:888−94.

[356] Castaneda-Bueno M, Cervantes LG, Vazquez N, Bobadilla NA, Uribe N, Alessi D, et al. In vivo activation of NCC by angiotensin II requires integrity of the WNK4-SPAK pathway. J Am Soc Nephrol 2011;22:102A.

[357] Sohara E, Rai T, Yang SS, Ohta A, Naito S, Chiga M, et al. Acute insulin stimulation induces phosphorylation of the Na-Cl co-transporter in cultured distal mpkDCT cells and mouse kidney. PLoS One 2011;6:e24277.

[358] Chavez-Canales M, Vazquez N, Arroyo JP, Castaneda-Bueno M, Ko B, Bobadilla NA, et al. Insulin is a positive modulator of NCC activity through a PI3K dependent mechanism. J Am Soc Nephrol 2010;21:64A.

[359] Fraser SA, Gimenez I, Cook N, Jennings I, Katerelos M, Katsis F, et al. Regulation of the renal-specific Na$^+$-K$^+$-2Cl$^-$ co-transporter NKCC2 by AMP-activated protein kinase (AMPK). Biochem J 2007;405:85−93.

[360] Hannemann A, Flatman PW. Phosphorylation and transport in the Na-K-2Cl co-transporters, NKCC1 and NKCC2A, compared in HEK-293 cells. PLoS One 2011;6:e17992.

[361] Carmosino M, Rizzo F, Ferrari P, Torielli L, Ferrandi M, Bianchi G, et al. NKCC2 is activated in Milan hypertensive rats contributing to the maintenance of salt-sensitive hypertension. Pflugers Arch 2011;462:281−91.

[362] Mutig K, Kahl T, Saritas T, Godes M, Persson P, Bates J, et al. Activation of the bumetanide-sensitive Na$^+$,K$^+$,2Cl$^-$-co-transporter NKCC2 is facilitated by Tamm-Horsfall protein in a chloride-sensitive manner. J Biol Chem 2011;286:30200−10.

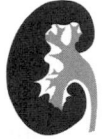

Sodium and Chloride Transport: Proximal Nephron

Alan M. Weinstein

Department of Physiology and Biophysics, Weill Medical College of Cornell University, New York, NY, USA

INTRODUCTION

The principal function of the proximal tubule is the reabsorption of some two-thirds to three-quarters of the glomerular filtrate. This means, primarily, reabsorption of Na^+, Cl^-, HCO_3^-, and in smaller quantities potassium, phosphate, and various filtered organic compounds. In view of the copious glomerular filtrate, proximal reabsorption plays a crucial role in the maintenance of fluid and electrolyte balance of the body. In particular, modern hypertension research has considered it essential to identify proximal tubule Na^+ transporters, and understand the signals and second messengers that regulate these transporters. Proximal tubular transport is energized by the metabolic reactions within the proximal tubular epithelium, either directly by ATP-driven "ion pumps" (primary active transport) or indirectly by the coupling of solute fluxes to Na-transport (secondary active transport). The workload to this epithelium is prescribed by the glomerular filtration rate (GFR), which can vary several-fold within the course of a day, so that the ensemble of epithelial transport systems are also asked to modulate their function responsively, and in a coordinated manner.

All segments of isolated proximal tubules are capable of reabsorbing the same solutes when perfused *in vitro*. Quantitatively, however, marked differences exist along the tubule; reabsorption of sodium, water, glucose, and bicarbonate in the early proximal tubule is about three-fold greater than that in the mid-portion of the convoluted proximal tubule, and nearly ten times that of the straight segment of the tubule. Furthermore, *in vivo*, the transtubular concentration gradients of the luminal solutes, as well as the electrical potential of the lumen, change as one moves from early- to late-proximal tubule. In the earliest part of the proximal tubule, preferential reabsorption of organic solutes (glucose and amino acids, etc.) and of sodium bicarbonate, lactate, acetate, phosphate, and citrate occurs. Consequently, the luminal concentration of these solutes is reduced in the remaining portion of the proximal tubule. Alterations in solute reabsorption have been inferred in a number of disorders of proximal tubule, and have been of particular interest to workers seeking to understand how changes in urine composition alter the propensity to kidney stone formation.

Historically, *in vivo* micropuncture and microperfusion was the experimental method that delineated proximal tubule transport properties, namely transepithelial fluxes and permeabilities. The next investigative focus was identification of specific transporters within luminal and peritubular cell membranes, and the experimental techniques have been diverse. Assessment of the cellular compartment was first done electrophysiologically, using conventional and ion-selective microelectrodes, and subsequently with pH- or cation-sensitive fluorescent dyes. More direct information about the membrane transporters derived from vesicle preparations enriched in fractions from luminal (brush border) or peritubular cell membranes. Patch-clamp techniques (whole-cell or excised patch) allowed the study of single membrane ion channels, but have had limited application to proximal tubule. A major advance came with molecular identification of the transporters, expressing these transporters in cells that are convenient for study, developing antibodies for location and quantification within tubular cell membranes, and examination of tubules from mice in which the transporter has been knocked-out.

Seldin and Giebisch's The Kidney, Fifth Edition.
DOI: http://dx.doi.org/10.1016/B978-0-12-381462-3.00033-1

Central to its role in body fluid homeostasis is the responsiveness of proximal tubule sodium transport to changes in GFR, as well as to neural and hormonal signals. In large measure, changes in sodium reabsorption that accompany changes in GFR may be understood in terms of transepithelial oncotic and hydrodynamic forces which impact on the tubule cells or on the paracellular pathway. Neurohumoral regulation of proximal tubule transport begins with a cellular signal, followed by transduction steps, which ultimately produce changes in transporter densities or kinetics within the cell membranes. The signaling pathways for the important neurohumoral regulators have been an object of intense investigation, although the insights have come slowly. This research program has had to contend with a number of cellular second messenger molecules, with a number of kinases and phosphatases, with identification of anchoring proteins that secure the local action of a signal, and with the cytoskeletal elements responsible for transporter traffic. Although much information is available, a facile description of the path from neurohumoral signal to transporter flux is not yet at hand.

The organization of this chapter starts with the description of whole tubule function: fluxes and the associated driving forces; and tubule permeabilities. Historically, this is the section with the oldest data, and the section that has undergone the least revision from earlier chapter versions. The next two sections are devoted to the description of the epithelial components: luminal and peritubular cell membrane transporters; the tight junction; and the lateral intercellular space. In view of the copious transepithelial solute fluxes, special attention will be given to the problem of matching luminal and peritubular transport fluxes, in order to avoid catastrophic perturbation of cell volume and composition. The last section describes the regulation of proximal transport, with emphasis on physical factors, and on the action of the two key regulatory molecules, angiotensin and dopamine.

EPITHELIAL FUNCTION

Net Fluxes

The filtered load of a solute to the proximal tubule is the product of the single nephron glomerular filtration rate (SNGFR) and the ultrafilterable concentration of the solute. For small nonelectrolyte species the ultrafilterable concentration is that in plasma water. For electrolytes, negatively-charged serum proteins produce a Donnan potential, which acts to decrease ultrafilterable Na^+ and increase Cl^- concentration with respect to that of plasma water.[556] In amphibian and mammalian proximal tubules, the net effect of proximal tubule transport is the reabsorption of the luminal solution, resulting in a diminished axial flow rate as one proceeds along the tubules. The systemic infusion of a substance, such as inulin, which is filtered at the glomerulus, not reabsorbed (or secreted) by the proximal tubule, and which may be assayed in aliquots of tubular fluid, permits the calculation of the net volume reabsorption by the tubule from the glomerulus to the point of sampling. Thus, in the rat superficial cortical nephrons, the tubular fluid (TF) inulin concentration at the end of the convoluted proximal tubules is twice that of plasma (P), indicating that half of the filtrate is reabsorbed proximally.[242] In the amphibian, *Necturus*, the TF/P ratio suggests that about one-third of the filtrate is reabsorbed by the proximal tubule,[600] and in certain fish, the net effect of proximal tubule transport is secretion of fluid into the lumen[88]; however, in view of translational considerations, only the mammalian kidney is considered in this chapter.

With micropuncture sampling of fluid from the proximal tubule, if a complete collection of tubule fluid is made, then the absolute transport rate by the nephron segment is known and can be expressed as a flux per unit area of epithelium (Table 33.1). Alternatively, one may perfuse dissected segments of tubule to directly

TABLE 33.1 Net Fluxes across Proximal Tubules

		Rat PCT	References	Rabbit PCT	References	Rabbit PST	References
SNGFR	(nl/min)	30	(a)	20	(c)		
PT diameter	(μm)	20	(a)	26	(d)	22	(g)
Length	(mm)	5.5	(a)	5.4	(c)	3.3	(h)
J_v	(nl/s/cm^2)	65	(b)	30	(e)	9.8	(g)
J_{Na}	(nEq/s/cm^2)	9.4	(b)	4.5	(e)	1.5	(g)
J_{Cl}		5.1	(b)			1.3	(g)
J_{HCO3}		2.7	(b)	1.7	(f)	0.2	(g)

(a)[242]; (b)[757]; (c)[152]; (d)[15]; (e)[388]; (f)[214]; (g)[597]; (h)[43].

establish the epithelial fluxes under well-defined luminal and peritubular conditions. One must then obtain an independent measure of SNGFR to estimate the fractional reabsorption. The advantage of this approach is that proximal nephron segments not accessible to micropuncture may be examined. For the data from the perfused proximal convoluted tubule of the rabbit shown in Table 33.1, the measured sodium flux, referred to a 5.4 mm segment of tubule, implies sodium reabsorption of 1.2 nEq/min. With a SNGFR of 20 nl/min, the filtered load of sodium is 2.9 nEq/min, so that the fractional reabsorption is predicted to be about 40%. In the instances of successful micropuncture of rabbit proximal tubule, the observed fractional reabsorption of sodium has been 50[152] and 45%.[762] This type of comparison is particularly important, in that it suggests a reasonably well-maintained transport capacity for tubules examined *in vitro*. When examined carefully, however, conditions *in vitro* can produce subtle differences from the tubule *in vivo*. As might be expected, dissection conditions of isolated rabbit proximal tubules can decrease the peritubular membrane electrical potential and increase cytosolic Na^+ concentration; however, they can also engender a peritubular membrane K^+ channel, not seen *in vivo*, and change the Na^+:HCO_3^- stoichiometry of the peritubular membrane co-transporter from 3:1 to 2:1.[490,492]

Unfortunately, attempts to present a concise tabulation of proximal transport (Table 33.1) must be tempered by an appreciation of internephron heterogeneity, and the structural changes along the individual tubule. In broad terms, two nephron populations have been identified: those with superficial cortical glomeruli, whose short loops of Henle turn at the outer–inner medullary border (about ⅔ of rat nephrons); and those with juxtamedullary glomeruli, whose long loops of Henle penetrate the inner medulla to variable extents. In many mammalian species, the juxtamedullary glomeruli are larger and have a greater SNGFR than the mid-cortical or superficial cortical nephrons.[556] In the rat, the filtration rate of juxtamedullary glomeruli has been measured by micropuncture collection of Henle limb fluid, and found to be about 1.5- to 2-fold that of superficial glomeruli.[286,344,512] In the rabbit, an indirect technique has given estimates confirming the disparity between superficial and juxtamedullary nephrons (e.g., 43 and 66 nl/min,[36]; 23 and 29 nl/min[43]). Comparisons of transport properties of superficial cortical and juxtamedullary proximal tubules are available.[78] Corresponding to the greater SNGFR of the juxtamedullary nephrons, there is a greater overall rate of volume and sodium reabsorption. Perfused tubule data from rabbit has indicated a relative magnitude of juxtamedullary-to-superficial Na^+ fluxes from 1.2-[341] to 2-fold[364] larger; the relative magnitude of HCO_3^-

fluxes is 2-fold larger.[342] Beyond this quantitative distinction, the relative importance of specific transport mechanisms may also differ between the two nephron populations.[342,468,634]

The capacity for volume transport gradually diminishes as one proceeds along the mammalian proximal nephron.[352] This occurs in association with morphologic changes at the electron-microscopic level that have prompted the division of mammalian proximal tubule into three segments[455] (Figure 33.1). The early proximal convoluted tubule, S1, is characterized by tall, densely-packed apical microvilli, numerous mitochondria, and an intricate pattern of folding and

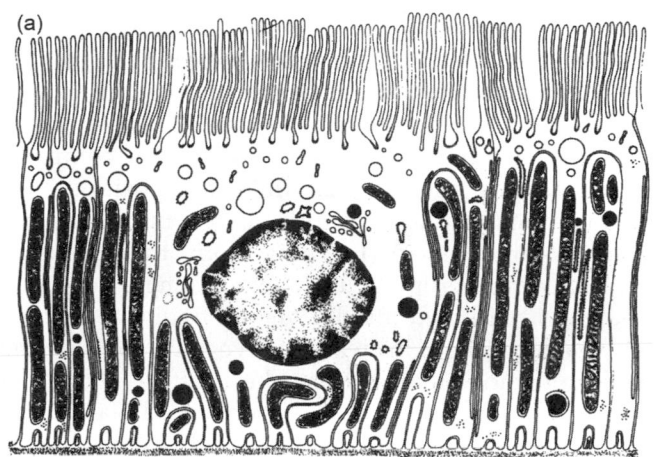

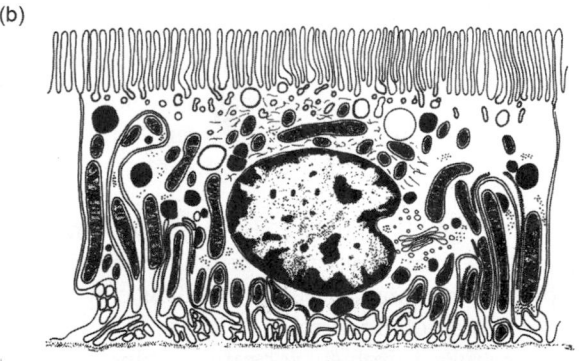

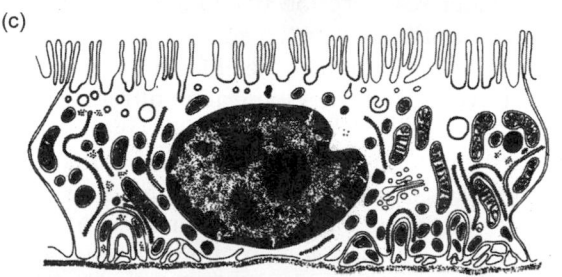

FIGURE 33.1 Proximal tubule cells within the: (a) S1; (b) S2; and (c) S3 segments of the rabbit nephron. (*From*[352], *with permission.*)

interdigitation of the lateral cell membranes.[739] There is a gradual transition to the S2 segment, which comprises the remainder of the proximal convoluted tubule and the very beginning of the proximal straight tubule. Here, there are fewer mitochondria and less amplification of membrane area. Finally, the proximal straight tubule, S3, shows a more cuboidal cell with fewer mitochondria and rare interdigitations. Welling and Welling[738] have compared the cell membrane areas in the S1 and S3 segments of rabbit proximal tubule, and found that for each segment, the apical and basolateral areas are nearly equal. In S1, however, the absorptive area of the cell is increased by membrane folding to 36 cm^2/cm^2 epithelium, whereas in S3 this value is 15 cm^2/cm^2 epithelium. The transport of solutes and water has been measured in dissected perfused segments of rabbit proximal tubule, and the spontaneous transport rate was substantially less in the proximal straight tubule than in convoluted segments[125,388] (Table 33.1). In the rat, microperfusion of proximal tubule segments *in vivo* (with comparable flow rates and luminal fluid composition) has demonstrated a lower volume reabsorption rate for segments more than 1−2 mm from the glomerulus.[165] Serial micropuncture along a single proximal tubule with filtered fluid flowing freely confirmed the sharp decline in reabsorptive flux of volume (sodium) and anions after the first 1−2 mm of tubule[426,427] (Figure 33.2). Comparison of Na^+ transport by perfused proximal straight tubules from superficial and juxtamedullary rabbit nephrons has demonstrated comparable reabsorptive rates. The respective convoluted tubule fluxes are two- and four-fold greater for Na^+,[45,364] with a similar proportionality for HCO_3^-.[708] Proximal convoluted tubule fluxes of glucose may be six-fold greater,[44] and of phosphate three-fold greater than those of proximal straight tubule.[530]

In rat and rabbit kidneys, the Na^+ concentration, and hence the total osmolality, remain relatively constant along the proximal tubule.[255,388] This constancy of tubule fluid osmolality implies "isotonic transport," and poses a special problem for rationalizing the forces at work in water reabsorption (*vide infra*). The fates of chloride and bicarbonate in the mammalian proximal tubule differ, however, in that the chloride rapidly rises to a level above that of the glomerular filtrate and the bicarbonate falls.[125,215,255,685] This shift in anion composition occurs early in the proximal tubule, that is to say, within the S1 segment. This is referred to as "preferential bicarbonate reabsorption," and has received much attention as a clue to transport activity at the cellular level. The key features of the compositional changes in tubular fluid during its passage through the mammalian proximal tubule are illustrated in

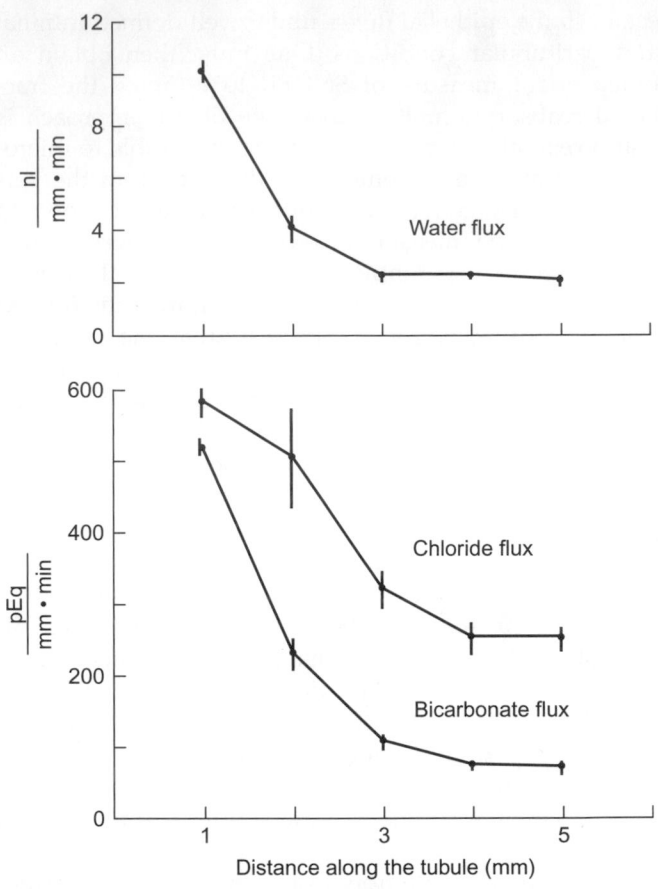

FIGURE 33.2   Reabsorption of water, bicarbonate, and chloride along the rat proximal convoluted tubule. (*From*[427].)

Figure 33.3.[552] The tubular fluid/plasma (TF/P) concentration ratio of several solutes is plotted as a function of proximal tubular length. TF/P inulin rises to approximately 2.0, indicating water reabsorption. Glucose and amino acids are rapidly reabsorbed so that at 25% proximal tubular length their concentrations decline to some 10% of the filtrate concentration. Preferential bicarbonate reabsorption lowers the bicarbonate concentration of tubular fluid to approximately 5−8 mM. Along the initial portion of the proximal tubule, the chloride concentration is increased by reabsorption of water.[28] In the initial segment, the transepithelial voltage is lumen negative,[46,220] due to the electrogenic nature of co-transport of sodium with glucose or amino acids.[221,387] As the concentration of these solutes declines and that of chloride rises, the polarity of the transepithelial electrical potential difference changes to lumen positive values.[46,220] This voltage is, at least in part, a diffusion potential, generated by the chloride and bicarbonate concentration gradients, and the greater permeability of the tubular wall to chloride than to bicarbonate.

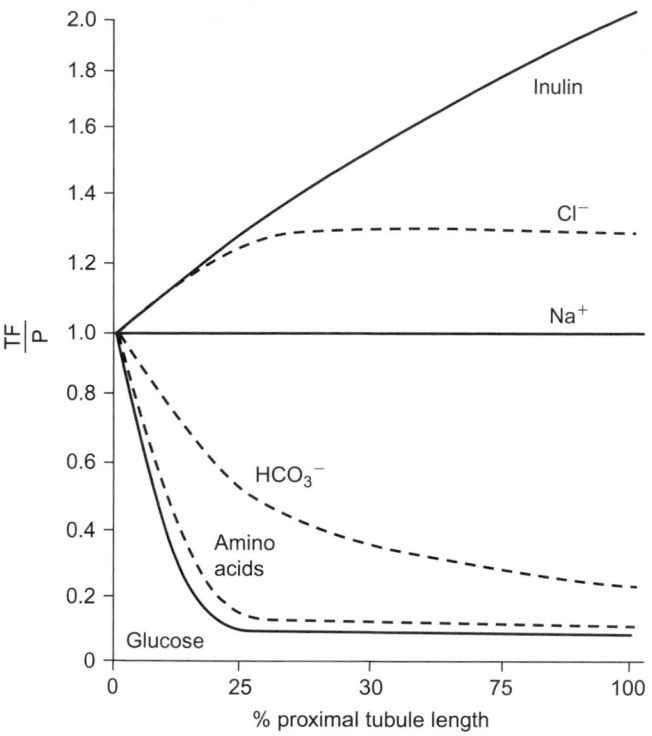

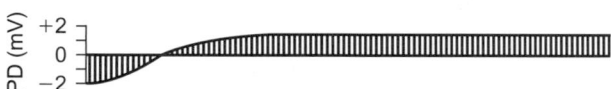

FIGURE 33.3   **Compositional changes in proximal tubule fluid along the mammalian nephron.** *(From[552], with permission.)*

Transport Forces

To attribute mechanisms to epithelial transport, fluxes must be resolved in terms of responsible driving forces, specifically hydrostatic or osmotic pressure, solute concentration gradients, electrical potential or metabolic energy. The transepithelial volume flow, J_v (ml/s · cm^2 epithelium), is a function of hydrostatic and osmotic driving forces:

$$J_v = L_p \left[\Delta p - RT \sum_1^n \sigma_i \Delta c_i \right] = (RTL_p) \left[\frac{\Delta p}{RT} - \sum_1^n \sigma_i \Delta c_i \right]$$

$$= \overline{v}_w P_f \left[\frac{\Delta p}{RT} - \sum_1^n \sigma_i \Delta c_i \right]$$

(33.1)

Here the water permeability of the epithelium is represented either by the coefficient L_p (ml/s · cm^2 · mmHg), by RTL_p (ml/s · cm^2 · Osm) or by P_f (cm/s), where RT is the product of the gas constant and absolute temperature (1.93×10^4 mmHg/Osm at 37°C), and $\overline{v}_w$ is the partial molar volume of water (0.018 ml/mmol). In Eq. (33.1) the osmotic effect of any

species is incorporated in the reflection coefficient, σ_i, ($0.0 \leq \sigma_i \leq 1.0$). For $\sigma_i = 1.0$, the species exerts a full osmotic effect, and the epithelium is an ideal semipermeable membrane. When $\sigma_i = 0.0$, the species exerts no osmotic force. To determine the reflection coefficient for a specific solute, the change in the transepithelial volume flow produced by a transepithelial concentration gradient, Δc_i, is compared to the volume flow produced by an equal concentration gradient of an impermeant species. The ratio of these two volume flows is just the reflection coefficient, σ_i.

To represent solute transport, J_i (mmol/s · cm^2), the epithelial flux equation is of the form:

$$J_i = J_v(1 - \sigma_i)\,\overline{c}_i + \sum_{j=1}^n L_{ij} \Delta \overline{\mu}_j^c =$$

$$J_v(1 - \sigma_i)\,\overline{c}_i + \sum_{j=1}^n L_{ij}[RT\Delta \ln(c_j) + z_j F \Delta \psi]$$

(33.2)

in which the first term is a convective flux in which a mean concentration appears:

$$\overline{c}_i = \frac{\Delta c_i}{\Delta \ln(c_i)} \approx 0.5 \cdot \left[c_i(l) + c_i(p) \right]$$

in which $c_i(l)$ and $c_i(p)$ designate luminal and plasma concentrations. It is a consequence of thermodynamic theory (Onsager symmetry) that the reflection coefficient, σ_i, from Eq. (33.1) also appears in Eq. (33.2) for convective solute drag. This formalizes the intuitive notion that the smaller solutes, which are least osmotically effective, are more likely to be entrained in the volume flow. The second term in Eq. (33.2) represents electrodiffusive solute flux, namely the flux of solute i as a function of the electrochemical potential differences, $\Delta \overline{\mu}_j^c$, of all of the solutes under consideration. Expansion of this potential is shown in the rightmost expression, in which RT is the product of gas constant and absolute temperature (2.57 J/mmol at 37°C), z_i is the valence of solute j, F is the Faraday (96.5 C/mEq), and $\Delta \psi$ is the electrical potential difference across the epithelium. It is also a consequence of Onsager symmetry that the coefficients $L_{ij} = L_{ji}$ (mmol^2/J · s cm^2). When the coefficient L_{ij} is positive (for i≠j), then a reabsorptive driving force on solute i will also promote reabsorption of solute j, so that this coefficient may be considered to represent co-transport of the two solutes. Such co-transport obviously arises when a common carrier transports the two species, but may also occur as a result of intraepithelial convective flows.[730]

Some of the most precise experimental measurements that can be made are those of electrical potentials and currents. In the absence of solute-solute interaction, the transepithelial solute flux is written:

$$J_i = J_v(1 - \sigma_i)\,\bar{c}_i + L_{ii}\left[RT\Delta\ln(c_i) + z_iF\Delta\psi\right] =$$
$$J_v(1 - \sigma_i)\,\bar{c}_i + P_i\left[\Delta c_i + \frac{z_iF}{RT}\bar{c}_i\Delta\psi\right] \quad (33.3)$$

where $RTL_{ii}/\bar{c}_i = P_i$ (cm/s) is the conventional solute permeability. Equation (33.3) has generally been the starting point for the application of electrophysiology to characterize proximal tubule. For example, if luminal and peritubular solutions have equal ionic concentrations ($\Delta c_i = 0$), and there is zero volume flow, then application of an electrical potential difference ($\Delta\psi$) produces a change in ionic current:

$$I_i = z_iFJ_i = P_i\left(\frac{z_i^2F^2}{RT}\right)\bar{c}_i\Delta\psi = g_i\Delta\psi \quad (33.4)$$

in which g_i (S/cm^2) is the partial ionic conductance of species i. The total epithelial electrical conductance, $g = \Sigma g_i$, or the epithelial electrical resistance, $R = 1/g$, thus provides a measure of the sum of the ionic permeabilities. When the luminal and peritubular solutions are unequal, the open-circuit potential, in the absence of net transepithelial volume flow ($J_v = 0$), gives useful information about the relative ionic permeabilities. In this case, the sum of all ionic currents is zero ($0 = \Sigma I_i$), so that the transepithelial electrical potential is:

$$\Delta\psi = -\sum_{i=1}^{n}\frac{g_i}{g}\frac{RT}{z_iF}\,\Delta\ln(c_i) \quad (33.5)$$

If, for example, the only concentration differences across the epithelium are equal and opposite anion gradients (such as chloride and bicarbonate), Eq. 33.5)

shows that the difference in ionic conductances determines the magnitude of the transepithelial "diffusion potential."

Table 33.2 is a compilation of the permeability properties of the proximal tubules of rat and rabbit. Again, the inclination to present such tabulation must be tempered by acknowledgement of variation of the permeabilities along the nephron, and of differences between superficial and juxtamedullary nephrons. With respect to water permeability, it has been suggested that there is a decline in L_p from the S1 to the S2 segment of the rat tubule.[432] Nevertheless, the water permeability remains at least as large in the straight segment as in the convoluted segment.[598] With respect to solute permeabilities, an increase in the electrical conductance of the rat proximal tubule has been observed as one moves from the earliest to the latest accessible segments.[620] Experiments in perfused rabbit tubules suggest that the increase in total conductance is due to an increase in the chloride permeability.[343] Comparison of tubule permeabilities indicates that juxtamedullary proximal convoluted tubules[82,84,164,343] and proximal straight tubules[330,364,708,713] are more cation selective than the superficial proximal tubule segments. Comparison of permeabilities of K$^+$[764] and of Cl$^-$,[713] between rabbit juxtamedullary and superficial proximal straight tubules suggests that the increase in cation selectivity derives from an absolute increase in juxtamedullary nephron cation permeability, with little difference in anion permeability.

There is no doubt that proximal tubule metabolism is required for transport to proceed at its normal rate. In the absence of ionic concentration gradients across the epithelium, reabsorption still proceeds and cooling or poisoning with metabolic inhibitors

TABLE 33.2   Permeabilities of Proximal Tubules

	Rat PCT	References	Rabbit PCT	References	Rabbit PST	References
$L_p \times 10^8$ ml/s·cm^2·mmHg	22.6	(a)	32.6		48.5	
P_f cm/s	0.24		0.35	(b)	0.52	(e)
σ(Na)	0.7	(a)			0.9–1.0	(b)
σ(Cl)	0.43	(a)			0.78–0.95	(b)
σ(HCO$_3$)	1.0	(a)			0.97	(b)
P(Na) $\times 10^5$ cm/s	24.7	(a)	4.0–11.9	(b)	2.3–2.6	(b)
P(K)	27.1	(a)				
P(Cl)	21.2	(a)	1.9–6.5	(b)	5.6–7.3	(b)
P(HCO$_3$)	6.7	(a)	1.3–2.3	(c,d)	0.4–2.0	(b)
Resistance ohm·cm^2	5	(a)	7.0	(b)	8.2	(b)

(a)[672]; (b)[595]; (c)[313]; (d)[713]; (e)[598].

abolishes transport. A generally accepted treatment of active transport by the proximal tubule has been that of Frömter[215] in which Eq. (33.2) is extended by inclusion of a term for metabolically driven transport, J_i^a:

$$J_i = J_v(1 - \sigma_i)\,\bar{c}_i + \sum_{j=1}^{n} L_{ij}\Delta\bar{\mu}_j^c + J_i^a \qquad (33.6)$$

or in the absence of coupled fluxes

$$J_i = J_v(1 - \sigma_i)\bar{c}_i + P_i\left[\Delta c_i + \frac{z_i F}{RT}\bar{c}_i\Delta\psi\right] + J_i^a \qquad (33.7)$$

It may also occur that water flux is linked to metabolic reactions in a way that reabsorption proceeds in the absence of transepithelial driving forces. This flux, J_v^a, has been termed "active water transport," and, by analogy with Eq. (33.6), Eq. (33.1) for transepithelial volume flow has been written[267,731]:

$$J_v = L_p\left[\Delta p - RT\sum_{1}^{n}\sigma_i\Delta c_i\right] + J_v^a \qquad (33.8)$$

A derivation of J_v^a from considerations of the internal structure of the tubule epithelium will be indicated in the section on the paracellular pathway.

THE TRANSCELLULAR PATHWAY

Cytosolic Concentrations

In the foregoing, proximal tubule transport has been treated from the perspective of the epithelium as a homogeneous entity, with reflection coefficients and permeabilities inferred from the transepithelial fluxes produced by changes in luminal and peritubular solutions. Over the last decades, however, a more microscopic view of proximal tubule transport has evolved. Crucial to this perspective were the observations that the intercellular tight junctions could serve as a low resistance route for transepithelial ion permeation.[223,758] This defines a "paracellular pathway" for fluxes, across the tight junction, into the lateral intercellular space, and out across the basement membrane to the peritubular capillaries. The "transcellular pathway" enters the cell cytosol via the luminal membrane and exits across the basal cell surface or across the lateral cell membrane into the lateral intercellular space. To discern solute transport across individual cell membranes, one must be able to monitor changes in intracellular concentrations.[110] Historically, the first estimates of cell ion content derived from chemical analysis of tissue. Difficulties with this method include the inaccuracy associated with the subtraction of the extracellular contribution to the total, as well as the

limitation of examining the concentration at only a single point in time. An additional concern arises when one tries to estimate transmembrane chemical potential differences, if some of the cell ion content is bound or sequestered, and thus not available to the "transport pool." Somewhat akin to the chemical assay has been the application of the electron probe to determine cell solutes. With the small beam of this technique, true intracellular sampling can be ensured, although the estimate of cell water is indirect and an important source of uncertainty. Nuclear magnetic resonance (NMR) spectroscopy has been used as a nondestructive method for measuring intracellular sodium of proximal tubules in suspension.[278,396] Unfortunately, only a portion of the cell sodium is "visible" by NMR, and additional steps must be taken to estimate the total pool.[111] One fruitful technique for probing the cell interior has been the use of microelectrodes capable of penetrating the cell membrane, presumably without destroying the functional integrity of the cell. The electrodes may record the electrical potential of the cytosol or, when fashioned with a substance that reacts selectively with an ion, the cytosolic electrochemical potential of the selected ion species. Although technically challenging, these measurements provide precisely the information necessary for establishing the driving forces for ionic fluxes.[219,370] Subsequently, ion-sensitive fluorescent dyes were developed, and these could be loaded into proximal tubule cells and used to monitor continuous changes in pH,[7] calcium[174] or chloride.[329,395]

Despite the technical difficulty of studying the small cells of mammalian proximal tubules, a reasonably complete picture of the intracellular milieu is available (Table 33.3). In the rat, the intracellular potential has been found to be −76 mV.[189] Good agreement has been reported for the cell sodium concentration estimated electrophysiologically (17.5 mmol/l)[782] and with the electron probe (20.3 mmol/l).[61] Potassium is actively accumulated above its electrochemical equilibrium.[141,189]

TABLE 33.3a Ion Activities in Rat Proximal Tubule

	Cell Conc.	Cell Activity	Capillary Conc.	Electrochemical Potential Difference (cell-capillary)[‡]
	(mM)	(mM)	(mM)	(J/mmol)
Na[+]	17.5	13 (a)	145	−12.8
K[+]	113	82 (b)	4	1.3
Cl[−]	18	13 (c)	118	2.5
HCO[−3]	17 (d)	12	25	6.3
PD		−76 mV (b)		

[‡]$RT = 2.57\ J/mmol$; (a)[781] (b)[189]; (c)[139]; (d)[7].

TABLE 33.3b   Ion Activities in Rabbit Proximal Tubule

	Cell Conc.	Cell Activity	Capillary Conc.	Electrochemical Potential Difference (cell-capillary)[‡]
	(mM)	(mM)	(mM)	(J/mmol)
Na^+	44 (e)	32	145	−9.0
K^+	68	49 (f)	5	0.8
Cl^-	25	18 (g)	118	1.9
HCO_3^-	16 (h)	12	25	4.7
PD		−61 mV (i)		

[‡]$RT = 2.57\ J/mmol$; (e)[278]; (f)[90]; (g)[335]; (h)[590]; (i)[70].

Although an early investigation suggested passive distribution of chloride across the proximal tubule,[639] subsequent work established cellular chloride uptake against a potential gradient.[139] The mechanism underlying this elevation of cytosolic chloride will be considered below. At this point, it suffices to acknowledge that the potential hill for chloride is linked via several anion exchangers to the bicarbonate potential. In turn, the elevation of cytosolic bicarbonate is regulated and maintained well above the equilibrium value (1.4 mmol/L) by a number of transport processes, including Na^+/H^+ exchange and metabolically driven proton extrusion from the cell (H^+-ATPase).[9,576]

It has also been possible to impale cells of the isolated perfused rabbit proximal tubule. The intracellular potentials of the proximal convoluted and proximal straight tubules were first found to be −51 and −47 mV respectively,[89] and subsequent determinations have been confirmatory (−50 mV[590]; −61 mV,[70]). In the proximal straight tubule, the cell potassium activity is higher than its electrical equilibrium. Both the cell potassium activity and the cell potential fall (depolarize) with ouabain-inhibition of the peritubular Na^+, K^+-ATPase.[90] As in the rat, the chloride activity is elevated above equilibrium, and there is good agreement between the electrophysiologic determination (18 mmol/L)[335] and that found using a fluorescent dye (21 mmol/L).[395] The intracellular pH of rabbit proximal tubules in suspension was first investigated using a radiolabeled weak organic acid. Under control conditions, the cells were found to be alkaline, 7.51, becoming acid with the application of ouabain, 7.42.[96] Subsequent determinations have revealed the pH to be lower (7.22,[590]), and thus more akin to that found in the rat proximal tubule.

Luminal Membrane

General Properties

Important information about membrane permeabilities and species-species interactions has been obtained from studies in vesicle suspensions prepared from proximal tubule brush border. The water permeability of the luminal membrane was assessed by the response of vesicle volume (light scattering) to an osmotic shock.[682,683,688] Corresponding to the approximate doubling of transepithelial water permeability from proximal convoluted tubule to proximal straight tubule of the rabbit (Table 33.2), is the observation of a comparable increase in water permeability of luminal membranes from these two segments.[680] Critical insight into the mechanism of water transport came with the discovery of an integral membrane protein (designated AQP-1), which serves as a water channel, or aquaporin, and is the principal water pathway for luminal and peritubular membranes of proximal tubule (reviewed by [2]). Consistent with the membrane water permeability measurements, the abundance of AQP-1 along the proximal tubule doubles as one moves from S2 to S3 segments.[449] In mice, the importance of AQP-1 for proximal tubule water flux was demonstrated with the study of S2 segments from AQP-1 knockout mice, whose water permeability (P_f) was about 20% that of wild-type mice.[794] Additional vesicle studies indicated that across the luminal membrane, solute−water interaction appears to be minimal, with a reflection coefficient for NaCl of 1.0.[523,681,682] This is consistent with absence of solute permeation through AQP-1, when expressed and studied in oocytes.[2] Thus, in the application of Eq. (33.6) to the luminal membrane, the terms for convective solute flux may be ignored.

Electrophysiological investigation of proximal tubule revealed that luminal membrane electrical resistance (260 ohm · cm^2) is between one and two orders of magnitude greater than the total epithelial resistance[217,218] (Table 33.2). The impact of altering luminal ionic composition on intracellular potential suggested that the potassium permeability of the luminal cell membrane was much greater than the sodium permeability, and that the chloride permeability was negligible.[216] These observations provided strong evidence that sodium entry into proximal tubule cells is coupled to the entry or exit of other solute species. Direct examination of the conductive channels within this membrane using the patch-clamp technique has been possible only to a limited extent. In the first successful attempt, Gögelein and Greger[250] identified a channel in the luminal membrane of rabbit proximal convoluted tubule, which showed a greater conductance to K^+ than to Na^+. Luminal K^+ channels have also been identified in patch-clamp studies of primary culture of rabbit S1 proximal tubule.[471] Additional K^+ channels have been identified immunohistochemically in the luminal cell membrane of mammalian proximal tubule, including the voltage-gated channel KCNA10,[776] and the voltage-dependent K^+ channel complex, KCNE1/ KCNQ1.[678] Both are thought to play a role in stabilizing the membrane potential against the depolarizing effect of Na^+-dependent uptake of glucose and amino acids (*vide infra*). This role for luminal K^+ channels received confirmation in microperfusion and electrophysiological investigation of proximal tubules from homozygous kcnq1 knockout mice.[679]

Luminal membrane sodium channels ($P_{Na}/P_K \geq 19$ and blocked by amiloride) have been found in a patch-clamp study of the rabbit proximal straight tubule.[251] This result anticipated the observation of voltage-sensitive, amiloride-blockable sodium entry across luminal membrane vesicles of this tubule segment,[340] and across the luminal membrane of cultured LLC-PK1 cells.[132] The LLC-PK1 cell line is derived from pig kidney, and is thought to resemble S3 proximal tubule. A later study of the S3 segment of rat proximal tubule demonstrated a luminal membrane conductance which could be inhibited by micromolar concentrations of amiloride, and which could be enhanced by a low-sodium diet or mineralocorticoid injection.[756] Under conditions of enhanced channel expression, the mRNA which encodes for the ENaC sodium channel could be detected in these proximal tubule cells. It is natural to surmise that the capacity of the proximal straight tubule of the rabbit to reabsorb sodium in the absence of a co-transported solute[599] might be a consequence of such channels.

Chloride channels have also been identified within proximal tubule cell membranes. In the mammalian kidney, an interesting finding has been the appearance of a chloride conductance after addition of cyclic AMP[424] or by modulating cytosolic production of cyclic AMP.[425] These observations, made in a preparation of brush border membrane vesicles, were confirmed in a patch-clamp study of the luminal membrane of proximal tubule cells in primary culture,[168,577,653] and parallels observations in other epithelia. Under the cellular conditions of Table 33.3, one would expect such a channel to be a pathway for Cl^- secretion; however, in the presence of a lumen-to-blood chloride gradient, application of cyclic AMP induces a reabsorptive transcellular chloride flux, which can be inhibited by luminal application of a chloride channel blocker.[702] The physiologic role of this chloride channel in proximal tubule function remains to be delineated.

Sodium-Glucose Co-Transport

The first sodium entry pathway to receive intensive study was its coupled transport with glucose. Considerable insight had been derived from intestinal and renal preparations, and the description of co-transport that emerged received confirmation as molecular biology provided expression and study of these transporters in other cells.[305,765,766,767] The co-transport of glucose with sodium was demonstrated in vesicles prepared from luminal membranes of rabbit[23] and rat[372] proximal tubules. In the presence of a sodium gradient (medium to vesicle), vesicle glucose concentration rises to levels above that in the medium, and then slowly equilibrates with the ambient concentration. This glucose uptake, which carries a net positive current, can be enhanced by short-circuiting the vesicle membrane.[62] Conversely, glucose gradients (medium to vesicles) may be used to drive vesicle sodium concentration transiently well above that of the bathing solution.[310] In the intact epithelium, the presence of glucose and sodium in the luminal perfusate depolarizes the luminal cell membrane.[217,452,586] Examining rat proximal tubule *in vivo*, Samarzija et al.[586] observed that the magnitude of luminal membrane depolarization is diminished by lowering either the luminal glucose or sodium concentrations, by depolarizing the luminal membrane, or by elevating the cell glucose concentration. In short, reabsorptive flux of the Na^+-glucose pair is dependent upon the electrochemical potentials for each species across the luminal membrane. These qualitative features of Na^+-dependent glucose flux could be captured using a linear nonequilibrium thermodynamic model of the co-transporter.[729]

Kinetic studies of glucose uptake across luminal membrane have been presented within the framework of carrier-mediated transport, characterized by a maximal transport rate and a luminal glucose concentration for which transport is half-maximal (K_m). When Turner and Silverman examined sodium-dependent uptake of glucose into vesicles prepared from dog renal cortex, their data suggested the presence of two such carrier sites.[671] In their preparation a high-velocity, low-affinity site had a $K_m = 4.5$ mmol/L, while the second site had a low velocity and high affinity ($K_m = 0.2$ mmol/L). The possibility was suggested that these two carriers might correspond to different sites of glucose uptake along the nephron. In pursuit of this issue, Turner and Moran[638,668] prepared vesicles from both the outer cortex and outer medulla of rabbit kidney. Here, the low-affinity carrier localized to the outer cortical region (presumably containing S1 and S2 segments of the proximal tubule), and the high affinity carrier localized to the outer medullary vesicles (presumably containing S3 segments). Corresponding to the affinity difference is the determination of a 1:1 (glucose:Na^+) stoichiometry of the cortical co-transporter,[316,669] and a 1:2 stoichiometry of the high affinity carrier.[670] More direct studies, localizing glucose uptake, were performed in isolated segments of rabbit proximal tubule by Barfuss and Schafer.[44] Their data were compatible with a single high-capacity carrier in the proximal convoluted tubule ($J_{max} = 1800$ pmol/s·cm^2 and $K_m = 1.7$ mmol/L), and low-capacity, high-affinity transporters in the proximal straight tubule ($J_{max} = 170-270$ pmol/s·cm^2 and $K_m = 0.35-0.70$). Thus, these experiments presented a coherent picture of a system of proximal glucose transport which would, under normal conditions, deliver only negligible quantities of glucose to the distal nephron. It should be noted that Na$^+$-glucose co-transport appears in cultured cell systems, and its identification was useful in establishing the similarity of the LLC-PK1 cell line to proximal tubule.[549] As in the straight tubule, the stoichiometry of glucose:Na$^+$ is 1:2.[417,476] Co-transport was also identified in primary cultures of proximal tubule cells,[153,777] again as high-affinity with 1:2 stoichiometry,[5,584] although electrophysiological study of one preparation suggested a lower affinity transporter.[74]

An important step in the study of Na$^+$-glucose co-transport came with the cloning of the gene for the intestinal co-transporter, SGLT1 (or, using the Human Genome Organization nomenclature, SoLute Carrier SLC5A1).[304] When this co-transporter was expressed in amphibian oocytes[328] or in mammalian cells,[102] it had high glucose affinity and kinetics indicating 1:2 stoichiometry. Early on, the availability of the intestinal transporter allowed identification of antigenic similarity with renal brush border proteins.[793] Subsequent *in situ* hybridization studies localized SGLT1 to the S3 segment of proximal tubule, precisely the site suggested by the kinetic data.[413] Prior to the cloning of this transporter, a number of detailed mathematical representations of Na$^+$ co-transport had been developed.[306,367,557,667] In each of these models, the co-transport of glucose and sodium was represented as a series of reactions: substrate binding to carrier; translocation of loaded carrier; unbinding at the opposite membrane face; and cycle completion by translocation of empty carrier. Expression of SGLT1 in oocytes enabled more extensive electrophysiological investigation and reformulation of a more secure model. Steady-state experiments revealed several salient features of the transporter: solute binding affinity is asymmetric, comparing inside and outside of the carrier; translocation of empty carrier is an important rate-limiting step and sensitive to the transmembrane PD; and solute-binding is not sufficiently rapid as to be considered at equilibrium with respect to translocation.[146,521,522] This expression system also enabled time-dependent studies to directly examine individual potential-dependent steps within the transport cycle. These have been useful in confirming charge of the unloaded carrier and identifying similarity in kinetics of SGLT1 from human, rat, and rabbit.[302,437,520] More recently, Loo and co-workers have focused on SGLT1 structure, and specifically characterization of the external sugar-binding domain.[311,439]

The cloning of SGLT1 also yielded insights not suspected from earlier studies, namely that protons could substitute for sodium in the transport of glucose,[312] and that in the translocation of two Na$^+$ and one glucose, SGLT1 also transports over 200 water molecules.[438,469] This degree of water transport may be important with respect to intestinal function, but in the kidney these fluxes through SGLT1 will be tiny. The discrepancy between the limited abundance of SGLT1 and the high capacity for glucose transport of cortical brush border membrane vesicles was readily apparent.[519] Homology screening revealed a gene which encoded for a second Na$^+$-glucose co-transporter, SGLT2 (SLC5A2), expressed in kidney, for which the stoichiometry is 1:1 and which, by *in situ* hybridization, localizes to the S1 segment of proximal tubule.[353] More detailed kinetic studies indicated that SGLT2 is the low-affinity, high-capacity system identified in kinetic studies.[784] When SGLT2 is expressed in oocytes and studied electrophysiologically, a kinetic scheme similar to that for SGLT1 could be developed to represent this transporter.[445] While still other sodium-glucose co-transporters have been identified, any significance with respect to renal transport remains to be established.

Sodium/Proton Exchange

From a quantitative perspective, the most important sodium flux across the luminal cell membrane is the Na$^+$/H$^+$ counter-transporter.[622] The Na$^+$/H$^+$ exchanger was securely established by Murer et al.,[494] using a suspension of vesicles composed predominately of luminal membrane. Their basic observation was that a sodium concentration gradient from suspension medium to vesicle interior resulted in acidification of the medium. This effect required the presence of intact vesicles, but was undisturbed when electrical potential differences between the vesicle interior and the medium were eliminated. Further, a suspension medium alkaline, with respect to vesicle interior, stimulated sodium uptake by the vesicles. These results were confirmed in rabbit proximal tubule vesicles by Kinsella and Aronson (Figure 33.4)[374], who further demonstrated alkalinization of the vesicle interior by the inwardly directed sodium gradient. This counter-transport is reversibly inhibited by amiloride,[375] and proceeds with a Na$^+$:H$^+$ stoichiometry of 1:1.[376] Following those early observations, kinetics of the proximal tubule luminal membrane Na$^+$/H$^+$ antiporter were studied intensively.[20,270,480] Vesicle preparations revealed a transport site that bound a single Na^{+}[714] with an affinity roughly one-tenth that of the external Na$^+$ concentration, and with competitive binding by H$^+$ or NH$_4$$^+$.[24,375] Studies of the antiporter at lower temperatures indicated that Na$^+$ uptake and H$^+$ extrusion occurred in a sequential ("ping-pong")

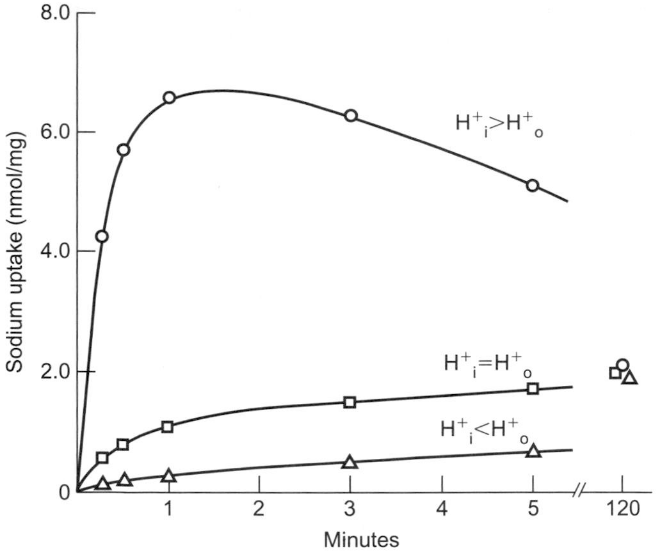

FIGURE 33.4 **Effect of proton gradients on sodium uptake by luminal membrane vesicles prepared from rabbit renal cortex.** Low internal pH ($H_i^+ > H_o^+$) enhances; and elevated internal pH; ($H_i^+ < H_o^+$) retards sodium entry, relative to the rate of entry in the absence of pH gradients. The vesicles were prepared in sodium-free medium and uptake was measured in solutions containing 1 mM Na^+. (From[374], with permission.)

fashion, with H^+ transport likely to be the rate-limiting step.[513,514] The effect of intracellular pH is more complex, with cytosolic alkalosis shutting off Na^+/H^+ exchange more sharply than a simple substrate depletion effect.[22] Cytosolic pH appears to have little impact on the Na^+ affinity of the antiporter,[377] but rather modifies the turnover rate.[514] With respect to the kinetic properties of this transporter, the information gained from renal brush border membrane vesicles has generally received confirmation in studies of isolated proximal tubule cell suspensions,[97,504] and in vesicles prepared from established cell lines[482] or from primary culture of proximal tubule cells.[209,652]

In mammalian proximal tubule, comparison of brush border and basolateral membrane vesicle showed that the Na^+/H^+ exchanger is primarily within the luminal cell membrane.[338] In the intact tubule, Schwartz[616] presented evidence for the direct coupling of Na^+ and H^+ fluxes, showing that ouabain inhibition of the peritubular Na,K-ATPase, presumably raising cell sodium concentration, could run the luminal Na^+/H^+ exchanger in reverse. Examination of vesicles from cortical and outer medullary regions of the kidney indicated that the Na^+/H^+ exchanger is present along both convoluted and straight segments of proximal tubule.[339,483] More direct evidence for the presence of the luminal membrane Na^+/H^+ exchanger in the S3 segment was offered by Kurtz.[400] Using tubules whose cells had been loaded with the

pH-sensitive fluorescent dye, BCECF, he found acidification of the cell interior with removal of luminal sodium. Nevertheless, the vesicle studies indicated that the maximal Na^+/H^+ exchange rate was lower in the outer medullary population, suggesting a lower density of the transporter in straight proximal tubules.[339] This also received confirmation by Baum,[52] who perfused both convoluted and straight proximal tubules with BCECF-loaded cells. Comparing the impact of changes in luminal sodium on intracellular pH, he concluded that, relative to the convoluted segment, the straight tubule had a 30% capacity for Na^+/H^+ exchange.

In the molecular era, the Na^+/H^+ exchangers came to be recognized as a family of transport proteins, NHE-, with the luminal membrane exchanger of proximal tubule identified as NHE3 (SLC9A3). The gene for NHE3 was cloned and sequenced,[511,662] and the product identified immunocytochemically in the brush border membrane.[99] Kinetic studies of the NHE3 in expression systems generally confirmed the properties noted a decade earlier in the membrane preparations.[510,663] With respect to the Na^+/H^+ exchange activity of the peritubular membrane, the NHE1 isoform was identified in basolateral membrane vesicles and in immunohistochemical staining of rabbit proximal tubule.[100] Failure to detect NHE3 protein in proximal straight tubule prompted speculation that another NHE isoform may be operative in this segment.[12] More generally, even in tubule segments in which NHE3 was abundant, the magnitude of the Na^+/H^+ flux that actually traversed this isoform was uncertain. Based on the observation that the inhibitor profile of rat brush border vesicle Na^+/H^+ exchange was identical to the inhibitor profile of NHE3 in expression systems, it was concluded that NHE3 was the sole exchanger within the luminal cell membrane.[700] That view was quickly amended with the development of the NHE3 knockout mouse, in which proximal microperfusion revealed rates for Na^+ and HCO_3^- reabsorption of 25% and 40% compared with wild-type.[610] In subsequent *in vivo* microperfusion studies, residual Na^+ reabsorption was found to be slightly greater, 60%[443] and 45%.[703] When the proximal tubules from knockout mice were dissected, loaded with BCECF, and perfused *in vitro*, the magnitude of luminal Na^+/H^+ exchange could be assessed as the change in intracellular pH in response to restoration of luminal Na^+.[151] In those experiments, the Na^+-dependent proton secretion in knockout tubules was about 50% of the wild-type, and completely inhibitable by amiloride. The magnitude of NHE3 flux was also assessed in rat proximal tubules perfused *in vivo*, in which a specific NHE3 inhibitor reduced Na^+ reabsorption by 30%[676] and 40%.[700] These values are likely to be underestimates of the NHE3 flux, in view of the fact that amiloride inhibition was only 50%.[700] In sum, it seems safe to attribute about half of the luminal membrane Na^+/H^+ exchange to NHE3. With respect to the molecular identity of the residual transport, both NHE2 knockout[151] and specific inhibitor studies[700] have eliminated NHE2 as a candidate. Goyal and co-workers identified NHE8, within kidney cortex[258] and expressed on proximal tubule brush border.[257] Its quantitative role in luminal Na^+/H^+ exchange remains to be defined.

Regarding the functional importance of the luminal membrane Na^+/H^+ exchanger in the proximal nephron, two caveats are in order. It is important to distinguish total HCO_3^- reabsorption from the Na^+-dependent portion of HCO_3^- reabsorption. The luminal membrane contains an H^+-ATPase,[120] and amiloride block of the Na^+/H^+ transporter has been used to identify a significant component of proton secretion via the H^+-ATPase.[41,319,400,537] The second caveat is that total Na^+-dependent proton secretion may be considerably greater than tubular HCO_3^- reabsorption. Preisig and Rector[538] microperfused rat proximal convoluted with a late proximal solution, low in bicarbonate and high in chloride. In this situation, where net bicarbonate absorption was virtually absent, amiloride still inhibited 44% of NaCl reabsorption. These findings were taken as evidence for the importance of parallel pathways through the luminal membrane for Na^+ (via the Na^+/H^+ exchanger) and for Cl^- (via a Cl^- base exchanger) in the net reabsorption of NaCl. The implication of such a scheme is that the net flux of Na^+ across the Na^+/H^+ transporter can well exceed the total reabsorptive bicarbonate flux. The first mathematical model of NHE3 was based on a scheme of Na^+-binding, translocation, and release, H^+-binding, translocation, and release, and also included competing NH_4^+-binding, translocation, and release.[734] In this model, all binding was assumed to be rapid (equilibrium), and affinity coefficients were assumed to be symmetric with respect to internal and external faces of the transporter. With one additional assumption, namely the inclusion of an internal modifier site which enhances translocation in response to cytosolic acidification, the kinetic behavior described in vesicle studies could be represented. When this simulation of NHE3 was incorporated into a mathematical model of rat proximal tubule, Na^+/H^+ exchange functioned directly to reabsorb luminal $NaHCO_3$, and in parallel with a luminal membrane Cl^-/base exchanger, yielded net NaCl reabsorption. An additional prediction of this kinetic model was that Na^+/NH_4^+ exchange via NHE3 is the most important mechanism for ammonia secretion by proximal tubule. This comported with conclusions from tubules *in vitro*, that ammonia secretion from cellular ammoniagenesis could be blocked by inhibition of NHE3.[496] Both experiment and model cast doubt on an earlier scheme of diffusive NH_3 secretion and trapping in acidic luminal fluid. With respect to NHE function, more sensitive experimental techniques have revealed nonlinearities. Fuster et al. used a pH-sensitive electrode to determine bath pH gradient in the immediate neighborhood of proton-transporting cells; from the gradient magnitude and the cell shape, they calculated the transmembrane proton flux.[231] When this methodology was applied to cells expressing NHE1 (and to a lesser extent NHE3), it was found that NHE turnover rate as a function of external Na^+ became sigmoidal.[232] Their observations were consistent with NHE schemes in which two "monomers" functioned cooperatively to yield a functional transport stoichiometry of $2Na^+$ for $2H^+$. The study demonstrated the power of an electrophysiological technique to examine an electroneutral transporter; whether the observations have a physiologic correlate in kidney tubule function, remains uncertain.

Chloride/Base Exchange

To enter the cell across the luminal membrane, chloride must be transported up an electrochemical potential gradient (Table 33.3); either co-transport with luminal Na^+ or exchange for cytosolic base, is energetically feasible. In the rat, Lucci and Warnock[444] found that furosemide inhibited two-thirds of the fluid transport when the luminal perfusion was a high-chloride, low-bicarbonate solution. In view of the ability of a known inhibitor of erythrocyte anion exchange (SITS) to also inhibit proximal volume reabsorption, Lucci and Warnock suggested that NaCl transport occurred via parallel luminal Na^+/H^+ and Cl^-/OH^- (or Cl^-/HCO_3^-) exchangers. Warnock and his colleagues supported this hypothesis with the demonstration of pH-gradient driven, electroneutral Cl^- fluxes across brush border membrane vesicles.[709,711,712] Similar conclusions were drawn by Liedtke and Hopfer,[421] whose study of luminal membrane vesicles from rat small intestine indicated that coupled Na^+-Cl^- co-transport was unlikely. Their work also indicated an inhibitory effect of furosemide on the Cl^-/OH^- exchanger.[422] Absence of Na^+-Cl^- co-transport was also a consistent finding in vesicles prepared from brush border membranes of the mammalian kidney.[493,623] In the straight proximal tubule of rabbit, a Cl^- microelectrode study has failed to detect Na^+-dependent luminal chloride entry.[335] Although a number of reports confirmed the presence of a Cl^-/OH^- exchanger in renal brush border membrane vesicles,[129,144,637] the absence of quantitatively significant flux through such an exchanger was indicated by others.[138,337,580,623] Methodological concerns relating to vesicle experiments were raised on both sides of this issue. When Schwartz[617] perfused rabbit proximal convoluted tubules with a sodium-free acidic fluid, there was no significant effect of luminal Cl⁻ on the appearance of bicarbonate within the luminal fluid.

Critical insight into luminal chloride transport came with the work of Karniski and Aronson,[355] who demonstrated a chloride-formate (Cl^-/HCO_2^-) exchanger in brush border membrane vesicles from the rabbit. In their experiments, a formate gradient could drive transmembrane chloride flux, and a chloride gradient could drive formate flux. This process was electroneutral and could be blocked by the anion exchange inhibitor, DIDS. Most significantly, they found (Figure 33.5) that while a pH gradient only slightly enhanced chloride uptake, this same gradient in the presence of a physiologic concentration of formate could drive substantial chloride flux. To account for this formate effect, they suggested that a backflux of formic acid, down its concentration gradient, from the acidic bath to the alkaline vesicle interior, would serve to constantly resupply the Cl^-/HCO_2^- exchanger. Karniski and Aronson proposed that in the intact tubule, the concurrent operation of Cl^-/HCO_2^- and Na^+/H^+ exchangers, along with backdiffusion of formic acid, would yield a net flux of NaCl across the luminal cell membrane. Subsequently,

this mechanism was refined, with the identification of a luminal membrane HCO_2^-/OH^- exchanger, which could recycle secreted formate back into the cell.[585] (By virtue of its inhibitor profile, this anion exchanger is distinct from the Cl^-/HCO_2^- antiporter.) One point of difficulty with the overall scheme was the subsequent finding that the diffusional permeability of the luminal membrane to formic acid was far too low to sustain a flux comparable to the estimated chloride flux.[535] An effort was made to rationalize this discrepancy mathematically, by considering the possibility of formic acid accumulation within an unstirred layer defined by the brush border. It was found, however, that with realistic diffusion coefficients, the microvilli were sufficiently short that no significant differences of formic acid concentration could develop between the bulk luminal solution and that near the cell membrane.[393,394] At this time, the possibility of a microdomain of low pH adjacent to the luminal membrane in which the formic acid to formate concentration ratio is enhanced remains the least secure element of this proposed mechanism.

Acknowledging points of uncertainty, a scheme emerged in which Cl^-/base exchange in proximal tubule is effected by two or more anion exchangers functioning in parallel[21] (Figure 33.6). To pursue this scheme further, a candidate protein for the Cl^-/HCO_2^- antiporter was sought and purified from brush border membrane vesicles.[642] Of uncertain significance was the observation that when reconstituted into phospholipid vesicles, this protein could also mediate direct Cl^-/HCO_3^- exchange.[641] The effect of formate has been examined in intact tubules, with cells containing BCECF, in which luminal chloride is able to acidify the cell in the presence (but not the absence) of formate.[8,51] It must also be acknowledged that one protocol which could detect formate stimulation of Cl^-/base exchange in superficial proximal convoluted tubules failed to detect it in tubules from juxtamedullary nephrons.[634] There has also been the observation of a negative formate effect in a study of proximal straight tubule,[402] again raising the possibility of nephron heterogeneity with respect to the mechanism of chloride entry. In their search for chloride entry mechanisms, Karniski and Aronson[356] also demonstrated a Cl^-/oxalate exchanger within brush border vesicles, on a carrier distinct from that for Cl^-/HCO_2^-. The subsequent finding of luminal membrane pathways for oxalate recycling, either in exchange for SO_4^{2-} or OH^-,[398] supported the possibility that the Cl^-/oxalate exchanger may also be an important route for luminal membrane Cl^- entry (Figure 33.6). Aronson and colleagues[398,698] envisioned the possibility that three carriers in parallel, Cl^-/oxalate and oxalate/SO_4^{2-} antiporters plus the $2Na^+-SO_4^{2-}$ co-transporter, would effect luminal entry of NaCl.

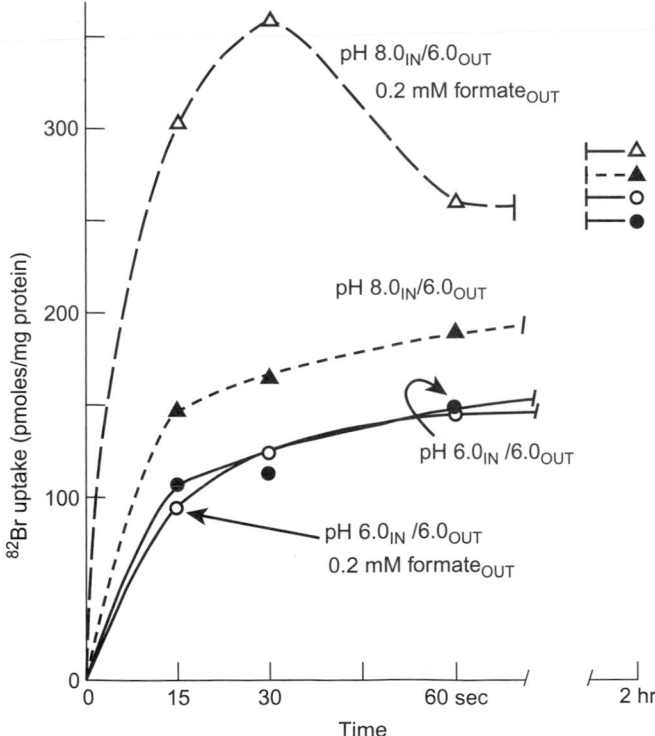

FIGURE 33.5 Effect of formate and a pH gradient on $^{82}Br^-$ **uptake by luminal membrane vesicles prepared from rabbit renal cortex.** While a pH gradient (8.0–6.0) only slightly enhances $^{82}Br^-$ transport, this same gradient in the presence of 0.2 mM formate produces a substantial increase in uptake, with an overshoot above the equilibrium concentration. (*From*[355].)

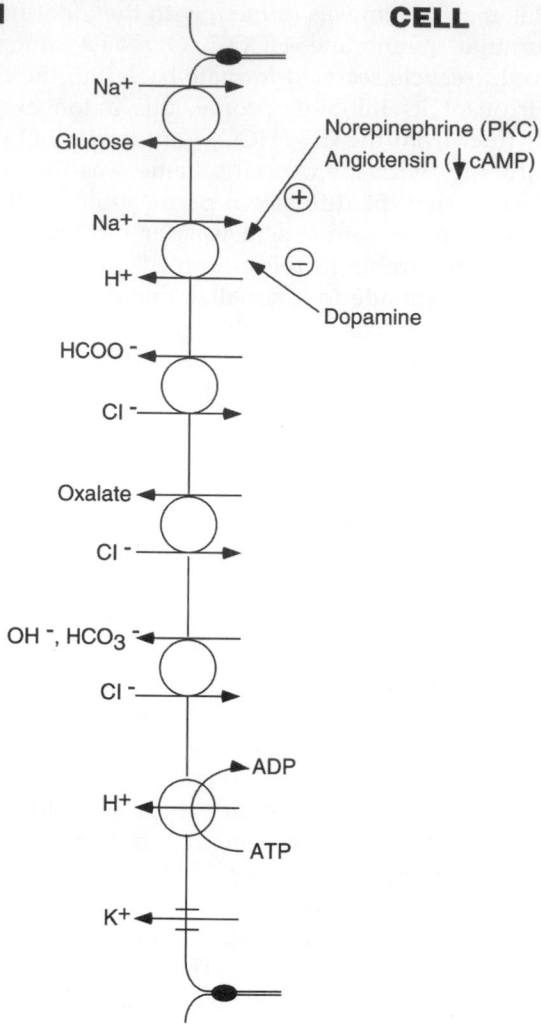

LUMEN   **CELL**

FIGURE 33.6   Transport pathways across the luminal cell membrane of the mammalian proximal tubule.

Confirmation of the importance of luminal chloride/base exchangers came with measurements of fluxes in intact proximal tubules. When any segment of rabbit proximal tubule (S1–S3) was perfused with an acidic (high Cl⁻, low HCO_3^-) solution, there was a substantial impact of formate to stimulate volume (NaCl) reabsorption[603,604] In perfusions with a relatively alkaline solution (such as an ultrafiltrate of plasma) there was no such enhancement, presumably due to the limited recycling of formate. In reviewing these observations, Berry and Rector[83] pointed out that the pH-dependence of formic acid permeation effectively prioritizes proximal anion reabsorption along the tubule, HCO_3^- taking precedence over Cl⁻. The increased volume reabsorption observed with formate was subsequently found to occur in association with an increase in cell volume, thus supporting the transcellular route for the increment in chloride flux.[601] With perfusion of proximal tubules of the intact rat kidney, both luminal formate

and oxalate enhance NaCl reabsorption from an acidic, high-chloride, luminal solution.[698,699,706] The ability of a chloride channel blocker, DPC, within the peritubular perfusate, to block the formate and oxalate effects is additional evidence that the increment in NaCl flux is transcellular.

Molecular identification of luminal membrane anion transporters has focused attention on the SLC26 family of anion exchangers.[178,489] Of the members in this family, the SLC26A4 transporter (pendrin) was demonstrated to be a Cl⁻/formate exchanger when expressed in *Xenopus* oocytes,[619] and its mRNA was identified in rat kidney cortex.[645] The protein, however, was not detected immunohistochemically in mouse proximal tubule brush border.[381] Furthermore, in pendrin knockout mice, Cl⁻/formate exchange in brush border membrane vesicles was normal, and microperfusion of proximal tubules showed normal formate stimulation of volume reabsorption.[357] The transporter SLC26A6 (CFEX, PAT1) could also mediate Cl⁻/formate exchange in oocytes, and the protein was expressed in brush border of mouse proximal tubules.[381] Further study of SCL26A6 revealed that it had a broad transport capacity, which included Cl⁻/oxalate, Cl⁻/HCO_3^-, and Cl⁻/OH⁻.[148,772] The observation that low concentrations of oxalate could inhibit Cl⁻/HCO_3^- exchange led Jiang et al.[345] to surmise that the primary function of SLC26A6 in proximal tubule was as the luminal Cl⁻/oxalate exchanger. This prediction was borne out in a study of mice deficient in SLC26A6.[705] The mice had normal serum electrolytes and normal proximal tubule volume reabsorption under control conditions; oxalate stimulation of proximal volume flux was absent. These knockout mice showed only a tendency toward deficient formate stimulation of volume reabsorption, so that at this time, the identity of the Cl⁻/formate exchanger(s) remains uncertain.

Suspicion that formate may have other effects on proximal transport, beyond luminal anion exchange, was raised in a mathematical model of rat proximal convoluted tubule which included representation of luminal membrane Cl⁻/HCO_2^- exchange.[733] Simulation of formate addition reproduced the observed cell swelling and increase in cytosolic chloride concentration; however, the density of the chloride/formate exchanger had virtually no effect on overall NaCl reabsorption along the tubule. In similar simulations, the density of the Na^+/H^+ exchanger had a powerful impact on NaCl reabsorption, indicating that for the model tubule, sodium reabsorption was rate-limiting for NaCl flux. Subsequent experimental examination of mice deficient in NHE3 found that formate stimulation of proximal sodium (volume) and chloride reabsorption was absent, although oxalate stimulation was entirely preserved.[704] These workers surmised that, in the normal tubule, there might be a functional coupling between NHE3 and the Cl^-/formate exchanger. A direct study of the formate effect on NHE3 function was undertaken by Petrovic et al.[528] In the absence of CO_2/HCO_3^-, addition of formate to the bath and lumen of mouse microperfused kidney proximal tubule caused intracellular alkalinization, with cell pH increasing from baseline level 7.17 to 7.55. Removal of sodium from the lumen or addition of EIPA completely prevented the alkalinization. It was concluded that formate stimulates the apical Na^+/H^+ exchanger NHE3 in kidney proximal tubule, and that formate stimulation of chloride reabsorption could be indirect and secondary to activation of NHE3. An intriguing possibility is that the Cl^-/formate exchanger may be acting as a formate receptor to modulate NHE3.[528] In a subsequent study, deletion of the Slc26a6 anion exchanger from the S3 mouse proximal tubule diminished NHE3 activity, despite comparable protein abundance.[527]

Peritubular Membrane

General Properties

The cell sodium content reflects the balance among conductive, coupled, and metabolically driven fluxes across both luminal and peritubular cell membranes. In the rat, the potassium-to-sodium permeability ratio is about 20:1,[215] and the electrical resistance of this membrane is 90 ohm $\cdot$ cm^2, roughly a third of the luminal membrane.[217] A similar apportionment of electrical resistance appears in the proximal convoluted tubule of the rabbit, where the peritubular and luminal resistances are 39 and 118 ohm $\cdot$ cm^2.[410] In the straight proximal tubule of the rabbit, Bello-Reuss[70] has found the peritubular sodium conductance undetectable. In the first successful application of a patch pipette to the peritubular membrane of rabbit proximal tubule, only a potassium channel was clearly identified.[250] With respect to convective sodium fluxes across this membrane, all the data are negative with one exception. Welling et al.[740,742] applied an osmotic shock to the peritubular surface of isolated rabbit tubules and recorded the change in cell volume. A comparison of the effect of raffinose and NaCl indicated a reflection coefficient, $\sigma_{NaCl} = 0.5$, suggesting that water flow across this membrane would carry significant quantities of NaCl. This surprising result did not receive confirmation, however, in two subsequent studies of basolateral membrane vesicles. Using either light-scattering[682] or a fluorescent indicator[523] to assess vesicle volume, salt reflection coefficients of 1.0 were obtained. Subsequent experiments in whole tubule preparations, with optical measurement of cell volume[284] or using a fluorescent indicator[635] indicated $\sigma_{NaCl} = 1.0$, implying no NaCl flowed convectively across the peritubular membrane.

Sodium Bicarbonate Co-transport

Co-transport of sodium with bicarbonate is an important pathway for sodium and the principal pathway for bicarbonate exit across the peritubular membrane in both amphibian and mammalian proximal nephron.[9,109,534] The delineation of this coupled transport followed from the careful examination of bicarbonate exit from the salamander proximal tubule by Boron and Boulpaep.[108] Using pH and Na^+-sensitive microelectrodes, they observed that a reduction in peritubular bicarbonate concentration led to a decline in cytosolic pH, a peritubular depolarization, and a decline in cell sodium activity. Further, a reduction in peritubular sodium also led to a decline in cytosolic pH and, in contrast to the expectation from a conductive Na^+ pathway, peritubular depolarization. All of these effects could be blocked by the anion transport inhibitor, SITS. These results suggested the operation of a coupled Na^+ and HCO_3^- co-transporter, with the exit of at least two bicarbonate ions for each sodium. In the salamander, the electrochemical gradient of bicarbonate across the peritubular membrane was sufficient to drive sodium exit from the cell, if the stoichiometry were 2:1 or greater (HCO_3^-:Na^+). Subsequent study of the *Necturus* proximal tubule confirmed the presence of substantial voltage-sensitive HCO_3^- exit across the peritubular membrane,[454] which was later shown to be coupled to Na^+ and HCO_3^- transport.[441] Here, it was suggested that the stoichiometry might well be 3:1. With regard to the issue of HCO_3^-:Na^+ stoichiometry, one interesting set of observations in *Necturus* was the finding that when functioning in the normal reabsorptive direction, this ratio was 3:1, but when bath conditions were changed to reverse the flux direction, the ratio changed to 2:1.[531] This suggested an asymmetry with respect to the affinities of the substrates, perhaps secondary to the conformational changes of the transporter during the translocation step.

In rat proximal tubule, experiments using conventional microelectrodes indicated that elimination of bicarbonate from the perfused peritubular capillaries produced a large instantaneous depolarization.[225] In this early work, the investigators attributed the depolarization to a conductive bicarbonate pathway and estimated (Eq. (33.5)) that nearly half the peritubular membrane conductance might be mediated by bicarbonate. Electrophysiologic study of the perfused straight proximal tubule of the rabbit also disclosed a steady-state depolarization with removal of peritubular bicarbonate.[70,89] In that work, however, the depolarization was attributed to a pH-dependent decrease in peritubular membrane K^+ conductance, and thus a decreased contribution of the K^+ potential to the overall membrane potential. The rat proximal tubule was then re-examined, and still the results indicated that the immediate depolarization produced by peritubular bicarbonate removal did not depend upon changes in membrane K^+ conductance.[123,124] This depolarization was inhibited by SITS, but a clear implication of Na^+ in the bicarbonate exit step was not confirmed. Within a short period of time, a number of investigators securely established the presence of $Na^+-HCO_3^-$ co-transport in the peritubular membrane of the mammalian kidney. Sasaki et al.[590] using pH-sensitive microelectrodes, demonstrated that in the straight proximal tubule of rabbit, elimination of bath sodium resulted in cellular acidification and peritubular depolarization, an effect that was partially blocked by SITS. Biagi and Sohtell[91,92] used conventional microelectrodes to document a peritubular depolarization with sodium removal in both convoluted and straight proximal segments. The effect was substantially blocked by SITS, and attributed to coupled HCO_3^- transport. Yoshitomi et al.[781] re-examined the rat proximal tubule, now using both Na^+-sensitive and pH-sensitive microelectrodes. Removal of peritubular sodium or bicarbonate led to the expected depolarization, acidification, and decrease in cell sodium activity. When these investigators compared the (SITS-inhibitable) depolarization with either 10-fold reductions of peritubular Na^+ or HCO_3^- (equal changes in chemical potential) they found that the impact of the bicarbonate removal was three-fold greater. They concluded that the $HCO_3^-:Na^+$ stoichiometry was 3:1. In an independent set of experiments, sudden reduction in peritubular bicarbonate produced peritubular HCO_3^- and Na^+ fluxes (estimated from cell size and buffering power), which confirmed the 3:1 coupling ratio.[781]

The peritubular bicarbonate pathway in the rat proximal tubule was also investigated using fluorescence of intracellular BCECF to monitor changes in cytosolic pH.[7] In this first use of BCECF in the rat, Alpern was able to document SITS-inhibitable acidification of the cell with reduction of peritubular sodium. When BCECF was used to detect pH changes along the nephron, the transporter was identified in the S3 segment, but in clearly reduced capacity compared with S2.[52,238] Abuladze et al.,[1] used BCECF to quantify $Na^+-HCO_3^-$ transport capacity in all three proximal tubule segments from both cortical and juxtamedullary rabbit kidneys. They reported S1 fluxes three- to five-fold greater than those of S2, and S2 fluxes eight-fold greater than those of S3. Examination of isolated basolateral membrane vesicles prepared from rabbit[4,263] and rat kidney[264] permitted the kinetics of the transporter to be studied in relative isolation. By determining driving force equilibrium across this

transporter, Soleimani et al.[644] confirmed that three negative charges were carried for each sodium. Subsequently, the co-transported species were identified as one HCO_3^- plus one CO_3^{2-}.[640] Identification of the transported species was also pursued electrophysiologically. In rabbit proximal tubules in vitro, under "standard" conditions, the stoichiometry of peritubular $HCO_3^-:Na^+$ flux through this co-transporter was 2:1, and insensitive to carbonic anhydrase inhibition. However, with perfusion conditions more closely approximating those in vivo, the stoichiometry shifted to 3:1, and was sensitive to carbonic anhydrase inhibition. This change in transport was interpreted as a shift of the transported species from $2HCO_3^--Na^+$ to $CO_3^{2-}-HCO_3^--Na^+$, as in vivo[490,492,625] Gross and Hopfer[273] studied the $Na^+-HCO_3^-$ co-transporter in a cell line derived from the S1 segment of rat proximal tubule, grown to confluence on filters. When the luminal cell membrane of this artificial epithelium was permeabilized with amphotericin, cytosolic solute concentrations were identified with those of the luminal solution, and the stilbene-sensitive transepithelial current with current through the $Na^+-HCO_3^-$ co-transporter. Data from this preparation indicated a 3:1 flux stoichiometry,[273] and provided information with which to construct a detailed kinetic model for this transporter.[274,275]

The $Na^+-HCO_3^-$ co-transporter (SLC4A4) was cloned first from Ambystoma kidney,[573] and then from human[127] and rat kidneys.[128,572] Denoted akNBC, hkNBC, and rkNBC respectively, all three co-transporters are comprised of 1035 amino acids, and structural comparisons have been presented.[571,643] Using antibody developed against rNBC, the protein was demonstrated in rat proximal tubule in an exclusively basolateral pattern, with intense staining in S1, rapid decline in S2, and no detectable staining in S3.[607] Staining in Ambystoma proximal tubule was also basolateral, but considerably weaker. Immunohistochemistry at the electron microscopic level confirmed these findings.[460] When rkNBC was expressed in Xenopus oocytes, transporter function could be studied electrophysiologically, and the stoichiometry of HCO_3^- to Na^+ fluxes was found to be 2:1.[184,618] It was concluded that the function of this transporter in mammalian cells in vivo was clearly different from its function in oocytes. The conundrum was sharpened with experiments in artificial epithelia derived from mouse proximal tubule or collecting duct, each deficient in NBC. In these two mammalian cells, transfected kNBC showed 3:1 or 2:1 stoichiometry for proximal and collecting duct cells, respectively.[271] Important insight came from, Müller-Berger et al.[491] who examined rkNBC in oocytes electrophysiologically, and found that with elevation of cytosolic calcium concentration, there was a relatively slow (30 second) activation of the NBC conductance, plus a shift in stoichiometry from 2:1 to 3:1. They understood that such events in the proximal tubule *in vivo* would constitute a switch from zero (or secretory) peritubular HCO_3^- flux to brisk HCO_3^- reabsorption. This switch was deciphered by Gross et al.,[272] working with the artificial mouse proximal tubule epithelium transfected with kNBC. They found that addition of cAMP caused a shift in stoichiometry from the basal 3:1 to 2:1, and this was PKA-dependent. Replacing the single PKA phosphorylation site of the transfected transporter eliminated the stoichiometric shift.

Chloride Transporters

In early electrophysiologic investigation of both amphibian[276,636] and mammalian[70,124,133] proximal tubules, peritubular chloride conductance appeared to be virtually absent or at least negligible. In proximal convoluted tubules of the rabbit, perfused *in vitro*, peritubular application of a chloride channel blocker had no effect on NaCl reabsorption.[53] Welling and O'Neil[744] found that in rabbit proximal straight tubule the conductive chloride pathway in peritubular membrane could account for about 6% of the total membrane conductance. However, after cell swelling induced by a 150 mOsmol hypotonic osmotic shock, the chloride conductance increased to 20% of the total peritubular membrane conductance. Using quantitative video microscopy, the volume of rabbit proximal convoluted tubules was unaffected by changes in peritubular chloride concentration. However, prior hypotonic cell swelling rendered the cell volume sensitive to peritubular chloride concentration, and this effect was eliminated by application of a chloride channel blocker.[602] Peritubular chloride channel blockers have also been effective in blunting the changes in the membrane electrical potential following a change in peritubular chloride concentration.[626] Further electrophysiologic study of rabbit convoluted tubule during osmotic shock estimated the fractional chloride conductance to increase from 3% to a maximum of 16%, with relaxation to 8%. During these same experiments, the fractional conductance of the $Na^+-3HCO_3^-$ pathway declined from 41 to 16%, with little change in the absolute conductance through this pathway. Data from such experiments provide enough information to estimate the reabsorptive flux of chloride through the peritubular channels. If one assumes that the peritubular membrane has an electrical resistance of 100 ohm $\cdot$ cm^2,[410] equivalently a conductance of 10 mS/cm^2, then the conductance of the $Na^+-3HCO_3^-$ pathway is about 5 mS/cm^2, as is the maximal chloride conductance after the osmotic shock. With reference to Table 33.3b, the cytosolic chloride electrochemical potential across this channel is about 2 J/mmol or 20 mV. Multiplication by the steady-state chloride conductance of the swollen cell, 2.5 mS/cm^2, yields a chloride current of 50 nA or 0.5 nmol/s $\cdot$ cm^2. This estimate may be compared with the overall transepithelial sodium flux of late proximal convoluted tubule at 4.5 nmol/s $\cdot$ cm^2. Thus, the conductive chloride flux is not insignificant, and yet it cannot be the whole story. Further, concern over the magnitude of the osmotic shocks used in these experiments prompted re-examination with smaller perturbations by Breton et al.[117] When the cell volumes increased by only 20–25%, the peritubular chloride conductance increased by only 3–4-fold from control. Another important observation from the study of Breton et al.[117] was that the time course of chloride channel activation was delayed with respect to the time course of cell swelling, suggesting perhaps a chemical modification of the channel, rather than an immediate stretch-activated response. As in the luminal membrane, increases in cytosolic cAMP also activate a chloride channel within the peritubular membrane of rabbit[627,628] and rat.[702]

From the considerations above, peritubular chloride fluxes must also occur as electroneutral-coupled transport with other ions. Guggino and associates[277,436] examined chloride transport across the peritubular membrane of *Necturus* proximal tubule, using Cl$^-$- and pH-sensitive microelectrodes. They found that following either removal of peritubular Cl$^-$ or increase of cytosolic Cl$^-$, exit of chloride from the cell was substantially blunted by removal of either peritubular Na$^+$ or HCO$_3^-$. This chloride exit was inhibited by SITS. In view of the electroneutral nature of the process, they proposed a coupled transport mechanism in which intracellular Cl$^-$ was exchanged for Na$^+$ and 2 HCO$_3^-$ from the peritubular side (Figure 33.7). Such coupled transport systems had been established in invertebrate neurons.[576] Other studies of chloride permeation of the peritubular membrane of amphibian proximal tubule suggested a Cl$^-$/HCO$_3^-$ exchanger that was independent of sodium,[188,783] although such a transporter would mediate chloride uptake by the cell. In the mammalian proximal tubule, peritubular Cl$^-$/HCO$_3^-$ exchange had been suspected from peritubular capillary perfusion studies in the rat.[119,673] More convincing evidence for the presence of Na$^+$-dependent Cl$^-$/HCO$_3^-$ exchange in the peritubular membrane of rat proximal tubule came from experiments of Alpern and Chambers.[10] In these tubules loaded with BCECF, restoration of peritubular capillary chloride produced cellular acidification. This acidification did not occur in the absence of ambient (luminal and peritubular) Na$^+$, and was blocked by SITS. Consistent with these findings was the observation[264] that in basolateral membrane vesicles from rat renal cortex, an oppositely directed Cl$^-$ gradient (inside to outside) stimulated

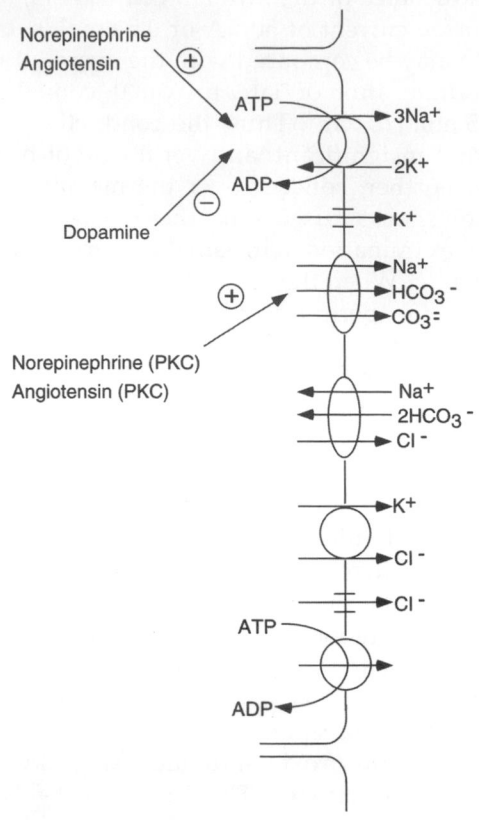

FIGURE 33.7 Transport pathways across the basolateral cell membrane of the mammalian proximal tubule.

HCO_3^--dependent Na^+ uptake. In vesicles from the rabbit, in which Cl^- uptake was assayed, it was found to be enhanced by an outwardly directed HCO_3^- gradient, and further stimulated by the addition of a Na^+ gradient.[145] In a Cl^- microelectrode study of rabbit proximal convoluted tubule, Ishibashi et al.[333] found that removal of either HCO_3^- or Na^+ from the peritubular bath increased cytosolic Cl^-, an effect inhibited by SITS, and which was interpreted as confirmation of Na^+-dependent Cl^-/HCO_3^- exchange. A subsequent examination of the rate of decline of cell Cl^- following perturbations of the peritubular bath suggested that this transporter was the dominant pathway for peritubular Cl^- exit.[334]

Examination of the straight proximal tubule of the rabbit has not yielded consistent findings regarding the Na^+-dependence of Cl^-/HCO_3^- exchange. Sasaki and his associates, using pH-sensitive microelectrodes, first found a small cellular alkalinization with the removal of peritubular chloride.[591] Subsequent study with a Cl^--sensitive electrode demonstrated a substantial increase in intracellular chloride with reduction of peritubular bicarbonate, an effect that was blunted by the complete removal of sodium and blocked by SITS.[593] Using

straight proximal tubules containing BCECF, Kurtz[401] found a peritubular Cl^-/HCO_3^- exchanger that could function in the absence of Na^+. A basolateral Cl^-/HCO_3^- exchanger in this segment was also identified by Nakhoul et al.,[500] but its Na^+-dependence could not be defined. A microelectrode study of the S3 segment of the rabbit was performed by Kondo and Frömter,[390] who observed that removal of bath Cl^- decreased intracellular Cl^-, alkalinized the cell, and produced no change in cytosolic Na^+. This effect was blocked by peritubular SITS. Further, reduction of peritubular HCO_3^- increased cell Cl^-, so that a strong case was advanced for the presence of a Na^+-independent Cl^-/HCO_3^- exchanger in the peritubular membrane. With reference to Table 33.3b, this exchanger must mediate chloride uptake by the cell. A cycle of this exchanger in association with a cycle of a luminal or peritubular Na^+/H^+ transporter would yield net cellular uptake of NaCl, and could increase the volume of the tubule cell. Indeed, the peritubular Cl^-/HCO_3^- exchanger has been implicated in the recovery of cell volume after shrinkage in a hyperosmolar medium.[434,435,570]

Electrically silent chloride exit across the peritubular membrane may also occur as co-transport of KCl.[710] This transport mechanism had been proposed in connection with studies of *Necturus* gallbladder by Reuss and his associates[559,560] as a means of rationalizing the necessary Cl^- exit with the low membrane chloride conductance, and was confirmed with the demonstration that intracellular chloride activity could be made to vary with variation in the basolateral potassium concentration.[163,558] With respect to the mammalian proximal tubule, beyond the need for Cl^- exit, the brisk influx of K^+ via the Na-K-ATPase mandates substantial peritubular K^+ exit. For the rat proximal tubule, it was estimated that the conductive pathway was inadequate to account completely for this exit, so that in the construction of a mathematical model of this epithelium a peritubular KCl co-transporter was incorporated.[727] The first evidence for the proximal tubule KCl co-transporter came with the experiments of Eveloff and Warnock[198] on rabbit renal basolateral membrane vesicles. Here, K^+ or Cl^- gradients drove uptake of the other species in a voltage-independent manner. These findings received support with observations of furosemide-sensitive cell volume decrease in rabbit proximal straight tubule,[743] and furosemide-sensitive K^+ exit in proximal tubule suspensions.[30,391] In proximal straight tubule, Sasaki et al.[589] used both K^+- and Cl^--sensitive microelectrodes to demonstrate the mutual interaction of K^+ and Cl^- across the peritubular membrane. This interaction was independent of membrane electrical potential, and independent of Na^+. These findings received confirmation in the proximal convoluted tubule, examined with Cl^--sensitive microelectrodes by Ishibashi et al.,[333] although in this work, coupled KCl exit appeared to be insensitive to furosemide. A subsequent electrophysiological investigation also failed to detect furosemide-sensitive coupled K^+ and Cl^- fluxes.[626] At the molecular level, four KCl co-transporters have been identified within the SLC12 family (SLC12A4-7), also known as KCC1-4.[303,487] Cloning and expression of KCC1 was achieved by Gillen et al.,[246] who reported that it was widely expressed; KCC3 and KCC4 were cloned by Mount et al.,[488] who noted a more selective expression, including kidney for both.

Na,K-ATPase

Metabolically driven sodium extrusion from the cell and potassium uptake are effected by the Na,K-ATPase situated exclusively within the peritubular cell membrane.[358,403] The biophysical properties of this pump were a key focus of early investigations of epithelial transport.[249,348–350] The functional transport unit of the Na,K-ATPase consists of an alpha-subunit bound to cytoplasmic structural proteins[485] and an externally protruding beta-subunit. Although there are three isoforms for the alpha-subunit, only a single isoform (α_1) appears to be expressed in proximal tubule.[467,666] The beta-subunit appears to function as a molecular chaperone, targeting insertion of the transporter.[237] Together the alpha–beta unit spans the peritubular membrane and contains, within its interior, cation-binding sites. A gamma-subunit to the Na,K-ATPase exists within kidney, and has been identified as one member of the FXYD family of proteins with wide ranging organ distribution.[27,234,237] The role of the gamma-subunit remains uncertain, although it has been suggested that it may function to limit transport during hypoxia or other tissue stress.[25,26] The most widely held scheme[350] for the operation of the pump envisions a cycle which begins with an E1 state, in which ATP is bound to the alpha-subunit and the cation-binding sites are open to the cytoplasmic surface for the binding of 3-Na^+ ions. With the binding of Na^+, ADP is released, leaving a phosphorylated unit in which the cations are initially inaccessible to either membrane face (occluded). A conformational change in the transport unit brings it to the E2 state, in which the cationic-binding sites are open to the external surface. At this point the release of Na^+ is followed by the binding of 2 K^+ ions, and with hydrolysis of the phosphate bond, these K^+ ions are occluded. Binding of ATP is associated with the conformational transition back to the E1 state, and release of K^+ into the cytoplasm. Stoichiometry of the Na,K-ATPase was first established in nonrenal systems,[249,379,503] and this was confirmed in oxygen utilization experiments in whole kidney[371] or in tubule suspensions.[298,299] A suspension of rabbit renal cortical tubules was examined, using NMR to monitor Na^+ transport from the cell and a K^+-electrode in the suspending medium to determine K^+ uptake, and it was demonstrated that over nearly an order of magnitude of Na,K-ATPase turnover, the Na:K stoichiometry remained 3:2.[29] By virtue of this stoichiometry, the Na,K-ATPase generates a net outward current across the peritubular membrane; pump inhibition with ouabain induces prompt depolarization of the peritubular membrane in rat proximal tubule.[222]

Development of a microassay system for Na, K-ATPase by Schmidt and Dubach[605,606] permitted the first estimate of enzyme activity within individual tubule segments. Subsequently, Morel and his colleagues developed a simpler assay and identified the distribution of Na,K-ATPase along the nephron.[180,360] They found comparable distribution in rat, rabbit, and mouse, with substantially greater concentration of ATPase in proximal convoluted tubule than in the straight segment. Garg et al.[233] found Na,K-ATPase activities of the S1, S2, and S3 segments of rabbit proximal tubule to be 17.5, 6.7, and 3.8 pmol ATP/s·cm tubule. Under conditions of the assay, maximal hydrolytic activity of the enzyme was determined, so that maximal Na^+ transport is three times these values. Corresponding to the transport activity of the Na, K-ATPase, there is a free energy change of 28.6 J/mmol (Table 33.3) or 6.8 cal/mmol, a figure compatible with the free energy of hydrolysis of ATP of 13–14 cal/mmol.[686] El Mernissi and Doucet[195] quantified ouabain-binding sites of rabbit PCT, and found 0.109 pmol/cm or 25×10^6 sites/cell. Thus, the ATPase activity of 10 pmol/s·cm would correspond to about 100 cycles/s of a single Na,K-ATPase unit. The actual rate of sodium transport by the Na,K-ATPase is usually less than maximal enzyme activity, and is dependent upon the levels of intracellular Na^+, peritubular K^+, and intracellular ATP. Of these three factors, in proximal tubule *in vivo*, cytosolic Na^+ concentration is the most important regulator of pump activity.[348,359] The half-maximal enzyme activation occurs at 31 mmol/l,[249,647] a level which is comparable to normal intracellular chemical concentrations. The physiological correlate to this biochemical data is the observation in *Necturus* proximal tubule that the rate of sodium transport responds to variations in the cytosolic sodium concentrations (Figure 33.8).[650] This suggested that under normal conditions the luminal cell membrane is the rate-limiting step for sodium transport. With respect to peritubular K^+, half-maximal ATPase activation occurs at concentrations under 1.0 mmol/l.[249,647] In lysed membrane preparations, the half-maximal saturation of ATPase activity, with respect to ATP, occurs at 0.4 mmol/l.[348,648] Thus, at normal levels of intracellular ATP (1–3 mmol/l) there should be little change in the rate of hydrolysis with variation of

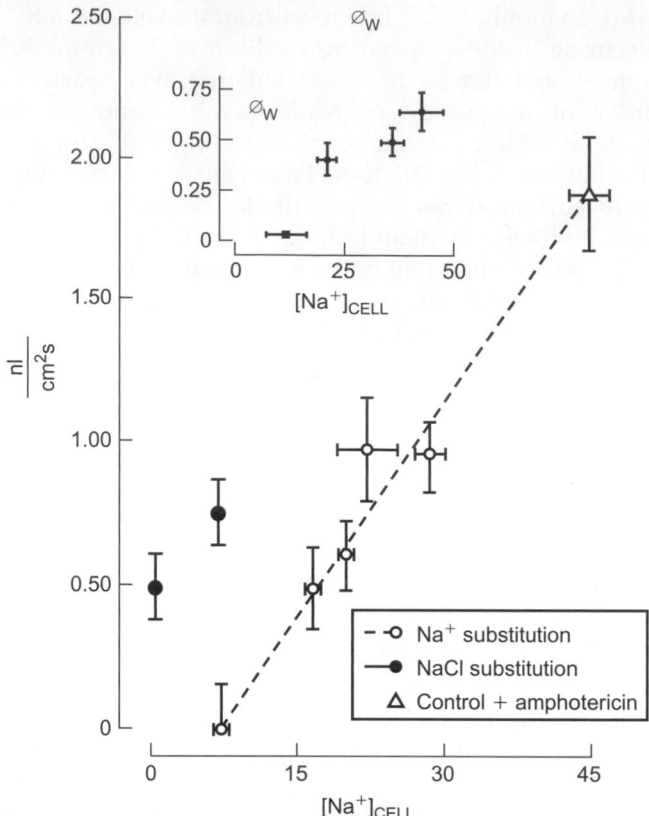

FIGURE 33.8 Transepithelial water flow, Φ_w, (or, equivalently, transepithelial sodium flux) is plotted as a function of intracellular sodium concentration in *Necturus* proximal tubules. Intracellular sodium is decreased from the control value (30 mM) by substitution of luminal Na^+ with tetramethylammonium (or substitution of luminal NaCl with mannitol — see inset); sodium is increased above control by the luminal application of amphotericin. (*From*[650], *with permission.*)

the ATP concentration. Nevertheless, in the intact tubule, partial inhibition of mitochondrial respiration produced proportional declines in cellular ATP and transport.[279] In a more extensive study, Soltoff and Mandel[646,648] found a linear correlation between cellular respiration and ion transport spanning a range of cellular ATP concentrations of 0–4 mmol/l. Thus, in the intact cell, it appears that ATP concentration can serve as an intermediary between transport and metabolism.

Coordination of Entry and Exit

Under normal circumstances, there may be several-fold variations in glomerular filtration rate to which the proximal tubule responds with nearly proportional changes in sodium reabsorption (*vide infra*). Although the mechanism underlying this glomerulotubular balance is not completely understood, the wide swings in the transcellular fluxes of sodium and bicarbonate pose

a threat to the proximal tubule cell, with respect to maintaining a viable cell volume and pH. Such challenges are not unique to proximal tubule, but threaten all transporting epithelial cells, particularly the gastro-intestinal epithelia, which experience swings in sodium-dependent glucose and amino acid uptake. In part, the kinetic response of Na,K-ATPase to cell Na^+ concentration will increase Na^+ exit (Figure 33.8), but this is generally insufficient to provide cellular homeostasis. Schultz and associates have emphasized the need for peritubular exit pathways to keep pace with luminal entry in order to preserve the integrity of cell composition and cell volume.[611,612,613] Beyond this, considerable attention has focused on the positive correlation between the potassium permeability of the peritubular membrane and the rate of epithelial sodium transport.[66,169] Increasing peritubular potassium conductance beyond enhancing potassium exit, should be expected to hyperpolarize the membrane, thus enhancing chloride and bicarbonate exit as well. The critical experimental observations were made in the epithelium of the small intestine of *Necturus*, from recordings with conventional and K^+-selective micro-electrodes.[262,280] It was found that with the addition of alanine to the luminal solution there was a prompt depolarization of the cell interior in association with a doubling of sodium reabsorption. Over a period of several minutes the K^+ conductance of the basolateral membrane increased, repolarizing the cell and further enhancing sodium transport. The parallel response of peritubular K^+-conductance with reabsorptive Na^+ flux was subsequently documented in frog proximal tubule, following the application of phenylalanine to the tubule lumen,[473,474] and in the mammalian proximal tubule with luminal application of glucose and alanine.[67,408,409] Direct examination of the K^+ channel of the peritubular membrane via patch-clamp has shown that the increase in K^+-conductance with luminal application of organics is the result of an increase in the open probability of this channel.[65] Thus, attention focused on identifying the signal by which luminal solute entry could activate these channels. The two principal candidates for modulators of peritubular exit have been cell volume and coupling of the Na, K-ATPase activity with K^+-channel open probability (pump-leak parallelism) via cytosolic ATP concentration. The signaling and transport effectors for cell volume regulation have been extensively reviewed.[406,407]

Examination of *Necturus* small intestine indicated that both increased sodium transport and hypotonic cell swelling had similar impact on the basolateral membrane. These observations led to the proposal that a transport-associated increase in cell volume might mediate the enhanced K^+-conductance found with increased Na^+ reabsorption.[412] It had been known since the experiments of MacRobbie and Ussing[446] that frog skin epithelium could volume-regulate. When the skin was placed in a hypotonic bathing solution, the initial swelling of the epithelial cells was followed by a gradual restoration of cell volume, presumably with the loss of cell solute. A critical observation was that hypotonic swelling of the toad urinary bladder was associated with increased basolateral membrane conductance.[210] In his analysis of cell volume regulation, Ussing[675] articulated the hypothesis that cell swelling was associated with the appearance or activation of both K^+ and Cl^- channels within the basolateral cell membrane, and loss of KCl via these pathways. With respect to proximal tubule, there has been considerable attention focused on the response of the peritubular membrane to increases in cell volume.[197,481,692] It was first noted in proximal tubules from the rabbit that exposure to a hypotonic solution was followed by a "volume regulatory decrease" (VRD).[170] This VRD was associated with a loss of cytosolic potassium.[261] In both *Necturus*[440] and rabbit tubules[378] cell swelling enhances peritubular K^+-conductance. Further, Kirk et al.[380] made the important observation that proximal tubule VRD occurred during isotonic swelling, where cell volume increased as a result of enhanced luminal Na^+ entry (rather than a hypotonic shock).

Proposed mechanisms of volume-induced K^+-conductance have included the direct effect of stretch on the K^+ channel or a volume-driven increase in cytosolic Ca^{2+}, with secondary channel activation. Patch-clamp studies have demonstrated stretch-activated K^+ channels within the peritubular membrane of amphibian proximal tubule,[362,582] as well as stretch-activated nonselective cation channels, which are permeable to Ca^{2+}.[207,208] In frog proximal tubule cells subjected to Na^+-alanine uptake, there is also evidence for stretch-activated anion channels.[475,567] In the mammalian tubule, stretch-activated K^+ channels have not been identified; however, it was observed that hypotonic cell swelling resulted in a rise in cytosolic calcium concentration.[462–464] This finding, in association with the appearance of Ca^{2+}-activated K^+ channels during hypotonic shock,[363] supplied a plausible mechanism for the increase in peritubular membrane K^+ permeability. In these studies (proximal straight tubules of the rabbit), blocking the rise in cytosolic calcium eliminated the hypotonic VRD. Questions were raised, however, by experiments in proximal convoluted tubule,[116] which indicated that VRD persists despite elimination of the rise in cell calcium. Most germane to the problem of coordinating entry and exit is the observation that when proximal convoluted tubules are exposed to luminal glucose and alanine, there is no significant increase in cytosolic calcium.[63] The importance of this result is the demonstration of differences in the cellular response to

hypotonic swelling, and that due to enhanced luminal entry. Indeed, even in amphibian tubules, differences between hypotonic and isotonic VRD have been discerned, with Na^+-coupled alanine uptake the VRD is independent of external Ca^{2+}.[486] Critical insight into the coupling of transport to peritubular K^+ permeability came with the discovery that the peritubular K^+ channel open probability was decreased by increases in cytosolic ATP concentration in the physiological range.[664] With application of luminal glucose and alanine to rabbit proximal convoluted tubule, sodium transport increased, cytosolic ATP decreased, and peritubular K^+ conductance increased in proportion to the decrease in ATP.[64,664] When ATP was applied exogenously, this effect of luminal organics to increase peritubular K^+ conductance was eliminated.[664] Conversely, application of an inhibitor of the Na,K-ATPase increased cytosolic ATP concentration, and thus decreased the open probability of the peritubular K^+ channel.[322]

One question which received relatively little attention in these investigations, was whether the observed changes in peritubular membrane K^+ permeability were sufficient to rationalize the observed volume homeostasis. Contributing to this homeostatic effect is the impact of increased K^+ permeability to hyperpolarize the peritubular membrane, and thus augment chloride and bicarbonate exit. These events are complicated by the fact that peritubular hyperpolarization will also enhance luminal entry via the Na^+-glucose cotransporter, and cytosolic acidification (increased peritubular HCO_3^- exit) will enhance luminal entry via the Na^+/H^+ exchanger. The quantitative issue of the sufficiency of the documented pump-leak parallelism to maintain cell volume was examined in a mathematical model of proximal tubule.[735] In those calculations, it was found that with realistic bounds on the electrical conductance of the peritubular membrane, variation of K^+ permeability by itself does not provide adequate homeostasis for proximal tubule. Satisfactory volume regulation was achieved, however, when the activity of the peritubular Na^+–$3HCO_3^-$ co-transporter was allowed to vary directly in response to changes in the rate of luminal Na^+/H^+ exchange. Evidence for the coordination of these two transporters will be considered below. There are data regarding the anion lost in association with K^+ during cell swelling, and it appears to show some variability among species. In *Necturus*[440] and mouse tubules,[691] omission of bicarbonate impairs VRD and cell swelling is associated with enhanced peritubular HCO_3^- conductance.[690] In the straight proximal tubule of rabbit, however, removal of chloride impaired VRD, while omission of bicarbonate or the application of SITS had no inhibitory effect.[743] In the proximal convoluted tubule of the rabbit, hypotonic swelling increases both K^+-conductance and Cl^--conductance of the peritubular cell membrane.[744,745] An intriguing examination of cell volume was undertaken in primary culture of mouse proximal tubule cells, comparing wild-type with knockouts of the peritubular K^+ channel, KCNE1.[47] The wild-type cells showed VRD with the appearance of swelling-induced K^+ and Cl^- channels; the knockouts showed neither K^+ nor Cl^- currents during swelling. When knockout cells were transfected with KCNE1, both swelling-activated K^+ and Cl^- currents were restored. These experiments demonstrated a close functional linkage between the two channels allowing a coordinated response to a volume challenge.

THE PARACELLULAR PATHWAY

The Lateral Intercellular Space

It had long been recognized that certain epithelia, such as gallbladder or small intestine, could transport water from lumen to blood against an adverse osmotic gradient. Curran[167] and Durbin[185] hypothesized that metabolically-driven salt transport into an intraepithelial compartment could drive transepithelial water flow, if the membranes bounding this compartment had suitable permeability properties. Subsequently, several groups of investigators[244,674,746] proposed that the space between the basolateral cell membrane and the basement membrane qualifies as the "middle compartment" within the epithelium. Salt transport into the interspace across the lateral cell membrane would

induce an osmotic water flow across this membrane. Accumulation of salt and water within the interspace would then generate local hydrostatic pressure, sufficient to drive this solution out across the permeable basement membrane and connective tissue. This proposal identifies the lateral intercellular space as part of the pathway for the bulk of transepithelial water flow. Morphologic observations on gall bladder,[366,660] intestine,[752] Necturus proximal tubule,[76,456,457] and the isolated perfused rabbit proximal tubule[659] have all been confirmatory, showing interspace dilatation with reabsorptive flow and interspace collapse with cessation or reversal of flow.

It is also a secure finding that along the length of the proximal tubule the luminal sodium concentration differs little, if at all, from that in peritubular blood. This means that water reabsorption must occur in a constant proportion to sodium reabsorption. Windhager et al.[759] demonstrated that in Necturus proximal tubule the sodium flux drives the net water reabsorption. These investigators introduced into the tubule lumen solutions isosmotic with plasma, but with varying sodium concentration, in order to obtain a wide range of values for the sodium flux. Over the course of the experiment, the luminal osmolality did not change, indicating a negligible external driving force in the passive movement of water. Nevertheless, a plot of the net water flux as a function of the net sodium flux shows a line, the slope of which indicates that transport occurred isotonically (Figure 33.9a). A similar series of experiments was performed in rat proximal convoluted tubule by Morel and Murayama.[484] They again verified

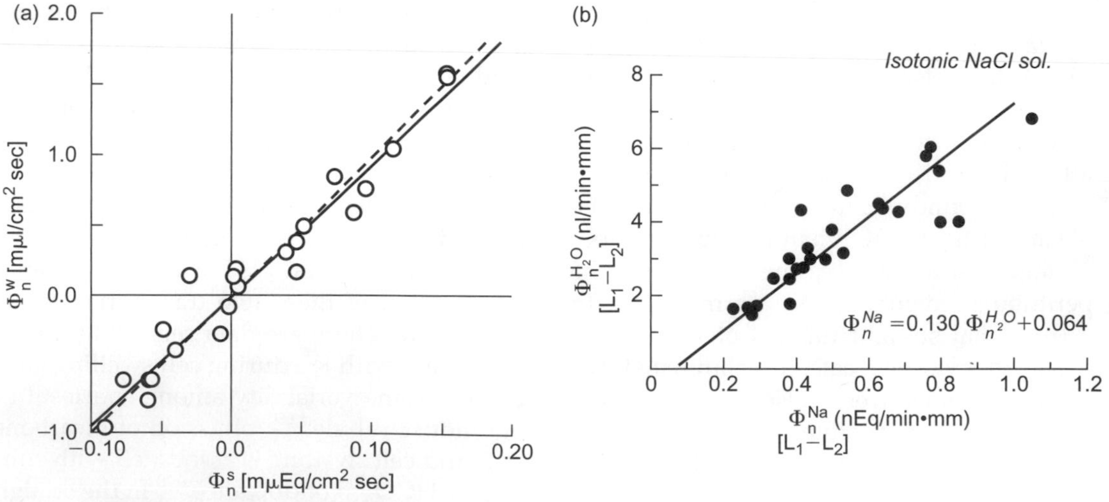

FIGURE 33.9 (a) Correlation of net solute flux, Φ_n^s, and net water flux, Φ_n^w, across the perfused proximal tubule of *Necturus*. The least squares line of regression for the data points (solid line) is not statistically different from the line through the origin (dashed line), whose slope is that for isotonic water reabsorption. (*From[759], with permission.*) (b) Correlation of net sodium flux, Φ_n^{Na}, and net water flux, Φ_n^{H2O}, occurring between two collection sites (L1 and L2) of a perfused rat proximal tubule. The line of regression for the data points (solid line) indicates isotonic transport of sodium. (*From[484], with permission.*)

over a wide range of luminal sodium concentrations (and sodium fluxes) that the flux of sodium determined the flow of water. Further, the water flow occurred so as to maintain the lumen isotonic to plasma (Figure 33.9b).

The dependence of isotonic water reabsorption on sodium reabsorption has been referred to as "coupled water transport" to distinguish it from water flux referable to a demonstrable transepithelial osmotic gradient. This coupled water transport has been rationalized in an analysis of the lateral intercellular space as an intraepithelial middle compartment.[731,736,737] As in Figure 33.10, the lateral interspace is represented with a tight junction (J_A), basement membrane (J_B), and lateral cell membranes (J_L). A reference osmolality, C_0, is assumed (such as that of the blood), and the osmolalities of the interspace, $C_0 + C_E$, of the lumen and cell interior, $C_0 + C_M$, and of the peritubular solution, $C_0 + C_S$, are written in terms of increments above or below the reference. Each membrane, α, (α = A, B or L) has water and solute permeabilities $L_{p\alpha}$ and H_α, and a reflection coefficient σ_α. Transmembrane fluxes for volume and solute are denoted by $J_{v\alpha}$ and $J_{s\alpha}$. Assumptions may be made which simplify the analysis, but which maintain most of the important features of the lateral interspace model: (1) the tight junction is relatively impermeable, $L_{pA} = H_A = 0$; (2) the lateral cell membrane is relatively solute impermeable, $H_L = 0$, and $\sigma_L = 1$; but (3) there is fixed solute transport across the lateral membrane at a rate, N; and (4) the reflection coefficient for the interspace basement membrane and underlying tissue is zero, $\sigma_B = 0$. With these assumptions the transport equations for each membrane may be written, for volume and solute flows:

$$J_v = J_{vL} = L_{pL}[(P_M - P_E) + RT(C_E - C_M)] = J_{vB} = L_{pB}[(P_E - P_S)]$$
$$(33.9)$$

$$J_s = J_{sL} = N = J_{sB} = J_{vB}C_0 + H_B(C_E - C_S) \qquad (33.10)$$

where P_M, P_E, and P_S are the hydrostatic pressures in the respective compartments. The equalities, $J_v = J_{vL} = J_{vB}$ and $J_s = J_{sL} = J_{sB}$, reflect the fact that in the steady-state, mass entry across the lateral membrane must be equal to that leaving the channel mouth. It

may be noted that an additional approximation has been introduced into Eq. (33.10), in which the reference concentration, C_0, is identified as the mean basement membrane concentration.

When the mass balance relations are used to eliminate the unknowns P_E and C_E, from Eqs (33.10) and (33.11), one obtains an expression for transepithelial volume flow:

$$J_v = L_p(P_M - P_S) + RTL_p\left(C_S - C_M + \frac{N}{H_B}\right) \qquad (33.11)$$

in which the epithelial water permeability, L_p, is given by the expression:

$$L_p = \frac{L_{pLB}H_B}{H_B + RTL_{pLB}C_0} \quad \text{where } L_{pLB} = \frac{L_{pL}L_{pB}}{L_{pL} + L_{pB}} \qquad (33.12)$$

Equation (33.12) describes the volume flow of the whole epithelial model in terms of the permeability parameters of the component membranes. It shows the volume flow to be a linear function of the pressure and osmolality of the bathing solutions. When there are exactly equal bathing media ($C_M = C_S = P_M = P_S = 0$), there is still transepithelial volume flow:

$$J_v^a = RTL_p\frac{N}{H_B} = RTL_p\hat{C} \qquad (33.13)$$

This "active water transport," referenced in Eq. (33.9), thus arises naturally as a component of volume flow driven by intraepithelial solute–solvent coupling, i.e., the empirically described "coupled water transport." It increases with larger rates of solute transport and decreases when there is little solute trapping by the basement membrane (large H_B). The virtual concentration, $\hat{C} = N/H_B$, represents the strength of transport of the epithelium, in that volume flow just ceases when the osmolality of the luminal solution is raised by this amount. For a proximal tubule model one must also verify isotonic transport. In approximate terms, this means that only a small decrement in luminal osmolality is required for the reabsorbate tonicity to be equal to that of the peritubular fluid. Formally, one seeks the osmotic deviation, C^*, such that if

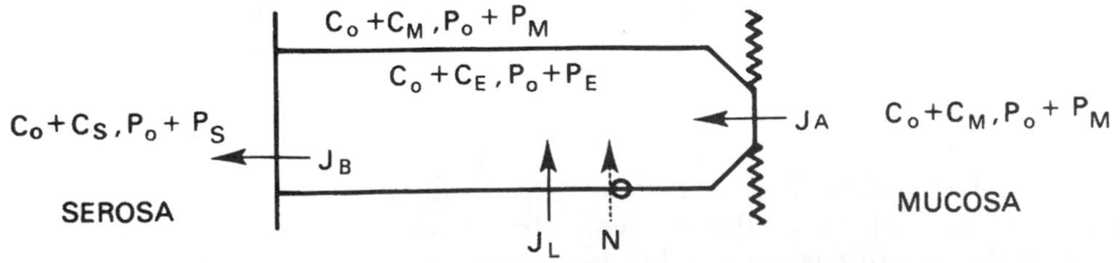

FIGURE 33.10 **Schematic representation of the lateral intercellular space.** The cell and mucosal medium are assumed to be at the same osmolality and pressure. (From[736], with permission.)

$C_S \approx C_0$, and $C_M \approx C_0 - C^*$, then $J_s/J_v \approx C_0$. This corresponds to solving the equation:

$$C_0 = \frac{J_s}{J_v} = \frac{N}{RTL_p(\hat{C} + C_s - C_M)} = \frac{N}{RTL_p(\hat{C} + C^*)} \quad (33.14)$$

which has the solution:

$$C^* = \frac{N}{RTL_{pLB}C_0} \quad (33.15)$$

When the luminal osmolality is decreased by the amount C*, transport is isotonic to plasma. Provided C* is at most a few mOsm/l, there will be no experimentally-detectable difference between lumen and blood. Transport is generally considered isotonic if C* is within 2% of C_0. It should also be noted that isotonic transport depends only upon the water permeabilities of the epithelial membranes. The notion of solute trapping within the interspace, which was crucial to uphill water transport, is really unimportant in the dynamics of isotonic transport.

Perhaps one of the confusing features of transport isotonicity is that the relevant membrane permeabilities may be quite different from the whole epithelial water permeability that is actually measured. The expression for L_p (Eq. (33.12)) shows that both water permeabilities and solute trapping effects are involved. Intuitively, this corresponds to the fact that water flow across the lateral membrane, driven by a hypotonic lumen, will tend to dilute the interspace and hence, negate some of the osmotic flow. The interspace dilution will be smaller for larger basement membrane permeabilities. This "intraepithelial solute polarization" effect is an inescapable feature of the lateral interspace. The expression for L_p may be rewritten:

$$\frac{L_p}{L_{pLB}} = \frac{1}{1 + \hat{C}/C^*} \quad (33.16)$$

which shows that to the extent that an epithelium can transport against a gradient (large $\hat{C}$), and yet reabsorb water isotonically (small C*), the observed epithelial L_p must be substantially smaller than the cell membrane water permeabilities.

In Table 33.4, this model is applied to the data of Tables 33.1 and 33.2 for proximal tubules of rat and rabbit. The upper panel shows rates of isotonic reabsorption, along with the measured water permeabilities. For the rat, two values for L_p are given, corresponding to the older[672] and later determinations.[536] A value for the equilibrium deviation from isotonicity (C*) has been assumed to be at 2% of the ambient osmolality. At least in the rat, this is comparable to experimental determinations.[265,432] The quantities in the lower panel of the table are derived from the

TABLE 33.4   Application of the Interspace Model to Proximal Tubule

		Rat PCT	Rat PCT	Rabbit PCT
J_s	(nOsm/s · cm²)	19	19	9.0
J_v	(nl/s · cm²)	65	65	30
$RTL_p \times 10^4$	(cm/s · Osm)	44	22	63
P_f	(cm/s)	0.24	0.12	0.35
c*	(mOsm/L)	6	6	6
$RTL_{LB} \times 10^4$	(cm/s · Osm)	105	105	50
$\hat{c}$	(mOsm/L)	8	23	—
$J_v{}^a$	(nl/s · cm²)	35	51	
$H_B \times 10^4$	(cm/s)	24	8.3	—

experimental data using the model equations. The estimate of cell membrane water permeability required for isotonic transport, RTL_{pLB}, is just J_v/C^*. If the value of RTL_{pLB} computed for the rabbit tubule is referred to the luminal and lateral cell membranes in series, each of 36 cm²/cm²,[738] then one obtains a unit membrane water permeability, consistent with direct estimates, using rapid video techniques.[136,741] In theory, the AQP1 knockout mouse, deficient in water channels from both luminal and peritubular cell membranes, provides a pure decrease in the parameter RTL_{pLB}. The experimental observations in this knockout were an overall epithelial water permeability (L_p) about 22% that of wild-type (Schnermann et al., 1998), and luminal hypotonicity (C*) about four-fold greater than wild-type.[677] In terms of the model developed here, and with the assumption that active Na⁺ transport is little changed in the knockout mouse, the change in C* should reflect a 78% reduction in L_{pLB}. The fact that the fractional change in overall L_p is comparable indicates that in the mouse, one would expect little intraepithelial solute polarization, and thus little capacity for water reabsorption against an adverse osmotic gradient. The discrepancy between the overall epithelial water permeability and that of the cell membranes in series, allows the calculation of the strength of transport, $\hat{C}$ in Eq. (33.13).

Williams and Schafer[754] have emphasized that the middle compartment need not be the true lateral interspace, but could actually be the cortical interstitial space. In their model of rat proximal tubule, the salt permeability of the peritubular capillary corresponds to the term H_B used here. With estimates of cell membrane water permeability and capillary solute permeability comparable to those of the first column in Table 33.4, they also predicted that solute polarization would reduce the epithelial L_p to about 50% of that of the cell membranes. For the rat, the discrepancy between L_p and L_{pLB} requires that active water transport be substantial, i.e., from 55–80% of the isotonic flux (Table 33.4). In the more detailed models of proximal tubule epithelium which have been developed there is considerable disagreement in the estimates of coupled water flux, ranging from predominant[323,324,583,657] to negligible.[14,595,707,753] In a simulation of the rat proximal tubule, in which both isotonic transport and the whole epithelial L_p were reproduced faithfully, coupled water flux was estimated to be about two-thirds of the isotonic transport rate.[727] This corresponded to a strength of transport of 23 mOsm/l of NaCl. There are few experimental studies examining uphill water transport by the proximal tubule. Bomsztyk and Wright[105] reported that in rat tubules, microperfused with a low bicarbonate (10 mEq/l) luminal solution, an additional 30 mmol/L of mannitol was required within the lumen to nullify volume reabsorption. Although the interpretation of this experiment was complicated by the presence of several forces favoring water reabsorption (anion gradients and protein oncotic forces), the findings suggested a substantial component of solute-linked water reabsorption by the rat proximal tubule. Green et al.[267] examined the doubly perfused rat proximal tubule, specifically with the aim of determining the presence of active water transport. Using low bicarbonate solutions in both tubule and capillary perfusions, an isotonic luminal solution yielded reabsorptive water flux of 1 nl/mm · min. Varying only the luminal NaCl concentration allowed the determination of volume flux as a linear function of the transepithelial salt gradient (Figure 33.11). Regression analysis indicated that a luminal osmolality between 13 and 29 mosm/l (depending on peritubular protein concentration) greater than in peritubular blood would be required to null volume reabsorption. These experiments document active water transport by rat proximal tubule, quantitatively close to model predictions, and thus provide support for solute–solvent coupling within the lateral intercellular space.

The interspace outlet permeability, H_B, is a parameter of critical importance. It directly determines the strength of transport (Eq. (33.13)), and when this solute permeability is sufficiently small ($H_B < RTL_{pLB}C_0$) it is dominant in determining the epithelial L_p (Eq. (33.12)). Persson and Spring[525] examined the subepithelial tissue of *Necturus* gallbladder and found that it has only about twice the resistivity of free solution. They argue, therefore, that any important limitation to solute exit from the interspace must derive from the small area of the lateral interspace as it abuts the basement membrane. More recent experiments using photoactivation of caged fluorescent dyes have indicated that solute

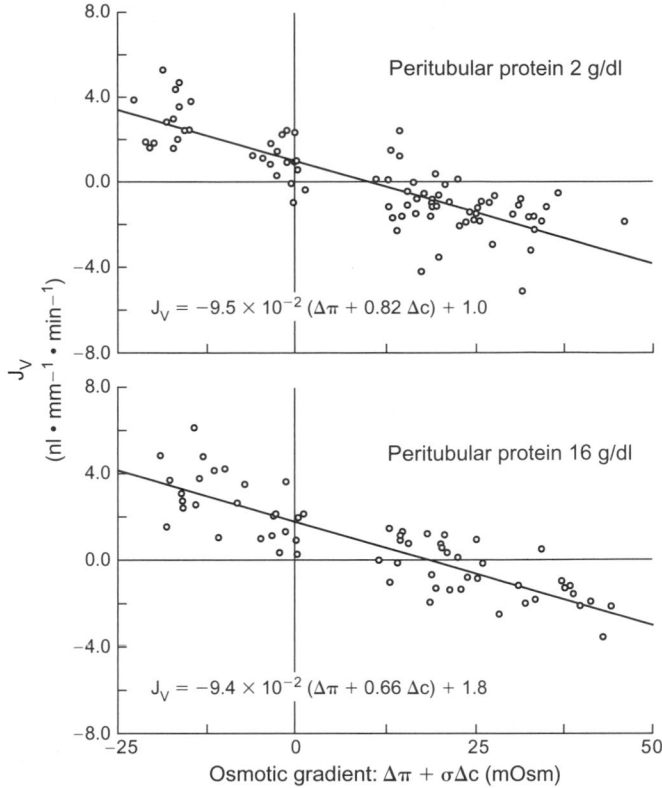

FIGURE 33.11 Volume flux as a function of transepithelial osmotic driving force in rat proximal tubules, in which both lumen and peritubular capillaries have been perfused. Each point corresponds to a single tubule perfusion. The abcissa is the transepithelial osmotic driving force, $\Delta\pi + \sigma\Delta C$; the ordinate is the measured volume flux, J_v. For each protein concentration, the line shown is the graph of Eq. (33.1), so that the ordinate intercept, $J_v{}^a$, is the coupled water transport (water flux in the absence of a transepithelial driving force.) The abcissa intercept is the concentration of the luminal impermeant required to null volume reabsorption. (*From[267], with permission.*)

diffusion within the lateral interspace is comparable to that in free solution.[770] Such had been the assumption in analytical estimates of the electrical resistance of the interspace fluid of proximal tubule from ultrastructural data. Mathias,[453] using data from the rabbit[739] estimated interspace resistance at about 4% that of tight junction, and Maunsbach and Boulpaep[458] calculated 4–21% of epithelial resistance may be attributed to the interspace. Welling et al.[740] have indicated that beyond the limitations of interspace width, interdigitating cellular elements at the base of the interspace may provide the most important barrier to mass exit. With reference to Table 33.4, Eq. (33.13) defines the outlet permeability required by the model ($H_B = N/\hat{C} = J_s/\hat{C}$). For the rat, H_B is predicted to be $8.3–24 \times 10^{-4}$ cm/s. When interpreted as an electrical resistance (Eq. (33.4)), this is 0.4–1.1 ohm · cm^2, and is not incompatible with the whole epithelial resistance of 5–10 ohm · cm^2.

The Tight Junction

The tight junction of the proximal tubule provides a low resistance pathway between the luminal solution and the lateral intercellular space. Morphologically, the tight junctions have been identified with the "zonula occludentes," visualized in electron microscopy, in which there is no detectable space between the epithelial cells. Freeze-fracture techniques indicated the fibrillar structure of these junctions, with relatively few fibrils present in the junctions of the proximal tubule.[156,539] In epithelia with greater electrical resistance, there are, correspondingly, a greater number of fibrils.[155,156] The TJ strands may be viewed as chains of particles, with typical spacing of these particles, as seen in freeze-fracture electron micrographs, being in the order of 20 nm.[509] The structural composition of these strands has been deciphered slowly.[477,608] Occludin was the first of the transmembrane proteins to be associated with the tight junction,[228] and to be implicated in a functional role in junctional permeability.[461] An important advance came with the identification of claudin-1 and claudin-2 within the junctional strands.[226,229] When claudin-2 was introduced into the Madin–Darby canine kidney (MDCK) cells, a conversion from a very "tight" junction to a "leaky" junction was observed.[227] This suggested that claudin-2 could be responsible for the leakiness of the MDCK epithelium and the formation of pores between apposing TJ strands. Indeed, when the claudins expressed in MDCK cells are selectively modified, the paracellular conductance of small electrolytes can be modulated, including the anion/cation selectivity preference.[159] The sodium conductance of tight junctions containing claudin-2 can also be modulated by changes in ambient calcium concentration.[785,786] Claudin-2 exists throughout the proximal tubule, and in a contiguous early segment of the thin descending limb of long-looped nephrons in mouse kidney.[196] In mice with deletion of the claudin-2 gene, the proximal tubules have a 2.5-fold increase in electrical resistance, due to a decrease in tight junctional Na^+ permeability.[495] Although these mice have normal renal function, they do excrete a Na^+ infusion more rapidly than wild-type mice. Of note, the high Na^+ permeability of proximal tubules appears as a maturational event, and is not present in the neonatal period in which natriuresis figures prominently.[57,546] Apparently, claudin-2 expression of proximal tubule is subject to modulation by changes in metabolic status, and in the rat is downregulated during metabolic acidosis.[37] If the impact of decreased claudin-2 is to increase distal NaCl delivery, this might be expected to enhance the distal nephron functions of K^+ and net acid excretion.

Like proximal tubule, other leaky epithelia (gallbladder, small intestine) also transport large volumes of salt solutions isotonically, and this encouraged speculation as to the function of the tight junction in isotonic water transport. A number of mathematical simulations of proximal tubule addressed this issue,[323,324,583,651,657,736,737] but have simply not provided an answer as to why electrical leakiness should correlate with the ability to transport isotonically. The fraction of reabsorptive water flow which actually traverses the tight junction is also unknown. Arguments in favor of transjunctional water flow in proximal tubules have included: substantial solvent drag of ionic species[16,106,224,266,308,361,596]; the appearance of streaming potentials with the application of an impermeant osmotic agent[164,221,661]; and ionic permeabilities roughly in proportion to their mobility in free solution.[392] None of these findings, however, provides proof of tight junctional water flow. Either streaming potentials or solvent drag can come as the result of a solute polarization effect within the interspace. With solute polarization, water flux across the cell and through the lateral interspace alters interspace ion concentrations, thus promoting either a diffusion potential or diffusive flux across the tight junction. For a true streaming potential, water flux across the tight junction must be present and carry either an anion or cation preferentially. This issue was addressed by Tripathi and Boulpaep[661] in their measurements of streaming potentials across the proximal tubule of *Ambystoma*. With the application of peritubular sucrose, a lumen-positive potential appeared, consistent with either a streaming potential or interspace NaCl depletion (and an anion-selective junction). When ambient chloride was replaced by cyclamate, the junction became cation-selective and its total conductance substantially decreased. Repeat application of peritubular sucrose produced the same lumen-positive potential, now inconsistent with a diffusion potential. With respect to the solvent drag measurements, it is undisputed that intraepithelial solute polarization may produce an overall reflection coefficient that is substantially less than that of the cell and tight junction, taken in parallel. The question is thus a quantitative one, as to whether one could construct a model of proximal tubule with just the right solute polarization to yield realistic reflection coefficients as well as a proper L_p. So far, this does not appear possible. For the rat, the data of Frömter et al.[224] were used to determine composite interspace models for this epithelium.[730] It was found that all of the acceptable interspace models required substantial tight junction convective chloride flux.

An apparently direct argument for tight junctional water flux in rabbit tubules came from Whittembury and associates,[135,253,748] whose estimate of the water permeability of the peritubular cell membrane indicated a transcellular water permeability less than the overall epithelial L_p. The unit membrane water permeability obtained with this technique has received confirmation in a vesicle preparation,[687,689] although higher values have also been obtained.[683] Strong evidence for tight junction water flow was also obtained in the rat, with observation of substantial convective entrainment of sucrose, despite relatively small diffusional flux.[747] The small diffusive component effectively rules out interspace solute polarization as a confounding factor. Nevertheless, an objection had been raised by Rector and Berry,[80,553] who presented calculations based on pore theory which indicated that the tight junctions were not large enough to allow passage of a significant fraction of transepithelial water flow. Subsequently, Preisig and Berry[536] measured the permeation of sucrose and mannitol across the rat proximal tubule. Applying the Renkin equations to their data, they computed the dimensions of the "sucrose pore," and indicated that it could be responsible for at most 2% of the tubule water permeability. It was acknowledged, however, that a smaller paracellular pore that did not admit the sucrose molecule could account for up to one-third of the water permeability. An important contribution to this discussion came with the suggestion of Fraser and Baines[213] that the tight junction might be more realistically represented as a fiber matrix, rather than as a collection of pores. The critical feature of the fiber matrix equations is that for a given solute permeability, the water permeability can be substantially greater than that predicted from the Renkin equations. It was demonstrated that this formulation was compatible with the known permeabilities of rat proximal tubule.[213] Alternatively, Guo et al.[281] reproduced a pore-theoretic representation of the tight junction, utilizing two pores to fit the mannitol and sucrose data of Preisig and Berry.[536] In this model, the two pores were given anatomic correlates: the small pore was referred to gaps in the apposition of claudins molecules, while the large pore corresponded to breaks within a strand, occupying about 2% of its length. With these dimensions, tight junction water permeability was predicted to be about 21% of transepithelial water permeability.

With the tight junction established as a route for reabsorptive solute flux, a hypothesis was advanced that the junction might be an important site for the regulation of proximal sodium reabsorption. Lewy and Windhager found that in rats, both with and without acutely elevated renal venous pressure, there was a direct correlation between single nephron filtration fraction and proximal tubule sodium reabsorption.[418] Given that lower filtration fractions would result in reduced protein oncotic pressure within the peritubular capillaries, they surmised that this would lead to reduced capillary uptake of fluid from the renal interstitium and lateral intercellular space and, hence, elevated interspace pressure. This, in turn, would result in increased backflux of the sodium, already transported into the interspace, that is, backflux across the tight junction into the lumen. At the time of this proposal, attention had focused on intrarenal mechanisms responsible for the natriuresis of extracellular fluid volume expansion with saline.[187,383,384] Dirks et al.[173] had shown that proximal tubule sodium reabsorption was depressed following saline expansion. In the dog, the ability to reverse the natriuresis with infusion of hyperoncotic albumin indicated that peritubular oncotic pressure could influence sodium reabsorption, and Earley and his associates[186,451] had proposed that renal interstitial pressure might be an intermediate variable. Subsequent micropuncture experiments in the rat documented enhancement of proximal sodium reabsorption by peritubular protein.[113,114,385] In particular, the depression of proximal tubule sodium reabsorption which occurs with saline infusion could be reversed by perfusion of the efferent arteriole with a solution whose protein concentration is comparable to that under control conditions.[115,649] It has been well-documented that changes in the ambient protein concentration alter sodium reabsorption by the perfused proximal tubule. In the isolated perfused rabbit proximal tubule, Imai and Kokko found enhancement of sodium reabsorption with increasing concentrations of protein in the bathing solution.[331] In the absence of peritubular colloid, the permeability of the tubule to sucrose was increased. In the rat kidney, Green et al.[269] studied proximal tubule volume reabsorption when albumin was present in varying concentrations in luminal or peritubular capillary perfusates. Figure 33.12 shows the asymmetry (luminal versus peritubular protein) and the non-linearity of the reabsorptive enhancement by peritubular colloid. This implies that the colloid effect is not a simple oncotic force, such as might be reckoned using Eq. (33.1) and the known water permeability. It does suggest that the increase in peritubular capillary albumin changes the "state" of the epithelium to make active sodium transport more efficient at driving volume reabsorption. A comparable asymmetric effect of protein on salt reabsorption was also documented in rabbit proximal convoluted tubule in vitro.[332]

It is a tenet of the backflux hypothesis that the action of peritubular protein is mediated through an effect on renal interstitial pressure and hence, pressures within lateral intercellular spaces. In substantiation of this point, decreases in peritubular capillary oncotic pressure, which occur with saline volume expansion, result in increases in renal interstitial pressure (as least as assessed by renal subcapsular pressures).[515,516,548,629]

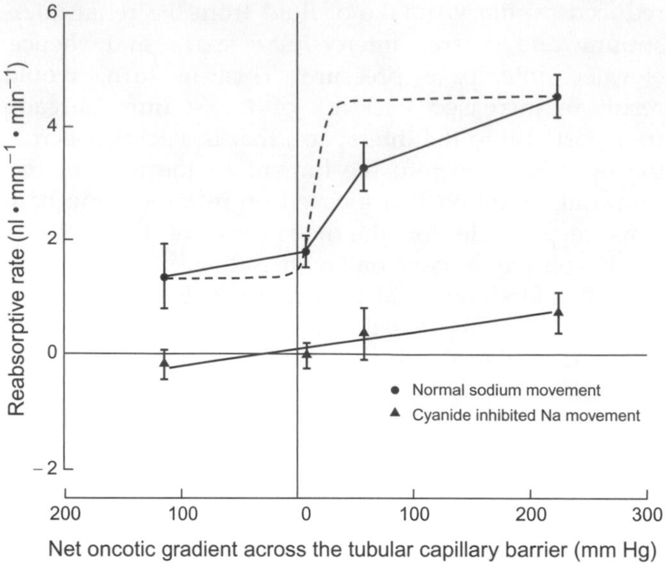

FIGURE 33.12 **Effects of transtubular oncotic pressure gradients on volume reabsorption by rat proximal tubule**. Both tubule lumen and peritubular capillaries are perfused with identical Ringer's solutions to which variable amounts of albumin have been added. In the tubules perfused with cyanide (lower curve) spontaneous sodium reabsorption has ceased and the effect of oncotic pressure is blunted. *(From[269], with permission.)* The dashed curve represents the prediction of an interspace model in which the tight junction is compliant. *(From[732].)*

Prevention of this rise in interstitial pressure by applying a renal artery clamp also prevents the fall in absolute proximal reabsorption associated with saline expansion.[212,327] Further, the deliberate increase of renal interstitial pressure by the instillation of fluid decreases proximal sodium reabsorption and produces a natriuresis.[260,287] Morphologic examination of the proximal tubule of the rat[75,140] has shown progressive dilation of the lateral intercellular space, as well as opening of the interspace at the tubule basement membrane, with increments of saline volume expansion. The precise mechanism of sodium "backflux" across the tight junction remains to be delineated. One possibility is that with increased interstitial pressure there is junctional widening and diffusion of sodium from interspace to lumen. A small decrease in epithelial electrical resistance has been documented with saline-loading in the rat.[621] In the rat, mannitol injected into the proximal tubule does not permeate and is completely recovered in the urine. However, with massive saline diuresis, as with renal venous constriction or elevated ureteral pressure, a significant fraction of the mannitol traversed the tubular epithelium into the systemic circulation.[442] Similarly, sucrose infused into the systemic circulation may permeate the proximal tubule epithelium during periods of renal vein constriction.[42] Perhaps the strongest objection to the view that sodium diffuses back

across widened junctions is that, at least in the rat proximal tubule, the electrodiffusive force on sodium is likely to be in the reabsorptive direction. A second possibility is that backflux of sodium across the tight junction occurs by convective flow. The tight junctions of the leaky epithelia are very sensitive to hydrostatic pressures applied from the contraluminal side. In rabbit gallbladder[684] and *Necturus* proximal tubule,[259,301] contraluminal pressures drive substantially greater volume flow across the epithelium than an equal luminal pressure. In *Necturus*, volume expansion decreases the proximal tubule NaCl reflection coefficient.[77] In these experiments, it is likely that junctional structure is distorted, forming relatively large pores with negligible sieving of solute, as both salt and water return to the lumen. Indeed, in the meticulous study of van Os et al.[684] on the rabbit gallbladder, serosal pressures drove water back into the lumen at a rate 30-fold greater than would have been predicted from the osmotic water permeability of this epithelium. This occurred with little change in diffusional solute permeability. These investigators suggested that their results were most compatible with a serosal pressure effect of opening up relatively large water channels at a small number of junctional loci. Convective backflux across the tight junction of rat proximal tubule has been invoked by Ramsey et al.[550] to explain their observation that the luminal appearance of lanthanum deposited within the renal interstitium is enhanced during saline volume expansion.

The mathematical model of the lateral interspace, set out in the previous section, cannot represent the peritubular oncotic effects on sodium reabsorption considered above.[728] However, when this model is extended by inclusion of a compliant tight junction, a regulatory effect of peritubular Starling forces can be simulated.[732] In this case, tight junction "compliance" signifies that both junctional salt and water permeability increase, and the salt reflection coefficient decreases in response to small pressure differences from lateral interspace to tubule lumen. Although these compliance properties were completely empirical, they provided a model in which decreases in peritubular protein (which increased interspace hydrostatic pressure) opened the tight junction, and produced a secretory salt flux. This backflux was a combination of both diffusive and convective terms, and did not specifically require either component to dominate. When this model was used to simulate the experiments of, Green et al.[269] the model predictions were consistent with the observed reabsorption. The predicted fluxes appear as the dashed curve in Figure 33.12. In this model of the tight junction, once the interspace pressure falls below that of the lumen, the junction is closed and junctional properties are fixed. The consequence of junction closure in the simulation of Figure 33.12 is that beyond a certain value of peritubular protein, one expects little influence of peritubular Starling forces on volume reabsorption. In this light, it is not surprising that a number of investigators found no significant influence of peritubular protein on proximal reabsorption,[40,161,315] and even interstitial Starling forces could correlate poorly with sodium transport.[103,472,665] Consistent with this view are the observations by Ott et al.[516] that in the dog, hyperoncotic albumin infusion increased proximal reabsorption only in the previously volume-expanded group. In the isolated perfused proximal tubule of the rabbit, several reports have indicated a lack of effect of peritubular bath protein on paracellular permeability.[79,82,410] Pirie and Potts[529] explored the influence of pressure gradients in this preparation. They found that elevations in intraluminal hydrostatic pressures abolished the effect of peritubular protein to enhance sodium reabsorption. Although they did not offer a specific explanation for their data, the present considerations might suggest that with higher luminal pressures, the tight junction always stayed closed.

REGULATION OF PROXIMAL NaCl TRANSPORT

Convergence on NHE3

Considerable attention has been given to understanding proximal sodium reabsorption in relation to neural and hormonal signals, and to changes in glomerular filtration rate. The luminal membrane Na^+/H^+ exchanger is responsible for both $NaHCO_3$ reabsorption and a substantial component of $NaCl$ reabsorption. This, along with the fact that luminal entry is rate-limiting for transcellular sodium flux, renders the antiporter ideally suited as a regulatory site for proximal reabsorption. Indeed, a coherent picture has emerged in which every signal that regulates proximal Na^+ reabsorption converges on NHE3. A remarkable diversity of pathways has been identified as proximate modifiers of the antiporter.[176,177,243,270,300,478,717] Regulatory signals to NHE3 converge on the carboxy-terminal tail of the transporter, and Donowitz and Li[176] have organized the NHE3 binding partners and signals anatomically, according to their position on this tail (Figure 33.13). Of these, the most important is inhibition by cAMP-dependent phosphorylation of the antiporter by protein kinase A (PKA).[351,479,722] Liu and Cogan[430] examined bicarbonate reabsorption by the S1 segment of rat proximal tubule following a variety of maneuvers designed to affect cellular cAMP concentration. When luminal appearance of cAMP is used as a measure of

cytosolic concentration, the correlation with bicarbonate transport over nearly a 10-fold range is striking (Figure 33.14). The acute nature of these experimental maneuvers must be emphasized, since the impact of chronic stimulation by cAMP is different.[131] Beyond cAMP effects, NHE3 activity is also phosphorylated acutely by the calcium—phospholipid-dependent protein kinase, PKC,[354,470,720,721,750] by direct signals from G-proteins,[6] and perhaps by a tyrosine kinase.[247] Beyond transporter phosphorylation, rapid regulation of sodium reabsorption via NHE3 is achieved through cellular machinery that makes NHE3 physically available within the brush border membrane, including insertion and retrieval of transporter from subapical vesicle pools.[104,199,307,790] Ultimately, chronic NHE3 regulation must be referable to the protein synthetic machinery.[317,130,248]

Of the signals that impact NHE3 flux, the first to be studied was the decrease in Na^+/H^+ exchange via cAMP-dependent phosphorylation, initially as a consequence of parathyroid hormone (PTH)-binding. This signal pathway is critical to the action of angiotensin II and dopamine, and will be considered below. The PTH effect was documented in isolated perfused proximal tubules,[171,293] and paralleled the effect of cAMP when examined in tubule suspensions[174] or brush border membrane vesicles.[351] A major advance came with the identification of a protein cofactor, NHERF-1 (NHE regulatory factor), which is required for cAMP phosphorylation of NHE3.[723,726,792] Ultimately, a number of such regulatory proteins have been identified whose role has come to be recognized as scaffolding molecules, for which transporter-binding occurs by virtue of their tertiary structure, termed PDZ domains.[93,175,176,716] The OK cell is a proximal tubule cell line from opossum kidney that expresses NHE3 and NHERF-1, and which displays cAMP-dependent inhibition of NHE3. This cell served as a preparation in which to demonstrate the physical link between NHE3 and NHERF-1, as well as a link between NHERF-1 and ezrin.[405] Ezrin is a protein kinase A (PKA) anchoring protein, as well as a linking molecule to the actin cytoskeleton. The scheme that emerged was that of a multiprotein signal complex, in which NHERF and ezrin brought PKA and NHE3 into proximity[718,724] (Figure 33.13). Supporting this picture in the intact kidney was immunocytochemical co-localization of NHE3, NHERF-1, and ezrin within the brush border of rat proximal tubule.[693] Although mice with homozygous deficiency of NHERF-1 show normal electrolytes, brush border membrane vesicles from these mice showed no effect of cAMP to inhibit NHE3 activity, despite normal protein levels of NHE3, PKA, and ezrin.[632,725] Cultured proximal tubule cells from these mice display absent regulation of NHE3 by

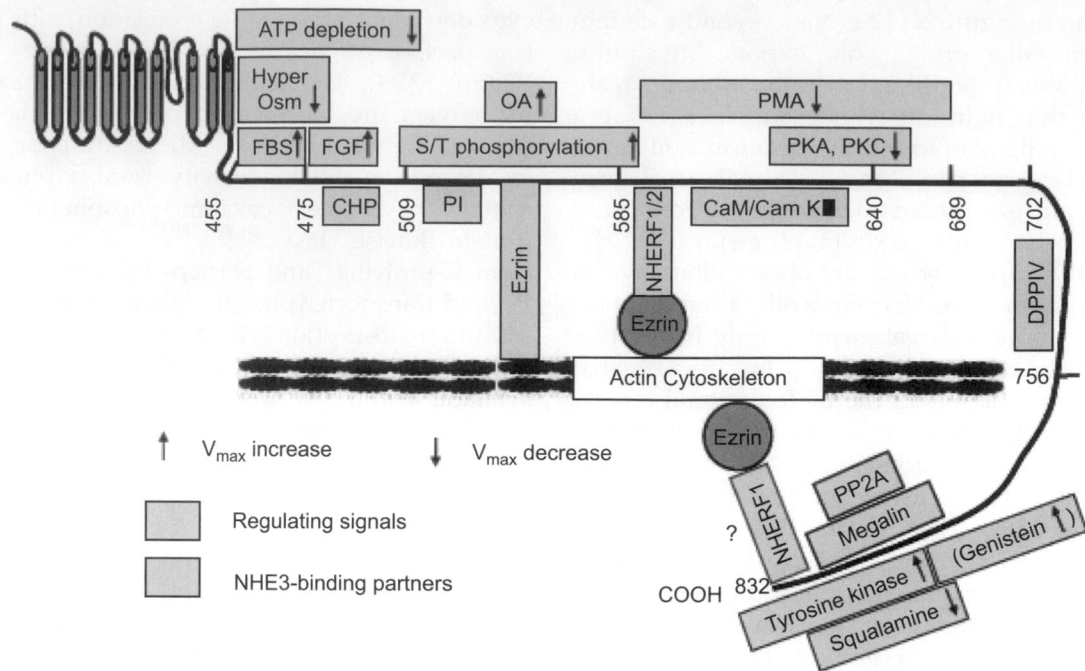

FIGURE 33.13   **NHE3 organization, including COOH-terminal domains involved in acute regulation and binding partners.** Shown above the COOH terminus in blue are sites of action of regulatory stimuli defined by the truncations, which abolish the specific regulatory effects. The direction of the arrow indicates acute stimulation or inhibition of NHE3 activity. Below the COOH terminus in yellow are listed associating proteins and the areas of their binding sites on NHE3. *(From[176].)* See color section at the end of the book.

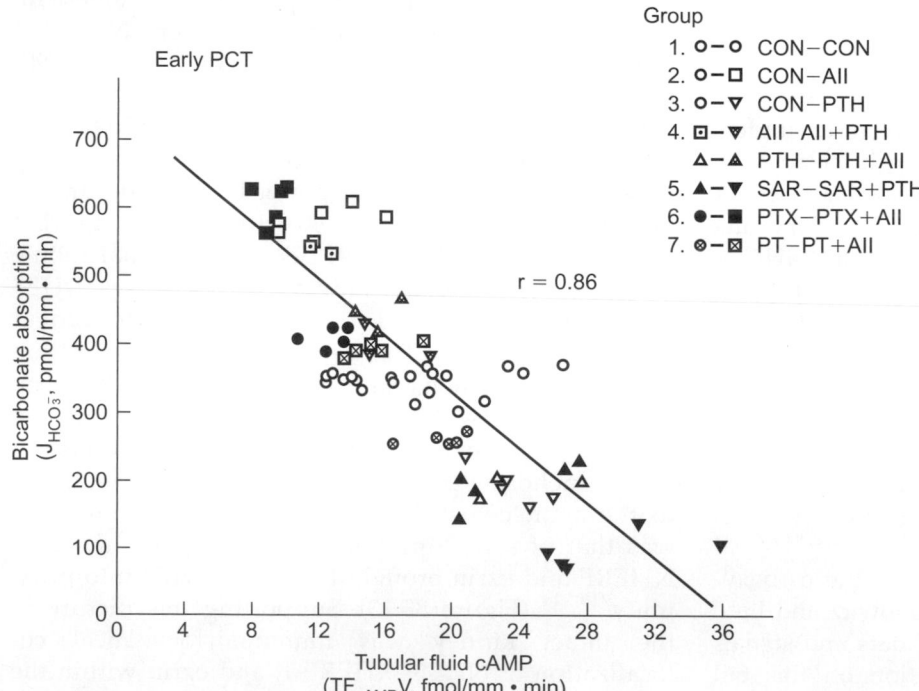

FIGURE 33.14   **Relationship of bicarbonate absorption to tubular fluid cAMP delivery in the early S1 segment of PCT.** A variety of maneuvers have been used to alter cellular content of cAMP, including parathyroidectomy (PTX) or infusion of angiotensin II (AII), parathyroid hormone (PTH), saralasin (SAR) or pertussis toxin (PT). *(From[430].)*

PTH, which could be restored via transfection with adenovirus containing the gene for NHERF-1.[166] Although NHERF-1 binds to the proximal tubule luminal membrane Na$^+$-phosphate co-transporter, NaPi-2a, and although NaPi-2a is downregulated by PTH, the NHERF-1 role in this context may be quite different from its NHE3 paradigm. In the case of NaPi-2a, NHERF-1 affects trafficking,[632] but there is no evidence that NHERF-1 is involved in the PTH-induced cAMP-dependent phosphorylation of this transporter.[93,94]

Beyond chemical modification of a fixed contingent of microvillous Na^+/H^+ exchangers, there is regulation of the NHE3 density within the luminal membrane.[466,633] An early observation in cultured proximal tubule cells was that PTH perturbed actin filament structure and caused microvillous shortening, events not replicated with application of cAMP alone.[252] Subsequently, density-gradient centrifugation of cell homogenates permitted examination of distinct membrane vesicle populations from rat proximal tubule suspension. It was found that PTH treatment resulted in migration of Na^+/H^+ exchange activity from one fraction to another, and then disappeared.[307] With the availability of NHE3-specific antibody, the distinction between Na^+/H^+ activity and NHE3 abundance could be made. Using vesicles prepared from the kidneys of parathyroidectomized rats treated acutely with PTH, it was found that within minutes of treatment Na^+/H^+ activity decreased, and phosphorylated NHE3 appeared. Over the course of hours, brush border NHE3 antigen declined, and this could be blocked by pretreating the animals with colchicine.[199] The ability of PTH to couple to adenylate cyclase appears to be critical to its ability to provoke NHE3 redistribution.[790] Events in vivo were mimicked in OK cells in which PTH induced a rapid phosphorylation of membrane-bound NHE3 and a parallel decrease in function, and then a slower retrieval of the cell surface transporter into an endocytic pathway.[160] Disruption of the actin cytoskeleton in proximal tubule suspension produced an increase in NHE3 abundance in luminal membrane vesicles prepared from these tubules.[142] A precise role, however, for the actin cytoskeleton in the regulation of NHE3 function has been elusive. Beyond transporter retrieval, the state of cellular actin fibers has been implicated in modulation of PKA phosphorylation of NHE3, consistent with its physical association with the NHERF–ezrin complex.[399,654] An additional complication is that the retrieval destination of apical transporters may be transporter-dependent. Whereas PTH in vivo produces transfer to endosomes of the luminal membrane sodium–phosphate transporter, the destination of NHE3 appears to be a reserve compartment at the base of the microvilli.[774] In addition, NHE3 is also internalized in association with megalin to a distinct vesicle compartment[98,101]; this appears to be critical to the action of the proximal tubule to reabsorb and process luminal proteins in OK cells and in mouse.[240,241] The kinetics of insertion and retrieval of NHE3 are clearly altered in consequence to demands for proximal Na^+ conservation (see below), although precise mechanisms remain uncertain, due in part to the uncertainty of extrapolation from cell culture preparations to tubules in vivo.

Modulation of the Na,K-ATPase

All of the regulatory signals that impact on the luminal Na^+/H^+ exchanger also modulate the Na, K-ATPase.[204] Early study of the action of PTH in OK cells identified the release of inositol triphosphate (IP3) and diacyl glycerol, along with an increase in cytosolic Ca^{2+}. In intact proximal tubule cells and basolateral membrane vesicles, it was possible to confirm the IP3 release.[320] With this information, it was natural to focus on the role of protein kinase C (PKC) in mediating the PTH-induced decrease in proximal Na^+ reabsorption. Baum and Hays[55] were first to examine the effect of PKC activation on PCT transport, and demonstrated inhibition of bicarbonate, chloride, and glucose transport by rabbit tubules in vitro. This global effect on multiple solutes was consistent with inhibition of the Na,K-ATPase, and this was the finding of Bertorello and Aperia,[85] who determined maximal Na,K-ATPase activity in rat proximal tubules preincubated with a PKC activator. The logical connection of these portions of the story was the demonstration that PTH inhibited maximal Na,K-ATPase activity in tubules in which cytosolic Na^+ was elevated by the ionophore, monensin.[562] This stimulation also occurred when a truncated PTH analog was used, which had no PKA activity, so that the Na,K-ATPase inhibition was dissociated from cAMP generation. These observations were supported by the finding in intact tubules that the PTH effect on Na,K-ATPase is eliminated by inhibition of PKC with staurosporine[594] or with calphostin.[508] Interest has focused on the structural correlates of Na,K-ATPase regulation, and these have been depicted by Feraille and Doucet[204] (Figure 33.15). The first observation is that regulatory phosphorylation occurs on the alpha-subunit, which can be phosphorylated by both PKA and PKC.[86] There is a single PKA phosphorylation site at a serine within the last cytoplasmic loop, while PKC phosphorylation occurs on the N-terminal cytoplasmic tail.[68,205] The rate of alpha chain phosphorylation by PKC was influenced by the ionic environment, enhancing with K^+ and diminishing with Na^+, suggesting preference for the E2 over the E1 conformation.[205] The converse of this observation has also been reported, namely that PKC phosphorylation impacts on the conformational equilibrium of the enzyme, favoring the E1-Na state.[433] Although an inhibitory effect of PKC phosphorylation had been reported[86], Feschenko and Sweadner[206] found no effect of alpha-subunit phosphorylation on Na,K-ATPase kinetics, neither on maximal velocity nor Na^+ affinity. They concluded that the regulatory impact of PKC must derive from the cellular environment, and other signals.

One complicating aspect of the PTH effect on proximal tubule Na,K-ATPase is the interaction with the

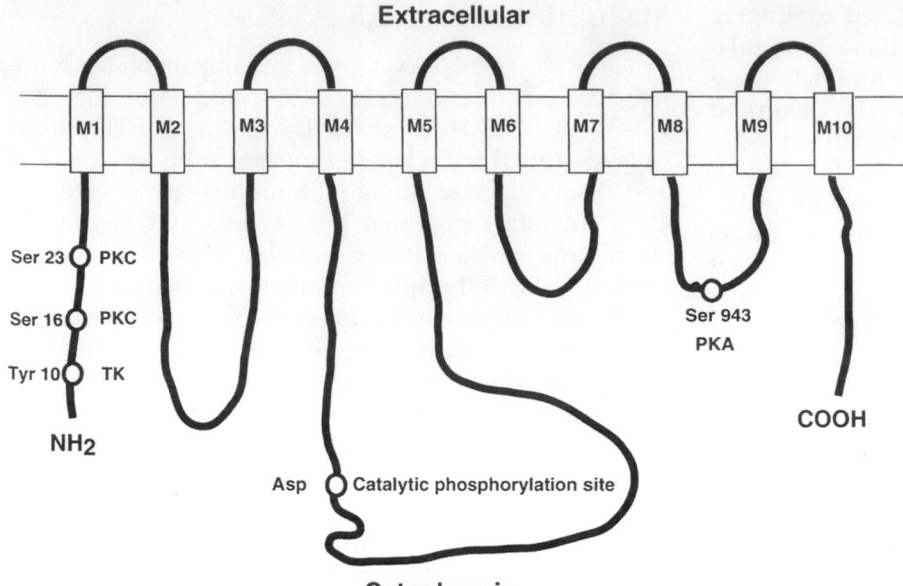

Extracellular

Ser 23 ○ PKC
Ser 16 ○ PKC
Tyr 10 ○ TK

NH₂

Ser 943
PKA

COOH

Asp ○ Catalytic phosphorylation site

Cytoplasmic

FIGURE 33.15 Transmembrane looping of the alpha subunit of the Na, K-ATPase, with localization of phosphorylated amino acids. The PKA site is located at serine-943; PKC sites are on the NH₂ cytoplasmic tail. The aspartate residue within the M4—M5 loop is phosphorylated during the catalytic cycle of the pump. (From[204].)

cytochrome P450 pathway. Ribeiro et al.[561] demonstrated that PTH released arachidonic acid in proximal tubule suspension, that a specific inhibitor of P450 prevented the inhibitory effect of PTH on the Na, K-ATPase, and that the effects of 20-hydroxyeicosatetraenoic acid (20-HETE) and PTH on the Na,K-ATPase were not additive. These observations were extended by Ominato et al.[508] working with rat proximal tubules, who showed that inhibition of cytochrome P450 not only blocked the PTH effect, but also Na,K-ATPase inhibition by activators of PKC, as well as inhibition by a PKC catalytic fragment. These workers drew the conclusion that the P450 product was an effector for PKC on the Na,K-ATPase. A slightly different conclusion was reached by Nowicki et al.[506] working in a cultured cell line (COS cells), who observed that 20-HETE had no effect on Na,K-ATPase in the absence of PKC, and that inhibitors of PKC (or mutation of the PKC catalytic site) eliminated the 20-HETE effect. These workers drew the conclusion that the P450 product was an effector for PKC on the Na,K-ATPase. A second complicating aspect of the regulation of Na,K-ATPase is the interaction with the cell's endocytic machinery. In proximal tubule cells in suspension, dopamine treatment caused phosphorylation of the alpha-subunit of Na,K-ATPase, decreasing its activity and resulting in its appearance in endosomes.[150] Dopamine-induced phosphorylation was blocked by PKC inhibition. In OK cells, phosphorylation of the alpha-subunit and its uptake into endosomes could be prevented with either PKC inhibition or by transfection with an alpha-subunit lacking the PKC phosphorylation site.[150]

Complexity of PKC modulation of the Na,K-ATPase became apparent with microperfusion studies of rat

proximal tubules by Liu and Cogan, and their observation that Na⁺ and HCO₃⁻ reabsorption was stimulated by PKC activation and depressed by PKC inhibition.[431] Wang and Chan[697] sharpened this picture with their report of a time-dependent effect of PKC activation on microperfused rat proximal tubules, with early stimulation (0 to 10 minutes) yielding to late inhibition after 25 to 35 minutes of perfusion. In rat proximal tubule cells in suspension, Feraille et al.[203] examined the effect of PKC activation on Na,K-ATPase activity, and reproduced prior observations that with standard incubation conditions PKC activation inhibited Na,K-ATPase activity. However, the thrust of their report was that in a well-oxygenated preparation, PKC was stimulatory due to an increase in Na⁺-affinity. Enhancement of the transport activity occurred in parallel with phosphorylation of the alpha-subunit of the Na,K-ATPase.[137] In contrast to the findings of Chibalin et al.[150], Efendiev et al.[191] reported that in OK cells, PKC activation increased Na,K-ATPase activity by recruiting new transporters to the cell membrane. With regard to the inhibitory or stimulatory effect of PKC on the Na,K-ATPase, Efendiev et al.[192] have focused attention on cytosolic Na⁺ concentration to act as a switch. Working in OK cells, they manipulated cell Na⁺ using the ionophore monensin, and used rubidium uptake to assay Na,K-ATPase activity in intact tubules. They found that PKC activation stimulated the pump at low cell [Na⁺], had no effect at estimated [Na⁺] around 12 mM, and was inhibitory at cell [Na⁺] greater than 16 mM. The inhibition, but not the stimulation, was abrogated with P450 inhibition. This work was extended by experiments in rat proximal tubules in which the phosphorylation of the PKC site of the alpha-subunit was measured.[326] It was found that at the normally low cell Na^+, the sites were largely phosphorylated, and only at abnormally high cell Na^+ were they dephosphorylated and susceptible to the action of PKC. In more recent studies in OK cells, fluorescence microscopy of tagged alpha-subunits has demonstrated an impact of increased cytosolic Na^+ to traffic Na,K-ATPase to endosomes adjacent to the cell membrane.[154] Whether this represents trafficking of transporter to or from the plasma membrane may depend upon other neuro-humoral factors.

Neural and Humoral Factors

Renal Nerves

Renal sympathetic nerves have long been known to modulate proximal tubule sodium transport, and are perhaps the most important regulator.[172,256] Denervation of the rat kidney reduced proximal reabsorption by 40% in the absence of any change in single nephron glomerular filtration.[71] Stimulation of the sympathetic nerves can increase reabsorption by 30%, again without change in filtration.[73] In the isolated perfused convoluted proximal tubule of the rabbit (but not the straight portion) both alpha and beta catecholamines enhance sodium transport.[69] Similar stimulation by both adrenergic agonists is observed in the doubly microperfused rat tubule.[719] In the perfused mammalian tubule, norepinephrine increases both bicarbonate and chloride transport.[60] Nord and his associates[505] found that in a suspension of tubule cells from the rabbit, sodium uptake was enhanced by alpha agonists and blocked by ethylisopropylamiloride, thus suggesting alpha stimulation of brush border Na^+/H^+ exchange. Subsequently, Wong et al.[761] demonstrated that in the microperfused S1 segment of rat proximal tubule, both acute renal denervation or acute alpha-1 blockade reduce chloride reabsorption by 40%, while manipulation of alpha-2 activity had little impact. The effect of alpha-1 blockade could be eliminated by pre-activation of PKC, suggesting that the calcium–phospholipid-dependent kinase was the important signaling pathway for renal sympathetic activity. In view of the increase in cellular cAMP with beta adrenergic agonists, the mechanism by which beta agonists enhance proximal sodium reabsorption must be indirect, and the evidence implicates NHERF: activated beta-2 receptor binds NHERF, and thus prevents cAMP-dependent downregulation of NHE3. When binding was prevented with a mutated beta receptor, the PKA-dependent decrease in NHE3 flux was also prevented.[292] A coordinated effect of sympathetic activity on luminal and peritubular cell membranes was suggested by the observation that PKC activation also enhanced activity of the peritubular $Na^+-3HCO_3^-$ co-transporter.[578] Of greater significance with respect to luminal-peritubular coordination is the observation that norepinephrine also increases the activity of the Na,K-ATPase.[60,87] The effect on the sodium pump, however, is more likely mediated by a phosphatase, since PKC is inhibitory here.[19,314,419]

Angiotensin

Angiotensin II has been intensely studied as a regulator of proximal sodium transport.[158,295,296,541,614] In the intact animal, selective blockade of angiotensin II is diuretic, so it appears that under normal conditions there is tonic stimulation of the proximal tubule.[771] In physiologic doses, it enhances Na^+ reabsorption in rat[297] or rabbit tubules,[615] and the stimulatory effect appears to be more pronounced in the S1 segment.[429] Specific receptors for angiotensin exist on both luminal[121] and peritubular membranes,[122] and the hormone effect may be achieved from either side of the cell.[429] Distinguished on the basis of inhibitor binding, several distinct receptor types have been identified on proximal tubule, each with affinity for angiotensin in the nanomolar range.[181,190] In intact rat tubules, the most prominent effect of angiotensin, in picomolar concentrations, is the stimulation of $NaHCO_3$ reabsorption via Na^+/H^+ exchange,[429] and this is mediated by binding to AT1 receptors.[543,763] In a suspension of proximal tubule cells, angiotensin II enhances both Na^+ uptake and cell pH recovery after an acid-load.[581] The increase in tubular reabsorption due to angiotensin is correlated with the inhibition of cAMP generation,[430] and these findings are reproduced in cultured proximal tubule cells transfected with the AT1 angiotensin receptor.[656]

While systemic angiotensin concentrations may be in the 0.01–0.1 nM range, luminal concentrations are 100-fold higher[624] due to tubular synthesis and secretion of angiotensin.[112,532] Microperfusion studies, combining luminal perfusion of angiotensin with simultaneous inhibition of local synthesis, have confirmed the stimulation of transport starting in the picomolar range.[58,540] However, over a broad range of luminal concentrations (0.01–10.0 nM) these workers found the stimulatory effect of luminal angiotensin to be relatively flat. With respect to the peritubular action of angiotensin, inhibition of Na^+ transport becomes apparent at concentrations above 0.1 nM as an attenuation of the stimulation seen at lower doses. Inhibition may dominate at concentrations greater than 100 nM,[296] and may involve binding to an AT2 receptor.[291] In vivo, AT1 blockade has been used to reveal an effect of peritubular angiotensin II, metabolized to angiotensin III, which then binds to the AT2 receptor to decrease Na^+ reabsorption.[517,518] Pursuit of the signaling pathway underlying the inhibitory effect of angiotensin has indicated formation (via phospholipase A2) of an epoxygenase metabolite of arachidonic acid.[181,294,318,448,575]

Microperfusion experiments have also revealed a coordinated action of luminal angiotensin and renal nerve activity. In volume-contracted animals, proximal reabsorption is brisk, additional luminal angiotensin adds little, and luminal AT1 antagonism has a dramatic inhibitory effect on reabsorption; in volume-expanded animals, there is only a small impact of luminal AT1 inhibition, while luminal angiotensin sharply increases volume reabsorption.[542] Quan and Baum[544] made the observation that when renal nerves were cut luminal perfusion of an angiotensin converting enzyme inhibitor (enalaprilat) failed to decrease proximal volume reabsorption, although the tubule remained sensitive to the stimulatory effect of directly applied luminal angiotensin. Conversely, stimulation of renal nerves conferred enalaprilat-sensitivity to proximal reabsorption.[545] These studies suggested that renal nerves amplified their signal to enhance proximal sodium reabsorption by switching on the local angiotensin synthetic machinery. A mysterious aspect of luminal angiotensin signaling is the luminal angiotensin concentration maintained well above that needed for maximal stimulation. One explanation that has been advanced is that in such a system, regulation of transport might be determined by AT1 receptor density.[389] Indeed, metabolic acidosis increases proximal tubule AT1 expression, and thus increases the effect of angiotensin to stimulate proximal ammoniagenesis.[498] In OK cells, both AT1 receptor expression[39] and NHE3 activity[230] are increased by insulin. The significance of the proximal AT1 receptor to total body Na^+ balance is suggested by the demonstration of Gurley et al.[283] that mice with AT1 knockout restricted to proximal tubule have decreased proximal tubule Na^+ reabsorption and are relatively hypotensive.

With respect to specific proximal tubule transporters, angiotensin is pleiotropic. Beyond the effect of decreasing cAMP to increase NHE3 flux, there is evidence that angiotensin can act to increase NHE3 membrane density in intact tubules.[415] It is likely that the increase in NHE3 activity contributes to the observed increase in NH_4^+ secretion by perfused mouse proximal tubule, although the increased NH_4^+ production in perfused S3 segments is evidence for a more global angiotensin action.[497] Within proximal tubules of rats with renovascular hypertension, there is increased expression of the Na^+-glucose co-transporter (SGLT2), which is blunted by AT1 inhibition.[59] Additionally, angiotensin augments proximal acidification by the luminal membrane H^+-ATPase, at least in part through transporter insertion.[694] Indeed in vivo, ACE inhibition produces translocation of an array of luminal transport proteins, including NHE3, NHERF,

ezrin, and the H^+-ATPase, from tip to base of brush border microvilli,[414] and this translocation is reversed by direct infusion of angiotensin II.[564] In the picomolar to nanomolar concentration range, angiotensin stimulates HCO_3^- exit via the peritubular Na^+–$3HCO_3^-$ co-transporter,[162,193,239] perhaps via a pathway which activates PKC,[579] and perhaps by increasing the membrane content of this transporter.[565] Within the concentration range of angiotensin that stimulates proximal reabsorption, there is increased peritubular Na, K-ATPase[235]; this occurs promptly and with changes in the phosphorylation of the Na,K-ATPase.[778] There is also increased peritubular K^+ conductance.[162] Despite enhancement of peritubular exit pathways, the net effect of angiotensin on cytosolic Na^+ concentration is an increase.[555]

Dopamine

The proximal tubule is also the target of natriuretic signals, and dopamine is the most important.[17,134,787] Among the key early observations were findings that urinary dopamine could derive from circulating L-DOPA,[34] that on balance, the whole kidney synthesized dopamine (consuming DOPA), with tubular secretion providing the bulk of urinary dopamine,[38] and that proximal tubules could be a source for this excreted dopamine.[35] Within proximal tubule, conversion from DOPA to dopamine is due to the enzyme L-amino acid decarboxylase (L-AADC), and the importance of the local generation of dopamine was underscored by the demonstration that maximal L-AADC activity was modulated by dietary salt intake.[631] In mice, in which proximal tubule AADC has been knocked-out, urinary dopamine is dramatically reduced, and the animals show elevated blood pressure (compared with wild-type) when on a normal- or high-salt diet.[791] Proximal tubules are a target for the locally generated dopamine. Dopamine inhibits sodium reabsorption in the isolated perfused straight tubule,[72] and in tubule suspensions.[411] In proximal convoluted tubules (in vitro), however, dopamine decreased sodium reabsorption only in tubules in which transport had been stimulated by norepinephrine,[56] consistent with the observation in vivo that a DA-1 agonist is not natriuretic in a denervated kidney.[325] RNA message for the DA-1 dopamine receptor was demonstrated in proximal tubule,[773] and subsequently the protein was identified on both luminal and peritubular cell membranes.[507]

As with angiotensin, dopamine impacts on transporters of both luminal and peritubular cell membranes, most notably but not exclusively NHE3 and the Na, K-ATPase. Studies of dopamine action via the DA-1 receptor have implicated a number of second messenger systems, but principally cAMP-PKA targeting

NHE3 and Ca^{2+}-PKC targeting the Na,K-ATPase.[17] When renal cortical tissue was incubated with dopamine or DA-1 agonists, Na^+/H^+ exchange in brush border membrane vesicles decreased, and this could be blocked by inhibition of either adenylate cyclase or PKA.[200] Use of OK cells permitted direct demonstration that dopamine (via DA-1) and PKA phosphorylated NHE3 on identical sites.[749] In large measure, the decrease in Na^+/H^+ exchange reflects a dopamine-mediated decrease in NHE3 within the luminal cell membrane.[32] This conclusion was based on experiments in which mouse cortical slices were treated with dopamine, and brush border membrane vesicles assayed for NHE3 activity and antigen. A prior observation had been made in OK cells that dopamine produced endocytosis of NHE3 in a PKA-dependent manner.[321] Development of antibodies recognizing NHE3 phosphorylated at PKA target sites, confirmed the effect of dopamine to increase phosphorylation at those sites, and permitted the observation that in the rat *in vivo*, NHE3 phosphorylation shifted from microvilli to a subapical location.[386] With respect to other luminal transporters, dopamine also induces internalization of the Na^+-phosphate co-transporter,[31] and this effect involves participation of NHERF.[715] The impact of dopamine on the Na,K-ATPase was demonstrable as a decrease of enzyme activity in microdissected tubules[18] or as a decrease in oxygen consumption by proximal tubules in suspension in which cell Na^+ was kept high by nystatin permeabilization.[630] The dopamine-mediated decrease in proximal tubule cellular Na,K-ATPase activity has been shown to occur in association with endocytosis of the enzyme, and blocking the endocytosis with an actin stabilizer eliminated the decrease in enzyme activity.[149] An early event in the endocytic process is PKC-dependent phosphorylation of the alpha-subunit of the Na,K-ATPase.[150] An early observation in rat proximal tubule was that, like ouabain, dopamine produced an increase in tubule diameter.[18] Subsequent study of rabbit PST with Na^+-sensitive fluorescent dye demonstrated a prompt rise in cell Na^+ in response to dopamine.[397] This indicates that with inhibition of both Na^+ entry and exit pathways, on balance, the effect of dopamine on the Na, K-ATPase dominates. In an electrophysiologic study, dopamine also blunted peritubular HCO_3^- exit via the Na^+–$3HCO_3^-$ co-transporter.[397]

The DA-1 receptor density is regulated, and consistent with the physiology, there is an inverse relationship with AT1 angiotensin receptor density. Early observations included the findings that in cell culture (LLCPK) dopamine recruits its own DA-1 receptor to the cell membrane[118]; and in rats, dopamine downregulates the AT1 receptor.[147] In a primary culture of rat proximal tubule cells, application of a dopamine agonist increased DA-1 density, decreased AT1 density, and eliminated the angiotensin-elicited increase in cytosolic Ca^{2+} (Figure 33.16).[368] In these same cells, angiotensin decreased the DA-1 density, and blunted the dopamine-agonist-induced increase in cAMP. The dopaminergic decrease in AT1 density was also observed in a primary culture of human proximal tubule cells.[245] Complementing these observations, the proximal tubule AADC knockout mouse showed increased renal AT1 mRNA expression.[791] Another aspect of dopamine receptor physiology, which may have direct translational impact, is "desensitization" of the DA1 receptor by phosphorylation.[201] In proximal tubule, the G-protein-coupled receptor kinase 4 (GRK4) is the principal kinase to phosphorylate the DA1 receptor, thus diminishing the dopamine effect. The critical observation is that in primary cultures of human proximal tubule, cells derived from hypertensive patients show decreased responsiveness to dopamine agonists and increased DA-1 phosphorylation.[587] These observations may be understood in light of the later demonstration that cells from hypertensive patients have substantially greater GRK activity.[202] Furthermore, a GRK4 mutation identified in human hypertension produced hypertension in a transgenic mouse.[202] Renal interstitial infusion of GRK4 antisense oligonucleotides decreased GRK4 expression, decreased DA-1 phosphorylation, and mitigated the blood pressure rise of spontaneously hypertensive rats.[588]

Nitric Oxide (NO)

Nitric oxide provides a paracrine signal from renal nerves or renal endothelial cells to affect proximal tubule Na^+ transport.[420] Due to its short half-life and difficulty in measurement, the impact of NO has been assessed indirectly, in experiments in which NO synthase (NOS) has been inhibited or NO donors have been infused, so that renal tubular dose–response for NO is not available. In whole animals, infusion of a NOS inhibitor at a dose which does not increase arterial blood pressure or glomerular filtration, leads to a reduction in sodium excretion.[404,450] Majid et al.[450] found that with NOS inhibition, urinary Na^+ excretion failed to increase as a function of renal perfusion pressure, and this prompted them to propose that NO may be a mediator of the pressure-natriuresis response (see below). When the NO donor, sodium nitroprusside (SNP), was added to tubule lumen or to peritubular capillaries, it decreased proximal Na^+ reabsorption.[194] Wu et al.[768] added the observation that when NOS inhibition increased proximal sodium reabsorption, the effect could be abrogated by transection of renal nerves; the NOS inhibition effect was reproduced with specific inhibition of neuronal NOS. With renal nerve stimulation, proximal Na^+ reabsorption increased, but

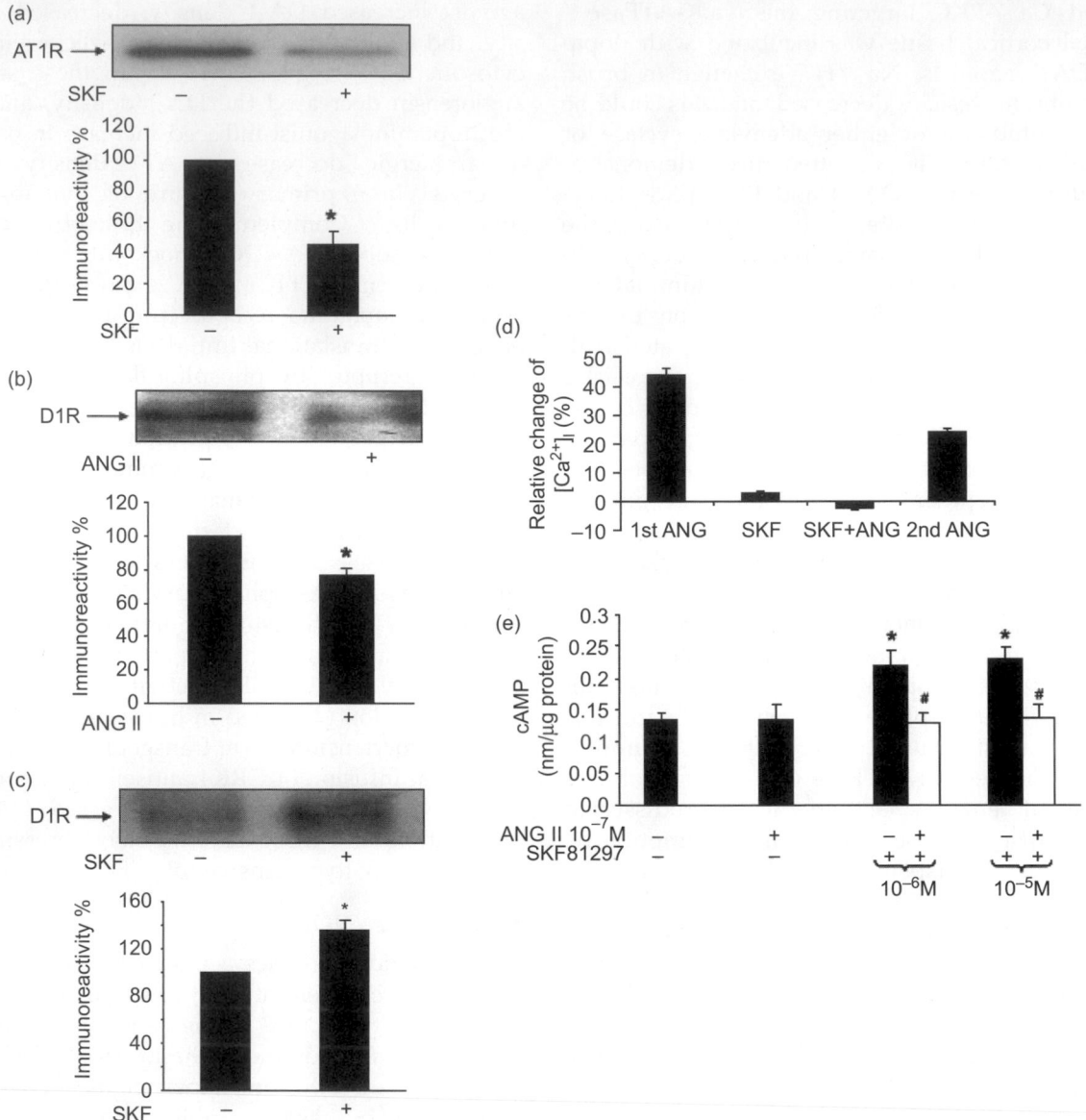

FIGURE 33.16   **Effects of ANG II and the DA-1 receptor (D1R) activating ligand, SKF81297, acting singly and in combination on renal proximal tubule (RPT) cells in culture**. (a)–(c): Cell surface expression of receptors was studied using biotinylation and densitometric quantification of bands. (a) Effect of SKF81297 on the abundance of cell surface membrane angiotensin receptor (AT1R); (b) effect of ANG II on the abundance of cell surface membrane D1R; (c) effect of SKF81297 on the abundance of cell surface membrane D1R. (d)–(e) SKF81297 abolishes the ANG II-mediated calcium response and ANG II abolishes the SKF81297-mediated cAMP response. (d) Treatment-induced change in the $[Ca^{2+}]i$ level was calculated as the percent change in the $[Ca^{2+}]_i$ value before and after each treatment. (e) Renal cortical slices were exposed to ANG II alone or SKF81297 alone or pretreated with ANG II and then treated with both ANG II and SKF81297 and cAMP levels were measured in the tissue lysates. (*P 0.05 vs. control. #P 0.05 vs. respective SKF81297-treated groups.) (*From*[368].)

not in the presence of neuronal NOS inhibition.[769] At apparent odds with the natriuretic effect of NO are rat micropuncture findings that NOS inhibition decreased proximal sodium reabsorption (an effect blocked by renal nerve transection or infusion of an alpha 2 adrenergic blocker)[658] or the observation that peritubular capillary perfusion with agents promoting NO release increased Na^+-dependent luminal proton secretion.[13] Consistent with these results, mice with deficient neuronal NOS showed defective proximal $NaHCO_3$ reabsorption.[701] Pertinent to such discordant findings are the observations of Wang,[696] who observed a dose-dependent effect of tubule perfusion with SNP, in which low dose increased and high dose decreased proximal Na^+ and HCO_3^- reabsorption; perfusion with a NOS inhibitor decreased reabsorption, consistent with the enhancing effect of low-dose SNP. One possible reconciliation has been the suggestion that the variable impact of NO on proximal tubule Na^+ transport may be contingent on cytosolic cAMP concentration.[236]

With respect to mechanism, proximal tubule epithelial cells do not contain RNA message for constitutive nitric oxide synthases (endothelial or neuronal NOS), but have abundant message for guanylate cyclase.[655] In primary culture, rat proximal tubule cells showed little cGMP production in response to NO inducers, but co-incubation with bovine pulmonary endothelial cells rendered the cells sensitive, and resulted in a sharp increase in cGMP, a decrease in Na,K-ATPase activity, and a decrease in vectorial Na^+ transport from apical to basal surfaces.[423] Carey and associates have offered the perspective that renal interstitial cGMP mediates the action of NO. Infusion of cGMP into the renal interstitium produces natriuresis in the whole kidney; infusion of an NO donor increases the interstitial cGMP concentration, and blocking the production of cGMP by administration of a soluble guanylate cyclase inhibitor completely blocked the natriureteic effect of NO.[346] In a follow-up to this observation, human proximal tubule cells in culture were found to contain soluble guanylate cyclase, and it was demonstrated that stimulation by NO produced cGMP that was secreted into the culture medium.[592] Of interest, in these experiments application of an NO donor resulted in a decrease in cell Na^+ content, consistent with a dominance of an inhibitory effect on Na^+ entry pathways.[592] A recent study has implicated a tyrosine kinase (Src) as a downstream mediator of the cGMP effect.[501]

Volume Expansion and Pressure Natriuresis

The influence of physical factors on the paracellular pathway does not preclude important effects of volume expansion on the cell itself. This was the supposition of, Robson et al.[566] who reported depression of glucose reabsorption in the kidney of the volume-expanded rat. This view found support in a whole organ tracer study, which failed to discern increased glucose backflux during volume expansion.[309] Proximal micropuncture documented decreased capacity for glucose reabsorption during volume expansion,[33] and a correlation of sodium and glucose reabsorption under the influence of albumin infusion.[365] The microperfusion study of Boonjarern et al.[107] demonstrated decreased reabsorptive flux of labeled glucose in the presence of volume expansion. The case for a cellular effect of peritubular protein has also been presented by Berry and associates, working with isolated tubules, and finding depression of chloride reabsorption with removal of bath protein.[81] The evidence was strengthened in subsequent experiments in which transepithelial concentration gradients were adjusted to virtually eliminate electro-diffusive forces across the epithelium. In that study, the increase of peritubular protein from 6 to 10 gm/dl still produced a 42% increase in NaCl reabsorption.[54] Consistent with these findings, micropuncture of the volume-expanded rat has also indicated a greater depression of proximal reabsorption of NaCl than $NaHCO_3$.[95,157] Pursuing this issue in another coupled transport system, Pitts et al. found that prior volume expansion of the rabbit depressed phosphate transport in straight proximal tubule removed and perfused over 90 minutes.[530] In the same study, prior volume expansion also depressed Na^+-coupled phosphate transport in brush border membrane vesicles.

There has been considerable effort to define the cellular impact of volume expansion. Electron probe analysis of rat kidney suggested that cell Na^+ concentration increases following saline infusion.[285] When the kidney from the volume-expanded rat is protected from physical factors using an arterial snare, the increase in cell Na^+ is eliminated.[554] These findings were interpreted as most consistent with a decrease in Na,K-ATPase activity during volume expansion. "Pressure natriuresis," in which systemic arterial pressure is increased, has been an important model with which to examine the acute impact of physical factors on proximal sodium reabsorption.[502,574] In these animals, renal autoregulation maintains a relatively constant renal blood flow and glomerular filtration rate, but renal sodium excretion increases in association with an increase in renal interstitial hydrostatic pressure.[369] In prior studies, Kinoshita and Knox[373] had shown that the decrease of proximal sodium reabsorption that normally follows increased renal interstitial pressure could be eliminated by blocking prostaglandin synthesis. In pressure natriuresis during block of prostaglandin synthesis with indomethacin, renal interstitial hydrostatic pressure still increases, but sodium and lithium reabsorption are no longer decreased.[254] Complementing this observation is the finding that with a directly applied increase in interstitial hydrostatic pressure, treatment with indomethacin eliminated the increase in tight junctional lanthanum permeability.[551] Although physical factors are involved, these results are best rationalized by an impact on the cell, rather than a direct tight junction effect.

To delineate cellular events following volume expansion, membrane fractions were obtained from kidneys undergoing pressure natriuresis, and examined for content of NHE3 and Na,K-ATPase.[789] This study revealed that acute hypertension prompted the retrieval of luminal membrane transporters (change in membrane fraction in which transport activity appeared), and a sharp reduction in the the activity of Na,K-ATPase. The retrieval of NHE3 was prompt (within 5 minutes of acute hypertension), reversible (within 20 minutes), and concurrent with the acute changes in lithium clearance.[788] With respect to the Na, K-ATPase, the decrease in activity was not accompanied by any loss of immunoreactivity of its subunits within the membrane fractions. Immunohistochemical staining of NHE3 plus confocal microscopy permitted the visual demonstration that with acute hypertension NHE3 redistributed from the brush border into the base of the microvilli, confirming the inference from the membrane fraction analysis (Figure 33.17). Complementing these structural changes, functional changes in luminal membrane Na^+/H^+ exchange could be identified *in vivo*. When proximal tubule cells were loaded with BCECF, cytosolic pH could be monitored continuously during luminal microperfusion, specifically the time course of cellular acidification following luminal Na^+ removal. Within 20 minutes of acute hypertension, the Na^+-dependent change in cytosolic pH was reduced 52% from control.[780] When brush border membrane vesicles were examined both for NHE3 protein and for Na^+/H^+ exchange activity, it was found that despite retrieval (change in membrane fraction), the activity per transporter remained constant.[774] Thus, in contrast to the changes in Na, K-ATPase activity, the reduction in Na^+/H^+ activity could not be attributed to kinetic modification of the NHE3 transporter. The chronic analog to pressure natriuresis is a high-salt diet, and in this model there was reduction in Na,K-ATPase activity, with no change in α1-subunit density.[524] Following 3 weeks of high salt, young rats showed retrieval of luminal membrane NHE3 and NaPi2 and peritubular membrane Na,K-ATPase.[775] With acute volume contraction, however, transporter kinetics do appear to change, since the increase in lithium reabsorption is not accompanied by the appearance of new NHE3.[416] Over time, however, chronic volume contraction does increase NHE3

message in proximal tubule.[211] McDonough[465] has provided a summary scheme of the impact of extracellular fluid volume or blood pressure on proximal tubule transporter expression (Figure 33.18).

The signals from interstitium to tubule have also been pursued in more detail, and there is evidence that arachidonic acid metabolites of cytochrome P450 are implicated. Acknowledging the prior identification of eicosanoids (specifically 20-hydroxyeicosatetraenoic acid, 20-HETE) as inhibitors of Na,K-ATPase, Zhang et al.[788] sought evidence for their role as mediators of pressure natriuresis. They examined pressure natriuresis in rats pretreated with cobalt chloride to blunt cytochrome P450 metabolism, and found that this treatment blocked the pressure-associated increase in lithium clearance. This occurred in association with failure of NHE3 retrieval from brush border vesicles, and failure of Na,K-ATPase activity to decrease within its membrane fraction.[788] These findings received support with the observation that proximal convoluted tubule contains abundant cytochrome P450 4A isoforms.[336] Furthermore, rabbit proximal straight tubules in suspension produce 20-HETE, and when 20-HETE production is inhibited in an isolated perfused tubule, volume reabsorption is enhanced.[547] Using a specific inhibitor of eicosanoid formation, Dos Santos et al.[179] re-examined pressure natriuresis in pretreated rats. In these animals, 20-HETE excretion was nearly eliminated, and the pressure-induced increase in sodium excretion and lithium clearance was substantially blunted. This occurred in association with blunted retrieval of NHE3 from brush border and blunted decrease in Na,K-ATPase activity.[179] A more specific inhibitor of 20-HETE formation reproduced these results, although it was emphasized that about half of the increase in pressure-induced Na^+ excretion persisted.[755] It must be acknowledged that this work leaves unanswered the identity of the signal from

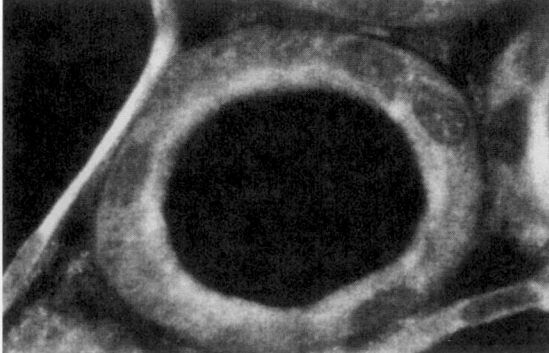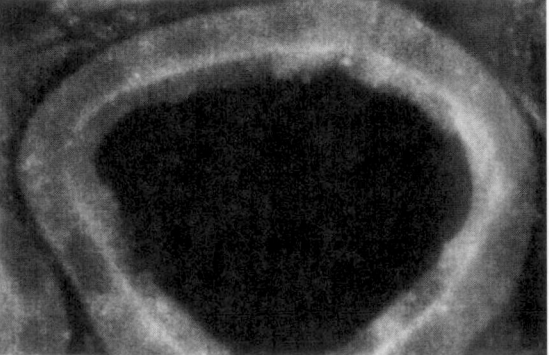

FIGURE 33.17 Effect of acute hypertension on NHE3 distribution in rat proximal tubules. Panels show NHE3 immunofluoresence under control conditions (left), and after 20 minutes of acute hypertension. Under control conditions, NHE3 appears along microvilli; with pressure natriuresis, there is redistribution of the exchanger to base of the brush border. *(From[779].)*

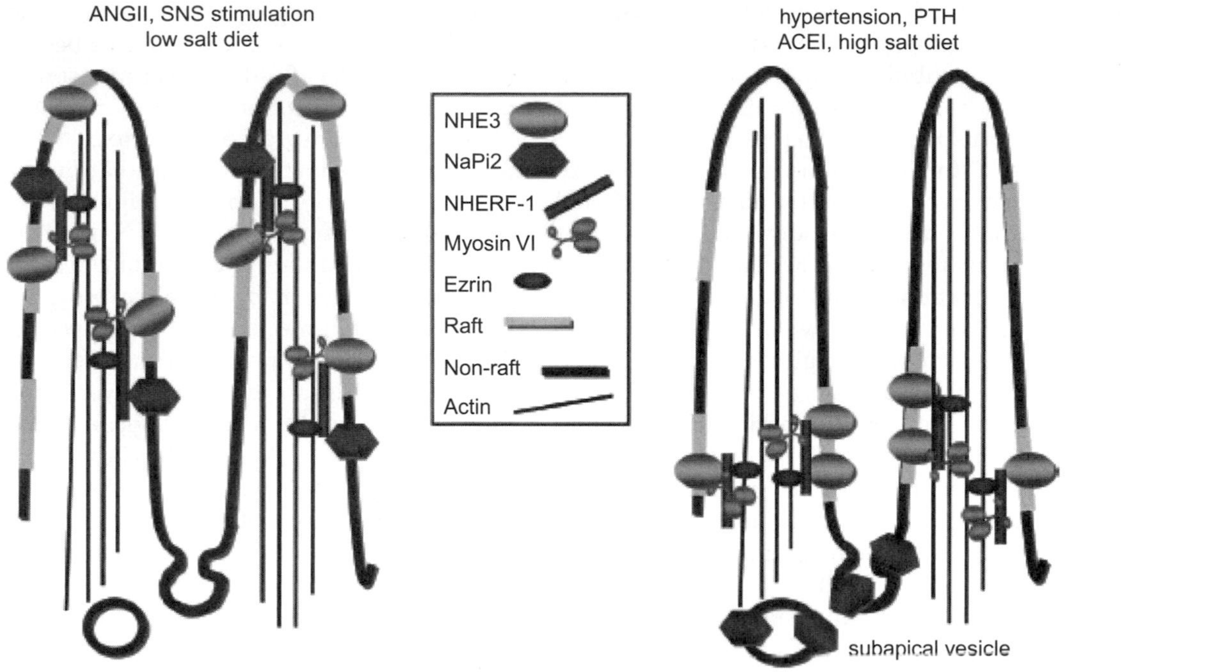

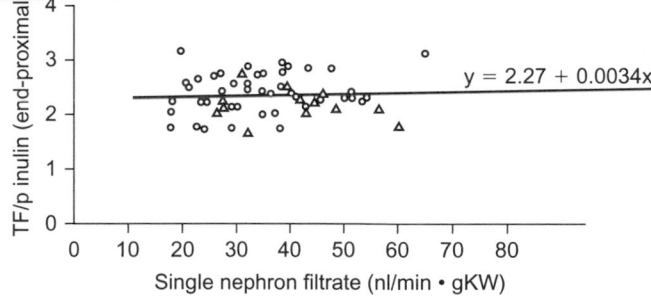

FIGURE 33.18 **Schematic representing response of renal PT sodium transporters NaPi2 and NHE3 to natriuretic and antinatriuretic stimuli.** With ANG II and sympathetic nerve stimulation, both NaPi2 and NHE3 are located in the body of the microvilli, NHE3 along with NHERF-1 and ezrin. With elevated perfusion pressure, ACEI or PTH, NHE3, and NaPi2 are translocated out of the body of the microvilli; NHE3 remains in a domain at the base of the microvilli, while NaPi2 moves to subabpical endosomes. (From[465].)

interstitial hydrostatic pressure to cell. A role for NO was examined in the rat, but NOS inhibition blunted transmission of renal perfusion pressure to the interstitium, so that the failure to observe pressure natriuresis may simply have been a consequence of low interstitial pressure.[499] More recently, renal interstitial cyclic GMP concentration was found to increase with renal perfusion pressure, and guanylyl cyclase inhibition blunted the pressure-associated decrease in proximal Na$^+$ reabsorption.[347] Leaving cGMP systhesis intact, but blocking cellular secretion of cGMP with intrarenal probenecid, also eliminated pressure natriuresis.[3] This action of extracellular cGMP to decrease Na$^+$ transport appeared to be tonic, in the sense that intrarenal infusion of phosphodiesterase decreased renal Na$^+$ excretion.[3]

Glomerulotubular Balance

In response to spontaneous variations in glomerular filtration rate, the rate of proximal tubule reabsorption varies proportionally. This "glomerulotubular balance" was apparent in the first micropuncture examination of mammalian kidney,[695] and was demonstrated elegantly by Schnermann et al.,[609] with their finding that over a four-fold change in GFR, the accessible rat proximal tubule reabsorbed roughly 40% of the filtered load (Figure 33.19). Although glomerulotubular balance may

FIGURE 33.19 **End-proximal tubular fluid was sampled from rat nephrons and plotted as a function of SNGFR.** With spontaneous variation in SNGFR over a four-fold range there is virtually no change in the fractional water reabsorption. (From[609], with permission.)

prevent solute loss following GFR increases, perhaps its most important effect is to preserve distal delivery of sodium (permitting distal regulation of acid and potassium excretion) in times of low GFR. The mechanisms underlying balanced tubular reabsorption include both peritubular capillary effects and luminal factors.[242,290,751] Peritubular oncotic forces are generally recognized as a major force in the maintenance of balanced tubular reabsorption.[187] Any increase in filtration fraction must result in an increased peritubular protein concentration, and thus, enhanced proximal reabsorption. Experimental maneuvers which distort this oncotic force (such as saline infusion or albumin administration) disrupt glomerulotubular balance. Nevertheless, in a mathematical model comprised of glomerulus, proximal tubule, peritubular capillary, and interstitium, simulation of only the filtration fraction effect on tubular transport failed to reproduce glomerulotubular balance.[732] In simulations of glomerular arteriolar resistance changes, it was found that fractional changes in proximal sodium reabsorption were smaller than the fractional changes in GFR. This derived from the fact that the variation in GFR came as a result of changes in glomerular plasma flow, as well as in filtration fraction. In order to achieve glomerulotubular balance, there must be a mechanism by which alterations in plasma flow, independent of peritubular Starling forces, can influence proximal reabsorption.

Perhaps the most important factor underlying perfusion–absorption balance is a direct effect of axial flow velocity on reabsorption.[751] Such "perfusion–absorption balance" has been found to influence the transport of glucose,[382] bicarbonate[11,143,428] and chloride.[268,760] One of the best illustrations of this phenomenon is the micropuncture data of Chan et al.[143] shown in Figure 33.20, in which a three-fold increase in luminal perfusion rate (with trivial changes in luminal HCO_3^- concentration)

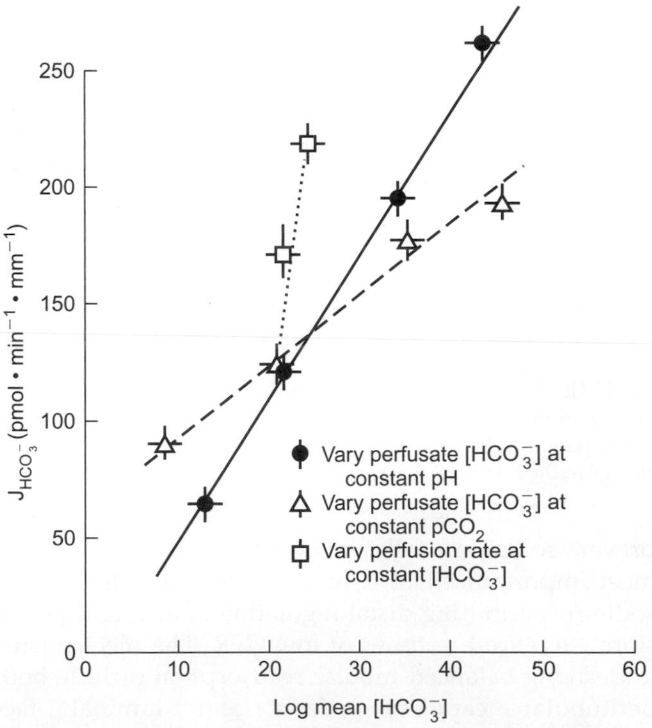

FIGURE 33.20 Net bicarbonate reabsorption, J_{HCO3}, by perfused rat proximal tubule as a function of mean luminal bicarbonate concentration. At a constant pCO_2, bicarbonate transport varies linearly with the transepithelial concentration gradient (dashed line). Elevation of pCO_2 enhances, and depression of pCO_2 diminishes, bicarbonate reabsorption (solid line). There is a steep dependence of J_{HCO3} on luminal flow rate. (From[143], with permission.)

produced a doubling of the rate of bicarbonate reabsorption. More pronounced effects have been reported with "native" tubular fluid, in comparison with artificial microperfusion solutions, suggesting the presence of a filtered, transport-promoting factor.[49,288] It may also be the case that reductions (rather than increases) in luminal flow are more faithfully followed by proportional changes in transport.[48,289,526,569] Nevertheless, the range over which modulation of luminal flow produces proportional changes in proximal reabsorption is broad.[568] The underlying mechanism for flow-dependent reabsorption has been a point of controversy. One perennial consideration is an unstirred layer effect within the brush border.[563] Morphological observations of Maunsbach et al.[459] demonstrated that lower tubule flow rates are associated with diminished tubule distention and a compaction of the brush border microvilli. Nevertheless, model calculations indicate it unlikely that there is any appreciable convective stirring within this pile,[50] neither should the diffusion barrier between the bulk luminal fluid and the cell membrane pose any significant hindrance to Na^+/H^+ exchange.[394] An intriguing mechanism for flow-dependent transport gained support from two studies, using very different methodologies, which both suggested that increases in axial flow velocity recruit new transporters into the luminal membrane. Preisig[533] loaded rat proximal tubule cells with the pH-indicator BCECF and examined recovery from an acute acid-load in vivo (ammonium pulse). With increases in luminal flow rate, the pH recovery mediated by Na^+/H^+ exchange was enhanced. Maddox et al.[447] subjected rats to acute changes in vascular volume in order to obtain hydropenic, euvolemic, and volume-expanded groups, with respective grouping according to decreased, normal, and increased GFR. When brush border membrane vesicles were prepared from each of these groups, and Na^+/H^+ kinetic parameters assessed, it was found that the V_{max} determinations stratified in parallel with GFR.

Guo et al.[282] proposed that the brush border microvilli serve as the sensor for axial flow along the proximal tubule. In that hypothesis, the drag force on each microvillus produces torque on an actin filament core, and this force is transmitted to the underlying cytoskeleton. The close spacing and uniform height of the microvilli allowed a precise calculation of that torque, and using the known bending moment for an actin filament, the Young's modulus for a microvillus was estimated. This yielded the prediction that for microvilli 2.5 μm in height, the tip deflection under axial flows of 30 nl/min would be about 4 nm, in effect depicting the microvilli as a set of stiff bristles that would retain their configuration through the physiological range of flows.[282] In a subsequent analysis, a simplified equation for microvillous torque was derived which has

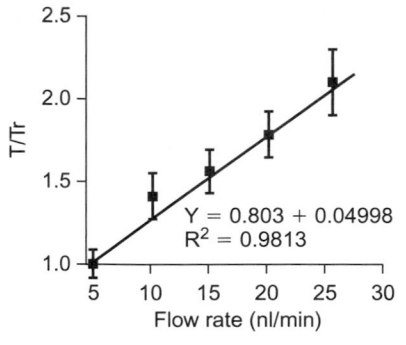
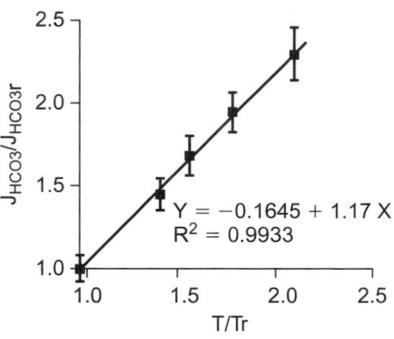

FIGURE 33.21 **Impact of luminal flow rate on bicarbonate reabsorption (J_{HCO3}) in mouse proximal tubules perfused *in vitro*.** The panel on the left shows the computed microvillous torque, T, at each flow, relative to the torque when perfusion is at 5 nl/min (T_r.) In the right panel, the observed J_{HCO3} is plotted as a function of the relative torque. (*From* [183], *with permission.*)

been useful for assessment of experimental data.[182] The essence of that derivation was identifying microvillous drag with the force on the tubular fluid:

$$D \cdot N = \frac{dp}{dz} \cdot \pi \cdot R^2 \qquad (33.17)$$

where D is the drag per microvillus, N is the number of microvilli per unit length of tubule, p is luminal hydrostatic pressure, z is axial length, and R is the tubule radius from center-line to microvillus tip. Assuming Poiseuille flow:

$$\frac{dp}{dz} = 8\mu Q / \pi R^4 \qquad (33.18)$$

where Q is luminal flow rate and μ is the tubule fluid viscosity. This provides the estimate of microvillous drag:

$$D \cdot N = 8\mu Q / R^2 \qquad (33.19)$$

and for a microvillus of height, L, the torque, T, is:

$$T \cdot N = 8\mu Q L / R^2 \qquad (33.20)$$

Since the number of microvilli, N, is not easily obtained, Eq. (33.20) is most useful in comparing two experimental trials in which flow is varied and the assumption is made that neither N nor L change with the experimental conditions:

$$\frac{T}{T_r} = \left[\frac{\mu Q}{\mu_r Q_r} \right] \cdot \left[\frac{R_r^2}{R^2} \right] \qquad (33.21)$$

in which the subscript "r" denotes a reference flow. This equation reveals the microvillous torque to vary directly with luminal flow and fluid viscosity, and inversely as the square of the luminal radius.

Du et al.[182] applied a slightly more detailed version of Eq. (33.21) to analyze the first experimental study of flow-dependent volume reabsorption, J_v, in isolated perfused mouse proximal tubules. The key finding of that work was that fractional changes in perfusion were greater than the fractional changes in J_v, but when changes in luminal diameter were included in the calculation, the fractional change in microvillous torque and J_v were identical. Furthermore, luminal

fluid viscosity increased J_v at constant perfusion rate. And finally, disruption of the cytoskeleton with cytochalasin D eliminated the perfusion-dependent increase in J_v. Du et al.[183] subsequently re-examined flow-dependent transport in mouse proximal tubule, with measurement of HCO_3^- reabsorption, J_{HCO3}. Over a five-fold variation of luminal perfusion rate, there was a predicted two-fold variation in microvillous torque, which scaled identically with the reabsorption (Figure 33.21). Du et al.[182] also reconsidered the data of Burg and Orloff,[126] widely cited as a negative effect of flow on proximal sodium reabsorption in isolated perfused rabbit proximal convoluted tubule. Burg and Orloff had observed that a three-fold increase in tubule perfusion rate produced a 37% increase in volume reabsorption, a value that did not achieve statistical significance. However, they also noted that with the highest flow, there was a 41% increase in tubule diameter. Du et al. estimated that these changes of flow and diameter would yield a 43% increase in microvillous torque, certainly compatible with the observed impact on J_v. In sum, it appears that rabbit proximal tubules were more distensible than mouse tubules, so that perfusion-dependent changes in luminal diameter precluded large deviations in microvillous torque. At present, the cellular signals from torque to Na^+/H^+ exchange remain to be delineated.

PERSPECTIVE

Sodium reabsorption along the proximal tubule refers to a multiplicity of processes, occurring in series and in parallel along a heterogeneous epithelium. Sodium transport cannot be considered out of context of the secretion of protons or the reabsorption of chloride, bicarbonate, potassium, calcium, and organic solutes. Furthermore, the precise interrelationship of these coupled transport processes depends upon the location along the proximal tubule, as well as upon physiologic parameters external to the nephron, such as plasma composition or extracellular volume status of the organism.

One focus of this chapter has been on the biophysics of transport, namely identification of the transporters and the driving forces for their fluxes. The feasibility of such an approach was due to the development of experimental technology, which permitted examination of cell membranes and recording of intracellular composition. With these tools, the first order of business had been definition and localization of the transporters. More recent molecular methods enhanced this aspect of tubule physiology by providing means to visualize a transporter within proximal tubule, and to distinguish biochemical modifications or changes in membrane density. The ability to clone and express transporters in high density in otherwise quiet systems (in which flux through the pathway of interest dominates) has yielded advances in the definition of transport kinetics.

The second order of business has been identifying important regulatory factors. This means an understanding of how changes in cell volume or composition translate into alterations of sodium reabsorption, and of the key neurohumoral signals and physical factors which modulate transport. The complexity of this task is in part technical, insofar as cellular transport machinery may involve an assembly of interacting proteins that are not fully recovered in convenient expression systems. Furthermore, the overall impact on sodium transport by one hormone may depend upon the state of activation of the other systems. Nevertheless, one recurring theme in descriptions of transport regulation has been the targeting of both luminal and peritubular membranes in a coordinated fashion.

Enrichment of our perspective of proximal tubule function must ultimately confer a quantitative understanding of its roles in pathologic states of the organism. Traditionally, this has focused on secondary renal response to disorders of extracellular volume homeostasis, such as edema forming states. It is entirely likely, however, that a role for proximal tubule may come to be identified in primary pathogenesis, as perhaps in volume-dependent hypertension. One anticipates, as a consequence of such information, that therapeutic intervention, which seeks to alter renal sodium transport, will be achieved with greater accuracy and greater safety.

Acknowledgment

This work was supported by National Institute of Diabetes and Digestive and Kidney Disease Grant 1-RO1-DK-29857.

References

[1] Abuladze N, Lee I, Newman D, Hwang J, Pushkin A, Kurtz I. Axial heterogeneity of sodium-bicarbonate co-transporter expression in the rabbit proximal tubule. Am J Physiol 1998;274: F628–33.

[2] Agre P, Preston GM, Smith BL, Jung JS, Raina S, Moon C, et al. Aquaporin CHIP: the archetypal molecular water channel. Am J Physiol 1993;265:F463–76.

[3] Ahmed F, Kemp BA, Howell NL, Siragy HM, Carey RM. Extracellular renal guanosine cyclic 3'5'-monophosphate modulates nitric oxide- and pressure-induced natriuresis. Hypertension 2007;50:958–63.

[4] Akiba T, Alpern RJ, Eveloff J, Calamina J, Warnock DG. Electrogenic sodium/bicarbonate co-transport in rabbit renal cortical basolateral membrane vesicles. J Clin Invest 1986;78:1472–8.

[5] Alavi N, Spangler RA, Jung CY. Sodium-dependent glucose transport by cultured proximal tubule cells. Biochim Biophys Acta 1987;899:9–16.

[6] Albrecht FE, Xu J, Moe OW, Hopfer U, Simonds WF, Orlowski J, et al. Regulation of NHE3 activity by G protein subunits in renal brush-border membranes. Am J Physiol 2000;278:R1064–73.

[7] Alpern RJ. Mechanism of basolateral membrane $H^+/OH^-/HCO3^-$ transport in the rat proximal convoluted tubule. A sodium-coupled electrogenic process. J Gen Physiol 1985;86:613–36.

[8] Alpern RJ. Apical membrane chloride/base exchange in the rat proximal convoluted tubule. J Clin Invest 1987;79:1026–30.

[9] Alpern RJ. Cell mechanisms of proximal tubule acidification. Physiol Rev 1990;70:79–114.

[10] Alpern RJ, Chambers M. Basolateral membrane Cl/HCO3 exchange in the rat proximal convoluted tubule. Na-dependent and-independent modes. J Gen Physiol 1987;89:581–98.

[11] Alpern RJ, Cogan MG, Rector Jr FC. Flow dependence of proximal tubular bicarbonate absorption. Am J Physiol 1983;245: F478–84.

[12] Amemiya M, Loffing Lötscher M, Kaissling B, Alpern RJ, Moe OW. Expression of NHE-3 in the apical membrane of rat renal proximal tubule and thick ascending limb. Kid Int 1995;48:1206–15.

[13] Amorena C, Castro AF. Control of proximal tubule acidification by the endothelium of the peritubular capillaries. Am J Physiol 1997;272:R691–4.

[14] Andreoli TE, Schafer JA. Volume absorption in the pars recta. III Luminal hypotonicity as a driving force for isotonic volume absorption. Am J Physiol 1978;234:F349–55.

[15] Andreoli TE, Schafer JA, Troutman SL. Perfusion rate-dependence of transepithelial osmosis in isolated proximal convoluted tubules: estimation of the hydraulic conductance. Kidney Int 1978;14:263–9.

[16] Andreoli TE, Schafer JA, Troutman SL, Watkins ML. Solvent drag component of Cl^- flux in superficial proximal straight tubules: evidence for a paracellular component of isotonic fluid absorption. Am J Physiol 1979;237:F455–62.

[17] Aperia AC. Intrarenal dopamine: a key signal in the interactive regulation of sodium metabolism. Ann Rev Physiol 2000;62:621–47.

[18] Aperia A, Bertorello A, Seri I. Dopamine causes inhibition of Na^+-K^+-ATPase activity in rat proximal convoluted tubule segments. Am J Physiol 1987;252:F39–45.

[19] Aperia A, Ibarra F, Svensson L-B, Klee C, Greengard P. Calcineurin mediates alpha-adrenergic stimulation of Na^+-K^+-ATPase activity in renal tubule cells. Proc Natl Acad Sci 1992;89:7394–7.

[20] Aronson PS. Kinetic properties of the plasma membrane Na^+-H^+ exchanger. Ann Rev Physiol 1985;47:545–60.

[21] Aronson PS, Giebisch G. Mechanisms of chloride transport in the proximal tubule. Am J Physiol 1997;273:F179–92.

[22] Aronson PS, Nee J, Suhm MA. Modifier role of internal H in activating the Na^+-H^+ exchanger in renal microvillus membrane vesicles. Nature 1982;299:161–3.

[23] Aronson PS, Sacktor B. The Na^+ gradient-dependent transport of D-glucose in renal brush border membranes. J Biol Chem 1975;250:6032–9.

[24] Aronson PS, Suhm MA, Nee J. Interaction of external H^+ with the Na^+–H^+ exchanger in renal microvillus membrane vesicles. J Biol Chem 1983;258:6767–71.

[25] Arystarkhova E, Donnet C, Muñoz-Matta A, Specht SC, Sweadner KJ. Multiplicity of expression of FXYD proteins in mammalian cells: dynamic exchange of phospholemman and g-subunit in response to stress. Am J Physiol 2007;292: C1179–91.

[26] Arystarkhova E, Sweadner KJ. Splice variants of the gamma subunit (FXYD2) and their significance in regulation of the Na, K-ATPase in kidney. J Bioenerg Biomembr 2005;37:381–6.

[27] Arystarkhova E, Wetzel RK, Sweadner KJ. Distribution and oligomeric association of splice forms of Na^+-K^+-ATPase regulatory g-subunit in rat kidney. Am J Physiol 2002;282: F393–407.

[28] Atherton JC. Comparison of chloride concentration and osmolality in proximal tubular fluid peritubular capillary plasma and systemic plasma in the rat. J Physiol (Lond) 1977;273: 765–73.

[29] Avison MJ, Gullans SR, Ogino T, Giebisch G, Shulman RG. Measurement of Na^+-K^+ coupling ratio of Na^+-K^+-ATPase in rabbit proximal tubules. Am J Physiol 1987;253:C126–36.

[30] Avison MJ, Gullans SR, Ogino T, Giebisch G. Na^+ and K^+ fluxes stimulated by Na^+-coupled glucose transport: evidence for a Ba^{2+}-insensitive K^+ efflux pathway in rabbit proximal tubules. J Membr Biol 1988;105:197–205.

[31] Bacic D, Capuano P, Baum M, Zhang J, Stange G, Biber J, et al. Activation of dopamine D1-like receptors induces acute internalization of the renal Na^+/phosphate co-transporter NaPi-IIa in mouse kidney and OK cells. Am J Physiol Renal Physiol 2005;288:F740–7.

[32] Bacic D, Kaissling B, McLeroy P, Zou L, Baum M, Moe OW. Dopamine acutely decreases apical membrane Na/H exchanger NHE3 protein in mouse renal proximal tubule. Kidney Int 2003;64:2133–41.

[33] Baines AD. Effect of extracellular fluid volume expansion on maximum glucose reabsorption rate and glomerular tubular balance in single rat nephrons. J Clin Invest 1971;50: 2414–25.

[34] Baines AD, Chan W. Production of urine free dopamine from DOPA: a micropuncture study. Life Sci 1980;26:253–9.

[35] Baines AD, Drangova R, Hatcher C. Dopamine production by isolated glomeruli and tubules from rat kidneys. Can J Physiol Pharmacol 1985;63:155–8.

[36] Baines AD, deRouffignac C. Functional hetereogeneity of nephrons. II. Filtration rates, intraluminal flow velocities and fractional water reabsorption. Pf Arch 1969;308:260–76.

[37] Balkovetz DF, Chumley P, Amlal H. Downregulation of claudin-2 expression in renal epithelial cells by metabolic acidosis. Am J Physiol 2009;297:F604–11.

[38] Ball SG, Gunn IG, Douglas IHS. Renal handling of dopa dopamine norepinephrine and epinephrine in the dog. Am J Physiol 1982;242:F56–62.

[39] Banday AA, Siddiqui AH, Menezes MM, Hussain T. Insulin treatment enhances AT1 receptor function in OK cells. Am J Physiol 2005;288:F1213–9.

[40] Bank N, Aynedjian HS. Failure of changes in intracapillary pressures to alter proximal fluid reabsorption. Kidney Int 1984;26:275–82.

[41] Bank N, Aynedjian HS, Mutz BF. Proximal bicarbonate absorption independent of Na^+-H^+ exchange: effect of bicarbonate load. Am J Physiol 1989;256:F577–82.

[42] Bank N, Yarger WE, Aynedjian HS. A microperfusion study of sucrose movement across the rat proximal tubule during renal vein constriction. J Clin Invest 1971;50:294–302.

[43] Bankir L, de Rouffignac C. Anatomical and functional heterogeneity of nephrons in the rabbit: Microdissection studies and SNGFR measurements. Pflügers Arch 1976;366: 89–93.

[44] Barfuss DW, Schafer JA. Differences in active and passive glucose transport along the proximal nephron. Am J Physiol 1981;240:F322–32.

[45] Barfuss DW, Schafer JA. Rate of formation and composition of absorbate from proximal nephron segments. Am J Physiol 1984;247:F117–29.

[46] Barratt LJ, Rector Jr. FC, Kokko JP, Seldin DW. Factors governing the transepithelial potential difference across the proximal tubule of the rat kidney. J Clin Invest 1974;53:454–64.

[47] Barriere H, Rubera I, Belfodil R, Tauc M, Tonnerieux N, Poujeol C, et al. Swelling-activated chloride and potassium conductance in primary cultures of mouse proximal tubules. Implication of KCNE1 protein. J Membr Biol 2003;193 (3):153–70.

[48] Bartoli E, Conger JD, Earley LE. Effect of intraluminal flow on proximal tubular reabsorption. J Clin Invest 1973;52:843–9.

[49] Bartoli E, Earley LE. Importance of ultrafilterable plasma factors in maintaining tubular reabsorption. Kidney Int 1973;3:142–50.

[50] Basmadjian D, Dykes DS, Baines AD. Flow through brushborders and similar protuberant wall structures. J Membr Biol 1980;56:183–90.

[51] Baum M. Effect of luminal chloride on cell pH in rabbit proximal tubule. Am J Physiol 1988;254:F677–83.

[52] Baum M. Axial heterogeneity of rabbit proximal tubule luminal H^+ and basolateral HCO_3^- transport. Am J Physiol 1989;256: F335–41.

[53] Baum M, Berry CA. Evidence for neutral transcellular NaCl transport and neutral basolateral chloride exit in the rabbit proximal convoluted tubule. J Clin Invest 1984;74: 205–11.

[54] Baum M, Berry CA. Peritubular protein modulates neutral active NaCl absorption in rabbit proximal convoluted tubule. Am J Physiol 1985;248:F790–5.

[55] Baum M, Hays SR. Phorbol myristate acetate and dioctanoylglycerol inhibit transport in rabbit proximal convoluted tubule. Am J Physiol 1988;254:F9–14.

[56] Baum M, Quigley R. Inhibition of proximal convoluted tubule transport by dopamine. Kidney Int 1998;54:1593–600.

[57] Baum M, Quigley R. Maturation of rat proximal tubule chloride permeability. Am J Physiol 2005;289:R1659–64.

[58] Baum M, Quigley R, Quan A. Effect of luminal angiotensin II on rabbit proximal convoluted tubule bicarbonate absorption. Am J Physiol 1997;273:F595–600.

[59] Bautista R, Manning R, Martinez F, Avila-Casado M, Soto V, Medina A, et al. Angiotensin II-dependent increased expression of Na^+-glucose co-transporter in hypertension. Am J Physiol 2004;286:F127–33.

[60] Beach RE, Schwab SJ, Brazy PC, Dennis VW. Norepinephrine increases Na^+-K^+-ATPase and solute transport in rabbit proximal tubules. Am J Physiol 1987;252:F215–20.

[61] Beck FX, Dorge A, Rick R, Schramm M, Thurau K. Effect of potassium adaptation on the distribution of potassium sodium and chloride across the apical membrane of renal tubular cells. Pflügers Arch 1987;409:477–85.

[62] Beck JC, Sacktor B. Energetics of the Na^+-dependent transport of D-glucose in renal brush border membrane vesicles. J Biol Chem 1975;250:8674–80.

[63] Beck JS, Breton S, Laprade R, Giebisch G. Volume regulation and intracellular calcium in the rabbit proximal convoluted tubule. Am J Physiol 1991;260:F861–7.

[64] Beck JS, Breton S, Mairbäurl H, Laprade R, Giebisch G. Relationship between sodium transport and intracellular ATP in isolated perfused rabbit proximal convoluted tubule. Am J Physiol 1991;261:F634–9.

[65] Beck JS, Hurst AM, Lapointe J-Y, Laprade R. Regulation of basolateral K channels in proximal tubule studied during continuous microperfusion. Am J Physiol 1993;264:F496–501.

[66] Beck JS, Laprade R, Lapointe J-Y. Coupling between transepithelial Na transport and basolateral K conductance in renal proximal tubule. Am J Physiol 1994;266:F517–27.

[67] Beck JS, Potts DJ. Cell swelling, co-transport activation and potassium conductance in isolated perfused rabbit kidney proximal tubules. J Physiol 1990;425:369–78.

[68] Beguin P, Beggah AT, Chibalin AV, Burgener-Kairuz P, Jaisser F, Mathews PM, et al. Phosphorylation of the NaK-ATPase alpha-subunit by protein kinase A and C in vitro and in intact cells. J Biol Chem 1994;269(39):24437–45.

[69] Bello-Reuss E. Effect of catecholamines on fluid reabsorption by the isolated proximal convoluted tubule. Am J Physiol 1980;238:F347–52.

[70] Bello-Reuss E. Electrical properties of the basolateral membrane of the straight portion of the rabbit proximal renal tubule. J Physiol (Lond) 1982;326:49–63.

[71] Bello-Reuss E, Colindres RE, Pastoriza-Munoz E, Mueller RA, Gottschalk CW. Effects of acute unilateral renal denervation in the rat. J Clin Invest 1975;56:208–17.

[72] Bello-Reuss E, Higashi Y, Kaneda Y. Dopamine decreases fluid reabsorption in straight portions of rabbit proximal tubule. Am J Physiol 1982;242:F634–40.

[73] Bello-Reuss E, Trevino DL, Gottschalk CW. Effect of renal sympathetic nerve stimulation on proximal water and sodium reabsorption. J Clin Invest 1976;57:1104–7.

[74] Bello-Reuss E, Weber MR. Electrophysiological studies on primary cultures of proximal tubule cells. Am J Physiol 1986;251: F490–8.

[75] Bengele HH, Evan AP. The effects of Ringer-Locke or blood infusions on the lateral intercellular spaces of the rat proximal tubule. Anat Rec 1975;182:201–14.

[76] Bentzel CJ, Parsa B, Hare DK. Osmotic flow across proximal tubule of *Necturus*: correlation of physiologic and anatomic studies. Am J Physiol 1969;217:570–80.

[77] Bentzel CJ, Reczek PR. Permeability changes in *Necturus* proximal tubule during volume expansion. Am J Physiol 1978;234: F225–34.

[78] Berry CA. Heterogeneity of tubular transport processes in nephron. Ann Rev Physiol 1982;44:181–201.

[79] Berry CA. Lack of effect of peritubular protein on passive NaCl transport in the rabbit proximal tubule. J Clin Invest 1983;71:268–81.

[80] Berry CA. Water permeability and pathways in the proximal tubule. Am J Physiol 1983;245:F279–94.

[81] Berry CA, Cogan MG. Influence of peritubular protein on solute absorption in the rabbit proximal tubule. A specific effect on NaCl transport. J Clin Invest 1981;68:506–16.

[82] Berry CA, Rector Jr. FC. Relative sodium-to-chloride permeability in the proximal convoluted tubule. Am J Physiol 1978;235:F592–604.

[83] Berry CA, Rector Jr. FC. Electroneutral NaCl absorption in the proximal tubule: mechanisms of apical Na-coupled transport. Kidney Int 1989;36:403–11.

[84] Berry CA, Warnock DG, Rector Jr. FC. Ion selectivity and proximal salt reabsorption. Am J Physiol 1978;235:F234–45.

[85] Bertorello A, Aperia A. Na+-K+-ATPase is an effector protein for protein kinase C in renal proximal tubule cells. Am J Physiol 1989;256:F370–3.

[86] Bertorello A, Aperia A, Walaas SI, Nairn AC, Greengard P. Phosphorylation of the catalytic subunit of Na+,K+-ATPase inhibits the activity of the enzyme. Proc Natl Acad Sci 1991;88:11359–62.

[87] Bertorello AM, Katz AI. Short-term regulation of renal Na-K-ATPase activity: Physiological relevance and cellular mechanisms. Am J Physiol 1993;265:F743–55.

[88] Beyenbach KW. Secretory NaCl and volume flow in renal tubules. Am J Physiol 1986;250:R753–63.

[89] Biagi B, Kubota T, Sohtell M, Giebisch G. Intracellular potentials in rabbit proximal tubules perfused *in vitro*. Am J Physiol 1981;240:F200–10.

[90] Biagi B, Sohtell M, Giebisch G. Intracellular potassium activity in the rabbit proximal straight tubule. Am J Physiol 1981;241: F677–86.

[91] Biagi BA, Sohtell M. pH sensitivity of the basolateral membrane of the rabbit proximal tubule. Am J Physiol 1986;250: F261–6.

[92] Biagi BA, Sohtell M. Electrophysiology of basolateral bicarbonate transport in the rabbit proximal tubule. Am J Physiol 1986;250:F267–72.

[93] Biber J, Gisler SM, Hernando N, Murer H. Protein/protein interactions (PDZ) in proximal tubules. J Membr Biol 2005;203:111–8.

[94] Biber J, Gisler SM, Hernando N, Wagner CA, Murer H. PDZ interactions and proximal tubular phosphate reabsorption. Am J Physiol 2004;287:F871–5.

[95] Bichara M, Paillard M, Corman B, de-Rouffignac C, Leviel F. Volume expansion modulates NaHCO3 and NaCl transport in the proximal tubule and Henle's loop. Am J Physiol 1984;247: F140–50.

[96] Bichara M, Paillard M, Leviel F, Gardin J-P. Hydrogen transport in rabbit kidney proximal tubules – Na:H exchange. Am J Physiol 1980;238:F445–51.

[97] Bidet M, Tauc M, Merot J, Vandewalle A, Poujeol P. Na+-H+ exchanger in proximal cells isolated from rabbit kidney. I Functional characteristics. Am J Physiol 1987;253:F935–44.

[98] Biemesderfer D, Nagy T, DeGray B, Aronson PS. Specific association of megalin and the Na+/H+ exchanger isoform NHE3 in the proximal tubule. J Biol Chem 1999;274(25):17518–24.

[99] Biemesderfer D, Pizzonia J, Abu-Alfa A, Exner M, Reilly R, Igarashi P, et al. NHE3: a Na+/H+ exchanger isoform of renal brush border. Am J Physiol 1993;265:F736–42.

[100] Biemesderfer D, Reilly RF, Exner M, Igarashi P, Aronson PS. Immunocytochemical characterization of Na+-H+ exchanger isoform NHE-1 in rabbit kidney. Am J Physiol 1992;263:F833–40.

[101] Biemesderfer D, DeGray B, Aronson PS. Active (9.6 S) and inactive (21 S) oligomers of NHE3 in microdomains of the renal brush border. J Biol Chem 2001;276:10161–7.

[102] Birnir B, Lee H-S, Hediger MA, Wright EM. Expression and characterization of the intestinal Na+/glucose co-transporter in COS-7 cells. Biochim Biophys Acta 1990;1048:100–4.

[103] Blantz RC, Tucker BJ. Determinants of peritubular capillary fluid uptake in hydropenia and saline and plasma expansion. Am J Physiol 1975;228:1927–35.

[104] Bloch RD, Zikos D, Fisher KA, Schleicher L, Oyama M, Cheng J-C, et al. Activation of proximal tubular Na+-H+ exchange by angiotensin II. Am J Physiol 1992;263:F135–43.

[105] Bomsztyk K, Wright FS. Effects of transepithelial fluid flux on transepithelial voltage and transport of calcium sodium chloride and potassium by renal proximal tubule. Kidney Int 1982;21:269 [Abstr.]

[106] Bomsztyk K, Wright FS. Dependence of ion fluxes on fluid transport by rat proximal tubule. Am J Physiol 1986;250:F680–9.

[107] Boonjarern S, Leski ME, Kurtzman NA. Effects of extracellular volume expansion on the tubular reabsorption of glucose. Pflügers Arch 1976;366:67–71.

[108] Boron WF, Boulpaep EL. Intracellular pH regulation in the renal proximal tubule of the salamander: Basolateral HCO_3^- transport. J Gen Physiol 1983;81:53–94.

[109] Boron WF, Boulpaep EL. The electrogenic Na/HCO_3 co-transporter. Kidney Int 1989;36:392–402.

[110] Boron WF, Sackin H. Measurement of intracellular ionic composition and activities in renal tubules. Ann Rev Physiol 1983;45:483–96.

[111] Boulanger Y, Vinay P, Boulanger M. NMR monitoring of intracellular sodium in dog and rabbit kidney tubules. Am J Physiol 1987;253:F904–11.

[112] Braam B, Mitchell KD, Fox J, Navar LG. Proximal tubular secretion of angiotensin II in rats. Am J Physiol 1993;264:F891–8.

[113] Brenner BM, Falchuk KH, Keimowitz RI, Berliner RW. The relationship between peritubular capillary protein concentration and fluid reabsorption by the renal proximal tubule. J Clin Invest 1969;48:1519–31.

[114] Brenner BM, Troy JL. Postglomerular vascular protein concentration: evidence for a causal role in governing fluid reabsorption and glomerulotubular balance by the renal proximal tubule. J Clin Invest 1971;50:336–49.

[115] Brenner BM, Troy JL, Daugharty TM. On the mechanism of inhibition in fluid reabsorption by the renal proximal tubule of the volume-expanded rat. J Clin Invest 1971;50:1596–602.

[116] Breton S, Beck JS, Cardinal J, Giebisch G, Laprade R. Involvement and source of calcium in volume regulatory decrease of collapsed proximal convoluted tubule. Am J Physiol 1992;263:F656–64.

[117] Breton S, Marsolais M, Lapointe JY, Laprade R. Cell volume increases of physiologic amplitude activate basolateral K and Cl conductances in the rabbit proximal convoluted tubule. J Am Soc Nephrol 1996;7:2072–87.

[118] Brismar H, Asghar M, Carey RM, Greengard P, Aperia A. Dopamine-induced recruitment of dopamine D1 receptors to the plasma membrane. Proc Natl Acad Sci 1998;95:5573–8.

[119] Brisolla-Diuana A, Amorena C, Malnic G. Transfer of base across the basolateral membrane of cortical tubules of rat kidney. Pflügers Arch 1985;405:209–15.

[120] Brown D, Hirsch S, Gluck S. Localization of proton-pumping ATPase in rat kidney. J Clin Invest 1988;82:2114–26.

[121] Brown GP, Douglas JG. Angiotensin II binding sites on isolated rat renal brush border membranes. Endocrinology 1982;111:1830–6.

[122] Brown GP, Douglas JG. Angiotensin II binding sites in rat and primate isolated renal tubular basolateral membranes. Endocrinology 1983;112:2007–14.

[123] Burckhardt B-Ch, Cassola AC, Frömter E. Electrophysiological analysis of bicarbonate permeation across the peritubular cell membrane of rat kidney proximal tubule. II Exclusion of HCO_3^- effects on other ion permeabilities and of coupled electroneutral HCO_3^- transport. Pflügers Arch 1984;401:43–51.

[124] Burckhardt B-Ch, Sato K, Frömter E. Electrophysiological analysis of bicarbonate permeation across the peritubular cell membrane of rat kidney proximal tubule. I Basic observations. Pflügers Arch 1984;401:34–42.

[125] Burg MB, Green N. Bicarbonate transport by isolated perfused rabbit proximal convoluted tubules. Am J Physiol 1977;233:F307–14.

[126] Burg MB, Orloff J. Control of fluid absorption in the renal proximal tubule. J Clin Invest 1968;47:2016–24.

[127] Burnham CE, Amlal H, Wang Z, Shull GE, Soleimani M. Cloning and functional expression of a human kidney Na^+:HCO_3^- co-transporter. J Biol Chem 1997;272:19111–4.

[128] Burnham CE, Flagella M, Wang Z, Amlal H, Shull GE, Soleimani M. Cloning renal distribution and regulation of the rat Na^+:HCO_3^- co-transporter. Am J Physiol 1998;274:F1119–26.

[129] Burnham C, Munzesheimer C, Rabon E, Sachs G. Ion pathways in renal brush border membranes. Biochem Biophys Acta 1982;685:260–72.

[130] Cano A, Baum M, Moe OW. Thyroid hormone stimulates the renal Na/H exchanger NHE3 by transcriptional activation. Am J Physiol 1999;276(1 Pt 1):C102–8.

[131] Cano A, Preisig P, Alpern RJ. Cyclic adenosine monophosphate acutely inhibits and chronically stimulates Na/H antiporter in OKP cells. J Clin Invest 1993;92:1632–8.

[132] Cantiello HF, Scott JA, Rabito CA. Conductive Na^+ transport in an epithelial cell line (LLC-PK\d1\u) with characteristics of proximal tubular cells. Am J Physiol 1987;252:F590–7.

[133] Cardinal J, Lapointe J-Y, Laprade R. Luminal and peritubular ionic substitutions and intracellular potential of the rabbit proximal convoluted tubule. Am J Physiol 1984;247:F352–64.

[134] Carey RM. Theodore Cooper Lecture. Renal dopamine system: Paracrine regulator of sodium homeostasis and blood pressure. Hypertension 2001;38:297–302.

[135] Carpi-Medina P, Gonzalez E, Whittembury G. Cell osmotic water permeability of isolated rabbit proximal convoluted tubules. Am J Physiol 1983;244:F554–63.

[136] Carpi-Medina P, Lindemann B, Gonzalez E, Whittembury G. The continuous measurement of tubular volume changes in response to step changes in contraluminal osmolality. Pflügers Arch 1984;400:343–8.

[137] Carranza ML, Feraille E, Favre H. Protein kinase C-dependent phosphorylation of Na^+-K^+-ATPase alpha-subunit in rat kidney cortical tubules. Am J Physiol 1996;271:C136–43.

[138] Cassano G, Stieger B, Murer H. Na/H and Cl/OH exchange in rat jejunal and rat proximal tubular brush border membrane vesicles. Pflügers Arch 1984;400:309–17.

[139] Cassola AC, Mollehauer M, Frömter E. The intracellular chloride activity of rat kidney proximal tubular cells. Pflügers Arch 1983;399:259–65.

[140] Caulfield JB, Trump BF. Correlation of ultrastructure with function in the rat kidney. Am J Pathol 1962;40:199–218.

[141] Cemerikic D, Wilcox CS, Giebisch G. Intracellular potential and K^+ activity in rat kidney proximal tubular cells in acidosis and K^+ depletion. J Membr Biol 1982;69:159–65.

[142] Chalumeau C, du Cheyron D, Defontaine N, Kellermann O, Paillard M, Poggioli J. NHE3 activity and trafficking depend on the state of actin organization in proximal tubule. Am J Physiol 2001;280:F283–90.

[143] Chan YL, Biagi B, Giebisch G. Control mechanisms of bicarbonate transport across the rat proximal convoluted tubule. Am J Physiol 1982;242:F532–43.

[144] Chen P-Y, Illsley NP, Verkman AS. Renal brush-border chloride transport mechanisms characterized using a fluorescent indicator. Am J Physiol 1988;254:F114–20.

[145] Chen P-Y, Verkman AS. Sodium-dependent chloride transport in basolateral membrane vesicles isolated from rabbit proximal tubule. Biochemistry 1988;27:655–60.

[146] Chen XZ, Coady MJ, Jackson F, Berteloot A, Lapointe JY. Thermodynamic determination of the Na^+:glucose coupling ratio for the human SGLT1 co-transporter. Biophys J 1995;69:2405–14.

[147] Cheng H, Becker BN, Harris RC. Dopamine decreases expression of type-1 angiotensin II receptors in renal proximal tubule. J Clin Invest 1996;97:2745−52.

[148] Chernova MN, Jiang L, Friedman DJ, Darman RB, Lohi H, Kere J, et al. Functional comparison of mouse slc26a6 anion exchanger with human SLC26A6 polypeptide variants. J Biol Chem 2005;280(9):8564−80.

[149] Chibalin AV, Katz AI, Berggren PO, Bertorello AM. Receptor-mediated inhibition of renal Na$^+$-K$^+$-ATPase is associated with endocytosis of its alpha and beta subunits. Am J Physiol 1997;273:C1458−65.

[150] Chibalin AV, Pedemonte CH, Katz AI, Feraille E, Berggren PO, Bertorello AM. Phosphorylation of the catalyic alpha-subunit constitutes a triggering signal for Na$^+$,K$^+$-ATPase endocytosis. J Biol Chem 1998;273(15):8814−9.

[151] Choi JY, Shah M, Lee MG, Schultheis PJ, Shull GE, Muallem S, Baum M. Novel amiloride-sensitive sodium-dependent proton secretion in the mouse proximal convoluted tubule. J Clin Invest 2000;105:1141−6.

[152] Chonko AM, Osgood RW, Nickel AE, Ferris TF, Stein JH. The measurement of nephron filtration rate and absolute reabsorption in the proximal tubule of the rat kidney. J Clin Invest 1975;56:232−5.

[153] Chung SD, Alavi N, Livingston D, Hiller S, Taub M. Characterization of primary rabbit kidney cultures that express proximal tubule functions in a hormonally defined medium. J Cell Biol 1982;95:118−26.

[154] Cinelli AR, Efendiev R, Pedemonte CH. Trafficking of Na-K-ATPase and dopamine receptor molecules induced by changes in intracellular sodium concentration of renal epithelial cells. Am J Physiol 2008;295:F1117−25.

[155] Claude P. Morphological factors influencing transepithelial permeability: a model for the resistance of the zonula occludens. J Membr Biol 1978;39:219−32.

[156] Claude P, Goodenough DA. Fracture faces of zonulae occludentes from "tight" and "leaky" epithelia. J Cell Biol 1973;58:390−400.

[157] Cogan MG. Volume expansion predominantly inhibits proximal reabsorption of NaCl rather than NaHCO$_3$. Am J Physiol 1983;245:F272−5.

[158] Cogan MG. Angiotensin II: a powerful controller of sodium transport in the early proximal tubule. Hypertension 1990;15:451−8.

[159] Colegio OR, van Itallie CM, McCrea HJ, Rahner C, Anderson JM. Claudins create charge-selective channels in the paracellular pathway between epithelial cells. Am J Physiol 2002;283:C142−7.

[160] Collazo R, Fan L, Hu MC, Zhao H, Wiederkehr MR, Moe OW. Acute regulation of Na$^+$/H$^+$ exchanger NHE3 by parathyroid hormone via NHE3 phosphorylation and dynamin-dependent endocytosis. J Biol Chem 2000;275(41):31601−8.

[161] Conger JD, Bartoli E, Earley LE. A study in vivo of peritubular oncotic pressure and proximal tubular reabsorption in the rat. Clin Sci Mol Med 1976;51:379−92.

[162] Coppola S, Frömter E. An electrophysiological study of angiotensin II regulation of Na-HCO$_3$ co-transport and K conductance in renal proximal tubules. I. Effect of picomolar concentrations. Pflügers Arch 1994;427:143−50.

[163] Corcia A, Armstrong WMcD. KCl co-transport: a mechanism for basolateral chloride exit in Necturus gallbladder. J Membr Biol 1983;76:173−82.

[164] Corman B. Streaming potentials and diffusion potentials across rabbit proximal convoluted tubule. Pflügers Arch 1985;403:156−63.

[165] Corman B, Roinel N, de Rouffignac C. Water reabsorption capacity of the proximal convoluted tubule: a microperfusion study on rat kidney. J Physiol 1981;316:379−92.

[166] Cunningham R, Steplock D, Wang F, Huang H, Xiaofei E, Shenolikar S, et al. Defective parathyroid hormone regulation of NHE3 activity and phosphate adaptation in cultured NHERF-1$^{-/-}$ renal proximal tubule cells. J Biol Chem 2004;279 (36):37815−21.

[167] Curran PF. Na Cl and water transport by rat ileum in vitro. J Gen Physiol 1960;43:1137−48.

[168] Darvish N, Winaver J, Dagan D. Diverse modulations of chloride channels in renal proximal tubules. Am J Physiol 1994;267:F716−24.

[169] Dawson DC, Richards NW. Basolateral K conductance: role in regulation of NaCl absorption and secretion. Am J Physiol 1990;259:C181−95.

[170] Dellasega M, Grantham JJ. Regulation of renal tubule cell volume in hypotonic media. Am J Physiol 1973;224: 1288−94.

[171] Dennis VW. Influence of bicarbonate on parathyroid hormone-induced changes in fluid absorption by the proximal tubule. Kidney Int 1976;10:373−80.

[172] DiBona GF. Neural regulation of renal tubular sodium reabsorption and renin secretion. Fed Proc 1985;44:2816−22.

[173] Dirks JH, Cirksena WJ, Berliner RW. The effect of saline infusion on sodium reabsorption by the proximal tubule of the dog. J Clin Invest 1965;44:1160−70.

[174] Dolson GM, Hise MK, Weinman EJ. Relationship among parathyroid hormone cAMP, and calcium on proximal tubule sodium transport. Am J Physiol 1985;249:F409−16.

[175] Donowitz M, Cha B, Zachos NC, Brett CL, Sharma A, Tse CM, et al. NHERF family and NHE3 regulation. J Physiol 2005;567:3−11.

[176] Donowitz M, Li X. Regulatory binding partners and complexes of NHE3. Physiol Rev 2007;87:825−72.

[177] Donowitz M, Mohan S, Zhu CX, Chen T, Lin R, Cha B, et al. NHE3 regulatory complexes. J Exp Biol 2009;212:1638−46.

[178] Dorwart MR, Shcheynikov N, Yang D, Muallem S. The solute carrier 26 family of proteins in epithelial ion transport. Physiology 2008;23:104−14.

[179] Dos Santos EA, Dahly-Vernon AJ, Hoagland KM, Roman RJ. Inhibition of the formation of EETs and 20-HETE with 1-aminobenzotriazole attenuates pressure natriuresis. Am J Physiol 2004;287:R58−68.

[180] Doucet A, Katz AI, Morel F. Determination of Na-K-ATPase activity in single segments of the mammalian nephron. Am J Physiol 1979;237:F105−13.

[181] Douglas JG, Hopfer U. Novel aspect of angiotensin receptors and signal transduction in the kidney. Ann Rev Physiol 1994;56:649−69.

[182] Du Z, Duan Y, Yan Q, Weinstein AM, Weinbaum S, Wang T. Mechanosensory function of microvilli of the kidney proximal tubule. Proc Natl Acad Sci 2004;101:13068−73.

[183] Du Z, Yan Q, Duan Y, Weinbaum S, Weinstein AM, Wang T. Axial flow modulates proximal tubule NHE3 and H-ATPase activities by changing microvillous bending moments. Am J Physiol 2006;290:F289−96.

[184] Ducoudret O, Diakov A, Muller-Berger S, Romero MF, Frömter E. The renal Na-HCO$_3$-co-transporter expressed in Xenopus laevis oocytes: inhibition by tenidap and benzamil and effect of temperature on transport rate and stoichiometry. Pflügers Arch 2001;442:709−17.

[185] Durbin RP. Osmotic flow of water across permeable cellulose membranes. J Gen Physiol 1960;44:315−26.

[186] Earley LE, Martino JA, Friedler RM. Factors affecting sodium reabsorption by the proximal tubule as determined during blockade of distal sodium reabsorption. J Clin Invest 1966;45:1668−84.

[187] Earley LE, Schrier RW. Intrarenal control of sodium excretion by hemodynamic and physical factors. In: Orloff J, Berliner RW, editors. Handbook of physiology. section 8:renal physiology. Washington DC: American Physiological Society; 1973. p. 721–62.

[188] Edelman A, Bouthier M, Anagnostopoulos T. Chloride distribution in the proximal convoluted tubule of *Necturus* kidney. J Membr Biol 1981;62:7–17.

[189] Edelman A, Curci S, Samarzija I, Frömter E. Determination of intracellular K^+ activity in rat kidney proximal tubular cells. Pflügers Arch 1978;378:37–45.

[190] Edwards RM, Alyar N. Angiotensin II receptor subtypes in the kidney. J Am Soc Nephrol 1993;3:1643–52.

[191] Efendiev R, Bertorello AM, Pressley TA, Rousselot M, Feraille E, Pedemonte CH. Simultaneous phosphorylation of Ser11 and Ser18 in the alpha-subunit promotes the recruitment of $Na(^+),K(^+)$-ATPase molecules to the plasma membrane. Biochemistry 2000;39:9884–92.

[192] Efendiev R, Bertorello AM, Zandomeni R, Cinelli AR, Pedemonte CH. Agonist-dependent regulation of renal Na^+, K^+-ATPase activity is modulated by intracellular sodium concentration. J Biol Chem 2002;277(13):11489–96.

[193] Eiam-Ong S, Hilden SA, Johns CA, Madias NE. Stimulation of basolateral $Na^+–HCO_3^-$ co-transporter by angiotensin II in rabbit renal cortex. Am J Physiol 1993;265:F195–203.

[194] Eitle E, Hiranyachattada S, Wang H, Harris PJ. Inhibition of proximal tubular fluid absorption by nitric oxide and atrial natriuretic peptide in rat kidney. Am J Physiol 1998;274: C1075–80.

[195] El Mernissi G, Duocet A. Quantitation of [u³dH]ouabain binding and turnover of Na-K-ATPase along the rabbit nephron. Am J Physiol 1984;247:F158–67.

[196] Enck AH, Berger UV, Yu AS. Claudin-2 is selectively expressed in proximal nephron in mouse kidney. Am J Physiol 2001;281:F966–74.

[197] Eveloff JL, Warnock DG. Activation of ion transport systems during cell volume regulation. Am J Physiol 1987;252: F1–10.

[198] Eveloff J, Warnock DG. K-Cl transport systems in rabbit renal basolateral membrane vesicles. Am J Physiol 1987;252:F883–9.

[199] Fan L, Wiederkehr MR, Collazo R, Wang H, Crowder LA, Moe OW. Dual mechanisms of regulation of Na/H exchanger NHE-3 by parathyroid hormone in rat kidney. J Biol Chem 1999;274(16):11289–95.

[200] Felder RA, Campbell T, Albrecht F, Jose PA. Dopamine inhibits Na^+-H^+ exchanger activity in renal BBMV by stimulation of adenylate cyclase. Am J Physiol 1990;259:F297–303.

[201] Felder RA, Jose PA. Mechanisms of disease: the role of GRK4 in the etiology of essential hypertension and salt sensitivity. Nature Clin Prac 2006;2:637–50.

[202] Felder RA, Sanada H, Xu J, Yu P, Wang Z, Watanabe H, et al. G protein-coupled receptor kinase 4 gene variants in human essential hypertension. Proc Natl Acad Sci 2002;99:3872–7.

[203] Feraille E, Carranza ML, Buffin-Meyer B, Rousselot M, Doucet A, Favre H. Protein kinase C-dependent stimulation of Na^+-K^+-ATPase in rat proximal convoluted tubule. Am J Physiol 1995;268:C1277–83.

[204] Feraille E, Doucet A. Sodium–potassium–adenosinetriphosphatase-dependent sodium transport in the kidney: hormonal control. Physiol Rev 2001;81:345–418.

[205] Feschenko MS, Sweadner KJ. Conformation-dependent phosphorylation of NaK-ATPase by protein kinase A and protein kinase C. J Biol Chem 1994;269(48):30436–44.

[206] Feschenko MS, Sweadner KJ. Phosphorylation of Na,K-ATPase by protein kinase C at Ser18 occurs in intact cells but does not result in direct inhibiton of ATP hydrolysis. J Biol Chem 1997;272:17726–33.

[207] Filipovic D, Sackin H. A calcium-permeable stretch-activated cation channel in renal proximal tubule. Am J Physiol 1991;260:F119–29.

[208] Filipovic D, Sackin H. Stretch- and volume-activated channels in isolated proximal tubule cells. Am J Physiol 1992;262: F857–70.

[209] Fine LG, Sakhrani LM. Proximal tubular cells in primary culture. Miner Electrolyte Metab 1986;12:51–7.

[210] Finn AL, Reuss L. Effects of changes in the composition of the serosal solution on the electrical properties of the toad urinary bladder epithelium. J Physiol 1975;250:541–58.

[211] Fisher KA, Lee SH, Walker J, Dileto-Fang C, Ginsberg L, Stapleton SR. Regulation of proximal tubule sodium/hydrogen antiporter with chronic volume contraction. Am J Physiol 2001;280:F922–6.

[212] Fitzgibbons JP, Gennari FJ, Garfinkel HB, Cortell S. Dependence of saline-induced natriuresis upon exposure of the kidney to the physical effects of extracellular fluid volume expansion. J Clin Invest 1974;54:1428–36.

[213] Fraser WD, Baines AD. Application of a fiber-matrix model to transport in renal tubules. J Gen Physiol 1989;94:863–79.

[214] Friedman PA, Figueiredo JF, Maack T, Windhager EE. Sodium–calcium interactions in the renal proximal convoluted tubule of the rabbit. Am J Physiol 1981;240:F558–68.

[215] Frömter E. Electrophysiology and isotonic fluid absorption of proximal tubules of mammalian kidney. In: Thurau K, editor. Kidney and urinary tract physiology MTP international reviews of science physiology series I, vol. 6. Baltimore: University Park Press; 1974. p. 1–38.

[216] Frömter E. Magnitude and significance of the paracellular shunt path in rat kidney proximal tubule. In: Kramer M, Lauterbach F, editors. Intestinal permeation, vol. 4. Amsterdam: Excerpta Medica; 1977. p. 393–405.

[217] Frömter E. Solute transport across epithelia: what can we learn from micropuncture studies on kidney tubules? J Physiol (Lond) 1979;288:1–31.

[218] Frömter E. Electrophysiological analysis of rat renal sugar and amino acid transport. Pflügers Arch 1982;393:179–89.

[219] Frömter E. Viewing the kidney through microelectrodes. Am J Physiol 1984;247:F695–705.

[220] Frömter E, Gessner K. Free-flow potential profile along rat kidney proximal tubule. Pflügers Arch 1974;351:69–83.

[221] Frömter E, Gessner K. Active transport potentials membrane diffusion potentials and streaming potentials across rat kidney proximal tubule. Pflügers Arch 1974;351:85–98.

[222] Frömter E, Gessner K. Effect of inhibitors and diuretics on electrical potential differences in rat kidney proximal tubule. Pflügers Arch 1975;357:209–24.

[223] Frömter E, Muller CW, Wick T. Permeability properties of the proximal tubular epithelium of the rat kidney studied with electrophysiological methods. In: Giebisch G, editor. Electrophysiology of epithelial cells. FK Schattauer Verlag Stuttgart; 1971. p. 119–48.

[224] Frömter E, Rumrich G, Ullrich KJ. Phenomenologic description of Na^+, Cl^-, and HCO_3^- absorption from proximal tubules. Pflügers Arch 1973;343:189–220.

[225] Frömter E, Sato K. Electrical events in active H^+/HCO_3^- transport across rat kidney proximal tubular epithelium. In: Kasbeker DK, Sachs G, Rehm WS, editors. Gastric hydrogen ion secretion. New York: Marcel Dekker; 1976. p. 382–403.

[226] Furuse M, Fujita K, Hiiragi T, Fujimoto K, Tsukita S. Claudin-1 and -2: novel integral membrane proteins localizing at tight

junctions with no sequence similarity to occludin. J Cell Biol 1998;141:1539–50.

[227] Furuse M, Furuse K, Sasaki H, Tsukita S. Conversion of zonulae occludentes from tight to leaky strand type by introducing claudin-2 into Madin–Darby canine kidney I cells. J Cell Biol 2001;153:263–72.

[228] Furuse M, Hirase T, Itoh M, Nagafuchi A, Yonemura S, Tsukita S, et al. Occludin: a novel integral membrane protein localizing at tight junctions. J Cell Biol 1993;123:1777–88.

[229] Furuse M, Sasaki H, Fujimoto K, Tsukita S. A single gene product claudin-1 or -2, reconstitutes tight junction strands and recruits occludin in fibroblasts. J Cell Biol 1998;43:391–401.

[230] Fuster DG, Bobulescu IA, Zhang J, Wade J, Moe OW. Characterization of the regulation of renal Na$^+$/H$^+$ exchanger NHE3 by insulin. Am J Physiol 2007;292:F577–85.

[231] Fuster D, Moe OW, Hilgemann DW. Lipid- and mechanosensitivities of sodium/hydrogen exchangers analyzed by electrical methods. Proc Natl Acad Sci 2004;101:10482–7.

[232] Fuster D, Moe OW, Hilgemann DW. Steady-state function of the ubiquitous mammalian Na/H exchanger (NHE1) in relation to dimmer coupling models with 2Na/2H stoichiometry. J Gen Physiol 2008;132:465–80.

[233] Garg LC, Knepper MA, Burg MB. Mineralocorticoid effects on Na-K-ATPase in individual nephron segments. Am J Physiol 1981;240:F536–44.

[234] Garty H, Karlish SJD. Role of FXYD proteins in ion transport. Annu Rev Physiol 2006;68:431–59.

[235] Garvin JL. Angiotensin stimulates bicarbonate transport and Na$^+$/K$^+$-ATPase in rat proximal straight tubules. J Am Soc Nephrol 1991;1:1146–52.

[236] Garvin JL, Herrera M, Ortiz Pa. Clinical implications. Annu Rev Physiol 2011;73:359–76.

[237] Geering K. FXYD proteins: new regulators of Na-K-ATPase. Am J Physiol 2006;290:F241–50.

[238] Geibel J, Giebisch G, Boron WF. Basolateral sodium-coupled acid–base transport mechanisms of the rabbit proximal tubule. Am J Physiol 1989;257:F790–7.

[239] Geibel J, Giebisch G, Boron WF. Angiotensin II stimulates both Na$^+$/H$^+$ exchange and Na$^+$/HCO$_3^-$ co-transport in the rabbit proximal tubule. Proc Natl Acad Sci 1990;87:7917–20.

[240] Gekle M, Serrano OK, Drumm K, Mildenberger S, Freudinger R, Gassner B, et al. NHE3 serves as a molecular tool for cAMP-mediated regulation of receptor-mediated endocytosis. Am J Physiol 2002;283:F549–58.

[241] Gekle M, Völker K, Mildenberger S, Freudinger R, Shull GE, Wiemann M. NHE3 Na$^+$/H$^+$ exchanger supports proximal tubular protein reabsorption in vivo. Am J Physiol 2004;287:F469–73.

[242] Gertz KH, Boylan JW. Glomerular-tubular balance. In: Orloff J, Berliner RW, editors. Handbook of physiology. section 8: renal physiology. Washington DC: American Physiological Society; 1973. p. 763–90.

[243] Gesek FA, Schoolwerth AC. Hormonal interactions with the proximal Na$^+$-H$^+$ exchanger. Am J Physiol 1990;258:F514–21.

[244] Giebisch G, Windhager EE. Renal tubular transfer of sodium chloride and potassium. Am J Med 1964;36:643–69.

[245] Gildea JJ, Wang X, Jose PA, Felder RA. Differential D1 and D5 receptor regulation and degradation of the angiotensin type 1 receptor. Hypertension 2008;51:360–6.

[246] Gillen CM, Brill S, Payne JA, Forbush III B. Molecular cloning and functional expression of the K-Cl co-transporter from rabbit, rat, and human. A new member of the cation-chloride co-transporter family. J Biol Chem 1996;271:16237–44.

[247] Girardi AC, Knauf F, Demuth HU, Aronson PS. Role of dipeptidyl peptidase IV in regulating activity of Na$^+$/H$^+$ exchanger isoform NHE3 in proximal tubule cells. Am J Physiol 2004;287:C1238–45.

[248] Girardi AC, Titan SMO, Malnic G, Reboucas NA. Chronic effect of parathyroid hormone on NHE3 expression in rat renal proximal tubules. Kidney Int 2000;58:1623–31.

[249] Glynn IM, Karlish SJD. The sodium pump. Annu Rev Physiol 1975;37:13–55.

[250] Gögelein H, Greger R. Single channel recordings from basolateral and apical membranes of renal proximal tubules. Pflügers Arch 1984;401:424–6.

[251] Gögelein H, Greger R. Na$^+$ selective channels in the apical membrane of rabbit late proximal tubules (pars recta). Pflügers Arch 1986;406:198–203.

[252] Goligorsky MS, Menton DN, Hruska KA. Parathyroid hormone-induced changes of the brush border topography and cytoskeleton in cultured renal proximal tubular cells. J Membr Biol 1986;92:151–62.

[253] Gonzalez E, Carpi-Medina P, Whittembury G. Cell osmotic water permeability of isolated rabbit proximal straight tubules. Am J Physiol 1982;242:F321–30.

[254] Gonzalez-Campoy JM, Long C, Roberts D, Berndt TJ, Romero JC, Knox FG. Renal interstitial hydrostatic pressure and PGE$_2$ in pressure natriuresis. Am J Physiol 1991;260:F643–9.

[255] Gottschalk CW. Renal tubular function: lessons from micropuncture. The harvey lectures series 58. New York and London: Academic Press; 1963. p. 99–124

[256] Gottschalk CW. Renal nerves and sodium excretion. Ann Rev Physiol 1979;41:229–40.

[257] Goyal S, Mentone S, Aronson PS. Immunolocalization of NHE8 in rat kidney. Am J Physiol 2005;288:F530–8.

[258] Goyal S, Vanden Heuvel G, Aronson PS. Renal expression of novel Na$^+$/H$^+$ exchanger isoform NHE8. Am J Physiol 2003;284:F467–73.

[259] Grandchamp A, Boulpaep EL. Pressure control of sodium reabsorption and intercellular backflux across proximal kidney tubule. J Clin Invest 1974;54:69–82.

[260] Granger JP, Haas JA, Pawlowska D, Knox FG. Effect of direct increases in renal interstitial hydrostatic pressure on sodium excretion. Am J Physiol 1988;254:F527–32.

[261] Grantham JJ, Lowe CM, Dellasega M, Cole BR. Effect of hypotonic medium on K and Na content of proximal renal tubules. Am J Physiol 1977;232:F42–9.

[262] Grasset E, Gunter-Smith P, Schultz SG. Effects of Na-coupled alanine transport on intracellular K activities and the K conductance of the basolateral membranes of Necturus small intestine. J Memb Biol 1983;71:89–94.

[263] Grassl SM, Aronson PS. Na$^+$/HCO$_3^-$ co-transport in basolateral membrane vesicles isolated from rabbit renal cortex. J Biol Chem 1986;261(19):8778–83.

[264] Grassl SM, Holohan PD, Ross CR. HCO$_3^-$ transport in basolateral membrane vesicles isolated from rat renal cortex. J Biol Chem 1987;262:2682–7.

[265] Green R, Giebisch G. Luminal hypotonicity: a driving force for fluid absorption from the proximal tubule. Am J Physiol 1984;246:F167–74.

[266] Green R, Giebisch G. Reflection coefficients and water permeability in rat proximal tubule. Am J Physiol 1989;257:F658–68.

[267] Green R, Giebisch G, Unwin R, Weinstein AM. Coupled water transport by rat proximal tubule. Am J Physiol 1991;261:F1046–54.

[268] Green R, Moriarty RJ, Giebisch G. Ionic requirements of proximal tubular fluid reabsorption: flow dependence of fluid transport. Kidney Int 1981;20:580–7.

[269] Green R, Windhager EE, Giebisch G. Protein oncotic pressure effects on proximal tubular fluid movement in the rat. Am J Physiol 1974;226:265—76.

[270] Grinstein S, Rothstein A. Mechanisms of regulation of the Na$^+$/H$^+$ exchanger. J Membr Biol 1986;90:1—12.

[271] Gross E, Hawkins K, Abuladze N, Pushkin A, Cotton CU, Hopfer U, et al. The stoichiometry of the electrogenic sodium bicarbonate co-transporter NBC1 is cell-type dependent. J Physiol 2001;531:597—603.

[272] Gross E, Hawkins K, Pushkin A, Sassani P, Dukkipati R, Abuladze N, et al. Phosphorylation of Ser(982) in the sodium bicarbonate co-transporter kNBC1 shifts the HCO$_3^-$:Na$^+$ stoichiometry from 3:1 to 2:1 in murine proximal tubule cells. J Physiol 2001;537:659—65.

[273] Gross E, Hopfer U. Activity and stoichiometry of Na$^+$:HCO$_3^-$ co-transport in immortalized renal proximal tubule cells. J Membr Biol 1996;152:245—52.

[274] Gross E, Hopfer U. Voltage and cosubstrate dependence of the Na-HCO$_3$ co-transporter kinetics in renal proximal tubule cells. Biophys J 1998;75:810—24.

[275] Gross E, Hopfer U. Effects of pH on kinetic parameters of the Na-HCO$_3$ co-transporter in renal proximal tubule. Biophys J 1999;76:3066—75.

[276] Guggino WB, Boulpaep EL, Giebisch G. Electrical properties of chloride transport across the *Necturus* proximal tubule. J Membr Biol 1982;65:185—96.

[277] Guggino WB, London R, Boulpaep EL, Giebisch G. Chloride transport across the basolateral cell membrane of the *Necturus* proximal tubule: dependence on bicarbonate and sodium. J Membr Biol 1983;71:227—40.

[278] Gullans SR, Avison MJ, Ogino T, Giebisch G, Shulman RG. NMR measurements of intracellular sodium in the rabbit proximal tubule. Am J Physiol 1985;249:F160—8.

[279] Gullans SR, Brazy PC, Soltoff SP, Dennis VW, Mandel LJ. Metabolic inhibitors: effects on metabolism and transport in the proximal tubule. Am J Physiol 1982;243:F133—40.

[280] Gunter-Smith PJ, Grasset E, Schultz SG. Sodium-coupled amino acid and sugar transport by *Necturus* small intestine. An equivalent electrical circuit analysis of a rheogenic co-transport system. J Memb Biol 1982;66:25—39.

[281] Guo P, Weinstein AM, Weinbaum S. A dual-pathway ultrastructural model for the tight junction of rat proximal tubule epithelium. Am J Physiol 2003;285:F241—57.

[282] Guo P, Weinstein AM, Weinbaum S. A hydrodynamic mechanosensory hypothesis for brush border microvilli. Am J Physiol 2000;279:F698—712.

[283] Gurley SB, Riquier-Brison ADM, Schnermann J, Sparks MA, Allen AM, Haase VH, et al. AT1A angiotensin receptors in the renal proximal tubule regulate blood pressure. Cell Metab 2011;13:469—75.

[284] Gutierrez AM, Gonzalez E, Echevarria M, Hernandez CS, Whittembury G. The proximal straight tubule (PST) basolateral cell membrane water channel: selectivity characteristics. J Membr Biol 1995;143:189—97.

[285] Györy AZ, Beck F, Rick R, Thurau K. Electron microprobe analysis of proximal tubule cellular Na Cl and K element concentrations during acute mannitol-saline volume expansion in rats: evidence for inhibition of the Na pump. Pflügers Arch 1985;403:205—9.

[286] Haas JA, Granger JP, Knox FG. Effect of renal perfusion pressure on sodium reabsorption from proximal tubules of superficial and deep nephrons. Am J Physiol 1986;250:F425—9.

[287] Haas JA, Granger JP, Knox FG. Effect of intrarenal volume expansion on proximal sodium reabsorption. Am J Physiol 1988;255:F1178—82.

[288] Häberle DA, Shiigai T. Flow-dependent volume reabsorption in the proximal convolution of the rat kidney — the role of glomerular-born tubular fluid for the maintenance of glomerulotubular balance. In: Vogel HG, Ullrich KJ, editors. New aspects of renal function. Amsterdam: Excerpta Medica; 1978. p. 198—206.

[289] Häberle DA, Shiigai TT, Maier G, Schiffl H, Davis JM. Dependency of proximal tubular fluid transport on the load of glomerular filtrate. Kidney Int 1981;20:18—28.

[290] Häberle DA, von Baeyer H. Characteristics of glomerulotubular balance. Am J Physiol 1983;244:F355—66.

[291] Haithcock D, Jiao H, Cui XL, Hopfer U, Douglas JG. Renal proximal tubular AT2 receptor: signaling and transport. J Am Soc Nephrol 1999;10(Suppl. 11):S69—74.

[292] Hall RA, Premont RT, Chow CW, Blitzer JT, Pitcher JA, Claing A, et al. The beta2-adrenergic receptor interacts with the Na$^+$/H$^+$-exchanger regulatory factor to control Na$^+$/H$^+$ exchange. Nature 1998;392(6676):626—30.

[293] Hamburger RJ, Lawson NL, Schwartz JH. Response to parathyroid hormone in defined segments of proximal tubule. Am J Physiol 1976;230:286—90.

[294] Han HJ, Park SH, Koh HJ, Taub M. Mechanism of regulation of Na$^+$ transport by angiotensin II in primary renal cells. Kidney Int 2000;57:2457—67.

[295] Harris PJ. Regulation of proximal tubule function by angiotensin. Clin Exp Pharmacol Physiol 1992;19:213—22.

[296] Harris PJ, Navar LG. Tubular transport responses to angiotensin. Am J Physiol 1985;248:F621—30.

[297] Harris PJ, Young JA. Dose-dependent stimulation and inhibition of proximal tubular sodium reabsorption by angiotensin II in the rat kidney. Pflügers Arch 1977;367:295—7.

[298] Harris SI, Balaban RS, Mandel LJ. Oxygen consumption and cellular ion transport: evidence for adenosine triphosphate to O$_2$ ratio near 6 in intact cell. Science 1980;208:1148—50.

[299] Harris SI, Patton L, Barrett L, Mandel LJ. (Na$^+$,K$^+$)-ATPase kinetics within the intact renal cell. J Biol Chem 1982;257:6996—7002.

[300] Hayashi H, Szaszi K, Grinstein S. Multiple modes of regulation of Na$^+$/H$^+$ exchangers. Ann NY Acad Sci 2002;976:248—58.

[301] Hayslett JP. Effect of changes in hydrostatic pressure in peritubular capillaries on the permeability of the proximal tubule. J Clin Invest 1973;52:1314—9.

[302] Hazama A, Loo DD, Wright EM. Presteady-state currents of the rabbit Na$^+$/glucose co-transporter (SGLT1). J Membr Biol 1997;155:175—86.

[303] Hebert SC, Mount DB, Gamba G. Molecular physiology of cation-coupled Cl$^-$ co-transport: the SCL12 family. Pflügers Arch 2004;447:580—93.

[304] Hediger MA, Coady MJ, Ikeda TS, Wright EM. Expression cloning and cDNA sequencing of the Na$^+$/glucose co-transporter. Nature 1987;330:379—81.

[305] Hediger MA, Rhoads DB. Molecular physiology of sodium—glucose co-transporters. Physiol Rev 1994;74:993—1026.

[306] Heinz E, Weinstein AM. The overshoot phenomenon in co-transport. Biochim Biophys Acta 1984;776:83—91.

[307] Hensley CB, Bradley ME, Mircheff AK. Parathyroid hormone-induced translocation of Na-H antiporters in rat proximal tubules. Am J Physiol 1989;257:C637—45.

[308] Hierholzer K, Kawamura S, Seldin DW, Kokko JP, Jacobson HR. Reflection coefficients of various substrates across superficial and juxtamedullary proximal convoluted segments of rabbit nephrons. Mineral Electrolyte Metab 1980;3:172—80.

[309] Higgins Jr. JT, Meinders AE. Quantitative relationship of renal glucose and sodium reabsorption during ECF expansion. Am J Physiol 1975;229:66—71.

[310] Hilden SA, Sacktor B. D-glucose-dependent sodium transport in renal brush border membrane vesicles. J Biol Chem 1979;254:7090–6.

[311] Hirayama BA, Loo DDF, Díez-Sampedro A, Leung DW, Meinild A, Lai-Bing M, et al. Sodium-dependent reorganization of the sugar-binding site of SGLT1. Biochemistry 2007;46:13391–406.

[312] Hirayama BA, Loo DD, Wright EM. Protons drive sugar transport through the Na$^+$/glucose co-transporter (SGLT1). J Biol Chem 1994;269:21407–10.

[313] Holmberg C, Kokko JP, Jacobson HR. Determination of chloride bicarbonate permeabilities in proximal convoluted tubules. Am J Physiol 1981;241:F386–94.

[314] Holtback U, Eklof AC. Mechanism of FK 506/520 action on rat renal proximal tubular Na$^+$,K$^+$-ATPase activity. Kidney Int 1999;56:1014–21.

[315] Holzgreve H, Schrier RW. Variation of proximal tubular reabsorptive capacity by volume expansion and aortic constriction during constancy of peritubular capillary protein concentration in rat kidney. Pflügers Arch 1975;356:73–86.

[316] Hopfer J, Groseclose R. The mechanism of Na$^+$-dependent D-glucose transport. J Biol Chem 1980;255:4453–62.

[317] Horie S, Moe O, Tejedor A, Alpern RJ. Preincubation in acid medium increases Na/H antiporter activity in cultured renal proximal tubule cells. Proc Natl Acad Sci 1990;87:4742–5.

[318] Houillier P, Chambrey R, Achard JM, Froissart M, Poggioli J, Paillard M. Signaling pathways in the biphasic effect of angiotensin II on apical Na/H antiport activity in proximal tubule. Kid Int 1996;50:1496–505.

[319] Howlin KJ, Alpern RJ, Rector Jr. FC. Amiloride inhibition of proximal tubular acidification. Am J Physiol 1985;248:F773–8.

[320] Hruska KA, Moskowitz D, Esbrit P, Civitelli R, Westbrook S, Huskey M. Stimulation of inositol trisphosphate and diacylglycerol production in renal tubular cells by parathyroid hormone. J Clin Invest 1987;79:230–9.

[321] Hu MC, Fan L, Crowder LA, Karim-Jimenez Z, Murer H, Moe OW. Dopamine acutely stimulates Na$^+$/H$^+$ exchanger (NHE3) endocytosis via clathrin-coated vesicles: dependence on protein kinase A-mediated NHE3 phosphorylation. J Biol Chem 2001;276(29):26906–15.

[322] Hurst AM, Beck JS, Laprade R, Lapointe J-Y. Na$^+$ pump inhibition downregulates an ATP-sensitive K$^+$ channel in rabbit proximal convoluted tubule. Am J Physiol 1993;264:F760–4.

[323] Huss RE, Marsh DJ. A model of NaCl and water flow through paracellular pathways of renal proximal tubules. J Membr Biol 1975;23:305–47.

[324] Huss RE, Stephenson JL. A mathematical model of proximal tubule absorption. J Membr Biol 1979;47:377–99.

[325] Ibarra F, Aperia A, Svensson L-B, Eklöf A-C, Greengard P. Bidirectional regulation of Na$^+$,K$^+$-ATPase activity by dopamine and an alpha-adrenergic agonist. Proc Natl Acad Sci 1993;90:21–4.

[326] Ibarra FR, Cheng SX, Agren M, Svensson LB, Aizman O, Aperia A. Intracellular sodium modulates the state of protein kinase C phosphorylation of rat proximal tubule Na$^+$,K$^+$-ATPase. Acta Physiol Scand 2002;175:165–71.

[327] Ichikawa I, Brenner BM. Mechanism of inhibition of proximal tubule fluid reabsorption after exposure of the rat kidney to the physical effects of expansion of extracellular fluid volume. J Clin Invest 1979;64:1466–74.

[328] Ikeda TS, Hwang E-S, Coady MJ, Hirayama BA, Hediger MA, Wright EM. Characterization of a Na$^+$/glucose co-transporter cloned from rabbit small intestine. J Membr Biol 1989;110:87–95.

[329] Illsley NP, Verkman AS. Membrane chloride transport measured using a chloride-sensitive fluorescent probe. Biochemistry 1987;26:1215–9.

[330] Imai M. Functional heterogeneity of the descending limbs of Henle's loop. II. Interspecies differences among rabbits, rats, and hamsters. Pf Arch 1984;402:393–401.

[331] Imai M, Kokko JP. Effect of peritubular protein concentration on reabsorption of sodium and water in isolated perfused proximal tubules. J Clin Invest 1972;51:314–25.

[332] Imai M, Kokko JP. Transtubular oncotic pressure gradients and net fluid transport in isolated proximal tubules. Kidney Int 1974;6:138–45.

[333] Ishibashi K, Rector Jr. FC, Berry CA. Chloride transport across the basolateral membrane of rabbit proximal convoluted tubules. Am J Physiol 1990;258:F1569–78.

[334] Ishibashi K, Rector Jr. FC, Berry CA. Role of Na-dependent Cl/HCO$_3$ exchange in basolateral Cl transport of rabbit proximal tubules. Am J Physiol 1993;264:F251–8.

[335] Ishibashi K, Sasaki S, Yoshiyama N. Intracellular chloride activity of rabbit proximal straight tubule perfused *in vitro*. Am J Physiol 1988;255:F49–56.

[336] Ito O, Alonso-Galicia M, Hopp KA, Roman RJ. Localization of cytochrome P-450 4A isoforms along rat nephron. Am J Physiol 1998;274:F395–404.

[337] Ives HE, Chen P-Y, Verkman AS. Mechanism of coupling between Cl$^-$ and OH$^-$ transport in renal brush-border membranes. Biochim Biophys Acta 1986;863:91–100.

[338] Ives HE, Yee VJ, Warnock DG. Asymmetric distribution of the Na$^+$/H$^+$ antiporter in the renal proximal tubule epithelial cell. J Biol Chem 1983;258(22):13513–6.

[339] Jacobsen C, Kragh-Hansen U, Sheikh MI. Na$^+$-H$^+$ exchange in luminal-membrane vesicles from rabbit proximal convoluted and straight tubules in response to metabolic acidosis. Biochem J 1986;239:411–6.

[340] Jacobsen C, Rigaard-Petersen H, Sheikh MI. Demonstration of Na$^+$-selective channels in the luminal-membrane vesicles isolated from pars recta of rabbit proximal tubule. FEBS-Lett 1988;236:95–9.

[341] Jacobson HR. Characteristics of volume reabsorption in rabbit superficial and juxtamedullary proximal convoluted tubules. J Clin Invest 1979;63:410–8.

[342] Jacobson HR. Effects of CO$_2$ and acetazolamide on bicarbonate and fluid transport in rabbit proximal tubules. Am J Physiol 1981;240:F54–62.

[343] Jacobson HR, Kokko JP. Intrinsic differences in various segments of the proximal convoluted tubule. J Clin Invest 1976;57:818–25.

[344] Jamison RL. Intrarenal heterogeneity. The case for two functionally dissimilar populations of nephrons in the mammalian kidney. Am J Med 1973;54:281–9.

[345] Jiang Z, Grichtchenko II, Boron WF, Aronson PS. Specificity of anion exchange mediated by mouse slc26a6. J Biol Chem 2002;277(37):33963–7.

[346] Jin X, Siragy HM, Carey RM. Renal interstitial cGMP mediates natriuresis by direct tubule mechanism. Hypertension 2001;38:309–16.

[347] Jin XH, McGrath HE, Gildea JJ, Siragy HM, Felder RA, Carey RM. Renal interstitial guanosine cyclic 3′,5′-monophosphate mediates pressure-natriuresis via protein kinase G. Hypertension 2004;43:1133–9.

[348] Jorgensen PL. Sodium and potassium ion pump in kidney tubules. Physiol Rev 1980;60:864–917.

[349] Jorgensen PL. Structure, function and regulation of NaK-ATPase in the kidney. Kidney Int 1986;29:10–20.

[350] Jorgensen PL, Andersen JP. Structural basis for E_1-E_2 conformational transitions in NaK-pump and Ca-pump proteins. J Membr Biol 1988;103:95—120.

[351] Kahn AM, Dolson GM, Hise MK, Bennett SC, Weinman EJ. Parathyroid hormone and dibutyryl cAMP inhibit Na$^+$-H$^+$ exchange in renal brush border vesicles. Am J Physiol 1985;248:F212—8.

[352] Kaissling B, Kriz W. Structural analysis of the rabbit kidney. Berlin: Springer-Verlag; 1979. pp.1-121

[353] Kanai Y, Lee W, You G, Brown D, Hediger MA. The human kidney low affinity Na$^+$/glucose co-transporter SGLT2. Delineation of the major renal reabsorptive mechanism for D-glucose. J Clin Invest 1994;93:397—404.

[354] Karim ZG, Chambrey R, Chalumeau C, Defontaine N, Warnock DG, Paillard M, et al. Regulation by PKC isoforms of Na$^{(+)}$/H$^{(+)}$ exchanger in luminal membrane vesicles isolated from cortical tubules. Am J Physiol 1999;277:F773—8.

[355] Karniski LP, Aronson PS. Chloride/formate exchange with formic acid recycling: a mechanism of active chloride transport across epithelial membranes. Proc Natl Acad Sci USA 1985;82 (18):6362—5.

[356] Karniski LP, Aronson PS. Anion exchange pathways for Cl$^-$ transport in rabbit renal microvillus membranes. Am J Physiol 1987;253:F513—21.

[357] Karniski LP, Wang T, Everett LA, Green ED, Giebisch G, Aronson PS. Formate-stimulated NaCl absorption in the proximal tubule is independent of the pendrin protein. Am J Physiol 2002;283:F952—6.

[358] Kashgarian M, Biemesderfer D, Caplan M, Forbush III B. Monoclonal antibody to NaK-ATPase: Immunocytochemical localization along nephron segments. Kidney Int 1985;28:899—913.

[359] Katz AI. Renal Na-K-ATPase: its role in tubular sodium and potassium transport. Am J Physiol 1982;242:F207—19.

[360] Katz AI, Doucet A, Morel F. Na-K-ATPase activity along the rabbit rat and mouse nephron. Am J Physiol 1979;237: F114—20.

[361] Kaufman JS, Hamburger RJ. Passive potassium transport in the proximal convoluted tubule. Am J Physiol 1985;248: F228—32.

[362] Kawahara K. A stretch-activated K$^+$ channel in the basolateral membrane of *Xenopus* kidney proximal tubule cells. Pflügers Arch 1990;415:624—9.

[363] Kawahara K, Ogawa A, Suzuki M. Hyposmotic activation of Ca-activated K channels in cultured rabbit kidney proximal tubule cells. Am J Physiol 1991;260:F27—33.

[364] Kawamura S, Imai M, Seldin DW, Kokko JP. Characteristics of salt and water transport in superficial and juxtamedullary straight segments of proximal tubules. J Clin Invest 1975;55: 1269—77.

[365] Kawamura J, Mazumdar DC, Lubowitz H. Effect of albumin infusion on renal glucose reabsorption in the rat. Am J Physiol 1977;232:F286—90.

[366] Kaye GI, Wheeler HO, Whitlock RT, Lane N. Fluid transport in the rabbit gallbladder. J Cell Biol 1966;30:237—68.

[367] Kessler M, Semenza G. The small intestinal Na$^+$-D-glucose co-transporter: an asymmetric gated channel (or pore) responsive to Dy. J Membr Biol 1983;76:27—56.

[368] Khan F, Zelenin SS, Holtbäck U, Scott L, Aperia A. Negative reciprocity between angiotensin II type 1 and dopamine D1 receptors in rat renal proximal tubule cells. Am J Physiol 2008;295:F1110—6.

[369] Khraibi AA, Haas JA, Knox FG. Effect of renal perfusion pressure on renal interstitial hydrostatic pressure in rats. Am J Physiol 1989;256:F165—70.

[370] Khuri RN. Electrochemistry of the nephron. In: Giebisch G, editor. Membrane transport in biology. Vol. IV: transport organs. Berlin: Springer-Verlag; 1979. p. 47—96.

[371] Kinne R. Metabolic correlates of tubular transport. In: Giebisch G, editor. Membrane transport in biology. Vol. IV: transport organs. Berlin: Springer-Verlag; 1979. p. 529—62.

[372] Kinne R, Murer H, Kinne-Saffran E, Thees M, Sachs G. Sugar transport by renal plasma membrane vesicles. J Membr Biol 1975;21:375—95.

[373] Kinoshita Y, Knox FG. Role of prostaglandins in proximal tubule sodium reabsorption: response to elevated renal interstitial hydrostatic pressure. Circ Res 1989;64:1013—8.

[374] Kinsella JL, Aronson PS. Properties of the Na$^+$-H$^+$ exchanger in renal microvillus membrane vesicles. Am J Physiol 1980;238: F461—9.

[375] Kinsella JL, Aronson PS. Amiloride inhibition of the Na$^+$-H$^+$ exchanger in renal microvillus membrane vesicles. Am J Physiol 1981;241:F374—9.

[376] Kinsella JL, Aronson PS. Determination of the coupling ratio for Na$^+$-H$^+$ exchange in renal microvillus membrane vesicles. Biochim Biophys Acta 1982;689:161—4.

[377] Kinsella JL, Cujdik T, Sacktor B. Kinetic studies on the stimulation of Na$^+$- H$^+$ exchange activity in renal brush border membranes isolated from thyroid hormone-treated rats. J Membrane Biol 1986;91:183—91.

[378] Kirk KL, DiBona DR, Schafer JA. Regulatory volume decrease in perfused proximal nephron: evidence for a dumping of cell K$^+$. Am J Physiol 1987;252:F933—42.

[379] Kirk KL, Halm DR, Dawson DC. Active sodium transport by turtle colon via an electrogenic Na-K exchange pump. Nature 1980;287:237—9.

[380] Kirk KL, Schafer JA, DiBona DR. Cell volume regulation in rabbit proximal straight tubule perfused *in vitro*. Am J Physiol 1987;252:F922—32.

[381] Knauf F, Yang CL, Thomson RB, Mentone SA, Giebisch G, Aronson PS. Identification of a chloride-formate exchanger expressed on the brush border membrane of renal proximal tubule cells. Proc Natl Acad Sci 2001;98:9425—30.

[382] Knight TF, Senekjian HO, Sansom SC, Weinman EJ. Proximal tubule glucose efflux in the rat as a function of delivered load. Am J Physiol 1980;238:F499—503.

[383] Knox FG, Haas JA. Factors influencing renal sodium reabsorption in volume expansion. Rev Physiol Biochem Pharm 1982;92:75—113.

[384] Knox FG, Mertz JI, Burnett Jr. JC, Haramati A. Role of hydrostatic and oncotic pressures in renal sodium reabsorption. Circ Res 1983;52:491—500.

[385] Knox FG, Schneider EG, Willis LR, Strandhoy JW, Ott CE. Effect of volume expansion on sodium excretion in the presence and absence of increased delivery from superficial proximal tubules. J Clin Invest 1973;52:1642—6.

[386] Kocinsky HS, Girardi ACC, Biemesderfer D, Nguyen T, Mentone S, Orlowski J, et al. Use of phosph-specific antibodies to determine the phosphorylation of endogenous Na$^+$/H$^+$ exchanger NHE3 at PKA consensus sites. Am J Physiol 2005;289:F249—58.

[387] Kokko JP. Proximal tubule potential difference: dependence on glucose HCO3- and amino acids. J Clin Invest 1973;52:1362—7.

[388] Kokko JP, Burg MB, Orloff J. Characteristics of NaCl and water transport in the renal proximal tubule. J Clin Invest 1971;50:69—76.

[389] Kolb RJ, Woost PG, Hopfer U. Membrane trafficking of angiotensin receptor type-1 and mechanochemical signal transduction in proximal tubule cells. Hypertension 2004;44:352—9.

[390] Kondo Y, Frömter E. Evidence of chloride/bicarbonate exchange mediating bicarbonate efflux from S3 segments of rabbit renal proximal tubule. Pflügers Arch 1990;415:726–33.

[391] Kone BC, Brady HR, Gullans SR. Coordinated regulation of intracellular K^+ in the proximal tubule: Ba^{2+} blockade down-regulates the Na^+,K^+-ATPase and up-regulates two K^+ permeability pathways. Proc Natl Acad Sci 1989;86:6431–5.

[392] Kottra G, Frömter E. Functional properties of the paracellular pathway in some leaky epithelia. J Exp Biol 1983;106:217–29.

[393] Krahn TA, Aronson PS, Weinstein AM. Weak acid permeability of a villous membrane: formic acid transport across rat proximal tubule. Bull Math Biol 1994;56:459–90.

[394] Krahn TA, Weinstein AM. Acid/base transport in a model of the proximal tubule brush border: impact of carbonic anhydrase. Am J Physiol 1996;270:F344–55.

[395] Krapf R, Berry CA, Verkman AS. Estimation of intracellular chloride activity in isolated perfused rabbit proximal convoluted tubules using a fluorescent indicator. Biophys J 1988;53:955–62.

[396] Kumar AM, Spitzer A, Gupta RK. 23Na NMR spectroscopy of proximal tubule suspensions. Kidney Int 1986;29:747–51.

[397] Kunimi M, Seki G, Hara C, Taniguchi S, Uwatoko S, Goto A, et al. Dopamine inhibits renal $Na^+:HCO_3^-$ co-transporter in rabbits and normotensive rats but not in spontaneously hypertensive rats. Kid Int 2000;57:534–43.

[398] Kuo S-M, Aronson PS. Pathways for oxalate transport in rabbit renal microvillus membrane vesicles. J Biol Chem 1996;271:15491–7.

[399] Kurashima K, D'Souza S, Szaszi K, Ramjeesingh R, Orlowski J, Grinstein S. The apical Na^+/H^+ exchanger isoform NHE3 is regulated by the actin cytoskeleton. J Biol Chem 1999;274 (42):29843–9.

[400] Kurtz I. Apical Na^+/H^+ antiporter and glycolysis-dependent H^+-ATPase regulate intracellular pH in the rabbit S3 proximal tubule. J Clin Invest 1987;80:928–35.

[401] Kurtz I. Basolateral membrane Na^+/H^+ antiport $Na^+/base$ co-transport and Na^+-independent $Cl^-/base$ exchange in the rabbit S3 proximal tubule. J Clin Invest 1989;83:616–22.

[402] Kurtz I, Nagami G, Yanagawa N, Li L, Emmons C, Lee I. Mechanism of apical and basolateral Na^+-independent $Cl^-/$ base exchange in the rabbit superficial proximal straight tubule. J Clin Invest 1994;94:173–83.

[403] Kyte J. Immunoferritin determination of the distribution of (Na^+,K^+) ATPase over the plasma membranes of renal convoluted tubules. II. Proximal segment. J Cell Biol 1976;68: 304–18.

[404] Lahera V, Salom MG, Miranda-Guardiola F, Moncada S, Romero JC. Effects of NG-nitro-L-arginine methyl ester on renal function and blood pressure. Am J Physiol 1991;261: F1033–7.

[405] Lamprecht G, Weinman EJ, Yun CH. The role of NHERF and E3KARP in the cAMP-mediated inhibition of NHE3. J Biol Chem 1998;273(45):29972–8.

[406] Lang F, Busch GL, Ritter M, Völkl H, Waldegger S, Gulbins E, et al. Functional significance of cell volume regulatory mechanisms. Physiol Rev 1998;78:247–306.

[407] Lang F, Busch GL, Völkl H. The diversity of volume regulatory mechanisms. Cell Physiol Biochem 1998;8:1–45.

[408] Lapointe J-Y, Duplain M. Regulation of basolateral membrane potential after stimulation of Na^+ transport in proximal tubules. J Membr Biol 1991;120:165–72.

[409] Lapointe J-Y, Garneau L, Bell PD, Cardinal J. Membrane cross-talk in the mammalian proximal tubule during alterations in transepithelial sodium transport. Am J Physiol 1990;258: F339–45.

[410] Lapointe J-Y, Laprade R, Cardinal J. Transepithelial and cell membrane electrical resistances of the rabbit proximal convoluted tubule. Am J Physiol 1984;247:F637–49.

[411] Laradi A, Sakhrani LM, Massry SG. Effect of dopamine on sodium uptake by renal proximal tubule cells of rabbit. Miner Electrolyte Metab 1986;12:303–7.

[412] Lau KR, Hudson RL, Schultz SG. Cell swelling increases a barium-inhibitable potassium conductance in the basolateral membrane of *Necturus* small intestine. Proc Natl Acad Sci 1984;81:3591–4.

[413] Lee WS, Kanai Y, Wells RG, Hediger MA. The high affinity $Na^+/glucose$ co-transporter. Re-evaluation of function and distribution of expression. J Biol Chem 1994;269:12032–9.

[414] Leong PKK, Devillez A, Sandberg MB, Yang LE, Yip DKP, Klein JB, et al. Effect of ACE inhibition on proximal tubule sodium transport. Am J Physiol 2006;290:F854–63.

[415] Leong PK, Yang LE, Holstein-Rathlou NH, McDonough AA. Angiotensin II clamp prevents the second step in renal apical NHE3 internalization during acute hypertension. Am J Physiol 2002;283:F1142–50.

[416] Leong PK, Yang LE, Lin HW, Holstein-Rathlou NH, McDonough AA. Acute hypotension induced by aortic clamp vs. PTH provokes distinct proximal tubule Na^+ transporter redistribution patterns. Am J Physiol 2004;287:R878–85.

[417] Lever JE. A two sodium ion/D-glucose symport mechanism: Membrane potential effect on phlorizin binding. Biochemistry 1984;23:4697–702.

[418] Lewy JE, Windhager EE. Peritubular control of proximal tubular fluid reabsorption in the rat kidney. Am J Physiol 1968;214:943–54.

[419] Li D, Xian S, Cheng J, Fisone G, Caplan MJ, Ohtomo Y, et al. Effects of okadaic acid calyculin A, and PDBu on state of phosphorylation of rat renal Na^+-K^+-ATPase. Am J Physiol 1998;275:F863–9.

[420] Liang M, Knox FG. Production and functional roles of nitric oxide in the proximal tubule. Am J Physiol 2000;278: R1117–24.

[421] Liedtke CM, Hopfer U. Mechanism of Cl^- translocation across small intestinal brush-border membrane. I. Absence of Na^+–Cl^- co-transport. Am J Physiol 1982;242:G263–71.

[422] Liedtke CM, Hopfer U. Mechanism of Cl^- translocation across small intestinal brush-border membrane. II. Demonstration of Cl^- OH^- exchange and Cl^- conductance. Am J Physiol 1982;242:G272–80.

[423] Linas SL, Repine JE. Endothelial cells regulate proximal tubule epithelial cell sodium transport. Kidney Int 1999;55: 1251–8.

[424] Lipkowitz MS, Abramson RG. Modulation of the ionic permeability renal cortical brush-border membranes by cAMP. Am J Physiol 1989;257:F769–76.

[425] Lipkowitz MS, London RD, Beck JC, Abramson RG. Hormonal regulation of rat renal proximal tubule brush-border membrane ionic permeability. Am J Physiol 1992;263:F144–51.

[426] Liu F-Y, Cogan MG. Axial heterogeneity in the rat proximal convoluted tubule. I. Bicarbonate chloride and water transport. Am J Physiol 1984;247:F816–21.

[427] Liu F-Y, Cogan MG. Axial heterogeneity of bicarbonate chloride and water transport in the rat proximal convoluted tubule. J Clin Invest 1986;78:1547–57.

[428] Liu F-Y, Cogan MG. Flow dependence of bicarbonate transport in the early (S1) proximal convoluted tubule. Am J Physiol 1988;254:F851–5.

[429] Liu F-Y, Cogan MG. Angiotensin II stimulation of hydrogen ion secretion in the rat early proximal tubule. Modes of action mechanism and kinetics. J Clin Invest 1988;82:601–7.

[430] Liu F-Y, Cogan MG. Angiotensin II stimulates early proximal bicarbonate absorption in the rat by decreasing cyclic adenosine monophosphate. J Clin Invest 1989;84:83–91.

[431] Liu F, Cogan MG. Role of protein kinase C in proximal bicarbonate absorption and angiotensin signaling. Am J Physiol 1990;258:F927–33.

[432] Liu F-Y, Cogan MG, Rector Jr FC. Axial heterogeneity in the rat proximal convoluted tubule. II Osmolality and osmotic water permeability. Am J Physiol 1984;247:F822–6.

[433] Logvinenko NS, Dulubova I, Fedosova N, Larsson SH, Nairn AC, Esmann M, et al. Phosphorylation by protein kinase C of serine-23 of the alpha-1 subunit of rat Na^+,K^+-ATPase affects its conformational equilibrium. Proc Natl Acad Sci 1996;93:9132–7.

[434] Lohr JW, Grantham JJ. Isovolumetric regulation of isolated S2 proximal tubules in anisotonic media. J Clin Invest 1986;78:1165–72.

[435] Lohr JW, Sullivan LP, Cragoe Jr. EJ, Grantham JJ. Volume regulation determinants in isolated proximal tubules in hypertonic medium. Am J Physiol 1989;256:F622–31.

[436] London R, Cohen B, Guggino WB, Giebisch G. Regulation of intracellular chloride activity during perfusion with hypertonic solutions in the Necturus proximal tubule. J Membr Biol 1983;75:253–8.

[437] Loo DD, Hazama A, Supplisson S, Turk E, Wright EM. Relaxation kinetics of the Na^+/glucose co-transporter. Proc Natl Acad Sci 1993;90:5767–71.

[438] Loo DD, Zeuthen T, Chandy G, Wright EM. Co-transport of water by the Na^+/glucose co-transporter. Proc Natl Acad Sci 1996;93:13367–70.

[439] Loo DDF, Hirayama BA, Karakossian MH, Meinild A, Wright EM. Conformational dynamics of hSGLT1 during Na^+/glucose co-transport. J Gen Physiol 2006;128:701–20.

[440] Lopes AG, Guggino WB. Volume regulation in the early proximal tubule of the Necturus kidney. J Memb Biol 1987;97:117–25.

[441] Lopes AG, Siebens AW, Giebisch G, Boron WF. Electrogenic Na/HCO_3 co-transport across basolateral membrane of isolated perfused Necturus proximal tubule. Am J Physiol 1987;253:F340–50.

[442] Lorentz Jr. WB, Lassiter WE, Gottschalk CW. Renal tubular permeability during increased intrarenal pressure. J Clin Invest 1972;51:484–92.

[443] Lorenz JN, Schultheis PJ, Traynor T, Shull GE, Schnermann J. Micropuncture analysis of single-nephron function in NHE3-deficient mice. Am J Physiol 1999;277:F447–53.

[444] Lucci MS, Warnock DG. Effects on anion-transport inhibitors on NaCl reabsorption in the rat superficial proximal convoluted tubule. J Clin Invest 1979;64:570–9.

[445] Mackenzie B, Loo DDF, Panayotova-Heiermann M, Wright EM. Biophysical characteristics of the pig kidney Na^+/glucose co-transporter SGLT2 reveal a common mechanism for SGLT1 and SGLT2. J Biol Chem 1996;271:32678–83.

[446] MacRobbie EAC, Ussing HH. Osmotic behavior of the epithelial cells of frog skin. Acta Physiol Scand 1961;53:348–65.

[447] Maddox DA, Fortin SM, Tartini A, Barnes WD, Gennari FJ. Effect of acute changes in glomerular filtration rate on Na^+/H^+ exchange in rat renal cortex. J Clin Invest 1992;89:1296–303.

[448] Madhun ZT, Goldthwait DA, McKay D, Hopfer U, Douglas JG. An epoxygenase metabolite of arachidonic acid mediates angiotensin II-induced rises in cytosolic calcium in rabbit proximal tubule epithelial cells. J Clin Invest 1991;88:456–61.

[449] Maeda Y, Smith BL, Agre P, Knepper MA. Quantification of aquaporin-CHIP water channel protein in microdissected renal tubules by fluorescence-based ELISA. J Clin Invest 1995;95:422–8.

[450] Majid DSA, Williams A, Navar LG. Inhibition of nitric oxide synthesis attenuates pressure-induced natriuretic responses in anesthetized dogs. Am J Physiol 1993;264:F79–87.

[451] Martino JA, Earley LE. Demonstration of a role of physical factors as determinants of the natriuretic response to volume expansion. J Clin Invest 1967;46:1963–78.

[452] Maruyama T, Hoshi T. The effect of D-glucose on the electrical potential profile across the proximal tubule of newt kidney. Biochim Biophys Acta 1972;282:214–25.

[453] Mathias RT. Epithelial water transport in a balanced gradient system. Biophys J 1985;47:823–36.

[454] Matsumura Y, Cohen B, Guggino WB, Giebisch G. Electrical effects of potassium and bicarbonate on proximal tubule cells of Necturus. J Membr Biol 1984;79:145–52.

[455] Maunsbach AB. Ultrastructure of the proximal tubule. In: Orloff J, Berliner RW, editors. Handbook of physiology. section 8: renal physiology. Washington DC: American Physiological Society; 1973. p. 31–80.

[456] Maunsbach AB, Boulpaep EL. Hydrostatic pressure changes related to paracellular shunt ultrastructure in proximal tubule. Kidney Int 1980;17:732–48.

[457] Maunsbach AB, Boulpaep EL. Paracellular shunt ultrastructure and changes in fluid transport in Necturus proximal tubule. Kidney Int 1983;24:610–9.

[458] Maunsbach AB, Boulpaep EL. Quantitative ultrastructure and functional correlates in proximal tubule of Ambystoma and Necturus. Am J Physiol 1984;246:F710–24.

[459] Maunsbach AB, Giebisch GH, Stanton BA. Effects of flow rate on proximal tubule ultrastructure. Am J Physiol 1987;253:F582–7.

[460] Maunsbach AB, Vorum H, Kwon TH, Nielsen S, Simonsen B, Choi I, et al. Immunoelectron microscopic localization of the electrogenic Na/HCO_3 co-transporter in rat and Ambystoma kidney. J Am Soc Nephrol 2000;11:2179–89.

[461] McCarthy KM, Skare IB, Stankewich MC, Furuse M, Tsukita S, Rogers RA, et al. Occludin is a functional component of the tight junction. J Cell Sci 1996;109:2287–98.

[462] McCarty NA, O'Neil RG. Dihydropyridine-sensitive cell volume regulation in proximal tubule: the calcium window. Am J Physiol 1990;259:F950–60.

[463] McCarty NA, O'Neil RG. Calcium-dependent control of volume regulation in renal proximal tubule cells: i. Swelling-activated Ca^{2+} entry and release. J Membr Biol 1991;123:149–60.

[464] McCarty NA, O'Neil RG. Calcium-dependent control of volume regulation in renal proximal tubule cells: II. Roles of dihydropyridine-sensitive and -insensitive Ca^{2+} entry pathways. J Membr Biol 1991;123:161–70.

[465] McDonough AA. Mechanisms of proximal tubule sodium transport regulation that link extracellular fluid volume and blood pressure. Am J Physiol 2010;298:R851–61.

[466] McDonough AA, Biemesderfer D. Does membrane trafficking play a role in regulating the sodium/hydrogen exchanger isoform 3 in the proximal tubule? Curr Opin Nephrol Hypertens 2003;12:533–41.

[467] McDonough AA, Magyar CE, Komatsu Y. Expression of Na^+-K^+-ATPase alpha- and beta-subunits along rat nephron: isoform specificity and response to hypokalemia. Am J Physiol 1994;267:C901–8.

[468] McKeown J, Brazy PC, Dennis VW. Intrarenal heterogeneity for fluid phosphate and glucose absorption in the rabbit. Am J Physiol 1979;234:F312–8.

[469] Meinild AK, Klaerke DA, Loo DDF, Wright EM, Zeuthen T. The human Na^+-glucose co-transporter is a molecular water pump. J Physiol 1998;508:15–21.

[470] Mellas J, Hammerman MR. Phorbol ester-induced alkalinization of canine renal proximal tubular cells. Am J Physiol 1986;250:F451–9.

[471] Merot J, Bidet M, Le Maout S, Tauc M, Poujeol P. Two types of K$^+$ channels in the apical membrane of rabbit proximal tubule in primary culture. Biochem Biophys Acta 1989;978:134–44.

[472] Mertz JJ, Haas JA, Berndt TJ, Burnett Jr. JC, Knox FG. Effects of bradykinin on renal interstitial pressures and proximal tubule reabsorption. Am J Physiol 1984;247:F82–5.

[473] Messner G, Koller A, Lang F. The effect of phenylalanine on intracellular pH and sodium activity in proximal convoluted tubule cells of the frog kidney. Pflügers Arch 1985;404:145–9.

[474] Messner G, Oberleithner H, Lang F. The effect of phenylalanine on the electrical properties of proximal tubule cells in the frog kidney. Pflügers Arch 1985;404:138–44.

[475] Millar ID, Robson L. Na$^+$-alanine uptake activates a Cl$^-$ conductance in frog renal proximal tubule cells via nonconventional PKC. Am J Physiol 2001;280:F758–67.

[476] Misfeldt DS, Sanders MJ. Transepithelial transport in cell culture: Stoichiometry of Na/phlorizin binding and Na/D-glucose co-transport. A two-step two-sodium model of binding and translocation. J Membr Biol 1982;70:191–8.

[477] Mitic LL, Anderson JM. Molecular architecture of tight junctions. Annu Rev Physiol 1998;60:121–42.

[478] Moe OW. Acute regulation of proximal tubule apical membrane Na/H exchanger NHE-3: role of phosphorylation protein trafficking and regulatory factors. J Am Soc Nephrol 1999;10:2412–25.

[479] Moe OW, Amemiya M, Yamaji Y. Activation of protein kinase A acutely inhibits and phosphorylates Na/H exchanger NHE-3. J Clin Invest 1995;96:2187–94.

[480] Montrose MH, Murer H. Kinetics of Na$^+$/H$^+$ exchange. In: Grinstein S, editor. Na$^+$-H$^+$ Exchange. Boca Raton FL: CRC Press; 1988. p. 57–75.

[481] Montrose-Rafizadeh C, Guggino WB. Cell volume regulation in the nephron. Ann Rev Physiol 1990;52:761–72.

[482] Moran A, Biber J, Murer H. A sodium–hydrogen exchange system in isolated apical membrane from LLC-PK1 epithelia. Am J Physiol 1986;251:F1003–8.

[483] Moran A, Stange G, Murer H. Sodium–hydrogen exchange system in brush border membranes from cortical and medullary regions of the proximal tubule. Biochem Biophys Res Commun 1989;163:269–75.

[484] Morel F, Murayama Y. Simultaneous measurement of unidirectional and net sodium fluxes in microperfused rat proximal tubules. Pflügers Arch 1970;320:1–23.

[485] Morrow JS, Cianci CD, Ardito T, Mann AS, Kashgarian M. Ankyrin links fodrin to the alpha subunit of NaK-ATPase in Madin–Darby canine kidney cells and in intact renal tubule cells. J Cell Biol 1989;108:455–65.

[486] Mounfield PR, Robson L. The role of Ca^{2+} in volume regulation induced by Na$^+$-coupled alanine uptake in single proximal tubule cells isolated from frog kidney. J Physiol 1998;510:145–53.

[487] Mount DB, Gamba G. Renal potassium–chloride co-transporters. Curr Opin Nephrol Hypertens 2001;10:685–91.

[488] Mount DB, Mercado A, Song L, Xu J, George Jr AL, Delpire E, et al. Cloning and characterization of KCC3 and KCC4, new members of the cation–chloride co-transporter gene family. J Biol Chem 1999;274:16355–62.

[489] Mount DB, Romero MF. The SLC26 gene family of multifunctional anion exchangers. Pflügers Arch 2004;447:710–21.

[490] Muller-Berger S, Coppola S, Samarzija I, Seki G, Frömter E. Partial recovery of in vivo function by improved incubation conditions of isolated renal proximal tubule. I. Change of

[491] Muller-Berger S, Ducoudret O, Diakov A, Frömter E. The renal Na-HCO$_3$-co-transporter expressed in Xenopus laevis oocytes: change in stoichiometry in response to elevation of cytosolic Ca^{2+} concentration. Pflügers Arch 2001;442:718–28.

[492] Muller-Berger S, Nesterov VV, Frömter E. Partial recovery of in vivo function by improved incubation conditions of isolated renal proximal tubule. II. Change of Na-HCO$_3$ co-transport stoichiometry and of response to acetazolamide. Pflügers Arch 1997;434:383–91.

[493] Murer H, Burckhardt G. Membrane transport of anions across epithelia of mammalian small intestine and kidney proximal tubule. Rev Physiol Biochem Pharmacol 1983;96:1–51.

[494] Murer H, Hopfer U, Kinne R. Sodium/proton antiport in brush-border-membrane vesicles isolated from rat small intestine and kidney. Biochem J 1976;154:597–604.

[495] Muto S, Hata M, Taniguchi J, Tsuruoka S, Moriwaki K, Saitou M, et al. Claudin-2-deficient mice are defective in the leaky and cation-selective paracellular permeability properties of renal proximal tubules. Proc Natl Acad Sci 2010;107:8011–6.

[496] Nagami GT. Luminal secretion of ammonia in the mouse proximal tubule perfused in vitro. J Clin Invest 1988;81:159–64.

[497] Nagami GT. Enhanced ammonia secretion by proximal tubules from mice receiving NH$_4$Cl: role of angiotensin II. Am J Physiol 2002;282:F472–7.

[498] Nagami GT, Chang JA, Plato ME, Santamaria R. Acid loading in vivo and low pH in culture increase angiotensin receptor expression: Enhanced ammoniagenic response to angiotensin II. Am J Physiol 2008;295:F1864–70.

[499] Nakamura T, Alberola AM, Salazar FJ, Saito Y, Kurashina T, Granger JP, et al. Effects of renal perfusion pressure on renal interstitial hydrostatic pressure and Na$^+$ excretion: role of endothelium-derived nitric oxide. Nephron 1998;78:104–11.

[500] Nakhoul NL, Chen LK, Boron WF. Intracellular pH regulation in rabbit S3 proximal tubule: Basolateral Cl-HCO$_3$ exchange and Na-HCO$_3$ co-transport. Am J Physiol 1990;258:F371–81.

[501] Nascimento NRF, Kemp BA, Howell NL, Gildea JJ, Santos CF, Harris TE, et al. Role of Src family kinase in extracellular renal cyclic guanosine 3′,5′-monophosphate- and pressure-induced natriuresis. Hypertension 2011;58:107–13.

[502] Navar LG, Majid DSA. Interactions between arterial pressure and sodium excretion. Curr Opin Nephrol Hyperten 1996;5:64–71.

[503] Nielsen R. A 3 to 2 coupling of the Na-K pump responsible for the transepithelial Na transport in frog skin disclosed by the effect of Ba. Acta Physiol Scand 1979;107:189–91.

[504] Nord EP, Goldfarb D, Mikhail N, Moradeshagi P, Hafezi A, Vaystub S, et al. Characteristics of the Na$^+$-H$^+$ antiporter in the intact renal proximal tubular cell. Am J Physiol 1986;250: F539–50.

[505] Nord EP, Howard MJ, Hafezi A, Moradeshagi P, Vaystub S, Insel PA. Alpha 2 adrenergic agonists stimulate Na$^+$-H$^+$ antiport activity in the rabbit renal proximal tubule. J Clin Invest 1987;80:1755–62.

[506] Nowicki S, Chen SL, Aizman O, Cheng XJ, Li D, Nowicki C, et al. 20-Hydroxyeicosa-tetraenoic acid (20-HETE) activates protein kinase C. Role in regulation of rat renal Na$^+$,K$^+$-ATPase. J Clin Invest 1997;99:1224–30.

[507] O'Connell DP, Botkin SJ, Ramos SI, Sibley DR, Ariano MA, Felder RA, et al. Localization of dopamine D1A receptor protein in rat kidneys. Am J Physiol 1995;268:F1185–97.

[508] Ominato M, Satoh T, Katz AI. Regulation of Na-K-ATPase activity in the proximal tubule: role of the protein kinase C pathway and of eicosanoids. J Membr Biol 1996;152:235–43.

[509] Orci L, Humbert F, Brown D, Perrelet A. Membrane ultrastructure in urinary tubules. In: Bourne GH, Danielli JF, Jeon KW, editors. International review of cytology, vol. 73. New York: Academic; 1981. p. 183−242.

[510] Orlowski J. Heterologous expression and functional properties of amiloride high affinity (NHE-1) and low affinity (NHE-3) isoforms of the rat Na/H exchanger. J Biol Chem 1993;268:16369−77.

[511] Orlowski J, Kandasamy RA, Shull GE. Molecular cloning of putative members of the Na/H exchanger gene family. cDNA cloning deduced amino acid sequence and mRNA tissue expression of the rat Na/H exchanger NHE-1 and two structurally related proteins. J Biol Chem 1992;267:9331−9.

[512] Osgood RW, Reineck HJ, Stein JH. Effect of hyperoncotic albumin on superficial and juxtamedullary nephron sodium transport. Am J Physiol 1979;237:F34−7.

[513] Otsu K, Kinsella JL, Koh E, Froehlich JP. Proton dependence of the partial reactions of the sodium-proton exchanger in renal brush border membranes. J Biol Chem 1992;267:8089−96.

[514] Otsu K, Kinsella JL, Sacktor B, Froehlich JP. Transient state kinetic evidence for an oligomer in the mechanism of Na^+-H^+ exchange. Proc Natl Acad Sci 1989;86:4818−22.

[515] Ott CE. Effect of saline expansion on peritubule capillary pressures and reabsorption. Am J Physiol 1981;240:F106−10.

[516] Ott CE, Haas JA, Cuche J-L, Knox FG. Effect of increased peritubule protein concentration on proximal tubule protein concentration on proximal tubule reabsorption in the presence and absence of extracellular volume expansion. J Clin Invest 1975;55:612−20.

[517] Padia SH, Howell NL, Siragy HM, Carey RM. Renal angiotensin type 2 receptors mediate natriuresis via angiotensin III in the angiotensin II type 1 receptor-blocked rat. Hypertension 2006;47:537−44.

[518] Padia SH, Kemp BA, Howell NL, Fournie-Zaluski M-C, Roques BP, Carey RM. Conversion of renal angiotensin II to angiotensin III is critical for AT2 receptor-mediated natriuresis in rats. Hypertension 2008;51:460−5.

[519] Pajor AM, Hirayama BA, Wright EM. Molecular evidence for two renal Na^+/glucose co-transporters. Biochim Biophys Acta 1992;1106:216−20.

[520] Panayotova-Heiermann M, Loo DD, Wright EM. Kinetics of steady-state currents and charge movements associated with the rat Na^+/glucose co-transporter. J Biol Chem 1995;270:27099−105.

[521] Parent L, Supplisson S, Loo DDF, Wright EM. Electrogenic properties of the cloned Na^+/glucose co-transporter: I. Voltage-clamp studies. J Membrane Biol 1992;125:49−62.

[522] Parent L, Supplisson S, Loo DDF, Wright EM. Electrogenic properties of the cloned Na^+/glucose co-transporter: II. A transport model under nonrapid equilibrium conditions. J Membrane Biol 1992;125:63−79.

[523] Pearce D, Verkman AS. NaCl reflection coefficients in proximal tubule apical and basolateral membrane vesicles. Measurement by induced osmosis and solvent drag. Biophys J 1989;55:1251−9.

[524] Periyasamy SM, Liu J, Tanta F, Kabak B, Wakefield B, Malhotra D, et al. Salt loading induces redistribution of the plasmalemmal Na/K-ATPase in proximal tubule cells. Kid Int 2005;67:1868−77.

[525] Persson B, Spring KR. Permeability properties of the subepithelial tissues of *Necturus* gallbladder. Biochim Biophys Acta 1984;772:135−9.

[526] Peterson OW, Gushwa LC, Blantz RC. An analysis of glomerular−tubular balance in the rat proximal tubule. Pflügers Arch 1986;407:221−7.

[527] Petrovic S, Barone S, Wang Z, McDonough AA, Amlal H, Soleimani M. Slc2616 (PAT1) deletion downregulates the apical Na^+/H^+ exchanger in the straight segment of the proximal tubule. Am J Nephrol 2008;28:330−8.

[528] Petrovic S, Barone S, Weinstein AM, Soleimani M. Activation of the apical Na^+/H^+ exchanger NHE3 by formate: a basis of enhanced fluid and electrolyte reabsorption by formate in the kidney. Am J Physiol 2004;287:F336−46.

[529] Pirie SC, Potts DJ. The effect of peritubular protein upon fluid reabsorption in rabbit proximal convoluted tubules perfused *in vitro*. J Physiol 1983;337:429−40.

[530] Pitts TO, McGowan JA, Chen TC, Silverman M, Rose ME, Puschett JB. Inhibitory effects of volume expansion performed *in vivo* on transport in the isolated rabbit proximal tubule perfused *in vitro*. J Clin Invest 1988;81:997−1003.

[531] Planelles G, Thomas SR, Anagnostopoulos T. Change of apparent stoichiometry of proximal-tubule $Na^{(+)}$-HCO_3^- co-transport upon experimental reversal of its orientation. Proc Natl Acad Sci 1993;90:7406−10.

[532] Pohl M, Kaminski H, Castrop H, Bader M, Himmerkus N, Bleich M, et al. Intrarenal renin angiotensin system revisited. Role of megalin-dependent endocytosis along the proximal nephron. J Biol Chem 2010;285:41935−46.

[533] Preisig PA. Luminal flow rate regulates proximal tubule H-HCO3 transporters. Am J Physiol 1992;262:F47−54.

[534] Preisig PA, Alpern RJ. Basolateral membrane H-OH-HCO3 transport in the proximal tubule. Am J Physiol 1989;256: F751−65.

[535] Preisig PA, Alpern RJ. Contributions of cellular leak pathways to net NaHCO3 and NaCl absorption. J Clin Invest 1989;83:1859−67.

[536] Preisig PA, Berry CA. Evidence for transcellular osmotic water flow in rat proximal tubules. Am J Physiol 1985;249:F124−31.

[537] Preisig PA, Ives HE, Cragoe Jr. EJ, Alpern RJ, Rector Jr FC. Role of the Na^+/H^+ antiporter in rat proximal tubule bicarbonate absorption. J Clin Invest 1987;80:970−8.

[538] Preisig PA, Rector Jr FC. Role of Na^+-H^+ antiport in rat proximal tubule NaCl absorption. Am J Physiol 1988;255:F461−5.

[539] Pricam C, Humbert F, Perrelet A, Orci L. A freeze-etch study of the tight junctions of the rat kidney tubules. Lab Invest 1974;30:286−91.

[540] Quan A, Baum M. Endogenous production of angiotensin II modulates rat proximal tubule transport. J Clin Invest 1996;97:2878−82.

[541] Quan A, Baum M. Regulation of proximal tubule transport by angiotensin II Semin. Nephrol 1997;17:423−30.

[542] Quan A, Baum M. Endogenous angiotensin II modulates rat proximal tubule transport with acute changes in extracellular volume. Am J Physiol 1998;275:F74−8.

[543] Quan A, Baum M. Effect of luminal angiotensin II receptor antagonists on proximal tubule transport. Am J Hypertension 1999;12:499−503.

[544] Quan A, Baum M. The renal nerve is required for regulation of proximal tubule transport by intraluminally produced ANG II. Am J Physiol 2001;280:F524−9.

[545] Quan A, Baum M. Renal nerve stimulation augments effect of intraluminal angiotensin II on proximal tubule transport. Am J Physiol 2002;282:F1043−8.

[546] Quigley R, Baum M. Developmental changes in rabbit proximal straight tubule paracellular permeability. Am J Physiol 2002;283:F525−31.

[547] Quigley R, Baum M, Reddy KM, Griener JC, Falck JR. Effects of 20-HETE and 19(S)-HETE on rabbity proximal straight tubule volume transport. Am J Physiol 2000;278:F949−53.

[548] Quinn MD, Marsh DJ. Peritubular capillary control of proximal tubule reabsorption in the rat. Am J Physiol 1979;236:F478−87.

III. FLUID AND ELECTROLYTE REGULATION AND DYSREGULATION

[549] Rabito CA, Ausiello DA. Na$^+$-dependent sugar transport in a cultured epithelial cell line from pig kidney. J Membr Biol 1980;54:31−8.

[550] Ramsey CR, Berndt T, Knox FG. Effect of volume expansion on the paracellular flux of lanthanum in the proximal tubule. J Am Soc Nephrol 1998;9:1147−52.

[551] Ramsey CR, Berndt TJ, Knox FG. Indomethacin blocks enhanced paracellular backflux in proximal tubules. J Am Soc Nephrol 2002;13:1449−54.

[552] Rector Jr FC. Sodium bicarbonate and chloride absorption by the proximal tubule. Am J Physiol 1983;244:F461−71.

[553] Rector Jr. FC, Berry CA. Role of the paracellular pathway in reabsorption of solutes and water by proximal convoluted tubule of the mammalian kidney. In: Bradley SE, Purcell EF, editors. The paracellular pathway. New York: Josiah Macy Jr. Foundation; 1982. p. 135−57.

[554] Reddy S, Gyory AZ, Bostrom T, Dyne M, Salipan-Moore N, Field MJ, et al. Proximal tubular cell electrolytes during volume expansion in the rat. J Physiol 1994;481:217−22.

[555] Reilly AM, Harris PJ, Williams DA. Am J Physiol 1995;269:F374−80.

[556] Renkin EM, Gilmore JP. Glomerular filtration. In: Orloff J, Berliner RW, editors. Handbook of physiology. section 8: renal physiology. Washington DC: American Physiological Society; 1973. p. 185−248.

[557] Restrepo D, Kimmich GA. Kinetic analysis of mechanism of intestinal Na$^+$-dependent sugar transport. Am J Physiol 1985;248:C498−509.

[558] Reuss L. Basolateral KCl co-transport in a NaCl-absorbing epithelium. Nature 1983;305:723−6.

[559] Reuss L. Electrical properties of the cellular transepithelial pathway in Necturus gallbladder. III. Ionic permeability of the basolateral cell membrane. J Membr Biol 1979;47:239−59.

[560] Reuss L, Weinman SA, Grady TP. Intracellular K$^+$ activity and its relation to basolateral membrane ion transport in Necturus gallbladder epithelium. J Gen Physiol 1980;76:33−52.

[561] Ribeiro CMP, Dubay GR, Falck JR, Mandel LJ. Parathyroid hormone inhibits Na$^+$-K$^+$-ATPase through a cytochrome P-450 pathway. Am J Physiol 1994;266:F497−505.

[562] Ribeiro CP, Mandel LJ. Parathyroid hormone inhibits proximal tubule Na$^+$-K$^+$-ATPase activity. Am J Physiol 1992;262:F209−16.

[563] Richardson IW, Licko V, Bartoli E. The nature of passive flows through tightly folded membranes. J Membr Biol 1973;11:293−308.

[564] Riquier-Brison ADM, Leong PKK, Pihakaski-Maunsbach K, McDonough AA. Angiotensin II stimulates trafficking of NHE3, NaPi2, and associated proteins into the proximal tubule microvilli. Am J Physiol 2010;298:F177−86.

[565] Robey RB, Ruiz OS, Espiritu DJ, Ibanez VC, Kear FT, Noboa OA, et al. Angiotensin II stimulation of renal epithelial cell Na/HCO$_3$ co-transport activity: a central role for Src family kinase/classic MAPK pathway coupling. J Membr Biol 2002;187:135−45.

[566] Robson AM, Srivastava PL, Bricker NS. The influence of saline loading on renal glucose reabsorption in the rat. J Clin Invest 1968;47:329−35.

[567] Robson L, Hunter M. Stimulation of Na$^+$-alanine co-transport activates a voltage-dependent conductance in single proximal tubule cells isolated from frog kidney. J Physiol 1999;517:193−200.

[568] Romano G, Favret G, Damato R, Bartoli E. Proximal reabsorption with changing tubular fluid inflow in rat nephrons. Exp Physiol 1998;83:35−48.

[569] Romano G, Favret G, Federico E, Bartoli E. The effect of intra-luminal flow rate on glomerulotubular balance in the proximal tubule of the rat kidney. Exp Physiol 1996;81:95−105.

[570] Rome L, Grantham J, Savin V, Lohr J, Lechene C. Proximal tubule volume regulation in hyperosmotic media: Intracellular K$^+$, Na$^+$, and Cl$^-$. Am J Physiol 1989;257:C1093−100.

[571] Romero MF, Boron WF. Electrogenic Na$^+$/HCO$_3^-$ co-transporters: Cloning and physiology. Ann Rev Physiol 1999;61:699−723.

[572] Romero MF, Fong P, Berger UV, Hediger MA, Boron WF. Cloning and functional expression of rNBC, an electrogenic Na$^{(+)}$-HCO$_3^{(-)}$ co-transporter from rat kidney. Am J Physiol 1998;274:F425−32.

[573] Romero MF, Hediger MA, Boulpaep EL, Boron WF. Expression cloning and characterization of a renal electrogenic Na$^+$/HCO$_3^-$ co-transporter. Nature 1997;387:409−13.

[574] Romero JC, Knox FG. Mechanisms underlying pressure-related natriuresis: the role of the renin−angiotensin and prostaglandin systems. Hypertension 1988;11:724−38.

[575] Romero MF, Hopfer U, Madhun ZT, Zhou J, Douglas JG. Angiotensin II mediated signaling mechanisms and electrolyte transport in the rabbit proximal tubule. Renal Physiol Biochem 1991;14:199−207.

[576] Roos A, Boron WF. Intracellular pH. Physiol Reviews 1981;61:296−434.

[577] Rubera I, Tauc M, Bidet M, Poujeol C, Cuiller B, Watrin A, et al. Chloride currents in primary cultures of rabbit proximal and distal convoluted tubules. Am J Physiol 1998;275:F651−63.

[578] Ruiz OS, Arruda JAL. Regulation of the renal Na−HCO$_3$ co-transporter by cAMP and Ca-dependent protein kinases. Am J Physiol 1992;262:F560−5.

[579] Ruiz OS, Qiu Y-Y, Wang L-J, Arruda JAL. Regulation of the renal Na−HCO$_3$ co-transporter: IV. Mechanisms of the stimulatory effect of angiotensin II. J Am Soc Nephrol 1995;6:1202−8.

[580] Sabolic J, Burckhardt G. Proton pathways in rat renal brush border and basolateral membranes. Biochim Biophys Acta 1983;734:210−20.

[581] Saccomani G, Mitchell KD, Navar LG. Angiotensin II stimulation of Na$^+$-H$^+$ exchange in proximal tubule cells. Am J Physiol 1990;258:F1188−95.

[582] Sackin H. Stretch-activated potassium channels in renal proximal tubule. Am J Physiol 1987;253:F1253−62.

[583] Sackin H, Boulpaep EL. Models for coupling of salt and water transport. J Gen Physiol 1975;66:671−733.

[584] Sakhrani LM, Badie-Dezfooly B, Trizna W, Mikhail N, Lowe AG, Taub M, et al. Transport and metabolism of glucose by renal proximal tubular cells in primary culture. Am J Physiol 1984;246:F757−64.

[585] Saleh AM, Rudnick H, Aronson PS. Mechanism of H$^+$-coupled formate transport in rabbit renal microvillus membranes. Am J Physiol 1996;271:F401−7.

[586] Samarzija I, Hinton BT, Frömter E. Electrophysiological analysis of rat renal sugar and amino acid transport. II. Dependence on various transport parameters and inhibitors. Pflügers Arch 1982;393:190−7.

[587] Sanada H, Jose PA, Hazen-Martin D, Yu P, Xu J, Bruns DE, et al. Dopamine-1 receptor coupling defect in renal proximal tubule cells in hypertension. Hypertension 1999;33:1036−42.

[588] Sanada H, Yatabe J, Midorikawa S, Katoh T, Hashimoto S, Watanabe T, et al. Amelioration of genetic hypertension by suppression of renal G protein-coupled receptor kinase type 4 expression. Hypertension 2006;47:1131−9.

[589] Sasaki S, Ishibashi K, Yoshiyama N, Shiigai T. KCl co-transport across the basolateral membrane of rabbit renal proximal straight tubules. J Clin Invest 1988;81:194−9.

[590] Sasaki S, Shiigai T, Takeuchi J. Intracellular pH in the isolated perfused rabbit proximal straight tubule. Am J Physiol 1985;249:F417—23.

[591] Sasaki S, Shiigai T, Yoshiyama N, Takeuchi J. Mechanism of bicarbonate exit across basolateral membrane of rabbit proximal straight tubule. Am J Physiol 1987;252:F11—8.

[592] Sasaki S, Siragy HM, Gildea JJ, Felder RA, Carey RM. Production and role of extracellular guanosine cyclic 3′,5′ monophosphate in sodium uptake in human proximal tubule cells. Hypertension 2004;43:286—91.

[593] Sasaki S, Yoshiyama N. Interaction of chloride and bicarbonate transport across the basolateral membrane of rabbit proximal straight tubule. Evidence for sodium coupled chloride/bicarbonate exchange. J Clin Invest 1988;81:1004—11.

[594] Satoh T, Cohen HT, Katz AI. Different mechanisms of renal Na-K-ATPase regulation by protein kinases in proximal and distal nephron. Am J Physiol 1993;265:F399—405.

[595] Schafer JA, Andreoli TE. Perfusion of isolated mammalian renal tubules. In: Giebisch G, editor. Membrane transport in biology. Vol. IV: transport organs. Berlin: Springer-Verlag; 1979. p. 473—528.

[596] Schafer JA, Patlak CS, Andreoli TE. A component of fluid absorption linked to passive ion flows in the superficial pars recta. J Gen Physiol 1975;66:445—71.

[597] Schafer JA, Patlak CS, Andreoli TE. Fluid absorption and active and passive ion flows in the rabbit superficial pars recta. Am J Physiol 1977;233:F154—67.

[598] Schafer JA, Patlak CS, Troutman SL, Andreoli TE. Volume absorption in the pars recta. II. Hydraulic conductivity coefficient. Am J Physiol 1978;234:F340—8.

[599] Schafer JA, Troutman SL, Watkins ML, Andreoli TE. Volume absorption in the pars recta. I. "Simple" active Na$^+$ transport. Am J Physiol 1978;234:F332—9.

[600] Schatzmann HJ, Windhager EE, Solomon AK. Single proximal tubules of the *Necturus* kidney. II. Effect of 2,4-dinitrophenol and ouabain on water reabsorption. Am J Physiol 1958;195:570—4.

[601] Schild L, Aronson PS, Giebisch G. Effects of apical membrane Cl$^-$-formate exchange on cell volume in rabbit proximal tubule. Am J Physiol 1990;258:F530—6.

[602] Schild L, Aronson PS, Giebisch G. Basolateral transport pathways for K$^+$ and Cl$^-$ in rabbit proximal tubule: effects on cell volume. Am J Physiol 1991;260:F101—9.

[603] Schild L, Giebisch G, Karniski L, Aronson PS. Chloride transport in the mammalian proximal tubule. Pflügers Arch 1986;407(Suppl. 2):S156—9.

[604] Schild L, Giebisch G, Karniski LP, Aronson PS. Effect of formate on volume reabsorption in the rabbit proximal tubule. J Clin Invest 1987;79:32—8.

[605] Schmidt U, Dubach UC. Activity of (Na$^+$,K$^+$)-stimulated adenosinetriphosphatase in the rat nephron. Pflügers Arch 1969;306:219—26.

[606] Schmidt U, Schmid H, Funk B, Dubach UC. The function of Na-K-ATPase in single portions of the rat nephron. Ann NY Acad Sci 1974;242:489—500.

[607] Schmitt BM, Biemesderfer D, Romero MF, Boulpaep EL, Boron WF. Immunolocalization of the electrogenic Na$^+$—HCO$_3^-$ co-transporter in mammalian and amphibian kidney. Am J Physiol 1999;276:F27—38.

[608] Schneeberger EE, Lynch RD. Structure, function and regulation of cellular tight junctions. Am J Physiol 1992;262:L647—61.

[609] Schnermann J, Wahl M, Liebau G, Fischbach H. Balance between tubular flow rate and net fluid reabsorption in the proximal convolution of the rat kidney. Pflügers Arch 1968;304:90—103.

[610] Schultheis PJ, Clarke LL, Meneton P, Miller ML, Soleimani M, Gawenis LR, et al. Renal and intestinal absorptive defects in mice lacking the NHE3 Na$^+$/H$^+$ exchanger. Nature Genetics 1998;19:2282—5.

[611] Schultz SG. Homocellular regulatory mechanisms in sodium-transporting epithelia: Avoidance of extinction by "flush-through". Am J Physiol 1981;241:F579—90.

[612] Schultz SG. Membrane cross-talk in sodium-absorbing epithelial cells. In: Seldin DW, Giebisch G, editors. Chap. 11 in the kidney. Physiology and pathophysiology. New York: Raven Press; 1992. p. 287—99.

[613] Schultz SG, Hudson RL, Lapointe JY. Electrophysiological studies of sodium co-transport in epithelia: toward a cellular model. Ann NY Acad Sci 1985;456:127—35.

[614] Schuster VL. Effects of angiotensin on proximal tubular reabsorption. Fed Proc 1986;45:1444—7.

[615] Schuster VL, Kokko JP, Jacobson HR. Angiotensin II directly stimulates sodium transport in rabbit proximal convoluted tubules. J Clin Invest 1984;73:507—15.

[616] Schwartz GJ. Na$^+$-dependent H$^+$ efflux from proximal tubule: evidence for reversible Na$^+$-H$^+$ exchange. Am J Physiol 1981;241:F380—5.

[617] Schwartz GJ. Absence of Cl$^-$—OH$^-$ or Cl$^-$—HCO$_3^-$ exchange in the rabbit renal proximal tubule. Am J Physiol 1983;245:F462—9.

[618] Sciortino CM, Romero MF. Cation and voltage dependence of rat kidney electrogenic Na($^+$)—HCO$_3$($^-$) co-transporter rkNBC, expressed in oocytes. Am J Physiol 1999;277:F611—23.

[619] Scott DA, Karniski LP. Human pendrin expressed in *Xenopus laevis* oocytes mediates chloride/formate exchange. Am J Physiol 2000;278:C207—11.

[620] Seely JF. Variation in electrical resistance along length of rat proximal convoluted tubule. Am J Physiol 1973;225:48—57.

[621] Seely JF. Effects of peritubular oncotic pressure on rat proximal tubule electrical resistance. Kidney Int 1973;4:28—35.

[622] Seifter JL, Aronson PS. Properties and physiologic roles of the plasma membrane sodium—hydrogen exchanger. J Clin Invest 1986;78:859—64.

[623] Seifter JL, Knickelbein R, Aronson PS. Absence of Cl-OH exchange and NaCl transport in rabbit renal microvillus membrane vesicles. Am J Physiol 1984;247:F753—9.

[624] Seikaly MG, Arant Jr. BS, Seney Jr. FD. Endogenous angiotensin concentrations in specific intrarenal fluid compartments of the rat. J Clin Invest 1990;86:1352—7.

[625] Seki G, Coppola S, Yoshitomi K, Burckhardt BC, Samarzija I, Muller-Berger S, et al. On the mechanism of bicarbonate exit from renal proximal tubular cells. Kidney Int 1996;49:1671—7.

[626] Seki G, Taniguchi S, Uwatoko S, Suzuki K, Kurokawa K. Evidence for conductive Cl$^-$ pathway in the basolateral membrane of rabbit renal proximal tubule S3 segment. J Clin Invest 1993;92:1229—35.

[627] Seki G, Taniguchi S, Uwatoko S, Suzuki K, Kurokawa K. Activation of the basolateral Cl$^-$ conductance by cAMP in rabbit renal proximal tubule S3 segments. Pflügers Arch 1995;430:88—95.

[628] Seki G, Yamada H, Taniguchi S, Uwatoko S, Suzuki K, Kurokawa K. Mechanism of anion permeation in the basolateral membrane of isolated rabbit renal proximal tubule S3 segment. Am J Physiol 1997;272:C837—46.

[629] Selen G, Persson AEG. Hydrostatic and oncotic pressures in the interstitium of dehydrated and volume expanded rats. Acta Physiol Scand 1983;117:75—81.

[630] Seri I, Kone BC, Gullans SR, Aperia A, Brenner BM, Ballerman BJ. Locally formed dopamine inhibits Na$^+$-K$^+$-ATPase activity in rat renal cortical tubule cells. Am J Physiol 1988;255:F666—73.

[631] Seri I, Kone BC, Gullans SR, Aperia A, Brenner BM, Ballerman BJ. Influence of Na$^+$ intake on dopamine-induced inhibition of renal cortical Na$^+$-K$^+$-ATPase. Am J Physiol 1990;258:F52−60.

[632] Shenolikar S, Voltz JW, Minkoff CM, Wade JB, Weinman EJ. Targeted disruption of the mouse NHERF-1 gene promotes internalization of proximal tubule sodium-phosphate co-transporter type IIa and renal phosphate wasting. Proc Natl Acad Sci 2002;99:11470−5.

[633] Shenolikar S, Weinman EJ. NHERF: targeting and trafficking membrane proteins. Am J Physiol 2001;280:F389−95.

[634] Sheu J-N, Quigley R, Baum M. Heterogeneity of chloride/base exchange in rabbit superficial and juxtamedullary proximal convoluted tubules. Am J Physiol 1995;268:F847−53.

[635] Shi L-B, Fushimi K, Verkman AS. Solvent drag measurement of transcellular and basolateral membrane NaCl reflection coefficient in kidney proximal tubule. J Gen Physiol 1991;98:379−98.

[636] Shindo T, Spring KR. Chloride movement across the basolateral membrane of proximal tubule cells. J Membr Biol 1981;58:35−42.

[637] Shiuan D, Weinstein SW. Evidence for electroneutral chloride transport in rabbit renal cortical brush border membrane vesicles. Am J Physiol 1984;247:F837−47.

[638] Silverman M. Glucose reabsorption in the kidney. Can J Physiol Pharmacol 1981;59:209−24.

[639] Sohtell M. Electrochemical forces for chloride transport in the proximal tubules of the rat kidney. Acta Physiol Scand 1978;103:363−9.

[640] Soleimani M, Aronson PS. Ionic mechanism of Na$^+$−HCO$_3^-$ co-transport in rabbit renal basolateral membrane vesicles. J Biol Chem 1989;264(31):18302−8.

[641] Soleimani M, Bizal GL. Functional indentity of a purified proximal tubule anion exchange protein: Mediation of chloride/formate and chloride/bicarbonate exchange. Kid Int 1996;50:1914−21.

[642] Soleimani M, Bizal GL, Anderson CC. A protein with anion exchange properties found in the kidney proximal tubule. Kid Int 1993;44:565−73.

[643] Soleimani M, Burnham CE. Na$^+$:HCO$_3^-$ co-transporters (NBC): cloning and characterization. J Membr Biol 2001;183:71−84.

[644] Soleimani M, Grassi SM, Aronson PS. Stoichiometry of Na$^+$−HCO$_3^-$ co-transport in basolateral membrane vesicles isolated from rabbit renal cortex. J Clin Invest 1987;79:1276−80.

[645] Soleimani M, Greeley T, Petrovic S, Wang Z, Amlal H, Kopp P, et al. Pendrin: an apical Cl$^-$/OH$^-$/HCO$_3^-$ exchanger in the kidney cortex. Am J Physiol 2001;280:F356−64.

[646] Soltoff SP, Mandel LJ. Active ion transport in the renal proximal tubule. I. Transport and metabolic studies. J Gen Physiol 1984;84:601−22.

[647] Soltoff SP, Mandel LJ. Active ion transport in the renal proximal tubule. II. Ionic dependence of the Na pump. J Gen Physiol 1984;84:623−42.

[648] Soltoff SP, Mandel LJ. Active ion transport in the renal proximal tubule. III. The ATP dependence of the Na pump. J Gen Physiol 1984;84:643−62.

[649] Spitzer A, Windhager EE. Effect of peritubular oncotic pressure changes on proximal tubular fluid reabsorption. Am J Physiol 1970;218:1188−93.

[650] Spring KR, Giebisch G. Kinetics of Na$^+$ transport in *Necturus* proximal tubule. J Gen Physiol 1977;70:307−28.

[651] Spring KR. A parallel path model for *Necturus* proximal tubule. J Membr Biol 1973;13:323−52.

[652] Stanton RC, Mendrick DL, Rennke HG, Seifter JL. Use of monoclonal antibodies to culture rat proximal tubule cells. Am J Physiol 1986;251:C780−6.

[653] Suzuki M, Morita T, Hanaoka K, Kawaguchi Y, Sakai O. A Cl$^-$ channel activated by parathyroid hormone in rabbit renal proximal tubule cells. J Clin Invest 1991;88:735−42.

[654] Szaszi K, Kurashima K, Kaibuchi K, Grinstein S, Orlowski J. Role of the cytoskeleton in mediating cAMP-dependent protein kinase inhibition of the epithelial Na$^+$/H$^+$ exchanger NHE3. J Biol Chem 2001;276(44):40761−8.

[655] Terada Y, Tomita K, Nonoguchi H, Marumo F. Polymerase chain reaction localization of constitutive nitric oxide synthase and soluble guanylate cyclase messenger RNAs in microdissected rat nephron segments. J Clin Invest 1992;90:659−65.

[656] Thekkumkara TJ, Cookson R, Linas SL. Angiotensin (AT1A) receptor-mediated increases in transcellular sodium transport in proximal tubule cells. Am J Physiol 1998;274:F897−905.

[657] Thomas SR, Mikulecky DC. A network thermodynamic model of salt and water flow across the kidney proximal tubule. Am J Physiol 1978;235:F638−48.

[658] Thomson SC, Vallon V. Alpha-2-adrenoceptors determine the response to nitric oxide inhibition in the rat glomerulus and proximal tubule. J Am Soc Nephrol 1995;6:1482−90.

[659] Tisher CC, Kokko JP. Relationship between peritubular oncotic pressure gradients and morphology in isolated proximal tubules. Kidney Int 1974;6:146−56.

[660] Tormey JM, Diamond JM. The ultrastructural route of fluid transport in rabbit gall bladder. J Gen Physiol 1967;50:2031−60.

[661] Tripathi S, Boulpaep EL. Cell membrane water permeabilities and streaming currents in *Ambystoma* proximal tubule. Am J Physiol 1988;255:F188−203.

[662] Tse C-M, Brant SR, Walker MS, Pouyssegur J, Donowitz M. Cloning and sequencing of a rabbit cDNA encoding an intestinal and kidney-specific Na$^+$/H$^+$ exchanger isoform (NHE-3). J Biol Chem 1992;267:9340−6.

[663] Tse C-M, Levine SA, Yun CHC, Brant SR, Pouyssegur J, Montrose MH, et al. Functional characteristics of a cloned epithelial Na$^+$/H$^+$ exchanger (NHE3): resistance to amiloride and inhibition by protein kinase C. Proc Natl Acad Sci 1993;90:9110−4.

[664] Tsuchiya K, Wang W, Giebisch G, Welling PA. ATP is a coupling modulator of parallel NaK-ATPase-K-channel activity in the renal proximal tubule. Proc Natl Acad Sci 1992;89:6418−22.

[665] Tucker BJ, Blantz RC. Determinants of proximal tubular reabsorption as mechanisms of glomerulotubular balance. Am J Physiol 1978;235:F142−50.

[666] Tumlin JA, Hoban CA, Medford RM, Sands JM. Expression of Na-K-ATPase alpha- and beta-subunit mRNA and protein isoforms in the rat nephron. Am J Physiol 1994;266:F240−5.

[667] Turner RJ. Quantitative studies of co-transport systems: models and vesicles. J Membr Biol 1983;76:1−15.

[668] Turner RJ, Moran A. Further studies of proximal tubular brush border membrane D-glucose transport heterogeneity. J Membr Biol 1982;70:37−45.

[669] Turner RJ, Moran A. Heterogeneity of sodium-dependent D-glucose transport sites along the proximal tubule: evidence from vesicle studies. Am J Physiol 1982;242:F406−14.

[670] Turner RJ, Moran A. Stoichiometric studies of the renal outer cortical brush border membrane D-glucose transporter. J Membr Biol 1982;67:73−80.

[671] Turner RJ, Silverman M. Sugar uptake into brush border vesicles from dog kidney. II. Kinetics. Biochim Biophys Acta 1978;511:470−86.

[672] Ullrich KJ. Permeability characteristics of the mammalian nephron. In: Geiger SR, Orloff J, Berliner RW, editors. Handbook of physiology. section 8: renal physiology. Washington DC: American Physiological Society; 1973. p. 377−98.

[673] Ullrich KJ, Papavassiliou F. Contraluminal bicarbonate transport in the proximal tubule of the rat kidney. Pflügers Arch 1987;410:501–4.

[674] Ullrich KJ, Rumrich G. Direkte Messung der Waserpermabilitat corticaler Nephronabschnitte bei Verschiedenen Diuresezustanden. Pflügers Arch 1963;351:35–48.

[675] Ussing HH. Volume regulation of frog skin epithelium. Acta Physiol Scand 1982;114:363–9.

[676] Vallon V, Schwark JR, Richter K, Hropot M. Role of Na$^{(+)}$/H$^{(+)}$ exchanger NHE3 in nephron function: Micropuncture studies with S3226, an inhibitor of NHE3. Am J Physiol 2000;278:F375–9.

[677] Vallon V, Verkman AS, Schnermann J. Luminal hypotonicity in proximal tubules of aquaporin-1-knockout mice. Am J Physiol 2000;278:F1030–3.

[678] Vallon V, Grahammer F, Richter K, Bleich M, Lang F, Barhanin J, et al. Role of KCNE1-dependent K$^+$ fluxes in mouse proximal tubule. J Am Soc Nephrol 2001;12:2003–11.

[679] Vallon V, Grahammer F, Volkl H, Sandu CD, Richter K, Rexhepaj R, et al. KCNQ1-dependent transport in renal and gastrointestinal epithelia. Proc Natl Acad Sci 2005;102:17864–9.

[680] Van der Goot F, Corman B. Axial heterogeneity of apical water permeability along rabbit kidney proximal tubule. Am J Physiol 1991;260:R186–91.

[681] Van der Goot FG, Podevin RA, Corman BJ. Water permeabilities and salt reflection coefficients of luminal basolateral and intracellular membrane vesicles isolated from rabbit kidney proximal tubule. Biochim Biophys Acta 1989;986:332–40.

[682] Van der Goot F, Ripoche P, Corman B. Determination of solute reflection coefficients in kidney brush-border membrane vesicles by light scattering: influence of the refractive index. Biochim Biophys Acta 1989;979:272–4.

[683] van Heeswijk MPE, van Os CH. Osmotic water permeabilities of brush border and basolateral membrane vesicles from rat renal cortex and small intestine. J Membr Biol 1986;92:183–93.

[684] van Os CH, Wiedner G, Wright EM. Volume flows across gallbladder epithelium induced by small hydrostatic and osmotic gradients. J Membr Biol 1979;49:1–20.

[685] Vari RC, Ott CE. In vivo proximal tubular fluid-to-plasma chloride concentration gradient in the rabbit. Am J Physiol 1982;242:F575–9.

[686] Veech RL, Lawson JWR, Cornell NW, Krebs HA. Cytosolic phosphorylation potential. J Biol Chem 1979;254:6538–47.

[687] Verkman AS. Mechanisms of regulation of water permeability in renal epithelia. Am J Physiol 1989;257:C837–50.

[688] Verkman AS, Dix JA, Seifter JL. Water and urea transport in renal microvillus membrane vesicles. Am J Physiol 1985;248:F650–5.

[689] Verkman AS, Ives HE. Water permeability and fluidity of renal basolateral membranes. Am J Physiol 1986;250:F633–43.

[690] Völkl H, Lang F. Electrophysiology of cell volume regulation in proximal tubules of the mouse kidney. Pflügers Arch 1988;411:514–9.

[691] Völkl H, Lang F. Ionic requirement for regulatory cell volume decrease in renal straight proximal tubules. Pflügers Arch 1988;412:1–6.

[692] Völkl H, Paulmichl M, Lang F. Cell volume regulation in renal cortical cells. Renal Physiol Biochem 1988;11:158–73.

[693] Wade JB, Welling PA, Donowitz M, Shenolikar S, Weinman EJ. Differential renal distribution of NHERF isoforms and their colocalization with NHE3, ezrin and ROMK. Am J Physiol 2001;280:C192–8.

[694] Wagner CA, Giebisch G, Lang F, Geibel JP. Angiotensin II stimulates vesicular H$^+$-ATPase in rat proximal tubular cells. Proc Natl Acad Sci 1998;95:9665–8.

[695] Walker AM, Bott PA, Oliver J, MacDowell MC. The collection and analysis of fluid from single nephrons of the mammalian kidney. Am J Physiol 1941;134:580–95.

[696] Wang T. Nitric oxide regulates HCO$_3^-$ and Na$^+$ transport by a cGMP-mediated mechanism in the kidney proximal tubule. Am J Physiol 1997;272:F242–8.

[697] Wang T, Chan YL. Time- and dose-dependent effects of protein kinase C on proximal bicarbonate transport. J Membr Biol 1990;117:131–9.

[698] Wang T, Egbert Jr. AL, Abbiati T, Aronson PS, Giebisch G. Mechanisms of stimulation of proximal tubule chloride transport by formate and oxalate. Am J Physiol 1996;271:F446–50.

[699] Wang T, Giebisch G, Aronson PS. Effects of formate and oxalate on volume absorption in rat proximal tubule. Am J Physiol 1992;263:F37–42.

[700] Wang T, Hropot M, Aronson PS, Giebisch G. Role of NHE isoforms in mediating bicarbonate reabsorption along the nephron. Am J Physiol 2001;281:F1117–22.

[701] Wang T, Inglis FM, Kalb RG. Defective fluid and HCO$_{(3)}^{(-)}$ absorption in proximal tubule of neuronal nitric oxide synthase-knockout mice. Am J Physiol 2000;279:F518–24.

[702] Wang T, Segal AS, Giebisch G, Aronson PS. Stimulation of chloride transport by cAMP in rat proximal tubules. Am J Physiol 1995;268:F204–10.

[703] Wang T, Yang CL, Abbiati T, Schultheis PJ, Shull GE, Giebisch G, et al. Mechanism of proximal tubule bicarbonate absorption in NHE3 null mice. Am J Physiol 1999;277:F298–302.

[704] Wang T, Yang CL, Abbiati T, Shull GE, Giebisch G, Aronson PS. Essential role of NHE3 in facilitating formate-dependent NaCl absorption in the proximal tubule. Am J Physiol 2001;281:F288–92.

[705] Wang Z, Wang T, Petrovic S, Tuo B, Riederer B, Barone S, et al. Renal and intestinal transport defects in Slc26a6-null mice. Am J Physiol 2005;288:C957–65.

[706] Wareing M, Green R. Effect of formate and oxalate on fluid reabsorption from the proximal convoluted tubule of the anaesthetized rat. J Physiol 1994;477:347–54.

[707] Warner RR, Lechene C. Isosmotic volume reabsorption in rat proximal tubule. J Gen Physiol 1980;76:559–86.

[708] Warnock DG, Burg MB. Urinary acidification: CO$_2$ transport by the rabbit proximal straight tubule. Am J Physiol 1977;232:F20–5.

[709] Warnock DG, Eveloff J. NaCl entry mechanisms in the luminal membrane of the renal tubule. Am J Physiol 1982;242:F561–74.

[710] Warnock DG, Eveloff J. K-Cl co-transport systems. Kidney Int 1989;36:412–7.

[711] Warnock DG, Yee VJ. Neutral NaCl co-transport in the proximal tubule: evidence for the parallel exchanger model. Clin Res 1981;29:479A [Abstr.]

[712] Warnock DG, Yee VJ. Chloride uptake by brush border membrane vesicles isolated from rabbit renal cortex. J Clin Invest 1981;67:103–15.

[713] Warnock DG, Yee VJ. Anion permeabilities of the isolated perfused rabbit proximal tubule. Am J Physiol 1982;242:F395–405.

[714] Warnock DG, Reenstra WW, Yee VJ. Na$^+$/H$^+$ antiporter of brush border vesicles: studies with acridine orange uptake. Am J Physiol 1982;242:F733–9.

[715] Weinman EJ, Biswas R, Steplock D, Douglass TS, Cunningham R, Shenolikar S. Sodium-hydrogen exchanger regulatory factor 1 (NHERF-1) transduces signals that mediate dopamine inhibition of sodium–phosphate co-transport in mouse kidney. J Biol Chem 2010;285:13454–60.

[716] Weinman EJ, Cunningham R, Wade JB, Shenolikar S. The role of NHERF-1 in the regulation of renal proximal tubule

sodium-hydrogen exchanger 3 and sodium-dependent phosphate co-transporter 2a. J Physiol 2005;567:27−32.

[717] Weinman EJ, Dubinsky W, Shenolikar S. Regulation of the renal Na$^+$-H$^+$ exchanger by protein phosphorylation. Kidney Int 1989;36:519−25.

[718] Weinman EJ, Minkoff C, Shenolikar S. Signal complex regulation of renal transport proteins: NHERF and regulation of NHE3 by PKA. Am J Physiol 2000;279:F393−9.

[719] Weinman EJ, Sansom SC, Knight TF, Senekjian HO. Alpha and beta adrenergic agonists stimulate water absorption in the rat proximal tubule. J Membr Biol 1982;69:107−11.

[720] Weinman EJ, Shenolikar S. Protein kinase C activates the renal apical membrane Na$^+$/H$^+$ exchanger. J Membr Biol 1986;93:133−9.

[721] Weinman EJ, Shenolikar S. Regulation of the renal brush border membrane Na$^+$/H$^+$ exchanger. Ann Rev Physiol 1993;55:289−304.

[722] Weinman EJ, Shenolikar S, Kahn AM. cAMP-associated inhibition of Na$^+$-H$^+$ exchanger in rabbit kidney brush-border membranes. Am J Physiol 1987;252:F19−25.

[723] Weinman EJ, Steplock D, Shenolikar S. CAMP-mediated inhibition of the renal brush border membrane Na$^+$-H$^+$ exchanger requires a dissociable phosphoprotein cofactor. J Clin Invest 1993;92:1781−6.

[724] Weinman EJ, Steplock D, Shenolikar S. Acute regulation of NHE3 by protein kinase A requires a multiprotein signal complex. Kidney Int 2001;60(2):450−4.

[725] Weinman EJ, Steplock D, Shenolikar S. NHERF-1 uniquely transduces the cAMP signals that inhibit sodium−hydrogen exchange in mouse renal apical membranes. FEBS Lett 2003;536:141−4.

[726] Weinman EJ, Steplock D, Wang Y, Shenolikar S. Characterization of a protein cofactor that mediates protein kinase A regulation of the renal brush border membrane Na$^+$-H$^+$ exchanger. J Clin Invest 1995;95:2143−9.

[727] Weinstein AM. A nonequilibrium thermodynamic model of the rat proximal tubule epithelium. Biophys J 1983;44:153−70.

[728] Weinstein AM. Transport by epithelia with compliant lateral intercellular spaces: Asymmetric oncotic effects across the rat proximal tubule. Am J Physiol 1984;247:F848−62.

[729] Weinstein AM. Glucose transport in a model of the rat proximal tubule epithelium. Math Biosci 1985;76:87−115.

[730] Weinstein AM. Convective paracellular solute flux: a source of ion−ion interaction in the epithelial transport equations. J Gen Physiol 1987;89:501−18.

[731] Weinstein AM. Modeling the proximal tubule: complications of the paracellular pathway. Am J Physiol 1988;254:F297−305.

[732] Weinstein AM. Glomerulotubular balance in a mathematical model of the proximal nephron. Am J Physiol 1990;258:F612−26.

[733] Weinstein AM. Chloride transport in mathematical model of the rat proximal tubule. Am J Physiol 1992;263:F784−98.

[734] Weinstein AM. Performance of a kinetically defined Na$^+$/H$^+$ antiporter within a mathematical model of the rat proximal tubule. J Gen Physiol 1995;105:617−41.

[735] Weinstein AM. Coupling of entry to exit by peritubular K$^+$-permeability in a mathematical model of the rat proximal tubule. Am J Physiol 1996;271:F158−68.

[736] Weinstein AM, Stephenson JL. Models of coupled salt and water transport across leaky epithelial. J Membr Biol 1981;60:1−20.

[737] Weinstein AM, Stephenson JL, Spring KR. The coupled transport of water. In: Bonting SL, de Pont JJHHM, editors. Membrane Transport. Amsterdam: Elsevier/North-Holland Biomedical Press; 1981. p. 311−51.

[738] Welling LW, Welling DJ. Surface areas of brush border and lateral cell walls in the rabbit proximal nephron. Kidney Int 1975;8:343−8.

[739] Welling LW, Welling DJ. Shape of epithelial cells and intracellular channels in the rabbit proximal nephron. Kidney Int 1976;9:385−94.

[740] Welling LW, Welling DJ, Holsapple JW, Evan AP. Morphometric analysis of distinct microanatomy near the base of proximal tubule cells. Am J Physiol 1987;22:F126−40.

[741] Welling LW, Welling DJ, Ochs TJ. Video measurement of basolateral membrane hydraulic conductivity in the proximal tubule. Am J Physiol 1983;245:F123−9.

[742] Welling LW, Welling DJ, Ochs TJ. Relative osmotic effects of raffinose KCl and NaCl across basolateral cell membrane. Am J Physiol 1990;259:F594−7.

[743] Welling PA, Linshaw MA. Importance of anion in hypotonic volume regulation of rabbit proximal straight tubule. Am J Physiol 1988;255:F853−60.

[744] Welling PA, O'Neil RG. Ionic conductive properties of rabbit proximal straight tubule basolateral membrane. Am J Physiol 1990;258:F940−50.

[745] Welling PA, O'Neil RG. Cell swelling activates basolateral membrane Cl and K conductances in rabbit proximal tubule. Am J Physiol 1990;258:F951−62.

[746] Whitlock RT, Wheeler HO. Coupled transport of solute and water across rabbit gallbladder epithelium. J Clin Invest 1964;48:2249−65.

[747] Whittembury G, Malnic G, Mello-Aires M, Amorena C. Solvent drag of sucrose during absorption indicates paracellular water flow in the rat kidney proximal tubule. Pflügers Arch 1988;412:541−7.

[748] Whittembury G, Pas-Aliaga A, Biondi A, Carpi-Medina P, Gonzalez E, Linares H. Pathways for volume flow and volume regulation in leaky epithelia. Pflügers Arch 1985;405:S17−22.

[749] Wiederkehr MR, Di Sole F, Collazo R, Quinones H, Fan L, Murer H, et al. Characterization of acute inhibition of Na/H exchanger NHE-3 by dopamine in opossum kidney cells. Kidney Int 2001;59:197−209.

[750] Wiederkehr MR, Zhao H, Moe OW. Acute regulation of Na/H exchanger NHE3 activity by protein kinase C: role of NHE3 phosphorylation. Am J Physiol 1999;276:C1205−17.

[751] Wilcox CS, Baylis C. Glomerular−tubular balance and proximal regulation. In: Seldin DW, Giebisch G, editors. The kidney. Physiology and pathophysiology. New York: Raven Press; 1985. p. 985−1012.

[752] Williams AW. Electron microscopic changes associated with water absorption in the jejunum. Gut 1963;4:1−7.

[753] Williams Jr. JC, Schafer JA. A model of osmotic and hydrostatic pressure effects on volume absorption in the proximal tubule. Am J Physiol 1987;253:F563−75.

[754] Williams JC, Schafer JA. Cortical interstitium as a site for solute polarization during tubular absorption. Am J Physiol 1988;254:F813−23.

[755] Williams JM, Sarkis A, Lopez B, Ryan RP, Flasch AK, Roman RJ. Elevations in renal interstitial hydrostatic pressure and 20-hydroxyeicosatetraenoic acid contribute to pressure natriuresis. Hypertension 2007;49:687−94.

[756] Willmann JK, Bleich M, Rizzo M, Schmidt-Hieber M, Ullrich KJ, Greger R. Amiloride-inhibitable Na$^+$ conductance in rat proximal tubule. Pflügers Arch 1997;434:173−8.

[757] Windhager EE. Sodium chloride transport. In: Giebisch G, editor. Membrane transport in biology. Vol. IV transport organs. Berlin: Springer-Verlag; 1979. p. 145−214.

[758] Windhager EE, Boulpaep EL, Giebisch G. Electrophysiological studies on single nephrons. Proceedings of the 3rd

international congress of nephrology. Washington: Karger Basel; 1967. pp. 35—47

[759] Windhager EE, Whittembury G, Oken DE, Schatzmann HJ, Solomon AK. Single proximal tubules of the *Necturus* kidney. III. Dependence of H_2O movement on NaCl concentration. Am J Physiol 1959;197:313—8.

[760] Wong KR, Berry CA, Cogan MG. Flow dependence of chloride transport in rat S1 proximal tubules. Am J Physiol 1995;269: F870—5.

[761] Wong KR, Berry CA, Cogan MG. Alpha-1 adrenergic control of chloride transport in the rat S1 proximal tubule. Am J Physiol 1996;270:F1049—56.

[762] Wong NL, Whiting SJ, Mizgala CL, Quamme GA. Electrolyte handling by the superficial nephron of the rabbit. Am J Physiol 1986;250:F590—5.

[763] Wong PS, Johns EJ. The receptor subtype mediating the action of angiotensin II on intracellular sodium in rat proximal tubules. Br J Pharm 1998;124:41—6.

[764] Work J, Troutman SL, Schafer JA. Transport of potassium in the rabbit pars recta. Am J Physiol 1982;242:F226—37.

[765] Wright EM. The intestinal Na^+/glucose co-transporter. Ann Rev Physiol 1993;55:575—89.

[766] Wright EM. Renal $Na^{(+)}$-glucose co-transporters. Am J Physiol 2001;280:F10—8.

[767] Wright EM, Loo DDF, Panayotova-Heiermann M, Lostao MP, Hirayama BH, Mackenzie B, et al. Active sugar transport in eukaryotes. J Exp Biol 1994;196:197—212.

[768] Wu XC, Harris PJ, Johns EJ. Nitric oxide and renal nerve-mediated proximal tubular reabsorption in normotensive and hypertensive rats. Am J Physiol 1999;277:F560—6.

[769] Wu XC, Johns EJ. Nitric oxide modulation of neurally induced proximal tubular fluid reabsorption in the rat. Hypertension 2002;39:790—3.

[770] Xia P, Bungay PM, Gibson CC, Kovbasnjuk ON, Spring KR. Diffusion coefficients in the lateral intercellular spaces of Madin—Darby canine kidney cell epithelium determined with caged compounds. Biophys J 1998;74:3302—12.

[771] Xie M-H, Liu F-Y, Wong PC, Timmermans PBMWM, Cogan MG. Proximal nephron and renal effects of DuP 753, a nonpeptide angiotensin II receptor antagonist. Kidney Int 1990;38:473—9.

[772] Xie Q, Welch R, Mercado A, Romero MF, Mount DB. Molecular characterization of the murine Slc26a6 anion exchanger: functional comparison with Slc26a1. Am J Physiol 2002;283:F826—38.

[773] Yamaguchi I, Jose PA, Mouradian MM, Canessa LM, Monsma Jr. FJ, Sibley DR, et al. Expression of dopamine D1A receptor gene in proximal tubule of rat kidneys. Am J Physiol 1993;264: F280—5.

[774] Yang LE, Maunsbach AB, Leong PK, McDonough AA. Differential traffic of proximal tubule Na^+ transporters during hypertension or PTH: NHE3 to base of microvilli vs. NaPi2 to endosomes. Am J Physiol 2004;287:F896—906.

[775] Yang LE, Sandberg MB, Can AD, Pihakaski-Maunsbach K, McDonough AA. Effects of dietary salt on renal Na + transporter subcellular distribution, abundance, and phosphorylation status. Am J Physiol 2008;295:F1003—16.

[776] Yao X, Tian S, Chan HY, Biemesderfer D, Desir GV. Expression of KCNA10, a voltage-gated K channel in glomerular endothelium and at the apical membrane of the renal proximal tubule. J Am Soc Nephrol 2002;13:2831—9.

[777] Yau C, Rao L, Silverman M. Sugar uptake into a primary culture of dog kidney proximal tubular cells. Can J Physiol Pharmacol 1985;63:417—26.

[778] Yingst DR, Massey KJ, Rossi NF, Mohanty MJ, Mattingly RR. Angiotensin II directly stimulates activity and alters the phosphorylation of Na-K-ATPase in rat proximal tubule with a rapid time course. Am J Physiol 2004;287:F713—21.

[779] Yip KP, Tse CM, McDonough AA, Marsh DJ. Redistribution of Na^+/H^+ exchXer isoform NHE3 in proximal tubules induced by acute and chronic hypertension. Am J Physiol 1998;275:F565—75.

[780] Yip KP, Wagner AJ, Marsh DJ. Detection of apical $Na^{(+)}$/H $^{(+)}$ exchanger activity inhibition in proximal tubules induced by acute hypertension. Am J Physiol 2000;279: R1412—8.

[781] Yoshitomi K, Burckhardt BC, Frömter E. Rheogenic sodium-bicarbonate co-transport in the peritubular cell membrane of rat renal proximal tubule. Pflügers Arch 1985;405:360—6.

[782] Yoshitomi K, Frömter E. How big is the electrochemical potential difference of Na^+ across rat renal proximal tubular cell membranes *in vivo*?. Pflügers Arch 1985;405(Suppl. 1):S121—6.

[783] Yoshitomi K, Hoshi T. Intracellular Cl^- activity of the proximal tubule of *Triturus* kidney: dependence on extracellular ionic composition and transmembrane potential. Am J Physiol 1983;245:F359—66.

[784] You G, Lee W, Barros EJG, Kanai Y, Huo T, Khawaja S, et al. Molecular characterization of Na^+-coupled glucose transporters in adult and embryonic rat kidney. J Biol Chem 1995,270:29365—71.

[785] Yu AS, Cheng MH, Angelow S, Günzel D, Kanzawa SA, Schneeberger EE, et al. Molecular basis for cation selectivity in claudin-2-based paracellular pores: identification of an electrostatic interaction site. J Gen Physiol 2009;133:111—27.

[786] Yu ASL, Cheng MH, Coalson RD. Calcium inhibits paracellular sodium conductance through claudin-2 by competitive binding. J Biol Chem 2010;285:37060—9.

[787] Zeng C, Jose PA. Dopamine receptors. Important antihypertensive counterbalance agains hypertensive factors. Hyptertension 2011;57:11—7.

[788] Zhang Y, Magyar CE, Norian JM, Holstein-Rathlou NH, Mircheff AK, McDonough AA. Reversible effects of acute hypertension on proximal tubule sodium transporters. Am J Physiol 1998;274:C1090—100.

[789] Zhang Y, Mircheff AK, Hensley CB, Magyar CE, Warnock DG, Chambrey R, et al. Rapid redistribution and inhibition of renal sodium transporters during acute pressure natriuresis. Am J Physiol 1996;270:F1004—14.

[790] Zhang Y, Norian JM, Magyar CE, Holstein-Rathlou NH, Mircheff AK, McDonough AA. *In vivo* PTH provokes apical NHE3 and NaPi2 redistribution and Na-K-ATPase inhibition. Am J Physiol 1999;276:F711—9.

[791] Zhang M, Yao B, Wang S, Fan X, Wu G, Yang H, et al. Intrarenal dopamine deficiency leads to hypertension and decreased longevity in mice. J Clin Invest 2011;121:2845—54.

[792] Zizak M, Lamprecht G, Steplock D, Tariq N, Shenolikar S, Donowitz M, et al. cAMP-induced phosphorylation and inhibition of Na^+/H^+ exchanger 3 (NHE3) are dependent on the presence but not the phosphorylation of NHE regulatory factor. J Biol Chem 1999;274:24753—8.

[793] Hirayama BA, Wong HC, Smith CD, Hagenbuch BA, Hediger MA, Wright EM. Intestinal and renal Na^+/glucose cotransporters share common structures. Am J Physiol 1991;261: C296—304.

[794] Schnermann J, Chou C, Ma T, Traynor T, Knepper MA, Verkman AS. Defective proximal tubular fluid reabsorption in transgenic aquaporin-1 null mice. Proc Natl Acad Sci 1998;95:9660—4.

III. FLUID AND ELECTROLYTE REGULATION AND DYSREGULATION

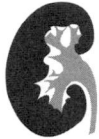

Sodium Chloride Transport in the Loop of Henle, Distal Convoluted Tubule, and Collecting Duct

Gerardo Gamba[1], Wenhui Wang[2] and Laurent Schild[3]

[1]Molecular Physiology Unit, Department of Nephrology and Mineral Metabolism, Instituto Nacional de Ciencias Médicas y Nutrición Salvador Zubirán, and Instituto de Investigaciones Biomédicas, Universidad Nacional Autónoma de México, Mexico City, Mexico

[2]Department of Pharmacology, New York Medical College, Valhalla, NY, USA

[3]Département de Pharmacologie et de Toxicologie, Université de Lausanne, Lausanne, Switzerland

INTRODUCTION

In this chapter we review the transport of ions by the loop of Henle, distal convoluted tubule, the connecting tubule, and the collecting duct. We will place special emphasis on the cellular and molecular mechanisms responsible for Na^+ transport in these regions, as well as the factors that regulate Na^+ transport.

ANATOMIC CONSIDERATIONS

The mammalian loop of Henle contains the descending thin limb, the ascending thin limb, and the thick ascending limb. The thin descending segment begins in the outer medulla after a gradual transition from the pars recta, and ends at the hairpin turn at the tip of Henle's loop. The thin ascending limb begins at the tip of Henle's loop and ends with its abrupt transition to the thick ascending limb. Loops of Henle that arise from superficial or midcortical nephrons may lack a thin ascending limb. In these short loops, thick limbs generally begin at, or slightly before, the hairpin turn (for a detailed discussion see Chapter 20).

The thick ascending limbs of Henle (TAL) of long looped nephrons begin at the boundary between the inner and outer medulla. The TAL of short looped nephrons does not extend as far into the medulla and may, in fact, be entirely cortical. The TAL extends up into the cortex, where it abuts the glomerulus of origin for that nephron and forms the macula densa part of the juxtaglomerular apparatus. The TAL is composed of two parts: a medullary portion and a cortical portion. The ratio of medullary to cortical TAL for a given nephron is a function of the depth of the glomerulus of the nephron such that superficial nephrons have primarily cortical thick limbs, while juxtamedullary nephrons possess primarily medullary thick limbs.

The distal nephron is divided into three segments: the distal convoluted tubule (DCT); the connecting tubule (CNT); and the collecting duct (CD). These segments are clearly delineated in the rabbit, but in many species the transition between segments is gradual. Therefore, distal tubule segments are most accurately defined by their respective cell types. The DCT begins about 50–100 μm beyond the macula densa, and is lined by a single type of cell: the DCT cell. Na^+-K^+-ATPase activity is particularly high in the basolateral membrane of this segment. The CNT forms a transition zone between the DCT and the cortical CD (CCD). In superficial nephrons, a single CNT drains the DCT into the collecting duct. The CNTs of deep nephrons, however, form arcades that ascend through the cortex draining several DCTs into a CCD. The CNT contains two types of cells: the CNT cell, exclusive to the CNT; and the intercalated cell, also found in the CD.

The collecting duct begins at or slightly before the confluence of two or more connecting tubules, and may be divided into three main parts: the CCD; the outer medullary collecting duct (OMCD); and the inner medullary collecting duct (IMCD). The CCD consists of at least three cell types: principal cells, responsible for Na^+ and K^+ transport; and two types of intercalated cells, responsible for H^+ and HCO_3^- transport. In the rabbit, principal cells account for 65–75% of cells in the CCD. The OMCD can be divided into two regions based on location: the outer stripe and the inner stripe. Approximately 80–90% of cells within the OMCD are principal cells. However, as will be discussed later, the functional properties of principal cells in the OMCD differ from those of the CCD. The IMCD extends from the junction between the inner and outer medulla to the tip of the papilla. The IMCD has been divided into three subsegments based on functional differences, including Na^+ transport. Intercalated cells account for about 10% of all cells in the initial portion of the IMCD, but are absent from the terminal IMCD.

Na^+ TRANSPORT IN THE LOOP OF HENLE

The loop of Henle is responsible for absorbing 25 to 40% of the filtered sodium load. Moreover, the dissociation of salt and water absorption by the loop of Henle is ultimately responsible for the capacity of the kidney either to concentrate or to dilute the urine. The active absorption of NaCl in the water-impermeable TAL serves both to dilute the urine and supply the energy for the single effect of countercurrent multiplication.

Salt Transport by Thin Descending and Thin Ascending Segments

There is morphologic and functional evidence of interspecies and inter- and intranephron heterogeneity in the thin loop segments. The morphologic characteristics of the loop of Henle are covered in detail in Chapter 20 of this volume. Generally, loops of Henle can be divided into two groups: long loops and short loops.[150] The thin descending limb of short loop nephrons is a simple, flat epithelium with few organelles and deep junctional complexes. The thin descending limbs of long loop nephrons are heterogeneous. The upper segment of these thin limbs has a larger diameter and thicker epithelium than short loops. The cells in this region have complicated basolateral interdigitations and apical microvilli, but shallow junctional complexes consist of a single junctional strand. These characteristics are most pronounced in rodents, while in rabbits and humans the upper portion of the thin descending limb has a simpler organization with less extensive interdigitation and deeper junctional complexes.

The lower portion of the thin descending limb consists of flat, noninterdigitating cells with a few apical microvilli and with junctional complexes of intermediate depth. There is little interspecies variability in this portion of the descending limb. The thin ascending limb, present only in long loop nephrons, consists of very flat cells connected by very shallow junctional complexes.

According to the passive models for urinary concentration (see Chapter 40), the thin descending limb should have very high water permeability such that the tubular fluid is concentrated by water abstraction rather than solute entry. *In vitro* microperfusion studies have confirmed that upper and lower portions of mammalian descending limbs are very permeable to water[149,150,176,219] (Table 34.1). The passive models also require the thin ascending limb to be rather impermeable to water, highly permeable to sodium chloride, and only modestly permeable to urea. As indicated in Table 34.1, *in vitro* microperfusion studies of thin ascending limb segments have demonstrated that these requirements are, in fact, satisfied.

The permeability of thin descending limb segments to sodium and chloride has been measured in hamsters, rats, and rabbits. In hamsters and rats, the upper portion of long looped descending limbs has a higher sodium permeability and higher P_{Na}/P_{Cl} ratio than do descending limbs of short looped nephrons. In contrast, there is little difference in P_{Na}/P_{Cl} between long and short loop nephrons in rabbits.[149,150] These results are consistent with the morphologic evidence of greater heterogeneity in rats and hamsters than in rabbits. The pathways for transepithelial movement of sodium and chloride in the descending limb are not defined.

The formation of dilute urine begins in the thin ascending limb of Henle. Fluid from the thin ascending limb is more dilute than fluid obtained from the descending limb at the same level. The decrease in osmolality is due primarily to a fall in the NaCl content of the luminal fluid. The mechanism for NaCl transport across the thin ascending limb epithelium is incompletely understood. Measurements of salt dilution potentials in microperfused thin ascending limb segments reveal them to be chloride selective, with P_{Cl}/P_{Na} ratios of 2.2 to 3.5 in rats and hamsters; segments perfused and bathed with symmetric solutions do not generate a spontaneous transepithelial voltage and do not show net transport of solute (reviewed in [150]). These observations have been interpreted to indicate that salt transport *in vivo* results from passive electrodiffusion rather than active transport. Although driven by passive electrochemical gradients, Cl^- movement across the TAL proceeds through a transcellular, and regulated, pathway. $^{36}Cl^-$ flux ratios and salt dilution voltages indicate that the Cl^- pathway discriminates among anions and is saturable.[150]

TABLE 34.1   Permeability Properties of Thin Limb of Henle Segments

| | P$_f$ (10^{-3}cm/sec) | P$_{Na}$ (10^{-5}cm/sec) | P$_{Cl}$ (10^{-5}cm/sec) | P$_{Na}$/P$_{Cl}$ | | P$_{urea}$(10^{-5}cm/sec) |
				SDL	LDL$_u$	
DESCENDING LIMB						
Rabbit	240–250	1.61	–	0.75	0.76	1.5
Rat	227	34–47	–	0.61	5.0	
Hamster SDL	285	4.2	1.3	0.68	–	7.4
Hamster LDL$_u$	403	45.6	4.2	–	4–6	1.5
ASCENDING LIMB						
Rabbit	0	25.5	117	0.29		6.7
Rat	2.5	67.9	183.7	0.43		23.0
Hamster	3	87.6	196	0.47		18.5

Table from Reeves, W. B., and Andreoli, T. E. (2008). Sodium chloride transport in the loop of Henle, distal convoluted tubule, and collecting duct. In "The Kidney: Physiology and Pathophysiology," 4th edn, 849–888, Alpern, R. J., and Hebert, S. C. (eds.). Elsevier.
Note: P$_{Na}$ and P$_{Cl}$ determined from isotope flux measurements. P$_{Na}$/P$_{Cl}$ determined from salt dilution voltages.
LDL$_u$: upper portion of long loop descending limb; P$_f$: osmotic water permeability; SDL: short loop descending limb.

NaCl Absorption in Thick Ascending Limb

General Features

Rocha and Kokko[257] and Burg and Green[33] first demonstrated the salient characteristics of salt absorption in rabbit medullary and cortical TAL segments, respectively. First, net salt absorption resulted in a lumen-positive transepithelial voltage (Ve, mV), which could be abolished by furosemide, and in dilution of the luminal fluid. Second, the transport of Cl$^-$ under these circumstances occurred against both electrical and chemical gradients, and hence involved an active transport process. Third, both net chloride absorption and the transepithelial voltage depended on (Na$^+$, K$^+$)-ATPase activity, present in large amounts along the basolateral membrane of this segment. A final curious feature of the TAL is that this segment is a "hybrid epithelium" possessing a very low permeability to water, yet a high ionic conductance (Table 34.2). The ionic conductance determined from the fluxes of ^{22}Na$^+$ and ^{36}Cl$^-$ is approximately 20–50 mS/cm^2, and is cation selective (P$_{Na}$/P$_{Cl}$ = 2–6). This high electrical conductance is unusual among epithelia with low water permeabilities.

Table 34.2 presents a summary of the important transport properties of the rabbit, mouse, and rat TAL which are relevant to the concentrating and diluting functions of this nephron segment. A low permeability to water is required for the TAL to function as a diluting segment. Hebert et al.,[138,140] and subsequently Hebert[132] demonstrated that the apical cell membrane constitutes the major barrier to transcellular water flow in this segment.

Studies of the electrophysiologic (Table 34.3) and biochemical properties of intact, isolated, perfused thick limb segments, and of apical and basolateral membranes of thick limb cells have provided insights into the specific transport mechanisms involved in salt absorption, and the origin of the lumen-positive transepithelial voltage in this nephron segment.[107,108,110–113,135,138–140] A model for salt absorption by the TAL, which integrates the results of these studies, is shown in Figure 34.1. Net Cl$^-$ absorption by the TAL is a secondary active transport process. Luminal Cl$^-$ entry into the cell is mediated by an electroneutral Na$^+$-K$^+$-2Cl$^-$ co-transport process driven by the favorable electrochemical gradient for sodium entry. More specifically, the net driving force for the entry of Cl$^-$ into the cell is determined by the sum of the chemical gradients for Na$^+$, K$^+$, and Cl$^-$. Since the Na$^+$ gradient is maintained by the continuous operation of the basolateral membrane (Na$^+$,K$^+$)-ATPase pump, apical entry of Cl$^-$ via the co-transporter ultimately depends on the operation of the basolateral (Na$^+$,K$^+$)-ATPase. Accordingly, maneuvers that inhibit ATPase activity, such as removal of K$^+$ from or addition of ouabain to, peritubular solutions leads to dissipation of the Na$^+$ gradient and subsequent inhibition of apical membrane Cl$^-$ entry.[138,257]

In contrast to the electroneutral entry of Cl$^-$ across the apical membrane, the majority of Cl$^-$ efflux across the basolateral membrane proceeds through conductive pathways.[135,142,276] A favorable electrochemical gradient for Cl$^-$ efflux through dissipative pathways has been demonstrated by Greger et al.[110] in the rabbit cTAL. In this study, an intracellular Cl$^-$ activity of 22 mM, measured using single Cl$^-$-selective microelectrodes, was substantially above the equilibrium value (5 mM) predicted from the intracellular voltage. Intracellular Cl$^-$ is maintained at concentrations above electrochemical

TABLE 34.2   Transport Properties of Cortical and Medullary Thick Ascending Limb of Henle

	VTe (mV)	Pf (µm/sec)	PNa (µm/sec)	PCl (µm/sec)	JCl (pEq/cm2/sec)
RABBIT					
cTAL	3–10	11	0.28	0.14	2500
mTAL	3–7	0	0.63	0.11	5600
MOUSE					
cTAL	8–12		0.63	0.51	5200
mTAL					
−ADH	5	6–23	0.23	0.10	3000
+ADH	10	6–23	0.25	0.12	10,900
RAT					
cTAL	7–8	0			8405
mTAL	5–6	0			9300

Table from Reeves, W. B., and Andreoli, T. E. (2008). Sodium chloride transport in the loop of Henle, distal convoluted tubule, and collecting duct. In "The Kidney: Physiology and Pathophysiology," 4th edn, 849–888, Alpern, R. J., and Hebert, S. C. (eds.). Elsevier.
Note: Values of J_{Cl} for rat were calculated assuming an inner tubule diameter of 20 µm.
J_{Cl}: chemically determined net rate of Cl^- absorption; P_f: osmotic water permeability; P_{Na}, P_{Cl}: isotopically determined Na^+ and Cl^- permeabilities; V_{Te}: transepithelial voltage (lumen positive).

TABLE 34.3   Basal Electrophysiologic Parameters of Thick Ascending Limb Segments

	Ve (mV)	Ge	Gc (mS/cm^2)	Gs	Va (mV)	Vbl	Ra/Rb
Rabbit cTAL	4–8	33	12	21	76	−69	2.0
Mouse mTAL	3–7	70–100	45–50	40–60	55.4	−50.7	1.2
Mouse cTAL	7–14	88	39	49			
Hamster mTAL	4.0	934				−72	

Table from Reeves, W. B., and Andreoli, T. E. (2008). Sodium chloride transport in the loop of Henle, distal convoluted tubule, and collecting duct. In "The Kidney: Physiology and Pathophysiology," 4th edn, 849–888, Alpern, R. J., and Hebert, S. C. (eds.). Elsevier.
G_c: transcellular conductance; G_e: transepithelial conductance; G_s: paracellular conductance; V_a: apical membrane voltage; V_{bl}: basolateral membrane voltage; V_c: transepithelial voltage; R_a/R_b: apical to basolateral membrane resistance.

equilibrium by the continued entry of Cl^- via the apical Na^+-K^+-$2Cl^-$ co-transporter. Blocking Cl^- entry through this pathway with furosemide or substitution of extracellular Cl^- by gluconate, caused the intracellular Cl^- activity to fall to a value close to its equilibrium.[110] In addition to electrodiffusive efflux of Cl^- across the basolateral membrane, a component of electroneutral KCl co-transport has been proposed in some species,[112] and the the K^+-Cl^- co-transporter, KCC4, has been shown to be present at the TAL basolateral membrane.[25]

In addition, according to the model in Figure 34.1, the potassium that enters TAL cells via the Na^+-K^+-Cl^- co-transporter recycles, to a large extent, across the apical membrane by way of a K^+ conductive pathway. This apical K^+ recycling serves several purposes. First, it ensures a continued supply of luminal potassium in order to sustain Na^+-K^+-Cl^- co-transport. Without recycling, the luminal K^+ concentration would fall rapidly as a consequence of K^+ entry via Na^+-K^+-Cl^- co-

transport, and would limit net NaCl absorption. Second, the apical membrane potassium current provides a pathway for net potassium secretion by the TAL, which is an active process, ultimately driven by the (Na^+,K^+)-ATPase, proceeding in the face of a lumen-positive transepithelial potential. Third, under open circuit conditions, the transcellular and paracellular pathways form a current loop in which the currents traversing the two pathways are of equal size but opposite direction. The potassium current from cell to lumen polarizes the lumen and causes an equivalent current to flow from lumen to bath through the paracellular pathway.[113] Since the paracellular pathway is cation-selective ($P_{Na}/P_{Cl} = 2$–6), the majority of the current through the paracellular pathway is carried by sodium moving from the lumen to the interstitium. This paracellular absorption of sodium increases the efficiency of sodium transport by the TAL. With reference to Figure 34.1, for each

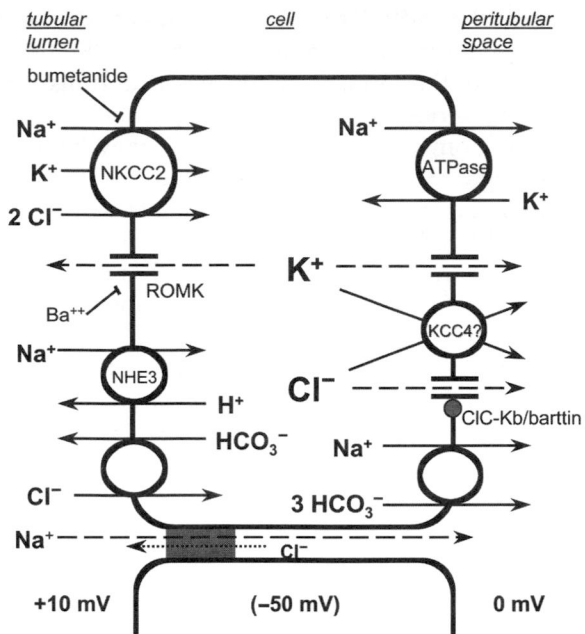

FIGURE 34.1 **A model depicting the major pathways involve in NaCl absorption mechanism by the thick ascending limb.** Dashed lines indicate passive movements down electrochemical gradient. *From Reeves, W. B., and Andreoli, T. E. (2008). Sodium chloride transport in the loop of Henle, distal convoluted tubule, and collecting duct. In "The Kidney: Physiology and Pathophysiology," 4th edn, 849–888, Alpern, R. J., and Hebert, S. C. (eds.). Elsevier.*

Na^+ transported through the cell — and requiring utilization of ATP — one Na^+ is transported through the paracellular pathway without any additional expenditure of energy. Finally, the apical K^+ current satisfies the continuity requirement imposed by a high degree of conductive Cl^- efflux across basolateral membranes.[135,214] A small component of sodium transport by the TAL (5–10%) is accounted for by sodium bicarbonate absorption.[105] Sodium bicarbonate absorption is thought to be mediated by an apical membrane amiloride-sensitive Na^+/H^+ exchanger and a basolateral membrane electrogenic $3Na^+/(HCO_3^-)$ co-transporter.[105] The following sections will describe the individual components of the mechanism for TAL salt transport (Figure 34.1) in greater detail.

Apical Na⁺-K⁺-Cl⁻ Co-Transport

The predominant mode for Cl^- entry into the TAL cell is via a Na^+-K^+-$2Cl^-$ co-transporter.[107,135,138] A characteristic feature of this transporter is its sensitivity to inhibition by furosemide, bumetanide, and other 5-sulfamoylbenzoic acid derivatives.[253] The first demonstration of dependence on luminal sodium for Cl^- absorption was reported by Greger in isolated perfused rabbit cortical TAL segments.[107] Moreover, a requirement for luminal potassium has been demonstrated for sodium and chloride absorption in both mouse medullary[135] and

rabbit[111] cortical thick ascending segments perfused *in vitro*. As a result of these studies, it is now recognized that Cl^- absorption in the TAL generally depends on the simultaneous presence of Na^+ and K^+ (or NH_4) in the lumen.

Measurement of isotope flux into TAL cells or membrane vesicles prepared from the inner stripe of outer medulla have delineated further the ionic requirements and stoichiometry of $1Na^+$-$1K^+$-$2Cl^-$ co-transport.[34,171,174] There is a general agreement that the co-transporter in the thick ascending limb conforms to this stoichiometry under most experimental conditions. However, under certain circumstances, which will be discussed below, apical membrane NaCl entry may be independent of luminal potassium. Early work suggested differences in apparent affinity constant for chloride along TAL[71,108,147,174] which suggested axial heterogeneity in the properties of the Na^+-K^+-$2Cl^-$ co-transporter, because Greger,[108] and Hus-Citharel and Morel[147] examined the cortical TAL, while Koenig et al.[174] and Burnham et al.[34] prepared membranes from the medulla. An axial heterogeneity in the regulation of co-transporter activity as the thick limb ascends from the medulla into the cortex might be anticipated. This is explained by differences in affinity constant for ions of axially distributed along TAL of alternatively spliced variants of the Na^+-K^+-$2Cl^-$ co-transporter.

SLC12A1 gene encodes for the absorptive form of the co-transporter, referred to as BSC1 or NKCC2, located exclusively at the apical membrane of TAL, simultaneously cloned by Gamba et al.[94] and Payne et al.[241] Molecular biology of this gene is extensively discussed in Chapter 32. Inactivating mutations in the *SLC12A1* gene is the cause of Bartter syndrome type I. This syndrome, characterized by hypokalemia, metabolic alkalosis, hyperaldosteronism, and low blood pressure, results from a defect in salt absorption by the TAL, providing strong support for the conclusion that NKCC2 is responsible for apical Na^+-K^+-$2Cl^-$ co-transport in the thick ascending limb.[92] The NKCC2 cDNA encodes a protein containing ~ 1100 amino acids and having a predicted molecular weight of 115–120 kDa.[92] The observed molecular weight, however, is approximately 150 kDa due to extensive glycosylation. Hydropathy analysis of the amino acid sequence predicts a protein having 12 putative transmembrane spanning domains (TM). Six isoforms of NKCC2 have been identified that are results of alternative splicing in the 5′ and 3′ regions of the NKCC2 gene. Three 5′ splice products, termed A, B, and F, are expressed in all mammalian species.[92] These variants differ only in a 96 bp region, which encodes the amino acids forming half of the second TM and interconnecting segment between TM2 and 3. The isoforms show differential expression within the thick ascending limb. Using RT-PCR, Yang et al.[345] examined the distribution of NKCC2 isoforms in single nephron segments. The A isoform was found in both the cortical and medullary TAL, the B isoform was restricted to the cortical TAL, while the F isoform was present in the medullary, but not cortical, TAL and, to a lesser extent, in the outer medullary collecting duct. Altough the three variants mediate Na^+-K^+-$2Cl^-$ co-transport, they have different transport properties. The A and B isoforms have higher affinities for Na^+, K^+, and Cl^- than the F isoform. The A isoform appears to have a greater transport capacity than the other isoforms[244] (see Figure 32.3 of Chapter 32). Thus, the presence of the A and F isoform in the medullary thick ascending limb could account for the observed high rates of NaCl transport relative to the cortical segment (Table 34.2), while the expression of the A and B isoforms in the cortical thick ascending limb may subserve the ability to achieve lower luminal NaCl concentrations in that segment. As discussed with detail in Chapter 32, difference in affinity for ions among the NKCC2 variants B and F has been attributed to only six residues within these exons.

There is experimental evidence that the apical co-transporter in TAL might operate as a simple NaCl symporter under certain conditions. Eveloff and co-workers have reported potassium-independent, furosemide-sensitive NaCl transport in isolated rabbit TAL cells and membrane vesicles prepared from TAL cells.[71] Potassium dependence of the co-transporter might be subject to physiologic regulation. Eveloff and Calamia[72] have shown that under isotonic conditions the chloride-dependent, furosemide-sensitive component of sodium uptake is independent of potassium, but that under hypertonic conditions the sodium uptake becomes K^+-dependent. Sun et al.[301] have also reported that, in perfused mouse medullary TAL segments, basal sodium chloride transport was K^+-independent, but that upon stimulation of salt transport by ADH NaCl transport became dependent on luminal K^+. The NKCC2 variants at the carboxyl terminal domain help to explain this discrepancy. Alternative splicing at the 3′ end of NKCC2 produces additional isoforms with either long (C9) or short (C4) carboxy-termini.[221] Under isotonic conditions, the truncated (C4) isoforms do not mediate Na^+-K^+-$2Cl^-$ co-transport. Under hypotonic conditions, however, the C4 isoforms mediate K^+-independent NaCl co-transport, which is inhibited by cAMP[243] and may account for the K^+-independent NaCl transport noted in earlier studies.[72,301] Of note, the C4 isoform inhibit the transport activity of the full-length (C9) isoforms when the two are co-expressed,[245] and this inhibition is relieved by cAMP.[245] The inhibition of C9 NKCC2 isoforms by C4 isoforms suggests a physical interaction between these proteins. Biochemical studies have

established that NKCC2 exists as a dimer.[295] Thus, it is possible that different combinations of NKCC2 isoforms within the dimer could produce transporters with a wide variety of functional properties. Moreover, the subunit composition of the dimers may be a point of physiologic regulation. Alternatively, the C4 isoform could alter membrane trafficking or stability of the C9 isoform. The C4 isoform resides predominantly in subapical vesicles rather than the cell membrane.[245] Meade et al.[209] found that co-expression of the C4 isoform reduced the abundance of C9 isoform in *Xenopus* oocyte membranes. The reduction in cell surface C9 isoform was reflected by a commensurate reduction in bumetanide-sensitive Rb uptake. The inhibitory effect of C4 on C9 cell surface localization could be prevented by cAMP or by disruption of microtubules, suggesting that C4 alters the trafficking of C9 in or out of the apical membrane.

Evidence for a model of two distinct binding sites for Cl^- with differing affinities follows from studies of Forbush and Palfrey[80] on ^{3}H-bumetanide binding to renal medullary membranes. In these studies, Na^+, K^+, and Cl^- were all required for bumetanide to bind to canine renal medullary membranes. The K_a values for sodium and potassium were 2 mM and 1 mM, respectively. The effect of Cl^- concentration on bumetanide binding was biphasic. At low concentrations (<5 mM), Cl^- enhanced ^{3}H-bumetanide-binding. These data are consistent with a model in which the binding of Cl^- to a high-affinity site exposes a second lower-affinity site that may be occupied either by bumetanide or by the second Cl^-. However, functional studies using chimeras constructed between the ubiquitously expressed Na^+-K^+-$2Cl^-$ co-transporter NKCC1 encoded by *SLC12A2* gene and NKCC2, as well as in wild-type and mutant variants A, B, and F of NKCC2, revealed that changes in chloride affinity are not paralleled by changes in bumetanide affinity, and *vice versa*, questioning the competition of chloride and bumetanide for a single-binding site (see Chapter 32 on NaCl co-transporters).

The binding of ions to the co-transporter is thought to be ordered and cooperative.[185] Thus, sodium binds to the co-transporter first, and promotes binding of a Cl^- and then K^+. Binding of K^+ to its site, in turn, promotes binding of the second Cl^- to the co-transporter. Once fully occupied, the co-transporter—ion complex translocates to the internal surface of the cell membrane, where debinding occurs in the same order. The full reaction sequence of binding and debinding results in inward Na^+/K^+/$2Cl^-$ transport. Partial reactions permit K^+/K^+ and Na^+/Na^+ exchange.

Apical Potassium (K) Channels

Studies of isolated, perfused, thick limb segments have established that the predominant, and perhaps only, conductance across the apical membrane is to potassium.[113,136] Blockade of the apical K conductance by luminal barium in mouse medullary thick ascending limb (mTAL) decreases the transepithelial electrical conductance (G_e) by roughly 50%, while increasing the apical-to-basolateral membrane resistance ratio (Ra/Rb) from 1.9 to 12.9.[135] Moreover, changes in the luminal K⁺ concentration produce essentially Nernstian changes in the apical membrane electrical potential.[135] Electrophysiological studies demonstrated that the apical membrane K⁺ conductance is sufficient to recycle the potassium uptake via the Na⁺-K⁺-2Cl⁻ co-transporter.

The properties of the apical membrane K⁺ conductance have been studied in plasma membrane vesicles prepared from outer renal medulla.[34,252] Conductive K⁺ fluxes in these vesicles can be measured by loading the vesicles with a high concentration of potassium, and then removing the potassium from the external solutions. Tracer amounts of $^{86}Rb^+$ are then added to the extravesicular solutions to begin uptake. Under these conditions, the outwardly directed K⁺ gradient creates an inside-negative diffusion potential that drives $^{86}Rb^+$ uptake into the vesicles. Burnham et al.[34] and Reeves et al.[252] were thus able to demonstrate barium-sensitive $^{86}Rb^+$ flux in membranes from rabbit outer medulla. The Rb⁺ flux was conductive as judged by its inhibition via collapse of the intravesicular voltage or by measurement of intravesicular voltage using voltage-sensitive dyes. The $K_{0.5}$ value for barium inhibition of Rb⁺ flux was 50–100 μM.[34] The barium-sensitive Rb⁺ flux was also dependent on the calcium activity within the vesicles.[34] Moreover, in reconstituted proteoliposomes prepared from porcine outer medulla, the calcium dependence of the K⁺ conductance was modulated by a high-affinity ($K_{0.5} = 0.1$ nM) calmodulin-binding site.[173]

The patch-clamp technique has identified two types of apical K⁺ channels in the TAL, a low-conductance (35 pS) K⁺ channel and an intermediate-conductance (70 pS) K⁺ channel in the apical membrane of the TAL. The 35 pS K⁺ channel is observed in the apical membrane of rabbit,[327] rat,[325] and mouse.[202] Moreover, exposure of the cytoplasmic surface of the patch to ATP inhibited channel activity. In addition to the 35 pS K⁺ channel, Bleich et al.[23] and Wang[325] described an intermediate conductance (60–70 pS) K⁺ channel in rat TAL segments. Like the low conductance K⁺ channel, the 70 pS K⁺ channel was inhibited by ATP and barium.[325] In addition, the channel activity was voltage-dependent with depolarization increasing its activity; the channel could be blocked by quinine, verapamil, and diltiazem, and was inhibited at low cytosolic pH. The activities of both the intermediate and low conductance K⁺ channels are increased by high dietary potassium.[200] An overview regarding regulation of

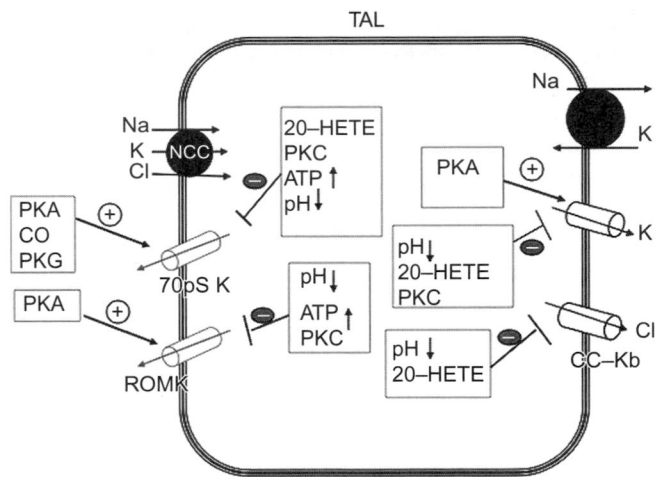

FIGURE 34.2 A cell scheme illustrating the inhibitory and stimulatory factors for regulation of apical and basolateral ion channels.

apical K⁺ channels in the TAL is summarized in Figure 34.2, and detailed information can also be found in the review articles.[141,329]

An ATP-dependent K⁺ channel was cloned from rat kidney by Ho et al.[143] This channel, termed ROMK (Renal Outer Medullary K⁺ channel), is the prototype for a large family of inward rectifying K⁺ channels (K_{IR} channels). K_{IR} channels have two transmembrane spanning domains, intracellular N- and C-termini, and an extracellular helical domain between the two transmembrane domains. Structural studies of other K_{IR} channels have established that the channels exist as heteromers of four K_{IR} subunits.[230,231,307] The extracellular helical domain appears to form the outer vestibule and selectivity filter of the channel, while the second transmembrane domain lines the pore cavity.

ROMK⁺ channels have three alternatively spliced forms and they are ROMK2 (Kir1.1b), ROMK3 (Kir1.1c),[26,350] and ROMK6 (Kir1.1d).[178] The encoded ROMK proteins differ at the beginning of the N-terminus; ROMK2 has the shortest N-terminus[177] and splicing adds either 19 or 26 amino acids for ROMK1 or ROMK3, respectively. Relative ROMK mRNA abundance measured by competitive PCR has shown that ROMK2 and ROMK3 are much more abundant than ROMK1 or ROMK6 in rat kidney.[17] Moreover, single-nephron PCR analysis indicated that ROMK1 is expressed in the collecting duct, while both ROMK2 and ROMK3 are expressed in the medullary and cortical thick ascending limb.[26] Immunolocalization of ROMK proteins, using antibodies that recognized all three isoforms, revealed apical membrane localization in the medullary and cortical thick ascending limb, the late distal tubule, the connecting tubule, and the cortical collecting duct.[210,341] Oddly, the expression of ROMK in the thick limb was heterogeneous, with some cells lacking demonstrable staining. In contrast, the expression of the Na^+-K^+-$2Cl^-$ co-transporter was uniform within the TAL.[341] This implies that apical K^+ recycling by the ROMK-positive cells may be sufficient to supply K^+ for Na^+-K^+-$2Cl^-$ transport in the ROMK-negative cells.

The 35 pS channel conductance of ROMK corresponds to the low conductance K^+ channel described by Wang et al.[325] The current–voltage relations exhibit weak inward rectification, which is due to blocking of the channel by intracellular Mg^{2+} or polyamines.[177] The activity of this channel is modulated by intracellular pH and by intracellular ATP, through both phosphorylation-dependent and phosphorylation-independent pathways.[141] The maintenance of ROMK$^+$ channel activity requires protein kinase A (PKA)-mediated phosphorylation and deletion of any two of three PKA-phosphorylation sites inactivates ROMK.[203] Phosphorylation of ROMK affects both channel activity (P_o) and the number of functional channels in the plasma membrane.[346] In addition, PKA-induced phosphorylation of ROMK enhances the sensitivity of the ROMK$^+$ channel to phosphatidylinositol phosphates (PIP2).[189]

Nucleotides have both inhibitory and stimulatory effects on ROMK activity. At micromolar concentrations, ATP stimulates ROMK activity via PKA-mediated phosphorylation and production of PIP_2.[329] Millimolar concentrations of ATP inhibit ROMK activity.[326,328] The inhibition by ATP can be relieved by increasing concentrations of ADP or by PIP_2.[198] Certain other members of the K_{IR} family are also inhibited by ATP. The ATP sensitivity of these channels—for example, $K_{IR}6.2$—is endowed by the association of regulatory subunits.[51] These regulatory subunits, such as the sulfonylurea receptor (SUR) and CFTR,[3,151] belong to the ABC gene family which is characterized by nucleotide-binding domains. The sulfonylurea receptor, together with $K_{IR}6.2$, forms the glibenclamide-sensitive, ATP-sensitive K^+ channel that controls insulin secretion by pancreatic β-cells.[151] The K_{IR}/SUR channels are more sensitive to inhibition by ATP than those of heterologously expressed ROMK$^+$ channels. In addition, the native 35 pS K^+ channel, but not the heterologously expressed ROMK$^+$ channel, is inhibited by glibenclamide.[324] These observations have prompted the search for regulatory subunits for the ROMK$^+$ channel. Both SUR2B[18] and CFTR[216] are expressed in the thick ascending limb and collecting duct, making them candidates for ROMK regulation. In transfection studies, co-expression of ROMK with either SUR2B[305] or CFTR[208,264] dramatically increases both the nucleotide dependence and glibenclamide sensitivity of ROMK. Immunoprecipitation studies confirmed that one of the ROMK isoforms, ROMK2, physically interacts with SUR2B.[305] The role of CFTR in

regulating the native ROMK$^+$ channels has been further suggested by the finding that PKA-induced regulation of ATP sensitivity of the native 35 pS K^+ channel is compromised in CFTR knockout mice.[199] Figure 34.3 is a cartoon illustrating the current view regarding the composition of the native ATP-sensitive K^+ channel in the apical membrane of the TAL.

The electrophysiologic properties of the ROMK channels have strongly suggested that ROMK is the native 35 pS K^+ channel expressed in the thick ascending limb.[47,233,329] In support of this view, no low-conductance K^+ channels were detected by patch-clamp analysis in ROMK knockout mice.[201] Moreover, deleting the gene product encoding ROMK also abolished the expression of intermediate conductance K^+ channels in the thick ascending limb.[200] It has been proposed that the intermediate conductance channel may be a heteromeric protein containing ROMK and other, as yet unidentified, subunits. The notion that one of the ROMK channels is the predominant channel responsible for apical K^+ recycling in the thick ascending limb is strongly supported by the finding of mutations in the ROMK gene in some families with Bartter syndrome.[290] Thus, the presence of ROMK mutations as a cause of Bartter syndrome indicates the important role of ROMK in net salt absorption by the thick ascending limb.

Basolateral Potassium (K) Channels

Basolateral K^+ channels in the TAL play an important role in the regulation of transepithelial transport.[98,141] They are responsible for generating basolateral membrane potential which is essential for Cl diffusion across the basolateral membrane in the TAL. Activation of basolateral K^+ channels in the TAL is expected to hyperpolarize the basolateral cell membrane, thereby augmenting the driving force for Cl exit across the basolateral membrane. In contrast, decreasing basolateral K^+ channel activity depolarizes the cell membrane potential, thereby diminishing the driving force for Cl^- exit across the basolateral membrane. Consequently, inhibition of Cl^- exit leads to an increase in intracellular Cl^- concentration which decreases the activity of NKCC2, probably via inhibiting WNK3-SPAK.[247]

The physiological importance of the basolateral K^+ channels in maintaining transepithelial membrane transport in the TAL and distal nephron is best demonstrated in SeSAME disease (Seizures, Sensorineural deafness, Ataxia, Mental retardation, and Electrolyte imbalance). This disease is the result of defective gene product encoding KCNJ10, an inwardly-rectifying K^+ channel,[281] which is also expressed in the basolateral membrane of TAL and distal nephron.[183] The renal phenotypes of SeSAME disease are hypokalemia, metabolic alkalosis, and hypomagnesemia. Presumably, defective basolateral K^+ channels cause membrane potential depolarization,

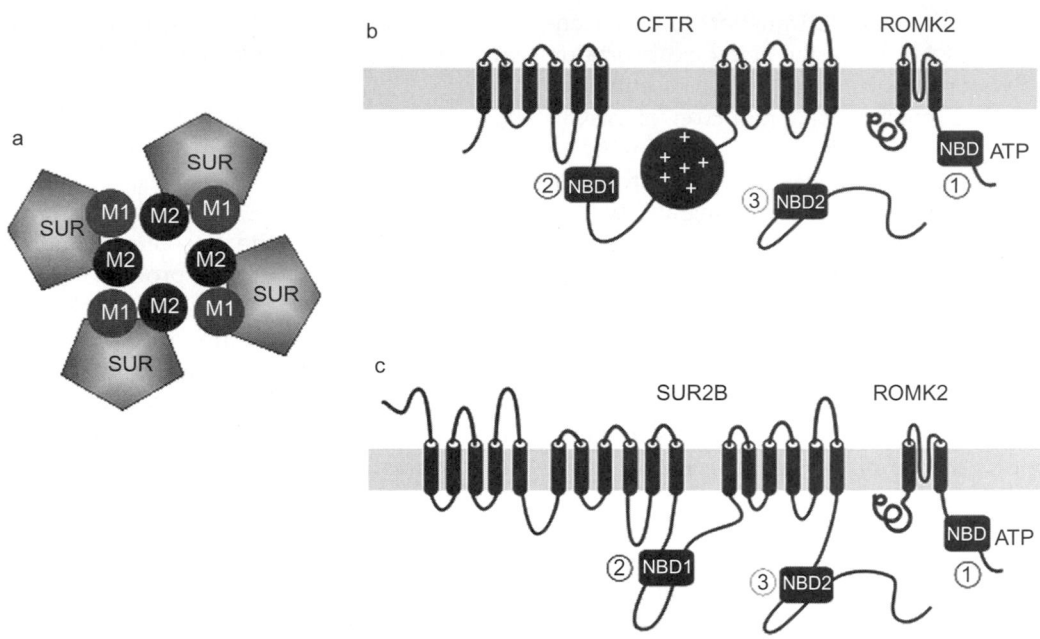

FIGURE 34.3 Assembly of the native ATP-sensitive K channels in the TAL with ATP-binding cassette [ABC] proteins. (a) The proposed hetero-octameric complex forming the native ATP-sensitive K channels in the TAL with four K_{IR} subunits and four sulfonylurea receptor [SUR] subunits. (b) The topology of CFTR and ROMK channels proposed to form kidney K_{ATP} channels. A single nucleotide-binding domain [NBD, 1] is present on the C-terminus of ROMK while two NBDs [numbered 2 and 3] are found on CFTR. (c) The topology of the sulfonylurea receptor, SUR2B, and ROMK proposed to form kidney K_{ATP} channels.

thereby decreasing Cl$^-$ diffusion across the basolateral membrane. Consequently, an increase in intracellular Cl$^-$ concentrations results in the inhibition of the apical Na entry through NKCC2, thereby suppressing Na absorption and diminishing the lumen-positive potential in the TAL. A decrease in the lumen-positive potential results in inhibition of magnesium absorption through the paracellular pathway in the TAL.[134] Also, the inhibition of Na absorption in the TAL increases Na delivery to the distal nephron, accordingly stimulating Na absorption in the expanse of K$^+$ in the connecting tubule and causing K$^+$-wasting. Therefore, an alteration in the basolateral K$^+$ channel activity in the TAL has a significant effect on transepithelial transport not only in the TAL, but also in the distal nephron segment.

Patch-clamp experiments demonstrated that an inwardly-rectifying 50 pS K$^+$ channel[119,238] and a Na$^+$ and Cl$^-$ activated 140–180 pS K$^+$ channel[240] are present in the basolateral membrane of the TAL. The 50 pS K$^+$ channel is highly-expressed, and may be the main K$^+$ channel in the basolateral membrane of the TAL. The regulation of the 50 pS K$^+$ channels has been intensively studied and several factors, including protein kinase A (PKA), 20-hydroxyeicosatetraenoic acid (20-HETE), and external Ca^{2+}, have been identified to modulate the 50 pS K$^+$ channels (Figure 34.2). Arachidonic acid inhibits the basolateral 50 pS K$^+$ channels in the TAL through the CYP-omega-hydroxylase-dependent

metabolism, and 20-HETE mediates the effect of arachidonic acid on the K$^+$ channel.[115,119] Also, raising the external Ca^{2+} inhibited the basolateral 50 pS K$^+$ channels in the TAL by a PKC-dependent mechanism.[179] Two lines of evidence suggest that the effect of the external Ca^{2+} on the basolateral 50 pS K$^+$ channels was the result of stimulating the Ca^{2+}-sensing receptor (CaSR) which is expressed in the TAL[133]: (1) the inhibitory effect of raising the external Ca^{2+} on the 50 pS K$^+$ channels was observed only in cell-attached patches, but not in excised patches; (2) the effect of raising external Ca^{2+} on the 50 pS K$^+$ channel was absent in the presence of the CaSR antagonist. It is possible that the CaSR might directly interact with the basolateral 50 pS K$^+$ channels in the TAL. This speculation is supported by reports from several studies. First, the basolateral 50 pS K$^+$ channels in the TAL might represent heterotetramers made of Kir4.1/Kir5.1, because the basolateral K$^+$ channels in the distal tubules with similar biophysical properties to those of the 50 pS K$^+$ channel in the TAL are composed of Kir4.1 and Kir5.1.[183,197] Second, immunostaining experiments demonstrated that Kir4.1 and Kir5.1 were expressed in the basolateral membrane of the TAL.[254,306] Finally, the study using immunoprecipitation performed in the cells transiently transfected with Kir4.1 and the CaSR has demonstrated that Kir4.1 was associated with the CaSR.[144] The regulation of the basolateral 50 pS K$^+$ channel by the external Ca^{2+} should play a role in the modulation of transepithelial Na transport and concentrating ability in the TAL. Since the active reabsorption of NaCl⁻ in the water-impermeable TAL is essential for urinary concentrating mechanism, inhibition of NaCl⁻ reabsorption in the TAL should result in a decrease in concentrating ability. Indeed, it has been reported that hypercalcemia impairs urinary concentrating ability.[99]

Because the activity of the basolateral K^+ channels is regulated by the external Ca^{2+}/Mg^{2+} concentrations at a physiologically relevant range (1 to 2 mM), the CaSR-mediated regulation of the membrane transport in the TAL is mainly through controlling the basolateral K^+ channel activity. Figure 34.4 is a cell scheme illustrating the role of basolateral K^+ channels in mediating the effect of stimulation of the CaSR on Na^+ and divalent cation transport in the TAL. Under physiological conditions, the basolateral K^+ channels maintain the cell membrane potential such that it could sustain a constant Cl^- diffusion across the basolateral membrane. An increase in the external Ca^{2+} (hypercalcemia) activates the CaSR, thereby inhibiting basolateral K^+ channels and decreasing the driving force for Cl^- diffusion across the basolateral membrane. Inhibition of Cl^- exit is expected to lead to hyperpolarization of transepithelial voltage (V_{te}). A less positive V_{te} would diminish the reabsorption of Na^+ and divalent cations such as Ca^{2+} and Mg^{2+}. Indeed, it has been reported

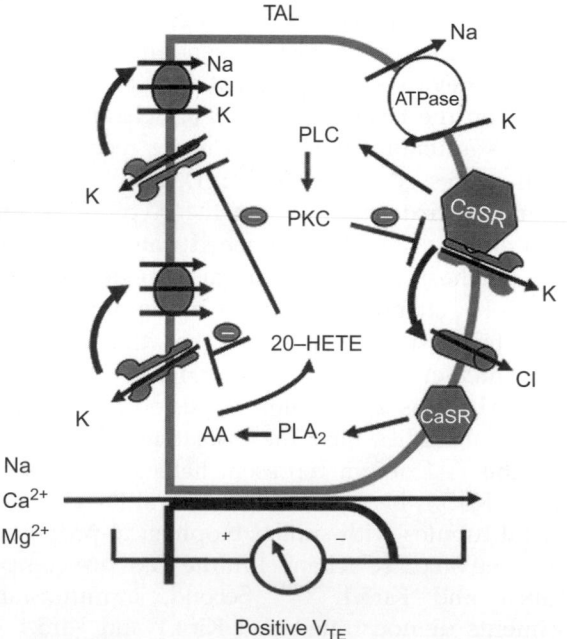

FIGURE 34.4   A cell scheme illustrating the role of stimulation of Ca^{2+} ensing receptor (CaSR) in regulation of apical and basolateral K channels, thereby affecting the transepithelial transport of Na and divalent cations. (Abbreviations: PLC: phospholipase C; PLA2: phospholipase A2; PKC: protein kinase C; 20-HETE: 20-hydroxyeicosatetraenoic acid.)

that an increase in plasma Ca^{2+}/Mg^{2+} level enhanced urinal Ca^{2+}/Mg^{2+} excretion.[249,250]

Basolateral Membrane Cl⁻ Channel and Transporter

Cl⁻ CHANNEL

Cl^- exit across the basolateral membrane of TAL cells is largely conductive, proceeding down its electrochemical gradient through Cl^--selective channels in the basolateral membrane. The notion that basolateral Cl^- transport is electrogenic first derived from observations that, in the mouse medullary TAL and rabbit cTAL,[138] net Cl^- absorption accounts for about 90% of the equivalent short-circuit current. Measurements of the basolateral membrane voltage by Greger and Schlatter[112] confirmed that reductions in bath chloride concentration depolarized the basolateral membrane, while reductions in intracellular chloride concentration produced by blocking Cl^- entry with furosemide hyperpolarized the basolateral membrane. Both sets of observations are consistent with the presence of a Cl^- conductance in the basolateral membrane. Consistent with the view that basolateral Cl^- transport is via chloride channels, a variety of compounds known to block Cl^- channels also inhibit salt absorption in TAL segments. Wangemann et al.[121] have catalogued the electrophysiologic effects, relative potencies, and structure−function relations of over 200 such compounds. The major effects of these agents, when present in the peritubular bathing solutions, are inhibition of transepithelial voltage, inhibition of the equivalent short circuit current, and hyperpolarization of the basolateral membrane.

Application of the patch-clamp technique to the TAL has established that Cl^- channels are present in the basolateral membrane of TAL cells. Paulais and Teulon detected a 40 pS anion selective channel ($P_{Cl}/P_{Na} = 20$) in the basolateral membrane of collagenase treated mouse cortical TAL segments.[121] The I−V relations of the channel were linear in both the cell-attached and excised configurations. The open probability of the channel in the cell-attached state was voltage-dependent, increasing as the membrane was depolarized. In the excised patch configuration, the open probability was no longer voltage-dependent. Greger et al. described a Cl^- channel in the basolateral membrane of rat TAL segments.[109] This channel also has a conductance of about 40 pS, but rather than having a linear I−V relation, this channel exhibits outward rectification. The open probability increases with depolarization in both the cell-attached and -excised patch configuration. A low conductance Cl^- channel (8−10 pS) having linear I−V relations has also been detected in the basolateral membrane of TAL cells.[121,120,118] The activity of this channel is increased following incubation with cAMP-dependent protein kinase and ATP,[120] and is inhibited by 20-HETE acid, a Cyp-ω-hydroxylase-dependent metabolite of arachidonic acid.[118]

Evidence for Cl$^-$ channels in the TAL also comes from studies of Cl$^-$ flux in renal medullary membrane vesicles. Since TALs comprise approximately 70% of the volume in the inner stripe of outer medulla, vesicles prepared from this region should be predominantly derived from this segment. ^{36}Cl$^-$ flux into vesicles from rabbit outer medulla[16] is electrogenic, cation-independent, inhibitable by chloride channel blockers, and has a low activation energy ($E_a = 6.4$ kcal/mole), characteristic of transport through a channel. Moreover, when vesicles from rabbit outer medulla were incorporated into planar lipid bilayers, chloride channel activity was demonstrated.[251] These channels were anion selective ($P_{Cl}/P_K = 10$) and had a single-channel conductance of 80—90 pS in 320 mM KCl solution. The I—V relations in symmetric solution were linear, and in asymmetric solutions the I—V relations conformed to the Goldman—Hodgkin—Katz equation. The open probability of this channel was voltage-dependent, increasing activity with depolarizing voltages. These channels are also seen in vesicles made from highly purified suspensions of mouse thick ascending limb.[337]

Molecular cloning has demonstrated the basolateral Cl$^-$ channels are composed of ClC-K1 and ClC-K2,[2,166,311] members of a large number of the ClC family of channels.[155] ClC-K1 and ClC-K2 are expressed exclusively within the rat kidney. In the human, the two corresponding channels are denoted hCLC-Ka and hCLC-Kb, and are located contiguously on chromosome 1.[265] Due to the high degree of sequence similarity between hCLC-Ka and hCLC-Kb, it is not certain which of the human channels correspond to ClC-K1 versus ClC-K2, although the distribution of ClC-K2 along the nephron most closely matches that of hClC-Kb.[304] Zimniak and colleagues[351] have cloned cDNA from rabbit renal outer medulla, named rbClC-Ka, which shares 80% homology to the rat ClC-K1 and ClC-K2. The distribution of rbClC-Ka along the nephron resembles that of ClC-K2 rather than ClC-K1.[351] Several lines of evidence support the view that ClC-K2 (or the probable human homolog hCLC-Kb) is the channel that mediates chloride efflux across the basolateral membrane of the thick ascending limb. First, using polymerase chain reaction amplification of single tubule segments, the ClC-K2 and rbClC-Ka channels were shown to be expressed primarily in the thick ascending limb and the collecting duct.[2,351] Second, immunohistochemical studies using an antibody against the rbClC-Ka channel revealed predominantly basolateral staining in the medullary and cortical thick ascending limb.[338] Similar results were obtained by Vandewalle

and colleagues using an antibody that recognized both CLC-K1 and CLC-K2.[314] Finally, and most compelling, is the identification of mutations in hCLC-Kb in patients with neonatal Bartter syndrome.[289] Thus, as was the case for the NKCC2 and ROMK proteins, linkage of ClC-Kb to Bartter syndrome establishes the importance of its gene product in transepithelial NaCl transport. Activating mutations of CLC-Kb have also been reported.[153] Specifically, substitution of threonine by serine at position 481 of CLC-Kb results in a dramatic increase in Cl$^-$ currents, without a change in channel selectivity or cell surface expression. The T481S polymorphism is relatively common in the general population, particularly in African populations. Among Caucasians, the presence of the T481S polymorphism was associated with higher systolic and diastolic blood pressures, and a higher prevalence of hypertension.[154] Thus, ClC-Kb is an attractive candidate gene for certain forms of essential hypertension, particularly salt-sensitive hypertension. Additional studies in different populations will be required to determine the significance of these ClC-Kb polymorphisms.

To form functional Cl$^-$ channels in thick ascending limb requires not only CLC-K2/hCLC-Kb, but also a subunit, named barttin.[21] Lost function of mutation of barttin is responsible for a form of Bartter syndrome accompanied by sensorineural deafness.[21] Barttin is believed to act, at least in part, by increasing the cell surface expression of ClC-Kb.[70]

KCl SYMPORTER

Some uncertainty remains regarding the role of basolateral electrochemical KCl symport in net Cl$^-$ efflux across that membrane. In the rabbit cortical TAL, Greger and Schlatter[239] concluded that KCl symport accounted for about one-third of basolateral Cl$^-$ efflux. This conclusion is based on the following observations: an increase in the K$^+$ concentration or decrease in the Cl$^-$ concentration of the basolateral solution depolarized the basolateral membrane; bath barium depolarized the basolateral membrane and abolished the K$^+$-induced changes in V_{bl}; and barium had no discernible effect on the transepithelial resistance or fractional resistance of the basolateral membrane. The lack of an effect of barium on resistance persuaded the investigators to propose that a barium-sensitive KCl co-transporter was present.[112] Alternatively, these data are compatible with parallel conductive pathways for K$^+$ and Cl$^-$. The absence of a barium effect on transepithelial resistance could be due to an offsetting increase in basolateral Cl$^-$ conductance or to changes in basolateral membrane resistance below the experimental limits of detection. A cloned KCl co-transporter, KCC4, is present in the basolateral membrane of the thick ascending limb.[316] However, its physiologic role in thick ascending limb function is not known.

Synchronous Na^+/H^+: Cl^-/HCO_3^- Exchange

An additional form of apical membrane NaCl entry has been observed in the mouse cTAL. Friedman and Andreoli[83] found that net Cl^- absorption and the trans-epithelial voltage were doubled when CO_2 and HCO_3^- were added to the external solutions bathing cTAL segments. Since the (CO_2 HCO_3^-)-stimulated rate of NaCl absorption did not result in net CO_2 transport, and could be abolished by the lipophilic carbonic anhydrase inhibitor ethoxyzolamide or by the luminal addition of the anion exchange inhibitor SITS or DIDS, it was proposed that the apical membrane of the mouse cTAL contains parallel, near-synchronous Na^+/H^+: Cl^-/HCO_3^- exchangers in addition to a Na^+-K^+-Cl^- co-transporter. Subsequent studies have shown that, like the mouse mTAL, the apical membrane of the mouse cTAL contains a potassium conductance, and that both the (CO_2 HCO_3^-)-dependent and (CO_2 HCO_3^-)-independent components of NaCl absorption require luminal potassium.[84,82] Thus, the cation exchange process may proceed as (Na^+, K^+)/2 H^+. Both the (CO_2 HCO_3^-)-dependent and -independent components of NaCl absorption in mouse cTAL segments were equally susceptible to inhibition by luminal bumetanide ($K_i = 5-8 \times 10-7$ M).[82] Addition of CO_2 and HCO_3^- to the bathing solutions has no effect on net NaCl transport in either rabbit cTAL or mouse mTAL. Both the rat and mouse mTAL do contain Na^+/H^+ exchangers in their apical membranes. However, in these segments, Na^+/H exchange plays a role in net HCO_3^- transport and cell pH regulation, rather than transcellular NaCl absorption.[104,168]

Bicarbonate and Ammonium Transport

Medullary and cortical TAL segments from the rat absorb bicarbonate and acidify the luminal fluid.[105] The rates of bicarbonate absorption measured in *in vitro* perfused TAL segments account for most of the filtered bicarbonate that is reabsorbed by the loop of Henle *in vivo*.[104] The rate of sodium bicarbonate absorption in the rat TAL is, however, only a small fraction (5–10%) of total sodium absorption by this segment. Thus, while bicarbonate transport by the TAL may play an important role in urinary acidification in some species, bicarbonate transport has little impact on net salt balance or free water excretion. There is considerable species variation in the rates of bicarbonate absorption by the TAL. No significant bicarbonate transport was detected in mouse and rabbit TAL.[83,105]

In the rabbit, this correlates with the absence of carbonic anhydrase activity in the TAL.[95]

The mechanism of bicarbonate absorption by the rat TAL has been reviewed.[105,38] Transcellular bicarbonate absorption results from proton secretion across the apical membrane and bicarbonate reabsorption across the basolateral membrane. The apical proton secretion occurs primarily by NaH exchange. Evidence for functional apical Na^+/H^+ exchange has been presented for the rat[104,180] and mouse TAL.[83,167] In these segments, acidification of luminal fluid is sodium-dependent and amiloride-sensitive. Moreover, removal of luminal sodium or luminal amiloride results in cytoplasmic acidification. As noted above, the NHE3 isoform of the Na^+/H^+ exchanger is expressed in the apical membrane of the thick ascending limb.[6] NHE3 expression in the TAL is increased by chronic metabolic acidosis, providing a mechanism for enhanced HCO_3^- absorption in this setting. An apical membrane H-ATPase may also contribute to bicarbonate absorption in the TAL.[105] Inhibition of the Na^+-K^+-Cl^- co-transporter by furosemide stimulates bicarbonate absorption in the rat TAL. Thus, this transporter is not directly involved in bicarbonate absorption. Rather, the reduction in cell Na^+ activity that attends inhibition of Na^+-K^+-Cl^- co-transport provides a greater driving force for apical Na^+/H^+ exchange.

Krapf[180] has demonstrated that base efflux across the basolateral membrane of perfused rat TAL segments occurs as $Na^+(HCO_3^-)$ co-transport. This process is electrogenic (probable stoichiometry $1Na^+$:$3HCO_3^-$), sodium-dependent, Cl^--independent, and SITS-sensitive. $Na^+(HCO_3^-)$ co-transport has been demonstrated in mouse medullary TAL as well. In the mouse, the apical Na^+/H^+ exchanger and basolateral $Na^+(HCO_3^-)$ co-transporter play a role in cell pH regulation, rather than transcellular bicarbonate transport.

Origin of Transepithelial Voltage

The spontaneous, lumen-positive transepithelial potential that accompanies net NaCl absorption is, in principle, the sum of at least two terms: an electrogenic voltage arising from rheogenic cellular pathways; and a zero-current dilution voltage referable to salt accumulation in intercellular spaces during salt absorption. Given the cation selectivity of the paracellular pathway ($P_{Na}/P_{Cl} \sim 2-6$), an accumulation of Na^+ in the lateral intracellular space mediated by the (Na^+, K^+)-ATPase could create a lumen-positive diffusion potential across the junctional complex. As discussed earlier, the lumen-positive potential arising from rheogenic cellular transport serves to drive a proportion of net sodium reabsorption through the paracellular pathway.

However, this paracellular sodium absorption will be diminished by the extent to which paracellular diffusion potential accounts for the spontaneous transepithelial voltage, V_e. Thus, it is pertinent to consider the relative contributions of both electrogenic and diffusion potentials to the total transepithelial voltage.

Hebert and Andreoli[136] assessed the possible contributions of a paracellular diffusion potential to V_e in the mouse TAL. The conductance of the paracellular pathway, G_s, was measured by blocking the transcellular conductance with 20 mM Ba^{2+} in the lumen. The junctional complexes were then disrupted by the imposition of large osmotic gradients produced by the addition of urea to the luminal perfusate. Using the value of G_s in the presence of 800 mM luminal urea as an estimate of the ionic conductance of the lateral interspace, exclusive of the junctional complex, Hebert and Andreoli[136] calculated that, during net NaCl transport, the maximal rise in NaCl concentration in the lateral interspace was 10 mEq/liter, and that the resulting dilution potential was less than 1 mV. These results are consistent with the notion that virtually all of the transepithelial voltage is the result of rheogenic transcellular processes.

Specifically, because the apical membrane is exclusively conductive to potassium, and because the Na$^+$K$^+$2Cl$^-$ co-transporter is electroneutral, the apical membrane voltage, V_a, will approximate the K$^+$ equilibrium voltage, E_K. The basolateral membrane voltage, V_{bl}, in contrast, is a function of several conductive pathways; examples include K$^+$ and Cl$^-$ channels, Na$^+$HCO$_3^-$ symport, (Na$^+$, K$^+$)-ATPase. Of these, Cl$^-$ is likely the most important conductive species across the basolateral membrane. V_{bl}, therefore, will be greater than E_{Cl}, but less that E_K, and hence less than V_a (Table 34.3). The lumen-positive V_e then is the result of differing conductance characteristics of the apical and basolateral membranes. The exact value of V_e will be determined by the relative magnitude of the basolateral K$^+$ and Cl$^-$ conductances, and the currents passing through the apical and basolateral membranes.

According to these arguments, the electrogenic nature of V_e should allow for a significant fraction of net sodium absorption to proceed via the paracellular pathway. Indeed, for a constant stoichiometry of the Na$^+$K$^+$-2Cl$^-$ entry, the ratio of net Cl$^-$ absorption to paracellular sodium absorption should have a value of 2. The rate of net paracellular Na$^+$ absorption depends on a variety of factors, such as V_e, G_s, and P_{Na}/P_{Cl}, which vary considerably from tubule to tubule. When each of these variables was measured in the same tubule, however, the ratio of net Cl$^-$ absorption to paracellular Na$^+$ absorption was reasonably constant at 2.4 ± 0.3.[136] Thus, the stoichiometry of Na$^+$K$^+$-2Cl$^-$ entry may be constant under those experimental conditions, that is, ADH stimulated mTAL segments, and the variables G_e, G_s, and P_{Na}/P_{Cl} are related in a given tubule in such a way as to maintain the net Cl$^-$ to paracellular Na$^+$ ratio at 2.

Coupling of Substrate Utilization to Ion Transport

Transepithelial NaCl absorption accounts for the single largest expenditure of energy by TAL cells. Inhibition of the (Na$^+$,K$^+$)-ATPase by ouabain reduces O$_2$ consumption by rabbit,[42,71] rat,[309] and mouse[168] TAL segments by 50%. The effect of ouabain on O$_2$ consumption can be mimicked by either furosemide or by removal of Na$^+$ or Cl$^-$ from the bath solutions.[42,71] This suggests that about one-half of the total cellular ATP supply is consumed by the basolateral membrane (Na$^+$,K$^+$)-ATPase pump, and that this pump operates almost exclusively for the purpose of transepithelial NaCl transport.

TAL segments utilize a variety of metabolic substrates including D-glucose, D-mannose, butyrate, β-OH-butyrate, acetoacetate, lactate, acetate, and pyruvate to support the high ATP requirement imposed by salt transport.[339] Uchida and Endou[310] determined the ability of various substrates to maintain cellular ATP concentrations in microdissected mouse TAL segments. In mTAL segments, glucose, lactate, and β-hydroxybutyrate all conserved cellular ATP content equally well. In the cTAL, lactate and β-hydroxybutyrate increased cellular ATP more than did glucose. Wittner et al. reported that in the absence of exogenous substrate, NaCl transport fell by 73% in 10 minutes in rabbit cTAL.[339] Chamberlin and Mandel[43] assessed the ability of various endogenous and exogenous substrates to support oxidative metabolism in suspensions of rabbit mTAL segments. Unlike the findings in rabbit cTAL, the mTAL suspensions maintained 85% of their basal O$_2$ consumption in the absence of exogenous substrates. Inhibitors of glycolysis, fatty acid oxidation, and amino acid oxidation reduced O$_2$ consumption, indicating that glucose, fatty acids, and amino acids all serve as endogenous substrates capable of supporting oxidative metabolism when the availability of exogenous substrate is limited.[43]

Therefore, the TAL, particularly the medullary portion, relies almost exclusively on oxidative metabolism as its source of energy. However, the mTAL resides in an oxygen-poor environment. The oxygen tension in the outer medulla is about 10 mmHg.[186] Apparently, like the cTAL, the O$_2$ affinity of the mTAL is sufficiently high that oxidative metabolism is maintained even at low oxygen pressures. Nonetheless, the high oxygen requirement in an oxygen-poor environment might predispose the mTAL to injury if oxygen delivery falls or salt transport requirements increase. Brezis and co-workers have shown that the medullary TAL is, in fact, exquisitely susceptible to hypoxic injury.[30] Maneuvers that diminish TAL salt transport, such as furosemide, exert a marked protective effect against hypoxic injury.[31]

Regulation of Salt Absorption in TAL

The rate of salt absorption by the thick ascending limb is modulated by physical factors, such as luminal flow rate and the composition and osmolality of luminal and peritubular fluids, and hormones, such as vasopressin and glucagon, which exert their effects through interactions with specific cellular receptor proteins. The regulation of TAL salt transport is characterized by considerable interspecies variation, as well as intranephron heterogeneity. It is worth noting, again, that the cortical and medullary portions of the TAL have different transport properties (Table 34.2) and subserve different functions. Salt absorption in both segments creates luminal fluid dilution and the potential for free water excretion; however, only salt absorption by the medullary TAL enriches the medullary interstitial osmolality and enhances urinary concentrating power. Given these differences, it is not surprising that the rates of transport in the medullary and cortical TAL are modulated quite differently. A good example of both species and intranephronal heterogeneity is the effect of antidiuretic hormone on TAL transport.

Antidiuretic Hormone

The ADH affects NaCl absorption in the ascending limb of Henle, and thereby regulates the countercurrent multiplication process. Support for this contention was provided by the demonstration, in some species, of an ADH-induced increase in adenylate cyclase

activity[40,55] and protein kinase activity[65] in the medullary, but not cortical, portions of the TAL.

Table 34.4 summarizes the effects of ADH on salt transport in *in vitro* microperfused medullary TAL segments of mouse, rat, and rabbit. Hall and Varney[123] established that ADH increased the lumen-positive transepithelial voltage and the net rate of tracer Cl$^-$ absorption in the mouse medullary TAL. Several laboratories have confirmed these effects of ADH on the transepithelial voltage and unidirectional Cl$^-$ flux in the mouse, and have demonstrated that the effect of ADH on NaCl transport was restricted to the medullary portion of this segment.[138,270,276,338] Moreover, the maximal stimulation of the transepithelial voltage in the mouse medullary TAL occurred at hormone concentrations of approximately 20 pg/ml or 10 μU/ml, found during states of antidiuresis.[138] A similar increase in transepithelial voltage can be obtained in the mouse medullary TAL, but not the cortical TAL, by the addition of cAMP analogs or forskolin, a nonhormonal activator of adenylate cyclase to the peritubular media.[138] In contrast, ADH, even at peritubular concentrations of 250 μU/ml, has no effect on V_e in the mouse cortical TAL.[138] Taken together, these results indicate that the mouse medullary TAL and cortical TAL are functionally heterogeneous with respect to the effect of ADH on net NaCl absorption, and that stimulation of net NaCl absorption in the mouse medullary TAL by ADH is mediated by cAMP. The effect of ADH in TAL does not seem to be contant in all species. ADH causes a variable increase in cyclic AMP production in the rabbit TAL, but pharmacologic concentrations of ADH had no effects on either the transepithelial voltage or tracer Cl$^-$ efflux in this species.[270] ADH or the V_2 selective analog dDAVP increased NaCl absorption from the TAL on homozygous Brattleboro (central diabetes insipidus) rats.[340] In humans evidence is limited. Studies in pump-perfused human kidneys rejected for transplantation have shown ADH-sensitive adenylate cyclase activity in collecting ducts, but not in TAL segments.[40,263] Since the ability of humans to elaborate concentrated urine is limited compared to the mouse, the failure of ADH to increase cAMP in the human TAL is consistent with Morel's suggestion that the response of medullary TAL segments to ADH correlates directly with urinary concentrating ability.[217]

Mechanisms of ADH Affect on TAL

The mechanism whereby ADH stimulates salt transport in the medullary TAL has been studied most extensively in the mouse. The effects of ADH in this segment are mediated predominantly through interaction of the hormone with the vasopressin V_2 receptor coupled to adenylate cyclase. Thus, ADH stimulates

TABLE 34.4 Effects of ADH on NaCl Transport by Thick Ascending Limb Segments

Species	ADH	V_e (mV)	J_{NaCl} (pmol/sec/cm^2)
Mouse	−	5	2600
	+	11	10,800
Rat	−	2.4–3.3	4825
	+	3.6–4.7	7770
Rabbit	−	3–7	6400
	+	3–7	Unchanged

Table from Reeves, W. B., and Andreoli, T. E. (2008). Sodium chloride transport in the loop of Henle, distal convoluted tubule, and collecting duct. In "The Kidney: Physiology and Pathophysiology," 4th edn, 849–888, Alpern, R. J., and Hebert, S. C. (eds.). Elsevier.

adenylate cyclase activity in the TAL,[217] and cAMP analogs and forskolin[139] mimic the effects of ADH on transport in this segment. Cholera toxin stimulates salt transport in the TAL, indicating that the V$_2$ receptor is coupled to the catalytic subunit of adenylate cyclase by a stimulatory guanine nucleotide-binding protein, G$_s$. The catalytic subunit of adenylate cyclase may, in turn, be influenced by calmodulin. Takaichi and Kurokawa[302] have shown that calmodulin inhibitors inhibited ADH-sensitive cAMP production in isolated mouse medullary TAL segments. Likewise, Ausiello and Hall[13] showed that the addition of exogenous calmodulin stimulated ADH-sensitive cAMP production by LLC PK$_1$ cells.

Table 34.5 lists the effects of ADH on several electrophysiologic parameters of mouse medullary TAL segments perfused *in vitro*. The approximate doubling of the equivalent short-circuit current results from an increase in the transepithelial voltage[135,138,214] and an increase of roughly 20% in the transepithelial conductance. Moreover, the ADH-induced increase in transepithelial conductance, G$_e$, is referable to an increase in the barium-sensitive or transcellular conductance, G$_c$. ADH has no effect on the magnitude or permselectivity of the paracellular conductance, G$_s$ (Table 34.5).

ADH increases both the apical and basolateral membrane conductance.[135,214] The apical membrane of TAL cells is, as noted previously, predominantly K$^+$ conductive. In the presence of luminal furosemide to block K$^+$ uptake via the Na$^+$-K$^+$-2Cl$^-$ co-transporter, mouse TAL segments exhibit net K$^+$ secretion that is increased by ADH.[135] Because the electrochemical driving force for K$^+$ secretion is presumably constant in the presence of furosemide, it was suggested that the increase in K$^+$ secretion was due to an increase in apical membrane K$^+$ conductance.[135] In support of this notion, using membrane vesicles prepared from rabbit outer medulla, Reeves et al.[252] demonstrated that *in vitro* exposure to cAMP-dependent protein kinase and ATP specifically enhanced barium-sensitive rates of ^{86}Rb$^+$ uptake. This finding has been confirmed in subsequent work that examined the effects of phosphorylation on the activity of ROMK channels. ROMK is phosphorylated by cAMP-dependent protein kinase at a number of sites,[342] and this phosphorylation increases the activity of the channel.[208]

The ADH-induced increase in transepithelial NaCl absorption can be blocked by luminal furosemide, and therefore represents an increase in apical Na$^+$-K$^+$-2Cl$^-$ co-transport activity. The mechanism whereby ADH increases apical co-transport activity is unclear. Sun et al.[301] demonstrated that in isolated perfused mouse TAL segments, ADH changed the stoichiometry of NaCl entry from 1Na$^+$:1Cl$^-$ to 1Na$^+$:1 K$^+$:2Cl$^-$. This change in stoichiometry, accompanied by apical K$^+$ recycling, could create a lumen-positive potential to drive Na$^+$ reabsorption via the paracellular pathway. Phosphorylation of the cloned Na$^+$-K$^+$-2Cl$^-$ co-transporter NKCC2 by cAMP-dependent protein kinase does not appear to directly increase co-transporter activity. However, phosphorylation may influence co-transporter activity by modulating the interactions between NKCC2 isoforms. As noted above, an isoform with a truncated C-terminus, denoted C4, can inhibit the activity of the full-length NKCC2.[245] However, the inhibition by the C4 isoform can be relieved by phosphorylation by cAMP-dependent protein kinase.[245,209] Thus, ADH may increase apical Na$^+$-K$^+$-2Cl$^-$ entry by releasing NKCC2 from tonic inhibition by truncated isoforms. Of note, the short C4 variant is expressed in medullary TAL, but not in cortical TAL,[221] providing a potential explanation for the lack of ADH effect on cortical TAL discussed above. Chronic exposure to ADH may increase apical Na$^+$-K$^+$-2Cl$^-$ entry by increasing the abundance of NKCC2.[64]

The predominant portion of the ADH-induced increase in cellular conductance is accounted for by an increase in the basolateral membrane Cl$^-$ conductance.[135,214] Two mechanisms have been suggested for the hormone-dependent increase in basolateral Cl$^-$ conductance. Schlatter and Greger[276] proposed that the ADH-induced increase in intracellular cAMP results in a direct increase in chloride channel activity. Such a mechanism has been amply demonstrated in Cl$^-$ secreting epithelia, such as the trachea and intestine. In support of their proposal, Schlatter and Greger demonstrated that cAMP and ADH elicited a fall in the fractional resistance of the basolateral membrane in mouse medullary TAL segments, even when cell Cl$^-$ activity was kept at low levels by blocking apical Cl$^-$ entry with furosemide.[276] Likewise, using patch-clamp analysis, Paulais and Teulon[239] found that preincubation of mouse cortical TAL segments with forskolin or cAMP analogs increased the number of Cl$^-$

TABLE 34.5 Effects of ADH on Electrophysiologic Parameters in Mouse Medullary TAL Segments

ADH (μU/ml)	V$_e$ (mV)	G$_e$ (mS/cm^2)	G$_c$ (mS/cm^2)	G$_s$ (mS/cm^2)	V$_a$ (mV)	V$_{bl}$ (mV)	R$_a$/R$_b$
0	5.6	103.7	45.1	58.6	54.4	− 50.7	1.2
250	10.3	121.3	60.2	61.0	47.3	− 38.9	2.2

Table from Reeves, W. B., and Andreoli, T. E. (2008). Sodium chloride transport in the loop of Henle, distal convoluted tubule, and collecting duct. In "The Kidney: Physiology and Pathophysiology," 4th edn, 849–888, Alpern, R. J., and Hebert, S. C. (eds.). Elsevier.

channels observed in basolateral membrane patches. It is now known that NKCC2 is sensitive to intracellular chloride concentration: chloride depletion activates the co-transporter by inducing phosphorylation of key amino terminal domain threonines of the co-transporter by a pathway involving the soluble kinases WNK3 and SPAK.[247] Additionaly, elimination of TAL basolateral chloride channels in Bartter's type III and IV reduces salt reabsorption by TAL, producing the disease. Thus, one mode of regulation of NKCC2 can be achieved by modulating intracellular chloride concentration in TAL.

Alternatively, ADH might enhance Cl^- conductance indirectly by increasing apical membrane Cl^- entry.[135] According to this proposal, an ADH-dependent activation of apical membrane Na^+-K^+-$2Cl^-$ co-transporter and K^+ channels leads to an increase in intracellular Cl^- activity, and a subsequent increase in basolateral Cl^- conductance. In support of this view, Molony et al.[214] found, also in mouse medullary TAL, that the ADH-dependent rise in cellular and basolateral conductance were much lower when Cl^- entry was inhibited by furosemide than in control conditions. Studies of Cl^- channels incorporated from basolaterally enriched renal medullary membrane vesicles into planar lipid bilayers have demonstrated several properties of these channels that may account for an intracellular Cl^- concentration-dependent rise in basolateral Cl^- conductance.[251,336] First, the activity of the Cl^- channels is increased with membrane depolarization evidently due to the basolateral membrane depolarization that follows ADH stimulation of TAL segments.[251] Second, Cl^- channels in the vesicles behave like Goldman rectifiers, so that increases in intracellular Cl^- cause an increase in the outward single-channel conductance.[251] Third, channel activity is dependent on the intracellular Cl^- concentration, such that increases in Cl^- over the range 2−50 mM result in large increases in the open time probability of these Cl^- channels.[336] In this respect, it should be recognized that the time-averaged conductance of a basolateral Cl^- channel is given by the product $g_{Cl}P_o$, where g_{Cl} is unit channel conductance and P_o is open time probability.

Thus, an ADH-dependent increase in apical Cl^- entry could stimulate basolateral Cl^- conductance to a far greater extent than expected from simple Goldman rectification. In that connection, at least two laboratories have found, in mTAL segments, that reducing intracellular Cl^- with luminal furosemide produced a three-fold reduction in basolateral Cl^- conductance.[214,276]

Modulation of ADH Effect on TAL Segments

Several factors, such as prostaglandins, peritubular calcium concentration, and peritubular osmolality, have been demonstrated to modulate the actions of ADH on NaCl absorption in the TAL (see the review articles by Hebert and Molony).[135,212] In isolated mouse and rabbit TAL segments, increases in peritubular osmolality, induced by adding urea or impermeant solutes such as mannitol, rapidly and reversibly inhibit the ADH-stimulated rate of net Cl^- absorption. Peritubular hypertonicity results in a prompt reduction in the transepithelial voltage and in the cellular conductance.[213] Molony and Andreoli determined that hypertonicity inhibits the basolateral membrane chloride conductance.[212] The antagonizing effect on ADH-induced stimulation of net Cl transport is not due to decreasing cAMP, because application of either ADH or cAMP is unable to reverse the hypertonicity-mediated effect. Thus, increasing the absolute magnitude of interstitial osmolality provides a negative feedback signal that can reduce ADH-dependent salt absorption by the mTAL.

PGE_2 also plays a role in modulating the effect of ADH on NaCl absorption in the mTAL (see Molony's review article [212]). In the mouse mTAL, PGE_2 abolished the effect of ADH on transepithelial voltage and on net NaCl absorption, while it had no effect on NaCl salt absorption in the absence of ADH. Likewise, reported biochemical studies in the mTAL[226] indicate that PGE_2 has no effect on cellular cAMP concentrations in the absence of ADH, and that PGE_2 markedly inhibits the ADH-dependent stimulation of cytosolic cAMP concentrations. The TAL, particularly in the macula densa, expresses COX-2.[130] COX-2 expression in these cells may be coupled to renin secretion. Thus, COX-2 expression is increased by salt restriction, diuretics, and in Bartter syndrome all conditions characterized by hyperreninemia.[46] In addition to PGE_2, 20-HETE may also modulate the effect of cAMP on Na^+ transport in the TAL. McGiff and co-workers[207] demonstrated that 20-HETE inhibits NaCl transport in the TAL by a mechanism involving inhibition of the apical K^+ channel[323] and the Na^+-K^+-$2Cl^-$ co-transporter.[69] Moreover, high 20-HETE concentration inhibits the effect of cAMP on the apical K^+ channels in the rat TAL.[116]

Hypercalcemia often results in an ADH-resistant urinary concentrating defect, that is, nephrogenic diabetes insipidus. At least part of this concentrating defect results from the inhibition of ADH-stimulated cAMP production in the TAL by calcium. Takaichi and Kurokawa demonstrated that high ambient calcium inhibited cAMP production stimulated by forskolin, indicating that the inhibition probably involved the catalytic subunit of adenylate cyclase. Preincubation of tubule segments with pertussis toxin abolishes the effect of hypercalcemia on cAMP generation, indicating that the inhibition of cAMP generation is mediated through activation of G_i.[303] The effects of hypercalcemia on cAMP production are mediated by a G-protein-coupled CaSR present on the basolateral membrane of

TAL cells.[133] As discussed above, stimulation of CaSR also inhibits the apical 70 pS and basolateral 50 pS K channels.[117,179] Consequently, activation of CaSR is expected to alter NaCl absorption, thereby affecting the concentrating mechanism.[137]

Intracellular Mechanisms for NKCC2 modulation in TAL

The physiological pathways for NKCC2 regulation have begun to be uncovered. The rate of salt reabsorption by TAL depends on the amount of NKCC2 protein expressed in the apical membrane at any given time; that is, the protein half-life in the plasma membrane. As shown in Figure 34.5, the amount of NKCC2 is the result of a dynamic process involving exocytosis and endocytosis mechanisms. Stimulators of NKCC2, such as cAMP (vasopressin, PTH, glucagon or β-adrenergic stimulation) promote exocytosis over endocytosis. Electron microscopy analysis of mouse TAL[100] and biotinylation of rat TAL apical membrane[232] demonstrated that only between 3–5% of total NKCC2 is present in the apical membrane in basal conditions. Vasopressin stimulates trafficking of NKCC2 towards the plasma membrane in *Xenopus* oocytes,[209] in mouse TAL,[100] and in rat TAL,[232] by a process that is modulated by the vesicle-associated membrane proteins VAMP2 and VAMP3. Exocytosis of NKCC2 is a continuous dynamic process that is further activated by cAMP, via protein kinase A (PKA).[9] Because PKA inhibition does not completely prevent cAMP-induced increase of NKCC2 presence in the apical membrane, it is possible that cAMP also inhibits endocytosis. Two amino acid residues of NKCC2 become phosphorylated by PKA, Ser126 and Ser874, but the exact consequence of this is not known.[122] Endocytosis of NKCC2 occurs also

constitutively in TAL. A fraction recycles toward the apical membrane and another fraction undergoes degradation. Inhibition of endocytosis by cholesterol depletion completely block NKCC2 retrieval from the membrane, increasing NKCC2 presence and chloride transport by TAL.[9] Supporting this view, it has been shown that part of NKCC2 is associated with lipid rafts.[331]

Inhibitors of NKCC2 such as nitric oxide, through the eNOS synthase,[246] atrial natriuretic peptide, and endothelin affect trafficking of the co-transporter, mainly through a cGMP-dependent activation of phosphodiestarese 2 (PDE2) that in turn degradates cAMP (Figure 34.5). The intracellular mechanism for other NKCC2 inhibitors such as 20-HETE and PGE₂ is not extensively known,[8] but can be achieved at least in part by modulating the ADH effect in TAL. PGE₂ for instance, in the *in vitro* mouse mTAL PGE₂ has no effect on NaCl salt absorption when ADH is absent.[246] In the presence of ADH, PGE₂ reduces the ADH-dependent values for transepithelial voltage and net NaCl absorption to ADH-independent values, by what appears to be inhibition of ADH-stimulated generation of cAMP in the mTAL by activating G_i. Hypercalcemia reduces TAL salt reabsorption by a calcium-induced inhibition of NKCC2 and ROMK vía calcium sensing receptor activation of G_i.[93]

Adrenergic Agents

Adenylate cyclase activity stimulated by β-adrenergic receptors is present in the rat, but not rabbit, TAL.[41] Likewise, β-adrenoceptors have been detected along the rat TAL by autoradiographic localization. The physiologic effects of adrenergic agents have been tested in micropunctures and *in vitro* microperfusion studies. DiBona and Sawin[58] demonstrated an enhancement of loop NaCl absorption during low-frequency renal nerve stimulation. Acute renal denervation, on the other hand, depressed NaCl absorption by the loop of Henle.[19]

Mineralocorticoids

There is controversy regarding mineralocorticoid effects on TAL. Some evidence suggests that aldosterone influences NaCl transport in the TAL (reviewed in [59]). First, clearance studies indicate that aldosterone increases free water clearance in adrenalectomized animals, consistent with an increase in NaCl absorption by the TAL. Second, nuclear mineralocorticoid receptors are present in both the medullary and cortical portions of the TAL of rat and rabbit, although it is known that the presence of mineralocorticoid receptors is no guarantee of being a specific target site of aldosterone. The mechanism of aldosterone actions are discussed in Chapter 35. Third, aldosterone appears to modulate the

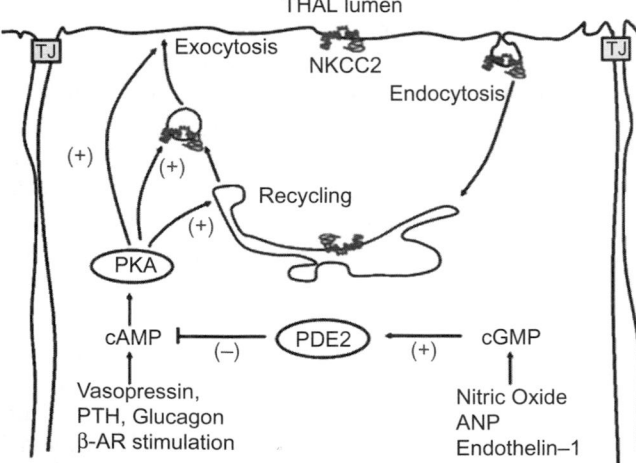

FIGURE 34.5 Physiological regulatory pathways of NKCC2 in thick ascending limbs of Henle's loop (TALs). *From ref. [8].*

activity of certain transport-related enzymes in the TAL. Specifically, adrenalectomy reduces the activity of (Na^+,K^+)-ATPase in the rabbit TAL. The activity of these enzymes can be restored to almost normal by aldosterone, but not by dexamethasone. In the adrenal-intact mouse, pharmacologic doses of mineralocorticoid increased (Na^+,K^+)-ATPase activity of mTAL segments by 25%. Finally, *in vivo* and *in vitro* microperfusion studies have demonstrated effects of aldosterone on TAL sodium transport. Adrenalectomy inhibited loop of Henle sodium absorption by 33–50%. Aldosterone, but not dexamethasone, increased sodium transport to control levels. Also in the rat medullary TAL, adrenalectomy decreases $NaHCO_3$ absorption by 33%. However, other studies have failed to show an effect of mineralocorticoids on (Na^+,K^+)-ATPase activity in the TAL (also reviewed in [59]). Additionally, a recent study shows that aldosterone administration on adernalectomized rats had no effect on NKCC2 expression.[313]

Na^+ TRANSPORT IN DISTAL CONVOLUTED TUBULE

General Characteristics

The DCT absorbs roughly 10% of the filtered sodium load.[255] Fluid enters the DCT with a sodium concentration of 25–30 mM, but salt is added along the initial 20% of the DCT, so that the sodium concentration averages 50 mM at a point 200–300 μm from the macula densa. From there, tubular sodium concentration decreases along the DCT to a value of approximately 30 mM at the end.[279] Tubular fluid to plasma sodium ratios as low as 0.10 have been observed during stationary microperfusion.[255] This finding, together with the presence of the lumen-negative potential difference (see subsequent discussion), establishes clearly the active nature of sodium absorption in this segment.

Sodium absorption by the DCT is load-dependent. That is, over a wide range of delivery rates, the proportion of sodium absorbed by the DCT remains constant at 80%.[255] At high tubular fluid flow rates, the fall in luminal sodium concentration along the tubule is attenuated; thus, more sodium is available to distal sodium absorptive sites at high flow rates than at low flow rates. Sodium absorption in the rat DCT has been reported to be 25–30 $pEq/mm^2/sec$, that is, about one-third of the rate occurring in the PCT. However, rates comparable to those in the PCT have been reported in isolated perfused DCT.[52,53,66]

Electophysiologic Considerations

The electrophysiologic and transport properties of the DCT and CNT are summarized in Table 34.6. The transepithelial voltage in the earliest loops of the DCT, measured with fine tip electrodes, ranges from 9 to 19 mV, lumen-negative. Small lumen-positive voltages, 3.7 to 5.7 mV, have been measured both in micropuncture experiments, by using low resistance micropuncture electrodes, and in isolated, perfused early DCT segments (reviewed in [255]). When the composition of the luminal perfusate resembled distal tubular fluid, i.e., having a low NaCl concentration (see earlier discussion), the lumen voltage tended to be slightly positive, whereas when tubules were perfused with solutions resembling plasma, i.e., high NaCl concentration, the lumen voltage was negative. The lumen-negative potential measured with high NaCl solutions was abolished by luminal amiloride, an inhibitor of epithelial sodium channels. The positive voltage under *in vivo* conditions is a salt dilution potential arising from the differential permeability of the DCT to Na^+ and Cl^-, while the lumen-negative potential under symmetric solutions reflects active Na^+ reabsorption via amiloride-sensitive sodium channels (see subsequent discussion).

The transepithelial electrical potential in the late DCT of rats measured *in vivo* ranges from 37 to 60 mV. Values in isolated rabbit DCT and CNT segments perfused with symmetric solutions are less negative, 5 to 30 mV.[114,286,347] The voltage can be inhibited by peritubular ouabain or luminal amiloride,[347] and is quite sensitive to changes in perfusion pressure and flow rate, decreasing with high pressures or flow rates.

The transepithelial resistance of the rat DCT decreases from 337 $\Omega\text{-}cm^2$ in the early DCT to 135 $\Omega\text{-}cm^2$ in the late DCT.[255] Hypotonic luminal fluids increase, and hypertonic perfusates decrease, the transepithelial resistance with respect to isotonic luminal fluid. Somewhat lower electrical resistances have been found in isolated perfused rabbit DCT[114,347] and CNT.[4]

Intracellular microelectrode analysis of rabbit DCT cells has yielded conflicting results. Yoshitomi et al.[347] found evidence for both K^+ and Na^+ conductive pathways in the apical membrane and K^+ and Cl^- conductive pathways in the basolateral membrane. The apical membrane accounted for 80% of the total cellular resistance. In contrast, Velazquez et al.[319] found the apical membrane to comprise over 99% of the cellular resistance, and could not detect any Na^+ or K^+ conductances in that membrane. Perhaps some of this discrepancy could have arisen from the examination of different portions of the DCT in the two laboratories. Ellison et al. have demonstrated that sodium reabsorption in the early DCT is largely mediated by a thiazide-sensitive, neutral NaCl co-transporter, while sodium absorption in the late DCT involves an amiloride-sensitive electrogenic pathway.[66] Thus, Yoshitomi et al.[347] may have described the late DCT and Velazquez et al.[319] the early DCT.

TABLE 34.6 Electrophysiologic and Transport Properties of DCT

	V_t (mV)	R_t ($\Omega - cm^2$)	V_{bl} (mV)	fRa	J_{Na} (pmol/mm/min)	J_{Cl} (pmol/mm/min)
Rat DCT	+8 to −19	81–382	−57 to −65		128–258	285
Rabbit DCT	−2 to −40	22–116	−78 to −84	0.78–0.99	82	
Rabbit CNT	−4 to −27	29–31	−71 to −83		62–121	405

Table from Reeves, W. B., and Andreoli, T. E. (2008). Sodium chloride transport in the loop of Henle, distal convoluted tubule, and collecting duct. In "The Kidney: Physiology and Pathophysiology," 4th edn, 849–888, Alpern, R. J., and Hebert, S. C. (eds.). Elsevier.

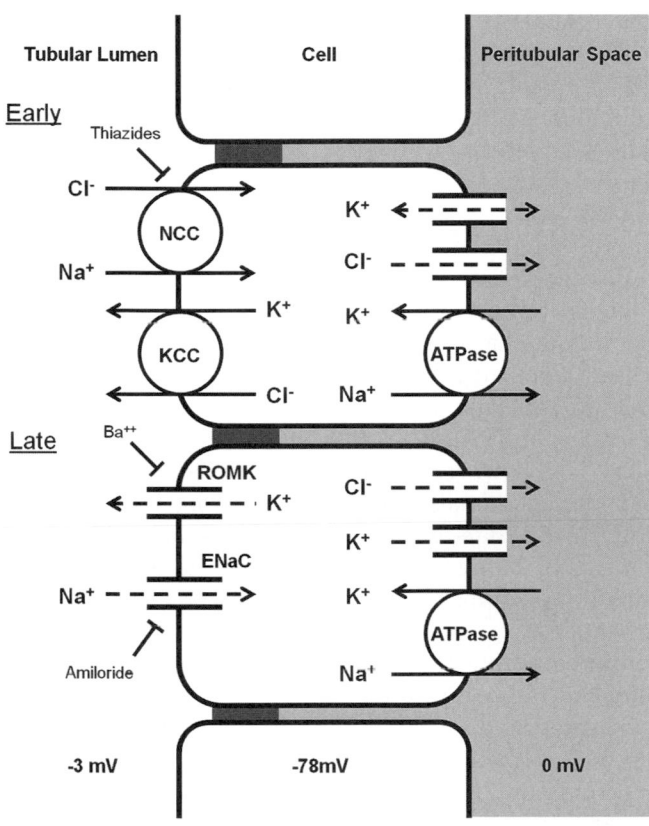

FIGURE 34.6 **Model of NaCl absorption by cells of the early (DCT1) and late (DCT2) convoluted tubule.** *Modified from Reeves, W. B., and Andreoli, T. E. (2008). Sodium chloride transport in the loop of Henle, distal convoluted tubule, and collecting duct. In "The Kidney: Physiology and Pathophysiology," 4th edn, 849–888, Alpern, R. J., and Hebert, S. C. (eds.). Elsevier.*

Mechanism of Na$^+$ Absorption

The available evidence permits the delineation of certain facets of Na$^+$ absorption in the DCT. A general model for these mechanisms is presented in Figure 34.6. Central among these are the characteristics discussed in the following subsections.

APICAL NaCl CO-TRANSPORT

The absorption of sodium and chloride in the early DCT is mutually dependent.[319] Sodium absorption is a function of the luminal chloride concentration, and chloride absorption is a function of the luminal sodium concentration. The half-maximal concentrations of both sodium and chloride are 10 mM.[319] Furthermore, the intracellular Cl$^-$ activity is above its electrochemical equilibrium, such that Cl$^-$ entry into the cell must involve active transport. The early distal tubule is the site of action of thiazide diuretics.[53,66,286]

A thiazide-sensitive neutral NaCl co-transporter (TSC) was cloned from the flounder urinary bladder using an expression cloning strategy.[95] A homologous transporter, NCC (SLC12A3) was subsequently cloned from the mammalian kidney.[94] NCC and NKCC2 are members of the same family of solute transporters and share considerable sequence homology (see Chapter 32). NCC transports NaCl with a 1:1 stoichiometry, is K-independent, and is inhibited by thiazide diuretics.[215] NCC is expressed in the apical membrane of early DCT cells (or DCT1) and extends, in most species, into the late DCT (or DCT2) (reviewed in [92,255,278]). In addition, mutations in the NCC gene are the cause of Gitelman syndrome that mimics the effects of thiazide diuretics.[92] Full discussion on NCC molecular physiology is presented in Chapter 32.

APICAL CONDUCTIVE SODIUM CHANNELS

The entry of sodium into the late rat DCT cell[52] is inhibited by amiloride, a sodium channel blocker. A sodium channel in the apical membrane would serve to depolarize the membrane and create the observed lumen-negative transepithelial potential. This transepithelial voltage, in turn, is a driving force for passive chloride reabsorption. Sodium channel subunits have been found by immunolocalization in the late DCT in mouse and rat kidney.[255,278]

BASOLATERAL ELECTROGENIC Na$^+$ PUMP

The voltage (V_{bl}) across the basolateral membrane of the *Amphiuma*[333] and rabbit[114,347] DCT is 60 to 90 mV. A reduction in the luminal sodium concentration causes V_{bl} to depolarize, while increases in the sodium concentration hyperpolarize V_{bl}. In addition, V_{bl} depolarizes after ouabain treatment. These observations are consistent with the notion that apical sodium entry stimulates the electrogenic (Na^+, K^+)-ATPase system in the basolateral membrane.

BASOLATERAL POTASSIUM CHANNELS

The basolateral membrane of DCT cells contains a large, barium-sensitive potassium conductance.[114] Patch-clamp studies of the basolateral membrane of DCT cells have identified three different potassium channels. Two of the channels have similar conductances (50—60 pS) and kinetics, and both are blocked by barium. The third channel is seen less frequently, has a conductance of 80 pS, and is not blocked by barium. A basolateral potassium channel Kir4.1/KCNJ10 which has been localized to the basolateral membrane of DCT when mutated causes the SeSAME/EAST syndrome characterized by epilepsy, ataxia, sensorineural deafness, and renal salt-losing nephropathy similar to Gitelman's disease.[254,281] Inactivating mutations of this channel prevent the K^+ efflux of the basolateral membrane, presumably increasing the intracellular K^+ concentration that inhibits the basolateral Na^+, K^+-ATPase.

BASOLATERAL CHLORIDE CHANNELS

Microelectrode studies by Yoshitomi et al.[347] provided evidence for a chloride conductive pathway in the basolateral membrane of rabbit DCT cells. Likewise, Gesek and Friedman[97] found evidence for basolateral membrane Cl^- channels in cultured mouse DCT cells. Specifically, inhibition of apical Cl^- entry with thiazide diuretics resulted in a fall in intracellular Cl^- activity and a hyperpolarization of the membrane voltage.[97] The thiazide-induced hyperpolarization could be abolished by either a reduction in the extracellular Cl^- concentration or by NPPB, a Cl^- channel blocker,[97] suggesting that a Cl^- channel accounts for the basolateral Cl^- conductance. The single-channel properties of Cl^- channels in DCT cells have not been reported, but now it is known that CLC-Kb chloride channels are present in DCT basolateral membrane.[283] The basolateral Cl^- conductance was increased by parathyroid hormone, presumably acting via cAMP.[97]

Regulation of NaCl Transport in DCT

Na^+ DELIVERY

As noted earlier, NaCl reabsorption in the DCT is dependent on the delivered load of NaCl. Chronic increases in the delivery of NaCl to the DCT can be achieved using furosemide to inhibit NaCl reabsorption in the thick ascending limb. The DCT responds to such a maneuver with an increase in the capacity for NaCl transport,[67] and increased expression of NCC,[1] as well as marked ultrastructural changes in the DCT cell. These morphologic changes include an increase in the size of the DCT cell, an increase in the basolateral membrane surface area, and an increase in the size of mitochondria.[67,159] Hypertrophy of DCT is also seen in Bartter's mice due to knockout of ROMK,[37] and in BAC transgenic mice harboring two alleles of WNK4 containing the pseudohypoaldosteronism type II (PHAII) type mutation Q562E.[184] Thus, it is likely that DCT hypertrophy is due to either an increase in sodium entry into the DCT cell or activation of the renin—angiotensin system (see discussion below). In addition, an increase in dietary sodium alone, which increases distal NaCl delivery but not distal Na^+ absorption or activation of the renin—angiotensin—aldosterone system, does not, in the rat, result in an increase in cell height.[67] Moreover, inhibition of NaCl entry into DCT cells with chronic thiazide treatment resulted in a loss of cell height, loss of normal polarity, and apoptosis of the DCT cells.[191]

STEROID HORMONES

The presence of both mineralocorticoid and glucocorticoid receptors in the DCT has been demonstrated by immunohistochemistry and by hormone-binding. In addition, adrenalectomy resulted in a decrease in (Na^+, K^+)-ATPase activity in the DCT.[59] Microperfusion studies of superficial distal tubules (containing both DCT and CNT), however, demonstrated an increase in sodium transport in animals receiving aldosterone infusions.[59,317] Both the thiazide-sensitive and thiazide-insensitive components of sodium transport were increased by aldosterone.[317] The former may reflect neutral NaCl co-transport in the DCT, while the latter reflects electrogenic sodium absorption in the late DCT or CNT. Aldosterone infusion also resulted in large increases in NCC protein,[1,169,258,317] and phosphorylation in amino-terminal domain regulatory threonines[313] (see Chapter 32). These findings establish NCC as an aldosterone-regulated transporter, a situation that occurs in DCT2 that is considered to be part of the aldosterone sensitive distal nephron.[11] Aldosterone increases of NCC expression do not seem to be due to an increased transcription rate of the SLC12A3 gene encoding NCC.[1,218] Instead, it has been observed that NCC expression in the plasma membrane is regulated by ubiquitylation via the HECT-E3 ubiquitin ligase Nedd4-2, which in turn is modulated by phosphorylation by the serum glucocorticoid kinase 1 (Sgk1),[10] similar to what occurs with ENaC. Thus, aldosterone regulation of NCC appears to be, at least in part, through the Sgk1-Nedd4-2 pathway. Interestingly, in some families with PHAII, an inherited form of salt-sensitive hypertension in humans also known as Familial Hyperkalemic Hypertension or Gordon's syndrome, it results from mutations in Cullin 3 and KLHL3 proteins, which are part of a RING-type E3 ubiquitin ligase complex which presumably modulates NCC activity by ubiquitilation processes.[29,196]

Glucocorticoids increase (Na$^+$,K$^+$)-ATPase activity following adrenalectomy in the DCT. This effect was not blocked by spironolactone, a mineralocorticoid receptor antagonist, suggesting that glucocorticoids were acting via glucocorticoid receptors rather than mineralocorticoid receptors.[59] In addition, dexamethasone infusions increased thiazide-sensitive NaCl transport and [^{3}H]metolazone-binding sites in adrenalectomized rats.[317] Nonetheless, the role of glucocorticoids in the physiologic regulation of sodium transport in the DCT remains unclear.

Gonadal steroid hormones may also influence NaCl transport in the DCT. Chen et al.[45] first reported gender differences in the density of thiazide receptors, and in the natriuretic response to thiazides in rats. Female rats had higher levels of thiazide-binding sites in the renal cortex than males. The levels in females fell following ovariectomy, while levels rose in males following orchiectomy. Moreover, the increase in urinary sodium excretion caused by thiazides was greater in females than in males, suggesting that the differences in thiazide-binding sites were reflective of differences in thiazide-sensitive salt transport *in vivo*. Likewise, using antibodies against the cloned thiazide-sensitive NaCl co-transporter (NCC), Verlander et al.[320] found that estrogen treatment increased NCC expression in the DCT. These results are consistent with the view that male sex hormones (e.g., testosterone) may downregulate NCC expression and salt transport, while estrogens increase NCC expression and salt transport in the DCT.

PROTEIN KINASES

Studies of PHAII have yielded additional insights into the regulation of NCC function. PHAII is the phenotypic opposite of Gitelman syndrome, and is characterized by hypertension, hyperkalemia, and metabolic acidosis. The disorder is largely corrected by thiazide diuretics. These features suggested that an increase in NCC activity may be involved in the pathogenesis of PHAII. Positional cloning demonstrated that PHAII in some families is caused by mutations in either of two serine-threonine kinases, WNK1 and WNK4,[334] and more recently the whole exomes sequencing strategy revealed that Cullin 3 and KLHL3[29,196] are responsible for the disease in WNK-negative families. Subsequent studies have shown that WNK4 acts to inhibit NCC-mediated NaCl transport, likely by reducing cell surface expression of NCC[35,334,343] and that effect of WNK4 turns into activation by the PHAII type mutations,[184,334,344] resulting in higher rates of NaCl transport. It has been observed that a switch of WNK4 from inhibiting to activating NCC can be achieved by angiotensin II,[266] suggesting that NCC activation by angiotensin II,[267] which is independent of the presence of aldosterone,[313] is a WNK4-dependent process. In this regard, it has been shown that WNK4-induced phosphorylation of the downstream kinase SPAK/OSR1 is modulated by calcium concentration,[225] and that phosphorylation of SPAK and NCC in the presence of a low-salt diet or angiotensin II infusion is abrogated in WNK4 total knockout mice,[39] supporting the proposal that angiotensin II signaling via the Gα_q-coupled AT1 receptor that increases intracellular calcium could be a modulator of the WNK4 type of effect on NCC. WNK4 also affects the activity of apical ROMK channels: wild-type WNK4 inhibits ROMK and the PHAII mutant WNK4 further reduces the activity of the channels, helping to explain the hyperkalemia of PHAII patients.[157] Recent observation also shows that angiotensin II-induced inhibition of ROMK channels[330] is at least in part dependent on the presence of WNK4.[349] Thus, it is possible that PHAII type mutations in WNK4 are of the gain-of-function type, mimicking the effect of angiotensin II on NCC and ROMK activity on DCT-CD. WNK4 also affects the Cl$^-$ permeability of the paracellular pathway.[156] The mechanism whereby WNK1 produces PHAII is less well-defined. Yang et al.[343] found that WNK1 does not directly affect NCC activity, but modulates the inhibition of NCC by WNK4. They propose that mutations that increase the activity of WNK1 prevent WNK4 from inhibiting NCC-mediated transport. Although not causing disease, WNK3 is also a powerful modulator of NCC activity. Wild-type WNK3 activates NCC, while the catalytically inactive WNK3 inhibits NCC.[256] Activity of NCC is also modulated by protein phosphatase 4.[101] (For an extensive review on NCC regulation see Chapter 32.)

Na$^+$ TRANSPORT IN THE CONNECTING TUBULE AND COLLECTING DUCT

The transport of Na$^+$ in the connecting tubule and the collecting duct is responsible for the final adjustments of renal Na$^+$ excretion. These tubular segments share in common an electrogenic Na$^+$ transport mediated by the epithelial sodium channel (ENaC), and sensitivity to aldosterone.

The Connecting Tubule

The connecting tubule connects the distal convoluted tubule (DCT) with the cortical collecting duct (CCD). Developmentally, the DCT originates from the metanephric blastema, whereas the CCD arises from the ureteric bud. The origin of the CNT is not clear, since the CNT shares some transport characteristics with both the late DCT and the downstream CCD.[14] This suggests that the CNT is a hybrid tubular segment that develops at the border of the two adjoining segments, the DCT and the CCD.[278] The transition between the late distal convoluted tubule (DCT2) and the CNT is gradual in the mouse, rat, and human kidney.[190] In the mouse kidney, the CNT represents more than 8% of the fractional renal tubular volume, compared to 12% for the DCT and 4% for the CCD.[194]

The distal convolutions of superficial nephrons comprising the late DCT, the CNT, and the initial collecting tubule, are accessible by micropuncture. The importance of the CNT in Na$^+$ absorption was evaluated in a number of *in vivo* experiments. Microperfusion studies of the late distal convoluted tubule show that more than 90% of the Na$^+$ delivery in the DCT is reabsorbed in the DCT2 and the CNT by an amiloride-sensitive Na$^+$ transport.[52,205] In the rabbit isolated and perfused CNT, Na$^+$ absorption measured by net ^{22}Na fluxes is 3−4-fold higher than in the CCD under similar conditions.[4] Furthermore, patch-clamp studies in microdissected CNTs from the cortical labyrinth show that the amiloride-sensitive current was 4−5-fold higher than that measured in the CCD of the same animal.[88] From these experiments it was estimated that the maximal Na$^+$ transport capacity of the CNT allows the reabsorption of 10% of the filtered load of Na$^+$. Thus, the CNT represents a major site for the regulation of distal Na$^+$ reabsorption. Recent genetic experiments using homologous recombination in the mouse to invalidate ENaC specifically in the DCT2 and the CNT, provided direct evidence that the CNT plays a critical role for the maintenance of the Na$^+$ and K$^+$ homeostasis.[50]

In the CNT, a significant fraction of Na$^+$ absorption is associated with K$^+$ secretion. Patch-clamp and immunolocalization studies identified the presence of the inward rectifier Kir1 channel ROMK at the apical membrane as the major channel.[87,210,318] The density of active ROMK channels was found to be higher in the CNT compared to CCD, consistent with the idea that the CNT is an important site for K$^+$ secretion in the distal nephron. However, the density of active ROMK channels in the CNT was independent of the K$^+$ diet. This suggests that the increased K$^+$ secretion under a high-K$^+$ diet is primarily due to an increase in the driving force for K$^+$ efflux across the apical membrane, due to the upregulation of the apical Na$^+$ conductance.

The connecting tubule contains CNT-specific cells and intercalated cells; the specific CNT cells represent 70−80% of the epithelial lining in the CNT, and are the site for Na$^+$ absorption and K$^+$ secretion; the remainder of the epithelial lining consists of the intercalated cells that mediate acid−base balance.[61,158,170,204] Under a standard Na$^+$ diet, the epithelial sodium channel (ENaC) is detected by immunohistochemistry at the apical membrane of CNT specific cells.[193] ENaC is

highly selective for Na$^+$ ions with a P$_{Na}$/P$_K$ >100, and a single channel conductance g$_{Na}$ of 4 to 5 pS.[36] ENaC is blocked by submicromolar concentrations of amiloride, and by triamterene at higher concentrations. ENaC is expressed in other epithelial tissues such as the lungs, the colon, salivary glands, and sweat ducts. The channel is constitutively open; analysis of the ENaC gating kinetics suggests two different gating modes, one with a high (>0.75), the other with low (<0.25) open probability.[236] Transitions between these gating modes are influenced by factors such as membrane voltage or Na ions; hyperpolarization or a low extracellular Na favors the high open probability gating mode. By contrast, an acute increase in extracellular or intracellular Na$^+$ reduces the ENaC openings and channel current.[234,235,236] These regulatory mechanisms, termed self-inhibition and feedback inhibition respectively, are likely important to prevent a massive entry of Na$^+$ ions into the cell when luminal Na$^+$ concentration is high.[7,48] Other intracellular factors associated with cellular stress such as a decrease in pH, an increase in oxidative stess or a rise in Ca^{2+} ions decrease channel open probability.[48,162,234] ENaC is not mechanosensitive.[236]

Cloning by functional expression revealed that the ENaC channel consists of three homologous α-, β-, and γ-subunits that all are required for the full expression and activity of the channel at the cell surface.[36] The ENaC subunits share 30% homology at the amino acid level; each subunit is made of two transmembrane α helices and a large extracellular domain that represents more than half of the mass of the protein; the amino- and carboxy-termini are facing the cytosolic side of the membrane. The recent crystalization of an ortholog of ENaC, the Acid Sensing Ion Channel 1 (ASIC1), confirms this membrane topology and provides a high-resolution structure of the homologous subunits that constitute the channel core.[152] Based on homology models and functional data, the second transmembrane α helix is lining the ENaC pore and comprises important functional domains controlling ion flux through the pore: they include sequentially from outside, an extracellular gate, the amiloride- and triamterene-binding site, and further downstream the selectivity filter.[102,163,164,165] The cytosolic N-terminus of ENaC comprises a functional domain made of conserved cysteines that control ENaC gating; the C-terminus of ENaC subunits is characterized by conserved proline residues involved in ENaC interactions with cytosolic regulatory proteins.[242,296]

ENaC is activated by soluble proteases including trypsin, chymotrypsin, kallikrein or elastase. In addition, ENaC activity is significantly increased *in vitro* when co-expressed with membrane-attached serine proteases, such as the GPI-anchored proteases CAP-1 (an ortholog of the human prostasin) or CAP-2 (an ortholog of the human transmembrane protease serine 4 (TRPMSS4)).[49,129,312,322] In heterologous expression systems and in the kidney, the α and the γ ENaC subunit are found as a high and a low molecular weight forms, the latter resulting from ENaC cleavage by endogenous proteases.[89,68,89,129,145,206] The active α and γ ENaC at the cell surface is predominantly in its cleaved form. The α and γ ENaC have both canonical cleavage sequences for furin-like proteases in their extracellular domain. Furin is an endoprotease, a member of the subtilisin-like proprotein convertase family that cleaves precursor proteins along their secretory pathway from the trans-Golgi network to the apical surface. The molecular mechanism of ENaC maturation and activation by endoproteases is not yet completely understood.

The ROMK are expressed at the apical membrane of specific CNT cells.[15,87,210] Big K channels (BK channels) or maxi-K channels have been shown to account for K⁺ secretion in the late distal tubule; the co-expression of these high-conductance Ca^{2+}-activated K channels (BK channels) with ENaC in CNT cells remains controversial.[15] From patch-clamp studies it seems that BK channels are restricted to the apical membrane of the intercalated cells.[237]

At the basolateral membrane, the Na/K-ATPase is responsible for pumping Na⁺ out of the cell in exchange with K⁺; the Na/K-ATPase activity as measured by pump current and ATP hydrolysis is higher in the CNT than in the CCD, consistent with the idea that the CNT transports more Na⁺ and K⁺ than the downstream segments.[161]

These membrane transporters provide a transcellular route for electrogenic Na⁺ reabsorption and K⁺ secretion in the CNT cells. ENaC at the apical membrane represents the entry step for Na⁺ ions along a favorable electrochemical gradient; the resulting depolarization of the apical membrane provides a favorable driving force for K⁺ secretion. The electrical coupling in the Na⁺ and K⁺ transport across the apical membrane, and the direct coupling of the Na⁺ and K⁺ transport by the basolateral Na/K pump, indicates that Na⁺ absorption in the CNT directly affects K⁺ secretion, and that these two ion transports are closely linked.

The Collecting Ducts

THE CORTICAL COLLECTING DUCT

The Na⁺ and the K⁺ transports in the CCD have been largely studied and differ from those in the CNT, more quantitatively than qualitatively. Table 34.7 summarizes the electrophysiologic and transport properties of CCD. The electrogenic Na⁺ absorption mediated by ENaC generates a lumen-negative transepithelial voltage (V) in the CCD that varies widely according to the mineralocorticoid status of animals.[106,269] This lumen-negative voltage in mammalian CCD segments is abolished by ouabain,[106,125] luminal amiloride,[300] and luminal sodium deletion.[300] However, the lumen-negative transepithelial potential in the rabbit CCD is seven times less negative compared with the CNT.[148]

The membrane transporters involved in Na⁺ absorption and K⁺ secretion in the CCD principal cells are essentially the same as in the CNT cells (see Figure 34.7). Immunohistochemical studies have shown that, under standard salt diet, the abundance of ENaC at the apical membrane decreases from the late DCT and CNT to the CCD, further supporting the idea that the CNT is a major site for ENaC-mediated Na⁺ absorption in the aldosterone distal nephron.[192,193] By contrast to the CNT, the selective invalidation of ENaC in the mouse CCD using homologous recombination does not result in any alteration in Na⁺ and K⁺ homeostasis, even under restricted dietary Na⁺ intake.[261] This suggests that the absence of ENaC in the CD can be compensated, at least in part, by an increase in ENaC activity in the CNT.

From isolated and perfused rat CCD, the major fraction of Na⁺ absorption in the CCD is electrogenic and mediated by ENaC; no evidence was found supporting the contribution of a thiazide-sensitive electroneutral NaCl co-transport in Na⁺ absorption.[260] Recent studies, however, have reported that a significant fraction of Na⁺ absorption in the mouse and rat CCD is electroneutral, insensitive to luminal amiloride, but sensitive to thiazides.[187] Microperfusion studies in different

TABLE 34.7 Electrophysiologic and Transport Properties of CCD

	V_t (mV)	R_t (Ω/cm²)	V_{bl} (mV)	fRa	J_{Na} (pmol/mm/min)	J_{Cl} (pmol/mm/min)
Rabbit CCD	−2 to −27	86–133	−73 to −85	0.31−0.53	5.7−24.3	− 3.4 to 4.0
Rat CCD	−1 to −5	51−64	−77 to −83	0.76−0.84	− 2.3 to 0.2	

Table from Reeves, W. B., and Andreoli, T. E. (2008). Sodium chloride transport in the loop of Henle, distal convoluted tubule, and collecting duct. In "The Kidney: Physiology and Pathophysiology," 4th edn, 849–888, Alpern, R. J., and Hebert, S. C. (eds.). Elsevier.
Note: Intracellular data from principal cells only.

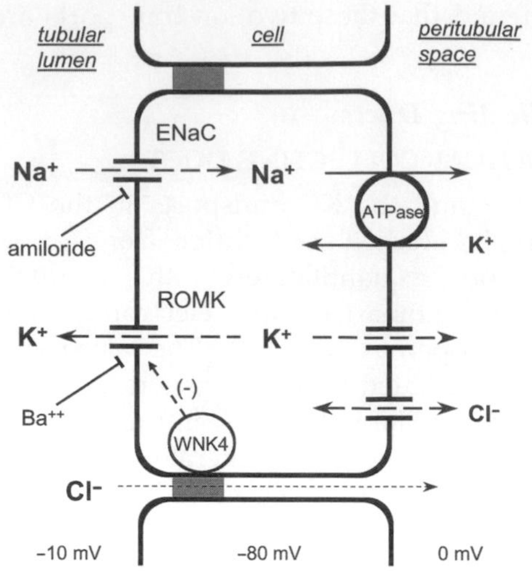

FIGURE 34.7   Model of salt transport by the principal cell of the cortical collecting duct. *From Reeves, W. B., and Andreoli, T. E. (2008). Sodium chloride transport in the loop of Henle, distal convoluted tubule, and collecting duct. In "The Kidney: Physiology and Pathophysiology," 4th edn, 849–888, Alpern, R. J., and Hebert, S. C. (eds.). Elsevier.*

genetically-engineered mouse models under a low-Na^+ diet concluded that this electroneutral Na^+ and Cl^- absorption results from the parallel operation of two bicarbonate transporters, a Na^+-dependent Cl/HCO_3^- exchanger and the anion exchanger pendrin. This amiloride-insensitive Na^+ transport pathway likely occurs through the intercalated cells.

THE OUTER MEDULLARY COLLECTING DUCT

The transport properties of the outer medullary collecting duct (OMCD) have been studied by *in vitro* perfusion of isolated tubule segments. The functional properties of the OMCD differ depending on the location of the segment within the outer medulla. Table 34.8 summarizes the electrophysiologic and transport properties of OMCD. Segments within the outer stripe of the outer medulla ($OMCD_o$) exhibit electrophysiologic properties resembling those of the cortical collecting duct, with an electrogenic apical Na^+ entry and a lumen-negative transepithelial voltage.[175] Compared to the CCD, the $OMCD_o$ displays a less-negative transepithelial voltage, much lower ionic permeabilities, and a lower rate of active reabsorption of Na^+.[298,299] In the collecting ducts extending into the medulla, principal cells that mediate Na^+ and K^+ transport in the CCD are progressively replaced by cells with electrical properties similar to intercalated cells of the CCD lacking a demonstrable Na^+ or K^+ conductance in the apical membrane.[175] Within the inner stripe of outer medulla ($OMCD_i$), principal cells are virtually absent and no net Na^+ absorption occurs.[298,299]

THE INNER MEDULLARY COLLECTING DUCT

The analysis of salt transport by the IMCD has been confounded by problems of axial tubule heterogeneity, species variability, and differences in experimental approaches. Studies examining IMCD function *in vivo* have yielded markedly different results than *in vitro* studies of isolated perfused tubules. Table 34.9 summarizes the electrophysiologic and transport properties of IMCD. *In vivo* microcatheterization studies and microperfusion studies have demonstrated that the IMCD reabsorbs about 80% of the sodium delivered to it[182,293] while, with one exception,[182] little sodium transport could be observed in IMCD tubules perfused *in vitro*.[268,294]

ENaC AND THE MAINTENANCE OF Na^+ BALANCE

ENaC represents the main transport pathway for Na^+ absorption in the CNT and the collecting duct. The role of ENaC in the maintenance of Na^+ homeostasis and extracellular body fluid is supported by genetic studies of rare monogenic diseases that identified functional mutations of ENaC associated with changes in Na^+ and K^+ balance, in plasma levels of aldosterone, and in blood pressure.

The pseudohypoaldosteronism type 1 (PHA-1) is characterized in the first week of life by severe dehydration, hyponatremia, hyperkalemia, and acidosis.[44] There are two clinically distinct forms of PHA-1: an autosomal recessive form that affects multiple organs (systemic form), including kidneys, colon, salivary glands, and sweat ducts (but not the skin or inner ear, for instance); and an autosomal dominant form that is restricted to the kidneys. Patients with the systemic form of PHA-1 have mutations in α, β, and γ ENaC subunits.[44] Mutations in the α, β or γ ENaC genes include nonsense, frameshift or missense mutations leading to different degrees of channel loss-of-function; the severity of the syndrome correlates usually with the extent to which ENaC activity is reduced. The autosomal dominant form of PHA-1 is caused by mutations of the mineralocorticoid receptors.[96] A variety of genetic mouse models recapitulate PHA-1 in which the constitutive inactivation of the genes encoding either the α, β or γ ENaC subunits leads to a severe renal phenotype of increased sodium excretion, hyperkalemia, metabolic acidosis, and elevated plasma aldosterone levels.[146]

Pseudoaldosteronism or Liddle's syndrome is an autosomal dominant form of salt-sensitive hypertension with early onset of elevated blood pressure during adolescence; the elevated blood pressure is usually associated with hypokalemia, metabolic alkalosis, low plasma aldosterone, and suppressed plasma renin activity.[28] The elevated blood pressure in Liddle's

TABLE 34.8 Electrophysiologic and Transport Properties of Rabbit OMCD

	V$_t$ (mV)	R$_t$ (Ω/cm^2)	V$_{bl}$ (mV)	fRa	J$_{Na}$ (pmol/mm/min)	J$_{Cl}$ (pmol/mm/min)
Outer OMCD	−2 to −11	233−272	−65	0.81	7.9	−1.4
Inner OMCD	+2 to +48	294−534	−24 to −36	0.96−0.99	1.5	−9.8

Table from Reeves, W. B., and Andreoli, T. E. (2008). Sodium chloride transport in the loop of Henle, distal convoluted tubule, and collecting duct. In "The Kidney: Physiology and Pathophysiology," 4th edn, 849−888, Alpern, R. J., and Hebert, S. C. (eds.). Elsevier.

TABLE 34.9 Electrophysiologic and Transport Properties of Rat IMCD

	V$_t$ (mV)	R$_t$ (Ω/cm^2)	V$_{bl}$ (mV)	fRa	J$_{Na}$ (pmol/mm/min)	J$_{Cl}$ (pmol/mm/min)
Initial IMCD	−2 to 0	73	−51	0.94	10	
Terminal IMCD	0	148	−81	0.99	54−92	72

Table from Reeves, W. B., and Andreoli, T. E. (2008). Sodium chloride transport in the loop of Henle, distal convoluted tubule, and collecting duct. In "The Kidney: Physiology and Pathophysiology," 4th edn, 849−888, Alpern, R. J., and Hebert, S. C. (eds.). Elsevier.

syndrome can be normalized under salt restriction and amiloride treatment. Based on these clinical evidences, G.W. Liddle postulated that the syndrome was *"a disorder in which the renal tubules transport ions with such abnormal facility that the end result simulates that of a mineralocorticoid excess"*.[188] The mutation identified in the index case is a 45 amino acid deletion in the cytosolic C-terminus of the β ENaC subunit.[287] Subsequent genetic analysis of other Liddle's syndrome families revealed corresponding missense or deletion mutations in the C-terminus of the γ ENaC subunit, but none in the α-subunit.[127,128] These mutations allowed the identification of a conserved proline-rich motif (a canonical PxxY motif) in the C-termini β and γ ENaC subunits as the common target for the mutations causing Liddle's syndrome.[275,292]

ENaC channels carrying mutations associated with Liddle's syndrome exhibit an increased ENaC activity *in vitro* and *in vivo*, consistent with Liddle's hypothesis.[12,54,274] These ENaC gain of function mutations result in both, an increased number of active channels at the cell surface, and a higher open probability.[79]

REGULATION OF Na$^+$ TRANSPORT

The regulation of Na$^+$ absorption mediated by ENaC is quite similar in the CNT and the collecting duct. Factors that directly modulate ENaC activity at the cell surface include extracellular or intracellular Na$^+$, membrane potential, serine proteases, as already mentioned. Certainly the most relevant ENaC regulation for the fine tuning of Na$^+$ absorption in the CNT and CCD is the control of ENaC activity by hormones such as aldosterone and vasopressin.

ALDOSTERONE

The effects and the mechanisms of action of aldosterone are reviewed in detail in Chapter 35, and are discussed here briefly. The major renal target for aldosterone action is ENaC in the DCT2, in the CNT-specific cells, and in the principal cells of the CCD.[62,75] The DCT2, CNT, and CCD are renal tubular segments that share the expression of the mineralocorticoid receptor (MR) and the enzyme 11β-steroid dehydrogenase type 2 (11βHSD2).[14,181,332] Aldosterone, but also glucocorticoids like cortisol, bind[5] with high affinity the cytoplasmic mineralocorticoid receptor. *In vivo* the specificity of aldosterone versus cortisol for the mineralocorticoid effects is due to the selective degradation of glucocorticoids, but not mineralocorticoids, by the 11βHSD2.[91] Which is high in CCD segments, and protects the MR from being activated by glucocorticoids[27,227] (see Figure 34.8). Illustrating the important role of this enzyme in preventing the activation of the mineralocorticoid receptor by glucocorticoids, the genetic deficiency of 11βHSD2 produces a syndrome of apparent mineralocorticoid excess (AME), which resembles hyperaldosteronism (hypertension, hypokalemia, metabolic alkalosis), except for the fact that aldosterone levels are low.[222,335] The clinical manifestations result from the stimulation of mineralocorticoid receptors by circulating cortisol.

Aldosterone increases the rates of Na$^+$ absorption and K$^+$ secretion in these nephron segments[269,273,282] (see Figure 34.8). An increase in the Na$^+$ permeability of the apical membrane occurs within a few hours of exposure. In the aldosterone-sensitive distal nephron (DCT2, CNT) and the CCD, aldosterone increases the

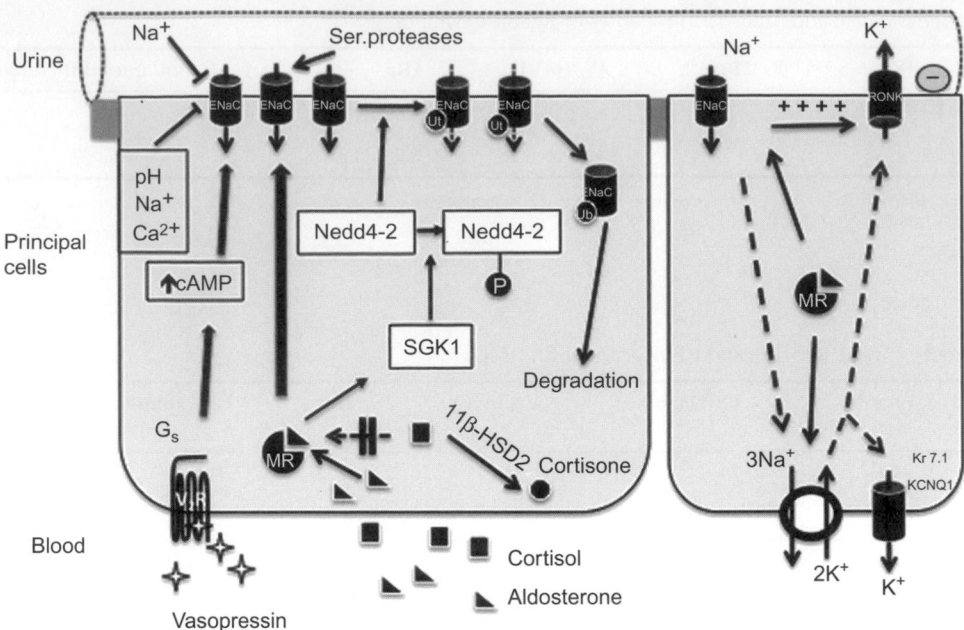

FIGURE 34.8   ENaC regulation and Na$^+$ absorption in the connecting tubule and the collecting duct. Na$^+$ absorption and K$^+$ secretion mediated by ENaC and ROMK, respectively, are coupled electrically at the apical membrane, and by the Na/K-ATPase at the basolateral membrane. Aldosterone regulates both ENaC and the Na/K-ATPase. Aldosterone and vasopressin increase the number of newly synthesized ENaC at the cell surface. The ubiquitin ligase Nedd4-2 controls the stability of ENaC at the cell surface. ENaC is activated by serine proteases.

biosynthesis of αENaC whereas the β and γ ENaC subunits are constitutively expressed.[86,195] The upregulation of the synthesis of αENaC by aldosterone leads to an increase in the expression of active, cleaved forms of ENaC channels at the cell surface.[85]

It is not clear whether the increase in the biosynthesis of αENaC is sufficient for triggering the trafficking of the multimeric αβγ ENaC channels at the cell surface or whether specific aldosterone-induced regulators of ENaC trafficking and stabilization at the apical membrane are required. For a constitutively active channel such as ENaC, the stability and the density of active channels at the cell surface is the most important determinant in the regulation of Na$^+$ absorption in the distal nephron. Measured by patch-clamp techniques in the amphibian distal nephron cell line A6, the half-life of ENaC activity at the cell surface was estimated at around three hours.[348] The molecular determinants of the ENaC half-life at the cell surface are not completely understood. Ubiquitylation is an important post-translational modification that determines ENaC stability at the cell surface. Ubiquitylation is a general process that labels proteins with ubiquitin to target the ubiquitylated proteins for endocytosis and/or degradation. Nedd4-2 is a protein ubiquitin ligase that catalyses the monoubiquitylation of β and γ ENaC subunits after binding specifically of the enzyme to conserved PY motifs in their cytosolic C-terminus of ENaC[259,296] (see Figure 34.8). The ubiquitylated ENaC

at the cell surface undergoes clathrin-mediated endocytosis and degradation. *In vitro*, Nedd4-2 efficiently suppresses ENaC activity. Mutations in the cytosolic PY motifs of ENaC subunits are associated with Liddle's syndrome and prevent the interaction between Nedd4-2 and ENaC; the resulting defect in ENaC ubiquitylation leads to the retention of active channels at the cell surface.[274,79] Deubiquitylation enzymes such as Usp2-45 increase ENaC activity *in vitro*.[262]

In vitro experiments support the idea that aldosterone stabilizes ENaC at the cell surface by inhibiting ENaC ubiquitylation and endocytosis.[297] A number of ENaC regulatory proteins are induced by aldosterone, such as the phosphatidylinositide 3′-kinase(PI3K)-dependent kinase SGK-1 (serum- and glucocorticoid-regulated kinase 1) or the 14-3-3 scaffolding protein.[56,73] The SGK-1 kinase (serum- and glucocorticoid-regulated kinase 1), increases the abundance of the active ENaC at the cell surface.[321,346] SGK-1 was shown to phosphorylate Nedd4-2, promoting the interaction between Nedd4-2 and the 14-3-3 scaffolding protein; this interaction prevents the Nedd4-2 dependent ubiquitylation of ENaC[56] (Figure 34.8). These studies, performed *in vitro* in heterologous expression systems or in cortical collecting duct cell lines, identify Nedd4-2 as a critical convergence point for the regulation of ENaC at the cell surface. In addition to the SGK1/Nedd4-2 pathway, a number of kinases have been reported to modulate ENaC activity *in vitro*. Activation of the Raf-1-MAPK/ERK kinases inhibits the cell surface expression of ENaC by stimulating the interaction between Nedd4-2 and ENaC.[74,229,284]

Mouse models in which genes contributing to the aldosterone-signaling pathway have been invalidated, only partially confirm the data obtained *in vitro* in heterologous expression systems. Mice deficient in the mineralocorticoid receptor (MR) have a normal prenatal development, but die soon after birth from dehydration and hyperkalemia. This severe PHA-1 phenotype confirms the roles of the MR, and the Na⁺ transporters ENaC and NCC, in maintaining Na⁺ and K⁺ homeostasis.[20] However, the severity of the MR knockout phenotype contrasts with the mild renal phenotype of the mice lacking the aldosterone-induced protein SGK1.[76] The SGK1 deficient mice show a higher natriuresis compared to wt mice only under a low-Na⁺ diet, and this higher natriuresis is not related to decreased ENaC activity.[76] Furthermore, under chronic aldosterone treatment, ENaC activity is identical in the SGK1 deficient mice and the wt littermates. This suggests that *in vivo* SGK1 is not central for the long-term regulation of ENaC by aldosterone; in addition, SGK1 could regulate other Na⁺ transporters such as NCC located upstream of ENaC.[10]

Mice carrying Liddle's mutation in the SCNN1B gene encoding a deletion of the C-terminus of β ENaC recapitulate Liddle's syndrome under a high-salt diet.[248] These mice with a defective interaction between ENaC and Nedd4-2 represent an informative model to evaluate the contribution of Nedd4-2 in the regulation of ENaC by aldosterone. In addition to the Liddle's phenotype including hypervolemia, elevated blood pressure, hypokalemia, metabolic alkalosis, these mice retain their ability to respond to aldosterone.[54] The knockout of the Nedd4-2 gene in mice results in an elevated blood pressure associated with low plasma aldosterone levels; these effects correlate with an increase in the expression of α and β ENaC, but also NCC.[24,285] These mice also remain sensitive to aldosterone. From these *in vivo* data it appears that neither SGK1 nor Nedd4-2 appear to be limiting in the signaling pathway of aldosterone for stimulating ENaC at the cell surface.

VASOPRESSIN

Exposure of rat CCD *in vitro* to antidiuretic hormone results in a sustained stimulation of a apical electrogenic Na⁺ transport,[272] as shown by the increase in the transepithelial potential, a depolarization of the apical membrane, and an increase the apical Na⁺ conductance of the tubule.[277] These changes are entirely reversed by luminal amiloride, consistent with Na⁺ absorption mediated by ENaC. These effects of ADH on ENaC are mediated by binding to vasopressin type 2 receptors (V2R) expressed in the CCD and CNT, activation of the adenylate cyclase, and by the generation of intracellular cAMP[32,77,220,224,272] (see Figure 34.8). In humans, a reduction in renal Na⁺ excretion starts to be observed when the urine osmolality reaches a certain threshold.[223] This suggest that the effect of vasopressin on Na⁺ reabsorption likely requires higher concentrations than for the effect on water reabsorption.[273] The effects of ADH on Na⁺ transport in the rat CCD are synergistic to aldosterone.[131]

It is not clear how vasopressin and the generation of intracellular c-AMP upregulate ENaC and stimulate ENaC-mediated Na⁺ absorption *in vivo* in the CCD. *In vivo* ADH increases both the number of active channels and the open probability.[32] In MDCK cells, c-AMP increases the amiloride-sensitive short-circuit current (I_{SC}) proportionally with the number of ENaC channels at the cell surface, indicating that an increase in active ENaC density can account for the upregulation of the ENaC-mediated Na⁺ absorption by vasopressin.[220] In COS cells, c-AMP-dependent phosphorylation and inhibition of Nedd4-2 could be demonstrated that would lead to an increased ENaC stability at the cell surface.[291] Of course, the Nedd4-2 pathway mediating both the vasopressin and aldosterone effects on ENaC cannot explain their synergistic stimulation of Na⁺ transport in the distal nephron and the collecting duct.

In addition to its short-term regulation of water and Na⁺ absorption in the CCD, vasopressin has long-term transcriptional effects. Chronic vasopressin treatment increases the expression of β and γ ENaC expression in the CCD, with a concommittent increase in Na⁺ transport.[63,228] However, no detectable change in the surface expression of the ENaC subunits could be observed.[271] An increase in the Isc and Na⁺ transport could be demonstrated after long-term treatment with vasopressin, which was only partially inhibited by amiloride.[60] Thus, the contribution of ENaC in mediating the chronic effects of vasopressin remains unclear, and probably does not simply result from effects on ENaC transcription or trafficking at the cell surface.

INSULIN

The direct effects of insulin on renal Na⁺ excretion is difficult to evaluate, because of its secondary effects on plasma glucose or potassium that are difficult to control precisely.

In humans and rats maintained euglycemic, insulin decreased urinary Na⁺ excretion.[57,172] This effect on Na⁺ excretion was abrogated when K⁺ was infused to correct for hypokalemia.[81] Using a euglycemic insulin-clamp technique, insulin does not change renal Na⁺ excretion[258] in rats when both plasma glucose and K⁺ levels are precisely controlled.

However, insulin and IGF-1 receptors are expressed in the mammalian renal tubular system including the collecting duct.[124] The effect of insulin on Na^+ transport appears tissue-specific. Insulin stimulates ENaC-mediated Na^+ transport in the frog skin,[280] toad urinary bladder[288] or in vitro in A6 cells[22] or in a mammalian CCD cell line.[103] In mammalian isolated and perfused CCD, insulin failed to increase Na^+ transport.[315] IGF-1 is under the control of growth hormone (GH). Both GH and IGF-1 induces fluid and Na^+ retention in humans.[126,211] In acromegalic rats, evidence supports that the IGF1-induced increase amiloride-sensitive Na^+ absorption accounts for renal Na^+ retention.[160]

Insulin increases Na/K-ATPase pump activity.[78] Evidence supporting upregulation of ENaC-mediated Na^+ absorption after acute insulin treatment has been reported.[308] However, a patch-clamp study failed to demonstrate an effect of insulin on whole cell amiloride-sensitive Na^+ conductance in rat CCD, whereas ROMK conductance and Na^+-pump current were clearly increased.[90] It is conceivable that under both euglycemic and normokalemic conditions insulin primarily increases K^+ secretion via ROMK; the resulting hyperpolarization of the apical membrane increases the driving force for Na^+ absorption through ENaC channels. This effect is expected to be small and can be compensated by other Na^+ transporters along the nephron so that Na excretion remains unchanged.

References

[1] Abdallah JG, Schrier RW, Edelstein C, Jennings SD, Wyse B, Ellison DH. Loop diuretic infusion increases thiazide-sensitive Na^+/Cl^- co-transporter abundance: role of aldosterone. J Am Soc Nephrol 2001;12:1335–41.

[2] Adachi S, Uchida S, Ito H, Hata M, Hiroe M, Marumo F, et al. Two isoforms of a chloride channel predominantly expressed in thick ascending limb of Henle's loop and collecting ducts of rat kidney. J Biol Chem 1994;269:17677–83.

[3] Aguilar-Bryan L, Nichols CG, Wechsler SW, Clement IV JP, Boyd III AE, Gonzalez G, et al. Cloning of the b cell high-affinity sulfonylurea receptor: a regulator of insulin secretion. Science 1995;268:423–6.

[4] Almeida AJ, Burg MB. Sodium transport in the rabbit connecting tubule. Am J Physiol 1982;243:F330–4.

[5] Alvarez dlR ZP, Naray-Fejes-Toth A, Fejes-Toth G, Canessa CM. The serum and glucocorticoid kinase sgk increases the abundance of epithelial sodium channels in the plasma membrane of Xenopus oocytes. J Biol Chem 1999;274:37834–9.

[6] Amemiya M, Loffing J, Lotscher M, Kaissling B, Alpern RJ, Moe OW. Expression of NHE-3 in the apical membrane of rat renal proximal tubule and thick ascending limb. Kidney Int 1995;48:1206–15.

[7] Anantharam A, Tian Y, Palmer LG. Open probability of the epithelial sodium channel is regulated by intracellular sodium. J Physiol 2006;574:333–47.

[8] Ares GR, Caceres PS, Ortiz PA. Molecular regulation of NKCC2 in the thick ascending limb. Am J Physiol Renal Physiol 2011;301:F1143–59.

[9] Ares GR, Ortiz PA. Constitutive endocytosis and recycling of NKCC2 in rat thick ascending limbs. Am J Physiol Renal Physiol 2010;299:F1193–202.

[10] Arroyo JP, Lagnaz D, Ronzaud C, Vazquez N, Ko BS, Moddes L, et al. Nedd4-2 modulates renal Na^+-Cl^- Co-transporter via the aldosterone-SGK1-Nedd4-2 pathway. J Am Soc Nephrol 2011;22:1707–19.

[11] Arroyo JP, Ronzaud C, Lagnaz D, Staub O, Gamba G. Aldosterone paradox: differential regulation of ion transport in distal nephron. Physiology (Bethesda) 2011;26:115–23.

[12] Auberson M, Hoffmann-Pochon N, Vandewalle A, Kellenberger S, Schild L. Epithelial Na^+ channel mutants causing Liddle's syndrome retain ability to respond to aldosterone and vasopressin. Am J Physiol Renal Physiol 2003;285:F459–71.

[13] Ausiello DA, Hall D. Regulation of vasopressin-sensitive adenylate cyclase by calmodulin. J Biol Chem 1981;256:9796–8.

[14] Bachmann S, Bostanjoglo M, Schmitt R, Ellison DH. Sodium transport-related proteins in the mammalian distal nephron – distribution, ontogeny and functional aspects. Anat Embryol (Berl) 1999;200:447–68.

[15] Bailey MA, Cantone A, Yan Q, MacGregor GG, Leng Q, Amorim JB, et al. Maxi-K channels contribute to urinary potassium excretion in the ROMK-deficient mouse model of Type II Bartter's syndrome and in adaptation to a high-K diet. Kidney Int 2006;70:51–9.

[16] Bayliss JM, Reeves WB, Andreoli TE. Cl^- transport in basolateral renal medullary vesicles: I. Cl^- transport in intact vesicles. J Membr Biol 1990;113:49–56.

[17] Beesley AH, Hornby D, White SJ. Regulation of distal nephron K^+ channels (ROMK) mRNA expression by aldosterone in rat kidney. J Physiol 1998;509:629–34.

[18] Beesley AH, Qureshi IZ, Giesberts AN, Parker AJ, White SJ. Expression of sulphonylurea receptor protein in mouse kidney. Pflugers Arch 1999;438:1–7.

[19] Bencsath P, Szenasi G, Takacs L. Water and electrolyte transport in Henle's loop and distal tubule after renal sympathectomy in the rat. Am J Physiol 1985;249:F308–14.

[20] Berger S, Bleich M, Schmid W, Cole TJ, Peters J, Watanabe H, et al. Mineralocorticoid receptor knockout mice: pathophysiology of Na^+ metabolism. Proc Natl Acad Sci USA 1998;95:9424–9.

[21] Birkenhager R, Otto E, Schurmann MJ, Vollmer M, Ruf EM, Maier-Lutz I, et al. Mutation of BSND causes bartter syndrome with sensorineural deafness and kidney failure. Nat Genet 2001;29:310–4.

[22] Blazer-Yost BL, Esterman MA, Vlahos CJ. Insulin-stimulated trafficking of ENaC in renal cells requires PI 3-kinase activity. Am J Physiol Cell Physiol 2003;284:C1645–53.

[23] Bleich M, Schlatter E, Greger R. The luminal K^+ channel of the thick ascending limb of Henle's loop. Pflgers Arch 1990;415:449–60.

[24] Boase NA, Rychkov GY, Townley SL, Dinudom A, Candi E, Voss AK, et al. Respiratory distress and perinatal lethality in Nedd4-2-deficient mice. Nat Commun 2011;2:287.

[25] Boettger T, Hubner CA, Maier H, Rust MB, Beck FX, Jentsch TJ. Deafness and renal tubular acidosis in mice lacking the K-Cl co-transporter Kcc4. Nature 2002;416:874–8.

[26] Boim MA, Ho K, Shuck ME, Bienkowski MJ, Block JH, Slightom JL, et al. ROMK inwardly rectifying ATP-sensitive K^+ channel. II. Cloning and distribution of alternative forms. Am J Physiol 1995;268:F1132–40.

[27] Bonvalet JP, Doignon I, Blot-Chabaud M, Pradelles P, Farman N. Distribution of 11 beta-hydroxysteroid dehydrogenase along the rabbit nephron. J Clin Invest 1990;86:832–7.

[28] Botero-Velez M, Curtis JJ, Warnock DG. Brief report: Liddle's syndrome revisited. A disorder of sodium reabsorption in the distal tubule. N Engl J Med 1994;330:178−81.

[29] Boyden LM, Choi M, Choate KA, Nelson-Williams CJ, Farhi A, Toka HR, et al. Mutations in kelch-like 3 and cullin 3 cause hypertension and electrolyte abnormalities. Nature 2012;482:98−102.

[30] Brezis M, Rosen S, Silva P, Epstein FH. Selective vulnerability of the medullary thick ascending limb to anoxia in the isolated perfused rat kidney. J Clin Invest 1984;73:182−90.

[31] Brezis M, Rosen S, Silva P, Epstein FH. Transport activity modifies thick ascending limb damage in the isolated perfused kidney. Kidney Int 1984;25:65−72.

[32] Bugaj V, Pochynyuk O, Stockand JD. Activation of the epithelial Na$^+$ channel in the collecting duct by vasopressin contributes to water reabsorption. Am J Physiol Renal Physiol 2009;297: F1411−8.

[33] Burg MB, Green N. Function of the thick ascending limb of Henle's loop. Am J Physiol 1973;224:659−68.

[34] Burnham C, Karlish SJD, Jorgensen PL. Identification and reconstitution of a Na$^+$/K$^+$/Cl$^-$ co-transporter and K$^+$ channel from lumninal membranes of red outer medulla. Biochim Biophys Acta 1985;821:461−9.

[35] Cai H, Cebotaru V, Wang YH, Zhang XM, Cebotaru L, Guggino SE, et al. WNK4 kinase regulates surface expression of the human sodium chloride co-transporter in mammalian cells. Kidney Int 2006;69:2162−70.

[36] Canessa CM, Schild L, Buell G, Thorens B, Gautshi I, Horisberger JD, et al. Amiloride-sensitive epithelial Na$^+$ channel is made of three homologous subunits. Nature 1994;367:463−7.

[37] Cantone A, Yang X, Yan Q, Giebisch G, Hebert SC, Wang T. Mouse model of type II Bartter's syndrome. I. Upregulation of thiazide-sensitive Na-Cl co-transport activity. Am J Physiol Renal Physiol 2008;294:F1366−72.

[38] Capasso G, Unwin R, Rizzo M, Pica A, Giebisch G. Bicarbonate transport along the loop of Henle: molecular mechanisms and regulation. J Nephrol 2002;15(Suppl. 5):S88−96.

[39] Castaneda-Bueno M, Cervantes LG, Vazquez N, Bobadilla NA, Uribe N, Alessi D, et al. In vivo activation of NCC by angiotensin II requires integrity of the WNK4-SPAK pathway. J Am Soc Nephrol 2011;22:102A.

[40] Chabardes D, Gagnan-Brunette M, Imbert-Teboul M, Gontcharevskaia O, Montegut M, Clique A, et al. Adenylate cyclase responsiveness to hormones in various portions of the human nephron. J Clin Invest 1980;65:439−48.

[41] Chabardes D, Imbert-Teboul M, Montegut M, Clique A, Morel F. Catecholamine sensitive adenylate cyclase activity in different segments of the rabbit nephron. Pflugers Arch 1975;361:9−15.

[42] Chamberlin ME, LeFurgey A, Mandel LJ. Suspension of medullary thick ascending limb tubules from the rabbit kidney. Am J Physiol 1984;247:F955−64.

[43] Chamberlin ME, Mandel LJ. Substrate support of medullary thick ascending limb oxygen consumption. Am J Physiol 1986;251(Renal. 20):F758−63.

[44] Chang SS, Grunder S, Hanukoglu A, Rosler A, Mathew PM, Hanukoglu I, et al. Mutations in subunits of the epithelial sodium channel cause salt wasting with hyperkalaemic acidosis, pseudohypoaldosteronism type 1. Nat Genet 1996;12: 248−53.

[45] Chen Z, Vaughn DA, Fanestill DD. Influence of gender on renal thiazide diuretic receptor density and response. J Am Soc Nephrol 1994;5:1112−9.

[46] Cheng HF, Harris RC. Cyclooxygenases, the kidney, and hypertension. Hypertension 2004;43:525−30.

[47] Choe H, Zhou H, Palmer LG, Sackin H. A conserved cytoplasmic region of ROMK modulates pH sensitivity, conductance, and gating. Am J Physiol (Renal Physiol) 1997;273: F516−29.

[48] Chraibi A, Horisberger JD. Na self inhibition of human epithelial Na channel: temperature dependence and effect of extracellular proteases. J Gen Physiol 2002;120:133−45.

[49] Chraibi A, Vallet V, Firsov D, Hess SK, Horisberger JD. Protease modulation of the activity of the epithelial sodium channel expressed in Xenopus oocytes. J Gen Physiol 1998;111: 127−38.

[50] Christensen BM, Perrier R, Wang Q, Zuber AM, Maillard M, Mordasini D, et al. Sodium and potassium balance depends on alphaENaC expression in connecting tubule. J Am Soc Nephrol 2010;21:1942−51.

[51] Clement JP, Kunjilwar K, Gonzalez G, Schwanstecher M, Panten U, Aguilar-Bryan L, et al. Association and stoichiometry of K$_{ATP}$ channel subunits. Neuron 1997;18:827−38.

[52] Costanzo LS. Comparison of calcium and sodium transport in early and late rat distal tubules: effect of amiloride. Am J Physiol (Renal Fluid Electrolyte Physiol) 1984;246:F937−45.

[53] Costanzo LS. Localization of diuretic action in microperfused rat distal tubules: Ca and Na transport. Am J Physiol (Renal Fluid Electrolyte Physiol) 1985;248:F527−35.

[54] Dahlmann A, Pradervand S, Hummler E, Rossier BC, Frindt G, Palmer LG. Mineralocorticoid regulation of epithelial Na$^+$ channels is maintained in a mouse model of Liddle's syndrome. Am J Physiol Renal Physiol 2003;285:F310−8.

[55] de Rouffignac C, Elalouf JM. Hormonal regulation of chloride transport in the proximal and distal nephron. Annu Rev Physiol 1988;50:123−40.

[56] Debonneville C, Flores SY, Kamynina E, Plant PJ, Tauxe C, Thomas MA, et al. Phosphorylation of Nedd4-2 by Sgk1 regulates epithelial Na(+) channel cell surface expression. EMBO J 2001;20:7052−9.

[57] DeFronzo RA, Cooke CR, Andres R, Faloona GR, Davis PJ. The effect of insulin on renal handling of sodium, potassium, calcium, and phosphate in man. J Clin Invest 1975;55:845−55.

[58] DiBona GF, Sawin LL. Effect of renal nerve stimulation on NaCl and H$_2$O transport in Henle's loop of the rat. Am J Physiol 1982;243:F576−80.

[59] Dietl P, Good D, Stanton B. Adrenal corticosteroid action on the thick ascending limb. Semin Nephrol 1990;10:350−64.

[60] Djelidi S, Fay M, Cluzeaud F, Escoubet B, Eugene E, Capurro C, et al. Transcriptional regulation of sodium transport by vasopressin in renal cells. J Biol Chem 1997;272:32919−24.

[61] Dorup J. Ultrastructure of distal nephron cells in rat renal cortex. J Ultrastruct Res 1985;92:101−18.

[62] Doucet A, Katz AI. Mineralocorticoid receptors along the nephron: [^{3}H]aldosterone binding in rabbit tubules. Am J Physiol 1981;241:F605−11.

[63] Ecelbarger CA, Kim GH, Terris J, Masilamani S, Mitchell C, Reyes I, et al. Vasopressin-mediated regulation of epithelial sodium channel abundance in rat kidney. Am J Physiol Renal Physiol 2000;279:F46−53.

[64] Ecelbarger CA, Kim GH, Wade JB, Knepper MA. Regulation of the abundance of renal sodium transporters and channels by vasopressin. Exp Neurol 2001;171:227−34.

[65] Edwards RM, Jackson BA, Dousa TP. Protein kinase activity in isolated tubules of rat renal medulla. Am J Physiol 1980;238: F269−78.

[66] Ellison DH, Velazquez H, Wright FS. Thiazide-sensitive sodium chloride co-transport in early distal tubule. Am J Physiol (Renal Fluid Electrolyte Physiol) 1987;253:F546−54.

[67] Ellison DH, Velazquez H, Wright FS. Adaptation of the distal convoluted tubule of the rat. Structural and functional effects of dietary salt intake and chronic diuretic infusion. J Clin Invest 1989;83:113–26.

[68] Ergonul Z, Frindt G, Palmer LG. Regulation of maturation and processing of ENaC subunits in the rat kidney. Am J Physiol Renal Physiol 2006;291:F683–93.

[69] Escalante B, Erlij D, Falck JR, McGiff JC. Effect of cytochrome P450 arachidonate metabolites on ion transport in rabbit kidney loop of Henle. Science 1991;251:799–802.

[70] Estevez R, Boettger T, Stein V, Birkenhager R, Otto E, Hildebrandt F, et al. Barttin is a Cl$^-$ channel b-subunit crucial for renal Cl$^-$ reabsorption and inner ear K$^+$ secretion. Nature 2001;414:558–61.

[71] Eveloff J, Bayerdorffer E, Silva P, Kinne R. Sodium–chloride transport in the thick ascending limb of Henle's looop. Oxygen consumption studies in isolated cells. Pfl_gers Arch 1981;389:263–70.

[72] Eveloff J, Calamia J. Effect of osmolarity on cation fluxes in medullary thick ascending limb cells. Am J Physiol (Renal Fluid Electrolyte Physiol) 1986;250:F176–80.

[73] Fakitsas P, Adam G, Daidie D, van Bemmelen MX, Fouladkou F, Patrignani A, et al. Early aldosterone-induced gene product regulates the epithelial sodium channel by deubiquitylation. J Am Soc Nephrol 2007;18:1084–92.

[74] Falin RA, Cotton CU. Acute downregulation of ENaC by EGF involves the PY motif and putative ERK phosphorylation site. J Gen Physiol 2007;130:313–28.

[75] Farman N, Bonvalet JP. Aldosterone binding in isolated tubules. III. Autoradiography along the rat nephron. Am J Physiol 1983;245:F606–14.

[76] Fejes-Toth G, Frindt G, Naray-Fejes-Toth A, Palmer LG. Epithelial Na$^+$ channel activation and processing in mice lacking SGK1. Am J Physiol Renal Physiol 2008;294:F1298–305.

[77] Fenton RA, Brond L, Nielsen S, Praetorius J. Cellular and subcellular distribution of the type-2 vasopressin receptor in the kidney. Am J Physiol Renal Physiol 2007;293:F748–60.

[78] Feraille E, Rousselot M, Rajerison R, Favre H. Effect of insulin on Na$^+$,K$^{(+)}$-ATPase in rat collecting duct. J Physiol 1995;488 (Pt 1):171–80.

[79] Firsov D, Schild L, Gautschi I, Merillat AM, Schneeberger E, Rossier BC. Cell surface expression of the epithelial Na channel and a mutant causing Liddle syndrome: a quantitative approach. Proc Natl Acad Sci USA 1996;93:15370–5.

[80] Forbush IB, Palfrey HC. [^{3}H]Bumetanide binding to membranes isolated from dog kidney outer medulla. Relationship to the Na,K,Cl co-transport system. J Biol Chem 1983;258:11787–92.

[81] Friedberg CE, Koomans HA, Bijlsma JA, Rabelink TJ, Dorhout Mees EJ. Sodium retention by insulin may depend on decreased plasma potassium. Metabolism 1991;40:201–4.

[82] Friedman PA. Bumetanide inhibition of [CO$_2$ + HCO$_3$]-dependent and -independent equivalent electrical flux in renal cortical thick ascending limbs. J Pharmacol Exp Ther 1986;238:407–14.

[83] Friedman PA, Andreoli TE. CO$_2$-stimulated NaCl absorption in the mouse renal cortical thick ascending limb of Henle. Evidence for synchronous Na$^+$/H$^+$ and Cl$^-$/HCO$_3^-$ exchange in apical plasma membranes. J Gen Physiol 1982;80:683–711.

[84] Friedman PA, Andreoli TE. Effects of (CO$_2$ + HCO$_3^-$) on electrical conductance in cortical thick ascending limbs. Kidney Int 1986;30:325–31.

[85] Frindt G, Ergonul Z, Palmer LG. Surface expression of epithelial Na channel protein in rat kidney. J Gen Physiol 2008;131:617–27.

[86] Frindt G, Masilamani S, Knepper MA, Palmer LG. Activation of epithelial Na channels during short term Na deprivation. Am J Physiol Renal Physiol 2001;280:F112–8.

[87] Frindt G, Palmer LG. Apical potassium channels in the rat connecting tubule. Am J Physiol Renal Physiol 2004;287:F1030–7.

[88] Frindt G, Palmer LG. Na channels in the rat connecting tubule. Am J Physiol Renal Physiol 2004;286:F669–74.

[89] Frindt G, Palmer LG. Surface expression of sodium channels and transporters in rat kidney: effects of dietary sodium. Am J Physiol Renal Physiol 2009;297:F1249–55.

[90] Frindt G, Palmer LG. Effects of insulin on Na and K transporters in the rat CCD. Am J Physiol Renal Physiol 2012;302(10):F1227–33.

[91] Funder JW, Pearce PT, Smith R, Smith AI. Mineralocorticoid action: target tissue specificity is enzyme, not receptor, mediated. Science 1988;242:583–5.

[92] Gamba G. Molecular physiology and pathophysiology of the electroneutral cation-chloride co-transporters. Physiol Rev 2005;85:423–93.

[93] Gamba G, Friedman PA. Thick ascending limb: the Na$^{(+)}$:K$^{(+)}$:2Cl$^{(-)}$ co-transporter, NKCC2, and the calcium-sensing receptor, CaSR. Pflugers Arch 2009;458:61–76.

[94] Gamba G, Miyanoshita A, Lombardi M, Lytton J, Lee WS, Hediger MA, et al. Molecular cloning, primary structure and characterization of two members of the mammalian electroneutral sodium-(potassium)-chloride co-transporter family expressed in kidney. J Biol Chem 1994;269:17713–22.

[95] Gamba G, Saltzberg SN, Lombardi M, Miyanoshita A, Lytton J, Hediger MA, et al. Primary structure and functional expression of a cDNA encoding the thiazide-sensitive, electroneutral sodium-chloride co-transporter. Proc Natl Acad Sci USA 1993;90:2749–53.

[96] Geller DS, Rodriguez-Soriano J, Vallo BA, Schifter S, Bayer M, Chang SS, et al. Mutations in the mineralocorticoid receptor gene cause autosomal dominant pseudohypoaldosteronism type I. Nat Genet 1998;19:279–81.

[97] Gesek FA, Friedman PA. Mechanism of calcium transport stimulated by chlorothiazide in mouse distal convoluted tubule cells. J Clin Invest 1992;90:429–38.

[98] Giebisch G. Physiological roles of renal potassium channels. Semin Nephrol 1999;19:458–71.

[99] Gill Jr JR, Bartter FC. On the impairment of renal concentrating ability in prolonged hypercalcemia and hypercalciuria in man. J Clin Invest 1961;40:716–22.

[100] Gimenez I, Forbush B. Short term stimulation of the renal Na-K-Cl co-transporter (NKCC2) by vasopressin involves phosphorylation and membrane translocation of the protein. J Biol Chem 2003;278:26946–51.

[101] Glover M, Mercier ZA, Figg N, O'Shaughnessy KM. The activity of the thiazide-sensitive Na$^{(+)}$-Cl co-transporter is regulated by protein phosphatase PP4. Can J Physiol Pharmacol 2010;88:986–95.

[102] Gonzales EB, Kawate T, Gouaux E. Pore architecture and ion sites in acid-sensing ion channels and P2X receptors. Nature 2009;460:599–604.

[103] Gonzalez-Rodriguez E, Gaeggeler HP, Rossier BC. IGF-1 vs insulin: respective roles in modulating sodium transport via the PI-3 kinase/Sgk1 pathway in a cortical collecting duct cell line. Kidney Int 2007;71:116–25.

[104] Good DW. Sodium-dependent bicarbonate absorption by cortical thick ascending limb of rat kidney. Am J Physiol (Renal Fluid Electrolyte Physiol) 1985;248-17:F821–9.

[105] Good DW. Bicarbonate absorption by the thick ascending limb of Henle's loop. Semin Nephrol 1990;10:132–8.

[106] Grantham JJ, Kurg MB, Obloff J. The nature of transtubular Na and K transport in isolated rabbit renal collecting tubules. J Clin Invest 1970;49:1815—26.

[107] Greger R. Chloride reabsorption in the rabbit cortical thick ascending limb of the loop of Henle. A sodium dependent process. Pflugers Arch 1981;390:38—43.

[108] Greger R. Coupled transport of Na$^+$ and Cl$^-$ in the thick ascending limb of Henle's loop of rabbit nephron. Scand Audiol Suppl 1981;14(Suppl):1—15.

[109] Greger R, Bleich M, Schlatter E. Ion channels in the thick ascending limb of Henle's loop. Renal Physiol Biochem 1990;13:37—50.

[110] Greger R, Oberleithner H, Schlatter E, Cassola AC, Weidtke C. Chloride activity in cells of isolated perfused cortical thick ascending limbs of rabbit kidney. Pflugers Arch 1983;399:29—34.

[111] Greger R, Schlatter E. Presence of luminal K$^+$, a prerequisite for active NaCl transport in the cortical thick ascending limb of Henle's loop of rabbit kidney. Pflugers Arch 1981;392:92—4.

[112] Greger R, Schlatter E. Properties of the basolateral membrane of the cortical thick ascending limb of Henle's loop of rabbit kidney. A model for secondary active chloride transport. Pflugers Arch 1983;396:325—34.

[113] Greger R, Schlatter E. Properties of the lumen membrane of the cortical thick ascending limb of Henle's loop of rabbit kidney. Pflugers Arch 1983;396:315—24.

[114] Greger R, Velazquez H. The cortical thick ascending limb and early distal convoluted tubule in the urinary concentrating mechanism. Kidney Int 1987;31:590—6.

[115] Gu RM, Wang WH. Arachidonic acid inhibits K channels in basolateral membrane of the thick ascending limb. Am J Physiol Renal Physiol 2002;283:F407—14.

[116] Gu RM, Wei Y, Jiang H, Balazy M, Wang WH. The role of 20-HETE in mediating the effect of dietary K intake on the apical K channels in the mTAL. Am J Physiol Renal Physiol 2001;280:F223—30.

[117] Gu RM, Wei Y, Jiang HL, Lin DH, Sterling H, Bloom P, et al. K depletion enhances the extracellular Ca^{2+}-induced inhibition of the apical K channels in the mTAL of rat kidney. J Gen Physiol 2002;119:33—44.

[118] Gu RM, Yang L, Zhang Y, Wang L, Kong S, Zhang C, et al. CYP-omega-hydroxylation-dependent metabolites of arachidonic acid inhibit the basolateral 10 pS chloride channel in the rat thick ascending limb. Kidney Int 2009;76:849—56.

[119] Gu R, Wang J, Zhang Y, Li W, Xu Y, Shan H, et al. Adenosine stimulates the basolateral 50 pS K channels in the thick ascending limb of the rat kidney. AJP-Renal Physiol 2007;293:F299—305.

[120] Guinamard R, Chraibi A, Teulon J. A small-conductance Cl$^-$ channel in the mouse thick ascending limb that is activated by ATP and protein kinase A. J Physiol 1995;485:97—112.

[121] Guinamard R, Paulais M, Teulon J. Inhibition of a small-conductance cAMP-dependent Cl$^-$ channel in the mouse thick ascending limb at low internal pH. J Physiol 1996;490:759—65.

[122] Gunaratne R, Braucht DW, Rinschen MM, Chou CL, Hoffert JD, Pisitkun T, et al. Quantitative phosphoproteomic analysis reveals cAMP/vasopressin-dependent signaling pathways in native renal thick ascending limb cells. Proc Natl Acad Sci USA 2010;107:15653—8.

[123] Hall DA, Varney DM. Effect of vasopressin on electrical potential difference and chloride transport in mouse medullary thick ascending limb of Henle's loop. J Clin Invest 1980;66:792—802.

[124] Hammerman MR, Miller SB. The growth hormone insulin-like growth factor axis in kidney revisited. Am J Physiol 1993;265:F1—14.

[125] Hanley MJ, Kokko JP, Gross JB, Jacobson HR. Electrophysiologic study of the cortical collecting tubule of the rabbit. Kidney Int 1980;17:74—81.

[126] Hansen TK, Moller J, Thomsen K, Frandsen E, Dall R, Jorgensen JO, et al. Effects of growth hormone on renal tubular handling of sodium in healthy humans. Am J Physiol Endocrinol Metab 2001;281:E1326—32.

[127] Hansson JH, Nelson-Williams C, Suzuki H, Schild L, Shimkets R, Lu Y, et al. Hypertension caused by a truncated epithelial sodium channel gamma subunit: genetic heterogeneity of Liddle syndrome. Nat Genet 1995;11:76—82.

[128] Hansson JH, Schild L, Lu Y, Wilson TA, Gautschi I, Shimkets R, et al. A de novo missense mutation of the beta subunit of the epithelial sodium channel causes hypertension and Liddle syndrome, identifying a proline-rich segment critical for regulation of channel activity. Proc Natl Acad Sci USA 1995;92:11495—9.

[129] Harris M, Firsov D, Vuagniaux G, Stutts MJ, Rossier BC. A novel neutrophil elastase inhibitor prevents elastase activation and surface cleavage of the epithelial sodium channel expressed in Xenopus laevis oocytes. J Biol Chem 2007;282:58—64.

[130] Harris RC, McKanna JA, Akai Y, Jacobson HR, Dubois RN, Breyer MD. Cyclooxygenase-2 is associated with the macula densa of rat kidney and increases with salt restriction. J Clin Invest 1994;94:2504—10.

[131] Hawk CT, Li L, Schafer JA. AVP and aldosterone at physiological concentrations have synergistic effects on Na$^+$ transport in rat CCD. Kidney Int Suppl 1996;57:S35—41.

[132] Hebert SC. Hypertonic cell volume regulation in mouse thick limbs. I. ADH dependency and nephron heterogeneity. Am J Physiol 1986;250:C907—19.

[133] Hebert SC. Extracellular calcium-sensing receptor: implications for calcium and magnesium handling in the kidney. Kidney Int 1996;50:2129—39.

[134] Hebert SC. Bartter syndrome. Curr Opin Nephrol Hypertens 2003;12:527—32.

[135] Hebert SC, Andreoli TE. Effects of antidiuretic hormone on cellular conductive pathways in mouse medullary thick ascending limbs of Henle: II. Determinants of the ADH-mediated increases in transepithelial voltage and in net Cl$^-$ absorption. J Membr Biol 1984;80:221—33.

[136] Hebert SC, Andreoli TE. Ionic conductance pathways in the mouse medullary thick ascending limb of Henle. The paracellular pathway and electrogenic Cl$^-$ absorption. J Gen Physiol 1986;87:567—90.

[137] Hebert SC, Brown EM. The scent of an ion: calcium-sensing and its roles in health and disease. Curr Opin Nephrol Hypertens 1996;5:45—53.

[138] Hebert SC, Culpepper RM, Andreoli TE. NaCl transport in mouse medullary thick ascending limbs. I. Functional nephron heterogeneity and ADH-stimulated NaCl co-transport. Am J Physiol (Renal Fluid Electrolyte Physiol) 1981;241:F412—31.

[139] Hebert SC, Culpepper RM, Andreoli TE. NaCl transport in mouse medullary thick ascending limbs. II. ADH enhancement of transcellular NaCl cotrasport; origin of transepithelial volatge. Am J Physiol (Renal Fluid Electrolyte Physiol) 1981;241:F432—42.

[140] Hebert SC, Culpepper RM, Andreoli TE. NaCl transport in mouse medullary thick ascending limbs. III. Modulation of ADH efect by peritubular osmolality. Am J Physiol (Renal Fluid Electrolyte Physiol) 1981;241:F443—51.

[141] Hebert SC, Desir G, Giebisch G, Wang W. Molecular diversity and regulation of renal potassium channels. Physiol Rev 2005;85:319—71.

[142] Hebert SC, Friedman PA, Andreoli TE. Effects of antidiuretic hormone on cellular conductive pathways in mouse medullary thick ascending limbs of Henle: I. ADH increases transcellular conductance pathways. J Membr Biol 1984;80:201–19.

[143] Ho K, Nichols CG, Lederer WJ, Lytton J, Vassilev PM, Kanazirska MV, et al. Cloning and expression of an inwardly rectifying ATP-regulated potassium channel. Nature 1993;362:31–8.

[144] Huang C, Sindic A, Hill CE, Hujer KM, Chan KW, Sassen M, et al. Interaction of the Ca^{2+}-sensing receptor with the inwardly rectifying potassium channels Kir4.1 and Kir4.2 results in inhibition of channel function. AJP—Renal Physiol 2007;292:F1073–81.

[145] Hughey RP, Mueller GM, Bruns JB, Kinlough CL, Poland PA, Harkleroad KL, et al. Maturation of the epithelial Na^+ channel involves proteolytic processing of the alpha- and gamma-subunits. J Biol Chem 2003;278:37073–82.

[146] Hummler E, Barker P, Talbot C, Wang Q, Verdumo C, Grubb R, et al. A mouse model for the renal salt-wasting syndrome pseudohypoaldosteronism. Proc Natl Acad Sci USA 1997;94:11710–5.

[147] Hus-Citharel A, Morel F. Coupling of metabolic CO_2 production to ion transport in isolated rat thick ascending limbs and collecting tubules. Pflugers Arch 1986;407:421–7.

[148] Imai M. The connecting tubule: a functional subdivision of the rabbit distal nephron segments. Kidney Int 1979;15:346–56.

[149] Imai M, Hayashi M, Araki M. Functional heterogeneity of the descending limbs of Henle's loop. I. Internephron heterogeneity in the hamster kidney. Pflugers Arch 1984;402:385–92.

[150] Imai M, Taniguchi J, Tabei K. Function of thin loops of Henle. Kidney Int 1987;31:565–79.

[151] Inagaki N, Gonoi T, Clement IV JP, Namba N, Inazawa J, Gonzalez G, et al. Reconstitution of I_{ATP}: an inward rectifier subunit plus the sulfonylurea receptor. Science 1995;270:1166–70.

[152] Jasti J, Furukawa H, Gonzales EB, Gouaux E. Structure of acid-sensing ion channel 1 at 1.9 A resolution and low pH. Nature 2007;449:316–23.

[153] Jeck N, Waldegger P, Doroszewicz J, Seyberth H, Waldegger S. A common sequence variation of the CLCNKB gene strongly activates ClC-Kb chloride channel activity. Kidney Int 2004;65:190–7.

[154] Jeck N, Waldegger S, Lampert A, Boehmer C, Waldegger P, Lang PA, et al. Activating mutation of the renal epithelial chloride channel ClC-Kb predisposing to hypertension. Hypertension 2004;43:1175–81.

[155] Jentsch TJ, Stein V, Weinreich F, Zdebik AA. Molecular structure and physiological function of chloride channels. Physiol Rev 2002;82:503–68.

[156] Kahle KT, MacGregor GG, Wilson FH, Van Hoek AN, Brown D, Ardito T, et al. Paracellular Cl^- permeability is regulated by WNK4 kinase: insight into normal physiology and hypertension. Proc Natl Acad Sci USA 2004;101:14877–82.

[157] Kahle KT, Wilson FH, Leng Q, Lalioti MD, O'Connell AD, Dong K, et al. WNK4 regulates the balance between renal NaCl reabsorption and K^+ secretion. Nat Genet 2003;35:372–6.

[158] Kaissling B. Ultrastructural characterization of the connecting tubule and the different segments of the collecting duct system in the rabbit kidney. Curr Probl Clin Biochem 1977;8:435–46.

[159] Kaissling B, Stanton BA. Adaptation of distal tubule and collecting duct to increased sodium delivery. I. Ultraestructure. Am J Physiol (Renal Fluid Electrolyte Physio) 1988;255:F1256–68.

[160] Kamenicky P, Viengchareun S, Blanchard A, Meduri G, Zizzari P, Imbert-Teboul M, et al. Epithelial sodium channel is a key mediator of growth hormone-induced sodium retention in acromegaly. Endocrinology 2008;149:3294–305.

[161] Katz AI, Doucet A, Morel F. Na-K-ATPase activity along the rabbit, rat, and mouse nephron. Am J Physiol 1979;237:F114–20.

[162] Kellenberger S, Gautschi I, Pfister Y, Schild L. Intracellular thiol-mediated modulation of epithelial sodium channel activity. J Biol Chem 2005;280:7739–47.

[163] Kellenberger S, Gautschi I, Schild L. A single point mutation in the pore region of the epithelial Na^+ channel changes ion selectivity by modifying molecular sieving. Proc Natl Acad Sci USA 1999;96:4170–5.

[164] Kellenberger S, Gautschi I, Schild L. An external site controls closing of the epithelial Na^+ channel ENaC. J Physiol 2002;543:413–24.

[165] Kellenberger S, Gautschi I, Schild L. Mutations in the epithelial Na^+ channel ENaC outer pore disrupt amiloride block by increasing its dissociation rate. Mol Pharmacol 2003;64:848–56.

[166] Kieferle S. Two highly homologous members of the ClC chloride channel family in both rat and human kidney. Proc Natl Acad Sci USA 1994;91:6943–7.

[167] Kikeri D, Azar S, Sun A, Zeidel ML, Hebert SC. $Na^{(+)}$-H^+ antiporter and $Na^{(+)}$-$(HCO_3^-)n$ symporter regulate intracellular pH in mouse medullary thick limbs of Henle. Am J Physiol 1990;258:F445–56.

[168] Kikeri D, Azar S, Sun A, Zeidel ML, Hebert SC. Na^+-H^+ antiporter and Na^+-$(HCO_3^-)_n$ symporter regulate intracellular pH in mouse medullary thick limbs of Henle. Am J Physiol (Renal Fluid Electrolyte Physiol) 1990;258-27:F445–56.

[169] Kim GH, Masilamani S, Turner R, Mitchell C, Wade JB, Knepper MA. The thiazide-sensitive Na-Cl co-transporter is an aldosterone-induced protein. Proc Natl Acad Sci USA 1998;95:14552–7.

[170] Kim J, Kim YH, Cha JH, Tisher CC, Madsen KM. Intercalated cell subtypes in connecting tubule and cortical collecting duct of rat and mouse. J Am Soc Nephrol 1999;10:1–12.

[171] Kinne R, Kinne-Saffran E, Scholermann B, Schutz H. The anion specificity of the sodium-potassium-chloride co-transporter in rabbit kidney outer medulla: studies on medullary plasma membranes. Pflugers Arch 1986;407(Suppl. 2):S168–73.

[172] Kirchner KA. Insulin increases loop segment chloride reabsorption in the euglycemic rat. Am J Physiol 1988;255:F1206–13.

[173] Klaerke DA, Petersen J, Jorgensen PL. Purification of Ca^{2+}-activated K^+ channel protein on calmodulin affinity columns after detergent solubilization of luminal membranes from outer medulla. FEBS Lett 1987;216:211–6.

[174] Koenig B, Ricapito S, Kinne R. Chloride transport in the thick ascending limb of Henle's loop: potassium dependence and stoichiometry of the NaCl co-transport system in plasma membrane vesicles. Pflugers Arch 1983;399:173–9.

[175] Koeppen BM. Conductive properties of the rabbit outer medullary collecting duct: inner stripe. Am J Physiol 1985;248:F500–6.

[176] Kokko JP. Sodium chloride and water transport in the descending limb of Henle. J Clin Invest 1970;49:1838–46.

[177] Kondo C, Isomoto S, Matsumoto S, Yamada M, Horio Y, Yamashita S, et al. Cloning and functional expression of a novel isoform of ROMK inwardly rectifying ATP-dependent K^+ channel, ROMK6 (Kir1.1f). FEBS Lett 1996;399:122–6.

[178] Kondo C, Isomoto S, Matsumoto S, Yamada M, Horio Y, Yamashita S, et al. Cloning and functional expression of a novel isoform of ROMK inwardly rectifying ATP-dependent K^+ channel, ROMK6 (Kir1.1f). FEBS Lett 1996;399:122–6.

[179] Kong S, Zhang C, Li W, Wang L, Luan H, Wang WH, et al. Stimulation of Ca^{2+}-sensing receptor inhibits the basolateral 50-pS K channels in the thick ascending limb of rat kidney.

Biochimica et Biophysica Acta (BBA)—Mol Cell Res 2012;1823: 273—81.

[180] Krapf R. Basolateral membrane H/OH/HCO$_3$ transport in the rat cortical thick ascending limb. Evidence for an electrogenic Na/HCO$_3$ co-transporter in parallel with a Na/H antiporter. J Clin Invest 1988;82:234—41.

[181] Krozowski Z, MaGuire JA, Stein-Oakley AN, Dowling J, Smith RE, Andrews RK. Immunohistochemical localization of the 11 beta-hydroxysteroid dehydrogenase type II enzyme in human kidney and placenta. J Clin Endocrinol Metab 1995;80:2203—9.

[182] Kudo LH, van Baak AA, Rocha AS. Effect of vasopressin on sodium transport across inner medullary collecting duct. Am J Physiol 1990;258:F1438—47.

[183] Lachheb S, Cluzeaud F, Bens M, Genete M, Hibino H, Lourdel S, et al. Kir4.1/Kir5.1 channel forms the major K$^+$ channel in the basolateral membrane of mouse renal collecting duct principal cells. AJP—Renal Physiol 2008;294:F1398—407.

[184] Lalioti MD, Zhang J, Volkman HM, Kahle KT, Hoffmann KE, Toka HR, et al. Wnk4 controls blood pressure and potassium homeostasis via regulation of mass and activity of the distal convoluted tubule. Nat Genet 2006;38:1124—32.

[185] Lauf PK, McManus TJ, Haas M, Forbush IB, Duhm J, Flatman PW, et al. Physiology and biophysics of chloride and cation co-transport across cell membranes. Fed Proc 1987;46:2377—94.

[186] Leichtweiss HP, Lubbers DW, Weiss CH, Baumgartl H, Reschke W. The oxygen supply of the rat kidney: measurement of intrarenal pO$_2$. Pflugers Arch 1969;309:328—49.

[187] Leviel F, Hubner CA, Houillier P, Morla L, El Moghrabi S, Brideau G, et al. The Na$^+$-dependent chloride-bicarbonate exchanger SLC4A8 mediates an electroneutral Na$^+$ reabsorption process in the renal cortical collecting ducts of mice. J Clin Invest 2010;120:1627—35.

[188] Liddle GW, Bledsoe T, Coppage Jr WS. A familial renal disorder simulating primary aldosteronism but with negligible aldosterone secretion. Trans Assoc Am Phys 1963;76:199—213.

[189] Liou HH, Zhou SS, Huang CL. Regulation of ROMK1 channel by protein kinase A via a phosphatidylinositol 4,5-bisphosphate-dependent mechanism. Proc Natl Acad Sci USA 1999;96:5820—5.

[190] Loffing J, Kaissling B. Sodium and calcium transport pathways along the mammalian distal nephron: from rabbit to human. Am J Physiol Renal Physiol 2003;284:F628—43.

[191] Loffing J, Loffing-Cueni D, Hegyi I, Kaplan MR, Hebert SC, Hir ML, et al. Thiazide treatment of rats provokes apoptosis in distal tubule cells. Kidney Int 1996;50:1180—90.

[192] Loffing J, Loffing-Cueni D, Macher A, Hebert SC, Olson B, Knepper MA, et al. Localization of epithelial sodium channel and aquaporin-2 in rabbit kidney cortex. Am J Physiol Renal Physiol 2000;278:F530—9.

[193] Loffing J, Pietri L, Aregger F, Bloch-Faure M, Ziegler U, Meneton P, et al. Differential subcellular localization of ENaC subunits in mouse kidney in response to high- and low-Na diets. Am J Physiol Renal Physiol 2000;279:F252—8.

[194] Loffing J, Vallon V, Loffing-Cueni D, Aregger F, Richter K, Pietri L, et al. Altered renal distal tubule structure and renal Na$^+$ and Ca^{2+} handling in a mouse model for Gitelman's syndrome. J Am Soc Nephrol 2004;15:2276—88.

[195] Loffing J, Zecevic M, Feraille E, Kaissling B, Asher C, Rossier BC, et al. Aldosterone induces rapid apical translocation of ENaC in early portion of renal collecting system: possible role of SGK. Am J Physiol Renal Physiol 2001;280:F675—82.

[196] Louis-Dit-Picard H, Barc J, Trujillano D, Miserey-Lenkei S, Bouatia-Naji N, Pylypenko O, et al. KLHL3 mutations cause

familial hyperkalemic hypertension by impairing ion transport in the distal nephron. Nat Genet 2012;44:456—60.

[197] Lourdel S, Paulais M, Cluzeaud F, Bens M, Tanemoto M, Kurachi Y, et al. An inward rectifier K$^+$ channel at the basolateral membrane of the mouse distal convoluted tubule: similarities with Kir4-Kir5.1 heteromeric channels. J Physiol 2002;538:391—404.

[198] Lu M, Hebert SC, Giebisch G. Hydrolyzable ATP and PIP$_2$ modulate the small conductance K$^+$ channel in apical membranes of rat cortical collecting duct (CCD). J Gen Physiol 2002;120:603—15.

[199] Lu M, Leng Q, Egan ME, Caplan MJ, Boulpaep E, Giebisch G, et al. CFTR is required for PKA-regulated ATP sensitivity of Kir1.1 potassium channels in mouse kidney. J Clin Invest 2006;116:797—807.

[200] Lu M, Wang T, Yan Q, Wang W, Giebisch G, Hebert SC. ROMK is required for expression of the 70pS K channel in the thick ascending limb. Am J Physiol Renal Physiol 2004;286: F490—5.

[201] Lu M, Wang T, Yan Q, Yang X, Dong K, Knepper MA, et al. Absence of small-conductance K$^+$ channel (SK) activity in apical membranes of thick ascending limb and cortical collecting duct in ROMK (Bartter's) knockout mice. J Biol Chem 2002;277:37881—7.

[202] Lu M, Wang W. Two types of K$^+$ channels are present in the apical membrane of the thick ascending limb of the mouse kidney. Kidney Blood Press Res 2000;23:75—82.

[203] MacGregor GG, Xu J, McNicholas CM, Giebisch G, Hebert SC. Partially active channels produced by PKA site mutation of the cloned renal K$^+$ channel ROMK2. Am J Physiol (Renal Physiol) 1998;275:F415—22.

[204] Madsen KM, Verlander JW, Tisher CC. Relationship between structure and function in distal tubule and collecting duct. J Electron Microsc Tech 1988;9:187—208.

[205] Malnic G, Klose RM, Giebisch G. Microperfusion study of distal tubular potassium and sodium transfer in rat kidney. Am J Physiol 1966;211:548—59.

[206] Masilamani S, Kim GH, Mitchell C, Wade JB, Knepper MA. Aldosterone-mediated regulation of ENaC alpha, beta, and gamma subunit proteins in rat kidney. J Clin Invest 1999;104: R19—23.

[207] McGiff JC. Cytochrome P-450 metabolism of arachidonic acid. Annu Rev Pharmacol Toxicol 1991;31:339—69.

[208] McNicholas CM, Guggino WB, Schwiebert EM, Hebert SC, Giebisch G, Egan ME. Sensitivity of a renal K$^+$ channel (ROMK2) to the inhibitory sulfonylurea compound, glibenclamide, is enhanced by co-expression with the ATP-binding cassette transporter cystic fibrosis transmembrane regulator. Proc Natl Acad Sci USA 1996;93:8083—8.

[209] Meade P, Hoover RS, Plata C, Vazquez N, Bobadilla NA, Gamba G, et al. cAMP-dependent activation of the renal-specific Na$^+$-K$^+$-2Cl$^-$ co-transporter is mediated by regulation of co-transporter trafficking. Am J Physiol Renal Physiol 2003;284:F1145—54.

[210] Mennitt PA, Wade JB, Ecelbarger CA, Palmer LG, Frindt G. Localization of ROMK channels in the rat kidney. J Am Soc Nephrol 1997;8:1823—30.

[211] Moller J, Jorgensen JO, Marqversen J, Frandsen E, Christiansen JS. Insulin-like growth factor I administration induces fluid and sodium retention in healthy adults: possible involvement of renin and atrial natriuretic factor. Clin Endocrinol (Oxf) 2000;52:181—6.

[212] Molony DA, Reeves WB, Andreoli TE. Na$^+$:K$^+$:2Cl$^-$ co-transport and the thick ascending limb. Kidney Int 1989;36:418—26.

[213] Molony DA, Reeves WB, Andreoli TE. Na$^+$:K$^+$:2Cl$^-$ co-transport and the thick ascending limb. Kidney Int 1989;36:418–26.

[214] Molony DA, Reeves WB, Hebert SC, Andreoli TE. ADH increases apical Na$^+$,K$^+$,2Cl$^-$ entry in mouse medullary thick ascending limbs of Henle. Am J Physiol (Renal Fluid Electrolyte Physiol) 1987;252:F177–87.

[215] Monroy A, Plata C, Hebert SC, Gamba G. Characterization of the thiazide-sensitive Na$^{(+)}$-Cl$^{(-)}$ co-transporter: a new model for ions and diuretics interaction. Am J Physiol Renal Physiol 2000;279:F161–9.

[216] Morales MM, Carroll TP, Morita T, Schwiebert EM, Devuyst O, Wilson PD, et al. Both the wild type and a functional isoform of CFTR are expressed in kidney. Am J Physiol (Renal Fluid Electrolyte Physiol) 1996;270:F1038–48.

[217] Morel F, Imbert-Teboul M, Chabardes D. Distribution of hormone-dependent adenylate cyclase in the nephron and its physiological significance. Annu Rev Physiol 1981;43:569–81.

[218] Moreno G, Merino A, Mercado A, Herrera JP, Gonzalez-Salazar J, Correa-Rotter R, et al. Electronuetral Na-coupled co-transporter expression in the kidney during variations of NaCl and water metabolism. Hypertension 1998;31:1002–6.

[219] Morgan T, Berliner RW. Permeability of the loop of Henle, vasa recta, and collecting duct to water, urea, and sodium. Am J Physiol 1968;215:108–15.

[220] Morris RG, Schafer JA. cAMP increases density of ENaC subunits in the apical membrane of MDCK cells in direct proportion to amiloride-sensitive Na$^{(+)}$ transport. J Gen Physiol 2002;120:71–85.

[221] Mount DB, Baekgard A, Hall AE, Plata C, Xu J, Beier DR, et al. Isoforms of the Na-K-2Cl transporter in murine TAL: I. Molecular characterization and intrarenal localization. Am J Physiol (Renal Physiol) 1999;276:F347–58.

[222] Mune T, Rogerson FM, Nikkila H, Agarwal AK, White PC. Human hypertension caused by mutations in the kidney isozyme of 11 beta-hydroxysteroid dehydrogenase. Nat Genet 1995;10:394–9.

[223] Musch W, Hedeshi A, Decaux G. Low sodium excretion in SIADH patients with low diuresis. Nephron Physiol 2004;96:11–8.

[224] Mutig K, Paliege A, Kahl T, Jons T, Muller-Esterl W, Bachmann S. Vasopressin V2 receptor expression along rat, mouse, and human renal epithelia with focus on TAL. Am J Physiol Renal Physiol 2007;293:F1166–77.

[225] Na T, Wu G, Peng JB. Disease-causing mutations in the acidic motif of WNK4 impair the sensitivity of WNK4 kinase to calcium ions. Biochem Biophys Res Commun 2012;419:293–8.

[226] Nakao A, Allen ML, Sonnenberg WK, Smith WL. Regulation of cAMP metabolism by PGE$_2$ in cortical and medullary thick ascending limb of Henle's loop. Am J Physiol (Cell Physiol) 1989;256-25:C652–7.

[227] Naray-Fejes-Toth A, Watlington CO, Fejes-Toth G. 11 beta-Hydroxysteroid dehydrogenase activity in the renal target cells of aldosterone. Endocrinology 1991;129:17–21.

[228] Nicco C, Wittner M, diStefano A, Jounier S, Bankir L, Bouby N. Chronic exposure to vasopressin upregulates ENaC and sodium transport in the rat renal collecting duct and lung. Hypertension 2001;38:1143–9.

[229] Nicod M, Michlig S, Flahaut M, Salinas M, Fowler JN, Horisberger JD, et al. A novel vasopressin-induced transcript promotes MAP kinase activation and ENaC downregulation. EMBO J 2002;21:5109–17.

[230] Nishida M, MacKinnon R. Structural basis of inward rectification. cytoplasmic pore of the G protein-gated inward rectifier GIRK1 at 1.8 Å resolution. Cell 2002;111:957–65.

[231] Nishida M, Cadene M, Chait BT, MacKinnon R. Crystal structure of a Kir3.1-prokaryotic Kir channel chimera. EMBO J 2007;26:4005–15.

[232] Ortiz PA. cAMP increases surface expression of NKCC2 in rat thick ascending limbs: role of VAMP. Am J Physiol Renal Physiol 2006;290:F608–16.

[233] Palmer LG, Choe H, Frindt G. Is the secretory K channel in the rat CCT ROMK? Am J Physiol (Renal Fluid Electrolyte Physiol) 1997;273:F404–10.

[234] Palmer LG, Frindt G. Effects of cell Ca and pH on Na channels from rat cortical collecting tubule. Am J Physiol 1987;253:F333–9.

[235] Palmer LG, Frindt G. Conductance and gating of epithelial Na channels from rat cortical collecting tubule. Effects of luminal Na and Li. J Gen Physiol 1988;92:121–38.

[236] Palmer LG, Frindt G. Gating of Na channels in the rat cortical collecting tubule: effects of voltage and membrane stretch. J Gen Physiol 1996;107:35–45.

[237] Palmer LG, Frindt G. High-conductance K channels in intercalated cells of the rat distal nephron. Am J Physiol Renal Physiol 2007;292:F966–73.

[238] Paulais M, Lourdel S, Teulon J. Properties of an inwardly rectifying K$^+$ channel in the basolateral membrane of mouse TAL. Am J Physiol Renal Physiol 2002;282:F866–76.

[239] Paulais M, Teulon J. cAMP-activated chloride channel in the basolateral membrane of the thick ascending limb of the mouse kidney. J Membr Biol 1993;113:253–60.

[240] Paulais M, Lachheb S, Teulon J. A Na$^+$- and Cl$^-$-activated K$^+$ channel in the thick ascending limb of mouse kidney. J Gen Physiol 2006;127:205–15.

[241] Payne JA, Forbush IB. Alternatively spliced isoforms of the putative renal Na-K-Cl co-transporter are differentially distributed within the rabbit kidney. Proc Natl Acad Sci USA 1994;91:4544–8.

[242] Pfister Y, Gautschi I, Takeda AN, van Bemmelen M, Kellenberger S, Schild L. A gating mutation in the internal pore of ASIC1a. J Biol Chem 2006;281:11787–91.

[243] Plata C, Meade P, Hall AE, Welch RC, Vazquez N, Hebert SC, et al. Alternatively spliced isoform of the apical Na-K-Cl co-transporter gene encodes a furosemide sensitive Na-Cl co-transporter. Am J Physiol Renal Physiol 2001;280:F574–82.

[244] Plata C, Meade P, Vazquez N, Hebert SC, Gamba G. Functional properties of the apical Na$^+$-K$^+$-2Cl$^-$ co-transporter isoforms. J Biol Chem 2002;277:11004–12.

[245] Plata C, Mount DB, Rubio V, Hebert SC, Gamba G. Isoforms of the Na-K-2Cl co-transporter in murine TAL. II. Functional characterization and activation by cAMP. Am J Physiol (Renal Physiol) 1999;276:F359–66.

[246] Plato CF, Stoods BA, Wang D, Garvin JL. Endogenous nitric oxide inhibits chloride transport in the thick ascending limb. Am J Physiol (Renal Physiol) 1999;276:F159–63.

[247] Ponce-Coria J, San Cristobal P, Kahle KT, Vazquez N, Pacheco-Alvarez D, los Heros P, et al. Regulation of NKCC2 by a chloride-sensing mechanism involving the WNK3 and SPAK kinases. Proc Natl Acad Sci 2008;105:8458–63.

[248] Pradervand S, Wang Q, Burnier M, Beermann F, Horisberger JD, Hummler E, et al. A mouse model for Liddle's syndrome. J Am Soc Nephrol 1999;10:2527–33.

[249] Quamme GA. Effect of hypercalcemia on renal tubular handling of calcium and magnesium. Can J Physiol Pharmacol 1982;60:1275–80.

[250] Quamme GA, de Rouffignac C. Epithelial magnesium transport and regulation by the kidney. Front Biosci 2000;5:D694–711.

[251] Reeves WB, Andreoli TE. Cl⁻ transport in basolateral renal medullary vesicles: II. Cl⁻ channels in planar lipid bilayers. J Membr Biol 1990;113:57–65.

[252] Reeves WB, McDonald GA, Mehta P, Andreoli TE. Activation of K⁺ channels in renal medullary vesicles by cAMP-dependent protein kinase. J Membr Biol 1989;109:65–72.

[253] Reeves WB, Molony DA. The physiology of loop diuretic action. Semin Nephrol 1988;8:225–33.

[254] Reichold M, Zdebik AA, Lieberer E, Rapedius M, Schmidt K, Bandulik S, et al. KCNJ10 gene mutations causing EAST syndrome (epilepsy, ataxia, sensorineural deafness, and tubulopathy) disrupt channel function. Proc Natl Acad Sci 2010;107:14490–5.

[255] Reilly RF, Ellison DH. Mammalian distal tubule: physiology, pathophysiology, and molecular anatomy. Physiol Rev 2000;80:277–313.

[256] Rinehart J, Kahle KT, De Los HP, Vazquez N, Meade P, Wilson FH, et al. WNK3 kinase is a positive regulator of NKCC2 and NCC, renal cation-Cl⁻ co-transporters required for normal blood pressure homeostasis. Proc Natl Acad Sci USA 2005;102:16777–82.

[257] Rocha AS, Kokko JP. Sodium chloride and water transport in the medullary thick ascending limb of Henle. Evidence for active chloride transport. J Clin Invest 1973;52:612–23.

[258] Rossetti L, Klein-Robbenhaar G, Giebisch G, Smith D, DeFronzo R. Effect of insulin on renal potassium metabolism. Am J Physiol 1987;252:F60–4.

[259] Rotin D, Schild L. ENaC and its regulatory proteins as drug targets for blood pressure control. Curr Drug Targets 2008;9:709–16.

[260] Rouch AJ, Chen L, Troutman SL, Schafer JA. Na⁺ transport in isolated rat CCD: effects of bradykinin, ANP, clonidine, and hydrochlorothiazide. Am J Physiol 1991;260:F86–95.

[261] Rubera I, Loffing J, Palmer LG, Frindt G, Fowler-Jaeger N, Sauter D, et al. Collecting duct-specific gene inactivation of alphaENaC in the mouse kidney does not impair sodium and potassium balance. J Clin Invest 2003;112:554–65.

[262] Ruffieux-Daidie D, Poirot O, Boulkroun S, Verrey F, Kellenberger S, Staub O. Deubiquitylation regulates activation and proteolytic cleavage of ENaC. J Am Soc Nephrol 2008;19:2170–80.

[263] Ruggles BT, Murayama N, Werness JL, Gapstur SM, Bentley MD, Dousa TP. The vasopressin-sensitive adenylate cyclase in collecting tubules and in thick ascending limb of Henle's loop of human and canine kidney. J Clin Endocrinol Metab 1985;60:914–21.

[264] Ruknudin A, Schulze DH, Sullivan SK, Lederer WJ, Welling PA. Novel subunit composition of a renal epithelial K_ATP channel. J Biol Chem 1998;273:14165–71.

[265] Saito-Ohara F. Assignment of the genes encoding the human chloride channels, CLCNKA and CLCNKB, to 1p36 and of CLCN3 to 4q32[ndash]q33 by in situ hybridization. Genomics 1996;36:372–4.

[266] San Cristobal P, Pacheco-Alvarez D, Richardson C, Ring AM, Vazquez N, Rafiqi FH, et al. Angiotensin II signaling increases activity of the renal Na-Cl co-transporter through a WNK4-SPAK-dependent pathway. Proc Natl Acad Sci USA 2009;106:4384–9.

[267] Sandberg MB, Maunsbach AB, McDonough AA. Redistribution of distal tubule Na⁺-Cl⁻ co-transporter (NCC) in response to a high-salt diet. Am J Physiol Renal Physiol 2006;291:F503–8.

[268] Sands JM, Nonoguchi H, Knepper MA. Hormone effects on NaCl permeability of rat inner medullary collecting duct. Am J Physiol 1988;255:F421–8.

[269] Sansom SC, O'Neil RG. Mineralocorticoid regulation of apical cell membrane Na⁺ and K⁺ transport of the cortical collecting duct. Am J Physiol 1985;248:F858–68.

[270] Sasaki S, Imai M. Effects of vasopressin on water and NaCl transport across the in vitro perfused medullary thick ascending limb of Henle's loop of mouse, rat, and rabbit kidneys. Pflugers Arch 1980;383:215–21.

[271] Sauter D, Fernandes S, Goncalves-Mendes N, Boulkroun S, Bankir L, Loffing J, et al. Long term effects of vasopressin on the subcellular localization of ENaC in the renal collecting system. Kidney Int 2006;69:1024–32.

[272] Schafer JA, Troutman SL. cAMP mediates the increase in apical membrane Na⁺ conductance produced in rat CCD by vasopressin. Am J Physiol 1990;259:F823–31.

[273] Schafer JA, Troutman SL, Schlatter E. Vasopressin and mineralocorticoid increase apical membrane driving force for K⁺ secretion in rat CCD. Am J Physiol 1990;258:F199–210.

[274] Schild L, Canessa CM, Shimkets RA, Gautschi I, Lifton RP, Rossier BC. A mutation in the epithelial sodium channel causing Liddle disease increases channel activity in the Xenopus laevis oocyte expression system. Proc Natl Acad Sci USA 1995;92:5699–703.

[275] Schild L, Lu Y, Gautschi I, Schneeberger E, Lifton RP, Rossier BC. Identification of a PY motif in the epithelial Na channel subunits as a target sequence for mutations causing channel activation found in Liddle syndrome. EMBO J 1996;15:2381–7.

[276] Schlatter E, Greger R. cAMP increases the basolateral Cl⁻ conductance in the isolated perfused medullary thick ascending limb of Henle's loop of the mouse. Pflugers Arch 1985;405:367–76.

[277] Schlatter E, Schafer JA. Electrophysiological studies in principal cells of rat cortical collecting tubules. ADH increases the apical membrane Na⁺-conductance. Pflugers Arch 1987;409:81–92.

[278] Schmitt R, Ellison DH, Farman N, Rossier BC, Reilly RF, Reeves WB, et al. Developmental expression of sodium entry pathways in rat nephron. Am J Physiol 1999;276:F367–81.

[279] Schnermann J, Briggs J, Schubert G. In situ studies of the distal convoluted tubule in the rat. I. Evidence for NaCl secretion. Am J Physiol 1982;243:F160–6.

[280] Schoen HF, Erlij D. Insulin action on electrophysiological properties of apical and basolateral membranes of frog skin. Am J Physiol 1987;252:C411–7.

[281] Scholl UI, Choi M, Liu T, Ramaekers VT, Usler MG, Grimmer J, et al. Seizures, sensorineural deafness, ataxia, mental retardation, and electrolyte imbalance (SeSAME syndrome) caused by mutations in KCNJ10. Proc Natl Acad Sci 2009;106:5842–7.

[282] Schwartz GJ, Burg MB. Mineralocorticoid effects on cation transport by cortical collecting tubules in vitro. Am J Physiol 1978;235:F576–85.

[283] Seyberth HW. An improved terminology and classification of Bartter-like syndromes. Nat Clin Pract Nephrol 2008;4:560–7.

[284] Shi H, Asher C, Chigaev A, Yung Y, Reuveny E, Seger R, et al. Interactions of beta and gamma ENaC with Nedd4 can be facilitated by an ERK-mediated phosphorylation. J Biol Chem 2002;277:13539–47.

[285] Shi PP, Cao XR, Sweezer EM, Kinney TS, Williams NR, Husted RF, et al. Salt-sensitive hypertension and cardiac hypertrophy in mice deficient in the ubiquitin ligase Nedd4-2. Am J Physiol Renal Physiol 2008;295:F462–70.

[286] Shimizu T, Yoshitomi K, Nakamura M, Imai M. Site and mechanism of action of trichlormethiazide in rabbit distal nephron segments perfused in vitro. J Clin Invest 1988;82:721–30.

[287] Shimkets RA, Warnock DG, Bositis CM, Nelson-Williamns C, Hansson JH, Schambelan M, et al. Liddle's syndrome:

heritable human hypertension caused by mutations in the beta subunit of the epithelial sodium channel. Cell 1994;79:407–14.

[288] Siegel B, Civan MM. Aldosterone and insulin effects on driving force of Na^+ pump in toad bladder. Am J Physiol 1976;230:1603–8.

[289] Simon DB, Bindra RS, Mansfield TA, Nelson-Williams C, MendonOa E, Stone R, et al. Mutations in the chloride channel gene, CLCNKB, cause Bartter's syndrome type III. Nat Genet 1997;17:171–8.

[290] Simon DB, Karet FE, Rodriguez-Soriano J, Hamdan JH, DiPietro A, Trachtman H, et al. Genetic heterogeneity of Bartter's syndrome revealed by mutations in the K^+ channel, ROMK. Nat Genet 1996;14:152–6.

[291] Snyder PM, Olson DR, Kabra R, Zhou R, Steines JC. cAMP and serum and glucocorticoid-inducible kinase (SGK) regulate the epithelial $Na^{(+)}$ channel through convergent phosphorylation of Nedd4-2. J Biol Chem 2004;279:45753–8.

[292] Snyder PM, Price MP, McDonald FJ, Adams CM, Volk KA, Zeiher BG, et al. Mechanism by which Liddle's syndrome mutations increase activity of a human epithelial Na^+ channel. Cell 1995;83:969–78.

[293] Sonnenberg H, Honrath U, Wilson DR. Effects of amiloride in the medullary collecting duct of rat kidney. Kidney Int 1987;31:1121–5.

[294] Stanton BA. Characterization of apical and basolateral membrane conductances of rat inner medullary collecting duct. Am J Physiol 1989;256:F862–8.

[295] Starremans PG, Kersten FF, van den Heuvel LP, Knoers NV, Bindels RJ. Dimeric architecture of the human bumetanide-sensitive Na-K-Cl Co-transporter. J Am Soc Nephrol 2003;14:3039–46.

[296] Staub O, Abriel H, Plant P, Ishikawa T, Kanelis V, Saleki R, et al. Regulation of the epithelial Na^+ channel by Nedd4 and ubiquitination. Kidney Int 2000;57:809–15.

[297] Staub O, Gautschi I, Ishikawa T, Breitschopf K, Ciechanover A, Schild L, et al. Regulation of stability and function of the epithelial Na^+ channel (ENaC) by ubiquitination. EMBO J 1997;16:6325–36.

[298] Stokes JB. Ion transport by the cortical and outer medullary collecting tubule. Kidney Int 1982;22:473–84.

[299] Stokes JB. Na and K transport across the cortical and outer medullary collecting tubule of the rabbit: evidence for diffusion across the outer medullary portion. Am J Physiol 1982;242:F514–20.

[300] Stoner LC, Burg MB, Orloff J. Ion transport in cortical collecting tubule; effect of amiloride. Am J Physiol 1974;227:453–9.

[301] Sun A, Grossman EB, Lombardi M, Hebert SC. Vasopressin alters the mechanism of apical Cl^- entry from Na^+:Cl^- to Na^+:K^+:$2Cl^-$ co-transport in mouse medullary thick ascending limb. J Membr Biol 1991;120:83–94.

[302] Takaichi K, Kurokawa K. AVP-sensitive cAMP production is dependent on calmodulin in both MTAL and MCT. Am J Physiol 1988;255:F834–40.

[303] Takaichi K, Kurokawa K. Inhibitory guanosine triphophate-binding protein-mediated regulation of vasopressin action in isolated single medullary of mouse kidney. J Clin Invest 1988;82:1437–44.

[304] Takeuchi Y, Uchida S, Marumo F, Sasaki S. Cloning, tissue distribution, and intrarenal localization of ClC chloride channels in human kidney. Kidney Int 1995;48:1497–503.

[305] Tanemoto M, Vanoye CG, Dong K, Welch R, Abe T, Hebert SC, et al. Rat homolog of sulfonylurea receptor 2B determines glibenclamide sensitivity of ROMK2 in Xenopus laevis oocyte. Am J Physiol Renal Physiol 2000;278:F659–66.

[306] Tanemoto M, Abe T, Onogawa T, Ito S. PDZ binding motif-dependent localization of K^+ channel on the basolateral side in distal tubules. Am J Physiol-Renal Physiol 2004;287:F1148–53.

[307] Tao X, Avalos JL, Chen J, MacKinnon R. Crystal structure of the eukaryotic strong inward-rectifier K^+ channel Kir2.2 at 3.1 Å resolution. Science 2009;326:1668–74.

[308] Tiwari S, Nordquist L, Halagappa VK, Ecelbarger CA. Trafficking of ENaC subunits in response to acute insulin in mouse kidney. Am J Physiol Renal Physiol 2007;293:F178–85.

[309] Trinh-Trang-Tan MM, Bouby MM, Coutaud C, Bankir L. Quick isolation of rat medullary thick ascending limbs. Pflugers Arch 1986;407:228–34.

[310] Uchida S, Endou H. Substrate specificity to maintain cellular ATP along the mouse nephron. Am J Physiol (Renal Fluid Electrolyte Physiol) 1988;255-24:F977–83.

[311] Uchida S, Sasaki S, Nitta K, Uchida K, Horita S, Nihei H, et al. Localization and functional characterization of rat kidney-specific chloride channel, ClC-K1. J Clin Invest 1995;95:104–13.

[312] Vallet V, Chraibi A, Gaeggeler HP, Horisberger JD, Rossier BC. An epithelial serine protease activates the amiloride-sensitive sodium channel. Nature 1997;389:607–10.

[313] van der LN, Lim CH, Fenton RA, Meima ME, Jan Danser AH, Zietse R, et al. Angiotensin II induces phosphorylation of the thiazide-sensitive sodium chloride co-transporter independent of aldosterone. Kidney Int 2011;79:66–76.

[314] Vandewalle A, Cluzeaud F, Bens M, Kieferle S, Steinmeyer K, Jentsch TJ. Localization and induction by dehydration of ClC-K chloride channels in the rat kidney. Am J Physiol (Renal Fluid Electrolyte Physiol) 1997;272:F678–88.

[315] Vehaskari VM, Hering-Smith KS, Moskowitz DW, Weiner ID, Hamm LL. Effect of epidermal growth factor on sodium transport in the cortical collecting tubule. Am J Physiol 1989;256: F803–9.

[316] Velazquez H, Silva T. Cloning and localization of KCC4 in rabbit kidney: expression in distal convoluted tubule. Am J Physiol-Renal Physiol 2003;285:F49–58.

[317] Velazquez H, Bartiss A, Bernstein P, Ellison DH. Adrenal steroids stimulate thiazide-sensitive NaCl transport by rat renal distal tubules. Am J Physiol (Renal Fluid Electrolyte Physiol) 1996;270:F211–9.

[318] Velazquez H, Ellison DH, Wright FS. Chloride-dependent potassium secretion in early and late renal distal tubules. Am J Physiol 1987;253:F555–62.

[319] Velazquez H, Good DW, Wright FS. Mutual dependence of sodium and chloride absorption by renal distal tubule. Am J Physiol (Renal Fluid Electrolyte Physiol) 1984;247:F904–11.

[320] Verlander JM, Tran TM, Zhang L, Kaplan MR, Hebert SC. Estradiol enhances thiazide-sensitive NaCl co-transporter density in the apical plasma membrane of the distal convoluted tubule in ovariectomized rats. J Clin Invest 1998;101:1661–9.

[321] Verrey F, Fakitsas P, Adam G, Staub O. Early transcriptional control of ENaC (de)ubiquitylation by aldosterone. Kidney Int 2008;73:691–6.

[322] Vuagniaux G, Vallet V, Jaeger NF, Pfister C, Bens M, Farman N, et al. Activation of the amiloride-sensitive epithelial sodium channel by the serine protease mCAP1 expressed in a mouse cortical collecting duct cell line. J Am Soc Nephrol 2000;11:828–34.

[323] Wang MH, Brand-Schieber E, Zand BA, Nguyen X, Falck JR, Balu N, et al. Cytochrome P450-derived arachidonic acid metabolism in the rat kidney: characterization of selective inhibitors. J Pharmacol Exp Ther 1998;284:966–73.

[324] Wang T, Wang WH, Klein-Robbenhaar G, Giebisch G. Effects of a novel K_{ATP} channel blocker on renal tubule function and K channel activity. J Pharmacol Exp Ther 1995;273:1382–9.

[325] Wang W. Two types of K$^+$ channel in TAL of rat kidney. Am J Physiol (Renal Fluid Electrolyte Physiol) 1994;267-36: F599−605.

[326] Wang W, Giebisch G. Dual effect of adenosine triphosphate on the apical small conductance K$^+$ channel of the rat cortical collecting duct. J Gen Physiol 1991;98:35−61.

[327] Wang W, White S, Geibel J, Giebisch G. A potassium channel in the apical membrane of rabbit thick ascending limb of Henle's loop. Am J Physiol (Renal Fluid Electrolyte Physiol) 1990;258-27:F244−53.

[328] Wang WH, Giebisch G. Dual modulation of renal ATP-sensitive K$^+$ channel by protein kinases A and C. Proc Natl Acad Sci USA 1991;88:9722−5.

[329] Wang WH, Hebert SC, Giebisch G. Renal K channels: structure and function. Ann Rev Physiol 1997;59:413−36.

[330] Wei Y, Zavilowitz B, Satlin LM, Wang WH. Angiotensin II inhibits the ROMK-like small conductance K channel in renal cortical collecting duct during dietary potassium restriction. J Biol Chem 2007;282:6455−62.

[331] Welker P, Boehlick A, Mutig K, Salanova M, Kahl T, Schlueter H, et al. Renal Na-K-Cl co-transporter activity and vasopressin-induced trafficking are lipid raft-dependent. Am J Physiol Renal Physiol 2008;295:F789−802.

[332] Whorwood CB, Ricketts ML, Stewart PM. Epithelial cell localization of type 2 11 beta-hydroxysteroid dehydrogenase in rat and human colon. Endocrinology 1994;135:2533−41.

[333] Wiederholt M, Hansen LL. *Amphiuma* kidney as a model for distal tubular transport studies. Contrib Nephrol 1980;19: 28−32.

[334] Wilson FH, Kahle KT, Sabath E, Lalioti MD, Rapson AK, Hoover RS, et al. Molecular pathogenesis of inherited hypertension with hyperkalemia: the Na-Cl co-transporter is inhibited by wild-type but not mutant WNK4. Proc Natl Acad Sci USA 2003;100:680−4.

[335] Wilson RC, Krozowski ZS, Li K, Obeyesekere VR, Razzaghy-Azar M, Harbison MD, et al. A mutation in the HSD11B2 gene in a family with apparent mineralocorticoid excess. J Clin Endocrinol Metab 1995;80:2263−6.

[336] Winters CJ, Reeves WB, Andreoli TE. Cl$^-$ channels in basolateral renal medullary membranes: III. Determinants of single-channel activity. J Membr Biol 1990;118:269−78.

[337] Winters CJ, Reeves WB, Andreoli TE. Cl$^-$ channels in basolateral renal medullary vesicles: V. Comparison of basolateral mTALH Cl$^-$ channels with apical Cl$^-$ channels from jejunum and trachea. J Membr Biol 1992;128:27−39.

[338] Winters CJ, Zimniak L, Reeves WB, Andreoli TE. Cl$^-$ channels in basolateral renal medullary membranes XII. Anti-rbClC-Ka antibody blocks MTAL Cl$^-$ channels. AJP−Renal Physiol 1997;273:F1030−8.

[339] Wittner M, Weidtke C, Schlatter E, diStefano A, Greger R. Substrate utilization in the isolated perfused cortical thick ascending limb of rabbit nephron. Pflugers Arch 1984;402: 52−62.

[340] Work J, Galla JH, Booker BB, Schafer JA, Luke RG. Effect of ADH on chloride reabsorption in the loop of Henle of the Brattleboro rat. Am J Physiol 1985;249:F698−703.

[341] Xu JZ, Hall AE, Peterson LN, Bienkowski MJ, Eessalu TE, Hebert SC. Localization of the ROMK protein on apical membranes of rat kidney nephron segments. Am J Physiol (Renal Physiol) 1997;273:F739−48.

[342] Xu ZC, Yang Y, Hebert SC. Phosphorylation of the ATP-sensitive, inwardly rectifying K$^+$ channel, ROMK, by cyclic AMP-dependent protein kinase. J Biol Chem 1996;271:9313−9.

[343] Yang CL, Angell J, Mitchell R, Ellison DH. WNK kinases regulate thiazide-sensitive Na-Cl co-transport. J Clin Invest 2003;111:1039−45.

[344] Yang SS, Morimoto T, Rai T, Chiga M, Sohara E, Ohno M, et al. Molecular pathogenesis of pseudohypoaldosteronism Type II: generation and analysis of a Wnk4(D561A/ +) knockin mouse model. Cell Metab 2007;5:331−44.

[345] Yang T, Huang YG, Singh I, Schnermann J, Briggs JP. Localization of bumetanide- and thiazide-sensitive Na-K-Cl co-transporters along the rat nephron. Am J Physiol (Renal Fluid Electrolyte Physiol) 1996;271:F931−9.

[346] Yoo D, Kim BY, Campo C, Nance L, King A, Maouyo D, et al. Cell surface expression of the ROMK (Kir 1.1) channel is regulated by the aldosterone-induced kinase, SGK-1, and protein kinase A. J Biol Chem 2003;278:23066−75.

[347] Yoshitomi K, Shimizu T, Taniguchi J, Imai M. Electrophysiological characterization of rabbit distal convoluted tubule cell. Pflugers Arch 1989;414:457−63.

[348] Yu L, Helms MN, Yue Q, Eaton DC. Single-channel analysis of functional epithelial sodium channel (ENaC) stability at the apical membrane of A6 distal kidney cells. Am J Physiol Renal Physiol 2008;295:F1519−27.

[349] Yue P, Sun P, Lin DH, Pan C, Xing W, Wang W. Angiotensin II diminishes the effect of SGK1 on the WNK4-mediated inhibition of ROMK1 channels. Kidney Int 2011;79:423−31.

[350] Zhou H, Chepilko S, Schutt W, Choe H, Palmer LG, Sackin H. Mutations in the pore region of ROMK enhance Ba^{2+} block. Am J Physiol 1996;271:C1949−56.

[351] Zimniak L, Winters CJ, Reeves WB, Andreoli TE. Cl$^-$ channels in basolateral renal medullary vesicles X. Cloning of a Cl$^-$ channel from rabbit outer medulla. Kidney Int 1995;48:1828−36.

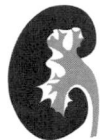

Mineralocorticoid Action in the Aldosterone Sensitive Distal Nephron

Olivier Staub[1] and Johannes Loffing[2]

[1]Department of Pharmacology & Toxicology, University of Lausanne, Lausanne, Switzerland
[2]Institute of Anatomy, University of Zurich, Zurich, Switzerland

INTRODUCTION

The kidney of vertebrates plays a major role in the homeostasis of the extracellular fluid. Despite large changes in water and salt intake, the kidney is able to maintain the extracellular osmolarity and volume within very narrow margins. Such fine control requires specific factors or hormones. In 1952, Simpson and Tait identified aldosterone as the most potent Na^+-retaining factor in mammals. When the Na^+-retaining activity of the newly identified steroid hormone was compared to that of cortisol (or corticosterone), aldosterone was found to be 3000-fold more potent *in vivo*. Aldosterone differs from cortisol (or corticosterone) by the presence of an aldehyde group in position 18 on the second ring. Thus, an apparently minimal change in the structure of the steroid confers on the molecule a strikingly different biological activity (see review in [1]). During the evolution of vertebrates, aldosterone appeared about 300 million years ago with amphibians, which were the first vertebrates to adapt to a dry, terrestrial environment.[2] The three most important and conserved functions of aldosterone are to promote Na^+ reabsorption and K^+ and H^+ secretion across certain "tight" epithelia — that is, epithelia which display a high transepithelial electrical resistance and an amiloride-sensitive, electrogenic Na^+ transport. In mammals, such epithelia are found in the distal part of the nephron, the bladder, the distal part of the intestine (mainly the surface epithelium of distal colon and rectum), and the ducts of exocrine glands (salivary, mammary, and sweat glands). In the mammalian kidney, the Na^+ and K^+ responses are localized in the segment-specific cells of the aldosterone-sensitive distal nephron (ASDN),

while acid secretion is mediated via intercalated cells. The main goal of this chapter is to provide an overview on the renal tubular sites that respond to aldosterone, and to highlight the underlying cellular and molecular mechanisms by which aldosterone controls sodium, potassium, and extracellular fluid homeostasis. The chapter is revised and updated from its previous version established by our colleagues François Verrey, Edith Hummler, Laurent Schild, and Bernard Rossier that appeared in the fourth edition of this book.

The Aldosterone Sensitive Distal Nephron (ASDN)

Each day, the glomeruli of the human kidney filter about 1.5 kg of NaCl out of the blood into the primary urine. However, usually less than 1% of the filtered NaCl is finally excreted. Thus, most of it is reabsorbed along the renal tubular system, which is composed by serial arrangement of the proximal tubule (PCT and PST), the thin limb (TL), the thick ascending limb (TAL), the distal convoluted tubule (DCT), the connecting tubule (CNT), and the collecting duct (CD) (Figure 35.1). While the bulk of Na^+ reabsorption occurs in the proximal tubule (PT) and the TAL, the final regulation of Na^+ excretion takes place in the so-called Aldosterone-Sensitive Distal Nephron (ASDN) which extends from the late portion of the DCT (also called DCT-2) to the end of the collecting duct (IMCD) in the renal papilla.[3] The three ASDN segments differ in their histotopographical localization and epithelial structure. The DCT and CNT are located in the cortical labyrinth, while the CD extends from the

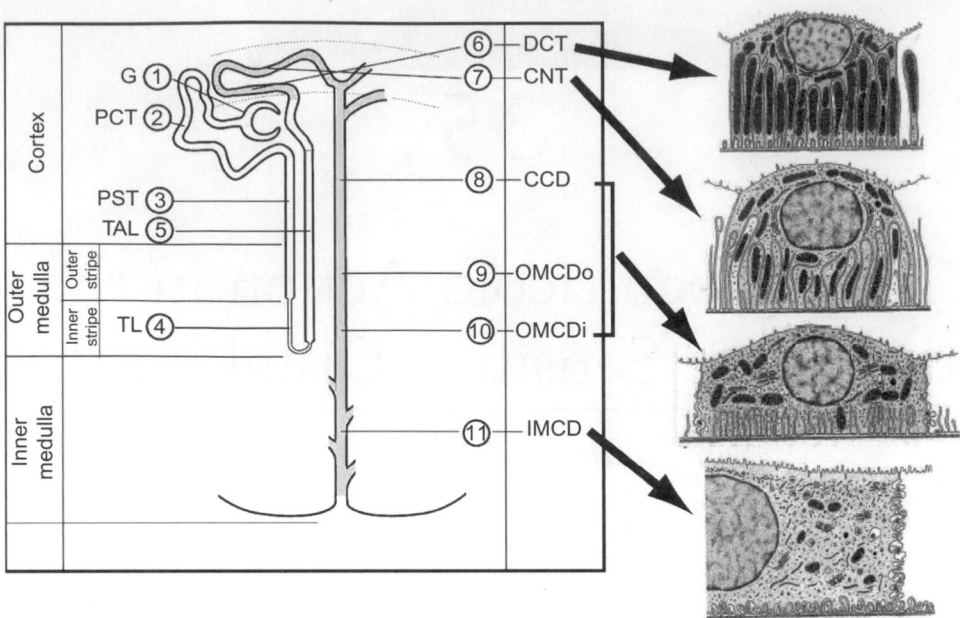

FIGURE 35.1   Schematic representation of the renal tubule system. On the right (see arrows): a distal convoluted tubule (DCT) cell, a connecting tubule (CNT) cell, a principal cell of the cortical and outer medullary collecting duct, and a principal cell of the inner medullary collecting duct (G: glomerulus; PCT: proximal convoluted tubule; PST: proximal straight tubule; TL: thin limb; TAL: thick ascending limb; DCT: distal convoluted tubule; CNT: connecting tubule; CCD: cortical collecting duct; OMCD: outer medullary collecting duct; IMCD: inner medullary collecting duct). The aldosterone-sensitive distal nephron (ASDN) comprises the late DCT, the CNT and the collecting duct. (*Adapted from Kriz, R. W., and Kaissling, B. (2000). Structural organization of the mammalian kidney. In "The Kidney," Vol. 1, 3rd edn, 587–654, Seldin, D. W., and Giebisch, G. (eds.). Lippincott Williams & Wilkins, Philadelphia.*)

medullary rays in the renal cortex down to the renal medulla until its opening on the tip of the renal papilla. DCT cells have an apical localized cell nucleus and numerous mitochondria that are densely stuffed into the interdigitating basolateral membrane infoldings. The CNT cells are usually less tall than the DCT cells, have less mitochondria and a basal membranous labyrinth that is predominantly formed by membrane infoldings. The CCD cells are even smaller, and are characterized by a basal thin rim of mitochondria-free membrane infoldings. The medullary CD is formed by cuboidal cells that have few cell organelles (Figure 35.1). Membrane infoldings and mitochondrial density progressively decrease from DCT to CCD, in parallel with a reduction in the abundance and activity of the Na^+,K^+-ATPase,[4] suggesting different ion transport rates along the ASDN. In fact, recordings of transepithelial Na^+ fluxes in isolated rabbit CNTs[5,6] and rat CCDs,[7,8] indicate at least a 10-fold higher Na^+ transport rate in the CNT than in the CCD (600–120 versus 0.2 to 24 pmoles Na^+/min/mm). The rates of Na^+ transport in OMCD and IMCD are generally low,[9] but Na^+ channels are also expressed in the OMCD and IMCD, and can be activated, at least to some extent, by aldosterone.[10]

Although the sequence of tubule portions appears to be quite similar in mammals, subtle species differences

in the structural and functional organization of the ASDN have to be taken into account if functional data from different nephron portions and species are compared.[11] For example, rabbits have morphologically well-defined sharp transitions from DCT to CNT and from CNT to CD, while the segment transitions in rats, mice, and humans are gradual. These morphological differences are reflected by the distribution pattern of ion- and water-transporting proteins. In rabbits, the sharp transitions from DCT to CNT and from CNT to CCD coincide with the immediate replacement of the DCT-specific NaCl co-transporter (NCC) by the epithelial Na^+ channel (ENaC), and the abrupt onset of aquaporin-2 (AQP2) expression.[12] In contrast, in rats, mice, and humans NCC and ENaC overlap in the late DCT (DCT2), and AQP2 extends into the connecting tubule.[11,13]

Despite the above-mentioned segmental and species differences, all ASDN cells in common express high levels of the mineralocorticoid receptor (MR), the glucocorticoid receptor (GR), the enzyme 11-beta-hydroxysteroid-dehydrogenase type 2 (11β-HSD2), and the epithelial Na^+ channel (ENaC)[3] (Figure 35.2). The MR and the GR are hormone-activated transcription factors that can bind both mineralocorticoid and glucocorticoid hormones, although with different affinities. While the MR is a high-affinity receptor (K_d for

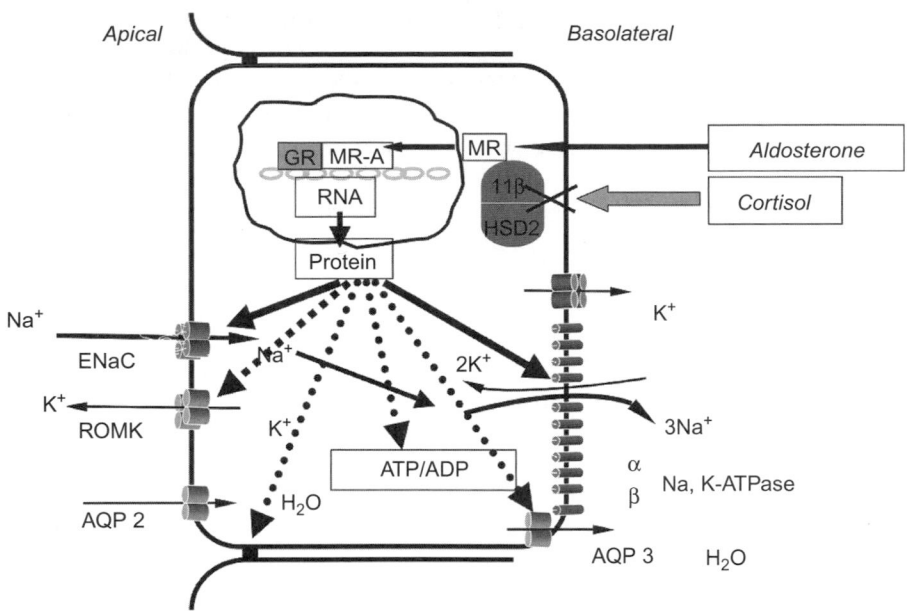

FIGURE 35.2 **Model of the mechanism of aldosterone action in an epithelial target cell.** Aldosterone crosses the plasma membrane and binds to its high affinity mineralocorticoid receptor (MR) and/or the low affinity glucocorticoid receptor (GR). Cortisol is metabolized by the 11βHSD-2 into inactive metabolites with a very low affinity for MR and GR. The complex translocates to the nucleus, where it undergoes interaction with promoter regions of target genes, activating or repressing their transcriptional activity. Induced or repressed proteins mediate an increase in transepithelial sodium transport by the activation of pre-existing transport proteins (ENaC, Na,K-ATPase), and a further accumulation of transport proteins and other elements of the sodium transport machinery. Possible effects on ROMK, tight junction proteins, mitochondria, and water transport proteins (AQP 3) are indicated with dotted arrows. *(From Verrey, F., Hummler, E., Schild, L., and Rossier, B. C. (2008). Mineralocorticoid action in the aldosterone-sensitive distal nephron. In "Seldin and Giebisch's The Kidney," Vol. 1, 4th edn., 889–924. Elsevier Inc.)*

aldosterone and cortisol in the range from 0.5 to 3 nM), the GR has a more than 10 times lower affinity for these steroids (K_d in the range from 20 to 65 nM).[14] The corticosteroid levels in the plasma (cortisol in humans and corticosterone in rats) are usually far above these K_d values, and exceed the plasma concentrations of aldosterone 100–1000-fold. Under these conditions, mineralocorticoid specificity is thought to be conferred to the ASDN cells by their high expression of 11β-HSD2 that rapidly hydrolyzes the physiological corticosteroids to inactive metabolites.[15] Upon hormone binding, the receptors are thought to homo- or heterodimerize and to translocate to the cell nucleus, where they modulate a transcriptional program that modulates the expression of ENaC, the Na$^+$,K$^+$-ATPase, and of regulatory proteins that control the activity of these Na$^+$-reabsorbing proteins.

Na$^+$ transport across the ASDN cells occurs in two steps. Na$^+$ uptake from the lumen into the cells is mediated by ENaC, while Na$^+$ exit across the basolateral plasma membrane depends on the Na$^+$,K$^+$-ATPase. The activity of ENaC and the Na$^+$,K$^+$-ATPase is electrogenic, and generates a transepithelial electrochemical gradient that drives paracellular Cl$^-$ reabsorption and transcellular K$^+$ secretion. The apical K$^+$ secretion is thought to occur via secretory K$^+$ channels

such as the renal outer medulla K$^+$ channel (ROMK) and the flow-dependent maxi-K (BK) channel.[16–19] Immunohistochemical studies revealed that ROMK is highly abundant in the DCT, CNT, and CD cells,[20,21] where it becomes activated and redistributed to the apical plasma membrane in response to an increased dietary K$^+$ intake.[22] Likewise, a high-K$^+$ diet appears to stimulate the BK channel. In rabbits, it increases the mRNA expression of the α-, β2-, and β4-subunits,[23] and in rats it elevates the electrical activity in CCD cells.[24] In contrast to ROMK, the BK channel is not only present in the segment-specific ASDN cells, but also in intercalated cells.[17] Intercalated cells may not only secrete but also reabsorb K$^+$ via their apical H$^+$, K$^+$-ATPase.[25] Thereby, intercalated cells may help to modulate the interdependence of ENaC-mediated Na$^+$ reabsorption and K$^+$ secretion via apical K$^+$ channels. A close link between the function of intercalated and segment-specific ASDN cells is also indicated by the fact that, in all species investigated so far, the appearance of intercalated cells in the early ASDN coincides precisely with the onset of functional ENaC expression.[11] Moreover, several recent studies on various rodent models further supported the idea of a functional cooperation between ASDN and intercalated cells. The ASDN has at least two types of intercalated cells.[26,27] The acid-secreting type-A intercalated cells have the vacuolar H^+-ATPase in the apical plasma membrane and the Cl^-/HCO_3^- anion exchanger AE1 in the basolateral plasma membrane, whereas the bicarbonate-excreting type-B intercalated cells have the H^+-ATPase in the basolateral plasma membrane, and are characterized by the abundance of the Cl^-/HCO_3^- exchanger pendrin in the apical membrane, which may contribute to a combined transcellular reabsorption of Na^+ (via ENaC) and Cl^- (via pendrin). In fact, experiments in pendrin-deficient mice indicated that bicarbonate secretion via the type-B intercalated cells is necessary for normal ENaC expression and activity.[28,29] Consistent with this view, the mice are prone to develop arterial hypotension when placed on an NaCl-deficient diet, and they are protected from hypertension under mineralocorticoid treatment.[30,31] Pendrin may not only cooperate with ENaC, but also with the Na^+-dependent chloride-bicarbonate exchanger SLC4A8,[32] which may account for the previously reported thiazide-sensitive NaCl reabsorption in the renal collecting system. Experiments in SLC4A8- and NCC-deficient mice indicated that about 40−70% of collecting duct Na^+-absorption involve SLC4A8.[32] Similar to ENaC, the thiazide-sensitive electroneutral Na^+ reabsorption, as well as SLC4A8, appear to be stimulated by aldosterone.[27] Na^+ reabsorption via ENaC may not only interfere with K^+, H^+, and Cl^- handling of the ASDN cells, but also with transepithelial water reabsorption. The ENaC activity generates an osmotic gradient that likely favors the vasopressin-dependent transepithelial water reabsorption via the water channels AQP2 in the apical and AQP3 and AQP4 in the basolateral plasma membrane of the segment-specific ASDN cells. Although there are some indications that aldosterone directly controls the expression and activity of ROMK,[33−35] BK,[36] pendrin,[31,37] SLC4A8,[32] AQP2,[38,39] and AQP3,[40] the functional significance of these regulations compared with the indirect effects mediated via enhanced activity of ENaC and Na^+,K^+-ATPase are still unclear. Nevertheless, the various cell types and ion transport pathways with manifold possible interactions likely contribute significantly to the complexity of ion handling along the ASDN which may allow adaptation of urinary ion excretion precisely to homeostatic needs. Details on the regulation of K^+ channels, pendrin, SLC4A8, and aquaporins are given in several excellent recent reviews.[16,17,26,27,37,41−43]

Aldosterone Action in Non-ASDN Cells

A huge variety of studies have been aimed at localizing MR and GR along the mammalian nephron.

Ligand-binding studies and RNAase protection assays on microdissected nephron portions, as well as autoradiography, *in situ* hybridization and immunohistochemistry on kidney sections, revealed a very high abundance of MR and GR along the classical ASDN.[44] Moreover, these studies indicated that the MR, the GR, and 11β-HSD2 are expressed in nephron segments and cell types that are considered not to be classical targets for aldosterone, including glomerular mesangial cells, podocytes, and proximal tubules (reviewed in [15]). Using a set of highly specific MR antibodies,[45] Ackerman et al. recently confirmed that the MR is expressed along the entire distal tubule, including the TAL and the entire DCT.[46] MR expression in the TAL is in line with studies describing a profound stimulatory effect of aldosterone on TAL Na^+ transport,[47] but contrasts with other reports that did not reveal any effect of the mineralocorticoid on the expression and activity of the Na^+,K^+-ATPase and K^+ transport in the TAL of adrenalectomized rabbits and rats, respectively.[48−50] Likewise, there is considerable evidence that aldosterone stimulates NaCl co-transport in the DCT. Velazquez et al. demonstrated that adrenalectomy lowers the electroneutral Na^+ transport activity (corresponding to NCC activity) in the DCT, and that this effect can be fully restored to normal when aldosterone and/or glucocorticoids are replaced.[51] Consistent with a stimulatory role of aldosterone on the DCT, immunoblotting and immunohistochemistry on rat kidneys showed that dietary Na^+ restriction, which stimulates endogenous aldosterone production, as well as exogenous aldosterone application, increases the abundance and phosphorylation of NCC in the DCT.[52−56] Frindt and Palmer used *in vivo* cell surface biotinylation to show in the rat that dietary Na^+ restriction does also increase the cell surface abundance of NCC.[57] Conversely, dietary Na^+-loading removes NCC from the plasma membrane, indicating that aldosterone may affect the trafficking of NCC as well.[58] Interestingly, the increase in NCC protein abundance and phosphorylation was significantly lower when MR was blocked by spironolactone.[53,59] Although the effect of spironolactone points to an MR-mediated transcriptional response, changes in plasma aldosterone do not appear to directly affect NCC mRNA expression, indicating that mineralocorticoids elicit their effects on NCC abundance via enhanced translation and/or reduced degradation of the protein.[55] In fact, there is increasing evidence that NCC protein abundance might be controlled by ubiquitylation, and hence by altered protein stability.[60−63] Aldosterone is also known to stimulate renal H^+ excretion. The intercalated cells in the ASDN play an important role for renal acid−base handling. However, so far it is unclear whether aldosterone directly affects renal acid secretion via activation of the H^+-ATPase in intercalated cells or indirectly via activation of ENaC-dependent Na^+ transport in principal cells, which increases the electrochemical driving force for H^+ secretion by intercalated cells. Functional studies on isolated collecting ducts indicated that aldosterone rapidly stimulates intercalated cells via non-genomic pathways that may involve PKC and PKA signaling,[64] and perhaps require the vasopressin V1 receptor.[65] Nevertheless, it is uncertain whether the observed effects depend on a yet-unknown putative membrane-bound corticosteroid-binding receptor or the classical MR. Although expression of the MR in intercalated cells was long disputed, a recent immunohistochemical study established rather strong expression of the MR, not only in the ASDN segment-specific cells, but also in all subtypes of intercalated cells.[46] However, this study did also provide evidence that the rather low expression levels of the 11β-HSD2 in TAL, early DCT, and intercalated cells, makes it unlikely that aldosterone has significant direct genomic effects on these cell types in the physiological context of several-fold higher plasma levels of corticosterone than aldosterone. Nevertheless, mineralocorticoid-selectivity might be conferred to the MR also in an 11β-HSD2-independent way by a functional preference of the receptor to aldosterone, as indicated in cell culture assays[66] and in vivo experiments.[67] Moreover, MR expression in TAL, early DCT, and intercalated cells may become relevant in patients with pharmacological (e.g., by spironolactone) or genetic (i.e., PHA-1) MR inactivation. Under these conditions, the loss of MR function in these cells may contribute to the salt-losing phenotype with hyperkalemia and metabolic acidosis.[68]

SODIUM TRANSPORT REGULATION BY ALDOSTERONE: PHYSIOLOGICAL AND BIOPHYSICAL MECHANISMS

Epithelial Na^+ transport is a two-step process that comprises: (1) facilitated transport — driven by an electrochemical potential difference — across the apical membrane (from urine to cell); and (2) active transport — driven by metabolic energy — across the basolateral membrane (from cell to interstitium).[69] In the ASDN, the apical-membrane entry step is mediated by Na^+-selective amiloride-sensitive ion channels,[70] while the exit step is catalyzed by Na^+, K^+-ATPase, the ouabain-sensitive Na^+ pump.[71,72] The aldosterone-dependent electrogenic transepithelial Na^+ transport has been studied in a great variety of in vitro, ex vivo, and in vivo models.[73,74] The different models revealed different baseline and maximal transport rates in response to aldosterone. In the toad urinary bladder, "basal" transport rates, measured by the short-circuit current method, are around $5–10 \mu A/cm^2$[75] and aldosterone produces a 2- to 5-fold increase in transport. In the rat colon, basal transport rates through amiloride-sensitive channels are very low, while tissues stimulated in vivo by adrenal steroids can have rates of $500–1000 \mu A/cm^2$.[76] Isolated, perfused rat cortical collecting ducts express no measurable net Na^+ fluxes when the animals are maintained on normal diets. When animals are placed on a low-Na^+ diet (to elevate endogenous aldosterone levels) or injected with mineralocorticoids, Na^+ reabsorption is as high as 30 pmoles/min-mm, which corresponds to $\sim 100 \mu A/cm^2$.[7,8] These values match well the amiloride-sensitive current measured by cell attached patches of mouse CCD cells.[77]

Aldosterone and the Epithelial Sodium Channel ENaC

The apical entry of Na^+ involves the low conductance, highly selective (Na^+ over K^+), and amiloride-sensitive epithelial Na^+ channel[78,79] (ENaC). ENaC was cloned from rat distal colon by functional expression in Xenopus oocytes. The channel is composed of three homologous subunits denoted α-, β-, and γ-ENaC, which share 30 to 40% identity at the level of their amino acid sequences. In addition to these three well-characterized ENaC subunits, a fourth EnaC subunit, δ-ENaC, has been cloned from a human kidney cDNA library.[80] However, this subunit has been described so far only in humans, and its relevance for transepithelial Na^+ reabsorption in the ASDN is unclear. When the three classical α-, β-, and γ-ENaC subunits are co-expressed in Xenopus laevis oocytes, the subunits form a channel with functional characteristics similar to the channel identified by Palmer in the rat CCD, with a low 5 pS conductance (for Na^+), a high selectivity ratio of Na^+ over K^+ (>20), and a high sensitivity for amiloride with a K_i in the submicromolar range. In the Xenopus oocyte expression system, the co-expression of all three ENaC subunits is required for maximal cell surface abundance and activity of the channel.[81] The subunit stoichiometry of the active channel is not finally resolved. Various technical approaches suggested models with four, eight or nine subunits.[82] Recently, the crystal structure of the closely related acid-sensing ion channel isoform ASIC1$_A$ has been reported, and points to a trimeric oligomerization of the channel.[83,84] However, this trimeric model still awaits further confirmation by establishing the crystal structure of ENaC itself.

ENaC is expressed in several organs including the kidney, the colon, the salivary and sweat glands.

ENaC-mediated Na$^+$ transport helps to adjust Na$^+$ excretion in the urine, feces, and sweat. In lung and airways, ENaC activity is important for alveolar liquid clearance and regulation of mucous fluidity. In the taste buds of the tongue, ENaC is likely involved in salt tasting, whereas ENaC expression in the eye and inner ear may help to control the ionic composition of the aqueous humor and the endolymph, respectively.[82] In the kidney the distribution of ENaC is fully compatible with its involvement in aldosterone-dependent Na$^+$ transport. Morphological and functional studies on rodent and human kidneys[11,13] clearly showed that the ENaC subunits are highly abundant along the entire ASDN, starting in the late DCT (DCT2), and extending through the CNT down to the medullary CD. In the ASDN cells, increased plasma aldosterone levels induced either by dietary Na$^+$ restriction or by exogenous application appear to stimulate ENaC mainly by three mechanisms. First, aldosterone increases the abundance of the α-ENaC mRNA and protein, without much affecting the mRNAs encoding for the β- and γ-subunits.[85–87] In contrast, the β- and γ-subunit mRNAs are upregulated in the colon by aldosterone, while the α-subunit mRNA is expressed constitutively.[85,86,88] Second, aldosterone induces the appearance of low molecular weight forms of α- and γ-ENaC, which are thought to represent proteolytically activated channel subunits.[89–91] Recently, Frindt and co-workers performed cell surface biotinylation experiments on rat kidneys perfused with biotin in situ. These experiments showed that feeding a low-Na$^+$ diet or the infusion of aldosterone for one week increases the cell surface pool of cleaved α- and γ-ENaC, but not β-ENaC subunits at the cell surface.[92] Third, aldosterone causes a redistribution of ENaC channel subunits from intracellular storage compartments to the apical plasma membrane. In fact, the subcellular localization of ENaC along the axis of the ASDN changes drastically with altered plasma aldosterone levels in response to altered dietary Na$^+$ intake.[90,93] In rodents kept under a high dietary Na$^+$ intake with low plasma aldosterone levels, ENaC subunits are barely detectable at the luminal membrane, and are found almost exclusively at intracellular sites. On a standard dietary Na$^+$ intake with moderate plasma aldosterone levels, ENaC subunits are traceable at the luminal membrane in the late DCT and the early CNT, but in downstream segments (i.e., late CNT and CD), particularly β- and γ-ENaC are found almost exclusively at intracellular sites.[93] Only the α-EnaC-subunit was reported to have a more pronounced apical localization and can be found at the apical plasma membrane in CNT and CD.[94] In response to dietary Na$^+$ restriction, the apical abundance of ENaC subunits drastically increases due to a translocation of channel subunits from intracellular compartments to the apical plasma membrane.[59,90,93,95,96] Nevertheless, the axial gradient for apical ENaC prevails, and the apical localization of ENaC subunits remains more prominent in early ASDN than in late ASDN.[12,97] The activation and apical translocation of ENaC occurs rapidly (within hours), suggesting that they are relevant for the renal adaptation to day-to-day variations of Na$^+$ intake.[3,89,98] Likewise, injection of aldosterone in adrenalectomized rats induces a rapid (within 2 hours) induction of α-ENaC-subunit expression along the ASDN which is followed by a translocation of all three ENaC subunits to the apical plasma membrane (Figure 35.3). Again, the apical shift occurs predominantly in the early and not in the late ASDN, although the induction of α-ENaC was seen to be similar along the entire segment.[3] Based on previous studies in Xenopus laevis A6 cells, it has been proposed that the induction of α-ENaC might be a prerequisite for full assembly of ENaC in the ER and its subsequent delivery to the cell surface.[99] However, in the kidney in vivo the induction of α-ENaC protein by aldosterone is rather small[90] and, at least in the CCD, not necessarily followed by an apical redistribution of all three ENaC subunits.[3] Moreover, apical targeting of ENaC apparently occurs even without previous α-ENaC induction.[100] Likewise, when ENaC activity was assessed as whole-cell amiloride-sensitive current, ENaC activity in rat CCD was drastically increased within 15 hours of salt restriction, and thus in a timeframe in which no changes in the abundance of ENaC mRNA or protein could be detected.[89] Thus, the induction of α-ENaC alone cannot account for the apical targeting of ENaC. Other co-stimulatory factors are needed. One of these factors was proposed to be the serum- and glucocorticoid-regulated kinase (Sgk1). Sgk1 is a member of the PKB/Akt family of serine/threonine kinases, and is rapidly induced by aldosterone in ASDN model epithelia in vitro, as well as in the kidney in vivo.[3,101–103] Likewise, prolonged dietary Na$^+$ restriction increases Sgk1 mRNA expression in the kidney.[104] Co-expression of ENaC with Sgk1 in heterologous expression systems profoundly increases ENaC-mediated Na$^+$-currents, most likely by an accelerated insertion-rate of ENaC into the plasma membrane.[105] Consistently, the induction of Sgk1 by aldosterone precedes the apical translocation of ENaC in ASDN cells in vitro and Sgk1-deficient mice (Table 35.1) show mild urinary Na$^+$-wasting that becomes aggravated on dietary Na$^+$ restriction.[106] At least part of the effects of Sgk1 on ENaC cell surface abundance is mediated by an Sgk1-dependent phosphorylation of the ubiquitin-protein ligase Nedd4-2. Nedd4-2 phosphorylation blocks the interaction of this ligase with the C-terminus of ENaC subunits, and thereby presumably prevents

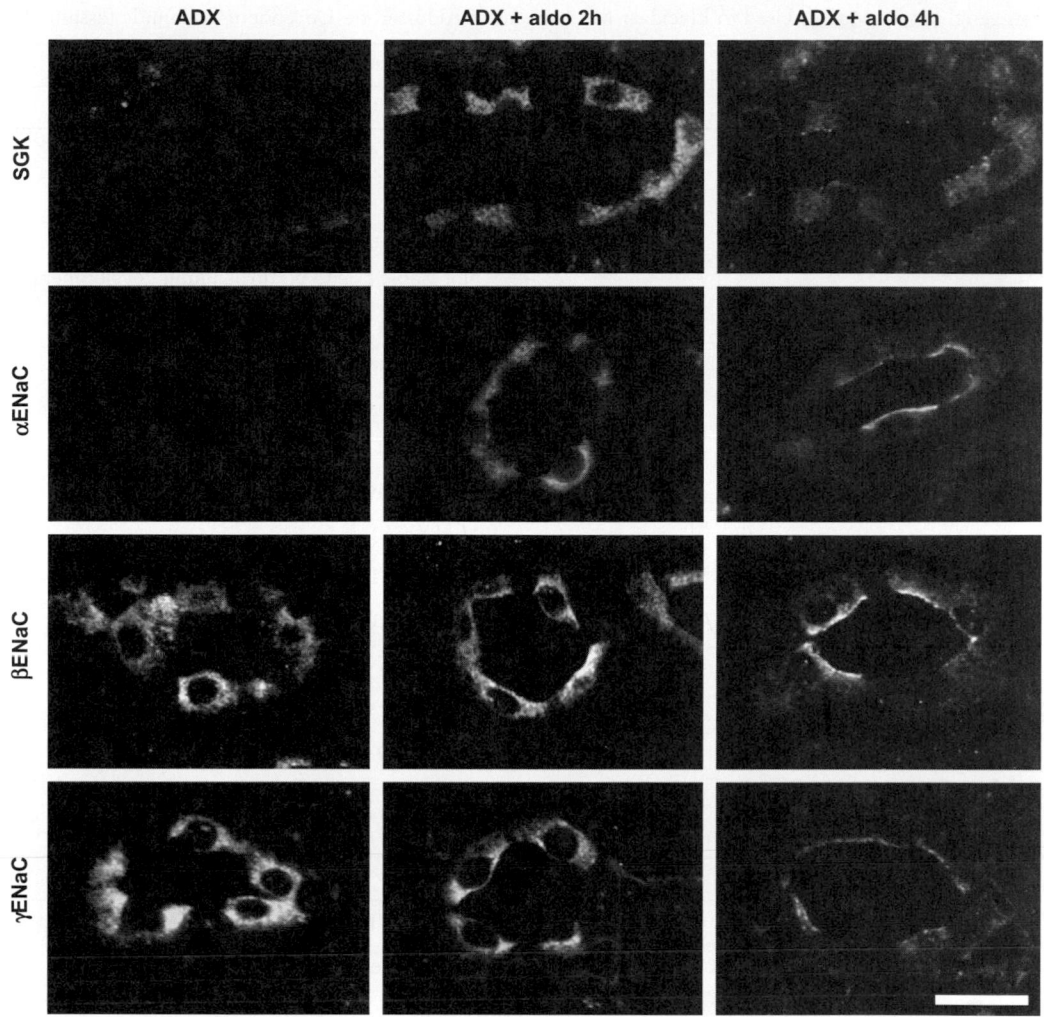

FIGURE 35.3 CNT profiles in kidney from ADX rats, 2 and 4 hours after aldosterone injection. Immunofluorescence with rabbit antisera against α-, β-, and γ-ENaC, and the serum-and-glucocorticoid-induced kinase (SGK1) on cryostat sections is shown. Unstained cells in the CNT epithelium are intercalated cells. Aldosterone induces a rapid induction of SGK1 and α-ENaC (at 2 hours) that precedes the apical translocation of all three ENaC subunits from intracellular sites towards the apical plasma membrane (at 4 hours). *(Adapted from Loffing, J., et al. (2001).[3])*

Nedd4-2-induced ubiquitylation and subsequent endocytosis and degradation of ENaC subunits.[107–109] Interestingly, immunohistochemical studies showed that the Nedd4-2 abundance increases along the ASDN, which is inverse to the axial gradient of apical ENaC abundance, and further supports the idea that Nedd4-2 is a negative regulator of ENaC cell surface abundance.[110]

Patch-clamp studies corroborated the immunohistochemically traceable axial gradient of the apical localization of ENaC.[111] The ASDN segments isolated from rats kept on a standard lab chow exhibited no amiloride-sensitive currents at the single channel level, whereas CNTs and CDs isolated from rats with elevated plasma aldosterone levels revealed significant single channel ENaC currents (Figure 35.4). Mice appear to have sizeable ENaC whole-cell currents

already on a standard diet, which further increase when animals are kept on low dietary Na^+ intake.[112] In general, amiloride-sensitive currents decrease in the following order: CNT > initial CD > CD.[113] These findings on apical ENaC localization and activity are consistent with previous studies on microperfused rat tubules,[7] and on isolated rabbit tubules[5] that established several times higher Na^+ transport rates in early ASDN (i.e., DCT and CNT) than in further downstream ASDN segments (i.e., CD). The axial gradient of ENaC also parallels the progressive decrease of the basolateral Na^+, K^+-ATPase activity along the ASDN.[4] Taken together, these data clearly indicate that the aldosterone-dependent adaptation of renal Na^+ excretion to dietary Na^+ intake occurs through ENaC, predominantly in the early ASDN, while the late ASDN gets recruited only under high plasma

TABLE 35.1 Transgenic Mouse Models Used to Elucidate Mechanisms of Aldosterone-Dependent Sodium/Potassium Transport

Strain	Phenotype	References
	Signaling Cascade	
MR − / −	Severe PHA-1	187,189
MR − / −, CNT/CD-specific (MRlox/lox AQP2Cre)	Mild PHA-1	116
MR − / −, CNT/CD-specific, inducible (MRlox/lox AQP2CreERT2)	Mild PHA-1	190
GR − / −	Not viable due to perturbed lung development	192
GR − / −, distal tubule-specific (GRlox/lox KspCre)	Slightly elevated blood pressure	194
GR overexpression, CD-specific (hGR Hoxb7-tetON2)	Mild renal sodium retention	193
Mutation GR knockin (hGRM604L)	Increased sensitivity to glucocorticoids	276
11-b HSD2 − / −	Severe AME	199
11-b HSD2 + / −	Salt-sensitive hypertension	277
Sgk1 − / −	Mild PHA1	106,278,279
Sgk1 − / − (Sgk1lox/lox c-TgCMVcre)	Mild PHA1	232
Sgk1 − / −, renal tubule-specific (Sgk1lox/lox Pax8/LC1)	Mild PHA1	233
Nedd4-2 − / −	Salt-sensitive hypertension	229
Nedd4-2 − / −	Not viable due to respiratory distress	231
Nedd4-2 − / −	Cystic fibrosis-like lung phenotype	230
Nedd4-2 − / −, renal tubule-specific (Nedd4-2lox/lox Pax8/LC1)	NCC upregulation	60
CHIF − / −	Mild renal and colon defect in Na/K transport	264
	ENaC	
α-ENaC − / −	Not viable due to respiratory distress	132
α-ENaC − / −, CD-specific (α-ENaClox/lox Hoxb7Cre)	No obvious phenotype	95
α-ENaC − / −, CNT/CD-specific (α-ENaClox/lox AQP2Cre)	Mild PHA-1	115
Transgenic α-ENaC − / − Tg	Mild PHA-1	133
Mutation β-ENaCm/m	Mild PHA-1	139
Mutation γ-ENaCL/L	Liddle's syndrome, salt-sensitive hypertension	77,127,128,280
β-ENaC − / −	Severe PHA-1	136
β-ENaC + / −	Very mild PHA-1	281
γ-ENaC − / −	Severe PHA-1	135

aldosterone levels. Using whole-cell current data, and considering the anatomical length of the two segments, Frindt and Palmer estimated that the Na$^+$ transport capacity of the CNT is at least 10 times higher than that of the CD.[113]

The importance of the early ASDN versus late ASDN for the maintenance of Na$^+$ balance was highlighted by the development of a mouse model with targeted inactivation of α-ENaC in the collecting duct.[95] These mice survive well and are able to maintain Na$^+$ and K$^+$ balance, even when challenged by salt restriction or K$^+$-loading (Figure 35.5a). Moreover, these mice show a normal urinary acidification in response to furosemide and thiazide treatment,[114] suggesting that functional expression of ENaC in the CNT is sufficient for maintaining ion homeostasis. In contrast, mice with targeted inactivation of α-ENaC in CD and CNT show symptoms of renal salt-wasting (Figure 35.5b). Already under control conditions, the mice have significantly higher urinary Na$^+$ excretion and increased plasma aldosterone levels. With dietary Na$^+$ restriction, the mice start to decompensate and exhibited at day 15 a more than 12% reduction in body weight and exceedingly high plasma aldosterone levels (~20,000 pg/ml in knockout

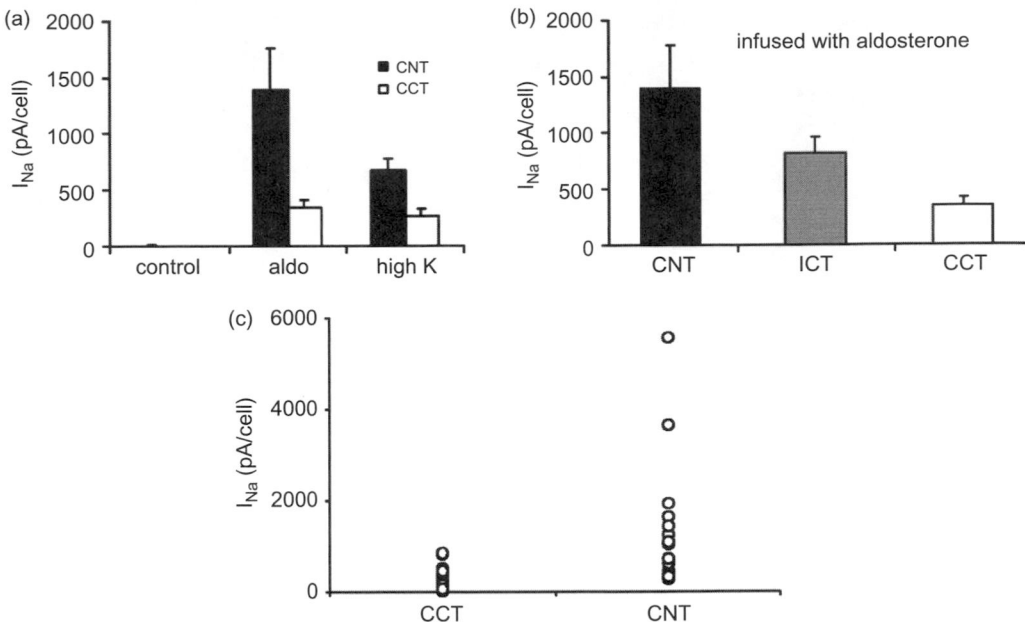

FIGURE 35.4   Sodium transport in CNT and principal cells of the ASDN (I_{Na}). (a) I_{Na} in CNT and cortical collecting tubule (CCT) of control rats fed a normal (control) diet, aldosterone treated rats fed a normal diet or rats fed a high-K diet. (b) I_{Na} in cells of CNT, initial collecting tubule (ICT), and CCT of aldosterone-treated rats. (c) Individual values of I_{Na} in CCT and CNT cells of aldosterone-treated rats. *(From Frindt, G., and Palmer, L.G. (2004).[113])*

mice versus ~1200 pg/ml in control mice). Moreover, the mice show hyperkalemia, that worsens with dietary K$^+$-loading. Furthermore, the mice are polyuric, consistent with the idea that ENaC is important not only for renal Na$^+$ and K$^+$ handling, but also for the control of water reabsorption.[115]

Similar to this CNT and CD α-ENaC knockout model, mice with targeted deletion of the MR in the CD and CNT, but intact MR expression and ENaC regulation in early CNT and DCT2, show impaired Na$^+$ balance (Figure 35.6). Although these mice develop normally under a standard diet, they continuously lose body weight and show signs of severe extracellular volume contraction under a low-Na$^+$ diet.[116] These studies did also show that the MR is crucial for the increased expression of αENaC and apical targeting of all three ENaC subunits in response to dietary Na$^+$ restriction. Interestingly, these observations in mice with genetic deletion of the MR contrast with findings in rodents with pharmacological inhibition of the MR. In rats, blockade of the MR by spironolactone does not prevent the apical translocation of ENaC in response to dietary Na$^+$ restriction.[100] Likewise, the combined inhibition of the MR and GR by spironolactone and RU486 does not block the induction of αENaC and ENaC trafficking induced by aldosterone-infusion.[117] Together with the observation that the severe symptoms of pseudohypoaldosteronism in MR-deficient mice can be improved by glucocorticoid treatment,[118] and that mice with CNT/CD-specific MR-deficiency have a milder

phenotype than mice with CNT/CD-specific deletion of αENaC, the data point to some redundancies in the MR and GR-dependent signaling pathways that control ENaC function.

ENaC-Related Genetic Diseases Underline Pathophysiological Relevance

The discovery that rare monogenic diseases caused by mutations in the genes encoding the ENaC subunits cause defects in the control of Na$^+$ balance and blood pressure provided direct evidence for the implication of this channel in these processes.[119] Remarkably, these diseases represent on the one hand, a gain-of-function phenotype (Liddle's syndrome), and on the other hand a loss-of-function disease (pseudohypoaldosteronism type I or PHAI).

LIDDLE'S SYNDROME

Liddle's syndrome is a rare disorder (pseudoaldosteronism) described first by G. W. Liddle in a family in which multiple siblings had early onset of severe hypertension associated with hypokalemia.[120] Urinary excretion of aldosterone was low in these patients, and no effects of spironolactone on blood pressure could be demonstrated. By contrast, administration of the Na$^+$ channel-blocker triamterene, together with restriction of salt intake, tended to normalize blood pressure. These clinical features suggested that hypertension was due to excessive aldosterone-independent Na$^+$ reabsorption in the distal nephron, due to the constitutive

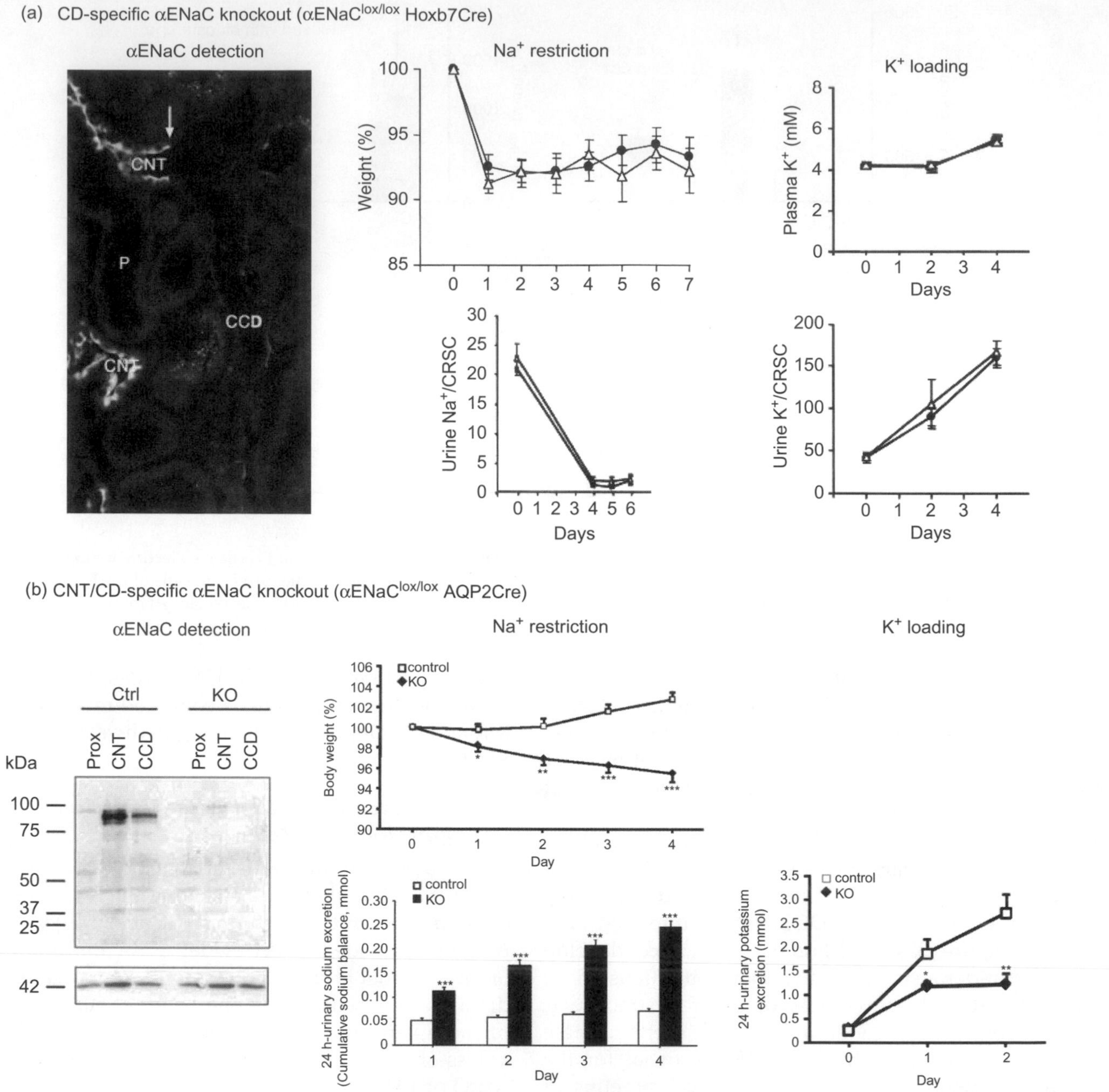

(a)   CD-specific αENaC knockout (αENaC$^{lox/lox}$ Hoxb7Cre)

(b) CNT/CD-specific αENaC knockout (αENaC$^{lox/lox}$ AQP2Cre)

FIGURE 35.5   Different phenotype of mice with targeted deletion of α-ENaC in the CD only (a) or in the CD and CD (b). Left panels (a) and (B): Detection of α-ENaC by immunohistochemistry (a) or immunoblotting (b) confirms the efficient deletion of α-ENaC in the targeted segments in the mouse models. Middle panels (a) and (b): On dietary Na$^+$ restriction, MR$^{lox/lox}$ Hoxb7Cre mice do not lose more body weight than control mice, while MR$^{lox/lox}$ AQP2Cre mice lose more body weight than controls. Moreover, MR$^{lox/lox}$ AQP2Cre mice do not retain Na$^+$ from the urine as efficently as control mice. Right panels (a) and (b): MR$^{lox/lox}$ Hoxb7Cre mice tolerate dietary K$^+$-loading without any differences from control mice with respect to plasma K$^+$ levels and fractional urinary K$^+$ excretion. In contrast, MR$^{lox/lox}$ AQP2Cre mice become hyperkalemic (Serum K$^+$ 7.7 ± 0.8 mM vs. 5.2 ± 0.2 mM in controls) and excrete less K$^+$ with their urine than control mice. *(Adapted from (a) Rubera, I., et al. (2003).[95]; and (b) from Christensen, B. M., et al. (2010)[115].)*

activation of ENaC. Despite the low plasma aldosterone in these patients, they still responded to aldosterone injections by further decreasing their renal Na$^+$ excretion.

The pedigree of the original kindred described by Liddle was in the meantime extended, clearly demonstrating the autosomal dominant inheritance of the disease.[121] A candidate gene approach was used to

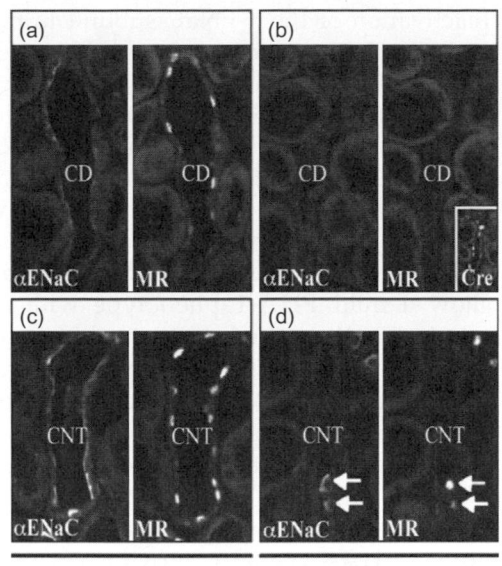

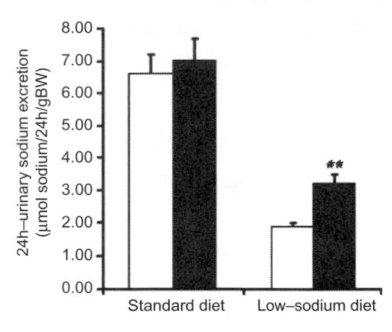

Diet	Plasma Aldosterone (pg/ml)	
	Controls	MR^AQP2Cre
Standard	430 ± 82 (7)	5195 ± 701 (11)[b]
Low-sodium (3 d)	1083 ± 154 (10)[c]	10500 ± 990 (9)[b,c]
Low-sodium (10 d)	3167 ± 423 (3)[c]	19719 ± 1667 (8)[b,c]

FIGURE 35.6 **Renal sodium wasting in transgenic mice with CNT- and CD-specific deletion of the MR (MR^AQPcre mice).** (a)–(d) Immunofluorescent detection of α-ENaC and MR in collecting ducts (CD) and connecting tubules (CNT) of control mice and of MR^AQPcre mice kept for 10 days on a low-NaCl diet. Deletion of the MR goes along with a loss of detectable α-ENaC levels. In only a few CNT cells with inefficient MR-targeting, does α-ENaC remain detectable at the cell surface (arrows). Insert in panel (b) shows expression of the Cre recombinase in the CCD of the transgenic mouse. While the rate of urinary Na⁺ excretion does not differ between the groups on a standard diet, MR^AQPcre mice cannot lower their urinary Na⁺ excretion as efficiently as control mice when kept for 9 days on dietary Na⁺ restriction (white bars: control mice; black bars: MR^AQPcre mice). Consistent with mild pseudohypoaldosteronism type 1, MR^AQPcre mice have higher plasma aldosterone levels than control mice on standard and low-sodium diets. *(Adapted from Ronzaud, C., et al. (2007).[116])*

identify mutations causing this rare Mendelian form of hypertension.[122] Complete linkage of the Liddle's syndrome to a locus encoding the β-subunit of ENaC, and analysis of the β gene revealed various mutations in the cytoplasmic C-terminus: deletion or frameshift mutations leading to truncation of a major portion of the C-terminus; and missense mutations in a highly-conserved proline-rich domain.[122–124] A deletion of the C-terminus in the γ-subunit has also been identified as a cause of Liddle's syndrome, whereas no mutations in the α-subunit have been linked to this disorder.[125] Expression of these β- and γ-ENaC variants, together with α-subunits in the *Xenopus* oocyte system, revealed a significant increase in ENaC channel activity at the cell surface, consistent with the initial postulate that these hyperactive channel mutants lead to an excessive Na⁺ reabsorption and hypertension.[126]

To elucidate the causal relationship between dietary salt intake, genetically-determined salt handling by the kidney, and hypertension, a mouse model for Liddle's syndrome was developed by introducing the R566stop mutation at the β-ENaC allele ("knockin" strategy).[127] Interestingly, with a normal-salt diet, mice carrying the β-ENaC mutated L/L allele remain normotensive, despite evidence of hypervolemia and increased Na⁺ reabsorption in the large intestine.

Moreover, plasma pH, Na⁺, K⁺, Cl⁻ or HCO₃⁻ concentrations were not significantly affected.[127] However, these mice manifested the classical Liddle's phenotype with higher blood pressure, metabolic alkalosis, and hypokalemia, accompanied by cardiac and renal hypertrophy in response to a high-salt diet. Moreover, evidence for impaired ENaC internalization was demonstrated *in vivo*, as the increase in urinary Na⁺ excretion upon short time (6–12 hours) salt repletion following 1 week of a low-salt diet is significantly delayed in Liddle mice, despite the presence of lower circulating aldosterone concentrations.[128] Isolated perfused CCDs from Liddle mice exhibit higher transepithelial potential differences, and confluent primary cultures of CCDs microdissected from their kidneys exhibit significant lower transepithelial electrical resistance and higher negative potential differences, consistent with an overall increased ENaC activity.[128] Interestingly, mineralocorticoid upregulation of ENaC expression and function is still maintained in Liddle mice that show a remarkable high sensitivity to aldosterone *in vitro*[129] and *in vivo*.[77] Renal CD cells from Liddle mice exhibit hyperactive apical vasopressin-regulated CFTR Cl⁻ conductance that could contribute to the enhanced NaCl reabsorption observed in the distal nephron of patients with Liddle's syndrome. In summary, in the Liddle mouse, dysfunction of ENaC in the kidney is demonstrated before onset of arterial hypertension that argues in favor of the kidney hypothesis proposed by Liddle.[120]

PSEUDOHYPOALDOSTERONISM TYPE 1

Pseudohypoaldosteronism type 1 (PHA-1) is characterized by dehydration, hyponatremia, hyperkalemia and metabolic acidosis, despite elevated plasma aldosterone concentration and plasma renin activity. The association of renal Na^+-wasting, hyperkalemia, and failure to respond to mineralocorticoids suggest a defective Na^+ reabsorption in the distal nephron. There are two forms of PHA-1, an inherited recessive disease characterized by a culminant clinical presentation in the neonatal period persisting in adulthood,[130] and an autosomal dominant or sporadic form which is milder and remits with age.[68] Genetic investigations of kindred with the recessive PHA-1 revealed deletion or missense mutations in each of the three ENaC subunits, resulting in decreased channel function when expressed in Xenopus oocytes. Linkage of PHA-1 to loss-of-function ENaC variants further supports the critical role ENaC in aldosterone regulation of Na^+ reabsorption.

Constitutive gene inactivation studies for all three subunits of ENaC (α-, β-, and γ-, encoded by *Scnn1a*, *Scnn1b*, and *Scnn1g*, respectively) revealed a crucial role for each subunit in the survival of the animal (see for review [131]). Constitutive inactivation of the mouse αENaC gene locus leads to severe respiratory distress with neonatal death, demonstrating the crucial role of ENaC in lung liquid clearance at birth.[132] The αENaC knockout neonates died so rapidly from their lung phenotype that they did not manifest any electrolyte disturbances. However, mice with a genetic rescue by reintroducing the αENaC-subunit under the control of a heterologous (cytomegalovirus) promoter demonstrated the importance of precise regulation of ENaC in the kidney.[133] The transgenic rescued mice had sufficient basal Na^+ absorptive capacity to clear lung liquid and survive the early neonatal period, but developed a severe PHA-1 like phenotype with renal salt-wasting, metabolic acidosis, high aldosterone levels, growth retardation, and increased early mortality.[134] In contrast to the αENaC knockout mice, mice with constitutive inactivation of βENaC and γENaC revealed severe early renal dysfunction.[135,136] Urinary Na^+-wasting, K^+ retention, and increased plasma aldosterone concentrations go along with failure to thrive and early postnatal deaths (see for review [137,138]). It seems that low residual ENaC activity in these mice is sufficient to circumvent the neonatal lung phenotype, consistent with the assumption that $\alpha\beta$- and $\alpha\gamma$-subunit combinations can establish some ENaC activity in airway epithelia.

Inactivation of the γ-ENaC-subunit in mice resulted in early death (at 36 hours after birth) of the mice, mainly due to disturbed total body electrolyte balance.[135] In the course of generating a mouse model for Liddle's syndrome by the insertion of a stop codon corresponding to residue R566 in human β-ENaC, together with the selection marker neomycin, mice were obtained with a partial disruption of the β-ENaC gene locus (β-ENaCm/m).[139] Under a normal-salt diet, these mice show a mild PHA-1 phenotype with reduced ENaC activity and elevated plasma aldosterone levels, but develop an acute PHA-1 with continuous weight loss, hyperkalemia, and decreased blood pressure when kept under a low-salt diet.

In summary, although the onset and severity of PHA-1 symptoms vary in these models, the renal phenotype of these mice corresponds well to the human PHA-1 phenotype (with salt-wasting, hyperkalemia, and metabolic acidosis), revealing the important implication of ENaC in Na^+, K^+ homeostasis.

Aldosterone and K^+ Secretion

The ASDN of mammals also plays a critical role in the maintenance of K^+ homeostasis. In this nephron segment, Na^+ reabsorption through ENaC is electrically coupled with K^+ secretion: increasing the Na^+ influx depolarizes the apical membrane and increases the driving force for K^+ secretion into the lumen, and *vice versa* (see Figure 35.2). Pathophysiological conditions where Na^+ absorption is increased in the ASDN (hyperaldosteronism, pseudoaldosteronism) are associated with hypokalemia; conversely, ENaC loss-of-function in PHA-1 results in a loss of Na^+ absorption in the ASDN and hyperkalemia (see above). Consistently, mice with constitutive inactivation of β- and γ-ENaC show renal Na^+-wasting and elevated plasma aldosterone level that goes along with renal K^+ retention and hyperkalemia.[135,136] While mice lacking the α-ENaC subunit die soon after birth due to respiratory insufficiency related to impaired alveolar fluid clearance,[132] mice with targeted inactivation of α-ENaC in the CNT and CD survive, and show not only renal salt-wasting, but also hyperkalemia,[115] further confirming the critical role of ENaC for Na^+ and K^+ homeostasis.

The K^+ secretion in the ASDN is mediated by a K^+ conductive pathway in the apical membrane of principal cells. Small conductance inwardly rectifying K^+ channels, termed SK channels, account for most of the apical conductance of principal cells.[140–142] These SK channels have been identified at the molecular level and are the product of the ROMK channel gene. Moreover, the large, Ca^{2+}-activated K^+ channel (BK), present in intercalated and/or principal cells, is thought to contribute to K^+ secretion along the ASDN.[17]

Experiments in mice deficient for either ROMK or the α-subunit of BK suggest that the channels may compensate for each other.[143,144] The functional role and the regulation of these channels in the kidney have been the topic of several recent reviews,[16,18,19,145] and are also extensively addressed in a separate chapter in this book. Therefore, we will here only briefly touch the possible impact of aldosterone on renal K^+ secretion via these channels.

High dietary K^+ intake and elevated plasma K^+ concentrations increase aldosterone secretion by the zona glomerulosa of the adrenal gland and stimulate urinary K^+ excretion. This raises the question of whether aldosterone has a primary effect on K^+ secretion, via genomic effects on principal cells of the ASDN. However, although some studies indicated that aldosterone may directly affect the activity of the renal secretory K^+ channels,[33−36] there is no strong evidence that aldosterone at physiological concentrations increases the apical K^+ conductance of principal cells in the CCD in vivo.[146] In fact, rats fed with a low-Na^+ diet have a high plasma level of aldosterone and show a large increase in the density of active ENaC channels in the apical membrane of principal cells, but the density of ROMK channels remains unchanged.[147] Recently, Fodstad and co-workers described that the established mouse CCD cell line (mCCD(cl1)) expresses ROMK mRNA and a robust Ba^{2+}- and tertiapin-Q sensitive K^+ conductance in the apical membrane.[148] Overnight exposure to 100 nM aldosterone did not significantly change the K^+ conductance, but it increased the amiloride-sensitive Na^+ transport. Surprisingly, in this cell model the mRNA levels of all ROMK isoforms measured by qRT-PCR were even decreased by 15−45%, further supporting the idea that aldosterone does not directly stimulate ROMK.

Nevertheless, a high dietary K^+ intake increases both the activity of ENaC and of ROMK (Figure 35.4). Interestingly, the kaliuretic response to dietary K^+ occurs very rapidly, and even before plasma K^+ and aldosterone levels are elevated. Moreover, renal kaliuresis can be clearly dissociated from renal Na^+ handling (for review see [145,149]). In a recent study, Frindt and Palmer addressed the question of whether the concomitant activation of ENaC is required for enhanced urinary K^+ excretion. Rats were kept on different K^+ diets, and then infused via osmotic minipumps with a constant dose of amiloride which was supposed to block more than 98% of Na^+ transport through ENaC. Measurements of urinary K^+ excretion indicated that on a control diet (0.6% KCl), distal nephron K^+ secretion completely depends on ENaC, while on a high-K^+ diet (10% KCl) an increasing fraction of K^+ excretion is independent of Na^+ channels.[150]

Taken together, the current evidence suggests that the activation of ENaC by aldosterone is sufficient to increase the driving force for K^+ secretion, leading to an increase in kaliuresis, without upregulating K^+ channels. In contrast, a high-K^+ diet increases the density of active ROMK channels, suggesting the presence of kaliuretic factors that control K^+ secretion, independently of aldosterone.[145,149]

Aldosterone and the Na^+,K^+-ATPase

For efficient transepithelial sodium reabsorption, apical Na^+ entry via ENaC has to be matched by Na^+ extrusion across the basolateral plasma membrane via the Na^+,K^+-ATPase. Consistently, the activity of the Na^+,K^+-ATPase is also regulated by aldosterone (for a review see [151,152]). Briefly, it was already shown 30 years ago that aldosterone induced augmentation of Na^+,K^+-ATPase in the CCD of adrenalectomized rats after 1 to 3 hours of aldosterone infusion.[153,154] In non-adrenalectomized animals, aldosterone also induced the Na^+ pump, but the response was delayed and observable between 2 days and 1 week.[48] In the rabbit CCD, Sansom and O'Neil observed a doubling in the basolateral membrane conductance after 24 hours of the mineralocorticoid DOCA (deoxycorticosterone acetate) treatment, which could be accounted for by a rise in basolateral K^+ and Cl^- conductance.[155] Moreover, morphometric studies revealed a significant increase in the basal side surface area of the rabbit CCD principal cells, which can be correlated with an increase in single cell capacitance.[156,157] However, these changes in cell surface area could only partially account for the increase in basolateral membrane conductance. It is not clear in these cases whether the mineralocorticoid-induced increase in basolateral membrane conductance is a direct effect of the hormone or secondary to an increase in Na^+ entry into the cell.

As discussed in,[151] it is likely that the early effects involve activation and/or translocation to the basolateral membrane of pre-existing Na^+,K^+-ATPases, whereas the late effects are caused by de novo synthesis of the Na^+,K^+-ATPase. Indeed, it has been shown both in adrenalectomized rats and in mpkCCD$_{cl4}$ cells that infusion or treatment for 2 to 3 hours with aldosterone strongly increases the cell surface abundance of Na^+,K^+-ATPase, whereas the total cellular pool was only affected later.[152,158,159] It was shown by the same researchers that Sgk1 is able to increase the cell surface expression of Na^+,K^+-ATPase,[160] providing a potential mechanism of how aldosterone may regulate the pump. However, it remains open if the kinase regulates Na^+,K^+-ATPase by direct phosphorylation or not.

Hence, aldosterone is able to modify Na^+,K^+-ATPase activity by increasing the number of Na^+,K^+-ATPase at the basolateral membrane, likely by translocating pre-existing pumps to the surface (short-term regulation), and by increasing the de novo synthesis of Na^+,K^+-ATPases. Moreover, aldosterone is also able to increase the basolateral membrane surface. The cellular and molecular mechanisms that are involved in this regulation are only vaguely known, and may involve Sgk1.

SODIUM TRANSPORT REGULATION BY ALDOSTERONE: CELLULAR AND MOLECULAR MECHANISMS

Non-Genomic Actions of Aldosterone

Aldosterone, similar to many other steroid hormones, has two fundamentally different mechanisms of action, namely rapid, non-genomic effects that are different from the classical and delayed genomic effects, involving MR and GR and the induction of a complex translational/transcriptional response.[161,162] The non-genomic effects of aldosterone on intracellular signaling pathways have been demonstrated in a variety of animal and human cell types, including those localized in the classical mineralocorticoid target organs.[161,162] These effects are characterized by short latencies of seconds or minutes, and do not involve changes in gene expression mediated by the transcriptional role of the MR.[163] They may involve MR itself and being sensitive to MR antagonists such as spironolactone or eplerenone or being independent of MR. The existence of an alternative receptor with high affinity for aldosterone has been postulated, which may be membrane-bound or representing a signaling molecule within the cell. Recently it has been shown that aldosterone signals independently of MR through GPR-30, an intracellular G-protein-coupled receptor localized in the endoplasmic reticulum, leading to extracellular related kinase (ERK) activation and apoptosis, and to myosin light chain phosphorylation.[164,165] It will be important to determine the role of GPR-30 in the ASDN, where its presence has been reported.[166]

The non-genomic effects involve the activation of protein kinase pathways, including mitogen activated protein (MAP) kinases, protein kinase D1 (PKD1), and protein kinase C (PKC).[162] Interestingly, PKCα (a PKC isoform) directly binds in vitro aldosterone via its C2 domain, leading to its autophosphorylation. Hence, PKCα may represent an intracellular aldosterone receptor distinct from the classical MR. PKC signaling is an illustrative example of cross-talk between non-genomic and genomic pathways, as demonstrated in cultured rat cortical collecting duct cells, in which transepithelial Na^+ transport may be stimulated in the early phase by PKCα and independent of MR, whereas the late phase requires genomic action via MR.[167] Also involved in short non-genomic activation of ENaC may

be PKD1 that appears to regulate subcellular localization of αENaC in M1 CCD cells.[168] Together, the number of different non-genomic effects of aldosterone that have been described, the lack of physiological targets in many cases, as well as the potentially diverse modes of action, do not allow us to draw a unifying conclusion. However, it is likely that non-genomic actions and genomic actions of aldosterone interfere in some instances with each other for the control of physiological functions.

Genomic Actions of Aldosterone

Mineralocorticoid Receptor (MR) and Glucocorticoid Receptor (GR)

As discussed above, both MR and GR act as aldosterone receptors, having different affinities to aldosterone. MR is the high-affinity type 1 receptor (K_d approximately 0.5 to 2 nmol/l), and GR is the low-affinity type 2 receptor (K_d approximately 14 to 60 nmol/l).[169] On the other hand, the glucocorticosteroid hormone cortisol (corticosterone in rodents) binds to MR with high affinity similar to that of aldosterone, and with a higher affinity to GR.[14,170] Cell-specific hormone and receptor specificity-conferring mechanisms discussed below are necessary to explain the differences in the response to mineralocorticoids and glucocorticoids at the systemic and organ levels.[161,171,172] It is important to note that the precise role of these two receptors (MR versus GR), the extent of their functional overlap, and the role of specificity-conferring mechanism are not fully-understood, and the analysis of MR/GR-modified animals may help to clarify these issues.

The clinical importance of the MRs was demonstrated in patients carrying mutations in the gene leading to an autosomal dominant form of pseudohypoaldosteronism, a disease that remits with age.[68] Moreover, various heterozygous loss-of-function mutations in the human MR (hMR) gene have been identified and characterized, including frameshift, nonsense, and missense mutations, and gene deletions.[173,174] In contrast, a constitutive active mutation in MR (S810L) has been found in patients with an early-onset hypertension that is markedly exacerbated in females during pregnancy.[175] This mutation alters the receptor specificity, and renders progesterone and other steroids lacking 21-hydroxyl groups, normally MR antagonists, to potent agonists of the receptor. Biochemical studies revealed that the S810L mutation induces a change in the receptor conformation, which increases the steroid—receptor complex stability, contributing to the agonistic action.[176,177]

MR and GR belong to the nuclear receptor superfamily that includes other steroid hormone receptors, including the thyroid hormone, retinoic acid, vitamin D. These nuclear receptors are modular proteins harboring different conserved domains.[178] The N-terminal domain is the less conserved among nuclear receptors, both in size and sequence, and represents in the case of MR almost half of the protein. This region contains a ligand-independent activation function, which is important for interaction with transcriptional co-regulators, and for intramolecular interactions with the ligand-binding domain (LBD) that lies at the C-terminus.[14,172] This latter domain is complex, as it harbors regions involved in formation of the ligand-binding pocket, interaction with heat shock proteins, dimerization, and a ligand-dependent activation function, which interacts with transcriptional co-regulators. The centrally located DNA-binding domain (DBD) is the most conserved region of the receptor. It folds into two zinc fingers, in which one zinc atom is tetra-coordinated by four cysteines. The core DBD contains two α-helices; the first one, or recognition helix, binds to the major groove of DNA making contacts with specific bases. This domain also contains segments involved in receptor homo- and heterodimerization. Putative nuclear localization signals are localized in the C-terminal part of the DBD and the beginning of the hinge region. Acting as enhancers or repressors of transcription, steroid receptors target specific DNA sequences; these hormone-responsive elements (HREs) then confer inducibility/repressibility to the genes by the corresponding hormone.[172]

In the absence of a ligand, the corticosteroid receptors and possibly all other members of the steroid receptor gene family are primarily localized in the cytosol and associated to a heat shock protein complex, which includes Hsp90, Hsp70, p23, p48, FK-binding protein 51, 52, 59 immunophilins or cyclophillin 40[171,179] (Figure 35.7). This maintains the receptors in an inactive, but ligand binding-competent and stable conformation. Recently it was suggested that this complex also binds via FKB52 to the motor protein dynein, promoting MR translocation into the nucleus.[180] Thereby, the classical concept that MR dissociates from the complex in order to translocate through the nuclear pore was challenged by showing that MR-Hsp90 cross-linked complexes accumulate in the nucleus in an aldosterone-dependent fashion (Figure 35.7). Hsp90 also stabilizes the MR, as inhibition of Hsp90 with the geldanamycin analog 17-AAG (17-Allylamino-17-demethoxygeldanamycin) promotes rapid ubiquitylation by the CHIP (carboxyl terminus of Hsc70-interacting protein) ubiquitin-protein ligase and consequent proteasomal degradation.[181] It was suggested that treatment with 17-AAG may represent an interesting and alternative pharmacological tool to interfere with MR activation. Activation of the receptor by the binding of an agonist or some antagonists results in receptor dimerization. After nuclear translocation, the dimerized receptors will bind to the corresponding hormone-responsive elements and alter the transcription of target gene(s), as do classical sequence-specific transcription factors.[171]

Once activated and translocated to the nucleus, MR and GR associate with and recruit a complex co-activator and co-repressor machinery, involving numerous proteins[171,179] (Figure 35.7). In the case of MR, these include the transcription co-activators SRC-1, SRC-1e, and PGC-1, the histone acetylase CBP/p300, the helicase RHA, and the Pol II elongation factor ELL. The latter one represents an MR-specific transcriptional co-regulator of MR. Similar complexes are also recruited by the GR.[182] Moreover, co-repressors of the steroid receptors are recruited as well. They include SMRT and NCoR, the apoptosis-controlling DAXX and the sumo ligase PIAS that has been shown to sumoylate MR, causing inhibition of transcription activation of MR.[179] Besides sumoylation, both MR and GR become modified by numerous post-translational modifications (PTMs). These modifications involve phosphorylation, ubiquitylation, and acetylation at various sites. For many of these PTMs the functional consequences have not yet been clearly established, nor have the specific sites been determined.

There are, beside aldosterone, other high-affinity ligands for MR which do not produce the same effects, including progesterone, spironolactone, and other antagonists.[183,184] The working hypothesis to explain this specific differential response is the following: (1) agonists bind to and produce a conformational change which fully activates the receptor and elicits the maximal biologic response; (2) partial agonists fully occupy the receptor, but afford incomplete activation and thus a partial response; and (3) antagonists fully occupy the receptor, but are not able to induce a conformational change necessary for binding to target DNA and transactivation.[185] In the latter case it is assumed that MR (or GR), upon antagonist binding, translocates into the nucleus and recruit instead of the transactivation a transrepression machinery, including the co-repressors described above.[172,186]

Specific aldosterone binding, immunochemical staining, and messenger RNA detection have identified MR in classical mineralocorticoid target tissues such as kidney, gut, and sweat glands, and also in skin, brain, pituitary, and heart.[171,172] In kidney, aldosterone appears to control Na$^+$ reabsorption across the entire distal nephron from DCT to the IMCD. Indeed, presence of MR and GR protein in the distal nephron has been demonstrated.[46] Both MR and GR are expressed in the TAL, DCT, CNT, CD, and in intercalated cells.[46] The GR is found additionally in proximal tubule cells. In the study by Ackermann et al.,[46] the concept of ligand-dependent translocation into the nucleus of GR and MR

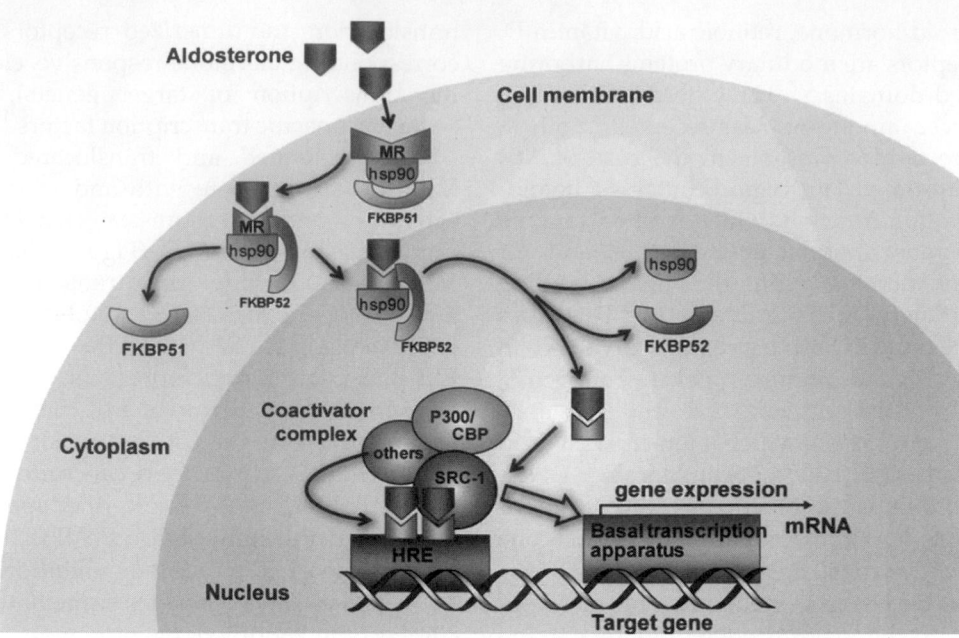

FIGURE 35.7   Model of MR transcriptional activation. In the non-stimulated state, MR is localized to the cytosol, where it is compexed to a number of proteins, including Hsp90, FKB51, FKB52, and other proteins. Upon binding to aldosterone, FKB51 dissociates, and MR/Hsp90/FKB52 translocate into the nucleus. There the complex dissociates, and MR will associate with a co-activator complex including SRC-1/P300/CBP and other proteins, and stimulate a complex transcriptional response. *(Reproduced with permission from Yang, J., and Fuller, P. J., (2012).[179])* See color section at the end of the book.

was nicely confirmed, although important differences between GR and MR were revealed (see below).

KO and Transgenic Mouse Models of MR and GR

Several mouse models have been generated to study the role of the MR and the GR for ENaC regulation and the control of ion homeostasis (Table 35.1). Mice in which the mineralocorticoid receptor (MR) was inactivated developed severe symptoms of pseudohypoaldosteronism with failure to thrive, weight loss, severe Na^+ and water loss, and highly stimulated renin–angiotensin system.[187] At day 10 after birth, these $MR^{-/-}$ mice die, since they are not able to compensate for Na^+ loss. Interestingly, amiloride-sensitive Na^+ reabsorption is reduced, but the abundance of the mRNAs encoding ENaC and Na^+,K^+-ATPase is unchanged in the kidney, indicating that regulation of Na^+ reabsorption via MR may not be achieved by transcriptional control of ENaC and Na^+,K^+-ATPase. In $MR^{-/-}$ mice, expression of the renin–angiotensin–aldosterone system (RAAS) is highly stimulated. The changes in mRNA levels of the components of the RAAS in 8-day-old $MR^{-/-}$ mice were not apparent in the heterozygous $MR^{+/-}$ mice. However, these animals have an increased urinary Na^+ loss, three-fold increase in Na^+ fractional excretion, and a modest compensatory stimulation of the circulating RAAS, revealed by a three-fold increase in renin, angiotensin II, and aldosterone levels compared with those in $MR^{+/+}$. This suggests a modest neonatal Na^+ loss,

compatible with survival in the $MR^{+/-}$ mice. This mild Na^+ loss exhibited by these heterozygous mice is similar to the phenotype observed in patients with autosomal dominant pseudohypoaldosteronism type I.[68] In patients with a heterozygous defect in the MR gene, a modest form of neonatal renal salt-wasting, with hyperkalemia and acidosis, was observed. The disease remits with age, indicating the crucial importance of aldosterone-dependent Na^+ reabsorption in the postnatal period, and its decreasing role with age.[188] Daily injections of β methasone, a synthetic glucocorticoid, from day 5 after birth onward prolonged the survival of $MR^{-/-}$ mice, suggesting that an activated GR can partially but not completely compensate for the loss of MR function.[188] Daily subcutaneous injections of NaCl from day 5 after birth until weaning and continued oral NaCl supply lead to the survival of MR knockout mice.[189] This NaCl rescue proves that neonatal MR knockout mice die because they are not able to compensate for their renal Na^+ loss. Injections of isotonic NaCl solution enabled the animals to live through a critical phase of life, after which they adapt their salt and water intake to their persisting renal salt-wasting. Mice in which tissue-specific deletion of the MR has been achieved in the late CNT and CD by Cre recombinase under the control of the AQP2 promotor (either constitutive or inducible by tamoxifen), develop normally and show unchanged Na^+ balance under standard conditions and highly elevated aldosterone levels. When kept under low Na^+ diet, mice

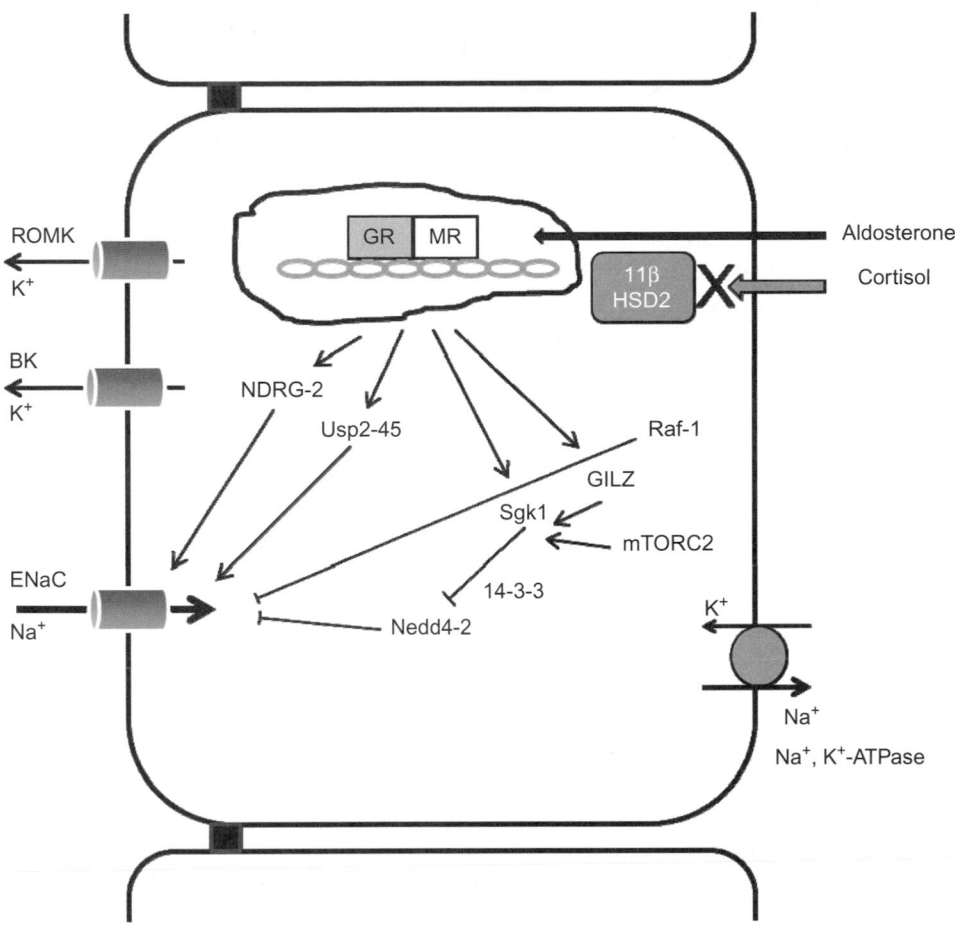

FIGURE 35.8   Model of the aldosterone-signaling cascade in the principal cells of CD/CCD. Upon binding of MR to the promotor regions of aldosterone-induced proteins (e.g., Sgk1, Usp2-45, NDRG-2, GILZ, 14-3-3β), transcription/translation leads to increased levels of these proteins. Sgk1, which is part of the ERC complex (comprising also Nedd4-2, GILZ and Raf-1), is activated by PI-3 kinase/mTORC2, stabilized by GILZ, and phosphorylates the ubiquitin-protein ligase Nedd4-2 on specific sites. 14-3-3β binds to these sites and interferes with binding and ubiquitylation of ENaC by Nedd4-2, causing reduced internalization and degradation of ENaC.

lose bodyweight due to Na^+ and water loss. The data indicate that the loss of MR in the late CNT and CD can be compensated by increased aldosterone levels, likely causing an increased MR-dependent Na^+ reabsorption in the DCT 2 and early CNT and/or activation of MR-independent sodium-retaining mechanisms in late CNT and CD.[116,190]

Constitutive hMR overexpression in all MR-expressing tissues, notably the kidney and heart, led to both renal and mild cardiac alterations compatible with hypokalemic nephropathies, despite normal K^+ serum levels.[191]

Inactivation of the GR *in vivo* resulted in perinatal death due to respiratory failure.[192] Lung maturation was severely retarded and RNA encoding ENaC was diminished, which may cause insufficient fluid clearance of the lung at birth. That the GR may play a role in the control of Na^+ handling along the ASDN can be deduced from the observation that mice with a conditional overexpression of the human GR in the CD show some signs of enhanced ENaC activation with renal

Na^+ retention.[193] However, mice with targeted deletion of the GR in the entire distal nephron do not reveal any overt phenotype, suggesting that the MR can largely compensate for the loss of the GR along the ASDN.[194]

11β-HSD2 and Molecular Determinants of Mechanisms Conferring Specificity

Aldosterone is present at low concentration in the extracellular fluid (in the order of $10^{-10}-10^{-8}$ mol/l). It can diffuse (or eventually be transported) through the plasma membrane of all cells, but may encounter a specific receptor only in target cells. The free MR and GR are localized mostly in the cytosol.[46] At the cellular level, the action of aldosterone is initiated by its binding to the MR, and under certain conditions also to the GR. However, the major glucocorticoid in humans is cortisol; in the plasma, 95% is bound to plasma proteins, in particular to the corticosteroid-binding globulin (CBG).[195] In comparison, the plasma level of aldosterone, the main mineralocorticoid hormone, is much lower (two orders of magnitude) than that of cortisol or corticosterone. Thus, the glucocorticoids, which have a similar high affinity for the MR as aldosterone, would be expected to occupy the high-affinity type I sites of MR. Indeed, even the "effective" free concentration of aldosterone, which in contrast to the natural glucocorticoids has no specific carrier plasma protein, is lower than that of glucocorticoids. However, glucocorticoids do normally not occupy MR or GR at a significant extent in aldosterone target epithelia. As described below, this is essentially due to the expression of a crucial protection mechanism represented by the 11β-hydroxysteroid dehydrogenase type 2 (11β-HSD2), which catalyzes the conversion of the active 11-hydroxycorticosteroids (cortisol and corticosterone) to 11-oxocorticosteroids (cortisone or 11-dehydrocorticosterone) that have a much lower affinity for the corticosteroid receptors.[15,196] Consequently, this mechanism allows aldosterone to occupy MR but also GR. Along the ASDN, 11β-HSD2 and MR may not only share the cellular, but also the subcellular localization. The 11β-HSD2 is thought to be restricted to the endoplasmic reticulum[197] that spans as a membranous labyrinth throughout almost the entire cytoplasm of the cells. In the non-activated state, MR may localize in direct vicinity to the 11β-HSD2, either outside or even inside the ER.[198] This close co-localization likely contributes to the efficient protection from cortisol activation. The crucial role of 11β-HSD2 for preventing the occupation of the MR by endogenous glucocorticoids is underlined by the fact that mutations of its gene or inhibition of its function by licorice (glycyrrhenetic acid) produces a syndrome of apparent mineralocorticoid excess (AME) with salt retention, arterial hypertension, and hypokalemic alkalosis.[196] Genetic inactivation of 11β-HSD2s in the mouse confirmed the crucial role of the enzyme in the protection of the MR (and GR) from circulating glucocorticoids, and allowed further study of the molecular and cellular mechanisms leading to the characteristic pathophysiology of AME.[199] About 50% of the 11β-HSD2 knockout mice die early after birth, showing muscle weakness, reduced suckling, intestinal ileus, and possible cardiac arrest, which are all likely due to the severe hypokalemia.[200] Also, the surviving knockouts exhibit hypokalemia with hypochloremia, hypotonic polyuria, and marked arterial hypertension. They further show striking histological changes, with marked hyperplasia and hypertrophy of the distal nephron, consistent with persistent MR activation, leading to the AME disease phenotype with severe electrolyte imbalances.[199] The structural changes to the ASDN cells might be irreversible, and hence may explain why suppression of endogenous glucocorticoid production does not always reverse the phenotype in AME patients.[200,201]

The utmost importance of 11β-HSD2 for the regulation of the renal corticosteroid receptors was also demonstrated by immunohistochemical studies on rat kidneys.[46] In the 11β-HSD2-positive cells of the ASDN, the MR and GR were found to be localized to the cell nuclei under control conditions. Under a high dietary Na^+ intake, when aldosterone plasma levels are low, the GR but not the MR was removed from the cell nuclei. The differential response was suggested to be the result of the different affinities of both receptors to corticosteroids. In the presence of low plasma aldosterone levels, the activity of the 11β-HSD2 is likely high enough to lower the intracellular corticosterone levels sufficiently to protect the low-affinity GR, but not the high-affinity MR, from glucocorticoid-binding and nuclear translocation. Consistently in adrenalectomized rats (having no endogenous gluco- and mineralocorticoids), any nuclear localization of the MR and GR was lacking. Infusion of low dose of corticosterone translocated the MR to the cell nucleus of all distal tubules cells, but the GR only translocated in those cells that have little or no 11β-HSD2 expression. Only when corticosterone was infused at high level, were both MR and GR located to the cell nuclei in all ASDN cells. These findings were interpreted to indicate that the 11β-HSD2 protects primarily the GR, and not the MR, from activation and translocation to the cell nuclei in the ASDN cells.[46] The separate regulation of MR and GR trafficking may allow for a differential control of MR and GR homo- and heterodimerization, which might be decisive for the induced and/or repressed transcriptional program,[44] and hence may contribute to the complexity of corticosteroid effects along the ASDN.

Other Specificity-Conferring Mechanisms

Two distinct molecular mechanisms are widely accepted to define the actions of nuclear receptors on gene expression: (1) the classic mechanisms involving transactivation and transrepression via interaction with cognate DNA-binding sites (e.g., HREs); and (2) mechanisms of transcription interference and synergy mediated by protein—protein interactions between corticosteroid receptors and other transacting factors. Transcriptional synergy, functionally defined as a more-than-additive increase in gene transcription conferred by multiple transacting factors or multiple linked cis-acting DNA response elements, can result from cooperative binding of transacting factors to linked enhancers, cooperative recruitment of transcription initiation complexes, and regulation of sequential steps in transcription initiation.[183] The relevance of the distinct properties of synergy of MR and GR is highlighted by the fact that in the MR, the N-terminal domain NTD and the ligand-binding domain (LBD) do interact in an aldosterone-dependent manner. This interaction is not observed in the GR, and is antagonized by the antagonists spironolactone and eplerenone, and surprisingly, by cortisol.[172] The precise regions involved in this interaction are not known. However, the N-terminal region of MR contains so-called synergy control (SC) motifs whose disruption selectively increased MR activity at GRE multimers.[202] Possibly of relevance, the SCs correspond also to sites that are modified by sumoylation. Although mutations of the sumoylation sites do not interfere with the NTD/LBD interaction, direct and distinguishable inhibitory roles for SUMO isoforms in the control of transcriptional synergy have been demonstrated,[203] although the mechanistic basis for SUMO1 synergy inhibition remains to be determined (see for review[172,204]).

In addition to the major role played by the prereceptor protective mechanisms, the nature of the cellular responses to aldosterone or glucocorticoid is determined to a large extent by the type and the state of the target cell. Indeed, the set of genes regulated by a given activated receptor is cell-specific. This is due to the fact that much more than a single regulatory protein has to bind to a gene to activate its transcription. An intracellular receptor can activate a gene only if an appropriate cell type-specific combination of other gene regulatory proteins is expressed. This opens the possibility of interaction at several levels. As mentioned above, protein–protein interactions play a central role in the establishment of pre-initiation complexes. Thus, the structural differences of the MR and GR, in particular at the level of their amino-terminal domains, certainly allow them to undergo receptor-specific interactions. These interactions, in turn, might selectively modulate the transregulatory action of the receptors, independent of their common DNA-binding properties. Considerable efforts have been made to identify ligand-specific interacting and/or transactivation proteins. RNA helicase A (RHA) has been found to mediate transactivation of MR only in the presence of aldosterone, but not of cortisol; it was speculated that the NTD/LBD interaction may be affected.[172] On the other hand, differential expression and regional distribution of steroid receptor co-activators SRC-1 and SRC-2 in brain and pituitary have been found, and two splice variants of the steroid receptor co-activator-1 (SRC-1), 1a and 1e, can differ significantly in certain cell populations.[205,206] Thus, each cell might have its specific pattern of co-activators which might be involved in cell-specific responses to corticosteroids in a promoter- and ligand-dependent way. Finally, PTMs may also modify the transcriptional effects of MR. Recently it has been shown that cyclin-dependent kinase 5 does modify the MR transcriptional response. However, it is not known to date if aldosterone and cortisol induce different modifications of MR, which

might contribute to the differential effects of the two corticosteroids.[172]

How Does Transcriptional Regulation Lead to Transport Regulation?

This question has interested many scientists over the last five decades. Until recently, the epithelial Na^+ channel (ENaC) and the Na^+ pump (Na^+,K^+-ATPase) were recognized as the two main transport proteins mediating Na^+ reabsorption in the ASDN, although the thiazide-sensitive Na^+,Cl^--co-transporter NCC may also be involved (see discussion above). Here we will focus on ENaC and the pump, which were primarily investigated in this context. Starting at the level of Na^+ transport effectors, this approach has permitted definition of different phases of aldosterone action: an early phase, characterized by an activation of pre-existing proteins; and a late phase, during which new structural proteins are accumulated. Another approach to the mechanism of aldosterone action starts from the transcriptional event, with the identification of aldosterone-regulated gene products.[207,208] These are then further investigated at the level of their potential involvement in the physiological action of the hormone. Using new powerful techniques to analyze differential gene expression, aldosterone-regulated gene products were identified, as discussed below. It is believed that there are still many important aldosterone-regulated gene products that remain to be identified.

ENaC Activation: Transcriptional Induction and Regulation

Aldosterone directly controls ENaC transcription at the level of the α-subunit gene.[209] The mRNA of this subunit was correspondingly shown to increase in the ASDN of adrenalectomized rats within 2 hours of aldosterone treatment, and on long-term treatment.[3,210] This effect can account for the accumulation of the α-subunit in ASDN cells that was also observed within 2 hours of aldosterone treatment and in the long-term.[3,90] Interestingly, at the protein level aldosterone not only increases the amount of α-ENaC, but also induces a cleavage of γ-ENaC.[90]

Although the induction of αENaC and the apical translocation of all three ENaC-subunits are well visible 2 and 4 hours after aldosterone treatment, transepithelial Na^+ reabsorption and K^+ secretion start earlier, being measurable already within 30 min of treatment.[211] Thus, the early aldosterone response must also involve the activation of pre-existing but previously silent channels. In this regard, ubiquitylation of ENaC (i.e., the modification with ubiquitin[212]) is an important aldosterone-regulated mechanism that has been shown to control channel surface expression and function.[213] Indeed, experiments have indicated that the ubiquitin-protein ligase Nedd4-2 ubiquitylates ENaC on Lys residues in the NH_2-terminal tails of ENaC-subunits.[214–217] The enzyme binds to PY motifs of the COOH-terminal tails of β- and γ-ENaC via WW protein–protein interaction domains,[214,215,218] and ubiquitylates the channel.[217] Interestingly, missense mutations causing deletion of the PY motifs in β- and γ-ENaC characteristic of Liddle's syndrome lead to an increase in cell surface ENaC expression, and also to an increase in its open probability (P_o), a condition leading to Na^+ retention, low K^+, and hypertension.[119,137,219] The control of ENaC by ubiquitylation appears to be regulated at several levels. First, dietary Na^+, likely via aldosterone action, controls Nedd4-2 expression in the ASDN. A high-salt diet increases Nedd4-2 expression, whereas a low-salt diet decreases it,[110] likely by interfering with excess Na^+ uptake via ENaC. Second, aldosterone has been shown to induce the expression of Sgk1 kinase[220] and the deubiquitylating enzyme Usp2-45.[221,222] In the former case, Sgk1 phosphorylates Nedd4-2, creating a binding site for 14-3-3 proteins.[107,216] By binding to Nedd4-2, 14-3-3 proteins mask the ENaC interacting motif of Nedd4-2, and thus prevent ENaC ubiquitylation and downregulation. This short cascade represents the first direct link between the aldosterone-regulated transcriptional activity of the MR and the function of ENaC that was demonstrated[220,223] (Figure 35.8). Besides acting via Nedd4-2, Sgk1 has been shown to act in concert via other mechanisms: (1) it may phosphorylate a consensus phosphorylation site on the C-terminus of α-ENaC close to the second transmembrane domain.[224] It is noteworthy, though, that this site is not conserved in *Xenopus laevis* ENaC, indicating that this mode of regulation has evolved lately in evolution; (2) it relieves the transcriptional repression by Dot1a-Af9 of the channel subunit,[225] consequently stimulating aldosterone-induced transcription of α-ENaC.

Usp2-45 was identified in a microarray screen of aldosterone early induced transcripts of the CCD.[221] This deubiquitylating enzyme was then shown to deubiquitylate ENaC, to interact both with ENaC and Nedd4-2, and to promote ENaC activity, activation by cleavage and cell surface expression.[226–228] The *in vivo* physiological relevance of Usp2-45 in ENaC regulation, however, remains to be demonstrated. Moreover, it is important to note that the Sgk1-Nedd4-2 pathway is not the only link between aldosterone and ENaC function. This has been indicated by results of experiments performed with mpkCCD cells expressing Liddle's-type ENaC that cannot bind Nedd4-2 and still responds to aldosterone, as did mutant mice expressing an ENaC β-subunit with the Liddle's mutation.[77,129]

Several mouse models deficient for Nedd4-2[60,229–231] and Sgk1[106,232,233] have been created (Table 35.1). Nedd4-2 knockout models have a relatively mild renal phenotype. They show normal Na^+ and K^+ balance, normal[229] or decreased[60] aldosterone, and salt-sensitive hypertension (Figure 35.9). They display increased ENaC protein levels, and in at least one model there were significantly increased NCC levels.[60] Therefore it is likely that Nedd4-2 is not only involved in ENaC regulation, but also in regulation of NCC. Two Nedd4-2 KO models have been shown to have a lung phenotype, with defective ENaC regulation.[230,231] The Sgk1 knockout mice generated by Wulff et al. and Fejes-Toth et al. are total knockouts, whereas the third model by Faresse et al. is an inducible, nephron-specific inactivation of Sgk1. They all display normal Na^+ and K^+ balance when kept under normal-salt diet, but have higher aldosterone levels, indicating a problem in the handling of Na^+ and K^+ (Figure 35.10). Under a low-salt diet, the knockout mice were unable to sufficiently upregulate NaCl reabsorption, despite excessive elevation of plasma aldosterone concentrations, and reduced and maintained apical ENaC translocation.[106,233] Intriguingly, although I_{Na} (measured by whole cell patch-clamping in the CD) was elevated, the proteolytic processing of γENaC is reduced in Sgk1 KO mice, even under conditions were aldosterone is induced.[232] These findings suggest that Sgk1 is required for processing of ENaC, but is not necessary for aldosterone-induced ENaC activation. The Sgk1 knockout models also revealed that Sgk1 is not only involved in ENaC regulation, but also controls the expression of NCC.[232,233] This control of NCC by Sgk1 appears to involve different regulatory pathways, and may act via Nedd4-2 phosphorylation[60,233] or via WNK kinases.[234–237]

Nedd4-2 has been associated through genome-wide studies with essential hypertension (for a recent review see [238]). On the other hand, the contribution of Sgk1 and Usp2-45 to hypertension has remained uncertain.[239–241]

The major part of the ENaC protein faces the extracellular milieu like a receptor, and evidence has accumulated during recent years that furin-mediated cleavage within the extracellular loop appears to be part of the maturation process of α- and γ-ENaC.[242] Yet luminal protease-mediated ENaC activation systems have also been suggested to play an important regulatory role in the function of ENaC. Originally this hypothesis was formulated from the model kidney cell line A6, when a cDNA that encodes a protease that activates ENaC by increasing its P_o was identified.[243] This channel-activating protease (CAP-1) and related

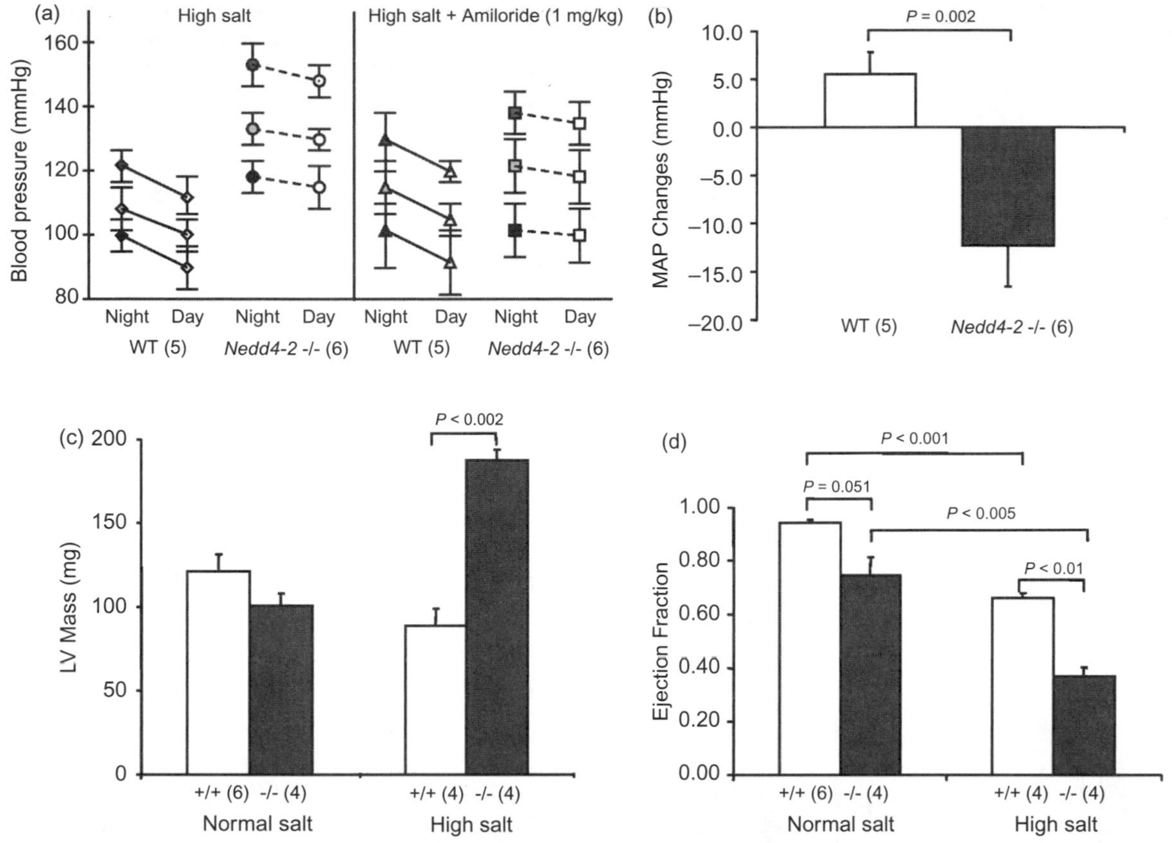

FIGURE 35.9 **Salt-sensitive arterial hypertension, cardiac hypertrophy, and reduced cardiac function in Nedd4-2$^{-/-}$ mice.** Top: Arterial blood pressure (bp) was recorded continuously by radiotelemetry in wild-type (WT) and Nedd4-2$^{-/-}$ mice that were kept for at least two weeks on a high-salt diet (Systolic bp: red symbols; diastolic bp: blue symbols; mean Bp: green symbols). Subsequent daily injections of amiloride for 12 days lowered arterial blood pressure in Nedd4-2$^{-/-}$, but not in WT mice (a), which was most evident when mean arterial pressure (MAP) values before and after amiloride treatment were plotted (b). Bottom: Left ventricular (LV) mass and cardiac ejection fraction in Nedd4-2$^{+/+}$ and Nedd4-2$^{-/-}$ mice kept for 8 to 10 months on normal or a high-salt diet. Heart weights and cardiac ejection fraction were determined by postmortem gravimetry and intravital echocardiography, respectively. (*Adapted from Shi, P. P., et al. (2008).*[229]) See color section at the end of the book.

proteases have been shown to be highly-expressed in ENaC expressing tissues, like kidney and intestine, in which protease inhibitors have also been shown to decrease Na$^+$ channel activity (for a review see [244]). The finding that proteolytic events modulate ENaC activity from the extracellular side is supported by the observation made in different cell lines that the application of protease inhibitors decreases, and the addition of proteases increases, Na$^+$ channel activity. As of yet, the actual mechanism by which this pathway leads to channel activation has not been elucidated. One report suggests that this ENaC-activating mechanism is induced by aldosterone. It was observed that urinary CAP1/prostasin was augmented by aldosterone in rats and humans.[245] Interestingly, proteolysis of ENaC by furin/extracellular proteases may be regulated by ubiquitylation of Nedd4-2. Indeed, it has been shown in transfected cells that ENaC channels with Liddle's mutations (inactivation of PY-motifs, the binding

motifs for Nedd4-2) display a higher degree of proteolytic cleavage,[246] similar to co-expression of the deubiquitylating enzyme Usp2-45.[226,227] In view of the fact that proteases have been shown to primarily affect P$_o$, these observations may explain the observed effect of Liddle's mutations on both cell surface expression and P$_o$.[219] These observations have to be confirmed *in vivo*. It is noteworthy, however, that in Sgk1 knockout mice, the proteolytic processing of γ-ENaC appears to be defective, compatible with the role of Sgk1 in Nedd4-2-dependent ENaC regulation.[232]

ENaC has also been found to be regulated by lipid-based signaling pathways involving phosphoinositides, such as phosphatidylinositol 4,5-biphosphate (PIP$_2$), and phosphatidylinositol 3,4,5-triphosphate (PIP$_3$).[247] PIP$_2$ is required for ENaC-gating, and is likely to bind directly to the channel. It is important to note that P2Y$_2$ receptors interfere with ENaC activity by stimulating the metabolism of PIP$_2$. Evidence for such regulation is

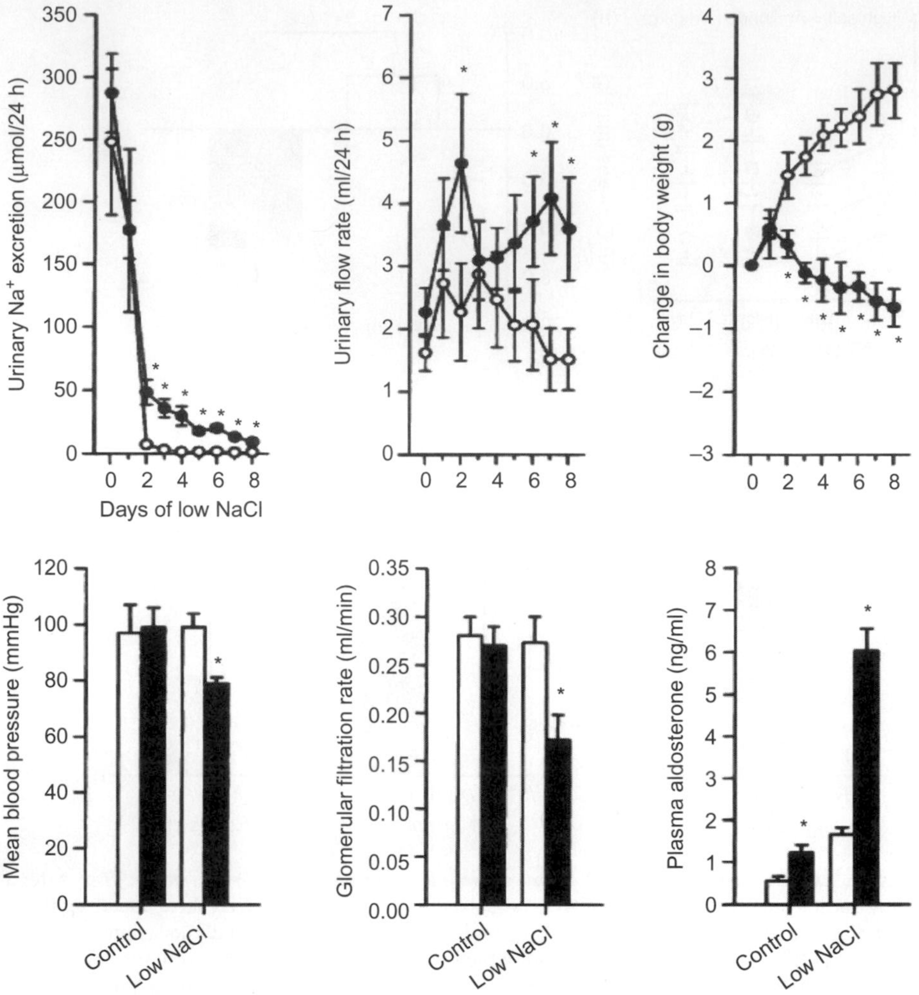

FIGURE 35.10 Deficient adaptive response to low-Na intake in Sgk1$^{-/-}$ mice. (Top) Urinary excretion of Na$^+$ and water, and change in body weight in response to a low-NaCl diet assessed in metabolic cages. (Bottom) Mean arterial blood pressure, glomerular filtration rate, and plasma aldosterone concentration in mice on the control diet and after feeding 3 days of a low-NaCl diet. Filled circles and bars indicate Sgk1$^{+/+}$ mice, open circles and bars indicate Sgk1$^{-/-}$ mice (*p 0.05 vs Sgk1$^{+/+}$mice). (Adapted from Wulff, P., et al. (2002).[106])

provided by P2Y$_2$ receptor null mice that are hypertensive with increased ENaC activity.[248] PIP$_3$ is thought to affect ENaC by several mechanisms: (1) PIP$_3$ may directly increase the P$_o$ of ENaC expressed in CHO cells, and the aldosterone-induced protein K-Ras[249,250] may act by localizing the PIP$_3$-producing enzyme phosphatidylinositol-3OH kinase PI3-K close to the channel[251,252]; (2) PI-3K and PIP$_3$ may acutely stimulate ENaC open probability, likely by direct binding to ENaC[247,253]; (3) another important role for PIP$_3$ in this context is its role as activator of the PDK kinases (e.g., mSIN1/mTORC2 complex) that in turn activate aldosterone-inducible Sgk1.[220,254] As discussed above, Sgk1 positively affects ENaC by the inhibition of the ubiquitin-protein ligase Nedd4-2, and eventually also by direct phosphorylation of α-ENaC.[220]

Identification of Aldosterone-Regulated RNAs by Gene Expression Profiling

The aim of this section is to mention additional aldosterone-regulated gene products that support the pleiotropic action of aldosterone. Some of these gene products were identified because they were considered as candidates for aldosterone regulation, and therefore the impact of the hormone on their expression was directly tested. Others were identified in the context of screening procedures for aldosterone-regulated mRNAs.[208] This was the case for the two gene products discussed above, Sgk1 and Usp2-45.[222]

Besides ENaC and Na$^+$,K$^+$-ATPase, three gene products clearly involved in NaCl reabsorption were identified due to their role in controlling the ion balance in the ASDN. First, two epithelial transporters were shown to be upregulated in vivo by mineralocorticoids in the long-term: the thiazide-sensitive Na$^+$,Cl$^-$-co-transporter NCC of DCT segment-specific cells; and the Cl$^-$/HCO$_3$-exchanger pendrin expressed in type B-intercalated cells.[31,52] Both transporters participate at the NaCl reabsorption, and might be upregulated by indirect mechanisms. The third candidate involved in NaCl transport and shown to be induced by aldosterone is the regulatory protein WNK1. This latter effect was shown in a cell culture model to be mediated rapidly by activated MR.[255] It will be interesting to verify the *in vivo* regulation of WNK1, the role of which appears to be the control of the balance between partially overlapping Na$^+$, K$^+$, and Cl$^-$ reabsorption.[256,257] The EGF receptor is an additional regulatory protein, the expression of which was shown in kidney cells to be induced by aldosterone. Interestingly, this receptor has been implicated in the signaling of non-genomic actions of aldosterone, and might play a role in the pathological actions of aldosterone.[258]

Progressively, molecular biology methods have become available that have started to allow the identification of regulated gene products. First, the group of Garty cloned a cDNA-encoding CHIF, a protein that is induced by aldosterone in the colon and belongs to the FXYD family of small Na$^+$,K$^+$-ATPase regulatory proteins.[259–261] Interestingly, CHIF is also localized to the distal part of the ASDN, and increases the apparent affinity of the Na$^+$,K$^+$-ATPase for Na$^+$.[262,263] CHIF-deficient mice have a rather mild phenotype pointing to some defects in renal and colonic Na$^+$ and K$^+$ transport when stressed by low-Na$^+$ or high-K$^+$ intake. The findings were consistent with a dysregulation of the Na$^+$-K$^+$-ATPase as the common denominator.[264]

Moreover, Spindler and colleagues used a differential display PCR approach to compare cDNA fragments generated from RNA of control and aldosterone-treated A6 epithelia.[249] They showed that only a small proportion of the mRNA ($< 0.5\%$) was significantly regulated within the lag period of aldosterone action, and hence potentially involved in its early effect. One of the regulated gene products was a splice variant of a *Xenopus* K-*ras*. Functional experiments in *Xenopus* oocytes showed that this small G-protein activates ENaC at the cell surface.[250] The connection of K-*Ras* with PIP$_3$-mediated ENaC activation has been described above.

Another aldosterone-regulated gene product that has been identified by subtractive hybridization is NDRG2.[265] When co-expressed with ENaC, it has been shown to potentiate ENaC activity.[266] Moreover, it is a potential target of Sgk1.[267] Its potential physiological role in the context of Na$^+$ transport remains to be established.

Some gene screens were performed by SAGE (Serial Analysis of Gene Expression) or gene array analysis on kidney-derived cultured cells.[208] The major limitation of these studies was the large number of genes normally repressed *in vivo* that are expressed in cultured cells, some of which are sensitive to corticosteroids. Nonetheless, some interesting gene products were identified. One of them is the strongly upregulated GILZ, a gene product identified in mpkCCD cells by SAGE analysis.[268] Its induction has been verified in kidney, but its functional role has not yet been unraveled.[269] Interestingly, GILZ has been shown recently

to be part of the ENaC regulatory complex (ERC), which also comprises the ENaC inhibitory proteins Raf-1 and Nedd4-2, as well as Sgk1.[270] In this context, GILZ is able to regulate ENaC via Sgk1 stabilization by decreasing its endoplasmic reticulum-mediated degradation.[271] Moreover, GILZ deficient mice show subtle deficiencies in water and Na$^+$ handling.[272]

In IMCD-3 cells, a series of aldosterone-regulated gene products (1 hour treatment) was identified. Sgk1 was one of the most highly-regulated ones. Moreover, genes involved in circadian rhythm were identified, and it was then shown that the circadian rhythm plays an essential role in ion and water homeostasis, and that Per1, part of the basic circadian regulatory machinery, is involved in α-ENaC regulation.[273–275] It will be timely to obtain a more complete list of the gene products regulated by aldosterone in target cells. It can be envisaged that most of them participate in signaling cascades, directly affecting the function of the cellular machinery for Na$^+$ reabsorption and K$^+$ secretion.

CONCLUSION

Since the identification of aldosterone as a major hormone that controls extracellular Na$^+$, K$^+$ and fluid homeostasis, tremendous progress has been made in the identification of the cellular and molecular mechanisms by which this hormone mediates its actions, in particular in the kidney. Structural and functional studies allowed us to define the renal tubule segments forming the aldosterone-sensitive distal nephron (ASDN) and to address their contribution to the adaptation of the kidneys to varying functional needs. The main receptors (e.g., MR, GR), specificity conferring mechanisms (e.g., 11-α-HSD2), and effectors (e.g., ENaC, NCC, and Na$^+$,K$^+$-ATPase) have been cloned and studied in various *in vitro* and *in vivo* settings. Rare human genetic diseases related to mutations in these proteins were unraveled, and mouse models mimicking the human phenotypes have been generated. Together, these studies further underlined the utmost importance of the ASDN for ion homeostasis and blood pressure control. However, we have just started to identify the homeostatic signals and mechanisms that ensure the efficient cooperation of the different ASDN segments and cell types, which ensure an independent regulation of renal Na$^+$, K$^+$, proton, and fluid excretion. Co-expression of the MR, the GR, and additional alternative receptors in the same ASDN cells may add significantly to the complexity of genomic and non-genomic corticosteroid actions along the ASDN. The mild phenotype of Sgk1, Nedd4-2, and CHIF deficient mice points to a rather extensive and redundant signaling cascade. The rapid advancement of molecular and physiological techniques, together with the increasing availability of genetic mouse models with conditional deletion or overexpression of the receptors and certain regulatory molecules will allow us to further unravel the complex control of the aldosterone-dependent control of renal ion homeostasis. As even subtle dysfunction within the underlying regulatory cascades may already predispose to human diseases such as salt-sensitive hypertension, further research is needed.

Acknowledgment

We are grateful to Drs. Edith Hummler, Bernard Rossier, Laurent Schild, and François Verrey for having established with the previous edition(s) of this chapter a solid base to build on. Moreover, we thank Drs. Dominique Loffing-Cueni, Caroline Ronzaud, and Nourdine Faresse for critically reading the manuscript. We also thank Mr. Jean-Claude Broillet for having established the Reference Databank.

References

[1] Simpson ER, Mason JI. Molecular Aspects of Biosynthesis of Adrenal Steroids. Oxford: Pergamon; 1979.

[2] Studer RA, Person E, Robinson-Rechavi M, Rossier BC. Evolution of the epithelial sodium channel and the sodium pump as limiting factors of aldosterone action on sodium transport. Physiol Genomics 2011;43:844–54.

[3] Loffing J, Zecevic M, Feraille E, Kaissling B, Asher C, Rossier BC, et al. Aldosterone induces rapid apical translocation of ENaC in early portion of renal collecting system: possible role of SGK. Am J Physiol Renal Physiol 2001;280:F675–82.

[4] Katz AI, Doucet A, Morel F. Na-K-ATPase activity along the rabbit, rat, and mouse nephron. Am J Physiol 1979;237:F114–20.

[5] Almeida AJ, Burg MB. Sodium transport in the rabbit connecting tubule. Am J Physiol 1982;243:F330–4.

[6] Shareghi GR, Stoner LC. Calcium transport across segments of the rabbit distal nephron in vitro. Am J Physiol 1978;235:F367–75.

[7] Tomita K, Pisano JJ, Knepper MA. Control of sodium and potassium transport in the cortical collecting duct of the rat. Effects of bradykinin, vasopressin, and deoxycorticosterone. J Clin Invest 1985;76:132–6.

[8] Reif MC, Troutman SL, Schafer JA. Sodium transport by rat cortical collecting tubule. Effects of vasopressin and desoxycorticosterone. J Clin Invest 1986;77:1291–8.

[9] Stokes JB. Ion transport by the cortical and outer medullary collecting tubule. Kidney Int 1982;22:473–84.

[10] Frindt G, Ergonul Z, Palmer LG. Na channel expression and activity in the medullary collecting duct of rat kidney. Am. J Physiol Renal Physiol 2007;292:F1190–6.

[11] Loffing J, Kaissling B. Sodium and calcium transport pathways along the mammalian distal nephron: from rabbit to human. Am J Physiol Renal Physiol 2003;284:F628–43.

[12] Loffing J, Loffing-Cueni D, Macher A, Hebert SC, Olson B, Knepper MA, et al. Localization of epithelial sodium channel and aquaporin-2 in rabbit kidney cortex. Am J Physiol Renal Physiol 2000;278:F530–9.

[13] Bachmann S, Bostanjoglo M, Schmitt R, Ellison DH. Sodium transport-related proteins in the mammalian distal nephron — distribution, ontogeny and functional aspects. Anat Embryol 1999;200:447–68.

[14] Arriza JL, Weinberger C, Cerelli G, Glaser TM, Handelin BL, Housman DE, et al. Cloning of human mineralocorticoid receptor complementary DNA: structural and functional kinship with the glucocorticoid receptor. Science 1987;237:268–75.

[15] Odermatt A, Kratschmar DV. Tissue-specific modulation of mineralocorticoid receptor function by 11beta-hydroxysteroid dehydrogenases: an overview. Mol Cell Endocrinol 2012;350:168–86.

[16] Wang WH, Giebisch G. Regulation of potassium (K) handling in the renal collecting duct. Pflug Arch Eur J Phy 2009;458:157–68.

[17] Holtzclaw JD, Grimm PR, Sansom SC. Role of BK channels in hypertension and potassium secretion. Curr Opin Nephrol Hypertens 2011;20:512–7.

[18] Rodan AR, Cheng CJ, Huang CL. Recent advances in distal tubular potassium handling. Am J Physiol Renal Physiol 2011;300:F821–7.

[19] Welling PA, Ho K. A comprehensive guide to the ROMK potassium channel: form and function in health and disease. Am J Physiol Renal Physiol 2009;297:F849–63.

[20] Mennitt PA, Wade JB, Ecelbarger CA, Palmer LG, Frindt G. Localization of ROMK channels in the rat kidney. J Am Soc Nephrol: JASN 1997;8:1823–30.

[21] Xu JZ, Hall AE, Peterson LN, Bienkowski MJ, Eessalu TE, Hebert SC. Localization of the ROMK protein on apical membranes of rat kidney nephron segments. Am J Physiol 1997;273:F739–48.

[22] Wade JB, Fang L, Coleman RA, Liu J, Grimm PR, Wang T, et al. Differential regulation of ROMK (Kir1.1) in distal nephron segments by dietary potassium. Am J Physiol Renal Physiol 2011;300(6):F1385–93.

[23] Najjar F, Zhou H, Morimoto T, Bruns JB, Li HS, Liu W, et al. Dietary K^+ regulates apical membrane expression of maxi-K channels in rabbit cortical collecting duct. Am J Physiol Renal Physiol 2005;289:F922–32.

[24] Li D, Wei Y, Babilonia E, Wang Z, Wang WH. Inhibition of phosphatidylinositol 3-kinase stimulates activity of the small-conductance K channel in the CCD. Am J Physiol Renal Physiol 2006;290:F806–12.

[25] Gumz ML, Lynch IJ, Greenlee MM, Cain BD, Wingo CS. The renal H^+-K^+-ATPases: Physiology, regulation, and structure. Am J Physiol Renal Physiol 2010;298:F12–21.

[26] Wagner CA, Mohebbi N, Capasso G, Geibel JP. The anion exchanger pendrin (SLC26A4) and renal acid–base homeostasis. Cell Physiol Biochem 2011;28:497–504.

[27] Eladari D, Hubner CA. Novel mechanisms for NaCl reabsorption in the collecting duct. Curr Opin Nephrol Hypertens 2011;20:506–11.

[28] Kim YH, Pech V, Spencer KB, Beierwaltes WH, Everett LA, Green ED, et al. Reduced ENaC protein abundance contributes to the lower blood pressure observed in pendrin-null mice. Am J Physiol Renal Physiol 2007;293:F1314–24.

[29] Pech V, Pham TD, Hong S, Weinstein AM, Spencer KB, Duke BJ, et al. Pendrin modulates ENaC function by changing luminal HCO3. J Am Soc Nephrol: JASN 2010;21:1928–41.

[30] Wall SM, Kim YH, Stanley L, Glapion DM, Everett LA, Green ED, et al. NaCl restriction upregulates renal Slc26a4 through subcellular redistribution: role in Cl^- conservation. Hypertension 2004;44:982–7.

[31] Verlander JW, Hassell KA, Royaux IE, Glapion DM, Wang ME, Everett LA, et al. Deoxycorticosterone upregulates PDS (Slc26a4) in mouse kidney: role of pendrin in mineralocorticoid-induced hypertension. Hypertension 2003;42:356–62.

[32] Leviel F, Hubner CA, Houillier P, Morla L, El Moghrabi S, Brideau G, et al. The Na^+-dependent chloride-bicarbonate

exchanger SLC4A8 mediates an electroneutral Na$^+$ reabsorption process in the renal cortical collecting ducts of mice. J Clin Invest 2010;120:1627–35.

[33] Yoo D, Kim BY, Campo C, Nance L, King A, Maouyo D, et al. Cell surface expression of the ROMK (Kir 1.1) channel is regulated by the aldosterone-induced kinase, SGK-1, and protein kinase A. J Biol Chem 2003;278:23066–75.

[34] Beesley AH, Hornby D, White SJ. Regulation of distal nephron K$^+$ channels (ROMK) mRNA expression by aldosterone in rat kidney. J Physiol 1998;509(Pt 3):629–34.

[35] Wald H, Garty H, Palmer LG, Popovtzer MM. Differential regulation of ROMK expression in kidney cortex and medulla by aldosterone and potassium. Am J Physiol 1998;275:F239–45.

[36] Estilo G, Liu W, Pastor-Soler N, Mitchell P, Carattino MD, Kleyman TR, et al. Effect of aldosterone on BK channel expression in mammalian cortical collecting duct. Am J Physiol Renal Physiol 2008;295:F780–8.

[37] Rozenfeld J, Efrati E, Adler L, Tal O, Carrithers SL, Alper SL, et al. Transcriptional regulation of the pendrin gene. Cell Physiol Biochem 2011;28:385–96.

[38] de Seigneux S, Nielsen J, Olesen ET, Dimke H, Kwon TH, Frokiaer J, et al. Long-term aldosterone treatment induces decreased apical but increased basolateral expression of AQP2 in CCD of rat kidney. Am J Physiol Renal Physiol 2007;293: F87–99.

[39] Hasler U, Mordasini D, Bianchi M, Vandewalle A, Feraille E, Martin PY. Dual influence of aldosterone on AQP2 expression in cultured renal collecting duct principal cells. J Biol Chem 2003;278:21639–48.

[40] Kwon TH, Nielsen J, Masilamani S, Hager H, Knepper MA, Frokiaer J, et al. Regulation of collecting duct AQP3 expression: response to mineralocorticoid. Am J Physiol Renal Physiol 2002;283:F1403–21.

[41] Wang WH, Yue P, Sun P, Lin DH. Regulation and function of potassium channels in aldosterone-sensitive distal nephron. Curr Opin Nephrol Hypertens 2010;19:463–70.

[42] Kwon TH, Nielsen J, Moller IIB, Fenton RA, Nielsen S, Frokiaer J. Aquaporins in the kidney. Handb Exp Pharmacol 2009;95–132.

[43] Boone M, Deen PM. Physiology and pathophysiology of the vasopressin-regulated renal water reabsorption. Pflug Arch Eur J Phy 2008;456:1005–24.

[44] Farman N, Rafestin-Oblin ME. Multiple aspects of mineralocorticoid selectivity. Am J Physiol Renal Physiol 2001;280:F181–92.

[45] Gomez-Sanchez CE, de Rodriguez AF, Romero DG, Estess J, Warden MP, Gomez-Sanchez MT, et al. Development of a panel of monoclonal antibodies against the mineralocorticoid receptor. Endocrinology 2006;147:1343–8.

[46] Ackermann D, Gresko N, Carrel M, Loffing-Cueni D, Habermehl D, Gomez-Sanchez C, et al. *In vivo* nuclear translocation of mineralocorticoid and glucocorticoid receptors in rat kidney: differential effect of corticosteroids along the distal tubule. Am J Physiol Renal Physiol 2010;299:F1473–85.

[47] Stanton BA. Regulation by adrenal corticosteroids of sodium and potassium transport in loop of Henle and distal tubule of rat kidney. J Clin Invest 1986;78:1612–20.

[48] El Mernissi G, Chabardes D, Doucet A, Hus-Citharel A, Imbert-Teboul M. Le Bouffant F, Montegut M, Siaume S, and Morel F. Changes in tubular basolateral membrane markers after chronic DOCA treatment. Am J Physiol 1983;245:F100–9.

[49] Garg LC, Knepper MA, Burg MB. Mineralocorticoid effects on Na-K-ATPase in individual nephron segments. Am J Physiol 1981;240:F536–44.

[50] Tsuruoka S, Muto S, Taniguchi J, Suzuki M, Imai M. Effects of glucocorticoid and mineralocorticoid on potassium transport in

the rat medullary thick ascending limb of Henle's loop. Kidney Int 1995;47:802–10.

[51] Velazquez H, Bartiss A, Bernstein P, Ellison DH. Adrenal steroids stimulate thiazide-sensitive NaCl transport by rat renal distal tubules. Am J Physiol 1996;270:F211–9.

[52] Kim GH, Masilamani S, Turner R, Mitchell C, Wade JB, Knepper MA. The thiazide-sensitive Na-Cl co-transporter is an aldosterone-induced protein. P Natl Acad Sci USA 1998; 95:14552–7.

[53] Chiga M, Rai T, Yang SS, Ohta A, Takizawa T, Sasaki S, et al. Dietary salt regulates the phosphorylation of OSR1/SPAK kinases and the sodium chloride co-transporter through aldosterone. Kidney Int 2008;74(11):1403–9.

[54] Vallon V, Schroth J, Lang F, Kuhl D, Uchida S. Expression and phosphorylation of the Na$^+$-Cl$^-$ co-transporter NCC *in vivo* is regulated by dietary salt, potassium, and SGK1. Am J Physiol Renal Physiol 2009;297:F704–12.

[55] Masilamani S, Wang X, Kim GH, Brooks H, Nielsen J, Nielsen S, et al. Time course of renal Na-K-ATPase, NHE3, NKCC2, NCC, and ENaC abundance changes with dietary NaCl restriction. Am J Physiol Renal Physiol 2002;283:F648–57.

[56] van der Lubbe N, Lim CH, Fenton RA, Meima ME, Jan Danser AH, Zietse R, et al. Angiotensin II induces phosphorylation of the thiazide-sensitive sodium chloride co-transporter independent of aldosterone. Kidney Int 2011;79:66–76.

[57] Frindt G, Palmer LG. Surface expression of sodium channels and transporters in rat kidney: effects of dietary sodium. Am J Physiol Renal Physiol 2009;297:F1249–55.

[58] Sandberg MB, Maunsbach AB, McDonough AA. Redistribution of distal tubule Na$^+$-Cl$^-$ co-transporter (NCC) in response to a high-salt diet. Am J Physiol Renal Physiol 2006;291:F503–8.

[59] Nielsen J, Kwon TH, Frokiaer J, Knepper MA, Nielsen S. Maintained ENaC trafficking in aldosterone-infused rats during mineralocorticoid and glucocorticoid receptor blockade. Am J Physiol Renal Physiol 2007;292:F382–94.

[60] Arroyo JP, Lagnaz D, Ronzaud C, Vazquez N, Ko BS, Moddes L, et al. Nedd4-2 modulates renal Na$^+$-Cl$^-$ co-transporter via the aldosterone-SGK1-Nedd4-2 pathway. J Am Soc Nephrol: JASN 2011;22:1707–19.

[61] Ko B, Kamsteeg EJ, Cooke LL, Moddes LN, Deen PM, Hoover RS. RasGRP1 stimulation enhances ubiquitination and endocytosis of the sodium-chloride co-transporter. Am J Physiol Renal Physiol 2010;299:F300–9.

[62] Louis-Dit-Picard H, Barc J, Trujillano D, Miserey-Lenkei S, Bouatia-Naji N, Pylypenko O, et al. KLHL3 mutations cause familial hyperkalemic hypertension by impairing ion transport in the distal nephron. Nat Genet 2012;44:456–60.

[63] Boyden LM, Choi M, Choate KA, Nelson-Williams CJ, Farhi A, Toka HR, et al. Mutations in kelch-like 3 and cullin 3 cause hypertension and electrolyte abnormalities. Nature 2012; 482:98–102.

[64] Winter C, Kampik NB, Vedovelli L, Rothenberger F, Paunescu TG, Stehberger PA, et al. Aldosterone stimulates vacuolar H(+)-ATPase activity in renal acid-secretory intercalated cells mainly via a protein kinase C-dependent pathway. Am J Physiol Cell Physiol 2011;301:C1251–61.

[65] Izumi Y, Hori K, Nakayama Y, Kimura M, Hasuike Y, Nanami M, et al. Aldosterone requires vasopressin V1a receptors on intercalated cells to mediate acid-base homeostasis. J Am Soc Nephrol JASN 2011;22:673–80.

[66] Lombes M, Kenouch S, Souque A, Farman N, Rafestin-Oblin ME. The mineralocorticoid receptor discriminates aldosterone from glucocorticoids independently of the 11 beta-hydroxysteroid dehydrogenase. Endocrinology 1994;135:834–40.

[67] Gomez-Sanchez EP, Venkataraman MT, Thwaites D, Fort C. ICV infusion of corticosterone antagonizes ICV-aldosterone hypertension. Am J Physiol 1990;258:E649—53.

[68] Geller DS, Rodriguezsoriano J, Boado AV, Schifter S, Bayer M, Chang SS, et al. Mutations in the mineralocorticoid receptor gene cause autosomal dominant pseudohypoaldosteronism type I. Nat Genet 1998;19:279—81.

[69] Koefoed-Johnson V, Ussing HH. The nature of the frog skin potential. Acta Physiol Scand 1958;42:298—308.

[70] Lindemann B, Van Driessche W. Sodium-specific membrane channels of frog skin are pores: current fluctuations reveal high turnover. Science 1977;195:292—4.

[71] Horisberger JD. The Na,K-ATPase: Structure-Function Relationship. Austin,TX: R.G. Landes Company; 1994.

[72] Jorgensen PL. Structure, function and regulation of Na,K-ATPase in the kidney. Kidney Int 1986;29:10—20.

[73] Rossier BC. Mechanisms of action of mineralocorticoid hormones. Endocr Res 1989;15:203—26.

[74] Handler JS. Use of cultured epithelia to study transport and its regulation. J Exp Biol 1983;106:55—69.

[75] Geering K, Claire M, Gaeggeler H-P, Rossier BC. Receptor occupancy vs induction of Na-K-ATPase and Na^+ transport by aldosterone. Am J Physiol 1985;248:C102—8.

[76] Will PC, Cortright RN, DeLisle RC, Douglas JG, Hopfer U. Regulation of amiloride-sensitive electrogenic sodium transport in the rat colon by steroid hormones. Am J Physiol 1985;248:G124—32.

[77] Dahlmann A, Pradervand S, Hummler E, Rossier BC, Frindt G, Palmer LG. Mineralocorticoid regulation of epithelial Na^+ channels is maintained in a mouse model of Liddle's syndrome. Am J Physiol Renal Physiol 2003;285:F310—8.

[78] Canessa CM, Horisberger J-D, Rossier BC. Epithelial sodium channel related to proteins involved in neurodegeneration. Nature 1993;361:467—70.

[79] Canessa CM, Schild L, Buell G, Thorens B, Gautschi I, Horisberger J-D, et al. Amiloride-sensitive epithelial Na^+ channel is made of three homologous subunits. Nature 1994; 367:463—7.

[80] Waldmann R, Champigny G, Bassilana F, Voilley N, Lazdunski M. Molecular cloning and functional expression of a novel amiloride- sensitive Na^+ channel. J Biol Chem 1995; 270:27411—4.

[81] Firsov D, Gautschi I, Mérillat A-M, Rossier BC, Schild L. The heterotetrameric architecture of the epithelial sodium channel (ENaC). EMBO J 1998;17:344—52.

[82] Loffing J, Schild L. Functional domains of the epithelial sodium channel. J Am Soc Nephrol: JASN 2005;16:3175—81.

[83] Jasti J, Furukawa H, Gonzales EB, Gouaux E. Structure of acid-sensing ion channel 1 at 1.9 Å resolution and low pH. Nature 2007;449:316—23.

[84] Gonzales EB, Kawate T, Gouaux E. Pore architecture and ion sites in acid-sensing ion channels and P2X receptors. Nature 2009;460:599—604.

[85] Asher C, Wald H, Rossier BC, Garty H. Aldosterone-induced increase in the abundance of Na^+ channel subunits. Am J Physiol 1996;271:C605—11.

[86] Escoubet B, Coureau C, Bonvalet JP, Farman N. Noncoordinate regulation of epithelial Na channel and Na pump subunit mRNAs in kidney and colon by aldosterone. Am J Physiol 1997;272:C1482—91.

[87] Ono S, Kusano E, Muto S, Ando Y, Asano Y. A low-Na^+ diet enhances expression of mRNA for epithelial Na^+ channel in rat renal inner medulla. Pflug Arch Eur J Phy 1997;434:756—63.

[88] Renard S, Voilley N, Bassilana F, Lazdunski M, Barbry P. Localization and regulation by steroids of the alpha, beta and gamma subunits of the amiloride-sensitive Na^+ channel in colon, lung and kidney. Pflug Arch Eur J Phy 1995;430:299—307.

[89] Frindt G, Masilamani S, Knepper MA, Palmer LG. Activation of epithelial Na channels during short-term Na deprivation. Am J Physiol Renal Physiol 2001;280:F112—8.

[90] Masilamani S, Kim GH, Mitchell C, Wade JB, Knepper MA. Aldosterone-mediated regulation of ENaC alpha, beta, and gamma subunit proteins in rat kidney. J Clin Invest 1999;104: R19—23.

[91] Ergonul Z, Frindt G, Palmer LG. Regulation of maturation and processing of ENaC subunits in the rat kidney. Am J Physiol Renal Physiol 2006;291:F683—93.

[92] Frindt G, Ergonul Z, Palmer LG. Surface expression of epithelial Na channel protein in rat kidney. J Gen Physiol 2008;131:617—27.

[93] Loffing J, Pietri L, Aregger F, Bloch-Faure M, Ziegler U, Meneton P, et al. Differential subcellular localization of ENaC subunits in mouse kidney in response to high- and low-Na diets. Am J Physiol 2000;279:F252—8.

[94] Hager H, Kwon TH, Vinnikova AK, Masilamani S, Brooks HL, Frokiaer J, et al. Immunocytochemical and immunoelectron microscopic localization of alpha-, beta-, and gamma-ENaC in rat kidney. Am J Physiol Renal Physiol 2001;280:F1093—106.

[95] Rubera I, Loffing J, Palmer LG, Frindt G, Fowler-Jaeger N, Sauter D, et al. Collecting duct-specific gene inactivation of aENaC in the mouse kidney does not impair sodium and potassium balance. J Clin Invest 2003;112:554—65.

[96] Dijkink L, Hartog A, Deen PM, van Os CH, Bindels RJ. Time-dependent regulation by aldosterone of the amiloride-sensitive Na^+ channel in rabbit kidney. Pflug Arch Eur J Phy 1999;438:354—60.

[97] Sauter D, Fernandes S, Goncalves-Mendes N, Boulkroun S, Bankir L, Loffing J, et al. Long-term effects of vasopressin on the subcellular localization of ENaC in the renal collecting system. Kidney Int 2006;69:1024—32.

[98] Frindt G, McNair T, Dahlmann A, Jacobs-Palmer E, Palmer LG. Epithelial Na channels and short-term renal response to salt deprivation. Am J Physiol Renal Physiol 2002;283:F717—26.

[99] May A, Puoti A, Gaeggeler H-P, Horisberger J-D, Rossier BC. Early effect of aldosterone on the rate of synthesis of the epithelial sodium channel a subunit in A6 renal cells. J Am Soc Nephrol 1997;8:1813—22.

[100] Nielsen J, Kwon TH, Masilamani S, Beutler K, Hager H, Nielsen S, et al. Sodium transporter abundance profiling in kidney: effect of spironolactone. Am J Physiol Renal Physiol 2002;283:F923—33.

[101] Chen S, Bhargava A, Mastroberardino L, Meijer OC, Wang J, Buse P, et al. Epithelial sodium channel regulated by aldosterone-induced protein sgk. P Natl Acad Sci USA 1999;96:2514—9.

[102] Shigaev A, Asher C, Latter H, Garty H, Reuveny E. Regulation of sgk by aldosterone and its effects on the epithelial Na(+) channel. Am J Physiol 2000;278:F613—9.

[103] Naray-Fejes-Toth A, Canessa CM, Cleaveland ES, Aldrich G, Fejes-Toth G. sgk is an aldosterone-induced kinase in the renal collecting duct. J Biol Chem 1999;274:16973—8.

[104] Hou J, Speirs HJ, Seckl JR, Brown RW. Sgk1 gene expression in kidney and its regulation by aldosterone: spatio-temporal heterogeneity and quantitative analysis. J Am Soc Nephrol: JASN 2002;13:1190—8.

[105] Alvarez de la Rosa D, Zhang P, Naray-Fejes-Toth A, Fejes-Toth G, Canessa CM. The serum and glucocorticoid kinase sgk increases the abundance of epithelial sodium channels in the plasma membrane of Xenopus oocytes. J Biol Chem 1999;274:37834—9.

[106] Wulff P, Vallon V, Huang DY, Volkl H, Yu F, Richter K, et al. Impaired renal Na($^+$) retention in the sgk1-knockout mouse. J Clin Invest 2002;110:1263−8.

[107] Debonneville C, Flores SY, Kamynina E, Plant PJ, Tauxe C, Thomas MA, et al. Phosphorylation of Nedd4-2 by Sgk1 regulates epithelial Na(+) channel cell surface expression. EMBO J 2001;20:7052−9.

[108] Snyder PM, Olson DR, Thomas BC. Serum and glucocorticoid-regulated kinase modulates Nedd4-2-mediated inhibition of the epithelial Na$^+$ channel. J Biol Chem 2002;277:5−8.

[109] Rauh R, Dinudom A, Fotia AB, Paulides M, Kumar S, Korbmacher C, et al. Stimulation of the epithelial sodium channel (ENaC) by the serum- and glucocorticoid-inducible kinase (Sgk) involves the PY motifs of the channel but is independent of sodium feedback inhibition. Pflug Arch Eur J Phy 2006;452 (3):290−9.

[110] Loffing-Cueni D, Flores SY, Sauter D, Daidie D, Siegrist N, Meneton P, et al. Dietary sodium intake regulates the ubiquitin-protein ligase nedd4-2 in the renal collecting system. J Am Soc Nephrol: JASN 2006;17:1264−74.

[111] Frindt G, Silver RB, Windhager EE, Palmer LG. Feedback regulation of Na channels in rat CCT. II. Effects of inhibition of Na entry. Am J Physiol 1993;264:F565−74.

[112] Nesterov V, Dahlmann A, Bertog M, Korbmacher C. Trypsin can activate the epithelial sodium channel (ENaC) in microdissected mouse distal nephron. Am J Physiol Renal Physiol 2008;295(4):F1052−62.

[113] Frindt G, Palmer LG. Na channels in the rat connecting tubule. Am J Physiol Renal Physiol 2004;286:F669−74.

[114] Kovacikova J, Winter C, Loffing-Cueni D, Loffing J, Finberg KE, Lifton RP, et al. The connecting tubule is the main site of the furosemide-induced urinary acidification by the vacuolar H($^+$)-ATPase. Kidney Int 2006;70(10):1706−16.

[115] Christensen BM, Perrier R, Wang Q, Zuber AM, Maillard M, Mordasini D, et al. Sodium and potassium balance depends on alphaENaC expression in connecting tubule. J Am Soc Nephrol: JASN 2010;21:1942−51.

[116] Ronzaud C, Loffing J, Bleich M, Gretz N, Grone HJ, Schutz G, et al. Impairment of sodium balance in mice deficient in renal principal cell mineralocorticoid receptor. J Am Soc Nephrol: JASN 2007;18:1679−87.

[117] Nielsen J, Kwon TH, Frokiaer J, Knepper MA, Nielsen S. Lithium-induced NDI in rats is associated with loss of alpha-ENaC regulation by aldosterone in CCD. Am J Physiol Renal Physiol 2006;290:F1222−33.

[118] Schulz-Baldes A, Berger S, Grahammer F, Warth R, Goldschmidt I, Peters J, et al. Induction of the epithelial Na$^+$ channel via glucocorticoids in mineralocorticoid receptor knockout mice. Pflug Arch Eur J Phy 2001;443:297−305.

[119] Lifton RP, Gharavi AG, Geller DS. Molecular mechanisms of human hypertension. Cell 2001;104:545−56.

[120] Liddle GW, Bledsoe T, Coppage Jr. WS. A familial renal disorder simulating primary aldosteronism but with negligible aldosterone secretion. Trans Assoc Am Physicians 1963;76:199−213.

[121] Botero-Velez M, Curtis JJ, Warnock DG. Brief report: Liddle's syndrome revisited − a disorder of sodium reabsorption in the distal tubule. N Engl J Med 1994;330:178−81.

[122] Shimkets RA, Warnock DG, Bositis CM, Nelson-Williams C, Hansson JH, Schambelan M, et al. Liddle's syndrome: Heritable human hypertension caused by mutations in the b subunit of the epithelial sodium channel. Cell 1994;79:407−14.

[123] Hansson JH, Schild L, Lu Y, Wilson TA, Gautschi I, Shimkets R, et al. A *de novo* missense mutation of the beta subunit of the epithelial sodium channel causes hypertension and Liddle syndrome, identifying a proline-rich segment critical

for regulation of channel activity. P Natl Acad Sci USA 1995;92:11495−9.

[124] Tamura H, Schild L, Enomoto N, Matsui N, Marumo F, Rossier BC, et al. Liddle disease caused by a missense mutation of beta subunit of the epithelial sodium channel gene. J Clin Invest 1996;97:1780−4.

[125] Hansson JH, Nelson-Williams C, Suzuki H, Schild L, Shimkets RA, Lu Y, et al. Hypertension caused by a truncated epithelial sodium channel gamma subunit: Genetic heterogeneity of Liddle syndrome. Nat Genet 1995;11:76−82.

[126] Schild L, Canessa CM, Shimkets RA, Warnock DG, Lifton RP, Rossier BC. A mutation in the epithelial sodium channel causing Liddle's disease increases channel activity in the *Xenopus laevis* oocyte expression system. Proc Nat Acad Sci USA 1995;92:5699−703.

[127] Pradervand S, Wang Q, Burnier M, Beermann F, Horisberger JD, Hummler E, et al. A mouse model for Liddle's syndrome. J Am Soc Nephrol 1999;10:2527−33.

[128] Pradervand S, Vandewalle A, Bens M, Gautschi I, Loffing J, Hummler E, et al. Dysfunction of the epithelial sodium channel expressed in the kidney of a mouse model for Liddle syndrome. J Am Soc Nephrol 2003;14:2219−28.

[129] Auberson M, Hoffmann-Pochon N, Vandewalle A, Kellenberger S, Schild L. Epithelial Na$^+$ channel mutants causing Liddle's syndrome retain ability to respond to aldosterone and vasopressin. Am J Physiol 2003;285:F459−71.

[130] Chang SS, Grunder S, Hanukoglu A, Rosler A, Mathew PM, Hanukoglu I, et al. Mutations in subunits of the epithelial sodium channel cause salt wasting with hyperkalaemic acidosis, pseudohypoaldosteronism type 1. Nat Genet 1996; 12:248−53.

[131] Hummler E. Implication of ENaC in salt-sensitive hypertension. J Steroid Biochem Mol Biol 1999;69:385−90.

[132] Hummler E, Barker P, Gatzy J, Beermann F, Verdumo C, Schmidt A, et al. Early death due to defective neonatal lung liquid clearance in aENaC-deficient mice. Nat Genet 1996; 12:325−8.

[133] Hummler E, Barker P, Talbot C, Wang Q, Verdumo C, Grubb BR, et al. A mouse model for the renal salt-wasting syndrome pseudohypoaldosteronism. P Natl Acad Sci USA 1997; 94:11710−5.

[134] Kerem E, Bistritzer T, Hanukoglu A, Hofmann T, Zhou ZQ, Bennett W, et al. Pulmonary epithelial sodium-channel dysfunction and excess airway liquid in pseudohypoaldosteronism. Nengl J Med 1999;341:156−62.

[135] Barker PM, Nguyen MS, Gatzy JT, Grubb B, Norman H, Hummler E, et al. Role of gammaENaC subunit in lung liquid clearance and electrolyte balance in newborn mice. Insights into perinatal adaptation and pseudohypoaldosteronism. J Clin Invest 1998;102:1634−40.

[136] McDonald FJ, Yang B, Hrstka RF, Drummond HA, Tarr Jr DE, Stokes MP, et al. Disruption of the beta subunit of the epithelial Na$^+$ channel in mice: Hyperkalemia and neonatal death associated with a pseudohypoaldosteronism phenotype. Proc Nat Acad Sci USA 1999;96:1727−31.

[137] Bonny O, Hummler E. Dysfunction of epithelial sodium transport: from human to mouse. Kidney Int 2000;57:1313−8.

[138] Bonny O, Rossier BC. Disturbances of Na/K balance: Pseudohypoaldosteronism revisited. J Am Soc Nephrol: JASN 2002;13:2399−414.

[139] Pradervand S, Barker PM, Wang Q, Ernst SA, Beerman F, Grubb BR, et al. Salt restriction induces pseudohypoaldosteronism type 1 in mice expressing low levels of the a-subunit of the amiloride-sensitive epithelial sodium channel. Proc Natl Acad Sci USA 1999;96:1732−7.

[140] Frindt G, Palmer LG. Apical potassium channels in the rat connecting tubule. Am J Physiol Renal Physiol 2004;287:F1030–7.

[141] Frindt G, Palmer LG. Low-conductance K channels in apical membrane of rat cortical collecting tubule. Am J Physiol 1989;256:F143–51.

[142] Wang WH, Schwab A, Giebisch G. Regulation of small-conductance K^+ channel in apical membrane of rat cortical collecting tubule. Am J Physiol 1990;259:F494–502.

[143] Rieg T, Vallon V, Sausbier M, Sausbier U, Kaissling B, Ruth P, et al. The role of the BK channel in potassium homeostasis and flow-induced renal potassium excretion. Kidney Int 2007; 72:566–73.

[144] Bailey MA, Cantone A, Yan Q, MacGregor GG, Leng Q, Amorim JB, et al. Maxi-K channels contribute to urinary potassium excretion in the ROMK-deficient mouse model of Type II Bartter's syndrome and in adaptation to a high-K diet. Kidney Int 2006;70:51–9.

[145] Youn JH, McDonough AA. Recent advances in understanding integrative control of potassium homeostasis. Annu Rev Physiol 2009;71:381–401.

[146] Palmer LG, Frindt G. Aldosterone and potassium secretion by the cortical collecting duct. Kidney Int 2000;57:1324–8.

[147] Gray DA, Frindt G, Palmer LG. Quantification of K^+ secretion through apical low-conductance K channels in the CCD. Am J Physiol Renal Physiol 2005;289:F117–26.

[148] Fodstad H, Gonzalez-Rodriguez E, Bron S, Gaeggeler H, Guisan B, Rossier BC, et al. Effects of mineralocorticoid and K^+ concentration on K^+ secretion and ROMK channel expression in a mouse cortical collecting duct cell line. Am J Physiol Renal Physiol 2009;296:F966–75.

[149] Palmer LG, Frindt G. Na^+ and K^+ transport by the renal connecting tubule. Curr Opin Nephrol Hypertens 2007;16:477–83.

[150] Frindt G, Palmer LG. K + secretion in rat kidney: Na^+-channel-dependent and independent mechanisms. Am J Physiol Renal Physiol 2009;297(2):F389–96.

[151] Feraille E, Doucet A. Sodium-potassium-adenosinetriphospha-tase-dependent sodium transport in the kidney: Hormonal control. Physiol Rev 2001;81:345–418.

[152] Feraille E, Mordasini D, Gonin S, Deschenes G, Vinciguerra M, Doucet A, et al. Mechanism of control of Na,K-ATPase in principal cells of the mammalian collecting duct. Ann N Y Acad Sci 2003;986:570–8.

[153] El Mernissi G, Doucet A. Short-term effects of aldosterone and dexamethasone on Na-K-ATPase along the rabbit nephron. Pflug Arch Eur J Phy 1983;399:147–51.

[154] El Mernissi G, Doucet A. Specific activity of Na-K-ATPase after adrenalectomy and hormone replacement along the rabbit nephron. Pflug Arch Eur J Phy 1984;402:258–63.

[155] Sansom SC, O'Neil RG. Effects of mineralocorticoids on transport properties of cortical collecting duct basolateral membrane. Am J Physiol 1986;251:F743–57.

[156] Kashgarian M, Ardito T, Hirsch DJ, Hayslett JP. Response of collecting tubule cells to aldosterone and potassium loading. Am J Physiol 1987;253:F8–14.

[157] Wade JB, O'Neil RG, Pryor JL, Boulpaep EL. Modulation of cell membrane area in renal collecting tubules by corticosteroid hormones. J Cell Biol 1979;81:439–45.

[158] Summa V, Mordasini D, Roger F, Bens M, Martin PY, Vandewalle A, et al. Short term effect of aldosterone on Na,K-ATPase cell surface expression in kidney collecting duct cells. J Biol Chem 2001;276:47087–93.

[159] Verrey F, Summa V, Heitzmann D, Mordasini D, Vandewalle A, Feraille E, et al. Short-term aldosterone action on Na,K-ATPase surface expression: role of aldosterone-induced SGK1? Ann N Y Acad Sci 2003;986:554–61.

[160] Zecevic M, Heitzmann D, Camargo SM, Verrey F. SGK1 increases Na,K-ATP cell-surface expression and function in Xenopus laevis oocytes. Pflug Arch Eur J Phy 2004;448:29–35.

[161] Funder JW. Minireview: Aldosterone and mineralocorticoid receptors: past, present, and future. Endocrinology 2010;151:5098–102.

[162] Dooley R, Harvey BJ, Thomas W. Non-genomic actions of aldosterone: from receptors and signals to membrane targets. Mol Cell Endocrinol 2012;350:223–34.

[163] Thomas W, Harvey BJ. Mechanisms underlying rapid aldosterone effects in the kidney. Annu Rev Physiol 2011;73:335–57.

[164] Gros R, Ding Q, Sklar LA, Prossnitz EE, Arterburn JB, Chorazyczewski J, et al. GPR30 expression is required for the mineralocorticoid receptor-independent rapid vascular effects of aldosterone. Hypertension 2011;57:442–51.

[165] Wendler A, Albrecht C, Wehling M. Nongenomic actions of aldosterone and progesterone revisited. Steroids 2012; 77:1002–6.

[166] Hofmeister MV, Damkier HH, Christensen BM, Olde B, Fredrik Leeb-Lundberg LM, Fenton RA, et al. 17beta-Estradiol induces nongenomic effects in renal intercalated cells through G protein-coupled estrogen receptor 1. Am J Physiol Renal Physiol 2012;302:F358–68.

[167] Le Moellic C, Ouvrard-Pascaud A, Capurro C, Cluzeaud F, Fay M, Jaisser F, et al. Early nongenomic events in aldosterone action in renal collecting duct cells: PKCalpha activation, mineralocorticoid receptor phosphorylation, and cross-talk with the genomic response. J Am Soc Nephrol: JASN 2004;15:1145–60.

[168] McEneaney V, Dooley R, Yusef YR, Keating N, Quinn U, Harvey BJ, et al. Protein kinase D1 modulates aldosterone-induced ENaC activity in a renal cortical collecting duct cell line. Mol Cell Endocrinol 2010;325:8–17.

[169] Hellal-Levy C, Couette B, Fagart J, Souque A, Gomez-Sanchez C, Rafestin-Oblin M. Specific hydroxylations determine selective corticosteroid recognition by human glucocorticoid and mineralocorticoid receptors. FEBS Lett 1999;464:9–13.

[170] Arriza JL, Simerly RB, Swanson LW, Evans RM. The neuronal mineralocorticoid receptor as a mediator of glucocorticoid response. Neuron 1988;1:887–900.

[171] Viengchareun S, Le Menuet D, Martinerie L, Munier M, Pascual-Le Tallec L, Lombes M. The mineralocorticoid receptor: insights into its molecular and (patho)physiological biology. Nucl Recept Signal 2007;5:e012.

[172] Fuller PJ, Yao Y, Yang J, Young MJ. Mechanisms of ligand specificity of the mineralocorticoid receptor. J Endocrinol 2012;213:15–24.

[173] Hubert EL, Teissier R, Fernandes-Rosa FL, Fay M, Rafestin-Oblin ME, Jeunemaitre X, et al. Mineralocorticoid receptor mutations and a severe recessive pseudohypoaldosteronism Type 1. J Am Soc Nephrol: JASN 2011;22(11):1997–2003.

[174] Riepe FG. Clinical and molecular features of type 1 pseudohypoaldosteronism. Horm Res 2009;72:1–9.

[175] Geller DS, Farhi A, Pinkerton N, Fradley M, Moritz M, Spitzer A, et al. Activating mineralocorticoid receptor mutation in hypertension exacerbated by pregnancy. Science 2000;289:119–23.

[176] Fagart J, Huyet J, Pinon GM, Rochel M, Mayer C, Rafestin-Oblin ME. Crystal structure of a mutant mineralocorticoid receptor responsible for hypertension. Nat Struct Mol Biol 2005;12:554–5.

[177] Huyet J, Pinon GM, Fay MR, Rafestin-Oblin ME, Fagart J. Structural determinants of ligand binding to the mineralocorticoid receptor. Mol Cell Endocrinol 2012;350:187–95.

[178] McKenna NJ. Discovery-driven research and bioinformatics in nuclear receptor and coregulator signaling. Biochim Biophys Acta 2011;1812:808−17.

[179] Yang J, Fuller PJ. Interactions of the mineralocorticoid receptor − within and without. Mol Cell Endocrinol 2012;350:196−205.

[180] Galigniana MD, Erlejman AG, Monte M, Gomez-Sanchez C, Piwien-Pilipuk G. The hsp90-FKBP52 complex links the mineralocorticoid receptor to motor proteins and persists bound to the receptor in early nuclear events. Mol Cell Biol 2010; 30:1285−98.

[181] Faresse N, Ruffieux-Daidie D, Salamin M, Gomez-Sanchez CE, Staub O. Mineralocorticoid receptor degradation is promoted by Hsp90 inhibition and the ubiquitin-protein ligase CHIP. Am J Physiol Renal Physiol 2010;299:F1462−72.

[182] Revollo JR, Cidlowski JA. Mechanisms generating diversity in glucocorticoid receptor signaling. Ann N Y Acad Sci 2009; 1179:167−78.

[183] Rupprecht R, Arriza JL, Spengler D, Reul JM, Evans RM, Holsboer F, et al. Transactivation and synergistic properties of the mineralocorticoid receptor: relationship to the glucocorticoid receptor. Mol Endocrinol 1993;7:597−603.

[184] Yang J, Chang CY, Safi R, Morgan J, McDonnell DP, Fuller PJ, et al. Identification of ligand-selective peptide antagonists of the mineralocorticoid receptor using phage display. Mol Endocrinol 2011;25:32−43.

[185] Fagart J, Wurtz JM, Souque A, Hellal-Levy C, Moras D, Rafestin-Oblin ME. Antagonism in the human mineralocorticoid receptor. EMBO J 1998;17:3317−25.

[186] Pascual-Le Tallec L, Lombes M. The mineralocorticoid receptor: a journey exploring its diversity and specificity of action. Mol Endocrinol 2005;19:2211−21.

[187] Berger S, Bleich M, Schmid W, Cole TJ, Peters J, Watanabe H, et al. Mineralocorticoid receptor knockout mice − pathophysiology of Na + metabolism. P Natl Acad Sci USA 1998; 95:9424−9.

[188] Berger S, Bleich M, Schmid W, Greger R, Schutz G. Mineralocorticoid receptor knockout mice: lessons on Na+ metabolism. Kidney Int 2000;57:1295−8.

[189] Bleich M, Warth R, Schmidt-Hieber M, Schulz-Baldes A, Hasselblatt P, Fisch D, et al. Rescue of the mineralocorticoid receptor knock-out mouse. Pflug Arch Eur J Phy 1999; 438:245−54.

[190] Ronzaud C, Loffing J, Gretz N, Schutz G, Berger S. Inducible renal principal cell-specific mineralocorticoid receptor gene inactivation in mice. Am J Physiol Renal Physiol 2011;300: F756−60.

[191] Le Menuet D, Viengchareun S, Muffat-Joly M, Zennaro MC, Lombes M. Expression and function of the human mineralocorticoid receptor: lessons from transgenic mouse models. Mol Cell Endocrinol 2004;217:127−36.

[192] Cole TJ, Blendy JA, Monaghan AP, Krieglstein K, Schmid W, Aguzzi A, et al. Targeted disruption of the glucocorticoid receptor gene blocks adrenergic chromaffin cell development and severely retards lung maturation. Genes Dev 1995; 9:1608−21.

[193] Nguyen Dinh Cat A, Ouvrard-Pascaud A, Tronche F, Clemessy M, Gonzalez-Nunez D, Farman N, et al. Conditional transgenic mice for studying the role of the glucocorticoid receptor in the renal collecting duct. Endocrinology 2009; 150:2202−10.

[194] Goodwin JE, Zhang J, Velazquez H, Geller DS. The glucocorticoid receptor in the distal nephron is not necessary for the development or maintenance of dexamethasone-induced hypertension. Biochem Biophys Res Commun 2010;394:266−71.

[195] Hammond GL, Smith CL, Goping IS, Underhill DA, Harley MJ, Reventos J, et al. Primary structure of human corticosteroid binding globulin, deduced from hepatic and pulmonary cDNAs, exhibits homology with serine protease inhibitors. P Natl Acad Sci USA 1987;84:5153−7.

[196] Ferrari P. The role of 11beta-hydroxysteroid dehydrogenase type 2 in human hypertension. Biochim Biophys Acta 2010;1802:1178−87.

[197] Naray-Fejes-Toth A, Fejes-Toth G. Extranuclear localization of endogenous 11beta-hydroxysteroid dehydrogenase-2 in aldosterone target cells. Endocrinology 1998;139:2955−9.

[198] Odermatt A, Arnold P, Frey FJ. The intracellular localization of the mineralocorticoid receptor is regulated by 11beta-hydroxysteroid dehydrogenase type 2. J Biol Chem 2001; 276:28484−92.

[199] Kotelevtsev Y, Brown RW, Fleming S, Kenyon C, Edwards CR, Seckl JR, et al. Hypertension in mice lacking 11beta-hydroxysteroid dehydrogenase type 2. J Clin Invest 1999;103:683−9.

[200] Holmes MC, Kotelevtsev Y, Mullins JJ, Seckl JR. Phenotypic analysis of mice bearing targeted deletions of 11beta-hydroxysteroid dehydrogenases 1 and 2 genes. Mol Cell Endocrinol 2001;171:15−20.

[201] Paterson JM, Seckl JR, Mullins JJ. Genetic manipulation of 11beta-hydroxysteroid dehydrogenases in mice. Am J Physiol Regul Integr Comp Physiol 2005;289:R642−52.

[202] Iniguez-Lluhi JA, Pearce D. A common motif within the negative regulatory regions of multiple factors inhibits their transcriptional synergy. Mol Cell Biol 2000;20:6040−50.

[203] Holmstrom S, Van Antwerp ME, Iniguez-Lluhi JA. Direct and distinguishable inhibitory roles for SUMO isoforms in the control of transcriptional synergy. P Natl Acad Sci USA 2003;100:15758−63.

[204] Bhargava A, Pearce D. Mechanisms of mineralocorticoid action: determinants of receptor specificity and actions of regulated gene products. Trends Endocrinol Metab 2004;15:147−53.

[205] Meijer OC, Kalkhoven E, van der Laan S, Steenbergen PJ, Houtman SH, Dijkmans TF, et al. Steroid receptor coactivator-1 splice variants differentially affect corticosteroid receptor signaling. Endocrinology 2005;146:1438−48.

[206] Meijer OC, Steenbergen PJ, De Kloet ER. Differential expression and regional distribution of steroid receptor coactivators SRC-1 and SRC-2 in brain and pituitary. Endocrinology 2000;141:2192−9.

[207] Verrey F. Transcriptional control of sodium transport in tight epithelial by adrenal steroids. J Membr Biol 1995;144:93−110.

[208] Firsov D. Revisiting sodium and water reabsorption with functional genomics tools. Curr Opin Nephrol Hypertens 2004;13:59−65.

[209] Mick VE, Itani OA, Loftus RW, Husted RF, Schmidt TJ, Thomas CP. The alpha-subunit of the epithelial sodium channel is an aldosterone-induced transcript in mammalian collecting ducts, and this transcriptional response is mediated via distinct cis-elements in the 5′-flanking region of the gene. Mol Endocrinol 2001;15:575−88.

[210] MacDonald P, MacKenzie S, Ramage LE, Seckl JR, Brown RW. Corticosteroid regulation of amiloride-sensitive sodium-channel subunit mRNA expression in mouse kidney. J Endocrinol 2000;165:25−37.

[211] Horisberger JD, Diezi J. Effects of mineralocorticoids on Na + and K + excretion in the adrenalectomized rat. Am J Physiol 1983;245:F89−99.

[212] Weissman AM, Shabek N, Ciechanover A. The predator becomes the prey: regulating the ubiquitin system by ubiquitylation and degradation. Nat Rev Mol Cell Biol 2011;12:605−20.

[213] Staub O, Gautschi I, Ishikawa T, Breitschopf K, Ciechanover A, Schild L, et al. Regulation of stability and function of the epithelial Na$^+$ channel (ENaC) by ubiquitination. EMBO J 1997;16:6325−36.

[214] Abriel H, Loffing J, Rebhun JF, Pratt JH, Horisberger J-D, Rotin D, et al. Defective regulation of the epithelial Na$^+$ channel (ENaC) by Nedd4 in Liddle's syndrome. J Clin Invest 1999;103:667−73.

[215] Kamynina E, Debonneville C, Bens M, Vandewalle A, Staub O. A novel mouse Nedd4 protein suppresses the activity of the epithelial Na$^+$ channel. FASEB J 2001;15:204−14.

[216] Bhalla V, Daidie D, Li H, Pao AC, Lagrange LP, Wang J, et al. Serum- and glucocorticoid-regulated kinase 1 regulates ubiquitin ligase neural precursor cell-expressed, developmentally down-regulated protein 4-2 by inducing interaction with 14-3-3. Mol Endocrinol 2005;19:3073−84.

[217] Rotin D, Staub O. Role of the ubiquitin system in regulating ion transport. Pflug Arch Eur J Phy 2010;461:1−21.

[218] Staub O, Dho S, Henry P, Correa J, Ishikawa T, McGlade J, et al. WW domains of Nedd4 bind to the proline-rich PY motifs in the epithelial Na$^+$ channel deleted in Liddle's syndrome. EMBO J 1996;15:2371−80.

[219] Firsov D, Schild L, Gautschi I, Mérillat A-M, Schneeberger E, Rossier BC. Cell surface expression of the epithelial Na$^+$ channel and a mutant causing Liddle syndrome: a quantitative approach. Proc Nat Acad Sci Usa 1996;93:15370−5.

[220] Loffing J, Flores SY, Staub O. Sgk kinases and their role in epithelial transport. Annu Rev Physiol 2006;68:461−90.

[221] Fakitsas P, Adam G, Daidie D, van Bemmelen MX, Fouladkou F, Patrignani A, et al. Early aldosterone-induced gene product regulates the epithelial sodium channel by deubiquitylation. J Am Soc Nephrol: JASN 2007;18:1084−92.

[222] Verrey F, Fakitsas P, Adam G, Staub O. Early transcriptional control of ENaC (de)ubiquitylation by aldosterone. Kidney Int 2008;73:691−6.

[223] Staub O, Verrey F. Impact of Nedd4 proteins and serum glucocorticoid-induced kinases on epithelial Na$^+$ transport in the distal nephron. J Am Soc Nephrol: JASN 2005;16:3167−74.

[224] Diakov A, Korbmacher C. A novel pathway of epithelial sodium channel activation involves a serum- and glucocorticoid-inducible kinase consensus motif in the C terminus of the channel's alpha-subunit. J Biol Chem 2004;279:38134−42.

[225] Zhang W, Xia X, Reisenauer MR, Rieg T, Lang F, Kuhl D, et al. Aldosterone-induced Sgk1 relieves Dot1a-Af9-mediated transcriptional repression of epithelial Na channel alpha. J Clin Invest 2007;117:773−83.

[226] Ruffieux-Daidie D, Poirot O, Boulkroun S, Verrey F, Kellenberger S, Staub O. Deubiquitylation regulates activation and proteolytic cleavage of ENaC. J Am Soc Nephrol: JASN 2008;19:2170−80.

[227] Ruffieux-Daidie D, Staub O. Intracellular ubiquitylation of the epithelial Na$^+$ channel controls extracellular proteolytic channel activation via conformational change. J Biol Chem 2011;286:2416−24.

[228] Oberfeld B, Ruffieux-Daidie D, Vitagliano JJ, Pos KM, Verrey F, Staub O. Ubiquitin-specific protease 2-45 (Usp2-45) binds to epithelial Na$^+$ channel (ENaC)-ubiquitylating enzyme Nedd4-2. Am J Physiol Renal Physiol 2011;301:F189−96.

[229] Shi PP, Cao XR, Sweezer EM, Kinney TS, Williams NR, Husted RF, et al. Salt-sensitive hypertension and cardiac hypertrophy in mice deficient in the ubiquitin ligase Nedd4-2. Am J Physiol Renal Physiol 2008;295:F462−70.

[230] Kimura T, Kawabe H, Jiang C, Zhang W, Xiang YY, Lu C, et al. Deletion of the ubiquitin ligase Nedd4L in lung epithelia causes cystic fibrosis-like disease. P Natl Acad Sci USA 2011;108(8):3216−21.

[231] Boase NA, Rychkov GY, Townley SL, Dinudom A, Candi E, Voss AK, et al. Respiratory distress and perinatal lethality in Nedd4-2-deficient mice. Nat Commun 2011;2:287.

[232] Fejes-Toth G, Frindt G, Naray-Fejes-Toth A, Palmer LG. Epithelial Na$^+$ channel activation and processing in mice lacking SGK1. Am J Physiol Renal Physiol 2008;294:F1298−305.

[233] Faresse N, Lagnaz D, Debonneville A, Ismailji A, Maillard M, Fejes-Toth G, et al. Inducible kidney-specific Sgk1 knockout mice show a salt-losing phenotype. Am J Physiol Renal Physiol 2012;302:F977−85.

[234] Ring AM, Leng Q, Rinehart J, Wilson FH, Kahle KT, Hebert SC, et al. An SGK1 site in WNK4 regulates Na$^+$ channel and K$^+$ channel activity and has implications for aldosterone signaling and K$^+$ homeostasis. Proc Nat Acad Sci Usa 2007;104:4025−9.

[235] Rozansky DJ, Cornwall T, Subramanya AR, Rogers S, Yang YF, David LL, et al. Aldosterone mediates activation of the thiazide-sensitive Na-Cl co-transporter through an SGK1 and WNK4 signaling pathway. J Clin Invest 2009;119:2601−12.

[236] Xu BE, Stippec S, Chu PY, Lazrak A, Li XJ, Lee BH, et al. WNK1 activates SGK1 to regulate the epithelial sodium channel. P Natl Acad Sci USA 2005.

[237] Heise CJ, Xu BE, Deaton SL, Cha SK, Cheng CJ, Earnest S, et al. Serum and glucocorticoid-induced kinase (SGK) 1 and the epithelial sodium channel are regulated by multiple with no lysine (WNK) family members. J Biol Chem 2010;285:25161−7.

[238] Rossier BC, Schild L. Epithelial sodium channel: Mendelian versus essential hypertension. Hypertension 2008;52:595−600.

[239] Vallon V, Lang F. New insights into the role of serum- and glucocorticoid-inducible kinase SGK1 in the regulation of renal function and blood pressure. Curr Opin Nephrol Hypertens 2005;14:59−66.

[240] Riepe FG, Holterhus PM. Exclusion of serum- and glucocorticoid-induced kinase 1 (SGK1) as a candidate gene for genetically heterogeneous renal pseudohypoaldosteronism Type I in eight families. Am J Nephrol 2007;27:164−9.

[241] Jin HS, Hong KW, Lim JE, Hwang SY, Lee SH, Shin C, et al. Genetic variations in the sodium balance-regulating genes ENaC, NEDD4L, NDFIP2 and USP2 influence blood pressure and hypertension. Kidney Blood Press Res 2010;33:15−23.

[242] Hughey RP, Bruns JB, Kinlough CL, Harkleroad KL, Tong Q, Carattino MD, et al. Epithelial sodium channels are activated by furin-dependent proteolysis. J Biol Chem 2004;279:18111−4.

[243] Vallet V, Chraibi A, Gaeggeler H-P, Horisberger J-D, Rossier BC. An epithelial serine protease activates the amiloride-sensitive sodium channel. Nature 1997;389:607−10.

[244] Rossier BC, Stutts MJ. Activation of the epithelial sodium channel (ENaC) by serine proteases. Annu Rev Physiol 2009;71:361−79 [250]

[245] Narikiyo T, Kitamura K, Adachi M, Miyoshi T, Iwashita K, Shiraishi N, et al. Regulation of prostasin by aldosterone in the kidney. J Clin Invest 2002;109:401−8.

[246] Knight KK, Olson DR, Zhou R, Snyder PM. Liddle's syndrome mutations increase Na$^+$ transport through dual effects on epithelial Na$^+$ channel surface expression and proteolytic cleavage. P Natl Acad Sci USA 2006;103:2805−8.

[247] Pochynyuk O, Bugaj V, Stockand JD. Physiologic regulation of the epithelial sodium channel by phosphatidylinositides. Curr Opin Nephrol Hypertens 2008;17:533−40.

[248] Rieg T, Bundey RA, Chen Y, Deschenes G, Junger W, Insel PA, et al. Mice lacking P2Y2 receptors have salt-resistant hypertension and facilitated renal Na$^+$ and water reabsorption. FASEB J 2007;21(13):3717−26.

[249] Spindler B, Mastroberardino L, Custer M, Verrey F. Characterization of early aldosterone-induced RNAs identified in A6 kidney epithelia. Pflügers Arch 1997;434:323–31.

[250] Mastroberardino L, Spindler B, Forster I, Loffing J, Assandri R, May A, et al. Ras pathway activates epithelial Na$^+$ channel and decreases its surface expression in Xenopus oocytes. Mol Biol Cell 1998;9:3417–27.

[251] Staruschenko A, Pochynyuk OM, Tong Q, Stockand JD. Ras couples phosphoinositide 3-OH kinase to the epithelial Na$^+$ channel. Biochim Biophys Acta 2005;1669:108–15.

[252] Staruschenko A, Patel P, Tong Q, Medina JL, Stockand JD. Ras activates the epithelial Na(+) channel through phosphoinositide 3-OH kinase signaling. J Biol Chem 2004;279: 37771–8.

[253] Staruschenko A, Pochynyuk O, Vandewalle A, Bugaj V, Stockand JD. Acute regulation of the epithelial Na$^+$ channel by phosphatidylinositide 3-OH kinase signaling in native collecting duct principal cells. J Am Soc Nephrol: JASN 2007;18: 1652–61.

[254] Lu M, Wang J, Ives HE, Pearce D. mSIN1 protein mediates SGK1 protein interaction with mTORC2 protein complex and is required for selective activation of the epithelial sodium channel. J Biol Chem 2011;286:30647–54.

[255] Naray-Fejes-Toth A, Snyder PM, Fejes-Toth G. The kidney-specific WNK1 isoform is induced by aldosterone and stimulates epithelial sodium channel-mediated Na$^+$ transport. P Natl Acad Sci USA 2004;101:17434–9.

[256] Hoorn EJ, Nelson JH, McCormick JA, Ellison DH. The WNK kinase network regulating sodium, potassium, and blood pressure. J Am Soc Nephrol: JASN 2011;22:605–14.

[257] Arroyo JP, Ronzaud C, Lagnaz D, Staub O, Gamba G. Aldosterone paradox: differential regulation of ion transport in distal nephron. Physiology (Bethesda) 2011;26:115–23.

[258] Grossmann C, Gekle M. Interaction between mineralocorticoid receptor and epidermal growth factor receptor signaling. Mol Cell Endocrinol 2012;350:235–41.

[259] Attali B, Latter H, Rachamim N, Garty H. A corticosteroid-induced gene expressing an "IsK-like" K$^+$ channel activity in Xenopus oocytes. Proceedings of the National Academy of Sciences of the Unites States of America 1995;92:6092–6.

[260] Geering K, Beguin P, Garty H, Karlish S, Fuzesi M, Horisberger JD, et al. FXYD proteins: new tissue- and isoform-specific regulators of Na,K-ATPase. Ann N Y Acad Sci 2003;986:388–94.

[261] Sweadner KJ, Arystarkhova E, Donnet C, Wetzel RK. FXYD proteins as regulators of the Na,K-ATPase in the kidney. Ann N Y Acad Sci 2003;986:382–7.

[262] Beguin P, Crambert G, Guennoun S, Garty H, Horisberger JD, Geering K. CHIF, a member of the FXYD protein family, is a regulator of Na,K-ATPase distinct from the gamma-subunit. EMBO J 2001;20:3993–4002.

[263] Capurro C, Coutry N, Bonvalet JP, Escoubet B, Garty H, Farman N. Cellular localization and regulation of CHIF in kidney and colon. Am J Physiol 1996;271:C753–62.

[264] Goldschmidt I, Grahammer F, Warth R, Schulz-Baldes A, Garty H, Greger R, et al. Kidney and colon electrolyte transport in CHIF knockout mice. Cell Physiol Biochem 2004;14:113–20.

[265] Boulkroun S, Fay M, Zennaro MC, Escoubet B, Jaisser F, Blot-Chabaud M, et al. Characterization of rat NDRG2 (N-Myc downstream regulated gene 2), a novel early mineralocorticoid-specific induced gene. J Biol Chem 2002;277: 31506–15.

[266] Wielputz MO, Lee IH, Dinudom A, Boulkroun S, Farman N, Cook DI, et al. (NDRG2) stimulates amiloride-sensitive Na + currents in Xenopus laevis oocytes and fisher rat thyroid cells. J Biol Chem 2007;282:28264–73.

[267] Murray JT, Campbell DG, Morrice N, Auld GC, Shpiro N, Marquez R, et al. Exploitation of KESTREL to identify NDRG family members as physiological substrates for SGK1 and GSK3. Biochem J 2004;384:477–88.

[268] Robert-Nicoud M, Flahaut M, Elalouf JM, Nicod M, Salinas M, Bens M, et al. Transcriptome of a mouse kidney cortical collecting duct cell line: effects of aldosterone and vasopressin. P Natl Acad Sci USA 2001;98:2712–6.

[269] Muller OG, Parnova RG, Centeno G, Rossier BC, Firsov D, Horisberger JD. Mineralocorticoid effects in the kidney: correlation between alphaENaC, GILZ, and Sgk-1 mRNA expression and urinary excretion of Na(+) and K(+). J Am Soc Nephrol 2003;14:1107–15.

[270] Soundararajan R, Melters D, Shih IC, Wang J, Pearce D. Epithelial sodium channel regulated by differential composition of a signaling complex. P Natl Acad Sci USA 2009;106:7804–9.

[271] Soundararajan R, Wang J, Melters D, Pearce D. Glucocorticoid-induced Leucine zipper 1 stimulates the epithelial sodium channel by regulating serum- and glucocorticoid-induced kinase 1 stability and subcellular localization. J Biol Chem 2010;285:39905–13.

[272] Suarez PE, Rodriguez EG, Soundararajan R, Merillat AM, Stehle JC, Rotman S, et al. The glucocorticoid-induced leucine zipper (gilz/tsc22d3-2) gene locus plays a crucial role in male fertility. Mol Endocrinol 2012;26(6):1000–13.

[273] Gumz ML, Stow LR, Lynch IJ, Greenlee MM, Rudin A, Cain BD, et al. The circadian clock protein Period 1 regulates expression of the renal epithelial sodium channel in mice. J Clin Invest 2009;119:2423–34.

[274] Nikolaeva S, Pradervand S, Centeno G, Zavadova V, Tokonami N, Maillard M, et al. The circadian clock modulates renal sodium handling. J Am Soc Nephrol: JASN 2012; 23:1019–26.

[275] Firsov D, Tokonami N, Bonny O. Role of the renal circadian timing system in maintaining water and electrolytes homeostasis. Mol Cell Endocrinol 2012;349:51–5.

[276] Zhang J, Ge R, Matte-Martone C, Goodwin J, Shlomchik WD, Mamula MJ, et al. Characterization of a novel gain of function glucocorticoid receptor knock-in mouse. J Biol Chem 2009;284:6249–59.

[277] Bailey MA, Craigie E, Livingstone DE, Kotelevtsev YV, Al-Dujaili EA, Kenyon CJ, et al. Hsd11b2 haploinsufficiency in mice causes salt sensitivity of blood pressure. Hypertension 2011;57:515–20.

[278] Huang DY, Wulff P, Volkl H, Loffing J, Richter K, Kuhl D, et al. Impaired regulation of renal K$^+$ elimination in the sgk1-knockout mouse. J Am Soc Nephrol: JASN 2004;15:885–91.

[279] Lang F, Vallon V. Serum- and glucocorticoid-inducible kinase 1 in the regulation of renal and extrarenal potassium transport. Clin Exp Nephrol 2012;16:73–80.

[280] Pradervand S, Wang Q, Burnier M, Beermann F, Horisberger JD, Hummler E, et al. A mouse model for Liddle's syndrome. J Am Soc Nephrol: JASN 1999;10:2527–33.

[281] Cao XR, Shi PP, Sigmund RD, Husted RF, Sigmund CD, Williamson RA, et al. Mice heterozygous for beta-ENaC deletion have defective potassium excretion. Am J Physiol Renal Physiol 2006;291:F107–15.

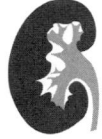

Inherited Disorders of Renal Salt Homeostasis: Insights from Molecular Genetics Studies

Ute I. Scholl and Richard P. Lifton

Departments of Genetics and Internal Medicine, Howard Hughes Medical Institute,
Yale University School of Medicine, New Haven, CT, USA

INTRODUCTION

Approaches to Identify Genes and Mutations that Contribute to Human Disease

The regulation of blood pressure is fantastically complex, with contributions from the brain, heart, vasculature, adrenal, and kidney. In the face of such complexity, it has been very difficult to identify the rate-limiting steps in the determination of long-term blood pressure from physiologic analysis alone. In this setting, human genetics has proven highly informative, because the finding of mutations in specific genes that result in significant effects on blood pressure can establish a causal link between specific genes, their biochemical pathways, and blood pressure.[1]

There are a number of approaches to the discovery of human disease genes. One approach is to search for rare mutations with large effects on the trait. In the most extreme form these are so-called Mendelian traits, in which the presence of rare mutations produces a distinctive trait, and the transmission of that trait can be followed through families based on the clinical features. These traits generally follow a few simple patterns of inheritance. Autosomal dominant traits are produced by the inheritance of one mutated copy of a gene. As a result, such traits are commonly transmitted from an affected parent to half of their offspring, and multi-generational pedigrees with many affected subjects can sometimes be found. Dominant mutations can either be gain-of-function — in which the mutant gene has function not present in the normal gene — or less often loss of biochemical function, with a large effect produced by a 50% reduction in gene dosage. Dominant mutations that drastically impair reproductive fitness are commonly found as *de novo* mutations; new mutations found in affected index cases that are absent in their biological parents. Autosomal recessive traits require the inheritance of mutations in the genes on both chromosomes. Typical recessive pedigrees show affected subjects among a single sibship in a family, with parents being clinically unaffected and one in four of their offspring being affected. The mutations that cause autosomal recessive traits typically result in loss of biochemical function. Mutations on the X-chromosome produce distinctive patterns of transmission, since males have only one copy of this chromosome. As a result, these traits are never transmitted from affected fathers to their sons, and loss-of-function traits are found far more frequently among males than females. Other patterns of Mendelian transmission are much less frequent.

The development of complete genetic maps of the human genome identified extensive variations in DNA sequence, allowing the comparison of the inheritance of every segment of every chromosome to the inheritance of the Mendelian trait in families. With sufficient numbers of informative individuals and families, the chromosomal location of disease genes can be mapped, and genes in the linked interval can be searched for mutations. The finding of independent mutations that show specificity for the trait, and which significantly segregate with the trait in pedigrees, provides evidence that a gene responsible for the trait has been identified.

Seldin and Giebisch's The Kidney, Fifth Edition.
DOI: http://dx.doi.org/10.1016/B978-0-12-381462-3.00036-7

To date, genes and their corresponding mutations that underlie more than 3000 human disease traits have been identified by this approach. The strength of Mendelian genetics has been that the identified mutations directly identify the gene whose function is altered, and is causal to the trait. A second strength is that because the effect size is typically very large, robust inferences about the effect of implicated genes on the trait are possible.

A second general approach to genetic analysis is genetic association. This approach has historically sought to determine whether specific common variants are found with significantly different frequency among cohorts of patients contrasting for specific phenotypes. Early efforts typically used candidate gene approaches, and commonly produced false-positive results. The development of dense maps containing millions of common variants called single nucleotide polymorphisms (SNPs) across the human genome, coupled with the ability to genotype these inexpensively, has led to large-scale genome-wide association studies (GWAS). These studies have allowed careful matching of genetic backgrounds of cases and controls, as well as rigorous statistical thresholds for significance. More than 1200 robust associations of common sequence variations with disease have been established using this approach. Strengths of the approach are the ability to find effects that are common in the population. These have been highly informative in diseases for which Mendelian forms have not been found. Weaknesses are that the common variants are most often not in genes, and consequently identifying the genes whose expression might be altered can be difficult to establish. Also, effect sizes are typically very small, changing disease risk by ~20%. As a result, new biological inferences are frequently difficult to immediately discern from these studies. Nonetheless, these studies can provide leads for diseases that have not yielded productive results from Mendelian studies.

Most recently, the ability to inexpensively sequence whole genomes or whole exomes (all the exons of protein-coding genes) has provided new opportunities for disease gene discovery. Classes of Mendelian traits that were previously intractable, such as diseases caused predominantly by *de novo* mutations, can now be solved. Moreover, one can anticipate that searches for rare variants with moderate effect size − less than typical Mendelian traits, but much larger than GWAS signals − are likely to be discovered by sequencing large cohorts of cases and controls.

Insight into Human Blood Pressure Variation from Genetic Studies

In the past 20 years, molecular genetic studies of rare Mendelian diseases featuring extreme forms of hyper- and hypotension have greatly contributed to our understanding of renal salt handling, and its role in blood pressure regulation.[1] Despite the complexity of blood pressure regulation, which is influenced by diverse mechanisms including the neuronal, cardiovascular, and endocrine systems, many if not all of the genes thus far identified ultimately directly or indirectly affect renal salt reabsorption. Specifically, genes whose products increase renal salt reabsorption cause hypertension, while genes diminishing renal salt reabsorption result in hypovolemia, and sometimes life-threatening hypotension. Increased salt reabsorption is accompanied by water reabsorption to maintain normal concentrations of Na^+, leading to increased intravascular volume, increased venous blood return to the heart, and increased cardiac output via the Frank−Starling mechanism. Blood pressure then rises according to Ohm's law. These findings have implicated renal salt handling as a key element of long-term blood pressure homeostasis.

Nonetheless, hemodynamic patterns among hypertensive patients, even among those with primary increases in renal salt homeostasis, show increased systemic vascular resistance (SVR) with normal cardiac output. An explanation for this has been provided by Hall and Guyton, who have shown that tissues regulate their perfusion by increasing or decreasing vascular resistance according to metabolic demand. Dogs given aldosterone initially show expanded intravascular volume and increased cardiac output, but within weeks evolve to a state of high SVR and normal cardiac output.[2] These findings establish that one cannot infer the initiating cause of hypertension from steady-state hemodynamic profiles.

Overview of Renal Salt Homeostasis

The kidneys filter about 180 liters of plasma per day, containing ~1.5 kg of salt; ~99.5% of the filtered salt load must be reabsorbed on a typical Western diet to maintain sodium homeostasis (Figure 36.1). The bulk of this reabsorption (50−60%) occurs in the proximal tubule, driven by the basolateral Na^+/K^+-ATPase and apical Na^+/H^+ exchanger, as well as co-transporters that couple uptake of glucose, amino acids, and other solutes to the favorable gradient for Na^+ reabsorption. Approximately 30% of the filtered load is reabsorbed in the thick ascending limb of Henle (TAL) via the $Na^+/K^+/2Cl^-$ co-transporter NKCC2, the target of loop diuretics, and ~7−10% in the distal convoluted tubule (DCT) via the thiazide-sensitive Na-Cl co-transporter NCC. The fine-tuning of renal salt reabsorption (~2−5%) occurs in the connecting tubule (CNT) and cortical collecting duct (CCD), and is predominantly mediated by the epithelial sodium channel

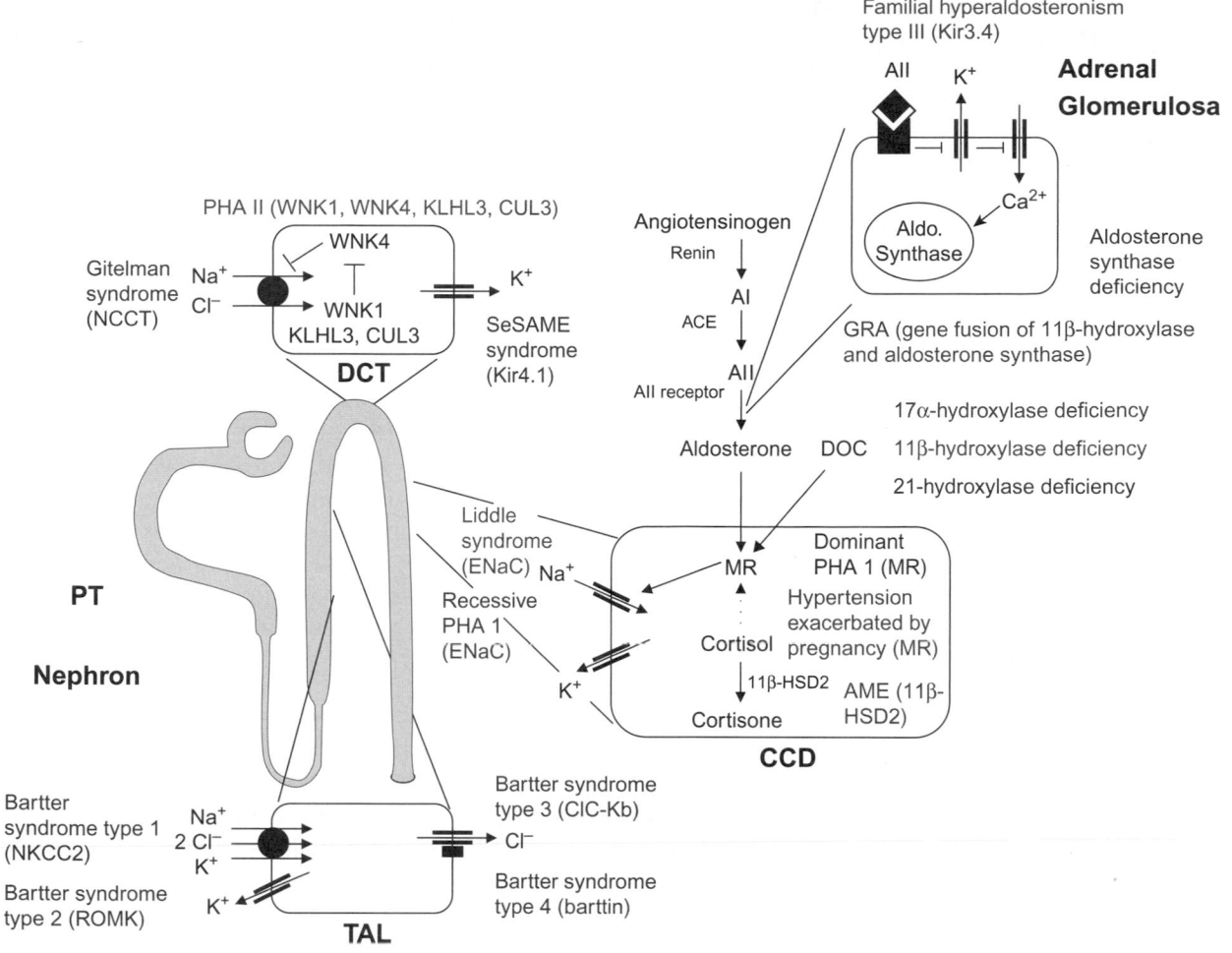

FIGURE 36.1 Diagram of the nephron and the renin–angiotensin–aldosterone system. Shown are key molecular pathways mutated in Mendelian forms of hypertension (red) and hypotension (blue). See text for details (AI: angiotensin I; AII: angiotensin II; ACE: angiotensin converting enzytme; Aldo. Synthase: aldosterone synthase; AME: apparent mineralocorticoid excess; CCD: cortical collecting duct; DOC: desoxycortisone; GRA: glucocorticoid remediable aldosteronism; MR: mineralocorticoid receptor; 11β-HSD2: 11β-hydroxysteroid dehydrogenase-2; PHAI: pseudohypoaldosteronism type 1; PHA II: pseudohypoaldosteronism type II; PT: proximal tubule; TAL: thick ascending limb of Henle). See color section at the back of the book *(adapted from ref. [1])*.

(ENaC), the target of the potassium-sparing diuretic amiloride. Many of the tubular channels, transporters, and regulators involved in these processes of salt reabsorption are affected by loss- and/or gain-of-function mutations that will be discussed in this chapter.

A major regulatory pathway that modulates renal salt reabsorption is the renin–angotensin–aldosterone system (Figure 36.1). In response to intravascular volume depletion or reduced delivery of salt to the thick ascending limb of Henle, the juxtaglomerular apparatus of the kidney secretes the active form of the aspartyl protease renin. Active renin cleaves angiotensinogen that is produced by the liver and constitutively circulates in the blood; this cleavage produces the decapeptide angiotensin I (AI), which is then cleaved by the angiotensin-converting enzyme (ACE), resulting in the octapeptide angiotensin II (AII). Angiotensin II binds to a specific G-protein-coupled receptor in adrenal glomerulosa (the type 1 angiotensin II receptor or AT1 receptor). This binding results in the activation of signaling cascades leading to adrenal glomerulosa membrane depolarization, activation of voltage-gated calcium channels, calcium influx, and increased synthesis of the steroid hormone aldosterone. Aldosterone, an effector of this pathway, communicates a signal for increased salt reabsorption to the kidney: it binds to the mineralocorticoid receptor (MR), a nuclear hormone receptor located in cells of the DCT, CNT, and principal cells of the CCD (the so-called aldosterone-sensitive distal nephron), leading to increased salt reabsorption via ENaC, and also the NCC (see above). The renin–angiotensin–aldosterone (RAA) pathway is not only mutated in genetic disorders of salt homeostasis, but is also the target of multiple pharmacologic approaches in the treatment of hypertension, including renin inhibitors, ACE inhibitors, angiotensin receptor blockers, and aldosterone antagonists.

This chapter covers the genetic disorders that modulate blood pressure by altering renal salt reabsorption, as well as the insights into physiological mechanisms of blood pressure regulation derived from these discoveries.

GENETIC DISORDERS CAUSING HYPERTENSION

Mendelian forms of hypertension are rare among the general hypertensive population. Clues to the deduction that a patient may have an underlying Mendelian cause of hypertension generally come from the age of onset, the family history, and distinctive biochemical features. Hypertension is very uncommon in the first decade of life, and unusual before the age of 18; however, this is a typical finding among subjects with Mendelian hypertension. Consequently, Mendelian diseases should be considered in patients with early onset hypertension, and should be ruled out if there is also a family history of early onset hypertension. Other diseases that can cause hypertension in young subjects, such as structural renal defects and other causes of renal insufficiency, should be ruled out as well. Hypertension can be very severe, but this is not invariably the case. Biochemical findings that are most helpful in pointing to a diagnosis are plasma renin activity, aldosterone levels (best measured in 24 hour urine specimens), and serum/plasma electrolyte values. It is important to note that patients with aldosteronism need not have hypokalemia, and the absence of this finding should not be taken to exclude a disorder caused by increased aldosterone or increased activity of the mineralocorticoid receptor. An algorithm that is helpful in the evaluation of these patients is shown in Figure 36.2.

Disorders of the Renin—Angiotensin—Aldosterone System

Mutations that Increase Activation of the Mineralocorticoid Receptor

A number of genes have been identified in which mutation results in hypertension due to increased activation of the mineralocorticoid receptor (MR). These include diseases caused by mutations that lead to renin-independent production of aldosterone, as well as diseases in which steroids other than aldosterone can activate MR.

MUTATIONS RESULTING IN INCREASED ALDOSTERONE SECRETION

GLUCOCORTICOID-REMEDIABLE ALDOSTERONISM (FAMILIAL HYPERALDOSTERONISM TYPE I) Glucocorticoid-Remediable Aldosteronism (GRA) is an autosomal dominant disease featuring hypertension with inappropriate aldosterone secretion despite suppression of the renin—angiotensin system.[3] Patients typically present with hypertension in the first two decades of life, and are found to have elevated

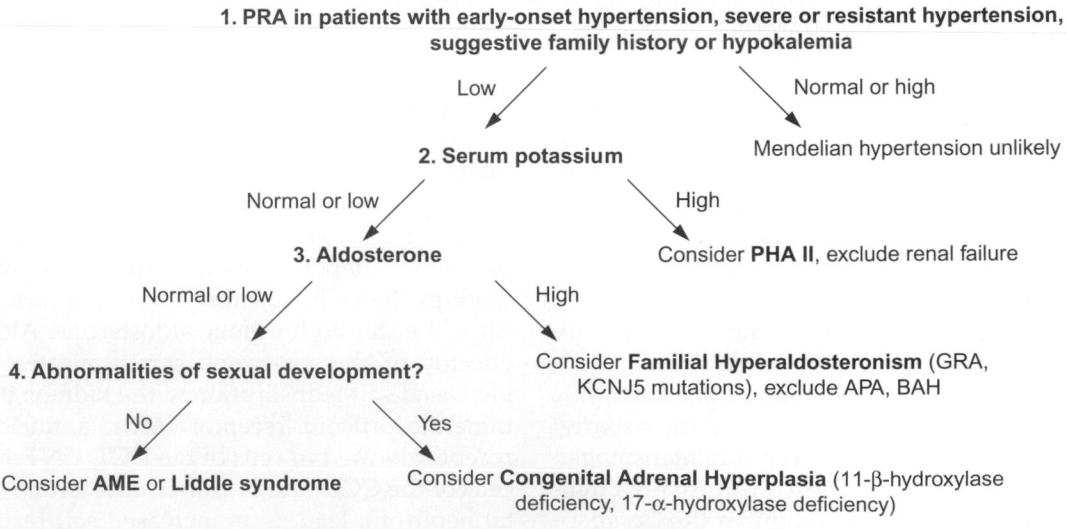

Evaluation for Mendelian Hypertension

FIGURE 36.2   **A diagnostic approach to Mendelian hypertension.** (PRA: plasma renin activity; PHAII: pseudohypoaldosteronism type II; GRA: glucocorticoid remediable aldosteronism; APA: aldosterone-producing adenoma; BAH: bilateral adrenal hyperplasia; AME: apparent mineralocorticoid excess.)

Adrenal Steroid Synthesis

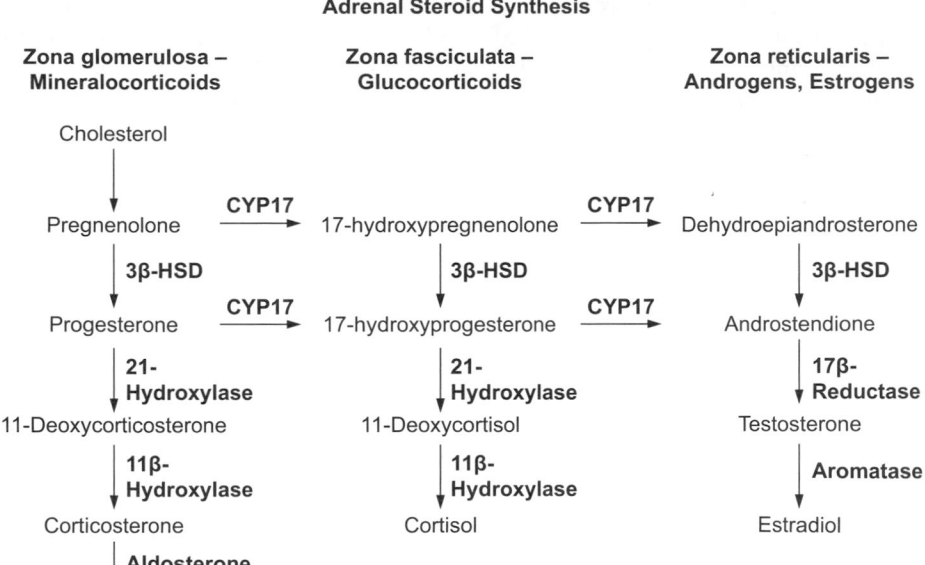

FIGURE 36.3 **Adrenal steroid synthesis.** Hormone synthesis in the adrenal cortex occurs in distinct compartments: aldosterone is synthesized in the outermost zona glomerulosa; cortisol in adrenal fasciculata; and sexual steroids in the innermost zona reticularis. Enzymes required for biosynthesis are noted (3β-HSD: 3β-hydroxysteroid dehydrogenase).

aldosterone secretion despite suppressed plasma renin activity, indicating autonomous production of aldosterone. Hypertension is often severe, and affected subjects are at a markedly increased risk of cerebral hemorrhage at young ages.[4] Hypokalemia and metabolic alkalosis are variable associated findings.[5,6] Consistent with autosomal dominant transmission, the family history is usually positive, with one parent and about half of siblings and offspring having early diagnosis of hypertension, and there is a frequent history of early cerebral hemorrhage.

Unlike normal individuals, aldosterone secretion in GRA shows sustained increase with administration of the cortisol secretagogue ACTH. Moreover, affected subjects produce so-called hybrid steroids, 18-hydroxy- and 18-oxocortisol, which are present in negligible amounts in normal subjects. These hybrid steroids have hydroxylation at C-17, characteristic of metabolism by 17-alpha hydroxylase (CYP17 gene) in the adrenal fasciculata, and oxidation at C-18, characteristic of metabolism by aldosterone synthase, which is normally confined to the adrenal glomerulosa[7,8] (Figure 36.3). Suppression of cortisol secretion from the adrenal gland by administration of exogenous glucocorticoids also causes rapid and sustained suppression of aldosterone secretion, a finding that does not occur in normal individuals.[3] These features suggest that aldosterone in GRA is produced in the adrenal fasciculata under the control of ACTH, rather than in adrenal glomerulosa under the control of the normal secretagogue angiotensin II (Ang II).

Analysis of linkage in a large GRA kindred demonstrated complete linkage of early hypertension to

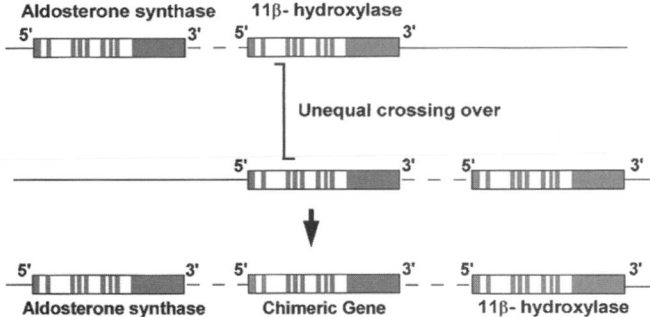

FIGURE 36.4 **Unequal crossing-over recombination between aldosterone synthase and 11-β hydroxylase causes GRA.** Shown is the segment of chromosome 8 that contains the two highly homologous genes. Unequal crossing-over between these two genes produces a chromosome with normal copies of aldosterone synthase and 11-β hydroxylase, and a third chimeric gene between them that fuses 5′ regulatory sequences from 11-β hydroxylase to coding sequences of aldosterone synthase, conferring aldosterone synthase function on the encoded gene product (*reproduced with permission from ref. [1]*).

chromosome 8q, which contains the gene aldosterone synthase (CYP11B2) and the closely related gene steroid 11-β hydroxylase (CYP11B1). These two genes recently evolved from a common ancestor, and are highly similar at the DNA sequence level. Patients with GRA prove uniformly to have mutations that result from unequal crossing-over recombination between these two homologous genes (Figure 36.4). This recombination event produces two mutant chromosomes, one with normal copies of aldosterone synthase and 11-β hydroxylase, and a third chimeric gene between them that fuses 5′ regulatory sequences from 11-β hydroxylase to coding sequences of aldosterone synthase.[9,10] This is the mutation uniformly found in patients with GRA. The other mutant chromosome has no normal gene, and only a single hybrid gene that fuses 5′ sequences from aldosterone synthase to a coding sequence that produces 11-β hydroxylase enzymatic activity. This mutation is found in some patients with 11-β hydroxylase deficiency. These events occur in pre-meiotic germ cell development, hence only one is transmitted to a zygote. All of these recombination events seen in GRA occur upstream of exon 5,[10] with the result that the hybrid genes in patients with GRA include the two amino acids in exons 5 and 6 that are critical for the resulting enzyme having aldosterone synthase rather than 11-β hydroxylase activity.[11] These hybrid genes bear the 5′ regulatory elements of 11-β hydroxylase, and are consequently expressed in adrenal fasciculata under the control of ACTH, but encode aldosterone synthase enzymatic activity. As a consequence, aldosterone secretion in these patients is constitutive, driven by ACTH and the maintenance of normal cortisol levels. The renin—angiotensin system is suppressed, but this fails to turn off aldosterone production. These mutations thus account for the ectopic production of aldosterone in adrenal fasciculata and its control by ACTH, and explain the resulting hypertension.

GRA should be suspected by the finding of hypertension in young individuals with elevated aldosterone level (best measured in 24 hour urine samples), despite suppressed plasma renin activity, particularly if there is a history of early hypertension among first degree relatives. Hypokalemia and metabolic alkalosis are common but by no means invariant, and the absence of these findings should not be used to exclude the diagnosis.[5] Molecular genetic testing by either Southern blotting[9] or PCR[12] provides a sensitive and specific means for establishing the diagnosis. Because of the autosomal dominant transmission, there are frequently many affected members among extended families of index cases, and case finding can be performed by sequential sampling, testing all first degree relatives of affected subjects, then all first degree relatives of positive cases in subsequent rounds. Sampling in these families is likely to prevent morbidity and mortality from uncontrolled hypertension and early cerebral hemorrhage. Because of the availability of genetic screening, determination of urinary levels of hybrid steroids or dexamethasone suppression test is no longer recommended.[13] Of note, family screening has demonstrated that not all individuals carrying the gene fusion are hypertensive,[14] and first degree relatives of patients with confirmed GRA should be genetically screened even in the absence of hypertension.[15]

Treatment options for GRA include use of mineralocorticoid receptor antagonists (spironolactone or eplerenone), amiloride or triamterene (which inhibit the epithelial sodium channel that drives both hypertension and hypokalemic alkalosis in GRA). Exogenous glucocorticoids can be used to shut down aldosterone production from the adrenal fasciculata. Careful attention to dosage in children is essential to maintain normal growth and to avoid glucocorticoid side-effects. Potassium-wasting diuretics such as hydrochlorothiazide and furosemide should be used with caution, because of the risk of severe hypokalemia.[13,15]

ALDOSTERONE-PRODUCING ADRENAL ADENOMA AND FAMILIAL HYPERALDOSTERONISM DUE TO KCNJ5 MUTATIONS Aldosterone-producing adenoma, also known as Conn's syndrome,[16] is a common cause of severe hypertension, found in about 5% of patients in hypertension referral clinics worldwide, and in about half of patients diagnosed with primary aldosteronism.[17] Patients typically present with worsening hypertension, and are found to have elevated serum and 24 hour urinary aldosterone levels in conjunction with suppressed plasma renin activity, consistent with these tumors having renin-independent aldosterone secretion. Hypokalemia and metabolic alkalosis are frequent, but not invariant findings. The finding of an adrenal mass by CT scan with increased aldosterone levels in ipsilateral adrenal vein plasma is considered diagnostic, and removal of these tumors corrects or improves blood pressure in the large majority of patients.[13]

Exome sequencing of four aldosterone-producing adrenal adenomas (APAs) and matched blood DNA enabled identification of somatic mutations in the tumors.[18] The results showed a low somatic mutation rate, with only 2—5 somatic mutations per tumor. Surprisingly, the K^+ channel encoded by KCNJ5 was mutated in two of these tumors. Examination of this channel in 22 tumors identified somatic KCNJ5 mutations in 8 tumors, and either of the same two mutations were found in all, substituting arginine for glycine at position 151 or arginine for leucine at position 168. These two positions lie in or abut the highly conserved K^+ channel selectivity filter that enables these channels to allow passage of K^+ but not other ions through the channel pore.[19,20] Electrophysiologic studies demonstrated that these mutations cause markedly increased Na^+ conductance of the mutant channel, sufficient to depolarize the cell.

These findings explain the pathogenesis of APA in these tumors. The normal adrenal glomerulosa cell is hyperpolarized owing to constitutively open K^+ channels.[21,22] Angiotensin II signaling results in closure of these channels,[23,24] resulting in depolarization and activation of voltage-gated calcium channels, which raises intracellular calcium. Hyperkalemia produces the same results, potentially via increased frequency of depolarizing membrane potential oscillations.[25] Increased intracellular Ca^{2+} is the acute signal for increased expression of aldosterone synthase and other rate-limiting steps in aldosterone biosynthesis. Chronic signaling provides the stimulus for increased cell replication.[26] Thus, these single mutations can explain both the cell-autonomous aldosterone secretion and cell proliferation that are the hallmarks of these benign tumors.

Subsequent work has confirmed these findings. The study of 287 tumors by Björklund et al. found the G151R or L168R mutations in 47% of APAs, and a markedly higher prevalence of these mutations among women with APA (63%) than men (22%). Only one additional mutation (E145Q) was found in two cases.[26a] Similar findings were observed by Boulkroun et al., who found either of these two mutations in 34% of all APAs with a similar bias for female subjects.[27] These tumors are more prevalent among younger individuals, and tend to be slightly larger compared to non-KCNJ5-mutant tumors.

In addition to these mutations causing APAs, they also account for a rare inherited form of primary aldosteronism. In 2008, Geller et al. reported a father and two daughters with a new familial form of severe early-onset hypertension due to primary aldosteronism.[28] Hypertension in these patients was diagnosed between the ages of 4 and 7 years; it was resistant to aggressive antihypertensive therapy, including spironolactone and amiloride. There was massive adrenocortical hyperplasia. Hybrid steroids 18-oxocortisol and 18-hydroxycortisol were elevated, however, in clear contrast to patients with GRA, there was a significant increase in aldosterone levels upon dexamethasone administration, and affected subjects did not have the gene fusion characteristic of GRA. Due to unrelenting hypertension, all three subjects underwent bilateral adrenalectomy in childhood, demonstrating massive adrenal hyperplasia (with paired adrenal weights up to 81 g, normal is less than 12 g) and diffuse hyperplasia of the zona fasciculata by light microscopy (with transitional zone morphology by electron microscopy). Screening of candidate genes revealed no pathogenic mutations.

Affected members of this family proved to have a T158A mutation in KCNJ5 which also modified channel selectivity, resulting in Na^+ conductance.[18] In this case, since the mutation is present in every cell, rather than acquired somatically by a single cell, every cell in the adrenal glomerulosa is receiving the signal for aldosterone production and cell proliferation, accounting for the massive adrenal hyperplasia and severe aldosteronism at young ages. This Mendelian form of disease provides strong evidence that these single mutations are sufficient for cell proliferation and constitutive aldosterone secretion.

Subsequent studies have identified additional families with early severe aldosteronism and mutations in KCNJ5. Most interestingly, these include two different mutations at the same amino acid — G151 — that result in markedly different phenotypes. One of these inherited mutations is G151R, the same mutation found as a somatic mutation in APA. Patients with inherited G151R[29] mutations develop massive adrenocortical hyperplasia, have difficult-to-control hypertension, and virtually invariably come to bilateral adrenalectomy for control of hypertension, similar to the T158A mutation described above. The other mutation is G151E. Patients with this mutation also present with early hypertension and aldosteronism; however, they do not develop adrenal hyperplasia, are typically responsive to antihypertensive therapy, and do not come to adrenalectomy.[29-31] Most interestingly, the milder human phenotype resulting from G151E is associated with a much more severe electrophysiologic phenotype. G151E results in dramatically greater Na^+ conductance than G151R. The consequence of this is markedly increased sodium-dependent lethality. This suggests a model in which cells expressing the G151E mutation differentiate from a stem cell pool, produce aldosterone as they are born, but die rapidly, preventing development of hyperplasia. Their continuous renewal from a stem cell pool provides a long-term source for excessive aldosterone production, and a milder hypertension than in subjects with the G151R mutation.

This phenotype of primary aldosteronism without adrenal hyperplasia due to KCNJ5 mutation is as yet unique to the G151E mutation, while massive adrenal hyperplasia requiring adrenalectomy has also been reported with another KCNJ5 mutation, I157S.[32]

While KCNJ5 mutations unequivocally explain the pathogenesis of a large fraction of APAs and a rare form of familial hypertension, the role of the wild-type channel in human adrenal function is less clear. Its activation by dopamine, an inhibitor of aldosterone secretion,[18,33] suggests that the normal role of this channel might be to hyperpolarize cells, contributing to inhibition of aldosterone secretion.

Primary aldosteronism due to mutations in aldosterone synthase and KCNJ5 both produce constitutive secretion of aldosterone and hypertension. Patients with KCNJ5 mutations tend to present in the first several years of life with severe hypertension, while those with GRA are more frequently, though not exclusively, diagnosed later in the first or second decade. Consistent with greater disease severity among KCNJ5 families and impaired reproductive fitness, no families with more than four affected members have been reported to date, while a number of large, multigenerational families with more than 20 members with GRA have been studied.

MUTATIONS CAUSING IMPAIRED CORTISOL BIOSYNTHESIS AND INCREASED MINERALOCORTICOIDS

CONGENITAL ADRENAL HYPERPLASIA DUE TO 11-β-HYDROXYLASE DEFICIENCY Congenital adrenal hyperplasia (CAH) is a recessive disease, featuring cortisol deficiency caused by inherited defects of enzymes required for cortisol biosynthesis in the adrenal gland. Affected patients have increased ACTH levels due to impaired feedback inhibition, which stimulates excessive production of steroids proximal to the impaired step in cortisol biosynthesis. Precursor steroids can have androgenic effects, and female patients may present with virilization. In the most common form of CAH (21-hydroxylase deficiency), impaired synthesis of mineralocorticoids leads to salt-wasting (see below), while other defects can result in accumulation of precursors which have mineralocorticoid effects, leading to hypertension.

The most common form of congenital adrenal hyperplasia associated with hypertension is 11-β-hydroxylase deficiency[34] (Figure 36.3). Affected females may present with ambiguous genitalia at birth or with menstrual irregularities and hirsutism in adolescence or adulthood, while male subjects may present with penile enlargement or precocious puberty. Hypertension and hypokalemia are variable associated features, and are thought to occur due to the accumulation of 11-deoxycorticosterone, a moderately potent mineralocorticoid. However, there is no clear correlation between 11-deoxycorticosterone levels, the degree of virilization and the presence of hypertension. Renin and aldosterone are typically low.[35–37]

In most cases, 11-β-hydroxylase deficiency is caused by recessive point mutations that cause loss-of-function of CYP11B1, although loss-of-function mutations due to the reciprocal product of unequal crossing-over between aldosterone synthase and 11-β-hydroxylase found in GRA (see above) can also produce loss-of-function mutations (in this case there is a chromosome that only expresses 11-β hydroxylase in adrenal glomerulosa).[38]

11-β-hydroxylase deficiency should be suspected in female infants with ambiguous genitalia and male infants with penile enlargement. In the late onset form, hirsutism and menstrual irregularities in female patients and precocious puberty in boys may be the only signs of presentation. The abnormal hormone profile, in particular the finding of elevated basal and ACTH-stimulated 11-deoxycortisol concentrations, is diagnostic. Treatment with exogenous glucocorticoids

suppresses ACTH secretion and the accumulation of precursor steroids. Precursor steroids should be monitored, and glucocorticoid dosage has to be carefully adjusted to avoid growth inhibition in children and exogenous Cushing's syndrome. Persistent hypertension may require additional treatment with aldosterone antagonists or amiloride.

CONGENITAL ADRENAL HYPERPLASIA DUE TO 17-α-HYDROXYLASE DEFICIENCY 17-α-hydroxylase deficiency[39] is a rare cause of congenital adrenal hyperplasia. Patients typically present in adolescence with lack of pubertal development. Genetic females have primary amenorrhea and do not develop secondary sexual characteristics; genetic males typically have complete pseudohermaphroditism with female external genitalia and intra-abdominal testes, although ambiguous genitalia have been reported. Hypertension is a common finding, and may be associated with hypokalemia.[40]

17-α-hydroxylase deficiency is caused by mutations in CYP17.[41] The encoded enzyme is expressed in adrenal gland and gonads, and has both 17-hydroxylase and 17,20-lyase activities (Figure 36.3). Most patients with CYP17 mutations thus have combined deficiencies of both enzymatic functions, although isolated deficiency of 17,20-lyase activity has been reported.[42] Hydroxylation at carbon 17 of the steroid nucleus is required for cortisol production, and in its absence normal activation of the glucocorticoid receptor is not achieved. In addition, 17,20-lyase activity is needed for the generation of androgen and estrogen precursors from cortisol precursors.

Patients with CYP17 mutations consequently have cortisol deficiency leading to elevated ACTH levels, as well as androgen and estrogen deficiency, accounting for sexual infantilism and pseudohermaphroditism. Hypertension is caused by activation of the mineralocorticoid receptor (MR) due to increased levels of 11-deoxysteroids (corticosterone, 11-deoxycorticosterone, and 18-hydroxy-deoxycorticosterone), similar to the mechanism of hypertension in 11-β-hydroxylase deficiency. As a result, renin and aldosterone are typically suppressed.

The diagnosis is based on the clinical presentation and characteristic hormone profile, and treatment relies on replacement of glucocorticoids and sex steroids, the latter starting in adolescence.

Mutations that Impair Conversion of Cortisol to Cortisone: Syndrome of Apparent Mineralocorticoid Excess

The syndrome of apparent mineralocorticoid excess (AME)[43] is an autosomal recessive disease featuring severe hypertension presenting in the first decade of life. It is associated with suppression of both the renin—angiotensin system and aldosterone secretion. Hypokalemia and metabolic alkalosis are common associated findings. The hypertension can be mitigated with antagonists of the mineralocorticoid receptor, which suggested the presence of a new circulating mineralocorticoid; however, such a molecule was not found. Instead, a defect in cortisol metabolism was identified in affected patients, causing reduced conversion of cortisol to cortisone, with a consequently increased half-life of cortisol.[44]

How this defect in cortisol metabolism resulted in hypertension remained unclear until the cloning and subsequent purification of the mineralocorticoid receptor (MR).[45] *In vitro*, cortisol binds and activates MR as well as aldosterone does,[46] while cortisol is normally a weak mineralocorticoid *in vivo*. This discrepancy is explained by the presence in many aldosterone-responsive cells of an enzyme, steroid 11-β hydroxysteroid dehydrogenase type 2 (11βHSD2), that "protects" MR from cortisol by converting cortisol to cortisone. Cortisone has negligible ability to activate MR. The finding of homozygous loss-of-function mutations in 11βHSD2 in AME provided proof of the relevance of this mechanism *in vivo*.[47] These findings fully explain the pathophysiology of AME, and are confirmed by the recapitulation of AME in mice deficient for 11βHSD2.[48]

AME should be suspected in young individuals with hypertension, suppressed PRA, and low aldosterone levels. AME shares these clinical features with Liddle syndrome (see below); however, Liddle syndrome is autosomal dominant, and affected subjects consequently commonly have one parent with early severe hypertension, and may have other relatives in earlier generations or other branches of the pedigree with similar findings. In contrast, AME is suggested by the absence of disease in earlier generations and the presence of parental consanguinity. The diagnosis of AME can typically be made by genetic testing involving sequencing of 11βHSD2. Abnormal cortisol:cortisone ratios can also establish the diagnosis.[49]

Inhibitors of the mineralocorticoid receptor, such as spironolactone or eplerenone, or inhibitors of the epithelial sodium channel, such as amiloride or triamterene, are treatment options in AME. Eplerenone has recently been suggested for prevention of strokes even in the absence of hypertension; however, the utility of this approach is not established.[50]

Intriguingly, exuberant ingestion of natural licorice produces a clinically similar syndrome owing to the effects of a metabolite of glycyrrhetinic acid — derived from glycyrrhizic acid in licorice — which inhibits 11βHSD2.[51] Carbenoxolone, a drug once used for peptic/gastric ulcer disease, has similar effects.

In the presence of 11βHSD2, elevated levels of cortisol are required to achieve activation of the mineralocorticoid receptor (by exceeding the capacity of 11βHSD2 to metabolize cortisol).[1] Hypertension can therefore occur in states of glucocorticoid excess, such as ectopic ACTH syndrome, Cushing's disease due to a pituitary tumor, iatrogenic Cushing's syndrome or cortisol-producing adenomas.

Mutations in the Mineralocorticoid Receptor

HYPERTENSION EXACERBATED IN PREGNANCY

As discussed above, binding of aldosterone to the mineralocorticoid receptor causes increased renal salt reabsorption by raising the activity of the epithelial sodium channel ENaC, which results in elevated blood pressure. Geller and colleagues identified an as-yet unique family with early onset of typically severe hypertension associated with suppressed PRA, negligible aldosterone levels, and variable hypokalemia and alkalosis; this trait segregated as an autosomal dominant trait in a large extended family.[52,53] A striking clinical feature among affected women was marked exacerbation of hypertension in pregnancy, requiring early delivery for poorly controlled hypertension and marked hypokalemia. Analysis of linkage in this large kindred localized the disease gene to the segment of chromosome 4 that harbors the mineralocorticoid receptor. This gene proved to have a novel missense mutation in the ligand-binding domain, S810L, which precisely co-segregated with the disease phenotype in the kindred.

The clinical features suggested that this mutation results in an activated receptor, despite the absence of aldosterone. *In vitro* studies demonstrated that this is the case: the mutant receptor shows partial constitutive activity in the absence of ligand. In addition, however, the mutation altered the specificity of the receptor such that some steroids lacking 21-hydroxyl groups, which normally fail to activate MR, are now potent agonists. One of these new agonists is progesterone, a steroid whose level increases dramatically in pregnancy. Cortisone is another molecule that can more weakly activate the mutant receptor, suggesting that this cortisol metabolite may play a constitutive role. The crystal structure of the mutant mineralocorticoid receptor was solved,[54] suggesting that progesterone-induced MR S810L activation is caused by a network of contacts at the A-ring, created by L810.

Mutations that Cause Hypertension without Activation of MR

Mineralocorticoids impart their renal effects by modulating the expression and activity of ion transporters and channels. Mutations in several genes have been identified that cause hypertension without activation of MR.

LIDDLE SYNDROME Liddle syndrome[55] is an autosomal dominant trait featuring hypertension with variable hypokalemia and alkalosis. While these features recapitulate the phenotype of the diseases with mineralocorticoid excess discussed above, there are no circulating mineralocorticoids in patients with Liddle syndrome. Hypertension is responsive to treatment with blockers of the epithelial sodium channel ENaC (amiloride or triamterene), but not to spironolactone.

Genetic studies identified rare mutations in subunits of ENaC as the cause of Liddle syndrome[56,57] (Figures 36.5 and 36.6). ENaC is composed of subunits encoded by three homologous genes, alpha, beta, and gamma[58]; each has cytoplasmic amino and carboxy termini, and traverses the plasma membrane twice.[59] Virtually all mutations that cause Liddle syndrome eliminate a sequence required for removal of the channel from the cell surface by clathrin-coated pit-mediated endocytosis. This internalization sequence, PPPXY (where X is variable among different ENaC subunits) is present in the carboxy terminus of each subunit.

Disease causing mutations introduce premature termination codons after the second transmembrane domain and before the PPPXY sequence, or alternatively produce missense mutations at one of the cognate positions of the internalization motif.[56,57,60] These mutations result in reduced clearance and prolonged half-life of the channel at the cell surface[61–63] (Figure 36.6). Nedd4 was subsequently identified as having domains that specifically bind the PPPXY domains in ENaC, and contribute to its clearance from the cell surface.[64] This protein contains ubiquitin-ligase domains, suggesting that ubiquitination and subsequent degradation plays a role in ENaC regulation. The likely candidate for this regulation in human kidney is Nedd4-2.[65] Together, these findings suggest that mutations in ENaC in Liddle syndrome impair binding of Nedd4 to the mutant channel, and prevent ubiquitination and degradation. In addition to the mutations deleting or altering the PY motif, a mutation in the extracellular domain of γ-ENaC has been reported as causing an increased open probability of the channel.[66] Consistent with these genetic findings, renal transplantation can cure the hypertension of Liddle syndrome.[67]

A mouse model of Liddle syndrome[68] does not develop hypertension or hypokalemic alkalosis on a standard diet, despite increased ENaC activity. However, a Liddle phenotype develops when these animals are fed a high-salt diet.

Liddle syndrome should be suspected in patients with early hypertension and suppressed PRA and aldosterone levels; hypokalemia and metabolic alkalosis are supportive, but not essential findings. As discussed above, these features are shared with AME. A family history of hypertension consistent with

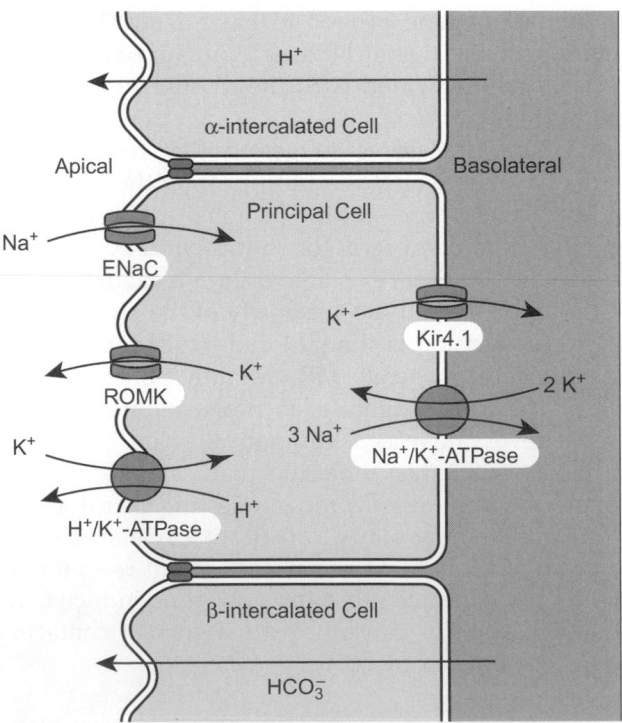

FIGURE 36.5 Salt reabsorption in the cortical collecting duct. Na$^+$ reabsorption in the principal cells of the cortical collecting duct is dependent on aldosterone and happens via ENaC. The resulting lumen-negative potential promotes K$^+$ secretion via ROMK and H$^+$ secretion.

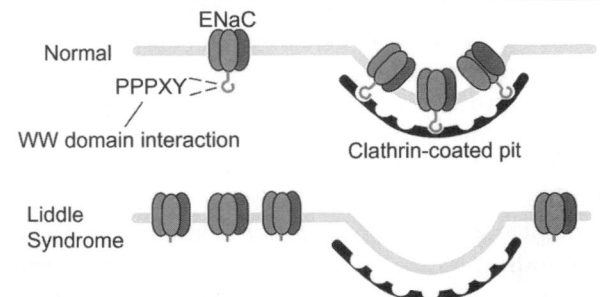

FIGURE 36.6 Increased surface expression of the epithelial sodium channel ENaC causes Liddle syndrome. The β- and γ-subunits of the channel contain a PPPXY motif in the cytoplasmic C-terminus. In normal individuals, binding of Nedd4-2 (not shown) leads to internalization in clathrin-coated pits. Channels are then either degraded or recycled back to the membrane. ENaC lacking the PPPXY motif in Liddle syndrome does not interact with Nedd4-2, and as a result is retained at the membrane. This causes increased Na$^+$ reabsorption and hypertension in affected individuals *(reproduced with permission from ref. [1]).*

autosomal dominant transmission, however, is suggestive of Liddle syndrome. Genetic testing is recommended. Treatment with amiloride or triamterene can correct hypertension and hypokalemia.

THE SYNDROME OF HYPERTENSION WITH HYPERKALEMIA (PSEUDOHYPOALDOSTERONISM TYPE II)

Aldosterone is secreted in two distinct physiologic conditions: volume depletion and hyperkalemia. Restoration of normal intravascular volume in the former condition requires increased salt and water reabsorption, while K^+ secretion must be increased in the latter state. How the kidney achieves these alternative results has been obscure. Classical explanations have suggested that this is a result of alterations in fluid flow and/or delivery of salt to the distal nephron. The notion that this is an incomplete explanation comes from a disease in which the kidney appears to be unable to use aldosterone to direct K^+ secretion, but instead constitutively activates salt reabsorption. This disease, referred to as pseudohypoaldosteronism type II (also known as syndrome of hyperkalemia with hypertension, Gordon syndrome) invariably features hyperkalemia, and has variable levels of hypertension and distal renal tubular acidosis. Aldosterone levels are normal to slightly elevated, and plasma renin activity is suppressed. Serum K^+ levels are virtually always greater than 5.0 mM without therapy, and can be greater than 7.0 mM. The disease was first described in 1964 by Paver and Pauline, who reported a 15-year-old boy with blood pressure 180/120 mmHg, serum potassium 7.0−8.2 mM, but normal glomerular filtration, and suppressed PRA and normal aldosterone.[69] Since early descriptions, the disease has been recognized to be familial, initially described as an autosomal dominant trait.[70−72]

Subsequent studies have demonstrated that K^+ cannot be corrected by supplemental aldosterone; however, both hypertension and hyperkalemia can be corrected by elimination of chloride intake or by low doses of thiazide diuretics.[70,73] These findings have suggested that increased activity of the thiazide-sensitive Na-Cl co-transporter may play a role in this disease.

Analysis of genetic linkage in families followed by molecular studies identified mutations in two members of a novel family of serine-threonine kinases, PRKWNK1 and PRKWNK4, as causes of PHAII[74] (Figure 36.7). Mutations in WNK4 were novel missense mutations that predominantly clustered in a short acidic domain of unknown function in the protein. Mutations in WNK1 were large deletions of 20,000 to 40,000 base pairs in the first intron of WNK1 that caused increased expression of WNK1 mRNA. These genes were both found to be expressed

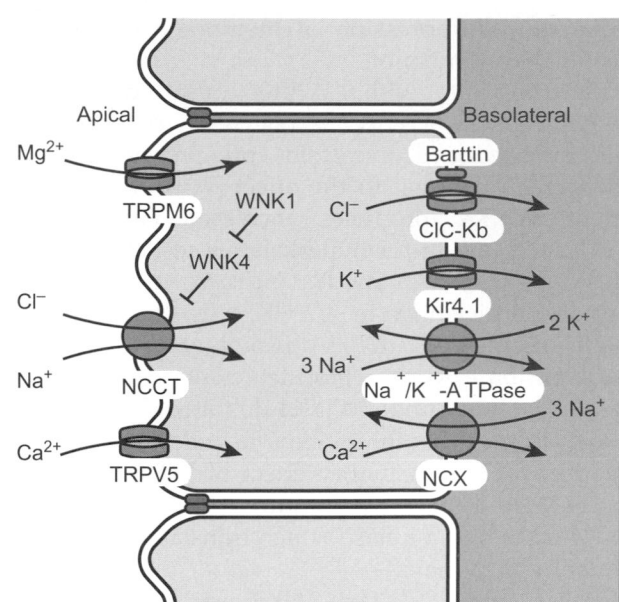

FIGURE 36.7 **Salt reabsorption in the distal convoluted tubule.** Salt reabsorption is driven by the activity of the Na^+/K^+-ATPase on the basolateral suface. K^+ entering the cell via the sodium pump recirculates through Kir4.1 ("pump leak coupling"). NaCl enters the cell via NCCT following the favorable Na^+ gradient, and Cl^- exits via basolateral ClC-Kb channels. The basolateral NCX transporter uses the Na^+ gradient for Ca^{2+} reabsorption. Ca^{2+} enters on the apical site via the TRPV5 channel. On the apical surface, Mg^{2+} enters the cell via TRPM6. The molecular identity of a putative basolateral Mg^{2+} transporter is unknown. NCCT activity is regulated by the WNK1 and WNK4 protein kinases.

in the distal convoluted tubule and collecting duct of the kidney.

At the time of this discovery, the normal and disease-related functions of WNK1 and WNK4 were entirely unknown. Much subsequent work has been done to determine the roles these WNK kinases play in physiology.[74−82] It appears that both play a role in coordinating the functions of diverse electrolyte flux pathways, and that a key function in the kidney is to regulate the balance between Na-Cl reabsorption and K^+ secretion. The WNK kinases regulate ion transport by several mechanisms, among them phosphorylation via intermediary kinases (SPAK, OSR1, and SGK1), and regulation of protein trafficking.[81]

Early studies addressed the role of WNK4 in the regulation of NCCT using the oocyte expression system.[75,83] Co-expression of NCCT with WT-WNK4 resulted in inhibition of thiazide-sensitive Na^+ uptake due to reduced surface expression. This effect was completely abrogated when a mutation seen in PHA II (Q562E) or kinase-dead WNK4 was used, suggesting that NCCT inhibition is lost in patients with PHA II, causing hypertension. Subsequent studies in mammalian cells suggested that this inhibitory WNK4 effect is mediated by suppression of membrane delivery via lysosomal accumulation.[84]

Co-expression with WNK4 also dramatically reduces ROMK activity in oocytes,[76] by interaction with an endocytic scaffold protein, intersectin.[85] However, in contrast to the effect on NCCT, PHA II-mutant WNK4 produces increased inhibition of ROMK, accounting for hyperkalemia in PHA II. While WT WNK4 led to a modest increase of paracellular chloride permeability in MDCK cells, this effect was greatly augmented in PHA II-mutant WNK4, which may contribute to the chloride retention observed in PHA II.[77,78] In addition, WNK4 inhibited ENaC activity in oocytes, and this inhibition was relieved by PHA II mutations.[86] The inhibitory effect of WNK4 on ENaC and ROMK appears to require phosphorylation of WNK4 by SGK1, a kinase which translates aldosterone effects in the kidney.[87]

Similar studies as for WNK4 were performed for WNK1. While a direct effect of WNK1 on NCCT was not identified, a long isoform of WNK1 (L-WNK1) inhibits WNK4 (which inhibits NCCT, see above), and a kidney-specific isoform (KS-WNK1) inhibits L-WNK1.[75] In addition, L-WNK1 inhibits ROMK, an effect reversed by KS-WNK1 and synergistic with, but not dependent on, the WNK4 effect on ROMK[88]; L-WNK1 also activates ENaC.[89] Finally, similar to WNK4, WNK1 increases paracellular chloride flux.[90] ATII, which is produced in volume depletion, appears to be an upstream regulator of WNK4, attenuating its inhibitory effect on NCCT and thus stimulating salt reabsorption via NCCT. In contrast, the inhibitory effect of WNK4 of ROMK is retained. These findings suggest that PHA II mutations mimic a state of volume depletion with increased angiotensin II levels.[91]

Regulation of several additional proteins (e.g., TRP channels, SLC26A6) by WNK1 and WNK4 kinases has been reported, and studies of the related kinase WNK3 has revealed a role in regulation of NKCC, as well as KCC co-transporters.[92]

Taken together, *in vitro* studies suggest a key role of the WNK kinases in a functional switch among three states governing the balance between salt reabsorption and K^+ secretion. In a basal equilibrium state, both NaCl reabsorption and K^+ secretion are inhibited by the WNK kinases. In the setting of low intravascular volume, AII signaling inhibits WNK4's inhibition of NCC, but increases inhibition of ROMK; this effect is mimicked by PHA II mutations, accounting for constitutive NaCl reabsorption and hyperkalemia seen in affected patients. In a third state, hyperkalemia leads to increased aldosterone production by the adrenal gland and, potentially via SGK, to increased ROMK activity and increased ENaC activity, with sustained inhibition of electroneutral salt reabsorption via NCCT.[80]

Animal models have confirmed the role of WNK1 and WNK4 in generating hyperkalemia and hypertension. A transgenic mouse model carrying an additional copy of PHA II-mutant WNK4 shows hypertension, hyperkalemia, and hypercalciuria and, in addition, increased mass of the distal convoluted tubule and increased NCCT expression. In contrast, an additional copy of WT WNK4 leads to decreased DCT mass and reduced NCCT abundance.[79] A knockout mouse model of WNK4 displays a phenotype similar to Gitelman syndrome (see below), with increased plasma renin activity, and decreased NCC activity.[93] Deletion of the first WNK1 intron as found in PHA II in mice leads to ubiquitous ectopic KS-WNK1 expression, as well as overexpression of L-WNK1 in the DCT,[94] which explains increased activity of NCCT through alleviation of WNK4 inhibition.

Importantly, mutations in WNK1 and WNK4 explained only about 15% of families with PHA II. Exome sequencing of unrelated PHA II cases led to the identification of two additional genes for PHA II, which together account for nearly all of the remaining cases.[95,96] These two genes are partners in a ubiquitin ligase complex. Cullin 3 (CUL3) is a scaffold that serves to assemble a complex containing a RING E-3 ubiquitin ligase and one of many BTB domain-containing proteins that target specific proteins for ubiquitination. One of these BTB domain proteins is Kelch-like 3 (KLHL3). KLHL3 has a C-terminal BTB domain, and an N-terminal kelch domain, a six-bladed propeller that is likely used to bind and target proteins for ubiquitination. Surprisingly, different families showed either autosomal dominant or autosomal recessive transmission of mutations in KLHL3. Recessive mutations are distributed throughout the protein, and include typical loss-of-function mutations such as premature termination mutations. In contrast, dominant mutations cluster at positions in the kelch domain that are clustered at parts of the domain inferred to be involved in target binding. Because these dominant mutations produce a phenotype very similar to that caused by homozygous loss-of-function mutations in KLHL3, the dominant mutations likely have a dominant-negative effect.

The mutations in CUL3 that cause PHA II all cause skipping of exon 9, resulting in an in-frame deletion of 57 amino acids between the BTB-binding and RING-binding domains. These mutations are all dominant, and nearly all appear to be *de novo* mutations. Because these mutations phenocopy recessive loss-of-function mutations in KLHL3, it is inferred that these CUL3 mutations selectively prevent ubiquitination at targets bound by KLHL3. While CUL3 is ubiquitously expressed, KLHL3 is selectively expressed in the distal nephron.

Comparison of the phenotypes of patients with mutations in these different genes reveals strong genotype—phenotype correlations. Patients with CUL3 mutations have the most severe hyperkalemia, are nearly always hypertensive at young ages, and commonly have acidosis. Patients with recessive and dominant KLHL3 mutations have intermediate phenotypic severity, and those with WNK1 and WNK4 mutations often have only hyperkalemia without hypertension at early ages, and do not uniformly develop hypertension at later ages. The molecular mechanisms that link mutations in KLHL3 and CUL3 to PHA II are presently unknown; however, it is highly likely that these mutations will intersect with the WNK/NCC/ROMK pathway.

GENETIC DISORDERS CAUSING RENAL SALT LOSS

Several Mendelian disorders can cause renal salt loss, leading to signs and symptoms ranging from mild polyuria and salt craving to life-threatening hypotension and shock. A diagnostic approach to these diseases is suggested in Figure 36.8.

Disorders of the Renin—Angiotensin—Aldosterone System

Mutations Affecting Circulating Mineralocorticoid Levels

MUTATIONS RESULTING IN CONGENITAL HYPOALDOSTERONISM

Congenital hyper-reninemic hypoaldosteronism is a rare autosomal recessive disorder.[97,98] Affected patients present in infancy with salt-wasting, leading to severe dehydration, failure to thrive and growth retardation, as well as hyponatremia and hyperkalemia. Aldosterone is low despite elevated renin. These features are a clinical mirror image of the states of primary aldosteronism described above.

Genetic studies identified mutations in the aldosterone synthase gene (CYP11B2) as the cause of congenital hypoaldosteronism.[99,100] Aldosterone synthase catalyzes both 18-hydroxylation of corticosterone, and the subsequent conversion of the 18-hydroxyl group to an aldehyde (Figure 36.3). Several mutations, including nonsense, missense, and frameshift mutations, affect the 18-hydroxylase activity of the enzyme; as a result, levels of 18-hydroxycorticosterone are low in these patients. In other cases, specific missense mutations can abolish 18-oxidase activity, while 18-hydroxylase activity remains intact or is only slightly reduced. These patients consequently have elevated levels of 18-hydroxycortisone.[99]

Not all patients with hyper-reninemic hypoaldosteronism, however, have mutations at the CYP11B2 locus. Kayes-Wandover et al.[101] described four unrelated kindreds (two consanguineous) without evidence of such mutations; linkage to the CYP11B2 locus could be excluded in the two consanguineous families, suggesting genetic heterogeneity. The underlying gene defect of this disorder, termed familial hyper-reninemic hypoaldosteronism type 2, remains to be established.

CONGENITAL ADRENAL HYPERPLASIA DUE TO STEROID 21-HYDROXYLASE DEFICIENCY

Steroid 21-hydroxylase deficiency is an autosomal recessive disease. It accounts for the vast majority of the cases of congenital adrenal hyperplasia (CAH), and is one of the most common Mendelian diseases.

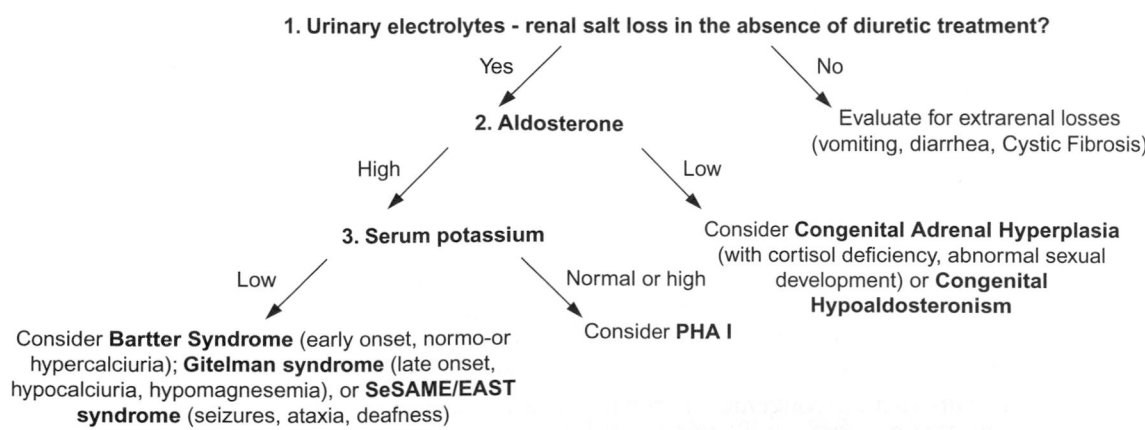

FIGURE 36.8 A diagnostic approach to Mendelian hypotension and renal salt loss. (PHA I: pseudohypoaldosteronism type I.)

21-hydroxylase catalyzes the 21-hydroxylation of progesterone, and is a required step in the biosynthesis of both cortisol and aldosterone (Figure 36.3).

Three subforms of the disease are recognized: patients with the salt-losing form of classic CAH are severely affected and present at birth or in infancy with cortisol and mineralocorticoid deficiency; females typically have ambiguous genitalia and virilization. In the simple virilizing form of classic CAH, high ACTH levels are sufficient to produce adequate levels of glucocorticoids and mineralocorticoids at the expense of increased adrenal androgen synthesis, resulting in virilization. Finally, patients with the late-onset or nonclassic form may present in childhood, adolescence or even adulthood with premature pubarche and accelerated bone age; female patients develop hirsutism, infertility or irregular menstrual cycles.

The salt-losing form of classic CAH has an estimated incidence of ~1/23,000 live births, and is due to mutations in 21-hydroxylase (CYP21A gene) in almost all cases.[102] Girls with this condition present as neonates with masculinization. Salt-losing adrenal crisis, with vomiting, dehydration, hypotension, hypoglycemia, and electrolyte abnormalities (hyponatremia and hyperkalemia) typically occurs in the first or second week of life, and these can be the only presenting symptoms in boys. When untreated, adrenal crisis can lead to shock, cardiac arrhythmia, and neonatal death.[103]

CYP21A mutations causing salt-losing CAH often arise from unequal crossing-over between the functional CYP21A gene and a non-functional pseudogene located in close proximity[104]; the mutated enzyme typically shows complete loss-of-function. 21-hydroxylase deficiency is recognized clinically in patients with ambiguous genitalia or adrenal crisis, or in newborn screening programs; the diagnosis is based on elevated levels of 17-hydroxyprogesterone. Genetic testing is available, and can be supplemental for prenatal diagnosis, genetic counseling or ambiguous cases. Prenatal therapy with exogenous glucocorticoids can prevent or ameliorate virilization in female children, but is only recommended in a research setting due to potential side-effects.[105] If the child is known to be at risk, treatment is started as early as the mother knows she is pregnant, and stopped if the child is found to be male or unaffected by prenatal screening. Treatment after birth includes glucocorticoid and mineralocorticoid replacement, as well as salt supplementation in infants, and potentially feminizing surgery.[105]

RARE CAUSES OF SALT-WASTING CONGENITAL ADRENAL HYPERPLASIA

Very rare causes of salt-wasting congenital adrenal hyperplasia include 3-β-HSD 2 deficiency[106] and StAR deficiency[107] in lipoid adrenal hyperplasia. In both diseases, severe adrenal insufficiency with deficiency of gluco- and mineralocorticoids occurs at neonatal age or in infancy; genetically male patients typically have abnormalities of sexual development at birth, with female external genitalia in StAR deficiency.

Mutations in Genes Expressed in the Kidney that Cause Salt-Wasting

PSEUDOHYPOALDOSTERONISM TYPE I

Pseudohypoaldosteronism Type I (PHA I) is a rare genetic syndrome whose features include renal salt-wasting, hyperkalemia, hyponatremia, and metabolic acidosis despite elevated renin and aldosterone levels.[52,108] The disease presents as either an autosomal dominant or autosomal recessive trait. The recessive form appears to be uniformly severe, and requires life-long salt supplementation. The dominant form is clinically more variable at birth, and typically largely resolves after the first years of life with the ability to self-select a high-salt diet.

AUTOSOMAL RECESSIVE PSEUDOHYPOALDO-STERONISM TYPE I (PHAI) Infants with autosomal recessive PHA I frequently present with life-threatening episodes of hypovolemia, sometimes leading to neonatal death. Affected subjects have marked renal salt-wasting and striking hyperkalemia (as high as 12 mM), and renal tubular acidosis despite drastic elevations of PRA and aldosterone. There is also salt-wasting from salivary and sweat glands, as well as the colon. These patients require life-long sodium supplementation and often chronic treatment with resin-binding agents for hyperkalemia. Frequent pulmonary infections somewhat reminiscent of cystic fibrosis have been reported in some patients,[109] and markedly increased ciliary clearance of lung water has been reported.[110]

Genetic studies led to identification of recessive loss-of-function mutations in the alpha, beta or gamma subunits of the epithelial Na^+ channel (ENaC) in virtually all affected subjects.[111,112] Functional studies in *Xenopus* oocytes confirmed loss of channel activity. In summary, these findings demonstrated that mutations in all ENaC subunits can cause PHA I. All the features of this disease are explained by loss of ENaC function. Loss of ENaC function results in dramatic salt-wasting, leading to activation of the renin—angiotensin system; however, because ENaC is absent, this fails to adequately augment salt reabsorption in the kidney. Impaired salt absorption in the colon may also contribute to disease severity. K^+ and H^+ secretion are also markedly impaired, owing to loss the lumen-negative potential resulting from loss of ENaC, causing hyperkalemia and acidosis.

These findings have been confirmed in animal studies. Mice deficient for the β- and γ-subunits show a phenotype characteristic of PHA I, with early death due to Na^+-wasting and K^+ retention,[113,114] and a PHA I-like phenotype is observed in α-ENaC knockout mice with transgenic expression of rat α-ENaC for rescue.[115] α-ENaC knockout mice show early postnatal demise with a mean survival of 24 hours postnatally due to respiratory distress,[116] suggesting a role of the mouse channel in pulmonary liquid clearance after birth that is apparently not observed at birth in humans but is found later in life.[110,117]

AUTOSOMAL DOMINANT PHA I Autosomal dominant PHA I has a milder phenotype that typically largely resolves in the early years of life. Patients may be asymptomatic or can present with renal salt-wasting and mild-to-moderate hyperkalemia and acidosis.[118,119] NaCl supplementation can typically be discontinued after early childhood, as the disease remits with age. Geller et al.[118] identified heterozygous mutations in the mineralocorticoid receptor gene in five kindreds with autosomal dominant PHA I. All mutations were inferred to be loss-of-function, inferred to cause diminished ENaC activity, with resulting salt loss. Since Na^+ reabsorption via ENaC is required for the lumen-negative potential that drives K^+ and H^+ secretion in the cortical collecting duct, diminished ENaC activity can cause hyperkalemic acidosis in these kindreds. The improvement with age is consistent with a decreasing requirement for aldosterone action in older children, presumably due to increasing salt intake and a self-selected high-salt diet after infancy. Adult carriers show no abnormalities of serum and urinary electrolytes or blood pressure, but consistently demonstrate markedly elevated serum aldosterone levels, consistent with homeostasis being achieved by compensating for the reduced level of MR by increased aldosterone levels.[119]

A case of autosomal recessive PHA I due to mutations in the mineralocorticoid receptor was recently reported — a newborn with very severe PHA I who was compound heterozygous for S166X and W806X deletions.[120] Within her family, carriers of the S166X mutation had typical autosomal dominant PHA I, while carriers of the W806X mutation were clinically asymptomatic, but had elevated renin and aldosterone levels.

A mouse model of PHA 1 shows increased renin and aldosterone, but develops normally in the heterozygous state. The homozygous knockout is lethal,[121] but can be rescued by subcutaneous NaCl injection before weaning.[122]

Mutations Affecting Renal Ion Channels, Transporters and their Regulators

Thick Ascending Limb of Henle

BARTTER SYNDROME

Bartter syndrome is a rare autosomal recessive disorder.[123] Patients may present at various ages with a variety of signs and symptoms. Renal salt-wasting is the key underlying primary problem, causing polyuria and subsequent polydipsia. In severe cases, patients present antenatally with polyhydramnios[124] (due to intrauterine polyuria), and affected subjects are often born prematurely. Renal salt-wasting, typically severe, leads to volume depletion, activation of the renin—angiotensin—aldosterone system and subsequent hypokalemic alkalosis; growth and mental development are impaired in some patients.[125] Hypercalciuria and nephrocalcinosis[126] are frequently found and can cause end-stage renal disease; deafness has been observed in a subset of patients.[127]

Early physiologic studies localized defective salt reabsorption in patients with Bartter syndrome to the loop of Henle[128] (Figure 36.9), and the finding of elevated levels of prostaglandins enabled treatment with inhibitors of prostaglandin synthesis.[129–131] The spectrum of clinical presentations and the underlying

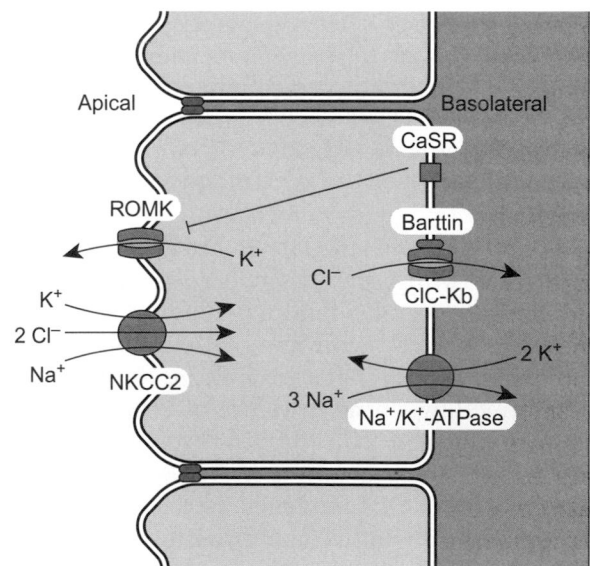

FIGURE 36.9 Salt reabsorption in the thick ascending limb of Henle's loop. Salt reabsorption is driven by the activity of the Na^+/K^+-ATPase on the basolateral suface. Na^+, Cl^-, and K^+ enter the cell on the apical surface via NKCC2 following the favorable gradient established by the sodium pump. While K^+ recirculates through ROMK, Cl^- is reabsorbed on the basolateral surface via ClC-Kb and its accessory subunit barttin. ROMK is inhibited by the calcium-sensing receptor (CaSR).

pathophysiology of this disorder was elucidated by the identification of the underlying genetic defects.

MUTATIONS IN NKCC2 CAUSE BARTTER SYNDROME TYPE I Recessive loss-of-function mutations in NKCC2, the bumetanide-sensitive Na-K-2Cl co-transporter (product of the SLC12A1 gene) were identified among a subset of patients with Bartter syndrome[132] (now Bartter syndrome type I). Affected index cases had all been born prematurely with poly-hydramnios, and presented as neonates with hypokalemia and hyper-reninemic hyperaldosteronism; all had hypercalciuria. These clinical findings were consistent with the observation that pharmacologic inhibitors of NKCC2 produce similar electrolyte abnormalities. Loss of Na-Cl reabsorption in the TAL leads to massive salt-wasting, with activation of the renin—angiotensin system, and defense of intravascular volume by increased ENaC activity, which causes increased K^+ loss via increased lumen-negative potential in the connecting tubule and collecting duct. NCKK2 activity leads to reabsorption of two Cl^- and one Na^+ ions; the K^+ that enters across the apical membrane returns to the lumen via the K^+ channel ROMK. This results in a lumen-positive potential, which provides the electrical driving force for paracellluar calcium and magnesium reabsorption in the TAL. It is thus not surprising that loss of NKCC2 function results in hypercalciuria. Surprisingly, however, Mg^{2+} levels remain normal with little renal Mg^{2+} loss, suggesting compensation in other nephron segments. A knockout mouse model of NKCC2[133] generally recapitulated the features of Bartter syndrome (salt loss, dehydration, failure to thrive, response to treatment with indomethacin, and hypercalciuria).

MUTATIONS IN ROMK CAUSE BARTTER SYNDROME TYPE II Following the discovery of mutations in NKCC2, Simon et al. identified nine additional kindreds with Bartter syndrome without mutations in NKCC2, and excluded genetic linkage to this locus in several, providing strong evidence of genetic heterogeneity and indicating that additional loci accounted for many cases of Bartter syndrome.[134]

In the TAL, NKCC2 mediates apical sodium, potassium, and chloride influx using the favorable sodium gradient established by the basolateral Na^+/K^+-ATPase. Because luminal K^+ levels are low in the TAL compared to Na^+ and Cl^-, a role for the apical "recycling" of K^+ was speculated to be important for normal salt reabsorption in the TAL.[135,136] This was proven to be true by the finding of recessive loss-of-function mutations in the renal outer medullary K^+ channel (ROMK, product of the KCNJ1 gene), the apical K^+ channel of the TAL, in a subset of patients with Bartter

syndrome (now referred to as Bartter syndrome type II).[134] These findings not only identified ROMK as a second disease locus in Bartter syndrome, but also established a key role of this apical potassium channel in renal salt reabsorption. Interestingly, ROMK is not only expressed in the thick ascending limb, but also in the cortical collecting duct, where it mediates apical potassium secretion (see above) driven by the lumen-negative potential established by reabsorption of Na^+ via ENaC. As found by Simon et al.,[134] and further elaborated by Peters et al.[137] and Finer et al.,[138] due to this defect in apical potassium secretion, serum potassium levels in patients with mutations in ROMK are significantly higher than in patients with NKCC2 mutations. Moreover, these patients typically present with hyperkalemia at birth. The development of relatively mild hypokalemia later in life indicates the presence of an alternative potassium-secreting channel with delayed maturation, likely the BK potassium channel.[139,140] A mouse model of Bartter syndrome with mutation in ROMK generally recapitulates the human phenotype.[141]

These findings define ROMK as a very promising target for the development of saluretic or antihypertensive agents with an adverse effect profile preferable over that of the common loop diuretics, limiting hypokalemia; such agents are currently under development.

MUTATIONS IN CLCNKB CAUSE BARTTER SYNDROME TYPE III Screening of 66 Bartter syndrome kindreds found mutations in NKCC2 and ROMK in only 22 kindreds.[142] This suggested the presence of at least one additional disease gene, supported by exclusion of linkage to either of the known genes by homozygosity mapping in 10 of 11 consanguineous kindreds. In the model of channels and transporters mediating salt reabsorption in the TAL outlined above, sodium enters via NKCC2 and exits via the Na^+/K^+-ATPase, while K^+ enters the cell via NKCC2 and returns to the lumen via ROMK. However, for net NaCl reabsorption, a basolateral exit pathway for chloride entering via NKCC2 is required. This exit had been suggested to be mediated by the chloride channels ClC-K1 and ClC-K2 in rat kidney[143,144] and their human homologs ClC-Ka (CLCNKA gene) and ClC-Kb (CLCNKB gene).[145] These two genes are closely linked, with CLCNKA located at 5′ of CLCNKB. Genetic analysis revealed linkage to this chromosome interval among Bartter syndrome families without mutation in NKCC2 and ROMK. Further analysis revealed deletions, missense, splice site, and premature termination mutations in the CLCNKB gene in affected members of 17 kindreds. Several of the deletions arose via unequal crossing-over between CLCNKB and CLCNKA. No point mutations were identified in the CLCNKA gene.

In contrast to the findings in patients with NKCC2 and ROMK mutations, hypercalciuria was variable, and none of the kindreds initially reported demonstrated nephrocalcinosis. Strikingly, there is a wide range of presentations in these patients, from severe volume depletion in the neonatal period to late-onset presentation. Hypomagnesemia[146] (see below) has been described in a few of these kindreds, but not to the extent generally seen in Gitelman syndrome. A possible explanation for this overlapping phenotype may be found in the expression of ClC-Kb, which is not restricted to the thick ascending limb of Henle, but extends into the distal convoluted tubule; the milder phenotype in some kindreds may be due to residual function of the mutant channel or partially compensating activity of the ClC-Ka channel in the thick ascending limb.

MUTATIONS IN BSND OR COMBINED MUTATIONS IN CLCNKA AND CLCNKB CAUSE BARTTER SYNDROME WITH SENSORINEURAL DEAFNESS (TYPE IV)

Patients with Bartter syndrome type IV[127] typically present early with polyhydramnios and prematurity, as well as polyuria and renal saltloss after birth. This subtype is clinically distinguished from other forms of Bartter syndrome by the presence of sensorineural deafness. Genetic studies[147,148] led to the identification of a novel gene, named BSND (Bartter syndrome with sensorineural deafness), which had recessive loss-of-function mutations in 11 kindreds with this phenotype.[148] The novel disease gene and its product, named barttin, were found to be expressed in human and mouse kidney, as well as stria vascularis of the cochlea and dark cells of the vestibular organ. In stria vascularis, a set of channels and transporters highly similar to that mediating salt reabsorption in the thick ascending limb is responsible for potassium secretion into the endolymph and generation of the endocochlear potential, effects that are essential for normal hearing. Barttin was found to be an accessory subunit of ClC-Ka and ClC-Kb chloride channels required for surface insertion of the channel.[149] Most BSND missense mutations reduced current compared to WT when co-expressed with the chloride channels. Barttin co-localized with ClC-K channels on the basolateral surface of thin and thick ascending limb of Henle and more distal segments, including intercalated cells of the cortical collecting duct. The more severe renal phenotype of patients with BSND mutations compared to patients with CLCNKB mutation is likely caused by an additional effect on the ClC-Ka channel. In the inner ear, ClC-Ka can compensate for loss of ClC-Kb function in patients with CLCNKB mutations, while mutations in BSND abrogate basolateral chloride conductance in this epithelium, leading to sensorineural deafness.

Accordingly, combined CLCNKA and CLCNKB mutations can cause Bartter syndrome and sensorineural deafness[150,151]; a condition sometimes referred to as Bartter syndrome type IVb. Isolated mutations in CLCNKA have not been described so far; a knockout ClC-K1 mouse model has diabetes insipidus,[152] which may clinically be less apparent than the salt loss observed with CLCNKB mutations. A constitutional BSND knockout mouse model manifests severe dehydration and early postnatal lethality, while inner-ear-specific disruption causes profound congenital hearing loss and subtle vestibular symptoms.[153]

MUTATIONS IN THE CALCIUM-SENSING RECEPTOR CAUSE BARTTER SYNDROME TYPE V

The calcium-sensing receptor (CaSR) is a G-protein-coupled receptor, which, by sensing extracellular calcium, regulates both PTH secretion from the parathyroid and renal calcium reabsorption. Activating mutations in CaSR cause the syndrome of autosomal dominant hypoparathyroidism,[154] characterized by hypocalcemia, hypomagnesemia, and low serum PTH. A small number of these patients demonstrate features of Bartter syndrome (hyper-reninemic hyperaldosteronism and hypokalemia due to volume depletion),[155,156] potentially due to inhibition of apical ROMK channels[157] and inhibition of paracellular Na^+, Ca^{2+}, and Mg^{2+} reabsorption in the thick ascending limb. Although this disease clearly differs from Bartter syndrome, and the primary manifestation is hypocalcemia rather than salt loss, it is sometimes referred to as Bartter syndrome type V.

In summary, the identification of the genes mutated in subsets of Bartter syndrome has suggested a detailed classification, including clinically relevant features such as transient hyperkalemia in patients with Bartter syndrome type II that had not been recognized previously. This classification is now preferred over the the traditional distinction of "hyperprostaglandin E syndrome" in patients with early onset, severe salt loss, and increased urinary prostaglandin production, and "classic Bartter syndrome" with later onset and milder phenotype.[158]

The clinical diagnosis of Bartter syndrome is based on the presence of renal salt loss in infancy or childhood (high urinary chloride excretion in the absence of diuretic treatment), hyperaldosteronism, and hypokalemic alkalosis in the absence of hypertension. Urinary calcium is typically elevated, but can be normal in some patients with Cl^- channel mutations. Serum Mg^{2+} may be normal or slightly low, but does not typically reach the extremely low values seen in Gitelman syndrome (see below). Other causes of hypokalemia, such as vomiting and treatment with diuretics, should be excluded. Genetic testing is available.

Genotype—phenotype correlations can suggest the underlying mutant gene from the clinical presentation. Patients with ROMK mutations are distinguished by typically having hyperkalemia in the neonatal period, and evolve to hypokalemia that is less severe than that seen in other patients. Patients with CLCNKB mutations are least likely to have hypercalciuria and nephrocalcinosis, and account for most patients with mild disease, as can be seen with a few particular mutations.[159] Patients with sensorineural deafness have either BSND or combined CLCNKA/CLCNKB mutations. Patients without these distinguishing features are enriched for NKCC2 mutations.

Prostaglandin synthesis inhibitors (NSAIDs) are an important part of the therapeutic regimen in Bartter syndrome. While the exact mechanism of increased prostaglandin synthesis in these patients remains unclear, prostaglandin E2 can exacerbate renal salt-wasting.[160] Monitoring for nephrotoxicity and gastrointestinal side-effects is important. Severe volume depletion requires intravenous fluids, and a life-long high-salt diet is encouraged. Potassium supplementation is often needed, and magnesium supplementation is occasionally also needed. Potassium-sparing diuretics to limit renal K^+ loss can be used if necessary; however, these must be used with caution as they will exacerbate renal salt loss in these patients. Therapy with growth hormone can be considered in patients with growth retardation. As expected for a genetic disease affecting the kidney, renal transplantation is curative. Transplantation is usually limited to patients who proceed to end-stage renal failure, although pre-emptive transplantation has been reported.[161]

Salt-Wasting Due to Mutations Affecting Salt Reabsorption in the Distal Convoluted Tubule

GITELMAN SYNDROME

Gitelman syndrome is an autosomal recessive disorder. The clinical features typically include renal salt-wasting, elevated levels of PRA and aldosterone, hypokalemia, metabolic alkalosis, hypomagnesemia, and hypocalciuria.[162,163] The clinical distinction from Bartter syndrome is usually obvious. While Bartter syndrome patients typically present in the first year of life (mean age 0.8 years), often with severe volume depletion, Gitelman patients typically present later (mean age 10.5 years) with symptoms that are less obviously due to volume depletion, but often related to hypokalemia and/or hypomagnesemia. The urinary calcium:creatinine ratio in Bartter syndrome is typically ≥ 0.4 mmol/mmol, hypocalciuria is characteristic of Gitelman syndrome (ratio ≤ 0.1 mmol/mmol). Mean plasma magnesium is considerably lower in Gitelman patients (mean 0.54 mmol/L versus 0.82 mmol/L in

Bartter syndrome), and seizures or tetanic episodes have been described in several cases.[163] While adult patients with Bartter syndrome are very uncommon, adult Gitelman syndrome patients are not rare, and women with Gitelman syndrome successfully complete pregnancy in many cases.

Clinical studies localized salt loss in Gitelman syndrome to the distal convoluted tubule (Figure 36.7), and demonstrated a reduced response to intravenous administration of a thiazide diuretic.[164] The thiazide-sensitive carrier, NCC, had been cloned from flounder bladder and rat kidney,[165,166] but not from human. To study NCC as a disease gene in Gitelman syndrome, Simon et al.[167] cloned and characterized the human gene; they isolated DNA from members of 12 kindreds with Gitelman syndrome and genotyped markers spanning the NCC locus, demonstrating linkage of Gitelman syndrome and NCC. Affected kindred members all had mutations in NCC, including splice site mutations and premature termination codons. The findings demonstrated that Gitelman syndrome is caused by mutations in NCCT. Many additional patients and mutations have been reported since; for example Ji et al. found 91 different mutations in 246 alleles among 123 patients with Gitelman syndrome.[168] In a single large kindred comprising more than 200 subjects segregating mutations in NCC, virtually complete penetrance of hypokalemia, alkalosis, and hypocalciuria was seen among subjects with two mutant NCC alleles, and these subjects had lower blood pressure than others in the pedigree, despite consuming significantly more salt.[206] Heterozygotes were intermediate in salt consumption and blood pressure.

While Gitelman syndrome is a much milder disease than Bartter syndrome, these patients are not asymptomatic — common complaints include salt craving, musculoskeletal symptoms such as cramps, muscular weakness, and aches, as well as fatigue, generalized weakness, polydipsia, and polyuria.[169]

The finding of mutations in NCC clearly explains renal salt loss in patients with Gitelman syndrome — apical NaCl entry in DCT is impaired, leading to reduced salt reabsorption with concomitant water loss, activation of the renin—angiotensin—aldosterone system and upregulation of ENaC activity in the collecting duct. This again accounts for hypokalemic alkalosis in these patients. It is less clear, however, why these patients develop hypomagnesemia and hypocalciuria, similar to patients treated with thiazide diuretics. Hypocalciuria has been attributed to increased proximal calcium reabsorption[170]; however, the exact physiologic mechanism of this effect is still a matter of debate. Hypomagnesemia was linked to decreased expression of the apical TRPM6 channel in DCT,[171] which mediates magnesium reabsorption and is mutated in another rare Mendelian syndrome, hypomagnesemia with secondary hypocalcemia. This may be due to the decreased mass of the distal convoluted tubule observed with NCC deficiency or thiazide treatment.[172,173]

The above results from human studies have been confirmed in a knockout mouse model of NCCT[172] featuring hypomagnesemia and hypocalciuria. While hypokalemia and hyperaldosteronism were absent on a normal rodent diet, a marked reduction in plasma potassium occured upon low-potassium diet, and was accompanied by polyuria, polydipsia, and hyperaldosteronism.[174]

Although genetic testing is available, the diagnosis of Gitelman syndrome can be made reliably in typical cases in adolescents and adults on the basis of elevated PRA and aldosterone with hypokalemic alkalosis, hypomagnesemia, hypocalciuria, and evidence of renal salt loss in the absence of diuretic treatment or abuse. Because this clinical picture is virtually identical to that seen with use of thiazide diuretics, affected patients are often suspected of surreptitiously taking these medications. Genetic studies can be helpful in this situation.

Therapeutic options include electrolyte supplements (although magnesium supplementation can be particularly challenging) and potassium-sparing diuretics, although the latter can worsen volume depletion. Treatment with NSAIDs is generally not recommended, because these patients typically do not show elevated prostaglandin production.

SeSAME/EAST SYNDROME

A novel autosomal-recessive genetic disorder featuring renal salt loss was recently independently described as SeSAME (seizures, sensorineural deafness, ataxia, mental retardation, and electrolyte imbalance)[175] and EAST (epilepsy, ataxia, sensorineural deafness, tubulopathy)[176] syndrome. The renal features of this disorder resemble Gitelman syndrome, with persistent hypokalemic alkalosis due to activation of the renin–angiotensin–aldosterone system and variable hypomagnesemia, as well as hypocalciuria. Patients typically present in infancy with recurrent seizures; brain MRI is normal. More severe sensorineural hearing loss may be apparent in neonatal screening, while milder cases may go unnoticed until late childhood. Speech and motor delay are associated features, and may in part be due to ataxia. Genome-wide linkage analysis in three informative kindreds demonstrated complete linkage of SeSAME to a single segment on chromosome 1q23, and the Kir4.1 inward rectifier potassium channel (encoded by the *KCNJ10* gene) was identified as a candidate gene within the interval. Kir4.1 is expressed in kidney, inner ear, and brain; a knockout mouse model shows seizures, sensorineural deafness, and ataxia.[177–179] Screening of five

affected subjects from four kindreds revealed homozygous or compound heterozygous mutations that segregated with the disease; this included a nonsense mutation and five missense mutations at conserved residues, which were inferred to be loss-of-function.[175] Similar findings were reported by Böckenhauer et al.[176] in two consanguineous families. In addition, they demonstrated electrophysiologic loss of channel function in mutant channels, and confirmed expression of Kir4.1 in the distal convoluted tubule, connecting tubule, and early cortical collecting duct. Analysis of the previously established knockout mouse model revealed polyuria, elevated urinary sodium concentration, and low urinary calcium concentration.

Seizures in patients with KCNJ10 mutations are likely due to loss of the channel's function in "spatial buffering",[180,181] i.e., glial uptake of excess potassium ions released during neuronal activity, followed by release at domains with low extracellular potassium concentration, a process that normally prevents neuronal hyperexcitability. Likewise, deafness is accounted for by expression of the channel in the stria vascularis, where it is essential for the generation of the endocochlear potential.[182]

The renal abnormalities in SeSAME/EAST syndrome are likely due to loss of basolateral potassium recycling which is required for maximal activity of the sodium pump ("pump leak coupling"[183]). Na^+/K^+-ATPase activity, which drives NaCl reabsorption via NCC, increases K^+ entry, which is inferred to be mitigated by return across the basolateral membrane via Kir4.1 activity. In the absence of this function, the accumulation of potassium in the cell limits Na^+/K^+-ATPase activity, and hence NaCl reabsorption in the DCT, and is inferred to cause hypomagnesemia and hypocalciuria due to impaired NCC function, analogous to Gitelman syndrome (see above). Subsequent studies have identified several additional families with SeSAME/EAST syndrome.[184–186] The diagnosis of this syndrome is based on the unique clinical findings. Genetic testing is available.

Treatment options include anticonvulsives and hearing aids to prevent further language delay. Potassium and, where required, magnesium supplementation and potassium-sparing diuretics are used to treat the electrolyte abnormalities in SESAME/EAST syndrome.

GENETIC STUDIES OF ESSENTIAL HYPERTENSION IN THE GENERAL POPULATION

The above considerations largely focus on rare genetic diseases with extreme phenotypes. The identification of the underlying defects had made an invaluable contribution to our current concept of renal salt handling, and to the identification of novel physiological pathways. The results of these studies unequivocally link increased renal salt reabsorption to hypertension, and renal salt loss to sometimes life-threatening hypotension.

While Mendelian diseases of blood pressure homeostasis are extremely rare, hypertension affects more than one billion people worldwide[187] and contributes to more than seven million deaths each year.[188,189] However, despite the early recognition from twin and family studies that blood pressure is influenced by genetic mechanisms,[190,191] with ~60% heritability of hypertension,[192] the genes involved are still largely unknown.

The genetic contribution to common diseases could, in theory, be based on common genetic variants (defined by an allelic frequency of more than 5%). Such variants are identified in genome-wide association studies (GWAS), where a large number of polymorphic markers is genotyped in affected subjects and controls to identify those associated with the disease. Many large GWAS studies on hypertension have been reported,[193,194] with the most recent large meta-analysis evaluating 2.5 million single nucleotide polymorphisms (SNPs) in 69,395 individuals, with replication in up to 133,661 individuals, all of European ancestry.[15] The authors identified 29 independent SNPs at 28 loci that were significantly associated with systolic blood pressure (SBP), diastolic blood pressure (DBP) or both. However, these variants are typically of very small effect size, less than 1 mmHg on systolic blood pressure, and the 29 SNPs reported collectively account for only 0.9% of the phenotypic variance for SBP and DBP. Even including an estimated another 116 variants with similar effect size that did not achieve statistical significance, only ~2.2% of the variance could be explained.

These considerations suggest that only a small fraction of heritability of blood pressure in the general population is explained by common variants, and raise the possibility that a greater fraction of heritability is based on rare variants with larger effect size. Such hypothetical variants are not amenable to analysis by GWAS due to their small allelic frequency. However, their proposed larger effect could well be due to alterations in similar pathways as in Mendelian diseases of blood pressure regulation, i.e., genes involved in renal salt homeostasis. To test this hypothesis, Ji et al. resequenced three target genes, encoding NCC, NKCC2, and ROMK implicated in Bartter and Gitelman syndrome, respectively (see above) in 3125 members of the Framingham Heart Study population (1985 unrelated subjects and 1140 kindred members), all with careful and systematic blood pressure measurements

at regular intervals.[168] From the frequency of the homozygous recessive state for Gitelman and Bartter syndrome, it was expected that heterozygous loss-of-function mutations should be present in about 1−2% of the population. Sequencing of these three genes in this cohort identified 23 subjects with 10 mutations that were previously known loss-of-function mutations or null alleles. Another 19 variants in 25 subjects were found at positions that are completely conserved from flies and worms to humans, strongly suggesting that these are functionally significant. Importantly, these functional mutations are all rare in the population, with allele frequencies less than 1 in 2000. Blood pressure in carriers of mutations in any of the three genes was significantly reduced at ages 40, 50, and 60 years compared to either non-carrier members of the cohort or non-carrier siblings, with a mean 9 mmHg reduction in systolic blood pressure at age 60. Mutation carriers were significantly protected from hypertension (59% risk reduction compared to non-carriers at age 60).

The development of next generation sequencing techniques and the dropping cost of this technology now enables genome-wide and unbiased analysis of rare variants by means of whole genome sequencing or, for reasons of cost effectiveness, whole exome sequencing, in large cohorts. It is expected that ongoing studies will provide new insights into the contribution of rare variants to blood pressure homeostasis, although large sample sizes will be required.[195]

NEW INSIGHTS INTO BASIC PHYSIOLOGY, PREVENTION, AND THERAPEUTICS FROM GENETIC STUDIES

The molecular genetic studies described above have collectively made a number of tangible contributions to our understanding of electrolyte homeostasis and blood pressure regulation. One element in renal physiology that was difficult to predict *a priori* was the physiologic consequence of eliminating specific transport pathways. For example, it was known that ENaC mediates the reabsorption of only a few percent of the filtered sodium load, and clinically used inhibitors of this channel have modest effects on salt balance and blood pressure. It consequently came as a surprise that genetic deficiency of any of the ENaC subunits results in profound renal salt-wasting with severe hyperkalemia and acidosis.[111,112] Affected subjects are extremely ill from birth onward, and typically require massive salt supplementation as well as treatment for hyperkalemia. These findings indicate that ENaC is constitutively active in the absence of an activated renin−angiotensin system, and is required for maintenance of normal salt balance; its absence cannot be reasonably compensated by increasing the activity of other nephron segments. These findings also left no doubt that ENaC activity is absolutely required for normal K^+ and H^+ ion secretion, since severe hyperkalemia and acidosis results in the absence of ENaC activity. In contrast, loss of activity of the target for thiazide diuretics, NCC, has a far more subtle effect on salt balance, despite the fact that NCC normally accounts for reabsorption of a far greater fraction of the filtered salt load.[167] Similarly, the effects of loss of ROMK on net salt and K^+ balance were quite unpredictable from physiologic studies alone.[134] Would loss of ROMK produce hyperkalemia owing to its normal role in K^+ secretion in the distal nephron or hypokalemia due to K^+-wasting from the TAL? The finding that loss of ROMK results in dramatic salt-wasting but only mild hypokalemia, much less severe than that seen with loss of NKCC2, suggests that inhibitors of ROMK might be of particular clinical benefit as antihypertensive diuretic agents.

Second, this work has firmly established the key role of altered renal salt balance in the determination of long-term blood pressure in humans. All mutations that increase salt reabsorption raise blood pressure, while those that reduce salt reabsorption lower blood pressure. Despite diverse effects on K^+, pH, Mg^{2+}, and Ca^{2+} handling, the vector for salt reabsorption dictates the direction of blood pressure. This has implications for control of blood pressure in the general population (see below). These findings underscore the observation that other known sufficient causes of hypertension also modulate renal salt handling. Renovascular hypertension caused by stenosis of one or both renal arteries decreases renal blood flow and thereby causes activation of the RAA system and increased renal salt reabsorption; renal blood flow is likewise reduced in aortic coarctation and pheochromocytoma, again leading to increased renal renin secretion. The same final common pathway is activated by primary aldosteronism with increased aldosterone production from the adrenal gland and by licorice intoxication. Finally, in ESRD, the kidney is unable to eliminate excess volume, leading to hypertension.

Third, this work has uncovered entirely new physiology that was not previously anticipated. Specifically, the role of the WNK kinases in the regulation of the balance between salt reabsorption and K^+ secretion, revealed by genetic studies,[74] has identified a new layer of regulatory physiology in which these kinases are orchestrating the activity of diverse flux pathways to allow appropriate responses to diverse environmental perturbations. Moreover, the realization of the yin and yang relationship between Na-Cl reabsorption and K^+ secretion produced by the WNK kinase pathway provides an explanation for the long-recognized blood pressure-lowering effect of increased dietary potassium—increased K^+ secretion must occur at the expense of reduced Na-Cl reabsorption, accounting for the observed reduction in blood pressure.[196-199] The recent identification of the CUL3-KLHL3 ubiquitin ligase pathway[95,96] will extend this developing paradigm in the coming years.

Perhaps the most important implication of this work is the recognition that modulation of salt balance can modulate blood pressure across the entire spectrum seen in the human population. For example, genetic loss of ENaC function results in life-threatening hypotension, while gain of ENaC function results in early and often severe hypertension. The finding that modulation of activity of single genes in this pathway can dial blood pressure across the entire spectrum seen in the human population reveals the power of this system. These findings provide the basic science foundation that suggests that reduction of dietary salt intake might be beneficial in lowering blood pressure in the general population. This idea has been supported by recent studies showing that even a modest 25% reduction in dietary salt results in clinically significant blood pressure reduction, and that larger reductions in salt intake have proportionally larger effects.[196,200] Goldman and colleagues[201] have estimated that such a 25% reduction in dietary salt intake would be expected to dramatically reduce the number of strokes, myocardial infarctions, all cause deaths, and healthcare costs. The Institute of Medicine has released a study suggesting that such a 25% reduction in salt intake could be approached by reducing salt in processed foods and restaurant meals.[202] Programs to reduce dietary salt have been implemented in a number of countries worldwide.

These insights also have implications for the control of hypertension among patients with end-stage renal disease (ESRD), who have a particularly high prevalence of hypertension. Interestingly, a retrospective cross-sectional study in patients on hemodialysis suggested that a traditional treatment protocol lowering "dry weight" (weight at the end of dialysis) until optimal blood pressure is achieved and limiting dietary salt intake to 5—6 g per day may lead to similar control of hypertension as treatment with antihypertensive drugs, yet better outcome in terms of left ventricular (LV) hypertrophy, LV function, and intradialytic hypotension.[203] Other studies demonstrated that longer, slower dialysis to remove more salt and volume enabled drastic reduction in the prevalence of hypertension.[204,205]

Lastly, these findings provide insight into the potential for new antihypertensive diuretic agents and rational combination therapy. It is striking that patients genetically deficient for the thiazide target (NCC) dramatically increase their dietary salt intake.[206] This suggests that activation of the renin—angiotensin system secondary to salt-wasting contributes to the drive to eat more salt as an adaptive response to volume depletion. Thus, the effects of diuretics are inherently blunted without blockade of compensatory activation of the renin—angotensin system.

The effects of loss-of-function mutations in specific genes provide an excellent proxy for both the magnitude of effect that could be achieved by pharmacologic inhibition of a target, as well as insight into potential mechanism-based adverse effects. It is interesting that loss of the thiazide target, NCC, has a modest effect on blood pressure compared to the effect of loss-of-function mutation in many other genes in the salt reabsorption pathway. The largest loss-of-function effects on blood pressure are seen with targets in the thick ascending limb and collecting duct. Among these, hyper- and hypokalemia are quite severe with most targets, including hypokalemia with mutations in NKCC2, CLCNKB, and BSND, and severe hyperkalemia with loss-of-function mutations in ENaC. These findings might limit the ability to push inhibition at these targets to high enough levels to achieve desired blood pressure lowering. In contrast, ROMK, which produces salt-wasting similar to that seen with mutations in NKCC2, the target of furosemide, produces much less hypokalemia, suggesting that one might achieve very large reductions in salt balance with little effect on K^+. Moreover, heterozygotes for ROMK mutations show significant reductions in blood pressure,[168] suggesting that graded effects can be achieved with dose modification. These findings suggest that ROMK inhibitors, plus inhibition of the renin—angiotensin system, could provide greater blood pressure lowering with fewer side-effects than current treatment regimens, and that ROMK inhibitors may also be of benefit in congestive heart failure. This speculation will require substantial empiric validation to determine the potential value of such agents.

References

[1] Lifton RP, Gharavi AG, Geller DS. Molecular mechanisms of human hypertension. Cell 2001;104:545—56.

[2] Montani JP, Mizelle HL, Adair TH, Guyton AC. Regulation of cardiac output during aldosterone-induced hypertension. J Hypertens Suppl 1989;7:S206—7.

[3] Sutherland DJ, Ruse JL, Laidlaw JC. Hypertension, increased aldosterone secretion and low plasma renin activity relieved by dexamethasone. Can Med Assoc J 1966;95:1109—19.

[4] Litchfield WR, Anderson BF, Weiss RJ, Lifton RP, Dluhy RG. Intracranial aneurysm and hemorrhagic stroke in glucocorticoid-remediable aldosteronism. Hypertension 1998;31:445—50.

[5] Rich GM, Ulick S, Cook S, Wang JZ, Lifton RP, Dluhy RG. Glucocorticoid-remediable aldosteronism in a large kindred: clinical spectrum and diagnosis using a characteristic biochemical phenotype. Ann Intern Med 1992;116:813—20.

[6] Litchfield WR, Coolidge C, Silva P, Lifton RP, Fallo F, Williams GH, et al. Impaired potassium-stimulated aldosterone production: a possible explanation for normokalemic glucocorticoid-remediable aldosteronism. J Clin Endocrinol Metab 1997;82:1507—10.

[7] Chu MD, Ulick S. Isolation and identification of 18-hydroxycortisol from the urine of patients with primary aldosteronism. J Biol Chem 1982;257:2218—24.

[8] Ulick S, Chu MD, Land M. Biosynthesis of 18-oxocortisol by aldosterone-producing adrenal tissue. J Biol Chem 1983;258:5498—502.

[9] Lifton RP, Dluhy RG, Powers M, Rich GM, Cook S, Ulick S, et al. A chimaeric 11 beta-hydroxylase/aldosterone synthase gene causes glucocorticoid-remediable aldosteronism and human hypertension. Nature 1992;355:262—5.

[10] Lifton RP, Dluhy RG, Powers M, Rich GM, Gutkin M, Fallo F, et al. Hereditary hypertension caused by chimaeric gene duplications and ectopic expression of aldosterone synthase. Nat Genet 1992;2:66—74.

[11] Pilon C, Mulatero P, Barzon L, Veglio F, Garrone C, Boscaro M, et al. Mutations in CYP11B1 gene converting 11beta-hydroxylase into an aldosterone-producing enzyme are not present in aldosterone-producing adenomas. J Clin Endocrinol Metab 1999;84:4228—31.

[12] Jonsson JR, Klemm SA, Tunny TJ, Stowasser M, Gordon RD. A new genetic test for familial hyperaldosteronism type I aids in the detection of curable hypertension. Biochem Biophys Res Commun 1995;207:565—71.

[13] Funder JW, Carey RM, Fardella C, Gomez-Sanchez CE, Mantero F, Stowasser M, et al. Case detection, diagnosis, and treatment of patients with primary aldosteronism: an endocrine society clinical practice guideline. J Clin Endocrinol Metab 2008;93:3266—81.

[14] Fallo F, Pilon C, Williams TA, Sonino N, Morra Di Cella S, Veglio F, et al. Coexistence of different phenotypes in a family with glucocorticoid-remediable aldosteronism. J Hum Hypertens 2004;18:47—51.

[15] Ehret GB, Munroe PB, Rice KM, Bochud M, Johnson AD, Chasman DI, et al. Genetic variants in novel pathways influence blood pressure and cardiovascular disease risk. Nature 2011;478:103—9.

[16] Conn JW, Louis LH. Primary aldosteronism: a new clinical entity. Trans Assoc Am Physicians 1955;68:215—31, discussion, 231—213.

[17] Rossi GP, Bernini G, Caliumi C, Desideri G, Fabris B, Ferri C, et al. A prospective study of the prevalence of primary aldosteronism in 1,125 hypertensive patients. J Am Coll Cardiol 2006;48:2293—300.

[18] Choi M, Scholl UI, Yue P, Bjorklund P, Zhao B, Nelson-Williams C, et al. K^+ channel mutations in adrenal aldosterone-producing adenomas and hereditary hypertension. Science 2011;331:768—72.

[19] Heginbotham L, Lu Z, Abramson T, MacKinnon R. Mutations in the K^+ channel signature sequence. Biophys J 1994;66:1061—7.

[20] Tao X, Avalos JL, Chen J, MacKinnon R. Crystal structure of the eukaryotic strong inward-rectifier K^+ channel Kir2.2 at 3.1 Å resolution. Science 2009;326:1668—74.

[21] Enyeart JJ, Xu L, Danthi S, Enyeart JA. An ACTH- and ATP-regulated background K^+ channel in adrenocortical cells is TREK-1. J Biol Chem 2002;277:49186—99.

[22] Czirjak G, Enyedi P. TASK-3 dominates the background potassium conductance in rat adrenal glomerulosa cells. Mol Endocrinol 2002;16:621—9.

[23] Lotshaw DP. Characterization of angiotensin II-regulated K$^+$ conductance in rat adrenal glomerulosa cells. J Membr Biol 1997;156:261—77.

[24] Brauneis U, Vassilev PM, Quinn SJ, Williams GH, Tillotson DL. ANG II blocks potassium currents in zona glomerulosa cells from rat, bovine, and human adrenals. Am J Physiol 1991;260:E772—9.

[25] Hu C, Rusin CG, Tan Z, Guagliardo NA, Barrett PQ. Zona glomerulosa cells of the mouse adrenal cortex are intrinsic electrical oscillators. J Clin Invest 2012;122(6):2046—53.

[26] Spat A, Hunyady L. Control of aldosterone secretion: a model for convergence in cellular signaling pathways. Physiol Rev 2004;84:489—539.

[26a] Akerström T, Crona J, Delgado Verdugo A, Starker LF, Cupisti K, Willenberg HS, et al. Comprehensive Re-Sequencing of Adrenal Aldosterone Producing Lesions Reveal Three Somatic Mutations near the KCNJ5 Potassium Channel Selectivity Filter. PLoS One 2012;7:e41926.

[27] Boulkroun S, Beuschlein F, Rossi GP, Golib-Dzib JF, Fischer E, Amar L, et al. Prevalence, clinical, and molecular correlates of KCNJ5 mutations in primary aldosteronism. Hypertension 2012;59:592—8.

[28] Geller DS, Zhang J, Wisgerhof MV, Shackleton C, Kashgarian M, Lifton RP. A novel form of human Mendelian hypertension featuring nonglucocorticoid-remediable aldosteronism. J Clin Endocrinol Metab 2008;93:3117—23.

[29] Scholl UI, Nelson-Williams C, Yue P, Grekin R, Wyatt RJ, Dillon MJ, et al. Hypertension with or without adrenal hyperplasia due to different inherited mutations in the potassium channel KCNJ5. Proc Natl Acad Sci USA 2012;109:2533—8.

[30] Mulatero P, Tauber P, Zennaro MC, Monticone S, Lang K, Beuschlein F, et al. KCNJ5 mutations in European families with nonglucocorticoid remediable familial hyperaldosteronism. Hypertension 2012;59:235—40.

[31] Mussa A, VCamilla R, Monticone S, Porta F, Tessaris D, Verna F, et al. Polyuric-polydipsic syndrome in a pediatric case of nonglucocorticoid remediable familial hyperaldosteronism. Endocr J 2012;59:497—502.

[32] Charmandari E, Sertedaki A, Kino T, Merakou C, Hoffman DA, Hatch MM, et al. A novel point mutation in the KCNJ5 gene causing primary hyperaldosteronism and early-onset autosomal dominant hypertension. J Clin Endocrinol Metab 2012;97:E1532-9.

[33] Pivonello R, Ferone D, de Herder WW, de Krijger RR, Waaijers M, Mooij DM, et al. Dopamine receptor expression and function in human normal adrenal gland and adrenal tumors. J Clin Endocrinol Metab 2004;89:4493—502.

[34] Tannin GM, Agarwal AK, Monder C, New MI, White PC. The human gene for 11 beta-hydroxysteroid dehydrogenase. Structure, tissue distribution, and chromosomal localization. J Biol Chem 1991;266:16653—8.

[35] Zachmann M, Tassinari D, Prader A. Clinical and biochemical variability of congenital adrenal hyperplasia due to 11 beta-hydroxylase deficiency. A study of 25 patients. J Clin Endocrinol Metab 1983;56:222—9.

[36] Rosler A, Leiberman E, Sack J, Landau H, Benderly A, Moses SW, et al. Clinical variability of congenital adrenal hyperplasia due to 11 beta-hydroxylase deficiency. Horm Res 1982;16:133—41.

[37] Cerame BI, New MI. Hormonal hypertension in children: 11beta-hydroxylase deficiency and apparent mineralocorticoid excess. J Pediatr Endocrinol Metab 2000;13:1537—47.

[38] Portrat S, Mulatero P, Curnow KM, Chaussain JL, Morel Y, Pascoe L. Deletion hybrid genes, due to unequal crossing over

between CYP11B1 (11beta-hydroxylase) and CYP11B2(aldosterone synthase) cause steroid 11beta-hydroxylase deficiency and congenital adrenal hyperplasia. J Clin Endocrinol Metab 2001;86:3197—201.

[39] Biglieri EG, Herron MA, Brust N. 17-hydroxylation deficiency in man. J Clin Invest 1966;45:1946—54.

[40] Costa-Santos M, Kater CE, Auchus RJ. Two prevalent CYP17 mutations and genotype-phenotype correlations in 24 Brazilian patients with 17-hydroxylase deficiency. J Clin Endocrinol Metab 2004;89:49—60.

[41] Kagimoto M, Winter JS, Kagimoto K, Simpson ER, Waterman MR. Structural characterization of normal and mutant human steroid 17 alpha-hydroxylase genes: molecular basis of one example of combined 17 alpha-hydroxylase/17,20 lyase deficiency. Mol Endocrinol 1988;2:564—70.

[42] Geller DH, Auchus RJ, Mendonca BB, Miller WL. The genetic and functional basis of isolated 17,20-lyase deficiency. Nat Genet 1997;17:201—5.

[43] New MI, Levine LS, Biglieri EG, VPareira J, Ulick S. Evidence for an unidentified steroid in a child with apparent mineralocorticoid hypertension. J Clin Endocrinol Metab 1977;44:924—33.

[44] Ulick S, Levine LS, Gunczler P, Zanconato G, Ramirez LC, Rauh W, et al. A syndrome of apparent mineralocorticoid excess associated with defects in the peripheral metabolism of cortisol. J Clin Endocrinol Metab 1979;49:757—64.

[45] Arriza JL, Weinberger C, Cerelli G, Glaser TM, Handelin BL, Housman DE, et al. Cloning of human mineralocorticoid receptor complementary DNA: structural and functional kinship with the glucocorticoid receptor. Science 1987;237:268—75.

[46] Krozowski ZS, Funder JW. Renal mineralocorticoid receptors and hippocampal corticosterone-binding species have identical intrinsic steroid specificity. Proc Natl Acad Sci USA 1983;80:6056—60.

[47] Mune T, Rogerson FM, Nikkila H, Agarwal AK, White PC. Human hypertension caused by mutations in the kidney isozyme of 11 beta-hydroxysteroid dehydrogenase. Nat Genet 1995;10:394—9.

[48] Kotelevtsev Y, Brown RW, Fleming S, Kenyon C, Edwards CR, Seckl JR, et al. Hypertension in mice lacking 11beta-hydroxysteroid dehydrogenase type 2. J Clin Invest 1999;103:683—9.

[49] Palermo M, Delitala G, Mantero F, Stewart PM, Shackleton CH. Congenital deficiency of 11beta-hydroxysteroid dehydrogenase (apparent mineralocorticoid excess syndrome): diagnostic value of urinary free cortisol and cortisone. J Endocrinol Invest 2001;24:17—23.

[50] Knops NB, Monnens LA, Lenders JW, Levtchenko EN. Apparent mineralocorticoid excess: time of manifestation and complications despite treatment. Pediatrics 2011;127:e1610—4.

[51] Stewart PM, Wallace AM, Valentino R, Burt D, Shackleton CH, Edwards CR. Mineralocorticoid activity of liquorice: 11-beta-hydroxysteroid dehydrogenase deficiency comes of age. Lancet 1987;2:821—4.

[52] Geller DS. Pseudohypoaldosteronism Type 1 and Hypertension Exacerbated in Pregnancy. In: Lifton RP, Somlo S, Giebisch GH, Seldin DW, editors. *Genetic diseases of the kidney*. burlington. London, San Diego, New York: Elsevier; 2009. p. 301—12.

[53] Geller DS, Farhi A, Pinkerton N, Fradley M, Moritz M, Spitzer A, et al. Activating mineralocorticoid receptor mutation in hypertension exacerbated by pregnancy. Science 2000;289:119—23.

[54] Fagart J, Huyet J, Pinon GM, Rochel M, Mayer C, Rafestin-Oblin ME. Crystal structure of a mutant mineralocorticoid receptor responsible for hypertension. Nat Struct Mol Biol 2005;12:554—5.

[55] Liddle GW, Bledsoe T, Coppage WS. A familial renal disorder stimulating primary aldosteronism but with negligible aldosterone secretion. Trans Assoc Am Physicians 1963;76:199—213.

[56] Shimkets RA, Warnock DG, Bositis CM, Nelson-Williams C, Hansson JH, Schambelan M, et al. Liddle's syndrome: heritable human hypertension caused by mutations in the beta subunit of the epithelial sodium channel. Cell 1994;79:407–14.

[57] Hansson JH, Nelson-Williams C, Suzuki H, Schild L, Shimkets R, Lu Y, et al. Hypertension caused by a truncated epithelial sodium channel gamma subunit: genetic heterogeneity of Liddle syndrome. Nat Genet 1995;11:76–82.

[58] Canessa CM, Schild L, Buell G, Thorens B, Gautschi I, Horisberger JD, et al. Amiloride-sensitive epithelial Na$^+$ channel is made of three homologous subunits. Nature 1994;367:463–7.

[59] Canessa CM, Merillat AM, Rossier BC. Membrane topology of the epithelial sodium channel in intact cells. Am J Physiol 1994;267:C1682–90.

[60] Hansson JH, Schild L, Lu Y, Wilson TA, Gautschi I, Shimkets R, et al. A *de novo* missense mutation of the beta subunit of the epithelial sodium channel causes hypertension and Liddle syndrome, identifying a proline-rich segment critical for regulation of channel activity. Proc Natl Acad Sci USA 1995;92:11495–9.

[61] Snyder PM, Price MP, McDonald FJ, Adams CM, Volk KA, Zeiher BG, et al. Mechanism by which Liddle's syndrome mutations increase activity of a human epithelial Na$^+$ channel. Cell 1995;83:969–78.

[62] Schild L, Canessa CM, Shimkets RA, Gautschi I, Lifton RP, Rossier BC. A mutation in the epithelial sodium channel causing Liddle disease increases channel activity in the *Xenopus laevis* oocyte expression system. Proc Natl Acad Sci USA 1995;92:5699–703.

[63] Firsov D, Schild L, Gautschi I, Merillat AM, Schneeberger E, Rossier BC. Cell surface expression of the epithelial Na channel and a mutant causing Liddle syndrome: a quantitative approach. Proc Natl Acad Sci USA 1996;93:15370–5.

[64] Staub O, Dho S, Henry P, Correa J, Ishikawa T, McGlade J, et al. WW domains of Nedd4 bind to the proline-rich PY motifs in the epithelial Na$^+$ channel deleted in Liddle's syndrome. EMBO J 1996;15:2371–80.

[65] Kamynina E, Debonneville C, Bens M, Vandewalle A, Staub O. A novel mouse Nedd4 protein suppresses the activity of the epithelial Na$^+$ channel. FASEB J 2001;15:204–14.

[66] Hiltunen TP, Hannila-Handelberg T, Petajaniemi N, Kantola I, Tikkanen I, Virtamo J, et al. Liddle's syndrome associated with a point mutation in the extracellular domain of the epithelial sodium channel gamma subunit. J Hypertens 2002;20:2383–90.

[67] Botero-Velez M, Curtis JJ, Warnock DG. Brief report: liddle's syndrome revisited – a disorder of sodium reabsorption in the distal tubule. N Engl J Med 1994;330:178–81.

[68] Pradervand S, Wang Q, Burnier M, Beermann F, Horisberger JD, Hummler E, et al. A mouse model for Liddle's syndrome. J Am Soc Nephrol 1999;10:2527–33.

[69] Paver WK, Pauline GJ. Hypertension and hyperpotassaemia without Renal disease in a young male. Med J Aust 1964;2:305–6.

[70] Farfel Z, Iaina A, Rosenthal T, Waks U, Shibolet S, Gafni J. Familial hyperpotassemia and hypertension accompanied by normal plasma aldosterone levels: possible hereditary cell membrane defect. Arch Intern Med 1978;138:1828–32.

[71] Farfel Z, Rosenthal T, Shibolet S, Iaina A, Gafni J. Familial hyperkalemia and hypertension. Harefuah 1976;90:468–70.

[72] Lee MR, Morgan DB. Familial hyperkalaemia responsive to benzothiadiazine diuretic. Lancet 1980;1:879.

[73] Schambelan M, Sebastian A, Rector Jr FC. Mineralocorticoid-resistant renal hyperkalemia without salt wasting (type II pseudohypoaldosteronism): role of increased renal chloride reabsorption. Kidney Int 1981;19:716–27.

[74] Wilson FH, Disse-Nicodeme S, Choate KA, Ishikawa K, Nelson-Williams C, Desitter I, et al. Human hypertension caused by mutations in WNK kinases. Science 2001;293:1107–12.

[75] Yang CL, Angell J, Mitchell R, Ellison DH. WNK kinases regulate thiazide-sensitive Na-Cl co-transport. J Clin Invest 2003;111:1039–45.

[76] Kahle KT, Wilson FH, Leng Q, Lalioti MD, O'Connell AD, Dong K, et al. WNK4 regulates the balance between renal NaCl reabsorption and K$^+$ secretion. Nat Genet 2003;35:372–6.

[77] Kahle KT, Macgregor GG, Wilson FH, Van Hoek AN, Brown D, Ardito T, et al. Paracellular Cl$^-$ permeability is regulated by WNK4 kinase: insight into normal physiology and hypertension. Proc Natl Acad Sci USA 2004;101:14877–82.

[78] Yamauchi K, Rai T, Kobayashi K, Sohara E, Suzuki T, Itoh T, et al. Disease-causing mutant WNK4 increases paracellular chloride permeability and phosphorylates claudins. Proc Natl Acad Sci USA 2004;101:4690–4.

[79] Lalioti MD, Zhang J, Volkman HM, Kahle KT, Hoffmann KE, Toka HR, et al. Wnk4 controls blood pressure and potassium homeostasis via regulation of mass and activity of the distal convoluted tubule. Nat Genet 2006;38:1124–32.

[80] Kahle KT, Ring AM, Lifton RP. Molecular physiology of the WNK kinases. Annu Rev Physiol 2008;70:329–55.

[81] Hoorn EJ, Nelson JH, McCormick JA, Ellison DH. The WNK kinase network regulating sodium, potassium, and blood pressure. J Am Soc Nephrol 2011;22:605–14.

[82] Kahle KT, Wilson FH, Lifton RP. The Syndrome of Hypertension and Hyperkalemia (Pseudohypoaldosteronism Type II): WNK Kinases regulate the balance between renal salt reabsorption and potassium secretion. In: Lifton RP, Somlo S, Giebisch G, Seldin DW, editors. Genetic diseases of the kidney. Burlington, London, San Diego, New York: Elsevier; 2009. p. 313–29.

[83] Wilson FH, Kahle KT, Sabath E, Lalioti MD, Rapson AK, Hoover RS, et al. Molecular pathogenesis of inherited hypertension with hyperkalemia: the Na-Cl co-transporter is inhibited by wild-type but not mutant WNK4. Proc Natl Acad Sci USA 2003;100:680–4.

[84] Subramanya AR, Liu J, Ellison DH, Wade JB, Welling PA. WNK4 diverts the thiazide-sensitive NaCl co-transporter to the lysosome and stimulates AP-3 interaction. J Biol Chem 2009;284:18471–80.

[85] He G, Wang HR, Huang SK, Huang CL. Intersectin links WNK kinases to endocytosis of ROMK1. J Clin Invest 2007;117:1078–87.

[86] Ring AM, Cheng SX, Leng Q, Kahle KT, Rinehart J, Lalioti MD, et al. WNK4 regulates activity of the epithelial Na$^+$ channel *in vitro* and *in vivo*. Proc Natl Acad Sci USA 2007;104:4020–4.

[87] Ring AM, Leng Q, Rinehart J, Wilson FH, Kahle KT, Hebert SC, et al. An SGK1 site in WNK4 regulates Na$^+$ channel and K$^+$ channel activity and has implications for aldosterone signaling and K$^+$ homeostasis. Proc Natl Acad Sci USA 2007;104:4025–9.

[88] Lazrak A, Liu Z, Huang CL. Antagonistic regulation of ROMK by long and kidney-specific WNK1 isoforms. Proc Natl Acad Sci USA 2006;103:1615–20.

[89] Xu BE, Stippec S, Chu PY, Lazrak A, Li XJ, Lee BH, et al. WNK1 activates SGK1 to regulate the epithelial sodium channel. Proc Natl Acad Sci USA 2005;102:10315–20.

[90] Ohta A, Yang SS, Rai T, Chiga M, Sasaki S, Uchida S. Overexpression of human WNK1 increases paracellular chloride permeability and phosphorylation of claudin-4 in MDCKII cells. Biochem Biophys Res Commun 2006;349:804–8.

[91] San-Cristobal P, Pacheco-Alvarez D, Richardson C, Ring AM, Vazquez N, Rafiqi FH, et al. Angiotensin II signaling increases activity of the renal Na-Cl co-transporter through a WNK4-SPAK-dependent pathway. Proc Natl Acad Sci USA 2009;106:4384–9.

[92] McCormick JA, Ellison DH. The WNKs: atypical protein kinases with pleiotropic actions. Physiol Rev 2011;91:177—219.

[93] Castaneda-Bueno M, Cervantes-Perez LG, Vazquez N, Uribe N, Kantesaria S, Morla L, et al. Activation of the renal Na$^+$:Cl$^-$ co-transporter by angiotensin II is a WNK4-dependent process. Proc Natl Acad Sci USA 2012;109:7929—34.

[94] Delaloy C, Elvira-Matelot E, Clemessy M, Zhou XO, Imbert-Teboul M, Houot AM, et al. Deletion of WNK1 first intron results in misregulation of both isoforms in renal and extrarenal tissues. Hypertension 2008;52:1149—54.

[95] Boyden LM, Choi M, Choate KA, Nelson-Williams CJ, Farhi A, Toka HR, et al. Mutations in kelch-like 3 and cullin 3 cause hypertension and electrolyte abnormalities. Nature 2012;482:98—102.

[96] Louis-Dit-Picard H, Barc J, Trujillano D, Miserey-Lenkei S, Bouatia-Naji N, Pylypenko O, et al. KLHL3 mutations cause familial hyperkalemic hypertension by impairing ion transport in the distal nephron. Nat Genet 2012;44:456—60.

[97] Peter M, Fawaz L, Drop SL, Visser HK, Sippell WG. Hereditary defect in biosynthesis of aldosterone: aldosterone synthase deficiency 1964-1997. J Clin Endocrinol Metab 1997;82:3525—8.

[98] Ulick S, Gautier E, Vetter KK, Markello JR, Yaffe S, Lowe CU. An aldosterone biosynthetic defect in a salt-losing disorder. J Clin Endocrinol Metab 1964;24:669—72.

[99] Pascoe L, Curnow KM, Slutsker L, Rosler A, White PC. Mutations in the human CYP11B2 (aldosterone synthase) gene causing corticosterone methyloxidase II deficiency. Proc Natl Acad Sci USA 1992;89:4996—5000.

[100] Mitsuuchi Y, Kawamoto T, Miyahara K, Ulick S, Morton DH, Naiki Y, et al. Congenitally defective aldosterone biosynthesis in humans: inactivation of the P-450C18 gene (CYP11B2) due to nucleotide deletion in CMO I deficient patients. Biochem Biophys Res Commun 1993;190:864—9.

[101] Kayes-Wandover KM, Tannin GM, Shulman D, Peled D, Jones KL, Karaviti L, et al. Congenital hyperreninemic hypoaldosteronism unlinked to the aldosterone synthase (CYP11B2) gene. J Clin Endocrinol Metab 2001;86:5379—82.

[102] White PC, New MI, Dupont B. HLA-linked congenital adrenal hyperplasia results from a defective gene encoding a cytochrome P-450 specific for steroid 21-hydroxylation. Proc Natl Acad Sci USA 1984;81:7505—9.

[103] Bongiovanni AM, Root AW. The adrenogenital syndrome. N Engl J Med 1963;268:1283—9 contd

[104] Higashi Y, Yoshioka H, Yamane M, Gotoh O, Fujii-Kuriyama Y. Complete nucleotide sequence of two steroid 21-hydroxylase genes tandemly arranged in human chromosome: a pseudogene and a genuine gene. Proc Natl Acad Sci USA 1986;83:2841—5.

[105] Speiser PW, Azziz R, Baskin LS, Ghizzoni L, Hensle TW, Merke DP, et al. Congenital adrenal hyperplasia due to steroid 21-hydroxylase deficiency: an Endocrine Society clinical practice guideline. J Clin Endocrinol Metab 2010;95:4133—60.

[106] Rheaume E, Simard J, Morel Y, Mebarki F, Zachmann M, Forest MG, et al. Congenital adrenal hyperplasia due to point mutations in the type II 3 beta-hydroxysteroid dehydrogenase gene. Nat Genet 1992;1:239—45.

[107] Lin D, Sugawara T, Strauss JF 3rd, Clark BJ, Stocco DM, Saenger P, et al. Role of steroidogenic acute regulatory protein in adrenal and gonadal steroidogenesis. Science 1995;267:1828—31.

[108] Cheek DB, Perry JW. A salt wasting syndrome in infancy. Arch Dis Child 1958;33:252—6.

[109] Hanukoglu A, Bistritzer T, Rakover Y, Mandelberg A. Pseudohypoaldosteronism with increased sweat and saliva electrolyte values and frequent lower respiratory tract infections mimicking cystic fibrosis. J Pediatr 1994;125:752—5.

[110] Kerem E, Bistritzer T, Hanukoglu A, Hofmann T, Zhou Z, Bennett W, et al. Pulmonary epithelial sodium-channel dysfunction and excess airway liquid in pseudohypoaldosteronism. N Engl J Med 1999;341:156—62.

[111] Chang SS, Grunder S, Hanukoglu A, Rosler A, Mathew PM, Hanukoglu I, et al. Mutations in subunits of the epithelial sodium channel cause salt wasting with hyperkalaemic acidosis, pseudohypoaldosteronism type 1. Nat Genet 1996;12:248—53.

[112] Strautnieks SS, Thompson RJ, Gardiner RM, Chung E. A novel splice-site mutation in the gamma subunit of the epithelial sodium channel gene in three pseudohypoaldosteronism type 1 families. Nat Genet 1996;13:248—50.

[113] McDonald FJ, Yang B, Hrstka RF, Drummond HA, Tarr DE, McCray Jr PB, et al. Disruption of the beta subunit of the epithelial Na$^+$ channel in mice: hyperkalemia and neonatal death associated with a pseudohypoaldosteronism phenotype. Proc Natl Acad Sci USA 1999;96:1727—31.

[114] Barker PM, Nguyen MS, Gatzy JT, Grubb B, Norman H, Hummler E, et al. Role of gammaENaC subunit in lung liquid clearance and electrolyte balance in newborn mice. Insights into perinatal adaptation and pseudohypoaldosteronism. J Clin Invest 1998;102:1634—40.

[115] Hummler E, Barker P, Talbot C, Wang Q, Verdumo C, Grubb B, et al. A mouse model for the renal salt-wasting syndrome pseudohypoaldosteronism. Proc Natl Acad Sci USA 1997;94:11710—5.

[116] Hummler E, Barker P, Gatzy J, Beermann F, Verdumo C, Schmidt A, et al. Early death due to defective neonatal lung liquid clearance in alpha-ENaC-deficient mice. Nat Genet 1996;12:325—8.

[117] Huppmann S, Lankes E, Schnabel D, Buhrer C. Unimpaired postnatal respiratory adaptation in a preterm human infant with a homozygous ENaC-alpha unit loss-of-function mutation. J Perinatol 2011;31:802—3.

[118] Geller DS, Rodriguez-Soriano J, Vallo Boado A, Schifter S, Bayer M, Chang SS, et al. Mutations in the mineralocorticoid receptor gene cause autosomal dominant pseudohypoaldosteronism type I. Nat Genet 1998;19:279—81.

[119] Geller DS, Zhang J, Zennaro MC, Vallo-Boado A, Rodriguez-Soriano J, Furu L, et al. Autosomal dominant pseudohypoaldosteronism type 1: mechanisms, evidence for neonatal lethality, and phenotypic expression in adults. J Am Soc Nephrol 2006;17:1429—36.

[120] Hubert EL, Teissier R, Fernandes-Rosa FL, Fay M, Rafestin-Oblin ME, Jeunemaitre X, et al. Mineralocorticoid receptor mutations and a severe recessive pseudohypoaldosteronism type 1. J Am Soc Nephrol 2011;22:1997—2003.

[121] Berger S, Bleich M, Schmid W, Cole TJ, Peters J, Watanabe H, et al. Mineralocorticoid receptor knockout mice: pathophysiology of Na$^+$ metabolism. Proc Natl Acad Sci USA 1998;95:9424—9.

[122] Bleich M, Warth R, Schmidt-Hieber M, Schulz-Baldes A, Hasselblatt P, Fisch D, et al. Rescue of the mineralocorticoid receptor knock-out mouse. Pflugers Arch 1999;438:245—54.

[123] Bartter FC, Pronove P, Gill Jr JR, Maccardle RC. Hyperplasia of the juxtaglomerular complex with hyperaldosteronism and hypokalemic alkalosis. A new syndrome. Am J Med 1962;33:811—28.

[124] Rodrigues Pereira R, Hasaart T. Hydramnios and observations in Bartter's syndrome. Acta Obstet Gynecol Scand 1982;61:477—8.

[125] Simopoulos AP. Growth characteristics in patients with Bartter's syndrome. Nephron 1979;23:130—5.

[126] Matsumoto J, Han BK, Restrepo de Rovetto C, Welch TR. Hypercalciuric Bartter syndrome: resolution of nephrocalcinosis with indomethacin. AJR Am J Roentgenol 1989;152:1251−3.

[127] Landau D, Shalev H, Ohaly M, Carmi R. Infantile variant of Bartter syndrome and sensorineural deafness: a new autosomal recessive disorder. Am J Med Genet 1995;59:454−9.

[128] Chaimovitz C, Levi J, Better OS, Oslander L, Benderli A. Studies on the site of renal salt loss in a patient with Bartter's syndrome. Pediatr Res 1973;7:89−94.

[129] Fichman MP, Telfer N, Zia P, Speckart P, Golub M, Rude R. Role of prostaglandins in the pathogenesis of Bartter's syndrome. Am J Med 1976;60:785−97.

[130] Verberckmoes R, van Damme BB, Clement J, Amery A, Michielsen P. Bartter's syndrome with hyperplasia of renomedullary cells: successful treatment with indomethacin. Kidney Int 1976;9:302−7.

[131] Gill Jr JR, Frolich JC, Bowden RE, Taylor AA, Keiser HR, Seyberth HW, et al. Bartter's syndrome: a disorder characterized by high urinary prostaglandins and a dependence of hyperreninemia on prostaglandin synthesis. Am J Med 1976;61:43−51.

[132] Simon DB, Karet FE, Hamdan JM, DiPietro A, Sanjad SA, Lifton RP. Bartter's syndrome, hypokalaemic alkalosis with hypercalciuria, is caused by mutations in the Na-K-2Cl co-transporter NKCC2. Nat Genet 1996;13:183−8.

[133] Takahashi N, Chernavvsky DR, Gomez RA, Igarashi P, Gitelman HJ, Smithies O. Uncompensated polyuria in a mouse model of Bartter's syndrome. Proc Natl Acad Sci USA 2000;97:5434−9.

[134] Simon DB, Karet FE, Rodriguez-Soriano J, Hamdan JH, DiPietro A, Trachtman H, et al. Genetic heterogeneity of Bartter's syndrome revealed by mutations in the K$^+$ channel, ROMK. Nat Genet 1996;14:152−6.

[135] Hebert SC. An ATP-regulated, inwardly rectifying potassium channel from rat kidney (ROMK). Kidney Int 1995;48:1010−6.

[136] Giebisch G. Renal potassium channels: an overview. Kidney Int 1995;48:1004−9.

[137] Peters M, Jeck N, Reinalter S, Leonhardt A, Tonshoff B, Klaus GG, et al. Clinical presentation of genetically defined patients with hypokalemic salt-losing tubulopathies. Am J Med 2002;112:183−90.

[138] Finer G, Shalev H, Birk OS, Galron D, Jeck N, Sinai-Treiman L, et al. Transient neonatal hyperkalemia in the antenatal (ROMK defective) Bartter syndrome. J Pediatr 2003;142: 318−23.

[139] Satlin LM. Postnatal maturation of potassium transport in rabbit cortical collecting duct. Am J Physiol 1994;266:F57−65.

[140] Satlin LM, Palmer LG. Apical K$^+$ conductance in maturing rabbit principal cell. Am J Physiol 1997;272:F397−404.

[141] Lorenz JN, Baird NR, Judd LM, Noonan WT, Andringa A, Doetschman T, et al. Impaired renal NaCl absorption in mice lacking the ROMK potassium channel, a model for type II Bartter's syndrome. J Biol Chem 2002;277:37871−80.

[142] Simon DB, Bindra RS, Mansfield TA, Nelson-Williams C, Mendonca E, Stone R, et al. Mutations in the chloride channel gene, CLCNKB, cause Bartter's syndrome type III. Nat Genet 1997;17:171−8.

[143] Vandewalle A, Cluzeaud F, Bens M, Kieferle S, Steinmeyer K, Jentsch TJ. Localization and induction by dehydration of ClC-K chloride channels in the rat kidney. Am J Physiol 1997;272:F678−88.

[144] Adachi S, Uchida S, Ito H, Hata M, Hiroe M, Marumo F, et al. Two isoforms of a chloride channel predominantly expressed in thick ascending limb of Henle's loop and collecting ducts of rat kidney. J Biol Chem 1994;269:17677−83.

[145] Kieferle S, Fong P, Bens M, Vandewalle A, Jentsch TJ. Two highly homologous members of the ClC chloride channel family in both rat and human kidney. Proc Natl Acad Sci USA 1994;91:6943−7.

[146] Jeck N, Konrad M, Peters M, Weber S, Bonzel KE, Seyberth HW. Mutations in the chloride channel gene, CLCNKB, leading to a mixed Bartter−Gitelman phenotype. Pediatr Res 2000;48:754−8.

[147] Brennan TM, Landau D, Shalev H, Lamb F, Schutte BC, Walder RY, et al. Linkage of infantile Bartter syndrome with sensorineural deafness to chromosome. Am J Hum Genet 1998;62:355−61.

[148] Birkenhager R, Otto E, Schurmann MJ, Vollmer M, Ruf EM, Maier-Lutz I, et al. Mutation of BSND causes Bartter syndrome with sensorineural deafness and kidney failure. Nat Genet 2001;29:310−4.

[149] Estevez R, Boettger T, Stein V, Birkenhager R, Otto E, Hildebrandt F, et al. Barttin is a Cl$^-$ channel beta-subunit crucial for renal Cl- reabsorption and inner ear K$^+$ secretion. Nature 2001;414:558−61.

[150] Schlingmann KP, Konrad M, Jeck N, Waldegger P, Reinalter SC, Holder M, et al. Salt wasting and deafness resulting from mutations in two chloride channels. N Engl J Med 2004;350:1314−9.

[151] Nozu K, Inagaki T, Fu XJ, Nozu Y, Kaito H, Kanda K, et al. Molecular analysis of digenic inheritance in Bartter syndrome with sensorineural deafness. J Med Genet 2008;45:182−6.

[152] Matsumura Y, Uchida S, Kondo Y, Miyazaki H, Ko SB, Hayama A, et al. Overt nephrogenic diabetes insipidus in mice lacking the CLC-K1 chloride channel. Nat Genet 1999;21:95−8.

[153] Rickheit G, Maier H, Strenzke N, Andreescu CE, De Zeeuw CI, Muenscher A, et al. Endocochlear potential depends on Cl$^-$ channels: mechanism underlying deafness in Bartter syndrome IV. EMBO J 2008;27:2907−17.

[154] Pearce SH, Williamson C, Kifor O, Bai M, Coulthard MG, Davies M, et al. A familial syndrome of hypocalcemia with hypercalciuria due to mutations in the calcium-sensing receptor. N Engl J Med 1996;335:1115−22.

[155] Vargas-Poussou R, Huang C, Hulin P, Houillier P, Jeunemaitre X, Paillard M, et al. Functional characterization of a calcium-sensing receptor mutation in severe autosomal dominant hypocalcemia with a Bartter-like syndrome. J Am Soc Nephrol 2002; 13:2259−66.

[156] Watanabe S, Fukumoto S, Chang H, Takeuchi Y, Hasegawa Y, Okazaki R, et al. Association between activating mutations of calcium-sensing receptor and Bartter's syndrome. Lancet 2002;360:692−4.

[157] Hebert SC, Brown EM, Harris HW. Role of the Ca$(^{2+})$-sensing receptor in divalent mineral ion homeostasis. J Exp Biol 1997;200:295−302.

[158] Seyberth HW, Koniger SJ, Rascher W, Kuhl PG, Schweer H. Role of prostaglandins in hyperprostaglandin E syndrome and in selected renal tubular disorders. Pediatr Nephrol 1987;1:491−7.

[159] Rodriguez-Soriano J, Vallo A, Perez de Nanclares G, Bilbao JR, Castano L. A founder mutation in the CLCNKB gene causes bartter syndrome type III in Spain. Pediatr Nephrol 2005;20: 891−6.

[160] Reinalter SC, Jeck N, Brochhausen C, Watzer B, Nusing RM, Seyberth HW, et al. Role of cyclooxygenase-2 in hyperprostaglandin E syndrome/antenatal Bartter syndrome. Kidney Int 2002;62:253−60.

[161] Chaudhuri A, Salvatierra Jr O, Alexander SR, Sarwal MM. Option of pre-emptive nephrectomy and renal transplantation for Bartter's syndrome. Pediatr Transplant 2006;10:266−70.

[162] Gitelman HJ, Graham JB, Welt LG. A new familial disorder characterized by hypokalemia and hypomagnesemia. Trans Assoc Am Physicians 1966;79:221–35.

[163] Bettinelli A, Bianchetti MG, Girardin E, Caringella A, Cecconi M, Appiani AC, et al. Use of calcium excretion values to distinguish two forms of primary renal tubular hypokalemic alkalosis: bartter and Gitelman syndromes. J Pediatr 1992;120:38–43.

[164] Sutton RA, Mavichak V, Halabe A, Wilkins GE. Bartter's syndrome: evidence suggesting a distal tubular defect in a hypocalciuric variant of the syndrome. Miner Electrolyte Metab 1992;18:43–51.

[165] Gamba G, Miyanoshita A, Lombardi M, Lytton J, Lee WS, Hediger MA, et al. Molecular cloning, primary structure, and characterization of two members of the mammalian electroneutral sodium-(potassium)-chloride co-transporter family expressed in kidney. J Biol Chem 1994;269:17713–22.

[166] Gamba G, Saltzberg SN, Lombardi M, Miyanoshita A, Lytton J, Hediger MA, et al. Primary structure and functional expression of a cDNA encoding the thiazide-sensitive, electroneutral sodium-chloride co-transporter. Proc Natl Acad Sci USA 1993;90:2749–53.

[167] Simon DB, Nelson-Williams C, Bia MJ, Ellison D, Karet FE, Molina AM, et al. Gitelman's variant of Bartter's syndrome, inherited hypokalaemic alkalosis, is caused by mutations in the thiazide-sensitive Na-Cl co-transporter. Nat Genet 1996;12:24–30.

[168] Ji W, Foo JN, O'Roak BJ, Zhao H, Larson MG, Simon DB, et al. Rare independent mutations in renal salt handling genes contribute to blood pressure variation. Nat Genet 2008;40:592–9.

[169] Cruz DN, Shaer AJ, Bia MJ, Lifton RP, Simon DB. Gitelman's syndrome revisited: an evaluation of symptoms and health-related quality of life. Kidney Int 2001;59:710–7.

[170] Nijenhuis T, Vallon V, van der Kemp AW, Loffing J, Hoenderop JG, Bindels RJ. Enhanced passive Ca^{2+} reabsorption and reduced Mg^{2+} channel abundance explains thiazide-induced hypocalciuria and hypomagnesemia. J Clin Invest 2005;115:1651–8.

[171] Schlingmann KP, Weber S, Peters M, Niemann Nejsum L, Vitzthum H, Klingel K, et al. Hypomagnesemia with secondary hypocalcemia is caused by mutations in TRPM6, a new member of the TRPM gene family. Nat Genet 2002;31:166–70.

[172] Schultheis PJ, Lorenz JN, Meneton P, Nieman ML, Riddle TM, Flagella M, et al. Phenotype resembling Gitelman's syndrome in mice lacking the apical Na^+-Cl^- co-transporter of the distal convoluted tubule. J Biol Chem 1998;273:29150–5.

[173] Loffing J, Loffing-Cueni D, Hegyi I, Kaplan MR, Hebert SC, Le Hir M, et al. Thiazide treatment of rats provokes apoptosis in distal tubule cells. Kidney Int 1996;50:1180–90.

[174] Morris RG, Hoorn EJ, Knepper MA. Hypokalemia in a mouse model of Gitelman's syndrome. Am J Physiol Renal Physiol 2006;290:F1416–20.

[175] Scholl UI, Choi M, Liu T, Ramaekers VT, Hausler MG, Grimmer J, et al. Seizures, sensorineural deafness, ataxia, mental retardation, and electrolyte imbalance (SeSAME syndrome) caused by mutations in KCNJ10. Proc Natl Acad Sci USA 2009;106:5842–7.

[176] Bockenhauer D, Feather S, Stanescu HC, Bandulik S, Zdebik AA, Reichold M, et al. Epilepsy, ataxia, sensorineural deafness, tubulopathy, and KCNJ10 mutations. N Engl J Med 2009;360:1960–70.

[177] Djukic B, Casper KB, Philpot BD, Chin LS, McCarthy KD. Conditional knock-out of Kir4.1 leads to glial membrane depolarization, inhibition of potassium and glutamate uptake, and enhanced short-term synaptic potentiation. J Neurosci 2007;27:11354–65.

[178] Kofuji P, Ceelen P, Zahs KR, Surbeck LW, Lester HA, Newman EA. Genetic inactivation of an inwardly rectifying potassium channel (Kir4.1 subunit) in mice: phenotypic impact in retina. J Neurosci 2000;20:5733–40.

[179] Neusch C, Rozengurt N, Jacobs RE, Lester HA, Kofuji P. Kir4.1 potassium channel subunit is crucial for oligodendrocyte development and in vivo myelination. J Neurosci 2001;21:5429–38.

[180] Olsen ML, Sontheimer H. Functional implications for Kir4.1 channels in glial biology: from K^+ buffering to cell differentiation. J Neurochem 2008;107:589–601.

[181] Chever O, Djukic B, McCarthy KD, Amzica F. Implication of Kir4.1 channel in excess potassium clearance: an in vivo study on anesthetized glial-conditional Kir4.1 knock-out mice. J Neurosci 2010;30:15769–77.

[182] Rozengurt N, Lopez I, Chiu CS, Kofuji P, Lester HA, Neusch C. Time course of inner ear degeneration and deafness in mice lacking the Kir4.1 potassium channel subunit. Hear Res 2003;177:71–80.

[183] Koefoed-Johnsen V, Ussing HH. The nature of the frog skin potential. Acta Physiol Scand 1958;42:298–308.

[184] Reichold M, Zdebik AA, Lieberer E, Rapedius M, Schmidt K, Bandulik S, et al. KCNJ10 gene mutations causing EAST syndrome (epilepsy, ataxia, sensorineural deafness, and tubulopathy) disrupt channel function. Proc Natl Acad Sci USA 2010;107:14490–5.

[185] Freudenthal B, Kulaveerasingam D, Lingappa L, Shah MA, Brueton L, Wassmer E, et al. KCNJ10 mutations disrupt function in patients with EAST syndrome. Nephron Physiol 2011;119:40–8.

[186] Thompson DA, Feather S, Stanescu HC, Freudenthal B, Zdebik AA, Warth R, et al. Altered electroretinograms in patients with KCNJ10 mutations and EAST syndrome. J Physiol 2011;589:1681–9.

[187] Kearney PM, Whelton M, Reynolds K, Muntner P, Whelton PK, He J. Global burden of hypertension: analysis of worldwide data. Lancet 2005;365:217–23.

[188] WHO. Global health risks - mortality and burden of disease attributable to selected major risks. Geneva: WHO; 2009.

[189] Chobanian AV, Bakris GL, Black HR, Cushman WC, Green LA, Izzo Jr JL, et al. The seventh report of the joint national committee on prevention, detection, evaluation, and treatment of high blood pressure: the jnc 7 report. Jama 2003;289:2560–72.

[190] Feinleib M, Garrison RJ, Fabsitz R, Christian JC, Hrubec Z, Borhani NO, et al. The NHLBI twin study of cardiovascular disease risk factors: methodology and summary of results. Am J Epidemiol 1977;106:284–5.

[191] Longini Jr IM, Higgins MW, Hinton PC, Moll PP, Keller JB. Environmental and genetic sources of familial aggregation of blood pressure in Tecumseh, Michigan. Am J Epidemiol 1984;120:131–44.

[192] Kupper N, Willemsen G, Riese H, Posthuma D, Boomsma DI, de Geus EJ. Heritability of daytime ambulatory blood pressure in an extended twin design. Hypertension 2005;45:80–5.

[193] Newton-Cheh C, Johnson T, Gateva V, Tobin MD, Bochud M, Coin L, et al. Genome-wide association study identifies eight loci associated with blood pressure. Nat Genet 2009;41:666–76.

[194] Levy D, Ehret GB, Rice K, Verwoert GC, Launer LJ, Dehghan A, et al. Genome-wide association study of blood pressure and hypertension. Nat Genet 2009;41:677–87.

[195] Tennessen JA, Bigham AW, O'Connor TD, Fu W, Kenny EE, Gravel S, et al. Evolution and functional impact of rare coding variation from deep sequencing of human exomes. Science 2012;337:64–9.

[196] Sacks FM, Svetkey LP, Vollmer WM, Appel LJ, Bray GA, Harsha D, et al. Effects on blood pressure of reduced dietary

sodium and the dietary approaches to stop hypertension (dash) diet. Dash-sodium collaborative research group. N Engl J Med 2001;344:3—10.

[197] Cappuccio FP, MacGregor GA. Does potassium supplementation lower blood pressure? A meta-analysis of published trials. J Hypertens 1991;9:465—73.

[198] Whelton PK, He J, Cutler JA, Brancati FL, Appel LJ, Follmann D, et al. Effects of oral potassium on blood pressure. Meta-analysis of randomized controlled clinical trials. Jama 1997;277:1624—32.

[199] Geleijnse JM, Kok FJ, Grobbee DE. Blood pressure response to changes in sodium and potassium intake: a metaregression analysis of randomised trials. J Hum Hypertens 2003;17:471—80.

[200] He FJ, Marciniak M, Visagie E, Markandu ND, Anand V, Dalton RN, et al. Effect of modest salt reduction on blood pressure, urinary albumin, and pulse wave velocity in white, black, and Asian mild hypertensives. Hypertension 2009;54:482—8.

[201] Bibbins-Domingo K, Chertow GM, Coxson PG, Moran A, Lightwood JM, Pletcher MJ, et al. Projected effect of dietary salt reductions on future cardiovascular disease. N Engl J Med 2010;362:590—9.

[202] McGuire S. Institute of Medicine. Strategies to reduce sodium intake in the United States. Adv Nutr, 1. Washington, DC: The National Academies Press 2010;49—50.

[203] Kayikcioglu M, Tumuklu M, Ozkahya M, Ozdogan O, Asci G, Duman S, et al. The benefit of salt restriction in the treatment of end-stage renal disease by haemodialysis. Nephrol Dial Transplant 2009;24:956—62.

[204] Chazot C, Charra B, Laurent G, Didier C, Vo Van C, Terrat JC, et al. Interdialysis blood pressure control by long haemodialysis sessions. Nephrol Dial Transplant 1995;10:831—7.

[205] Culleton BF, Walsh M, Klarenbach SW, Mortis G, Scott-Douglas N, Quinn RR, et al. Effect of frequent nocturnal hemodialysis vs conventional hemodialysis on left ventricular mass and quality of life: a randomized controlled trial. Jama 2007;298:1291—9.

[206] Cruz DN, Simon DB, Nelson-Williams C, Farhi A, Finberg K, Burleson L, et al. Mutations in the Na-Cl co-transporter reduce blood pressure in humans. Hypertension 2001;37:1458—64.

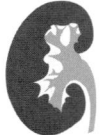

Natriuretic Hormones

David L. Vesely

University of South Florida Cardiac Hormone Center, and James A. Haley Veterans Medical Center,
Tampa, FL, USA

INTRODUCTION

Cardiac, Renal, Intestinal, and Adrenal Hormones which Enhance Sodium Excretion

Hormones which enhance sodium excretion, i.e., natriuretic peptide hormones, are very important for the maintenance of extracellu/lar fluid volume within a narrow range, despite wide variations in dietary sodium intake. This regulation occurs through a complex interplay of the antinatriuretic renin—angiotensin—aldosterone system and the antinatriuretic renal sympathetic system, which help to conserve sodium when sodium intake is low, and the natriuretic hormones, which enhance sodium excretion whenever sodium excess occurs. Several of the cardiac natriuretic hormones (Figure 37.1) directly inhibit aldosterone secretion[14,46,124,195,214,354,375] and/or indirectly inhibit aldosterone secretion by inhibiting renin release from the kidney to help regulate extracellular fluid volume.[39,104,149,197,214,404] This chapter will concentrate on the natriuretic hormones (cardiac, intestinal, renal, and adrenal) in normal renal physiology, their synthesis, secretion, biologic effects, pathophysiological changes with hypertension and renal diseases, and potential for treating diseases such as acute renal failure.

HISTORY OF ATRIAL (CARDIAC) NATRIURETIC PEPTIDE HORMONES

In 1628, Harvey[147] first correctly described the heart as a pump or a muscular organ that contracts in rhythm, pushing blood first to the lungs for oxygenation and then through the peripheral vascular system, bringing oxygen and nutrients to every cell in the body. It was another 350 years before the heart was established as an endocrine gland with its main physiologic targets being the kidney and vasculature.[366] The history of experimentation leading to defining the cardiac natriuretic peptide hormonal system (the first of the natriuretic hormonal systems) has followed two pathways: anatomical and physiological.

History of Cardiac Hormones: Anatomical Studies

Atrial Granule Structure

Shortly before Henry and colleagues[150] reported their observation that balloon distention of atria caused a diuresis, in 1955 Kisch,[188] utilizing electron microscopy, described dense granules that were located in the atria, but not in the ventricles of mammals. The presence of these dense granules in the cytoplasm of atrial cardiac myocytes, but not in the ventricles of the heart, was rapidly confirmed by others utilizing electron microscopy.[28,156,268] Jamieson and Palade[164] demonstrated that such granules are present in cardiocytes of the atria of all mammals, including humans, and were the first, in 1964, to suggest that these granules resemble other granules that release polypeptide hormones.[164] These granules are usually adjacent to one or occasionally both poles of the nucleus, and are interspersed among the voluminous elements of the Golgi complex and within close proximity to the mitochondria,[164] and are influenced by salt intake reduction.[218,269]

Ultrastructural cytochemistry has shown that these granules consist of proteins.[151] They incorporate both [^{3}H]-leucine and [^{3}H]-fructose in a pattern identical to other endocrine-secreting cells, with protein synthesis

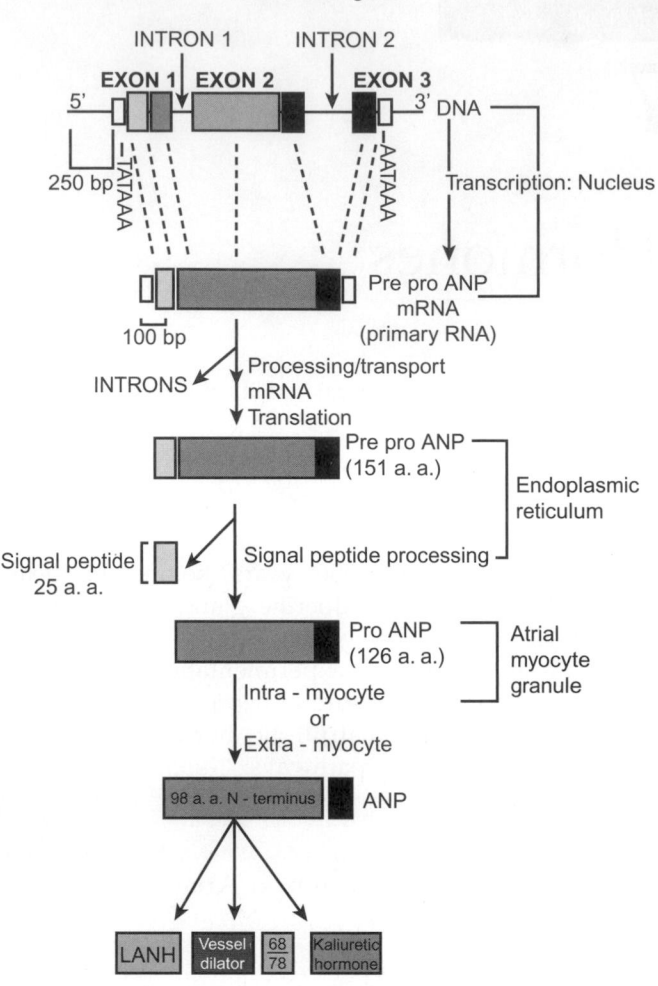

FIGURE 37.1   Structure of the atrial natriuretic peptide prohormone (proANP) gene. Four peptide hormones (e.g., atrial natriuretic peptide (ANP), long-acting natriuretic peptide (LANP), vessel dilator, and kaliuretic peptide) are synthesized by this gene. Each of these peptide hormones have biological effects, such as natriuresis and diuresis, mediated via the kidney[24,72,73,124,126,201,329,350,376,437] (a.a.: amino acids; LANH: long-acting natriuretic hormone (a different nomenclature for LANP). *(With permission, from ref. [366].)*

occurring in the Golgi complex.[155] The ultrastructural features of the specific granules of different species are similar, in that they display an amorphous core and a limiting membrane, and generally measure 300–500 nm.[68,70,164] The size and number of these granules vary among species, and generally are inversely related to size. Thus, atrial myocytes from large animals such as cows contain fewer and smaller granules than myocytes from small rodents such as rats.[70] In the rat there are up to 600 spherical, electron-opaque granules per cell.[70,164]

Atrial Extracts and Natriuresis

In 1922, Banting and Best[20] utilized what is now considered a classic endocrinological technique in their discovery of insulin. They pulverized pancreas with buffer, filtered the crude tissue extract, and found that it produced hypoglycemia in an experimental dog.[20] In 1981, deBold and colleagues,[69] utilizing a similar approach, infused the supernatants of extracts of rat cardiac atria and rat ventricles into other rats, and found that the rat atria extracts, but not the extracts from the rat ventricles, caused dramatic diuresis and natriuresis, with urine flow increasing 10-fold, and sodium and chloride excretion increasing 30-fold. This simple but elegant experiment led to the discovery of atrial peptides that have the most potent endogenous natriuretic activity of any substance yet described.[349] Atrial natriuretic peptide(s) isolated from these atrial extracts has been found to be a two-fold stronger natriuretic producing agent than furosemide (Lasix®), which is one of the most potent natriuretic producing drugs utilized in clinical medicine today.)[349] Other investigators quickly confirmed this natriuretic action,[110] as well as the ability of atrial extracts to cause vasodilation.[63,419] It was rapidly demonstrated that these effects were at least partially due to a peptide(s).[70,349] Further investigation revealed that the atrial extracts have significantly more natriuresis and diuresis than pure synthetic ANP, suggesting that other peptide hormones with natriuretic properties were in these atrial extracts.[75,123,140]

History of Cardiac Hormones: Physiological Studies

Association of Heart and Renal Function

In 1847, Harthshorne suggested that the heart possessed volume receptors capable of sensing the "fullness of bloodstream" induced by whole-body immersion, which he clearly recognized had a diuretic effect.[146] This observation received little further notice until 1935, when John Peters of Yale University made the same proposal that "the fullness of the bloodstream may provoke the diuretic response on the part of the kidney".[262] This concept then received experimental verification when it was shown that expansion of blood volume increases urine flow.[29,118,263,264,441] Peters also suggested that the diuretic response was secondary to the ability of the heart, or something very near the heart, to "sense the fullness of the bloodstream".[262]

Balloon Distention of Atria

Experimental evidence of an association between cardiac atria and renal function was provided in

1956 by Henry et al.,[150] who observed that balloon distention of the left atrium in anesthetized dogs was associated with an increase in urine flow. Because the renal response to left atrial distention could not be elicited after the cervical vagi had been cooled to block nerve conduction, Henry and colleagues[150,151] concluded that stretch receptors in the left atrium must be present. This finding was later extended to the right atrium.[117] In their reports, Henry et al.[150,151] noted the diuresis, but did not investigate whether it was associated with increased salt excretion (natriuresis). It is well-established now, however, that balloon distention of the cardiac atria causes natriuresis as well as diuresis.[121,123,213] Evidence that animals with denervated hearts or denervated kidneys may also respond to an atrial pressure increase to produce diuresis[209] suggests a hormonal pathway between the heart and the kidney. At least part of this hormonal pathway involves hormones made in the heart.

The "Third Factor"

With respect to a possible hormonal agent causing natriuresis and diuresis, de Wardener and colleagues[73] demonstrated in 1961 that saline infusion produced an increase in urine flow and sodium excretion in anesthetized dogs independent of changes in glomerular filtration rate (GFR), which was decreased, and even in the presence of high circulating levels of aldosterone. These experiments gave rise to the popular concept of an unidentified "third factor," a term coined by Levinsky and Lalone.[206] The other two factors were aldosterone and GFR-affected sodium excretion. The search for this third factor soon focused on a possible hormonal mediator that came to be known as "natriuretic hormone." Although this mediator (or mediators) from plasma or urine of volume-expanded humans or animals that causes natriuresis when injected into animals[37] was never chemically identified, the evidence points toward this third factor having a peptide structure(s), because acid hydrolysis characteristically inactivated this substance.[149] The "third factor" that was sought for decades now appears to be a family of peptide hormones termed "atrial natriuretic peptides" (ANPs), so named since they are found in their highest concentrations in the atria of the heart, have natriuretic properties, and are peptides. The third factor(s) also has the ability to inhibit Na^+,K^+-ATPase in the kidney.[149] Some of the natriuretic peptide hormones synthesized in the heart fill all of the criteria of being the "third factor(s)." Atrial natriuretic peptide (ANP) does not inhibit Na^+,K^+-ATPase,[51,139,270] so it would not fulfill the criteria of being the "third factor." Three of the other peptide hormones synthesized

by the ANP prohormone gene (Figure 37.1), namely long-acting natriuretic peptide, vessel dilator, and kaliuretic peptide, however, do inhibit renal Na^+, K^+-ATPase[51,139] and fill all of the criteria of being the "third factor(s)" that researchers have sought since the 1960s.

Family of Cardiac Natriuretic Peptide Hormones

At first it was thought that a single peptide was found in atrial extracts, but further investigation revealed a sophisticated endocrine system in the atria (and other tissues including the kidney) in which the atrial natriuretic peptide (ANP) prohormone gene synthesized four peptide hormones[23,368,369,370] (Figure 37.1), and two other genes were present, as reviewed below. The three other peptide hormones synthesized by the ANP prohormone gene — long-acting natriuretic peptide, vessel dilator, and kaliuretic peptide — were first demonstrated to have biologic effects in 1987,[389] and one of their mechanisms of action, via intracellular messenger cyclic GMP, was also elucidated in 1987.[373] Fifth and sixth members of the natriuretic peptide family were identified in 1988, i.e., brain natriuretic peptide (BNP) isolated from a porcine brain cDNA library,[332] and urodilatin, a peptide formed by differential processing of ANP prohormone in the kidney, which was first found in opossum urine.[205,240,315] A seventh member of this family was identified in 1990 in brain tissue and termed C-type natriuretic peptide (CNP).[333] A possible eighth member, DNP, was first described in 1992 from the venom of the green mamba snake.[316]

FAMILY OF CARDIAC NATRIURETIC HORMONES: SYNTHESIS OF THREE PROHORMONES

This family of cardiac peptide hormones has been designated atrial natriuretic peptides (ANPs), also known as atrial natriuretic hormones (ANHs). These peptide hormones are synthesized by three different genes,[94,116,205,216,240,290,426] and then stored as three different prohormones (126 amino acid (a.a.) ANP, 108 a. a. BNP, and 103 a.a. CNP prohormones).[205,366] In healthy adults, the main site of ANP prohormone synthesis is the atrial myocyte with its mRNA being 30−50-fold higher in the atria than that observed in the ventricle,[114] but it is also synthesized in a variety of other tissues including the kidney.[114,393] The different organs that synthesize the ANPs in the approximate order that they contribute to the synthesis of ANPs are listed in Table 37.1.

TABLE 37.1   Site of Synthesis, Molecular Weight, and Hemodynamic and Natriuretic Properties of Natriuretic Peptides

	Molecular Weight (kDa)	Site of Synthesis	MAP	Diuresis	Natriuresis
LANP	3508	Atria, ventricle, GI, lung, kidney, brain, adrenal	↓	↑	↑
Vessel dilator	3878	Atria, ventricle, GI, lung, kidney, brain, adrenal	↓	↑	↑
Kaliuretic peptide	2184	Atria, ventricle, GI, lung, brain, adrenal	↓	↑	—[a]
ANP	3078	Atria, ventricle, GI, lung, kidney, brain, adrenal	↓	↑	↑
Urodilatin	3503	Kidney	↓	↑	↑
BNP	3462	Atria, ventricle, brain, adrenal	↓	↑	↑
CNP	2198	Endothelium, CNS	↓	↑	—
DNP	4191	Atria, ventricle	↓	↑	↑
Adrenomedullin	6029	Adrenal, kidney	↓	↑	↑

[a]*No significant effect.*

Note: The sites of synthesis are listed in approximate order in which they contribute to synthesis.

ANP: atrial natriuretic peptide; BNP: brain natriuretic peptide; CNP: C-type natriuretic peptide; CNS: central nervous system; DNP: *Dendroaspis* natriuretic peptide; GI:, gastrointestinal tract; ANP: long-acting natriuretic peptide; MAP: mean arterial pressure.

(*With permission, from ref. [368].*)

CARDIAC PEPTIDE HORMONES ORIGINATING FROM ATRIAL NATRIURETIC PEPTIDE PROHORMONE

Within the 126 a.a. ANP prohormone encoded by a single gene are four peptide hormones (Figure 37.1) with blood pressure lowering, natriuretic, diuretic, and/or kaliuretic (i.e., potassium excreting) properties in both animals[24,77,78,140,141,220,389,405,433,434] and humans.[379–382] These peptide hormones, numbered by their a.a. sequences beginning at the N-terminal end of the ANP prohormone, consist of the first 30 a.a. of the prohormone (proANP 1–30, long-acting natriuretic peptide [LANP]); a.a. 31–67 (proANP 31–67, vessel dilator); a.a. 79–98 (proANP 79–98, kaliuretic peptide); and a.a. 99–126 (ANP) (Figure 37.1). These peptide hormones which were each discovered before BNP and CNP were named for their most prominent biologic effects rather than the tissue they were first found in, because these peptides are synthesized in many tissues.[114,369,393] Brain natriuretic peptide, so named because it was first found in porcine brain cDNA, for example, is actually present in the heart in 10-fold higher concentrations than in the brain.[52,140,212,344] Each of the four peptide hormones from the ANP prohormone circulate in healthy humans, with LANP and vessel dilator concentrations in plasma being 15–20-fold higher than ANP and 100-fold higher than BNP.[18,72,102,103,160,391,420,421]

BNP and CNP Prohormones

The BNP and CNP genes, on the other hand, appear to synthesize only one peptide hormone each within their respective prohormones, that is, BNP and

CNP.[22,93,116,199,200,428] The pro BNP gene and its regulation are reviewed in the section on BNP prohormone gene. The biologic effects of BNP and CNP are reviewed in sections on BNP, "Biologic Effects" and CNP, "Circulating Concentrations and Biologic Effects."

ORIGINATION OF PEPTIDE HORMONES FROM PROHORMONES

More than one peptide hormone originating from the same prohormone is common with respect to the synthesis of hormones.[366] Adrenocorticotropin (ACTH), for example, is derived from a prohormone that contains four known peptide hormones.[366] α-MSH, which has natriuretic properties,[157,158] originates from this same prohormone. ACTH, similar to vessel dilator, originates from the middle of its prohormone. The middle of their respective prohormones is the most common origin of hormones with calcitonin, glucagon, vasoactive intestinal peptide, gastrin, cholecystokinin, and substance P, as well as ACTH and vessel dilator.[366] Several hormones, such as vasopressin (antidiuretic hormone (ADH)), oxytocin, pancreatic polypeptide, angiotensin, and gastrin-releasing peptide, originate from the N-terminus of their respective prohormones,[366] as does long-acting natriuretic peptide (proANF 1–30). The origin of hormones from the C-terminus of their respective prohormones like ANP, BNP, and CNP is less common, with somatostatin, inhibin, and parathyroid hormone (PTH) being the only known C-terminal prohormone-derived peptides.[366] In the case of PTH, 84 of the 90 a.a. in its prohormone are considered to be the C-terminal "active" hormone; thus, it is not a small C-terminal-derived prohormone peptide, but rather nearly the intact PTH prohormone that serves as the actual peptide hormone.

MOLECULAR BIOLOGY OF THE CARDIAC NATRIURETIC HORMONAL SYSTEM

ProANP Gene

The gene encoding the synthesis of atrial natriuretic peptide prohormone (proANP) consists of three exon (coding) sequences separated by two intron (intervening) sequences which encode for a mature mRNA transcript approximately 900 bases long[135,171,172,244,251,275,321,440] (Figure 37.1). Translation of human ANP prohormone mRNA results in a 151 a. a. preprohormone.[135,244,251,321] Exon 1 encodes the 5'-untranslated region, the hydrophobic signal peptide (leader segment), and the first 16 a.a. of the ANP prohormone (first 16 a.a. of long-acting natriuretic peptide).[133,135,244,251,321] The signal peptide, which is important for the translocation of the precursor peptide from the ribosome into the rough endoplasmic reticulum,[244,249] is cleaved from the preprohormone (151 a.a.) in the endoplasmic reticulum (Figure 37.1). The resulting 126 a.a. prohormone is the storage form for the four atrial natriuretic peptide hormones in tissues and the major constituent of the atrial granules.[27,135,244,251] The first 16 a.a. of this prohormone encoded by exon 1 are, after proteolytic processing of the ANP prohormone, also the first 16 a.a. of long-acting natriuretic peptide (LANP) (Figure 37.1). Exon 3 encodes for the terminal tyrosine (a.a. 126 of the ANP prohormone) in humans, and terminal three a.a. (Try-Arg-Arg) in rat, rabbit, cow, and mouse.[133,135,244,251,321] Deletion of this terminal tyrosine residue encoded by exon 3 does slightly affect the binding of ANP, but does not appear to contribute to biologic activity, as there is no apparent decrease in biologic activity when this terminal tyrosine is not present.[313] Exon 2 encodes for the rest of the prohormone (a.a. 17–125 in humans).[135,244,251,321]

There is considerable homology in the proANP gene among species, particularly in the encoding and 5' flanking sequences.[93,251,406] The proANP gene has many features common to all eukaryotic genes,[27,33,242,276,382] including a TATTA box (T=thymine; A=adenine), intervening sequences bounded by GT-AG splicing signals (G=guanine), and a consensus sequence found in promoted regions. An interesting feature of the human proANP gene is a consensus sequence for a putative glucocorticoid hormone regulatory element in the second intron.[115,260,321]

The amino acid sequence of the whole ANP prohormone synthesized by the above gene is strikingly homologous among many species with differences clustered at the extreme carboxy terminal end of the prohormone, i.e., where ANP is formed.[15,120,148,173,175,183,202,216,242,244,251,252,406,450] In each species, the C-terminus is distinguished from the rest of the prohormone by forming a 17 a.a. ring structure via the joining by a disulfide bond between two cysteine residues (105 and 121 of the prohormone), as schematically shown in Figure 37.2. The ring structure originally was believed to be absolutely necessary for biologic activity,[64,152] but linear forms (same amino acids in linear form) without a ring structure have since been shown also to have biologic activity.[30] For full natriuretic and vasorelaxant activity, the Phe-Arg-Tyr (a.a. 124–126) at the COOH-terminus[64] and a.a. 99–104 of the NH2-terminus of ANP are necessary.[34] In the dog, it appears that deletion of a.a. 99–102 of prohormone does not affect natriuresis, but deletion of a.a. 103 and 104 decreases natriuretic activity 10-fold.[34] Twenty of 30 a.a. in long-acting natriuretic peptide (Figure 37.2) are exactly the same in the five above species, and another six of the remaining 10 amino acids are exactly the same in four out of the five species.[15,93,94,119,321] Only three a.a. (33, 42, and 43 of the prohormone) are not the same in vessel dilator (Figure 37.2) in the majority of the five species.[119,174,251,321,406] Kaliuretic peptide has a highly-conserved sequence among the aforementioned five species, with 16 of its 20 a.a. (Figure 37.2) being the same in all five.[15,93,94,119,174,321]

BNP

This extraordinary conservation among species of LANP, vessel dilator, and kaliuretic peptide is not observed in the BNP prohormone, where there is a marked difference in amino acid sequence homology among species.[93,113,199,290,332]

Tissue-Specific Expression of ProANP Gene

In healthy adult animals and humans, the atrial myocyte is the main site of the ANP prohormone synthesis, but it is also synthesized in a variety of other tissues.[114,128,129,271,273] ProANP gene expression is 30–50 times higher in the atria of the heart than in extraatrial tissues.[114] The expression of this gene has been found in kidney, gastrointestinal tract (antrum of stomach, small and large intestine), lung, aorta, central nervous system, anterior pituitary, and hypothalamus.[114,128,129,272,273] An example of where the

Natriuretic Peptides

LANP	Asn-Pro-Met-Tyr-Asn-Ala-Val-Ser-Asn-Ala-Asp-Leu-Met-Asp-Phe-Lys-Asn-Leu-Leu-Asp-His-Leu-Glu-Glu-Lys-Met-Pro-Leu-Glu-Asp
Vessel dilator	Glu-Val-Val-Pro-Pro-Gln-Val-Leu-Ser-Glu-Pro-Asn-Glu-Glu-Ala-Gly-Ala-Ala-Leu-Ser-Pro-Leu-Pro-Glu-Val-Pro-Pro-Trp-Thr-Gly-Glu-Val-Ser-Pro-Ala-Gln-Arg
Kaliuretic peptide	Ser-Ser-Asp-Arg-Ser-Ala-Leu-Leu-Lys-Ser-Lys-Leu-Arg-Ala-Leu-Leu-Thr-Ala-Pro-Arg
ANP	Ser-Leu-Arg-Arg-Ser-Ser-Cys-Phe-Gly-Gly-Arg-Met-Asp-Arg-Ile-Gly-Ala-Gln-Ser-Gly-Leu-Gly-Cys-Asn-Ser-Phe-Arg-Tyr
Urodilatin	Thr-Ala-Pro-Arg-Ser-Leu-Arg-Arg-Ser-Ser-Cys-Phe-Gly-Gly-Arg-Met-Asp-Arg-Ile-Gly-Ala-Gln-Ser-Gly-Leu-Gly-Cys-Asn-Ser-Phe-Arg-Tyr
BNP	Ser-Pro-Lys-Met-Val-Gln-Gly-Ser-Gly-Cys-Phe-Gly-Arg-Lys-Met-Asp-Arg-Ile-Ser-Ser-Ser-Ser-Gly-Leu-Gly-Cys-Lys-Val-Leu-Arg-Arg-His
CNP	Gly-Leu-Ser-Lys-Gly-Cys-Phe-Gly-Leu-Lys-Leu-Asp-Arg-Ile-Gly-Ser-Met-Ser-Gly-Leu-Gly-Cys
DNP	Glu-Val-Lys-Tyr-Asp-Pro-Cys-Phe-Gly-His-Lys-Ile-Asp-Arg-Ile-Asn-His-Val-Ser-Asn-Leu-Gly-Cys-Pro-Ser-Leu-Arg-Asp-Pro-Arg-Pro-Asn-Ala-Pro-Ser-Thr-Ser-Ala
Adrenomedullin	Tyr-Arg-Gln-Ser-Met-Asn-Asn-Phe-Gln-Gly-Leu-Arg-Ser-Phe-Gly-Cys-Arg-Phe-Gly-Thr-Cys-Thr-Val-Gln-Lys-Leu-Ala-His-Gln-Ile-Tyr-Gln-Phe-Thr-Asp-Lys-Asp-Lys-Asp-Asn-Val-Ala-Pro-Arg-Ser-Lys-Ile-Ser-Pro-Gln-Gly-Tyr

FIGURE 37.2   Amino acid sequences of the natriuretic peptides. Each of the sequences are human sequences except for *Dendroaspis* natriuretic peptide (DNP), whose sequence is only known in the snake. The brackets illustrate the location of cysteine bridges that help to form a ring structure in a number of these peptides (BNP: brain natriuretic peptide; CNP: C-type natriuretic peptide). *(With permission, from ref. [370].)*

proANP gene synthesized peptides localized in the kidney is illustrated in Figure 37.3.

Mechanisms of Action of Gene Products (i.e., Cardiac Hormones and Urodilatin) of ProANP Gene

Part of the intracellular mechanism of action(s) of the four peptide hormones encoded by the proANP gene is that after they bind to their specific receptors they enhance membrane-bound guanylyl cyclase to cause an increase in the intracellular messenger cyclic GMP[50,409,429](Figure 37.4). Cyclic GMP then stimulates a cyclic GMP-dependent, protein kinase that phosphorylates protein(s) in the cell, producing physiologic effects (Figure 37.4). Cyclic GMP mediates the vasodilation of each of the cardiac hormones.[250,373,419] The receptors for ANP that mediate ANPs biologic effects (e.g., ANP-A and -B receptors) are interesting, in that they contain guanylyl cyclase and a protein kinase in the receptors themselves[82,194,369](Figure 37.5). The NPR-A receptor has a 441 a.a. extracellular portion that binds ANP which, in turn, activates the catalytic portion of guanylyl cyclase in the cell (Figure 37.5). The protein kinase in this receptor has an inhibitory

influence on guanylyl cyclase until this receptor is activated by ANP or BNP.[82,369] There is a 21 a.a. portion of this receptor which attaches this receptor to the membrane (Figure 37.5). The natriuresis secondary to the ANP is thought to also be mediated by cyclic GMP.[34] Vessel dilator, LANP, and kaliuretic peptide's mechanisms of action of producing a natriuresis is via enhancing the synthesis of prostaglandin E_2, which in turn inhibits $Na^+ - K^+$-ATPase in the kidney,[51,139] which ANP does not do.[45,51,270] Vessel dilator and kaliuretic peptide's homodynamic effects via vasodilation of blood vessels are, however, mediated by cyclic GNP.

PROCESSING OF ATRIAL NATRIURETIC PEPTIDE PROHORMONE IN KIDNEY

ANP prohormone processing is different in the kidney compared to other tissues, resulting in an additional four a.a. added to the N-terminus of ANP (proANP 95–126, urodilatin (Figure 37.2)), a peptide first identified in opossum urine.[315] Thus, in the kidney, the identical four a.a. from the C-terminus of kaliuretic peptide are added to ANP to form the peptide urodilatin (Figure 37.2). At first, urodilatin was thought not to circulate,[231,315] and that it was not a

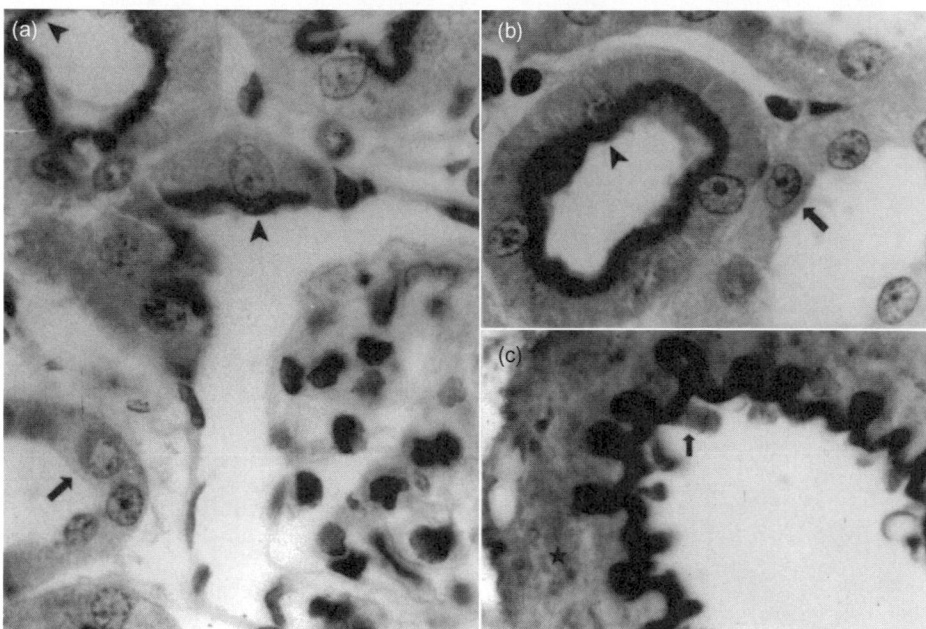

FIGURE 37.3 Vessel dilator immunoperoxidase staining in the rat kidney reveals strong staining of the sub-brush border of proximal convoluted tubules (arrowheads in a and b), including a proximal tubule in (a) originating directly from the top left portion of the glomerulus. The interstitial artery (c) had strong proANF (31–67) staining of the elastica with moderate staining of endothelial cells (arrow) and media (*). The distal tubules and collecting ducts (arrows in a and b) had weak staining with no demonstrable staining in some of the collecting ducts cells (Magnification×940). (*With permission, from ref. [281].*)

hormone. To be defined as a hormone, a given protein has to be synthesized in a tissue or organ, circulate in the bloodstream, and have biologic effects in another tissue or organ.[366] With a very sensitive radioimmunoassay, it appears that urodilatin does circulate, but in such low concentrations (9–12 pg/ml) that it may not be physiologically relevant.[392] Since urodilatin constitutes less than 1% of the circulating natriuretic hormones, its physiologic importance as a circulating hormone is very limited, with over 99% of the physiologic natriuretic effects being from the other natriuretic hormones. Urodilatin, however, may have paracrine functions, and may mediate the effects of one of the other natriuretic hormones (ANP).[392] Infusion of ANP increases the circulating concentration of urodilatin, suggesting that some ANP effects may be mediated by urodilatin.[392] Infusion of long-acting natriuretic peptide, vessel dilator, and kaliuretic peptide, on the other hand, do not affect the circulating concentration of urodilatin in healthy humans.[392]

REGULATION OF ATRIAL NATRIURETIC PEPTIDE PROHORMONE GENE

Enhancement of ProANP Gene Expression

Stretch

Mechanical stretch, or more specifically tension, delivered across the atrial wall is a potent activator of proANP gene expression and/or secretion.[74,76,408] In animals, an increase of sodium intake results in

an increased release of the ANP prohormone peptides.[78,80,403]

Thyroid Hormones

Thyroid hormones thyroxine (T_4) and triiodothyronine (T_3) increase proANP gene expression.[13,198] The increase in proANP mRNA in hypothyroidism when treated with thyroid hormone is paralleled by the increase in circulating concentrations of the gene products of this synthesis — vessel dilator, LANP, and ANP — in persons with hypothyroidism treated with thyroid hormone.[400]

The changes in proANP mRNA in both hypothyroidism and hyperthyroidism parallel very closely the circulating concentrations of vessel dilator, LANP, and ANP in humans, which are decreased in hypothyroidism and increased in hyperthyroidism.[400,438,439] When the hyperthyroid subjects were treated with the antithyroid drug propylthiouracil (PTU) the circulating concentrations of LANP, vessel dilator, and ANP decreased 50% after one week of treatment, with a simultaneous 50% decrease in serum triiodothyronine (T_3) levels.[400]

Glucocorticoids

Dexamethasone, at a dose of 1 mg/day, increases proANP mRNA levels in both atria and ventricles of the rat approximately two-fold.[115] There is negative feedback between cortisol and the gene products of proANP gene expression in that the cardiac hormones vessel dilator, LANP, kaliuretic hormone, and ANP decrease the circulating concentration of

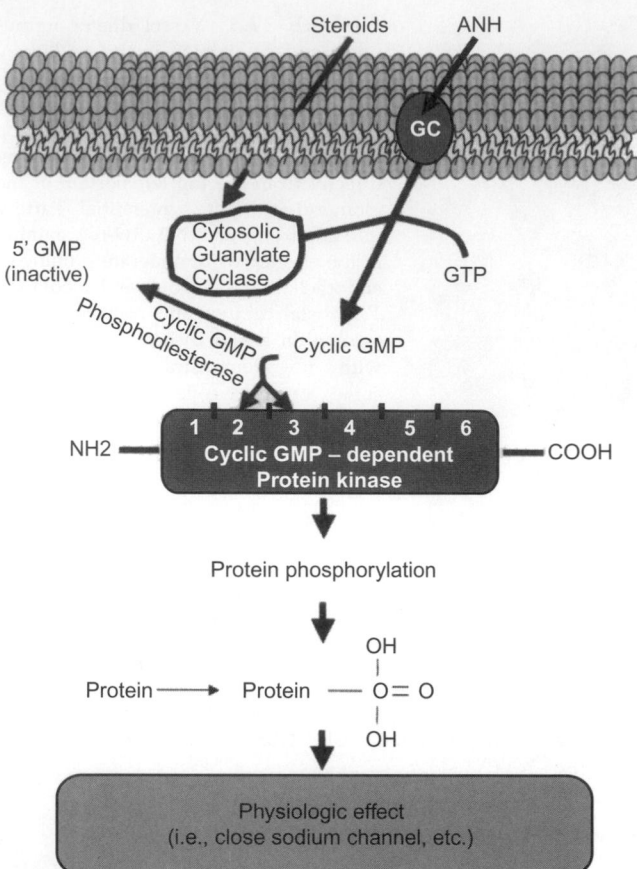

FIGURE 37.4 Atrial natriuretic hormone (ANH) stimulates a membrane-bound guanylate cyclase. Steroid hormones, on the other hand, diffuse through the cell to enhance the activity of a cytosolic guanylate cyclase. When either membrane-bound or soluble guanylate cyclase is activated, the intracellular messenger, cyclic 3'5'-guanosine monophosphate (cyclic GMP) is generated from guanosine triphosphate (GTP). Cyclic GMP then stimulates cyclic GMP-dependent protein kinase, which, in turn, phosphorylates proteins within the cell producing a biologic effect. Cyclic GMP is metabolized to an inactive 5'-GMP within the cell by cyclic GMP phosphodiesterase. *(With permission, from ref. [366].)*

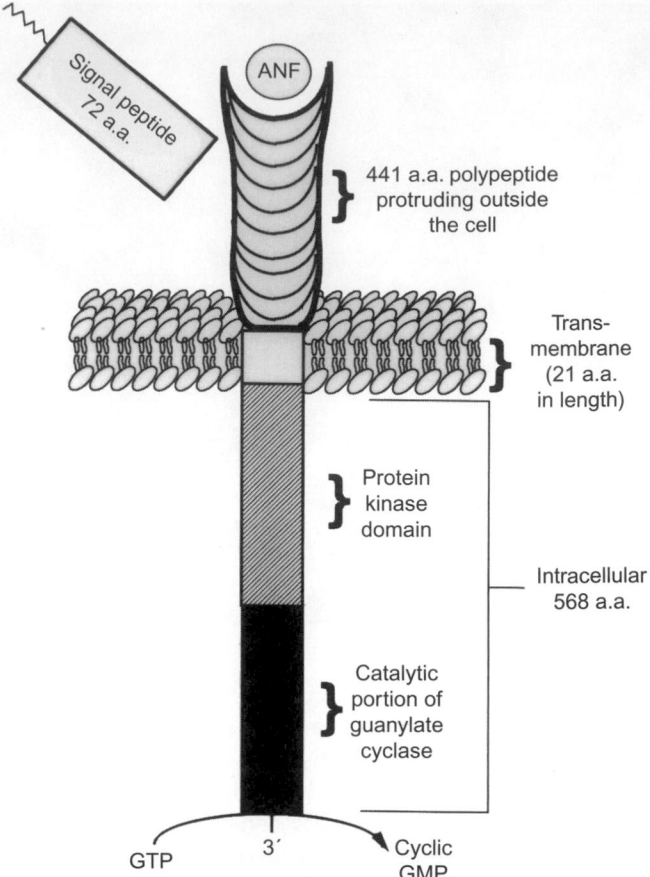

FIGURE 37.5 Structure of atrial natriuretic peptide (ANP or NPR)-A (active) receptor. The 441 amino acid (a.a.) extracellular portion of the receptor binds ANP, which activates the catalytic prrtion of guanylate cyclase within the cell. The protein kinase within this receptor has an inhibitory influence on guanylate cyclase until the receptor is activated by ANP. *(With permission, from ref. [366].)*

cortisol.[398] This decrease in cortisol is due, at least in part, to these cardiac hormones decreasing the circulating concentration of the hypothalamic peptide corticotrophin-releasing hormone (CRH), with a resultant decrease in ACTH, which stimulates the production of cortisol.[398]

Mineralocorticoids

Administration of mineralocorticoids to animals causes transient fluid and sodium retention. Despite continued administration of a mineralocorticoid, animals return to sodium balance within a few days, a phenomenon termed "mineralocorticoid escape." To investigate the role of ANP in mineralocorticoid

escape, Ballerman et al.[19] administered DOCA to rats in sodium balance, and found plasma ANP levels and atrial proANP mRNA content increased in rats retaining sodium in response to DOCA. After "escape" from the mineralocorticoid-induced sodium retention, plasma ANP levels returned to baseline and relative atrial proANP mRNA content remained moderately elevated.[19] This increase in proANP mRNA probably resulted from the secondary cardiovascular effects of the steroids (e.g., increased intravascular volume), rather than from a direct effect of the mineralocorticoids on the ANP-secreting cell, as DOCA has no direct effect on proANP mRNA in ANP-expressing neonatal cardiocytes.[113,115]

Vasoconstrictive Peptides

Several vasoconstrictive peptides, including endothelin, norepinephrine, and angiotensin II, stimulate proANP transcription and secretion.[290,294,295] The cardiac hormones, in turn, affect endothelin in a negative-feedback manner.[376]

Calcium

Primary cultures of neonatal rat cardiocytes exposed for 24 hours to 2 mM $CaCl_2$ in the culture media increase proANP messenger RNA three-fold, and increase secretion of ANP prohormone into the media three-fold.[201] When these cardiocytes were treated with the calcium channel-blocking agents diltiazem, nifedipine or verapamil, both proANP synthesis and secretion decreased to 25–40% of control values.[201]

TRANSGENIC KNOCKOUT AND/OR MICE OVEREXPRESSING ATRIAL NATRIURETIC PEPTIDE PROHORMONE GENE

Transgenic mice with an 11 base-pair deletion in exon 2 of the proANP gene (Figure 37.1) have increased blood pressure in homologous ($^{-/-}$) mice of 8–23 mmHg compared to wild-type ($^{+/+}$) mice.[168] Exon 2 of the proANP gene encodes for vessel dilator, kaliuretic peptide, and ANP (Figure 37.2). Exon 2 homozygote mutants have no circulating ANP, and they become hypertensive when fed a standard diet.[168] Heterozygotes ($^{+/-}$) with this base pair deletion in exon 2 are salt-sensitive and become hypertensive (systolic blood pressure increases 27 mmHg) on a high-salt (8%) diet.[168] Mice that overexpress the proANP gene, on the other hand, become hypotensive.[331]

HUMAN DISEASES WITH UPREGULATION OF ATRIAL NATRIURETIC PEPTIDE PROHORMONE GENE

Cerebrovascular Disease (Stroke and Hypertension)

A genetic linkage study followed 22,071 male physicians, all of whom had no history of stroke, from 1982 to 1999.[293] DNA extracted from peripheral white blood cells of those individuals who had a subsequent stroke revealed that, when compared to those without strokes, these individuals had a molecular variant in exon 1 of the proANP gene that was associated with a two-fold ($p < 0.01$) increased risk of stroke.[293] The individuals who had cerebrovascular accident (stroke) had significantly ($p < 0.001$) higher systolic and diastolic blood pressures than the persons who did not have a stroke.[293] This molecular variant of the proANP gene

was found to be an independent risk factor (in addition to hypertension) for a cerebrovascular accident. This molecular variant was found to be responsible for a valine-to-methionine transposition in long-acting natriuretic peptide (LANP), i.e., the only peptide hormone synthesized by exon 1.[366] (Exon 1 does not encode for ANP.) In the 16 a.a. of LANP encoded by exon 1 there is only one valine, which is at position 7 of LANP (Figure 37.2).[370] Residue #7 (amino acid #7 of the ANP prohormone) is highly-conserved among different species.[15,93,94,119,321] In this human study there was no defect in the structure or expression of the proBNP gene.[293] In humans, blood pressure and the cardiac hormones correlate throughout the 24-hour period in a circadian relationship.[329,330] There is evidence to suggest that long-acting natriuretic peptide reflects salt sensitivity in hypertension-prone individuals, even before they develop hypertension.[228]

LANP and Stroke

Long-acting natriuretic peptide (LANP) has potent vasodilatory properties in both animals[389] and humans.[381,382] Antisera to LANP (to block the biologic activity of this peptide hormone) results in a significant increase in mean arterial pressure from 112 ± 12 mmHg to 131 ± 9 mmHg in normotensive animals, and exacerbates hypertension in spontaneously hypertensive rats (SHR) from 140 ± 10 mmHg to 159 ± 9 mmHg.[79] These antisera data indicate an important physiological role for long-acting natriuretic peptide in the regulation of arterial pressure.[79] In the brain of stroke-prone rats, the expression ANP prohormone gene (which synthesizes LANP) is significantly reduced.[291] There were no mutations in the BNP gene, and no differences in BNP gene expression between stroke-prone and stroke-resistant animals.[291,292]

Further evidence of the importance of the peptide hormones synthesized by the ANP prohormone gene derives from studies in mice with the ANP prohormone gene knocked-out: all develop salt-sensitive hypertension within one week leading to stroke.[168] The BNP gene does not upregulate to prevent hypertension and/or stroke when the proANP gene is knocked-out.[168] Downregulation of the proANP gene in the brain in stroke-prone SHRs has further been found to co-segregate with the occurrence of early strokes in their F_2 descendants.[291]

Natriuretic Peptide Hormones and Hypertension

The original hypothesis for hypertension was that there was a defect in the production of the blood pressure-lowering cardiac hormones.[12,334] Experimental evidence revealed that, rather than being decreased, these blood pressure lowering cardiac hormones are elevated in the circulation in an apparent attempt to overcome the elevated blood pressure.[12,227,334,371] ANP increases in essential hypertension[12,334] and in persons with pheochromocytomas.[371] The hypertension associated with pheochromocytomas is characterized by increased circulating concentrations of vessel dilator and long-acting natriuretic peptide (LANP), as well as ANP.[372] Each of these blood pressure lowering hormones increase further with surgical manipulation-induced increases in blood pressure, and then these peptides return to normal after surgical removal of the pheochromocytomas and lowering of blood pressure.[371,372] The hypertension of obesity also is associated with increased circulating concentrations of ANP which decreases into the normal range with weight reduction-induced decrease in high blood pressure.[227]

In pregnancy, cardiac hormones increase in each trimester with the plasma volume expansion which accompanies a normal pregnancy.[229] ANP, vessel dilator, and LANP increase dramatically with the hypertension of pre-eclampsia, compared to their circulating concentrations in healthy pregnant women.[230] If one knocks-out the ANP prohormone gene that synthesizes the four cardiac hormones (Figure 37.1), within one week the animals develop salt-sensitive hypertension[168] while, on the other hand, transgenic mice overexpressing the ANP prohormone gene develop hypotension.[331] In addition to directly vasodilating vasculature, kaliuretic peptide and ANP inhibit the release of the potent vasoconstrictive peptide endothelin which is produced by the vascular endothelium.[376]

Congestive Heart Failure

In congestive heart failure (CHF), proANP gene expression is upregulated.[83,274,350] The increase in proANP gene expression is, however, not in the atria of the heart, but rather in the ventricle of the heart.[83,273,274,350] In persons with CHF, there is no defect in the production of the peptides from the ANP prohormone, but rather each are increased in the bloodstream in an attempt by the heart to overcome abnormal sodium and water retention by releasing more of these peptides that cause sodium and water excretion.[379,380,420] Vessel dilator and LANP increase in direct proportion to the severity of CHF, as classified by the New York Heart Association (NYHA).[420] The ANP-clearance receptor pathway is not linked to the avid sodium retention and/or to the renal ANP resistance observed in CHF.[32]

Cirrhosis with Ascites

Another salt- and water-retaining state, cirrhosis with ascites, is characterized by increased circulating concentration of the cardiac hormones, and with a 4.1-fold ventricular (but not atrial) increased steady-state proANP messenger RNA.[273] Although the liver expresses proANP messenger RNA, there is no upregulation of proANP gene expression in the liver when ascites develops.[272] Rather, the upregulation of this gene is only in the ventricle of the heart.[272]

LOCALIZATION OF ATRIAL NATRIURETIC PEPTIDE PROHORMONE GENE ON CHROMOSOMES

The proANP gene is located on the distal short arm of chromosome 1 in band 1P36 in humans and on chromosome 4 in mice.[366]

BRAIN NATRIURETIC PEPTIDE PROHORMONE GENE

The BNP gene is comprised of three exons separated by two introns, similar to the proANP gene in Figure 37.1.[113,345] Regulation of the BNP gene is controlled at the transcriptional level by several cis-acting regulatory elements in the proximal promoter, and the transcription factors that associate with them.[26,44,138,345] The cardiac specific transcription factor GATA 4 plays a major role directing basal activity of the BNP gene promoter.[44,138] GATA 4 is a nuclear mediator of mechanical stretch-activated BNP gene,[266] and might function as a central integrator of regulatory activity controlled by other transcription factors, such as GATA 6,[44] the neuron restricted silencer element-binding factor,[249] and YY1 the embryonic development protein.[26] Several of these factors interact synergistically with GATA 4, in both a physical and a functional sense, to stimulate BNP gene transcription.[44,249] Both the proANP and proBNP genes are activated in cardiac hypertrophy.[113,138] The GATA 4 transcription factor activates the proANP gene, as well as the proBNP gene.[113,138,266]

In healthy animals, cardiac BNP mRNA is mainly of atrial origin, that is, 10–50-fold more abundant than in ventricles.[52,140,212,344] In early left ventricular (LV) dysfunction, BNP mRNA markedly increases in the left atrium, but remains below or just barely at the level of detection in the ventricles.[212] The majority of investigations have found no increase in BNP mRNA in the ventricles in congestive heart failure,[140,212] which is exactly the opposite of ANP prohormone gene expression which increases in the ventricle but not in the atria in sodium and water-retaining states.[83,274,350] Likewise, with streptotocin-induced diabetes BNP mRNA doubles in atria, without any change in ventricular myocardium BNP mRNA.[52] BNP gene knockout mice do not develop hypertension or hypertrophy[343] as ANP prohormone knockout mice do.[168] BNP knockout mice exhibit cardiac fibrosis as the only known effect of the BNP gene being knocked-out.[343] These knockout studies suggest that regulation of blood pressure is contributed to by the cardiac hormones synthesized by the proANP gene, but not by BNP.

SECRETION OF CARDIAC NATRIURETIC PEPTIDES

The main physiological stimulus to secretion of these peptide hormones to control blood volume appears to be an increase in pressure in the atria.[74,76,264,294,295,408] An increase of 4 to 6 mmHg in the atria releases the four cardiac hormones from the ANP prohormone.[76] These peptide hormones, in turn, decrease the volume returning to the heart secondary to their causing a diuresis and natriuresis.[76,220,405] Rapid heart rates at 125 beats/min and higher release the cardiac hormones into the circulation.[247] Both atrial and ventricular arrhythmias with heart rates of 125 beats/min and higher release these peptide hormones and increase the circulating concentrations of these cardiac hormones in humans.[246] Hypoxia and a variety of humoral factors (endothelin, glucocorticoids, acetylcholine, adrenergic agonists) have been suggested as contributing to release, but the majority of these humoral factors' effects are to increase the ANP prohormone gene synthesis, as outlined previously, rather than release *per se*.[294,295] With respect to hyperosmolarity, the threshold for ANP release is as low as 10 mOsmol/kg H_2O and this is regulated by a crosstalk between sarcolemmal L-type Ca^2 channel and the sarcoplasmic Ca^2 release.[167] ANP, vessel dilator, LANP, and kaliuretic peptide have a feedback mechanism whereby they inhibit their own and each other's release.[381] CNP also inhibits ANP release.[203]

BIOLOGIC EFFECTS OF THE CARDIAC NATRIURETIC HORMONES AND THEIR MECHANISMS OF ACTION

ANP

Vasodilation

The original report by deBold et al.[69] where crude atrial extracts cause diuresis and natriuresis also indicated that these extracts could decrease mean arterial pressure. Crude atrial extracts were then shown to possess vasorelaxant activity in isolated aortic segments.[5,63,111] When synthetic ANP became available, it was demonstrated that the pure form of ANP could also cause vasodilation *in vitro*.[112,191,312,374,419] Both crude[5] and synthetic[107] ANP decrease total peripheral resistance. Large central arteries (aorta and renal) relax, whereas more distal (ear and basilar) arteries are refractory to nanomalor concentrations of ANP.[283,366] Pulmonary, femoral, and iliac arteries are intermediate in their response to ANP.[366] One exception to small arteries not responding well upon the addition of ANP is the carotid arteries, which respond well.[283] In general, veins do not appear to vasodilate with the addition of ANP as well as arteries do, but ANP has been shown to relax peripheral veins in addition to aortic rings.[312]

ANP produces a dose-dependent reduction in systemic blood pressure in humans.[413] The immediate blood pressure lowering of 5.5 mmHg in 2 minutes with 100 µg ANP intravenously has been associated with a sensation of facial flushing in four of six human subjects, suggesting acute vasodilation of skin.[366] ANP elicits greater blood pressure-lowering properties in spontaneously hypertensive rats than in normotensive rats.[366] A greater response in hypertensive versus normotensive subjects is also true for most, if not all, antihypertensive agents.

MECHANISM OF ANP-INDUCED VASODILATION

The vasodilation observed with ANP is endothelium-independent.[317,373,419] It is mediated by cyclic GMP, which is increased after enhancement of membrane-bound guanylyl cyclase by ANP.[250,373,419] Cyclic GMP itself has been demonstrated to cause vasodilation.[282,317,419] The vasorelaxation with ANP appears to be independent of calcium[373,419] and cyclic AMP, with no change in cyclic AMP occurring during the same period of time that cyclic GMP increases.[373,419] With respect to calcium, ANP can increase cyclic GMP and cause vasodilation with no calcium in the incubation media,[250,373,409,419] but possible shifts of calcium already in the vasculature are still being debated. The ANP-induced relaxation of contracted vasculature is not blocked by adrenergic antagonists,[111] cholinergic antagonists[111] or indomethacin,[111] the latter suggesting that this vasodilation is not mediated by prostaglandins.

Natriuresis

ANP-induced natriuresis[8,105,259,327] appears to have a dependence on renal vasodilation, since ligation of the renal artery eliminates ANP-induced natriuresis.[328]

ANP has been shown to directly increase renal blood flow in dogs.[39] Redistribution of renal blood flow to the proximal[144] and distal[181] tubules has been reported as contributing to the natriuretic effects. The proximal tubule contains guanylyl cyclase, and cyclic GMP produced by this enzyme increases amiloride-sensitive [22]Na uptake in the phosphorylated brush border membranes of the proximal tubule, suggesting that the ANP intracellular mediator, cyclic GMP, directly stimulates the Na—H antiporter in the proximal tubule.[134]

ANP and Site of Action in Kidney

The renal actions of ANP are complex. Hemodynamic effects of pharmacologic doses of exogenous ANP constrict efferent and dilate afferent arterioles[219]; the resultant increase in glomerular capillary hydrostatic pressure could increase the glomerular filtration rate (GFR).[56,105] Physiologic doses of ANP, however, do not increase GFR.[105,259,327] The circulating physiological concentration of ANP is below the concentration of ANP that has been found necessary to increase GFR.[259,327] Early micropuncture and microcatheterization studies suggested a late distal nephron site of action, but functional studies of ANP in the inner medullary collecting duct (IMCD) indicate that it is a major target site of ANP action in the tubule.[433,435] Binding studies indicated specific binding sites for ANP on IMCD cells.[366] ANP increases cGMP accumulation in isolated cells from this segment in a concentration-dependent manner.[433] ANP also inhibits oxygen consumption in IMCD cells, indicative of inhibition of sodium transport.[435] This inhibition occurs through a cGMP-mediated effect on an amiloride-sensitive sodium channel.[433,435]

A proximal tubular site of action has been suggested from studies showing that ANP inhibits angiotensin II-stimulated proximal sodium reabsorption at very low concentrations (as low as 10^{-12} mol/L).[109,145] In the cortical collecting ducts, ANP inhibits tubular water transport by antagonizing the action of vasopressin.[81] ANP has been localized by immunoperoxidase and immunofluorescence methods to the sub-brush border of the pars convuluta and pars recta proximal tubule, as well as the distal tubule.[281,297] These studies indicate that ANP may have widespread actions on tubular function.

ANP Inhibits the Renin—Aldosterone System

Atrial natriuretic peptide has been found to be a potent *in vivo* and *in vitro* inhibitor of aldosterone secretion via a direct effect on aldosterone secretion from the zona glomerular cells of adrenal cortex,[14,46,124,195,214,354,375] and indirectly through

inhibition of renin release from the juxtaglomerular cells of the kidney.[39,104,149,197,214,404] The mechanism of the inhibition of renin release by ANP appears to involve cyclic GMP, as this inhibition is duplicated by permeable analogs of cyclic GMP.[149,197]

Cardiac Peptide Hormones: LANP, Vessel Dilator, and Kaliuretic Peptide

Vasodilation

LANP, vessel dilator, and kaliuretic peptide cause vasodilation of vasculature that is endothelium-independent,[373] and similar to ANP endothelium-independent vasodilation of vasculature.[317,374,419] The amount of vasodilation *in vitro* with these cardiac peptide hormones is similar to that observed with addition of ANP.[373] When infused over 2 hours at the same 100 ng/kg of body weight/per minute concentration, vessel dilator and ANP were found to decrease blood pressure from an average of 145 to 124 mmHg ($p < 0.05$), and from 143 to 123 mmHg ($p < 0.05$), respectively.[220] Long-acting natriuretic peptide lowered blood pressure from a mean of 138 to 122 mmHg ($p < 0.05$), whereas kaliuretic peptide decreased blood pressure from a mean of 155 to 138 mmHg ($p < 0.05$).[220] Blood pressure did not change in the control animals throughout the 120-minute pre-experimental period or during the 120-minute experimental period.[220] Similar to ANP, the mechanism of vasodilating vasculature for these hormones is mediated by cyclic GMP.[373] The enhancement of guanylyl cyclase by the cardiac hormones is calcium-independent in vasculature.[373]

Cardiac Hormones: LANP, Vessel Dilator, and Kaliuretic Peptide

Natriuresis Mechanism of Action

Comparison of the relative natriuretic and diuretic potencies of the same dose in 100 ng/kg of body weight per minute of vessel dilator, revealed that LANP and ANP have significant natriuretic properties in healthy humans, but kaliuretic peptide enhancement of the urinary sodium excretion rate was not significant.[382] The natriuretic properties of vessel dilator are especially impressive in light of the fact that ANP has been found to be a more potent natriuretic and diuretic agent than furosemide,[349] and that vessel dilator has equally potent natriuretic effects[376,380,382] and circulates normally at a 17-fold higher concentration than ANP and 100-fold higher than BNP.[72,102,103,113,126,145,160,390,391,420] This 17-fold higher circulating concentration is found both during unstimulated conditions and with release secondary to physiological stimuli, such as head-out water immersion where the atria are stretched releasing these peptides.[390,391] Vessel dilator's biologic effects also last significantly longer than ANP (greater than 6 hours versus 30 minutes).[376,380,382] Vessel dilator and ANP, with nearly equal abilities to enhance sodium excretion, are markedly different, however, with respect to potassium excretion.[382] Vessel dilator is the only one of the four cardiac peptide hormones from the ANP prohormone that does not significantly enhance potassium excretion.[220,382] This potassium-sparing effect of vessel dilator makes it distinctly different from ANP, LANP, and kaliuretic peptide. Kaliuretic peptide does not significantly enhance the fractional excretion of sodium (FE_{Na}), but it is the only natriuretic peptide that significantly enhances the fractional excretion of potassium (FE_k) in healthy humans. (Fractional excretion of sodium or potassium is the percentage of glomerular-filtered sodium or potassium that is excreted into the urine.[382])

The natriuretic effects of long-acting natriuretic peptide, kaliuretic peptide, and vessel dilator have different mechanism(s) of action from ANP, in that they inhibit renal Na^+,K^+-ATPase secondary to their ability to enhance the synthesis of prostaglandin E_2,[51,139] which ANP does not do.[51,139,270] ANP, BNP, and CNP effects in the kidney are thought to be mediated by cyclic GMP.[34,140,294,368]

Cardiac Hormones: Localization within the Kidney

Immunohistochemical studies have localized vessel dilator (Figure 37.3) and long-acting natriuretic peptide as well as ANP to the sub-brush border of the pars convuluta and pars recta of the proximal tubules of animal[281] and human[297] kidneys. Immunofluorescent studies reveal that each of these peptides has a strong inclination for the perinuclear region in both the proximal and distal tubules.[281,297]

LANP, Vessel Dilator, and Kaliuretic Peptide: Renin–Aldosterone System

Kaliuretic hormone and long-acting natriuretic peptide (LANP) are potent inhibitors of the circulating concentrations of aldosterone in healthy humans.[375] Kaliuretic peptide and LANP effects on decreasing plasma aldosterone levels last for at least 3 hours after their infusions have stopped, while ANP no longer has any effect on plasma aldosterone concentrations within 30 minutes of infusion cessation.[375] Vessel dilator does not appear to have direct effects on aldosterone synthesis, but is a potent inhibitor (66%) of plasma renin activity.[404] Thus, the four cardiac hormones from the ANP prohormone gene act as endogenous antagonists

of the vasoconstrictor and salt-and-water-retaining systems (e.g., the renin—angiotensin—aldosterone system, vasopressin,[81] and endothelin[351,376]) in the body's defense against blood pressure elevation and plasma volume expansion via direct vasodilator, diuretic, and natriuretic properties. These four cardiac hormones' multiple biologic effects are illustrated in Figure 37.6. It is important to note in this illustration with respect to the kidney, that these peptide hormones also increase protein excretion (albumin, B2 microglobulin)[226,394,395] and phosphate reabsorption,[144] as well as cause a natriuresis and diuresis.

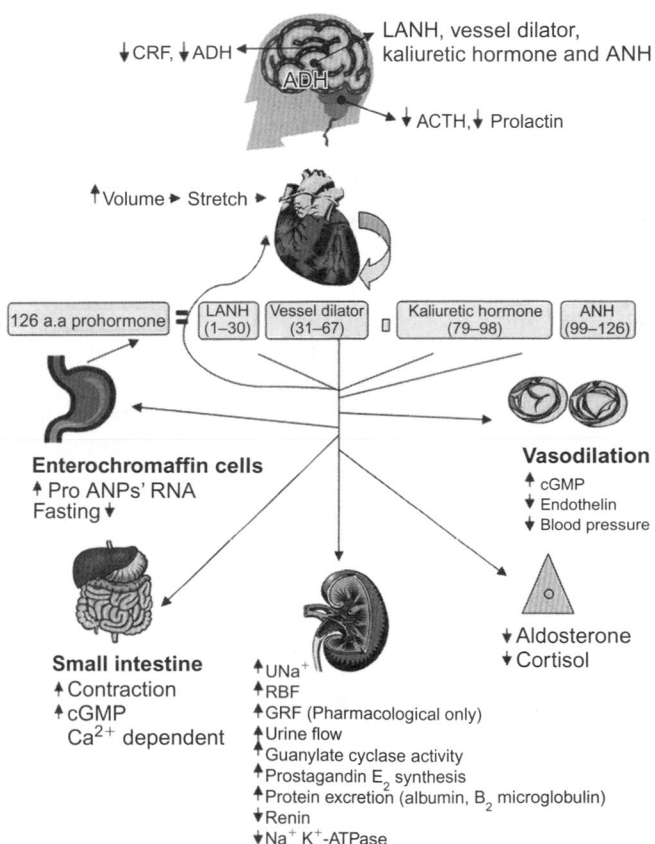

FIGURE 37.6 Long-acting natriuretic hormone (LANH or LANP), vessel dilator, kaliuretic hormone, and atrial natriuretic hormone (ANH or ANP) are released with increased volume, which causes stretching of the atrium of the heart. The biological effects of these peptide hormones include vasodilation mediated via enhancing guanylate cyclase activity with a resultant increase in the intracellular messenger cyclic GMP and inhibiting the vasoconstrictive peptide endothelin. ANPs cause a natriuresis mediated (except for ANH) by their enhancing the synthesis of prostaglandin E2, which, in turn, inhibits renal Na^+,K^+-ATPase. These peptide hormones also reduce circulating cortisol, aldosterone, and/or plasma renin activity. ANPs decrease corticotrophin-releasing factor (CRF) and antidiuretic hormone (ADH) from the hypothalamus as well as decrease the circulating concentration of adenocorticotropin (ACTH) and prolactin from the anterior pituitary. They increase protein excretion by the kidney.[394,395] (*With permission, from ref. [369].*)

Kidney Hormone: Urodilatin

Vasodilation

Urodilatin has vasodilatory effects similar to those of ANP.[309,315] This would be expected, since the ANP prohormone post-translational processing in the kidney results in an additional four a.a. from kaliuretic peptide being added to the N-terminus of ANP (proANP 95–126, urodilatin)[205,240,315] (Figure 37.2). The rest of the amino acids in urodilatin are identical, and in the same sequence as those in ANP (Figure 37.2). Urodilatin and ANP have identical ring structures formed with cysteine-to-cysteine bonding (Figure 37.2). The four a.a. added to form urodilatin are the same four a.a. present in the C-terminus of kaliuretic peptide in other tissues, but in the kidney the ANP prohormone is cleaved between a.a. 94 and 95 rather than between a.a. 98 and 99 to form urodilatin.[315] Urodilatin is not formed in the heart or in other tissues except the kidney.[205] Urodilatin at first was thought not to be a hormone, in that it was thought that it did not circulate,[315] but sensitive assays revealed that it circulates at very low concentrations (9–12 pg/ml).[392] Infusion of ANP increases the circulating concentration of urodilatin, suggesting that some ANP effects may be mediated by urodilatin.[392] Infusion of long-acting natriuretic peptide, vessel dilator, and kaliuretic peptide, on the other hand, do not affect the circulating concentration of urodilatin in healthy humans.[392]

Urodilatin: Natriuresis

Urodilatin has natriuretic and diuretic effects similar to ANP,[309] and since it has an identical amino acid sequence and ring structure as ANP one would expect it to bind to the same receptors and have similar biologic effects as ANP. It does bind to the same receptor and has similar biologic effects as ANP.

Localization of Urodilatin in Kidney

Immunohistochemical studies have localized urodilatin to the distal tubule with no evidence of urodilatin in the proximal tubule.[281] ANP messenger-RNA studies have confirmed that the ANP prohormone is synthesized in the kidney.[137] The amount of the ANP prohormone present in the kidney, however, is only 1/190th of that produced in the atria of the heart.[274] These studies taken together suggest that since urodilatin is found mainly in the distal nephron,[137,281,288] and since it is part of the ANP prohormone,[278,315,369] synthesis of the ANP prohormone may take place in the distal nephron.[137,281,288] The ANP prohormone gene is present and can be expressed in the kidney.[137,274] This gene is upregulated within the kidney in early renal failure in diabetic animals,[324] and in the remnant kidney of rats with 5/6 reduced renal mass.[347] Within the kidney, in addition to urodilatin, the ANP prohormone gene synthesizes LANP, vessel dilator, and a shortened form of kaliuretic peptide, but not ANP per se.[130,369]

Urodilatin and Renin–Aldosterone System

Urodilatin does not affect renin or aldosterone concentrations.[88]

BNP and CNP

BNP: Biologic Effects

Brain natriuretic peptide (BNP) is a 32 a.a. peptide in humans (45 a.a. in rat) with similar diuretic and natriuretic effects and a short half-life as ANP[332] (Figure 37.2). BNP half-life is 100-fold shorter than the half-lives of vessel dilator and LANP.[4,199,332,333,366] BNP has remarkable sequence homology to ANP with only four a.a. being different in the 17 a.a. ring structure formed by a disulfide bond common to both peptides[199,200,290,294,332] (Figure 37.2). Although BNP was named[332] for where it was first isolated (porcine brain), the main source of its synthesis and secretion is the heart (10-fold greater than brain)[65,140,199,205,294,344] (Table 37.1). As with ANP, the highest levels of BNP are found in the atria of the heart.[140,344] BNP levels in the atria, however, are less than 1% of ANP levels.[344] The immunoreactive level of BNP in the ventricles is only 1% of BNP concentration in the atria; in brief, 99% of BNP is found in the atria.[344] BNP, however, has been termed a "ventricular" peptide, based on ventricular BNP mRNA levels being similar to those in the atria with ventricles being much larger than the atria,[240] but as above, 99% of BNP is in the atria rather than the ventricles.[344]

The 108 a.a. BNP prohormone is processed in the heart to yield a biologic functioning BNP consisting of a.a. 77–108 of the BNP prohormone (in humans) and a biologically inactive N-terminus of the BNP prohormone (a.a. 1–76 of prohormone), both of which circulate.[199] BNP circulating concentration is less than 20% of ANP.[140] The sequence homology of BNP differs appreciably across species (both in size and a.a. sequence).[93,199,240,344] The major circulating form varies substantially among species, being 26, 45, and 32 a.a. in pig, rat, and human, respectively.[113,199] The marked sequence variability of BNP explains in part variations in its biologic activity in different species. The peptide hormones from the ANP prohormone, on the other hand, have remarkable homology across different species.[15,93,94,116,120,321] Mice overexpressing the BNP gene, where the circulating concentration of BNP is 10- to 100-fold higher than in healthy mice, have less glomerular hypertrophy and mesangial expansion with intraglomerular cells than healthy mice 16 weeks after both received renal ablation.[179] This mouse model of subtotal renal ablation, however, also has significantly increased ANP concentrations,[254,303,378] which may also have contributed to the effects attributed to BNP in the BNP-gene overexpressing mice.[179]

CNP: Circulating Concentrations and Biologic Effects

C-type natriuretic peptide (CNP) is a 22 a.a. peptide with remarkable similarity to ANP and BNP in its amino acid sequence, but lacks the carboxy-terminal tail of ANP and BNP[21,22,333] (Figure 37.2). CNP was found originally in the brain, but more recent studies suggest that it is also present in the heart[176] and kidney.[222,223,342] The amount of CNP in the heart, however, is very low and only small amounts are present in plasma.[176] Two CNP molecules, 22 and 53 a.a. in length, have been identified in plasma.[22,55] Each is derived from a single CNP prohormone, with the 22 a.a. form contained in the carboxy-terminal portion of the 53 a.a. form. The 22 a.a. form predominates in plasma, and is more potent than the 53 a.a. form in humans.[21,22,55,333] The plasma concentration of CNP is very low, with some authors reporting that CNP is not normally detectable but becomes detectable only in renal failure[304] and congestive heart failure.[176] CNP is present in the human kidney.[223,342] CNP has been found to have little effect on renal vasoconstriction.[430] Although CNP has been reported to have natriuretic effects in some animals, when infused in humans at physiological concentrations and in concentrations that reached four- to ten-fold above those observed in disease states, CNP did not affect renal function.[21] Thus, in healthy humans CNP had no effect on renal hemodynamics, systemic hemodynamics, intrarenal sodium handling, sodium excretion or plasma levels of renin and aldosterone.[21] Even when CNP was increased 60-fold in human plasma there were no significant hemodynamic or natriuretic effects.[159] The authors of this study concluded that it is unlikely that CNP has any endocrine role in circulatory physiology.[159] There is one study in humans where infusion of CNP to increase CNP plasma levels 550-fold above normal caused a 1.5-fold increase in urine volume and sodium excretion.[161] With this very high plasma concentration of CNP, both ANP and BNP also increased 2.4-fold,[161] which may have been the cause of the natriuresis and diuresis observed that was not observed in any other study with CNP.[21,159] Each of these studies suggests that CNP does not contribute physiologically to any natriuresis or diuresis in healthy humans.[21,159,161] The main site of CNP synthesis is vascular endothelium, and CNP acts as a paracrine endothelium-derived hyperpolarizing factor (EDHF) via activation of NPR-C

receptor and the opening of a G-protein-gated inwardly rectifying K channel (GIRK) in mesenteric resistance arteries to mediate vasodilation.[47] In conduit vessels, on the other hand, CNP induces relaxation via a cyclic GMP-dependent mechanism.[47]

Adrenal Natriuretic Peptides, Adrenomedullin and Proadrenomedullin N-Terminal 20 Peptide: Biologic Effects

Adrenomedullin (ADM), a 52 a.a. peptide with one intramolecular disulfide bond (Figure 37.2) originally isolated from an extract of a pheochromocytoma,[189] also has a range of biologic properties similar to the cardiac hormones, but these properties are less pronounced than those of the cardiac hormones[170,189,190,301] (Table 37.1). Infusion of ADM lowers blood pressure and produces diuresis and natriuresis.[170,189,301] Adrenomedullin causes a long-lasting hypotension accompanied by increased heart rate as a side-effect.[257] ANP, but not LANP, vessel dilator or kaliuretic hormone, increases the circulating concentration of adrenomedullin three- to four-fold, suggesting that some of the reported effects of ANP may be mediated via adrenomedullin.[374] However, the natriuresis and diuresis secondary to ANP were much larger than has ever been observed with adrenomedullin,[374] suggesting that ADM does not mediate all of the natriuretic and diuretic effects of ANP. Adrenomedullin is a larger peptide than any of the cardiac hormones, with its main site of synthesis being in the adrenal (Table 37.1), but isolated renal cells also have the ability to synthesize adrenomedullin secondary to stimulation by vasopressin via V2 receptors.[301,306] Since vasopressin (antidiuretic hormone, ADH) inhibits a diuresis these findings are opposed to findings that ADM causes a diuresis.[170,189,301] Adrenomedullin is part of a peptide family that shares structural similarity with calcitonin gene-related peptides and amylin, which share biologic effects and some cross-reactivity between receptors.[89,301,305] The adrenomedullin prohormone at its N-terminal end contains another biologically active peptide with vasodilating properties known as proadrenomedullin N-terminal 20 peptide (PAMP).[90,302] Whether more PAMP or adrenomedullin is produced depends on alternate splicing of its prohormone by the enzyme peptidylglycine C-amidating monooxygenase.[53,170,190,301,302] Adrenomedullin exerts its actions through G-protein-coupled membrane receptors linked to adenylyl cyclase, resulting in an increase in cellular cyclic AMP[301] as opposed to the cardiac hormones (ANP, BNP, LANP, vessel dilator, and kaliuretic peptide) whose second messenger is cyclic GMP.[373,409,419] Proadrenomedullin is thought not to act via either cyclic AMP or cyclic GMP, but rather via potassium channels, which eventually exert a presympathetic inhibition of sympathetic nerves innervating blood vessels.[302]

Dendroaspis Natriuretic Peptide: Biologic Effects

Dendroaspis natriuretic peptide (DNP) is the newest of the natriuretic peptides (Figure 37.2). This peptide was isolated from the venom of the green mamba snake *Dendroaspis angusticeps*.[316] This venom also contains several polypeptide toxins that block cholinergic receptors to cause paralysis.[316] DNP-like peptide has been reported to be present in human plasma and in heart atria.[310] In plasma, DNP concentration is very low at 6 pg/ml, which is 0.5% of the circulating cardiac hormones.[310] This peptide has a 17 a.a. disulfide ring structure similar to ANP, BNP, and CNP (Figure 37.2), and causes a natriuresis and diuresis in dogs.[210] Infusion of DNP does not cause any significant change in the circulating levels of ANP, BNP, or CNP.[210]

Richards et al.[286] have questioned whether DNP actually exists in humans and mammals, since it has not been characterized by high-pressure liquid chromatography linked to immunoassay, followed by purification and analysis to establish the human amino acid sequence, as has been done with the aforementioned cardiac hormones. The gene for DNP has not been cloned in the snake or in any mammal as has been done for each of the other natriuretic peptides.[286] Richards et al.[286] suggest that DNP may be "snake BNP," since BNP varies markedly in amino acid sequence among species (and the BNP sequence in this snake is unknown). The peptides from the ANP prohormone are markedly conserved among species,[15,93,94,116,119,321] and one would not suspect that DNP is one of these peptides as their amino acid sequences are markedly different from DNP. Further experimentation with the studies discussed previously suggested by Richards et al.[286] should give one more insight with respect to this peptide.

Guanylin, Lymphoguanylin, Renoguanylin, and Uroguanylin: Biologic Effects

Guanylin, a 15 a.a. peptide,[62] isolated from rat intestine, and uroguanylin, a 16 a.a. peptide originally isolated from opossum urine,[99,143] are peptides which are structurally and functionally similar to bacterial heat-stable enterotoxins produced by strains of pathogenic *Escherichia coli* intestinal bacteria.[82] Traveler's diarrhea is the result of these enterotoxins interacting with a membrane-bound guanylyl cyclase-C (GC-C receptor)

on the luminal surface of enterocytes.[82] The resulting increase in cyclic GMP phosphorylates the cystic fibrosis transmembrane conductance regulator (CFTR), leading to an efflux of chloride into the intestinal lumen.[287] Cyclic GMP in the intestine inhibits Na$^+$ absorption mediated by apical Na$^+$/H$^+$ exchange, and activates protein kinase G II.[326] Guanylin and uroguanylin, which have similar structures to this enterotoxin, have a similar mechanism of action in the intestine via the same GC-C receptor.[100,101] These peptides have been identified in the intestine in different locations, with guanylin in the colon but not the proximal intestine, and uroguanylin expressed in the proximal intestine but not in the colon.[91,97,99,142] These intestinal peptides have natriuretic properties.[62,99] The observation of renal expression of guanylin and uroguanylin mRNA[62,99] suggests renal synthesis and a local paracrine action of these peptides in a manner analogous to the ANP prohormone gene products. Wang et al.[412] showed that intravenous and intraluminal administration of uroguanylin in the kidney affects tubuloglomerular feedback, but it failed to cause a natriuresis and diuresis in rats at up to 100 nmol/kg/h intravenously, which was less than other supraphysiologic concentrations used previously[41,136] to cause a natriuresis. The uroguanylin dose used by Wang et al.[412] was still, however, a pharmacologic dose which resulted in higher uroguanylin concentrations in rat blood and urine than physiological concentrations which are in the femtomolar range.[106] Rats fed a high-salt diet had higher uroguanylin and cGMP concentrations in the urine; however, the plasma concentration of uroguanylin was not increased, which argues against uroguanylin being an endocrine hormone in the kidney.[106]

Renoguanylin is a peptide hormone similar to guanylin and uroguanylin that has, thus far, been only found in Japanese eels.[432] In the eel it has been proposed that renoguanylin may be involved in osmol regulation, but this has not been proven at present.[432] Renoguanylin was not as prominent in the kidney and intestine of the eel as guanylin and uroguanylin.[432] Renoguanylin has not been found in mammals or humans and may be unique to the Japanese eel and fish.[432] Lymphoguanylin is a 109 a.a polypeptide expressed in spleen and lymphoid tissues of opossum.[98] The 109 a.a polypeptide shares 84% and 40% of its residues with prouroguanylin and proguanylin, respectively.[98] Lymphoguanylin is less potent than uroguanylin or guanylin in intestinal bioassay, and has reduced efficacy for activation of OK-GC receptor in the kidney.[98] 100 μM of lymphoguanylin stimulates cGMP production in renal cells only five-fold, compared to 206-fold with uroguanylin and 88-fold with guanylin.[98] A serine-7 analog of lymphoguanylin has natriuretic properties in *ex vivo* rat kidneys and increases cyclic GMP 1000-fold more than the native lymphoguanylin.[96]

The inactive precursor of uroguanylin, i.e., prouroguanylin, is delivered to the kidney as an unprocessed propeptide,[277] and is processed to its active natriuretic form exclusively within the renal tubules.[277] The proximal convoluted tubule is thought to be the target for the uroguanylin natriuretic response.[87] Renal uroguanylin messenger RNA expression is also highest in proximal tubules, while guanylin is expressed mainly in the collecting ducts.[271] Salt-loading (1% NaCl in drinking water) for three days increases uroguanylin mRNA expression by 1.8-fold, but has no effect on guanylin expression.[271] The synthesis of these peptides by renal tubule epithelium may contribute to local control of renal function and adaptation to dietary salt.[271]

Both guanylin and uroguanylin elicit natriuretic responses from the kidney.[40,95,136] Both guanylin and uroguanylin exist in conformationally distinct A and B type topoisomers.[222,238,239] Topoisomer uroguanylin B has natriuretic activity in the kidney,[239] while the uroguanylin A in high concentration antagonizes the natriuretic action of the B form.[239] Uroguanylin knockout mice have an impaired ability to excrete an enteral load of NaCl, primarily due to an inappropriate increase in renal Na^+ reabsorption.[211] Further, there appears to be an interaction between guanylin, uroguanylin, and the cardiac hormone natriuretic peptide system, in that pretreatment with ANP (0.03 nM) enhances guanylin and uroguanylin's natriuretic activity when ANP is present in low dose.[304] When pharmacological doses of ANP or urodilatin are utilized they clearly inhibit uroguanylin-induced natriuresis.[304]

The GC-C receptor with which the heat-stable enterotoxin, uroguanylin, and guanylin interact in the intestine was cloned from intestinal cDNA libraries.[82] It exhibits 55% identity to NPR-A and NPR-B receptors in the catalytic region, 39% identity in the protein kinase domain, but only 10% identity in the extracellular region.[82] Within the kidneys, heat-stable enterotoxin, uroguanylin, and guanylin bind chiefly to apical membranes of proximal tubule cells,[91,100] also a site of CFTR expression.[60]

Two different guanylyl cyclase signaling receptors have been identified, one in kidney (OK-GC) and one in the intestine (GC-C), that are activated by the guanylin peptides.[101] Uroguanylin and guanylin regulate transport in mouse renal cortical collecting ducts independent of guanylyl cyclase C receptor,[325] and in guanylyl cyclase C-receptor deficient mice renal effects are retained,[325] strongly suggesting that GC-C is not the mediator of uroguanylin or guanylin effects in the kidney.

ANP Prohormone System and Expression in Gastrointestinal Tract

Almost 37 years ago it was noted that an oral load of sodium resulted in a natriuresis that was greater than the same amount of sodium chloride given intravenously, suggesting that the gastrointestinal tract monitors and responds to oral sodium-load.[204] Guanylin and uroguanylin may respond to this oral sodium-load in the colon and proximal intestine, respectively, but the stomach is an earlier monitor of this sodium-load. Immunoreactive cardiac hormones, ANP prohormone, and mRNA are present in the proximal stomach and antrum.[84,128,129,132] ANP prohormone gene expression and gene products LANP and ANP have been localized to the enterochromaffin cells in the lower portion of antropyloric glands of the stomach.[129] Fasting for 72 hours in adult rats results in a significant ($p < 0.05$) decrease in the levels of ANP prohormone messenger RNA, and a decrease in immunoreactive long-acting natriuretic peptide and ANP to <33% of that of fed rats.[129] In humans, food intake increases the excretion of LANP, vessel dilator, and ANP into the urine, suggesting an interaction between the cardiac hormones synthesized in the gastrointestinal tract and the kidneys.[384] A fluid load of Coca-Cola© rapidly (in 15 minutes) decreases the excretion of LANP, vessel dilator, and ANP into the urine, allowing more of these peptides which cause a diuresis to be present to respond to the fluid load.[384] In the stomach, cholinergic neurons inhibit, and pituitary adenylate cyclase-activating polypeptide neurons stimulate, ANP secretion, suggesting that there is also neuronal control of their secretion from the stomach.[127] ANPs are present not only in the stomach, but throughout the gastrointestinal tract (small intestine) and colon,[122,393,407] as opposed to guanylin and uroguanylin, which are present only in specific portions of the gastrointestinal tract.[91,97,99,142] Guanylyl cyclases A and B, which ANP, BNP, and CNP interact with, are present in the gastrointestinal tract,[280] as well as guanylyl cyclase-C which guanylin and uroguanylin enhance.[100] ANPs also appear to have effects within the gastrointestinal track itself.[17] ANP increases the spontaneous phasic contractions of longitudinal music two- to four-fold over a concentration range of 10 pm to 1000 mM, which was associated with a three-fold increase in cyclic GMP.[17] Vessel dilator and LANP also increase these spontaneous place contractions, which are additive with ANP.[17] The ANPs appear to act as neurotransmitters in the gastrointestinal tract to move water and feces through the gastrointestinal tract via increased force of contraction of the longitudinal muscles[17] until feces reaches the anal sphincter which ANP has been shown to relax to expel the contents of the gastrointestinal tract.[17,63]

Melanocyte-Stimulating Hormones

Melanocyte-stimulating hormones (MSHs) are small peptides of three different primary sequences (α-, β-, and γ-MSH), derived from the precursor prohormone pro-opiomelanocortin (POMC), which also gives rise to ACTH. Thus, MSHs, like ANPs, are from a prohormone containing four peptide hormones when proteolytically processed.[157,158] Each of the MSH peptides is natriuretic when infused in experimental animals.[49,157,158,253] The mechanisms of action of the MSHs are different from those of the cardiac hormones, in that MSH works via intracellular cyclic AMP rather than cyclic GMP.[388] The MSH-induced natriuresis does not appear to be a direct effect on the kidney, but rather via an interaction with renal nerves to inhibit sodium reabsorption, as prior renal denervation completely prevents the natriuresis secondary to MSH.[49]

Ouabain-Like Factors

Ouabain-like factors (factors that circulate and by definition inhibit Na^+,K^+-ATPase) have been sought for decades. Utilizing a very sensitive radioimmunoassay to ouabain, E. P. Gomez-Sanchez et al. determined that ouabain itself does not circulate in human or rat plasma, as a peak corresponding to ouabain was not found on high pressure liquid chromatography.[125] In most samples, they found only very low levels of an ouabain-like substance was present.[125] As outlined previously, vessel dilator, long-acting natriuretic peptide, and kaliuretic peptide are circulating peptide hormones[72,102,103,160,391,420,421] that inhibit the ouabain site on renal Na^+-K^+-ATPase.[51,139] ANP does not inhibit renal Na^+-K^+-ATPase,[51,139,270] and therefore would not be the "third factor" or an ouabain-like factor. Since the other three peptide hormones fulfill all the characteristic of the "third factor," they may actually be the "ouabain-like factors" that have been sought. Since LANP, vessel dilator, and kaliuretic peptide circulate at 100-fold higher levels than this substance, the volume-expanded substance(s) that do the majority of inhibiting of Na^+-K^+-ATPase at the ouabain site on the Na^+-K^+-ATPase are LANP, vessel dilator, and kaliuretic peptide, rather than some substance structurally similar to ouabain which, if it circulates, is present in extremely low levels in the circulation.[125]

NATRIURETIC PEPTIDE RECEPTORS A, B, AND C

Atrial natriuretic peptides, after moving via the circulation to their respective target tissues, mediate their action(s) at the cellular level by first binding to high-affinity specific receptors on the cell surface (Figure 37.4), which results in the intracellular generation of cyclic GMP via activation of the enzyme guanylyl cyclase which resides in the cytosolic domain of these membrane receptors as an integral part of these receptors.[50,82,194] Guanylyl cyclase (also termed guanylate cyclase) catalyzes the formation of the intracellular messenger cyclic 3′,5′-guanosine monophosphate (cyclic GMP).[373,409,419]

The area in the kidney with the most ANP-binding sites is the glomeruli, followed by proximal tubules and then inner medullary collecting ducts.[194] With respect to ANP, BNP, and CNP receptors, cDNA cloning has shown three types of natriuretic peptide receptors (NPR): NPR-A; NPR-B; and NPR-C.[50,82,194,199,240] Only NPR-A and NPR-B exhibit the intracellular guanylyl cyclase (GC) catalytic domain (Figure 37.4), whereas the third receptor, NPR-C, contains no guanylyl cyclase domain.[82,194,240] NPR-A and NPR-B, which bind ANP, BNP, and CNP, are structurally similar and contain a ligand-binding extracellular domain,[194] a protein kinase-like domain, and a guanylyl cyclase domain[50,82,194] (Figure 37.4). Upon ligand biding, a change in receptor conformation allows cytosolic factors to interact with the kinase-like domain, leading to activation of guanylyl cyclase and the consequent generation of cGMP, the second messenger of the cardiac hormones. The NPR-A receptor binds ANP, BNP, CNP, and urodilatin with a rank order of selectivity being ANP = urodilatin > BNP > CNP.[50,82,194,240] The order is reversed for NPR-B receptor (CNP >> ANP > BNP). NPR-B is structurally similar to the NPR-A receptor, with 74% homology at the cytoplasmic domain, but only 44% homology in the extracellular-binding domain, which may explain the difference in ligand specificities of the two guanylyl cyclase receptors.[50,194]

NPR-A mRNA is expressed mainly in the kidney, in the glomeruli, renal vasculature, proximal tubules, and in the IMCD.[19,50,194] The distribution of NPR-B overlaps to some extent with that of the NPR-A, and is found in the kidney, vasculature, and brain. In vascular endothelium and smooth muscle, NPR-B is more abundant than NPR-A. Compared to the NPR-A receptor, low levels of the NPR-B receptor are present in the kidney.[34,221]

Number of ANP Receptors per Cell

The number of ANP receptors per cell varies with the cell type.[19,71,152] Smooth muscle vasculature appears to be the target cell most richly endowed with ANP receptors.[152] The reported number of receptors in vascular smooth muscle cells has ranged from 18,400 binding sites per cell to 500,000.[366] Comparison of a variety of cultured cells revealed 310,000, 80,000, 50,000, 14,000, and 3,000 sites per cell for vascular smooth muscle, lung fibroblasts, adrenal cortex, aortic endothelial cells, and Leydig cells of the testis, respectively.[366] Twelve thousand ANP-binding sites per cell have been found in kidney glomerular mesangial cells; markedly less than in other vascular areas, but the receptors in the mesangial cells exhibited as high affinity as other vascular areas for ANP.[19]

Inverse Relationship of Change in Number of ANP Receptors with Circulating ANP Concentrations

The number of ANP receptors varies with fluid status, and inversely with the circulating ANP concentration.[366] Deprivation of water decreases the circulating ANP concentration and augments receptor number in both kidney and adrenal gland.[366] Rats fed a low-salt diet for 2 weeks exhibit "upregulation" of glomerular ANP receptor density, whereas animals fed a high-salt diet have a decreased receptor density.[366] The decrease in total ANP receptors, at least after salt-loading, is due exclusively to a decrease in the NPR-C receptor, rather than the NPR-A receptor.[366]

Structure of NPR-A Receptor

The structure of the NPR-A receptor is illustrated in Figure 37.5. This structure was elucidated using complimentary DNA (cDNA) encoding a 115 kDa human natriuretic peptide receptor (NPR)-active (A or functional) receptor that possesses guanylyl cyclase activity.[50,82,194] The NPRA receptor has 1029 a.a., a 32 a.a. signal sequence followed by at 441 a.a. extracellular domain (i.e., projecting from the cell).[50,82,194] This extracellular portion of the NPR-A receptor is 33% homologous to the 60 kDa NPR-C receptor.[82,194] This extracellular portion of the receptor is the binding site for ANP, BNP, and CNP. A 21 a.a. transmembrane portion of the receptor "anchors" the receptor to the membrane. Inside the cell (intracellular domain) there is a 568 a.a. cytoplasmic portion of the receptor with homology (23%) to the protein kinase family (protein kinase domain) being next to the membrane,[50,82,194] followed by a large guanylyl cyclase catalytic portion of the receptor (Figure 37.5) that is 42% homologous to cytoplasmic guanylyl cyclase.[50,82,194] The kinase domain binds ATP, but lacks true kinase activity. Rather, it functions to inhibit the guanylyl cyclase domain. If the kinase domain is "knocked-out,"

guanylyl cyclase continuously functions. The molecular weight of this receptor is 114,426.[50]

The guanylyl cyclase portion of human and rat NPR-A receptors are 90% identical throughout their sequences.[50,82] The similar amino acid sequence between the NPR-C receptor[82,194,240] and the extracellular portion of the NPR-A receptor reflect a common function shared between them — they both bind ANP, BNP, and CNP.

NPR-C (Clearance) Receptor

Cross-linking studies revealed that in addition to the high molecular weight receptors for ANP, BNP, and CNP there was also a low molecular weight 60 kDa receptor that appeared to be a subunit of the high molecular weight receptor.[82,194,240] This 60 kDa receptor was found not to contain guanylyl cyclase or to mediate any of the known effects of ANP, such as natriuresis or diuresis.[82,194,215]

Structure of NPR Clearance Receptor

The NPR-C receptor is similar structurally outside the cell to the NPR-A receptor, with 496 a.a. compared to the 441 a.a. projecting from the cell for the NPR-A receptor.[82,194,215] They have a similar single short transmembrane-spanning region, but where the two receptors markedly differ is inside the cell. The NPR-C receptor has only a very short 37 a.a. tail into the cytoplasm of the cell as compared to the large 568 a.a. portion in the cell for the NPR-A receptor.[50,82,194,215] Neither the protein kinase domain nor the guanylyl cyclase catalytic site is present in the NPR-C receptor. That the NPR-C receptor is not linked to a second messenger system explains its inability to cause vasodilation, diuresis or natriuresis.[50,82,194,215] The order of binding to the NPR-C receptor is ANP > CNP > BNP. The NPR-C receptor is the most abundant receptor of the natriuretic receptors, accounting for more than 95% of the total receptor population, and is located at high density in kidney, vascular endothelium, smooth muscle cells, and the heart.[82,194,215]

Vessel Dilator and LANP Receptors

Vessel dilator and long-acting natriuretic peptide do not bind to the NPR-A, B or C receptors, but rather have their own specific receptors.[365,372,378,397] Vessel dilator, LANP, and kaliuretic peptide, on the other hand, are linear peptide hormones, and one would not expect binding to the above NPR-A, -B, and -C receptors which require a ring structure for binding[50,82,194,215,240] which ANP, BNP, and CNP have.[372,378]

LANP Receptor

Long-acting natriuretic peptide (LANP), as well as ANP, binds specifically to smooth muscle membranes,[378] placental membranes,[365] distal nephrons,[397] proximal tubules,[397] and renal cortical and medullary membranes.[397] ANP and vessel dilator inhibit ^{125}I-labeled LANP-binding somewhat at concentrations above which these peptide hormones are known to circulate, i.e., 10^{-6} M for ANP and 10^{-7} M for vessel dilator. Scatchard analysis of the LANP-binding data resulted in a straight line,[378] suggesting that these smooth muscle cells contain a single class of high-affinity binding sites for LANP with an equilibrium dissociation constant (K_d) of 0.11 nM. The binding capacity (maximal binding, B_{max}) for LANP was 2.57 fmol/10^6 cells, and the number of binding sites was calculated to be 1548 per cell.[378]

Vessel Dilator Receptor

Vessel dilator also binds specifically to smooth muscle membranes,[378] proximal tubules,[397] distal nephrons,[397] placental membranes,[365] and renal cortical and medullary membranes[397] at a site distinct from the binding of ANP to membranes. The binding of this peptide hormone could be inhibited by concentrations (10^{-4} to 10^{-7} M) of ANP, LANP, insulin, and ACTH, which are far in excess of their respective circulating concentrations.[378] Scatchard analysis of the vessel dilator-binding data resulted in a straight line,[378] suggesting that smooth muscles contain a single class of high-affinity binding sites for vessel dilator with an equilibrium dissociation constant (K_d) of 4 nM. B_{max} for vessel dilator was 59.9 fmol/10^6 cells, and the number of binding sites was calculated to be 36,087 per cell.[378]

DEGRADATION OF NATRIURETIC PEPTIDES BY KIDNEY

The inactivation of the ANP, BNP, and CNP occurs via two pathways: binding to clearance receptors and enzymatic degradation. The clearance receptor (NPR-C)[32,50,82,194,240] clears ANP, BNP, and CNP through receptor-mediated uptake, internalization, and lysosomal hydrolysis with rapid and efficient recycling of internalized receptors to the cell surface. Enzymatic degradation of ANP, BNP, and CNP takes place in the lung, liver, and kidney, and the main enzyme responsible for this degradation is neutral endopeptidase (NEP-24.11).[34,411] NEP, originally referred to as enkephalinase because of its ability to degrade opioid peptides in the brain, was subsequently shown to be identical to a well-characterized zinc metallopeptidase present in the kidney.[411] This zinc metalloproteinase

hydrolyzes internal peptide bonds of polypeptides, rather than those adjacent to their N- or C-terminal ends. NEP has a ubiquitous tissue distribution and multiple functions, sharing structural similarities with various metallopeptidases, including aminopeptidase ACE, and carboxypeptidases A, B, and E.[411] NEP is most abundant in the brush borders of the proximal tubules of the kidney, where it rapidly degrades filtered ANP, thus preventing ANP from reaching more distal luminal receptors.[411] In the case of ANP, NEP-24.11 cleaves the Cys[105]–Phe[106] bond to disrupt the ring structure and inactivate the peptide. NEP 24.11 is a nonspecific enzyme that also cleaves enkephalins, endothelin, substance P, kinins, neurotensin, insulin B chain, angiotensin, calcitonin gene-related peptide, and adrenomedullin, as well as ANP, BNP, and CNP. With respect to ANPs in humans,[411] ANP and CNP are preferred substrates for NEP as opposed to BNP with the Cys–Phe bond of human BNP being relatively insensitive to enzymatic cleavage.[411]

INFLUENCE OF ACUTE RENAL FAILURE ON CIRCULATING CONCENTRATION OF CARDIAC HORMONES

Each of the cardiac hormones from the ANP prohormone (vessel dilator, ANP, LANP, and kaliuretic peptide),[12,18,48,56,103,160,193,243,300,395,396,420,421] BNP,[39,43,58,108,199,200] and CNP[22,159,161,348] increase in the circulation (mainly from the heart ventricle[83,115,271]) in salt- and water-retaining states such as renal failure and congestive heart failure, compared to their concentrations in healthy individuals, in an apparent attempt to overcome the salt and water retention via their natriuretic and diuretic properties.[379,380] The disease state associated with the highest circulating concentrations of the cardiac natriuretic peptides is renal failure.[102,103,307,417,421] One would suspect that cardiac natriuretic peptides are higher in renal failure versus Class IV New York Heart Association congestive heart failure patients, because of the added pathophysiology of decreased degradation of these peptides with the decreased functioning renal parenchyma.[421] Franz et al.,[103] however, have shown that there is an increased excretion of the cardiac natriuretic peptides in renal failure, and that the increase in vessel dilator excretion occurs even before serum creatinine levels begin to rise. The circulating concentrations of the cardiac hormones in chronic renal failure appear to reflect volume status.[193,236,284,422] Despite increased circulating concentrations of cardiac hormones in sodium-retaining disease states, the kidney retains sodium and is hyporesponsive to ANP, LANP, and BNP.[35,199,277,352,379] The mechanism for the attenuated renal response to these natriuretic peptides is multifactoral and includes renal hypoperfusion, activation of the renin–angiotensin–aldosterone and the sympathetic nervous systems.[34,140,235]

Influence of Renal Failure on other Natriuretic Peptides

Adrenomedullin,[90,305,346] guanylin,[187] and uroguanylin[185,186] increase in renal failure and/or experimental nephrotic syndrome.

HEMODIALYSIS

Cardiac Hormones Synthesized by ANP Prohormone Gene

The circulating concentrations of the cardiac hormones have been suggested as possible indicators of when to perform dialysis in persons with chronic renal failure.[193,236,284,307,422] Other data, however, suggest that ANPs are not useful to predict when hemodialysis is necessary.[29] Hemodialysis lowers the circulating concentration of cardiac hormones by 34%–42%, with the amount of decrease appearing to be related to volume status of the patients.[193,417,422] Hemodialysis does not return the levels of ANP to those of healthy adults,[193,416,417,422] and it does not reduce circulating concentrations of vessel dilator and LANP.[422] Part of the reason for the difference in hemodialysis effects on the cardiac hormones is that less than 1.5% of vessel dilator and LANP cross the dialysis membrane, compared to 15% to 25% of ANP crossing hemodialysis membranes.[422] Hemodialysis using cellulose-triacetate dialyzers reduces plasma levels of these peptides in acute renal failure more than hemodialysis therapy with polysulfone dialyzers.[102]

BNP

Hemodialysis has been reported both to lower,[200] and to have no effect on circulating BNP levels.[49] Before dialysis in persons with chronic renal failure (CRF), plasma BNP levels have no relationship to serum creatinine or mean blood pressure.[192] In CRF patients whose plasma BNP levels decrease with dialysis, this decrease correlates with the degree of postural blood pressure drop, but there is no correlation with the fall in serum creatinine.[200] In none of the studies of BNP and dialysis[39,58,192,200] has BNP ever returned its circulating concentration to that of healthy individuals. With volume repletion after hemodialysis there is an exaggerated release of ANP, but changes in BNP are small and without any correlation with either atrial or ventricular volume.[58]

Adrenomedullin and Proadrenomedullin N-Terminal 20 Peptide

Both adrenomedullin and proadrenomedullin N-terminal 20 peptide (PAMP) increase in chronic renal failure.[90,305,346] Hemodialysis decreases these peptides to near-control levels, with PAMP being 2.17 ± 0.18 fmol/ml versus 1.64 ± 0.12 fmol/ml for controls.[346]

Guanylin and Uroguanylin

Both guanylin and uroguanylin are increased in persons with impaired renal function.[168,169] Hemodialysis with EVAL membranes decreases guanylin concentrations after one hour of dialysis, but the plasma levels after hemodialysis with PC membranes show no change.[187]

RENAL TRANSPLANTATION

Successful transplantation of functioning kidneys decreases the markedly elevated circulating levels of cardiac hormones in persons with acute renal failure to those of healthy individuals.[265,279] Nonfunctioning renal allografts continue to have elevated circulating concentrations of the cardiac hormones.[265,279] Post renal transplant, it takes seven days for ANP and 10 days for vessel dilator to return to normal.[265] This suggests that the allograft kidney does not fully function immediately with respect to clearing these peptides. The half-life of ANP in healthy persons is only 2.5–3.5 minutes.[4,366] If the transplanted kidneys began to function immediately, one would have expected the circulating concentration of ANP to have decreased to the normal range within 24 hours (360 half-lives). Vessel dilator has a 20-fold longer half-life compared to that of ANP,[4,366] which may explain why it takes three more days for this peptide hormone to normalize in the circulation after successful renal transplantation. If one gives ANP (via infusion) at the time of renal transplant, this does not appear to have any beneficial effect on the outcome of the renal allograft.[303] It is important to note that the elevated circulating cardiac hormones in heart failure also normalize with successful heart transplantation.[416]

ATRIAL NATRIURETIC PEPTIDE PROHORMONE GENE EXPRESSION IN INVERTEBRATES AND PLANTS

In addition to proANP gene being present in mammals and vertebrates, where lower vertebrates such as the frog have an identical proANP gene,[296] blue crabs and oysters have been demonstrated to have the proANP gene in their hearts.[273,367] The proANP gene in oysters and blue crabs can be upregulated by increasing salinity in the external environment, such as when the animal moves from freshwater to seawater.[273,402] This change in environmental salinity also modulates end-product concentrations of this gene expression, that is, the cardiac hormones.[256] Environmental salinity also modulates ANP in the teleost fish *Gila atraria*.[415] Seawater trout have higher concentrations of ANP, vessel dilator, and LANP than freshwater trout to help them maintain volume homeostasis in a higher salt environment.[59] Even the most primitive heart in the animal kingdom contains the atrial natriuretic peptide hormonal system.[386] Diving is a modulator of ANP in lower animals, with diving increasing ANP in freshwater diving turtles[16] similar to whole body immersion in humans.[390,391,396]

Although a gene in the animal kingdom expressing a peptide hormonal system in plants had never been demonstrated previously, there is now evidence for a proANP-like gene in plants.[401] Southern blots of English ivy (*Hedera helix*) genomic DNA revealed that the proANP gene sequence was present in its roots, stems, and leaves.[401] In plants, ANPs enhance the flow of water up stems to flowers and leaves, a process that is at least partially due to increasing the rate of transpiration (loss of water from the leaves) via opening the stomatal pores in leaves.[367,387] These peptides are present even in *Euglena*, a single-cell, flagellated, chlorophyll-containing plant without leaves, stems or roots.[387] The oldest existing trees on Earth, the *Metasequoia*, which exist only in China, contain the ANP prohormone and ANP.[427] These peptide hormones are also found in single-cell animals, such as paramecium.[385] In single cell organisms, these peptides appear to help maintain the internal volume of the cell.[385] The demonstration of the proANP gene sequences and expression of the ANP-like gene in plants suggests that plants and animals may have evolved much more similarly than previously thought.[387]

PROTECTIVE AND THERAPEUTIC EFFECTS OF CARDIAC AND RENAL HORMONES IN ACUTE RENAL FAILURE

ANP and Urodilatin

Animals

Acute renal failure (ARF) develops in 2–5% of all patients admitted to tertiary care hospitals.[154,423] The underlying cause is a renal insult (acute tubular necrosis) in 60% of patients.[154,423] When dialysis was

introduced in the mid-1940s, the mortality resulting from severe ARF was approximately 50%.[154] This poor prognosis has not improved, with mortality now in the 40–80% range in oliguric ARF.[9,31,66,153,154,308,423] The occurrence of ARF in the hospital increases the relative risk of dying by 6.2-fold, and the length of hospitalization by 10 days.[277]

Several of the cardiac hormones have been investigated as possible treatment(s) for ARF. Atrial natriuretic peptide (ANP) had encouraging results in early studies of ARF in animals.[57,208] The infusion of ANP[57,208,219,236,240,245,254,278,308,322,378,379] or urodilatin[232,314,323] in rat models of ischemic ARF attenuated renal tissue damage and preserved glomerular filtration rate. Nakamoto et al.[241] and Shaw et al.[322] were able to shorten the course of renal artery cross-clamping-induced ARF in rats with ANP. Conger et al.[57] found marked improvement in GFR in a rat renal artery-clamp model when ANP-III (0.2 μg/kg/min) was given intravenously immediately after clamp release in combination with dopamine sufficient to maintain mean arterial pressure above 100 mmHg. In the rat, ANP had no effect on GFR when given intravenously, but did have a GFR effect when given directly into the renal artery for four hours.[322] The inability of ANP to increase GFR when given intravenously could be restored if dopamine was given simultaneously.[57] In the dog, the improvement in renal perfusion only lasted for a short period after a 180-minute infusion of ANP.[245] When ANP was given by intra-aortic bolus on days 1 and 2 after the above infusion, there was no significant improvement in renal perfusion on those days.[245] Thus, in animals the improvement in renal failure with ANP was only of short duration and depended upon whether ANP was given intravenously or directly into the artery.[57,245,322]

Humans

The administration of 0.2 μg of ANP/kg of body weight^{-1}/min^{-1} for 24 hours to humans with ARF revealed that ANP did not cause significant improvement, and did not reduce the need for dialysis or reduce mortality.[7,207] ANP infusions were associated with decreased survival in the nonoliguric ARF subjects (75% of subjects).[7] The usefulness of ANP for treatment is hampered by its short half-life of 2.5 minutes,[4,366] and by its very short duration of action.[57,208,214,220,278,382] Of 504 ARF patients treated with ANP, 46% developed hypotension, which would further limit its usefulness in ARF.[7] Urodilatin has also been associated with severe hypotension and bradycardia, when given as a potential treatment of congestive heart failure.[184] ANP is now considered more harmful than helpful with respect to the treatment of acute renal failure.[35] When ANP was given before and during radiocontrast study in 247 patients with chronic renal failure, no beneficial effect was found.[196] Urodilatin has been suggested as a possible treatment of renal failure,[231,314,315] but in double-blind phase II trials in acute renal failure patients, urodilatin has been found to have no beneficial effect.[232]

Vessel Dilator

Vessel dilator appears to be the cardiac hormone with the most promising therapeutic potential in ARF. Vessel dilator ($0.3\,\mu g/kg^{-1}/min^{-1}$ via intraperitoneal pump) decreases blood urea nitrogen (BUN) and serum creatinine from $162 \pm 4\,mg/dl$ and $8.17 \pm 0.5\,mg/dl$, respectively, to $53 \pm 17\,mg/dl$ and $0.98 \pm 0.12\,mg/dl$ in acute renal failure animals, where ARF was established for 2 days (after vascular clamping) before vessel dilator was given.[54] At day 6 of ARF, mortality decreased to 14% with vessel dilator from 88% without vessel dilator.[54] The ARF animals that did not receive vessel dilator had moderate (25%−75% of all tubules involved) to severe (>75% of all tubules necrotic) acute tubular necrosis by day 8 after their ischemic event (Figure 37.7b). As shown in Figure 37.7b, the nuclei in the tubules of these animals were almost completely destroyed, and the tubules were filled with sludge. The destruction of the tubules included both the proximal and distal tubules, with the proximal tubules being more severely affected (Figure 37.7b). The glomerulus of the ARF animals was spared compared to the renal tubules, with glomerulus appearing to be normal in the ARF animals (Figure 37.7a and 37.7b).

The addition of vessel dilator after renal failure had been present for two days resulted in a marked improvement in the renal histology (Figure 37.7c), with scores ranging from 0 (no tubular necrosis) to 1 + (<5% of the tubules involved).[54] The nuclei of the ischemic tubules regenerated secondary to vessel dilator (Figure 37.7c). When the kidneys were examined at day 8 of renal failure, the brush borders of the proximal tubules of the ARF animals treated with vessel dilator were present (Figure 37.7c), which was similar to the proximal tubules of healthy animals (Figure 37.7a). In the ARF animals not treated with vessel dilator, the brush borders of the tubules were destroyed (Figure 37.7b). The glomeruli of vessel dilator-treated ARF animals also appeared normal (Figure 37.7c). It is important to note that the animals treated with vessel dilator who had a significant increase in survival had nonoliguric renal failure.[54] As noted previously, nonoliguric renal failure subjects treated with ANP had a decreased survival and it was the nonoliguric renal failure subjects who did not

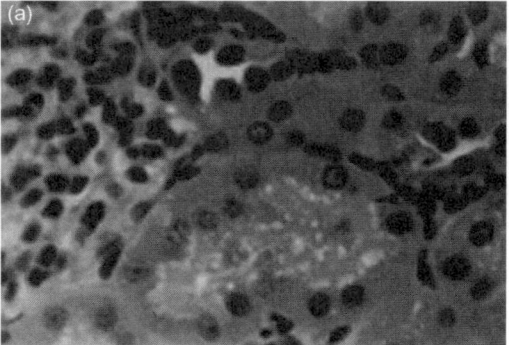
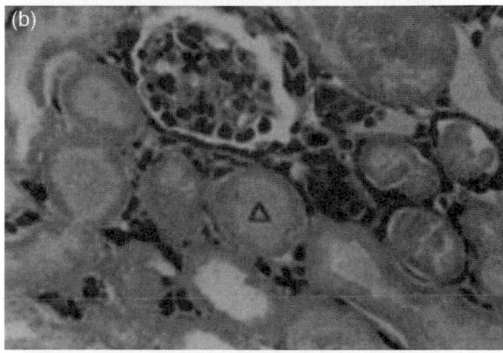
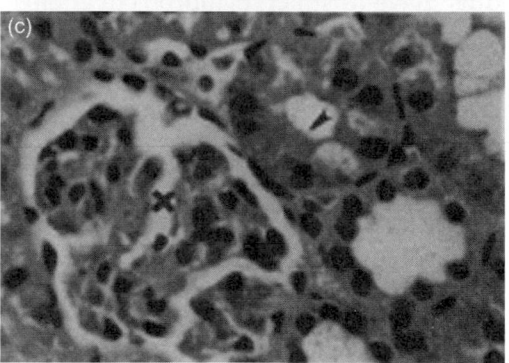

FIGURE 37.7 **Renal histology of healthy Sprague−Dawley rat.** (a) with intact proximal tubular brush border (arrowhead). (b) ARF rat at day 8 with marked tubular necrosis (open triangle) and without intact brush border present (>75% of tubules are necrotic). The glomerulus (x) appears to be normal. (c) ARF rat treated with vessel dilator from days 2 to 5 of ARF with kidney examined after day 8 of ARF reveals brush border to be present in proximal tubule (arrowhead). No tubules are necrotic in this ARF animal treated with vessel dilator. The glomerulus (x) is intact (Magnification of hematoxylin and eosin: $\times 426$ (a) and (c); and $\times 320$ (b); ARF: acute renal failure). *(With permission, from ref. [54].)*

respond to ANP.[7] Vessel dilator, LANP, and kaliuretic peptide, as opposed to ANP, BNP, and urodilatin, have never caused a hypotensive episode when given to either healthy animals or humans[220,381,382] or when given to humans with sodium and water retention.[243,379,380]

The ability of vessel dilator to reverse ischemic ARF is consistent with the important concept that the pathophysiology of ischemic ARF is due to a sublethal and reversible injury to renal tubular cells.[31,234] Part of the improvement by vessel dilator may be due to its ability to cause intrarenal vasodilation, as it is a strong vasodilator.[389] The reason why vessel dilator has greater beneficial effects than ANP, BNP, CNP, and urodilatin in acute renal failure appears due, at least in part, to its ability to cause the endogenous synthesis of renoprotective prostaglandin E_2 (PGE_2)[6,180,414] which ANP, BNP, CNP, and urodilatin do not do.[51,139]

A suggestion that PGE_2 is renoprotective (by maintaining glomerular hemodynamics) is reinforced by the observation that cyclooxygenase inhibitors in congestive heart failure and volume depletion states augment the reduction in RBF and GFR.[92,410] There is a dramatic decrease with prostaglandins in the outer medulla perfusion following ischemic injury,[178] a region of renal tissue which normally operates "on the verge of ischemia".[36] Prostaglandins have a favorable effect on blood flow distribution to this region.[237] In addition, prostaglandins have distinct cytoprotective effects and improve microvascular permeability in ischemic ARF.[42,180] Prostaglandins are not stored in the kidney, but rather have to be synthesized acutely secondary to a stimulating agent such as vessel dilator[51,139] in order for prostaglandins to have a positive beneficial effect in renal failure.

Adrenomedullin

There is evidence that ADM is renoprotective in Dahl salt-sensitive rats, in that when perfused for seven days the glomerular injury score is 54% less ($p < 0.05$) than in untreated Dahl salt-sensitive rats.[248] The adrenomedullin treated salt-sensitive rats, however, had considerably more ($p < 0.01$) glomerular sclerosis and anteriolar sclerosis and atrophic tubules after treatment than the control Dahl salt-resistant rats.[248]

BNP

BNP has not been investigated as a treatment of acute renal failure, but one would expect that BNP, similar to ANP, will have blunted or no effects in ARF compared to its effects in healthy animals.[7,207,245]

CNP

CNP increases in the circulation in ARF,[348] but its effects in acute renal failure are unknown. As discussed above, CNP has no natriuretic effects in healthy humans.[21,47,161]

DNP

DNP has been evaluated in persons with end-stage renal disease on dialysis and was found not to correlate ($p = 0.62$) with echocardiographic left ventricular mass index (LVMI), while ANP and BNP did correlate with LVMI of these end-stage renal patients.[43] DNP has not been investigated with respect to its possible therapeutic effects in renal failure.

TREATMENT OF OTHER DISEASES WITH ABNORMAL BLOOD VOLUME

Congestive Heart Failure

As part of the adaptive response to the pathophysiology of congestive heart failure, cardiac hormones increase in circulation.[32,38,83,108,176,177,273,350,368,379,380,418] The rationale for treatment of the pathophysiology of CHF with cardiac hormones (which are already increased in the circulation) is based upon other hormonal systems, where if one gives pharmacological rather than physiological concentrations of a hormone one often can overcome a defect in the target organ with respect to a particular hormone. In congestive heart failure, the pathophysiology with respect to atrial natriuretic peptides appears to be in the target organ(s) — the kidney has a diminished response to some of the atrial peptides — rather than the heart not producing enough of the respective hormones.[366] When ANP was investigated for possible treatment of CHF pathophysiology, it was found to have a markedly attenuated natriuretic response.[56,104,255,318] High-dose administration of ANP produces little or no diuresis or natriuresis in humans with CHF.[56] Synthetic brain natriuretic peptide (Nesteride®) in CHF individuals causes a small increase in urine volume (90 ± 38 versus 67 ± 27 ml/hr).[217] There is no significant natriuresis[3] or diuresis[166,233] with Nesteride® infusion in humans with CHF. In CHF animals, BNP has had no significant natriuretic or diuretic effects.[199] BNP can cause significant hypotension, however, in CHF subjects[3,233] with an incidence of 27% reported with 0.06 μg/kg/min dose.[233] Urodilatin infusion in CHF animals, likewise, causes significantly less natriuresis and diuresis compared to healthy animals.[1]

Vessel dilator, when given intravenously for 60 minutes to NYHA Class III CHF subjects, increases urine flow two- to 13-fold, which is still increased three hours after its infusion is stopped.[380] In CHF subjects, vessel dilator infusion enhances sodium excretion levels three- to four-fold, and the fractional excretion of sodium (FE_{Na}) six-fold, which are still significantly ($p < 0.01$) elevated 3 hours later.[380] Vessel dilator simultaneously decreases systemic vascular resistance 24%, pulmonary vascular resistance 25%, pulmonary capillary wedge pressure 33%, and central venous pressure 27%, while simultaneously increasing cardiac output 34%, cardiac index 35%, and stroke volume index 24% in individuals with CHF.[380] There were no side-effects with infusion of vessel dilator in CHF subjects, and specifically none of the CHF subjects became hypotensive as with BNP and ANP.[380] The natriuretic and diuretic effects of vessel dilator to help reverse the pathophysiology of CHF are as potent (not decreased or blunted) in persons with CHF as those observed in healthy persons.[380]

Long-acting natriuretic peptide (LANP) maximally increases urine flow and natriuresis only two-fold in persons with CHF[379] compared to four- to five-fold increase in urine flow and three- to eight-fold increase in natriuresis in healthy individuals.[382]

ANTIPROLIFERATIVE AND ANTI-CANCER PROPERTIES OF CARDIAC NATRIURETIC HORMONES

In blood vessels, ANP inhibits smooth muscle cell proliferation (hyperplasia) as well as smooth muscle cell growth (hypertrophy).[2,162,163,431] Atrial natriuretic peptide has growth-regulatory properties in a variety of other tissues including brain, bone, myocytes, red blood cell precursors, and endothelial cells.[10,11,143,169,261,431] In the kidney, ANP causes antimitogenic and antiproliferative effects in glomerular mesangial cells via inhibiting DNA synthesis.[10,11,169] The newest discovered property of the cardiac hormones, urodilatin, CNP, and DNP is their ability to inhibit the growth of cancers *in vitro* and *in vivo*.[361,362,377] The first cancer studied both *in vitro* and *in vivo* was human pancreatic adenocarcinomas, which have the lowest five-year survival rate of all common cancers.[267,424] The five-year survival rate of persons with adenocarcinoma of the pancreas is 1%.[267,424] The median survival is four months.[267,424] Current cancer chemotherapy and surgery prolong survival by a few months, but the abovementioned survival rates are for persons treated with surgery and/or currently available cancer chemotherapeutic agents.[267,424]

The four cardiac hormones from the ANP prohormone (Figure 37.1) decrease the number, i.e., eliminate up to 97% of human pancreatic, kidney, prostate, colon, breast, and ovarian adenocarcinoma cells,[131,355,356,357,361,362] angiosarcoma of the heart cells,[363] melanomas,[358] medullary thyroid carcinomas,[85] glioblastomas of brain,[359] as well as small-cell,[364] and squamous cell lung carcinoma cells[360] within 24 hours.

There was a 97.4%, 87%, 88%, and 89% ($p < 0.001$ for each) decrease (i.e., elimination) of human prostate adenocarcinoma cells secondary to vessel dilator, long-acting natriuretic peptide, kaliuretic peptide, and ANP, respectively, within 24 hours at their 1 mM concentrations, without any proliferation in the three days following this decrease.[355] When utilized with these four cardiac hormones respective antibodies, their ability to decrease the number of prostate cancer cells was completely blocked, indicating that their effects were specific, i.e., not due to some other hormone or substance.[355] Atrial natriuretic peptide reduces the number of hepatoblastoma cells in culture.[285]

BRAIN NATRIURETIC PEPTIDE AND C-NATRIURETIC HAVE LESS SIGNIFICANT ANTI-CANCER EFFECTS

Dose–response investigations indicate that brain natriuretic peptide (BNP) has no anti-cancer effects at any concentration.[131,355–357,364] The addition of BNP for 24 hour results in a 1%, 2%, and 4% (all non-significant) decrease in renal carcinoma cell numbers at its 1, 10, and 100 μM concentrations.[356] C-natriuretic peptide (CNP) has anti-cancer effects, but only at 100-fold higher concentrations than that observed for the four cardiac hormones synthesized by the proANP gene.[356,364] With exposure to CNP for 24 hours there was a 1% (n.s.), 7% (n.s.), and 10% ($p = 0.04$) decrease in renal carcinoma cell numbers at its 1, 10, and 100 μM concentrations.[356] Similar results were found at 48, 72, and 96 hours exposure to BNP and CNP.[356]

THE KIDNEY HORMONE URODILATIN ALSO HAS ANTI-CANCER EFFECTS

One might expect that urodilatin may have anti-cancer effects, as this peptide has identical a.a. to ANP and identical a.a. to the four terminal a.a. of kaliuretic peptide, both of which have anti-cancer effects. Urodilatin decreases the number of renal carcinoma cells by 66% at its 100 μM concentration, while ANP and kaliuretic peptide with the same amino acids at this same concentration eliminated 70% and 74% of the renal carcinoma cells in 24 hours.[356] Urodilatin, vessel dilator, LANP, kaliuretic peptide, and ANP each at their 1 μM concentrations inhibit DNA synthesis when incubated with the human renal carcinoma cells for 24 hours by 65%, 84%, 70%, 74%, and 77%, respectively ($p < 0.001$).[356]

CARDIAC NATRIURETIC HORMONES ELIMINATE UP TO 80% OF HUMAN PANCREATIC ADENOCARCINOMAS IN VIVO

When the four cardiac hormones from the proANP gene each at $3\,nM\,min^{-1}\,kg^{-1}$ body weight were infused subcutaneously for 28 days in athymic mice bearing human pancreatic adenocarcinomas, ANP eliminated 80% of the human pancreatic cancers.[383] Vessel dilator, LANP, and kaliuretic peptide eliminated the primary pancreatic cancers in 33%, 20%, and 14% of their respective treatment groups.[383] In none of the animals in which the pancreatic adenocarcinomas were eliminated in the primary site did a single animal ever have a recurrence in the primary site during its normal lifespan.[383] One ANP-treated animal developed a metastatic lesion, and this lesion was eliminated with treatment with vessel dilator.[383] Even in the treated animals which did not have total elimination of their human pancreatic adenocarcinoma, their tumor volume decreased to less than 10% (and with vessel dilator to less than 2%) of that of the untreated animals both during treatment and in a 12-month follow-up period.[383]

CARDIAC HORMONES ELIMINATE TWO-THIRDS OF HUMAN BREAST CANCERS IN VIVO WITHOUT ANY SURGERY

It was estimated that in 2009 there were 194,280 new cases of breast cancer and 40,610 deaths from breast cancer in the United States.[165] Breast cancer is the second leading cause of death from cancer in women, and the leading cause of death in women aged 40 to 55 in the United States.[258] Breast cancer is the leading cause of cancer death in women worldwide.[258] The number of new cases of breast cancer worldwide was estimated to be 1.05 million, with 370,000 deaths in 2000.[258]

Vessel dilator, LANP, kaliuretic peptide, and ANP eliminated 67%, 50%, 67%, and 33% of the human breast adenocarcinomas in athymic mice when infused subcutaneously for 28 days $3\,nM\,min^{-1}\,kg^{-1}$ body weight.[399] There was no recurrence of the breast cancers in the primary site, and no metastasis except in the ANP-treated group[399] (Table 37.2).

CARDIAC AND KIDNEY HORMONES ELIMINATE UP TO 86% OF HUMAN SMALL-CELL LUNG CANCERS IN MICE IN VIVO

Cancer of the lung and bronchus is the leading cause of cancer death in both men and women in the United

TABLE 37.2 Cardiac Hormones Ability to Eliminate Human Cancer Growing in Athymic Mice

	Breast Cancer	Pancreatic Adenocarcinoma	Small-cell Lung Cancer
VDL	67%	33%	71%
LANP	50%	20%	86%
ANP	33%	80%	43%
KP	67%	14%	57%

The numbers in each column are the percentages of human cancers which are eliminated and never recur in the primary site in athymic mice when treated with each of the cardiac hormones for 28 days at 3 nM/kg body weight/minute. Abbreviations: VDL: vessel dilator; LANP: long acting natriuretic peptide; ANP: atrial natriuretic peptide; KP: kaliuretic peptide.

States, with an estimated 88,900 deaths in men and 70,490 deaths in women in 2009.[165] The same trend is seen in many other countries.[353] In the current management of small-cell lung cancers, the majority of patients are treated first with chemotherapy plus radiotherapy, but with this combination survival is only 20% with limited disease and 0% survival with more extensive disease at three years.[182,353]

Long-acting natriuretic peptide, vessel dilator, kaliuretic peptide, ANP, and urodilatin eliminated 86%, 71%, 57%, 43% ($p < 0.001$ for each of the cardiac hormones), and 25% ($p < 0.05$; urodilatin) of the human small-cell lung carcinomas.[86] One vessel dilator-treated small-cell lung carcinoma animal developed a large tumor ($8,428\,mm^3$ volume) on treatment, and this tumor was eliminated utilizing atrial natriuretic peptide and then long-acting natriuretic peptide each for four weeks sequentially.[86]

ANTI-CANCER MECHANISM WITHIN CANCER CELLS OF THE CARDIAC HORMONES

The Ras mitogen-activated protein kinase (MAPK)/extracellular signal-related kinase (ERK) kinase-(MEK)-ERK cascade (Figure 37.8), hereafter referred to as the Ras-MAPK pathway, is the prototypical signal transduction pathway in cancer.[224,313] This pathway is aberrantly activated in many types of neoplasms, including prostate and breast cancer, with this activation being associated with a poor prognosis.[224,313] The integral role of the Ras-MEK-ERK pathway in mediating multiple hallmarks of cancer has suggested that the different kinases in this pathway may be targets for the treatment of cancer.[225,289,319,320]

Ras

Structural alteration in the GTPase Ras occur in 25 to 30% of human cancers, which allows them to relay

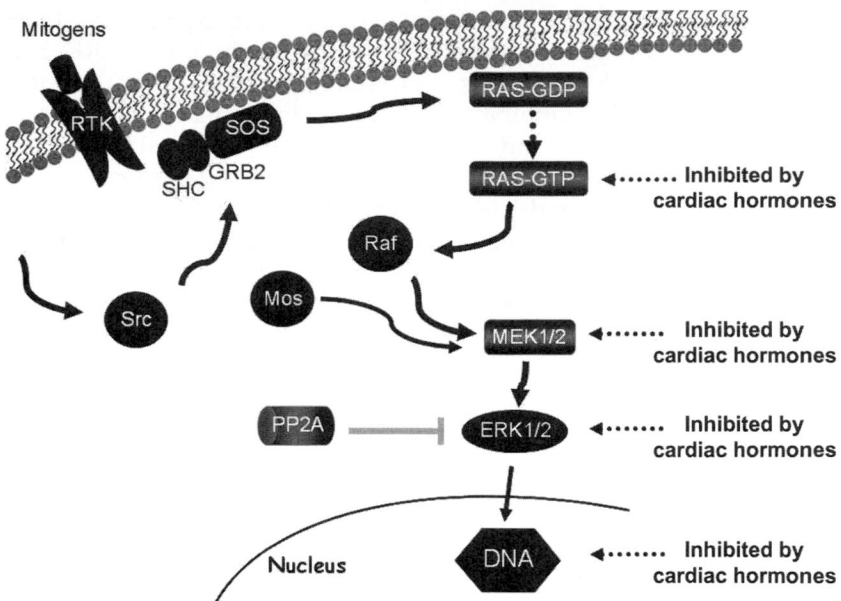

FIGURE 37.8 **Mitogens such as epidermal growth factor bind to their tyrosine kinase receptor (RTK) to convert inactive Ras-GTP mainly via SHC to active Ras-GTP.** Cardiac hormones inhibit up to 98% of 5 metabolic targets (kinases) important in cancer cell growth, i.e., Ras-GTP, MEK 1/2 kinases, and ERK 1/2 kinases of the Ras-MEK 1/2-ERK 1/2 kinase cascade in cancer cells. They are also strong inhibitors (up to 91%) of DNA synthesis within cancer cells. The cardiac hormones also block mitogens such as epidermal growth factor's ability to stimulate the conversion of Ras-GDP to Ras-GTP. [442]

mitogen signals in a ligand-independent manner, thereby obviating the need for ligand activation of growth factor receptors that occurs in normal cells.[225,319] Attempts to target Ras by perturbing its interaction with either Son of Sevenless gene (SOS) or growth factor receptor-bound 2 (GRB2) (Figure 37.8) have not yielded viable drug development candidates, largely because of the inherent difficulties of disrupting protein–protein interactions with drug-like molecules.[319] Several drug discovery programs have also been devoted to finding inhibitors of farnesyltransferase as a means to prevent the membrane localization of Ras.[319] Despite the successful identification of several chemical leads that effectively inhibited this prenylation enzyme, tumor cells, however, have proved generally to be impervious to the action of this class of inhibitors.[319]

Vessel dilator and kaliuretic peptide decrease the activation of Ras-GTP over a concentration range of $0.01\,\mu M$ to $1\,\mu M$.[335] Vessel dilator and kaliuretic peptide (each $1\,\mu M$) inhibit the activation of Ras by 95% ($p < 0.001$) and 90% ($p < 0.001$), respectively. At $0.01\,\mu M$ of kaliuretic peptide, the maximal inhibition was 95%. The inhibition of Ras lasted for 48 to 72 hours secondary to both peptides.[335] Their ability to inhibit Ras was inhibited by cyclic GMP antibody, and cyclic GMP itself inhibited Ras phosphorylation (89%; $p = 0.0015$).[335]

ANP and long-acting natriuretic peptide (each $0.1\,\mu M$) inhibited the phosphorylation of Ras 90% ($p < 0.0001$) and 83% ($p < 0.0001$), respectively.[336] At $0.01\,\mu M$ of long-acting natriuretic peptide, the maximal inhibition was 89%, which occurred within 5 minutes.

Both peptide hormones inhibited the activation of Ras for 3 to 4 hours.[336] Their ability to inhibit Ras was inhibited by cyclic GMP antibody and cyclic GMP itself inhibited Ras phosphorylation (72%; $p = 0.009$).[336] Thus, ANP, vessel dilator, kaliuretic peptide, and long-acting natriuretic peptide inhibit the activation of Ras via cyclic GMP as part of their anti-cancer mechanism(s) of action.[335,336]

MEK 1/2 Kinases

The prototype member of the MEK kinases, designated MAP kinase kinase (MKK-1)/or MEK-1, specifically phosphorylates the MAP kinase regulatory threonine and tyrosine residues present in the Thr-Glu-Tyr motif of ERK 1/2[61,425] (Figure 37.8). A second MEK family member, i.e., MEK-2, resembles MEK-1 at its substrate specificity, but is seven residues longer than MEK-1 with the amino acid sequence of MEK-2 being 81% identical to MEK-1.[425]

Vessel dilator and kaliuretic peptide decrease the activation of MEK 1/2 (Figure 37.8) over a concentration range of $0.01\,\mu M$ to $10\,\mu M$.[339] Vessel dilator and kaliuretic peptide (each $10\,\mu M$) inhibited the phosphorylation of MEK 1/2 kinase 98% ((Figure 37.9, $p < 0.0001$) and 81% ($p < 0.001$), respectively.[339] The inhibition of MEK 1/2 lasted for at least two hours, where it was maximal, secondary to both peptides.[339] Their ability to inhibit MEK 1/2 was inhibited by cyclic GMP antibody, and cyclic GMP itself inhibited MEK 1/2 phosphorylation, indicating that cyclic GMP is important for mediating these cardiac hormones' effects.[339]

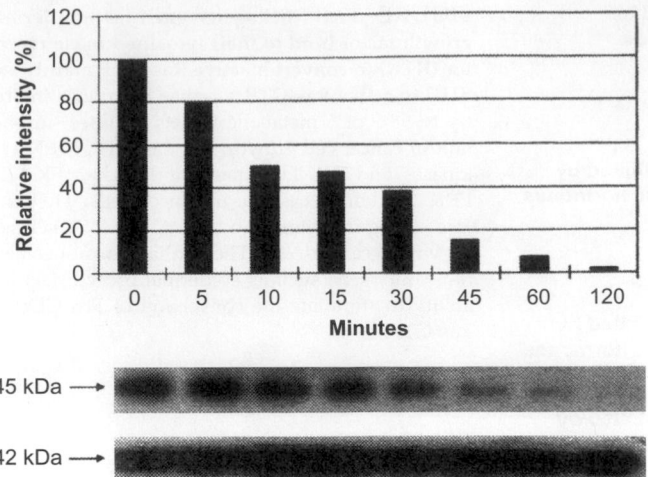

FIGURE 37.9 Vessel dilator at 10 μM inhibits 98% of the phosphorylation of mitogen-activated protein kinase kinase (MEK 1/2), which was maximal at two hours and significant at $p < 0.00001$ when evaluated by analysis of variance (ANOVA). MEK 1/2 is at 45 kDa while B-actin (loading control) is at 42 kDa. The relative intensity in the bar graphs is a comparison against untreated MEK 1/2 (100% intensity). (*Reprinted from Anticancer Res.* **27**, 1387–1392, 2007.)

ANP and long-acting natriuretic peptide decreased the activation of MEK 1/2 over a concentration range of 0.01 μM to 10 μM.[340] Long-acting natriuretic peptide and atrial natriuretic peptide (each 10 μM) inhibited the phosphorylation of MEK 1/2 kinase 97% ($p < 0.00001$) and 88% ($p < 0.00001$), respectively.[340] The inhibition of MEK 1/2 was maximal at two hours, and ceased by four hours secondary to both peptides.[340] The ability of peptides to inhibit MEK 1/2 was inhibited by cyclic GMP antibody, and cyclic GMP itself inhibited MEK 1/2 phosphorylation by 93%,[340] indicating that cyclic GMP is an important mediator of the cardiac natriuretic peptides' effects on MEK 1/2 kinase.

Cardiac Hormones Inhibit Activation of ERK 1/2 Kinases

Extracellular-signal regulated kinase (ERK) 1/2 is a mitogen-activated protein kinase (MAP kinase) important for the growth of cancer(s).[67,311] Growth factors such as epidermal growth factor (EGF), fibroblast growth factor, platelet derived growth factor, and vascular endothelial growth factor (VEGF) after binding to their specific receptor tyrosine kinases work via ERK 1/2 kinase to cause proliferation.[311]

Vessel dilator and kaliuretic peptide decrease the activation of ERK 1/2 over a concentration range of 0.01 μM to 1 μM. Vessel dilator and kaliuretic peptide (each 1 μM) inhibit the phosphorylation of ERK 1/2 kinases 96 and 70% ($p < 0.001$), respectively.[337] Both

have significant effects within five minutes at their 0.01 μM concentrations.[337] The inhibition of ERK 1/2 lasted for at least two hours secondary to both. Their ability to inhibit ERK 1/2 was inhibited by cyclic GMP antibody, and cyclic GMP itself inhibited ERK 1/2 phosphorylation.[337]

ANP and LANP, likewise, decrease the activation of ERK 1/2 over a concentration range of 0.01 μM to 10 μM[297d]. ANP and LANP's maximal inhibition of the phosphorylation of ERK 1/2 kinase were 94 and 88% ($p < 0.0001$), respectively.[338] Their ability to inhibit ERK 1/2 was inhibited by cyclic GMP antibody, and cyclic GMP itself inhibited ERK 1/2 phosphorylation, suggesting that cyclic GMP mediates their effects of inhibition the phosphorylation of ERK 1/2.[338]

Growth promoting hormones such as insulin and epidermal growth factor (EGF) work as mitogens via ERK 1/2 (mitogen-activated) protein kinase (MAP kinase) to cause growth.[67,311] Insulin (1 μM) and EGF (10 ng/ml) each enhance the phosphorylation of ERK 1/2 by 66%.[341] This enhanced phosphorylation of ERK 1/2 by EGF and insulin was decreased down to 10%, 8%, 27%, and 13% above non-stimulated ERK 1/2 by vessel dilator, kaliuretic peptide, LANP, and ANP.[341]

CARDIAC HORMONES' MECHANISM OF ACTION: INHIBITION OF DNA SYNTHESIS

Vessel dilator, LANP, kaliuretic peptide, and ANP each at their 1 μM concentrations inhibit DNA synthesis when incubated with pancreatic adenocarcinoma cells for 24 hours by 91%, 84%, 86%, and 83%, respectively ($p < 0.001$ for each).[361] One of the known mediators[369,409] of these peptide hormones' mechanism(s) of action, i.e., cyclic GMP, inhibited DNA synthesis in these adenocarcinoma cells by 51%.[361] These four cardiac hormones inhibit DNA synthesis by 80–91% in all human cancer cell lines.[85,131,355–359,361,364] Thus, after inhibiting ERK 1/2, DNA synthesis (a further or final step in the Ras-ERK 1/2 pathway) is inhibited within the nucleus. The ability of these peptide hormones to inhibit DNA synthesis is specifically mediated by the intracellular mediator cyclic GMP, as when a cyclic GMP antibody is incubated with the cardiac hormones they are unable to inhibit DNA synthesis.[131]

LOCALIZATION OF CARDIAC HORMONES TO THE NUCLEUS OF PANCREATIC ADENOCARCINOMAS

All four of these cardiac hormones synthesized by the ANP gene localize to the nucleus of human pancreatic adenocarcinomas by immunocytochemical evaluation, where they can inhibit DNA synthesis.[298,299] These are the first antigrowth peptide hormones that have been demonstrated to localize to the nucleus of cancers, and all four cardiac hormones localized to the nucleus.[298,299] These four cardiac hormones also localize to the capillaries growing into the human cancers, and the cytoplasm and fibroblasts within the tumors.[298,299]

SUMMARY AND FUTURE DIRECTIONS

Cardiac natriuretic peptides are synthesized both in the kidney and the heart,[130,271,347] and have some of their most potent biologic effects, such as natriuresis and diuresis, in the kidney.[24,27,78,139,141,220,405,434] Vessel dilator, via its ability to ameliorate acute renal failure and enhance tubule regeneration in acute tubular necrosis,[54] may prove useful in the future for the treatment of acute renal failure. BNP and adrenomedullin, with their effects in glomerular hypertrophy[179] and glomerular injury,[248] respectively, may be useful for the treatment of renal glomerular diseases. Since BNP, ANP, and adrenomedullin do not appear to help tubular diseases such as acute tubular necrosis, the major cause of acute renal failure,[154,423] their therapeutic potential in acute tubular necrosis appears limited. Future studies with these peptide hormones in humans with acute renal failure and/or glomerular diseases are necessary to determine whether the findings in animal models of ARF are applicable to the treatment of humans with acute renal failure.

Future research will concentrate on these cardiac hormones in humans with acute renal failure and renal cancer. With respect to side-effects, there have been no side-effects when infused for 28 days in athymic mice.[86,399] These cardiac hormones have been infused for one hour in 50 healthy humans and 50 humans with congestive heart failure, and one person had a marked decrease in blood pressure with ANP which was immediately corrected with 0.9% saline.[380,382] There have been no side-effects with the other three cardiac hormones in humans,[380,382] suggesting that they will be safe to treat persons with acute tubular necrosis and renal cancer and other cancers.

References

[1] Abassi ZA, Powell JR, Golomb E, Keiser HR. Renal and systemic effects of urodilatin in rats with high-output heart failure. Am J Physiol 1992;262:F615–21.

[2] Abell TJ, Richards AM, Ikram H, Espiner EA, Yandle T. Atrial natriuretic factor inhibits proliferation of vascular smooth muscle cells stimulated by platelet derived growth factor. Biochem Biophys Res Commun 1989;160:1392–6.

[3] Abraham WT, Lowes BD, Ferguson DA, Odom J, Kim JK, Robertson AD, et al. Systemic hemodynamic, neurohormonal, and renal effects of a steady-state infusion of human brain natriuretic peptide in patients with hemodynamically decompensated heart failure. J Card Fail 1998;4:37–44.

[4] Ackerman BH, Overton RM, McCormick MT, Schocken DD, Vesely DL. Disposition of vessel dilator and long-acting natriuretic peptide in healthy humans after a one-hour infusion. J Pharmacol Exp Therap 1997;282:603–8.

[5] Ackermann U, Irizawa TG, Milojevie S, Sonnennberg H. Cardiovascular effects of atrial extracts in anesthetized rats. Can J Physiol Pharmacol 1984;62:819–26.

[6] Agmon Y, Peleg H, Greenfeld Z, Rosen S, Brezis M. Nitric oxide and prostanoids protect the renal outer medulla from radiocontrast toxicity in the rat. J Clin Invest 1994;94:1069–75.

[7] Allgren RL, Marbury TC, Rahman SN, Weisberg LS, Fenves AZ, Lafayette RA, et al. Anaritide in acute tubular necrosis. N Engl J Med 1997;336:828–34.

[8] Anderson JV, Donckier J, Payne NN, Beacham H, Stater JDH, Bloom SR. Atrial natriuretic peptide: evidence as a natriuretic hormone at physiological plasma concentrations in man. Clin Sci 1987;72:305–12.

[9] Anderson RJ, Schrier RW. Acute renal failure. In: Schrier RW, editor. Diseases of the Kidney and Urinary Tract. 7th ed. Philadelphia: Lippincott, Williams & Wilkins; 2001. p. 1093–136.

[10] Appel RG. Growth inhibitory activity of atrial natriuretic factor in rat glomerular mesangial cells. FEBS Lett 1988;238:135–8.

[11] Appel RG. Growth-regulatory properties of atrial natriuretic factor. Am J Physiol 1992;262:F911–8.

[12] Arendt R, Gerbes A, Ritter D, Stangl E, Bach P, Zahringer J. Atrial natriuretic factors in plasma of patients with arterial hypertension, heart failure or cirrhosis of the liver. J Hypertens 1986;4(Suppl. 2):131–5.

[13] Argentin S, Drouin J, Nemer M. Thyroid hormone stimulates rat pro-natriodilatin mRNA levels in primary cardiocyte cultures. Biochem Biophys Res Commun 1987;146:1336–41.

[14] Atarashi K, Mulrow PJ, Franco-Saenz R, Snajdar R, Rapp J. Inhibition of aldosterone production by an atrial extract. Science 1984;224:992–4.

[15] Atlas SA, Kleinert HD, Camargo MJ, Januszewicz A, Sealey JE, Laragh JH, et al. Purification, sequencing and synthesis of natriuretic and vasoactive rat atrial peptide. Nature 1984;309:717–9.

[16] Baeyens DA, Price E, Winters CJ, Vesely DL. Diving increases atrial natriuretic factor-like peptide in fresh water diving turtles. Comp Physiol Biochem 1989;94 A:515–8.

[17] Baeyens DA, Walters JM, Vesely DL. Atrial natriuretic factor increases the magnitude of duodenal spontaneous phasic contractions. Biochem Biophys Res Commun 1988;155:1437–43.

[18] Baker BJ, Wu WL, Winters CJ, Dinh H, Wyeth R, Sallman AL, et al. Exercise increases the circulating concentration of the N-terminus of the atrial natriuretic factor prohormone in normal humans. Am Heart J 1991;122:1395–402.

[19] Ballerman BJ, Bloch KD, Seidman JG, Brenner BM. Atrial natriuretic peptide transcription, secretion and glomerular receptor activity during mineralocorticoid escape in the rat. J Clin Invest 1986;78:840–3.

[20] Banting FG, Best CH. The internal secretion of the pancreas. J Lab Clin Med 1922;7:251–61.

[21] Barletta G, Lazzeri C, Vecchiarino S, Del Bene R, Messeri G, Dello Sbarba A, et al. Low-dose C-type natriuretic peptide does not affect cardiac and renal function in humans. Hypertension 1988;31:802–8.

[22] Barr CS, Rhodes P, Struthers AD. C-type natriuretic peptide. Peptides 1996;17:1243–51.

[23] Beltowski J, Wojcicka G. Regulation of renal tubular transport by cardiac natriuretic peptides: two decades of research. Med Sci Monit 2002;8:RA39—52.

[24] Benjamin BA, Peterson TV. Effects of proANF-(31-67) on sodium excretion in conscious monkeys. Am J Physiol Regul Integr Comp Physiol 1995;269:R1351—5.

[25] Benoist C, Chambon P. In vivo sequence requirements of the SV40 early promoter region. Nature 1981;290:304—10.

[26] Bhalla SS, Robitaille L, Nemer M. Cooperative activation by GATA-4 and YY1 of the cardiac B-type natriuretic peptide promoter. J Biol Chem 2001;276:11439—45.

[27] Bloch KD, Scott JA, Zisfein JB, Fallon JT, Margolis NN, Seidman CE, et al. Biosynthesis and secretion of proatrial natriuretic factor by cultured rat cardiocytes. Science 1985;230:1168—71.

[28] Bompiani GD, Rouiller CH, Hatt PY. Le tissue de conduction du coeur chez le rat. Etude au microscope electronique. I. Le tronc commun du faisceau de His et les cellules claires de L'oreillette droite. Arch Mal Coeur 1959;52:1257—74.

[29] Borst JGG. The maintenance of an adequate cardiac output by the regulation of the urinary excretion of water and sodium chloride; an essential factor in the genesis of edema. Acta Med Scand 1948;130(Suppl. 207):1—71.

[30] Bovy PR, O'Neal JM, Olins GM, Patton DR, Mehta PP, McMahon EG, et al. A synthetic linear decapeptide binds to the atrial natriuretic peptide receptors and demonstrates cyclase activation and vasorelaxant activity. J Biol Chem 1989;264: 20309—13.

[31] Brady HR, Brenner BM, Clarkson MR, Lieberthal W. Acute renal failure. In: Brenner M, editor. Brenner & Rector's the kidney. 6th ed. Philadelphia: WB Saunders; 2000. p. 1201—62.

[32] Brandt RB, Redfield MM, Aarhus LL, Lewicki JA, Burnett Jr JC. Clearance receptor-mediated control of atrial natriuretic factor in experimental congestive heart failure. Am J Physiol 1994;266: R936—43.

[33] Breathnach R, Chambon P. Organization and expression of eukaryotic split genes coding for proteins. Am Rev Biochem 1981;50:349—83.

[34] Brenner BM, Ballermann BJ, Gunning ME, Zeidel ML. Diverse biological actions of atrial natriuretic peptide. Physiol Rev 1990;70:665—99.

[35] Brenner RM, Chertow GM. The rise and fall of atrial natriuretic peptide for acute renal failure. Curr Opin Nephrol Hypertens 1997;6:474—6.

[36] Brezis M, Rosen S, Silva P, Epstein FH. Renal ischemia: a new perspective. Kidney Int 1984;26:375—83.

[37] Bricker NS, Klahr S, Purkerson M, Schultze RG, Avioli LV, Binge SJ. In vitro assay for a humoral substance present during volume expansion and uremia. Nature 1968;219:1058—9.

[38] Buckley MG, Sethi D, Markandu ND, Sagnella GA, Singer DR, MacGregor GA. Plasma concentrations and comparisons of brain natriuretic peptide and atrial natriuretic peptide in normal subjects, cardiac transplant recipients and patients with dialysis-independent or dialysis-dependent chronic renal failure. Clin Sci 1992;83:437—44.

[39] Burnett Jr JC, Granger JP, Opgenorth TJ. Effects of synthetic atrial natriuretic factor on renal function and renin release. Am J Physiol 1984;247:F863—6.

[40] Carrithers SL, Ott CE, Hill MJ, Johnson BR, Cai W, Chang JJ, et al. Guanylin and uroguanylin induce natriuresis in mice lacking guanylyl cyclase-C receptor. Kidney Int 2004;65: 40—53.

[41] Carrithers SL, Hill MJ, Johnson BR, O'Hara SM, Jackson BA, Ott CE, et al. Renal effects of uroguanylin and guanylin in vivo. Braz J Med Biol Res 1999;32:1137—44.

[42] Casey KF, Machiedo GW, Lyons MJ, Slotman GJ, Novak RT. Alteration of postischemic renal pathology by prostaglandin infusion. J Surg Res 1980;29:1—10.

[43] Cataliotti A, Malatino LS, Jougasaki M, Zoccali C, Castellino P, Giacone G, et al. Circulating natriuretic peptide concentrations in patients with end-state renal disease: role of brain natriuretic peptide as a biomarker for ventricular remodeling. Mayo Clin Proc 2001;76:1111—9.

[44] Charron F, Paradis P, Bronchain O, Nemer G, Nemer M. Cooperative interaction between GATA-4 and GATA-6 regulates myocardial gene expression. Mol Cell Biol 1999;19: 4355—65.

[45] Charlton JA, Baylis PH. Lack of inhibition of vasopressin-stimulated Na^+K^+-ATPase by atrial natriuretic factor in rat renal medullary thick ascending limb of Henle's loop. Cell Biochem Funct 1990;8:25—9.

[46] Chartier L, Schiffrin E, Thibault G. Effect of atrial natriuretic factor (ANF)-related peptides on aldosterone secretion by adrenal glomerulosa cells: critical role of the intramolecular disulphide bond. Biochem Biophys Res Commun 1984;122: 171—4.

[47] Chauhan SD, Nilsson H, Ahluwalia A, Hobbs AJ. Release of C-type natriuretic peptide accounts for the biological activity of endothelium-derived hyperpolarizing factor. Proc Natl Acad Sci USA 2003;100:1426—31.

[48] Chen JH, Tsai JH, Lai YH, Hwang SJ. Plasma atrial natriuretic peptide in patients with chronic renal failure. J Formos Med Assoc 1990;89:645—50.

[49] Chen XW, Ying WZ, Valentin JP, Ling KT, Lin SY, Wiedemann E, et al. Mechanism of the natriuretic action of γ-melanocyte-stimulating hormone. Am J Physiol 1997;272: R1946—53.

[50] Chinkers M, Garbers DL, Chang MS, Lowe DG, Chin HM, Goeddel DV, et al. A membrane form of guanylate cyclase is an atrial natriuretic peptide receptor. Nature 1989;338:78—83.

[51] Chiou S, Vesely DL. Kaliuretic peptide: the most potent inhibitor of Na^+-K^+-ATPase of the atrial natriuretic peptides. Endocrinology 1995;136:2033—9.

[52] Christoffensen C, Goetz JP, Bartles ED, Larsen MD, Ribel U, Rehfeld JF, et al. Chamber-dependent expression of brain natriuretic peptide and its mRNA in normal and diabetic pig heart. Hypertension 2002;40:54—60.

[53] Chun TH, Itoh H, Ogawa Y, Tamura N, Takaya K, Igaki T, et al. Shear stress augments expression of C-type natriuretic peptide and adrenomedullin. Hypertension 1997; 29:1296—302.

[54] Clark LC, Farghaly H, Saba SR, Vesely DL. Amelioration with vessel dilator of acute tubular necrosis and renal failure established for 2 days. Am J Physiol 2000;278:H1555—64.

[55] Clavell AL, Stingo AJ, Wei CM, Heublein DM, Burnett Jr. JC. C-type natriuretic peptide: a selective cardiovascular peptide. Am J Physiol 1993;264:R290—5.

[56] Cody RJ, Atlas SA, Laragh JH, Kubo SH, Covit AB, Ryman KS, et al. Atrial natriuretic factor in normal subjects and heart failure patients: plasma levels and renal, hormonal, and hemodynamic responses to peptide infusion. J Clin Invest 1986;78: 1362—74.

[57] Conger JD, Falk SA, Yuan BH, Schrier RW. Atrial natriuretic peptide and dopamine in a rat model of ischemic acute renal failure. Kidney Int 1989;35:1126—32.

[58] Corboy JC, Walker RJ, Simmonds MB, Wilkins GT, Richards AM, Espiner EA. Plasma natriuretic peptides and cardiac volume during acute changes in intravascular volume in haemodialysis patients. Clin Sci 1994;87:679—84.

[59] Cousins KL, Farrell AP, Sweeting RM, Vesely DL, Keen JE. Release of atrial natriuretic factor prohormone peptides 1-30,

31-67, and 99-126 from fresh-water and sea-water acclimated perfused trout (*Oncorhynchus mykiss*) hearts. J Exp Biol 1997;200:1351−62.

[60] Crawford I, Maloney PC, Zeitlin PL, Guggino WB, Hyde SC, Turley H, et al. Immunocytochemical localization of the cystic fibrosis gene product CFTR. Proc Natl Acad Sci USA 1991;88:9262−6.

[61] Crews CM, Alessandrini A, Erikson RL. The primary structure of MEK, a protein kinase that phosphorylates the ERK gene product. Science 1992;258:478−80.

[62] Currie MG, Fok KF, Kato J, Moore RJ, Hamra FK, Duffin KL, et al. Guanylin: an endogenous activator of intestinal guanylate cyclase. Proc Natl Acad Sci USA 1992; 89:947−51.

[63] Currie MG, Geller DM, Cole BR, Boylan JG, Yu Sheng W, Holmberg SW, et al. Bioactive cardiac substances: potent vasorelaxant activity in mammalian atria. Science 1983;221: 71−3.

[64] Currie MG, Geller DM, Cole BR, Siegel NR, Fox KF, Adams SP, et al. Purification and sequence analysis of bioactive atrial peptides. Science 1984;223:67−9.

[65] Dagnino L, Lavigne JP, Nemer M. Increased transcripts for B-type natriuretic peptide in spontaneously hypertensive rats: quantitative polymerase chain reaction for atrial and brain natriuretic peptide transcripts. Hypertension 1992;20: 690−700.

[66] Davidman M, Olson P, Kohen J, Leither T, Kjellstrand C. Iatrogenic renal disease. Arch Intern Med 1991;151:1809−12.

[67] Davis RJ. Signal transduction by the JNK group of Map kinases. Cell 2000;103:239−52.

[68] Debold AJ. Heart atria granularity effects changes in water-−electrolyte balance. Proc Soc Exp Biol Med 1979;161:508−11.

[69] Debold AJ, Borenstein HB, Veress AT, Sonnenberg H. A rapid and potent natriuretic response to intravenous injections of atrial myocardial extracts in rats. Life Sci 1981;28: 89−94.

[70] DeBold AJ, Salerno TA. Natriuretic activity of extracts obtained from hearts of different species and from various rat tissues. Can J Physiol Pharmacol 1983;61:127−30.

[71] De Lean A, Gutkowska J, McNicoll N, Schiller PW, Cantin M, Genest J. Characterization of specific recepors for atrial natriuretic factor in bovine adrenal zona glomerulosa. Life Sci 1984;35:2311−8.

[72] De Palo EF, Woloszczuk W, Meneghetti M, DePalo CB, Nielsen HB, Secher NH. Circulating immunoreactive proANP (1-30) and proANP (31-67) in sedentary subjects and athletes. Clin Chem 2000;46:843−7.

[73] de Wardener HE, Mills IH, Clapham WF, Hayter CJ. Studies on the efferent mechanism of sodium diuresis which follows administration of intravenous saline in the dog. Clin Sci 1961;21:249−58.

[74] Dietz JR. Release of natriuretic factor from rat heart−lung preparation by atrial distension. Am J Physiol 1984;247: R1093−6.

[75] Dietz JR, Landon CS, Nazian SJ, Vesely DL, Gower Jr. WR. Effects of cardiac hormones on arterial pressure and sodium excretion in NPRa knockout mice. Exp Biol Med 2004;229: 813−8.

[76] Dietz JR, Nazian SJ, Vesely DL. Release of ANF, proANF 1-98, and proANF 31-67 from isolated rat atria by atrial distention. Am J Physiol 1991;260:H1774−8.

[77] Dietz JR, Scott DY, Landon CS, Nazian SJ. Evidence supporting a physiological role for pro ANP (1-30) in the regulation of renal excretion. Am J Physiol 2001;280:R1510−7.

[78] Dietz JR, Vesely DL, Gower Jr WR, Nazian SJ. Secretion and renal effects of ANF prohormone peptides. Clin Exp Pharmacol Physiol 1995;22:115−20.

[79] Dietz JR, Vesely DL, Gower Jr WR, Landon CS, Lee S, Nazian SJ. Neutralization of proANP 1-30 exacerbates hypertension in spontaneously hypertensive rat (SHR). Clin Exp Pharm Physiol 2003;30:627−31.

[80] Dietz JR, Vesely DL, Nazian SJ. The effect of changes in sodium intake on atrial natriuretic factor (ANF) and peptides derived from the N-terminus of the ANF prohormone in the rat. Proc Soc Exp Biol Med 1992;200:44−8.

[81] Dillingham MA, Anderson RJ. Inhibition of vasopressin action by atrial natriuretic factor. Science 1986;250:F963−6.

[82] Drewett JG, Garbers DL. The family of guanylyl cyclase receptors and their ligands. Endocr Rev 1994;15:135−62.

[83] Edwards BS, Ackerman DM, Lee ME, Reeder GS, Wold LE, Burnett JC. Identification of atrial natriuretic factor within ventricular tissue in hamsters and humans with congestive heart failure. J Clin Invest 1988;81:82−6.

[84] Ehrenreich H, Sinowatz R, Schulz RM, Arendt RM, Goebel FD. Immunoreactive atrial natriuretic peptide (ANP) in endoscopic biopsies of human gastrointestinal tract. Res Exp Med 1989;189:421−5.

[85] Eichelbaum EJ, Vesely BA, Alli AA, Sun Y, Gower Jr WR, Vesely DL. Four cardiac hormones decrease up to 82% of human medullary thyroid carcinoma cells within 24 hours. Endocrine 2006;30:325−32.

[86] Eichelbaum EJ, Sun Y, Alli AA, Gower Jr WR, Vesely DL. Cardiac hormones and urodilatin eliminate up to 86% of human small-cell lung carcinomas in mice. Eur J Clin Invest 2008;38:562−70.

[87] Elitsur N, Lorenz JN, Hawkins JA, Rudolph JA, Witte D, Yang LE, et al. The proximal convoluted tubule is a target for the uroguanylin-regulated natriuretic response. J Pediatr Gastroenterol Nutr 2006;43:S74−81.

[88] Elsner D, Muders F, Muntze A, Kromer EP, Forssmann WG, Riegger G. Efficacy of prolonged infusion of urodilatin [ANP 95-126] in patients with congestive heart failure. Am Heart J 1995;129:766−73.

[89] Entzeroth M, Doods HN, Wieland HA, Wiene W. Adrenomedullin mediates vasodilation via CGRP1 receptors. Life Sci 1995;56:PL19−25.

[90] Eto T, Washimine H, Kato J, Kitamura K, Yamamoto Y. Adrenomedullin and proadrenalmedullin N-terminal 20 peptide in impaired renal function. Kidney Int Suppl 1996;55:S148−9.

[91] Fan X, Hamra FK, Freeman RH, Eber SL, Krause WJ, Lin RW, et al. Uroguanylin: cloning of preprouroguanylin cDNA, mRNA expression in the intestine and heart and isolation of uroguanylin and prouroguanylin from plasma. Biochem Biophys Res Commun 1996;219:457−62.

[92] Fink MP, Mac Vittie TJ, Casey LC. Effects of nonsteroidal anti-inflammatory drugs on renal function in septic dogs. J Surg Res 1984;36:516−25.

[93] Flynn TG. Past and current perspectives on the natriuretic peptides. Proc Soc Exp Biol Med 1996;213(2):98−104.

[94] Flynn TG, deBold ML, deBold AJ. The amino acid sequence of an atrial peptide with potent diuretic and natriuretic properties. Biochem Biophys Res Commun 1983;117:859−65.

[95] Fonteles MC, Greenberg RN, Monteiro HAS, Currie MG, Forte LR. Natriuretic and kaliuretic activities of guanylin and uroguanylin in the isolated perfused rat kidney. Am J Physiol 1998;44: F191−7.

[96] Fonteles MC, Carrithers SL, Monteiro HSA, Carvalho AF, Coelho GR, Greenberg RN, et al. Renal effects of serine-7 analog of lymphoguanylin in *ex vivo* rat kidney. Am J Physiol Renal Physio 2001;280:F207−13.

[97] Forte LR. Uroguanylin: cloning of preprouroguanylin cDNA, mRNA expression in intestine and heart and isolation of

uroguanylin and prouroguanylin from plasma. Biochem Biophys Res Commun 1996;219:457−62.

[98] Forte LR, Eber SL, Fan X, London RM, Rowland LM, Chin DT, et al. Lymphoguanylin: cloning characterization of a unique member of the guanylin peptide family. Endocrinology 1999;140:1800−6.

[99] Forte LR, Fan S, Hamra FK. Salt and water homeostasis: uroguanylin is a circulating peptide hormone with natriuretic activity. Am J Kidney Dis 1996;28:296−304.

[100] Forte LR, Krause WJ, Freeman RH. *Escherichia coli* enterotoxin receptors: localization in opossum kidney, intestine, and testis. Am J Physiol 1989;257:F874−81.

[101] Forte LR, London RM, Freeman RH, Krause WJ. Guanylin peptides: renal actions mediated by cyclic GMP. Am J Physiol Renal Physiol 2000;278:F180−91.

[102] Franz M, Woloszczuk W, Horl WH. N-terminal fragments of the proatrial natriuretic peptide in patients before and after hemodialysis treatment. Kidney Int 2000;58:374−8.

[103] Franz M, Woloszczuk W, Horl WH. Plasma concentration and urinary excretion of N-terminal proatrial natriuretic peptides in patients with kidney diseases. Kidney Int 2001;59: 1928−34.

[104] Freeman RH, David JO, Vari RC. Renal response to atrial natriuretic factor in conscious dogs with caval constriction. Am J Physiol 1985;248:R495−500.

[105] Freid TA, Osgood RW, Stein JH. Tubular site(s) of action of atrial natriuretic peptide in rat. Am J Physiol 1988;255:F313−6.

[106] Fukae H, Kinoshita H, Fujimoto S, Kita T, Nakazato M, Eto T. Changes in urinary levels and renal expression of uroguanylin on low or high salt diets in rats. Nephron 2002;92: 373−8.

[107] Fukioka S, Tamaki T, Fukui K, Ikahara T, Abe Y. Effects of a synthetic human atrial natriuretic polypeptide on regional blood flow in rats. Eur J Pharmacol 1985;109:301−4.

[108] Fyhrquist F, Tikkanen I, Totterman KJ, Hynynen M, Tikkanen T, Andersson S. Plasma atrial natriuretic peptide in health and disease. Eur Heart J 1987;8(Suppl. B):117−22.

[109] Garcia NH, Garvin JL. ANF and angiotensin II interact via kinases in the proximal straight tubule. Am J Physiol 1995;268: F730−5.

[110] Garcia R, Cantin M, Thibault G, Ong H, Genest J. Relationship of specific granules to the natriuretic and diuretic activity of rat atria. Experientia 1982;38:1071−3.

[111] Garcia R, Thibault G, Cantin M, Genest J. Effect of a purified atrial natriuretic factor on rat and rabbit vascular strips and vascular beds. Am J Physiol 1984;247:R34−9.

[112] Garcia R, Thibault G, Nutt RF, Cantin M, Genest J. Comparative vasoactive effects of native and synthetic atrial natriuretic factor (ANF). Biochem Biophys Res Commun 1984;119:685−8.

[113] Gardner DG. Natriuretic peptides: markers or modulators of cardiac hypertrophy. Trends Endo Metab 2003;14:411−6.

[114] Gardner DG, Deschepper CT, Ganong WF, Hane S, Fiddes J, Baxter JD, et al. Extra-atrial expression of the gene for atrial natriuretic factor. Proc Natl Acad Sci USA 1986;83:6697−701.

[115] Gardner DG, Gertz BJ, Deschepper CF, Kim DY. Gene for the rat atrial natriuretic peptide is regulated by glucocorticoids *in vitro*. J Clin Invest 1988;82:1275−81.

[116] Gardner DG, Kovacic-Milivojevic BK, Garmai M. Molecular biology of the natriuretic peptides. In: Vesely DL, editor. Atrial natriuretic peptides. Trivandrum, India: Research Signpost; 1997. p. 15−38.

[117] Gauer OH, Henry JP, Seiker HO. Cardiac receptors and fluid volume control. Progr Cardiovasc Dis 1961;4:1−26.

[118] Gauer OH, Henry JP. Circulatory basis of fluid volume control. Physiol Rev 1963;43:423−81.

[119] Geller DM, Currie MG, Siegel NR, Fok KF, Adams SP, Needleman P. The sequence of an atriopeptigen: a precursor of the bioactive atrial peptides. Biochem Biophys Res Commun 1984;121:802−7.

[120] Geller DM, Currie MG, Wakitani K, Cole BR, Adams SP, Fok KF, et al. Atriopeptins: a family of potent biologically active peptides derived from mammalian atria. Biochem Biophys Res Commun 1984;120:333−8.

[121] Gillespie DJ, Sandberg RL, Koike TI. Dual effect of left atrial receptors on the excretion of sodium and water in the dog. Am J Physiol 1973;255:706−10.

[122] Godellas CV, Gower Jr WR, Fabri PJ, Knierim TH, Giordano AT, Vesely DL. Atrial natriuretic factor (ANF) − a possible new gastrointestinal regulatory peptide. Surgery 1991;110: 1022−7.

[123] Goetz KL, Bond GC, Bloxham DD. Atrial receptors and renal function. Physiol Rev 1975;55:157−205.

[124] Goodfriend TL, Elliott ME, Atlas SA. Actions of synthetic atrial natriuretic factor on bovine adrenal glomerulosa. Life Sci 1984;35:1675−82.

[125] Gomez-Sanchez EP, Foecking MF, Sellers D, Blankenship MS, Gomez-Sanchez CE. Is circulating ouabain-like compound quabain? Am J Hypertens 1994;7:647−50.

[126] Gower Jr WR, Chiou S, Skolnick K, Vesely DL. Molecular forms of circulating atrial natriuretic peptides in human plasma and their metabolites. Peptides 1994;15:861−7.

[127] Gower WR, Dietz JR, McCuen RW, Fabri PJ, Lerner EA, Schubert ML. Regulation of atrial natriuretic peptide secretion by cholinergic and PACAP neurons of the gastric antrum. Am J Physiol 2003;284:G68−74.

[128] Gower Jr WR, Dietz JR, Vesely DL, Finley CL, Skolnick KA, Fabri PJ, et al. Atrial natriuretic peptide gene expression in the rat gastrointestinal tract. Biochem Biophys Res Commun 1994;202:562−70.

[129] Gower Jr WR, Salhab KF, Foulis WL, Pillai N, Bund JR, Vesely DL, et al. Regulation of atrial natriuretic peptide gene expression in gastric antrum by fasting. Am J Physiol 2000;278: R770−80.

[130] Gower Jr WR, San Miguel GI, Carter GM, Hassan I, Farese RV, Vesely DL. Atrial natriuretic prohormone gene expression in cardiac and extracardiac tissues of diabetic Goto-Kakizaki rats. Mol Cell Biochem 2003;252:263−71.

[131] Gower Jr WR, Vesely BA, Alli AA, Vesely DL. Four peptides decrease human colon adenocarcinoma cell number and DNA synthesis via guanosine 3′,5′-cyclic monophosphate. Int J Gastrointestinal Cancer 2005;36:77−87.

[132] Gower Jr WR, Vesely DL. The gastrointestinal natriuretic peptide system. Trends Comp Biochem Physiol 2000;6:125−38.

[133] Grammer RT, Fukumi H, Inagami T, Misono KS. Rat atrial natriuretic factor. Purification and vasorelaxant activity. Biochem Biophys Res Commun 1983;116:696−703.

[134] Green M, Ruiz OS, Kear F, Arruda JA. Dual effect of cyclic GMP on renal brush border Na-H antiporter. Proc Soc Exp Biol Med 1991;198:846−51.

[135] Greenberg BD, Bencen GH, Seilhamer JJ, Lewicki JA, Fiddes JC. Nucleotide sequence of the gene encoding human ANF precursor. Nature 1984;312:656−8.

[136] Greenberg RN, Hill M, Crytzer J, Krause WJ, Eber SL, Hamra FK, et al. Comparison of effects of uroguanylin, guanylin, and *Escherichia coli* heat-stable entertoxin STa in mouse intestine and kidney: evidence that uroguanylin is an intestinal natriuretic hormone. J Invest Med 1997;45:276−82.

[137] Greenwald JE, Needleman P, Wilkins MR, Schreiner GF. Renal synthesis of atriopeptin-like protein in physiology and pathophysiology. Am J Physiol 1991;260:F602−7.

[138] Grepin C, Dagino L, Robitaille L, Haberstroh L, Antakly T, Nemer M. A hormone-encoding gene identifies a pathway for cardiac but not skeletal muscle gene transcription. Mol Cell Biol 1994;14:3115−29.

[139] Gunning ME, Brady HR, Otuechere G, Brenner BM, Zeidel ML. Atrial natriuretic peptide (31−67) inhibits Na^+ transport in rabbit inner medullary collecting duct cells: role of prostaglandin E_2. J Clin Invest 1992;89:1411−7.

[140] Gunning ME, Brenner BM. Natriuretic peptides and the kidney: current concepts. Kidney Int 1992;42(Suppl. 38): S127−33.

[141] Habibullah AA, Villarreal D, Freeman RH, Dietz JR, Vesely DL, Simmons JC. Atrial natriuretic peptide fragments in dogs with experimental heart failure. Clin Exp Pharmacol Physiol 1995;22:130−5.

[142] Hamra FK, Forte LR, Eber SL, Pidhorodeckyj NV, Krause WJ, Freeman RH, et al. Uroguanylin: structure and activity of a second endogenous peptide that stimulates intestinal guanylate cyclase. Proc Natl Acad Sci USA 1993;90:10464−8.

[143] Harma F, Hagiwara H, Inoue A, Yamaguchi A, Yokose S, Furuya M, et al. cGMP produced in response to ANP and CNP regulates proliferation and differentiation of osteoblastic cells. Am J Physiol 1996;270:C1311−8.

[144] Hammond TG, Haramati A, Knox FG. Synthetic atrial natriuretic factor decreases renal tubular phosphate reabsorption in rats. Am J Physiol 1985;249:F315−8.

[145] Harris PJ, Thomas D, Morgan TO. Atrial natriuretic peptide inhibits angiotensin-stimulated proximal tubular sodium and water reabsorption. Nature 1987;326:697−8.

[146] Harthshorne H. Water versus hydrotherapy. Philadelphia: Lloyd P. Smith Press; 1847.

[147] Harvey W. Exercitatio de motu cordis et sanguinis animalibus. Leake CD [trans], Francofurti guilielem fitzeri, 1628. Springfield, IL: Charles C. Thomas; 1928.

[148] Hayashida H, Miyata T. Sequence similarity between epidermal growth factor precursor and atrial natriuretic factor precursor. FEBS Lett 1985;185:125−8.

[149] Henrich WL. Southwestern Internal Medicine Conference: renal sodium excretion and atrial natriuretic factor. Am J Med Sci 1986;291:199−208.

[150] Henry JP, Gauer OH, Reeves JL. Evidence of the atrial location of receptors influencing urine flow. Circ Res 1956;4:85−90.

[151] Henry JP, Pearce JW. The possible role of cardiac atrial stretch receptors in the induction of changes in urine flow. J Physiol 1956;131:572−85.

[152] Hirata Y, Tomita M, Takada S, Yoshimi H. Vascular receptor binding activities and cyclic GMP responses by synthetic human and rat atrial natriuretic peptides (ANP) and receptor down-regulation by ANP. Biochem Biophys Res Commun 1985;128:538−46.

[153] Hock R, Anderson RJ. Prevention of drug-induced nephrotoxicity in the intensive care unit. J Crit Care 1995;10:33−43.

[154] Hou SH, Bushinsky DA, Wish JB, Cohen JJ, Harrington JT. Hospital acquired renal insufficiency: a prospective study. Am J Med 1983;74:243−8.

[155] Huet M, Benchimol S, Berlinguet JC, Castonguay Y, Cantin M. Cytochimie ultrastructurale des cardiocytes de l'oreillette humaine. IV. Digestion des granules specifiques par less proteases. J Microsc 1974;21:147−58.

[156] Huet M, Cantin M. Ultrastructural cytochemistry of atrial muscle cells. II. Characterization of the protein content of specific granules. Lab Invest 1974;30:525−32.

[157] Humphreys MH. Gamma-MSH, sodium metabolism, and salt sensitive hypertension. Am J Physiol 2004;286:R417−30.

[158] Humphreys MH, Lin SY. Peptide hormones and the control of sodium excretion. Hypertension 1988;11:397−410.

[159] Hunt PJ, Richards AM, Espiner EA, Nicholls ME, Yandle TG. Bioactivity and metabolism of C-type natriuretic peptide in normal man. J Clin Endocrinol Metab 1994;78:1428−35.

[160] Hunter EFM, Kelly PA, Prowse C, Woods FJ, Lowry PJ. Analysis of peptides derived from pro atrial natriuretic peptide that circulate in man and increase in heart disease. Scand J Clin Lab Invest 1998;58:205−16.

[161] Igaki T, Itoh H, Suga S, Hama N, Ogawa Y, Komatsu Y, et al. C-type natriuretic peptide in chronic renal failure and its action in humans. Kidney Int 1996;49(Suppl. 55):S144−7.

[162] Itoh H, Pratt RE, Dzau VJ. Atrial natriuretic polypeptide inhibits hypertrophy of vascular smooth muscle cells. J Clin Invest 1990;86:1690−7.

[163] Itoh H, Pratt RE, Ohno M, Dzau VJ. Atrial natriuretic polypeptide as a novel antigrowth factor of endothelial cells. Hypertension 1992;19:758−61.

[164] Jamieson JD, Palade GE. Specific granules in atrial muscle cell. J Cell Biol 1964;23:151−62.

[165] Jemal A, Siegel R, Ward E, Hao Y, Xu J, Thun MJ. Cancer Statistics, 2009. Ca Cancer J Clin 2009;59:225−49.

[166] Jensen KT, Eiskjaer H, Carstens J, Pedersen EB. Renal effects of brain natriuretic peptide in patients with congestive heart failure. Clin Sci 1999;96:5−15.

[167] Jin JY, Wen JF, Li D, Cho KW. Osmoregulation of atrial myocytic ANP release: osmotransduction via cross-talk between L-type Ca^2 channel and SR Ca^2 release. Am J Physiol 2004;287: R1101−9.

[168] John SWM, Krege JH, Oliver PM, Hagaman JR, Hodgkin JB, Pang SC, et al. Genetic decreases in atrial natriuretic peptide and salt-sensitive hypertension. Science 1995;267:679−81.

[169] Johnson A, Lermioglu F, Garg UC, Morgan-Boyd R, Hassid A. A novel biological effect of atrial natriuretic hormone: inhibition of mesangial cell mitogenesis. Biochem Biophys Res Commun 1988;152:893−7.

[170] Jougasaki M, Burnett Jr JC. Adrenomedullin: potential in physiology and pathophysiology. Life Sci 2000;66:855−72.

[171] Kangawa K, Fukuda A, Kubota I, Hayashi Y, Matsuo H. Identification in rat atrial tissue of multiple forms of natriuretic polypeptides of about 3,000 daltons. Biochem Biophys Res Commun 1984;121:585−91.

[172] Kangawa K, Fukuda A, Matsuo H. Purification and complete amino acid sequence of rat atrial natriuretic polypeptides of 5,000 daltons. Biochem Biophys Res Commun 1984;119: 933−40.

[173] Kangawa K, Fukuda A, Matsuo H. Structural identification of beta- and gamma-human atrial natriuretic polypeptides (β- and γ-ANP). Nature 1985;313:397−400.

[174] Kangawa K, Matsuo H. Purification and complete amino acid sequence of alpha-human atrial natriuretic polypeptide (alpha-hANP). Biochem Biophys Res Commun 1984;118:131−9.

[175] Kangawa K, Tawaragi Y, Oikawa S, Mizuno A, Sakuragawa Y, Nakazato M, et al. Identification rat gamma atrial natriuretic polypeptide and characterization of the cDNA encoding its precursor. Nature 1984;312:152−5.

[176] Karla PR, Anker SD, Struthers AD, Coats AJS. The role of C-natriuretic peptide in cardiovascular medicine. Eur Heart J 2001;22:997−1007.

[177] Kalra PR, Clague JR, Bolger AP, Anker SD, Poole-Wilson PA, Struthers AD, et al. Myocardial production of C-type natriuretic peptide in chronic heart failure. Circulation 2003;107: 571−3.

[178] Karlberg L, Norlen BJ, Ojteg G, Wolgast M. Impaired medullary circulation in postischemic acute renal failure. Acta Physiol Scand 1983;118:11—7.

[179] Kasahara M, Mukoyama M, Sugawara A, Makino H, Suganami T, Ogawa Y, et al. Ameliorated glomerular injury in mice over expressing brain natriuretic peptide with renal ablation. J Am Soc Nephrol 2000;11:1691—701.

[180] Kaufman Jr RP, Anner H, Kobzik L, Valeri CR, Shepro D, Hechtman HB. Vasodilator prostaglandins (PG) prevent renal damage after ischemia. Ann Surg 1987;205:195—8.

[181] Keeler R. Atrial natriuretic factor has a direct, prostaglandin-independent action on kidneys. Can J Physiol Pharmacol 1982;60:1078—82.

[182] Kelley MJ, Johnson BE. Molecular biology of lung cancer. In: Mendelsohn J, Howley PM, Israel MA, Liotta LA, editors. The molecular basis of cancer. 2nd ed. Philadelphia: W.B. Saunders Company; 2001. p. 260—87.

[183] Kennedy BP, Marsden JJ, Flynn TG, DeBold AJ, Davies PL. Isolation and nucleotide sequence of a cloned cardionatrin cDNA. Biochem Biophys Res Commun 1984;122:1076—82.

[184] Kentsch M, Drummer C, Gerzer R, Muller-Esch G. Severe hypotension and bradycardia after continuous intravenous infusion of urodilatin (ANP 95-126) in a patient with congestive heart failure. Eur J Clin Invest 1995;25:281—3.

[185] Kikuchi M, Fujimoto S, Fukae H, Kinoshita H, Kita T, Nakazato M, et al. Role of uroguanylin, a peptide with natriuretic activity, in rats with experimental nephrotic syndrome. J Am Soc Nephrol 2005;16(2):392—7.

[186] Kinoshita H, Fujimoto S, Fukae H, Yokota N, Hisanaga S, Nakazato M, et al. Plasma and urine levels of uroguanylin, a new natriuretic peptide, in nephrotic syndrome. Nephron 1999;81:160—4.

[187] Kinoshita H, Nakazato M, Yamaguchi H, Matsukura S, Fujimoto S, Eto T. Increased plasma guanylin levels in patients with impaired renal function. Clin Nephrol 1997;47:28—32.

[188] Kisch B. Studies in comparative electron microscopy of the heart. II. Guinea pig and rat. Exp Med Surg 1955;13:404—28.

[189] Kitamura K, Kangawa K, Kawamoto M, Ichiki Y, Nakamura S, Matsuo H, et al. Adrenomedullin: a novel hypotensive peptide isolated from human pheochromocytoma. Biochem Biophys Res Commun 1993;192:553—60.

[190] Kitamura K, Kangawa K, Matsuo H, Eto T. Adrenomedullin: implications for hypertension research. Drugs 1995;49:485—95.

[191] Kleinert HD, Maack T, Atlas SA, Januszewicz A, Sealey JE, Laragh JH. Atrial natriuretic factor inhibits angiotensin-, norepinephrine-, and potassium-induced vascular contractility. Hypertension 1984;6(Suppl. I):I143—7.

[192] Kohse KP, Feifel K, Mayer-Wehrstein R. Differential regulation of brain and atrial natriuretic peptides in hemodialysis patients. Clin Nephrol 1993;40:83—90.

[193] Kojima S, Inoue I, Hirata Y, Kimura G, Saito F, Kawano Y, et al. Plasma concentrations of immunoreactive-atrial natriuretic polypeptide in patients on hemodialysis. Nephron 1987;46:45—8.

[194] Koller KJ, Goeddel DV. Molecular biology of natriuretic peptides and their receptors. Circulation 1992;86:1081—8.

[195] Kudo T, Baird A. Inhibition of aldosterone production in the adrenal glomerulosa by atrial natriuretic factor. Nature 1984;312:756—7.

[196] Kurnik BR, Allgren RL, Genter FC, Solomon RJ, Bates ER, Weisberg LS. Prospective study of atrial natriuretic peptide for the prevention of radiocontrast-induced nephropathy. Am J Kidney Dis 1998;31:674—80.

[197] Kurtz A, Della Bruna R, Pfeilschifter J, Taugner R, Bauer C. Atrial natriuretic peptide inhibits renin release from juxtaglomerular cells by cGMP-mediated process. Proc Natl Acad Sci USA 1986;83:4769—73.

[198] Ladenson PW, Bloch KD, Seidman JG. Modulation of atrial natriuretic factor by thyroid hormone: messenger ribonucleic acid and peptide levels in hypothyroid, euthyroid, and hyperthyroid rat atria and ventricles. Endocrinology 1988;123:652—7.

[199] Lainchbury J, Richards AM, Nicholls MG. Brain natriuretic peptide in heart failure. In: Vesely DL, editor. Atrial natriuretic peptides. Trivandrum, India: Research Signpost; 1997. p. 151—8.

[200] Lang CC, Choy AM, Henderson IS, Coutie WJ, Struthers AD. Effect of haemodialysis on plasma levels of brain natriuretic peptide in patients with chronic renal failure. Clin Sci 1992;82:127—31.

[201] La Pointe MC, Deschepper CF, Wu J, Gardner DG. Extracellular calcium regulates expression of the gene for atrial natriuretic factor. Hypertension 1990;15:20—8.

[202] Lazure C, Seidah NG, Chretien M, Thibault G, Garcia R, Cantin M, et al. Atrial pronatriodilatin: a precursor for natriuretic factor and cardiodilatin. FEBS Lett 1984;172:80—6.

[203] Lee SJ, Kim SZ, Cui X, Kim SH, Lee KS, Chung YJ, et al. C-type natriuretic peptide inhibits ANP secretion and atrial dynamics in perfused atria: NPR-B-cGMP signaling. Am Heart J 2000;278:H208—21.

[204] Lennane RJ, Peart WS, Carey RM, Shaw J. A comparison on natriuresis after oral and intravenous sodium loading in sodium-depleted rabbits: evidence for a gastrointestinal or portal monitor of sodium intake. Clin Sci Mol Med 1975;49:433—6.

[205] Levin ER, Gardner DG, Samson WK. Natriuretic peptides. N Engl J Med 1998;339:321—8.

[206] Levinsky NG, Lalone RC. Mechanism of sodium diuresis after saline infusion in the dog. J Clin Invest 1963;42:1261—8.

[207] Lewis J, Salem MM, Chertow GM, Weisberg LS, McGrew F, Marbury TC, et al. Atrial natriuretic factor in oliguric acute renal failure. Anaritide Acute Renal Failure Study Group. Am J Kidney Dis 2000;36:767—74.

[208] Lieberthal W, Sheridan AM, Valeri CR. Protective effect of atrial natriuretic factor and mannitol following renal ischemia. Am J Physiol 1990;258:F1266—72.

[209] Linden RJ, Sreeharan N. Humoral nature of the urine response to stimulation of atrial receptors. Q J Exp Physiol 1981;66:431—8.

[210] Lisy O, Jougasaki M, Heublein DM, Schirger JA, Chen HH, Wennberg PW, et al. Renal actions of synthetic dendroaspis natriuretic peptide. Kidney Int 1999;56:502—8.

[211] Lorenz JN, Nieman M, Sabo J, Sanford LP, Hawkins JA, Elitsur N, et al. Uroguanylin knockout mice have increased blood pressure and impaired natriuretic response to enteral NaCl load. J Clin Invest 2003;112:1244—54.

[212] Luchner A, Stevens TL, Borgeson DD, Redfield M, Wei CM, Porter JG, et al. Differential atrial and ventricular expression of myocardial BNP during evaluation of heart failure. Am J Physiol 1998;274:H1684—9.

[213] Lydtin H, Hamilton WF. Effect of acute changes in left atrial pressure on urine flow in unanesthetized dogs. Am J Physiol 1964;207:503—36.

[214] Maack T, Marion DN, Camargo MJ, Kleinert HD, Laragh JH, Vaughan Jr ED, et al. Effects of auriculin (atrial natriuretic factor) on blood pressure, renal function, and the renin—aldosterone system in dogs. Am J Med 1984;77:1069—75.

[215] Maack T, Suzuki M, Almedida FA, Nussenzveig D, Scarborough RW, McEnroe GA, et al. Physiological role of silent receptors of atrial natriuretic factor. Science 1987;238:675—8.

[216] Maki M, Takayanagi R, Misono KS, Pandy KN, Tibbetts C, Inagami T. Structure of rat atrial natriuretic factor precursor deduced for cDNA sequence. Nature 1984;309:722–4.

[217] Marcus LS, Hart D, Packer M, Yushak M, Medina N, Danziger RS, et al. Hemodynamic and renal excretory effects of human brain natriuretic peptide infusions in patients with congestive heart failure. A double-blind, placebo-controlled, randomized crossover trial. Circulation 1996;94:3184–9.

[218] Marie JP, Guillemont H, Hatt PY. Le degree de granulation des cardiocytes auriculaires. Etude planimetrique au cours de differents apports d'eau et de sodium chez le rat. Pathol Biol 1976;24:549–54.

[219] Marin-Grez M, Fleming JT, Steinhausen M. Atrial natriuretic peptide causes pre-glomerular vasodilatation and post-glomerular vasoconstriction in rat kidney. Nature 1986;324:473–6.

[220] Martin DR, Pevahouse JB, Trigg DJ, Vesely DL, Buerkert JE. Three peptides from the ANF prohormone NH_2-terminus are natriuretic and/or kaliuretic. Am J Physiol 1990;258: F1401–8.

[221] Marttila M, Puhakka J, Luodonpaa M, Vuolteenaho O, Ganten L, Ruskoaho H. Augmentation of BNP gene expression in atria by pressure overload in transgenic rats harboring human renin and angiotensinogen genes. Blood Press 1999;8:308–16.

[222] Marx UC, Klodt J, Meyer M, Gerlach H, Rosch P, Forsmann WG, et al. One peptide, two topologies: structure and interconversion dynamics of human uroguanylin isomers. J Pept Res 1998;2:229–40.

[223] Mattingly MT, Brandt RR, Heublein DM, Wei CM, Nir A, Burnett Jr JC. Presence of C-type natriuretic peptide in human kidney and urine. Kidney Int 1994;46:744–7.

[224] McCubrey JA, Steelman LS, Chappell WH, Abrams SL, Wong EWT, Chang F, et al. Roles of the Raf/MEK/ERK pathway in cell growth, malignant transformation and drug resistance. Biochim Biophys Acta 2007;1773:1263–84.

[225] McCubrey JA, Milella M, Tafuri A, Martelli AM, Lunghi P, Bonati A, et al. Targeting the Raf/MEK/ERK pathway with small-molecule inhibitors. Curr Opin Investig Drugs 2008;9:614–30.

[226] McMurray J, Seidenlin PH, Howey JEA, Balfour DJ, Struthers AD. The effect of atrial natriuretic factor on urinary albumin and beta-2-microglobulin excretion in man. Hypertension 1988;6:783–6.

[227] McMurray RW, Vesely DL. Weight reduction decreases atrial natriuretic factor and blood pressure in obese patients. Metabolism 1989;38:1231–7.

[228] Melander O, Frandsen E, Groop L, Hulthen UL. Plasma proANP 1-30 reflects salt sensitivity in subjects with hereditary for hypertension. Hypertension 2002;39:996–9.

[229] Merkouris RW, Miller FC, Catanzarite V, Rigg LA, Quirk Jr JG, Vesely DL. Increase in the plasma levels of the N-terminal and C-terminal portions of the prohormone of atrial natriuretic factor in normal pregnancy. Am J Obstet Gynecol 1990;162: 859–64.

[230] Merkouris RW, Miller FC, Catanzarite V, Quirk Jr JG, Rigg LA, Vesely DL. The N-terminal and C-terminal portions of the atrial natriuretic factor prohormone increase during preeclampsia. Am J Obstet Gynecol 1991;164:1197–202.

[231] Meyer M, Richter R, Forssmann WG. Urodilatin a natriuretic peptide with clinical implications. Eur J Med Res 1998;3: 103–10.

[232] Meyer M, Pfarr E, Schirmer G, Uberbacher HJ, Schope K, Bohm E, et al. Therapeutic use of the natriuretic peptide ularitide in acute renal failure. Ren Fail 1999;21:85–100.

[233] Mills RM, LeJemtel TH, Horton DP, Liang C, Lang R, Silver MA, et al. Sustained hemodynamic effects of an infusion of nesiritide (human b-type natriuretic peptide) in heart failure: a randomized, double-blind, placebo-controlled clinical trial. Natrecor Study Group. J Am Coll Cardiol 1999;34: 155–62.

[234] Molitoris BA, Meyer C, Dahl R, Geerdes A. Mechanism of ischemia-enhanced aminoglycoside binding and uptake by proximal tubule cells. Am J Physiol 1993;264:F907–16.

[235] Morgan DA, Peuler JD, Koepke JP, Mark AL, DiBona GF. Renal sympathetic nerves attenuate the natriuretic effects of atrial peptide. J Lab Clin Med 1989;114:538–44.

[236] Morrissey EC, Wilner KD, Barager RR, Ward DM, Ziegler MG. Atrial natriuretic factor in renal failure and posthemodialytic postural hypotension. Am J Kidney Dis 1988;12: 510–5.

[237] Moskowitz PS, Korobkin M, Rambo ON. Diuresis and improved renal hemodynamics produced by prostaglandin E_1 in the dog with norepinephrine-induced acute renal failure. Invest Radiol 1975;10:284–99.

[238] Moss NG, Fellner RC, Qian X, Yu SJ, Li Z, Nakazato M, et al. Uroguanylin, an intestinal natriuretic peptide, is delivered to the kidney as an unprocessed propeptide. Endocrinology 2008;149:4486–98.

[239] Moss NG, Riguera DA, Solinga RM, Kessler MM, Zimmer DP, Arendshorst WJ, et al. The natriuretic peptide uroguanylin elicits physiologic actions through 2 distinct topoisomers. Hypertension 2009;53:867–76.

[240] Nakao K, Ogawa Y, Suga S, Imura H. Molecular biology and biochemistry of the natriuretic peptide system. I. Natriuretic peptides. J Hypertens 1992;10:907–12.

[241] Nakamoto M, Shapiro JI, Shanley PF, Chan L, Schrier RW. In vitro and in vivo protective effect of atriopeptin III on ischemic acute renal failure. J Clin Invest 1987;80:698–705.

[242] Nakayama K, Ohkubo H, Hirose T, Inayama S, Nakanishi S. mRNA sequence for human cardiodilatin-atrial natriuretic factor precursor and regulation of precursor mRNA in rat atria. Nature 1984;310:699–701.

[243] Nasser A, Dietz JR, Siddique M, Patel H, Khan N, Antwi EK, et al. Effects of kaliuretic peptide on sodium and water excretion in persons with congestive heart failure. Am J Cardiol 2001;88:23–9.

[244] Nemer M, Chamberland M, Sirois D, Argentin J, Drouin RA, Dixon RA, et al. Gene structure of human cardiac hormone precursor, pronatriodilatin. Nature 1984;312:654–6.

[245] Neumayer HH, Blossei N, Seherr-Thohs U, Wagner K. Amelioration of postischaemic acute renal failure in conscious dogs by human atrial natriuretic peptide. Nephrol Dial Transplant 1990;5:32–8.

[246] Ngo L, Bissett JK, Winters CJ, Vesely DL. Plasma prohormone atrial natriuretic peptides 1-98 and 31-67 increase with supraventricular and ventricular arrhytmias. Am J Med Sci 1990;300:71–7.

[247] Ngo L, Wyeth RP, Bissett JK, Hester WL, Newton MT, Sallman AL, et al. Prohormone atrial natriuretic peptides 1-30, and 99-126 increase in proportion to right ventricular pacing rate. Am Heart J 1989;118:893–900.

[248] Nishikimi T, Mori Y, Kobayashi N, Tadokoro K, Wang X, Akimoto K, et al. Renoprotective effect of chronic adrenomedullin infusion in Dahl salt-sensitive rats. Hypertension 2002;39:1077–82.

[249] Ogawa E, Saito Y, Kuwahara K, Harada M, Miyamoto Y, Hamana I, et al. Fibronectin signaling stimulates BNP gene transcription by inhibiting neuron-restrictive silencer element-dependent repression. Cardiovasc Res 2002;53:451–9.

[250] Ohlstein EH, Berkowitz BA. Cyclic guanosine monophosphate mediates vascular relaxation induced by atrial natriuretic factor. Hypertension 1985;7:306–10.

[251] Oikawa S, Imai M, Inuzuka C, Tawaragi Y, Nakazato H, Matsuo H. Structure of dog and rabbit precursors of atrial natriuretic polypeptides deduced from nucleotide sequence of cloned cDNA. Biochem Biophys Res Commun 1985;132:892—9.

[252] Oikawa S, Imai M, Ueno A, Tanaka S, Noguchi T, Nakazato H, et al. Cloning and sequence analysis of cDNA encoding a precursor for human atrial natriuretic peptide. Nature 1984;309:724—6.

[253] Orias R, McCann SM. Natriuresis induced by alpha and beta melanocyte stimulating hormones in rats. Endocrinology 1972;90:700—6.

[254] Ortola FV, Ballermann BJ, Brenner BM. Endogenous ANP augments fractional excretion of Pi, Ca, and Na in rats with reduced renal mass. Am J Physiol 1988;255:F1091—7.

[255] Palmer BF, Alpern RJ. Pathogenesis of edema formation in the nephrotic syndrome. Kidney Int 1997;59:521—7.

[256] Palmer PA, Friedl FE, Giordano AT, Vesely DL. Alteration of environmental salinity modulates atrial natriuretic peptides' concentrations in heart, and hemolymph of the oyster, *Crassostrea virginica*. Comp Biochem Physiol 1994;108A:589—97.

[257] Parkes DG. Cardiovascular actions of adrenomedullin in conscious sheep. Am J Physiol 1995;268:H2574—8.

[258] Parkin DM. Global cancer statistics in the year 2000. Lancet Oncol 2001;2:533—43.

[259] Paul RV, Kirk KA, Navar LG. Renal autoregulation and pressure natriuresis during ANF-induced diuresis. Am J Physiol 1987;253:F424—31.

[260] Payvar F, DeFranco D, Firestone G, Edgar B, Wrange O, O'Kret S, et al. Sequence specific binding of glucocorticoid receptor to MMTV DNA at sites within and upstream of the transcribed region. Cell 1983;35:381—92.

[261] Pedram A, Razandi M, Hu RM, Levin ER. Vasoactive peptides modulate vascular endothelial cell growth factor production and endothelial cell proliferation and invasion. J Biol Chem 1997;272:17097—103.

[262] Peters JP. Body water: the exchange of fluids in man. Springfield, IL: Charles C Thomas; 1935.

[263] Pettersson A, Hedner J, Hedner T. Renal interaction between sympathetic activity and ANP in rats with chronic heart failure. Acta Physiol Scand 1989;135:487—92.

[264] Pettersson A, Hedner J, Ricksten SE, Towle AC, Hedner T. Acute volume expansion as a physiological stimulus for the release of atrial natriuretic peptides in the rat. Life Sci 1986;38:1127—33.

[265] Pevahouse JB, Flanigan WJ, Winters CJ, Vesely DL. Normalization of elevated circulating N-terminal and C-terminal atrial natriuretic factor prohormone concentrations by renal transplantation. Transplantation 1992;53:1375—7.

[266] Pikkarainen S, Tokola H, Majalahti-Palviainen T, Kerkela R, Hautala N, Bahalla SS, et al. GATA-4 is a nuclear mediator of mechanical stretch-activated hypertrophic program. J Biol Chem 2003;278:23807—16.

[267] Pitchumoni CS. Pancreatic disease. In: Stein JH, editor. Internal Medicine. St. Louis, MO: Mosby; 1998. p. 2233—47.

[268] Poche R. Electronenmikroskopische untersuchuwgen des liopfuscin im herzmuskel des menschen. Zbl Allg Path Anat 1957;96:395.

[269] Poche R. Submikroskopische beitrage zur pathologie der herzmuskelzelle bei phosphorvergiftung. Hypertrophie, atrophie und kaliummangel. Virchows Arch 1958;331:165—248.

[270] Pollock DM, Mullins MM, Banks RO. Failure of atrial myocardial extract to inhibit renal Na$^+$-K$^+$-ATPase. Renal Physiol 1983;6:295—9.

[271] Potthast R, Ehler E, Sheving LA, Sindic A, Schlatter E, Kuhn M. High salt intake increases uroguanylin expression in mouse kidney. Endocrinology 2001;142:3087—97.

[272] Poulos JE, Gower Jr WR, Fontanet HL, Kalmus GW, Vesely DL. Cirrhosis with ascites: increased atrial natriuretic peptide gene expression in rat ventricle. Gastroenterology 1995;108:1496—503.

[273] Poulos JE, Gower Jr WR, Friedl FE, Vesely DL. Atrial natriuretic peptide gene expression within invertebratic hearts. Gen Comp Endocrinol 1995;100:61—8.

[274] Poulos JE, Gower Jr WR, Sullebarger JT, Fontanet HL, Vesely DL. Congestive heart failure: increased cardiac and extracardiac atrial natriuretic peptide gene expression. Cardiovasc Res 1996;32:909—19.

[275] Proudfoot N. The end of the message. Nature 1982;298:516—7.

[276] Proudfoot NT, Brownlee GG. 3' non-coding region sequences in eukaryotic messenger RNA. Nature 1976;263:211—4.

[277] Qian X, Moss NG, Fellner RC, Goy MF. Circulating prouroguanylin is processed to its active natriuretic form exclusively within the renal tubules. Endocrinology 2008;149:4499—509.

[278] Rahman SN, Kim GE, Mathew AS, Goldberg CA, Allgren R, Schrier RW, et al. Effects of atrial natriuretic peptide in clinical acute renal failure. Kidney Int 1994;45:1731—8.

[279] Raine AE, Anderson JV, Bloom SR, Morris PJ. Plasma atrial natriuretic factor and graft function in renal transplant recipients. Transplantation 1989;48:796—800.

[280] Rambotti MG, Giambanco I, Spreca A. Detection of guanylate cyclases A and B stimulated by natriuretic peptides in gastrointestinal tract of rat. Histochem J 1996;29:117—26.

[281] Ramirez G, Saba SR, Dietz JR, Vesely DL. Immunocytochemical localization of proANF1-30, proANF 31-67, and atrial natriuretic factor in the kidney. Kidney Int 1992;41:334—41.

[282] Rapoport RM. Cyclic guanosine monophosphate inhibition of contraction may be mediated through inhibition of phosphatidylinositol hydrolysis in rat aorta. Circ Res 1986;58:407—10.

[283] Rapoport RM, Ginsburg R, Waldman SA, Murad F. Effects of atriopeptins on relaxation and cyclic GMP levels in human coronary artery *in vitro*. Eur J Pharmacol 1986;124:193—6.

[284] Rascher W, Tulassay T, Lang RE. Atrial natriuretic peptide in plasma of volume-overloaded children with chronic renal failure. Lancet 1985;2:303—5.

[285] Rashed HM, Su H, Patel TB. Atrial natriuretic peptide inhibits growth of hepatoblastoma (HEP G2) cells by means of activation of clearance receptors. Hepatology 1993;17:677—84.

[286] Richards AM, Lainchbury JG, Nicholls MG, Cameron AV, Yandle TG. *Dendroaspis* natriuretic peptide: endogenous or dubious? Lancet 2002;359:5—6.

[287] Riordan JR. The cystic fibrosis transmembrane conductance regulator. Annu Rev Physiol 1993;55:609—30.

[288] Ritter D, Chao J, Needleman P, Tetens E, Greenwald JE. Localization, synthetic regulation, and biology of renal atriopeptin-like prohormone. Am J Physiol 1992;263:F503—9.

[289] Roberts PJ, Der CJ. Targeting the RAF-MEK-ERK mitogen-activated protein kinase cascade for the treatment of cancer. Oncogene 2007;26:3291—310.

[290] Rosenzweig A, Seidman CE. Atrial natriuretic factor and related peptide hormones. Annu Rev Biochem 1991;60:229—55.

[291] Rubattu S, Gilberti R, Ganten U, Volpe M. A differential brain atrial natriuretic peptide expression co-segregates with occurrence of early strokes in the stroke prone phenotype of spontaneously hypertensive rat. J Hypertens 1999;17:1849—52.

[292] Rubattu S, Lee-Kirsch MA, DePaolis P, Giliberti R, Gigante B, Lombardi A, et al. Altered structure, regulation, and function

of the gene encoding the atrial natriuretic peptide in stroke prone spontaneously hypertensive rat. Cir Res 1999;85:900−5.

[293] Rubattu S, Ridker P, Stampfer MJ, Volpe M, Henekens CH, Lindpaintner K. The gene encoding atrial natriuretic peptide and the risk of human stroke. Circulation 1999;100:1722−6.

[294] Ruskoaho H. Atrial natriuretic peptide: synthesis, release, and metabolism. Pharmacol Rev 1992;44:479−602.

[295] Ruskoaho H, Leskinen H, Magga J, Tashinen P, Mantymaa P, Vuolteenaho O, et al. Mechanisms of mechanical load-induced atrial natriuretic peptide secretion: role of endothelin, nitric oxide, and angiotensin II. J Mol Med 1997;75:876−85.

[296] Ryu H, Cho KW, Kim SH, Kim SZ, Oh SH, Hwang YH, et al. Frog lymph heart synthesizes and stores immune reactivate atrial natriuretic peptide. Gen Comp Endocrinol 1992;87: 171−7.

[297] Saba SR, Ramirez G, Vesely DL. Immunocytochemical localization of ProANF 1-30, ProANF 31-67, atrial natriuretic factor and urodilatin in the human kidney. Am J Nephrol 1993;13: 85−93.

[298] Saba SR, Garces AH, Clark LC, Gower Jr WR, Vesely DL. Immunocytochemical localization of atrial natriuretic peptide, vessel dilator, long acting natriuretic peptide, and kaliuretic peptide in human pancreatic adenocarcinomas. J Histochem Cytochem 2005;53:989−95.

[299] Saba SR, Vesely DL. Cardiac natriuretic peptides: hormones with anti-cancer effects that localize to nucleus, cytoplasm, endothelium and fibroblasts of human cancers. Histol Hitopathol 2006;21:775−83.

[300] Sagnella GA, Saggar-Malik AK, Buckley MG, Markandu ND, Eastwood JB, MacGregor GA. Association between atrial natriuretic peptide and cyclic GMP in hypertension and in chronic renal failure. Clin Chem Acta 1998;275:9−18.

[301] Samson WK. Adrenomedullin and the control of fluid and electrolyte homeostasis. Annu Rev Physiol 1999;61:363−89.

[302] Samson WK. Proadrenomedullin-derived peptides. Front Neuroendocrinol 1998;19:100−17.

[303] Sands JM, Neylan JF, Olson RA, O'Brien DP, Whelchel JD, Mitch WE. Atrial natriuretic factor does not improve the outcome of cadaveric renal transplantation. J Am Soc Nephrol 1991;1:1081−6.

[304] Santos-Neto MS, Carvalho AF, Monteiro HS, Forte LR, Fonteles MC. Interaction of atrial natriuretic peptide, urodilatin, guanylin and uroguanylin in the isolated perfused rat kidney. Regul Pept 2006;136:14−22.

[305] Sato K, Hirata Y, Imai T, Iwashita M, Mariuo F. Characterization of immunoreactive adrenomedullin in human plasma and urine. Life Sci 1995;57:189−94.

[306] Sato K, Imai T, Iwashina M, Marumo F, Hirata Y. Secretion of adrenomedullin by renal tubular cell lines. Nephron 1998;78:9−14.

[307] Saxenhofer H, Gnadinger MP, Weidmann P, Shaw S, Schohn D, Hess C, et al. Plasma levels and dialysance of atrial natriuretic peptide in terminal renal failure. Kidney Int 1987;32:554−61.

[308] Schafferhans K, Heidbreder E, Grimm D, Heidland A. Norepinephrine-induced acute renal failure: beneficial effects of atrial natriuretic factor. Nephron 1986;44:240−4.

[309] Schermuly RT, Weissmann N, Enke B, Ghofrani HA, Forssmann WG, Grimminger F, et al. Urodilatin, a natriuretic peptide stimulating guanylate cyclase, and the phosphodiesterase five inhibitor dipyridamole attenuate experimental pulmonary hypertension. Am J Respir Cell Mol Biol 2001;25: 219−25.

[310] Schirger JA, Heublein DM, Chen HH, Lisy O, Jougasaki M, Wennberg PW, et al. Presence of Dendroaspis natriuretic peptide-like immunoreactivity in human plasma and its increase during human heart failure. Mayo Clin Proc 1999;74:126−30.

[311] Schlessinger J. Cell signaling by receptor tyrosine kinases. Cell 2000;103:211−25.

[312] Schnermann J, Marin-Grez M, Briggs JP. Filtration pressure response to infusion of atrial natriuretic peptides. Pflugers Arch 1986;406:237−9.

[313] Scholl FA, Dumesic PA, Khavan PA. Effects of active MEK 1 expression in vivo. Cancer Lett 2005;230:1−8.

[314] Schramm L, Heidbreder E, Schaar J, Lopau K, Zimmermann J, Gotz R, et al. Toxic acute renal failure in the rat: effects of diltiazem and urodilatin on renal function. Nephron 1994;68: 454−61.

[315] Schulz-Knappe P, Forssmann K, Herbst F, Hock D, Pipkorn R, Forssmann WG. Isolation and structural analysis of "urodilatin," a new peptide of the cardiodilatin-(ANP)-family, extracted from human urine. Klin Wochenschr 1988;66: 752−9.

[316] Schweitz H, Vigne P, Moinier D, Frelin C, Lazdunski M. A new member of the natriuretic peptide family is present in the venom of the green mamba (Dendroaspis augusticeps). J Biol Chem 1992;267:13928−32.

[317] Scivoletto R, Carcalho MHC. Cardionatrin causes vasodilation in vitro which is not dependent on the presence of endothelial cells. Eur J Pharmacol 1984;101:143−5.

[318] Scriven TA, Burnett Jr JC. Effects of synthetic atrial natriuretic peptide on renal function and renin release in acute experimental heart failure. Circulation 1985;72:892−7.

[319] Sebolt-Leopold JS. Advances in the development of cancer therapeutics directed against the Ras mitogen-activated protein kinase pathway. Clin Can Res 2008;14:3651−6.

[320] Sebolt-Leopold JS, Herrera R. Targeting the mtogen-activated protein kinase casecade to treat cancer. Nature Rev Cancer 2004;4:937−47.

[321] Seidman C, Bloch KD, Klein KA, Smith JA, Seidman JG. Nucleotide sequences of the human and mouse atrial natriuretic factor genes. Science 1984;226:1206−9.

[322] Shaw SG, Weidmann P, Hodler J, Zimmermann A, Paternostro A. Atrial natriuretic peptide protects against ischemic renal failure in the rat. J Clin Invest 1987;80:1232−7.

[323] Shaw SG, Weidmann P, Zimmermann A. Urodilatin not nitroprusside, combined with dopamine reverses ischemic acute renal failure. Kidney Int 1992;42:1153−9.

[324] Shin SJ, Lee YJ, Tan MS, Hsieh TJ, Tsai JH. Increased atrial natriuretic peptide mRNA expression in the kidney of diabetic rats. Kidney Int 1997;51:1100−5.

[325] Sindic A, Velic A, Basoglu C, Hirsch JR, Edemir B, Kuhn M, et al. Uroguanylin and guanylin regulate transport of mouse cortical collecting duct independent of guanylate cyclase C. Kidney Int 2005;68:1008−17.

[326] Sindic A, Schlatter E. Mechanisms of action or uroguanylin and guanylin and their role in salt handling. Nephrol Dial Transplant 2006;21:3007−12.

[327] Soejima H, Grekin RJ, Briggs JP, Schnermann J. Renal response of anesthetized rats to low-dose infusion of atrial natriuretic peptide. Am J Physiol 1988;255:R449−55.

[328] Sosa RE, Volpe M, Marion DN, Atlas SA, Laragh JH, Vaughn Jr ED, et al. Relationship between renal hemodynamic and natriuretic effects of atrial natriuretic factor. Am J Physiol 1986;250:F520−4.

[329] Sothern RB, Vesely DL, Kanabrocki EL, Bremner FW, Third JLAC, Boles MA, et al. Blood pressure and atrial natriuretic peptides correlate throughout the day. Am Heart J 1995;129:907−16.

[330] Sothern RB, Vesely DL, Kanabrocki EL, Hermida RC, Bremner FW, Third JLAC, et al. Temporal (circadian) and functional relationship between atrial natriuretic peptides and blood pressure. Chronobiol Int 1995;12:106−20.

[331] Steinhelper ME, Cochrane KL, Field LJ. Hypotension in transgenic mice expressing atrial natriuretic factor fusion genes. Hypertension 1990;16:301−7.

[332] Sudoh T, Kangawa K, Minamino W, Matsuo H. A new natriuretic peptide in porcine brain. Nature 1988;332:78−81.

[333] Sudoh T, Minamino N, Kangawa K, Matsuo H. C-type natriuretic peptide (CNP): a new member of the natriuretic peptide family identified in porcine brain. Biochem Biophys Res Commun 1990;168:863−70.

[334] Sugawara A, Nakao K, Sakamoto M, Morii N, Yamada T, Itoh H, et al. Plasma concentration of atrial natriuretic polypeptide in essential hypertension. Lancet 1985;2:1426−7.

[335] Sun Y, Eichelbaum EJ, Skelton IV WP, Lenz A, Regales N, Wang H, et al. Vessel dilator and kaliuretic peptide inhibit Ras in human prostate cancer cells. Anticancer Res 2009;29:971−5.

[336] Sun Y, Eichelbaum EJ, Lenz A, Skelton IV WP, Wang H, Vesely DL. Atrial natriuretic peptide and long-acting natriuretic peptide inhibit Ras in human prostate cancer cells. Anticancer Res 2009;29:1889−93.

[337] Sun Y, Eichelbaum EJ, Wang H, Vesely DL. Vessel dilator and kaliuretic peptide inhibit activation of ERK 1/2 in human prostate cancer cells. Anticancer Res 2006;26:3217−22.

[338] Sun Y, Eichelbaum EJ, Wang H, Vesely DL. Atrial natriuretic peptide and long acting natriuretic peptide inhibit ERK 1/2 in prostate cancer cells. Anticancer Res 2006;26:4143−8.

[339] Sun Y, Eichelbaum EJ, Wang H, Vesely DL. Vessel dilator and kaliuretic peptide inhibit MEK 1/2 activation in human prostate cancer cells. Anticancer Res 2007;27:1387−92.

[340] Sun Y, Eichelbaum EJ, Wang H, Vesely DL. Atrial natriuretic peptide and long acting natriuretic peptide inhibit MEK 1/2 activation in human prostate cancer cells. Anticancer Res 2007;27:3813−8.

[341] Sun Y, Eichelbaum EJ, Wang H, Vesely DL. Insulin and epidermal growth factor activation of ERK 1/2 and DNA synthesis is inhibited by four cardiac hormones. J Cancer Mol 2007;3:113−20.

[342] Suzuki E, Hirata Y, Hayakawa H, Omata M, Kojima M, Kangawa K, et al. Evidence for C-type natriuretic peptide production in the rat kidney. Biochem Biophys Res Commun 1993;192:532−8.

[343] Tamura N, Ogawa Y, Chusho H, Nakamura K, Nakao K, Suda M, et al. Cardiac fibrosis in mice lacking brain natriuretic peptide. Proc Natl Acad Sci USA 2000;97:4239−44.

[344] Tateyama H, Hino J, Minamino N, Kangawa K, Ogihara T, Matsuo H. Characterization of immunoreactive brain natriuretic peptide in human cardiac atrium. Biochem Biophys Res Commun 1990;166:1080−7.

[345] Thueauf DJ, Hanford DS, Glembotski CC. Regulation of rat brain natriuretic peptide transcription. Potential role for GATA-related transcription factors in myocardial gene expression. J Biol Chem 1994;269:17772−5.

[346] Tokura T, Kinoshita H, Fujimoto S, Kitamura K, Eto T. Plasma levels of proadrenomedullin N-terminal 20 peptide and adrenomedullin in patients undergoing hemodialysis. Nephron Clin Pract 2003;95:C67−72.

[347] Totsune K, Mackenzie HS, Totsune H, Troy JL, Lytton J, Brenner BM. Upregulation of atrial natriuretic peptide gene expression in remnant kidney of rats with reduced renal mass. J Am Soc Nephrol 1998;9:1613−7.

[348] Totsune K, Takahashi, Murakami O, Satoh F, Sone M, Mouri T. Elevated plasma C-type natriuretic peptide concentrations in patients with chronic renal failure. Clin Sci 1994;87:319−22.

[349] Trippodo NC, MacPhee AA, Cole FE, Blakesley HL. Partial chemical characterization of a natriuretic substance in rat atrial heart tissue. Proc Soc Exp Biol Med 1982;170:502−8.

[350] Tsuchimochi H, Yazaki Y, Ohno H, Takanashi R, Takaku F. Ventricular expression of atrial natriuretic peptide. Lancet 1987;2:336−7.

[351] Valentin JP, Gardner DG, Wiedemann E, Humphreys MH. Modulation of endothelin effects on blood pressure and hematocrit by atrial natriuretic peptide. Hypertension 1991;17:864−9.

[352] Valentin JP, Ying WZ, Couser WG, Humphreys MH. Extra renal resistance to atrial natriuretic peptide in rats with experimental nephrotic syndrome. Am J Physiol 1998;274:F556−63.

[353] Vaporciyan AA, Kies M, Stevens C, Komaki R, Roth JA. Cancer of the lung. In: Kufe DW, Pollock RE, Weichselbaum RR, Bast RC, Gansler TS, Holland JR, Frei III E, editors. Cancer medicine. 6th ed. Hamilton, Ontario, BC: Decker Inc.; 2003. p. 1385−445.

[354] Vari RC, Freeman RH, Davis JO, Villarreal D, Verburg KM. Effect of synthetic atrial natriuretic factor on aldosterone secretion in the rat. Am J Physiol 1986;251:R48−52.

[355] Vesely BA, Alii AA, Song S, Gower Jr WR, Sanchez-Ramos J, Vesely DL. Four peptide hormones specific decrease (up to 97%) of human prostate carcinoma cells. Eur J Clin Invest 2005;35:700−10.

[356] Vesely BA, Eichelbaum EJ, Alli AA, Sun Y, Gower Jr WR, Vesely DL. Urodilatin and four cardiac hormones decrease human renal carcinoma cell number. Eur J Clin Invest 2006;36:810−9.

[357] Vesely BA, Eichelbaum EJ, Alii AA, Sun Y, Gower Jr WR, Vesely DL. Four cardiac hormones cause cell death in 81% of human ovarian adenocarcinoma cells. Cancer Therapy 2007;5:97−104.

[358] Vesely BA, Eichelbaum EJ, Alii AA, Sun Y, Gower Jr WR, Vesely DL. Four cardiac hormones cause cell death of melanoma cells and inhibit their DNA synthesis. Am J Med Sci 2007;334:342−9.

[359] Vesely BA, Eichelbaum EJ, Alii AA, Sun Y, Gower Jr WR, Vesely DL. Four cardiac hormones eliminate 4-fold more human glioblastoma cells than green mamba snake peptide. Cancer Lett 2007;254:94−101.

[360] Vesely BA, Fitz SR, Gower Jr WR, Vesely DL. Vessel dilator: most potent of the atrial natriuretic peptides in decreasing the number and DNA synthesis of squamous lung cancer cells. Cancer Lett 2006;232:226−31.

[361] Vesely BA, McAfee Q, Gower Jr WR, Vesely DL. Four peptides decrease the number of human pancreatic adenocarcinoma cells. Eur J Clin Invest 2003;33:998−1005.

[362] Vesely BA, Song S, Sanchez-Ramos J, Fitz SR, Solivan SM, Gower Jr WR, et al. Four peptide hormones decrease the number of human breast adenocarcinoma cells. Eur J Clin Invest 2005;35:60−9.

[363] Vesely BA, Alli A, Song S, Sanchez-Ramos J, Fitz SR, Gower Jr WR, et al. Primary malignant tumors of the heart: four cardiovascular hormones decrease the number and DNA synthesis of human angiosarcoma cells. Cardiology 2006;105:226−33.

[364] Vesely BA, Song S, Sanchez-Ramos J, Fitz SR, Alli A, Solivan SM, et al. Five cardiac hormones decrease the number of human small-cell cancer cells. Eur J Clin Invest 2005;35:388−98.

[365] Vesely DL. Aprotinin blocks the binding of pro atrial natriuretic peptides 1−30, 31−67, and 99−126 to human placental membranes. Am J Obstet Gynecol 1991;165:567−73.

[366] Vesely DL. Atrial natriuretic hormones. Englewood Cliffs, NJ: Prentice Hall; 1992.

[367] Vesely DL. Atrial natriuretic peptides within invertebrates and plants. Trends Comp Biochem Physiol 1998;4:89−103.

[368] Vesely DL. Atrial natriuretic peptides in pathophysiological diseases. Cardiovasc Res 2001;51:647−58.

[369] Vesely DL. Atrial natriuretic peptide prohormone gene expression: hormones and diseases that upregulate its expression. IUBMB Life 2002;53:153−9.

[370] Vesely DL. Natriuretic peptides and acute renal failure. Am J Physiol 2003;285:F167−77.

[371] Vesely DL, Arnold WC, Winters CJ, Sallman AL, Rico DM. Increased circulating concentration of atrial natriuretic factor in persons with pheochromocytomas. Clin Exp Hypertens [A] 1989;11:353−69.

[372] Vesely DL, Arnold WC, Winters CJ, Sallman AL, Rico DM. Increased circulating concentration of the N-terminus of the atrial natriuretic prohormone in persons with pheochromocytomas. J Clin Endocrinol Metab 1990;71:1138−46.

[373] Vesely DL, Bayliss JM, Sallman AL. Human prepro atrial natriuretic factors 26−55 56−92 and 104−123 increase renal guanylate cyclase activity. Biochem Biophys Res Commun 1987;143:186−93.

[374] Vesely DL, Blankenship M, Douglass MA, McCormick MT, Rodriguez-Paz G, Schocken DD. Atrial natriuretic peptide increases adrenomedullin in the circulation of healthy humans. Life Sci 1996;59:243−54.

[375] Vesely DL, Chiou S, Douglass MA, McCormick MT, Rodriguez-Paz G, Schocken DD. Kaliuretic peptide and long acting natriuretic peptide as well as atrial natriuretic factor inhibit aldosterone secretion. J Endocrinol 1995;146: 373−80.

[376] Vesely DL, Chiou S, Douglass MA, McCormick MT, Rodriguez-Paz G, Schocken DD. Atrial natriuretic peptides negatively and positively modulate circulating endothelin in humans. Metabolism 1996;45:315−9.

[377] Vesely DL, Clark LC, Garces AH, McAfee QW, Soto J, Gower Jr. WR. Novel therapeutic approach for cancer using four cardiovascular hormones. Eur J Clin Invest 2004;34: 674−82.

[378] Vesely DL, Cornett LE, McCleod SL, Nash AA, Norris JS. Specific binding sites for prohormone atrial natriuretic peptides 1−30, 31−67, and 99−126. Peptides 1990;11:193−7.

[379] Vesely DL, Dietz JR, Parks JR, Antwi EA, Overton RM, McCormick MT, et al. Comparison of vessel dilator and long acting natriuretic peptide in the treatment of congestive heart failure. Am Heart J 1999;138:625−32.

[380] Vesely DL, Dietz JR, Parks JR, Baig M, McCormick MT, Cintron G, et al. Vessel dilator enhances sodium and water excretion and has beneficial hemodynamic effects in persons with congestive heart failure. Circulation 1998;98: 323−9.

[381] Vesely DL, Douglass MA, Dietz JR, Giordano AT, McCormick MT, Rodriguez-Paz G, et al. Negative feedback of atrial natriuretic peptides. J Clin Endocrinol Metab 1994;78:1128−34.

[382] Vesely DL, Douglass MA, Dietz JR, Gower Jr WR, McCormick MT, Rodriguez-Paz G, et al. Three peptides from the atrial natriuretic factor prohormone amino terminus lower blood pressure and produce diuresis, natriuresis, and/or kaliuresis in humans. Circulation 1994;90:1129−40.

[383] Vesely DL, Eichelbaum EJ, Sun Y, Alli AA, Vesely BA, Luther SL, et al. Elimination of up to 80% of human pancreatic adenocarcinomas in athymic mice by cardiac hormones. In Vivo 2007;21:445−52.

[384] Vesely DL, Giordano AT. Food intake and body positional change alter the circadian rhythm of atrial natriuretic peptides excretion into human urine. Chronobiol Int 1991;8: 373−84.

[385] Vesely DL, Giordano AT. Atrial natriuretic factor-like peptide and its prohormone within single cell organisms. Peptides 1992;13:177−82.

[386] Vesely DL, Giordano AT. The most primitive heart in the animal kingdom contains the atrial natriuretic peptide hormonal system. Comp Biochem Physiol 1992; 101C:325−9.

[387] Vesely DL, Gower Jr WR, Giordano AT. Atrial natriuretic peptides throughout the plant kingdom: enhancement of solute flow by peptides from the N-terminus of the atrial natriuretic factor prohormone. Am J Physiol 1993;265:E465−77.

[388] Vesely DL, Hadley ME. Calcium requirements for melanophore-stimulating hormone action on melanophores. Science 1971;173:923−5.

[389] Vesely DL, Norris JS, Walters JM, Jespersen RR, Baeyens DA. Atrial natriuretic prohormone peptides 1−30, 31−67 and 79−98 vasodilate the aorta. Biochem Biophys Res Commun 1987;148:1540−8.

[390] Vesely DL, Norsk P, Gower Jr WR, Chiou S, Epstein M. Release of kaliuretic peptide during immersion-induced central hypervolemia in healthy humans. Proc Soc Exp Biol Med 1995;209:20−6.

[391] Vesely DL, Norsk P, Winters CJ, Rico DM, Sallman AL, Epstein M. Increased release of the N-terminal and C-terminal portions of the prohormone of atrial natriuretic factor during immersion-induced central hypervolemia in normal humans. Proc Soc Exp Biol Med 1989;192:230−5.

[392] Vesely DL, Overton RM, Blankenship M, McCormick MT, Schocken DD. Atrial natriuretic peptide increases urodilatin in the circulation. Am J Nephrol 1998;18:204−13.

[393] Vesely DL, Palmer PA, Giordano AT. Atrial natriuretic factor prohormone peptides are present in a variety of tissues. Peptides 1992;13:165−70.

[394] Vesely DL, Perez-Lamboy GI, Schocken DD. Long acting natriuretic peptide, vessel dilator, and kaliuretic peptide enhance urinary excretion of β_2 microglobulin. Metabolism 2000;49: 1592−7.

[395] Vesely DL, Perez-Lamboy GI, Schocken DD. Long acting natriuretic peptide, vessel dilator, and kaliuretic peptide enhance urinary excretion rate of β_2 microglobulin in congestive heart failure patients. J Cardiac Failure 2001;7:55−63.

[396] Vesely DL, Preston R, Gower Jr WR, Chiou S, Epstein M. Increased release of kaliuretic peptide during immersion-induced central hypervolemia in cirrhotic humans. Am J Nephrol 1996;16:128−37.

[397] Vesely DL, Sallman AL, Bayliss JM. Specific binding sites for pro atrial natriuretic factors 1−30, 31−67, and 99−126 on distal nephrons, proximal tubules, renal cortical and medullary membranes. Renal Physiol Biochem 1992;15:23−32.

[398] Vesely DL. San Miguel GI, Hassan I, Schocken DD. Atrial natriuretic hormone, vessel dilator, long acting natriuretic hormone, and kaliuretic hormone decrease the circulating concentrations of corticotropin releasing hormone, corticotropin and cortisol. J Clin Endocrinol Metab 2001;86:4244−9.

[399] Vesely DL, Vesely BA, Eichelbaum EJ, Sun Y, Alli AA, Gower Jr. WR. Four cardiac hormones eliminate up to two-thirds of human breast cancers in athymic mice. In Vivo 2007;21:973−8.

[400] Vesely DL, Winters CJ, Sallman AL. Prohormone atrial natriuretic peptides 1−30 and 31−67 increase in hyperthyroidism and decrease in hypothyroidism. Am J Med Sci 1989;297: 209−15.

III. FLUID AND ELECTROLYTE REGULATION AND DYSREGULATION

[401] Vesely MD, Gower Jr WR, Perez-Lamboy GI, Overton RM, Graddy L, Vesely DL. Evidence for an atrial natriuretic peptide-like gene in plants. Exp Biol Med 2001;226:61–5.

[402] Vesely MD, Vesely DL. Environmental upregulation of atrial natriuretic peptide gene in the living fossil, *Limulus polyphemus.* Biochem Biophys Res Commun 1999;254:751–6.

[403] Villarreal D, Freeman RH, Reams GP. Natriuretic peptides and salt sensitivity: endocrine cardiorenal integration in heart failure. Congest Heart Fail 2002;8:29–36.

[404] Villarreal D, Freeman RH, Taraben A, Reams GP. Modulation of renin secretion by atrial natriuretic factor prohormone fragment 31–67. Am J Med Sci 1999;318:330–5.

[405] Villarreal D, Reams GP, Taraben A, Freeman RH. Hemodynamic and renal effects of proANF 31-67 in hypertensive rats. Proc Soc Exp Biol Med 1999;221:166–70.

[406] Vlasuk G, Miller J, Beneen G, Lewicki J. Structure and analysis of the bovine atrial natriuretic peptide precursor gene. Biochem Biophys Res Commun 1986;136:396–403.

[407] Vuolteenaho O, Arjama O, Vakkuri O, Madsniemi T, Nikkila L, Kangas J, et al. Atrial natriuretic peptide (ANP) in rat gastrointestinal tract. FEBS Lett 1988;233:79–82.

[408] Vuolteenaho O, Leskinen H, Magga J, Taskinen P, Mantymaa P, Leppaluoto J, et al. Regulation of atrial natriuretic peptide synthesis and secretion. In: Vesely DL, editor. Atrial natriuretic peptides. Trivandrum, India: Research Signpost; 1997. p. 39–52.

[409] Waldman SA, Rapoport RM, Murad F. Atrial natriuretic factor selectively activates particulate guanylate cyclase and elevates cyclic GMP in rat tissues. J Biol Chem 1984;259:14332–4.

[410] Walshe JJ, Venuto RC. Acute oliguric renal failure induced by indomethacin: possible mechanism. Ann Intern Med 1979;91:47–9.

[411] Walter T, Stepan H, Pankow K, Becker M, Schultheiss HP, Sein WE. Biochemical analysis of neutral endopeptidase activity reveals independent catabolism of atrial and brain natriuretic peptide. J Biol Chem 2004;385:179–84.

[412] Wang T, Kawabata M, Haneda M, Takabatake T. Effects of uroguanylin, an intestinal natriuretic peptide, on ubuloglomerular feedback. Hypertens Res 2003;26:557–82.

[413] Weidmann P, Hasler L, Gnadinger MP, Lang RE, Uehlinger DE, Shaw S, et al. Blood levels and renal effects of atrial natriuretic peptide in normal man. J Clin Invest 1986;77:734–42.

[414] Werb R, Clark WF, Lindsay RM, Jones EO, Turnbull DI, Linton AL. Protective effect of prostaglandin [PGE$_2$] in glycerol-induced acute renal failure in rats. Clin Sci Mol Med 1978;55:505–7.

[415] Westenfelder C, Birch FM, Baranowski RL, Rosenfeld MJ, Shiozawa DK, Kablitz C. Atrial natriuretic factor and salt adaptation in the teleost fish *Gila atraria.* Am J Physiol 1988;255:F1281–6.

[416] Weston MW, Cintron GB, Giordano AT, Vesely DL. Normalization of circulating atrial natriuretic peptides in cardiac transplant recipients. Am Heart J 1994;127:129–42.

[417] Wilkins MR, Wood JA, Adu D, Lote CJ, Kendall MJ, Michael J. Change in plasma immunoreactive atrial natriuretic peptide during sequential ultrafiltration and haemodialysis. Clin Sci 1986;71:157–60.

[418] Williamson JR, Holmberg SW, Chang K, Marvel J, Sutera SP, Needleman P. Mechanisms underlying atriopeptin-induced increases in hematocrit and vascular permeation in rats. Circ Res 1989;64:890–9.

[419] Winquist RJ, Faison EP, Waldman SA, Schwartz K, Murad F, Rapoport RM. Atrial natriuretic factor elicits an endothelium independent relaxation and activates particulate guanylate cyclase in vascular smooth muscle. Proc Natl Acad Sci USA 1984;81:7661–4.

[420] Winters CJ, Sallman AL, Baker BJ, Meadows J, Rico DM, Vesely DL. The N-terminus and a 4000 molecular weight peptide from the mid portion of the N-terminus of the atrial natriuretic factor prohormone each circulate in humans and increase in congestive heart failure. Circulation 1989;80:438–49.

[421] Winters CJ, Sallman AL, Meadows J, Rico DM, Vesely DL. Two new hormones: prohormone atrial natriuretic peptides 1–30 and 31–67 circulate in man. Biochem Biophys Res Commun 1988;150:231–6.

[422] Winters CJ, Vesely DL. Change in plasma immunoreactive N-terminus, C-terminus, and 4000 dalton mid portion of atrial natriuretic factor prohormone with hemodialysis. Nephron 1991;58:17–22.

[423] Woolf AS, Mansell MA, Hoffbrand BI, Cohen SL, Moult PJ. The effect of low dose intravenous 99–126 atrial natriuretic factor infusion in patients with chronic renal failure. Postgrad Med J 1989;65:362–6.

[424] Wolff RA, Abbruzzese JL, Evans DB. Neoplasms of the exocrine pancreas. In: Holland JF, Frei III E, editors. Cancer medicine. London: BC Decker Inc; 2000. p. 1436–74.

[425] Wu J, Harrison JK, Dent P, Lynch KR, Weber MJ, Sturgill TW. Identification and characterization of a new mammalian mitogen-activated protein kinase kinase MKK-2. Mol Cell Biol 1993;13:4539–48.

[426] Yamanaka M, Greenberg B, Johnson L, Seilhamer J, Brewer M, Friedemann T, et al. Cloning and sequence analysis of the cDNA for the rat atrial natriuretic factor precursor. Nature 1984;309:719–22.

[427] Yang Q, Gower Jr WR, Li C, Chen P, Vesely DL. Atrial natriuretic-like peptide and its prohormone within Metasequoia. Proc Soc Exp Biol Med 1999;221:188–92.

[428] Yokota N, Bruneau BG, Fernandez BE, Kuroski de Bold ML, Piazza LA, Eid H, et al. Dissociation of cardiac hypertrophy, myosin heavy chain isoform expression, and natriuretic peptide production in DOCA-salt rats. Am J Hypertens 1995;8:301–10.

[429] Yonemaru M, Ishii K, Murad F, Raffin TA. Atriopeptin-induced increases in endothelial permeability are associated with elevated cGMP levels. Am J Physiol 1992;263:L363–9.

[430] Yoshida K, Yamagata T, Tomura Y, Suzuki-Kusaba M, Yoshida M, Hisa H, et al. Effects of c-type natriuretic peptide on vasoconstriction in dogs. Eur J Pharmacol 1997;338:131–4.

[431] Yu SM, Hung LM, Lin CC. CGMP-elevating agents suppress proliferation of vascular smooth muscle cells by inhibiting the activation of epidermal growth factor signaling pathway. Circulation 1997;95:1269–77.

[432] Yuge S, Inoue K, Hyodo S, Takei Y. A novel guanylin family (guanylin, uroguanylin, and renoguanylin) in eels: possible osmoregulartory hormones in intestine and kidney. J Biol Chem 2003;278:22726–33.

[433] Zeidel ML. Renal actions of atrial natriuretic peptide: regulation of collecting duct sodium and water transport. Annu Rev Physiol 1990;52:747–59.

[434] Zeidel ML. Regulation of collecting duct Na$^+$ reabsorption by ANP 31–67. Clin Exp Pharmacol Physiol 1995;22:121–4.

[435] Zeidel ML, Kikeri D, Silva P, Burrowes M, Brenner BM. Atrial natriuretic peptides inhibit conductive sodium uptake by

rabbit inner medullary collecting duct cells. J Clin Invest 1988;82:1067−74.

[436] Zhang PL, Mackenzie HS, Troy KL, Brenner BM. Effects of natriuretic peptide receptor inhibition on remnant kidney function in rats. Kidney Int 1994;46:414−20.

[437] Zietse R, Schalekamp MA. Effect of synthetic human atrial natriuretic peptide (102−126) in nephrotic syndrome. Kidney Int 1988;34:717−24.

[438] Zimmerman RS, Gharib H, Zimmerman D, Heublein D, Burnett Jr JC. Atrial natriuretic peptide in hypothyroidism. J Clin Endocrinol Metab 1987;64:353−5.

[439] Zimmerman RS, Trippodo NC, MacPhee AA, Martinez AZ, Barbee RW. High-dose atrial natriuretic factor enhances

albumin escape from the systemic but not the pulmonary circulation. Circ Res 1990;67:461−8.

[440] Zivin RA, Condra JH, Dixon R, Seidah NG, Chreitien M, Nemer M, et al. Molecular cloning and characterization of DNA sequences encoding rat and human ANF. Proc Natl Acad Sci USA 1984;81:6325−9.

[441] Zuidema GD, Clarke NP, Reeves JL, Gauer OH, Henry JP. Influence of moderate changes in blood volume on urine flow. Am J Physiol 1956;186:89−92.

[442] Ying Sun, Ehrentraud J. Eichelbaum, Anne Lenz, Hai Wang, David L. Vesely. Epidermal growth factor's activation of Ras is inhibited by four cardiac hormones. European Journal of Clinical Investigation, 2010;40(5):408−13.

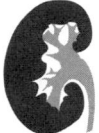

Pathophysiology of Sodium Retention and Wastage

Biff F. Palmer[1], Robert J. Alpern[2] and Donald W. Seldin[1]

[1]Department of Internal Medicine, Division of Nephrology, University of Texas Southwestern Medical Center, Dallas, TX, USA

[2]Office of the Dean, Yale University School of Medicine, New Haven, CT, USA

INTRODUCTION

Extracellular fluid (ECF) volume is determined by the balance between sodium intake and renal excretion of sodium. Under normal circumstances, wide variations in salt intake lead to parallel changes in renal salt excretion, such that ECF volume is maintained within narrow limits. This relative constancy of ECF volume is achieved by a series of afferent sensing systems, central integrative pathways, and renal and extrarenal effector mechanisms acting in concert to modulate sodium excretion by the kidney.

In the major edematous states, effector mechanisms responsible for sodium retention behave in a more-or-less nonsuppressible manner, resulting in either subtle or overt expansion of ECF volume. In some instances, an intrinsic abnormality of the kidney leads to primary retention of sodium, resulting in expansion of ECF volume. In other instances, the kidney retains sodium secondarily as a result of an actual or sensed reduction in effective circulatory volume.

Renal sodium wastage can be defined as the inability of the kidney to conserve sodium to such an extent that continued loss of sodium into the urine leads to contraction of intravascular volume and hypotension. Renal sodium wastage occurs in circumstances where renal sodium transport is pharmacologically interrupted (administration of diuretics), where the integrity of renal tubular function is breached (tubulointerstitial renal disease) or when mineralocorticoid activity or tubular responsiveness are diminished or absent.

SODIUM INTAKE AND SODIUM BALANCE

Under normal circumstances, renal excretion of sodium is regulated so that balance is maintained between intake and output, and ECF volume is stabilized. A subject maintained on a normal-sodium diet is in balance when body weight is constant, and sodium intake and output are equal. When the diet is abruptly decreased, a transient negative sodium balance ensues. A slight contraction of ECF volume signals activation of sodium-conserving mechanisms, which lead to decreases in urinary sodium excretion. After a few days, sodium balance is achieved and ECF volume and weight are stabilized, albeit at a lower value. If sodium intake is increased to the previous normal values, transient positive sodium balance leads to expansion of ECF volume, thereby suppressing those mechanisms that enhanced sodium reabsorption. A new steady-state is reached when ECF volume has risen sufficiently so that sodium excretion now equals intake (Figure 38.1). In both directions a steady-state is achieved, whereby sodium intake equals output, while ECF volume is expanded during salt loads and shrunk during salt restriction. The kidney behaves as though ECF volume is the major regulatory element modulating sodium excretion.

The major edematous states — congestive heart failure, cirrhosis of the liver, and nephrotic syndrome — depart strikingly from those constraints. These states are characterized by persistent renal salt retention despite progressive expansion of ECF volume.

Seldin and Giebisch's The Kidney, Fifth Edition.
DOI: http://dx.doi.org/10.1016/B978-0-12-381462-3.00038-0

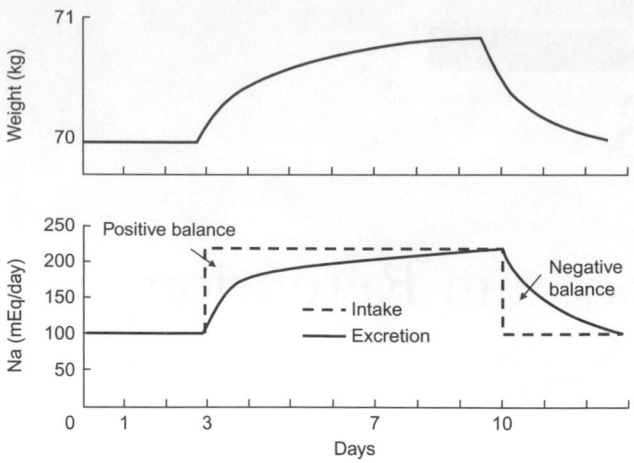

FIGURE 38.1 Changes in body weight in response to abrupt changes in dietary salt demonstrating the ability of a normal subject to maintain salt balance with only minimal changes in extracellular fluid volume.

Unrelenting sodium reabsorption is not the result of diminished sodium intake or even in most cases diminished plasma volume, as dietary salt is adequate and total ECF and plasma volumes are expanded. Renal sodium excretion no longer parallels changes in ECF volume; rather, the kidney behaves as if sensing a persistent low-volume stimulus. Some critical component of ECF volume remains underfilled.

PRIMARY AND SECONDARY EDEMA

A common feature of the major edematous states is persistent renal salt retention despite progressive expansion of both plasma and ECF volume. Two themes have been proposed to explain the persistent salt retention that characterizes the major edematous states: salt retention may be a primary abnormality of the kidney or a secondary response to some disturbance in circulation.

Primary edema (overflow, overfill, nephritic) refers to expansion of ECF volume and subsequent edema formation consequent to a primary defect in renal sodium excretion. Increased ECF volume and expansion of its subcompartments result in manifestations of a well-filled circulation. Hypertension and increased cardiac output are commonly present. The mechanisms normally elicited in response to an underfilled circulation are suppressed (↓renin−angiotensin−aldosterone, ↓ antidiuretic hormone (ADH), ↓activity of sympathetic nerves, ↓circulating catecholamines). Acute post-streptococcal glomerulonephritis and acute or advanced chronic kidney disease are disorders in which edema formation is primary in origin.

Secondary edema (underfill) results from the response of normal kidneys to actual or sensed underfilling of the circulation. In this form of edema, a primary disturbance within the circulation secondarily triggers renal mechanisms for sodium retention. Those systems that normally serve to defend the circulation are activated (rises in renin−angiotensin−aldosterone, ADH, activity of sympathetic nerves, and circulating catecholamines). The renal response in underfill edema is similar to that in normal subjects placed on a low-salt diet, that is, low fractional excretion of sodium, increased filtration fraction, and prerenal azotemia. Despite these similarities, a number of critical features distinguish these two states: (1) sodium balance is positive in underfill edema while salt-restricted normal subjects are in balance; and (2) administration of salt to sodium-restricted normals transiently expands ECF volume, after which sodium excretion equals intake, whereas in underfill edema, ECF volume expands progressively consequent to unyielding salt retention; and features of an underfilled circulation persist in underfill edema, while the circulation is normalized in normals.

The circulatory compartment that signals persistent activation of sodium-conserving mechanisms in secondary edema is not readily identifiable. Cardiac output may be high (arteriovenous shunts) or low (dilated cardiomyopathy). Similarly, plasma volume may be increased (arteriovenous shunts and heart failure) or decreased (some cases of nephrotic syndrome). The body fluid compartment ultimately responsible for signaling a volume-regulatory reflex leading to renal sodium retention is effective arterial blood volume (EABV). EABV identifies that critical component of arterial blood volume, actual or sensed, that regulates sodium reabsorption by the kidney.[184] In both normal circumstances and the major edematous states, the magnitude of EABV is the major determinant of renal salt and water handling.

CONCEPT OF EFFECTIVE ARTERIAL BLOOD VOLUME

In order to explain adequately persistent sodium retention in underfill edema, two cardinal features must exist. First, there must be a persistent low-volume stimulus sensed by the kidney that is then translated into persistent, indeed often unrelenting, retention of sodium despite adequate salt intake and overexpansion of ECF volume. Second, there must be a disturbance in those forces that partition retained fluid into the various subcompartments of the ECF space, resulting in an inability to terminate the low-volume stimulus. The first feature can be ascribed to a shrunken EABV, a feature common to all major edematous states. The second feature can be attributed to a disruption in Starling forces, which normally dictate the distribution of fluid within the extracellular compartment. A disturbance in the circulation exists such that retained fluid is unable to restore EABV but rather is sequestered, resulting in edema formation.

Fluctuations in EABV are modulated by two key determinants: (1) filling of the arterial tree (normally determined by venous return and cardiac output); and (2) peripheral resistance (a factor influenced by compliance of the vasculature and degree of arteriolar runoff). A reduction in EABV can be the result of decreased arterial blood volume owing to low cardiac output, as in congestive heart failure. Conversely, EABV can be reduced in the face of increased arterial blood volume when there is excessive peripheral runoff, as seen in arteriovenous shunting and vasodilation. Increased compliance of the arterial vasculature in which arterial blood volume is reduced relative to the holding capacity of the vascular tree results in decreased EABV. For example, administration of salt to a subject with a highly compliant or "slack" circulation (as in pregnancy or cirrhosis) results in a sluggish natriuretic response, in contrast to a high resistance or "tight" circulation (as in primary aldosteronism or accelerated hypertension) in which salt administration causes prompt natriuresis.

Under normal circumstances, EABV is well-correlated with ECF volume. Figure 38.1 depicts the relationship between subcompartments of ECF volume and renal sodium excretion in both normal and edematous states. Under normal circumstances, subcompartments of ECF volume freely communicate in response to changes in dietary sodium, such that expansion or shrinkage of these compartments occurs in concert (Figure 38.2, states 1A and 1B). In steady-state conditions, sodium intake and output are in balance; the set point at which balance is attained is dictated by salt intake.

By contrast, major edematous states are characterized by a shrunken EABV, which cannot be filled despite expansion of one or more subcompartments. No longer is EABV well-correlated with total ECF volume and salt intake. Due to a disturbance in the forces that normally partition fluid into the various subcompartments of ECF space, EABV remains contracted even though total ECF volume is greatly expanded. Activation of sodium-conserving mechanisms persists, despite plentiful salt intake. Such derangements in fluid distribution can be categorized as disturbances in Starling forces within the interstitial space, between interstitial space and vascular tree, and disturbances within the circulation. These disturbances are summarized next.

1. *Trapped fluid* (Figure 38.2, state 2A). In the first type of disturbance, fluid is trapped within a pathologic compartment such that it cannot contribute to effective extracellular volume, that is, volume capable of filling interstitial and vascular spaces. Decrease in effective extracellular volume leads to decreases in total blood volume, arterial blood volume, and EABV, and renal sodium retention is stimulated. Retention of salt and water cannot re-expand effective extracellular volume, as fluid is sequestered into an abnormal fluid compartment behind the "Starling block" within the interstitial space. Such spacing of fluid into inflamed tissue, vesicles and bullae, peritonitis, necrotizing pancreatitis, rhabdomyolysis, and burns functionally behaves as if lost from the body.

2. *Reduced oncotic pressure.* A reduction in the circulating level of albumin can lead to a second type of fluid maldistribution. Decreased plasma oncotic pressure allows fluid to translocate from the vascular compartment to the interstitial space. Reductions in total blood volume, arterial blood volume, and EABV lead to sodium retention. The retained salt and water, owing to a "Starling block" across the capillary bed, leaks into the interstitial space.

3. *Vascular disturbances* (Figure 38.2, states 2B and 2C). A third type of fluid distributory disturbance results from abnormalities within the circulation, and can be of two types. The prototypical example of the first type is congestive heart failure. A failing ventricle results in decreased cardiac output and high diastolic intraventricular pressures. Venous return is impeded, with consequent reductions in arterial blood volume and EABV. Sodium retention is stimulated, but arterial blood volume and EABV remain contracted due to a circulatory block across the heart. In consequence, venous volume expands and leads to transudation of fluid into the interstitial space. The second type of circulatory abnormality that leads to fluid maldistribution is exemplified by arteriovenous shunting (e.g., Paget's disease, beriberi, thyrotoxicosis, anemia, cirrhosis). Widespread shunting through multiple small arteriovenous communications results in increased venous return, thereby augmenting cardiac output and arterial filling. However, arterial runoff and vasodilation lead to underperfusion of some critical area in the microcirculation. The circulatory block lies between the arterial blood volume and EABV.

What distinguishes secondary edematous states from the normal circumstance is an inability to expand EABV owing to Starling or circulatory blocks within the extracellular space. Normally, the system of

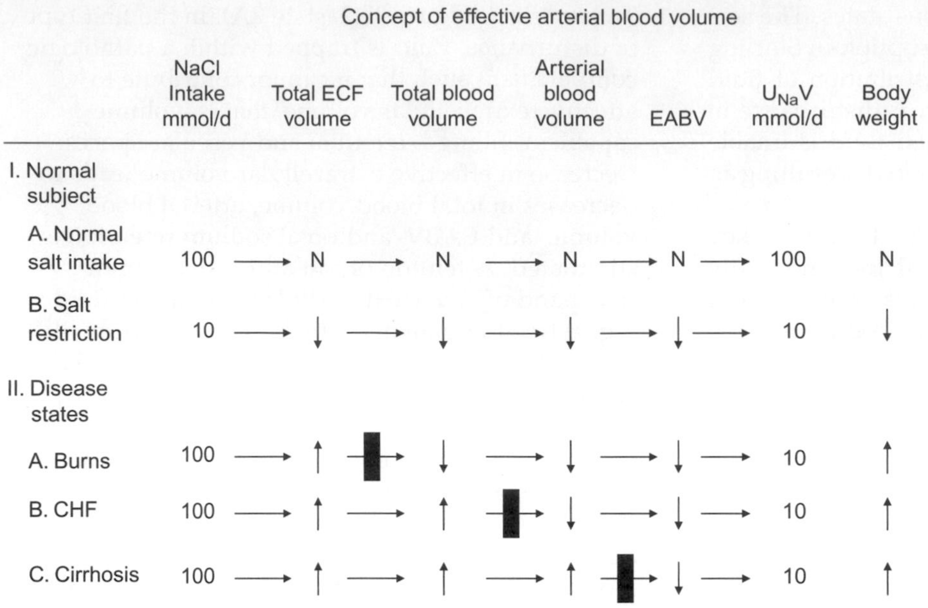

Concept of effective arterial blood volume

	NaCl Intake mmol/d	Total ECF volume	Total blood volume	Arterial blood volume	EABV	$U_{Na}V$ mmol/d	Body weight
I. Normal subject							
A. Normal salt intake	100	→ N →	N →	N →	N →	100	N
B. Salt restriction	10	→ ↓ →	↓ →	↓ →	↓ →	10	↓
II. Disease states							
A. Burns	100	→ ↑ ▮	↓ →	↓ →	↓ →	10	↑
B. CHF	100	→ ↑ →	↑ ▮	↓ →	↓ →	10	↑
C. Cirrhosis	100	→ ↑ →	↑ →	↑ ▮	↓ →	10	↑

FIGURE 38.2 Concept of effective arterial blood volume and effect of fluid distributory disturbances on sodium balance and sodium excretion.

volume regulation behaves as an open system, such that fluctuations in one compartment are quickly translated into parallel changes in other compartments; total ECF volume and EABV are closely related. In contrast, volume regulation in underfill edema can be regarded as clamped; EABV remains shrunken despite expansion of the subcompartments of the extracellular space. EABV becomes dissociated from total ECF volume; salt retention becomes unrelenting and salt administration cannot re-expand the contracted EABV.

The reader is referred to the fourth edition of this book, in which a comprehensive discussion is provided on the afferent and efferent mechanisms involved in the regulation of extracellular fluid volume under normal circumstances. An overview of renal sodium handling in each segment of the nephron was also provided in that discussion. In this edition, the chapter will focus exclusively on the pathophysiology of the major edematous and salt-wasting states.

CONGESTIVE HEART FAILURE

The fundamental abnormality underlying congestive heart failure is an inability of the heart to maintain its function as a pump. As a result, a series of complex compensatory reflexes are initiated that serve to defend the circulation. The renal response to a failing myocardium is retention of salt and water resulting in expansion of ECF volume. If myocardial dysfunction is mild, expansion of ECF volume leads to increased left ventricular end-diastolic volume, which raises cardiac output according to the dictates of the Frank–Starling principle. In this state of compensated congestive heart failure, salt intake and output come into balance, but at the expense of an expanded ECF volume. Further deterioration in ventricular function leads to further renal retention of salt and water. There is progressive expansion of ECF volume and features of a congested circulation become manifest: peripheral edema, engorged neck veins, and pulmonary edema. Despite massive overexpansion of ECF volume, the kidneys behave as though they were responding to a low-volume stimulus. In subsequent sections, a detailed analysis of the afferent and efferent regulatory limbs in congestive heart failure will be provided.

Afferent Sensing Mechanisms in Congestive Heart Failure

Low and High Pressure Baroreceptors

A characteristic feature in many forms of congestive heart failure is increased stretch and transmural pressure within the cardiac atria. These alterations would normally provide afferent signals that suppress sympathetic outflow and decrease the release of renin and ADH, and ultimately result in a diuretic and natriuretic response. In congestive heart failure, this afferent signaling mechanism is markedly perturbed. Despite the presence of venous congestion and elevated cardiac filling pressures, sympathetic nervous activity and serum concentrations of renin and ADH are increased and urinary salt excretion is blunted. Both clinical and experimental studies are consistent with a decrease in sensitivity of the pressure-sensitive receptors in the cardiac atria.

Increased renal sympathetic nerve activity in cardiac failure has also been attributed to impaired arterial baroreceptor function. High pressure baroreceptors in the carotid sinus and aortic arch normally exert a tonic inhibitory effect on central nervous system sympathetic outflow. Although the precise mechanism for the sympathoexcitation is not known, a sustained reduction in arterial pressure is unlikely to be the sole explanation, since arterial pressure is usually normal in congestive heart failure. Rather, sympathetic tone becomes insensitive to manipulations that normally suppress or enhance its activity. For example, infusion of nitroprusside increases both the heart rate and the circulating norepinephrine levels in normal subjects, whereas equivalent hypotensive doses in subjects with congestive heart failure elicit a blunted response.[149] Similarly, patients with heart failure show less bradycardia when arterial pressure is raised by infusion of phenylephrine. Such alterations in baroreflex function may result from abnormalities peripherally or alterations in central autonomic regulatory centers.

Several observations suggest angiotensin II may contribute to the depressed baroreflex sensitivity in heart failure. Angiotensin II has been shown to upwardly reset the arterial baroreflex control of heart rate in the rabbit, independent of a change in arterial pressure.[20] In the rat, increased levels of endogenous angiotensin II produced by changes in dietary salt intake tonically increase the basal level of renal sympathetic nerve activity, and upwardly reset the arterial baroreflex control of renal sympathetic nerve activity.[36] In experimental models, administration of an angiotensin II receptor blocker can reverse these changes and improve the sensitivity of the arterial baroreflex mechanism. Interestingly, captopril administered to patients with congestive heart failure restores the normal hemodynamic response to postural tilt and infusion of vasoconstrictive agents.[30]

Cardiac Output

A reduction in cardiac output has been suggested as the afferent signal that leads to Na retention in heart failure. When cardiac output is reduced by constriction of the abdominal or thoracic vena cava, urinary sodium excretion is typically decreased.[166,186] Restoring cardiac output to normal by autologous blood transfusion ameliorates renal salt retention, despite persistently elevated venous and hepatic pressures.[166] By contrast, rats with small-to-moderate myocardial infarctions have normal capacities to increase cardiac output in response to volume loads, and yet renal sodium excretion remains blunted in these animals. Even when cardiac output is increased above normal, as with the creation of an arteriovenous fistula in dogs, clinical findings of ascites and peripheral and pulmonary edema develop.[218] Despite increased cardiac output, levels of renin, aldosterone, and ANP are high.[202]

Thus, the signal which initiates renal salt retention in congestive heart failure cannot originate solely from a decrease in cardiac output.

Other Sensors

Other afferent sensing mechanisms potentially active in congestive heart failure include intrahepatic baroreceptors and mechanoreceptors within the kidney. Chemosensitive receptors that respond to changing levels of metabolic breakdown products may participate in sensing of ECF volume. One such sensing mechanism may relate to the cardiac sympathetic afferent reflex. The reflex begins with sympathetic afferent fibers that respond to changes in cardiac pressure and dimension or substances that may accumulate in ischemia or heart failure. The reflex is excitatory in nature, such that activation of the afferent fibers leads to increased central sympathetic outflow. In summary, a contracted EABV serves as the afferent signal that elicits activation of effector mechanisms resulting in sodium retention. As with other edematous disorders, the exact volume compartment that comprises EABV has not been elucidated (Figure 38.3).

Effector Mechanisms in Congestive Heart Failure

Nephron Sites of Renal Sodium Retention

Renal sodium handling in the setting of congestive heart failure is similar to that which occurs in an otherwise normal individual who is volume-depleted. Activation of effector mechanisms lead to alterations in renal hemodynamics and tubular transport mechanisms that culminate in renal salt retention.

Renal hemodynamics in congestive heart failure are characterized by reduced renal plasma flow and a well-preserved glomerular filtration rate, such that filtration fraction is typically increased. In a rat model of myocardial infarction, Hostetter et al.[75] found a positive correlation between the decline in renal plasma flow and the degree to which left ventricular function was impaired. The glomerular filtration rate remained well-preserved as a result of an increased filtration fraction, except in animals with a severely compromised left ventricle. When examined at the level of the single nephron, these hemodynamic changes were found to be the result of a disproportionate increase in efferent arteriolar vasoconstriction and increased glomerular capillary hydraulic pressure.[76] Treatment with an angiotensin-converting enzyme inhibitor caused a decline in filtration fraction and efferent arteriolar resistance, suggesting an important role for angiotensin II in mediating efferent arteriolar constriction.

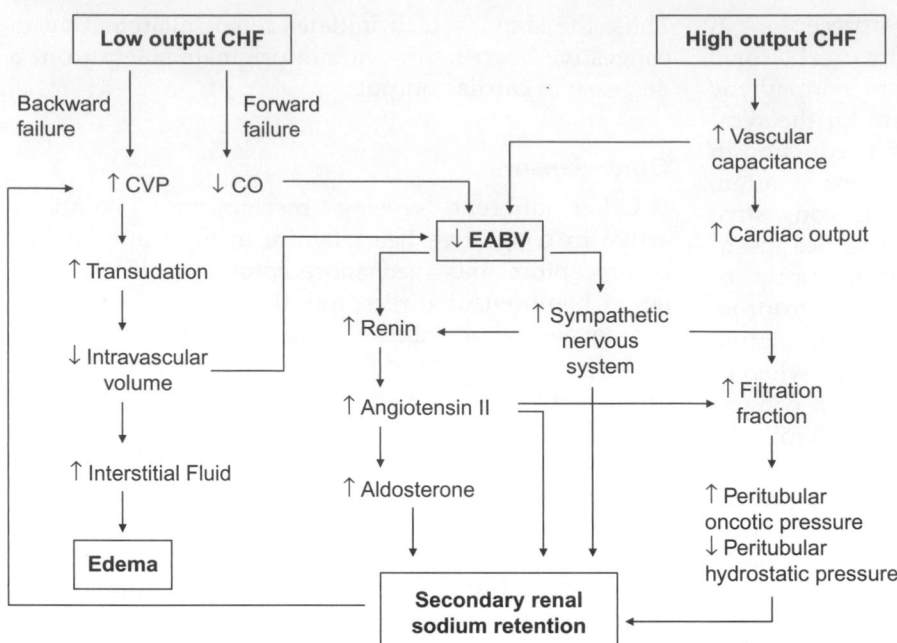

FIGURE 38.3 Summary of pathways leading to renal sodium retention in low- and high-output congestive heart failure (CO: cardiac output; EABV: effective arterial blood volume; CVP: central venous pressure).

Changes in glomerular and proximal tubular function in heart failure are similar to those that result from infusion of angiotensin II or norepinephrine. Angiotensin II, catecholamines, and renal nerves are all capable of increasing both the afferent and the efferent arteriolar tone, but predominantly act on the latter. These changes serve to maintain glomerular filtration rate near normal as renal plasma flow declines secondary to impaired cardiac function. As cardiac function progressively declines and the reduction in renal plasma flow becomes severe, the glomerular filtration rate will begin to fall. At this point there is an inadequate rise in filtration fraction, because efferent arteriolar vasoconstriction can no longer offset the intense afferent arteriolar constriction. Higher plasma catecholamines and further increases in sympathetic nerve activity acting to provide circulatory stability result in greater constriction of the afferent arteriole, such that glomerular plasma flow and transcapillary hydraulic pressure are reduced. In this setting, the glomerular filtration rate becomes dependent on afferent arteriolar flow.

These observations are similar to what has been observed in human subjects with varying degrees of left ventricular function.[119] As left ventricular function declines, the glomerular filtration rate is initially maintained by an increased filtration fraction. However, in patients with severely depressed left ventricular function, a progressive decline in renal blood flow becomes associated with a fall in glomerular filtration rate due to an inadequate rise in filtration fraction. In this setting, administration of an ACE inhibitor can result in a further lowering of the glomerular filtration rate, even though systemic arterial pressure remains fairly constant.[151]

Both experimental and clinical studies support the proximal nephron as a major site of increased sodium reabsorption in the setting of congestive heart failure. In human subjects, clearance techniques have primarily been employed to demonstrate the contribution of the proximal nephron. For example, infusion of mannitol was shown to increase free water excretion to a greater extent in patients with congestive heart failure as compared to normal controls. Since mannitol inhibits fluid reabsorption proximal to the diluting segment, it was inferred that enhanced free water clearance was reflective of augmented delivery of Na from the proximal tubule to the diluting segment.[10] In dogs with an arteriovenous fistula, there is a failure to escape from the Na-retaining effects of deoxycorticosterone acetate. In addition, these animals do not develop hypokalemia in contrast to normal controls.[82] The absence of hypokalemia in the setting of mineralocorticoid excess is best explained by decreased delivery of Na to the distal nephron due to enhanced proximal Na reabsorption. Alterations in peritubular hydrostatic and oncotic forces, as well as direct effects of various neurohormonal effectors, account for enhanced proximal sodium and water absorption in this setting.[76]

Clearance and micropuncture studies are also consistent with enhanced sodium reabsoption in the distal tubule in states of congestive heart failure. The loop of Henle has been identified as a site of enhanced sodium reabsoption in dogs with chronic vena cava obstruction[112] and rats with an arteriovenous fistula.[193]

Renin—Angiotensin—Aldosterone System

The renin—angiotensin—aldosterone system is activated when the heart fails as a pump.[139] Components of this system serve to compensate for decreased cardiac output by stabilizing the circulation and expanding ECF volume.

Several mechanisms are activated in the setting of a failing myocardium which serve to increased renin release. Diminished pressure in the afferent arteriole enhances renin release via a baroreceptor mechanism, the sensitivity of which is heightened consequent to augmented baseline sympathetic nerve activity.[94] Enhanced salt and water reabsorption in the proximal tubule and loop of Henle diminishes sodium chloride concentration at the macula densa, providing a stimulatory signal for renin release by way of the tubuloglomerular feedback mechanism. Finally, increased sympathetic nerve activity directly enhances renin release via stimulation of β-adrenergic receptors on the juxtaglomerular cells.

Renin acts on angiotensinogen synthesized in the liver and elsewhere to produce the decapeptide, angiotensin I. Angiotensin I is converted to angiotensin II by the angiotensin-converting enzyme present in the lungs, kidney, and blood vessels throughout the circulation.

Angiotensin II plays a pivotal role in glomerular and proximal tubule function in models of congestive heart failure (Figure 38.4). By selectively increasing efferent arteriolar tone, adjustments in the glomerular and postglomerular circulatory network favor net reabsorption in the proximal tubule. Increased filtration fraction leads to increased peritubular oncotic pressure, and in combination with decreased peritubular hydrostatic pressure net sodium reabsorption is enhanced. Angiotensin II also stimulates salt and water reabsorption through a direct effect on proximal tubular cells.[70,187] Increased efferent arteriolar resistance increases glomerular capillary hydrostatic pressure, mitigating any fall in GFR that would otherwise occur from decreased renal blood flow. In clinical, as well as experimental, models of heart failure, administration of ACE inhibitors improves renal blood flow and increases urinary sodium excretion, consistent with important angiotensin II-mediated effects on the renal microvasculature.[44]

Angiotensin II also contributes to renal salt and water retention through effects mediated by increased renal sympathetic nerve activity. As previously mentioned, angiotensin II decreases the sensitivity of the baroreflex mechanism such that a higher pressure is required to decrease central sympathetic outflow. In addition, angiotensin II directly stimulates sympathetic outflow at the level of the central nervous system.

Chronic administration of an ACE inhibitor to patients with congestive heart failure reduces central sympathetic outflow and improves the sympathoinhibitory response to baroreflex stimulation.[65]

Angiotensin II also influences renal salt and water handling in the distal nephron, primarily through stimulatory effects on aldosterone release in the adrenal gland.[183] Aldosterone acts primarily on the collecting duct to promote tubular reabsorption of sodium. Aldosterone-stimulated sodium reabsorption generates a luminal-negative voltage that secondarily enhances excretion of hydrogen and potassium ions. The magnitude of potassium secretion will depend on the volume and composition of filtrate reaching the collecting duct. In this regard, patients with heart failure rarely manifest hypokalemia and alkalosis, despite oversecretion of mineralocorticoid, unless distal sodium delivery is increased by use of a diuretic. In the absence of diuretic therapy, distal delivery of sodium is low due to enhanced proximal reabsorption mediated by angiotensin II, sympathetic nerves, and peritubular physical factors. Thus, although plasma renin and aldosterone levels are frequently elevated in heart failure, there is conflicting data as to the importance of aldosterone in mediating renal salt retention.[43,71,206]

Conflicting data regarding the importance of the renin—angiotensin—aldosterone system in the generation of cardiac edema is best resolved when analyzed with respect to severity of heart failure. The initial response to constriction of the pulmonary artery or thoracic inferior vena cava in dogs is a reduction in blood pressure, and increases in renin and aldosterone levels. During this acute phase there is avid renal sodium retention,[206] and stability of blood pressure is critically dependent on circulating angiotensin II. Over several days plasma volume and body weight increase, while renin, aldosterone, and sodium balance return to control values. During the acute phase, administration of a converting enzyme inhibitor results in hypotension, while no effect on blood pressure is observed during this chronic phase. If plasma renin and aldosterone fail to decrease due to severe impairment of cardiac output, then converting enzyme inhibitor-induced hypotension persists.

A similar pattern is seen in dogs with an arteriovenous fistula.[202] In the early phase of this high-output cardiac failure model, significant elevations in renin and aldosterone levels occur, and renal sodium retention is marked. Several days later, after development of peripheral edema and ascites, renin and aldosterone levels return to baseline and daily sodium excretion begins to match dietary intake.

A similar relationship between the renin—angiotensin—aldosterone system and stage and

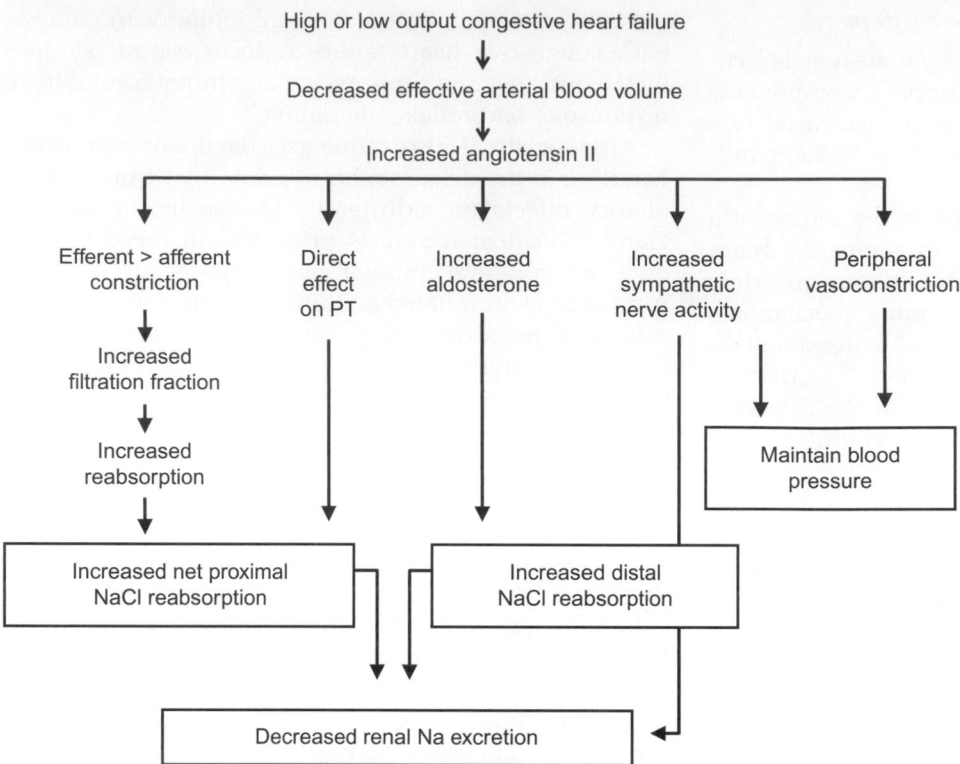

FIGURE 38.4 Pathways by which angiotensin II regulates renal sodium excretion in response to a decrease in effective arterial blood volume.

severity of congestive heart failure exists in humans.[43] This relationship may explain why renal function improves in some patients treated with ACE inhibitors, whereas renal function deteriorates in others.[152] In subjects whose renal function worsens after administration of the drug, there is a greater fall in mean right atrial pressure, left ventricular filling pressure, mean arterial pressure, and systemic vascular resistance as compared to subjects with stable renal function. In addition, plasma renin activity increases to a greater extent. These changes suggest a more contracted EABV and greater dependency of systemic vascular resistance on circulating angiotensin II in patients with ACE inhibitor-induced renal dysfunction.

In summary, during severe decompensated left ventricular failure, decreased EABV elicits release of renin with consequent activation of angiotensin II and aldosterone. Acutely, increased circulating levels of angiotensin II serve to maintain systemic blood pressure and augment renal sodium reabsorption. Salt retention is the result of hemodynamic and direct effects of angiotensin II at the level of the proximal tubule, and enhanced sodium reabsorption in the distal nephron primarily mediated by increased aldosterone. As ECF volume expands, renin, angiotensin II, and aldosterone become suppressed, although not necessarily to normal levels. Maintenance of systemic blood pressure is more dependent on volume rather than angiotensin II. Sodium balance is now achieved, but at the expense of

increased steady-state ECF volume. ACE inhibitor therapy is not associated with deleterious effects on renal function at this stage of the disease. Should further deterioration in cardiac function ensue, persistent activation of the renin—angiotensin—aldosterone system may result, such that systemic blood pressure remains dependent on circulating angiotensin II despite expansion of ECF volume. In this setting, ACE inhibitor therapy can precipitate hypotension and significant reductions in the glomerular filtration rate. One has to consider this sequential change in renin to volume dependency of mean arterial blood pressure in attempting to predict net renal and hemodynamic effects of converting enzyme inhibition.[156,194]

Sympathetic Nervous System

The sympathetic nervous system is activated in congestive heart failure. Plasma norepinephrine levels are elevated, and concentrations correlate with the degree of left ventricular dysfunction.[111] Direct nerve recordings demonstrate a direct relationship between central sympathetic nerve outflow and left ventricular filling pressures.[109]

Increased sympathetic tone influences renal reabsorption of salt and water by indirect, as well as direct, mechanisms (Figure 38.5). Glomerular hemodynamics are affected similarly to that produced by angiotensin II. In addition, sympathetic nerves directly stimulate

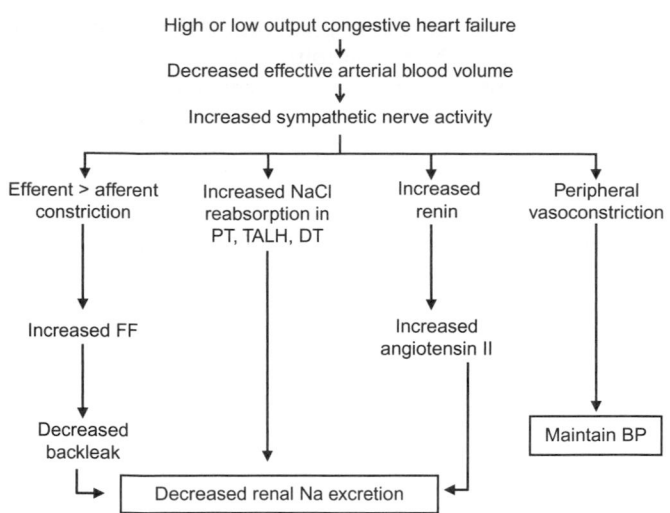

FIGURE 38.5 **Pathways by which sympathetic nerves regulate renal sodium excretion in response to a decrease in effective arterial blood volume.**

tubular reabsorption of salt and water in both the proximal and the distal nephron.

Increased sympathetic nerve activity stimulates renin release. The subsequent formation of angiotensin II provides a positive feedback loop leading to further increases in sympathetic nerve activity. Angiotensin II sensitizes tissues to the actions of catecholamines, and acts synergistically with renal nerves in modulating renal blood flow.[158]

Arginine Vasopressin

Increased circulating levels of AVP is a characteristic finding in patients with congestive heart failure.[172] The nonosmotic release of AVP plays an important role in the development of hyponatremia, which in turn is a well-defined predictor of mortality in heart failure patients. In experimental heart failure, there is

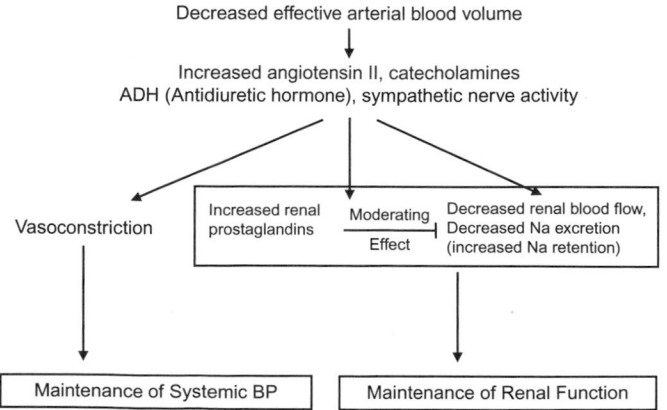

FIGURE 38.6 **Renal prostaglandins moderate the effect of various effector mechanisms, thereby allowing renal function to be well-maintained in the setting of increased systemic vasoconstrictor input.**

upregulation of the mRNA for vasopressin in the hypothalamus.[91] In addition, there is increased expression of the mRNA and the protein for the aquaporin-2 water channel.[216] In a rat model of heart failure, selective antagonism of the V-2 receptor is associated with a significant improvement in free water clearance.[216] Administration of a V-2 receptor antagonist to patients with congestive heart failure is associated with a significant reduction in body weight and improvement in dyspnea, but has not been shown to reduce mortality.[173]

Prostaglandins

Increased production of prostaglandins plays an important role in maintaining circulatory homeostasis in congestive heart failure. In response to decreases in cardiac output, neurohumoral vasoconstrictor forces (i.e., the renin—angiotensin—aldosterone system, the neurosympathoadrenal axis) participate in the maintenance of systemic arterial pressure, and result in increased total peripheral vascular resistance. These same vasoconstrictors stimulate the renal production of vasodilatory prostaglandins, such that the rise in renal vascular resistance is less than that seen in the periphery. Vasodilatory prostaglandins function in a counter-regulatory role, attenuating the fall in renal blood flow and glomerular filtration rate that would otherwise occur if vasoconstrictor forces were left unopposed.[154]

Renal prostaglandins also serve to moderate salt and water retention that would otherwise occur in the setting of unopposed activation of effector mechanisms such as angiotensin II, aldosterone, renal sympathetic nerves, and ADH.[154] The importance of prostaglandins in modulating renal hemodynamics, sodium excretion, and circulatory homeostasis progressively increases in proportion to the severity of the heart failure (Figure 38.6).

Natriuretic Peptides

Circulating atrial natriuretic peptide (ANP) and brain natriuretic peptide (BNP) are circulating hormones which are primarily synthesized in the cardiac atria and ventricles respectively. The synthesis and release of these peptides provide a mechanism whereby cardiac atria and ventricles serve both an afferent and efferent function in the control of ECF volume. Levels of ANP are elevated and correlate with the severity of disease in humans and experimental animals with heart failure.[29,168]

The natriuretic and vasodilatory properties of ANP suggest that this peptide plays an important counter-regulatory role in congestive heart failure. However, attempts to use ANP therapeutically in congestive heart failure have produced disappointing results.[29,95] ANP infused in patients with heart failure causes only a minimal change in fractional sodium excretion and urine flow rates, as compared to the robust response in normal controls.[29] The mechanism of renal nonresponsiveness in heart failure is not entirely clear. A downregulation of receptors due to sustained exposure to high levels of ANP or altered intrarenal hemodynamics are possibilities. Decreased delivery of sodium to the distal nephron where ANP normally exerts its natriuretic effect is also a likely cause of resistance. While ANP levels are uniformly elevated in congestive heart failure, potentially beneficial natriuretic properties are overwhelmed by more powerful antinatriuretic effector mechanisms.

Similar to ANP, plasma levels of BNP are elevated in congestive heart failure, and in proportion to the severity of systolic and diastolic dysfunction.[153] Infusion of BNP is associated with a significant reduction in pulmonary capillary wedge pressure, pulmonary artery pressure, right atrial pressure, and mean arterial pressure, as well as an increase in cardiac index. These hemodynamic benefits are accompanied by significant increases in urinary volume and sodium excretion, in some but not all studies.[131,133] Infusion of BNP can be associated with hypotension, particularly when given with other vasodilators. Measurement of plasma BNP levels is often utilized as a diagnostic tool to differentiate between cardiac versus other causes of pulmonary congestion. In addition, BNP levels can be used as a prognostic indicator and a marker reflecting the degree of cardiac dysfunction.

Endothelin and Nitric Oxide

Circulating levels of endothelin are increased in congestive heart failure, and correlate positively with the degree of myocardial dysfunction. Studies in which endothelin antagonists have been administered suggest this substance may play a role in the pathophysiology of cardiac failure.[130,172] In a randomized, double-blind study of human subjects with heart failure, infusion of an ETa and ETb receptor blocker (bosentan) was associated with a reduction in right atrial pressure, pulmonary artery pressure, pulmonary capillary wedge pressure, and mean arterial pressure.[93] In a dog model of heart failure,[204] ETa blockade alone lead to a reduction in cardiac filling pressures and increased cardiac output. These hemodynamic changes were associated with an increase in GFR and renal plasma flow, as well as increased urinary sodium excretion. By contrast, administration of an ETb receptor blocker caused an increase in cardiac filling pressures and a decrease in cardiac output, suggesting endogenous endothelins adversely effect cardiac hemodynamics and cause fluid retention, primarily through ETa receptors.

Nitric oxide production is increased in congestive heart failure.[210] Increased release of nitric oxide from resistance vessels may partly antagonize neurohumoral vasoconstrictor forces. Inhibiting nitric oxide production in heart failure patients causes a significant increase in pulmonary and systemic vascular resistance, as well as a decline in cardiac output. In the renal vasculature, nitric oxide production is also increased; however, the renal vasodilatory response to nitric oxide is impaired.[2] Administration of an angiotensin receptor antagonist restores nitric oxide-mediated renal vasodilation, suggesting angiotensin II plays a contributory role in this defect.[1]

CIRRHOSIS

Renal sodium excretion is normally regulated so that extracellular fluid (ECF) volume is maintained within normal limits. Any maneuver that increases ECF volume will lead to a prompt and sustained natriuresis until the volume returns to normal. In patients with cirrhosis, this homeostatic mechanism becomes deranged such that large increases in ECF volume are accompanied by continued renal salt retention, resulting in edema and ascites formation.

Presinusoidal Versus Postsinusoidal Obstruction and Ascites Formation

In patients with cirrhosis, the kidneys are normal but are signaled to retain salt in an unrelenting manner. The critical event in the generation of this signal is development of hepatic venous outflow obstruction. In the normal state, the portal circulation is characterized by high flow, low pressure, and low resistance. The imposition of a resistance into this high-flow vasculature will uniformly raise portal pressure, but development of ascites is critically dependent on location of the resistance. Conditions associated with presinusoidal vascular obstruction, such as portal vein thrombosis and schistosomiasis, raise portal pressure but are not generally associated with ascites. By contrast, hepatic diseases such as Laennec's cirrhosis and Budd Chiari syndrome cause early postsinusoidal vascular obstruction, and are associated with marked degrees of salt retention, anasarca, and ascites. Thus, during the development of the cirrhotic process, ascites will accumulate primarily when the pathologic process is associated with hepatic venous outflow obstruction and sinusoidal hypertension.

This distinction between presinusoidal and postsinusoidal obstruction can best be explained by comparing the characteristics of fluid exchange in capillaries of the splanchnic bed versus those in the hepatic sinusoids. The intestinal capillaries are similar to those in the peripheral tissues, in that they have continuous membranes with small pores such that a barrier exists, preventing plasma proteins from moving into the interstitial space. An increase in capillary hydrostatic pressure will cause the movement of a protein-poor fluid to enter the interstitial compartment and decrease the interstitial protein concentration. Interstitial protein concentration is further reduced by an acceleration in lymph flow that is stimulated by the fluid movement. As a result, the interstitial oncotic pressure falls, and the plasma oncotic pressure remains unchanged. The net oncotic force therefore rises and offsets the increase in hydrostatic force, providing a buffer against excessive fluid filtration. The fall in intestinal lymph protein concentration is maximal at relatively low pressures, and is much greater than that observed from the cirrhotic liver.[8,213] Thus, the increase in net oncotic force associated with dilution of the interstitial protein and accelerated lymph flow contribute to the protection against ascites in patients whose only abnormality is portal hypertension.

The situation across the liver sinusoids is quite different. Hepatic sinusoids, unlike capillaries elsewhere in the body, are extremely permeable to protein. As a result, colloid osmotic pressure exerts little influence on movement of fluid. Rather, direction of fluid movement is determined almost entirely by changes in sinusoidal hydraulic pressure. Thus, efflux of protein-rich filtrate into the space of Disse is critically dependent on hepatic venous pressures. Obstruction to hepatic venous outflow will lead to large increments in the formation of hepatic lymph and flow through the thoracic duct. Unlike the intestinal capillaries, there is little or no restriction in the movement of protein into the interstitium, such that the protein concentration of hepatic lymph will quickly approach that of plasma.[64] As a result, no significant oncotic gradient develops between plasma and the interstitium at high sinusoidal pressures and flow.

When sinusoidal pressure increases to such a degree that hepatic lymph formation exceeds the capacity of the thoracic duct to return fluid to the circulation, interstitial fluid weeps off the liver into the peritoneal space and forms ascites. Lymph formation in the setting of cirrhosis can be more than 20-fold greater than that which occurs under normal circumstances.[213] Whereas in normal humans 1–1.5 liters/day of lymph are returned to the circulation, subjects with cirrhosis, even without ascites, may have lymph flow through the thoracic duct as high as 15–20 liters/day.[212] The predominance of hepatically-produced lymph to overall lymph production is illustrated by studies in experimental animals with cirrhosis. Barrowman and Granger[8] found a 29-fold increase in hepatic lymph flow, while only a three-fold increase was noted in the splanchnic lymphatics. Eleven of 19 animals had normal flows of intestinal lymph, while all the cirrhotic animals had increased flows in liver lymph.

Conditions associated with the rapid onset of postsinusoidal obstruction, such as acute right-sided congestive heart failure and Budd–Chiari syndrome, initially give rise to ascitic fluid that has a high protein concentration that may even approach that of plasma. This high protein concentration is reflective of the liver being the predominant source of the ascitic fluid. However, over time the protein content of ascites in these conditions begins to decrease. Witte et al.[214] measured the total protein in ascitic, pleural, and peripheral edema fluid in acute and chronic heart failure patients. In the setting of acute heart failure, the mean concentration of protein in ascitic fluid was approximately 5 g/dl. By contrast, the protein concentration in ascitic fluid of chronic congestive heart failure patients was 2.7 g/dl. A lower protein concentration is also typical of conditions such as Laennec's cirrhosis, in which postsinusoidal obstruction develops slowly.

Two phenomena contribute to this change in ascitic fluid protein concentration. If the hepatic sinusoids are subject to an increased hydrostatic pressure for a long period of time, they begin to assume the anatomic and functional characteristics of capillaries found elsewhere in the body, a process referred to as capillarization.[181] This change leads to a decrease in albumin permeability, such that oncotic forces begin to play some role in hepatic lymph formation. At the same time, hypoalbuminemia develops secondary to decreased hepatic synthesis, as well as dilution secondary to ECF volume expansion. As a result, the protein content of hepatic lymph, although still high, falls to approximately 50–55% of plasma values.[213]

The second factor contributing to the lower ascitic protein concentration is the superimposition of portal hypertension. Early in the development of portal hypertension when plasma protein concentration is normal only minimal amounts of ascitic fluid are derived from the splanchnic bed, due to the buffering effect of increased net oncotic force opposing fluid filtration. Extremely high hydrostatic pressures are required to produce significant amounts of ascitic fluid in the setting of normal plasma protein concentrations. By contrast, less and less hydrostatic pressure is required for the formation of ascitic fluid, as the plasma albumin concentration decreases and the net osmotic force declines. In this setting, the splanchnic bed begins to make a greater contribution to the generation of ascites, and the fluid is characterized by a low protein concentration.[9]

The development of portal hypertension is also associated with changes in the splanchnic circulation that secondarily lead to increased lymph production in the splanchnic bed. The importance of the splanchnic lymphatic pool in the generation of ascites is reflected by the fact that in most instances ascitic fluid is transudative and characterized by a protein concentration of approximately 2.5 g/dl. Classically, portal hypertension was considered to be the sole result of increased resistance to portal venous flow. However, studies in experimental models suggest that increased portal venous flow resulting from generalized splanchnic arteriolar vasodilation also plays a role in the genesis of increased portal pressure.[19,203] This vasodilation leads to changes in the splanchnic microcirculation that may predispose to increased filtration of fluid. For example, an acute elevation of venous pressure in the intestine normally elicits a myogenic response that leads to a reduction in blood flow. This decrease in flow is thought to serve a protective role against the development of bowel edema. However, in chronic portal hypertension this myogenic response is no longer present. In this setting, arteriolar resistance is reduced, such that capillary pressure and filtration are increased.[12,174] The loss of this autoregulatory mechanism may account for the greater increase in intestinal capillary pressure and lymph flow seen under conditions of chronic portal hypertension when compared to acute increases in portal pressure of the same magnitude.[102] The potential causes of splanchnic arteriolar vasodilation are discussed below.

The importance of portal hypertension in the pathogenesis of ascites is highlighted by several observations. First, patients with ascites have significantly higher portal pressures as compared to those without ascites.[143] Although the threshold for ascites development is not clearly defined, it is unusual for ascites to develop with a pressure below 12 mmHg. Gines found that only 4 of 99 cirrhotic patients with ascites had a portal pressure <12 mmHg, as estimated by hepatic venous wedged pressure.[63] Second, portal pressure correlates inversely with urinary sodium excretion.[143] Third, maneuvers designed to reduce portal pressure are known to have a favorable effect on the development of ascites. For example, surgical portosystemic shunts used in the treatment of variceal bleeding reduce portal pressure, and are associated with a lower probability of developing ascites during follow-up.[29] Both side-to-side and end-to-side portocaval anastomosis have been shown effective in the management of refractory ascites in cirrhosis. Recent studies also suggest that reducing portal pressure with a transjugular intrahepatic portasystemic shunt has a beneficial effect on ascites.[148]

In summary, ascites develops when the production of lymph from either or both the hepatic sinusoids and the splanchnic circulation exceeds the transport capacity of the lymphatics. In this setting, fluid will begin to weep from the surface of the liver and the splanchnic capillary bed, and accumulate as ascites. The final protein concentration measured in the peritoneal fluid is determined by the sum of the two contributing pools of fluid; one relatively high in protein originating in the liver and the other, a low protein filtered across splanchnic capillaries. Hepatic venous outflow obstruction leading to increased sinusoidal pressure and portal hypertension are the major determinants of whether lymph production will be of a magnitude sufficient for ascitic fluid to accumulate. Increased sinusoidal pressure is also related to the subsequent development of renal salt retention. The mechanism by which sinusoidal hypertension signals the kidney to retain sodium is discussed in the following section.

Afferent Limb of Sodium Retention: Overfill Versus Underfill Mechanisms

Classical Underfill Mechanism for Renal Salt Retention

The mechanism by which hepatic venous outflow obstruction leads to sufficiently high sinusoidal pressures for ascites formation is controversial. The classical (underfill) theory predicts that the degree of hepatic venous outflow obstruction is sufficient in the presence of normal splanchnic perfusion to perturb the balance between rates of hepatic lymph formation and thoracic duct flow, thereby resulting in the formation of ascites. Both increased sinusoidal and portal venous pressures, in conjunction with hypoalbuminemia, cause formation of ascites in the presence of normal splanchnic perfusion. The formation of ascites, however, occurs at the expense of decreased intravascular volume. In consequence, a low venous filling pressure and a low cardiac output activate baroreceptor mechanisms, resulting in renal salt retention. According to this formulation, development of ascites is the primary event that leads to an underfilled circulation and subsequent renal salt retention.

The failure of measured hemodynamic parameters to satisfy predictions of the classical theory has raised questions regarding its validity. As originally conceived, it was predicted that extrasplanchnic plasma volume would be decreased, and that cardiac output would be low. When measured, however, these values have rarely been low. In fact, measurements have indicated that total plasma volume is usually elevated in cirrhotic patients. Similarly, cardiac output is rarely low, but tends to vary from normal to very high. In addition, studies performed in animal models of cirrhosis have found that sodium retention precedes the formation of ascites, suggesting that salt retention is a cause and not a consequence of ascites formation.

Overfill Mechanism for Renal Salt Retention

The incompatibility of measured hemodynamic parameters and timing of renal salt retention with the classical theory of ascites has led others to propose the overflow theory.[118] Once again, hepatic disease with venous outflow obstruction is viewed as a prerequisite for development of increased sinusoidal and portal pressures. In contrast to the classical theory, however, normal splanchnic perfusion fails to raise sinusoidal pressure sufficiently to cause ascites formation. Rather, venous outflow obstruction signals renal sodium retention independent of diminished intravascular volume. Salt retention, in turn, increases plasma volume, cardiac output, and splanchnic perfusion, thus raising sinusoidal and portal pressures sufficiently to culminate in translocation of fluid into the interstitial space and eventually the peritoneum. The combination of portal hypertension and increased arterial volume would lead to overflow ascites formation. This hypothesis is supported by the positive correlation between plasma volume and hepatic venous pressure, and the persistence of increased plasma volume after portacaval anastomosis. Moreover, patients with ascites have significantly higher portal pressure than patients without ascites, and portal pressure correlates inversely with urinary sodium excretion.[63]

Additional evidence linking hepatic venous outflow obstruction directly to renal sodium retention comes from studies performed in dogs fed the potent hepatotoxin dimethylnitrosamine.[115–117] The pathophysiologic disturbances and histologic changes that develop over a 6–8-week period are similar in nature to those seen in Laennec's cirrhosis. In this model, sodium retention and increases in plasma volume precede formation of ascites by about 10 days.[115] In order to exclude the possibility that the increase in plasma volume was solely due to an increased splanchnic plasma volume, repeat measurements were obtained after ligation of the superior and inferior mesenteric arteries, the celiac axis, and portal vein. In this way, any contribution of the splanchnic circulation could be excluded. These studies clearly showed that extrasplanchnic plasma volume was elevated at a time when dogs were in positive sodium balance. To further prove that extrasplanchnic plasma volume was increased, end-to-side portacaval shunts were placed prior to inducing cirrhosis.[117] This maneuver was designed to prevent any increase in splanchnic plasma volume. In these studies, evidence of salt retention preceded the formation of ascites, and was accompanied by a parallel increase in plasma volume.

In another series of studies using this same model, hemodynamic parameters were monitored during control, precirrhotic, and postcirrhotic sodium balance periods.[116] Sodium retention was found to precede any detectable change in cardiac output or peripheral vascular resistance. Once ascites developed, plasma volume increased further, and this was associated with increased cardiac output and a fall in peripheral vascular resistance. It was concluded that initiation of sodium retention and plasma volume expansion was not dependent on alterations in systemic hemodynamics. This conclusion has been corroborated in the canine model of hepatic cirrhosis induced by bile duct ligation,[197] as well as in rats made cirrhotic with carbon tetrachloride inhalation and oral phenobarbital.[123]

The pathway by which primary renal sodium retention would be linked to venous outflow obstruction in the overfill theory is not clear. Convincing evidence does exist for the presence of an intrahepatic sensory network composed of osmoreceptors, ionic receptors, and baroreceptors. Studies in which hepatic venous pressure is raised have demonstrated increases in hepatic afferent nerve activity.[113,114,197] Furthermore, a neural reflex pathway linking hepatic venous congestion and augmented sympathetic nerve activity has been identified.[104] In addition, acute constriction of the portal vein in dogs results in renal sodium and water retention in the innervated unilateral kidney, while these effects are abolished in the contralateral denervated kidney.[2] In addition to a neural mechanism, there may also be a hormonal system by which the liver and kidney can communicate. Hepatically-produced cAMP has been proposed to be a component of such a system.[6] Circulating cAMP is known to inhibit proximal salt and water absorption, as well as to contribute to the regulation of glomerular filtration rate. According to this hypothesis, decreased circulating cAMP levels as a result of liver disease could secondarily lead to renal salt retention and impaired renal function.

In summary, the overfill hypothesis is supported by a number of observations that indicate sodium retention precedes development of ascites in the absence of hemodynamic factors known to lead to salt retention. Moreover, high cardiac output coupled with increased plasma volume argues strongly for increased arterial blood volume, a finding seemingly incompatible with the underfill theory. Against such an analysis, however, is that mechanisms that sense arterial volume physiologically may be more sensitive than methods used to measure it. It should be noted that while statistically insignificant, there was a fall in blood pressure at the time of positive sodium balance in the dimethylnitrosamine model. This decrease may have been of sufficient magnitude to signal renal salt retention.[116] Since cardiac output was unchanged, total peripheral resistance may have decreased. Similarly, patients with hepatic cirrhosis and ascites behave as if they are effectively volume-depleted. Despite an increase in cardiac output and plasma volume, arterial pressure is typically low. This fall in systemic blood pressure is consistent with an underfilled arterial vascular compartment. Thus, the distinction between classical and overflow theories better rests on the measurement of effective arterial blood volume (EABV).

Use of EABV to Distinguish Underfill and Overfill Mechanisms of Renal Salt Retention

The classical (underfill) theory predicts that EABV is low in patients with ascites, and is the afferent mechanism signaling renal salt retention. The overflow theory predicts that EABV is expanded due to primary salt retention. While EABV cannot be measured directly, assessing the level of activation of neurohumoral effectors known to be regulated by EABV can be considered a measure of it. In this regard, levels of renin, aldosterone, ADH, and norepinephrine can serve as markers reflective of the magnitude of the EABV.

When renin and aldosterone values have been measured in patients with cirrhosis, values have varied from low to high. It is important, however, to consider these levels in the context of whether ascites is present or not. In the absence of ascites, subjects are in sodium balance, and renin and aldosterone levels are normal.[171] In the presence of ascites, mean renin and aldosterone levels are elevated, but individual values are often still normal.[4,63] This observation seems in conflict with the classical theory, as all patients with ascites who are in positive sodium balance should have decreased EABV and high aldosterone levels. However, not all patients with ascites are retaining sodium. In fact, some patients are in balance such that sodium intake equals output. Thus, in examining the mechanism of sodium retention in cirrhosis with ascites, neurohumoral effectors such as renin, aldosterone, ADH, and sympathetic nerve activity should be considered with respect to the rate of sodium excretion. When examined in this fashion, a significant inverse relationship is found between urinary sodium excretion and neurohumoral markers, suggesting the presence of a contracted EABV.

One component of the circulation that appears to be contributing to the overall decrease in EABV is the central circulation. Indirect measurements demonstrate that central blood volume is reduced, while noncentral blood volume is expanded.[140] In fact, the size of central and arterial blood volume is inversely correlated with sympathetic nervous system activity, suggesting that unloading of central arterial baroreceptors is responsible for enhanced sympathetic activity. This conclusion is supported by studies using the technique of head-out water immersion (HWI).[49,50] In this technique, subjects are seated and immersed in a water bath up to their necks. This technique results in redistribution of

ECF volume from the interstitial space into the vasculature, with a sustained increase in central blood volume. The central volume expansion is comparable to that induced by infusion of 2 liters of isotonic saline.[50] Such a maneuver would be expected to raise both the EABV and the hepatic sinusoidal pressure. The classical theory would predict that HWI would lead to decreases in renin, aldosterone, ADH, and norepinephrine concentrations in response to expansion of EABV. Since renin levels correlate with wedged hepatic vein pressures, the overfill theory would predict further rises in renin and other hormonal systems consequent to initiation of a sinusoidal pressure-sensitive hepatorenal reflex. When HWI was performed in a heterogeneous group of patients with cirrhosis, the natriuretic response was variable, but suppression of renin and aldosterone levels was uniform.[52] In a more homogenous group of patients characterized by impaired ability to excrete water and sodium, HWI was shown consistently to suppress plasma AVP, renin, aldosterone, and norepinephrine, as well as to increase sodium and water excretion.[17,146]

Taken together, the multiplicity of data support the presence of decreased EABV in patients with decompensated cirrhosis, and is most consistent with an underfill mechanism of renal salt retention (Figure 38.7). Since blockade of endogenous vasoconstrictor systems in patients with cirrhosis and ascites leads to marked arterial hypotension, activation of these systems function to contribute to the maintenance of arterial pressure. At least one component of the decrease in EABV may be due to an underfilled central circulation. As discussed in the following paragraphs, increased perfusion of arteriovenous communications, systemic vasodilation, and increased perfusion of the splanchnic bed are important factors in the genesis of an underfilled circulation. In addition, these factors play a major role in the hyperdynamic circulation that is typical of patients with chronic liver disease.

Hyperdynamic Circulation in Cirrhosis

Arteriovenous Communications

The characteristic circulatory changes observed in animal, as well as clinical, studies of cirrhosis consist of increased cardiac output, low mean arterial pressures, and low peripheral vascular resistance. The most attractive explanation for a contracted EABV in the setting of such a hyperdynamic circulation assigns a pivotal role to increased vascular capacitance.[92] An increased vascular holding capacity out of proportion to plasma volume results in an underfilled circulation and decreased EABV. One factor that may account for increased vascular capacitance and a hyperdynamic

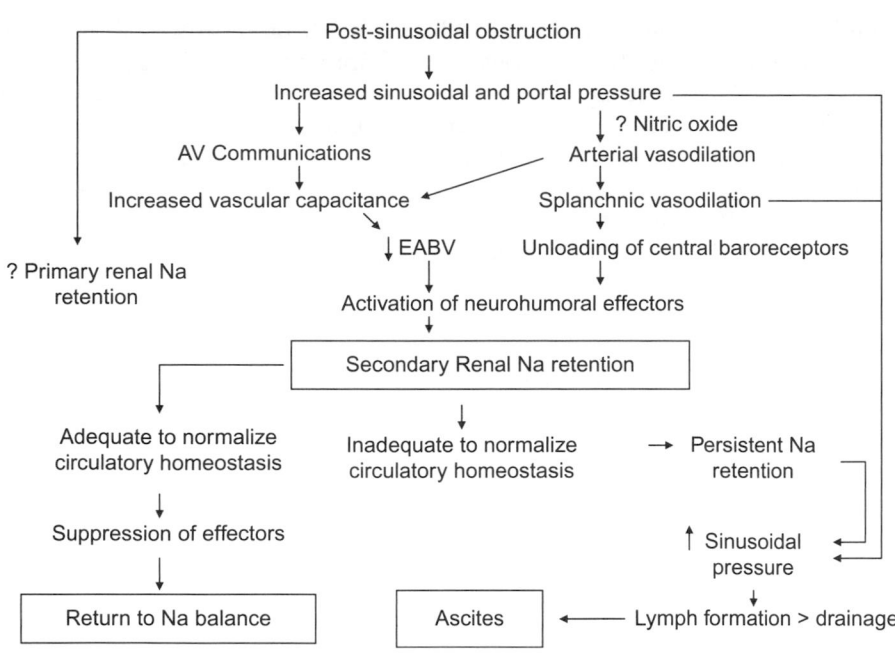

FIGURE 38.7 **Unified theory of ascites formation: a modified underfill mechanism.**

circulation is the formation of widespread arteriovenous communications.[15] In cirrhotics, arteriovenous fistula formation has been identified in the pulmonary, mesenteric, and upper and lower extremity circulations. In addition, increased blood flow has been measured in muscle and skin of the upper extremity not attributable to increased oxygen consumption, anemia or thiamine deficiency.[97] Postmortem injection demonstrated intense proliferation of small arteries in the splenic vasculature of patients with cirrhosis.[129]

The hemodynamic changes and salt retention that occur with an arteriovenous fistula are reminiscent of what occurs in cirrhotic humans.[48] With an open fistula, peripheral vascular resistance falls, cardiac output increases, and diastolic and mean blood pressures fall. The proportionately greater increase in vascular capacitance over cardiac output results in a contracted EABV. Consequent sodium retention expands ECF volume, raises venous filling pressure, and further increases cardiac output until balance is achieved between cardiac output and lowered peripheral resistance. At this point, sodium intake equals excretion, EABV is normalized, and the patient is in balance.

In cirrhosis, a similar imbalance occurs between plasma volume and vascular capacitance, such that EABV remains contracted and renal sodium retention is stimulated. In contrast to a simple arteriovenous fistula, however, several factors are present in cirrhosis that make sodium balance more difficult to achieve. First, these patients often have impaired cardiovascular function.[15] Diminished venous return consequent to tense ascites or cardiomyopathy from alcohol or malnutrition may limit increases in cardiac output.

Furthermore, depression of left ventricular function in response to increased afterload suggests subclinical cardiac disease, despite elevated forward output.[120] Second, retained sodium does not remain in the vascular space and lead to increased venous return. Rather, retained sodium becomes sequestered within the abdomen as ascites. Third, increased vascular permeability may further impair the ability of retained sodium to expand EABV. Peripheral arterial vasodilation in cirrhotic rats is associated with increased vasopermeability to albumin, electrolytes, and water.[25] Examination of interstitial fluid dynamics by means of a subcutaneous plastic capsule reveals substantial increases in interstitial fluid volume early in cirrhosis before the appearance of ascites or peripheral edema.[179] Such capillary leakage impedes filling of the intravascular compartment and prevents replenishment of a contracted EABV.

Primary Arterial Vasodilation

Arteriovenous fistulas and formation or hyperdynamic perfusion of pre-existing capillary beds are changes that develop as cirrhosis progresses. Nevertheless, salt retention occurs early in the cirrhotic process before these anatomic changes are fully-established. Since sodium retention antedates the formation of overt ascites and portosystemic shunting, peripheral arterial vasodilation has been proposed to be a primary event in the initiation of sodium and water retention in cirrhosis.[185] In this manner, a decreased EABV and increased vascular capacitance could still be the signal for renal salt retention, even in the earliest stages of liver injury. The peripheral arterial vasodilation hypothesis is supported by several studies in animal models.[209] In rats with partial ligation of the portal vein, evidence of a reduced systemic vascular resistance precedes the onset of renal salt retention. In addition, a direct correlation has been found between the onset of decreased arterial pressure and renal sodium retention in spontaneously hypertensive rats with experimental cirrhosis.[123] As opposed to the classical underfilling theory, the arterial vascular underfilling would not be the result of a reduction in plasma volume, which in fact is increased, but rather to a disproportionate enlargement of the arterial tree secondary to arterial vasodilation. In the rat with carbon tetrachloride-induced cirrhosis, the fall in peripheral vascular resistance and hyperdynamic circulatory state precede ascites formation, suggesting that generalized vasodilation is indeed an early finding with hepatic injury.[56]

Perhaps the best evidence to date in support of an underfilled circulation due to arterial vasodilation comes from human studies of HWI accompanied by infusion of a vasoconstrictor. HWI is associated with increased perfusion of the central circulation, however, urinary excretion rates of salt and water improve, but do not normalize with this procedure alone.[17] Since systemic vascular resistance falls during HWI, it was proposed that further vasodilation may prevent complete restoration of EABV in subjects already peripherally vasodilated. Infusion of a vasoconstrictor will increase peripheral vascular resistance, but will do little to improve an underfilled central circulation. Predictably, infusion of norepinephrine alone into cirrhotic subjects fails to significantly increase urinary sodium excretion.[188] By contrast, when norepinephrine is infused during HWI so as to increase central perfusion and at the same time attenuate the fall in systemic vascular resistance, sodium excretion increases significantly. In six subjects with decompensated cirrhosis, this combined maneuver was found to increase urinary sodium excretion to an amount that when extrapolated over a 24-hour period was greater than sodium intake.[188] These results are consistent with the hypothesis that arterial vasodilation causes an abnormal distribution of the total blood volume, such that effective central blood volume is reduced.

SPLANCHNIC ARTERIAL VASODILATION

As alluded to earlier, arterial vasodilation is particularly marked in the splanchnic arteriolar bed.[80,180,203] Increasing degrees of splanchnic vasodilation contribute to the fall in mean arterial pressure and unloading of baroreceptors in the central circulation.[32,135] As a result, central afferent sensors signal the activation of neurohumoral effectors, which in turn decrease perfusion of other organs, but in particular in the kidney. The importance of splanchnic vasodilation in the

genesis of renal ischemia has been indirectly illustrated by the response to ornipressin, an analog of AVP that is a preferential splanchnic vasoconstrictor.[67,110] The administration of ornipressin to patients with advanced cirrhosis leads to correction of many of the systemic and renal hemodynamic abnormalities that are present. These include an elevation in mean arterial pressure, reductions in plasma renin activity and norepinephrine concentration, and increases in renal blood flow, glomerular filtration rate, and urinary sodium excretion and volume. Similar benefits have been reported with the combined use of octreotide and midodrine.[85]

ROLE OF NITRIC OXIDE IN ARTERIAL VASODILATION

The underlying cause of arterial vasodilation, particularly in the early stages of cirrhosis, has not been fully-elucidated, but a great deal of attention has been focused on humoral factors.[79] There is an increasing body of experimental and preliminary human evidence suggesting that increased nitric oxide production may be an important factor in this process. In both experimental models and in human subjects with cirrhosis, increased production of nitric oxide can be demonstrated.[176,192,207] In the cirrhotic rat, evidence of increased production is already present when the animals begin to retain sodium, and antedates the appearance of ascites.[11] Administration of nitric oxide synthase inhibitor L-NMMA to cirrhotic human subjects improves the vasoconstrictor response to noradrenaline, suggesting that overproduction of nitric oxide is an important mediator of the impaired responsiveness of the vasculature to circulating vasoconstrictors.[24] In addition, this same inhibitor administered in low doses has been shown to correct the hyperdynamic circulation in cirrhotic rats.[147] In a more recent study utilizing this same model, normalization of nitric oxide production was associated with a marked natriuretic and diuretic response, as well as a reduction in the degree of ascites in cirrhotic rats.[132]

The precise mechanism for increased nitric oxide production in cirrhosis is not known, but may be mediated at least in part via the release of tumor necrosis factor-alpha.[121] In experimental models of hepatic disease, for example, the administration of anti-TNF-alpha antibodies or an inhibitor of nitric oxide synthesis results in increases in splanchnic and total vascular resistance, an elevation in the mean arterial pressure, and a reduction in cardiac output toward or, with nitric oxide inhibition, to normal.[121,147] Similarly, blocking the signaling events induced by TNF and nitric oxide production, via inhibition of protein tyrosine kinase, ameliorates the hyperdynamic abnormalities in rats with cirrhosis and portal hypertension.[122] Studies in cirrhotic humans with an increased cardiac output and systemic vasodilatation have shown evidence of enhanced nitric oxide production, a finding compatible with the experimental observations. Portosystemic shunts and decreased reticuloendothelial cell function may allow intestinal bacteria and endotoxin to enter the systemic circulation, providing a potential stimulus for tumor necrosis factor-alpha and/or nitric oxide production.

It is not yet known with certainty whether the endothelial (eNOS) or the inducible (iNOS) isoform is primarily responsible for increased production of nitric oxide. The hyperdynamic circulatory state of cirrhosis may impose a shear stress on the vascular endothelium, thus providing a stimulus for the upregulation of eNOS.[134,207] On the other hand, increased activity of nitric oxide synthase in polymorphonuclear cells and monocytes (cells that primarily contain iNOS) in cirrhotic human subjects suggest the inducible isoform may also play a role in increased production.[134]

In summary, an underfill mechanism appears to explain the bulk of experimental, as well as clinical, findings in established cirrhosis (Figure 38.7). Less certain are mechanisms responsible for sodium retention that precede the development of ascites. The overfill theory invokes the presence of a hepatorenal reflex sensitive to subtle rises in intrahepatic pressure mediating initiation of renal salt retention. However, the finding of decreased peripheral vascular resistance, even at this early stage, suggests diminished arterial filling.[116] Early peripheral arterial vasodilation and later formation of anatomic shunts lead to disproportionate increases in vascular capacitance with subsequent contraction of EABV, thereby signaling renal salt retention.[59,103,141] While it is conceivable that both overfill mechanisms and underfill mechanisms may be operative at different stages of disease, the multiplicity of data both clinical and experimental can be assimilated into an underfill theory.

Concept of Balance in Cirrhosis

In the earliest stages of cirrhosis when arterial vasodilation is moderate and the lymphatic system is able to return increased lymph production to the systemic circulation, renal sodium and water retention are sufficient to restore EABV and thereby suppress neurohumoral effectors. Balance is re-established such that sodium intake equals sodium excretion, but at the expense of an increased ECF volume. As liver disease progresses, this sequence of arterial underfilling followed by renal salt retention is repeated. As long as the EABV can be restored to near normal levels the activation of effector mechanisms will be moderated,

and balance will be achieved albeit at ever-increasing levels of ECF volume (Figure 38.8). Eventually, lymph production will begin to exceed the drainage capacity of the lymphatic system. At this stage of the disease renal salt retention becomes less efficient at restoring EABV, as retained fluid is sequestered in the peritoneal cavity as ascites. At the same time arterial underfilling is more pronounced, particularly as splanchnic arteriolar vasodilation becomes more prominent. Activation of neurohumoral effectors is magnified, resulting in more intense renal salt retention. Even at this stage of the disease cirrhotic patients with ascites eventually re-establish salt balance. The terminal stages of the cirrhotic process are characterized by extreme arterial underfilling. At this time there is intense and sustained activation of neurohumoral effectors. As a result, renal salt retention is nearly complete as the urine becomes virtually devoid of sodium. The vasoconstrictor input focused in on the kidney is of such a degree that renal failure begins to develop.

Effector Mechanisms in Cirrhosis

Nephron Sites of Renal Sodium Retention

Salt retention and impaired free water clearance are characteristic disturbances in renal function in cirrhotic patients. Evidence is available to support an important role for proximal and distal nephron segments in mediating enhanced sodium reabsorption.

PROXIMAL NEPHRON

Indirect evidence supporting enhanced proximal salt reabsorption comes from studies in human cirrhotic subjects in which infusion of mannitol or saline improves free water clearance.[27,182] Increased proximal

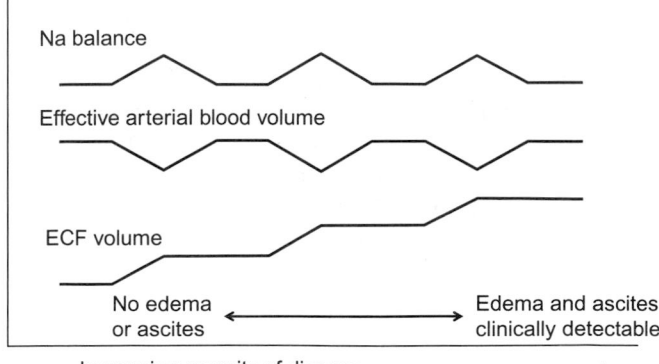

Concept of balance in cirrhosis

FIGURE 38.8 **As liver disease progressively worsens, salt balance is continually re-established as total extracellular fluid (ECF) volume increases.** Early in the disease process the increase in ECF volume is not clinically detectable. With more severe disease, peripheral edema and ascites are readily apparent.

tubular salt reabsorption leads to decreased delivery of filtrate to the distal diluting segments, thereby impairing free water formation. Presumably, by restoring distal delivery of filtrate, mannitol and saline infusions result in increased solute free water formation. Similar increases in free water clearance occur when central hypervolemia is induced by HWI. The increase in urine sodium is accompanied by increased K excretion, suggesting enhanced distal delivery of sodium. Increased water excretion seen in response to HWI, combined with simultaneous infusion of norepinephrine, is also consistent with baseline enhanced proximal sodium reabsorption in decompensated cirrhotics.[188]

Experimental models of cirrhosis have provided more direct assessment of nephron function. Micropuncture studies in rats made cirrhotic by ligation of the common bile duct demonstrated increases in both the proximal tubule solute reabsorption and filtration fraction.[5] Enhanced proximal reabsorption was attributed to increased peritubular oncotic pressure. In a dog model of cirrhosis,[136] intrarenal administration of the vasodilator acetylcholine was found to ameliorate the blunted natriuretic response to saline infusion. In this model, sodium reabsorption was enhanced in both the proximal and the diluting segments of the nephron.[16]

DISTAL NEPHRON

Clinical and experimental evidence also supports an important role for distal nephron sodium retention in cirrhosis. In cirrhotic patients manifesting a sluggish natriuretic response to HWI, phosphate clearance was found similar to a group who demonstrated an appropriate increase in urinary sodium excretion.[53] Since phosphate clearance was used as a marker of proximal sodium reabsorption, it was concluded that distal sodium reabsorption contributed importantly to renal sodium retention in patients with a sluggish natriuretic response. The results of a prospective, double-blind study comparing the diuretic response of furosemide to spironolactone in cirrhotic patients with ascites suggest that salt absorption in the cortical collecting tubule is enhanced.[161] When administered furosemide, only 11 of 21 patients exhibited a diuresis, while 18 of 19 patients responded to spironolactone. Furthermore, 10 patients who failed to respond to furosemide demonstrated a diuretic response to spironolactone. Furosemide inhibits sodium reabsorption in the loop of Henle, thereby increasing delivery to the collecting duct. All patients treated with furosemide had increases in the rate of potassium excretion, including the 11 patients who failed to increase urinary sodium excretion. These results, combined with the clinical effectiveness of spironolactone in treatment of cirrhotic

ascites, suggest enhanced salt absorption in the aldosterone-sensitive cortical collecting tubule.[7]

In summary, clinical and experimental studies suggest an important role for proximal, as well as distal, nephron sites mediating renal salt retention in cirrhosis. The relative contribution of different nephron sites to impaired salt and water excretion may depend on the degree to which systemic hemodynamics are altered. With each stage of advancing liver disease there becomes a greater contraction of the EABV. In the earliest stages of liver disease, enhanced proximal reabsorption limits distal delivery of solute in a manner analogous to a nonedematous subject with intravascular volume depletion. If distal delivery can be normalized at this early stage, distal nephron sites may continue to reabsorb sodium avidly, and therefore appear as the primary site responsible for ECF volume expansion. With severe reductions in EABV, presumably the proximal nephron becomes the dominant site of fluid reabsorption, such that the contribution of the distal nephron becomes much less apparent.

Sympathetic Nervous System

The sympathetic nervous system has been shown to contribute importantly to abnormalities in body fluid homeostasis in cirrhosis. Studies in rats made cirrhotic by ligating the common bile duct suggest that increased renal nerve activity is a major factor in the progressive salt retention that occurs in these animals.[35,37] In this model, baseline renal nerve activity is increased, and fails to decrease appropriately in response to intravenous saline. Renal denervation significantly improves the impaired ability to excrete an oral or intravenous salt-load. In addition, renal denervation has been shown to normalize the attenuated diuretic and natriuretic response to the intravenous administration of ANP.[96] In chronic metabolic studies, renal denervation also leads to a significant improvement in the positive cumulative sodium balance. The cause of increased renal nerve activity is multifactorial. Impaired aortic and cardiopulmonary baroreceptor regulation, as well as[175] abnormalities in hepatic NaCl-sensitive receptors and their immediate intrahepatic afferent connections, have been implicated as a cause of heightened autonomic activity.

Studies in human cirrhotic subjects are more indirect, but also suggest an important role for the sympathetic nervous system. Levels of norepinephrine in patients with cirrhosis are high, and are inversely correlated with urinary sodium excretion.[18] In addition, direct measurement of peripheral nerve firing rates show evidence of increased central sympathetic activity. Patients characterized by impaired ability to excrete water loads have plasma levels of norepinephrine that correlate positively with levels of ADH, aldosterone, and plasma renin activity.[18]

Decreased EABV leads to baroreceptor-mediated activation of sympathetic nerve activity, with subsequent enhancement of proximal salt reabsorption. The subsequent decrease in sodium delivery to the diluting segment, in addition to nonosmotic release of ADH, contributes to the inability to maximally excrete waterloads. Increased renal nerve activity also contributes to enhanced distal sodium reabsorption through activation of the renin—angiotensin—aldosterone system.

In addition to stimulating renal salt and water retention, activation of the sympathetic nervous system serves as a compensatory response to cirrhosis-induced vasodilation. Increased renal nerve activity contributes to increased renal vascular resistance, and is one of several factors responsible for the progressive decline in renal function which occurs as patients develop the hepatorenal syndrome.[38,51]

In summary, the sympathetic nervous system is activated under conditions of decompensated cirrhosis. Overactivity of this system is the result of a contracted EABV. In addition, there is impaired regulation of sympathetic outflow due to abnormalities in several afferent sensing mechanisms. Increased renal nerve activity contributes to the cumulative salt retention that accompanies advancing liver disease. In addition, activation of sympathetic outflow plays an important compensatory role in maintaining vascular tone in the setting of decreased vascular resistance.

Aldosterone

In patients with cirrhosis and ascites, plasma concentrations of aldosterone are frequently elevated. Although aldosterone metabolism is impaired in liver disease, secretion rates are greatly elevated, and are the major cause of elevated levels.[177] The relationship between hyperaldosteronism and sodium retention is not entirely clear. Several studies have provided evidence that argues against an important role of aldosterone in mediating salt retention in cirrhosis. For example, patients treated with an aldosterone synthesis inhibitor do not necessarily exhibit a natriuretic response.[177] In one study, renal salt excretion and changes in plasma renin and aldosterone levels were examined in 11 patients with ascites subjected to 5 days of high-salt intake. In patients with normal suppression of renin and aldosterone, salt retention and weight gain occurred to the same extent as patients who had persistent hypersecretion of renin and aldosterone.[28] In addition, cirrhotic patients in positive sodium balance, as compared to controls with matched sodium excretion, have increased fractional distal sodium reabsorption despite lower plasma aldosterone levels. In 16 cirrhotic patients subjected to HWI, plasma

renin activity and plasma aldosterone levels were found to decrease promptly. Despite suppression of the hormones, however, half of the patients manifested a blunted or absent natriuretic response.[52] In another group of cirrhotic patients with ascites and edema, HWI induced a significant natriuresis despite acute administration of desoxycorticosterone, suggesting that enhanced sodium reabsorption can occur independently of increased mineralocorticoid activity.

By contrast, other studies suggest aldosterone is an important factor in the pathogenesis of sodium retention in patients with cirrhosis. For example, adrenalectomy or administration of a competitive inhibitor of aldosterone increases urinary sodium excretion.[45] Patients who fail to manifest a diuretic response to furosemide tend to have higher renin and aldosterone levels and lower urinary sodium concentrations prior to treatment.[16] Inability of furosemide to increase urinary sodium in these patients may result from reabsorption of delivered sodium in the collecting tubule under the influence of aldosterone. Similarly, patients with the highest renin and aldosterone levels are those who fail to diurese in response to HWI.[52,144,145]

As with the conflicting data regarding the role of the proximal and distal nephron in salt retention discussed previously, the degree to which systemic hemodynamics and EABV are impaired may explain some of the conflicting data noted above. It is possible that in patients with the greatest contraction of EABV, intense proximal sodium reabsorption limits distal delivery to such an extent that the contribution of aldosterone to increase salt absorption is difficult to detect. By contrast, with less impairment in EABV, distal delivery is better maintained, and the contribution of aldosterone to renal sodium retention is more obvious.

Alternatively, acquired inhibition of 11β-hydroxysteroid dehydrogenase type 2 may be of importance in the salt retention that occurs in some patients with cirrhosis of the liver. Bile acids which can accumulate in the setting of chronic liver disease have been shown to inhibit the activity of 11β-hydroxysteroid dehydrogenase type 2.[195] Such an effect would allow cortisol-mediated stimulation of the mineralocorticoid receptor, and potentially explain aldosterone-independent salt retention in the distal nephron in liver cirrhosis. Studies in the bile duct ligation and carbon tetrachloride models of chronic liver disease are consistent with a component of cortisol-mediated stimulation of the mineralocorticoid receptor.[195] In these models there is decreased activity of 11β-hydroxysteroid dehydrogenase type 2 that is temporally related to increased ENaC abundance in the apical membrane of the cortical collecting duct. These changes are most pronounced in the sodium-retaining stage of disease.

Prostaglandins

Prostaglandins function in a protective role in decompensated cirrhosis. Similar to other hypovolemic states, prostaglandins act to maintain renal blood flow and GFR by ameliorating pressor effects of angiotensin II and sympathetic nerves.[154] These agents counterbalance the salt retaining effects of these effectors and mitigate the impairment in free water clearance mediated by AVP. Administration of prostaglandin inhibitors can partially correct excessive hyperreninemia and hyperaldosteronism, and restore the pressor response to angiotensin II.

Kallikrein–Kinin System

Urinary kallikrein activity is increased in cirrhotic patients with ascites and preserved GFR, while urinary activity decreases in association with impaired renal function.[160] The correlation between renal plasma flow and GFR suggests that the renal kallikrein–kinin system may contribute to maintenance of renal hemodynamics in cirrhosis.

At the level of the renal tubule, bradykinin has been shown to exhibit a natriuretic effect. However, bradykinin also is a potent peripheral vasodilator, and can cause microvascular leakage. In cirrhosis, these later effects could exacerbate an already contracted EABV, and cause further salt retention. MacGilchrist et al.[127] studied the effects of kinin inhibition by systemically infusing aprotinin (a strong inhibitor of tissue kallikrein) into a group of patients with cirrhosis. This infusion was associated with a doubling of urinary sodium excretion, and an increase in renal plasma flow and GFR. This beneficial effect on renal function in the setting of kinin inhibition was attributed to an improvement in systemic hemodynamics as systemic vascular resistance increased. Similarly, administration of a bradykinin receptor antagonist to cirrhotic rats normalized renal sodium retention, and reduced the activity of the renin–angiotensin–aldosterone system.[211] Inhibiting bradykinin-induced microvascular leakage and lessening the degree of vascular underfilling was felt to be the mechanism of the beneficial effect.

Natriuretic Peptides

The role of ANP in the pathogenesis of edema in hepatic cirrhosis remains undefined. While atrial ANP content was reduced in cirrhotic rats, most data indicate ANP levels are either normal or elevated in cirrhotic humans.[81,190] Elevated levels are the result of increased cardiac release rather than just impaired clearance. The cause of the high levels is not understood, because atrial pressure is normal and central blood volume is reduced. Stimulating the endogenous release of ANP induces a natriuretic response in some patients with cirrhosis, while other patients are insensitive.[190] However, both groups of patients exhibited an increase in urinary cGMP, suggesting that the kidney is still capable of responding to ANP even in the absence of a natriuretic effect.[190]

Several potential mechanisms may account for ANP resistance in cirrhosis. This resistance could be the result of a defect intrinsic to the kidney or could be the result of altered systemic hemodynamics leading to activation of more potent sodium-retaining mechanisms.[128] With regards to the first possibility, an altered density of glomerular ANP-binding sites has been demonstrated in the bile duct-ligated rat model of cirrhosis.[62] In addition, ANP resistance was found in the isolated perfused kidney taken from sodium avid rats with cirrhosis induced by carbon tetrachloride.[157] In the chronic caval dog model of cirrhosis, intrarenal infusion of bradykinin restored ANP responsiveness to previously resistant animals, suggesting that an intrarenal deficiency of kinins could be a contributing factor.[108]

Other studies have focused on systemic hemodynamics as a cause of ANP resistance. With each stage of advancing liver disease there becomes a greater reduction in EABV. Since ANP resistance tends to occur with more severe and advanced disease, it is possible that ANP resistance is directly related to the impairment in EABV. Decreased EABV is associated with enhanced proximal reabsorption of solute. As a result, ANP resistance may be due to decreased delivery of salt to the site where ANP exerts its natriuretic effect. In support of this possibility, ANP resistance could be restored in cirrhotic rats by infusions of vasopressors so as to normalize arterial pressure, and presumably improve the decrease in EABV.[124] In human cirrhotics, ANP responsiveness can be markedly improved when distal sodium delivery is increased by administration of mannitol.[143]

Circulating brain natriuretic peptide (BNP) levels are also increased in patients with cirrhosis.[107] Infusion of BNP at a dose that elicits an increase in GFR, renal plasma flow, and urinary sodium excretion in normal controls has no effect in cirrhotic humans. The infusion is associated with an increase in urinary cGMP, as well as a fall in plasma aldosterone levels, suggesting that the peptide is capable of interacting with its receptor in these patients. As with ANP, the lack of natriuretic response to BNP may be due to overactivity of other antinatriuretic factors, as well as decreased delivery of sodium to its tubular site of action.

Adrenomedullin is a peptide with vasodilatory properties that is highly expressed in cardiovascular tissues. Increased circulating levels that correlate with severity of disease have been described in patients with cirrhosis.[57] Urodilatin is a natriuretic factor that is exclusively synthesized within the kidney. Unlike other natriuretic factors, levels are not increased in patients with cirrhosis.[178]

Endothelin

Increased circulating levels of endothelin have been reported in cirrhosis.[142] The stimulus and pathophysiologic significance of these levels is not known with certainty. The peptide may play a role in the renal vasoconstriction seen in the hepatorenal syndrome.[63,142]

Therapeutic Implications for Treatment of Salt Retention in Cirrhosis

Renal salt retention is the most common abnormality of renal function in chronic liver disease. Whenever urinary sodium excretion falls to an amount less than dietary salt intake ECF volume will begin to expand and eventually lead to the development of ascites and peripheral edema. The approach to the treatment of the cirrhotic patient with ascites is to alter sodium balance in such a way that urinary sodium excretion exceeds dietary salt intake.

In the earliest stages of the disease, urinary sodium excretion is plentiful and negative salt balance can be achieved by simply lowering dietary sodium intake. As the disease advances, neurohumoral effectors become more activated, initially resulting in more intense renal salt retention and later in a progressive decline in renal function. Eventually, the filtered load of sodium becomes completely reabsorbed by the tubule, such that the final urine becomes virtually devoid of salt. If some component of the filtered load reaches the collecting duct or beyond spironolactone will be effective in increasing urinary sodium excretion. Once sodium reabsorption is complete proximal to the collecting duct then thiazides, and later loop diuretics, will have to be added to spironolactone in order to increase urinary sodium excretion. Eventually, the filtered load is completely reabsorbed proximal to the thick ascending loop of Henle. At this point the patient is resistant to the effects of diuretics, and requires more invasive procedures such as repetitive large-volume paracentesis in order to remain in salt balance. In the terminal stages of the disease, the glomerular filtration rate falls to such a degree that oliguria, azotemia, and eventually uremia are present, and the patient is clinically diagnosed with hepatorenal syndrome (Figure 38.9). Vasoconstrictive input focused on the kidney is severe. The renal failure is functional in nature, however, since restoration of near normal renal function can be obtained following a liver transplant.

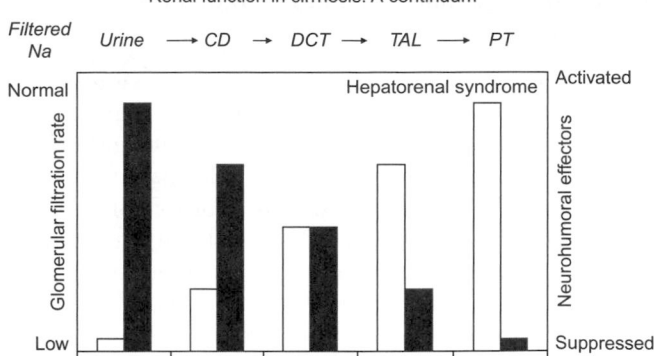

FIGURE 38.9 **The fall in glomerular filtration rate (solid bars) and activation of neurohumoral effectors (open bars) can be viewed as a continuum that varies according to severity of the underlying cirrhotic process.** As the disease advances, the urinary Na concentration falls. The filtered load of Na is completely reabsorbed at progressively more proximal sites along the nephron. A patient with hepatorenal syndrome is merely at the end of this continuum, when the glomerular filtration rate has fallen sufficiently to cause significant azotemnia.

NEPHROTIC SYNDROME

The development of edema is one of the cardinal features of nephrotic syndrome. The mechanism of its formation is not entirely understood. The classical view of edema formation in nephrotic syndrome describes the process as an underfill mechanism. According to this theory, urinary loss of protein results in hypoalbuminemia and decreased plasma oncotic pressure. As a result, plasma water translocates from the intravascular space into the interstitial space. When the magnitude of this transudation is sufficiently great, clinically detectable edema develops. Reduction in intravascular volume elicits activation of effector mechanisms that signal renal salt and water retention in an attempt to restore plasma volume. The renal response leads to further dilution of plasma protein concentration, thereby exaggerating the already reduced plasma oncotic pressure and further enhancing edema formation. In order for this formulation of edema genesis to be true, three critical predictions must be satisfied: (1) blood and plasma volume must be reduced during accumulation of edema; (2) measurement of neurohumoral effectors should reflect activation consequent to contraction of effective arterial blood volume; and (3) maneuvers that increase plasma volume into the normal range should result in a natriuretic response. As discussed below, these predictions are satisfied in some patients, especially those with minimal-change nephrotic syndrome, whereas the majority of nephrotic patients fail to conform to this conceptual model.

Blood and Plasma Volume in Nephrotic Syndrome

The classical view of edema formation assigns a pivotal role to decreased plasma volume serving as the afferent mechanism signaling renal salt and water retention. When measured directly, plasma volume has indeed been low in a variable proportion of patients with nephrotic syndrome.[106,138,198] Even in patients judged to be normovolemic, an exaggerated fall in plasma volume has been observed when nephrotic patients go from the recumbent to the standing position.[46,84] This orthostatic reduction in plasma volume can be profound and may, in part, explain the development of acute oliguric renal failure and hypovolemic shock that has been reported in patients with nephrotic syndrome.[191]

Most studies, however, have failed to find a consistent reduction in blood and plasma volume in patients with nephrotic syndrome.[39,47,61,100] In a survey of 10 studies, plasma volume measurements were analyzed in 217 nephrotic patients.[40] In only one-third of patients was plasma volume reduced, whereas it was normal in 42% and increased in 25%. It has been suggested that conflicting measurements of plasma volume in patients with nephrotic syndrome can be reconciled by separating patients according to histologic class.[137] In this regard, one study compared the volume status of four patients with minimal change disease to that in five patients with membranous or membranoproliferative lesions.[137] In patients with minimal change disease, plasma volume was decreased and plasma renin activity and aldosterone levels were increased. By contrast, plasma volume was either normal or increased and plasma renin activity was suppressed in the latter group. These authors concluded that edema formation in minimal change disease was primarily the result of decreased effective circulatory volume inciting secondary renal salt retention. By contrast, patients with more distorted glomerular architecture were felt to have a primary defect in renal salt excretion, leading secondarily to an expanded plasma volume and eventually formation of edema.

Other studies have failed to find such a correlation between histology and plasma volume measurements. Even in patients with untreated minimal change disease, plasma volume has been found to be increased.[40] In order to avoid potential methodologic problems, a recent study first established a reference frame for blood volume that was normalized to lean body mass, and measured directly from plasma volume and red cell volume in otherwise normal children.[205] Blood volume measurements in children with nephrotic syndrome due to minimal change disease, as well as other histologic lesions, were all found to be within this defined normal range. Following successful therapy with steroids, patients with minimal change disease demonstrate a fall in plasma volume and blood pressure, and an increase in plasma renin activity.[40] These changes are exactly the opposite of what one would expect if arterial underfilling were the proximate cause of renal salt retention. Finally, a large study of nephrotic patients, including 35 patients with minimal change disease, found virtually all patients have normal or increased plasma and blood volume.[60]

Neurohumoral Markers of Effective Circulatory Volume

Measurements of plasma renin activity and aldosterone concentration have been utilized as a method to indirectly differentiate primary sodium retention from an underfill mechanism of edema formation in nephrotic patients. Elevated values would be expected if blood volume was decreased, while suppressed values would occur in the setting of primary renal sodium retention and blood volume expansion. In this regard, plasma renin activity values collated from nine studies were found to be normal or low in 64 of 123 patients investigated.[39] Plasma aldosterone levels were also decreased in the majority of these patients. When measured with respect to salt intake or urinary sodium excretion, no consistent relationship was found. While some studies have found elevated plasma renin activity and aldosterone concentrations in patients with minimal change diseases, others have not.[69,137] In a study examining plasma renin activity with respect to blood volume, no relationship was found in either patients with minimal change disease or those with histologic lesions on light microscopy.[61] Although a higher proportion of patients with minimal change disease have elevated plasma renin and aldosterone levels as compared to those with histologic glomerular lesions, these values tend to overlap.[61,69] Thus, measurement of various elements of the renin–angiotensin–aldosterone axis suggests that an underfill mechanism may mediate renal sodium retention in some but not all patients with nephrotic syndrome.

Effects of Manipulations to Expand Central Blood Volume

Another approach utilized to investigate the pathogenesis of sodium retention in the nephrotic syndrome has been to examine renal sodium handling and hormonal indices of effective circulatory volume in response to expansion of the intravascular blood volume. This has been primarily achieved by infusing albumin or expanding central blood volume by head-out body water immersion (HWI).[34,87] The classical view of nephrotic edema would predict that expansion of the intravascular volume should correct renal salt and water retention. In children with minimal change disease, infusion of albumin has been reported to decrease plasma renin activity, arginine vasopressin (AVP), aldosterone, and catecholamines.[169,196] In association with these hormonal changes, there was a significant increase in the glomerular filtration rate, urine flow, and sodium excretion. In a less homogenous group of adult patients with nephrotic syndrome, baseline blood volumes were found to be low when expressed per kilogram wet weight.[199] Plasma AVP was inversely correlated with blood volume and failed to decrease in response to a water-load. When blood volume was expanded with 20% albumin, plasma levels of AVP fell, accompanied by an augmented water diuresis. It was concluded that a contracted blood volume was responsible for the nonosmotic release of AVP. By contrast, other studies have found either no or only a minimal increase in urinary sodium excretion in response to infusion of albumin. In one study, infusion of hyperoncotic albumin in quantities sufficient to expand blood volume by 35% resulted in only a modest natriuretic response.[100] In order to exclude the possibility that the blunted natriuretic response was due to an increase in peritubular colloid osmotic pressure, similar studies have been performed utilizing a prolonged infusion of iso-oncotic albumin. This maneuver was similarly accompanied by only a modest increase in sodium excretion, such that the patients remained in positive salt balance.[167] Studies utilizing HWI to expand blood volume have likewise produced conflicting results. Expansion of central blood volume by HWI in children with minimal change disease resulted in decreased levels of AVP, aldosterone, noradrenaline and plasma renin activity.[169,170] These changes were accompanied by significant increases in urine flow and sodium excretion. Similarly, adult patients with a variety of histologic lesions subjected to HWI were found to have significant increases in urinary sodium excretion.[13,105] By contrast, a more recent study in 10 patients with a variety of underlying glomerular diseases found only a blunted natriuretic response to HWI.[165] While ANP levels rose to the same extent in control and nephrotic subjects, suggesting equivalent degrees of volume expansion, peak urinary sodium excretion and urine flow in the nephrotic patients were one-third that in the control group.

A number of other observations also question the pivotal role assigned to hypoalbuminemia and reduced plasma oncotic pressure in the initiation of edema formation.[3,83,84] For example, reducing plasma protein concentration in humans[3] or experimental animals[83,84]

with plasmapheresis results in either no change or actually increases plasma volume. In addition, patients with congenital analbuminemia demonstrate no disturbance in water and electrolyte balance, and do not necessarily develop edema. Despite the reduction in plasma oncotic pressure, these patients exhibit an exaggerated natriuretic response when administered isotonic saline.

In summary, available data would argue for a contracted plasma volume as the afferent mechanism initiating sodium retention in some but not all patients with nephrotic syndrome. Rather, some component of primary renal sodium retention appears to be operative in nephrotic syndrome with histologic glomerular lesions, as well as in many patients with minimal change disease (Table 38.1). Studies in experimental animals also suggest a defect intrinsic to the nephrotic kidney as the mechanism responsible for salt retention in nephrotic syndrome. In the rat model of unilateral proteinuric renal disease induced by infusing puromycin aminonucleoside (PAN) into one kidney, diminished urinary sodium excretion was confined to the proteinuric kidney, despite the fact that each kidney shared the same systemic milieu.[77] In kidneys taken from rats previously exposed to PAN and then perfused in vitro, less sodium was excreted as compared to kidneys taken from control rats. Utilizing this experimental design, the defect in renal salt excretion was found to be localized to the kidney, as systemic and circulating factors were eliminated.

In some patients, primary salt retention and an underfill mechanism of edema formation may coexist. For example, in the earliest stages of a glomerular disease salt retention by the kidney may be primary in origin. As hypoalbuminemia develops and becomes progressively severe, plasma volume may fall and result in an element of superimposed secondary salt retention. The coexistence of these two mechanisms

TABLE 38.1 Evidence for Primary Renal Sodium Retention in the Nephrotic Syndrome

Blood volume is often normal or increased.

Blood pressure is often increased.

Renin activity and aldosterone levels are not uniformly increased.

Onset of natriuresis during recovery precedes rise in plasma protein concentration.

Sodium excretion is modest in response to HWI or albumin infusion.

Experimental models.

Sodium retention in a unilateral nephrosis model is confined to the diseased kidney.

Kidneys taken from nephrotic animals and perfused in vitro retain Na.

may account for the lack of uniformity in hemodynamic, as well as hormonal and neurocirculatory, profiles in patients with nephrotic syndrome.

Peripheral Capillary Mechanisms of Edema Formation

The presence of normal or increased plasma volume in the setting of a decreased serum albumin concentration is difficult to reconcile with the classical view of edema formation in the nephrotic syndrome. These findings can best be explained by examining the alterations that are known to occur in transcapillary exchange mechanisms in the setting of hypoproteinemia. Fluid movement within the capillary bed between intravascular and interstitial spaces is determined by the balance of Starling forces between these two compartments:

$$J_v = K_f[(P_c - P_i) - (\Pi_c - \Pi_i)]$$

where J_v is fluid flux along the length of a capillary, K_f is the ultrafiltration coefficient, P_c is capillary hydrostatic pressure, P_i is interstitial hydrostatic pressure, Π_c is capillary oncotic pressure, and Π_i is interstitial oncotic pressure. On the arterial side of the capillary, the net hydrostatic pressure gradient $P_c - P_i$ (ΔP) exceeds the net colloid osmotic pressure gradient $\Pi_c - \Pi_i$ ($\Delta\Pi$), resulting in net filtration of fluid into the interstitial space. Due to an axial fall in capillary hydrostatic pressure, the balance of Starling forces at the venous end of the capillary ($\Delta\Pi > \Delta P$) favors net reabsorption of fluid back into the capillary. In some tissues, net hydrostatic pressure exceeds opposing net colloid osmotic pressure throughout the length of the capillary, such that filtration occurs along its entire length. Net ultrafiltrate is returned to the circulation via lymphatic flow, such that in steady-state conditions total body capillary flux is equal to lymph flow; interstitial and intravascular volume remain stable and edema formation does not occur.

Absence of compensatory mechanisms would predict that small changes in ΔP, $\Delta\Pi$ or K_f would lead to increased fluid transudation and result in clinically detectable edema. However, the poor correlation between plasma albumin concentration and the presence or absence of edema suggests that counter-regulatory adjustments do occur in those forces that govern fluid exchange between the intravascular and interstitial space (Table 38.2). One such factor relates to compliance characteristics of the interstitium.[68] Under normal circumstances, interstitial pressure ranges from 6 mmHg to 10 mmHg. Due to the noncompliant nature of this compartment, small increases in interstitial volume result in large increases in interstitial pressure.

TABLE 38.2 Edema Defense Mechanisms which Limit Excessive Capillary Fluid Filtration

Increased interstitial hydrostatic pressure.
Increased lymph flow.
Decreased interstitial oncotic pressure.
Decreased permeability of the capillary to protein.

Such increases in P_i act to oppose further transudation of fluid, and provide an initial defense against the formation of edema. Increased interstitial pressure leads to the development of a second factor that also protects against edema formation, namely, increased lymphatic flow. Lymph flow can increase many-fold under conditions of augmented net capillary fluid filtration. In patients with edema resulting from heart failure or nephrosis, the disappearance rate of a subcutaneous injection of ^{131}I-albumin is markedly enhanced consistent with increased lymphatic flow.[73]

A third factor that minimizes fluid filtration is a reduction in interstitial oncotic pressure.[54] In normal human plasma, colloid oncotic pressure (COP) is about 24 mmHg, and interstitial COP is about 12 mmHg, creating a transcapillary COP gradient of about 12 mmHg.[84] Since transcapillary fluid flux consists primarily of a protein-free ultrafiltrate, interstitial protein concentration tends to become diluted. In addition, increased lymphatic flow removes fluid and protein from the interstitial space, and returns both to the vascular compartment thereby further reducing interstitial oncotic pressure. Body albumin pools are redistributed such that a greater fraction than normal is located in the vascular compartment.[84] As hypoalbuminemia develops in the nephrotic syndrome, the COP of the interstitial fluid space falls in parallel with the COP of plasma.[74,99,101] Nephrotic patients studied both in remission and in relapse demonstrate almost equivalent changes in the COP of plasma and the interstitium at all levels of serum albumin.[101] The maintenance of the net COP gradient within the normal range mitigates this potential driving force for transudation of fluid into the interstitial space. A final factor that favors decreased fluid filtration is a change in the permeability of the capillary. Under conditions of hypoalbuminemia, the intrinsic permeability of the capillary to protein tends to decrease, thereby increasing Π_c along the capillary.[215]

In summary, the reduction in serum oncotic pressure that accompanies the nephrotic syndrome would be predicted to alter Starling forces in a direction favoring net flux of fluid across the capillary bed. Despite this alteration, however, fluid tends not to accumulate within the interstitium in response to hypoalbuminemia, because of the activation of a series of defense mechanisms that serve to oppose those forces favoring fluid movement from the intravascular space. These edema-preventing factors include increased interstitial hydrostatic pressure, accelerated lymphatic flow, a parallel decline in plasma and interstitial oncotic pressure, and decreased capillary permeability to protein. However, in the setting of ongoing primary renal salt retention, these buffering mechanisms become exhausted and clinically apparent edema may become evident. This occurs because salt retention leads to increases in capillary hydrostatic pressure at the very time defense mechanisms normally employed to prevent edema have been maximized. In the hypoproteinemic patient without salt retention, edema-preventing factors may be sufficient to protect against the development of edema. Thus, edema formation in the nephrotic syndrome results from the combined effects of primary salt retention coupled with exhausted defenses against edema (Figure 38.10).

The changes in mean arterial pressure and blood volume as a function of varying extracellular fluid volume in hypoalbuminemic nephrotic patients as compared to normoalbuminemic chronic renal-failure patients illustrate these principles.[98] In hypoalbuminemic patients with nephrotic syndrome, expansion of the extracellular fluid volume leads to immediate translocation of fluid into the extravascular space, as evidenced by little change in mean arterial pressure or blood volume. Presumably, factors that serve to prevent edema are already maximized, and are overwhelmed by increases in capillary hydrostatic pressure that occur as a result of extracellular fluid volume expansion. By contrast, normoalbuminemic patients with chronic renal failure develop an increase in mean arterial pressure and blood volume as extracellular fluid volume expands. In these patients, more of the fluid is retained in the vascular tree due to activation of edema preventing factors. At some point of extracellular fluid volume expansion, these factors would also become overwhelmed and clinically detectable edema would develop.

Mechanism of Salt Retention in Nephrotic Syndrome

The bulk of experimental and clinical data implicate a tubular mechanism as the primary cause of salt retention in the nephrotic syndrome. Both experimental and clinical studies implicate the distal nephron as the site responsible for sodium retention. Utilizing clearance techniques, proximal sodium handling was assessed during diuretic-induced distal tubular blockade using chlorothiazide and ethacrynic acid.[66] Nephrotic patients exhibited a greater natriuretic response than controls, suggesting that distal nephron sites were responsible for enhanced sodium reabsorption. Measurement of tubular glucose handling has been used as a marker of proximal sodium reabsorption.[198] In a group of nephrotic patients, glucose titration curves revealed a reduced threshold for glucose reabsorption, further suggesting diminished proximal sodium reabsorption.

In volume-expanded rats with autologous immune complex nephritis, a model that resembles membranous nephropathy, micropuncture, and clearance methodology were used to study the site of sodium retention.[14] Absolute proximal sodium reabsorption was decreased in nephrotic rats, while sodium delivery to the late distal tubule of superficial nephrons was comparable in control as well as nephrotic animals. Since fractional excretion of sodium was significantly lower in nephrotic versus control rats, the collecting duct was suggested as a possible site of altered handling of sodium. Enhanced sodium reabsorption in juxtamedullary nephrons not accessible to micropuncture could not be excluded. In the rat model of unilateral proteinuric renal disease induced by infusing PAN into one kidney, diminished urinary sodium excretion was confined to the proteinuric kidney.[77] Since sodium delivery to the initial portion of the collecting duct was similar to the control kidney, increased sodium reabsorption at the collecting duct must have been the primary site of salt retention.

Studies using immunocytochemical analysis are consistent with the distal nephron being a major site for sodium retention in nephrotic syndrome.[33,41,89,90,125] The activity of the $Na^+ - K^+$-ATPase is increased in the colleting duct in the puromycin aminonucleoside rat model of nephrosis. There is also increased expression and targeting of the epithelial sodium channel (ENaC) in the connecting tubule and collecting duct in these animals, as well as those made nephrotic through injection of $HgCl_2$.

Neurohumoral Control of Enhanced Tubular Sodium Excretion

Renin–Angiotensin–Aldosterone

Studies demonstrating increased sodium retaining activity in the urine of nephrotic patients lead early investigators to suggest that aldosterone might play an important role in mediating sodium retention in the nephrotic syndrome.[126] In rats made nephrotic with PAN, juxtaglomerular cell granularity was found to vary directly with the degree of sodium retention. In this same model, prior adrenalectomy prevented sodium retention that otherwise occurred in nephrotic

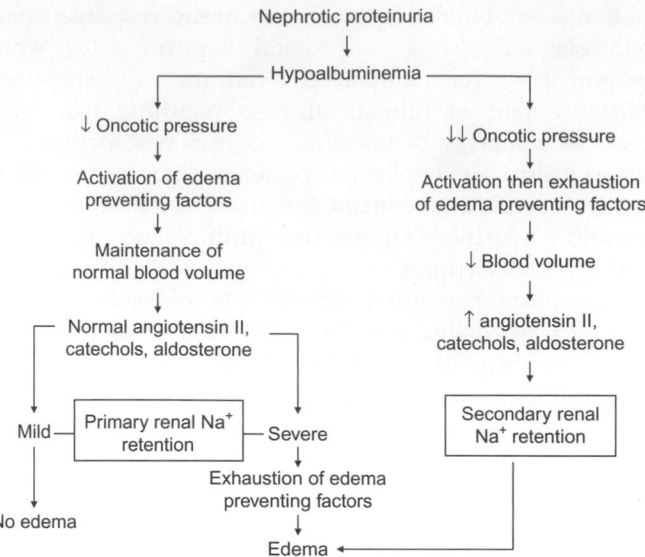

FIGURE 38.10   **The left side of the figure depicts the mechanism of edema formation in most patients with nephrotic syndrome.** An important variable that helps to explain the poor correlation between serum albumin concentration and the presence or absence of edema is the degree of primary renal Na retention. With severe Na retention by the kidney, edema-preventing factors become exhausted and edema becomes clinically apparent, even when the serum albumin concentration is only mildly depressed. In the setting of mild renal Na retention, these factors remain adequate to prevent edema formation, even in the presence of severe hypoalbuminemia. **The right side of the figure depicts the classical view of edema formation in which low blood volume serves as the signal for secondary renal Na retention.** This mechanism of edema formation is most commonly present in children with minimal change disease. In some patients, both mechanisms of edema formation may be operative. For example, early in the nephrotic syndrome, blood volume is normal and only primary renal Na retention is present. With worsening hypoalbuminemia, blood volume may begin to fall and result in a component of superimposed secondary renal Na retention.

controls with intact capacity to secrete aldosterone.[86] When plasma renin activity and aldosterone concentrations were measured in a large group of nephrotic patients placed on a low-sodium diet values varied widely, although a negative correlation was found between urinary sodium and plasma aldosterone concentration.[61] In a study of five nephrotic patients placed on a high-salt diet for 8 days, plasma renin activity and plasma aldosterone levels were similar in both nephrotic subjects and control subjects.[189] Administration of the aldosterone antagonist, spironolactone, on day 4 of the study resulted in an increase in urinary sodium excretion in the nephrotic patients, while no change was observed in the control group. Since aldosterone exerts salt-retaining effects on the distal nephron, a site implicated in formation of nephrotic edema, excess aldosterone activity is an attractive explanation for observed salt retention.

Most data, however, fail to confirm an important role for aldosterone. In patients spontaneously retaining sodium, measurements of plasma renin activity and aldosterone concentration may be either low or high.[21,23] This disassociation is also seen during steroid-induced remission of nephrotic syndrome. In four patients with minimal change disease, plasma renin and aldosterone concentrations fell during steroid-induced diuresis, but once in remission these hormones returned to the same plasma concentrations observed when edema was present.[137] Studies involving administration of either saralasin or converting enzyme inhibitors also fail to support an important role for the renin—angiotensin—aldosterone system in mediating salt retention.[22,23,42] In nephrotic patients selected for high plasma renin activity, captopril administration also failed to prevent sodium retention, despite producing marked reductions in plasma aldosterone.[22] In the unilateral model of PAN-induced nephrosis, infusion of saralasin led to substantial increases in total kidney and single-nephron GFR of the perfused kidney, but urinary sodium excretion remained unchanged.[77] This observation lends support for an intrarenal mechanism of salt retention independent of changes in GFR or activation of the renin—angiotensin—aldosterone system.

Sympathetic Nervous System

Increased plasma and urinary catecholamine concentrations have been found in patients with nephrotic syndrome.[88,150] The role of renal sympathetic nerve activity in mediating salt retention in nephrotic syndrome has been studied in rats made nephrotic by injection of adriamycin. An impaired ability to excrete an acute oral or intravenous isotonic saline-load was improved by bilateral renal denervation.[35] In response to acute infusion of saline, efferent renal sympathetic-nerve activity decreased to a lesser extent than that in control rats. Metabolic balance studies carried out over 26 days revealed an overall decrease in cumulative sodium balance only in those nephrotic rats with bilateral renal denervation.[72] Given the evidence for a distal nephron site of sodium reabsorption in nephrotic syndrome, it is noteworthy that beta-adrenergic stimulation of rabbit cortical collecting tubules enhances chloride transport.[78]

Other studies show enhanced sodium retention in nephrotic syndrome cannot be entirely explained by sympathetic nervous system activity. In kidneys taken from rats previously exposed to puromycin aminonucleoside and perfused *in vitro* so as to remove extrinsic neural factors, urinary sodium excretion is decreased as compared to kidneys taken from control animals.[58] Similarly, bilateral renal denervation does not correct the blunted natriuretic response to volume expansion in the adriamycin model of nephrosis.[200]

Atrial Natriuretic Peptide

Levels of ANP are reported to be normal or slightly elevated in patients with nephrotic syndrome.[196] In animal models of nephrotic syndrome, renal responsiveness to ANP has generally been found to be blunted.[162] In contrast, infusion of synthetic human ANP to nephrotic patients results in increased sodium and water excretion, similar to that in normal subjects. Infusion of albumin in children with nephrotic syndrome resulted in a rise in ANP levels that closely correlated with urinary sodium excretion. However, other studies have found a blunted natriuretic response to ANP in nephrotic patients.[162] It has been proposed that enhanced distal sodium reabsorption in the nephrotic syndrome may, in part, be due to resistance of the collecting duct to the natriuretic actions of ANP.[159,163] The cellular basis of this resistance does not appear to be an abnormality in ANP binding to its receptor. Rather, the mechanism appears to be an inability to generate adequate amounts of the intracellular cGMP as a result of heightened activity of intracellular cGMP phosphodiesterase.[201]

In summary, edema formation in the majority of patients with nephrotic syndrome can best be explained by an overfill mechanism. The maintenance of a normal plasma volume in the setting of hypoalbuminemia is the result of a series of edema preventing factors that act to both oppose fluid filtration across the capillary wall, and to return fluid back into the vascular tree. The single most important variable in determining whether these factors are sufficient to prevent edema formation is the degree of renal salt retention. The variability in renal salt retention explains the poor correlation between the presence or absence of edema and the serum albumin concentration. In patients with severe hypoalbuminemia and no edema, renal salt retention is likely to be minimal, such that edema preventing factors are sufficient in preventing excessive fluid filtration across the capillary wall. By contrast, edematous patients with near normal serum albumin concentration are more likely to have avid renal salt retention, such that the factors opposing fluid filtration become exhausted. The defect in renal salt excretion has not been precisely localized, but appears to reside in the distal nephron. The exact mechanism underlying this defect is unknown.

SODIUM-WASTAGE

Renal salt-wastage may be defined as persistent inappropriate renal loss of sodium from the body

sufficient in magnitude to result in shrinkage of extracellular fluid volume causing azotemia, hypotension, and when extreme, circulatory collapse. When evaluating the relationship between urine sodium excretion and dietary intake, the initial status of the extracellular fluid volume must be taken into consideration before concluding renal salt-wasting is present. For example, renal salt-wasting should not be considered present when urine sodium excretion greatly exceeds dietary intake in edematous patients placed on a low salt diet. In this instance, negative salt balance is an appropriate response to correct the volume-expanded state. As extracellular fluid volume normalizes, the natriuresis will stop and sodium balance will be re-established. By contrast, the imposition of a salt-restricted diet to a euvolemic patient with chronic kidney disease may result in negative salt balance, and contraction of extracellular fluid volume below normal limits. Even though the cumulative amount of sodium lost from the body may be far less than in the diuresing edematous patient, renal salt-wasting is considered present since the reduction of extracellular fluid volume has fallen below normal. In this setting, worsening azotemia and hypotension may be present. The critical feature of renal salt-wasting is the continued shrinkage of extracellular fluid volume below the lower limit of normal as a result of ongoing natriuresis. Disorders of renal salt-wasting can be divided into intrinsic disorders of the kidney and disorders of efferent mechanisms that regulate renal sodium handling.

Intrinsic Renal Disease

Chronic Kidney Disease

Patients with advanced chronic kidney disease may exhibit mild renal salt-wastage when subjected to rigid dietary sodium restriction. The pathogenesis of salt-wastage is related to the adaptive increase in perfusion of remaining viable nephrons, as total nephron mass progressively declines. Accompanying nephron hyperperfusion is a large increase in solute-load. This solute-load exceeds the reabsorptive capacity of remaining nephrons, resulting in increased excretion of salt and water. The nephrons of patients with chronic kidney disease are continuously undergoing an osmotic diuresis of solutes, including urea and the sodium salts of acids.

Studies by Coleman et al.[31] support an important role of osmotic diuresis in hyperfiltering nephrons in the genesis of salt-wastage in chronic kidney disease. In these experiments, patients with chronic kidney disease are placed on a low sodium diet and then subjected to a water diuresis. As urine volume increases, the urine sodium concentration falls to a minimum value and thereafter remains fixed. At this point, urine sodium excretion increases in parallel with further increases in urine flow rates. In salt-restricted normal participants subjected to a water diuresis combined with mannitol diuresis, the urine sodium concentration at which flow dependence of urine sodium excretion commences is greater compared to the level during water diuresis alone. These data indicate that an osmotic diuresis is at least in part responsible for the mild salt-wastage observed in patients with chronic kidney disease.

Clinical evidence of salt-wastage in most patients with chronic kidney disease is typically only found when dietary salt restriction is extreme. Patients ingesting dietary sodium of 10–15 mEq/day require a much longer period of time to establish salt balance compared to normals, and in many patients salt balance is never achieved. A persistent negative sodium balance leads to volume depletion, weight loss, relative hypotension, and worsening azotemia. In most instances, these findings are seen during the course of an intercurrent illness when salt intake is abruptly stopped or markedly reduced.

There are several reports in the literature in which renal salt-wastage is more severe.[26] Most of these cases have been described in patients with what appears to be chronic tubulointerstitial disease accompanied by cystic transformation of the renal medulla. In these unusual cases, urine sodium excretion is of such a magnitude that contraction of extracellular fluid volume develops in the setting of normal salt intake. Medullary cystic disease is an autosomal recessive disorder with cystic changes in corticomedullary and medullary regions of the kidney in which renal salt-wastage can be severe.

Acute Renal Failure

Transient renal salt-wastage is often seen in patients during the recovery phase of acute tubular necrosis. The magnitude of the natriuresis is a function of the amount of salt and water retained as the renal failure developed. Massive salt-wasting leading to volume-depletion and cardiovascular collapse is not a feature of this disorder. Some degree of salt-wastage is often seen following the relief of urinary obstruction. The excretion of retained urea and other solutes contribute to an osmotic diuresis and account for the natriuresis. However, persistent salt-wastage after these solutes are cleared does not typically occur.

Renal Tubular Disorders

Proximal or type II renal tubular acidosis is associated with renal salt-wastage owing to the loss of sodium bicarbonate into the urine. Defective proximal acidification leads to a large increase in distal sodium bicarbonate delivery that is subsequently lost into the urine. The bicarbonaturic effect will continue until the serum bicarbonate concentration falls to a level that matches the reabsorptive capacity of the proximal nephron, at which point sodium-wastage will cease. As a result, salt-wastage is transient in this disorder, but nevertheless causes mild volume-depletion from inappropriate renal salt loss.

Distal or type I renal tubular acidosis is also characterized by a mild form of renal salt-wastage. The defect in distal acidification leads to the development of a hyperchloremic metabolic acidosis. Systemic acidosis impairs proximal salt reabsorption, resulting in mild sodium-wastage.[55]

Bartter's and Gitelman's syndromes are characterized by renal salt-wastage due to genetic defects in ion transporters involved in sodium reabsorption. In Bartter's syndrome, impaired salt transport is localized to the thick ascending limb, while in Gitelman's syndrome the defect is localized to the distal convoluted tubule.

A variety of drugs can cause renal salt-wastage as a result of tubular injury. This injury can be due to direct toxic effects of the drug, as with Cis-platinum, aminoglycosides, and amphotericin B or be the result of acute tubulointerstitial nephritis, as reported with methicillin and trimethoprim/sulfamethoxazole.

Disorders of Effector Mechanisms that Regulate Renal Sodium Transport

Decreased Mineralocorticoid Activity

Mineralocorticoid activity plays an important role in renal sodium conservation. Decreased activity and renal resistance to mineralocorticoids are causes of renal sodium-wastage.[217] The most clinically relevant form of mineralocorticoid deficiency results from primary diseases of the adrenal cortex. These diseases may either be acquired or congenital in origin. Subnormal aldosterone secretory rates lead to decreased reabsorption of sodium chloride in the cortical collecting tubule of the kidney. The kidney is fundamentally intact and the cortical collecting tubule cell responds normally to exogenously administered mineralocorticoids.

Renal salt-wastage is a hallmark of Addison's disease, in which patients may demonstrate severe volume-depletion and cardiovascular collapse. Addison's disease results from progressive adrenocortical destruction, leading to deficiencies in glucocorticoid and mineralocorticoid activity. These patients present with anorexia, vomiting, abdominal pain, weight loss, weakness, and salt craving. Physical examination reveals generalized hyperpigmentation, particularly in skin folds and the axillae, as well as bluish-grey hyperpigmentation of the lingual and buccal mucosa. Orthostatic hypotension is very common, indicative of volume depletion. Laboratory examination reveals increased blood urea nitrogen-to-creatinine ratio characteristic of prerenal azotemia and elevated urinary sodium concentration. Hyponatremia, hyperkalemia, and hyperchloremic metabolic acidosis are the characteristic electrolyte abnormalities.

Isolated aldosterone deficiency accompanied by normal glucocorticoid production occurs in association with hyporeninism, as an inherited biosynthetic defect, during protracted heparin administration, and postoperatively following the removal of an aldosterone secreting adenoma. These patients have an inadequate ability to release aldosterone during salt restriction. In severe cases, salt-wastage may be present on a normal salt intake.

Mineralocorticoid Unresponsiveness

Defective transport of sodium may also result from abnormalities in tubular responsiveness to aldosterone. Disorders in which there is a resistance to aldosterone have been localized to abnormalities in the mineralocorticoid receptor, and to postreceptor defects in the epithelial sodium channel (ENaC).[217]

Pseudohypoaldosteronism type I is an inherited disorder of salt-wasting that presents in infancy. The autosomal dominant form of this disease has been linked to functional mutations in the mineralocorticoid receptor. Renal salt-wasting in these patients tends to be mild, and spontaneously improves as patient's age. A second form of the disease is inherited in an autosomal recessive fashion, and is caused by inactivating mutations in either the alpha- or beta-subunits of the epithelial sodium channel in the collecting duct. The clinical manifestations are more severe in this form of the disease. Patients present in infancy with severe unrelenting salt-wasting, hyperkalemia, and hyperchloremic metabolic acidosis, and a failure to survive syndrome. In addition to renal manifestations, patients also display frequent respiratory tract illnesses caused by an increase in the volume of airway secretions.

Cerebral Salt-Wasting

The concept of a CSW syndrome was first introduced by Peters and colleagues in 1950 in a report describing three patients with neurological disorders who presented with hyponatremia, clinical evidence of volume depletion, and renal sodium-wasting without an obvious disturbance in the pituitary–adrenal axis.[164] These findings were subsequently confirmed in additional patients with widely varying forms of cerebral disease.[208] The mechanism by which cerebral disease leads to renal salt-wasting is poorly-understood. The most probable process involves disruption of

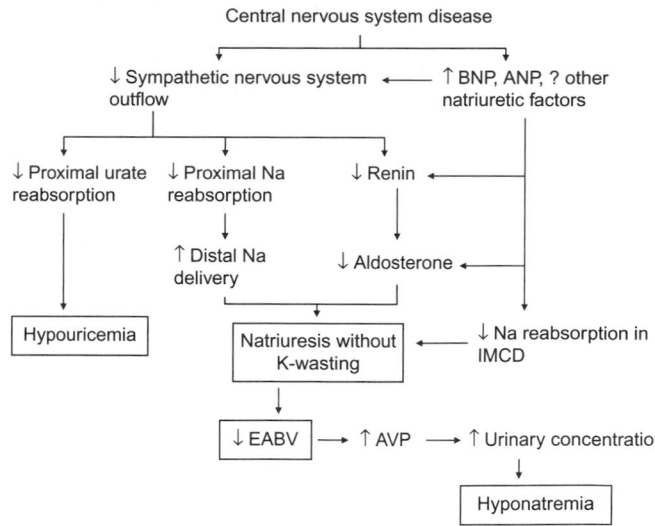

FIGURE 38.11 **The pathophysiology of cerebral salt-wasting.** Conditions associated with increased urinary sodium excretion in the setting of volume contraction would be expected to result in renal potassium-wasting, because of increased delivery of sodium to the cortical collecting duct in the setting of increased aldosterone levels. The lack of renal potassium-wasting in CSW can be accounted for by the failure of aldosterone to increase in spite of low extracellular fluid volume (ANP: atrial natriuretic peptide; AVP: arginine vasopressin; BNP: brain natriuretic peptide; CSW: cerebral salt-wasting; EABV: effective arterial blood volume; IMCD: inner medullary collecting duct).

neural input into the kidney and/or central elaboration of a circulating natriuretic factor (Figure 38.11).

CSW should be considered in patients with central nervous system disease who develop hyponatremia and otherwise meet the clinical criteria for a diagnosis of SIADH, but have a volume status that is inconsistent with that diagnosis. Unlike patients with SIADH who are volume-expanded, patients with CSW show evidence of negative salt balance and reductions in plasma, as well as total blood volume.[155] The onset of this disorder is typically seen within the first 10 days following a neurosurgical procedure or after a definable event, such as a subarachnoid hemorrhage or stroke. CSW has been described in other intracranial disorders, such as carcinomatous or infectious meningitis and metastatic carcinoma.

References

[1] Abassi ZA, Gurbanov K, Mulroney SE, Potlog C, Opgenorth TJ, Hoffman A, et al. Impaired nitric oxide–mediated renal vasodilation in rats with experimental heart failure: role of angiotensin II. Circulation 1997;96:3655–64.

[2] Anderson RJ, Cronin RE, McDonald KM, Schrier RW. Mechanisms of portal hypertension-induced alterations in renal hemodynamics, renal water excretion, and renin secretion. J Clin Invest 1976;58:964–70.

[3] Anderson SB, Rossing N. Metabolism of albumin and G-globulin during albumin infusions and plasmapheresis. Scand J Clin Lab Invest 1967;20:183–4.

[4] Arroyo V, Bosch J, Mauri M, et al. Renin, aldosterone and renal hemodynamics in cirrhosis with ascites. Eur J Clin Invest 1979;9:69–73.

[5] Bank N, Aynedjian HS. A micropuncture study of renal salt and water retention in chronic bile duct obstruction. J Clin Invest 1975;55:994–1002.

[6] Bankir L, Martin H, Dechaux M, Ahloulay M. Plasma Camp: a hepatorenal link influencing proximal reabsorption and renal hemodynamics? Kidney Int 1997;51(Suppl. 59):S50–6.

[7] Bansal S, Lindenfeld J, Schrier RW. Sodium retention in heart failure and cirrhosis: potential role of natriuretic doses of mineralocorticoid antagonist? Circ Heart Fail 2009;2:370–6.

[8] Barrowman JA, Granger DN. Effects of experimental cirrhosis on splanchnic microvascular fluid and solute exchange in the rat. Gastroenterology 1984;87:165–72.

[9] Battin DL, Ali S, Shahbaz AU, Massie JD, Munir A, Davis Jr RC, et al. Hypoalbuminemia and lymphocytopenia in patients with decompensated biventricular failure. Am J Med Sci 2010;339:31–5.

[10] Bell NH, Schedl HP, Bartter FC. An explanation for abnormal water retention and hypoosmolality in congestive heart failure. Am J Med 1964;36:351–60.

[11] Bennett WM, Bagby GC, Antonovic JN, Porter GA. Influence of volume expansion on proximal tubular sodium reabsorption in congestive heart failure. Am Heart 1973;85:55–64.

[12] Benoit JN, Granger DN. Intestinal microvascular adaptation to chronic portal hypertension in the rat. Gastroenterology 1988;94:471–6.

[13] Berlyne GM, Sutton J, Brown C, Feinroth M, Adler AJ, Friedman EA. Renal salt and water handling in water immersion in the nephrotic syndrome. Clin Sci 1981;61:605–10.

[14] Bernard DB, Alexander EA, Couser WG, Levinsky NG. Renal sodium retention during volume expansion in experimental nephrotic syndrome. Kidney Int 1978;14:478–85.

[15] Better O. Renal and cardiovascular dysfunction in liver disease. Kidney Int 1986;29:598–607.

[16] Better OS, Massry SG. Effect of chronic bile duct obstruction on renal handling of salt and water. J Clin Invest 1972;51:402–11.

[17] Bichet DG, Groves BM, Schrier RW. Mechanisms of improvement of water and sodium excretion by immersion in decompensated cirrhotic patients. Kidney Int 1983;24:788–94.

[18] Bichet DG, Van Putten VJ, Schrier RW. Potential role of increased sympathetic activity in impaired sodium and water excretion in cirrhosis. N Engl J Med 1982;307:1552–7.

[19] Bosch J, Enriquez R, Groszmann RJ, Storer EH. Chronic bile duct ligation in the dog: hemodynamic characterization of a portal hypertensive model. Hepatology 1983;3:1002–7.

[20] Brooks VL, Ell KR, Wright RM. Pressure-independent baroreflex resetting produced by chronic infusion of angiotensin II in rabbits. Am J Physiol 1993;265:H1275–82.

[21] Brown EA, Markandu ND, Roulston JE, Jones BE, Squires M, MacGregor GA. Is the renin–angiotensin–aldosterone system involved in the sodium retention in the nephrotic syndrome. Nephron 1982;32:102–7.

[22] Brown EA, Markandu ND, Sagnella GA, Jones BE, MacGregor GA. Lack of effect of captopril on the sodium retention of the nephrotic syndrome. Nephron 1984;37:43–8.

[23] Brown EA, Markandu ND, Sagnella GA, Squires M, Jones BE, MacGregor GA. Evidence that some mechanism other than the rennin system causes sodium retention in nephrotic syndrome. Lancet 1982;2:1237–9.

[24] Campillo B, Chabrier P-E, Pelle G, Sediame S, Altan G, Fouet P, et al. Inhibition of nitric oxide synthesis in the forearm arterial bed of patients with advanced cirrhosis. Hepatology 1995;22:1423–9.

[25] Caramelo C, Fernandez-Munoz D, Santos JC, Blanchart A, Rodriguez-Puyol D, Lopez-Novoa JM, et al. Effect of volume expansion on hemodynamics, capillary permeability and renal function in conscious, cirrhotic rats. Hepatology 1986;6:129–34.

[26] Chagnac A, Zevin D, Weinstein T, Hirsh J, Levi J. Combined tubular dysfunction in medullary cystic disease. Arch Intern Med 1986;146:1007–9.

[27] Chiandussi L, Bartoli E, Arras S. Reabsorption of sodium in the proximal renal tubule in cirrhosis of the liver. Gut 1978;19:497–503.

[28] Chonko AM, Bay WH, Stein J, Ferris TF. The role of renin and aldosterone in the salt retention of edema. Am J Med 1977;63:881–9.

[29] Cody RJ, Atlas SA, Laragh JH, Kubo SH, Covit AB, Ryman KS, et al. Atrial natriuretic factor in normal subjects and heart failure patients. J Clin Invest 1986;78:1362–74.

[30] Cody RJ, Franklin KW, Kluger J, Laragh JH. Mechanisms governing the postural response and baroreceptor abnormalities in chronic congestive heart failure: effect of acute and long-term converting enzyme inhibition. Circulation 1982;66:135–42.

[31] Coleman AJ, Arias M, Carter NW, Rector FC, Seldin DW. The mechanism of salt wastage in chronic renal disease. J Clin Invest 1966;45:1116–25.

[32] Colombato L, Albillos A, Groszmann R. The role of blood volume in the development of sodium retention in portal hypertensive rats. Gastroenterology 1996;110:193–8.

[33] de Seigneux S, Kim SW, Hemmingsen SC, Frokiaer JNielsen S. Increased expression but not targeting of ENaC in adrenalectomized rats with PAN-induced nephrotic syndrome. Am J Physiol Renal Physiol 2006;291:F208–17.

[34] Dharmaraj R, Hari P, Bagga A. Randomized cross-over trial comparing albumin and furosemide infusions in nephrotic syndrome. Pediatr Nephrol 2009;24:775–82.

[35] DiBona GF, Herman PJ, Sawin LL. Neural control of renal function in edema-forming states. Am J Physiol 1988;254:R1017–24.

[36] DiBona GF, Jones SY, Sawin LL. Effect of endogenous angiotensin II on renal nerve activity and its arterial baroreflex regulation. Am J Physiol 1996;271:R361–7.

[37] DiBona GF, Sawin LL. Role of renal nerves in sodium retention of cirrhosis and congestive heart failure. Am J Physiol 1991;260:R298–305.

[38] DiBona GF. Renal neural activity in hepatorenal syndrome. Kidney Int 1984;25:841–53.

[39] Dorhout Mees EJ, Geers AB, Koomans HA. Blood volume and sodium retention in the nephrotic syndrome: a controversial pathophysiological concept. Nephron 1984;36:201–11.

[40] Dorhout Mees EJ, Roos JC, Boer P, Yoe EH, Simatupang TA. Observations on edema formation in the nephrotic syndrome in adults with minimal lesions. Am J Med 1979;67:378–84.

[41] Doucet A, Favre G, Deschenes G. Molecular mechanism of edema formation in nephrotic syndrome: therapeutic implications. Pediatr Nephrol 2007;22:1983–90.

[42] Dusing R, Vetter H, Kramer HJ. The renin–angiotensin–aldosterone system in patients with nephrotic syndrome: effects of 1-sar-8 ala-angiotensin II. Nephron 1980;25:187–92.

[43] Dzau VJ, Colucci WS, Hollenberg NK, Williams GH. Relation of the renin–angiotensin–aldosterone system to clinical state in congestive heart failure. Circulation 1981;63:645–51.

[44] Dzau VJ, Colucci WS, Williams GH, Curfman G, Meggs L, Hollenberg NK. Sustained effectiveness of converting enzyme

inhibition in patients with severe congestive heart failure. N Engl J Med 1980;302:1373—9.

[45] Eggert RC. Spironolactone diuresis in patients with cirrhosis and ascites. BMJ 1970;4:401—3.

[46] Eisenberg S. Postural changes in plasma volume in hypoalbuminemia. Arch Intern Med 1963;112:544—9.

[47] Eisenberg S. Blood volume in persons with the nephrotic syndrome. Am J Med Sci 1968;255:320—6.

[48] Epstein FH, Post RS, McDowell M. The effect of an arteriovenous fistula on renal hemodynamics and electrolyte excretion. J Clin Invest 1953;32:233—41.

[49] Epstein M. Cardiovascular and renal effects of head-out water immersion in man. Circ Res 1976;39:619—28.

[50] Epstein M. Deranged sodium homeostasis in cirrhosis. Gastroenterology 1979;76:622—35.

[51] Epstein M, Berk DP, Hollenberg NK, Adams DF, Chalmers TC, Abrams HL, et al. Renal failure in the patient with cirrhosis. The role of active vasoconstriction. Am J Med 1970;49:175—85.

[52] Epstein M, Levinson R, Sancho J, Haber E, Re R. Characterization of the renin—aldosterone system in decompensated cirrhosis. Circ Res 1977;41:818—29.

[53] Epstein M, Ramachandran M, De Nunzio AG. Interrelationship of renal sodium and phosphate handling in cirrhosis. Miner Electrolyte Metab 1982;7:305—15.

[54] Fadnes HO, Pape JF, Sundsfjord JA. A study on oedema mechanism in nephrotic syndrome. Scand J Clin Lab Invest 1986;46:533—8.

[55] Faroqui S, Sheriff S, Amlal H. Metabolic acidosis has dual effects on sodium handling by rat kidney. Am J Physiol Renal Physiol 2006;291:F322—31.

[56] Fernandez-Munoz D, Caramelo C, Santos JC, Blanchart A, Hernando L, Lopez-Novoa JM. Systemic and splanchnic hemodynamic disturbances in conscious rats with experimental liver cirrhosis without ascites. Am J Physiol 1985;249:G316—20.

[57] Fernandez-Rodriguez C, Prada I, Prieto J, Montuenga LM, Elssasser T, Quiroga J, et al. Circulating adrenomedullin in cirrhosis: relationship to hyperdynamic circulation. J Hepatol 1998;98:250—6.

[58] Firth JD, Raine AEG, Ledingham JGG. Abnormal sodium handling occurs in the isolated perfused kidney of the nephrotic rat. Clin Sci 1989;76:387—95.

[59] Garcia-Tsao G, Bosch J. Management of varices and variceal hemorrhage in cirrhosis. N Engl J Med 2010;362:823—32.

[60] Geers AB, Koomans HA, Boer P, Dorhout Mees EJ. Plasma and blood volumes in patients with the nephrotic syndrome. Nephron 1984;38:170—3.

[61] Geers AB, Koomans HA, Roos JC, Boer P, Dorhout Mees EJ. Functional relationships in the nephrotic syndrome. Kidney Int 1984;26:324—30.

[62] Gerbes AL, Kollenda MC, Vollmar AM, Reichen J, Vakil N, Scarborough RM. Altered density of glomerular binding sites for atrial natriuretic factor in bile duct-ligated rats with ascites. Hepatology 1991;13:562—6.

[63] Gines P, Fernandez-Esparrach G, Arroyo V, Rodes J. Pathogenesis of ascites in cirrhosis. Semin Liver Dis 1997;17:175—89.

[64] Granger DN, Miller T, Allen R, Parker RE, Parker JC, Taylor AE. Permselectivity of cat liver blood—lymph barrier to endogenous macromolecules. Gastroenterology 1979;77:103—9.

[65] Grassi G, Cattaneo BM, Seravalle G, Lanfranchi A, Pozzi M, Morganti A, et al. Effects of chronic ACE inhibition on sympathetic nerve traffic and baroreflex control of circulation in heart failure. Circulation 1997;96:1173—9.

[66] Grausz H, Lieberman R, Earley LE. Effect of plasma albumin on sodium reabsorption in patients with nephrotic syndrome. Kidney Int 1972;1:47—54.

[67] Guevara M, Gines P, Fernandez-Esparrach G, Sort P, Salmeron JM, Jimenez W, et al. Reversibility of hepatorenal syndrome by prolonged administration of ornipressin and plasma volume expansion. Hepatology 1988;27:35—41.

[68] Guyton AC. Interstitial fluid pressure II. Pressure volume curves of the interstitial space. Circ Res 1965;16:452—60.

[69] Hammond TG, Whitworth JA, Saines D, Thatcher R, Andrews J, Kincaid-Smith P. Renin—angiotensin—aldosterone system in nephrotic syndrome. Am J Kidney Dis 1984;4:18—23.

[70] Harris PJ, Young JA. Dose-dependent stimulation and inhibition of proximal tubular sodium reabsorption by angiotensin II in the rat kidney. Pflugers Arch 1977;367:295—7.

[71] Hensen J, Abraham WT, Durr JA, Schrier RW. Aldosterone in congestive heart failure: analysis of determinants and role in sodium retention. Am J Nephrol 1991;11:441—6.

[72] Herman PJ, Sawin LL, DiBona GF. Role of renal nerves in renal sodium retention of nephrotic syndrome. Am J Physiol 1989;256:F823—9.

[73] Hollander W, Reilly P, Burrows BA. Lymphatic flow in human subjects as indicated by the disappearance of 131I-labeled albumin from the subcutaneous tissue. J Clin Lab Invest 1989;40:222—3.

[74] Hommel E, Mathiesen ER, Aukland K, Parving HH. Pathophysiological aspects of edema formation in diabetic nephropathy. Kidney Int 1990;38:1187—92.

[75] Hostetter TH, Pfeffer JM, Pfeffer MA, Dworkin LD, Braunwald E, Brenner BM. Cardiorenal hemodynamics and sodium excretion in rats with myocardial infarction. Am J Physiol 1983;245:H98—103.

[76] Ichikawa I, Pfeffer JM, Pfeffer MA, Hostetter TH, Brenner BM. Role of angiotensin II in the altered renal function of congestive heart failure. Circ Res 1984;55:669—75.

[77] Ichikawa I, Rennke HG, Hoyer JR, Badr KF, Schor N, Troy JL, et al. Role for intrarenal mechanisms in the impaired salt excretion of experimental nephrotic syndrome. J Clin Invest 1983;71:91—103.

[78] Iino Y, Troy JL, Brenner BM. Effects of catecholamines on electrolyte transport in cortical collecting tubule. J Membr Biol 1981;61:67—73.

[79] Iwakiri Y. The molecules: mechanisms of arterial vasodilatation observed in the splanchnic and systemic circulation in portal hypertension. J Clin Gastroenterol 2007;41(Suppl. 3):S288—94.

[80] Iwao T, Toyonaga A, Sato M, Oho K, Sakai T, Tayama C, et al. Effect of posture-induced blood volume expansion on systemic and regional hemodynamics in patients with cirrhosis. J Hepatol 1997;27:484—91.

[81] Jimenez W, Martinez-Pardo A, Arroyo V, Gaya J, Rivera F, Rodes J. Atrial natriuretic factor: reduced cardiac content in cirrhotic rats with ascites. Am J Physiol 1986;250:F749—52.

[82] Johnston CI, Davis JO, Robb CA, Mackenzie JW. Plasma renin in chronic experimental heart failure and during renal sodium "escape" from mineralocorticoids. Circ Res 1968;22:113—25.

[83] Joles JA, Koomans HA, Kortlandt W, Boer P, Dorhout Mees EJ. Hypoproteinemia and recovery from edema in dogs. Am J Physiol 1988;254:F887—94.

[84] Joles J, Rabelink T, Braam B, Koomans HA. Plasma volume regulation: defenses against edema formation (with special emphasis on hypoproteinemia). Am J Nephrol 1993;13:399—412.

[85] Kalambokis G, Economou M, Fotopoulos A, Al Bokharhii J, Pappas C, Katsaraki A, et al. The effects of chronic treatment with octreotide versus octreotide plus midodrine on systemic hemodynamics and renal hemodynamics and function in nonazotemic cirrhotic patients with ascites. Am J Gastroenterol 2004;99:1—7.

[86] Kalant N, Das Gupta D, Despointes R, Giroud CJP. Mechanisms of edema in experimental nephrosis. Am J Physiol 1962;202:91–6.

[87] Kapur G, Valentini RP, Imam AA, Mattoo TK. Treatment of severe edema in children with nephrotic syndrome with diuretics alone: a prospective study. Clin J Am Soc Nephrol 2009;4:907–13.

[88] Kelsch RC, Light GS, Oliver WJ. The effect of albumin infusion upon plasma norepinephrine concentration in nephrotic children. J Lab Clin Med 1972;79:516–25.

[89] Kim SW, Frokiaer J, Nielsen S. Pathogenesis of oedema in nephrotic syndrome: role of epithelial sodium channel. Nephrology (Carlton) 2007;12(Suppl. 3):S8–10.

[90] Kim SW, de Seigneux S, Sassen MC, Lee J, Kim J, Knepper MA, et al. Increased apical targeting of renal ENaC subunits and decreased expression of 11betaHSD2 in HgCl2-induced nephrotic syndrome in rats. Am J Physiol Renal Physiol 2006;290:F674–87.

[91] Kim JK, Michel J-B, Soubrier F, Durr J, Corvol P, Schrier RW. Arginine vasopressin gene expression in chronic cardiac failure in rats. Kidney Int 1990;38:818–22.

[92] Kim MY, Baik SK. Hyperdynamic circulation in patients with liver cirrhosis and portal hypertension. Korean J Gastroenterol 2009;54:143–8.

[93] Kiowski W, Sutsch G, Hunziker P, Müller P, Kim J, Oechslin E, et al. Evidence for endothelin-1-mediated vasoconstriction in severe chronic heart failure. Lancet 1995;346:732–6.

[94] Kirchheim HR, Finke R, Hackenthal E, Lowe W, Persson P. Baroreflex sympathetic activation increases threshold pressure for the pressure-dependent renin release in conscious dogs. Pflugers Arch 1985;405:127–35.

[95] Koepke JP, DiBona GF. Blunted natriuresis to atrial natriuretic peptide in chronic sodium-retaining disorders. Am J Physiol 1987;252:F865–71.

[96] Koepke JP, Jones S, DiBona GF. Renal nerves mediate blunted natriuresis to atrial natriuretic peptide in cirrhotic rats. Am J Physiol 1987;252:R1019–23.

[97] Kontos HA, Shapiro W, Mauck HP, Patterson Jr JL. General and regional circulatory alterations in cirrhosis of the liver. Am J Med 1964;37:526–35.

[98] Koomans HA, Braam B, Geers AB, Roos JC, Dorhout Mees EJ. The importance of plasma protein for blood volume and blood pressure homeostasis. Kidney Int 1986;30:730–5.

[99] Koomans HA, Geers AB, Dorhout Mees EJ, Kortland W. Lowered tissue-fluid oncotic pressure protects the blood volume in the nephrotic syndrome. Nephron 1986;42:317–22.

[100] Koomans HA, Geers AB, Meiracker AH, Roos JC, Boer P, Dorhout Mees EJ. Effects of plasma volume expansion on renal salt handling in patients with the nephrotic syndrome. Am J Nephrol 1984;4:227–34.

[101] Koomans HA, Kortlandt W, Geers AB, Dorhout Mees EJ. Lowered protein content of tissue fluid in patients with the nephrotic syndrome: observations during disease and recovery. Nephron 1985;40:391–5.

[102] Korthuis RJ, Kinden DA, Brimer GE, Slattery KA, Stogsdill P, Granger DN. Intestinal capillary filtration in acute and chronic portal hypertension. Am J Physiol 1988;254:G339–45.

[103] Kashani A, Landaverde C, Medici V, Rossaro L. Fluid retention in cirrhosis: pathophysiology and management. QJM 2008;101:71–85.

[104] Kostreva DR, Castaner A, Kampine JP. Reflex effects of hepatic baroreceptors on renal and cardiac sympathetic nerve activity. Am J Physiol 1980;238:R390–4.

[105] Krishna GG, Danovitch K, Danovitch GM. Effects of water immersion on renal function in the nephrotic syndrome. Kidney Int 1982;21:395–401.

[106] Kumagai H, Onoyama K, Iseki K, Omae T. Role of renin angiotensin aldosterone on minimal change nephrotic syndrome. Clin Nephrol 1985;23:229–35.

[107] La Villa G, Riccardi D, Lazzeri C, Cassini Raggi V, Dello Sbarba A, Tosti Guerra C, et al. Blunted natriuretic response to low-dose brain natriuretic peptide infusion in nonazotemic cirrhotic patients with ascites and avid sodium retention. Hepatology 1995;22:1745–50.

[108] Legault L, Cernacek P, Levy M, Maher E, Farber D. Renal tubular responsiveness to atrial natriuretic peptide in sodium-retaining chronic caval dogs: a possible role for kinins and luminal actions of the peptide. J Clin Invest 1992;90:1425–35.

[109] Leimbach WN, Wallin BG, Victor RG, Aylward PE, Sundlof G, Mark AL. Direct evidence from intraneural recordings for increased central sympathetic outflow in patients with heart failure. Circulation 1986;73:913–9.

[110] Lenz K, Hortnagl H, Druml W, Reither H, Schmid R, Schneewiess B, et al. Ornipressin in the treatment of functional renal failure in decompensated liver cirrhosis. Gastroenterology 1991;101:1060–7.

[111] Levine TB, Francis GS, Goldsmith SR, Simon AB, Cohn JN. Activity of the sympathetic nervous system and renin–angiotensin system assessed by plasma hormone levels and their relation to hemodynamic abnormalities in congestive heart failure. Am J Cardiol 1982;49:1659–66.

[112] Levy M. Effects of acute volume expansion and altered hemodynamics on renal tubular function in chronic caval dogs. J Clin Invest 1972;51:922–34.

[113] Levy M, Wexler MJ. Sodium excretion in dogs with low-grade caval constriction: role of hepatic nerves. Am J Physiol 1987;253:F672–8.

[114] Levy M, Wexler MJ. Hepatic denervation alters first-phase urinary sodium excretion in dogs with cirrhosis. 1987;253:F664–71.

[115] Levy M. Sodium retention and ascites formation in dogs with experimental portal cirrhosis. Am J Physiol 1977;233:F572–85.

[116] Levy M, Allotey JB. Temporal relationships between urinary salt retention and altered systemic hemodynamics in dogs with experimental cirrhosis. J Lab Clin Med 1978;92:560–9.

[117] Levy M, Wexler MJ. Renal sodium retention and ascites formation in dogs with experimental cirrhosis but without portal hypertension or increased splanchnic vascular capacity. J Lab Clin Med 1978;91:520–36.

[118] Lieberman FL, Denison EK, Reynolds TB. The relationship of plasma volume, portal hypertension, ascites, and renal sodium retention in cirrhosis: the overflow theory of ascites formation. Ann NY Acad Sci 1978;170:202–11.

[119] Ljungman S, Laragh JH, Cody RJ. Role of the kidney in congestive heart failure: relationship of cardiac index to kidney function. Drugs 1990;39(Suppl. 4):10–21.

[120] Limas CJ, Guiha NH, Lekagul O, Cohn JN. Impaired left ventricular function in alcoholic cirrhosis with ascites. Circulation 1974;69:755–60.

[121] Lopez-Talavera JC, Merrill WM, Groszmann RJ. Tumor necrosis factor a: a major contributor to the hyperdynamic circulation in prehepatic portal-hypertensive rats. Gastroenterology 1995;108:761–7.

[122] Lopez-Talavera JC, Levitzki A, Martinez M, Gazit A, Esteban R, Guardia J. Tyrosine kinase inhibition ameliorates the hyperdynamic state and decreases nitric oxide production in cirrhotic rats with portal hypertension and ascites. J Clin Invest 1997;100:664–70.

[123] Lopez C, Jimenez W, Arroyo V, Claria J, La Villa G, Asbert M, et al. Temporal relationship between the decrease in arterial pressure and sodium retention in conscious spontaneously

hypertensive rats with carbon tetrachloride-induced cirrhosis. Hepatology 1991;13:585—9.

[124] Lopez C, Jimenez W, Arroyo V, La Villa G, Gaya J, Claria J, et al. Role of altered systemic hemodynamics in the blunted renal response to atrial natriuretic peptide in rats with cirrhosis and ascites. J Hepatology 1989;9:217—26.

[125] Lourdel S, Loffing J, Favre G, Paulais M, Nissant A, Fakitsas P, et al. Hyperaldosteronemia and activation of the epithelial sodium channel are not required for sodium retention in puromycin-induced nephrosis. J Am Soc Nephrol 2005;16:3642—50.

[126] Luetscher JA, Johnson BB. Observations on the sodium-retaining corticoid (aldosterone) in the urine of children and adults in relation to sodium balance and edema. J Clin Invest 1954;33:1441—6.

[127] MacGilchrist A, Craig KJ, Hayes PC, Cumming AD. Effect of the serine protease inhibitor, aprotinin, on systemic haemodynamics and renal function in patients with hepatic cirrhosis and ascites. Clin Sci 1994;87:329—35.

[128] Maher E, Cernacek P, Levy M. Heterogeneous renal responses to atrial natriuretic factor II. Cirrhotic dogs. Am J Physiol 1989;257:R1068—74.

[129] Manenti F, Williams R. Injection studies of the splenic vasculature in portal hypertension. Gut 1966;7:175—80.

[130] Mann JF, Green D, Jamerson K, Ruilope LM, Kuranoff SJ, Littke T, et al. Avosentan for overt diabetic nephropathy. J Am Soc Nephrol 2010;21:527—35.

[131] Marcus LS, Hart D, Packer M, Yushak M, Medina N, Danziger RS, et al. Hemodynamic and renal excretory effects of human brain natriuretic peptide infusion in patients with congestive heart failure: a double-blind, placebo-controlled, randomized crossover trial. Circulation 1996;94:3184—9.

[132] Martin P-Y, Ohara M, Gines P, Xu DL, St John J, Niederberger M, et al. Nitric oxide synthase (NOS) inhibition for one week improves renal sodium and water excretion in cirrhotic rats with ascites. J Clin Invest 1998;101:235—42.

[133] Martin P-Y, Schrier RW. Sodium and water retention in heart failure: pathogenesis and treatment. Kidney Int 1997;51(Suppl. 59):S57—61.

[134] Martin P, Gines P, Schrier R. Nitric oxide as a mediator of hemodynamic abnormalities and sodium and water retention in cirrhosis. N Engl J Med 1998;339:533—41.

[135] Mejias M, Garcia-Pras E, Tiani C, Miquel R, Bosch J, Fernandez M. Beneficial effects of sorafenib on splanchnic, intrahepatic, and portocollateral circulations in portal hypertensive and cirrhotic rats. Hepatology 2009;49:1245—56.

[136] Melman A, Massry SG. Role of renal vasodilation in the blunted natriuresis of saline infusion in dogs with chronic bile duct obstruction. J Lab Clin Med 1977;89:1053—65.

[137] Meltzer J, Keim HJ, Laragh JH, Sealey JE, Jan KM, Chien S. Nephrotic syndrome: vasoconstriction and hypervolemic types indicated by renin-sodium profiling. Ann Intern Med 1979;91:688—96.

[138] Metcoff J, Janeway CA. Studies on the pathogenesis of nephrotic edema. J Pediatr 1961;58:640—85.

[139] Metlauer B, Rouleau JL, Bichet D, Juneau C, Kortas C, Barjon JN, et al. Sodium and water excretion abnormalities in congestive heart failure. Ann Intern Med 1986;105:161—7.

[140] Moller S, Henriksen JH. Circulatory abnormalities in cirrhosis with focus on neurohumoral aspects. Semin Nephrol 1997;17:505—19.

[141] Moller S, Henriksen JH, Bendtsen F. Ascites: pathogenesis and therapeutic principles. Scand J Gastroenterol 2009;44:902—11.

[142] Moore K, Wendon J, Frazer M, Karani J, Williams R, Badr K. Plasma endothelin immunoreactivity in liver disease and the hepatorenal syndrome. N Engl J Med 1992;327:1774—8.

[143] Morali GA, Tobe SW, Skorecki KL, Blendis LM. Refractory ascites: modulation of atrial natriuretic factor unresponsiveness by mannitol. Hepatology 1992;16:42—8.

[144] Nicholls KM, Shapiro MD, Groves BS, Schrier RW. Factors determining renal response to water immersion in nonexcretor cirrhotic patients. Kidney Int 1986;30:417—21.

[145] Nicholls KM, Shapiro MD, Kluge R, Chung HM, Bichet DG, Schrier RW. Sodium excretion in advanced cirrhosis: effect of expansion of central blood volume and suppression of plasma aldosterone. Hepatology 1986;6:235—8.

[146] Nicholls KM, Shapiro MD, Van Putten VJ, Kluge R, Chung HM, Bichet DG, et al. Elevated plasma norepinephrine concentrations in decompensated cirrhosis. Circ Res 1985;56:457—61.

[147] Niederberger M, Martin P-Y, Gines P, Morris K, Tsai P, Xu DL, et al. Normalization of nitric oxide production corrects arterial vasodilation and hyperdynamic circulation in cirrhotic rats. Gastroenterology 1995;109:1624—30.

[148] Ochs A, Rossle M, Haag K, Hauenstein KH, Deibert P, Siegerstetter V, et al. The transjugular intrahepatic portosystemic stent-shunt procedure for refractory ascites. N Engl J Med 1995;332:1192—7.

[149] Olivari MT, Levine TB, Cohn JN. Abnormal neurohormonal response to nitroprusside infusion in congestive heart failure. J Am Coll Cardiol 1983;2:411.

[150] Oliver WJ, Kelsch RC, Chandler JP. Demonstration of increased catecholamine excretion in the nephrotic syndrome. Proc Soc Exp Biol Med 1967;125:1176—80.

[151] Packer M, Lee WH, Kessler PD. Preservation of glomerular filtration in human heart failure by activation of the renin—angiotensin system. Circulation 1986;74:766—74.

[152] Packer M, Lee WH, Medina N, Yushak M, Kessler PD. Functional renal insufficiency during long-term therapy with captopril and enalapril in severe chronic heart failure. Ann Intern Med 1987;106:346—54.

[153] Palazzuoli A, Gallotta M, Quatrini I, Nuti R. Natriuretic peptides (BNP and NT-proBNP): measurement and relevance in heart failure. Vasc Health Risk Manag 2010;6:411—8.

[154] Palmer BF. Renal complications associated with use of nonsteroidal anti-inflammatory agents. J Invest Med 1995;43:516—33.

[155] Palmer BF. Hyponatremia in patients with central nervous system disease: SIADH or CSW. Trends Endocrinol Metab 2003;14:182—743.

[156] Palmer BF. Renal dysfunction complicating treatment of hypertension. N Engl J Med 2002;347:1256—61.

[157] Panos MZ, Gove C, Firth JD, Raine AE, Ledingham JG, Westaby D, et al. Impaired natriuretic response to atrial natriuretic peptide in the isolated kidney of rats with experimental cirrhosis. Clin Sci 1990;79:67—71.

[158] Pelayo JC, Ziegler MG, Blantz RC. Angiotensin II in adrenergic-induced alterations in glomerular hemodynamics. Am J Physiol 1984;247:F799—807.

[159] Pelayo JC, Ziegler MG, Jose PA, Blantz RC. Renal denervation in the rat: analysis of glomerular and proximal tubular function. Am J Physiol 1983;244:F70—7.

[160] Perez-Ayuso RM, Arroyo V, Camps J, Rimola A, Costa J, Gaya J, et al. Renal kallikrein excretion in cirrhosis with ascites: relationship to renal hemodynamics. Hepatology 19844:247—252.

[161] Perez-Ayuso RM, Arroyo V, Planas R, Gaya J, Bory F, Rimola A, et al. Randomized comparative study of efficacy of furosemide versus spironolactone in nonazotemic cirrhosis with ascites. Gastroenterology 1983;84:961—8.

[162] Perico N, Remuzzi G. Edema of the nephrotic syndrome: the role of the atrial peptide system. Am J Kidney Dis 1993;22:355—66.

[163] Perico N, Remuzzi G. Renal handling of sodium in the nephrotic syndrome. Am J Nephrol 1993;13:413—21.

[164] Peters JP, Welt LG, Sims EA, Orloff J, Needham J. Salt-wasting syndrome associated with cerebral disease. Trans Assoc Am Physicians 1950;63:57—64.

[165] Peterson C, Madson B, Perlman A, Chan AY, Myers BD. Atrial natriuretic peptide and the renal response to hypervolemia in nephrotic humans. Kidney Int 1988;34:825—31.

[166] Priebe HJ, Heimann JC, Hedley-White J. Effects of renal and hepatic venous congestion on renal function in the presence of low and normal cardiac output in dogs. Circ Res 1980;47:883—90.

[167] Rabelink T, Bijlsma J, Koomans H. Iso-oncotic volume expansion in the nephrotic syndrome. Clin Sci 1993;84:627—32.

[168] Raine AE, Erne P, Burgisser E, Muller FB, Bolli P, Burkart F, et al. Atrial natriuretic peptide and atrial pressure in patients with congestive heart failure. N Engl J Med 1986;315:533—7.

[169] Rascher W, Tulassay T. Hormonal regulation of water metabolism in children with nephrotic syndrome. Kidney Int 1987;32:583—9.

[170] Rascher W, Tulassay T, Seyberth HW, Himbert U, Lang U, Scharer K. Diuretic and hormonal response to head-out water immersion in nephrotic syndrome. J Pediatr 1986;109:609—14.

[171] Rector WG, Hossack KF. Pathogenesis of sodium retention complicating cirrhosis: is there room for diminished "effective" arterial blood volume? Gastroenterology 1988;95:1658—63.

[172] Rehsia NS, Dhalla NS. Potential of endothelin-1 and vasopressin antagonists for the treatment of congestive heart failure. Heart Fail Rev 2010;15:85—101.

[173] Reilly T, Schork MR. Vasopressin antagonists: pharmacotherapy for the treatment of heart failure. Ann Pharmacother 2010;44:680—7.

[174] Resch M, Wiest R, Moleda L, Fredersdorf S, Stoelcker B, Schroeder JA, et al. Alterations in mechanical properties of mesenteric resistance arteries in experimental portal hypertension. Am J Physiol Gastrointest Liver Physiol 2009;297:G849—57.

[175] Rodriguez-Martinez M, Sawin LL, DiBona GF. Arterial and cardiopulmonary baroreflex control of renal nerve activity in cirrhosis. Am J Physiol 1995;268:R117—29.

[176] Ros J, Jimenez W, Lamas S, Claria J, Arroyo V, Rivera F, et al. Nitric oxide production in arterial vessels of cirrhotic rats. Hepatology 1995;21:554—60.

[177] Rosoff L, Zia P, Reynolds T, Horton R. Studies of renin and aldosterone in cirrhotic patients with ascites. Gastroenterology 1975;69:698—705.

[178] Salo J, Jimenez W, Kuhn M, Ginès A, Ginès P, Fernández-Esparrach G, et al. Urinary excretion of urodilatin in patients with cirrhosis. Hepatology 1996;24:1428—32.

[179] Sanz E, Caramelo C, Lopez-Novoa JM. Interstitial dynamics in rats with early stage experimental cirrhosis of the liver. Am J Physiol 1989;256:F497—503.

[180] Sato S, Ohnishi K, Sugita S, Okuda K. Splenic artery and superior mesenteric artery blood flow: nonsurgical Doppler US measurement in healthy subjects and patients with chronic liver disease. Radiology 1987;164:347—52.

[181] Schaffner F, Popper H. Capillarization of hepatic sinusoids in man. Gastroenterology 1963;44:239—42.

[182] Schedl HP, Bartter FC. An explanation for an experimental correction of the abnormal water diuresis in cirrhosis. J Clin Invest 1960;39:248—61.

[183] Schrier RW, Masoumi A, Elhassan F. Aldosterone: role in edematous disorders, hypertension, chronic renal failure, and metabolic syndrome. Clin J Am Soc Nephrol 2010;5:1132—40.

[184] Schrier RW. Decreased effective blood volume in edematous disorders: what does this mean? J Am Soc Nephrol 2007;18:2028—31.

[185] Schrier RW. Pathogenesis of sodium and water retention in high-output and low-output cardiac failure, nephrotic syndrome, cirrhosis, and pregnancy. N Engl J Med 1988;319 (1065—1072):1127—34.

[186] Schrier RW, Humphreys MH, Ufferman RC. Role of cardiac output and the autonomic nervous system in the antinatriuretic response to acute constriction of the thoracic superior vena cava. Circ Res 1971;29:490—8.

[187] Schuster VL, Kokko JP, Jacobson HR. Angiotensin II directly stimulates sodium transport in rabbit proximal convoluted tubules. J Clin Invest 1984;73:507—15.

[188] Shapiro MD, Nicholls KM, Groves BM, Kluge R, Chung HM, Bichet DG, et al. Interrelationship between cardiac output and vascular resistance as determinants of effective arterial blood volume in cirrhotic patients. Kidney Int 1985;28:206—11.

[189] Shapiro MD, Hasbargen J, Hensen J, Schrier RW. Role of aldosterone in the sodium retention of patients with nephrotic syndrome. Am J Nephrol 1990;10:44—8.

[190] Skorecki KL, Leung WM, Campbell P, Warner LC, Wong PY, Bull S, et al. Role of atrial natriuretic peptide in the natriuretic response to central volume expansion induced by head-out water immersion in sodium-retaining cirrhotic subjects. Am J Med 1988;85:375—82.

[191] Smith JD, Hayslett JP. Reversible renal failure in the nephrotic syndrome. Am J Kidney Dis 1992;19:201—13.

[192] Sogni P, Garnier P, Gadano A, Moreau R, Dall'Ava-Santucci J, Dinh-Xuan AT, et al. Endogenous pulmonary nitric oxide production measured from exhaled air is increased in patients with severe cirrhosis. J Hepatol 1995;23:471—3.

[193] Stumpe KO, Solle H, Klein H, Kruck . Mechanism of sodium and water retention in rats with experimental heart failure. Kidney Int 1973;4:309—17.

[194] Suki WN. Renal hemodynamic consequences of angiotensin-converting enzyme inhibition in congestive heart failure. Arch Intern Med 1989;149:669—73.

[195] Thiesson HC, Jensen B, Bistrup C, Ottosen PD, McNeilly AD, Andrew R, et al. Renal sodium retention in cirrhotic rats depends on glucocorticoid-mediated activation of mineralocorticoid receptor due to decreased renal beta 11beta-HSD-2 activity. Ann J Physiol Integr Comp Physiol 2007;292:R625—36.

[196] Tulassay T, Rascher W, Lang RE, Seyberth HW, Scharer K. Atrial natriuretic peptide and other vasoactive hormones in nephrotic syndrome. Kidney Int 1987;31:1391—5.

[197] Unikowsky B, Wexler MJ, Levy M. Dogs with experimental cirrhosis of the liver but without intrahepatic hypertension do not retain sodium or form ascites. J Clin Invest 1983;72:1594—604.

[198] Usberti M, Federico S, Cianciaruso B, Costanzo R, Russo D, Andreucci VE. Relationship between serum albumin concentration and tubular reabsorption of glucose in renal disease. Kidney Int 1983;16:546—51.

[199] Usberti M, Federico S, Meccariello S, Cianciaruso B, Balletta M, Pecoraro C, et al. Role of plasma vasopressin in the impairment of water excretion in nephrotic syndrome. Kidney Int 1984;25:422—9.

[200] Valentin J, Qiu C, Muldowney WP, Ying WZ, Gardner DG, Humphreys MH. Cellular basis for blunted volume expansion natruresis in experimental nephrotic syndrome. J Clin Invest 1992;90:1302—12.

[201] Valentin J, Ying W, Sechi LA, Ling KT, Qiu C, Couser WG, et al. Phosphodiesterase inhibitors correct resistance to

natriuretic peptides in rate with Heymann nephritis. J Am Soc Nephrol 1996;7:582—93.

[202] Villareal D, Freeman RH, Davis JO, Verburg KM, Vari RC. Atrial natriuretic factor secretion in dogs with experimental high-output heart failure. Am J Physiol 1987;252:H692—6.

[203] Vorobioff J, Bredfeldt JE, Groszmann RJ. Increased blood flow through the portal system in cirrhotic rats. Gastroenterology 1984;87:1120—6.

[204] Wada A, Tsutamoto T, Fukai D, Ohnishi M, Maeda K, Hisanaga T, et al. Comparison of the effects of selective endothelin ETA and ETB receptor antagonists in congestive heart failure. J Am Coll Cardiol 1997;30:1385—92.

[205] Walle J, Donckerwolcke R, Boer P, van Isselt HW, Koomans HA, Joles JA. Blood volume, colloid osmotic pressure and F-cell ratio in children with the nephrotic syndrome. Kidney Int 1996;49:1471—7.

[206] Watkins L, Burton JA, Haber E, Cant JR, Smith FW, Barger AC. The renin—angiotensin—aldosterone system in congestive heart failure in conscious dogs. J Clin Invest 1976;57: 1606—17.

[207] Weigert AL, Martin P-Y, Schrier RW. Vascular hyporesponsiveness in cirrhotic rats: role of different nitric oxide synthase isoforms. Kidney Int 1997;52(Suppl. 61):S41—4.

[208] Welt LG, Seldin DW, Nelson WP, German WJ, Peters JP. Role of the central nervous system in metabolism of electrolytes and water. Arch Intern Med 1952;90:355—78.

[209] Wiest R. Splanchnic and systemic vasodilation: the experimental models. J Clin Gastroenterol 2007;41(Suppl. 3):S272—87.

[210] Winlaw DS, Smythe GA, Keogh AM, Schwens CG, Spratt PM, Macdonald PS. Increased nitric oxide production in heart failure. Lancet 1994;344:373—4.

[211] Wirth KJ, Bickel M, Hropot M, Gunzler V, Heitsch H, Ruppert D, et al. The bradykinin B2 receptor antagonist Icatibant (HOE 140) corrects avid Na retention in rats with CCL4-induced liver cirrhosis: possible role of enhanced microvascular leakage. Eur J Pharmacol 1997;337:45—53.

[212] Witte MH, Witte CL, Dumont AE. Progress in liver disease: physiological factors involved in the causation of cirrhotic ascites. Gastroenterology 1971;61:742—50.

[213] Witte MH, Witte CL, Dumont AE. Estimated net transcapillary water and protein flux in the liver and intestine of patients with portal hypertension from hepatic cirrhosis. Gastroenterology 1981;80:265—72.

[214] Witte CL, Witte MH, Dumont AE, Cole WR, Smith JR. Protein content in lymph and edema fluids in congestive heart failure. Circulation 1969;40:623—30.

[215] Wraight EP. Capillary permeability of protein as a factor in the control of plasma volume. J Physiol 1974;237:39.

[216] Xu D-L, Martin P-Y, Ohara St M, John J, Pattison T, Meng X, et al. Upregulation of aquaporin-2 water channel expression in chronic heart failure rat. J Clin Invest 1997;99:1500—5.

[217] Zennaro M-C, Lombes M. Mineralocorticoid resistance. Trends Endocrinol Metab 2004;15:264—70.

[218] Zucker IH, Earle AM, Gilmore JP. The mechanism of adaptation of left atrial stretch receptors in dogs with chronic congestive heart failure. J Clin Invest 1977;60:323—31.

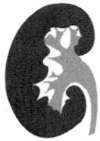

Physiology and Pathophysiology of Hypertension

John E. Hall[1], Joey P. Granger[2] and Michael E. Hall[2]

[1]Department of Physiology and Biophysics, University of Mississippi Medical Center, MS, USA

[2]Department of Physiology and Biophysics and Department of Medicine, University of Mississippi Medical Center, MS, USA

INTRODUCTION

Hypertension is the leading risk factor for cardiovascular deaths, causing approximately 7.6 million premature deaths per year worldwide.[1] Over 1 billion people including more than 50 million Americans have hypertension, making it the most common chronic disease.[1,2] Blood pressure (BP) typically rises with age and in the United States, approximately 50% of people 60–69 years old and 75% of people 70 years and older have hypertension.[1] In non-industrialized populations, however, BP does not rise with aging and only a small fraction of the population develops hypertension. This suggests that environmental factors play a major role in causing hypertension, and that a rise in BP with aging is not inevitable when these conditions are absent.

A direct positive relationship between BP and cardiovascular disease CVD risk has been observed in men and women of all ages, races, ethnic groups, and countries, regardless of other risk factors for CVD.[2] Observational studies indicate that death from CVD increases progressively as BP rises above 115 mmHg systolic and 75 mmHg diastolic pressure.[2] For every 20 mmHg systolic or 10 mmHg diastolic increase in BP there is a doubling of mortality from ischemic heart disease and stroke in all age groups from 40 to 89 years old.[3]

Despite major advances in our understanding of its pathophysiology, and the availability of many drugs that can effectively reduce BP in most hypertensive subjects, hypertension is still poorly-controlled in most countries, including the United States, and continues to be the most important modifiable risk factor for CVD.

BLOOD PRESSURE CLASSIFICATION FOR HYPERTENSION TREATMENT

BP is a variable, quantitative trait with a normal distribution slightly skewed toward higher BPs. Although there is no clear level of BP where cardiovascular or renal disease begins to occur, a definition of hypertension is useful for treatment decisions. A commonly used BP classification was proposed in 2003 by the Seventh Report of the United States Joint National Committee on Prevention, Detection, Evaluation, and Treatment of High BP JNC 7 and is now widely used.[4]

According to these criteria, normal BP is defined as a systolic BP <120 mmHg and a diastolic BP <80 mmHg. Persons with a systolic BP between 120–139 mmHg or diastolic BP between 80–89 mmHg are designated as having *prehypertension*. Hypertension is further characterized by two stages: Stage 1, the milder (systolic 140–159 mmHg and/or diastolic 90–99 mmHg) and most common form of hypertension, accounts for approximately 80% of hypertension. Stage 2 hypertension includes those with systolic BP ≥160 mmHg and/or diastolic BP ≥100 mmHg. Isolated systolic hypertension is defined as systolic BP of ≥140 mmHg and diastolic BP <90 mmHg.

Using these definitions, and including those taking antihypertensive medications, approximately 24% of the adult population in the United States has hypertension.[4] This percentage varies with: 1) race, being higher in blacks 32% and lower in whites 23% and Mexican Americans 23%; 2) age, because systolic BP rises throughout life in the United States, as well as in most industrialized countries, whereas diastolic BP rises until age 55–60 years; 3) gender, with hypertension being more prevalent in men than in premenopausal women, after menopause women have BPs that are nearly the same as in men; 4) geographic patterns, with hypertension being more prevalent in the Southeastern United States; and 5) socioeconomic status, which is inversely related to the prevalence of hypertension.

Primary hypertension accounts for about 95% of all cases of hypertension, and is usually defined as elevated BP for which an obvious secondary cause (e.g., renovascular disease, aldosteronism, pheochromocytoma or gene mutations) cannot be determined. Although primary hypertension is a heterogeneous disorder, some of the main risk factors are known. For example, overweight and obesity may account for as much as 65–75% of the risk for primary hypertension. Other factors, such as sedentary lifestyle, excess consumption of alcohol or sodium chloride, and low potassium intake are also thought to contribute to increased BP in many patients.[5] This review discusses basic concepts of BP control and pathophysiological changes that may cause primary hypertension, as well as selected forms of genetic and secondary hypertension.[5,6]

BASIC PHYSIOLOGY OF BLOOD PRESSURE REGULATION

BP regulation depends on integrated actions of multiple cardiovascular, renal, neural, endocrine, and local tissue control systems. Although hypertension is usually considered as a disorder of the average level at which BP is regulated, there is increasing interest in other measures of BP, including peak arterial pressure, BP variability, nighttime and daytime BP, and responses of BP to stress, which may affect cardiovascular risk.

The complex local control, hormonal, neural, and renal systems that regulate BP are often discussed in terms of how they influence cardiac function or vascular resistance because of the well-known formula: *mean arterial pressure = cardiac output × total peripheral resistance*. This conceptual framework, with the addition of factors that influence vascular capacity and transcapillary fluid exchange, is adequate to explain short-term BP regulation, but not chronic hypertension.[5,7] Two additional concepts are useful when considering chronic BP regulation: 1) BP control mechanisms are time-dependent; and 2) renal excretion of water and electrolytes play a key role in long-term BP regulation.

Blood Pressure Control Systems are Time-Dependent

Figure 39.1 shows the maximum feedback gains of major BP controllers following a sudden disturbance,

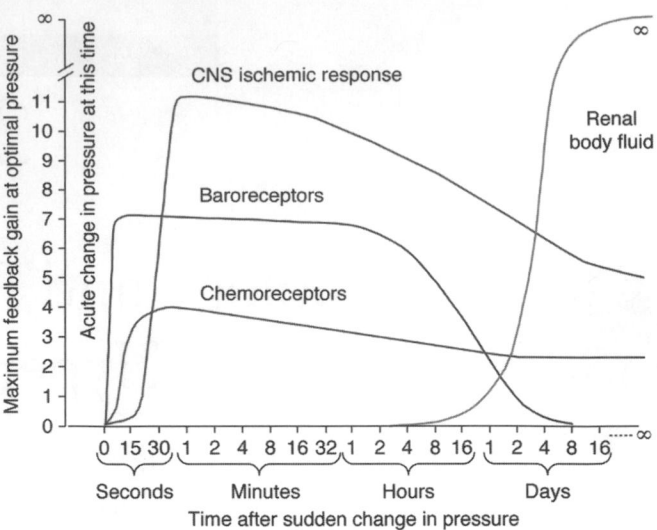

FIGURE 39.1 Time-dependency of blood pressure control mechanisms. Approximate maximum feedback gains of various blood pressure control mechanisms at different time intervals after the onset of a disturbance to arterial pressure.

as might occur with rapid blood loss. Three important neural control systems begin to function powerfully within a few seconds: 1) the arterial baroreceptors, which detect changes in BP and send appropriate autonomic reflex signals back to the heart and blood vessels to return the BP toward normal; 2) the chemoreceptors, which detect changes in oxygen or carbon dioxide in the blood and initiate autonomic feedback responses that influence BP; and 3) the central nervous system, which responds within a few seconds to ischemia of the vasomotor centers in the medulla, especially when BP falls below about 50 mmHg. Each of these nervous control mechanisms works rapidly and has potent effects on BP. Also note, however, that the feedback gains of these systems decrease with time, as disturbances of BP are maintained.

Within a few minutes or hours after a BP disturbance, additional control systems react, including: 1) a shift of fluid from the interstitial spaces into the blood in response to decreased BP or a shift of fluid out of the blood into the interstitial spaces in response to increased BP; 2) the renin–angiotensin–aldosterone system RAAS which is activated when BP falls too low and is suppressed when BP increases above normal; 3) multiple vasodilator systems not shown in the figure that are suppressed when BP decreases and stimulated when BP rises above normal.

Most of the BP regulators are *proportional* control systems. This means that they can correct a BP abnormality only part of the way back toward the normal level, but never all the way back. The arterial baroreceptor reflex system, for example, has a feedback gain of approximately 2.0 during acute changes in BP, and

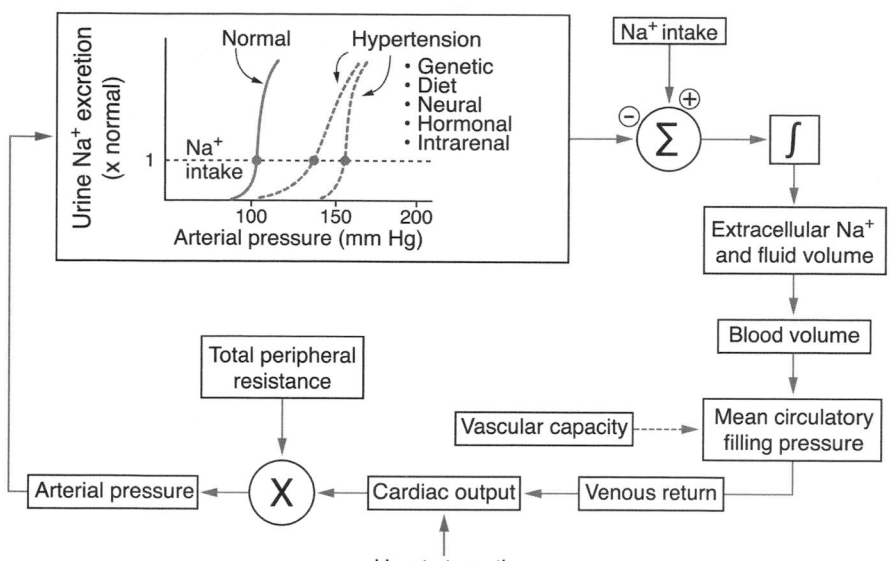

FIGURE 39.2 Block diagram showing the basic elements of the renal—body fluid feedback mechanism for long-term regulation of arterial pressure.

therefore buffers about two-thirds of a sudden change in the BP. The renal—body fluid feedback system, however, is the one BP control system with *near infinite feedback gain* if it is given enough time to operate.[7]

The Renal—Body Fluid Feedback Mechanism for Long-Term BP Regulation

Figure 39.2 shows the basic components of the renal—body fluid feedback mechanism. Extracellular fluid volume is determined by the balance between intake and excretion of salt and water by the kidneys. Even a temporary imbalance between intake and output can lead to a change in extracellular volume, and potentially a change in BP. Under steady-state conditions there must be a precise balance between intake and output of salt and water; otherwise, there would be continued accumulation or loss of fluid leading to circulatory collapse within a few days. A key component of this mechanism for regulating salt and water balance is *pressure natriuresis*—the effects of increased BP to raise sodium excretion.[5] Under many conditions this mechanism stabilizes BP. For example, when BP is increased above the renal set-point, because of increased TPR or increased cardiac pumping ability, this also tends to increase sodium excretion, via pressure natriuresis, if the effectiveness of pressure natriuresis is not impaired (Figure 39.3). As long as fluid excretion exceeds intake, extracellular fluid volume will continue to decrease, reducing venous return and cardiac output, until BP returns to normal and fluid balance is re-established.

An important feature of pressure natriuresis is that it continues to operate until BP returns to the original set-point. Another key aspect of pressure natriuresis is

that various neurohumoral systems can amplify or blunt the pressure natriuresis mechanism.[5] For example, increases in sodium intake are associated with only small changes in BP in many people. One reason for this insensitivity of BP to changes in salt intake is decreased formation of antinatriuretic hormones such as angiotensin II and aldosterone, which enhance the effectiveness of pressure natriuresis and allow sodium balance to be maintained with minimal increases in BP. On the other hand, excessive activation of these antinatriuretic systems reduces the effectiveness of pressure natriuresis, necessitating greater increases in BP to maintain sodium balance.

In all forms of human or experimental hypertension studied thus far, there is a shift of pressure natriuresis toward higher BPs. In some cases, impaired pressure natriuresis is caused by *intrarenal* disturbances that reduce glomerular filtration rate GFR or increase tubular reabsorption. In other instances, impaired pressure natriuresis is caused by *extrarenal* factors, such as increased activity of the SNS or antinatriuretic hormones that reduce the kidney's ability to excrete sodium and eventually raise BP.

Vasoconstrictors May Decrease Extracellular Volume Despite Impairing Renal-Pressure Natriuresis

Some forms of hypertension, especially those associated with increased levels of vasoconstrictors such as norepinephrine, are associated with reduced rather than increased extracellular fluid volume. How can the hypertension in these instances be attributed to impaired renal pressure natriuresis when there is no evidence of sodium retention? Consider the physiological changes caused by infusion of a powerful

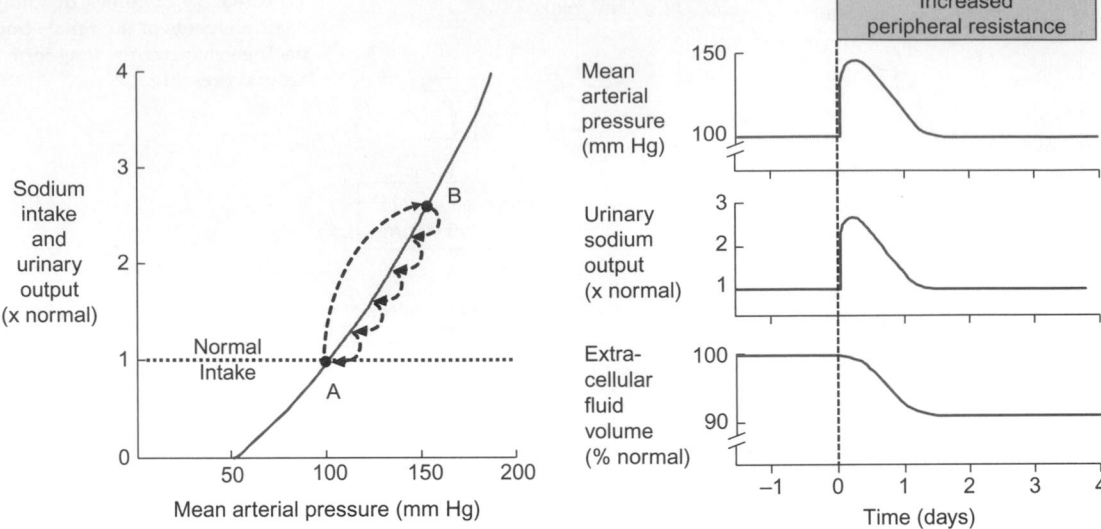

FIGURE 39.3   Long-term effects of increased total peripheral resistance (TPR), such as that caused by closure of a large arteriovenous fistula, with no change in the renal pressure natriuresis relationship. BP is initially increased from point A to point B, but elevated BP cannot be sustained because sodium excretion exceeds intake, reducing extracellular fluid volume until BP returns to normal and sodium balance is re-established.[10]

vasoconstrictor such as norepinephrine. Chronic iv infusion of norepinephrine causes mild hypertension associated with an initial increase in sodium excretion as BP rises.[8] After several days, sodium excretion returns to normal but extracellular fluid volume is reduced. On the other hand, if norepinephrine is infused directly into the renal artery at a low dose so that its effect on other vascular beds is minimal or if renal perfusion pressure is servo-controlled and prevented from increasing during iv norepinephrine infusion there is significant sodium retention, demonstrating a direct antinatriuretic effect on the kidneys, as well as development of hypertension.[5,8]

Figure 39.4 shows the relationship between BP and sodium excretion caused by a powerful vasoconstrictor, such as norepinephrine, which has a relatively weak antinatriuretic action. The antinatriuretic effect shifts pressure natriuresis to higher BPs, but because norepinephrine has a weak antinatriuretic effect, compared to its peripheral vasoconstrictor effect, BP initially increases above the renal set-point for sodium balance and causes transient natriuresis. After a few days, extracellular fluid volume decreases and BP stabilizes at a point where sodium intake and output are balanced. The sodium retaining actions are obscured by peripheral vasoconstriction which raises BP above the renal set-point at which sodium balance is maintained, causing increased renal excretion and decreased extracellular fluid volume. However, the maintenance of high BP chronically depends on the changes in renal function that shift pressure natriuresis to higher BPs.

RENAL MECHANISMS OF HYPERTENSION

Commonly used measurements of kidney function, such as GFR, renal blood flow, serum creatinine, and sodium excretion, are often within the normal range in hypertensive patients, at least prior to renal damage due to prolonged high BP. On the other hand, increased TPR is found in many hypertensive patients, leading to emphasis on peripheral vasoconstriction as a cause of increased BP. However, increased TPR may be an autoregulatory response to increased BP, and may not cause sustained hypertension in the absence of impaired pressure natriuresis.

Almost all forms of experimental hypertension and all monogenic forms of human hypertension discovered thus far are caused by insults to the kidneys that alter renal hemodynamics or tubular reabsorption. For example, constriction of the renal arteries e.g., Goldblatt hypertension, compression of the kidneys e.g., perinephritic hypertension or administration of sodium-retaining hormones (e.g., mineralocorticoids or angiotensin II) are all associated with either initial reductions in renal blood flow and GFR or increases in renal tubular reabsorption prior to development of hypertension. Likewise, in all known monogenic forms of human hypertension there is impaired renal excretory function caused by mutations that increase renal sodium reabsorption or activity of antinatriuretic hormones. As BP rises, the initial changes are obscured by compensations that restore kidney function toward

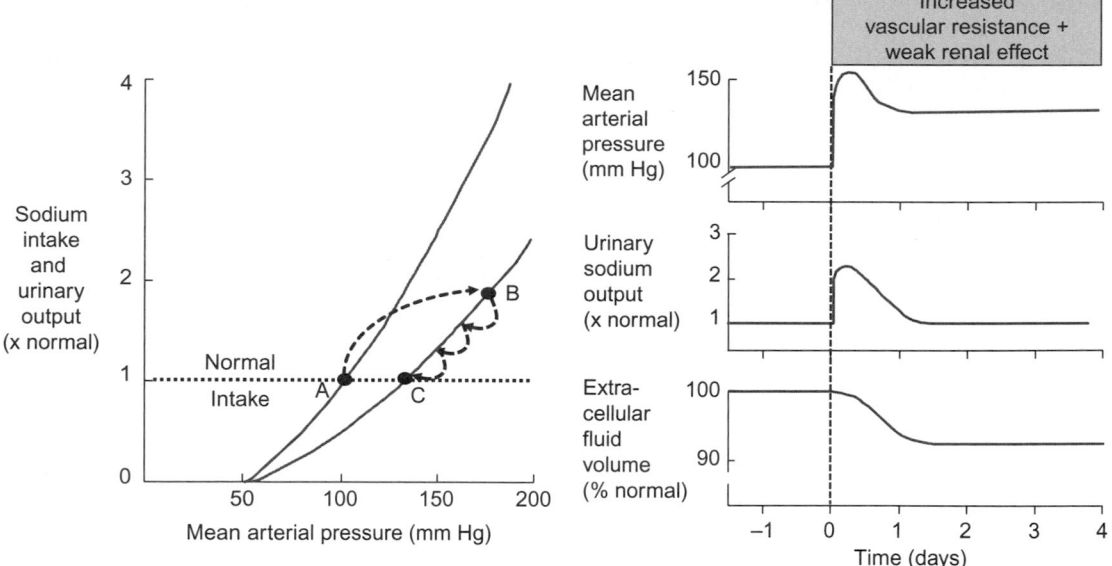

FIGURE 39.4 **Long-term effects of norepinephrine, a vasoconstrictor that has a relatively weak effect to impair pressure natriuresis.** The normal curve (blue) is compared with the vasoconstrictor curve (red line). Initially the vasoconstrictor raises BP (from point A to point B) above the renal set point for sodium balance. Increased BP, however, causes a transient natriuresis and decreases extracellular fluid volume until BP eventually stabilizes at a level (point C) at which sodium intake and output are balanced at a reduced extracellular fluid volume.[10] See color section at the back of the book.

normal. The rise in BP then initiates a cascade of cardiovascular changes, including increased TPR that may be more striking than the initial kidney disturbance. For this reason, the importance of renal dysfunction in causing hypertension has often been underestimated.

Although specific abnormalities of kidney function are difficult to identify in most patients with primary hypertension, one aspect of kidney function that is invariably abnormal is renal pressure natriuresis.[9,10] Maintenance of a normal sodium excretion equal to sodium intake despite elevated BP, which would normally cause natriuresis and diuresis, indicates that pressure natriuresis is reset in hypertensive subjects.

Some types of renal abnormalities that cause chronic hypertension include: 1) increased preglomerular resistance; 2) decreased glomerular capillary filtration coefficient; 3) reduced numbers of functional nephrons; and 4) increased tubular reabsorption (Figure 39.5). As discussed below, some of these abnormalities cause blood pressure to be more sensitive to changes in dietary salt intake (salt-sensitive), whereas other renal abnormalities may cause hypertension that is relatively insensitive to changes in salt intake (salt-insensitive).

Generalized Increases in Preglomerular Resistance Cause Salt-Insensitive Hypertension

Examples of a generalized increase in preglomerular resistance are those caused by suprarenal aortic coarctation or constriction of one renal artery and

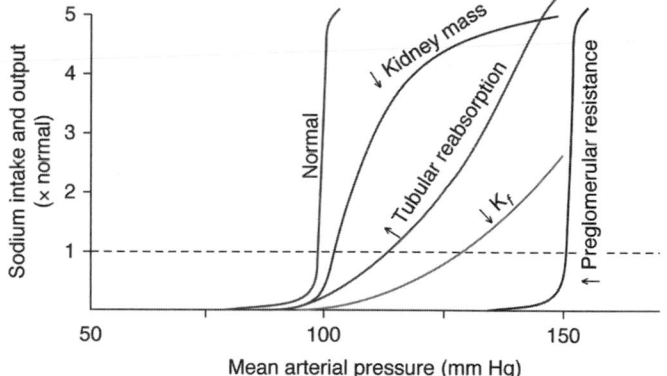

FIGURE 39.5 **Steady-state relationships between BP, sodium excretion, and sodium intake for subjects with normal kidneys and four general types of renal dysfunction that cause hypertension:** decreased kidney mass; increased reabsorption in distal and collecting tubules; reductions in glomerular capillary filtration coefficient (K_f); and increased preglomerular resistance. Note that increased preglomerular resistance causes *salt-insensitive* hypertension, whereas the other renal abnormalities cause *salt-sensitive* hypertension.

removal of the contralateral kidney (e.g., 1-kidney, 1-clip Goldblatt hypertension). After renal artery constriction or aortic coarctation, renal blood flow, GFR, and sodium excretion are initially reduced, and there is a rapid rise in renin secretion. Renal blood flow and GFR may return to near normal if autoregulatory mechanisms are not impaired, and if constriction is not so severe that it reduces renal perfusion pressure below the autoregulatory range ~65–70 mmHg. Even if GFR is not fully autoregulated, sodium excretion returns to normal and sodium balance is re-established within a few days. If sodium and fluid intakes are normal, renin secretion also returns to normal in the established phase of hypertension. At this point, most indices of renal function are nearly normal, including BP distal to the stenosis if the constriction is not too severe.[11]

Homogeneous increases in preglomerular resistance typically cause salt-insensitive rather than salt-sensitive hypertension. One of the main reasons that increased salt intake does not greatly exacerbate this form of hypertension is that after BP increases sufficiently to restore renal perfusion pressure and renin secretion to nearly normal, the RAAS is fully capable of appropriate suppression during high salt intake. As discussed later, the ability to effectively modulate RAAS activity is critical for preventing salt-sensitivity of BP.

Functional or pathologic increases in preglomerular resistance at other sites besides the main renal arteries, such as the interlobular arteries or afferent arterioles, could also increase BP through the same mechanisms activated by clipping the renal artery. For example, structural increases in afferent arteriolar resistance (e.g., nephrosclerosis or functional increases in resistance caused by excessive activation of the SNS) could also cause hypertension through the same mechanisms as constriction of the main renal artery. Some patients with primary hypertension have essentially the same characteristics seen in 1-kidney, 1-clip Goldblatt hypertension, including nearly normal GFR and plasma renin activity, a parallel shift of pressure natriuresis to higher BP, and a relatively salt-insensitive form of hypertension.[5,11] Also, drug therapies that decrease preglomerular resistance, such as calcium channel blockers, cause a parallel shift of pressure natriuresis toward lower BP.[6] Thus, primary hypertension in some patients may be caused by functional or pathologic increases in preglomerular resistance. This is almost certainly the case in patients who have severe atherosclerotic lesions in the renal blood vessels.

Non-Homeogeneous Increases in Preglomerular Resistance Cause Salt-Sensitive Hypertension

In 2-kidney, 1-clip Goldblatt hypertension or in patients with a stenosis in only one renal artery, there is a non-homogeneous increase in preglomerular resistance, with ischemia occurring in nephrons of the clipped/stenotic kidney, while nephrons in the contralateral nonstenotic kidney have normal or increased single-nephron blood flow and GFR. The underperfused clipped kidney secretes large amounts of renin, whereas the untouched kidney secretes little renin.[6,12]

In the 2-kidney, 1-clip model, the glomeruli of the untouched kidney are subject to the full effects of increased BP. With prolonged hypertension, pathologic changes in the untouched kidney may further impair renal function. At this stage, removal of the clipped kidney only partially normalizes BP. However, removal of the contralateral untouched kidney and unclipping the stenotic kidney usually normalizes BP if the underperfusion of the clipped kidney is not too severe and ischemic injury has not occurred. Thus, chronic exposure to high BP in the untouched kidney may cause pathological changes that increase the severity of hypertension.

Non-homogeneous increases in preglomerular resistance may also cause salt-sensitivity of BP. The main reason is that the underperfused nephrons secrete large amounts of renin, whereas the remaining nephrons are overperfused and have reduced renin secretion.[5,6] In both cases, the nephrons have impaired ability to adequately suppress renin secretion during high salt intake, and BP becomes more salt-sensitive.

Some patients with essential hypertension may have non-homogenous nephrosclerosis within each kidney, providing another clinical counterpart to the 2-kidney, 1-clip Goldblatt model of hypertension. In these instances, the combined effects of hypertension and hyperfiltration in non-ischemic nephrons may eventually damage the nephrons that were not initially ischemic, leading to progressive nephron loss.

Reduced Glomerular Capillary Filtration Coefficient

Decreased glomerular capillary filtration coefficient K_f initially lowers GFR and sodium excretion, while stimulating renin release and causing vasodilation of afferent arterioles via macula densa feedback.[5,6] The sodium retention and increased angiotensin II formation raise BP, which helps to normalize GFR and renin release. After these compensations, the main persistent abnormalities of kidney function are reduced filtration fraction, increased glomerular hydrostatic pressure, and increased renal blood flow. Unfortunately, compensatory increases in BP and glomerular hydrostatic pressure, which offset a fall in K_f and restore sodium excretion to normal, may also cause further glomerular injury, loss of glomeruli, further reductions in K_f, and additional increases in BP.

The clinical counterparts of this sequence may be found in hypertension caused by glomerulonephritis or by other conditions that cause thickening and damage to the glomerular capillary membranes, such as chronic diabetes mellitus.

Nephron Loss Increases Salt-Sensitivity

Surgical removal of large amounts of the kidney, to the point that uremia occurs, rarely cause much hypertension as long as sodium intake is normal.[6,9,13] In this case, GFR and tubular reabsorption capability are proportionally reduced so that balance between filtration and reabsorption are maintained without major changes in BP. Reducing the number of nephrons, however, makes the kidneys susceptible to additional challenges of sodium homeostasis. For example, hypertension associated with excess mineralocorticoids is more severe after reducing kidney mass. Likewise, high sodium intake is accompanied by larger BP increases when kidney mass is reduced.[6]

Nephron loss also initiates compensatory changes that may damage the surviving nephrons. For example, renal vasodilation and increased single nephron GFR, over long periods of time, may lead to glomerulosclerosis and reductions in K_f. These pathologic changes, in addition to loss of functional nephrons, may further impair pressure natriuresis and cause hypertension. Thus, even though hypertension may not begin with nephron loss, chronic elevations in glomerular pressure and other metabolic abnormalities often associated with hypertension may cause progressive nephron loss that amplifies the hypertension and makes BP salt-sensitive.

Partial renal infarction causes high renin hypertension. In contrast to the effects of surgical removal of kidney mass, loss of nephrons because of ischemia or infarction of renal tissue usually causes marked hypertension, even with normal salt intake. The so-called *5/6 ablation* model is produced by removing one kidney and obstructing two of the three branches of the renal artery of the remaining kidney. In this model, hypertension develops even without high salt intake because of ischemia of the surviving nephrons, activation of the RAAS, and immune-mediated renal injury.[14] This hypertension model has non-homogeneous areas of renal ischemia with characteristics similar to that described for the 2-kidney, 1-clip Goldblatt model. The clinical counterpart of this model occurs with partial renal infarction caused by septic emboli, thrombus, trauma or sometimes after corrective surgery for renal artery stenosis.

Increased Renal Tubular Sodium Reabsorption

Hypertension caused by increased *distal* or *collecting tubular reabsorption* is exacerbated by increased salt intake. Increased reabsorption at sites beyond the macula densa elicits increased sodium chloride delivery to the macula densa which, in turn, suppresses renin secretion,[5,10] sometimes to very low levels, which prevents further suppression of angiotensin II formation during high sodium intake, making BP salt-sensitive.

An increase in *proximal* or *loop of Henle* tubular reabsorption, however, may result in a salt-insensitive hypertension. Increased proximal tubular reabsorption tends to increase renin secretion, and elicits a compensatory renal vasodilation that raises GFR and renal plasma flow in response to reduced macula densa NaCl delivery. However, as hypertension develops, macula densa NaCl delivery and renin secretion return to nearly normal, and the RAAS may be fully capable of responding to increased salt intake. Therefore, high salt intake may be accompanied by appropriate suppression of angiotensin II formation, which permits sodium balance to be maintained with only small increases in BP.[10] Nevertheless, pressure natriuresis is shifted to higher BP.

A feature of hypertension caused by increased tubular reabsorption is that it may initially be associated with extracellular volume-expansion. However, volume-expansion and increased cardiac output usually subside because of pressure natriuresis, and TPR increases secondarily to increased BP. When increased tubular reabsorption is also associated with marked peripheral vasoconstriction, such as occurs with very high levels of angiotensin II, the degree of volume-expansion depends on the relative effects of the vasoconstrictor on peripheral and renal blood vessels.[5] With severe peripheral vasoconstriction and decreased vascular capacitance, relatively small amounts of volume retention can lead to substantial hypertension.

Significance of Salt-Sensitive Hypertension

Many factors are associated with salt-sensitivity of BP. Older individuals are usually more salt-sensitive than young people, and African Americans are often more salt-sensitive than whites. However, there are exceptions to these generalizations and considerable heterogeneity exists in the BP responses to increased salt intake.

Genetic factors independent of ethnicity have been linked to salt-sensitivity of BP, especially monogenic disorders that increase distal and collecting tubule sodium reabsorption or that increase secretion of sodium-retaining hormones.[15] Also, diabetes mellitus, renal diseases that cause nephron loss, and abnormalities of the RAAS are associated with increased salt-sensitivity of BP.[5] Many of these examples share two common pathways to salt-sensitivity: 1) loss of functional nephrons as discussed previously or 2) reduced responsiveness of the RAAS.

Figure 39.6 shows the importance of changes in angiotensin II formation in maintaining BP relatively constant during wide variations in salt intake. In dogs with a fully-functional RAAS, only small increases in

BP were associated with a 100-fold increase in sodium intake.[16,17] However, when angiotensin II was prevented from being suppressed as sodium intake was raised, BP became salt-sensitive. After blockade of angiotensin II formation, BP was also salt-sensitive, although maintained at lower levels.[17] Thus, a major function of the RAAS is to permit wide variations in sodium intake and excretion without large fluctuations in BP.

As discussed previously, focal nephrosclerosis or patchy preglomerular vasoconstriction, as occurs with renal infarction, leads to increased renin secretion in ischemic nephrons and very low levels of renin release by overperfused nephrons.[6] Thus, in ischemic and overperfused nephrons, the ability to suppress renin secretion during high salt intake is impaired. Another cause of reduced responsiveness of the RAAS is increased distal and collecting tubular sodium reabsorption, as occurs with mineralocorticoid excess or mutations that increase distal and collecting tubule reabsorption (e.g., Liddle syndrome). In these conditions, excess sodium retention causes almost complete suppression of renin secretion, resulting in an inability to further decrease renin release during high sodium intake. Consequently, BP becomes very salt-sensitive.

Salt-Sensitive Subjects May Have Greater Target Organ Injury

Some studies suggest that salt-sensitivity predicts hypertensive target organ injury. Salt-sensitive hypertension may be associated with glomerular hyperfiltration and increased glomerular hydrostatic pressure

that is further amplified by the hypertension[5]; together the hypertension and renal hyperfiltration may promote glomerular injury and cause loss of nephron function. Clinical studies support this concept, and demonstrate that salt-sensitive individuals typically have increased glomerular pressure and albumin excretion when given a salt-load, whereas salt-resistant individuals have lower glomerular pressure and less urinary albumin excretion.[18]

There is also evidence that salt-sensitive subjects may die earlier than individuals who are salt-resistant. Weinberger et al. studied individuals for more than 20 years and found that normotensive individuals with increased salt-sensitivity died almost at the same rate as hypertensive individuals, and much faster than salt-resistant individuals who were normotensive.[19] Whether this increased mortality was related to BP effects of salt or to other effects is still unclear. It is also not known whether long-term high salt intake may cause a person who is initially salt-insensitive to become salt-sensitive as a consequence of gradual renal injury.

NEURAL AND HORMONAL MECHANISMS OF HYPERTENSION

The following sections discuss the multiple neural, hormonal, and autacoid mechanisms that alter renal pressure natriuresis, and their potential roles in hypertension.

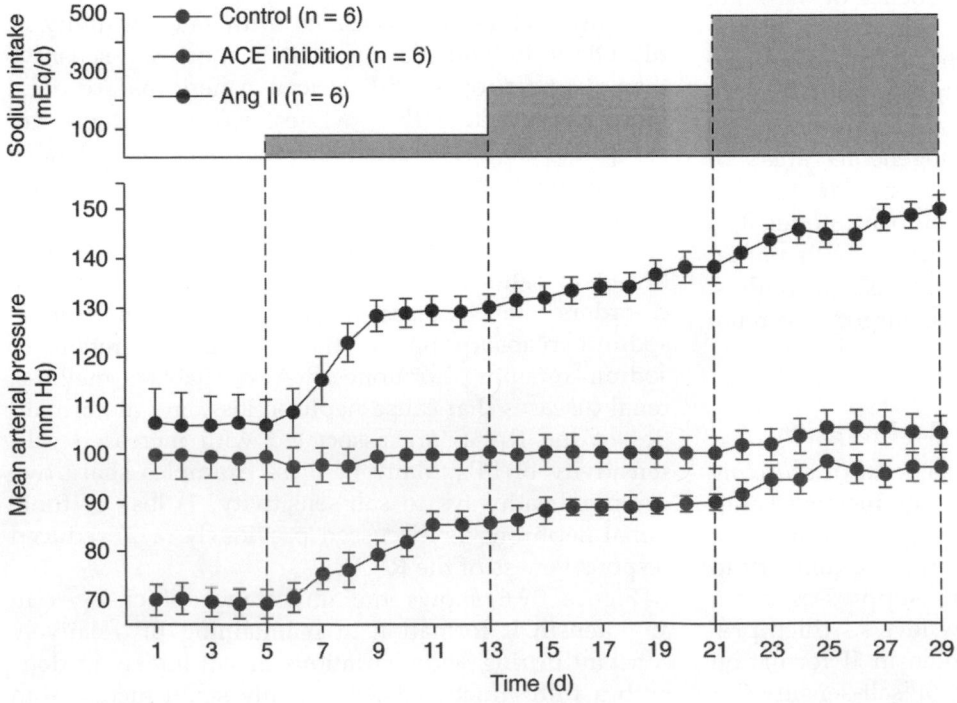

FIGURE 39.6 Changes in mean arterial pressure during chronic changes in sodium intake in normal control dogs, after ACE inhibition, or after angiotensin II infusion (5 ng/kg/min) to prevent angiotensin II from being suppressed when sodium intake was raised ref. [17].

The Sympathetic Nervous System SNS

Activation of the SNS can raise BP within a few seconds by causing vasoconstriction, increased cardiac pumping capability, and increased heart rate. Conversely, sudden inhibition of SNS activity can decrease BP to as low as half normal in less than a minute. Therefore, changes in SNS activity, caused by various reflex mechanisms, central nervous system ischemia or by activation of higher centers in the brain, provide powerful and rapid moment-to-moment regulation of BP.

The SNS also plays an important role in long-term regulation of BP and in the pathogenesis of hypertension by activation of the renal sympathetic nerves.[20] There is extensive innervation of the renal blood vessels, the juxtaglomerular apparatus, and the renal tubules, and overactivation of these nerves causes sodium retention, increased renin secretion, and impaired renal pressure natriuresis.[20] Even mild increases of the renal sympathetic nerve activity (RSNA) stimulate renin secretion and sodium reabsorption in multiple segments of the nephron, including the proximal tubule, the loop of Henle, and more distal segments.[20] Thus, the renal nerves provide a mechanism by which the various autonomic reflexes and central nervous system (CNS) centers contribute to long-term BP regulation.

Multiple studies have shown that renal denervation reduces BP in some experimental models of hypertension.[20] For example, renal denervation attenuates hypertension in (SHR)[20] as well as in obese hypertensive dogs.[21] Renal denervation also delays or attenuates increased BP in other forms of experimental hypertension, although some studies have not found an important role for the renal nerves in various forms of secondary hypertension.[5]

Human primary hypertension, especially when associated with obesity, is often associated with increased RSNA.[22] Bilateral renal denervation in humans, using a percutaneous, catheter-based radiofrequency method to selectively ablate the nerves that run along the renal arteries, reduced BP in patients who were resistant to the usual antihypertensive drugs.[23,24] Moreover, reductions in BP were sustained for up to two years of follow-up, suggesting the absence of substantial nerve fiber regrowth. However, longer follow-up periods will be needed to determine if the renal nerves eventually regrow and reinitiate increased BP, as observed in experimental animal models of renal denervation.

Although the mechanisms that activate renal sympathetic nerves in primary hypertension or in most experimental models are still unclear, we will briefly discuss two that have attracted the interest of many researchers.

Resetting of Baroreceptor Reflexes in Hypertension

The importance of the arterial baroreceptors in buffering moment-to-moment changes in BP is clearly evident in baroreceptor-denervated animals in which there is extreme BP variability associated with normal daily activities.[25] After baroreceptor denervation, BP increases to very high levels or falls to low levels with normal daily activities, although the average 24-hour BP is not markedly altered. However, some studies suggest that the baroreceptors are relatively unimportant in chronic regulation of BP, because they tend to reset within a few days after a change in BP.[25] To the extent that resetting of baroreceptors occurs, this would attenuate their potency in long-term control of BP.

Other experimental studies suggest that the baroreceptors do not completely reset and may contribute to chronic BP regulation. With prolonged increases in BP, the baroreflexes may contribute to *reductions* in renal sympathetic activity, and promote sodium and water excretion.[26] This, in turn, may attenuate the rise in BP. Thus, impairment of baroreflexes may cause increased lability of BP in hypertension, and fail to attenuate the rise in BP caused by other disturbances.

Currently, there is little evidence that primary disturbances of baroreceptor function play a major role in *causing* chronic hypertension. However, experimental studies in dogs indicate that chronic electrical stimulation of carotid sinus baroreceptors reduces BP in some forms of experimental hypertension.[26] In humans with hypertension resistant to drug treatment, electrical stimulation of baroreceptors also reduced BP.[26] These observations are consistent with the hypothesis that strong activation of baroreceptors can have long-term influences on BP. However, this finding does not necessarily imply that impaired baroreflexes actually *cause* chronic hypertension. The primary role of arterial baroreceptors in hypertension, as in normotension, appears to be buffering of rapid deviations in BP from the set-point determined by renal pressure natriuresis.

Obesity Causes Chronic SNS Activation

Excess weight gain appears to be a major cause of human primary hypertension, and one key mechanism that links obesity with increased BP is SNS activation.[10] Obese persons have elevated SNS activity in various tissues, including the kidneys.[10,22] Studies in experimental animals and humans indicate that combined α-and β-adrenergic blockade markedly attenuates obesity-associated hypertension.[10] Moreover, renal sympathetic efferent nerves mediate much of the chronic effects of SNS activation on BP in obesity, as bilateral renal denervation greatly attenuates sodium retention and hypertension in obese dogs.[10] Thus, obesity increases renal sodium reabsorption, impairs pressure natriuresis, and causes hypertension in part by increasing RSNA. The mechanisms for SNS activation in obesity have not been fully-elucidated, as discussed in more detail later in this chapter.

The Renin−Angiotensin−Aldosterone System (RAAS)

The RAAS is perhaps the body's most powerful hormone system for regulating BP, as evidenced by the effectiveness of various RAAS blockers in treating hypertension. Although the RAAS has many components, its most important effects on BP are exerted by angiotensin II, a powerful vasoconstrictor that maintains BP in conditions associated with blood volume depletion, sodium depletion or circulatory depression e.g., heart failure. The long-term effects of angiotensin II on BP, however, are closely intertwined with volume homeostasis through direct and indirect effects on the kidneys.

Blockade of the RAAS, with angiotensin II receptor blockers ARBs, angiotensin converting enzyme ACE inhibitors or mineralocorticoid receptor MR antagonists, increases renal excretory capability so that sodium balance is maintained at reduced BP.[5,6] However, blockade of the RAAS also makes BP salt-sensitive.[16] Thus, effectiveness of RAAS blockers in lowering BP is greatly diminished by high salt intake; conversely, reducing sodium intake or addition of a diuretic improves effectiveness of RAAS blockers in reducing BP.

Inappropriately high levels of angiotensin II reduce renal excretory capability and impair pressure natriuresis, thereby necessitating increased BP to maintain sodium balance. The mechanisms that mediate the potent antinatriuretic effects of angiotensin II include direct and indirect effects to increase tubular reabsorption, as well as renal hemodynamic effects.[16]

Angiotensin II Stimulates Renal Sodium Reabsorption

Angiotensin II increases renal sodium reabsorption through stimulation of aldosterone secretion, by direct effects on epithelial transport, and by hemodynamic effects. Angiotensin II-mediated constriction of efferent arterioles reduces renal blood flow and peritubular capillary hydrostatic pressure, and increases peritubular colloid osmotic pressure as a result of increased filtration fraction.[16] These changes, in turn, increase the driving force for fluid reabsorption across tubular epithelial cells. Reductions in renal medullary blood flow caused by efferent arteriolar constriction or by direct effects of angiotensin II on the vasa recta may also

enhance reabsorption in the loop of Henle and collecting ducts.[16]

Angiotensin II also directly stimulates tubular sodium reabsorption. This effect occurs at low angiotensin II concentrations, and is mediated by actions on the luminal and basolateral membranes.[16,27] In proximal tubules, angiotensin II stimulates the $Na^+−H^+$ exchanger on luminal membranes and increases sodium−potassium ATPase activity, as well as sodium bicarbonate co-transport on basolateral membranes[13,27] (Figure 39.7). These effects are partly mediated by inhibition of adenyl cyclase and increased phospholipase C activity.

Angiotensin II also stimulates sodium reabsorption in the loop of Henle, macula densa, and distal nephron segments. At physiologic concentrations, angiotensin II increases loop of Henle bicarbonate reabsorption and stimulates $Na^+−K^+−2Cl$ transport in the medullary thick ascending loop of Henle.[5,16] In the distal parts of the nephron, angiotensin II stimulates multiple ion transporters, including H^+-ATPase activity, as well as epithelial sodium channel activity in the cortical collecting ducts.[5,16]

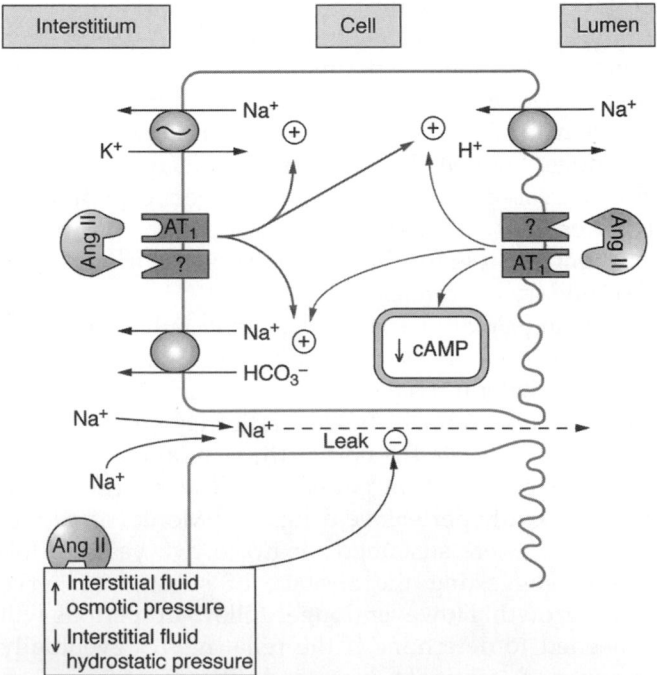

FIGURE 39.7 Angiotensin II increases proximal tubular reabsorption by binding to receptors on the luminal and basolateral membranes and stimulating Na^+/H^+ antiporter, Na^+/HCO_3 co-transport, and Na^+/K^+ adenosine triphosphatase (ATPase) activity. Angiotensin II also increases reabsorption by increasing interstitial fluid colloid osmotic pressure and decreasing interstitial fluid hydrostatic pressure.

Renal hemodynamic Effects of Angiotensin II

Angiotensin II is a powerful renal vasoconstrictor, but in most physiological conditions the constriction is confined mainly to postglomerular efferent arterioles. For example, efferent arteriolar constriction by angiotensin II acts in concert with other autoregulatory mechanisms, such as tubuloglomerular feedback (TGF) and myogenic activity, to prevent excessive reductions in GFR when kidney perfusion is threatened.[16] In these cases, administration of ARBs or ACE inhibitors may reduce GFR further, even though renal blood flow is preserved. Impairment of GFR after RAS blockade is caused, in part, by inhibition of the constrictor effects of angiotensin II on efferent arterioles, as well as reduced BP.[16]

The relatively weak constrictor action of angiotensin II on preglomerular vessels is due partly to protection of these vessels by autacoid mechanisms, such as prostaglandins or endothelial-derived nitric oxide NO.[16] When the ability of the kidney to produce these autacoids is impaired by treatment with nonsteroidal anti-inflammatory drugs (NSAIDS) or by chronic vascular disease (e.g., atherosclerosis) angiotensin II may reduce GFR by constricting afferent arterioles.

ANGIOTENSIN II MAY CONTRIBUTE TO GLOMERULAR INJURY IN OVERPERFUSED KIDNEYS

Although blockade of angiotensin II vasoconstrictor of efferent arterioles may cause a further decline of GFR in ischemic nephrons, RAAS blockade may be beneficial when nephrons are hyperfiltering, especially if angiotensin II is not appropriately suppressed. For example, in diabetes mellitus and in certain forms of hypertension associated with glomerulosclerosis and nephron loss, angiotensin II blockade, by decreasing efferent arteriolar resistance and BP, lowers glomerular hydrostatic pressure and attenuates glomerular hyperfiltration.[16] Thus, RAAS blockers are more effective than other antihypertensive agents in preventing glomerular injury, even with similar reductions in BP.[28,29]

DOES ANGIOTENSIN II CAUSE TARGET ORGAN INJURY INDEPENDENT OF INCREASED BP?

Angiotensin II has been suggested to cause injury to the kidneys and other organs through direct actions, in addition to its hemodynamic effects. Although RAAS blockers may provide greater renal protection than other antihypertensive drugs, decreases in glomerular hydrostatic pressure because of efferent arteriolar vasodilation may have contributed to these beneficial effects. In studies where BP was measured accurately, using 24-hour telemetry, the renal protective effects of angiotensin II blockade appeared to be largely a result of reduced BP.[30]

An observation that is difficult to reconcile with the concept that ANG II directly mediates target organ injury, independent of BP, is the finding that physiologic activation of the RAAS is not associated with vascular or renal injury as long as the BP is not elevated. For example, sodium depletion does not cause renal, cardiac or vascular injury, despite marked increases in renal angiotensin II levels. Also, the clipped kidney in 2-kidney, 1-clip Goldblatt hypertension is exposed to high angiotensin II levels, but is protected from increased BP by the clip on the renal artery and has no visible injury as long as the stenosis is not too severe. However, the nonclipped kidney, exposed to lower angiotensin II concentrations but higher BP, has marked focal segmental glomerular sclerosis, as well as tubulointerstitial changes characteristic of hypertension.[31]

Convincing evidence in this controversial area of research comes from the observations of Coffman and colleagues who studied the effects of chronic angiotensin II infusion in normal wild-type mice, in wild-type mice that received transplanted kidneys from AT1 receptor knockout mice, and in AT1 receptor knockout mice that received transplanted kidneys from normal wild-type mice.[32] Chronic angiotensin II infusion in normal wild-type mice increased BP and caused cardiac hypertrophy and fibrosis. However, in wild-type mice that received transplanted kidneys from AT1 receptor knockout mice (i.e., AT1 receptors were present in the heart and other organs, but not in the kidneys), angiotensin II infusion did not chronically raise BP or cause cardiac hypertrophy and fibrosis. In AT1 receptor knockout mice that received transplanted kidneys from normal wild-type mice (i.e., AT1 receptors were present only in the kidneys and not in the heart or other organs), angiotensin II infusion caused chronic hypertension, as well as cardiac hypertrophy and fibrosis.[32] These observations indicate that: 1) the renal effects of angiotensin II, and not the peripheral vascular or other non-renal effects, mediate chronic increases in BP; and 2) in the absence of hypertension, angiotensin II does not cause cardiac hypertrophy or fibrosis. Thus, the hemodynamic effects appear to account for most of the target organ injury that occurs in angiotensin II-dependent hypertension, and the effects of angiotensin II to raise BP are due to its renal actions, not to extrarenal effects, such as peripheral vasoconstriction or central nervous system effects.

Aldosterone

Aldosterone is also a powerful sodium-retaining hormone, and consequently has important effects on renal pressure natriuresis and BP regulation. The primary sites of actions of aldosterone on sodium reabsorption are the principal cells of the distal tubules, cortical collecting tubules, and collecting ducts where aldosterone stimulates sodium reabsorption and potassium secretion. Aldosterone binds to intracellular mineralocorticoid receptors (MRs) and activates transcription by target genes which, in turn, stimulate synthesis or activation of the Na^+-K^+-ATPase pump on the basolateral epithelial membrane and activation of amiloride-sensitive sodium channels on the luminal epithelial membrane.[33] These effects are termed *genomic*, because they are mediated by gene transcription and require 60–90 minutes to occur after aldosterone administration.

Aldosterone also exerts rapid *nongenomic* effects on the cardiovascular and renal systems.[33] Aldosterone increases the sodium current in principal cells of the cortical collecting tubule through activation of the amiloride-sensitive channel, and stimulates the Na^+-H^+ exchanger a few minutes after application.[33] In vascular smooth muscle cells, aldosterone stimulates sodium influx by activating the Na^+-H^+ exchanger in less than 4 minutes. Acute aldosterone administration may rapidly reduce forearm blood flow in humans, although some investigators have found no change or an increase in blood flow.[33] The putative membrane receptor and the cell-signaling mechanisms responsible for these rapid actions of aldosterone have not been identified, especially with physiologic levels of aldosterone. Thus, the importance of the nongenomic effects of aldosterone on long-term regulation of BP is still unclear.

The overall effects of aldosterone on pressure natriuresis are similar to those observed for angiotensin II. With low sodium intake, increased aldosterone helps prevent sodium loss and reductions in BP. Conversely, during high sodium intake, suppression of aldosterone prevents excessive sodium retention and attenuates increased BP. Excess aldosterone secretion reduces the slope of pressure natriuresis so that BP becomes salt-sensitive. Consequently, increasing plasma aldosterone six-to ten-fold causes marked hypertension when sodium intake is normal or elevated, but there is very little effect on BP when sodium intake is low.[5]

The role of aldosterone and MR activation in human hypertension is a topic of renewed interest in recent years. Hyperaldosteronism may be more common than previously believed, especially in patients with hypertension that are resistant to treatment with the usual antihypertensive medications. For example, the prevalence of primary aldosteronism is reported to be almost 20% among patients referred to specialty clinics for resistant hypertension. Many of these patients, however, are overweight or obese.[34]

There is also emerging evidence that MR antagonism may provide an important therapeutic tool for reducing BP and preventing target organ injury in hypertension[34]; for example, antagonism of MR attenuated sodium retention, hypertension, and glomerular hyperfiltration in obese dogs fed a high-fat diet even though plasma aldosterone concentration was only slightly elevated.[35] However, even mild increases of plasma aldosterone may increase BP when accompanied by high sodium intake and volume-expansion, because aldosterone greatly enhances salt-sensitivity of BP.

In obese, insulin-resistant patients there may be enhanced sensitivity to the effects of aldosterone because of increased abundance of epithelial sodium channels ENaCs, which would amplify the effects of MR activation on sodium reabsorption and BP. It is also possible that glucocorticoids may contribute to MR activation in obese, insulin-resistant patients.

Endothelin

Endothelin-1 ET-1 is derived from a 203 amino acid peptide precursor, preproendothelin, which is cleaved after translation to form proendothelin. A converting enzyme cleaves proendothelin to produce the 21 amino acid peptide, endothelin. ET-1 receptor-binding sites have been identified throughout the body, with the greatest numbers of receptors in the kidneys and lungs.[36,37] ET-1 can either elicit a hypertensive effect by activating endothelin type A (ET_A) receptors or an antihypertensive effect via endothelin type B (ET_B) receptor activation in the kidneys.[36,37] Thus, the ability of ET-1 to influence BP regulation is highly dependent on where ET-1 is produced, and which ET receptor type is activated (Figure 39.8).

ET-1 Elicits a Hypertensive Effect by Activating ET_A Receptors in the Kidneys

Endothelin-1 produces renal and systemic vasoconstriction, impairs renal pressure natriuresis, and increases BP via ET_A receptor activation.[36,37] ET-1 exerts multiple actions via ET_A receptor activation that, if sustained chronically, could contribute to the development of hypertension and progressive renal injury. ET-1 decreases GFR and renal plasma flow through stimulation of vascular smooth muscle and mesangial cell contraction.[36,37] Long-term effects of ET-1 on the kidneys include stimulation of mesangial cell proliferation and extracellular matrix deposition, as well as vascular smooth muscle hypertrophy in renal resistance vessels.[36,37] Expression of ET-1 is greatly enhanced in several animal models of severe hypertension with renal vascular hypertrophy, and in models of

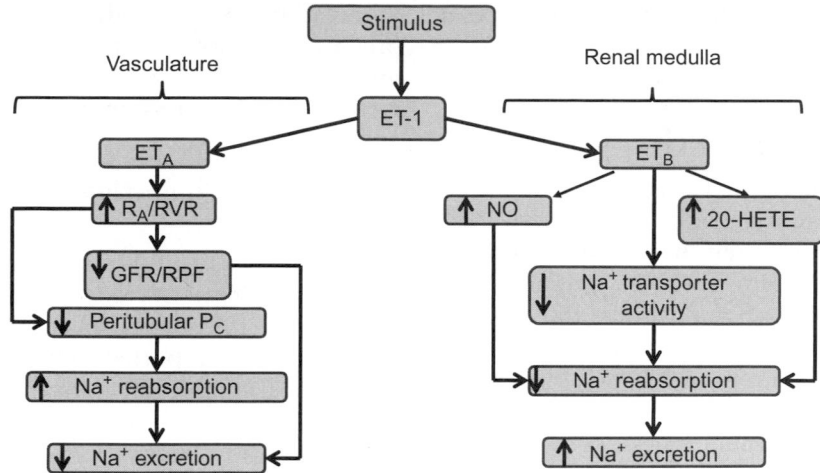

FIGURE 39.8 Summary of the pro- and antihypertensive actions of endothelin-1 (ET-1). The ability of ET-1 to influence blood pressure and renal pressure natriuresis is highly dependent on where ET-1 is produced, and which renal ET receptor type is activated. ET-1 can elicit a prohypertensive anti-natriuretic effect by activating ET_A receptors in the kidneys. Activation of renal ET_A receptors increases renal vascular resistance (RVR), which decreases renal plasma flow (RPF) and glomerular filtration rate (GFR), and enhances sodium reabsorption by decreasing peritubular capillary hydrostatic pressure (Pc). The net effect of renal ET_A receptor activation is decreased sodium excretion and increased BP. Conversely, ET-1 can elicit an antihypertensive natriuretic effect via ET_B receptor activation. Activation of the renal ET_B receptor leads to enhanced synthesis of nitric oxide (NO) and 20-HETE, and suppression of the renin—angiotensin system. The net effect of renal ET_B receptor activation is increased sodium excretion and decreased BP.

progressive renal injury.[36,37] Treatment with endothelin receptor antagonists attenuated the hypertension and small artery morphologic changes, and improved kidney function in these models.[36,37]

ET-1 Elicits an Antihypertensive Effect by Activating ET_B Receptors in the Kidneys

ET_B receptor activation by ET-1 causes vasodilation, enhances renal pressure natriuresis, and decreases BP. While much attention has been given to ET_A receptor activation, several studies indicate an important antihypertensive role for ET_B receptor.[37] The most compelling evidence comes from reports that transgenic mice deficient in ET_B receptors develop salt-sensitive hypertension, and that pharmacologic antagonism of ET_B receptors produces hypertension in rats.[36–38]

Because ET_B receptors are located on multiple cell types throughout the body, including endothelial cells and renal epithelial cells, both intrarenal and extrarenal mechanisms could theoretically mediate the hypertension produced by chronic disruption of ET_B receptors. Bagnall et al. reported that ablation of ET_B receptors exclusively from endothelial cells produced endothelial dysfunction, but did not cause hypertension.[39] In contrast to models of total ET_B receptor ablation, the BP response to a high-salt diet was unchanged in endothelial cell-specific $ET_{A/B}$ receptor knockouts compared to control mice.[37,40,41] These findings suggest that ET_B receptors in non-endothelial cells are important for BP regulation. Supporting this concept are the findings that collecting duct ET_B knockout mice on a

normal-sodium diet were hypertensive and a high-sodium diet worsened the hypertension.[40,41] Moreover, collecting duct ET_B knockout mice on a normal-sodium diet were hypertensive, and a high-sodium diet worsened the hypertension.[37,40,41] These findings provide strong evidence that the intrarenal effect of ET_B receptor activation on the collecting duct is an important physiologic regulator that increases renal sodium excretion and reduces BP.

ET-1 Plays an Important Role in Experimental Salt-Sensitive Hypertension

Dahl salt-sensitive (DS) rats placed on a high-sodium diet have impaired pressure natriuresis and develop hypertension and progressive renal injury. ET-1, acting via an ET_A receptor, may play a role in mediating renal injury in DS hypertension. Prepro-ET-1 mRNA and vascular responsiveness to ET-1 are increased in the renal cortex of DS rats compared with Dahl salt-resistant (DR) rats, and a positive correlation between ET-1 generation in the renal cortex and the extent of glomerulosclerosis has been reported in DS hypertensive rats.[42] Acute infusion of a nonselective ET_A-ET_B receptor antagonist directly into the renal interstitium improved renal hemodynamic and excretory function in DS rats, but not in DR rats.[43] Moreover, chronic blockade of ET_A receptors attenuated hypertension and proteinuria, and ameliorated glomerular and tubular damage associated with high-salt intake in DS rats. An important unanswered question is whether these beneficial effects of ET_A blockade are mediated through lower BP or through direct renal mechanisms.

Role of Endothelin in Human Hypertension

Bosentan, a combined ET_A-ET_B receptor antagonist, lowered BP in a large, double-blind, clinical trial, indicating that the endothelin system helps maintain BP in human hypertension.[44,45] However, the magnitude of the BP reduction by bosentan was almost the same as that observed in normotensive humans. This observation suggests that endothelin probably may not play a major role in raising BP in most patients with essential hypertension, although bosentan blocks both ET_A and ET_B receptors and antagonism of the antihypertensive ET_B receptor may have masked an important role of endothelin on BP via ET_A receptor activation. In another study, six weeks of darusentan, a selective ET_A receptor antagonist, lowered systolic and diastolic BP.[44] Bakris et al.[46] and Weber et al.[47] also showed that darusentan reduced mean 24 hour systolic BP more than placebo in patients with treatment-resistant hypertension. There are currently no clinical studies that directly compare selective and mixed ET receptor antagonism in the treatment of hypertension, although both approaches clearly reduce BP. Moreover, clinical studies examining the effect of selective ET_A receptor antagonism in humans with salt-sensitive hypertension are lacking. Therefore, the importance of ET-1 in human essential hypertension deserves further investigation.[37,45]

Nitric Oxide

Release of nitric oxide NO by the vascular endothelium and renal tubular cells plays a major role in regulating renal hemodynamics and tubular function.[48–50] Long-term inhibition of NO synthase causes impaired renal pressure natriuresis and sustained hypertension.[48–50] The renal mechanisms whereby reduction in NO synthesis impairs pressure natriuresis can be divided into hemodynamic and tubular components, each of which may be modulated by processes that are intrinsic or extrinsic to the kidneys Figure 39.9. For example, reduced NO synthesis may decrease renal sodium excretory function by increasing renal vascular resistance directly or by enhancing responsiveness to vasoconstrictors such as angiotensin II or norepinephrine.[49,50] Reductions in NO synthesis also increase renal sodium reabsorption via direct effects on tubular transport, and through changes in intrarenal physical factors, such as renal interstitial hydrostatic pressure (RIHP) and medullary blood flow. Inhibition of NO synthesis reduces RIHP and urinary sodium excretion.[49,50]

Stimulation of NO production normalizes the blunted pressure natriuretic response in DS rats as a result of improvement in the kidney's ability to generate increased RIHP in response to increased BP.[49,50]

Impaired NO Production Produces Salt-Sensitive Hypertension

Increased renal NO production, as evidenced by increased urinary excretion of NO metabolites or the NO second messenger, cyclic guanosine mono-phosphate, has been reported to be essential for the maintenance of normotension during a dietary salt challenge. Prevention of this increase in renal NO production resulted in salt-sensitive hypertension.[48–51]

There is also evidence that NO-induced vasodilation is impaired in many models of hypertension, and in some vascular beds in human essential hypertension.[52,53] The extent to which these effects are secondary to hypertension or reflect important mechanisms for the etiology of hypertension remains unclear. NO activity does not increase with increasing dietary salt-loading in the Dahl salt-sensitive DS hypertensive rats as it does in normotensive Dahl salt-resistant DR rats; furthermore, chronic administration of L-arginine prevents hypertension during dietary salt-loading in the DS rat, but has no effect on BP in DR rats.[54] We have shown that injections of L-arginine will prevent the development of hypertension in DS rats, even during prolonged exposure to an 8% sodium diet.[49,50] This is

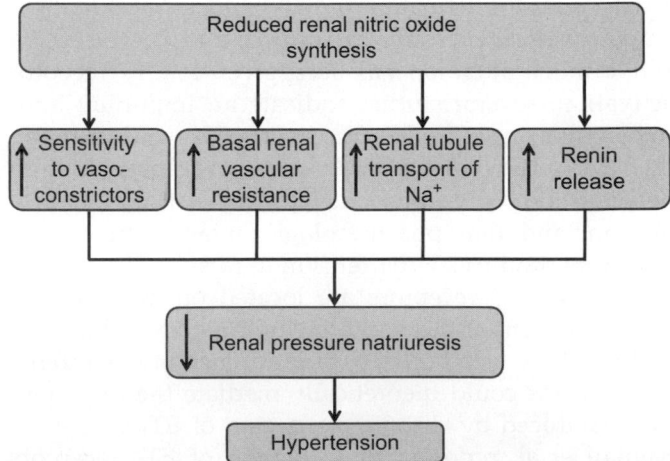

FIGURE 39.9 **Renal mechanisms whereby reduced nitric oxide (NO) synthesis decreases pressure natriuresis and increases BP.** Decreased endothelial-derived nitric oxide (EDNO) synthesis impairs renal sodium excretory function by increasing basal renal vascular resistance, enhancing the renal vascular responsiveness to vasoconstrictors such as angiotensin II or norepinephrine, or activating the renin–angiotensin system. Reductions in NO synthesis also impair sodium excretory function, either by directly increasing tubular reabsorption or by altering intrarenal physical factors, such as renal interstitial hydrostatic pressure or medullary blood flow.

not the case in all models of hypertension, even when individual tissues from these animals show impaired NO responses. Thus, in 2-kidney, 1-clip renovascular hypertension, inhibitors of NO synthesis result in an exaggerated increase in BP and vascular resistance compared to normotensive rats, but L-arginine does not prevent hypertension. Similarly, in the DOCA salt-hypertensive model, L-arginine administration improves agonist-induced NO release, but has no effect on BP.[48–50]

Because of the central role of the kidney in sustaining changes in BP, it is reasonable to postulate that the long-term increases in BP induced by inhibition of NO synthase in normal animals, as well as the reduction in blood pressure induced by NO agonists in DS rat, should be associated with changes in the relationship between renal perfusion pressure and urinary sodium excretion. This has been confirmed in several studies.[48–50] In normal animals, the acute intrarenal administration of the NO synthesis inhibitor NG nitro L-arginine methyl ester L-NAME significantly reduces the natriuresis and diuresis usually induced by increases in renal perfusion pressure. Chronic NO synthase inhibition also blunts the chronic renal function curve measured during changes in sodium intake.[48–50] Stimulation of NO production by L-arginine supplementation has also been reported to alter BP and enhance renal pressure natriuresis. Chronic L-arginine supplementation in DS rats maintained on a high-sodium diet normalizes the blunted pressure natriuresis relationship which usually characterizes these hypertensive-prone animals.[48–50,54] Thus, alterations in NO production or release can have important effects on renal pressure natriuresis.

Role of NO in Human Hypertension

There is also evidence that NO synthesis is impaired in vascular beds in human primary hypertension.[52] The extent to which these changes are secondary to increased BP or reflect important mechanisms for the pathogenesis of hypertension, however, remains unclear. NO deficiency can occur by multiple mechanisms, including altered NOS enzyme expression, NO scavenging or NOS enzyme inhibition by endogenous inhibitors. Recent studies have implicated the endogenous NO synthase inhibitor asymmetric dimethylarginine ADMA in the pathogenesis of hypertension.[55,56] While there is a strong correlation between ADMA levels and severe cardiovascular events and mortality, only a few clinical studies have shown a relationship between high BP and high plasma ADMA concentrations.[55,56] However, when hypertension and renal disease are present, increased plasma ADMA is observed. Thus, it appears that the observed increase in ADMA during hypertension may be secondary to chronic kidney disease.[52,54–56]

Oxidative Stress

Recent studies suggest that reactive oxygen species (ROS) may play a role in the initiation and progression of cardiovascular dysfunction associated with hypertension.[57–59] In many forms of hypertension, increased ROS appear to be derived mainly from nicotinamide adenine dinucleotide phosphate (NADPH) oxidases, which could serve as a trigger for uncoupling endothelial nitrous oxide synthase NOS by oxidants. Four members of the NADPH oxidase Nox enzyme family have been identified as important sources of ROS in the vasculature: Nox1, Nox2, Nox4, and Nox5.[57,59] Multiple factors control the expression and activity of these enzymes and of their regulatory subunits, such as p22phox, p47phox, Noxa1, and p67phox.[57,59] Several physical, hormonal, and local autocoid factors are known to be important stimuli for the production of ROS. For example angiotensin II, aldosterone, ET-1, and sodium intake all enhance production of ROS.[57,59] Moreover, BP-induced endothelial damage is also associated with increased production of ROS. Thus, in many forms of hypertension, the elevation in ROS production may be secondary to the increased BP.

ROS produced by migrating inflammatory cells and/or vascular cells cause endothelial dysfunction, increased renal tubule sodium transport, cell growth and migration, inflammatory gene expression, and stimulation of extracellular matrix formation.[57,59] ROS, by affecting vascular and renal tubule function, can also impair renal pressure natriuresis, alter systemic hemodynamics, and raise BP[60–62] (Figure 39.10).

There is growing evidence that supports a role for ROS in various animal models of hypertension, especially salt-sensitive models.[60–62] The DS rat, for example, has increased vascular and renal superoxide production, and increased levels of H_2O_2. Renal expression of superoxide dismutase is decreased in the kidneys of DS rats, and long-term administration of Tempol, a superoxide dismutase mimetic, significantly decreases BP and attenuates renal damage.[62] Another salt-sensitive model, the stroke-prone SHR, has elevated levels of superoxide and decreased plasma antioxidant capacity.[60–62] Superoxide production is also increased in the deoxycorticosterone acetate (DOCA)-salt hypertensive rat, and treatment with apocynin, a nicotinamide adenine dinucleotide phosphate NADPH oxidase inhibitor, decreases BP.[60–62] ROS also appears to play an important role in chronic angiotensin II hypertension. Angiotensin II is a potent stimulator of

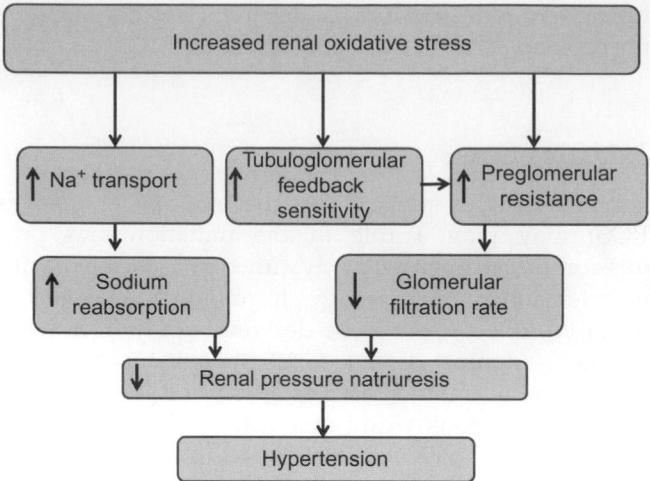

FIGURE 39.10 Renal mechanisms whereby ROS impair pressure natriuresis and increase BP. An increase in renal oxidative stress impairs renal pressure natriuresis by increasing renal vascular resistance or enhancing tubuloglomerular feedback, both of which decrease the glomerular filtration rate. Renal oxidative stress also reduces sodium excretion by direct effects to increase renal tubular reabsorption.

NADPH oxidase, and long-term administration of Tempol significantly decreases the chronic BP response to angiotensin II.[60–62]

Despite the fact that elevated ROS plays an important role in many experimental models of hypertension, antioxidant therapy has failed to lower BP in clinical studies.[63] An imbalance between total oxidant production and the antioxidant capacity in human primary hypertension has been reported to occur in some, but not all, studies. Equivocal findings in humans are partly due to the difficulty of assessing oxidative stress in clinical studies. Measurement of ROS in tissues represents a challenge, because of their low levels and relatively short half-lives.[64] Most human studies have found that chronic antioxidant therapy with vitamin E and C supplementation has little effect on BP. However, a major shortcoming of clinical trials using vitamin E and C is the lack of verification that antioxidant treatment actually decreased ROS.[63]

Inflammatory Cytokines and the Immune System

While inflammation and the immune system activation were first associated with hypertension over four decades ago, it has become increasingly evident over the last few years that inflammatory cytokines and the immune system play an important role in the progression of various models of experimental and genetic hypertension.[65–68]

Increased Inflammatory Cytokines in Hypertension

Plasma levels of proinflammatory cytokines correlate with increased BP in human hypertension, and in some experimental animal models of hypertension.[65,67] Moreover, several studies have demonstrated that chronic increases in plasma cytokines, comparable to concentrations observed in hypertension associated with pre-eclampsia, cause significant increases in BP.[69,70] A two-fold elevation in the plasma levels of Tumor Necrosis Factor alpha (TNF-α) significantly increased BP and renal vascular resistance in pregnant rats.[69,70] These studies are consistent with the hypothesis that increasing plasma levels of cytokines may contribute to pregnancy-induced hypertension. Etanercept, a selective TNF-α inhibitor, was not only effective in lowering BP, but also in dampening the ET-1 transcript that is typically observed in response to placental ischemia in pregnant rats.[69,70] Whether etanercept and other cytokine inhibitors would have beneficial effects in pre-eclamptic women remains unknown, because elevated levels of cytokines and exaggerated inflammatory responses have been reported in some studies.

Lee and co-workers[71] found that hypertension caused by chronic angiotensin II excess may depend, at least in part, on the presence of Interleukin-6 (IL-6). Mice with knockout of IL-6 had significantly lower BP than wild-type mice during two weeks of angiotensin II infusion. Although these findings demonstrate a significant role for IL-6 in mediating the chronic hypertensive response to angiotensin II in mice, the importance of inflammatory cytokines in the pathogenesis and progression of the various forms of human hypertension is unclear, and is currently an area of active investigation.

Several recent studies have demonstrated that T-cells play an important role in the progression of hypertension. Harrison and colleagues proposed that hypertensive stimuli lead to renal injury, neoantigen formation, and eventual T-cell activation within the kidney.[67,68,72] T-cell-derived signals promote entry of other inflammatory cells such as macrophages, which result in renal vasoconstriction and increased sodium reabsorption, thereby increasing the severity of the hypertension.[68] Supporting this concept is a recent report that RAG-1$^{-/-}$ mice, which lack T-cells and B-cells, do not develop the degree of hypertension in response to angiotensin II infusion as the wild-type mice, an observation that was attributed to lack of T-cells. Moreover, chronic angiotensin II infusion was associated with a greater number of activated T-cells, as well as increased Rantes, a chemotaxic protein, in the vasculature and perivascular fat.[67,68,72] These observations were confirmed by Crowley et al.[73] using a model very similar to the RAG-1$^{-/-}$ mice. They reported that angiotensin II hypertension, renal injury, left ventricular hypertrophy, and cardiac fibrosis were prevented in mice lacking T-cells. While these findings in experimental models of hypertension are intriguing, the importance of the immune system in the pathogenesis of essential hypertension in humans remains to be determined.

Eicosanoids

The kidneys produce several types of prostaglandins with multiple functions, including prostacyclin, thromboxane, 20-hydroxyeicosatetraenoic acid 20-HETE, and epoxyeicosatetraenoic acids (EETs), all of which have been reported to influence renal pressure natriuresis and BP. However, the major renal prostaglandin controlling sodium excretion is probably PGE_2.[74] The largest production of PGE_2 occurs in the renal medulla, with decreasing synthesis in the cortex. PGE_2 is synthesized and released, not stored. Once released, PGE_2 inhibits sodium reabsorption by several mechanisms, including direct effects on the renal tubules.

Even though long-term administration of PG synthesis inhibitors has very little effect on volume and/or BP regulation under normal physiologic conditions, renal PGs may be important in pathophysiologic states associated with enhanced activity of the RAAS. *In vitro* and *in vivo* studies indicate that renal PGs protect the preglomerular vessels from excessive angiotensin II-induced vasoconstriction. In the absence of this protective mechanism, the renal vasculature could be exposed to the potent vasoconstrictor actions of angiotensin II in various conditions, such as sodium and volume depletion. This could, in turn, lead to significant impairment of renal hemodynamics and excretory function.

Inhibitors of the COX-2 enzyme reduce pressure natriuresis, cause vasoconstriction, and increase BP.[74–76] There are at least two distinct cyclooxygenases—COX-1 and COX-2. COX-1 is called the *constitutive enzyme*, because of its wide tissue distribution, whereas COX-2 has been termed as *inducible*, because of its more restricted basal expression and its upregulation by inflammatory and/or proliferative stimuli. Based on the concept that COX-1 performs cellular housekeeping functions for normal physiologic activity and COX-2 acts at inflammatory sites, it was initially hypothesized that the BP and renal effects of nonsteroidal anti-inflammatory drugs might be linked to COX-1 inhibition.[74] However, experimental and clinical evidence indicates that COX-2 metabolites may also play a role in the regulation of vascular and renal function under various physiologic and pathophysiologic conditions.[74–76]

Selective COX-2 inhibitors were designed to minimize gastrointestinal complications of traditional NSAIDs—adverse effects attributed to suppression of COX-1-derived PGE_2 and prostacyclin. However, randomized controlled clinical trials of inhibitors of COX-2 indicate that such compounds may elevate the risk of hypertension, myocardial infarction, and stroke, possibly by removing the protective action of prostacyclin in counteracting thrombogenesis, hypertension, and atherogenesis.[75,76]

Eicosanoids produced by cytochrome P450 monooxygenase metabolism of arachidonic acid alter vascular function and renal pressure natriuresis. In addition to the PGs generated via the COX pathway, other eicosanoids that affect vascular function and/or renal sodium transport are produced by cytochrome P450 CYP monooxygenase metabolism of arachidonic acid. CYP enzymes metabolize arachidonic acid primarily to 20-HETE and EETs. 20-HETE is a potent vasoconstrictor that may regulate vascular tone and contribute to the autoregulation of renal blood flow. 20-HETE also inhibits sodium reabsorption in the proximal tubule and thick ascending limb of the loop of Henle.[77,78] Therefore, the ability of 20-HETE to influence BP regulation and renal pressure natriuresis is highly dependent on where 20-HETE is produced. The effect of 20-HETE to inhibit sodium transport tends to lower BP, whereas its vasoconstrictor effects on the renal vasculature and glomerulus tend to lower glomerular filtration rate, promote sodium retention, and increase BP (Figure 39.11).

Compelling evidence suggests that the renal production of CYP metabolites of arachidonic acid is altered in genetic and experimental models of hypertension, and contributes to the resetting of pressure natriuresis and increased BP.[77,78] Studies in humans also suggest that CYP metabolites may play a role in sodium homeostasis. Urinary 20-HETE excretion is regulated by salt intake, and is differentially regulated in salt-sensitive versus salt-resistant individuals.[79,80] Moreover, there appears to be a strong negative relationship between 20-HETE excretion and body mass index BMI, suggesting that some factor related to obesity may be responsible for decreased synthesis or excretion of this eicosanoid.[79,80] These observations support the possibility that attenuated renal production of 20-HETE could impair pressure natriuresis in human hypertension, especially when associated with obesity. However, further mechanistic studies are needed to test the importance of 20-HETE in human hypertension.

Atrial Natriuretic Peptide (ANP)

ANP is a 28 amino acid peptide synthesized and released from atrial cardiocytes in response to stretch.

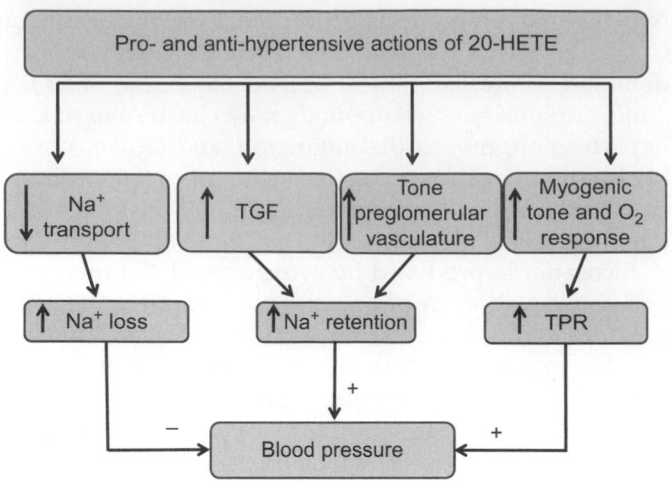

FIGURE 39.11 **Summary of the pro- and antihypertensive actions of 20-HETE. 20-HETE produced in the renal tubules which inhibits sodium transport and lowers BP.** In the renal vasculature and glomerulus, 20-HETE is a constrictor that lowers glomerular filtration rate, promotes sodium retention, and increases BP. In the peripheral circulation, 20-HETE increases vascular tone and increases BP (TGF: tubuloglomerular feedback; TPR: total peripheral resistance).

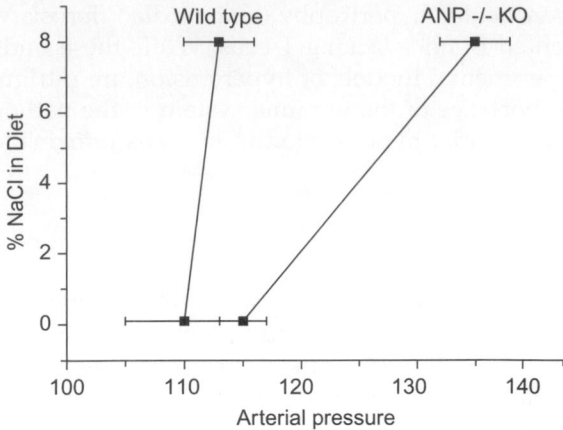

FIGURE 39.12 **Effect of atrial natriuretic peptide (ANP) receptor knockout on the chronic pressure natriuresis relationship.**[83]

ANP reduces vascular resistance, while enhancing sodium excretion through extrarenal and intrarenal mechanisms. ANP increases GFR, but has little effect on renal blood flow. However, an increase in GFR is not a prerequisite for ANP to enhance sodium excretion. ANP may also inhibit renal tubular sodium reabsorption directly by inhibiting active tubular sodium transport or indirectly via alterations in medullary blood flow, physical factors, and inhibiting formation of antinatriurectic hormones such as angiotensin II and aldosterone.

Plasma levels of ANP are elevated in numerous physiologic conditions associated with enhanced sodium excretion. Acute blood volume expansion consistently elevates circulating ANP. Some investigators report that chronic increases in dietary sodium intake also raise circulating levels of ANP.[81] Infusions of exogenous ANP at rates that result in physiologically relevant plasma concentrations, comparable to those observed during volume-expansion, elicit significant natriuresis, especially in the presence of other natriuretic stimuli, such as high renal perfusion pressure. Long-term physiologic elevations in plasma ANP also enhance pressure natriuresis and reduce BP.[82]

Transgenic mice overexpressing ANP are hypotensive relative to their wild-type littermates, whereas mice harboring functional disruptions of the ANP or NPR-A genes are hypertensive.[81,83] ANP gene knockout mice develop a salt-sensitive form of hypertension (Figure 39.12) in association with failure to adequately

suppress the RAAS.[83] While these findings suggest that genetic deficiencies in ANP or its receptors could play a role in the pathogenesis of salt-sensitive hypertension, the importance of this system in the pathogenesis of human hypertension remains unclear.

PRIMARY ESSENTIAL HYPERTENSION

Human primary essential hypertension appears to be largely a modern disorder associated with industrialization and the ready availability of food. Nearly all studies of Westernized, industrialized populations have demonstrated that BP, and therefore the prevalence of hypertension, rises with age.[84] Hunter-gatherers living in non-industrialized societies, however, rarely develop hypertension or age-related increases in systolic and mean pressures.[84] Thus, environmental factors appear to play a major role in raising BP in most patients with primary hypertension. However, it is likely that genetic variation contributes to differences in baseline BP that result in the normal distribution of BP in a population. When hypertension-producing environmental factors are added to the population baseline BP, the normal distribution is shifted toward higher BP; variations in the impact of environmental factors appear to flatten the BP curve and cause greater variability in BP of the population.

What elements of industrialized societies cause BP to increase in the majority of people as they age? How do they affect the physiologic controllers of BP? One factor that is clearly important is resetting of renal pressure natriuresis to higher BPs.[10] In some cases, this resetting may be related to increased renal sodium reabsorption, because of abnormalities intrinsic to the kidneys or altered neurohumoral control of the kidneys.[10] In other instances, resetting of pressure natriuresis may be associated with renal vasoconstriction and reductions in GFR, as a result of intrarenal mechanisms or nervous and hormonal mechanisms.[10] However, many of these initial changes in kidney function are difficult to discern after hypertension is established, because increased BP often returns renal function to normal. Experimental, clinical, and population studies suggest one of the key factors that affect BP is excess weight gain.

Overweight and Obesity are Major Risk Factors for Primary Hypertension

The prevalence of obesity has risen dramatically in the past 2–3 decades, and is now the most important public health problem in many industrialized countries, including the United States. Current estimates indicate that more than 1 *billion* people in the world are overweight or obese.[85] In the United States, more than 65% of adults are overweight, and one-third of the adult population is obese with a BMI greater than 30.[86] Population studies show that the relationship between BMI and systolic and diastolic BP is nearly linear in diverse populations throughout the world. Risk estimates from the Framingham Heart Study, for example, suggest that approximately 78% of primary hypertension in men and 65% in women can be ascribed to excess weight gain.[87] Clinical studies also indicate that weight loss is effective in reducing BP in most hypertensive subjects, and that weight loss, if it can be achieved, is effective in primary prevention of hypertension.[88]

If excess weight gain is a major cause of hypertension, why are some obese persons not hypertensive (i.e., BP greater than 140/90 mmHg)? Perhaps this is not so surprising if one considers that excess weight gain shifts the normal frequency distribution of BP toward higher levels. Although obesity increases the probability that a person's BP will register in the hypertensive range, not all obese people will have BPs greater than 140/90 mmHg. However, obese individuals who are classified as "normotensive" have higher BP than they would at a lower body weight. Thus, weight loss lowers BP in "normotensive" as well as "hypertensive" obese subjects.[5] Although the importance of obesity as a cause of hypertension is well-established, the physiologic mechanisms by which excess weight gain alters renal function and raises BP are only beginning to be elucidated.

Obesity is associated with extracellular fluid volume expansion, as well as increased tissue blood flow and cardiac output.[10] Studies in experimental animals and in humans indicate that blood flow is increased in many tissues, including the heart, kidneys, gastrointestinal tract, and skeletal muscles.[10] Some of the increased flow is caused by growth of skeletal muscle and organs in response to increased workload and the metabolic demands associated with obesity. However, obesity also causes functional vasodilation, perhaps as a consequence of an increased metabolic rate, higher oxygen consumption, and accumulation of vasodilator metabolites. This vasodilation occurs despite mild activation of the RAAS and SNS. Although resting blood flows are increased in many tissues, there appears to be reduced blood flow "reserve" during exercise or during reactive hyperemia in obese, compared to lean, individuals.[10] Cardiac reserve is also reduced in obesity, despite higher resting cardiac outputs.

Increased renal tubular sodium reabsorption and impaired pressure natriuresis play a major role in initiating the rise in BP associated with excess weight gain. At least three mechanisms are important in altering renal function in obesity hypertension (Figure 39.13): 1) increased SNS activity; 2) activation of the RAAS; and 3) physical compression of the kidneys by fat accumulation within and around the kidneys, and by increased abdominal pressure.

SNS Activation in Obesity Hypertension

Several observations indicate that increased SNS activity contributes to obesity hypertension[10]: 1) SNS activation, especially renal sympathetic activity, is increased in obese subjects; 2) pharmacologic blockade of adrenergic activity lowers BP to a greater extent in obese, compared to lean, individuals; and 3) renal denervation markedly attenuates sodium retention and hypertension associated with a high-fat diet in experimental animals.

Administration of α-and β-adrenergic blockers or clonidine, a drug that stimulates central α-2 receptors and reduces SNS activity, prevents most of the rise in BP in obese dogs fed a high-fat diet.[10,89] In obese hypertensive patients, combined α-and β-adrenergic blockade for one month reduced ambulatory BP significantly more in obese than in lean essential hypertensive patients.[10] These findings suggest that increased adrenergic activity contributes importantly to the development and maintenance of obesity hypertension in experimental animals and in humans.[10,89] The renal sympathetic nerves mediate most, if not all, of the chronic effects of SNS activation on BP in obesity. Bilateral renal denervation greatly attenuated sodium retention and hypertension in obese dogs fed a high-fat diet.[10]

Obesity does not cause mass activation of the SNS. Instead, increased SNS activity in various tissues is modest, and appears to be differentially controlled in obesity. For example, cardiac sympathetic activity does

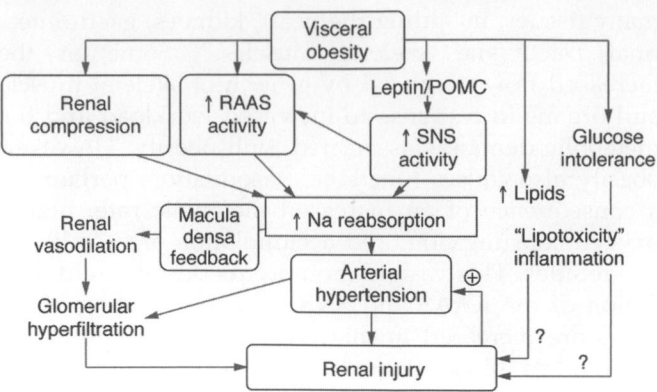

FIGURE 39.13 Summary of mechanisms by which obesity causes hypertension and renal injury. Visceral obesity increases BP by activation of the sympathetic nervous system (SNS), the renin—angiotensin—aldosterone system (RAAS), and by physical compression of the kidneys from the fat surrounding the kidneys. SNS activation may be caused by, in large part, the effects of leptin, which acts on proopiomelanocortin (POMC) neurons in the hypothalamus and brainstem. Obesity-induced hypertension and glomerular hyperfiltration may cause renal injury, especially when combined with dyslipidemia and hyperglycemia. Renal injury then exacerbates the hypertension and makes it more difficult to control.

not appear to be substantially elevated, whereas renal and skeletal muscle SNS activity is usually increased in obese subjects.[90–92] Obesity-induced SNS activation is usually not sufficient to cause vasoconstriction in most tissues, such as skeletal muscle or the kidneys, but does contribute to renin secretion and increased renal tubular sodium reabsorption.[60]

Several potential mediators of SNS activation in obesity have been suggested, including: 1) hyperinsulinemia; 2) angiotensin II; 3) increased levels of free fatty acids; 4) impaired baroreceptor reflexes; 5) activation of chemoreceptor-mediated reflexes associated with sleep apnea; and 6) cytokines released from adipocytes i.e., "adipokines" such as leptin, TNF-α and IL-6. Although these mechanisms have been reviewed previously,[5,6,10] there is little direct evidence to support cause-and-effect relationships for most of these factors and obesity-induced SNS activation.

Leptin—Melanocortin Activation May Mediate SNS Activation in Obesity

A promising candidate for linking obesity with hypertension is hyperleptinemia (Figure 39.14). Leptin, released from adipocytes in proportion to the degree of adiposity, acts on the hypothalamus and other regions of the brain to reduce appetite and increase SNS activity. In rodents, leptin increases sympathetic activity and BP.[10,93] Moreover, the hypertensive effects of leptin are enhanced when NO synthesis is inhibited,[10] as often occurs in obese subjects with endothelial dysfunction.

Additional support for leptin as a potential mechanism of obesity hypertension is the finding that leptin-deficient, obese mice and obese mice with mutations of the leptin receptor usually have little or no increase in BP compared to their lean controls.[89] Similar results have been found in obese children with leptin gene mutations who have early onset morbid obesity, but normal BP and impaired SNS activity.[94] Furthermore, children with leptin gene mutations did not have hypertension, despite having many other characteristics of the metabolic syndrome, including severe insulin resistance, hyperinsulinemia, and hyperlipidemia.[94] These observations suggest that the functional effects of leptin may be critical in linking obesity with SNS activation and hypertension.[89]

Leptin's stimulatory effect on SNS activity appears to be mediated by interactions with other hypothalamic factors, especially the proopiomelanocortin POMC pathway (Figure 39.14). In mice with leptin receptors deleted specifically in POMC neurons, leptin's hypertensive effects were completely abolished.[95] Also, pharmacological antagonism of melanocortin 3/4 receptors MC3/4R completely prevented leptin's chronic BP effects,[89] and the chronic hypertensive effects of leptin were absent in MC4R knockout mice.[89] These observations indicate that leptin's chronic BP effects are mediated almost entirely by activation of POMC neurons which, in turn, release α-melanocyte-stimulating hormone α-MSH, leading to activation of MC4R and increased SNS activity.[89]

A study in humans also suggests that MC4R activation may contribute to obesity-induced hypertension. The prevalence of hypertension is lower in MC4R-deficient humans compared to obese control subjects, despite severe obesity and associated metabolic disorders.[96] Moreover, subcutaneous administration of an MC4R agonist for seven days significantly increased BP. Thus, in humans and rodents, chronic activation of MC4R raises BP, and the presence of a functional MC4R system appears to be necessary for obesity and hyperleptinemia to increase SNS activity and BP.[96]

RAAS Activation in Obesity

Obese subjects, especially those with visceral obesity, often have mild-to-moderate increases in plasma renin activity PRA, angiotensinogen, ACE activity, angiotensin II, and aldosterone levels.[5] Activation of the RAAS occurs despite sodium retention, volume expansion, and hypertension, all of which normally tend to suppress renin secretion and angiotensin II formation.

An important role for angiotensin II in stimulating renal sodium reabsorption and in mediating obesity hypertension is supported by studies in experimental animals demonstrating that angiotensin II receptor blockade or ACE inhibition markedly attenuates

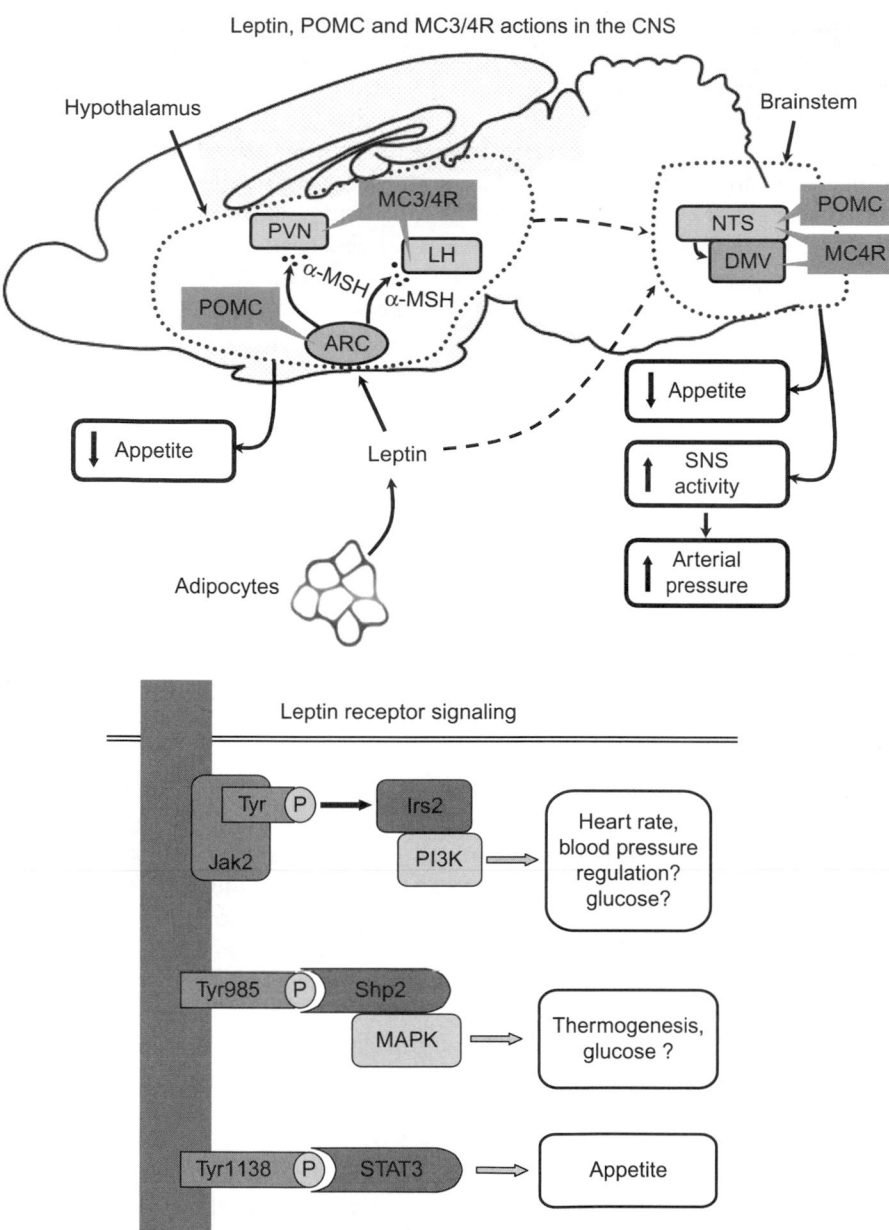

Leptin, POMC and MC3/4R actions in the CNS

Leptin receptor signaling

FIGURE 39.14 **Possible links among leptin and its effects on the hypothalamus, sympathetic activation, and hypertension.** Within the hypothalamus, one of the key pathways of leptin's action on appetite, SNS activity, and BP is stimulation of the proopiomelanocortin (POMC) neurons in the arcuate nucleus (ARC). These neurons send projections to the paraventricular nucleus (PVN) and lateral hypothalamus, releasing α-melanocyte-stimulating hormone (α-MSH), which then acts as an agonist for melanocortin 4 receptors (MC4R). These neurons, in turn, send projections to the nucleus of the solitary tract (NTS) to effect changes in appetite, SNS activity, and blood pressure. Leptin also suppresses the NPY/AGRP neurons, but their role in controlling SNS activity and BP are still unclear. Leptin—melanocortin activation in distinct areas of the brain and through multiple intracellular signaling pathways may differentially regulate appetite, energy expenditure, and BP (LH: lateral hypothalamus; RSNA: renal sympathetic nerve activity).

sodium retention, volume expansion, and increased BP during the development of obesity.[5,6,97] Whether the effects of angiotensin II to raise BP in obesity are due primarily to direct actions on the kidneys or stimulation of aldosterone secretion is unclear. The direct renal sodium-retaining effects of angiotensin II are well-known, as are the effects of angiotensin II to stimulate aldosterone secretion.

Although smaller clinical trials have clearly shown that both ARBs and ACE inhibitors are effective in lowering BP in obese hypertensive patients, there have been no large-scale clinical studies comparing the effectiveness of RAAS blockers in obese and lean hypertensive patients.

Activation of the RAAS may also contribute to the glomerular injury and nephron loss associated with obesity. By constricting efferent arterioles, increased angiotensin II formation exacerbates the rise in glomerular hydrostatic pressure caused by systemic arterial hypertension.[5] Studies in type II diabetic patients, who are usually overweight or obese, clearly indicate that ACE inhibitors or ARBs slow the progression of renal disease.[28,98] Thus, ARBs and ACE inhibitors may be particularly useful in obese patients, especially those with diabetes and renal disease.

Mineralocorticoid Receptor (MR) Activation in Obesity Hypertension

Studies in experimental animals and in humans suggest that antagonism of MR may provide an important therapeutic tool not only for lowering BP, but also for attenuating target organ injury in obesity hypertension. Antagonism of MR in obese dogs markedly attenuated sodium retention, hypertension, and glomerular hyperfiltration.[35] The observation that MR antagonism attenuated glomerular hyperfiltration may also have important implications for renal protection in obesity, although there are no studies, to our knowledge, that have directly tested this in non-diabetic obese humans. Administration of MR antagonists also provides significant antihypertensive benefit in resistant obese patients.[34] Reductions in BP caused by MR antagonism in obese patients with resistant hypertension occurred despite concurrent therapy with ACE inhibitor or ARB, calcium channel blocker, and thiazide diuretic, suggesting that MR activation in obesity can occur independently of angiotensin II-mediated stimulation of aldosterone secretion.

Visceral Obesity May Cause Renal Compression

Visceral obesity initiates several changes that lead to compression of the kidneys, increased intrarenal pressures, impaired renal pressure natriuresis, and hypertension.[10] Intra-abdominal pressure rises in proportion to abdominal diameter, reaching levels as high as 35–40 mmHg in some individuals.[5] In addition, retroperitoneal adipose tissue often encapsulates the kidney and penetrates the renal hilum into the renal medullary sinuses in obese dogs as well as in obese humans, causing additional compression and increased intrarenal pressures.[99]

Obesity also causes changes in renal medullary histology and increased extracellular matrix that exacerbate intrarenal compression and hypertension.[97] Increased intrarenal hydrostatic pressure may, in turn, cause compression of the loops of Henle and vasa recta, thereby increasing tubular sodium and water reabsorption. Although these physical changes in the kidneys cannot account for the initial increase in BP that occurs with rapid weight gain, they may help to explain why abdominal obesity is much more closely associated with hypertension than subcutaneous obesity.[97]

Kidney Injury in Obesity Hypertension

Obesity has not been widely recognized as a major risk factor for ESRD, and is not included as a cause of kidney failure in renal data registries. However, the impact of obesity on renal disease is clear when one considers that diabetes and hypertension, both of which are closely associated with excess weight gain, account for more than 70% of ESRD. Moreover, the rapid rise in the prevalence of ESRD in the past two decades has paralleled increasing obesity and diabetes.[97] Although most of the increasing prevalence of ESRD has been attributed to the increase in type II diabetes, patients with diabetes are usually hypertensive, and the increased BP likely contributes to renal injury.

Population studies indicate that obesity is a major cause of renal disease, even after adjustment for hypertension, diabetes or pre-existing renal disease. In a retrospective analysis of adults who were followed for 15–35 years, the rate of ESRD increased in a stepwise manner as BMI increased.[100] This relationship was not affected by BP or diabetes, and the analysis was adjusted for age, sex, race, education level, smoking status, history of myocardial infarction, serum cholesterol level, proteinuria, hematuria, and serum creatinine level. Thus, observational studies suggest that obesity may be an important risk factor for renal disease through other mechanisms in addition to hypertension and diabetes.

Obesity may also amplify the effect of other primary renal insults, even those that are usually considered to be relatively benign, such as unilateral nephrectomy. Praga and co-workers[101] reported that of patients with a BMI greater than 30 who had undergone unilateral nephrectomy, 92% developed proteinuria or renal insufficiency, whereas only 12% of patients with a BMI less than 30 developed these disorders. Similar findings have also been reported for patients with immunoglobulin A nephropathy.[102] These observations suggest that obesity exacerbates the loss of kidney function in patients with pre-existing glomerulopathies, and that weight loss may lessen the impact of renal injury from other causes.

Animals placed on a high-fat diet for only a few weeks also have significant structural changes in the kidneys, including enlargement of the Bowman space, glomerular cell proliferation, increased mesangial matrix, and increased expression of glomerular TGF-β.[103] These early changes occur with only modest hypertension, only mild metabolic abnormalities, and may be the precursors of more severe renal injury as obesity is sustained. Obese patients often develop proteinuria, frequently in the nephrotic range, that is followed by progressive loss of kidney function.[97] The most common types of renal lesions observed in renal biopsies of obese subjects are focal and segmental glomerular sclerosis and glomerulomegaly.

The gradual loss of kidney function, as well as the hypertension and diabetes that commonly coexist with obesity, may lead to progressive impairment of pressure natriuresis, salt-sensitivity, and greater increases in BP. Thus, renal injury in obese subjects not only exacerbates the hypertension, but also makes BP more difficult to control with antihypertensive drugs. The mechanisms of obesity-induced renal injury are not fully-understood, but likely involve a combination of hemodynamic and metabolic abnormalities.

As discussed previously, obesity causes marked glomerular hyperfiltration and preglomerular vasodilation that permits greater transmission of the increased BP to the glomerular capillaries. These renal hemodynamic changes, along with the metabolic abnormalities, such as hyperglycemia and hyperlipidemia, exacerbate the effects of increases in BP to cause renal injury. A synergistic relationship may exist between the metabolic abnormalities and increased glomerular pressure in causing chronic renal vascular disease and nephron loss, similar to the synergistic effects of hypertension, diabetes, and dyslipidemia in increasing the risk for coronary artery disease and myocardial infarction. However, there are no large-scale studies that have tested this idea.

How Does "Metabolic Syndrome" Relate to Primary Hypertension?

Dyslipidemia, hyperinsulinemia, and hyperglycemia often occur concurrently with hypertension, leading to the proposal of a unique pathophysiologic condition that is often called the *metabolic syndrome*. Definitions of the metabolic syndrome have been proposed by the World Health Organization WHO,[104] the Third Report of the National Cholesterol Education Program's Adult Treatment Panel ATP III,[105] and other organizations.[104] All of these definitions include disordered glucose homeostasis or measures of insulin resistance, dyslipidemia, hypertension, and obesity.

Recent analyses of the metabolic syndrome have questioned whether insulin resistance and hyperinsulinemia are the underlying causes of this complex cluster of cardiovascular risk factors.[104,106] Chronic hyperinsulinemia, in the absence of obesity, does not raise BP in dogs or humans.[107] Multiple studies in humans have also shown that chronic insulin treatment does not raise BP in patients with type 1 or type 2 diabetes, and patients with severe hyperinsulinemia as a result of insulinoma are not hypertensive.[107] Taken together, these observations suggest that hyperinsulinemia *per se* is insufficient to cause chronic hypertension.

Insulin resistance has been proposed to cause hypertension independent of hyperinsulinemia. However, there are several disorders associated with severe insulin resistance and hyperinsulinemia in humans and experimental animal models that are not linked with hypertension. In mice, mutations of the leptin gene or the leptin receptor or mutations of the MC4-R, cause severe insulin resistance and many characteristics of the metabolic syndrome, but BP is not increased compared to wild-type controls.[5,89] Likewise, humans with leptin gene or MC4R mutations have severe insulin resistance, but no indication of SNS activation or hypertension.[94,96] These observations do not support a direct role for insulin resistance in causing hypertension.

Several reports indicate that agents that increase insulin sensitivity, such as the thiazolidinediones, also lower BP. However, these drugs influence expression of multiple genes by binding to the peroxisome proliferator-activated receptor-γ (PPARγ), a nuclear receptor. Thiazolidinediones may also inhibit L-type calcium channels, and they reduce BP in renovascular hypertension that is not associated with insulin resistance or hyperinsulinemia.[5,108] Therefore, it appears that the BP-lowering effects of these drugs are related to other actions besides improvement of insulin sensitivity.

Abnormalities of glucose and lipid metabolism associated with insulin resistance may, over many years, lead to athereosclerosis and vascular injury, and in this way contribute indirectly to increased BP, especially if the renal blood vessels and glomeruli are damaged. Progressive loss of kidney function could contribute to salt-sensitivity of BP and gradual development of hypertension. Thus, the metabolic disturbances associated with severe insulin resistance may exacerbate hypertension by causing renal injury, although the importance of these effects, in the absence of diabetes, is still unclear.

Although insulin resistance and hypertension are often closely correlated, much of the available evidence suggests that this association is largely a consequence of obesity which causes both insulin resistance and high BP through parallel mechanisms. There is little doubt that obesity, especially visceral obesity, is a major cause of the entire cluster of CVD risk factors associated with the metabolic syndrome.[104,107] Importantly, all of the disorders associated with the metabolic syndrome can usually be reversed by weight loss.

GENETIC CAUSES OF HYPERTENSION

Success in identifying genes that contribute importantly to human primary hypertension has been limited mainly to identification of monogenic forms of hypertension. When one considers the complexity of the multiple neural, hormonal, renal, and vascular mechanisms that contribute to short-term and long-term BP regulation, it is perhaps not surprising that finding a few variant genes alleles to account for a major portion of BP variation has been challenging. The complexity of the problem is compounded by the likelihood that BP variation is caused not only by single-gene variants, but also by polymorphic genetic differences, complex interactions among several genes, and interaction among genetic and environmental factors. The finding that hypertension does not often occur in populations living in non-industrialized regions of the world suggests that environmental influences play a major role in common forms of hypertension.

What is the evidence that gene variants play a major role in human primary hypertension? Multiple studies provide evidence that the closer the genetic relatedness, the greater the similarity of BP.[109] For monozygotic twins (with genetic similarity of 100%), the correlation coefficient for systolic BP has ranged from 0.5 to 0.8 (average: 0.6), for dizygotic twins it has ranged from 0.19 to 0.46 (average: 0.35), and for non-twin siblings (genetic similarity of around 50%) the correlation coefficient has averaged around 0.23. There is also a better correlation of BP values in biologic children than in adopted children. However, the importance of shared family environment is also evident from the BP correlations observed in genetically unrelated adopted siblings.

Comprehensive familial analyses that include other relatives in addition to twins suggest that environment may contribute to as much as 30% of BP variance, and genetic factors may contribute 40 to 50% of BP variance.[109] However, despite the use of sophisticated mathematical models for these calculations, the possibility of nonlinear gene–environmental interactions makes it difficult to quantify the precise roles of genes and environment in BP variation.

Hypertension has been suggested to result from additive effects of multiple variant genes acting in concert to elevate BP. Each gene variant is presumed to have a relatively weak impact on BP, but may produce significant hypertension when they act together in the presence of the necessary environmental conditions. This *polygenic* model also applies to other complex diseases such as diabetes or cancer, where multiple genes and environmental factors may play a role in the development of the disease.

Although the hypertension research literature is replete with studies showing associations of gene polymorphisms and BP, the genetic alterations that contribute to primary hypertension remain unknown.[109] Most of these genetic studies have produced mixed results, even for widely studied polymorphisms such as the ACE insertion/deletion and angiotensinogen polymorphisms.[110] Polymorphisms and mutations in other genes such as α-adducin, atrial natriuretic factor, the insulin receptor, β$_2$-adrenergic receptor, calcitonin gene-related peptide, angiotensinase C, renin-binding protein, endothelin-1 precursor, G-protein β$_3$-subunit have also been associated with the development of hypertension in some studies[110]; however, all of these polymorphisms show weak associations, if any, with BP, and many of the early studies

showing statistically significant associations have not been confirmed. Large-scale genome-wide association studies (GWAS) in which hundreds of thousands of common genetic variants are genotyped and analyzed for blood pressure association have shown limited success in identifying genes that contribute to hypertension. At best, the gene variations discovered thus far explain only a tiny part of the BP variation found in humans.[111]

Monogenic Disorders that Cause Hypertension

Table 39.1 shows some of the monogenic disorders that are associated with high BP. An interesting feature of these genetic disorders is that they all affect electrolyte transport in the renal tubule or the synthesis and/or activity of RAAS hormones. In all monogenic hypertensive disorders thus far, the final common pathway to hypertension appears to be increased sodium reabsorption and volume expansion. Monogenic hypertension, however, is rare, and all of the known forms together account for less than 1% of human hypertension.

Familial Hyperaldosteronism Type I

Also called *glucocorticoid remediable aldosteronism (GRA)*, familial hyperaldosteronism type I (FH-I) is inherited as an autosomal dominant trait caused by a chimeric gene derived from a meiotic mismatch and unequal crossing between the promoter of the 11β-hydroxylase *CYP11B1* controlled by the structural portion of the aldosterone synthase gene *CYP11B2*.[15] This causes aldosterone secretion to be abnormally regulated by adrenocorticotrophic hormone (ACTH). Because ACTH is suppressed by glucocorticoids, administration of excess glucocorticoids is effective in reducing aldosterone secretion in patients with FH-I.

Patients with FH-I exhibit many of the same characteristics as those with primary aldosteronism, including high aldosterone, hypokalemia, volume expansion, metabolic alkalosis, and low renin. Although some patients with FH-I have severe hypertension, others have only moderate hypertension or may even be normotensive. This wide range of BP could be related to variable expression of the chimeric gene or to other differences in genetic background that would place the inherited BP in the low or normal range in the absence of the FH-I mutation. The final BP could therefore be the combined result of the low or normal inherited BP, the hypertensive effect of the FH-I mutation, and other environmental factors, such as salt intake. Patients with FH-I respond well to thiazide diuretics, as well as spironolactone.

TABLE 39.1 Known Genetic Causes of Hypertension

Genetic Disorder	Age of Onset	Pattern of Inheritance	Aldosterone Level	Serum Potassium Level	Treatment[a]
FH-I (GRA)[b]	2nd or 3rd decade	Autosomal dominant	High	Decreased in 50% of cases; marked decrease with thiazides	Glucocorticoids
FH-II[c]	Middle age	Autosomal dominant	High	Low to normal	Spironolactone, eplerenone
DOC oversecretion due to CAH[c,d]	Childhood	Autosomal recessive	Low	Low to normal	Glucocorticoids
Activating MR mutation exacerbated by pregnancy[e]	2nd or 3rd decade	Unknown	Low	Low to normal	Delivery of fetus
AME2[c,f]	Childhood	Autosomal recessive	Low	Low to normal	Spironolactone, dexamethasone
Liddle's syndrome[g]	3rd decade	Autosomal dominant	Low	Low to normal	Amiloride, triamterene
Gordon's syndrome[h]	2nd or 3rd decade	Autosomal dominant	Low	High	Thiazide diuretic, low-sodium diet

[a]Treatment for underlying mechanisms; other forms of treatment, including different antihypertensive medications, might be needed to adequately control BP.
[b]Familial hyperaldosteronism.
[c]Excess production of non-aldosterone mineralocorticoids.
[d]Congenital adrenal hyperplasia, DOC-producing tumors.
[e]Increased activity of MR
[f]Apparent mineralocorticoid excess caused by either licorice ingestion or ectopic ACTH secretion.
[g]Increased activity of sodium channels.
[h]Increased activity of NaCl co-transporter in the distal tubule.
ACTH: adrenocorticotropic hormone; AME: apparent mineralocorticoid excess; CAH: congenital adrenal hyperplasia; DOC: deoxycorticosterone; FH-I: familial hyperaldosteronism type I; FH-II: familial hyperaldosteronism type II; GRA: glucocorticoid-remediable aldosteronism; MR: mineralocorticoid receptor.

Familial Hyperaldosteronism Type II

Familial hyperaldosteronism type II (FH-II) is a rare disease in which hypertension is caused by excessive aldosterone secretion that is not suppressed by glucocorticoid administration, distinguishing it from FH-I.[112] Patients with FH-II have the same clinical symptoms as patients with primary hyperaldosteronism caused by bilateral adrenal hyperplasia. The genetic abnormality causing FH-II has been localized to chromosome 7p22.[112] Although hypertension in FH-II is unresponsive to glucocorticoids, spironolactone is effective in reducing BP and correcting the metabolic disturbances.

Congenital Adrenal Hyperplasia and Excess Deoxycorticosterone Secretion

This disorder describes a group of syndromes caused by defects in cortisol biosynthesis. Congenital adrenal hyperplasia is an autosomal recessive disorder. When 21-hydroxylase CYP21A2 is deficient, the most common cause of congenital adrenal hyperplasia, patients are normotensive.[112] When 11β-hydroxylase CYP11B1 and 17β-hydroxylase CYP17 are deficient, production of deoxycorticosterone, which has mineralocorticoid activity, is increased, leading to hypertension. Defects in CYP11B1 and CYP17 cause inhibition of cortisol production with a subsequent reduction in

feedback inhibition of ACTH secretion by the anterior pituitary and hypothalamus. Increased ACTH secretion then stimulates production of steroid precursors proximal to the blocked step, leading to excessive levels of deoxycorticosterone.

Both forms of congenital adrenal hyperplasia are associated with early-onset hypertension and hypokalemia. Signs of androgen excess distinguish the two disorders: 11β-hydroxylase deficiency causes virilization in girls and precocious puberty in boys, whereas 17α-hydroxylase deficiency causes sex hormone deficiency, primary amenorrhea, and delayed sexual development in girls, and ambiguous genitalia in boys. Genetic diagnosis of both conditions relies on testing for mutations that either severely depress or abolish enzyme activity. Both conditions can be effectively treated by administering glucocorticoids that normalize ACTH secretion and ACTH-mediated build-up of cortisol precursors proximal to the enzymatic deficiency, including deoxycorticosterone.

Liddle's Syndrome

This is an autosomal dominant form of monogenic hypertension that results from mutations in the amiloride-sensitive ENaC. Several mutations that result in the elimination of 45–75 amino acids from the cytoplasmic carboxyl terminus of β- or γ-subunits of the channel have been reported. Mutations that increase ENaC activity, in turn, cause excessive distal and collecting tubule sodium reabsorption and hypertension.[15,112]

Liddle's syndrome is characterized by early-onset hypertension with hypokalemia and suppression of renin and aldosterone. Decreased aldosterone and lack of responsiveness to MR antagonists differentiates this syndrome from primary aldosteronism. Both hypertension and hypokalemia vary in severity, depending on salt intake, and can be treated with amiloride or triamterene, specific inhibitors of ENaC.

Apparent Mineralocorticoid Excess (AME)

AME is an autosomal recessive form of monogenic hypertension that results from a mutation in the renal-specific isoform of the 11β-hydroxysteroid dehydrogenase 2 gene.[15,112] This enzyme normally converts cortisol to the inactive metabolite cortisone and "protects" the MR from being activated by cortisol. This is important, because the renal epithelial MR receptor in the distal and collecting tubules has a similar affinity for aldosterone and cortisol, while cortisol concentrations are normally much higher than aldosterone. Deficiency of 11β-hydroxysteroid dehydrogenase 2 allows the tubular MR to be occupied and activated by cortisol, causing sodium retention and volume expansion, low renin, low aldosterone, and a form of hypertension that is salt-sensitive.

A non-genetic form of the AME syndrome is found in persons ingesting large amounts of licorice which contains glycyrrhetinic acid, an inhibitor of the enzyme 11β-hydroxysteroid dehydrogenase. Both forms of apparent mineralocorticoid excess are effectively treated with MR antagonists, such as spironolactone or eplerenone.

Pseudohypoaldosteronism Type II

Also called *Gordon's syndrome*, pseudohypoaldosteronism type II is a rare Mendelian form of hypertension that is salt-sensitive and associated with hyperkalemia, hyperchloremia, metabolic acidosis, and suppressed renin and aldosterone levels. The disorder is caused by mutations in two genes encoding the serine/threonine protein kinases, WNK1 and WNK4.[113]

The phenotypes of excessive salt retention and hypertension are caused by loss of normal inhibition or constitutive activation of the renal tubular NaCl co-transporter by mutant WNK1 or WNK4 genes. WNK4 normally inhibits NaCl co-transporter activity, and loss-of-function mutations therefore increase NaCl reabsorption and cause hypertension. WNK1 does not regulate NaCl co-transporter activity directly, but exerts an indirect effect through suppression of WNK4 inhibition of the NaCl transporter. Therefore, gain-of-function mutations of WNK1 result in highly active NaCl co-transporter, volume expansion, and hypertension with characteristics similar to those caused by loss-of-function mutations of WNK4.[113]

Hyperkalemia is a major feature of pseudohypoaldosteronism type II[112] and may be due, in part, to decreased NaCl delivery to the cortical collecting tubules, which limits their secretion of potassium. Mutant WNKs may also cause hyperkalemia by inhibiting activity of renal outer medullary potassium (ROMK) channels, the major potassium secretory channels in the distal nephron. The fact that hyperkalemia is invariably present in pseudohypoaldosteronism type II is often used to distinguish it from other monogenic forms of hypertension.

Thiazide diuretics, which inhibit distal nephron NaCl reabsorption, are especially effective in reducing BP and correcting hyperkalemia in patients with pseudohypoaldosteronism type II. Because NaCl co-transporter activity is regulated by luminal salt delivery, decreased NaCl intake also reduces activity of the transporter, and therefore attenuates volume-expansion and hypertension in patients with pseudohypoaldosteronism type II syndrome. Therefore, BP in Gordon's syndrome is highly salt-sensitive.

Mineralocorticoid Receptor Activating Mutation

This monogenic disorder is caused by a substitution of leucine for serine at codon 810 of the MR.[15] This mutation alters the shape and specificity of the MR, and eliminates the usual requirement for the 21-hydroxyl group of aldosterone to interact with the MR. This explains why other steroids, such as progesterone, activate the MR and why spironolactone, which is normally an antagonist of the MR, acts as an agonist for the MR in this disorder. Thus, treatment of these patients with spironolactone or increased levels of progesterone worsens the sodium retention, hypokalemia, and hypertension.

SECONDARY CAUSES OF HYPERTENSION

In a small fraction of patients, the clinical features, history, and physical examination point to a specific cause of increased BP, and the hypertension is therefore said to be *secondary*. Some types of secondary hypertension have a genetic basis, whereas others are caused by cardiovascular diseases and target organ injury associated with various disorders such as diabetes and kidney disease, and in some instances hypertension can be caused by drugs or treatments that patients receive. Table 39.2 lists some of the most frequently-diagnosed causes of secondary hypertension, although we discuss only a few of the more common types.

TABLE 39.2 Some Secondary Causes of Hypertension

A. Renal parenchymal disease
- Acute and chronic glomerulonephritis
- Chronic nephritis e.g., pyelonephritis, radiation
- Polycystic disease
- Diabetic nephropathy
- Hydronephrosis
- Neoplasms

B. Renovascular
- Renal artery stenosis/compression
- Intrarenal vasculitis
- Suprarenal aortic coarctation

C. Renoprival renal failure, loss of kidney tissue

D. Endocrine disorders
- Renin-producing tumors
- Cushing syndrome
- Primary aldosteronism
- Pheochromocytoma adrenal or extraadrenal chromaffin tumors
- Acromegaly

E. Pregnancy-induced hypertension

F. Sleep apnea

G. Increased intracranial pressure brain tumors, encephalitis

H. Hormones and drugs (partial list)
- Glucocorticoids
- Mineralocorticoids
- Sympathomimetics
- Tyramine-containing foods and monoamine oxidase inhibitors
- Estrogen (e.g., oral contraceptive pills)
- Apparent mineralocorticoid excess (e.g., licorice)
- Nonsteroidal anti-inflammatory drugs
- Cyclosporine
- Excess alcohol use
- Drug abuse (e.g., amphetamines, cocaine)

Renovascular Hypertension

Renovascular hypertension, although accounting for only 2–3% of all hypertension, is one of the most common causes of secondary hypertension. The pathophysiology of renovascular hypertension is due to an initial reduction in renal perfusion that occurs as a result of stenosis of the main renal artery, one of its branches or stenosis/injury of other smaller preglomerular blood vessels and glomeruli. The majority of renal vascular lesions reflect either fibromuscular dysplasia or atherosclerosis.[114] The predominant lesion found in the main renal artery or its branches in patients older than 50 years of age is atherosclerotic disease. More subtle functional constriction or structural changes in smaller blood vessels (e.g., afferent arterioles, glomeruli) are difficult to detect clinically, but can contribute to increased BP.

Renovascular hypertension can be unilateral or bilateral, and can result in a homogeneous or non-homogeneous ischemia of nephrons. As discussed earlier in the chapter, there are some important differences in the pathophysiology of homogeneous compared to non-homogenous impairments of renal perfusion. Experimental counterparts of these two clinical forms of renovascular hypertension can be found in the 1-kidney, 1-clip and the 2-kidney, 1-clip models of Goldblatt hypertension, respectively.

Renal Artery Stenosis in a Single Remaining Kidney or Aortic Coarctation above Both Renal Arteries

Renal artery constriction or aortic coarctation, if severe enough to reduce renal perfusion pressure below the range of autoregulation (approximately 70 mmHg), initially decreases renal blood flow, GFR, and sodium excretion, while increasing renin secretion. However, if the stenosis is not too severe, sodium excretion returns to normal, and if sodium intake is normal and adequate volume is available, renin secretion also returns to nearly normal in the established phase of hypertension.[9,115] At this point, the hypertension is stable, and most indices of renal function are relatively normal, including pressure distal to the stenosis.

Increased angiotensin II accounts for much of the rapid increase in BP after stenosis of the renal artery or suprarenal aortic coarctation. However, even after blocking the RAAS, BP still increases although more slowly until renal perfusion pressure returns to nearly normal. This increase in renal perfusion pressure, at the expense of systemic arterial hypertension, permits normal excretion of sodium and water to be maintained. As long as the sodium intake is normal, activation of the RAAS serves mainly to increase the rate at which BP is elevated. In the established phase of hypertension, blockade of the RAAS causes only small reductions in BP, similar to the decreases observed in normal subjects after angiotensin II blockade.[5]

The importance of volume-expansion in elevating BP in 1-kidney, 1-clip Goldblatt hypertension or suprarenal aortic coarctation depends on the sodium intake. With normal-or high-sodium intake, significant volume-expansion occurs, whereas a low-sodium diet converts this model of hypertension to one that is highly angiotensin II-dependent. When the stenosis is severe and adequate renal perfusion cannot be restored even with increased systemic BP, renin secretion continues to increase, as does BP, leading eventually to malignant hypertension and renal failure. Thus, the ability to return renal perfusion pressure to normal or nearly normal, by volume retention or activation of the RAAS, is critical to maintaining homeostasis when there is stenosis of a single remaining kidney. The same sequence occurs when there are widespread homogeneous increases in preglomerular resistance caused by bilateral renal artery stenosis or aortic coarctation above both renal arteries.[11]

Non-Homogeneous Increases in Renal Vascular Resistance or Unilateral Renal Artery Stenosis in Patients with two Kidneys

As discussed previously, non-homogeneous increases in preglomerular resistance can occur as a result of stenosis of one renal artery and normal perfusion of the contralateral kidney. Also, patchy increases in preglomerular resistance within the kidneys, with some nephrons being underperfused and others having normal or increased blood flow, can cause hypertension with characteristics similar to those found in the 2-kidney, 1-clip form of Goldblatt hypertension. These forms of hypertension all have underperfusion of some nephrons, and normal or increased blood flow in adjacent nephrons or in the nonstenotic kidney.

In experimental models with unilateral renal artery stenosis, the increase in BP is less predictable if the contralateral kidney does not become injured because of the hypertension. In this situation, underperfused nephrons or the entire underperfused kidney in the case of a unilateral renal artery stenosis are exposed to reduced perfusion pressure, secrete increased amounts of renin, and excrete less sodium and water than kidneys with normal blood flow. In contrast, the non-ischemic nephrons or nonstenotic kidney are exposed to increased renal perfusion pressure, causing renin secretion to fall to low levels and increasing sodium excretion above normal. However, even with increased perfusion pressure, the function of the non-ischemic nephrons or unclipped, nonstenotic kidney is impaired because of high circulating angiotensin II, which exerts an antinatriuretic effect and helps to sustain hypertension.

The higher BPs experienced by the nonstenotic kidney may eventually cause nephron damage which then maintains increased BP, even after correction of the stenosis in the other kidney. However, correction of the stenosis plus nephrectomy of the non-stenotic kidney may normalize BP if the stenosis is not so severe that it causes vascular rarefaction and permanent injury to the stenotic kidney.[5,6]

Administration of ACE inhibitors or ARBs as a treatment for renovascular hypertension may improve the structure and function of the non-stenotic kidney, but can in severe cases produce serious reductions in GFR and shrinkage of the stenotic kidney, resulting in fibrosis and further deterioration of its function. This is partly a result of the fall in BP, which may reduce renal perfusion pressure distal to the lesion to below the range of autoregulation. Blockade of angiotensin II also causes vasodilation of efferent arterioles which contributes to a decline in GFR in the stenotic kidney. In some patients with severe renal vascular lesions, administration of ACE inhibitors or ARBs may cause severe decreases in renal function, especially when there is also volume-depletion because of concomitant use of diuretics. Therefore, renal function should be monitored frequently after administration of RAS inhibitors in patients suspected of having renovascular hypertension. Fortunately, these effects appear to be reversible upon cessation of ACE inhibition or ARB, and in many patients the beneficial effects of angiotensin II blockade to reduce BP can be achieved without precipitating further loss of kidney function.

Adrenal Cortex Hypertension

Aldosterone normally exerts nearly 90% of the mineralocorticoid activity of the adrenocortical secretions. However, cortisol can also provide a significant amount of mineralocorticoid activity in some conditions. Aldosterone's mineralocorticoid activity is about 3000 times greater than that of cortisol, but the plasma concentration of cortisol is nearly 2000 times that of aldosterone. Normally, the renal MR is protected from activation by cortisol by 11β-HSD2, which converts active cortisol into inactive cortisone. However, when activity of this enzyme is reduced or when cortisol levels are very high, the MR can be activated by cortisol.

Primary Aldosteronism (Conn Syndrome)

Primary aldosteronism, also called *Conn Syndrome*, results from hypersecretion of aldosterone in the absence of a known stimulus. The excess aldosterone secretion almost always comes from the adrenal cortex, and is usually associated with a solitary adenoma or bilateral hyperplasia of the adrenal cortex. *Secondary aldosteronism* refers to increased aldosterone secretion caused by a known stimulus, such as high levels of angiotensin II. This is the most common form of aldosteronism, and occurs in various conditions associated with increased renin secretion and angiotensin II formation, such as congestive heart failure, sodium depletion or renal artery stenosis.[116]

Primary aldosteronism can occur as a result of an aldosterone-producing adenoma (APA) or because of unilateral or bilateral adrenal hyperplasia.[117] The effects of excess aldosterone were discussed earlier, but the most important actions with regard to BP regulation are increased sodium reabsorption and increased potassium secretion by the renal tubules. This leads to extracellular fluid volume-expansion, hypertension, decreased renin secretion, hypokalemia, and metabolic alkalosis. Most of these effects are highly salt-sensitive, and low sodium intake can greatly attenuate the hypertension and hypokalemia.

Adrenal adenomas and bilateral adrenal hyperplasia account for more than 95% of primary aldosteronism. However, in most studies of unselected patients, the classic form of primary aldosteronism was found in less than 1% of hypertensive patients. Some adrenal glands in patients with primary aldosteronism may have varying degrees of hyperplasticity, and the term *idiopathic hyperaldosteronism* (IHA) was coined to describe this condition. Clinically, APA and IHA are difficult to distinguish, although patients with APA often have more severe hypertension and hypokalemia compared to those with IHA.

The measurement of the aldosterone–renin ratio has been used in an attempt to define more subtle cases of primary aldosteronism.[34,117] This approach has led to the suggestion that excess aldosterone secretion may account for as much as 5 to 10% of essential hypertension. However, there is still debate about whether patients with increased aldosterone–renin ratio truly have primary aldosteronism. In many of these patients, the main reason for the increased aldosterone–renin ratio is the low level of renin, rather than excess aldosterone secretion.[116]

"ESCAPE" FROM SODIUM RETENTION DURING HYPERALDOSTERONISM

Although aldosterone is a powerful sodium-retaining hormone, sodium excretion eventually returns to match sodium intake, even in patients with very high levels of aldosterone. This "escape" from sodium retention is secondary to increased extracellular fluid volume and pressure natriuresis.[118] Thus, after the extracellular fluid volume increases 5–15% above normal, BP also increases 15–25 mmHg, and the elevated BP returns the renal output of salt and water to normal, despite the excess aldosterone. The importance of pressure natriuresis in permitting aldosterone escape has been demonstrated experimentally by servo-controlling renal perfusion pressure; when renal perfusion pressure was servo-controlled, aldosterone infusion caused continued sodium retention and progressive increases in cumulative sodium balance and extracellular fluid volume, resulting in severe circulatory congestion and edema.[118] Failure of the kidneys to escape from aldosterone-induced sodium retention also occurs in patients with heart failure who, because of a severely weakened heart, cannot increase BP sufficiently to re-establish salt and water balance.

Cushing Syndrome Glucocorticoid Excess

Cushing syndrome is characterized by excess secretion of glucocorticoids, with hypertension occuring in approximately 80% of patients.[119] The hypertension with cortisol excess is often difficult to control, morbidity is substantial, and risk for death is largely a result of cardiovascular events, including heart attack and stroke.

Cushing syndrome can be caused by administration of excess cortisol (e.g., for treatment of various inflammatory disorders) or by oversecretion of endogenous cortisol. The most common cause of endogenous cortisol excess is overproduction of ACTH from a pituitary adenoma, a condition referred to as *Cushing disease*. The increased ACTH causes adrenal hyperplasia and stimulates cortisol secretion. Cushing disease can also occur as a result of ectopic secretion of ACTH by tumors outside the pituitary, such as an abdominal carcinoma.

ACTH-independent hypercortisolism can also occur as a result of adenomas of the adrenal cortex. Primary overproduction of cortisol by the adrenal glands, independent of ACTH, accounts for approximately 20–25% of Cushing syndrome, and is usually associated with suppressed ACTH caused by cortisol-induced feedback inhibition of ACTH secretion by the anterior pituitary gland. Administration of large doses of dexamethasone, a synthetic glucocorticoid, can distinguish between ACTH-dependent and ACTH-independent Cushing syndrome. In patients with overproduction of cortisol because of an ACTH-secreting pituitary adenoma or hypothalamic–pituitary dysfunction, even large doses of dexamethasone usually do not suppress ACTH secretion. In contrast, patients with primary adrenal overproduction of cortisol ACTH-independent usually have low or undetectable levels of ACTH. However, the dexamethasone test may occasionally give an incorrect diagnosis, because some ACTH-secreting pituitary tumors respond to dexamethasone with suppression of ACTH secretion.

Glucocorticoids modulate many cell processes, and the precise mechanisms by which hypercortisolism causes hypertension are incompletely-understood. One potential mechanism is activation of the MR; the high levels of cortisol in Cushing syndrome may simply overwhelm the ability of renal 11β-HSD2 to convert active cortisol into inactive cortisone at the MR receptor, so that cortisol stimulates the MR and causes sodium retention, volume-expansion, hypertension, and hypokalemia. High levels of cortisol may also increase the responsiveness to various pressor stimuli, including angiotensin II and norepinephrine.[120]

Studies in experimental animals suggest that excess cortisol may also raise BP through mechanisms that may be at least partially independent of activation of classical glucocorticoid receptor or MR.[120] Most of the available evidence, however, suggests that sodium retention may play a key role, although the precise mechanisms that lead to sodium retention are incompletely-understood.

Pheochromocytoma

Pheochromocytoma is a rare form of secondary hypertension occurring in approximately 0.05% of hypertensive patients.[116] Although rare, pheochromocytoma can provoke fatal hypertensive crises if unrecognized and untreated. Pheochromocytoma can arise from neuroectodermal chromaffin cells, which are part of the sympathoadrenal system. The chromaffin cells have the capacity to synthesize and store catecholamines, and are normally found mainly in the adrenal medulla. Although most chromaffin cell tumors are found in the adrenal medulla, as many as 15 to 30% may be extra-adrenal, located along the sympathetic chain or, rarely, in other sites.[116]

The symptoms and severity of hypertension associated with pheochromocytoma vary depending on the secretory pattern and amount of catecholamines released.[121] With tumors that continuously release large amounts of catecholamines, there may be sustained hypertension with few paroxysms or sudden bursts of very high BP. Tumors that are less active may have cyclical release of catecholamine stores that induce paroxysms of hypertension.

The clinical presentation also depends on whether the predominant catecholamine secreted is norepinephrine or epinephrine. Norepinephrine produces α-adrenergically-mediated vasoconstriction with diastolic hypertension, whereas epinephrine produces β-adrenergically-mediated systolic hypertension and tachycardia, along with sweating, tremors, and flushing. Patients with predominantly epinephrine-secreting tumors sometimes have hypertension alternating with hypotension, and approximately 5% of patients with pheochromocytoma remain normotensive.[116]

Pheochromocytoma patients often have decreased blood volume, consistent with the potent vasoconstrictor effects of norepinephrine. This observation, and the finding that chronic excess catecholamines often increase sodium excretion, could be interpreted as evidence that the hypertensive effects of catecholamines are unrelated to any impairment of renal function. However, the natriuretic effect of catecholamines and volume contraction appear to be secondary to peripheral vasoconstriction, decreased vascular capacitance, and increased BP, which causes pressure natriuresis.[10] Chronic intrarenal infusion of norepinephrine causes sodium retention and sustained hypertension, indicating important direct effects of catecholamines on the kidney to cause hypertension.

Although a high level of circulating catecholamine is the ultimate cause of hypertension in pheochromocytoma, BP is often only modestly correlated with the level of plasma catecholamines. However, the periodic burst of catecholamine release may cause moderate-to-severe hypertension, and lead to target organ injury. Consequently, diagnosis and effective treatment of pheochromocytoma are essential.

Pre-eclampsia

Pre-eclampsia occurs in approximately 5−7% of all pregnancies, with significantly higher rates in certain subpopulations. It remains one of the leading causes of maternal and fetal morbidity and mortality.[122,123] Disease manifestations, including hypertension, proteinuria, and edema, typically occur after 20 weeks of gestation.[69,123−126]

Pre-eclampsia is postulated to occur in two distinct phases: an early maternally asymptomatic phase in which abnormalities of vascular remodeling lead to placental insufficiency and hypoxia; and a later symptomatic phase characterized by widespread maternal endothelial dysfunction. The direct result of the failure to remodel the maternal arteries is that the placenta becomes severely hypoxic. In response, the placenta produces several factors that are released into the maternal circulation, and elicit many of the symptoms characteristic of pre-eclampsia. Several pathways which have been recently elucidated include altered angiogenic balance, increased maternal inflammation/immunological dysfunction, suppression of NO production, enhanced endothelin-1 production, and the creation of harmful ROS, as shown in Figure 39.15.

Multiple Placental Factors Cause Endothelial Dysfunction

One of the most intensely studied pathways activated by placental ischemia is abnormal circulating levels of pro-and antiangiogenic factors. Experimental reductions in vascular endothelial growth factor (VEGF), a protein necessary for the maintenance of endothelial cell health, result in hypertension, proteinuria, and glomerular endotheliosis, all common symptoms of pre-eclampsia.[123] In pre-eclampsia, VEGF and placental growth factor (PLGF) are antagonized by soluble fms-like tyrosine kinase-1 (sFlt-1), an inducible splice variant of the VEGF receptor flt-1 which binds to circulating VEGF and renders it unavailable for receptor binding.[123] Thus, sFlt-1 effectively acts as a competitive inhibitor of VEGF. In pre-eclamptic patients, circulating sFlt-1 levels increase significantly, sometimes well before pre-eclampsia symptoms develop. Furthermore, several models of experimental pre-eclampsia demonstrate elevated production of sFlt-1, and concomitant decreases in the amount of bioavailable VEGF.[123] Finally, administration of VEGF in these models has been shown to attenuate the associated hypertension.[123−126]

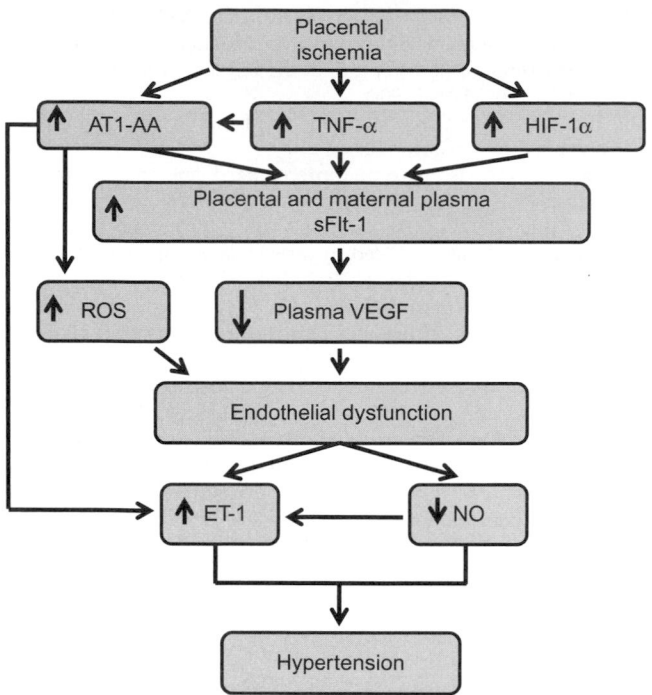

FIGURE 39.15 Mechanisms linking placental ischemia and hypertension during pre-eclampsia. (AT1-AA: angiotensin 1 receptor auto antibody; TNF-α: tumor necrosis factor-α; HIF-1α: hypoxia inducible factor-1α; ROS: reactive oxygen species; VEGF: vascular endothelial growth factor; sFlt-1: soluble fms-like tyrosine kinase-1; PlGF: placental growth factor; sEng: soluble endoglin; ET-1: endothelin-1; NO: nitric oxide.)

Another major pathway activated by the ischemic placenta is maternal inflammation. Even during normal pregnancy there is a heightened maternal inflammatory response. In pre-eclampsia, however, this seems to be exaggerated.[70] Inflammatory cytokines, such as IL-6 and TNF-α, are increased in pre-eclamptic women. Administration of either cytokine in pregnant rodents induces a gestational hypertension, similar to that seen in placental ischemia models. Administration of the soluble TNF-α receptor Etanercept in a rodent model of placental ischemia blunted the hypertension through ET-1 suppression, implicating TNF-α as an important link between placental ischemia and endothelial dysfunction.[70]

The maternal immune component of pre-eclampsia also includes circulating agonistic autoantibodies to the angiotensin type 1 receptor AT1-AA.[124] Besides its proposed role in the activation of the AT1 receptor, there appears to be a significant correlation between AT1-AA levels and the production of sFlt-1. Infusion of the purified antibody into pregnant rodents leads to gestational hypertension similar to that seen in placental ischemia models. This effect can be blocked by concurrent infusion of a synthetic heptapeptide which mimics the antibody's natural epitope on the AT1 receptor.[124]

Another important factor implicated in the characteristic maternal endothelial dysfunction associated with pre-eclampsia is elevated levels of the signaling peptide endothelin-1 ET-1.[126] The preponderance of published studies indicate that there is no significant increase in circulating endothelin in pre-eclamptic women compared to non-pregnant controls; however, local tissue levels of preproET-1 are elevated in women with pre-eclampsia.[126] One interesting aspect of ET-1 in pre-eclampsia is that increased vascular and renal ET-1 production have been shown to result from several independent mechanistic pathways, suggesting that it is a central connecting agent in the pathologies associated with these models.[126]

While an effective treatment for pre-eclampsia remains elusive, improved understanding of the mechanisms underlying the disease pathology offer new targets for intervention. Continued research into these molecular and physiological pathways should prove illuminating in the search for a treatment for pre-eclampsia.

Acknowledgments

Our research was supported by grants from the National Heart, Lung and Blood Institute. We thank Stephanie Lucas for expert assistance in preparing this chapter.

References

[1] Lloyd-Jones D, Adams R, Carnethon M, De SG, Ferguson TB, Flegal K, et al. Heart disease and stroke statistics—2009 update: a report from the American Heart Association Statistics Committee and Stroke Statistics Subcommittee. Circulation 2009;119: e21–181.

[2] Lawes CM, Vander HS, Rodgers A. Global burden of blood-pressure-related disease, 2001. Lancet 2008;371:1513–8.

[3] Lewington S, Clarke R, Qizilbash N, Peto R, Collins R. Age-specific relevance of usual blood pressure to vascular mortality: a meta-analysis of individual data for one million adults in 61 prospective studies. Lancet 2002;360:1903–13.

[4] Chobanian AV, Bakris GL, Black HR, Cushman WC, Green LA, Izzo Jr JL, et al. Seventh report of the joint national committee on prevention, detection, evaluation, and treatment of high blood pressure. Hypertension 2003;42:1206–52.

[5] Hall JE, Granger JP, Jones DW, Hall ME. Pathophysiology of hypertension. In: Fuster V, Walsh RA, Harrington RA, editors. Hurst's the heart. McGraw-Hill, Inc; 2011. p. 1549–84.

[6] Hall JE, Granger JP, do Carmo JM, da Silva AA, Dubinion J, George E, et al. Hypertension: physiology and pathophysiology. In: Pollock DM, Garvin JL, editors. Comprehensive physiology-renal physiology; 2012. [In Press].

[7] Guyton AC, Coleman TG, Granger HJ. Circulation: overall regulation. Annu Rev Physiol 1972;34:13–46.

[8] Hall JE, Mizelle HL, Woods LL, Montani JP. Pressure natriuresis and control of arterial pressure during chronic norepinephrine infusion. J Hypertens 1988;6:723–31.

[9] Guyton AC. Arterial pressure and hypertension. Circulatory physiology III. Philadelphia: WB Saunders; 1980.

[10] Hall JE. The kidney, hypertension, and obesity. Hypertension 2003;41:625–33.

[11] Hall JE. Renal function in one-kidney, one-clip hypertension and low renin essential hypertension. Am J Hypertens 1991;4:523S–33S.

[12] Hall JE, Guyton AC, Brands MW. Pressure–volume regulation in hypertension. Kidney Int Suppl 1996;55:S35–41.

[13] Hall JE, Granger JP. Regulation of fluid and electrolyte balance in hypertension: role of hormones and peptides. In: Battegay EJ, Lip GHY, Bakris GL, editors. Hypertension: principles and practice. Boca Raton: Taylor & Francis; 2005. p. 121–42.

[14] Norman Jr. RA, Galloway PG, Dzielak DJ, Huang M. Mechanisms of partial renal infarct hypertension. J Hypertens 1988;6:397–403.

[15] Lifton RP, Gharavi AG, Geller DS. Molecular mechanisms of human hypertension. Cell 2001;104:545–56.

[16] Hall JE. Control of sodium excretion by angiotensin II: intrarenal mechanisms and blood pressure regulation. Am J Physiol 1986;250:R960–72.

[17] Hall JE, Guyton AC, Smith Jr MJ, Coleman TG. Blood pressure and renal function during chronic changes in sodium intake: role of angiotensin. Am J Physiol 1980;239:F271–80.

[18] Campese VM. Salt sensitivity in hypertension. Renal and cardiovascular implications. Hypertension 1994;23:531–50.

[19] Weinberger MH, Fineberg NS, Fineberg SE, Weinberger M. Salt sensitivity, pulse pressure, and death in normal and hypertensive humans. Hypertension 2001;37:429–32.

[20] DiBona GF. Neural control of the kidney: past, present,and future. Hypertension 2003;41:621–4.

[21] Kassab S, Kato T, Wilkins FC, Chen R, Hall JE, Granger JP. Renal denervation attenuates the sodium retention and hypertension associated with obesity. Hypertension 1995;25:893–7.

[22] Esler M, Straznicky N, Eikelis N, Masuo K, Lambert G, Lambert E. Mechanisms of sympathetic activation in obesity-related hypertension. Hypertension 2006;48:787–96.

[23] DiBona GF, Esler M. Translational medicine: the antihypertensive effect of renal denervation. Am J Physiol Regul Integr Comp Physiol 2010;298:R245–53.

[24] Krum H, Sobotka P, Mahfoud F, Bohm M, Esler M, Schlaich M. Device-based antihypertensive therapy: therapeutic modulation of the autonomic nervous system. Circulation 2011;123:209–15.

[25] Cowley Jr AW. Long-term control of arterial blood pressure. Physiol Rev 1992;72:231–300.

[26] Lohmeier TE, Iliescu R. Chronic lowering of blood pressure by carotid baroreflex activation: mechanisms and potential for hypertension therapy. Hypertension 2011;57:880–6.

[27] Hall JE, Brands MW, Henegar JR. Angiotensin II and long-term arterial pressure regulation: the overriding dominance of the kidney. J Am Soc Nephrol 1999;10(Suppl. 12):S258–65.

[28] Brenner BM, Cooper ME, de ZD, Keane WF, Mitch WE, Parving HH, et al. Effects of losartan on renal and cardiovascular outcomes in patients with type 2 diabetes and nephropathy. N Engl J Med 2001;345:861–9.

[29] Lewis EJ, Hunsicker LG, Bain RP, Rohde RD. The effect of angiotensin-converting-enzyme inhibition on diabetic nephropathy. The collaborative study group. N Engl J Med 1993;329:1456–62.

[30] Griffin KA, Abu-Amarah I, Picken M, Bidani AK. Renoprotection by ACE inhibition or aldosterone blockade is blood pressure-dependent. Hypertension 2003;41:201–6.

[31] Eng E, Veniant M, Floege J, Fingerle J, Alpers CE, Menard J, et al. Renal proliferative and phenotypic changes in rats with two-kidney, one-clip Goldblatt hypertension. Am J Hypertens 1994;7:177–85.

[32] Crowley SD, Gurley SB, Herrera MJ, Ruiz P, Griffiths R, Kumar AP, et al. Angiotensin II causes hypertension and cardiac hypertrophy through its receptors in the kidney. Proc Natl Acad Sci USA 2006;103:17985–90.

[33] Fuller PJ, Young MJ. Mechanisms of mineralocorticoid action. Hypertension 2005;46:1227–35.

[34] Calhoun DA. Is there an unrecognized epidemic of primary aldosteronism? Pro. Hypertension 2007;50:447–53.

[35] de Paula RB, da Silva AA, Hall JE. Aldosterone antagonism attenuates obesity-induced hypertension and glomerular hyperfiltration. Hypertension 2004;43:41–7.

[36] Granger JP, Abram S, Stec D, Chandler D, LaMarca B. Endothelin, the kidney, and hypertension. Curr Hypertens Rep 2006;8:298–303.

[37] Kohan DE, Rossi NF, Inscho EW, Pollock DM. Regulation of blood pressure and salt homeostasis by endothelin. Physiol Rev 2011;91:1–77.

[38] Gariepy CE, Ohuchi T, Williams SC, Richardson JA, Yanagisawa M. Salt-sensitive hypertension in endothelin-B receptor-deficient rats. J Clin Invest 2000;105:925–33.

[39] Bagnall AJ, Kelland NF, Gulliver-Sloan F, Davenport AP, Gray GA, Yanagisawa M, et al. Deletion of endothelial cell endothelin B receptors does not affect blood pressure or sensitivity to salt. Hypertension 2006;48:286–93.

[40] Ge Y, Bagnall A, Stricklett PK, Strait K, Webb DJ, Kotelevtsev Y, et al. Collecting duct-specific knockout of the endothelin B receptor causes hypertension and sodium retention. Am J Physiol Renal Physiol 2006;291:F1274–80.

[41] Ge Y, Bagnall A, Stricklett PK, Webb D, Kotelevtsev Y, Kohan DE. Combined knockout of collecting duct endothelin A and B receptors causes hypertension and sodium retention. Am J Physiol Renal Physiol 2008;295:F1635–40.

[42] Kassab S, Miller MT, Novak J, Reckelhoff J, Clower B, Granger JP. Endothelin-A receptor antagonism attenuates the hypertension and renal injury in Dahl salt-sensitive rats. Hypertension 1998;31:397–402.

[43] Kassab S, Novak J, Miller T, Kirchner K, Granger J. Role of endothelin in mediating the attenuated renal hemodynamics in Dahl salt-sensitive hypertension. Hypertension 1997;30:682–6.

[44] Krum H, Viskoper RJ, Lacourciere Y, Budde M, Charlon V. The effect of an endothelin-receptor antagonist, bosentan, on blood pressure in patients with essential hypertension. Bosentan hypertension investigators. N Engl J Med 1998;338:784–90.

[45] Prasad VS, Palaniswamy C, Frishman WH. Endothelin as a clinical target in the treatment of systemic hypertension. Cardiol Rev 2009;17:181–91.

[46] Weber MA, Black H, Bakris G, Krum H, Linas S, Weiss R, et al. A selective endothelin-receptor antagonist to reduce blood pressure in patients with treatment-resistant hypertension: a randomised, double-blind, placebo-controlled trial. Lancet 2009;374:1423–31.

[47] Bakris GL, Lindholm LH, Black HR, Krum H, Linas S, Linseman JV, et al. Divergent results using clinic and ambulatory blood pressures: report of a darusentan-resistant hypertension trial. Hypertension 2010;56:824–30.

[48] Cowley Jr. AW, Mori T, Mattson D, Zou AP. Role of renal no production in the regulation of medullary blood flow. Am J Physiol Regul Integr Comp Physiol 2003;284:R1355–69.

[49] Granger JP, Alexander BT. Abnormal pressure-natriuresis in hypertension: role of nitric oxide. Acta Physiol Scand 2000;168:161–8.

[50] Schnackenberg C, Patel AR, Kirchner KA, Granger JP. Nitric oxide, the kidney and hypertension. Clin Exp Pharmacol Physiol 1997;24:600–6.

[51] O'Conner PM, Cowley Jr AW. Modulation of pressure-natriuresis by renal medullary reactive oxygen species and nitric oxide. Curr.Hypertens.Rep 2010;12:86—92.

[52] Baylis C. Nitric oxide deficiency in chronic kidney disease. Am J Physiol Renal Physiol 2008;294:F1—9.

[53] Rajapakse NW, Mattson DL. Role of L-arginine in nitric oxide production in health and hypertension. Clin Exp Pharmacol Physiol 2009;36:249—55.

[54] Chen PY, Sanders PW. L-arginine abrogates salt-sensitive hypertension in Dahl/Rapp rats. J Clin Invest 1991;88:1559—67.

[55] Boger RH. Asymmetric dimethylarginine ADMA and cardiovascular disease: insights from prospective clinical trials. Vasc Med 2005;10(Suppl. 1):S19—25.

[56] Matsuoka H, Itoh S, Kimoto M, Kohno K, Tamai O, Wada Y, et al. Asymmetrical dimethylarginine, an endogenous nitric oxide synthase inhibitor, in experimental hypertension. Hypertension 1997;29:242—7.

[57] Lassegue B, Griendling KK. NADPH oxidases: functions and pathologies in the vasculature. Arterioscler Thromb Vasc Biol 2010;30:653—61.

[58] Rodrigo R, Gonzalez J, Paoletto F. The role of oxidative stress in the pathophysiology of hypertension. Hypertens Res 2011;34:431—40.

[59] Taniyama Y, Griendling KK. Reactive oxygen species in the vasculature: molecular and cellular mechanisms. Hypertension 2003;42:1075—81.

[60] Cowley Jr AW. Renal medullary oxidative stress, pressure-natriuresis, and hypertension. Hypertension 2008;52:777—86.

[61] Garvin JL, Ortiz PA. The role of reactive oxygen species in the regulation of tubular function. Acta Physiol Scand 2003;179:225—32.

[62] Manning Jr. RD, Meng S, Tian N. Renal and vascular oxidative stress and salt-sensitivity of arterial pressure. Acta Physiol Scand 2003;179:243—50.

[63] Pechanova O, Simko F. Chronic antioxidant therapy fails to ameliorate hypertension: potential mechanisms behind. J Hypertens Suppl 2009;27:S32—6.

[64] Dikalov S, Griendling KK, Harrison DG. Measurement of reactive oxygen species in cardiovascular studies. Hypertension 2007;49:717—27.

[65] Chae CU, Lee RT, Rifai N, Ridker PM. Blood pressure and inflammation in apparently healthy men. Hypertension 2001;38:399—403.

[66] Dzielak DJ. Immune mechanisms in experimental and essential hypertension. Am J Physiol 1991;260:R459—67.

[67] Harrison DG, Guzik TJ, Goronzy J, Weyand C. Is hypertension an immunologic disease? Curr Cardiol Rep 2008;10:464—9.

[68] Harrison DG, Guzik TJ, Lob HE, Madhur MS, Marvar PJ, Thabet SR, et al. Inflammation, immunity, and hypertension. Hypertension 2011;57:132—40.

[69] LaMarca BD, Gilbert J, Granger JP. Recent progress toward the understanding of the pathophysiology of hypertension during preeclampsia. Hypertension 2008;51:982—8.

[70] LaMarca BD, Ryan MJ, Gilbert JS, Murphy SR, Granger JP. Inflammatory cytokines in the pathophysiology of hypertension during preeclampsia. Curr Hypertens Rep 2007;9:480—5.

[71] Lee DL, Sturgis LC, Labazi H, Osborne Jr JB, Fleming C, Pollock JS, et al. Angiotensin II hypertension is attenuated in interleukin-6 knockout mice. Am J Physiol Heart Circ Physiol 2006;290: H935—40.

[72] Guzik TJ, Hoch NE, Brown KA, McCann LA, Rahman A, Dikalov S, et al. Role of the T cell in the genesis of angiotensin II induced hypertension and vascular dysfunction. J Exp Med 2007;204:2449—60.

[73] Crowley SD, Song YS, Lin EE, Griffiths R, Kim HS, Ruiz P. Lymphocyte responses exacerbate angiotensin II-dependent hypertension. Am J Physiol Regul Integr Comp Physiol 2010;298:R1089—97.

[74] Cheng HF, RC. Harris. Cyclooxygenases, the kidney, and hypertension. Hypertension 2004;43:525—30.

[75] Grosser T, Fries S, FitzGerald GA. Biological basis for the cardiovascular consequences of COX-2 inhibition: therapeutic challenges and opportunities. J Clin Invest 2006;116:4—15.

[76] Snowden S, Nelson R. The effects of nonsteroidal anti-inflammatory drugs on blood pressure in hypertensive patients. Cardiol Rev 2011;19:184—91.

[77] Roman RJ. P-450 metabolites of arachidonic acid in the control of cardiovascular function. Physiol Rev 2002;82:131—85.

[78] Williams JM, Murphy S, Burke M, Roman RJ. 20-hydroxyeicosatetraeonic acid: a new target for the treatment of hypertension. J Cardiovasc Pharmacol 2010;56:336—44.

[79] Laffer CL, Laniado-Schwartzman M, Wang MH, Nasjletti A, Elijovich F. 20-HETE and furosemide-induced natriuresis in salt-sensitive essential hypertension. Hypertension 2003;41:703—8.

[80] Laffer CL, Laniado-Schwartzman M, Wang MH, Nasjletti A, Elijovich F. Differential regulation of natriuresis by 20-hydroxyeicosatetraenoic acid in human salt-sensitive versus salt-resistant hypertension. Circulation 2003;107:574—8.

[81] Melo LG, Steinhelper ME, Pang SC, Tse Y, Ackermann U. ANP in regulation of arterial pressure and fluid-electrolyte balance: lessons from genetic mouse models. Physiol Genomics 2000;3:45—58.

[82] Granger JP, Opgenorth TJ, Salazar J, Romero JC, Burnett Jr JC. Long-term hypotensive and renal effects of atrial natriuretic peptide. Hypertension 1986;8:II112—6.

[83] Melo LG, Veress AT, Chong CK, Pang SC, Flynn TG, Sonnenberg H. Salt-sensitive hypertension in ANP knockout mice: potential role of abnormal plasma renin activity. Am J Physiol 1998;274:R255—61.

[84] Whelton PK. Epidemiology of hypertension. Lancet 1994;344:101—6.

[85] Yach D, Stuckler D, Brownell KD. Epidemiologic and economic consequences of the global epidemics of obesity and diabetes. Nat Med 2006;12:62—6.

[86] Ogden CL, Carroll MD, Curtin LR, McDowell MA, Tabak CJ, Flegal KM. Prevalence of overweight and obesity in the United States, 1999—2004. JAMA 2006;295:1549—55.

[87] Garrison RJ, Kannel WB, Stokes III J, Castelli WP. Incidence and precursors of hypertension in young adults: the framingham offspring study. Prev Med 1987;16:235—51.

[88] Stevens VJ, Obarzanek E, Cook NR, Lee IM, Appel LJ, Smith WD, et al. Long-term weight loss and changes in blood pressure: results of the Trials of hypertension prevention, phase II. Ann Intern Med 2001;134:1—11.

[89] Hall JE, da Silva AA, do Carmo JM, Dubinion J, Hamza S, Munusamy S, et al. Obesity-induced hypertension: role of sympathetic nervous system, leptin, and melanocortins. J Biol Chem 2010;285:17271—6.

[90] Esler M. The sympathetic system and hypertension. Am J Hypertens 2000;13:99S—105S.

[91] Grassi G, Seravalle G, Cattaneo BM, Bolla GB, Lanfranchi A, Colombo M, et al. Sympathetic activation in obese normotensive subjects. Hypertension 1995;25:560—3.

[92] Rumantir MS, Vaz M, Jennings GL, Collier G, Kaye DM, Seals DR, et al. Neural mechanisms in human obesity-related hypertension. J Hypertens 1999;17:1125—33.

[93] Shek EW, Brands MW, Hall JE. Chronic leptin infusion increases arterial pressure. Hypertension 1998;31:409—14.

III. FLUID AND ELECTROLYTE REGULATION AND DYSREGULATION

[94] Ozata M, Ozdemir IC, Licinio J. Human leptin deficiency caused by a missense mutation: multiple endocrine defects, decreased sympathetic tone, and immune system dysfunction indicate new targets for leptin action, greater central than peripheral resistance to the effects of leptin, and spontaneous correction of leptin-mediated defects. J Clin Endocrinol Metab 1999;84:3686–95.

[95] do Carmo JM, da Silva AA, Cai Z, Lin S, Dubinion JH, Hall JE. Control of blood pressure, appetite, and glucose by leptin in mice lacking leptin receptors in proopiomelanocortin neurons. Hypertension 2011;57:918–26.

[96] Greenfield JR, Miller JW, Keogh JM, Henning E, Satterwhite JH, Cameron GS, et al. Modulation of blood pressure by central melanocortinergic pathways. N Engl J Med 2009;360:44–52.

[97] Hall JE, Crook ED, Jones DW, Wofford MR, Dubbert PM. Mechanisms of obesity-associated cardiovascular and renal disease. Am J Med Sci 2002;324:127–37.

[98] Lewis EJ, Hunsicker LG, Clarke WR, Berl T, Pohl MA, Lewis JB, et al. Renoprotective effect of the angiotensin-receptor antagonist irbesartan in patients with nephropathy due to type 2 diabetes. N Engl J Med 2001;345:851–60.

[99] Hall JE, Henegar JR, Dwyer TM, Liu J, da Silva AA, Kuo JJ, et al. Is obesity a major cause of chronic kidney disease? Adv Ren Replace Ther 2004;11:41–54.

[100] Hsu CY, McCulloch CE, Iribarren C, Darbinian J, Go AS. Body mass index and risk for end-stage renal disease. Ann Intern Med 2006;144:21–8.

[101] Praga M, Hernandez E, Herrero JC, Morales E, Revilla Y, Diaz-Gonzalez R, et al. Influence of obesity on the appearance of proteinuria and renal insufficiency after unilateral nephrectomy. Kidney Int 2000;58:2111–8.

[102] Bonnet F, Deprele C, Sassolas A, Moulin P, Alamartine E, Berthezene F, et al. Excessive body weight as a new independent risk factor for clinical and pathological progression in primary IgA nephritis. Am J Kidney Dis 2001;37:720–7.

[103] Hall JE, Jones DW, Henegar J, Dwyer TW, Kuo J. Obesity hypertension, and renal disease. In: Eckel RH, editor. Obesity: mechanisms and clinical management. Philadelphia: Lippincott, Williams & Wilkins; 2003. p. 273–300.

[104] Alberti KG, Eckel RH, Grundy SM, Zimmet PZ, Cleeman JI, Donato KA, et al. Harmonizing the metabolic syndrome: a joint interim statement of the International diabetes federation task force on epidemiology and prevention; national heart, lung, and blood institute; american heart association; world heart federation; international atherosclerosis society; and international association for the study of obesity. Circulation 2009;120:1640–5.

[105] Executive summary of the third report of the national cholesterol education program ncep expert panel on detection, evaluation, and treatment of high blood cholesterol in adults adult treatment panel III. JAMA 2001;285:2486–97.

[106] Kahn R, Buse J, Ferrannini E, Stern M. The metabolic syndrome: time for a critical appraisal—joint statement from the american diabetes association and the european association for the study of diabetes. Diabetes Care 2005;28:2289–304.

[107] Hall JE, Summers RL, Brands MW, Keen H, Alonso-Galicia M. Resistance to metabolic actions of insulin and its role in hypertension. Am J Hypertens 1994;7:772–88.

[108] Kurtz TW, Gardner DG. Transcription-modulating drugs: a new frontier in the treatment of essential hypertension. Hypertension 1998;32:380–6.

[109] Cui J, Hopper JL, Harrap SB. Genes and family environment explain correlations between blood pressure and body mass index. Hypertension 2002;40:7–12.

[110] Luft FC. Geneticism of essential hypertension. Hypertension 2004;43:1155–9.

[111] Kurtz TW. Genome-wide association studies will unlock the genetic basis of hypertension: con side of the argument. Hypertension 2010;56:1021–5.

[112] Garovic VD, Hilliard AA, Turner ST. Monogenic forms of low-renin hypertension. Nat Clin Pract Nephrol 2006;2:624–30.

[113] McCormick JA, Ellison DH. The WNKs: atypical protein kinases with pleiotropic actions. Physiol Rev 2011;91:177–219.

[114] Garovic VD, Textor SC. Renovascular hypertension and ischemic nephropathy. Circulation 2005;112:1362–74.

[115] Bianchi G, Tenconi LT, Lucca R. Effect in the conscious dog of constriction of the renal artery to a sole remaining kidney on haemodynamics, sodium balance, body fluid volumes, plasma renin concentration and pressor responsiveness to angiotensin. Clin Sci 1970;38:741–66.

[116] Kaplan NM. Clinical hypertension. Philadelphia: Lippincott, William & Wilkins; 2002, p. 89–92.

[117] Young Jr WF. Minireview: primary aldosteronism—changing concepts in diagnosis and treatment. Endocrinology 2003;144:2208–13.

[118] Hall JE, Granger JP, Smith Jr MJ, Premen AJ. Role of renal hemodynamics and arterial pressure in aldosterone "escape". Hypertension 1984;6:I183–92.

[119] Fallo F, Paoletta A, Tona F, Boscaro M, Sonino N. Response of hypertension to conventional antihypertensive treatment and/or steroidogenesis inhibitors in Cushing's syndrome. J Intern Med 1993;234:595–8.

[120] Whitworth JA, Mangos GJ, Kelly JJ. Cushing, cortisol, and cardiovascular disease. Hypertension 2000;36:912–6.

[121] Goldstein DS, Eisenhofer G, Flynn JA, Wand G, Pacak K. Diagnosis and localization of pheochromocytoma. Hypertension 2004;43:907–10.

[122] Ilekis JV, Reddy UM, Roberts JM. Preeclampsia—a pressing problem: an executive summary of a National Institute of Child Health and Human Development workshop. Reprod Sci 2007;14:508–23.

[123] Powe CE, Levine RJ, Karumanchi SA. Preeclampsia, a disease of the maternal endothelium: the role of antiangiogenic factors and implications for later cardiovascular disease. Circulation 2011;123:2856–69.

[124] George EM, Granger JP. Recent insights into the pathophysiology of preeclampsia. Expert Rev Obstet Gynecol 2010;5:557–66.

[125] George EM, Granger JP. Mechanisms and potential therapies for preeclampsia. Curr Hypertens Rep 2011;13:269–75.

[126] George EM, Palei AC, Granger JP. Endothelin as a final common pathway in the pathophysiology of preeclampsia: therapeutic implications. Curr Opin Nephrol Hypertens 2012;21:157–62.

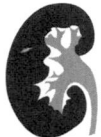

Physiology and Pathophysiology of Diuretic Action

David H. Ellison

Oregon Health & Science University & VA Medical Center, Portland, OR, USA

INTRODUCTION

The term *diuretic* derives from the Greek *diouretikos*, meaning "to promote urine." Although infusion of saline or ingestion of water would therefore qualify as being diuretic, the term *diuretic* usually connotes a drug that can reduce the extracellular fluid (ECF) volume by increasing urinary solute or water excretion. The term aquaretic has sometimes been applied to drugs that increase excretion of solute free water, distinguishing them from traditional diuretics, which increase solute and water together. The clinical picture of ECF volume expansion leading to edema or "dropsy" (from the Latin, *hydrops*) has been recognized since the earliest days of recorded history. Ancient Egyptians referred to "flooding of the heart," and the Hippocratic Corpus later suggested specific remedies for dropsical patients, although their results are not noted. In 1553, Paracelsus recorded the first truly effective form of therapy for dropsy, inorganic mercury (Calomel). Inorganic mercury remained the mainstay of diuretic treatment until the beginning of this century.

In 1919, the ability of organic mercurial antisyphilitics to effect diuresis was discovered by Vogl, then a medical student. This observation led to the development of effective organic mercurial diuretics, drugs that were used commonly until the 1960s. In 1937, the antimicrobial, sulfanilamide, was found to cause metabolic acidosis in patients. Carbonic anhydrase had been discovered in 1932; it was know that sulfanilamide inhibited this enzyme. Pitts demonstrated that sulfanilamide inhibited Na bicarbonate reabsorption in dogs, and Schwartz showed that sulfanilamide could induce diuresis in patients with congestive heart failure who were resistant to organic mercurial diuretics. Soon, more potent sulfonamide-based carbonic anhydrase inhibitors were developed, but these drugs suffered from side-effects and limited potency. Nevertheless, a group at Sharp & Dohme Inc. was stimulated by these developments to explore the possibility that modification of sulfonamide-based drugs could lead to drugs that enhanced Na *chloride* rather than Na *bicarbonate* excretion. The result of this program was the synthesis of chlorothiazide and its marketing in 1957. This drug ushered in the modern era of diuretic therapy, and revolutionized the clinical treatment of edema.

The search for more potent classes of diuretics continued, based on the structure of chlorothiazide and sulonamyl derivatives. This led to the development of ethacrynic acid and furosemide in the United States and Germany, respectively. The safety and efficacy of these drugs led them to replace the organic mercurials as drugs of first choice for severe and resistant edema. Spironolactone, marketed in 1961, was developed after the properties and structure of aldosterone had been established, and steroidal analogs of aldosterone were found to have aldosterone-blocking activity. Triamterene was initially synthesized as a folic acid antagonist, but was found to have diuretic and K-sparing activity.

The availability of safe, effective, and relatively inexpensive diuretic drugs has made it possible to treat edematous disorders and hypertension effectively. Driven by clinical need, however, the development of effective diuretic drugs generated specific ligands that interact with Na and Cl transport proteins in the kidney. In the 1990s, these ligands were used to identify and clone the Na and Cl transport proteins that mediate the bulk of renal Na and Cl reabsorption.

Seldin and Giebisch's The Kidney, Fifth Edition.
DOI: http://dx.doi.org/10.1016/B978-0-12-381462-3.00040-9

The diuretic-sensitive transport proteins that have been cloned include the sodium hydrogen exchanger (NHE) family of proteins, the bumetanide-sensitive Na-K-2Cl co-transporters, the thiazide-sensitive Na-Cl co-transporter, and the epithelial Na channel. The information derived from molecular cloning has also permitted identification of inherited human diseases that are caused by mutations in these transport proteins. The phenotypes of several of these disorders resemble the manifestations of chronic diuretic administration. The recognition, for example, that Gitelman's syndrome results from mutation of the thiazide-sensitive Na-Cl co-transporter, has spurred interest in determining how blockade or dysfunction of this transport protein leads to magnesium-wasting. Thus, the development of clinically useful diuretics permitted identification, and later cloning, of specific ion transport pathways. The molecular cloning then helped to define mechanisms of diuretic action and diuretic side-effects, permitting the development of specific antibodies and probes, and of animals in which diuretic-sensitive transport pathways have been "knocked-out." Many primarily historical references included in prior editions of this book have been omitted here. The interested reader is referred to prior editions for more complete references and details.[1]

Diuretic-Sensitive Salt Transport

In a normal human kidney, approximately 23 moles of NaCl are filtered in 150 liters of fluid each day. Approximately 6−10 grams of salt (102−170 mEq NaCl) are consumed each day by individuals on a typical Western diet. To maintain balance, renal NaCl excretion must be approximately 92−160 mmol/day (the difference owing to nonrenal losses). Such calculations imply that 99.2% of the filtered NaCl load is reabsorbed by kidney tubules each day (the fractional sodium excretion, FE_{Na}, is 0.8%). Sodium, chloride, and water reabsorption along the nephron is driven by the metabolic energy in ATP. The ouabain-sensitive Na/K-ATPase is expressed at the basolateral cell membrane of nearly all Na transporting epithelial cells along the nephron. This pump maintains large ion gradients across the plasma membrane, with the intracellular Na concentration maintained low and the intracellular K concentration maintained high. Because the pump is electrogenic, and because it is associated with a K channel, renal epithelial cells have a voltage across the plasma membrane oriented with the inside negative relative to the outside.

The combination of the low intracellular Na concentration and the plasma membrane voltage generates a large electrochemical gradient favoring Na entry from lumen or interstitium. Specific diuretic-sensitive Na transport pathways are expressed at the apical surface of cells along the nephron, permitting vectorial transport of Na from lumen to blood (see Figure 40.1). Along the proximal tubule, where approximately two-thirds of filtered Na is reabsorbed, a major component of Na reabsorption is exchanged for H^+ via an isoform of the Na/H exchanger (NHE3) at the apical membrane. Along the thick ascending limb, where approximately 20−25% of filtered Na is reabsorbed, an isoform of the Na-K-2Cl co-transporter (NKCC2) is expressed at the apical membrane. Along the distal convoluted tubule (DCT), where approximately 5% of filtered Na is reabsorbed, the thiazide-sensitive Na-Cl co-transporter (NCC) is expressed. The DCT comprises two subsegments, the DCT1 (or "early DCT") and the DCT2 (or "late DCT"). Along the DCT1, the NCC is the predominant Na transporter. Along the connecting tubule and cortical collecting duct, where approximately 3% of filtered Na is reabsorbed, isoforms of the amiloride-sensitive epithelial Na channel are expressed (ENaC). DCT2 cells express both NCC and ENaC. Together, these apical Na transport pathways along the nephron form the molecular targets for diuretic action.

This chapter will discuss the physiological and pharmacological bases for diuretic action in the kidney. Although some aspects of clinical diuretic usage will be discussed, we have emphasized physiological principles and mechanisms of action. Several recent texts provide detailed discussions of diuretic treatment of clinical conditions.[2] Extensive discussions of diuretic pharmacokinetics are also available.[3] The influence of renal disease on diuretic drug usage is discussed in the following chapter of this volume.

One classification of diuretic drugs is based on the primary nephron site of action. Such a scheme emphasizes that drugs of more than one chemical class can affect the same ion transport mechanism. Although most diuretic drugs have actions on more than one nephron segment, most owe their clinical effects primarily to their ability to inhibit Na transport by one particular nephron segment. An exception is the osmotic diuretics. Although these drugs were initially believed to inhibit solute and water flux primarily along the proximal tubule, subsequent studies have revealed effects in multiple segments. Other diuretics, however, will be classified according to their primary site of action.

OSMOTIC DIURETICS

Osmotic diuretics are substances that are freely filtered at the glomerulus, but are poorly reabsorbed (see Figure 40.2). The pharmacological activity of drugs in

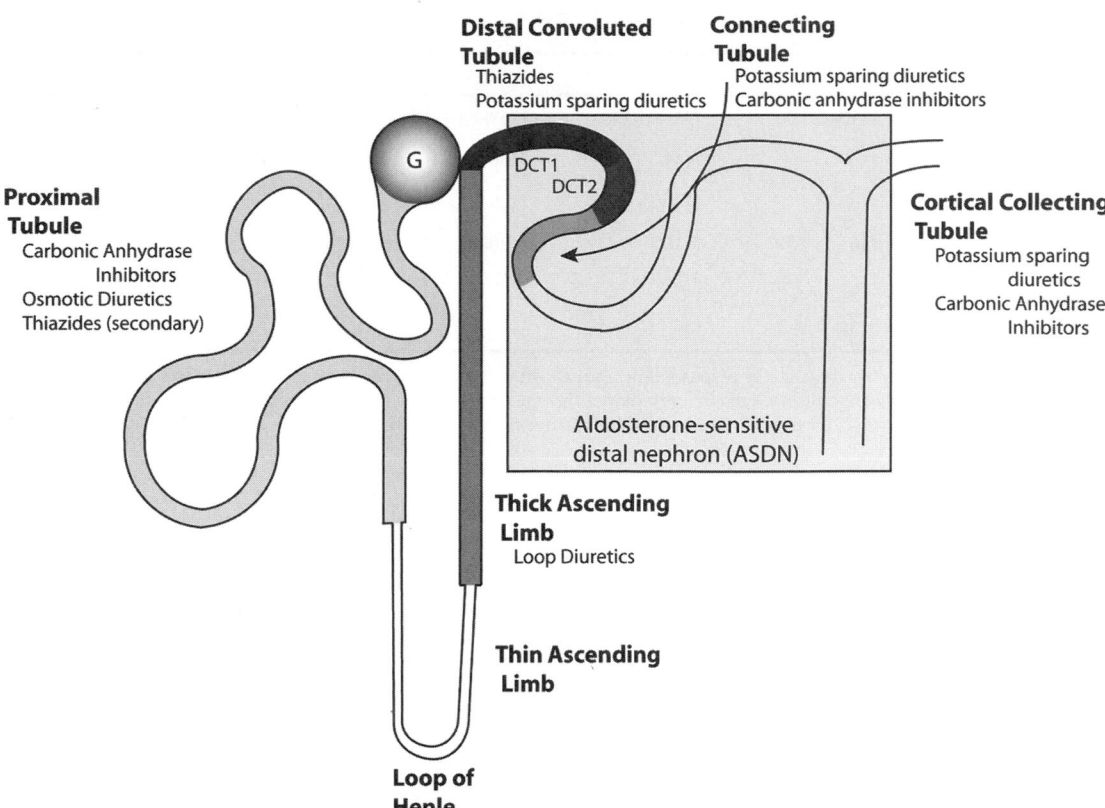

FIGURE 40.1 Sites of diuretic action along the nephron. Carbonic anhydrase inhibitors reduce Na reabsorption along the proximal tubule (light gray). Loop diuretics inhibit Na and Cl transport along the thick ascending limb of the Loop of Henle (medium gray). Distal convoluted tubule diuretics (thiazides and others) inhibit Na and Cl transport primarily along the distal convoluted tubule (DCT1 and the DCT2, as shown), with a secondary effect along the collecting duct, under some conditions. Potassium-sparing diuretics inhibit electrogenic Na transport along the aldosterone-sensitive distal nephron, which is indicated by the gray box.

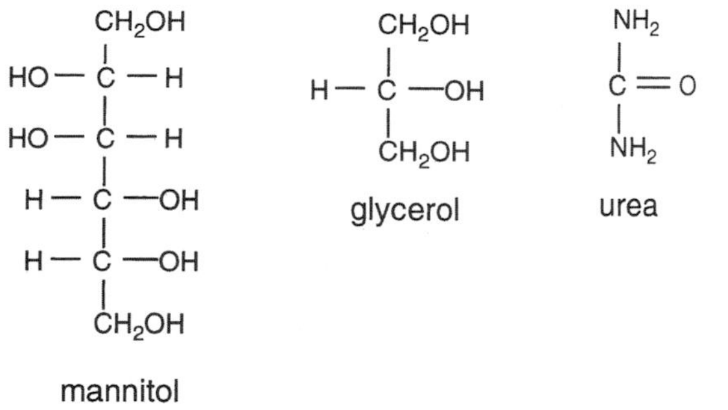

FIGURE 40.2 Structures of osmotic diuretics.

this group depends entirely on the osmotic pressure exerted by the drug molecules in solution, and not on interaction with specific transport proteins or enzymes. Mannitol is the prototypical osmotic diuretic. Its diuretic effect is not due to interactions with receptors or renal transporters, but rather it is due to more complex mechanisms that involve osmotic effects on tubule epithelium and reduction of the medullary interstitial osmolality. Because the relationship between the

magnitude of effect and concentration of osmotic diuretic in solution is linear, all agents used clinically are small molecules. Other agents considered in this class include urea, sorbitol, and glycerol.

Urinary Electrolyte Excretion

Although osmotic agents do not act directly on transport pathways, the rate of transport of ions is affected. Following the infusion of mannitol, the excretion of sodium, potassium, calcium, magnesium, bicarbonate, and chloride is increased (see Table 40.1). The fractional reabsorption rates for sodium and water are reduced substantially following the infusion of mannitol. Reabsorption of magnesium and calcium are also reduced in the proximal tubule and loop of Henle, and phosphate reabsorption is inhibited slightly along the proximal tubule. In addition to increasing electrolyte excretion, mannitol infusion increases cortical and medullary blood flow, and has a variable effect on GFR. The most pronounced effect observed with mannitol is a brisk diuresis and natriuresis.

TABLE 40.1 Effects of Diuretics on Electrolyte Excretion

	Na	Cl	K	Pi	Ca	Mg
Osmotic diuretics	↑(10–25%)	↑(15–30%)	↑(6%)	↑(5–10%)	↑(10–20%)	↑(>20%)
Carbonic anhydrase inhibitors	↑(6%)	↑(4%)	↑(60%)	↑(>20%)	↑ or ⇔ (<5%)	↑(<5%)
Loop diuretics	↑(30%)	↑(40%)	↑(60–100%)	↑(>20%)	↑(>20%)	↑(>20%)
DCT diuretics	↑(6–11%)	↑(10%)	↑(200%)	↑(>20%)	↓	↑(5–10%)
Na channel blockers	↑(3–5%)	↑(6%)	↓(8%)	⇔	⇔	↓
Spironolactone	↑(3%)	↑(6%)	↓	⇔	⇔	↓

Figures indicate approximate maximal fractional excretions of ions following acute diuretic administration in maximally effective doses. ↑ indicates that the drug increases excretion; ↓ indicates that the drug decreases excretion; ⇔ indicates that the drug has little or no direct effect on excretion. During chronic treatment, effects often wane (Na excretion), may increase (K excretion during DCT diuretic treatment) or may reverse as with uric acid (not shown). For references that support this table, please see[1].

Mechanism of Action

The mechanisms by which mannitol produces a diuresis are thought to be secondary to: (1) an increase in osmotic pressure in the proximal tubule fluid and loop of Henle, thereby retarding the passive reabsorption of water; and (2) an increase in renal blood flow and washout of the medullary tonicity.

Mannitol is freely filtered at the glomerulus, and its presence in the tubule fluid minimizes passive water reabsorption primarily by the proximal tubule and by the thin limbs of the loop of Henle. Normally, within the proximal tubule, sodium reabsorption creates an osmotic gradient for water reabsorption. When an osmotic diuretic is administered, however, the osmotic force of the nonreabsorbable solute in the lumen opposes the osmotic force produced by sodium reabsorption. Isoosmolality of the tubule fluid is preserved, because molecules of mannitol replace sodium ions reabsorbed. Sodium reabsorption eventually stops, however, because the luminal sodium concentration is reduced to a point where a limiting gradient is reached. Surprisingly, mincropuncture experiments showed that mannitol has a greater effect on inhibiting Na and water reabsorption in the loop of Henle than in the proximal tubule. Within the loop of Henle the site of action of mannitol appears to be restricted to the thin descending limb, resulting in a decrease in reabsorption of Na and water. In the thick ascending limb, reabsorption of Na will continue in proportion to its delivery to this segment. The sum of net transport in the thin and thick limbs will determine the net effect of mannitol in the loop of Henle. Further downstream in the collecting duct, mannitol also reduces sodium and water reabsorption.

Renal Hemodynamics

During the administration of mannitol, its molecules diffuse from the bloodstream into the interstitial space.

In the interstitial space, the increased osmotic pressure draws water from the cells to increase ECF volume. This effect increases total renal plasma flow. Cortical blood flow and medullary blood flow are both increased following mannitol infusion. Single nephron GFR, on the other hand, increases in the cortex and decreases in the medulla, this action on the medulla washes out the medullary osmotic gradient by reducing papillary sodium and urea content. The mechanisms that contribute to the increase in renal blood flow include a decrease in hematocrit and blood viscosity, and the release of vasoactive agents. Experimental studies indicate that the osmotic effect of mannitol to increase water movement from intracellular to extracellular space leads to a decrease in hematocrit and in blood viscosity. This fact contributes to a decrease in renal vascular resistance and increase in renal blood flow. Both prostacyclin (PGI_2) synthesis and atrial natriuretic peptide could mediate the effect of mannitol on renal blood flow. The vasodilatory effect of mannitol is reduced when the recipient is pretreated with indomethacin or meclofenamate, suggesting that PGI_2 is involved in the vasodilatory effect.

The effect of mannitol on GFR has been variable, but most studies indicate that the overall effect of mannitol is to increase GFR.[4] Whereas mannitol increased cortical and medullary blood flow, it increased cortical but decreased medullary single nephron GFR. The mechanisms by which mannitol reduces the GFR of deep nephrons are not known, but it has been postulated that mannitol reduces efferent arteriolar pressure. Micropuncture studies examining the determinants of GFR in superficial nephrons have demonstrated that the increase in single nephron GFR is owing to an increase in single nephron plasma flow, and a decrease in oncotic pressure. Alterations in renal hemodynamics contribute to the diuresis observed following administration of mannitol. An increase in medullary blood flow rate reduces medullary tonicity primarily by decreasing papillary sodium and urea content, and increasing urine flow rate.

Pharmacokinetics

Mannitol is not readily absorbed from the intestine;[4] therefore it is routinely administered intravenously. Following infusion, mannitol distributes in ECF with a volume of distribution of approximately 16 liters; its excretion is almost entirely by glomerular filtration.[5] Of the filtered load, less than 10% is reabsorbed by the renal tubule, and a similar quantity is metabolized, probably in the liver. With normal GFR, plasma half-life is approximately 2.2 hours.

Clinical Use

Mannitol is often used prophylactically to help prevent acute kidney injury (AKI) in the setting of rhabdomyolysis,[4] although some controlled studies have not confirmed benefit.[6] It was previously used for prophylaxis from contrast-induced nephropathy, but appears of no benefit here, and is of potential harm.[7] In the past, it was also used to treat established AKI, but its use here has also fallen from favor, as convincing evidence of benefit has been lacking.

Mannitol is used for short-term reduction of intraocular pressure. By increasing the osmotic pressure, mannitol reduces the volume of aqueous humor and the intraocular pressure by extracting water. Mannitol also decreases cerebral edema and the increase in intracranial pressure associated with trauma, tumors, and neurosurgical procedures, where its benefits are most clearly established.[8] Mannitol is used perioperatively in patients undergoing cardiopulmonary bypass surgery. The beneficial effects may be related to its osmotic activity reducing intravenous fluid requirement,[9] and its ability to act as a free radical antioxidant.[10] Mannitol and other osmotic agents have been used in the treatment of dialysis disequilibrium syndrome.[11,12] This syndrome is characterized acute symptoms immediately following hemodialysis. Most significant symptoms are attributable to disorders of the central nervous system, such as headache, nausea, blurred vision, confusion, seizure, coma, and death. Rapid removal of small solutes such as urea during dialysis of patients who are markedly azotemic is associated with the development of an osmotic gradient for water movement into brain cells producing cerebral edema and neurologic dysfunction. Dialysis disequilibrium syndrome can be minimized by slow solute removal and raising plasma osmolality with saline or mannitol.

Adverse Effects

In patients with reduced cardiac output, an increase in extracellular volume induced by mannitol infusion may lead to pulmonary edema. Intravenous administration of mannitol increases cardiac output and pulmonary capillary wedge pressures. Acute and prolonged administration of mannitol leads to different electrolyte disturbances. Acute overzealous use or the accumulation of mannitol leads to dilutional metabolic acidosis and hyponatremia. Accumulation of mannitol also produces hyperkalemia, as a result of an increase in plasma osmolality. An increase in plasma osmolality increases potassium movement from intracellular to extracellular fluid from bulk solute flow, and increases the electrochemical gradient for potassium secretion. Prolonged administration of mannitol can lead to urinary losses of sodium and potassium, leading to volume-depletion, hypernatremia (as urinary loss of sodium is invariably less than water), and hypokalemia. Marked accumulation of mannitol in patients can lead to reversible AKI that appears to be due to vasoconstriction and tubular vacuolization. Mannitol-induced AKI usually occurs when large cumulative doses of $\sim 295\,g$ are given to patients with previously compromised renal function.[6]

PROXIMAL TUBULE DIURETICS

(Carbonic Anhydrase Inhibitors)

Through the development of carbonic anhydrase inhibitors, important compounds were discovered that have utility as therapeutic agents, and as research tools. Carbonic anhydrase inhibitors (CAI) have a limited therapeutic role as diuretic agents, because of weak natriuretic properties. They are used primarily to reduce intraocular pressure in glaucoma, and to enhance bicarbonate excretion in metabolic alkalosis. CAIs have been useful in the development of other diuretic agents, such as thiazide and loop diuretics, and have been instrumental in elucidating transport function in proximal and distal nephron segments. Structures of carbonic anhydrase inhibitors are shown in Figure 40.3.

Urinary Electrolyte Excretion

Through their effects on carbonic anhydrase in the proximal tubule, CAIs increase bicarbonate excretion by 25–30% (see Table 40.1). Chronic CAI administration, however, causes only a modest natriuresis, despite the magnitude of carbonic anhydrase-dependent proximal Na reabsorption. Several factors account for this. First, carbonic anhydrase is required for reabsorption of HCO_3^-, whereas about two thirds of the proximal Na^+ reabsorption is accompanied by Cl^-. Second, some proximal HCO_3^- reabsorption persists

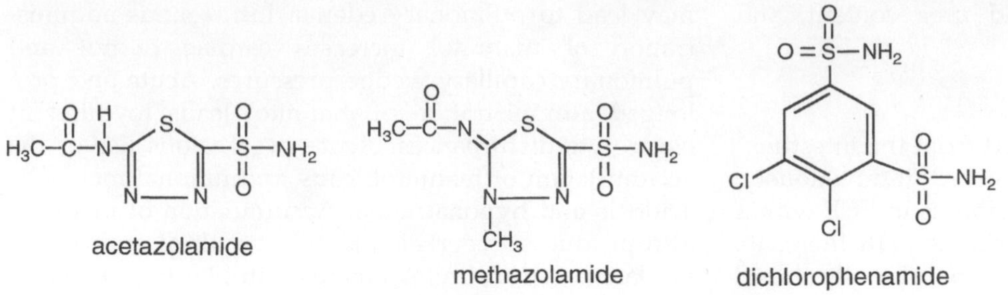

FIGURE 40.3 Structures of carbonic anhydrase inhibitors.

even after apparently full inhibition of carbonic anhydrase. Third, some of the HCO_3^- that is delivered from the proximal tubule can be reabsorbed at more distal sites. Fourth, the metabolic acidosis that develops limits the filtered load to HCO_3^-, and thereby curtails the natriuresis. Fifth, the increased delivery of filtered Na^+ to the macula densa elicits a tubuloglomerular feedback (TGF)-induced reduction in the GFR. Micropuncture studies of mice with deletion of the proximal Na^+/H^+ exchanger, NHE3, also show that inhibition of proximal Na reabsorption is largely balanced by reduced GFR,[13] suggesting that the reduction of GFR with CAI use contributes importantly to limiting their natriuretic potency.

The effecs of CAI on calcium excretion are complex. Proximal tubule calcium and phosphate reabsorption are inhibited by acetazolamide, partly because sodium and calcium reabsorption are closely linked within this segment.[14] Yet fractional calcium excretion is often unchanged or reduced, because distal calcium reabsorption is stimulated[15] and because luminal bicarbonate promotes calcium reabsorption. Over the longer-term, however, CAI can increase urinary calcium excretion and predispose to nephrocalcinosis and kidney stone formation.[16] In contrast, phosphate appears to escape distal reabsorption following acetazolamide administration, resulting in an increase in fractional excretion of phosphate by $\sim 3\%$.[17] Although proximal tubule magnesium transport is inhibited by CAI, fractional excretion is either unchanged or is increased as a result of variable distal reabsorption.[17]

Acetazolamide increases potassium excretion.[17] Although a direct effect of acetazolamide has not been established, it is likely that several indirect effects could contribute to the observed kaliuresis. Carbonic anhydrase inhibition could block proximal tubule potassium reabsorption and increase delivery to the distal tubule, but the reported effects of carbonic anhydrase inhibition on proximal tubule transport have been conflicting. Whereas CAI decreases proximal tubule sodium, bicarbonate, and water absorption during both free flow micropuncture and microperfusion, the effects of CAI on *proximal* tubule potassium transport have been less consistent. In free flow

micropuncture studies, carbonic anhydrase inhibition did not affect proximal tubule potassium reabsorption, whereas net potassium transport was reduced during proximal perfusion *in vivo*.[18] The effect of acetazolamide on the proximal tubule ion transport does, however, facilitate an increase in tubular fluid flow rate and delivery to the distal nephron of sodium bicarbonate. This effect is thought to increase the concentration of nonreabsorbable anions, creating an increase in lumen-negative voltage and an increase in flow rate,[19] factors known to increase potassium secretion by the distal tubule.

Most diuretics have some CAI action.[20] This contributes to the weak inhibition of proximal reabsorption by furosemide and chlorothiazide, and to the relaxation of vascular smooth muscle cells by high-dose furosemide Goldfarb diuretics.[20]

Mechanism of Action

In the kidney, CAI likely acts via three distinct, but related mechanisms (see Figure 40.4). First, they inhibit the hydration of CO_2 within cells, thereby reducing the generation of substrate for H^+ and HCO_3^- transporters; second, they reduce the dehydration of carbonic acid to CO_2 and H_2O in the luminal compartment, thereby inhibiting continued H^+ secretion; finally, intracellular CA appears to associate with several membrane transport proteins, and may affect their activity more directly. These actions take place along the nephron, but actions along the proximal tubule and collecting duct are especially important. The biochemical, morphological, and functional properties of carbonic anhydrase have been reviewed previously.[21] Carbonic anhydrase (CA), a metalloenzyme containing one zinc atom per molecule, is important in sodium bicarbonate reabsorption and hydrogen ion secretion by renal epithelial cells.

CA is expressed by many tissues, including erythrocytes, kidney, gut, ciliary body, choroid plexus, and glial cells. Although at least 15 isoforms of CA have been identified,[21] two play predominant roles in renal acid−base homeostasis: CAII and CAIV. CAII is widely expressed, comprising the enzyme expressed by red blood cells and a variety of secretory and absorptive

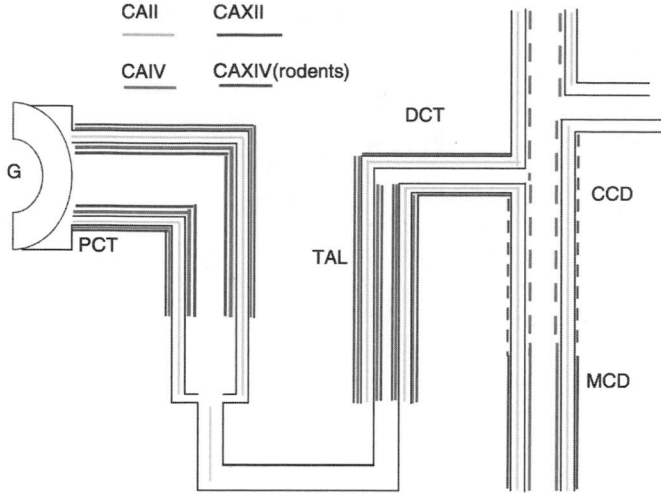

FIGURE 40.4 Localization of CA isoforms along the nephron. CAII (yellow stripe) is expressed within the cytoplasm of virtually all nephron segments with the exception of the loop of Henle and the thin ascending limb. CAIV (green stripe) is both apically and basolaterally expressed in the S1 and S2 segments of the proximal tubule and the thick ascending limb. In the distal nephron CAIV is expressed exclusively on the luminal (apical) surface of a-intercalated cells of the CCD and acid secreting cells of the medullary collecting duct. CAXII (blue stripe) is found on the basolateral membrane of S1and S2 segments of the proximal tubule and the thick ascending limb. In the distal nephron, CAXII is located in distal convoluted tubules, principal cells of the CCD, and the medullary collecting duct of some species. In rodent species CAXIV is expressed on the luminal surface of cells in the S1 and S2 segments of the proximal tubule and the thick ascending limb. *(Figure 40 from ref. [21], with permission.)* See color section at the back of the book.

epithelia. In the kidney, CAII is a cytoplasmic protein expressed, comprising 95% of renal CA.[21] It is present in proximal tubule cells and intercalated cells of the aldosterone-sensitive distal nephron (ASDN)[21](see Figure 40.4). In rodents, carbonic anhydrase XIV is expressed at the luminal border of the cells of the proximal tubule, thick ascending limb (TAL) of the loop of Henle, and α-intercalated cells of the ASDN,[22] but its role in other species is not as clear.[21]

Carbonic anhydrase (CA) catalyzes the reversible hydration of CO_2 according to the reaction:

$$H^+ + HCO_2^- \leftrightarrow H_2CO_2 \leftrightarrow CO_2 + H^+$$

CO_2 gas dissolves in water and is in equilibrium with the acid H_2CO_3. The Henderson—Hasselbalch equation relates pH, HCO_3^- concentration, and partial pressure of CO_2 gas in physiologic solutions:

$$pH = 6.1 + \log_{10}\frac{(HCO_3^-)}{0.03 \times pCO_2}$$

The uncatalyzed hydration of CO_2 is relatively slow, whereas the turnover number for CAII is in the order of $10^6\ s^{-1}$.

Type IV carbonic anhydrase is bound to renal cortical membranes, comprising up to 5% of the overall activity in kidney, and is sensitive to sulfonamides.[23,24] Type IV carbonic anhydrase, expressed on basolateral and luminal plasma membranes of proximal tubule cells and luminal membrane of intercalated cells,[25] catalyzes the dehydration of intraluminal carbonic acid generated from secreted protons.

Evidence for the physiological importance of carbonic anhydrase is apparent, as a deficiency of CAII leads to a renal acidification defect resulting in renal tubular acidosis.[26] Furthermore, metabolic acidosis leads to an adaptive increase in both CAII and CAIV mRNA expression in kidney,[27] suggesting the importance of both carbonic anhydrase isoforms in this disorder.

Carbonic anhydrase, which is associated with the brush border, prevents H^+ from accumulating in tubule fluid, and secondarily permits the continued secretion of H^+ (see Figure 40.5). Carbon dioxide rapidly diffuses from the lumen into the cell across the apical membrane. Within the cell, H is secreted into the tubule lumen via Na/H exchange, and perhaps other pathways such as H-ATPase. Following H secretion, OH^- formed combines with CO_2, forming HCO_3, which exits the basolateral membrane via $Na(HCO_3)_3$ co-transport.[28] Thus, in the early proximal tubule, the net effect of the process described results in the isosmotic reabsorption of $NaHCO_3$. The lumen chloride concentration increases, because water continues to be reabsorbed producing a lumen-positive potential. These axial changes provide an electrochemical gradient for transport of chloride via paracellular and transcellular pathways. The latter pathway for chloride likely involves a chloride—base exchanger operating in parallel with a Na/H proton exchanger.[29] The dual operation of these parallel exchangers results in net transepithelial NaCl absorption.

The participation of a membrane-bound component of carbonic anhydrase was first suggested by Rector, Carter, and Seldin.[30] The observation that carbonic anhydrase inhibitors produced an acid disequilibrium pH in the proximal tubule suggested that luminal fluid was normally in contact with carbonic anhydrase. Disequilibrium pH refers to the difference between the pH of tubule fluid *in situ* (in this case during infusion of carbonic anhydrase inhibitors), and the pH achieved after the tubule fluid is allowed to reach chemical equilibrium at known pCO_2. Thus, when carbonic anhydrase is present, the pH measured *in situ* should be the same as the pH measured at equilibrium (in other words, CA should make the HCO_3 dissociate into CO_2 and H_2O very rapidly). When carbonic anhydrase is inhibited by the administration of CAI, the dissociation of HCO_3 to OH and CO_2 is slow, allowing H to accumulate in the lumen, and reducing pH.

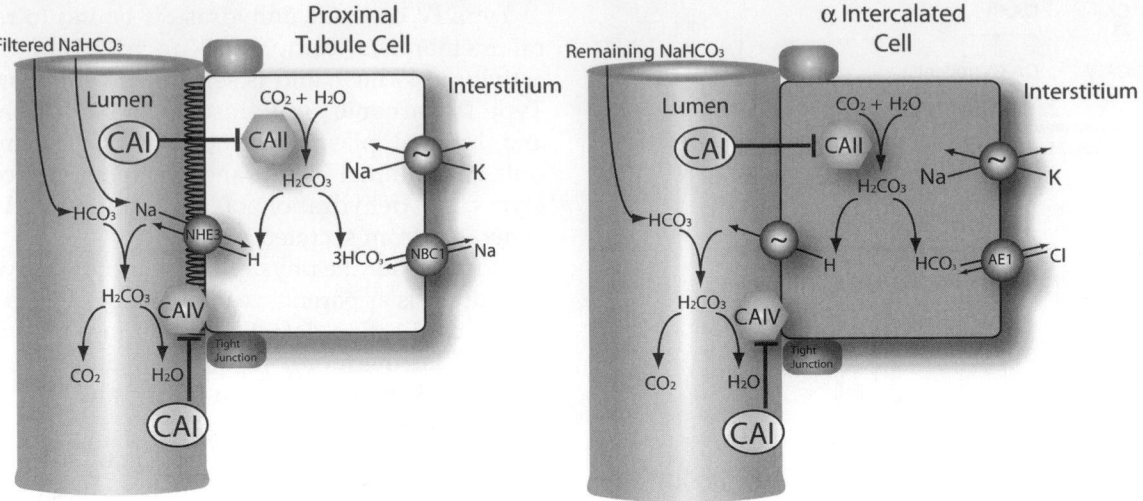

FIGURE 40.5   Mechanisms of carbonic anhydrase inhibitors in the proximal tubule. Water and CO_2 form carbonic acid (H_2CO_3) inside proximal cells. Carbonic anhydrase inside the cell (isoform II, CAII) catalyzes the formation of HCO_3 from OH and CO_2. Bicarbonate leaves the cell via the Na,HCO_3 co-transporter (see text). A second pool of carbonic anhydrase (isoform IV, CAIV) is located in the brush border. This participates in disposing of luminal carbonic acid, formed by the combination of filtered bicarbonate and secreted protons. Both pools of carbonic anhydrase are inhibited by acetazolamide and other carbonic anhydrase inhibitors (see text for details).

The demonstration of an acid disequilibrium pH provided physiological evidence in support of previous histochemical findings that a fraction of enzymatic activity was present in the tubule lumen. Although the cytoplasmic carbonic anhydrase constitutes the majority of enzyme activity in kidney, it is believed that the membrane bound carbonic anhydrase plays a significant role in bicarbonate reabsorption by the proximal tubule. Studies addressing this question have employed CAIs that differ in their ability to penetrate proximal tubule cell membranes. Benzolamide is charged at normal pH and is relatively impermeant, whereas acetazolamide enters the cell relatively easily. Both intravenous and intratubular administration of benzolamide resulted in an acid disequilibrium pH, indicating that luminal carbonic anhydrase inhibition contributes to bicarbonate absorption. Furthermore, proximal tubular perfusion of benzolamide resulted in 90% inhibition of bicarbonate reabsorption. Despite near equal efficacy in inhibiting proximal tubule bicarbonate reabsorption, benzolamide lowered tubular fluid pH, whereas acetazolamide increased tubular fluid pH. These results suggest that the site of action of benzolamide is at the luminal membrane, whereas the site of action of acetazolamide is within the cell. Inhibition of luminal carbonic anhydrase causes lumen pH to decrease, because of the continued secretion of hydrogen ions and its accumulation in the tubular lumen. In contrast, acetazolamide does not produce an acid disequilibrium pH.[31] The conclusion that tubular fluid was in direct contact with membrane carbonic anhydrase was substantiated by the use of dextran-bound carbonic anhydrase inhibitor. In proximal tubules perfused *in vivo*, Lucci et al.[32] determined that dextran-bound inhibitors, which inhibit only luminal carbonic anhydrase, decreased proximal tubule bicarbonate absorption by approximately 80%, and reduced lumen pH. Although these studies establish the importance of luminal carbonic anhydrase, they also support a role for intracellular carbonic anhydrase, and as acetazolamide is the only CAI used for its renal properties, suggesting that cytoplasmic CA is the predominant drug target in humans.

Following administration of carbonic anhydrase inhibitors, proximal tubule bicarbonate reabsorption is inhibited variably between 35 and >85%. As suggested from the sites of expression along the nephron (see Figure 40.4), however, additional sites of action of carbonic anhydrase inhibitors include proximal straight tubule or loop of Henle, distal tubule, collecting tubule, and papillary collecting duct.

As noted, CAII may participate more directly in facilitating net bicarbonate and, perhaps, NaCl reabsorption. CAII has been shown to associate with several proximal transporters, including the basolateral bicarbonate exit transport system, kNBC1,[33] the apical Cl/base exchanger, SCL26A6,[34] and the basolateral Na/H exchanger, NHE1,[35] by binding to their respective carboxyl-terminal tails, associations that may be physiologically relevant.[36] Thus, CAIs may act both directly on transporters and via inhibition of substrate production.[37,38]

In α-intercalated cells (see Figure 40.5) within the DCT2, connecting tubule, and collecting duct, CA facilitates acid secretion that is mediated by a vacuolar H adenosinetriphosphatase (H-ATPase)[39] H-K-ATPase, and the blood group protein RhCG at the apical membrane;[40] RhCG is now known to be an important contributor to renal ammonia secretion.[41-43] The anion exchanger (AE3) at the basolateral cell membrane participates importantly in bicarbonate reabsorption. As for the proximal tubule, both membrane-associated and cytosolic forms of CA likely contribute to distal acidification. Individuals with CAII deficiency display both proximal and distal acidification defects,[44] confirming a role for this enzyme in the distal nephron. Yet, luminal administration of acetazolamide produced an acid disequilibrium pH in the outer medullary collecting duct, suggesting contribution a of luminal carbonic anhydrase as well.[45] In subsequent studies, a membrane-impermeant carbonic anhydrase inhibitor reduced bicarbonate absorption, thus confirming the presence of membrane-bound carbonic anhydrase in the outer medullary collecting duct.[46] The K_i for inhibition of bicarbonate absorption was $5\,\mu M$, consistent with the inhibition of Type IV carbonic anhydrase.

Like the proximal tubule, where CAII association with solute transporters may contribute to their regulation and activity, CAII has been shown to associate with CAII at the basolateral membrane,[47,48] and inhibition of CA nearly completely blocked the bicarbonate transport induced by transfection of cells with AE1.

Effects of CAI on renal calcium transporters have also been examined. In mice, acetazolamide increased urinary pH and urinary calcium excretion, in association with a reduced TRPV5 abundance. Similar changes were induced by loading with NH_4Cl, but not by treatment with $NaHCO_3$, suggesting that they were the result of systemic acidosis, and not high urine pH. The importance of TRPV5 in these processes was confirmed by showing that acetazolamide did not alter urinary calcium excretion in TRPV5 knockout mice.[49] These studies suggest that the hypercalciuria and tendency to stone formation induced by CAI is the result of systemic acidosis.

Renal Hemodynamics

Inhibition of carbonic anhydrase produces an acute decrease in GFR by activating TGF.[18] Systemic infusion of acetazolamide resulted in a 30% decrease in GFR. Distally measured single nephron glomerular filtration rate (SNGFR) was reduced by 23% during acetazolamide infusion, whereas proximally measured SNGFR was not affected. These results indicated that acetazolamide blocked activated TGF, which in turn reduced GFR. Similar results were observed following infusion of benzolamide.[50] Sar-ala8-angiotensin I, an angiotensin II antagonist, prevented the decrease in SGNFR,

suggesting the involvement of local angiotensin II in response to benzolamide.[50]

Pharmacokinetics

Acetazolamide is well-absorbed from the gastrointestinal (GI) tract. More than 90% of the drug is plasma protein-bound. The highest concentrations are found in tissues that contain large amounts of carbonic anhydrase (e.g., renal cortex, red blood cells). Renal effects are noticeable within 30 minutes, and are usually maximal at 2 hours. Acetazolamide is not metabolized, but is excreted rapidly by glomerular filtration and proximal tubular secretion. The half-life is approximately 5 hours, and renal excretion is essentially complete in 24 hours.[5] In comparison, methazolamide is absorbed more slowly from the GI tract, and its duration of action is long, with a half-life of approximately 14 hours.

Adverse Effects

Generally, carbonic anhydrase inhibitors are well-tolerated, with infrequent serious adverse effects. Side-effects of carbonic anhydrase inhibitors may arise from the continued excretion of electrolytes. Significant hypokalemia and metabolic acidosis may develop. In elderly patients with glaucoma treated with acetazolamide (250 mg to 1000 mg/day), metabolic acidosis was a frequent finding in comparison to a control group.[51] Acetazolamide is also associated with nephrocalcinosis and nephrolithiasis, due to its effects on urine pH facilitating stone formation.[52] Premature infants treated with furosemide and acetazolamide are particularly susceptible to nephrocalcinosis, presumably due to the combined effect of an alkaline urine and hypercalciuria.[53] Other adverse effects include drowsiness, fatigue, CNS depression, and parathesias. Bone marrow suppression has been reported.[51,54]

Clinical Use

The popularity of carbonic anhydrase inhibitors as diuretics has waned, principally because more effective agents are available, but in specific settings these drugs remain useful. In general, tolerance to the natriuretic effects of CAI develops rapidly, and renders them relatively ineffective in treatment of edema. Daily use produces systemic acidemia from an increase in urinary excretion of bicarbonate. Nevertheless, acetazolamide can be administered for short-term therapy, usually in combination with other diuretics to patients who are resistant or who do not respond adequately to other agents. The rationale for using a combination of diuretic agents is based on the summation of their effect at different sites along the nephron.[55]

The major indication for the use of acetazolamide as a diuretic agent is in the treatment of patients with metabolic alkalosis that is accompanied by edematous states or chronic obstructive lung disease.[56] In patients with cirrhosis, congestive heart failure or nephrotic syndrome, aggressive diuresis with loop diuretics promotes intravascular chloride and volume-depletion, secondary hyperaldosteronism, and renal insufficiency, conditions that promote metabolic alkalosis. Administration of sodium chloride to correct the metabolic alkalosis may exacerbate edema. Acetazolamide can improve metabolic alkalosis by decreasing proximal tubule bicarbonate reabsorption and distal proton secretion, thereby increasing the fractional excretion of bicarbonate. An increase in urinary pH (>7.0) indicates enhanced bicarbonaturia. However, it should be noted that potassium-depletion should be corrected prior to acetazolamide use, as acetazolamide will increase potassium excretion. The time-course of acetazolamide effect is rapid. In critically ill patients on ventilators, following the correction of fluid and electrolyte disturbances, intravenous acetazolamide produced an initial effect within 2 hours, and a maximum effect in 15 hours.[57]

Acetazolamide was used to treat chronic open-angle glaucoma, but its popularity has been limited by side-effects and limited efficacy. The high bicarbonate concentration in aqueous humor is carbonic anhydrase-dependent, and oral carbonic anhydrase inhibition can be used to reduce aqueous humor formation. Dorzolamide is a topical CAI that is in clinical use to treat glaucoma.

Acute mountain sickness usually occurs in sojourners who ascend to heights greater than 2500–3000 feet. Symptoms occur within the 12–72 hours, and are characterized by a symptom complex consisting of headache, nausea, dizziness, and breathlessness. Carbonic anhydrase inhibitors improve symptoms and arterial oxygenation.[58–60]

The administration of acetazolamide has been used in the treatment of familial hypokalemic periodic paralysis,[61,62] a disorder characterized by intermittent episodes of muscle weakness and flaccid paralysis. Its efficacy may be related to a decrease in influx of potassium as a result of a decrease in plasma insulin and glucose[63] or to metabolic acidosis. Carbonic anhydrase inhibitors can also be used as an adjunct treatment of epilepsy,[64] pseudotumor cerebri,[65] and central sleep apnea.[66]

By increasing urinary pH, acetazolamide has been used effectively in certain clinical conditions. Acetazolamide is used to treat cystine and uric acid stones by increasing their solubility in urine. Acetazolamide, in combination with sodium bicarbonate infusion, is also used to treat salicylate toxicity.

Salicylates are weak acids (pK_a 3.0), therefore their ionic and nonionic forms exist in equilibrium. They are excreted primarily by the kidney through secretion via the organic anion transport pathway in the proximal tubule. Acetazolamide and sodium bicarbonate infusions increase urinary pH, thereby favoring formation of a nondiffusible nonionic form of salicylate, thus increasing excretion of salicylates.[67]

LOOP DIURETICS

The loop diuretics inhibit sodium and chloride transport along the loop of Henle. Although these drugs also impair ion transport by proximal and distal tubules under some conditions, these effects probably contribute little to their action clinically. Although the predominant natriuretic effects result from blockade of NKCC2, the apical transporter of the TAL, other effects may result from blockade of NKCC1, the more widely-expressed form. The affinity of loop diuretics for the two classes of transporter appears to be similar;[68] differential selectivity for the renal isoform during topical use is likely the result of the concentration of secreted drug within the tubule lumen, leading to a higher concentration adjacent to TAL cells. The role of NKCC1 inhibition in pharmacological actions of loop diuretics is discussed below. The loop diuretics available in the United States include furosemide, bumetanide, torsemide, and ethacrynic acid (see Figure 40.6). Organic mercurial diuretics also inhibit ion transport along the loop of Henle, but these drugs are of historical interest, as they are no longer available for clinical use.

Urinary Electrolyte and Water Excretion

Loop diuretics increase the excretion of water, Na, K, Cl, phosphate, magnesium, and calcium (see Table 40.1). The dose–response relationship between loop diuretic and urinary Na and Cl excretion is sigmoidal (see Figure 40.7). The steep dose–response relationship in the therapeutic range has led many to refer to these as "threshold" drugs.[3] Loop diuretics have the highest natriuretic and chloriuretic potency of any class of diuretics; they can increase Na and Cl excretion to more than 25% of the filtered load. Following oral water-loading, the administration of a loop diuretic decreases free water clearance (C_{H2O}) and increases osmolar clearance, although the urine always remains dilute. This effect contrasts with that of osmotic diuretics, in which increases in osmolar clearance are associated with increase in C_{H2O}. During water deprivation, loop diuretics impair the reabsorption of solute free water (T^C_{H2O}). Loop diuretics may induce a "negative"

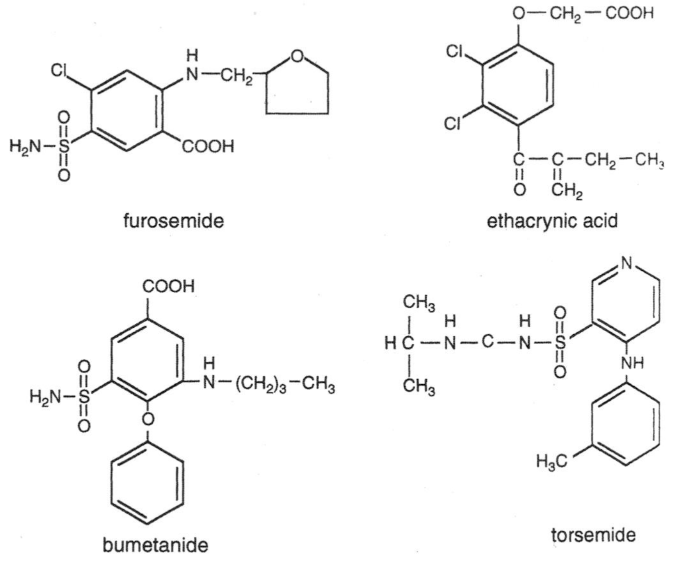

FIGURE 40.6 Structures of loop diuretics.

T_{H2O}^C, even during water deprivation. During maximal loop diuretic action, the urinary Na concentration is usually between 75–100 mM.[69] Because urinary K concentrations during furosemide-induced natriuresis remain low, the clearance of electrolyte free water (C_{H2O}) is increased when loop diuretics are administered during conditions of water diuresis or water deprivation.[69]

Mechanisms of Action

Na and Cl Transport

The predominant effect of loop diuretic drugs is to inhibit the electroneutral Na-K-2Cl co-transporter at the apical surface of thick ascending limb cells. The loop of Henle, defined as the region between the last surface proximal segment and the first surface distal segment, reabsorbs from 20–50% of the filtered Na-and Cl-load (see Figure 40.1); approximately 10–20% is reabsorbed by thick ascending limb cells. The model in Figure 40.8 shows key components of Na, K, and Cl transport pathways in a thick ascending limb cell. Although mechanisms of Na and Cl transport are discussed more thoroughly in other chapters in this volume, some important points deserve emphasis. First, as in other nephron segments, the Na/K-ATPase at the basolateral cell membrane maintains the intracellular Na concentration low (approximately 10-fold lower than interstitial) and the K concentration high (approximately 20-fold higher than interstitial). Potassium channel(s) in the basolateral cell membrane permit K to diffuse out of the cell, rendering the cell membrane voltage oriented with the intracellular surface negative,

relative to extracellular fluid.[70] A chloride channel in the basolateral cell membrane[71] and a barium-sensitive K channel permit Cl to exit the cell.

The transporter inhibited by loop diuretics is one member of the cation-chloride co-transporter family.[72] The cation-chloride co-transporters are part of the amino acid, polyamine, organocation (APC) superfamily.[73] This Na-K-2Cl co-transporter of the thick ascending limb, NKCC2 (formerly called the bumetanide-sensitive co-transporter, BSC1), is encoded by the gene *SLC12A1*. It is a protein with 12 putative membrane-spanning domains that is expressed at the apical membrane of thick ascending limb[74] and macula densa (MD) cells.[75] It lies in parallel with a K channel (ROMK, Kir 1.1) that permits potassium to recycle from the cell to the lumen.[76] Along the thick ascending limb, the asymmetrical orientation of channels (apical versus basolateral), and the action of the Na/K-ATPase and Na-K-2Cl co-transporter, combine to create a transepithelial voltage oriented with the lumen-positive, with respect to the interstitium. This lumen-positive potential drives paracellular absorption of Na, Ca, and Mg. The paracellular component of Na reabsorption comprises as much as 50% of the total transepithelial Na transport by thick ascending limb cells[77]; it should be noted, however, that both the transcellular and the paracellular components of Na transport are inhibited by loop diuretics, the former directly and the latter indirectly; this is because loop diuretics reduce the magnitude of the transepithelial voltage, which normally drives paracellular transport. The thick ascending limb is virtually impermeable to water. The combination of solute absorption and water impermeability leads to dilution of tubule fluid.

Until recently, models of ion- and diuretic-binding to NKCC2 were largely inferential. One model of Na-K-2Cl co-transport, based on the ionic requirements for transport, postulates that ion-binding sites on the transporter must be occupied sequentially, first by Na, then by chloride, then by potassium, and finally by a second chloride.[78] Loop diuretics are organic anions that bind to the NKCC2 from the luminal surface. Early studies showed that [³H] bumetanide binds to membranes that express the NKCC proteins. Optimal binding requires the presence of all three transported species, and binding and inhibition is competed by Cl⁻.[79] Binding of bumetanide is also known to be a relatively slow process, and bumetanide becomes "occluded" with Na, K, and Cl.[80] Studies using chimeric NKCC molecules investigated sites of bumetanide-binding and interactions with ions by determining effects on ion transport of heterologously expressed NKCC proteins. Using this approach, it was shown that changes in amino acids that affected bumetanide-binding are not the same as those affecting the kinetics of ion translocation, and it

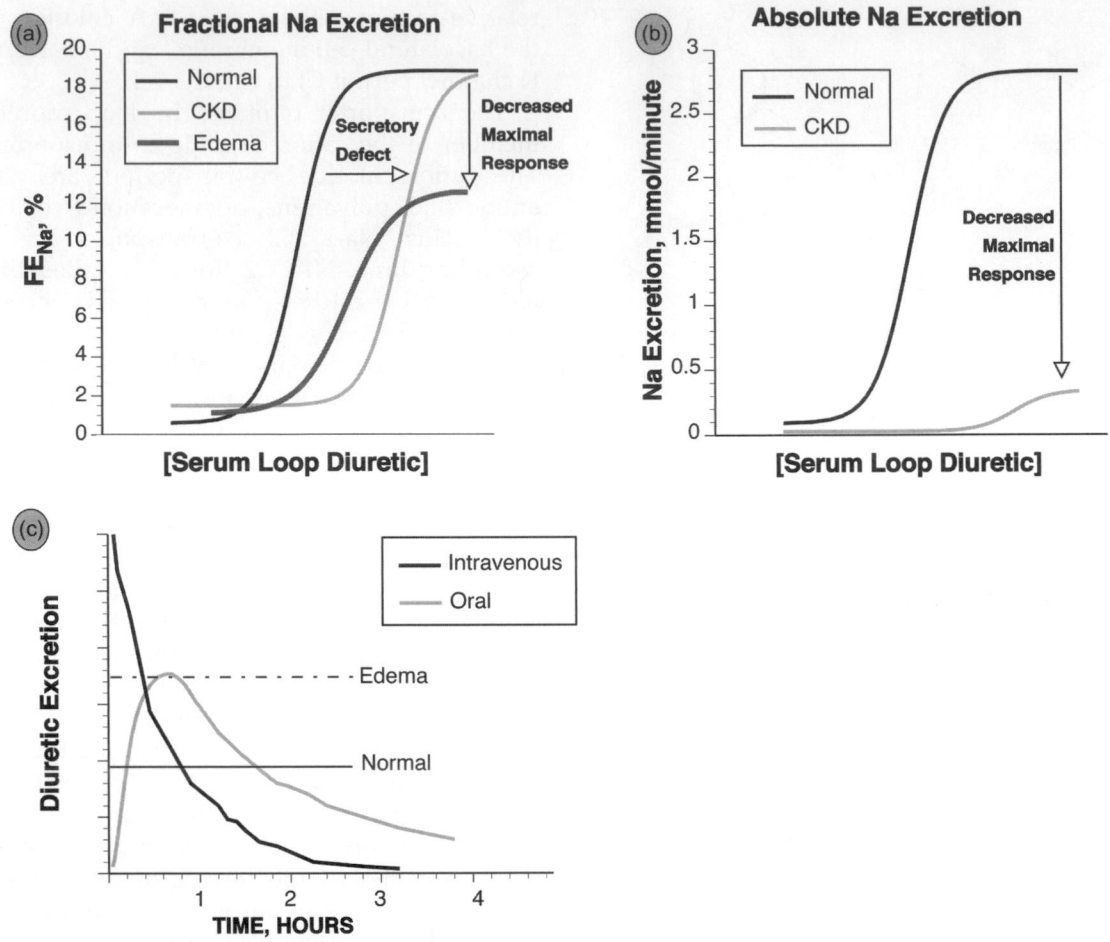

FIGURE 40.7 **Dose—response curve for loop diuretics.** Panel a shows the fractional Na excretion (FE_{Na}) as a function of loop diuretic concentration. Compared with normal patients, patients with chronic renal failure (CKD) show a rightward shift in the curve, owing to impaired diuretic secretion. The maximal response is preserved when expressed as FE_{Na}, but when expressed as absolute Na excretion, (Panel b), maximal natriuresis is reduced in patients with CKD. Patients with edema demonstrate a rightward and downward shift, even when expressed as FE_{Na} (Panel a). Panel c compares the response to intravenous and oral doses of loop diuretics. In a normal individual (Normal), an oral dose may be as effective as an intravenous dose, because the time above the natriuretic threshold (indicated by the "normal" line) is approximately equal. If the natriuretic threshold increases (as indicated by the dashed line, from an edematous patient), then the oral dose may not provide a high enough serum level to elicit natriuresis.

was suggested that bumetanide- and Cl-binding did not occur to the same site.[81,82]

More recently, however, a substantial advance in understanding mechanisms of ion transport and diuretic action has been made possible by solution of the crystal structure of two members of the APC super-family.[83-86] The insights derived recently permitted Forbush and colleagues[73] to perform homology-based modeling of NKCC1, and to use cysteine mutagenesis of putative pore and binding regions to investigate function. While the work utilized NKCC1, the ubiquitous form, rather than NKCC2, the apical form from TAL, it is likely that the structural insights apply, at least in part. The results suggest that functionally important residues in transmembrane segment 3 (TM3) face the translocation pathway; in contrast to past

results in which effects of mutations on affinity were modest, mutations of residues in TM3 led to large changes in inhibitor affinities. Three mutations led to dramatic alterations, one (M382) at the extracellular entry port, and two (F372 and I371) at the inner end of the proposed pore. The investigators suggested, therefore, that loop diuretics bind within the translocating pore, and that the binding site may be near its inner surface. The work also identified a mutation that produces a virtually bumetanide-insensitive NKCC, but which retains some furosemide sensitivity. This work appears to help resolve some discrepancies, and confirm that loop diuretics interact with vital ion transporting segments of the protein.

Although direct inhibition of ion transport is the most important natriuretic action of loop diuretics,

Mechanistic Model

Proposed Structure with Diuretic Binding Site

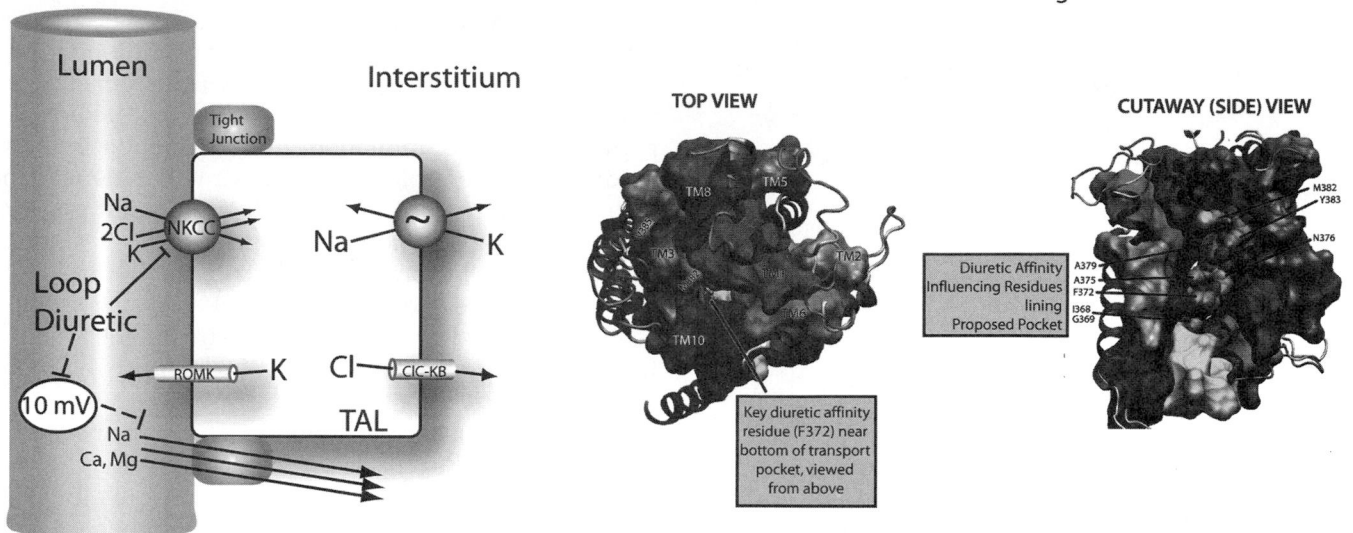

FIGURE 40.8 Mechanisms of loop diuretic action and proposed NKCC1 structure. Left panel: Na and Cl are reabsorbed across the apical membrane via the loop diuretic-sensitive Na-K-2Cl co-transporter, NKCC2. Note that the transepithelial voltage along the thick ascending limb is oriented with the lumen-positive relative to interstitium. This transepithelial voltage drives a component of Na (and calcium and magnesium) reabsorption via the paracellular pathway (the "tight junction," shown). Loop diuretics block the NKCC2 directly, thereby reducing the magnitude of the transepithelial voltage, and reducing Na, K, Cl, Mg, and Ca reabsorption. Right panel: Proposed structure of NKCC1. On the left, a view from above shows the translocation pocket, where residue F372, which lies nears its bottom, can be seen through the open pocket. On the right, a cutaway view into transmembrane segment 3, showing pore-lining residues colored blue and labeled. *(Structural models are adapted from J. Biol. Chem. (2012). Mar 21. (Epub ahead of print) PMID: 22437837, with permission.)* See color section at the back of the book.

other actions may contribute to natriuresis. Thick ascending limb cells have been shown to produce prostaglandin E_2 following stimulation with furosemide[87] or low luminal NaCl concentration.[88] Blockade of cyclooxygenase reduces the effects of furosemide to inhibit loop segment chloride transport in rats[89]; prostaglandin E_2, but not I_2, can restore this effect.[90] Animals defective in PGE_2 receptors also demonstrate blunted natriuresis, compared with wild-type animals,[91] indicating an important role for PGE_2 in loop diuretic-induced natriuresis. Increases in renal prostaglandins may contribute to the hemodynamic effects of loop diuretics, described below.

Ca and Mg Transport

Loop diuretics increase the excretion of the divalent cations, calcium and magnesium. This effect to increase calcium excretion is used to advantage when furosemide is added to saline to treat hypercalcemia,[92] although this approach is no longer recommended routinely[93] (see below). Although a component of magnesium and calcium absorption by thick ascending limbs may be active (especially when circulating PTH levels are high[94]), a large component of their absorption is passive and paracellular, driven by the transepithelial voltage. As described above, active NaCl transport by thick ascending limb cells leads to a transepithelial voltage, oriented in the lumen-positive direction. The paracellular pathway in the thick ascending limb is cation selective; expression of claudins 16 and 19 appear to play dominant roles.[95–97] The positive voltage in the lumen, relative to interstitium, drives calcium and magnesium absorption through the paracellular pathway; because these are divalent cations, the electrical driving force is double that for Na. Loop diuretics, by blocking the activity of the Na-K-2Cl co-transporter at the apical membrane of thick ascending limb cells, reduce the transepithelial voltage, impairing passive calcium and magnesium absorption.

Renin Secretion

In addition to enhancing Na and Cl excretion, effects that result directly from inhibiting Na and Cl transport, loop diuretics also stimulate renin secretion. A portion of this effect results from contraction of the ECF volume and a reduction of blood pressure (see below), but loop diuretics also stimulate renin secretion by inhibiting NaCl uptake by macula densa cells (see Figure 40.9). Macula densa cells sense the NaCl concentration in the lumen of the thick ascending limb, because NaCl enters the cell across the apical membrane.[98] High luminal NaCl concentrations in the

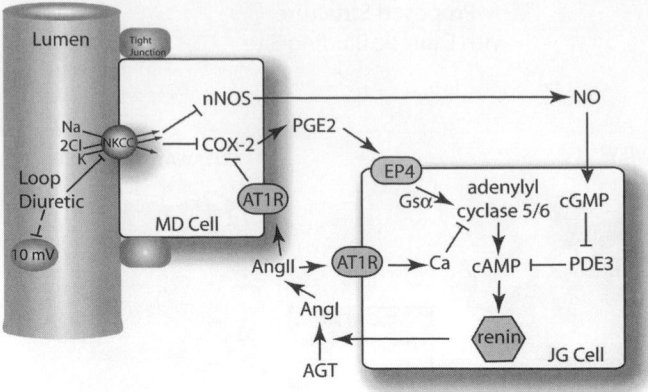

FIGURE 40.9 Regulation of renin secretion by diuretics. A macula densa (MD) cell is shown expressing NKCC2 at its apical surface, in parallel with a K channel. Movement of NaCl across the apical membrane inhibits production of nitric oxide (NO) via nitric oxide synthase I (nNOS). When loop diuretics inhibit NaCl uptake, nitric oxide is produced and diffuses to the extraglomerular mesangium or directly to juxtaglomerular (JG) cells, where it increases cGMP. cGMP inhibits phosphodiesterase 3 (PDE$_3$) which metabolizes cAMP to 5" AMP. cAMP stimulates renin secretion. NaCl entry across the apical membrane also inhibits cyclooxygenase (COX-2). When loop diuretics block NaCl entry, COX-2 produces prostaglandin E$_2$ (PGE$_2$), which acts via Gsα to stimulate adenylyl cyclase, thereby increasing cAMP and renin.

region of the macula densa lead to two distinct but related effects. First they activate the TGF response, which suppresses the GFR. Second, they inhibit renin secretion. The relation between these two effects is complex and has been reviewed,[98] but both appear to be controlled, at least in part, by NaCl movement across the apical membrane.

The pathways mediating Na and Cl uptake into macula densa cells are similar to those expressed by adjacent TAL cells. These include the loop diuretic-sensitive Na-K-2Cl co-transporter at the apical surface. Under normal conditions, an increase in luminal NaCl concentration in the thick ascending limb raises the NaCl concentration inside macula densa cells. Because the activity of the basolateral Na/K-ATPase is lower in macula densa cells than in surrounding thick ascending limb cells,[99] the cell NaCl concentration is much more dependent on luminal NaCl concentration than in TAL cells.[100] When luminal and macula densa cell NaCl concentrations decline, COX-2 activity and expression are induced; this leads to the production of PGE$_2$, which diffuses to juxtaglomerular cells. There, PGE$_2$ activates EP4 receptors, resulting in Gsα-mediated activation of adenylyl cyclase. This process, in turn, increases the concentration of cyclic AMP, which eventually stimulates renin secretion.[98]

The constitutive (neuronal) isoform of nitric oxide synthase (NOS I) is expressed by macula densa cells,

but not substantially by other cells in the kidney. Nitric oxide produced by macula densa cells has a paracrine effect to increase cAMP in adjacent juxtaglomerular cells (Figure 40.9). In these cells, nitric oxide increases cellular concentrations of cGMP, which inhibit phosphodiesterase 3.[101] Inhibition of phosphodiesterase 3 permits cAMP accumulation. Renin secretion induced by dietary NaCl depletion or furosemide is dependent on an intact nitric oxide system,[102] although it appears that basal renin secretion is not.

The second isoform of cyclooxygenase, COX-2, is also highly expressed by macula densa cells; its expression is increased by loop diuretic treatment.[88,103–105] Blockade of prostaglandin synthesis either by nonspecific cyclooxygenase inhibitors or by specific COX-2 blockers[106] reduces the renin secretory response to loop diuretics. Current views suggest that loop diuretics, like low luminal NaCl delivery, stimulate renin secretion by macula densa cells by activating COX-2, leading to PGE$_2$ production. PGE$_2$ stimulates EP4 receptors leading to renin synthesis.[107]

RENAL HEMODYNAMICS AND OXYGENATION

Most classes of diuretic reduce glomerular filtration; in contrast, loop diuretics tend to preserve GFR and renal blood flow, although GFR and RPF can decline when ECF volume contracts. NKCC1 is expressed by many cells, including vascular smooth muscle cells,[108] where it appears to contribute to vasoconstriction. The ability of loop diuretics to inhibit NKCC1, therefore, would suggest that the hemodynamic effect of loop diuretics in the kidney should consist of vasodilatation. In addition, a reduction of renal vascular resistance should result from the well-known blockade of TGF mechanism by loop diuretics, discussed below. In several species, an effect of loop diuretics to increase renal blood flow and dilate renal vessels has been observed in studies in humans[69] and dogs.[109,110] In contrast, in the majority of studies in the rat, furosemide led to a ~10–20% reduction of RBF.[111,112] In the rodent, the renal hemodynamic effects of NKCC inhibition may be unrelated to the primary actions of the diuretic on tubular and vascular functions, but to result from secondary effects on RBF activated by the diuretic. In addition, loop diuretics are known to rapidly stimulate renin secretion and prostaglandin formation, so that differences in the response of these regulatory systems to the diuretic could cause species-specific responses. Oppermann and colleagues[112] found that furosemide dilated glomerular afferent arterioles, when perfused *in vitro*, as expected from a direct effect to inhibit NKCC1, but rather led to a 50% reduction in total renal blood flow and a 27% reduction in superficial blood flow. Notably, mice in which NKCC1 was knocked-out responded with qualitatively similar reductions in renal blood flow. These workers suggested that the effects on renal blood flow may have resulted from increased angiotensin II production, production of vasoconstrictor prostaglandins or intrarenal pressure changes consequent to diuresis.

Changes in renal hemodynamics are associated with changes in renal oxygen consumption and tissue oxygenation. Most studies in animals show that renal oxygen consumption declines and renal oxygen tension increases, especially in the medulla.[113,114] This information was used to suggest that loop diuretics might be beneficial in preventing or treating AKI; although this prediction was not borne out by clinical trials (see below), it is clear that loop diuretics do increase renal medullary oxygen tension, both in animals and in humans, as detected by BOLD MRI.[115,116]

Another factor that may contribute to the tendency of loop diuretics to maintain GFR and renal plasma flow despite volume contraction is their effect on the TGF system. The sensing mechanism that activates TGF involves NaCl transport across the apical membrane of macula densa cells by NKCC2 (see Figure 40.9). Under normal conditions when the luminal concentration of NaCl reaching the macula densa rises (as during volume expansion) GFR decreases via TGF. To a large degree, the TGF-mediated decrease in GFR results from afferent arteriolar constriction.[98] Although the mechanisms by which ion transport across the apical membrane of macula densa cells translates to afferent arteriolar vasoconstriction are unclear, they appear to involve the production of adenosine (an afferent arteriolar vasoconstrictor) and an increase in mesangial and smooth muscle cell calcium concentrations.[98] ATP release from macula densa cells[117] leads to the extracellular formation of adenosine by ecto-5'-nucleotidase. The fact that TGF is blunted in animals where ecto-5'-nucleotidase and A1 receptors are pharmacologically inhibited, and in A1 receptor and ecto-5'-nucleotidase knockout mice, supports the importance of adenosine formation and activation of adenosine A1 receptors in mediating TGF.[118-121] In a manner analogous to the effects on renin secretion, loop diuretic drugs block TGF by blocking the sensing step. In the absence of direct effects to inhibit NaCl uptake by macula densa cells, loop diuretics would be expected to suppress GFR and RPF, because they increase NaCl delivery (this action explains the effects of CAI and distal convoluted tubule diuretics on TGF[18]). Instead, blockade of NaCl uptake actually inhibits the TGF, despite increased delivery, permitting GFR and RPF to be maintained.

Systemic Hemodyanamics

Acute intravenous administration of loop diuretics tends to increase venous capacitance.[122] Most studies suggest that this effect results from stimulation of prostaglandin synthesis by the kidney.[123,124] Other studies, however, suggest that loop diuretics have effects in peripheral vascular beds as well[125] or may stimulate nitric oxide production.[126] Pickkers and co-workers examined the local effects of furosemide in the human forearm. Furosemide had no effect on arterial vessels, but did cause dilation of veins, an effect that was dependent on local prostaglandin production.[127] As noted above, there is increasing interest in the role of NKCC1 in maintaining vascular smooth muscle tone. Some,[128,129] but not other,[130] investigators have reported that NKCC1 knockout leads to basal hypotension; although NKCC1 inhibition may contribute to vasodilation under some circumstances, the plasma diuretic concentration needed for this effect is probably rare in clinical practice, for reasons noted above.

Although venodilation and improvements in cardiac hemodynamics frequently result from intravenous therapy with loop diuretics, the hemodynamic response to intravenous loop diuretics is more complex. Johnston et al. reported that low-dose furosemide increased venous capacitance, but that higher doses did not.[131] It was suggested that furosemide-induced renin secretion may generate angiotensin II-induced vasoconstriction. This vasoconstrictor might overwhelm the prostaglandin-mediated vasodilatory effects in some patients. In two series, 1–1.5 mg/kg furosemide boluses, administered to patients with chronic congestive heart failure, resulted in transient *deteriorations* in hemodyanamics (during the first hour), with a decline in stroke volume index, an increase in left ventricular filling pressure,[132,133] and exacerbation of congestive heart failure symptoms. These changes were attributed to activation of both the sympathetic nervous system and the renin—angiotensin system by the diuretic drug. Evidence for a role of the renin—angiotensin system in the furosemide-induced deterioration in systemic hemodynamics includes the temporal association between its activation and hemodynamic deterioration,[132,133] and the ability of angiotensin I-converting enzyme inhibitors to prevent much of the pressor effect.[132,133] Other studies have shown that acute loop diuretic administration frequently produces a transient decline in cardiac output; whether diuretic administration increases or decreases left atrial pressure acutely may depend primarily on the state of underlying sympathetic nervous system and renin—angiotensin axis activation. Interestingly, these complex interactions between prior physiological state and hemodynamic response to loop diuretics in humans parallel the

TABLE 40.2   Pharmacokinetics of Loop Diuretics

	Bioavailability, % Oral Dose Absorbed	Healthy	Kidney Disease	Liver Disease	HF
Furosemide	50% (range: 10–100%)	1.5–2	2.8	2.5	2.7
Bumetanide	80–100%	1	1.6	2.3	1.3
Torsemide	80–100%	3–4	4–5	8	6

Data from ref. [72].
Elimination half-life: h; HF: heart failure.

complex interactions postulated to explain the paradoxical effects of loop diuretics in mice.[112]

Pharmacokinetics

The three loop diuretics that are used most commonly, furosemide, bumetanide, and torsemide, are absorbed quickly after oral administration, reaching peak concentrations within 0.5–2 hours (see Table 40.2). Furosemide absorption is slower than the rate of elimination in normal subjects; thus, the time to reach peak serum level is slower for furosemide than for bumetanide and torsemide. This phenomenon is called "absorption-limited kinetics".[3] The bioavailability of loop diuretics varies from 50 to 90% (Table 40.2), with furosemide having the lowest, and most variable oral bioavailability. For this reason, when changing a patient from intravenous to oral furosemide, the dose is frequently doubled to account for its limited oral bioavailability.[3] The half-lives of the loop diuretics available in the United States vary, but all are relatively short (ranging from approximately 1 hour for bumetanide to 3–4 hours for torsemide). The half-lives of muzolimine, xipamide, and ozolinone, none of which is available in the United States, are 6–15 hours.

Loop diuretics are organic anions that circulate tightly bound to albumin (>95%); thus their volumes of distribution are small, except during extreme hypoproteinemia.[134] Approximately 50% of an administered dose of furosemide is excreted unchanged into the urine. The remainder appears to be eliminated by glucuronidation, probably by the kidney. Bumetanide and torsemide are both metabolized by the liver, and also excreted unchanged by the kidney. These differences mean that furosemide kinetics are affected by renal disease, whereas bumetanide and torsemide kinetics tend not to be; this has clinical implications, discussed below.[135]

Clinical Use

Indications for loop diuretic use are given in Table 40.3. They are used commonly to treat the edematous conditions, heart failure, cirrhosis of the liver, and nephrotic syndrome. In addition, a variety of other electrolyte, fluid, and acid–base disorders can respond to loop diuretic therapy. Essentials of diuretic treatment of disease are the focus of other reviews, and will not be discussed here. The interested reader is referred to other sources for information.[2,55,136]

Loop diuretics are commonly used in the treatment of AKI. Diuretics might be thought to reduce the severity of AKI by preventing tubule obstruction and decreasing oxygen consumption,[114] as discussed above, but studies have failed to demonstrate convincingly that diuretics affect rates of renal recovery rate of patients with established AKI.[137]

Adverse Effects

There are at least three types of adverse effects of loop diuretics. The first and most common effects result directly from the effects of these drugs on renal electrolyte and water excretion. The second are toxic effects of the drugs that are dose-related and predictable. The third are idiosyncratic allergic drug reactions.

Loop diuretics are frequently administered to treat edematous expansion of the ECF volume. Edema usually results from a decrease in the "effective" arterial blood volume. Thus, zealous diuretic usage or the development of complicating illnesses can lead to excessive contraction of the ECF volume. This can be manifested by orthostatic hypotension, renal dysfunction or evidence of sympathetic overactivity. Although patients suffering from heart failure usually require diuretic therapy, the combination of diuretics and angiotensin-converting enzyme inhibitors can exacerbate prerenal azotemia. High diuretic doses or extreme dietary NaCl restriction may predispose to renal dysfunction during therapy with diuretics and angiotensin-converting enzyme inhibitors or angiotensin-receptor blockers for heart failure.[138,139] In this case, renal failure often abates when the diuretic dose is reduced or the dietary NaCl intake is liberalized, permitting continued administration of the ACE inhibitor.

Other patients at increased risk for relative contraction of the ECF volume during loop diuretic therapy include elderly patients,[140] patients with pre-existing renal insufficiency,[141] patients with right-sided heart failure or pericardial disease, and concomitant use of non-steroidal anti-inflammatory drugs.[142,133]

Disorders of Na and K concentration are among the most frequent adverse effects of loop diuretics. Hyponatremia may be less common with loop diuretics than with distal convoluted tubule diuretics (DCT diuretics; see below), but it still may occur. Its pathogenesis is usually multifactorial, but involves the effect of loop diuretics to impair the clearance of solute-free water. Additional factors that may contribute include

TABLE 40.3 Indications for Diuretic Drugs

I. INDICATIONS FOR OSMOTIC DIURETICS

A. Prevention of rhabdomyolysis
B. To reduce intraocular or intracranial pressure

II. INDICATIONS FOR CARBONIC ANHYDRASE INHIBITORS

A. Glaucoma
B. Acute mountain sickness
C. Metabolic alkalosis
D. Cystinuria
E. Resistant Edema (used in combination with other diuretics)
F. Pseudotumor cerebri

III. INDICATIONS FOR LOOP DIURETICS

A. Edematous Conditions
   1. Congestive Heart Failure
   2. Cirrhotic Ascites
   3. Nephrotic Syndrome
B. Hypercalcemia (now recommended only as second line treatment)
C. Hyperkalemia
D. Hyponatremia (with saline)
E. Hyperkalemic, hyperchloremic metabolic acidosis (Type 4 RTA)
F. Hypermagnesemia
G. Intoxications
H. Hypertension
I. AKI

IV. INDICATIONS FOR DISTAL CONVOLUTED TUBULE DIURETICS

A. Hypertension
B. Edematous Conditions
   1. Heart Failure
   2. Cirrhotic Ascites
   3. Nephrotic Syndrome
C. Prevention of recurrent nephrolithiasis
D. Nephrogenic Diabetes Insipidus
E. Osteoporosis
F. Hypoparathyroidism
G. Diuretic Resistance (used in combination with other diuretics)

V. INDICATIONS FOR POTASSIUM-SPARING DIURETICS

A. Cirrhotic Ascites
B. Lithium-induced diabetes insipidus
C. Prevention of hypokalemia (owing to potassium-wasting diuretics)
D. Prevention of hypomagnesemia (owing to potassium-wasting diuretics)
E. Diuretic Resistance (used in combination with other diuretics
F. Heart Failure with systolic dysfunction
G. Resistant hypertension
H. Aldosteronism

VI. INDICATIONS FOR AQUARETICS

A. Euvolemic hyponatremia
B. Hypervolemic hyponatremia

the non-osmotic release of arginine vasopressin,[144] hypokalemia, and hypomagesemia.[145] Conversely, loop diuretics have been used to treat hyponatremia when combined with hypertonic saline, in the setting of the syndrome of inappropriate ADH secretion.[146,147] In contrast, the combination of loop diuretics and angiotensin I-converting enzyme inhibitors has been reported to correct hyponatremia in the setting of heart failure, presumably in part owing to improved cardiac function.[148]

Hypokalemia occurs commonly during therapy with loop diuretics, although the magnitude is smaller than the magnitude of hypokalemia induced by diuretics that act in the DCT (loop diuretics, 0.3 mM versus DCT diuretics, 0.5–0.9 mM[149,150]). Loop diuretics increase the delivery of potassium to the distal tubule, because they block potassium reabsorption via the Na-K-2Cl co-transporter. In rats, approximately half the excreted potassium is delivered to the "early" distal tubule. During furosemide infusion, the delivery of potassium to the "early" distal tubule rose to 28% of the filtered load.[151] Thus, it appears that a large component of the effect of loop diuretics to increase potassium excretion acutely reflects their ability to block potassium reabsorption by the thick ascending limb. By increasing flow to the aldosterone-sensitive distal nephron, loop diuretics will also stimulate potassium secretion by activating flow-dependent maxi-K (BK) channels.[152] Nevertheless, during chronic diuretic therapy, when urinary flow has returned to or close to baseline, the degree of potassium-wasting correlates best with volume contraction and serum aldosterone levels.[153] These data suggest that, under chronic conditions, the predominant effect of loop diuretics to stimulate potassium excretion results from their tendency to increase mineralocorticoid hormones, while simultaneously increasing distal Na and water delivery.

Metabolic alkalosis is very common during chronic treatment with loop diuretics. Loop diuretics cause metabolic alkalosis via several mechanisms. First, they increase urine volume; the elaborated urine is bicarbonate-free, but contains Na and Cl. This leads to contraction of the ECF around a fixed amount of bicarbonate buffer; a phenomenon known as "contraction alkalosis." This probably contributes only slightly to the metabolic alkalosis that commonly accompanies chronic loop diuretic treatment. Loop diuretics directly inhibit transport of Na and Cl into thick ascending limb cells. In some species, these cells also express an isoform of the Na/H exchanger at the apical surface. When Na entry via the Na-K-2Cl co-transporter is blocked by a loop diuretic, the decline in intracellular Na activity will stimulate H secretion via the Na/H exchanger.[154–156] Loop diuretics also stimulate the renin–angiotensin–aldosterone pathway, both directly and indirectly, as discussed above. Aldosterone directly stimulates H secretion by the medullary collecting tubule,[157] but more importantly increases the magnitude of the transepithelial voltage in the cortical collecting duct. This effect stimulates H secretion via the electrogenic H-ATPase present at the apical membrane of α-intercalated cells. Loop diuretics frequently cause hypokalemia, which may contribute to metabolic alkalosis by increasing ammonium production,[158] stimulating bicarbonate reabsorption by proximal tubules,[159] and increasing the activity of the H/K-ATPase in the distal nephron.[160] Finally, contraction of the ECF volume stimulates Na/H exchange in the proximal tubule, and may reduce the filtered load of bicarbonate. All of these factors may contribute to the metabolic alkalosis observed during chronic loop diuretic treatment.

Ototoxicity is the most common toxic effect of loop diuretics that is unrelated to their effects on the kidney. Deafness, which is usually temporary but can be permanent, was reported shortly after the introduction of loop diuretics.[161] It appears likely that all loop diuretics cause ototoxicity, because ototoxicity can occur during use of chemically dissimilar drugs, such as furosemide and ethacrynic acid. The mechanism of ototoxicity remains unclear, although the stria vascularis, which is responsible for maintaining endolymphatic potential and ion balance, appears to be a primary target for toxicity.[162] Loop diuretics reduce the striatal potential from +80 mV to −10 to −20 mV within minutes of application.[163] A characteristic finding in loop diuretic ototoxicity is strial edema. This suggests that toxicity involves inhibition of ion fluxes.[162] Ikeda and Morizono detected functional evidence for the presence of a Na-K-2Cl co-transporter in the basolateral membrane of marginal cells.[164] According to the model proposed by these investigators, marginal cells resemble secretory cells in other organ systems, with a Na-K-2Cl co-transporter and Na/K-ATPase at the basolateral cell membrane and channels for K and Cl at the apical surface. According to this model, loop diuretic-induced shrinkage of marginal cells results from inhibition of cell Na, K, and Cl uptake across the basolateral cell membrane.

The ototoxic effects of loop diuretics appear to be related to their ability to inhibit NKCC1. This protein has been localized in the lateral wall of the cochlea, using specific antibodies[165] and RT-PCR.[166] Mice lacking the secretory isoform of the Na-K-2Cl co-transporter are profoundly deaf.[167,168] Loop diuretics cause loss of outer hair cells in the basal turn of the cochlea, rupture of endothelial layers, cystic formation in the stria vascularis, and marginal cell edema in the stria vascularis.[163]

Ototoxicity appears to be related to the peak serum concentration of loop diuretic, and therefore tends to occur during rapid drug infusion of high doses. This is likely to be related to the need to attain levels in the plasma that typically are only achieved in the renal tubule, for inhibition of NKCC1 to occur. For this reason, this complication is most common in patients with uremia,[169] where higher loop diuretic doses are frequently administered. It is recommended that furosemide infusion be no more rapid than 4 mg/minute, to avoid this complication.[169] In addition to renal failure, infants, patients with cirrhosis, and patients receiving aminoglycosides or cisplatin may be at increased risk.[169]

DISTAL CONVOLUTED TUBULE DIURETICS

The first orally active drug that inhibited Na and Cl transport along the DCT was chlorothiazide. Chlorothiazide was developed when chemical modification of sulfonamide-based CA inhibitors resulted in substances that increased NaCl, rather than $NaHCO_3$, excretion. The development of modified CA inhibitors that increased NaCl excretion preferentially was recognized immediately as significant, because ECF contains predominantly NaCl rather than $NaHCO_3$, and acidosis limited the effectiveness of CA inhibitors. Subsequent development led to a wide variety of benzothiadiazide (thiazide) diuretics (see Figure 40.10); all are analogs of 1,2,4-benzothiadiazine-1,1-dioxide. Other structurally related non-thiazide diuretics include the quinazolinones (such as metolazone) and substituted benzopehenone sulfonamide (such as chlorthalidone). Although there was some confusion initially about the site of their action along the nephron, molecular identification of their target ion transporter permitted delineation of their predominant site of action as the DCT. Recent studies, however, suggest an additional site of action along the collecting duct. Based upon the common site at which both true thiazide and "thiazide-like" diuretics inhibit ion transport, it is reasonable to refer to this class of drugs as *distal convoluted tubule diuretics*, in analogy with the *loop diuretics*.

Urinary Electrolyte and Water Excretion

Acute administration of these drugs increases the excretion of Na, K, Cl, HCO_3, phosphate, and urate, although the increases in HCO_3, phosphate, and urate excretion are probably related primarily to CA inhibition (see below). As such, the effects of DCT diuretics to increase HCO_3, phosphate, and urate excretion may vary, depending on the CA inhibiting potency of the

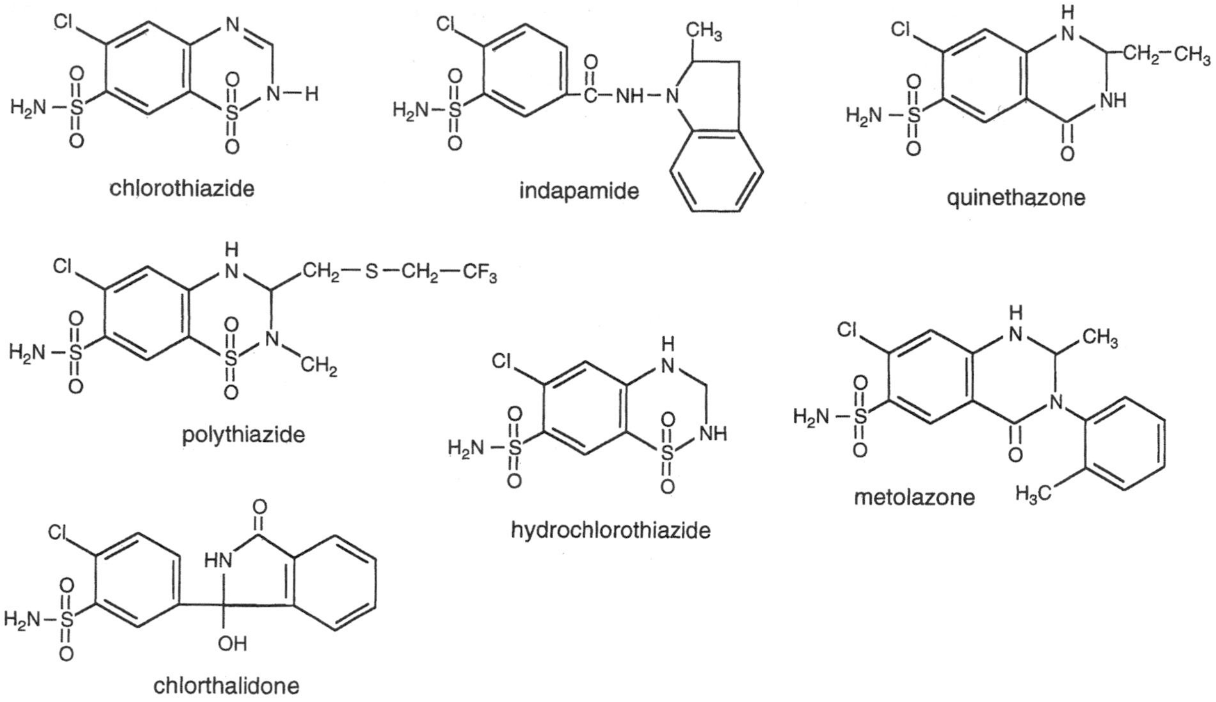

FIGURE 40.10 Structures of DCT diuretics.

DCT diuretic. Chronically, as contraction of the ECF volume occurs, uric acid excretion declines and hyperuricemia can occur. Further, any initial excretion of bicarbonaturia ceases, whereas continuing losses of chloride without bicarbonate and ECF volume contraction may lead to metabolic alkalosis. In contrast to loop and proximally acting diuretics, DCT diuretics tend to reduce urinary calcium excretion. Although the effects on urinary calcium excretion can be variable during acute administration,[170] these drugs uniformly lead to calcium retention when administered chronically, and also lead to positive calcium balance in humans.[171]

DCT diuretics inhibit the clearance of solute-free water (C_{H2O}) when administered during water diuresis. This effect is similar to that of loop diuretics, and originally led to the mistaken inference that they act along the thick ascending limb. In contrast to loop diuretics, however, DCT diuretics do not limit free water reabsorption during antidiuresis.

Mechanism of Action

Na AND WATER TRANSPORT IN THE PROXIMAL TUBULE

DCT diuretics are related chemically to CA inhibitors, and most retain significant CA-inhibiting potential. As discussed above, CA inhibitors interfere indirectly with the activity of NHE3 in the proximal tubule. Although this effect of DCT diuretics may be useful when these drugs are administered acutely (as during intravenous chlorothiazide administration), it probably contributes little to the overall natriuresis during chronic use. Yet this effect may play a role in the tendency for DCT diuretics to reduce the GFR and activate the TGF mechanism.[18] The relative CA inhibiting potency (shown in parentheses, compared with hydrochlorothiazide) of some commonly used DCT diuretics is chlorthalidone (67) >benthiazide (50) >polythiazide (40) >chlorothiazide (14) >hydrochlorothiazide (1) >bendroflumethiazide (0.07).[172]

NaCl ABSORPTION IN THE DISTAL NEPHRON

The predominant site at which DCT diuretics inhibit ion transport is the DCT. Although clearance studies had identified one site of thiazide action as the cortical diluting segment, and a second site as the proximal tubule, micropuncture studies pinpointed the primary site of action as the superficial "distal tubule".[173] This region of the nephron, which lies between the macula densa and the confluence with another nephron to form the cortical collecting duct, is morphologically heterogenous. It comprises a short stretch of post macula densa thick ascending limb, the DCT, the connecting tubule, and the initial portion of the cortical collecting duct. When this morphological heterogeneity became evident, experiments were designed to determine the site of thiazide action more precisely. Microperfusion experiments in rats indicated that thiazide diuretics inhibit Na and Cl transport along the "early" portion of the distal tubule,[174,175] a segment known to contain predominantly DCT cells.[176]

Although microperfusion data from rats indicated that thiazide diuretics inhibit Na transport in the DCT, the transition along the distal nephron segments in rats is gradual. For several years, therefore, it was impossible to attribute thiazide-sensitive Na-Cl transport to a specific cell type in the rat. In contrast, rabbit distal nephron segments have abrupt transitions. *In vitro* studies suggested that thiazide-sensitive Na-Cl co-transport is present in connecting tubules instead of DCTs,[177,178] but Velázquez and Greger obtained indirect evidence for thiazide-sensitive transport in rabbit DCTs.[179] Molecular cloning[180] permitted definitive identification of DCT cells as the only sites of thiazide-sensitive Na-Cl co-transporter expression in both rat and rabbit.[181–183] Friedman and colleagues developed a clonal cell line from immunodissected mouse thick ascending limb and DCT cells that expresses thiazide-sensitive transport.[184] Molecular studies identified the DCT as the site of thiazide-sensitive Na-Cl co-transport in this species, as well.[185]

In 1984, Velázquez and colleagues reported the mutual dependence of Na and Cl transport in the superficial rat distal tubule.[186] The same year, Stokes reported evidence that a directly-coupled thiazide-sensitive Na-Cl co-transporter is expressed in the urinary bladder of the Winter Flounder.[187] Gamba et al. cloned this protein[180] and detected homologous mRNA in mammalian kidney. The same group cloned a rat form of the thiazide-sensitive Na-Cl co-transporter.[188] Mouse, human, and rabbit forms were cloned shortly thereafter;[189–191] the gene is *SLC12A3*; it is a member of the cation-chloride co-transporter family, which includes NKCC1 and NKCC2. This transport protein was previously termed the TSC (thiazide-sensitive co-transporter), and the NCCT (sodium chloride co-transporter), but most investigators prefer the term NCC (sodium chloride co-transporter), for its analogy with NKCC. At the molecular level, the NCC is expressed only by DCT cells in all mammalian species examined to date. In humans, rats, and mice, expression of NCC also extends into a transitional segment, referred to as the "late" DCT or DCT-2, which shares properties of the distal convoluted and connecting tubules.[181,185]

Evidence for thiazide action in other nephron segments has also been obtained, however. *In vivo* catheterization experiments demonstrated a component of thiazide-sensitive Na transport in medullary collecting tubules of rats.[192] Some,[193] but not other[194] investigators have detected thiazide-sensitive Na-Cl transport in rat cortical collecting ducts perfused *in vitro*. In those experiments, pretreatment of animals with mineralocorticoid hormones was necessary to elicit the thiazide-

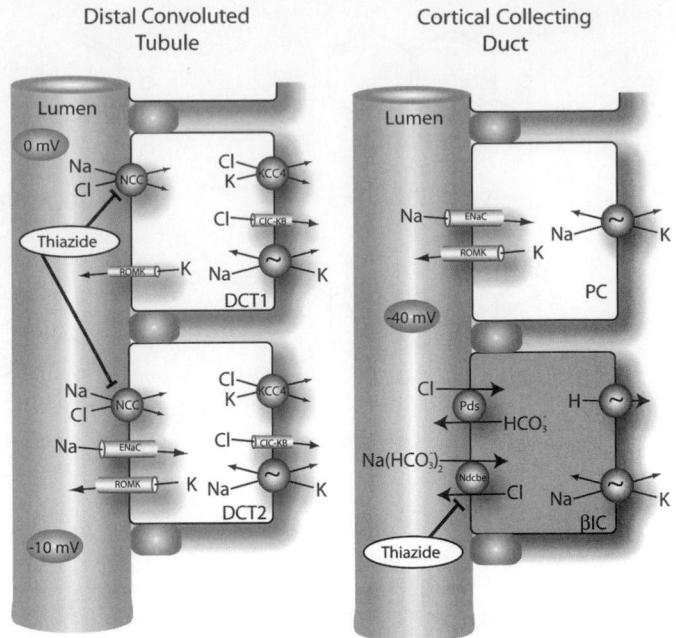

FIGURE 40.11   Mechanisms of thiazide diuretics. The left panel shows the mechanism of action of thiazide diuretics in the DCT. Two types of DCT cells have been identified; referred to here as DCT1 and DCT2. Na and Cl are reabsorbed across the apical membrane of DCT1 cells only via the thiazide-sensitive Na-Cl co-transporter. This transport protein is also expressed by DCT2 cells, where Na can also cross through the epithelial Na channel, ENaC (see text for details). Thus, the transepithelial voltage along the DCT-1 is near to 0 mV, whereas it is lumen-negative along the DCT-2. The right panel shows recently established mechanisms of action of thiazide diuretics along the collecting duct, in the presence of aldosterone stimulation. Here Na is reabsorbed in exchange for K by principal cells (PC), but in beta type intercalated cells (βIC) Na reabsorption occurs via a Na-dependent chloride bicarbonate exchanger (Ndcbe). This occurs in parallel with the action of pendrin (Pds) to achieve net NaCl reabsorption. The Ndcbe appears to be sensitive to thiazide diuretics.

sensitive Na and Cl transport. Eladari and colleagues[195] detected an effect of DCT diuretics on NaCl excretion in NCC knockout mice; these mice lack NCC entirely, and therefore the observed effect must be related to NCC-independent pathways. They also found that collecting ducts from animals exposed to aldosterone reabsorbed Na and Cl in a thiazide-sensitive manner. They went on to show that this transport was dependent on the Na-dependent chloride bicarbonate transporter (NDCBE) and on pendrin (SLC26A4), transport proteins expressed by intercalated cells. While this work deserves verification, it strongly suggests that DCT diuretics may have important effects on net NaCl transport within segments other than the DCT. A model of NaCl transport by DCT cells and a proposed model for NaCl transport by intercalated cells in the collecting duct are shown in Figure 40.11.

Like loop diuretics, DCT diuretics, including the thiazides, are organic anions that bind to the transport protein from the luminal surface. Results of studies to determine the mechanism by which DCT diuretics interact with the transport protein have varied, depending on the methods employed, and in a manner that resembles those described above concerning loop diuretics and NKCC. Before the transport protein was identified at the molecular level, Fanestil and colleagues showed that [^{3}H] metolazone binds avidly to kidney membrane proteins; its binding is inhibited competitively by Cl^-, suggesting that Cl^- and diuretic compete for the same binding site.[196,197] These results are reminiscent of those that utilized [^{3}H] bumetanide to study properties of the NKCC proteins and were used to develop a kinetic model for the NCC.[198] More recently, Gamba and colleagues have expressed chimeras of the NCC in *Xenopus* oocytes and determined thiazide affinity based on transport inhibition. The results suggest a more complicated picture. They conclude that thiazide diuretic affinity is conferred by transmembrane segments 8–12, whereas transmembrane segments 1–7 affect chloride affinity. Both segments are involved in determining Na$^+$ affinity.[199] These data suggest that that the affinity of thiazide diuretics for binding to the transport protein is in a region distinct from that which participates in Cl^- transport. As was the case for NKCC, however, it seems likely that the recent data concerning the crystal structure of APC transporters, coupled with molecular modeling, will provide new information concerning potential binding sites that can then be tested empirically.[73]

Calcium and Magnesium Transport

When administered chronically, DCT diuretics reduce calcium excretion. This effect has been utilized clinically to reduce the risk of recurrent calcium nephrolithiasis (see below). As noted above, acute administration of DCT diuretics has a variable effect on calcium excretion, sometimes leading to increases in calcium excretion. This probably reflects the CA-inhibiting capacity of these drugs, because CA inhibitors increase urinary calcium excretion acutely. Ca reabsorption by proximal tubules is functionally coupled to sodium reabsorption (see Figure 40.12); drugs that inhibit proximal Na reabsorption also inhibit proximal calcium reabsorption. During chronic treatment, however, the filtered calcium-load decreases, owing to the hemodynamic effects discussed below, and the proximal calcium reabsorption increases, owing to ECF volume contraction.

Mechanisms and sites responsible for the hypocalciuric effects of DCT diuretics have been quite controversial.[200] Early micropuncture and microperfusion studies showed that DCT diuretics stimulate Ca reabsorption along the DCT costanzo.[201,202] Three potential

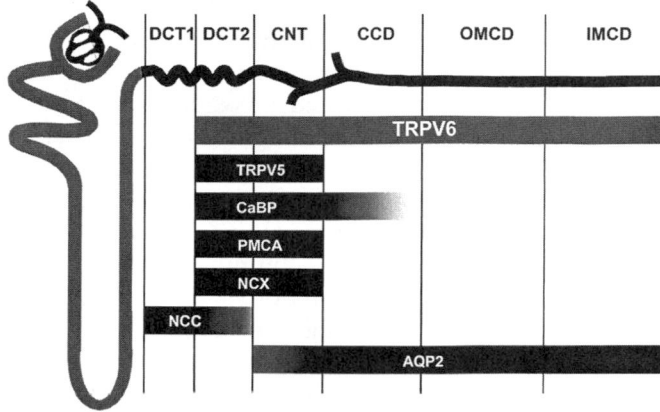

	Reabsorption					
	Proximal	TAL	DCT1	DCT2	CNT	Exc
CAI	↓	↔	↔	↓	↓	↑*
Loop	↑	↓	↔	↓	↓	↑*
DCT	↑	?↑	↔	↑	↑	↓↓
K-sparing	↔	↔	↔	↔	↑	↓

FIGURE 40.12 **Summary of diuretic effects on calcium excretion and sites of calcium transport protein expression.** Top panel: Effects of diuretics, including carbonic anhydrase inhibitors (CAI), loop diuretics (Loop), distal convoluted tubule diuretics (DCT), and K-sparing diuretics on calcium reabsorption along the proximal tubule, the thick ascending limb (TAL), the distal convoluted tubule (segments 1, DCT1, and 2, DCT2), and connecting tubule (CNT). Also shown are effects of these diuretics on urinary excretion (Exc). As noted by *, effects of CAI and loop diuretics to increase urinary calcium excretion may be inhibited when moderate depletion of the ECF volume increases reabsorption further along the proximal tubule. CAIs have been shown to reduce the abundance of TRPV5, as discussed in text. Effects of DCT diuretics on transport along TAL are speculative.[212] Bottom panel: Sites of expression of calcium-transporting proteins, including TRPV5 and -6, the calcium-binding proteins (CaBP), the plasma membrane Ca ATPase (PMCA), the Na/Ca exchanger (NCX). It also shows sites of NCC and AQP expression. Note the concurrence of expression within the DCT2 and CNT. *(Bottom panel from Nijenhuis, T., et al. (2003). J. Am. Soc. Nephrol. 14 (11); 2731–2740, with permission.)*

and non-redundant mechanisms were postulated to account for this.[203] First, blockade of luminal NaCl entry should reduce the tubule cell [Na$^+$] sufficiently to enhance the basolateral Na$^+$/Ca^{2+} exchange.[202] A low cellular Na concentration provides part of the driving force for basolateral calcium exit via the 3Na/Ca exchanger. Second, thiazides reduce cell [Cl^-] concentration, which should hyperpolarize the membrane voltage (making the interior of the cell more negative, electrically). Hyperpolarization should enhance calcium absorption, because the 3Na/Ca exchanger is electrogenic, so transport (in the reabsorptive direction) should be stimulated, and the transient receptor potential channel subfamily V, member 5 (TRPV5) channel, which is expressed at the apical membrane of DCT and connecting tubule cells, may be stimulated.[204,205]

More recently, the role of proximal tubular processes has been re-emphasized. In one study[206] thiazides were found to reduce Ca^2 excretion, even when the major calcium reabsorptive pathway of the distal nephron, TRPV5, was deleted genetically. TRPV5 deletion produced a marked rise in urinary calcium excretion at baseline, but hydrochlorothiazide still reduced urine calcium excretion in these animals, albeit to levels which were quite high. A prominent role for ECF volume contraction and enhanced proximal reabsorption is consistent with older data suggesting that thiazides stimulate proximal reabsorption of Ca^2.[207] Yet, there are several reasons to consider that a distal effect also contributes importantly. First, HCTZ induced a profound hypocalciuria in parvalbumin knockout mice, without increasing NaCl excretion.[208] This argues that ECF volume depletion is not a prerequisite for DCT diuretic-induced hypocalciuria. Second, saline infusion does not normalize urinary calcium excretion, either in humans with Gitelman syndrome,[209] in whom NCC is dysfunctional or in mice with the kinase SPAK deleted, in whom the abundance and phosphorylation of NCC is missing.[210] One difference may be related to species and dose. Animals such as the TRPV5 knockout animals, often display evidence of marked ECF volume-depletion in response to thiazide treatment (as indicated by hemoconcentration and weight loss), whereas ECF volume, at least at steady-state, is typically normal in people treated with DCT diuretics clinically. Most recently, it was shown that individuals with Gitelman syndrome have evidence of activated NaCl transport along the TAL.[211] It has been suggested on this basis that increased solute transport along the TAL might then contribute to increased calcium reabsorption there, as transepithelial voltage should vary directly with solute transport.[212]

DCT diuretics also increase urinary magnesium excretion when administered chronically, and can cause hypomagnesemia,[213,214] although the acute effects of DCT diuretics are more variable. Magnesium transport across the apical membrane of DCT cells is mediated, largely, by the transient receptor potential channel, TRPM6.[215] Chronic treatment of rats with hydrochlorothiazide reduced the abundance of this transport protein, a finding that is mimicked by genetic disruption of the NCC.[206] Thus, thiazides may induce magnesium-wasting, at least in part, by reducing the abundance of the apical magnesium channel. These data are consistent with findings from NCC knockout animals, and from results of chronic thiazide treatment of rats. In NCC knockout animals, the DCT1 is atrophic,[216] an effect that appears to be mimicked by chronic thiazide infusion.[217] Inasmuch as this segment

normally expresses TRPM6 at high levels, such atrophy may explain the reduced TRPM6 expression and magnesium-wasting. This finding, however, may also account for the relatively mild effects of DCT diuretics on magnesium homeostasis in humans. The effects of DCT diuretics to cause apoptosis and atrophy of parts of the DCT may be a species-specific phenomenon[218]; thiazide treatment of humans has not been reported to cause substantial tubule disruption.

Other effects of DCT diuretics have been suggested to contribute to magnesium-wasting. Dai et al. proposed that magnesium is transported across the apical membrane of DCT cells by a hyperpolarization-activated magnesium channel.[219] They found that DCT diuretics stimulated magnesium uptake into DCT cells by reducing the intracellular activity of chloride, hyperpolarizing the membrane voltage, and activating magnesium channels. These magnesium channels are sensitive to dihydropyridines, but appear to be distinct from calcium channels. Amiloride was found to have similar effects on magnesium uptake.[220] The importance of these channels in renal magnesium homeostasis, however, is unclear, as molecular and genetic studies have suggested the key role played by TRPM6.[221]

Quamme proposed that magnesium-wasting in Gitelman"s syndrome (and by analogy during DCT diuretic treatment) results from hypokalemia and from hyperaldosteronism.[222] Ellison suggested that distal magnesium transport is dependent on the transepithelial voltage. In this case, thiazide diuretics, by increasing aldosterone concentrations and blocking electroneutral Na reabsorption, would enhance the luminal negativity. This would inhibit magnesium reabsorption.[203] The mechanisms of drugs that cause distal depolarization, such as amiloride magnesium,[223–225] or that block mineralocorticoid receptors (MR), such as spironolactone,[226,227] remain to be defined.

Renal Hemodynamics

DCT diuretics increase renal vascular resistance and decrease the GFR when given acutely. Okusa et al.[18] showed that intravenous chlorothiazide reduced the GFR by 16% when measured as whole kidney clearance or by micropuncture of a superficial distal tubule. In contrast, however, when flow to the macula densa was blocked and the SNGFR was measured by micropuncture of a proximal tubule, intravenous chlorothiazide had no effect on GFR. These data indicate that diuretic-induced stimulation of the TGF system mediates the effect of DCT diuretics on GFR; DCT diuretics are known to increase the concentration of Na in luminal fluid entering the superficial distal tubule. It is assumed that a change in the tubule fluid ion concentration mediates this effect.

During chronic treatment with DCT diuretics, contraction of the ECF volume develops, thereby increasing solute and water reabsorption by the proximal tubule. This effect reduces the distal Na delivery to levels that are lower than under control conditions. In view of the fact that the initial suppression of GFR resulted from TGF, initiated by distal NaCl delivery, the GFR usually returns close to control values during chronic treatment with DCT diuretics.[228,229] Thus, when used chronically, DCT diuretics lead to a state of very mild ECF volume contraction, increased fractional proximal reabsorption, and relatively preserved glomerular filtration.

When administered acutely, the effect of DCT diuretics on renin secretion is variable. If urinary NaCl losses are replaced, these drugs tend to suppress renin secretion, probably by increasing NaCl delivery to the macula densa.[18] In contrast, during chronic administration, renin secretion increases both because solute delivery to the macula densa declines, and because volume-depletion activates the vascular mechanism for renin secretion.[102]

Pharmacokinetics

DCT diuretics are organic anions that circulate in a highly protein-bound state. As with loop diuretics, the amount reaching the tubule fluid by filtration across the glomerular basement membrane is small; the predominant route of entry into tubule fluid is by secretion via the organic anion secretory pathway in the proximal tubule. DCT diuretics are rapidly absorbed, reaching peak concentrations within 1.5 to 4 hours.[3] The amount of administered drug that reaches the urine varies greatly (for a review see [3]), as does the half-life. Short-acting DCT diuretics include bendroflumethiazide, hydrochlorothiazide, tizolemide, and trichlormethiazide. Medium-acting DCT diuretics include chlorothiazide, hydroflumethiazide, indapamide, and mefruside. Long-acting DCT diuretics include chlorthalidone, metolazone, and polythiazide.[3] The clinical effects of the differences in half-life are increasingly being appreciated. The incidence of hypokalemia may be higher in patients taking the longer-acting drugs such as chlorthalidone,[149,230] but it also appears that longer-acting drugs, and especially chlorthalidone, have greater antihypertensive efficacy.[231]

Clinical Use

Indications for the use of DCT diuretics are listed in Table 40.3. Many details of DCT diuretic use are available in other reviews[2,55,232] and will not be discussed here. DCT diuretics are used most commonly to treat essential hypertension. Despite a great deal of recent debate about their potential complications in the setting of essential hypertension, DCT diuretics continue to be recommended as drugs of first choice in the treatment of hypertension.[233] DCT diuretics are also used commonly to treat edematous conditions, although they are frequently perceived as being less effective than loop diuretics. Although the maximal effect of loop diuretics to increase urinary Na, Cl, and water excretion is greater than that of DCT diuretics, Leary and colleagues have shown that the cumulative effects of DCT diuretics on urinary Na and Cl excretion are greater than those of once daily furosemide.[234] Although these studies were conducted in normal volunteers, they may extend to patients with mild cases of edema. In addition, DCT diuretics have proved useful to treat edematous patients who have become resistant to loop diuretics. In this case, the addition of a DCT diuretic to a regimen that includes a loop diuretic frequently increases urinary Na and Cl excretion dramatically (see below).

DCT diuretics have become drugs of choice to reduce the recurrence of risk for kidney stones in patients with idiopathic hypercalciuria.[235] As noted, these drugs decrease urine calcium excretion, and in randomized controlled trials they significantly reduced recurrence rates of calcium stones by more than 50% during three-year periods, as compared with placebo. Long-acting agents like chlorthalidone and indapamide are effective with once-daily doses, whereas twice-daily doses are recommended for hydrochlorothiazide.

The ability of DCT diuretics to reduce urinary calcium excretion suggests that these drugs may prevent bone loss. Some,[236,237] but not all,[238,239] epidemiological studies suggested that DCT diuretics reduce the risk of hip fracture and osteoporosis. Clinical trials have confirmed that thiazide diuretics reduce the loss of cortical bone and may prevent hip fracture, although the effect seems modest, and does not persist once the drug has been discontinued.[240–242]

DCT diuretics are also employed to treat nephrogenic diabetes insipidus, causing a paradoxical decrease in urinary volume flow rate. This action of DCT diuretics results from the combination of actions. The best-studied effects include the induction of mild ECF volume contraction, owing to diuretic-induced natriuresis, suppression of GFR, owing largely to diuretic-induced activation of the TGF, and reduced distal water delivery. Such a mechanism would require depletion of the ECF volume, a requirement that has been documented in several studies.[229,243] The human DCT, like the thick ascending limb, is nearly impermeable to water.[244] Solute reabsorption by the thiazide-sensitive Na-Cl co-transporter therefore contributes directly to urinary dilution; thus, blocking Na-Cl co-transport reduces urinary diluting capacity. More recently, DCT diuretics have been shown to alter the abundance of water and salt transport pathways in the distal nephron. Kim and colleagues used a rat model of lithium-induced diabetes insipidus. They showed a lithium-induced decrease in aquaporin expression that could be reversed, partially, by DCT diuretics.[245] Another report showed that DCT diuretics enhance water absorption in IMCD from normal rats (in the absence of ADH) and from Brattleboro rats, and that HCTZ-stimulated water permeability was blocked partially by PGE_2.[246]

Adverse Effects

Electrolyte disorders, such as hypokalemia, hyponatremia, and hypomagnesemia, are common side-effects of DCT diuretics. A measurable fall in serum K concentration is nearly universal in patients given DCT diuretics, but most patients do not become frankly hypokalemic.[230] In the Allhat study, the largest controlled antihypertensive trial, mean plasma K concentrations were 0.3 mM lower in patients randomized to cholorthalidone, compared with amoldipine (which has little effect on K metabolism). The clinical significance of diuretic-induced hypokalemia continues to be debated.[247,248] Unlike the loop diuretics, DCT diuretics do not influence K transport directly.[249,250] Instead, they increase K excretion indirectly. DCT diuretics increase tubule fluid flow in the connecting tubule and collecting duct, the predominant sites of K secretion along the nephron. Increased flow stimulates K secretion both via flow-dependent potassium channels[152] and by diluting luminal potassium.[251] In addition, DCT diuretic-induced ECF volume contraction activates the renin—angiotensin—aldosterone system, further stimulating K secretion. Evidence for the central role of aldosterone in diuretic-induced hypokalemia includes the observation that hypokalemia is somewhat more common during treatment with long-acting DCT diuretics, such as chlorthalidone, than with short-acting DCT diuretics, such as hydrochlorothiazide or with the very-short-acting loop diuretics.[149] Another reason that DCT diuretics may produce more potassium-wasting than loop diuretics is the differences in effects on calcium transport. As discussed above, loop diuretics inhibit calcium transport by the thick ascending limb, increasing distal calcium delivery. In contrast, DCT diuretics stimulate calcium transport, reducing calcium delivery to sites of potassium secretion. Okusa and colleagues[252,253] showed that high luminal concentrations of calcium inhibit ENaC in the distal nephron, thereby inhibiting potassium secretion. DCT diuretics also increase urinary magnesium excretion and can lead to hypomagnesemia, as discussed above. Hypomagnesemia may cause or contribute to the hypokalemia observed under these conditions.[254] Some

studies suggest that maintenance magnesium therapy can prevent or attenuate the development of hypokalemia,[255,256] but this has not been supported universally.

Diuretics have been reported to contribute to more than 50% of all hospitalizations for serious hyponatremia. Hyponatremia is especially common during treatment with DCT diuretics,[257] compared with other classes of diuretics, and the disorder is potentially life-threatening. Several factors contribute to DCT diuretic-induced hyponatremia. First, as discussed above, DCT diuretics inhibit solute transport in the terminal portion of the "diluting segment," the DCT. This impairs the ability to excrete free water. Second, DCT diuretics can reduce the GFR, primarily by activating the TGF system. This limits solute delivery to the diluting segment, and impairs free water clearance. Third, DCT diuretics lead to volume-contraction, which increases proximal tubule solute and water reabsorption, further restricting delivery to the "diluting segment." Fourth, hyponatremia has been correlated with the development of hypokalemia in patients receiving DCT diuretics,[258] suggesting total cation depletion. Finally, susceptible patients may be stimulated to consume water during therapy with DCT diuretics; although the mechanisms are unclear, this may contribute importantly to the sudden appearance of hyponatremia that can occur during DCT diuretic therapy. Of note, one report suggests that patients who are predisposed to develop hyponatremia during treatment with DCT diuretics will demonstrate an acute decline in serum sodium concentration in response to a single dose of the drug.[259] Recent studies suggest that female gender, advanced age, and low body mass are risk factors for thiazide-induced hyponatremia.[260,261]

DCT diuretics frequently cause metabolic alkalosis. The mechanisms are similar to those described above for loop diuretics, except that DCT diuretics do not stimulate Na/H exchange in the TAL.

DCT diuretics cause several disturbances of endocrine glands. Glucose intolerance has been a recognized complication of DCT diuretic use since the 1950s. This complication appears to be dose-related.[262,263] The pathogenesis of DCT diuretic-induced glucose intolerance remains unclear, but several factors have been suggested to contribute. First, diuretic-induced hypokalemia may alter insulin secretion by the pancreas, via effects on the membrane voltage of pancreatic β-cells. When hypokalemia was prevented by oral potassium supplementation, the insulin response to hyperglycemia normalized, suggesting an important role for hypokalemia.[264] Hypokalemia may also interfere with insulin-mediated glucose uptake by muscle, but most patients demonstrate relatively normal insulin sensitivity.[265] Yet others have suggested that hypokalemia is not likely the only factor, as individuals with familial

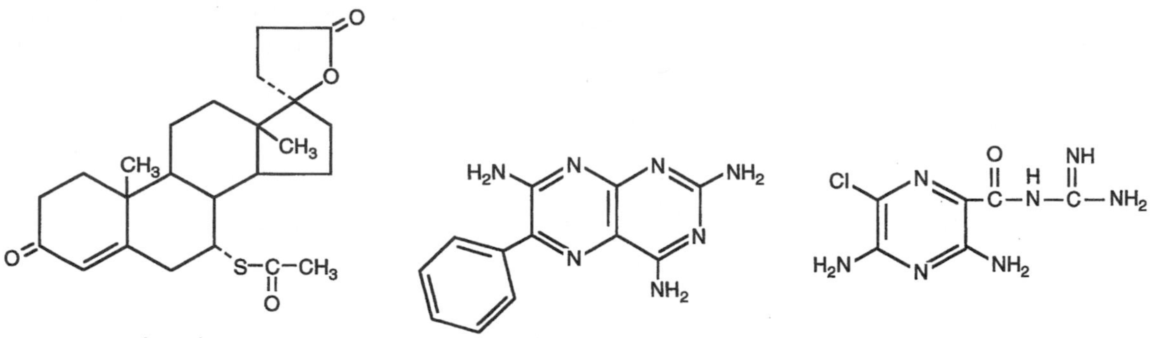

FIGURE 40.13   Structure of collecting duct diuretics.

hyperkalemic hypertension who are treated with DCT diuretics can manifest impaired glucose tolerance, despite normal-to-high serum potassium.[218] Other factors may contribute to glucose intolerance as well. Volume-depletion may stimulate catecholamine secretion, but volume-depletion during therapy with DCT diuretics is usually very mild. DCT diuretics directly activate calcium-activated potassium channels that are expressed by pancreatic β-cells, perhaps contributing to the hyperglycemia.[266] Activation of these channels is known to inhibit insulin secretion.

DCT diuretics increase levels of total cholesterol, total triglyceride, and LDL cholesterol. These drugs reduce the HDL.[265] Definitive information about the mechanisms by which DCT diuretics alter lipid metabolism is not available, but many of the mechanisms that affect glucose homeostasis have been suggested to contribute. Hyperlipidemia, like hyperglycemia, is a dose-related side-effect, and one that wanes with chronic diuretic use. In several recent large clinical studies, the effect of low-dose DCT diuretic treatment on serum LDL was not significantly different from placebo.[267] In the ALLHAT study, mean cholesterol concentrations were higher in the group randomized to chlorthalidone, but the absolute differences at two and four years were 2–3 mg/dl.

POTASSIUM-SPARING DIURETICS

Diuretic drugs that act primarily along the aldosterone-sensitive distal nephron (which includes the DCT2, the connecting tubule, and the collecting duct) comprise three pharmacologically distinct groups: aldosterone antagonists (spironolactone); pteridines (triamterene); and pyrazinoylguanidines (amiloride, see Figure 40.13). The site of action for all diuretics of this class is the segment of the nephron that begins within the DCT. It has been recognized increasingly

that the DCT2 and the connecting tubule play especially important roles in modulating renal Na and K balance in response to aldosterone.[268] Because of the ability to minimize the normal tendency of diuretic drugs to increase potassium excretion, these drugs are considered "potassium-sparing." Acute diuretic activity is weak, because fractional sodium reabsorption in the collecting tubule usually does not exceed 3% of the filtered load. For this reason, potassium-sparing drugs are ordinarily used in combination with thiazides or loop diuretics, often in a single preparation, to restrict potassium losses and sometimes augment diuretic action. However, in certain conditions potassium-sparing diuretics are used as first line agents (see Table 40.2). For example, spironolactone is used in the treatment of edema in patients with cirrhosis,[269] and amiloride or triamterene is used as a first line treatment of Liddle's syndrome.[270]

Urinary Electrolyte Excretion

Amiloride, triamterene, and spironolactone are weak natriuretic agents (see Table 40.1). Their major effect is to diminish potassium excretion. Additionally, these three diuretic agents decrease hydrogen ion secretion by the ASDN. Evidence that spironolactone decreases hydrogen ion excretion comes from the finding of metabolic acidosis associated with mineralocorticoid deficiency, and the finding that spironolactone produces metabolic acidosis in patients with cirrhosis who have mineralocorticoid excess. In rats, the administration of amiloride and triamterene has been shown to inhibit urinary acidification. A common mechanism is likely to be involved in mediating the effects of all three diuretic agents on hydrogen ion secretion. These drugs reduce the voltage across the distal epithelium, which is oriented in the lumen-negative direction; they thus decrease the gradient for hydrogen ion secretion (see Figure 40.14).

Distal Convoluted Tubule

Connecting & Collecting Tubule

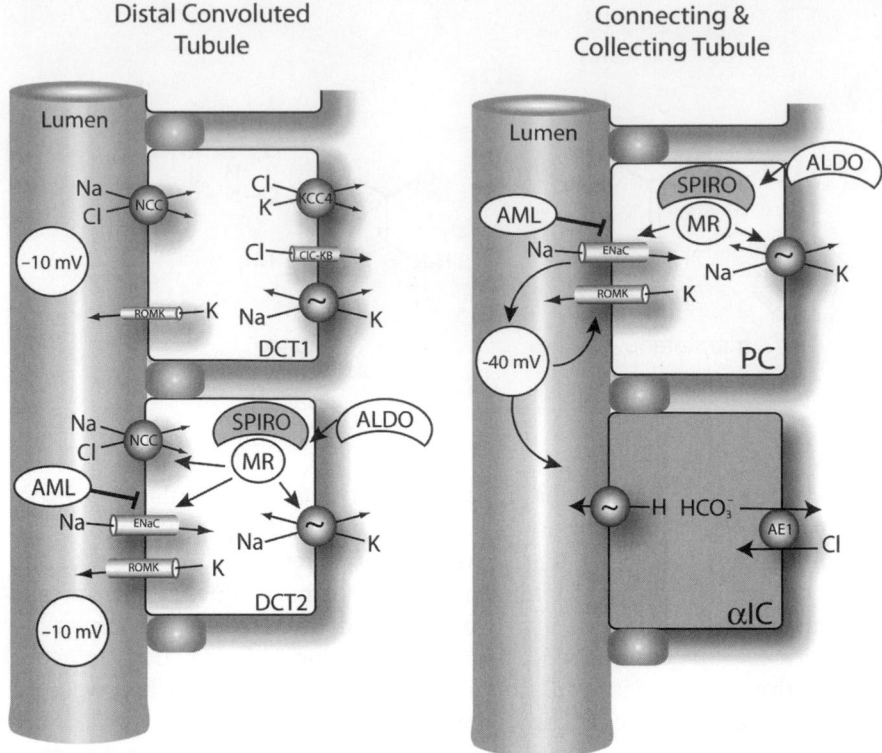

FIGURE 40.14 **Mechanisms of potassium-sparing diuretics.** Amiloride (AML, and triamterene, not shown) block ENaC directly, as discussed in the text. This occurs in the DCT2 and in the connecting and collecting tubules. Blockade reduces the magnitude of the transepithelial voltage, which secondarily inhibits K secretion and H secretion. Spironolactone (and eplerenone, not shown) act by blocking mineralocorticoid receptors (MR), impeding aldosterone's (ALDO) ability to bind. These drugs, therefore, only act when aldosterone levels are elevated. DCT1 and DCT2 cells are shown (PC: principal cell; βIC: beta intercalated cell).

Clearance studies in rats have demonstrated that amiloride produces a decrease in calcium excretion.[202] In these studies, amiloride produced both a decrease in the calcium clearance/Na clearance ratio (C_{Ca}/C_{Na}), as well as a decrease in the fractional excretion of calcium. The effect of triamterene on clearance of calcium was less clear, although it did decrease the C_{Ca}/C_{Na} ratio. *In vivo* microperfusion of rat distal tubules demonstrated that the effect of chlorothiazide on calcium absorption was enhanced when amiloride was added, suggesting that amiloride also increased calcium absorption by the distal tubule.[175] Furthermore, *in vitro* perfusion of connecting tubules has shown that amiloride stimulates calcium absorption.[271] Amiloride is believed to stimulate calcium absorption through its ability to block sodium channels, thereby hyperpolarizing the apical membrane.[94] Hyperpolarization of the apical membrane stimulates calcium entry through epithelial calcium channels TRPV5 (see DCT diuretics, above). Amiloride has also been reported to reduce magnesium excretion,[214,272] and to prevent the development of hypomagesemia during therapy with a DCT diuretic (see above).

Mechanism of Action

The site of action of potassium-sparing diuretics is ASDN (see Figure 40.1 and above). The ASDN comprises the second part of the DCT, the DCT2, where amiloride-sensitive Na channels intermingle with NCC at the apical membrane.[176] It also includes the connecting tubule, a segment that may play the dominant role in regulating urinary K excretion. Finally, it comprises the cortical and medullary collecting tubules. The connecting and collecting tubules are composed of two cell types; although they appear to have separate functions, some information has suggested that the view that principal cells are responsible for the transport of sodium, potassium, and water, whereas intercalated cells are primarily responsible for the secretion of hydrogen or bicarbonate ions, is oversimplified. The apical membrane of principal cells expresses separate channels that permit selective conductive transport of sodium and potassium (Figure 40.14). The mechanism by which sodium reabsorption occurs is through conductive sodium channels (for a review see [273]). The low intracellular sodium concentration as a result of the basolateral Na,K-ATPase generates a favorable electrochemical gradient for sodium entry through sodium channels. Because sodium channels are present only in the apical membrane of principal cells, sodium conductance depolarizes the apical membrane, resulting in an asymmetric voltage profile across the cell. This effect produces a lumen-negative transepithelial potential difference. The lumen-negative potential difference, together with a high intracellular-to-lumen potassium concentration gradient, provides the driving force for potassium secretion.

Sodium is the principal extracellular cation whose conductance across the principal cell of the collecting duct is amiloride-sensitive, and is regulated by the activity and apical membrane expression of the epithelial sodium channel (ENaC).[274,275] The functional channel comprises at least three homologous subunits, α, β, γ. The biophysical characteristics of ENaC include a low single channel conductance of ~ 5 pS, long open and closed times, a high Na^+ to K^+ selectivity ratio of $>100:1$, and it is inhibited by submicromolar concentrations of amiloride.[276] Although inferential work suggested several different stoichiometries,[277,278] the crystal structure of the structurally-related acid sensing channel, ASIC, provides strong support for a heterotrimeric model, in which one of each subunit is present.[279,280,283]

Although the crystal structure should permit clearer insights into the site of ENaC blockade by amiloride, a great deal of information has already accumulated. Amiloride and other large cations block apical Na^+ channels in a voltage-dependent manner, suggesting that amiloride block occurs within the pore of these channels.[281] Schild et al.[282] found that mutations at equivalent positions in all three subunits reduce the efficacy of amiloride block. When cysteine residues were introduced at these sites, they were susceptible to chemical modification by methanethiosulfonate compounds from the extracellular space,[283] suggesting that amiloride gains entry to and binds within the channel pore. If this is confirmed, it is strikingly similar to the new model for loop diuretic binding to NKCC1.[73]

Kleyman and colleagues[283] describe two potential models for ENaC structure. Mutation of sites within the proposed selectivity tract and an upstream site one helical turn away alters the efficacy of amiloride block. In one model, these sites face the pore lumen, but lie on the cytosolic side of the most constricted part. The selectivity tract lies one turn further toward the cytosol. In the other model, these sites lie near the extracellular entry of the most constricted part of the pore. It was suggested that the requirement for amiloride addition to the extracellular side of the membrane for inhibition is more consistent with the latter configuration, but these issues should be clarified now that relevant crystal structures are becoming available.

This group further suggested that the glycines at β525 and γ537 (the greek letters correspond to the ENaC subunits), and the tolerance of a wide variety of substitutions for serine α583, indicate that these residues probably do not interact directly with amiloride, but instead affect the shape of the amiloride-binding pocket. They proposed a model for amiloride-binding where the pyrazine ring is positioned at the αSer583/βGly525/γGly537 site, and the guanidinium group is positioned at the outer mouth of the selectivity tract.[284]

As the ASIC crystal structure is not in the open-state likely to bind to the diuretic, it is not surprising that the pore models do not allow for amiloride to interact with the channel at these sites, and that neither model is fully consistent with functional data. Both models are based on structures of ASIC1 in a nonconducting state, and amiloride blocks ENaC in the open state. It is likely, however, that progress in unraveling what has been a difficult question concerning the mechanisms of amiloride association with the channel will now be more rapid, and should resolve these confusing issues.

The amount of sodium and potassium present in the final urine is tightly controlled by aldosterone action on cells of the ASDN. Extensive studies have demonstrated that, in epithelia, aldosterone produces an early increase in sodium conductance,[285,286] followed by a sustained increase in transepithelial sodium transport. As a result, transepithelial sodium transport is increased, an effect that depolarizes the apical membrane (see Figure 40.14). An increase in the lumen negative potential in turn enhances potassium secretion through conductive potassium channels located in the apical membrane. The cellular mechanisms that are responsible for these events have been extensively studied and reviewed.[287,288] The effects of aldosterone are largely mediated through a classical genomic effect through action on MR. Nongenomic actions in extrarenal tissues are likely to occur, but appear less prominent in the kidney.[287–289] Genomic actions of aldosterone are initiated by penetration of the hormone through the basolateral membrane of principal cells and attachment to a cytosolic MR, a heterotrimeric 8–9 s complex of proteins. This receptor complex includes the steroid-binding protein and heat shock proteins (HSP). Binding of aldosterone to this complex stimulates the release of HSPs, leading to the translocation of the receptor-aldosterone complex to the nucleus. The function of HSPs is not clear. It is thought that they facilitate anchoring of unbound steroid receptors to the cytoskeleton, maintaining a high-affinity conformation.[290] Evidence also indicates that released HSP90 stimulates calcineurin, a protein phosphatase that regulates sodium transport, in a transcription-independent process.[291] This binding and translocation sequence leads to production of proteins called *aldosterone-induced proteins* (AIPs)[292] that regulate sodium flux.[293] These AIPs regulate channel activity.[292,294] Although signaling pathways for aldosterone in the ASDN remain incompletely understood, a central role for serum and glucocorticoid-regulated kinase (sgk1) is generally inferred.[289] Sgk is regulated at the level of transcription by corticosteroids, including aldosterone,[295,296] and in turn is known to phosphorylate Nedd4 ubiquitin ligases.[297] Serum and glucocorticoid-regulated kinase modulates Nedd4–2-mediated inhibition of the epithelial Na$^+$ channel. Nedd4−2 phosphorylation induces serum and glucocorticoid-regulated kinase (SGK) ubiquitination and degradation,[298] and prolongs the surface expression and activity of ENac. The reader is referred to other chapters in these volumes for a more thorough discussion of aldosterone signaling.

SPIRONOLACTONE AND EPLERENONE

Spirolactones are compounds that have the principal effect of blocking aldosterone action.[299,300] One of these, spironolactone (Figure 40.13), is an analog of aldosterone that is extensively metabolized. Spironolactone is converted by deacylation to 7α-thiospironolactone or by diethioacetylation to canrenone.[300] The appearance of active metabolites means that the physiological effects of spironolactone outlast the half-life of the parent drug (see below). In the kidney, spironolactone and its metabolites enter target cells from the peritubular side, and compete for binding to cytosolic MRs. In studies using radiolabeled spironolactone or aldosterone, [^{3}H]-spironolactone-receptor complexes were found to be excluded from the nucleus. In contrast, [^{3}H]-aldosterone-receptor complexes were detected in the nucleus.[301] These results are consistent with the proposal that aldosterone antagonists block the translocation of MRs to the nucleus. The mechanism by which aldosterone antagonists block nuclear localization of antagonist-receptor complexes is not known, however, it has been suggested that they destabilize MRs, facilitating proteolysis.[302] As discussed previously MRs, like other steroid receptors, contain a steroid-binding unit associated with other cellular components including HSP90, in its inactive state. Steroid-binding produces dissociation of HSP90 from the steroid-binding unit, uncapping the DNA-binding sites. Spironolactone facilitates the release of HSP90, and in combination with rapid dissociation of ligand, could lead to degradation of the receptor.[302]

A newer aldosterone receptor antagonist, eplerenone, is also a competitive antagonist of the aldosterone receptor. Replacing the 17alpha-thoacetyl group of spironolactone with a carbomethoxy group confers improved selectivity for aldosterone receptors, and negligible activity at the cytochrome P450 enzyme,[303] but 10−20-fold lower affinity for its receptor.[304] Eplerenone has a slightly longer half-life of 3.5 hours compared to spironolactone, but it does not produce important metabolites; thus, the apparent effective half-life of eplerenone is shorter than that of spironolactone, in clinical use. *In vitro* receptor-binding studies have revealed that the affinity of eplerenone is approximately 10- to 20-fold less than the affinity of spironolactone for the MR.

Spironolactone induces a mild increase in sodium excretion (1−2%), and a decrease in potassium and hydrogen ion excretion.[305,306] Its effect depends on the presence of aldosterone, as spironolactone is ineffective in adrenalectomized animals, and in patients with Addison"s disease or patients on a high-salt diet. In cortical collecting tubules perfused *in vitro*, spironolactone added to the bath solution reduced the aldosterone-induced lumen-negative transepithelial voltage. By blocking sodium absorption in the collecting tubule, a decrease in lumen-negative potential reduces the driving force for passive sodium and hydrogen ion secretion (see Figure 40.14). It is likely that the mechanism of eplerenone action on Na and K transport along the ASDN is identical.

AMILORIDE AND TRIAMTERENE

Amiloride and triamterene (see Figure 40.13) differ structurally, but both are organic cations that use the same primary site of action (see Figure 40.14). Triamterene is an aminopteridine chemically related to folic acid, and amiloride is a pyrazinoylguanidine. Systemically administered amiloride results in an increase in sodium excretion and a decrease in potassium excretion.[151] Their actions on sodium and potassium transport, unlike spironolactone, are independent of aldosterone. Systemically administered amiloride produced a small increase in sodium excretion, and a much larger decrease in potassium excretion. Sampling of tubule fluid from the distal tubule demonstrated an inhibition of the normal rise in the tubule fluid-to-plasma potassium ratio. These results indicated that amiloride decreased distal tubule potassium secretion. Experiments employing *in vivo* microperfusion of distal tubules[250,307] and *in vitro* perfusion of isolated cortical collecting tubules[308,309] demonstrated that luminally administered amiloride reduced sodium absorption and potassium secretion. Similar results were obtained following *in vivo* microperfusion with benazamil,[253] a more potent amiloride analog that is not available for use clinically. The mechanism by which amiloride decreases potassium secretion is due to its effect in blocking sodium conductance in the apical membrane of distal tubule and collecting tubule cells (see Figure 40.14), thereby decreasing the electrochemical gradient for potassium secretion.

In high concentrations (>100 μM), amiloride interacts nonspecifically with different transporters, enzymes, and receptors, however, at concentrations of 0.05 to 0.5 μM, amiloride interacts specifically with sodium channels. Furthermore, aromatic substitutions on the guanidinium moiety render the molecule even more potent (IC$_{50}$ 10−20-fold lower than amiloride).[310,311]

Clearance and free-flow micropuncture studies using triamterene demonstrated results similar to studies with amiloride,[151] although the mechanism of action is not as clearly defined. In earlier studies of rabbit cortical collecting tubules perfused *in vitro*, triamterene produced a gradual, reversible inhibition of the potential difference after a latent period of 10 minutes, suggesting a mechanism different from amiloride. Recent studies, however, suggest that triamterene binds to the epithelial sodium channel, and thus has a mechanism of action similar to amiloride.[312]

Pharmacokinetics

Spironolactone is poorly soluble in aqueous fluids. Bioavailability of an oral dose is approximately 90% in some, but not all, commercial preparations. The drug is rapidly metabolized in the liver into a number of metabolites. Until recently, canrenone was thought to be the major metabolite of spironolactone.[299,313] This conclusion was based on fluorometric assays. Assays of spironolactone and its metabolites by the use of high performance liquid chromatography (HPLC), however, demonstrated that fluorometrically measured levels of canrenone overestimated true canrenone levels.[314] Using HPLC, the predominant metabolite, 7α-methylspironolactone,[315] is responsible for roughly 80% of the potassium-sparing effect. Spironolactone and its metabolites are extensively bound to plasma protein (98%). In normal volunteers, taking spironolactone (100 mg/day) for 15 days, the mean half-lives for spironolactone, canrenone, 7-thiomethylspironolactone, and 6β-hydroxy-7α-thiomethylspironolactone were 1.4, 16.5, 13.8, and 15 hours, respectively. Thus, although unmetabolized spironolactone is present in serum, it has a rapid elimination time. The onset of action is extremely slow, with peak response sometimes occurring 48 hours or more after the first dose; effects gradually wane over a period of 48 to 72 hours. Spironolactone is used in cirrhotic patients to induce a natriuresis. In these patients, pharmacokinetic studies indicate that the half-lives of spironolactone and its metabolites are increased. The half-lives for spironolactone, canrenone, 7α-thiomethylspironolactone, and 6β-hydroxy-7α-thiomethylspironolactone are 9, 58, 24, and 126 hours respectively.[316]

Less information concerning pharmacokinetics is available for amiloride and triamterene. Amiloride is rapidly absorbed, and reaches peak serum concentrations after approximately 4 hours. Its elimination half-life is 17−26 hours, with 40−60% appearing in the urine unchanged.[3] Both amiloride and triamterene are organic cations that are secreted into proximal tubule fluid by an organic cation transporter, in a manner analogous to secretion of loop and DCT diuretics by the organic anion transporter.

Clinical Use

The uses of potassium-sparing diuretics are broadening, as negative effects of aldosterone in human disease are discovered. Traditionally, an important indication for potassium-sparing diuretics is to prevent or attenuate K losses that are consequent to administration of DCT or loop diuretics.[317]

MR antagonists become effective natriuretics in patients with high circulating aldosterone levels, such as in primary (adrenal adenoma or bilateral adrenal hyperplasia)[318] or secondary hyperaldosteronism (congestive heart failure, cirrhosis, nephrotic syndrome). Spironolactone is especially appropriate for the treatment of cirrhosis with ascites, a condition invariably associated with secondary hyperaldosteronism. In comparison to loop or thiazide diuretics, spironolactone is equivalent or more effective.[319] The reason for this observation could be related to the differences in the mechanism of drug action, including the fact that MR antagonists do not require secretion by transporters to reach their sites of action. A combination of loop diuretic in addition to spironolactone is considered to be the best combination between safety and efficacy in cirrhotic patients with resistant edema (ratio of 40 mg furosemide to 100 mg spironolactone[320]).

Although its acute natriuretic action is weak, MR antagonists lower blood pressure and are often quite effective in the control of resistant hypertension.[321] Spironolactone or eplerenone is also indicated for the treatment of mineralocorticoid hypertension. Several controlled randomized studies have shown benefits of MR blockade on outcomes in patients with heart failure. A discussion of these indications is beyond the scope of this chapter, but it has been suggested that these beneficial effects are independent of effects of these drugs on the kidney.[322]

Triamterene or amiloride is generally used in combination with potassium-wasting diuretics (thiazide or loop diuretics), especially when maintenance of normal serum potassium concentrations is clinically important. In addition, amiloride (or triamterene) has also been used as initial therapy in potassium-wasting states, such as primary hyperaldosteronism,[323,324] Liddle's[325] or Gitelman's syndrome.[326] Amiloride has been used in the treatment of lithium-induced nephrogenic diabetes insipidus. The efficacy of amiloride in this disorder relates to the ability of amiloride to block collecting duct sodium channels, a pathway which lithium uses to gain entry into cells.[327]

Adverse Effects

The most serious adverse reaction encountered during therapy with spironolactone and eplerenone is hyperkalemia.[328] Serum potassium should be monitored periodically, even when the drug is administered with a potassium-wasting diuretic. Patients at highest risk are those with low GFRs, and those individuals who take potassium supplements concurrently. In patients with cirrhosis and ascites treated with spironolactone, hyperchloremic metabolic acidosis can develop independent of changes in renal function. Unwanted antiandrogenic and progestational side-effects of spironolactone include gynecomastia, decreased libido, and impotence in men. Women may develop menstrual irregularities, hirsutism or swelling and tenderness of the breast. These troublesome side-effects were the impetus for developing eplerenone. In subjects receiving eplerenone for heart failure, the incidence of gynecomastia and impotence among men was similar to placebo.[329] These differences in side-effects are likely related to eplerenone's greater selectivity for the MR versus androgen and progesterone receptors. Spironolactone-induced agranulocytosis has also been reported.[330]

Triamterene and amiloride may cause hyperkalemia. The risk of hyperkalemia is highest in patients with limited renal function (e.g., renal insufficiency, diabetes, and elderly patients). Additional complications included elevated blood urea nitrogen and uric acid, glucose intolerance, and GI disturbances. Triamterene induces crystalluria or cylinduria,[331] and may contribute to or initiate formation of renal stones[332] and AKI when combined with nonsteroidal anti-inflammatory agents.[333,334] The drugs are contraindicated in patients with hyperkalemia, individuals taking potassium supplements in any form, and in patients with severe renal failure with progressive oliguria.

AQUARETICS (VASOPRESSIN RECEPTOR ANTAGONISTS)

Urinary Electrolyte Excretion

Vasopressin-receptor antagonists are nonpeptide molecules that competitively inhibit one or more of the human vasopressin receptors V1a, V1b or V2. Conivaptan is a combined V1a/V2-receptor antagonist for intravenous use, whereas tolvaptan, mozavaptan, and lixivaptan are orally active V2-selective receptor antagonists. All of these agents cause a free water diuresis without appreciable natriuresis or kaliuresis, and they are therefore sometimes referred to as "aquaretics." This effect is mainly attributed to inhibition of the V2-receptor in the collecting duct, which prevents vasopressin from recruiting AQP2 water channels to increase water reabsorption. Therefore, vasopressin-receptor antagonists can be used to treat hypervolemic or euvolemic hyponatremia, in which increased vasopressin is considered "inappropriate."

Mechanism of Action

The effects of arginine vasopressin (AVP, also called antidiuretic hormone, ADH) are mediated by two major receptor subtypes: V_1- and V_2. V_1 receptors are expressed in many cell types, including vascular smooth muscle (V_{1a}) and adenohypophysis (V_{1b}). V_2-vasopressin receptors are expressed in kidney and seminal vesicles. V_2 receptors have been localized to principal cells of the connecting tubule, cortical and medullary collecting duct. Binding of AVP to V_2-vasopressin receptors in collecting duct cells results in water reabsorption. Many clinical disorders such as cirrhosis, congestive heart failure, and syndrome of inappropriate antidiuretic hormone secretion (SIADH) are associated with high levels of AVP that prevent appropriate water excretion, resulting in hyponatremia.

Nonpeptide vasopressin receptor antagonists (conivaptan and tolvaptan) are now available for clinical use in the United States; they are indicated to treat euvolemic and hypervolemic hyponatremia. Conivaptan is a benzazepine derivative and the first combined vasopressin V1aR/V2R antagonist.[335] This agent displaces a selective vasopressin V1aR antagonist in a dose-dependent manner from rat liver membranes; the IC_{50} was 2.2 ± 0.1 nmol/L. The agent also caused a concentration-dependent displacement of a vasopressin V2R antagonist from renal medullary membranes, and the IC_{50} of the binding affinity was 0.4 ± 0.1 nmol/L.[336] Oral conivaptan given for seven days in normotensive rats caused a dose-dependent aquaresis, with no effect on specific blood pressure.[337] When administered to healthy volunteers orally, conivaptan effects were observed after two hours including a seven-fold increase in the urinary flow rate, and a decrease in urinary osmolality from 600 mOsm/kg to <100 mOsm/kg. Plasma osmolality increased from 283 ± 1.3 mOsm/kg to 289 ± 1.7 mOsm/kg.[336]

Clinical Use

In double-blind, randomized, placebo-controlled clinical trials conivaptan was shown to increase serum Na concentrations in a variety of settings.[336] Although conivaptan was originally discovered as an orally active V1a/V2 antagonist, it was developed for intravenous application. In one study it was given intravenously by continuous infusion over four days at doses of 40 mg/day and 80 mg/day following a loading dose of 20 mg intravenously on the first day. During the study, patients adhered to fluid restriction of 2 L/day. In the group of patients receiving high-dose conivaptan (80 mg/day), the treatment increased the serum sodium concentration significantly from a baseline of 125 mmol/L to 134 mmol/L.[336] These data suggest that conivaptan is an efficient therapy of hyponatremia and is safe. Unfortunately, infusion side-effects, including infusion site reactions are quite common.

At present, some 20 clinical trials have tested these agents against placebo or conventional therapy in patients with liver cirrhosis, heart failure or hyponatremia secondary to SIADH.[338] In all trials, vasopressin-receptor angatonists effectively raised serum sodium and helped to correct hyponatremia. In addition, a positive effect on some secondary endpoints was observed, including improved mental condition and reductions in body weight, dyspnea, and ascites.[339–341] Unfortunately, these effects have not led to improvements in most hard endpoints. The Efficacy of Vasopressin Antagonist in Heart Failure Outcome Study with Tolvaptan (EVEREST), which included 4133 patients hospitalized for heart failure, did not show a beneficial effect on the primary outcomes of death or rehospitalization for heart failure.[339] Thus, vasopressin-receptor antagonists appear effective in the correction of hyponatremia, but have not yet shown an effect on primary outcomes.

GENERAL PRINCIPLES OF DIURETIC ACTION

When a diuretic drug (other than an aquaretic) is first administered to a normal individual, urinary sodium and chloride excretion rates increase. The magnitude of the increase is determined by the nature of the drug, the dose, the gastrointestinal absorption, the delivery to the kidney, entry into tubule fluid (for diuretics that act from the tubule lumen), and the physiological state of the individual. Except for diuretics that act predominantly in the proximal tubule, such as the CA inhibitors, the maximal natriuretic potency of a diuretic can be predicted from its site of action. Table 40.1 shows that loop diuretics can increase fractional Na excretion to 30%, DCT diuretics can increase it to 9%, and Na channel blockers can increase it to 3% of the filtered load. Because CA inhibitors enhance excretion of Na with bicarbonate rather than chloride, and because they induce adaptive processes that are described more fully below, the maximal natriuretic potency of CA inhibitors is much lower than would be predicted from their site of action. The dose–response curve for diuretic action has been best characterized for loop diuretics. In this case, the relationship is sigmoidal (see Figure 40.7), when the fractional Na excretion is plotted versus the urinary diuretic concentration.[136] Most diuretics act from the luminal surface. Therefore, the best external indicator of diuretic drug concentration at the active site is the urinary diuretic concentration.

The bioavailability of diuretic drugs varies widely, between classes of drugs, between different drugs of the same class, and even between days of the week with the same drug. The bioavailability of loop diuretics ranges from 10–100% (mean of 50% for furosemide, 80–100% for bumetanide and torsemide (see Table 40.2). Limited bioavailability can usually be overcome by appropriate dosing, but some drugs, such as furosemide, are variably absorbed, making precise titration difficult.[136] Although the bioavailability predicts that oral furosemide should be half as potent as intravenous furosemide, the relationship is not simple, and depends on the clinical state of the individual. For example, the amount of Na excreted during 24 hours is similar when furosemide is administered to a normal individual by mouth or by vein (see Figure 40.7). Yet the total amount of furosemide excreted in the urine during the same period is approximately half as great following oral compared with intravenous administration.[342,343] This paradox results from the fact that oral furosemide absorption is slower than its clearance, leading to "absorption-limited" kinetics. Thus, effective serum furosemide concentrations persist longer when the drug is given by mouth, because a reservoir in the gastrointestinal tract continues to supply furosemide to the body. This relationship holds for a normal individual (Figure 40.7), but not necessarily for a patient who suffers from an edematous disorder. In this case, a higher serum drug level may be needed to elicit natriuresis, and the lower serum drug level achieved by oral treatment may be inadequate to reach the natriuretic threshold. For this reason, it is customary to double the furosemide dose when changing from intravenous to oral therapy.[136] Variations in bioavailability may lead to increased hospitalizations for patients with congestive heart failure treated with furosemide, compared to a drug such as torsemide that is more completely absorbed, but this remains to be established in larger studies.[344]

A third factor that determines the maximal natriuresis following diuretic drug administration is drug delivery to its active site. Most diuretics, including the loop diuretics, DCT diuretics, and amiloride, act from the luminal surface. Thus, to be effective, these drugs must be delivered into tubule fluid by glomerular filtration or by tubular secretion. Although most diuretics are small molecules, most circulate tightly bound to protein and reach tubule fluid primarily by secretion. When serum albumin concentrations are very low, the volume of diuretic distribution increases,[134] but this factor may not be as important in causing diuretic resistance as believed previously.[345] Nevertheless, when serum albumin concentrations are less than 2 g/L, reduced diuretic delivery to the kidney may play a role in resistance.[346–349]

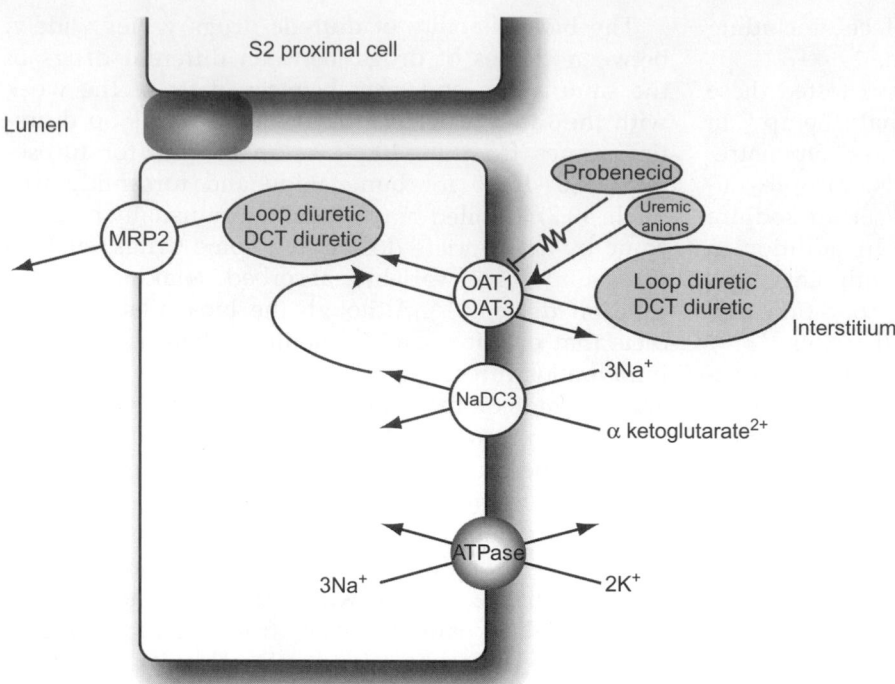

FIGURE 40.15 Mechanisms of diuretic secretion by proximal tubule cells. Cell diagram of the S2 segment of the proximal tubule, showing secretion of anionic diuretic, including loop diuretics and DCT diuretics. Peritubular uptake by an organic anion transporter (primarily OAT1, although OAT3 may play a smaller role) is in exchange for α-ketoglutarate. α-Ketoglutarate is brought into the cell by the Na-dependent cation transporter, NaDC-3. Luminal secretion can be via a voltage-dependent pathway or in exchange for luminal hydroxyl (OH⁻) or urate. A portion of the luminal transport traverses the multidrug resistance protein-2 (MRP-2).[412]

Loop and DCT diuretics are organic anions that circulate bound to albumin, and reach tubule fluid primarily via organic anion secretory pathways in the proximal tubule.[350] Four isoforms of organic anion transporters (OATs) have been cloned and are expressed in the kidney.[351,352] Peritubular uptake by an OAT is a tertiary active process (see Figure 40.15). Energy derives from the basolateral Na$^+$,K$^+$-ATPase that provides a low intracellular [Na$^+$] that drives an uptake of Na$^+$ coupled to a-ketoglutarate (aKG$^-$) to maintain a high intracellular level of aKG$^-$. This, in turn, drives a basolateral OA$^-$/aKG$^-$ countertransporter. OAT translocates diuretics into the proximal tubule cell where they can be sequestered in intracellular vesicles. They are secreted across the luminal membrane by a voltage-driven OAT,[353] and by a countertransporter in exchange for urate or OH$^-$.[352] OAT1 is expressed on the basolateral membrane of the S2 segment of the proximal tubule. Genetic OAT1 causes dramatically impaired renal organic anion secretion, and also furosemide resistance.[354] Thus, OAT1 plays a central role in mediating loop diuretic secretion by proximal cells. Albumin has been reported to stimulate renal organic anion secretion directly, in a dose-dependent manner, up to a maximum when the concentration reaches 1 g/dl.[355]

Endogenous and exogenous substances may compete with diuretics for secretion into tubule fluid and affect diuretic response. Uremic anions,[356] non-steroidal anti-inflammatory drugs,[357] probenecid[358] and penicillins all inhibit loop and DCT diuretic secretion into tubule fluid. Under some conditions, this may predispose to diuretic resistance, because the concentration of drug achieved in tubule fluid does not exceed the diuretic threshold. For example, in chronic kidney disease, diuretic delivery into the urine is reduced. This shifts the diuretic dose−response curve to the right, requiring a higher dose to achieve maximal effect (see Figure 40.7). Surprisingly, however, probenecid *increases* the natriuretic effects of chlorothiazide and furosemide when administered to normal individuals.[358,359] This effect results from the probenecid-induced impairment in renal diuretic clearance, which prolongs the effective half-life, permitting diuresis to continue over a longer period of time. Thus, achieving sufficient levels, the effect of a secretory inhibitor will be to increase the natriuretic response, owing to a prolonged half-life. In contrast, in a patient whose dose is near to the diuretic threshold, impairments of secretion can lead to achievement of sub-threshold levels in tubule fluid, and to diuretic resistance.

Amiloride and triamterene are organic cations that reach tubule fluid via organic cation secretory pathways in the proximal tubule. Movement of cationic diuretics from cell to lumen occurs, at least in part, via an organic cation/H exchanger, which is coupled functionally to the apical Na/H exchanger.[350] Creatinine, cimetidine, trimethoprim, quinidine, quinine, atropine, ofloxacin, morphine, and paraquat are all secreted by this pathway.[350] Cimetidine has been shown to inhibit the secretion of amiloride.[360]

A fourth factor that may influence diuretic effectiveness is protein-binding in tubule fluid. Diuretic drugs are normally bound to proteins in the plasma, but not once they are secreted into tubule fluid. This reflects the normally low protein concentrations in tubule fluid. In contrast, when serum proteins such as albumin are filtered in appreciable quantities, diuretic drugs will interact with them.[361] This protein—drug interaction appears to inhibit the ability of the diuretic to interact with luminal transport proteins. Kirchner and colleagues showed that adding albumin to diuretic-containing fluid used to perfuse rat loops of Henle reduced the effects of the loop diuretic by approximately 50%. This effect was specific for albumin, since IgG did not mimic it,[362] and the effect could be prevented by adding inhibitors of protein-binding such as warfarin or sulfisoxizole.[363] The role of this process in human diuretic resistance, however, has been questioned, as protein-binding inhibitors do not increase diuretic efficacy in proteinurinc humans.[364] Although the reasons for the discrepant results between animal models and humans are unclear, it seems unlikely that urinary albumin-binding to diuretics is an important contributor to diuretic resistance.

Patients given diuretic drugs to treat edematous conditions all manifest some diuretic resistance (see Figure 40.7). This is evident in the shift to the right and downward in the dose—response curve for a loop diuretic.

DIURETIC ADAPTATIONS AND DIURETIC RESISTANCE

Although the clinically useful diuretic drugs all increase urinary solute and water excretion, the goal of diuretic therapy of edema is to reduce the ECF volume. This usually requires an increase in urinary solute and water excretion, but such an increase is not sufficient to effect ECF volume contraction by itself. Furthermore, any initial increase in daily urinary NaCl and water excretion begins to wane after several days of diuretic treatment. That is because of specific renal adaptations that occur during diuretic therapy. When diuretic adaptation becomes manifest once the desired ECF volume has been attained, it is clinically useful and prevents progressive ECF volume contraction. When these same processes develop prior to achieving the desired ECF volume, they would be viewed as contributing to diuretic resistance. Because specific therapeutic approaches can be devised to overcome these adaptations, an understanding of renal adaptations to diuretic treatment is crucial for understanding diuretic treatment of edema. For the purposes of this discussion, diuretic adaptations will be classified as *immediate*, *short-term*, and *chronic*. Immediate adaptations limit the intrinsic potency of diuretic drugs; these occur during the initial diuretic-induced natriuresis, and generally result from intrinsic renal processes. Short-term adaptations occur after the initial effect of the diuretic drug has worn off, and may result from both systemic and intrarenal processes. Chronic adaptations occur only when diuretic drugs have been administered during a long period of time (days to weeks). Because diuretic resistance is most commonly observed in patients who have received high doses of loop diuretics during long periods of time, these chronic adaptations may be especially relevant to the phenomenon of diuretic resistance in patients.

Immediate Adaptations

About 25 moles of sodium are filtered every day by the kidneys in a normal human. Because dietary salt intake on a Western diet is typically 110—260 mmol daily, approximately 3 pounds of salt (17 moles = 1 kg NaCl) must be reabsorbed every day by the renal tubules to maintain salt balance. As discussed above, all sodium chloride reabsorption along the mammalian nephron is driven by the action of Na/K-ATPase, which is present along the basolateral cell membrane of most renal epithelial cells. Transepithelial sodium transport occurs because apical transport pathways permit Na to move down its electrochemical gradient from tubule lumen to cell, often coupled to the movement of other ions across the same membrane. Most diuretics drugs act by inhibiting apical Na transport pathways. Because apical Na transport pathways are nephron segment-specific, each class of diuretic inhibits Na transport *predominantly* along a single segment of the nephron (see Figure 40.1). The axial organization of renal tubules, and the nephron segment-specific inhibition of salt transport by diuretics, means that diuretics have both direct effects and indirect effects on solute transport along the nephron.

When NaCl reabsorption along the thick ascending limb is inhibited by loop diuretics, the NaCl concentration in fluid that enters the distal tubule is greatly increased. In one study, the Na concentration in fluid entering the distal tubule of rats rose from 42 to 140 mM during acute loop diuretic infusion.[151] The higher luminal NaCl concentration increased Na absorption along the distal tubule (from 148 to 361 pmol/minute), because NaCl transport varies directly with the luminal NaCl concentration. Further, loop diuretics have little or no effect on ion transport along the distal tubule.[250] The bulk of the increased NaCl transport along the distal tubule appears to result from enhanced transcellular transport via the thiazide-sensitive Na-Cl co-transporter. In microperfused rat distal tubules, raising the luminal NaCl concentration two-fold increased transepithelial Na transport by a factor of 3; this increase could be blocked entirely by luminal chorothiazide.[365] The dependence of transepithelial NaCl transport on luminal NaCl concentration probably results from a dependence of the thiazide-sensitive Na-Cl co-transporter on extracellular Na and Cl concentrations,[180] although effects to increase the abundance of NCC may also be involved.

This first level of adaptation to diuretic drugs occurs *during* the period of diuretic-induced natriuresis; this is the compensatory increase in NaCl reabsorption along segments that are not targets of diuretic action. The *net* effect of acute diuretic administration on urinary Na and Cl excretion, therefore, reflects the sum of effects in the diuretic-sensitive segment (inhibition of NaCl reabsorption) and in diuretic-insensitive segments (secondary stimulation of NaCl reabsorption). Although the most clinically important example of this form of adaptation involves loop diuretics, these compensatory processes occur during administration of most classes of diuretics. The importance of compensatory processes to blunt the acute effects of diuretics is exemplified by CA inhibitors, which inhibit Na transport across cells of the proximal tubule. Because a large portion of the Na that is rejected by the proximal tubule during CA inhibitor administration is reabsorbed along the loop of Henle and distal tubule, only a fraction escapes into the urine. CA inhibitors, therefore, are drugs of only modest potency. Blockade of immediate adaptive processes enhances the effects of the administered diuretic, as when loop diuretics are combined with CA inhibitors, acutely. A similar phenomenon has been observed in animals lacking NHE3, the apical Na/H exchanger of the proximal tubule.[13] These animals exhibit minimal salt-wasting, owing to compensatory processes.

Short-Term Adaptations (Post-Diuretic NaCl Retention)

The half-life of most diuretics (especially the loop diuretics) is relatively short. Thus, serum diuretic concentrations are often below the natriuretic threshold during a portion of each day, except when the drugs are infused constantly. This second type of adaptive response to diuretic administration occurs after the peak natriuresis has occurred, and is most prominent when the drug concentration in plasma and tubular fluid declines below the diuretic threshold. In this situation, diuretic is no longer present in tubule fluid to inhibit renal Na reabsorption and a period of NaCl retention, often termed "post-diuretic NaCl retention" begins (see Figure 40.16). The net effect of the diuretic drug during 24 hours, therefore, results from a period of natriuresis (when NaCl transport is inhibited by the

diuretic), and a period of anti-natriuresis (when the drug concentration is low, before the next dose is given).

Mechanisms that contribute to post-diuretic NaCl retention have been investigated intensively and may be grouped into three classes: first, factors that result from changes in ECF volume; second, factors that result from diuretic-induced increases in distal sodium, chloride, and fluid delivery; and third, factors that result from direct effects of diuretic drugs on tubule transport processes. One signal initiating NaCl retention in the post-diuretic period is the change in ECF volume and the change in "effective" arterial blood volume. Evidence indicating a central role for changes in ECF volume includes the observation that post-diuretic NaCl retention can be prevented by administering Na, K, and Cl at rates sufficient to equal diuretic induced losses.[366] This observation does not, however, exclude a contributory role for mechanisms that occur independent of changes in ECF volume, as will be discussed below.

Diuretic drugs have effects on vascular and ECF volume within minutes of administration, both because of their ability to increase renal Na and Cl excretion, and because they have direct vascular effects. These changes activate a number of physiological control systems, which tend to favor NaCl retention and act to attenuate further NaCl loss. Important contributors to ECF volume-dependent NaCl retention have been discussed above, and include changes in the GFR, activation of the renin–angiotensin–aldosterone system, stimulation of efferent renal sympathetic nerves, suppression of atrial natriuretic peptide secretion, and suppression of renal prostaglandin secretion. Post-diuretic NaCl retention has been shown to occur in humans whether dietary NaCl intake is high or low, suggesting that true ECF volume *depletion* may not be essential. Some *decline* in ECF volume, however, was shown to be necessary for secondary NaCl retention during furosemide-induced natriuresis in rats. In rats given furosemide continuously, the secondary decline in NaCl excretion was associated with a 25% decline in GFR, suggesting that decreases in filtered NaCl-load contribute to short-term adaptations to diuretic treatment.[367] In normal humans, changes in GFR were reported to be statistically insignificant during post-diuretic NaCl retention, suggesting a decline in filtered Na does not contribute.[368] Although a statistically significant decline in GFR can be observed in the post-diuretic period when the data from several subgroups are pooled,[368] the magnitude of this effect is small, and increases in NaCl reabsorption rather than declines in GFR probably play the larger role.

One mechanism that may mediate a decline in GFR after loop diuretic drug concentrations decline may be

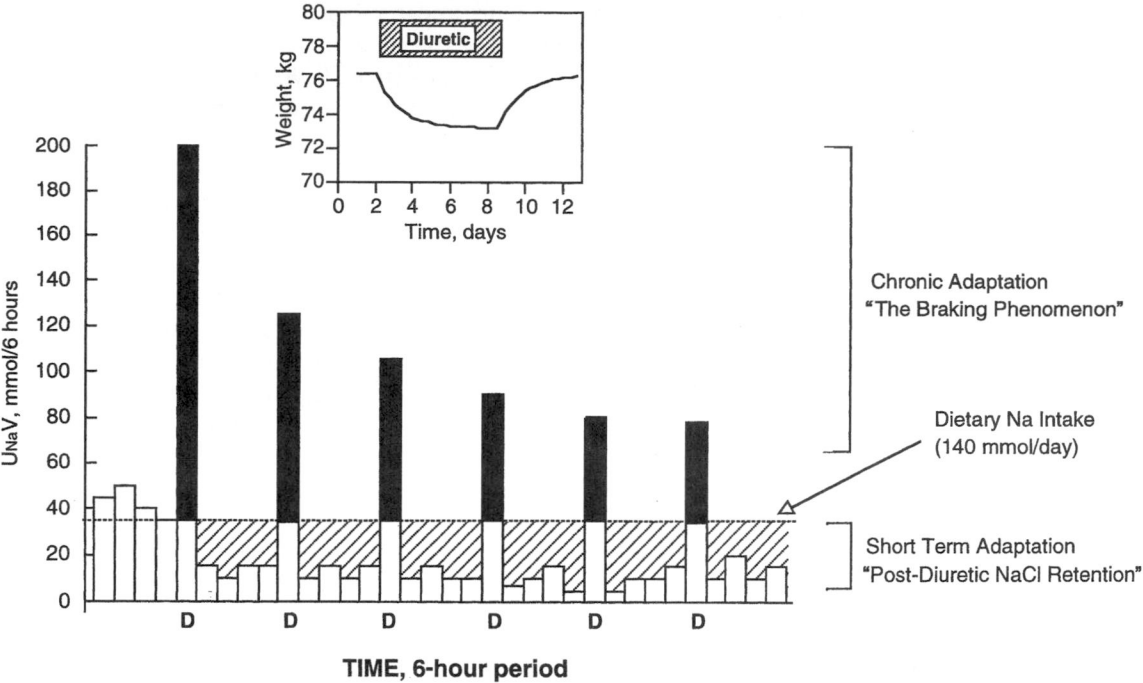

FIGURE 40.16 **Effects of diuretics on urinary Na excretion and ECF volume.** Inset: Effect of diuretic on body weight, an index of ECF volume. Note that steady-state is reached within 6—8 days, despite continued diuretic administration. Main graph: Effects of loop diuretic on urinary Na excretion. Bars represent six-hour periods before (in Na balance) and after doses of loop diuretic (D). The dotted line indicates dietary Na intake. The solid portion of bars indicates the amount by which Na excretion exceeds intake during natriuresis. The hatched areas indicate the amount of positive Na balance after the diuretic effect has dissipated. Net Na balance during 24 hours is the difference between the hatched area (post-diuretic NaCl retention) and the solid area (diuretic-induced natriureisis). Chronic adaptation is indicated by progressively smaller peak natriuretic effects (the "braking phenomenon"), and is mirrored by a return to neutral balance, as indicated in the inset, where the solid and hatched areas are equal. As discussed in the text, chronic adaptation requires ECF volume depletion.

activation of the TGF system. Loop diuretics block this system directly by interfering with Na and Cl uptake by macula densa cells, as discussed above. Thus, loop diuretics tend to maintain the GFR higher than would be expected in the absence of diuretic action. When the diuretic concentration declines, and the inhibitory effects at the macula densa wane, the TGF system is poised to respond again to NaCl delivery and to suppress the GFR, thus contributing to post-diuretic NaCl retention.

Diuretic drugs stimulate the renin—angiotensin—aldosterone axis via mechanisms described above and in Figure 40.9. The renin—angiotensin—aldosterone axis contributes importantly to renal NaCl homeostasis, but evidence for an important role of these hormones in post-diuretic NaCl retention has been mixed. In normal volunteers, post-diuretic NaCl retention was unaffected by the angiotensin-converting enzyme inhibitor captopril[369] given in doses sufficient to block furosemide-induced changes in angiotensin II and aldosterone levels. Further, in those studies, diuretic-induced changes in blood pressure were similar with or without captopril, suggesting that hypotension did not mediate the NaCl retention in the ACE inhibitor group. These

data indicate that post-diuretic NaCl retention *can* occur without activation of the renin—angiotensin—aldosterone system; they do not indicate, however, that stimulation of the renin—angiotensin—aldosterone axis has no role in post-diuretic NaCl retention when it occurs. An important role for the renin—angiotensin—aldosterone axis is implied by comparing the effects of volume removal via loop diuretics and hemofiltration. In one study, diuresis of patients with heart failure led to a larger increase in renin than did removal of the same fluid using an ultrafiltration device.[370,371] Yet this effect was not supported by more recent studies.[372]

Stimulation of alpha adrenergic renal nerves enhances NaCl reabsorption. Petersen et al. showed that systemic α-1 blockade attenuated the secondary reduction in NaCl excretion that occurs during short-term furosemide-induced volume-depletion in rats.[373] They concluded that stimulation of α-1 adrenoceptors on proximal tubules contributed to the compensatory response to short-term furosemide infusion. In humans, however, administration of prazosin, in doses that block the pressor response to α-adrenergic agonists, does not prevent post-diuretic NaCl retention. Even when both prazosin and captopril are administered concurrently, to block both the renin—angiotensin—aldosterone axis and the effects of renal nerve activity, post-diuretic NaCl retention may occur ([374]; although in this case, furosemide did reduce mean arterial pressure significantly). Thus, ECF volume-dependent stimulation of α-1 adrenergic receptors, especially along the proximal tubule, may contribute to post-diuretic NaCl retention.

Diuretic-induced decrements in ECF volume have been shown to be associated with suppression of atrial natriuretic peptide secretion. These changes occur following diuretic administration in both normal individuals, and in patients with nephrotic syndrome,[375] chronic glomerulonephritis, and essential hypertension. In some studies, atrial natriuretic peptide concentrations have declined before significant changes in extracellular or blood volume occur; in these cases it has been suggested that furosemide-induced changes in venous capacitance may underlie the effect.

The studies discussed above in which post-diuretic NaCl retention occurred despite blockade of several effector mechanisms raise the possibility that changes in ECF volume are not required for post-diuretic NaCl retention to occur. Wilcox and colleagues investigated acute effects of the loop diuretic bumetanide in the absence of ECF volume-depletion. Na, K, Cl, and water were administered to volunteers during loop diuretic administration to balance electrolyte losses completely. When changes in ECF volume were prevented, post-diuretic NaCl retention did not occur, indicating that decrements in ECF volume do play a critical role in post-diuretic NaCl retention. A volume-independent component of adaptation may also contribute to NaCl retention, however. When volunteers were challenged with a 100 mmol NaCl-load with or without prior diuretic treatment, differences were observed. The NaCl-load was excreted fully within two days under control conditions; after pretreatment with bumetanide, however, much less of the administered load was excreted during the subsequent two days.[366] This result occurred despite complete replacement of water and electrolyte losses induced by the loop diuretic. These results suggest that there are subtle but physiologically significant effects of diuretic administration, even in the short-term, that favor NaCl retention in the absence of changes in ECF volume status (see below).

In normal individuals, diuretic administration strongly activates the control systems discussed above; in edematous individuals, however, one or more of these control systems may be active at baseline, having contributed to the pathological accumulation of extracellular volume. The role of these control systems in the adaptive response to diuretic may, therefore, be different in normal and edematous individuals.

One mechanism by which diuretic drugs may increase the tendency for NaCl retention directly without changes in ECF volume involves diuretic-induced *activation* of ion transporters within the diuretic sensitive nephron segment. The cation chloride co-transporters, such as the NKCC2, are phosphorylated and activated by low intracellular chloride concentrations[376]; because loop diuretics reduce the Cl concentration in cells of the thick ascending limb, pre-existing transporters should be activated leading to increased NaCl transport capacity. This increase will be unmasked once the luminal concentration of loop diuretic declines. Ecelbarger et al.[377] reported evidence that furosemide administration activates NKCC2 via more than one mechanism. Five days of furosemide infusion led to a 50—100% increase in abundance of NKCC2, and also to an upward mobility shift of 9 kDa in apparent molecular mass. These results were interpreted as suggesting that furosemide blockade of apical NaCl uptake led to both increased expression and "modification" of NKCC2. As phosphorylation of NKCC2 regulates its activity, one possibility is that loop diuretic blockade activates the transporter via phosphorylation.

A similar mechanism has been reported to occur along the distal tubule during short-term administration of thiazide diuretics. Within 60 minutes of thiazide administration, the number of thiazide-sensitive Na-Cl co-transporters in kidney cortex (measured as the number of [^{3}H]metolazone binding sites) increases substantially.[378] The techniques used to estimate the number of transporters in these experiments do not permit one to determine whether the increased number reflects insertion of pre-existing transporters from a subapical storage pool or activation of transporters that are present but inactive in the apical membrane. It is now clear that a subapical pool of NCC shuttles to and from the apical membrane in response to physiological perturbation.[379] An increase in the number of activated ion transporters at the apical membrane would be expected to increase the transport capacity, so that when diuretic concentrations decline, increased Na and Cl transport would result.

Another mechanism by which diuretic drugs may enhance the tendency to NaCl retention directly involves stimulation of transport pathways in nephron segments that lie distal to the target of diuretic action (segments that are insensitive to the diuretic drug). For example, the number of metolazone-binding sites increases within 60 minutes after a loop diuretic has been administered.[378] Because NCC is expressed by nephron segments that do not express loop diuretic-sensitive pathways, the increased NCC is believed to result from increases in salt and water delivery to DCT cells (discussed in more detail below).

Post-diuretic NaCl retention can have major effects on the clinical efficacy of diuretic drugs. The half-life of most loop diuretics is short, so that NaCl retention can occur during 18 hours per day, if the drug is administered once daily (see Figure 40.16). If dietary NaCl intake is low, then post-diuretic NaCl retention does not compensate for the drug-induced NaCl losses, and NaCl balance becomes negative (the desired therapeutic response). If, on the other hand, dietary NaCl intake is high, then post-diuretic NaCl retention can compensate entirely for the initial NaCl losses during the period of drug action. When dietary NaCl intake is high, therefore, salt balance may be neutral, even from the first day of diuretic therapy,[368] despite impressive increases in urine volume after each dose of diuretic. This is one reason that dietary NaCl intake is a key determinant of diuretic efficacy, especially for the short-acting loop diuretics.

Chronic Adaptations (The "Braking" Phenomenon)

When diuretics reduce ECF volume effectively, NaCl balance gradually returns to neutral, despite continued diuretic administration[368,380] (see Figure 40.16). This "braking phenomenon" occurs when the magnitude of natriuresis following each diuretic dose declines. Several factors, acting in concert, may participate in chronic adaptation. A critical factor that is necessary for the braking phenomenon to occur is a decline in the ECF volume. Wilcox and co-workers showed that the magnitude of each diuretic-induced natriuresis declined during ECF volume-depletion of humans consuming a low-NaCl diet. In contrast, when dietary NaCl intake was high, ECF volume-depletion did not occur, and the magnitude of diuretic-induced natriuresis did not decline.[368,380] Relative or absolute ECF volume contraction limits NaCl excretion by reducing the amount of NaCl that is filtered, and by increasing the amount of NaCl that is reabsorbed. In experimental animals, declines in renal blood flow occur during chronic diuretic treatment. Declines in GFR are usually modest, however, unless volume depletion is extreme or unles renal perfusion is compromised by drugs or physical factors such as renal artery stenosis. The effects of diuretics on glomerular filtration and renal blood flow are not caused primarily by changes in mean arterial pressure, as the renal autoregulatory response tends to maintain GFR and renal blood flow relatively constant when arterial pressure changes. Instead, ECF volume contraction itself leads to decrements in renal blood flow and GFR; because renal blood flow declines proportionately more than GFR, ECF volume-contraction increases the filtration fraction (GFR/RPF).

The role of the proximal tubule in diuretic adaptation has been documented clearly in rats treated chronically with thiazide diuretics, and in animals and humans treated with loop diuretics. In the case of thiazide treatment, micropuncture studies showed that hydrochlorothiazide initially inhibited Na and Cl absorption along both the proximal tubule (by inhibiting CA) and the distal tubule (by inhibiting Na-Cl co-transport) of rats.[228] After 7−10 days of treatment, however, ECF volume-contraction led to increases in proximal solute reabsorption, thereby limiting delivery of Na and Cl to the distal sites of thiazide action. During the chronic phase of treatment, inhibition of NaCl transport along the distal nephron (the predominant site of thiazide action) counterbalanced the reduction in distal NaCl delivery; under these conditions, at steady-state, urinary NaCl was equal to dietary NaCl intake.[228] Loop diuretics such as furosemide have also been shown to inhibit Na and Cl absorption by the proximal tubule, although the mechanism is unclear. But, as with DCT diuretics, chronic treatment with loop diuretics leads to ECF volume-contraction and enhanced proximal NaCl reabsorption.[381] That effects on proximal absorption require decrements in ECF volume was shown by comparing NaCl delivery out of the proximal tubule during furosemide administration, with and without volume replacement. Only when the ECF volume was permitted to decline was proximal absorption stimulated.[367] Many of the same effector systems that participate in post-diuretic NaCl retention also may participate in chronic adaptations to diuretic drugs.

Physical Factors

A rise in filtration fraction increases the protein oncotic pressure in peritubular capillaries (more protein free filtrate is formed per ml of blood flow, thereby contracting the plasma volume around a constant amount of serum protein). The increased peritubular oncotic pressure increases solute and fluid reabsorption, especially in the proximal tubule. ECF volume contraction also enhances proximal solute and fluid reabsorption by decreasing the renal interstitial pressure during chronic diuretic treatment.

Sympathetic Renal Nerve Activity

Efferent sympathetic nerves innervate the renal vasculature, the macula densa, and essentially all segments of the nephron. Stimulation of sympathetic nerves reduces urinary NaCl excretion by reducing renal blood flow, by stimulating renin release at the macula densa, by stimulating tubule NaCl reabsorption along the nephron, and by interacting with hormonal modulators of NaCl transport. Renal nerves may contribute to NaCl retention in edematous disorders, and renal nerve activity is stimulated when furosemide is administered either to normal or volume-depleted animals.[382] Yet experimental models of chronic diuretic administration have failed to substantiate a central role for renal nerve activity in adaptive processes. Chronic sympathectomy or blockade of α-1 receptors inhibits the compensatory increase in proximal NaCl reabsorption that occurs during furosemide-induced ECF volume-depletion, but these maneuvers did not enhance the natriuretic response to furosemide.[383] This indicates that the inhibition of proximal solute reabsorption which occurs secondary to adrenergic blockade is compensated by increased reabsorption distally. Use of systemic pharmacological sympathetic blockade to study the role of renal nerves in diuretic adaptation is limited because of drug-induced systemic hypotension, but Petersen and DiBona showed that even anatomical renal denervation in normal rats does not abrogate the compensatory response to chronic furosemide administration.[384] Although it seems clear that renal nerves do not play a critical role in mediating compensation to chronic diuretic use in normal humans and animals, the consistent observation that diuretics do stimulate renal nerve activity suggests that renal nervous activity may contribute to diuretic adaptation in some patients. In patients suffering from edematous disorders, distal Na reabsorption may already be stimulated; denervation in this situation might lead to significant impairment in adaptation to diuretic drugs.

Renin–Angiotensin–Aldosterone

A third factor participating in chronic adaptation to diuretic drugs is the renin–angiotensin–aldosterone system. Renin acts on angiotensinogen to generate angiotensin I, which is converted to angiotensin II by converting enzyme. Angiotensin II stimulates aldosterone secretion from the adrenal cortex; aldosterone stimulates salt reabsorption by the distal nephron. Recent studies indicate that, in addition to stimulating Na transport by ENaC of the collecting duct, as discussed above, mineralocorticoid hormones stimulate Na transport by the thiazide-sensitive Na-Cl co-transporter of the DCT.[191,385–387] In addition, however, angiotensin II directly stimulates Na reabsorption along both the proximal and distal tubule by stimulating Na/H exchange activity.[388] Thus, diuretic drugs frequently result in stimulation of the renin–angiotensin–aldosterone system, and the Na retention that occurs during diuretic treatment may result in part from this. As is the case with renal nerves, it has been difficult to show conclusively that the renin–angiotensin–aldosterone system plays a critical role in chronic adaptation to diuretic drugs. Yet as with renal nerves, the systemic effects of inhibition of the system, either with angiotensin I-converting enzyme inhibitor, angiotensin II receptor blockers or competitive aldosterone blockers make it difficult to exclude a role for this hormonal system in the compensation to diuretic therapy.

Epithelial Hypertrophy and Hyperplasia

Other factors that can enhance renal NaCl reabsorptive capacity are structural and functional changes in the nephron itself. When a diuretic is administered, solute delivery to segments that lie distal to the site of diuretic action increase, leading to load-dependent increases in solute reabsorption, as discussed above.[389] When solute delivery and solute reabsorption increase chronically, epithelial cells undergo both hypertrophy and hyperplasia (see Figure 40.17). Infusion of furosemide into rats continuously for seven days increased the percentage of renal cortical volume occupied by distal nephron cells. DCT cell volume increased by nearly 100%, with accompanying increases in luminal membrane area per length of tubule, in basolateral membrane area per length of tubule, and in mitochondrial volume per cell.[365,390,391] Chronic loop diuretic administration increases the Na/K-ATPase activity in the distal convoluted and cortical collecting tubules[392,393](see Figure 40.17), and increases the number of thiazide-sensitive Na-Cl co-transporters, measured as the maximal number of binding sites for [^{3}H] metolazone.[181,385] In one study, chronic furosemide treatment increased expression of mRNA encoding the thiazide-sensitive Na-Cl co-transporter, as detected by in situ hybridization[181](see Figure 40.18). In another study, however, mRNA expression of the thiazide-sensitive Na-Cl co-transporter, as well as ouabain-sensitive Na/K-ATPase, were not affected by chronic furosemide infusion, when detected by Northern analysis.[394] Distal tubule cells that express high levels of transport proteins and are hypertrophic have a higher Na and Cl transport capacity than normal tubules. Compared with tubules from normal animals, tubules of animals treated chronically with loop diuretics can absorb Na and Cl up to three times more rapidly than control animals, even when salt and water delivery are fixed by microperfusion (Figure 40.18). When distal tubules are presented with high NaCl-loads, as occurs during loop diuretic administration in vivo, Na and Cl absorption rates approach those commonly observed only in the proximal tubule.[365] Chronic treatment of rats with loop diuretics also results in significant hyperplasia of cells along the distal nephron. Whereas mitoses of renal tubule epithelial cells are infrequent in adult kidneys, distal tubules from animals treated with furosemide chronically demonstrate prominent mitoses; increased synthesis of DNA in these cells was confirmed by showing increases in labeling of DCT cells with bromodeoxyurindine and proliferating cell nuclear antigen.[395]

The diuretic-induced signals that initiate changes in distal nephron structure and function are poorly-

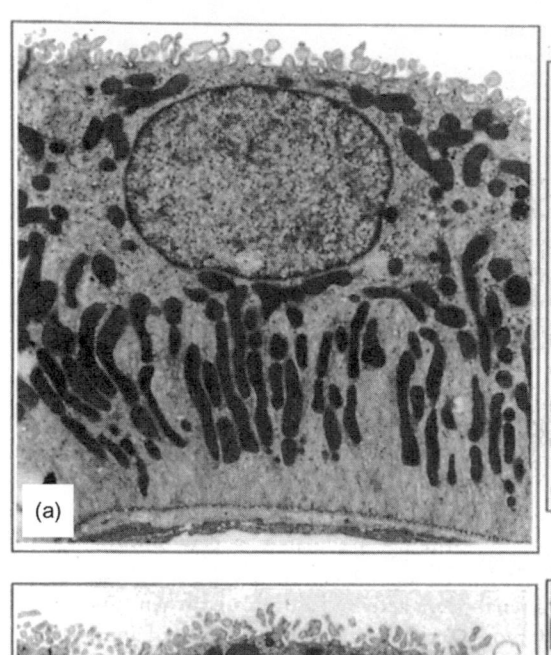

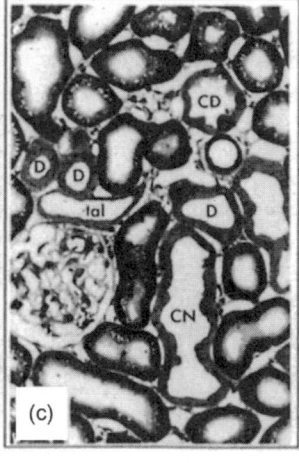

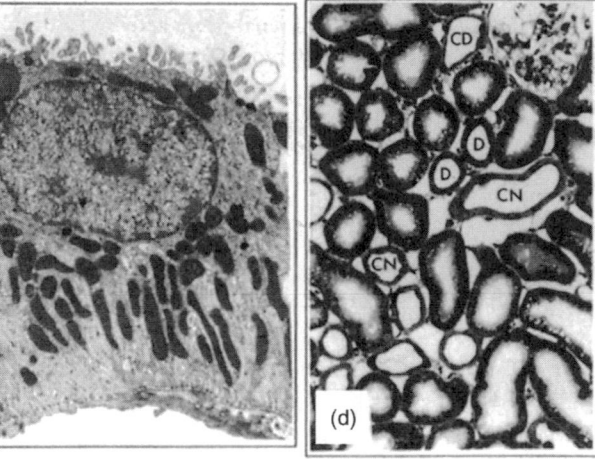

FIGURE 40.17 Effects of chronic loop diuretic administration on distal convoluted tubule cells of rats. Rats received furosemide continuously for seven days. Panels (a) and (b): Electron micrographs (×10,000) of distal convoluted tubule cells from control- and furosemide-infused animals respectively. Note that furosemide increases the size of the cell, the size of the nucleus, the amount of mitochondrial volume, and the amount of basolateral membrane area. Panels (c) and (d): Photomicrographs of kidney cortices from control and furosemide infused animals respectively (×480) (*D*: distal convoluted tubule; *CN*: connecting tubule; *CD*: cortical collecting duct: *tal*: thick ascending limb). Note thickening of the epithelium in all distal segments. *(Photomicrographs are used with permission from ref. [365].)*

understood.[389] Several factors, acting in concert, may contribute to these changes; these include diuretic-induced increases in Na and Cl delivery to distal segments, effects of ECF volume depletion on systemic hormone secretion and renal nerve activity, and local effects of diuretics on autocrine and paracrine secretion. Increased production of angiotensin II or increased secretion of aldosterone resulting from increases in renin activity may contribute to hypertrophy and hyperplasia. Angiotensin is a potent mitogen; angiotensin II receptors have not been localized definitively to DCT cells, but recent functional studies do suggest that DCT cells express angiotensin II receptors.[396] Beck et al.[397] showed that angiotensin I-converting enzyme inhibitors do not prevent loop diuretic-induced hypertrophy of DCT cells. Yet the hypertrophy during angiotensin I-converting enzyme inhibition is one that results from lengthening of kidney tubules; in their absence the hypertrophy results from thickening of the tubular cells.

Aldosterone also promotes growth of responsive tissues under some circumstances[398]; when salt delivery to the collecting duct is increased in the presence of high levels of circulating aldosterone, principal cell hypertrophy develops; when salt delivery is high in the absence of aldosterone secretion, hypertrophy is absent. This indicates that aldosterone plays a permissive role in the development of cellular hypertrophy in this aldosterone-responsive renal epithelium. Aldosterone does affect ion transport by cells of the DCT,[185,190,399,400] and aldosterone almost certainly contributes to adaptations along the cortical collecting tubule. Yet hypertrophy of DCT cells has been shown to occur during chronic loop diuretic infusion, even when changes in circulating mineralocorticoid, glucocorticoid, and vasopressin levels are prevented.[391]

One intriguing hypothesis is that cellular ion concentrations regulate epithelial cell growth directly.[401] Increases in Na uptake across the apical plasma

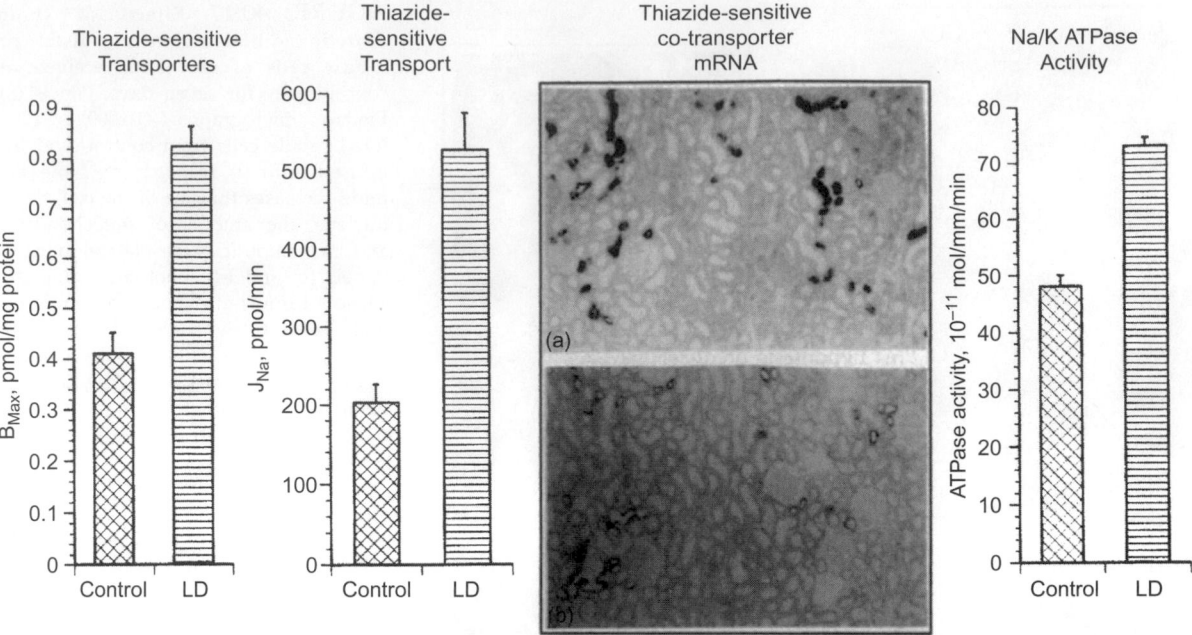

FIGURE 40.18 **Effects of continuous loop diuretic infusion on rat kidney.** Loop diuretic infusion increased the number of thiazide-sensitive Na-Cl co-transporters,[378] the rate of thiazide-sensitive Na transport along the distal tubule,[365] the abundance of thiazide-sensitive Na-Cl co-transporter mRNA (a: furosemide-treated kidney cortex; b: control kidney cortex). *(Ref. [181], used with permission)*, and Na/K-ATPase activity along the distal convoluted tubule. *(Data from ref. [392].)*

membrane precede cell growth in the TAL during treatment with ADH,[402] in principal cells of the CCT during treatment with mineralocorticoid hormones,[403,404] and in the DCT during treatment with loop diuretics.[365,398] Although the cause of the increased Na uptake varies, changes in the intracellular Na concentration appear to precede growth in each example. This hypothesis predicts that blockade of apical Na entry would lead to atrophy of epithelial cells. Chronic treatment of rats with DCT diuretics reduces activity of Na/K-ATPase and Na transport capacity of DCT segments,[405,406] but these experiments are complicated by other structural effects of chronic DCT diuretic treatment, discussed below. Regardless of the proximate stimulus for DCT cell growth, recent experiments have shown that immunoreactivity for insulin-like growth factor-1 (IGF-1), and for an IGF-binding protein (IGFBP-1), increases during chronic treatment of rats with loop diuretics.[407] The changes in IGF-1 expression appeared not to result from changes in IGF-1 mRNA expression, but rather appeared to reflect post-transcriptional events. IGFBP-1 mRNA was increased by three-fold 18 hours after loop diuretic treatment was initiated. IGF-1 has been shown to participate in regeneration of injured or ischemic renal tissue, and promotes cell proliferation and differentiation *in vitro*; whether these changes in IGF expression mediate the effects of diuretics on distal nephron structure remains to be established.

Morphological changes in the distal nephron during loop diuretic administration are not restricted to Na reabsorbing cells. Chronic diuretic infusion stimulates selective hypertrophy of type-B intercalated-cells.[408] Type-B intercalated-cells secrete bicarbonate and express apical Cl/HCO$_3$ exchangers and basolateral H-ATPase pumps; chronic bumetanide infusion increased the number of apical microvilli in Type-B cells, increased the basolateral cell membrane area, and led to marked cytoplasmic and basolateral labeling for H-ATPase. Type-A cells, which normally mediate acid secretion, were small; H-ATPase was distributed primarily within intracellular tubulovesicles in the tubules of treated animals. The authors concluded that the structural changes in intercalated cells resulted from increased distal chloride delivery, because serum pH and electrolyte concentrations were not affected by the diuretic treatment. Increased distal chloride delivery might be expected to enhance Cl/HCO$_3$ exchange, increasing transepithelial solute transport, stimulating cell growth via mechanisms similar to those discussed above. These effects are likely to contribute to the profound metabolic alkalosis that can complicate aggressive treatment with loop diuretics.

Chronic diuretic administration has structural effects not only on nephron segments that lie distal to the site of diuretic action, but also on the nephron segments that are directly inhibited by the drugs themselves.

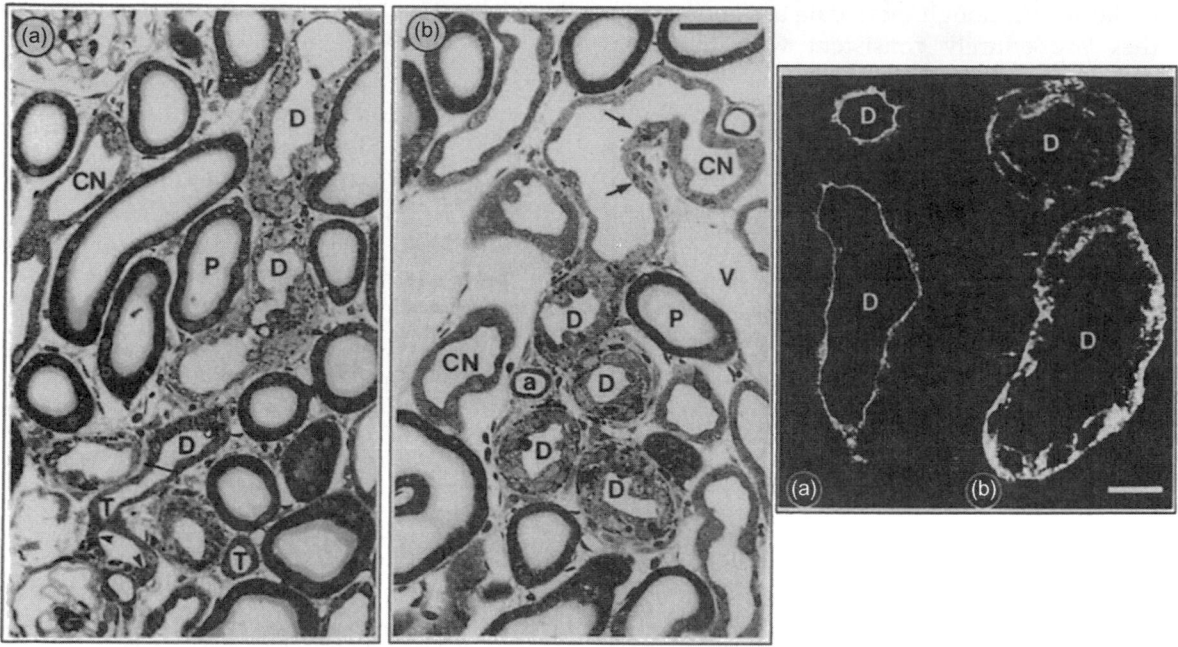

FIGURE 40.19 **Effects of continuous DCT diuretic treatment on the structure of distal convoluted tubules.** Panels a and b at the left show photomicrograph of kidney cortex from animals treated chronically with thiazide diuretics; note extreme hyperplasia and dysmorphology of distal segments (compare normal distal convoluted tubules in Figure 40.16, above) (T: thick ascending limb; D: distal convoluted tubule; CN: connecting tubule; CD: collecting duct; P: proximal tubule; a: arteriole). Double arrow indicates transition from thick ascending limb to distal convoluted tubule; note normal morphology of the thick ascending limb. Panels a and b on the right show immunostaining for the thiazide-sensitive Na-Cl co-transporter from control rats (a) and rats infused with a thiazide continuously for 10 days (b). Note that the normal apical localization of the transporter immunoreactivity (a) is distributed throughout the cytoplasm in animals exposed to diuretics chronically (b). *(From ref. [217]. Used with permission.)*

Within hours of furosemide administration to rats, autophagocytic vacuoles develop in thick ascending limb cells.[409] Following seven days of furosemide treatment of rats, the cell height of thick ascending limb cells was significantly reduced.[365] Chronic treatment of rabbits with loop diuretics decreased Na/K-ATPase activity in medullary thick ascending limb cells by approximately one-third.[410] These results are consistent with an effect of transepithelial ion transport to stimulate "work hypertrophy" and blockade of transepithelial transport to stimulate "disuse atrophy." When DCT diuretics are administered chronically, Na/K-ATPase activity in the DCT is reduced,[406] and the capacity of DCT cells to reabsorb Na and Cl declines.[405] Yet chronic administration of DCT diuretics, like genetic disruption of the thiazide-sensitive Na-Cl co-transporter,[216] to rats leads to profound changes in cellular morphology; the DCT epithelium becomes disordered, DCT cells undergo apoptosis and necrosis, and interstitial fibrosis occurs (see Figure 40.19). Chronic treatment also leads to the disappearance of normal polarization of thiazide-sensitive Na-Cl co-transporter proteins. Under normal conditions, immunoreactivity for the thiazide-sensitive Na-Cl co-transporter is restricted to the apical membrane and to a small subapical pool of

vesicles (see Figure 40.19). During chronic treatment with DCT diuretics, the protein is distributed uniformly throughout the cell. Surprisingly, based on the severe morphological degenerative changes in tubular morphology, chronic thiazide administration results in an *increase* in the density of [³H] metolazone-binding sites (functional thiazide-sensitive transporters) in kidney cortex,[406] despite a decline in mRNA expression for the transporter.[395] These results demonstrate that chronic thiazide administration regulates the thiazide-sensitive transporter in a complex way. Further studies are necessary to determine the mechanisms involved.

Although experimental data concerning structural and functional responses of the distal nephron to chronic treatment with diuretic drugs come predominantly from studies employing experimental animals, Loon et al.[411] reported that chronic treatment with loop diuretics in humans enhanced ion transport rates in the distal tubule. They estimated the transport capacity of the DCT as the portion of Na and Cl reabsorption that could be inhibited by thiazide diuretics. When furosemide was administered to volunteers for one month, the enhancement in sodium excretion that occurred resulting from dose of a thiazide diuretic was significantly larger. Although these data are necessarily indirect, they are entirely consistent with the data derived from experimental animals given loop diuretics chronically. The ECF volume-independent component of NaCl retention that occurs following loop diuretic administration[366] may also reflect changes in distal nephron structure and function.

Acknowledgments

Work in the author's laboratory has been supported by a Merit Review from the Department of Veterans Affairs, by a Grand-In-Aid from American Heart Association, by a Scherbenske Award from the American Society of Nephrology, and by an RO1 from the National Institutes of Health. The author thanks Mark Okusa, the coauthor of the previous version of this text, for much of the research that led to this update.

References

[1] Okusa MD, Ellison DH. Physiology and pathophysiology of diuretic action. In: Alpern RJ, Hebert SC, editors. The kidney: physiology and pathophysiology. 4th ed. Amsterdam: Elsevier; 2008. p. 1051–984.

[2] Ellison DH, Hoorn EJ, Wilcox CS. Diuretics. In: Taal MW, Chertow GM, Marsden PA, Skorecki K, Yu AS, Brenner BM, editors. Brenner and Rector's the kidney. 9th ed. Philadelphia: Elsevier; 2012. p. 1879–916.

[3] Brater DC. Diuretic pharmacokinetics and pharmacodynamics. In: Seldin DW, Giebisch G, editors. Diuretic agents: clinical physiology and pharmacology. San Diego: Academic Press; 1997. p. 189–208.

[4] Better OS, Rubinstein I, Winaver JM, Knochel JP. Mannitol therapy revisited (1940–1997). Kidney Int 1997;51:886–94.

[5] Weiner IM. Diuretics and other agents employed in the mobilization of edema fluid. In: Gilman AG, Rall TW, Nies AS, Taylor AS, editors. The pharmacological basis of therapuetics. 8th ed. New York: Pergamon Press; 1990. p. 713–42.

[6] Homsi E, Barreiro MF, Orlando JM, Higa EM. Prophylaxis of acute renal failure in patients with rhabdomyolysis. Ren Fail 1997;19(2):283–8.

[7] Majumdar SR, Kjellstrand CM, Tymchak WJ, Hervas-Malo M, Taylor DA, Teo KK. Forced euvolemic diuresis with mannitol and furosemide for prevention of contrast-induced nephropathy in patients with CKD undergoing coronary angiography: a randomized controlled trial. Am J Kidney Dis 2009;54(4):602–9.

[8] Hinson HE, Stein D, Sheth KN. Hypertonic saline and mannitol therapy in critical care neurology. J Intensive Care Med. 2011; epub ahead of print.

[9] Jenkins IR, Curtis AP. The combination of mannitol and albumin in the priming solution reduces positive intraoperative fluid balance during cardipulmonary bypass. Perfusion 1995;10:301–5.

[10] England MD, Cavaroocchi NC, O'Brien JF, Solis E, Pluth JR, Orszulak TA, et al. Influence of antioxidants (mannitol and allopurinol) on oxygen free radical generation during and after cardiopulmonary bypass. Circulation 1986;74:134–7.

[11] Arieff AI. Dialysis disequilibrium syndrome: current concepts on pathogenesis and prevention. Kidney Int 1994;45:629–35.

[12] Gong G, Lindberg J, Abrams J, Whitaker WR, Wade CE, Gouge S. Comparison of hypertonic saline solutions and dextran in dialysis-induced hypotension. J Am Soc Nephrol 1993;3: 1808–12.

[13] Lorenz JN, Schultheis PJ, Traynor T, Shull GE, Schnermann J. Micropuncture analysis of single-nephron function in NHE3-deficient mice. Am J Physiol 1999;277(3 Pt 2):F447–53.

[14] Bomsztyk K, George JP, Wright FS. Effects of luminal fluid anions on calcium transport by proximal tubule. Am J Physiol 1984;246:F600–8.

[15] Beck LH, Goldberg M. Effects of acetazolamide and parathyroidectomy on renal transprot of sodium, calcium and phosphate. Am J Physiol 1973;224:1136–42.

[16] Higashihara E, Nutahara K, Takeuchi T, Shoji N, Araie M, Aso Y. Calcium metabolism in acidotic patients induced by carbonic anhydrase inhibitors: responses to citrate. J Urol 1991;145(5): 942–8.

[17] Puschett JB, Winaver J. Efects of diuretics on renal function. In: Windhager EE, editor. Handbook of physiology section 8: renal physiology. New York: Oxford University Press; 1992. p. 2335–406.

[18] Okusa MD, Erik A, Persson G, Wright FS. Chlorothiazide effect on feedback-mediated control of glomerular filtration rate. Am J Physiol 1989;257:F137–44.

[19] Good DW, Wright FS. Luminal influences on potassium secretion: sodium concentration and fluid flow rate. Am J Physiol 1979;236:F192–205.

[20] Puscas I, Coltau M, Baican M, Pasca R, Domuta G. The inhibitory effect of diuretics on carbonic anhydrases. Res Commun Mol Pathol Pharmacol 1999;105(3):213–36.

[21] Purkerson JM, Schwartz GJ. The role of carbonic anhydrases in renal physiology. Kidney Int 2007;71(2):103–15.

[22] Kaunisto K, Parkkila S, Rajaniemi H, Waheed A, Grubb J, Sly WS. Carbonic anhydrase XIV: luminal expression suggests key role in renal acidification. Kidney Int 2002;61(6):2111–8.

[23] Eveloff J, Swenson ER, Maren TH. Carbonic anhydrase activity of brush border and plasma membraens prepared from rat kidney cortex. Biochem Pharmacol 1979;28:1434–7.

[24] Maren TH. Current status of membrane-bound carbonic anhydrase. Ann NY Acad Sci 1980;341:246–58.

[25] Lonnerholm G, Wistrand PJ. Membrane-bound carbonic anhydrase CA IV in the human kidney. Acta Physiol Scand 1991;141: 231–4.

[26] Sly WS, Whyte MP, Sundaram V, Tashian RE, Hewett-Emmett D, Guibaud P, et al. Carbonic anhydrase II deficiency in 12 families with the autosomal recessive syndrome of osteopetrosis with renal tubular acidosis and cerebral calcification. N Engl J Med 1985;313:139–45.

[27] Tsuruoka S, Kittelberger AM, Schwartz GJ. Carbonic anhydrase II and IV mRNA in rabbit nephron segments: stimulation during metabolic acidosis. Am J Physiol 1998;274(2 Pt 2): F259–67.

[28] Moe OW, Preisig PA, Alpern RJ. Cellular model of proximal tubule NaCl and $NaHCO_3$ absorption. Kidney Int 1990;38: 605–11.

[29] Aronson PS. Role of SLC26A6-mediated Cl–oxalate exchange in renal physiology and pathophysiology. J Nephrol 2010;23 (Suppl. 16):S158–64.

[30] Rector Jr. FC, Carter NW, Seldin DW. The mechanism of bicarbonate reabsorption in the proximal and distal tubules of the kidney. J Clin Invest 1965;44:278–90.

[31] Lucci MS, Pucacco LR, DuBose Jr. TD, Kokko JP, Carter NW. Direct evaluation of acidification by rat proximal tubule: role of carbonic anhydrase. Am J Physiol 1980;238:F372–9.

[32] Lucci MS, Tinker JP, Weiner I, DuBose Jr. TD. Function of proximal tubule carbonic anhydrase defined by selective inhibition. Am J Physiol 1983;245:F443–9.

[33] Gross E, Pushkin A, Abuladze N, Fedotoff O, Kurtz I. Regulation of the sodium bicarbonate co-transporter kNBC1

function: role of Asp(986), Asp(988) and kNBC1-carbonic anhydrase II binding. J Physiol 2002;544(Pt 3):679–85.

[34] Alvarez BV, Kieller DM, Quon AL, Markovich D, Casey JR. Slc26a6: a cardiac chloride-hydroxyl exchanger and predominant chloride-bicarbonate exchanger of the mouse heart. J Physiol 2004;561(Pt 3):721–34.

[35] Li X, Alvarez B, Casey JR, Reithmeier RA, Fliegel L. Carbonic anhydrase II binds to and enhances activity of the Na$^+$/H$^+$ exchanger. J Biol Chem 2002;277(39):36085–91.

[36] Soleimani M, Xu J. SLC26 chloride/base exchangers in the kidney in health and disease. Semin Nephrol 2006;26(5):375–85.

[37] Soleimani M, Aronson PS. Effects of acetazolamide on Na$^+$-HCO$_3^-$ co-transport in basolateral membrane vesicles isolated from rabbit renal cortex. J Clin Invest 1989;83:945–51.

[38] Sasaki S, Marumo F. Effects of carbonic anhydrase inhibitors on basolateral base transport of rabbit proximal straight tubule. Am J Physiol 1989;257:F947–52.

[39] Brown D, Hirsch S, Gluck S. An H$^+$-ATPase in opposite plasma membrane domains in kidney epithelial cell subpopulations. Nature 1988;331:622–4.

[40] Wagner CA, Devuyst O, Bourgeois S, Mohebbi N. Regulated acid–base transport in the collecting duct. Pflugers Arch: Eur J Phy 2009;458(1):137–56.

[41] Biver S, Belge H, Bourgeois S, Van Vooren P, Nowik M, Scohy S, et al. A role for Rhesus factor Rhcg in renal ammonium excretion and male fertility. Nature 2008;456(7220):339–43.

[42] Lee HW, Verlander JW, Bishop JM, Igarashi P, Handlogten ME, Weiner ID. Collecting duct-specific Rh C glycoprotein deletion alters basal and acidosis-stimulated renal ammonia excretion. Am J Physiol Renal Physiol 2009;296(6):F1364–75.

[43] Weiner ID, Verlander JW. Role of NH$_3$ and NH$_4^+$ transporters in renal acid–base transport. Am J Physiol Renal Physiol 2011;300(1):F11–23.

[44] Sato S, Zhu XL, Sly WS. Carbonic anhydrase isozymes IV and II in urinary membranes from carbonic anhydrase II-deficient patients. Proc Natl Acad Sci USA 1990;87(16):6073–6.

[45] Star RA, Burg MB, Knepper MA. Luminal disequilibrium pH and ammonia transport in outer medullary collecting duct. Am J Physiol 1987;29984:26980–8021.

[46] Shuichi T, Schwartz GJ. HCO$_3^-$ absorption in rabbit outer medullary collecting duct: role of luminal carbonic anhydrase. Am J Physiol 1998;274:F139–47.

[47] Sterling D, Reithmeier RA, Casey JR. Carbonic anhydrase: in the driver's seat for bicarbonate transport. Jop 2001;2(4 Suppl.):165–70.

[48] Sterling D, Reithmeier RA, Casey JR. A transport metabolon. functional interaction of carbonic anhydrase II and chloride/bicarbonate exchangers. J Biol Chem 2001;276(51):47886–94.

[49] Nijenhuis T, Renkema KY, Hoenderop JG, Bindels RJ. Acid–base status determines the renal expression of Ca^{2+} and Mg^{2+} transport proteins. J Am Soc Nephrol 2006;17(3):617–26.

[50] Tucker BJ, Blantz RC. Studies on the mechanism of reduction in glomerular filtration rate after benzolamide. Pflugers Arch 1980;388:211–6.

[51] Johnson T, Kass MA. Hematologic reactions to carbonic anhydrase inhibitors. Am J Opthal 1986;101:410–8.

[52] Paisley KE, Tomson CR. Calcium phosphate stones during long-term acetazolamide treatment for epilepsy. Postgrad Med J 1999;75(885):427–8.

[53] Stafstrom CE, Gilmore HE, Kurtin PS. Nephrocalcinosis complicating medical treatment of posthemorrhagic hydrocephalus. Pediatr Neurol 1992;8:179–82.

[54] Werblin TP, Pollack IP, Liss RA. Blood dyscrasias in patients suing methazolamide (Neptazane) for glaucoma. Opthalmology 1980;87:350–4.

[55] Ellison DH, Wilcox CS. Diuretics: use in edema and the problem of resistance. In: Brady HR, Wilcox CS, editors. Therapy in nephrology and hypertension. London: Saunders; 2003. p. 955–76.

[56] Kassamali R, Sica DA. Acetazolamide: a forgotten diuretic agent. Cardiol Rev 2011;19(6):276–8.

[57] Marik PE, Kussman BD, Lipman J, Kraus P. Acetazolamide in the treatment of metabolic alkalosis in critically ill patients. Heart Lung 1991;20:455–9.

[58] Fiore DC, Hall S, Shoja P. Altitude illness: risk factors, prevention, presentation, and treatment. Am Fam Physician 2010;82(9):1103–10.

[59] Gertsch JH, Lipman GS, Holck PS, Merritt A, Mulcahy A, Fisher RS, et al. Prospective, double-blind, randomized, placebo-controlled comparison of acetazolamide versus ibuprofen for prophylaxis against high altitude headache: the Headache Evaluation at Altitude Trial (HEAT). Wilderness Environ Med 2010;21(3):236–43.

[60] Seupaul RA, Welch JL, Malka ST, Emmett TW. Pharmacologic prophylaxis for acute mountain sickness: a systematic shortcut review. Ann Emerg Med 2011;59(4):307–17.

[61] Resnick JS, Engle WK, Griggs RC, Stam AC. Acetazolamide prophylaxis in hypokalemic periodic paralysis. N Engl J Med 1968;278:582–6.

[62] Grissom CK, Roach RC, Sarnquist FH, Hackett PH. Acetazolamide in the treatment of acute mountain sickenss: clinical efficacy and effect on gas. Ann Intern Med 1992;116:461–5.

[63] Johnsen T. Effect upon serum insulin, glucose and potassium concentrations of acetazolamide during attacks of familial periodic hypokalemic paralysis. Acta Neurol Scand 1977;56:533–41.

[64] Reiss WG, Oles KS. Acetazolamide in the treatment of seizures. Ann Pharmacother 1996;30:514–9.

[65] Shoeman JF. Childhood pseudotumor cerebri: clinical and intracranial pressure response to acetazolamide and furosemide treatment in a case series. J Child Neurol 1994;9:130–4.

[66] Shore ET, Millman EP. Central sleep apnea and acetazolamide therapy. Arch Intern Med 1983;143:1278–80.

[67] Prescott LF, Balali-Mood M, Critchley JA, Johnstone AF, Proudfoot AT. Diuresis or urinary alkalinization for salicylate poisoning? British Med J 1982;285:1383–6.

[68] Hannaert P, Alvarez-Guerra M, Pirot D, Nazaret C, Garay RP. Rat NKCC2/NKCC1 co-transporter selectivity for loop diuretic drugs. Naunyn–Schmiedeberg's Arch Pharmacol 2002;365(3):193–9.

[69] Puschett JB, Goldberg M. The acute effects of furosemide on acid and electrolyte excretion in man. J Lab Clin Med 1968;71:666–77.

[70] Paulais M, Lachheb S, Teulon JA. Na$^+$- and Cl$^-$-activated K$^+$ channel in the thick ascending limb of mouse kidney. J Gen Physiol 2006;127(2):205–15.

[71] Vandewalle A, Cluzeaud F, Bens M, Kieferle S, Steinmeyer K, Jentsch TJ. Localization and induction by dehydration of ClC-K chloride channels in the rat kidney. Am J Physiol 1997;272(5 Pt 2):F678–88.

[72] Shankar SS, Brater DC. Loop diuretics: from the Na-K-2Cl transporter to clinical use. Am J Physiol 2003;284(1):F11–21.

[73] Somasekharan S, Tanis J, Forbush B. Loop diuretic and ion binding residues revealed by scanning mutagenesis of transmembrane helix 3 (TM3) of the Na-K-Cl Co-transporter (NKCC1). J Biol Chem 2012.

[74] Kaplan MR, Plotkin MD, Lee WS, Xu ZC, Lytton J, Hebert SC. Apical localization of the Na-K-Cl co-transporter, rBSC1, on rat thick ascending limbs. Kidney Int 1996;49:40–7.

[75] Obermuller N, Kunchaparty S, Ellison DH, Bachmann S. Expression of the Na-K-2Cl co-transporter by macula densa and thick ascending limb cells of rat and rabbit nephron. J Clin Invest 1996;98(3):635–40.

[76] Ho K, Nichols CG, Lederer WJ, Lytton J, Vassilev PM, Kanazirska MV, et al. Cloning and expression of an inwardly rectifying ATP-regulated potassium channel. Nature 1993;362 (6415):31–8.

[77] Hebert SC, Reeves WB, Molony DA, Andreoli TE. The medullary thick limb: function and modulation of the single-effect multiplier. Kidney Int 1987;31:580–8.

[78] Lytle C, McManus TJ, Haas M. A model of Na-K-2Cl co-transport based on ordered ion binding and glide symmetry. Am J Physiol 1998;274:C299–309.

[79] Haas M, McManus TJ. Bumetanide inhibits (Na + K + 2Cl) co-transport at a chloride site. Am J Physiol 1983;245:C235–40.

[80] Moore ML, George JN, Turner RJ. Anion dependence of bumetanide binding and ion transport by the rabbit parotid Na($^+$)-K ($^+$)-2Cl$^-$ co-transporter: evidence for an intracellular anion modifier site. Biochem J 1995;309(Pt 2):637–42.

[81] Isenring P, Jacoby SC, Chang J, Forbush B. Mutagenic mapping of the Na-K-Cl co-transporter for domains involved in ion transport and bumetanide binding. J Gen Physiol 1998;112(5): 549–58.

[82] Gagnon E, Bergeron MJ, Brunet GM, Daigle ND, Simard CF, Isenring P. Molecular mechanisms of Cl$^-$ transport by the renal Na($^+$)-K($^+$)-Cl$^-$ co-transporter. Identification of an intracellular locus that may form part of a high affinity Cl($^-$)-binding site. J Biol Chem 2004;279(7):5648–54.

[83] Kowalczyk L, Ratera M, Paladino A, Bartoccioni P, Errasti-Murugarren E, Valencia E, et al. Molecular basis of substrate-induced permeation by an amino acid antiporter. Proc Natl Acad Sci USA 2011;108(10):3935–40.

[84] Gao X, Zhou L, Jiao X, Lu F, Yan C, Zeng X, et al. Mechanism of substrate recognition and transport by an amino acid antiporter. Nature 2010;463(7282):828–32.

[85] Fang Y, Jayaram H, Shane T, Kolmakova-Partensky L, Wu F, Williams C, et al. Structure of a prokaryotic virtual proton pump at 3.2 Å resolution. Nature 2009;460(7258):1040–3.

[86] Shaffer PL, Goehring A, Shankaranarayanan A, Gouaux E. Structure and mechanism of a Na$^+$-independent amino acid transporter. Science 2009;325(5943):1010–4.

[87] Miyanoshita A, Terada M, Endou H. Furosemide directly stimulates prostaglandin E2 production in the thick ascending limb of Henle's loop. J Pharmacol Exp Ther 1989;251:1155–9.

[88] Peti-Peterdi J, Komlosi P, Fuson AL, Guan Y, Schneider A, Qi Z, et al. Luminal NaCl delivery regulates basolateral PGE2 release from macula densa cells. J Clin Invest 2003;112(1): 76–82.

[89] Kirchner KA. Prostaglandin inhibitors alter loop segment chloride uptake during furosemide diuresis. Am J Physiol 1985;248:F698–704.

[90] Kirchner KA, Martin CJ, Bower JD. Prostaglandin E2 but not I2 restores furosemide response in indomethacin-treated rats. Am J Physiol 1986;250:F980–5.

[91] Nusing RM, Treude A, Weissenberger C, Jensen B, Bek M, Wagner C, et al. Dominant role of prostaglandin E2 EP4 receptor in furosemide-induced salt-losing tubulopathy: a model for hyperprostaglandin E syndrome/antenatal Bartter syndrome. J Am Soc Nephrol 2005;16(8):2354–62.

[92] Bilezikian JP. Management of hypercalcemia. J Clin Endocrin Metab 1993;77:1445–9.

[93] LeGrand SB, Leskuski D, Zama I. Narrative review: furosemide for hypercalcemia: an unproven yet common practice. Ann Intern Med 2008;149(4):259–63.

[94] Friedman PA. Codependence of renal calcium and sodium transport. Annu Rev Physiol 1998;60:179–97.

[95] Hou J, Renigunta A, Gomes AS, Hou M, Paul DL, Waldegger S, et al. Claudin-16 and claudin-19 interaction is required for their assembly into tight junctions and for renal reabsorption of magnesium. Proc Natl Acad Sci USA 2009;106(36):15350–5.

[96] Hou J, Goodenough DA. Claudin-16 and claudin-19 function in the thick ascending limb. Curr Opin Nephrol Hypertens 2010;19(5):483–8.

[97] Hou J, Shan Q, Wang T, Gomes AS, Yan Q, Paul DL, et al. Transgenic RNAi depletion of claudin-16 and the renal handling of magnesium. J Biol Chem 2007;282(23):17114–22.

[98] Schnermann J, Homer W. Smith Award lecture. The juxtaglomerular apparatus: from anatomical peculiarity to physiological relevance. J Am Soc Nephrol 2003;14(6):1681–94.

[99] Schnermann J. Juxtaglomerular cell complex in the regulation of renal salt excretion. Am J Physiol 1998;274:R263–79.

[100] Lapointe J-Y, Laamarti A, Hurst AM, Fowler BC, Bell PD. Activation of Na:2Cl:K co-transport by luminal chloride in macula densa cells. Kidney Int 1995;47:752–7.

[101] Kurtz A, Gotz KH, Hamann M, Wagner C. Stimulation of renin secretion by nitric oxide is mediated by phosphodiesterase 3. Proc Natl Acad Sci USA 1998;95:4743–7.

[102] Schnermann J, Briggs JP. Synthesis and secretion of renin in mice with induced genetic mutations. Kidney Int 2012;81(6): 529–38.

[103] Harris RC, McKanna JA, Akai Y, Jacobson HR, Dubois RN, Breyer MD. Cyclooxygenase-2 is associated with the macula densa of rat kidney and increases with salt restriction. J Clin Invest 1994;94(6):2504–10.

[104] Komhoff M, Jeck ND, Seyberth HW, Grone HJ, Nusing RM, Breyer MD. Cyclooxygenase-2 expression is associated with the renal macula densa of patients with Bartter-like syndrome [In Process Citation]. Kidney Int 2000;58(6):2420–4.

[105] Mann B, Hartner A, Jensen BL, Kammerl M, Kramer BK, Kurtz A. Furosemide stimulates macula densa cyclooxygenase-2 expression in rats. Kidney Int 2001;59(1):62–8.

[106] Harding P, Sigmon DH, Alfie ME, Huang PL, Fishman MC, Beierwaltes WH, et al. Cyclooxygenase-2 mediates increased renal renin content induced by low-sodium diet. Hypertension 1997;29:297–302.

[107] Facemire CS, Nguyen M, Jania L, Beierwaltes WH, Kim HS, Koller BH, et al. A major role for the EP4 receptor in regulation of renin. Am J Physiol Renal Physiol 2011;301(5): F1035–41.

[108] Orlov SN. NKCC1 as a regulator of vascular tone and a novel target for antihypertensive therapeutics. Am J Physiol Heart Circ Physiol 2007;292(5):H2035–6.

[109] Gerber JG, Nies AS. Furosemide-induced vasodilation: importance of the state of hydration and filtration. Kidney Int 1980;18(4):454–9.

[110] Patak RV, Fadem SZ, Rosenblatt SG, Lifschitz MD, Stein JH. Diuretic-induced changes in renal blood flow and prostaglandin E excretion in the dog. Am J Physiol 1979;236(5):F494–500.

[111] Dobrowolski L, Bdzynska B, Sadowski J. Differential effect of frusemide on renal medullary and cortical blood flow in the anaesthetised rat. Exp Physiol 2000;85(6):783–9.

[112] Oppermann M, Hansen PB, Castrop H, Schnermann J. Vasodilatation of afferent arterioles and paradoxical increase of renal vascular resistance by furosemide in mice. Am J Physiol Renal Physiol 2007;293(1):F279–87.

[113] Brezis M, Agmon Y, Epstein FH. Determinants of intrarenal oxygenation. I. Effects of diuretics. Am J Physiol Renal, Fluid Electrolyte Physiol 1994;267:F1059–62.

[114] Heyman SN, Rosen S, Epstein FH, Spokes K, Brezis ML. Loop diuretics reduce hypoxic damage to proximal tubules of the isolated perfused rat kidney. Kidney Int 1994;45(4):981−5.

[115] Kusakabe Y, Matsushita T, Honda S, Okada S, Murase K. Using BOLD imaging to measure renal oxygenation dynamics in rats injected with diuretics. Magn Reson Med Sci 2010;9(4): 187−94.

[116] Warner L, Glockner JF, Woollard J, Textor SC, Romero JC, Lerman LO. Determinations of renal cortical and medullary oxygenation using blood oxygen level-dependent magnetic resonance imaging and selective diuretics. Invest Radiol 2011;46(1):41−7.

[117] Bell PD, Lapointe JY, Sabirov R, Hayashi S, Peti-Peterdi J, Manabe K, et al. Macula densa cell signaling involves ATP release through a maxi anion channel. Proc Natl Acad Sci U S A 2003;100(7):4322−7.

[118] Sun D, Samuelson LC, Yang T, Huang Y, Paliege A, Saunders T, et al. Mediation of tubuloglomerular feedback by adenosine: evidence from mice lacking adenosine 1 receptors. Proc Natl Acad Sci U S A 2001;98(17):9983−8.

[119] Thomson S, Bao D, Deng A, Vallon V. Adenosine formed by 5′-nucleotidase mediates tubuloglomerular feedback. J Clin Invest 2000;106(2):289−98.

[120] Vallon V, Richter K, Huang DY, Rieg T, Schnermann J. Functional consequences at the single-nephron level of the lack of adenosine A1 receptors and tubuloglomerular feedback in mice. Pflugers Arch 2004;448(2):214−21.

[121] Brown R, Ollerstam A, Johansson B, Skott O, Gebre-Medhin S, Fredholm B, et al. Abolished tubuloglomerular feedback and increased plasma renin in adenosine A1 receptor-deficient mice. Am J Physiol Regul Integr Comp Physiol 2001;281(5): R1362−7.

[122] Dikshit K, Vyden JK, Forrester JS, Chatterjee K, Prakash R, Swan HJC. Renal and extrarenal hemodynamic effects of furosemide in congestive heart failure after acute myocardial infarction. N Engl J Med 1973;288:1087−90.

[123] Mukherjee SK, Katz MA, Michael UF, Ogden DA. Mechanisms of hemodynamic actions of furosemide: differentiation of vascular and renal effects on blood pressure in functionally anephric hypertensive patients. Am Heart J 1981;101:313−8.

[124] Bourland WA, Day DK, Williamson HE. The role of the kidney in the early nondiuretic action of furosemide to reduce elevated left atrial pressure in the hypervolemic dog. J Pharmacol Exp Ther 1977;202:221−9.

[125] Schmieder RE, Messerli FH, deCarvalho JGR, Husserl FE. Immediate hemodynamic response to furosemide in patients undergoing chronic hemodialysis. Am J Kidney Dis 1987;9: 55−9.

[126] Costa MA, Loria A, Elesgaray R, Balaszczuk AM, Arranz C. Role of nitric oxide pathway in hypotensive and renal effects of furosemide during extracellular volume expansion. J Hypertens 2004;22(8):1561−9.

[127] Pickkers P, Dormans TP, Russel FG, Hughest AD, Thien T, Schaper N, et al. Direct vascular effects of furosemide in humans. Circulation 1997;96:1847−52.

[128] Meyer JW, Flagella M, Sutliff RL, Lorenz JN, Nieman ML, Weber CS, et al. Decreased blood pressure and vascular smooth muscle tone in mice lacking basolateral Na($^+$)-K($^+$)-2Cl ($^−$) co-transporter. Am J Physiol Heart Circ Physiol 2002;283(5): H1846−55.

[129] Wall SM, Knepper MA, Hassell KA, Fischer MP, Shodeinde A, Shin W, et al. Hypotension in NKCC1 null mice: role of the kidneys. Am J Physiol Renal Physiol 2006;290(2):F409−16.

[130] Kim SM, Eisner C, Faulhaber-Walter R, Mizel D, Wall SM, Briggs JP, et al. Salt sensitivity of blood pressure in NKCC1-

[131] Johnston GD, Nicholls DP, Leahey WJ. The dose−response characteristics of the acute non-diuretic peripheral vascular effects of frusemide in normal subjects. Br J Clin Pharmacol 1984;18:75−81.

[132] Francis GS, Siegel RM, Goldsmith SR, Olivari MT, Levine B, Cohn JN. Acute vasoconstrictor response to intravenous furosemide in patients with chronic congestive heart failure. Ann Intern Med 1985;103:1−6.

[133] Goldsmith SR, Francis G, Cohn JN. Attenuation of the pressor response to intravenous furosemide by angiotensin converting enzyme inhibition in congestive heart failure. Am J Cardiol 1989;64:1382−5.

[134] Inoue M, Okajima K, Itoh K, Ando Y, Watanabe N, Yasaka T, et al. Mechanism of furosemide resistance in analbuminemic rats and hypoalbuminemic patients. Kidney Int 1987;32: 198−203.

[135] Brater DC. Disposition and response to bumetanide and furosemide. Am J Cardiol 1986;57(2):20A−5A.

[136] Brater DC. Diuretic therapy. N Engl J Med 1998;339:387−95.

[137] Nigwekar SU, Waikar SS. Diuretics in acute kidney injury. Semin Nephrol 2011;31(6):523−34.

[138] Packer M, Lee WH, Medina N, Yushak M, Kessler PD. Functional renal insufficiencey during long-term therapy with captopril and enalapril in severe congestive heart failure. Ann Intern Med 1987;106:346−54.

[139] Packer M. Identification of risk factors predisposing to the development of functional renal insufficiency during treatment with converting-enzyme inhibitors in chronic heart failure. Cardiology 1989;76(Suppl. 2):50−5.

[140] Smith WE, Steele TH. Avoiding diuretic related complications in older patients. Geriatrics 1983;38:117−9.

[141] Kaufman AM, Levitt MF. The effect of diuretics on systemic and renal hemodynamics in patients with renal insufficiency. Am J Kidney Dis 1985;5:A71−8.

[142] Heerdink ER, Leufkens HG, Herrings RMC, Ottervanger JP, Stricker BHC, Bakker A. NSAIDs associated with increased risk of congestive heart failure in elderly patients taking diuretics. Arch Intern Med 1998;158:1108−12.

[143] Huerta C, Castellsague J, Varas-Lorenzo C, Garcia Rodriguez LA. Nonsteroidal anti-inflammatory drugs and risk of ARF in the general population. Am J Kidney Dis 2005;45(3): 531−9.

[144] Bichet DG, Van Putten VJ, Schrier RW. Potential role of increased sympathetic activity in impaired sodium and water excretion in cirrhosis. N Engl J Med 1982;307:1552−7.

[145] Dyckner T, Webster PO. Magnesium treatment of diuretic-induced hyponatremia with a preliminary report on a new aldosterone antagonist. J Am Coll Nutr 1982;1:149−53.

[146] Schrier RW. New treatments for hyponatremia. N Engl J Med 1978;298:214−5.

[147] Hantman D, Rossier B, Zohlman R, Schrier RW. Rapid correction of hyponatremia in the syndrom of inappropriate secretion of antidiuretic hormone: an alternative treatment to hypertonic saline. Ann Intern Med 1973;78:870−5.

[148] Dzau VJ, Hollenberg NK. Renal response to captopril in severe heart failure: role of furosemide in natriuresis and reversal of hyponatremia. Ann Intern Med 1984;100: 777−82.

[149] Ram CV, Garrett BN, Kaplan NM. Moderate sodium restriction and various diuretics in the treatment of hypertension. Arch Intern Med 1981;141(8):1015−9.

[150] Palmer BF. Potassium disturbances associated with the use of diuretics. San Diego: Academic Press; 1997. p. 571−583.

deficient mice. Am J Physiol Renal Physiol 2008;295(4): F1230−8.

III. FLUID AND ELECTROLYTE REGULATION AND DYSREGULATION

[151] Hropot M, Fowler NB, Karlmark B, Giebisch G. Tubular action of diuretics: distal effects on electrolyte transport and acidification. Kidney Int 1985;28:477–89.

[152] Sansom SC, Welling PA. Two channels for one job. Kidney Int 2007;72(5):529–30.

[153] Wilcox CS, Mitch WE, Kelly RA, Freidman PA, Souney PF, et al. Factors affecting potassium balance during frusemide administration. Clin Sci 1984;67:195–203.

[154] Good DW. Sodium-dependent bicarbonate absorption by cortical thick ascending limb of rat kidney. Am J Physiol 1985;248: F821–9.

[155] Knepper MA, Good DW, Burg MB. Ammonia and bicarbonate transport by rat cortical collecting ducts perfused *in vitro*. Am J Physiol 1985;249:F870–7.

[156] Oberleithner H, Lang F, Messner G, Wang W. Mechanism of hydrogen ion transport in the diluting segment of frog kidney. Pflügers Arch 1984;402:272–80.

[157] Stone DK, Seldin DW, Kokko JP, Jacobson HR. Mineralocorticoid modulation of rabbit medullary collecting duct acidification. J Clin Invest 1983;72:77–83.

[158] Han KH. Mechanisms of the effects of acidosis and hypokalemia on renal ammonia metabolism. Electrolyte Blood Press 2011;9(2):45–9.

[159] Aronson PS, Giebisch G. Effects of pH on potassium: new explanations for old observations. J Am Soc Nephrol 2011;22 (11):1981–9.

[160] Wingo CS, Straub SG. Active proton secretion and potassium absorption in the rabbit outer medullary collecting duct. Functional evidence for proton-potassium-activated adenosine triphosphatase. J Clin Invest 1989;84:361–5.

[161] Maher JF, Schreiner GF. Studies on ethacrynic acid in patients with refractory edema. Ann Intern Med 1965;62:15–29.

[162] Ikeda K, Oshima T, Hidaka H, Takasaka T. Molecular and clinical implications of loop diuretic ototoxicity. Hear Res 1997;107:1–8.

[163] Ryback LP. Ototoxicity of loop diuretics. Otolaryngol Clin N Am 1993;26:829–44.

[164] Ikeda K, Morizono T. Electrochemical profiles for monvalent ions in the stria vascularis: cellular model of ion transport mechanisms. Hear Res 1989;39:279–86.

[165] Mizuta K, Adachi M, Iwasa KH. Ultrastructural localization of the Na-K-Cl co-transporter in the lateral wall of the rabbit cochlear duct. Hear Res 1997;106(1–2):154–62.

[166] Hidaka H, Oshima T, Ikeda K, Furukawa M, Takasaka T. The Na-K-Cl co-transporters in the rat cochlea: RT-PCR and partial sequence analysis. Biochem Biophys Res Comm 1996;220: 425–30.

[167] Flagella M, Clarke LL, Miller ML, Erway LC, Giannella RA, Andringa A, et al. Mice lacking the basolateral Na-K-2Cl co-transporter have impaired epithelial chloride secretion and are profoundly deaf. J Biol Chem 1999;274(38):26946–55.

[168] Delpire E, Lu J, England R, Dull C, Thorne T. Deafness and imbalance associated with inactivation of the secretory Na-K-2Cl co-transporter. Nat Genet 1999;22(2):192–5.

[169] Star RA. Ototoxicity. San Diego: Academic Press; 1997 [p. 637642]

[170] Eknoyan G, Suki WN, Martinez-Maldonado M. Effect of diuretics on urinary excretion of phosphate, calcium, and magnesium in thyroparathyroidectomized dogs. J Lab Clin Med 1970;76:257–66.

[171] Bolland MJ, Ames RW, Horne AM, Orr-Walker BJ, Gamble GD, Reid IR. The effect of treatment with a thiazide diuretic for 4 years on bone density in normal postmenopausal women. Osteoporos Int 2007;18(4):479–86.

[172] Friedman PA, Hebert SC. Site and mechanism of diuretic action. San Diego: Academic Press; 1997 [p. 75-111]

[173] Kunau Jr. RT, Weller DR, Webb HL. Clarification of the site of action of chlorothiazide in the rat nephron. J Clin Invest 1975;56(2):401–7.

[174] Ellison DH, Velázquez H, Wright FS. Thiazide sensitive sodium chloride co-transport in the early distal tubule. Am J Physiol 1987;253:F546–54.

[175] Costanzo LS. Localization of diuretic action in microperfused rat distal tubules: Ca and Na transport. Am J Physiol 1985;248: F527–35.

[176] Reilly RF, Ellison DH. Mammalian distal tubule: physiology, pathophysiology, and molecular anatomy. Physiol Rev 2000;80 (1):277–313.

[177] Imai M, Nakamura R. Function of distal convoluted and connecting tubules studied by isolated nephron fragments. Kidney Int 1982;22:465–72.

[178] Shimizu T, Yoshitomi K, Nakamura M, Imai M. Site and mechanism of action of trichlormethiazide in rabbit distal nephron segments perfused *in vitro*. J Clin Invest 1988;82:721–30.

[179] Velázquez H, Greger R. Electrical properties of the early distal convoluted tubules of the rabbit kidney. Renal Physiol 1986;55.

[180] Gamba G, Saltzberg SN, Lombardi M, Miyanoshita A, Lytton J, Hediger MA, et al. Primary structure and functional expression of a cDNA encoding the thiazide-sensitive, electroneutral sodium-chloride co-transporter. Proc Natl Acad Sci USA 1993;90:2749–53.

[181] Obermuller N, Bernstein P, Velazquez H, Reilly R, Moser D, Ellison DH, et al. Expression of the thiazide-sensitive Na-Cl co-transporter in rat and human kidney. Am J Physiol 1995;269 (6 Pt 2):F900–10.

[182] Bachmann S, Velazquez H, Obermuller N, Reilly RF, Moser D, Ellison DH. Expression of the thiazide-sensitive Na-Cl co-transporter by rabbit distal convoluted tubule cells. J Clin Invest 1995;96(5):2510–4.

[183] Plotkin MD, Kaplan MR, Verlander JW, Lee W-S, Brown D, Poch E, et al. Localization of the thiazide sensitive Na-Cl co-transporter, rTSC1, in the rat kidney. Kidney Int 1996;50: 174–83.

[184] Pizzonia JH, Gesek FA, Kennedy SM, Coutermarsh BA, Bacskai BJ, Friedman PA. Immunomagnetic separation, primary culture, and characterization of cortical thick ascending limb plus distal convoluted tubule cells from mouse kidney. In Vitro Cell Dev Biol 1991;27A:409–16.

[185] Campean V, Kricke J, Ellison D, Luft FC, Bachmann S. Localization of thiazide-sensitive Na($^+$)-Cl($^-$) co-transport and associated gene products in mouse DCT. Am J Physiol 2001;281(6):F1028–35.

[186] Velázquez H, Good DW, Wright FS. Mutual dependence of sodium and chloride absorption by renal distal tubule. Am J Physiol 1984;247:F904–11.

[187] Stokes JB. Sodium chloride absorption by the urinary bladder of the winter flounder: a thiazide-sensitive electrically neutral transport system. J Clin Invest 1984;74:7–16.

[188] Miyanoshita A, Gamba G, Lytton J, Lombardi M, Brenner BM, Hebert SC. Primary structure and functional expression of the rat renal thiazide-sensitive Na$^+$:Cl$^-$ co-transporter. Proc 12th Int Congr Nephrol 1993:110.

[189] Simon DB, Nelson-Williams C, Bia MJ, Ellison D, Karet FE, Molina AM, et al. Gitelman's variant of Bartter's syndrome, inherited hypokalaemic alkalosis, is caused by mutations in the thiazide-sensitive Na-Cl co-transporter. Nat Genet 1996;12(1):24–30.

[190] Velázquez H, Naray-Fejes-Toth A, Reilly RF, Ellison DH. NaCl co-transporter and 11-b- hydroxysteroid dehydrogenase are coexpressed in rabbit distal convoluted tubule. FASEB J 1996;: A368.

[191] Bostanjoglo M, Reeves WB, Reilly RF, Velazquez H, Robertson N, Litwack G, et al. 11Beta-hydroxysteroid dehydrogenase, mineralocorticoid receptor, and thiazide-sensitive Na-Cl co-transporter expression by distal tubules. J Am Soc Nephrol 1998;9(8):1347–58.

[192] Wilson DR, Honrath U, Sonnenberg H. Thiazide diuretic effect on medullary collecting duct function in the rat. Kidney Int 1983;23:711–6.

[193] Terada Y, Knepper MA. Thiazide-sensitive NaCl absorption in rat cortical collecting duct. Am J Physiol Renal, Fluid Electrolyte Physiol 1990;259:F519–28.

[194] Rouch AJ, Chen L, Troutman SL, Schafer JA. Na$^+$ transport in isolated rat CCD: effects of bradykinin, ANP, clonidine, and hydrochlorothiazide. Am J Physiol Renal, Fluid Electrolyte Physiol 1991;260:F86–95.

[195] Leviel F, Hubner CA, Houillier P, Morla L, El Moghrabi S, Brideau G, et al. The Na$^+$-dependent chloride-bicarbonate exchanger SLC4A8 mediates an electroneutral Na$^+$ reabsorption process in the renal cortical collecting ducts of mice. J Clin Invest 2010;120(5):1627–35.

[196] Beaumont K, Vaughn DA, Fanestil DD. Thiazide diuretic drug receptors in rat kidney: identification with [^{3}H]Metolazone. Proc Natl Acad Sci 1988;85:2311–4.

[197] Tran JM, Farrell MA, Fanestil DD. Effect of ions on binding of the thiazide-type diuretic metolazone to kidney membrane. Am J Physiol 1990;258:F908–15.

[198] Chang H, Fujita T. A kinetic model of the thiazide-sensitive Na-Cl co-transporter. Am J Physiol 1999;:276.

[199] Moreno E, San Cristobal P, Rivera M, Vazquez N, Bobadilla NA, Gamba G. Affinity defining domains in the Na-Cl co-transporter: different location for Cl$^-$ and thiazide binding. J Biol Chem 2006;281(25):17266–75.

[200] Reilly RF, Huang CL. The mechanism of hypocalciuria with NaCl co-transporter inhibition. Nat Rev Nephrol 2011;7(11): 669–74.

[201] Costanzo LS, Weiner IM. On the hypocalciuric action of chlorothiazide. J Clin Invest 1974;54:628–37.

[202] Costanzo LS, Windhager EE. Calcium and sodium transport by the distal convoluted tubule of the rat. Am J Physiol 1978;235:F492–506.

[203] Ellison DH. Divalent cation transport by the distal nephron: insights from Bartter's and Gitelman's syndromes. Am J Physiol 2000;279(4):F616–25.

[204] den Dekker E, Hoenderop JG, Nilius B, Bindels RJ. The epithelial calcium channels, TRPV5 & TRPV6: from identification towards regulation. Cell Calcium 2003;33(5-6):497–507.

[205] Friedman PA. Calcium transport in the kidney. Curr Opin Nephrol Hypertens 1999;8(5):589–95.

[206] Nijenhuis T, Vallon V, van der Kemp AW, Loffing J, Hoenderop JG, Bindels RJ. Enhanced passive Ca^{2+} reabsorption and reduced Mg^{2+} channel abundance explains thiazide-induced hypocalciuria and hypomagnesemia. J Clin Invest 2005;115(6):1651–8.

[207] Porter RH, Cox BG, Heaney D, Hostetter TH, Stinebaugh BJ, Suki WN. Treatment of hypoparathyroide patients with chlorthalidone. N Engl J Med 1978;298:577–81.

[208] Belge H, Gailly P, Schwaller B, Loffing J, Debaix H, Riveira-Munoz E, et al. Renal expression of parvalbumin is critical for NaCl handling and response to diuretics. Proc Natl Acad Sci U S A 2007;104(37):14849–54.

[209] Cheng CJ, Shiang JC, Hsu YJ, Yang SS, Lin SH. Hypocalciuria in patients with Gitelman syndrome: role of blood volume. Am J Kidney Dis 2007;49(5):693–700.

[210] McCormick JA, Mutig K, Nelson JH, Saritas T, Hoorn EJ, Yang C-L, et al. A SPAK isoform switch modulates renal salt transport and blood pressure. Cell Metab 2011;14(3):352–64.

[211] Favre GA, Nau V, Kolb I, Vargas-Poussou R, Hannedouche T, Moulin B. Localization of tubular adaptation to renal sodium loss in Gitelman syndrome. Clin J Am Soc Nephrol 2012;7(3): 472–8.

[212] Ellison DH. Adaptation in gitelman syndrome: "we just want to pump you up.". Clin J Am Soc Nephrol 2012;7(3):379–82.

[213] Dai LJ, Ritchie G, Kerstan D, Kang HS, Cole DE, Quamme GA. Magnesium transport in the renal distal convoluted tubule. Physiol Rev 2001;81(1):51–84.

[214] Douban S, Brodsky MA, Whang DD. Significance of magnesium in congestive heart failure. Am Heart J 1996;132:664–71.

[215] Voets T, Nilius B, Hoefs S, van der Kemp AW, Droogmans G, Bindels RJ, et al. TRPM6 forms the Mg^{2+} influx channel involved in intestinal and renal Mg^{2+} absorption. J Biol Chem 2004;279(1):19–25.

[216] Loffing J, Vallon V, Loffing-Cueni D, Aregger F, Richter K, Pietri L, et al. Altered renal distal tubule structure and renal Na($^+$) and Ca($^{2+}$) handling in a mouse model for Gitelman's syndrome. J Am Soc Nephrol 2004;15(9):2276–88.

[217] Loffing J, Loffing-Cueni D, Hegyi I, Kaplan MR, Hebert SC, Le Hir M, et al. Thiazide treatment of rats provokes apoptosis in distal tubule cells. Kidney Int 1996;50(4):1180–90.

[218] Ellison DH, Loffing J. Thiazide effects and adverse effects: insights from molecular genetics. Hypertension 2009;54(2): 196–202.

[219] Dai LJ, Friedman PA, Quamme GA. Cellular mechanisms of chlorothiazide and potassium depletion on Mg^{2+} uptake in mouse distal convoluted tubule cells. Kidney Int 1997;51: 1008–17.

[220] Dai LJ, Friedman PA, Quamme GA. Mechanisms of amiloride stimulation of Mg^{2+} uptake in immortalized mouse distal convoluted tubule cells. Am J Physiol 1997;F249–56.

[221] Dimke H, Hoenderop JG, Bindels RJ. Molecular basis of epithelial Ca^{2+} and Mg^{2+} transport: insights from the TRP channel family. J Physiol 2011;589(Pt 7):1535–42.

[222] Quamme GA. Renal magnesium handling: new insights in undertsanding old problems. Kidney Int 1997;52:1180–95.

[223] Dyckner T, Wester P-O, Widman L. Amiloride prevents thiazide-induced intracellular potassium and magnesium losses. Acta Med Scand 1988;224:25–30.

[224] Murdoch DL, Forrest G, Davies DL, McInnes GT. A comparison of the potassium and magnesium-sparing properties of amiloride and spironolactone in diuretic-treated normal subjects. Br J Clin Pharmacol 1993;35(4):373–8.

[225] Wazny LD, Brophy DF. Amiloride for the prevention of amphotericin B-induced hypokalemia and hypomagnesemia. Ann Pharmacother 2000;34(1):94–7.

[226] Stergiou GS, Mayopoulou-Symvoulidou D, Mountokalakis TD. Attenuation by spironolactone of the magnesiuric effect of acute frusemide administration in patients with liver cirrhosis and ascites. Miner Electrolyte Metab 1993;19(2):86–90.

[227] Gao X, Peng L, Adhikari CM, Lin J, Zuo Z. Spironolactone reduced arrhythmia and maintained magnesium homeostasis in patients with congestive heart failure. J Card Fail 2007;13(3): 170–7.

[228] Walter SJ, Shirley DG. The effect of chronic hydrochlorothiazide administration on renal function in the rat. Clin Sci (Lond) 1986;70(4):379–87.

[229] Earley LE, Orloff J. The mechanism of antidiuresis associated with the administration of hydrochlorothiazide to patients with vasopressin-resistant diabetes insipidus. J Clin Invest 1962;41:1988–97.

[230] Siegel D, Hulley SB, Black DM, Cheitlin MD, Sebastian A, Seeley DG, et al. Diuretics, serum and intracellular electrolyte levels, and ventricular arrhythmias in hypertensive men. JAMA 1992;267:1083–9.

[231] Kountz DS, Goldman A, Mikhail J, Ezer M. Chlorthalidone: the forgotten diuretic. Postgrad Med 2012;124(1):60–6.

[232] Ellison DH, Wilcox CS. Diuretics. In: Brenner BM, editor. Brenner and Rector's the kidney. 2008. p. 1646–78.

[233] Appel LJ. The verdict from ALLHAT – thiazide diuretics are the preferred initial therapy for hypertension. JAMA 2002;288 (23):3039–42.

[234] Leary WP, Reyes AJ. Renal excretory actions of diuretics in man: correction of various current errors and redefinition of basic concepts. In: Reyes AJ, Leary WP, editors. Clinical pharmacology and therapeutic uses of diuretics. 153rd ed. Stuttgart: GustavFischer Verlag; 1988. p. 153–66.

[235] Worcester EM, Coe FL. Clinical practice. Calcium kidney stones. N Engl J Med 2010;363(10):954–63.

[236] Ray WA, Griffin MR, Downey W, Melton III LJ. Long-term use of thiazide diuretics and risk of hip fracture. Lancet 1989;1: 687–90.

[237] Felson DT, Sloutskis D, Anderson JJ, Anthony JM, Kiel DP. Thiazide diuretics and the risk of hip fracture. Results from the Framingham study. JAMA 1991;265:370–3.

[238] Cauley JA, Cummings SR, Seeley DG, Black D, Browner W, Kuller LH, et al. Effects of thiazide diuretic therapy on bone mass, fractures, and falls. Ann Intern Med 1993;118:666–73.

[239] Heidrich FE, Stergachis A, Gross KM. Diuretic drug use and the risk for hip fracture. Ann Intern Med 1991;115:1–6.

[240] Reid IR, Ames RW, Orr-Walker BJ, Clearwater JM, Horne AM, Evans MC, et al. Hydrochlorothiazide reduces loss of cortical bone in normal postmenopausal women: a randomized controlled trial. Am J Med 2000;109(5):362–70.

[241] Rejnmark L, Vestergaard P, Pedersen AR, Heickendorff L, Andreasen F, Mosekilde L. Dose-effect relations of loop- and thiazide-diuretics on calcium homeostasis: a randomized, double-blinded Latin-square multiple cross-over study in postmenopausal osteopenic women. Eur J Clin Invest 2003;33(1): 41–50.

[242] Schoofs MW, van der Klift M, Hofman A, de Laet CE, Herings RM, Stijnen T, et al. Thiazide diuretics and the risk for hip fracture. Ann Intern Med 2003;139(6):476–82.

[243] Janjua NR, Jonassen TE, Langhoff S, Thomsen K, Christensen S. Role of sodium depletion in acute antidiuretic effect of bendroflumethiazide in rats with nephrogenic diabetes insipidus. J Pharmacol Exp Ther 2001;299(1):307–13.

[244] Biner HL, Arpin-Bott MP, Loffing J, Wang X, Knepper M, Hebert SC, et al. Human cortical distal nephron: distribution of electrolyte and water transport pathways. J Am Soc Nephrol 2002;13(4):836–47.

[245] Kim GH, Lee JW, Oh YK, Chang HR, Joo KW, Na KY, et al. Antidiuretic effect of hydrochlorothiazide in lithium-induced nephrogenic diabetes insipidus is associated with upregulation of aquaporin-2, Na-Cl co-transporter, and epithelial sodium channel. J Am Soc Nephrol 2004;15(11):2836–43.

[246] Cesar KR, Magaldi AJ. Thiazide induces water absorption in the inner medullary collecting duct of normal and Brattleboro rats. Am J Physiol 1999;277(5 Pt 2):F756–60.

[247] Moser M. Diuretics should continue to be one of the preferred initial therapies in the management of hypertension: the

argument for. J Clin Hypertens (Greenwich) 2005;7(2):111–6 [quiz 21-2].

[248] Sica DA. Diuretics should continue to be one of the preferred initial therapies in the management of hypertension: the argument against. J Clin Hypertens (Greenwich) 2005;7(2):117–20 [quiz 21-2].

[249] Velázquez H, Wright FS. Control by drugs of renal potassium handling. Ann Rev Pharmacol Toxicol 1986;26:293–309.

[250] Velázquez H, Wright FS. Effects of diuretic drugs on Na, Cl, and K transport by rat renal distal tubule. Am J Physiol 1986;250:F1013–23.

[251] Wright FS. Flow-dependent transport processes: filtration, absorption, secretion. Am J Physiol 1982;243:F1–11.

[252] Okusa MD, Velazquez H, Ellison DH, Wright FS. Luminal calcium regulates potassium transport by the renal distal tubule. Am J Physiol 1990;258(2 Pt 2):F423–8.

[253] Okusa MD, Velazquez H, Wright FS. Effect of Na-channel blockers and lumen Ca on K secretion by rat renal distal tubule. Am J Physiol 1991;260(3 Pt 2):F459–65.

[254] Huang CL, Kuo E. Mechanism of hypokalemia in magnesium deficiency. J Am Soc Nephrol 2007;18(10):2649–52.

[255] Odvina CV, Mason RP, Pak CY. Prevention of thiazide-induced hypokalemia without magnesium depletion by potassium-magnesium-citrate. Am J Ther 2006;13(2):101–8.

[256] Dorup I, Skajaa K, Thybo NK. Oral magnesium supplementation restores the concentrations of magnesium, potassium and sodium-potassium pumps in skeletal muscle of patients receiving diuretic treatment. J Intern Med 1993;233:117–23.

[257] Leung AA, Wright A, Pazo V, Karson A, Bates DW. Risk of thiazide-induced hyponatremia in patients with hypertension. Am J Med 2011;124(11):1064–72.

[258] Fichman MP, Vorherr H, Kleeman CR, Telfer N. Diuretic-induced hyponatremia. Ann Intern Med 1971;75:853–63.

[259] Friedman E, Shadel M, Halkin H, Farfel Z. Thiazide-induced hyponatremia: reproducibility by single dose rechallenge and an analysis of pathogenesis. Ann Intern Med 1989;110:24–30.

[260] Chow KM, Szeto CC, Wong TY, Leung CB, Li PK. Risk factors for thiazide-induced hyponatraemia. QJM 2003;96(12):911–7.

[261] Chow KM, Kwan BC, Szeto CC. Clinical studies of thiazide-induced hyponatremia. J Natl Med Assoc 2004;96(10):1305–8.

[262] Harper R, Ennis CN, Heaney AP, Sheridan B, Gormley M, Atkinson AB, et al. A comparison of the effects of low- and conventional-dose thiazide diuretic on insulin action in hypertensive patients with NIDDM. Diabetologia 1995;38:853–9.

[263] Carlsen JE, Kober L, Torp-Pedersen C, Johansen P. Relation between dose of bendrofluazide, antihypertensive effect, and adverse biochemical effects. BMJ (Clinical Research Ed.) 1990;300:975–8.

[264] Helderman JH, Elahi D, Andersen DK, Raizes GS, Tobin JD, Shocken D, et al. Prevention of the glucose intolerance of thiazide diuretics by maintenance of body potassium. Diabetes 1983;32(2):106–11.

[265] Toto RA. Metabolic derangements associated with diuretic use: insulin resistance, dyslipidemia, hyperuricemia, and anti-adronergic effects. In: Seldin DW, Giebisch G, editors. Diuretic agents: clinical physiology and pharmacology. San Diego: Academic Press; 1997. p. 621–36.

[266] Pickkers P, Schachter M, Hughes AD, Feher MD, Sever PS. Thiazide-induced hyperglycaemia: a role for calcium-activated potassium channels? Diabetologia 1996;39:861–4.

[267] Grimm Jr RH, Flack JM, Granditis GA. Treatment of Mild Hypertension Study (TOMHS) Research Group. Long-term effects on plasma lipids of diet and drugs to treat hypertension. JAMA 1996;275:1549–56.

[268] Meneton P, Loffing J, Warnock DG. Sodium and potassium handling by the aldosterone-sensitive distal nephron: the pivotal role of the distal and connecting tubule. Am J Physiol Renal Physiol 2004;287(4):F593—601.

[269] Perez-Ayuso RM, Arroyo V, Planas R, Gaya J, Bory F, Rimola A, et al. Randomized comparative study of efficacy of furosemide versus spironolactone in nonazotemic cirrhosis with ascites. Relationship between the diuretic response an the activity of the renin—aldosterone system. Gastroenterology 1983;84: 961—8.

[270] Casavola V, Guerra L, Reshkin SJ, Jacobson KA, Verrey F, Murer H. Effect of adenosine on Na$^+$ and Cl$^-$ curents in A6 monolayers. Receptor localization and messenger involvement. J Membrane Biol 1996;151:237—45.

[271] Shimizu T, Nakamura M, Yoshitomi K, Imai M. Interaction of trichlormethiazide or amiloride with PTH in stimulating Ca^{2+} absorption in rabbit CNT. Am J Physiol 1991;261:F36—43.

[272] Bundy JT, Connito D, Mahoney MD, Pontier PJ. Treatment of idiopathic renal magesium wasting with amiloride. Am J Nephrol 1995;15:75—7.

[273] Schild L. The epithelial sodium channel: from molecule to disease. Rev Physiol Biochem Pharmacol 2004;151:93—107.

[274] Canessa CM, Horisberger J-D, Rossier BC. Epithelial sodium channel related to proteins involved in neurodegeneration. Nature 1993;361:467—70.

[275] Canessa CM, Schild L, Buell G, Thorens B, Gatuschi I, Horisberger J-D, et al. Amiloride-sensitive epithelial Na$^+$ channel is made of three homologous subunits. Nature 1994;367:463—7.

[276] Kellenberger S, Schild L. Epithelial sodium channel/degenerin family of ion channels: a variety of functions for a shared structure. Physiol Rev 2002;82(3):735—67.

[277] Kosari F, Sheng S, Li J, Mak DO, Foskett JK, Kleyman TR. Subunit stoichiometry of the epithelial sodium channel. J Biol Chem 1998;273(22):13469—74.

[278] Firsov D, Gautschi I, Merillat AM, Rossier BC, Schild L. The heterotetrameric architecture of the epithelial sodium channcl (ENaC). EMBO J 1998;17(2):344—52.

[279] Jasti J, Furukawa H, Gonzales EB, Gouaux E. Structure of acid-sensing ion channel 1 at 1.9 Å resolution and low pH. Nature 2007;449(7160):316—23.

[280] Canessa CM. Structural biology: unexpected opening. Nature 2007;449(7160):293—4.

[281] Palmer LG. Voltage-dependent block by amiloride and other monovalent cations of apical Na channels in the toad urinary bladder. J Membr Biol 1984;80(2):153—65.

[282] Grunder S, Jaeger NF, Gautschi I, Schild L, Rossier BC. Identification of a highly conserved sequence at the N-terminus of the epithelial Na$^+$ channel alpha subunit involved in gating. Pflugers Arch 1999;438(5):709—15.

[283] Kashlan OB, Kleyman TR. ENaC structure and function in the wake of a resolved structure of a family member. Am J Physiol Renal Physiol 2011;301(4):F684—96.

[284] Sheng S, Perry CJ, Kashlan OB, Kleyman TR. Side chain orientation of residues lining the selectivity filter of epithelial Na$^+$ channels. J Biol Chem 2005;280(9):8513—22.

[285] Verrey F, Pearce D, Pfeiffer R, Spindler B, Mastroberardino L, Summa V, et al. Pleiotropic action of aldosterone in epithelia mediated by transcription and post-transcription mechanisms. Kidney Int 2000;57(4):1277—82.

[286] Loffing J, Zecevic M, Feraille E, Kaissling B, Asher C, Rossier BC, et al. Aldosterone induces rapid apical translocation of ENaC in early portion of renal collecting system: possible role of SGK. Am J Physiol 2001;280(4):F675—82.

[287] Gründer S, Rossier BC. A reappraisal of aldosterone effects on kidney: new insights provided by epithelial sodium channel cloning. Curr Opin Nephrol Hypertens 1997;6:35—9.

[288] Funder JW. The nongenomic actions of aldosterone. Endocr Rev 2005;26(3):313—21.

[289] Fourkiotis VG, Hanslik G, Hanusch F, Lepenies J, Quinkler M. Aldosterone and the kidney. Horm Metab Res 2012;44 (3):194—201.

[290] Pratt WB. The role of heat shock proteins in regulating the function, folding, and trafficking of the glucocorticoid receptor. J Biol Chem 1993;268:21455—8.

[291] Tumlin JA, Lea JP, Swanson CE, Smith CL, Edge SS, Someren JS. Aldosterone and dexamethasone stimulate calcineurin activity through a transcription-independent mechanism involving steroid receptor-associated heat shock proteins. J Clin Invest 1997;99(6):1217—23.

[292] Verrey F. Transcriptional control of sodium transport in tight epithelia by adrenal steroids. J Membrane Biol 1995;144: 93—110.

[293] Rogerson FM, Brennan FE, Fuller PJ. Mineralocorticoid receptor binding, structure and function. Mol Cell Endocrinol 2004;217(1-2):203—12.

[294] Rokaw MD, Benos DJ, Palevsky PM, Cunningham SA, West ME, Johnson JP. Regulation of a sodium channel-associated G-protein by aldosterone. J Biol Chem 1996;271(8):4491—6.

[295] Chen SY, Bhargava A, Mastroberardino L, Meijer OC, Wang J, Buse P, et al. Epithelial sodium channel regulated by aldosterone-induced protein sgk. Proc Natl Acad Sci U S A 1999;96 (5):2514—9.

[296] Naray-Fejes-Toth A, Canessa C, Cleaveland ES, Aldrich G, Fejes-Toth G. sgk is an aldosterone-induced kinase in the renal collecting duct. Effects on epithelial Na$^+$ channels. J Biol Chem 1999;274(24):16973—8.

[297] Snyder PM, Olson DR, Thomas BC. Serum and glucocorticoid-regulated kinase modulates Nedd4-2-mediated inhibition of the epithelial Na$^+$ channel. J Biol Chem 2002;277(1):5—8.

[298] Zhou R, Snyder PM. Nedd4-2 phosphorylation induces serum and glucocorticoid-regulated kinase (SGK) ubiquitination and degradation. J Biol Chem 2005;280(6):4518—23.

[299] Shackleton CR, Wong NLM, Sutton RA. Distal (potassium-sparing) diuretics. In: Dirks JH, Sutton RAL, editors. Diuretics physiology, pharmacology and clinical use. 1st ed. Philadelphia: W.B. Saunders; 1986. p. 117—34.

[300] Fanestil DD. Mechanism of action of aldosterone blockers. Sem Nephrol 1988;8:249—63.

[301] Marver D, Stewart J, Funder JW, Feldman D, Edelman IS. Renal aldosterone receptors: studies with [^{3}H]aldosterone and the antimineralocorticoid [^{3}H]spirolactone (SC26304). Proc Natl Acad Sci 1974;71:1431—5.

[302] Couette B, Lombes M, Baulieu E-E, Rafestin-Oblin M-E. Aldosterone antagonists destablilize the mineralocorticoid receptor. Biochem J 1992;282:697—702.

[303] Delyani JA. Mineralocorticoid receptor antagonists: the evolution of utility and pharmacology. Kidney Int 2000;57(4): 1408—11.

[304] de Gasparo M, Joss U, Ramjoue HP, Whitebread SE, Haenni H, Schenkel L, et al. Three new epoxy-spirolactone derivatives: characterization in vivo and in vitro. J Pharmacol Exp Ther 1987;240(2):650—6.

[305] Liddle GW. Aldosterone antagonists and triamterene. Ann NYAcad Sci 1966;134:466—70.

[306] Kagawa CM. Blocking the renal electrolyte effects of mineralocorticoids with an orally active steroidal spirolactone. Endocrinology 1960;65:125—32.

[307] Costanzo LS. Comparison of calcium and sodium transport in early and late rat distal tubules: effect of amiloride. Am J Physiol 1984;246:F937−45.

[308] Stokes JB. Ion transport by the cortical and outer medullary collecting tubule. Kidney Int 1982;22:473−84.

[309] Stoner LC, Burg MB, Orloff J. Ion transport in cortical collecting tubule; effect of amiloride. Am J Physiol 1974;227:453−9.

[310] Garty H, Benos D. Characteristics and regulatory mechanisms of the amiloride-blockable Na$^+$ channel. Physiol Reviews 1988;68:309−73.

[311] Cassin S, Vogh B. Effect of Hydrochlorothiazide on renal blood flow and clearance of para-aminohippurate and creatinine. Proc Soc Exp Biol Med 1966;122:970−3.

[312] Busch AE, Suessbrich H, Kunzelmann K, Hipper A, Greger R, Waldegger S, et al. Blockade of epithelial Na$^+$ channels by triamterene-underlying mechanisms and molecular basis. Pflugers Arch 1996;432:760−6.

[313] Karim A. Spironolactone: disposition, metabolism, pharmacodynamics and bioavailability. Drug Metab Rev 1978;8:151−88.

[314] Merkus FWHM, Overdiek JWPM, Cilissen J, Zuidema J. Pharmacokinetics of spironolactone after a single dose: evaluation of the true canrenone serum concentrations during 24 hours. Clin Exp Hypertens 1983;([[A]5):249−69.

[315] Gardiner P, Schrode K, Quinlan D, Martin BK, Boreham DR, Rogers MS, et al. Spironolactone metabolism: steady-state serum levels of the sulfur-containing metabolites. J Clin Pharmacol 1989;29:342−7.

[316] Sungaila I, Bartle WR, Walker SE, DeAngelis C, Uetrecht J, Pappas C, et al. Spironolactone pharmacokinetics and pharmacodynamics in patients with cirrhotic ascites. Gastroenterology 1992;102:1680−5.

[317] Widmer P, Maibach R, Kunzi UP, Capaul R, Mueller U, Galeazzi R, et al. Diuretic-related hypokalaemia: the role of diuretics, potassium supplements, glucocorticoids and beta 2-adrenoceptor agonists. Results from the comprehensive hospital drug monitoring programme, Berne (CHDM). Eur J Clin Pharmacol 1995;49(1-2):31−6.

[318] Brown JJ, Davies DL, Ferriss JB, Fraser R, Haywood E, Lever AF, et al. Comparison of surgery and prolonged spironolactone therapy in patients with hypertension, aldosterone excess, and low plasma renin. Br Med J 1972;2:729−34.

[319] Laffi G, La Villa G, Carloni V, Foschi M, Bartoletti L, Quartini M, et al. Loop diuretic therapy in liver cirrhosis with ascites. J Cardiovasc Pharmacol 1993;22(Suppl. 3):S51−8.

[320] Runyon BA. Practice Guidelines Committee AAftSoLD. Management of adult patients with ascites due to cirrhosis. Hepatology 2004;39(3):841−56.

[321] Chapman N, Dobson J, Wilson S, Dahlof B, Sever PS, Wedel H, et al. Effect of spironolactone on blood pressure in subjects with resistant hypertension. Hypertension 2007;49(4):839−45.

[322] Rossignol P, Menard J, Fay R, Gustafsson F, Pitt B, Zannad F. Eplerenone survival benefits in heart failure patients post-myocardial infarction are independent from its diuretic and potassium-sparing effects. Insights from an EPHESUS (Eplerenone Post-Acute myocardial infarction heart failure efficacy and survival study) substudy. J Am Coll Cardiol 2011;58(19):1958−66.

[323] Griffing GT, Cole AG, Aurecchia SA, Sindler BH, Komanicky P, Melby JC. Amiloride for primary hyperaldosteronism. Clin Pharmacol Ther 1982;31:56−61.

[324] Ganguly A, Weinberger MH. Triamteren-thiazide combination: alternative therapy for primary aldosteronism. Clin Pharmacol Ther 1981;30:246−50.

[325] Botero-Velez M, Curtis JJ, Warnock DG. Brief report: Liddle's syndrome revisited − a disorder of sodium reabsorption in the distal tubule. N Engl J Med 1994;174:178−8078.

[326] Okusa MD, Bia MJ. Bartter's syndrome. In: Foa PP, Cohen MP, editors. Endocrinology and metabolism. 1st ed. New York: Springer-Verlag; 1987. p. 231−63.

[327] Kortenoeven ML, Li Y, Shaw S, Gaeggeler HP, Rossier BC, Wetzels JF, et al. Amiloride blocks lithium entry through the sodium channel thereby attenuating the resultant nephrogenic diabetes insipidus. Kidney Int 2009;76(1):44−53.

[328] Juurlink DN, Mamdani MM, Lee DS, Kopp A, Austin PC, Laupacis A, et al. Rates of hyperkalemia after publication of the Randomized Aldactone Evaluation Study. N Engl J Med 2004;351(6):543−51.

[329] Pitt B, Remme W, Zannad F, Neaton J, Martinez F, Roniker B, et al. Eplerenone, a selective aldosterone blocker, in patients with left ventricular dysfunction after myocardial infarction. N Engl J Med 2003;348(14):1309−21.

[330] Whitling AM, Pergola PE, Sang JL, Talbert RL. Spironolactone-induced agranulocytosis. Ann Pharmacother 1997;31:582−5.

[331] Perazella MA. Crystal-induced acute renal failure. Am J Med 1999;106(4):459−65.

[332] Carr MC, Prien Jr. EL, Babayan RK. Triamterene nephrolithiasis: renewed attention is warranted. J Urol 1990;144:1339−40.

[333] Weinberg MS, Quigg RJ, Salant DJ, Bernard DB. Anuric renal failure precipitated by indomethacin and triamterene. Nephron 1985;40:216−8.

[334] Favre L, Glasson P, Vallotton MB. Reversible acute renal failure from combined triamterene and indomethacin: a study in healthy subjects. Ann Intern Med 1982;96:317−20.

[335] Tahara A, Tomura Y, Wada KI, Kusayama T, Tsukada J, Takanashi M, et al. Pharmacological profile of YM087, a novel potent nonpeptide vasopressin V1A and V2 receptor antagonist, in vitro and in vivo. J Pharmacol Exp Ther 1997;282(1):301−8.

[336] Palm C, Pistrosch F, Herbrig K, Gross P. Vasopressin antagonists as aquaretic agents for the treatment of hyponatremia. Am J Med 2006;119(7 Suppl. 1):S87−92.

[337] Risvanis J, Naitoh M, Johnston CI, Burrell LM. In vivo and in vitro characterisation of a nonpeptide vasopressin V(1 A) and V(2) receptor antagonist (YM087) in the rat. Eur J Pharmacol 1999;381(1):23−30.

[338] Hoorn EJ, Zietse R. Hyponatremia and mortality: how innocent is the bystander? Clin J Am Soc Nephrol 2011;6(5):951−3.

[339] Konstam MA, Gheorghiade M, Burnett Jr. JC, Grinfeld L, Maggioni AP, Swedberg K, et al. Effects of oral tolvaptan in patients hospitalized for worsening heart failure: the EVEREST Outcome Trial. Jama 2007;297(12):1319−31.

[340] Schrier RW, Gross P, Gheorghiade M, Berl T, Verbalis JG, Czerwiec FS, et al. Tolvaptan, a selective oral vasopressin V2-receptor antagonist, for hyponatremia. N Engl J Med 2006;355(20):2099−112.

[341] Cardenas A, Gines P, Marotta P, Czerwiec F, Oyuang J, Guevara M, et al. Tolvaptan, an oral vasopressin antagonist, in the treatment of hyponatremia in cirrhosis. J Hepatol 2012;56(3):571−8.

[342] Kelly MR, Cutler RE, Forrey AW, Kimpel BM. Pharmacokinetics of orally administered furosemide. Clin Pharmacol Ther 1973;15:178−86.

[343] Branch RA, Roberts CJC, Homeida M, Levine D. Determinants of response to frusemide in normal subjects. Br J Clin Pharmacol 1977;4:121−7.

[344] Murray MD, Deer MM, Ferguson JA, Dexter PR, Bennett SJ, Perkins SM, et al. Open-label randomized trial of torsemide

compared with furosemide therapy for patients with heart failure. Am J Med 2001;111(7):513—20.

[345] Brater DC, Chalasani N, Gorski JC, Horlander JCS, Craven R, Hoen H, et al. Effect of albumin-furosemide mixtures on response to furosemide in cirrhotic patients with ascites. Trans Am Clin Climatol Assoc 2001;112:108—15 [discussion 16]

[346] Fliser D, Zurbruggen I, Mutschler E, Bischoff I, Nussberger J, Franek E, et al. Coadministration of albumin and furosemide in patients with the nephrotic syndrome [In Process Citation]. Kidney Int 1999;55(2):629—34.

[347] Blendis L, Wong F. Intravenous albumin with diuretics: protean lessons to be learnt? [editorial; comment] J Hepatol 1999;30(4):727—30.

[348] Gentilini P, Casini-Raggi V, Di Fiore G, Romanelli RG, Buzzelli G, Pinzani M, et al. Albumin improves the response to diuretics in patients with cirrhosis and ascites: results of a randomized, controlled trial. J Hepatol 1999;30(4):639—45.

[349] Na KY, Han JS, Kim YS, Ahn C, Kim S, Lee JS, et al. Does albumin preinfusion potentiate diuretic action of furosemide in patients with nephrotic syndrome? J Korean Med Sci 2001;16(4):448—54.

[350] Kirchner KA. Impairment of diuretic secretion. In: Seldin DW, Giebisch G, editors. Diuretic agents: clinical physiology and pharmacology. San Diego: Academic Press; 1997. p. 259—70.

[351] Uwai Y, Saito H, Hashimoto Y, Inui KI. Interaction and transport of thiazide diuretics, loop diuretics, and acetazolamide via rat renal organic anion transporter rOAT1. J Pharmacol Exp Ther 2000;295(1):261—5.

[352] Sweet DH, Bush KT, Nigam SK. The organic anion transporter family: from physiology to ontogeny and the clinic. Am J Physiol 2001;281(2):F197—205.

[353] Krick W, Wolff NA, Burckhardt G. Voltage-driven p-aminohippurate, chloride, and urate transport in porcine renal brush-border membrane vesicles. Pflugers Arch 2000;441(1):125—32.

[354] Eraly SA, Vallon V, Vaughn DA, Gangoiti JA, Richter K, Nagle M, et al. Decreased renal organic anion secretion and plasma accumulation of endogenous organic anions in OAT1 knockout mice. J Biol Chem 2006;281(8):5072—83.

[355] Beseghir K, Mosig D, Roch-Ramel F. Facilitation by serum albumin of renal tubular secretion of organic anions. Am J Physiol 1989;256:F475—84.

[356] Rose H, O'Malley K, Pruitt A. Depression of renal clearance of furosemide in man by azotemia. Clin Pharmacol Ther 1976;21:141—6.

[357] Chennavasin P, Seiwell R, Brater DC. Pharmacokinetic-dynamic analysis of the indomethacin-furosemide interaction in man. J Pharmacol Exp Ther 1980;215:77—81.

[358] Brater DC. Increase in diuretic effect of chlorothiazide by probenecid. Clin Pharmacol Ther 1978;23:259—65.

[359] Chennavasin P, Seiwell R, Brater DC, Liang WM. Pharmacodynamic analysis of the furosemide-probenecid interaction in man. Kidney Int 1979;16:187—95.

[360] Somogyi AA, Hovens CM, Muirhead MR, Bochner F. Renal tubular secretion of amiloride and its inhibition by cimetidine in humans and in an animal model. Drug Metab Dispos 1989;17(2):190—6.

[361] Voelker JR, Jameson DM, Brater DC. In vitro evidence that urine composition affects the fraction of active furosemide in the nephrotic syndrome. J Pharmacol Exp Ther 1989;250:772—8.

[362] Kirchner KA, Voelker JR, Brater DC. Intratubular albumin blunts the response to furosemide: a mechanism for diuretic resistance in the nephrotic syndrome. J Pharmacol Exp Ther 1990;252:1097—101.

[363] Kirchner KA, Voelker JR, Brater DC. Binding inhibitors restore furosemide potency in tubule fluid containing albumin. Kidney Int 1991;40:418—24.

[364] Agarwal R, Gorski JC, Sundblad K, Brater DC. Urinary protein binding does not affect response to furosemide in patients with nephrotic syndrome. J Am Soc Nephrol 2000;11(6):1100—5.

[365] Ellison DH, Velazquez H, Wright FS. Adaptation of the distal convoluted tubule of the rat. Structural and functional effects of dietary salt intake and chronic diuretic infusion. J Clin Invest 1989;83(1):113—26.

[366] Almeshari K, Ahlstrom NG, Capraro FE, Wilcox CS. A volume-independent component to postdiuretic sodium retention in humans. J Am Soc Nephrol 1993;3:1878—83.

[367] Christensen S, Steiness E, Christensen H. Tubular sites of furosemide natriuresis in volume-replaced and volume-depleted conscious rats. J Pharmacol Exp Ther 1986;239:211—8.

[368] Wilcox CS, Mitch WE, Kelly RA, Skorecki K, Meyer TW, Friedman PA, et al. Response of the kidney to furosemide: I. Effects of salt intake and renal compensation. J Lab Clin Med 1983;102:450—8.

[369] Kelly RA, Wilcox CS, Mitch WE, Meyer TW, Souney PF, Rayment CM, et al. Response of the kidney to furosemide. II. Effect of captopril on sodium balance. Kidney Int 1983;24:233—9.

[370] Agostoni P, Marenzi G, Lauri G, Perego G, Schianni M, Sganzerla P, et al. Sustained improvement in functional capacity after removal of body fluid with isolated ultrafilration in chronic cardiac insufficiency: failure of furosemide to provide the same result. Am J Med 1994;96:191—9.

[371] Marenzi G, Lauri G, Grazi M, Assanelli E, Campodonico J, Agostoni P. Circulatory response to fluid overload removal by extracorporeal ultrafiltration in refractory congestive heart failure. J Am Coll Cardiol 2001;38(4):963—8.

[372] Costanzo MR, Guglin ME, Saltzberg MT, Jessup ML, Bart BA, Teerlink JR, et al. Ultrafiltration versus intravenous diuretics for patients hospitalized for acute decompensated heart failure [See comment] J Am Coll Card 2007;49(6):675—83.

[373] Petersen JS, Shalmi M, Abildgaard U, Christensen S. Alpha-1 blockade inhibits compensatory sodium reabsorption in the proximal tubules during furosemide-induced volume contraction. J Pharmacol Exp Ther 1991;258:42—8.

[374] Wilcox CS, Guzman NJ, Mitch WE, Kelly RA, Maroni BJ, Souney PF, et al. Na$^+$,K$^+$ and BP homeostasis in man during furosemide: effects of prozosin and captopril. Kidney Int 1987;31:135—41.

[375] Jespersen B, Jensen L, Sorensen SS, Pedersen EB. Atrial natriuretic factor, cyclic 3',5'-guanosine monophosphate and prostaglandin E2 in liver cirrhosis: relation to blood volume and changes in blood volume after furosemide. Eur J Clin Invest 1990;20:632—41.

[376] Isenring P, Jacoby SC, Payne JA, Forbush III B. Comparison of Na-K-Cl co-transporters. J Biol Chem 1998;273:11295—301.

[377] Ecelbarger CA, Terris J, Hoyer JR, Nielsen S, Wade JB, Knepper MA. Localization and regulation of the rat renal Na$^+$-K$^+$-2Cl$^-$ co-transporter, BSC-1. Am J Physiol Renal, Fluid Electrolyte Physiol 1996;271:F619—28.

[378] Chen ZF, Vaughn DA, Beaumont K, Fanestil DD. Effects of diuretic treatment and of dietary sodium on renal binding of 3H-metolazone. J Am Soc Nephrol 1990;1:91—8.

[379] Sandberg MB, Maunsbach AB, McDonough AA. Redistribution of distal tubule Na$^+$-Cl$^-$ co-transporter (NCC) in response to a high-salt diet. Am J Physiol Renal Physiol 2006;291(2):F503—8.

[380] Ellison DH. Diuretic resistance: physiology and therapeutics. Sem Nephrol 1999;19(6):581–97.

[381] Stein JH, Osgood RW, Boonjarern S, Cox JW, Ferris TF. Segmental sodium reabsorption in rats with mild and severe volume depletion. Am J Physiol 1974;227:351–9.

[382] DiBona GF, Sawin LL. Renal nerve activity in conscious rats during volume expansion and depletion. Am J Physiol 1985;248:F15–23.

[383] Petersen JS, Shalmi M, Lam HR, Christensen S. Renal response to furosemide in conscious reats: effects of acute instrumentation and peripheral sympathectomy. J Pharmacol Exp Ther 1991;258:1–7.

[384] Petersen JS, DiBona GF. Effects of renal denervation on sodium balance and renal function during chronic furosemide administration in rats. J Pharmacol Exp Ther 1992;262:1103–9.

[385] Chen Z, Vaughn DA, Blakeley P, Fanestil DD. Adrenocortical steroids increase renal thiazide diuretic receptor density and response. J Am Soc Nephrol 1994;5:1361–8.

[386] Bernstein PL, Velázquez H, Bartiss A, Reilly RF, Desir GV, Kunchaparty S, et al. Adrenal steroids stimulate thiazide-sensitive Na-Cl co-transport by rat distal tubules. J Am Soc Nephrol 1994:282.

[387] Velázquez H, Náray-Fejes-Tóth A, Silva T, Andújar E, Reilly RF, Desir GV, et al. The distal convoluted tubule of the rabbit coexpresses NaCl co-transporter and 11b-hydroxysteroid dehydrogenase. Kidney Int 1998;54:464–72.

[388] Wang T, Giebisch G. Angiotensin II regulates bicarbonate and fluid transport in the early and late distal tubule in rat kidney. J Am Soc Nephrol 1994:673.

[389] Kim GH. Long-term adaptation of renal ion transporters to chronic diuretic treatment. Am J Nephrol 2004;24(6):595–605.

[390] Kaissling B, Bachmann S, Kriz W. Structural adaptation of the distal convoluted tubule to prolonged furosemide treatment. Am J Physiol 1985;248:F374–81.

[391] Kaissling B, Stanton BA. Adaptation of distal tubule and collecting duct to increased sodium delivery. I. Ultrastructure. Am J Physiol 1988;255:F1256–68.

[392] Scherzer P, Wald H, Popovtzer MM. Enhanced glomerular filtration and Na⁺-K⁺-ATPase with furosemide administration. Am J Physiol 1987;252:F910–5.

[393] Wald H, Scherzer P, Popovtzer MM. Na, K-ATPase in isolated nephron segments in rats with experimental heart failure. Circ Res 1991;68:1051–8.

[394] Moreno G, Merino A, Mercado A, Herrera JP, Gonzalez-Salazar J, Correa-Rotter R, et al. Electroneutral Na-coupled cotransporter expression in the kidney during variations of NaCl and water metabolism. Hypertension 1998;31(4):1002–6.

[395] Loffing J, Le Hir M, Kaissling B. Modulation of salt transport rate affects DNA synthesis in vivo in rat renal tubules. Kidney Int 1995;47:1615–23.

[396] Wang T, Giebisch G. Effects of angiotensin II on electrolyte transport in the early and late distal tubule in rat kidney. Am J Physiol Renal, Fluid Electrolyte Physiol 1996;271:F143–9.

[397] Beck FX, Ohno A, Muller E, Seppi T, Pfaller W. Inhibition of angiotensin-converting enzyme modulates structural and functional adaptation to loop diuretic-induced diuresis. Kidney Int 1997;51:36–43.

[398] Kaissling B, Stanton BA. Structure-function correlation in electrolyte transporting epithelia. In: Seldin DW, Giebisch G, editors. The kidney: physiology and pathophysiology. 2nd ed. New York: Raven Press, Ltd; 1992. p. 779–801.

[399] Kim GH, Masilamani S, Turner R, Mitchell C, Wade JB, Knepper MA. The thiazide-sensitive Na-Cl co-transporter is an aldosterone-induced protein. Proc Natl Acad Sci U S A 1998;95 (24):14552–7.

[400] Velazquez H, Bartiss A, Bernstein P, Ellison DH. Adrenal steroids stimulate thiazide-sensitive NaCl transport by rat renal distal tubules. Am J Physiol 1996;270(1 Pt 2):F211–9.

[401] Stanton BA, Kaissling B. Regulation of renal ion transport and cell growth by sodium. Am J Physiol 1989;257:F1–10.

[402] Bouby N, Bankir L, Trinh-Trang-Tan MM, Minuth WW, Kriz W. Selective ADH-induced hypertrophy of the medullary thick ascending limb in Brattleboro rats. Kidney Int 1985;28: 456–66.

[403] Petty KJ, Kokko JP, Marver D. Secondary effect of aldosterone on Na-K ATPase activity in the rabbit cortical collecting tubule. J Clin Invest 1981;68:1514–21.

[404] Kaissling B. Structural adaptation to altered electrolyte metabolism by cortical distal segments. Fed Proc 1985;44:2710–6.

[405] Morsing P, Velazquez H, Wright FS, Ellison DH. Adaptation of distal convoluted tubule of rats. II. Effects of chronic thiazide infusion. Am J Physiol 1991;261(1 Pt 2):F137–43.

[406] Garg LC, Narang N. Effects of hydrochlorothiazide on Na-K-ATPase activity along the rat nephron. Kidney Int 1987;31: 918–22.

[407] Kobayashi S, Clemmons DR, Nogami H, Roy AK, Venkatachalam MA. Tubular hypertrophy due to work load induced by furosemide is associated with increses of IGF-1 and IGFBP-1. Kidney Int 1995;47:818–28.

[408] Kim J, Welch WJ, Cannon JK, Tisher CC, Madsen KM. Immunocytochemical response of type A and type B intercalated cells to increased sodium chloride delivery. Am J Physiol Renal, Fluid Electrolyte Physiol 1992;262:F288–302.

[409] Bahro M, Gertig G, Pfeifer U. Short-term stimulation of cellular autophagy by furosemide in the thick ascending limb of Henle's loop in the rat kidney. Cell Tissue Res 1988;253:625–9.

[410] Grossman EB, Hebert SC. Modulation of Na-K-ATPase activity in the mouse medullary thick ascending limb of Henle: effects of mineralocorticoids and sodium. J Clin Invest 1988;81: 885–92.

[411] Loon NR, Wilcox CS, Unwin RJ. Mechanism of impaired natriuretic response to furosemide during prolonged therapy. Kidney Int 1989;36:682–9.

[412] Burckhardt BC, Burckhardt G. Transport of organic anions across the basolateral membrane of proximal tubule cells. Rev Physiol Biochem Pharmacol 2003;146:95–158.

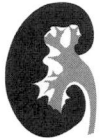

Aquaporin Water Channels in Mammalian Kidney

Søren Nielsen[1], Tae-Hwan Kwon[2], Henrik Dimke[3], Martin Skøtt[4] and Jørgen Frøkiær[5]

[1]Water and Salt Research Center, Department of Biomedicine, University of Aarhus, Aarhus, Denmark
[2]Department of Biochemistry and Cell Biology, School of Medicine, Kyungpook National University, Taegu, Korea
[3]Department of Biomedicine, University of Aarhus, Aarhus, Denmark; The Samuel Lunenfeld Research Institute, Mt. Sinai Hospital, Toronto, Ontario, Canada
[4]Department of Biomedicine, University of Aarhus, Aarhus, Denmark
[5]Water and Salt Research Center, Department of Clinical Physiology, Aarhus University Hospital-Skejby, Aarhus, Denmark

INTRODUCTION

Water is the most abundant component of all cells, and the ability to absorb and release water is considered a fundamental process of life. Plasma membranes serve as selective barriers that control the solute composition of the cell and regulate the entry of ions, small uncharged solutes, and even water. Epithelial tissues have apical and basolateral plasma membranes that constitute serial barriers that regulate the transepithelial movement of solutes and water, thereby contributing to the homeostasis of multicellular organisms. Identification and characterization of the molecular entities responsible for the function of biologic membranes have been long-standing goals of physiologists; however, the molecular identity of water transporters remained unknown until less than two decades ago.

Because water can slowly diffuse through lipid bilayers, all biologic membranes exhibit some degree of water permeability. Nevertheless, observations made in multiple laboratories indicated that specialized membrane water-transport molecules must exist in tissues with distinctively high water permeability (see review [1]). For example, the water permeability of red cell membranes is higher than that of many other cell types or artificial lipid bilayers, and the activation energy of this process is equivalent to the diffusion of water in solution, $E_a < 5$ kcal/mol.[2] In addition, reversible inhibition by $HgCl_2$ and a subset of organomercurials suggested that the water transporter is a membrane protein (see review [3]). Further evidence that a membrane protein is involved in water transport was provided by the observation that some epithelial tissues exhibit changes in water permeability on a timescale that is not compatible with changes in lipid composition.

Kidneys are the major determinant of body water and electrolyte composition. Thus, comprehending the mechanisms of water transport is essential to understanding mammalian kidney physiology and water balance. Because of its importance to human health, water permeability has been particularly well-characterized in the mammalian kidney (see review [4]). Approximately 180 L/day of glomerular filtrate is generated in an average adult human, the majority of this is reabsorbed by the highly water-permeable proximal tubules and descending thin limbs of Henle's loop. The ascending thin limbs and thick limbs are relatively impermeable to water, and empty into renal distal tubules and ultimately into the collecting ducts. The collecting ducts are extremely important clinically in water-balance disorders, because they are the chief site

Seldin and Giebisch's The Kidney, Fifth Edition.
DOI: http://dx.doi.org/10.1016/B978-0-12-381462-3.00041-0

of regulation of water reabsorption. Basal epithelial water permeability in collecting duct principal cells is low, but the water permeability can become exceedingly high when stimulated with vasopressin (also known as ADH, antidiuretic hormone). In this regard, the toad urinary bladder behaves like the collecting duct, and it has served as an important model of vasopressin-regulated water permeability. Stimulation of this epithelium with vasopressin produces an increase in water permeability in the apical membrane, which coincides with the redistribution of intracellular particles to the cell surface.[5–8] These particles were believed to contain water channels.

DISCOVERY OF AQUAPORIN-1 (AQP1)

The molecular identity of membrane water channels long proved elusive. Attempts to purify water channel proteins from native tissues or to isolate water channel cDNAs by expression cloning, were unproductive (see review [9]). This may be explained by the physical characteristics of water, a simple molecule not amenable to chemical modification such as introduction of chemical cross-linking groups or labels. In addition, $HgCl_2$ was known to inhibit membrane water channels, a property potentially useful in the identification of the water channel proteins. However, because the agent reacts with free sulfhydryls in other proteins, its inhibitory effect on water channels is not specific. This circumstance led to the mistaken identification of the band 3 anion exchanger as a molecular water channel.[10] In addition, the diffusional permeability of all biologic membranes results in high background permeability, and frustrated efforts to clone cDNAs for water channels by functional expression.

The recognized characteristics of membrane water channels led to chance identification of the first known water channel. In the process of isolating the 32 kDa bilayer-spanning polypeptide component of the red cell Rh blood group antigen,[11] a 28 kDa polypeptide was partially co-purified.[12] Initial studies demonstrated that the 28 kDa polypeptide comprised hydrophobic amino acids and exhibited an unusual detergent solubility, which facilitated purification and biochemical characterization. The 28 kDa polypeptide was found to exist as an oligomeric protein with physical dimensions of a tetramer; a unique N-terminal amino acid sequence was identified[13] which permitted cDNA cloning.[14] Also of note, radiation inactivation studies of water permeability by renal vesicles yielded a target size of 30 kDa.[15] Because the 28 kDa polypeptide was found to be abundant in red cells, renal proximal tubules, and descending thin limbs,[12] it was suggested that this protein might be the sought-after water

channel. Although this protein was first known as "CHIP28" (channel-like integral protein of 28 kDa), the need for a functionally relevant name was recognized. The name "aquaporin" was coined. After recognition of related proteins with similar functions, this name was formally proposed for the emerging family of water channels now known as the aquaporins.[16] Thus, CHIP28 was designated aquaporin-1 (symbol AQP1). The Human Genome Nomenclature Committee has embraced this nomenclature for all related proteins,[17] and presently a total of 13 such related proteins have been identified in mammals.

The measurement of the movement of water across cell membranes poses a unique experimental challenge. Unlike ion conductances, which may be measured electrophysiologically, or solute transport, which may be measured with radioactive substrates, transmembrane water movement in cells relies on determination of changes in cell volume in response to an osmotic driving force. The *Xenopus laevis* oocyte expression system was used to search for water channel RNAs, because these cells are known to exhibit remarkably low membrane water permeability.[18,19] Oocytes injected with cRNA encoding AQP1 exhibit remarkably high osmotic water permeability ($P_f \sim 200 \times 10^{-17}$ cm/s), causing the cells to swell rapidly and eventually rupture in hyposmotic buffer.[20] In contrast, control oocytes not injected with AQP1 cRNA exhibited less than one tenth of this permeability.

Oocyte studies demonstrated that AQP1 behaves like the water channels in native cell membranes.[20] Osmotically-induced swelling of oocytes expressing AQP1 occurs with a low activation energy, and is reversibly inhibited by $HgCl_2$. Moreover, AQP1 oocytes fail to demonstrate any measurable increase in membrane current. Although these early studies demonstrated only swelling of oocytes, it was predicted that the direction of water flow through AQP1 is determined by the orientation of the osmotic gradient. Thus, AQP1 oocytes swell in hyposmolar buffers but shrink in hyperosmolar buffers.[21]

To confirm that the interpretation of the oocyte studies was correct, highly purified AQP1 protein from human red cells was reconstituted with pure phospholipids into proteoliposomes, which were compared with simple vesicles (liposomes) by rapid transfer to hyperosmolar buffer.[22] These studies permitted determination of the unit water permeability, which had an astonishingly high value ($P_f \sim 3 \times 10^9$ water molecules subunit^{-1} sec^{-1}). Moreover, the water permeability is reversibly inhibited by $HgCl_2$, and exhibits low activation energy. Several of these studies have been confirmed by using red cell membranes partially depleted of other proteins,[23] and attempts to demonstrate permeation by other small solutes or even protons showed that AQP1 is water selective.[24] Together, these studies indicated that AQP1 is both necessary and sufficient to explain the well-recognized membrane water permeability of the red cell, and suggested that AQP1 or similar proteins could be the long-sought-after epithelial water channels of the nephron and collecting ducts.

STRUCTURE AND FUNCTION OF AQUAPORINS

General Structure of AQP1

The availability of pure AQP1 protein in milligram quantities and the simple functional assay in oocytes led to rapid advances in the understanding of the molecular structure of AQP1. Hydropathy analysis of the deduced amino acid sequence of AQP1 predicted that the protein resides primarily within the lipid bilayer,[14] a feature in agreement with initial studies of red cell AQP1.[12,13] As previously described for the homolog major intrinsic protein from lens (MIP, now referred to as AQP0), the polypeptide contains an internal repeat (Figure 41.1), with the N- and C-terminal halves being sequence-related, and each containing the signature motif Asn-Pro-Ala (NPA),[25,26] suggesting ancestral gene duplication.[14] When evaluated by

hydropathy analysis, six bilayer-spanning domains, five connecting loops (A—E), and intracellular N-and C-termini are predicted. Attenuated total reflection-FTIR (Fourier Transform InfraRed spectroscopy) of highly-purified red cell AQP1 reconstituted into membrane crystals demonstrated a lack of beta structure in AQP1, indicating the existence of tilted alpha helices.[27]

The two homologous domains equivalent to the N-and C-termini halves of the protein each consist of three transmembrane helices that are thought to be oppositely orientated in the lipid bilayer.[28] A system was adapted for analyzing the structure of AQP1 after minimally perturbing the molecule by adding peptide epitopes at various sites. It was important that the epitope did not destroy function, and could be localized to intracellular or extracellular sites with antibodies and by selective proteolysis of intact membranes or inside-out membrane vesicles. These studies demonstrated that loop C resides at the extracellular surface of the oocytes and the intracellular location of loop D as well as the N-and C-termini. Moreover, the obverse symmetry of the N-and C-terminal halves of the molecule was confirmed[29] (Figure 41.1).

Loops B and E

Loops B and E encompass the two NPA motifs, and are the most conserved regions in the major intrinsic protein family. The loops exhibit significant hydrophobicity, suggesting association with the lipid bilayer.[14] Subsequent studies implicated loops B and E as a structural component of the aqueous pathway. Experiments expressing AQP1 in *Xenopus* oocytes led to the observation that Cys[189] in loop E is the site of mercurial inhibition.[30,31] Site-directed mutagenesis experiments in oocytes revealed that substitution of Cys[189] with a serine residue eliminates $HgCl_2$ sensitivity and increases osmotic water permeability, while substitution with larger amino acids residues prevents facilitated water transport.[30] These results suggest that water transport and selectivity in AQP1 is somehow dependent on the steric properties of Cys[189]. In accordance with the internal repeat theory, Ala[73] located in loop B, the equivalent to Cys[189] in loop E, was investigated. By creating double mutants expressing Cys[189] as a serine and Ala[73] as a cysteine, the $HgCl_2$ sensitivity and osmotic water permeability were restored.[32] These results suggested that loops B and E were arranged in a symmetrical fashion, and underlined that these loops were functionally essential for water permeability. This line of inquiry lead to the "hourglass" model,[32] in which these domains overlap midway between the leaflets of the bilayer, creating a constitutively open, narrow aqueous pathway (Figure 41.2).

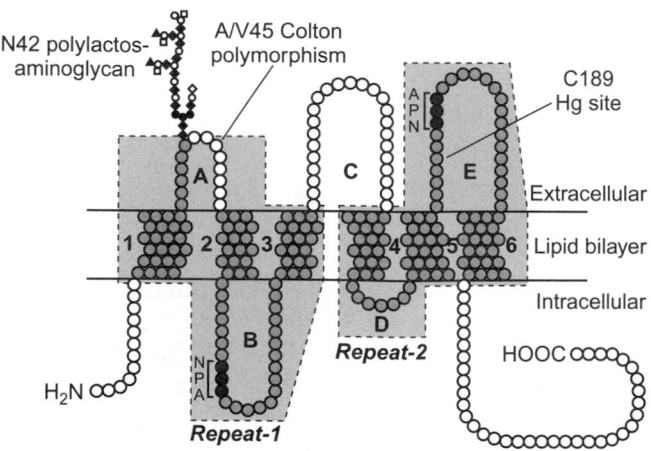

FIGURE 41.1 Proposed membrane topology of AQP1 subunit. Each molecule subunit spans the plasma membrane six times with the N- and C-termini in the cytoplasmic space. Extracellular and intracellular loops are labeled A—E.[32] Loop A contains an attachment site for a polylactosaminoglycan at asparagine-42 and the Co blood group polymorphism at alanine/valine-45.[100] The aquaporin signature motif asparagine-proline-alanine (NPA) is present in the loop Band E. Loop E also contains the site of mercury inhibition at cysteine-189. The amino acid sequences of C-termini of the known aquaporins are not conserved, and are sufficiently immunogenic to permit preparation of specific polyclonal antibodies to each aquaporin (see text) *(reproduced and modified from ref. [370], with permission).*

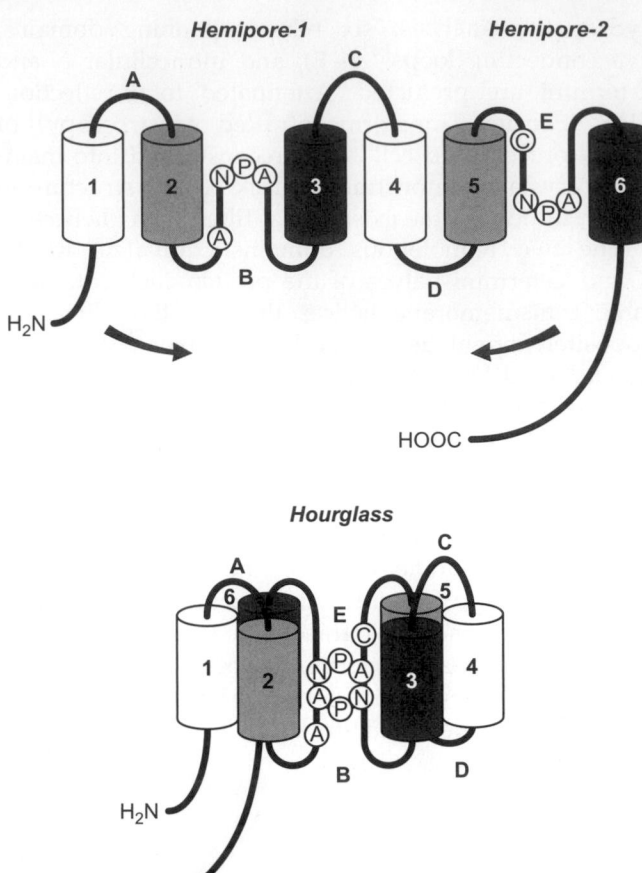

FIGURE 41.2   Hourglass model of aquaporin-1 (AQP1) structure. Bilayer spans 1–3 (Repeat-l) and spans 4–6 (Repeat-2) are sequence-related, and are oriented in obverse symmetry. Loop B and loop E are believed to dip into the bilayer and emerge from the same side (top). When folded together, loops B and E form a single aqueous pathway (the "hourglass"), flanked by the site of mercury inhibition at cysteine189 (bottom) *(reproduced and modified from ref. [32], with permission)*.

Tetrameric Organization

Early biophysical characterization of AQP1 suggested that the protein formed multisubunit oligomers.[13] Rotary and unidirectionally shadowed freeze-fracture electron microscopic analyses of AQP1 protein from human red cell membranes reconstituted in proteoliposomes provided detailed molecular insights. AQP1 had an oligomeric structure, consisting of four subunits surrounding a central depression. These tetrameric structures were also seen in highly water-permeable nephron segments expressing native AQP1.[33] Although the oligomerization of AQP1 is still not understood in detail, all studies indicate that the protein is a tetramer composed of functionally-independent aqueous pores.[15,30,32,34]

Structural Analyses and Molecular Dynamics of Aquaporins

By reconstituting the highly-purified red cell AQP1 into membranes under controlled conditions, membrane crystals were produced with AQP1 in highly uniform lattices. These membranes appeared as flat sheets or as large, resealed vesicles in which the AQP1 protein was found to fully retain water permeability.[35] Thus, the opportunity to define the structure of AQP1 in a biologically-active state became possible. Electron microscopic studies by multiple groups permitted the elucidation of the protein at increasing levels of resolution. By performing high-resolution electron microscopic evaluation of negatively-stained membranes at a series of tilts, a three-dimensional view was obtained.[36] Image projections revealed the presence of multiple bilayer-spanning domains, and atomic force microscopy further defined the orientation and extramembranous dimensions of AQP1.[37] Electron crystallographic analysis of cryopreserved specimens has been undertaken at tilts of up to 60°. These analyses revealed the three-dimensional structure of AQP1 at increasing resolutions, down to 3.8 Å.[38–46] X-ray crystallographic analysis has added further information about the structure of AQP1. Using the above method, the structure of AQP1 has been determined down to a resolution of 2.2 Å.[47] In contrast to the previous studies, the high resolution enables observation of water molecules in transit through the channel. Based on combined efforts, a detailed picture of AQP1s tertiary structure could be formed.

As earlier studies indicated, the AQP1 monomers form a tetrameric cluster. The model shows an extension of the tetramer from the extracellular plane, while the intracellular surfaces form a shallow depression. The N-termini from one monomer is closely situated near the C-termini of the neighboring monomer. The gap formed by the four monomers narrows from 8.5 Å down to 3.5 Å. The residues surrounding the gap are hydrophobic, suggesting an interaction with a hydrophobic molecule.[43] So, despite the monomeric formation of a central cavity, the tetrameric structure does not support the transport of water. This is in agreement with earlier observations, suggesting that each monomer is capable of facilitating water transport.

The dimensions of each monomer are 40 Å across and 60 Å long, as reported by Sui et al.[47] (Figure 41.3). The monomer is composed of six bilayer-spanning alpha helices surrounding a central density. The C loop located on the extracellular surface connects the N-and C-termini halves of the protein. Part of the central density represents the B and E loops, which appear as two short α-helix structures not permeating the

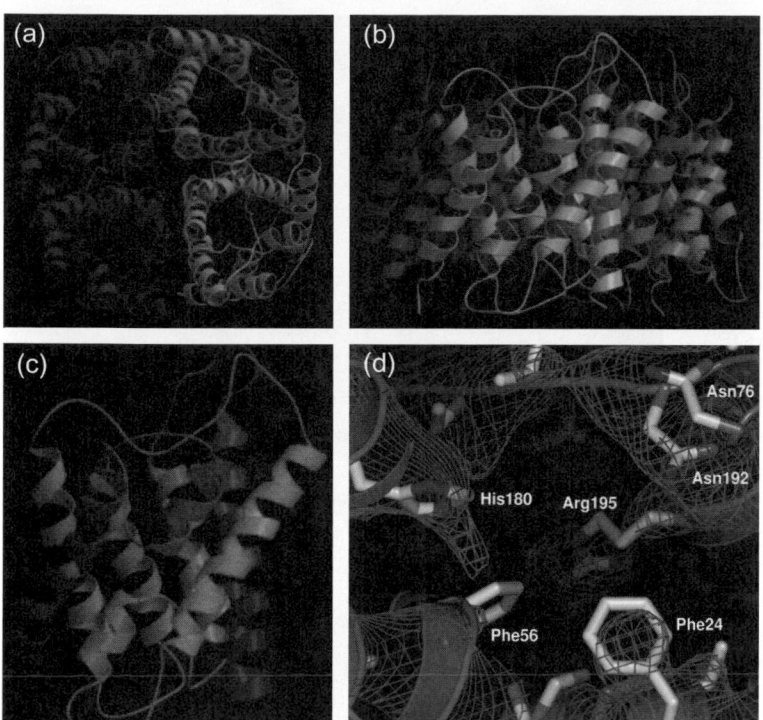

FIGURE 41.3 (a)–(b): Structure of the human AQP1 tetramer, viewed from the top (a) and side (b). (c): Structure of the human AQP1 monomer. (d): Model of the central pore region of human AQP1-EM3 structure (pdb code 1H6I [371] together with the 3.8 Å resolution EM potential map rendered at 1.0s.[43] Several residues critical for AQP1 facilitated water transport are marked (*reproduced and modified with permission from ref. [372]*).

membrane[42] (Figure 41.3). This organization is strikingly similar to the proposed hourglass arrangement of the B and E loops.[32] The NPA containing loops are located on opposite sides of the membrane, juxtapositional to each other, interacting through their NPA motifs. The central density is composed of an extracellular and intracellular vestibule, separated by a narrow pore. The extracellular vestibule is approximately 15 Å at its widest.[47] Following the extracellular vestibule towards the lipid bilayer, a decrease in diameter occurs and the pore becomes exceedingly small.[43,47] The constriction site (also referred to as the aromatic/arginine constriction) is located 20 Å from the beginning of the extracellular vestibule, and is composed of several highly-conserved residues in conventional aquaporins. The constriction site is approximately 2.8 Å wide, about the diameter of a water molecule.[47] After the constriction site the pore continues for 20 Å, a region termed the "selectivity filter".[47] The selectivity filter is slightly wider and part of the region is formed by the helical loops B and E.[43,47] This locates the asparagine residues in the NPA motifs within the selectivity filter.[43,47] Additionally, Cys[189] in loop E protrudes into the pore, confirming earlier studies, suggesting that HgCl$_2$ sensitivity was due to steric hindrance of water movement through the pore.[32,43,47] Following the pore towards the intracellular vestibule, the diameter increases again, reaching 15 Å[47] (Figure 41.3).

Using molecular dynamic simulations, de Groot and Grubmüller obtained time-resolved, atomic resolution models of water transport through AQP1.[48] From the extracellular vestibule, water molecules enter the constriction site, composed of side chains from the aromatic Phe[56] and His[180], and the charged Arg[195]. This conformation situates the water molecule, allowing hydrogen bonding with the polar residues, thereby reducing hydrogen bonding between water molecules. In addition, electrostatic repulsion by Arg[195] suggests that the constriction site is the main site for exclusion of protons (hydronium ions) and other ions.[48] This is further supported by mutagenic analysis of the residues in the constriction site, showing permeation of urea, glycerol, and ammonia in AQP1 when altered. Moreover, replacing Arg[195] with a valine residue appears to facilitate proton transport.[49] Passing onward through the hydrophobic selectivity filter, exposed polar moieties mainly consisting of backbone carbonyls, lead the water molecules towards the NPA motifs. The water molecule transiently reorientates to bond with the two asparagines residues of the NPA motifs, and is led out of the selectivity filter towards the intracellular vestibule, again by hydrogen bonding with a few selected backbone carbonyls. Hence, the selectivity filter encompassing the highly-conserved NPA motifs appears to serve mainly as a filter for size,[48] while the ar/R constriction is a major checkpoint for solute amd ion permeability. The *Escherichia coli* aquaglyceroporin (GlpF) selectively facilitates glycerol transport over that of water.[50] Evaluation of differences between AQP1 and GlpF using molecular dynamic simulations revealed a larger selectivity filter in GlpF. Moreover, the preference for glycerol could be explained by what de Groot and Grubmüller describe as a glycerol-mediated "induced fit" gating motion (i.e., glycerol transport serves as the prime mechanism for water exclusion).[48]

Structural characterizations of crystallized human AQP2 in two-dimensional protein–lipid arrays by atomic force microscopy and electron crystallography have revealed the structure of AQP2 at a resolution of 4.5 Å in the membrane plane.[51] As with AQP1, AQP2 is found in a tetrameric assembly in the lipid bilayer.[51,52] The AQP2 monomer shows structural features similar to those earlier reported for AQP1,[51] while structural variation is found around the tetramer's axis.[51,53]

The structure of AQP0 has also been determined down to a resolution of 2.2 Å.[54,55] The water conductance of AQP0 is much lower than that reported for AQP1,[56] possibly due to highly-conserved tyrosine residues in AQP0 imposing further constriction on the channel.[55] The constriction site is smaller than that in AQP1, and the selectivity filter is also narrower.[54,55] Molecular dynamics studies suggest that water movement is facilitated by AQP0 due to thermal motions of certain side chains, although this builds up a free energy barrier, possibly contributing to the lower permeability of AQP0.[57] The extensive analyses of the structure of various AQP isoforms have provided detailed insight into the molecular basis for transmembrane water transport. Future studies aimed at defining the distinct structure of other members, including aquaglyceroporins such as AQP7 and AQP9 that appear to be involved in metabolism rather than water transport may provide further insights. Several studies have also been aimed at identifying novel aquaporin blockers. Although some progress has been reported so far, only a few compounds, including related tetraammonium compounds, have shown selective effects on AQPs.[58–60] Copper[61] and nickel[62] also significantly block aquaporins. Over the past five years the overall structural concepts of aquaporins have been confirmed.[63–74]

DISTRIBUTION OF AQP1 IN KIDNEY AND OTHER TISSUES

Well before recognition of its function, the red cell AQP1 protein was known to be expressed at high levels in the proximal convoluted tubules and descending thin limbs of kidney.[12] This was confirmed with polyclonal rabbit antiserum,[75] and was defined in rat and human kidney with affinity-purified immunoglobulin specific for the N- and C-terminal domains of

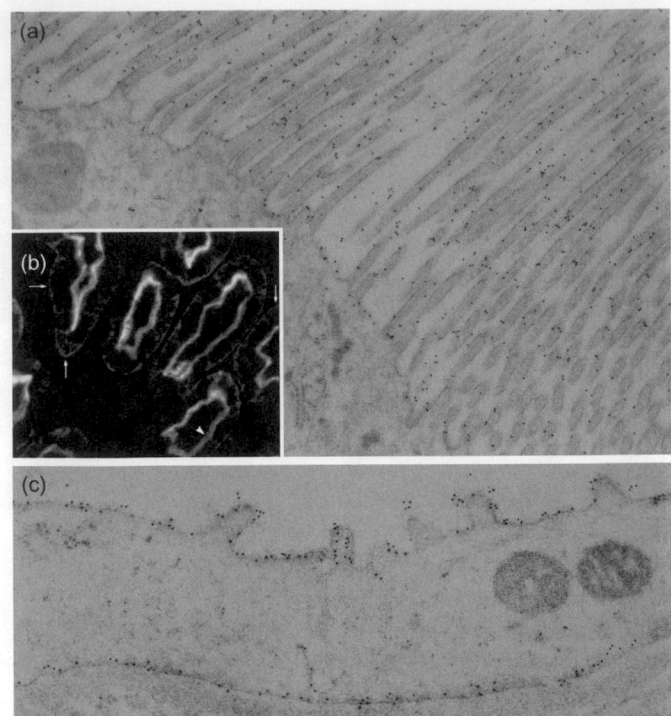

FIGURE 41.4 Distribution of aquaporin 1 (AQP1) in kidney. Ultrathin cryosections of rat renal cortex and inner medulla stained with anti-immunogold AQP1. (a): Strong labeling is present over the apical brush border of S3 section of proximal tubule. (b): Strong labeling is present over apical and basolateral membrane of thin descending limb of Henle's loop (*reproduced and modified from ref. [77], with permission*).

AQP1.[76,77] In all studies, AQP1 was demonstrated to be constitutively present in the apical plasma membranes (i.e., the brush borders), and in basolateral membranes of S2 and S3 segment proximal tubules (Figure 41.4). Quantitative immunoblotting indicated that AQP1 makes up 0.9% of total membrane protein from rat renal cortex and 4% of brush border proteins.[77] Enzyme-Linked Immunosorbent Assay (ELISA) measurements of microdissected tubules revealed that proximal tubules contain approximately 20 million copies of AQP1 per cell.[78] Additionally, AQP1 is found in the plasma membrane of glomerular mesangial cells in humans, although not in rat.[76,77,79] Other immunohistochemical and immunogold electron microscopic studies have demonstrated AQP1 in multiple capillary endothelia throughout the body,[80–82] including the renal vasa recta.[83] AQP1 is also abundant in peribronchiolar capillary endothelium, where expression is induced by glucocorticoids,[80,84] apparently acting through the classic glucocorticoid response elements in the *AQP1* gene.[85] In addition, AQP1 has been defined in multiple water-permeable epithelia including choroid plexus, peritoneal mesothelial cells,[86] fetal membranes,[87] at multiple locations in eye, including ciliary epithelium, lens epithelium, and corneal endothelium,[81,88,89] and in hepatobiliary epithelium,[90] pancreatic interlobular ducts,[91] heart and skeletal muscle,[92] gall bladder,[93] salivary glands,[94] inner ear,[95] and several other organs including the nervous system (see review [96]). AQP1 has also been localized in tumor cells and their vasculature.[97] Developmental expression of AQP1 is complex: transient expression occurs in some tissues before birth; expression in other tissues is subsequent to birth; constitutive life-long expression is found in other tissues.[84,98,99]

AQP1 DEFICIENCY

Humans have been identified who totally lack the AQP1 protein. The human *AQP1* gene was localized to chromosome 7p14 and the Co blood group antigens were previously linked to 7p, suggesting a molecular relationship. It was determined that the Co blood group antigen results from an Ala/Val polymorphism at the extracellular surface of red cell AQP1[100] (Figure 41.1). Although the International Blood Group Referencing Laboratory in Bristol, England, has detailed phenotyping information on millions of donors worldwide, only six individuals had been shown to lack Co. Most of these Co-null individuals are women who developed anti-Co during pregnancy. Three of these Co-null individuals were found to have mutations in the *AQP1* gene.[101] Although the exceedingly rare blood group phenotype makes them impossible to match for blood transfusion, it was surprising that none of them exhibited any other obvious severe clinical phenotype. The extreme rarity of the Co-null state may reflect an important developmental role, resulting in reduced fetal survival; however, the frequency of the heterozygous state is unknown. Detailed studies of the urinary concentrating ability of Co-null individuals revealed a marked inability of the individuals to concentrate urine to more than 400 mOsm/l, even in the presence of dehydration or dDAVP treatment, revealing a significant urinary concentrating defect.[102] Moreover, Co-null individuals display reduced pulmonary vascular permeability.[103]

The development of *AQP1* gene knockout mice has provided further insights into the role of AQP1 in renal water homeostasis. AQP1-null (AQP1$^{-/-}$) mice appeared moderately polyuric under basal conditions. However, AQP1$^{-/-}$ animals exhibited an extreme degree of polyuria and polydipsia when undergoing water deprivation, including rapid hyperosmolar extracellular fluid volume depletion.[104] Additionally, AQP1$^{-/-}$ mice failed to respond appropriately to vasopressin, suggesting that renal water conservation and urinary concentration is highly dependent on AQP1 protein.[104] Detailed classic *in vivo* and *in vitro* physiological evaluation of proximal tubules from the AQP1$^{-/-}$ mice established that transepithelial water permeability was reduced by 80%, and led to an approximate 50% decrease in proximal tubule fluid reabsorption.[105] The apparent differences in transepithelial water permeability and proximal tubule fluid reabsorption are likely dependent on the generation of a hypotonic filtrate in proximal tubules of AQP1$^{-/-}$ mice.[106] Despite these observations, distal fluid delivery in AQP1$^{-/-}$ remained unchanged, due to a compensatory reduction in single nephron glomerular filtration.[105] When blunting the TGF response, and thereby the compensatory reduction in glomerular filtration observed in AQP1$^{-/-}$ mice, ambient urine osmolalities and urinary flow rates appeared no different from normal AQP1$^{-/-}$ mice, probably due to distal tubular compensatory mechanisms.[107] The impaired proximal fluid reabsorption observed in AQP1$^{-/-}$ mice, albeit with normal distal fluid delivery, suggests that the polyuric phenotype largely depends on a concentrating defect impairing collecting duct water reabsorption

Studies using isolated perfused thin descending limbs have revealed that the osmotic water permeability of the type II thin descending limbs (outer medullary thin descending limbs from long loop nephron) is decreased by 90% relative to wild-type values in kidneys from AQP1 knockout mice.[108] Additionally, earlier observations using freeze-fracture electron microscopic techniques showed a remarkably high density of intramembrane particles in the thin descending limb of rat, which has been attributed to the tetrameric assembled AQP1 subunits.[33] In the thin descending limb of AQP1$^{-/-}$ mice, the abundance and size of these intramembrane particles was markedly reduced.[108] Moreover, the distribution of AQP1 in the vasa recta suggests a role in microvascular exchange, hence affecting urinary concentration. In the presence of a NaCl gradient, osmotic water permeability was almost eliminated in the descending vasa recta of AQP1$^{-/-}$ mice, leading to a predicted reduction in medullary interstitial osmolality and likely an impairment of countercurrent multiplication.[109] Additional studies using adenoviral gene delivery restored AQP1 protein expression in the proximal tubule epithelia and renal microvessels of AQP1$^{-/-}$ knockout mice, albeit not in the descending thin limbs. The adenovirus-treated mice showed slight restoration of the concentrating defect during water deprivation, probably due to reinsertion of AQP1 water channels in the vasa recta, although urinary concentrating ability was still highly insufficient in comparison to wild-type mice.[110] In conclusion, the severe concentrating defect seen in the AQP1$^{-/-}$ mice primarily results from impaired water absorption in the thin descending limb, underlining the necessity for a constitutively high water permeability in this segment for a functional countercurrent multiplication system.

ADDITIONAL FUNCTIONS OF AQP1

AQP1 is generally believed to be a constitutively active, water-selective pore. Nonetheless, some observations contradict this. A small degree of permeation by glycerol has been seen in oocytes which may represent opening of an unidentified leak pathway,[111] and the biologic significance remains unclear.[21] Forskolin was reported to induce a cation current in AQP1-expressing oocytes,[112] but multiple other scientific groups have failed to reproduce this effect.[113] Although small changes in water permeability by oocytes expressing a bovine homolog of AQP1 have also been ascribed to vasopressin and atrial natriuretic peptide, the significance is uncertain.[114] Likewise, secretin-induced membrane trafficking has been noted in isolated cholangiocytes[115,116]; however, this awaits confirmation by immunoelectron microscopy. Permeation of AQP1 by CO_2 has also been evaluated. Rates of pH change are about 40% higher in oocytes expressing AQP1[117] than in control oocytes. Although the background permeation of lipid bilayers by CO_2, as well as oxygen, ammonia, nitric oxide, and other gases, may be high,[118] the potential physiological relevance of AQP1 permeation by gases warrants more study (see review [119]). Additionally, AQP1 appears to play a role in cell migration.[120] AQP1$^{-/-}$ mice implanted with tumor cells show reduced tumor vascularity and growth, thus leading to improved survival in comparison to wild-type mice. Moreover, *in vitro* analysis of endothelial cells isolated from AQP1$^{-/-}$ mice showed marked impairment in cell migration.[120] In primary cultures of proximal tubule cells from AQP1$^{-/-}$ mice, *in vitro* cell migration was impaired compared to AQP1$^{+/+}$ mice. Furthermore, in an ischemia–reperfusion model of acute renal tubular injury, AQP1$^{-/-}$ mice showed more severe pathological changes, including more prominent tubule degeneration.[121] Thus, although the evidence that AQP1 functions as a water channel is incontrovertible, the possibility of yet undiscovered transport functions cannot be excluded.

AQUAPORINS IN KIDNEY

The first functional definition of one member of a protein family often prompts a search for related proteins. This has certainly been the case for the aquaporins, and the homology cloning approach has been undertaken by multiple laboratories whose combined efforts have expanded the aquaporin family membership list. Homology cloning has most frequently been undertaken by using polymerase chain amplification with degenerate oligonucleotide primers.[122] Thirteen mammalian aquaporins are now known, and they form at least two subgroups: water-selective channels (orthodox aquaporins) and channels permeated by water, glycerol, and other small molecules (aquaglyceroporins). Given the large potential for confusion, the Human Genome Organization has established an Aquaporin Nomenclature System,[117] accessible by internet (http://www.gene.ucl.ac.uk/nomenclature). Of the known aquaporins, eight are expressed in mammalian kidney (Table 41.1). Soon after AQP1 was discovered to be a water channel, AQP2 was identified in renal collecting duct,[123] where it is regulated by vasopressin and is involved in multiple clinical disorders (Table 41.2). AQP3 was identified in kidney and other tissues, and was found to be permeated by glycerol and water.[124–126] AQP4, a $HgCl_2$-insensitive water channel is most abundantly expressed in brain, and is present in kidney collecting duct in the basolateral plasma membrane of principal and IMCD cells and in other tissues, but it is not inhibited by mercury.[127,128] AQP6 was identified at the cDNA level and found to be localized in intracellular vesicles in the collecting duct intercalated cells in the kidney.[129–131] AQP7 is permeated by water and glycerol.[132,133] First cloned from testis,[132] AQP7 is present in segment 3 proximal tubule brush border membranes, where it facilitates glycerol and water transport.[134] AQP8 is a $HgCl_2$-sensitive water channel found in intracellular domains of proximal tubule and collecting duct cells[135,136]; however, its function remains unclear. AQP11 is found in the cytoplasm of renal proximal tubule cells.[137] The exact function is not established, although deletion of the *AQP11* gene produces a severe phenotype with renal vacuolization and cyst formation.[137]

Localization and Function of AQP2, AQP3, AQP4, AQP6, AQP7, AQP8, and AQP11 in Kidney

The amino acid sequences of the N-and C-termini of the different aquaporins are not closely related, and specific polyclonal antibodies can be raised in rabbits immunized with synthetic peptides conjugated to carrier proteins such as keyhole limpet hemocyanin. As with AQP1, these antibodies have permitted localization of the other aquaporins in kidney by immunocytochemistry, immunoelectron microscopy, and single

TABLE 41.1 Aquaporins in Kidney

AQP	Localization (renal)	Subcellular Distribution	Regulation	Localization (extrarenal)
AQP1	S2, S3 segments of proximal tubules	Apical and basolateral plasma membranes	Glucocorticoids (peribronchiolar capillary endothelium)	Multiple tissues, including capillary endothelia, choroids plexus, ciliary and lens epithelium, etc.
AQP2	Collecting duct principal cells	Intracellular vesicles, apical plasma membrane	Vasopressin stimulates short-term exocytosis long-term biosynthesis	Epididymis
AQP3	Collecting duct principal cells	Basolateral plasma membrane	Vasopressin stimulates long-term biosynthesis	Multiple tissues, including airway basal epithelia, conjunctiva, colon
AQP4	Collecting duct principal cells	Basolateral plasma membrane	Dopamine, protein kinase C	Multiple tissues, including central nervous system astroglia, ependyma, airway surface epithelia
AQP6	Collecting duct intercalated	Intracellular vesicles	Rapidly gated	Unknown
AQP7	S3 proximal tubules	Apical plasma membrane	Insulin (adipose tissue)	Multiple tissues, including adipose tissue, testis, and heart
AQP8	Proximal tubule, collecting duct cells	Intracellular domains	Unknown	Multiple tissues, including gastronintestinal tract, testis, and airways
AQP11	Proximal tubule	Intracellular domains	Unknown	Multiple tissues, including liver, testes, and brain

AQP, aquaporin.

tubule microdissection combined with ELISA (Figure 41.5).

Three aquaporins (AQP2, AQP3, and AQP4) are expressed in the collecting duct principal cells and the connecting tubule segment, sites where vasopressin regulates epithelial water permeability. AQP2 is located in the apical plasma membrane and small intracellular vesicles of collecting duct principal cells[138] (Figure 41.6). ELISA measurements of microdissected rat collecting ducts have revealed that AQP2 is an extremely abundant protein in the collecting duct, with more than six million copies per cell throughout the collecting duct system.[139] Additional studies using the single-tubule ELISA method and immunocytochemistry demonstrated co-localization of AQP2 and V2 vasopressin receptor expression on connecting tubule arcades, suggesting that regulated water transport may occur in the arcades of the cortical labyrinth in addition to the collecting duct.[139,140] Additionally, AQP2 has been identified in the basolateral membranes of connecting tubules and inner medullary collecting ducts.[141]

The apical plasma membrane is the rate-limiting barrier for transepithelial water transport across the collecting duct principal cell, and is the site where vasopressin regulates water permeability.[142] Localization of AQP2 in the apical plasma membrane suggested that it is the target for vasopressin-regulated collecting duct water permeability (Figure 41.6). This conclusion was firmly established by multiple studies. A direct correlation between AQP2 expression and

collecting duct water permeability has been demonstrated in Brattleboro rats, which lack circulating vasopressin owing to a mutation in the gene encoding vasopressin precursor protein.[143] Likewise, human patients with mutations in the *AQP2* gene manifest severe vasopressin-resistant nephrogenic diabetes insipidus,[144] demonstrating the requirement for AQP2 in collecting duct water transport. Lack of functional AQP2 expression in mice, by generation of *AQP2* gene knockouts, produces a severe concentration defect, resulting in early postnatal death.[145,146] Moreover, morphological changes including renal medullary atrophy and dilation of the collecting ducts is observed in these mice.[145,146] Generation of AQP2$^{-/-}$ knockouts selectively in the collecting ducts, but not in the connecting tubule segments, rescues mice from the lethal phenotype; however, body weight, urinary production, and the response to water deprivation is still severely impaired.[145] Additionally, in a tamoxifen-inducible mouse model of AQP2 gene deletion, adult mice present with severe polyuria, a marked urinary concentration defect, and develop mild renal damage.[147] Together these studies demonstrate the pivotal role of AQP2 in urinary concentration.

AQP3 is localized in a large variety of organs and highly-expressed in the kidney. AQP3 was originally cloned from rat kidney,[124−126] and when expressed in *Xenopus* oocytes it facilitated glycerol transport (discussed below) and increased HgCl$_2$-sensitive osmotic water permeability.[148−150] Moreover, channel-gating is

TABLE 41.2 Water-balance Disorders Associated with Aquaporin Abnormalities

---

Congenital defects

Central diabetes insipidus

Mutation in gene encoding vasopressin (Brattleboro rat)

Nephrogenic diabetes insipidus

Mutations in gene encoding V_2 receptor (human, X-linked)

Mutations in gene encoding aquaporin-2 (human, dominant and recessive)

Partial concentration defects

Targeted disruption of gene encoding aquaporin-1 (mouse)

Targeted disruption of gene encoding aquaporin-4 (mouse)

Acquired defects

Lithium treatment

Hypokalemia

Hypercalcemia

Postobstructive nephropathy, unilateral or bilateral

Conditions with water retention

Congestive heart failure

Hepatic cirrhosis

Nephritic syndrome

Pregnancy

Other conditions

Syndrome of inappropriate vasopressin secretion

Primary polydipsia

Chronic renal failure

Acute renal failure

Low-protein diet

Age-induced reduction in renal concentration

---

regulated by protons and copper.[61,150] AQP4 was found to be expressed in several tissues with high abundance in the brain. In oocyte expression studies, the protein increased osmotic water permeability in a $HgCl_2$-insensitive manner.[127,149]

AQP3 and AQP4 are also present in the connecting tubule and collecting duct principal cells; however, the sites where they are expressed do not overlap with the expression of AQP2 in most portions of the collecting duct.[140,151–153] AQP3 and AQP4 are restricted to the basolateral plasma membranes of collecting duct principal cells, where they are presumed to permit water entry into the interstitium. Although both are basolateral water channels, they are distributed differently along the collecting duct system, with the greatest abundance of AQP3 in cortical and outer medullary collecting ducts, and the greatest abundance of AQP4 in inner medullary collecting duct.[153] AQP4 is also found in basolateral membranes of proximal tubule S3 segments, although only in mice.[154] Using freeze-fracture electron microscopy, orthogonal arrays of intramembrane particles (OAP) were demonstrated in the basolateral membranes of the proximal tubule S3 segment in $AQP4^{+/+}$, but not in $AQP4^{-/-}$, mice.[154] AQP4 is expressed in two splice isoforms, the M1 and M23 splice variants. The M23-AQP4 appears to be the OAP-forming water channel when expressed in LLC-PK1 cells. When organized in OAPs, a significantly higher single-channel water permeability coefficient is observed in comparison to the non-AOP forming M1-AQP4.[141,155] Shuttling of AQP3 or AQP4 is not expected to occur, as the predominant fraction is found in the plasma membrane (short- and long-term regulation of these aquaporins will be discussed later). Sodium restriction or aldosterone infusion in normal and Brattleboro rats greatly increases the abundance of AQP3, while AQP3 abundance is markedly reduced during aldosterone deficiency, suggesting a direct effect of aldosterone on collecting duct AQP3 expression.[156] AQP4 appears to be regulated by PKC and dopamine, where stimulation by these factors decreases water permeability in AQP4 transfected cells.[157]

Deletion of the *AQP3* gene induces polyuria and polydipsia and a marked reduction in osmotic water permeability in the basolateral plasma membrane of the cortical collecting duct.[148] Moreover, urinary osmolality is reduced in $AQP3^{-/-}$ mice and they fail to respond appropriately to dDAVP, thus presenting with a urinary concentrating defect.[148] Targeted disruption of AQP4 in mice results in a 75% reduction in the osmotic water permeability of the inner medullary collecting duct.[158] However, phenotypically the $AQP4^{-/-}$ mice appeared grossly normal, presenting with a very mild urinary concentrating defect.[159] In double $AQP3^{-/-}/AQP4^{-/-}$-knockout mice, concentrating ability was only slightly more impaired than in the $AQP3^{-/-}$ mice.[148] It should be noted that the localization of AQP2 in basolateral membranes in both the connecting tubule and inner medullary collecting duct raises the possibility that the observed effect is partly compensated by this mechanism.[141]

AQP6 vesicles reside in subapical vesicles within intercalated cells of the collecting duct, where it is co-expressed with the V-type H^+-ATPase.[131,160] AQP6 appears functionally distinct from other known aquaporins. Oocyte expression studies have revealed low water permeability of AQP6 during basal conditions, while in the presence of $HgCl_2$ a rapid increase in water permeability and ion conductance is observed.

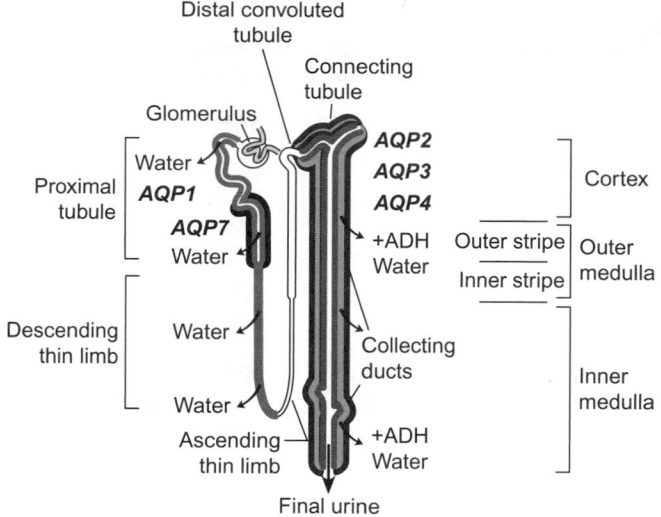

FIGURE 41.5 **Sites of aquaporin (AQP1) expression in kidney and segmental water-transport function.** Proximal nephron: AQP1 is present in apical and basolateral plasma membranes of proximal tubules and thin descending limbs. AQP6 is present in intracellular vesicles of collecting duct intercalated cells. AQP7 is present in proximal tubules. Distal nephron: aquaporins are not present in ascending limbs. Collecting duct: AQP2 is present in intracellular vesicles and apical plasma membranes of principal cells; AQP3 and AQP4 are present in basolateral membranes. AQP6 is present in intracellular vesicles in type A intercalated cells.

Additionally, reductions in pH (below 5.5) quickly and reversibly increase anion conductance and water permeability in AQP6 expressing oocytes.[160] Subsequent studies have shown that the channel is permeable to halides, with the highest permeability to NO_3^-,[160,161] while the ionic selectivity becomes less specific after the addition of $HgCl_2$.[162] Moreover, when Asn^{60}, a residue unique in mammalian AQP6, is converted to glycine, a highly-conserved residue in other mammalian aquaporins, anionic permeability is abolished and osmotic water permeability is increased during basal conditions.[163]

AQP7 is a member of the aquaglyceroporin family, and was originally cloned from rat testis.[132] Additionally, AQP7 is expressed in several organs, including adipose tissue and kidney.[132,164] In the kidney, AQP7 localizes to the brush border membrane of the proximal tubule S3 segment.[165,166] Expression of AQP7 in *Xenopus* oocytes showed that AQP7 facilitated the transport of glycerol and urea in addition to water.[132] The development of AQP7 knockout mice has aided understanding of the physiological role of AQP7. Glycerol excretion is markedly increased in $AQP7^{-/-}$ mice, suggesting a role for AQP7 in facilitating proximal tubular glycerol transport, and possibly renal gluconeogenesis (discussed below).[134] In terms of water transport, $AQP7^{-/-}$ mice experience only a slight reduction in proximal tubule membrane water permeability, and AQP7/AQP1 double knockout mice showed only a slightly more severe urinary concentrating defect than $AQP1^{-/-}$ mice during water deprivation.[134] Additionally, evaluation of the channels' permeability to urea in $AQP7^{-/-}$ mice revealed no change in urinary urea excretion or urea accumulation in the papilla, indicating a less prominent physiological role in urea transport.[134] Expression of AQP7 in *Xenopus* oocytes increases the permeability to arsenite, thereby providing a possible route for arsenite uptake in mammalian cells[167]; the physiological role of these observations awaits further investigation.

Cloning of the murine AQP8 water channel[136,168,169] revealed its presence in many organs, including the kidney.[135,136,168,169] In kidney, AQP8 localizes to intracellular domains of proximal tubule and collecting duct cells.[135] Expression of AQP8 in *Xenopus* oocytes increased $HgCl_2$-sensitive osmotic water permeability. Additionally, oocyte expression of AQP8 showed permeability to urea.[136] Targeted deletion of the *AQP8* gene produced a mild phenotype in $AQP8^{-/-}$ mice, with no obvious changes in renal parameters.[170] Subsequent studies have suggested that AQP8 facilitates NH_3 transport in *Xenopus* oocytes[171,172] and in ammonia transport-deficient yeast.[173] In $AQP8^{-/-}$ mice, ammonia-loading mildly reduced hepatic ammonia accumulation and increased renal ammonia excretion,[174] indicating that AQP8 does not play a significant physiological role in facilitated NH_3 transport.

Recently a new aquaporin was cloned from rat testis, namely AQP11.[168] This AQP has only one NPA motif, and shares low similarity with the conventional aquaporins. AQP11 is most abundantly expressed in the testis, kidney, and liver.[168] In the kidney, the AQP11 protein localizes to the cytoplasm of the renal proximal tubules.[137] While lack of plasma membrane expression of the AQP11 protein in *Xenopus* oocytes greatly impaired measurements of transport,[137] targeted deletion of the *AQP11* gene in mice resulted in a severe phenotype with vacuolization and cyst formation in the proximal tubule. The $AQP11^{-/-}$ mice died of renal failure and kidneys were polycystic. The cyst epithelia contained vacuoles, and the $AQP11^{-/-}$ mice also presented with a proximal tubular endosomal acidification defect.[137]

AQUAGLYCEROPORINS

AQP3, AQP7, and AQP9 constitute a subgroup of aquaporins with a broader permeation range that includes glycerol, hence the name "aquaglyceroporins." AQP3, which transports water and glycerol, was cloned by three groups at the same time.[124–126] The

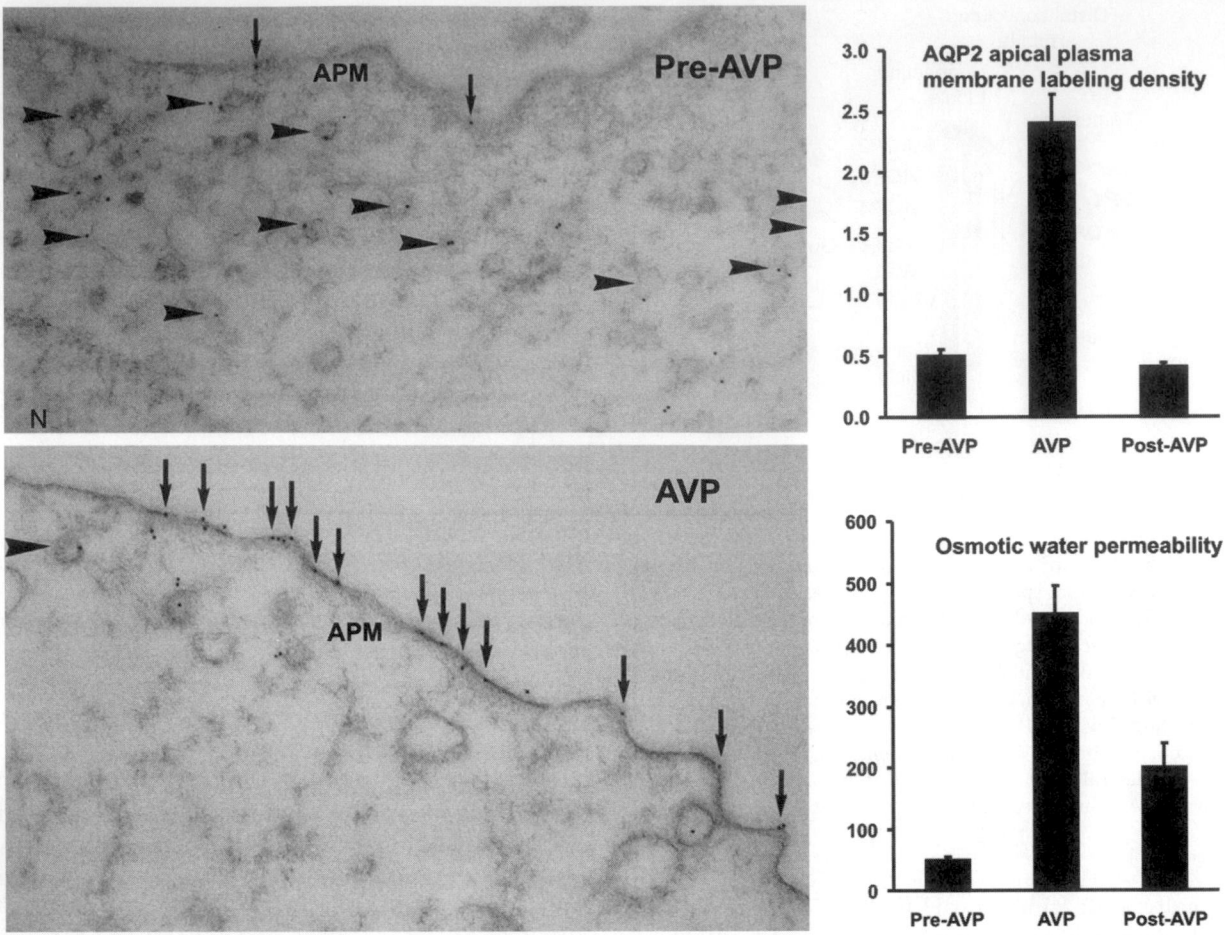

FIGURE 41.6   **Vasopressin-induced trafficking of aquaporin 2 (AQP2) in isolated, perfused rat collecting duct and resulting changes in water permeability.** Anti-AQP2 immunogold electron microscopy of ultrathin cryosections of isolated rat collecting duct fixed before exposure to arginine vasopressin (pre-AVP, top left), and after exposure (AVP, bottom left). Note intracellular AQP2 (arrowheads) and plasma membrane AQP2 (small arrows). Quantification of AQP2 labeling density before, during or after vasopressin exposure (top right). Quantification of osmotic water permeability of isolated collecting duct (bottom right) (Nucleus: N; mitochondrion: M; × 50,000) *(reproduced and modified from ref. [182], with permission).*

distribution at multiple sites, including the kidney collecting duct principal cells, airway epithelia, skin, urinary bladder, and secretory glands, suggests several functions.[151,152,175] AQP3-null mice exhibit a nephrogenic diabetes insipidus phenotype; however, human mutants have not yet been reported. AQP7 is also permeated by water and glycerol, and is localized to the apical brush border of the proximal tubules, especially to the S3 segment. Recent studies have indicated that AQP7 may play a role in glycerol metabolism by showing adaptation to fasting by glycerol transport through AQP7 in adipose tissue.[176] AQP7$^{-/-}$ mice have a significantly lower plasma glycerol concentration than wild-type mice, and impaired adipocytic glycerol release in response to a β3 receptor stimulation.[176] Moreover, AQP7$^{-/-}$ mice experience severe hypoglycemia, but show normal hepatic gluconeogenesis during fasting, indicative of defective adipocytic glycerol

transport in these mice.[176] Glycerol excretion is also markedly increased in AQP7$^{-/-}$ mice, suggesting a role for AQP7 in facilitating proximal tubular glycerol transport.[134] AQP9, which is expressed in the liver but not in kidney,[177−179] is permeated by a range of solutes including glycerol and urea.[180] Recently, it has been demonstrated that expression of AQP9 in liver was induced up to 20-fold in rats fasted for 24−96 hours, and that AQP9 levels gradually declined after re-feeding.[181] This indicates that the liver takes up glycerol for gluconeogenesis through AQP9 during starvation.

VASOPRESSIN REGULATION OF KIDNEY AQUAPORINS

Of all the aquaporins, AQP2 has invoked the largest interest by nephrologists, because it is expressed in principal cells of the renal collecting duct, where it is the primary target for short-term regulation of collecting duct water permeability.[182-184] AQP2 and AQP3 are also regulated either directly or indirectly by vasopressin through long-term effects that alter the abundance of these water-channel proteins in collecting duct cells.[138,143,151,185-187]

Short- and Long-Term Regulation of Water Permeability in the Collecting Duct

Two modes of vasopressin-mediated regulation of water permeability have been identified in the renal collecting duct. Both involve regulation of the AQP2 water channel. Short-term regulation is the widely recognized process by which vasopressin rapidly increases water permeability of principal cells by binding to vasopressin V2-receptors at the basolateral membranes, a response measurable within 5 to 30 minutes after increasing peritubular vasopressin concentration.[188,189] It is believed that vasopressin, acting through a cyclic adenosine monophosphate (cAMP) cascade, causes intracellular AQP2 vesicles to fuse with the apical plasma membrane, which increases the number of water channels in the apical plasma membrane (Figures 41.6 and 41.7). Long-term regulation of collecting duct water permeability is seen when circulating vasopressin levels are increased for 24 hours or more, resulting in an increase in the maximal water permeability of the collecting duct epithelium.[185] This response is a consequence of an increase in the abundance of AQP2 water channels per cell in the collecting duct,[138,143] apparently due to increased transcription of the *AQP2* gene (Figure 41.7).

Short-Term Regulation of AQP2 by Vasopressin-Induced Trafficking

The final concentration of the urine depends on the medullary osmotic gradient built up by the loop of Henle, and the water permeability of the collecting ducts through the cortex and medulla (see review [190]). Collecting duct water permeability is regulated by vasopressin, and it has been suspected for many years on the basis of indirect biophysical evidence that the vasopressin-induced increase in water permeability depended on the appearance of specific water channels in the apical plasma membrane of the vasopressin-responsive cells. Molecular actions of vasopressin to increase epithelial water permeability were first demonstrated in the 1950s and early 1960s in the skin and urinary bladder of amphibia.[191,192] Direct demonstrations that vasopressin rapidly increases water permeability of isolated

collecting ducts were made during the next few years.[193,194] These studies, undertaken with *in vitro* preparations, showed that vasopressin applied to the basolateral aspect of the collecting duct cells directly increased transepithelial osmotic water permeability within minutes. Kinetic studies in isolated perfused inner medullary collecting ducts revealed an increase in osmotic water permeability after only 40 seconds of incubation at 37°C, and half of the maximal water permeability was reached within 10 minutes.[189,195] cAMP has been implicated in the regulatory process, because direct application of cAMP analogs to the collecting duct was found to mimic the short-term effects of vasopressin.[193]

Multiple studies with affinity-purified polyclonal antibodies to AQP2 have unequivocally established that AQP2 is specifically involved in vasopressin-induced increases of renal collecting duct water permeability. Soon after isolation of the AQP2 cDNA and generation of specific antibodies,[123] immunoperoxidase microscopy and immunoelectron microscopy clearly demonstrated that principal cells within renal collecting ducts contain abundant AQP2 in the apical plasma membranes and in subapical vesicles.[138,143] These studies strongly supported the "shuttle hypothesis" originally proposed more than a decade earlier.[196] This hypothesis proposed that water channels can shuttle between an intracellular reservoir in subapical vesicles and the apical plasma membrane, and that vasopressin alters water permeability by regulating the shuttling process.[8] Shuttling of AQP2 was directly demonstrated in isolated perfused tubule studies.[182] In these studies, water permeability of isolated perfused collecting ducts was measured before or after stimulation with vasopressin, and the tubules were fixed directly for immunoelectron microscopic examination (Figure 41.6). Vasopressin stimulation resulted in a markedly decreased immunogold labeling of intracellular AQP2, accompanied by a five-fold increase in the appearance of AQP2 immunogold particles in the apical plasma membrane. This redistribution was associated with an increase in osmotic water permeability of similar magnitude. These findings were reproduced *in vivo* by injecting rats with vasopressin, which also caused redistribution of AQP2 to the apical plasma membrane of collecting duct principal cells.[183,197] In contrast to the effect of vasopressin treatment, removal of vasopressin led to a reappearance of AQP2 in intracellular vesicles, and a decline in osmotic water permeability in the isolated perfused collecting duct system[182,186] (Figure 41.6). Moreover, the off-set response to vasopressin has been examined *in vivo* by acute treatment of rats with vasopressin-V_2-receptor antagonist[198,199] or acute water-loading (to reduce endogenous vasopressin levels[200]). These treatments (both reducing

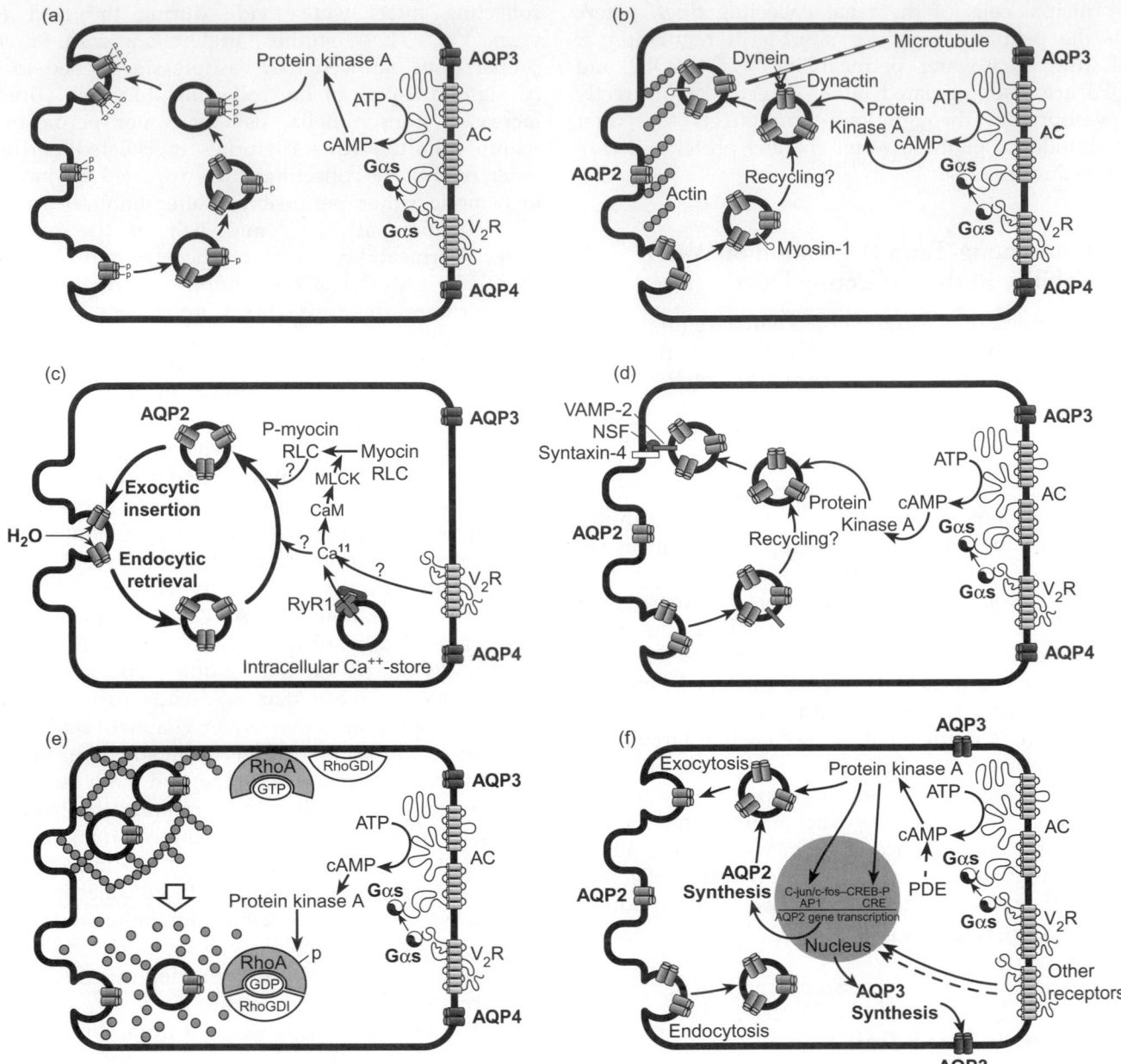

FIGURE 41.7   Regulation of AQP2 trafficking (Panels a–e), and expression (Panel F) in collecting duct principal cells. (a):Vasopressin binding to basolateral G-protein-linked V2-receptor stimulates adenylyl cyclase (AC); cyclic adenosine monophosphate (cAMP) activates protein kinase A to phosphorylate AQP2 in intracellular vesicles; phosphorylated AQP2 is exocytosed to the apical plasma membrane, resulting in increased apical membrane water permeability. (b): Overview of cytoskeletal elements, which may be involved in AQP2-trafficking. AQP2-containing vesicles may be transported along microtubules by dynein/dynactin. The cortical actin web may act as a barrier to fusion with the plasma-membrane. (c): Intracellular calcium signaling and AQP2-trafficking. Increases in intracellular Ca^{2+} concentration may arise from stimulation of the V2 receptor. The existence and potential role of other receptors and pathways, e.g., VACM-1, in Ca^{2+} mobilization is still uncertain. The downstream targets of the calcium signal are unknown, and conflicting data exist on the importance of a rise in intracellular Ca^{2+} for the hydrosmotic response to vasopressin. (d): Vesicle-targeting receptors and AQP2-trafficking. AQP2 vesicles dock at the apical membrane by association of VAMP-2 with syntaxin-4 targets in the presence of NSF; the exact role of these remains to be established. (e): Changes in the actin cytoskeleton associated with AQP2-trafficking to the plasma membrane. Inactivation of RhoA by phosphorylation and increased formation of RhoARhoGDI complexes seem to control the dissociation of actin fibers seen after vasopressin stimulation. (f): Specifically, cAMP participates in the long-term regulation of AQP2 by increasing the levels of the catalytic subunit of PKA in the nuclei, which is thought to phosphorylate transcription factors such as CREB-P (Cyclic AMP Responsive Element Binding Protein) and C-Jun/c-Fos. Binding of these factors are thought to increase gene transcription of AQP2, resulting in synthesis of AQP2 protein which in turn enters the regulated trafficking system. In parallel, AQP3 and AQP4 synthesis and trafficking to the basolateral plasma membrane takes place. Importantly, AQP2 regulation can be modified by a number of hormones including dopamine, ANP, PGE2, and adrenergic hormones. See text for details (Vasopressin-V2-receptors: V2R; adenylyl cyclase: AC; cAMP and protein kinase A: PKA) *(redrawn and modified from ref. [190]).*

vasopressin action) resulted in a prominent internalization of AQP2 from the apical plasma membrane to intracellular subapical vesicles, further underscoring the role of AQP2 trafficking in the regulation of collecting duct water permeability and the reversibility of AQP2 trafficking to the plasma membrane.

The quantity of AQP2 in the apical plasma membrane is determined by the relative rates of exocytosis and endocytosis. Both processes occur continuously, and their relative rates are regulated to effect changes in water permeability. Kinetic evidence indicates that vasopressin regulates both endocytosis and exocytosis of apical water channels.[195,201] These conclusions are supported by multiple earlier experiments with fluid-phase markers, which assessed rates of internalization of the apical plasma membrane.[202–204] Intravenous injection of horseradish peroxidase was followed by uptake of the material into intracellular vesicles and multivesicular bodies by collecting duct principal cells.[202] When compared with normal rats, the rate of uptake by vasopressin-deficient Brattleboro rats was much lower; however, this difference was lost after administration of vasopressin, presumably reflecting an effect of vasopressin in accelerating exocytosis, followed by a secondary increase in the rate of endocytosis to re-establish the steady-state. These observations were supported by studies with fluorescein-labeled dextrans,[203] which confirmed that vasopressin enhances the rate of endocytosis of the apical plasma membrane under steady-state conditions. In apparent contrast, removal of vasopressin from isolated perfused rabbit cortical collecting ducts also was accompanied by increased endocytosis of horseradish peroxidase from the lumen, and it was suggested that water channels would also be internalized at an increased rate.[204] Similar results were obtained in isolated rat inner medullary collecting duct, which showed that vasopressin washout was associated with increased appearance of albumin-gold or cationic ferritin in small apical vesicles and multivesicular bodies.[205] Presumably this response reflects a direct effect of vasopressin to decrease the intrinsic rate of endocytosis and is reversed on vasopressin removal. Therefore, it appears that two factors affect the rate of endocytosis of the apical plasma membrane of collecting duct principal cells: (1) vasopressin directly decelerates endocytosis by unknown mechanisms; and (2) vasopressin indirectly accelerates the rate of endocytosis by stimulating exocytosis and increasing the total amount of apical plasma membrane. The latter effect is believed to be slower than the former, resulting in a biphasic decline in water permeability on vasopressin removal.[195,201] Other studies have demonstrated that apical endocytosis is most rapid

at about 3 to 5 minutes after vasopressin washout from isolated perfused inner medullary collecting ducts,[205] corresponding to the period of the most rapid decrease in transepithelial water permeability.[195,201] Thus, the results taken together strongly suggest that vasopressin directly regulates both endocytosis and exocytosis of AQP2. Presumably the net increase in water permeability seen in response to vasopressin is due both to direct stimulation of exocytosis and to direct inhibition of endocytosis.

Several groups have now successfully reconstituted the AQP2 delivery system using cultured cells transfected with either wild-type AQP2 or AQP2 tagged with a marker protein or a fluorescent protein.[206–211] Using such cultured cells stably transfected with AQP2, it has been shown that AQP2 trafficking occurs from vesicles to the apical plasma membrane, albeit in some cases to the basolateral plasma membrane, as well as retrieval and subsequent trafficking back to the surface upon repeated stimulation. This recycling of AQP2 also occurs in LLC-PK1 cells in the continued presence of cycloheximide, preventing *de novo* AQP2 synthesis. Despite remaining uncertainties, a working model for collecting duct water permeability permits molecular insight into this process (Figure 41.7). The short-term effects of vasopressin-enhanced water permeability are explained by the redistribution of AQP2 to the apical plasma membrane in collecting duct principal cells. Acting through the V2 receptor, vasopressin stimulates adenylyl cyclase; the elevated levels of intracellular cAMP activate protein kinase A (PKA), causing a redistribution of AQP2 from intracellular vesicles to the apical plasma membrane by inducing exocytosis of AQP2 vesicles, and by inhibiting endocytosis of AQP2 from the apical membrane. The net increase of AQP2 in the apical plasma membrane increases the water permeability. In the pre-antidiuretic state, the apical membrane is the rate-limiting barrier for transepithelial water transport, because AQP3 and AQP4 are abundant in the basolateral plasma membrane. Thus, increasing the water permeability of the apical plasma membrane by insertion of AQP2 water channels results in an increase in transepithelial osmotic water permeability. Whereas the general model is now well-established, the molecular details explaining how an elevation in intracellular cAMP levels regulates trafficking of AQP2 to the apical plasma membrane and back remain uncertain. Serine at position 256, in the carboxyl-terminal tail of AQP2, is apparently a substrate for protein kinase A, and regulation of exocytosis and endocytosis of AQP2 is expected to involve phosphorylation and dephosphorylation of AQP2,[208,212,213] and of ancillary proteins involved in the trafficking processes. This question will likely be a major focus of future research.

Signal Transduction Pathways Involved in Vasopressin Regulation of AQP2 Trafficking

The signal transduction pathways have been described thoroughly in previous reviews.[190,214–217] cAMP levels in collecting duct principal cells are increased by binding of vasopressin to V_2-receptors.[218,219] The synthesis of cAMP by adenylate cyclase is stimulated by a V_2-receptor coupled heterotrimeric GTP-binding protein, G_s. G_s interconverts between an inactive GDP-bound form and an active GTP-bound form, and the vasopressin-V_2-receptor complex catalyzes the exchange of GTP for bound GDP on the ∀-subunit of G_s. This causes release of the ∀-subunit, G_s∀-GTP, which subsequently binds to adenylate cyclase, thereby increasing cAMP production. Protein kinase A is a multimeric protein which is activated by cAMP, and consists in its inactive state of two catalytic subunits and two regulatory subunits. When cAMP binds to the regulatory subunits, these dissociate from the catalytic subunits, resulting in activation of the kinase activity of the catalytic subunits.

AQP2 contains a consensus site for PKA phosphorylation (RRQS) in the cytoplasmic COOH terminus at Ser[256].[123] Recent studies using ^{32}P labeling or using an antibody specific for phosphorylated AQP2 showed a very rapid phosphorylation of AQP2 (within 1 minute) in response to vasopressin-treatment of slices of the kidney papilla.[220] This is compatible with the time-course of vasopressin-stimulated water permeability of kidney collecting ducts.[189] As described above, PKA-induced phosphorylation of AQP2 apparently does not change the water conductance of AQP2 significantly. Importantly, it was recently demonstrated that vasopressin or forskolin treatment failed to induce translocation of AQP2 when Ser[256] was substituted by an alanine (S256A) in contrast to a significant regulated trafficking of wild-type AQP2 in LLC-PK1 cells.[208] A parallel study by Sasaki and colleagues also demonstrated the lack of cAMP-mediated exocytosis of mutated (S256A) AQP2 transfected into LLC-PK1 cells.[221] Thus, these studies indicate a specific role of PKA-induced phosphorylation of AQP2 for regulated trafficking. To explore this further, an antibody was designed that exclusively recognizes AQP2 which is phosphorylated in the PKA consensus site (Ser256). In normal rats phosphorylated AQP2 (Ser256) is present in intracellular vesicles and apical plasma membrane, indicating that it is constitutively phosphorylated even in low circulating vasopressin states.[222,223] In contrast, phosphorylated AQP2 is mainly located in intracellular vesicles in Brattleboro rats, as shown by immunocytochemistry and immunoblotting using membrane fractionation.[222] Importantly, dDAVP treatment of Brattleboro rats caused a marked redistribution of phosphorylated AQP2 (Ser256) to the apical plasma membrane, which is in agreement with an important role of PKA phosphorylation in this trafficking.[222] Conversely, treatment with V_2-receptor antagonist induced a marked decrease in the abundance of phosphorylated AQP2 (Ser256),[222] likely due to reduced PKA activity and/or increased dephosphorylation of AQP2, e.g., by increased phosphatase activity. Moreover, the necessity for the Ser[256] phosphorylation in AQP2-regulated urine concentration is underlined by the recent identification of this site as being spontaneously mutated in congenital progressive hydronephrosis (cph).[224] The spontaneous conversion of the serine phosphorylated site (Ser 256) to leucine in the cytoplasmic tail of the AQP2 protein in cph-mice prevents its phosphorylation at Ser[256], and inhibits the subsequent accumulation of AQP2 on the apical membrane of the collecting duct principal cells. This causes polydipsia, polyuria, and a severe urinary concentration defect leading to hydronephrosis and obstructive nephropathy in these mice. Recently, three previously unknown phosphorylation sites in the C-terminus of AQP2 were identified (S261, S264, and S269) by using liquid chromatography coupled to mass spectrometry neutral loss scanning.[225] During basal conditions, AQP2 phosphorylated on Ser[261] is approximately 24-fold more abundant than Ser[256] phosphorylated AQP2. During administration of dDAVP a decrease in Ser261 phosphorylation was observed, while AQP2 phosphorylated on Ser256, Ser264, and Ser269 increased.[225,226] It is clear that phosphorylation of AQP2 is required for cell surface expression; however, it is still unclear how phosphorylation of AQP2 (S256, S261, S264, S269) induces apical trafficking of AQP2. One possibility is that phosphorylation of AQP2 directly influences an interaction between AQP2-containing vesicles and the cell cytoskeleton, microtubules or accessory cross-linking proteins. Indeed, S256 is important for a direct interaction of AQP2 with 70 kDa heat-shock proteins.[227] Alternatively, phosphorylation could prevent endocytosis of AQP2, leading to accumulation at the cell surface.

Prostaglandin E_2 (PGE_2) has been known to inhibit vasopressin-induced water permeability by reducing cAMP levels. Zelenina et al.[228] investigated the effect of PGE_2 on PKA phosphorylation of AQP2 in rat kidney papilla, and the results suggest that the action of prostaglandins are associated with retrieval of AQP2 from the plasma membrane, but this appears to be independent of AQP2 phosphorylation by PKA.[228] In contrast, a recent study revealed the effect of selective

E-prostanoid receptor agonists on the vasopressin-independent targeting of AQP2.[229] *In vitro*, PGE2 and selective agonists for the E-prostanoid receptors EP2 or EP4 all increased trafficking and AQP2 phosphorylation (Ser264) in MDCK cells. *In vivo*, a V2R antagonist caused a severe urinary concentrating defect in rats, which was greatly alleviated by treatment with a selective agonist for the EP2 receptor.[229] Further studies are still needed on the effects of PGE2 on urine concentration.

Phosphorylation of AQP2 by other kinases, e.g., protein kinase C or casein kinase II, may potentially participate in regulation of AQP2 trafficking. Angiotensin II-induced activation of protein kinase C could be, at least in part, involved in the AQP2 trafficking/expression.[207,230,231] S256 is also a substrate for Golgi casein kinase 2, which is required for the Golgi transition of AQP2.[232] Additionally, the phosphatase inhibitor okadaic acid induces increased AQP2 expression at the cell surface, even in the presence of the PKA inhibitor H89 and S256A AQP2 mutants (that lack S256 phosphorylation) which are able to accumulate at the cell surface after treatment with cholesterol-depleting agents.[233] Phosphorylation of other cytoplasmic or vesicular regulatory proteins may also be involved. These issues remain to be investigated directly.

Involvement of the Cytoskeleton and Ca^{2+} in AQP2 Trafficking

The cytoskeleton has been shown to be involved in AQP2 trafficking in the kidney collecting duct. In particular, the microtubular network has been implicated in this process, since chemical disruption of microtubules inhibits the increase in permeability both in the toad bladder and in the mammalian collecting duct.[234,235] Thus, AQP2 vesicles may be transported along microtubules on their way to the apical plasma membrane. The microtubule-based motor protein dynein and the associated protein Arp1, which is part of the protein complex dynactin, were found by immunoblotting to be among the proteins associated with AQP2 vesicles from rat inner medulla. Immunoelectron microscopy further supported the presence of both AQP2 and dynein on the same vesicles.[236] Moreover, both vanadate (a non-specific inhibitor of ATPases) and EHNA (a specific inhibitor of dynein) inhibit the antidiuretic response in toad bladder[237,238] and kidney collecting duct.[239] Thus, it is likely that dynein may drive the microtubule-dependent delivery of AQP2-containing vesicles to the apical plasma membrane.

Actin filaments are also involved in the hydrosmotic response.[240–245] Recently evidence was provided that the myosin light chain kinase (MLCK) pathway,

through calmodulin-mediated calcium activation of MLCK, leads to phosphorylation of myosin regulatory light chain and non-muscle myosin 2 motor activity.[246] Studies in isolated perfused rat inner medullary collecting ducts showed the MLCK inhibitors ML-7 and ML-9 reduce the vasopressin-induced increase in water permeability,[246] indicating that MLCK may be a downstream target for the vasopressin-induced Ca^{2+} signal.

The intracellular Ca^{2+} concentration has been shown to increase upon stimulation of isolated perfused rat inner medullary collecting ducts with vasopressin or dDAVP.[247] These observations have been followed by a number of studies on the role of Ca^{2+} in the vasopressin-induced increase in water permeability. Vasopressin or 8–4-chlorophenylthio-cAMP induced a marked increase in intracellular $[Ca^{2+}]$ in isolated perfused IMCD, and BABTA blocked the rise in intracellular $[Ca^{2+}]$ and co-contaminantly led to inhibition of the vasopressin-induced increase in tubular water permeability.[248] Moreover, blocking calmodulin with W7 or trifluoperazine also inhibited the effect of vasopressin on tubular water permeability, and inhibited the vasopressin-induced AQP2 plasma membrane targeting in primary cultured IMCD cells.[248] Removing Ca^{2+} from both bath and lumen in isolated perfused tubules did not affect the vasopressin-induced Ca^{2+} signal, indicating that Ca^{2+} was released from an intracellular source. This was further supported by the observations that ryanodine inhibited the Ca^{2+} signal in perfused IMCDs and inhibited AQP2 accumulation in the plasma membrane in primary cultured IMCD cells. In addition, RyR1 ryanodine receptor was localized to rat IMCD by immunohistochemistry.[248] Ryanodine receptors are generally known to mediate a positive feedback and release Ca^{2+} from intracellular stores in response to an initial rise in intracellular $[Ca^{2+}]$. Thus, it is likely that another mechanism is responsible for the initialization of the rise in intracellular $[Ca^{2+}]$. Further studies revealed that vasopressin or dDAVP elicited oscillations in intracellular $[Ca^{2+}]$ in isolated perfused rat IMCD.[249] The results on isolated perfused IMCDs indicate that an intracellular increase in $[Ca^{2+}]$ is an obligate component of the vasopressin response leading to increased AQP2 expression in the apical plasma membrane. However, it should be mentioned that there is a discrepancy between the results from primary cultured IMCD cells[250] and isolated perfused IMCD tubules[248] with regard to the role of intracellular $[Ca^{2+}]$ in vasopressin-induced AQP2 trafficking. Consistent with this, Lorenz et al.[250] demonstrated that AQP2 shuttling is evoked neither by AVP-dependent increase of $[Ca^{2+}]$ nor by AVP-independent increase of $[Ca^{2+}]$ in primary cultured IMCD cells from rat kidney, although clamping of intracellular $[Ca^{2+}]$ below resting levels inhibits AQP2 exocytosis. Further studies are required to clarify this discrepancy, which may be related to altered expression levels of vasopressin receptors and/or AQP2 or other elements in the AQP2 trafficking system.

Mechanism of AQP2 Trafficking by Targeting Receptors

The mechanism by which AQP2 vesicles are targeted to the apical plasma membrane and the mechanism by which cAMP controls docking and fusion of vesicles is a current area of active investigation. Considerable insight into this problem has been obtained from previous studies of regulated exocytosis of synaptic vesicles, which involve the actions of multiple proteins.[251,252] Vesicle-targeting receptors (often referred to as "SNAREs") are believed to induce specific interaction of vesicles with membrane sites. Vesicle-targeting receptors associated chiefly with translocating vesicles are known as "VAMPs" (vesicle associated membrane proteins, also referred to as "synaptobrevins") and "synaptotagmins." Two other families of membrane proteins are believed to serve as receptors in target membranes: the "syntaxins" and SNAP-25 homologs. Several of these SNAREs have been found in the renal collecting duct.[253-260]

Syntaxins are 30 to 40 kDa integral membrane proteins. Syntaxins have a one bilayer-spanning domain near the C-terminus, so the majority of the protein resides in the cytoplasm. Syntaxins are widely distributed among mammalian tissues. It has been established that syntaxin-4 is expressed in the mammalian collecting duct by studies using polyclonal antibodies raised to conjugated peptides specific for individual syntaxins, and this has been confirmed by reverse transcription polymerase chain reaction.[258] Immunolocalization studies have demonstrated that syntaxin-4 is predominantly located in the apical plasma membrane of collecting duct principal cells, where AQP2 is targeted in response to vasopressin.

VAMPs are believed to induce specific docking of vesicles by interacting directly with syntaxins in the target plasma membrane (Figure 41.7). Although their primary amino acid sequences are not related to syntaxins, VAMPs also have a single bilayer-spanning domain near the C-terminus, and the majority of the protein resides in the cytoplasm. Three VAMP isoforms were initially identified[261]: VAMP-1; VAMP-2; and VAMP-3 (also referred to as "cellubrevin"), and subsequently several additional homologs have been cloned.[262] VAMP-2 and VAMP-3 have been localized in principal cells of renal collecting duct.[253-260] Double-labeling immunoelectron microscopy revealed that AQP2 and VAMP-2 reside in the same intracellular vesicles in collecting duct principal cells.[260] Furthermore, AQP2 vesicles isolated by differential centrifugation were found to contain VAMP-2.[254,257]

At this time, several putative vesicle-targeting proteins are known to reside in collecting duct principal cells. VAMP-2 resides in AQP2 intracellular vesicles, and syntaxin-4 resides in the apical plasma membrane. *In vitro* binding assays have documented that VAMP-2 binds syntaxin-4 with high affinity, but VAMP-2 has not been shown to interact with syntaxin-3 or syntaxin-2.[263,264] Thus, VAMP-2 and syntaxin-4 are likely participants in the targeting of AQP2 vesicles to the apical plasma membrane; however, a functional role for these targeting proteins remains to be formally demonstrated. A third SNARE protein, SNAP-23, has also been identified in principal cells of the collecting duct.[255] Although considered a target-membrane SNARE (t-SNARE), SNAP-23 is present both in AQP2-containing vesicles and in the apical plasma membrane of principal cells. VAMP-2, syntaxin-4, and SNAP-23 may potentially form a complex with the N-ethylmaleimide-sensitive factor (NSF). Finally, synaptotagmin VIII, a calcium-insensitive homolog, was identified in collecting duct principal cells,[256] and may potentially also play a role in vesicle targeting.

Recently, LC-MS/MS-based proteomic analysis of immunoisolated AQP2-containing intracellular vesicles from rat inner medullary collecting duct revealed that AQP2-containing vesicles are heterogeneous, and that intracellular AQP2 resides chiefly in endosomes, trans-Golgi network, and rough endoplasmic reticulum.[265] Vasopressin-stimulated exocytosis of AQP2 vesicles involves several steps including: (1) translocation of vesicles from a diffuse distribution throughout the cell to the apical region of the cell; (2) translocation of AQP2 across the apical part of the cell composed of a dense filamentous actin network; (3) priming of vesicles for docking; (4) docking of vesicles; and (5) fusion of vesicles with the apical plasma membrane. Theoretically, each of these steps could be a target for regulation by vasopressin. If the SNARE proteins are involved in the vasopressin-induced trafficking of AQP2 to the apical plasma membrane, the regulatory mechanism might involve selective phosphorylation of one of the SNARE proteins or an ancillary protein that binds to them, possibly via protein kinase A or calmodulin-dependent kinase II. Although the SNARE proteins are recognized as potential targets for phosphorylation,[266-268] there is presently no evidence for phosphorylation in the collecting duct. As noted above, however, AQP2 itself appears to be a target for PKA-mediated phosphorylation at a serine in position 256.[212] The phosphorylation does not modify the single channel water permeability of AQP2,[213] and instead the phosphorylation is believed to play a critical role in regulation of AQP2 trafficking to the plasma membrane.[208,221] The establishment of a role for these SNARE proteins in regulated trafficking of AQP2 will most likely depend on the preparation of targeted knockouts for each of these genes in the collecting duct.

Long-Term Regulation of Aquaporin Expression

It has been known for more than 40 years that urinary concentrating ability is regulated through a long-term conditioning effect of sustained increases in vasopressin levels exerted over a period of days.[269] The physiological and molecular basis for long-term conditioning of urinary concentrating ability is still being investigated. Water restriction causes a large, stable increase in water permeability of inner medullary collecting ducts dissected from rat kidneys and perfused *in vitro*.[185] Thus, water permeability of the tubules from water-restricted rats became five-fold greater than that measured in well-hydrated rats by a mechanism independent of the short-term action of vasopressin. Other studies confirmed that water restriction enhances the vasopressin-independent water permeability of collecting ducts,[270,271] and increases vasopressin-stimulated water permeability.[272] This contrasts with the lack of an observed increase in urea permeability in water-restricted rats.[185] These studies provided the firm conclusion that restriction of water intake for 24 hours or longer leads to a marked increase in the water-reabsorbing capacity of the renal collecting duct epithelium.

Further studies with anti-peptide antibodies have documented that the conditioned increase in water permeability is associated with increased expression of aquaporin proteins in collecting duct principal cells. Specifically, the increased water permeability that occurs in response to water restriction is accompanied by significant increases in the levels of AQP2 and AQP3 proteins in rat collecting ducts.[138,151,195] Water restriction for 24 to 48 hours resulted in an approximately five-fold increase in AQP2 protein in the rat renal inner medulla when measured by immunoblotting[138,195] and by immunostaining.[199] This increase paralleled the increase in water permeability in response to water restriction.[185]

A direct role for vasopressin in AQP2 expression has been established by multiple studies. Continuous infusion of arginine vasopressin into Brattleboro rats for 5 days resulted in a three-fold increase in AQP2 expression and a three-fold increase in water permeability of inner medullary collecting ducts.[143] When the time-course of AQP2 expression in inner medullary collecting duct was studied, it was found that 5 days of vasopressin infusion were required to reach maximal AQP2 levels in Brattleboro rats.[139]

Vasopressin is believed to be essential for evoking AQP2 expression, because Brattleboro rats totally lack circulating vasopressin fail to exhibit increased expression of AQP2 protein after long-term water restriction.[273] Moreover, administration of a selective V2-receptor antagonist blocked the increase in AQP2 expression usually seen with thirsting in normal rats,[199] whereas administration of the V2-selective agonist dDAVP (1-desamino-8-D-arginine vasopressin) to rats elicited a large increase in renal AQP2 mRNA[274] and AQP2 protein abundance.[275] The question of hyperosmolar induction of AQP2 during thirsting has been raised; however, five-day infusion of arginine vasopressin increased AQP2 comparably in renal cortex and medulla. This indicates that the vasopressin-induced expression of AQP2 is not critically dependent on increased osmolality or ionic strength in the tissue surrounding the collecting ducts.[187] Thus, it has been clearly established that the major increase in AQP2 water channel expression elicited by restriction of water intake is due to vasopressin binding to the V2 receptor in collecting duct principal cells. However, studies of the mechanism of escape from the antidiuretic effects of vasopressin[275,276] make it clear that AQP2 expression is regulated by other factors in addition to vasopressin (see later).

AQP3 protein expression also has been found to parallel AQP2 expression. A marked increase in AQP3 protein expression was observed in rats in response to restriction of water intake[151] and after a five-day infusion of arginine vasopressin.[187] These conditions did not lead to observed changes in AQP1 or AQP4 protein expression.[153,187] Thus, it is concluded that long-term circulation of high vasopressin levels is associated with an adaptive increase in maximal water permeability in collecting ducts, apparently due a selective increase in the expression of both AQP2 and AQP3 in the principal cells of the collecting duct. However, immunoelectron microscopy has demonstrated that AQP3 is predominantly present in the basolateral plasma membranes with little labeling of intracellular vesicles.[151] This suggests that AQP3 is not regulated by vesicular trafficking (in contrast to the findings with AQP2[182]). Moreover, there are several examples where there is a decoupling of AQP2 and AQP3 expression, suggesting that other factors in addition to vasopressin may regulate one or other of the aquaporins. This is seen in conditions such as hepatic cirrhosis,[277] vasopressin-escape,[275] low-protein diet,[278] and restriction of NaCl intake.[156]

The adaptive changes in AQP2 and AQP3 expression are believed to be due to transcriptional regulation of these genes. Increased AQP2 mRNA was found in the inner medullae of water-restricted rats,[279] and in response to infusion of dDAVP.[274,275] All of these studies indicate that the long-term upregulation of AQP2 expression in the rat kidney is due to elevation of the levels of AQP2 mRNA. Vasopressin-induced increase in AQP2 mRNA expression could reflect either increased gene transcription or reduced transcript degradation. Examination of the 3′-untranslated region of the AQP2 mRNA has not revealed the presence of recognizable mRNA stabilization motifs, and it is presumed that vasopressin directly increases *AQP2* gene transcription; however, no direct evidence supports this presumption. Transcriptional regulation would most likely occur through the vasopressin-induced increases in intracellular cyclic AMP that activates protein kinase A in collecting duct cells. Examination of the 5′-flanking region of the *AQP2* gene revealed a putative cAMP-response element (CRE), which may play a role in the vasopressin-induced increase in AQP2 expression.[280] Attempts to demonstrate expression of AQP2 promoter-luciferase reporter constructs have been undertaken in cultured renal epithelial cells and suggest that the putative CRE can drive increased expression of the *AQP2* gene; however, the inability of the cell line to express AQP2 protein limits the interpretation.[281–283]

As with AQP2, AQP3 mRNA levels were induced by infusion with the selective V2 agonist dDAVP.[275] Examination of the 5′-flanking DNA of AQP3 failed to reveal a CRE; however, Sp1 and AP2 cis-regulatory elements are present,[284] and these are known to be associated with cyclic AMP-mediated transcriptional regulation of other genes. A previous study revealed that AQP2 is ubiquitinated with one UbLys63-linked poly-Ub chain at K270 of AQP2 and lysosomal degradation was extensive for ubiquitinated AQP2.[285] The degradation pathways, therefore, balance the abundance of proteins which play an important role in body water homeostasis.[186]

DYSREGULATION OF RENAL AQUAPORINS IN WATER BALANCE DISORDERS

In a variety of conditions renal water handling is disturbed. Over the past decade, the role of changes in the expression and/or function of aquaporins have been investigated in a range of these conditions, including genetic defects or acquired defects showing a decreased renal responsiveness to vasopressin (acquired nephrogenic diabetes insipidus). The importance of aquaporins playing an essential role for regulation of renal water balance has been established (Table 41.2), and the following text represents extracted and updated information reported in previous reviews by the authors or other investigators.[190,286–288]

URINARY CONCENTRATING DEFECTS

Inherited Diabetes Insipidus

There are two significant inherited forms of diabetes insipidus (DI): central and nephrogenic. In central (or neurogenic) DI, there is a defect of vasopressin production. Central DI is rarely hereditary in man, but usually occurs as a consequence of head trauma or diseases in the hypothalamus or pituitary gland. The Brattleboro rat provides an excellent model of this condition. These animals have a total or near-total lack of vasopressin production.[289,290] Consequently, Brattleboro rats have substantially decreased expression levels of vasopressin-regulated AQP2 compared with the parent strain (Long Evans), and the AQP2 deficit was reversed by chronic vasopressin infusion, suggesting that patients lacking vasopressin are likely to have decreased AQP2 expression.[143] The subsequent work showing that expression of AQP3 is also regulated by vasopressin implies that the expression levels of these water channels will also be decreased in patients with CDI. The most important denominator is the deficiency of AQP2 trafficking to the apical membrane. These deficits are likely to be the most important causes of the polyuria from which these patients suffer, which will be reversed by desmopressin treatment. The second form of DI is called nephrogenic diabetes insipidus (NDI), and is caused by the inability of the kidney to respond to vasopressin stimulation. The most common hereditary cause (in 95% of cases) is an X-linked disorder associated with mutations of the V2 vasopressin receptor (AVPR2) making the collecting duct cells insensitive to vasopressin.[291] Although there is no direct evidence, it is likely that this form of NDI will be associated with decreased expression of AQP2, since the cells are unable to respond to circulating vasopressin.[292] This will compound the lack of AQP2 trafficking. Consistent with this, urinary AQP2 levels are very low in patients with X-linked NDI.[196,293] However, since the amount of AQP2 in the urine appears to be determined largely by the response of the collecting duct cells to vasopressin[294] rather than their content of AQP2, the data must be interpreted with caution with respect to predicting AQP2 expression levels. More rarely (in 5% of cases), congenital diabetes insipidus (CNDI) is inherited in an autosomal recessive fashion which is not due to mutations in the gene encoding the V2 vasopressin receptor, but these patients have been found to possess mutations in both alleles of the *AQP2* gene, and the sites of point mutations were observed at functionally important sites in the water transport pathway.[144,295–298] Since these patients manifest a particularly severe form of diabetes insipidus, the critical role of AQP2 in renal water conservation was established. It is believed that these mutations lead to abnormal intracellular routing of the expressed protein.[299] More than 155 mutations in the vasopressin receptor gene have been recognized to cause CNDI. Functional analysis has been carried out for over 79 of these mutations.[300] The analyses have revealed four different types of mutant receptors. The most common is impaired intracellular trafficking, which is seen in up to 70% of cases.[300] The remaining types include reduced ligand-binding capacity, failure to generate cAMP, and defects in the synthesis of stable mRNA.[301] Only five of the 155 known mutations cause partial CNDI (D85N, R104C, G201D, P322S, and S329R). Recently, a different kindred was identified with a dominant form of nephrogenic diabetes insipidus, and biochemical evaluations revealed that the mutation in the cytoplasmic C-terminus blocked the trafficking of AQP2 vesicles to the cell surface.[302] Thus, intracellular trafficking of vesicles containing products of the mutant allele and the product of the normal allele may be misdirected. It is not known if these individuals suffer a more or less severe clinical defect, and recently it was shown that the ligand-binding and signal transduction capability are dependent on localization of the amino acid variation, suggesting that striking divergences at the level of receptor functionality may thus underlie similar clinical phenotypes in CNDI.[303–305]

Acquired Nephrogenic Diabetes Insipidus

Acquired abnormalities of AQP2 expression have been implicated in multiple clinical disorders associated with abnormal water balance (Table 41.2). The role of vasopressin-regulated AQP2 has been established in a number of rat models with acquired NDI. In many of these conditions the kidney is unable to handle water, due to an impaired responsiveness to vasopressin; in the following text the most important of these condtions are described.

Lithium-Induced NDI

Lithium is a major therapeutic agent used to treat bipolar disorder (also referred to as "manic depressive disease") which affects approximately 1% of the US population.[306] However, lithium treatment is associated with a variety of renal side-effects, including nephrogenic diabetes insipidus (NDI, i.e., a pronounced vasopressin-resistant polyuria and inability to concentrate urine),[307,308] increased urinary sodium excretion,[309] and distal renal tubular acidosis.[310] Patients who have been treated with lithium manifest a slow recovery of urinary concentrating ability when treatment is discontinued. In rats treated with lithium

for 4 weeks, AQP2 and AQP3 levels were progressively reduced to approximately 5% of levels in control rats.[307,308] AQP2 downregulation was paralleled by a progressive development of severe polyuria.[307,308] Quantitative immunoelectron microscopy of AQP2 labeling in the inner medullary collecting duct principal cells showed that there was a reduction of AQP2 in the apical plasma membrane, as well as in the basolateral plasma membrane and intracellular vesicles. Reduction in AQP2 (and AQP3) expression may be induced by a lithium-dependent impairment in the production of cAMP in collecting duct principal cells,[309,311] indicating that inhibition of cAMP production may in part be responsible for the reduction in AQP2 expression, as well as the inhibition of targeting to the plasma membrane in response to lithium treatment. This is consistent with the presence of a cAMP-responsive element in the 5′-untranslated region of the AQP2 gene,[281,282] and with the demonstration that mice with inherently low cAMP levels have low expression of AQP2 ($DI^{+/+}$ severe mouse).[312] Lithium treatment is also associated with a concomitant increase in urinary sodium excretion, which is likely to play a role in the polyuria. It has also been demonstrated that chronic lithium treatment induces a marked decrease in protein abundance of epithelial sodium channel β- and γ-ENaC in the cortex and outer medulla, whereas the other renal sodium transporters upstream from the connecting tubule are unchanged.[313] This was also revealed by immunocytochemistry showing an almost complete absence of β-ENaC and γ-ENaC labeling in cortical and outer medullary collecting duct. This suggests a reduced responsiveness to aldosterone and vasopressin in these specific renal tubule segments, and that dysregulation of ENaC subunits is likely to play a role in the development of natriuresis and partly in the decreased urinary concentrating ability in rats with lithium-induced NDI.[314] Additional studies have identified proteins with altered abundance in the inner medullary collecting ducts (IMCD) of lithium-treated rats and their possible cellular function.[315,316] Moreover, it has been shown that prostaglandins, in lithium-treated mpkCCD cells, dcreases APQ2 protein stability by increasing its lysosomal degradation, indicating that *in vivo* paracrine-produced prostaglandins might have a role in lithium-induced NDI via this mechanism.[317]

Hypokalemia and Hypercalcemia

Hypokalemia and hypercalcemia are also associated with polyuria due to a vasopressin-resistant urinary concentrating defect. Rat models of these conditions are valuable tools to study the molecular defects. Treating rats with a potassium-deficient diet for 4 days induced a significant hypokalemia which was associated with downregulation of AQP2 expression and polyuria.[318] Likewise, hypercalcemia induced in rats by oral treatment for 7 days with dihydrotachysterol produced a urinary concentrating defect and polyuria which was also associated with downregulaion of AQP2.[319,320] Thus, both hypokalemia and hypercalcemia are associated with downregulation of AQP2 expression, and immunolocalization studies of AQP2 demonstrated similar features. In addition to the downregulation of AQP2, expression of Na-K-2Cl co-transporter in the thick ascending limb was decreased in both conditions,[321,322] suggesting that reduced sodium and chloride reabsorption in the thick ascending limb, and hence decreased medullary hyperosmolality, could also partly contribute to the polyuria and decreased urinary concentration in hypokalemia and hypercalcemia. Thus, these studies in part describe the underlying molecular defects involved in the development of the polyuria in these conditions.

Urinary Tract Obstruction

Another serious condition seen in both children and adults is urinary tract obstruction which is associated with complex changes in renal function involving marked alterations in both glomerular and tubular function and bilateral urinary tract obstruction (BUO) which may result in long-term impairment of the ability to concentrate urine.[323] BUO for 24 hours in rats is associated with markedly reduced expression of AQP2, AQP3, AQP4, and AQP1.[324−327] In addition, BUO is associated with marked downregulation of key sodium transporters and urea transporters.[328] Following release of the obstruction, there is a marked polyuria, during which period AQP2 and AQP3 levels remain downregulated up to two week after release, providing an explanation at the molecular level for the observed post-obstructive polyuria. In a number of studies BUO has been demonstrated to be associated with COX2 induction and cellular infiltration of the renal medulla.[292,329−331] Using specific COX2 inhibition to rats subjected to BUO it was demonstrated that this treatment prevents downregulation of AQP2 and several sodium transporters located to the proximal tubule and mTAL.[329,330] Also, increased expression and activity of the P2Y2, EP1, and EP3 receptors have been suggested to play important roles in post-obstructive polyuria.[332] Moreover, specific inhibition of the AT1 receptor in rats subjected to BUO prevented AVP2R downregulation of NaPi2 in the PT, BSC-1 in the mTAL, and AQP2/pS256-AQP2 in the CD three days after release of BUO,[134,333] confirming that the renin−angiotensin system plays an important role for the pathophysiological changes in urinary tract obstruction.

In contrast to BUO conditions, unilateral ureteral obstruction is not associated with changes in the absolute excretion of sodium and water since the non-obstructed kidney compensates for the reduced ability of the obstructed kidney to excrete solutes.[328,334] These studies demonstrated a profound downregulation of AQP1, AQP2, AQP3, and AQP4, and pAQP2 levels in the obstructed kidney, suggesting that local factors play a major role.

Renal Failure

Renal failure, both acute and chronic, is associated with polyuria and a urinary concentrating defect, and in both cases there is a wide range of glomerular and tubular abnormalities that contribute to the overall renal dysfunction. Ischemia and reperfusion (I/R)-induced experimental acute renal failure (ARF) in rats is a model that is widely used. In this model there are structural alterations in the renal tubule, in association with an impaired urinary concentration.

ARF is associated with defects both in collecting duct water reabsorption and proximal tubule water reabsorption, as well as defects in solute handling.[335−337] Using the isolated tubule microperfusion model, it was demonstrated that water reabsorption in the proximal tubule and cortical collecting duct was significantly reduced following ischemia,[335] and no differences in either basal or vasopressin-induced cAMP levels in outer or inner medulla in rats with ARF were demonstrated,[338] supporting the view that there are defects in collecting duct water reabsorption. Consistent with these findings, it was demonstrated that AQP2 and AQP3 expression in the collecting duct, as well as AQP1 expression in the proximal tubule, are significantly reduced in response to ARF.[339,340] The decreased levels of aquaporins were associated with impaired urinary concentration in rats with both oliguric or nonoliguric ARF. The reduced expression of AQP1−3 and the reduced urinary concentration capacity was significantly prevented by co-treatment with alpha-melanocyte-stimulating hormone (α-MSH), which is an anti-inflammatory cytokine that inhibits both neutrophil and nitric oxide pathways.[340] This finding indicates that decreased levels of aquaporins in both the proximal tubule and collecting duct in post-ischemic kidneys may play a significant role in the impaired urinary concentration. Recently it was also demonstrated that hemorrhagic shock-induced acute renal failure is associated with decreased expression of collecting duct water channel AQP2 and AQP3,[341] and that erythropoietin treatment (single or combined with α-MSH) in rats with I/R-induced ARF, which is known to prevent caspase-3, -8, and -9 activation *in vivo* and reduces apoptotic cell death,[342] prevents or reduces the urinary concentrating defects and downregulation of AQP expression levels.[341] Consistent with this, it was demonstrated that NF-kappaB activation is of importance for the downregulation of AQP2 channel and vasopressin V2-receptor expression during sepsis in a cecal ligation and puncture (CLP) mouse model of ARF, and that NF-kappaB inhibition ameliorates sepsis-induced ARF in the CLP model.[343]

Patients with advanced chronic renal failure (CRF) have urine which remains hypotonic to plasma despite the administration of supramaximal doses of vasopressin.[344] This vasopressin-resistant hyposthenuria specifically implies abnormalities in collecting duct water reabsorption in CRF patients. Recent observations demonstrated virtual absence of V2 receptor mRNA in the inner medulla of CRF rat kidneys,[345] providing evidence for significant defects in the collecting duct water permeability. Consistent with these observations, it has shown both decreased collecting duct water channel AQP2 and AQP3 expression and a vasopressin-resistant downregulation of AQP2 in a 5/6 nephrectomy-induced CRF rat model.[346]

WATER RETENTION

Congestive Heart Failure

Retention of sodium and water is a common and clinically important complication of congestive heart failure (CHF). Two studies have examined the changes in renal AQP expression in rats with CHF induced by ligation of the left coronary artery[347,348] to test if upregulation of AQP2 expression and targeting may play a role in the water retention in CHF. Both studies demonstrated that renal water retention in severe CHF in rats is associated with dysregulation of AQP2 in the renal collecting duct principal cells, involving both an increase in the AQP2 expression and a marked redistribution of AQP2 to the apical plasma membrane.[347,348] Rats with severe CHF had significantly elevated left ventricular end-diastolic pressures (LVEDP), and had reduced plasma sodium concentrations.[347] Immunoblotting revealed a three-fold increase in AQP2 expression compared with sham operated animals. These changes were associated with elevated LVEDP or hyponatremia, since animals with normal LVEDP and plasma sodium did not have increased AQP2 levels compared with sham operated controls.[347] Furthermore, this study showed an increased plasma membrane targeting, providing an explanation for the increased permeability of the collecting duct and an increase in water reabsorption. This may provide an explanation for excess free water retention in severe CHF, and for the development of hyponatremia. In parallel, the other study showed upregulation of both AQP2 protein and AQP2 mRNA levels in kidney inner medulla and cortex in rats with CHF.[348] These rats had significantly decreased cardiac output and, importantly, increased plasma vasopressin levels. Furthermore, in this study administration of V2 antagonist OPC 31260 was associated with a significant increase in diuresis, a decrease in urine osmolality, a rise in plasma osmolality, and a significant reduction in AQP2 protein and AQP2 mRNA levels compared with untreated rats with CHF. Consistent with this, treatment of V2-receptor antagonist in human patients and rats with heart failure is associated with a dose-related increase in water excretion and a decrease in urinary AQP2 excretion.[349,350] Moreover, it has been shown in patients with CHF that treatment with furosemide increases the urinary excretion of AQP2, free water clearance, and sodium exceretion.[351]

Hepatic Cirrhosis

Hepatic cirrhosis is another chronic condition associated with water retention.[352] It has been suggested that an important pathophysiological factor in the impaired ability to excrete water could be increased levels of plasma vasopressin. However, unlike CHF, the changes in expression of AQP2 protein levels vary considerably between different experimental models of hepatic cirrhosis. Several studies have examined the changes in renal AQP expression in rats with cirrhosis induced by common bile duct ligation (CBDL).[277,353,354] The rats displayed impaired vasopressin-regulated water reabsorption despite normal plasma vasopressin levels. Consistent with this, semiquantitative immunoblotting showed a significant decrease in AQP2 expression in rats with hepatic cirrhosis.[277,353] In addition, the expression levels of AQP3 and AQP4 were downregulated in CBDL rats. This may predict a reduced water permeability of the collecting duct in this model[277]; hence, renal water reabsorption in the collecting duct is decreased in rats with compensated liver cirrhosis. In contrast, Fujita et al.[274] demonstrated that hepatic cirrhosis induced by intraperitoneal administration of carbon tetrachloride (CCl4) was associated with a significant increase in both AQP2 protein levels and AQP2 mRNA expression. Interestingly, AQP2 mRNA expression correlated with the amount of ascites, suggesting that AQP2 may play a role in the abnormal water retention followed by the development of ascites in hepatic cirrhosis.[355] In a different model of CCl4-induced cirrhosis, using CCl4 inhalation, AQP2 expression was not increased.[356] There was, however, evidence for increased trafficking of AQP2 to the plasma membrane, consistent with the presence of elevated levels of vasopressin in the plasma. Interestingly, there was a marked increase in AQP3 expression that is likely to be due to increased vasopressin levels. The pattern of increased AQP3 expression without upregulation of AQP2 is consistent with previous findings observed in the vasopressin escape,[276] suggesting that the lack of increase in AQP2 expression could be a result of a normal compensatory response related to the escape phenomenon. Although the explanation for the differences between cirrhosis induced by CBDL and CCl₄ administration remains to be determined, it is well-known that the dysregulation of body water balance depends on the severity of cirrhosis.[357–360] CBDL results in a compensated cirrhosis characterized by peripheral vasodilation and increased cardiac output, whereas cirrhosis induced by 12 weeks of CCl₄ administration may be associated with the late state of decompensated liver cirrhosis characterized by sodium retention, edema, and ascites.[358,359,361] Thus, the downregulation of AQP2 observed in milder forms of cirrhosis (i.e., in a compensated stage without water retention) may represent a compensatory mechanism to prevent development of water retention. In contrast, the increased levels of vasopressin seen in severe "noncompensated" cirrhosis with ascites may induce an inappropriate upregulation of AQP2 that would in turn participate in the development of water retention. Recent studies have shown a prominent role for AQP1 in angiogenesis, fibrosis, and portal hypertension after bile duct ligation in wild-type and AQP1 knockout mice.[362]

Experimental Nephrotic Syndrome

Nephrotic syndrome is characterized by extracellular volume expansion with excessive renal salt and water reabsorption. The underlying mechanisms of salt and water retention are poorly-understood; however, they can be expected to be associated with dysregulation of solute transporters and water channels.[359] In contrast to congestive heart failure and liver cirrhosis, a marked downregulation of AQP2 and AQP3 expression was demonstrated in rats with PAN-induced and adriamycin-induced nephrotic syndrome.[363–365] The reduced expression of collecting duct water channels could represent a physiologically appropriate response to extracellular volume expansion. The signal transduction involved in this process is not clear, but circulating vasopressin levels are high in rats with PAN-induced nephrotic syndrome. Thus, the marked downregulation of AQP2 in experimental nephrotic syndrome may

share similarities with the downregulation of AQP2 in water-loaded dDAVP-treated rats that escape from the action of vasopressin.[275,276]

SIADH and Vasopressin Escape

Hyponatremia, defined as a serum sodium less than 135 mmol/L, is one of the most commonly encountered electrolyte disorders of clinical medicine.[366] The predominant cause of hyponatremia is an inappropriate secretion of vasopressin relative to serum osmolality or the "syndrome of inappropriate antidiuretic hormone secretion" (SIADH).[367] SIADH occurs most frequently in association with vascular, infectious or neoplastic abnormalities in the lung or central nervous system. In an experimental rat model of SIADH it was shown that AQP2 mRNA expression and AQP2 protein expression were increased in the collecting duct.[274] Thus, increased expression of AQP2 in the collecting duct accounts for the water retention and hyponatremia in SIADH.

The degree of hyponatremia is limited by a process that counters the water-retaining action of vasopressin, namely "vasopressin escape." Vasopressin escape is characterized by a sudden increase in urine volume with a decrease in urine osmolality independent of high circulating vasopressin levels. The onset of escape coincided temporally with a marked decrease in renal AQP2 protein, as measured by immunoblotting, as well as decreased mRNA expression, as assessed by Northern blotting.[276] In contrast to AQP2, there were no decreases in renal expression of AQP1, AQP3, and AQP4.[276] These results suggest that escape from vasopressin-induced antidiuresis is attributable, at least in part, to a selective vasopressin-independent decrease in AQP2 expression in the renal collecting duct.[368,369]

Acknowledgments

Support for this chapter was partially provided by funds from the Danish National Research Foundation, The European Commission, the Danish Medical Research Council, Novo Nordic Foundation, Karen Elise Jensen Foundation and the National Institutes of Health. Portions of the text were previously published in abridged form and are reproduced and modified with permission.[122] Moreover, the authors gratefully acknowledge the major contributions from Peter Agre and Mark Knepper, who together with SN authored a previous version of this chapter.

References

[1] Finkelstein A. Water movement through lipid bilayers, pores, and plasma membranes: theory and reality. New York: John Wiley & Sons; 1987.
[2] Solomon AK. Characterization of biological membranes by equivalent pores. J Gen Physiol 1968;51(Suppl).

[3] Macey RI. Transport of water and urea in red blood cells. Am J Physiol 1984;246:C195—203.

[4] Knepper MA, Wade JB, Terris J, Ecelbarger CA, Marples D, Mandon B, et al. Renal aquaporins. Kidney Int 1996;49:1712—7.

[5] Bourguet J, Chevalier J, Hugon JS. Alterations in membrane-associated particle distribution during antidiuretic challenge in frog urinary bladder epithelium. Biophys J 1976;16:627—39.

[6] Brown D, Orci L. Vasopressin stimulates formation of coated pits in rat kidney collecting ducts. Nature 1983;302:253—5.

[7] Kachadorian WA, Wade JB, DiScala VA. Vasopressin: induced structural change in toad bladder luminal membrane. Science 1975;190:67—9.

[8] Wade JB, Stetson DL, Lewis SA. ADH action: evidence for a membrane shuttle mechanism. Ann N.Y Acad Sci 1981;372:106—17.

[9] Agre P, Preston GM, Smith BL, Jung JS, Raina S, Moon C, et al. The archetypal molecular water channel. Am J Physiol 1993;265:F463—76.

[10] Solomon AK, Chasan B, Dix JA, Lukacovic MF, Toon MR, Verkman AS. The aqueous pore in the red cell membrane: band 3 as a channel for anions, cations, nonelectrolytes, and water. Ann NY Acad Sci 1983;414:97—124.

[11] Agre P, Saboori AM, Asimos A, Smith BL. Purification and partial characterization of the Mr 30,000 integral membrane protein associated with the erythrocyte Rh(D) antigen. J Biol Chem 1987;262:17497—503.

[12] Denker BM, Smith BL, Kuhajda FP, Agre P. Identification, purification, and partial characterization of a novel Mr 28,000 integral membrane protein from erythrocytes and renal tubules. J Biol Chem 1988;263:15634—42.

[13] Smith BL, Agre P. Erythrocyte Mr 28,000 transmembrane protein exists as a multisubunit oligomer similar to channel proteins. J Biol Chem 1991;266:6407—15.

[14] Preston GM, Agre P. Isolation of the cDNA for erythrocyte integral membrane protein of 28 kilodaltons: member of an ancient channel family. Proc Natl Acad Sci USA 1991;88:11110—4.

[15] Van Hoek AN, Hom ML, Luthjens LH, de J, Dempster JA, van Os CH. Functional unit of 30 kDa for proximal tubule water channels as revealed by radiation inactivation. J Biol Chem 1991;266:16633—5.

[16] Agre P, Sasaki S, Chrispeels MJ. Aquaporins: a family of water channel proteins. Am J Physiol 1993;265:F461.

[17] Agre P. Molecular physiology of water transport: aquaporin nomenclature workshop. Mammalian aquaporins. Biol Cell 1997;89:255—7.

[18] Fischbarg J, Kuang KY, Vera JC, Arant S, Silverstein SC, Loike J, et al. Glucose transporters serve as water channels. Proc Natl Acad Sci USA 1990;87:3244—7.

[19] Zhang RB, Logee KA, Verkman AS. Expression of mRNA coding for kidney and red cell water channels in Xenopus oocytes. J Biol Chem 1990;265:15375—8.

[20] Preston GM, Carroll TP, Guggino WB, Agre P. Appearance of water channels in Xenopus oocytes expressing red cell CHIP28 protein. Science 1992;256:385—7.

[21] Meinild AK, Klaerke DA, Zeuthen T. Bidirectional water fluxes and specificity for small hydrophilic molecules in aquaporins 0—5. J Biol Chem 1998;273:32446—51.

[22] Zeidel ML, Ambudkar SV, Smith BL, Agre P. Reconstitution of functional water channels in liposomes containing purified red cell CHIP28 protein. Biochemistry 1992;31:7436—40.

[23] Van Hoek AN, Verkman AS. Functional reconstitution of the isolated erythrocyte water channel CHIP28. J Biol Chem 1992;267:18267—9.

[24] Zeidel ML, Nielsen S, Smith BL, Ambudkar SV, Maunsbach AB, Agre P. Ultrastructure, pharmacologic inhibition, and transport selectivity of aquaporin channel-forming integral protein in proteoliposomes. Biochemistry 1994;33:1606—15.

[25] Pao GM, Wu LF, Johnson KD, Hofte H, Chrispeels MJ, Sweet G, et al. Evolution of the MIP family of integral membrane transport proteins. Mol Microbiol 1991;5:33—7.

[26] Wistow GJ, Pisano MM, Chepelinsky AB. Tandem sequence repeats in transmembrane channel proteins. Trends Biochem Sci 1991;16:170—1.

[27] Cabiaux V, Oberg KA, Pancoska P, Walz T, Agre P, Engel A. Secondary structures comparison of aquaporin-1 and bacteriorhodopsin: a fourier transform infrared spectroscopy study of two-dimensional membrane crystals. Biophys J 1997;73:406—17.

[28] Reizer J, Reizer A, Saier Jr MH. The MIP family of integral membrane channel proteins: sequence comparisons, evolutionary relationships, reconstructed pathway of evolution, and proposed functional differentiation of the two repeated halves of the proteins. Crit Rev Biochem Mol Biol 1993;28:235—57.

[29] Preston GM, Jung JS, Guggino WB, Agre P. Membrane topology of aquaporin CHIP. Analysis of functional epitope-scanning mutants by vectorial proteolysis. J Biol Chem 1994;269:1668—73.

[30] Preston GM, Jung JS, Guggino WB, Agre P. The mercury-sensitive residue at cysteine 189 in the CHIP28 water channel. J Biol Chem 1993;268:17—20.

[31] Zhang R, Van Hoek AN, Biwersi J, Verkman AS. A point mutation at cysteine 189 blocks the water permeability of rat kidney water channel CHIP28k. Biochemistry 1993;32:2938—41.

[32] Jung JS, Preston GM, Smith BL, Guggino WB, Agre P. Molecular structure of the water channel through aquaporin CHIP. The hourglass model. J Biol Chem 1994;269:14648—54.

[33] Verbavatz JM, Brown D, Sabolic I, Valenti G, Ausiello DA, Van Hoek AN, et al. Tetrameric assembly of CHIP28 water channels in liposomes and cell membranes: a freeze-fracture study. J Cell Biol 1993;123:605—18.

[34] Shi LB, Skach WR, Verkman AS. Functional independence of monomeric CHIP28 water channels revealed by expression of wild-type mutant heterodimers. J Biol Chem 1994;269:10417—22.

[35] Walz T, Smith BL, Zeidel ML, Engel A, Agre P. Biologically active two-dimensional crystals of aquaporin CHIP. J Biol Chem 1994;269:1583—6.

[36] Walz T, Smith BL, Agre P, Engel A. The three-dimensional structure of human erythrocyte aquaporin CHIP. EMBO J 1994;13:2985—93.

[37] Walz T, Tittmann P, Fuchs KH, Muller DJ, Smith BL, Agre P, et al. Surface topographies at subnanometer-resolution reveal asymmetry and sidedness of aquaporin-1. J Mol Biol 1996;264:907—18.

[38] Cheng A, Van Hoek AN, Yeager M, Verkman AS, Mitra AK. Three-dimensional organization of a human water channel. Nature 1997;387:627—30.

[39] Jap BK, Li H. Structure of the osmo-regulated H₂O-channel, AQP-CHIP, in projection at 3.5 Å resolution. J Mol Biol 1995;251:413—20.

[40] Li H, Lee S, Jap BK. Molecular design of aquaporin-1 water channel as revealed by electron crystallography. Nat Struct Mol Biol 1997;4:263—5.

[41] Mitra AK, Van Hoek AN, Wiener MC, Verkman AS, Yeager M. The CHIP28 water channel visualized in ice by electron crystallography. Nat Struct Biol 1995;2:726—9.

[42] Mitsuoka K, Murata K, Walz T, Hirai T, Agre P, Heymann JB, et al. The structure of aquaporin-1 at 4.5-Å resolution reveals short [alpha]-helices in the center of the monomer. J Struct Biol 1999;128:34—43.

[43] Murata K, Mitsuoka K, Hirai T, Walz T, Agre P, Heymann JB, et al. Structural determinants of water permeation through aquaporin-1. Nature 2000;407:599—605.

[44] Ren G, Cheng A, Reddy V, Melnyk P, Mitra AK. Three-dimensional fold of the human AQP1 water channel determined at 4 Å resolution by electron crystallography of two-dimensional crystals embedded in ice. J Mol Biol 2000;301:369–87.

[45] Ren G, Reddy VS, Cheng A, Melnyk P, Mitra AK. Visualization of a water-selective pore by electron crystallography in vitreous ice. Proc Natl Acad Sci USA 2001;98:1398–403.

[46] Walz T, Hirai T, Murata K, Heymann JB, Mitsuoka K, Fujiyoshi Y, et al. The three-dimensional structure of aquaporin-1. Nature 1997;387:624–7.

[47] Sui H, Han BG, Lee JK, Walian P, Jap BK. Structural basis of water-specific transport through the AQP1 water channel. Nature 2001;414:872–8.

[48] de Groot BL, Grubmuller H. Water permeation across biological membranes. mechanism and dynamics of aquaporin-1 and GlpF. Science 2001;294:2353–7.

[49] Beitz E, Wu B, Holm LM, Schultz JE, Zeuthen T. Point mutations in the aromatic/arginine region in aquaporin 1 allow passage of urea, glycerol, ammonia, and protons. Proc Nat Acad Sci 2006;103:269–74.

[50] Maurel C, Reizer J, Schroeder JI, Chrispeels MJ, Saier Jr. MH. Functional characterization of the *Escherichia coli* glycerol facilitator, GlpF, in *Xenopus* oocytes. J Biol Chem 1994;269:11869–72.

[51] Schenk AD, Werten PJL, Scheuring S, de Groot BL, Muller SA, Stahlberg H, et al. The 4.5 Å structure of human AQP2. J Mol Biol 2005;350:278–89.

[52] Werten PJL, Hasler L, Koenderink JB, Klaassen CHW, de Grip WJ, Engel A, et al. Large-scale purification of functional recombinant human aquaporin-2. FEBS Lett 2001;504:200–5.

[53] Fotiadis D, Suda K, Tittmann P, Jeno P, Philippsen A, Muller DJ, et al. Identification and structure of a putative Ca^{2+}-binding domain at the C terminus of AQP1. J Mol Biol 2002;318:1381–94.

[54] Gonen T, Sliz P, Kistler J, Cheng Y, Walz T. Aquaporin-0 membrane junctions reveal the structure of a closed water pore. Nature 2004;429:193–7.

[55] Harries WEC, Akhavan D, Miercke LJW, Khademi S, Stroud RM. The channel architecture of aquaporin 0 at a 2.2-Å resolution. Proc Nat Acad Sci 2004;101:14045–50.

[56] Mulders SM, Preston GM, Deen PMT, Guggino WB, Os CH, Agre P. Water channel properties of major intrinsic protein of lens. J Biol Chem 1995;270:9010–6.

[57] Han BG, Guliaev AB, Walian PJ, Jap BK. Water transport in AQP0 aquaporin. Molecular dynamics studies. J Mol Biol 2006;360:285–96.

[58] Brooks HL, Regan JW, Yool AJ. Inhibition of Aquaporin-1 water permeability by tetraethylammonium: involvement of the loop E pore region. Mol Pharmacol 2000;57:1021–6.

[59] Detmers FJM, de Groot BL, Muller EM, Hinton A, Konings IBM, Sze M, et al. Quaternary ammonium compounds as water channel blockers. Specificity, potency, and site of action. J Biol Chem 2006;281:14207–14.

[60] Verkman AS. Applications of aquaporin inhibitors. Drug News Perspect 2001;14:412.

[61] Zelenina M, Tritto S, Bondar AA, Zelenin S, Aperia A. Copper inhibits the water and glycerol permeability of aquaporin-3. J Biol Chem 2004;279:51939–43.

[62] Zelenina M, Bondar AA, Zelenin S, Aperia A. Nickel and extracellular acidification inhibit the water permeability of human aquaporin-3 in lung epithelial cells. J Biol Chem 2003;278:30037–43.

[63] Agemark M, Kowal J, Kukulski W, Norden K, Gustavsson N, Johanson U, et al. Reconstitution of water channel function and 2D-crystallization of human aquaporin 8. Biochim Biophys Acta 2012;1818:839–50.

[64] Berthaud A, Manzi J, Perez J, Mangenot S. Modeling detergent organization around aquaporin-0 using small angle X-ray scattering. J Am Chem Soc 2012;134(24):10080–8.

[65] Crane JM, Rossi A, Gupta T, Bennett JL, Verkman AS. Orthogonal array formation by human aquaporin-4: examination of neuromyelitis optica-associated aquaporin-4 polymorphisms. J Neuroimmunol 2011;236:93–8.

[66] Fischer G, Kosinska-Eriksson U, ponte-Santamaria C, Palmgren M, Geijer C, Hedfalk K, et al. Crystal structure of a yeast aquaporin at 1.15 angstrom reveals a novel gating mechanism. PLoS Bio 2009;7:e1000130.

[67] Fujiyoshi Y. Electron crystallography for structural and functional studies of membrane proteins. *J Electron Microsc* (Tokyo) 2011;60(Suppl. 1):S149–59.

[68] Ho JD, Yeh R, Sandstrom A, Chorny I, Harries WE, Robbins RA, et al. Crystal structure of human aquaporin 4 at 1.8 Å and its mechanism of conductance. Proc Natl Acad Sci USA 2009;106:7437–42.

[69] Horsefield R, Norden K, Fellert M, Backmark A, Tornroth-Horsefield S, Terwisscha van Scheltinga AC, et al. High-resolution x-ray structure of human aquaporin 5. Proc Natl Acad Sci USA 2008;105:13327–32.

[70] Jiang Y. Expression and functional characterization of NPA motif-null aquaporin-1 mutations. IUBMB Life 2009;61:651–7.

[71] Strand L, Moe SE, Solbu TT, Vaadal M, Holen T. Roles of aquaporin-4 isoforms and amino acids in square array assembly. Biochemistry 2009;48:5785–93.

[72] Wolburg H, Wolburg-Buchholz K, Fallier-Becker P, Noell S, Mack AF. Structure and functions of aquaporin-4-based orthogonal arrays of particles. Int Rev Cell Mol Biol 2011;287:1–41.

[73] Wree D, Wu B, Zeuthen T, Beitz E. Requirement for asparagine in the aquaporin NPA sequence signature motifs for cation exclusion. FEBS J 2011;278:740–8.

[74] Yakata K, Tani K, Fujiyoshi Y. Water permeability and characterization of aquaporin-11. J Struct Biol 2011;174:315–20.

[75] Sabolic I, Valenti G, Verbavatz JM, Van Hoek AN, Verkman AS, Ausiello DA, et al. Localization of the CHIP28 water channel in rat kidney. Am J Physiol 1992;263:C1225–33.

[76] Maunsbach AB, Marples D, Chin E, Ning G, Bondy C, Agre P, et al. Aquaporin-1 water channel expression in human kidney. J Am Soc Nephrol 1997;8:1–14.

[77] Nielsen S, Smith B, Christensen EI, Knepper MA, Agre P. CHIP28 water channels are localized in constitutively water-permeable segments of the nephron. J Cell Biol 1993;120:371–83.

[78] Maeda Y, Smith BL, Agre P, Knepper MA. Quantification of aquaporin-CHIP water channel protein in microdissected renal tubules by fluorescence-based ELISA. J Clin Invest 1995;95:422–8.

[79] Bedford JJ, Leader JP, Walker RJ. Aquaporin expression in normal human kidney and in renal disease. J Am Soc Nephrol 2003;14:2581–7.

[80] King LS, Nielsen S, Agre P. Aquaporin-1 water channel protein in lung: ontogeny, steroid-induced expression, and distribution in rat. J Clin Invest 1996;97:2183–91.

[81] Nielsen S, Smith BL, Christensen EI, Agre P. Distribution of the aquaporin CHIP in secretory and resorptive epithelia and capillary endothelia. Proc Natl Acad Sci USA 1993;90:7275–9.

[82] Schnitzer JE, Oh P. Aquaporin-1 in plasma membrane and caveolae provides mercury-sensitive water channels across lung endothelium. Am J Physiol 1996;270:H416–22.

[83] Pallone TL, Kishore BK, Nielsen S, Agre P, Knepper MA. Evidence that aquaporin-1 mediates NaCl-induced water flux across descending vasa recta. Am J Physiol 1997;272:F587–96.

[84] King LS, Nielsen S, Agre P. Aquaporins in complex tissues. I. Developmental patterns in respiratory and glandular tissues of rat. Am J Physiol 1997;273:C1541–8.

[85] Moon C, King LS, Agre P. Aqp1 expression in erythroleukemia cells: genetic regulation of glucocorticoid and chemical induction. Am J Physiol 1997;273:C1562–70.

[86] Lai, KN., Li, FG., Yui, LH., Tang, S., Tsang, AWL., Chan, DTM, et al., Expression of aquaporin-1 in human peritoneal mesothelial cells and its upregulation by glucose in vitro. J Am Soc Nephrol 12:1036–45.

[87] Mann SE, Ricke EA, Yang BA, Verkman AS, Taylor RN. Expression and localization of aquaporin 1 and 3 in human fetal membranes. Am J Obstet Gynecol 2002;187:902–7.

[88] Hasegawa H, Lian SC, Finkbeiner WE, Verkman AS. Extrarenal tissue distribution of CHIP28 water channels by *in situ* hybridization and antibody staining. Am J Physiol 1994;266:C893–903.

[89] Stamer WD, Snyder RW, Smith BL, Agre P, Regan JW. Localization of aquaporin CHIP in the human eye: implications in the pathogenesis of glaucoma and other disorders of ocular fluid balance. Invest Ophthalmol Vis Sci 1994;35:3867–72.

[90] Roberts SK, Yano M, Ueno Y, Pham L, Alpini G, Agre P, et al. Cholangiocytes express the aquaporin CHIP and transport water via a channel-mediated mechanism. Proc Natl Acad Sci USA 1994;91:13009–13.

[91] Ko SBH, Naruse S, Kitagawa M, Ishiguro H, Furuya S, Mizuno N, et al. Aquaporins in rat pancreatic interlobular ducts. AJP-Gastrointest Liver Physiol 2002;282:G324–31.

[92] Au CG, Cooper ST, Lo HP, Compton AG, Yang N, Wintour EM, et al. Expression of aquaporin 1 in human cardiac and skeletal muscle. J Mol Cell Cardiol 2004;36:655–62.

[93] Calamita G, Ferri D, Bazzini C, Mazzone A, Botta G, Liquori G, et al. Expression and subcellular localization of the AQP8 and AQP1 water channels in the mouse gall-bladder epithelium. Biol Cell 2005;97(6):415–23.

[94] Gresz V, Kwon TH, Hurley PT, Varga G, Zelles T, Nielsen S, et al. Identification and localization of aquaporin water channels in human salivary glands. AJP-Gastrointest Liver Physiol 2001;281:G247–54.

[95] Huang D, Chen P, Chen S, Nagura M, Lim DJ, Lin X. Expression patterns of aquaporins in the inner ear: evidence for concerted actions of multiple types of aquaporins to facilitate water transport in the cochlea. Hear Res 2002;165:85–95.

[96] Takata K, Matsuzaki T, Tajika Y. Aquaporins: water channel proteins of the cell membrane. Prog Histochem Cytochem 2004;39:1–83.

[97] Endo M, Jain RK, Witwer B, Brown D. Water channel (aquaporin 1) expression and distribution in mammary carcinomas and glioblastomas. Microvasc Res 1999;58:89–98.

[98] Bondy C, Chin E, Smith BL, Preston GM, Agre P. Developmental gene expression and tissue distribution of the CHIP28 water-channel protein. Proc Natl Acad Sci USA 1993;90:4500–4.

[99] Smith BL, Baumgarten R, Nielsen S, Raben D, Zeidel ML, Agre P. Concurrent expression of erythroid and renal aquaporin CHIP and appearance of water channel activity in perinatal rats. J Clin Invest 1993;92:2035–41.

[100] Smith BL, Preston GM, Spring FA, Anstee DJ, Agre P. Human red cell aquaporin CHIP. I. Molecular characterization of ABH and Colton blood group antigens. J Clin Invest 1994;94:1043–9.

[101] Preston GM, Smith BL, Zeidel ML, Moulds JJ, Agre P. Mutations in aquaporin-1 in phenotypically normal humans without functional CHIP water channels. Science 1994;265: 1585–7.

[102] King LS, Choi M, Fernandez PC, Cartron JP, Agre P. Defective urinary concentrating ability due to a complete deficiency of aquaporin-1. N Engl J Med 2001;345:175–9.

[103] King LS, Nielsen S, Agre P, Brown RH. Decreased pulmonary vascular permeability in aquaporin-1-null humans. Proc Natl Acad Sci 2002;99:1059–63.

[104] Ma T, Yang B, Gillespie A, Carlson EJ, Epstein CJ, Verkman AS. Severely impaired urinary concentrating ability in transgenic mice lacking aquaporin-1 water channels. J Biol Chem 1998;273:4296–9.

[105] Schnermann J, Chou CL, Ma T, Traynor T, Knepper MA, Verkman AS. Defective proximal tubular fluid reabsorption in transgenic aquaporin-1 null mice. Proc Natl Acad Sci USA 1998;95:9660–4.

[106] Vallon V, Verkman AS, Schnermann J. Luminal hypotonicity in proximal tubules of aquaporin-1-knockout mice. AJP-Renal Physiol 2000;278:F1030–3.

[107] Hashimoto S, Huang Y, Mizel D, Briggs J, Schnermann J. Compensation of proximal tubule malabsorption in AQP1-deficient mice without TGF-mediated reduction of GFR. Acta Physiol Scand 2004;181:455–62.

[108] Chou CL, Knepper MA, Hoek AN, Brown D, Yang B, Ma T, et al. Reduced water permeability and altered ultrastructure in thin descending limb of Henle in aquaporin-1 null mice. J Clin Invest 1999;103:491–6.

[109] Pallone TL, Edwards A, Ma T, Silldorff EP, Verkman AS. Requirement of aquaporin-1 for NaCl-driven water transport across descending vasa recta. J Clin Invest 2000;105:215–22.

[110] Yang B, Tonghui MA, Dong JY, Verkman AS. Partial correction of the urinary concentrating defect in aquaporin-1 null mice by adenovirus-mediated gene delivery. Human Gene Therapy 2000;11:567–75.

[111] Abrami L, Tacnet F, Ripoche P. Evidence for a glycerol pathway through aquaporin 1 (CHIP28) channels. Pflugers Arch 1995;430:447–58.

[112] Yool AJ, Stamer WD, Regan JW. Forskolin stimulation of water and cation permeability in aquaporin 1 water channels. Science 1996;273:1216–8.

[113] Agre P, Lee MD, Devidas S, Guggino WB. Aquaporins and ion conductance. Science 1997;275:1490.

[114] Patil RV, Saito I, Yang X, Wax MB. Expression of aquaporins in the rat ocular tissue. Exp Eye Res 1997;64:203–9.

[115] Marinelli RA, Pham L, Agre P, LaRusso NF. Secretin promotes osmotic water transport in rat cholangiocytes by increasing aquaporin-1 water channels in plasma membrane. Evidence for a secretin-induced vesicular translocation of aquaporin-1. J Biol Chem 1997;272:12984–8.

[116] Marinelli RA, Tietz PS, Pham LD, Rueckert L, Agre P, LaRusso NF. Secretin induces the apical insertion of aquaporin-1 water channels in rat cholangiocytes. AJP-Gastrointest Liver Physiol 1999;276:G280–6.

[117] Nakhoul NL, Davis BA, Romero MF, Boron WF. Effect of expressing the water channel aquaporin-1 on the CO_2 permeability of *Xenopus* oocytes. Am J Physiol 1998;274:C543–8.

[118] Reuss L. Focus on "Effect of expressing the water channel aquaporin-1 on the CO_2 permeability of *Xenopus* oocytes". Am J Physiol 1998;274:C297–8.

[119] Cooper GJ, Zhou Y, Bouyer P, Grichtchenko II, Boron WF. Transport of volatile solutes through AQP1. J Physiol Online 2002;542:17–29.

[120] Saadoun S, Papadopoulos MC, Hara-Chikuma M, Verkman AS. Impairment of angiogenesis and cell migration by targeted aquaporin-1 gene disruption. Nature 2005;434:786−92.

[121] Hara-Chikuma M, Verkman AS. Aquaporin-1 facilitates epithelial cell migration in kidney proximal tubule. J Am Soc Nephrol 2006;17:39−45.

[122] Agre P, Bonhivers M, Borgnia MJ. The aquaporins, blueprints for cellular plumbing systems. J Biol Chem. 1998;273: 14659−62.

[123] Fushimi K, Uchida S, Hara Y, Hirata Y, Marumo F, Sasaki S. Cloning and expression of apical membrane water channel of rat kidney collecting tubule. Nature 1993;361:549−52.

[124] Echevarria M, Windhager EE, Tate SS, Frindt G. Cloning and expression of AQP3, a water channel from the medullary collecting duct of rat kidney. Proc Natl Acad Sci USA 1994;91:10997−1001.

[125] Ishibashi K, Sasaki S, Fushimi K, Uchida S, Kuwahara M, Saito H, et al. Molecular cloning and expression of a member of the aquaporin family with permeability to glycerol and urea in addition to water expressed at the basolateral membrane of kidney collecting duct cells. Proc Natl Acad Sci USA 1994;91:6269−73.

[126] Ma T, Frigeri A, Hasegawa H, Verkman AS. Cloning of a water channel homolog expressed in brain meningeal cells and kidney collecting duct that functions as a stilbene-sensitive glycerol transporter. J Biol Chem 1994;269:21845−9.

[127] Hasegawa H, Ma T, Skach W, Matthay MA, Verkman AS. Molecular cloning of a mercurial-insensitive water channel expressed in selected water-transporting tissues. J Biol Chem. 1994;269:5497−500.

[128] Jung JS, Bhat RV, Preston GM, Guggino WB, Baraban JM, Agre P. Molecular characterization of an aquaporin cDNA from brain: candidate osmoreceptor and regulator of water balance. Proc Natl Acad Sci USA 1994;91:13052−6.

[129] Ma T, Frigeri A, Skach W, Verkman AS. Cloning of a novel rat kidney cDNA homologous to CHIP28 and WCH-CD water channels. Biochem Biophys Res Commun 1993;197: 654−9.

[130] Ma T, Yang B, Kuo WL, Verkman AS. cDNA cloning and gene structure of a novel water channel expressed exclusively in human kidney: evidence for a gene cluster of aquaporins at chromosome locus 12q13. Genomics 1996;35:543−50.

[131] Yasui M, Kwon TH, Knepper MA, Nielsen S, Agre P. Aquaporin-6. An intracellular vesicle water channel protein in renal epithelia. Proc Natl Acad Sci 1999;96:5808−13.

[132] Ishibashi K, Kuwahara M, Gu Y, Kageyama Y, Tohsaka A, Suzuki F, et al. Cloning and functional expression of a new water channel abundantly expressed in the testis permeable to water, glycerol, and urea. J Biol Chem. 1997;272:20782−6.

[133] Kuriyama H, Kawamoto S, Ishida N, Ohno I, Mita S, Matsuzawa Y, et al. Molecular cloning and expression of a novel human aquaporin from adipose tissue with glycerol permeability. Biochem Biophys Res Commun 1997;241:53−8.

[134] Sohara E, Rai T, Miyazaki Ji, Verkman AS, Sasaki S, Uchida S. Defective water and glycerol transport in the proximal tubules of AQP7 knockout mice. AJP-Renal Physiol 2005;289: F1195−200.

[135] Elkjar ML, Nejsum LN, Gresz V, Kwon TH, Jensen UB, Frokiar J, et al. Immunolocalization of aquaporin-8 in rat kidney, gastrointestinal tract, testis, and airways. AJP-Renal Physiol 2001;281:F1047−57.

[136] Ma T, Yang B, Verkman AS. Cloning of a novel water and urea-permeable aquaporin from mouse expressed strongly in colon, placenta, liver, and heart. Biochem Biophys Res Commun 1997;240:324−8.

[137] Morishita Y, Matsuzaki T, Hara-chikuma M, Andoo A, Shimono M, Matsuki A, et al. Disruption of aquaporin-11 produces polycystic kidneys following vacuolization of the proximal tubule. Mol Cell Biol 2005;25:7770−9.

[138] Nielsen S, DiGiovanni SR, Christensen EI, Knepper MA, Harris HW. Cellular and subcellular immunolocalization of vasopressin- regulated water channel in rat kidney. Proc Natl Acad Sci USA 1993;90:11663−7.

[139] Kishore BK, Terris JM, Knepper MA. Quantitation of aquaporin-2 abundance in microdissected collecting ducts: axial distribution and control by AVP. Am J Physiol 1996;271: F62−70.

[140] Coleman RA, Wu DC, Liu J, Wade JB. Expression of aquaporins in the renal connecting tubule. AJP-Renal Physiol 2000;279: F874−83.

[141] Christensen BM, Wang W, Frokiar J, Nielsen S. Axial heterogeneity in basolateral AQP2 localization in rat kidney: effect of vasopressin. AJP-Renal Physiol 2003;284:F701−17.

[142] Flamion B, Spring KR. Water permeability of apical and basolateral cell membranes of rat inner medullary collecting duct. Am J Physiol 1990;259:F986−99.

[143] DiGiovanni SR, Nielsen S, Christensen EI, Knepper MA. Regulation of collecting duct water channel expression by vasopressin in Brattleboro rat. Proc Natl Acad Sci USA 1994;91:8984−8.

[144] Deen PM, Verdijk MA, Knoers NV, Wieringa B, Monnens LA, van Os CH, et al. Requirement of human renal water channel aquaporin-2 for vasopressin-dependent concentration of urine. Science 1994;264:92−5.

[145] Rojek A, Fuchtbauer EM, Kwon TH, Frokiar J, Nielsen S. Severe urinary concentrating defect in renal collecting duct-selective AQP2 conditional-knockout mice. Proc Natl Acad Sci 2006;103(15):6037−42.

[146] Yang B, Gillespie A, Carlson EJ, Epstein CJ, Verkman AS. Neonatal mortality in an aquaporin-2 knock-in mouse model of recessive nephrogenic diabetes insipidus. J Biol Chem 2001;276:2775−9.

[147] Yang B, Zhao D, Qian L, Verkman AS. Mouse model of inducible nephrogenic diabetes insipiduc produced by floxed aquaporin-2 gene deletion. AJP-Renal Physiol 2006;291(2): F465−72.

[148] Ma T, Song Y, Yang B, Gillespie A, Carlson EJ, Epstein CJ, et al. Nephrogenic diabetes insipidus in mice lacking aquaporin-3 water channels. Proc Natl Acad Sci 2000;97: 4386−91.

[149] Yang B, Verkman AS. Water and glycerol permeabilities of aquaporins 1−5 and MIP determined quantitatively by expression of epitope-tagged constructs in Xenopus oocytes. J Biol Chem 1997;272:16140−6.

[150] Zeuthen T, Klaerke DA. Transport of water and glycerol in aquaporin 3 is gated by H$^+$. J Biol Chem 1999;274:21631−6.

[151] Ecelbarger CA, Terris J, Frindt G, Echevarria M, Marples D, Nielsen S, et al. Aquaporin-3 water channel localization and regulation in rat kidney. Am J Physiol 1995;269:F663−72.

[152] Frigeri A, Gropper MA, Turck CW, Verkman AS. Immunolocalization of the mercurial-insensitive water channel and glycerol intrinsic protein in epithelial cell plasma membranes. Proc Natl Acad Sci USA 1995;92:4328−31.

[153] Terris J, Ecelbarger CA, Marples D, Knepper MA, Nielsen S. Distribution of aquaporin-4 water channel expression within rat kidney. Am J Physiol 1995;269:F775−85.

[154] van Hoek AN, Ma T, Yang B, Verkman AS, Brown D. Aquaporin-4 is expressed in basolateral membranes of proximal tubule S3 segments in mouse kidney. AJP-Renal Physiol 2000;278:F310−6.

[155] Silberstein C, Bouley R, Huang Y, Fang P, Pastor-Soler N, Brown D, et al. Membrane organization and function of M1 and M23 isoforms of aquaporin-4 in epithelial cells. AJP-Renal Physiol 2004;287:F501−11.

[156] Kwon TH, Nielsen J, Masilamani S, Hager H, Knepper MA, Frokiar J, et al. Regulation of collecting duct AQP3 expression: response to mineralocorticoid. AJP-Renal Physiol 2002;283: F1403−21.

[157] Zelenina M, Zelenin S, Bondar AA, Brismar H, Aperia A. Water permeability of aquaporin-4 is decreased by protein kinase C and dopamine. AJP-Renal Physiol 2002;283:F309−18.

[158] Chou CL, Ma T, Yang B, Knepper MA, Verkman AS. Fourfold reduction of water permeability in inner medullary collecting duct of aquaporin-4 knockout mice. Am J Physiol 1998;274: C549−54.

[159] Ma T, Yang B, Gillespie A, Carlson EJ, Epstein CJ, Verkman AS. Generation and phenotype of a transgenic knockout mouse lacking the mercurial-insensitive water channel aquaporin-4. J Clin Invest 1997;100:957−62.

[160] Yasui M, Hazama A, Kwon TH, Nielsen S, Guggino WB, Agre P. Rapid gating and anion permeability of an intracellular aquaporin. Nature 1999;402:184−7.

[161] Ikeda M, Beitz E, Kozono D, Guggino WB, Agre P, Yasui M. Characterization of aquaporin-6 as a nitrate channel in mammalian cells. Requirement of pore-lining residue threonine 63. J Biol Chem 2002;277:39873−9.

[162] Hazama A, Kozono D, Guggino WB, Agre P, Yasui M. Ion permeation of AQP6 water channel protein. Single-channel recordings after Hg^{2+} activation. J Biol Chem 2002;277: 29224−30.

[163] Liu K, Kozono D, Kato Y, Agre P, Hazama A, Yasui M. From the cover. Conversion of aquaporin 6 from an anion channel to a water-selective channel by a single amino acid substitution. Proc Natl Acad Sci 2005;102:2192−7.

[164] Kishida K, Kuriyama H, Funahashi T, Shimomura I, Kihara S, Ouchi N, et al. Aquaporin adipose, a putative glycerol channel in adipocytes. J Biol Chem 2000;275:20896−902.

[165] Ishibashi K, Imai M, Sasaki S. Cellular localization of aquaporin 7 in the rat kidney. Nephron Exp Nephrology 2000;8:252−7.

[166] Nejsum LN, Elkjaer M-L, Hager H, Frokiaer J, Kwon TH, Nielsen S. Localization of aquaporin-7 in rat and mouse kidney using RT-PCR, immunoblotting, and immunocytochemistry. Biochem Biophys Res Commun 2000;277:164−70.

[167] Liu Z, Shen J, Carbrey JM, Mukhopadhyay R, Agre P, Rosen BP. Arsenite transport by mammalian aquaglyceroporins AQP7 and AQP9. Proc Natl Acad Sci 2002;99:6053−8.

[168] Ishibashi K, Kuwahara M, Kageyama Y, Tohsaka A, Marumo F, Sasaki S. Cloning and functional expression of a second new aquaporin abundantly expressed in testis. Biochem Biophys Res Commun 1997;237:714−8.

[169] Koyama Y, Yamamoto T, Tani T, Nihei K, Kondo D, Funaki H, et al. Expression and localization of aquaporins in rat gastrointestinal tract. Am J Physiol 1999;276:C621−7.

[170] Yang B, Song Y, Zhao D, Verkman AS. Phenotype analysis of aquaporin-8 null mice. AJP-Cell Physiol 2005;288:C1161−70.

[171] Holm LM, Jahn TP, Moller AL, Schjoerring JK, Ferri D, Klaerke DA, et al. NH_3 and NH_4^+ permeability in aquaporin-expressing Xenopus oocytes. Pflugers Arch 2005;450:415−28.

[172] Liu KF, Nagase HF, Huang CG, Calamita G, Agre P. Purification and functional characterization of aquaporin-8. Biol Cell 2006;98(3):153−61.

[173] Jahn TP, Moller ALB, Zeuthen T, Holm LM, Klaerke DA, Mohsin B, et al. Aquaporin homologues in plants and mammals transport ammonia. FEBS Lett 2004;574:31−6.

[174] Yang B, Zhao D, Solenov E, Verkman AS. Evidence from knockout mice against physiologically significant aquaporin-8 facilitated ammonia transport. AJP-Cell Physiol 2006;291(3): C417−423.

[175] Nielsen S, King LS, Christensen BM, Agre P. Aquaporins in complex tissues. II. Subcellular distribution in respiratory and glandular tissues of rat. AJP-Cell Physiol 1997;273:C1549−61.

[176] Maeda N, Funahashi T, Hibuse T, Nagasawa A, Kishida K, Kuriyama H, et al. Adaptation to fasting by glycerol transport through aquaporin 7 in adipose tissue. Proc Natl Acad Sci 2004;101:17801−6.

[177] Ishibashi K, Kuwahara M, Gu Y, Tanaka Y, Marumo F, Sasaki S. Cloning and functional expression of a new aquaporin (AQP9) abundantly expressed in the peripheral leukocytes permeable to water and urea, but not to glycerol. Biochem Biophys Res Commun 1998;244:268−74.

[178] Ko SB, Uchida S, Naruse S, Kuwahara M, Ishibashi K, Marumo F, et al. Cloning and functional expression of rAOP9L a new member of aquaporin family from rat liver. Biochem Mol Biol Int 1999;47:309−18.

[179] Tsukaguchi H, Weremowicz S, Morton CC, Hediger MA. Functional and molecular characterization of the human neutral solute channel aquaporin-9. AJP-Renal Physiol 1999;277: F685−96.

[180] Tsukaguchi H, Shayakul C, Berger UV, Mackenzie B, Devidas S, Guggino WB, et al. Molecular characterization of a broad selectivity neutral solute channel. J Biol Chem 1998;273: 24737−43.

[181] Carbrey JM, Gorelick-Feldman DA, Kozono D, Praetorius J, Nielsen S, Agre P. Aquaglyceroporin AQP9. Solute permeation and metabolic control of expression in liver. Proc Natl Acad Sci 2003;100:2945−50.

[182] Nielsen S, Chou CL, Marples D, Christensen EI, Kishore BK, Knepper MA. Vasopressin increases water permeability of kidney collecting duct by inducing translocation of aquaporin-CD water channels to plasma membrane. Proc Natl Acad Sci USA 1995;92:1013−7.

[183] Sabolic I, Katsura T, Verbavatz JM, Brown D. The AQP2 water channel: effect of vasopressin treatment, microtubule disruption, and distribution in neonatal rats. J Membr Biol 1995;143: 165−75.

[184] Yamamoto T, Sasaki S, Fushimi K, Ishibashi K, Yaoita E, Kawasaki K, et al. Vasopressin increases AQP-CD water channel in apical membrane of collecting duct cells in Brattleboro rats. AJP-Cell Physiol 1995;268:C1546−51.

[185] Lankford SP, Chou CL, Terada Y, Wall SM, Wade JB, Knepper MA. Regulation of collecting duct water permeability independent of cAMP-mediated AVP response. Am J Physiol 1991;261: F554−66.

[186] Lee YJ, Lee JE, Choi HJ, Lim JS, Jung HJ, Baek MC, et al. E3 ubiquitin-protein ligases in rat kidney collecting duct: response to vasopressin stimulation and withdrawal. Am J Physiol-Renal Physiol 2011;301:F883−96.

[187] Terris J, Ecelbarger CA, Nielsen S, Knepper MA. Long-term regulation of four renal aquaporins in rats. Am J Physiol 1996;271:F414−22.

[188] Kuwahara M, Verkman AS. Pre-steady-state analysis of the turn-on and turn-off of water permeability in the kidney collecting tubule. J Membr Biol 1989;110:57−65.

[189] Wall SM, Han JS, Chou CL, Knepper MA. Kinetics of urea and water permeability activation by vasopressin in rat terminal IMCD. Am J Physiol 1992;262:F989−98.

[190] Nielsen S, Frokiar J, Marples D, Kwon TH, Agre P, Knepper MA. Aquaporins in the Kidney. From molecules to medicine. Physiol Rev 2002;82:205−44.

III. FLUID AND ELECTROLYTE REGULATION AND DYSREGULATION

[191] Hays RM, Leaf A. Studies on the movement of water through the isolated toad bladder and its modification by vasopressin. J Gen Physiol 1962;45:905—19.

[192] Koefoed-Johnsen V, Ussing HH. The contributions of diffusion and flow to the passage of D2O through living membranes; effect of neurohypophyseal hormone on isolated anuran skin. Acta Physiol Scand 1953;28:60—76.

[193] Grantham JJ, Burg MB. Effect of vasopressin and cyclic AMP on permeability of isolated collecting tubules. Am J Physiol 1966;211:255—9.

[194] Morgan T, Berliner RW. Permeability of the loop of Henle, vasa recta, and collecting duct to water, urea, and sodium. Am J Physiol 1968;215:108—15.

[195] Nielsen S, Knepper MA. Vasopressin activates collecting duct urea transporters and water channels by distinct physical processes. Am J Physiol 1993;265:F204—13.

[196] Kanno K, Sasaki S, Hirata Y, Ishikawa S, Fushimi K, Nakanishi S, et al. Urinary excretion of aquaporin-2 in patients with diabetes insipidus. N Eng J Med 1995;332:1540—5.

[197] Marples D, Knepper MA, Christensen EI, Nielsen S. Redistribution of aquaporin-2 water channels induced by vasopressin in rat kidney inner medullary collecting duct. Am J Physiol 1995;269:C655—64.

[198] Christensen BM, Marples D, Jensen UB, Frokiaer J, Sheikh-Hamad D, Knepper M, et al. Acute effects of vasopressin V2-receptor antagonist on kidney AQP2 expression and subcellular distribution. AJP-Renal Physiol 1998;275:F285—97.

[199] Hayashi M, Sasaki S, Tsuganezawa H, Monkawa T, Kitajima W, Konishi K, et al. Expression and distribution of aquaporin of collecting duct are regulated by vasopressin V2 receptor in rat kidney. J Clin Invest 1994;94:1778—83.

[200] Saito T, Ishikawa SE, Sasaki S, Fujita N, Fushimi K, Okada K, et al. Alteration in water channel AQP-2 by removal of AVP stimulation in collecting duct cells of dehydrated rats. AJP-Renal Physiol 1997;272:F183—91.

[201] Knepper MA, Nielsen S. Kinetic model of water and urea permeability regulation by vasopressin in collecting duct. Am J Physiol 1993;265:F214—24.

[202] Brown D, Weyer P, Orci L. Vasopressin stimulates endocytosis in kidney collecting duct principal cells. Eur J Cell Biol 1988;46:336—41.

[203] Lencer WI, Brown D, Ausiello DA, Verkman AS. Endocytosis of water channels in rat kidney: cell specificity and correlation with in vivo antidiuresis. Am J Physiol 1990;259:C920—32.

[204] Strange K, Willingham MC, Handler JS, Harris Jr HW. Apical membrane endocytosis via coated pits is stimulated by removal of antidiuretic hormone from isolated, perfused rabbit cortical collecting tubule. J Membr Biol 1988;103:17—28.

[205] Nielsen S, Muller J, Knepper MA. Vasopressin- and cAMP-induced changes in ultrastructure of isolated perfused inner medullary collecting ducts. Am J Physiol 1993;265:F225—38.

[206] Deen PM, van Aubel RA, Van Lieburg AF, van Os CH. Urinary content of aquaporin 1 and 2 in nephrogenic diabetes insipidus. J Am Soc Nephrol 1996;7:836—41.

[207] Katsura T, Ausiello DA, Brown D. Direct demonstration of aquaporin-2 water channel recycling in stably transfected LLC-PK1 epithelial cells. AJP-Renal Physiol 1996;270:F548—53.

[208] Katsura T, Gustafson CE, Ausiello DA, Brown D. Protein kinase A phosphorylation is involved in regulated exocytosis of aquaporin-2 in transfected LLC-PK1 cells. Am J Physiol 1997;272:F817—22.

[209] Katsura T, Verbavatz J, Farinas J, Ma T, Ausiello DA, Verkman AS, et al. Constitutive and regulated membrane expression of aquaporin 1 and aquaporin 2 water channels in stably transfected LLC-PK1 epithelial cells. Proc Natl Acad Sci 1995;92:7212—6.

[210] Valenti G, Frigeri A, Ronco PM, D'Ettorre C, Svelto M. Expression and functional analysis of water channels in a stably AQP2-transfected human collecting duct cell line. J Biol Chem 1996;271:24365—70.

[211] Frische S, Kwon TH, Frokiaer J, Nielsen S. Aquaporin-2 trafficking. In: Boles E, Kramer R, editors. Molecular mechanisms controlling transmembrane transport. Berlin: Springer; p. 353—77.

[212] Kuwahara M, Fushimi K, Terada Y, Bai L, Marumo F, Sasaki S. cAMP-dependent phosphorylation stimulates water permeability of aquaporin-collecting duct water channel protein expressed in Xenopus oocytes. J Biol Chem 1995;270:10384—7.

[213] Lande MB, Jo I, Zeidel ML, Somers M, Harris Jr. HW. Phosphorylation of aquaporin-2 does not alter the membrane water permeability of rat papillary water channel-containing vesicles. J Biol Chem 1996;271:5552—7.

[214] Knepper M, Nielsen S, Chou CL, DiGiovanni, SR, Mechanism of vasopressin action in the renal collecting duct. Semin Nephrol 14:302—21.

[215] Kwon TH, Nielsen J, Moller HB, Fenton RA, Nielsen S, Frokiaer J. Aquaporins in the kidney. Handb Exp Pharmacol 2009;190:95—132.

[216] Moeller HB, Olesen ET, Fenton RA. Regulation of the water channel aquaporin-2 by posttranslational modification. AJP-Renal Physiol 2011;300:F1062—73.

[217] Nedvetsky PI, Tamma G, Beulshausen S, Valenti G, Rosenthal W, Klussmann E. Regulation of aquaporin-2 trafficking. Handb Exp Pharmacol 2009;190:133—57.

[218] Edwards RM, Jackson BA, Dousa TP. ADH-sensitive cAMP system in papillary collecting duct: effect of osmolality and PGE2. Am J Physiol 1981;240:F311—8.

[219] Kurokawa K, Massry SG. Interaction between catecholamines and vasopressin on renal medullary cyclic AMP of rat. Am J Physiol 1973;225:825—9.

[220] Nishimoto G, Zelenina M, Li D, Yasui M, Aperia A, Nielsen S, et al. Arginine vasopressin stimulates phosphorylation of aquaporin-2 in rat renal tissue. Am J Physiol 1999;276:F254—9.

[221] Fushimi K, Sasaki S, Marumo F. Phosphorylation of serine 256 is required for cAMP-dependent regulatory exocytosis of the aquaporin-2 water channel. J Biol Chem 1997;272:14800—4.

[222] Christensen BM, Zelenina M, Aperia A, Nielsen S. Localization and regulation of PKA-phosphorylated AQP2 in response to V (2)-receptor agonist/antagonist treatment. Am J Physiol Renal Physiol 2000;278:F29—42.

[223] Moeller HB, Praetorius J, Rutzler MR, Fenton RA. Phosphorylation of aquaporin-2 regulates its endocytosis and protein—protein interactions. Proc Natl Acad Sci USA 2010;107:424—9.

[224] McDill BW, Li SZ, Kovach PA, Ding L, Chen F. Congenital progressive hydronephrosis (cph) is caused by an S256L mutation in aquaporin-2 that affects its phosphorylation and apical membrane accumulation. Proc Natl Acad Sci 2006;103:6952—7.

[225] Hoffert JD, Pisitkun T, Wang G, Shen RF, Knepper MA. Quantitative phosphoproteomics of vasopressin-sensitive renal cells. Regulation of aquaporin-2 phosphorylation at two sites. Proc Natl Acad Sci 2006;103:7159—64.

[226] Hoffert JD, Fenton RA, Moeller HB, Simons B, Tchapyjnikov D, McDill BW, et al. Vasopressin-stimulated increase in phosphorylation at Ser269 potentiates plasma membrane retention of aquaporin-2. J Biol Chem 2008;283:24617—27.

[227] Lu HAJ, Sun TX, Matsuzaki T, Yi XH, Eswara J, Bouley R, et al. Heat shock protein 70 interacts with aquaporin-2 and regulates its trafficking. J Biol Chem 2007;282:28721—32.

[228] Zelenina M, Christensen BM, Palmer J, Nairn AC, Nielsen S, Aperia A. Prostaglandin E(2) interaction with AVP: effects on AQP2 phosphorylation and distribution. Am J Physiol Renal Physiol 2000;278:F388—94.

[229] Olesen ET, Rutzler MR, Moeller HB, Praetorius HA, Fenton RA. Vasopressin-independent targeting of aquaporin-2 by selective E-prostanoid receptor agonists alleviates nephrogenic diabetes insipidus. Proc Natl Acad Sci USA 2011;108: 12949—54.

[230] Kwon TH, Nielsen J, Knepper MA, Frokiaer J, Nielsen S. Angiotensin II AT1 receptor blockade decreases vasopressin-induced water reabsorption and AQP2 levels in NaCl-restricted rats. AJP-Renal Physiol 2005;288:F673—84.

[231] Lee YJ, Song IK, Jang KJ, Nielsen J, Frokiaer J, Nielsen S, et al. Increased AQP2 targeting in primary cultured IMCD cells in response to angiotensin II through AT1 receptor. Am J Physiol-Renal Physiol 2007;292:F340—50.

[232] Procino G, Carmosino M, Marin O, Brunanti AM, Contri A, Pinna LA, et al. Ser-256 phosphorylation dynamics of aquaporin 2 during maturation from the endoplasmic reticulum to the vesicular compartment in renal cells. FASEB J 2003;17(13): 1886—8.

[233] Lu H, Sun TX, Bouley R, Blackburn K, McLaughlin M, Brown D. Inhibition of endocytosis causes phosphorylation (S256)-independent plasma membrane accumulation of AQP2. AJP-Renal Physiol 2004;286:F233—43.

[234] Phillips ME, Taylor A. Effect of nocodazole on the water permeability response to vasopressin in rabbit collecting tubules perfused *in vitro*. J Physiol 1989;411:529—44.

[235] Phillips ME, Taylor A. Effect of colcemid on the water permeability response to vasopressin in isolated perfused rabbit collecting tubules. J Physiol 1992;456:591—608.

[236] Marples D, Schroer TA, Ahrens N, Taylor A, Knepper MA, Nielsen S. Dynein and dynactin colocalize with AQP2 water channels in intracellular vesicles from kidney collecting duct. Am J Physiol 1998;274:F384—94.

[237] de Sousa RC, Grosso A. Vanadate blocks cyclic AMP-induced stimulation of sodium and water transport in amphibian epithelia. Nature 1979;279:803—4.

[238] Marples D, Barber B, Taylor A. Effect of a dynein inhibitor on vasopressin action in toad urinary bladder. J Physiol 1996;490 (Pt 3):767—74.

[239] Shaw S, Marples D. N-ethylmaleimide causes aquaporin-2 trafficking in the renal inner medullary collecting duct by direct activation of protein kinase A. Am J Physiol Renal Physiol 2005;288:F832—9.

[240] Dibona DR. Cytoplasmic involvement in ADH-mediated osmosis across toad urinary bladder. Am J Physiol 1983;245: C297—307.

[241] Ding GH, Franki N, Condeelis J, Hays RM. Vasopressin depolymerizes F-actin in toad bladder epithelial cells. Am J Physiol 1991;260:C9—16.

[242] Kachadorian WA, Ellis SJ, Muller J. Possible roles for microtubules and microfilaments in ADH action on toad urinary bladder. Am J Physiol 1979;236:F14—20.

[243] Muller J, Kachadorian WA. Aggregate-carrying membranes during ADH stimulation and washout in toad bladder. Am J Physiol 1984;247:C90—8.

[244] Pearl M, Taylor A. Actin filaments and vasopressin-stimulated water flow in toad urinary bladder. Am J Physiol 1983;245: C28—39.

[245] Wade JB, Kachadorian WA. Cytochalasin B inhibition of toad bladder apical membrane responses to ADH. Am J Physiol. 1988;255:C526—30.

[246] Chou CL, Christensen BM, Frische S, Vorum H, Desai RA, Hoffert JD, et al. Non-muscle myosin II and myosin light chain kinase are downstream targets for vasopressin signaling in the renal collecting duct. J Biol Chem 2004;279:49026—35.

[247] Star RA, Nonoguchi H, Balaban R, Knepper MA. Calcium and cyclic adenosine monophosphate as second messengers for vasopressin in the rat inner medullary collecting duct. J Clin Invest 1988;81:1879—88.

[248] Chou CL, Yip KP, Michea L, Kador K, Ferraris JD, Wade JB, et al. Regulation of aquaporin-2 trafficking by vasopressin in the renal collecting duct. Roles of ryanodine-sensitive Ca^{2+} stores and calmodulin. J Biol Chem 2000;275:36839—46.

[249] Yip KP. Coupling of vasopressin-induced intracellular Ca^{2+} mobilization and apical exocytosis in perfused rat kidney collecting duct. J Physiol 2002;538:891—9.

[250] Lorenz D, Krylov A, Hahm D, Hagen V, Rosenthal W, Pohl P, et al. Cyclic AMP is sufficient for triggering the exocytic recruitment of aquaporin-2 in renal epithelial cells. EMBO Rep 2003;4:88—93.

[251] Bajjalieh SM, Scheller RH. The biochemistry of neurotransmitter secretion. J Biol Chem 1995;270:1971—4.

[252] Sollner T, Whiteheart SW, Brunner M, Erdjument-Bromage H, Geromanos S, Tempst P, et al. SNAP receptors implicated in vesicle targeting and fusion. Nature 1993;362:318—24.

[253] Franki N, Macaluso F, Schubert W, Gunther L, Hays RM. Water channel-carrying vesicles in the rat IMCD contain cellubrevin. Am J Physiol 1995;269:C797—801.

[254] Harris Jr HW, Zeidel ML, Jo I, Hammond TG. Characterization of purified endosomes containing the antidiuretic hormone-sensitive water channel from rat renal papilla. J Biol Chem 1994;269:11993—2000.

[255] Inoue T, Nielsen S, Mandon B, Terris J, Kishore BK, Knepper MA. SNAP-23 in rat kidney: colocalization with aquaporin-2 in collecting duct vesicles. Am J Physiol 1998;275:F752—60.

[256] Kishore BK, Wade JB, Schorr K, Inoue T, Mandon B, Knepper MA. Expression of synaptotagmin VIII in rat kidney. Am J Physiol 1998;275:F131—42.

[257] Liebenhoff U, Rosenthal W. Identification of Rab3-, Rab5a- and synaptobrevin II-like proteins in a preparation of rat kidney vesicles containing the vasopressin-regulated water channel. FEBS Lett 1995;365:209—13.

[258] Mandon B, Chou CL, Nielsen S, Knepper MA. Syntaxin-4 is localized to the apical plasma membrane of rat renal collecting duct cells: possible role in aquaporin-2 trafficking. J Clin Invest 1996;98:906—13.

[259] Mandon B, Nielsen S, Kishore BK, Knepper MA. Expression of syntaxins in rat kidney. Am J Physiol 1997;273:F718—30.

[260] Nielsen S, Marples D, Birn H, Mohtashami M, Dalby NO, Trimble M, et al. Expression of VAMP-2-like protein in kidney collecting duct intracellular vesicles. Colocalization with aquaporin-2 water channels. J Clin Invest 1995;96: 1834—44.

[261] Sudhof TC, De CP, Niemann H, Jahn R. Membrane fusion machinery: insights from synaptic proteins. Cell 1993;75:1—4.

[262] Advani RJ, Bae HR, Bock JB, Chao DS, Doung YC, Prekeris R, et al. Seven novel mammalian SNARE proteins localize to distinct membrane compartments. J Biol Chem 1998;273: 10317—24.

[263] Calakos N, Bennett MK, Peterson KE, Scheller RH. Protein—protein interactions contributing to the specificity of intracellular vesicular trafficking. Science 1994;263:1146—9.

[264] Pevsner J, Hsu SC, Braun JE, Calakos N, Ting AE, Bennett MK, et al. Specificity and regulation of a synaptic vesicle docking complex. Neuron 1994;13:353—61.

[265] Barile M, Pisitkun T, Yu MJ, Chou CL, Verbalis MJ, Shen RF, et al. Large scale protein identification in intracellular aquaporin-2 vesicles from renal inner medullary collecting duct. Mol Cell Proteomics 2005;4:1095–106.

[266] Foster LJ, Yeung B, Mohtashami M, Ross K, Trimble WS, Klip A. Binary interactions of the SNARE proteins syntaxin-4, SNAP23, and VAMP-2 and their regulation by phosphorylation. Biochemistry 1998;37:11089–96.

[267] Risinger C, Bennett MK. Differential phosphorylation of syntaxin and synaptosome-associated protein of 25 kDa (SNAP-25) isoforms. J Neurochem 1999;72:614–24.

[268] Shimazaki Y, Nishiki T i, Omori A, Sekiguchi M, Kamata Y, Kozaki S, et al. Phosphorylation of 25-kDa synaptosome-associated protein. Possible involvement in protein kinase c-mediated regulation of neurotransmitter release. J Biol Chem 1996;271:14548–53.

[269] Jones RV, De Wardener HE. Urine concentration after fluid deprivation or pitressin tannate in oil. Br Med J 1956;1 (4961):271–4.

[270] Han JS, Maeda Y, Ecelbarger C, Knepper MA. Vasopressin-independent regulation of collecting duct water permeability. Am J Physiol 1994;266:F139–46.

[271] Wade JB, Nielsen S, Coleman RA, Knepper MA. Long-term regulation of collecting duct water permeability: freeze-fracture analysis of isolated perfused tubules. Am J Physiol 1994;266:F723–30.

[272] Flamion B, Spring KR, Abramow M. Adaptation of inner medullary collecting duct to dehydration involves a paracellular pathway. Am J Physiol 1995;268:F53–63.

[273] Chou CL, DiGiovanni SR, Mejia R, Nielsen S, Knepper MA. Oxytocin as an antidiuretic hormone. I. Concentration dependence of action. Am J Physiol 1995;269:F70–7.

[274] Fujita N, Ishikawa SE, Sasaki S, Fujisawa G, Fushimi K, Marumo F, et al. Role of water channel AQP-CD in water retention in SIADH and cirrhotic rats. Am J Physiol 1995;269: F926–31.

[275] Ecelbarger CA, Nielsen S, Olson BR, Murase T, Baker EA, Knepper MA, et al. Role of renal aquaporins in escape from vasopressin-induced antidiuresis in rat. J Clin Invest 1997;99:1852–63.

[276] Ecelbarger CA, Chou CL, Lee AJ, DiGiovanni SR, Verbalis JG, Knepper MA. Escape from vasopressin-induced antidiuresis: role of vasopressin resistance of the collecting duct. Am J Physiol 1998;274:F1161–6.

[277] Fernandez-Llama P, Turner R, Dibona G, Knepper MA. Renal expression of aquaporins in liver cirrhosis induced by chronic common bile duct ligation in rats. J Am Soc Nephrol 1999;10:1950–7.

[278] Sands JM, Naruse M, Jacobs JD, Wilcox JN, Klein JD. Changes in aquaporin-2 protein contribute to the urine concentrating defect in rats fed a low-protein diet. J Clin Invest 1996;97:2807–14.

[279] Ma T, Hasegawa H, Skach WR, Frigeri A, Verkman AS. Expression, functional analysis, and in situ hybridization of a cloned rat kidney collecting duct water channel. Am J Physiol 1994;266:C189–97.

[280] Uchida S, Sasaki S, Fushimi K, Marumo F. Isolation of human aquaporin-CD gene. J Biol Chem 1994;269:23451–5.

[281] Hozawa S, Holtzman EJ, Ausiello DA. cAMP motifs regulating transcription in the aquaporin 2 gene. Am J Physiol 1996;270: C1695–702.

[282] Matsumura Y, Uchida S, Rai T, Sasaki S, Marumo F. Transcriptional regulation of aquaporin-2 water channel gene by cAMP. J Am Soc Nephrol 1997;8:861–7.

[283] Yasui M, Zelenin SM, Celsi G, Aperia A. Adenylate cyclase-coupled vasopressin receptor activates AQP2 promoter via a dual effect on CRE and AP1 elements. Am J Physiol 1997;272: F443–50.

[284] Inase N, Fushimi K, Ishibashi K, Uchida S, Ichioka M, Sasaki S, et al. Isolation of human aquaporin 3 gene. J Biol Chem 1995;270:17913–6.

[285] Kamsteeg EJ, Hendriks G, Boone M, Konings IBM, Oorschot V, van der Sluijs P, et al. Short-chain ubiquitination mediates the regulated endocytosis of the aquaporin-2 water channel. Proc Natl Acad Sci 2006;103:18344–9.

[286] Agre P, King LS, Yasui M, Guggino WB, Ottersen OP, Fujiyoshi Y, et al. Aquaporin water channels—from atomic structure to clinical medicine. J Physiol Online 2002;542:3–16.

[287] Nielsen S, Knepper MA, Kwon T-H, Frokiaer J. Regulation of water balance. Urine concentration and dilution. In: Schrier RW, editor. Diseases of the Kidney and Urinary Tract. Philadelphia, Lippincott Willialms & Wilkins; 2004. p. 109–34.

[288] Robben JH, Knoers NV, Deen PM. Cell biological aspects of the vasopressin type-2 receptor and aquaporin 2 water channel in nephrogenic diabetes insipidus. AJP-Renal Physiol 2006;291: F257–70.

[289] Babey M, Kopp P, Robertson GL. Familial forms of diabetes insipidus: clinical and molecular characteristics. Nat Rev Endocrinol 2011;7:701–14.

[290] Schmale H, Ivell R, Breindl M, Darmer D, Richter D. The mutant vasopressin gene from diabetes insipidus (Brattleboro) rats is transcribed but the message is not efficiently translated. EMBO J 1984;3(13):3289–93.

[291] Bichet DG. Vasopressin receptors in health and disease. Kidney Int 1996;49:1706–11.

[292] Jensen AM, Bae EH, Fenton RA, Noregaard R, Nielsen S, Kim SW, et al. Angiotensin II regulates V2 receptor and pAQP2 during ureteral obstruction. Am J Physiol-Renal Physiol 2009;296:F127–34.

[293] Deen PM, van Aubel RA, Van Lieburg AF, van Os CH. Urinary content of aquaporin 1 and 2 in nephrogenic diabetes insipidus. J Am Soc Nephrol 1996;7(6):836–41.

[294] Wen H, Frokiaer J, Kwon TH, Nielsen S. Urinary excretion of aquaporin-2 in rat is mediated by a vasopressin-dependent apical pathway. J Am Soc Nephrol 1999;10:1416–29.

[295] Moon SS, Kim HJ, Choi YK, Seo HA, Jeon JH, Lee JE, et al. Novel mutation of aquaporin-2 gene in a patient with congenital nephrogenic diabetes insipidus. Endocrine J 2009;56: 905–10.

[296] Mulders SM, Knoers NV, Van Lieburg AF, Monnens LA, Leumann E, Wuhl E, et al. New mutations in the AQP2 gene in nephrogenic diabetes insipidus resulting in functional but misrouted water channels. J Am Soc Nephrol 1997;8:242–8.

[297] Oksche A, Moller A, Dickson J, Rosendahl W, Rascher W, Bichet DG, et al. Two novel mutations in the aquaporin-2 and the vasopressin V2 receptor genes in patients with congenital nephrogenic diabetes insipidus. Hum Genet 1996;98:587–9.

[298] Van Lieburg AF, Verdijk MA, Knoers VV, van Essen AJ, Proesmans W, Mallmann R, et al. Patients with autosomal nephrogenic diabetes insipidus homozygous for mutations in the aquaporin 2 water-channel gene. Am J Hum Genet 1994;55: 648–52.

[299] Deen PM, Croes H, van Aubel RA, Ginsel LA, van Os CH. Water channels encoded by mutant aquaporin-2 genes in nephrogenic diabetes insipidus are impaired in their cellular routing. J Clin Invest 1995;95:2291–6.

[300] Morello JP, Salahpour A, Petaja-Repo UE, Laperriere A, Lonergan M, Arthus MF, et al. Association of calnexin with

wild type and mutant AVPR2 that cause nephrogenic diabetes insipidus. Biochemistry 2001;40:6766—75.

[301] Knoers NV, van Os CH. Molecular and cellular defects in nephrogenic diabetes insipidus. Curr Opin Nephrol Hypertens 1996;5:353—8.

[302] Mulders SM, Bichet DG, Rijss JP, Kamsteeg EJ, Arthus MF, Lonergan M, et al. An aquaporin-2 water channel mutant which causes autosomal dominant nephrogenic diabetes insipidus is retained in the Golgi complex. J Clin Invest 1998;102:57—66.

[303] Faerch M, Christensen JH, Corydon TJ, Kamperis K, de ZF, Gregersen N, et al. Partial nephrogenic diabetes insipidus caused by a novel mutation in the AVPR2 gene. Clin Endocrinol(Oxf) 2008;68:395—403.

[304] Faerch M, Christensen JH, Rittig S, Johansson JO, Gregersen N, de ZF, et al. Diverse vasopressin V2 receptor functionality underlying partial congenital nephrogenic diabetes insipidus. AJP-Renal Physiol 2009;297:F1518—25.

[305] Faerch M, Corydon TJ, Rittig S, Christensen JH, Hertz JM, Jendle J. Skewed X-chromosome inactivation causing diagnostic misinterpretation in congenital nephrogenic diabetes insipidus. Scand J Urol Nephrol 2010;44:324—30.

[306] Timmer RT, Sands JM. Lithium intoxication. J Am Soc Nephrol 1999;10:666—74.

[307] Kwon T-H, Laursen UH, Marples D, Maunsbach AB, Knepper MA, Frokiaer J, et al. Altered expression of renal AQPs and Na$^{(+)}$ transporters in rats with lithium-induced NDI. Am J Physiol Renal Physiol 2000;279:F552—64.

[308] Marples D, Christensen S, Christensen EI, Ottosen PD, Nielsen S. Lithium-induced downregulation of aquaporin-2 water channel expression in rat kidney medulla. J Clin Invest 1995;95:1838—45.

[309] Christensen S, Kusano E, Yusufi AN, Murayama N, Dousa TP. Pathogenesis of nephrogenic diabetes insipidus due to chronic administration of lithium in rats. J Clin Invest 1985;75:1869—79.

[310] Kim YH, Kwon TH, Christensen BM, Nielsen J, Wall SM, Madsen KM, et al. Altered expression of renal acid—base transporters in rats with lithium-induced NDI. AJP-Renal Physiol 2003;285:F1244—57.

[311] Wilting I, Baumgarten R, Movig KL, Laarhoven J, Apperloo AJ, Nolen WA, et al. Urine osmolality, cyclic AMP and aquaporin-2 in urine of patients under lithium treatment in response to water loading followed by vasopressin administration. Eur J Pharmacol 2007;566:50—7.

[312] Frokiaer J, Marples D, Valtin H, Morris JF, Knepper MA, Nielsen S. Low aquaporin-2 levels in polyuric DI$^{+/+}$ severe mice with constitutively high cAMP-phosphodiesterase activity. AJP-Renal Physiol 1999;276:F179—90.

[313] Nielsen J, Kwon TH, Praetorius J, Kim YH, Frokiaer J, Knepper MA, et al. Segment-specific ENaC downregulation in kidney of rats with lithium-induced NDI. AJP-Renal Physiol 2003;285: F1198—209.

[314] Christensen BM, Zuber AM, Loffing J, Stehle JC, Deen PM, Rossier BC, et al. ENaC-mediated lithium absorption promotes nephrogenic diabetes insipidus. J Am Soc Nephrol 2011;22: 253—61.

[315] Nielsen J, Hoffert JD, Knepper MA, Agre P, Nielsen S, Fenton RA. Proteomic analysis of lithium-induced nephrogenic diabetes insipidus. Mechanisms for aquaporin 2 downregulation and cellular proliferation. Proc Natl Acad Sci 2008;105:3634—9.

[316] Nielsen J, Kwon TH, Christensen BM, Frokiaer J, Nielsen S. Dysregulation of renal aquaporins and epithelial sodium

[317] Kortenoeven ML, Schweer H, Cox R, Wetzels JF, Deen PM. Lithium reduces aquaporin-2 transcription independent of prostaglandins. Am J Physiol-Cell Physiol 2012;302: C131—40.

[318] Marples D, Frokiaer J, Dorup J, Knepper MA, Nielsen S. Hypokalemia-induced downregulation of aquaporin-2 water channel expression in rat kidney medulla and cortex. J Clin Invest 1996;97:1960—8.

[319] Earm JH, Christensen BM, Frokiaer J, Marples D, Han JS, Knepper MA, et al. Decreased aquaporin-2 expression and apical plasma membrane delivery in kidney collecting ducts of polyuric hypercalcemic rats. J Am Soc Nephrol 1998;9: 2181—93.

[320] Sands JM, Flores FX, Kato A, Baum MA, Brown EM, Ward DT, et al. Vasopressin-elicited water and urea permeabilities are altered in IMCD in hypercalcemic rats. AJP-Renal Physiol 1998;274:F978—85.

[321] Elkjar ML, Kwon TH, Wang W, Nielsen J, Knepper MA, Frokiar J, et al. Altered expression of renal NHE3, TSC, BSC-1, and ENaC subunits in potassium-depleted rats. AJP-Renal Physiol 2002;283:F1376—88.

[322] Wang W, Li C, Kwon TH, Miller RT, Knepper MA, Frokiaer J, et al. Reduced expression of renal Na$^+$ transporters in rats with PTH-induced hypercalcemia. AJP-Renal Physiol 2004;286: F534—45.

[323] Zeidel M, Pirtskhalaishvili G. Urinary tract obstruction. In: Brenner BM, editor. The kidney. Philadelphia: Saunders; 2004. p. 1867—94.

[324] Frokiaer J, Marples D, Knepper MA, Nielsen S. Bilateral ureteral obstruction downregulates expression of vasopressin-sensitive AQP-2 water channel in rat kidney. Am J Physiol 1996;270:F657—68.

[325] Kim SW, Cho SH, Oh BS, Yeum CH, Choi KC, Ahn KY, et al. Diminished renal expression of aquaporin water channels in rats with experimental bilateral ureteral obstruction. J Am Soc Nephrol 2001;12:2019—28.

[326] Li C, Wang W, Kwon TH, Isikay L, Wen JG, Marples D, et al. Downregulation of AQP1, -2, and -3 after ureteral obstruction is associated with a long-term urine-concentrating defect. AJP-Renal Physiol 2001;281:F163—71.

[327] Stodkilde L, Norregaard R, Fenton RA, Wang G, Knepper MA, Frokiar J. Bilateral ureteral obstruction induces early downregulation and redistribution of AQP2 and phosphorylated AQP2. Am J Physiol-Renal Physiol 2011;301:F226—35.

[328] Li C, Wang W, Knepper MA, Nielsen S, Frokiar J. Downregulation of renal aquaporins in response to unilateral ureteral obstruction. AJP-Renal Physiol 2003;284:F1066—79.

[329] Cheng X, Zhang H, Lee HL, Park JM. Cyclooxygenase-2 inhibitor preserves medullary aquaporin-2 expression and prevents polyuria after ureteral obstruction. J Urol 2004.

[330] Norregaard R, Jensen BL, Li C, Wang W, Knepper MA, Nielsen S, et al. COX-2 inhibition prevents downregulation of key renal water and sodium transport proteins in response to bilateral ureteral obstruction. AJP-Renal Physiology 2005;289: F322—33.

[331] Norregaard R, Jensen BL, Topcu SO, Diget M, Schweer H, Knepper MA, et al. COX-2 activity transiently contributes to increased water and NaCl excretion in the polyuric phase after release of ureteral obstruction. Am J Physiol-Renal Physiol 2007;292:F1322—33.

[332] Zhang Y, Kohan DE, Nelson RD, Carlson NG, Kishore BK. Potential involvement of P2Y2 receptor in diuresis of

postobstructive uropathy in rats. AJP-Renal Physiol 2010;298: F634—42.

[333] Jensen AM, Li C, Praetorius HA, Norregaard R, Frische S, Knepper MA, et al. Angiotensin II mediates downregulation of aquaporin water channels and key renal sodium transporters in response to urinary tract obstruction. AJP-Renal Physiol 2006;291(5):F1021—32.

[334] Frokiaer J, Christensen BM, Marples D, Djurhuus JC, Jensen UB, Knepper MA, et al. Downregulation of aquaporin-2 parallels changes in renal water excretion in unilateral ureteral obstruction. Am J Physiol 1997;273:F213—23.

[335] Hanley MJ. Isolated nephron segments in a rabbit model of ischemic acute renal failure. Am J Physiol 1980;239: F17—23.

[336] Tanner GA, Sloan KL, Sophasan S. Effects of renal artery occlusion on kidney function in the rat. Kidney Int 1973;4: 377—89.

[337] Venkatachalam MA, Bernard DB, Donohoe JF, Levinsky NG. Ischemic damage and repair in the rat proximal tubule: differences among the S1, S2, and S3 segments. Kidney Int 1978;14: 31—49.

[338] Anderson RJ, Gordon JA, Kim J, Peterson LM, Gross PA. Renal concentration defect following nonoliguric acute renal failure in the rat. Kidney Int 1982;21:583—91.

[339] Fernandez-Llama P, Andrews P, Turner R, Saggi S, Di Mari J, Kwon T-H, et al. Role of collecting duct aquaporins in polyuria of post-ischemic acute renal failure in rats. J Am Soc Nephrol 1999;10:1658—68.

[340] Kwon T-H, Frokiaer J, Fernandez-Llama P, Knepper MA, Nielsen S. Reduced abundance of aquaporins in rats with bilateral ischemia-induced acute renal failure: prevention by alpha-MSH. Am J Physiol 1999;277:F413—27.

[341] Gong H, Wang W, Kwon TH, Jonassen T, Frokiaer J, Nielsen S. Reduced renal expression of AQP2, p-AQP2 and AQP3 in haemorrhagic shock-induced acute renal failure. Nephrol Dialysis Transplant 2003;18:2551—9.

[342] Sharples EJ, Patel N, Brown P, Stewart K, Mota-Philipe H, Sheaff M, et al. Erythropoietin protects the kidney against the injury and dysfunction caused by ischemia-reperfusion. J Am Soc Nephrol 2004;15:2115—24.

[343] Hocherl K, Schmidt C, Kurt B, Bucher M. Inhibition of NF-kappaB ameliorates sepsis-induced downregulation of aquaporin-2/V2 receptor expression and acute renal failure *in vivo*. AJP-Renal Physiol 2010;298:F196—204.

[344] Tannen RL, Regal EM, Dunn MJ, Schrier RW. Vasopressin-resistant hyposthenuria in advanced chronic renal disease. N Engl J Med 1969;280:1135—41.

[345] Teitelbaum I, McGuinness S. Vasopressin resistance in chronic renal failure. Evidence for the role of decreased V2 receptor mRNA. J Clin Invest 1995;96:378—85.

[346] Kwon T-H, Frokiaer J, Knepper MA, Nielsen S. Reduced AQP1, -2, and -3 levels in kidneys of rats with CRF induced by surgical reduction in renal mass. Am J Physiol 1998;275: F724—41.

[347] Nielsen S, Terris J, Andersen D, Ecelbarger C, Frokiaer J, Jonassen T, et al. Congestive heart failure in rats is associated with increased expression and targeting of aquaporin-2 water channel in collecting duct. Proc Natl Acad Sci USA 1997;94: 5450—5.

[348] Xu DL, Martin PY, Ohara M, St.John J, Pattison T, Meng X, et al. Upregulation of aquaporin-2 water channel expression in chronic heart failure rat. J Clin Invest 1997;99: 1500—5.

[349] Lutken SC, Kim SW, Jonassen T, Marples D, Knepper MA, Kwon TH, et al. Changes of renal AQP2, ENaC, and NHE3 in

experimentally induced heart failure: response to angiotensin II AT1 receptor blockade. Am J Physiol-Renal Physiol 2009;297: F1678—88.

[350] Martin PY, Abraham WT, Lieming X, Olson BR, Oren RM, Ohara M, et al. Selective V2-receptor vasopressin antagonism decreases urinary aquaporin-2 excretion in patients with chronic heart failure. J Am Soc Nephrol 1999;10: 2165—70.

[351] Starklint J, Bech JN, Nyvad O, Jensen P, Pedersen EB. Increased urinary aquaporin 2 excretion in response to furosemide in patients with chronic heart failure. Scandinavian J Clinical Lab Invest 2006;66:55—66.

[352] Portincasa P, Palasciano G, Svelto M, Calamita G. Aquaporins in the hepatobiliary tract. Which, where and what they do in health and disease? European J Clin Invest 2008;38:1—10.

[353] Jonassen TE, Nielsen S, Christensen S, Petersen JS. Decreased vasopressin-mediated renal water reabsorption in rats with compensated liver cirrhosis. Am J Physiol 1998;275: F216—25.

[354] Jonassen TE, Promeneur D, Christensen S, Petersen JS, Nielsen S. Decreased vasopressin-mediated renal water reabsorption in rats with chronic aldosterone-receptor blockade. Am J Physiol Renal Physiol 2000;278:F246—56.

[355] Asahina Y, Izumi N, Enomoto N, Sasaki S, Fushimi K, Marumo F, et al. Increased gene expression of water channel in cirrhotic rat kidneys. Hepatology 1995;21: 169—73.

[356] Fernandez-Llama P, Jimenez W, Bosch-Marce M, Arroyo V, Nielsen S, Knepper MA. Dysregulation of renal aquaporins and Na-Cl co-transporter in CCl4-induced cirrhosis. Kidney Int 2000;58:216—28.

[357] Esteva-Font C, Baccaro ME, Fernández-Llama P, Sans L, Guevara M, Ars E, et al. Aquaporin-1 and aquaporin-2 urinary excretion in cirrhosis: relationship with ascites and hepatorenal syndrome. Hepatology 2006;44:1555—63.

[358] Gines P, Berl T, Bernardi M, Bichet DG, Hamon G, Jimenez W, et al. Hyponatremia in cirrhosis: from pathogenesis to treatment. Hepatology 1998;28:851—64.

[359] Kim SW, Schou UK, Peters CD, de Seigneux S, Kwon TH, Knepper MA, et al. Increased apical targeting of renal epithelial sodium channel subunits and decreased expression of type 2 11beta-hydroxysteroid dehydrogenase in rats with CCl4-induced decompensated liver cirrhosis. J Am Soc Nephrol 2005;16:3196—210.

[360] Wood LJ, Massie D, McLean AJ, Dudley FJ. Renal sodium retention in cirrhosis: tubular site and relation to hepatic dysfunction. Hepatology 1988;8:831—6.

[361] Levy M, Wexler MJ. Hepatic denervation alters first-phase urinary sodium excretion in dogs with cirrhosis. Am J Physiol 1987;253:F664—71.

[362] Huebert RC, Jagavelu K, Hendrickson HI, Vasdev MM, Arab JP, Splinter PL, et al. Aquaporin-1 promotes angiogenesis, fibrosis, and portal hypertension through mechanisms dependent on osmotically sensitive microRNAs. Am J Pathol 2011;179:1851—60.

[363] Apostol E, Ecelbarger CA, Terris J, Bradford AD, Andrews P, Knepper MA. Reduced renal medullary water channel expression in puromycin aminonucleoside: induced nephrotic syndrome. J Am Soc Nephrol 1997;8:15—24.

[364] Fernandez-Llama P, Andrews P, Ecelbarger CA, Nielsen S, Knepper M. Concentrating defect in experimental nephrotic syndrome: altered expression of aquaporins and thick ascending limb Na$^+$ transporters. Kidney Int 1998;54: 170—9.

[365] Fernandez-Llama P, Andrews P, Nielsen S, Ecelbarger CA, Knepper MA. Impaired aquaporin and urea transporter expression in rats with adriamycin-induced nephrotic syndrome. Kidney Int 1998;53:1244—53.

[366] Flear CT, Gill GV, Burn J. Hyponatraemia: mechanisms and management. Lancet 1981;2:26—31.

[367] Bartter FC, Schwartz WB. The syndrome of inappropriate secretion of antidiuretic hormone. Am J Med 1967;42: 790—806.

[368] Ishikawa S, Saito T, Saito T, Kasono K, Funayama H. Pathophysiological role of aquaporin-2 in impaired water excretion. In: Neumann ID, editor. Progress in brain research

advances in vasopressin and oxytocin—from genes to behaviour to disease. Elsevier; 2008. p. 581—8.

[369] Verbalis JG. Whole-body volume regulation and escape from antidiuresis. Am J Med 2006;119:S21—9.

[370] Heymann JB, Agre P, Engel A. Progress on the structure and function of aquaporin 1. J Struct Biol 1998;121:191—206.

[371] de Groot BL, Engel A, Grubmuller H. A refined structure of human aquaporin-1. FEBS Lett 2001;504:206—11.

[372] de Groot BL, Engel A, Grubmuller H. The structure of the aquaporin-1 water channel. A comparison between cryo-electron microscopy and X-ray crystallography. J Mol Biol 2003;325:485—93.

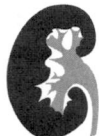

Thirst and Vasopressin

Gary L. Robertson

The Feinberg School of Medicine, Northwestern University, Chicago, IL, USA

INTRODUCTION

Thirst and the antidiuretic hormone, arginine vasopressin, are the principal elements of a powerful homeostatic system that regulates the "effective" osmotic pressure of body fluids. This variable, usually referred to as "tonicity," must be important for survival since mechanisms to regulate it are found throughout the animal kingdom, and abnormalities in humans can have adverse effects, especially on central nervous function. However, it is less clear why it is important. It may be that regulating the *tonicity* of body fluids is mainly an indirect way to minimize changes in the *volume* of water within cells, particularly those of the brain.[1] It may also be that tight control of intracellular water and solute concentrations is necessary for optimum function of the cell.[2]

The tonicity of body fluids is regulated primarily by raising or lowering total body water to keep it in balance with solute. In a healthy adult, about 55 to 60% of body weight is water.[3] It is slightly lower in women than men, owing to differences in body fat. About two-thirds of body water is intracellular. The rest is in the extracellular space, where it is subdivided further between the interstitial and intravascular (plasma) compartments in a ratio of about 3:1. Thus, a human weighing 70 kg contains about 39 L of water, of which 26 L is intracellular, 10 L is interstitial fluid, and 3 L is plasma.

A change in total body water results in a proportionate change in the volume of all compartments, providing the solute content of the compartments does not also change. The reason is that almost all cell membranes are penetrated by channels composed of aquaporin proteins[4] that permit the passive diffusion of water selectively in response to an osmotic gradient. In contrast, these membranes resist the passage of sodium, potassium, and most other solutes by actively pumping them in or out of the cell (see Chapter 2).

Thus, a change in the amount of water in one compartment creates an osmotic gradient that results in a rapid flow of water from one compartment to the other, thereby restoring osmotic equilibrium and redistributing the change in volume in a similar proportion to each compartment. Thus, a reduction in the water content of the extracellular compartment due, for example, to increased perspiration, increases the tonicity and reduces the volume of the intracellular and extracellular compartments in equal proportion. A rise in total body water has the opposite but equivalent effect on the tonicity and volume of the two compartments.

In contrast, the volume of extracellular and intracellular water changes in opposite directions if the *amount* of osmotically effective solute in either compartment changes, but total body water does not. Osmotically effective solutes are those, such as sodium and its anions, which do not equilibrate readily across cell membranes. Thus, if the *amount* of sodium and its anions in extracellular fluid increases, the effective osmotic pressure or "tonicity" of this fluid also increases, resulting in a rapid osmotically-driven inflow of water from the intracellular compartment until osmotic equilibrium is re-established. The net effect is again an increase in the osmotic pressure of both compartments, but at a level lower than if the shift of water had not occurred. In fact, because of this shift, the effect on plasma sodium *concentration* of adding a given amount of sodium to the extracellular compartment is the same as if the sodium was distributed throughout total body water. In this circumstance, however, the volume of extracellular fluid increases, while that of intracellular fluid decreases. A reduction in the amount of sodium in extracellular fluid has opposite effects.

Because sodium and its anions normally make up 95% of all solutes, and nearly 100% of osmotically effective solute in extracellular fluid, the measurement of either plasma sodium or osmolarity probably

Seldin and Giebisch's The Kidney, Fifth Edition.
DOI: http://dx.doi.org/10.1016/B978-0-12-381462-3.00042-2

provides an accurate estimate of the "tonicity" or effective osmotic pressure of both the intracellular and extracellular fluids. Urea and glucose contribute little if anything because, normally, they are present in relatively low molar concentrations, and can enter or leave cells very rapidly. In the absence of insulin, however, glucose becomes osmotically effective because it enters cells much more slowly. In that situation, hyperglycemia induces a shift of water from the intracellular to extracellular space, and the tonicity of body fluids is determined much more reliably by measuring plasma osmolarity than plasma sodium. In intracellular fluid (ICF), the major solutes are potassium and its anions, but others including proteins, polyols, and some as yet unidentified solutes are also present.[2]

Body water is in a constant state of flux, owing to obligatory unregulated losses and gains produced by physical activity, the environment, diet, and the metabolism of fat. The rate of evaporative water loss from skin and lungs can vary markedly, depending on ambient temperature and physical activity, but it amounts to at least 10 mL/kg a day (0.7 L in a 70 kg human), even at rest in a comfortably cool environment.[5] The rate of solute-free water loss in urine is tightly regulated by vasopressin but, in humans, it cannot be reduced below a certain minimum required to excrete the load of sodium, chloride, potassium, urea, and other waste solutes derived from the diet and metabolism. This load varies with the diet, but is usually about 700 mosmols a day. Since humans cannot increase their urine osmolarity much above 1400 mosmols/L, the amount of urine required to carry this solute load is at least 7 ml/kg a day (0.5 L a day in a 70 kg human) even under conditions of maximum antidiuresis. The total daily obligatory water loss in a healthy adult is, therefore, at least 17 mL/kg (1.2 L in a 70 kg human), and may be much more at times depending on diet, activity, and temperature. Normally, this loss does not result in dehydration because it is replaced by an equivalent intake of water. Much of the intake is incidental to other physiological needs. About 7 mL/kg (0.5 L in a 70 kg human) comes from water in food, and about 4 mL/kg (0.3 L/day in a 70 kg human) is derived from metabolism of fat. The rest is consumed as beverages with meals in response to various influences,[6] including a slight increase in plasma osmolarity and thirst induced by adsorption of salt and other solutes in food. Thus, water balance is usually maintained at relatively low levels of urine output and discretionary fluid intake. Alterations in this basic state bring into play corrective changes in water excretion and/or intake under control of the antidiuretic and thirst mechanisms.

VASOPRESSIN AND RELATED PEPTIDES

Chemistry

Arginine vasopressin (AVP) is a nonapeptide containing an intrachain disulfide bridge and a tripeptide tail on which the terminal-carboxyl is amidated[7] (Figure 42.1). Substitution of lysine for arginine in position 8 yields lysine vasopressin (LVP), the antidiuretic hormone found exclusively in pigs and other members of the suborder Suina.[8] Vasopressin is structurally similar to oxytocin, another nonapeptide hormone found in the posterior pituitary of all mammals Oxytocin differs chemically from vasopressin by the substitution of isoleucine for

FIGURE 42.1 The primary amino acid structures of oxytocin, vasopressin and desmopressin.

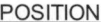

POSITION

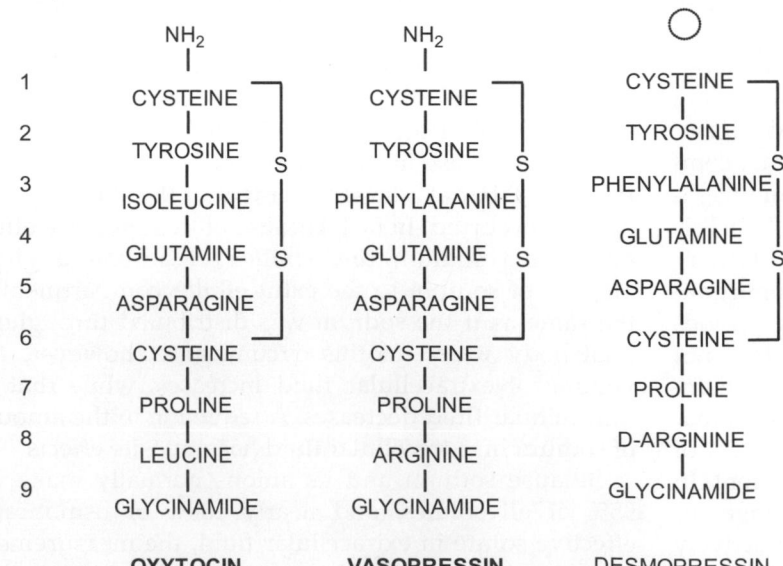

phenylalanine at position 3, and of leucine for arginine at position 8.[7] Desmopressin is a potent synthetic analog of vasopressin used therapeutically because of its longer half-life and reduced effects on smooth muscle.

ANATOMY

Vasopressin and oxytocin are produced and stored in large amounts by magnocellular neurons in the hypothalamic neurohypophyseal tract.[9–14] These neurons arise bilaterally in the supraoptic and paraventricular nuclei of the hypothalamus, project medially to merge in the pituitary stalk, and continue through the diaphragm sella into the sella turcica, where they form the posterior lobe of the pituitary (Figure 42.2). Microscopically, the posterior pituitary appears as a densely interwoven network of capillaries, pituicytes,

and large nonmyelinated neurons containing many electron-dense secretory granules. The neurons terminate as bulbous enlargements on capillary networks at many different levels throughout the stalk and body of the neurohypophysis. In healthy adults and children, the posterior pituitary usually appears as a hyperintense signal or "bright spot" on T-l weighted magnetic resonance images (MRI) of the brain.[15] The origin of this signal is still unknown, but it appears to be closely related to the content or turnover of vasopressin, and is almost invariably absent not only in patients with the pituitary form of diabetes insipidus, but also in many of those with nephrogenic diabetes insipidus (unpublished data). Vasopressin is also present in the suprachiasmatic nucleus and parvocellular neurons that originate in the paraventricular nucleus and project to the portal veins, anterior pituitary, and many other areas of the brain.[11,13] Oxytocin is also present in

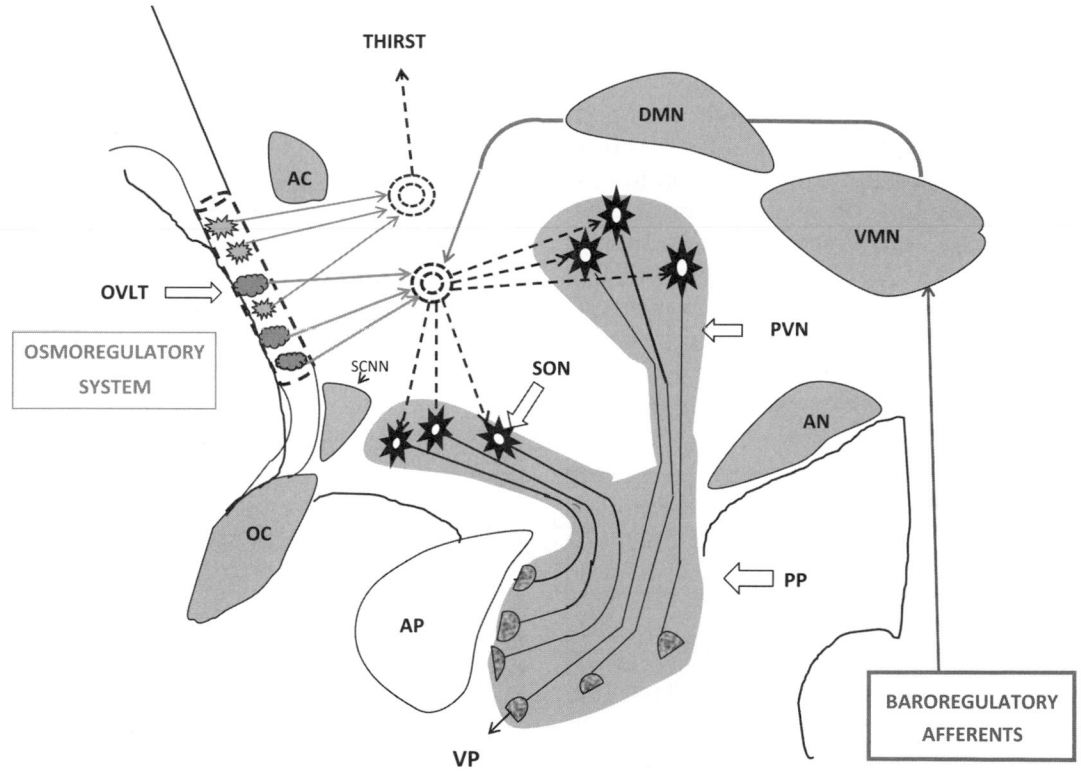

FIGURE 42.2 Schematic diagram of the hypothalamic–neurohypophyseal tract and areas that osmoregulate thirst and vasopressin secretion. The supraoptic nucleus (SON), paraventricular nucleus (PVN) and posterior pituitary are shaded red. The origin and course of the magnocellular neurons that form the tract and posterior pituitary are indicated in black. The green and blue icons represent the osmoreceptors that regulate vasopressin secretion and thirst, respectively. They appear to be in distinct but overlapping areas within in the organum vasculosum of the lamina terminalis (OVLT). The vasopressin osmoreceptors probably do not project directly to the SON or PVN but, as indicated by the black concentric circle with broken borders, appear to interact somewhere with ascending input from the baroregulatory system before the integrated signal is relayed to the magnocellular neurons in the SON and PVN. Signals from the thirst osmoreceptors probably follow a similar path to integration with baroregulatory input before projecting onwards to of the cerebral cortex. Other nearby landmarks shown include the anterior commissure (AC), optic chiasm (OC), suprachiasmatic nucleus (SCM), anterior pituitary (AP) and arcuate nucleus (AC). The ventral medial nucleus (VMN) and dorsal medial nucleus (DMN) probably transmit afferent input from the baroregulatory system. Not shown are the parvocellular vasopressinergic neurons which project to many other areas of brain including the SCM and portal venous system of the AP. See color section at the end of the book.

many parvocellular neurons of brain,[11–14] as well as in the uterus, prostate, and other peripheral tissues.[16]

The hypothalamic neurohypophyseal tract is supplied with blood by branches of the superior and inferior hypophyseal arteries that arise from the posterior communicating and intracavernous portions of the internal carotids.[9] In the body of the neurohypophysis, the arterioles break up into the aforementioned capillary networks that drain directly into the jugular vein by way of the sellar, cavernous, and lateral venous sinuses. In the stalk or infundibulum, the primary capillary networks coalesce into another system, the portal veins, which perfuse the anterior pituitary before discharging into the systemic circulation.

BIOSYNTHESIS

Vasopressin is synthesized as part of a protein precursor composed of a signal peptide at its amino terminus, vasopressin, the vasopressin-binding protein, neurophysin II, and a glycosylated peptide, copeptin, at its carboxyl-terminus[17,18] (Figure 42.3). During or after translocation to the endoplasmic reticulum, the signal peptide is removed and the N-terminus of the vasopressin moiety binds to a pocket in the neurophysin moiety. The prohormone then folds, forms a number of intrachain disulfide bridges, and dimerizes, before moving through the Golgi and into the neurosecretory granules where it is transported down the axon and further processed to yield amidated vasopressin, neurophysin, and

copeptin.[19] Vasopressin and its neurophysin are stored in nerve terminals as insoluble complexes which dissociate completely after release into the systemic circulation.[20] Biosynthesis of vasopressin appears to be accelerated by stimuli, such as dehydration or hypertonic saline infusion,[21] which increase secretion. However, this compensatory response develops slowly, and may not completely offset the increased rate of release because pituitary stores of the hormone are severely depleted by a strong, sustained secretory stimulus such as prolonged water deprivation.[22]

The gene encoding the vasopressin—neurophysin precursor in humans is located distally on the short arm of chromosome 20 (20p13).[23] It contains three exons which code, respectively, for: (1) the signal peptide, vasopressin, a dipeptide link, and the N-terminal variable portion of neurophysin; (2) the middle, highly-conserved part of neurophysin; and (3) the C-terminal, variable portion of neurophysin, a peptide link and the glycopeptide, copeptin[24] (Figure 42.3). The 5′ untranslated region upstream of the transcription start site also has many conserved sequences, suggesting a role in regulation of gene expression.[25,26] Dehydration or osmotic stimulation increases expression of the vasopressin gene in the supraoptic nucleus,[27,28] whereas adrenal insufficiency or febrile stress does so in parts of the paraventricular nucleus.[28] In contrast, sustained hypoosmolarity inhibits expression.[29] The vasopressin genes in rats,[30] cows,[31] and mice[32] are similar to those in humans, but have several substitutions at either end of the highly-conserved central portion of the neurophysin moiety.

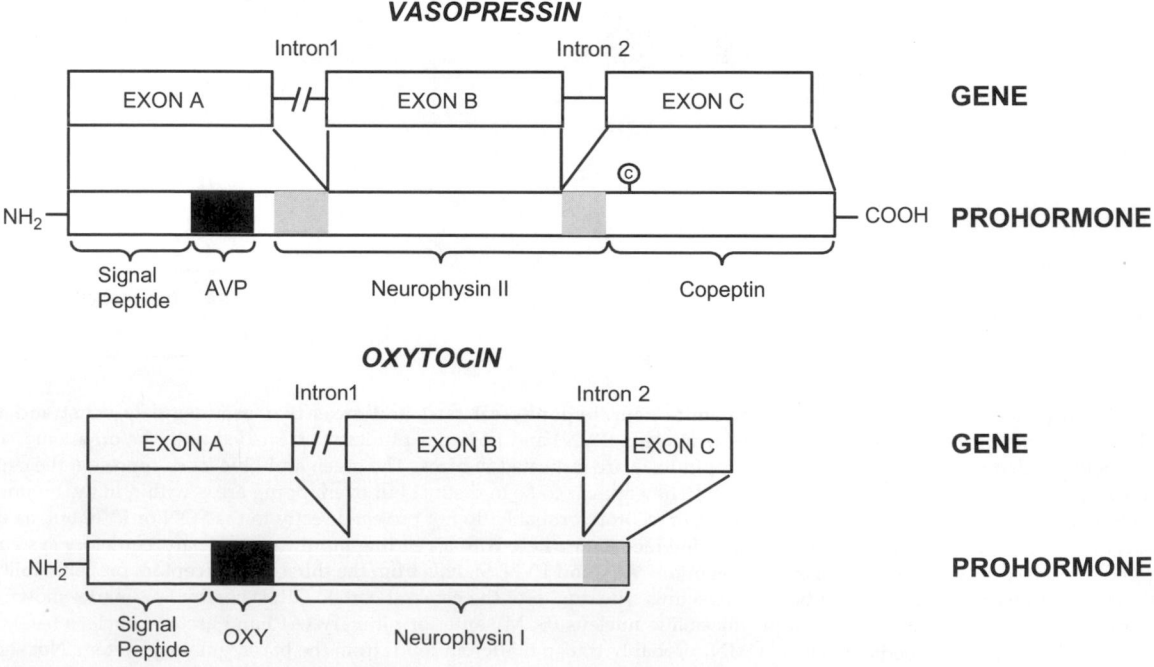

FIGURE 42.3   **Structure of the genes and the protein prohormones of vasopressin and oxytocin.**

The oxytocin gene is closely linked to the vasopressin gene on chromosome 20 with an intergenic region of only 11 kilobases.[24,33] However, the two genes are transcribed from opposite DNA strands, implying a tail-to-tail orientation, differ significantly in putative regulatory regions,[25] and are expressed in mutually-exclusive sets of neurons.[34] The oxytocin gene also differs significantly from the vasopressin gene, in that it does not contain a copeptin encoding sequence in exon 3.[25] Expression of the oxytocin gene in brain and some peripheral tissues is promoted by gonadal steroids.[16]

neurons, dissociates from the hormone at the concentrations and pH present in plasma.[42] Binding of vasopressin to other plasma proteins has not been demonstrated. However, it does attach to platelets.[43] It is unclear whether or not the platelet-bound vasopressin represents a store of the hormone in equilibrium with free plasma vasopressin. However, the bound and unbound fractions of vasopressin do not appear to track together, at least during acute changes in secretion.[44] Oxytocin is also co-secreted with its neurophysin.[16]

SECRETION

Vasopressin- and oxytocin-containing secretory granules are released from the terminals of magnocellular neurohypophysial neurons by a process of calcium-mediated exocytosis that is triggered by action potentials generated in the cell bodies of the supraoptic or paraventricular nucleus.[35] Many different neurotransmitters or neuromodulators including, possibly, vasopressin itself, can stimulate or inhibit this activity.[36,37] However, it is not yet known which, if any, of them are important in the regulation of secretion in health or disease. Secretory activity may also be influenced by the many glial cells in close proximity to the dendrites of the vasopressin cell bodies in the supraoptic nucleus.[38]

Vasopressin as well as the neurophysin and copeptin moieties with which it is associated are released into capillaries scattered throughout all levels of the posterior pituitary.[39–41] From there, they travel via the cavernous sinus to the subclavian vein, and thence to the inferior vena cava, heart, and general circulation. Neurophysin, which binds vasopressin in magnocellular

ASSAY

The measurement of vasopressin at physiologic levels in plasma presents an unusual combination of concerns that must be addressed with exceptional care.[45] One problem is the large amount of hormone bound to platelets (see above). Because of it, vasopressin must be assayed not in serum, but in plasma that has been harvested very carefully to avoid contamination with platelets or fragments thereof.

A second problem is the fastidious requirements of the vasopressin assay itself. It must be unusually sensitive, because the hormone normally circulates and acts at very low concentrations. In healthy, normally hydrated, recumbent humans, the plasma concentration of "free" vasopressin is usually between 0.5 and 2.5 pg/mL ($\sim 10^{-12}$ M), an amount sufficient to concentrate the urine (Figure 42.4a). Basal levels in other mammals are similar. The assay must also be very specific, because plasma also contains oxytocin, a nonapeptide that is structurally similar to vasopressin but has different biologic effects. The only practical method now available

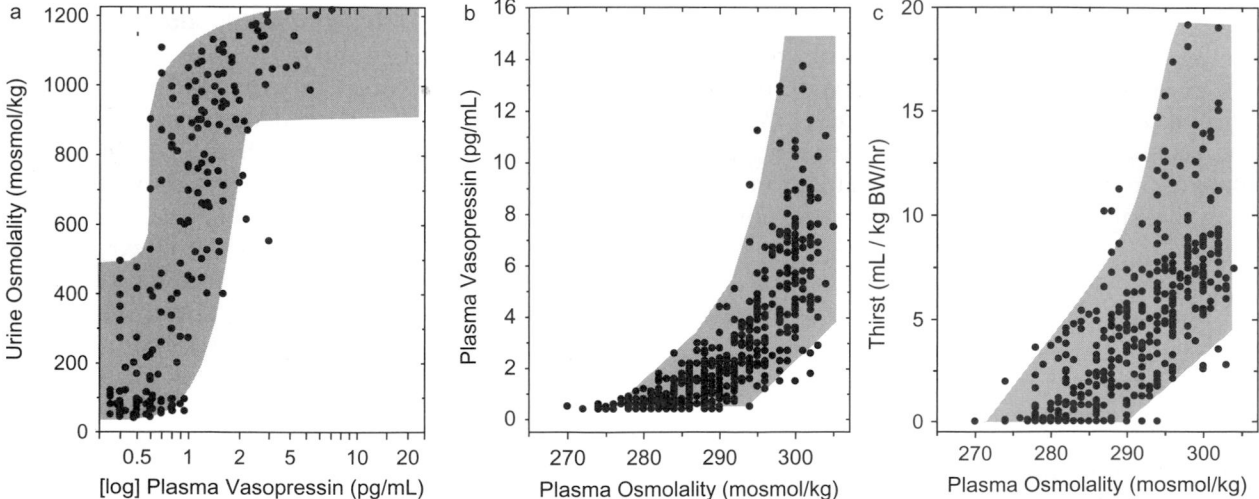

FIGURE 42.4 Relationship of urine osmolality to plasma vasopressin (a), plasma vasopressin to plasma osmolality (b), and thirst to plasma osmolality (c) in healthy adults in various states of water balance.

that can meet both requirements is radioimmunoassay. However, it too presents unusual problems, because vasopressin is relatively small and weakly antigenic. To complicate matters, most, if not all, the vasopressin antisera generated to date are susceptible to non-specific interference by one or more other unidentified components of plasma. Moreover, the characteristics and abundance of this interference can vary with the antiserum and type of anticoagulant used to prevent the blood from clotting. Consequently, vasopressin must be extracted from plasma, even if the antiserum employed is sensitive enough to detect the hormone at physiologic levels in unconcentrated extracts. Unfortunately, there is no one extraction method that is suitable for all assays. Therefore, the extraction method, as well as the anticoagulant, must be selected and tailored for the particular antiserum being used.

A third problem for vasopressin assays is the lack of a universal reference standard. Judging from the advertised biologic potencies, those available vary by as much as two-fold in purity, and unknown values reported in weight usually are not corrected for these differences. Therefore, unless the purity or potency of the standards is specified, it is impossible to compare absolute values reported by different laboratories unless they use the same standard, antiserum, and extraction technique.

The radioimmunoassay of vasopressin in urine would appear to be much easier than plasma, because the concentrations in urine are usually much higher, and interference by other substances is much less. However, urine samples must usually be diluted or concentrated to a constant solute concentration (preferably hypotonic), because some antisera are affected by high concentrations of salt or urea. Also, to adjust for the effect of changes in antidiuresis *per se*, the total amount of vasopressin in a urine sample must be expressed as a function of the length of time over which the sample was collected or of the amount of a solute such as creatinine that is excreted at a relatively constant rate. Finally, although changes in urinary excretion of vasopressin usually parallel the changes in plasma, this relationship can be distorted by changes in glomerular filtration or solute clearance.[45]

REGULATION

Osmotic

The most important determinant of vasopressin secretion under physiologic conditions is the "tonicity" or effective osmotic pressure of body water.[46] This influence is mediated by a group of cells known collectively as osmoreceptors,[47] that are located near but separate from the supraoptic nucleus, in or near a part of the anterior hypothalamus known as the organum vasculosum lamina terminalis[48−54] (Figure 42.2). Unlike the neurohypophysis, which receives its blood supply from a branch of the internal carotid artery, the area containing the osmoreceptors is supplied by small perforating branches of the anterior cerebral or communicating arteries.[9] Thus, the interruption of these perforators (or damage to the anterior hypothalamus by other diseases or experimental lesions) can eliminate the osmoregulation of vasopressin secretion, without affecting the neurohypophysis or its response to hemodynamic or other nonosmotic stimuli.[55,56] This dissociation indicates that the osmoregulation of vasopressin is mediated not by the magnocellular neurons that make the hormone, but by afferent inputs from osmosensitive cells located in other, anatomically discrete areas of the anterior hypothalamus. It is not yet known exactly how many such areas there are, whether they contain inhibitory as well as stimulatory elements, how they integrate with other regulatory afferents or how they communicate with vasopressin-producing neurons. Therefore, it may be more appropriate to refer to them as an osmoregulatory system.

The functional properties of the system that osmoregulates vasopressin resemble those of a discontinuous or "set-point" receptor (Figure 42.4b). Thus, in healthy adults and children, plasma vasopressin is very low or undetectable (<0.5 pg/mL) when plasma osmolarity is below a certain minimum or threshold level. Above that "set-point," plasma vasopressin increases steeply in direct proportion with the increase in plasma osmolality. The slope of the line describing this relationship indicates that, on average, a rise in plasma osmolality of 1% increases plasma vasopressin by 1 pg/mL, an amount sufficient to significantly alter urinary concentration and flow (Figure 42.4).

The functional properties of the osmoregulatory system are similar in men and non-pregnant women,[57,58] as well as in blacks and whites.[59] Within each group, however, they vary considerably from person to person.[58] Individual differences in the slope or sensitivity of the response are particularly large, varying as much as 10-fold. Differences in the apparent threshold or set-point are smaller, but still range from 274 to 293 mosmoles/L. These individual differences are constant over time, and appear to be determined largely by genetic factors.[58] However, neither the sensitivity or the set-point is totally immutable, because they can be altered by a variety of conditions, drugs, and hormones (see below).

It is uncertain whether the threshold concept accurately represents the operation of the osmoreceptor at its most fundamental level. The relation of plasma vasopressin to plasma osmolarity in the population as a whole appears to be slightly curvilinear[60-62] (Figure 42.4). This curvilinearity could be due simply to individual variation, since there as a positive correlation between slope and threshold, i.e., the higher the threshold the steeper the slope. It is also possible, however, that the stimulation of vasopressin secretion is self-amplifying.[44] At present, however, the precision and reproducibility of the vasopressin assays at the low levels present under basal conditions are insufficient to determine if the best fit of the relationship is linear or exponential. It is also possible that vasopressin secretion reflects the balance of inhibitory as well as stimulatory inputs from a bimodal osmoregulatory system, because patients and animals with adipsic hypernatremia due to destruction of the osmoreceptors may lose the capacity to osmotically suppress, as well as to stimulate, vasopressin secretion.[54,55,57,63] As a practical matter, however, the concept of an osmotic threshold remains, for the present, a valid and useful way of describing many aspects of normal and abnormal osmoregulatory function in the intact animal.

It is also uncertain whether vasopressin is secreted continuously or episodically in response to osmotic stimulation. When nonosmotic stimuli such as posture, activity, and blood pressure are controlled, infusion of hypertonic saline in humans almost always produces a smooth progressive increase in systemic venous plasma vasopressin that correlates very closely with the increase in plasma osmolality.[45,58,64-67] However, samples obtained from experimental animals nearer the source of the hormone, for example, from the internal jugular vein, exhibit large fluctuations in plasma vasopressin during osmotic stimulation.[68] Whether these fluctuations reflect an intrinsic property of the neurohypophysis or the osmoreceptors, or are artifacts of the experimental conditions is unknown. Irregular phasic firing of the neurosecretory neurons has been observed by unit recording techniques during stimulation,[69] but this activity is unlikely to be related to episodic fluctuations in plasma vasopressin because the discharge cycles have a much shorter periodicity and are not synchronized from cell to cell.

The system that osmoregulates vasopressin secretion is not equally sensitive to all the solutes in plasma and extracellular fluid.[70-72] The most potent stimuli are sodium and its anions, the solutes that ordinarily account for more than 95% of measured plasma osmolarity. However, certain sugars, such as mannitol and sucrose, are also very effective when infused intravenously. In fact, particle-for-particle, mannitol is as potent as sodium chloride.[72] In contrast, an increase in plasma osmolarity produced by infusion of urea or glucose causes little or no increase in plasma

vasopressin in healthy adults.[70-72] Thus, the concentration of sodium and its anions is the principal, if not the only, determinant of osmotically-mediated vasopressin secretion under normal conditions. The basic mechanism by which the osmoregulatory system senses changes in the plasma concentration of sodium and its anions has not been completely established. On the basis of studies in dogs, Verney proposed that the osmoreceptor is stimulated when its intracellular volume is reduced by an osmotically driven efflux of water.[47] If so, solutes that enter the osmoreceptor cells slowly or not at all would be "effective" stimuli, whereas those that penetrate rapidly would have little or no effect. This theory is consistent with the observations that vasopressin secretion is stimulated similarly by infusing hypertonic saline or mannitol, both of which are excluded from cells. In addition, vasopressin is not stimulated by a rise in plasma osmolarity produced by rapid infusion of hypertonic glucose, a solute which enters cells rapidly in the presence of insulin. If anything, the hyperglycemic hyperosmolarity produced by infusion of hypertonic glucose suppresses plasma vasopressin, probably because it also lowers the plasma concentration of sodium salts by inducing an osmotically driven efflux of water from the intracellular to the extracellular compartment. This disparity suggests that, in the presence of insulin, glucose enters osmoreceptor cells even more rapidly than many other cells of the body.

Another theory posits that the osmoreceptors are actually sodium receptors located on the brain side of the blood–brain barrier.[70,73] It is consistent with the observed effects of hypertonic mannitol infusion, because this solute does not cross the blood–brain barrier and, as a consequence, causes an osmotically driven efflux of water from brain that probably raises the extracellular concentration of sodium in that organ. However, the sodium receptor theory is not consistent with the relatively small rise in plasma vasopressin produced by an acute rise in plasma urea,[72] because this solute also crosses the blood–brain barrier slowly and, as a consequence, reduces brain water and raises brain extracellular sodium concentration much like mannitol. This singular disparity indicates that most, if not all, of the osmoreceptors are probably located outside the blood–brain barrier, and that another factor, most likely the solute permeability of the osmoreceptor cell itself, determines the solute-specificity of the system. This concept is also consistent with two other observations: (1) the osmoregulatory system appears to be located in or near the organum vasculosum lamina terminalis, a region of the anterior hypothalamus that is known to lack a blood–brain barrier; and (2) a severe deficiency of insulin sensitizes the osmoreceptors to stimulation by hyperglycemia,[74] presumably by decreasing its permeability to glucose. It is not yet known, however, what distinguishes the cells of the osmoregulatory system from all the others whose volume and solute concentrations are similarly affected by changes in the extracellular concentration of sodium and its anions.

NON-OSMOTIC

Hemodynamic

An acute decrease of blood pressure or blood volume increases plasma vasopressin by an amount that is roughly proportional to the degree of hypotension or hypovolemia.[75–77] However, the stimulus–response relationship follows a distinctly exponential pattern (Figure 42.5). Small decreases in blood pressure or volume of 5 to 10% usually have little or no perceptible effect on plasma vasopressin, whereas decreases of 20 to 30% result in plasma hormone levels many times those required to produce maximum antidiuresis. Acute orthostasis, which decreases "effective" blood volume by 10 to 15%, usually doubles plasma vasopressin. In rats, chronic or sustained hypovolemia of 24 to 48 hours duration has even less effect on vasopressin, even though pituitary stores of the hormone

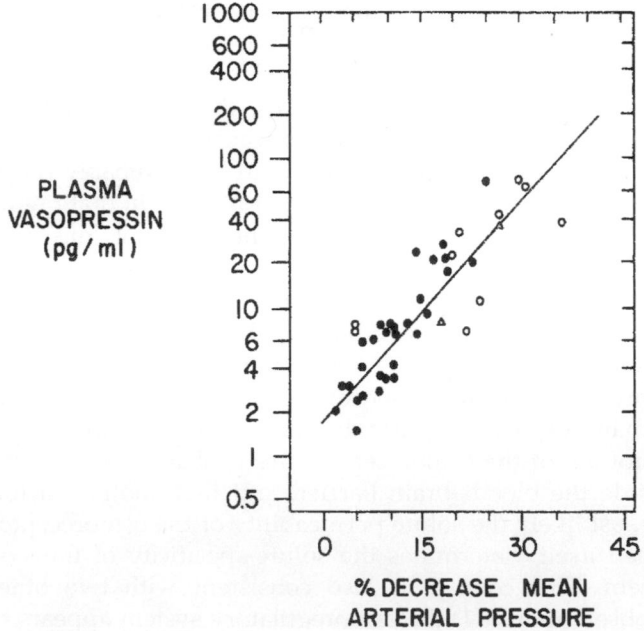

FIGURE 42.5 Relationship between plasma vasopressin and percentage decrease in arterial pressure in healthy adults. Hypotension was produced by infusion of a ganglionic blocker (filled symbols) or phlebotomy followed by orthostasis (open symbols). Note that plasma vasopressin is plotted on a log scale.

are undiminished.[78] This suggests that chronic stimulation selectively desensitizes the volume control mechanism.

The effects of acute hypovolemia on vasopressin secretion appear to be mediated largely by neuronal afferents that arise in pressure-sensitive receptors in the left side of the heart[79] and project by way of the vagus and glossopharyngeal nerves to primary synapses on the nuclei of the solitary tracts in the medulla. From there, signals ascend to the hypothalamus via postsynaptic pathways that appear to be mediated in part by a highly selective opioid neurotransmitter of the kappa subclass in the lateral parabrachial nucleus.[80–83] The vasopressin response to acute hypotension is mediated by neurogenic afferents that arise in high-pressure receptors in the aorta and carotid sinus, and project via the vagus and glossopharyngeal nerves, presumably, to the nuclei of the solitary tracts.[84,85] From there, pathways that are at least partly noradrenergic[86] ascend to the hypothalamus. At least for part of their length, these ascending pathways are separate from those that mediate the vasopressin response to hypovolemia, because they are not blocked by opioid antagonists that abolish the response to hypovolemia.[80,81,83]

Acute hypervolemia or hypertension can inhibit vasopressin secretion.[87–90] However, the increase in blood volume or pressure required is relatively large, and the inhibition of AVP is slight. The pathways that mediate the hemodynamic inhibition have not been fully-elucidated, and they may be the same as those that mediate stimulation. Interruption of primary vagal afferents eliminates the effect of hemodynamic stimuli, but also results in an acute rise in basal vasopressin secretion.[91,92] This suggests that the baroregulatory afferents tonically inhibit vasopressin secretion under basal, normovolemic, and normotensive conditions. If so, the slight decrease in vasopressin produced by acute hypervolemia and hypertension may be simply enhancement of this tonic inhibitory effect. Likewise, the increase in vasopressin produced by acute hypovolemia or hypotension could result from a reduction in basal inhibition of secretion. The effect of a *chronic* increase in blood volume or pressure is largely undefined. The osmoregulation of vasopressin secretion appears to be normal in patients with uncomplicated essential hypertension,[93,94] but may be inhibited slightly in primary hyperaldosteronism,[95] suggesting that chronic expansion of the blood volume has an effect opposite to that of hypovolemia.

Changes in blood volume or pressure large enough to affect vasopressin secretion do not interfere with osmoregulation of the hormone. Instead, they appear to act by shifting the set of the system in such a way as to increase or decrease the effect on vasopressin of a given osmotic stimulus.[46,75,96-98] This means that the osmoregulatory and baroregulatory systems, although different in location and function, ultimately converge and act upon the same population of neurosecretory neurons[46,99] (Figure 42.2). Exactly how and where this integration occurs is unknown.

Emetic

Nausea is an extremely potent stimulus for vasopressin secretion in humans.[100] The pathways that mediate this effect have not been defined, but they probably involve the chemoreceptor trigger zone in the area postrema of the medulla. The effect on vasopressin is instantaneous and extremely potent. Increases of 100 to 500 times basal levels are not unusual, even when the nausea is transient and unaccompanied by vomiting or changes in blood pressure. Pretreatment with fluphenazine, haloperidol or promethazine in doses sufficient to prevent nausea completely abolish the vasopressin response.[100] The inhibitory effect of these dopamine antagonists is specific for emetic stimuli, because they do not alter the vasopressin response to osmotic or hemodynamic stimuli. Water-loading blunts, but does not abolish, the effect of nausea on vasopressin release, suggesting that osmotic and emetic influences interact in a manner similar to osmotic and hemodynamic pathways. The effect of emetic stimuli is also species-dependent. Whereas emetics such as apomorphine, cholecystokinin, lithium chloride, and copper sulfate stimulate the secretion of vasopressin but not oxytocin in humans[100,101] and monkeys,[102] they increase the secretion of oxytocin but have little effect on vasopressin in rodents.[103]

Emetic stimuli probably mediate many pharmacologic and pathologic effects on vasopressin secretion. These include not only apomorphine,[100] but also high doses of morphine,[104] nicotine,[105] alcohol,[100] cholecystokinin,[101,102] and motion sickness.[106] They may also be responsible, at least in part, for the increases in vasopressin secretion that have been observed with intravenous cyclophosphamide,[107] acute hypoxia,[108] diabetic ketoacidosis,[109] vasovagal syncope,[110] and hyperemesis gravidarum.[111] Because nausea and vomiting are frequent side-effects of many other drugs and diseases, additional examples of nausea-induced vasopressin secretion doubtlessly will be observed. The potency and ubiquity of emetic stimuli create special problems for research studies of vasopressin secretion in animals and unconscious subjects, because the occurrence of nausea is difficult to ascertain except by verbal report.

OTHER INFLUENCES

Glucopenia

Acute insulin-induced hypoglycemia also stimulates vasopressin release in proportion to the decrease in plasma glucose.[112] The rate of decrease in glucose is probably the critical determinant, however, because the increase in plasma vasopressin is not sustained even when the hypoglycemia persists.[113] The receptor and pathway that mediate this effect are unknown. They are probably separate from those that mediate the effects of other recognized stimuli, because hypoglycemia stimulates vasopressin secretion in patients who have selectively lost the capacity to respond to osmotic, hemodynamic or emetic stimuli.[112] However, the vasopressin response is accentuated by dehydration and abolished by water-loading,[113] indicating that hypoglycemic stimuli probably act in concert with osmotic influences even though the osmoreceptors *per se* are unnecessary for the response. The effect of hypoglycemia is not due to nonspecific stress, because it can occur in the absence of symptoms and is more pronounced in rats, a species in which vasopressin secretion appears to be unaffected by pain and other noxious stimuli. The variable that actually triggers the release of vasopressin may be an intracellular deficiency of glucose or one of its metabolites, because 2-deoxyglucose is also an effective stimulus.[114,115]

Angiotensin

The renin—angiotensin system has also been implicated in the control of vasopressin secretion.[116] The precise site and mechanism of action have not been defined, but one or more central receptors seem likely, because angiotensin II is most effective when injected directly into brain ventricles or cranial arteries.[117] The magnitude of the vasopressin response may depend on the concurrent osmotic stimulus.[118,119] This dependency may account for the failure of some investigators to demonstrate stimulation by peripherally administered angiotensin.[120] However, if angiotensin is directly involved in the physiologic control of vasopressin, it is more likely that produced by the renin—angiotensin system of the brain.[121]

Stress

Nonspecific stress caused by pain, emotion or physical exercise has long been thought to release vasopressin.[122] However, it has never been determined whether this effect is mediated by a specific pathway or is secondary to other stress-induced stimuli, such as the severe hypotension and/or nausea that often accompanys the vasovagal reaction to pain or fear. In rats and humans, stresses severe enough to activate the pituitary adrenal axis and sympathetic nervous system do not stimulate an increase in plasma vasopressin unless they also lower blood pressure or alter blood volume.[123,124] If anything, stress seems to transiently suppress plasma vasopressin, possibly as a consequence of an acute rise in blood pressure or activation of other inhibitory input.[125] However, stresses of various types have been found to stimulate the release of vasopressin (as well as corticotropin releasing hormone) from parvocellular neurons which project to portal veins of the anterior pituitary and appear to play a role in the regulation of ACTH secretion.[126]

Temperature

Environmental temperature can also influence plasma vasopressin. In healthy adults, exposure to cold for a relatively short period of time depresses plasma vasopressin, and heat has the opposite effect.[127,128] These changes are independent of changes in plasma osmolality, but they cannot as yet be divorced from changes in effective blood volume or blood pressure. Experimentally-induced hypothermia or fever in animals is also associated with changes in plasma vasopressin,[129–131] but the effects seem to vary, possibly as a function of the species, the dose of endotoxin administered or the time interval. Thus, it is still uncertain how exogenous or endogenous changes in temperature effect vasopressin secretion by magnocellular neurons.

Oropharynx

Drinking can also inhibit vasopressin secretion, even before it produces a detectable decrease in plasma osmolarity or sodium.[132–134] This effect does not depend on the water reaching the stomach, and is unrelated to changes in blood pressure or blood volume. It may depend on the volume or temperature of the fluid ingested because, in humans at least, small volumes of water (100 mL) at room temperature are less inhibitory than larger volumes (700–1200 mL) or small amounts of ice. Thus, the inhibition may be mediated by neural afferents that originate in taste, temperature or other sensory receptors in the oropharynx. Inhibition of vasopressin by oropharyngeal receptors is rapid and transient. This may explain why it is not associated with a concurrent decrease in urine concentration. The rapidity of the decrease is also unexplained, since it appears to exceed the rate at which vasopressin is cleared from plasma under steady-state conditions (see below).

Age

Normal aging also appears to alter the osmoregulation of vasopressin secretion in humans, but the nature of the change is controversial.[135–138] Some find that the vasopressin response to an osmotic stimulus is enhanced, but others report no change or a decreased response. These differences are unexplained, and may represent individual variation in the impact of aging on various components of the osmoregulatory and other interacting control systems. Histologic studies of the human brain show variable changes in the suprachiasmitic nucleus and other vasopressin-containing parvocellular pathways, but no decrease in the number of large cell bodies in the supraoptic and paraventricular nucleus.[12,139] MRI studies indicate that the posterior pituitary bright spot is diminished or absent more often in the elderly than in the young,[140] but this decrease can be due either to atrophy of the gland or to more rapid turnover of vasopressin due, for example, to decreased fluid intake or decreased renal effect of the hormone. Aging does not seem to impair the ability to osmotically suppress vasopressin secretion and dilute the urine, but it does diminish the capacity to excrete a water-load, because of the large age-related reduction in glomerular filtration rate.[141] The capacity to maximally concentrate the urine also diminishes with age, but this may also be due largely to renal factors.[142]

Gender, Pregnancy, the Menstrual Cycle, and Gonadal Hormones

The effects of gender on the osmoregulation of vasopressin secretion are complex and unsettled. There appears to be little or no difference between adult human males and non-gravid females,[57,58] but pregnancy results in a relatively large reduction in the osmotic threshold for vasopressin release in rats as well as in humans.[143,144] Downward resetting of the osmostat also occurs during the luteal phase of the human menstrual cycle,[66,145] but the shift is small relative to that in pregnancy and is smaller even than the range of individual variation in men and non-gravid women.[58] The cause of the resetting is uncertain, but it may be mediated by relaxin,[144] an increase in estrogens[67] or chorionic gonadotropin,[65] since they also lower the set of the osmostat in humans. Progesterone appears to have no effect.[146] In rats, large doses of estrogen seem to have a different effect than in humans, since they enhance the slope or sensitivity of the vasopressin response to plasma osmolality, but do not significantly alter its set-point.[143]

TABLE 42.1 Drugs and Hormones that Affect Vasopressin Secretion

Stimulatory	Inhibitory
Acetycholine	Fluphenazine
Morphine (high doses)	Haloperidol
Epinephrine	Promethazine
Histamine	Oxilorphan
Bradykinin	Butorphanol
Prostaglandins	Opiods (κ and δ agonists)
β-Endorphin	Morphine (low doses)
Cyclophosphamide	Alcohol
Vincristine	Carbamazepine
Lithium	? Glucocorticoids
? Chlorpropamide	? Phenytoin
? Clofibrate	
? Corticotropin-releasing factor	

Drugs and Other Hormones

Many drugs and hormones also influence vasopressin secretion (Table 42.1). Those that stimulate, such as histamine, bradykinin, prostaglandin, β-endorphin, and high doses of morphine, have not been studied sufficiently to define their mechanisms of action, but may act by decreasing blood pressure or producing nausea. Vincristine may have a direct toxic effect on the neurohypophysis or peripheral neurons involved in the regulation of vasopressin secretion. Lithium, which antagonizes the antidiuretic effect of vasopressin, also increases secretion of the hormone. This effect is independent of changes in water balance, and appears to result from an increase in sensitivity of the osmoregulatory system.[147] The stimulatory effects of chlorpropamide and clofibrate are still controversial, and a mechanism of action has not been proposed.

Inhibitors such as the dopaminergic antagonists fluphenazine, haloperidol, and promethazine probably act by suppressing the emetic center, because they inhibit the vasopressin response to nausea but not to osmotic or hemodynamic stimuli. Antihistamines inhibit the vasopressin response to dehydration[148] which is largely an osmotic stimulus, indicating that some part of the osmoregulatory afferents may be histaminergic. Many opiates are also inhibitory. They include oxilorphan and butorphanol, the KAPPA agonists U50488[149] leu-morphin and U62066E, as well as low doses of morphine. In the case of morphine and butorphanol,[150] the inhibition is due to an increase in the osmotic threshold for vasopressin release, and is

independent of changes in blood volume or pressure. The mechanism of the resetting has not been completely defined. However, it would appear to be due to the agonist properties of these opiates, because it can be blocked by naloxone.[150,151] The inhibitory effect of alcohol[136] may also be mediated in part by endogenous opiates, because it is also due to upward resetting of the osmostat and can be partly reversed by treatment with naloxone.[152] Carbamazepine inhibits vasopressin secretion by diminishing the sensitivity of the osmoregulatory system.[153] This effect is not dependent on changes in blood volume or blood pressure, and suggests that the ability of carbamazepine to produce antidiuresis in patients with neurogenic (pituitary) diabetes insipidus is due to an independent action on the kidney. The regulation of oxytocin secretion has not been studied extensively, partly because of the limited availability of reliable assays. However, it appears to be stimulated by gonadal steroids, as well as by labor and parturition.[16]

DISTRIBUTION AND CLEARANCE

After release into the systemic circulation, vasopressin distributes quickly into a space approximating extracellular fluid volume.[45,154] The mixing phase is followed by a second, slower decline that presumably reflects the metabolic or irreversible phase of clearance. It has a half-life of 10 to 30 minutes. Thus, the total clearance rate of vasopressin ranges from about 10 to 20 mL/kg body weight per minute. The metabolic clearance rate increases markedly during pregnancy, reaching a level three- to four-fold greater than normal by the third trimester.[155] Smaller animals, such as rats, also clear vasopressin much more rapidly because their cardiac output is much higher relative to body weight and surface area.[154] Although many tissues have the capacity to inactivate vasopressin *in vitro*, most metabolism *in vivo* appears to occur in liver and kidney.[154] In pregnancy, vasopressin is also degraded by a vasopressinase produced by the placenta.[155]

Some vasopressin is excreted intact in the urine. The amount can vary considerably depending on the overall rate of solute excretion,[45] but it is never more than a fraction of total irreversible clearance. In healthy, normally hydrated adults, the urinary clearance of vasopressin ranges from 0.1 to 0.6 mL/kg/min. The mechanisms involved in the excretion of vasopressin have not been defined, but the hormone is probably filtered at the glomerulus and variably reabsorbed at one or more sites along the tubule. The latter process seems to be influenced by the reabsorption of sodium and chloride in the proximal nephron, because the urinary clearance rate of vasopressin varies by as much as

20-fold in direct relationship to the clearance rate of total solute.[45] Thus, changes in urinary vasopressin excretion do not provide a reliable guide to changes in plasma vasopressin unless glomerular filtration or solute clearance rates are constant and normal.

ACTIONS

The biologic effects of vasopressin are mediated by three subtypes of a heptahelical transmembranous receptor coupled to guanine nucleotide-binding (GNB) proteins. Two of the receptors, V1a and V1b, activate phospholipase via GBN–protein coupling. The third, V2, activates adenyl cyclase and increases cyclic-AMP, also via GBN–protein coupling.[156,157] The genes encoding these receptors are located on different chromosomes: V1a on 12q14–15; V1b on 1q32; and V2 on Xq28. Among humans of different ethnic backgrounds, the gene encoding V1a receptors shows considerable polymorphism in the upstream regulatory regions and intron–exon junctions.[158] The anatomic distribution and sensitivity of the three receptors also differs. V1a receptors are found mainly in liver, platelets, the central nervous system, and vascular/gastrointestinal smooth muscle. V1b receptors are found mainly in the ACTH-producing cells of the anterior pituitary, but may also be in other areas of the brain. The V2 receptors are expressed in the distal and collecting tubules of the kidney. The V2 receptors bind vasopressin at very low plasma concentrations (10^{-12} M), and mediate the effect of the hormone on urinary concentration and flow. The V1 receptors, in contrast, are stimulated by vasopressin only at concentrations much higher than those found in plasma under physiological conditions. Thus, their role in other possible physiological functions of this hormone in the periphery is uncertain but unlikely. However, the relative insensitivity of the V1 receptors may not prevent them from acting as neurotransmitters in the brain, the anterior pituitary or other areas where locally high concentrations of the hormone may be produced in synapses with little or no dilution.

The biologic effects of oyxtocin are also mediated by a 7-transmembrane domain receptor coupled to GNB protein.[157] It is encoded by a gene on chromosome 3p25-26 and expressed in uterine smooth muscle, as well as other sites that vary according to the species and the effect of gonadal steroids. The oxytocin receptor is less specific than those for vasopressin, and can be activated by the latter at concentrations only tenfold higher than oxytocin.

Numerous peptide and non-peptide agonists and antagonists of the vasopressin and oxytocin receptors have been, and are still being, developed.[159] One peptide, a V2-selective agonist known generically as desmopressin, has been used for decades to treat the vasopressin-deficient form of diabetes insipidus, and recently also enuresis in children and nocturia in adults. Several non-peptides, antagonists with variable specificity for the V2 receptor, are now being used to treat certain types of hyponatremia resulting from osmotically inappropriate antidiuresis.[160] Non-peptide antagonists for the V1 or oxytocin receptors are now in various stages of development and testing. They may prove to be very helpful in determining if these receptors play a significant role in physiology or pathophysiology. The results of such studies should be interpreted with caution, however, because the receptor specificity and activity of many agonists and antagonists differ considerably, especially between species.[159]

RENAL ACTIONS

The principal, if not the only, clearly documented physiological role of peripherally secreted vasopressin in humans is to decrease urine output by increasing urine concentration. This antidiuretic effect is achieved by binding to G-protein-coupled V2 receptors located on the basal surface of principal cells in the distal and collecting tubules of the kidney (Figure 42.6). Binding to these receptors activates adenyl cyclase and increases intracellular cyclic AMP which, in turn, results in phosphorylation of aquaporin-2, one of a large family of proteins that self-associate to form water channels in other tissues of the body.[4] Aquaporin-2 is encoded by a gene on chromosome 12q13, and expressed almost exclusively in the collecting ducts of the cortex and inner/outer medulla of the kidney. It self-associates to form homotetramers that when phosphorylated are routed to the apical (luminal) surface of the principal cells and inserted through the membrane. There, they function as channels that selectively permit some of the water in dilute tubular fluid to back-diffuse across the membrane into the cell, and then out again into the body through channels formed on the basolateral side by aquaporin 3 and aquaporin 4.[161–164] This process of reabsorption is driven by the hyperosmolar gradient created in the renal medulla by the countercurrent mechanism of the kidney (see Chapter 43). Since water is reabsorbed without solute, the fluid that remains is decreased in volume and increased in concentration, by an amount proportional to the level of vasopressin stimulation and the number of water channels inserted through the apical surface of the cell.

The maximum antidiuresis achievable in healthy adult humans usually occurs at a plasma vasopressin concentration of about 2 to 3 pg/mL (Figure 42.4).

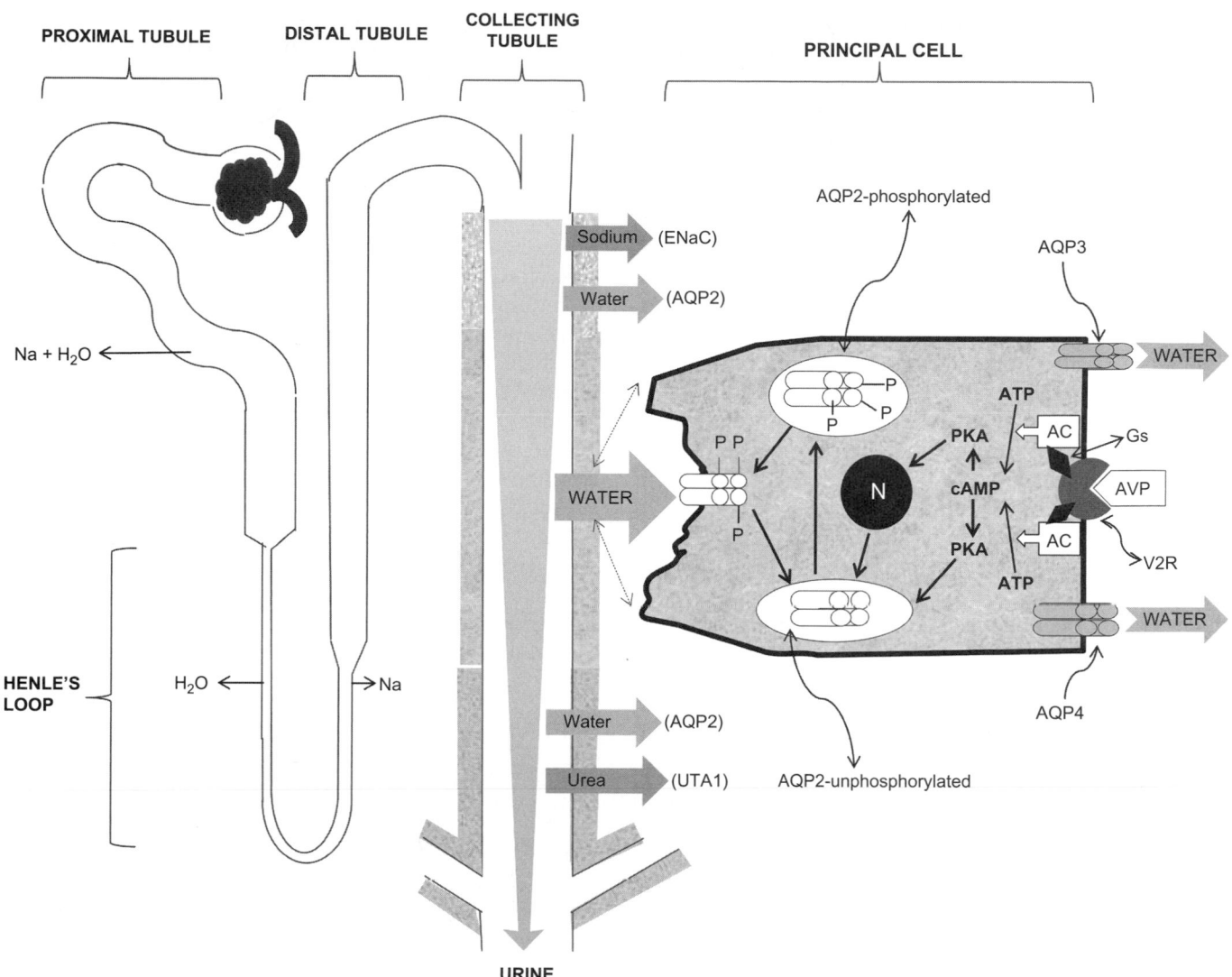

FIGURE 42.6   Schematic diagram of renal nephron and a principal cell of the collecting tubule. In healthy adults, the glomerulus filters about 180 L a day of ultrafiltrate with an osmolarity and sodium concentration approximating that of plasma. Water and sodium chloride are reabsorbed from the filtrate in the proximal tubule, Henle's loop, and the distal tubule, reducing the volume and the osmolarity of the fluid that enters the collecting tubules to about 15 L/day and 60 mosmols/L, respectively. In the absence of vasopressin action most, if not all, of this dilute fluid passes unmodified through the collecting tubules and is excreted as urine because the luminal (apical) surface of the principal cells that line the collecting tubules are impermeable to water and solute. This condition is known as a water diuresis. In the presence of vaso-pressin (AVP), the apical and basal lateral surfaces of the principal cells become permeable to water, allowing it to back-diffuse through the cell down the hyperosmotic gradient formed by the countercurrent mechanism in the renal medulla. As a consequence, the fluid that remains in the collecting tubules to be excreted as urine is more concentrated and less voluminous. Under conditions of maximal antidiuresis, the osmo-larity can reach 1200–1400 mosmols/L, and the volume can be as low as 0.5 to 0.7 L/day. The increase in water permeability of the principal cell occurs by a series of intracellular reactions that begin with binding of AVP to a V2 receptor (V2R) on the basal surface, activation of adenyl cyclase (AC) via coupling of G-protein (◇) and conversion of adenosine triphosphate (ATP) to cyclic adenosine monophosphate (cAMP), which activates protein kinase A (PKA). The PKA has two effects. First, it causes the phosphorylation of preformed tetramers of aquaporin-2 (AQP2) which are stored in vesicles just below the apical surface of the cell. This phosphorylation, indicated in the diagram by −P, directs the tetramers to the apical surface of the cell, where they are inserted and function as channels allowing the passage of water into the cells and out the baso-lateral side through water channels formed by aquaporin 3 and 4 (AQP3 and AQP4). This process of reabsorption of water is driven by the hyperosmotic gradient created in the renal medulla by the countercurrent system.

It usually results in a urine osmolality of 1000 to 1200 mosmols/L, and a rate of excretion as low as 0.5 to 0.7 ml/min. By reducing the amount of urine needed to excrete urea and other waste solutes, this antidiure-tic mechanism serves to minimize the amount of water that must be ingested to prevent dehydration. Rats and many other mammals are capable of even greater levels of antidiuresis, largely because their renal papilla are longer and, consequently, able to generate greater levels of hypertonicity in the medulla. The level of antidiuresis produced in humans by a given level of plasma vasopressin also varies considerably, depending on the rate of solute excretion as well as, probably, the abundance of aquaporin channels available for insertion, and the rate at which they are removed from the membrane and recycled for later use. The factors that determine the abundance of water channels remain to be fully-defined, but probably include the level of prior vasopressin stimulation because the hormone also stimulates the synthesis of aquaporin-2. This may partly explain why antidiuretic response to vasopressin or desmopressin observed after a prolonged deficiency of the hormone (e.g., in pituitary diabetes insipidus or primary polydipsia) is blunted for several hours.[165] The variables that influence the removal of water channels from the membrane have not been fully-defined, but may include prostaglandin, dopamine, and hypertonicity itself.[163]

Vasopressin also has two other effects on the kidney that enhance its antidiuretic effects. One is to stimulate the activity of a urea transporter (UTA1) in the inner medullary collecting duct.[166,167] This effect, which is also mediated by V2 receptors and cyclic AMP, replenishes the concentration of urea in the renal medulla, thereby helping to maintain the hypertonic gradient generated by the countercurrent mechanism. The other renal effect of vasopressin is to stimulate the readsorption of sodium through an epithelial sodium channel (ENaC) in the collecting duct.[168] This also helps to reinforce the medullary concentration gradient. It does not appear to result in a sustained increase in total body sodium, probably because there is a compensatory decrease in proximal readsorption of sodium.

In the absence of vasopressin stimulation, the apical surfaces of the principal cells, as well as the tight junctions between them, are impermeable to water because the aquaporin-2 water channels remain in vesicles within the cell. As a consequence, the large volume of dilute filtrate that normally issues from the ascending limb of Henle's loop passes unmodified through the collecting ducts to be excreted as urine. In this condition, known as a water diuresis, the osmolarity of urine approximates 40 to 60 mosmols/L (Figure 42.4a), and the rate of excretion may be as high 10–15 mL/min. The excretion of water at this rate normally provides an effective barrier to over-hydration, since it suffices to offset all but the most pathologically excessive rates of water intake.

EXTRARENAL ACTIONS

Apart from its actions on the kidney, vasopressin has been investigated extensively for other effects that might be mediated via V1a or V1b receptors in the periphery or brain. These studies have yet to provide convincing evidence for a significant role in human physiology. However, they suggest that the V1 receptors may mediate certain pharmacologic or *in vitro* effects of the hormone on vascular resistance[169,170] or platelet aggregation,[171] and may also mediate the effects of parvocellular vasopressinergic neurons in brain to modulate various types of complex social behavior[172–174] or the effect of stress on ACTH secretion.[126,175]

The actions attributed to oxytocin are numerous,[16] but their role in human physiology or pathophysiology is not yet fully-defined. Most relate to sexual activity or reproduction, earning oxytocin the sobriquet of "the hormone of love." In the periphery, it stimulates contraction of smooth muscle in reproductive tissues, especially the uterus and mammary glands. However, it is not yet clear whether those effects are essential or only supportive for birth and nursing. In the brain, it has also been implicated in the genesis of various sexual behaviors and social bonding, in addition to regulation of temperature and cardiovascular function.

THIRST

The regulation of fluid intake is an indispensable part of the homeostatic system that regulates the tonicity of body fluids. It ensures that obligatory losses of water through urination, perspiration, and respiration are always replaced promptly and completely. This protection is provided by the thirst mechanism. Thirst may be defined as the subjective sensation of a desire or need for water. It is sometimes associated with feelings of dry mouth, headache or irritability, but these symptoms are not specific to thirst since they also have other causes. It must also be distinguished from cultural, social, psychological, medical, and other motivations to drink. Its vital importance is shown dramatically by the episodes of severe and sometimes fatal hypertonic dehydration that occur in patients who lack the sensation of thirst due to pathology in the anterior hypothalamus.[54] The opposite risk — that of hypotonic overhydration due to too much fluid intake — is not as great, because the mechanisms for suppressing vasopressin and excreting excess water can normally offset all but the most pathologically extreme polydipsia. However, excretory capacity can be impaired by a decrease in urinary solute load or a non-osmotic stimulus to vasopressin secretion. Therefore, the mechanism for regulating fluid intake also seems to include an inhibitory component that operates by producing a sense of satiation or distaste for water.

ANATOMY

The parts of the brain that mediate the conscious awareness of thirst and satiation have not been fully-defined. Studies using functional magnetic resonance imaging or positron emission tomography of the brain in healthy adults have shown that thirst is associated with activation in several areas, including the anterior wall of the third ventricle, anterior cingulate cortex, parahippocampal gyrus, inferior and middle frontal gyrus, insula, and cerebellum.[176] The difficulty with such findings, however, is that the sensation of thirst probably activates many brain areas involved in secondary feelings, thoughts or responses such as anxiety, discomfort or physical movement induced by feelings of thirst. To differentiate these secondary areas of arousal from those that mediate the consciousness of thirst *per se*, it will be necessary to employ a variety of other unpleasant stimuli as controls[177] or study the effect of discrete strokes or other ablative lesions in different brain areas.

REGULATION

Osmotic

Like the secretion of vasopressin, thirst is regulated primarily by the tonicity or effective osmotic pressure of body fluids.[54] This effect is also mediated via hypothalamic osmoreceptors that appear to be anatomically distinct from, but intermingled with, those that regulate vasopressin[178-180] (Figure 42.2). Their functional properties also seem to be similar to the vasopressin osmoreceptors, in that the intensity of thirst increases steeply in direct proportion to plasma osmolarity (Figure 42.4). The only difference is that the threshold for initiation of thirst seems to be set slightly higher than that for the initiation of vasopressin secretion.[54,58] In healthy adults, the level of plasma osmolality at which thirst begins averages about 287 mosmols/L, but varies from person to person over a range from 277 to 294 mosmols/L. In each individual, the the osmotic threshold for thirst tends to be about 4 mosmols/kg higher than that for vasopressin release. Therefore, thirst is not experienced until plasma osmolality rises to a level at which plasma vasopressin is high enough to maximally concentrate the urine. In other respects, the thirst osmoreceptors behave much like those for vasopressin secretion. They have the same solute specificity, since increases in plasma osmolality produced by infusion of hypertonic saline or mannitol are dipsogenic, whereas those resulting from infusions of hypertonic urea or glucose are not.[71,72] Their sensitivity — that is, the intensity of the thirst produced by a given rise in plasma osmolality — also differs significantly from person to person, and these differences also appear to be genetically determined.[58] However, one or both properties also can be altered by changes in blood volume,[181] pregnancy,[144] the menstrual cycle,[66] and human chorionic gonadotrophin.[65]

OTHER INFLUENCES

Hemodynamic

Anecdotal evidence indicates that thirst can also be stimulated by severe reductions in blood volume or blood pressure. The pathways that mediate this effect have not been defined, but are probably the same as those that mediate the effects on vasopressin (see above). In rats, a hypovolemia-induced increase in angiotensin II may also play an important role (see below), but such an effect has not been convincingly documented in humans. Also like vasopressin, moderate reductions in blood volume lower the osmotic threshold for thirst, but do not otherwise interfere with continued operation of the osmoregulatory system.[181]

Angiotensin

In rats and some other animals, angiotensin II stimulates water intake, particularly when injected into the lateral ventricles or other areas of brain.[180] Presumably, the increased intake is due to thirst, although some other type of inducement cannot be excluded. In humans, the dipsogenic effect of angiotensin II has not been investigated.

Glucopenia

Although anecdotal evidence suggests that thirst can also be induced by acute, insulin-induced hypoglycemia, controlled studies are lacking. However, it is clear that an intracellular deficiency of glucose produced by administration of 2-deoxy-glucose stimulates thirst as well as vasopressin release.[115]

Oropharynx

Like vasopressin secretion, thirst is also inhibited rapidly and transiently by the act of drinking *per se*.[182] The characteristics of this effect are similar to those for vasopressin (see above). They appear to be independent of osmotic and hemodynamic influences as well as the solute content of the fluid, but may be influenced by its volume or temperature. The inhibition of thirst is extremely rapid and nearly complete, decreasing the sensation to near zero in a matter of minutes.

However, it is also transient, lasting no more than 10 to 15 minutes, well short of the time required to absorb enough water to begin reducing the osmotic stimulus. Thus, thirst begins to increase again before undergoing a second decline due to absorption of the water and lowering of plasma osmolality. This timing is consistent with the temporal dissociation between the drinking-induced decrease of PET and MRI activity in the anterior cingulated cortex and the anterior hypothalamus (organum vasculosum lamina terminalis).[176] It may also explain why drinking in response to a strong osmotic stimulus often occurs in two or more bouts separated by 15 to 30 minutes.

Eating

It is common knowledge documented by observational studies that most of the water ingested each day is drunk in association with meals.[183] The finding that the amount of liquid drunk with each meal correlates with its estimated protein and carbohydrate content, and not with its estimated sodium content, lead to a theory that eating *per se* is a major independent stimulus to thirst unrelated to osmotic stimulation.[184] However, in healthy adults allowed to eat, drink, and ambulate at will, there appear to be slight increases in plasma osmolality and decreases in plasma protein during meals. Thus, it is not yet certain if drinking with meals is due to osmotically-induced thirst or to some other stimulus, such as taste or cultural habit.

Aging

In contrast to vasopressin secretion, the sensation of thirst and the drinking response to dehydration is diminished among the elderly.[185] The reason, however, is controversial. One theory holds that the sensitivity of the response is decreased due to loss of the potentiating effect of the mild volume depletion that occurs during dehydration. Others find that the decrease in thirst is due largely to upward resetting of the thirst osmostat, with little or no decrease in sensitivity. Compared to healthy young adults, however, there does not appear to be any change in the amount of fluid consumed in response to a given level of thirst or in the rapidity and extent of thirst suppression by oropharyngeal influences.

EFFECTS

Thirst induces the ingestion of water or other fluids in amounts proportional to the strength of the osmotic stimulus.[58] The water is absorbed from the gastrointestinal tract within 30 to 45 minutes, and is carried by blood throughout the body, distributing rapidly between ECF and ICF in a ratio of about 1:2. Thus, it dilutes all body fluid equally. The total amount of fluid drunk at one time, commonly referred to as a "bout" of drinking, is usually less than the amount required to restore tonicity to normal. This pause in drinking may be due to rapid inhibition of thirst by neural pathways arising in oropharyngeal receptors (see above). However, the inhibition is of short duration (10 to 15 minutes), and soon gives way to a return of thirst and drinking until enough water is absorbed to lower plasma osmolality to basal levels. These bouts may be repeated 2 or 3 times for up to 2 to 3 hours, until the hypertonicity is completely eliminated.

Hypotonicity often induces feelings of satiation which help to prevent further overhydration by producing a conscious aversion to drinking water. In humans, it occurs less often and less strongly than the sensation of thirst, but seems to result in negative "thirst" ratings and a marked reduction of spontaneous fluid intake after induction of plasma hypotonicity either by water-loading or repeat administration of high doses of the V2 agonist, desmopressin.[186]

VASOPRESSIN AND THIRST IN OSMOREGULATION

Vasopressin and thirst act in concert to control the tonicity of body fluids by raising or lowering body water to keep the concentration of osmotically effective solutes within a very narrow range. This control must be exerted largely, if not completely, by the osmoregulatory system because fluctuations in plasma osmolarity rarely exceed 1–2%, a change in body water too small to activate the baroregulatory system. The upper and lower limits of plasma osmolarity and sodium are determined by the osmotic thresholds for thirst and vasopressin secretion, because the very large increases in water intake or excretion that normally occur at these thresholds present almost insurmountable barriers to further dehydration or overhydration. Thus, even patients with a severe polyuria due to a deficiency of vasopressin maintain plasma osmolarity and sodium within normal limits simply by drinking more, while those with severe polydipsia do the same by rapidly increasing urine output. However, because the set of the thirst and vasopressin osmostats differs appreciably from person to person, the level at which plasma osmolarity is maintained also differs among healthy adults. This difference is reflected in the normal laboratory values for plasma osmolarity and sodium concentration which, depending on the laboratory methods employed, range from about 270 to 295 mosmols/L

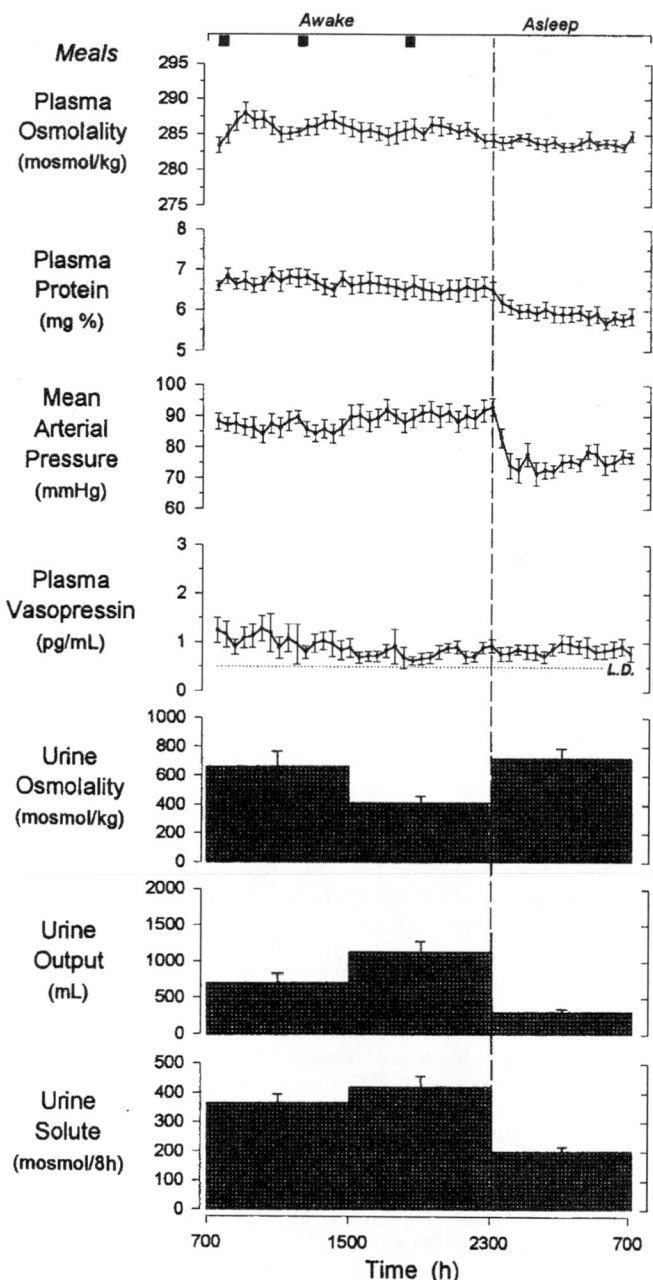

FIGURE 42.7 **Circadian variations in antidiuretic function and related variables in healthy young adults.** Each value is the mean ± SEM of 9 subjects (4 females and 5 males) on *ad libitum* intake of food and water. The three closed squares at the top indicate meals. Fluid intake, which is not shown, averaged 3.1 liters a day. It occurred in equal amounts during the two periods of the day (7 am to 3 pm, and 3 pm to 11 pm), usually with meals. *(From Robertson, G. L., Rittig, S., and Kovacs, L. (1993). Unpublished.)*

elicits a prompt change in vasopressin secretion and urine production, as well as in thirst and water intake. Consequently, the osmolality of plasma and other body fluids within each person rarely deviates by more than 3 to 5 mosmols/kg (1–1.5%), even in the face of large variations in insensible water loss and dietary solute load. In humans, the operation of this elegant osmoregulatory system is subject to changes in blood pressure or volume induced by posture and sleep. However, these influences do not seen to affect osmoregulation, probably because the system that mediates hemodynamic influences on thirst and/or vasopressin is relatively insensitive to normal fluctuations in blood pressure and volume, and even large changes produce only transient small changes in the set of the osmoregulatory system. Thus, plasma osmolarity, plasma vasopressin and urine osmolarity are relatively constant in the course of a normal day (Figure 42.7).

References

[1] Verbalis JG. Brain volume regulation in response to changes in osmolality. Neuroscience 2010;168:862–70.

[2] Ho SN. Intracellular water homeostasis and the mammalian cellular osmotic stress response. J Cell Phsiol 2006;206(1):9–15.

[3] Jaffrin MY, Morel H. Body fluid volume measurements by impedance: a review if bioimpedance spectroscopy (BIS) and bioempedance analysis (BIA) methods. Med Eng Phys 2008;30 (10):1257–69.

[4] Kruse E, Uehlein N, Kaldenhoff R. The Aquaporins. Genome Biol 2006;7:206.

[5] Adolph EF. In: Visscher MB, Bronk DW, Landis EM, et al., editors. Physiology of man in the desert. New York: Hafner; 1969.

[6] Kraly FS. Effects of eating on drinking. In: Ramsay DJ, Booth DA, editors. Thirst. London, UK: Springer-Verlag; 1991. p. 296–312.

[7] Du Vigneaud V. Hormones of the posterior pituitary gland: oxytocin and vasopressin. In: Du Vigneaud V, Bing RJ, Oncley JL, editors. The harvey lectures 1954–55. Orlando: Academic Press; 1956. p. 1–24.

[8] Sawyer W. Evolution of antidiuretic hormones and functions. Am J Med 1967;42:678–86.

[9] Haymaker W. Hypothalamo–pituirary neural pathways and the circulatory systems of the pituitary. In: Haymaker W, et al., editors. The hypothalamus. Springfield, IL: Charles C Thomas; 1969. p. 219.

[10] Scharrer E, Scharrer B. Hormones produced by neurosecretory cells. Recent Prog Horm Res 1954;10:183–240.

[11] Schwaab DE. Neurohypophysial peptides in the human hypothalamus in relation to development, sexual differentiation, aging and disease. Regul Pept 1993;45:143–7.

[12] Schwaab DE. Aging of the human hypothalamus. Horm Res 1995;43:8–11.

[13] Sofroniew MY, Weindl A, Schrell U, Wetzstein R. Immunohistochemistry of vasopressin, oxytocin and neurophysin in the hypothalamus and extrahypothalamic regions of the human and primate brain. Acta Histochem 1981;34(Suppl.):79–95.

[14] Zimmerman EA. The organization of oxytocin and vasopressin pathways. In: Martin JB, Reichlin S, Bick KL, editors. Neurosecretion and brain peptides. New York: Raven Press; 1981. p. 63–75.

and 133 to 145 mmols/L, respectively. Within each person, however, these values are maintained even more tightly about half-way between his or her own setpoint for thirst and vasopressin secretion. From that point, even a tiny increase or decrease in tonicity resulting from a change in water or sodium balance

[15] Fujisawa I. Magnetic resonance imaging of the hypothalamic–neurohypophyseal system. J Neuroendocrinol 2004;16:297–302.

[16] Tom JN, Assinder SJ. Oxytocin in health and disease. Internat J Biochem Cell Biol 2010;42(2):202–5.

[17] Schmale H, Fehr S, Richter D. Vasopressin synthesis: from gene to peptide hormone. Kidney Int Suppl 1987;21:S8–13.

[18] Brownstein MJ, Russell JT, Gainer H. Synthesis, transport and release of posterior pituitary hormones. Science 1980;207:373–8.

[19] Breslow E. The conformation and functional domains of neurophysins. In: Gross P, Richter D, Robertson GL, editors. Vasopressin. Paris: John Libbey Eurotext; 1993. p. 143–55.

[20] Breslow E. The neurophysins. Adv Enzymol 1974;40:271–333.

[21] Sachs H, Fawcett P, Takabatake Y, Portanova R. Biosynthesis and release of vasopressin and neurophysin. Recent Prog Horm Res 1969;25:447–91.

[22] Moses AM, Miller M. Accumulation and release of pituitary vasopressin in rats heterozygous for hypothalamic diabetes insipidus. Endocrinology 1970;86:34–41.

[23] Rao VV, Loffler C, Battey J, Hansmann I. The human gene for oxytocin neurophysin I (OXT) is physically mapped to chromosome 20p13 by in situ hybridization. Cytogenet Cell Genet 1992;61:271–3.

[24] Sausville E, Carney D, Battey J. The human vasopressin gene is linked to the oxytocin gene and is selectively expressed in a cultured lung cancer cell line. J Biol Chem 1985;260:10236–41.

[25] Richter D. Molecular events in expression of vasopressin and oxytocin and their cognate receptors. Am J Physiol 1988;255:F207.

[26] Iwasaki Y, Oiso Y, Saito H, Majzoub JA. Positive and negative regulation of the rat vasopressin gene promoter. Endocrinology 1997;138(12):5266–74.

[27] Zingg HH, Lefebvre D, Almazang G. Regulation of vasopressin gene expression in rat hypothalamic neurons; response to osmotic stimulation. J Biol Chem 1986;261(28):12956–9.

[28] Ueta Y, Fujihara H, Dayanithi G, Kawata M, Murphy D. Specific Expression of optically active reporter gene in arginine vasopressin-secreting neurosecretory cells in the hypothalamic–neurohypophyseal system. J Neuroendocrinol 2008;20(6):660–4.

[29] Robinson AG, Roberts MM, Evron WA, Verbalis JG, Sherman TG. Hyponatremia in rats induces downregulation of vasopressin synthesis. J Clin Invest 1990;86:1023–9.

[30] Ivell R, Richter D. Structure and comparison of the oxytocin and vasopressin genes from rat. Proc Nat Acad Sci USA 1984;81:2006–10.

[31] Ruppert S, Scherer G, Schutz G. Recent gene conversion involving bovine vasopressin and oxytocin precursor genes suggested by the nucleotide sequence. Nature 1984;308:554–7.

[32] Hara Y, Battey J, Gainer H. Structure of mouse vasopressin and oxytocin genes. Mol Brain Res 1990;8:319–24.

[33] Mohr E, Schmitz E, Richter D. A single rat genomic DNA fragment encodes both the oxytocin and vasopressin genes separated by 11 kilobases and oriented in opposite transcriptional directions. Biochimie 1988;70:649–54.

[34] Mohr E, Bahnsen U, Kiessling C, Richter D. Expression of the vasopressin and oxytocin genes in rats occurs in mutually exclusive sets of hypothalamic neurons. FEBS Lett 1988;242:144–8.

[35] Dayanithi G, Viero C, Shibuya I. The role of calcium in the action and release of vasopressin and ocytocin from CNS neurons/terminals to the heart. J Physiol Pharmacol 2008;59(S8):7–26.

[36] McDonald NA, Kuzmiski JB, Naderi N, SDchwab Y, Pittman QJ. Endogenous modulators of synaptic transmission: cannabinoid regulation in the supraoptic nucleus. Prog Brain Res 2008;170:129–36.

[37] Engel PA, Rowe JW, Minnaker KL, Robertson GL. Effect of exogenous vasopressin on vasopressin release. Am J Physiol 1984;246(9):E202–7.

[38] Panatier A. Glial cells: indispensable partners of hypothalamic magnocellular neurone. J Neuroendocrinol 2009;21:665–72.

[39] Jochberger S, Dorler J, Luckner G, Mayr VD, Wenzel V, Ulmer H, et al. The vasopressin and copeptin response to infection, severe sepsis and septic shock. Crit Care Med 2009;37(2):476–82.

[40] Szinnai G, Morgenthaler NG, Berneis K, Struck J, Muller B, Keller U, et al. Changes in plasma copeptin, the C-terminal portion of arginine vasopressin during water deprivation and excess in healthy subjects. J Clin Endocrinol Metab 2007;92(10):3973–8.

[41] Seif SM, Robinson AG. Localization and release of neurophysins. Ann Rev Physiol 1978;40:45–76.

[42] Breslow E. Chemistry and biology of the neurophysins. Ann Rev Biochem 1979;48:251–74.

[43] Preibisz JJ, Sealey JE, Laragh JH, Cody RJ, Weksler BB. Plasma and platelet vasopressin in essential hypertension and congestive heart failure. Hypertension 1983;5(SI):I1129–38.

[44] Bichet DG, Arthus MF, Barjon JM, Lonergan M, Kortas C. Human platelet fraction arginine vasopressin. Potential physiologic role. J Clin Invest 1987;79(3):881–7.

[45] Robertson GL. Vasopressin function in health and disease. Recent Prog Horm Res 1977;33:333–85.

[46] Robertson GL, Athar S, Shelton RL. Osmotic control of vasopressin function. In: Andreoli TE, Grantham JJ, Rector Jr RC, editors. Disturbances in body fluid osmolality. Bethesda, MD: American Physiological Society; 1977. p. 125–48.

[47] Verney EB. The antidiuretic hormone and the factors which determine its release. Proc R Soc Lond (Biol) 1947;135:25–106.

[48] Gardiner TW, Verbalis G, Stricker EM. Impaired secretion of vasopressin and oxytocin in rats after lesions of nucleus medianus. Am J Physiol 1985;249:R681–8.

[49] Jewell PA, Verney EB. An experimental attempt to determine the site of the neurohypophyseal osmoreceptors in the dog. Philos Trans R Soc Lond (Biol) 1957;240:197–324.

[50] Mangiapane ML, Thrasher TN, Keil LC, Simpson JB, Ganong WF. Deficits in drinking and vasopressin secretion after lesions of the nucleus medianus. Neuroendocrinology 1983;37:73–7.

[51] Peck JW, Blass EM. Localization of thirst and antidiuretic osmoreceptors by intracranial injections in rats. Am Physiol 1975;228:1501–9.

[52] McKinley MJ, Mathai ML, McAllen RM, McClear RC, Miselis RR, Pennington GL, et al. Vasopressin secretion: osmotic and hormonal regulation by the lamina terminalis. J Neuroendocrinol 2004;16:340–7.

[53] Van Germert M, Miller M, Carey RJ, Moses AM. Polyuria and impaired ADH release following medial preoptic lesioning in the rat. Am Physiol 1975;228:1293–7.

[54] Robertson GL. Disorders of thirst in man. In: Ramsay D, editor. Thirst: physiological and psychological aspects. London: Springer-Verlag; 1991. p. 453–75.

[55] Robertson GL. Physiopathology of ADH secretion. In: Tolis G, Labrie F, Martin JB, et al., editors. Clinical neuroendocrinology: a pathophysiological approach. New York: Raven Press; 1979. p. 247–60.

[56] Halter JB, Goldberg AP, Robertson GL, Porte Jr. D. Selective osmoreceptor dysfunction in the syndrome of chronic hypernatremia. J Clin Endo Metab 1977;44:609–16.

[57] Robertson GL, Shelton RL, Athar S. The osmoregulation of vasopressin. Kidney Int 1976;10:25–37.

[58] Zerbe RL, Miller JZ, Robertson GL. The reproducibility and heritability of individual differences in osmoregulatory function in normal humans. J Lab Clin Med 1991;117:51–9.

[59] Hancock ML, Bichet DG, Eckert JG, Bankir L, Wagner MA, Pratt JH. Race, sex and the redulation of urine osmolarity: observations made during water deprivation. Am J Physiol Regul Integr Comp Phsiol 2010;299:R977—80.

[60] Moses AM. Is there an osmotic threshold for vasopressin release? Am J Physiol 1978;234:E339—40.

[61] Rodbard D, Munson PJ. Editorial comment. Am J Physiol 1978;234:E340—2.

[62] Weitzman RE, Fisher DA. Log—linear relationship between plasma arginine vasopressin and plasma osmolality. Am J Physiol 1977;233:E37—40.

[63] Robertson GL. Physiology of ADH secretion. Kidney Int 1987;32:S20—6.

[64] Baylis PH, Robertson GL. Plasma vasopressin response to hypertonic saline infusion to assess posterior pituitary function. J Roy Soc Med 1980;73:255—60.

[65] Evbuomwan IO, Davison JM, Baylis PH, Murdoch AP. Altered osmotic thresholds for arginine vasopressin secretion and thirst during superovulation and in the ovarian hyperstimulation syndrome (OHSS): relevance to the pathophysiology of OHSS. Fertil Steril 2001;75:933—41.

[66] Vokes TJ, Weiss NM, Schreiber J, Gaskill MB, Robertson GL. Osmoregulation of thirst and vasopressin during normal menstrual cycle. Am J Physiol 1988;254:R641—7.

[67] Stachenfeld NS, Keefe DL. Estrogen effects on osmotic regulation of AVP and fluid balance. Am J Physiol 2002;283(4):E711—21.

[68] Weitzman RE, Fisher DA, DiStefano III JH, Bennett CM. Episodic secretion of arginine vasopressin. Am J Physiol 1977;233:E32—6.

[69] Armstrong W. Morphological and electrophysiological classification of hypothalamic supraoptic neurons. Prog Neurobiol 1995;47(4—5):291—339.

[70] McKinley MJ, Denton DA, Weisinger RS. Sensors for antidiuresis and thirst — osmoreceptors or CSF sodium detectors? Brain Res 1978;141:89—103.

[71] Thrasher TN, Brown CJ, Keil LC, Ramsay DJ. Thirst and vasopressin release in the dog: an osmoreceptor or sodium receptor mechanism? Am J Physiol 1980;238:R333—9.

[72] Zerbe RL, Robertson GL. Osmoregulation of thirst and vasopressin secretion in human subjects: effect of various solutes. Am J Physiol 1983;224:E607—14.

[73] Olsson K, Kolmodin R. Dependence of basic secretion of antidiuretic hormone on cerebrospinal fluid (Na). Acta Physiol Scand 1974;91:286—8.

[74] Vokes T, Aycinena PR, Robertson GL. Effect of insulin on osmoregulation of vasopressin. Am J Physiol 1987;252:E538—48.

[75] Robertson GL. Thirst and vasopressin function in normal and disordered states of water balance. J Lab Clin Med 1983;101 (3):351—71.

[76] Wade CE, Keil LC, Ramsay DJ. Role of volume and osmolality in the control of plasma vasopressin in dehydrated dogs. Neuroendocrinology 1983;37:349—53.

[77] Zerbe RL, Henry D, Robertson GL. Vasopressin response to orthostatic hypotension: etiological and clinical implications. Am J Med 1983;74:265—71.

[78] Iwasaki Y, Gaskill MB, Robertson GL. Adaptive resetting of the volume control of vasopressin secretion during sustained hypovolemia. Am J Physiol 1995;268:R349—57.

[79] Goetz KL, Wang BC, Sundet WD. Comparative effects of cardiac receptors and sinoaortic baroreceptors on elevations of plasma vasopressin and renin activity elicited by haemorrhage. J Physiol (Lond) 1984;879:440—5.

[80] Iwasaki Y, Gaskill MB, Robertson GL. The effect of selective opioid antagonists on vasopressin secretion in the rat. Endocrinology 1994;134:55—62.

[81] Iwasaki Y, Gaskill MB, Boss CA, Robertson GL. The effect of the non-selective opioid antagonist diprenorphine on vasopressin secretion in the rat. Endocrinology 1994;134:48—54.

[82] Iwasaki Y, Gaskill MB, Fu R, Saper CB, Robertson GL. Opioid antagonist diprenorphine microinjected in parabrachial nucleus selectively inhibits vasopressin response ro hypovolemic stimuli in the rat. J Clin Invest 1993;92:2230—9.

[83] Robertson GL, Oiso Y, Vokes TP, Gaskill MB. Diprenorphine inhibits selectively the vasopressin response to hypovolemic stimuli. Trans Assoc Am Physicians 1985;98:322—33.

[84] Kirchheim HR. Systemic arterial baroreceptor reflexes. Physiol Rev 1976;56:100—76.

[85] Lee M, Thrasher TN, Keil LC, Ramsay DJ. Cardiac receptors, vasopressin, and corticosteroid release during arterial hypotension in dogs. Am J Physiol 1986;251:R614—20.

[86] Sawchenko PE, Swanson LW. Central noradrenergic pathways for the integration of hypothalamic neuroendocrine and autonomic responses. Science 1981;214:685—7.

[87] Berl T, Cadnapaphornachai P, Harbottle JA, Schrier RW. Mechanism of suppression of vasopressin during alpha-adrenergic stimulation with norepinephrine. J Clin Invest 1974;53:219—27.

[88] Billman GE, Keyl MJ, Dickey DT, Kern DC, Keil LC, Stone HL. Hormonal and renal response to plasma volume expansion in the primate Macaca mulatta. Am J Physiol 1983;244:H201—5.

[89] Jhamandas JH, Renaud LP. Neurophysiology of a central baroreceptor pathway projecting to hypothalamic vasopressin neurons. Can J Neurol Sci 1987;14:17—24.

[90] Shimamoto K, Miyahara M. Effect of norepinephine infusion on plasma vasopressin levels in normal human subjects. Clin Endocrinol Metab 1976;43:201—4.

[91] Schrier RW, Bed T, Harbottle JA. Mechanism of the antidiuretic effect associated with interruption of parasympathetic pathways. J Clin Invest 1972;51:2613—20.

[92] Thames MD, Schmid PG. Cardiopulmonary receptors with vagal afferents tonically inhibit ADH release in the dog. Am J Physiol 1979;237:H299—304.

[93] Ando T, Shimamoto K, Nakahashi Y, Nishitani T, Hosoda S, Ishida H, et al. Plasma antidiuretic hormone levels in patients with normal and low renin essential hypertension and secondary hypertension. Endocrinol Jpn 1983;30(4):567—70.

[94] Robertson GL, Ganguly A. Osmoregulation and baroregulation of plasma vasopressin in essential hypertension. J Cardiovasc Pharmacol 1986;8:S87—91.

[95] Ganguly A, Robertson GL. Elevated threshold for vasopressin release in primary aldosteronism. Clin Res 1980;28:330A (abstr).

[96] Moses AM, Miller M, Streeten DHP. Quantitative influence of blood volume expansion on the osmotic threshold for vasopressin release. Clin Endocrinol Metab 1967;27:655—62.

[97] Robertson GL, Athar S. The interaction of blood osmolality and blood volume in regulating plasma vasopressin in man. J Clin Endocrinol Metab 1976;42:613—20.

[98] Stricker EM, Verbalis JG. Interaction of osmotic and volume stimuli in regulation of neurohypophyseal secretion in rats. Am J Physiol 1986;250:R267—75.

[99] Kannan H, Yagi K. Supraoptic neurosecretory neurons: evidence for the existence of converging inputs both from carotid baroreceptors and osmoreceptors. Brain Res 1978;145:385—90.

[100] Rowe JW, Shelton RL, Helderman JH, Vestal RE, Robertson GL. Influence of the emetic reflex on vasopressin release in man. Kidney Int 1979;16:729—35.

[101] Miaskiewicz SL, Stricker EM, Verbalis JG. Neurohypophyseal secretion in response to cholecystokinin but not meal-induced

gastric distension in humans. J Clin Endocrinol Metab 1989;68:837—43.

[102] Verbalis JG, Richardson DW, Stricker EM. Vasopressin release in response to nausea-producing agents and cholecystokinin ip monkeys. Am J Physiol 1987;252:R749—53.

[103] McCann MJ, Verbalis JG, Stricker EM. LiCI and CCK inhibit gastric emptying and feeding and stimulate OT secretion in rats. Am J Physiol 1989;256:R463—8.

[104] Duke HN, Pickford M, Watt JA. The antidiuretic effect of morphine: its site and mode of action in the hypothalamus of the dog. Q J Exp Physiol 1951;36:149—58.

[105] Cates JE, Garrod O. The effect of nicotine on urinary flow in diabetes insipidus. Clin Sci 1951;10:145—60.

[106] Eversmann T, Guttsmann M, Uhlich E, Ulbrecht G, von Werder K, Scriba PC. Increased secretion of growth hormone, prolactin, antidiuretic hormone and cortisol induced by the stress of motion sickness. Aviat Space Environ Med 1978;49:53—7.

[107] Steele TH, Serpick AA, Block JB. Antidiuretic response to cyclophosphamide in man. J Pharmacol Exp Ther 1973;185:245—53.

[108] Heyes M, Farber MO, Manfredi F, Robertson GL, Fineberg NS, Manfredi F. Acute effects of hypoxia on renal and endocrine function in normal man. Am J Physiol 1982;243:R265—70.

[109] Zerbe RL, Vinicor F, Robertson GL. Plasma vasopressin in uncontrolled diabetes mellitus. Diabetes 1979;28:503—8.

[110] Wiggins RC, Basar I, Slater JD, Forsling M, Ramage CM. Vasovagal hypotension and vasopressin release. Clin Endocrinol 1977;6:387—93.

[111] Coutinho EM. Oxytocic and antidiuretic effects of nausea in women. Am J Obstet Gynecol 1969;105:127—31.

[112] Baylis PH, Zerbe RL, Robertson GL. Arginine vasopressin response to insulin-induced hypoglycemia in man. J Clin Endocrinol Metab 1981;53:935—40.

[113] Baylis PH, Robertson GL. Rat vasopressin response to insulin induced hypoglycemia. Endocrinology 1980;107:1975—9.

[114] Baylis PH, Robertson GL. Vasopressin response to 2-deoxy-d-glucose in the rat. Endocrinology 1980;107:1970—4.

[115] Thompson DA, Cambell RG, Lilavivat U, Welle SL, Robertson GL. Increased thirst and plasma arginine vasopressin levels during 2-deoxy_d-glucose-induced glucoprivation in humans. J Clin Invest 1981;67:1083—93.

[116] Mouw D, Bonjour JP, Malvin RL, Vander A. Central action of angiotensin in stimulating ADH release. Am J Physiol 1971;220:239—42.

[117] Keil Le, Summy-Long J, Severs WE. Release of vasopressin by angiotensin II. Endocrinology 1975;96:1063—5.

[118] Shimizu K, Share L, Claybaugh JR. Potentiation of angiotensin II of the vasopressin response to an increasing plasma osmolality. Endocrinology 1973;93:42—50.

[119] Yamaguchi K, Koike M, Hama H. Plasma vasopressin response to peripheral administration of angiotensin in conscious rats. Am J Physiol 1985;248:R249—56.

[120] Cadnapaphornachai P, Boykin J, Harbottle JA, McDonald KM, Schrier RW. Effect of angiotensin II on renal water excretion. Am J Physiol 1975;228:155—9.

[121] McKinley MJ, Allen AM, Mathai ML, May C, McCallen RM. Brain angiotensin and body fluid homeostasis. Jpn J Physiol 2001;51:281—9.

[122] Rydin H, Verney EB. The inhibition of water-diuresis by emotional stress and by muscular exercise. Q J Exp Physiol 1938;27:373—4.

[123] Edelson JT, Robertson GL. The effect of the cold pressor test on vasopressin secretion in man. Psychoneuroendocrinology 1986;11:307—16.

[124] Keil LC, Severs WE. Reduction of plasma vasopressin levels of dehydrated rats following acute stress. Endocrinology 1977;100:30—8.

[125] Engelmann M, Ludwig M. The activity of the hypothalamo—eurohypophysial system in response to acute stressor exposure: neuroendocrine and electrophysiological observations. Stress 2004;7(2):91—6.

[126] Aguilera G, Subburaju S, Young S, Chen J. The parvocellular vasopressinergic system and responsiveness of the hypothalamic pituitary adrenal axis during chronic stress. Prog Brain Res 2008;170:29—39.

[127] Segar WE, Moore WW. The regulation of antidiuretic hormone release in man. J Clin Invest 1968;47:2143—51.

[128] Takamata A, Mack GW, Stachenfeld MS, Nadel ER. Body temperature modification of osmotically induced vasopressin secretion and thirst in humans. Am J Physiol 1995;269:R874—80.

[129] Kasting NW, Mazurek MF, Martin JB. Endotoxin increases vasopressin release independently of known phsysiologic stimuli. Am J Physiol 1985;248:E420—4.

[130] Parrott RF, Vellucci SV, Goode JA, Lloyd DM, Forsling ML. Interrelated adrenocortical and neurohypophyseal responses associated with fever in endotoxin treated pigs. Am J Physiol 1997;273:R1046—52.

[131] Giusti-Piava A, Branco LGS, deCastro M, Autunes-Rodriguez J, Carnio EC. Role of nitric oxide in thermoregulation during septic shock: involvement of vasopressin. Pflugers Archiv-European J Physiol 2003;447(2):175—80.

[132] Davison JM, Shiells EA, Philips PR, Lindheimer MD. Suppression of AVP release by drinking despite hypertonicity during and after gestation. Am J Physiol 1988;254:F588—92.

[133] Geelen G, Keil LC, Kravik SE, Wade CE, Thrasher TN, Barnes PR, et al. Inhibition of plasma vasopressin after drinking in dehydrated humans. Am J Physiol 1984;247:R968—71.

[134] Thompson CJ, Burd JM, Baylis PH. Acute suppression of plasma vasopressin and thirst after drinking in hypernatremic humans. Am J Physiol 1987;252:RI138—42.

[135] Bevilacqua M, Norbiato G, Chebat E, Raggi U, Cavaiani P, Guzzetti R, et al. Osmotic and nonosmotic control of vasopressin release in the elderly: effect of metoclopramide. J Clin Endocrinol Metab 1987;65(6):1243—7.

[136] Helderman JH, Vestal RE, Rowe JW, Tobin JD, Andres R, Robertson GL. The response of arginine vasopressin to intravenous ethanol and hypertonic saline in man: the impact of aging. J Gerontol 1978;33:39—47.

[137] Ledingham JGG, Crowe MJ, Forsling ML, Phillips PA, Rolls BJ. Effects of aging on vasopressin secretion, water excretion and thirst in man. Kidney Int 1987;32(Suppl. 21):S90—2.

[138] Miller M. Fluid and electrolyte homeostasis in the elderly: physiological changes of ageing and clinical consequences. Baillieres Clin Endocrinol Metab 1997;11:367—87.

[139] Hofman MA. Lifespan changes in the human hypothalamus. Exp Gerontol 1997;32(4—5):559—75.

[140] Terano T, Seya A, Tamura Y, Yoshida S, Hirayama T. Characteristics of the pituitary gland in elderly subjects from magnetic resonance images: relationship to pituitary hormone secretion. Clin Endocrinol 1996;45:273—9.

[141] Crowe MJ, Forsling MJ, Rolls BJ, Phillips PA, Ledingham JG, Smith RF. Altered water excretion in healthy elderly men. Age Ageing 1987;16:285—93.

[142] Rowe JW, Andres R, Tobin JD, Norris AH, Shock NW. The effect of age on creatinine clearance in men: a cross-sectional and longitudinal study. J Geront 1976;31:155—63.

[143] Barron WM. Water metabolism and vasopressin secretion during pregnancy. Baillieres Clin Obstet Gynaecol 1987;1:853—71.

[144] Lindheimer MD, Davison JM. Osmoregulation, the secretion of arginine vasopressin and its metabolism during pregnancy. Eur J Endocrinol 1995;132:133–43.

[145] Spruce BA, Baylis PH, Burd J, Watson MJ. Variation of osmoregulation of arginine vasopressin during the human menstrual cycle. Clin Endocrinol 1985;22:37–42.

[146] Calzone WL, Silva C, Keefe DL. Progesterone does not alter osmotic regulation of AVP. Am J Physiol 2001;281(6): R2011–20.

[147] Gold PW, Robertson GL, Post RM, Stachenfeld NS. The effect of lithium on the osmoregulation of arginine vasopressin secretion. J Clin Endocrinol Metab 1983;56:295–9.

[148] Kjaer A, Knigge U, Jorgensen H, Warberg J. Dehydration induced vasopressin secretion in humans: involvement of the histaminergic system. Am J Physiol 2000;279(6):E1305–10.

[149] Oiso Y, Iwasaki Y, Kondo K, Takatsuki K, Tomita A. Effect of the opioid kappa-receptor agonist U50488H on the secretion of arginine vasopressin. Neuroendocrinology 1988;48:658–62.

[150] Miller M. Role of endogenous opioids in neurohypophyseal function of man. J Clin Endocrinol Metab 1980;50:1016–20.

[151] van Wimersma Greidanus TB, Thody TJ, Verspaget H, de Rotte GA, Goedemans HJ, Croiset G, et al. Effects of morphine and β endorphin on basal and elevated plasma levels of alpha-MSH and vasopressin. Life Sci 1979;24:579–86.

[152] Oiso Y, Robertson GL. Role of endogenous opiates in mediating ethanol-induced suppression of vasopressin. Endocrinology 1982;751:267 (abstr)

[153] Gold PW, Robertson GL, Ballenger JC, Kaye W, Chen J, Rubinow DR, et al. Carbamazepine diminishes the sensitivity of the plasma arginine vasopressin response to osmotic stimulation. J Clin Endocrinol Metab 1983;57:952–7.

[154] Lausen HD. Metabolism of the neurohypophysial hormones. In: Geige SR, editor. Handbook of physiology, section 7. Endocrinology Vol. IV, Part 1. Bethesda, MD: American Physiological Society; 1974. p. 287–393.

[155] Davison JM, Sheills EA, Barron WM, Robinson AG, Lindheimer MD. Changes in the metabolic clearance of vasopressin and in plasma vasopressinase throughout human pregnancy. J Clin Invest 1989;83:1313–8.

[156] Birnbaumer M. Vasopressin receptors. Trends Endocrinol Metab 2000;11(1):406–10.

[157] Maybauer MO, Maybauer DM, Enkhbaatar P, Traber DL. Physiol Vasopressin Recept 2008;22(2):253–63.

[158] Thibonnier M. Genetics of vasopressin receptors. Curr Hypertens Rep 2004;6:21–6.

[159] Manning M, Stoev S, Chini B, Durroux T, Mouillac B, Guillon G. Peptide and non-peptide agonists and antagonists for the vasopressin and oxytocin V1a, V1b, V2 and OT receptors: research tools and potential therapeutic agents. Prog Brain Res 2008;170:473–512.

[160] Robertson GL. Vaptans for the treatment of hyponatremia. Nat Rev Endocrinol 2011;7(3):151–61.

[161] Sasaki S, Noda Y. Aquaporin-2 protein dynamics within the cell. Curr Opin Nephrol Hypertens 2007;16:348–52.

[162] Fenton RA, Moeller HB. Recent discoveries in vasopressin-regulated aquaporin-2 trafficking. Prog Brain Res 2008;170: 571–9.

[163] Brown D, Hasler U, Nunes P, Bouley R, Lu HAJ. Phosphorylation events and modulation of aquaporin 2 cell surface expression. Curr Opin Nephrol Hypertens 2008;17:491–8.

[164] Hoffert JD, Chou C, Knepper MA. Aquaporin-2 in the "-omics" era. J Biol Chem 2009;284(22):14683–7.

[165] Zerbe RL, Robertson GL. A comparison of plasma vasopressin measurements with a standard indirect test in the differential diagnosis of polyuria. N Engl J Med 1981;305:1539–46.

[166] Yang B, Bankir L. Urea and urine concentrating ability: new insights from studies in mice. Am J Physiol 2005;288: F881–96.

[167] Fenton RA. Essential role of vasopressin regulated urea transport processes in the mammalian kidney. Pfluger Arch-Eur J Physiol 2009;458:169–77.

[168] Bankir L, Bichet DG, Bouby N. Vasopressin V2 receptors, ENaC and sodium reabsorption: a risk factor for hypertension. Am J Physiol Renal Physiol 2010;299:F917–28.

[169] Voelckel WG, Covertino VA, Lurie KG, Karlbauer A, Schochl H, Lindner KH, et al. Vasopressin for hemorrhagic shock management: revisiting the potential value in civilian and combat casualty care. J Trauma 2010;69:S69–74.

[170] Oliver JA, Landry DW. Endogenous and exogenous vasopressin in shock. Curr Opin Crit Care 2007;13:376–82.

[171] Tomasiak M, Stelmach H, Rusak T, Ciborowski M, Radziwon P. Vasopressin acts on platelets to generate procoagulant activity. Blood Coagul Fibrinolysis 2008;19:615–24.

[172] Caldwell HK, Lee HJ, Macbeth AH, Young WH. Vasopressin: behavioral roles of an "original" neuropeptide. Prog Neurobiol 2008;84(1):1–24.

[173] Heinrichs M, Domes G. Neuropeptides and social behavior: effects of oxytocin and vasopressin in humans. Prog Brain Res 2008;170:337–50.

[174] Donaldson ZR, Young LJ. Oxytocin, vasopressin and the neurogenetics of sociality. Science 2008;322(5903):900–4.

[175] Serradeil-Le Gal C, Wagnon J, Tonnerre B, Roux R, Garcia G, Griebel G, et al. An overview of SSR149415, a selective non-peptide vasopressin V1b receptor antagonist for the treatment of stress related disorders. CNS Drug Rev 2005;11(1):53–68.

[176] Egan G, Silk T, Zamarripa F, Williams J, Federico P, Cunnington R, et al. Neural correlates of the emergence of consciousness of thirst. Proc Nat Acad Sci USA 2003;100 (25):15241–6.

[177] Farrel MJ, Egan GF, Zamarripa F, Shade R, Blair-West J, Fox P, et al. Unique, common and interacting cortical correlates of thirst and pain. Proc Soc Nat Acad Sci USA 2006;103(7):2416–21.

[178] Andersson B. Regulation of water intake. Physiol Rev 1978;58:582–603.

[179] Erickson S, Simon-Oppermann C, Simon E, Gray DA. Occlusion of rostroventral 3rd ventricle abolishes drinking but not AVP release in response to central osmotic stimulation. Brain Res 1988;448(1):121–7.

[180] McKinley MJ, Cairns MJ, Denton DA, Egan C, Mathai ML, Uschakov A, et al. Physiological and pathophysiological influences on thirst. Physiol Behav 2004;81(5):795–803.

[181] Weiss NM, Conder ML, Robertson GL. The effect of hypovolemia on the osmoregulation of thirst and AVP. Clin Res 1984;32:786A.

[182] Figaro MK, Mack GW. Control of fluid intake in dehydrated humans: role of oropharyngeal stimulation. Am J Physiol 1997;272:R1740–6.

[183] DeCastro JM. A microregulatory analysis of spontaneous fluid intake by humans: evidence that the amount of fluid ingestion and its timing is governed by feeding. Physiol Behav 1988;43:705–14.

[184] DeCastro JM. The relation of spontaneous macronutrient and sodium intake with fluid ingestion and thirst in humans. Physiol Behav 1991;49:513–9.

[185] Kenney WL, Chiu P. Influence of age on thirst and fluid intake. Med Sci Sports Exerc 2001;33(9):1524–32.

[186] Kovacs L, Rittig S, Robertson GL. Effects of sustained antidiuretic treatment on plasma sodium concentration and body water homeostasis in healthy humans on *ad libitum* fluid intake. Clin Res 1991;40:165A (abst).

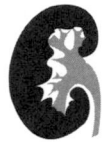

The Urine Concentrating Mechanism and Urea Transporters

Jeff M. Sands[1] and Harold E. Layton[2]

[1]Renal Division, Department of Medicine, Emory University School of Medicine, Atlanta, GA, USA

[2]Department of Mathematics, Duke University, Durham, NC, USA

The ability to vary water excretion is essential for mammals, which generally do not have continuous access to water, but must maintain a nearly constant blood plasma osmolality. Mammals, therefore, need a mechanism that allows them to regulate water loss to closely match water intake. In addition, because sodium and its anions are the principal osmotic constituents of blood plasma, and plasma sodium concentration must be kept nearly constant, water loss must be regulated by a mechanism that decouples water and sodium. These critical regulatory capabilities are provided by the kidney's urine concentrating mechanism: when water intake is large enough to dilute blood plasma, urine more dilute than plasma is produced to concentrate the plasma; when water intake is so small that blood plasma is concentrated, urine more concentrated than plasma is produced to dilute the plasma. In both cases, the rate of sodium excretion is small and varies little; indeed, the total solute excretion rate varies little (Figure 43.1).

Urine osmolality varies widely in response to changes in water intake. Following a prolonged period without water intake, such as occurs when an individual sleeps, human urine osmolality may rise to ~1200 mOsm/kg H_2O, about four times plasma osmolality (~290 mOsm/kg H_2O). However, following the ingestion of large quantities of water, such as commonly occurs at breakfast, urine osmolality may decrease rapidly. Humans (and other mammalian species) are able to dilute their urine to ~50 mOsm/kg H_2O. Such large and rapid changes in osmolality require that the cells of the inner medulla have adaptive mechanisms (e.g., osmolytes) to protect them from osmotic damage.

Maximum urine osmolality varies widely among mammalian species. The long-nosed bat *Leptonycteris sanborni* can concentrate only to about 350 mOsm/kg H_2O, while the Australian hopping mouse *Notomys alexis* can concentrate to nearly 9400 mOsm/kg H_2O.[1] Primates can typically concentrate their urines from ~1000 to 2000 mOsm/kg H_2O.[1-3] Beluga whales and bottle-nosed dolphins, which have access only to hypertonic ocean water (~1000 mOsm/kg H_2O), can concentrate urine up to ~1800 mOsm/kg H_2O.[4] Most laboratory data relevant to the urine concentrating mechanism have been obtained from rabbits or rodents that can achieve higher maximum urine osmolalities than humans: the European rabbit can concentrate to ~1400 mOsm/kg H_2O, whereas the eastern cotton tail can concentrate to ~3300 mOsm/kg H_2O; rats to ~3000 mOsm/kg H_2O; mice and hamsters to ~4000 mOsm/kg H_2O; and chinchillas to ~7600 mOsm/kg H_2O.[1,4,5]

Regardless of maximum concentrating ability, the kidneys of all mammals maintain an osmotic gradient that increases from the cortico-medullary boundary to the tip of the medulla (papillary tip). This osmotic gradient is sustained even in diuresis, although it is diminished in magnitude relative to antidiuresis.[6,7] The major constituent of the osmotic gradient in the outer medulla is NaCl; in the inner medulla, the major constituents are NaCl and urea.[6,7] The cortex is nearly isotonic to plasma, while the papillary tip is hypertonic to plasma and, in antidiuresis, has osmolality similar to urine.[5] The major urinary solutes are sodium and potassium accompanied by univalent anions and by urea; urea is the predominant solute in urine during antidiuresis.[6,7] The sodium, potassium, and urea concentrations in rat plasma, papillary tissue, and urine,

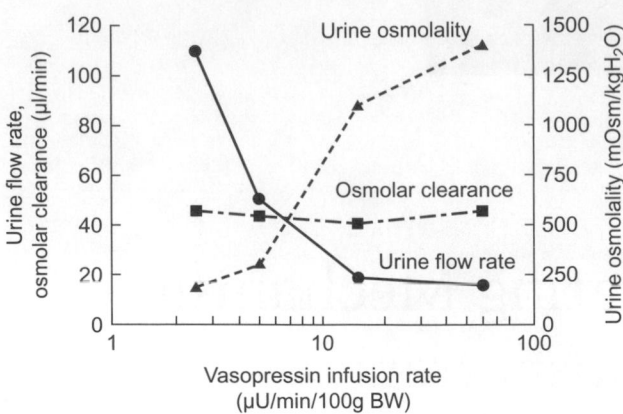

FIGURE 43.1 Independent control of water and solute excretion. Rats were infused with exogenous vasopressin and given a water-load (4% of body weight) to suppress endogenous vasopressin secretion. Vasopressin infusion causes a significant decrease in urine flow rate (left axis, circles) and increase in urine osmolality (right axis, triangles), but has little effect on osmolar clearance (left axis, squares). *(Figure is modified, with permission, from reference [232], using data from reference [450].)*

TABLE 43.1 Plasma, Papilla, and Urine Composition During Diuresis and Antidiuresis in Rats

A. Diuresis (urine flow/animal = 192:l/min)

Component	Plasma	Papilla	Urine
Na$^+$ (mEq/l)	138	159	5.4
K$^+$ (mEq/l)	6.0	66.0	5.9
Urea (mM)	4.5	34.1	22.6
Osmolality (mOsm/kg H$_2$O)	304	572	59

B. Antidiuresis (urine flow/animal = ~5:l/min)

Component	Plasma	Papilla	Urine
Na$^+$ (mEq/l)	145	417	148
K$^+$ (mEq/l)	6.7	102	140
Urea (mM)	4.4	605	946
Osmolality (mOsm/kg H$_2$O)	314	1832	1805

The data given in this table is from tables and figures in references [6,36,454].

during both diuresis and antidiuresis, are given in Table 43.1.

The mechanisms responsible for the separate control of water and sodium excretion are largely located in the renal medulla, where the nephron segments and vasa recta are arranged in complex but specific anatomic relationships, both in terms of which segments connect to which segments, and in terms of three-dimensional configuration. The production of concentrated urine involves complex interactions among the nephron segments and vasculature. In the outer medulla, thick ascending limbs of the loop of Henle

actively absorb NaCl, diluting the luminal fluid and providing NaCl to increase the osmolality of the medullary interstitium, pars recta, descending limbs, collecting ducts, and vasculature. The countercurrent configuration of nephron segments and vessels allows the generation of a medullary osmolality gradient along the cortico-medullary axis. In the inner medulla, osmolality continues to increase, but the source of the concentrating effect remains controversial. However, the most widely accepted mechanism remains passive absorption of NaCl, in excess of solute secretion, from thin ascending limbs of the loops of Henle.[8,9]

KIDNEY STRUCTURE

The structural organization of the mammalian kidney is discussed in detail elsewhere in this book. This section, based in large measure on key studies (e.g.,[10–12]), summarizes features that are pertinent to the urine concentrating mechanism.

In most mammals studied, the kidney contains short looped and long-looped nephrons; both have loops of Henle that are arranged in a hairpin configuration (Figure 43.2). They differ in two important aspects: the loops of short-looped nephrons turn near the inner-outer medullary border and lack a thin ascending limb, whereas the loops of long-looped nephrons extend into the inner medulla and contain a thin ascending limb. Thin ascending limbs are found only in the inner medulla, and their transition to thick ascending limbs defines the inner–outer medullary border. Thus, only thick ascending limbs are found in the outer medulla, regardless of the type of loop. Some mammalian kidneys, e.g., human kidneys, have nephrons whose loops of Henle do not reach into the medulla; these nephrons are called cortical nephrons. Tubular fluid flows from thick ascending limbs of both short and long looped nephrons to distal convoluted tubules. Several distal tubules merge to form cortical collecting ducts that descend through the cortex and then become medullary collecting ducts that pass through the outer medulla. The collecting ducts merge along the entire length of the inner medulla, ultimately forming the ducts of Bellini, which open into the renal pelvis at the papillary tip.

Small mammals, such as rodents, have unipapillate kidneys. In these mammals, the papilla is an inverted pyramid-shaped portion of the innermost inner medulla; the papilla descends into the renal pelvis. Larger mammals (including humans) have multipapillate kidneys in which each papilla descends into a renal calyx. The renal pelvis is formed from the merging of these calyces. In all mammals, urine exits through the ducts of Bellini into the renal pelvis.

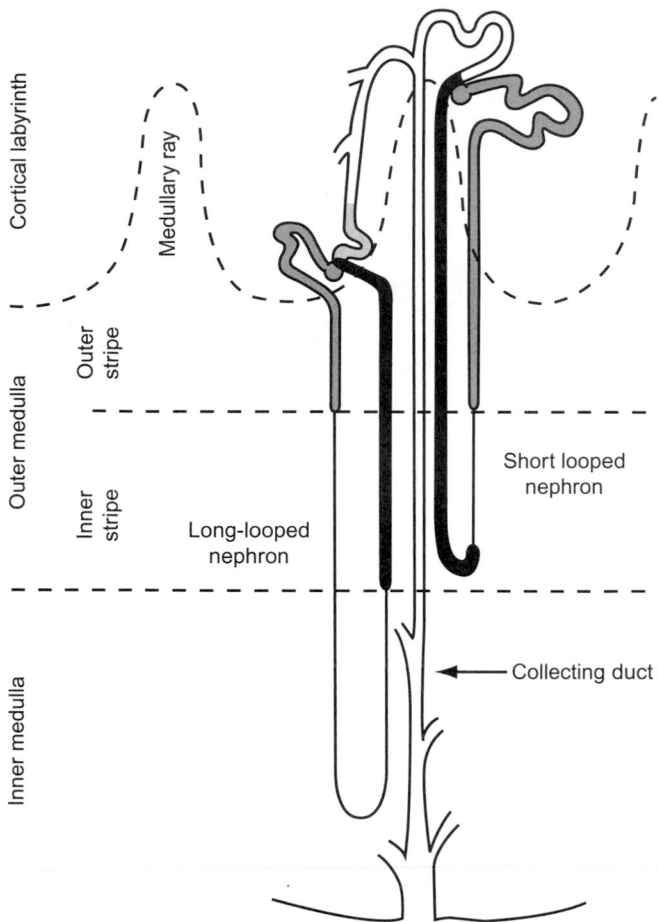

FIGURE 43.2 Basic structure of mammalian kidney. Diagram shows both a long-looped and a short-looped nephron. Glomeruli are shown as circles, proximal tubules are hatched, thin limbs of Henle's loop are lines, thick ascending limbs of Henle's loops are solid, distal convoluted tubules are stippled, and collecting duct system is open. *(Reproduced with permission, from reference [232].)*

The pelvis, which connects to the ureter, is bounded by two epithelia: the papillary surface epithelium lining the surface of the papilla, and a ureteral-type epithelium extending from the ureter up into the renal pelvic fornices.[13–16]

The descending and ascending vasa recta, which provide the blood supply for the medulla, are arranged roughly in parallel. Although their configuration is similar to the hair-pin configuration of the loops of Henle, there is an important anatomic difference: the tubular segments that make up the loops of Henle are contiguous, whereas the descending and ascending vasa recta are separated by capillary plexuses. Blood enters the medulla through descending vasa recta, passes through capillary plexuses located at various depths within the medulla, and then enters ascending vasa recta. Vascular bundles, which are aggregations of both descending and ascending vasa recta, form in the

outer stripe, but become much more prominent in the inner stripe. Lemley and Kriz have proposed using the vascular bundle (see detail, Figure 43.3) as the histotopographical core around which the various outer medullary tubule structures are arranged.[10–12,17]

Studies of inner medullary structure by Kriz and co-workers,[10–12,17] and recent studies by Pannabecker and Dantzler,[18,19] found that the inner medullary collecting ducts (IMCDs) in the inner medullary base form clusters that coalesce along the cortico–medullary axis. Using immunohistochemical labeling and computer-assisted reconstruction, Pannabecker, Dantzler, and colleagues have elucidated new detail of the functional architecture of the rat inner medulla (see recent review [20]). A computerized reconstruction of the inner medullary portion of several long-looped nephrons from rats is shown in Figure 43.4, in which antibodies to the water channel aquaporin-1 (AQP1, shown in red) and the chloride channel ClC-K1 (shown in green)[18] are used to label the thin descending and ascending limbs of the loops of Henle, respectively (reviewed in [20]). In the base of the inner medulla, thin descending limbs are predominantly present at the periphery of these clusters, and appear to form an asymmetric ring around each collecting duct cluster. In thin descending limbs of loops of Henle that turn within the upper first millimeter of the inner medulla, no AQP1 was detected. In contrast, there are three discernible functional subsegments in thin descending limbs of loops of Henle that turn below the first millimeter: the upper 40% expresses AQP1, whereas the lower 60% do not. ClC-K1, a marker of the thin ascending limb-type epithelium, is first detected in the final ~165 micrometers of the thin descending limb, as well as in the contiguous thin ascending limb. Thus, ClC-K1 is detected before the bend of the loops of Henle. This finding is consistent with previous morphological studies demonstrating that the descending limb to ascending limb transition occurs before the loop bend. In addition, a substantial portion of the inner medullary thin descending limbs of long-looped nephrons did not express either AQP1 or ClC-K1, as indicated in gray in Figure 43.4a.

In contrast, thin ascending limbs are distributed relatively uniformly among collecting ducts and thin descending limbs. In Munich-Wistar rats, Pannabecker and Dantzler[19] identified three population groups of loops of Henle, distinguished by thin ascending limb position at the base of the inner medulla and by differing loop length. Group 1 loops, having thin ascending limbs that are interposed between collecting ducts, reach a mean length of 700 μm into the inner medulla; Group 2 loops, having thin ascending limbs that are adjacent to just one collecting duct, reach 1500 μm and Group 3 loops, having thin ascending limbs that lie more than a half-tubule diameter from a collecting

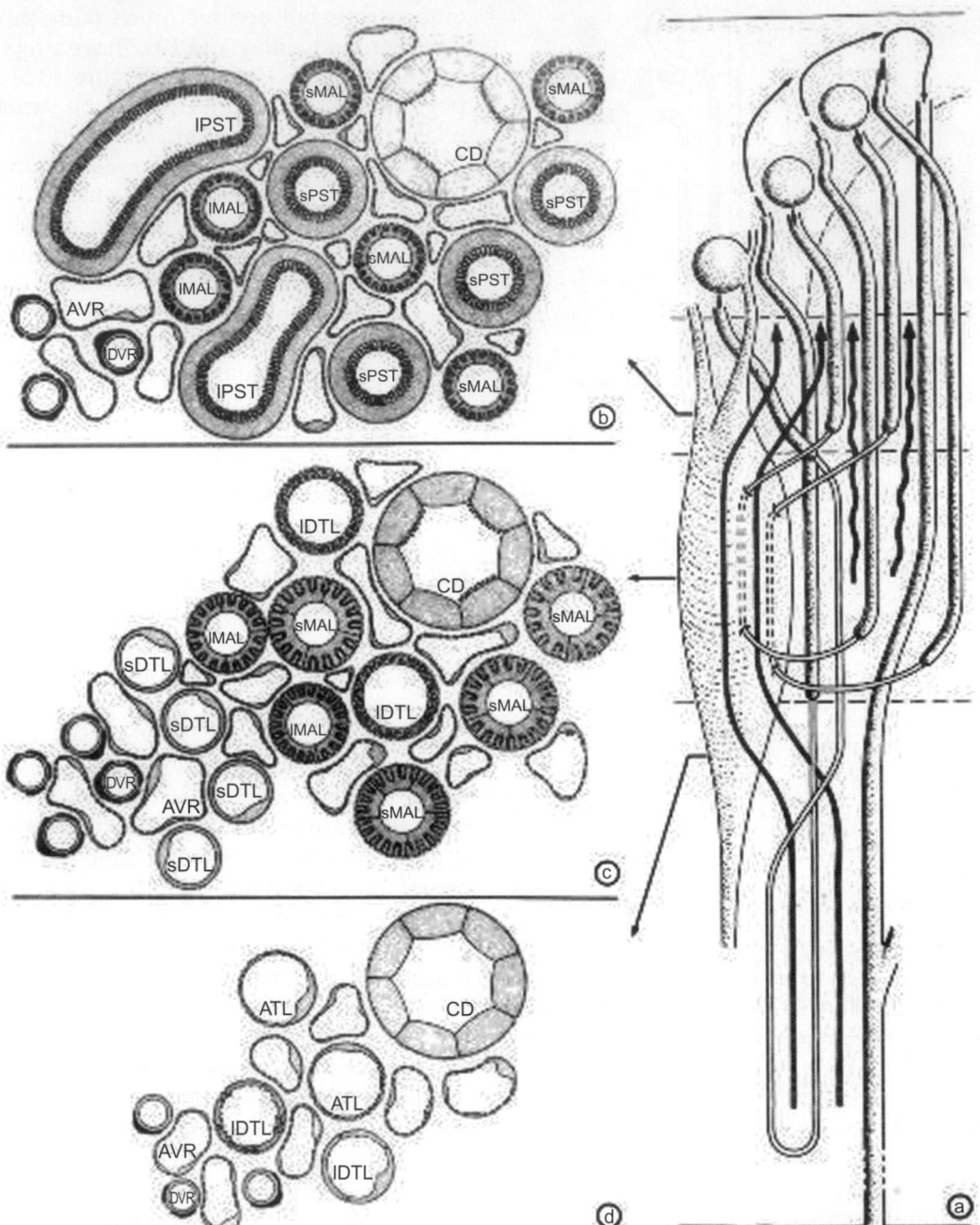

FIGURE 43.3   Lemley and Kriz model of the architectural organization of the rat renal medulla. Shown are a schematic longitudinal section (a); and cross-sections through the outer stripe of the outer medulla (b); inner stripe of the outer medulla (c); and the inner medulla (IM) (d). In (a) 1 long and 2 short loops of Henle, the collecting duct, and a vascular bundle (shown in three-dimensional solid form) are shown. The vascular bundle contains ascending vasa recta (AVR) originating from the inner medulla (AVRIM, long, bold-face arrows) and the descending limbs of the short-looped nephrons (sDTL). Ascending vasa recta originating from the inner stripe (AVRIS, bold, wavy arrows) ascend directly within the interbundle region. In the cross-sections (b)–(d), the relationships of 4 short and 2 long loops of Henle are shown with the collecting duct (CD) and vasa recta. (b) In the outer stripe, the proximal straight tubules (PST) and medullary thick ascending limbs of long-looped nephrons (lMAL) are located among the AVRIM near the vascular bundle. Located at a distance from the vascular bundle are the collecting ducts (CD) and the PSTs, and thick ascending limbs from short looped nephrons (sMAL). These structures are surrounded by AVRIS and the true capillaries (smaller unlabeled structures). (c) In the inner stripe, the core of a vascular bundle contains AVR and descending vasa recta (DVR), whereas sDTL are found among the AVRIM in the periphery. In the interbundle region, the thin descending limbs of long looped nephrons (lDTL) and CD run together with thick ascending limbs of short looped nephrons (sMAL); the lMAL are found bordering the vascular bundle. (d) In this section through the upper IM, a vascular bundle is still discernible, but AVR are already present throughout the cross-section. The CD is distant from the vascular bundle. Between the bundle and the CD are lDTL (with different wall structures corresponding to upper and lower part epithelia) and ascending limbs of long looped nephrons (ATL) (Abbreviations: AVR and DVR: ascending and descending vasa recta; CD: collecting duct; DTL: descending thin limb; MAL: medullary thick ascending limb; PST: proximal straight tubule (pars recta); subscripts s and l: short-looped and long-looped nephrons, respectively; OS, IS, and IM: outer and inner stripe of the outer medulla and inner medulla, respectively). *(Reproduced with permission, from reference [12].)*

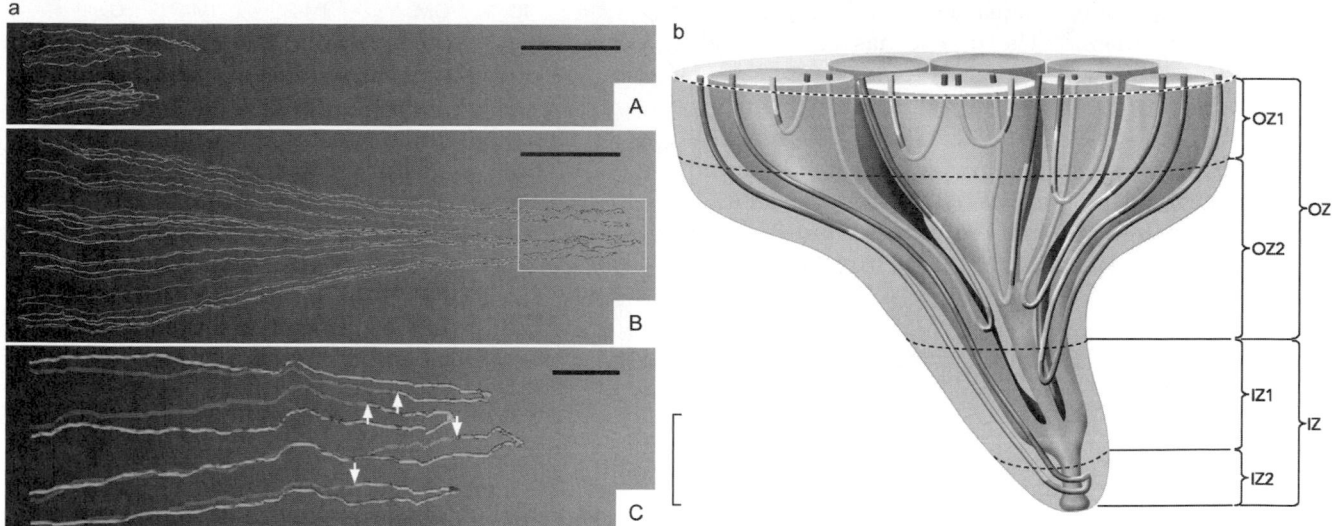

FIGURE 43.4 (a) Computer-assisted reconstruction of loops of Henle from rat inner medulla showing expression of aquaporin-1 (AQP1; red) and ClC-K1 (green); gray regions (B-crystallin) express undetectable levels of AQP1 and ClC-K1. Loops are oriented along the corticopapillary axis, with the left edge of each image nearer the base of the inner medulla. Panel A: Thin limbs that have their bends within the first millimeter beyond the outer–inner medullary boundary. Descending segments lack detectable AQP1. ClC-K1 is expressed continuously along the prebend segment and the thin ascending limb. Panel B: Loops that have their bends beyond the first millimeter of the inner medulla. AQP1 is expressed along the initial 40% of each thin descending limb, and is absent from the remainder of each loop. ClC-K1 is expressed continuously along the prebend segment and the thin ascending limb. Boxed area is enlarged in panel C. Panel C: Enlargement of near-bend regions of 4 thin limbs from box in panel B. ClC-K1 expression, corresponding to thin descending limb prebend segment, begins, on average, 165 μm before the loop bend (arrows). Scale bars, 500 μm (panels A and B); and 100 μm (panel C). *(Reproduced with permission, from reference [20].)* (b) Based on computer-assisted functional anatomy reconstructions that included immunolabeling of key transporters along the limbs of long loops of Henle, Pannabecker et al.[21] have proposed that the inner medulla of the rat can be considered to have four four zones (or subsections): (1) an outer-most zone (OZ1), about 1 mm thick, that lies just below the OM and in which loops labeling for little or no AQP1 have their bends; (2) a larger outer zone (OZ2), 2 to 2.5 mm in thickness that lies just below OZ1 that has well-organized CD clusters and tubules where loop bends turn within central portions of the clusters; (3) an outer inner zone (IZ1) where the organization of CD clusters diminishes, and all vasa recta are fenestrated; and (4) an inner-most zone (IZ2) where CD clusters can no longer be distinguished, where all vasa recta are fenestrated, and where many loops of Henle have transversely-running segments that wrap alongside CDs. The two inner zones combined are 1.5 to 2 mm thick. Representative collecting duct clusters are shown in blue; intercluster tissue is orange. AQP1-positive and AQP1-negative descending thin limbs are shown in red and yellow, respectively. Prebend segments and ascending thin limbs are shown in green. This color scheme differs from that of Figure 43.4A only by the use of yellow rather than gray for AQP-1 negative descending thin limbs. *(Reproduced with permission from [21].)* See color section at the back of the book.

duct, reach 2200 μm. As collecting ducts coalesce and shorter loops disappear, the originating portions of longer thin ascending limbs run alongside the collecting ducts for substantial distances (a more detailed description of inner medullary loop subgroups was given in [20]).

Moreover, Pannabecker et al.[20,21] proposed that the inner medulla has at least four distinguishable zones (axial subsections) that can be differentiated by the variable characteristics of vasa recta and loops of Henle. The four zones are illustrated in Figure 43.4b. Three countercurrent systems were hypothesized to exist within these zones: (1) an intercluster system within the CD clusters where most of the work of concentrating is conducted in and around nodal spaces that are surrounded by IMCDs, thin ascending limbs, and AVR; (2) an extracluster system in the outerzones (outer 3 to 3.5 mm) that serves to carry water absorbed from water-permeable

portions of descending limbs back to the OM via AVR; and (3) a papillary system in the inner zones where the highest concentrations are attained with the aid of direct interactions between transversely-running segments of loops of Henle and collecting ducts.

Distinct types of interstitium are found in the vascular bundle in the outer medulla, in the interbundle region of the outer medulla, and in the inner medulla.[12] These interstitia may play an important role in medullary solute and water transfer, especially in the inner medulla, where interstitial cells are interspersed in a gelatinous matrix of acid mucopolysaccharides, which is largely devoid of any capillary plexuses, laterally flowing capillaries or lymphatics.[12,22,23] Thus, the inner medullary interstitium should greatly slow lateral bulk flow of solutes and water.

The number of nephrons found in mammals, and thus the number of loops of Henle, varies over many orders of magnitude, increasing sub-linearly with increasing body mass.[24] The mouse has about 12,400 nephrons per kidney[24]; rat, 30,000—40,000[24,25]; rabbit, 230,000[24,25]; human, 0.3—1.4 million[26,27]; elephant, 7.5 million[24]; and fin whale, 192 million.[27] In contrast, medullary thickness in mammals varies from 3 to 25 mm, thus indicating that maximum loop of Henle length varies over about an order of magnitude[4]; proximal tubule diameter changes little from rat to fin whale, increasing by a factor of about 1.3.[27,28]

Although loops of Henle of variable length are found in all mammals, most mammals are thought to have both short- and long-looped nephrons. Exceptions include the dog, with all long loops,[29] and the mountain beaver *Aplodontia rufa*, which has thick ascending limbs only, and has a renal medulla that corresponds to the outer medulla of other mammals.[30] Generally, however, there are more short-looped than long looped nephrons, and the long-looped nephrons tend to exhibit substantial variation in the depth reached within the inner medulla. Measurements in the rabbit[31] and rat[25,32] indicate that the decrease in loop of Henle and collecting duct population in the inner medulla is approximately exponential, with most loops of Henle turning back in the outer portion of the inner medulla, and with collecting ducts converging to a few ducts of Bellini. A similar pattern is seen in the medullary cones of the avian kidney[33] which, like the mammalian kidney, is able to produce a concentrated urine, although only to osmolalities of about twice that of blood plasma.[34]

The pattern of decrease in the tubule populations of the rat renal medulla[25,32] is portrayed in Figure 43.5, which gives curves approximating loop and collecting duct population as a function of normalized medullary depth. About 38,000 loops and 7300 collecting ducts extend through most of the outer medulla.[25] About 28—33% of the loops of Henle in rat have thin ascending limbs and reach into the inner medulla.[10,29] The populations of loops of Henle and collecting ducts both decline rapidly, but the loop population decreases more rapidly, so that the loop and collecting duct populations are more nearly equal in the papilla. In human, about $\frac{1}{7}$ of the loops of Henle reach into the inner medulla.[27]

Figure 43.5 also portrays the concentration of urea, the sum of the concentrations of sodium and its anions, and the osmolality, as a function of medullary depth, as determined in tissue slices harvested from vasopressin-treated Wistar rats.[6,35,36] The experimental data points indicated in Figure 43.5 are connected by natural cubic splines which generate smooth curves; these curves have shapes supported by other studies in rat.[37,38] Osmolality increases by a factor of about 2 in the outer medulla, and by an additional factor of 3

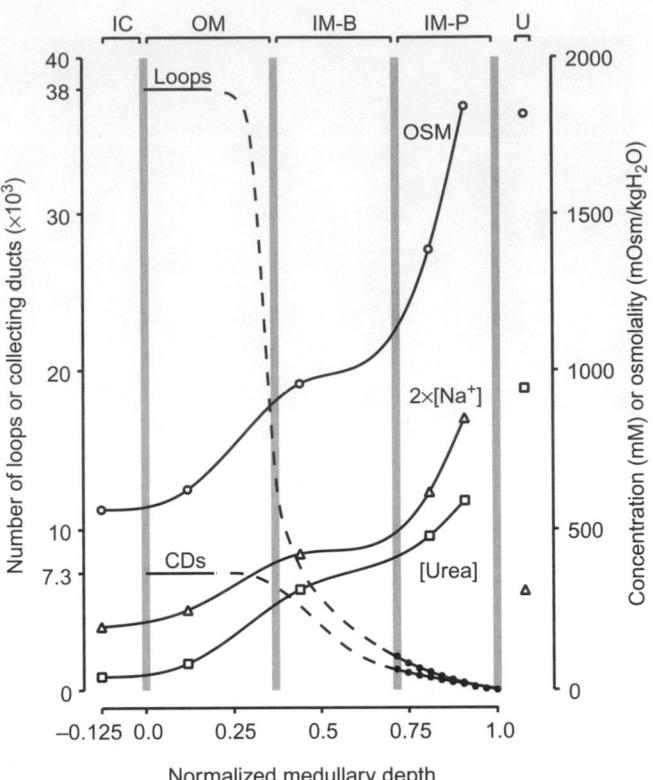

FIGURE 43.5 Loop of Henle and collecting duct population in rat (scale at left) as a function of normalized medullary depth; also, tissue osmolality, concentration of urea, and concentration of sodium plus its anion (scale at right). Loop of Henle and collecting duct populations decrease in inner medulla because loops turn back and collecting ducts merge. The osmolality gradient is larger in the outer medulla and papilla than in the outer part of the inner medulla. The gradient is largest in the papilla, where the osmolality and concentration profiles appear to increase exponentially. The shape of the sodium profile has been corroborated by electron microprobe measurements[38] (Key: IC: inner cortex; OM: outer medulla; IM: outer part (base) of inner medulla; P: papilla or inner part (tip) of inner medulla; U: urine). Figure based on published data. Curves connecting data points are natural cubic splines, computed by standard algorithms.[451] Dashed curve segments are interpolations without supporting measurements. Tubule populations in papilla are from reference[32]; tubule populations in outer medulla are based on estimates in reference.[25] Concentrations and osmolalities are from tissue slices and urine samples collected 4.5 hours after onset of vasopressin infusion at 15 μU/min/100 g body weight. Data is from Figure 5 in reference[36] and Figures 1, 3, and 9 in reference[6]; slice locations were given in reference.[35] The osmolality reported in the inner cortex seems high relative to the reported plasma concentration of 314 mOsm/kg H₂O. The osmolality and concentration profiles, as drawn in reference[6], apparently do not take into account relative distances between tissue sample sites.

in the inner medulla, where urea makes a substantive contribution. As can be inferred from the values for urine (U) in Figure 43.5, sodium is largely carried by flow in the loops of Henle and vasculature, while urea makes up a large portion of the solute in collecting duct flow. Potassium has a tissue concentration of about 80–100 mM along the medulla, but it makes a larger contribution (~150 mM) to urine.[6,36]

The osmolality increase along the outer medulla arises from the vigorous transepithelial transport of NaCl from thick ascending limbs into the surrounding interstitium. This effect is believed to be augmented by a process of countercurrent multiplication, described in a subsequent section (*vide infra*). However, as shown in Figure 43.5, the osmolality gradient is largest in the papilla, even though only a small fraction of the loops, tubules, and vasa recta reach into the papilla, and even though the population of tubules and vessels is rapidly decreasing there. The remarkable capacity for generating high osmolalities in so small a volume (~0.5% of total kidney volume[22]) has thus far resisted a generally satisfactory explanation.

TRANSPORT PROPERTIES OF INDIVIDUAL NEPHRON SEGMENTS

This section will review the water, urea, and sodium permeability values measured in isolated perfused tubules in nephron segments involved in producing concentrated or dilute urine. Thin limb segments are difficult to perfuse, and most measurements involving different species have been made by different laboratories. Thus, some caution must be used in comparing these values. Tables 43.2–43.5 contain values obtained from animals receiving food and water *ad libitum*; representative values were chosen since space does not permit citing every original manuscript.

In the past two decades, many of the proteins which mediate water, urea, and sodium transport in nephron segments important for urinary concentration and dilution have been cloned (Figure 43.6). The water channels (called aquaporins) and sodium transporters are discussed in detail elsewhere in this book. The urea transport proteins and their role in the long-term regulation of the urine concentrating mechanism are discussed later in this chapter.

In general, the water, urea, and sodium transport proteins are highly specific. Reflection coefficients are not included in Tables 43.2–43.5, since the specificity of these transport proteins appears to eliminate a molecular basis for solvent drag and suggests that the reflection coefficients should be 1.

THIN DESCENDING LIMB

Thin descending limbs are conventionally divided into types I, II, and III: types I and II are located in the outer medulla in short and long looped nephrons, respectively, while type III limbs are located in the

TABLE 43.2 Permeability Properties in Thin Descending Limb Nephron Segments[a]

	Species			
	Chinchilla	Rat	Rabbit	Hamster
THIN DESCENDING LIMB TYPE I				
Na[b]			0–2 [65;64;66c]	4.8[58]
Urea[b]		13[63c]	1–2[60,62c]	8[58]
Water[d]		2295[44c]	2420[64c]	3257[58]
Na$^+$/K$^+$-ATPase[e]		2–5[67,68c]	2–4[67c]	
THIN DESCENDING LIMB TYPE II				
Na[b]			1[64–66c]	23–66[58,59]
Urea[b]	3[57]	0[61]	1[60,62c]	3[58,59]
Water[d]	2600[42,49]	2295[79c]	2315[64c]	5378[58]
Na$^+$/K$^+$-ATPase[e]		2–5[67,68c]	2–4[67c]	
THIN DESCENDING LIMB TYPE III				
Na[b]	29[57]			4[59]
Urea[b]	17–29[52,57]	13[63c]		13[59]
Water[d]	1550[42,49]	2295[79c]		1693[59]
Na$^+$/K$^+$-ATPase[e]		3[68]		
THIN DESCENDING LIMB TYPE III DISTAL (PAPILLARY SUBSEGMENT)				
Na[b]	74[57]			
Urea[b]	48[57]			
Water[d]	60[42,49]			

[a]References are in supercripted.
[b]units: 10^{-5} cm/sec.
[c]Subsegment not specified, thus cannot differentiate between thin descending limb subtypes.
[d]units: μm/sec.
[e]units: pmol/mm/min.

inner medulla.[39,40] The osmotic water permeability of thin descending limb subtypes that express aquaporin 1 (AQP1) water channels[41] is extremely high in all species studied[42–45] (Table 43.2). AQP1, a constitutively active water channel, is present in both the apical and basolateral plasma membranes in sufficient abundance to account for the measured rates of transepithelial water transport.[46] Transgenic mice lacking the AQP1 channel (which is also found in proximal tubule and descending vasa recta), were found to have greatly impaired urine concentrating capability, which was attributed in large measure to defective water absorption from the proximal tubules and descending limbs, which may lead to an overloading of available concentrating capacity.[47,48]

The chinchilla has an additional inner medullary subsegment (type II distal) in the deepest 20% of the

TABLE 43.3 Permeability Properties in Ascending Limb Nephron Segments[a]

	Species			
	Chinchilla	Rat	Rabbit	Mouse
THIN ASCENDING LIMB				
Na[b]	238[57]	80[79]	26[80]	55–88[79,82]
Urea[b]	171[57]	14–23[63,79]	7[80]	19[79]
Water[c]	0–8[42,49]	25[79]	13[80]	29[79]
Na$^+$/K$^+$-ATPase[d]		2–4[67,68]	3[67]	
MEDULLARY THICK ASCENDING LIMB				
Na[b]			6[94,430]	2[455]
Cl[b]			1[94]	1[455]
Urea[b]		1.4 (outer stripe)[98]	1[99]	
		0.6–0.9 (inner stripe)[98]		
Water[c]			0[94]	23[456]
K[b]			1[457]	
PD[e]		2–3[458]	3–7[94,459,460]	
Na$^+$/K$^+$-ATPase[d]		41–139 (outer stripe)[95]	41–124[67]	62[67]
		260 (inner stripe)[95]		
CORTICAL THICK ASCENDING LIMB				
Na[b]		1[461]	3[462]	
Cl[b]		1[461]	1[462]	
Urea[b]		1.5[98]	2[463]	
Water[c]			0[94]	23[456]
PD[e]			3–7[92,462]	
Na$^+$/K$^+$-ATPase[d]		83–133[95]	16–31[67]	61[67]

[a]References are superscripted.
[b]units: 10^{-5} cm/sec.
[c]units: μm/sec.
[d]units: pmol/mm/sec.
[e]PD: transepithelial potential difference, mV.

TABLE 43.4 Permeability Properties in Cortical and Outer Medullary Collecting Duct Segments[a]

	Species	
	Rat	Rabbit
CORTICAL COLLECTING DUCT		
Na[b]		0.1[464]
K[b]		1–2[464,465]
Cl[b]		2–5[108,464]
Urea[b] ± [c] AVP	1[98,104]	0–1[100,466]
Water[d] − AVP	17–43[101,102]	4–13[225,467,468]
+ AVP	389–994[101,102,469]	166–280[225,467,468,470]
Na$^+$/K$^+$-ATPase[e]	13–81[67,68,95]	12–23[67,471–474]
OUTER MEDULLARY COLLECTING DUCT		
Na[b]		0.39[465]
K[b]		0.59[465]
Cl[b]		0.5[475]
Urea[b]	3.5[102]	0.3[99]
Water[d] −AVP		14[99,110]
+ AVP		445[99,110]
Na$^+$/K$^+$-ATPase[e]	11–41[95,68]	8–19[67,471,472,474]

[a]References are superscripted;
[b]units: 10^{-5} cm/sec.
[c]± AVP: value unchanged by AVP; − AVP: no vasopressin; + AVP: with vasopressin.
[d]units: μm/sec;
[e]units: pmol/mm/min.

longest loops of Henle.[42] This subsegment has low osmotic water permeability[42,49] and lacks AQP1.[50] The Munich-Wistar rat has a similar subsegment in the deepest 60% of the longest loops[51,52] and also a prebend segment of ∼164 μm in length that labels for the ClC-K1 chloride transporter, but not for AQP1.[18] Avian loops of Henle appear to have similar pre-bend segments.[53] The pre-bend segments may be functionally important as a site of NaCl absorption.[52,54–56]

Urea permeability varies in different portions of the thin descending limb (Table 43.2). Urea permeability is relatively low in types I and II thin descending limbs.[57–62] Urea permeability is higher in type III thin descending limbs,[52,57,59,63] and is quite high in the chinchilla type III distal thin descending limb.[57] The reflection coefficient for urea is close to 1 in thin descending limbs.[58,64]

Sodium permeability is relatively low in rabbit types I and II[64–66] and hamster types I and III thin descending limbs,[58,59] but is relatively high in hamster type II and chinchilla types III and III distal thin descending limbs.[57–59] Na$^+$/K$^+$-ATPase activity is very low in all thin descending limb segments in which it has been measured.[67,68] Rabbit types I and II thin descending limbs have a NaCl reflection coefficient that is close to 1.[64] However, the measured NaCl reflection coefficient is heterogeneous in hamster: 0.83 in type II and 0.99 in type III thin descending limbs.[58,69]

The perfused tubule studies reviewed above provide important information about the transport properties of

TABLE 43.5 Permeability Properties in Inner Medullary Collecting Duct Subsegments[a]

	Species		
	Rat	Rabbit	Hamster
INITIAL INNER MEDULLARY COLLECTING DUCT – IMCD₁			
Urea[b] ± [c]AVP	2–5[102,104,114,118]	1[104]	8–9[116]
Sodium-Urea[d]	0[115,118]		
Water[e] − AVP	16–81[102,117,476]		
+AVP	148–460[102,117,476]		534[116]
Na⁺/K⁺-ATPase[f]	18–42[68]		
TERMINAL INNER MEDULLARY COLLECTING DUCT – IMCD₂			
Na[b]	1[124]		2[116]
K[b]	4[123]		
Cl[b]	1–2[123,124]		
Urea[b] −AVP	15–46[102,104,114,120,476]	12[104]	12[116]
+AVP	69–93[102,114,120]		32[116]
+Hypertonic bath:	120–143[119,121]		
+Hypertonic bath and AVP:	163–190[119,121]		
Sodium-Urea[g]	0–1[115,118]		
Water[e] − AVP	70–333[102,117,476]		
+AVP	208–749[102,117,476]		646[116]
Na⁺/K⁺-ATPase[f]	12–40[68]		
TERMINAL INNER MEDULLARY COLLECTING DUCT - IMCD₃			
Na[b]	1[124]		
Urea[b] − AVP	39–49[104,114]	13[104]	
+AVP	110[114]		
Sodium-Urea[g]	−9[115]		
Water[e] − AVP	43–145[102,117]		
+AVP	389–749[102,117]		
Na⁺/K⁺-ATPase[f]	8–17[68]		
PAPILLARY SURFACE EPITHELIUM			
Chloride[b] ± AVP	2–3[127]		
Urea[b] ± AVP	1[104]		
Water[d] ± AVP	14[127]		

[a]*References are superscripted.*
[b]*units: 10^{-5} cm/sec.*
[c] *± AVP: value unchanged by AVP; − AVP: no vasopressin; + AVP: with vasopressin.*
[d]*sodium-urea co-transport, units: pmol/mm/min.*
[e]*units: μm/sec.*
[f]*units: pmol/mm/min.*
[g]*sodium-urea counter-transport, units: pmol/mm/min; + : urea absorption; − : urea secretion.*

the individual nephron segments comprising the descending limb of the loop of Henle. In contrast, micropuncture studies provide *in vivo* information about the concentrations of solute within the portions of the descending limb that are accessible to micropuncture: comparisons can be made between the composition of tubular fluid near the ends of those proximal convoluted tubules that are accessible on the cortical surface and the composition of fluid in the bends of the longest loops of Henle near the papillary tip. Since proximal tubules on the surface of the kidney originate from superficial glomeruli, and the loops of Henle which reach the papillary tip generally originate from juxtamedullary nephrons, it is not possible, currently, to compare fluid samples taken from cortical and medullary sites in a single nephron. Thus, the validity of this comparison depends upon the assumption that the composition and delivery of solute and water to the beginning of the superficial and juxtamedullary descending limbs are similar. In addition, papillary micropuncture requires the removal of the ureter, which also reduces maximum urinary concentrating ability by a mechanism that is not completely understood.[70–72] Thus, micropuncture studies are limited to studies performed during moderate, not maximal, antidiuretic conditions.

In the rat, osmolality increases along the length of the descending limb. Water removal accounts for 90% of this increase in osmolality in Brattleboro rats that are not treated with vasopressin.[73] When Brattleboro rats are treated with vasopressin, there is an increase in the osmotic pressure of the descending limb fluid and in the volume of water absorbed from the descending limb.[73] This rise in descending limb fluid osmolality results from water extraction (60%), and from urea addition (40%).[72,73] The delivery of urea to the end of the thin descending limb averages 550% of the filtered load of urea.[72] Thus, urea is either secreted into the descending limb fluid[74] or there is a major difference between the filtered load of urea in superficial versus juxtamedullary glomeruli. When urea is infused into rats fed a low-protein diet, both water extraction from the descending limb and urinary concentrating ability are significantly increased.[75]

In hamster, ~65% of the osmotically active solute in fluid obtained near the bend of the loop of Henle is due to sodium (plus a univalent anion), while ~20% is due to urea.[70] Since only ~10% of the filtered load of water reaches the bend of the loop of Henle, the high luminal fluid sodium concentration results primarily from water extraction from the descending limb.[70] Both sodium and inulin concentrations increase along the length of the hamster descending limb, showing that water is extracted from the descending limb fluid.[76,77] As in the rat, significant amounts of urea are added to the descending limb fluid.

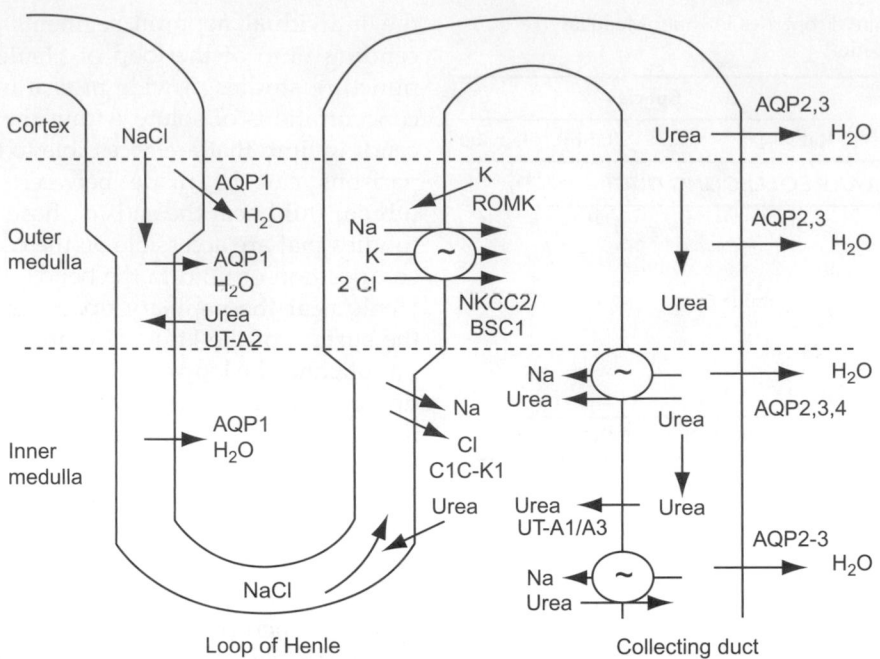

FIGURE 43.6   Location and identities of the water, urea, and sodium transport proteins involved in the passive mechanism hypothesis for countercurrent multiplication in the inner medulla.[8,9] The major kidney regions are shown on the left. NaCl is actively absorbed across the thick ascending limb by the apical membrane $Na^+-K^+-2Cl^-$ co-transporter (NKCC2, BSC1), and the basolateral membrane Na^+/K^+-ATPase (not shown). K^+ is recycled through an apical membrane ROMK channel. Water is absorbed across the descending limb by AQP1 water channels in both apical and basolateral plasma membranes. In the presence of vasopressin, water is absorbed across the apical plasma membrane of the collecting duct by AQP2 water channels. Water is absorbed across the basolateral plasma membrane by AQP3 water channels in the cortical and outer medullary collecting duct, and by both AQP3 and AQP4 water channels in the inner medullary collecting duct (IMCD). Urea is concentrated within the collecting duct lumen (by water absorption) until it reaches the terminal IMCD where it is absorbed by the UT-A1 and UT-A3 urea transporters. According to the passive mechanism hypothesis (see text), the fluid which enters the thin ascending limb from the contiguous thin descending limb has a higher NaCl and a lower urea concentration than the inner medullary interstitium, resulting in passive NaCl absorption and dilution of the fluid within the thin ascending limb. Also shown are 2 active urea transport pathways: a Na^+-urea counter-transporter is expressed in the terminal IMCD of normal rats and is upregulated by water diuresis[115]; a Na^+-urea co-transporter is expressed in the initial IMCD of hypercalcemic rats or rats fed a low-protein diet but not from rats fed a normal protein diet[423,118,358] (Abbreviations: AQP: aquaporin; UT: urea transporter).

Psammomys obesus, a desert rodent, feeds on halophilic plants which provide water along with large quantities of NaCl. In these animals, tubular fluid flow rate decreases by 1.7-fold along the descending limb, while osmotic pressure increases four-fold.[37,78] Water removal accounts for 40% of the increase and solute addition accounts for 60% under moderate NaCl-loading conditions.[37] Unlike the rat, NaCl is the principal solute added to descending limb fluid[37]; urea is added but is much less important than in the rat. In *Psammomys* which are producing more highly concentrated urine (although still less concentrated than can be achieved by the intact animal), NaCl addition accounts for nearly 80% of the rise in osmolality.[37]

Thin Ascending Limb

The thin ascending limb (Table 43.3) has an extremely low osmotic water permeability in all species studied,[42,49,79,80] and no aquaporin proteins have been detected (reviewed in [81]). Although the thin ascending limb has a urea permeability that is lower than its NaCl permeability,[57,63,79,82] it is significantly higher than the value that mathematical models indicate is required for the effective operation of the hypothesized passive mechanism (*vide infra*). While this is true in all species, it is especially true in chinchilla.[52,57]

The thin ascending limb has a very low level of Na^+/K^+-ATPase activity[67,68] that would not support a significant rate of active sodium transport.[83] However, some *in vivo* studies have found evidence for active sodium transport in thin ascending limbs.[72,77] The thin ascending limb has a high passive NaCl permeability.[57,63,79,80,82] Chloride transport occurs transcellularly via the ClC-K1 chloride channel, which is present in both the apical and basolateral plasma membranes.[84] Vasopressin increases chloride transport in thin ascending limbs,[85] and water deprivation increases the mRNA abundance of ClC-K1.[86] Transgenic mice lacking the ClC-K1 transporter were found to have greatly reduced urine concentrating capability, which was attributed to defective chloride transport in the thin ascending limb.[87] Sodium transport is thought to occur paracellularly, since no apical plasma membrane sodium transport pathway has been demonstrated.[88,89]

When rabbit thin ascending limbs are perfused *in vitro* with concentration gradients of NaCl and urea that simulate *in vivo* conditions (NaCl gradient from lumen-to-bath and a urea gradient from bath-to-lumen), they are able to dilute their luminal fluid by purely passive means. Perfusing rabbit thin ascending limbs *in vitro* with solutions whose osmolality is increased from 290 to 600 mOsm/kg H_2O by adding NaCl to the perfusate and urea to the bath (to mimic the higher concentration of NaCl in the tubule lumen and the higher urea concentration in the medullary interstitium) reduces collected fluid osmolality to 70% of perfusate osmolality, suggesting that it may be possible to dilute the luminal fluid within thin ascending limbs without active transport *in vivo*.[80]

Heterogeneity in Thin Limbs of Long Loops

Pannabecker et al.[18] investigated inner medullary functional structure in Munich-Wistar rats by means of computer-assisted three-dimensional reconstructions of cross-sections in which tubules were identified and labeled by direct immunofluorescence of antibodies raised against specific transport proteins. The reconstructions indicate that thin descending limbs of Henle's loops that have bends within the first millimeter below the outer–inner medullary boundary lack the water transporter AQP1. Thin descending limbs of loops that have bends beyond the first millimeter express AQP1 for about the first 40% of their length below the outer–inner medullary boundary, but beyond that point lack AQP1 expression. Expression of ClC-K1 chloride channels begins abruptly with a prebend segment of length ~165 μm, and ClC-K1 expression continues uniformly along the entire length of thin ascending limbs. Co-localization of AQP1 and ClC-K1 was not found in any loop of Henle segment. Preliminary sections show no evidence of expression of the urea transporters UT-A1, UT-A2 or UT-A4 in thin limbs below the first millimeter of the inner medulla.[54] These observations are generally consistent with expression patterns indicated in other immunocytochemical studies in rat.[43,90] However, Mejia and Wade[91] found in Sprague-Dawley rats that ~30% of thin descending limbs that reached deep into the papilla labeled for AQP1 (in Brattleboro rats, ~11%); and Wade et al.[90] found co-labeling of a UT-A urea transport protein and AQP1 in thin descending limbs in the base of the inner medulla of Brattleboro rats (these limbs may correspond to the longer population identified by Pannabecker et al.[18]).

Thick Ascending Limb

Both the medullary and cortical portions of the thick ascending limb (Table 43.3) have osmotic water permeabilities that are essentially zero, and neither subsegment expresses aquaporin proteins (reviewed in [81]). Thus, the primary mechanism for diluting the luminal fluid in thick ascending limbs is net absorption of solute, particularly NaCl. NaCl is actively absorbed by the Na^+-K^+-$2Cl^-$ co-transporter (NKCC2, BSC1) in the apical plasma membrane, and the sodium pump (Na^+/K^+-ATPase) in the basolateral plasma membrane. The thick ascending limb from short looped nephrons can lower the concentration of NaCl in the luminal fluid at loop bend from ~300 to ~117−40 mM at the cortico−medullary border,[92,93] while the cortical thick ascending limb can lower the concentration of NaCl to ~32 mM.[94] However, the medullary portion has the capacity to absorb more NaCl than the cortical portion, as evidenced by the higher Na^+/K^+-ATPase activity in the medullary thick ascending limb.[67,95] The regulation of NaCl absorption in the thick ascending limb is discussed in detail in Chapter 34.

Vasopressin increases NaCl absorption in medullary and cortical thick ascending limbs in mouse.[96,97] This response is consistent with vasopressin's role in urinary concentration, and suggests that vasopressin can increase or maintain concentrating ability by increasing NaCl absorption across thick ascending limbs. However, vasopressin does not increase NaCl absorption in human and canine, and only weakly stimulates absorption in rabbit medullary thick ascending limbs.[96]

Urea permeability in the medullary thick ascending limb is lower than in the cortical thick ascending limb.[98,99] In rat, the transition to a higher urea permeability occurs between the inner and outer stripe portions of the medullary thick ascending limb, while in rabbit it occurs between outer medulla and cortex.[98] Urea permeability in the thick ascending limb could permit dilution of tubular fluid by passive urea absorption or increase urea concentration in the thick ascending limb by secretion.

Cortical Collecting Duct

The cortical collecting duct has an extremely low osmotic water permeability (Table 4) in the absence of vasopressin.[100−102] Vasopressin significantly increases the osmotic water permeability by a factor of 10 to 100 in both rat[101,102] and rabbit.[100] Arachidonic acid metabolites, produced by cytochrome P450, inhibit vasopressin-stimulated osmotic water permeability by a post-cyclic AMP (cAMP) mechanism[103]; the mechanism by which vasopressin increases osmotic water permeability is discussed in detail in Chapter 41 on Water Channels.

The cortical collecting duct has a low urea permeability that is unaffected by vasopressin.[98,104] Thus, vasopressin-induced water absorption will increase the urea concentration within the lumen of the cortical collecting duct, and also the osmolality, provided that there is no significant net absorption of solutes.

The cortical collecting duct is the major site for aldosterone-mediated sodium absorption and potassium secretion.[105] Vasopressin also stimulates sodium absorption in the cortical collecting duct.[106] Sodium is actively absorbed via the epithelial sodium channel (ENaC) in the apical plasma membrane of principal cells,[107] and sodium absorption is responsible for the generation of a lumen-negative voltage.[105] Sodium exits the principal cell via Na^+/K^+-ATPase in the basolateral plasma membrane.[67,95] Chloride is transported by both paracellular and transcellular pathways. Chloride absorption is primarily passive in rabbit, although some evidence for chloride absorption against an electrochemical gradient exists.[108] Active chloride absorption occurs in rat, and is stimulated by vasopressin and inhibited by bradykinin.[109]

Outer Medullary Collecting Duct

Few permeability measurements exist for the rat outer medullary collecting duct (Table 43.4). In rabbit, the outer medullary collecting duct has a low osmotic water permeability which is increased 20- or 30-fold by vasopressin.[99,110] The urea permeability is low in the outer medullary collecting duct in both rat and rabbit.[98,99]

Inner Medullary Collecting Duct

The inner medullary collecting duct (IMCD) was originally divided into three subsegments: $IMCD_1$; $IMCD_2$; and $IMCD_3$.[111] Subsequent studies showed that the inner medullary collecting duct could generally be viewed as consisting of two morphologically and functionally distinct subsegments: the initial IMCD (corresponding to the $IMCD_1$) and the terminal IMCD (corresponding to the $IMCD_2$ and $IMCD_3$).[102,104,112,113] However, some recent studies have found functional differences between the $IMCD_2$ and $IMCD_3$.[114,115] Histologically, the rat initial IMCD (or $IMCD_1$) contains 90% principal cells and 10% intercalated cells[112]; the rat terminal IMCD (or $IMCD_2$ and $IMCD_3$) contains a unique cell type, the IMCD cell.[113] Most of the permeability values available for IMCD subsegments are from the rat (Table 43.5).

In the absence of vasopressin, the initial IMCD has a low osmotic water permeability which is increased 10- to 30-fold by vasopressin.[102,116,117] Urea permeability is low in the initial IMCD, and is unaffected by vasopressin.[102,104,114,116,118] The initial IMCD from normal rats does not show any active urea transport.[115,118,119]

The terminal IMCD has a higher basal (no vasopressin) osmotic water permeability than other portions of the collecting duct.[102,116,117] Vasopressin can rapidly increase osmotic water permeability by a factor of 10.[102,117] The terminal IMCD also has a higher basal urea permeability than other portions of the collecting duct.[102,104,114,116,120] Vasopressin and hypertonicity can each increase urea permeability by a factor of 4–6, and together they can increase urea permeability by a factor of 10.[102,116,119–121] Although early studies suggested a urea reflection coefficient of less than 1, more recent studies which re-measured the urea reflection coefficient and explicitly measured the dissipation of the imposed urea gradient, showed that the urea reflection coefficient equals 1.[50,122] The $IMCD_2$ subsegment from normal rats does not show any active urea transport.[115,118] However, active urea secretion, which is completely dependent upon luminal sodium, is present in the $IMCD_3$ from normal rats, suggesting that sodium absorption may be coupled to urea secretion.[115]

Sodium and chloride permeabilities are low in the terminal IMCD.[116,123,124] Micropuncture studies indicate substantial rates of NaCl absorption from the IMCD, but perfused tubule studies have been unable to detect it.[124–126]

Papillary Surface Epithelium

Only a few permeability coefficients have been measured across the papillary surface epithelium, and these have been measured only in rabbit (Table 43.5). The urea and osmotic water permeabilities are low and unaffected by vasopressin.[104,127] The basal chloride permeability is higher than that of the terminal IMCD, and is inhibited by vasopressin.[127] The apical membrane of the papillary surface epithelial cell, which faces the urinary space, expresses a $Na^+-K^+-Cl^-$ co-transporter that is stimulated by vasopressin and inhibited by bumetanide.[15] The basolateral membrane contains a potassium conductive pathway in rat and rabbit.[128,129]

GENERAL FEATURES OF URINARY CONCENTRATION AND DILUTION

Countercurrent Multiplication Hypothesis

Since the late 1950s, the countercurrent multiplication hypothesis has been the generally accepted explanation for the generation of the osmolality gradient along the cortico–medullary axis in both the outer and inner medullas.[130] This hypothesis holds that, at each level of the medulla, a small osmolality difference between tubular fluid flows in ascending and descending limbs is multiplied by the countercurrent flow configuration to establish a large axial osmolality difference. The principle of countercurrent multiplication is illustrated in Figure 43.7. The loop shown in the figure panels may be identified with a short loop of Henle: the left channel is analogous to the descending limb, whereas the right channel is analogous to the thick ascending limb. The channels are separated by a water-impermeable barrier. Vertical arrows indicate flow down the left channel and flow up the right channel. Left-directed horizontal arrows indicate active transport of solute from the right channel to the left channel. The numbers within channels indicate local fluid osmolality. Successive panels represent the time course of the multiplication process.

Panel (a) of Figure 43.7 illustrates a loop with isosmolar fluid throughout. In panel (b), an active transport mechanism has pumped enough solute to establish a 20 mOsm/kg H$_2$O osmolality difference between the ascending and descending flows at each level. This small difference, transverse to the flow, is called the "single effect." Panel (c) illustrates the osmolality values after the fluid has advected (or carried) the solute half-way down the left channel and half-way up the right channel. In panel (d), the active transport mechanism has re-established a 20 mOsm/kg H$_2$O osmolality difference, and the luminal fluid near the bend of the loop has attained a higher osmolality than in panel (a). By successive iterations of this process, a progressively higher osmolality is attained at the loop bend, and a large osmolality difference is generated along the flow direction. This is illustrated in panel (e), where the osmolality at the loop bend is nearly 300 mOsm/kg H$_2$O above the osmolality of the fluid entering the loop. Thus, the "single effect" of a 20 mOsm/kg H$_2$O difference has been multiplied axially down the length of the loop by the process of countercurrent multiplication.

In the outer medulla, countercurrent multiplication is believed to occur in the short loops of Henle by a process that is similar to that shown in Figure 43.7. The tubular fluid of the proximal tubule that enters the outer medulla is isotonic to plasma (about 290 mOsm/kg H$_2$O). That fluid is concentrated, as it passes through the pars recta and the thin descending limb, by osmotically driven water absorption; the absorption is driven by vigorous active transport of NaCl from the thick ascending limbs. At the bend of the loop of Henle, the tubular fluid osmolality attains an osmolality about twice that of blood plasma. Because the thick ascending limbs are nearly impermeable to water, its tubular fluid is diluted by NaCl absorption as it flows toward the cortex, so that the fluid emerging from this segment is hypoosmotic to blood plasma.

Countercurrent multiplication in the outer medulla, however, differs in important ways from the process illustrated in Figure 43.7. In some of the most completely studied mammals, the descending and ascending limbs do not abut one another[131]; therefore, solute is not directly transported from ascending limbs to descending limbs. Rather, NaCl is pumped from thick ascending limbs to the interstitium, raising the osmolality of the interstitial fluid and the blood flowing through the vasa recta and capillaries. The increased interstitial osmolality withdraws water from thin descending limbs, and some NaCl may diffuse into thin descending limbs, thus raising the osmolality of descending limb fluid. The NaCl absorbed from ascending limbs and the water absorbed from descending limbs is carried to the cortex by the vasa recta, which, somewhat like the loops of Henle, are arranged in a countercurrent configuration. Thus, a large axial osmolality difference, from the cortico—medullary boundary to the boundary of the inner and outer medulla, is established in the loops of Henle, the vasculature, and the interstitium.

In addition, Figure 43.7 does not represent the flow in the collecting ducts. Some of the water and solute in thick ascending limb tubular fluid delivered to the

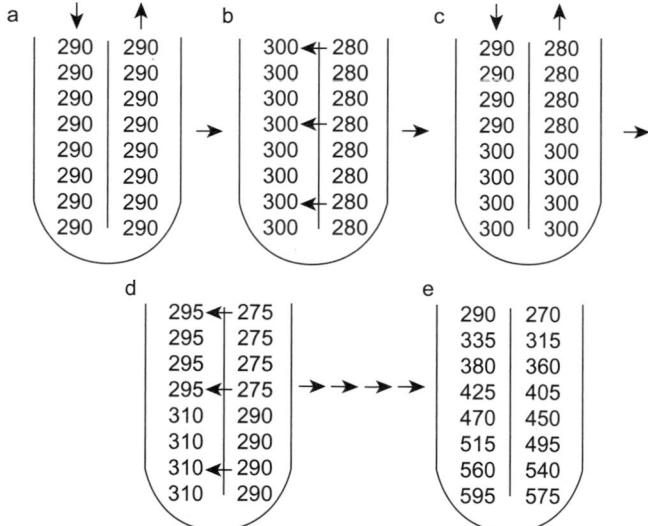

FIGURE 43.7 Countercurrent multiplication of a single effect. Panel (a): Process begins with isosmolar fluid throughout both channels. Panel (b): Active solute transport establishes a 20 mOsm/kg H$_2$O transverse gradient (single effect) across the boundary separating the channels. Panel (c): Fluid flows half-way down the descending limb and up the ascending limb. Panel (d): Active transport reestablishes a 20 mOsm/kg H$_2$O transverse gradient. Note that the luminal fluid near the bend of the loop achieves a higher osmolality than loop-bend fluid in panel (b). Panel (e): As the processes in (c) and (d) are repeated, the bend of the loop achieves a progressively higher osmolality so that the final axial osmotic gradient far exceeds the transverse 20 mOsm/kg H$_2$O gradient generated at any level.

cortex re-enters the outer medulla in the collecting ducts, and in the presence of vasopressin, sufficient water is absorbed from the collecting ducts, as a consequence of the hyperosmotic medullary interstitium, to bring collecting duct flow to near osmotic equilibrium with the surrounding interstitium. Thus, a large axial osmolality difference, similar to that in the thin descending limb, is established in collecting duct fluid.

Finally, the discrete, sequential process represented in Figure 43.7 does not arise under normal physiological conditions. Rather, the axial osmolality difference, or gradient, is sustained in near steady-state, much as indicated in panel (e), with a bend osmolality that is limited primarily by the rate of active transport, the diffusive back-leak of NaCl into the thick ascending limb, the length of the loop, the rate of water absorption from collecting duct flow, and the dissipative effects of the vasculature.

In recent years, some reasons have emerged for skepticism of the countercurrent multiplication hypothesis as the explanation for the axial osmolality gradient in the outer medulla. Several laboratories have reported evidence for the absence of AQP1 in significant portions of the terminal thin desending limbs of short loops of Henle.[43,90,132] Moreover, two modeling studies[55,133] have suggested that the osmotic load that is put on the concentrating mechanism in the outer medulla may be increased by water-permeable descending limbs, relative to water-impermeable limbs, and thus may reduce or eliminate the hypothesized concentration advantage of water absorption from descending limbs of short loops.

The axial osmolality gradient in the inner medulla has also been generally believed to be generated by the countercurrent multiplication of a small transverse osmolality difference, presumably between thin ascending and thin descending limbs. However, evidence for significant active transport from thin ascending limbs is lacking, and experiments indicate that the thin ascending limbs are highly permeable to both NaCl and urea. Thus, the inner medullary single effect must arise from a mechanism different from that found in the outer medulla. The roles of the vasculature and collecting duct are considered below; a more detailed treatment of countercurrent multiplication, and in particular, the concentrating mechanism of the inner medulla, is given in a subsequent section (*vide infra*).

Countercurrent Exchange

The descending and ascending vasa recta are arranged in a counter-flow configuration connected by a capillary plexus. Vasa recta are freely permeable to water, sodium, and urea, and achieve osmotic equilibration through a combination of water absorption and solute secretion.[134] Descending vasa recta gain solute and lose water, while ascending vasa recta lose solute and gain water. The exchange of solute and water between the descending and ascending vasa recta and the surrounding interstitium is called "countercurrent exchange."

Efficient countercurrent exchange is essential for producing concentrated urine, because hypotonic fluid carried into the medulla and hypertonic fluid carried away from the medulla both tend to dissipate the cortico–medullary gradient of countercurrent multiplication. Thus, to minimize wasted work, fluid flowing through the vasa recta must achieve near osmotic equilibrium with the surrounding interstitium at each medullary level, and fluid entering the cortex from the ascending vasa recta must have an osmolality close to that of blood plasma. Conditions which decrease medullary blood flow, such as volume depletion, improve the efficiency of countercurrent exchange and urine concentrating ability by allowing more time for blood in the ascending vasa recta to lose solute and achieve osmotic equilibration.[134] Conversely, conditions which increase medullary blood flow, such as osmotic diuresis, impair the efficiency of countercurrent exchange and decrease urine concentrating ability.[134] For a detailed treatment of countercurrent exchange, see Chapter 24.

Role of the Collecting Duct

The collecting duct, under the control of vasopressin and other factors, is the nephron segment responsible for final control of water excretion. Whereas the osmolality gradient along the cortico–medullary axis, in both the outer and inner medulla, presumably arises from mechanisms that principally involve participation of the loops of Henle, and countercurrent exchange in the vasa recta minimizes the dissipative effect of vascular flow, the excretion of water requires another structural component, the collecting duct system, which starts in the cortex and ends at the papillary tip. In the absence of vasopressin, the cortical, outer medullary, and initial inner medullary portions of the collecting duct are nearly water-impermeable. (The terminal IMCD has a moderate water-permeability even in the absence of vasopressin (*vide supra*).) Since the fluid that leaves the thick ascending limb and enters the cortical collecting duct is dilute relative to plasma, excretion of dilute urine only requires that not much water be absorbed nor much solute be secreted along the collecting duct.

In the presence of vasopressin, the entire collecting duct becomes highly water-permeable. This process takes place in the following way. Plasma osmolality increases when a person or an animal becomes water depleted. Osmoreceptors in the hypothalamus, which can sense an increase of only 2 mOsm/kg H_2O, stimulate vasopressin secretion from the posterior pituitary. Vasopressin binds to V_2-receptors in the basolateral plasma membrane of principal and IMCD cells in the collecting duct, stimulates adenylyl cyclase to produce cAMP, activates protein kinase A (PKA), phosphorylates aquaporin-2 (AQP2) at serines 256, 261, 264, and 269, inserts AQP2 water channels into the apical plasma membrane, and increases water absorption across the collecting duct ([135–138] and reviewed in [81]). This regulated trafficking of AQP2 between subapical vesicles and the apical plasma membrane is the major mechanism for acute regulation of water absorption by vasopressin (reviewed in [81]). Wade and colleagues originally proposed the "membrane shuttle hypothesis," which proposes that water channels are stored in vesicles and inserted exocytically into the apical plasma membrane in response to vasopressin.[139] Since the cloning of AQP2, the shuttle hypothesis has been proven experimentally in rat inner medulla (reviewed in [81]). Subsequent studies have elucidated several signal transduction pathways that are involved in regulating AQP2 trafficking (insertion and retrieval of AQP2), the role of vesicle targeting proteins (SNAP/SNARE system), and the cytoskeleton (reviewed in [81]); these processes are discussed in more detail in Chapter 41.

Vasopressin-induced water permeability allows water to be absorbed across the collecting ducts at a sufficiently high rate for collecting duct tubular fluid to attain near osmotic equilibration with the hyperosmotic medullary interstitium; the absorbed water is returned to the systemic circulation via the ascending vasa recta. The majority of water is absorbed from collecting ducts in the cortex and outer medulla. Although the inner medulla has a higher osmolality than the outer medulla, its role in absorbing water from the collecting duct is important only when maximal water conservation is required. More water is actually absorbed across the IMCD during diuresis than antidiuresis, owing to the large transepithelial osmolality difference.[140]

URINE CONCENTRATING MECHANISM: HISTORY AND THEORY

Overview

The conceptual history of the urine concentrating mechanism may be divided into three periods. The first period, extending from 1942 through 1971, was inaugurated by the publication of a study by Kuhn and Ryffel,[141] who proposed that concentrated urine is produced by the countercurrent multiplication of a "single effect," and who constructed a working apparatus that exemplified the principles of countercurrent multiplication. During this first period, the theory of the countercurrent multiplication hypothesis was developed further, and experimental evidence accumulated that supported the hypothesis as the explanation for the concentrating mechanism of the outer medulla. In particular, active transport of NaCl from thick ascending limbs was identified as the source of the outer medullary single effect.[94,142]

The second period of conceptual history, extending from 1972 through 1992, was inaugurated by the simultaneous publication, by Kokko and Rector and by Stephenson, of papers proposing that a "passive mechanism" provides the single effect for countercurrent multiplication in the inner medulla.[8,9] According to the passive mechanism hypothesis, a net solute efflux from thin ascending limbs results from favorable transepithelial NaCl and urea gradients; these gradients arise from the separation of NaCl and urea, which is largely driven by the outer medullary concentrating mechanism. Although initially much experimental evidence appeared to support the passive mechanism, findings from many subsequent studies are difficult to reconcile with this hypothesis.[22,143,144] Moreover, mathematical models incorporating measured transepithelial permeabilities failed to predict a significant inner medullary concentrating effect.[52,145,146] The discrepancy between the consistently negative results from mathematical modeling studies and the very effective inner medullary concentrating effect has persisted through more than three decades. The discrepancy has helped to stimulate research on the transport properties of the renal tubules of the inner medulla and the formulation of several highly sophisticated mathematical models (notably,[147]), but no model study has resolved the discrepancy to the general satisfaction of experimentalists and modelers.

In the early 1990s, new hypotheses for the inner medullary concentrating mechanism began to receive serious consideration, and a third period of conceptual thought may be considered to have begun in 1993: in that year, Knepper and colleagues proposed a key role for the peristalsis of the papilla,[143,148] and in 1994 Jen and Stephenson[149] examined the principle of "externally driven" countercurrent multiplication, arising, e.g., by the net production of osmotically active particles in the interstitium. At about the same time, perfused tubule studies in chinchilla, which can produce very highly concentrated urine, provided evidence that the passive mechanism, as originally proposed, cannot explain the inner medullary concentrating mechanism.[57] Recent studies have sought to further develop hypotheses involving peristalsis,[150] the potential generation of osmotically active particles, especially lactate,[151,152] and the role of complex inner medullary anatomy and detailed transporter localization.[21,54,153] In 2004, evidence suggesting an absence of significant urea transport proteins in loops of Henle reaching deep into the medulla led to a reconsideration of hypotheses related to the passive mechanism.[54]

Countercurrent Multiplication Hypothesis

In 1942, Kuhn and Ryffel proposed that urine is concentrated by means of multiplication (or augmentation) of a single effect ("Vervielfältigung des Einzeleffektes").[141] More precisely, they suggested that a small osmotic pressure difference between flows in parallel renal tubules (the single effect) was multiplied by means of the countercurrent principle ("Gegenstromprinzip"), resulting in a large increase in osmotic pressure along the cortico—medullary axis (*vide supra*: Figure 43.7 and accompanying discussion). Kuhn and Ryffel, however, made no specific conjectures regarding which tubules or what transport properties were involved. To test their hypothesis, Kuhn and Ryffel constructed an apparatus that, by embodying the countercurrent principle and by employing phenol and sucrose solutions separated by selectively permeable membranes, was able to increase the concentration of the sucrose solution by a factor of 3.5. This apparatus suggested that three fundamental components are needed for a physiologically plausible mechanism for generating concentrated urine: (1) countercurrent flow; (2) a source of energy to sustain a single effect (in this case, potential energy in the form of the differing solutions); and (3) specific membrane permeability characteristics.

In a 1951 study, Hargitay and Kuhn[154] proposed the basic framework for the modern conception of the urine concentrating mechanism. They hypothesized that the loop of Henle is a biological realization of a hairpin counterflow system, that the loops of Henle would generate a cortico—medullary osmolality gradient, and that final urine concentration would be achieved by the osmotic withdrawal of water from collecting ducts. Their study, which included both a working apparatus and a mathematical model, confirmed that countercurrent multiplication could generate a significant axial concentration gradient. However, their apparatus relied on the transport of water across the separating membrane, and they employed a mechanical pressure as a driving force to sustain the single effect. The pressure required for a significant axial gradient (estimated at 550 mmHg) was judged by the authors to far exceed a pressure likely to be found *in vivo* (~120 mmHg). They proposed, as

an alternative, a single effect arising from water transport driven by a process of electro-osmosis ("Electroosmose"), which was hypothesized to arise from metabolic processes in epithelial cells. In 1959, a mathematical analysis by Kuhn and Ramel showed that active NaCl transport from ascending limbs could serve to provide the required single effect.[155]

The countercurrent multiplier hypothesis was bolstered by a 1951 study in which Wirz, Hargitay, and Kuhn used slices of renal tissue from hydropenic rats to demonstrate an osmotic pressure gradient, starting at approximately the cortico—medullary boundary, and increasing along the cortico—medullary axis to the papillary tip. In subsequent experimental studies, active transport of NaCl from thick ascending limbs was established as the driving force required to sustain the transepithelial osmolality difference needed for countercurrent multiplication in the outer medulla,[94,142] and the osmotic absorption of water from collecting ducts into the hypertonic interstitium was established as the ultimate process by which collecting duct fluid is concentrated in antidiuresis.[156] However, investigation of the inner medullary renal tubules revealed no active transport process that could generate a significant transepithelial osmolality difference.[63,130]

Concentrating Mechanism of the Outer Medulla

In the presence of vasopressin, the outer medullary concentrating mechanism is believed to operate as follows. Transepithelial active transport of NaCl, from the tubular fluid of thick ascending limbs and into the surrounding interstitium, raises the osmolality of interstitial fluid and promotes the osmotic absorption of water from the tubular fluid of nearby descending limbs and collecting ducts. Because of the absorption of fluid from descending limbs, the fluid delivered to the ascending limbs has a high NaCl concentration that favors the transepithelial transport of NaCl from ascending limb fluid. (There may also be some diffusion of NaCl into descending limb fluid.) NaCl transport dilutes the tubular fluid of thick ascending limbs, so that at each medullary level the fluid osmolality is less than that in the other tubules and in the vessels, and so that the fluid delivered to the cortex is dilute relative to blood plasma. The ascending limb fluid that enters the cortex is further diluted by active NaCl transport from cortical thick ascending limbs, so that its osmolality is less than the osmolality of blood plasma. In cortical collecting ducts, which are water-permeable in the presence of vasopressin, sufficient water is absorbed to return the collecting duct tubular fluid to isotonicity with blood plasma. This water absorption greatly reduces the load that is placed on the concentrating mechanism by the fluid that re-enters the medulla. In the absence of vasopressin, the collecting duct system, both in the cortex and outer medulla, is much less water-permeable, and even though some water is absorbed due to the very large osmotic pressure gradient, fluid that is dilute relative to plasma is delivered by the collecting ducts to the border of the outer and inner medulla.

This modern conceptual formulation of the outer medullary concentrating mechanism (which is very similar to the proposal of Hargitay and Kuhn as modified by Kuhn and Ramel[154,155]) is supported by recent mathematical modeling studies using parameters compatible with micropuncture and perfused tubule experiments.[52,133,157−160] In particular, the osmotic gradients in the outer medulla predicted by simulations are consistent with the gradients reported in tissue slice experiments, where osmolality is increased by a factor of 2−3.[37,161]

Mass Balance in the Renal Medulla

For the outer medullary gradient to be sustained in a steady-state, the water and solute flows in the tubules and vessels of the outer medulla and, therefore, the spatial distribution of water and solute, must remain nearly fixed (provided there are no significant metabolic solute sources or sinks). Thus, for any transverse slice of the medulla, say of a thickness extending from location X_1 to X_2, the directed sum of water flow rates in all tubules and vessels at X_1 must equal that at level X_2, and the directed sum of solute flow rates in all tubules and vessels at level X_1 must equal that at level X_2. This is the principle of steady-state mass balance (for an explicit mathematical formulation see reference[7]).

Global mass balance for the outer medulla is thought to be preserved as follows (the relatively small effects of long looped nephrons, of vasa recta reaching into the inner medulla, and of solutes other than NaCl are ignored here for simplicity). At the cortico−medullary boundary, the water flowing in ascending vasa recta exceeds that flowing in descending vasa recta, owing to water absorption from thin descending limbs and collecting ducts. In contrast, the water flow emerging from thick ascending limbs is significantly reduced relative to the flow entering descending limbs at the cortico−medullary boundary. The directed sum of these flows, plus flow entering collecting ducts at the cortico−medullary boundary results in a small net flow from the cortex into the outer medulla that nearly equals net water flow at the outer−inner medullary boundary.

Similarly, solute flows must be balanced. At the cortico−medullary boundary, the solute emerging from ascending vasa recta exceeds that flowing in descending vasa recta, owing to NaCl absorption from thick ascending limbs. In contrast, the solute flow emerging from thick ascending limbs is reduced (relative to flow entering descending limbs) by a larger fraction than the thick ascending limb fluid flow. The directed sum of these solute flows at the cortico−medullary boundary, plus solute flow entering collecting ducts at that boundary, results in a small net solute flow nearly equal to net solute flow at the inner−outer medullary boundary.

The ratio of NaCl to water in net flow across the cortico−medullary boundary, and the ratio of NaCl to water in collecting duct flow at the inner−outer medullary boundary, both depend on whether the animal is in a diuretic or antidiuretic state. In either case, a greater fraction of loop of Henle solute flow is absorbed, relative to water flow, in the outer medulla and, consequently, a greater fraction of water is delivered to the cortex, relative to solute. Consequently, dilute fluid is delivered by the thick ascending limbs to the cortex, and this fluid is further diluted by NaCl transport from the cortical thick ascending limb.

In diuresis, little water is absorbed from the cortical collecting ducts. Consequently, the net fluid absorbed into the cortical circulation (taking into account NaCl absorption from cortical thick ascending limbs) is concentrated relative to blood plasma, and the fluid re-entering the outer medulla in collecting ducts remains dilute relative to blood plasma. The low water permeability of the outer medullary collecting duct in diuresis will prevent any significant dilution of vasa recta flow, and thus prevent any significant reduction in the concentrating capacity of the countercurrent mechanism. Thus, combined with slightly concentrated flow from ascending vasa recta, the ultimate effect of fluid absorbed in the cortex will be to raise the osmolality of the systemic circulation. Moreover, owing to the dominating effect of hypotonic fluid flowing from the cortical collecting ducts into the outer medullary collecting ducts, the net fluid flow from the cortex to the outer medulla will be dilute relative to systemic plasma, and as a consequence of mass balance, the net fluid flow across the inner−outer medullary boundary will be dilute relative to blood plasma.

In antidiuresis, much water is absorbed from the water-permeable cortical collecting ducts. Consequently, the net fluid absorbed in the cortex, from fluid entering the cortex via the thick ascending limbs, is dilute relative to plasma, and its diluting effect on the cortex outweighs the concentrating effect of slightly hypertonic ascending vasa recta flow. Collecting duct fluid entering the outer medulla is isotonic to blood plasma, and relative to the case of diuresis, reduced in flow rate, so that the fluid absorbed from the now-permeable outer medullary collecting duct does not significantly reduce the concentrating capacity of the countercurrent mechanism. Thus, the ultimate effect of dilute fluid absorbed from the cortical collecting duct is to lower the osmolality of the systemic circulation. Moreover, owing to the dominating effect of dilute fluid emerging from the outer medullary thick ascending limbs into the cortex, the net flow from the cortex to the outer medulla will be concentrated relative to systemic blood plasma, and as a consequence of mass balance, the net flow of collecting duct fluid across the inner—outer medullary boundary will be concentrated relative to blood plasma.

Because the inner medullary concentrating effect remains elusive, and because the net generation of osmotically active molecules has been suggested as a possible source of the single effect for the inner medulla,[149,151,162] the role of the inner medullary concentrating mechanism has been ignored in our description of mass balance. However, a mass balance analysis similar to that given above for the outer medulla would apply to the inner medulla separately, and thus also to the whole medulla, according to most hypotheses for the inner medullary concentrating mechanism. (In the presence of oscillations in tubular flow mediated by the tubuloglomerular feedback mechanism[163] or in the presence of peristalsis of the papilla,[164] mass balance would have to be reformulated for time-averaged flows.) In any case, the overall effect of mass balance in the renal medulla, in diuresis, is that systemic blood plasma is concentrated by the production of urine that is dilute relative to plasma; in antidiuresis, blood plasma is diluted by the production of urine that is concentrated relative to plasma.

The Passive Mechanism Hypothesis for the Inner Medulla

Although active NaCl transport from thick ascending limbs was identified as the fundamental source of the outer medullary concentrating mechanism, isolated perfused tubule experiments in rabbits demonstrated that the thin ascending limb had no significant active NaCl transport,[63,94] but instead had relatively high permeabilities to sodium and urea, while being impermeable to water.[80] The inner medullary thin descending limb in rabbit, in contrast, was found to be highly water-permeable, but to have low sodium and urea permeabilities.[60,64] Moreover, evidence from some species showed that urea tended to accumulate in the inner medulla, with concentrations similar to those of NaCl,[6] and it had long been known that urea administration enhances maximum urine concentration in protein-deprived rats and humans.[165,166] Several models were published that sought to explain the inner

medullary concentrating mechanism,[167–171] but they failed to gain general acceptance.

In 1972, independent papers by Kokko and Rector and by Stephenson (appearing in the same volume of *Kidney International*) proposed that the concentrating effect in the inner medulla arises from a "passive mechanism".[8,9] The key components of the passive mechanism are represented in Figure 43.6. Active absorption of NaCl from the thick ascending limb, and the subsequent absorption of water from the cortical and outer medullary collecting ducts work together to increase the urea concentration of collecting duct fluid. Urea diffuses down its transepithelial concentration gradient from the highly urea-permeable terminal IMCD into the inner medullary interstitium; urea is trapped in the inner medulla by countercurrent exchange in the vasa recta (*vide supra*). The fluid entering the thin ascending limb has a high NaCl concentration relative to urea, and the thin ascending limb is hypothesized to have a high NaCl permeability relative to urea. In addition, due to accumulation of urea in the interstitium, the NaCl concentration in the thin ascending limb exceeds the NaCl concentration in the interstitium, and consequently NaCl diffuses down its concentration gradient into the interstitium. If the thin ascending limb has sufficiently low urea permeability, the rate of NaCl efflux from the ascending limb will exceed the rate of urea influx, resulting in the dilution of thin ascending limb fluid, and the flow of relatively dilute fluid up the thin ascending limb at each medullary level and into the thick ascending limb. Thus, dilute fluid is removed from the inner medulla, and mass balance requires that the osmolality of the inner medulla be progressively elevated along the tubules of the inner medulla. The elevated osmolality will draw water from the thin descending limbs, thus raising the NaCl concentration of the descending limb flow that enters thin ascending limbs. In addition, the elevated osmolality of the inner medulla will draw water from the water-permeable IMCD, raising the concentration of urea in collecting duct flow; accumulation of NaCl in the interstitium will tend to sustain a transepithelial urea concentration gradient favorable to urea absorption from the terminal IMCD.

Several matters are worthy of note. First, this process, described above in step-wise fashion, should be thought of as a continuous, steady-state process. Second, although the mechanism is characterized as "passive," it depends on the separation of NaCl and urea that is sustained by the active absorption of NaCl by thick ascending limbs. The separated high concentration flows of NaCl (in the loop of Henle) and of urea (in the collecting duct) constitute a source of potential energy that is used to effect a net transport of solute from the thin ascending limb. Thus, the laws of thermodynamics are not violated. Third, the description above speaks rather loosely of NaCl and urea as solutes having equal standing, but the atoms of NaCl are nearly completely dissociated, so that each NaCl molecule has nearly twice the osmotic effect of each urea molecule. This distinction must be represented in formal mathematical descriptions. Fourth, the passive mechanism hypothesis is very similar to the concentrating mechanism of the outer medulla, inasmuch as it depends on net solute absorption from the thin ascending limb to dilute thin ascending limb fluid and raise the osmolality of adjacent flows and structures. Finally, the concentrating effect is balanced, as in the outer medulla, by the dissipative effects of vascular flows, and by the production of a small amount of highly concentrated urine. These dissipative effects limit the achievable urine osmolality.

The passive mechanism hypothesis, as described above, closely follows the Kokko and Rector formulation,[8] which made use of key ideas set forth by Kokko in a largely experimental study.[60] Kokko and Rector acknowledged Niesel and Rosenbleck[169] for the proposal that urea absorbed from the IMCD contributes to the inner medullary osmolality gradient. Kokko and Rector presented the passive mechanism hypothesis conceptually, and although it was accompanied by a plausible set of solute fluxes, concentrations, and fluid flow rates that are consistent with the requirements of mass balance, their presentation did not include a mathematical treatment, and it did not demonstrate that measured loop of Henle permeabilities were consistent with the hypothesis. Stephenson's presentation of the passive hypothesis[9] included a more mathematical treatment, and it introduced the highly influential central core assumption (*vide infra*), but it also did not contain a mathematical reconciliation of tubular transport properties with the hypothesis.

The crucial test needed to confirm the passive mechanism hypothesis was an adequate mathematical representation of all the major components of the hypothesized mechanism, including tubular and vascular flows, transepithelial transport, tubular and vascular interactions, and medullary anatomy. The mathematical representation was needed to show that the magnitudes and distributions of the flow rates, transport rates, interactions, and structures, could produce a medullary gradient consistent with tissue slice experiments and measured urine osmolalities.

The Central Core Assumption

In the same paper that set forth the passive mechanism hypothesis,[9] Stephenson introduced the central core assumption, in which the interstitium and the vasculature are merged into a single compartment through which the renal tubules interact. Stephenson argued that if the vasa recta were sufficiently permeable to solutes and water, the vasa recta would serve as a nearly perfect countercurrent exchanger, in nearly complete osmotic equilibrium with each other, and with the interstitium, at each medullary level. In such a case, a very substantial simplification in conceptual and mathematical analysis could be obtained: the central core could be treated very much as an additional species of tubule, but serving a special role as the medium through which other tubules interact. Using the central core assumption, Stephenson was able to derive simplified mathematical expressions that not only aided the model analysis of the passive mechanism, but which were also general enough to permit extensive analysis in terms of fundamental quantities.[9,172–175]

The central core assumption, as illustrated by Stephenson, is represented in Figure 43.8. The upper panel depicts the interaction of the renal tubules with the central core. The lower panels show that the central core may be conceptualized as a single tubule through which the other tubules interact. The central core may be considered to carry, from the medulla to the cortex, the net water and solutes absorbed from the tubules.

The central core assumption has been examined in several theoretical studies,[176–178] all of which concluded that the assumption is a good approximation provided that vasa recta permeabilities are sufficiently high; experiments on vasa recta have tended to confirm the high permeabilities that are required for nearly ideal countercurrent exchange (see Chapter 24). The central core assumption has been used in a number of mathematical models and computer simulations.[10–12,17,23,52,54,55,159,178–181] However, models based on the central core assumption cannot incorporate the effects of the radial organization of medullary structures with respect to the vascular bundles in the outer medulla or with respect to the collecting duct clusters in the inner medulla, because that organization is likely to result in differing solute concentrations in the various interstitial spaces, tubules, and vessels as a function of their positions.[12,147]

Computer Simulations

Computer simulations of the urine concentrating mechanism are based on detailed mathematical models; the models consist of differential equations and algebraic relations that embody transepithelial transport processes and the requirements of water and solute mass balance. The degree of sophistication of these models has varied substantially in the number of molecular species represented, the degree of detail in

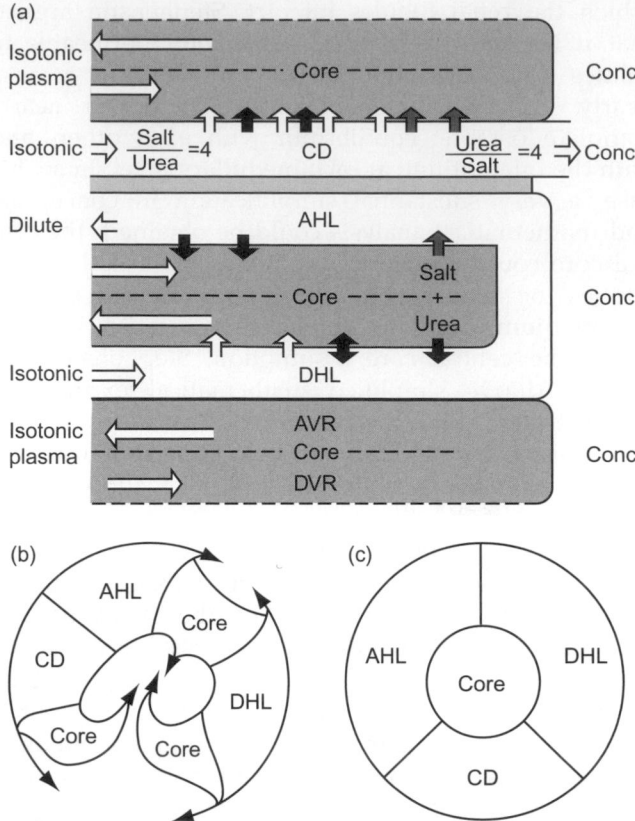

FIGURE 43.8 **Schematic representation of central core assumption, in which the interstitium and vasa recta (AVR, DVR) are merged into a single compartment (Core).** Upper panel (a) shows interaction of tubules with Core. Vertical arrows indicate transepithelial fluxes of NaCl (black), urea (hatched), and water (white); horizontal arrows indicate relative fluid flow. Water is absorbed from descending limb (DHL) into Core, urea enters DHL from Core, and NaCl may move in either direction. NaCl is absorbed from ascending limb (AHL) into Core, while urea enters AHL. Water, NaCl, and urea are absorbed from collecting duct (CD) into Core; as a result of differential absorption, salt/urea concentration reverses. Panel (b) shows Core from (a) being consolidated into a final cross-section (c), in which a single Core compartment interacts with AHL, DHL, and CD. *(Reproduced with permission, from reference [9].)*

the formulation of epithelial transport, the numbers of loops of Henle and collecting ducts, the representation of the vasculature, and the representation of three-dimensional connectivity. Because the mathematical models involve a large number of nonlinear equations, explicit solutions in terms of elementary functions cannot be obtained, and approximate solutions must be found by the methods of numerical analysis. Owing to the very large permeabilities measured in some renal tubules, and to orders-of-magnitude changes in the water and solute flow rates along the nephron, model solutions are difficult to approximate, and consequently a large amount of effort has been expended in the development of suitable numerical methods (see, e.g.,[20,133,153,157,182–186]). For comprehensive reviews of

models and simulations of the concentrating mechanism, including substantial mathematical detail, see[187,188].

The passive mechanism hypothesis was developed at about the same time that it was becoming practical for large-scale simulations to be conducted on digital computers. Indeed, a computer simulation by Stewart and collaborators[189,190] appeared in the same issue of *Kidney International* that contained the papers that set forth the passive mechanism hypothesis.[8,9] In the absence of active NaCl transport from thin ascending limbs, a significant inner medullary osmolality gradient was generated when loop urea permeabilities were set to 0.1×10^{-5} cm/s. But the gradient was greatly diminished when thin descending limb urea permeability was increased to 0.3×10^{-5} cm/s, a small value compared to measurements in all species examined (see Table 43.2). Thus, the addition of a small amount of urea to thin descending limb fluid resulted in a marked decrease in the inner medullary gradient. Moreover, the authors reported that: "Computer simulation confirmed that low sodium or high urea permeability in ascending limb or high sodium or urea permeability in descending limb, singly or in combination, virtually abolished the osmotic gradient in the inner medulla." These results were difficult to reconcile with experiments that had shown significant net urea addition to both thin descending and ascending limbs in the hamster.[76]

This early simulation immediately cast doubt on the passive mechanism hypothesis, and it reported a result that was confirmed in many subsequent simulations: the addition of urea to the loops of Henle reaching into the inner medulla tends to dissipate the transepithelial NaCl and urea gradients that are required for the successful operation of the passive mechanism (see, e.g.,[145,146,179,180,191,192]). Thus, for example, if the thin ascending limb is significantly urea-permeable, diffusion of urea from the interstitium into thin ascending limb fluid counterbalances the diluting effect of the diffusion of NaCl from ascending limb fluid into the interstitium. Consequently, fluid in the ascending limb tends to osmotic equilibrium with respect to surrounding interstitial fluid. Because thin ascending limb fluid is not dilute relative to fluid in tubules and vessels at the same level, there is no inner medullary single effect to be multiplied by means of the countercurrent flow configuration.

Figure 43.9, based on data from a simulation published in 1996,[52] shows results that are representative of most simulation studies. Medullary osmolality and concentrations of electrolytes and urea are given as flow-weighted averages, taken across all tubules at each medullary level. Figure 43.9 has been drawn so that it may be easily compared with Figure 43.5.

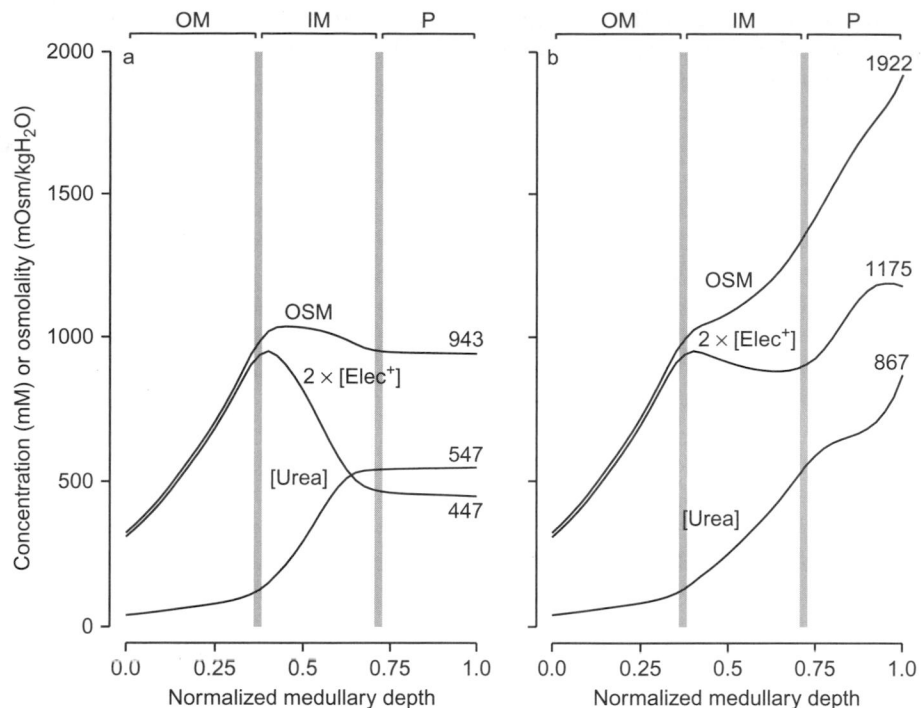

FIGURE 43.9 Concentration and osmolality profiles as a function of medullary depth from computer simulation by Layton et al.[52] Profiles represent flow-weighted averages across all tubules. Cation concentration [Elec$^+$] arose from Na$^+$, except in collecting ducts, where both Na$^+$ and K$^+$ were represented. Urine values are given at right of each panel. Profiles in panel (a) were computed from loop of Henle permeabilities based on measurements in chinchilla ([57]; see Tables 43.2 and 43.3). The non-increasing osmolality profile in the inner medulla is similar to that computed with lower permeability values from rabbit, rat, and hamster in a number of model studies (e.g., references[191,179,180,145,146]). Profiles in panel (b) were obtained when urea permeability ($\times 10^{-5}$ cm/s) was reduced from 16.8 to 1 in inner medullary descending limbs and from 170 to 1 in thin ascending limbs. Resulting profiles compare favorably with data from rat (cf. Figure 43.4), but despite greatly reduced urea permeabilities, model urine osmolality falls far short of 7600 mOsm/kg H$_2$O, the maximum concentrating capability of chinchilla.[1] Note that while tubular electrolytes (principally Na$^+$ and accompanying anions) account for most of the simulated osmolality in the outer medulla (in both panels (a) and (b)), the experimental results in Figure 43.4 show a large osmotic gap; this gap is mostly accounted for by large intracellular concentrations of K$^+$. *(The profiles in panels (a) and (b) were computed from data generated for cases designated V and I, respectively, in reference [52].)*

The simulation used loop and collecting duct distributions that are similar to those displayed in Figure 43.5, and the flow-weighted profiles in Figure 43.9 are roughly comparable to the tissue-slice profiles in Figure 43.5, although it must be kept in mind that Figure 43.5 includes the effects of intracellular fluid.

Panel (a) in Figure 43.9 shows results obtained using NaCl and urea permeabilities based on values measured in inner medullary thin descending and ascending limbs of chinchilla (see Tables 43.2 and 43.3). Owing to the significant entry of urea into descending and ascending limbs, no inner medullary gradient is generated. Moreover, the profile labeled as $2 \times$[Elec$^+$], arising mostly from sodium and its anions, fails to show an exponential rise as it does in Figure 43.5 and in electron microprobe experiments.[106] Parameter studies showed that loop urea permeabilities and descending limb NaCl permeability must all be reduced to the range of $1-5 \times 10^{-5}$ cm/s to elicit a significant concentrating effect.[52]

Panel (b) in Figure 43.9 shows profiles obtained when loop urea permeability and descending limb NaCl permeability were reduced to 1×10^{-287} cm/s. Ascending limb NaCl permeability remains high, 294×10^{-5} cm/s. With these parameters, simulation profiles are remarkably similar to those reported for the rat in Figure 43.5. However, the greatly reduced permeabilities used for urea and NaCl in descending limbs, and for urea in ascending limbs, are much smaller than those measured in rat (see Tables 43.2 and 43.3), and the urine osmolality obtained, 1922 mOsm/kg H$_2$O, is far smaller than the maximum urine osmolality obtained in chinchilla, 7600 mOsm/kg H$_2$O.[1,4,5]

In recent years, mathematical simulations of the urine concentrating mechanism have become increasingly comprehensive and sophisticated in the representation of tubular transport (e.g.,[158,159,162]) and medullary architecture.[52,55,133,147,153,157,193,194] This evolution is a consequence of the increasing body of experimental knowledge, faster computers with increased computational capacity, and the sustained failure of simulations to exhibit a significant inner medullary concentration gradient.

Stephenson and collaborators re-examined the passive mechanism hypothesis in a two-nephron central core model, in which the electrolyte concentrations for sodium, potassium, and chloride were represented, along with urea.[159] In a simulation using transport parameters from rabbit inner medulla, a significant inner medullary gradient could only be obtained when the urea permeabilities in both descending and ascending limbs had been reduced to less than 10^{-6} cm/s. For permeability values obtained from the hamster, both urea and electrolyte permeabilities needed to be greatly reduced, especially in thin descending limbs. Although it has been frequently suggested that a reduction in the urea reflection coefficient for the collecting duct epithelium could augment collecting duct osmolality by retaining urea in excess of fluid, this study showed that such a reduction was ineffective without a mechanism for generating a salt gradient in the core.

Layton and collaborators, in a series of papers, have sought to elucidate the role of the distributed loops of Henle.[52,55,180,195–197] These studies employ a model representation of the loops of Henle that allows the simulation of loops turning back at all levels of the inner medulla, while also representing the fluid flow and concentrations in individual loops.[195] Previously, models had typically used a small number of discrete loops (see, e.g.,[184]) or had employed shunts between a merged descending and ascending flow to represent the decreasing number of loops of Henle as a function of inner medullary depth (e.g.,[145]).

The distributed loop representation has been used to obtain several theoretical results. If solute is mostly absorbed near loop bends, then the loop distribution may allow a cascade effect that tends to increase the achievable concentration, provided, of course, that a net solute absorption can be obtained.[55,195] The concentrating effect can be further enhanced if solute is absorbed from a short, prebend segment of the descending limb with low water permeability[55] as has been detected in chinchilla,[42] and which may be present in other species (*vide supra*). Layton hypothesized that a cascade effect could allow the generation of an inner medullary osmolality gradient, despite large loop urea permeabilities, provided that the passive mechanism could operate near loop bends.[196,180] Average flow, taken over all thin ascending limbs at each medullary level, would be hypoosmotic relative to the flows in the surrounding tubules and vessels, due to the effect of more and more loops turning, as one proceeds from the papillary tip to the outer medulla. However, simulations using reported permeabilities in rat or chinchilla failed to support this hypothesis.[52,180]

Studies by Wexler and collaborators have sought to assess the role of preferential interactions among tubules and vessels.[147,160,162,194,198,199] Wexler, Kalaba, and Marsh introduced what has become known as the WKM model,[147,199] which was based on the organization of tubules around vascular bundles (Figure 43.3), and which therefore allowed both axial and radial concentration gradients. The preferential interaction of collecting ducts with both thick and thin ascending limbs was proposed as the key principle that allowed the generation of an inner medullary osmolality gradient. The preferential interaction with thick ascending limbs allowed highly concentrated collecting duct fluid to pass from the outer medulla to the inner medulla. The preferential interaction with thin ascending limbs allowed the passive mechanism to operate, since a urea-rich environment could be sustained around thin ascending limbs, and dissipative interaction of collecting ducts with thin descending limbs was diminished.

The WKM model drew criticism for some of its structural and transport assumptions.[32,176,200,201] Subsequent studies responded to these criticisms (with modified model assumptions), and acknowledged that preferential interactions are not sufficient to explain the inner medullary concentrating effect in the papilla.[160,162,198] Nonetheless, results from the WKM model and its successors have provided persuasive evidence that preferential interactions can be a significant factor in the degree of the outer and inner medullary concentrating effects. Moreover, the model structure permitted sensitivity testing as a function of interaction strength, and compared to other model studies, it allowed for a more accurate assessment of solute and water recycling pathways.

Two hypotheses closely related to the passive mechanism have been recently proposed by Layton et al.[54]; these hypotheses were motivated by the implications of recent studies in rat by Pannabecker et al..[18,19] One hypothesis is based directly on the principles of the passive mechanism: low urea permeabilities in thin limbs of Henle were assumed because no significant labeling for urea transport proteins was found in loops reaching deep into the inner medulla.[54] A second, more innovative hypothesis assumed very high urea loop of Henle permeabilities, but limited NaCl-permeability and zero water-permeability in thin descending limbs reaching deep into the inner medulla. Thus, in the innermost inner medulla, tubular fluid urea concentration in loops of Henle would nearly equilibrate with the local interstitial urea concentration; thin descending limb fluid osmolality would be raised by urea secretion; and substantial NaCl absorption would occur in the prebend segment and early thin ascending limb. Both hypotheses emphasize the role of the decreasing loop of Henle population, which facilitates a spatially distributed NaCl absorption along the inner medulla, from prebend segments and early thin ascending limbs. A distinctive aspect of both hypotheses is an emphasis on NaCl transport from the IMCDs as an important active transport process that separates NaCl from tubular fluid urea, and that indirectly drives water and urea absorption from the collecting ducts. Computer simulations for both hypotheses predicted urine osmolalities, flow, and concentrations consistent with urine from moderately antidiuretic rats. The critical dependence of the first hypothesis on low loop urea permeabilities is subject to the criticism that urea transport may be paracellular rather than transepithelial: that hypothesis depends on more conclusive experiments to determine urea transport properties in rat. The second hypothesis may contribute to understanding the concentrating mechanism in chinchilla, in which high loop urea permeabilities have been measured.[57]

Subsequently, a modeling study by Marcano et al.,[181] which was based on the principles of the passive mechanism, produced somewhat higher osmolalities than reported by Layton et al.,[54] but did not reach osmolalities as large as those found in highly-concentrating rats. A modeling study by Layton et al.[153] that sought to represent the interactions among tubules and vessels hypothesized by Pannabecker et al.[20] exhibited concentrating capability similar to that found by Marcano et al.[181] A second modeling study by Layton et al.[202] that represented the interactions hypothesized by Pannabecker et al.[20] set forth the hypothesis that plentiful urine flow rates in rats accompanied by high urine concentrations may arise, in some cases, from altered boundary conditions at the boundary of the inner and outer medulla. Such altered conditions may arise from hyperfiltration and from inner stripe hypertrophy that result from feeding urea (thus providing, in part, an explanation for for findings by Gamble et al.[166]) or from a high-protein diet, water restriction or the administration of antidiuretic hormone.[203]

Steady-State Alternatives to the Passive Mechanism

The passive mechanism hypothesis is a comprehensive explanation for a large body of experimental findings, including the dilution of thin ascending limb fluid without active transport,[80,204,205] a role for urea in the concentrating mechanism,[166] and the NaCl and urea permeabilities measured in loops of Henle from rabbit inner medulla (see Tables 43.2 and 43.3). However, the larger permeabilities measured in rat, hamster, and chinchilla, in conjunction with the results of numerous simulation studies, have provided little support for the hypothesis. Significant concentrations

of urea measured in long loops of Henle from rat and hamster[72,73,76] are generally consistent with studies reporting high loop urea permeabilities. In addition, some animals with high urine-concentrating ability, e.g., *Psammomys*, generate a medullary gradient that depends mostly on NaCl, with little medullary urea accumulation,[206] a result which suggests that, at least in some species, a mechanism differing from the passive mechanism is involved. Thus, while the passive mechanism hypothesis remains highly influential in both experimental and theoretical research, the accumulated evidence, from both experimental and mathematical studies, indicates that crucial elements are missing in our understanding of the inner medullary concentrating effect.

Alternatives to the original passive mechanism hypothesis have taken three forms. First, many simulation studies have attempted to show that a better representation of transepithelial transport or of medullary anatomy is required for the effective operation of the passive mechanism; some of these studies were summarized in the preceding section. Second, a number of steady-state mechanisms involving a single effect generated in either thin descending limbs or collecting ducts have been proposed. Third, several hypotheses which depend on the peristaltic contractions of the pelvic wall and their impact on the papilla have been proposed. The steady-state alternatives involving descending limbs or collecting ducts are considered directly below, within a general context of possible steady-state mechanisms; mechanisms involving peristalsis are considered in the subsequent subsection.

Based on the principle of mass balance, Knepper and colleagues have provided a systematic classification of possible steady-state concentrating models for the inner medulla.[7,148] The classification shows that a single effect for countercurrent multiplication can exist in any structure having axial flow. Thus, a single effect could be present in thin descending limbs, thin ascending limbs, collecting ducts, descending vasa recta or ascending vasa recta. The classification also shows that a concentrating single effect in an upward flowing stream (toward the cortex) would require a luminal osmolality less than that of the surrounding interstitium, whereas a single effect in a downward flowing stream would require a luminal osmolality exceeding that of the interstitium. Thus, for example, the active transport of NaCl from the thick ascending limbs of the outer medulla lowers the osmolality of the upward flowing luminal fluid relative to the surrounding interstitium; similarly the passive mechanism hypothesis proposes that diffusion of NaCl from thin ascending limbs renders luminal fluid hypoosmotic relative to the interstitium.

Several investigators have proposed a single effect in descending limbs arising from flow that is hyperosmotic relative to the interstitium. Bonventre and Lechene proposed that the equilibration of descending limb flow with a compartment rendered hyperosmotic by active NaCl transport from ascending limbs or active secretion of solute into descending limb produces a relatively hyperosmotic descending flow from the outer medulla into the inner medulla.[207] In a mathematical simulation, Lory showed that an inwardly-directed NaCl transport combined with a loop of Henle cascade could produce a significant concentrating effect.[208] Jen and Stephenson performed a general mathematical analysis of mechanisms involving a hyperosmotic descending limb flow, and concluded that such mechanisms, in theory, could generate a potent single effect.[149] Their claim was supported by a subsequent simulation study by Thomas and Wexler,[162] which represented an external osmotic driving force to extract water from descending limbs and collecting ducts; the driving force was hypothesized to arise from the accumulation of osmotically active particles in local vessels or capillaries as a consequence of osmolyte production. Layton and colleagues[52] suggested that a descending limb single effect is consistent with the high NaCl and urea permeabilities of chinchilla ascending limb: the ascending limb could function as an equilibrating segment in which high permeabilities reduce dissipative osmotic lag. However, despite the attractive features of a descending limb single effect, experimental support for a relatively hypertonic descending limb is lacking. Moreover, in most species examined, the NaCl and urea permeabilities in thin descending limbs are too high to sustain a significant transepithelial osmolality gradient in the papilla, where the concentrating effect is most pronounced.

A single effect in the IMCD would require that the osmolality of luminal flow exceed the osmolality of the surrounding interstitium. Rabinowitz proposed such a single effect, based on the assumption that the urea reflection coefficient for the collecting duct is significantly less than unity.[209] He showed that the resulting reduction in the osmotic effect of urea in the collecting duct could, in theory, result in a water flux from collecting duct to interstitium that would significantly raise the osmolality of collecting duct fluid. A number of investigators have proposed or analyzed this hypothesis, including Sanjana et al.,[210] Bonventre and Lechene,[207] Chandhoke et al.,[211] and Imai et al.[39] However, experimental studies indicate that the urea reflection coefficient in rat does not differ significantly from unity.[50,122]

Thomas[152] and Hervy and Thomas[151] have investigated the hypothesis that the concentrating mechanism of the inner medulla may be driven or aided by lactate accumulation in the rat papilla. Anaerobic glycolysis in the hypoxic inner medulla is a net source of osmoles, because two lactates are produced for each glucose molecule. The rate of production, however may not be sufficient to produce a general concentrating effect. Modeling studies[151] indicate that lactate produced from glucose by anaerobic glycolysis could concentrate tubular fluid in thin descending limbs and collecting ducts (thus producing descending flows in these tubules that are relatively hyperosmotic to flows in other structures at each medullary level), provided that the descending limbs and collecting ducts are impermeable to lactate, as appears to be the case from low lactate levels in urine. However, several conditions require experimental verification: sufficient lactate production, impermeability of thin descending limbs to lactate, and sufficient intramedullary lactate cycling by vascular countercurrent exchange. The lactate-based mechanism is attractive because it appears to be insensitive to thin descending limb urea permeability, and independent of a necessary role for urea. However, modeling results for this mechanism appear to produce subphysiological urine flow, and do not explain the experimentally observed urea gradient in rat.

Hypotheses Based on the Peristalsis of the Papilla

Regular, sustained peristaltic contractions of the smooth muscles of the renal pelvic wall have been observed in a number of mammalian species. In the unipapillate kidneys of hamsters and rats, peristaltic contractions are propagated from the fornices to the lower pelvis, and continue in synchrony down the ureter. In the multipapillate kidneys of both humans and pigs, peristaltic contractions pass from the fornices down the calyces surrounding each papilla, but contractions in calyces are not synchronized with each other or with the peristalsis of the ureter. For a comprehensive review of the anatomy, physiology, and peristalsis of the renal pelvic region, see [212].

In hamsters and rats, the rates of pelvic contractions are about 13/min and 25/min, respectively.[164,213] The contractions interrupt fluid flow by forcing the collecting ducts, loops of Henle, and capillaries of the papilla to collapse. In hamster, the contractions induce bolus flow down the papillary collecting duct, with a bolus speed of about 1.6 mm/second. At the low urine flow rates characteristic of antidiuresis, boluses are so short that, 1 mm from the papillary tip, collecting ducts may be collapsed up to 94% of the time.[164] Even so, large quantities of urea, electrolytes, and, especially, water are absorbed in the final millimeters of the collecting duct system. Indeed, about 50% of the water in a bolus passing through the final millimeter of the collecting duct is absorbed.[214]

The blood in the capillaries of the papilla undergoes complicated motion during a pelvic contraction.[213] As a peristaltic wave approaches, blood is trapped in the capillaries closest to the papillary tip, which are full and expanded. As the wave passes over, the capillaries empty, with blood moving up both the descending and ascending *vasa recta*; after the wave has passed, the capillaries refill. The fluid motion in the loops of Henle is much like that of blood in the capillaries: fluid is trapped at the turns of the loops, and may move retrograde up the descending and ascending limbs as the peristaltic wave passes.[215] A net orthograde flow through the capillaries and loops of Henle is ensured by glomerular filtration pressure.

During the rising urine flow rates that accompany the onset of diuresis, the peristalsis in hamsters and rats induces refluxes of urine over the papilla and up into the fornices.[213] These refluxes, called full refluxes, may bathe the papillary surface epithelium with urine that is hypoosmotic and that has a low urea concentration, relative to the medullary structures; thus, water may diffuse into the medulla, and urea may diffuse out. Experiments in hamsters suggest that full refluxes accelerate the transition to the diuretic state.[216] When urine flow is constant or decreasing, refluxes are sporadic and limited to the lower $50-100\,\mu$m of the papilla.[213]

Experiments have shown that the excision of the pelvic wall results in a substantial reduction in urine osmolality[217–219]; the reduction has been attributed to the disruption of pelvic urea recycling[219–221] or to the dissipative effect of medullary blood flow, increased by continuous flow[164] or by prostaglandin release.[217] However, no significant change in osmolality was found in urine samples from rats 5–40 minutes after the smooth muscles of the pelvic wall were paralyzed with a topical application of verapamil and dimethylsulfoxide.[218] In the same study, the excision of the pelvic wall dramatically reduced the osmolality gradient in the papilla, and the gradient was substantially reduced when the ureter was severed just beyond the papillary tip, a procedure that preserved pelvic peristalsis (and intermittent urine flow), but eliminated urine reflux.[218] These results were interpreted to mean that while an intact pelvic wall, continuous with the ureter, is required for the production of maximally concentrated urine, the pelvic contractions are not. However, some experiments suggest that the peristaltic contractions do play a direct role in the concentrating mechanism. When the pelvic wall in rats was removed, causing a 10% decrease/hour in urine osmolality, and peristalsis was then simulated by a mechanical system, the decrease was reduced to 5%/hour.[222] When the muscles of the pelvic wall in hamster were paralyzed by cauterization or by xylocaine, urine osmolality was

reduced by about 20% after one hour,[223] through a reduction in papillary sodium content.

Several studies have provided evidence of solute and water transport across the papillary surface epithelium. When the papillae of rats and gerbils were bathed in a solution containing ^{14}C-urea and ^{3}H-water, there was a marked tissue label for urea, increasing from cortex to inner medulla, and a smaller effect for water.[226] When the papilla was bathed *in vivo* with artificial solutions containing varying concentrations of urea, higher concentration of urea in the superfusate led to a higher osmolality in the urine that was collected as it emerged from the terminal IMCD.[220] Fluid collected from small catheters inserted far up into the fornices of the rat pelvis extracted fluid with concentrations of inulin and total solutes that were significantly lower than the concentrations in urine collected at the papillary tip.[227]

Recycling of urea from urine across the papillary surface epithelium has been proposed as a component of the inner medullary concentrating mechanism.[207,228] However, a comparison of ureteral urine and urine collected from the ducts of Bellini of hydropenic hamsters showed no significant differences in filtered water and urea,[229] and an analysis based on measured urea permeability and papillary surface area in rabbits suggests that urea transport across the papillary surface epithelium is negligible.[104]

The lack of a satisfactory explanation for the inner medullary concentrating effect has led to the formulation of hypotheses based on the peristaltic contractions of the smooth muscles of the pelvic wall. Layton proposed that the NaCl and urea concentrations in the tubular cells and interstitium undergo oscillations in tandem with the contractions.[196] Urea absorbed from boluses advancing down the collecting duct system would transiently, and substantially, increase urea concentration in collecting duct cells and in the interstitium. Immediately following passage of the peristaltic wave, NaCl absorbed from restored orthograde loop of Henle flow would significantly raise the interstitial NaCl concentration. The very large urea concentration encountered by loop flow would, perhaps, be sufficient to result in the transient operation of the passive mechanism near loop bends, raising interstitial osmolality. Consequently, water, in excess of solute, would be absorbed from the next bolus passing down the collecting duct, and a large urea gradient, resulting from increased interstitial NaCl, would favor urea absorption. However, as in the case of the steady-state formulation of the passive mechanism, the large permeabilities measured in chinchilla[57] suggest that rapid equilibration of NaCl and urea concentrations across thin ascending limbs would compromise this hypothesis.

Knepper and collaborators proposed that water may be driven out of thin descending limbs by the advancing peristaltic wave, thus concentrating tubular fluid and generating a single effect in descending limbs.[143,148] A sufficient net water flux might be achieved if the compliance of the papillary surface epithelium exceeds that of the thin descending limb, and if large enough pressures are attained by the compression wave. After the passage of the wave, solute would be absorbed in the relatively water-impermeable pre-bend segment, and in the early portion of the thin ascending limb, where NaCl and urea permeabilities are high. This hypothesis provides no explanation for the special role of urea in the production of high urine concentrations.[166]

Schmidt-Nielsen proposed that the contraction—relaxation cycle creates negative pressures in the interstitium that act to transport water, in excess of solute, from the collecting duct system.[230] According to this hypothesis, the compression wave would raise hydrostatic pressure in the collecting duct lumen, promoting a water flux into collecting duct cells. Because pressure would induce water flow through aquaporin water channels, without a commensurate solute flux, the remaining luminal fluid would be concentrated, relative to the contents of collecting duct cells and the surrounding interstitium. After the peristaltic wave had passed, the collecting ducts would be collapsed. The papilla, transiently lengthened and narrowed by the wave, would rebound, and a negative hydrostatic pressure would develop in the elastic interstitium, which is rich in glycosamine glycans and hyaluronic acid. The negative pressure would withdraw water from the collecting duct cells (through aquaporins) and into the vasa recta, which re-open during the relaxation phase of the contraction and carry reabsorbate toward the cortex. This hypothesis appears to provide no role for long loops of Henle, and it does not explain the large NaCl gradient generated in the papilla[6,106] or the special role of urea in producing concentrated urine.[166]

Knepper and colleagues[150] have recently hypothesized that hyaluronic acid, which is plentiful in the interstitium of the rat papilla, could serve as a mechano-osmotic transducer, i.e., that the intrinsic viscoelastic properties of hyaluronic acid could be utilized to transform the mechanical work of papillary peristalsis into osmotic work that could be used to concentrate urine. Three distinct concentrating mechanisms arising from peristalsis are proposed: (1) in the contraction phase, interstitial sodium activity would be reduced through the immobilization of cations by their pairing with fixed negative charges on hyaluronic acid. This would result in a lowered NaCl concentration in fluid that can be expressed from the interstitium, and that relatively dilute fluid would enter the ascending vasa recta. In the relaxation phase, water would be absorbed from descending thin limbs: (2) as a result of decreased interstitial pressure (previously proposed by Knepper and co-workers[143,148]); and (3) as a result of elastic forces exerted by the expansion of the elastic interstitial matrix arising from hyaluronic acid. If water is so absorbed, without proportionate solute, then the descending limb tubular fluid would be relatively concentrated relative to other flows.

All of the hypotheses summarized above involve complex, highly coordinated cycles, with critical combinations of permeabilities, flow rates, compliances, pressures, and frequencies of peristalsis. Moreover, a determination of the adequacy of these hypotheses would appear to require a comprehensive knowledge of the physical properties of the renal papilla, and a demonstration that the energy input of the contractions, plus any other sources of harnessed energy, is sufficient to account for the osmotic work performed. Thus, the evaluation of these hypotheses, whether by means of experiments or mathematical models, presents a daunting technical challenge.

OSMOPROTECTIVE OSMOLYTES

Since the osmolality in the renal medulla is able to vary rapidly over a wide range, medullary cells must be able to adapt to this unusual osmotic environment in order to survive.[207,231] One way for medullary cells to achieve osmotic balance would be for these cells to accumulate intracellularly the major osmotically active compounds (osmolytes) that are found extracellularly in the medullary interstitium and urine, i.e., NaCl and urea.[232] The problem with this approach is that NaCl and urea can perturb protein function.[231] If medullary cells accumulated such perturbing osmolytes to achieve osmotic balance, then it is likely that these cells would need to develop special mechanisms that would allow their proteins to function over a wide range of intracellular ionic compositions and/or in high concentrations of urea.

An alternative mechanism would be for medullary cells to accumulate osmotically active substances that do not alter protein function, i.e., non-perturbing osmolytes.[231,233,234] This second approach is actually employed by medullary cells (Figure 43.10). Medullary cells accumulate non-perturbing or "organic" osmolytes such as sorbitol, glycerophosphocholine, betaine, inositol, and taurine.[232,235–238] These organic osmolytes are divided into two general categories: compatible and counteracting osmolytes. Sorbitol, inositol, and taurine are the major compatible osmolytes, and have no effect on protein function. They are accumulated intracellularly to osmotically balance extracellular

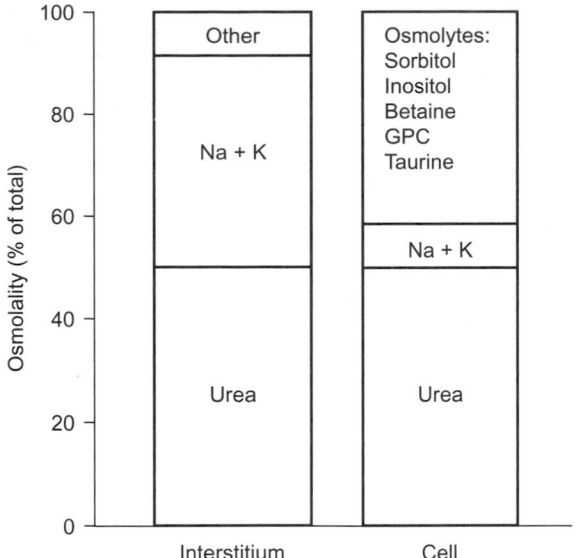

FIGURE 43.10 **Comparison of osmotic composition of the inner medullary interstitium and of cells in the inner medulla.** Sodium and potassium salts in the interstitium are balanced by compatible osmolytes (sorbitol, inositol, taurine). The denaturing effect of urea is balanced by counteracting osmolytes (betaine, glycerophosphocholine (GPC)). Data from references [452,453]. *(Figure is modified, with permission, from reference [232].)*

NaCl.[236,237,239] Glycerophosphocholine and betaine are the major counteracting osmolytes: in addition to being osmotically active, they have stabilizing effects on protein function and counteract the destabilizing effects of urea when they are accumulated intracellularly at a ratio of 1 mole of counteracting osmolyte to 2 moles of urea.[231,233,234,239,240,241]

In the medulla, organic osmolytes are regulated to respond to prolonged periods without water ingestion followed by short periods in which water is ingested.[236] During periods of antidiuresis, medullary cells maintain high intracellular concentrations of organic osmolytes to match extracellular osmolality. When water is ingested, these cells respond by rapidly losing osmolytes into the urine by increasing their cell membrane permeability to these osmolytes, thus decreasing intracellular osmolality.[236,237] However, the medullary cells continue osmolyte production during these short periods of diuresis. Although this continued osmolyte production may appear inefficient, it enables the cell to respond rapidly to the cessation of water ingestion. When water ingestion ceases, the cell's permeability to osmolyte efflux decreases, and intracellular osmolyte concentration is rapidly restored, since osmolyte production is maintained.[236,237] However, if the diuresis is prolonged (days), then osmolyte production is decreased in addition to the increase in cell permeability.[236,237] In this case, osmolyte concentration cannot be

restored rapidly, since the upregulation of osmolyte production requires an increase in the transcription of osmolyte genes and new protein synthesis.[236]

ROLE OF UREA

Urea plays a unique role in the urine concentrating mechanism. Its importance to the generation of a concentrated urine has been appreciated since 1934, when Gamble and colleagues described "an economy of water in renal function referable to urea".[166] Several studies show that maximal urine concentrating ability is decreased in protein-deprived animals and humans, and is restored by urea infusion.[75,165,166,242–246] This is the mechanism that has been proposed to explain why protein-restricted and malnourished humans are unable to concentrate their urine maximally. Recently, a UT-A1/UT-A3 knockout mouse,[144] a UT-A2 knockout mouse,[247] and a UT-B knockout mouse[248–250] were each shown to have urine concentrating defects. Thus, any solution to the question of how the inner medulla concentrates urine needs to take into account some effect derived from urea.

Facilitated Urea Transporters

Several early studies in dog and rat suggested that vasopressin could increase urea permeability across the IMCD.[63,251–253] Direct evidence was obtained in the 1980s, when three groups showed that vasopressin could increase passive urea permeability in isolated perfused rat IMCDs.[102,120,123] A specific facilitated or carrier-mediated urea transport process in rat and rabbit terminal IMCDs was first proposed in 1987.[102] The physiologic studies provided a functional characterization for a vasopressin-regulated urea transporter (reviewed in [254–258]). Two urea transporter genes have been cloned: the UT-A (*Scl14A2*) gene encodes 6 protein and 9 cDNA isoforms; the UT-B (*Scl14A1*) gene encodes two protein isoforms[259] (and reviewed in[260]) (Table 43.6). The UT-A gene was initially cloned from rat,[261] then from human and mouse.[262,263] It has two promoter elements: promoter I is upstream of exon 1 and drives the transcription of UT-A1, UT-A1b, UT-A3, UT-A3b, and UT-A4; promoter II is located within intron 12 and drives the transcription of UT-A2 and UT-A2b.[224,261]

The mouse UT-A promoter α, equivalent to the rat UT-A promoter I, has been further studied by the creation of transgenic mice in which 4.2 kb of the 5'-flanking region of the UT-A gene is linked to a β-galactosidase reporter gene.[264] This transgene is sufficient to drive IMCD-specific expression of β-galactosidase in terminal IMCDs.[264] The β-galactosidase transgene is regulated by both water restriction and

TABLE 43.6   Cloned Mammalian Urea Transporters

Gene	Isoform	Tissue Localization
Slc14A1	UT-B1	red blood cells, endothelial cells, descending vasa recta
	UT-B2	bovine rumen
Slc14A2	UT-A1/UT-A1b	inner medullary collecting duct, apical membrane
	UT-A2/UT-A2b	thin descending limb (also heart and liver)
	UT-A3/UT-A3b	inner medullary collecting duct, apical and basolateral membranes
	UT-A4	rat medulla (not detected in mouse)
	UT-A5	mouse testis (not expressed in kidney)
	UT-A6	human colon (not expressed in kidney)

The original references can be found in the following reviews or references: [254,255,257−259,477−479].

glucocorticoids, similar to the regulation of the endogenous UT-A promoter α.[263−266]

UT-A1 is the largest UT-A protein and is expressed in the apical plasma membrane of cells in the IMCD.[262,267,268] Urea transport by UT-A1 is stimulated by cAMP when expressed in *Xenopus* oocytes,[269−271] and by vasopressin in cells that are stably transfected with UT-A1, UT-A1-MDCK cells,[272−274] and UT-A1-mIMCD3 cells.[275] Western blots of inner medullary tip proteins show bands at both 117 and 97 kDa; both bands represent glycosylated versions of a non-glycosylated 84 kDa UT-A1 protein.[276] UT-A1 protein is most abundant in the inner medullary tip; only the 97 kDa protein is detected in the inner medullary base, and it is not detected in outer medulla or cortex.[268,277,278]

UT-A3 is also expressed in the IMCD,[279] although reports of its location have varied in different studies. Initial studies performed in rat detected UT-A3 staining in the apical plasma membrane and intracellular cytoplasmic vesicles of terminal IMCDs, but none in the basolateral plasma membrane.[268,280] Subsequent studies detected UT-A3 staining only in the IMCD basolateral plasma membrane in mouse IMCD, and in mUT-A3-MDCK cells.[281,282] The most recent study detected UT-A3 staining in the basolateral plasma membrane in rats, but in both the apical and basolateral plasma membranes in rats following vasopressin administration.[283] UT-A3 expression in the basolateral plasma membrane provides a mechanism for transepithelial urea transport in the IMCD, with UT-A1 in the apical plasma membrane and UT-A3 in the basolateral plasma membrane.

Urea transport by UT-A3 is stimulated by cAMP analogs when expressed in human embryonic kidney

(HEK) 293 cells or *Xenopus* oocytes in three studies,[269,279,284] but not in a fourth.[285] Vasopressin also stimulates urea transport via a PKA-dependent pathway in cells that are stably transfected with mouse UT-A3, mUT-A3-MDCK cells.[282]

UT-A2, the first urea transporter cloned,[286] is expressed in thin descending limbs.[90,267,268] Urea transport by UT-A2 is not stimulated by cAMP analogs when expressed in either *Xenopus* oocytes or human embryonic kidney HEK-293 cells.[270,271,279,286−289] UT-A4 is expressed in rat kidney medulla, although its exact location is unknown, and it has not been detected in mouse kidney.[248,263,269] Urea transport by UT-A4 is stimulated by cAMP analogs when expressed in HEK-293 cells.[279] UT-A5 and UT-A6 are expressed in testis and colon, respectively, but not in kidney.[284,290] In addition, there are three UT-A cDNA variants with alternative 3′-untranslated regions, but no difference in coding region, named UT-A1b, UT-A2b, and UT-A3b, respectively.[224]

The UT-B1 cDNA was initially cloned from a human erythroid cell line,[291] then from rodents.[249,292−294] UT-B1 protein is the Kidd antigen (in humans), and several mutations of the UT-B1/Kidd antigen gene exist[295−299]; red blood cells from these individuals also lack phloretin-sensitive facilitated urea transport.[300] The human UT-B gene encodes a single cDNA and a single protein[295]; both the N- and C-termini are located intracellularly.[296] However, in rat, two cDNA sequences that differ by only a few nucleotides at their 3′ end have been reported.[292,294] Whether the two cDNAs truly represent different rat UT-B1 isoforms, a polymorphism or a sequencing artifact is uncertain, since humans have only a single isoform. UT-B1 protein is detected as a broad band between 45−65 kDa in human red blood cells and 35−55 kDa in rodent red blood cells and kidney medulla.[249,301,302] UT-B1 protein and phloretin-inhibitable urea transport are present in descending vasa recta.[61,249,301−306]

Several studies have addressed the question of whether UT-B1 transports urea only, or water and urea.[249,307,308] Although red blood cells from a UT-B1/AQP1 double-knockout mouse show that UT-B1 can function as a water channel, the amount of water transported through UT-B1 under physiologic conditions is small (in comparison to AQP1), and is probably not physiologically significant to the urine concentrating mechanism.[250]

Rapid Regulation of Facilitated Urea Transport

The primary method for investigating the rapid regulation of urea transport has been perfusion of rat IMCDs. This method provides physiologically relevant functional data, although it cannot determine which urea transporter isoform is responsible for a specific functional effect in rat terminal IMCDs, since both UT-A1 and UT-A3 are expressed in this nephron segment. Vasopressin addition to the basolateral membrane of a rat terminal IMCD results in binding to V_2-vasopressin receptors, stimulating adenylyl cyclase, generating cAMP, and ultimately increasing facilitated urea permeability.[63,102,120,121,253,309,310] This effect occurs within minutes of adding vasopressin to the bath.[311] Oxytocin also increases urea permeability by binding to V_2-receptors and increasing cAMP production in rat terminal IMCDs.[312] Functional studies show that phloretin-inhibitable urea transport is present in both the apical and basolateral plasma membranes, with the apical membrane being the rate-limiting barrier for vasopressin-stimulated urea transport.[313] As discussed above, it is unclear whether UT-A3 is the basolateral membrane urea transporter.[280,281]

The acute stimulation of urea permeability by vasopressin occurs by an increase in the number of functional urea transporters (V_{max}), without a change in the transporter's affinity (K_m) for urea.[314] Adding vasopressin to the lumen of a perfused rat terminal IMCD also increases urea permeability by binding to luminal V_2-receptors.[315] However, when vasopressin is first added to the bath, adding vasopressin to the lumen inhibits urea permeability, suggesting that luminal vasopressin is a negative modulator of basolateral vasopressin on urea permeability in rat terminal IMCDs.[315]

One mechanism for rapid regulation is a vasopressin-stimulated increase in UT-A1 phosphorylation.[316] The deduced amino acid sequence for UT-A1 contains several consensus sites for phosphorylation by PKA, as well as by protein kinase C (PKC) and tyrosine kinase.[279] UT-A1 and UT-A3 have been identified in proteomic and cDNA array approaches as proteins that are phosphorylated by vasopressin in the inner medulla.[137,317–322] Vasopressin increases the phosphorylation of both the 117 and 97 kDa UT-A1 proteins in freshly isolated suspensions of rat IMCDs within 2 minutes,[316] and of the 67 and 44 kDa UT-A3 proteins.[283] Vasopressin also increases UT-A1 phosphorylation in UT-A1-MDCK cells[273,274] and UT-A1-mIMCD3 cells.[275] The time-course and dose–response for vasopressin-stimulated increases in UT-A1 phosphorylation is similar to the time-course and dose–response for vasopressin-stimulated increases in urea permeability in perfused rat terminal IMCDs.[309–311,316] Cyclic AMP, dDAVP (a V_2-selective agonist), and forskolin also increase UT-A1 phosphorylation, and PKA inhibitors block vasopressin or forskolin-stimulated UT-A1 phosphorylation in rat IMCD suspensions[316] and UT-A1-MDCK cells.[274]

Vasopressin/cAMP can stimulate Epac, exchange protein activated by cAMP,[323–328] in addition to stimulating PKA. Epac activation increases urea permeability in perfused rat terminal IMCDs, and increases UT-A1 phosphorylation in IMCD suspensions.[329]

Serine 486 was identified in a phosphoproteomic analysis as a potential vasopressin-stimulated phosphorylation site in UT-A1.[137] Serine 486 was identified in a second study, which also identified serine 499 as a second potential PKA phosphorylation site.[330] Using site-directed mutagenesis and transient transfection in heterologous expression systems, PKA was shown to phosphorylate UT-A1 at both serine 486 and serine 499.[330] Phospho-specific antibodies to serine 486 show that vasopressin increases UT-A1 phosphorylation at serine 486.[275,331] Phospho-serine 486-UT-A1 is detected primarily in the apical plasma membrane in rat IMCDs.[275] Recent work with chimera proteins of UT-A that attached the loop region of UT-A1 (aa 460–532) containing serines 486 and 499 to the UT-A2 protein, which normally lacks these amino acids, showed that this section conferred vasopressin sensitivity to UT-A2.[332]

A subsequent phosphoproteomic analysis showed that purified PKA could phosphorylate UT-A1 at serines 486 and 499; that analysis also showed that serine 84, which is present in both UT-A1 and UT-A3, could be phosphorylated by PKA.[317] In rat, vasopressin phosphorylates both UT-A1 and UT-A3 at serine 84, based upon studies utilizing a phospho-specific antibody to serine 84.[331] However, the equivalent site in mouse UT-A3, serine 85, was shown not to be a PKA phosphorylation site, based on site-directed mutagenesis.[284] The latter study also showed that serine 92 was not a PKA phosphorylation site.[284]

Another mechanism by which vasopressin rapidly increases urea transport is regulated trafficking or redistribution of UT-A1 between an intracellular compartment and the apical plasma membrane. In freshly isolated suspensions of rat IMCDs from normal rats, vasopressin increases the plasma membrane accumulation of UT-A1 and UT-A3.[283,333] However, in IMCDs from Brattleboro rats or two week water diuretic rats, vasopressin does not increase the plasma membrane accumulation of UT-A1.[333,334] (Brattleboro rats have central diabetes insipidus due to a congenital absence of vasopressin production in the hypothalamus.) When forskolin is used as the agonist, rather than vasopressin, it does increase the plasma membrane accumulation of UT-A1 in IMCDs from two week water diuretic rats.[333] Since chronically diuretic animals have a blunted cAMP response to vasopressin,[335–337] directly stimulating adenylyl cyclase with forskolin[337] may result in higher levels of cAMP production, which may result in an increase in UT-A1 accumulation in the plasma membrane.[333] Epac activation also increases UT-A1 plasma membrane accumulation in rat IMCD suspensions.[329]

Either vasopressin or forskolin increases UT-A1 apical plasma membrane accumulation in UT-A1-MDCK cells[272,333] and UT-A1-mIMCD3 cells.[275] Mutation of both serines 486 and 499, but not either one alone, eliminates the stimulation of UT-A1 apical plasma membrane accumulation and urea transport by vasopressin, indicating that at least one of these serines must be phosphorylated in order to increase apical plasma membrane accumulation and urea flux.[330] A phospho-specific antibody to S486-UT-A1 also showed that vasopressin increases UT-A1 accumulation in the apical plasma membrane, and that the S486-phospho-UT-A1 form is primarily detected in the apical plasma membrane.[275]

Vasopressin also increases UT-A3 accumulation in both the basolateral and apical plasma membranes in rat IMCDs.[283] In mUT-A3-MDCK cells, vasopressin stimulation for 10 minutes increases urea flux through transporters already in the basolateral plasma membrane.[338] Vasopressin stimulation for one hour increases UT-A3 localization in the basolateral plasma membrane and further increases urea flux in mUT-A3-MDCK cells.[338] The basal expression of UT-A3 in the basolateral plasma membrane involves PKC and calmodulin, while UT-A3 regulation by vasopressin involves a casein-kinase II-dependent pathway.[338]

UT-A1 is linked to the SNARE machinery via snapin in rat IMCDs, suggesting that the SNARE-SNAP vesicle trafficking mechanism may be functionally important for regulating urea transport.[339] UT-A1 also interacts with caveolin-1 in lipid rafts, providing another mechanism for UT-A1 regulation of UT-A1 activity within the plasma membrane.[340] Both UT-A1 and UT-A3 proteins can be ubiquitinated.[341,342] However, only UT-A1 has been rigorously shown to express ubiquitinated higher molecular weight forms by immunoprecipitation and Western analysis.[341] The ubiquitin ligase MDM2 mediates UT-A1 ubiquitination and degradation, providing another regulatory mechanism for UT-A1.[341] Finally, mutation of the two N-linked glycosylation sites in UT-A1 that are predicted to reside in extracellular domains, Asn 279 and Asn 742, reduces urea flux by reducing UT-A1 half-life and apical plasma membrane accumulation in MDCK cells.[272]

Increasing osmolality to high physiological values, either by adding NaCl or mannitol, in the absence of vasopressin, acutely increases urea permeability in rat terminal IMCDs,[119,121,343] suggesting that hyperosmolality is an independent stimulator of urea transport. When osmolality is increased and vasopressin is present, they have additive stimulatory effects on urea

permeability.[119,121,343,344] Hyperosmolality-stimulated urea permeability is inhibited by phloretin and the urea analog thiourea.[119] Kinetic studies show that hyperosmolality, like vasopressin, stimulates urea permeability by increasing V_{max} rather than reducing K_m.[119] However, hyperosmolality stimulates urea permeability via increases in intracellular calcium and activation of PKC,[345,346] whereas vasopressin stimulates urea permeability via increases in adenylyl cyclase.[310] Hypersomolality increases the phosphorylation and the plasma membrane accumulation of both UT-A1 and UT-A3, similar to vasopressin.[283,316,333,347] Thus, both hyperosmolality and vasopressin increase urea permeability by increasing V_{max}, but they do so via different second messenger pathways.

Active Urea Transporters

Functional evidence exists for two types of active urea transport in the rat collecting duct: sodium-urea co-transport and sodium-urea countertransport (reviewed in [255,256]). Although no sodium-dependent active urea transporter has been cloned to date, several sodium-coupled co-transporters (rabbit sodium-glucose co-transporters 1 and 3, human sodium-chloride-GABA co-transporter 1) behave as urea channels when expressed in *Xenopus* oocytes.[348,349]

LONG-TERM REGULATION OF UREA TRANSPORTERS

Vasopressin

Administering vasopressin to Brattleboro rats (which lack vasopressin) for 5 days decreases UT-A1 protein abundance in the inner medulla.[350,351] However, administering vasopressin for 12 days increases UT-A1 protein abundance.[350] This delayed increase in UT-A1 protein is consistent with the time-course for the increase in inner medullary urea content in Brattleboro rats following vasopressin administration.[352] In normal rats, suppressing endogenous vasopressin levels by two weeks of water diuresis also decreases UT-A1 protein abundance.[350] This time-course may be explained by analysis of UT-A promoter I, since the 1.3 kb that has been cloned does not contain a cAMP response element (CRE), and cAMP does not increase promoter activity.[261,265] However, promoter I does contain a tonicity enhancer (TonE) element, and hyperosmolality increases promoter activity.[261,265] Thus, vasopressin may increase UT-A1 indirectly after directly increasing the transcription of other genes, such as the Na-K-2Cl co-transporter NKCC2/BSC1 and the AQP2 water channel, which begin to increase inner medullary osmolality.[353,354] Consistent with this hypothesis, water restricting rats with primary polydipsia results in an increase in plasma vasopressin, but no increase in medullary osmolality or UT-A1 protein abundance.[355]

In Brattleboro rats, UT-A2 mRNA increases at both 4 and 72 hours after administering dDAVP, while UT-A1 mRNA is unchanged.[318] The dDAVP-stimulated increase in UT-A2 mRNA is consistent with the presence of a CRE in UT-A promoter II, and the stimulation of promoter II activity by cAMP.[261]

Administering either vasopressin or dDAVP for 6 hours reduces UT-B mRNA abundance in both the outer and inner medulla of Brattleboro rats.[356] In contrast, administering vasopressin or dDAVP for 5 days increases UT-B mRNA abundance in the inner stripe of the outer medulla and the inner medullary base, while it is still decreased in the inner medullary tip.[356] Administering dDAVP for 7 days to normal rats decreases UT-B protein abundance in the inner medulla.[302]

Low-Protein Diet

Feeding rats a low-protein diet for at least 2 weeks results in a decrease in the fractional excretion of urea,[246] induces the functional expression of vasopressin-stimulated urea permeability in the initial IMCD,[118,287,357] increases basal urea permeability in the IMCD$_3$,[358] and increases the abundance of the 117 kDa glycoprotein form of UT-A1 in the inner medulla.[351] The vasopressin-stimulated urea permeability in the initial IMCD from low-protein fed rats is stimulated by hyperosmolality and inhibited by phloretin and thiourea.[118,287] Thus, it has the same functional characteristics as the vasopressin-stimulated urea permeability which is normally expressed in the terminal IMCD.[287] Whether the mRNA abundance of UT-A1 or UT-A2 changes in the inner medulla of low-protein fed rats is controversial.[287,289,359] Varying dietary protein between 10 and 40% has no effect on UT-B mRNA abundance in any portion of the medulla in either normal or Brattleboro rats.[359]

Glucocorticoids

Glucocorticoids (dexamethasone) increase the fractional excretion of urea[360] and decrease UT-A promoter I activity, UT-A1 and UT-A3 mRNA abundances, UT-A1 protein abundance, and facilitated urea transport.[266,361,362] Mineralocorticoids (aldosterone) also decrease UT-A1 protein abundance in the inner medulla of adrenalectomized rats, and this decrease can be blocked by spironolactone, a mineralocorticoid-receptor antagonist.[361] In contrast, spironolactone does not block the decrease due to dexamethasone,[361] indicating that each steroid hormone works through its own receptor. Aldosterone-induced volume-expansion (with a high-NaCl diet) decreases both UT-A1 and UT-A3 protein abundance.[363]

Dahl salt-sensitive rats have increased abundances of UT-A1 and UT-A3 proteins in the inner medulla, and of facilitated urea transport in the terminal IMCD.[364] They also have an increased level of the corticosterone-inactivating enzyme 11-hydroxysteroid dehydrogenase type II.[364] Inactivating glucocorticoids by increasing 11-hydroxysteroid dehydrogenase type II would lessen the repression of UT-A promoter I activity, thereby increasing UT-A1 and UT-A3 transcription and abundance.

Diabetes Mellitus

Uncontrolled diabetes mellitus (induced by streptozotocin) causes an osmotic diuresis and increases urea excretion, corticosterone production, and plasma vasopressin levels.[365−367] UT-A1 protein abundance decreases at 3−5 days after inducing diabetes mellitus in the rat inner medulla, but not in adrenalectomized diabetic rats.[336,368] The decrease in UT-A1 protein abundance is restored by giving dexamethasone to adrenalectomized diabetic rats, indicating that glucocorticoids mediate the decrease in UT-A1 protein.[368]

In contrast, UT-A1 mRNA and protein are increased 10−21 days after diabetes mellitus is induced in normal rats.[336,369] UT-A1 protein did not increase in diabetic Brattleboro rats, indicating that vasopressin is necessary for this increase in UT-A1.[350] In addition, vasopressin did not increase UT-A1 phosphorylation in either Brattleboro rats or diabetic Brattleboro rats, indicating that vasopressin is necessary for the increase in UT-A1 protein abundance and phosphorylation that occurs at 10−21 days after diabetes is induced.[350] UT-A2 is also decreased in the streptozotocin-induced diabetic rat. The reason for the decrease is not known, but it appears to result from a post-translational alteration in protein abundance, since the message for UT-A2 in control and diabetic rats is not different.[369]

The increase in UT-A1 protein abundance in the inner medulla from diabetic rats is accompanied by a shift in the glycoprotein forms expressed in inner medullary tip versus base.[336,370,371] The base of the inner medulla, which normally expresses only the 97 kDa glycoprotein form of UT-A1, shows both 97 kDa and 117 kDa forms in the diabetic rat.[336,370,371] Vasopressin sensitivity is also changed in the diabetic rat inner medulla. In the normal rat, only urea transport in the inner medullary tip is subject to stimulation by vasopressin, whereas in the diabetic kidney, urea permeability in both the tip and the base are increased by vasopressin.[372] In addition, both UT-A1 and UT-A3 protein abundance increases in response to treatment of the diabetic rat with the angiotensin receptor-blocker candesartan, apparently to reduce the loss of solute during uncontrolled diabetes.[370]

A model of type 2 diabetes is the obese Zucker rat, which has a genetic mutation of the leptin-receptor gene that leads to obesity, insulin resistance, hypertension, and diabetes.[373] UT-A1 protein abundance is decreased in the obese Zucker rat when compared to the lean Zucker (non-diabetic) rat.[374] The decrease in UT-A1 protein abundance may be a response to the hypertension present in the obese Zucker rat, similar to the decrease in UT-A1 observed in normal Sprague-Dawley rats made hypertensive with angiotensin II.[375]

Angiotensin II

Angiotensin II does not affect basal (no vasopressin) facilitated urea permeability in rat terminal IMCDs.[346] However, it increases both vasopressin-stimulated urea permeability and UT-A1 phosphorylation via a PKC-mediated effect.[346] Thus, angiotensin II may play a physiologic role in the urine concentrating mechanism by augmenting the maximal urea permeability response to vasopressin. In the inner medulla of mice that lack tissue angiotensin-converting enzyme, and hence lack angiotensin II, UT-A1 protein abundance is decreased to 25% of the level in wild-type mice.[376,377] Administering angiotensin II to these mice for 2 weeks did not correct the reduction in UT-A1 protein, nor in urine concentrating ability.[377]

Osmolality

Renal medullary osmolality varies between diuresis and antidiuresis. The major solutes contributing to inner medullary osmolality are urea and NaCl. Urea-specific signaling pathways are present in mIMCD3 cells (reviewed in [378,379]). When the percentage of urea in total urinary solute is low, UT-A1 protein abundance increases.[380–383] The increase in UT-A1 may occur in order to restore inner medullary interstitial urea and urine concentrating ability.[380] In the outer medulla, UT-A2 and UT-B1 protein abundance increases when medullary interstitial urea concentration is high, such as during a urea-induced osmotic diuresis, but not during a NaCl- or glucose-induced osmotic diuresis.[380–383] During osmotic diuresis, the urinary urea and NaCl concentrations regulate UT-A1 and UT-A3 protein abundances, but in opposite directions.[384] This regulation involves the tonicity enhancer-binding protein,

Ton EBP, and appears to be an attempt to minimize changes in plasma osmolality and maintain water homeostasis.[384]

TonEBP, which is also named OREBP (osmotic response element binding protein) or NFAT5, is an essential regulator of urine concentrating ability.[385,386] Transgenic mice that overexpress a dominant-negative form of TonEBP have reduced urine osmolality, and UT-A1 and UT-A2 mRNA abundance.[386] In these mice, water deprivation or vasopressin administration increases urine osmolality and UT-A1 mRNA abundance, but not UT-A2 mRNA abundance.[386] TonEBP also stimulates the transcription of genes whose products drive cellular accumulation of organic osmolytes, such as aldose reductase.[385] Mice with genetic deletion of aldose reductase have a urine osmolality below 1000 mOsm/kg H_2O.[387] The urine concentrating defect was largely corrected in bitransgenic mice in which an aldose reductase transgene was knocked-in. These mice displayed a tendency toward increased UT-A1 expression that might contribute to the restoration of urine concentration.[387]

Electrolye Abnormalities

Hypercalcemia or hypokalemia reduce urine concentrating ability.[278,388–390] Basal urea permeability is increased in terminal IMCDs from hypercalcemic rats compared to normocalcemic control rats.[278] Consistent with this functional increase, the abundance of UT-A1 protein is also increased.[278] These changes may be regulated by a calcium-sensing receptor in the apical plasma membrane of cells in the terminal IMCD.[391] In a mouse model of autosomal dominant polycystic kidney disease (ADPKD) or a rat model of autosomal recessive PKD (ARPKD), treatment with a type 2 calcimimetic, R-568, results in hypocalcemia, polyuria, and minimal changes in UT-A1 protein abundance, with significant increases in UT-A1 seen only in the female ARPKD rats.[392]

A low-potassium diet reduces the abundance of UT-A1, UT-A3, and UT-B proteins in the inner medulla, but increases UT-A2 protein abundance in the outer medulla.[389] TonEBP protein abundance and nuclear distribution in the medulla are reduced by hypokalemia.[393] TonEBP downregulation contributes to the reduced expression of UT-A1 and UT-A2, although UT-A2 expression is transcriptionally reduced whereas UT-A1 is reduced post-transcriptionally.[393] In addition, UT-B1 expression is reduced, along with a decrease in mRNA abundance in response to hypokalemia.[393] Another study also found that feeding rats a low-potassium diet reduces the abundance of UT-A1, UT-A3, and UT-B1 proteins in the inner medulla.[389] However, this latter study found that hypokalemia increases UT-A2 protein abundance in the outer medulla.[389] The reason for the differing findings regarding UT-A2 in these studies is unclear.

Hypothyroidism

Hypothyroidism reduces urine concentrating ability, but does not alter UT-A1 or UT-A2 protein abundance in rats.[394] Water-restricting hypothyroid rats alters neither UT-A1 nor UT-A2 abundance.[394] Urine concentrating ability is reduced in normal aging (reviewed in [395]). UT-A1, UT-A3, and UT-B1 proteins are reduced in kidneys of aged rats.[396–398] A supra-physiologic dose of dDAVP increases UT-A1 and UT-B1 protein abundance and urine osmolality in aged rats, but not to the levels observed in younger rats.[399]

Purinergic P2Y2 Receptor

P2Y2 receptor activation in the IMCD tends to oppose the actions of vasopressin.[400] Urine concentrating ability, and UT-A1 and UT-A2 protein abundances, are higher in P2Y2-receptor knockout mice than in wild-type mice.[400] Vasopressin administration for 45 minutes or 5 days increases UT-A1 protein abundance in P2Y2-receptor knockout mice.[400] Vasopressin administration for 5 days increases UT-A2 protein abundance in both control and P2Y2 purinergic receptor-null mice,[400] suggesting a role for cAMP in the regulation of UT-A2. While acute treatment with PKA agonists did not increase UT-A2,[269] longer treatment times did upregulate UT-A2 protein abundance,[90,401] suggesting that cAMP may be involved in the long-term regulation, rather than in the acute response, for UT-A2.

Ureteral Obstruction

UT-A1, UT-A3, and UT-B1 protein abundances are reduced by bilateral or unilateral ureteral obstruction in rat inner medulla.[402] The abundance of all three urea transporters remained reduced at 2 weeks after release of bilateral ureteral obstruction.[402]

Lithium

Lithium causes nephrogenic diabetes insipidus and an inability to concentrate urine (reviewed in [403]). Lithium causes a marked reduction in inner medullary interstitial osmolality due to reductions in interstitial urea and NaCl concentrations.[404] Lithium-treated rats have marked reductions in AQP2, UT-A1, UT-A3, and UT-B1 proteins, and vasopressin-stimulated UT-A1 phosphorylation.[405–408] UT-A1 and UT-A3 protein abundances return to control levels 14 days after stopping lithium therapy.[405] A proteomic analysis shows that several proteins involved in various signaling cascades that have been implicated in urea transporter function and/or trafficking are altered after 14 days of lithium treatment.[409] However, immunohistochemistry shows that UT-A1 localization appears normal after recovery from lithium treatment,[405] indicating that the trafficking machinery remains intact. Surprisingly, lithium stimulates urea flux in UT-A1-MDCK cells, despite suppressing cAMP formation.[410] Lithium does not increase UT-A1 biotinylation, which suggests that the increased urea flux in UT-A1-MDCK cells is due to an alteration in cellular signaling, rather than the trafficking of UT-A1.[410]

Genetic Knockout of UT-B

Humans with genetic loss of Kidd antigen (UT-B1) are unable to concentrate their urine above 800 mOsm/kg H_2O, even following overnight water deprivation and exogenous vasopressin administration.[411] Mice with a genetic knockout of UT-B1 also have mildly reduced urine concentrating ability, which is not improved by urea loading.[249,412] UT-A1 and UT-A3 abundance unchanged in UT-B1 knockout mice, but UT-A2 protein abundance is increased.[248] Since UT-A2 mediates urea recycling through the thin descending limb, it may be upregulated to partially compensate for the loss of urea recycling through UT-B1, thereby contributing to the mild phenotype observed in humans lacking UT-B1/Kidd antigen, and in UT-B1 knockout mice.

Mathematical models of microcirculatory exchange between the descending and ascending vasa recta predict that the absence of UT-B1 will decrease the efficiency of small solute trapping within the renal medulla, thereby decreasing the efficiency of countercurrent exchange and urine concentrating ability.[413,414] Thus, UT-B1 protein expression in red blood cells and/or descending vasa recta is necessary for the production of maximally concentrated urine.[411–416]

UT-B1 knockout mice have an impaired ability to concentrate their urine, achieving a maximal urine osmolality of 2400 mOsm/kg H_2O, compared to 3400 in a wild-type mouse.[249] This is similar to the phenotype in humans lacking UT-B1, the Kidd antigen, who are unable to concentrate their urine above 800 mOsm/kg H_2O, even following overnight water deprivation and exogenous vasopressin administration.[411] These findings support the concept that urea transport in red blood cells is necessary to preserve the efficiency of countercurrent exchange.[115] Both red blood cells and perfused rat descending vasa recta exhibit phloretin-inhibitable urea transport and express

UT-B1 protein,[61,301,303–306] suggesting that UT-B1 mediates urea transport in red blood cells and descending vasa recta.

UT-A2 protein abundance is increased, while UT-A1 and UT-A3 abundance is unchanged in UT-B1 knockout mice.[248] UT-A2 may be upregulated to compensate for the loss of UT-B1, since both UT-A2 and UT-B1 are involved in urea recycling.[248] This may account for the mild phenotype observed in UT-B1 knockout mice, and in humans lacking UT-B1/Kidd antigen.

Genetic Knockout of UT-A1 and UT-A3

Genetic knockout of both UT-A1 and UT-A3 in mice results in reduced urine concentrating ability, reduced inner medullary interstitial urea content, and a lack vasopressin-stimulated or phloretin-inhibitable urea transport in the IMCD.[144,417] When these mice are fed a low-protein diet, they are able to concentrate their urine almost as well as wild-type mice fed a low-protein diet,[144,417] supporting the concept that IMCD urea transport contributes to urine concentrating ability by preventing urea-induced osmotic diuresis.[418] Inner medullary tissue urea content was markedly reduced following water restriction, but there was no measurable difference in NaCl content between UT-A1/UT-A3 knockout mice and wild-type mice.[144,417] This finding was initially interpreted as being inconsistent with the predictions of the passive mechanism hypothesis.[8,9,144,417,419,420] However, a mathematical modeling analysis of these same data concludes that the results found in the UT-A1/UT-A3 knockout mice are exactly what one would predict for the passive mechanism hypothesis.[20]

The UT-A1/UT-A3 knockout mice were used to revisit Gamble's classic study from 1934.[166] Urea and NaCl each induce an osmotic diuresis when given in large amounts, supporting the concept that the decrease in water excretion with mixtures of urea and NaCl added to the diet results from the separate abilities of these two solutes to induce osmotic diuresis, rather than to any specific interaction of urea and NaCl transport at the epithelial level.[421]

Genetic Knockout of UT-A2

UT-A2 knockout mice also have an impaired ability to concentrate urine.[247,419,422] The reduction in urine concentrating ability results from an impairment of urea recycling.[247,419,422]

Active Urea Transport

When urine concentrating ability is reduced, there are changes in active urea transport that follow one of two patterns.[115,118,357,358,423,424] The first pattern, which occurs in response to water diuresis, is upregulation of active urea secretion in the IMCD$_3$ and its induction in the IMCD$_2$. This increase in urea secretion will directly decrease urea content in the deep inner medulla. The second pattern, which occurs in response to a low-protein diet, hypercalcemia, and furosemide, is induction of active urea absorption in the IMCD$_1$ and inhibition of active urea secretion in the IMCD$_3$. This second pattern will increase urea delivery to the inner medullary base, thereby decreasing urea delivery to the inner medullary tip; the accompanying inhibition of active urea secretion in the IMCD$_3$ may prevent an even greater reduction in urea content in the deep inner medulla.

UREA RECYCLING

Several urea recycling pathways are believed to contribute to high urea concentrations within the inner medulla.[418,425,426] The major recycling pathway involves urea absorption from the terminal IMCD, mediated by UT-A1 and UT-A3, secretion into the thin descending limb, and, especially, the thin ascending limb (Figure 43.11). Collecting ducts and thin ascending limbs are nearly adjoining within much of the inner medulla.[12] The urea that enters the thin ascending limb is carried distally as the luminal fluid moves through several nephron segments having very low urea permeability until it reaches the urea-permeable terminal

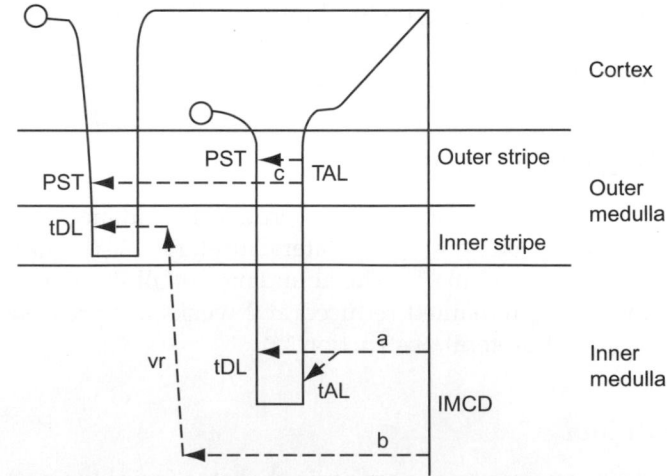

FIGURE 43.11   Urea recycling pathways in mammalian kidney. Diagram shows a short looped nephron (left) and a long looped nephron (right). Dashed lines labeled a, b, and c show urea recycling pathways (Abbreviations: PST: proximal straight tubule; tDL: thin descending limb of Henle's loop; tAL: thin ascending limb of Henle's loop; TAL: thick ascending limb of Henle's loop; IMCD: inner medullary collecting duct; vr: vasa recta). (*Figure is modified, with permission, from reference* [425].)

IMCD. Thus, urea is recycled from the terminal IMCD through the interstitium into the thin ascending limb, and back to the terminal IMCD.

Two other pathways for urea recycling may exist in the kidney.[425] One pathway is urea absorption from terminal IMCDs through ascending vasa recta and secretion into thin descending limbs of short looped nephrons[427] mediated by UT-A2[90] or into descending vasa recta mediated by UT-B1. The other pathway is urea absorption from cortical thick ascending limbs and secretion into proximal straight tubules.[425] All three urea recycling pathways would limit urea dissipation from the inner medulla where it is needed to increase interstitial osmolality.[425]

It must be emphasized that the terminal IMCD is the only portion of the collecting duct in which vasopressin increases urea permeability, even though the entire collecting duct is permeable to water when vasopressin is present. Water absorption from the cortical, outer medullary, and initial inner medullary collecting ducts concentrates urea within the collecting duct lumen. When the luminal fluid finally reaches the urea-permeable terminal IMCD, the luminal urea concentration is very high and exceeds that in vasa recta,[72,75,428,429] allowing urea to be rapidly absorbed into the deepest portion of the inner medullary interstitium where, in many studied mammals, it is needed to concentrate urine maximally.[102,192] This pattern of urea and water permeabilities separates the primary sites of urea and water absorption (Figure 43.6); water is primarily absorbed in the cortex and outer medulla where there is extensive vascularization with high blood flow, and the absorbed water can be returned to the circulation without diluting the deep inner medulla. Urea is principally absorbed in the deep inner medulla.[102,192]

Urea serves a second function in the medulla: it is the major source for excretion of nitrogenous waste; large quantities of urea need to be excreted daily. The kidney's ability to concentrate urea reduces the need to excrete water simply to remove nitrogenous waste. In addition, a high interstitial urea concentration is able to osmotically balance urea within the collecting duct lumen. If interstitial urea were unavailable to offset the osmotic effect of luminal urea destined for excretion, then the interstitial NaCl concentration would have to be much higher.[144,430]

DEVELOPMENT OF URINE CONCENTRATING ABILITY

Newborn mammals and birds are unable to concentrate their urine.[431−435] Rats and rabbits do not develop the ability to concentrate their urine maximally until 14−21 days after birth.[434,436−439] In rats, the increase in urine osmolality is paralleled by an increase in both medullary sodium and urea content.[440] In 10-day-old rats, neither urea- nor NaCl-loading enhances urine concentrating ability.[441] However, in 20-day-old rats, urea-loading significantly increases urine osmolality following water deprivation; NaCl loading has no effect.[441] The development of urine concentrating ability can be hastened by giving glucocorticoids to 10−17-day-old rats, but not to older rats.[440,442] Conversely, adrenalectomizing 16-day-old rats slows the development of urine concentrating ability and abolishes the increase in inner medullary sodium and urea concentrations that normally occurs at this age.[440]

In 1-day-old rats, the thin descending limb, thin ascending limb, and IMCD are all nearly water-impermeable.[433] At day 4, AQP1 mRNA is detected in the thin descending limb and water-permeability increases, however, it does not reach adult levels until day 14.[433] Even though AQP2 protein is detected starting at day 1, water-permeability remains low in the IMCD at day 7, but reaches adult levels at day 14.[368,433,443] However, AQP2 trafficking in the immature kidney responds normally to vasopressin[443] and AQP2 mRNA, and protein levels increase 24 hours after a single dose of betamethasone.[442]

In fetal rat kidney, UT-A protein is not detected and UT-B1 protein is weakly detected at embryonic age 20 days.[267] In 1-day-old rats, UT-A1, UT-A2, and UT-B1 proteins appear,[267] but the IMCD has a low urea permeability that is not stimulated by vasopressin.[433] At day 14, urea permeability becomes vasopressin-stimulatable and UT-A1 mRNA is detected, although the values are only one-third of adult levels.[433] UT-A1, UT-A2, and UT-B1 proteins increase progressively until adult levels are achieved at 21 days of age.[267] Thus, the time-course for the increases in UT-A1, UT-A2, and UT-B1 proteins coincides with the development of urine concentrating ability. On the basis of the functional implications of these findings, Lui et al.[433] proposed that the concentrating mechanism in newborn rats is similar to that in the avian kidney, which has very low descending limb water permeability, does not utilize urea, and can concentrate urine to only moderate levels; however, within about 14 days, the neonatal rat kidney more closely resembles the adult rat kidney.

In rabbits, the sodium concentration in cortex and medulla is similar regardless of age.[437] However, the medullary/cortical urea concentration ratio increases markedly between 14 and 21 days of age, coincident with the development of concentrated urine.[437] This increase in medullary/cortical urea concentration is primarily due to a reduction in cortical urea concentration, rather than an increase in medullary urea content.[437] However, in dogs, the developmental increase in urinary concentrating ability is due predominantly to an increase in the medullary sequestration of urea.[444]

Newborn humans also have an inability to concentrate their urine.[445] Infants fed a high-protein diet are able to increase their urine osmolality following water deprivation; infants given a diet in which the extra protein is replaced by NaCl achieve a lower urine osmolality.[445] Thus, even in infants, urea has a special role in the production of concentrated urine.[166,445]

Aldose reductase enzyme activity is absent in IMCDs from newborn rat pups (<12 hours old), but is present in 3-day-old pups and increases progressively up to 20 days of age; enzyme activity then decreases to adult levels.[434] Consistent with these functional measurements, aldose reductase mRNA cannot be detected, even by RT-PCR, in inner medullas from newborn rats (<12 hours old), but can be detected in 3-day-old pups.[434] Aldose reductase mRNA abundance peaks between 8–20 days after birth, then decreases to levels found in adult rats.[434,446] Thus, aldose reductase mRNA and enzyme activity are induced prior to urine concentrating ability during development.

TonEBP is detected in the kidney at fetal day 16, and its expression increases at fetal day 20 and at postnatal day 1.[447] At day 21, the adult pattern of TonEBP expression is achieved, along with the development of urine concentrating ability.[434,447] Thus, TonEBP expression precedes the expression of its target genes, UT-A1 and UT-A3, and UT-A promoter I is under the transcriptional control of TonEBP.[265,447] In mouse kidney, NKCC2/BSC1 is first detected at fetal day 14, TonEBP at day 15, UT-A at day 16–18, and UT-A immunoreactivity increases markedly after birth.[448] Neonatal mice treated with furosemide have reduced expression of both TonEBP and UT-A.[448] These findings support the hypothesis that hypertonicity produced by NKCC2/BSC1 activates TonEBP, which in turn increases the transcription of UT-A during development and early postnatal life in mice,[448] consistent with UT-A promoter I containing a TonE.[224,261]

KLF12 is a transcription factor that is expressed in the fetal kidney starting at day 15.[449] KLF12 is able to increase UT-A promoter I activity by binding to a CACCC motif.[449] Thus, UT-A1 is a target gene of KLF12, which may be involved in collecting duct maturation after birth.[449]

SUMMARY

Concentrated urine is produced in the renal medulla through the generation of an osmotic gradient extending from the cortico–medullary boundary to the papillary tip. In the outer medulla, the gradient is generated by active NaCl transport from the thick limbs, and the resulting increase in osmolality in the interstitium and in water-permeable tubules and vessels; the effectiveness of this transport is widely believed to be augmented by a countercurrent multiplication mechanism involving interactions between descending and ascending limbs of Henle. Although the passive mechanism, proposed by Kokko and Rector[8] and by Stephenson,[9] remains the most widely-accepted hypothesis for the generation of the inner medullary osmolality gradient, much of the evidence from perfused tubule and micropuncture studies, and from the UT-A1/UT-A3 knockout mouse[144] is either inconclusive or at variance with the passive mechanism. Moreover, the passive mechanism has not been supported by mathematical simulations using measured transepithelial transport parameters.

Nonetheless, there have been important recent advances in the understanding of key components of the urine concentrating mechanism, notably the identification and localization of key transport proteins for water, urea, and sodium, and the elucidation of the role and regulation of osmoprotective osmolytes. Continued experimental investigation of transepithelial transport and its regulation, both in normal animals and in genetically-engineered mice, a more complete understanding of the interaction of anatomy and transmural transport among tubules and vessels, and incorporation of the resulting information into mathematical simulations, may help to more fully elucidate the inner medullary concentrating mechanism.

Acknowledgments

This work was supported by National Institutes of Health grants R01-DK41707 (to JM Sands) and R01-DK42091 (to HE Layton).

References

[1] Beuchat CA. Body size, medullary thickness, and urine concentrating ability in mammals. Am J Physiol 1990;258:R298–308.

[2] Tisher CC. Relationship between renal structure and concentrating ability in the rhesus monkey. Am J Physiol 1971;220:1100–6.

[3] Tisher CC, Schrier RW, McNeil JS. Nature of urine concentrating mechanism in the macaque monkey. Am J Physiol 1972;223:1128–37.

[4] Beuchat CA. Structure and concentrating ability of the mammalian kidney: correlations with habitat. Am J Physiol 1996;271: R157–79.

[5] Knepper MA. Measurement of osmolality in kidney slices using vapor pressure osmometry. Kidney Int 1982;21:653–5.

[6] Hai MA, Thomas S. The time-course of changes in renal tissue composition during lysine vasopressin infusion in the rat. Pfluegers Arch 1969;310:297–319.

[7] Knepper MA, Stephenson JL. Urinary concentrating and diluting processes. In: Andreoli TE, Hoffman JF, Fanestil DD, Schultz SG, editors. Physiology of membrane disorders. 2nd ed. New York: Plenum; 1986. p. 713–26.

[8] Kokko JP, Rector FC. Countercurrent multiplication system without active transport in inner medulla. Kidney Int 1972;2:214—23.

[9] Stephenson JL. Concentration of urine in a central core model of the renal counterflow system. Kidney Int 1972;2:85—94.

[10] Kriz W. Der architektonische und funktionelle Aufbau der Rattenniere. Z Zellforsch 1967;82:495—535.

[11] Kriz W, Schnermann J, Koepsell H. The position of short and long loops of Henle in the rat kidney. Z Anat Entwicklungsgesch 1972;138:301—19.

[12] Lemley KV, Kriz W. Cycles and separations: the histotopography of the urinary concentrating process. Kidney Int 1987;31:538—48.

[13] Khorshid MR, Moffat DB. The epithelia lining the renal pelvis in the rat. J Anat 1974;118:561—9.

[14] Lacy ER, Schmidt-Nielsen B. Anatomy of the renal pelvis in the hamster. Am J Anat 1979;154:291—320.

[15] Sands JM, Knepper MA, Spring KR. Na-K-Cl co-transport in apical membrane of rabbit renal papillary surface epithelium. Am J Physiol 1986;251:F475—84.

[16] Silverblatt FJ. Ultrastructure of the renal pelvic epithelium of the rat. Kidney Int 1974;5:214—20.

[17] Kriz W, Bankir L. Structural organization of the renal medullary counterflow system. Fed Proc 1983;42:2379—85.

[18] Pannabecker TL, Abbott DE, Dantzler WH. Three-dimensional functional reconstruction of inner medullary thin limbs of Henle's loop. Am J Physiol Renal Physiol 2004;286:F38—45.

[19] Pannabecker TL, Dantzler WH. Three-dimensional lateral and vertical relationships of inner medullary loops of Henle and collecting ducts. Am J Physiol Renal Physiol 2004;287:F767—74.

[20] Pannabecker TL, Dantzler WH, Layton HE, Layton AT. Role of three-dimensional architecture in the urine concentrating mechanism of the rat renal inner medulla. Am J Physiol Renal Physiol 2008;295:F1271—85.

[21] Layton AT, Layton HE, Dantzler WH, Pannabecker TL. The mammalian urine concentrating mechanism: hypotheses and uncertainties. Physiology (Bethesda) 2009;24:250—6.

[22] Jamison RL, Kriz W. Urinary concentrating mechanism. Structure and function. New York: Oxford University Press; 1982.

[23] Kriz W, Lever AF. Renal countercurrent mechanisms: structure and function. Am Heart J 1969;78:101—18.

[24] Rytand DA. The number and size of mammalian glomeruli as related to kidney and body weight, with methods for their enumeration and measurement. Am J Anat 1938;62:507—20.

[25] Knepper MA, Danielson RA, Saidel GM, Post RS. Quantitative analysis of renal medullary anatomy in rats and rabbits. Kidney Int 1977;12:313—23.

[26] Nyengaard JR, Bendtsen TF. Glomerular number and size in relation to age, kidney weight, and body surface in normal man. AR 1992;232:194—201.

[27] Oliver J. Nephrons and kidneys: a quantitative study of developmental and evolutionary mammalian renal architectonics. New York: Harper and Row; 1968.

[28] Calder WAI, Braun EJ. Scaling of osmotic regulation in mammals and birds. Am J Physiol Regul Integr Comp Physiol 1983;244:R601—6.

[29] Sperber I. Studies on the mammalian kidney. Zool Bidrag Uppsala 1944;22:249—437.

[30] Pfeiffer EW, Nungesser WC, Iverson DA, Wallerius JF. The renal anatomy of the primitive rodent, *Aplodontia rufa*, and a consideration of its functional significance. AR 1960;137:227—35.

[31] Sasaki Y, Takahashi T, Suwa N. Quantitative structural analysis of the inner medulla of rabbit kidney. Tohoku J Exp Med 1969;98:21—32.

[32] Han JS, Thompson KA, Chou C-L, Knepper MA. Experimental tests of three-dimensional model of urinary concentrating mechanism. J Am Soc Nephrol 1992;2:1677—88.

[33] Casotti G, Lindberg KK, Braun EJ. Functional morphology of the avian medullary cone. Am J Physiol Regul Integr Comp Physiol 2000;279:R1722—30.

[34] Williams JB, Pacelli MM, Braun EJ. The effect of water deprivation on renal function in conscious unrestrained Gambel's quail (*Callipepla gambelli*). Physiol Zool 1991;64:1200—16.

[35] Atherton JC, Hai MA, Thomas S. The time course of changes in renal tissue composition during mannitol diuresis in the rat. J Physiol 1968;197:411—28.

[36] Atherton JC, Hai MA, Thomas S. Acute effects of lysine vasopressin injection (single and continuous) on urinary composition in the conscious water diuretic rat. Pfluegers Arch 1969;310:281—96.

[37] de Rouffignac C. The urinary concentrating mechanism. In: Kinne RKH, editor. Urinary concentrating mechanisms. comparative physiology. Basel: Karger; 1990. p. 31—102.

[38] Koepsell H, Nicholson WAP, Kriz W, Hohling HJ. Measurements of exponential gradients of sodium and chlorine in the rat kidney medulla using the electron microprobe. Pfluegers Arch 1974;350:167—84.

[39] Imai M, Taniguchi J, Tabei K. Function of thin loops of Henle. Kidney Int 1987;31:565—79.

[40] Kriz W, Bankir L. A standard nomenclature for structures of the kidney. Am J Physiol Renal Physiol 1988;254:F1—8.

[41] Preston GM, Carroll TP, Guggino WB, Agre P. Appearance of water channels in *Xenopus* oocytes expressing red cell CHIP28 protein. Science 1992;256:385—7.

[42] Chou C-L, Nielsen S, Knepper MA. Structural—functional correlation in chinchilla long loop of Henle thin limbs: a novel papillary subsegment. Am J Physiol Renal, Fluid Electrolyte Physiol 1993;265:F863—74.

[43] Nielsen S, Pallone T, Smith BL, Christensen EI, Agre P, Maunsbach AB. Aquaporin-1 water channels in short and long loop descending thin limbs and in descending vasa recta in rat kidney. Am J Physiol Renal,Fluid Electrolyte Physiol 1995;268: F1023—37.

[44] Nielsen S, Smith BL, Christensen EI, Knepper MA, Agre P. CHIP28 water channels are localized in constitutively water-permeable segments of the nephron. J Cell Biol 1993;120:371—83.

[45] Sabolic I, Valenti G, Verbavatz J-M, Van Hoek AN, Verkman AS, Ausiello DA, et al. Localization of the CHIP28 water channel in rat kidney. Am J Physiol Cell Physiol 1992;263: C1225—33.

[46] Maeda Y, Smith BL, Agre P, Knepper MA. Quantification of Aquaporin-CHIP water channel protein in microdissected renal tubules by fluorescence-based ELISA. J Clin Invest 1995;95:422—8.

[47] Ma TH, Yang BX, Gillespie A, Carlson EJ, Epstein CJ, Verkman AS. Severely impaired urinary concentrating ability in transgenic mice lacking aquaporin-1 water channels. J Biol Chem 1998;273:4296—9.

[48] Schnermann J, Chou CL, Ma TH, Traynor T, Knepper MA, Verkman AS. Defective proximal tubular fluid reabsorption in transgenic aquaporin-1 null mice. Proc Natl Acad Sci USA 1998;95:9660—4.

[49] Chou C-L, Knepper MA. *In vitro* perfusion of chinchilla thin limb segments: segmentation and osmotic water permeability. Am J Physiol Renal Physiol 1992;263:F417—26.

[50] Chou C-L, Sands JM, Nonoguchi H, Knepper MA. Urea-gradient associated fluid absorption with $s_{urea} = 1$ in rat terminal collecting duct. Am J Physiol 1990;258:F1173—80.

III. FLUID AND ELECTROLYTE REGULATION AND DYSREGULATION

[51] Dantzler WH, Evans KE, Pannabecker TL. Osmotic water permeabilities in specific segments of rat inner medullary thin limbs of Henle's loops (Abstract). FASEB J 2009;23: [970.3]

[52] Layton HE, Knepper MA, Chou C-L. Permeability criteria for effective function of passive countercurrent multiplier. Am J Physiol 1996;270:F9−20.

[53] Braun EJ, Reimer PR. Structure of avian loop of Henle as related to countercurrent multiplier system. Am J Physiol 1988;255: F500−12.

[54] Layton AT, Pannabecker TL, Dantzler WH, Layton HE. Two modes for concentrating urine in rat inner medulla. Am J Physiol Renal Physiol 2004;287:F816−39.

[55] Layton HE, Davies JM. Distributed solute and water reabsorption in a central core model of the renal medulla. Math Biosci 1993;116:169−96.

[56] Layton HE, Davies JM, Casotti G, Braun EJ. Mathematical model of an avian urine concentrating mechanism. Am J Physiol Renal Physiol 2000;279:1139−60.

[57] Chou C-L, Knepper MA. In vitro perfusion of chinchilla thin limb segments: urea and NaCl permeabilities. Am J Physiol Renal Physiol 1993;264:F337−43.

[58] Imai M, Hayashi M, Araki M. Functional heterogeneity of the descending limbs of Henle's loop. I. internephron heterogeneity in the hamster kidney. Pfluegers Arch 1984;402:385−92.

[59] Imai M, Taniguchi J, Yoshitomi K. Transition of permeability properties along the descending limb of long-loop nephron. Am J Physiol 1988;254:F323−8.

[60] Kokko JP. Urea transport in the proximal tubule and the descending limb of Henle. J Clin Invest 1972;51:1999−2008.

[61] Pallone TL, Work J, Myers RL, Jamison RL. Transport of sodium and urea in outer medullary descending vasa recta. J Clin Invest 1994;93:212−22.

[62] Stoner LC, Roch-Ramel F. The effects of pressure on the water permeability of the descending limb of Henle's loops of rabbits. Pfluegers Arch 1979;382:7−15.

[63] Morgan T, Berliner RW. Permeability of the loop of Henle, vasa recta, and collecting duct to water, urea, and sodium. Am J Physiol 1968;215:108−15.

[64] Kokko JP. Sodium chloride and water transport in the descending limb of Henle. J Clin Invest 1970;49:1838−46.

[65] Abramow M, Orci L. On the "tightness" of the rabbit descending limb of the loop of Henle-physiological and morphological evidence. Int J Biochem 1980;12:23−7.

[66] Rocha AS, Kokko JP. Membrane characteristics regulating potassium transport out of the isolated perfused descending limb of Henle. Kidney Int 1973;4:326−30.

[67] Katz AI. Distribution and function of classes of ATPases along the nephron. Kidney Int 1986;29:21−31.

[68] Terada Y, Knepper MA. Na+-K+-ATPase activities in renal tubule segments of rat inner medulla. Am J Physiol 1989;256: F218−23.

[69] Tabei K, Imai M. K transport in upper portion of descending limbs of long-loop nephron from hamster. Am J Physiol 1987;252:F387−92.

[70] Gottschalk CW, Mylle M. Micropuncture study of composition of loop of Henle fluid in desert rodents. Am J Physiol 1959;204:532−5.

[71] Horster M, Thurau K. Micropuncture studies on the filtration rate of single superficial and juxtamedullary glomeruli in the rat kidney. Pfluegers Arch 1968;301:162−81.

[72] Pennell JP, Lacy FB, Jamison RL. An in vivo study of the concentrating process in the descending limb of Henle's loop. Kidney Int 1974;5:337−47.

[73] Jamison RL, Buerkert J, Lacy FB. A micropuncture study of Henle's thin loop in brattleboro rats. Am J Physiol 1973;224:180−5.

[74] Bankir L, Trinh-Trang-Tan M-M. Urea and the kidney. In: Brenner BM, editor. Brenner and Rector's the kidney. 6th ed. Philadelphia: Saunders; 2000. p. 637−79.

[75] Pennell JP, Sanjana V, Frey NR, Jamison RL. The effect of urea infusion on the urinary concentrating mechanism in protein-depleted rats. J Clin Invest 1975;55:399−409.

[76] Marsh DJ. Solute and water flows in thin limbs of Henle's loop in the hamster kidney. Am J Physiol 1970;218:824−31.

[77] Marsh DJ, Azen SP. Mechanism of NaCl reabsorption by hamster thin ascending limb of Henle's loop. Am J Physiol 1975;228:71−9.

[78] Ito M, Oiso Y, Murase T, Kondo K, Saito H, Chinzei T, et al. Possible involvement of inefficient cleavage of preprovasopressin by signal peptidase as a cause for familial central diabetes insipidus. J Clin Invest 1993;91:2565−71.

[79] Imai M. Function of the thin ascending limbs of Henle of rats and hamsters perfused in vitro. Am J Physiol 1977;232:F201−9.

[80] Imai M, Kokko JP. Sodium, chloride, urea, and water transport in the thin ascending limb of Henle. J Clin Invest 1974;53:393−402.

[81] Nielsen S, Frokiaer J, Marples D, Kwon ED, Agre P, Knepper M. Aquaporins in the kidney: from molecules to medicine. Physiol Rev 2002;82:205−44.

[82] Kondo Y, Imai M. Effect of glutaraldehyde on renal tubular function. II. Selective inhibition of Cl− transport in the hamster thin ascending limb of Henle's loop. Pfluegers Arch 1987;408:484−90.

[83] Kondo Y, Abe K, Igarashi Y, Kudo K, Tada K, Yoshinaga K. Direct evidence for the absence of active Na+ reabsorption in hamster ascending thin limb of Henle's loop. J Clin Invest 1993;91:5−11.

[84] Uchida S, Sasaki S, Nitta K, Uchida K, Horita S, Nihei H, et al. Localization and functional characterization of rat kidney-specific chloride channel, ClC-K1. J Clin Invest 1995;95:104−13.

[85] Takahashi N, Kondo Y, Ito O, Igarashi Y, Omata K, Abe K. Vasopressin stimulates Cl− transport in ascending thin limb of Henle's loop in hamster. J Clin Invest 1995;95:1623−7.

[86] Uchida S, Sasaki S, Furukawa T, Hiraoka M, Imai T, Hirata Y, et al. Molecular cloning of a chloride channel that is regulated by dehydration and expressed predominantly in kidney medulla. J Biol Chem 1993;268:3821−4.

[87] Akizuki N, Uchida S, Sasaki S, Marumo F. Impaired solute accumulation in inner medulla of Clcnk1−/− mice kidney. Am J Physiol Renal Physiol 2001;280:F79−87.

[88] Koyama S, Yoshitomi K, Imai M. Effect of protamine on ion conductance of ascending thin limb of Henle's loop from hamsters. Am J Physiol 1991;261:F593−9.

[89] Takahashi N, Kondo Y, Fujiwara I, Ito O, Igarashi Y, Abe K. Characterization of Na+ transport across the cell membranes of the ascending thin limb of Henle's loop. Kidney Int 1995;47:789−94.

[90] Wade JB, Lee AJ, Liu J, Ecelbarger CA, Mitchell C, Bradford AD, et al. UT-A2: A 55 kDa urea transporter protein in thin descending limb of Henle's loop whose abundance is regulated by vasopressin. Am J Physiol 2000;278:F52−62.

[91] Mejia R, Wade JB. Immunomorphometric study of rat renal inner medulla. Am J Physiol Renal Physiol 2002;282:F553−7.

[92] Burg MB, Green N. Function of the thick ascending limb of Henle's loop. Am J Physiol 1973;224:659−68.

[93] Horster M. Loop of Henle functional differentiation: in vitro perfusion of the isolated thick ascending segment. Pfluegers Arch 1978;378:15−24.

[94] Rocha AS, Kokko JP. Sodium chloride and water transport in the medullary thick ascending limb of Henle. Evidence for active chloride transport. J Clin Invest 1973;52:612−23.

[95] Garg LC, Mackie S, Tisher CC. Effect of low potassium-diet on Na-K-ATPase in rat nephron segments. Pfluegers Arch 1982;394:113–7.

[96] Morel F, Imbert-Teboul M, Chabardes D. Distribution of hormone-dependent adenylate cyclase in the nephron and its physiologic significance. Annual Rev Physiol 1981;43:569–81.

[97] Wittner M, Di Stefano A, Mandon B, Roinel N, de Rouffignac C. Stimulation of NaCl reabsorption by antidiuretic hormone in the cortical thick ascending limb of Henle's loop of the mouse. Pfluegers Arch 1991;419:212–4.

[98] Knepper MA. Urea transport in isolated thick ascending limbs and collecting ducts from rats. Am J Physiol 1983;245:F634–9.

[99] Rocha AS, Kokko JP. Permeability of medullary nephron segments to urea and water: effect of vasopressin. Kidney Int 1974;6:379–87.

[100] Grantham JJ, Burg MB. Effect of vasopressin and cyclic AMP on permeability of isolated collecting tubules. Am J Physiol 1966;211:255–9.

[101] Reif MC, Troutman SL, Schafer JA. Sustained response to vasopressin in isolated rat cortical collecting tubule. Kidney Int 1984;26:725–32.

[102] Sands JM, Nonoguchi H, Knepper MA. Vasopressin effects on urea and H_2O transport in inner medullary collecting duct subsegments. Am J Physiol 1987;253:F823–32.

[103] Badr KF. Kidney and endocrine system. Part1: eicosanoids. In: Massry SG, Glassock RJ, editors. Book of nephrology. 3rd ed. Baltimore: Williams and Wilkins Co.; 1995. p. 182–91.

[104] Sands JM, Knepper MA. Urea permeability of mammalian inner medullary collecting duct system and papillary surface epithelium. J Clin Invest 1987;79:138–47.

[105] Grantham JJ, Burg MB, Orloff J. The nature of transtubular Na and K transport in isolated rabbit renal collecting tubules. J Clin Invest 1970;49:1815–26.

[106] Tomita K, Pisano JJ, Knepper MA. Control of sodium and potassium transport in the cortical collecting duct of the rat. Effects of bradykinin, vasopressin, and deoxycorticosterone. J Clin Invest 1985;76:132–6.

[107] Palmer LG, Frindt G. Amiloride-sensitive Na channels from the apical membrane of the rat cortical collecting tubule. Proc Natl Acad Sci USA 1986;83:2767–70.

[108] Hanley MJ, Kokko JP. Study of chloride transport across the rabbit cortical collecting tubule. J Clin Invest 1978;62:39–44.

[109] Tomita K, Pisano JJ, Burg MB, Knepper MA. Effects of vasopressin and bradykinin on anion transport by the rat cortical collecting duct. Evidence for an electroneutral sodium chloride transport pathway. J Clin Invest 1986;77:136–41.

[110] Horster MF, Zink H. Functional differentiation of the medullary collecting tubule: influence of vasopressin. Kidney Int 1982;22:360–5.

[111] Madsen KM, Tisher CC. Structural–functional relationship along the distal nephron. Am J Physiol 1986;250:F1–15.

[112] Clapp WL, Madsen KM, Verlander JW, Tisher CC. Intercalated cells of the rat inner medullary collecting duct. Kidney Int 1987;31:1080–7.

[113] Clapp WL, Madsen KM, Verlander JW, Tisher CC. Morphologic heterogeneity along the rat inner medullary collecting duct. Lab Invest 1989;60:219–30.

[114] Kato A, Naruse M, Knepper MA, Sands JM. Long-term regulation of inner medullary collecting duct urea transport in rat. J Am Soc Nephrol 1998;9:737–45.

[115] Kato A, Sands JM. Evidence for sodium-dependent active urea secretion in the deepest subsegment of the rat inner medullary collecting duct. J Clin Invest 1998;101:423–8.

[116] Imai M, Taniguchi J, Yoshitomi K. Osmotic work across inner medullary collecting duct accomplished by difference in

[117] Sands JM, Naruse M, Jacobs JD, Wilcox JN, Klein JD. Changes in aquaporin-2 protein contribute to the urine concentrating defect in rats fed a low-protein diet. J Clin Invest 1996;97:2807–14.

[118] Isozaki T, Verlander JW, Sands JM. Low protein diet alters urea transport and cell structure in rat initial inner medullary collecting duct. J Clin Invest 1993;92:2448–57.

[119] Gillin AG, Sands JM. Characteristics of osmolarity-stimulated urea transport in rat IMCD. Am J Physiol 1992;262:F1061–7.

[120] Kondo Y, Imai M. Effects of glutaraldehyde fixation on renal tubular function. I. Preservation of vasopressin-stimulated water and urea pathways in rat papillary collecting duct. Pfluegers Arch 1987;408:479–83.

[121] Sands JM, Schrader DC. An independent effect of osmolality on urea transport in rat terminal IMCDs. J Clin Invest 1991;88:137–42.

[122] Knepper MA, Sands JM, Chou C-L. Independence of urea and water transport in rat inner medullary collecting duct. Am J Physiol 1989;256:F610–21.

[123] Rocha AS, Kudo LH. Water, urea, sodium, chloride, and potassium transport in the in vitro perfused papillary collecting duct. Kidney Int 1982;22:485–91.

[124] Sands JM, Nonoguchi H, Knepper MA. Hormone effects on NaCl permeability of rat inner medullary collecting duct subsegments. Am J Physiol 1988;255:F421–8.

[125] Ullrich KJ, Papavassiliou F. Sodium reabsorption in the papillary collecting ducts of rats. Pfluegers Arch 1979;379:49–52.

[126] Weinstein AM. A mathematical model of the inner medullary collecting duct of the rat: pathways for Na and K transport. Am J Physiol Renal Physiol 1998;274:F841–55.

[127] Packer RK, Sands JM, Knepper MA. Chloride and osmotic water permeabilities of isolated rabbit renal papillary surface epithelium. Am J Physiol 1989;257:F218–24.

[128] Reeves WB. Conductive properties of papillary surface epithelium. Am J Physiol 1994;266:F259–65.

[129] Sands JM, Ivy EJ, Beeuwkes III R. Transmembrane potential difference of renal papillary epithelial cells. Effect of urea and DDAVP. Am J Physiol 1985;248:F762–6.

[130] Smith HW. The fate of sodium and water in the renal tubules. Bull NY Acad Med 1959;35:293–316.

[131] Kriz W. Structural organization of the renal medulla: comparative and functional aspects. Am J Physiol Regul Integr Comp Physiol 1981;241:R3–16.

[132] Zhai XY, Fenton RA, Andreasen A, Thomsen JS, Christensen AE. Aquaporin-1 is not expressed in descending thin limbs of short-loop nephrons. J Am Soc Nephrol 2007;18:2937–44.

[133] Layton AT, Layton HE. A region-based mathematical model of the urine concentrating mechanism in the rat outer medulla. I. Formulation and base-case results. Am J Physiol Renal Physiol 2005;289:F1346–66.

[134] Zimmerhackl BL, Robertson CR, Jamison RL. The medullary microcirculation. Kidney Int 1987;31:641–7.

[135] Fenton RA, Moeller HB, Hoffert JD, Yu MJ, Nielsen S, Knepper MA. Acute regulation of aquaporin-2 phosphorylation at Ser-264 by vasopressin. PNAS 2008;105:3134–9.

[136] Hoffert JD, Fenton RA, Moeller HB, Simons B, Tchapyjnikov D, McDill BW, et al. Vasopressin-stimulated increase in phosphorylation at Ser269 potentiates plasma membrane retention of aquaporin-2. J Biol Chem 2008;283:24617–27.

[137] Hoffert JD, Pisitkun T, Wang G, Shen R-F, Knepper MA. Quantitative phosphoproteomics of vasopressin-sensitive renal cells: regulation of aquaporin-2 phosphorylation at two sites. Proc Natl Acad Sci USA 2006;103:7159–64.

III. FLUID AND ELECTROLYTE REGULATION AND DYSREGULATION

[138] Hoffert JD, Pisitkun T, Wang GH, Shen RF, Knepper MA. Dynamics of aquaporin-2 serine-261 phosphorylation in response to short-term vasopressin treatment in collecting duct. Am J Physiol Renal Physiol 2007;292:F691−700.

[139] Wade JB, Stetson DL, Lewis SA. ADH action: evidence for a membrane shuttle mechanism. Annals NY Acad Sci 1981;372:106−17.

[140] Jamison RL, Buerkert J, Lacy FB. A micropuncture study of collecting tubule function in rats with hereditary diabetes insipidus. J Clin Invest 1971;50:2444−52.

[141] Kuhn W, Ryffel K. Herstellung konzentrierrter Lösungen aus verdünnten durch blosse Membranwirkung: ein Modellversuch zur Funktion der Niere. Hoppe-Seylers Z Physiol Chem 1942;276:145−78.

[142] Ullrich KJ, Schmidt-Nielsen B, O'Dell R, Pehling G, Gottschalk CW, Lassiter WE, et al. Micropuncture study of composition of proximal and distal tubular fluid in rat kidney. Am J Physiol 1963;204:527−31.

[143] Chou C-L, Knepper MA, Layton HE. Urinary concentrating mechanism: the role of the inner medulla. Semin Nephrol 1993;13:168−81.

[144] Fenton RA, Chou C-L, Stewart GS, Smith CP, Knepper MA. Urinary concentrating defect in mice with selective deletion of phloretin-sensitive urea transporters in the renal collecting duct. Proc Natl Acad Sci USA 2004;101:7469−74.

[145] Moore LC, Marsh DJ. How descending limb of Henle's loop permeability affects hypertonic urine formation. Am J Physiol 1980;239:F57−71.

[146] Wexler AS, Kalaba RE, Marsh DJ. Passive, one-dimensional countercurrent models do not simulate hypertonic urine formation. Am J Physiol 1987;253:F1020−30.

[147] Wexler AS, Kalaba RE, Marsh DJ. Three-dimensional anatomy and renal concentrating mechanism. I. Modelling results. Am J Physiol 1991;260:F368−83.

[148] Knepper MA, Chou C-L, Layton HE. How is urine concentrated by the renal inner medulla? Contrib Nephrol 1993;102:144−60.

[149] Jen JF, Stephenson JL. Externally driven countercurrent multiplication in a mathematical model of the urinary concentrating mechanism of the renal inner medulla. Bull Math Biol 1994;56:491−514.

[150] Knepper MA, Saidel GM, Hascall VC, Dwyer T. Concentration of solutes in the renal inner medulla: interstitial hyaluronan as a mechano-osmotic transducer. Am J Physiol Renal Physiol 2003;284:F433−46.

[151] Hervy S, Thomas SR. Inner medullary lactate production and urine-concentrating mechanism: a flat medullary model. Am J Physiol Renal Physiol 2003;284:F65−81.

[152] Thomas SR. Inner medullary lactate production and accumulation: a vasa recta model. Am J Physiol Renal Physiol 2000;279:F468−81.

[153] Layton AT, Pannabecker TL, Dantzler WH, Layton HE. Functional implications of the three-dimensional architecture of the rat renal inner medulla. Am J Physiol Renal Physiol 2010;298:F973−87.

[154] Hargitay B, Kuhn W. Das Multiplikationsprinzip als Grundlage der Harnkonzentrierung in der Niere. Z Elektrochem 1951;55:539−58.

[155] Vehaskari VM, Hering-Smith KS, Moskowitz DW, Weiner ID, Hamm LL. Effect of epidermal growth factor on sodium transport in the cortical collecting tubule. Am J Physiol 1989;256:F803−9.

[156] Morel F, Mylle M, Gottschalk CW. Tracer microinjection studies of effect of ADH on renal tubular diffusion of water. Am J Physiol 1965;209:179−87.

[157] Layton AT, Layton HE. A region-based mathematical model of the urine concentrating mechanism in the rat outer medulla. II. Parameter sensitivity and tubular inhomogeneity. Am J Physiol Renal Physiol 2005;289:F1367−81.

[158] Stephenson JL, Zhang Y, Eftekhari A, Tewarson RP. Electrolyte transport in a central core model of the renal medulla. Am J Physiol 1989;253:F982−97.

[159] Stephenson JL, Zhang Y, Tewarson RP. Electrolyte, urea, and water transport in a two-nephron central core model of the renal medulla. Am J Physiol 1989;257:F388−413.

[160] Wang X, Thomas SR, Wexler AS. Outer medullary anatomy and the urine concentrating mechanism. Am J Physiol 1998;274:F413−24.

[161] Macri P, Breton S, Marsolais M, Lapointe JY, Laprade R. Hypertonicity decreases basolateral K^+ and Cl^- conductances in rabbit proximal convoluted tubule. J Membr Biol 1997;155:229−37.

[162] Thomas SR, Wexler AS. Inner medullary external osmotic driving force in a 3D model of the renal concentrating mechanism. Am J Physiol 1995;269:F159−71.

[163] Holstein-Rathlou N-H, Marsh DJ. Oscillations of tubular pressure, flow, and distal chloride concentration in rats. Am J Physiol 1989;256:F1007−14.

[164] Reinking LN, Schmidt-Nielsen B. Peristaltic flow of urine in the renal papillary collecting ducts of hamsters. Kidney Int 1981;20:55−60.

[165] Epstein FH, Kleeman CR, Pursel S, Hendrikx A. The effect of feeding protein and urea on the renal concentrating process. J Clin Invest 1957;36:635−41.

[166] Gamble JL, McKhann CF, Butler AM, Tuthill E. An economy of water in renal function referable to urea. Am J Physiol 1934;109:139−54.

[167] Lever AF. The vasa recta and countercurrent multiplication. Acta Med Scand 1965;178:1−43.

[168] Niesel W, Röskenbleck H. Moglichkeiten der Konzentrierung von Stoffen biologischen Gegenstromsystemen. Pfluegers Arch 1963;276:555−67.

[169] Niesel W, Röskenbleck H. Konzentrierung von Lösungen unterschiedlicher Zusammensetzung durch alleinige Gegenstromdiffusion und Geggenstromosmose als möglicher Mechanismus der Harnkonzentrierung. Pfluegers Arch 1965;283:230−41.

[170] Niesel W, Röskenbleck H, Hanke P, Specht N, Heure L. Die gegenseitige Beeinflussung von Harnstoff, NaCl, KCl und Harnfluss bei der Bildung eines maximal konzentrierten Harns. Pfluegers Arch 1970;315:308−20.

[171] Pinter GG, Shohet JL. Origin of sodium concentration profile in the renal medulla. Nature 1963;200:955−8.

[172] Stephenson JL. Concentrating engines and the kidney. II. Multisolute central core systems. Biophys J 1973;13:546−67.

[173] Stephenson JL. Concentrating engines and the kidney. I. Central core model of the renal medulla. Biophys J 1973;13:512−45.

[174] Stephenson JL. Concentrating engines and the kidney. III. Canonical mass balance equation for multinephron models of the renal medulla. Biophys J 1976;16:1273−86.

[175] Stephenson JL. Concentrating engines and the kidney. IV. Mass balance in a single stage of a multistage model of the renal medulla. Math Biosci 1981;55:265−78.

[176] Jen JF, Wang H, Tewarson RP, Stephenson JL. Comparison of central core and radially separated models of renal inner medulla. Am J Physiol 1995;268:F693−7.

[177] Kellogg RB. Some singular perturbation problems in renal models. J Math Anal Appl 1987;128:214−40.

[178] Stephenson JL, Tewarson RP, Mejia R. Quantitative analysis of mass and energy balance in non-ideal models of the renal

counterflow system. Proc Natl Acad Sci USA 1974;71: 1618−22.

[179] Foster DM, Jacquez JA. Comparison using central core model of renal medulla of the rabbit and rat. Am J Physiol 1978;234: F402−14.

[180] Layton HE. Urea transport in a distributed loop model of the urine-concentrating mechanism. Am J Physiol 1990;258: F1110−24.

[181] Marcano M, Layton AT, Layton HE. Maximum urine concentrating capability in a mathematical model of the inner medulla of the rat kidney. Bull Math Biol 2010;72:314−39.

[182] Layton AT, Layton HE. An efficient numerical method for distributed-loop models of the urine concentrating mechanism. Math Biosci 2003;118:111−32.

[183] Layton HE, Pitman EB, Knepper MA. A dynamic numerical method for models of the urine concentrating mechanism. SIAM J Appl Math 1995;55:1390−418.

[184] Mejia R, Stephenson JL. Solution of a multinephron, multisolute model of the mammalian kidney by Newton and continuation methods. Math Biosci 1984;68:279−98.

[185] Tewarson RP, Wang H, Stephenson JL, Jen JF. Efficient computer algorithms for kidney modeling. Math Model Sci Comput 1993;1:164−71.

[186] Wexler AS, Marsh DJ. Numerical methods for three-dimensional models of the urine concentrating mechanism. Appl Math Comput 1991;45:219−40.

[187] Layton HE. Mathematical models of the mammalian urine concentrating mechanism. In: Layton HE, Weinstein AM, editors. Membrane transport and renal physiology. New York: Springer-Verlag; 2002. p. 233−72.

[188] Stephenson JL. Urinary concentration and dilution: models. In: Windhager EE, editor. Handbook of physiology: renal physiology. Bethesda: American Physiological Society; 1992. p. 1349−408.

[189] Stewart J, Luggen ME, Valtin H. A computer model of the renal countercurrent system. Kidney Int 1972;2:253−63.

[190] Stewart J, Valtin H. Computer simulation of osmotic gradient without active transport in renal inner medulla. Kidney Int 1972;2:264−70.

[191] Barrett GL, Packer JS, Davies JM. Sodium chloride, water and urea handling in the rat renal medulla: a computer simulation. Renal Physiol , Basel 1986;9:223−40.

[192] Chandhoke PS, Saidel GM. Mathematical model of mass transport throughout the kidney. Effects of nephron heterogeneity and tubular-vascular organization. Ann Biomed Eng 1981;9:263−301.

[193] Thomas SR. Cycles and separations in a model of the renal medulla. Am J Physiol Renal Physiol 1998;275:F671−90.

[194] Wang X, Wexler AS, Marsh DJ. The effect of solution non-ideality on membrane transport in three-dimensional models of the renal concentrating mechanism. Bull Math Biol 1994;56:515−46.

[195] Layton HE. Distribution of Henle's loops may enhance urine concentrating capability. Biophys J 1986;49:1033−40.

[196] Layton HE. Concentrating urine in the inner medulla of the kidney. Comments Theor Biol 1989;1:179−96.

[197] Layton HE. Distributed loops of Henle in a central core model of the renal medulla: where should the solute come out? Math Comput Modelling 1990;14:533−7.

[198] Wang XQ, Wexler AS. The effects of collecting duct active NaCl reabsorption and inner medulla anatomy on renal concentrating mechanism. Am J Physiol Renal, Fluid Electrolyte Physiol 1996;270:F900−11.

[199] Wexler AS, Kalaba RE, Marsh DJ. Three-dimensional anatomy and renal concentrating mechanism. II. Sensitivity results. Am J Physiol 1991;260:F384−94.

[200] Stephenson JL, Jen JF, Wang H, Tewarson RP. Convective uphill transport of NaCl from ascending thin limb of loop of Henle. Am J Physiol 1995;268:F680−92.

[201] Stephenson JL, Wang H, Tewarson RP. Effect of vasa recta flow on concentrating ability of models of renal inner medulla. Am J Physiol 1995;268:F698−709.

[202] Layton AT, Pannabecker TL, Dantzler WH, Layton HE. Hyperfiltration and inner stripe hypertrophy may explain findings by Gamble and co-workers. Am J Physiol Renal Physiol 2010;298:F962−72.

[203] Bankir L, Kriz W. Adaptation of the kidney to protein intake and to urine concentrating activity: similar consequences in health and CRF. Kidney Int 1995;47:7−24.

[204] Jamison RL. Micropuncture study of segments of thin loop of Henle in the rat. Am J Physiol 1968;215:236−42.

[205] Jamison RL, Bennett CM, Berliner RW. Countercurrent multiplication by the thin loops of Henle. Am J Physiol 1967;212:357−66.

[206] de Rouffignac C, Morel F. Micropuncture study of water, electrolytes and urea movements along the loop of Henle in *Psammomys*. J Clin Invest 1969;48:474−86.

[207] Bonventre JV, Lechene C. Renal medullary concentrating process: an integrative hypothesis. Am J Physiol 1980;239:F578−88.

[208] Lory P. Effectiveness of a salt transport cascade in the renal medulla: computer simulations. Am J Physiol 1987;252: F1095−102.

[209] Rabinowitz L. Discrepancy between experimental and theoretical urine-to-papilla osmotic gradient. J Appl Physiol 1970;29:389−90.

[210] Sanjana VF, Robertson CR, Jamison RL. Water extraction from the inner medullary collecting tubule system: a role for urea. Kidney Int 1976;10:139−48.

[211] Chandhoke PS, Saidel GM, Knepper MA. Role of inner medullary collecting duct NaC1 transport in urinary concentration. Am J Physiol 1985;18:F688−97.

[212] Schmidt-Nielsen B. Function of the pelvis. In: Kinne RKH, editor. Urinary concentrating mechanisms. Basel: Karger; 1990. p. 103−40.

[213] Schmidt-Nielsen B, Churchill M, Reinking LN. Occurrence of renal pelvic refluxes during rising urine flow rate in rats and hamsters. Kidney Int 1980;18:419−31.

[214] Schmidt-Nielsen B, Reinking LN. Morphometry and fluid reabsorption during peristaltic flow in hamster renal papillary collecting ducts. Kidney Int 1981;20:789−98.

[215] Schmidt-Nielsen B, Graves B. Changes in fluid compartments in hamster renal papilla due to peristalsis in the pelvic wall. Kidney Int 1982;22:613−25.

[216] Schmidt-Nielsen B. The renal pelvis. Kidney Int 1987;31:621−8.

[217] Chuang EL, Reineck HJ, Osgood RW, Kunau RT, Stein JH. Studies on the mechanism of reduced urinary osmolality after exposure of the renal papilla. J Clin Invest 1978;61:633−9.

[218] Oliver RE, Roy DR, Jamison RL. Urinary concentration in the papillary collecting duct of the rat. J Clin Invest 1982;69:157−64.

[219] Schütz W, Schnermann J. Pelvic urine composition as a determinant of inner medullary solute concentration and urine osmolality. Pfluegers Arch 1972;334:154−66.

[220] Bonventre JV, Karnovsky MJ, Lechene CP. Renal papillary epithelial morphology in antidiuresis and water diuresis. Am J Physiol 1978;235:F69−76.

[221] Bonventre JV, Roman RJ, Lechene C. Effect of urea concentration of pelvic fluid on renal concentrating ability. Am J Physiol 1980;239:F609−18.

[222] Reinking LN, Veale MC. Mechanical stimulation of renal pelvic wall peristalsis in the rat. Experientia 1984;40:540−1.

[223] Schmidt-Nielsen B, Graves B, MacDuffie H. Effect of peristaltic contractions of the renal papilla in hamsters, *Misocricetus auratus*. Bull MDIBL 1985;25:70–2.

[224] Bagnasco SM, Peng T, Nakayama Y, Sands JM. Differential expression of individual UT-A urea transporter isoforms in rat kidney. J Am Soc Nephrol 2000;11:1980–6.

[225] Ando Y, Jacobson HR, Breyer MD. Phorbol myristate acetate, dioctanoylglycerol, and phosphatidic acid inhibit the hydroosmotic effect of vasopressin on rabbit cortical collecting tubule. J Clin Invest 1987;80:590–3.

[226] Paxton WG, Runge M, Horaist C, Cohen C, Alexander RW, Bernstein KE. Immunohistochemical localization of rat angiotensin II AT$_1$ receptor. Am J Physiol Renal Physiol 1993;264:F989–95.

[227] Bargman J, Leonard SL, McNuly E, Robertson CR, Jamison RL. Examination of transepithelial exchange of water and solute in the rat renal pelvis. J Clin Invest 1984;74:1860–70.

[228] Lory P, Gilg A, Horster M. Renal countercurrent system: role of collecting duct convergence and pelvic urea predicted from a mathematical model. J Math Biol 1983;16:281–304.

[229] Marsh DJ, Martin CM. Lack of water or urea movement from pelvic urine to papilla in hydropenic hamsters. Miner Electrolyte Metab 1980;3:81–6.

[230] Schmidt-Nielsen B. The renal concentrating mechanism in insects and mammals: a new hypothesis involving hydrostatic pressures. Am J Physiol 1995;268:R1087–100.

[231] Yancey PH, Clark ME, Hand SC, Bowlus RD, Somero GN. Living with water stress: evolution of osmolyte systems. Science 1982;217:1214–22.

[232] Knepper MA, Rector Jr FC. Urinary concentration and dilution. In: Brenner BM, editor. The kidney. 5th ed. Philadelphia: W.B. Saunders Co.; 1996. p. 532–70.

[233] Burg MB. Role of aldose reductase and sorbitol in maintaining the medullary intracellular milieu. Kidney Int 1988;33:635–41.

[234] Burg MB, Kador PF. Sorbitol, osmoregulation, and the complications of diabetes. J Clin Invest 1988;81:635–40.

[235] Bagnasco SM, Balaban RS, Fales HM, Yang YM, Burg MB. Predominantly osmotically active organic solutes in rat and rabbit renal medullas. J Biol Chem 1986;261:5872–7.

[236] Garcia-Perez A, Burg MB. Renal medullary organic osmolytes. Physiol Rev 1991;71:1081–115.

[237] Sands JM. Regulation of intracellular polyols and sugars in response to osmotic stress. In: Strange K, editor. Cellular and molecular physiology of cell volume regulation. 1st ed. Boca Raton, FL: CRC Press, Inc; 1994. p. 133–44.

[238] Yancey PH, Burg MB. Distribution of major organic osmolytes in rabbit kidneys in diuresis and antidiuresis. Am J Physiol 1989;257:F602–7.

[239] Yancey PH. Osmotic effectors in kidneys of xeric and mesic rodents: corticomedullary distribution and changes with water availability. J Comp Physiol B 1988;158:369–80.

[240] Yancey PH, Burg MB. Counteracting effects of urea and betaine in mammalian cells in culture. Am J Physiol 1990;258:R198–204.

[241] Yancey PH, Somero GN. Methylamine osmoregulatory solutes of elasmobranch fishes counteract urea inhibition of enzymes. J Exp Zool 1980;212:205–13.

[242] Crawford JD, Doyle AP, Probst H. Service of urea in renal water conservation. Am J Physiol 1959;196:545–8.

[243] Hendrikx A, Epstein FH. Effect of feeding protein and urea on renal concentrating ability in the rat. Am J Physiol 1958;195:539–42.

[244] Klahr S, Alleyne GAO. Effects of chronic protein-calorie malnutrition on the kidney. Kidney Int 1973;3:129–41.

[245] Levinsky NG, Berliner RW. The role of urea in the urine concentrating mechanism. J Clin Invest 1959;38:741–8.

[246] Peil AE, Stolte H, Schmidt-Nielsen B. Uncoupling of glomerular and tubular regulations of urea excretion in rat. Am J Physiol Renal, Fluid Electrolyte Physiol 1990;258:F1666–74.

[247] Uchida S, Sohara E, Rai T, Ikawa M, Okabe M, Sasaki S. Impaired urea accumulation in the inner medulla of mice lacking the urea transporter UT-A2. Mol Cell Biol 2005;25:7357–63.

[248] Klein JD, Sands JM, Qian L, Wang X, Yang B. Upregulation of urea transporter UT-A2 and water channels AQP2 and AQP3 in mice lacking urea transporter UT-B. J Am Soc Nephrol 2004;15:1161–7.

[249] Yang B, Bankir L, Gillespie A, Epstein CJ, Verkman AS. Urea-selective concentrating defect in transgenic mice lacking urea transporter UT-B. J Biol Chem 2002;277:10633–7.

[250] Yang B, Verkman AS. Analysis of double knockout mice lacking aquaporin-1 and urea transporter UT-B. J Biol Chem 2002;277:36782–6.

[251] Jaenike JR. The influence of vasopressin on the permeability of the mammalian collecting duct to urea. J Clin Invest 1961;40:144–51.

[252] Morgan T. Permeability of the nephron to urea. In: Schmidt-Nielsen B, Kerr DWS, editors. Urea and the kidney. 1st ed. Amsterdam: Excerpta Medica Foundation; 1970. p. 186–92.

[253] Morgan T, Sakai F, Berliner RW. *In vitro* permeability of medullary collecting duct to water and urea. Am J Physiol 1968;214:574–81.

[254] Bagnasco SM. Gene structure of urea transporters. Am J Physiol Renal Physiol 2003;284:F3–10.

[255] Sands JM. Mammalian urea transporters. Annu Rev Physiol 2003;65:543–66.

[256] Sands JM. Molecular mechanisms of urea transport. J Membr Biol 2003;191:149–63.

[257] Sands JM. Renal urea transporters. Curr Opin Nephrol Hypertens 2004;13:525–32.

[258] Shayakul C, Hediger MA. The SLC14 gene family of urea transporters. Pfluegers Arch 2004;447:603–9.

[259] Stewart GS, Graham C, Cattell S, Smith TPL, Simmons NL, Smith CP. UT-B is expressed in bovine rumen: potential role in ruminal urea transport. Am J Physiol Regul Integr Comp Physiol 2005;289:R605–12.

[260] Sands JM, Layton HE. The urine concentrating mechanism and urea transporters. In: Alpern RJ, Hebert SC, editors. The kidney: physiology and pathophysiology. 4th ed. San Diego: Academic Press; 2008. p. 1143–78.

[261] Nakayama Y, Naruse M, Karakashian A, Peng T, Sands JM, Bagnasco SM. Cloning of the rat Slc14a2 gene and genomic organization of the UT-A urea transporter. Biochim Biophys Acta 2001;1518:19–26.

[262] Bagnasco SM, Peng T, Janech MG, Karakashian A, Sands JM. Cloning and characterization of the human urea transporter UT-A1 and mapping of the human *Slc14a2* gene. Am J Physiol Renal Physiol 2001;281:F400–6.

[263] Fenton RA, Cottingham CA, Stewart GS, Howorth A, Hewitt JA, Smith CP. Structure and characterization of the mouse UT-A gene (*Slc14a2*). Am J Physiol Renal Physiol 2002;282:F630–8.

[264] Fenton RA, Shodeinde A, Knepper MA. UT-A urea transporter promoter, UT-Aalpha, targets principal cells of the renal inner medullary collecting duct. Am J Physiol Renal Physiol 2006;290:F188–95.

[265] Nakayama Y, Peng T, Sands JM, Bagnasco SM. The TonE/TonEBP pathway mediates tonicity-responsive regulation of UT-A urea transporter expression. J Biol Chem 2000;275:38275–80.

[266] Peng T, Sands JM, Bagnasco SM. Glucocorticoids inhibit transcription and expression of the rat UT-A urea transporter gene. Am J Physiol Renal Physiol 2002;282:F853–8.

[267] Kim Y-H, Kim D-U, Han K-H, Jung JY, Sands JM, Knepper MA, et al. Expression of urea transporters in the developing rat kidney. Am J Physiol Renal Physiol 2002;282:F530—40.

[268] Nielsen S, Terris J, Smith CP, Hediger MA, Ecelbarger CA, Knepper MA. Cellular and subcellular localization of the vasopressin-regulated urea transporter in rat kidney. Proc Natl Acad Sci USA 1996;93:5495—500.

[269] Fenton RA, Stewart GS, Carpenter B, Howorth A, Potter EA, Cooper GJ, et al. Characterization of the mouse urea transporters UT-A1 and UT-A2. Am J Physiol Renal Physiol 2002;283: F817—25.

[270] Promeneur D, Rousselet G, Bankir L, Bailly P, Cartron JP, Ripoche P, et al. Evidence for distinct vascular and tubular urea transporters in the rat kidney. J Am Soc Nephrol 1996;7:852—60.

[271] Shayakul C, Steel A, Hediger MA. Molecular cloning and characterization of the vasopressin-regulated urea transporter of rat kidney collecting ducts. J Clin Invest 1996;98:2580—7.

[272] Chen G, Fröhlich O, Yang Y, Klein JD, Sands JM. Loss of N-linked glycosylation reduces urea transporter UT-A1 response to vasopressin. J Biol Chem 2006;281:27436—42.

[273] Fröhlich O, Klein JD, Smith PM, Sands JM, Gunn RB. Urea transport in MDCK cells that are stably transfected with UT-A1. Am J Physiol Cell Physiol 2004;286:C1264—70.

[274] Fröhlich O, Klein JD, Smith PM, Sands JM, Gunn RB. Regulation of UT-A1-mediated transepithelial urea flux in MDCK cells. Am J Physiol Cell Physiol 2006;291:C600—6.

[275] Klein JD, Blount MA, Fröhlich O, Denson CE, Tan X, Sim JH, et al. Phosphorylation of UT-A1 on serine 486 correlates with membrane accumulation and urea transport activity in both rat IMCDs and cultured cells. Am J Physiol Renal Physiol 2010;298:F935—40.

[276] Bradford AD, Terris J, Ecelbarger CA, Klein JD, Sands JM, Chou CL, et al. 97 and 117 kDa forms of the collecting duct urea transporter UT-A1 are due to different states of glycosylation. Am J Physiol Renal Physiol 2001;281:F133—43.

[277] Sands JM. Urea transport: it's not just "freely diffusible" anymore. NIPS 1999;14:46—7.

[278] Sands JM, Flores FX, Kato A, Baum MA, Brown EM, Ward DT, et al. Vasopressin-elicited water and urea permeabilities are altered in the inner medullary collecting duct in hypercalcemic rats. Am J Physiol Renal Physiol 1998;274:F978—85.

[279] Karakashian A, Timmer RT, Klein JD, Gunn RB, Sands JM, Bagnasco SM. Cloning and characterization of two new mRNA isoforms of the rat renal urea transporter: UT-A3 and UT-A4. J Am Soc Nephrol 1999;10:230—7.

[280] Terris JM, Knepper MA, Wade JB. UT-A3: localization and characterization of an additional urea transporter isoform in the IMCD. Am J Physiol Renal Physiol 2001;280:F325—32.

[281] Stewart GS, Fenton RA, Wang W, Kwon TH, White SJ, Collins VM, et al. The basolateral expression of mUT-A3 in the mouse kidney. Am J Physiol Renal Physiol 2004;286:F979—87.

[282] Stewart GS, King SL, Potter EA, Smith CP. Acute regulation of the urea transporter mUT-A3 expressed in a MDCK cell line. Am J Physiol Renal Physiol 2007;292:F1157—63.

[283] Blount MA, Klein JD, Martin CF, Tchapyjnikov D, Sands JM. Forskolin stimulates phosphorylation and membrane accumulation of UT-A3. Am J Physiol Renal Physiol 2007;293: F1308—13.

[284] Smith CP, Potter EA, Fenton RA, Stewart GS. Characterization of a human colonic cDNA encoding a structurally novel urea transporter, UT-A6. Am J Physiol Cell Physiol 2004;287: C1087—93.

[285] Shayakul C, Tsukaguchi H, Berger UV, Hediger MA. Molecular characterization of a novel urea transporter from kidney inner medullary collecting ducts. Am J Physiol Renal Physiol 2001;280:F487—94.

[286] You G, Smith CP, Kanai Y, Lee W-S, Stelzner M, Hediger MA. Cloning and characterization of the vasopressin-regulated urea transporter. Nature 1993;365:844—7.

[287] Ashkar ZM, Martial S, Isozaki T, Price SR, Sands JM. Urea transport in initial IMCD of rats fed a low-protein diet: functional properties and mRNA abundance. Am J Physiol 1995;268:F1218—23.

[288] Shayakul C, Knepper MA, Smith CP, DiGiovanni SR, Hediger MA. Segmental localization of urea transporter mRNAs in rat kidney. Am J Physiol 1997;272:F654—60.

[289] Smith CP, Lee W-S, Martial S, Knepper MA, You G, Sands JM, et al. Cloning and regulation of expression of the rat kidney urea transporter (rUT2). J Clin Invest 1995;96: 1556—63.

[290] Fenton RA, Howorth A, Cooper GJ, Meccariello R, Morris ID, Smith CP. Molecular characterization of a novel UT-A urea transporter isoform (UT-A5) in testis. Am J Physiol Cell Physiol 2000;279:C1425—31.

[291] Olives B, Neau P, Bailly P, Hediger MA, Rousselet G, Cartron JP, et al. Cloning and functional expression of a urea transporter from human bone marrow cells. J Biol Chem 1994;269:31649—52.

[292] Couriaud C, Ripoche P, Rousselet G. Cloning and functional characterization of a rat urea transporter: expression in the brain. Biochim Biophys Acta Gene Struct Expression 1996;1309:197—9.

[293] Sands JM, Timmer RT, Gunn RB. Urea transporters in kidney and erythrocytes. Am J Physiol 1997;273:F321—39.

[294] Tsukaguchi H, Shayakul C, Berger UV, Tokui T, Brown D, Hediger MA. Cloning and characterization of the urea transporter UT3. Localization in rat kidney and testis. J Clin Invest 1997;99:1506—15.

[295] Lucien N, Sidoux-Walter F, Olivès B, Moulds J, Le Pennec PY, Cartron JP, et al. Characterization of the gene encoding the human Kidd blood group urea transporter protein: evidence for splice site mutations in Jk_null individuals. J Biol Chem 1998;273:12973—80.

[296] Lucien N, Sidoux-Walter F, Roudier N, Ripoche P, Huet M, Trin-Trang-Tan MM, et al. Antigenic and functional properties of the human red blood cell urea transporter hUT-B1. J Biol Chem 2002;277:34101—8.

[297] Olivès B, Martial S, Mattei MG, Matassi G, Rousselet G, Ripoche P, et al. Molecular characterization of a new urea transporter in the human kidney. FEBS Lett 1996;386:156—60.

[298] Olivès B, Mattei M-G, Huet M, Neau P, Martial S, Cartron JP, et al. Kidd blood group and urea transport function of human erythrocytes are carried by the same protein. J Biol Chem 1995;270:15607—10.

[299] Sidoux-Walter F, Lucien N, Nissinen R, Sistonen P, Henry S, Moulds J, et al. Molecular heterogeneity of the Jk_null phenotype: expression analysis of the Jk(S291P) mutation found in Finns. Blood 2000;96:1566—73.

[300] Kimoto Y, Constantinou CE. Effects of [1-desamino-8-D-arginine]vasopressin and papaverine on rabbit renal pelvis. Eur J Pharmacol 1990;175:359—62.

[301] Timmer RT, Klein JD, Bagnasco SM, Doran JJ, Verlander JW, Gunn RB, et al. Localization of the urea transporter UT-B protein in human and rat erythrocytes and tissues. Am J Physiol Cell Physiol 2001;281:C1318—25.

[302] Trinh-Trang-Tan M-M, Bouby N, Kriz W, Bankir L. Functional adaptation of thick ascending limb and internephron heterogeneity to urine concentration. Kidney Int 1987;31:549—55.

III. FLUID AND ELECTROLYTE REGULATION AND DYSREGULATION

[303] Hu MC, Bankir L, Michelet S, Rousselet G, Trinh-Trang-Tan M-M. Massive reduction of urea transporters in remnant kidney and brain of uremic rats. Kidney Int 2000;58:1202–10.

[304] Pallone TL. Characterization of the urea transporter in outer medullary descending vasa recta. Am J Physiol 1994;267: R260–7.

[305] Pallone TL, Nielsen S, Silldorff EP, Yang S. Diffusive transport of solute in the rat medullary microcirculation. Am J Physiol Renal,Fluid Electrolyte Physiol 1995;269:F55–63.

[306] Xu Y, Olives B, Bailly P, Fischer E, Ripoche P, Ronco P, et al. Endothelial cells of the kidney vasa recta express the urea transporter HUT11. Kidney Int 1997;51:138–46.

[307] Sidoux-Walter F, Lucien N, Olivès B, Gobin R, Rousselet G, Kamsteeg EJ, et al. At physiological expression levels the Kidd blood group/urea transporter protein is not a water channel. J Biol Chem 1999;274:30228–35.

[308] Yang BX, Verkman AS. Urea transporter UT3 functions as an efficient water channel: direct evidence for a common water/ urea pathway. J Biol Chem 1998;273:9369–72.

[309] Nielsen S, Knepper MA. Vasopressin activates collecting duct urea transporters and water channels by distinct physical processes. Am J Physiol Renal,Fluid Electrolyte Physiol 1993;265: F204–13.

[310] Star RA, Nonoguchi H, Balaban R, Knepper MA. Calcium and cyclic adenosine monophosphate as second messengers for vasopressin in the rat inner medullary collecting duct. J Clin Invest 1988;81:1879–88.

[311] Wall SM, Suk Han J, Chou C-L, Knepper MA. Kinetics of urea and water permeability activation by vasopressin in rat terminal IMCD. Am J Physiol Renal Fluid Electrolyte Physiol 1992;262:F989–98.

[312] Chou C-L, DiGiovanni SR, Luther A, Lolait SJ, Knepper MA. Oxytocin as an antidiuretic hormone. II. Role of V_2 vasopressin receptor. Am J Physiol Renal Fluid Electrolyte Physiol 1995;269:F78–85.

[313] Star RA. Apical membrane limits urea permeation across the rat inner medullary collecting duct. J Clin Invest 1990;86:1172–8.

[314] Chou C-L, Knepper MA. Inhibition of urea transport in inner medullary collecting duct by phloretin and urea analogues. Am J Physiol 1989;257:F359–65.

[315] Nonoguchi H, Owada A, Kobayashi N, Takayama M, Terada Y, Koike J, et al. Immunohistochemical localization of V_2 vasopressin receptor along the nephron and functional role of luminal V_2 receptor in terminal inner medullary collecting ducts. J Clin Invest 1995;96:1768–78.

[316] Zhang C, Sands JM, Klein JD. Vasopressin rapidly increases the phosphorylation of the UT-A1 urea transporter activity in rat IMCDs through PKA. Am J Physiol Renal Physiol 2002;282: F85–90.

[317] Bansal AD, Hoffert JD, Pisitkun T, Hwang S, Chou CL, Boja ES, et al. Phosphoproteomic profiling reveals vasopressin-regulated phosphorylation sites in collecting duct. J Am Soc Nephrol 2010;21:303–15.

[318] Brooks HL, Ageloff S, Kwon TH, Brandt W, Terris JM, Seth A, et al. cDNA array identification of genes regulated in rat renal medulla in response to vasopressin infusion. Am J Physiol Renal Physiol 2003;284:F218–28.

[319] Hoorn EJ, Hoffert JD, Knepper MA. Combined proteomics and pathways analysis of collecting duct reveals a protein regulatory network activated in vasopressin escape. J Am Soc Nephrol 2005;16:2852–63.

[320] Uawithya P, Pisitkun T, Ruttenberg BE, Knepper MA. Transcriptional profiling of native inner medullary collecting duct cells from rat kidney. Physiol Genomics 2008;32:229–53.

[321] Yu MJ, Pisitkun T, Wang G, Aranda JF, Gonzales PA, Tchapyjnikov D, et al. Large-scale quantitative LC-MS/MS analysis of detergent-resistant membrane proteins from rat renal collecting duct. Am J Physiol Cell Physiol 2008;295: C661–78.

[322] Yu MJ, Pisitkun T, Wang G, Shen RF, Knepper MA. LC-MS/ MS analysis of apical and basolateral plasma membranes of rat renal collecting duct cells. Mol Cell Proteomics 2006;5:2131–45.

[323] Bos JL. Epac: a new cAMP target and new avenues in cAMP research. Nat Rev Mol Cell Biol 2003;4:733–8.

[324] Helms MN, Chen X-J, Ramosevac S, Eaton DC, Jain L. Dopamine regulation of amiloride-sensitive sodium channels in lung cells. Am J Physiol Lung Cell Mol Physiol 2006;291: L610–8.

[325] Honegger KJ, Capuano P, Winter C, Bacic D, Stange G, Wagner CA, et al. Regulation of sodium-proton exchanger isoform 3 (NHE3) by PKA and exchange protein directly activated by cAMP (EPAC). Proc Natl Acad Sci USA 2006;103:803–8.

[326] Laroche-Joubert N, Marsy S, Michelet S, Imbert-Teboul M, Doucet A. Protein kinase A-independent activation of ERK and H,K-ATPase by cAMP in native kidney cells. Role of Epac I. J Biol Chem 2002;277:18598–604.

[327] Li Y, Konings IBM, Zhao J, Price LS, de Heer E, Deen PMT. Renal expression of exchange protein directly activated by cAMP (Epac) 1 and 2. Am J Physiol Renal Physiol 2008;295: F525–33.

[328] Yip KP. Epac-mediated Ca^{2+} mobilization and exocytosis in inner medullary collecting duct. Am J Physiol Renal Physiol 2008;291:F882–90.

[329] Wang Y, Klein JD, Blount MA, et al. Epac regulation of the UT-A1 urea transporter in rat IMCDs. J Am Soc Nephrol 2009;20:2018–24.

[330] Blount MA, Mistry AC, Fröhlich O, Price SR, Chen G, Sands JM, et al. Phosphorylation of UT-A1 urea transporter at serines 486 and 499 is important for vasopressin-regulated activity and membrane accumulation. Am J Physiol Renal Physiol 2008;295:F295–9.

[331] Hwang S, Gunaratne R, Rinschen MM, Yu MJ, Pisitkun T, Hoffert JD, et al. Vasporessin increases phosphorylation of ser84 and ser486 in Slc14a2 collecting duct urea transporters. Am J Physiol Renal Physiol 2010;299:F559–67.

[332] Mistry AC, Mallick R, Klein JD, Sands JM, Froehlich O. Functional characterization of the central hydrophilic linker region of the urea transporter UT-A1: cAMP activation and snapin binding. Am J Physiol Cell Physiol 2010;298: C1431–7.

[333] Klein JD, Fröhlich O, Blount MA, Martin CF, Smith TD, Sands JM. Vasopressin increases plasma membrane accumulation of urea transporter UT-A1 in rat inner medullary collecting ducts. J Am Soc Nephrol 2006;17:2680–6.

[334] Inoue T, Terris J, Ecelbarger CA, Chou C-L, Nielsen S, Knepper MA. Vasopressin regulates apical targeting of aquaporin-2 but not of UT1 urea transporter in renal collecting duct. Am J Physiol 1999;276:F559–66.

[335] Cotte N, Balestre MN, Phalipou S, Hibert M, Manning M, Barberis C, et al. Identification of residues responsible for the selective binding of peptide antagonists and agonists in the V2 vasopressin receptor. J Biol Chem 1998;273:29462–8.

[336] Kim D-U, Sands JM, Klein JD. Changes in renal medullary transport proteins during uncontrolled diabetes mellitus in rats. Am J Physiol Renal Physiol 2003;285:F303–9.

[337] Seamon KB, Padgett W, Daly JW. Forskolin: unique diterpene activator of adenylate cyclase in membranes and intact cells. Proc Natl Acad Sci USA 1981;87:3363–7.

[338] Stewart GS, Thistlethwaite A, Lees H, Cooper GJ, Smith C. Vasopressin regulation of the renal UT-A3 urea transporter. Am J Physiol Renal Physiol 2009;296:F642–9.

[339] Mistry AC, Mallick R, Fröhlich O, Klein JD, Rehm A, Chen G, et al. The UT-A1 urea transporter interacts with snapin, a snare-associated protein. J Biol Chem 2007;282:30097–106.

[340] Feng X, Huang H, Yang Y, Fröhlich O, Klein JD, Sands JM, et al. Caveolin-1 directly interacts with UT-A1 urea transporter: the role of caveolae/lipid rafts in UT-A1 regulation at the cell membrane. Am J Physiol Renal Physiol 2009;296:F1514–20.

[341] Chen G, Huang H, Fröhlich O, Yang Y, Klein JD, Price SR, et al. MDM2 E3 ubiquitin ligase mediates UT-A1 urea transporter ubiquitination and degradation. Am J Physiol Renal Physiol 2008;295:F1528–34.

[342] Stewart GS, O'Brien JH, Smith CP. Ubiquitination regulates the plasma membrane expression of renal UT-A urea transporters. Am J Physiol Cell Physiol 2008;295:C121–9.

[343] Kudo LH, César KR, Ping WC, Rocha AS. Effect of peritubular hypertonicity on water and urea transport of inner medullary collecting duct. Am J Physiol Renal Fluid Electrolyte Physiol 1992;262:F338–47.

[344] Chou C-L, Sands JM, Nonoguchi H, Knepper MA. Concentration dependence of urea and thiourea transport pathway in rat inner medullary collecting duct. Am J Physiol 1990;258:F486–94.

[345] Gillin AG, Star RA, Sands JM. Osmolarity-stimulated urea transport in rat terminal IMCD: role of intracellular calcium. Am J Physiol 1993;265:F272–7.

[346] Kato A, Klein JD, Zhang C, Sands JM. Angiotensin II increases vasopressin-stimulated facilitated urea permeability in rat terminal IMCDs. Am J Physiol Renal Physiol 2000;279: F835–40.

[347] Blessing NW, Blount MA, Sands JM, Martin CF, Klein JD. Urea transporters UT-A1 and UT-A3 accumulate in the plasma membrane in response to increased hypertonicity. Am J Physiol Renal Physiol 2008;295:F1336–41.

[348] Leung DW, Loo DDF, Hirayama BA, Zeuthen T, Wright EM. Urea transport by co-transporters. J Physiol (Lond) 2000;528:251–7.

[349] Panayotova-Heiermann M, Wright EA. Mapping the urea channel through the rabbit Na^+-glucose co-transporter SGLT1. J Physiol (Lond) 2001;535:419–25.

[350] Kim D-U, Sands JM, Klein JD. Role of vasopressin in diabetes mellitus-induced changes in medullary transport proteins involved in urine concentration in Brattleboro rats. Am J Physiol Renal Physiol 2004;286:F760–6.

[351] Terris J, Ecelbarger CA, Sands JM, Knepper MA. Long-term regulation of collecting duct urea transporter proteins in rat. J Am Soc Nephrol 1998;9:729–36.

[352] Harrington AR, Valtin H. Impaired urinary concentration after vasopressin and its gradual correction in hypothalamic diabetes insipidus. J Clin Invest 1968;47:502–10.

[353] Igarashi P, Whyte DA, Nagami GT. Cloning and kidney cell-specific activity of the promoter of the murine renal Na-K-Cl co-transporter gene. J Biol Chem 1996;271:9666–74.

[354] Yasui M, Zelenin SM, Celsi G, Aperia A. Adenylate cyclase-coupled vasopressin receptor activates AQP2 promoter via a dual effect on CRE and AP1 elements. Am J Physiol Renal Physiol 1997;272:F443–50.

[355] Cadnapaphornchai MA, Summer SN, Falk S, Thurman JM, Knepper MA, Schrier RW. Effect of primary polydipsia on aquaporin and sodium transporter abundance. Am J Physiol Renal Physiol 2003;285:F965–71.

[356] Promeneur D, Bankir L, Hu MC, Trinh-Trang-Tan M-M. Renal tubular and vascular urea transporters: influence of antidiuretic hormone on messenger RNA expression in Brattleboro rats. J Am Soc Nephrol 1998;9:1359–66.

[357] Isozaki T, Gillin AG, Swanson CE, Sands JM. Protein restriction sequentially induces new urea transport processes in rat initial IMCDs. Am J Physiol 1994;266:F756–61.

[358] Kato A, Sands JM. Urea transport processes are induced in rat IMCD subsegments when urine concentrating ability is reduced. Am J Physiol 1999;276:F62–71.

[359] Hu MC, Bankir L, Trinh-Trang-Tan MM. mRNA expression of renal urea transporters in normal and Brattleboro rats: effect of dietary protein intake. Exp Nephrol 1999;7:44–51.

[360] Knepper MA, Danielson RA, Saidel GM, Johnston KH. Effects of dietary protein restriction and glucocorticoid administration on urea excretion in rats. Kidney Int 1975;8:303–15.

[361] Gertner R, Klein JD, Bailey JL, Kim DU, Luo XH, Bagnasco SM, et al. Aldosterone decreases UT-A1 urea transporter expression via the mineralocorticoid receptor. J Am Soc Nephrol 2004;15:558–65.

[362] Naruse M, Klein JD, Ashkar ZM, Jacobs JD, Sands JM. Glucocorticoids downregulate the rat vasopressin-regulated urea transporter in rat terminal inner medullary collecting ducts. J Am Soc Nephrol 1997;8:517–23.

[363] Wang X-Y, Beutler K, Nielsen J, Nielsen S, Knepper MA, Masilamani S. Decreased abundance of collecting duct urea transporters UT-A1 and UT-A3 with ECF volume expansion. Am J Physiol Renal Physiol 2002;282:F577–84.

[364] Fenton RA, Chou C-L, Ageloff S, Brandt W, Stokes III JB, Knepper M. Increased collecting duct urea transporter expression in Dahl salt-sensitive rats. Am J Physiol Renal Physiol 2003;285:F143–51.

[365] Brooks DD, Nutting DF, Crofton JT, Share L. Vasopressin in rats with genetic and streptozotocin-induced diabetes. Diabetes 1989;38:54–7.

[366] Mitch WE, Bailey JL, Wang X, Jurkovitz C, Newby DN, Price SR. Evaluation of signals activating ubiquitin-proteasome proteolysis in a model of muscle wasting. Am J Physiol Cell Physiol 1999;276:C1132–8.

[367] Trinder D, Phillips PA, Stephenson JM, Risvanis J, Aminian A, Adam W, et al. Vasopressin V_1 and V_2 receptors in diabetes mellitus. Am J Physiol Endocrinol Metab 1994;266:E217–23.

[368] Klein JD, Price SR, Bailey JL, Jacobs JD, Sands JM. Glucocorticoids mediate a decrease in the AVP-regulated urea transporter in diabetic rat inner medulla. Am J Physiol 1997;273:F949–53.

[369] Bardoux P, Ahloulay M, Le Maout S, Bankir L, Trinh-Trang-Tan MM. Aquaporin-2 and urea transporter-A1 are up-regulated in rats with type I diabetes mellitus. Diabetologia 2001;44:637–45.

[370] Blount MA, Sands JM, Kent KJ, Smith TD, Price SR, Klein JD. Candesartan augments compensatory changes in medullary transport proteins in the diabetic rat kidney. Am J Physiol Renal Physiol 2008;285:F1448–52.

[371] Klein JD, Kozlowski SD, Abi Antooun T, Sands JM. Adrenalectomy blocks the compensatory increases in UT-A1 and AQP2 in diabetic rat kidney. J Membr Biol 2006;212 (2):139–44.

[372] Pech V, Klein JD, Kozlowski SD, Wall SM, Sands JM. Vasopressin increases urea permeability in initial IMCDs from diabetic rats. Am J Physiol Renal Physiol 2005;289:F531–5.

[373] Van Zwieten PA, Kam KL, ijl AJ, Hendriks MGC, Beenen OHM, Pfaffendorf M. Hypertensive diabetic rats in pharmacological studies. Pharmacol Res 1996;33:95–105.

[374] Bickel CA, Knepper MA, Verbalis JG, Ecelbarger CA. Dysregulation of renal salt and water transport proteins in diabetic Zucker rats. Kidney Int 2002;61:2099–110.

III. FLUID AND ELECTROLYTE REGULATION AND DYSREGULATION

[375] Klein JD, Murrell BP, Tucker S, Kim Y-H, Sands JM. Urea transporter UT-A1 and aquaporin-2 proteins decrease in response to angiotensin II or norepinephrine-induced acute hypertension. Am J Physiol Renal Physiol 2006;291:F952—9.

[376] Esther Jr CR, Marrero MB, Howard TE, Machaud A, Corvol P, Capecchi MR, et al. The critical role of tissue angiotensin-converting enzyme as revealed by gene targeting in mice. J Clin Invset 1997;99:2375—85.

[377] Klein JD, Quach DL, Cole JM, Disher K, Mongiu AK, Wang X, et al. Impaired urine concentration and the absence of tissue ACE: the involvement of medullary transport proteins. Am J Physiol Renal Physiol 2002;283:F517—24.

[378] Berl T. On the adaptation of renal cells to hypertonicity. Am J Kidney Dis 2000;35:XLVII—L.

[379] Tian W, Cohen DM. Signaling and gene regulation by urea in cells of the mammalian kidney medulla. Comp Biochem Physiol A 2001;130:429—36.

[380] Kim D-U, Klein JD, Racine S, Murrell BP, Sands JM. Urea may regulate urea transporter protein abundance during osmotic diuresis. Am J Physiol Renal Physiol 2005;288:F188—97.

[381] Lam AK, Ko BC, Tam S, Morris R, Yang JY, Chung SK, et al. Osmotic response element-binding protein (OREBP) is an essential regulator of the urine concentrating mechanism. J Biol Chem 2004;279:48048—54.

[382] Leroy C, Basset G, Gruel G, Ripoche P, Trinh-Trang-Tan M-M, Rousselet G. Hyperosmotic NaCl and urea synergistically regulate the expression of the UT-A2 urea transporter in vitro and in vivo. Biochem Biophys Res Commun 2000;271:368—73.

[383] Lim SW, Han KH, Jung JY, Kim WY, Yang CW, Sands JM, et al. Ultrastructural localization of UT-A and UT-B in rat kidneys with different hydration status. Am J Physiol Regul Integr Comp Physiol 2006;290:R479—92.

[384] Kim YM, Kim WY, Lee HW, Kim J, Kwon HM, Klein JD, et al. Urea and NaCl regulate UT-A1 urea transporter in opposing directions via TonEBP pathway during osmotic diuresis. Am J Physiol Renal Physiol 2009;296:F67—77.

[385] Jeon US, Kim JA, Sheen MR, Kwon HM. How tonicity regulates genes: story of TonEBP transcriptional activator. Acta Physiol Scand 2006;187:241—7.

[386] Lam AKM, Ko BCB, Tam S, Morris R, Yang JY, Chung SK, et al. Osmotic response element-binding protein (OREBP) is an essential regulator of the urine concentrating mechanism. J Biol Chem 2004;279:48048—54.

[387] Yang JY, Tam WY, Tam S, Guo H, Wu X, Li G, et al. Genetic restoration of aldose reductase to the collecting tubules restores maturation of the urine concentrating mechanism. Am J Physiol Renal Physiol 2006;291:F186—95.

[388] Galla JH, Booker BB, Luke RG. Role of the loop segment in the urinary concentrating defect of hypercalcemia. Kidney Int 1986;29:977—82.

[389] Jung JY, Madsen KM, Han KH, Yang CW, Knepper MA, Sands JM, et al. Expression of urea transporters in potassium-depleted mouse kidney. Am J Physiol Renal Physiol 2003;285:F1210—24.

[390] Levi M, Peterson L, Berl T. Mechanism of concentrating defect in hypercalcemia. Role of polydipsia and prostaglandins. Kidney Int 1983;23:489—97.

[391] Sands JM, Naruse M, Baum M, Jo I, Hebert SC, Brown EM, et al. An apical extracellular calcium/polyvalent cation-sensing receptor regulates vasopressin-elicited water permeability in rat kidney inner medullary collecting duct. J Clin Invest 1997;99:1399—405.

[392] Wang X, Harris PC, Somlo S, Batlle D, Torres VE. Effect of calcium-sensing receptor activation in models of autosomal recessive or dominant polycystic kidney disease. Nephrol Dial Transplant 2009;24:526—34.

[393] Jeon US, Han K-H, Park SH, Lee SD, Sheen MR, Jung JY, et al. Downregulation of renal TonEBP in hypokalemic rats. Am J Physiol Renal Physiol 2007;293:F408—15.

[394] Cadnapaphornchai MA, Kim Y-W, Gurevich AK, Summer SN, Falk S, Thurman JM, et al. Urinary concentrating defect in hypothyroid rats: role of sodium, potassium, 2-chloride co-transporter, and aquaporins. J Am Soc Nephrol 2003;14:566—74.

[395] Sands JM. Urine-concentrating ability in the aging kidney. Sci Aging Knowledge Environ 2003;:24 [pe15]

[396] Combet S, Teillet L, Geelen G, Pitrat B, Gobin R, Nielsen S, et al. Food restriction prevents age-related polyuria by vasopressin-dependent recruitment of aquaporin-2. Am J Physiol Renal Physiol 2001;281:F1123—31.

[397] Preisser L, Teillet L, Aliotti S, Gobin R, Berthonaud V, Chevalier J, et al. Downregulation of aquaporin-2 and-3 in aging kidney is independent of V_2 vasopressin receptor. Am J Physiol Renal Physiol 2000;279:F144—52.

[398] Trinh-Trang-Tan MM, Geelen G, Teillet L, Corman B. Urea transporter expression in aging kidney and brain during dehydration. Am J Physiol Regul Integr Comp Physiol 2003;285: R1355—65.

[399] Combet S, Geffroy N, Berthonaud V, Dick B, Teillet L, Verbavatz JM, et al. Correction of age-related polyuria by dDAVP: molecular analysis of aquaporins and urea transporters. Am J Physiol Renal Physiol 2003;284:F199—208.

[400] Zhang Y, Sands JM, Kohan DE, Nelson RD, Martin CF, Carlson NG, et al. Potential role of purinergic signaling in urinary concentration in inner medulla: insights from P2Y2 receptor gene knockout mice. Am J Physiol Renal Physiol 2008;295: F1715—24.

[401] Verkman AS, Yang BX, Song YL, Manley GT, Ma TH. Role of water channels in fluid transport studied by phenotype analysis of aquaporin knockout mice. Exp Physiol 2000;85:233S—41S.

[402] Li C, Klein JD, Wang W, Knepper MA, Nielsen S, Sands JM, et al. Altered expression of urea transporters in response to ureteral obstruction. Am J Physiol Renal Physiol 2004;286: F1154—62.

[403] Timmer RT, Sands JM. Lithium intoxication. J Am Soc Nephrol 1999;10:666—74.

[404] Christensen S, Kusano E, Yusufi ANK, Murayama N, Dousa TP. Pathogenesis of nephrogenic diabetes insipidus due to chronic administration of lithium in rats. J Clin Invest 1985;75:1869—79.

[405] Blount MA, Sim JH, Zhou R, Martin CF, Lu W, Sands JM, et al. The expression of transporters involved in urine concentration recover differently after ceasing lithium treatment. Am J Physiol Renal Physiol 2010;298:F601—8.

[406] Klein JD, Gunn RB, Roberts BR, Sands JM. Down-regulation of urea transporters in the renal inner medulla of lithium-fed rats. Kidney Int 2002;61:995—1002.

[407] Marples D, Christensen S, Christensen EI, Ottosen PD, Nielsen S. Lithium-induced downregulation of Aquaporin-2 water channel expression in rat kidney medulla. J Clin Invest 1995;95:1838—45.

[408] Okusa MD, Crystal LJT. Clinical manifestations and management of acute lithium intoxication. Am J Med 1994;97:383—9.

[409] Nielsen J, Hoffert JD, Knepper MA, Agre P, Nielsen S, Fenton RA. Proteomic analysis of lithium-induced nephrogenic diabetes insipidus: mechanisms for aquaporin 2 down-regulation and cellular proliferation. PNAS 2008;105:3634—9.

[410] Fröhlich O, Aggarwal D, Klein JD, Kent KJ, Yang Y, Gunn RB, et al. Stimulation of UT-A1-mediated transepithelial urea flux in MDCK cells by lithium. Am J Physiol Renal Physiol 2008;294:F518—24.

[411] Sands JM, Gargus JJ, Fröhlich O, Gunn RB, Kokko JP. Urinary concentrating ability in patients with Jk(a-b-) blood type who lack carrier-mediated urea transport. J Am Soc Nephrol 1992;2:1689–96.

[412] Bankir L, Chen K, Yang B. Lack of UT-B in vasa recta and red blood cells prevents urea-induced improvement of urinary concentrating ability. Am J Physiol Renal Physiol 2004;286: F144–51.

[413] Edwards A, Pallone TL. Facilitated transport in vasa recta: theoretical effects on solute exchange in the medullary microcirculation. Am J Physiol Renal Physiol 1997;272:F505–14.

[414] Edwards A, Pallone TL. A multiunit model of solute and water removal by inner medullary vasa recta. Am J Physiol Heart Circ Physiol 1998;274:H1202–10.

[415] Macey RI. Transport of water and urea in red blood cells. Am J Physiol 1984;246:C195–203.

[416] Macey RI, Yousef LW. Osmotic stability of red cells in renal circulation requires rapid urea transport. Am J Physiol 1988;254:C669–74.

[417] Fenton RA, Flynn A, Shodeinde A, Smith CP, Schnermann J, Knepper MA. Renal phenotype of UT-A urea transporter knockout mice. J Am Soc Nephrol 2005;16:1583–92.

[418] Berliner RW, Levinsky NG, Davidson DG, Eden M. Dilution and concentration of the urine and the action of antidiuretic hormone. Am J Med 1958;24:730–44.

[419] Fenton RA, Knepper MA. Urea and renal function in the 21st century: insights from knockout mice. J Am Soc Nephrol 2007;18:679–88.

[420] Sands JM. Critical role of urea in the urine-concentrating mechanism. J Am Soc Nephrol 2007;18:670–1.

[421] Fenton RA, Chou CL, Sowersby H, Smith CP, Knepper MA. Gamble's "economy of water" revisited: studies in urea transporter knockout mice. Am J Physiol Renal Physiol 2006;291: F148–54.

[422] Fenton RA. Urea transporters and renal function: lessons from knockout mice. Curr Opin Nephrol Hypertens 2008;17: 513–8.

[423] Isozaki T, Lea JP, Tumlin JA, Sands JM. Sodium-dependent net urea transport in rat initial IMCDs. J Clin Invest 1994;94:1513–7.

[424] Kato A, Sands JM. Active sodium-urea counter-transport is inducible in the basolateral membrane of rat renal initial inner medullary collecting ducts. J Clin Invest 1998;102:1008–15.

[425] Knepper MA, Roch-Ramel F. Pathways of urea transport in the mammalian kidney. Kidney Int 1987;31:629–33.

[426] Lassiter WE, Gottschalk CW, Mylle M. Micropuncture study of net transtubular movement of water and urea in nondiuretic mammalian kidney. Am J Physiol 1961;200:1139–46.

[427] Valtin H. Structural and functional heterogeneity of mammalian nephrons. Am J Physiol 1977;233:F491–501.

[428] Imbert M, de Rouffignac C. Role of sodium and urea in the renal concentrating mechanism in Psammomys obesus. Pfluegers Arch 1976;361:107–14.

[429] Ullrich KJ, Rumrich G, Schmidt-Nielsen B. Urea transport in the collecting duct of rats on normal and low protein diet. Pfluegers Arch 1967;295:147–56.

[430] Aoshima T, Kajita M, Sekido Y, Kikuchi S, Yasuda I, Saheki T, et al. Novel mutations (H337R and 238-362del) in the CPS1 gene cause carbamoyl phosphate synthetase I deficiency. Hum Hered 2001;52:99–101.

[431] Calcagno PL, Rubin MI, Weintraub DH. Studies on the renal concentrating and diluting mechanisms in the premature infant. J Clin Invest 1954;33:91–6.

[432] Edelmann Jr CM, Barnett HL, Troupkou V. Renal concentrating mechanisms in newborn infants. Effect of dietary protein and water content, role of urea, and responsiveness to antidiuretic hormone. J Clin Invest 1960;39:1062–9.

[433] Liu W, Morimoto T, Kondo Y, Iinuma K, Uchida S, Imai M. "Avian-type" renal medullary tubule organization causes immaturity of urine-concentrating ability in neonates. Kidney Int 2001;60:680–93.

[434] Schwartz GJ, Zavilowitz BJ, Radice AD, Garcia-Perez A, Sands JM. Maturation of aldose reductase expression in the neonatal rat inner medulla. J Clin Invest 1992;90:1275–83.

[435] Winberg J. Determination of renal concentrating capacity in infants and children without renal disease. Acta Paediatr 1959;48:318–28.

[436] Falk G. Maturation of renal function in infant rats. Am J Physiol 1955;181:157–70.

[437] Forrest Jr JN, Stanier MW. Kidney composition and renal concentrating ability in young rabbits. J Physiol 1966;187:1–4.

[438] Heller H. Effects of dehydration on adult and newborn rats. J Physiol 1949;108:303–14.

[439] McCrory Jr WW. Developmental nephrology. Cambridge, MA: Harvard University Press; 1972.

[440] Rane S, Aperia A, Neroth P, Lundin S. Development of urinary concentrating capacity in weaning rats. Pediatr Res 1985;19:472–5.

[441] Trimble ME. Renal response to solute loading in infant rats: relation to anatomical development. Am J Physiol 1970;219:1089–97.

[442] Yasui M, Marples D, Belusa R, Eklof AC, Celsi G, Nielsen S, et al. Development of urinary concentrating capacity: role of aquaporin-2. Am J Physiol Renal, Fluid Electrolyte Physiol 1996;271:F461–8.

[443] Bonilla-Felix M, Jiang W. Aquaporin-2 in the immature rat: expression, regulation, and trafficking. J Am Soc Nephrol 1997;8:1502–9.

[444] Horster M, Valtin H. Postnatal development of renal function: micropuncture and clearance studies in the dog. J Clin Invest 1971;50:779–95.

[445] Edelmann Jr CM, Barnett HL, Troupkou V. Renal concentrating mechanisms in newborn infants. Effect of dietary protein and water content, role of urea, and responsiveness to antidiuretic hormone. J Clin Invset 1960;39:1062–9.

[446] Bondy CA, Lightman SL. Developmental and physiological regulation of aldose reductase mRNA expression in renal medulla. Mol Endocrinol 1989;3:1409–16.

[447] Han KH, Woo SK, Kim WY, Park SH, Cha JH, Kim J, et al. Maturation of TonEBP expression in developing rat kidney. Am J Physiol Renal Physiol 2004;287:F878–85.

[448] Lee HW, Kim WY, Song HK, Yang CW, Han KH, Kwon HM, et al. Sequential expression of NKCC2, TonEBP, aldose reductase, and urea transporter-A in developing mouse kidney. Am J Physiol Renal Physiol 2007;292:F269–77.

[449] Suda S, Rai T, Sohara E, Sasaki S, Uchida S. Postnatal expression of KLF12 in the inner medullary collecting ducts of kidney and its trans-activation of UT-A1 urea transporter promoter. Biochem Biophys Res Commun 2006;344:246–52.

[450] Atherton JC, Green R, Thomas S. Influence of lysine-vasopressin dosage on the time course of changes in renal tissue and urinary composition in the conscious rat. J Physiol 1971;213:291–309.

[451] Press WH, Teukolsky SA, Vetterling WT, Flannery BP. Numerical recipes in FORTRAN: the art of scientific computing. 2nd ed. New York: Cambridge University Press; 1992.

[452] Beck F, Dorge A, Rick R, Thurau K. Intra- and extracellular element concentrations of rat renal papilla in antidiuresis. Kidney Int 1984;25:397–403.

III. FLUID AND ELECTROLYTE REGULATION AND DYSREGULATION

[453] Beck F, Dorge A, Rick R, Thurau K. Osmoregulation of renal papillary cells. Pfluegers Arch 1985;405(Suppl. 1):S28−32.

[454] Atherton JC, Hai MA, Thomas S. The time course of changes in renal tissue composition during water diuresis in the rat. J Physiol 1968;197:429−43.

[455] Hebert SC, Culpepper RM, Andreoli TE. NaCl transport in mouse medullary thick ascending limbs. I. Functional nephron heterogeneity and ADH-stimulated NaCl co-transport. Am J Physiol 1981;241:F412−31.

[456] Hall DA, Varney DM. Effect of vasopressin on electrical potential differences and chloride transport in mouse medullary thick ascending limb of Henle's loop. J Clin Invest 1980;66:792−802.

[457] Shareghi GR, Agus ZS. Magnesium transport in the cortical thick ascending limb of Henle's loop of the rabbit. J Clin Invest 1982;69:759−69.

[458] Nonoguchi H, Tomita K, Marumo F. Effects of atrial natriuretic peptide and vasopressin on chloride transport in long- and short-looped medullary thick ascending limbs. J Clin Invest 1992;90:349−57.

[459] Imai M. Effect of bumetanide and furosemide on the thick ascending limb of Henle's loop of rabbits and rats perfused in vitro. Eur J Pharmacol 1977;41:409−16.

[460] Stokes JB. Effect of prostaglandin E₂ on chloride transport across the rabbit thick ascending limb of Henle. J Clin Invest 1979;64:495−502.

[461] Mason J, Gutsche H-U, Moore L, Müller-Suur R. The early phase of experimental acute renal failure. IV. The diluting ability of the short loops of Henle. Pfluegers Arch 1979;379:11−8.

[462] Burg MB, Bourdeau JE. Function of the thick ascending limb of Henle's loop. In: Vogel HG, Ullrich KJ, editors. New aspects of renal function. Amsterdam: Excerpta Medica; 1978. p. 91−102.

[463] Knepper MA. Urea transport in nephron segments from medullary rays of rabbits. Am J Physiol 1983;244:F622−7.

[464] Stoner LC, Burg MB, Orloff J. Ion transport in cortical collecting tubule effect of amiloride. Am J Physiol 1974;227:453−9.

[465] Stokes JB. Sodium and potassium transport across the cortical and outer medullary collecting tubule of the rabbit: evidence for diffusion across the outer medullary portion. Am J Physiol 1982;242:F514−20.

[466] Schafer JA, Andreoli TE. The effect of antidiuretic hormone on solute flows in mammalian collecting tubules. J Clin Invest 1972;51:1279−86.

[467] Kuwahara M, Berry CA, Verkman AS. Rapid development of vasopressin-induced hydroosmosis in kidney collecting tubules measured by a new fluorescence technique. Biophys J 1988;54:595−602.

[468] Schafer JA, Andreoli TE. Cellular constraints to diffusion. The effect of antidiuretic hormone on water flows in isolated mammalian collecting tubules. J Clin Invest 1972;51:1264−78.

[469] Nonoguchi H, Sands JM, Knepper MA. Atrial natriuretic factor inhibits NaCl and fluid absorption in cortical collecting duct of rat kidney. Am J Physiol 1989;256:F179−86.

[470] Lorenzen M, Frindt G, Taylor A, Windhager EE. Quinidine effect on hydrosmotic response of collecting tubules to vasopressin and cAMP. Am J Physiol 1987;252:F1103−11.

[471] Garg LC, Knepper MA, Burg MB. Mineralocorticoid effects on Na-K-ATPase in individual nephron segments. Am J Physiol 1981;240:F536−44.

[472] Katz AI, Doucet A, Morel F. Na-K-ATPase activity along the rabbit, rat and mouse nephron. Am J Physiol 1979;237:F114−20.

[473] O'Neil RG, Dubinsky WP. Micromethodology for measuring ATPase activity in renal tubules: mineralocorticoid influence. Am J Physiol 1984;247:C314−20.

[474] Schmidt U, Horster M. Na-K-activated ATPase: activity maturation in rabbit nephron segments dissected in vitro. Am J Physiol 1977;233:F55−60.

[475] Stokes JB, Ingram MJ, Williams AD, Ingram D. Heterogeneity of the rabbit collecting tubule: localization of mineralocorticoid hormone action to the cortical portion. Kidney Int 1981;20:340−7.

[476] Lankford SP, Chou C-L, Terada Y, Wall SM, Wade JB, Knepper MA. Regulation of collecting duct water permeability independent of cAMP-mediated AVP response. Am J Physiol Renal, Fluid Electrolyte Physiol 1991;261:F554−66.

[477] Sands JM, Layton HE. The physiology of urinary concentration: an update. Semin Nephrol 2009;29:178−95.

[478] Tickle P, Thistlethwaite A, Smith CP, Stewart GS. Novel bUT-B2 urea transporter isoform is constitutively activated. Am J Physiol Regul Integr Comp Physiol 2009;297:R323−9.

[479] Zhao HY, Tian W, Cohen DM. Rottlerin inhibits tonicity-dependent expression and action of TonEBP in a PKCd-independent fashion. Am J Physiol Renal Physiol 2002;282:F710−7.

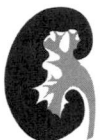

Hyponatremia

Richard H. Sterns[1], Stephen M. Silver[2] and J. Kevin Hix[3]

[1]Chief of Medicine, Rochester General Hospital, Professor of Medicine, University of Rochester
School of Medicine and Dentistry, Rochester, New York, USA

[2]Clinical Professor of Medicine, University of Rochester School of Medicine and Dentistry, Rochester, New York, USA

[3]Clinical Assistant Professor of Medicine, University of Rochester School of Medicine and Dentistry,
Rochester, New York, USA

THE PLASMA SODIUM CONCENTRATION AND BODY FLUID TONICITY

Sodium and its accompanying anions are the principle osmotically active solutes in extracellular fluid.[1,2] When extracellular osmolality is low, intracellular osmolality is equally low. Therefore, although there are exceptions (Table 44.1), hyponatremia is usually associated with hypoosmolality and dilution of all body fluids.[1,2,3]

When (as is usually the case) the concentration of non-permeant extracellular solutes other than sodium is very low, the plasma sodium concentration is a function of three variables, as indicated by the following equation:

$$Plasma[Na^+] \cong \frac{Exchangeable\ Na^+ + Exchangeable\ K^+}{Total\ body\ water}$$

(44.1)

Only the exchangeable fractions of sodium and potassium are included in the equation, because one-third of body sodium is bound to bone and osmotically inactive.[1] This relationship, which has been validated empirically,[3,4] indicates that the plasma (or serum) sodium concentration can be reduced by depletion of body cations, by an increase in body water or by a combination of these processes.[5] Recently, it has been emphasized that the original equation describing the relationship between the plasma sodium concentration, exchangeable sodium, exchangeable potassium, and total body water has an intercept that can be explained

theoretically.[6] The simplified form of the relationship Eq. (44.1), which omits the intercept, is useful conceptually, but should not be considered a completely accurate basis for predicting the effect of therapy on the plasma sodium concentration.

It is intuitively obvious that the extracellular sodium concentration should be proportional to the body's content of water and soluble sodium. The sodium concentration falls when the body retains water (without solute) or when there are net external losses of sodium (without water). The importance of intracellular potassium stores to the plasma sodium concentration is less obvious.[7,8] In potassium depletion, sodium ions move intracellularly as intracellular potassium is lost, balancing negative charges on intracellular macromolecules. Thus, external loss of exchangeable potassium causes an internal loss of extracellular sodium. Similarly, when intracellular potassium is replaced by hydrogen ions, rather than sodium or when it is lost with phosphate (an intracellular anion), the loss of osmotically active intracellular solute causes a redistribution of water from the intracellular to the extracellular fluid compartments, diluting extracellular sodium ions.

PHYSIOLOGIC CONTROL OF WATER EXCRETION

Osmotic Regulation

Controlled by changes in water intake, vasopressin secretion, and water excretion, the plasma sodium

TABLE 44.1 Causes of Non-Hypotonic Hyponatremia

Plasma Osmolality	Disorder	Pathogenesis
Normal	Pseudohyponatremia	Excess non-aqueous material decreases plasma water content; no change in ECF or ICF volume
	Hyperlipidemia	
	Multiple myeloma	
	Exogenous solutes	Expansion of ECF volume with non-sodium solutes and water; no change in ICF volume
	Isotonic IV mannitol	
	Irrigant absorption	
Increased	Hyperglycemia, hypertonic IV mannitol, and maltose containing IgG solutions	Initial expansion of ECF volume and shift of water out of cells; decrease in ICF volume

concentration is normally prevented from rising above 142 mEq/L or falling below 135 mEq/L. When the plasma sodium concentration changes by as little as 1% (with a corresponding change in plasma osmolality), cell volume receptors ("osmoreceptors") in the hypothalamus respond, relaying signals to vasopressin-secreting neurons located in the supraoptic and paraventricular nuclei whose axons terminate in secretory bulbs in the neurohypophysis.[9–11] The antidiuretic hormone, arginine vasopressin, which is released into the systemic circulation by the neurohypophysis, controls water excretion by the kidneys. The hormone activates V_2 receptors on the basolateral membrane of principal cells in the renal collecting duct, initiating a cyclic AMP-dependent process that culminates in increased production of water channels (aquaporin 2), and their insertion into the cells' luminal membranes.[12] The effect of vasopressin on water flow is inhibited by locally produced prostaglandin E_2, which is stimulated by vasopressin action on V_1 receptors.[13] Vasopressin's short half-life in the circulation and continuous shuttling of aquaporins between the collecting duct's cell membrane and cytosol allow rapid changes in urinary water excretion in response to changes in body fluid tonicity.

Vasopressin levels are normally unmeasurable when the plasma sodium concentration falls to approximately 135 mEq/L. Low levels of the hormone allow the excretion of large volumes of a maximally dilute urine (≈ 50 mOsm/kg) which reduces body water content and restores the plasma sodium concentration to normal. At higher plasma sodium levels, plasma vasopressin is directly related to the plasma sodium concentration, reaching levels that are high enough to promote the excretion of maximally concentrated urine (≈ 1200 mOsm/kg) at a plasma sodium concentration of approximately 142 mEq/L. A rising plasma sodium concentration also stimulates thirst. Ingested water is retained, returning the plasma sodium concentration back towards normal.

Hemodynamic Regulation

Under day-to-day conditions, vasopressin secretion, urinary free water excretion, and thirst respond primarily to changes in body fluid tonicity. Under pathologic conditions, osmotic control of vasopressin secretion and thirst can be overridden by hemodynamic stimuli.[14] In addition to input from osmoreceptors, the hypothalamic neurons that secrete vasopressin also receive neural input from baroreceptors in the great vessels, and volume receptors in the atria. When these receptors are stimulated by hypotension or by a major reduction in plasma volume, impulses are carried via cranial nerves IX and X to the hypothalamus. The thirst center in the hypothalamus responds to similar non-osmotic stimuli. Vasopressin and thirst responses to hypovolemia and hypotension lead to water retention, despite hypotonicity of body fluids. These hemodynamic responses can be regarded as back-up systems that serve to maintain arterial blood volume under emergency conditions, sacrificing tonicity to tissue perfusion. Although high levels of vasopressin occur in response to hypovolemia, under experimental conditions, a rather large stimulus is required; while plasma vasopressin is measurably increased by a 1% change in plasma osmolality, a 10% change in extracellular fluid volume is required to elicit the same response. However, these experimental findings are difficult to reconcile with clinical observations, suggesting that non-osmotic vasopressin secretion occurs with more subtle volume depletion.

HYPOTONIC HYPONATREMIA: CLASSIFICATION AND PATHOGENESIS

Traditionally, patients with hyponatremia are divided into categories according to their body sodium content and/or intravascular volume: low body sodium content (volume depletion); high body sodium content (edematous conditions) or normal body sodium content (euvolemic hyponatremia or SIADH).[15] Although this time-honored approach is often helpful to clinicians, intravascular volume and body sodium content do not always change in parallel (e.g., self-induced water intoxication), and some causes of hyponatremia (e.g., diuretic-induced and cerebral salt-wasting) may be difficult to classify by intravascular volume. Moreover, physiologic responses to extracellular volume expansion and contraction often create ambiguities in volume status. Thus, secondary water retention in response to volume depletion and secondary natriuresis in response to water overload may ultimately yield similar values for total body sodium and water (Figure 44.1).

Table 44.2 classifies hyponatremia by the physiologic mechanism underlying the electrolyte disturbance. As the plasma sodium concentration is proportional to the ratio of exchangeable cations and total body water, it follows that changes in sodium concentration are related to external balances of sodium, potassium, and water. However, because the plasma sodium concentration is normally maintained within a narrow physiologic range by control systems which regulate water balance, hypotonic hyponatremia can only occur if water excretion is impaired or overwhelmed. The various causes of hyponatremia are therefore divided according to the status of urinary water excretion. Disordered water balance is often accompanied by changes in cation balance, which also play a pivotal role in the pathogenesis of hyponatremia.

TABLE 44.2 Pathophysiologic Classification of Hypotonic Hyponatremia

Urine Diluting Ability	Cause of Hyponatremia
Unimpaired	Psychotic polydipsia
	Beer potomania
	Infantile water intoxication
Impaired: vasopressin-independent	Oliguric renal failure
	Tubular interstitial renal disease
	Diuretics
	Nephrogenic syndrome of antidiuresis[a]
Impaired: vasopressin-dependent	Hemodynamically-mediated
	Volume-depletion
	Spinal cord disease
	Congestive heart failure
	Cirrhosis
	Addison's disease[b]
	Cerebral salt-wasting[b]
	SIADH (see Table 44.3)

[a]Hereditary disorder of the V2 receptor with clinical features of SIADH, but with undetectable plasma vasopressin levels.
[b]Disorders with both hemodynamic and non-hemodynamic bases for vasopressin release.

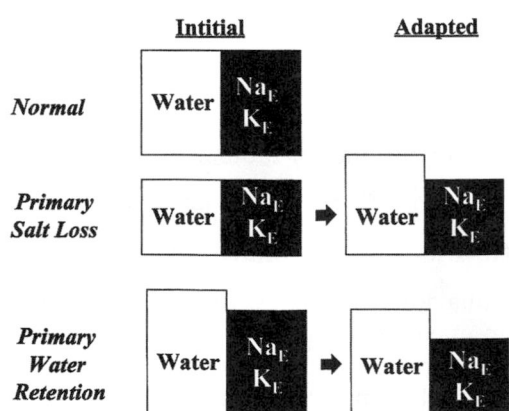

FIGURE 44.1 Body water and cation content in hyponatremia. When the primary disturbance is loss of salt water (middle figures), compensatory mechanisms are triggered—hemodynamically mediated thirst and vasopressin secretion—which result in secondary water retention. When the primary disturbance is pathologic secretion of vasopressin and water retention (bottom figures), compensatory mechanisms are triggered—increased secretion of atrial natriuretic peptide, decreased secretion of aldosterone, and pressure natriuresis—which result in secondary salt loss. Because of these adaptations, primary salt loss and primary water retention both result in near normal values for total body water and decreased body cation stores.

WATER INTOXICATION WITH MAXIMALLY DILUTE URINE

Pathophysiology

Rarely, fluid intake can overwhelm normal mechanisms for water excretion. In the absence of vasopressin, urine osmolality falls to approximately 50 mOsm/kg. A typical American diet provides a daily load of 600 to 900 milliosmoles of solute (electrolytes and urea) that must be excreted. At this rate of solute excretion, the volume of maximally dilute urine equals 12 to 18 liters per day or 500 to 750 ml/hour. Water intake can occasionally exceed this large excretory capacity. Patients with severe acute water intoxication are truly "waterlogged," and susceptible to pulmonary edema due to retained water.

Self-Induced Water Intoxication in Psychotic Polydipsia

Polydipsia and polyuria are extremely common among institutionalized patients with mental illness.[16–20] Many patients with polydipsia have frequent episodes of hyponatremia, which may present with seizures. About half the reported cases have had maximally dilute urine (urine osmolalities below 100 mOsm/kg) at presentation. In others, inappropriately concentrated urine was present immediately following seizures or in association with nausea,[19] but the rate of correction of hyponatremia indicates that the urine became dilute soon afterwards.

In most psychotic water drinkers, hyponatremia can be ascribed to a generalized dilution of body solutes by retained water; thus, body weight increases in proportion to the severity of hyponatremia. Patients gain weight and become hyponatremic during the course of the day, and then spontaneously diurese, normalizing their plasma sodium concentration and body weight during the night. Caregivers in psychiatric hospitals routinely monitor weight changes in patients who are habitual water drinkers to determine when access to water must be rigidly restricted to avoid severe symptomatic hyponatremia.

Agents that interfere with the ability to maximally dilute the urine (e.g., diuretics or carbamazepine) should be avoided in polydipsic patients, as they can precipitate a rapid onset of life-threatening hyponatremia.[21,22]

Water Intoxication in Infants

Acute water intoxication is common among infants who are given excessively dilute formula.[23,24] The hungry infant ingests large volumes of fluid leading to water retention, despite the excretion of maximally dilute urine. Once water is restricted, the plasma sodium concentration self-corrects as large volumes of urine are excreted.

Beer Drinkers Potomania

Alcoholics who eat little and subsist on large volumes of beer may also become hyponatremic while excreting maximally dilute urine.[25–27] Beer's low protein content and the protein-sparing effect of its carbohydrate result in profoundly reduced blood urea nitrogen concentrations and urinary urea excretion. The total daily excretion of urinary solute may be only 200 to 300 milliosmoles. Thus, even at a urine osmolality of 50 mOsm/kg, urine output is limited to 4 to 6 liters per day, an amount that fails to match the enthusiastic beer drinker's intake of electrolyte free water. A similar phenomenon has been reported in non-beer drinkers with a high fluid and low protein intake.[27,28] Volume-depletion from gastrointestinal losses, and transient vasopressin release caused by nausea or alcohol withdrawal, may further limit the beer drinker's

ability to excrete free water, contributing to the development and persistence of hyponatremia.[29]

VASOPRESSIN-INDEPENDENT DEFECTS IN WATER EXCRETION

Pathophysiology

Maximal free water excretion depends on adequate delivery of glomerular filtrate to the renal diluting segments (the ascending limb of the loop of Henle and the distal tubule), reabsorption of salt without water by the diluting segments to create hypotonic fluid within the tubular lumen, and a collecting duct that is relatively impermeable to water, so that the dilute tubular fluid formed "upstream" can be eliminated in the final urine. Hyponatremia occurs when water is taken in at a time when these mechanisms are not functioning normally.

Renal Failure

The most obvious cause of impaired water excretion is oliguric renal failure. Even when nonoliguric, patients with advanced renal failure have fixed isosthenuria, and are unable to excrete dilute urine despite normally suppressed vasopressin secretion. In the absence of renal failure, urinary dilution can still be impaired, despite low levels of vasopressin, by two mechanisms: (1) enhanced proximal reabsorption of the glomerular filtrate, limiting fluid delivery to the renal diluting segments (as in volume depletion, congestive heart failure, and cirrhosis)[30]; and (2) impaired sodium reabsorption in the renal diluting segments (by diuretics or tubular interstitial disease).[31]

Diuretic-Induced Hyponatremia

Both thiazides and loop diuretics interfere with the ability to maximally dilute the urine.[32] Thus, both classes of diuretic can lead to water intoxication in patients who habitually ingest extremely large volumes of water. Diuretics are one of the most important causes of hyponatremia.[33–37] Most cases are caused by thiazide or thiazide-like agents; loop diuretics are implicated much less commonly. Thiazides may be the sole factor responsible for causing hyponatremia, and they may also exacerbate hyponatremia in patients with disorders associated with SIADH.[36,38] The mechanism of thiazide-induced hyponatremia remains somewhat unclear; however, as for all causes of hyponatremia, water retention and/or cation depletion must be responsible. There is evidence that thiazides have a direct antidiuretic effect mediated by upregulation of aquaporin 2 (AQP2).[39]

Most cases of thiazide-induced hyponatremia have occurred in elderly small women who have been prescribed diuretics for the treatment of hypertension.[35,40–42] The impairment of renal diluting ability caused by thiazides is more pronounced in elderly people, especially those who have previously experienced thiazide-induced hyponatremia.[43] The predisposition of elderly women to severe hyponatremia may be explained by body size, in that small changes in body water and electrolyte content can lead to marked changes in serum sodium.

In susceptible individuals, the serum sodium may fall within hours of diuretic ingestion, and severe hyponatremia can develop in less than two days.[41,44–46] While in many cases the diuretic had been recently prescribed, in others thiazides had been used chronically without incident until, for some reason, water intake increased, dietary salt and protein intake decreased or an intercurrent illness led to "inappropriate" antidiuretic hormone secretion.[33,47] Mild hyponatremia often persists for a few weeks when diuretic therapy is withdrawn from patients with diuretic-induced hyponatremia,[48] apparently reflecting temporary "resetting" of the osmostat[49] or alternatively, slow restoration of depleted cation stores.

Although thiazide diuretics do not inhibit the ability to concentrate the urine, they do impair diluting ability in several ways[31,39,50–52]: inhibition of electrolyte transport at the cortical diluting sites; direct stimulation of vasopressin release; direct upregulation of AQP2; reduction of glomerular filtration; and enhancement of fractional proximal water reabsorption, reducing delivery to diluting sites.

Positive water balance during the onset of thiazide-induced hyponatremia and negative balance during its correction have been documented.[22,44,46] Some patients with thiazide-induced hyponatremia have low serum uric acid levels and high uric acid clearances (markers of volume expansion) which return to normal as the serum sodium normalizes.[36,53] Most affected patients drink large amounts of water, and the superimposed diuretic prevents urine output from keeping pace with water intake.[44]

Although increased total body water often contributes to the pathogenesis of thiazide-induced hyponatremia, there are many cases in which body weight decreased or remained the same during the fall in serum sodium.[41,54,55] In others, direct measurements of total body water in affected patients have been normal.[41] In these cases, other explanations for hyponatremia must be sought.

Negative cation balance plays a major role in the pathogenesis of diuretic-induced hyponatremia.

Rejected cations may be excreted at a total concentration which exceeds that of plasma, directly "desalinating" the plasma even in the absence of water intake.[44] Potassium depletion is an important factor in many cases; treatment of hypokalemia has been shown to increase the plasma sodium concentration with no change in body weight.[41] Magnesium repletion may act similarly, presumably through an effect on skeletal muscle Na-K-ATPase.[56] Surprisingly, despite negative cation balance, many patients appear to be euvolemic. Apparently, enough water is retained to offset the initial tendency toward hypovolemia. Once diuretics are withdrawn, urinary sodium excretion falls to very low levels.[41,46]

VASOPRESSIN-DEPENDENT DEFECTS IN WATER EXCRETION

Pathophysiology

Normally, in response to hypotonicity, vasopressin secretion is suppressed, the collecting duct is impermeable to water, and a maximally dilute urine is formed. In two large surveys of hospitalized patients with hyponatremia, over 90% of cases were associated with elevated vasopressin levels.[57,58] Vasopressin levels are rarely elevated into pathologic ranges, even in cases associated with ectopic secretion by tumors. Rather, vasopressin levels are inappropriately high relative to the plasma osmolality. Non-osmotic vasopressin secretion may be an adaptive response driven by hemodynamic stimuli or it may be "inappropriate" and independent of any of the usual physiologic mechanisms which regulate water excretion. Persistent vasopressin secretion despite hypoosmolality allows ingested or infused free water to be retained, causing hypotonic hyponatremia. Vasopressin-mediated hyponatremia is characterized by urine which is more concentrated (usually much more) than 100 mOsm/kg and which becomes more dilute after administration of a V2 receptor antagonist (see section "V_2-Receptor Antagonists").

Patients with inappropriate vasopressin secretion must take in water to become hyponatremic. In some cases, hyponatremia develops when electrolyte-free water is administered parenterally. More commonly, patients become hyponatremic while ingesting water. Theoretically, osmotic inhibition of thirst should prevent water ingestion when the ability to excrete water is impaired. However, patients with SIADH continue to drink despite plasma osmolalities below the normal osmotic threshold for thirst. Formal testing has shown that there is downward resetting of the osmotic threshold for thirst in SIADH, but that thirst responds to

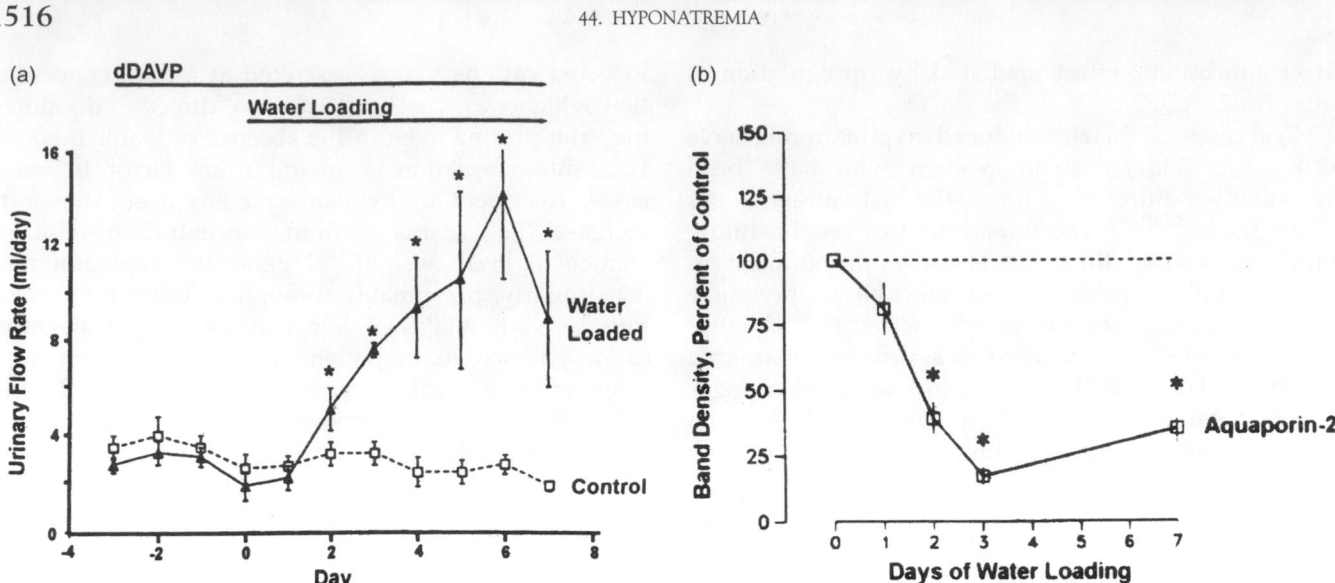

FIGURE 44.2   Vasopressin escape.[64] Panel (a) illustrates the gradual increase in urine flow rate (accompanied by a decrease in urine osmolality) that occurs when rats treated continuously with dDAVP are made hyponatremic with water-loading. The escape from the antidiuretic effect of vasopressin begins on the second day of water-loading. Panel (b) illustrates the levels of acquaporin 2 protein levels from kidney homogenates taken on each day of water-loading. Levels of acquaporin 2 protein decrease despite continued administration of vasopressin, and correlate with changes in urine volume.

osmotic stimulation and is suppressed by drinking around the lowered set-point.[59]

Escape from Vasopressin-Induced Water Retention

Experimentally, after several days of constant vasopressin infusion and constant water intake, there is an escape from the antidiuretic effect of vasopressin. With the onset of vasopressin escape, the urine becomes less concentrated, allowing water balance to be re-established at a new steady-state in which the plasma sodium concentration stabilizes at a level lower than normal. In experimental models, escape is temporally associated with a marked decrease in renal aquaporin-2 protein, accompanied by suppression of aquaporin-2 mRNA levels (Figure 44.2).[60] V2-receptor mRNA expression and binding are decreased, as is c-AMP production in response to vasopressin.[61] Plasma and urine aldosterone and mean arterial pressure are increased as are thiazide-sensitive Na-Cl co-transporter and ENaC proteins in the distal nephron that are known to be upregulated by aldosterone.[62] Inhibition of nitric oxide synthase or prostaglandin synthesis synergistically inhibit the escape phenomenon, supporting a role for nitric oxide and prostaglandins in mediating vasopressin escape.[63]

In conditions characterized by vasopressin-mediated water retention, (e.g., SIADH, congestive heart failure), renal escape from vasopressin-induced antidiuresis

(along with decreased water intake in some cases) permits patients with vasopressin-mediated hyponatremic states to manifest a relatively stable level of hyponatremia, despite continued water intake and continued presence of vasopressin.

HEMODYNAMIC CAUSES OF VASOPRESSIN-MEDIATED HYPONATREMIA

Pathophysiology

Hypovolemia, heart failure, and cirrhosis are the most common non-osmotic stimuli for antidiuretic hormone secretion.[64] In a series of 100 consecutive hospitalized patients with hypotonic hyponatremia, volume contraction (29%), advanced heart failure (25%), and liver cirrhosis (16%) were identified as the cause of hyponatremia in a high percentage of cases.[58] The hemodynamic abnormalities that stimulate vasopressin release in these conditions also promote sodium reabsorption by the renal tubules (mediated by aldosterone, increased sympathetic nervous system activity, peritubular Starling forces, etc.), causing both sodium and water retention. In volume-depletion, sodium retention serves to replace a sodium deficit; in heart failure and cirrhosis, sodium retention serves to compensate for the circulatory abnormality, but it also causes edema.

Volume-Depletion

Sodium and potassium losses associated with gastrointestinal fluids (or with urinary losses caused by osmotic or loop diuretics) do not directly lower the plasma sodium concentration, because these fluids are either hypotonic or isotonic. However, the intravascular volume-depletion caused by such losses is a hemodynamic stimulus for thirst and vasopressin secretion; as a result, ingested water is retained, lowering the plasma sodium concentration. Thus, hyponatremia in these conditions is associated with a reduced content of both total body cations and water. However, in many patients, compensatory water retention makes it difficult to detect the underlying volume depletion. Laboratory clues, including a low urine sodium concentration and elevated serum uric acid levels, can be helpful diagnostically.[65]

Spinal Cord Disease

Hyponatremia is very common after spinal cord injury, particularly among patients with complete quadriplegia.[66,67] Contributing factors include a large water intake (reflecting physician recommendations, angiotensin II-mediated thirst, and loss of pharyngeal and gastric satiety signals), and baroreceptor-mediated vasopressin release. One study showed normal osmoregulation of vasopressin secretion and excretion of a water-load when subjects were supine, but with the subjects in a sitting position, there was a reduced osmotic threshold and increased sensitivity for vasopressin release, and urine diluting ability and free water clearance were markedly impaired.[68]

Edematous Conditions

Severe hyponatremia can occur despite increased body sodium content if retained sodium is offset by a disproportionate increase in body water.

Congestive Heart Failure

Hyponatremia in heart failure stems from reduced cardiac output and blood pressure which stimulate vasopressin, catecholamines, and the renin—angiotensin—aldosterone axis.[64,69–71] Increased vasopressin levels have even been documented in patients with impaired left ventricular function before the onset of symptomatic heart failure.[72] Hyponatremic patients with congestive heart failure have higher levels of plasma renin activity, norepinephrine, epinephrine, and lower renal and hepatic plasma flows than normonatremic patients with an apparently similar degree of heart disease. Hyponatremia in heart failure is associated with a poor prognosis.[73]

Hepatic Cirrhosis

Cirrhosis is characterized by a hyperdynamic circulation with low blood pressure, low systemic vascular resistance, and high cardiac output.[74] Systemic vasodilatation causes relative underfilling of the arterial vascular compartment and neurohumoral responses similar to those that occur in response to a low cardiac output.[75] Activation of the renin—angiotensin—aldosterone axis and the sympathetic system, combined with non-osmotic release of vasopressin, results in renal water and sodium retention.[76,77] Escape from the sodium-retaining effect of aldosterone does not occur, and there is renal resistance to atrial natriuretic peptide. Although the pathogenesis of the peripheral arterial vasodilation is incompletely understood, increased vascular nitric oxide by the endothelium may play a role. In a rat model of cirrhosis, normalization of vascular nitric oxide production with a nitric oxide synthetase inhibitor corrects the hyperdynamic circulation, improves sodium and water excretion, and decreases neurohumoral activation.[74]

Peritoneovenous shunting of hyponatremic cirrhotic patients with refractory ascites improves cardiac output, renal plasma flow, and creatinine clearance, and results in an immediate diuresis and natriuresis with a decrease in urine osmolality and an increase in plasma sodium concentration associated with a small but significant decrease in plasma vasopressin levels.[74]

INAPPROPRIATE VASOPRESSIN SECRETION (SIADH)

Pathophysiology

Definitions

Non-osmotic release of vasopressin without a hemodynamic stimulus to account for it is considered "inappropriate".[78] When Bartter and Schwarz first described the syndrome of inappropriate antidiuretic hormone secretion (SIADH), they defined clinical criteria for the disorder which are still generally accepted: hypoosmolality and clinical euvolemia with a sodium-containing urine (>30 mmol/L) that is less than maximally dilute (>100 mOsm/kg) without recent diuretic use or impaired renal function. Schwarz and Bartter also excluded endocrine disorders—primary and secondary adrenal insufficiency and hypothyroidism—from this designation. We have not made this exclusion, because patients with undiagnosed endocrine disturbances may present with all the clinical features of SIADH. Indeed, the discovery of SIADH is often the presenting feature of a clinically important systemic disease. Abnormal vasopressin secretion may be caused by ectopic production of the hormone by tumors, from disordered secretion by the neurohypophysis or from increased sensitivity to the hormone (Table 44.3).

Patients with the syndrome of inappropriate antidiuretic hormone secretion (SIADH) retain ingested water, but they have no evidence of volume depletion and no tendency to form edema. Because of water retention, SIADH causes mild, subclinical volume-expansion, which is reflected by high uric acid clearance, a low plasma uric acid concentration, and urine sodium excretion which matches or exceeds sodium intake.[79,80] Clinicians make use of these characteristics to distinguish SIADH from hyponatremia caused by volume-depletion. The recently described syndrome of nephrogenic inappropriate antidiuresis (see section "Common Causes of SIADH") is discussed in this section because it exhibits clinical features of SIADH; in physiological terms, however, it is a cause of hyponatremia that is independent of vasopressin, as plasma vasopressin levels are undetectable (Table 44.2).[81]

Patterns of Vasopressin Secretion

In most patients with SIADH, vasopressin secretion has followed one of two basic patterns: "reset osmostat" or "vasopressin leak".[11,82] In the reset osmostat variant of SIADH, seen in patients with chronic, debilitating illness and in normal pregnancy, the urine can be diluted maximally, but at a lower set-point than normal.[49] Such patients are thus mildly hyponatremic, but unlike other patients with SIADH, their plasma sodium concentration is very stable and they do not require dietary water restriction or other measures used to treat chronic hyponatremia. In the vasopressin leak variant, the basal level of vasopressin is elevated and unresponsive to osmotic stimuli when the plasma osmolality is low, but the levels increase appropriately when the plasma osmolality increases above a threshold level. Less commonly, patients exhibit erratic vasopressin secretion which is unrelated to osmotic stimuli. In about 10% of patients who present with typical clinical manifestations of SIADH, plasma vasopressin levels are at a low basal level that fails to increase as plasma osmolality increases. Such a pattern would be expected if an antidiuretic factor other than vasopressin were produced or if the collecting tubules were hypersensitive to normal hormone levels.

Interplay of Water Retention and Cation Depletion in SIADH

In SIADH, increased intravascular volume decreases renin secretion and increases release of atrial natriuretic peptide. These volume and hormonal changes promote sodium excretion, despite a low serum sodium concentration. Natriuresis in SIADH blunts the increase in extracellular volume caused by water

TABLE 44.3   Causes of SIADH

Major Classification	Common Examples
Tumors	Small-cell lung cancer
	Head and neck tumors
Lung diseases	Pulmonary infection
	Hypoxia and hypercarbia
	Severe asthma
Neurologic disorders	Subarachnoid hemorrhage[a]
	Guillain-Barre syndrome[a]
	CNS infections
	Cerebral hemorrhage and infarction
	Brain tumors
Endocrine diseases	Hypothyroidism[a]
	Hypopituitarism
	Isolated ACTH deficiency
Medications	Arginine vasopressin and desmopressin acetate
	Amiodarone
	Chlorpropamide
	Carbamazepine and oxcarbazepine
	Cyclophosphamide
	Nonsteroidal anti-inflammatory agents; serotonin reuptake inhibitors
	Tricyclic antidepressants
	Vincristine
	3,4-methylenedioxymethamphetamine (ecstasy)
Hereditary	Nephrogenic syndrome of antidiuresis[b]
Miscellaneous, transitory causes	Surgery
	Pain and stress
	Nausea
	Alcohol withdrawal

[a]Disorders with both hemodynamic and non-hemodynamic bases for vasopressin release.
[b]Hereditary disorder of the V2 receptor with clinical features of SIADH, but with undetectable plasma vasopressin levels.

retention (Figure 44.1),[80,83] but it also exacerbates hyponatremia (Eq. (44.1)). Balance studies in a group of patients with SIADH showed that during a period of high water and low sodium intake, the plasma sodium concentration decreased by 8 mEq/L with no gain in weight and no increase in chloride space (a measure of extracellular fluid volume).[84] Negative sodium and potassium balances accounted for the stability of

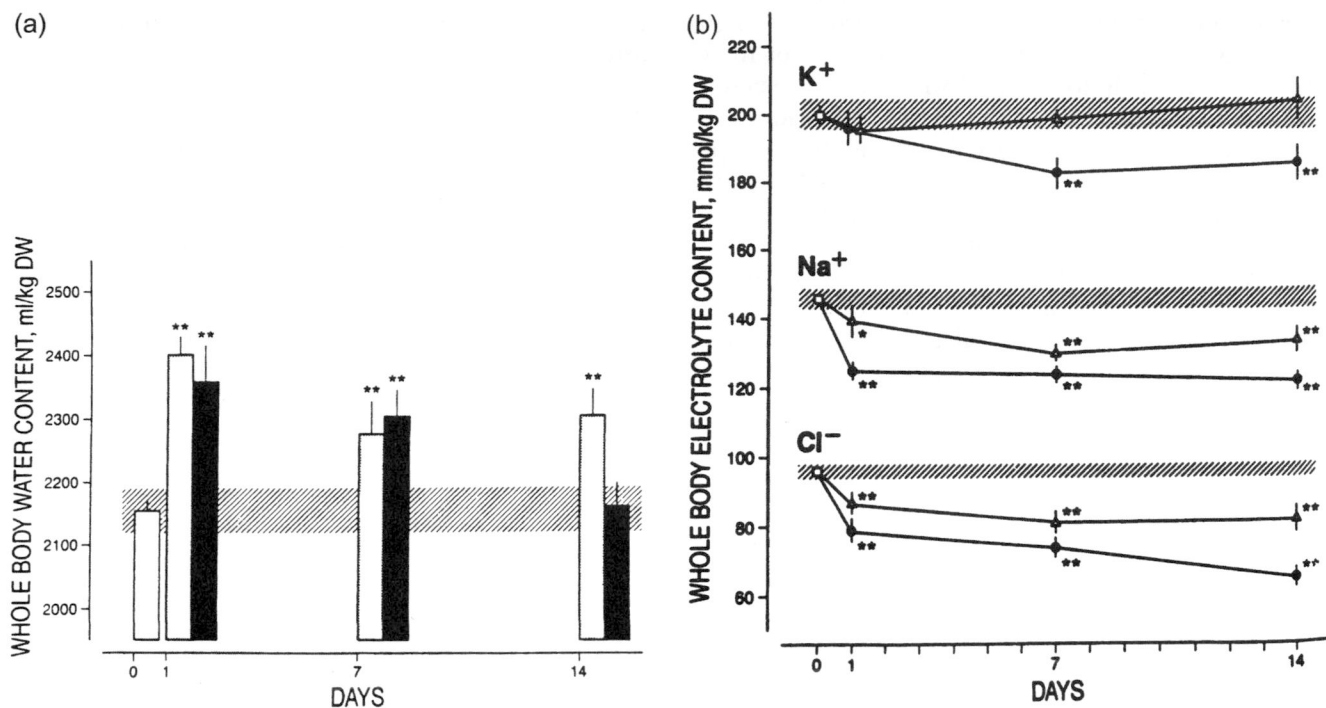

FIGURE 44.3   Body water content in experimental SIADH.[88] Panel (a) depicts measurements of body water content in rats made hyponatremic with dDAVP and a liquid diet. The open bar at the far left of the figure represents measurements obtained in normonatremic controls given no dDAVP. The black bars represent measurements obtained in animals made severely hyponatremic (plasma sodium 106 to 112 mmol/l) by giving dDAVP at 5 ng/hr; the gray bars represent measurements obtained in animals made less hyponatremic (plasma sodium 119 to 124 mmol/l) by giving dDAVP at 1 ng/hr. Body water content initially increases after the first day of hyponatremia at both doses of dDAVP, but falls to control levels after 14 days of severe hyponatremia. Panel (b) depicts whole body Na, K, and Cl measurements in the same experiment. Cation and chloride losses occur, beginning on the first day of hyponatremia, and are more severe in animals given the higher dose of dDAVP (with lower plasma sodium levels). Depletion of Na and Cl most likely represent adaptive responses to extracellular fluid volume expansion caused by retained water. Depletion of body K most likely represents a cell volume adaptive response.

extracellular volume, and for over 80% of the calculated solute loss. During a period of high sodium intake, over 600 mEq of sodium was retained (with only a small increase in weight and chloride space), fully accounting for the 11 mEq/L increase in serum sodium concentration.[84] In this study, there was a strong negative correlation between water intake and sodium balance, and between water intake and aldosterone secretory rate. Similar findings have been reported in studies in which pituitary extract was administered chronically to normal subjects.[83,85,86]

In an experimental model of SIADH produced by DDAVP and half-isotonic saline in the rat, hyponatremia was caused exclusively by negative balances of sodium and potassium; water balance, which was slightly negative, did not contribute to the decrease in sodium concentration.[87] Despite negative balances for sodium, chloride, and water, the extracellular volume (measured by inulin space) was not contracted, suggesting that water shifted from the intracellular to the extracellular space in response to the loss of intracellular solute (potassium and phosphate).

Similarly, direct measurements of body composition in a rat model of chronic SIADH showed that after 14 days of severe hyponatremia, body water content had returned to control levels[88] (Figure 44.3). Body sodium and chloride levels were reduced after one day of hyponatremia and were sustained for 14 days, and body potassium was significantly decreased after 7 days. Acutely, water retention was the major cause of hyponatremia, but solute depletion was primarily responsible when the electrolyte disturbance was sustained.

Urinary losses can directly lower the plasma sodium concentration when the concentration of sodium plus potassium in the urine is higher than the plasma sodium concentration. This can occur when high vasopressin levels (which concentrate the urine) and high rates of sodium and potassium excretion occur together. The excretion of hypertonic urine generates free water, in essence "desalinating" the plasma.[89]

Serum Bicarbonate Concentration in SIADH

In SIADH, the serum sodium and chloride concentrations are lowered by dilution, but the serum bicarbonate concentration is typically normal.[90,91] This finding has been explained by a direct effect of hyponatremia on the adrenal gland to increase aldosterone secretion, which then augments renal net acid excretion.[92] Patients with hyponatremia due to hypopituitarism have many features in common with patients with non-endocrine SIADH, but their serum bicarbonate concentrations are about 5 mmol/l lower. Consistent with the hypothesis that hyponatremia-induced hyperaldosteronism is responsible for the normal serum bicarbonate in classic SIADH, aldosterone levels are much lower in patients with ACTH deficiency than in patients with non-endocrine SIADH.[90]

Common Causes of SIADH

Tumors

The first cases of SIADH were described in patients with lung cancer.[78] Small-cell carcinoma of the lung remains a common cause of the syndrome; approximately 10 to 15% of these patients present with SIADH, whereas fewer than 1% of patients with non-small-cell lung cancer become hyponatremic.[93,94] Ectopic production of vasopressin appears to be responsible for most cases hyponatremia associated with small-cell carcinoma.[95,96] Arginine vasopressin, oxytocin, and neurophysins have been found by radioimmunoassay in tumors, and are produced by the vast majority of small-cell lung cancers; the quantity of vasopressin peptide is closely correlated with the presence of hyponatremia.[97-99] Atrial natriuretic peptide mRNA has also been detected in a high percentage of cell lines from patients with small-cell cancer.[100] Hyponatremia develops in approximately 3 to 7% of patients with head and neck cancer[94,101]; the mechanism for SIADH associated with these tumors is unknown. Although a number of other tumors can produce vasopressin, there are very few reports of hyponatremia associated with them.[94] SIADH may also emerge in patients with acute tumor lysis syndrome.[102,103]

Pulmonary Disease

Mild hyponatremia has long been recognized in patients with tuberculosis.[104,105] The mechanism for vasopressin release has not been determined, but hormone levels fall in response to water-loading, reflecting the reset osmostat variant of SIADH. Ectopic secretion of antidiuretic hormone was the presumptive cause of SIADH in a patient with central diabetes insipidus who developed pulmonary tuberculosis.[106] Tuberculosis-associated hyponatremia resolves within days to weeks of antituberculous therapy. Plasma vasopressin levels are typically elevated on admission in patients with bacterial pneumonia, and fall rapidly during treatment.[107] Hyponatremia is common,[108,109] and usually self-corrects relatively rapidly after a few days.[110] Abnormal vasopressin secretion in simple pneumonia is not attributable to hypovolemia, hypotension or abnormal PO_2 or PCO_2. An antidiuretic decapeptide ("pneumadin"), which rapidly increases arginine vasopressin (AVP) levels, has been isolated from rat and human lung.[111,112] Further study is needed to determine if the decapeptide mediates SIADH associated with pneumonia and other lung disorders. Acute respiratory failure (hypoxia and hypercarbia) and severe asthma are also associated with SIADH.[113,114]

Endocrine Disease

Hyponatremia is present in up to 88% of patients with Addison's disease, and in 28% of patients with isolated ACTH deficiency.[115] In Addison's disease, vasopressin is released in response to volume-depletion caused by mineralocorticoid deficiency, and altered hemodynamics caused by glucocorticoid deficiency. Glucocorticoids may also directly inhibit vasopressin release. Unlike Addison's disease, impaired water excretion in hypopituitarism is not associated with hyperkalemia, and it does not respond to volume replacement with isotonic saline so that hyponatremia in this condition has all the features of SIADH.[116-119] However, hyponatremia in patients with hypopituitarism is associated with a lower serum bicarbonate concentration than in patients with hyponatremia from other causes of SIADH (see section "Serum Bicarbonate Concentration in SIADH").[90] Impaired water excretion in hypopituitarism and in adrenalectomized mineralocorticoid replaced subjects is associated with elevated vasopressin levels; administration of a vasopressin V2 receptor-antagonist normalizes urinary water excretion in adrenalectomized mineralocorticoid replaced rats.[120] Inhibitory glucocorticoid receptors have been identified in the magnocellular neurons which secrete vasopressin, and these receptors are markedly increased under hypoosmolar conditions.[121-123] Hyponatremia with clinical features of SIADH has been described frequently in hypothyroidism; impaired water excretion can be corrected rapidly by the administration of thyroid hormone. However, it is unclear whether hemodynamic or intrarenal factors, rather than vasopressin, is responsible for impaired water excretion in this condition.[124,125]

Non-Diuretic Drugs

Arginine vasopressin used therapeutically in the treatment of gastrointestinal bleeding or in the management of septic shock, and the vasopressin analog desmopressin acetate (DDAVP), a pure V2 receptor-agonist used to treat diabetes insipidus, enuresis, and von Willebrand disease, may cause hyponatremia.[126,127] In addition, a growing number of drugs that are unrelated to vasopressin have been reported to cause hyponatremia. Most published reports involve thiazide and thiazide-like diuretics, chlorpropamide, carbamazepine, oxcarbantipsychotics, antidepressants, and nonsteroidal anti-inflammatory drugs.[128–130] Vincristine and vinblastine increase vasopressin release by unknown mechanisms, and hyponatremia associated with these agents is dose related.[128]

Several drugs associated with hyponatremia appear to increase the response of the collecting duct to circulating vasopressin.[128,131] Chlorpropamide has been the most thoroughly studied.[132] In addition to augmenting release of vasopressin from the neurohypophysis, chlorpropamide increases the number of vasopressin receptors on collecting tubule cells[133] and inhibits renal medullary synthesis of prostaglandin E$_2$, an agent which blunts the hydroosmotic effect of vasopressin by diminishing adenylate cyclase activity.[134–136] Inhibition of PGE$_2$ permits increased cAMP formation, enhancing the effect of the hormone. Nonsteroidal anti-inflammatory agents increase the hydroosmotic effect of vasopressin by a similar mechanism. Hyponatremia attributable solely to nonsteroidals has been rarely reported, but these commonly used drugs may exacerbate other causes of hyponatremia.[137,138]

Carbamazepine most commonly causes hyponatremia when it is given to subjects who habitually drink large volumes of water.[130,139] Carbamazepine increases water permeability of the distal inner medulary collecting duct in the absence of vasopressin, an effect that is cAMP-dependent and negated by a vasopressin V2 receptor-antagonist, implying an action on the V2 receptor–protein G complex.[140] Oxcarbazepine, which is enjoying increased use because of fewer drug interactions than carbamazepine, causes hyponatremia in 9% of patients with epiliepsy who are treated with the drug.[141]

Hyponatremia caused by cyclophosphamide may also be due to enhanced vasopressin action, but the mechanism for this effect has not yet been elucidated.[130] Cyclophosphamide's antidiuretic effect is delayed, with a time-course which parallels excretion of active metabolites of the drug.[142] Cyclophosphamide's antidiuretic effect may be enhanced by indomethacin.[143] There are many reports of SIADH associated with psychotropic drugs, including phenothiazines, monoamine oxidase inhibitors, and tricyclic antidepressants; causality has been most convincingly demonstrated with tricyclics.[144] More recently, a large number of cases of SIADH have been reported in patients taking serotonin reuptake inhibitors (SSRIs).[145–147] Prospective series in elderly patients

have shown that 12 to 40% became hyponatremic within two weeks of starting therapy with paroxetine.[147–149] All of these agents act centrally, and could conceivably affect vasopressin release directly. There is evidence that SSRIs may have a direct effect on water permeability of the inner medullary collecting duct, increasing AQP2 without changing vasopressin levels.[150] The recreational drug, 3,4-methylenedioxy-methamphetamine ("Ecstasy") has been associated with severe, and sometimes fatal, acute hyponatremia.[151] Ecstasy induces vasopressin secretion, and users of the drug who become hyponatremic typically manifest marked polydipsia.[152,153] Many cases of SIADH associated with amiodarone have been reported.[154–157]

Post-Operative SIADH

Vasopressin levels are elevated after operative procedures, and remain elevated for several days.[158] Administration of hypotonic fluid during this period of antidiuresis causes acute hyponatremia, with potentially disastrous consequences.

Urinary cation loss has been shown to play an important role in the pathogenesis of hyponatremia in patients with post-operative SIADH. In the post-operative period, it is common for physicians to infuse several liters of isotonic or hypotonic saline solutions, exceeding the intended replacement of third-space and external losses, and actually causing extracellular fluid volume-expansion. A balance study in women undergoing uncomplicated gynecological surgery showed that sodium plus potassium concentrations in the urine peaked at 295 ± 9 mEq/L, and remained hypertonic to plasma for the first 16 hours after induction of anesthesia[89](Figure 44.4). Because of the action of vasopressin and the natriuretic response to saline-induced volume-expansion, electrolyte-free water was generated, lowering the plasma sodium concentration despite infusion of isotonic saline. The infused saline was, in effect, "desalinated." A similar phenomenon occurs when patients with subarachnoid hemorrhage and "cerebral salt-wasting" are given large volumes of isotonic saline to protect cerebral perfusion.[159]

Neurologic Disorders and Cerebral Salt-Wasting

An association between hyponatremia and intracranial disease has been recognized since the 1950s, and hyponatremia has been reported in a wide variety of systemic diseases involving the CNS, including systemic lupus erythematosus, Guillain-Barre syndrome, meningitis, encephalitis, brain tumors, and brain abscesses.[160] Noting increased urinary sodium excretion in hyponatremic patients with neurologic disorders, Peters referred to the condition as "cerebral salt-wasting".[161] Once it was recognized that high rates

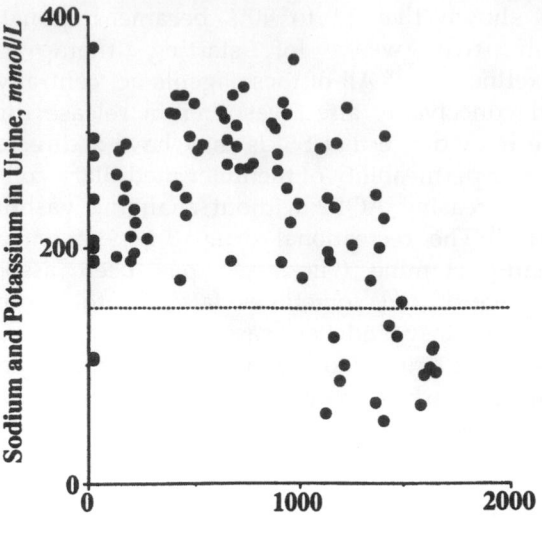

FIGURE 44.4 Urine electrolytes in post-operative SIADH.[89] The figure depicts the sum of urine sodium and potassium concentrations obtained post-operatively in 22 women undergoing uncomplicated gynecologic surgery and receiving infusions of 0.9% saline (sodium concentration 154 mmol/l) or lactated Ringer's solution (sodium concentration 130 mmol/l). The dotted line represents a urine cation concentration of 150 mmol/l, isotonic to normal plasma water. During the first 1000 minutes after the induction of anesthesia, urine cation concentrations were uniformly hypertonic to plasma, contributing to the genesis of hyponatremia. In samples obtained after 1000 minutes (from 16 to 24 hours), the urine remained hypertonic in some patients and became hypotonic in others. Hypotonic urine (below the dotted line) contributes to the correction of hyponatremia.

of urinary sodium excretion could be caused by unregulated secretion of antidiuretic hormone, most investigators ascribed hyponatremia in brain disease to SIADH, a syndrome which has been associated a wide array of central nervous system disorders, consistent with the multiple anatomic pathways leading to vasopressin secretion by hypothalamic neurons (Table 44.3).[162]

Cerebral salt-wasting was generally a forgotten term until the early 1980s, when a more concerted effort was made to understand the pathogenesis of hyponatremia in patients with intracranial disease (especially subarachnoid hemorrhage).[163,164] Reduced blood and plasma volume were found in most patients with intracranial disease who were presumed to have hyponatremia secondary to SIADH.[165–167] Prospective studies of patients with subarachnoid hemorrhage given maintenance fluids documented negative sodium balance, decreasing plasma volume, and increasing BUN among patients who became hyponatremic within a week of presentation.[164,168,169] A course consistent with cerebral salt-wasting was also observed in

patients with head injury, brain metastases, and hydrocephalus.[170–172]

Maintaining an adequate circulatory volume has important clinical implications, especially in subarachnoid hemorrhage, where volume depletion and fluid restriction have been reported to predispose to cerebral ischemia and infarction.[173,174] This finding, and evidence that volume-expansion protects against cerebral ischemic events in subarachnoid hemorrhage, has led to a general acceptance of "hypertensive, hypervolemic, hemodilutional" therapy for the disorder.[175–177] When such treatment is given, a high urine sodium concentration and hyponatremia are not reliable indicators of salt-wasting, because hyponatremia may be due to SIADH and the natriuresis may be a response to iatrogenic volume-expansion. In one study, a positive balance for sodium could be documented in most patients believed to have cerebral salt-wasting when calculations included all infusions from the time of first contact with medical or paramedical personnel.[178] High levels of catecholamines which are often associated with brain injury decrease venous capacitance and raise blood pressure, potentially increasing "effective arterial blood volume," and promoting a physiological natriuresis.[179]

A valid diagnosis of cerebral salt-wasting requires proof of urinary sodium losses, despite reduced effective arterial blood volume. Attempts to establish a diagnosis of hypovolemia have included clinical impressions, central venous pressure, and measurements of plasma and blood volume; none of these can define hypovolemia definitively.[180]

As in patients with SIADH, plasma vasopressin levels are increased and urine sodium concentrations are elevated, but the increased vasopressin secretion in cerebral salt-wasting has been attributed to volume-depletion caused by the primary salt-wasting. Investigation into the pathogenesis of cerebral salt-wasting has focused primarily on the relative roles of natriuretic hormones and vasopressin after subarachnoid hemorrhage.[181–183] Atrial natriuretic peptide (ANP) and brain natriuretic peptide (BNP) are both derived from cardiac tissue, and have natriuretic and aldosterone-inhibiting properties. Although BNP has been localized to the hypothalamus, it is primarily of cardiac origin. Cardiac release of ANP and BNP is regulated in part by the CNS, and brain injury may induce their release from cardiac tissue. Plasma ANP levels generally correlate with the presence and severity of blood in the ventricles and increased intracranial pressure.[182] In one study, however, plasma levels of BNP, but not ANP or vasopressin, were correlated with urinary sodium excretion,[184] and in a rat model of cerebral salt-wasting, ANP levels decreased and BNP levels did not change.[185] Jugular venous sampling in suspected cerebral salt-wasting did not support cerebral release of BNP.[186] It is thus unclear whether elevated natriuretic peptide levels are responsible for natriuresis in subarachnoid hemorrhage, and other factors, such altered sympathetic tone, depressed aldosterone levels, ouabain-like compound, and endothelin may contribute.[160,167,181,187] In fact, several studies have indicated that fludrocortisone may be effective in the treatment of cerebral salt-wasting.[188-191]

Regardless of the pathogenesis of renal salt-wasting in patients with subarachnoid hemorrhage, hyponatremia appears to be caused by vasopressin release that is independent of volume-depletion, and is thus "inappropriate." In a large prospective study of acute aneurysmal subarachnoid hemorrhage treated aggressively with isotonic saline (between 3 and 8 liters daily), hyponatremia developed in one-third of the patients within 4 to 6 days, despite positive fluid balance, increased blood volume, and suppressed plasma renin and aldosterone levels.[159] Plasma vasopressin was measured at concentrations of 1 to 4 pg/ml, despite plasma osmolalities at which the hormone should have been undetectable. Although plasma ANP levels were also increased in most patients, they did not correlate with serum sodium concentration. Thus, it is likely that both salt loss and SIADH contribute in varying degrees to the pathogenesis of hyponatremia after subarachnoid hemorrhage.

The true incidence of cerebral salt-wasting among patients with subarachnoid hemorrhage is probably low, and a clear distinction between this entity and SIADH in neurosurgical patients may not be important, because in either case the most effective treatment is intravenous hypertonic saline.[180]

Nephrogenic Syndrome of Inappropriate Antidiuresis

A gain-of-function mutation of the V2 receptor gene, named nephrogenic syndrome of antidiuresis (NSIAD), was first described in 2005.[81] Patients with this X-linked disease present with clinical and laboratory evaluations typical of SIADH, with undetectable plasma vasopressin levels. Missense mutations substituting cysteine or leucine for arginine on codon 137 cause constitutive activation of the vasopressin receptor, analogous to loss-of-function mutations found in patients with X-linked nephrogenic diabetes insipidus. Infants with NSIAD are at high risk for hyponatremia, because their diet consists primarily of liquid with little solute. However, the disease can escape detection until adulthood, and it should be suspected in young patients with a clinical diagnosis of idiopathic SIADH, especially if there is unresponsiveness to vasopressin antagonists. Female heterozygotes with skewed X-inactivation may develop spontaneous hyponatremia or an abnormal water-loading test.[192,193]

ADAPTATIONS TO HYPOTONIC HYPONATREMIA

Organic Osmolytes and Cell Volume Regulation

The osmotic challenges faced by hyponatremic patients are analogous to those faced by invertebrate organisms when they are exposed to a hypotonic environment. Throughout nature, cells respond to water stress in a similar manner. Water crosses cell membranes in response to osmotic forces, equalizing the activities of intracellular and extracellular solute. Cell volume is determined by the amount and concentration of intracellular solute. Since at equilibrium intracellular and extracellular osmolalities are equal, the relationship between cell volume and extracellular osmolality can be described by the following equation:

$$\text{Cell water} \approx \frac{\text{Cell solute content}}{\text{Extracellular osmolality}} \qquad (44.2)$$

Hypotonicity causes cells to swell initially as water diffuses into them, equalizing the osmolality of intracellular and extracellular fluids. Almost immediately, however, most cells begin to adjust their volume back towards normal.[194-196] This "volume regulatory decrease," is explained by reductions in cell solute content. The first response to osmotic stress is a loss of potassium. With time, loss of organic solutes dominate the response.

Most cells maintain relatively high concentrations of small, osmotically-active organic molecules known as "organic osmolytes." The major organic osmolytes found in nature are limited to a few classes of compounds—polyols, methylamines, and free amino acids—that are shared by diverse species. Organic osmolytes are non-perturbing solutes; unlike sodium and potassium, their intracellular concentrations may vary widely without affecting tertiary protein structure. Cells accumulate organic osmolytes under hypertonic conditions and lose them when confronted with hypotonicity. Several organic osmolytes are exported from swollen cells through a common channel, the volume-sensitive organic osmolyte/anion channel (VSOAC).[196,197] Osmolytes are transported into the cell by specific transporters, such as the sodium-myoinositol transporter (SMIT)[198] and the taurine transporter (TAUT).[199]

Cell volume control mechanisms could modify the relationship between the plasma sodium concentration and body water, sodium, and potassium content shown in Eq. (44.1). For example, if the intracellular fluid compartment were to lose 15% of its solute (exclusive of potassium) in response to cell swelling, the amount of water needed to lower the plasma sodium concentration would be reduced by one-third. Some balance studies in patients with very low plasma sodium concentrations have failed to fully account for the severity of hyponatremia, a finding that would be expected if there were substantial losses of organic osmolytes from body cells.

Brain Adaptations to Hyponatremia

The need for cell volume regulation is greatest in the brain, where the rigid calvarium limits the degree of tissue swelling that can be tolerated.[200,201] An increase in brain water content of more than about 5 to 10% is incompatible with life. Although the capillary endothelium that forms the blood–brain barrier has a limited permeability to ions and other solutes, it allows relatively rapid water movement into the brain. Therefore, an osmotic gradient between the brain and plasma can exist only transiently, and it is dissipated by water movement in less than one hour. Hydraulic conductivity of the capillaries which form the blood–brain barrier decreases in response to hypotonicity.[202] However, because the brain and plasma must eventually come into osmotic equilibrium, this adaptation can only postpone brain swelling. The brain's interstitial fluid compartment communicates with the spinal fluid through a series of extracellular channels. Bulk flow of fluid between the brain's interstitial space and the cerebrospinal fluid provides a rapid defense against osmotic brain swelling. Ultimately, protection against lethal cerebral edema depends on the ability of brain cells to reduce their solute content.

In experimental hyponatremia in the rat, depletion of brain sodium, potassium, and chloride accounts for about two-thirds of the adaptive decrease in brain osmolality, while approximately one-third is contributed by organic osmolyte losses. Within 24 hours of the onset of hyponatremia, diminished brain concentrations of myoinositol, glutamate, creatine/phosphocreatine, and taurine can be detected.[203] During sustained hyponatremia, these compounds, plus glycerophosphorylcholine and glutamine, continue to be lost from the brain for approximately three days.[204,205] Reduced concentrations of these solutes persist when animals are kept severely hyponatremic for as long as two weeks. The loss of organic osmolytes contributes substantially to both the early and late adaptations to hyponatremia. In rats whose serum sodium concentrations were reduced to 96 mmol/L in one day, brain water content increased by less than 5%; it was estimated that the increase would have been 11% had there been no losses of organic osmolytes.[203] After three days of hyponatremia, additional losses of brain solute further decrease the severity of brain edema; animals exhibit minimal neurologic findings despite serum sodium concentrations of 95 to 100 mmol/L.[206]

Magnetic resonance spectroscopy has provided evidence of reduced concentrations of organic osmolytes in the brains of patients with hyponatremia.[207] One study showed that the peak associated with inositol remained depressed for at least two weeks after correction of hyponatremia (Figure 44.5).[208] An adaptive response of the brain is evident among patients with chronic hyponatremia. Computed axial tomography and magnetic resonance images do not show evidence of brain edema, and neurologic symptoms may be subtle even in patients with serum sodium concentrations less than 110 mEq/L. Most patients with hyponatremia of this severity survive, and the few neurologic sequelae that occur appear to be caused by overzealous correction of hyponatremia, rather than the electrolyte disturbance itself.[36,209]

In contrast to chronic hyponatremia, patients who become severely hyponatremic in less than 48 hours develop headaches, vomiting, agitated delirium, and eventually stupor, seizures, and coma. The clinical syndrome in both humans and experimental animals is associated with cerebral edema which can be reversed by the administration of hypertonic saline. On occasion, acute hyponatremia can lead to respiratory arrest, transtentorial herniation, and death.[210–214] When large volumes of water are retained in a short period of time, the arterial sodium concentration (to which the brain is exposed) may be up to 4 mmol/l lower than the venous concentration (which is most commonly sampled for clinical sodium measurements).[215]

Age, Sex, and the Adaptation to Hyponatremia

Recently, a single group of investigators have reported on over 100 previously healthy patients who became hyponatremic 1–2 days after routine elective surgery, and who subsequently died or suffered permanent brain damage. Individual patients had serum sodium concentrations as high as 129 mEq/L when they developed respiratory arrest and brain herniation.[212–214] The most recent reports emphasize the frequent association of hyponatremic encephalopathy with neurogenic pulmonary edema[213] and terminal diabetes insipidus.[216] Remarkably, virtually all of the reported patients were women, usually of child-bearing age[214] or prepubescent children.[212] These findings led these authors to suggest that sex hormones alter

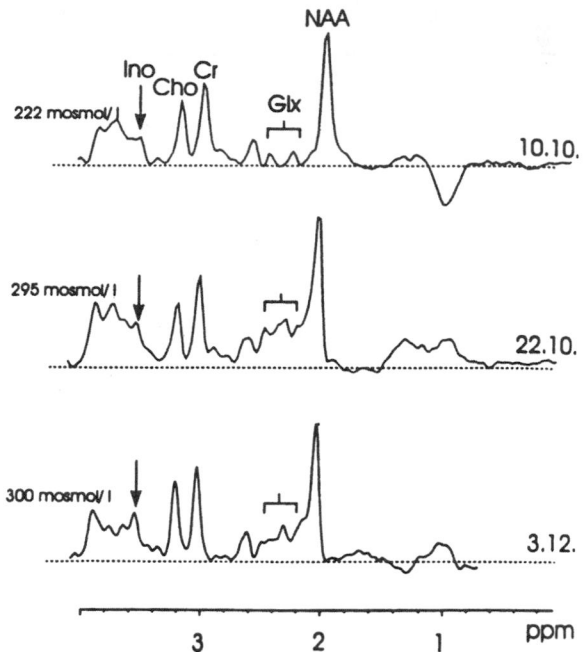

FIGURE 44.5 Brain organic osmolytes in human hyponatremia.[208] The figure depicts the results of magnetic resonance spectroscopy of the brain of a single patient before and after treatment of severe hyponatremia (plasma sodium 101 mmol/l, plasma osmolality 222 mosm/kg). The spectroscopy tracings were obtained on three different dates. The top tracing, taken on October 10, when the plasma osmolality was 222 mosm/l, shows an extremely low inositol peak (arrow). The middle tracing, taken on October 22, ten days after treatment of hyponatremia when the plasma osmolality was 295 mosm/l, shows an inositol peak that is still depressed. The bottom tracing, taken on December 3, 7 weeks after correction of hyponatremia shows a much higher inositol peak.

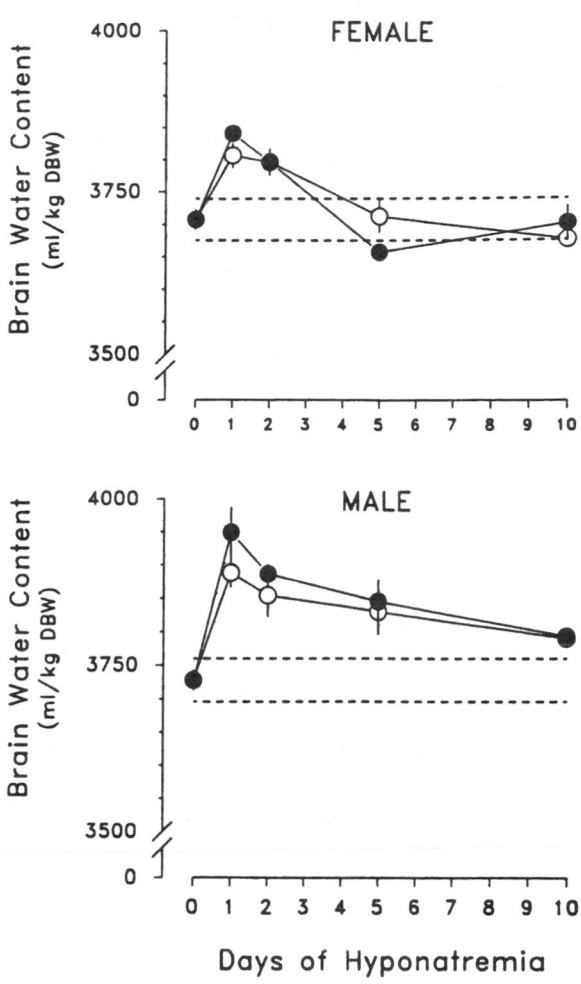

FIGURE 44.6 Brain water content in hyponatremic male and female rats.[219] The figure depicts measurements of brain water content obtained in male and female rats made hyponatremic with a liquid diet and either arginine vasopressin (solid circles) or dDAVP (open circles). Brain water contents are comparable in the two sexes, returning to or toward control values after ten days of hyponatremia.

the adaptive mechanisms that protect against brain edema in hyponatremia.[217]

The same investigators have used experimental models to test their hypothesis that hyponatremia causes more severe brain swelling in females than in males. The results of these studies are inconclusive. The investigators initially found that mortality from hyponatremia was markedly increased in adult female rats[218] (a finding that has not been reproduced by other laboratories[219]). They attributed excess mortality in females to lower levels of brain Na-K-ATPase (and thus a decreased ability to extrude brain sodium), and to increased susceptibility to vasopressin-induced vasoconstriction of the cerebral vasculature. *In vitro* studies showed that estrogens inhibit volume regulation in rat brain astrocyte culture.[220] However, measurements of brain water and solutes in whole brain by these and other investigators show comparable responses to hyponatremia in male and female animals[219] (Figure 44.6).

More recently, Arieff and co-workers reported that although brain water and electrolyte contents in

hyponatremic adult male and female rats do not differ, the brains of newborn rats paradoxically accumulate excess sodium in response to hyponatremia, unless the animals are pretreated with testosterone.[221] Silver and co-workers were unable to reproduce this provocative finding.[222]

Hypoxia and the Adaptation to Hyponatremia

Some investigators have emphasized the adverse effects of hypoxia in hyponatremic patients. According to this view, when brain damage complicates symptomatic hyponatremia, an hypoxic episode can usually be implicated.[223] Although it is likely that hypoxia is an important factor among patients with acute hyponatremia who die of cerebral edema, the role of hypoxia in the demyelinating brain lesions which complicate the treatment of chronic hyponatremia has not been proven (see section "Rapid Correction of Hyponatremia and Osmotic Demyelination").[224,225] Despite recurrent episodes of acute hyponatremia, hyponatremic seizures, respiratory arrests requiring endotracheal intubation, and rapid correction of hyponatremia (due to spontaneous diuresis), infants and psychotic patients with acute water intoxication rarely develop neurologic sequelae.[209]

Hyponatremic animals are more likely to die when exposed to hypoxia than normonatremic animals, and ischemic brain injury impairs the adaptive loss of brain sodium which protects against brain swelling in hyponatremia.[226] In addition, hyponatremia has been shown to lower levels of the antioxidants taurine, glutathione, and ascorbate in brain tissue, which could predispose to oxidant injury when a period of hypoxia is followed by reoxygenation.[227,228]

RAPID CORRECTION OF HYPONATREMIA AND OSMOTIC DEMYELINATION

Biochemical Effects of Rapid Correction of Hyponatremia

Adaptations that protect against brain swelling also predispose to injury when sustained hypotonicity is suddenly corrected. When the plasma sodium is returned to normal, cellular solutes lost in the adaptive phase must be recovered to prevent cellular dehydration. Electrolytes and glutamate quickly return to the brain after correction, but reaccumulation of other organic osmolytes requires several days, because it requires upregulation of sodium-dependent transport proteins.[229,230] The taurine transporter, SNAT2, may be particularly important because of its preferential localization on oligodendrocytes, the cells that are selectively damaged and lost when chronic hyponatremia is rapidly corrected.[231] After rapid correction of hyponatremia, solute-depleted brain cells are initially dehydrated. Brain electrolyte content then "overshoots," increasing to supernormal levels, possibly in compensation for the deficit in organic osmolyte content[225,232] (Figure 44.7).

Clinical Effect of Rapid Correction of Hyponatremia

In humans, correction of severe chronic hyponatremia by more than 10 mEq/L in 24 hours or 18 mEq/L in less than 48 hours is associated with a distinctive clinical disorder known as the "osmotic demyelination syndrome".[210,233–236] In typical cases of the syndrome,

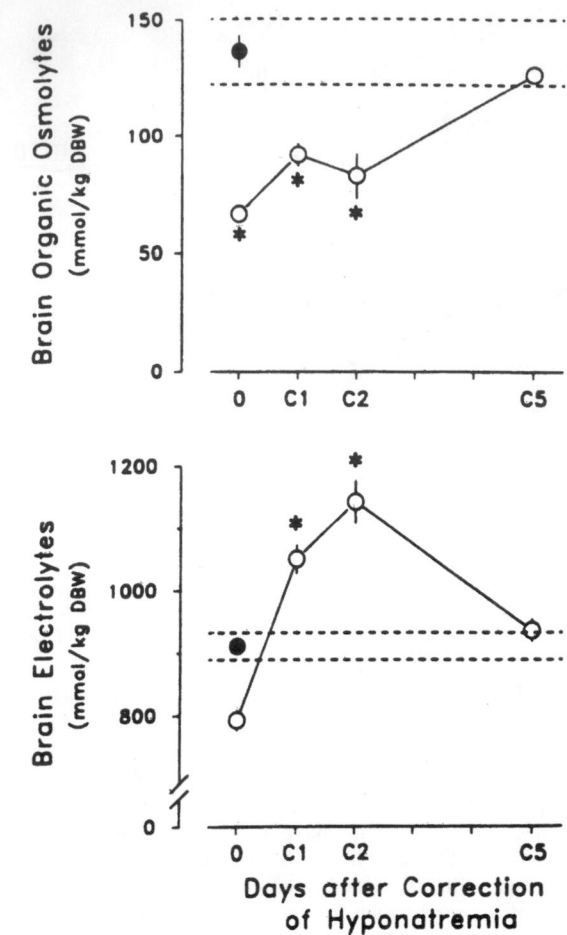

FIGURE 44.7 **Brain organic osmolytes and brain electrolytes after rapid correction of experimental hyponatremia.**[232] The figure depicts measurements of brain organic osmolytes (top panel) and brain electrolytes (bottom panel) made in rats made hyponatremic with dDAVP and a liquid diet and then corrected by withdrawal of dDAVP. Brain organic osmolytes remain significantly below normonatremic control levels (solid circle and dotted lines) on the first two days after correction (C1 and C2), and have not reached normal levels until five days after correction (C5). During the first two days after correction, brain electrolyte content "overshoots" exceeding control levels.

improvement of hyponatremic symptoms during correction of hyponatremia is followed within one to several days by gradual neurologic deterioration. Behavioral disturbances, seizures, movement disorders or akinetic mutism may emerge, and severe cases develop clinical features of a pontine disorder (pseudobulbar palsy, quadriparesis, and pseudocoma).

The clinical symptoms are associated with demyelinating brain lesions which can be demonstrated by magnetic resonance images.[237,238] The most characteristic lesions are located in the center of the pons ("central pontine myelinolysis"),[239,240] but histologically similar lesions are often found in a symmetrical distribution in extrapontine areas of the brain where there is a close admixture of gray and white matter.[234] The lesions are distinctly different from those caused by hypoxia, and they may develop without a preceding hypoxic insult.[209,235,236,241]

Patients with acute hyponatremia (e.g., infants and psychotic patients) usually tolerate rapid correction of hyponatremia without developing complications, and patients with liver disease (a disorder characterized by low levels of brain myoinositol,[242]) alcoholism, malnutrition, and potassium depletion[243] seem to be particularly susceptible to osmotic demyelination.

Experimental Models of Osmotic Demyelination

The osmotic demyelination syndrome has been reproduced in animal models in three different species by multiple laboratories.[206,244–248] These studies have confirmed the strong clinical impression that the disorder is caused by treatment of hyponatremia, rather than hyponatremia itself. Osmotic demyelination does not develop in animals with uncorrected or slowly-corrected hyponatremia. Rapid correction of chronic (three days), but not acute, hyponatremia produces a delayed onset of neurologic symptoms and brain lesions that are histologically similar to those seen in the human disease. Neurologic deterioration and histologic brain damage are preceded by pathologic evidence of blood–brain barrier disruption which can be demonstrated ultrastructurally as early as three hours, and by magnetic resonance imaging one day after rapid correction of hyponatremia.[249–251] After excessive correction of chronic hyponatremia, re-induction of hyponatremia when neurologic findings begin to appear improves survival and prevents the subsequent appearance of myelinolysis in rats, and this strategy has been successfully employed in isolated clinical case reports.[252–254]

Depletion of brain organic osmolytes is felt to play a key role in the blood–brain barrier disruption and demyelination that occurs after rapid correction of hyponatremia. In rats, measurements of organic osmolyte content in different areas of the brain after rapid correction of hyponatremia has shown that areas with the most severe demyelinating lesions are those with the least recovery of organic osmolytes.[255] It has been suggested that blood–brain barrier disruption can be explained by loss of organic osmolytes from brain capillary endothelial cells during the adaptation to hyponatremia with subsequent endothelial cell shrinkage after rapid correction. Blood–brain barrier disruption permits complement, and possibly other toxic plasma constituents, to enter the brain, which may explain the occurrence of progressive myelinolysis even after blood–brain integrity is restored.[249] Re-induction of hyponatremia following rapid correction prevents blood–brain barrier opening and microglial activation, and this can also be achieved by administering glucocorticoids; however, while therapeutic re-lowering of the serum sodium concentration reduced mortality after rapid correction, glucocorticoids did not, suggesting that the increased permeability seen in osmotic demyelination syndrome may not be a primary pathophysiological insult in this syndrome.[252]

Hyponatremic animals with uremia are relatively tolerant of rapid correction, with a lower incidence and severity of myelinolysis than non-uremic animals.[225,256] Resistance to myelinolysis in uremia is associated with more rapid reuptake of organic osmolytes, in particular myoinositol, following rapid correction of hyponatremia. In addition, rapidly corrected uremic animals do not exhibit the "overshoot" in brain sodium content seen in non-uremic animals. Normalization of brain myoinositol can be accelerated in non-uremic hyponatremic rats by administering myoinositol exogenously during rapid correction of the electrolyte disturbance.[257] Exogenous myoinositol improves survival and reduces mortality from rapid correction of chronic hyponatremia in rats.[258]

BONE DISEASE IN HYPONATREMIA

Even mild hyponatremia is associated with gait instability and an increased incidence of falls and fractures.[259,260] Hyponatremia-induced bone loss amplifies the risk of fracture. Three months of severe hyponatremia reduces bone mineral density by 30% in the rat, and is associated with decreased bone formation and increased bone resorption; cross-sectional human data showing that mild hyponatremia is associated with significantly increased odds of osteoporosis are consistent with the experimental data in rodents.[261]

TREATMENT OF HYPOTONIC HYPONATREMIA

Treatment Modalities

Water Restriction

Even with maximally-concentrated urine, evaporative water losses from the skin and lungs will lead to negative water balance and gradual correction of hyponatremia, regardless of the cause of the electrolyte disturbance. In patients whose ability to dilute the urine is intact (e.g., self-induced water intoxication) or can be restored to normal (e.g., by saline infusion in volume-depleted subjects), restriction of free water leads to a steady and sometimes rapid increase in the plasma sodium concentration. In patients with persistent defects in water excretion (e.g., SIADH caused by tumors), water restriction alone increases the plasma sodium concentration extremely slowly, and it will be totally ineffective if the concentrations of sodium plus potassium in the urine exceed that of plasma.[262]

Sodium Chloride

Assuming that free water intake is restricted, sodium chloride solutions increase the plasma sodium concentration as long as the electrolyte concentration of the solution exceeds that of the urine. As urine cation concentrations rarely exceed 400 mEq/L, 3% sodium chloride (513 mEq/L) is always an effective treatment for hyponatremia. Isotonic saline itself does little to increase the plasma sodium concentration, unless it provokes a water diuresis by eliminating a hemodynamic stimulus for vasopressin secretion caused by volume-depletion. In fact, large volumes of isotonic saline can exacerbate hyponatremia in patients with SIADH who excrete highly concentrated urine.[89] The rate of hypertonic saline infusion must be adjusted frequently in response to the observed increase in serum sodium concentration; predictive formulas are unreliable, because urinary water losses often increase during therapy, even in patients who appear to have euvolemic hyponatremia.[263,264]

Potassium Chloride

Given the relationship between the plasma sodium concentration and exchangeable sodium and potassium,[3,8] it follows that potassium repletion of hypokalemic hyponatremic subjects should increase the plasma sodium concentration. There is limited published experience validating this expectation in patients with diuretic-induced hyponatremia,[41] and in the authors' experience (unpublished observations) potassium effectively corrects hyponatremia, regardless of the cause of potassium depletion.

Loop Diuretics

By blocking sodium reabsorption in the ascending limb of the loop of Henle, loop diuretics impair the ability to maximally concentrate the urine, even in the presence of high levels of plasma vasopressin. Used alone or in combination with angiotensin-converting enzyme inhibitors, loop diuretics are effective in treating hyponatremia associated with edematous conditions.[265-267] In patients with SIADH, loop diuretics can be combined with 3% saline for the treatment of hyponatremic emergencies.[268] Traditionally, in this maneuver, urinary sodium losses are matched with infused saline. However, given the adaptive loss of sodium that occurs in SIADH, it may be more appropriate to allow sodium intake to exceed urinary losses. In patients with SIADH who require chronic outpatient

therapy, loop diuretics combined with oral salt tablets and potassium replacement (or concurrent therapy with a potassium sparing diuretic) are effective.

Demeclocycline

Demeclocycline is a tetracycline antibiotic which blocks the effect of vasopressin in the collecting duct. After a few days of therapy, demeclocycline induces a state of nephrogenic diabetes insipidus, which resolves within several days when the drug is stopped.[269] This side-effect of the antibiotic has been exploited in the long-term treatment of SIADH.[270,271] Demeclocycline is nephrotoxic in patients with heart failure and liver disease.[272,273]

Urea

Urea, administered orally in a daily dose of 0.5 g/kg body weight per day, increases urinary electrolyte free water losses, allowing liberalized fluid intake in patients with chronic hyponatremia due to SIADH, and other disorders such as congestive heart failure.[274,275] However, it tastes poorly and is contraindicated in liver and renal failure. Intravenous urea has also been effective in treating acute hyponatremia.[276] In experimental models, Soupart and Decaux have demonstrated that acute correction of chronic hyponatremia with urea decreases the risk of myelinolysis.[277] Although the mechanism of this protection is unknown, it has been speculated that urea enters the brain and then is cleared from the plasma more slowly than it is cleared from brain tissue,[278,279] thereby protecting against brain cell shrinkage after rapid correction. Experience with urea is much more extensive in Europe than in the United States.

V₂-Receptor Antagonists

Vasopressin antagonists, called "vaptans" because of the suffix applied to their generic names, block the binding of vasopressin to its renal receptor, preventing water reabsorption, decreasing urine osmololality, and increasing urine output. These agents induce a dose-related water diuresis lasting approximately six hours without a significant increase in urinary sodium or potassium excretion; therefore, vasopressin receptor-antagonists are sometimes called "aquaretics"[280-282] (Figure 44.8).

Tolvaptan (OPC-41061), and conivaptan (YM-087) have been approved by the United States Food and Drug Administration for the treatment of hyponatremia. Tolvaptan is selective for the vasopressin-2 (V2) receptor responsible for the antidiuretic actions of arginine vasopressin, conivaptan is active at both the V2 receptor and the V1a receptor responsible for the vasoconstricting properties of arginine vasopressin. Selective V2-antagonists have been shown to be

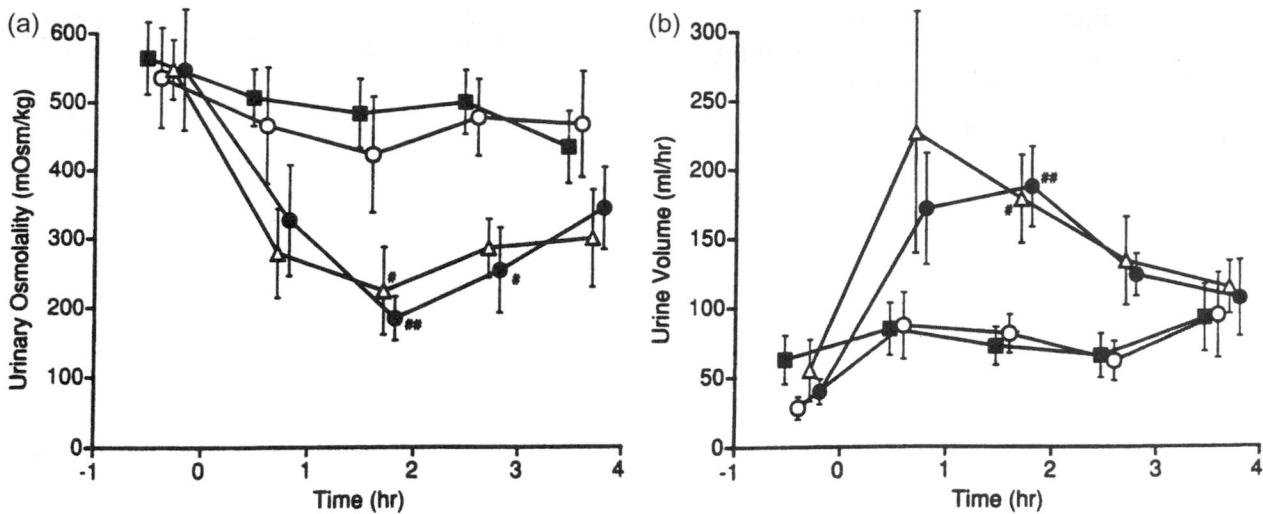

FIGURE 44.8 **Response to V2 receptor blocker in patients with SIADH.**[321] The figure depicts urine osmolality (panel a) and volume (panel b) in control subjects (closed squares) and in patients with SIADH given OPC-31260 intravenously in three doses: 0.1 mg/kg (open circles); 0.25 mg/kg (open triangles); 0.5 mg/kg (closed circles). The urine osmolality falls significantly below control values and urine volume increases significantly above control values after one hour at the two higher doses of the drug.

effective in correcting hyponatremia due to SIADH, cirrhosis, and heart failure in humans.[283-285] Conivaptan corrects hyponatremia in animal models of cirrhosis,[286] but it may be contraindicated in the human disease, because blockade of the V1a receptor may potentially provoke the hepatorenal syndrome. However, the dual receptor activity may be particularly useful in patients with CHF, because of load reduction from V1a receptor-blockade combined with reduced cardiac preload and increased sodium concentrations induced by V2 receptor antagonism.[287,288]

Because these agents cause a brisk and relatively prolonged water diuresis, V_2-receptor antagonists may risk overly rapid correction and osmotic demyelinization if they are used to treat severe chronic hyponatremia. Indeed, in an experimental model of chronic hyponatremia, increasing the plasma sodium concentration with a V_2-receptor antagonist was comparable to hypertonic saline in causing osmotic demyelination.[289]

Therapeutic Guidelines

The proper treatment of hyponatremia has been a controversial topic that has been extensively reviewed.[210,290,291] There is a general consensus that the dangers of cerebral edema and seizures mandate prompt and definitive treatment with one of the above modalities to ensure that the plasma sodium concentration begins to return to normal. Initial therapy in patients with acute hyponatremia or severe symptoms should probably begin with a bolus infusion of 1 to 2 ml/kg body weight of 3% saline, aiming for an increase of 1 to 2 mEq/L.[291-293] Therapy in all patients should be limited to avoid iatrogenic injury. Most investigators now agree that correction should not exceed 10 mEq/L in a single day or 18 mEq/L in two days, because these rates are sometimes harmful in susceptible patients, and have no proven advantage over more limited correction.[291,294] It should be emphasized that these are limits and not therapeutic goals; given the risks of severe neurological injury, and the danger of inadvertently "overshooting the mark" owing to an unexpected water diuresis, therapeutic regimens should be targeted at an increase of 6 to 8 mEq/L/day, with adjustments based on frequent measurements of the serum sodium concentration.[210,264,295]

Managing Unintentional Overcorrection

If a water diuresis occurs during therapy, sodium administration should be discontinued and, to avoid overcorrection, water losses should either be replaced or halted with the administration of desmopressin.[296,297] Alternatively, particularly in patients likely to have reversibly impaired ability to excrete dilute urine, desmopressin can be administered prophylactically, thereby maintain relatively constant urinary water losses while raising the serum sodium concentration with a concurrent infusion of 3% saline.[298]

Even with careful management, many patients experience a greater than intended increase in sodium concentration.[264,299] If this occurs, therapeutic re-lowering of the serum sodium concentration with a brief infusion of 5% dextrose in water, using desmopressin to prevent further water losses, has been shown to be well-tolerated in a small series and a few case reports.[296,297] As discussed previously, this strategy prevents osmotic demyelination and mortality in experimental models.[252]

NON-HYPOTONIC HYPONATREMIA

Pseudohyponatremia

Plasma is normally 93% water. Thus, a sodium concentration of 143 mEq/L in a sample of whole plasma reflects a sodium concentration of 154 mEq/L in plasma water (143/0.93 = 154). Physiologic saline solutions (e.g., 0.9% NaCl) were designed to reproduce the sodium concentration in plasma water.

Pseudohyponatremia is an exaggeration of the physiologic dilution of plasma sodium by non-aqueous material.[300] High concentrations of intravascular protein (as in multiple myeloma) or lipid "dilute" the plasma sodium concentration, but do not alter the solute concentrations of the intracellular or interstitial fluid compartments. Because the "diluent" in these conditions is non-aqueous, the sodium concentration of the aqueous portion of a plasma sample, as determined by an ion-specific electrode in undiluted serum or plasma, is normal.[301,302] Plasma osmolality, as measured by an osmometer, is also normal. Thus, hyponatremia associated with hyperlipidemia or hyperproteinemia can be considered artifactual, and is called "pseudo-hyponatremia." Laboratory determinations which depend on a diluting step yield artifactually low sodium concentrations in samples taken from patients with severe hyperlipidemia or plasma cell dyscrasias, even if the instrument employs an ion-specific electrode.[301,303] In these disorders, the plasma aliquot obtained for dilution contains less plasma water (and therefore less sodium) than normal; the sodium concentration in the diluted sample is thus artifactually reduced.

Hypertonic and Isotonic Hyponatremia

Pathophysiology

If non-permeant solutes other than sodium salts accumulate in the extracellular space, the extracellular fluid volume expands, reducing the concentration of the sodium normally present in this fluid compartment. Plasma osmolality varies, depending on the cause of the syndrome.

Retention of a sodium-free isotonic solution (e.g., infusion of isotonic mannitol in a patient with renal insufficiency who excretes the solute slowly) causes isotonic hyponatremia. Mannitol, a solute that is unable to permeate cell membranes, is confined to the extracellular space; the fluid infused with the solute is similarly confined.[304] Thus, the extracellular fluid expands, and the intracellular compartment is unaffected. Sodium-free hypotonic solutions containing impermeant solutes can be considered isotonic solutions to which water has been added; hyponatremia caused by these solutions is primarily extracellular, but plasma osmolality is slightly reduced and the intracellular compartment is slightly diluted.

Retention of a sodium-free hypertonic solution (e.g., infusion of hypertonic mannitol) causes hypertonic hyponatremia.[305] In this case, intracellular water is osmotically drawn to the extracellular fluid compartment, compounding the dilution of extracellular sodium caused by the infused diluent. Thus, the sodium concentration of the extracellular space is reduced, while the osmolality of both extracellular and intracellular fluid compartments is increased.[306] A similar phenomenon has been described after administration of IgG solutions containing maltose or sucrose.[307]

Hyperglycemia

Glucose normally contributes only 5 milliosmoles per liter to plasma osmolality. The osmotic importance of glucose increases dramatically in patients with diabetic hyperglycemia. As glucose cannot permeate most cell membranes without insulin, hyperglycemia attracts intracellular water to the extracellular space, causing hyponatremia despite hyperosmolality of both extracellular and intracellular fluid compartments. Several correction factors have been offered to quantify this relationship.[308] However, a precise correction factor is probably unobtainable, because in practice hyperglycemia develops, in part, from the ingestion of glucose with water and resolves, in part, from the urinary excretion of glucose with water.[309] In patients with oliguric kidney failure, whose hyperglycemia is corrected solely by metabolism, the change in serum sodium during correction of hyperglycemia averages 1.6 mEq/L per 100 mg/dl change in blood glucose, but with considerable variability.[310]

Irrigant Absorption Syndrome

Until recently, fluid used to irrigate the operative field during transurethral resection of the prostate (TURP) and hysteroscopy had to be electrolyte free.[311] To avoid hemolysis, isosmotic to slightly hypoosmotic solutions of mannitol, sorbitol or glycine have been utilized. Several liters of irrigant may be absorbed systemically during these procedures, causing profound hyponatremia.[312–314] There are fundamental

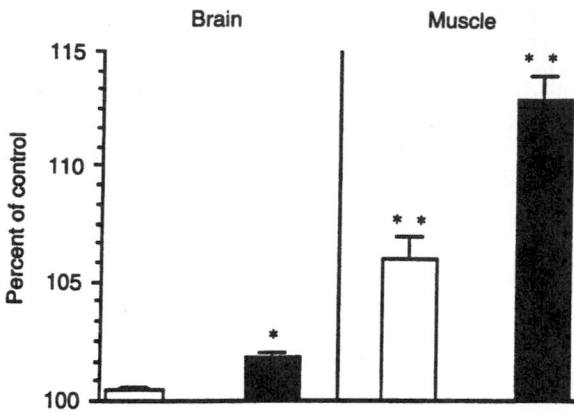

FIGURE 44.9 **Muscle and brain water contents in experimental irrigant absorption syndrome.**[318] The figure depicts measurements of brain and skeletal muscle tissue water contents, expressed as a percentage of normonatremic controls, made in ureter-ligated rats, two hours after infusion of intravenous infusion of isotonic mannitol (open bars) or glycine (black bars). Brain water content is only slightly higher after infusion of glycine than after infusion of mannitol (reflecting minimal but statistically significant penetration of the blood-brain barrier by glycine), and muscle water content is markedly higher in glycine infused animals, reflected the diffusion of glycine into muscle cells.

differences between irrigant absorption hyponatremia and post-operative hypotonic hyponatremia.

The most commonly used irrigant is 1.5% (200 mOsm/kg) glycine. Unlike patients dying of water intoxication, cerebral edema is not a prominent finding after systemic absorption of glycine irrigant and, in contrast to water intoxication, plasma osmolality is only mildly decreased despite severe hyponatremia.[315,316] Glycine and its metabolites, primarily serine and glucose, remain in the plasma for hours after absorption, contributing to plasma osmolality.[315,317]

Studies in experimental animals indicate that isosmotic (2.2%) glycine is initially confined to the extracellular space, markedly diluting the plasma sodium concentration without changing plasma osmolality.[318] As the amino acid enters skeletal muscle cells, carrying water with it, the plasma sodium concentration increases, but plasma osmolality remains constant, owing to increased plasma levels of glycine, serine, and other amino acids, urea, and glucose; in the absence of hypoosmolality brain water content increased only slightly because glycine did not enter the brain[318] (Figure 44.9). Toxicity from glycine or its metabolites, rather than hyponatremia, may contribute to the neurologic symptoms that develop after irrigant absorption. Glycine is a major inhibitory transmitter in retina, and visual hallucinations and transient blindness may occur even in the absence of hyponatremia after prostatectomy using glycine irrigant.[319] Plasma ammonia levels increase in glycine-infused animals

and in humans who have absorbed glycine irrigant.[315,320] In brain, ammonia is metabolized by glutamine synthase to form glutamine, which may serve to protect the brain from the effects of hyperammonemia in liver failure.[242] In animals infused with isosmotic glycine, increased brain glutamine may contribute to the small increase in brain water content which occurs.[318] Levels of ammonia, a major metabolite of glycine, have correlated with neurologic symptoms in some, but not all, studies.

Recently, new resectoscopes have become available which permit endoscopic surgery using isotonic saline. As their use becomes more widespread, it is likely that irrigant absorption syndromes, although fascinating, will be relegated to historical interest.[311]

Hyperosmolality without Hyponatremia

Increased concentrations of permeant solutes like urea or ethanol do not affect the distribution of water in body fluid compartments, and do not cause hyponatremia. However, these solutes increase the plasma osmolality and may cause diagnostic confusion if they are present in patients with hypotonic hyponatremia from other causes.

References

[1] Edelman IS, Leibman J. Anatomy of body water and electrolytes. Am J Med 1959;27:256–77.

[2] Gennari FJ. Current concepts. Serum osmolality. Uses and limitations. N Engl J Med 1984;310(2):102–5.

[3] Edelman IS, Leibman J, O'Meara MW, Birkenfeld LW. Interrelations between serum sodium concentrations, serum osmolality and total exchangeable sodium, total exchangeable potassium and total body water. J Clin Invest 1958;37:1236–56.

[4] Overgaard-Steensen C, Larsson A, Bluhme H, Tonnesen E, Frokiaer J, Ring T. Edelman's equation is valid in acute hyponatremia in a porcine model: plasma sodium concentration is determined by external balances of water and cations. Am J Physiol Regul Integr Comp Physiol 2010;298(1):R120–9.

[5] Rose BD. New approach to disturbances in the plasma sodium concentration. Am J Med 1986;81(6):1033–40.

[6] Nguyen MK, Kurtz I. New insights into the pathophysiology of the dysnatremias: a quantitative analysis. Am J Physiol Renal Physiol 2004;287(2):F172–80.

[7] Gowrishankar M, Chen CB, Mallie JP, Halperin ML. What is the impact of potassium excretion on the intracellular fluid volume: importance of urine anions. Kidney Int 1996;50(5):1490–5.

[8] Nguyen MK, Kurtz I. Role of potassium in hypokalemia-induced hyponatremia: lessons learned from the Edelman equation. Clin Exp Nephrol 2004;8(2):98–102.

[9] Antunes-Rodrigues J, de Castro M, Elias LL, Valenca MM, McCann SM. Neuroendocrine control of body fluid metabolism. Physiol Rev 2004;84(1):169–208.

[10] Baylis PH, Thompson CJ. Osmoregulation of vasopressin secretion and thirst in health and disease. Clin Endocrinol (Oxf) 1988;29(5):549–76.

[11] Robertson GL, Aycinena P, Zerbe RL. Neurogenic disorders of osmoregulation. Am J Med 1982;72(2):339–53.

[12] Kwon TH, Hager H, Nejsum LN, Andersen ML, Frokiaer J, Nielsen S. Physiology and pathophysiology of renal aquaporins. Semin Nephrol 2001;21(3):231–8.

[13] Raymond KH, Lifschitz MD. Effect of prostaglandins on renal salt and water excretion. Am J Med 1986;80(1A):22–33.

[14] Robertson GL, Ganguly A. Osmoregulation and baroregulation of plasma vasopressin in essential hypertension. J Cardiovasc Pharmacol 1986;8(Suppl. 7):S87–91.

[15] Narins RG, Jones ER, Stom MC, Rudnick MR, Bastl CP. Diagnostic strategies in disorders of fluid, electrolyte and acid–base homeostasis. Am J Med 1982;72(3):496–520.

[16] Illowsky BP, Kirch DG. New information on polydipsia and hyponatremia in psychiatric patients. Am J Psychiatry 1988;145 (8):1039.

[17] de Leon J. Polydipsia—a study in a long-term psychiatric unit. Eur Arch Psychiatry Clin Neurosci 2003;253(1):37–9.

[18] Illowsky BP, Kirch DG. Polydipsia and hyponatremia in psychiatric patients. Am J Psychiatry 1988;145(6):675–83.

[19] Kawai N, Baba A, Suzuki T, Shiraishi H. Roles of arginine vasopressin and atrial natriuretic peptide in polydipsia-hyponatremia of schizophrenic patients. Psychiatry Res 2001;101(1):39–45.

[20] Mercier-Guidez E, Loas G. Polydipsia and water intoxication in 353 psychiatric inpatients: an epidemiological and psychopathological study. Eur Psychiatry 2000;15(5):306–11.

[21] Beresford HR. Polydipsia, hydrochlorothiazide, and water intoxication. Jama 1970;214(5):879–83.

[22] Kennedy RM, Earley LE. Profound hyponatremia resulting from a thiazide-induced decrease in urinary diluting capacity in a patient with primary polydipsia. N Engl J Med 1970;282 (21):1185–6.

[23] Bruce RC, Kliegman RM. Hyponatremic seizures secondary to oral water intoxication in infancy: association with commercial bottled drinking water. Pediatrics 1997;100(6):E4.

[24] Keating JP, Schears GJ, Dodge PR. Oral water intoxication in infants. An American epidemic. Am J Dis Child 1991;145(9): 985–90.

[25] Fenves AZ, Thomas S, Knochel JP. Beer potomania: two cases and review of the literature. Clin Nephrol 1996;45(1):61–4.

[26] Harrow AS. Beer potomania. South Med J. 1995;88(5):602.

[27] Thaler SM, Teitelbaum I, Berl T. "Beer potomania" in non-beer drinkers: effect of low dietary solute intake. Am J Kidney Dis 1998;31(6):1028–31.

[28] Steiner RW. Physiology of beer or non-beer potomania. Am J Kidney Dis 1998;32(6):1123.

[29] Taivainen H, Laitinen K, Tahtela R, Kilanmaa K, Valimaki MJ. Role of plasma vasopressin in changes of water balance accompanying acute alcohol intoxication. Alcohol Clin Exp Res 1995;19(3):759–62.

[30] Harrington AR. Hyponatremia due to sodium depletion in the absence of vasopressin. Am J Physiol 1972;222(3):768–74.

[31] Loffing J. Paradoxical antidiuretic effect of thiazides in diabetes insipidus: another piece in the puzzle [comment]. J Am Soc Nephrol 2004;15(11):2948–50.

[32] Beermann B. Thiazides and loop-diuretics therapeutic aspects. Acta Med Scand Suppl 1986;707:75–8.

[33] Chow KM, Kwan BC, Szeto CC. Clinical studies of thiazide-induced hyponatremia. J Natl Med Assoc 2004;96(10):1305–8.

[34] Kone B, Gimenez L, Watson AJ. Thiazide-induced hyponatremia. South Med J. 1986;79(11):1456–7.

[35] Sonnenblick M, Friedlander Y, Rosin AJ. Diuretic-induced severe hyponatremia. Review and analysis of 129 reported patients. Chest 1993;103(2):601–6.

[36] Sterns RH. Severe symptomatic hyponatremia: treatment and outcome. A study of 64 cases. Ann Intern Med 1987;107(5): 656–64.

[37] Clayton JA, Rodgers S, Blakey J, Avery A, Hall IP. Thiazide diuretic prescription and electrolyte abnormalities in primary care. Br J Clin Pharmacol 2006;61(1):87–95.

[38] Jiang JY, Wong MC, Ali MK, Griffiths SM, Mercer SW. Association of antihypertensive monotherapy with serum sodium and potassium levels in Chinese patients. Am J Hypertens 2009;22(3):243–9.

[39] Kim GH, Lee JW, Oh YK, Chang HR, Joo KW, Na KY, et al. Antidiuretic effect of hydrochlorothiazide in lithium-induced nephrogenic diabetes insipidus is associated with upregulation of aquaporin-2, Na-Cl co-transporter, and epithelial sodium channel. J Am Soc Nephrol 2004;15(11):2836–43.

[40] Chow KM, Szeto CC, Wong TY, Leung CB, Li PK. Risk factors for thiazide-induced hyponatraemia. Qjm 2003;96(12):911–7.

[41] Fichman MP, Vorherr H, Kleeman CR, Telfer N. Diuretic-induced hyponatremia. Ann Intern Med. 1971;75(6):853–63.

[42] Greenberg A. Diuretic complications. Am J Med Sci. 2000;319 (1):10–24.

[43] Clark BA, Shannon RP, Rosa RM, Epstein FH. Increased susceptibility to thiazide-induced hyponatremia in the elderly. J Am Soc Nephrol 1994;5(4):1106–11.

[44] Ashraf N, Locksley R, Arieff AI. Thiazide-induced hyponatremia associated with death or neurologic damage in outpatients. Am J Med 1981;70(6):1163–8.

[45] Fadel S, Karmali R, Cogan E. Safety of furosemide administration in an elderly woman recovered from thiazide-induced hyponatremia. Eur J Intern Med 2009;20(1):30–4.

[46] Friedman E, Shadel M, Halkin H, Farfel Z. Thiazide-induced hyponatremia. Reproducibility by single dose rechallenge and an analysis of pathogenesis. Ann Intern Med 1989;110(1): 24–30.

[47] Booker JA. Severe symptomatic hyponatremia in elderly outpatients: the role of thiazide therapy and stress. J Am Geriatr Soc 1984;32(2):108–13.

[48] Hamburger S, Koprivica B, Ellerbeck E, Covinsky JO. Thiazide-induced syndrome of inappropriate secretion of antidiuretic hormone. Time course of resolution. Jama 1981;246(11):1235–6.

[49] DeFronzo RA, Goldberg M, Agus ZS. Normal diluting capacity in hyponatremic patients. Reset osmostat or a variant of the syndrome of inappropriate antidiuretic hormone secretion. Ann Intern Med 1976;84(5):538–42.

[50] Earley LE, Kahn M, Orloff J. The effects of infusions of chlorothiazide on urinary dilution and concentration in the dog. J Clin Invest 1961;40:857–66.

[51] Sonnenblick M, Algur N, Rosin A. Thiazide-induced hyponatremia and vasopressin release. Ann Intern Med 1989;110(9):751.

[52] Spital A. Diuretic-induced hyponatremia. Am J Nephrol. 1999;19(4):447–52.

[53] Sonnenblick M, Rosin AJ. Significance of the measurement of uric acid fractional clearance in diuretic induced hyponatraemia. Postgrad Med J 1986;62(728):449–52.

[54] Fuisz RE, Lauler DP, Cohen P. Diuretic-induced hyponatremia and sustained antidiuresis. Am J Med 1962;33:783–91.

[55] Januezewicz W, Heinemann H, Demartini F, Laragh J. A clinical study of the effects of hydrochlorothiazide on the renal excretion of electrolytes and free water. N Engl J Med 1959;261: 264–9.

[56] Dyckner T, Wester PO. Effects of magnesium infusions in diuretic induced hyponatraemia. Lancet 1981;1(8220 Pt 1): 585–6.

[57] Anderson RJ, Chung HM, Kluge R, Schrier RW. Hyponatremia: a prospective analysis of its epidemiology and the pathogenetic role of vasopressin. Ann Intern Med 1985;102(2):164–8.

[58] Gross PA, Pehrisch H, Rascher W, Schomig A, Hackenthal E, Ritz E. Pathogenesis of clinical hyponatremia: observations of

vasopressin and fluid intake in 100 hyponatremic medical patients. Eur J Clin Invest 1987;17(2):123—9.

[59] Smith D, Moore K, Tormey W, Baylis PH, Thompson CJ. Downward resetting of the osmotic threshold for thirst in patients with SIADH. Am J Physiol Endocrinol Metab 2004;287 (5):E1019—23.

[60] Ecelbarger CA, Nielsen S, Olson BR, Murase T, Baker EA, Knepper MA, et al. Role of renal aquaporins in escape from vasopressin-induced antidiuresis in rat. J Clin Invest 1997;99(8): 1852—63.

[61] Ecelbarger CA, Murase T, Tian Y, Nielsen S, Knepper MA, Verbalis JG. Regulation of renal salt and water transporters during vasopressin escape. Prog Brain Res 2002;139:75—84.

[62] Song J, Hu X, Khan O, Tian Y, Verbalis JG, Ecelbarger CA. Increased blood pressure, aldosterone activity, and regional differences in renal ENaC protein during vasopressin escape. Am J Physiol Renal Physiol 2004;287(5):F1076—83.

[63] Murase T, Tian Y, Fang XY, Verbalis JG. Synergistic effects of nitric oxide and prostaglandins on renal escape from vasopressin-induced antidiuresis. Am J Physiol Regul Integr Comp Physiol 2003;284(2):R354—62.

[64] Schrier RW, Gurevich AK, Cadnapaphornchai MA. Pathogenesis and management of sodium and water retention in cardiac failure and cirrhosis. Semin Nephrol 2001;21(2): 157—72.

[65] Chung HM, Kluge R, Schrier RW, Anderson RJ. Clinical assessment of extracellular fluid volume in hyponatremia. Am J Med 1987;83(5):905—8.

[66] Peruzzi WT, Shapiro BA, Meyer Jr PR, Krumlovsky F, Seo BW. Hyponatremia in acute spinal cord injury. Crit Care Med 1994;22(2):252—8.

[67] Sica DA, Midha M, Zawada E, Stacy W, Hussey R. Hyponatremia in spinal cord injury. J Am Paraplegia Soc 1990;13(4):78—83.

[68] Williams HH, Wall BM, Horan JM, Presley DN, Crofton JT, Share L, et al. Nonosmotic stimuli alter osmoregulation in patients with spinal cord injury. J Clin Endocrinol Metab 1990;71(6):1536—43.

[69] Oren RM. Hyponatremia in congestive heart failure. Am J Cardiol 2005;95(9A):2B—7B.

[70] Schrier RW. Pathogenesis of sodium and water retention in high-output and low-output cardiac failure, nephrotic syndrome, cirrhosis, and pregnancy (2). N Engl J Med 1988;319 (17):1127—34.

[71] Sica DA. Hyponatremia and heart failure: pathophysiology and implications. Congest Heart Fail 2005;11(5):274—7.

[72] Francis GS, Benedict C, Johnstone DE, Kirlin PC, Nicklas J, Liang CS, et al. Comparison of neuroendocrine activation in patients with left ventricular dysfunction with and without congestive heart failure. A substudy of the studies of left ventricular dysfunction (SOLVD). Circulation 1990;82(5):1724—9.

[73] Packer M, Lee WH, Kessler PD, Gottlieb SS, Bernstein JL, Kukin ML. Role of neurohormonal mechanisms in determining survival in patients with severe chronic heart failure. Circulation 1987;75(5 Pt 2):IV80—92.

[74] Martin PY, Gines P, Schrier RW. Nitric oxide as a mediator of hemodynamic abnormalities and sodium and water retention in cirrhosis. N Engl J Med 1998;339(8):533—41.

[75] Martin PY, Schrier RW. Pathogenesis of water and sodium retention in cirrhosis. Kidney Int Suppl 1997;59:S43—9.

[76] Epstein M. Derangements of renal water handling in liver disease. Gastroenterology 1985;89(6):1415—25.

[77] Gines P, Berl T, Bernardi M, Bichet DG, Hamon G, Jiminez W, et al. Hyponatremia in cirrhosis: from pathogenesis to treatment. Hepatology 1998;28(3):851—64.

[78] Schwartz WB, Bennett W, Curelop S, Bartter FC. A syndrome of renal sodium loss and hyponatremia probably resulting from inappropriate secretion of antidiuretic hormone. Am J Med 1957;23(4):529—42.

[79] Beck LH. Hypouricemia in the syndrome of inappropriate secretion of antidiuretic hormone. N Engl J Med 1979;301 (10):528—30.

[80] Maesaka JK, Batuman V, Yudd M, Salem M, Sved AF, Venkatesan J. Hyponatremia and hypouricemia: differentiation from SIADH. Clin Nephrol. 1990;33(4):174—8.

[81] Feldman BJ, Rosenthal SM, Vargas GA, Fenwick RG, Huang EA, Matsuda-Abedini M, et al. Nephrogenic syndrome of inappropriate antidiuresis [see comment] N Engl J Med 2005;352 (18):1884—90.

[82] Zerbe R, Stropes L, Robertson G. Vasopressin function in the syndrome of inappropriate antidiuresis. Annu Rev Med 1980;31:315—27.

[83] Wrong O. The relationship between water retention and electrolyte excretion following administration of anti-diuretic hormone. Clin Sci (Lond) 1956;15(3):401—8.

[84] Cooke CR, Turin MD, Walker WG. The syndrome of inappropriate antidiuretic hormone secretion (SIADH): pathophysiologic mechanisms in solute and volume regulation. Medicine (Baltimore) 1979;58(3):240—51.

[85] Jaenike JR, Waterhouse C. The renal response to sustained administration of vasopressin and water in man. J Clin Endocrinol Metab 1961;21:231—42.

[86] Leaf A, Bartter FC, Santos RF, Wrong O. Evidence in man that urinary electrolyte loss induced by pitressin is a function of water retention. J Clin Invest 1953;32(9):868—78.

[87] Gowrishankar M, Chen CB, Cheema-Dhadli S, Steele A, Halperin ML. Hyponatremia in the rat in the absence of positive water balance. J Am Soc Nephrol 1997;8(4):524—9.

[88] Verbalis JG. Pathogenesis of hyponatremia in an experimental model of the syndrome of inappropriate antidiuresis. Am J Physiol 1994;267(6 Pt 2):R1617—25.

[89] Steele A, Gowrishankar M, Abrahamson S, Mazer CD, Feldman RD, Halperin ML. Postoperative hyponatremia despite near isotonic saline infusion: a phenomenon of desalination. Ann Intern Med 1997;126(1):20—5.

[90] Decaux G, Musch W, Penninckx R, Soupart A. Low plasma bicarbonate level in hyponatremia related to adrenocorticotropin deficiency. J Clin Endocrinol Metab 2003;88(11): 5255—7.

[91] Graber M, Corish D. The electrolytes in hyponatremia. Am J Kidney Dis 1991;18(5):527—45.

[92] Cohen JJ, Hulter HN, Smithline N, Melby JC, Schwartz WB. The critical role of the adrenal gland in the renal regulation of acid—base equilibrium during chronic hypotonic expansion. Evidence that chronic hyponatremia is a potent stimulus to aldosterone secretion. J Clin Invest 1976;58(5):1201—8.

[93] List AF, Hainsworth JD, Davis BW, Hande KR, Greco FA, Johnson DH. The syndrome of inappropriate secretion of antidiuretic hormone (SIADH) in small-cell lung cancer. J Clin Oncol 1986;4(8):1191—8.

[94] Sorensen JB, Andersen MK, Hansen HH. Syndrome of inappropriate secretion of antidiuretic hormone (SIADH) in malignant disease. J Intern Med 1995;238(2):97—110.

[95] Johnson BE, Chute JP, Rushin J, Williams J, Le PT, Venzon D, et al. A prospective study of patients with lung cancer and hyponatremia of malignancy. Am J Respir Crit Care Med 1997;156(5):1669—78.

[96] Moses AM, Scheinman SJ. Ectopic secretion of neurohypophyseal peptides in patients with malignancy. Endocrinol Metab Clin North Am 1991;20(3):489—506.

III. FLUID AND ELECTROLYTE REGULATION AND DYSREGULATION

[97] Legros JJ, Geenen V, Carvelli T, Martens H, Andre M, Corhay JL, et al. Neurophysins as markers of vasopressin and oxytocin release. A study in carcinoma of the lung. Horm Res 1990;34(3-4):151−5.

[98] Maurer LH, O'Donnell JF, Kennedy S, Faulkner CS, Rist K, North WG. Human neurophysins in carcinoma of the lung: relation to histology, disease stage, response rate, survival, and syndrome of inappropriate antidiuretic hormone secretion. Cancer Treat Rep 1983;67(11):971−6.

[99] North WG, Friedmann AS, Yu X. Tumor biosynthesis of vasopressin and oxytocin. Ann N Y Acad Sci 1993;689:107−21.

[100] Gross AJ, Steinberg SM, Reilly JG, Bliss Jr DP, Brennan J, Le PT, et al. Atrial natriuretic factor and arginine vasopressin production in tumor cell lines from patients with lung cancer and their relationship to serum sodium. Cancer Res 1993;53(1):67−74.

[101] Ferlito A, Rinaldo A, Devaney KO. Syndrome of inappropriate antidiuretic hormone secretion associated with head neck cancers: review of the literature. Ann Otol Rhinol Laryngol 1997;106(10 Pt 1):878−83.

[102] Saintigny P, Chouahnia K, Cohen R, Pallier MC, Brechot JM, Morere JF, et al. Tumor lysis associated with sudden onset of syndrome of inappropriate antidiuretic hormone secretion. Clin Lung Cancer 2007;8(4):282−4.

[103] Vanhees SL, Paridaens R, Vansteenkiste JF. Syndrome of inappropriate antidiuretic hormone associated with chemotherapy-induced tumour lysis in small-cell lung cancer: case report and literature review. Ann Oncol 2000;11(8):1061−5.

[104] Hill AR, Uribarri J, Mann J, Berl T. Altered water metabolism in tuberculosis: role of vasopressin. Am J Med 1990;88(4):357−64.

[105] Sims EA, Welt LG, Orloff J, Needham JW. Asymptomatic hyponatremia in pulmonary tuberculosis. J Clin Invest 1950;29(11):1545−57.

[106] Lee P, Ho KK. Hyponatremia in pulmonary TB: evidence of ectopic antidiuretic hormone production. Chest 2010;137(1):207−8.

[107] Dreyfuss D, Leviel F, Paillard M, Rahmani J, Coste F. Acute infectious pneumonia is accompanied by a latent vasopressin-dependent impairment of renal water excretion. Am Rev Respir Dis 1988;138(3):583−9.

[108] Kennedy PG, Mitchell DM, Hoffbrand BI. Severe hyponatraemia in hospital inpatients. Br Med J 1978;2(6147):1251−3.

[109] Thomas TH, Morgan DB, Swaminathan R, Ball SG, Lee MR. Severe hyponatraemia. A study of 17 patients. Lancet 1978;1(8065):621−4.

[110] Dixon BS, Anderson RJ. Pneumonia and the syndrome of inappropriate antidiuretic hormone secretion: don't pour water on the fire. Am Rev Respir Dis 1988;138(3):512−3.

[111] Kosowicz J, Miskowiak B, Konwerska A, Tortorella C, Nussdorfer GG, Malendowicz LK. Tissue distribution of pneumadin immunoreactivity in the rat. Peptides 2003;24(2):215−20.

[112] Watson JD, Jennings DB, Sarda IR, Pang SC, Lawson B, Wigle DA, et al. The antidiuretic effect of pneumadin requires a functional arginine vasopressin system. Regul Pept 1995;57(2):105−14.

[113] Farber MO, Weinberger MH, Robertson GL, Fineberg NS, Manfredi F. Hormonal abnormalities affecting sodium and water balance in acute respiratory failure due to chronic obstructive lung disease. Chest 1984;85(1):49−54.

[114] Valli G, Fedeli A, Antonucci R, Paoletti P, Palange P. Water and sodium imbalance in COPD patients. Monaldi Arch Chest Dis 2004;61(2):112−6.

[115] Verbalis J. Hyponatremia: endocrinologic causes and consequences of therapy. Trends Endocrinol Metab 1992;3:1−7.

[116] Boykin J, DeTorrente A, Erikson A, Robertson G, Schrier R. Role of vasopressin in impaired water excretion of glucocorticoid deficiency. J Clin Invest 1978;62:738−44.

[117] Diederich S, Franzen NF, Bahr V, Oelkers W. Severe hyponatremia due to hypopituitarism with adrenal insufficiency: report on 28 cases. Eur J Endocrinol 2003;148(6):609−17.

[118] Oelkers W. Hyponatremia and inappropriate secretion of vasopressin (antidiuretic hormone) in patients with hypopituitarism. N Engl J Med 1989;321(8):492−6.

[119] Olchovsky D, Ezra D, Vered I, Hadani M, Shimon I. Symptomatic hyponatremia as a presenting sign of hypothalamic-pituitary disease: a syndrome of inappropriate secretion of antidiuretic hormone (SIADH)-like glucocorticosteroid responsive condition. J Endocrinological Invest 2005;28(2):151−6.

[120] Ishikawa S, Schrier R. Effect of arginine vasopressin antagonist on renal water excretion in glucocorticoid and mineralocorticoid deficient rats. Kidney Int 1982;22:587−93.

[121] Berghorn KA, Knapp LT, Hoffman GE, Sherman TG. Induction of glucocorticoid receptor expression in hypothalamic magnocellular vasopressin neurons during chronic hypoosmolality. Endocrinology 1995;136(2):804−7.

[122] Kiss JZ, Van Eekelen JA, Reul JM, Westphal HM, De Kloet ER. Glucocorticoid receptor in magnocellular neurosecretory cells. Endocrinology 1988;122(2):444−9.

[123] Papanek PE, Sladek CD, Raff H. Corticosterone inhibition of osmotically stimulated vasopressin from hypothalamic-neurohypophysial explants. Am J Physiol 1997;272(1 Pt 2):R158−62.

[124] Hanna FW, Scanlon MF. Hyponatraemia, hypothyroidism, and role of arginine-vasopressin. Lancet 1997;350(9080):755−6.

[125] Iwasaki Y, Oiso Y, Yamauchi K, Takatsuki K, Kondo K, Hasegawa H, et al. Osmoregulation of plasma vasopressin in myxedema. J Clin Endocrinol Metab 1990;70(2):534−9.

[126] Callreus T, Ekman E, Andersen M. Hyponatremia in elderly patients treated with desmopressin for nocturia: a review of a case series. Eur J Clin Pharmacol 2005;61(4):281−4.

[127] Kristeller JL, Sterns RH. Transient diabetes insipidus after discontinuation of therapeutic vasopressin. Pharmacotherapy 2004;24(4):541−5.

[128] Brater DC. Drug-induced electrolyte disorders and use of diuretics. In: Kokko JP, Tannen RL, editors. Fluids and electrolytes. 3rd ed. Philadelphia: WB Saunders; 1996. p. 693−728.

[129] Chan TY. Drug-induced syndrome of inappropriate antidiuretic hormone secretion. Causes, diagnosis and management. Drugs Aging 1997;11(1):27−44.

[130] Van Amelsvoort T, Bakshi R, Devaux CB, Schwabe S. Hyponatremia associated with carbamazepine and oxcarbazepine therapy: a review. Epilepsia 1994;35(1):181−8.

[131] Moses AM, Miller M. Drug-induced dilutional hyponatremia. N Engl J Med 1974;291(23):1234−9.

[132] Weissman PN, Shenkman L, Gregerman RI. Chlorpropamide hyponatremia: drug-induced inappropriate antidiuretic-hormone activity. N Engl J Med 1971;284(2):65−71.

[133] Hensen J, Haenelt M, Gross P. Water retention after oral chlorpropamide is associated with an increase in renal papillary arginine vasopressin receptors. Eur J Endocrinol 1995;132(4):459−64.

[134] Mendoza SA, Brown CFJ. Effect of chlorpropamide on osmotic water flow across toad bladder and the response to vasopressin, theophylline and cyclic AMP. J Clin Endocrinol Metab 1974;38:883−9.

[135] Webster B, Bain J. Antidiuretic effect and complications of chlorpropamide therapy in diabetes insipidus. J Clin Endocrinol Metab 1970;30(2):215—27.

[136] Zusman RM, Keiser HR, Handler JS. Inhibition of vasopressin-stimulated prostaglandin E biosynthesis by chlorpropamide in the toad urinary bladder. Mechanism of enhancement of vasopressin-stimulated water flow. J Clin Invest 1977;60:1348—53.

[137] Clive DM, Stoff JS. Renal syndromes associated with nonsteroidal anti-inflammatory drugs. N Engl J Med 1984;310:563—72.

[138] Petersson I, Nilsson G, Hansson BG, Hedner T. Water intoxication associated with non-steroidal anti-inflammatory drug therapy. Acta Med Scand 1987;221(2):221—3.

[139] Yassa R, Iskandar H, Nastase C, Camille Y. Carbamazepine and hyponatremia in patients with affective disorder. Am J Psychiatry 1988;145(3):339—42.

[140] de Braganca AC, Moyses ZP, Magaldi AJ. Carbamazepine can induce kidney water absorption by increasing aquaporin 2 expression. Nephrol Dial Transplant 2010;25(12):3840—5.

[141] Ortenzi A, Paggi A, Foschi N, Sabbatini D, Pistoli E. Oxcarbazepine and adverse events: impact of age, dosage, metabolite serum concentrations and concomitant antiepileptic therapy. Funct Neurol 2008;23(2):97—100.

[142] Spital A, Ristow S. Cyclophosphamide induced water intoxication in a woman with Sjogren's syndrome. J Rheumatol 1997;24(12):2473—5.

[143] Webberley MJ, Murray JA. Life-threatening acute hyponatraemia induced by low dose cyclophosphamide and indomethacin. Postgrad Med J 1989;65(770):950—2.

[144] Spigset O, Hedenmalm K. Hyponatremia in relation to treatment with antidepressants: a survey of reports in the world health organization data base for spontaneous reporting of adverse drug reactions. Pharmacotherapy 1997;17(2):348—52.

[145] Liu BA, Mittmann N, Knowles SR, Shear NH. Hyponatremia and the syndrome of inappropriate secretion of antidiuretic hormone associated with the use of selective serotonin reuptake inhibitors: a review of spontaneous reports. Cmaj 1996;155 (5):519—27.

[146] Spigset O. Adverse reactions of selective serotonin reuptake inhibitors: reports from a spontaneous reporting system. Drug Saf 1999;20(3):277—87.

[147] Woo MH, Smythe MA. Association of SIADH with selective serotonin reuptake inhibitors. Ann Pharmacother 1997;31 (1):108—10.

[148] Fabian TJ, Amico JA, Kroboth PD, Mulsant BH, Corey SE, Begley AE, et al. Paroxetine-induced hyponatremia in older adults: a 12-week prospective study. Arch Intern Med 2004;164 (3):327—32.

[149] Fabian TJ, Amico JA, Kroboth PD, Mulsant BH, Reynolds III CF, Pollock BG. Paroxetine-induced hyponatremia in the elderly due to the syndrome of inappropriate secretion of antidiuretic hormone (SIADH). J Geriatr Psychiatry Neurol 2003;16 (3):160—4.

[150] Moyses ZP, Nakandakari FK, Magaldi AJ. Fluoxetine effect on kidney water reabsorption. Nephrol Dial Transplant 2008;23 (4):1173—8.

[151] Hartung TK, Schofield E, Short AI, Parr MJ, Henry JA. Hyponatraemic states following 3,4-methylenedioxymethamphetamine (MDMA, "ecstasy") ingestion. QJM 2002;95(7): 431—7.

[152] Brvar M, Kozelj G, Osredkar J, Mozina M, Gricar M, Bunc M. Polydipsia as another mechanism of hyponatremia after "ecstasy" (3,4 methyldioxymethamphetamine) ingestion. Eur J Emerg Med 2004;11(5):302—4.

[153] Henry JA, Fallon JK, Kicman AT, Hutt AJ, Cowan DA, Forsling M. Low-dose MDMA ("ecstasy") induces vasopressin secretion. Lancet 1998;351(9118):1784.

[154] Aslam MK, Gnaim C, Kutnick J, Kowal RC, McGuire DK. Syndrome of inappropriate antidiuretic hormone secretion induced by amiodarone therapy. Pacing Clin Electrophysiol 2004;27(6 Pt 1):831—2.

[155] Ikegami H, Shiga T, Tsushima T, Nirei T, Kasanuki H. Syndrome of inappropriate antidiuretic hormone secretion (SIADH) induced by amiodarone: a report on two cases. J Cardiovasc Pharmacol Ther 2002;7(1):25—8.

[156] Odeh M, Schiff E, Oliven A. Hyponatremia during therapy with amiodarone. Arch Intern Med 1999;159(21):2599—600.

[157] Shavit E, Sherer Y. Hyponatremia induced by amiodarone therapy. Isr Med Assoc J 2007;9(7):564—5.

[158] Thomas TH, Morgan DB. Post-surgical hyponatraemia: the role of intravenous fluids and arginine vasopressin. Br J Surg 1979;66(8):540—2.

[159] Diringer MN, Wu KC, Verbalis JG, Hanley DF. Hypervolemic therapy prevents volume contraction but not hyponatremia following subarachnoid hemorrhage. Ann Neurol 1992;31(5): 543—50.

[160] Palmer BF. Hyponatremia in patients with central nervous system disease: SIADH versus CSW. Trends Endocrinol Metab 2003;14(4):182—7.

[161] Peters JP, Welt LG, Sims EA, Orloff J, Needham J. A salt-wasting syndrome associated with cerebral disease. Trans Assoc Am Physicians 1950;63:57—64.

[162] Kroll M, Juhler M, Lindholm J. Hyponatraemia in acute brain disease. J Intern Med 1992;232(4):291—7.

[163] Nelson PB, Seif S, Gutai J, Robinson AG. Hyponatremia and natriuresis following subarachnoid hemorrhage in a monkey model. J Neurosurg 1984;60(2):233—7.

[164] Nelson PB, Seif SM, Maroon JC, Robinson AG. Hyponatremia in intracranial disease: perhaps not the syndrome of inappropriate secretion of antidiuretic hormone (SIADH). J Neurosurg 1981;55(6):938—41.

[165] Nelson RJ. Blood volume measurement following subarachnoid haemorrhage. Acta Neurochir Suppl (Wien) 1990;47: 114—21.

[166] Solomon RA, Post KD, McMurtry III JG. Depression of circulating blood volume in patients after subarachnoid hemorrhage: implications for the management of symptomatic vasospasm. Neurosurgery 1984;15(3):354—61.

[167] Yamaki T, Tano-oka A, Takahashi A, Imaizumi T, Suetake K, Hashi K. Cerebral salt wasting syndrome distinct from the syndrome of inappropriate secretion of antidiuretic hormone (SIADH). Acta Neurochir (Wien) 1992;115(3-4):156—62.

[168] Kurokawa Y, Uede T, Ishiguro M, Honda O, Honmou O, Kato T, et al. Pathogenesis of hyponatremia following subarachnoid hemorrhage due to ruptured cerebral aneurysm. Surg Neurol 1996;46(5):500—7 [discussion 507-508]

[169] Wijdicks EF, Vermeulen M, ten Haaf JA, Hijdra A, Bakker WH, van Gijn J. Volume depletion and natriuresis in patients with a ruptured intracranial aneurysm. Ann Neurol 1985;18(2): 211—6.

[170] Ganong CA, Kappy MS. Cerebral salt wasting in children. The need for recognition and treatment. Am J Dis Child 1993;147 (2):167—9.

[171] Oster JR, Perez GO, Larios O, Emery WE, Bourgoignie JJ. Cerebral salt wasting in a man with carcinomatous meningitis. Arch Intern Med 1983;143(11):2187—8.

[172] Tanneau RA, Pennec YL, Jouquan J, Le Menn G. Cerebral salt wasting in elderly persons. Ann Intern Med 1987;107(1):120.

[173] Hasan D, Wijdicks EF, Vermeulen M. Hyponatremia is associated with cerebral ischemia in patients with aneurysmal subarachnoid hemorrhage. Ann Neurol 1990;27(1):106−8.

[174] Wijdicks EF, Vermeulen M, Hijdra A, van Gijn J. Hyponatremia and cerebral infarction in patients with ruptured intracranial aneurysms: is fluid restriction harmful? Ann Neurol 1985;17(2):137−40.

[175] Oropello JM, Weiner L, Benjamin E. Hypertensive, hypervolemic, hemodilutional therapy for aneurysmal subarachnoid hemorrhage. Is it efficacious? No. Crit Care Clin 1996;12 (3):709−30.

[176] Sivakumar V, Rajshekhar V, Chandy MJ. Management of neurosurgical patients with hyponatremia and natriuresis. Neurosurgery 1994;34(2):269−74 [discussion 274]

[177] Ullman JS, Bederson JB. Hypertensive, hypervolemic, hemodilutional therapy for aneurysmal subarachnoid hemorrhage. Is it efficacious? Yes. Crit Care Clin 1996;12(3):697−707.

[178] Carlotti AP, Bohn D, Rutka JT, Singh S, Berry WA, Sharman A, et al. A method to estimate urinary electrolyte excretion in patients at risk for developing cerebral salt wasting. J Neurosurg 2001;95(3):420−4.

[179] Singh S, Bohn D, Carlotti AP, Cusimano M, Rutka JT, Halperin ML. Cerebral salt wasting: truths, fallacies, theories, and challenges. Crit Care Med. 2002;30(11):2575−9.

[180] Sterns RH, Silver SM. Cerebral salt wasting versus SIADH: what difference? J Am Soc Nephrol 2008;19(2):194−6.

[181] Diringer MN. Neuroendocrine regulation of sodium and volume following subarachnoid hemorrhage. Clin Neuropharmacol 1995;18(2):114−26.

[182] Diringer MN, Lim JS, Kirsch JR, Hanley DF. Suprasellar and intraventricular blood predict elevated plasma atrial natriuretic factor in subarachnoid hemorrhage. Stroke 1991;22(5):577−81.

[183] McGirt MJ, Blessing R, Nimjee SM, Friedman AH, Alexander MJ, Laskowitz DT, et al. Correlation of serum brain natriuretic peptide with hyponatremia and delayed ischemic neurological deficits after subarachnoid hemorrhage. Neurosurgery 2004;54 (6):1369−73 discussion 1373−1364.

[184] Berendes E, Walter M, Cullen P, Prien T, Van Aken H, Horsthemke J, et al. Secretion of brain natriuretic peptide in patients with aneurysmal subarachnoid haemorrhage. Lancet 1997;349(9047):245−9.

[185] Kojima J, Katayama Y, Moro N, Kawai H, Yoneko M, Mori T. Cerebral salt wasting in subarachnoid hemorrhage rats: model, mechanism, and tool. Life Sci. 2005;76(20):2361−70.

[186] Powner DJ, Hergenroeder GW, Awili M, Atik MA, Robertson C. Hyponatremia and comparison of NT-pro-BNP concentrations in blood samples from jugular bulb and arterial sites after traumatic brain injury in adults: a pilot study. Neurocrit Care 2007;7(2):119−23.

[187] Wijdicks EF, Schievink WI, Burnett Jr. JC. Natriuretic peptide system and endothelin in aneurysmal subarachnoid hemorrhage. J Neurosurg 1997;87(2):275−80.

[188] Celik US, Alabaz D, Yildizdas D, Alhan E, Kocabas E, Ulutan S. Cerebral salt wasting in tuberculous meningitis: treatment with fludrocortisone. Ann Trop Paediatr 2005;25(4):297−302.

[189] Ishikawa SE, Saito T, Kaneko K, Okada K, Kuzuya T. Hyponatremia responsive to fludrocortisone acetate in elderly patients after head injury. Ann Intern Med 1987;106(2):187−91.

[190] Lee P, Jones GR, Center JR. Successful treatment of adult cerebral salt wasting with fludrocortisone. Arch Intern Med 2008;168(3):325−6.

[191] Papadimitriou DT, Spiteri A, Pagnier A, Bayle M, Mischalowski MB, Bourdat G, et al. Mineralocorticoid deficiency in post-operative cerebral salt wasting. J Pediatr Endocrinol Metab 2007;20(10):1145−50.

[192] Levtchenko EN, Monnens LA. Nephrogenic syndrome of inappropriate antidiuresis. Nephrol Dial Transplant 2010;25 (9):2839−43.

[193] Ranchin B, Boury-Jamot M, Blanchard G, Dubourg L, Hadj-Aissa A, Morin D, et al. Familial nephrogenic syndrome of inappropriate antidiuresis: dissociation between aquaporin-2 and vasopressin excretion. J Clin Endocrinol Metab 2010;95(9): E37−43.

[194] Hoffmann EK, Lambert IH, Pedersen SF. Physiology of cell volume regulation in vertebrates. Physiol Rev 2009;89(1): 193−277.

[195] McManus ML, Churchwell KB, Strange K. Regulation of cell volume in health and disease. N Engl J Med 1995;333(19): 1260−6.

[196] Strange K. Cellular volume homeostasis. Adv Physiol Educ 2004;28(1−4):155−9.

[197] Emma F, McManus M, Strange K. Intracellular electrolytes regulate the volume set point of the organic osmolyte/anion channel VSOAC. Am J Physiol 1997;272(6 Pt 1):C1766−75.

[198] Ibsen L, Strange K. In situ localization and osmotic regulation of the Na$^{(+)}$-myoinositol co-transporter in rat brain. Am J Physiol 1996;271(4 Pt 2):F877−85.

[199] Benrabh H, Bourre JM, Lefauconnier JM. Taurine transport at the blood−brain barrier: an in vivo brain perfusion study. Brain Res 1995;692(1-2):57−65.

[200] Gullans SR, Verbalis JG. Control of brain volume during hyperosmolar and hypoosmolar conditions. Annu Rev Med 1993;44:289−301.

[201] Mount DB. The brain in hyponatremia: both culprit and victim. Semin Nephrol 2009;29(3):196−215.

[202] Olson JE, Banks M, Dimlich RV, Evers J. Blood−brain barrier water permeability and brain osmolyte content during edema development. Acad Emerg Med 1997;4(7):662−73.

[203] Sterns RH, Baer J, Ebersol S, Thomas D, Lohr JW, Kamm DE. Organic osmolytes in acute hyponatremia. Am J Physiol 1993;264(5 Pt 2):F833−6.

[204] Thurston JH, Hauhart RE, Nelson JS. Adaptive decreases in amino acids (taurine in particular), creatine, and electrolytes prevent cerebral edema in chronically hyponatremic mice: rapid correction (experimental model of central pontine myelinolysis) causes dehydration and shrinkage of brain. Metab Brain Dis 1987;2(4):223−41.

[205] Verbalis JG, Gullans SR. Hyponatremia causes large sustained reductions in brain content of multiple organic osmolytes in rats. Brain Res 1991;567(2):274−82.

[206] Sterns RH, Thomas DJ, Herndon RM. Brain dehydration and neurologic deterioration after rapid correction of hyponatremia. Kidney Int 1989;35(1):69−75.

[207] Videen JS, Michaelis T, Pinto P, Ross BD. Human cerebral osmolytes during chronic hyponatremia. A proton magnetic resonance spectroscopy study. J Clin Invest 1995;95(2):788−93.

[208] Haussinger D, Laubenberger J, vom Dahl S, Ernst T, Bayer S, Langer M, et al. Proton magnetic resonance spectroscopy studies on human brain myoinositol in hypo-osmolarity and hepatic encephalopathy. Gastroenterology 1994;107(5): 1475−80.

[209] Sterns RH, Clark EC, Silver SM. Clinical consequences of hyponatremia and its correction. In: Seldin DW, Giebisch G, editors. Clinical disorders of water metabolism. New York: Raven Press; 1993. p. 225−36.

[210] Adrogue HJ, Madias NE. Hyponatremia. N Engl J Med 2000;342(21):1581−9.

[211] Arieff AI. Hyponatremia, convulsions, respiratory arrest, and permanent brain damage after elective surgery in healthy women. N Engl J Med 1986;314(24):1529−35.

[212] Arieff AI, Ayus JC, Fraser CL. Hyponatraemia and death or permanent brain damage in healthy children. Bmj 1992;304 (6836):1218–22.

[213] Ayus JC, Arieff AI. Pulmonary complications of hyponatremic encephalopathy. Noncardiogenic pulmonary edema and hypercapnic respiratory failure. Chest 1995;107(2):517–21.

[214] Ayus JC, Wheeler JM, Arieff AI. Postoperative hyponatremic encephalopathy in menstruant women. Ann Intern Med 1992;117(11):891–7.

[215] Shafiee MA, Charest AF, Cheema-Dhadli S, Glick DN, Napolova O, Roozbeh J, et al. Defining conditions that lead to the retention of water: the importance of the arterial sodium concentration. Kidney Int 2005;67(2):613–21.

[216] Fraser CL, Arieff AI. Fatal central diabetes mellitus and insipidus resulting from untreated hyponatremia: a new syndrome. Ann Intern Med 1990;112(2):113–9.

[217] Ayus JC, Achinger SG, Arieff A. Brain cell volume regulation in hyponatremia: role of sex, age, vasopressin, and hypoxia. Am J Physiol Renal Physiol 2008;295(3):F619–24.

[218] Fraser CL, Kucharczyk J, Arieff AI, Rollin C, Sarnacki P, Norman D. Sex differences result in increased morbidity from hyponatremia in female rats. Am J Physiol 1989;256(4 Pt 2): R880–5.

[219] Verbalis JG. Hyponatremia induced by vasopressin or desmopressin in female and male rats. J Am Soc Nephrol 1993;3(9): 1600–6.

[220] Fraser CL, Swanson RA. Female sex hormones inhibit volume regulation in rat brain astrocyte culture. Am J Physiol 1994;267 (4 Pt 1):C909–14.

[221] Arieff AI, Kozniewska E, Roberts TP, Vexler ZS, Ayus JC, Kucharczyk J. Age, gender, and vasopressin affect survival and brain adaptation in rats with metabolic encephalopathy. Am J Physiol 1995;268(5 Pt 2):R1143–52.

[222] Silver SM, Schroeder BM, Bernstein P, Sterns RH. Brain adaptation to acute hyponatremia in young rats. Am J Physiol 1999;276(6 Pt 2):R1595–9.

[223] Knochel JP. Hypoxia is the cause of brain damage in hyponatremia. Jama 1999;281(24):2342–3.

[224] Soupart A, Penninckx R, Stenuit A, Decaux G. Lack of major hypoxia and significant brain damage in rats despite dramatic hyponatremic encephalopathy. J Lab Clin Med 1997;130(2): 226–31.

[225] Soupart A, Silver S, Schrooeder B, Sterns R, Decaux G. Rapid (24-hour) reaccumulation of brain organic osmolytes (particularly myoinositol) in azotemic rats after correction of chronic hyponatremia. J Am Soc Nephrol 2002;13(6):1433–41.

[226] Ayus JC, Armstrong D, Arieff AI. Hyponatremia with hypoxia: effects on brain adaptation, perfusion, and histology in rodents. Kidney Int 2006;69(8):1319–25.

[227] Clark EC, Thomas D, Baer J, Sterns RH. Depletion of glutathione from brain cells in hyponatremia. Kidney Int 1996;49(2): 470–6.

[228] Siushansian R, Dixon SJ, Wilson JX. Osmotic swelling stimulates ascorbate efflux from cerebral astrocytes. J Neurochem 1996;66(3):1227–33.

[229] Lien YH, Shapiro JI, Chan L. Study of brain electrolytes and organic osmolytes during correction of chronic hyponatremia. Implications for the pathogenesis of central pontine myelinolysis. J Clin Invest 1991;88(1):303–9.

[230] Spector R, Lorenzo AV. Myoinositol transport in the central nervous system. Am J Physiol 1975;228(5):1510–8.

[231] Maallem S, Mutin M, Gonzalez-Gonzalez IM, Zafra F, Tappaz ML. Selective tonicity-induced expression of the neutral amino-acid transporter SNAT2 in oligodendrocytes in rat brain

[232] Verbalis JG, Gullans SR. Rapid correction of hyponatremia produces differential effects on brain osmolyte and electrolyte reaccumulation in rats. Brain Res 1993;606(1):19–27.

[233] Karp BI, Laureno R. Pontine and extrapontine myelinolysis: a neurologic disorder following rapid correction of hyponatremia. Medicine (Baltimore) 1993;72(6):359–73.

[234] Laureno R, Karp BI. Myelinolysis after correction of hyponatremia. Ann Intern Med 1997;126(1):57–62.

[235] Martin RJ. Central pontine and extrapontine myelinolysis: the osmotic demyelination syndromes. J Neurol Neurosurg Psychiatry 2004;75(Suppl. 3):iii22–8.

[236] Sterns RH, Riggs JE, Schochet Jr. SS. Osmotic demyelination syndrome following correction of hyponatremia. N Engl J Med 1986;314(24):1535–42.

[237] Miller GM, Baker Jr. HL, Okazaki H, Whisnant JP. Central pontine myelinolysis and its imitators: MR findings. Radiology 1988;168(3):795–802.

[238] Ruzek KA, Campeau NG, Miller GM. Early diagnosis of central pontine myelinolysis with diffusion-weighted imaging. AJNR Am J Neuroradiol 2004;25(2):210–3.

[239] Adams RD, Victor M, Mancall EL. Central pontine myelinolysis: a hitherto undescribed disease occurring in alcoholic and malnourished patients. AMA Arch Neurol Psychiatry 1959;81 (2):154–72.

[240] Norenberg MD, Leslie KO, Robertson AS. Association between rise in serum sodium and central pontine myelinolysis. Ann Neurol 1982;11(2):128–35.

[241] Sterns RH, Cappuccio JD, Silver SM, Cohen EP. Neurologic sequelae after treatment of severe hyponatremia: a multicenter perspective. J Am Soc Nephrol 1994;4(8):1522–30.

[242] Restuccia T, Gomez-Anson B, Guevara M, Alessandria C, Torre A, Alayrach ME, et al. Effects of dilutional hyponatremia on brain organic osmolytes and water content in patients with cirrhosis. Hepatology 2004;39(6):1613–22.

[243] Lohr JW. Osmotic demyelination syndrome following correction of hyponatremia: association with hypokalemia. Am J Med 1994;96(5):408–13.

[244] Illowsky BP, Laureno R. Encephalopathy and myelinolysis after rapid correction of hyponatraemia. Brain 1987;110(Pt 4): 855–67.

[245] Kleinschmidt-DeMasters BK, Norenberg MD. Rapid correction of hyponatremia causes demyelination: relation to central pontine myelinolysis. Science 1981;211(4486):1068–70.

[246] Kleinschmidt-DeMasters BK, Norenberg MD. Neuropathologic observations in electrolyte-induced myelinolysis in the rat. J Neuropathol Exp Neurol 1982;41(1):67–80.

[247] Laureno R. Central pontine myelinolysis following rapid correction of hyponatremia. Ann Neurol 1983;13(3):232–42.

[248] Verbalis JG, Martinez AJ. Neurological and neuropathological sequelae of correction of chronic hyponatremia. Kidney Int 1991;39(6):1274–82.

[249] Adler S, Martinez J, Williams DS, Verbalis JG. Positive association between blood–brain barrier disruption and osmotically-induced demyelination. Mult Scler 2000;6(1):24–31.

[250] Rojiani AM, Cho ES, Sharer L, Prineas JW. Electrolyte-induced demyelination in rats. 2. Ultrastructural evolution. Acta Neuropathol (Berl) 1994;88(4):293–9.

[251] Rojiani AM, Prineas JW, Cho ES. Electrolyte-induced demyelination in rats. 1. Role of the blood–brain barrier and edema. Acta Neuropathol (Berl) 1994;88(4):287–92.

[252] Gankam Kengne F, Soupart A, Pochet R, Brion JP, Decaux G. Re-induction of hyponatremia after rapid overcorrection of

hyponatremia reduces mortality in rats. Kidney Int 2009;76 (6):614−21.

[253] Oya S, Tsutsumi K, Ueki K, Kirino T. Reinduction of hyponatremia to treat central pontine myelinolysis. Neurology 2001;57 (10):1931−2.

[254] Soupart A, Ngassa M, Decaux G. Therapeutic relowering of the serum sodium in a patient after excessive correction of hyponatremia. Clin Nephrol 1999;51(6):383−6.

[255] Lien YH. Role of organic osmolytes in myelinolysis. A topographic study in rats after rapid correction of hyponatremia. J Clin Invest 1995;95(4):1579−86.

[256] Soupart A, Penninckx R, Stenuit A, Decaux G. Azotemia (48 h) decreases the risk of brain damage in rats after correction of chronic hyponatremia. Brain Res 2000;852(1):167−72.

[257] Silver SM, Schroeder BM, Sterns RH. Brain uptake of myoinositol after exogenous administration. J Am Soc Nephrol 2002;13(5):1255−60.

[258] Silver SM, Schroeder BM, Sterns RH, Rojiani A. Myoinositol administration improves survival and reduces myelinolysis after rapid correction of hyponatremia in rats. J Neuropathol Exp Neurol 2006;65:1−8.

[259] Gankam Kengne F, Andres C, Sattar L, Melot C, Decaux G. Mild hyponatremia and risk of fracture in the ambulatory elderly. QJM 2008;101(7):583−8.

[260] Renneboog B, Musch W, Vandemergel X, Manto MU, Decaux G. Mild chronic hyponatremia is associated with falls, unsteadiness, and attention deficits. Am J Med 2006;119(1):71.e71−8.

[261] Verbalis JG, Barsony J, Sugimura Y, Tian Y, Adams DJ, Carter EA, et al. Hyponatremia-induced osteoporosis. J Bone Miner Res. 2010;25(3):554−63.

[262] Chen S, Jalandhara N, Batlle D. Evaluation and management of hyponatremia: an emerging role for vasopressin receptor antagonists. Nat Clin Pract Nephrol 2007;3(2):82−95.

[263] Bhaskar E, Kumar B, Ramalakshmi S. Evaluation of a protocol for hypertonic saline administration in acute euvolemic symptomatic hyponatremia: a prospective observational trial. Indian J Crit Care Med 2010;14(4):170−4.

[264] Mohmand HK, Issa D, Ahmad Z, Cappuccio JD, Kouides RW, Sterns RH. Hypertonic saline for hyponatremia: risk of inadvertent overcorrection. Clin J Am Soc Nephrol 2007;2 (6):1110−7.

[265] Dzau VJ, Hollenberg NK. Renal response to captopril in severe heart failure: role of furosemide in natriuresis and reversal of hyponatremia. Ann Intern Med 1984;100(6):777−82.

[266] Elisaf M, Theodorou J, Pappas C, Siamopoulos K. Successful treatment of hyponatremia with angiotensin-converting enzyme inhibitors in patients with congestive heart failure. Cardiology 1995;86(6):477−80.

[267] Packer M, Medina N, Yushak M. Correction of dilutional hyponatremia in severe chronic heart failure by converting-enzyme inhibition. Ann Intern Med 1984;100(6):782−9.

[268] Hantman D, Rossier B, Zohlman R, Schrier R. Rapid correction of hyponatremia in the syndrome of inappropriate secretion of antidiuretic hormone. An alternative treatment to hypertonic saline. Ann Intern Med 1973;78(6):870−5.

[269] De Troyer A. Demeclocycline. Treatment for syndrome of inappropriate antidiuretic hormone secretion. Jama 1977;237 (25):2723−6.

[270] Forrest Jr JN, Cox M, Hong C, Morrison G, Bia M, Singer I. Superiority of demeclocycline over lithium in the treatment of chronic syndrome of inappropriate secretion of antidiuretic hormone. N Engl J Med 1978;298(4):173−7.

[271] Trump DL. Serious hyponatremia in patients with cancer: management with demeclocycline. Cancer 1981;47(12): 2908−12.

[272] Miller PD, Linas SL, Schrier RW. Plasma demeclocycline levels and nephrotoxicity. Correlation in hyponatremic cirrhotic patients. Jama 1980;243(24):2513−5.

[273] Perez-Ayuso RM, Arroyo V, Camps J, Jimenez W, Rodamilans M, Rimola A, et al. Effect of demeclocycline on renal function and urinary prostaglandin E2 and kallikrein in hyponatremic cirrhotics. Nephron 1984;36(1):30−7.

[274] Cauchie P, Vincken W, Decaux G. Urea treatment for water retention in hyponatremic congestive heart failure. Int J Cardiol 1987;17(1):102−4.

[275] Decaux G, Genette F. Urea for long-term treatment of syndrome of inappropriate secretion of antidiuretic hormone. Br Med J (Clin Res Ed) 1981;283(6299):1081−3.

[276] Reeder RF, Harbaugh RE. Administration of intravenous urea and normal saline for the treatment of hyponatremia in neurosurgical patients. J Neurosurg 1989;70(2):201−6.

[277] Soupart A, Stenuit A, Perier O, Decaux G. Limits of brain tolerance to daily increments in serum sodium in chronically hyponatraemic rats treated with hypertonic saline or urea: advantages of urea. Clin Sci (Lond) 1991;80 (1):77−84.

[278] Silver SM, DeSimone Jr. JA, Smith DA, Sterns RH. Dialysis disequilibrium syndrome (DDS) in the rat: role of the "reverse urea effect". Kidney Int 1992;42(1):161−6.

[279] Silver SM, Sterns RH, Halperin ML. Brain swelling after dialysis: old urea or new osmoles? Am J Kidney Dis 1996;28 (1):1−13.

[280] Costello-Boerrigter LC, Smith WB, Boerrigter G, Ouyang J, Zimmer CA, Orlandi C, et al. Vasopressin-2 receptor antagonism augments water excretion without changes in renal hemodynamics or sodium and potassium excretion in human heart failure. Am J Physiol Renal Physiol 2005.

[281] Rozen-Zvi B, Yahav D, Gheorghiade M, Korzets A, Leibovici L, Gafter U. Vasopressin receptor antagonists for the treatment of hyponatremia: systematic review and meta-analysis. Am J Kidney Dis 2010;56(2):325−37.

[282] Verbalis JG. Vasopressin V2 receptor antagonists. J Mol Endocrinol 2002;29(1):1−9.

[283] Gerbes AL, Gulberg V, Gines P, Decaux G, Gross P, VPA study group, et al. Therapy of hyponatremia in cirrhosis with a vasopressin receptor antagonist: a randomized double-blind multicenter trial. Gastroenterology 2003;124(4):933−9.

[284] Gheorghiade M, Gattis WA, O'Connor CM, Adams Jr KF, Elkayam U, Barbagelata A, et al. Effects of tolvaptan, a vasopressin antagonist, in patients hospitalized with worsening heart failure: a randomized controlled trial. Jama 2004;291 (16):1963−71.

[285] Wong F, Blei AT, Blendis LM, Thuluvath PJ. A vasopressin receptor antagonist (VPA-985) improves serum sodium concentration in patients with hyponatremia: a multicenter, randomized, placebo-controlled trial. Hepatology 2003;37(1): 182−91.

[286] Fernandez-Varo G, Ros J, Cejudo-Martin P, Cano C, Arroyo V, Rivera F, et al. Effect of the V1a/V2-AVP receptor antagonist, Conivaptan, on renal water metabolism and systemic hemodynamics in rats with cirrhosis and ascites. J Hepatol 2003;38(6): 755−61.

[287] Goldsmith SR. Current treatments and novel pharmacologic treatments for hyponatremia in congestive heart failure. Am J Cardiol 2005;95(9A):14B−23B.

[288] Udelson JE, Smith WB, Hendrix GH, Painchaud CA, Ghazzi M, Thomas I, et al. Acute hemodynamic effects of conivaptan, a dual V(1A) and V(2) vasopressin receptor antagonist, in patients with advanced heart failure. Circulation 2001;104(20): 2417−23.

[289] Verbalis JG, Martinez AJ. Determinants of brain myelinolysis following correction of chronic hyponatremia in rats. In: Jamison RL, Jaid S, editors. Vasopressin. Paris: John Libby; 1991. p. 539–47.

[290] Sterns RH. The treatment of hyponatremia: first, do no harm. Am J Med 1990;88(6):557–60.

[291] Sterns RH, Nigwekar SU, Hix JK. The treatment of hyponatremia. Semin Nephrol 2009;29(3):282–99.

[292] Hew-Butler T, Almond C, Ayus JC, et al. Consensus statement of the 1st international exercise-associated hyponatremia consensus development conference, cape town, South Africa 2005. Clin J Sport Med 2005;15(4):208–13.

[293] Hew-Butler T, Ayus JC, Kipps C, et al. Statement of the Second International Exercise-Associated Hyponatremia Consensus Development Conference, New Zealand, 2007. Clin J Sport Med 2008;18(2):111–21.

[294] Verbalis JG, Goldsmith SR, Greenberg A, Schrier RW, Sterns RH. Hyponatremia treatment guidelines 2007: expert panel recommendations. Am J Med 2007;120(11 Suppl. 1):S1–21.

[295] Sterns RH, Hix JK, Silver S. Treating profound hyponatremia: a strategy for controlled correction. Am J Kidney Dis 2010;56 (4):774–9.

[296] Perianayagam A, Sterns RH, Silver SM, Grieff M, Mayo R, Hix J, et al. DDAVP is effective in preventing and reversing inadvertent overcorrection of hyponatremia. Clin J Am Soc Nephrol 2008;3(2):331–6.

[297] Sterns RH, Hix JK. Overcorrection of hyponatremia is a medical emergency. Kidney Int 2009;76(6):587–9.

[298] Sterns RH, Hix JK, Silver S. Treating profound hyponatremia: a strategy for controlled correction. Am J Kidney Dis 2010.

[299] Pham PC, Chen PV, Pham PT. Overcorrection of hyponatremia: where do we go wrong? Am J Kidney Dis 2000;36(2):E12.

[300] Nguyen MK, Ornekian V, Butch AW, Kurtz I. A new method for determining plasma water content: application in pseudo-hyponatremia. Am J Physiol Renal Physiol 2007;292(5):F1652–6.

[301] Turchin A, Scifter JL, Seely EW. Clinical problem-solving. Mind the gap. N Engl J Med 2003;349(15):1465–9.

[302] Weisberg LS. Pseudohyponatremia: a reappraisal. Am J Med. 1989;86(3):315–8.

[303] Ladenson JH, Apple FS, Koch DD. Misleading hyponatremia due to hyperlipemia: a method-dependent error. Ann Intern Med 1981;95(6):707–8.

[304] Nissenson AR, Weston RE, Kleeman CR. Mannitol. West J Med. 1979;131(4):277–84.

[305] Yun JJ, Cheong I. Mannitol-induced hyperosmolal hyponatraemia. Int Med J. 2008;38(1):73.

[306] Spital A, Sterns RH. The paradox of sodium's volume of distribution. Why an extracellular solute appears to distribute over total body water. Arch Int Med 1989;149(6):1255–7.

[307] Palevsky PM, Rendulic D, Diven WF. Maltose-induced hyponatremia. Ann Int Med 1993;118(7):526–8.

[308] Roscoe JM, Halperin ML, Rolleston FS, Goldstein MB. Hyperglycemia-induced hyponatremia: metabolic considerations in calculation of serum sodium depression. Can Med Assoc J 1975;112(4):452–3.

[309] Davids MR, Edoute Y, Stock S, Halperin ML. Severe degree of hyperglycaemia: insights from integrative physiology. QJM 2002;95(2):113–24.

[310] Tzamaloukas AH, Ing TS, Siamopoulos KC, Rohrscheib M, Elisaf MS, Raj DS, et al. Body fluid abnormalities in severe hyperglycemia in patients on chronic dialysis: review of published reports. J Diabetes Complications 2008;22(1):29–37.

[311] Issa MM, Young MR, Bullock AR, Bouet R, Petros JA. Dilutional hyponatremia of TURP syndrome: a historical event in the 21st century. Urology 2004;64(2):298–301.

[312] Gonzales R, Brensilver JM, Rovinsky JJ. Posthysteroscopic hyponatremia. Am J Kidney Dis. 1994;23(5):735–8.

[313] Hahn RG. The transurethral resection syndrome. Acta Anaesthesiol Scand 1991;35(7):557–67.

[314] Henderson DJ, Middleton RG. Coma from hyponatremia following transurethral resection of prostate. Urology 1980;15(3):267–71.

[315] Agarwal R, Emmett M. The post-transurethral resection of prostate syndrome: therapeutic proposals. Am J Kidney Dis 1994;24(1):108–11.

[316] Campbell HT, Fincher ME, Sklar AH. Severe hyponatremia without severe hypoosmolality following transurethral resection of the prostate (TURP) in end-stage renal disease. Am J Kidney Dis 1988;12(2):152–5.

[317] Agraharkar M, Agraharkar A. Posthysteroscopic hyponatremia: evidence for a multifactorial cause. Am J Kidney Dis 1997;30(5):717–9.

[318] Silver SM, Kozlowski SA, Baer JE, Rogers SJ, Sterns RH. Glycine-induced hyponatremia in the rat: a model of postprostatectomy syndrome. Kidney Int 1995;47(1):262–8.

[319] Mizutani AR, Parker J, Katz J, Schmidt J. Visual disturbances, serum glycine levels and transurethral resection of the prostate. J Urol 1990;144(3):697–9.

[320] Istre O, Jellum E, Skajaa K, Forman A. Changes in amino acids, ammonium, and coagulation factors after transcervical resection of the endometrium with a glycine solution used for uterine irrigation. Am J Obstet Gynecol 1995;172(3):939–45.

[321] Saito T, Ishikawa S, Abe K, Kamoi K, Yamada K, Shimizu K, et al. Acute aquaresis by the nonpeptide arginine vasopressin (AVP) antagonist OPC-31260 improves hyponatremia in patients with syndrome of inappropriate secretion of antidiuretic hormone (SIADH). J Clin Endocrinol Metab 1997;82(4):1054–7.

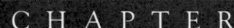

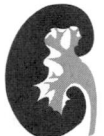

Hypernatremic States

Christopher J. Rivard, Wei Wang and Laurence Chan

University of Colorado Denver, Aurora, Colorado, USA

Hypernatremia can occur with normal, increased or decreased total body sodium content. In healthy individuals and in normal conditions, the plasma concentration of sodium ranges between 136 and 143 mEq/l of plasma, despite large individual variations in the intake of salt and water. The concentration is maintained at constant levels because of the homeostatic mechanism in the body. Claude Bernard was the first to appreciate that higher animals: "have really two environments: a *milieu exterieur* in which the organism is situated, and a *milieu interieur* in which the tissue elements live." The latter is the extracellular fluid (ECF) that bathes the cells of the body.[1,2,3] Maintenance of this consistency of plasma sodium and solute activity is the function of the thirst–neurohypophyseal–renal axis.[4,5] Thirst and urinary concentration are the main defenses against hyperosmolality, and hence hypernatremia. Hypernatremia is a relatively common problem, with prevalence in hospitalized patients of 0.5 to 2%. It is defined as plasma Na^+ concentration ($[Na^+]$) greater than 145 mEq/l. It can be produced by the administration of hypertonic sodium solutions or in almost all cases, by the loss of free water. Since $[Na^+]$ is an effective osmole, the increase in the plasma osmolality (P_{osm}) induced by hypernatremia creates an osmotic gradient that results in water movement out of the cells into the ECF. It is this cellular dehydration, particularly in the brain, that is primarily responsible for the neurologic symptoms associated with hypernatremia. A similar syndrome can be produced when the plasma osmolality is elevated by hyperglycemia. However, when hyperosmolality is due to the accumulation of cell-permeable solute, such as urea or ethanol, there is no water shift in the steady-state because osmotic equilibrium is reached by solute entering the cell.

REGULATION OF WATER HOMEOSTASIS

Significance of the Plasma Sodium Concentration

The total body water (about 60% of body weight in males and 50% in females) is distributed between the intracellular fluid (ICF, 60% of body water) and extracellular fluid (ECF, 40% of body water) spaces.[6–9] Flame photometry and, more recently, ion selective electrode technology have made the plasma sodium concentration one of the simplest and most frequently measured constituents of the body fluids. It is not always appreciated that a given concentration of the plasma sodium may be consistent with different functional states.[10,11] The plasma sodium is simply a concentration term, and as such reflects only the relative amounts of sodium and water present in the sample. The concentration is not a measure of total body sodium content.[12] It is determined empirically by the following relationship:

$$\text{Plasma } [Na^+] = \frac{\text{Total-body } Na^+ + \text{Total-body } K^+}{\text{Total-body water}}$$

$$(\text{Eq.45.1})$$

The relationship indicates the fact that hypernatremia can occur as a consequence of a decrease in total body water, an increase in total body sodium or a combination of these events. It gives no information regarding replacement or removal of sodium. When flame spectrophotometry is used to measure the amount of sodium in a plasma sample, substances such as plasma proteins, abnormally high glucose, and lipid can occupy a large fraction of the plasma volume and underestimate the actual sodium concentration. The

Seldin and Giebisch's The Kidney, Fifth Edition.
DOI: http://dx.doi.org/10.1016/B978-0-12-381462-3.00045-8

ionic composition of the plasma is measured as milliequivalents per liter of plasma. Only about 930 ml of each liter of plasma is water. The remaining 70 ml is occupied by the plasma proteins and, to a lesser degree, lipids. In the presence of hyperlipidemia or hyperproteinemia, the plasma water content may be less than 93%.

Generation of Hypernatremia

Since Na^+ and its accompanying anions are the major effective ECF osmoles, hypernatremia is a state of hyperosmolality. As a result of the fixed number of ICF particles, maintenance of osmotic equilibrium in hypernatremia results in ICF volume-contraction. The increase in the plasma osmolality induced by hypernatremia creates an osmotic gradient that results in water movement out of the cells into the ECF. A similar syndrome can be produced when plasma osmolality is elevated by hyperglycemia. When hyperosmolality is due to the accumulation of a cell-permeable solute, such as urea or ethanol, there is no water shift because osmotic equilibrium is reached by solute entry into cells. Therefore, both urea and ethanol are ineffective osmoles. Plasma osmolality can be measured directly by determining freezing point depression or vapor pressure.[13,14] Variable changes in the plasma sodium concentration occur with hyperglycemia. Since glucose enters cells slowly, an increase in the plasma glucose concentration raises effective plasma osmolality and causes water to move from the cells into the ECF. By dilution, this lowers the plasma Na^+ concentration. In theory, every 62 mg/dl increment in the plasma glucose concentration should draw enough water out of the cells to reduce the plasma Na^+ concentration by 1 mEq/l.[15,16]

The number of particles per gram of water determines the osmolality of a solution. Since sodium salts (particularly NaCl and $NaHCO_3$), glucose, and urea are primary extracellular osmoles, the plasma osmolality can be approximated from:

$$\text{Plasma osmolality } (P_{osm}) =$$
$$2 \times \text{Plasma } [Na^+] + \frac{[\text{Glucose}]}{18} + \frac{BUN}{2.8}$$
$$(\text{Eq.45.2})$$

where 2 reflects the osmotic contribution of the anion accompanying Na^+, and 18 and 2.8 represent the conversion of the plasma glucose concentration and blood urea nitrogen (BUN) from units of milligrams per deciliter (mg/dl) into millimoles per liter (mmol/l).

Although urea contributes to the absolute value of the P_{osm}, it does not act to hold water within the extracellular space because of its membrane permeability.

Therefore, urea is an ineffective osmole and does not contribute to the effective P_{osm}.

In general, the effective plasma osmolality can be calculated from or estimated from:

$$\text{Effective plasma osmolality} =$$
$$\text{Measured plasma osmolality} - \frac{BUN}{2.8}$$

or estimated from

$$\text{Effective plasma osmolality} =$$
$$2 \times \text{Plasma } [Na^+] + \frac{[\text{Glucose}]}{18} \qquad (\text{Eq.45.3})$$

Under normal circumstances, glucose and urea contribute less than 10 mOsm/kg H_2O, and the plasma Na^+ concentration is the main determinant of the plasma osmolality, the osmolality of body fluids can be estimated to be twice the plasma sodium concentration.[14]

The major ECF particles are Na^+ and its accompanying anions Cl^- and HCO_3^-; a high plasma sodium concentration is always associated with a high osmolality. This indicates that water is needed to restore isotonicity. The water deficit can be estimated from the plasma sodium level. The percentage increase in sodium concentration approximates the percentage decrease in total body water. The water deficit can be estimated by the equation:

$$\text{Water deficit} = \text{Total-body Water} \times \left(\frac{\text{Plasma } [Na^+]}{140} - 1 \right)$$
$$(\text{Eq.45.4})$$

Total body water varies with body size and fat content. It is approximately 60% of body weight in young men, 50% of body weight in old men and young women, and only 40% in elderly women.

DEFENSE MECHANISMS AGAINST WATER DEPLETION

Two primary mechanisms defend the body against water depletion and hyperosmolality of extracellular fluid space. These two defense mechanisms are the capacity of the kidney to excrete a concentrated urine, and stimulation of thirst to increase water intake. Each pathway is very effective and disturbance of the urinary concentrating mechanism alone generally does not cause hyperosmolality if the thirst mechanism is intact.

Control of ADH Secretion

Hypernatremia results in the stimulation of both the antidiuretic hormone (ADH) release and thirst by the hypothalamic osmoreceptors (Figure 45.1). Argenine vasopressin is the ADH in humans.[17] Argenine vasopressin binds to specific receptors on collecting ducts (V_2 receptors), which are coupled to cyclic AMP (cAMP) formation. The regulation of ADH release from the posterior pituitary is dependent primarily on two mechanisms: osmotic and nonosmotic pathways (Figure 45.2). The osmotic regulation of ADH is dependent on osmoreceptor cells in the anterior hypothalamus.[18] These cells, most likely by altering their volume, recognize changes in ECF osmolality. Cell volume is decreased readily by substances that are restricted to the ECF, such as hypertonic saline or hypertonic mannitol. These substances are effective in stimulating ADH release. In contrast, urea moves readily into cells, and therefore does not alter cell volume and does not effectively stimulate ADH release. A similar response pattern is evident when vasopressin release is studied in the hypothalamo—neurohypophyseal complex in organ culture. Specifically, sodium chloride, sucrose, and mannitol at 310 mOsm/kg H_2O cause a three-fold increase in argenine vasopressin release, while urea and glucose fail to stimulate vasopressin. These studies also support the view that the receptor responds to changes in osmolality rather than sodium. The effects of increased osmolality on vasopressin release are associated with a measurable increase in vasopressin precursor messenger RNA (mRNA) in the hypothalamus[19,20] and salt-loading increases vasopressin RNA in the pituitary.[21,22] Vasopressin release can also occur in the absence of changes in plasma osmolality.[23] Physical pain, emotional stress, hypoglycemia, and a decrease in blood pressure or blood volume are important nonosmotic stimuli for vasopressin release. A 7 to 10% decrement in blood pressure or blood volume causes the prompt release of vasopressin (Figure 45.2). Although there are considerable genetically-determined individual variations in both the threshold and sensitivity, a close correlation between argenine vasopressin and plasma osmolality has been demonstrated in subjects with various states of hydration (Figure 45.3).

The secretion of ADH generally begins when the plasma osmolality exceeds 275 to 285 mOsm/kg H_2O.

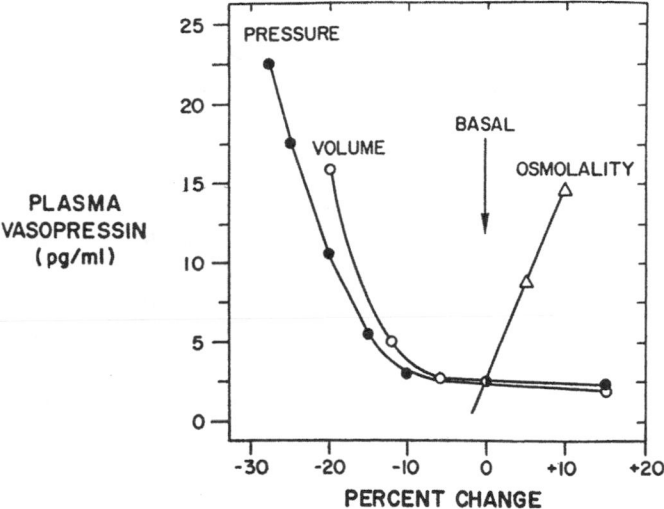

FIGURE 45.2 Osmotic and nonosmotic stimulation of arginine vasopressin release. (from ref. [90]).

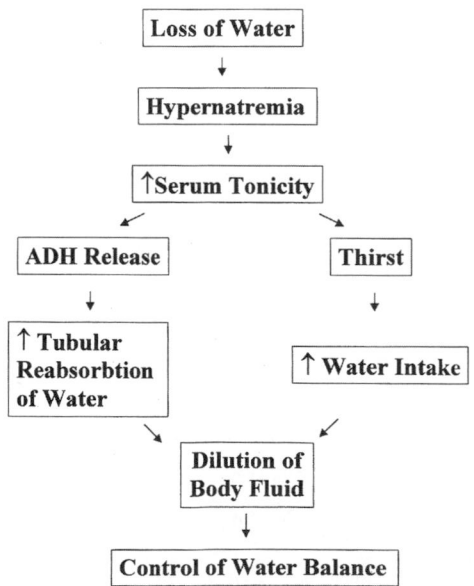

FIGURE 45.1 Regulation of water homeostasis: feedback loop for the stimulation of antidiuretic hormone (ADH) release and thirst. Hypernatremia results in an increase in the plasma osmolality, which enhances ADH secretion and thirst, resulting in water retention and a reduction in the plasma osmolality toward normal.

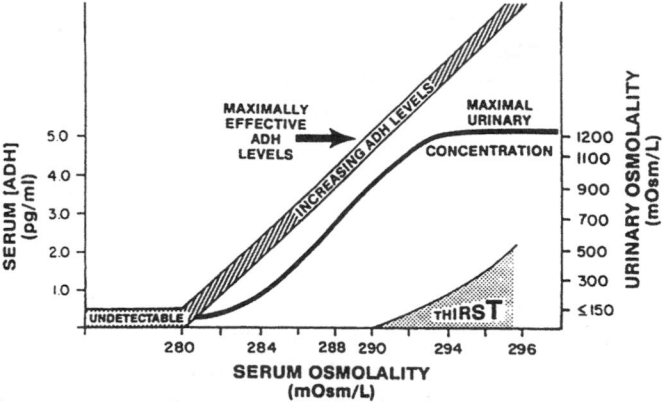

FIGURE 45.3 Antidiuretic hormone (ADH) levels, urinary osmolality, and thirst as functions of serum osmolality. (from ref. [188]).

The threshold for thirst appears to be approximately 10 mOsm/kg H_2O above that of vasopressin release. Prevention of a total body water deficit is thus largely dependent on water intake as modulated by thirst. The thirst center appears to be closely associated anatomically with the osmoreceptors in the region of the hypothalamus. Defects in thirst response may involve either organic or generalized central nervous system lesions, and can lead to severe water deficit even in the presence of a normal concentrating mechanism. The water deficit will occur more promptly if renal concentrating ability is also impaired.[24]

Thirst and the Maintenance of Hypernatremia

Thirst is, in fact, so effective that even patients with complete diabetes insipidus avoid hypernatremia by fluid intake in excess of 10 l/day.[25-27] Hypernatremia supervenes, therefore, only when hypotonic fluid losses occur in combination with a disturbance in water intake. This is most commonly seen in the aged with an alteration in level of consciousness, in the very young with inadequate access to water or in a rare subject with a primary disturbance in thirst.[28,29] Prevention of a total body water deficit is thus largely dependent on water intake as modulated by thirst. The thirst center appears to be closely associated anatomically with the osmoreceptors in the region of the hypothalamus. Defects in thirst response may involve either organic or generalized central nervous system lesions, and can lead to severe water deficit even in the presence of a normal concentrating mechanism.

In summary, persistent hypernatremia does not occur in normal subjects, because the ensuing rise in plasma osmolality stimulates both the releases of ADH, thereby minimizing further water loss and, more importantly, thirst. The associated increase in water intake then lowers the plasma sodium concentration back to normal. This regulatory system is so efficient that the plasma osmolality is maintained within a range of 1% to 2%, despite wide variations in sodium and water intake. Even patients with diabetes insipidus, who often have marked polyuria due to diminished ADH effect, maintain a near-normal plasma sodium concentration by appropriately increasing water intake. The net effect is that hypernatremia primarily occurs in those patients who cannot express thirst normally: infants and adults with impaired mental status.[30] The latter most often occurs in the elderly, who also appear to have diminished osmotic stimulation of thirst. A patient with a plasma sodium concentration of 150 mEq/l or more who is alert but not thirsty has, by definition, a hypothalamic lesion affecting the thirst center.

CELLULAR RESPONSE TO HYPERNATREMIA

Volume Regulation

When exposed to a change in extracellular osmolality, a cell shrinks or swells and subsequently exhibits either a regulatory volume increase or a regulatory volume decrease.[31-33] When exposed to hypertonicity, a cell loses water until the intracellular and extracellular osmolality are equal. Recovery of water is mediated by accumulation of inorganic and organic solutes known as osmolytes.[31,34] The principle inorganic osmolytes are Na^+, K^+, and Cl^-. The principle organic osmolytes may be classified into three general groups: polyols; methylamines; and amino acids.[35] A comparison of major and minor organic osmolytes for the kidney and brain are depicted in Table 45.1.

While hypernatremia in mammals affects all tissues, the greatest potential for harm is to the brain and kidney. Of these two organs, even modest changes in serum osmolality can have severe consequences to the brain, resulting in volume changes.[36] In the brain, acute hypernatremia is associated with a rapid decrease in water content and a corresponding increase in solute concentration.[32] In a study of rats by Cserr and co-workers,[37,38] acute hypernatremia (plasma Na^+ = 180 mEq/l) was accompanied by a prompt

TABLE 45.1 Organic Osmolytes in Kidney and Brain

Organic Osmolyte	Kidney [252-254]	Brain [32,33]
Major	Glutamate	Glutamate
	Glutamine	Glutamine
	Taurine	Taurine
	Myoinositol	Myoinositol
	Urea	Urea
	Alanine	Alanine
	Sorbitol	Aspartate
	GPC	Glycine
	Betaine	GABA
Minor	Val/Leu/Isoleu	Theonine
	Phosphocreatine	GPC
	Creatine	Betaine
		Choline
		Phosphocreatine
		Lysine
		Serine

GABA: γ-aminobutyric acid; GPC: glycerophosphorylcholine.

TABLE 45.2 Proposed Hypothesis for Cellular Osmoregulation in the Kidney

Name	Details	Reference
Compatible osmolyte principle	Cells accumulate high levels of polyols or certain amino acids that do not affect protein function in contrast to NaCl or KCl	255
Counteracting osmolyte principle	Cells accumulate methylamines (i.e., GPC or betaine) to attenuate the destabilizing effect of urea on protein structure	256,257
Constant transmembrane gradient	Cells maintain constant transmembrane gradients for sodium and potassium, thus the driving force for sodium gradient-coupled transport systems for organic and inorganic solutes	258,259

TABLE 45.3 Effect of Early Hypertonic Stress on Kidney Cell Function

General Function	Reference
DNA: Damage, inhibition of repair, dissociation of protein from chromatin, induction of p53	44,58,260,261,262
Metabolism, cell growth: Disruption of mitochondria function, cell cycle arrest, growth factor-dependent signaling inhibition, alteration in cytoskeletal structure, inhibition of protein translation	261,263−272
Secondary stress, apoptosis: Induction of secondary oxidative stress, apoptosis	261,265,273

decrease (7%) in total brain water content. The fall in water content was less than expected for simple osmotic behavior, indicating significant volume regulation had occurred. Moreover, the decrease in total brain water was the result of a fall in extracellular volume. Intracellular volume was not significantly changed at 30 and 90 minutes. The rapid regulatory volume increase was mediated by increases in Na^+, K^+, and Cl^-.[38] Most of these ions were derived from bulk flow of NaCl from cerebral spinal fluid (CSF). There was also a lesser contribution of electrolytes from the blood. During experimental hypernatremia in rabbits, intracellular brain water content also decreased by 12% at 1 hour and by 17% at 4 hours, accompanied by a corresponding increase in intracellular osmolality.[39] Most of the acute increase in brain osmolality was due to an increase in intracellular sodium and potassium concentration.[40] Although a substantial component of the increase in electrolyte concentration resulted from transcellular water loss, whole brain electrolyte content also increased, with the sodium content increasing from 268 ± 9 mm/kg dry weight in control animals to 321 ± 19 mmol/kg dry weight after 4 hours of hypernatremia. After sustained hypernatremia of 7 days duration, brain water and volume values were restored to normal. More prolonged hypernatremia results in accumulation of organic osmolytes to restore total brain water content to normal levels.[41−43]

In the kidney, the general mechanism for cellular osmoregulation in the face of hypertonic conditions involves the accumulation of organic rather than inorganic osmolytes. This strategy for the transport of organic rather than inorganic osmolytes across the cellular membrane has been explained in at least three hypothesized mechanisms, as detailed in Table 45.2. However, before mounting a coordinated osmoresponse, cells experience a "molecular mayhem"[44] due to the initial decrease in cellular volume, resulting in crowding of macromolecules and an increase in ionic osmolytes. These early changes in the cellular status, as well as the loss of water which can affect a variety of biochemical processes, can result in a variety of deleterious effects on normal cellular functions and viability, as depicted in Table 45.3.

Osmolytes

Organic molecules serve an important biologic function in the process of cellular osmoregulation.[4] When extracellular osmolality increases, organic molecules accumulate in the cells, thus maintaining cell volume and counteracting the perturbation of enzyme function and protein structure by high concentrations of inorganic ions and other molecules such as urea.[45] Lien and his co-workers[32] studied the effect of varying degrees and duration of hypernatremia on the concentrations of substances believed to be important idiogenic brain osmoles in rats using conventional biochemical assays, nuclear magnetic resonance spectroscopy, and high performance liquid chromatography. Idiogenic osmoles have been postulated to develop in the brain cells of patients suffering from chronic elevations in the osmolality of ECF. Moreover, the rapid correction of the osmolality in such patients is associated with the development of cerebral edema.

It has been known for more than 35 years that changes in intracellular brain sodium and potassium concentrations cannot account for all of the observed changes in brain osmolality that occur during chronic exposure to extracellular hypernatremia. The solutes that develop to maintain equality between extracellular and intracellular brain osmolality during this adaptation to hyperosmotic stress have been investigated by several groups. Arieff and his associates[46,47] have demonstrated that osmoles accumulated in the brain of chronic hypernatremic, but not in acute hypernatremic,

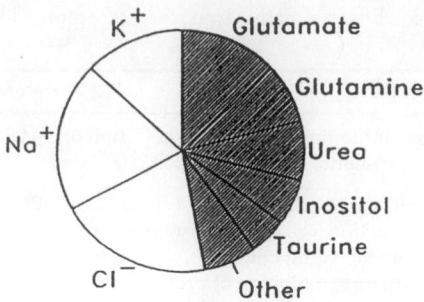

FIGURE 45.4 Relative changes in brain osmolytes in chronic hypernatremia. *(from ref. [32]).*

rabbits. Other investigators have shown that the level of amino acids and their derivatives, such as glutamine, taurine, and urea, rise in the brain of chronic hypernatremic animals, and account for about half of the increment of brain osmoles.[48] However, many of the idiogenic osmoles have not yet been characterized in brain tissue. Polyols and trimethylamines accumulate intracellularly in marine animals, plants, and bacteria when extracellular or environmental osmolality is significantly increased. In this study, it was found that the inorganic osmolytes account for 50% to 60% of the increase in solute content, whereas organic osmolytes account for the remainder during adaptation to chronic hypernatremia (Figure 45.4).

Recovery from chronic hypernatremia involves a small transient rise in brain water, which is restored to normal within 48 hours. With the exception of myoinositol, all the electrolytes and organic osmoles fall to normal levels within 24 to 48 hours. The cellular mechanisms responsible for the loss of intracellular organic osmolytes are poorly understood. *In vitro* studies of brain tissue found that cell swelling causes rapid loss of electrolytes and organic osmolytes. The losses of cellular K^+ and Cl^- are likely mediated by swelling-activated ion channels. Characterization of the organic osmolyte efflux pathways suggests that they represent pores or channels in the membrane that are permeable to Cl^-, as well as small organic salts. Roy and Banderali described a chloride channel that can transport small organic solutes, such as taurine and amino acids.[5] No specific inhibitors of the pathways are known. However, inhibitors of arachidonic acid metabolism are able to prevent activation of the efflux pathway, implicating eicosanoids in the signal transduction mechanism.

Lien et al.[32,33] reviewed previous studies to estimate the percentage of the osmolality that is still idiogenic. The contributions of electrolytes and other solutes to the changes in brain osmolality for various durations

and degrees of hypernatremia were reported in different studies (Table 45.4).

As a group, amino acids represent the major pool of brain organic osmolytes (20–30%); polyols and methylamines represent 7 to 10%. Taurine, a sulfonated amino acid, appears to be very important in neonatal brain volume regulation. Urea (8%–9%), unlike other osmolytes, is not preferentially accumulated intracellularly. Therefore, the vast majority of the total change in brain osmolality can be accounted for by changes in the concentrations of measured solutes. In other words, there are no significant idiogenic brain osmoles.[49,50]

Response to hypertonic conditions in the kidney depends on the cell type, as determined by presence along the nephron. Microdissection of kidney nephron segments for study is difficult; however, data may be obtained from *in vitro* studies of stable cell lines derived from specific nephron segments. An example of the heterogeneous nature of osmolyte accumulation in response to hypertonic stress in cells along the nephron is depicted in Figure 45.5.

While these data only summarize the changes in selected organic osmolytes, the data indicate that different cells accumulate different osmolytes when challenged to increasing extracellular tonicity. Proximal and distal tubule cells accumulate more myoinositol compared with inner medullary collecting duct cells, and the reverse is true for glycerophosphorylcholine (GPC) in collecting duct cells. The cells located in the inner medullary collecting duct (IMCD) cells are exposed to the greatest range in tonicity, and are therefore valuable in studying the effects of chronic hypertonicity on cellular accumulation of organic osmolytes. Figure 45.6 demonstrates that $IMCD_3$ cells accumulate varying amounts of different organic osmolytes in response to increasing levels of tonicity.

Of interest in these cells is the substantial accumulation of sorbitol at substantially high hypertonic conditions. Sorbitol plays an important role in the osmotic response, especially at high tonicity, because it is not required to be transported across the membrane in the face of a substantial concentration gradient, but rather is metabolized from glucose by the cellular protein aldose reductase (AR). Thus, within the same cell line of the kidney, substantial changes in the accumulation of specific osmolytes occur with increasing tonicity. In the kidney, further metabolism of sorbitol by sorbitol dehydrogenase (SDH) produces fructose (polyol pathway). Studies show that $IMCD_3$ cells chronically adapted to increasing levels of tonicity increase AR message, while at the same time decreasing message for SDH (Figure 45.7). This allows cells to accumulate the organic osmolyte sorbitol. During a reduction in tonicity, cells can export sorbitol from the cell via

TABLE 45.4 Published Experimental Models of Animals with Hypernatremia.

Duration	Animal Species	Changes of Osmolality (mmol/kg)	Contribution to Osmolality Change				Reference
			Na$^+$	K$^+$	Cl$^+$	Other Solutes	
ACUTE HYPERNATREMIA (HOURS)							
1	Rat	139	24	24	ND	Amino acids Urea	106
1	Rabbit	60	38	32	18	ND	47
2	Rat	101	ND	ND	ND	Urea	32,33
3	Rat	117	30	19	30	ND	43
4	Rat	55	ND	ND	ND	Amino acids	274
4	Rabbit	96	21	26	24	Amino acids	47
9	Rabbit	118	29	19	25	ND	49
CHRONIC HYPERNATREMIA (DAYS)							
3	Rat	74	ND	ND	ND	Polyols	275
4	Rat	83	ND	ND	ND	Amino acids	274
4	Mouse	80	19	26	ND	Amino acids Urea	48
5	Rat	50	ND	ND	ND	Amino acids Methylamines polyols	34
7	Rat	80	25	1	25	ND	43
7	Rabbit	80	8	5	15	Amino acids	47
		58	28	21	19	ND	
7	Rat	102	ND	ND	ND	Amino acids Methylamines Polyols urea	32,33

ND: no data.

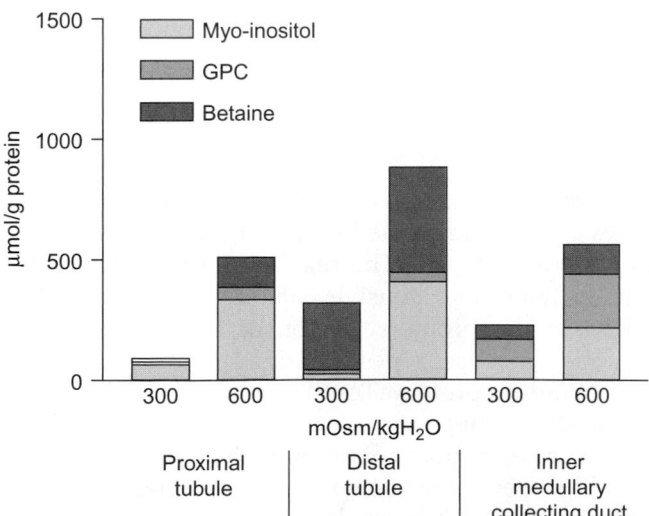

FIGURE 45.5 **Comparison of typical organic osmolytes accumulated in cell lines derived from the proximal tubule (LLC-PK1), distal tubule (thick ascending loop of Henle [TALH]), and inner medullary collecting duct (IMCD).** *(From ref. [250, 251]).*

sorbitol permease or by upregulation of SDH, thereby converting sorbitol to fructose with eventual recycling to glucose in the cell.

Accumulations of minor organic osmolytes in the kidney are similar to major organic osmolytes in demonstrating differential accumulation with increasing levels of hypertonicity. Figure 45.8 shows that, similar to major organic osmolytes, IMCD cells accumulate various amino acids as minor organic osmolytes to different levels in response to increasing extracellular tonicity. Glutamate and glutamine constitute the greatest level of accumulation.

Adaptation to Hypertonicity: *in Vivo* versus *in Vitro*

Interestingly, osmotic tollerance and adaptation is quite different in kidney tissues compared to cells grown *in vitro*. In the medulla of the kidney, cells routinely are bathed in hypertonic interstitum which

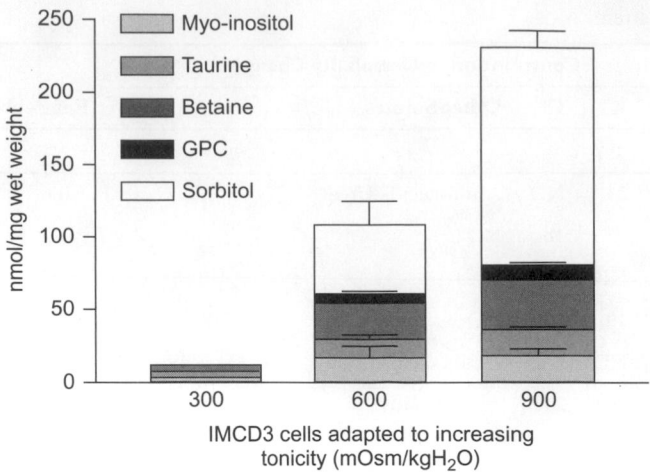

FIGURE 45.6 Comparison of relative changes in common organic osmolyte concentration in IMCD3 cells chronically adapted to increasing tonicity. *(from ref. [254]).*

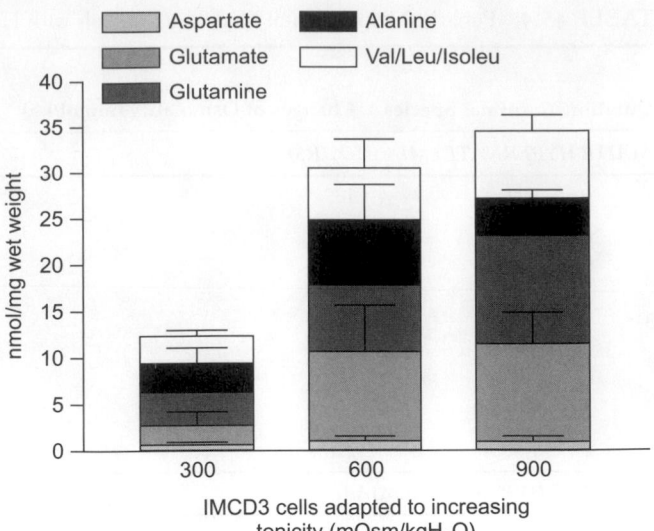

FIGURE 45.8 Selective accumulation of amino acids as minor organic osmolytes in inner medullary collecting duct cells at increasing extracelluar tonicity. *(from ref. [254]).*

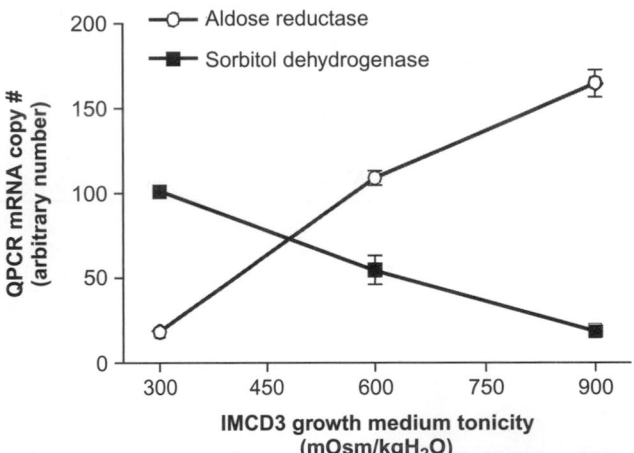

FIGURE 45.7 Changes in cellular message levels for aldose reductase and sorbitol dehydrogenase in IMCD3 cells in response to chronic adaptation to increasing tonicity.

Furthermore, they demonstrated that hormone additions, including insulin-like growth factor I, epidermal growth factor or vasopressin, and use of growth supports including porous media, collagen I, collagen IV, fibronectin, laminin or fibrillar collagen I, have no significant effect on cellular adaptation to acute increases in tonicity.[55] Rather, these researchers suggested that cells which demonstrate greater proliferative rates, and thus increased DNA replication, are more sensitive to acute changes in tonicity.[53,58] This level of sensitivity to acute changes in tonicity can be blunted if cells in culture are preadapted to moderate levels of tonicity.[53]

Regulation of Transcription in Response to Hypertonicity

Hypertonicity-induced stimulation of transcription plays an important role in the adaptation of renal cells to hypertonicity.[59,60] The regulatory sequence element named tonicity-responsive enhancer (TonE) has been found in the promoter region of a large number of osmotic response genes identified in Table 45.5. The TonE-binding protein (TonEBP) mediates the transcriptional stimulation in response to hypertonicity. These sequences have been found in the 52 flanking region of the aldose reductase gene in several species, suggesting a common mechanism by which tonicity response genes are regulated.[59,60] The TonEBP protein has been cloned by a number of researchers naming this protein nuclear factor of activated T-cell 5 (NFAT5),[61] NFAT-like protein 1 (NFATL1),[62] and osmotic response

reaches 1000 mOsm/kgH$_2$O or more during antidiuresis[51] without signs of cell injury.[52,53] However, cultured kidney cells including mouse IMCD3[54] and inner medullary epithelial cells[53,55] demonstrate substantial cell death with acute changes in media tonicity. For cultured cells, the rate at which cells are exposed to increases in tonicity plays an important role in adaptation and survival. Capasso and co-workers demonstrated that small increases of 50–100 mOsm/KgH$_2$O allow IMCD3 cells to be adapted to levels of 900 mOsm/KgH$_2$O or greater.[56,57] Extensive studies by Cai and co-workers determined a similar finding for mIM cells, in that a linear increase in culture tonicity allowed for better adaptation and survival.[53,55]

TABLE 45.5 Tonicity Enhancer Binding Protein (TonEBP) Target Genes

Target Gene			
Gene Name	Abbreviation	Function	Reference
Aldose reductase	AR	Conversion of glucose to sorbitol	78,276
Sodium/myoinositol co-transporter	SMIT	Transports myoinositol	78,277
Sodium/chloride/ betaine co-transporter	BGT1	Transport betaine	60,78
Urea transporter	UT-A	Vasopressin-regulated urea transporter	278
Taurine transporter	TauT	Specific amino acid transporter	279
Heat shock protein 70	HSP70−2	Molecular chaperone	77,280
Sodium-coupled neutral amino acid transporter-2	ATA2, SNAT2	Neutral amino acid transporter	281
Osmotic stress protein 94	Osp94	Putative molecular chaperone	282
Aquaporin 2	AQP2	Water channel	78,283

element-binding protein (OREBP).[63] TonEBP/NFAT5 belongs to the Rel family of transcription factors which includes NF-kB and the calcineurin binding NFATs.[64] This family is defined by the conserved Rel DNA-binding domain.[65] The DNA-binding domain of TonEBP/NFAT5 has the ability to encircle the DNA, which may allow for greater kinetic stability.[66] The TonEBP/NFAT5 DNA-binding domain requires dimerization similar to NF-kB proteins to bind to DNA. In addition, TonEBP/NFAT5 forms dimers only with itself and not with other members of the Rel family. It also has a stricter recognition sequence (TGGAAAC/A/T) as compared to other Rel proteins.

Regulation of TonEBP/NFAT5 transcriptional activity in response to hypertonicity involves: (1) nuclear translocation; (2) upregulation of transcriptional activity; and (3) enhanced synthesis. Under unstimulated conditions, TonEBP/NFAT5 proteins shuttle in and out of the nucleus. However, following exposure of cells to hypertonic conditions, essentially all of the TonEBP/NFAT5 protein is translocated to the nucleus. This trafficking of TonEBP/NFAT5 to the nucleus is regulated by both specific nuclear localization sequences (NLS) and specific nucleoporin complexes.[67] Under hypertonic conditions, Nucleoporin 88 is upregulated in IMCD3 cells, and acts in concert with other nucleoporins to form a complex which retains TonEBP/NFAT5 to the nucleus. Transcriptional activation of TonEBP/NFAT5 is via the hypertonicity-responsive C-terminal domain.[68,69] While TonEBP/NFAT5 is phosphorylated in response to hypertoncity, and phosphorylation correlates with increased transactivation activity, activation can also occur in the presence of increased tonicity without phosphorylation.[68] Various studies have identified a number of kinases to be involved in phosphorylation of TonEBP/NFAT5 including p38, Fyn, PKA, ATM, and PI3K.[70−73] Finally, TonEBP/NFAT5 is also regulated by increased synthesis, resulting in substantial increases in protein under hypertonic conditions.[69,74] Increased levels of TonEBP/NFAT5 mRNA under hypertonic conditions are in part due to enhanced stabilization of pre-existing mRNA mediated by the 5′UTR of the message.[75]

An alternative role for TonEBP/NFAT5 has slowly emerged as additional transcriptional targets are identified. Lee and co-workers have used microarray analysis to identify greater than 100 genes in which transcription was upregulated two-fold or greater under a moderate increase in tonicity.[76] While the conventional osmotic response targets were identified (see Table 45.5), non-osmolyte accumulating genes were identified including asporin, insulin-like growth factor-binding protein 5 and 7, and extracellular lysophospholipase D. While mice lacking TonEBP/NFAT5 demonstrate reduced embryo survival and substantial perinatal death, implicating renal defects,[77,78] embryonic lethality may not be renal in nature as the maintenance of the extracellular milieu of the developing embryo is dependent on the placenta, and not the developing kidney.[64] In fact, TonEBP/NFAT5 has been shown to be expressed in most developing organs of the mouse embryo.[79] Furthermore, Dressler and co-workers have shown that Pax-2 knockout mice, which fail to develop kidneys, do not suffer from embryonic lethality.[80] While the exact nature of TonEBP/NFAT5 involvement in embryonic organ development is still unknown, it is likely extremely important to embryo development.

Nuclear Magnetic Resonance Spectroscopy

Nuclear magnetic resonance (NMR) is a physical phenomenon of atomic nuclei that has many biochemical and biophysical applications.[81−83] The methodologies derived from NMR imaging enable the chemical identification of different molecules, kinetic analysis of suitable chemical reactions, studies of secondary and tertiary protein structure, and analysis of receptor−ligand interactions. It is this latter application that has become an important clinical tool. The application of spectroscopy, in concert with different imaging methods, ultimately may prove even more valuable than imaging alone in our understanding of the pathogenesis of different diseases. Bloch and Purcell first demonstrated NMR as a physical phenomenon, independently, in 1946. The fundamental basis of the NMR phenomenon is that nuclei have a quantum characteristic called spin, which because of the charged nature of the nucleus results in these nuclei having magnetic moments, and the net biological samples having magnetic moment in the direction of an applied external magnetic field (Bo). Transitions between the spin state aligned with and against the Bo field can be induced by a radiofrequency pulse, and sampled by radiofrequency antenna as free induction decay (FID). The FID can be transformed from a plot of magnetization-versus-time to a plot of magnetization-versus-frequency, also called an NMR spectrum, by a mathematical manipulation called a Fourier transformation. The frequency of the FID (υ) can be predicted by the knowledge of the nucleus under study and its gyromagnetic ratio (τ), and the magnitude of the Bo field by the following relationship:

$$\upsilon = \tau Bo / 2\pi \qquad (45.5)$$

The area under the resultant spectral peak is directly proportional to the quantity of nuclei existing free in solution in the sample being studied. This, in fact, is the basis of NMR imaging experiments. Spectroscopic methodologies make use of the fact that the chemical environment of a given nucleus placed in a Bo field will affect the effective magnetic field of a given nucleus (B_{eff}). This can be described by the chemical environment of a nucleus defining the density of the electron cloud about that nucleus, which tends to appose the Bo field. We can, therefore, describe a shielding constant σ that results from this electron cloud apposing the Bo field in the following equation:

$$B_{eff} = Bo \ (1 - \sigma) \qquad (45.6)$$

The magnitude of σ is usually small, and it is expressed in the dimensionless term of parts per million (ppm). This means that the spectrum acquired from a sample, containing the same nucleus in different chemical environments, will have multiple spectral peaks corresponding to these different chemical environments, allowing for chemical identification on the basis of the shielding constants of these nuclei, also known as chemical shift. Chemical shift, expressed in parts per million, is independent of the strength of the Bo field. Although other physical phenomena may be used in chemical identification (e.g., spin coupling, nuclear Overhauser effect), chemical shift is the primary method of chemical identification that has been used in NMR of living tissues.[81,82]

Figure 45.9 shows the H-1 NMR spectra of brain extract from normal and hypernatremic rats. The most prominent peaks represent N-acetylaspartate (2.02 ppm) and phosphocreatine (3.03 and 3.93 ppm). The peaks in the range of 2.0 to 2.5 ppm represent primarily amino acids, which have not been completely characterized yet. But it was evident that the peak area was larger in severe chronic hypernatremia than normal rat. The major peaks of polyols and trimethylamines were located between 3.1 and 3.9 ppm; GPC, 3.23; betaine, 3.26; myoinositol, 3.27, 3.57, 3.59, 3.61, and 4.06; and sorbitol, 3.85 ppm. We observed the increase of GPC, betaine, and myoinositol in severe chronic hypernatremia compared with normal rats. Sorbitol peak was not visualized in normal rats with severe chronic hypernatremia. The spectra of brain extracts from acute hypernatremia were similar to those of normal rats, and thus are not shown.[32]

Using clinical magnetic resonance imaging (MRI) and spectroscopy, Lee and his co-workers[84] examined an 18-month-old girl with severe dehydration and hypernatremia (plasma sodium concentration 195 mEq/l). A conventional 1.5 Tesla (1.5 T) Sigma General Electric magnetic resonance scanner was used. After MRI, quantitative proton NMR spectroscopy was performed in the parietal and occipital regions of the patient's cerebral cortex, revealing primarily white matter and gray matter, respectively. Spectra from the same regions in 50 healthy infants were also acquired. MRI revealed partial haloprosencephaly. Proton NMR spectroscopy of occipital gray matter and parietal white matter revealed several striking abnormalities (Figure 45.10). The principle abnormality was a reversal of the normal ratio of peak intensities between the neuronal metabolite N-acetylaspartate and the putative osmolyte myoinositol. The principle change was in the concentration of myoinositol, which was three times normal, whereas that of N-acetylaspartate was normal. Concentrations of choline and glutamine (plus glutamate) were also increased. The sequential spectra obtained during correction of the dehydration are shown (Figure 45.10).

The calculated concentrations of the five principle metabolites shown in the spectra of the infant's brain on days 4 to 36 are shown in Table 45.6. The direct determination of patterns of disordered cerebral organic osmolytes by proton NMR spectroscopy may be valuable in guiding therapy.[84,85]

NMR analyses of metabolic changes in the kidney in response to hypertonic stress have focused on specific cell lines and, in particular, the inner medullary collecting duct. Analysis of changes in organic osmolytes with respect to chronic adaptation of $IMCD_3$ cells to increasing tonicity from 300 to 900 mOsm/kg H_2O were studied by proton NMR, as shown in

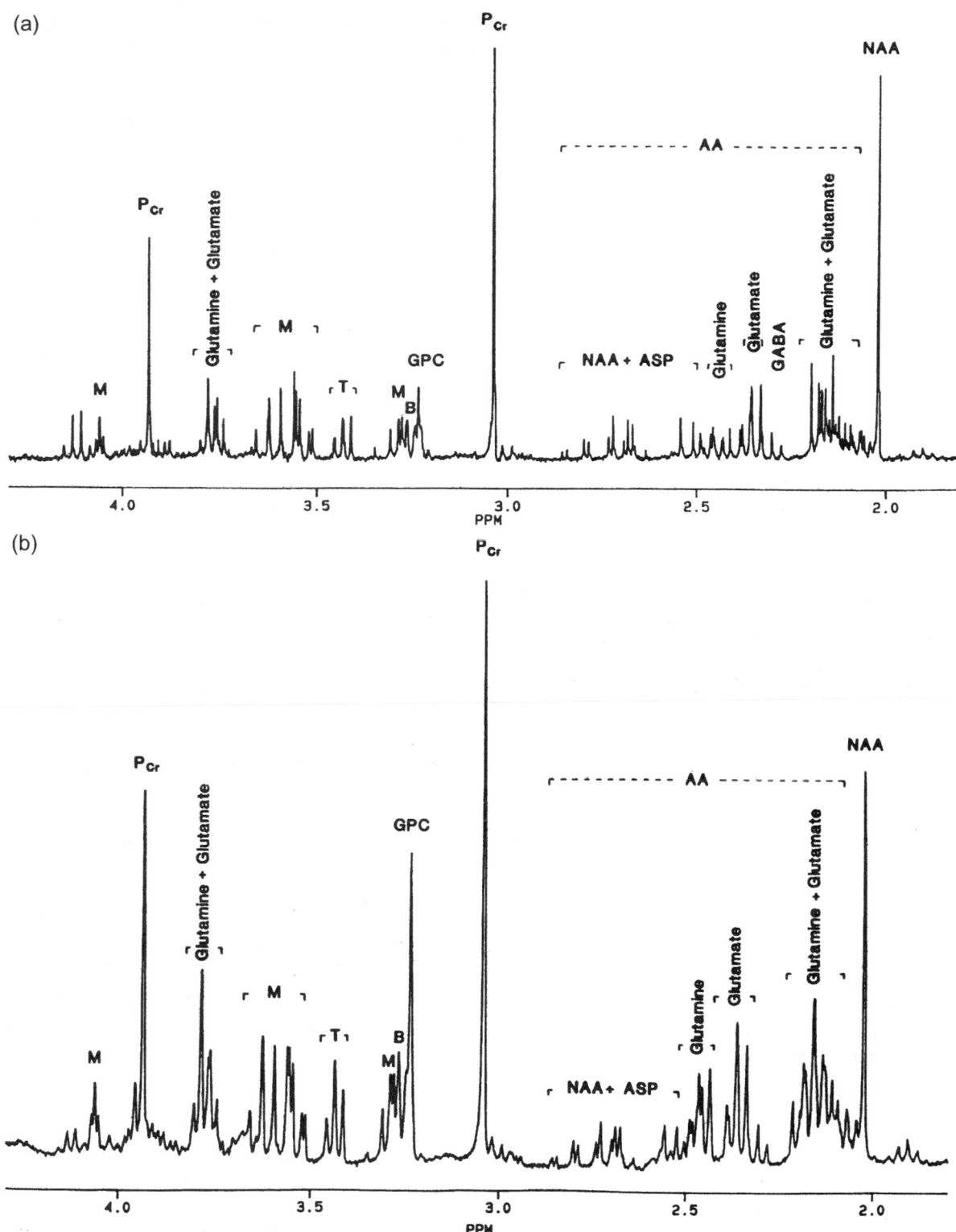

FIGURE 45.9 Proton nuclear magnetic resonance (NMR) spectra of brain extracts from normal rat (a) and severe chronic hypernatremic rat (b). These spectra are the sum of 128 transients and are referenced to trimethylsilylproprionate (TSP). Only peaks derived from glycerophosphoryl choline (GPC), betaine 67, myoinositol (M), amino acids (AA), phosphocreatine (PCr), and N-acetylaspartate (NAA) have been labeled. *(from ref. [32]).*

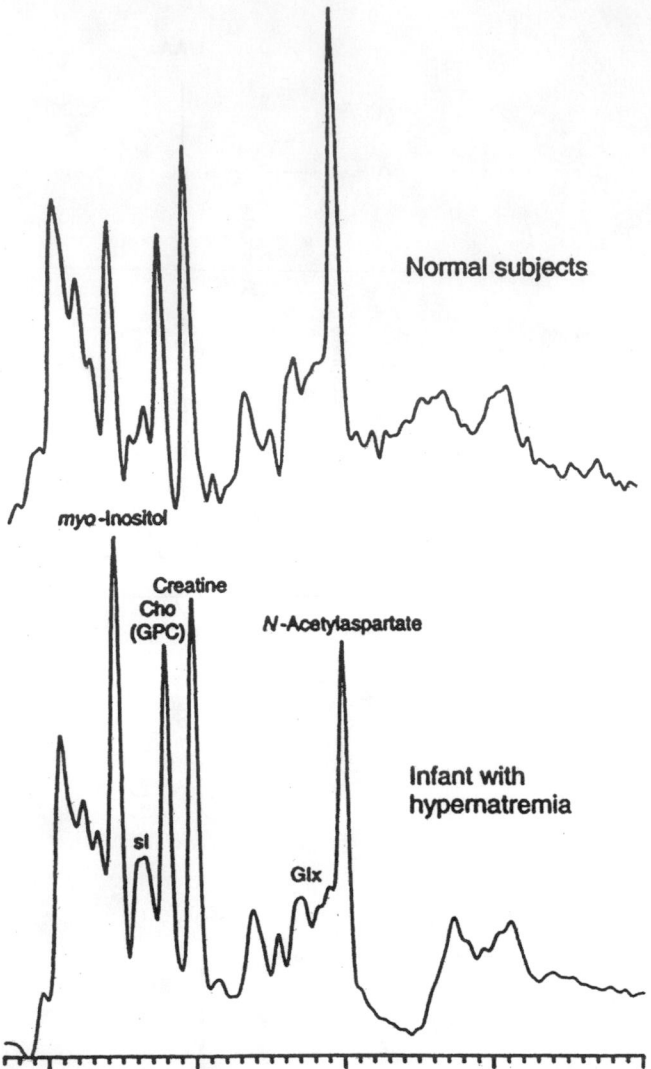

FIGURE 45.10 **Short-echo-time proton nuclear magnetic resonance (NMR) spectrum of cortical gray matter in an infant with severe dehydration.** The striking differences from normal in this patient were the apparent increase in myoinositol and the decrease in N-acetylaspartate. The increase in myoinositol was accompanied by increases in the concentrations of its stereoisomer, scyllo-inositol (sl), and choline-containing compounds (ho), especially glycerophosphoryl choline (GPC), glutamine plus glutamate (Glx), and creatine. *(from ref. [84]).*

Figure 45.11. Gross examination of NMR spectra demonstrates profound changes in nearly all organic osmolytes. Analysis of phosphorylated compounds can be determined by [86]P NMR, as shown in Figure 45.12. In a similar fashion, initial reflection indicates a substantial increase in GPC with more minor changes in GPE and PCr. While [86]P NMR has been used for analysis of nucleotide triphosphates (NTPs), possibly improved techniques involving HPLC-MS appear to provide for higher sensitivity, greater reproducibility, and throughput for analytical measurements.

ETIOLOGY OF HYPERNATREMIC STATES

Hypernatremia may be due to primary Na^+ gain or water deficit (Table 45.7). The two components of an appropriate response to hypernatremia are increased water intake stimulated by thirst, and the excretion of the minimum volume of maximally-concentrated urine reflecting ADH secretion in response to an osmotic stimulus.[87,88] Most cases of hypernatremia result from the loss of water. Since water is distributed between the ICF and the ECF in a 2:1 ratio, a given amount of solute-free water loss will result in a two-fold greater reduction in the ICF compartment than the ECF compartment. Sodium overload will result in hypernatremia with an increase in total body sodium, and the patient will have an increase in ECF. Water deficit, however, may occur with low or normal total body sodium.

Water deficit in excess of sodium deficit is associated with hypovolemic hypernatremia, and the patient will have low total body sodium. When hypernatremia is caused by pure water loss, the patient is euvolemic and the total body sodium remains normal. The causes of water losses in both of these settings may be renal or extrarenal. Renal losses of water may be a consequence of diabetes insipidus or osmotic diuresis. Diabetes insipidus will be discussed in more detail later in this chapter, in hypernatremia associated with normal total body sodium.

In the absence of increased water losses, hypernatremia can still develop (with normal total body sodium) if there is primary hypothalamic disease impairing thirst (called *hypodipsia*). Two different syndromes have been described, which are most often due to tumors, granulomatous diseases (such as sarcoidosis) or vascular disease. In the first, there is a defect in thirst, with or without concomitant diabetes insipidus. In this disorder, forced water intake is usually sufficient to maintain a normal plasma sodium concentration.[89,90] Other hypodipsic patients will not respond to water-loading, as the excess water will be excreted in the urine with little change in the plasma sodium concentration.[91,92]

Transient hypernatremia (in which the plasma sodium concentration can rise by 10 to 15 mEq/l within a few minutes) can be induced by severe exercise or seizures, which are also associated with the development of lactic acidosis. In this setting, the breakdown of glycogen into smaller, more osmotically active molecules (such as lactate) can increase the cell osmolality, thereby causing the osmotic movement of water into the cells. The plasma sodium concentration returns to normal within 5 to 15 minutes after the cessation of exertion.

TABLE 45.6 Results of Clinical Proton NMR Specteroscopy for Cerebral Osmometry of the Brain of an Infant with Hypernatremia and Normal Subjects

Metabolite	Normal Subjects	Study Patients (mmol)				
		Day 4	Day 7	Day 11	Day 22	Day 36
Myoinositol	6	18	13	13	11	10
Choline	1.5	3.3	2.6	2.7	2.7	2.5
Creatine	8	10	8	9	8	8
Glutamine plus glutamate	15	18	15	15	15	10
N-acetylaspartate	8	6	6	7	7	7
Total	38.5	55.3	44.6	46.7	43.7	37.5
Excess metabolite	0	+ 16.8	+ 6.1	+ 8.2	+ 5.2	− 1.0

From Lee, J.H., Arcinue, E., and Ross, B. D. (1994). Brief report: Organic osmolytes in the brain of an infant with hypernatremia (see comments). N. Engl. J. Med. **331**, 439–442, with permission.

Peak areas were converted to concentrations as previously described.[266] The T1 and T2 relaxation times of water and each metabolite were within the normal range given in that report, except for myoinositol, for which the value obtained in this study was 209 msec. As compared with a mean (± SD) of 301 ± 33 in the study by Ernst et al.[266]

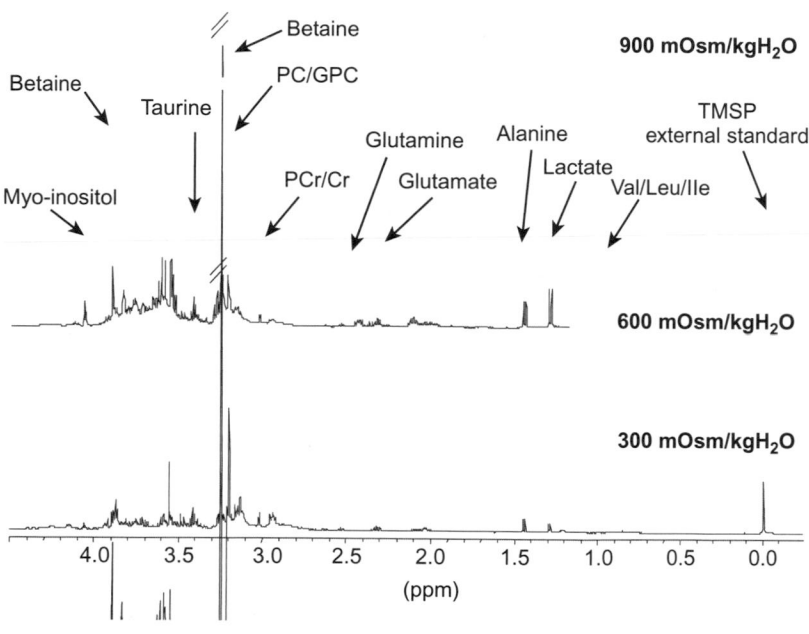

FIGURE 45.11 ¹H-nuclear magnetic resonance (NMR) spectra of PCA cell extracts. These spectra show the differences between cells cultivated in media containing 300 (bottom), 600 (middle), and 900 mOsm/kg H$_2$O (upper spectrum) (GPC: glycerophosphocholine; PC: phosphocholine; Cr: creatine; PCr: phosphocreatine; TMSP: trimethylsilyl propionic-2,2,3,3,-d4 acid).

CLASSIFICATION OF HYPERNATREMIA BASED ON TOTAL BODY SODIUM

Another clinical approach to the hypernatremic patient is based on the assessment of the ECF volume status and the total body sodium.

Hypernatremia in Patients with Low Total Body Sodium

Patients who sustain losses of both sodium and water, but with a relatively greater loss of water, are classified as having hypernatremia with low total body sodium. Signs of hypovolemia include orthostatic hypotension, tachycardia, flat neck veins, poor skin turgor, and dry mucous membranes. Isotonic sodium chloride should be given until systemic hemodynamics are stabilized.

The sources of free water loss that can lead to hypernatremia if intake is not increased include insensible water loss from the skin by evaporation and sweat, the loss of which is increased by fever, exercise, and exposure to high temperatures. Burns and infections will also increase the water loss. Some gastrointestinal losses, particularly osmotic diarrheas, will promote the

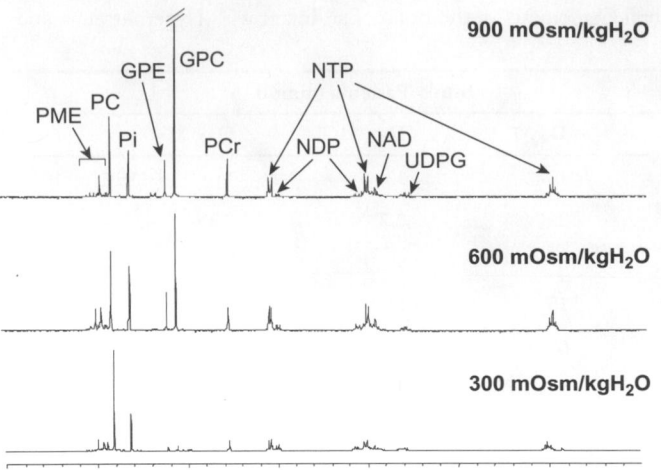

FIGURE 45.12 **^{31}P-nuclear magnetic resonance (NMR) spectra of PCA cell extracts.** These spectra show the differences between cells cultivated in media containing 300 (bottom), 600 (middle), and 900 mOsm/kg H_2O (upper spectrum) (PME: phosphomonoester; PC: phophocholine; Pi: inorganic phosphate; GPE: glycerophophoethanolamine; GPC: glycerophophocholine; PCr: phosphocreatine; NTP: nucleotide triphosphates; NDP: nucleotide diphosphates; NAD: nicotinamide adenine dinucleotide; UDPG: uridine diphosphosphate glucose).

TABLE 45.7 Etiology of Hypernatremic States

Water loss
Insensible
Increased sweating
Burns
Respiratory infections
Renal
Central diabetes insipidus
Nephrogenic diabetes insipidus
Osmotic diuresis
Gastrointestinal
Osmotic diarrhea
Hypothalamic
Primary hypodipsia
Reset osmostat due to volume expansion in primary mineralocorticoid excess
Water loss into cells
Seizures or severe exercise
Rhabdomyoluiss
Sodium overload
Administration of hypertonic NaCl or $NaHCO_3$
Ingestion of sodium

development of hypernatremia, because the sodium plus potassium concentration is less than that in the plasma.[93] Although primarily recognized in children, lactulose-induced diarrhea leading to hypernatremia appears to be common. Since the renal water- and sodium-conserving mechanisms operate normally in these patients, urinary osmolality is high (usually >800 mOsm/kg H_2O), and urinary sodium concentration is low (<10 mEq/l). An elevation in the plasma sodium concentration with diarrhea illness is particularly common in infants in whom fluid replacement with a relatively dilute solution can minimize the risk of hypernatremia. Decreased release of ADH or renal resistance to its effect causes the excretion of relatively dilute urine.[94,95] Most of these patients have a normal thirst mechanism. As a result, they typically present with polyuria and polydipsia, and at most a high-normal plasma sodium concentration. However, marked and symptomatic hypernatremia can occur if a central lesion impairs both ADH release and thirst, thereby preventing replacement of the urinary water losses.

An osmotic diuresis due to glucose, mannitol or urea causes an increase in urine output in which the sodium plus potassium concentration is well below that in the plasma, because of the presence of the nonreabsorbed organic solute. Patients with diabetic ketoacidosis or nonketotic hyperglycemia typically present with marked hyperosmolality, although the plasma sodium concentration may not be elevated due to hyperglycemia-induced water movement out of the cells. Hypotonic losses can also occur by the renal route during a loop diuretic-induced hypotonic diuresis or an osmotic diuresis with mannitol, glucose, glycerol or, more rarely, urea. Elderly patients with partial urinary tract obstruction can excrete large volumes of hypotonic urine.[96] The urine in these cases is hypotonic or isotonic, and the urinary sodium concentration is greater than 20 mEq/l. Since glucose and mannitol enhance osmotic water movement from the intracellular fluid to the ECF compartment, some of these patients may have a normal or even low serum sodium concentration, in spite of serum hypertonicity.

Hypernatremia in Patients with Normal Total Body Sodium

When hypernatremia is caused by pure water loss, total body sodium remains normal. Patients are usually euvolemic. The extrarenal sources of such water losses are the skin and the respiratory tract. A high environmental temperature, as well as a febrile or hypermetabolic states, can cause considerable water losses. If such hypotonic losses are not accompanied by appropriate water intake, hypernatremia supervenes. Urine osmolality is very high, reflecting an intact osmoreceptor—vasopressin—renal response. Urinary sodium concentration will vary according to the patient's sodium intake. This kind of hypernatremia has been reported in hepatic failure.[97] It was believed to occur due to total body water loss. The possible mechanisms include increased insensible losses, decreased access to water secondary to hepatic encephalopathy, and increased hypotonic losses in stool secondary to osmotic cathartics used for treatment of encephalopathy. Chronic alcoholic subjects with end-stage liver disease who present with fulminant liver failure and hepatic encephalopathy have a high mortality rate.[97,98] Patients with liver disease who develop hypernatremia are particularly susceptible to the development of cerebral demyelinating lesions.

Diabetes insipidus is a polyuric disorder characterized by high rates of electrolyte-free water excretion.[99] When these are not appropriately replaced, hypernatremia supervenes. The causes of central neurogenic diabetes insipidus are listed in Table 45.8. If the thirst mechanism is intact and water is available, patients with central diabetes insipidus do not develop hypernatremia, and thus have no symptoms except for the inconvenience associated with the marked polyuria and polydipsia. With concomitant hypodipsia, no access to water or an illness that precludes adequate water intake, however, severe and even life-threatening hypernatremia can supervene.

Hypernatremia secondary to nonosmotic urinary water loss is usually due to central or neurogenic diabetes insipidus characterized by impaired argenine vasopressin secretion or nephrogenic diabetes insipidus resulting from end-organ (renal) resistance to the actions of AVP. The most common cause of central diabetes insipidus is destruction of the neurohypophysis. This may occur as a result of trauma, neurosurgery, granulomatous disease, neoplasms, vascular accidents or infection. In many cases, central diabetes insipidus is idiopathic and may occasionally be hereditary. The familial form of the disease is inherited in an autosomal dominant fashion, and has been attributed to mutations in the propressophysin (argenine vasopressin precursor) gene.[100–104] Nephrogenic diabetes insipidus may be either inherited or acquired. Congenital nephrogenic diabetes insipidus I is an X-linked recessive trait due to mutations in the V2 receptor gene.[105–112] Mutations in the autosomal aquaporin-2 gene may also result in NDI.[113–118] The aquaporin-2 gene encodes the water channel protein whose membrane insertion is stimulated by AVP. The causes of sporadic nephrogenic diabetes insipidus are numerous, and include drugs (especially lithium),[119–126] hypercalcemia, hypokalemia, and conditions that impair medullary hypertonicity (e.g., papillary necrosis or osmotic diuresis).[127–131] Pregnant women, in the second or third trimester, may develop nephrogenic diabetes insipidus as a result of excessive elaboration of vasopressinase by the placenta.[132,133]

Congenital nephrogenic diabetes insipidus is a rare hereditary disorder in which the renal tubule is insensitive to vasopressin.[134] The disease manifests itself in the complete clinical form only in males and in a subclinical form in females, suggesting a sex-linked dominant inheritance with variable penetrance in the female. The gene responsible for the defect has, in fact, been mapped to region 28 on the long arm of the X-chromosome (Xq28). Although the disease is most probably inborn, the diagnosis is usually not made until the infant has hyposmolar urine with severe dehydration, hypernatremia, vomiting, and fever. Unlike some of the females, who have partial responsiveness to vasopressin, the male with the full-blown complete form of this disorder will not have hypertonic urine even in the face of severe dehydration. The impaired growth and occasional mental retardation that supervene in these cases are most likely due to repeated episodes of dehydration and hypernatremia, rather than being integral components of the disease. Hydronephrosis is also common in these patients, perhaps because of voluntary retention of large volumes of urine, with subsequent vesicoureteral reflux.[135]

Neither vasopressin nor other pharmacologic agents that potentiate its action or stimulate its release, such as chlorpropamide, are effective in concentrating the urine of patients with nephrogenic diabetes insipidus. An intact thirst mechanism is, therefore, indispensable for the maintenance of good hydration in children with this disorder, as is careful monitoring of fluid balance.

TABLE 45.8 Causes of Central Diabetes Insipidus (CDI)

Hereditary
Autosomal dominant
Autosomal recessive (Wolfram syndrome)
Acquired
Head trauma, skull fracture, and orbital trauma
Posthypophysectomy
Suprasellar and intrasellar tumors
Primary (suprasellar cyst, craniopharyngioma, pinealoma, meningioma, and glioma)
Metastatic (breast or lung cancer, leukemia, and lymphomas)
Granulomas
Sarcoid
Wegener granulomatosis
Tuberculosis
Syphilis
Histiocytosis
Eosinophilic granuloma
Hand–Schuller–Christian disease
Infections
Encephalitis
Meningitis
Guillain-Barre syndrome
Vascular
Cerebral aneurysm
Cerebral thrombosis or hemorrhage
Sickle cell disease
Postpartum necrosis (Sheehan syndrome)
Pregnancy (transient)

Since the excretion of solute requires further water losses, children with this disorder who need rehydration should receive hypotonic (2.5%) rather than isotonic (5%) glucose solutions. Glucosuria may occur with the latter solution, and thus aggravate fluid losses.

Limitation of oral solute intake (low-sodium diet) may also lead to a decrease in urine flow in patients with nephrogenic diabetes insipidus. Thiazide diuretics, which inhibit sodium reabsorption in the cortical diluting segment of the nephron, have met with some success in the management of these patients. The ability of thiazides to diminish sodium reabsorption in this water-impermeable portion of the nephron would itself decrease C_{H2O}, but not urine flow. It seems most likely that the decrease in urine flow is secondary to the sodium loss and ECF volume-contraction. ECF volume-depletion in turn decreases glomerular filtration rate (GFR), and increases proximal tubular sodium and water reabsorption. These secondary effects of the diuretic agent then decrease urine flow. The ECF volume-contraction can be maintained with a low sodium intake after discontinuance of the diuretic, so that the therapy still remains effective. The addition of amiloride to hydrochlorothiazide may provide added benefit.[136–139] Nonsteroidal anti-inflammatory agents have been found to be effective.

The acquired form of nephrogenic diabetes insipidus is much more common than the congenital form of the disease, but it is rarely severe.[140] While maximal concentrating ability is impaired in this disorder, the ability to elaborate a hypertonic urine is usually preserved. Nocturia, polyuria, and polydipsia may occur in this acquired form of nephrogenic diabetes insipidus, but the urine volumes are generally less (<3–4 l/day) than those observed with complete central diabetes insipidus, psychogenic water-drinking or congenital nephrogenic central diabetes insipidus. The more common causes of acquired nephrogenic diabetes insipidus are listed in Table 45.9.

A defect in renal concentrating capacity is a consistent accompaniment of most forms of advanced renal failure.[141,142] Thus, chronic renal failure constitutes a form of acquired nephrogenic diabetes insipidus. Advanced renal insufficiency of any cause can cause a vasopressin resistance associated with hypotonic urine. In some forms of kidney disease vasopressin unresponsiveness can occur at a stage when GFR is not markedly diminished. The occurrence of a profound diuresis in association with a concentrating defect in glomerular diseases of the kidney is rare and, in general, a close correlation exists between GFR and maximal urinary osmolality. The causes of the defect in renal concentrating capacity associated with chronic renal failure are probably multiple.[143–145] These

TABLE 45.9 Causes of Acquired Nephrogenic Diabetes Insipidus (NDI)

Chronic renal disease
Polycystic disease
Medullary cystic disease
Ureteral obstruction
Amyloidosis
Advanced renal failure of any etiology
Electrolyte disorders
Hypokalemia
Hypercalcemia
Drugs
Alcohol
Lithium
Demeclocycline
Glyburide
Amphotericin
Foscarnet
Sickle cell disease
Dietary abnormalities
Excessive water intake
Decreased sodium chloride intake
Decreased protein intake
Miscellaneous
Gestational diabetes insipidus

include: (1) a disruption of inner medullary structures or local alterations in medullary blood flow, as is seen in tubulointerstitial diseases, sickle cell disease,[146,147] and analgesic nephropathy; (2) impairment in sodium chloride transport out of the thick ascending limb of Henle's loop, a process that limits maximal interstitial tonicity; and (3) increase in solute excretion in the remaining few functioning nephrons, an adaptive response to the need to excrete the same solute load as the normal kidney.

Hypokalemia has long been known to cause polyuria as a consequence of a vasopressin-resistant renal concentrating defect.[40] A direct effect of hypokalemia on the collecting tubule is supported by studies in the toad bladder which show a decrease in cyclic AMP and vasopressin-stimulated water flow when potassium is removed from the bathing solution.[148] These findings suggest both a precyclic AMP and postcyclic AMP defect. The hypokalemia-induced resistance to vasopressin is associated with decreased cyclic AMP accumulation, apparently due to decreased adenylyl cyclase activity. Hypokalemia from any cause, such as diarrhea, chronic diuretic use or primary aldosteronism, may be associated with a urinary concentrating defect. The defect is generally reversible, but requires a longer time (1–3 months) than would be expected from a purely functional defect.

Hypercalcemia is another well-recognized cause of impaired urinary concentrating ability.[149–151] A decrement in medullary interstitial tonicity is clearly present with hypercalcemia, which may be related to diminished solute reabsorption in the thick ascending limb. This defect is associated with a decrement in AVP-stimulated adenylate cyclase in this nephron segment. The concentrating defect is, however, multifactorial, as the elaboration of hypotonic urine implies an intrinsic defect in the collecting tubule. In this regard, studies in isolated toad bladders, as well as papillary collecting ducts, reveal a decreased response to vasopressin in hypercalcemia.

Various pharmacologic agents have been found to impair the renal capacity to concentrate urine (Table 45.9). Ethanol and phenytoin (Dilantin) seem to exert their action by a central effect on vasopressin release.[152] Some hypoglycemic agents cause a diuresis by a mechanism probably unrelated to suppression of vasopressin release. The renal toxicity of amphotericin can manifest in the form of a concentrating defect.[153] Foscarnet, an agent increasingly employed in the treatment of cytomegalovirus (CMV) infection in patients with acquired immune deficiency syndrome (AIDS), has been described to cause a nephrogenic diabetes insipidus.[91,154]

The drugs most commonly associated with nephrogenic diabetes insipidus are demeclocycline and lithium.[119,120,122,123,125,155] Since it was first recognized as a cause of nephrogenic diabetes insipidus, demeclocycline has become the drug of choice for the treatment of the syndrome of inappropriate ADH secretion (SIADH). It has yet to be determined if demeclocycline reduces argenine vasopressin secretion. It is clear, however, that demeclocycline induces dose-dependent decreases in human renal medullary adenylate cyclase activity. Since the drug decreases not only vasopressin but also cyclic AMP-stimulated water flow, a postcyclic AMP defect may be operant.[156]

Lithium is the most common cause of nephrogenic diabetes insipidus. There is no evidence that lithium impairs vasopressin release. In terms of the mechanism of its renal action, lithium does not interfere with accumulation of medullary solutes. Thus, an intrinsic tubular defect is postulated. In this regard, lithium decreases vasopressin-stimulated water transport in the perfused cortical collecting duct. An inhibition in adenylate cyclase or in cyclic AMP generation is observed in human tissue and cultured cells exposed to the cation, as well as in animals chronically treated with lithium. More recently, a downregulation of the vasopressin-regulated water channel (aquaporin) has been described in lithium-treated rats.[157] It is of interest that the urinary aquaporin levels remained low after removal of lithium, in line with the slow recovery of concentrating ability seen in man.

A renal concentrating defect is a common accompaniment of sickle cell anemia and sickle cell trait.[146,158,159] Sickling of red blood cells in the hypertonic medullary interstitium with occlusion of the vasa recta appears to cause inner medullary and papillary damage. Microradioangiographic studies have failed to demonstrate vasa recta blood flow in patients with sickle cell disease. The resultant medullary ischemia may impair sodium chloride transport in the ascending limb, and thus diminish medullary tonicity. Transfusions of normal blood have been shown to restore renal concentrating capacity in children, thus indicating that the sickled red blood cells have a role in the defect. With more prolonged disease, medullary infarcts occur and the concentrating defect is no longer reversible with transfusions.

The syndrome of essential hypernatremia and hypodipsia has been described in patients with normal total body sodium. A partial list of causes of this hypodipsia-hypernatremia syndrome is shown in Table 45.10. These patients exhibit persistent hypernatremia not explained by any volume loss. There is absence or attenuation of thirst. The patient may also have partial diabetes insipidus and a normal renal response to ADH. This is due to a primary hypothalamic disease impairing thirst (called *hypodipsia*). Two different syndromes have been described, which are most often due to tumors, granulomatous diseases (such as sarcoidosis) or vascular disease. In the first, there is a defect in thirst, with or without concomitant diabetes insipidus. In this disorder, forced water intake is usually sufficient to maintain a normal plasma sodium concentration.[89,160] Other hypodipsic patients will not respond to water-loading, as the excess water will be excreted in the urine with little change in the plasma sodium concentration.[91,92] It had been postulated that these

TABLE 45.10 Causes of the Hypodipsia—Hypernatremia Syndrome

Ectopic pinealoma
Dysgerminoma/germinoma
Craniopharyngioma
Teratoma
Meningioma
Metastatic bronchial carcinoma
Eosinophilic granuloma
Hand—Schuller—Christian disease
Ganulomatous tumor
Hypothalamic neuronal degeneration
Subarachnoid hemorrhage
Posttraumatic carotid cavernous fistula
Microcephaly
Occult hydrocephalus
Head trauma
Aneurysectomy (anterior communicating artery)
Sarcoidosis

From Levi, M., and Berl, T. (1982). Water metabolism In "Current Nephrology," Vol 5, 37, Gonick, H. C. (ed.). Year Book Medical, Chicago.[130]

patients had a reset osmostat upward (called *essential hypernatremia*), so that the new high plasma sodium concentration was recognized as normal.[161,162] Thus, giving water will decrease ADH release, and the excess water will be excreted in dilute urine. It is now clear, however, that these patients have selective injury to the osmoreceptors, with ADH secretion being primarily governed by changes in volume.[163] Thus, the suppression of ADH release by water-loading in this setting is due to the associated mild volume expansion, rather than a fall in plasma osmolality. True resetting of the osmostat upwards has been described only in patients with primary mineralocorticoid excess (such as primary hyperaldosteronism). The plasma sodium concentration in these patients is usually between 143 and 147 mEq/l. It is presumed that the suppressive effect of chronic mild volume expansion on ADH release is responsible for the resetting. This appears to be due to a specific osmoreceptor defect resulting in nonosmotic regulation of argenine vasopressin release. These patients are characterized by persistent hypernatremia not explained by any apparent extracellular volume loss with a normal response to AVP. It has been proposed that these patients have a "resetting" of the osmoreceptor, since these patients tend to concentrate and dilute urine at inappropriately high levels of plasma osmolality.[164–169] However, using the regression analysis of plasma argenine vasopressin level versus plasma osmolality, it has been shown that in some of these patients the tendency to concentrate and dilute urine at inappropriately high levels of plasma osmolality is due solely to a marked reduction in sensitivity or gain of the osmoregulatory mechanism. In other patients, however, plasma argenine vasopressin levels fluctuate in a random manner, bearing no apparent relationship to changes in plasma osmolality. Such patients frequently display large swings in serum sodium concentration. It appears that most patients with essential hypernatremia fit one of these two patterns.[88,170] Hypodipsia can also occur in elderly patients without overt hypothalamic lesions, and can culminate in severe hypernatremia.[168,171] It has been suggested that a decrement in angiotensin II-mediated thirst existed in the elderly.[29,172]

Hypernatremia in Patients with Increased Total Body Sodium

Hypernatremia with increased total body sodium is the least common type of hypernatremia, and is usually due to exogenous administration of hypertonic sodium containing solutes (Table 45.11).[13] Acute and often marked hypernatremia (in which the plasma sodium concentration can exceed 175–200 mEq/l) can be induced by the administration of hypertonic sodium-containing solutions. Hypernatremia supervenes during resuscitative efforts with hypertonic sodium bicarbonate,[46,173] inadvertent intravascular infusion of hypertonic saline in therapeutic abortions, inadvertent dialysis against a high sodium concentration dialysate, sea water drowning, and even after ingestion of large quantities of sodium chloride tablets.[174–178] Accidental or nonaccidental salt poisoning has been reported in infants and young children, and in patients taking highly concentrated saline emetic or gargle.[174,179,180] The hypernatremia in this setting will correct spontaneously if renal function is normal, since the excess sodium will be rapidly excreted in the urine. This process can be facilitated by inducing a sodium and water diuresis with a loop diuretic, and then replacing the urine output with water. Too rapid correction should be avoided if the patient is asymptotic. Since the hypernatremia is generally very acute with little time for cerebral adaptation, these patients are less likely to develop cerebral edema during correction.[181,182] The degree of hyperosmolality is typically mild, unless the thirst mechanism is abnormal or access

TABLE 45.11 Therapeutic Hypertonic Solutions

Solute	Molecular Weight	Concentration (mg/dL%)	Osmolality (mosm/kg water)	Typical Container Size (ML)	Use
Sodium chloride	58.5	3	1026	500	Emergency teatment of hypotonic states; intra-amniotic instillation for therapeutic abortion
		5	1711	500	
		20	6845	250	
Sodium bicarbonate	84.0	5	1190	500	Treatment of metaboliuc acidosis, hyperkalemia, cardiopulmonary arrest
		7.5	1786	50	

From Morrison, G., and Singer, L. (1994). Hyperosmolal states. In "Clinical Disorders of Fluid and Electrolyte Metabolism," 646, Narins, R. G., (ed.). McGraw-Hill, New York.[187]

to water is limited. This occurs in infants, the physically handicapped, patients with impaired mental status, in the postoperative state, and in patients on ventilators. Patients with primary hyperaldosteronism and Cushing syndrome have slight, clinically unimportant elevations in serum sodium concentration. As expected, patients with hypernatremia and high total body sodium excrete generous quantities of the cation in the urine.

CLINICAL FEATURES IN HYPERNATREMIA

A complete history and physical examination will often provide clues as to the underlying cause of hypernatremia.[183,184] Relevant symptoms and signs include the absence or presence of thirst, diaphoresis, diarrhea, polyuria, and the features of ECF volume contraction.[185–188] The major symptoms of hypernatremia are neurologic and include altered mental status, weakness, neuromuscular irritability, focal neurologic deficits, and occasionally coma or seizures (Table 45.12). As a consequence of hypertonicity, water shifts out of cells, leading to a contracted ICF volume. A decreased brain cell volume is associated with an increased risk of subarachnoid or intracerebral hemorrhage.[189–192] Patients may also complain of polyuria or thirst. For unknown reasons, patients with polydipsia from CDI tend to prefer ice-cold water. The signs and symptoms of volume depletion are often present in patients with a history of excessive sweating, diarrhea or an osmotic diuresis.[132,183,193–197]

The severity of the clinical manifestations is related to the acuity and magnitude of the rise in plasma Na^+ concentration. Chronic hypernatremia is generally less symptomatic as a result of adaptive mechanisms designed to defend cell volume. Brain cells initially take up Na^+ and K^+ salts, later followed by accumulation of organic osmolytes, such as inositol. This serves to restore the brain ICF volume towards normal.

The signs and symptoms of hypernatremia are most likely related to a variety of anatomic derangements.

TABLE 45.12 Signs and Symptoms of Hypernatremia

Intense thirst
Irritability
Signs of volume depletion (variable)
Nausea or vomiting
Depression of sensorium
Seizures (unusual in adults)
Focal neurologic deficits
Muscle spasticity (unusual in adults)
Fever
Labored respiration

The most prominent manifestations of hyperosmolar disorders are of a neurologic nature.[198–204] The loss of volume and the shrinkage of brain cells associated with the hyperosmolar states causes tearing of cerebral vessels. In addition to these gross anatomic changes, the brain sustains alterations in the composition of water and solutes that may be of great importance in the pathophysiology of the symptoms of hypernatremia. These are responses designed to regulate volume and restore cell size. Thus, the water losses are not as severe as would be predicted. In the early phase, the entry of sodium and chloride into brain cells greatly mitigates the loss of water that would otherwise occur from ideal osmotic behavior. After 7 days of hypernatremia, brain water has returned to control levels as brain osmolality remains elevated. At this time idiogenic osmoles account for as much as 60% of the increase in intracellular osmolality. It now seems possible that some of these idiogenic osmoles are due to an increase in intracellular amino acids, particularly taurine. In addition, accumulation of osmolytes such as urea, glutamine, glycerolphosphorylcholine, and myoinositol has been documented in hypernatremic rats, as well as in human using NMR spectroscopy.

Measurement of urine volume and osmolality are essential in the evaluation of hypernatremia. The appropriate renal response to hypernatremia is the excretion of the minimum volume (500 ml/d) of maximally-concentrated urine (urine osmolality greater than 800 mOsm/kg H_2O). These findings suggest extrarenal or remote renal water loss or administration of hypertonic Na^+ salt solutions. The presence of a primary Na^+ excess can be confirmed by the presence of ECF volume expansion and natriuresis (urine Na^+ concentration usually greater than 100 mmol/l). Many causes of hypernatremia are associated with polyuria and a submaximal urine osmolality. The product of the urine volume and osmolality, i.e., the solute excretion rate, is helpful in determining the basis of the polyuria. To maintain a steady-state, total solute excretion must equal solute production. Individuals eating a normal diet generate approximately 600 mOsm/d. Therefore, daily solute excretion in excess of 750 mOsm/d defines an osmotic diuresis. This can be confirmed by measuring the urine glucose and urea. In general, both CDI and NDI present with polyuria and hypotonic urine (urine osmolality less than 250 mOsm/kg H_2O). The degree of hypernatremia is usually mild unless there is an associated thirst abnormality.

THERAPY FOR HYPERNATREMIA

The therapeutic goals are to stop ongoing water loss by treating the underlying cause, and to correct the

TABLE 45.13 Diagnosis and Therapeutic Approach to the Hypernatremic Patient

	Causes	Urinary		Therapies
		Tonicity	Na$^+$ (mEq/L)	

Hypovolemia
  Low total body
  Na$^+$, H$_2$O loss
	Renal loss
	  Osmotic or loop diuretics
	  Postobstruction
	  Intrinsic renal disease
		Iso-
		Hypo-
			>20	Hypotonic saline

	Extrarenal loss
	  Dermal
	  Sweating
	  Burns
	Gastrointestinal
	  Diarrhea
	  Fistulas
		Hyper-	<10	

Euvolemia
  Normal total body Na$^+$
  H$_2$O loss
	Renal loss
	  Diabetes insipidus
	  Nephrogenic
	  Central
	  Partial
	  Gestational
	  Hypodispsia
		Hypo-
		Iso-
		Hyper-
			Variable	Water replacement

	Extrarenal loss
	  Insensible losses
	  Respiratory
	  Dermal
		Hyper-	Variable	

Hypervolemia
  Increased total body Na$^+$
  Na$^+$ addition
	Primary hyperaldosteronism
	Cushing syndrome
	Hypertonic dialysate
	Hypertonic sodium bicarbonate
	Sodium chloride tablets
		Iso-
		Hyper-
			>20	Diuretics and water replacement

water deficit. The specific approach depends on the patient's ECF volume (Table 45.13). Reversal of hypernatremic state must be undertaken slowly to prevent neurological complications. Rapid correction may result in cerebral edema, seizure, and death.[183,205–211]

When the patient has low total body sodium, as evidenced by circulatory manifestations (e.g., orthostatic hypotension), isotonic sodium chloride should be given until systemic hemodynamics are stabilized. Thereafter, the hypernatremia can be treated with 0.45% sodium chloride or 5% dextrose. When the patient is hypervolemic and hypernatremic, the removal of excess sodium is the goal, which can be achieved either by administration of diuretics along with 5% dextrose or, if renal function is impaired, by dialysis. The euvolemic hypernatremic patient who has sustained pure water losses requires water replacement as a 5% dextrose infusion. The water deficit in this setting can be calculated based on the current sodium concentration and body weight, using the assumption that total body water is approximately 50 or 60% of body weight:

$$\text{Water deficit} = \text{Total-body water} \times \left(\frac{\text{Plasma } [\text{Na}^+]}{140} \right)$$

(45.7)

In addition to replacing the calculated water deficit, ongoing fluid losses should be replaced. In acute hypernatremia, repletion of the water deficit may be faster. The electrolytes accumulated in the brain during hypernatremia are rapidly extruded into the extracellular space during treatment, minimizing the risk of cerebral edema.[206] In contrast, rapid correction in chronic hypernatremia is potentially dangerous. In this case, a sudden decrease in osmolality could potentially cause a rapid shift of water into cells that have undergone osmotic adaptation. This would result in swollen brain cells, and increase the risk of seizures or permanent neurologic damage.[212] A slower rate of correction probably can prevent this sequence of events by allowing idiogenic osmoles time to be dissipated.

The plasma Na$^+$ concentration should be lowered by 0.5 mmol/L per hour, and by no more than 12 mmol/L over the first 24 hours. The safest route of administration of water is by mouth or via a nasogastric tube (or other feeding tube). Alternatively, 5% dextrose in water or half-isotonic saline can be given intravenously. The patient's neurological status should be monitored carefully throughout treatment. Deterioration of neurological status after an initial improvement suggests the development of cerebral edema, and mandates temporary discontinuation or slowing the rate of water replacement.

In patients with essential hypernatremia and the elderly with hypodipsia, 1 to 2 liters of water per day may need to be administered as a prescription. Chlorpropamide itself augments thirst, and its use with desmopressin in patients with adipsia has been proposed.

Patients with central diabetes insipidus do not develop hypernatremia if the thirst mechanism is intact and water is available. Hormonal replacement and pharmacologic agents are available for the treatment of central diabetes insipidus. In acute settings, such as after hypophysectomy, the aqueous vasopressin (Pitressin) preparation is preferable. Its short duration of action allows for more careful monitoring, and decreases the likelihood of complications such as water intoxication. In chronic settings, vasopressin tannate in oil (Pitressin Tannate) is potent and effective for 24 to 72 hours. It requires a deep subcutaneous or intramuscular injection by a fairly large-gauge needle, because of the viscosity of the oil vehicle. This material can cause sterile abscesses in some subjects, and on occasion be associated with resistance due to development of antibodies.[213-215] A modification of the natural vasopressin molecule to form desmopressin acetate (dDAVP) has resulted in a compound with prolonged antidiuretic activity (6–24 hours) and virtual elimination of vasopressor activity (antidiuretic to pressor ratio of approximately 2000:1) compared with the natural hormone argenine vasopressin (duration of action of 2–4 hours and antidiuretic to pressor ratio of 1:1[216-220]). Substitution of D-argenine for L-argenine at position 8 resulted in a peptide DAVP with diminished vasopressor activity, and deamination of the hemicysteine at position 1 gave rise to a second peptide, with enhanced antidiuretic to pressor activity and prolonged duration of action. dDAVP is administered intranasally in the dosage ranging from 10 to 20 μg every 8 to 12 hours.[221,222] Intranasal dDAVP is now the treatment of choice for central diabetes insipidus.

In some patients with partial central diabetes insipidus, drugs that stimulate argenine vasopressin secretion or enhance its action on the kidney have been useful. These include chlorpropamide, clofibrate, carbamazepine, and nonsteroidal anti-inflammatory drugs (NSAIDs).[223-226] Since, with very dilute urine of fixed osmolality, the urine volume is determined by the solute-load requiring excretion, a reduction of salt and protein in the diet will reduce the major urinary solutes, and thus the volume of urine necessary to accommodate their excretion.[14] A number of pharmacologic agents with antidiuretic properties are also used. Chlorpropamide (Diabinese) is the most commonly used. Its antidiuretic effects are manifested only if some

vasopressin is present, and it is therefore useful only in partial diabetes insipidus. In Brattleboro rats with diabetes insipidus, chlorpropamide augmented the antidiuretic responses to dDAVP. A trial of 250 mg every day or twice a day may be offered to patients with partial central diabetes insipidus and at least 7 days allowed for an effect to occur. The anticonvulsant carbamazepine (Tegretol) has also caused antidiuresis in subjects with diabetes insipidus. A combination of chlorpropamide and carbamazepine has been found to provide an effect that could be synergistic.[227,228] Clofibrate also has been used to treat partial central diabetes insipidus.

In patients with nephrogenic diabetes insipidus, the concentrating defect may be reversible by treating the underlying disorder or eliminating the offending drug. Symptomatic polyuria can be treated with a low-sodium diet and thiazide diuretics.[136] This induces mild volume-depletion, which leads to enhanced proximal reabsorption of salt and water, and decreased delivery to the site of action of AVP, the collecting duct. By impairing renal prostaglandin synthesis, NSAIDs potentiate argenine vasopressin action, and thereby increase urine osmolality and decrease urine volume.[229] Amiloride may be useful in patients with nephrogenic diabetes insipidus who need to be on lithium.[126,230] The nephrotoxicity of lithium requires the drug to be taken up into collecting duct cells via the amiloride-sensitive Na^+ channel.

CLINICAL STUDIES AND OUTCOME

The clinical outcome of patients with hypernatremia depends on the age of the patient and the rapidity with which the hypernatremic state was attained.[231-233] Acute hypernatremia is associated with a 40% mortality, whereas the mortality for chronic hypernatremia is about 10%. In children, the mortality of acute hypernatremia ranges between 10 and 70%, with a mean of approximately 45%. Unfortunately, even in survivors, neurologic sequelae are common, affecting as many as two-thirds of the children.[30,234-237] In adults, acute elevation of serum sodium above 160 mEq/l is associated with a 75% mortality, while the mortality in chronic cases is approximately 60%. Note, however, that in the adult, hypernatremia frequently occurs in the setting of serious underlying diseases, which may be the primary cause of the high mortality.[153,238-240]

Table 45.14 summarizes clinical studies of hypernatremia in adults that have been published over the past two decades. From these varied studies,[232,233,241-246] it is apparent that hypernatremia is a common disturbance, with an incidence ranging from less than 1% to more than 3%. The variation in incidence is, in part, a

TABLE 45.14 Published Clinical Series of Patients with Hypernatremia

Series reference	Definition [Na], mmol/L	N	Incidence	Age years, mean ± SD	Etiologic Factors	Mortality
Daggett et al. [242]	>154	20	0.12%	N/A	Diabetes mellitus (57%)	40%
					CNS disease (57%)	
Mahowald and Himmelstein [245]	>150	23	N/A	72 ± 12	Infection (224%)	52%
Himmelstein et al. [243]	>150	56	0.65−2.25	73 ± 15	Infection (174%)	46%
					Nursing home care (265%)	
Snyder et al. [246]	>148 age >205 years	162	1.1%	78 ± 9	Febrile illness infirmity	42%
					Nutritional supplementation post-operative state	
Bhatnagar and Weinkove [241]	>160	27	N/A	71.4	Poor intake (55%)	79%
					Increased insensible losses	
					Diuresis (100%)	
					Increased GI losses (241%)	
Long et al. [244]	>150	160	0.3%	76 median	Diuretics (193%)	54%
					Depressed sensorium 80%	
					Febrile illness (205%)	
					Mechanical ventilation (221%)	
Borra et al. [86]	>150	111	3.5%	On admission 83 ± 11	Infection (267%)	49%
					Malignancy (158%)	
				Hospital-acquired 76 ± 15	Diabetes mellitus (67%)	
Palevsky [232]	>150	103	On admission 0.2%	On admission 77 ± 17	On admission infection (190%)	41%
			Hospital-acquired 1.0%	Hospital-acquired 59 ± 19	Hospital-acquired fever (222%)	
					Mechanical ventilation (99%)	
					Enteral fluid loss (57%)	
					Mental status changes (255%)	

CNS: central nervous system; GI: gastrointestinal.

function of the populations at risk and the definition of hypernatremia used in various studies. The patient groups at increased risk for development of severe hypernatremia are listed in Table 45.15. Hypernatremia developing in nonhospitalized adults is predominantly a disease of the elderly,[86,245,247−249] is commonly a manifestation of underlying infection, and may reflect inadequate nursing care of patients in chronic care facilities. However, hospital-acquired hypernatremia occurs in a wider range of patients with an age distribution more similar to the general hospitalized population. The main factor contributing to the development of hypernatremia is the inability to control water intake in the setting of increased water losses. Pure water loss from diabetes insipidus rarely contributes to its development; more common etiologies of water loss include diuretic administration, solute diuresis, enteral fluid loss, and fever. The results from these clinical series

TABLE 45.15 Patient Groups at Increased Risk for Development of Severe Hypernatremia

Elderly patients
Hospitalized patients
Hypertonic infusions
Tube feedings
Osmotic diuretics
Lactulose
Mechanical ventilation
Patients with decreased baseline levels of consciousness
Patients with uncontrolled diabetes
Patients with underlying polyuric disorders

support the recommendation that the serum sodium concentration be corrected promptly, but gradually, over 48 to 72 hours.

References

[1] Peters JP. Water exchange. Physiol Rev 1944;24:40.

[2] Rose BD. New approach to disturbances in the plasma sodium concentration. Am J Med 1986;81:1033–40.

[3] Smith HW. From fish to philosopher. Boston: Little; 1953. p. 264

[4] Robertson GL, Aycinena P, Zerbe RL. Neurogenic disorders of osmoregulation. Am J Med 1982;72:339–53.

[5] Roy G, Banderali U. Channels for ions and amino acids in kidney cultured cells (MDCK) during volume regulation. J Exp Zool 1994;268:121–6.

[6] Abraham WT, Schrier RW. Body fluid volume regulation in health and disease. Adv Intern Med 1994;39:23–47.

[7] Berl T. The cAMP system in vasopressin-sensitive nephron segments of the vitamin D-treated rat. Kidney Int 1987;31:1065–71.

[8] Berl T, Anderson RJ, McDonald KM, Schrier RW. Clinical disorders of water metabolism. Kidney Int 1976;10:117–32.

[9] Gamble JL. Chemical anatomy, physiology and pathology of extracellular fluid: a lecture syllabus. Cambridge, Massachusetts: Harvard University Press; 1947.

[10] De Wardener HE, Herxheimer A. The effect of a high water intake on the kidney's ability to concentrate the urine in man. J Physiol 1957;139:42–52.

[11] Edelman IS, Leibman J, O'Meara MP, Birkenfeld LW. Interrelations between serum sodium concentration, serum osmolarity and total exchangeable sodium, total exchangeable potassium and total body water. J Clin Invest 1958;37:1236–56.

[12] Gault MH, Dixon ME, Doyle M, Cohen WM. Hypernatremia, azotemia, and dehydration due to high-protein tube feeding. Ann Intern Med 1968;68:778–91.

[13] Feig PU, McCurdy DK. The hypertonic state. N Engl J Med 1977;297:1444–54.

[14] Gennari FJ. Current concepts. Serum osmolality. Uses and limitations. N Engl J Med 1984;310:102–5.

[15] Shoker AS. Application of the clearance concept to hyponatremic and hypernatremic disorders: a phenomenological analysis. Clin Chem 1994;40:1220–7.

[16] Smithline N, Gardner Jr KD. Gaps—anionic and osmolal. JAMA 1976;236:1594–7.

[17] Verbalis JG. Disorders of body water homeostasis. Best Pract Res Clin Endocrinol Metab 2003;17:471–503.

[18] Gines P, Abraham WT, Schrier RW. Vasopressin in pathophysiological states. Semin Nephrol 1994;14:384–97.

[19] Majzoub JA, Rich A, van Boom J, Habener JF. Vasopressin and oxytocin mRNA regulation in the rat assessed by hybridization with synthetic oligonucleotides. J Biol Chem 1983;258:14061–4.

[20] Uhl GR, Zingg HH, Habener JF. Vasopressin mRNA in situ hybridization: localization and regulation studied with oligonucleotide cDNA probes in normal and Brattleboro rat hypothalamus. Proc Natl Acad Sci USA 1985;82:5555–9.

[21] Goldsmith C, Beasley HK, Whalley PJ, Rector Jr FC, Seldin DW. The effect of salt deprivation on the urinary concentrating mechanism in the dog. J Clin Invest 1961;40:2043–52.

[22] Murphy D, Levy A, Lightman S, Carter D. Vasopressin RNA in the neural lobe of the pituitary: dramatic accumulation in response to salt loading. Proc Natl Acad Sci USA 1989;86: 9002–5.

[23] Zerbe RL, Robertson GL. A comparison of plasma vasopressin measurements with a standard indirect test in the differential diagnosis of polyuria. N Engl J Med 1981;305:1539–46.

[24] Kumar S, Berl T. Sodium. Lancet 1998;352:220–8.

[25] Andersson B. Regulation of water intake. Physiol Rev 1978;58:582.

[26] Fitzsimons JT. Angiotensin, thirst, and sodium appetite: retrospect and prospect. Fed Proc 1978;37:2669–75.

[27] Fitzsimons JT. Thirst. Physiol Rev 1972;52:468–561.

[28] Phillips PA, Bretherton M, Johnston CI, Gray L. Reduced osmotic thirst in healthy elderly men. Am J Physiol 1991;261: R166–171.

[29] Phillips PA, Rolls BJ, Ledingham JG, Forsling ML, Morton JJ, Crowe MJ, et al. Reduced thirst after water deprivation in healthy elderly men. N Engl J Med 1984;311:753–9.

[30] Papadimitriou A, Kipourou K, Manta C, Tapaki G, Philippidis P. Adipsic hypernatremia syndrome in infancy. J Pediatr Endocrinol Metab 1997;10:547–50.

[31] Gullans SR, Verbalis JG. Control of brain volume during hyperosmolar and hypoosmolar conditions. Annu Rev Med 1993;44:289–301.

[32] Lien YH, Shapiro JI, Chan L. Effects of hypernatremia on organic brain osmoles. J Clin Invest 1990;85:1427–35.

[33] Lien YH, Shapiro JI, Chan L. Study of brain electrolytes and organic osmolytes during correction of chronic hyponatremia. Implications for the pathogenesis of central pontine myelinolysis. J Clin Invest 1991;88:303–9.

[34] Heilig CW, Stromski ME, Blumenfeld JD, Lee JP, Gullans SR. Characterization of the major brain osmolytes that accumulate in salt-loaded rats. Am J Physiol 1989;257:F1108–1116.

[35] Fishman RA, Chan PH. Changes in ammonia and amino acid metabolism induced by hyperosmolality in vivo and in vitro. Trans Am Neurol Assoc 1976;101:34–9.

[36] Verbalis JG. Brain volume regulation in response to changes in osmolality. Neuroscience 2010;168:862–70.

[37] Cserr HF, DePasquale M, Patlak CS. Regulation of brain water and electrolytes during acute hyperosmolality in rats. Am J Physiol 1987;253:F522–529.

[38] Cserr HF, DePasquale M, Patlak CS. Volume regulatory influx of electrolytes from plasma to brain during acute hyperosmolality. Am J Physiol 1987;253:F530–537.

[39] Ayus JC, Armstrong DL, Arieff AI. Effects of hypernatraemia in the central nervous system and its therapy in rats and rabbits. J Physiol 1996;492(Pt 1):243–55.

[40] Relman AS, Schwartz WB. The kidney in potassium depletion. Am J Med 1958;24:764–73.

[41] Chan PH, Fishman RA. Elevation of rat brain amino acids, ammonia and idiogenic osmoles induced by hyperosmolality. Brain Res 1979;161:293–301.

[42] Hochstenbach SL, Ciriello J. Plasma hypernatremia induces c-fos activity in medullary catecholaminergic neurons. Brain Res 1995;674:46–54.

[43] Holliday MA, Kalayci MN, Harrah J. Factors that limit brain volume changes in response to acute and sustained hyper- and hyponatremia. J Clin Invest 1968;47:1916—28.

[44] Proft M, Struhl K. MAP kinase-mediated stress relief that precedes and regulates the timing of transcriptional induction. Cell 2004;118:351—61.

[45] Yancey PH, Clark ME, Hand SC, Bowlus RD, Somero GN. Living with water stress: evolution of osmolyte systems. Science 1982;217:1214—22.

[46] Arieff AI, Guisado R. Effects on the central nervous system of hypernatremic and hyponatremic states. Kidney Int 1976;10:104—16.

[47] Arieff AI, Guisado R, Lazarowitz VC. The pathophysiology of hyperosmolar states. In: Andreoli TE, Grantham JJ, Rector FC, editors. Disturbances in body fluid osmolality. Baltimore: Williams & Wilkins; 1977. p. 227.

[48] Thurston JH, Hauhart RE, Dirgo JA. Taurine: a role in osmotic regulation of mammalian brain and possible clinical significance. Life Sci 1980;26:1561—8.

[49] Sotos JF, Dodge PR, Talbot NB. Studies in experimental hypertonicity. II. Hypertonicity of body fluids as a cause of acidosis. Pediatrics 1962;30:180—93.

[50] Soupart A, Penninckx R, Namias B, Stenuit A, Perier O, Decaux G. Brain myelinolysis following hypernatremia in rats. J Neuropathol Exp Neurol 1996;55:106—13.

[51] Beck FX, Burger-Kentischer A, Muller E. Cellular response to osmotic stress in the renal medulla. Pflugers Arch 1998;436: 814—27.

[52] Terada Y, Inoshita S, Hanada S, Shimamura H, Kuwahara M, Ogawa W, et al. Hyperosmolality activates Akt and regulates apoptosis in renal tubular cells. Kidney Int 2001;60:553—67.

[53] Zhang Z, Cai Q, Michea L, Dmitrieva NI, Andrews P, Burg MB. Proliferation and osmotic tolerance of renal inner medullary epithelial cells *in vivo* and in cell culture. Am J Physiol Renal Physiol 2002;283:F302—308.

[54] Rauchman MI, Nigam SK, Delpire E, Gullans SR. An osmotically tolerant inner medullary collecting duct cell line from an SV40 transgenic mouse. Am J Physiol 1993;265:F416—424.

[55] Cai Q, Michea L, Andrews P, Zhang Z, Rocha G, Dmitrieva N, et al. Rate of increase of osmolality determines osmotic tolerance of mouse inner medullary epithelial cells. Am J Physiol Renal Physiol 2002;283:F792—798.

[56] Capasso JM, Rivard CJ, Berl T. Long-term adaptation of renal cells to hypertonicity: role of MAP kinases and Na-K-ATPase. Am J Physiol Renal Physiol 2001;280:F768—776.

[57] Capasso JM, Rivard CJ, Enomoto LM, Berl T. Adaptation of murine inner medullary collecting duct (IMCD3) cell cultures to hypertonicity. Ann N Y Acad Sci 2003;986:410—5.

[58] Dmitrieva N, Michea L, Burg M. p53 Protects renal inner medullary cells from hypertonic stress by restricting DNA replication. Am J Physiol Renal Physiol 2001;281:F522—530.

[59] Miyakawa H, Woo SK, Chen CP, Dahl SC, Handler JS, Kwon HM. Cis- and trans-acting factors regulating transcription of the BGT1 gene in response to hypertonicity. Am J Physiol 1998;274: F753—761.

[60] Miyakawa H, Woo SK, Dahl SC, Handler JS, Kwon HM. Tonicity-responsive enhancer binding protein, a rel-like protein that stimulates transcription in response to hypertonicity. Proc Natl Acad Sci USA 1999;96:2538—42.

[61] Lopez-Rodriguez C, Aramburu J, Rakeman AS, Rao A. NFAT5, a constitutively nuclear NFAT protein that does not cooperate with Fos and Jun. Proc Natl Acad Sci USA 1999;96:7214—9.

[62] Trama J, Lu Q, Hawley RG, Ho SN. The NFAT-related protein NFATL1 (TonEBP/NFAT5) is induced upon T cell activation in a calcineurin-dependent manner. J Immunol 2000;165:4884—94.

[63] Ko BC, Turck CW, Lee KW, Yang Y, Chung SS. Purification, identification, and characterization of an osmotic response element binding protein. Biochem Biophys Res Commun 2000;270: 52—61.

[64] Aramburu J, Drews-Elger K, Estrada-Gelonch A, Minguillon J, Morancho B, Santiago V, et al. Regulation of the hypertonic stress response and other cellular functions by the rel-like transcription factor NFAT5. Biochem Pharmacol 2006;72:1597—604.

[65] Hogan PG, Chen L, Nardone J, Rao A. Transcriptional regulation by calcium, calcineurin, and NFAT. Genes Dev 2003;17:2205—32.

[66] Stroud JC, Lopez-Rodriguez C, Rao A, Chen L. Structure of a TonEBP-DNA complex reveals DNA encircled by a transcription factor. Nat Struct Biol 2002;9:90—4.

[67] Andres-Hernando A, Lanaspa MA, Rivard CJ, Berl T. Nucleoporin 88 (Nup88) is regulated by hypertonic stress in kidney cells to retain the transcription factor tonicity enhancer-binding protein (TonEBP) in the nucleus. J Biol Chem 2008;283:25082—90.

[68] Lee SD, Colla E, Sheen MR, Na KY, Kwon HM. Multiple domains of TonEBP cooperate to stimulate transcription in response to hypertonicity. J Biol Chem 2003;278:47571—7.

[69] Lopez-Rodriguez C, Aramburu J, Jin L, Rakeman AS, Michino M, Rao A. Bridging the NFAT and NF-kappaB families: NFAT5 dimerization regulates cytokine gene transcription in response to osmotic stress. Immunity 2001;15:47—58.

[70] Ferraris JD, Persaud P, Williams CK, Chen Y, Burg MB. cAMP-independent role of PKA in tonicity-induced transactivation of tonicity-responsive enhancer/ osmotic response element-binding protein. Proc Natl Acad Sci USA 2002;99:16800—5.

[71] Irarrazabal CE, Liu JC, Burg MB, Ferraris JD. ATM, a DNA damage-inducible kinase, contributes to activation by high NaCl of the transcription factor TonEBP/OREBP. Proc Natl Acad Sci USA 2004;101:8809—14.

[72] Ko BC, Lam AK, Kapus A, Fan L, Chung SK, Chung SS. Fyn and p38 signaling are both required for maximal hypertonic activation of the osmotic response element-binding protein/ tonicity-responsive enhancer-binding protein (OREBP/ TonEBP). J Biol Chem 2002;277:46085—92.

[73] Woo SK, Maouyo D, Handler JS, Kwon HM. Nuclear redistribution of tonicity-responsive enhancer binding protein requires proteasome activity. Am J Physiol Cell Physiol 2000;278: C323—330.

[74] Dahl SC, Handler JS, Kwon HM. Hypertonicity-induced phosphorylation and nuclear localization of the transcription factor TonEBP. Am J Physiol Cell Physiol 2001;280:C248—253.

[75] Cai Q, Ferraris JD, Burg MB. High NaCl increases TonEBP/ OREBP mRNA and protein by stabilizing its mRNA. Am J Physiol Renal Physiol 2005;289:F803—807.

[76] Lee SD, Choi SY, Lim SW, Lamitina ST, Ho SN, Go WY, et al. TonEBP stimulates multiple cellular pathways for adaptation to hypertonic stress: Organic osmolyte-dependent and -independent pathways. Am J Physiol Renal Physiol 2011.

[77] Go WY, Liu X, Roti MA, Liu F, Ho SN. NFAT5/TonEBP mutant mice define osmotic stress as a critical feature of the lymphoid microenvironment. Proc Natl Acad Sci USA 2004;101:10673—8.

[78] Lopez-Rodriguez C, Antos CL, Shelton JM, Richardson JA, Lin F, Novobrantseva TI, et al. Loss of NFAT5 results in renal atrophy and lack of tonicity-responsive gene expression. Proc Natl Acad Sci USA 2004;101:2392—7.

[79] Maouyo D, Kim JY, Lee SD, Wu Y, Woo SK, Kwon HM. Mouse TonEBP-NFAT5: expression in early development and alternative splicing. Am J Physiol Renal Physiol 09, 2002;282:F802—8.

[80] Dressler GR, Wilkinson JE, Rothenpieler UW, Patterson LT, Williams-Simons L, Westphal H. Deregulation of Pax-2

expression in transgenic mice generates severe kidney abnormalities. Nature 1993;362:65–7.

[81] Chan L. The current status of magnetic resonance spectroscopy–basic and clinical aspects. West J Med 1985;143:773–81.

[82] Chan L, Shapiro JI. Contributions of nuclear magnetic resonance to study of acute renal failure. Ren Fail 1989;11:79–89.

[83] Ross B, Freeman D, Chan L. Contributions of nuclear magnetic resonance to renal biochemistry. Kidney Int 1986;29:131–41.

[84] Lee JH, Arcinue E, Ross BD. Brief report: organic osmolytes in the brain of an infant with hypernatremia. N Engl J Med 1994;331:439–42.

[85] Schulman M. Organic osmolytes in the brain of an infant with hypernatremia. N Engl J Med 1994;331:1776–7.

[86] Borra SI, Beredo R, Kleinfeld M. Hypernatremia in the aging: causes, manifestations, and outcome. J Natl Med Assoc 1995;87:220–4.

[87] Perez GO, Oster JR, Robertson GL. Severe hypernatremia with impaired thirst. Am J Nephrol 1989;9:421–34.

[88] Robertson G. The physiopathology of ADH secretion. In: Tolis G, Labrie F, Martin J, editors. Clinical neuroendocrinology: a pathophysiological approach. New York: Ravens Press; 1979. p. 247.

[89] Robertson G. Disorders of thirst in man. In: Ramsay D, Booth D, editors. Thirst: physiological and psychological aspects. London: Springer-Verlag; 1991. p. 453.

[90] Robertson GL. Pathophysiology of water metabolism. In: Brenner BM, Rector FC, editors. The kidney. Philadelphia: Saunders; 1991. p. 677.

[91] Keuneke C, Anders HJ, Schlondorff D. Adipsic hypernatremia in two patients with AIDS and cytomegalovirus encephalitis. Am J Kidney Dis 1999;33:379–82.

[92] McIver B, Connacher A, Whittle I, Baylis P, Thompson C. Adipsic hypothalamic diabetes insipidus after clipping of anterior communicating artery aneurysm. BMJ 1991;303:1465–7.

[93] Shiau YF, Feldman GM, Resnick MA, Coff PM. Stool electrolyte and osmolality measurements in the evaluation of diarrheal disorders. Ann Intern Med 1985;102:773–5.

[94] Pollock AS, Arieff AI. Abnormalities of cell volume regulation and their functional consequences. Am J Physiol 1980;239: F195–205.

[95] Robertson GL. Antidiuretic hormone. Normal and disordered function. Endocrinol Metab Clin North Am 2001;30:671–94 vii

[96] Visser L, Devuyst O. Physiopathology of hypernatremia following relief of urinary tract obstruction. Acta Clin Belg 1994;49:290–5.

[97] Warren SE, Mitas JA, Swerdlin AH. Hypernatremia in hepatic failure. Jama 1980;243:1257–60.

[98] Kleeman CR, Rubini ME, Lamdin E, Epstein FH. Studies on alcohol diuresis. II. The evaluation of ethyl alcohol as an inhibitor of the neurohypophysis. J Clin Invest 1955;34:448–55.

[99] Chu HI, Liu SH, Yu TF. Water and electrolyte metabolism in diabetes insipidus. Proc Soc Exp Biol Med 1941;46:682.

[100] Birnbaumer M. The V2 vasopressin receptor mutations and fluid homeostasis. Cardiovasc Res 2001;51:409–15.

[101] Kinoshita K, Miura Y, Nagasaki H, Murase T, Bando Y, Oiso Y. A novel deletion mutation in the arginine vasopressin receptor 2 gene and skewed X chromosome inactivation in a female patient with congenital nephrogenic diabetes insipidus. J Endocrinol Invest 2004;27:167–70.

[102] McLeod JF, Kovacs L, Gaskill MB, Rittig S, Bradley GS, Robertson GL. Familial neurohypophyseal diabetes insipidus associated with a signal peptide mutation. J Clin Endocrinol Metab 1993;77:599AG.

[103] Merendino Jr JJ, Speigel AM, Crawford JD, O'Carroll AM, Brownstein MJ, Lolait SJ. Brief report: a mutation in the vasopressin V2-receptor gene in a kindred with X-linked nephrogenic diabetes insipidus. N Engl J Med 1993;328:1538–41.

[104] Miyakoshi M, Kamoi K, Murase T, Sugimura Y, Oiso Y. Novel mutant vasopressin-neurophysin II gene associated with familial neurohypophyseal diabetes insipidus. Endocr J 2004;51: 551–6.

[105] Bichet DG, Birnbaumer M, Lonergan M, Arthus MF, Rosenthal W, Goodyer P, et al. Nature and recurrence of AVPR2 mutations in X-linked nephrogenic diabetes insipidus. Am J Hum Genet 1994;55:278–86.

[106] Chan Seem CP, Dossetor JF, Penney MD. Nephrogenic diabetes insipidus due to a new mutation of the arginine vasopressin V2 receptor gene in a girl presenting with non-accidental injury. Ann Clin Biochem 1999;3(Pt 6):779–82.

[107] Holtzman EJ, Harris Jr HW, Kolakowski Jr LF, Guay-Woodford LM, Botelho B, Ausiello DA. Brief report: a molecular defect in the vasopressin V2-receptor gene causing nephrogenic diabetes insipidus. N Engl J Med 1993;328: 1534–7.

[108] Holtzman EJ, Kolakowski Jr LF, Geifman-Holtzman O, O'Brien DG, Rasoulpour M, Guillot AP, et al. Mutations in the vasopressin V2 receptor gene in two families with nephrogenic diabetes insipidus. J Am Soc Nephrol 1994;5:169–76.

[109] Kambouris M, Dlouhy SR, Trofatter JA, Conneally PM, Hodes ME. Localization of the gene for X-linked nephrogenic diabetes insipidus to Xq28. Am J Med Genet 1988;29:239–46.

[110] Knoers N, Monnens LA. A variant of nephrogenic diabetes insipidus: V2 receptor abnormality restricted to the kidney. Eur J Pediatr 1991;150:370–3.

[111] Knoers N, van der Heyden H, van Oost BA, Ropers HH, Monnens L, Willems J. Nephrogenic diabetes insipidus: close linkage with markers from the distal long arm of the human X chromosome. Hum Genet 1988;80:31–8.

[112] Rosenthal W, Seibold A, Antaramian A, Lonergan M, Arthus MF, Hendy GN, et al. Molecular identification of the gene responsible for congenital nephrogenic diabetes insipidus. Nature 1992;359:233–5.

[113] Asai T, Kuwahara M, Kurihara H, Sakai T, Terada Y, Marumo F, et al. Pathogenesis of nephrogenic diabetes insipidus by aquaporin-2 C-terminus mutations. Kidney Int 2003;64:2–10.

[114] Boccalandro C, De Mattia F, Guo DC, Xue L, Orlander P, King TM, et al. Characterization of an aquaporin-2 water channel gene mutation causing partial nephrogenic diabetes insipidus in a Mexican family: evidence of increased frequency of the mutation in the town of origin. J Am Soc Nephrol 2004;15:1223–31.

[115] de Mattia F, Savelkoul PJ, Kamsteeg EJ, Konings IB, van der Sluijs P, Mallmann R, et al. Lack of arginine vasopressin-induced phosphorylation of aquaporin-2 mutant AQP2-R254L explains dominant nephrogenic diabetes insipidus. J Am Soc Nephrol 2005;16(10):2872–80.

[116] Kamsteeg EJ, Bichet DG, Konings IB, Nivet H, Lonergan M, Arthus MF, et al. Reversed polarized delivery of an aquaporin-2 mutant causes dominant nephrogenic diabetes insipidus. J Cell Biol 2003;163:1099–109.

[117] Marr N, Bichet DG, Hoefs S, Savelkoul PJ, Konings IB, De Mattia F, et al. Cell-biologic and functional analyses of five new aquaporin-2 missense mutations that cause recessive nephrogenic diabetes insipidus. J Am Soc Nephrol 2002;13: 2267–77.

[118] Nielsen S, Frokiaer J, Marples D, Kwon TH, Agre P, Knepper MA. Aquaporins in the kidney: from molecules to medicine. Physiol Rev 2002;82:205–44.

[119] Baylis PH, Heath DA. Water disturbances in patients treated with oral lithium carbonate. Ann Intern Med 1978;88:607–9.

[120] Boton R, Gaviria M, Batlle DC. Prevalence, pathogenesis, and treatment of renal dysfunction associated with chronic lithium therapy. Am J Kidney Dis 1987;10:329–45.

[121] Christensen S, Kusano E, Yusufi AN, Murayama N, Dousa TP. Pathogenesis of nephrogenic diabetes insipidus due to chronic administration of lithium in rats. J Clin Invest 1985;75:1869–79.

[122] Cogan E, Abramow M. Inhibition by lithium of the hydroosmotic action of vasopressin in the isolated perfused cortical collecting tubule of the rabbit. J Clin Invest 1986;77:1507–14.

[123] Dousa TP. Interaction of lithium with vasopressin-sensitive cyclic AMP system of human renal medulla. Endocrinology 1974;95:1359–66.

[124] Forrest Jr JN, Cohen AD, Torretti J, Himmelhoch JM, Epstein FH. On the mechanism of lithium-induced diabetes insipidus in man and the rat. J Clin Invest 1974;53:1115–23.

[125] Goldberg H, Clayman P, Skorecki K. Mechanism of Li inhibition of vasopressin-sensitive adenylate cyclase in cultured renal epithelial cells. Am J Physiol 1988;255:F995–1002.

[126] Walker RG. Lithium nephrotoxicity. Kidney Int Suppl 1993;42:S93–98.

[127] Berl T, Linas SL, Aisenbrey GA, Anderson RJ. On the mechanism of polyuria in potassium depletion. The role of polydipsia. J Clin Invest 1977;60:620–5.

[128] Gutsche HU, Peterson LN, Levine DZ. In vivo evidence of impaired solute transport by the thick ascending limb in potassium-depleted rats. J Clin Invest 1984;73:908–16.

[129] Kim JK, Summer SN, Berl T. The cyclic AMP system in the inner medullary collecting duct of the potassium-depleted rat. Kidney Int 1984;26:384–91.

[130] Levi M, Peterson L, Berl T. Mechanism of concentrating defect in hypercalcemia. Role of polydipsia and prostaglandins. Kidney Int 1983;23:489–97.

[131] Peterson LN. Vitamin D-induced chronic hypercalcemia inhibits thick ascending limb NaCl reabsorption in vivo. Am J Physiol 1990;259:F122–129.

[132] Barron WM, Cohen LH, Ulland LA, Lassiter WE, Fulghum EM, Emmanouel D, et al. Transient vasopressin-resistant diabetes insipidus of pregnancy. N Engl J Med 1984;310:442–4.

[133] Siristatidis C, Salamalekis E, Iakovidou H, Creatsas G. Three cases of diabetes insipidus complicating pregnancy. J Matern Fetal Neonatal Med 2004;16:61–3.

[134] Robertson GL, McLeod JF, Zerbe RL. Vasopressin function in heritable forms of diabetes insipidus. In: Gross P, Richter D, Robertson GL, editors. Vasopressin. Paris: John Libbey Eurotext; 1993. p. 493–502.

[135] Carter RD, Goodman AD. Nephrogenic diabetes insipidus accompanied by massive dilatation of the kidneys, ureters and bladder. J Urol 1963;89:366–9.

[136] Alon U, Chan JC. Hydrochlorothiazide-amiloride in the treatment of congenital nephrogenic diabetes insipidus. Am J Nephrol 1985;5:9–13.

[137] Kirchlechner V, Koller DY, Seidl R, Waldhauser F. Treatment of nephrogenic diabetes insipidus with hydrochlorothiazide and amiloride. Arch Dis Child 1999;80:548–52.

[138] Konoshita T, Kuroda M, Kawane T, Koni I, Miyamori I, Tofuku Y, et al. Treatment of congenital nephrogenic diabetes insipidus with hydrochlorothiazide and amiloride in an adult patient. Horm Res 2004;61:63–7.

[139] Pattaragarn A, Alon US. Treatment of congenital nephrogenic diabetes insipidus by hydrochlorothiazide and cyclooxygenase-2 inhibitor. Pediatr Nephrol 2003;18:1073–6.

[140] Bichet DG. Nephrogenic diabetes insipidus. Am J Med 1998;105:431–42.

[141] Tannen RL, Regal EM, Dunn MJ, Schrier RW. Vasopressin-resistant hyposthenuria in advanced chronic renal disease. N Engl J Med 1969;280:1135–41.

[142] Teitelbaum I, McGuinness S. Vasopressin resistance in chronic renal failure. Evidence for the role of decreased V2 receptor mRNA. J Clin Invest 1995;96:378–85.

[143] Fine LG, Salehmoghaddam S. Water homeostasis in acute and chronic renal failure. Semin Nephrol 1984;4:289.

[144] Fine LG, Schlondorff D, Trizna W, Gilbert RM, Bricker NS. Functional profile of the isolated uremic nephron. Impaired water permeability and adenylate cyclase responsiveness of the cortical collecting tubule to vasopressin. J Clin Invest 1978;61:1519–27.

[145] Gabow PA, Kaehny WD, Johnson AM, Duley IT, Manco-Johnson M, Lezotte DC, et al. The clinical utility of renal concentrating capacity in polycystic kidney disease. Kidney Int 1989;35:675–80.

[146] Buckalew Jr VM, Someren A. Renal manifestations of sickle cell disease. Arch Intern Med 1974;133:660–9.

[147] Statius van Eps LW, Pinedo-Veels C, de Vries GH, de Koning J. Nature of concentrating defect in sickle-cell nephropathy. Microradioangiographic studies. Lancet 1970;1:450–2.

[148] Finn AL, Handler JS, Orloff J. Relation between toad bladder potassium content and permeability response to vasopressin. Am J Physiol 1966;210:1279–84.

[149] Beck N, Singh H, Reed SW, Murdaugh HV, Davis BB. Pathogenic role of cyclic AMP in the impairment of urinary concentrating ability in acute hypercalcemia. J Clin Invest 1974;54:1049–55.

[150] Goldfarb S, Agus ZS. Mechanism of the polyuria of hypercalcemia. Am J Nephrol 1984;4:69–76.

[151] Lins LE. Renal function in hypercalcemia. A clinical and experimental study. Acta Med Scand Suppl 1979;632:1–46.

[152] Gabow PA. Ethylene glycol intoxication. Am J Kidney Dis 1988;11:277–9.

[153] Douglas JB, Healy JK. Nephrotoxic effects of amphotericin B, including renal tubular acidosis. Am J Med 1969;46:154–62.

[154] Farese Jr RV, Schambelan M, Hollander H, Stringari S, Jacobson MA. Nephrogenic diabetes insipidus associated with foscarnet treatment of cytomegalovirus retinitis. Ann Intern Med 1990;112:955–6.

[155] Christensen S. Acute and chronic effects of vasopressin in rats with lithium-polyuria. Acta Pharmacol Toxicol (Copenh) 1976;38:241–53.

[156] Quintanilla AP. Pathophysiology of renal concentrating defects. Ann Clin Lab Sci 1981;11:300–7.

[157] Kanno K, Sasaki S, Hirata Y, Ishikawa S, Fushimi K, Nakanishi S, et al. Urinary excretion of aquaporin-2 in patients with diabetes insipidus. N Engl J Med 1995;332:1540–5.

[158] Ataga KI, Orringer EP. Renal abnormalities in sickle cell disease. Am J Hematol 2000;63:205–11.

[159] Pham PT, Pham PC, Wilkinson AH, Lew SQ. Renal abnormalities in sickle cell disease. Kidney Int 2000;57:1–8.

[160] Robertson G. Pathophysiology of water metabolism. In: Brenner B, editor. The kidney. Philadelphia: WB Saunders; 1996. p. 873–928.

[161] Hollenberg NK. Set point for sodium homeostasis: surfeit, deficit, and their implications. Kidney Int 1980;17:423–9.

[162] Hollenberg NK. Surfeit, deficit, and the set point for sodium homeostasis. Kidney Int 1982;21:883–4.

[163] Halter JB, Goldberg AP, Robertson GL, Porte Jr D. Selective osmoreceptor dysfunction in the syndrome of chronic hypernatremia. J Clin Endocrinol Metab 1977;44:609–16.

[164] Brezis M, Weiler-Ravell D. Hypernatremia, hypodipsia and partial diabetes insipidus: a model for defective osmoregulation. Am J Med Sci 1980;279:37–45.

[165] DeRubertis FR, Michelis MF, Beck N, Field JB, Davis BB. "Essential" hypernatremia due to ineffective osmotic and intact volume regulation of vasopressin secretion. J Clin Invest 1971;50:97–111.

[166] DeRubertis FR, Michelis MF, Davis BB. "Essential" hypernatremia. Report of three cases and review of the literature. Arch Intern Med 1974;134:889–95.

[167] Hammond DN, Moll GW, Robertson GL, Chelmicka-Schorr E. Hypodipsic hypernatremia with normal osmoregulation of vasopressin. N Engl J Med 1986;315:433–6.

[168] Miller PD, Krebs RA, Neal BJ, McIntyre DO. Hypodipsia in geriatric patients. Am J Med 1982;73:354–6.

[169] Moder KG, Hurley DL. Fatal hypernatremia from exogenous salt intake: report of a case and review of the literature. Mayo Clin Proc 1990;65:1587–94.

[170] Thompson CJ, Baylis PH. Thirst in diabetes insipidus: clinical relevance of quantitative assessment. Q J Med 1987;65: 853–62.

[171] Silver AJ. Aging and risks for dehydration. Cleve Clin J Med 1990;57:341–4.

[172] Yamamoto T, Harada H, Fukuyama J, Hayashi T, Mori I. Impaired arginine-vasopressin secretion associated with hypoangiotensinemia in hypernatremic dehydrated elderly patients. Jama 1988;259:1039–42.

[173] Mattar JA, Weil MH, Shubin H, Stein L. Cardiac arrest in the critically ill. II. Hyperosmolal states following cardiac arrest. Am J Med 1974;56:162–8.

[174] Ellis RJ. Severe hypernatremia from sea water ingestion during near-drowning in a hurricane. West J Med 1997;167: 430–3.

[175] Meadow R. Non-accidental salt poisoning. Arch Dis Child 1993;68:448–52.

[176] Reid DE, Frigoletto Fd J, Goodlin RC. Hypernatremia from intravascular saline infusion during therapeutic abortion. Jama 1972;220:1749.

[177] Sanderson NA, Katz MA. The fate of hypertonic saline administered during hemodialysis. Anna J 1994;21:162–9 [discussion 170].

[178] Williams DJ, Jugurnauth J, Harding K, Woolfson RG, Mansell MA. Acute hypernatraemia during bicarbonate-buffered haemodialysis. Nephrol Dial Transplant 1994;9:1170–3.

[179] Allerton JP, Strom JA. Hypernatremia due to repeated doses of charcoal-sorbitol. Am J Kidney Dis 1991;17:581–4.

[180] Peskind ER, Jensen CF, Pascualy M, Tsuang D, Cowley D, Martin DC, et al. Sodium lactate and hypertonic sodium chloride induce equivalent panic incidence, panic symptoms, and hypernatremia in panic disorder. Biol Psychiatry 1998;44: 1007–16.

[181] Ishikawa S, Sakuma N, Fujisawa G, Tsuboi Y, Okada K, Saito T. Opposite changes in serum sodium and potassium in patients in diabetic coma. Endocr J 1994;41:37–43.

[182] Kahn T. Hypernatremia with edema. Arch Intern Med 1999;159:93–8.

[183] Lin M, Liu SJ, Lim IT. Disorders of water imbalance. Emerg Med Clin North Am 2005;23:749–70, ix.

[184] Richman RA, Post EM, Notman DD, Hochberg Z, Moses AM. Simplifying the diagnosis of diabetes insipidus in children. Am J Dis Child 1981;135:839–41.

[185] Milles JJ, Spruce B, Baylis PH. A comparison of diagnostic methods to differentiate diabetes insipidus from primary polyuria: a review of 21 patients. Acta Endocrinol (Copenh) 1983;104:410–6.

[186] Moses AM, Streeten DH. Differentiation of polyuric states by measurement of responses to changes in plasma osmolality induced by hypertonic saline infusions. Am J Med 1967;42:368–77.

[187] Narins RG, Krishna GC. Disorders of water balance. In: Stein JH, editor. Internal Medicine. Boston: Little, Brown; 1987. p. 794.

[188] Narins RG, Riley Jr LJ. Polyuria: simple and mixed disorders. Am J Kidney Dis 1991;17:237–41.

[189] AlOrainy IA, O'Gorman AM, Decell MK. Cerebral bleeding, infarcts, and presumed extrapontine myelinolysis in hypernatraemic dehydration. Neuroradiology 1999;41:144–6.

[190] Finberg L, Luttrell C, Redd H. Pathogenesis of lesions in the nervous system in hypernatremic states. II. Experimental studies of gross anatomic changes and alterations of chemical composition of the tissues. Pediatrics 1959;23:46–53.

[191] Fiordalisi I. Central nervous system complications during hypernatremia and its repair. Arch Pediatr Adolesc Med 1994;148:539–40.

[192] Korkmaz A, Yigit S, Firat M, Oran O. Cranial MRI in neonatal hypernatraemic dehydration. Pediatr Radiol 2000;30:323–5.

[193] Dunger DB, Broadbent V, Yeoman E, Seckl JR, Lightman SL, Grant DB, et al. The frequency and natural history of diabetes insipidus in children with langerhans-cell histiocytosis. N Engl J Med 1989;321:1157–62.

[194] Durr JA, Hoggard JG, Hunt JM, Schrier RW. Diabetes insipidus in pregnancy associated with abnormally high circulating vasopressinase activity. N Engl J Med 1987;316:1070–4.

[195] Ford Jr SM. Transient vasopressin-resistant diabetes insipidus of pregnancy. Obstet Gynecol 1986;68:288–9.

[196] Weiss NM, Robertson GL. Water metabolism in endocrine disorders. Semin Nephrol 1984;4:303.

[197] Yap HY, Tashima CK, Blumenschein GR, Eckles N. Diabetes insipidus and breast cancer. Arch Intern Med 1979;139:1009–11.

[198] Hartfield DS, Loewy JA, Yager JY. Transient thalamic changes on MRI in a child with hypernatremia. Pediatr Neurol 1999;20:60–2.

[199] Hilliard TN, Marsh MJ, Malcolm P, Murdoch IA, Wood BP. Radiological case of the month. Sagittal sinus thrombosis in hypernatremic dehydration. Arch Pediatr Adolesc Med 1998;152:1147 [discussion 1148].

[200] Hochstenbach SL, Ciriello J. Effects of plasma hypernatremia on nucleus tractus solitarius neurons. Am J Physiol 1994;266: R1916–1921.

[201] Manelfe C, Louvet JP. Computed tomography in diabetes insipidus. J Comput Assist Tomogr 1979;3:309–16.

[202] Marks SL, Taboada J. Hypernatremia and hypertonic syndromes. Vet Clin North Am Small Anim Pract 1998;28:533–43.

[203] Riggs JE. Neurologic manifestations of electrolyte disturbances. Neurol Clin 2002;20:227–39, vii.

[204] Tareen N, Martins D, Nagami G, Levine B, Norris KC. Sodium disorders in the elderly [Erratum appears in J Natl Med Assoc. 2005 apr;97(4):446] J Natl Med Assoc 2005;97:217–24.

[205] De Petris L, Luchetti A, Emma F. Cell volume regulation and transport mechanisms across the blood–brain barrier: implications for the management of hypernatraemic states. Eur J Pediatr 2001;160:71–7.

[206] Meyers A. Fluid and electrolyte therapy for children. Curr Opin Pediatr 1994;6:303–9.

[207] Miller NL, Finberg L. Peritoneal dialysis for salt poisoning. Report of a case. N Engl J Med 1960;263:1347–50.

[208] Sterns RH, Baer J, Ebersol S, Thomas D, Lohr JW, Kamm DE. Organic osmolytes in acute hyponatremia. Am J Physiol 36, 1993;264:F833–8.

[209] Sterns RH, Riggs JE, Schochet Jr SS. Osmotic demyelination syndrome following correction of hyponatremia. N Engl J Med 1986;314:1535–42.

[210] Verbalis JG, Gullans SR. Rapid correction of hyponatremia produces differential effects on brain osmolyte and electrolyte reaccumulation in rats. Brain Res 1993;606:19–27.

[211] Vexler ZS, Ayus JC, Roberts TP, Fraser CL, Kucharczyk J, Arieff AI. Hypoxic and ischemic hypoxia exacerbate brain injury associated with metabolic encephalopathy in laboratory animals. J Clin Invest 1994;93:256−64.

[212] Hogan GR, Dodge PR, Gill SR, Pickering LK, Master S. The incidence of seizures after rehydration of hypernatremic rabbits with intravenous or ad libitum oral fluids. Pediatr Res 1984;18:340−5.

[213] Scherbaum WA, Bottazzo GF. Autoantibodies to vasopressin cells in idiopathic diabetes insipidus: evidence for an autoimmune variant. Lancet 1983;1:897−901.

[214] Seckl JR, Dunger DB. Diabetes insipidus. Current treatment recommendations. Drugs 1992;44:216−24.

[215] Vokes TJ, Gaskill MB, Robertson GL. Antibodies to vasopressin in patients with diabetes insipidus. Implications for diagnosis and therapy. Ann Intern Med 1988;108:190−5.

[216] Harris AS. Clinical experience with desmopressin: efficacy and safety in central diabetes insipidus and other conditions. J Pediatr 1989;114:711−8.

[217] Moses AM, Coulson R. Augmentation by chlorpropamide of 1-deamino-8-D-arginine vasopressin-induced antidiuresis and stimulation of renal medullary adenylate cyclase and accumulation of adenosine 3′,5′-monophosphate. Endocrinology 1980;106:967−72.

[218] Rado JP, Marosi J, Borbely L, Tako J. Individual differences in the antidiuretic response induced by DDAVP in diabetes insipidus. Horm Metab Res 1976;8:155−6.

[219] Redmond GP, Rothner AD, Hahn JF, Schumacher OP. Combined desmopressin (DDAVP) and chlorpropamide therapy for diabetes insipidus with absent thirst. Cleve Clin Q 1983;50:351−2.

[220] Robertson GL, Harris A. Clinical use of vasopressin analogues. Hosp Pract (Off Ed) 1989;24:114−8 126−118, 133 passim.

[221] Bichet DG, Razi M, Lonergan M, Arthus MF, Papukna V, Kortas C, et al. Hemodynamic and coagulation responses to 1-desamino[8-D-arginine] vasopressin in patients with congenital nephrogenic diabetes insipidus. N Engl J Med 1988;318:881−7.

[222] Cunnah D, Ross G, Besser GM. Management of cranial diabetes insipidus with oral desmopressin (DDAVP). Clin Endocrinol (Oxf) 1986;24:253−7.

[223] Becker DJ, Foley Jr TP. 1-deamino-8-D-arginine vasopressin in the treatment of central diabetes insipidus in childhood. J Pediatr 1978;92:1011−5.

[224] Durr JA, Hensen J, Ehnis T, Blankenship MS. Chlorpropamide upregulates antidiuretic hormone receptors and unmasks constitutive receptor signaling. Am J Physiol Renal Physiol 2000;278:F799−808.

[225] Froyshov I, Haugen HN. Chlorpropamide treatment in diabetes insipidus. Acta Med Scand 1968;183:397−400.

[226] Wales JK. Treatment of diabetes insipidus with carbamazepine. Lancet 1975;2:948−51.

[227] Orloff J, Burn MB. Vasopressin-resistant diabetes insipidus. In: Stanbury J, Wyngaarden JB, BFrederickson NS, editors. The metabolic basis of inherited disease. New York: McGraw-Hill; 1972. p. 1567.

[228] Rado JP. Combination of carbamazepine and chlorpropamide in the treatment of "hyporesponder" pituitary diabetes insipidus. J Clin Endocrinol Metab 1974;38:1−7.

[229] Libber S, Harrison H, Spector D. Treatment of nephrogenic diabetes insipidus with prostaglandin synthesis inhibitors. J Pediatr 1986;108:305−11.

[230] Finch CK, Kelley KW, Williams RB. Treatment of lithium-induced diabetes insipidus with amiloride. Pharmacotherapy 2003;23:546−50.

[231] Finberg L. Hypernatremic (hypertonic) dehydration in infants. N Engl J Med 1973;289:196−8.

[232] Palevsky PM. Hypernatremia. Semin Nephrol 1998;18:20−30.

[233] Palevsky PM, Bhagrath R, Greenberg A. Hypernatremia in hospitalized patients. Ann Intern Med 1996;124:197−203.

[234] Chilton LA. Prevention and management of hypernatremic dehydration in breast-fed infants. West J Med 1995;163:74−6.

[235] Cooper WO, Atherton HD, Kahana M, Kotagal UR. Increased incidence of severe breastfeeding malnutrition and hypernatremia in a metropolitan area. Pediatrics 1995;96:957−60.

[236] Crook M, Robinson R, Swaminathan R. Hypertriglyceridaemia in a child with hypernatraemia due to a hypothalamic tumour. Ann Clin Biochem 1995;32(Pt 2):226−8.

[237] Dunn K, Butt W. Extreme sodium derangement in a paediatric inpatient population. J Paediatr Child Health 1997;33:26−30.

[238] Bacic A, Gluncic I, Gluncic V. Disturbances in plasma sodium in patients with war head injuries. Mil Med 1999;164:214−7.

[239] Gowrishankar M, Sapir D, Pace K, Halperin ML. Profound natriuresis, extracellular fluid volume contraction, and hypernatremia with hypertonic losses following trauma. Geriatr Nephrol Urol 1997;7:95−100.

[240] Vullo-Navich K, Smith S, Andrews M, Levine AM, Tischler JF, Veglia JM. Comfort and incidence of abnormal serum sodium, BUN, creatinine and osmolality in dehydration of terminal illness. Am J Hosp Palliat Care 1998;15:77−84.

[241] Bhatnagar D, Weinkove C. Serious hypernatraemia in a hospital population. Postgrad Med J 1988;64:441−3.

[242] Daggett P, Deanfield J, Moss F, Reynolds D. Severe hypernatraemia in adults. Br Med J 1979;1:1177−80.

[243] Himmelstein DU, Jones AA, Woolhandler S. Hypernatremic dehydration in nursing home patients: an indicator of neglect. J Am Geriatr Soc 1983;31:466−71.

[244] Long CA, Marin P, Bayer AJ, Shetty HG, Pathy MS. Hypernatraemia in an adult in-patient population. Postgrad Med J 1991;67:643−5.

[245] Mahowald JM, Himmelstein DU. Hypernatremia in the elderly: relation to infection and mortality. J Am Geriatr Soc 1981;29:177−80.

[246] Snyder NA, Feigal DW, Arieff AI. Hypernatremia in elderly patients. A heterogeneous, morbid, and iatrogenic entity. Ann Intern Med 1987;107:309−19.

[247] Ayus JC, Arieff AI. Abnormalities of water metabolism in the elderly. Semin Nephrol 1996;16:277−88.

[248] Kugler JP, Hustead T. Hyponatremia and hypernatremia in the elderly. Am Fam Physician 2000;61:3623−30.

[249] Mandal AK, Saklayen MG, Hillman NM, Markert RJ. Predictive factors for high mortality in hypernatremic patients. Am J Emerg Med 1997;15:130−2.

[250] Grunewald RW, Kinne RK. Osmoregulation in the mammalian kidney: the role of organic osmolytes. J Exp Zool 1999;283:708−24.

[251] Nakanishi T, Balaban RS, Burg MB. Survey of osmolytes in renal cell lines. Am J Physiol 1988;255:C181−191.

[252] Garcia-Perez A, Burg MB. Renal medullary organic osmolytes. Physiol Rev 1991;71:1081−115.

[253] Ho SN. Intracellular water homeostasis and the mammalian cellular osmotic stress response. J Cell Physiol 2006;206:9−15.

[254] Klawitter J, Rivard CJ, Capasso JM, Almeida NE, Berl T, Chan L. Metabonomic analysis of the effects of adaptation to hypertonicity in inner medullary collecting duct (IMCD3) cells. JASN 2004;15:90A.

[255] Burg MB. Molecular basis of osmotic regulation. Am J Physiol 1995;268:F983−996.

[256] Burg MB. Coordinate regulation of organic osmolytes in renal cells. Kidney Int 1996;49:1684—5.

[257] Yancey PH, Burg MB. Counteracting effects of urea and betaine in mammalian cells in culture. Am J Physiol 1990;258: R198—204.

[258] Grunewald JM, Grunewald RW, Kinne RK. Ion content and cell volume in isolated collecting duct cells: effect of hypotonicity. Kidney Int 1993;44:509—17.

[259] Grunewald JM, Grunewald RW, Kinne RK. Regulation of ion content and cell volume in isolated rat renal IMCD cells under hypertonic conditions. Am J Physiol 1994;267: F13—19.

[260] Dmitrieva NI, Cai Q, Burg MB. Cells adapted to high NaCl have many DNA breaks and impaired DNA repair both in cell culture and *in vivo*. Proc Natl Acad Sci USA 2004;101:2317—22.

[261] Dmitrieva NI, Michea LF, Rocha GM, Burg MB. Cell cycle delay and apoptosis in response to osmotic stress. Comp Biochem Physiol A Mol Integr Physiol 2001;130:411—20.

[262] Kultz D, Chakravarty D. Hyperosmolality in the form of elevated NaCl but not urea causes DNA damage in murine kidney cells. Proc Natl Acad Sci USA 2001;98:1999—2004.

[263] Alexander MR, Tyers M, Perret M, Craig BM, Fang KS, Gustin MC. Regulation of cell cycle progression by Swe1p and Hog1p following hypertonic stress. Mol Biol Cell 2001;12:53—62.

[264] Belli G, Gari E, Aldea M, Herrero E. Osmotic stress causes a G1 cell cycle delay and downregulation of Cln3/Cdc28 activity in *Saccharomyces cerevisiae*. Mol Microbiol 2001;39:1022—35.

[265] Copp J, Wiley S, Ward MW, van der Geer P. Hypertonic shock inhibits growth factor receptor signaling, induces caspase-3 activation, and causes reversible fragmentation of the mitochondrial network. Am J Physiol Cell Physiol 2005;288: C403—415.

[266] Desai BN, Myers BR, Schreiber SL. FKBP12-rapamycin-associated protein associates with mitochondria and senses osmotic stress via mitochondrial dysfunction. Proc Natl Acad Sci USA 2002;99:4319—24.

[267] Di Ciano C, Nie Z, Szaszi K, Lewis A, Uruno T, Zhan X, et al. Osmotic stress-induced remodeling of the cortical cytoskeleton. Am J Physiol Cell Physiol 2002;283:C850—865.

[268] Escote X, Zapater M, Clotet J, Posas F. Hog1 mediates cell-cycle arrest in G1 phase by the dual targeting of Sic1. Nat Cell Biol 2004;6:997—1002.

[269] Fumarola C, La Monica S, Guidotti GG. Amino acid signaling through the mammalian target of rapamycin (mTOR) pathway: role of glutamine and of cell shrinkage. J Cell Physiol 2005;204:155—65.

[270] Michea L, Ferguson DR, Peters EM, Andrews PM, Kirby MR, Burg MB. Cell cycle delay and apoptosis are induced by high salt and urea in renal medullary cells. Am J Physiol Renal Physiol 2000;278:F209—218.

[271] Morley SJ, Naegele S. Phosphorylation of eukaryotic initiation factor (eIF) 4E is not required for *de novo* protein synthesis following recovery from hypertonic stress in human kidney cells. J Biol Chem 2002;277:32855—9.

[272] Naegele S, Morley SJ. Molecular cross-talk between MEK1/2 and mTOR signaling during recovery of 293 cells from hypertonic stress. J Biol Chem 2004;279:46023—34.

[273] Zhang Z, Dmitrieva NI, Park JH, Levine RL, Burg MB. High urea and NaCl carbonylate proteins in renal cells in culture and *in vivo*, and high urea causes 8-oxoguanine lesions in their DNA. Proc Natl Acad Sci USA 2004;101:9491—6.

[274] Lockwood AH. Acute and chronic hyperosmolality. Effects on cerebral amino acids and energy metabolism. Arch Neurol 1975;32:62—4.

[275] Lohr JW, McReynolds J, Grimaldi T, Acara M. Effect of acute and chronic hypernatremia on myoinositol and sorbitol concentration in rat brain and kidney. Life Sci 1988;43: 271—6.

[276] Ko BC, Ruepp B, Bohren KM, Gabbay KH, Chung SS. Identification and characterization of multiple osmotic response sequences in the human aldose reductase gene. J Biol Chem 1997;272:16431—7.

[277] Rim JS, Atta MG, Dahl SC, Berry GT, Handler JS, Kwon HM. Transcription of the sodium/myo-inositol cotransporter gene is regulated by multiple tonicity-responsive enhancers spread over 50 kilobase pairs in the 5'-flanking region. J Biol Chem 1998;273:20615—21.

[278] Nakayama Y, Peng T, Sands JM, Bagnasco SM. The TonE/TonEBP pathway mediates tonicity-responsive regulation of UT-A urea transporter expression. J Biol Chem 2000;275: 38275—80.

[279] Ito T, Fujio Y, Hirata M, Takatani T, Matsuda T, Muraoka S, et al. Expression of taurine transporter is regulated through the TonE (tonicity-responsive element)/TonEBP (TonE-binding protein) pathway and contributes to cytoprotection in HepG2 cells. Biochem J 2004;382:177—82.

[280] Woo SK, Lee SD, Na KY, Park WK, Kwon HM. TonEBP/NFAT5 stimulates transcription of HSP70 in response to hypertonicity. Mol Cell Biol 2002;22:5753—60.

[281] Trama J, Go WY, Ho SN. The osmoprotective function of the NFAT5 transcription factor in T cell development and activation. J Immunol 2002;169:5477—88.

[282] Kojima R, Randall JD, Ito E, Manshio H, Suzuki Y, Gullans SR. Regulation of expression of the stress response gene, Osp94: identification of the tonicity response element and intracellular signalling pathways. Biochem J 2004;380:783—94.

[283] Kasono K, Saito T, Tamemoto H, Yanagidate C, Uchida S, Kawakami M, et al. Hypertonicity regulates the aquaporin-2 promoter independently of arginine vasopressin. Nephrol Dial Transplant 2005;20:509—15.

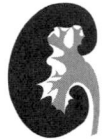

Polyuria and Diabetes Insipidus

Daniel G. Bichet

Hôpital du Sacré-Coeur de Montréal, Departments of Medicine and Physiology, University of Montreal, Montréal,
Québec, Canada

ARGININE VASOPRESSIN

Synthesis

Nonapeptides of the vasopressin family are the key regulators of water homeostasis in amphibia, reptiles, birds, and mammals. Since these peptides reduce urinary output, they are also referred to as antidiuretic hormones. Oxytocin and AVP (Figure 46.1) are synthesized in separate populations of magnocellular neurons of the supraoptic and paraventricular nuclei.[1] Oxytocin is most recognized for its key role in parturition and milk letdown in mammals.[2] The axonal projections of AVP- and oxytocin-producing neurons from supraoptic and paraventricular nuclei reflect the dual function of AVP and oxytocin as hormones and as neuropeptides, in that they project their axons to several brain areas, and to the neurohypophysis. The regulation of the release of AVP from the posterior pituitary is primarily dependent, under normal circumstances, on tonicity information relayed by central osmoreceptor neurons expressing TRPV1[3] (Figure 46.2) and peripheral osmoreceptor neurons expressing TRPV4.[4] AVP and its corresponding carrier, neurophysin II, are synthesized as a composite precursor by the magnocellular neurons of the supraoptic and paraventricular nuclei of the hypothalamus (for review see [5]). The precursor is packaged into neurosecretory granules and transported axonally in the stalk of the posterior pituitary. En route to the neurohypophysis, the precursor is processed into the active hormone. Pre-provasopressin has 164 amino acids, and is encoded by the 2.5 kb *AVP* gene located in chromosome region 20p13.[6,7] The *AVP* gene (coding for AVP and neurophysin II) and the *OXT* gene (coding for oxytocin and neurophysin I) are located in the same chromosome region, at a very short distance from each other (12 kb in humans) in head-to-head orientation.

Data from transgenic mouse studies indicate that the intergenic region between the *OXT* and the *AVP* genes contains the critical enhancer sites for cell-specific expression in the magnocellular neurons.[5] It is phylogenetically interesting to note that *cis* and *trans* components of this specific cellular expression have been conserved between the *Fugu* isotocin (the homolog of mammalian oxytocin) and rat oxytocin genes.[8] Exon 1 of the *AVP* gene encodes the signal peptide, AVP, and the NH$_2$-terminal region of neurophysin II. Exon 2 encodes the central region of neurophysin II, and exon 3 encodes the COOH-terminal region of neurophysin II and the glycopeptide. Provasopressin is generated by the removal of the signal peptide from pre-provasopressin, and from the addition of a carbohydrate chain to the glycopeptide (Figure 46.3). Additional post-translational processing occurs within neurosecretory vesicles during transport of the precursor protein to axon terminals in the posterior pituitary, yielding AVP, neurophysin II, and the glycopeptide. The AVP–neurophysin II complex forms tetramers that can self-associate to form higher oligomers.[9] Neurophysins should be seen as chaperone-like molecules facilitating intracellular transport in magnocellular cells. In the posterior pituitary, AVP is stored in vesicles. Exocytotic release is stimulated by minute increases in serum osmolality (hypernatremia, osmotic regulation), and by more pronounced decreases in extracellular fluid (hypovolemia, non-osmotic regulation). Oxytocin and neurophysin I are released from the posterior pituitary by the suckling response in lactating females.

Immunocytochemical and radioimmunologic studies have demonstrated that oxytocin and vasopressin are synthesized in separate populations of the supraoptic nuclei and the paraventricular nuclei neurons,[10,11] the central and vascular projections of which have

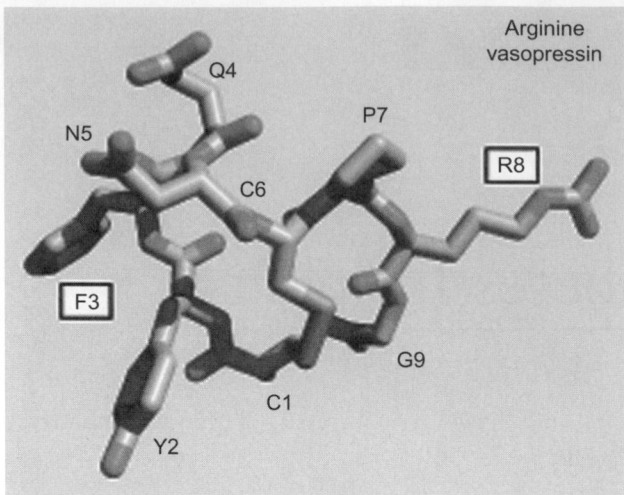
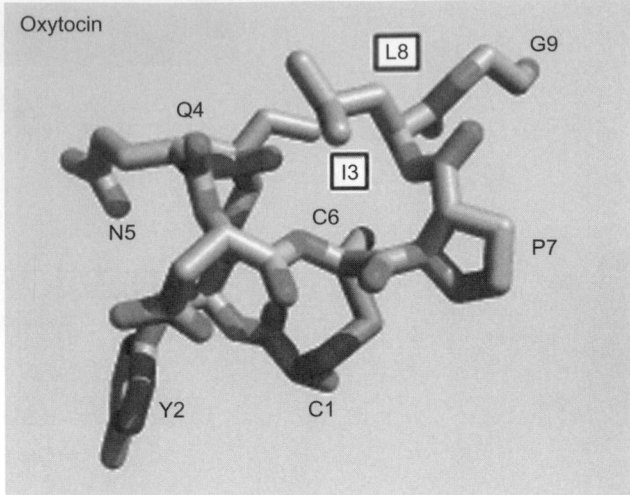

FIGURE 46.1   Contrasting structures of arginine-vasopressin (AVP) and oxytocin (OT). The peptides differ only by two amino acids (F3 → I3 and R8 → L8 in AVP and OT, respectively). *(The conformation of AVP was obtained from ref. [241]; and the conformation of OT was obtained from the Protein Data Bank (PDB Id 1XY1).)*

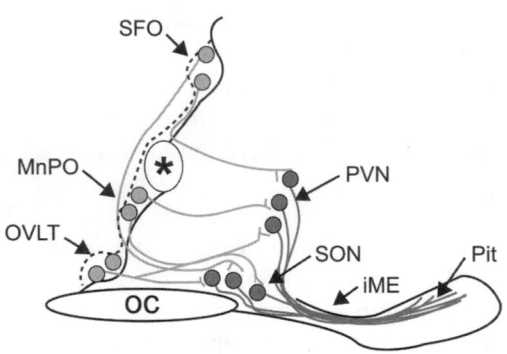

FIGURE 46.2   Schematic representation of the osmoregulatory pathway of the hypothalamus (sagittal section of midline of ventral brain around the 3rd ventricle in mice). Neurons (lightly filled circles) in the lamina terminalis (OVLT), median preoptic nucleus (MnPO) and subfornical organ (SFO) that are responsive to plasma hyptertonicity send efferent axonal projections (gray lines) to magnocellular neurons of the paraventricular (PVN) and supraoptic nuclei (SON). The OVLT is one of the brain circumventricular organs and is a key osmosensing site in the mammalian brain (*vide infra*). The processes (dark lines) of these magnocellular neurons form the hypothalamo–neurohypophysial pathway that courses in the median eminence to reach the posterior pituitary, where neurosecretion of vasopressin and oxytocin occurs. *(Modified from ref. [242].)*

been described in great detail.[12] Some cells express the *AVP* gene and other cells express the *OXT* gene. Immunohistochemical studies have revealed a second vasopressin neurosecretory pathway that transports high concentrations of the hormone to the anterior pituitary gland from parvocellular neurons to the hypophyseal portal system. In the portal system, the high concentration of AVP acts synergistically with corticotropin-releasing hormone (CRH) to stimulate adrenocorticotropic hormone (ACTH) release from the anterior pituitary. More than half of parvocellular neurons co-express both *CRH* and *AVP*. In addition, while passing through the median eminence and the hypophyseal stalk, magnocellular axons can also release AVP into the long portal system. Furthermore, a number of neuroanatomic studies have shown the existence of short portal vessels that allow communication between the posterior and anterior pituitary. Therefore, in addition to parvocellular vasopressin, magnocellular vasopressin is able to influence ACTH secretion.[13,14]

Mammals are Osmoregulators: the Cellular Perception of Tonicity to Stimulate Thirst and Vasopressin Release

Mammals are osmoregulators: they have evolved mechanisms that maintain extracellular fluid (ECF) osmolality near a stable value. Yet, although mammals strive to maintain a constant ECF osmolality, values measured in an individual can fluctuate around the set-point owing to intermittent changes in the rates of water intake and water loss (through evaporation or diuresis), and to variations in the rates of Na intake and excretion (natriuresis). In humans, for example, 40 minutes of strenuous exercise in the heat[15,16] or 24 hours of water deprivation[17] causes plasma osmolality to rise by more than 10 mosmol kg^{-1}. In a dehydrated individual, drinking the equivalent of two large glasses of water (~850 ml) lowers osmolality by approximately 6 mosmol kg^{-1} within 30minutes.[18] Similarly, ingestion of 13 g of salt increases plasma osmolality by approximately 5 mosmol kg^{-1} within 30 minutes.[19] Although osmotic perturbations larger than

Structure of the human vasopressin (AVP) gene and prohormone

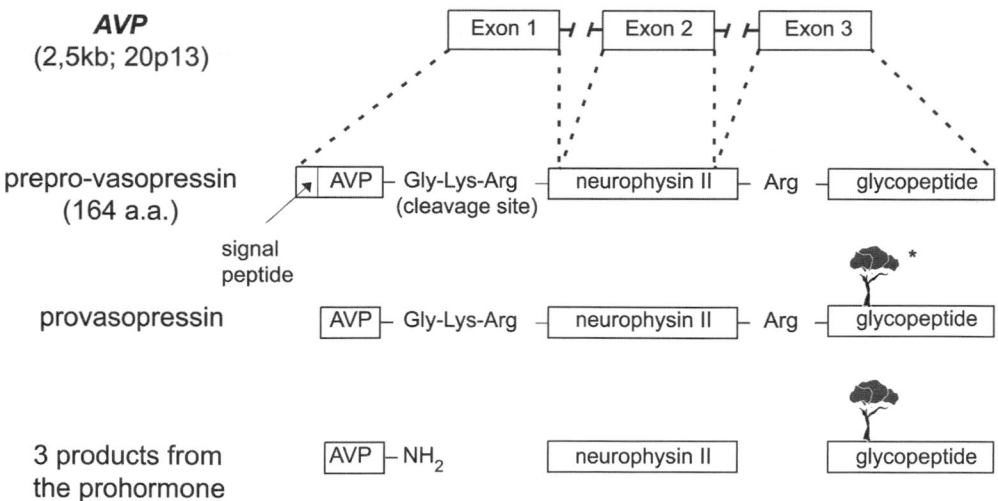

* addition of a carbohydrate chain

FIGURE 46.3 **Structure of the human vasopressin (AVP) gene and prohormone.** Cascade of vasopressin biosynthesis signal peptide; AVP, arginine-vasopressin; neurophysin; glycoprotein.

these can be deleterious to health, changes in the 1—3% range play an integral part in the control of body fluid homeostasis. Differences between the ECF osmolality and the desired set-point induce proportional homeostatic responses according to the principle of negative feedback.[3] ECF hyperosmolality stimulates the sensation of thirst to promote water intake, and the release of vasopressin to enhance water reabsorption in the kidney. By contrast, ECF hypoosmolality suppresses basal VP secretion in rats and humans.[20]

As summarized elegantly by Bourque,[3] early studies provided clear evidence that "cellular dehydration" (that is, cell shrinking) was required for thirst and vasopressin release to be stimulated during ECF hyperosmolality: these responses could be induced by infusions of concentrated solutions containing membrane-impermeable solutes, which extract water from cells, but not by infusions of solutes that readily equilibrate across the cell membrane (such as urea). Verney coined the term "osmoreceptor" to designate the specialized sensory elements. He further showed that these were present in the brain, and postulated that they might comprise "tiny osmometers" and "stretch receptors" that would allow osmotic stimuli to be "transmuted into electrical" signals.[21] Osmoreceptors are therefore defined functionally as neurons that are endowed with an intrinsic ability to detect changes in ECF osmolality, and it is now known that both cerebral and peripheral osmoreceptors contribute to the body fluid balance.

Although magnocellular neurons are themselves osmosensitive, they require input by glutamatergic afferents from the lamina terminalis to respond fully to osmotic challenges (Figure 46.2).

Hypertonicity is sensed by Organum Vasculosum Lamina Terminalis (OVLT) neurons expressing TRPV1 (Transient Receptor Potential Vanilloid-1, *vide infra*): OVLT serves as the brain's primary osmoreceptor area,[22] and neurons in this nucleus transduce hyperosmotic conditions into proportional increases in action-potential firing rate.[23] The information encoded by the electrical activity of these neurons is then relayed synaptically to diverse subsets of homeostatic effector neurons that induce appropriate osmoregulatory responses such as thirst, natriuresis, and antidiuretic hormone release.[3,24—27] The mechanical modulation of TRPV1 is well-demonstrated.[28]

Because the subfornical organ (SFO) and the organum vasculosum of the lamina terminalis (OVLT) lie outside the blood—brain barrier, they can integrate this information with endocrine signals borne by circulating hormones, such as angiotensin II (Ang-II), relaxin, and atrial natriuretic peptide (ANP). While circulating angiotensin II and relaxin excite both OT and vasopressin magnocellular neurons, ANP inhibits vasopressin neurons. The non-osmotic pathways are more physiologically described now as "osmoregulatory gain," since angiotensin II amplifies osmosensory transduction by enhancing the proportional relationship between osmolality, receptor potential, and action potential firing in rat supraoptic nucleus neurons[29] (Figure 46.4). Modifications in osmoregulatory gain induced by angiotensin explain why the changes in the

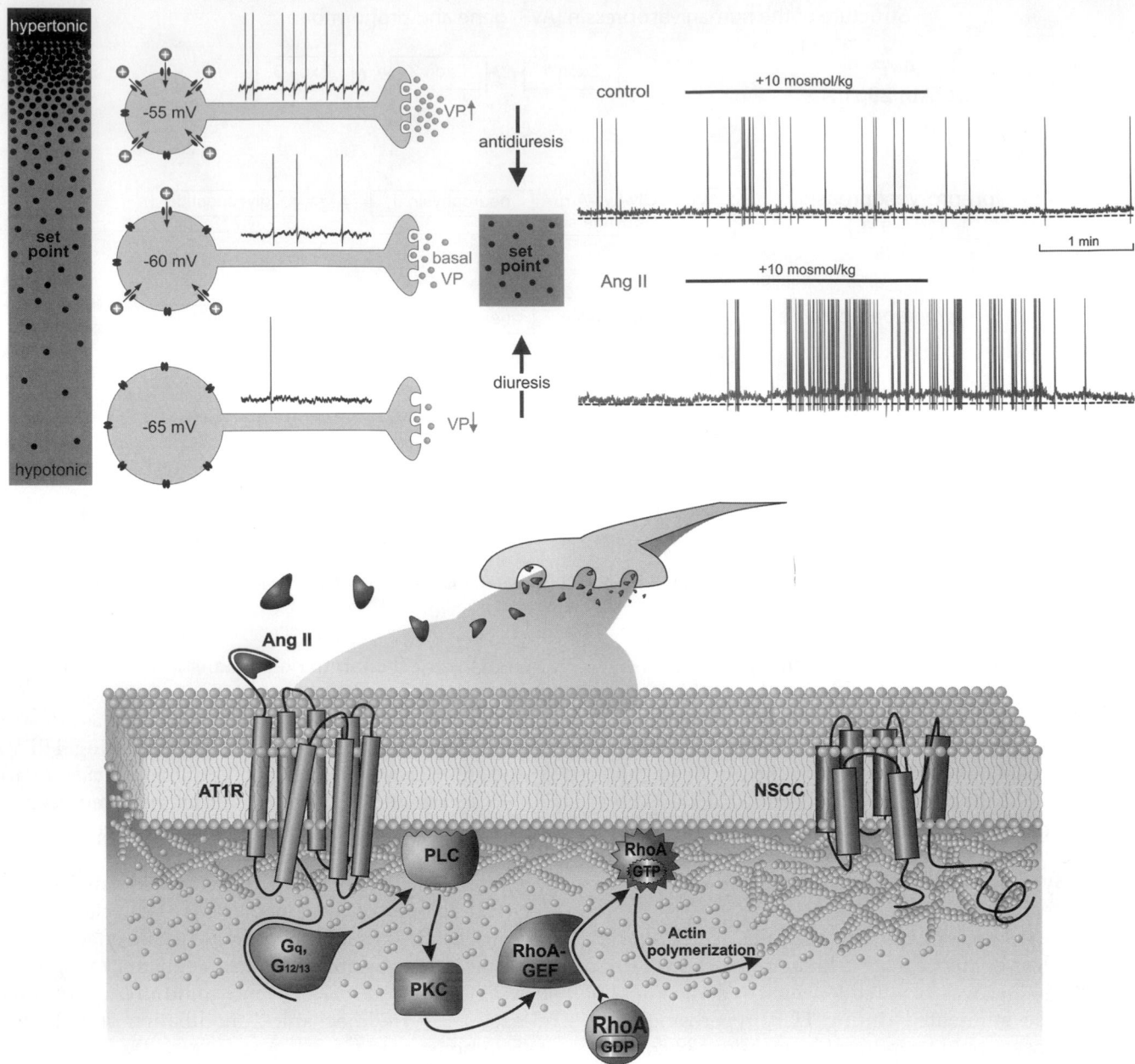

FIGURE 46.4 Upper left: Cell autonomous osmoreception in vasopressin neurons. Changes in osmolality cause inversely proportional changes in soma volume. Shrinkage activates nonselective cation channels (NSCCs) and the ensuing depolarization increases action potential firing rate and vasopressin (VP) release from axon terminals in the neurohypophysis. Increased VP levels in blood enhance water reabsorption by the kidney (antidiuresis) to restore extracellular fluid osmolality toward the set point. Hypotonic stimuli inhibit NSCCs. The resulting hyperpolarization and inhibition of firing reduces VP release and promotes diuresis. Upper right: Whole cell current clamp recordings from isolated MNCs (left) and averaged data from multiple cells show that the depolarizing and action potential firing responses induced by a hypertonic stimulus are significantly enhanced in the presence of 100 nM angiotensin II. Lower right: Hypothetical events mediating central angiotensin II enhancement of osmosensory gain. Angiotensin II released by afferent nerve terminals (e.g., during hypovolemia) binds to AT1 receptor (AT1R) coupled to G-proteins such as Gq or/and G12/13. Activated G-proteins signal through phospholipase C (PLC) and protein kinase C (PKC) to activate a RhoA-specific guanine nucleotide exchange factor (RhoA–GEF), such as p115RhoGEF or LARG (leukemia-associated Rho guanine–nucleotide exchange factor). Activation of RhoA–GEF converts inactive cytosolic RhoA (RhoA–GDP) into active, membrane-associated RhoA–GTP by promoting the exchange of GDP to GTP. ActivatedRhoA induces actin polymerization and increases submembrane F-actin density to enhance the mechanical gating of non-specific cation channels. (*With permission from ref. [243].*)

slope and threshold of the relationship between plasma osmolality and vasopressin secretion are potentiated by hypovolemia or hypotension, and are attenuated by hypervolemia or hypertension[30] (Figure 46.5).

The osmotic stimulation of AVP release by dehydration or hypertonic saline infusion, or both, is regularly used to test the AVP secretory capacity of the posterior pituitary. This secretory capacity can be assessed directly by comparing the plasma AVP concentration measured sequentially during a dehydration procedure with the normal values, and then correlating the plasma AVP with the urinary osmolality measurements obtained simultaneously[31] (Figure 46.6).

The AVP release can also be assessed indirectly by measuring plasma and urine osmolalities at regular intervals during the dehydration test.[32] The maximum urinary osmolality obtained during dehydration is compared with the maximum urinary osmolality obtained after the administration of vasopressin or 1-desamino-8-D-arginine vasopressin (dDAVP; Pitressin: 5 units subcutaneously (SQ) in adults; 1 unit SQ in children or dDAVP 1−4 mg intravenously over 5 to 10 minutes).

The nonosmotic stimulation of AVP release can be used to assess the vasopressin secretory capacity of the posterior pituitary in a rare group of patients with the essential hyponatremia and hypodipsia syndrome. Although some of these patients may have partial central diabetes insipidus, they respond normally to nonosmolar AVP release signals such as hypotension, emesis, and hypoglycemia.[33] In all other cases of suspected central diabetes insipidus, these nonosmotic stimulation tests will not give additional clinical information.[34]

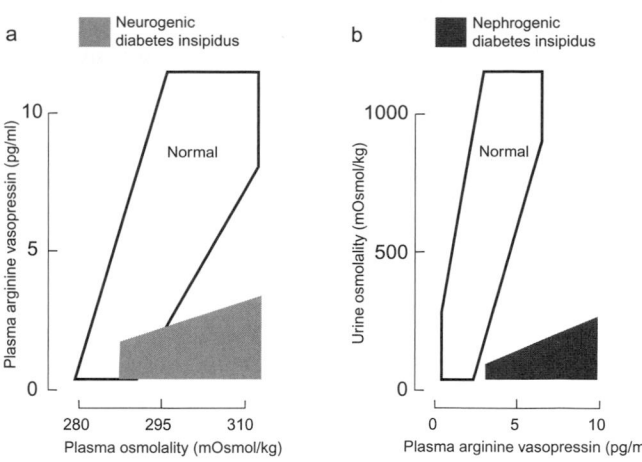

FIGURE 46.6 (a) Schematic diagram of the relationship between plasma arginine-vasopressin (AVP) and plasma osmolality during hypertonic saline infusion. In patients with neurogenic diabetes insipidus, plasma AVP is almost always subnormal relative to plasma osmolality. In contrast, patients with primary polydipsia or nephrogenic diabetes insipidus (NDI) have values within the normal range (light gray area). (b) Relationship between urine osmolality and plasma AVP during a dehydration test. Patients with NDI have hypotonic urine despite high plasma AVP. In contrast, patients with neurogenic diabetes insipidus or primary polydipsia have values within the normal range (dark gray area). *(from ref. [31].)*

Tonicity Information is Relayed by Central Osmoreceptor Neurons Expressing TRPV1 and Peripheral Osmoreceptor Neurons Expressing TRPV4

The osmotic regulation of the release of AVP from the posterior pituitary is primarily dependent, under normal circumstances, on tonicity information relayed by central osmoreceptor neurons expressing TRPV1,[3] and peripheral osmoreceptor neurons expressing TRPV4.[4]

The cellular basis for osmoreceptor potentials has been characterized using patch-clamp recordings and morphometric analysis in magnocellular cells isolated from the supraoptic nucleus of the adult rat. In these cells, stretch-inactivating cationic channels transduce osmotically evoked changes in cell volume into functionally relevant changes in membrane potential. In addition, magnocellular neurons also operate as intrinsic Na^+ detectors. The N-terminal variant of the transient receptor potential channel (TRPV1) is an osmotically activated channel expressed in the magnocellular cells producing vasopressin,[35] and in the circumventricular organs, the OVLT, and the SFO.[23] Since osmoregulation still operates in *Trpv1*$^{-/-}$ mice, other osmosensitive neurons or pathways must be able to compensate for loss of central osmoreceptor function.[23,35,36] Afferent neurons expressing the osmotically-activated ion channel, TRPV4, in the thoracic

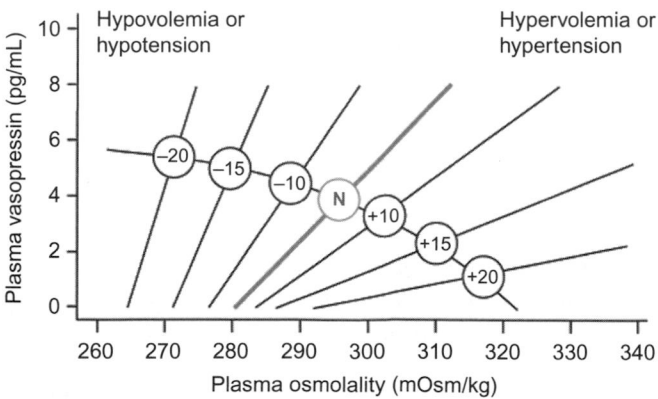

FIGURE 46.5 **Schematic representation of the relationship between plasma vasopressin and plasma osmolality in the presence of differing states of blood volume and/or pressure.** The line labeled N represents normovolemic normotensive conditions. Minus numbers to the left indicate percentage fall, and positive numbers to the right, percentage rise in blood volume or pressure. *(Data from Vokes, T. P., and Robertson, G. L. (1985) Physiology of secretion of vasopressin, In "Frontiers in Hormone Research: Diabetes Insipidus in Man," Vol. 13, 127−155, Czernichow, A. G. R. P., (ed.). S. Karger, Basel.[244])*

dorsal root ganglia that innervate hepatic blood vessels and detect physiological hypoosmotic shifts in blood osmolality have recently been identified.[4] In mice lacking the osmotically-activated ion channel, TRPV4, hepatic sensory neurons no longer exhibit osmosensitive inward currents, and activation of peripheral osmoreceptors *in vivo* is abolished. In a large cohort of human liver transplantees, who presumably have denervated livers, plasma osmolality is significantly elevated compared to healthy controls, suggesting the presence of an inhibitory vasopressin effect of hyponatremia, perceived in the portal vein from hepatic afferents.[4] TRPV1 (expressed in central neurons) and TRPV4 (expressed in peripheral neurons) thus appear to play entirely complementary roles in osmoreception. Lechner et al. have thus identified the primary afferent neurons that constitute the afferent arc of a well-characterized reflex in man and more recently also in rodents.[37] This reflex engages the sympathetic nervous system to raise blood pressure and stimulate metabolism.[38,39] Of clinical interest, it has already been demonstrated that orthostatic hypotension and postprandial hypotension respond to water drinking.[40−42] Moreover, water drinking in man can prevent neutrally-mediated syncope during blood donation or after prolonged standing.[43] Finally, water drinking is also associated with weight loss in overweight individuals.[44] Other peripheral sensory neurons expressing other mechanosensitive proteins may also be involved in osmosensitivity.[45]

Cellular Actions of Vasopressin

The neurohypophyseal hormone AVP has multiple actions, including the inhibition of diuresis, contraction of smooth muscle, platelet aggregation, stimulation of liver glycogenolysis, modulation of adrenocorticotropic hormone release from the pituitary, and central regulation of somatic and higher functions (thermoregulation, blood pressure, autonomic expression of fear, neurobiology of attachment).[46−48] These multiple actions of AVP could be explained by the interaction of AVP with at least three types of G-protein-coupled receptors: the V1a (vascular hepatic) and V1b (anterior pituitary) receptors act through phosphatidylinositol hydrolysis to mobilize calcium[49]; and the V2 (kidney) receptor is coupled to adenylate cyclase.[48]

The transfer of water across the principal cells of the collecting ducts is now known at such a detailed level that billions of molecules of water traversing the membrane can be represented; see useful teaching tools at http://www.mpibpc.gwdg.de/abteilungen/073/gallery.html and http://www.ks.uiuc.edu/research/aquaporins. The 2003 Nobel Prize in chemistry was awarded to Peter Agre and Roderick MacKinnon, who solved two complementary problems presented by the cell membrane: how does a cell let one type of ion through the lipid membrane to the exclusion of other ions; and how does it permeate water without ions? This contributed to a momentum and renewed interest in basic discoveries related to the transport of water, and indirectly to diabetes insipidus.[50,51] The first step in the action of AVP (synthesized by du Vigneaud, Nobel Prize in Chemistry 1955)[52] on water excretion is its binding to arginine vasopressin type-2 receptors (hereafter referred to as V2 receptors) on the basolateral membrane of the collecting duct cells (Figure 46.7). The human *AVPR2* gene that codes for the V2 receptor is located in chromosome region Xq28, and has three exons and two small introns.[53,54] The sequence of the cDNA predicts a polypeptide of 371 amino acids with seven transmembrane, four extracellular, and four cytoplasmic domains. The activation of the V2 receptor on renal collecting tubules stimulates adenylyl cyclase via the stimulatory G-protein (Gs) (1994 Nobel Prize in Physiology and Medicine to Rodbell and Gilman for signal transduction and G-proteins), and promotes the cyclic adenosine monophosphate (cAMP)-mediated incorporation of water channels into the luminal surface of these cells.[55] E. Sutherland and T. Rall isolated cyclic adenosine monophosphate in 1956, and Sutherland was awarded the Nobel Prize in Physiology or Medicine in 1971.[56] There are two ubiquitously expressed intracellular cAMP receptors: (1) the classical protein kinase A (PKA) that is a cAMP-dependent protein kinase; and (2) the recently discovered exchange protein directly activated by cAMP that is a cAMP-regulated guanine nucleotide exchange factor. Both of these receptors contain an evolutionarily-conserved cAMP-binding domain that acts as a molecular switch for sensing intracellular cAMP levels to control diverse biological functions.[57] Several proteins participating in the control of cAMP-dependent AQP2 trafficking have been identified; for example, A-kinase anchoring proteins tethering PKA to cellular compartments; phosphodiesterases regulating the local cAMP level; cytoskeletal components such as F-actin and microtubules; small GTPases of the Rho family controlling cytoskeletal dynamics; motor proteins transporting AQP2-bearing vesicles to and from the plasma membrane for exocytic insertion and endocytic retrieval; SNAREs inducing membrane fusions, hsc70, a chaperone important for endocytic retrieval. These processes are the molecular basis of the vasopressin-induced increase in the osmotic water permeability of the apical membrane of the collecting tubule.[58−60]

AVP also increases the water reabsorptive capacity of the kidney by regulating the urea transporter

Outer and inner medullary collecting duct

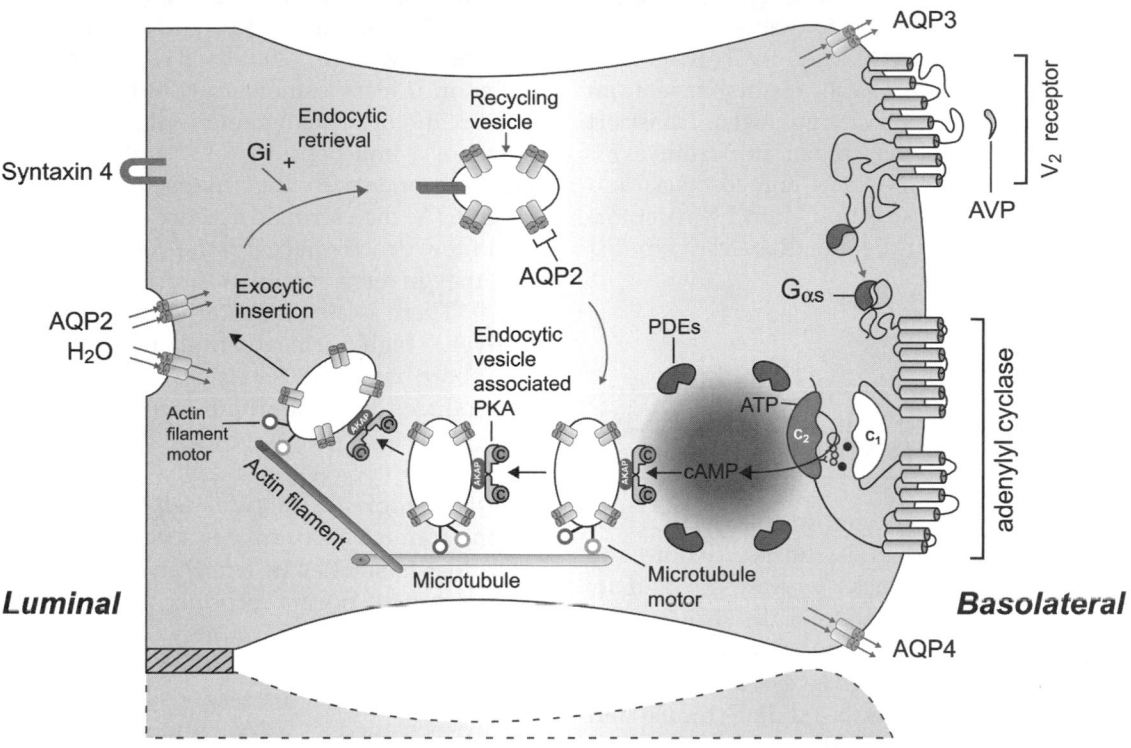

FIGURE 46.7 **Schematic representation of the effect of vasopressin (AVP) to increase water permeability in the principal cells of the collecting duct.** AVP is bound to the V2 receptor (a G-protein-linked receptor) on the basolateral membrane. The basic process of G-protein-coupled receptor signaling consists of three steps: a hepta-helical receptor that detects a ligand (in this case, AVP) in the extracellular milieu; a G-protein ($G_{\alpha s}$) that dissociates into a subunits bound to GTP and bg subunits after interaction with the ligand-bound receptor; and an effector (in this case, adenylyl cyclase) that interacts with dissociated G-protein subunits to generate small-molecule second messengers. AVP activates adenylyl cyclase, increasing the intracellular concentration of cAMP. The topology of adenylyl cyclase is characterized by two tandem repeats of six hydrophobic transmembrane domains separated by a large cytoplasmic loop, and terminates in a large intracellular tail. The dimeric structure (C_1 and C_2) of the catalytic domains is represented. Conversion of ATP to cAMP takes place at the dimer interface. Two aspartate residues (in C_1) coordinate two metal co-factors (Mg^{2+} or Mn^{2+}, represented here as two small black circles), which enable the catalytic function of the enzyme. Adenosine is shown as an open circle and the three phosphate groups (ATP) are shown as smaller open circles. Protein kinase A (PKA) is the target of the generated cAMP. The binding of cAMP to the regulatory subunits of PKA induces a conformational change, causing these subunits to dissociate from the catalytic subunits. These activated subunits (C) as shown here are anchored to an aquaporin-2 (AQP2)-containing endocytic vesicle via an A-kinase anchoring protein. The local concentration and distribution of the cAMP gradient is limited by phosphodiesterases (PDEs). Cytoplasmic vesicles carrying the water channels (represented as homotetrameric complexes) are fused to the luminal membrane in response to AVP, thereby increasing the water permeability of this membrane. The dissociation of the A-kinase anchoring protein from the endocytic vesicle is not represented. Microtubules and actin filaments are necessary for vesicle movement toward the membrane. When AVP is not available, AQP2 water channels are retrieved by an endocytic process, and water permeability returns to its original low rate. Aquaporin-3 (AQP3) and aquaporin-4 (AQP4) water channels are expressed constitutively at the basolateral membrane.

variants UT-A1/3, which are present in the inner medullary collecting duct, predominantly in its terminal part.[61] AVP also increases the permeability of principal collecting duct cells to sodium. In summary, as stated elegantly by Ward and colleagues,[62] in the absence of AVP stimulation, collecting duct epithelia exhibit very low permeabilities to sodium urea and water. These specialized permeability properties permit the excretion of large volumes of hypotonic urine formed during intervals of water diuresis. In contrast, AVP stimulation of the principal cells of the collecting ducts leads to selective increases in the permeability of the apical membrane to water (P_f), urea (P_{urea}), and Na (P_{Na}).

The actions of vasopressin in the distal nephron are possibly modulated by prostaglandin E2, nitric oxide,[63] and by luminal calcium concentration. PGE_2 is synthesized and released in the collecting duct, which expresses all four E-prostanoid receptors (EP1–4). Both EP2 and EP4 can signal via increased cAMP. Olesen et al. hypothesized that selective EP receptor stimulation could mimic the effects of vasopressin, and demonstrated that, at physiological levels, PGE_2 markedly increased apical membrane abundance and phosphorylation of AQP2 *in vitro* and *ex vivo*, leading to increased cell water permeability.[64] In their experiments, both EP2 and EP4 selective agonists were able to mimic these effects. Furthermore, an EP2-agonist was able to positively regulate urinary-concentrating mechanisms in an animal model of nephrogenic diabetes insipidus where AVPR2 receptors were blocked by Tolvaptan, a non-peptide V2-antagonist. These results reveal an alternative mechanism for regulating water transport in the collecting duct that has major importance for understanding whole body water homeostasis, and provide a rationale for investigations into EP receptor-agonist use in X-linked nephrogenic diabetes insipidus treatment.

THE BRATTLEBORO RAT WITH AUTOSOMAL RECESSIVE NEUROGENIC DIABETES INSIPIDUS

The animal model of diabetes insipidus that has been most extensively studied is the Brattleboro rat. Discovered in 1961, the rat lacks vasopressin and its neurophysin, whereas the synthesis of the structurally-related hormone oxytocin is not affected by the mutation.[65] Its inability to synthesize vasopressin is inherited as an autosomal recessive trait. Schmale and Richter[66] isolated and sequenced the vasopressin gene from homozygous Brattleboro rats, and found that the defect is due to a single nucleotide deletion of a G residue within the second exon encoding the carrier protein neurophysin (Figure 46.8). The shift in the reading frame caused by this deletion predicts a precursor with an entirely different C-terminus. The messenger RNA (mRNA) produced by the mutated gene encodes a normal AVP, but an abnormal NPII moiety[66] which impairs transport and processing of the AVP-NPII precursor and its retention in the endoplasmic reticulum of the magnocellular neurons where it is produced.[67,68] Homozygous Brattleboro rats may still demonstrate

deleted in Brattleboro rat

↓

```
GGA AGC GGA GGC CGC TGC GCT GCC     Rat
Gly Ser Gly Gly Arg Cys Ala Ala


GGG AGC GGG GGC CGC TGC GCC GCC     Human
Gly Ser Gly Gly Arg Cys Ala Ala
 62  63  64  65  66  67  68  69
```

FIGURE 46.8 Neurophysin II genomic and amino acid sequence showing the 1 bp (G) deleted in the Brattleboro rat. The human sequence (GenBank entry M11166) is also shown. It is almost identical to the rat prepro sequence. In the Brattleboro rat, G1880 is deleted with a resultant frameshift after 63 amino acids (amino acid-1 is the first amino acid of neurophysin II).

some V2 (*vide infra*) antidiuretic effects, since the administration of a selective non-peptide V2-antagonist (SR 121463 A, 10 mg/kg i.p.) induced a further increase in urine flow rate (200 to 354 ± 42 mL/24 h) and a decline in urinary osmolality (170 to 92 ± 8 mmol/kg).[69] This decline in urine osmolality following the administration of a non-peptide V2 receptor antagonist could also be secondary to the "inverse agonist" properties of SR121463A: the intrinsic activity or "tone," of the V2R would be deactivated by the SR121463A compound (for the inverse agonist properties of SR121463A see [70]). There is also an alternative explanation to this relatively high urine osmolality of 170 since, in Brattleboro rats, low levels of hormonally-active AVP are produced from alternate forms of AVP preprohormone. Due to a process called molecular misreading, one transcript contains a 2 bp deletion downstream from the single nucleotide deletion that restores the reading frame, and produces a variant AVP preprohormone that is smaller in length by one amino acid and differs from the normal product by only 13 amino acids in the neurophysin II moiety.[71] Oxytocin, which is present at enhanced plasma concentrations in Brattleboro rats, may be responsible for the antidiuretic activity observed.[72,73] Oxytocin is not stimulated by increased plasma osmolality in humans.

KNOCKOUT MICE WITH URINARY CONCENTRATION DEFECTS

A useful strategy to establish the physiological function of a protein is to determine the phenotype produced by pharmacological inhibition of protein function or by gene disruption. Transgenic knockout mice deficient in AQP1, AQP2, AQP3, AQP4, and CLCNK1, NKCC2, NFAT5, AVPR2 or AGT have been engineered.[74-83] Angiotensinogen (AGT)-deficient mice are characterized by both concentrating and diluting defects secondary to a defective renal papillary architecture.[80] The *Aqp3*, *Aqp4*, *Clcnk1*, and *Agt* knockout mice have no identified human counterparts. Of interest, *AQP1*-null individuals have no obvious symptoms.[84] Yang et al.[85] have generated an AQP2-T126M "conditional knock-in" model of NDI, to recapitulate the clinical features of the naturally occurring human AQP2 mutation T126M.[86] The conditional knock-in adult mice showed polyuria, urinary hypoosmolality, and ER retention of AQP2-T126M in the collecting duct. Screening of candidate protein folding "correctors" in AQP2-T126M-transfected kidney cells showed increased AQP2-T126M plasma membrane expression with the Hsp90 inhibitor 17-allylamino-17-demethoxygeldanamycin (17-AAG), a compound currently in clinical trials for tumor therapy. 17-AAG increased urine osmolality in the AQP2-T126M mice (without effect in AQP2 null mice), and partially rescued defective AQP2-T126M cellular processing. These proof-of-concept findings suggest the possibility of using existing drugs for therapy in some forms of NDI.

Mice lacking the AVPR2 receptor failed to thrive and died within the first week after birth due to hypernatremic dehydration.[83] Li et al.[87] generated mice in which the *Avpr2* gene could be conditionally deleted during adulthood by administration of 4-OH-tamoxifen. Adult mice displayed all characteristic symptoms of X-linked NDI, including polyuria, polydipsia, and resistance to the antidiuretic actions of vasopressin. Gene expression analysis suggested that activation of renal EP4 PGE_2 receptors might compensate for the lack of renal V2R activity in X-linked NDI mice, and both acute and chronic treatment of the mutant mice with a selective EP4 receptor agonist greatly reduced all major manifestations of XNDI. This beneficial effect is likely secondary to the intracellular generation of cAMP at the principal cell level by EP4 PGE_2 receptors.

As reviewed by Rao and Verkman,[88] extrapolation of data in mice to humans must be made with caution. For example, the maximum osmolality of mouse (< 3000 mOsm/kg H_2O) is much greater than that of human urine (1000 mOsmol/kg H_2O), and normal serum osmolality in mice is 330 to 345 mOsmol/kg H_2O, substantially greater than that in humans (280–290 mOsm/kg H_2O). Protein expression patterns, and thus the interpretation of phenotype studies, may also be species-dependent. For example, AQP4 is expressed in both proximal tubule and collecting duct in mouse, but only in collecting duct in rat and human.[88]

Ethylnitrosourea-mutagenized mice heterozygous for the F204V mutation in the *Aqp2* gene have been described,[89] and mice from the Jackson Laboratory with congenital progressive hydronephrosis bear the S256L mutation in *Aqp2* which affects its phosphorylation and apical membrane accumulation.[90,91]

QUANTITATING RENAL WATER EXCRETION

Diabetes insipidus is characterized by the excretion of abnormally large volumes of hypoosmotic urine (< 250 mmol/kg). This definition excludes osmotic diuresis, which occurs when excess solute is being excreted, as with glucose in the polyuria of diabetes mellitus. Other agents that produce osmotic diuresis are mannitol, urea, glycerol, contrast media, and loop diuretics. Osmotic diuresis should be considered when solute excretion exceeds 60 mmol/hour. The quantification of water excretion (free water clearance, osmolar clearance, free electrolyte water reabsorption, effective water clearance) is described elsewhere in this textbook.

CLINICAL CHARACTERISTICS OF DIABETES INSIPIDUS DISORDERS

Neurogenic Diabetes Insipidus

Common Forms

Failure to synthesize or secrete vasopressin normally limits maximal urinary concentration and, depending on the severity of the disease, causes varying degrees of polyuria and polydipsia. Experimental destruction of the vasopressin-synthesizing areas of the hypothalamus (supraoptic and paraventricular nuclei) causes a permanent form of the disease. Similar results are obtained by sectioning the hypophyseal hypothalamic tract above the median eminence. Sections below the median eminence, however, produce only transient diabetes insipidus. Lesions to the hypothalamic–pituitary tract are frequently associated with a three-stage response in experimental animals and in humans[92]: (1) an initial diuretic phase lasting from a few hours to 5 to 6 days; (2) a period of antidiuresis unresponsive to fluid administration (this antidiuresis is probably due to vasopressin release from injured axons and may last from a few hours to several days; because urinary dilution is impaired during this phase, continued water administration can cause severe hyponatremia); and (3) a final period of diabetes insipidus. The extent of the injury determines the completeness of the diabetes insipidus and, as already discussed, the site of the lesion determines whether the disease will be permanent.

Twenty-five percent of patients studied after transsphenoidal surgery developed spontaneous isolated hyponatremia, 20% developed diabetes insipidus, and 46% remained normonatremic. Normonatremia, hyponatremia, and diabetes insipidus were associated with increasing degrees of surgical manipulation of the posterior lobe and pituitary stalk during surgery.[93] Central diabetes insipidus observed after transphenoidal surgery is often transient, and only 2% of patients need long-term treatment with dDAVP.[94]

The causes of central diabetes insipidus in adults and in children are listed in Table 46.1.[95–98] Rare causes of central diabetes insipidus include leukemia, thrombotic thrombocytopenic purpura, pituitary apoplexy, sarcoidosis[99] and Wegener granulomatosis, xanthoma disseminatum,[100] septooptico dysplasia and agenesis of the corpus callosum,[101] metabolic anorexia nervosa, lymphocytic hypophysitis,[102] and necrotizing

TABLE 46.1 Etiology of Hypothalamic Diabetes Insipidus in Children and Adults

	Children (%)	Children and Young Adults (%)	Adults (%)
Primary brain tumor[a]	49.5	22.0	30.0
Before surgery	33.5		13.0
After surgery	16.0		17.0
Idiopathic (isolated or familial)	29.0	58.0	25.0
Histiocytosis	16.0	12.0	–
Metastatic cancer[b]	–		8.0
Trauma[c]	2.2	2.0	17.0
Postinfectious disease	2.2	6.0	–

*Data from Czernichow, P., Pomarede, R., Brauner, R., Rappaport, R. (1985). Neurogenic diabetes insipidus in children. In "Frontiers of Hormone Research," 190−20, Czernichow, P., and Robinson, A. G. (eds.). S. Karger, Basel, Switzerland[95]; Greger, N. G., Kirkland, R. T., Clayton, G. W., and Kirkland, J. L. (1986). Central diabetes insipidus. 22 years' experience. Am. J. Dis. Child **140**, 551−554[96]; Moses, A. M., Blumenthal, S. A., and Streeten, D. H. P. (1985). Acid−base and electrolyte disorders associated with endocrine disease: Pituitary and thyroid. In "Fluid, Electrolyte and Acid−Base Disorders," 851−892, Arieff, A. I., and de Fronzo, R. A., (eds.). Churchill Livingstone, New York[98]; Maghnie, M., Cosi, G., and Genovese, E., et al. (2000). Central diabetes insipidus in children and young adults. N. Engl. J. Med. **343**, 998−1007.[97]*
[a]Primary malignancy: craniopharyngioma, dysgerminoma, meningioma, adenoma, glioma, astrocytoma.
[b]Secondary: metastatic from lung or breast, lymphoma, leukemia, dysplastic pancytopenia.
[c]Trauma could be severe or mild.

infundibulo-hypophysitis.[103] Maghnie et al.[97] studied 79 patients with central diabetes insipidus: additional deficits in anterior pituitary hormones were documented in 61% of patients, a median of 0.6 years (range, 01−18.0 years) after the onset of diabetes insipidus. The most frequent abnormality was growth hormone deficiency (59%), followed by hypothyroidism (28%), hypogonadism (24%), and adrenal insufficiency (22%). Seventy-five percent of the patients with Langerhans cell histiocytosis had an anterior pituitary hormone deficiency that was first detected a median of 3.5 years after the onset of diabetes insipidus.[97] None of the patients with central diabetes insipidus secondary to *AVP* mutations developed anterior pituitary hormone deficiencies.

Rare Forms

AUTOSOMAL DOMINANT AND RECESSIVE NEUROGENIC DIABETES INSIPIDUS

Lacombe[104] and Weil[105] described a familial non-X-linked form of diabetes insipidus without any associated mental retardation. The descendants of the family described by Weil were later found to have autosomal dominant neurogenic diabetes insipidus.[106−108]

Hereditary neurogenic diabetes insipidus (OMIM 125700)[109] is a well-characterized entity, secondary to mutations in *AVP* (OMIM 192340).[109] Patients with autosomal dominant neurogenic diabetes insipidus retain some limited capacity to secrete AVP during severe dehydration, and the polyuropolydipsic symptoms usually appear after the first year of life,[110] when the infant's demand for water is more likely to be understood by adults. In hereditary neurohypophyseal diabetes insipidus, termed familial neurohypophyseal diabetes insipidus (FNDI), levels of AVP are insufficient, and patients show a positive response to treatment with dAVP. Growth retardation might be observed in untreated children with autosomal dominant FNDI.[111] Over 60 mutations in the prepro-arginine-vasopressin-neurophysin II *AVP* gene located on chromosome 20p13 have been reported in dominant FNDI (adFNDI). Knock-in mice heterozygous for a nonsense mutation in the AVP carrier protein neurophysin II showed progressive loss of AVP-producing neurons over several months correlated with increased water intake, increased urine output, and decreased urine osmolality. The data suggest that vasopressin mutants accumulate as fibrillar aggregates in the endoplasmic reticulum and cause cumulative toxicity to magnocellular neurons, explaining the later age-of-onset.[112,113] To date, recessive FNDI, with early polyuric manifestations, has only been described in three studies.[114−116] Very early (first week of life) polyuric states are usually nephrogenic, but we and others have observed autosomal recessive central diabetes insipidus patients with early polyuria, dehydration episodes responding to dDAVP with specific mutations of the AVP gene.[114−117] A study by Christensen[118] examined the differences in cellular trafficking between dominant and recessive AVP mutants, and found that dominant forms were concentrated in the cytoplasm, whereas recessive forms were localized to the tips of neurites. The expression of regulated secretory proteins such as granins and prohormones, including pro-vasopressin, generates granule-like structures in a variety of neuroendocrine cell lines due to aggregation in the trans-Golgi.[119] Co-staining experiments unambiguously distinguished between these granule-like structures and the accumulations by pathogenic dominant mutants formed in the ER, since the latter, but not the trans-Golgi granules, co-localized with specific ER markers.[112] As studies concerning both dominant and recessive FNDI accumulate, it is becoming evident that FNDI exhibits a variable age-of-onset, and this may be related to the cellular handling of the mutant AVP. This progressive toxicity, sometimes called a toxic gain-of-function, shares mechanistic pathways with other neurodegenerative diseases, such as Huntington's and Parkinson's.

Of interest, errors in protein folding represent the underlying basis for many inherited diseases[120–122] and are also pathogenic mechanisms for *AVP*, *AVPR2*, and *AQP2* mutants. Why AVP-misfolded mutants are cytotoxic to AVP-producing neurons is an unresolved issue. Protein misfolding, an "unfolded protein response" in cells, and the accumulation of excess misfolded protein leading to apoptotic cell death are well-documented for autosomal dominant retinitis pigmentosa.[123]

WOLFRAM SYNDROME

Wolfram syndrome, also known as DIDMOAD, is an autosomal recessive neurodegenerative disorder accompanied by insulin-dependent diabetes mellitus and progressive optic atrophy. The acronym DIDMOAD describes the following clinical features of the syndrome: *d*iabetes *i*nsipidus, *d*iabetes *m*ellitus, *o*ptic *a*trophy, and sensorineural *d*eafness. An unusual incidence of psychiatric symptoms has also been described in patients with this syndrome. These included paranoid delusions, auditory or visual hallucinations, psychotic behavior, violent behavior, organic brain syndrome typically in the late or preterminal stages of their illness, progressive dementia, and severe learning disabilities or mental retardation or both. Patients with Wolfram syndrome develop diabetes mellitus and bilateral optical atrophy mainly in the first decade of life, the diabetes insipidus is usually partial and of gradual onset, and the polyuria can be wrongly attributed to poor glycemic control. Furthermore, a severe hyperosmolar state can occur if untreated diabetes mellitus is associated with an unrecognized posterior pituitary deficiency. The dilatation of the urinary tract observed in the DIDMOAD syndrome may be secondary to chronic high urine flow rates and, perhaps, to some degenerative aspects of the innervation of the urinary tract. The gene responsible for Wolfram syndrome, located in chromosome region 4p16.1, encodes a putative 890 amino acid transmembrane protein referred as *wolframin*. Wolframin is an endoglycosidase H-sensitive glycoprotein, which localizes primarily in the endoplasmic reticulum of a variety of neurons, including neurons in the supraoptic nucleus and neurons in the lateral magnocellular division of the paraventricular nucleus.[124,125] Disruption of the *Wfs1* gene in mice cause progressive β-cell loss and impaired stimulus-secretion coupling in insulin secretion, but central diabetes insipidus is not observed in *Wfs*[−/−] mice.[126] Miner1, another endoplasmic reticulum protein, is causative in Wolfram syndrome 2[127] and WFS1 negatively regulates a key transcription factor involved in ER stress signalling.[128]

SYNDROME OF HYPERNATREMIA AND HYPODIPSIA

Some patients with the hypernatremia and hypodipsia syndrome may have partial central diabetes insipidus. These patients also have persistent hypernatremia that is not due to any apparent extracellular volume loss, absence or attenuation of thirst, and a normal renal response to AVP. In almost all the patients studied, the hypodipsia has been associated with cerebral lesions in the vicinity of the hypothalamus. It has been proposed that in these patients there is a "resetting" of the osmoreceptor, because their urine tends to become concentrated or diluted at inappropriately high levels of plasma osmolality. However, using the regression analysis of plasma AVP concentration versus plasma osmolality, it has been shown that in some of these patients the tendency to concentrate and dilute urine at inappropriately high levels of plasma osmolality is due solely to a marked reduction in sensitivity or a gain in the osmoregulatory mechanism.[129] This finding is compatible with the diagnosis of partial central diabetes insipidus. In other patients, however, plasma AVP concentrations fluctuate in a random manner, bearing no apparent relationship to changes in plasma osmolality. Such patients frequently display large swings in serum sodium concentration, and frequently exhibit hypodipsia. It appears that most patients with "essential hypernatremia" fit one of these two patterns (Figure 46.9). Both of these groups of patients consistently respond normally to nonosmolar AVP release signals, such as hypotension, emesis, hypoglycemia or all three. These

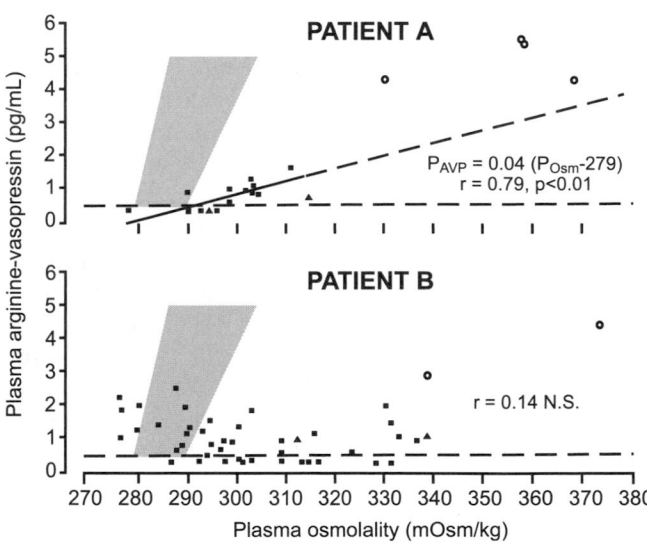

FIGURE 46.9   Plasma arginine vasopressin (PAVP) as a function of "effective" plasma osmolality(P_{Osm}) in two patients with adipsic hypernatremia. Open circles indicate values obtained on admission; filled squares indicate those obtained during forced hydration; filled triangles indicate those obtained after 1 to 2 weeks of ad libitum water intake; gray areas indicate range of normal values. *(From ref. [245].)*

observations suggest that: (1) the osmoreceptor may be anatomically, as well as functionally, separate from the nonosmotic efferent pathways and neurosecretory neurons for vasopressin, and a hypothalamic lesion may impair the osmotic release of AVP while the nonosmotic release of AVP remains intact; and (2) the osmoreceptor neurons that regulate vasopressin secretion are not synonymous with those that regulate thirst.

Hereditary Nephrogenic Diabetes Insipidus

In nephrogenic diabetes insipidus (NDI), the kidney is unable to concentrate urine despite normal or elevated concentrations of the antidiuretic hormone arginine vasopressin. In congenital NDI, the obvious clinical manifestations of the disease, that is polyuria and polydipsia, are present at birth and need to be immediately recognized to avoid severe episodes of dehydration. It is clinically useful to distinguish two types of hereditary NDI: a "pure" type characterized by loss of water only; and a complex type characterized by loss of water and ions. Patients who have congenital NDI and mutations in the *AVPR2* or *AQP2* genes have a pure NDI phenotype with loss of water but normal conservation of sodium, potassium, chloride, and calcium. Patients with inactivating mutations in genes (*SLC12A1*, *KCNJ1*, *CLCNKB*, *CLCNKA*, and *CLCNKB* in combination or *BSND*) that encode the membrane proteins of the thick ascending limb of the loop of Henle have a complex polyuropolydipsic syndrome with loss of water, sodium, chloride, calcium, magnesium, and potassium. Most (>90%) of pure congenital NDI patients have mutations in the *AVPR2* gene, the Xq28 gene coding for the vasopressin V2 (antidiuretic) receptor. In less than 10% of the families studied, congenital NDI has an autosomal recessive inheritance, and mutations have been identified in the *AQP2* gene located in chromosome region 12q13, that is, the vasopressin-sensitive water channel. When studied *in vitro*, most *AVPR2* mutations lead to receptors that are trapped intracellularly, and are unable to reach the plasma membrane. A minority of the mutant receptors reaches the cell surface, but is unable to bind AVP or to trigger an intracellular cAMP signal. Similarly, *AQP2* mutant proteins are trapped intracellularly and cannot be expressed at the luminal membrane. AVPR2 and AQP2-trafficking defects are correctable by chemical chaperones.

LOSS-OF-FUNCTION MUTATIONS OF *AVPR2*

X-linked NDI (OMIM 304800)[109] is secondary to *AVPR2* mutations, which result in a loss-of-function or dysregulation of the V2 receptor.[130] Males who have an *AVPR2* mutation have a phenotype characterized by early dehydration episodes, hypernatremia, and hyperthermia as early as the first week of life. Dehydration episodes can be so severe that they lower arterial blood pressure to a degree that is not sufficient to sustain adequate oxygenation to the brain, kidneys, and other organs. Mental and physical retardation and renal failure are the classical "historic" consequences of a late diagnosis and lack of treatment. Heterozygous females exhibit variable degrees of polyuria and polydipsia, because of skewed X-chromosome inactivation.[131,132]

Clinical Characteristics

The historic clinical characteristics include hypernatremia, hyperthermia, mental retardation, and repeated episodes of dehydration in early infancy.[133–136] Mental retardation, a consequence of repeated episodes of dehydration, was prevalent in the Crawford and Bode study,[133] in which only nine (11%) of 82 patients had normal intelligence. Early recognition and treatment of X-linked NDI with an abundant intake of water allows a normal lifespan with normal physical and mental development.[137] Two characteristics suggestive of X-linked NDI are the familial occurrence and the confinement of mental retardation to male patients. It is then tempting to assume that the family described in 1892 by McIlraith,[138] and discussed by Reeves and Andreoli[139] was an X-linked NDI family.

Crawford and Bode[133] clearly describe the early symptoms of the nephrogenic disorder and its severity in infancy. The first manifestations of the disease can be recognized during the first week of life. The infants are irritable, cry almost constantly and, although eager to suck, will vomit milk soon after ingestion unless prefed with water. The history given by the mothers often includes persistent constipation, erratic unexplained fever, and failure to gain weight. Although the patients characteristically show no visible evidence of perspiration, increased water loss during fever or in warm weather exaggerates the symptoms. Unless the condition is recognized early, children experience frequent bouts of hypertonic dehydration, sometimes complicated by convulsions or death; mental retardation is a frequent consequence of these episodes. The intake of large quantities of water, combined with the patient's voluntary restriction of dietary salt and protein intake, lead to hypocaloric dwarfism beginning in infancy. Frequently, lower urinary tract dilatation and obstruction, probably secondary to the large volume of urine produced,[140] develop in affected children. Dilatation of the lower urinary tract is also seen in primary polydipsic patients, and in patients with neurogenic diabetes insipidus.[141,142] Chronic renal insufficiency may occur by the end of the first decade of life, and could be the result of episodes of dehydration with thrombosis of the glomerular tufts.[133]

History

In 1989, we observed that the administration of dDAVP, a V2-receptor agonist, increased plasma cAMP concentrations in healthy subjects, but had no effect in 14 male patients with X-linked NDI.[143] Intermediate responses were observed in obligate carriers of the disease, corresponding to half of the normal receptor response. On the basis of these results, we predicted that the defective gene in these patients with X-linked NDI was likely to code for a defective V2 receptor.[143] Since that time, a number of experimental results have confirmed our hypothesis: (1) the NDI locus was mapped to the distal region of the long arm of the X-chromosome[144–147]; (2) the V2 receptor was identified as

a candidate gene for NDI[148]; (3) the human V2 receptor was cloned[53]; and (4) 214 putative disease-causing mutations have now been identified in the V2 receptor, and the list of mutations is still expanding[149,150] (Figure 46.10).

Population Genetics of AVPR2 Mutations

X-linked NDI is generally a rare disease in which the affected male patients do not concentrate their urine after administration of AVP.[151] Because this form is a rare, recessive X-linked disease, female individuals are unlikely to be affected, but heterozygous female individuals can exhibit variable degrees of polyuria and polydipsia because of skewed X-chromosome inactivation. In Quebec, the incidence of this disease among male individuals was estimated to be approximately 8.8 in 1,000,000 male live births.[131] A founder effect of two particular *AVPR2* mutations,[152] one in Ulster Scot immigrants (the Hopewell mutation, W71X), and one

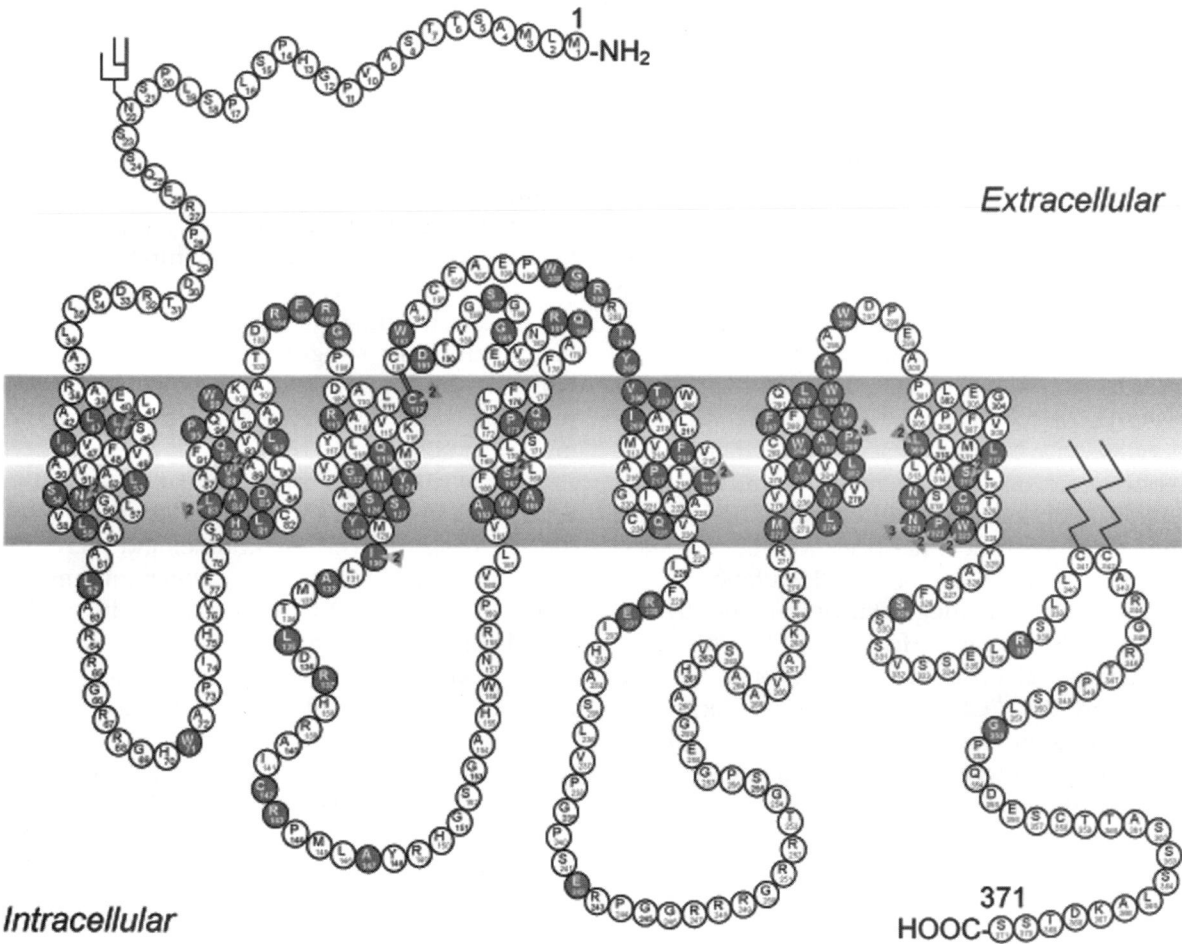

FIGURE 46.10 Schematic representation of the V2 receptor and identification of 193 putative disease-causing AVPR2 mutations. Predicted amino acids are shown as the one-letter amino acid code. A solid symbol indicates a codon with a missense or nonsense mutation; a number indicates more than one mutation in the same codon; other types of mutations are not indicated on the figure. There are 95 missense, 18 nonsense, 46 frameshift deletion or insertion, 7 inframe deletion or insertion, 4 splice-site, and 22 large deletion mutations, and one complex mutation.

in a large Utah kindred (the Cannon pedigree), result in an elevated prevalence of X-linked NDI in their descendants in certain communities in Nova Scotia, Canada, and Utah, United States.[117] These founder mutations have now spread all over the North American continent. We have identified the W71X mutation in 42 affected male individuals who reside predominantly in the Maritime Provinces of Nova Scotia and New Brunswick, and the L312X mutation in eight affected males who reside in the central United States. We know of 98 living affected male individuals of the Hopewell kindred, and 18 living affected male individuals of the Cannon pedigree.

We propose that all families with hereditary diabetes insipidus should have their molecular defect identified. The molecular identification underlying X-linked NDI is of immediate clinical significance, because early diagnosis and treatment of affected infants can avert the physical and mental retardation that results from repeated episodes of dehydration. Affected premature male infants may experience less severe polyuric symptoms, and may need only increased hydration during their first week without a need for hydrochlorothiazide treatment. Water should be offered every 2hours day and night, and temperature, appetite, and growth should be monitored. Admission to hospital may be necessary for continuous gastric feeding. The voluminous amounts of water kept in patients' stomachs will exacerbate physiological gastrointestinal reflux in infants and toddlers, and many affected boys frequently vomit. These young patients often improve with the absorption of an H_2 blocker, and with metoclopramide (which could induce extrapyramidal symptoms) or with domperidone, which seems to be better-tolerated and efficacious. As mentioned previously, all polyuric states (whether neurogenic, nephrogenic or psychogenic) can induce large dilatations of the urinary tract and bladder,[133,141,142] and bladder function impairment has been well-documented in patients who bear *AVPR2* or *AQP2* mutations.[153,154] Of interest, in mice with congenital progressive hydronephrosis (cph) homozygote for the S266L mutation (*Aqp2*) the congenital obstructive uropathy is likely a result of the polyuria.[90] Chronic renal failure secondary to bilateral hydronephrosis has been observed as a long-term complication in these patients. Renal and abdominal ultrasound should be done annually, and simple recommendations, including frequent urination and "double voiding" could be important to prevent these consequences.

Expression Studies

Classification of the defects of naturally occurring mutant human V2 receptors can be based on a similar scheme to that used for the LDL receptor. Mutations have been grouped according to the function and subcellular localization of the mutant protein whose cDNA has been transiently transfected in a heterologous expression system.[155] Using this classification, type 1 mutant V2 receptors reach the cell surface, but display impaired ligand binding and are consequently unable to induce normal cAMP production. The presence of mutant V2 receptors on the surface of transfected cells can be determined pharmacologically. By carrying out saturation-binding experiments using tritiated AVP, the number of cell surface mutant V2 receptors and their apparent binding affinity can be compared with that of the wild-type receptor. In addition, the presence of cell surface receptors can be assessed directly by using immunodetection strategies to visualize epitope-tagged receptors in whole-cell immunofluorescence assays.

Type 2 mutant receptors have defective intracellular transport. This phenotype is confirmed by carrying out, in parallel, immunofluorescence experiments on cells that are intact (to demonstrate the absence of cell surface receptors) or permeabilized (to confirm the presence of intracellular receptor pools). In addition, protein expression is confirmed by Western blot analysis of membrane preparations from transfected cells. It is likely that these mutant type 2 receptors accumulate in a pre-Golgi compartment, because they are initially glycosylated but fail to undergo glycosyl-trimming maturation.

Type 3 mutant receptors are ineffectively transcribed and lead to unstable mRNA, which are rapidly degraded. This subgroup seems to be rare, since Northern blot analysis of cells expressing mutant V2 receptors showed mRNA of normal quantity and molecular size.

Most of the *AVPR2* mutants that we and other investigators have tested are type 2 mutant receptors. They did not reach the cell membrane, and were trapped in the interior of the cell.[156–159] Other mutant G-protein-coupled receptors[160] and gene products that cause genetic disorders are also characterized by protein misfolding. Mutations that affect the folding of secretory proteins, integral plasma membrane proteins or enzymes destined to the endoplasmic reticulum, Golgi complex, and lysosomes result in loss-of-function phenotypes irrespective of their direct impact on protein function, because these mutant proteins are prevented from reaching their final destination.[161] Folding in the endoplasmic reticulum is the limiting step: mutant proteins which fail to correctly fold are retained initially in the endoplasmic reticulum and subsequently often degraded. Key proteins involved in the urine countercurrent mechanisms are good examples of this basic mechanism of misfolding. *AQP2* mutations responsible for autosomal recessive NDI are characterized by misrouting of the misfolded mutant proteins, and are trapped in the endoplasmic reticulum.[162] Mutants that encode other renal membrane proteins that are responsible for Gitelman syndrome,[163] Bartter syndrome,[164,165] and cystinuria[166] are also retained in the endoplasmic reticulum.

The *AVPR2* missense mutations are likely to impair folding and to lead to rapid degradation of the misfolded polypeptide, and not to the accumulation of toxic aggregates (as is the case for AVP mutants), because the other important functions of the principle cells of the collecting duct (where *AVPR2* is expressed) are entirely normal. These cells express the epithelial sodium channel (ENaC). Decreased function of this channel results in a sodium-losing state.[167] This has not been observed in patients with *AVPR2* mutations. By contrast, another type of conformational disease is characterized by the toxic retention of the misfolded protein. The relatively common Z mutation in a_1-antitrypsin deficiency not only causes retention of the mutant protein in the endoplasmic reticulum, but also affects the secondary structure by insertion of the reactive center loop of one molecule into a destabilized b sheet of a second molecule.[168] These polymers clog up the endoplasmic reticulum of hepatocytes and lead to cell death and juvenile hepatitis, cirrhosis, and hepatocarcinomas in these patients.[169]

If the misfolded protein/traffic problem that is responsible for so many human genetic diseases can be overcome, and the mutant protein transported out of the endoplasmic reticulum to its final destination, these mutant proteins could be sufficiently functional.[120] Therefore, using pharmacological chaperones or pharmacoperones to promote escape from the endoplasmic reticulum is a possible therapeutic approach.[121,156,161] We used selective nonpeptide V2 and V1 receptor-antagonists to rescue the cell-surface expression and function of naturally occurring misfolded human V2 receptors.[158] Because the beneficial effect of nonpeptide V2 antagonists could be secondary to prevention and interference with endocytosis, we studied the R137H mutant previously reported to lead to constitutive endocytosis.[170] We found that the antagonist did not prevent the constitutive b-arresting-promoted endocytosis.[156] These results indicate that, as for other *AVPR2* mutants, the beneficial effects of the treatment result from the action of the pharmacological chaperones. These studies were confirmed *in vitro* with the use of non-peptide V2 agonists.[171] In clinical studies, we administered a nonpeptide vasopressin antagonist SR49059 to five adult patients who have NDI and bear the del62-64, R137H, and W164S mutations. SR49059 significantly decreased urine volume and water intake and increased urine osmolality whereas sodium, potassium, and creatinine excretions and plasma sodium

levels were constant throughout the study.[156] This new therapeutic approach could be applied to the treatment of several hereditary diseases resulting from errors in protein folding and kinesis.[120,121]

Because most human gene-therapy experiments using viruses to deliver and integrate DNA into host cells are potentially dangerous,[172] other treatments are being actively pursued. Schöneberg and colleagues[173] used aminoglycoside antibiotics, because of their ability to suppress premature termination codons.[174] They demonstrated that geneticin, a potent aminoglycoside antibiotic, increased AVP-stimulated cAMP in cultured collecting duct cells prepared from E242X mutant mice. The urine concentrating ability of heterozygous mutant mice was also improved.

LOSS-OF-FUNCTION MUTATIONS OF AQP2 (OMIM 222000, 125800, 107777)

On the basis of desmopressin infusion studies and phenotypic characteristics of both male and female individuals who are affected with NDI, a non-X-linked form of NDI with a postreceptor (post-cAMP) defect was suggested.[109,175–177] A patient who presented shortly after birth with typical features of NDI, but who exhibited normal coagulation and normal fibrinolytic and vasodilatory responses to desmopressin, was shown to be a compound heterozygote for two missense mutations (R187C and S217P) in the *AQP2* gene.[178] To date, 46 putative disease-causing *AQP2* mutations have been identified in 52 NDI families (Figure 46.11). The oocytes of the African clawed frog (*Xenopus laevis*) have provided a most useful experimental system for studying the function of many channel proteins. This convenient expression system was key to the discovery of AQP1 by Agre,[179] because frog oocytes have very low permeability and survive even in freshwater ponds. Control oocytes are injected with water alone; test oocytes are injected with various quantities of synthetic transcripts from AQP1 or AQP2 DNA (cRNA). When subjected to a 20 mOsm osmotic shock, control oocytes have exceedingly low water permeability, but test oocytes become highly permeable to water. These osmotic water permeability assays demonstrated an absence or very low water transport for all of the cRNA with *AQP2* mutations. Immunofluorescence and immunoblot studies demonstrated that these recessive mutants were retained in the endoplasmic reticulum.

AQP2 mutations in autosomal recessive NDI, which are located throughout the gene, result in misfolded proteins that are retained in the endoplasmic reticulum. In contrast, the dominant mutations reported to date are located in the region that codes for the carboxyl-terminus of AQP2.[180–182] Dominant AQP2

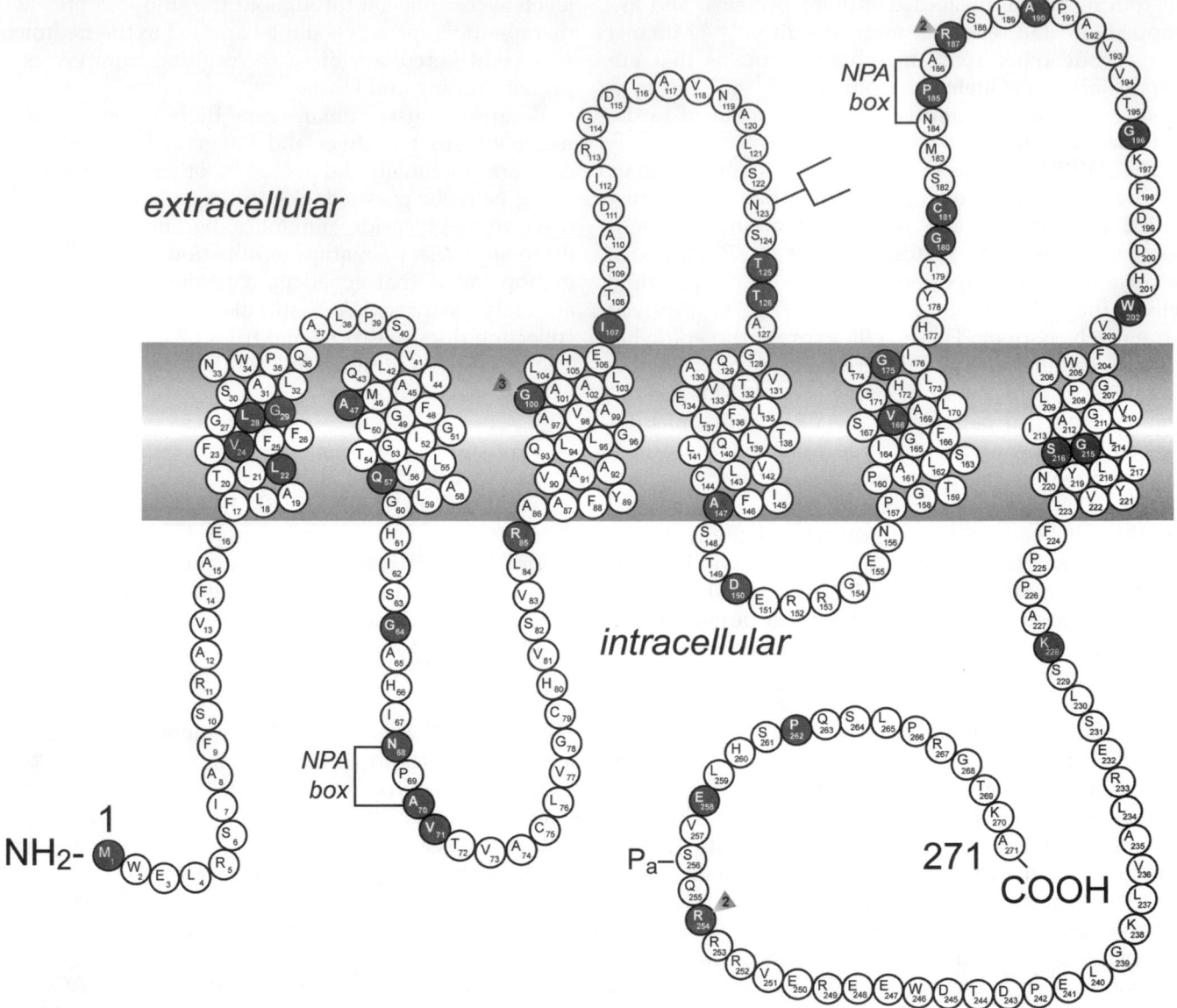

FIGURE 46.11 **A representation of the AQP2 protein and identification of 46 putative disease-causing AQP2 mutations.** A monomer is represented with six transmembrane helices. The location of the PKA phosphorylation site (Pa) is indicated. The extracellular, transmembrane, and cytoplasmic domains are defined according to *Deen, P. M., et al. (1994)*.[178] Solid symbols indicate the location of the mutations (for references, see Table 46.1): M1I; L22V; V24A; L28P; G29S; A47V; Q57P; G64R; N68S; A70D; V71M; R85X; G100X; G100V; G100R; I107D; 369delC; T125M; T126M; A147T; D150E; V168M; G175R; G180S; C181W; P185A; R187C; R187H; A190T; G196D; W202C; G215C; S216P; S216F; K228E; R254Q; R254L; E258K; and P262L. GenBank accession numbers—AQP2: AF147092, exon 1; AF147093, exons 2 through 4. NPA motifs and the N-glycosylation site are also indicated.

mutants form heterotetramers with wild-type AQP2 and are misrouted. Patients bearing these dominant mutations have a less severe phenotype compared to patients who are compound heterozygotes or homozygotes for recessive mutations: the patient and her daughter first described to bear the AQP2-E258K dominant mutation increased their urine osmolality to 350 mOsm/kg H_2O following dDAVP.[183] Also, the patient with a detailed phenotype described by Robertson and Kopp[184] increased her urine osmolality

to 220 mOsm/kg H_2O during a mildly hypertonic dehydration, to 258 mOsm/kg H_2O after dDAVP, and to 305 mOsm/kg H_2O after hydrochlorothiazide and indomethacin. This patient was found to be heterozygous for the R254Q mutation, possibly interfering with the S256 phosphorylation site.[185] In the mutant AQP2 (763−772) knock-in mice, Sohara et al. demonstrated a slight increase in urine osmolality following dehydration, but a marked increase after the administration of Rolipram, a phosphodiesterase 4 inhibitor.[186]

COMPLEX POLYUROPOLYDIPSIC SYNDROME

In contrast to a pure NDI phenotype, with loss of water but normal conservation of sodium, potassium, chloride, and calcium, in Bartter syndrome, patients' renal-wasting starts prenatally, and polyhydramnios often leads to prematurity. Bartter syndrome (OMIM 601678, 241200, 607364, and 602522) refers to a group of autosomal recessive disorders caused by inactivating mutations in genes (*SLC12A1*, *KCNJ1*, *CLCNKB*, *CLCNKA*, and *CLCNKB* in combination or *BSND*) that encode membrane proteins of the thick ascending limb of the loop of Henle (for review see [187,188]). Although Bartter syndrome and Bartter mutations are commonly used as a diagnosis, it is likely, as explained by Jeck et al.,[189] that the two patients with a mild phenotype originally described by Dr. Bartter had Gitelman syndrome, a thiazide-like, salt-losing tubulopathy with a defect in the distal convoluted tubule.[189] As a consequence, salt-losing tubulopathy of the furosemide-type is a more physiologically appropriate definition.

Thirty percent of the filtered sodium chloride is reabsorbed in the thick ascending limb of the loop of Henle through the apically expressed sodium–potassium–chloride co-transporter NKCC2 (encoded by the *SLC12A1* gene), which uses the sodium gradient across the membrane to transport chloride and potassium into the cell. The potassium ions must be recycled through the apical membrane by the potassium channel ROMK (encoded by the *KCNJ1* gene). In the large experience of Seyberth and colleagues,[190] who studied 85 patients with a hypokalemic salt-losing tubulopathy, all 20 patients with *KCNJ1* mutations (except one) and all 12 patients with *SLC12A1* mutations were born as preterm infants after severe polyhydramnios. Of note, polyhydramnios is never seen during a pregnancy that leads to infants bearing *AVPR2* or *AQP2* mutations. The most common causes of increased amniotic fluid include maternal diabetes mellitus, fetal malformations and chromosomal aberrations, twin-to-twin transfusion syndrome, rhesus incompatibility, and congenital infections.[191] Postnatally, polyuria was the leading symptom in 19 of the 32 patients. Renal ultrasound revealed nephrocalcinosis in 31 of these patients. These patients with complex polyuropolydipsic disorders are often poorly-recognized, and may be confused with pure NDI. As a consequence, congenital polyuria does not suggest automatically *AVPR2* or *AQP2* mutations, and polyhydramnios, salt-wasting, hypokalemia, and nephrocalcinosis are important clinical and laboratory characteristics that should be assessed. In patients with Bartter syndrome (salt-losing tubulopathy/furosemide-type), the dDAVP test will only indicate a partial type

of NDI. The algorithm proposed by Peters et al.[190] is useful, since most mutations in *SLC12A1* and *KCNJ1* are found in the carboxyl-terminus or in the last exon and, as a consequence, are amenable to rapid DNA sequencing.

Polyuria, polydipsia, electrolyte imbalance, and dehydration may also been seen in cystinosis, nephronophthisis, and apparent mineralocorticoid excess. Polyuria may be as mild as persistent enuresis and as severe as to contribute to death from dehydration and electrolyte abnormalities in infants with cystinosis who have acute gastroenteritis.[192] Nephronophthisis and apparent mineralocorticoid excess are also associated with low urine osmolality unresponsive to vasopressin.[193]

ACQUIRED NEPHROGENIC DIABETES INSIPIDUS

Acquired NDI is much more common than congenital NDI, but it is rarely as severe. The ability to produce hypertonic urine is usually preserved, even though there is inadequate concentrating ability of the nephron. Polyuria and polydipsia are therefore moderate (3−4 l/d).

The more common causes of acquired NDI are listed in Table 46.2. Lithium administration has become the most frequent cause; 54% of 1105 unselected patients on chronic lithium therapy developed NDI.[194] Nineteen percent of these patients had polyuria, as defined by a 24hour urine output exceeding 3 liters. The mechanism whereby lithium causes polyuria has been extensively studied. Lithium inhibits adenylyl cyclase in a number of cell types, including renal epithelia.[195,196] The dysregulation of aquaporin-2 expression is the result of cytotoxic accumulation of lithium which enters via the epithelial sodium channel (ENaC) on the apical membrane, and leads to the inhibition of signaling pathways that involve glycogen synthase kinase type 3 beta.[197] The concentration of lithium in urine of patients on well-controlled lithium therapy (i.e., 10 to 40 mOsmol/L) is sufficient to exert this effect. For patients on long-term lithium therapy, amiloride has been proposed to prevent the uptake of lithium in the collecting ducts, thus preventing the inhibitory effect of intracellular lithium on water transport.[198]

Primary Polydipsia

Primary polydipsia is a state of hypotonic polyuria secondary to excessive fluid intake. Primary polydipsia was extensively studied by Barlow and de Wardener in 1959[199]; however, the understanding of the

TABLE 46.2 Causes of Nephrogenic Diabetes Insipidus.

Narrow definition of NDI: water permeability of the collecting duct not increased by AVP

Congenital (idiopathic)

Hypercalcemia

Hypokalemia

Drugs:

    Lithium

    Nonpeptide vasopressin receptor (V2) antagonists

    Demeclocycline

    Amphotericin B

    Methoxyflurane

    Diphenylhydantoin

    Nicotine

    Alcohol

Broad definition of NDI: defective medullary countercurrent function

Renal failure, acute or chronic (especially interstitial nephritis or obstruction)

Medullary damage:

    Sickle-cell anemia and trait

    Amyloidosis

    Sjögren syndrome

    Sarcoidosis

    Hypercalcemia

    Hypokalemia

    Protein malnutrition

    Cystinosis

Modified from ref. [246]

pathophysiology of this disease has made little progress. Barlow and de Wardener[199] described seven women and two men who were compulsive water drinkers; their ages ranged from 48 to 59 years, except for one patient who was 24 years old. Eight of these patients had histories of previous psychological disorders, which ranged from delusions, depression, and agitation to frank hysterical behavior. The other patient appeared normal. The consumption of water fluctuated irregularly from hour to hour or from day to day; in some patients, there were remissions and relapses lasting several months or longer. In eight of the patients, the mean plasma osmolality was significantly lower than normal. Vasopressin tannate in oil made most of these patients feel ill; in one, it caused overhydration. In four patients, the fluid intake returned to normal

after electroconvulsive therapy or a period of continuous narcosis; the improvement in three was transient, but in the fourth it lasted two years. Polyuric female subjects might be heterozygous for *de novo* or previously unrecognized *AVPR2* mutations, may bear *AQP2* mutations, and may be classified as compulsive water drinkers.[200] Therefore, the diagnosis of compulsive water drinking must be made with care, and may represent our ignorance of yet undescribed pathophysiological mechanisms. Robertson[200] has described under the name "dipsogenic diabetes insipidus" a selective defect in the osmoregulation of thirst. Three studied patients had, under basal conditions of *ad libitum* water intake, thirst, polydipsia, polyuria, and high-normal plasma osmolality. They had a normal secretion of AVP, but osmotic threshold for thirst was abnormally low. These dipsogenic diabetes insipidus cases might represent up to 10% of all patients with diabetes insipidus.[200]

Diabetes Insipidus and Pregnancy

Pregnancy in a Patient Known to Have Diabetes Insipidus

An isolated deficiency of vasopressin without a concomitant loss of hormones in the anterior pituitary does not result in altered fertility, and with the exception of polyuria and polydipsia, gestation, delivery, and lactation are uncomplicated.[201] Patients may require increasing dosages of dDAVP. The increased thirst may be due to a resetting of the thirst osmostat.[202]

Increased polyuria also occurs during pregnancy in patients with partial NDI.[203] These patients may be obligatory carriers of the NDI gene[204] or may be homozygotes, compound heterozygotes or may have dominant AQP2 mutations.

Syndromes of Diabetes Insipidus that Begin during Gestation and Remit after Delivery

Barron et al.[205] described three pregnant women in whom transient diabetes insipidus developed late in gestation and subsequently remitted postpartum. In one of these patients, dilute urine was present despite high plasma concentrations of AVP. Hyposthenuria in all three patients was resistant to administered aqueous vasopressin. Because excessive vasopressinase activity was not excluded as a cause of this disorder, Barron et al. labeled the disease vasopressin-resistant, rather than NDI.

A well-documented case of enhanced activity of vasopressinase has been described in a woman in the third trimester of a previously uncomplicated pregnancy.[206] She had massive polyuria and markedly elevated plasma vasopressinase activity. The polyuria did not respond to large intravenous doses of AVP, but responded promptly to dDAVP, a vasopressinase-resistant analog of AVP. The polyuria disappeared with the disappearance of the vasopressinase. It is suggested that pregnancy may be associated with several different forms of diabetes insipidus, including central, nephrogenic, and vasopressinase mediated.[203,207,208]

Polyuria and Nocturia in Diabetes Insipidus, Nocturnal Polyuria in Enuretic Children

Polyuria could be constant during the day but also present at night: the urine is normally most concentrated in the morning due to lack of fluid ingestion overnight and increased vasopressin secretion during the late sleep period.[209] Neurons in the suprachiasmatic nucleus, the brain biological clock, send axonal projections toward the supraoptic nucleus, one of the hypothalamic nuclei producing vasopressin,[5] providing a possible anatomical substrate for the circadian modulation, an osmoregulatory gain during the late sleep period.[209] As a result, the first manifestation of a mild-to-moderate loss of concentrating ability is often nocturia. However, nocturia is not diagnostic of a defect in concentrating ability, since it can also be caused by other factors such as drinking before going to bed or, in men, by prostatic hypertrophy, which is characterized by urinary frequency rather than polyuria. Psychogenic polydipsic patients tend to ingest large amounts of fluid during the day but not at night, therefore nocturia is rarely seen in primary polydipsic patients.[199] The pattern of nocturnal polyuria in enuretic children is similar to that observed in acute sleep deprivation, and enuresis in children might be related to the failure of sleep to cause a reflex reduction in arterial pressure and urine production.[210,211]

INVESTIGATION OF A PATIENT WITH POLYURIA

Plasma sodium and osmolality are maintained within normal limits (136−143 mOsmol/l for plasma sodium; 275−290 mOsmol/kg for plasma osmolality) by a thirst−AVP−renal axis. Thirst and AVP release, both stimulated by increased osmolality, is a "double-negative" feedback system.[212] Even when the AVP component of this double-negative regulatory feedback system is lost, the thirst mechanism still preserves the plasma sodium and osmolality within the normal range, but at the expense of pronounced polydipsia and polyuria. Thus, the plasma sodium concentration or osmolality of an untreated patient with diabetes insipidus may be slightly greater than the mean normal value, but these small increases have no

diagnostic significance. Polyuric patients should be asked about their thirst and their way to quench it: cold water will quench thirst more effectively in severely polyuric and dehydrated patients, irrespective of their etiology (central versus nephrogenic). Primary polydipsic patients may tend to absorb large quantities of water, ice-cold or not. Glucose-induced osmotic diuresis is more frequent than any cause of non-osmotic polyuria. High plasma glucose levels with polyuria could also be observed in brain-dead patients with diabetes insipidus receiving glucose infusions at a rate exceeding 500 ml/hour, which corresponds to the maximum (25 g/hour) possibility for glucose metabolism. The polyuria observed in post-obstructive diuresis is appropriate, representing an attempt to excrete the fluid retained during the period of obstruction.[213]

Excepting the context of brain trauma, brain surgery or long-term lithium administration, where the diagnosis of polyuria is obvious, a logical approach to the patient with polyuria is to search for arguments supporting known causes of polyuric states. Such arguments may be: (1) morphological (brain magnetic resonance imaging), including the presence of a hypothalamic tumour or mass related to a granulomatous or inflammatory process; (2) hormonal, suggesting that the posterior pituitary involvement is not isolated, but rather is associated with other signs of anterior pituitary deficits; (3) systemic, with the presence of a generalized inflammatory process or pituitary metastasis; (4) hereditary, with other members of the family affected with central or nephrogenic diabetes insipidus.

An abrupt onset of polyuria in an adult would suggest acquired central diabetes insipidus. Magnetic resonance imaging of the hypothalamic structures and of the posterior pituitary should be obtained to assess the posterior pituitary normal "bright spot," a possible surrogate of the posterior pituitary vasopressin content, and any accompanying lesions. Clinical and biochemical indices of associated anterior pituitary/hormone deficiency should also be obtained,[97] since additional deficits in anterior pituitary hormones were documented in 61% of patients, a median of 0.6 years after the onset of diabetes insipidus. The most frequent abnormality was growth hormone deficiency (59%), followed by hypothyroidism (28%), hypogonadism (24%), and adrenal insufficiency (22%). Seventy-five percent of the patients with Langerhans cell histiocytosis had an anterior pituitary hormone deficiency that was first detected a median of 3.5 years after the onset of diabetes insipidus.

In this context, the dehydration test is rarely necessary, and is only recommended for patients with isolated polyuria, a normal pituitary stalk and hypothalamic region on magnetic resonance imaging, and with no familial history of polyuria. If plasma osmolality and/or sodium concentration under conditions of *ad libitum* fluid intake are above 295 mmol/kg and 143 mmol/L, the diagnosis of primary polydipsia is excluded.[214]

If severe polyuric symptoms and signs are documented, water should be restricted to only two to four hours during day time in infants, plasma sodium should be available every two hours during testing and should not exceed 145–148 in children and adults, since a maximal endogenous vasopressin stimulation (more than 3.5 pg/mL) should occur at this level with a maximal urine osmolality response (higher than 800 mOsm/kg H$_2$O). If delays of more than 60minutes are encountered to obtain plasma sodium or urine osmolalities during dehydration tests, these tests should be done in other institutions where almost immediate laboratory reports are obtained after blood samplings.

Theoretically, it should be relatively easy to differentiate between neurogenic diabetes insipidus, NDI, and primary polydipsia by comparing the osmolality of urine obtained during dehydration with that of urine obtained after the administration of dDAVP. Patients with neurogenic diabetes insipidus should reveal a rapid increase in urinary osmolality, whereas it should increase normally in response to moderate dehydration in patients with primary polydipsia. However, for several reasons, these distinctions may not be as clear as one might expect.[215] First, chronic polyuria resulting from any cause interferes with the maintenance of the medullary concentration gradient, and this "wash-out" effect diminishes the maximum concentrating ability of the nephron. The extent of the blunting varies in direct proportion to the severity of the polyuria. Hence, for any given basal urine output, the maximum urine osmolality achieved in the presence of saturating concentrations of AVP is depressed to the same extent in patients with primary polydipsia, neurogenic diabetes insipidus or NDI (Figure 46.12). Second, most patients with neurogenic diabetes insipidus maintain a small, but detectable, capacity to secrete AVP during severe dehydration, and urinary osmolality may then increase to greater than the plasma osmolality. Third, patients referred to as partial diabetes insipidus (either neurogenic or nephrogenic) and patients with acquired NDI have an incomplete response to AVP, and are able to concentrate their urine to varying degrees in a dehydration test. Finally, all polyuric states (whether neurogenic, nephrogenic or psychogenic) can induce large dilatations of the urinary tract and bladder.[141,142] As a consequence, the urinary bladder of these patients has an increased residual capacity, and changes in urinary osmolality induced by diagnostic maneuvers might be difficult to demonstrate.

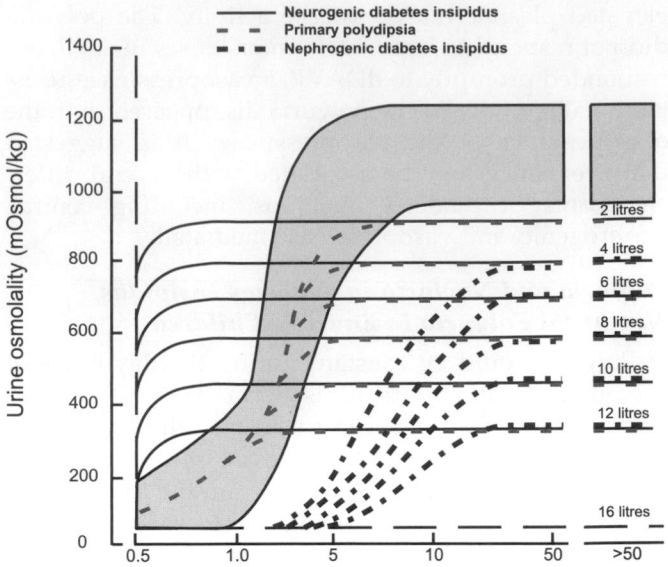

FIGURE 46.12 Schematic diagram of the relationship between urine osmolality and plasma vasopressin in patients with polyuria of diverse cause and severity. The shaded area represents the normal range. For each of the three categories of polyuria, the relationship is described by a family of sigmoid curves that differ in height. These differences in height reflect differences in maximum concentrating capacity due to "wash-out" of the medullary concentration gradient. They are proportional to the severity of the underlying polyuria (indicated in liters at the right-hand side of each plateau), and are largely independent of the cause. The three categories of diabetes insipidus differ principally in the submaximal or ascending portion of the dose–response curve. In patients with neurogenic diabetes insipidus, this part of the curve lies to the left of normal, reflecting increased sensitivity to the antidiuretic effects of very low concentrations of plasma vasopressin. In contrast, in patients with neurogenic diabetes insipidus, this part of the curve lies to the right of normal, reflecting decreased sensitivity to the antidiuretic effects of normal concentrations of plasma vasopressin. In primary polydipsia, this relationship is relatively normal. *(From ref. [215].)*

Indirect Tests for Diabetes Insipidus

The measurement of urinary osmolality after dehydration and dDAVP administration is usually referred to as "indirect testing," because AVP secretion is indirectly assessed through changes in urinary osmolalities.[32] The patient is maintained on a complete fluid-restriction regimen until urinary osmolality reaches a plateau, as indicated by an hourly increase of less than 30 mOsmol/kg for at least 3 successive hours. After measuring the plasma osmolality, 2 mg dDAVP are administered subcutaneously. Urinary osmolality is measured 30 and 60minutes later. The last urinary osmolality value obtained before the dDAVP injection, and the highest value obtained after the injection, are compared. In patients with severe neurogenic diabetes insipidus, urinary osmolality after dehydration is usually low (< 200 mOsmol/kg) and increases more than

50% after dDAVP administration. In patients with severe NDI, urinary osmolality after dehydration is also low (< 200 mOsmol/kg), but does not increase after dDAVP administration (<20%). Urinary osmolality increases to variable degrees (10% to 50%) after dDAVP administration to patients with partial neurogenic or partial nephrogenic diabetes insipidus. In patients with primary polydipsia, maximum urinary osmolality will be obtained after dehydration (>295 mOsmol/kg) and does not increase after dDAVP administration (<10%).

Alternatively, plasma sodium and plasma and urinary osmolalities can be measured at the beginning of the dehydration procedure and at regular intervals (usually hourly) thereafter, depending on the severity of the polyuria.[216] For example, an 8-year-old patient (body weight 31 kg) with a clinical diagnosis of congenital NDI (later found to bear an *AVPR2* mutation) continued to excrete large volumes of urine (300 ml/h) during a short 4hour dehydration test. During this time, the patient suffered from severe thirst, his plasma sodium was 155 mOsmol/l, plasma osmolality was 310 mOsmol/kg, and urinary osmolality was 85 mOsmol/kg. The patient received 1 mg of dDAVP intravenously and was allowed to drink water. Repeated urinary osmolality measurements demonstrated a complete urinary resistance to dDAVP. It would have been dangerous and unnecessary to prolong the dehydration further in this young patient. Thus, the usual prescription of overnight dehydration should not be used in patients, and especially children, with severe polyuria and polydipsia (more than 30 ml/kg body weight per day). Great care should be taken to avoid any severe hypertonic state, arbitrarily defined as plasma sodium greater than 155 mOsmol/l.

Direct Tests of Diabetes Insipidus

The two approaches of Zerbe and Robertson are used,[217] although they are expensive, time-consuming, and difficult to do on young patients. In the first approach, during the dehydration test, plasma is collected hourly and assayed for AVP. The results are plotted on a nomogram depicting the normal relationship between plasma sodium or osmolality and plasma AVP in normal individuals (Figure 46.6a). If the relationship goes below the normal range, the disorder is diagnosed as neurogenic diabetes insipidus.

In the second approach, NDI can be differentiated from primary polydipsia by analyzing the relationship between plasma AVP and urinary osmolality at the end of the dehydration period (Figure 46.6b). However, definitive differentiation might be impossible, because a normal or even supranormal AVP response to increased plasma osmolality occurs in polydipsic patients. None of the patients with psychogenic or other forms of severe polydipsia studied by Robertson showed any evidence of pituitary suppression.[215]

In a comparison of diagnoses based on indirect versus direct tests of AVP function in 54 patients with polyuria of diverse cause, Robertson[215] found that the indirect test was reliable only for patients with severe defects. Three patients with severe NDI, and 16 of 17 patients with severe neurogenic diabetes insipidus were accurately diagnosed. However, the error rate of the indirect test was about 50% in diagnosing partial neurogenic diabetes insipidus, partial NDI or primary polydipsia in patients who were able to concentrate their urine to varying degrees when water-deprived. The benefits of combined direct and indirect testing of AVP function have been discussed by Stern and Valtin.[218] The diagnosis of primary polydipsia remains one of exclusion, and the cause could be psychogenic[199] or inappropriate thirst.[200,219] Psychiatric patients with polydipsia and hyponatremia have unexplained defects in urinary dilution, the osmoregulation of water intake or the secretion of vasopressin.[148]

Therapeutic Trial of dDAVP

In selected patients with an uncertain diagnosis, a closely monitored therapeutic trial of dDAVP (10 mg intranasally twice a day for 2 to 3 days) may be used to distinguish partial NDI from partial neurogenic diabetes insipidus or primary polydipsia. If dDAVP at this dosage causes a significant antidiuretic effect, NDI is effectively excluded. If polydipsia and polyuria are abolished and plasma sodium does not go below the normal range, the patient probably has neurogenic diabetes insipidus. Conversely, if dDAVP causes a reduction in urine output without reduction in water intake and hyponatremia appears, the patient probably has primary polydipsia. Since fatal water intoxication is a remote possibility, the dDAVP trial should be closely monitored. The methods of differential diagnosis of diabetes insipidus are described in Table 46.3.

Carrier Detection, Perinatal Testing, and Early Treatment

The identification of mutations in the genes that cause hereditary diabetes insipidus allows the early diagnosis and management of at-risk members of families with identified mutations. We encourage physicians who follow families with autosomal neurogenic, X-linked, and autosomal NDI to recommend mutation analysis before the birth of an infant, because early diagnosis and treatment can avert the physical and mental retardation associated with episodes of

TABLE 46.3 Differential Diagnosis of Diabetes Insipidus.

1. Measure plasma osmolality and/or sodium concentration under conditions of *ad libitum* fluid intake. If plasma osmolality is >295 mOsmol/kg and sodium is >143 mOsmol/l, the diagnosis of primary polydipsia is excluded and the work-up should proceed to step (5) and/or (6) to distinguish between NDI and neurogenic diabetes insipidus. *Otherwise*:

2. Perform a dehydration test. If urinary concentration does not occur before plasma osmolality reaches 295 mOsmol/kg and/or sodium reaches 143 mOsmol/l, the diagnosis of primary polydipsia is again excluded and the work-up should proceed to step (5) and/or (6). *Otherwise*:

3. Determine the ratio of urine to plasma osmolality at the end of the dehydration test. If it is <1.5, the diagnosis of primary polydipsia is again excluded and the work-up should proceed to step (5) and/or (6). *Otherwise*:

4. Perform a hypertonic saline infusion with measurement of plasma AVP and osmolality at intervals during the procedure. If the relationship between these two variables falls below the normal range, the diagnosis of neurogenic diabetes insipidus is established. *Otherwise*:

5. Perform a dDAVP infusion test. If urine osmolality increases by <150 mOsmol/kg above the value obtained at the end of the dehydration test, the diagnosis of NDI is established. *Alternatively*:

6. Measure urine osmolality and plasma AVP at the end of the dehydration test. If the relationship falls below the normal range, the diagnosis of NDI is established.

Data from ref. [219].

dehydration. Diagnosis of X-linked NDI was accomplished by mutation testing of cultured amniotic cells ($n = 7$), chorionic villus samples ($n = 10$) or cord blood obtained at birth ($n = 57$) in 74 of our patients. Thirty-five males were found to bear mutant sequences, 22 males were not affected, and nine females were not carriers. These affected patients were immediately given abundant water intake, a low-sodium diet, and hydrochlorothiazide. They never experienced episodes of dehydration, and their physical and mental development is normal. Gene analysis is also important for the identification of nonobligatory female carriers in families with X-linked NDI. Most females heterozygous for a mutation in the V2 receptor do not have clinical symptoms: few are severely affected.[131,220,221] Mutation detection in families with inherited neurogenic diabetes insipidus provides a powerful clinical tool for early diagnosis and management of subsequent cases, especially in early childhood, when diagnosis is difficult and the clinical risks are the greatest.[222]

Neurogenic diabetes insipidus (central or Wolfram) is easily treated with dDAVP.[223] All complications of congenital NDI are prevented by an adequate water intake. Thus, patients should be provided with unrestricted amounts of water from birth to ensure normal development. In addition to a low-sodium diet, the use of diuretics (thiazides) or indomethacin may reduce urinary output. This advantageous effect has to be weighed against the side-effects of these drugs (thiazides: electrolyte disturbances; indomethacin: reduction of the glomerular filtration rate and gastrointestinal symptoms).

RADIOIMMUNOASSAY OF AVP AND OTHER LABORATORY DETERMINATIONS

Radioimmunoassay of AVP

Three developments were basic to the elaboration of a clinically useful radioimmunoassay for plasma AVP[224,225]: (1) the extraction of AVP from plasma with petrol-ether and acetone and the subsequent elimination of nonspecific immunoreactivity; (2) the use of highly-specific and sensitive rabbit antiserum; and (3) the use of a tracer (^{125}I-AVP) with high specific activity. These same extraction procedures are still widely used,[161,198,213,216] and commercial tracers (^{125}I-AVP) and antibodies are available. AVP can also be extracted from plasma by using Sep-Pak C18 cartridges.[226–228]

Blood samples collected in chilled 7 ml lavender-stoppered tubes containing ethylenediaminetetraacetic acid are centrifuged at 4°C, 1000 g (3000 rpm in a usual laboratory centrifuge), for 20minutes. This 20minute centrifugation is mandatory for obtaining platelet-poor plasma samples, because a large fraction of the circulating vasopressin is associated with the platelets in humans.[229,230] The tubes may be kept for 2hours on slushed ice before centrifugation. Plasma is then separated, frozen at $-20°C$ and extracted within 6 weeks of sampling. Details for sample preparation (Table 46.4) and assay procedure (Table 46.5) can be found in writings by Bichet and colleagues.[229,231] An AVP radioimmunoassay should be validated by demonstrating: (1) a good correlation between plasma sodium or osmolality and plasma AVP during dehydration and infusion of hypertonic saline solution (Figure 46.6); and (2) the inability to obtain detectable values of AVP in patients with severe central diabetes insipidus. Plasma AVP immunoreactivity may be elevated in patients with diabetes insipidus following hypothamic surgery.[232]

In pregnant patients, the blood contains high concentrations of cystine aminopeptidase, which can (*in vitro*) inactivate enormous quantities (ng mL^{-1} min^{-1}) of AVP. However, phenanthrolene effectively inhibits these cystine aminopeptidases (Table 46.6).

Aquaporin-2 Measurements

Urinary AQP2 excretion could be measured by radioimmunoassay[233] or quantitative Western analysis,[234] and could provide an additional indication of the responsiveness of the collecting duct to AVP.

TABLE 46.4 Arginine Vasopressin Measurements: Sample Preparation.

4°C − Blood in EDTA tubes
Centrifugation 1000 g × 20 min.
Plasma frozen − 20°C
Extraction:
2 mL acetone + 1 mL plasma
1000 g × 30 min 4°C
Supernatant + 5 mL of petrol-ether
1000 g × 20 min 4°C
Freeze − 80°C
Throw nonfrozen upper phase
Evaporate lower phase to dryness
Store desiccated samples at − 20°C

TABLE 46.5 Arginine Vasopressin Measurements: Assay Procedure

Day 1	Assay set-up 400 µL/tube (200 µL sample or standard + 200 µL of antiserum or buffer). Incubation 80 hours, 4°C
Day 4	^{125}I-AVP 100 µL/tube 1000 cpm/tube. Incubation 72 hours, 4°C
Day 7	Separation dextran + charcoal

Data from ref. [247].

TABLE 46.6 Measurements of Arginine Vasopressin Levels in Pregnant Patients.

1,10-phenanthroline monohydrate (Sigma) solubilized with several drops of glacial acetic acid
0.1 mL/10 mL of blood

Plasma Sodium, Plasma, and Urine Osmolality

Measurements of plasma sodium, plasma, and urinary osmolality should be immediately available at various intervals during dehydration procedures. Plasma sodium is easily measured by flame photometry or with a sodium-specific electrode.[235] Plasma and urinary osmolalities are also reliably measured by freezing point depression instruments with a coefficient of variation at 290 mmol/kg of less than 1%.

At variance with published data,[229,217] we have found that plasma and serum osmolalities are equivalent (i.e., similar values are obtained). Blood taken in heparinized tubes is easier to handle, because the plasma can be more readily removed after centrifugation. The tube used (green-stoppered tube) contains a minuscule concentration of lithium and sodium, which does not interfere with plasma sodium or osmolality measurements.

Frozen plasma or urinary samples can be kept for further analysis of their osmolalities, because the results obtained are similar to those obtained immediately after blood sampling, except in patients with severe renal failure. In the latter patients, plasma osmolality measurements are increased after freezing and thawing, but the plasma sodium values remain unchanged.

Plasma osmolality measurements can be used to demonstrate the absence of unusual osmotically active substances (e.g., glucose and urea in high concentrations, mannitol, ethanol).[236] With this information, plasma or serum sodium measurements are sufficient to assess the degree of dehydration and its relationship to plasma AVP. Nomograms describing the normal plasma sodium/plasma AVP relationship are equally as valuable as classic nomograms describing the relationship between plasma osmolality and effective osmolality (i.e., plasma osmolality minus the contribution of "ineffective" solutes: glucose and urea).

MAGNETIC RESONANCE IMAGING IN PATIENTS WITH DIABETES INSIPIDUS

Magnetic resonance imaging (MRI) permits visualization of the anterior and posterior pituitary glands and the pituitary stalk. The pituitary stalk is permeated by numerous capillary loops of the hypophyseal−portal blood system. This vascular structure also provides the principle blood supply to the anterior pituitary lobe, because there is no direct arterial supply to this organ. In contrast, the posterior pituitary lobe has a direct vascular supply. Therefore, the posterior lobe can be more rapidly visualized in a dynamic mode after administration of gadolinium (gadopentate dimeglumine) as contrast material during MRI. The posterior pituitary lobe is easily distinguished by a round, high-intensity signal (the posterior pituitary "bright spot") in the posterior part of the sella turcica on T1-weighted images. Loss of the pituitary hyperintense spot or bright spot on a T1-weighted MRI image reflects loss of functional integrity of the neurohypophysis, and is a non-specific indicator of neurohypophyseal diabetes insipidus regardless of the underlying cause.[97,237] It is now considered that the bright spot represents normal AVP storage in the posterior lobe of the pituitary, that the intensity is correlated with the amount of AVP, and that after 60 years of age the signal is often less intense, with irregularities in the normally smooth convex edge.[238,239] MRI is reported to be the best technique with which to evaluate the pituitary stalk and infundibulum in patients with idiopathic polyuria. A thickening or enlargement of the pituitary stalk may suggest an infiltrative process destroying the neurohypophyseal tract.[240]

TREATMENT

In most patients with complete hypothalamic diabetes insipidus, the thirst mechanism remains intact. Thus, hypernatremia does not develop in these patients, and they suffer only from the inconvenience associated with marked polyuria and polydipsia. If hypodipsia develops or access to water is limited, then severe hypernatremia can supervene. The treatment of choice for patients with severe hypothalamic diabetes insipidus is dDAVP, a synthetic, long-acting vasopressin analog with minimal vasopressor activity, but a large antidiuretic potency. The usual intranasal daily dose is between 5 and 20 mg. To avoid the potential complication of dilutional hyponatremia, which is exceptional in these patients as a result of an intact thirst mechanism, dDAVP can be withdrawn at regular intervals to allow the patients to become polyuric. Aqueous vasopressin (Pitressin) or dDAVP (4.0 mg/1 ml ampule) can be used intravenously in acute situations, such as after hypophysectomy or for the treatment of diabetes insipidus in the brain-dead organ donor. Pitressin tannate in oil and nonhormonal antidiuretic drugs are somewhat obsolete and now rarely used. For example, chlorpropamide (250–500 mg daily) appears to potentiate the antidiuretic action of circulating AVP, but troublesome side-effects of hypoglycemia and hyponatremia do occur.

The treatment of congenital NDI has been reviewed by Knoers and Monnens.[176] An abundant unrestricted water intake should always be provided, and affected patients should be carefully followed during their first years of life. Water should be offered every 2 hours day and night, and temperature, appetite, and growth should be monitored. The parents of these children easily accept setting their alarm clock every 2 hours during the night. Hospital admission may be necessary to allow continuous gastric feeding. A low-osmolar and low-sodium diet, hydrochlorothiazide (1–2 mg/kg/d) alone or with amiloride, and indomethacin (0.75–1.5 mg/kg) substantially reduce water excretion, and are helpful in the treatment of children. Many adult patients receive no treatment.

Acknowledgments

The author's work cited in this chapter was supported by the Canadian Institutes of Health Research, the Kidney Foundation of Canada, and the Fonds de la Recherche en Santé du Québec. We thank our co-workers, Marie-Françoise Arthus, Joyce Crumley, Mary Fujiwara, Michèle Lonergan, and Kenneth Morgan, and many colleagues who contributed families and ideas to our work.

References

[1] Richter D. Molecular events in the expression of vasopressin and oxytocin and their cognate receptors. Am J Physiol 1988;255:F207–19.

[2] Williams PD, Pettibone DJ. Recent advances in the development of oxytocin receptor antagonists. Curr Pharm Design 1996;2: 41–58.

[3] Bourque CW. Central mechanisms of osmosensation and systemic osmoregulation. Nat Rev Neurosci 2008;9:519–31.

[4] Lechner SG, Markworth S, Poole K, Smith ES, Lapatsina L, Frahm S, et al. The molecular and cellular identity of peripheral osmoreceptors. Neuron 2011;69:332–44.

[5] Burbach JP, Luckman SM, Murphy D, Gainer H. Gene regulation in the magnocellular hypothalamo–neurohypophysial system. Physiol Rev 2001;81:1197–267.

[6] Rao VV, Loffler C, Battey J, Hansmann I. The human gene for oxytocin-neurophysin I (OXT) is physically mapped to chromosome 20p13 by in situ hybridization. Cell Genet 1992;61:271–3.

[7] Sausville E, Carney D, Battey J. The human vasopressin gene is linked to the oxytocin gene and is selectively expressed in a cultured lung cancer cell line. J Biol Chem 1985;260:10236–41.

[8] Venkatesh B, Si-Hoe SL, Murphy D, Brenner S. Transgenic rats reveal functional conservation of regulatory controls between the Fugu isotocin and rat oxytocin genes. Proc Natl Acad Sci USA 1997;94:12462–6.

[9] Chen L, Rose JP, Breslow E, Yang D, Chang WR, Furey WFJ, et al. Crystal structure of a bovine neurophysin II dipeptide complex at 2.8 Angström determined from the single-wave length anomalous scattering signal of an incorporated iodine atom. Proc Natl Acad Sci USA 1991;88:4240–4.

[10] Swab D, Pool WC, Novelty F. Immunofluorescence of vasopressin and oxytocin in the rat hypothalamo–neurohypophyseal system. J Neural Transm 1975;36:195.

[11] Vandesande F, Dierickx K. Identification of the vasopressin producing and of the oxytocin producing neurons in the hypothalamic magnocellular neurosecretroy system of the rat. Cell Tissue Res 1975;164:153–62.

[12] Sofroniew M. Morphology of vasopressin and oxytocin neurones and their central and vascular projections, vol. 60. New York: Elsevier; 1983.

[13] Kalogeras KT, Nieman LN, Friedman TC, Doppman JL, Cutler GBJ, Chrousos GP, et al. Inferior petrosal sinus sampling in healthy human subjects reveals a unilateral corticotropin-releasing hormone-induced arginine vasopressin release associated with ipsilateral adrenocorticotropin secretion. J Clin Invest 1996;97:2045–50.

[14] Yanovski JA, Friedman TC, Nieman LK, Chrousos GP, Cutler Jr. GB, Doppman JL, et al. Inferior petrosal sinus AVP in patients with cushing's syndrome. Clin Endocrinol (Oxf) 1997;47:199–206.

[15] Edwards AM, Mann ME, Marfell-Jones MJ, Rankin DM, Noakes TD, Shillington DP. Influence of moderate dehydration on soccer performance: physiological responses to 45 min of outdoor match-play and the immediate subsequent performance of sport-specific and mental concentration tests. Br J Sports Med 2007;41:385–91.

[16] Saat M, Sirisinghe RG, Singh R, Tochihara Y. Effects of short-term exercise in the heat on thermoregulation, blood parameters, sweat secretion and sweat composition of tropic-dwelling subjects. J Physiol Anthropol Appl Human Sci 2005;24: 541–9.

[17] Shirreffs SM, Merson SJ, Fraser SM, Archer DT. The effects of fluid restriction on hydration status and subjective feelings in man. Br J Nutr 2004;91:951–8.

[18] Geelen G, Greenleaf JE, Keil LC. Drinking-induced plasma vasopressin and norepinephrine changes in dehydrated humans. J Clin Endocrinol Metab 1996;81:2131–5.

[19] Andersen LJ, Jensen TU, Bestle MH, Bie P. Gastrointestinal osmoreceptors and renal sodium excretion in humans. Am J Physiol Regul Integr Comp Physiol 2000;278:R287–94.

[20] Claybaugh JR, Sato AK, Crosswhite LK, Hassell LH. Effects of time of day, gender, and menstrual cycle phase on the human response to a water load. Am J Physiol Regul Integr Comp Physiol 2000;279:R966—73.

[21] Verney E. The antidiuretic hormone and the factors which determine its release. Proc R Soc London Ser B 1947;135:25—6.

[22] Ramsay DJ, Thrasher TN, Keil LC. The organum vasculosum laminae terminalis: a critical area for osmoreception. Prog Brain Res 1983;60:91—8.

[23] Ciura S, Bourque CW. Transient receptor potential vanilloid 1 is required for intrinsic osmoreception in organum vasculosum lamina terminalis neurons and for normal thirst responses to systemic hyperosmolality. J Neurosci 2006;26:9069—75.

[24] Denton DA, McKinley MJ, Weisinger RS. Hypothalamic integration of body fluid regulation. Proc Natl Acad Sci USA 1996;93:7397—404.

[25] Hollis JH, McKinley MJ, D'Souza M, Kampe J, Oldfield BJ. The trajectory of sensory pathways from the lamina terminalis to the insular and cingulate cortex: a neuroanatomical framework for the generation of thirst. Am J Physiol Regul Integr Comp Physiol 2008;294:R1390—401.

[26] Johnson AK. The sensory psychobiology of thirst and salt appetite. Med Sci Sports Exerc 2007;39:1388—400.

[27] McKinley MJ, Denton DA, Oldfield BJ, De Oliveira LB, Mathai ML. Water intake and the neural correlates of the consciousness of thirst. Semin Nephrol 2006;26:249—57.

[28] Ciura S, Liedtke W, Bourque CW. Hypertonicity sensing in organum vasculosum lamina terminalis neurons: a mechanical process involving TRPV1 but not TRPV4. J Neurosci 2011;31:14669—76.

[29] Zhang Z, Bourque CW. Amplification of transducer gain by angiotensin II-mediated enhancement of cortical actin density in osmosensory neurons. J Neurosci 2008;28:9536—44.

[30] Robertson GL, Athar S. The interaction of blood osmolality and blood volume in regulating plasma vasopressin in man. J Clin Endocrinol Metab 1976;42:613—20.

[31] Zerbe RL, Robertson GL. Disorders of ADH. Med North Am 1984;13:1570.

[32] Miller M, Dalakos T, Moses AM, Fellerman H, Streeten DH. Recognition of partial defects in antidiuretic hormone secretion. Ann Intern Med 1970;73:721—9.

[33] Bichet DG, Kluge R, Howard RL, Schrier RW. Hyponatremic states. In: Seldin DW, Giebisch G, editors. The kidney: physiology and pathophysiology. 2nd ed. New York: Raven Press; 1992. p. 1727—51.

[34] Baylis PH, Gaskill MB, Robertson GL. Vasopressin secretion in primary polydipsia and cranial diabetes insipidus. Q J Med 1981;50:345—58.

[35] Sharif Naeini R, Witty MF, Seguela P, Bourque CW. An N-terminal variant of Trpv1 channel is required for osmosensory transduction. Nat Neurosci 2006;9:93—8.

[36] Taylor AC, McCarthy JJ, Stocker SD. Mice lacking the transient receptor vanilloid potential 1 channel display normal thirst responses and central Fos activation to hypernatremia. Am J Physiol Regul Integr Comp Physiol 2008;294:R1285—93.

[37] McHugh J, Keller NR, Appalsamy M, Thomas SA, Raj SR, Diedrich A, et al. Portal osmopressor mechanism linked to transient receptor potential vanilloid 4 and blood pressure control. Hypertension 2010;55:1438—43.

[38] Boschmann M, Steiniger J, Franke G, Birkenfeld AL, Luft FC, Jordan J. Water drinking induces thermogenesis through osmosensitive mechanisms. J Clin Endocrinol Metab 2007;92: 3334—7.

[39] Tank J, Schroeder C, Stoffels M, Diedrich A, Sharma AM, Luft FC, et al. Pressor effect of water drinking in tetraplegic patients may be a spinal reflex. Hypertension 2003;41:1234—9.

[40] Jordan J, Shannon JR, Black BK, Ali Y, Farley M, Costa F, et al. The pressor response to water drinking in humans: a sympathetic reflex? Circulation 2000;101:504—9.

[41] Schroeder C, Bush VE, Norcliffe LJ, Luft FC, Tank J, Jordan J, et al. Water·drinking acutely improves orthostatic tolerance in healthy subjects. Circulation 2002;106:2806—11.

[42] Shannon JR, Diedrich A, Biaggioni I, Tank J, Robertson RM, Robertson D, et al. Water drinking as a treatment for orthostatic syndromes. Am J Med 2002;112:355—60.

[43] Claydon VE, Schroeder C, Norcliffe LJ, Jordan J, Hainsworth R. Water drinking improves orthostatic tolerance in patients with posturally related syncope. Clin Sci (Lond) 2006;110:343—52.

[44] Stookey JD, Constant F, Popkin BM, Gardner CD. Drinking water is associated with weight loss in overweight dieting women independent of diet and activity. Obesity (Silver Spring) 2008;16:2481—8.

[45] Coste B, Mathur J, Schmidt M, Earley TJ, Ranade S, Petrus MJ, et al. Piezo1 and Piezo2 are essential components of distinct mechanically activated cation channels. Science 2010;330: 55—60.

[46] Huber D, Veinante P, Stoop R. Vasopressin and oxytocin excite distinct neuronal populations in the central amygdala. Science 2005;308:245—8.

[47] Insel TR, Young LJ. The neurobiology of attachment. Nat Rev Neurosci 2001;2:129—36.

[48] Jard S. Mechanisms of action of vasopressin and vasopressin antagonists. Kidney Int Suppl 1988;26:S38—42.

[49] Nathanson MH, Moyer MS, Burgstahler AD, O'Carroll AM, Brownstein MJ, Lolait SJ. Mechanisms of subcellular cytosolic Ca^{2+} signaling evoked by stimulation of the vasopressin V1a receptor. J Biol Chem 1992;267:23282—9.

[50] Murata K, Mitsuoka K, Hirai T, Walz T, Agre P, Heymann JB, et al. Structural determinants of water permeation through aquaporin-1. Nature 2000;407:599—605.

[51] Tajkhorshid E, Nollert P, Jensen MO, Miercke LJ, O'Connell J, Stroud RM, et al. Control of the selectivity of the aquaporin water channel family by global orientational tuning. Science 2002;296:525—30.

[52] Ragnarsson U. The nobel trail of vincent du vigneaud. J Pept Sci 2007;13:431—3.

[53] Birnbaumer M, Seibold A, Gilbert S, Ishido M, Barberis C, Antaramian A, et al. Molecular cloning of the receptor for human antidiuretic hormone. Nature 1992;357:333—5.

[54] Seibold A, Brabet P, Rosenthal W, Birnbaumer M. Structure and chromosomal localization of the human antidiuretic hormone receptor gene. Am J Hum Genet 1992;51:1078—83.

[55] Raju TN. The Nobel chronicles. 1994: Alfred G Gilman (b 1941) and Martin Rodbell (1925—98). Lancet 2000;355:2259.

[56] Raju TN. The Nobel chronicles. 1971: Earl Wilbur Sutherland, Jr. (1915—74). Lancet 1999;354:961.

[57] Rehmann H, Wittinghofer A, Bos JL. Capturing cyclic nucleotides in action: snapshots from crystallographic studies. Nat Rev Mol Cell Biol 2007;8:63—73.

[58] Boone M, Deen PM. Physiology and pathophysiology of the vasopressin-regulated renal water reabsorption. Pflugers Arch 2008;456:1005—24.

[59] Nedvetsky PI, Tamma G, Beulshausen S, Valenti G, Rosenthal W, Klussmann E. Regulation of aquaporin-2 trafficking. Handb Exp Pharmacol 2009;:133—57.

[60] Nielsen S, Frokiaer J, Marples D, Kwon TH, Agre P, Knepper MA. Aquaporins in the kidney: from molecules to medicine. Physiol Rev 2002;82:205—44.

[61] Fenton RA, Shodeinde A, Knepper MA. UT-A urea transporter promoter, UT-A alpha, targets principal cells of the renal inner medullary collecting duct. Am J Physiol Renal Physiol 2006;290: F188—95.

[62] Ward DT, Hammond TG, Harris HW. Modulation of vasopressin-elicited water transport by trafficking of aquaporin2-containing vesicles. Annu Rev Physiol 1999;61:683—97.

[63] Morishita T, Tsutsui M, Shimokawa H, Sabanai K, Tasaki H, Suda O, et al. Nephrogenic diabetes insipidus in mice lacking all nitric oxide synthase isoforms. Proc Natl Acad Sci USA 2005;102:10616—21.

[64] Olesen ET, Rutzler MR, Moeller HB, Praetorius HA, Fenton RA. Vasopressin-independent targeting of aquaporin-2 by selective E-prostanoid receptor agonists alleviates nephrogenic diabetes insipidus. Proc Natl Acad Sci USA 2011;108: 12949—54.

[65] Valtin H, North WG, Edwards BR, Gellai M. Animal models of diabetes insipidus. Front Horm Res 1985;13:105—26.

[66] Schmale H, Richter D. Single base deletion in the vasopressin gene is the cause of diabetes insipidus in Brattleboro rats. Nature 1984;308:705—9.

[67] Richter D. Reflections on central diabetes insipidus: retrospective and perspectives. In: Gross P, Richter D, Robertson GL, editors. Vasopressin. Paris: John Libbey Eurotext; 1993. p. 3—14.

[68] Schmale H, Bahnsen U, Fehr S, Nahke D, Richter D, editors. Hereditary diabetes insipidus in man and rat. Paris: John Libbey Eurotext; 1991.

[69] Serradeil-Le Gal C, Lacour C, Valette G, Garcia G, Foulon L, Galindo G, et al. Characterization of SR 121463A, a highly potent and selective, orally active vasopressin V2 receptor antagonist. J Clin Invest 1996;98:2729—38.

[70] Jean-Alphonse F, Perkovska S, Frantz MC, Durroux T, Mejean C, Morin D, et al. Biased agonist pharmacochaperones of the AVP V2 receptor may treat congenital nephrogenic diabetes insipidus. J Am Soc Nephrol 2009;20:2190—203.

[71] Evans DA, De Bree FM, Nijenhuis M, Van Der Kleij AA, Zalm R, Korteweg N, et al. Processing of frameshifted vasopressin precursors. J Neuroendocrinol 2000;12:685—93.

[72] Balment RJ, Brimble MJ, Forsling ML. Oxytocin release and renal actions in normal and Brattleboro rats. Ann NY Acad Sci US 1982;394:241—53.

[73] Chou CL, DiGiovanni SR, Luther A, Lolait SJ, Knepper MA. Oxytocin as an antidiuretic hormone II. Role of V2 vasopressin receptor. Am J Physiol 269 (Renal Fluid Electrolyte Physiol 1995;38:F78—85.

[74] Chou CL, Knepper MA, Hoek AN, Brown D, Yang B, Ma T, et al. Reduced water permeability and altered ultrastructure in thin descending limb of Henle in aquaporin-1 null mice. J Clin Invest 1999;103:491—6.

[75] Lopez-Rodriguez C, Antos CL, Shelton JM, Richardson JA, Lin F, Novobrantseva TI, et al. Loss of NFAT5 results in renal atrophy and lack of tonicity-responsive gene expression. Proc Natl Acad Sci USA 2004;101:2392—7.

[76] Ma T, Song Y, Yang B, Gillespie A, Carlson EJ, Epstein CJ, et al. Nephrogenic diabetes insipidus in mice lacking aquaporin-3 water channels. Proc Natl Acad Sci USA 2000;97: 4386—91.

[77] Ma T, Yang B, Gillespie A, Carlson EJ, Epstein CJ, Verkman AS. Generation and phenotype of a transgenic knockout mouse lacking the mercurial-insensitive water channel aquaporin-4. J Clin Invest 1997;100:957—62.

[78] Ma T, Yang B, Gillespie A, Carlson EJ, Epstein CJ, Verkman AS. Severely impaired urinary concentrating ability in transgenic mice lacking aquaporin-1 water channels. J Biol Chem 1998;273:4296—9.

[79] Matsumura Y, Uchida S, Kondo Y, Miyazaki H, Ko SB, Hayama A, et al. Overt nephrogenic diabetes insipidus in mice lacking the CLC-K1 chloride channel. Nat Genet 1999;21: 95—8.

[80] Okubo S, Niimura F, Matsusaka T, Fogo A, Hogan BL, Ichikawa I. Angiotensinogen gene null-mutant mice lack homeostatic regulation of glomerular filtration and tubular reabsorption. Kidney Int 1998;53:617—25.

[81] Takahashi N, Chernavvsky DR, Gomez RA, Igarashi P, Gitelman HJ, Smithies O. Uncompensated polyuria in a mouse model of Bartter's syndrome. Proc Natl Acad Sci USA 2000;97: 5434—9.

[82] Yang B, Gillespie A, Carlson EJ, Epstein CJ, Verkman AS. Neonatal mortality in an aquaporin-2 knock-in mouse model of recessive nephrogenic diabetes insipidus. J Biol Chem 2001;276:2775—9.

[83] Yun J, Schoneberg T, Liu J, Schulz A, Ecelbarger CA, Promeneur D, et al. Generation and phenotype of mice harboring a nonsense mutation in the V2 vasopressin receptor gene. J Clin Invest 2000;106:1361—71.

[84] Preston GM, Smith BL, Zeidel ML, Moulds JJ, Agre P. Mutations in aquaporin-1 in phenotypically normal humans without functional CHIP water channels. Science 1994;265:1585—7.

[85] Yang B, Zhao D, Qian L, Verkman AS. Mouse model of inducible nephrogenic diabetes insipidus produced by floxed aquaporin-2 gene deletion. Am J Physiol Renal Physiol 2006;291: F465—72.

[86] Mulders SB, Knoers NVAM, van Lieburg AF, Monnens LAH, Leumann E, Wühl E, et al. New mutations in the AQP2 gene in nephrogenic diabetes insipidus resulting in functional but misrouted water channels. J Am Soc Nephrol 1997;8:242—8.

[87] Li JH, Chou CL, Li B, Gavrilova O, Eisner C, Schnermann J, et al. A selective EP4 PGE2 receptor agonist alleviates disease in a new mouse model of X-linked nephrogenic diabetes insipidus. J Clin Invest 2009;119:3115—26.

[88] Rao S, Verkman AS. Analysis of organ physiology in transgenic mice. Am J Physiol Cell Physiol 2000;279:C1—18.

[89] Lloyd DJ, Hall FW, Tarantino LM, Gekakis N. Diabetes insipidus in mice with a mutation in aquaporin-2. PLoS Genet 2005;1: e20.

[90] McDill BW, Li SZ, Kovach PA, Ding L, Chen F. Congenital progressive hydronephrosis (cph) is caused by an S256L mutation in aquaporin-2 that affects its phosphorylation and apical membrane accumulation. Proc Natl Acad Sci USA 2006;103: 6952—7.

[91] Moeller HB, Olesen ET, Fenton RA. Regulation of the water channel aquaporin-2 by posttranslational modification. Am J Physiol Renal Physiol 2011;300:F1062—73.

[92] Verbalis JG, Robinson AG, Moses AM, editors. Postoperative and post-traumatic diabetes insipidus, vol. 13. Basel: S. Karger; 1985.

[93] Olson BR, Gumowski J, Rubino D, Oldfield EH. Pathophysiology of hyponatremia after transsphenoidal pituitary surgery. J Neurosurg 1997;87:499—507.

[94] Nemergut EC, Zuo Z, Jane Jr. JA, Laws Jr. ER. Predictors of diabetes insipidus after transsphenoidal surgery: a review of 881 patients. J Neurosurg 2005;103:448—54.

[95] Czernichow P, Pomarede R, Brauner R, editors. Neurogenic diabetes insipidus in children, vol. 13. Basel: S. Karger; 1985.

[96] Greger NG, Kirkland RT, Clayton GW, Kirkland JL. Central diabetes insipidus. 22 years' experience. Am J Dis Child 1986;140:551—4.

[97] Maghnie M, Cosi G, Genovese E, Manca-Bitti ML, Cohen A, Zecca S, et al. Central diabetes insipidus in children and young adults. N Engl J Med 2000;343:998—1007.

[98] Moses AM, Blumenthal SA, Streeten DH, editors. Acid—base and electrolyte disorders associated with endocrine disease: pituitary and thyroid. New York: Churchill Livingstone; 1985.

[99] Fery F, Plat L, van de Borne P, Cogan E, Mockel J. Impaired counterregulation of glucose in a patient with hypothalamic sarcoidosis. N Engl J Med 1999;340:852–6.

[100] Odell WD, Doggett RS. Xanthoma disseminatum, a rare cause of diabetes insipidus. J Clin Endocrinol Metab 1993;76:777–80.

[101] Masera N, Grant DB, Stanhope R, Preece MA. Diabetes insipidus with impaired osmotic regulation in septo-optic dysplasia and agenesis of the corpus callosum. Arch Dis Child 1994;70:51–3.

[102] Imura H, Nakao K, Shimatsu A, Ogawa Y, Sando T, Fujisawa I, et al. Lymphocytic infundibuloneurohypophysitis as a cause of central diabetes insipidus. N Engl J Med 1993;329:683–9.

[103] Ahmed SR, Aiello DP, Page R, Hopper K, Towfighi J, Santen RJ. Necrotizing infundibulo-hypophysitis: a unique syndrome of diabetes insipidus and hypopituitarism. J Clin Endocrinol Metab 1993;76:1499–504.

[104] Lacombe UL. De la polydipsie. Thesis of Medicine, no. 99. Imprimerie et Fonderie de Rignoux. Paris; 1841.

[105] Weil A. Ueber die hereditare form des diabetes insipidus. Archives fur Pathologische Anatomie und Physiologie and fur Klinische Medicine (Virchow's Archives) 1884;95:70–95.

[106] Camerer JW. Eine ergänzung des Weilschen diabetes-insipidus-stammbaumes. Archiv für Rassen-und Gesellschaftshygiene Biologie 1935;28:382–5.

[107] Dölle W. Eine weitere ergänzung des Weilschen diabetes-insipidus-stammbaumes. Zeitschrift für Menschliche Vererbungs-und Konstitutionslehre 1951;30:372–4.

[108] Weil A. Ueber die hereditare form des diabetes insipidus. Deutches Archiv fur Klinische Medizin 1908;93:180–290.

[109] McKusick VA. Mendelian inheritance in man and its online version, OMIM. Am J Hum Genet 2007;80:588–604.

[110] Rittig R, Robertson GL, Siggaard C, Kovacs L, Gregersen N, Nyborg J, et al. Identification of 13 new mutations in the vasopressin-neurophysin II gene in 17 kindreds with familial autosomal dominant neurohypophyseal diabetes insipidus. Am J Hum Genet 1996;58:107–17.

[111] Brachet C, Birk J, Christophe C, Tenoutasse S, Velkeniers B, Heinrichs C, et al. Growth retardation in untreated autosomal dominant familial neurohypophyseal diabetes insipidus caused by one recurring and two novel mutations in the vasopressin-neurophysin II gene. Eur J Endocrinol 2011;164:179–87.

[112] Birk J, Friberg MA, Prescianotto-Baschong C, Spiess M, Rutishauser J. Dominant pro-vasopressin mutants that cause diabetes insipidus form disulfide-linked fibrillar aggregates in the endoplasmic reticulum. J Cell Sci 2009;122:3994–4002.

[113] Castino R, Davies J, Beaucourt S, Isidoro C, Murphy D. Autophagy is a prosurvival mechanism in cells expressing an autosomal dominant familial neurohypophyseal diabetes insipidus mutant vasopressin transgene. FASEB J 2005;19:1021–3.

[114] Abu Libdeh A, Levy-Khademi F, Abdulhadi-Atwan M, Bosin E, Korner M, White PC, et al. Autosomal recessive familial neurohypophyseal diabetes insipidus: onset in early infancy. Eur J Endocrinol 2009;162:221–6.

[115] Christensen JH, Kvistgaaard H, Knudsen J, Shaikh G, Tolmie J, Cooke S, et al. A novel deletion partly removing the avp gene causes autosomal recessive inheritance of early onset neurohypophyseal diabetes insipidus. Clin Genet 2011; epub ahead of print

[116] Willcutts MD, Felner E, White PC. Autosomal recessive familial neurohypophyseal diabetes insipidus with continued secretion of mutant weakly active vasopressin. Hum Mol Genet 1999;8:1303–7.

[117] Bichet DG, Arthus M-F, Lonergan M, Morgan K, Fujiwara TM. Hereditary central diabetes insipidus: Autosomal dominant and autosomal recessive phenotypes due to mutations in the prepro-AVP-NPII gene. J Am Soc Nephrol 1998;9:386A.

[118] Christensen JH, Siggaard C, Corydon TJ, Robertson GL, Gregersen N, Bolund L, et al. Differential cellular handling of defective arginine vasopressin (AVP) prohormones in cells expressing mutations of the AVP gene associated with autosomal dominant and recessive familial neurohypophyseal diabetes insipidus. J Clin Endocrinol Metab 2004;89:4521–31.

[119] Beuret N, Stettler H, Renold A, Rutishauser J, Spiess M. Expression of regulated secretory proteins is sufficient to generate granule-like structures in constitutively secreting cells. J Biol Chem 2004;279:20242–9.

[120] Cohen FE, Kelly JW. Therapeutic approaches to protein-misfolding diseases. Nature 2003;426:905–9.

[121] Ulloa-Aguirre A, Janovick JA, Brothers SP, Conn PM. Pharmacologic rescue of conformationally-defective proteins: implications for the treatment of human disease. Traffic 2004;5:821–37.

[122] Welch WJ, Howard M. Antagonists to the rescue. J Clin Invest 2000;105:853–4.

[123] Kennan A, Aherne A, Humphries P. Light in retinitis pigmentosa. Trends Genet 2005;21:103–10.

[124] Domenech E, Gomez-Zaera M, Nunes V. Study of the WFS1 gene and mitochondrial DNA in Spanish Wolfram syndrome families. Clin Genet 2004;65:463–9.

[125] Takeda K, Inoue H, Tanizawa Y, Matsuzaki Y, Oba J, Watanabe Y, et al. WFS1 (Wolfram syndrome 1) gene product: predominant subcellular localization to endoplasmic reticulum in cultured cells and neuronal expression in rat brain. Hum Mol Genet 2001;10:477–84.

[126] Ishihara H, Takeda S, Tamura A, Takahashi R, Yamaguchi S, Takei D, et al. Disruption of the WFS1 gene in mice causes progressive beta-cell loss and impaired stimulus-secretion coupling in insulin secretion. Hum Mol Genet 2004;13:1159–70.

[127] Conlan AR, Axelrod HL, Cohen AE, Abresch EC, Zuris J, Yee D, et al. Crystal structure of Miner1: the redox-active 2Fe-2S protein causative in Wolfram Syndrome 2. J Mol Biol 2009;392:143–53.

[128] Fonseca SG, Ishigaki S, Oslowski CM, Lu S, Lipson KL, Ghosh R, et al. Wolfram syndrome 1 gene negatively regulates ER stress signaling in rodent and human cells. J Clin Invest 2010;120:744–55.

[129] Howard RL, Bichet DG, Schrier RW. Hypernatremic and polyuric states. In: Seldin DW, Giebisch G, editors. The kidney: physiology and pathophysiology. 2nd ed. New York: Raven Press, Ltd; 1992. p. 1753–78.

[130] Fujiwara TM, Bichet DG. Molecular biology of hereditary diabetes insipidus. J Am Soc Nephrol 2005;16:2836–46.

[131] Arthus M-F, Lonergan M, Crumley MJ, Naumova AK, Morin D, De Marco L, et al. Report of 33 novel AVPR2 mutations and analysis of 117 families with X-linked nephrogenic diabetes insipidus. J Am Soc Nephrol 2000;11:1044–54.

[132] Nomura Y, Onigata K, Nagashima T, Yutani S, Mochizuki H, Nagashima K, et al. Detection of skewed X-inactivation in two female carriers of vasopressin type 2 receptor gene mutation. J Clin Endocrinol Metab 1997;82:3434–7.

[133] Crawford JD, Bode HH. Disorders of the posteriorpituitary in children. In: Gardner LI, editor. Endocrine and genetic diseases of childhood and adolescence. 2nd ed. Philadelphia: W.B. Saunders; 1975. p. 126–58.

[134] Forssman H. On the mode of hereditary transmission in diabetes insipidus. Nordisk Medicine 1942;16:3211–3.

[135] Waring AG, Kajdi L, Tappan V. Congenital defect of water metabolism. Am J Dis Child 1945;69:323–5.

[136] Williams RM, Henry C. Nephrogenic diabetes insipidus transmitted by females and appearing during infancy in males. Ann Int Med 1947;27:84–95.

[137] Niaudet P, Dechaux M, Trivin C, Loirat C, Broyer M. Nephrogenic diabetes insipidus: clinical and pathophysiological aspects. Adv Nephrol Necker Hosp 1984;13:247–60.

[138] McIlraith CH. Notes on some cases of diabetes insipidus with marked family and hereditary tendencies. Lancet 1892;2: 767–8.

[139] Reeves WB, Andreoli TE. Nephrogenic diabetes insipidus. In: Scriver CR, Beaudet AL, Sly WS, Valle D, editors. The metabolic basis of inherited disease. 7th ed. New York: McGraw-Hill; 1995. p. 3045–71.

[140] Streitz JMJ, Streitz JM. Polyuric urinary tract dilatation with renal damage. J Urol 1988;139:784–5.

[141] Boyd SD, Raz S, Ehrlich RM. Diabetes insipidus and nonobstructive dilatation of urinary tract. Urology 1980;16:266–9.

[142] Gautier B, Thieblot P, Steg A. Mégauretère, mégavessie et diabète insipide familial. Sem Hop 1981;57:60–1.

[143] Bichet DG, Razi M, Arthus M-F, Lonergan M, Tittley P, Smiley RK, et al. Epinephrine and dDAVP administration in patients with congenital nephrogenic diabetes insipidus. Evidence for a pre-cyclic AMP V2 receptor defective mechanism. Kidney Int 1989;36:859–66.

[144] Bichet DG, Hendy GN, Lonergan M, Arthus M-F, Ligier S, Pausova Z, et al. X-linked nephrogenic diabetes insipidus: from the ship hopewell to restriction fragment length polymorphism studies. Am J Hum Genet 1992;51:1089–102.

[145] Kambouris M, Dlouhy SR, Trofatter JA, Conneally PM, Hodes ME. Localization of the gene for X-linked nephrogenic diabetes insipidus to Xq28. Am J Med Genet 1988;29:239–46.

[146] Knoers N, van der Heyden H, van Oost BA, Monnens L, Willems J, Ropers HH. Three-point linkage analysis using multiple DNA polymorphic markers in families with X-linked nephrogenic diabetes insipidus. Genomics 1989;4:434–7.

[147] van den Ouweland AM, Knoop MT, Knoers VV, Markslag PW, Rocchi M, Warren ST, et al. Colocalization of the gene for nephrogenic diabetes insipidus (DIR) and the vasopressin type 2 receptor gene (AVPR2) in the Xq28 region. Genomics 1992;13:1350–2.

[148] Goldman MB, Luchins DJ, Robertson GL. Mechanisms of altered water metabolism in psychotic patients with polydipsia and hyponatremia. N Engl J Med 1988;318:397–403.

[149] Babey M, Kopp P, Robertson GL. Familial forms of diabetes insipidus: clinical and molecular characteristics. Nat Rev Endocrinol 2011;7:701–14.

[150] Spanakis E, Milord E, Gragnoli C. AVPR2 variants and mutations in nephrogenic diabetes insipidus: review and missense mutation significance. J Cell Physiol 2008;217:605–17.

[151] Bichet DG, Fujiwara TM. Nephrogenic diabetes insipidus. In: Scriver CR, Beaudet AL, Sly WS, editors. The metabolic and molecular basis of inherited disease. New York: McGraw Hill; 2001. p. 4181–204.

[152] Bichet DG, Arthus M-F, Lonergan M, Hendy GN, Paradis AJ, Fujiwara TM, et al. X-linked nephrogenic diabetes insipidus mutations in North America and the Hopewell hypothesis. J Clin Invest 1993;92:1262–8.

[153] Shalev H, Romanovsky I, Knoers NV, Lupa S, Landau D. Bladder function impairment in aquaporin-2 defective nephrogenic diabetes insipidus. Nephrol Dial Transplant 2004;19: 608–13.

[154] Ulinski T, Grapin C, Forin V, Vargas-Poussou R, Deschenes G, Bensman A. Severe bladder dysfunction in a family with ADH receptor gene mutation responsible for X-linked nephrogenic diabetes insipidus. Nephrol Dial Transplant 2004;19:2928–9.

[155] Hobbs HH, Russell DW, Brown MS, Goldstein JL. The LDL receptor locus in familial hypercholesterolemia: mutational analysis of a membrane protein. Annu Rev Genet 1990;24: 133–70.

[156] Bernier V, Lagace M, Lonergan M, Arthus MF, Bichet DG, Bouvier M. Functional rescue of the constitutively internalized V2 vasopressin receptor mutant R137H by the pharmacological chaperone action of SR49059. Mol Endocrinol 2004;18:2074–84.

[157] Hermosilla R, Oueslati M, Donalies U, Schonenberger E, Krause E, Oksche A, et al. Disease-causing V(2) vasopressin receptors are retained in different compartments of the early secretory pathway. Traffic 2004;5:993–1005.

[158] Morello JP, Salahpour A, Laperrière A, Bernier V, Arthus M-F, Lonergan M, et al. Pharmacological chaperones rescue cell-surface expression and function of misfolded V2 vasopressin receptor mutants. J Clin Invest 2000;105:887–95.

[159] Wuller S, Wiesner B, Loffler A, Furkert J, Krause G, Hermosilla R, et al. Pharmacochaperones post-translationally enhance cell surface expression by increasing conformational stability of wild-type and mutant vasopressin V2 receptors. J Biol Chem 2004;279:47254–63.

[160] Schoneberg T, Schulz A, Biebermann H, Hermsdorf T, Rompler H, Sangkuhl K. Mutant G-protein-coupled receptors as a cause of human diseases. Pharmacol Ther 2004;104: 173–206.

[161] Romisch K. A cure for traffic jams: small molecule chaperones in the endoplasmic reticulum. Traffic 2004;5:815–20.

[162] Tamarappoo BK, Verkman AS. Defective aquaporin-2 trafficking in nephrogenic diabetes insipidus and correction by chemical chaperones. J Clin Invest 1998;101:2257–67.

[163] Kunchaparty S, Palcso M, Berkman J, Velazquez H, Desir GV, Bernstein P, et al. Defective processing and expression of thiazide-sensitive Na-Cl co-transporter as a cause of Gitelman's syndrome. Am J Physiol 1999;277:F643–9.

[164] Hayama A, Rai T, Sasaki S, Uchida S. Molecular mechanisms of Bartter syndrome caused by mutations in the BSND gene. Histochem Cell Biol 2003;119:485–93.

[165] Peters M, Ermert S, Jeck N, Derst C, Pechmann U, Weber S, et al. Classification and rescue of ROMK mutations underlying hyperprostaglandin E syndrome/antenatal Bartter syndrome. Kidney Int 2003;64:923–32.

[166] Chillaron J, Estevez R, Samarzija I, Waldegger S, Testar X, Lang F, et al. An intracellular trafficking defect in type I cystinuria rBAT mutants M467T and M467K. J Biol Chem 1997;272: 9543–9.

[167] Bonnardeaux A, Bichet DG. Inherited disorders of the renal tubule. In: 9th ed. Taal MW, Marsden PA, Skorecki K, Yu ASL, Brenner BM, editors. Brenner & rector's the kidney, vol. 2. Philadelphia: Elsevier Saunders; 2012. p. 1584–625.

[168] Lomas DA, Evans DL, Finch JT, Carrell RW. The mechanism of Z alpha 1-antitrypsin accumulation in the liver. Nature 1992;357:605–7.

[169] Lawless MW, Greene CM, Mulgrew A, Taggart CC, O'Neill SJ, McElvaney NG. Activation of endoplasmic reticulum-specific stress responses associated with the conformational disease Z alpha 1-antitrypsin deficiency. J Immunol 2004;172:5722–6.

[170] Barak LS, Oakley RH, Laporte SA, Caron MG. Constitutive arrestin-mediated desensitization of a human vasopressin receptor mutant associated with nephrogenic diabetes insipidus. Proc Natl Acad Sci USA 2001;98:93–8.

[171] Robben JH, Kortenoeven ML, Sze M, Yae C, Milligan G, Oorschot VM, et al. Intracellular activation of vasopressin V2 receptor mutants in nephrogenic diabetes insipidus by nonpeptide agonists. Proc Natl Acad Sci USA 2009;106:12195–200.

[172] Glover DJ, Lipps HJ, Jans DA. Towards safe, non-viral therapeutic gene expression in humans. Nat Rev Genet 2005;6: 299–310.

[173] Sangkuhl K, Schulz A, Rompler H, Yun J, Wess J, Schoneberg T. Aminoglycoside-mediated rescue of a disease-causing nonsense mutation in the V2 vasopressin receptor gene in vitro and in vivo. Hum Mol Genet 2004;13:893–903.

[174] Mankin AS, Liebman SW. Baby, don't stop!. Nat Genet 1999;23:8–10.

[175] Brenner B, Seligsohn U, Hochberg Z. Normal response of factor VIII and von Willebrand factor to 1-deamino-8D-arginine vasopressin in nephrogenic diabetes insipidus. J Clin Endocrinol Metab 1988;67:191–3.

[176] Knoers N, Monnens LA. A variant of nephrogenic diabetes insipidus: V2 receptor abnormality restricted to the kidney. Eur J Pediatr 1991;150:370–3.

[177] Langley JM, Balfe JW, Selander T, Ray PN, Clarke JT. Autosomal recessive inheritance of vasopressin-resistant diabetes insipidus. Am J Med Genet 1991;38:90–4.

[178] Deen PM, Verdijk MA, Knoers NV, Wieringa B, Monnens LA, van Os CH, et al. Requirement of human renal water channel aquaporin-2 for vasopressin-dependent concentration of urine. Science 1994;264:92–5.

[179] Agre P. Aquaporin water channels (Nobel Lecture). Angew Chem Int Ed Engl 2004;43:4278–90.

[180] Kamsteeg EJ, Bichet DG, Konings IB, Nivet H, Lonergan M, Arthus MF, et al. Reversed polarized delivery of an aquaporin-2 mutant causes dominant nephrogenic diabetes insipidus. J Cell Biol 2003;163:1099–109.

[181] Kuwahara M, Iwai K, Ooeda T, Igarashi T, Ogawa E, Katsushima Y, et al. Three families with autosomal dominant nephrogenic diabetes insipidus caused by aquaporin-2 mutations in the C-terminus. Am J Hum Genet 2001;69:738–48.

[182] Marr N, Bichet DG, Lonergan M, Arthus MF, Jeck N, Seyberth HW, et al. Heteroligomerization of an Aquaporin-2 mutant with wild-type Aquaporin-2 and their misrouting to late endosomes/lysosomes explains dominant nephrogenic diabetes insipidus. Hum Mol Genet 2002;11:779–89.

[183] Mulders SM, Bichet DG, Rijss JPL, Kamsteeg E-J, Arthus M-F, Lonergan M, et al. An aquaporin-2 water channel mutant which causes autosomal dominant nephrogenic diabetes insipidus is retained in the Golgi complex. J Clin Invest 1998;102:57–66.

[184] Robertson GL, Kopp P. A novel dominant mutation of the aquaporin-2 gene resulting in partial nephrogenic diabetes insipidus. Global Conference Proceedings, NDI Foundation; April 26–28, 2002:7A.

[185] de Mattia F, Savelkoul PJ, Bichet DG, Kamsteeg EJ, Konings IB, Marr N, et al. A novel mechanism in recessive nephrogenic diabetes insipidus: wild-type aquaporin-2 rescues the apical membrane expression of intracellularly retained AQP2-P262L. Hum Mol Genet 2004;13:3045–56.

[186] Sohara E, Rai T, Yang SS, Uchida K, Nitta K, Horita S, et al. Pathogenesis and treatment of autosomal-dominant nephrogenic diabetes insipidus caused by an aquaporin 2 mutation. Proc Natl Acad Sci USA 2006;103:14217–22.

[187] Bichet DG. Nephrogenic diabetes insipidus: new developments. Nephrol Self-Assessment Progr 2004;3:187–91.

[188] Bichet DG, Fujiwara TM. Reabsorption of sodium chloride — lessons from the chloride channels. N Engl J Med 2004;350: 1281–3.

[189] Jeck N, Schlingmann KP, Reinalter SC, Komhoff M, Peters M, Waldegger S, et al. Salt handling in the distal nephron: lessons learned from inherited human disorders. Am J Physiol Regul Integr Comp Physiol 2005;288:R782–95.

[190] Peters M, Jeck N, Reinalter S, Leonhardt A, Tonshoff B, Klaus GG, et al. Clinical presentation of genetically defined patients with hypokalemic salt-losing tubulopathies. Am J Med 2002;112:183–90.

[191] Marek S, Tekesin I, Hellmeyer L, Komhoff M, Seyberth HW, Maier RF, et al. [Differential diagnosis of a polyhydramnion in hyperprostaglandin E syndrome: a case report]. Z Geburtshilfe Neonatol 2004;208:232–5.

[192] Gahl WA, Thoene JG, Schneider JA. Cystinosis. N Engl J Med 2002;347:111–21.

[193] Bockenhauer D, van't Hoff W, Dattani M, Lehnhardt A, Subtirelu M, Hildebrandt F, et al. Secondary nephrogenic diabetes insipidus as a complication of inherited renal diseases. Nephron Physiol 2010;116:p23–9.

[194] Boton R, Gaviria M, Batlle DC. Prevalence, pathogenesis, and treatment of renal dysfunction associated with chronic lithium therapy. Am J Kidney Dis 1987;10:329–45.

[195] Christensen S, Kusano E, Yusufi AN, Murayama N, Dousa TP. Pathogenesis of nephrogenic diabetes insipidus due to chronic administration of lithium in rats. J Clin Invest 1985;75:1869–79.

[196] Cogan E, Svoboda M, Abramow M. Mechanisms of lithium-vasopressin interaction in rabbit cortical collecting tubule. Am J Physiol 1987;252:F1080–7.

[197] Grunfeld JP, Rossier BC. Lithium nephrotoxicity revisited. Nat Rev Nephrol 2009;5:270–6.

[198] Christensen BM, Zuber AM, Loffing J, Stehle JC, Deen PM, Rossier BC, et al. alphaENaC-mediated lithium absorption promotes nephrogenic diabetes insipidus. J Am Soc Nephrol 2011;22:253–61.

[199] Barlow ED, de Wardener HE. Compulsive water drinking. Q J Med New Series 1959;28:235–58.

[200] Robertson GL. Dipsogenic diabetes insipidus: a newly recognized syndrome caused by a selective defect in the osmoregulation of thirst. Trans Assoc Am Physicians 1987;100:241–9.

[201] Amico JA. Diabetes insipidus and pregnancy. In: Czernichow AGRP, editor. Frontiers of hormone research. Basel: Karger; 1985. p. 266–77.

[202] Davison JM, Shiells EA, Philips PR, Lindheimer MD. Serial evaluation of vasopressin release and thirst in human pregnancy. Role of human chorionic gonadotrophin in the osmoregulatory changes of gestation. J Clin Invest 1988;81:798–806.

[203] Iwasaki Y, Oiso Y, Kondo K, Takagi S, Takatsuki K, Hasegawa H, et al. Aggravation of subclinical diabetes insipidus during pregnancy. N Engl J Med 1991;324:522–6.

[204] Forssman J. On hereditary diabetes insipidus, with special regard to a sex-linked form. Acta Med Scand 1945;159:1–196.

[205] Barron WM, Cohen LH, Ulland LA, Lassiter WE, Fulghum EM, Emmanouel D, et al. Transient vasopressin-resistant diabetes insipidus of pregnancy. N Engl J Med 1984;310:442–4.

[206] Durr JA, Hoggard JG, Hunt JM, Schrier RW. Diabetes insipidus in pregnancy associated with abnormally high circulating vasopressinase activity. N Engl J Med 1987;316:1070–4.

[207] Brewster UC, Hayslett JP. Diabetes insipidus in the third trimester of pregnancy. Obstet Gynecol 2005;105:1173–6.

[208] Hiett AK, Barton JR. Diabetes insipidus associated with craniopharyngioma in pregnancy. Obstet Gynecol 1990;76:982–4.

[209] Trudel E, Bourque CW. Central clock excites vasopressin neurons by waking osmosensory afferents during late sleep. Nat Neurosci 2010;13:467–74.

[210] Denton KM. In the arms of morpheus. Am J Physiol Renal Physiol 2012;302(2):F234–5.

[211] Mahler BT, Kamperis K, Schroeder M, Frokiaer J, Djurhuus JC, Rittig S. Sleep deprivation induces excess diuresis and natriuresis in healthy children. Am J Physiol Renal Physiol 2011;302 (2):F236–42.

[212] Leaf A. Nephrology forum: neurogenic diabetes insipidus. Kidney Int 1979;15:572–80.

[213] Bichet DG. Clinical manifestations and causes of nephrogenic diabetes insipidus. UpToDate, <www.uptodate.com>; 2011.

[214] Robertson GL. Diseases of the posterior pituitary. In: Felig D, Baxter JD, Broadus AE, editors. Endocrinology and metabolism. New York: McGraw-Hill; 1981. p. 251.

[215] Robertson GL. Diagnosis of diabetes insipidus. In: Czernichow AGRP, editor. Frontiers of hormone research, vol. 13. Basel: Karger; 1985. p. 176.

[216] Bichet D. Nephrogenic diabetes insipidus. In: Davison A, Cameron J, Grünfeld J, Kerr D, Ritz E, Winearls C, editors. Oxford textbook of clinical nephrology. New York: Oxford University Press; 2012, in press

[217] Zerbe RL, Robertson GL. A comparison of plasma vasopressin measurements with a standard indirect test in the differential diagnosis of polyuria. N Engl J Med 1981;305:1539–46.

[218] Stern P, Valtin H. Verney was right, but. N Engl J Med 1981;305:1581–2.

[219] Robertson GL. Differential diagnosis of polyuria. Annu Rev Med 1988;39:425–42.

[220] Oksche A, Dickson J, Schülein R, Seyberth HW, Müller M, Rascher W, et al. Two novel mutations in the vasopressin V2 receptor gene in patients with congenital nephrogenic diabetes insipidus. Biophys Biochem Res Com 1994;205:552–7.

[221] van Lieburg AF, Verdijk MAJ, Schoute F, Ligtenberg MJL, van Oost BA, Waldhauser F, et al. Clinical phenotype of nephrogenic diabetes insipidus in females heterozygous for a vasopressin type 2 receptor mutation. Hum Genet 1995; 96:70–8.

[222] Miller WL. Molecular genetics of familial central diabetes insipidus. J Clin Endocrinol Metab 1993;77:592–5.

[223] Bichet DG. Nephrogenic and central diabetes insipidus. In: Schrier RW, editor. Diseases of the kidney. 9th ed. New York: Lippincott Williams and Wilkins; 2012, in press.

[224] Robertson GL, Klein LA, Roth J, Gorden P. Immunoassay of plasma vasopressin in man. Proc Natl Acad Sci USA 1970;66: 1298–305.

[225] Robertson GL, Mahr EA, Athar S, Sinha T. Development and clinical application of a new method for the radioimmunoassay of arginine vasopressin in human plasma. J Clin Invest 1973;52:2340–52.

[226] Hartter E, Woloszczuk W. Radioimmunological determination of arginine vasopressin and human atrial natriuretic peptide after simultaneous extraction from plasma. J Clin Chem Clin Biochem 1986;24:559–63.

[227] LaRochelle Jr. FT, North WG, Stern P. A new extraction of arginine vasopressin from blood: the use of octadecasilyl-silica. Pflugers Arch 1980;387:79–81.

[228] Ysewijn-Van Brussel KA, De Leenheer AP. Development and evaluation of a radioimmunoassay for Arg8-vasopressin, after extraction with Sep-Pak C18. Clin Chem 1985; 31:861–3.

[229] Bichet DG, Arthus MF, Barjon JN, Lonergan M, Kortas C. Human platelet fraction arginine-vasopressin. Potential physiological role. J Clin Invest 1987;79:881–7.

[230] Preibisz JJ, Sealey JE, Laragh JH, Cody RJ, Weksler BB. Plasma and platelet vasopressin in essential hypertension and congestive heart failure. Hypertension 1983;5:I129–38.

[231] Bichet DG, Kortas C, Mettauer B, Manzini C, Marc-Aurele J, Rouleau JL, et al. Modulation of plasma and platelet vasopressin by cardiac function in patients with heart failure. Kidney Int 1986;29:1188–96.

[232] Seckl JR, Dunger DB, Bevan JS, Nakasu Y, Chowdrey C, Burke CW, et al. Vasopressin antagonist in early postoperative diabetes insipidus. Lancet 1990;335:1353–6.

[233] Kanno K, Sasaki S, Hirata Y, Ishikawa S, Fushimi K, Nakanishi S, et al. Urinary excretion of aquaporin-2 in patients with diabetes insipidus. N Engl J Med 1995;332:1540–5.

[234] Elliot S, Goldsmith P, Knepper M, Haughey M, Olson B. Urinary excretion of aquaporin-2 in humans: a potential marker of collecting duct responsiveness to vasopressin. J Am Soc Nephrol 1996;7:403–9.

[235] Maas AH, Siggaard-Andersen O, Weisberg HF, Zijlstra WG. Ion-selective electrodes for sodium and potassium: a new problem of what is measured and what should be reported. Clin Chem 1985;31:482–5.

[236] Gennari FJ. Current concepts. Serum osmolality. Uses and limitations. N Engl J Med 1984;310:102–5.

[237] De Buyst J, Massa G, Christophe C, Tenoutasse S, Heinrichs C. Clinical, hormonal and imaging findings in 27 children with central diabetes insipidus. Eur J Pediatr 2007;166:43–9.

[238] Cattin F, Bonneville F, Chayep C. Imagerie par resonance magnetique du diabete insipide. Feuillets de Radiologie 2005;45: 425–34.

[239] Fujisawa I. Magnetic resonance imaging of the hypothalamic-neurohypophyseal system. J Neuroendocrinol 2004;16: 297–302.

[240] Rappaport R. Magnetic resonance imaging in pituitary disease. Growth Genetics & Hormones 1995;11:1–5.

[241] Mouillac B, Chini B, Balestre M-N, Elands J, Trumpp-Kallmeyer S, Hoflack J, et al. The binding site of neuropeptide vasopressin V1a receptor. J Biol Chem 1995;270: 25771–7.

[242] Wilson Y, Nag N, Davern P, Oldfield BJ, McKinley MJ, Greferath U, et al. Visualization of functionally activated circuitry in the brain. Proc Natl Acad Sci USA 2002;99: 3252–7.

[243] Prager-Khoutorsky M, Bourque CW. Osmosensation in vasopressin neurons: changing actin density to optimize function. Trends Neurosci 2010;33:76–83.

[244] Vokes TP, Robertson GL. Physiology of secretion of vasopressin. In: Czernichow AGRP, editor. Frontiers in hormone research: diabetes insipidus in man, vol. 13. Basel: S. Karger; 1985. p. 127–55.

[245] Robertson G. The pathophysiology of ADH secretion. In: Tolis G, Labrie F, Martin JB, editors. Clinical neuroendocrinology: a pathophysiological approach. New York: Raven Press; 1979.

[246] Magner PO HM. Polyuria – a pathophysiological approach. Med North America 1987;15:2987–97.

[247] Davison JM, Gilmore EA, Durr J, Robertson GL, Lindheimer MD. Altered osmotic thresholds for vasopressin secretion and thirst in human pregnancy. Am J Physiol 1984;246: F105–9.

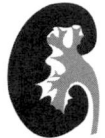

The Molecular Biology of Renal K⁺ Channels

WenHui Wang[1] and Chou-Long Huang[2]

[1]Department of Pharmacology, New York Medical College, Valhalla, NY, USA

[2]University of Texas, Southwestern Medical Center, Dallas, TX, USA

INTRODUCTION

Renal epithelial transport depends on the coordinated function of potassium channels with ion transporters (co-transporters, channels, and exchangers) and ion pumps in apical and basolateral membranes of distinct cell types along the nephron of the mammalian kidney. Potassium (K^+) channels are key members of this integrated transport system in renal epithelial cells. First, renal K^+ channels participate in generating cell membrane potential; since numerous transporters are electrogenic, changes in cell membrane potential could alter the transport rate of a given substance. Second, renal K^+ channels are involved in the volume regulation that is essential for preventing cell swelling or shrinking in the hypotonic or hypertonic environment. Third, renal K^+ channels play an important role in K^+ recycling which is essential for maintaining the function of several transport proteins, such as Na^+-K^+-ATPase. Finally, renal K^+ channels are extremely involved in K^+ secretion in the aldosterone-sensitive distal nephron (ASDN). Figure 47.1 is a scheme providing an overview regarding the role of K channels in different renal segments.

Since K^+ channels play such an important role in kidney function, understanding the structure and regulation of renal K^+ channels is essential to gaining insights into the molecular mechanisms of kidney potassium handling. In the past decades, the development of molecular biology and patch-clamp techniques has had a significant impact on the exploration of the molecular identity of some renal K^+ channels. This chapter summarizes our current understanding of the molecular identity of renal K^+ channels, and will specifically focus on the ROMK (Kir1; *KCNJ1*) channel. We will discuss similarities, as well as certain differences, in the properties of cloned K^+ channels compared to native K^+ channels expressed in the different nephron segments.

THE MOLECULAR BIOLOGY OF ROMK, A DISTAL K⁺ SECRETORY CHANNEL

Structure of Inward Rectifying K⁺ Channels and ROMK

The K^+ channel, *ROMK* (Kir1; *KCNJ1*[1]), belongs to a growing family of inwardly rectifying K^+ (Kir) channels[2] that are functionally characterized by high potassium selectivity and by either weak or strong inward rectification. To date, 16 Kir genes have been identified and classified into seven subfamilies (Kir1.x to Kir7.x). All Kir channels have a membrane topology consisting of two membrane-spanning domains (M1 and M2), an intervening H5 pore-forming region, and cytoplasmic amino (NH₂-) and carboxyl (COOH-)-terminal domains (Figure 47.2[3–5]). This membrane topology corresponds to the last two membrane spanning segments of the voltage-gated K^+ channels, suggesting a common ancestral origin.[6–8] The N- and C-terminal cytoplasmic regions of Kir channels provide regulatory domains (Figure 47.2) that can be phosphorylated by kinases,[9] and that interact with protons,[10–12] nucleotides,[13] and phosphoinositides.[14,15]

The three-dimensional structure of ROMK is not available, but it can be inferred from X-ray crystallographic structures of bacterial and eukaryotic K^+ channels. The first crystal structure of K^+ channel

Seldin and Giebisch's The Kidney, Fifth Edition.

DOI: http://dx.doi.org/10.1016/B978-0-12-381462-3.00047-1

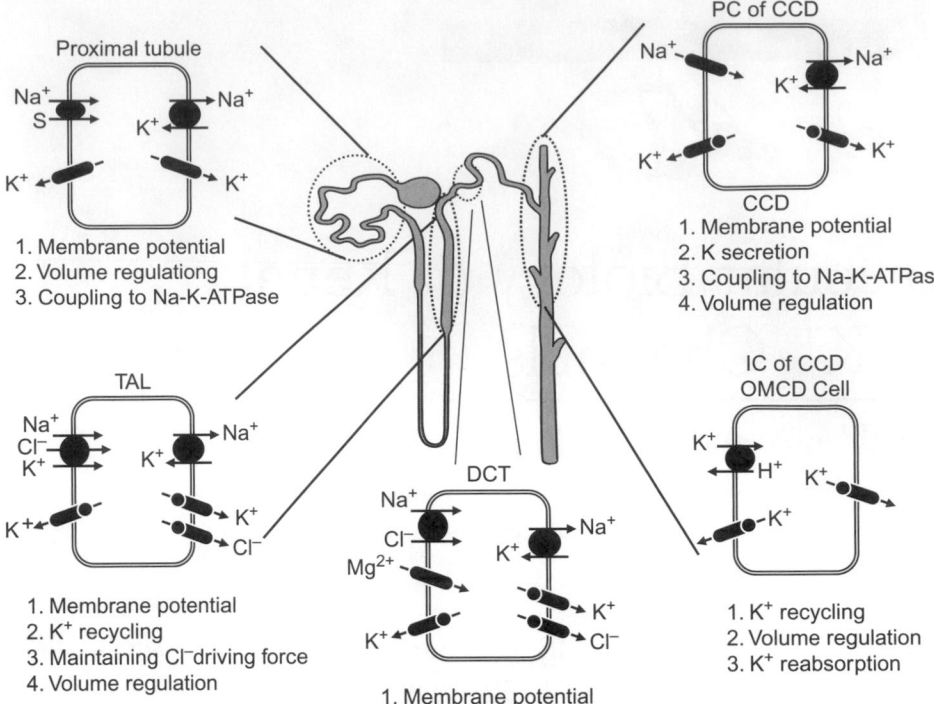

FIGURE 47.1 A cell model demonstrating the role of K channels in different renal segments.

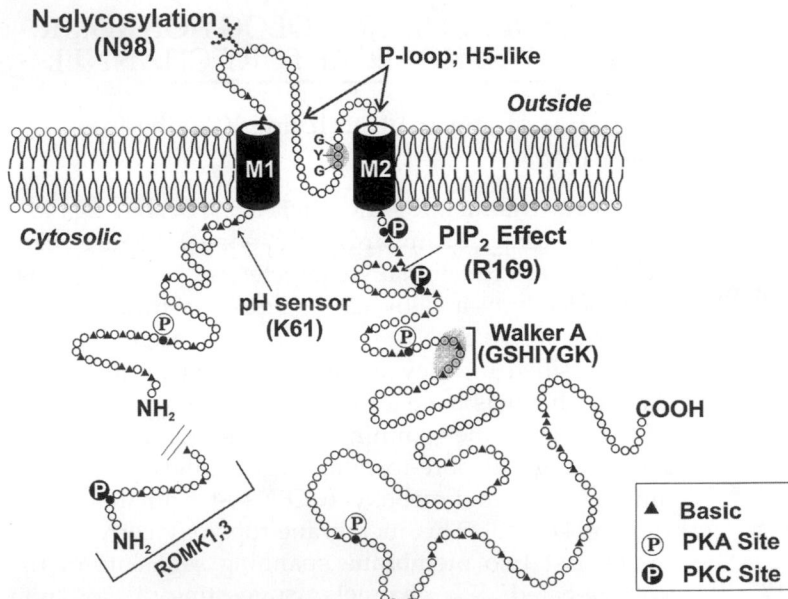

FIGURE 47.2 Topology of ROMK (Kir1.1) K⁺ channel. M1 and M2 represent the two membrane-spanning domains characterizing the inward-rectifier family of potassium channel. Some important functional sites are indicated. A short amphipathic segment in the M1-M2 linking segment in ROMK forms the pore-forming (P-loop) or H5 region. The canonical T-X-G-Y-G amino acid sequence found in all K⁺ channels is shown in the H5 segment. Numbering is based on amino acid sequence of ROMK2 (Kir1.1b).

determined is from *Streptomyces lividans* (KcsA).[16] Although not an inward rectifier K⁺ channel, KcsA shares the same membrane topology with Kir channels with two membrane-spanning M1 and M2 segments, a H5 pore-forming region, and N- and C-terminal cytoplasmic domains. The amino acid sequence of KcsA is similar to the corresponding region of other K⁺ channels, including vertebrate and invertebrate voltage-gated K⁺ channel, inward rectifier, and calcium-activated K⁺ channels. The crystal structure of KcsA reveals a tetramer with four identical subunits that encircle a central ion conduction pathway with four-fold symmetry (Figure 47.3). The M1 and M2 segments of each subunit form α-helices and are inserted into the

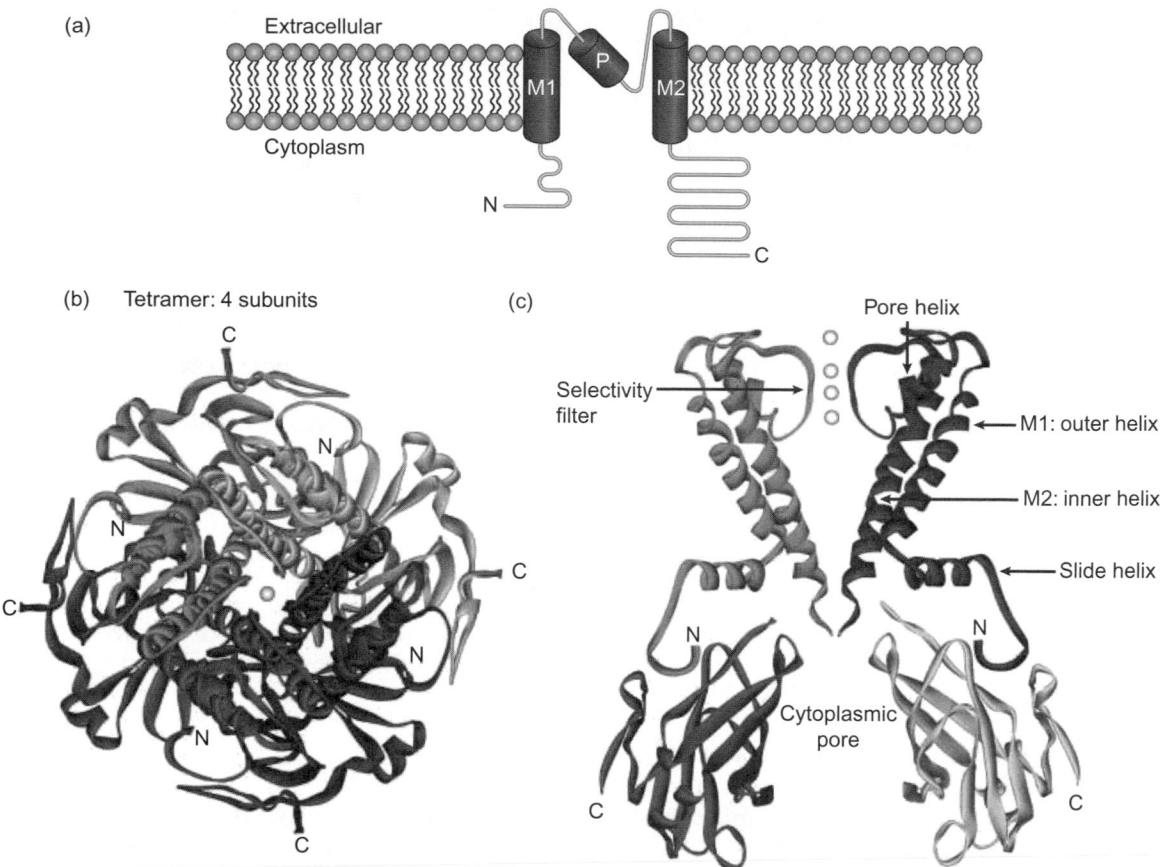

FIGURE 47.3 **Architecture of inwardly rectifying K (Kir) channels 276.** (a) A scheme of Kir channels: each subunit contains two transmembrane helices (M1 and M2), a channel pore (P), and both N- and C-termini. (b) The tetrameric structure of the KirBac1.1 channel4 (PDB ID:1P7B) viewed from the extracellular side. Each monomer is marked by red, green, yellow, and blue, respectively. The conduction pathway is indicated by a K ion (white). (c) Side view of two subunits of the KirBac1.1 illustrating the transmembrane domain (green and blue), the C-terminal domains of their neighbouring subunits (red and yellow) and K ions (white) in the selectivity filter. See color section at the back of the book.

tetramer such that M2 faces the central ion conduction pathway (termed inner helix), and M1 faces the lipid membrane (outer helix). Amino acids connecting M1 and M2 (from N to C) form the turret, a tilted pore helix that runs half-way through the membrane, and the selectivity filter bearing the Thr-X-Gly-Tyr-Gly (X is any amino acid) signature sequence of all K$^+$ channels. The inner helices are tilted with respect to the membrane, so that the subunits open like the petals of a flower facing the outside of the cell. Furthermore, the four inner helices pack against each other as a bundle near the intracellular aspect of the membrane, giving the appearance of an inverted teepee.

The ion conduction pathway (pore) of KcsA can be functionally divided into three parts that (from the outside of the cell) consist of the selectivity filter, a water-filled wide cavity near the middle of the membrane (the central cavity; ~10Å across), and the internal part of the pore made up of the anti-lipid facing amino acids of four inner helices. The selectivity filter (~12Å

in length) is the narrowest part of the pore, and is lined by four evenly spaced layers of carbonyl oxygen atoms from amino acids X-Gly-Tyr-Gly, and a single layer of hydroxyl oxygen atoms from amino acid threonine. K$^+$ ions dehydrate and enter the selectivity filter in single file. The five layers of oxygen atoms form four consecutive K$^+$ ion-binding sites to stabilize dehydrated K$^+$ ions in the filter, which compensates for the energy required for dehydration. Due to repulsion between closely spaced ions, K$^+$ ions occupy only two of the four binding sites at a given time, in either 1,3 or 2,4 configuration. These unique structural and energetic features contribute to the extremely high selectivity (~1000 to 1 for K$^+$ over Na$^+$) yet fast conduction rate (up to ~10^{8}ions/sec) of K$^+$ channels for K$^+$ ions.

The crossing of four inner helices of KcsA as a bundle near the intracellular aspect of the membrane creates a point of structural constraint between the membrane pore and the cytoplasm, referred to as bundle crossing. Structural comparison of KcsA with

Mthk, a bacterial calcium-activated K⁺ channel,[17] provides insights into how bundle crossing might function as an activation gate for K⁺ channels. In KcsA, the inner helices are straight and the diameter of bundle crossing is about 3.5Å, suggesting that the crystal structure of KcsA is in closed conformation. In contrast, the crystal structure of Mthk, which is solved in the presence of high (Ca^{2+}), thus likely in the open conformation, reveals that inner helices are bent at a hinge point and splayed open so that the bundle crossing does not form a barrier to the flow K⁺ ions between the central cavity and the cytoplasm. Thus, KcsA and Mthk structures likely represent closed and open pore conformations of many different K⁺ channels, including ROMK. Conservation of a glycine residue at the inner helix hinge point in most K⁺ channels supports this conclusion.

The structural studies of KcsA and Mthk do not include the cytoplasmic N- and C-terminal domains. The crystallographic structure of the bacterial inward rectifier K⁺ channel KirBac1.1, including the transmembrane and cytoplasmic domains, provides the first insight into the intracellular domains of Kir channels.[18] The structures of the intracellular domains of eukaryotic Kir channels are determined in two ways. One uses only the N- and C-terminal cytoplasmic domains connected by an artificial kinker for crystallographic studies.[19] The other determines the structures of cytoplasmic domains, together with the transmembrane domains, using either a chimeric channel containing the outer three quarters of the membrane domains of KirBac3.1 and the inner one quarter of the membrane domain and the intracellular N- and C-terminal domains of Kir3.1[20] or the native form of inward rectifier K⁺ channel from chicken (Kir2.2).[21] Overall, these studies reveal that the N-terminal cytoplasmic domain of one subunit interacts with the C-terminus of the adjacent subunit, and together form predominantly β-sheet structures. The four sets of associated N- and C-terminal domains assemble into a tetramer surrounding a water-filled cytoplasmic pore that extends coaxially from the transmembrane pore domain. Thus, the cytoplasmic pore extends the ion permeation pathway to ~60Å, nearly twice the length of the transmembrane pore. The apex of the cytoplasmic pore abutting the transmembrane domain is formed by a loop referred to as the "G-loop." In the crystal structures, the G-loops are in either a constricted or dilated conformation, likely representing closed and open states of the cytoplasmic pore, respectively.[19-21] Thus, Kir channels contain two regions along the length of ion conduction pathway that can adopt constricted or dilated conformation and function as the gates. One is the inner helix bundle crossing, and the other is the apex of the cytoplasmic pore formed by the G-loops.

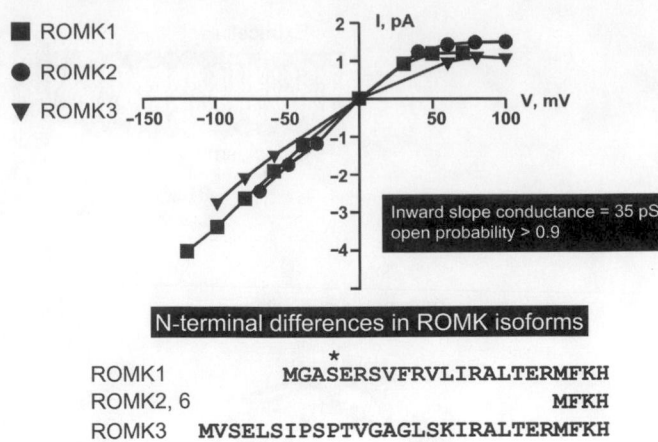

FIGURE 47.4 The ROMK splice variants. Current-voltage relationships for ROMK1, 2, and 3 are shown. Each of these variants has a similar I–V curve and calculated single channel conductance of ~35 pS. The open probability of these three channels is also similar and >0.9. ROMK1, 2, 3, and 6 N-terminal amino acid sequences are shown using the single letter notation for residues. ROMK2 and 6 have an identical amino acid sequence. ROMK1 and ROMK3 have 19 and 26 additional N-terminal amino acids, respectively, compared to ROMK2 or 6. The asterisk in the ROMK1 sequence indicates a functional PKC phosphorylation site.

Interestingly, the plasma-membrane facing surface of the cytoplasmic pore contains many positively charged amino acids known to be important for binding to membrane phosphatidylinositol-4,5-bisphosphate (PIP_2)[4,22] (see section on "Regulation of ROMK by PIP_2" below). Interaction between these amino acids and membrane PIP_2 may alter the conformation of the G-loop and the inner helix bundle crossing to activate the channel.[19,20]

ROMK Channel Isoforms

Following the cloning of ROMK1 (Kir1.1a) from rat kidney,[3] three additional alternatively spliced forms of this channel were isolated (Figures 47.2 and 47.4), and named ROMK2 (Kir1.1b), ROMK3 (Kir1.1c)[23,24] and ROMK6 (Kir1.1d).[25] The encoded ROMK proteins differ at the beginning of the N-terminus – ROMK2 (also rat ROMK6, which has the same amino acid sequence as ROMK2; Figure 47.4[25]) has the shortest N-terminus, and splicing adds either 19 or 26 amino acids for ROMK1 or ROMK3, respectively (see Figures 47.2 and 47.4). Relative ROMK mRNA abundance measured by competitive PCR has shown that ROMK2 and ROMK3 are much more abundant than ROMK1 or ROMK6 in rat kidney.[26] In addition, a novel set of ROMK proteins, about one-third the size of native ROMK, has been suggested to be formed from alternative splicing of the ROMK core exon.[27] The significance of these putative smaller channel proteins remains unclear. Six splice variants[28-30] have been identified in the human ROMK gene, *KCNJ1*, located on chromosome 11q24.[28] These six human transcripts apparently encode only three distinct polypeptides, two of which are similar to rat ROMK1 and ROMK2.[28] A rat homolog of the third human ROMK isoform has not been identified. Two ROMK homologs have also been cloned from human kidney, but their roles in renal function are unknown.[31]

ROMK Channel Localization

Rat ROMK1-3 are differentially expressed along the nephron from the thick ascending limb of Henle, TAL, to the outer medullary collecting duct, OMCD, (Figure 47.5[23,32]). The rat TAL and distal convoluted tubule, DCT, express ROMK2 and ROMK3 messenger RNA, while principal cells in the cortical collecting duct, CCD, express ROMK1 and ROMK2 transcripts (see Figure 47.5). The outer medullary collecting duct cells appear to express only ROMK1 transcripts. The general single channel properties of the ROMK1, 2, and 3 isoforms are similar, e.g., single channel conductance and open probability (Figure 47.4). Although the specific functional/regulatory consequences of the different isoforms have not been fully-elucidated, a serine at the fourth position in the extended N-terminus in ROMK1 has been shown to be required for sensitivity to arachidonic acid (Figures 47.2 and 47.4)[33] and protein kinase C[34] (see section on ROMK function below). Thus, ROMK1 may add distinct functional characteristics to ROMK channels. No specific role for the extended N-terminus of ROMK3 has yet been identified. Whether tetrameric ROMK channels are formed of different subunits (e.g., heterotetramers of ROMK2 and ROMK1 in the cortical collecting duct) or exist only as homotetramers is not known. Finally, ROMK transcripts are present in some other tissues,[3] including the early gravid uterus.[35] Roles for ROMK in these tissues have not been determined.

Antibody generated to sequences of ROMK shared by all isoforms has demonstrated an apical pattern of channel protein expression in rat TAL (including macula densa cells), DCT, and early CNT cells, and principal cells of the CCD and OMCD.[36-39] This localization is consistent with the ROMK channel providing a K$^+$ secretory pathway in these renal epithelia.

ROMK Channel Properties are Similar to the Distal (SK) K$^+$ Secretory Channel

The single channel characteristics and regulatory properties of ROMK channels expressed in *X. laevis* frog oocytes are virtually identical to those of the native ATP-sensitive, small conductance (SK) channels in TAL cells[40,41] (Figure 47.6) and principal cells in the CCD[42-48] (Figure 47.7). Similar kinetic characteristics of K$^+$, NH$_4^+$, and Tl$^+$ have been observed in the native secretory K$^+$ channel in the rat CCD and ROMK2 channels expressed in *X. laevis* oocytes,[49,50] leading Palmer and co-workers to conclude that the native SK and cloned ROMK channels were identical. A further characteristic of the low conductance secretory K$^+$ channel found in principal cells is a lack of sensitivity to external TEA$^+$.[42]

The general properties of ROMK channels expressed in *Xenopus* oocytes include: (1) weak inward rectification (Figure 47.4) that is dependent on the binding of cytosolic Mg^{2+} or other polyvalent cations to the channel pore[51-56]; (2) activation by protein kinase A-dependent phosphorylation processes[9,39,57,58]; (3) inhibition by high concentrations of MgATP[13]; (4) inhibition by slight reductions in cytosolic pH[59,60]; and (5) inhibition by arachidonic acid and protein kinase C.[33,34] When coupled with gene expression and protein localization studies, these functional similarities strongly suggest that ROMK makes up the pore-forming subunit of the renal distal SK potassium channel.[46,50]

Characteristics of the ROMK Channel Pore

CHANNEL KINETICS

ROMK channels are characterized by a high open probability (P$_o$) of greater than 0.9 for inward K$^+$ flux.[3,49,57,61] The high open probability results from one open state and two closed states. One closed state is very short (~1 ms; 99% frequency), and the other is longer (~40 ms) but very infrequent (~1%).[57,61] The infrequent closed state is due to blocking by divalent cations, as it can be abolished by EDTA.[61] Choe and

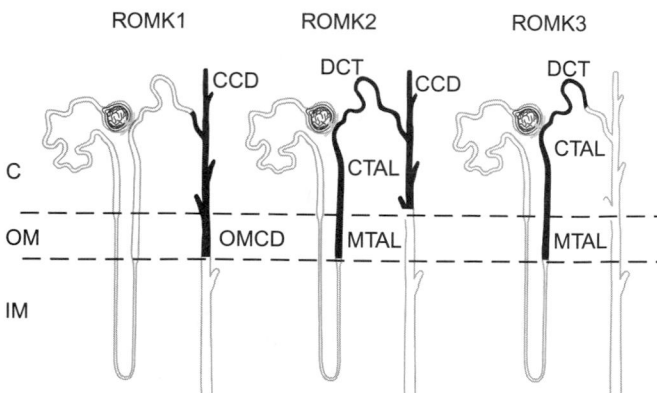

FIGURE 47.5 The distribution of the ROMK 1, 2, and 3 isoforms along the rat nephron. The shaded regions indicate the localization of ROMK transcripts and protein (CCD: cortical collecting duct; CTAL: cortical thick ascending limb; DCT: distal convoluted tubule; MTAL: medullary thick ascending limb; OMCD: outer medullary collecting duct). In the CCD and OMCD, ROMK is expressed only in principal cells.

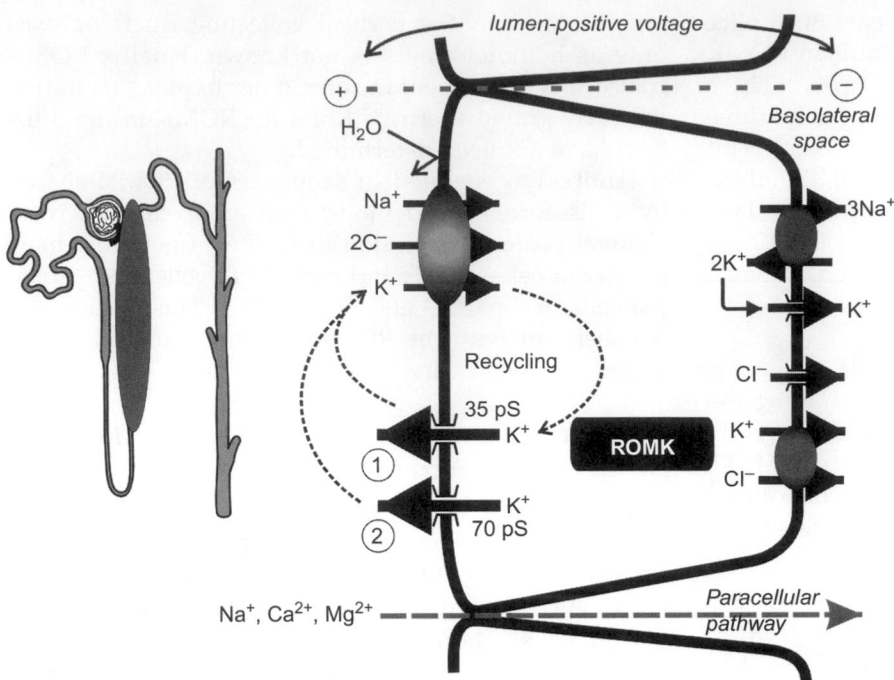

FIGURE 47.6 Model for ion transport in the thick ascending limb. The two types of apical K$^+$ channels are shown; 35 pS (also called the small K$^+$ or SK channel) and 70 pS channels. ROMK and SK functional and regulatory characteristics are essentially identical. It has been proposed that the 70 pS channel is also formed by ROMK in association with another channel subunit, but this remains to be demonstrated.

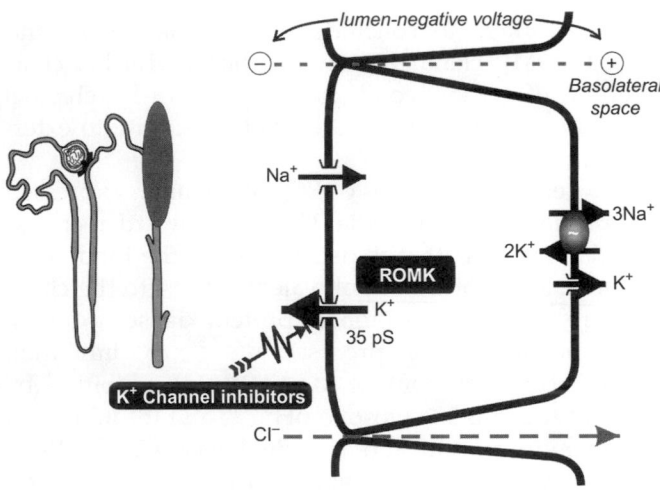

FIGURE 47.7 Model for ion transport by the principal cell in the collecting duct. The apical K$^+$ secretory channel in this cell is ROMK.

co-workers[61] have also suggested that the closed state of ROMK results from K$^+$ ions transiently blocking its own pathway. Such a model would not require large molecular motions, but rather small molecular oscillations.

CHANNEL RECTIFICATION

One of the fundamental characteristics of ROMK, as well as all Kir channels is inward rectification, the property of passing current more easily in the inward than in the outward direction (see Figure 47.4).

Although this seems to be contrary to the role of ROMK in K$^+$ secretion, the inward rectification observed with ROMK, and with the kidney K$^+$ secretory channel, is "weak." The term "weak" rectification refers to the ability of ROMK to actually pass outward current, albeit to a lesser extent than inward current. Many of the other Kir channels are "strong" rectifiers, and characteristically pass little outward current. The very high open probability of the ROMK channel, usually >0.9, may help make up for the rectification effect on K$^+$ secretion. In other words, although the outward conductance (ease of passing K$^+$ secretory current) is less than the inward conductance, the channels are open most of the time, and thus are able to secrete large amounts of K$^+$. We now know that inward rectification of ROMK is due to blocking of the channel pore by Mg^{2+}[55] or polyamines like spermine or spermidine from the intracellular side.[52,53] Thus, it is possible that variations in the cytosolic concentrations of these inorganic and organic cations could provide an important mechanism regulating outward (i.e., K$^+$ secretory current. It was suggested that the inhibition of outward K$^+$ fluxes through ROMK by Mg^{2+} may contribute to K$^+$-wasting in the setting of Mg^{2+} deficiency.[62] A subsequent study by Yang et al.[63] examining the regulation of ROMK expressed in *Xenopus* oocytes and the native channel by intracellular and extracellular Mg^{2+} supports this idea.

Kinetic studies of inward rectification by Mg^{2+} and polyamines indicate that the effect is voltage-dependent and depends on the extracellular

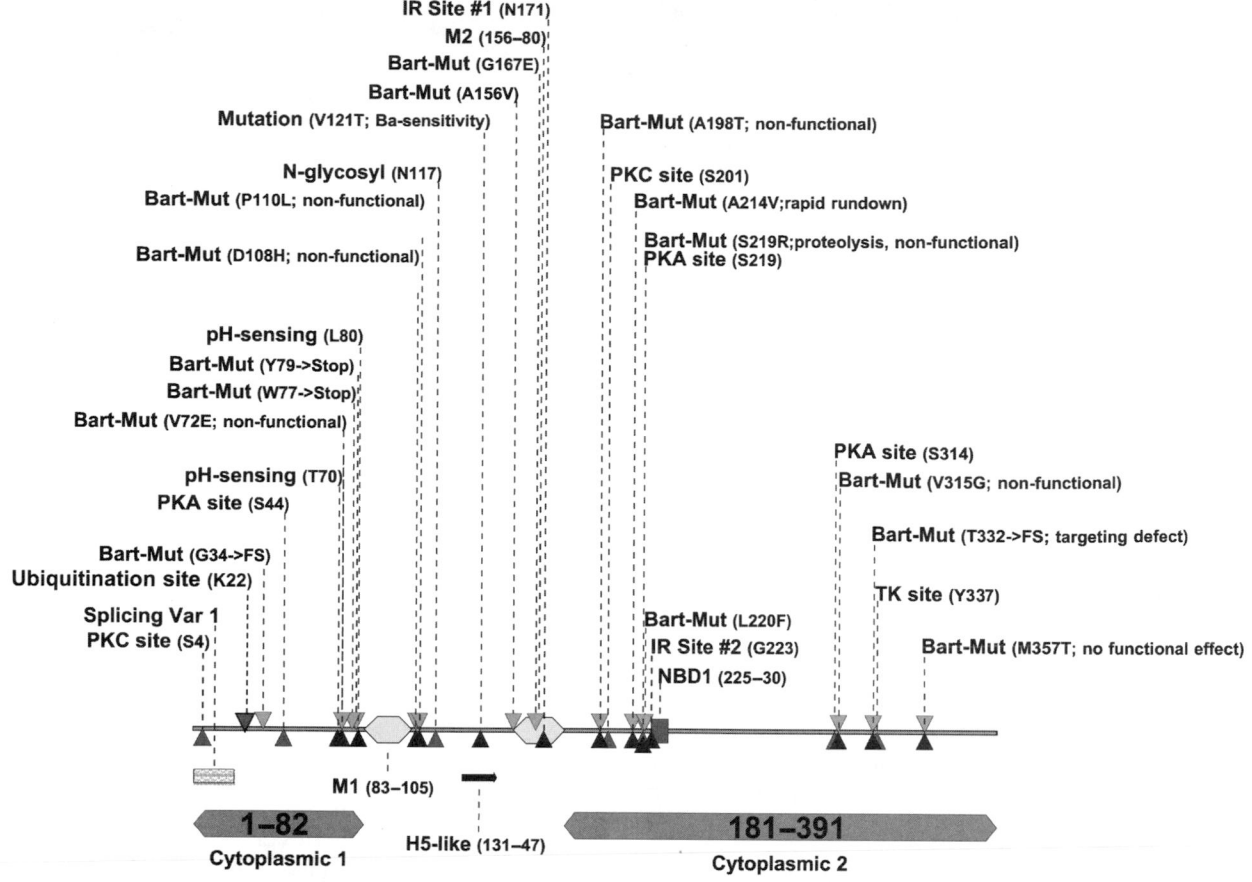

FIGURE 47.8 The major functional and regulatory sites, and the Bartter's mutations are shown in this schematic representation of ROMK1, Kir1.1a (see text for discussion).

concentration of K$^+$ (thus varies with the K$^+$ reversal potential in the constant intracellular (K$^+$)).[54,55,61,64,65] These findings suggest an interaction between permeant and blocking ions, and the presence of a variable energy well within the channel pore. The crystal structure of Kir revealing a long channel pore with multiple binding sites for K$^+$ and blocking ions is consistent with this idea.[19-21]

Electrophysiological studies have demonstrated the importance of the M2 segment and COOH-termini in determining the inward rectifying characteristics of inwardly rectifying K$^+$ channels.[54,56,66,67] Two residues are particularly important in determining whether the rectification is strong or weak. In strong inward rectifiers like IRK1 (Kir2.1),[5] a negatively charged residue, aspartic acid (D172 in IRK1), in the M2 membrane segment has been shown to be critical for strong inward rectification.[54,56] In ROMK the aspartate residue is replaced by asparagine (see Figure 47.8, IR Site #1, N171 in ROMK1), consistent with the weak rectification of this channel. A second residue located in the C-terminus has also been shown to be an important contributor to strong rectification in IRK1.[67] This

glutamate residue (E224 in IRK1) is replaced by a glycine residue in ROMK (see Figure 47.8; IR Site #2). This C-terminal glycine residue in ROMK is a part of the Walker A site that contributes to the nucleotide-binding interactions (see Figure 47.1, and IR Site #2 in Figure 47.8) in the nucleotide-binding domain (NBD; Figure 47.8), and thus serves a different gating function in ROMK. As expected from this model, exchange of the ROMK C-terminus with that on IRK1 produces strong rectification in oocytes injected with the mutant ROMK channel.[66] Consistent with the electrophysiological results, the crystal structure of Kir2.2 reveals that the inner helices line the central cavity and the internal half of the membrane pore, and the side chain of D172 points to the center of the central cavity.[21] The binding sites for Mg^{2+} in the crystal structure of Kir2.2 were examined by soaking the crystal with 10 mM Sr^{2+}, an electron dense mimic of Mg^{2+}. Three density peaks due to Sr^{2+} are observed in the crystal of Kir2.2: one in the central cavity corresponding to the position of D172 and two in the cytoplasmic pore, referred to as the upper ring and lower ring of charges, respectively. The upper ring of charges consists of E224 of IRK1 and an additional glutamate residue E229 from each of four subunits. The lower ring of charges consists of four D255, one from each subunit.[21]

Finally, two different extracts of venom have been suggested to specifically inhibit ROMK channels.[68,69] Both the snake toxin, δ-dendrotoxin,[68] the honey bee venom extract, tertiapin, and the modified compond, tertiapin-Q[69,70] appear to block ROMK activity by interacting with channel pore. Tertiapin-Q specifically blocks ROMK and Kir3.1, but not other Kir channels such as Kir4 and Kir5, and has been explored to estimate the density of ROMK channels in the CCD and CNT in response to dietary K⁺ intake.[71] A study, however, indicates that tertiapin-Q can also block MaxiK (or BK, *hSlo1*) Ca²⁺-activated K⁺ channels.[72] Thus, caution should be exercised when utilizing tertiapin-Q to define ROMK activity under the condition in which MaxiK channels are activated by flow.

Regulation of the ROMK K⁺ Channel

ROMK channel activity, like that of the native SK channel in TAL and principal cells, is regulated by a variety of factors that either activate or inhibit channel activity (Figure 47.9). The molecular mechanisms for these alterations in channel function are rapidly being identified.

PROTEIN KINASE A (PKA)

PKA-dependent phosphorylation processes activated by receptor-mediated events or alterations in cytosolic second messengers (e.g., cyclic AMP, cAMP) play important roles in regulating the native SK channel in principal cells of the CCD (Figure 47.10[45–48,73]). Phosphorylation-dephosphorylation processes also modulate the activity of the cloned ROMK K⁺ channel.[9,33,34,57,58] K⁺ channel activity in excised inside-out

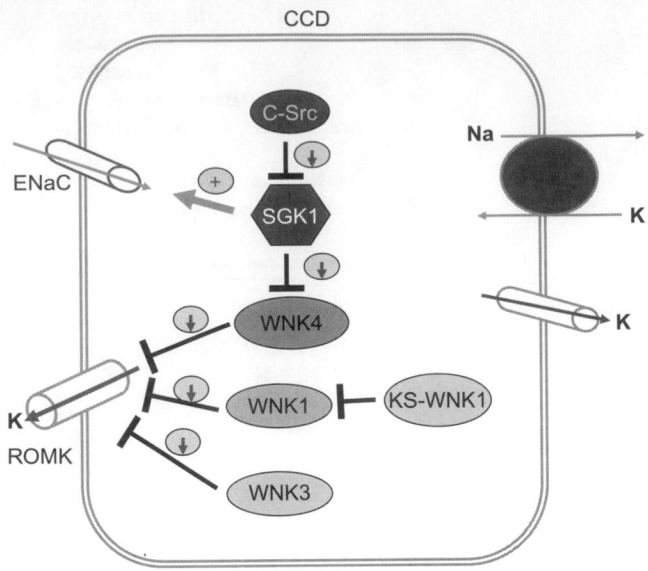

FIGURE 47.10 A cell model illustrating the mechanism by which ROMK channel activity is regulated by the interaction among c-Src, SGK1, and WNKs in the CCD.

patches of oocytes expressing ROMK requires activation by PKA-dependent phosphorylation processes.[58] Rundown or loss of ROMK channel activity in these patches occurs whenever phosphatase-mediated dephosphorylation activity is greater than phosphorylation (see also section on PIP₂ below for role of protein versus lipid kinases and phosphatases in the process of rundown and reactivation by MgATP).

The critical PKA phosphorylation sites are on the channel protein itself (see Figure 47.2). This has been demonstrated by several observations. First, ROMK protein expressed in HEK-293 cells can be phosphorylated by PKA.[9] Phosphopeptide analysis and mapping have shown three serine residues phosphorylated by PKA (one residue on the N-terminus (serine 25 in ROMK2) and two residues on the C-terminus (serine 200 and serine 294 in ROMK2)). Mutation of any single PKA phosphorylation site on ROMK2 reduces whole cell K⁺ currents by 35–40% in oocytes; mutation of two or more of the three sites produces non-functional channels.[9] This is consistent with the critical role of PKA phosphorylation in channel activation. Second, at the single channel level the N-terminal and C-terminal PKA phosphorylation sites alter the channel activity, albeit differently.[57] None of the mutations with serine residues replaced by alanine alters the single channel conductance. Each of the C-terminal PKA phosphorylation site mutations, however, reduces open probability (P₀) by about 40%, due to the appearance of a new long closed state. This reduction in P₀ is sufficient to account for the observed reduction in whole oocyte currents.[9] Replacing the N-terminal serine with alanine

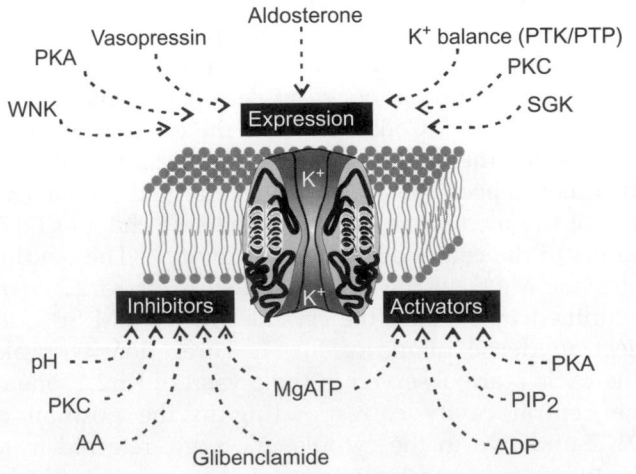

FIGURE 47.9 The major identified regulators of ROMK channels.

does not change P$_o$, but does reduce the probability of finding functioning channels by about 60%. The mechanism for this reduction in active channels is not known at present. The mechanism by which PKA increases ROMK channel activity may include stimulation of surface expression and enhance the effect of PIP$_2$ on ROMK channels. It has been shown that stimulation of PKA increases the sensitivity of ROMK channels to PIP$_2$ in *Xenopus* oocytes.[74] Also, a recent study demonstrates that mutation of serine residue 44 to aspartate increases the surface delivery of ROMK1 channels.[75] One of the fundamental characteristics of SK channels in principal cells and in the TAL is their activation by Gs-coupled receptors or by the addition of cyclic AMP.[46] AKAPs are A-Kinase Anchoring Proteins that bind PKA holoenzyme (catalytic plus regulatory subunits), and maintain the enzyme at specific intracellular sites.[76,77] Wang and co-workers reported that ROMK1 channels expressed in *X. laevis* oocytes could not be activated by cyclic AMP unless expressed with an isoform of AKAP, AKAP79.[78] On the other hand, findings that ROMK channels carrying PKA site mutations exhibit reduced current in *Xenopus* oocytes in the absence of AKAP79 suggests that ROMK can be phosphorylated without AKAP79.[78] The role of AKAP in the native tissue is not determined. Some studies suggested that the Na/H exchange regulatory protein 2 (NHERF-2) might act as an AKAP, because NHERF-2 interacts with ROMK channels[79] and facilitates the stimulatory effect of SGK1 on ROMK channels.[80]

ARACHIDONIC ACID (AA)

Like the native SK channel in the CCD,[81] ROMK1 channels expressed in *Xenopus* oocytes are sensitive to arachidonic acid (AA[33,34]). The effect of AA is specific, since other fatty acids failed to mimic the effect of AA.[33] However, AA has little-to-no effect on the other two ROMK family members, ROMK2 and ROMK3.[34] Since the amino acid sequences of the ROMK channels are identical, with the exception of the N-terminus, the role of the N-terminus in mediating the effect of AA is strongly suggested. This is supported by the demonstration that deletion of the initial 37 aa of ROMK1 abolished the effect of AA. Moreover, a serine residue at the fourth position within the N-terminus of ROMK1 has been shown to play a crucial role in the AA-mediated inhibition of ROMK1, since mutation of this serine residue to alanine abolished the effect of AA (Figures 47.1 and 47.3[34]). Since this serine residue is a putative PKC phosphorylation site,[3] and AA has been shown to activate PKC, the effect of AA may depend on stimulation of a membrane-bound PKC.

PROTEIN KINASE C (PKC)

Activation of PKC phosphorylation processes inhibits the apical SK channel in the CCD.[48] ROMK1, which is exclusively expressed in collecting ducts, has three potential PKC phosphorylation sites involving serine residues: one on the N-terminus; and two on the C-terminal end. ROMK2 and ROMK3 only have the two C-terminal PKC phosphorylation sites (see Figures 47.2 and 47.4). Using an *in vitro* phosphorylation assay, it was observed that serine residue 4 in the N-terminus and serine residue 201 in the C-terminus are two major PKC-induced phosphorylation sites. The effect of PKC on ROMK channels is complex. It was demonstrated that phosphorylation of either serine residue 4 or 201 is essential for ROMK1 export to the plasma membrane.[18] On the other hand, stimulation of PKC *in vivo* has been shown to inhibit ROMK channel activity. The N-terminal serine residue at the fourth position appears to be most important to PKC-mediated K$^+$ channel inhibition of ROMK1. Interestingly, this is the same residue critical for the inhibitory effect of arachidonic acid (see Figure 47.4). However, it is possible that PKC-induced inhibition of ROMK channels may be indirect, resulting from a decrease in PIP$_2$ content. It was demonstrated that stimulation of PKC decreases the PIP$_2$ level in the plasma membrane.[82] Because PIP$_2$ is essential for maintaining ROMK channels in the open state, decreases in PIP$_2$ levels may contribute to the PKC-induced inhibition.

WNKS (WITH NO LYSINE KINASE)

WNKs are a family of four serine/threonine protein kinases named WNK1–4.[83,84] Among them, WNK1, 3, and 4 are expressed in the distal nephron.[85–87] The discovery that mutations in WNK1 and WNK4 cause the autosomal-dominant hypertension and hyperkalemia known as pseudohypoaldosteronism type 2 (PHA2) led to extensive characterization of their properties and function.[88] Evidence indicates that the WNK family plays an important role in the regulation of ROMK channels.[22,87,89–92] WNK1, 3, and 4 inhibits the ROMK channel activity (Figure 47.10), and the effect of WNKs on ROMK is mediated by stimulation of clathrin-dependent endocytosis.[22,89] Intersectin, a scaffold protein containing two Eps15 homology domains and four or five tandem SH3 domains, interacts with WNK1 and 4, which is required for the regulation of clathrin-mediated endocytosis of ROMK by WNKs.[93] In addition, a clathrin adaptor protein, Autosomal Recessive Hypercholesterolemia (ARH), has been shown to interact with ROMK, and the interaction may be involved in the stimulation of endocytosis of ROMK by WNK1.[16] Dysregulation of ROMK by

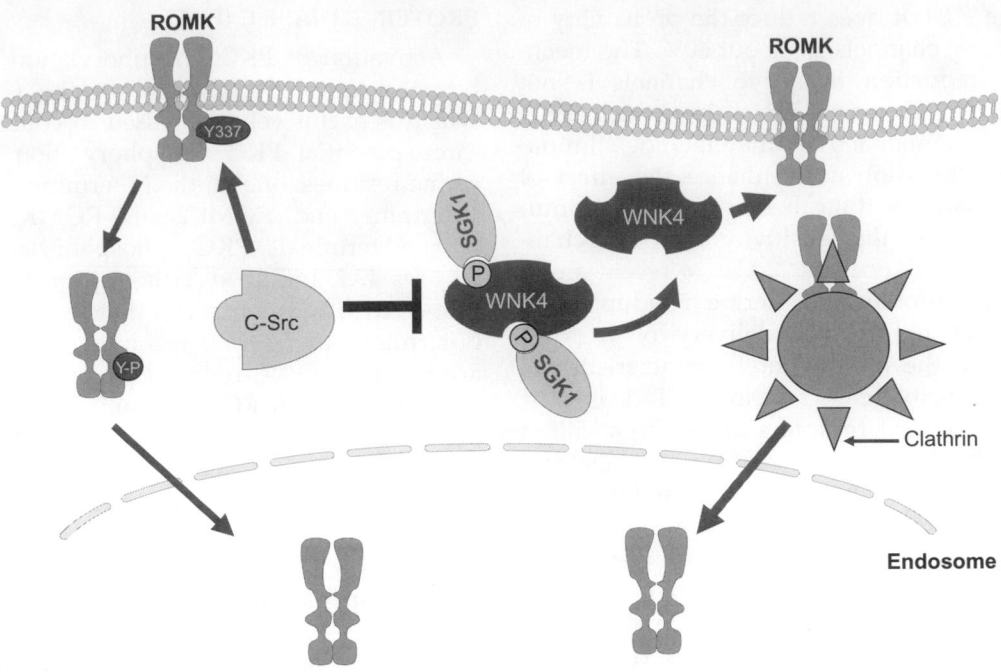

FIGURE 47.11   A cell model demonstrating the regulation of ROMK1 channel in the CCD by Src-family PTK, SGK1, and WNK4.

WNK1 and 4 may contribute to the hyperkalemia in PHA2.[94]

A kidney-specific splice form of WNK1 (KS-WNK1), in which an alternative 5′ exon replaces the first four exons of WNK1, is expressed in the distal nephron.[95] Unlike the long form of WNK, KS-WNK1 lacks kinase activity and, by itself, does not regulate ROMK channels. However, KS-WNK1 antagonizes the inhibitory effect of WNK1 on ROMK.[90,92] It has been reported that high K⁺ intake increases, whereas low K⁺ intake decreases, the expression of KS-WNK1, and that increased KS-WNK1 expression attenuates the inhibitory effect of WNK1 on ROMK channels.[90,92] Thus, the alteration of the ratio between the long and short form of WNK1 may be an important mechanism by which a dietary K⁺ intake regulates ROMK channel activity.

PROTEIN TYROSINE KINASE (PTK)

The ROMK channel is a substrate of PTK, and tyrosine residue 337 in the C-terminus of ROMK1 has been demonstrated to be a PTK phosphorylation site[95,97] (Figure 47.8). Tyrosine phosphorylation of ROMK is regulated by dietary K⁺ intake: a low K⁺ intake increases, whereas a high K⁺ intake decreases, tyrosine phosphorylation.[98] The regulation of tyrosine phosphorylation of ROMK by K⁺ diet is partially achieved by modulating the expression of Src family PTK in response to a dietary K⁺ intake. Low K⁺ increases, whereas a high K⁺ suppresses, the expression of Src family PTK.[99] Immunostaining has also demonstrated that c-Src, the most ubiquitously distributed member of Src family PTK, is present in the thick ascending limb, connecting tubule, and cortical collecting duct.[96] Also, CD63, a tetra-spanning protein, increases c-Src activity by stimulating c-Src phosphorylation in tyrosine residue 416, thereby enhancing the c-Src-induced inhibition of ROMK channels.[100]

Although the fate of tyrosine phosphorylated ROMK is not completely understood, the stimulation of tyrosine phosphorylation of ROMK1 facilitates channel internalization (Figure 47.11[97]). Because ROMK1 is exclusively expressed in the connecting tubule and CCD, this mechanism should play an important role in K balance during K restriction. However, the upstream signaling which stimulates PTK is still not known. K restriction has been shown to stimulate renin and the angiotensin II system.[101–103] Moreover, micropuncture studies have revealed that luminal perfusion of angiotensin II inhibited K secretion in the distal nephron.[104] Patch-clamp experiments have further demonstrated that angiotensin II downregulates ROMK channels in the CCD, and that such inhibition could be demonstrated only in the CCD from K-restricted rats.[105] In addition, two lines of evidence indicate that superoxide is a mediator of the effect of K diet on the Src family PTK: (1) low K intake stimulates superoxide anion levels; and (2) incubation of M-1 cells, a cultured mouse CCD principal cell, with hydrogen peroxide increases the expression of c-Src.[106] The notion that superoxide anion could serve as a second messenger of low K intake on the Src family PTK is also supported by the finding that suppression of superoxide anion attenuates the effect of low-K intake on c-Src expression, and diminishes the tyrosine phosphorylation of ROMK. Thus, superoxide and PTK pathway play important roles in maintaining K homeostasis.

ALDOSTERONE AND SERUM-GLUCOCORTICOID-INDUCED KINASE (SGK)

SGK1 has been reported to stimulate ROMK1 channels by facilitating the phosphorylation of ROMK channels at serine residue (Ser) 44, thereby enhancing the export of ROMK channels from the ER.[107,108] SGK1 also suppresses the effect of WNK4 on ROMK channels (Figure 47.10) through the phosphorylation of WNK4 at Ser 1169[91] and 1196.[109] Thus, the C-terminus containing Ser 1169 and 1196 was called the "switch-domain" for renal K secretion. Moreover, WNK1 has also been reported to stimulate SGK1 through PI3 kinase.[110] WNK1-induced activation of SGK1 could also play a role in mediating the effect of a high-K intake on K secretion. A large body of evidence suggests that SGK1 mediates, at least in part, the effect of aldosterone on renal K secretion.[91,111–113] For instance, the phenotype of SGK1 deletion is similar to MR knockout mice, and displays compromised renal K secretion in response to a high dietary K intake.[111] However, it is still not known whether the stimulatory effect of SGK on renal K secretion is the result of increased ENaC activity which in turn augments the electrochemical gradient for K secretion or due to a direct stimulation of ROMK channel insertion. It has shown that ROMK expression in the apical membrane of the TAL and CCD is actually increased rather than decreased in SGK null mice.[114] This suggests that the role of SGK in stimulating ROMK insertion may not be essential or can be replaced by other kinases, such as cAMP-dependent protein kinase A. A possible role of SGK in regulating renal K secretion by a daily dietary K intake has been suggested by the report that a high dietary K intake for 12hours stimulates SGK expression in the kidney.[115] Moreover, ROMK channel activity increased significantly in the CCD from rats on a high-K diet for only 6hours. Thus, SGK may regulate ROMK channel activity in the CT and CCD in response to a daily variation of dietary K intake.

INTERACTION OF PTK, SGK1, AND WNK4

As discussed above, WNK4 inhibits ROMK channels and K secretion in the CNT and the CCD. SGK1 reversed the inhibitory effect on ROMK channels by stimulation of WNK4 phosphorylation in serine residues 1169 and 1196. However, Wang and his associates have demonstrated that Src family PTK modulates the effect of SGK1 on WNK4, and abolishes the SGK1-induced phosphorylation of WNK4. Figure 47.11 is a model illustrating the role of the interaction among c-Src, SGK1, and WNK4 in regulating ROMK channels and K secretion. Activation of c-Src inhibits the SGK1-mediated phosphorylation of WNK4, thereby restoring the inhibitory effect of WNK4 on ROMK channels and K secretion.[116] The c-Src-dependent modulation of SGK1-WNK4 interaction may play a key role in preventing K loss during volume-depletion, and in stimulating K secretion during a high-K intake. Both volume-depletion and K secretion are expected to increase SGK1 expression. However, a high-K intake has been shown to suppress PTK activity, whereas volume-depletion does not inhibit PTK expression. Consequently, although a volume-depletion stimulates SGK1 activity, a high PTK activity blocks the effect of SGK1 and prevents K loss.

UBIQUITINATION

Ubiquitination plays an important role in the regulation of protein degradation and recycling by attaching ubiquitin molecules to lysine residues of substrate protein. Ubiquitination can further be classified into mono-ubiquitination by adding only one or two ubiquitin molecules to the substrate protein or polyubiquitination by attaching more than four ubiquitin molecules. The polyubiquitinated protein is subjected to degradation, whereas monoubiquitinated proteins are targeted to internalization and possibly recycling to the cell membrane. ROMK1 channel activity could be regulated by monoubiquitination, and the ubiquitin-binding site is on Lysine residue 22 on the N-terminus of ROMK1[117] (Figure 47.8). The physiological importance of monoubiquitination in the regulation of ROMK channel is still not clear. Because ROMK channel activity in the CCD decreases in response to stimulation of PTK, it would be interesting to determine whether monoubiquitination is required for the PTK-induced internalization of ROMK1 in the CCD. POSH (plenty of SH3) is an E3 ubiquitin ligase, and expression of POSH enhances the ubiquitination of ROMK, suggesting that POSH is involved in ubiquitination of ROMK channels.[118]

NUCLEOTIDES, THE CYSTIC FIBROSIS TRANSMEMBRANE CONDUCTANCE REGULATOR (CFTR), AND SULFONYLUREA RECEPTOR (SUR) PROTEINS

MgATP both activates and inhibits ROMK channels (Figure 47.9), with the net effect of nucleotide action being the integration of these opposite and complex events. Activation occurs by stimulation of PKA-mediated phosphorylation (see section on PKA, above) or by altering the generation of PIP$_2$ (,[15] and see section on regulation by PIP$_2$, below). These processes modulate channel-gating or plasma membrane channel density (e.g., by regulating trafficking of the channel to the

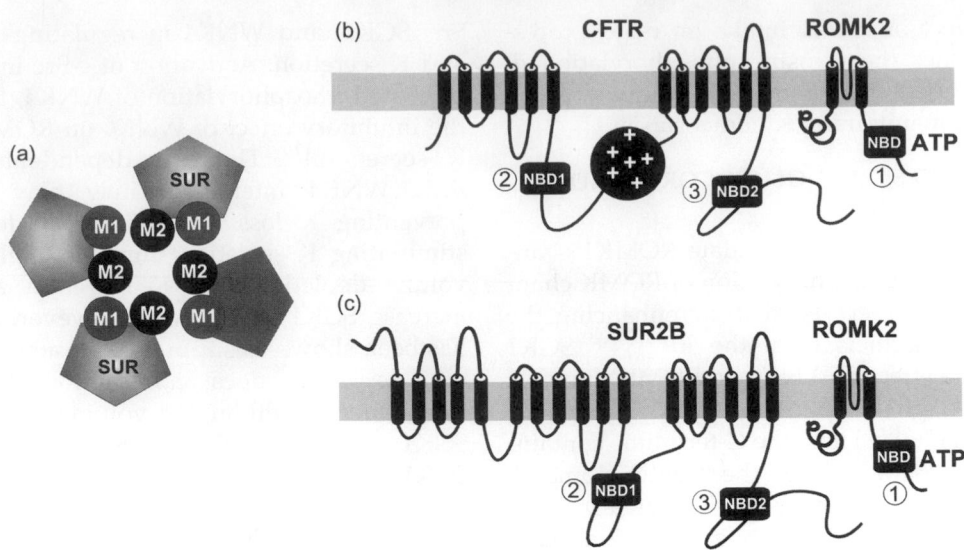

FIGURE 47.12   Assembly of K$_{ATP}$ and ROMK channels with ATP Binding Cassette (ABC) proteins. (a) The proposed hetero-octameric complex forming ATP-sensitive (K$_{ATP}$) channels with four K$_{IR}$ subunits and four sulfonylurea receptor (SUR) subunits. The M1 and M2 membrane segment arrangement is as shown in Figure 47.2a, with the M2 membrane segments lining the channel pore. (b) The topology of CFTR and ROMK channels proposed to form kidney K$_{ATP}$ channels. A single nucleotide-binding domain (NBD, 1) is present on the C-terminus of ROMK, while two NBDs (numbered 2 and 3) are found on CFTR. (c) The topology of the sulfonylurea receptor, SUR2B, and ROMK proposed to form kidney K$_{ATP}$ channels.

apical plasma membrane for the endoplasmic reticulum[75]). Inhibition of the SK secretory channel in CCD by MgATP[45] identifies this channel as belonging to a subgroup of Kir channels, referred to as ATP-sensitive or K$_{ATP}$ channels (the classical K$_{ATP}$ channels, Kir6.x; and Kir1.1 or ROMK channels[43,119]). The renal SK or K$_{ATP}$ channel is somewhat less sensitive to ATP than the pancreatic β-cell or other K$_{ATP}$ channels. As observed with other K$_{ATP}$ channels,[119,120] addition of MgADP to MgATP-inhibited ROMK channels relieves the ATP block.[13] Thus, changes in the cytosolic MgATP concentration or in the MgATP/ADP ratio, as may occur with alterations in the activity of Na$^+$-K$^+$-ATPase, could modulate ROMK channel activity. This may provide one mechanism for coupling basolateral Na$^+$-pump activity with apical K$^+$ secretion in the principal cells of the CCD.

Channel inhibition by Mg-ATP is incompletely understood; however, the mechanism likely involves both direct binding of MgATP to the ROMK protein at an unconventional nucleotide-binding site (NBD; Figure 47.2b) and interaction with CFTR. The direct binding of ATP to K$_{ATP}$ channels is supported by cross-linking of azido-ATP compounds to the channel proteins.[51,121,122] In addition, recent biochemical observations using fluorescent ATP analogs have shown that Mg-ATP can bind directly to K$_{ATP}$ channels, including ROMK.[51,123,124] Both N- and C-terminal segments form the nucleotide-binding site which is situated at a region modeled to be involved in channel

gating.[61,125,126] The crucial N-C-terminal interaction occurs between adjacent subunits; in other words, the nucleotide-binding site is intermolecular. As observed with other K$_{ATP}$ channels,[119,120] addition of ADP to ATP-inhibited ROMK channels relieved the ATP block.[13]

Only a few studies have found that ATP can inhibit ROMK when expressed alone in *X. laevis* oocytes,[12,13,127] suggesting that direct binding of MgATP to ROMK is insufficient for channel inhibition. Several studies have demonstrated that ROMK channels may interact with CFTR or sulfonylurea receptor type 2B (SUR2B) (Figure 47.12a), and that such interaction is required for ATP sensitivity.[128–130] Moreover, a characteristic of K$_{ATP}$ channels, including the renal SK channel, is their sensitivity to inhibition by sulfonylureas like glibenclamide.[119,131] The pancreatic β-cell K$_{ATP}$ channel is formed by two subunits; a pore-forming polypeptide, Kir6.2; and the sulfonylurea-binding protein, SUR1 (an ABC (ATP-Binding Cassette) protein family member like CFTR[132–134]) in a 4:4 ratio (see Figure 47.12a[135–137]). Kir6.2 provides the K$^+$ channel permeation pathway and ATP binding-inhibition site, while SUR is required for sulfonylurea binding, and for certain aspects of regulation by nucleotides (e.g., ADP effects[133,138,139]). Two lines of evidence suggest that CFTR-ROMK interaction may play a key role for the sensitivity of ROMK to sulfonylurea agents: (1) CFTR is expressed in the same apical regions as ROMK channels in the CTAL and CCD,[140] and a functional truncated hemi-CFTR is also expressed in the MTAL[141]; (2) glibenclamide- and Mg-ATP-sensitive whole cell K$^+$ currents in *X. laevis* oocytes are only observed when ROMK is co-expressed with CFTR.[127,142] In the kidney, glibenclamide induces natriuresis in rats,[143,144] and patch-clamp experiments have shown that 200 μM glibenclamide inhibits the apical SK channel in the rat TAL by about 60−70%.[40,145] The sensitivity of the SK channel in TAL to sulfonylureas is, however, much less than in other K$_{ATP}$ channels.[43] Thus, the ability of glibenclamide to inhibit the K$^+$ secretory channels in renal distal tubule suggests that a SUR-like protein is associated with this channel, and is involved in the sulfonylurea effect (Figure 47.12C). However, the role of CFTR in regulating ATP-sensitivity of ROMK channels is still not completely understood.[146] Because the regulation of ROMK channels by ATP required PKA-dependent phosphorylation of CFTR, ATP-sensitivity of ROMK might be the result of the PKA-phosphorylation state of CFTR, rather than direct ATP regulation.[146]

INTRACELLULAR pH AND EXTRACELLULAR K

Small reductions in cytosolic pH reversibly inhibit ROMK channel activity expressed in *X. laevis* oocytes,[10−12,60,147] and the SK channel in TAL and CCD.[45,47,48,148] Lysine at position 80 on the N-terminus of ROMK1 (K61 on ROMK2; see Figures 47.2 and 47.8) is primarily responsible for conferring this pH-sensitivity, as mutation of this residue abolished pH-dependency[10,11,149]; although later studies have suggested an alternative role of lysine-80 in the pH regulation of ROMK1.[150,151] The pH-dependent gating of ROMK is rapidly reversible as long as the exposure to low pH (6.0−7.0) is short. Longer exposure to low pH results in "irreversibility." Schulte and co-workers have recently provided an explanation for the latter. The pH-dependent conformational change in ROMK apparently exposes N- and C-terminal cysteine residues forming disulfide bridges that lock the protein in a closed conformation. The disulfide bridges can be broken by DTT (dithiothreitol), resulting in channel reopening.

Cytosolic pH can also alter ROMK channel activity in another way. The K$_{1/2}$ for inhibition of ROMK channel activity is not fixed, but can be modulated by altering cytosolic side pH. McNicholas and co-workers[12] found that decreasing the pH from 7.4 to 7.2 on the cytosolic face of excised patches from oocytes expressing ROMK2 reduced the K$_{1/2}$ for MgATP inhibition from about 2.5 mM to <0.5 mM, almost a 10-fold increase in affinity with this small acidification. This effect appears to be independent of the lysine residue implicated in pH-dependent regulation of ROMK channel activity,[10,11] indicating that another pH sensor may be present on ROMK. This notion is supported by

the report that the residues on the N-terminus of ROMK and the helix bundle crossing near the cytoplasmic end of the transmembrane pore have also been shown to modulate sensitivity to pH.[10,152] Relevant to the existence of multiple internal pH sensors is the finding that pH-dependent gating of ROMK1 is associated with conformational changes in both N- and C-termini.[147] The pH sensitivity of ROMK channels is controlled by extracellular K^{+}.[153,154] It has been shown that removal of extracellular K$^+$ inactivates ROMK channels which are closed by internal acidic pH. In the absence of extracellular K$^+$, intracellular alkalization fails to reactivate ROMK channels, and adding extracellular K$^+$ is required to reactivate ROMK channels. It has been suggested that internal pH-gating and external K$^+$-gating might act in the same amino acid (leucine residue 160 of ROMK2).[155] Acidification induces conformation changes, preventing K$^+$ access to the transmembrane pore from the cytoplasm.[152]

Not only affecting ATP sensitivity, change in pH also modulates the effect of polyamine block of ROMK channels. A negatively-charged glutamic acid residue in this C-terminal region (e.g., E224 in Kir2) has been shown to modulate block by Mg^{2+} or polyamines.[67] In addition, a histidine residue in Kir6.2 (H216, see Figure 47.2[156]) in a region corresponding to the Walker A site in ROMK, has been shown to mediate pH-dependent modulation of polyamine block of this K$_{ATP}$ channel. Thus, this region of the C-terminus of Kir channels is involved in a variety of different gating functions (ATP, pH, polyamines).[157]

PHOSPHOINOSITIDES

Phospholipids, particularly PIP$_2$, have been shown to modulate Kir channels including ROMK1.[14,15,158] Exposure of inside-out patches from oocytes expressing Kir6.2 to PIP$_2$ reduces the ATP-sensitivity of this K$_{ATP}$ channel, apparently by reducing the probability of ATP-binding to its receptor site.[158] Consequently, increasing concentrations of PIP$_2$ increase K$_{ATP}$ channel activity. PIP$_2$ interacts with the pore-forming subunit rather than the SUR subunit of K$_{ATP}$ channels, since PIP$_2$ modifies the ATP sensitivity of the C-terminal truncated Kir6.2 channel in the absence of SUR1.[158] ROMK, like many Kir channels, contains a high density of positively-charged amino acids just C-terminal to M2 (see Figure 47.2). Huang and co-workers[15] have shown that labeled phospholipid vesicles bind to a recombinant ROMK1 C-terminal fusion protein. These investigators implicated arginine 186 in the ROMK1 C-terminus (see Figure 47.2), as mutation of this residue to glutamine modified PIP$_2$ effects. Since PIP$_2$ is generated by ATP-dependent lipid kinases, Huang and co-workers have suggested that the stimulatory effect of MgATP may be due to the generation of PIP$_2$ by lipid kinases.[15] Interaction with PIP$_2$ in the membrane is likely a general mechanism for activating Kir channels (see section on the structure of Kir and ROMK above).

REGULATION OF ROMK EXPRESSION IN KIDNEY (K$^+$ INTAKE, MINERALOCORTICOIDS, VASOPRESSIN, Klotho)

Since K$^+$ homeostasis is mainly controlled by aldosterone and the potassium-load, it is not surprising that ROMK mRNA expression in rat kidney is regulated by aldosterone, K$^+$ adaptation, and vasopressin (see Figure 47.9). It is well-established that rats fed a high-K$^+$ diet adapt by upregulating renal K$^+$ secretion and excretion.[159] This results, at least in part, from an increase in the SK channel density in CCD.[160] Wald and co-workers[161] found that K$^+$ deficiency reduces ROMK mRNA expression in both cortex and medulla, while K$^+$-loading increases ROMK transcript slightly only in medulla. Moreover, several studies have shown that K$^+$ deficiency decreased ROMK expression in the plasma membrane of the collecting duct,[162,163] presumably by stimulating internalization including clathrin and syntaxin-1A-dependent endocytosis.[164,165] The specific ROMK isoforms that changed with potassium were not assessed. Moreover, Frindt and co-workers[166] found that ROMK transcript abundance by *in situ* hybridization in the CCD was not affected by a high-K$^+$ diet. Thus, the high-K$^+$ diet-induced increase in density of active SK channels in principal cells in the CCD is not due to increased abundance of ROMK mRNA. Rather, changes in ROMK protein abundance, channel activation or ROMK channel translocation to the membrane are potential mechanisms to account for the high-K$^+$ adaptation effect on SK channels in the principal cells.

Mineralocorticoids also regulate ROMK abundance. Adrenalectomy decreased ROMK mRNA abundance in cortex, but increased transcript abundance in the medulla.[161] In this latter study, K$^+$ deficiency in adrenalectomized rats reduced ROMK mRNA to control levels, suggesting that the hyperkalemia associated with adrenalectomy was the cause for the increased ROMK message in medulla. In another study, White and colleagues[26] showed that aldosterone administration by minipump to adrenal intact rats increased ROMK transcripts in whole kidney. In the latter study, the ROMK2, 3, and 6 isoforms were increased by the mineralocorticoid. This latter study would be consistent with mineralocorticoid-mediated regulation of ROMK mRNA abundance in cortex. However, the glucocorticoid-responsive element responsible for transcriptional regulation of ROMK by mineralocorticoid has never been identified in the promoter region of the RMOK gene, KCNJ1.

Vasopressin, via cyclic AMP, stimulates K$^+$ secretion in principal cells,[47] and activates the apical K$^+$ channels in TAL cells[40,167] (see Figure 47.6). Although the activation of PKA by cAMP would phosphorylate ROMK (or the SK channel), it remains to be shown whether this is sufficient to account for the stimulation of K$^+$ channel activity or whether additional mechanisms, such as channel insertion into the membrane, are required. As discussed above, PKA-anchoring proteins appear to be required for cAMP activation of ROMK currents in oocytes[78] (see Figure 47.10).

Klotho is an aging-suppressing protein which is expressed in several organs, including the kidney. The application of the Klotho's extracellular domain increases the surface expression of ROMK1, and enhances urinary K$^+$ excretion.[168] The mechanism by which Klotho increases the expression of ROMK in the plasma membrane is by eliminating terminal sialic acids from N-glycan of ROMK. Consequently, underlying disaccharide galactose-N-acetylglucosamine is exposed and binds to galectin-1, a ubiquitous galactoside-binding lectin. Binding of ROMK to galectin-1 inhibits the clathrin-dependent endocytosis of ROMK. The physiological role of endogenous Klotho in K$^+$ homeostasis is unknown.

Lessons from Bartter's Syndrome

Bartter's syndrome[169] comprises a set of autosomal recessive renal tubulopathies characterized by hypokalemic metabolic alkalosis, salt-wasting, hyperreninemia, and hyperaldosteronsim.[170-173] Antenatal Bartter's syndrome is the most severe form of the inherited disorders, and is characterized by hyperprostaglandinemia (PGE$_2$). Antenatal Bartter's syndrome is genetically heterogeneous, resulting from mutations in one of five genes.[174] Three of the Bartter's genes encode the major Na$^+$, K$^+$, Cl$^-$ transporters in the TAL: the SLC12A1 gene encoding the apical Na-K-2Cl co-transporter[175,176]; the CLCKB basolateral Cl$^-$ channel[177]; and the KCNJ1 apical K$^+$ recycling channel, ROMK (see mutations in Figure 47.8[178-180]). Mutations in two other genes also produce the Bartter's phenotype — barttin and the extracellular calcium-sensing receptor (CaSR). Barttin is a membrane protein that is required for trafficking of the ClCKb channel to the basolateral membrane of TAL cells, and loss-of-function mutations in barttin result in the absence of basolateral Cl$^-$ channel activity.[181] Gain-of function mutations in the CaSR result in inhibition of Na,K-ATPase, NKCC2, and apical 70 pS K channel activity.[174,182,183]

The effect of loss-of-function mutations in ROMK on TAL function can be understood, since apical K$^+$ recycling is crucial both to supplying K$^+$ to the Na-K-2Cl

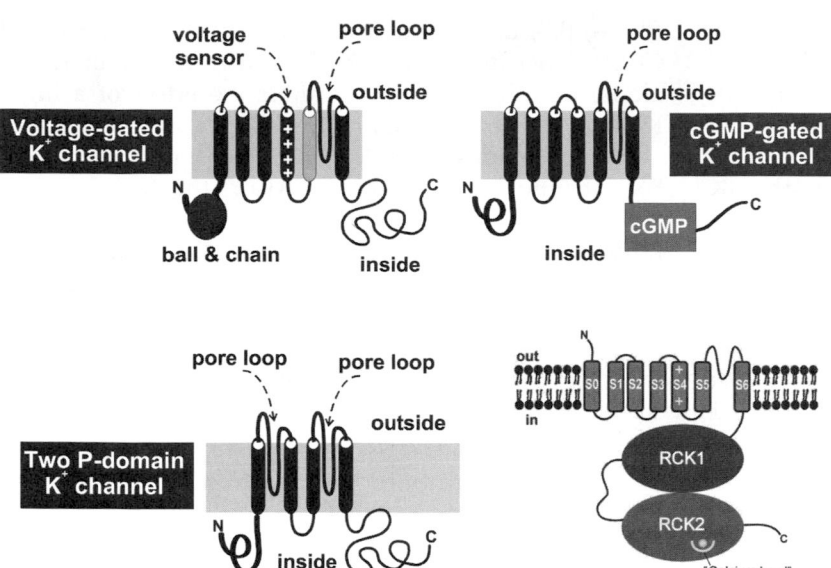

FIGURE 47.13 Proposed topologies of the voltage-gated, cyclic nucleotide-gated, two-P-domain K$^+$ channel and Ca^{2+}-activated BK channels expressed in mammalian kidney. The pore loops are indicated in each channel. Note the two pore loops for the two-P channel.

co-transporter, and to generation of the lumen-positive transepithelial voltage that drives 50% of the reabsorbed sodium through the paracellular pathway.[184,185] ROMK channels with some of the Bartter's mutations express either no or little function in *X. laevis* oocytes,[186–188] consistent with mutations in *KCNJ1* in Bartter's syndrome resulting in ROMK loss-of-function. Based on the location of the amino acid residue altered with certain KCNJ1 mutations (e.g., at or near phosphorylation sites or the nucleotide-binding site), the resultant ROMK channels would be expected to exhibit altered gating (see discussion above on "Regulation of the ROMK K$^+$ Channel"). A ROMK-deficient mouse has been developed and exhibits a Bartter's-like phenotype.[189,190]

While both human and mouse studies clearly demonstrate the importance of ROMK in TAL function, several questions regarding the resulting Bartter's phenotype remained. First, two types of apical K$^+$ channels have been observed in the rat TAL,[40] an SK channel with characteristics typical of ROMK and an intermediate conductance (~70 pS) channel that is similar only in some properties with ROMK. In rat TAL cells, however, the 70 pS channel predominates, so that mutations in the ROMK gene that generate inactive SK channels would only be expected to have minimal effect on the apical K$^+$ conductance of TAL cells. This has suggested that the intermediate conductance channel requires ROMK for function (e.g., either as a subunit or as a regulator). This possibility has been established by the absence of 70 pS K$^+$ channels in the TAL from ROMK null mice.[191] Second, ROMK comprises the apical K$^+$ secretory channel in principal cells of the CCD. Yet, Bartter's individuals with *KCNJ1*

mutations are hypokalemic. This is due to the impairment of NaCl and fluid reabsorption in TAL which leads to increased NaCl and fluid delivery to the distal nephron, which stimulates K$^+$ secretion via the alternative flow-stimulated Maxi-K channel[94] (see section on "Maxi-K Channel" below).

OTHER RENAL POTASSIUM CHANNELS

Several other K$^+$ channels have been cloned from kidney-derived cell lines or are found in mammalian kidney (Figure 47.13). Physiological roles for these channels are less-defined than that for ROMK.

Ca^{2+}-Activated Big-Conductance K$^+$ Channels (BK, Maxi-K Channel)

The BK channel is composed of a pore-forming α-subunit (*Slo* 1), and an accessory β-subunit.[192,193] BK channel activity has been detected at the apical membrane of both principal cell (PC) and intercalated cell (IC), basolateral membrane of PC in the CNT and CCD[194,195] and in the podocytes where the BK channels may be involved in regulating glomerular filtration rate.[196]

BK IN THE APICAL MEMBRANE

Microperfusion experiments have demonstrated that BK channels are involved in mediated K$^+$ secretion during increased dietary K$^+$ intake.[197] However, the observation that the deletion of the BK channel α-subunit does not affect the net K$^+$ excretion in mice fed with a high-K$^+$ diet suggests that HK-induced stimulation of

ROMK channel expression and high plasma aldosterone level can compensate for deleting BK channels on K$^+$ secretion.[198] Although the role of BK channels in mediating flow-stimulated K$^+$ secretion has been firmly established,[198–201] it is still not completely-understood whether IC or PC is responsible for mediating the BK-dependent K$^+$ secretion. Patch-clamp experiments have demonstrated that apical BK channel activity is higher in IC than those in PC.[195] However, because IC has a low Na-K-ATPase activity, it is still arguable whether BK channels in IC significantly contribute to K$^+$ secretion in the collecting duct.[202] A recent study performed in $Kcnmb4^{-/-}$ mice in which the BK β4-subunit is deleted suggests the role of BK channels in IC in mediating flow-dependent K$^+$ secretion. Holtzclaw et al. have demonstrated that renal K$^+$ excretion was compromised in response to a HK intake in mice lacking the BK β4-subunit which is expressed in the apical membrane of IC in the CNT and CCD.[203] Furthermore, immunocytochemical staining shows that a high-K$^+$ intake decreased IC size in wild-type, but not in $Kcnmb4^{-/-}$, mice. Moreover, the flow rate speed was higher in knockout mice than those of wild-type mice. It is suggested that the BK channel in IC plays a role in K$^+$ secretion through decreasing IC size and increasing luminal volume of the CNT and the CCD, thereby creating conditions more favorable for K$^+$ secretion.

BK CHANNEL IN THE BASOLATERAL MEMBRANE

Immunocytochemical staining shows that BK α- and β1-subunits are expressed in the basolateral membrane of PC in the CNT and CCD, and their expression is stimulated by Na$^+$ restriction. The physiological function of basolateral BK channels in PC is possibly responsible for hyperpolarizing the basolateral membrane, thereby increasing the driving force for Na$^+$ absorption. The notion is supported by the observation that BK-β1($^{-/-}$) mice ($Kcnmb1^{-/-}$) have a higher Na$^+$ clearance than those of wild-type mice in response to low Na$^+$ intake.[204] The impaired function of basolateral BK channels in PC also affects the renal K$^+$ secretion in $Kcnmb1^{-/-}$ mice in response to a high-K$^+$ intake.[205] $Kcnmb1^{-/-}$ mice on a high-K$^+$ diet are hypertensive, volume-expanded, and have reduced urinary K$^+$ and Na$^+$ clearances, an effect which can be treated with mineralocorticoids receptor antagonist. This suggests that the impaired K$^+$ secretion results from high aldosterone levels which stimulate Na$^+$ transport in $Kcnmb1^{-/-}$ mice.

Regulation of BK Channels
DIETARY K$^+$ INTAKE

Real-time PCR analysis has demonstrated that a high K$^+$ intake stimulates the mRNA transcription of BK α-, β2-, and β4-subunits, but not β1, in the rabbit CCD.[206] Because a low-Na$^+$ intake, which increases aldosterone levels, fails to mimic the effect of a high-K$^+$ intake on the mRNA level of BK α- β2-, and β4-subunits, it excludes the role of aldosterone in regulating BK channel expression.[207] Also, the patch-clamp experiments demonstrated that a high-K$^+$ intake stimulates the BK channel activity in PC of the CCD.[194] Since inhibition of P38 and ERK activates BK channels in PC, and a high-K$^+$ intake suppresses both MAPK,[194] p38, and ERK, MAPK may be involved in mediating the effect of a high-K$^+$ intake on BK channels.

PKA AND PKC

Patch-clamp study has demonstrated that PKA and PKC inhibit BK channel activity in the PC of the CCD.[208] The role of PKA and PKC in regulating the flow-stimulated BK-dependent K$^+$ secretion in the CCD is also shown in the isolated perfused rabbit CCD. PKA induced a tonical inhibition of BK channels or an associated regulatory protein in PC. However, PKA has no inhibitory effect on BK channel in IC. It is possible that BK channels in PC and IC may be the results of different splice variants which respond to PKA in different ways.

CYTOCHROME P450 (CYP) EPOXYGENASE

BK channels in the PC are activated by CYP-epoxygenase-dependent metabolism of arachidonic acid, an effect which is also mimicked by 11,12-epoxyeicosatrienoic acid (11,12-EET), a main product of CYP-epoxygenase-dependent metabolism in the kidney.[209] Because a high-K$^+$ intake increased 11,12-EET levels in the CCD and stimulated the expression of CYP2C44 homolog, a main CYP-epoxygenase in the kidney, 11,12-EET may play a role in stimulating BK channel-dependent K$^+$ secretion during a high-K$^+$ intake. This notion is also supported by the finding that inhibition of CYP-epoxygenase abolished the flow-stimulated and BK-dependent K$^+$ excretion in the isolated rabbit CCD.[209]

Other 6-TM Renal K$^+$ Channels

The voltage-gated K$^+$ (Kv) channels are expressed in the kidney, and their function in regulating epithelial transport is well-documented.

KCNQ1 CHANNEL

KCNQ1 forms a small conductance (2–10 pS) Kv channel in kidney, existing as a heteromultimeric complex with KCNE1 (minK). MinK has a single transmembrane segment and is highly-expressed at the apical membrane. KCNQ1 and KCNE1 have been

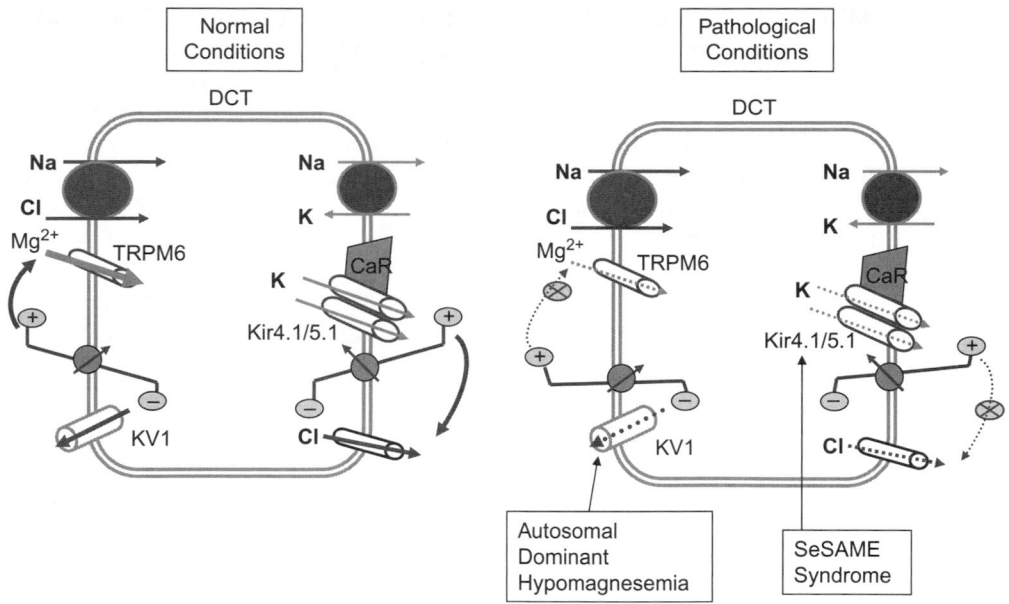

FIGURE 47.14 A cell model illustrating the role of Kv1 and Kir4.1/5.1 in regulating Mg^{2+} transport and transepithelial Cl^- transport in the DCT. SeSAME syndrome (for seizures, sensorineural deafness, ataxia, mental retardation and electrolyte imbalance).

extensively characterized in heart, where they play crucial roles in cardiac repolarization.[210–212] Mutations of these genes cause long QT syndrome. Immunostaining has demonstrated that voltage-gated K channels, such as ERG1 and KCNQ1, are expressed in the apical membrane of DCT and collecting duct.[213,214] The voltage-gated K^+ channels may prevent the membrane depolarization that occurs following stimulation of electrogenic Na^+-coupled transport of glucose or amino acids.[215] Accordingly, KCNE1 deficient mice exhibit a reduction in glucose and amino acid uptake, and defective volume regulation in the proximal tubule.[216] However, additional Kv channels and BK may also participate in stabilizing proximal tubule membrane potential during electrogenic Na^+ uptake.

KCNA1 FAMILY CHANNEL

A genetic study has revealed that voltage-gated K^+ channels (Kv1.1; KCNA1), which are expressed in the apical membrane of the DCT, play a role in regulating Mg^{2+} transport in the DCT.[217] A missense mutation in the Kv1.1 voltage-gated K channel caused human autosomal dominant hypomagnesemia. Figure 47.14 is a model illustrating the possible role of Kv1.1 in regulating Mg^{2+} transport in DCT. The activation of voltage-gated K channels is expected to hyperpolarize the apical membrane, thereby increasing the driving force for Mg^{2+} absorption through transient receptor potential cation channel 6 (TRPM6). Defective Kv1.1 channel function would impair the hyperpolarization of apical membrane potential, thereby decreasing the driving

force for transepithelial Mg^{2+} transport through TRPM6.

KCNA10 is found at the apical membrane of the proximal tubule.[218] The *KCNA10* gene is located on 1p11–13, and transcripts are expressed in kidney, heart, and aorta. KCNA10 has 58% amino acid identity with Kv1.3, which also resides at 1p11–13.[219] The predicted secondary structure is identical to that of other Shaker-related K^+ channels, including intracellular N- and C-termini, 6 transmembrane segments, a voltage sensor (S4), and a pore (P) region. Unlike Shaker proteins, however, KCNA10 contains a putative cyclic nucleotide (CN)-binding domain at the C-terminus, suggesting that protein function is regulated by cyclic nucleotides (Figure 47.13).

2-TM Renal K^+ Channel (Non-ROMK)

Kir4.1 (KCNJ10), Kir4.2 (KCNJ15), AND Kir5.1 (KCNJ16) CHANNELS

Heteromeric Kir4.1/Kir5.1 and/or Kir4.1/Kir5.1 channels form the basolateral small conductance K^+ channel in distal nephron segments.[220] The inward rectifier K^+ channel, Kir4.1, was originally identified from rat brain, and exhibits 53% amino acid identity to ROMK1.[221,222] The kidney also expresses Kir4.1 mRNA, and the channel protein has been immunolocalized to the basolateral membrane of distal nephron segments, including DCT, CNT, and CCD.[223] Internal protons decrease Kir4.1 K^+ current by reducing open probability, however, internal protons also increase channel conductance.[224] Mice with deletion of the Kir4.1 gene (KCN10) have been generated[225] but, due to early lethality in the neonatal stage, renal phenotype has not been examined.

Kir4.2 was originally cloned from human kidney and called Kir1.3.[31] While this study reported that Kir4.2 channels were not functional in X. laevis oocytes,[31] subsequent studies have shown that this protein forms inward rectifying K$^+$ channels that are inhibited by protein kinase C and internal protons.[220,226] Kir4.2 mRNA is found in human[31] and mouse[220] kidney, and in the latter species, specifically in the DCT.

The inward rectifier K$^+$ channel, Kir5.1, was also cloned from rat brain, but does not form functional K$^+$ channels by itself when expressed in X. laevis oocytes.[221] Kir5.1 mRNA is present in kidney,[221,227] and channel protein is abundantly expressed in PT, and in DCT and CCD segments,[228] where Kir4.1 is also expressed.[223] Recent studies have demonstrated that Kir4.1 or Kir4.2 can form heteromeric inward rectifying K$^+$ channels with Kir5.1 with distinct properties in the heterologous expression systems,[220,227,229] as well as in the native kidney.[227] The heteromeric interaction of Kir5.1 with other Kir K$^+$ channels is specific for Kir4.x channels, and requires a small region in the proximal COOH-terminus of Kir4.1.[229]

Patch-clamp experiments, immunocytochemical and molecular biological methods have confirmed the expression of several inwardly-rectifying K channels in the basolateral membrane.[204,230–233] Two lines of evidence suggest that Kir4.1/5.1 heterotetramers are the main type of K channels in the basolateral membrane in the ASDN: (1) the Kir4.1 protein is detected in the basolateral membrane of the DCT and the CCD[220,232]; and (2) the patch-clamp experiments have shown that Kir4.1/Kir5.1 channels form the major K channels in the basolateral membrane of principal cells (PC) in the CCD.[232] The most dramatic and specific effect of the Kir4.x-Kir5.1 assembly on K$^+$ channel function is the shift in the pKa for inhibition by internal protons from 6.0 to the physiologically relevant pKa of 7.4.[227,228,234,235] Internal pH sensitivity of Kir4.1-Kir5.1 is modulated by PIP$_2$,[236] similarly to Kir1.1 (ROMK).[237]

Kir4.1 has been shown to interact with Ca^{2+}-sensing receptor which inactivates the K channels.[238] Because Kir4.1 participates in generating the cell membrane potential, activation of Ca^{2+}-sensing receptor is expected to depolarize the membrane potential, thereby inhibiting transepithelial Na/Cl transport in the DCT. The importance of Kir4.1 in regulating membrane transport in the DCT is best demonstrated in patients with EAST (for epilepsy, ataxia, sensorineural deafness, and tubulopathy)[239] or SeSAME syndrome (for seizures, sensorineural deafness, ataxia, mental retardation and electrolyte imbalance).[240] The disease is caused by defective gene product encoding KCNJ10 (Kir4.1), which is expressed in a variety of tissues including in the basolateral membrane of the ASDN. The renal phenotypes of EAST/SeSAME syndrome are hypokalemia, metabolic alkalosis, and hypomagnesemia.[239,240] Figure 47.14 is a cell model illustrating the role of Kir4.1/5.1 in regulating NaCl transport in the DCT. Activation of Kir4.1/5.1 is expected to increase the negativity of basolateral membrane, thereby providing the driving force for Cl$^-$ exit across the basolateral membrane. In contrast, defective Kir4.1 depolarizes the basolateral membrane, thereby diminishing the driving force for Cl$^-$ exit across the basolateral membrane. Consequently, delivery of NaCl to the CNT and CCD is increased and leads to enhanced Na absorption in the CNT and CCD at the expense of K$^+$-wasting, resulting in hypokalemia and metabolic alkalosis. It was suggested that decreased basolateral membrane potential impairs Mg^{2+} absorption in the DCT, due to a compromised driving force for Mg^{2+}.[44]

Kir2.3 (KCNJ4) CHANNEL

In cortical collecting duct principal cells the maintenance of the negative membrane potential depends, at least in part, on the activity of an inwardly rectifying 18 pS K$^+$ channel. This basolateral K$^+$ channel has been suggested to be the inwardly rectifying K$^+$ channel, Kir2.3.[241] The kidney Kir2.3 was cloned from a mouse CCD cell line and its expression in kidney confirmed by Northern analysis.[241] When the MDCK cells were transfected with Kir2.3, the channel is expressed in the basolateral membrane,[242] and a basolateral sorting signal was identified at the COOH-terminal tail.[243,244] Kir 2.3 shares some biophysical properties with the native 18 pS K$^+$ channel, such as high open probability and channel conductance, 14.5 pS.[241]

Kir6.1 (KCNJ8) CHANNEL

Kir6.1 was originally cloned from a rat pancreatic islet cell cDNA library using Kir3.1 as a probe,[245] and belongs to the Kir6.x (ATP-sensitive; K$_{ATP}$) subfamily of inwardly rectifying K$^+$ channels.[2,246] Exogenous expression of Kir6.1 channels in X. laevis oocytes form ATP-sensitive channels only when co-expressed with a sulfonylurea receptor protein.[246,247] Although this inward rectifier is predominantly found in brain, heart, and vascular tissue, expression in kidney has been documented.[245,248] Kir6.1 has been localized to both mitochondria[249] and plasma membranes.[249,250] Upregulation of Kir6.1 mRNA has been observed following ischemic injury in rat kidney, consistent with the proposed role of K$_{ATP}$ channel activation in protection from ischemic damage (e.g., in the heart[251]). Recently, Kir6.1 was cloned from rabbit proximal tubule cDNA library, and expression of Kir6.1, SUR2A, and SUR2B in rabbit proximal tubule confirmed by PCR.[250] Functional studies in *X. laevis* oocytes suggested that Kir6.1 may form the basolateral ATP- and taurine-sensitive K$^+$ channel involved in the basolateral K$^+$ conductance of proximal tubules.[250] Adenylate kinase, which promotes phosphoryl transfer between ATP and ADP and associates with K$_{ATP}$ channels,[252] has been cloned from the rabbit proximal tubule library,[253] and may associate with Kir6.1 in these cells to promote metabolic sensing.

Kir7.1 (KCNJ13) CHANNEL

The inward rectifier K$^+$ channel, Kir7.1, was originally cloned from human brain cDNA libraries after searching the GenBank expressed sequence Tag (EST) database using Kir1.1 and Kir6.2.[254,255] The Kir7.1 K$^+$ channel displays unusual K$^+$ permeation properties, with a low single channel conductance of 50 fS, low sensitivity to blocking by external Ba^{2+} or Cs$^+$, and very low dependence of conductance on external K$^+$.[254–256] PCR and Western blot analyses have identified Kir7.1 transcripts and protein, respectively, in rat, guinea pig, and human kidney.[254,255,257,258] Expression of Kir7.1 along the rat nephron was demonstrated by Western blots of microdissected nephron segments,[258] which showed K$^+$ channel protein in TAL, DCT, CNT, CCD, OMCD, and IMCD.[258] Immunostaining localized Kir7.1 to basolateral membranes of DCT and principal cells.[258] In the guinea pig, Kir7.1 protein is expressed in basolateral membranes of proximal tubule and TAL cells.[257] In the CCD, Kir7.1 is expressed in principal cells, but not intercalated cells. The unique pore properties of Kir7.1 and its localization close to Na-K-ATPase suggested that this K$^+$ channel may be functionally coupled to Na-K-ATPase, and involved in K$^+$ recycling across basolateral membranes.[258,259]

The Two-Pore K$^+$ Channels (K$_t$)

In CNT and CCD, a double-pore K channel (KCNK1) is expressed in the apical membrane.[38,260–262] However, the physiological function of the two-pore K channels in the CNT or CCD is still not clear. The most recently-discovered class of K$^+$ channels is characterized by a topology containing two pores or P-loops. These channels are also appropriately referred to as the "two pore domain" (or K$_t$, two-P, TWIK-related) K$^+$ channels (e.g., see [263]). K$_t$ channels exhibit four membrane spanning domains consisting of two Kir-like domains that are linked in a single subunit (see Figure 47.13[263–269]). Structurally similar channels have been identified in the *C. elegans* genome project and

represent the most abundant class of K$^+$ channels in this species.[270] The TWIK-related channels, including TWIK-1,[263,264,266–269,271] TWIK-2,[265] TREK-1,[263,272,273] TASK-1,[263,274] and TASK-2,[263] are all expressed in mammalian kidney.[263]

Both TWIK-1[267] and TWIK-2[265] express weakly inward-rectifying K$^+$ channels that are inhibited by intracellular acidification. Transcripts for TWIK-1 are expressed in rabbit cortical TAL and collecting duct,[269] and TWIK-1 protein has been localized to the brush border of proximal convoluted tubules, intracellular and apical border of intercalated cells in the CCD, and in cortical and medullary TAL cells.[266] TREK-1 gives rise to mechanosensitive outward-rectifying K$^+$ currents that are activated by arachidonic acid and are inhibited by protein kinases A and C.[272,275] TASK channels exhibit noninactivating outward-rectifying K$^+$ currents that are very sensitive to external pH.[263,274] While the properties of TWIK-related K$^+$ channels do not fit with any of the known native K$^+$ channels in kidney, their widespread expression in mammalian and other organisms (e.g., *C. elegans*) suggests either that they have been missed in patch-clamp recording or that they associate with other (unidentified to date) subunits to produce pores with native channel properties.

SUMMARY AND CONCLUSIONS

While we have gained significant insights into the structural diversity of K$^+$ channels expressed in the mammalian kidney, many new channels will likely be identified in the near future. Likewise, electrophysiological studies continue to expand our database of physiologically and pharmacologically distinct K$^+$ channels. The exciting challenge is to identify which channel genes encode which native channels. Given that many K$^+$ channels are probably comprised of more than one subunit (e.g., the K$_{ATP}$ channels), this challenge is somewhat daunting, and will require many more years of investigation. Finally, we expect that new inherited disorders due to mutations in some of these channel genes (channelopathies) will be identified. These channelopathies will not only provide new insights into the physiological roles of K$^+$ channels, but will likely raise new questions as it has for ROMK mutations in Bartter's syndrome.

Acknowledgments

WHW is supported by DK54983 and CLH is supported by DK59530 from the National Institutes of Health.

References

[1] Hebert SC, Wang W-H. Structure and function of the low conductance K$_{ATP}$ channel, ROMK. Wien Klin Wochenschr 1997;109:471−6.

[2] Nichols CG, Lopatin AN. Inward rectifier potassium channels. Ann Rev Physiol 1997;59:171−91.

[3] Ho K, Nichols CG, Lederer WJ, Lytton J, Vassilev PM, Kanazirska MV, et al. Cloning and expression of an inwardly rectifying ATP-regulated potassium channel. Nature 1993;362:31−8.

[4] Jan LY, Jan YN. Cloned potassium channels from eukaryotes and prokaryotes. Ann Rev Neurosci 1997;20:91−123.

[5] Kubo Y, Baldwin TJ, Jan YN, Jan LY. Primary structure and functional expression of a mouse inward rectifier potassium channel. Nature 1993;362:127−33.

[6] Jan LY, Jan YN. Tracing the roots of ion channels. Cell 1992;715:715−8.

[7] Jan LY, Jan YN. Potassium channels and their evolving gates. Nature 1994;371:119−22.

[8] Jan LY, Jan YN. Voltage-gated and inwardly rectifying potassium channels. J Physiol 1997;505:267−82.

[9] Xu ZC, Yang Y, Hebert SC. Phosphorylation of the ATP-sensitive, inwardly rectifying K⁺ channel, ROMK, by cyclic AMP-dependent protein kinase. J Biol Chem 1996;271: 9313−9.

[10] Choe H, Zhou H, Palmer LG, Sackin H. A conserved cytoplasmic region of ROMK modulates pH sensitivity, conductance, and gating. Am J Physiol (Renal Physiol) 1997;273: F516−29.

[11] Fakler B, Schultz JH, Yang J, Schulte U, Brändle U, Zenner HP, et al. Identification of a titratable lysine residue that determines sensitivity of kidney potassium channels (ROMK) to intracellular pH. EMBO J 1996;15:4093−9.

[12] McNicholas CM, MacGregor GG, Islas LD, Yang Y, Hebert SC, Giebisch G. pH-dependent modulation of the cloned renal K⁺ channel, ROMK. Am J Physiol (Renal Physiol) 1998;275: F972−81.

[13] McNicholas CM, Yang Y, Giebisch G, Hebert SC. Molecular site for nucleotide binding on an ATP-sensitive renal K⁺ channel (ROMK2). Am J Physiol (Renal Fluid Electrolyte Physiol) 1996;271:F275−85.

[14] Hilgemann DW, Ball R. Regulation of cardiac Na⁺-Ca²⁺ exchange and K$_{ATP}$ potassium channels by PIP$_2$. Science 1996;273:956−9.

[15] Huang C-L, Feng S, Hilgemann DW. Direct activation of inward rectifier potassium channels by PIP$_2$ and its stabilization by Gbg. Nature 1998;391:803−6.

[16] Fang L, Ganuti R, Kim BY, Wade JB, Welling PA. The ARH adaptor protein regulates endocytosis of the ROMK potassium secretory channel in mouse kidney. J Clin Invest 2009;119: 3278−89.

[17] Jiang Y, Lee A, Chen J, Cadene M, Chalt B, MacKinnon R. The open pore conformation of potassium channels. Nature 2002;417:523−6.

[18] Lin DH, Sterling H, Lerea KM, Giebisch G, Wang WH. Protein kinase C (PKC)-induced phosphorylation of ROMK1 is essential for the surface expression of ROMK1 channels. J Biol Chem 2002;277:44332−8.

[19] Pegan S, Arrabit C, Zhou W, Kwiatkowski W, Collins A, Slesinger PA, et al. Cytoplasmic domain structures of Kir2.1 and Kir3.1 show sites for modulating gating and rectification. Nat Neurosci 2005;8:279−87.

[20] Nishida M, Cadene M, Chait BT, MacKinnon R. Crystal structure of a Kir3.1-prokaryotic Kir channel chimera. EMBO J 2007;26:4005−15.

[21] Tao X, Avalos JL, Chen J, MacKinnon R. Crystal structure of the eukaryotic strong inward-rectifier K⁺ Channel Kir2.2 at 3.1 + Å resolution. Science 2009;326:1668−74.

[22] Kahle KT, Wilson FH, Leng Q, Lalioti MD, O'Connell AD, Dong K, et al. WNK4 regulates the balance between renal NaCl reabsorption and K⁺ secretion. Nat Genet 2003;35:372−6.

[23] Boim MA, Ho K, Shuck ME, Bienkowski MJ, Block JH, Slightom JL, et al. ROMK inwardly rectifying ATP-sensitive K⁺ channel. II. Cloning and distribution of alternative forms. Am J Physiol 1995;268:F1132−40.

[24] Zhou H, Chepilko S, Schutt W, Choe H, Palmer LG, Sackin H. Mutations in the pore region of ROMK enhance Ba²⁺ block. Am J Physiol 1996;271:C1949−56.

[25] Kondo C, Isomoto S, Matsumoto S, Yamada M, Horio Y, Yamashita S, et al. Cloning and functional expression of a novel isoform of ROMK inwardly rectifying ATP-dependent K⁺ channel, ROMK6 (Kir1.1f). FEBS Lett 1996;399:122−6.

[26] Hornby AH, White D. SJ. Regulation of distal nephron K⁺ channels (ROMK) mRNA expression by aldosterone in rat kidney. J Physiol 1998;509:629−34.

[27] Beesley AH, Ortega B, White SJ. Splicing of a retained intron within ROMK K⁺ channel RNA generates a novel set of isoforms in rat kidney. Am J Physiol (Cell Physiol) 1999;276: C585−92.

[28] Bock JH, Shuck ME, Benjamin CW, Chee M, Bienkowski MJ, Slightom JL. Nucleotide sequence analysis of the human KCNJ1 potassium channel locus. Gene 1997;188:9−16.

[29] Shuck ME, Block JH, Benjamin CW, Tsai T-D, Lee KS, Slightom JL, et al. Cloning and characterization of multiple forms of the human kidney ROM-K potassium channel. J Biol Chem 1994;269:24261−70.

[30] Yano H, Philipson LH, Kugler JL, Tokuyama Y, Davis EM, Le Beau MM, et al. Alternative splicing of human inwardly rectifying K⁺ channel ROMK1 mRNA. Mol Pharmacol 1994;45: 854−60.

[31] Shuck ME, Piser TM, Block JH, Slightom JL, Lee KS, Bienkowski MJ. Cloning and characterization of two K⁺ inward rectifier (K$_{ir}$) 1.1 potassium channel homologs from human kidney (K$_{ir}$1.2 and K$_{ir}$1.3). J Biol Chem 1997;272:586−93.

[32] Lee W-S, Hebert SC. The ROMK inwardly rectifying ATP-sensitive K⁺ channel. I. Expression in rat distal nephron segments. Am J Physiol (Renal Fluid Electrolyte Physiol) 1995;268: F1124−31.

[33] Macica CM, Yang Y, Hebert SC, Wang W-H. Arachidonic acid inhibits the activity of the cloned renal K⁺ channel, ROMK1. Am J Physiol (Renal Fluid Electrolyte Physiol) 1996;40:F588−94.

[34] Macica CM, Yang Y, Lerea K, Hebert SC, Wang W. Role of the NH$_2$ terminus of the cloned renal K⁺ channel, ROMK1, in arachidonic acid-mediated inhibition. Am J Physiol (Renal Physiol) 1997;274:F175−81.

[35] Lundgren DW, Moore JJ, Chang SM, Collins PL, Chang AS. Gestational changes in the uterine expression of an inwardly rectifying K⁺ channel, ROMK. Proc Soc Exp Biol Med 1997;216:57−64.

[36] Kohda Y, Ding W, Phan E, Housini I, Wang J, Star RA, et al. Localization of the ROMK potassium channel to the apical membrane of distal nephron in rat kidney. Kidney Internat 1998;54:1214−23.

[37] Mennitt PA, Wade JB, Ecelbarger CA, Palmer LG, Frindt G. Localization of ROMK channels in the rat kidney. J Am Soc Nephrol 1997;8:1823−30.

[38] Palmer LG. Potassium secretion and the regulation of distal nephron K channels. Am J Physiol 1999;277:F821−5.

[39] Xu JZ, Hall AE, Peterson LN, Bienkowski MJ, Eessalu TE, Hebert SC. Localization of the ROMK protein on apical

membranes of rat kidney nephron segments. Am J Physiol (Renal Physiol) 1997;273:F739—48.

[40] Wang W. Two types of K$^+$ channel in TAL of rat kidney. Am J Physiol (Renal Fluid Electrolyte Physiol) 1994;267-36: F599—605.

[41] Wang W, White S, Geibel J, Giebisch G. A potassium channel in the apical membrane of rabbit thick ascending limb of Henle's loop. Am J Physiol (Renal Fluid Electrolyte Physiol) 1990;258-27:F244—53.

[42] Frindt G, Palmer LG. Low-conductance K channels in apical membrane of rat cortical collecting tubule. Am J Physiol (Renal Fluid Electrolyte Physiol) 1989;256-25:F143—51.

[43] Misler S, Giebisch G. ATP-sensitive potassium channels in physiology, pathophysiology, and pharmacology. Curr Opin Nephrol Hypertens 1992;1:21—33.

[44] Schlatter E, Lohrmann E, Greger R. Properties of the potassium conductances of principal cells of rat cortical collecting ducts. Pflügers Arch 1992;420:39—45.

[45] Wang W, Giebisch G. Dual effect of adenosine triphosphate on the apical small conductance K$^+$ channel of the rat cortical collecting duct. J Gen Physiol 1991;98:35—61.

[46] Wang W, Hebert SC, Giebisch G. Renal K$^+$ channels: structure and function. Ann Rev Physiol 1997;59:413—36.

[47] Wang W, Sackin H, Giebisch G. Renal potassium channels and their regulation. Annu Rev Physiol 1992;54:81—96.

[48] Wang WH, Giebisch G. Dual modulation of renal ATP-sensitive K$^+$ channel by protein kinases A and C. Proc Natl Acad Sci USA 1991;88:9722—5.

[49] Chepilko S, Zhou H, Sackin H, Palmer LG. Permeation and gating properties of a cloned renal K$^+$ channel. Am J Physiol 1995;268:C389—401.

[50] Palmer LG, Choe H, Frindt G. Is the secretory K channel in the rat CCT ROMK? Am J Physiol (Renal Fluid Electrolyte Physiol) 1997;273:F404—10.

[51] Dong K, Tang L, MacGregor GG, Leng Q, Hebert SC. Novel nucleotide-binding sites in ATP-sensitive potassium channels formed at gating interfaces. EMBO J 2005;24:1318—29.

[52] Ficker E, Taglialatela M, Wible BA, Henley CM, Brown AM. Spermine and spermidine as gating molecules for inward rectifier K$^+$ channels. Science 1994;266:1068—72.

[53] Lopatin AN, Makhina EN, Nichols CG. Potassium channel block by cytoplasmic polyamines as the mechanism of intrinsic rectification. Nature 1994;372:366—9.

[54] Lu Z, MacKinnon R. Electrostatic tuning of Mg^{2+} affinity in an inward-rectifier K$^+$ channel. Nature 1994;371:243—6.

[55] Nichols CG, Ho K, Hebert SC. Mg^{2+}-dependent inward rectification of ROMK1 potassium channels expressed in Xenopus oocytes. J Physiol 1994;476:399—409.

[56] Wible BA, Taglialatela M, Ficker E, Brown AM. Gating of inwardly rectifying K$^+$ channels localized to a single negatively charged residue. Nature 1994;371:246—9.

[57] MacGregor GG, Xu J, McNicholas CM, Giebisch G, Hebert SC. Partially active channels produced by PKA site mutation of the cloned renal K$^+$ channel ROMK2. Am J Physiol (Renal Physiol) 1998;275:F415—22.

[58] McNicholas CM, Wang W, Ho K, Hebert SC, Giebisch G. Regulation of ROMK1 K$^+$ channel activity involves phosphorylation processes. Proc Natl Acad Sci USA 1994;91:8077—81.

[59] Leipziger J, MacGregor GG, Cooper GJ, Xu J, Hebert SC, Giebisch G. PKA site mutations of ROMK2 channels shift the pH dependence to more alkaline values. Am J Physiol Renal Physiol 2000;279:F919—26.

[60] Tsai TD, Shuck ME, Thompson DP, Bienkowski MJ, Lee KS. Intracellular H$^+$ inhibits a cloned rat kidney outer medulla K$^+$ channel expressed in Xenopus oocytes. Am J Physiol 1995;268: C1173—8.

[61] Choe H, Sackin H, Palmer LG. Permeation and gating of an inwardly rectifying potassium channel. Evidence for a variable energy well. J Gen Physiol 1998;112:433—46.

[62] Huang CL, Kuo E. Mechanism of hypokalemia in magnesium deficiency. J Am Soc Nephrol 2007;18:2649—52.

[63] Yang L, Frindt G, Palmer LG. Magnesium modulates ROMK channel G comediated potassium secretion. J Am Soc Nephrol 2010;21:2109—16.

[64] Oliver D, Hahn H, Antz C, Ruppersberg JP, Fakler B. Interaction of permeant and blocking ions in cloned inward-rectifier K$^+$ channels. Biophys J 1998;74:2318—26.

[65] Spassova M, Lu Z. Coupled ion movement underlies rectification in an inward-rectifier K$^+$ channel. J Gen Physiol 1998;112: 211—21.

[66] Taglialatela M, Wible BA, Caporaso R, Brown AM. Specification of pore properties by the carboxyl terminus of inwardly rectifying K$^+$ channels. Science 1994;264:844—7.

[67] Yang J, Jan YN, Jan LY. Control of rectification and permeation by residues in two distinct domains in an inward rectifier K$^+$ channel. Neuron 1995;14:1047—54.

[68] Imredy JP, Chen C, MacKinnon R. A snake toxin inhibitor of inward rectifier potassium channel ROMK1. Biochemistry 1998;37:14867—74.

[69] Jin W, Lu Z. A novel high-affinity inhibitor for inward-rectifier K$^+$ channels. Biochemistry 1998;37:13291—9.

[70] Sackin H, Vasilyev A, Palmer LG, Krambis M. Permeant cations and blockers modulate pH gating of ROMK channels. Biophys J 2003;84:910—21.

[71] Frindt G, Palmer LG. Effects of dietary K on cell-surface expression of renal ion channels and transporters. Am J Physiol-Renal 2010;299:F890—7.

[72] Kanjhan R, Coulson EJ, Adams DJ, Bellingham MC. Tertiapin-Q blocks recombinant and native large conductance K channels in a use-dependent manner. J Pharmacol Exp Ther 2005;314: 1353—61.

[73] Wang WH, Giebisch G. The role of potassium and sodium channels in renal tubule electrolyte transport. Nippon Jinzo Gakkai Shi 1991;33:448—62.

[74] Liou HH, Zhou SS, Huang CL. Regulation of ROMK1 channel by protein kinase A via a phosphatidylinositol 4,5-bisphosphate-dependent mechanism. Proc Natl Acad Sci USA 1999;96: 5820—5.

[75] O'Connell AD, Leng Q, Dong K, MacGregor GG, Giebisch G, Hebert SC. Phosphorylation regulated ER retention signal in the ROMK potassium channel. Proc Natl Acad Sci USA 2005;102:9954—9.

[76] Faux MC, Scott JD. Molecular glue: kinase anchoring and scaffold proteins. Cell 1996;85:9—12.

[77] Pawson T, Scott JD. Signaling through scaffold, anchoring, and adaptor proteins. Science 1997;278:2075—80.

[78] Ali S, Chen X, Lu M, Xu J-C, Lerea KM, Hebert SC, et al. A kinase anchoring protein (AKAP) is required for mediating the effect of PKA on ROMK1. Proc Natl Acad Sci USA 1998;95: 10274—8.

[79] Yoo D, Flagg TP, Olsen O, Raghuram V, Foskett JK, Welling PA. Assembly and trafficking of a multiprotein ROMK (Kir1.1) channel complex by PDZ interactions. J Biol Chem 2004;279: 6863—73.

[80] Yun CC, Palmada M, Embark HM, Fedorenko O, Feng Y, Henke G, et al. The serum and glucocorticoid-inducible kinase SGK1 and the Na$^+$/II$^+$ exchange regulating factor NHERF2 synergize to stimulate the renal outer medullary K$^+$ channel ROMK1. J Am Soc Nephrol 2002;13:2823—30.

[81] Grantham JJ, Lowe CM, Dellasega M, Cole BR. Effect of hypotonic medium on K and Na content of proximal renal tubules. Am J Physiol (Renal Fluid Electrolyte Physiol) 1977;232:F42–9.

[82] Zeng WZ, Li XJ, Hilgemann DW, Huang CL. Protein kinase C inhibits ROMK1 channel activity via a phosphatidylinositol 4,5-bisphosphate-dependent mechanism. J Biol Chem 2003;278: 16852–6.

[83] Verissimo F, Jordan P. WNK kinases, a novel protein kinase subfamily in multi-cellular organisms. Oncogene 2001;20: 5562–9.

[84] Xu B, English JM, Wilsbacher JL, Stippec S, Goldsmith EJ, Cobb MH. WNK1, a novel mammalian serine/threonine protein kinase lacking the catalytic lysine in subdomain II. J Biol Chem 2000;275:16795–801.

[85] Kahle KT, Gimenez I, Hassan H, Wilson FH, Wong RD, Forbush B, et al. WNK4 regulates apical and basolateral Cl⁻ flux in extrarenal epithelia. P Natl Acad Sci 2004;101:2064–9.

[86] Kahle KT, Ring AM, Lifton RP. Molecular physiology of the WNK kinases. Ann Rev Physiol 2008;70:329–55.

[87] Leng Q, Kahle KT, Rinehart J, MacGregor GG, Wilson FH, Canessa CM, et al. WNK3, a kinase related to genes mutated in hereditary hypertension with hyperkaelemia, regulates the K⁺ channel ROMK1 (Kir1.1). J Physiol 2006;571:275–86.

[88] Wilson FH, Disse-Nicodeme S, Choate KA, Ishikawa K, Nelson-Williams C, Desitter I, et al. Human hypertension caused by mutations in WNK kinases. Science 2001;293: 1107–12.

[89] Cope G, Murthy M, Golbang AP, Hamad A, Liu CH, Cuthbert AW, et al. WNK1 affects surface expression of the ROMK potassium channel independent of WNK4. J Am Soc Nephrol 2006;17:1867–74.

[90] Lazrak A, Liu Z, Huang CL. Antagonistic regulation of ROMK by long and kidney-specific WNK1 isoforms. Proc Natl Acad Sci 2006;103:1615–20.

[91] Ring AM, Leng Q, Rinehart J, Wilson FH, Kahle KT, Hebert SC, et al. An SGK1 site in WNK4 regulates Na⁺ channel and K⁺ channel activity and has implications for aldosterone signaling and K⁺ homeostasis. Proc Natl Acad Sci 2007;104: 4025–9.

[92] Wade JB, Fang L, Liu J, Li D, Yang CL, Subramanya AR, et al. WNK1 kinase isoform switch regulates renal potassium excretion. Proc Nat Acad Sci 2006;103:8558–63.

[93] He G, Wang HR, Huang SK, Huang C-L. Intersectin links WNK kinase to endocytosis of ROMK1. J Clin Invest 2007;117:1078–87.

[94] Rodan AR, Huang CL. Distal potassium handling based on flow modulation of maxi-K channel activity. Curr Opin Nephrol Hypertens 2009;18(4):350–5.

[95] O'Reilly M, Marshall E, Speirs HJL, Brown RW. WNK1 a gene within a novel blood pressure control pathway, tissue-specifically generates radically different isoforms with and without a kinase domain. J Am Soc Nephrol 2003;14:2447–56.

[96] Lin DH, Sterling H, Yang B, Hebert SC, Giebisch G, Wang WH. Protein tyrosine kinase is expressed and regulates ROMK1 location in the cortical collecting duct. Am J Physiol Renal Physiol 2004;286:F881–92.

[97] Moral Z, Dong K, Wei Y, Sterling H, Deng H, Ali S, et al. Regulation of ROMK1 channels by protein-tyrosine kinase and -tyrosine phosphatase. J Biol Chem 2001;276:7156–63.

[98] Lin DH, Sterling H, Lerea KM, Welling P, Jin L, Giebisch G, et al. K depletion increases the protein tyrosine-mediated phosphorylation of ROMK. Am J Physiol Renal Physiol 2002;283:F671–7.

[99] Wei Y, Bloom P, Lin DH, Gu RM, Wang WH. Effect of dietary K intake on the apical small-conductance K channel in the CCD: role of protein tyrosine kinase. Am J Physiol Renal Physiol 2001;281:F206–12.

[100] Lin D, Kamsteeg EJ, Zhang Y, Jin Y, Sterling H, Yue P, et al. Expression of tetraspan protein CD63 activates protein-tyrosine kinase (PTK) and enhances the PTK-induced inhibition of ROMK channels. J Biol Chem 2008;283:7674–81.

[101] Ray PE, Suga SI, Liu XH, Huang X, Johnson RJ. Chronic potassium depletion induces renal injury, salt sensitivity, and hypertension in young rats. Kidney Int 2001;59:1850–8.

[102] Saikaley A, Bichet D, Kucharczyk J, Peterson LN. Neuroendocrine factors mediating polydipsia induced by dietary Na, Cl, and K depletion. Am J Physiol Regul Integr Comp Physiol 1986;251:R1071–7.

[103] Sealey JE, Clark I, Bull MB, Laragh JH. Potassium balance and the control of renin secretion. J. Clin. Invest 1970;49:2119–27.

[104] Wang T, Giebisch G. Effects of angiotensin II on electrolyte transport in the early and late distal tubule in rat kidney. Am J Physiol 1996;271:F143–9.

[105] Wei Y, Zavilowitz B, Satlin LM, Wang WH. Angiotensin II inhibits the ROMK-like small-conductance K channel in renal cortical collecting duct during dietary K restriction. J Biol Chem 2007;282:6455–62.

[106] Babilonia E, Wei Y, Sterling H, Kaminski P, Wolin MS, Wang WH. Superoxide anions are involved in mediating the effect of low K intake on c-Src expression and renal K secretion in the cortical collecting duct. J Biol Chem 2005;280:10790–6.

[107] O'Connell AD, Leng Q, Dong K, MacGregor GG, Giebisch G, Hebert SC. Phosphorylation-regulated endoplasmic reticulum retention signal in the renal outer-medullary K⁺ channel (ROMK). Proc Nat Acad Sci 2005;102:9954–9.

[108] Yoo D, Kim BY, Campo C, Nance L, King A, Maouyo D, et al. Cell surface expression of the ROMK (Kir 1.1) channel is regulated by the aldosterone-induced kinase, SGK-1, and protein kinase A. J Biol Chem 2003;278:23066–75.

[109] Rozansky DJ, Cornwall T, Subramanya AR, Rogers S, Yong-Feng Y, David LL, et al. Aldosterone mediates activation of the thiazide-sensitive Na-Cl co-transporter through an SGK1 and WNK4 signaling pathway. J Clin Invest 2009;119: 2601–12.

[110] Xu B, Stippec S, Lazrak A, Huang CL, Cobb MH. WNK1 activates SGK1 by a phosphatidylinositol 3-kinase-dependent and non-catalytic mechanism. J Biol Chem 2005;280:34218–23.

[111] Huang DY, Wulff P, Volkl H, Loffing J, Richter K, Kuhl D, et al. Impaired regulation of renal K⁺ elimination in the sgk1-knockout mouse. J Am Soc Nephrol 2004;15:885–91.

[112] Vallon V, Wulff P, Huang DY, Loffing J, Volkl H, Kuhl D, et al. Role of Sgk1 in salt and potassium homeostasis. Am J Physiol Regul Integr Comp Physiol 2005;288:R4–10.

[113] Verrey F, Summa V, Heitzmann D, Mordasini D, Vandewalle A, Feraille E, et al. Short-term aldosterone action on Na,K-ATPase surface expression: role of aldosterone-induced SGK1? Ann NY Acad Sci 2003;986:554–61.

[114] Huang DY, Wulff P, Volkl H, Loffing J, Richter K, Kuhl D, et al. Impaired regulation of renal K elimination in the sgk1-knockout mouse. JASN 2004;15:885–91.

[115] Palmer LG, Frindt G. Regulation of apical K channels in rat cortical collecting tubule during changes in dietary K intake. Am J Physiol 1999;277:F805–12.

[116] Yue P, Lin DH, Pan CY, Leng Q, Giebisch G, Lifton RP, et al. Src family protein tyrosine kinase (PTK) modulates the effect of SGK1 and WNK4 on ROMK channels. Proc Natl Acad Sci 2009;106:15061–6.

[117] Lin DH, Sterling H, Wang Z, Babilonia E, Yang B, Dong K, et al. ROMK1 channel activity is regulated by monoubiquitination. Proc Natl Acad Sci USA 2005;102:4306–11.

[118] Lin DH, Yue P, Pan CY, Sun P, Zhang X, Han Z, et al. POSH stimulates the ubiquitination and the clathrin-independent endocytosis of ROMK1 channels. J Biol Chem 2009;284: 29614—24.

[119] Ashcroft SJH, Ashcroft FM. Properties and functions of ATP-sensitive K-channels. Cell Signalling 1990;2:197—214.

[120] Kakei M, Kelly RP, Ashcroft SJH, Ashcroft FM. The ATP-sensitivity of K^+ channels in rat pancreatic B-cells is modulated by ADP. FEBS Lett 1986;208:63—6.

[121] Tanabe K, Tucker SJ, Ashcroft FM, Proks P, Kioka N, Amachi T, et al. Direct photoaffinity labeling of Kir6.2 by (g-^{32}P)ATP-(g)4- azidoanilide. Biochem Biophys Res Commun 2000;272: 316—9.

[122] Tanabe T, Tucker SJ, Matsuo M, Proks P, Ashcroft FM, Seino S, et al. Direct photoaffinity labeling of the Kir6.2 subunit of the ATP-sensitive K^+ channel by 8-azido-ATP. J Biol Chem 1999;274:3931—3.

[123] Dong K, Tang L, MacGregor GG, Hebert SC. Localization of the ATP/phosphatidylinositol 4,5 diphosphate-binding site to a 39-amino acid region of the carboxyl terminus of the ATP-regulated K^+ channel Kir1.1. J Biol Chem 2002;277: 49366—73.

[124] Vanoye CG, MacGregor GG, Dong K, Tang L, Buschmann AE, Hall AE, et al. The carboxyl termini of K_{ATP} channels bind nucleotides. J Biol Chem 2002;277:23260—70.

[125] Dabrowski M, Tarasov A, Ashcroft FM. Mapping the architecture of the ATP-binding site of the KATP channel subunit Kir6.2. J Physiol 2004;557:347—54.

[126] Doyle DA. Structural changes during ion channel gating. Trends Neurosci 2004;27:298—302.

[127] Ruknudin A, Schulze DH, Sullivan SK, Lederer WJ, Welling PA. Novel subunit composition of a renal epithelial K_{ATP} channel. J Biol Chem 1998;273:14165—71.

[128] Dong K, Xu J, Vanoye CG, Welch R, MacGregor GG, Giebisch G, et al. An amino acid triplet in the NH_2 terminus of rat ROMK1 determines interation with SUR2B. J Biol Chem 2001;276:44347—53.

[129] Lu M, Leng Q, Egan ME, Caplan MJ, Boulpaep E, Giebisch G, et al. CFTR is required for PKA-regulated ATP sensitivity of Kir1.1 potassium channels in mouse kidney. J Clin Invest 2006;116:797—807.

[130] McNicholas CM, Nason MW, Guggino WB, Schwiebert EM, Hebert S, Giebisch G, et al. The functional CFTR-NBF1 is required for ROMK2-CFTR interaction. Am J Physiol 1997;273: F843—8.

[131] Ashcroft SJH, Ashcroft FM. The sulfonylurea receptor. Biochim Biophys Acta 1992;1175:45—59.

[132] Aguilar-Bryan L, Nichols CG, Wechsler SW, Clement IV JP, Boyd III AE, González G, et al. Cloning of the b cell high-affinity sulfonylurea receptor: a regulator of insulin secretion. Science 1995;268:423—6.

[133] Babenko AP, Aguilar-Bryan L, Bryan J. A view of sur/KIR6.X, K_{ATP} channels. Ann Rev Physiol 1998;60:667—87.

[134] Bryan J, Aguilar-Bryan L. The ABCs of ATP-sensitive potassium channels: more pieces of the puzzle. COCB 1997;9:553—9.

[135] Clement JP, Kunjilwar K, Gonzalez G, Schwanstecher M, Panten U, Aguilar-Bryan L, et al. Association and stoichiometry of K_{ATP} channel subunits. Neuron 1997;18:827—38.

[136] Inagaki N, Gonoi T, Seino S. Subunit stoichiometry of the pancreatic b-cell ATP-sensitive K^+ channel. FEBS Letters 1997;409: 232—6.

[137] Lorenz E, Alekseev AE, Krapivinsky GB, Carrasco AJ, Clapham DE, Terzic A. Evidence for direct physical association between a K^+ channel (Kir6.2) and ATP-binding cassette protein (SUR1) which affects cellular distribution and kinetic behavior of an ATP-sensitive K^+ channel. Mol Cell Biol 1998;18:1652—9.

[138] Aguilar-Bryan L, Clement JP, Gonzalez G, Kunjilwar K, Babenko A, Bryan J. Toward understanding the assembly and structure of K_{ATP} channels. Physiol Rev 1998;78:227—45.

[139] Mikhailov MV, Proks P, Ashcroft FM, Ashcroft SJ. Expression of functionally active ATP-sensitive K-channels in insect cells using baculovirus. FEBS Lett 1998;429:390—4.

[140] Crawford I, Maloney PC, Zeitlin PL, Guggino WB, Hyde SC, Turley H, et al. Immunocytochemical localization of the cystic fibrosis gene product CFTR. Proc Natl Acad Sci USA 1991;88: 9262—6.

[141] Morales MM, Carroll TP, Morita T, Schwiebert EM, Devuyst O, Wilson PD, et al. Both the wild type and a functional isoform of CFTR are expressed in kidney. Am J Physiol (Renal Fluid Electrolyte Physiol) 1996;270:F1038—48.

[142] McNicholas CM, Guggino WB, Schwiebert EM, Hebert SC, Giebisch G, Egan ME. Sensitivity of a renal K^+ channel (ROMK2) to the inhibitory sulfonylurea compound, glibenclamide, is enhanced by co-expression with the ATP-binding cassette transporter cystic fibrosis transmembrane regulator. Proc Natl Acad Sci USA 1996;93:8083—8.

[143] Clark MA, Humphrey SJ, Smith MP, Ludens JH. Unique natriuretic properties of the ATP-sensitive K^+ channel blocker glyburide in concious rats. J Pharmacol Exp Ther 1993;165:933—7.

[144] Makita K, Takahashi K, Kerara A, Jacobson HR, Falck JR, Capdevila JH. Experimental and/or genetically controlled alterations of the renal microsomal cytochrome P450 epoxygenase induce hypertension in rats fed a high salt diet. J Clin Invest 1994;94:2414—20.

[145] Wang T, Wang W-H, Klein-Robbenhaar G, Giebisch G. Effects of glyburide on renal tubule transport and potassium-channel activity. Renal Physiol Biochem 1995;18:169—82.

[146] Lu M, Dong K, Egan ME, Giebisch GH, Boulpaep EL, Hebert SC. Mouse cystic fibrosis transmembrane conductance regulator forms cAMP-PKAG-regulated apical chloride channels in cortical collecting duct. Proc Natl Acad Sci 2010;107(13): 6082—7.

[147] Schulte U, Hahn H, Wiesinger H, Ruppersberg JP, Fakler B. pH-dependent gating of ROMK ($K_{ir}1.1$) channels involves conformational changes in both N and C termini. J Biol Chem 1998;273:34575—9.

[148] Schlatter E, Bleich M, Hirsch J, Greger R. pH-sensitive K^+ channels in the distal nephron. Nephrol Dial Trans 1993;8:488—90.

[149] Rapedius M, Haider S, Browner KF, Shang L, Sanson MSP, Baukroitz T, et al. Structural and functional analysis of the putative pH sensor in the Kir1.1 (ROMK) potassium channel. EMBO Rep 2006;7:611—6.

[150] Rapedius M, Fowler PW, Shang L, Sansom MSP, Tucker SJ, Baukrowitz T. H bonding at the helix-bundle crossing controls gating in Kir potassim channels. Neuron 2007;55(4):602—14.

[151] San Cristobal P, Pacheco-Alvarez D, Richardson C, Ring AM, Vazquez N, Rafiqi FH, et al. Angiotensin II signaling increases activity of the renal Na-Cl co-transporter through a WNK4-SPAK-dependent pathway. Proc Nat Acad Sci 2009;106: 4384—9.

[152] Zhang Y-Y, Sackin H, Palmer LG. Localization of the pH gate in Kir1.1 channels. Biophys J 2006;91:2901—9.

[153] Dahlmann A, Li M, Gao Z, McGarrigle D, Sackin H, Palmer LG. Regulation of Kir channels by intracellular pH and extracellular K^+: mechanisms of coupling. J Gen Physiol 2004;123: 441—54.

[154] Sackin H, Syn S, Palmer LG, Choe H, Walters DE. Regulation of ROMK by extracellular cations. Biophys J 2001;80:683—97.

[155] Sackin H, Nanazashvili M, Palmer LG, Krambis M, Walters DE. Structural locus of the pH gate in the Kir1.1 inward rectifier channel. Biophys J 2005;88:2597–606.

[156] Baukrowitz T, Tucker SJ, Schulte U, Benndorf K, Ruppersberg JP, Fakler B. Inward rectification in K$_{ATP}$ channels: a pH switch in the pore. EMBO J 1999;18:847–53.

[157] Leng Q, MacGregor GG, Dong K, Giebisch G, Hebert SC. Subunit-subunit interactions are critical for proton sensitivity of ROMK: evidence in support of an intermolecular gating mechanism. Proc Nat Acad Sci USA 2006;103:1982–7.

[158] Baukrowitz T, Schulte U, Oliver D, Herlitze S, Krauter T, Tucker SJ, et al. PIP$_2$ and PIP as determinants for ATP inhibition of K$_{ATP}$ channels. Science 1998;282:1141–4.

[159] Malnic G, Klose R, Giebisch G. Micropuncture study of renal potassium excretion in the rat. Am J Physiol 1964;206:674–86.

[160] Palmer LG, Antonian L, Frindt G. Regulation of apical K and Na channels and Na/K pumps in rat cortical collecting tubule by dietary K. J Gen Physiol 1994;104:693–710.

[161] Wald H, Garty H, Palmer LG, Popovtzer MM. Differential regulation of ROMK expression in kidney cortex and medulla by aldosterone and potassium. Am J Physiol 1998;275:F239–45.

[162] Chu PY, Quigley R, Babich V, Huang CL. Dietary potassium restriction stimulates endocytosis of ROMK channel in rat cortical collecting duct. Am J Physiol Renal Physiol 2003;285: F1179–87.

[163] Lin DH, Sterling H, Wang WH. The protein tyrosine kinase-dependent pathway mediates the effect of K intake on renal K secretion. Physiology (Bethesda) 2005;20:140–6.

[164] Sun TJ, Zeng WZ, Huang CL. Inhibition of ROMK potassium channel by syntaxin 1A. AJP - Renal Physiol 2005;288:F284–9.

[165] Zeng WZ, Babich V, Ortega B, Quigley R, White SJ, Welling PA, et al. Evidence for endocytosis of ROMK potassium channel via clathrin-coated vesicles. Am J Physiol Renal Physiol 2002;283:F630–9.

[166] Frindt G, Zhou H, Sackin H, Palmer LG. Dissociation of K channel density and ROMK mRNA in rat cortical collecting tubule during K adaptation. Am J Physiol 1998;274: F525–31.

[167] Reeves WB, McDonald GA, Mehta P, Andreoli TE. Activation of K$^+$ channels in renal medullary vesicles by cAMP-dependent protein kinase. J Membr Biol 1989;109:65–72.

[168] Cha SK, Hu MC, Kurosu H, Kuro-o M, Moe O, Huang CL. Regulation of renal outer medullary potassium channel and renal K$^+$ excretion by Klotho. Mol Pharmacol 2009;76:38–46.

[169] Bartter FC, Pronove P, Gill Jr JR, MacCardle RC, Diller E. Hyperplasia of the juxtaglomerular complex with hyperaldosteronoism and hypokalemic alkalosis. Am J Med 1962;33: 811–28.

[170] Asteria C. Molecular basis of Bartter's syndrome: new insights into correlation between genotype and phenotype. Eur J Endocrinol 1997;137:613–5.

[171] Guay-Woodford LM. Molecular insights into the pathogenesis of inherited renal tubular disorders. Curr Opin Nephrol Hypertens 1995;4:121–9.

[172] Karolyi L, Koch MC, Grzeschik KH, Seyberth HW. The molecular genetic approach to "Bartter's syndrome". J Mol Med 1998;76:317–25.

[173] Rodriguez-Soriano J. Bartter and related syndromes: the puzzle is almost solved. Pediatr Nephrol 1998;12:315–27.

[174] Hebert SC. Bartter syndrome. Curr Opin Nephrol Hypertens 2003;12:527–32.

[175] Simon DB, Karet FE, Hamdan JM, DiPietro A, Sanjad SA, Lifton RP. Bartter's syndrome, hypokalaemic alkalosis with hypercalciuria, is caused by mutations in the Na-K-2Cl cotransporter. NKCC2 Nat Genet 1996;13:183–8.

[176] Vargas-Poussou R, Feldmann D, Vollmer M, Konrad M, Kelly L, van den Heuvel LP, et al. Novel molecular variants of the Na-K-2Cl co-transporter gene are responsible for antenatal Bartter syndrome. Am J Hum Genet 1998;62:1332–40.

[177] Simon DB, Bindra RS, Mansfield TA, Nelson-Williams C, Mendonça E, Stone R, et al. Mutations in the chloride channel gene, CLCNKB, cause Bartter's syndrome type III. Nat Genet 1997;17:171–8.

[178] Karolyil L, Konrad M, Kockerling A, Ziegler A, Zimmermann DK, Roth B, et al. Mutations in the gene encoding the inwardly-rectifying renal potassium channel, ROMK, cause the antenatal variant of Bartter syndrome: evidence for genetic heterogeneity. Hum Mol Genet 1997;6:17–26.

[179] Simon DB, Karet FE, Rodriguez-Soriano J, Hamdan JH, DiPietro A, Trachtman H, et al. Genetic heterogeneity of Bartter's syndrome revealed by mutations in the K$^+$ channel, ROMK. Nat Geneti 1996;14:152–6.

[180] Vollmer M, Koehrer M, Topaloglu R, Strahm B, Omran H, Hildebrandt F. Two novel mutations of the gene for Kir 1.1 (ROMK) in neonatal Bartter syndrome. Pediatr Nephrol 1998;12:69–71.

[181] Estevez R, Boettger T, Stein V, Birkenhager R, Otto E, Hildebrandt F, et al. Barttin is a Cl$^-$ channel b-subunit crucial for renal Cl$^-$ reabsorption and inner ear K$^+$ secretion. Nature 2001;414:558–61.

[182] Vargas-Poussou R, Huang C, Hulin P, Houillier P, Jeunemaitre X, Paillard M, et al. Functional characterization of a calcium-sensing receptor mutation in severe autosomal dominant hypocalcemia with a Bartter-like syndrome. J Am Soc Nephrol 2002;13:2259–66.

[183] Watanabe S, Fukumoto S, Chang H, Takeuchi Y, Hasegawa Y, Okazaki R, et al. Association between activating mutations of calcium-sensing receptor and Bartter's syndrome. Lancet 2002;360:692–4.

[184] Bleich M, Schlatter E, Greger R. The luminal K$^+$ channel of the thick ascending limb of Henle's loop. Pflügers Arch 1990;415: 449–60.

[185] Greger R, Bleich M, Schlatter E. Ion channels in the thick ascending limb of Henle's loop. Renal Physiol Biochem 1990;13:37–50.

[186] Derst C, Konrad M, Köckerling A, Karschin A, Daut J, Seyberth HW. Mutations in the ROMK gene in antenatal Bartter syndrome are associated with impaired K$^+$ channel function. Biochem Biophys Res Comm 1997;230:641–5.

[187] Schwalbe RA, Bianchi L, Accili EA, Brown AM. Functional consequences of ROMK mutants linked to antenatal Bartter's syndrome and implications for treatment. Hum Mol Genet 1998;7:975–80.

[188] Schwalbe RA, Bianchi L, Accili EA, Brown AM. Functional consequences of ROMK mutants linked to antenatal Bartter's syndrome and implications for treatment. Hum Mol Genet 1998;7:975–80.

[189] Lorenz JN, Baird NR, Judd LM, Noonan WT, Andringa A, Doetschman T, et al. Impaired renal NaCl absorption in mice lacking the ROMK potassium channel, a model for type II Bartter's syndrome. J Biol Chem 2002;277:37871–80.

[190] Lu M, Wang T, Yan Q, Yang X, Dong K, Knepper MA, et al. Absence of small-conductance K$^+$ channel (SK) activity in apical membranes of thick ascending limb and cortical collecting duct in ROMK (Bartter's) knockout mice. J Biol Chem 2002;277:37881–7.

[191] Lu M, Wang T, Yan Q, Wang W, Giebisch G, Hebert SC. ROMK is required for expression of the 70 pS K channel in the thick ascending limb. Am J Physiol Renal Physiol 2004;286: F490–5.

[192] Lu R, Alioua A, Kumar Y, Eghbali M, Stefani E, Toro L. MaxiK channel partners: physiological impact. J Physiol 2006;570: 65—72.

[193] Salkoff L, Butler A, Ferreira G, Santi C, Wei A. High-conductance potassium channels of the SLO family. Nat Rev Neurosci 2006;7:921—31.

[194] Li DM, Wang ZJ, Sun P, Jin Y, Lin DH, Hebert SC, et al. Inhibition of mitogen-activated protein kinase stimulates the Ca^{2+}-dependent big conductance K channels (BK) in cortical collecting duct. Proc Natl Acad Sci USA 2006;103:19569—74.

[195] Palmer LG, Frindt G. High-conductance K channels in intercalated cells of the rat distal nephron. AJP - Renal Physiol 2007;292:F966—73.

[196] Morton MJ, Hutchinson K, Mathieson PW, Witherden IR, Saleem MA, Hunter M. Human podocytes possess a stretch-sensitive, Ca^{2+}-activated K^+ channel: potential implications for the control of glomerular filtration. J Am Soc Nephrol 2004;15:2981—7.

[197] Bailey MA, Cantone A, Yan QS, MacGregor GG, Leng Q, Amorim JB, et al. Maxi-K channels contribute to urinary potassium excretion in the ROMK-deficient mouse model of type II Bartter's syndrome and in adaptation to a high K diet. Kidney Int 2006;70:51—9.

[198] Rieg T, Vallon V, Sausbier M, Sausbier U, Kaissling B, Ruth P, et al. The role of the BK channel in potassium homeostasis and flow-induced renal potassium excretion. Kidney Int 2007;72:566—73.

[199] Liu W, Morimoto T, Woda C, Kleyman TR, Satlin LM. Ca^{2+} dependence of flow-stimulated K secretion in the mammalian cortical collecting duct. AJP - Renal Physiol 2007;293:F227—35.

[200] Taniguchi J, Imai M. Flow-dependent activation of maxi K^+ channels in apical membrane of rabbit connecting tubule. J Membr Biol 1998;164:35—45.

[201] Woda CB, Bragin A, Kleyman TR, Satlin LM. Flow-dependent K^+ secretion in the cortical collecting duct is mediated by a maxi-K channel. Am J Physiol Renal Physiol 2001;280: F786—93.

[202] Beck F-X, Dorge A, Giebisch G, Thurau K. Effect of diuretics on cell potassium transport: an electron microprobe study. Kidney Int 1990;37:1423—8.

[203] Holtzclaw JD, Grimm PR, Sansom SC. Intercalated cell BK-$\alpha/\beta4$ channels modulate sodium and potassium handling during potassium adaptation. J Am Soc Nephrol 2010;21:634—45.

[204] Grimm PR, Irsik DL, Liu L, Holtzclaw JD, Sansom SC. Role of BK $\beta1$ in Na^+ reabsorption by cortical collecting ducts of Na^+-deprived mice. AJP - Renal Physiol 2009;297:F420—8.

[205] Grimm PR, Irsik DL, Settles DC, Holtzclaw JD, Sansom S. Hypertension of Kcnmb1$^{-/-}$ is linked to deficient K secretion and aldosteronism. Proc Nat Acad Sci 2009;106:11800—5.

[206] Najjar F, Zhou H, Morimoto T, Bruns JB, Li HS, Liu W, et al. Dietary K^+ regulates apical membrane expression of maxi-K channels in rabbit cortical collecting duct. Am J Physiol Renal Physiol 2005;289:F922—32.

[207] Estilo G, Liu W, Pastor-Soler N, Mitchell P, Carattino MD, Kleyman TR, et al. Effect of aldosterone on BK channel expression in mammalian cortical collecting duct. AJP - Renal Physiol 2008;295:F780—8.

[208] Liu W, Wei Y, Sun P, Wang WH, Kleyman TR, Satlin LM. Mechanoregulation of BK channel activity in the mammalian cortical collecting duct: role of protein kinases A and C. AJP - Renal Physiol 2009;297:F904—15.

[209] Sun P, Liu W, Lin DH, Yue P, Kemp R, Satlin LM, et al. Epoxyeicosatrienoic acid (EET) activates the Ca^{2+}-dependent bid conductance K channel in the cortical collecting duct. J Am Soc Nephrol 2009;20:513—23.

[210] Barhanin J, Lesage F, Guillemare E, Fink M, Lazdunski M, Romey G. KvLQT1 and IsK (minK) proteins associate to form the I_{ks} cardiac potassium current. Nature 1996;384:78—80.

[211] Sanguinetti MC, Curran ME, Zou A, Shen J, Spector PS, Atkinson DL, et al. Coassembly of K_vLQT1 and minK (IsK) proteins to form cardiac I_{Ks} potassium channel. Nature 1996;384:80—3.

[212] Wang Q, Curran ME, Splawski I, Burn TC, Millholland JM, VanRaay TJ, et al. Positional cloning of a novel potassium channel gene: KVLQT1 mutations cause cardiac arrhythmias. Nat Genet 1996;12:17—23.

[213] Carrisoza R, Salvador C, Bobadilla N, Trujillo J, Escobar L. Expression and immunolocalization of ERG1 potassium channels in the rat kidney. Histochem Cell Biol 2010;133:189—99.

[214] Zheng W, Verlander JW, Lynch IJ, Cash M, Shao J, Stow LR, et al. Cellular distribution of the potassium channel KCNQ1 in normal mouse kidney. AJP - Renal Physiol 2007;292:F456—66.

[215] Vallon V, Grahammer F, Richter K, Bleich M, Lang F, Barhanin J, et al. Role of KCNE1-dependent K^+ fluxes in mouse proximal tubule. J Am Soc Nephrol 2001;12:2003—11.

[216] Millar ID, Hartley JA, Haigh C, Grace AA, White SJ, Kibble JD, et al. Volume regulation is defective in renal proximal tubule cells isolated from KCNE1 knockout mice. Exp Physiol 2004;89:173—80.

[217] Glaudemans B, van der Wijst J, Scola RH, Lorenzoni PJ, Heister A, van der Kemp AW, et al. A missense mutation in the Kv1.1 voltage-gated potassium channel-encoding gene KCNA1 is linked to human autosomal dominant hypomagnesemia. J Clin Invest 2009;119:936—42.

[218] Yao X, Tian S, Chan H-Y, Biemesderfer D, Desir GV. Expression of KCNA10, a voltage-gated K channel, in glomerular endothelium and at the apical membrane of the renal proximal tubule. J Am Soc Nephrol 2002;13(12):2831—9.

[219] Orias M, Bray-Ward P, Curran ME, Keating MT, Desir GV. Genomic localization of the human gene for KCNA10, a cGMP-activated K channel. Genomics 1997;42:33—7.

[220] Lourdel S, Paulais M, Cluzeaud F, Bens M, Tanemoto M, Kurachi Y, et al. An inward rectifier K^+ channel at the basolateral membrane of the mouse distal convoluted tubule: similarities with Kir4-Kir5.1 heteromeric channels. J Physiol 2002;538: 391—404.

[221] Bond CT, Pessia M, Xia XM, Lagrutta A, Kavanaugh MP, Adelman JP. Cloning and expression of a family of inward rectifier potassium channels. Receptors Channels 1994;2:183—91.

[222] Takumi T, Ishii T, Horio Y, Morishige K, Takahashi N, Yamada M, et al. A novel ATP-dependent inward rectifier potassium channel expressed predominantly in glial cells. J Biol Chem 1995;270:16339—46.

[223] Ito M, Inanobe A, Horio Y, Hibino H, Isomoto S, Ito H, et al. Immunologicalization of an inwardly rectifying K^+ channel, K_{AB}-2 (Kir4.1), in the basolateral membrane of renal distal tubular epithelia. FEBS Lett 1996;388:11—5.

[224] Yang Z, Jiang C. Opposite effects of pH on open-state probability and single channel conductance of kir4.1 channels. J Physiol 1999;520(Pt 3):921—7.

[225] Kofuji P, Ceelen P, Zahs KR, Surbeck LW, Lester HA, Newman EA. Genetic inactivation of an inwardly rectifying potassium channel (Kir4.1 subunit) in mice: phenotypic impact in retina. J Neurosci 2000;20:5733—40.

[226] Pearson WL, Dourado M, Schreiber M, Salkoff L, Nichols CG. Expression of a functional Kir4 family inward rectifier K^+ channel from a gene cloned from mouse liver. J Physiol 1999;514(Pt 3):639—53.

[227] Tanemoto M, Kittaka N, Inanobe A, Kurachi Y. *In vivo* formation of a proton-sensitive K^+ channel by heteromeric

subunit assembly of Kir5.1 with Kir4.1. J Physiol 2000;525(Pt 3): 587−92.

[228] Tucker SJ, Imbrici P, Salvatore L, D'Adamo MC, Pessia M. pH dependence of the inwardly rectifying potassium channel, Kir5.1, and localization in renal tubular epithelia. J Biol Chem 2000;275:16404−7.

[229] Konstas AA, Korbmacher C, Tucker SJ. Identification of domains which control the heteromeric assembly of Kir5.1/Kir4.0 potassium channels. Am J Physiol Cell Physiol 2003;284:C910−7.

[230] Gray DA, Frindt G, Zhang YY, Palmer LG. Basolateral K$^+$ conductance in principal cells of rat CCD. AJP - Renal Physiol 2005;288:F493−504.

[231] Grimm PR, Foutz RM, Brenner R, Sansom SC. Identification and localization of BK-beta subunits in the distal nephron of the mouse kidney. AJP - Renal Physiol 2007;293:F350−9.

[232] Lachheb S, Cluzeaud F, Bens M, Genete M, Hibino H, Lourdel S, et al. Kir4.1/Kir5.1 channel forms the major K$^+$ channel in the basolateral membrane of mouse renal collecting duct principal cells. AJP - Renal Physiol 2008;294:F1398−407.

[233] Lourdel S, Paulais M, Cluzeaud F, Bens M, Tanemoto M, Kurachi Y, et al. An inward rectifier K$^+$ channel at the basolateral membrane of the mouse distal convoluted tubles: similarities with Kir4-Kir5.1 heteromeric channels. J Physiol 2002;538:391−404.

[234] Pessia M, Imbrici P, D'Adamo MC, Salvatore L, Tucker SJ. Differential pH sensitivity of Kir4.1 and Kir4.2 potassium channels and their modulation by heteropolymerisation with Kir5.1. J Physiol 2001;532:359−67.

[235] Xu H, Cui N, Yang Z, Qu Z, Jiang C. Modulation of kir4.1 and kir5.1 by hypercapnia and intracellular acidosis. J Physiol 2000;524(Pt 3):725−35.

[236] Yang Z, Xu H, Cui N, Qu Z, Chanchevalap S, Shen W, et al. Biophysical and molecular mechanisms underlying the modulation of heteromeric Kir4.1-Kir5.1 channels by CO$_2$ and pH. J Gen Physiol 2000;116:33−45.

[237] Leung YM, Zeng WZ, Liou HH, Solaro CR, Huang CL. Phosphatidylinositol 4,5-bisphosphate and intracellular pH regulate the ROMK1 potassium channel via separate but interrelated mechanisms. J Biol Chem 2000;275:10182−9.

[238] Huang C, Sindic A, Hill CE, Hujer KM, Chan KW, Sassen M, et al. Interaction of the Ca^{2+}-sensing receptor with the inwardly rectifying potassium channels Kir4.1 and Kir4.2 results in inhibition of channel function. AJP - Renal Physiol 2007;292:F1073−81.

[239] Reichold M, Zdebik AA, Lieberer E, Rapedius M, Schmidt K, Bandulik S, et al. KCNJ10 gene mutations causing EAST syndrome (epilepsy, ataxia, sensorineural deafness, and tubulopathy) disrupt channel function. Proc Natl Acad Sci 2010;107:14490−5.

[240] Scholl UI, Choi M, Liu T, Ramaekers VT, Häusler MG, Grimmer J, et al. Seizures, sensorineural deafness, ataxia, mental retardation, and electrolyte imbalance (SeSAME syndrome) caused by mutations in KCNJ10. Proc Natl Acad Sci 2009;106:5842−7.

[241] Welling PA. Primary structure and functional expression of a cortical collecting duct K$_{ir}$ channel. Am J Physiol 1997;273: F825−36.

[242] Le Maout S, Brejon M, Olsen O, Merot J, Welling PA. Basolateral membrane targeting of a renal-epithelial inwardly rectifying potassium channel from the cortical collecting duct, CCD- IRK3, in MDCK cells. Proc Natl Acad Sci USA 1997;94: 13329−34.

[243] Le Maout S, Welling PA, Brejon M, Olsen O, Merot J. Basolateral membrane expression of a K$^+$ channel, Kir 2.3, is

directed by a cytoplasmic COOH-terminal domain. Proc Natl Acad Sci USA 2001;98:10475−80.

[244] Olsen O, Liu H, Wade JB, Merot J, Welling PA. Basolateral membrane expression of the Kir 2.3 channel is coordinated by PDZ interaction with Lin-7/CASK complex. Am J Physiol Cell Physiol 2002;282:C183−95.

[245] Inagaki N, Tsuura Y, Namba N, Masuda K, Gonoi T, Horie M, et al. Cloning and functional characterization of a novel ATP-sensitive potassium channel ubiquitously expressed in rat tissues, including pancreatic islets, pituitary, skeletal muscle, and heart. J Biol Chem 1995;270:5691−4.

[246] Seino S. ATP-sensitive potassium channels: a model of heteromultimeric potassium channel/receptor assemblies. Ann Rev Physiol 1999;61:337−62.

[247] Bryan J, Aguilar-Bryan L. Sulfonylurea receptors: ABC transporters that regulate ATP-sensitive K$^+$ channels. Biochim Biophys Acta 1999;1461:285−303.

[248] Erginel-Unaltuna N, Yang WP, Blanar MA. Genomic organization and expression of KCNJ8/Kir6.1, a gene encoding a subunit of an ATP-sensitive potassium channel. Gene 1998;211: 71−8.

[249] Suzuki M, Kotake K, Fujikura K, Inagaki N, Suzuki T, Gonoi T, et al. Kir6.1: a possible subunit of ATP-sensitive K$^+$ channels in mitochondria. Biochem Biophys Res Commun 1997;241: 693−7.

[250] Brochiero E, Wallendorf B, Gagnon D, Laprade R, Lapointe JY. Cloning of rabbit Kir6.1, SUR2A, and SUR2B: possible candidates for a renal K$_{ATP}$ channel. Am J Physiol Renal Physiol 2002;282:F289−300.

[251] Akao M, Otani H, Horie M, Takano M, Kuniyasu A, Nakayama H, et al. Myocardial ischemia induces differential regulation of K$_{ATP}$ channel gene expression in rat hearts. J Clin Invest 1997;100:3053−9.

[252] Carrasco AJ, Dzeja PP, Alekseev AE, Pucar D, Zingman LV, Abraham MR, et al. Adenylate kinase phosphotransfer communicates cellular energetic signals to ATP-sensitive potassium channels. Proc Natl Acad Sci USA 2001;98: 7623−8.

[253] Brochiero E, Coady MJ, Klein H, Laprade R, Lapointe JY. Activation of an ATP-dependent K$^+$ conductance in Xenopus oocytes by expression of adenylate kinase cloned from renal proximal tubules. Biochim Biophys Acta 2001;1510:29−42.

[254] Krapivinsky G, Medina I, Eng L, Krapivinsky L, Yang Y, Clapham DE. A novel inward rectifier K$^+$ channel with unique pore properties. Neuron 1998;20:995−1005.

[255] Partiseti M, Collura V, Agnel M, Culouscou JM, Graham D. Cloning and characterization of a novel human inwardly rectifying potassium channel predominantly expressed in small intestine. FEBS Lett 1998;434:171−6.

[256] Doring F, Derst C, Wischmeyer E, Karschin C, Schneggenburger R, Daut J, et al. The epithelial inward rectifier channel Kir7.1 displays unusual K$^+$ permeation properties. J Neurosci 1998;18:8625−36.

[257] Derst C, Hirsch JR, Preisig-Muller R, Wischmeyer E, Karschin A, Doring F, et al. Cellular localization of the potassium channel Kir7.1 in guinea pig and human kidney. Kidney Int 2001;59:2197−205.

[258] Ookata K, Tojo A, Suzuki Y, Nakamura N, Kimura K, Wilcox CS, et al. Localization of inward rectifier potassium channel Kir7.1 in the basolateral membrane of distal nephron and collecting duct. J Am Soc Nephrol 2000;11:1987−94.

[259] Nakamura N, Suzuki Y, Sakuta H, Ookata K, Kawahara K, Hirose S. Inwardly rectifying K$^+$ channel Kir7.1 is highly expressed in thyroid follicular cells, intestinal epithelial cells and choroid plexus epithelial cells: implication for a functional

coupling with Na$^+$,K$^+$-ATPase. Biochem J 1999;342(Pt 2): 329—36.

[260] Frindt G, Palmer LG. Apical potassium channels in the rat connecting tubule. Am J Physiol Renal Physiol 2004;287: F1030—7.

[261] Ho K. The ROMK-cystic fibrosis transmembrane conductance regulator connection: new insights into the relationship between ROMK and cystic fibrosis transmembrane conductance regulator channels. Curr Opin Nephrol Hypertens 1998;7:49—58.

[262] Satlin LM, Palmer LG. Apical K$^+$ conductance in maturing rabbit principal cell. Am J Physiol 1997;272:F397—404.

[263] Reyes R, Duprat F, Lesage F, Fink M, Salinas M, Farman N, et al. Cloning and expression of a novel pH-sensitive two pore domain K$^+$ channel from human kidney. J Biol Chem 1998;273:30863—9.

[264] Arrighi I, Lesage F, Scimeca J-C, Carle GF, Barhanin J. Structure, chromosome localization, and tissue distribution of the mouse *twik* K$^+$ channel gene. FEBS Lett 1998;425:310—6.

[265] Chavez RA, Gray AT, Zhao BB, Kindler CH, Mazurek MJ, Mehta Y, et al. TWIK-2, a new weak inward rectifing member of the tandem pore domain potassium channel family. J Biol Chem 1999;274:7887—92.

[266] Cluzeaud F, Reyes R, Escoubet B, Fay M, Lazdunski M, Bonvalet JP, et al. Expression of TWIK-1, a novel weakly inward rectifying potassium channel in rat kidney. Am J Physiol (Cell Physiol) 1998;275:C1602—9.

[267] Lesage F, Guillemare E, Fink M, Duprat F, Lazdunski M, Romey G, et al. TWIK-1 a ubiquitous human weakly inward rectifying K$^+$ channel with a novel structure. EMBO J 1996;15:1004—11.

[268] Lesage F, Guillemare E, Fink M, Duprat F, Lazdunski M, Romey G, et al. TWIK-1 a ubiquitous human weakly inward rectifying K$^+$ channel with novel structure. EMBO J 1996;15:1004—11.

[269] Orias M, Velazquez H, Tung F, Lee G, Desir GV. Cloning and localization of a double-pore K channel, KCNK1: exclusive expression in distal nephron segments. Am J Physiol 1997;273: F663—6.

[270] Wei A, Jegla T, Salkoff L. Eight potassium channel families revealed by the *C. elegans* genome project. Neuropharmacology 1996;35:805—29.

[271] Lesage F, Lauritzen I, Duprat F, Reyes R, Fink M, Heurteaux C, et al. The structure, function and distribution of the mouse TWIK-1K$^+$ channel. FEBS Lett 1997;402:28—32.

[272] Fink M, Duprat F, Lesage F, Reyes R, Romey G, Heurteaux C, et al. Cloning, functional expression and brain localization of a novel unconventional outward rectifier K$^+$ channel. EMBO J 1996;15:6854—62.

[273] Lesage F, Lazdunski M. Mapping of human potassium channel genes TREK-1 (*KCNK2*) and TASK (*KCNK3*) to chromosomes 1q41 and 2p23. Genomics 1998;51:478—9.

[274] Duprat F, Lesage F, Fink M, Reyes R, Heurteaux C, Lazdunski M. TASK a human background K$^+$ channel to sense external pH variations near physiological pH. EMBO J 1997;16: 5464—71.

[275] Patel AJ, Honore E, Maingret F, Lesage F, Fink M, Duprat F, et al. A mammalian two pore domain mechano-gated S-like K$^+$ channel. EMBO J 1998;17:4283—90.

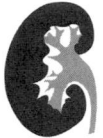

Extrarenal Potassium Metabolism

Vaibhav Sahni, Aleksandra Gmurczyk, Robert M. Rosa

The Feinberg School of Medicine, Northwestern University, Chicago, IL, USA

Internal potassium homeostasis is defined as the regulation of potassium distribution between the intracellular and extracellular fluid compartments, as distinct from the net gain or loss of potassium from the body. While the kidney plays the predominant role in maintaining external potassium balance, nonrenal tissues, especially muscle and liver, are quantitatively the most important organs involved in the regulation of internal potassium balance.

The ratio of potassium between intracellular and extracellular fluids is critically important, not only to the behavior of electrically excitable cells, such as muscle and nerve, but also to the vital processes of all living cells. The reason for this is that a major regulator of cell function is the transmembrane potential. The determinants of this membrane potential are described by the Goldman–Hodgkin–Katz equation, the most important term of which is the logarithm of the ratio of internal to external ionic activity of potassium.

Of the 3500 mEq of potassium found in the body of a 70 kg human, about 98% is confined to intracellular water (Figure 48.1). Of this, 80% is contained in muscle cells, at a concentration of about 150 mEq/liter. The remaining 2% of total body potassium (about 70 mEq) is located in the extracellular fluid (about 14 liters), where the normal concentration is 3.5–5.5 mEq/liter. The chief biological mechanism responsible for maintaining this 30-fold potassium gradient between cell water and extracellular fluid is the Na,K-ATPase pump, situated in the plasma membrane of all animal cells. A minor role is played by the inward transport of potassium coupled with sodium and chloride, via the Na–K–2Cl transporter in the plasma membrane of some cells. Transcellular distribution of potassium is also modulated by hormonal factors, such as insulin and catecholamines, by hydrogen ion balance, plasma osmolality, intracellular potassium content, and by factors that affect the passive movement of potassium through membrane channels, such as the level of intracellular calcium and pH (Table 48.1). Some of these factors, such as the activity of Na,K-ATPase and the distribution of hydrogen ions, may concurrently affect the potassium content of cells of the distal nephron, and thereby influence the external balance of potassium.

From a practical standpoint, a key determinant of transmembrane potential is the plasma potassium. Since the concentration of potassium inside cells far exceeds extracellular concentration, percentile changes in intracellular potassium are relatively small, even during extreme degrees of total body potassium surfeit, deficit or internal redistribution. The changes in extracellular potassium seen in diseased states are therefore much more likely to alter the membrane potential of cells than are concomitant changes in intracellular potassium. For this reason, a variety of mechanisms have evolved to preserve the extracellular concentration of potassium within the normal range.

If a moderate load of potassium (0.5 mEq/kg) is administered intravenously over 1 hour, about 40% of it is excreted into the urine at the end of that time. Within 3 hours, renal excretion is complete and the serum potassium, which initially increases by about 0.6 mEq/liter, returns to baseline.[1,2] The ability of the normal human kidney to excrete all of an oral load of potassium is more sluggish; while potassium excretion increases 6-10-fold within a few hours,[3–5] only about half of the load is excreted during the first 3–6 hours after it is ingested.[5–9] Of considerable interest, however, is recent evidence that is consistent with the existence of an unidentified "gut" and/or "hepatoportal factor" that senses potassium ingestion, and

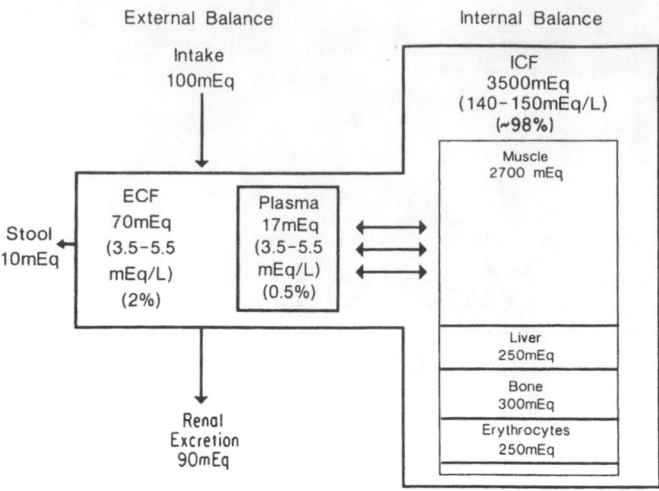

FIGURE 48.1 Internal potassium homeostasis in a 70 kg person. The potassium concentration in the extracellular fluid (ECF) depends on both the external balance (intake and output) and the internal balance (distribution between extracellular and intracellular fluid, ICF). Factors affecting internal balance are listed in Table 48.1. Note that the large ICF pool exists at a far greater K concentration than the small ECF pool; the ECF pool will therefore change more dramatically with changes in total body K or K distribution.

TABLE 48.1 Factors Affecting Internal Potassium Homeostasis

Factor	Effect on Potassium
Insulin	Enhanced cell uptake
β-Catecholamines	Enhanced cell uptake
α-Catecholamines	Impaired cell uptake
Acidosis	Impaired cell uptake and enhanced efflux[a]
Alkalosis	Enhanced cell uptake and reduced efflux[a]
External potassium balance	Loose correlation
Drugs	See text
Hyperosmolality	Enhance cell efflux

[a]*Degree varies with disturbance.*

rapidly initiates the process of renal potassium excretion in the absence of a significant change in plasma potassium concentration.[10,11]

Consumption of only 35 mEq of potassium by a 70 kg adult during an average meal (an amount equivalent to 1% of total body potassium) would, if confined exclusively to the extracellular space, raise the plasma potassium by 2.5 mEq/liter — enough to have pronounced effects on neuromuscular function. It is well-established, however, that a potassium load given to a normal human or dog has an apparent volume of distribution of 70–80% of body weight, somewhat greater than total body water,[6,12] instead of the 20% that represents extracellular fluid. In other words, only a small portion (about one quarter) of the 35 mEq of ingested potassium will normally remain in the extracellular compartment, raising the concentration of potassium in plasma by only about 0.6 mEq/liter. In contrast, a similar load of potassium administered to patients with deranged extrarenal potassium homeostasis may produce serious hyperkalemia.[13]

The cells also buffer plasma potassium during potassium depletion. In states of progressive potassium deficiency, as depletion worsens, a greater amount of potassium is lost from within cells to lessen the fall in external concentration, and to minimize the alteration in its intracellular to extracellular ratio.

These examples of potassium surfeit or deficit emphasize the critical role of internal potassium homeostasis in mitigating potentially dangerous changes in the plasma potassium. Disorders of the factors that mediate this adjustment thus may have substantial clinical importance and are the primary topic of this chapter.

POTASSIUM DEPLETION AND REPLETION

In many conditions, such as vomiting, diabetic ketoacidosis, and chronic renal failure, abnormalities of internal and external potassium homeostasis coexist. Just as internal potassium homeostasis can affect potassium uptake and excretion by the kidney, so changes in external potassium balance, by altering cellular potassium content, can independently influence internal potassium homeostasis.

Potassium Depletion

The idealized curvilinear relationship between total body potassium and the serum potassium concentration illustrated in Figure 48.2 is derived from several measurements in hypokalemic patients with positive potassium balance during replacement therapy,[14–16] and from unpublished data on hyperkalemic humans and animals.[17] In the early stages of depletion, extracellular potassium loss is proportionately greater than the loss of cellular potassium.[18] Nonetheless, since only a small fraction of total body potassium is extracellular, the quantity of potassium lost from the extracellular compartment is much smaller than that lost from inside cells.

In the early phases of hypokalemia (>2.5 mEq/liter), patients tend to display an almost linear relationship between total body potassium and the serum

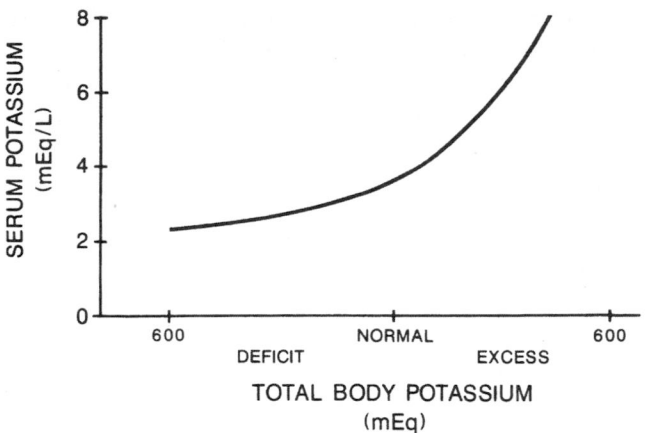

FIGURE 48.2 Idealized relationship between the serum potassium concentration and the body potassium content. *Reprinted with permission from ref. [17].*

potassium concentration. It has been observed that a change of 100–200 mEq in total body potassium (about 5%) is required to lower the serum potassium by 1.0 mEq/liter.[17] In such a situation, the extracellular potassium concentration would be expected to fall proportionately more (e.g., 4.0 to 3.0 mEq/liter) than the intracellular concentration (e.g., 140 to 133 mEq/liter). Because of the relationship of cell membrane potentials to the ratio of internal to external ionic activity of potassium, excessive extracellular potassium loss would be expected to hyperpolarize cells (resting membrane potential is increased). This expectation has been confirmed in studies of early potassium deficiency in both dogs[19] and humans.[20]

When potassium depletion becomes more severe, so that serum levels fall below about 2.5 mEq/liter, a further 1.0 mEq/liter fall will represent a much larger 200–400 mEq decrement in total body potassium (greater than 10%), reflecting a greater degree of potassium loss from within the cells[17,21] than occurred in the early phases of depletion. Decreased cell potassium content has, in fact, been observed in several tissues during severe hypokalemia.[15,22,23]

In severe potassium depletion cells tend to depolarize (resting membrane potential is decreased), at least in dogs[19] which, like humans, then develop weakness and muscle paralysis. Under conditions of chronic hypokalemia, however, there is also upregulation of the colonic form of H,K-ATPase (HKα2), which leads to enhanced potassium reabsorption from the gut.[24]

Potassium Repletion

During potassium repletion for severe hypokalemia, cellular potassium uptake is enhanced both in animals[25,26] and in humans[27]; that is, the administered

potassium has an increased volume of distribution; as potassium is gained by the body and the stores become higher, the cellular uptake of potassium decreases. In anuric humans, for example, the cellular uptake of a potassium-load decreases as total body potassium increases.[27] Extracellular potassium then tends to rise and membrane potential decreases.[28] The important therapeutic caveat in the late phases of correction of potassium depletion is that less potassium administration is required than in earlier phases to increase serum potassium, which may rise suddenly to unexpected, dangerously hyperkalemic levels.[29]

As reviewed extensively by Sterns et al.,[27] the serum potassium alone is, at best, an extremely rough guide for estimating potassium replacement therapy, presumably because other factors, such as acid–base status, influence it. A low serum potassium value (e.g., 3.0 mEq/liter) may be associated with a range of total body deficits spanning a few hundred millequivalents (Figure 48.2).

The exact mechanisms that produce this curvilinear relationship are uncertain. They may stem in part from impairment of the electrogenic sodium pump.[19,30,31] During potassium depletion in rats, skeletal muscle potassium loss is associated with a reduced capacity for Na-K pumping and a reversible decrease in the number of [³H] ouabain-binding sites.[32] A possible mechanism for suppression of the Na-K pump during potassium depletion is enhanced stimulation of alpha-adrenoreceptors[33] (see "Catecholamines"). In addition, even modest dietary potassium restriction provokes resistance to insulin-mediated cellular potassium uptake (see "Insulin").

INSULIN

The effect of insulin on potassium homeostasis was first demonstrated two years after its purification by Banting and Best. Harrop and Benedict,[34] and Briggs and Koechig[35] described the fall in serum potassium coincident with lowering of blood sugar when insulin was administered to diabetic patients, as well as in the non-diabetic human, dog, and rabbit. Later, there were reports of severe hypokalemia in insulin-treated patients with ketoacidosis who developed paralysis.[36]

Cellular Mechanism

The hypokalemic action of insulin derives from its capacity to cause net potassium uptake in skeletal muscle,[37–39] adipose tissue, and hepatic cells,[40–42] as well as other extrarenal sites.[43] This effect was formerly assumed to occur to preserve electrical neutrality when insulin-mediated glucose uptake produced intracellular anionic sugars[44,45] and deposited potassium as an accompaniment of glycogen in the liver.[46]

This classical hypothesis did not explain the clinical observation that sudden lowering of serum potassium could precede the fall in blood sugar in insulin-treated diabetic coma. Zierler[47] first noted that insulin's effect on potassium movement in rat muscle occurred even in the absence of glucose; its known effect to increase sodium efflux *in vitro* also occurred without glucose.[48] Furthermore, enhancement of potassium disposal in the intact animal was separable temporally from glucose uptake[49,50] and occurred at plasma insulin concentrations having no measurable influence on uptake of glucose *in vivo*.[51] Different receptor mechanisms for potassium and glucose transport appear to exist.[45]

In vitro, insulin is known to stimulate both potassium uptake[52,53] and sodium efflux[37,54] in frog and rat muscle preparations. Similar effects have been reported in rat adipose tissue,[55] hepatocytes,[56] and other cells.[57] Considerable evidence[45] suggests that following binding to cell surface receptors,[58] insulin accelerates monovalent cation transport by stimulating Na,K-ATPase, the sodium-potassium pump. Most convincing is the fact that both insulin-stimulated net sodium efflux and potassium influx are blocked by ouabain.[37,52,54,59] *In vitro*, addition of insulin to purified plasma membrane of skeletal muscle increases the activity of the Na,K-ATPase.[60] Little evidence is currently available on whether insulin affects potassium permeability or potassium channels in skeletal muscle cells. Insulin activation of sodium—hydrogen exchange sensitive to amiloride[61] does not appear to be important to sodium-pump-mediated potassium uptake.[62] In adipocytes, insulin-stimulated uptake of K^+ and Rb^+ is inhibited by bumetanide and by removal of Cl^- from the extracellular fluid, suggesting a primary action of insulin on the Na—K—2Cl co-transporter.[63] On the other hand, in skeletal muscle, insulin does not appear to activate the co-transport of K^+ with Na^+ and Cl^-.[64] There is evidence, however, that the serum and glucocorticoid-inducible kinase SGK1 participates in the different signaling pathways that mediate the hypokalemic effect of insulin.[65]

Stimulation of active sodium—potassium transport by Na,K-ATPase could be due to a *de novo* increase in the number of sodium pump sites or to allosteric activation of existing sites. The latter theory is consistent with the rapid activation of transport that occurs,[66] as well as with the lack of new ouabain-binding sites[67,68] after exposure to insulin *in vitro*.

At least three molecular forms of the Na,K-ATPase catalytic subunit have been identified, designated alpha1, alpha2, and alpha3. In both rat and human skeletal muscles, insulin mediates the Na,K-ATPase alpha1- and alpha2-subunit translocation into the plasma membrane via a phosphatidylinositol 3-kinase-dependent mechanism.[69] In liver, the effect of insulin can be accounted for by increased intracellular sodium concentration.[56] Insulin also activates a KCl co-transporter uptake system in a cultured cell line resembling skeletal muscle.[70]

It should be noted that insulin is known to produce hyperpolarization of cellular membranes, not only in skeletal muscle,[71,72] but in a variety of other tissues.[73,74] This rapid effect appears to precede measurable increases in intracellular potassium.[39] Although stimulation of Na,K-ATPase could account for insulin's hyperpolarizing effect,[75] failure of ouabain to block it, at least in some studies, suggests that changes in ion permeability may be responsible. The role of hyperpolarization in mediating insulin effects on cation transport is uncertain. The effect of insulin to stimulate active sodium and potassium transport in skeletal muscle is mimicked by insulin-like growth factor I (IGF-I).[76]

In Vivo Effects

Abundant evidence therefore exists that insulin increases net uptake of potassium ions by several tissues *in vitro*. Since skeletal muscle is well-documented to respond to insulin and is the major body reservoir for potassium, it is most likely the dominant site for insulin-stimulated extrarenal potassium disposal *in vivo*. Human forearm muscle (and adipose tissue) increases potassium uptake during arterial infusion[51] of insulin.

Wilde[77] noted over half-a-century ago that injected potassium rapidly disappeared from the blood of cats, but was followed by a secondary rise in serum potassium. Recent investigation suggests that, at least during insulin infusion, hepatic disposal plays an important role in potassium homeostasis in the first hour of exposure to insulin in humans.[78] Splanchnic uptake accounted for two-thirds of the fall in plasma potassium during euglycemic hyperinsulinemia. In the second hour, net splanchnic uptake reversed, and peripheral tissues became the dominant site of potassium disposal.

That the effect of insulin on extrarenal potassium homeostasis is dose related is well-established[79,80] (Figure 48.3). In normal subjects, neither intramuscular nor subcutaneous administration of insulin, which achieved plasma insulin levels of about $50 \mu U/ml$, decreased the plasma potassium.[81] Intravenous insulin injection, by comparison, produced 40-fold greater insulin levels, which were accompanied by a steady-state reduction in plasma potassium, with a maximal effect of about 30% occurring 50 minutes after insulin injection.

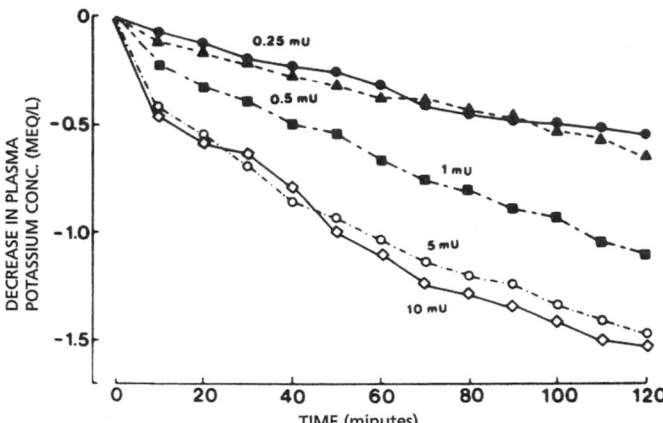

FIGURE 48.3   Dose-related effect of euglycemic hyperinsulinemia on plasma potassium concentration. Infusion of insulin at the doses shown produced plasma insulin levels of approximately 25, 50, 100, 500, and 1000 μU/ml above basal values. *Reprinted with permission from ref.* [79].

On the other hand, much smaller increments of insulin, about three-fold above basal values, either during constant venous[78,82] or intra-arterial infusion[49,51,83] also appear capable of augmenting potassium uptake *in vivo*.[27] Under conditions of prolonged potassium depletion, however, the expression of skeletal muscle Na,K-ATPase α2 isoform is decreased, which allows for enhanced efflux of potassium from muscle to the extracellular space.[84] Of particular interest is the observation that even modest dietary potassium restriction leads to a decrease in insulin-mediated cellular potassium uptake in rats in the absence of a fall in plasma potassium concentration.[85]

Clinical Implications

The relevance of these findings to a given clinical situation of exogenous potassium challenge will depend on the magnitude of potassium-load requiring disposal, and the elevation of insulin accompanying it. Following carbohydrate feeding, for example, increased liver uptake of potassium occurs.[46] Since peripheral venous insulin levels for 2 hours following oral glucose loading are elevated five-fold,[86] well within the range capable of augmenting potassium uptake, it seems likely that insulin contributes to the transient decrease in potassium that occurs after feeding.[87] Even basal circulating insulin levels may be essential to disposal of an acute potassium-load, since disposal is impaired when basal levels are decreased 50% by somatostatin.[88] The effect of carbohydrate meals to blunt or prevent hyperkalemia may be particularly important in anuric patients dependent on extracorporeal dialysis.[89]

During exogenous potassium challenge, the importance of insulin to potassium disposal by the intact organism deprived of endogenous insulin[90–93] or resistant to the actions of insulin[94] is well-established. As expected, supraphysiologic doses of exogenous insulin are capable of improving potassium tolerance.[92] Thus, for emergency treatment of hyperkalemia, the intravenous administration of insulin together with glucose is indicated, unless the patient is already hyperglycemic from diabetes in which case additional glucose is not warranted.

The ability of potassium-loading to stimulate the release of pancreatic insulin directly, in amounts sufficient to contribute to disposal of that potassium, is less clear. In pancreatic B-cells, ATP-sensitive K channels link cellular membrane potential to hormone secretion.[95] These channels control the transmembrane potential, and thereby the calcium channels that trigger glucose-induced insulin secretion.[96] Depolarization of the cell membrane (as expected with hyperkalemia) induces an increase in insulin secretion.[97] In humans[98] and intact dogs,[99–101] minor increments in blood potassium appear capable of triggering pancreatic insulin secretion. Since elevations in portal venous insulin far exceed those in the peripheral circulation when insulin release is stimulated,[100,102,103] it seems reasonable to conclude that, under conditions of significant hyperkalemia, induction of insulin release to promote potassium uptake does constitute a homeostatic feedback control system.

GLUCAGON

The effect of glucagon on extrarenal potassium disposal has been difficult to isolate, because the hormone also influences the secretion of insulin, epinephrine, and aldosterone. Administration of glucagon to cats does appear to mobilize potassium from the liver and produce a transient rise in arterial potassium levels.[104] In humans, the hyperkalemic response to the hormone appears to be only partly due to an epinephrine-like effect of glucagon to increase liver glycogenolysis.[105]

For example, aortic injection of glucagon in humans, which results in hepatic vein glucagon levels within the pathophysiologic range, causes a transient increment in hepatic vein potassium concentrations, but this precedes the slow rise in glucose in hepatic venous blood.[106] The specific source of the modest rise in hepatic venous potassium under these conditions has not been determined. Previous *in vitro* investigations using perfused rat liver suggest that glucagon releases potassium directly from the liver.[41,107] The effect would not appear to be due to diminished Na—K pump-mediated potassium uptake, since isolated rat hepatocytes exposed to glucagon actually undergo stimulation of this cation pump.[108]

Systemic infusion of glucagon to physiologic levels tends to elevate plasma potassium slightly by an extrarenal mechanism, at least when glucagon-induced insulin secretion is suppressed by somatostatin, both in normal subjects[105] and in diabetic subjects.[109] It is unclear whether hyperglucagonemia, which occurs in decompensated diabetes mellitus,[110] uremia,[111] and exhausting exercise[112] affect potassium homeostasis. In the dog, potassium-stimulated insulin release appears to be accompanied by a modest rise in circulating glucagon.[92,112]

CATECHOLAMINES

The observation of D'Silva[113] in 1934 that epinephrine lowers the serum potassium in cats has since acquired important physiologic and clinical relevance.[114–116] Although D'Silva emphasized the rapid rise in the serum potassium that followed a bolus injection of epinephrine (now felt to be a consequence of transient hepatic discharge of potassium by alpha-adrenergic stimulation),[117–119] of greater significance was the sustained "after-fall" in serum potassium that he observed. This secondary decrease in potassium was found to persist throughout a 1 hour infusion of epinephrine.[120]

Since epinephrine inhibited the renal excretion of potassium,[121,122] its late hypokalemic action was attributed to net uptake of potassium by extrarenal tissues. Indeed, *in vivo* limb studies in dogs[123] and humans,[124,125] as well as tissue analysis and ion flux studies, supported accelerated uptake of potassium, primarily in skeletal muscle,[126] but also in liver[126] and heart,[127] in response to epinephrine. *In vitro*, epinephrine was demonstrated to stimulate potassium uptake, as well as sodium efflux, by isolated skeletal muscle in both rats[128,129] and humans.[128] A similar effect was present in rat diaphragm,[130] cat cardiac muscle,[131] and frog sartorius muscle.[132]

Because epinephrine may influence insulin secretion, it was necessary to show that its hypokalemic effect was independent of insulin.[133,134] Independence from renin-mediated aldosterone release was established by the lowering of potassium despite nephrectomy.[135,136] Since extrarenal potassium disposal was impaired when nephrectomized rats were subjected to adrenalectomy or to chemical sympathectomy,[93] both circulating adrenomedullary epinephrine, as well as peripheral sympathetic nervous activity, appeared to be important sources of sympathetic influence on potassium.

Beta-Adrenergic Effects

Epinephrine stimulates both alpha- and beta-adrenergic receptors.[137] The conclusion that its hypokalemic action was a result of beta-adrenergic stimulation derived from experiments many years later employing beta-agonists and beta-antagonists.[119,123] Isoproterenol, a nonspecific beta-agonist, reproduced the prolonged hypokalemia earlier observed by D'Silva, and this effect was reversed by the beta-adrenergic-antagonist propranolol; likewise, epinephrine's effects on cation flux were blocked by beta-antagonists.[1,114]

Beta-agonists and -antagonists have been used to establish that the stimulating effect of catecholamines on potassium uptake is mediated by the beta2-receptor subtype.[138,139] Epinephrine's effect on potassium is prevented by the presence of nonselective beta-antagonists such as propranolol[1,115,123,131,141–143] and timolol,[144] as well as by the nonspecific alpha-beta blocker labetalol.[145] Less reversal occurs with the partially beta1-selective-antagonists metoprolol[146] and atenolol.[144] No effect on potassium appears to be produced by the more specific beta1-antagonist practolol.[131,147] In addition, the selective beta2-antagonists butoxamine[138,148] and ICI-118551[149,150] are able to block the hypokalemic action of beta-agonists.

Numerous studies of beta-agonists have revealed that several beta2-agonists, including salbutamol,[151–155] terbutaline,[136,156–158] fenoterol,[159] and ritodrine[156] lower potassium levels, unlike the beta1-agonist ITP,[131] which has no effect. These pharmacologic studies therefore provide strong support for beta2 mediation of adrenergic effects to enhance potassium disposal.

Mechanism of Action

The specific cellular mechanism by which cell surface beta2-receptor stimulation augments transcellular potassium uptake in affected tissues has been evaluated in detail. Compelling evidence exists to support the proposal of Clausen[114] that beta2-stimulation initiates cyclic AMP formation,[160] which leads to activation of the sodium pump (Na,K-ATPase), and therefore electrogenic sodium efflux accompanied by potassium uptake.[161] Beta receptors are known to stimulate adenylate cyclase,[38,160,162] enhancing conversion of intracellular ATP to cyclic AMP.[163] Linkage of beta receptors and cyclic AMP is supported by the ability of theophylline to potentiate the effect of epinephrine on cation transport and membrane potential,[114] as well as by the increase in membrane potential that dibutyryl cyclic AMP and theophylline produce in rat diaphragm muscle.[164] Epinephrine, in stimulating cation transport, is well known to produce hyperpolarization of membranes in skeletal muscle.[114]

The sodium pump of muscle cells and lipocytes is activated by cyclic AMP. For example, Na,K-ATPase activity in smooth muscle membrane fragments is enhanced by exposure to cyclic AMP.[165] The most compelling evidence that catecholamine-mediated potassium influx involves the beta-adrenergic system through activation of the sodium pump, however, are the demonstrations in a series of experiments that potassium influx occurs as active movement of the cation against its electrochemical gradient[166]; ouabain blocks the ability of epinephrine to promote potassium influx in rat soleus muscle[129]; epinephrine markedly increases the ouabain-sensitive 22Na efflux by stimulating the Na—K pump in frog skeletal muscle, and this effect is blocked by propranolol[167]; epinephrine produces membrane hyperpolarization and transient decreases in extracellular potassium and intracellular sodium, which is blocked by ouabain, in isolated rat soleus muscle and human intercostal muscle[128]; and isoproterenol directly stimulates the Na—K pump in isolated rabbit myocytes.[168] While the specific sequence of events linking beta-adrenergic stimulation to sodium pump activity has not been delineated, phosphorylation of some portion of the sodium pump after beta2-receptor stimulation is presumably involved.[166] Beta-adrenergic agents also stimulate the cellular uptake of potassium via the Na—K—2Cl transporter in the skeletal muscle membrane of rats.[64]

There are numerous clinical examples showing that enhanced exogenous or endogenous beta-adrenergic stimulation augments extrarenal potassium uptake in humans. Whether high potassium levels can stimulate secretion of endogenous adrenomedullary epinephrine, and thereby form a homeostatic feedback loop, remains unresolved. Supraphysiologic levels of potassium *in vitro* can cause the release of catecholamines from isolated chromaffin cells[169] and perfused adrenal glands,[170] possibly related to the membrane depolarizing effect of a high potassium level. Induction of tyrosine hydroxylase, the rate-limiting enzyme in catecholamine biosynthesis,[171] by extremely high levels of potassium has also been observed. Reports that intra-arterial injections of KCl augment catecholamine release in cats[172] and in the dogfish shark[173] suggest a potential role for potassium as a catecholamine secretagogue *in vivo*.

Although specific stimulation of catecholamine release by potassium is not yet established, it is clear that physiologic elevations of endogenous catecholamines do enhance potassium uptake. Similar to the pharmacologic doses of epinephrine used in earlier animal reports of its protective effect during potassium-loading,[120,131,174] as well as its ability to lower basal potassium,[175] relatively small doses[1,140] have also been shown to enhance extrarenal disposal of an acute

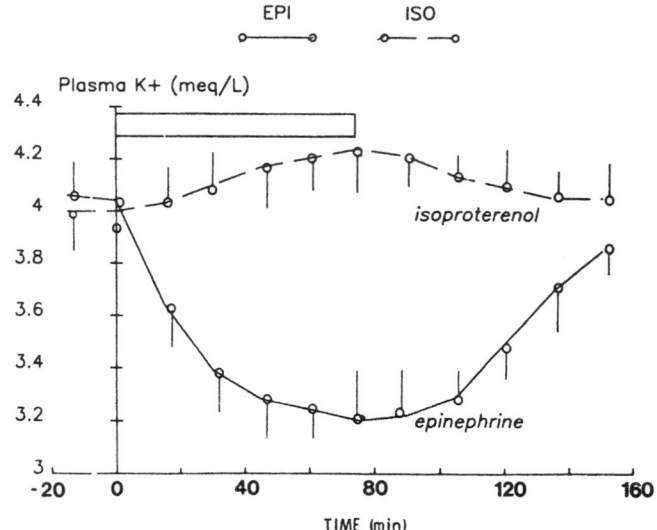

FIGURE 48.4 **Effect of epinephrine and isoproterenol infusions (long box) on the plasma potassium concentration.** The contrasting effects of the two beta-agonists probably are due to the relative beta2 selectivity of epinephrine at the dose given. Plasma epinephrine concentrations achieved by infusion were similar to those known to occur in myocardial infarction and other disorders. *Reprinted with permission from ref. [176].*

potassium-load. It has also been established that ambient potassium may be lowered when sustained epinephrine infusions[176] (Figure 48.4) elevate plasma concentrations of epinephrine to levels no higher than those observed in stressful conditions, such as myocardial infarction,[177] surgical stress,[178] and diabetic ketoacidosis.[179] By comparison, acute beta blockade does not appear to elevate fasting potassium levels,[176] suggesting that basal beta-adrenergic tone plays a limited role in potassium homeostasis in normal fasted individuals at rest.

It has recently been appreciated, however, that there are two common physiologic circumstances in which endogenous catecholamines could act to defend against increments in extracellular potassium concentration. The first of these is postprandial disposal of dietary potassium. Feeding is now known to be associated with stimulation of the sympathetic nervous system.[180] Since only half of the potassium ingested in a meal is normally excreted within 6 hours,[7] enhanced beta-adrenergic-mediated extrarenal potassium disposal may help to limit elevations of serum potassium in the immediate postprandial period. In conjunction with enhanced potassium uptake due to insulin release, this mechanism would be particularly important in subjects at risk for hyperkalemia for any reason.

The second circumstance is the dramatic effect of catecholamine release during vigorous exertion to moderate the acute physiological hyperkalemia of

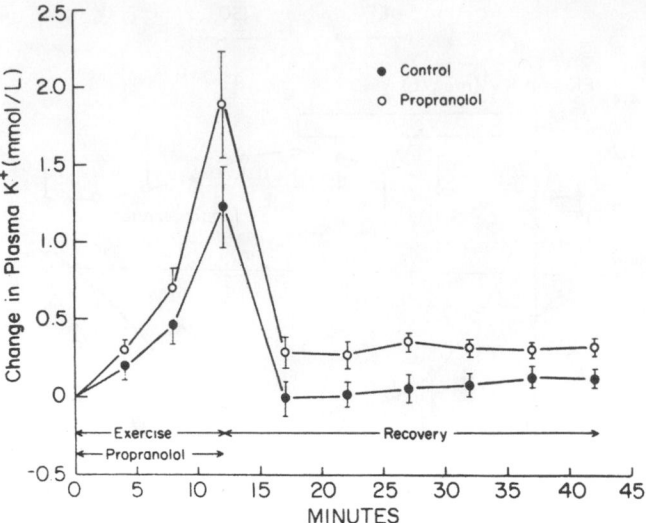

FIGURE 48.5 Effect of adrenergic blockade on the plasma potassium concentration during vigorous exercise and recovery. Beta-blockade with propranolol potentiated the rise of plasma potassium at peak exercise and prolonged its elevation during recovery. In the same subjects, alpha blockade with phentolamine was shown to lower the peak plasma potassium level, as well as the overall potassium curve. *Reprinted with permission from ref. [182].*

exercise. Catecholamines circulate at high levels during vigorous exercise, and the associated short-term elevation of potassium that is released into the circulation from working muscles is exaggerated by beta block-ade[181,182] (Figure 48.5), suggesting that endogenous beta-adrenergic activity does protect against extreme hyperkalemia during exhaustive exercise. In this context, it is of particular interest that training leads to upregulation of the content of the Na,K-ATPase,[183] which serves to mitigate the rise in extracellular potassium concentration relative to the work performed.[184] Another mechanism that might mitigate the rise in extracellular potassium seen during exercise is AMP-activated protein kinase. This cellular enzyme, which is normally stimulated by exercise or ischemia, has been demonstrated to produce a decrease in plasma potassium when stimulated chemically in the rat.[185] This decrease does not appear, however, to be mediated by the Na,K-ATPase, and may instead be secondary to diminished efflux of potassium from the intracellular compartment.

Alpha-Adrenergic Effects

The fact that opposing alpha- and beta-adrenergic influences have in the past been reported on smooth muscle tone,[186] glucoregulatory hormones,[187] presynaptic membrane receptors,[188] and changes in intracellular second messengers[160,189] suggests the role of alpha-adrenergic agonists in potassium homeostasis. As noted

previously, the early rise in extracellular potassium emphasized by D'Silva in 1934[113] was later attributed to alpha-mediated hepatic potassium release by the mixed alpha- and beta-agonist epinephrine.[119] This initial rise in potassium could be prevented by alpha blockade.[119] In addition, phenylephrine, a pure alpha-agonist, was observed to cause a sustained increase in potassium in dogs.[119,190]

When phenylephrine was infused into normal human subjects who were challenged with an intravenous potassium-load, the overall rise in plasma potassium was augmented by about 50%,[2] despite no change in insulin, renin, aldosterone or urinary potassium. In separate studies, addition of the alpha-antagonist phentolamine blocked the phenylephrine effect on potassium disposal. Neither alpha stimulation nor blockade appeared to affect the concentration of potassium in the absence of potassium-loading.

Other evidence suggests that the alpha effect might directly contribute to potassium homeostasis in certain circumstances. Alpha-receptor stimulation during vigorous exercise contributes to the acute rise in potassium that is maximal at peak exercise, and limits the dramatic fall due to potassium re-uptake during recovery.[182] Furthermore, during potassium depletion in rats, the sodium—potassium pump of skeletal muscle is suppressed by an increase in alpha-adrenergic activity mediated by nerves, an action that would mitigate the expected fall in plasma potassium concentration.[33] It is therefore speculated that enhanced alpha-agonist activity might act to preserve potassium similarly during a variety of acute illnesses, such as myocardial infarction[176] or delirium tremens,[191] where catecholamine stimulation of both beta- and alpha-receptors may coexist. Unopposed stimulation of alpha receptors may contribute to the impairment of potassium disposal caused by beta-receptor blockade.

Dopamine

The infusion of dopamine is known to augment glomerular filtration rate, renal plasma flow, osmolar clearance, sodium excretion,[192] and potassium excretion[193] in normal humans and animals. Levodopa, the metabolic precursor of dopamine, has also been reported to enhance renal potassium excretion,[194,195] and an increase in endogenous dopamine produced by protein feeding has been associated with augmented kaliuresis.[196] On the other hand, the dopamine antagonist metoclopramide also increases potassium excretion, an action ascribed to its blockade of tonic dopaminergic inhibition of aldosterone release.[197] Whether the dopaminergic system plays a role in extrarenal potassium homeostasis remains uncertain. Both dopamine and dobutamine lower plasma potassium when infused into anesthetized dogs, but only by a few tenths of a mEq per liter.[198] While some studies demonstrate enhanced extrarenal potassium uptake into cells following administration of metoclopramide,[199–201] others demonstrate no such effect of either metoclopramide[202–204] or the dopamine agonist bromocriptine.[202,203,205] The discrepancy between these studies may well be attributed, at least in part, to the fact that metoclopramide is a nonspecific antagonist of dopamine.[206] The determination of the role, if any, of the dopaminergic system in extrarenal potassium homeostasis must await studies employing specific dopamine antagonists.

Clinical Implications

The clinical significance of epinephrine-induced hypokalemia is underscored by reports of hypokalemia occurring during acute illnesses, such as myocardial infarction, as well as during medical treatment with beta-agonists.[207] Struthers et al.[144] discovered that when epinephrine infusion produced circulating epinephrine levels similar to those found after myocardial infarction, the serum potassium fell from 4.06 to 3.22 mEq/liter in normal volunteers. This ability of small doses of epinephrine to diminish potassium levels was confirmed by Brown et al.[176] In this context, the frequency of hypokalemia during acute myocardial infarction has been observed to be 8 to 30%.[208–211] Concomitant therapy with diuretics may further increase the frequency of hypokalemia during myocardial infarction,[212,213] as it appears to do in normal subjects who are experimentally infused with epinephrine.[214]

Because several studies have suggested that hypokalemia is an independent risk factor for cardiac arrhythmias in patients with acute myocardial infarction, these observations may have clinical relevance. A higher incidence of atrial fibrillation[215] and ventricular arrhythmias are reported in hypokalemic compared with normokalemic patients during infarction.[209,216] In one report,[210] ventricular tachycardia or fibrillation increased three-fold (to 35%), and hospital mortality doubled in hypokalemic patients with myocardial infarction.

It must be appreciated, however, that the hypokalemia reported during earlier studies of epinephrine infusion occurred when high concentrations of plasma epinephrine were sustained by infusion. Whether elevations of plasma epinephrine during acute myocardial infarction are similarly sustained, rather than transient,[177] is uncertain. The contribution of circulating epinephrine to the hypokalemia that may occur during this form of acute illness therefore remains hypothetical. Nonetheless, pharmacologic data do suggest that such acutely ill patients may be protected from the hypokalemia that is sometimes associated with myocardial infarction by the use of beta blockers.[142,143,217] Whether the beneficial effect of beta blockade reported in this setting is due to diminution in hypokalemia-related arrhythmias is not known. That hypokalemia is not more prevalent in the setting of acute myocardial infarction may, in part, be a consequence of a simultaneous elevation in plasma norepinephrine, suggesting alpha-receptor stimulation that might antagonize the effect of epinephrine on potassium homeostasis.

Transient lowering of potassium levels has also been reported in other acute medical conditions[218–221] in which catecholamines might stimulate beta-adrenergic receptors capable of increasing cellular uptake of potassium. Pharmacologic therapy employing beta2-agonists such as terbutaline, ritodrine, and salbutamol to prevent premature labor[151,155,156,158,222] may produce a substantial degree of hypokalemia. Administration of salbutamol and albuterol in the treatment of bronchospasm[153,223] may also produce unwanted hypokalemia. In this context, it is important to appreciate that administration of inhaled beta2-agonists to healthy volunteers in doses similar to those used by asthmatic patients during an acute attack has produced decrements of plasma potassium by as much as 0.9 mEq/liter.[159] These observations raise the disturbing possibility that such usage of these agents may be the explanation for the high incidence of sudden death in adolescent asthmatics.[224] Hypokalemia in this setting might be further exaggerated by the concomitant use of theophylline[225] or other methylxanthines.[226,227] Theophylline not only increases the level of circulatory catecholamines, but also enhances catechol stimulation of adenylate cyclase by blocking inhibitory adenosine receptors. Hypokalemia associated with elevated levels of epinephrine has also been reported in patients admitted for trauma,[228] and in normal subjects who received endotoxin.[229] Sepsis induced in rats, moreover, increases the activity of Na,K-ATPase.[230]

The clinical significance of the adrenergic nervous system in potassium balance is also evident in the well-established effect of beta-antagonists to elevate extracellular potassium concentration. An example is the acute effect of propranolol to exaggerate the hyperkalemia of vigorous exercise.[182] Some,[231–233] but not all,[234,235] investigators have reported a 10–15% increase in ambient plasma potassium during chronic beta blockade with nonselective agents. In addition, one study suggests that the serum potassium may rise above 6 mEq/liter in patients on nonselective beta-blockers at the time of open heart surgery.[236] Transient hyperkalemia has been reported after cyclosporine administration in patients on beta-blocking agents, but not when these are omitted.[237] Patients receiving succinylcholine anesthesia may also be at risk for the development of hyperkalemia.[238] Patients with end-stage renal failure on dialysis, moreover, regularly exhibit an increase in predialysis potassium of about 1 mEq/L when treated with propranolol.[239] Despite the clinical relevance of these studies describing an increase in extracellular potassium concentration in a variety of clinical conditions in patients receiving beta-blockers, it is important to realize that beta-blockers are unlikely to produce any significant increment in potassium concentration in subjects in whom the other mechanisms of potassium homeostasis are intact.

Since some studies do substantiate the anticipated absence of effect on potassium of cardioselective beta1-antagonists,[236,240,241] selected groups of patients at risk for hyperkalemia might be protected from significant elevations in potassium due to beta blockade by the use of such selective agents. Such patients include those with diabetes mellitus, hypoaldosteronism, and renal failure.

THYROID

Thyroid hormones enhance the activity of Na, K-ATPase in muscle cells,[242] accelerating the extrarenal disposal of potassium.[243] A portion of this effect can be ascribed to upregulation of beta-adrenergic receptors and an increase in beta-adrenergic responsiveness, but there appears to be a direct effect on cellular Na, K-ATPase as well.[243] Hypokalemic paralysis occasionally complicates thyrotoxicosis; in such cases urinary excretion of potassium is always low, reinforcing the hypothesis that the low serum potassium reflects a shift of potassium from the extracellular to the intracellular compartment rather than urinary losses of potassium. The hypokalemia and paralysis respond to the administration of beta-adrenergic-blocking agents.[244] This syndrome has been reported many times in Orientals, but is extremely rare in Caucasians and Blacks. It is not, moreover, associated with the inherited mutations in the calcium and sodium ion channels reported to cause familial hypokalemic periodic paralysis, but may in some cases be associated with a mutation in a channel mediating potassium efflux.[245] Hyperkalemia has been reported in hypothyroid dogs after exercise, but not in humans with hypothyroidism.[246]

ACID−BASE

Although acid−base balance affects potassium excretion by the kidney, shifts of potassium in and out of body cells are the initial way in which acid−base disturbances alter serum potassium. These movements are influenced by a variety of factors, including the changes in extracellular and intracellular pH, the degree of cellular buffering, the nature of the anion accompanying H^+, and the associated changes in hormonal and neural regulators of potassium uptake, including insulin and catecholamines.

The concentration of potassium in plasma tends to vary in the same direction as that of free hydrogen ions,[27,247−249] so that acidosis promotes hyperkalemia and alkalosis promotes hypokalemia. Since approximately 40% of the acid buffering capacity of the body is provided by intracellular proteins, largely in muscle cells,[250] and since potassium is the chief intracellular cation of muscle, the release of intracellular potassium is to be expected as a consequence of the intracellular buffering of hydrogen ions. Conversely, with repair of acidosis or during alkalosis, potassium will tend to move into cells. This exchange of K^+ for H^+ is not necessarily equimolar, and the routes across the plasma membrane that are responsible for such transfers have not been completely delineated. A simple reciprocal exchange of K^+ and H^+ via a single plasma membrane transporter has not been described in muscle cells.

Hydrogen Ion

The importance of pH in affecting internal potassium distribution during acidosis was demonstrated in early studies.[251−254] Fenn and Cobb[247] reported in 1934 that potassium exited from skeletal muscle *in vitro* when the bath pH was lowered, and moved into the tissue when blood at physiologic pH was substituted for acidic medium. They invoked the Donnan equilibrium to account for similarity in the intracellular to extracellular ratios of hydrogen and potassium ions, so that a decrease in that ratio produced by acidosis would be associated with a decrease in the ratio for potassium − that is, an increase in extracellular K^+. *In vivo* as well, an approximately linear relationship appears to exist between the potassium gradient and the pH gradient across muscle cell membranes, as predicted by the Donnan effect.[255,256] Nevertheless, the shifts in potassium observed in experimental situations are not always fully explained, either by the Donnan effect or by changes in membrane potential.[256,257]

Since the ratio Ki/Ke for skeletal muscle is approximately 30, the maintenance of a similar hydrogen ion ratio between intracellular and extracellular fluid would require an intracellular pH of approximately 5.92. However, intracellular pH is actually in the range of 6.9−7.0, so that the intracellular to extracellular proton ratio is only approximately 3 rather than 30. The major reason for this is the operation of the amiloride-sensitive $Na^+—H^+$ antiporter, which transports H^+ out of cells by a secondary active mechanism that ultimately derives its energy from ATP via the Na,K-ATPase of plasma membranes.

Moreover, the direction of the movement of potassium during acute acid—base disorders is not uniform among various tissues.[257] During acute respiratory acidosis, potassium moves out of the cells in muscle and liver, but into cardiac muscle. Yet, in both skeletal and cardiac muscle, the ratio of intracellular to extracellular hydrogen ion concentration falls. As will be seen subsequently, powerful evidence has been adduced under both *in vitro* and *in vivo* conditions suggesting that, in some circumstances, the ionic ratios of hydrogen and potassium can be dissociated and transmembrane fluxes of potassium change in the face of a stable pH gradient.

Inhibition of the sodium—potassium pump of plasma membranes by an acid pH contributes importantly to the relationship between acidosis and plasma potassium. In every case in which it has been measured, an increase in plasma potassium associated with systemic acidosis is accompanied by a fall in intracellular potassium. The optimal pH for mammalian Na,K-ATPase is 7.5—7.6, whereas intracellular pH of muscle is 6.9—7.2.[258] The effect of pH on the activity of the sodium—potassium pump is exerted from the intracellular, rather than the extracellular, side of the membrane.[259,260] In bladder epithelial cells, for example, a reduction of intracellular pH by 0.3 units, from pH 7.2 to 6.9, reduced pump activity to about 70% of that at pH 7.2. On the other hand, alkalinizing the cell interior to pH 7.5 led to a 35% increase in sodium-pump activity.[260]

In addition to a direct effect of pH on the sodium—potassium transport enzyme, an indirect mechanism might involve the linked operation of the Na-H antiporter and the Na,K-ATPase. An attractive mechanism to explain the shift of potassium out of cells that occurs in acidosis involves the linked operation of these two transporters. Both of these transporters are present in the plasma membranes of most cells, including skeletal muscle. Acidification of the extracellular fluid would be expected to slow the rate at which hydrogen ions leave the cell and sodium ions enter, via the Na-H antiporter. The resultant decrease in intracellular sodium concentration would slow the Na-K pump, reduce active uptake of potassium by cells, and increase the concentration of potassium in extracellular fluid. A prediction of this hypothesis is that amiloride, which blocks the Na-H antiporter, would prevent the hyperkalemia produced by acidosis. It is not yet known whether this is the case, but amiloride does block the extracellular acidosis produced by KCl infusions.[261]

Finally, intracellular acidosis appears to open ATP-sensitive potassium channels in skeletal muscle by reducing the degree of channel inhibition by ATP, an action that might accelerate efflux of K^+ from muscle cells during anoxia or extreme acidosis.[262]

Mineral Acids

Acute mineral acidosis, produced by infusing HCl or NH_4Cl, elevated plasma potassium by an average of 0.7 mEq/liter per 0.1 unit decrease in blood pH, in 14 different studies summarized by Adrogue and Madias.[257] The results of these studies were extremely variable, however, ranging from 0.24 to 1.67 mEq/liter per 0.1 pH unit.

One reason for the variability in these reports is that the effect of mineral acid infusions on plasma potassium depends on the duration of the acidosis.[27,254,263,264] Immediately following an acute acid infusion there is a marked fall in extracellular pH and bicarbonate, followed by a gradual rise over the next 2 hours or so, as tissue buffering and respiratory compensation moderate the initial changes in blood pH.[249,250,254,264] Plasma potassium begins to rise early in the course of the infusion and increases progressively as buffering takes place, so that its concentration does not change in parallel with the change in pH. Late in the course of an acute acid-load, when cell buffers have been exhausted and intracellular pH drops sharply, plasma potassium rises more steeply.

It might be expected that the hyperkalemic response to an acid-load would be influenced by the state of muscle potassium. Experimental potassium depletion induced by DOCA (mean plasma K^+ 1.9 mEq/liter) did indeed attenuate the increase in plasma potassium produced by metabolic acidosis, but did not prevent it, and the percentage rise in plasma potassium from baseline induced by NH_4Cl acid-loading was not significantly different from that of controls.[265]

Clinical observations on the endogenous mineral acidosis of uremia, due to retention of sulfate and phosphate, suggest that the change in potassium that is observed when acidosis is corrected is of the magnitude expected in experimental mineral acidosis.[17,266]

Organic Acids

That changes in acidity are not the sole determinant of the kalemic response to acidosis is indicated by the disparate effects which mineral acidosis and nonmineral acidosis have on potassium. In humans and animals, infusion of organic acids such as acetic, lactic or beta-hydroxybutyric acid produce far smaller elevations of potassium than hydrochloric acid.[264,267—270]

The prevailing hypothesis is that the anions of organic acids, either by readily penetrating the intracellular compartment,[257] by entering cells as intact molecules[271] or by being formed endogenously within cells,[272] minimize the necessity for potassium cations to leave cells in exchange for hydrogen ions.[273] The addition of HCl to rat diaphragms *in vitro* results in a loss of potassium from the muscle,[253] whereas when extracellular pH is lowered by addition of acetic acid, beta-hydroxybutyric acid or lactic acid, no shift of potassium out of the cell is observed.[271]

For similar degrees of clinical severity, less elevation of serum potassium occurs with endogenous organic acidosis encountered in ill patients than with mineral acidosis, although the correlation of pH and serum potassium in clinical states of organic acidosis is further complicated by prior total body potassium depletion, oliguric renal failure, hypercatabolism, and other factors.[273] Ketone acids, for example, stimulate the secretion of insulin by the normal pancreas, while suppressing the secretion of glucagon. Infusions of hydrochloric acid, on the other hand, do not stimulate insulin secretion, but enhance plasma glucagon,[102] which in turn tends to elevate the serum potassium. The sympathoadrenal system, which is strongly activated in most clinical states accompanied by organic acidosis (e.g., diabetic or alcoholic ketoacidosis, and the lactic acidosis of circulatory shock), plays an important role in minimizing hyperkalemia, because of the hypokalemic action of beta-adrenergic stimulation. Moderately severe potassium depletion (as occurs in diabetic ketoacidosis) itself attenuates the increase in plasma potassium induced by metabolic acidosis.[265]

Untreated severe diabetic ketoacidosis is characterized by marked deficits (200–300 mEq) in total body potassium,[274] owing primarily to coincident potassium losses from the gastrointestinal tract or kidneys. Despite these losses, hypokalemia is uncommon, present in only 4% of episodes in one series,[275] probably because of concomitant acidosis. Serum potassium is usually normal or elevated at presentation,[276] but falls during successful treatment. Hypokalemia during recovery from diabetic ketoacidosis is most prominent in patients who initially received sodium bicarbonate.

Since insulin plays a significant role in cellular shifts of potassium, lack of insulin is presumably important in promoting hyperkalemia during diabetic ketoacidosis,[277] as it is in patients with hyperosmolar nonketotic coma, who may have severe hyperkalemia without acidosis.[278]

Similar to uncontrolled diabetes, several factors in lactic acidosis complicate the effect of acidemia *per se* on serum potassium. These include volume-depletion, prerenal azotemia, hypercatabolism, concomitant diabetes, catecholamine effects, and external potassium imbalance.[279] Although severe hyperkalemia is unusual in lactic acidosis, Perez et al.[273] have pointed out the absence of detailed studies on potassium in this varied disorder. In experimental lactic acid infusion in animals,[270] and in uncomplicated post-seizure lactic acidosis in humans,[272,280,281] potassium does not increase with the appearance of acidosis. However, in other forms of lactic acidosis, such as those earlier encountered due to phenformin therapy in diabetes,[276] and in other forms not associated with tissue hypoxia, mild elevation of potassium may occur.[272] Renal insufficiency may be a contributing factor in such patients. Most patients with alcoholic ketoacidosis have a normal extracellular potassium concentration,[282,283] although there is significant variability. The effects of rarer forms of organic acidosis on internal potassium homeostasis have been reviewed elsewhere in detail.[273]

Respiratory Acidosis

The effect of acute respiratory acidosis in elevating plasma potassium is, in general, smaller in magnitude than that of metabolic acidosis, though some effect can usually be detected.[248,255,284,285] A rise varying from 0.06 to 0.3 mEq K^+/liter per 0.1 pH unit was detected in 22 studies of mild to moderate respiratory acidosis.[257] More severe experimental acidosis, provoked by inhaled concentrations of CO_2 as high as 30%, induce more pronounced hyperkalemia.[257] In anephric dogs, the initial effect on potassium is small, but after 2 hours respiratory acidosis may increase to the range observed in metabolic acidosis.[27] On the other hand, in *in vitro* experiments, when the extracellular medium bathing isolated rat diaphragms was acidified by raising the ambient CO_2 from 2 to 10%, no shift in potassium was observed,[271] consistent with the ability of carbonic acid to permeate cells, as do other organic acids. Chronic respiratory acidosis produced in dogs was not attended by hyperkalemia.[285]

The increase in serum potassium induced by severe respiratory acidosis in intact rats could be roughly approximated from the decrease in $(H^+)_i/(H^+)_o$, and was attributed to the importance of the Donnan effect in producing these changes.[255] In addition, it is very likely that sympathoadrenal stimulation plays a major role in modulating serum potassium during respiratory acidosis *in vivo*, since it is well-established that acute hypercapnia results in an intense sympathetic discharge and an increase in the plasma concentration of epinephrine.[257,286] Glycogenolysis induced by epinephrine probably contributes to the initial release of glucose and potassium from the liver with hypercapnia, noted by Fenn and Asano,[287] and the hypokalemic effect of beta-adrenergic stimulation is likely to blunt the movement of potassium out of skeletal muscle that would otherwise accompany acidosis. Probably for this reason, mild respiratory acidosis induced acutely in anesthetized patients was not found to elevate the plasma potassium,[288] although beta-adrenergic blockade produced marked hyperkalemia in hypercapneic animals.[289]

Bicarbonate

It has been suggested that the serum bicarbonate concentration, even at constant or "isohydric" pH, alters extrarenal potassium distribution and might account in part for the weak correlation between pH and serum potassium in many studies. Under conditions of constant blood pH, infusion of sodium bicarbonate appears to lower serum potassium,[257,290,291] and during acidosis in rats, potassium may correlate better with serum bicarbonate than with blood pH.[292] A similar correlation can be found in patients with hyperkalemia of diverse etiologies,[293] as well as in experimental acute ammonium chloride acidosis.[294] This has been taken to indicate that bicarbonate therapy, in addition to beneficially raising pH, corrects hyperkalemia directly, perhaps via intracellular transfer with the potassium cation.

Another explanation of the same data is that it is the quantity of acid buffered by cells, rather than the arterial pH, that governs the release of intracellular potassium. This would account for the fact that extracellular bicarbonate, rather than arterial pH, sometimes seems to exert an independent controlling influence on extracellular potassium. Effective buffering of an acid-load by intracellular and extracellular buffers, so as to produce a low serum bicarbonate and a normal arterial pH, involves the liberation of substantial amounts of potassium cations from intracellular proteins.[295] It can be inferred from the foregoing that alkali treatment of hyperkalemia should be most effective when the plasma bicarbonate is low and acidosis marked, and less so when plasma bicarbonate and pH are normal; this is indeed the case.[296] This result is also inherent in the finding that the changes in plasma potassium produced by metabolic alkalosis are smaller than those seen in metabolic acidosis.

Alkalosis

Metabolic and respiratory alkalosis are commonly associated with hypokalemia. In both, renal losses are important in initiating and perpetuating hypokalemia, but extrarenal adjustments are also involved. Acute alkalosis induced by infusions of sodium bicarbonate usually leads to a decrement in plasma potassium concentrations. The $\Delta(K)p/\Delta pH$ slope is usually smaller than that commonly observed in acute mineral acidosis, although the reported range is wide, from -0.09 to -0.42 mEq/liter per 0.1 pH unit.[257,297,298] The initial change is not attributable to kaliuresis. Acute respiratory alkalosis produces a comparable decrease in plasma potassium, although during voluntary overbreathing this fall may be counteracted by an increase in circulating norephinephrine which, as noted earlier, tends to increase plasma potassium.[299] It should be pointed out that most studies of extrarenal effects of metabolic alkalosis have involved the infusion of hypertonic solutions of sodium bicarbonate. Since hypertonicity itself promotes a rise in plasma potassium, this would tend to counteract any hypokalemic effect of alkalosis *per se*.

An intuitively appealing explanation for the extrarenal effect of alkalosis is replacement of H^+ associated with cellular buffers by potassium, in the reverse of the sequence discussed earlier by which acidosis releases intracellular potassium ions. Enhanced exchange of intracellular H^+ for extracellular Na^+ via the amiloride-sensitive Na^+-H^+ antiporter would accelerate cellular potassium accumulation by stimulating the Na, K-ATPase pump. In addition, intracellular alkalosis probably stimulates the sodium–potassium pump directly, as discussed earlier.

The combined effects of respiratory alkalosis on renal and extrarenal potassium handling commonly produce mild hypokalemia (around 3.0 mEq/liter) resistant to potassium replacement in hypocapneic patients who are artificially ventilated. Extreme hypocapneic alkalosis and hypokalemia, as seen in recently intubated patients who are overventilated, may produce serious cardiac arrhythmias.[300]

ALDOSTERONE

In addition to its action on the kidney to increase potassium excretion, aldosterone enhances potassium secretion into intestinal fluids and saliva. Aldosterone-induced colonic potassium secretion appears to occur through increased expression of luminal BK channels.[301] In chronic renal insufficiency, moreover, the colonic secretion of potassium is greatly enhanced.[302] In that sense, its effect on serum potassium can be said to have an extrarenal component. Aldosterone also has an independent action to accelerate renal acid excretion, and the consequent alkalosis itself has a secondary effect on cellular uptake of potassium. Apart from these mechanisms, there is no convincing evidence for a direct action of aldosterone to increase potassium uptake by muscle cells. For example, incubation of isolated rat diaphragms with aldosterone results in a loss, rather than a gain, of intracellular potassium.[303,304]

An extrarenal action of aldosterone has been suggested in the past, because of several lines of evidence. First, in experimental animals, hyperkalemia after adrenalectomy seemed not to be entirely accounted for by a positive balance of potassium.[305] Furthermore, the fall in plasma potassium accompanying the administration of mineralocorticoids was not necessarily associated with an increase in potassium excretion.[306–308] Interpretation of such data is complicated, because of the effect of adrenal medullary hormones on extrarenal potassium uptake, and the renal action of mineralocorticoids to retain sodium and excrete acid, resulting in expansion of extracellular fluid volume and alkalosis, both of which might secondarily lower serum potassium.

Long-term treatment of dogs by Young and Jackson[308] with high doses of aldosterone altered the relationship between plasma potassium and total body exchangeable potassium, so that at any level of exchangeable potassium, plasma potassium was lower than in untreated animals. In these experiments, however, mean plasma bicarbonate was significantly higher in aldosterone-treated dogs than in controls, leaving open the possibility that aldosterone-induced alkalosis influenced potassium distribution.

Bia et al.[135] gave intravenous potassium loads to adrenalectomized and nephrectomized rats, and found that the acute administration of aldosterone prior to infusing potassium blunted the hyperkalemia. The differences they observed, however, were small, and could have been completely accounted for by a modest increase in the potassium concentration of gastrointestinal secretions (e.g., an increase of 20 mEq/liter in 1 ml of intestinal fluid) caused by the known action of aldosterone to increase intestinal potassium secretion.

The role of mineralocorticoids in the disposition of an oral potassium-load was studied in anephric humans by Sugarman and Brown.[309] Anephric patients were given 0.5 mEq/kg of KCl after 72 hours of either mineralocorticoid treatment (10 mg DOCA daily) or spironolactone (300 mg daily). The rise in serum potassium was delayed by DOCA, but the difference from control experiments with spironolactone was most marked at 1 hour, much less pronounced at 2 and 3 hours, and not present at 24 hours, suggesting that the mineralocorticoid had delayed absorption of potassium from the gastrointestinal tract. Chronic administration of high doses of mineralocorticoids is said to diminish serum potassium slightly in anuric patients, perhaps because of an increase in stool potassium.[310]

Finally, Alexander and Levinsky[311] reported that chronic potassium-loading improved extrarenal disposal of an acute potassium-load given after a night's fast, an effect abolished by adrenalectomy and restored by chronic (but not acute) high-dose mineralocorticoid replacement. They postulated that chronic hyperaldosteronism acts directly by enhancing cellular uptake of an acute potassium-load.[311] Another interpretation was offered by Spital and Sterns.[26] These investigators showed that, when dietary potassium is withdrawn from rats previously fed a high-potassium diet, high rates of potassium excretion persist and "overshoot," causing these animals to become progressively more depleted of potassium than controls. This "paradoxical potassium depletion" is responsible, at least in part, for extrarenal potassium adaptation, by creating a sink of potassium-hungry cells that avidly take up potassium, and thereby blunt the increment in plasma potassium after an acute potassium-load. Hyperaldosteronism magnifies urinary potassium losses during fasting, and thus promotes potassium depletion, which in turn facilitates the uptake into muscle of an acute potassium-load.[312]

In summary, aldosterone and other mineralocorticoid hormones do accelerate the disposal of potassium, but probably not by a direct effect on muscle. The changes observed can be accounted for by the known actions of aldosterone on the renal and gastrointestinal transport of sodium and potassium, and the separate action of aldosterone to produce systemic alkalosis by enhancing acid excretion.

RENAL FAILURE

In states of mild-to-moderate chronic renal failure, the ability to excrete potassium is well maintained by an adaptive increase in the rate of fractional potassium excretion to levels near the maximal for subjects with normal renal function.[313,314] As renal function declines further, however, so does the ability to excrete potassium in a timely manner.[315] With advanced renal failure, potassium is retained longer[5] and dependence on extrarenal disposal becomes more critical.

Whether extrarenal potassium disposal is enhanced, normal or impaired in the setting of uremia remains controversial.[316] Studies in which an oral potassium load was given found that patients with chronic renal failure excreted only one quarter[9] to one-half[7,8] the amount of potassium excreted by subjects with normal renal function over a comparable period of time. Nonetheless, an exaggerated rise in serum potassium did not always occur.[7,9] Reports of impaired extrarenal disposal of an oral potassium-load in patients with chronic renal failure might be criticized, either because the patients had higher basal serum potassium concentrations or might have been more acidotic than the control subjects.[8,317,318] Another study that concluded that extrarenal potassium disposal was impaired in patients with chronic renal failure involved chronic rather than acute potassium-loading.[319] A more general criticism of studies administering oral potassium that might account for some of the discrepant conclusions, however, is the inherent difficulty of estimating the rate of gastrointestinal absorption of potassium in the setting of renal failure. With intravenous potassium-loading, however, most,[101,135,320] but not all[321] animal studies appear to show a discernible defect in extrarenal potassium disposal in the setting of renal failure. With rare exceptions,[320,322] however, these studies examined extrarenal potassium homeostasis immediately after acute nephrectomy, rather than in the uremic state.

If extrarenal potassium disposal is impaired in uremia, it cannot be a consequence of increased cellular potassium content or high total body potassium, since both are normal or low in this state.[323–328] Nor does there appear to be peripheral resistance to insulin-mediated potassium uptake,[329] despite the known resistance to the action of insulin on glucose metabolism in renal failure.[330] The chronic hyperinsulinemia of end-stage renal failure may afford some protection against hyperkalemia. Renin production, which might be expected to be suppressed in patients with end-stage renal disease, is normal or elevated in many patients. Furthermore, both hyperkalemia[27,331] and salt restriction[332] appear to stimulate aldosterone production adequately in the setting of chronic renal failure (in patients who do not have hyporeninemic hypoaldosteronism), and a lowering of the plasma potassium suppresses aldosterone secretion normally.[333]

Catecholamines circulate at increased levels in most,[334,335] but not all,[336] patients with renal failure. While it is likely that much, if not all, of this increase is a consequence of decreased renal excretion, the pressor and pulse responses to norepinephrine infusion have been reported to be impaired in renal failure.[334,336] Both intravenous[337] and inhaled[338] albuterol appear, however, to be effective and rapid therapeutic modalities to treat hyperkalemia in patients with advanced renal failure. If beta-adrenergic-mediated extrarenal potassium homeostasis is blunted in renal failure when compared with normal subjects,[339] it may well be in those whose endogenous plasma epinephrine levels are chronically elevated[340] or who are more acidemic. Contrarily, it should be appreciated that the administration of drugs that possess beta2-antagonist properties can produce significant hyperkalemia in patients with renal failure on dialysis.[239]

Impaired extrarenal disposal of potassium in uremia might conceivably be caused by high circulating levels of parathyroid hormone. Infusion of parathyroid hormone appears to impair extrarenal disposition of a potassium-load in nephrectomized rats,[341] an action ascribed to the enhancement of potassium efflux from cells produced by increasing intracellular calcium. Potassium tolerance in partially nephrectomized rats with chronic renal failure is improved by parathyroidectomy, and by administration of the calcium channel-blocker verapamil.[342]

Metabolic acidosis can impair cellular potassium uptake (see "Acid–Base"), and alkalinization has been demonstrated to reverse this effect in anuric patients.[318] Part of this effect of acidosis may be to diminish the activity of Na,K-ATPase, which has a pH optimum in the range of 7.5–7.6 in mammalian tissue.[258]

That the activity of the Na-K pump is impaired in the erythrocytes of some uremic subjects has been well-established.[343–349] The impairment is correlated with an increase in intracellular sodium of red blood cells. Also, the diminished pump activity is reversed when the red blood cells of uremic patients are incubated in normal plasma[344] or when the patients are dialyzed,[343,345,348,350] and the impairment is reproduced when normal erythrocytes are incubated in uremic plasma.[344,351] These studies suggest the presence of a circulating inhibitor of the Na-K pump in some uremics. Other investigators have reported a decrease in the number of pump sites, estimated by ouabain-binding, rather than in the activity of the pump (defined as the ion turnover rate per pump site) in the red blood cells of certain uremic patients.[352,353] Experimental uremia in rats decreases the Na,K-ATPase activity of skeletal muscle,[354] an effect reproduced by incubating normal muscle cells with uremic serum.[354] The excessive rise in plasma potassium exhibited by patients with chronic renal failure undergoing exercise is consistent, moreover, with an impairment in skeletal muscle Na,K-ATPase in humans with this condition,[355] although a higher baseline potassium concentration or a more acidotic state can be confounding variables in such studies.

MAGNESIUM

In a variety of clinical states, potassium-depletion accompanies magnesium-depletion. Among patients with hypokalemia, the coincidence of magnesium deficiency may range from less than 10%[356] to over 40%.[357,358] Clinical conditions with a high incidence of combined deficiencies in potassium and magnesium, such as diuretic administration, alcoholism, and diabetic ketoacidosis, generally involve a defect in renal conservation of potassium. Along with interest in the relationship between extrarenal magnesium and potassium balances[359] has come information on the relationship of their movements in and out of cells.[360]

Because potassium and magnesium are the principal intracellular cations, it is not surprising that an important physiologic relationship might exist between them. For each, reduced intracellular concentrations may exist in certain states of depletion, out of proportion to the reduction in serum levels.[361,362] Furthermore, a high correlation is found between magnesium and potassium concentrations in extrarenal tissues, such as skeletal muscle.[363] A deficiency of magnesium evokes potassium-depletion in animals and humans. In rats, however, serum potassium remains normal,[364] whereas in human subjects, hypokalemia is often observed.[357,361]

A specific effect of magnesium-depletion on potassium homeostasis can be deduced from experimental magnesium deficiency states in which magnesium deficiency is associated with renal potassium-wasting.[365] One proposed mechanism is of importance to their internal homeostasis, insofar as it would involve a direct effect of magnesium depletion on the ability of both renal and extrarenal cells to preserve their potassium.[359,366] It is known that experimental dietary magnesium depletion in rats results in loss of cellular potassium in cardiac as well as skeletal muscle.[367] Furthermore, during magnesium depletion in both animals[368] and humans,[365] the intracellular deficiency of potassium cannot be restored by provision of potassium alone; correction of the magnesium deficiency is required. Clinical combined depletion may play a role in cardiac arrhythmias seen in patients with alcoholism or on diuretics,[357,369] underscoring the importance of magnesium replacement in the correction of refractory hypokalemia and cellular potassium-depletion.

Two extrarenal mechanisms have been suggested: reduced Na,K-ATPase activity; and increased cell membrane permeability to potassium. Cellular potassium-depletion due to diminished active potassium uptake mediated by Na,K-ATPase might occur because this cation pump requires cellular magnesium.[258] Animal studies have shown that magnesium-depletion is associated with a reduced concentration of Na—K pump units in rat skeletal muscle.[370] Reduced ouabain-binding, indicative of a decreased number of Na—K pumps, has also been found in humans treated with diuretics who developed low muscle potassium concentrations associated with hypomagnesemia.[371] Additional data suggest that magnesium-depletion may also exert its effect on intracellular potassium through an impairment of the activity of the sodium-potassium pump *per se*, rather than on the number of pump sites per cell.[372]

The second proposed mechanism of potassium loss would involve effects of magnesium on membrane potassium channels. In mammalian heart cells and in a cultured insulin-secreting cell line investigated by the patch-clamp technique, physiologic concentrations of intracellular magnesium block outward current by inhibiting the opening of ATP-sensitive potassium channels.[373,374] Magnesium may therefore play an important role in the low conductance of the outward potassium current through these channels[375] under normal conditions. Such a direct effect of magnesium on potassium channels might result in cellular potassium-depletion during magnesium deficiency.

DRUGS

Medications are the primary etiologic factor in as many as one-third of cases of clinically significant hyperkalemia,[376–379] and are contributing factors in more than 60% of hyperkalemic episodes in hospitalized adults.[380] Potassium supplements, angiotensin-converting enzyme inhibitors, angiotensin-II receptor-antagonists, potassium-sparing diuretics, trimethoprim, pentamidine, heparin, and prostaglandin-suppressing drugs that induce hyporeninemic hypoaldosteronism account for most of these cases; relative to those, hyperkalemia due to drugs that alter internal potassium distribution would appear to be uncommon.[377,381] As is true for drug-induced hyperkalemia in general, the risk of significant hyperkalemia is substantially increased in patients with diabetes mellitus, renal insufficiency, hypoaldosteronism, and in the elderly. In most other cases, the rise in potassium is mild.[377]

Impaired Extrarenal Disposal

Hyperkalemia due to beta-adrenergic-blockers, the most common class of medications that elevate potassium by extrarenal mechanisms, was discussed in an earlier section. A small, transient increase in serum potassium usually occurs in patients given depolarizing muscle relaxants, such as succinylcholine.[382–385] Exaggerated increments, however, may occur in patients with central nervous system diseases, spinal cord injury, increased intracranial pressure, and a variety of other ailments.[379] In such pathological states, the acetylcholine receptors may be increased beyond the junctional area.[386] Because potassium efflux from muscle end plates occurs during normal depolarization, massive efflux of the cation from such sensitized muscle can account for the hyperkalemia noted in patients with neurologic motor deficits, tetanus or muscle damage.[387] Succinylcholine-induced hyperkalemia may also be seen with neuroleptic malignant syndrome[388] and skeletal muscle metastasis of a rhabdomyosarcoma.[389] Why burn patients and those with intracranial lesions not involving upper motor neurons[384] are also at risk is less apparent. In patients at risk, succinylcholine should be used with caution and in the smallest dose possible, and with pretreatment by nondepolarizing muscle relaxants.[387]

Muscle cell breakdown may also result in hyperkalemia in patients who develop myositis due to the HMG-CoA reductase inhibitor, lovastatin.[390] Such reactions are more likely when lovastatin is administered in combination with gemfibrozil, cyclosporine, and nicotinic acid.[391] HMG-CoA reductase inhibitors are commonly used in patients already predisposed to hyperkalemia due to diabetes mellitus or renal insufficiency.

Arginine HCl, in doses used for the correction of metabolic alkalosis, may increase serum potassium.[392] When this cationic amino acid is taken up by cells, potassium is displaced into the extracellular fluid. Hyperkalemia is more likely in patients with renal failure[393] who are unable to excrete this endogenous potassium-load, and in those with liver failure who are unable to metabolize the administered arginine normally.[394] The magnitude of potassium rise in normal subjects is under 1 mEq/liter[392]; it is not closely correlated with pH, and may occur in patients before correction of the alkalosis is accomplished.[394] Lysine HCl may also increase serum potassium levels. The antifibrinolytic agent epsilon aminocaproic acid (Amicar) has been reported to cause hyperkalemia as well,[395] although the mechanism underlying this effect is unclear.

Trivial increments in potassium may also occur at therapeutic or mildly toxic levels of cardiac glycosides.[396,397] Blockade of Na,K-ATPase-mediated potassium uptake with normal doses of digitalis has minimal effect on the serum potassium, since glycoside binding to skeletal muscle, the major body reservoir of potassium, is limited. At toxic concentrations of digitalis, however, such as following massive overdose, marked hyperkalemia is well-described and indicates a poor prognosis.[398,399] The toxic concentration of digitalis also prevents standard treatment of the hyperkalemia with calcium. Although no significant effect to retard potassium disposal in normal subjects with therapeutic digitalis levels has been published, it is likely that such an effect may exacerbate hyperkalemia in patients at risk. In patients with renal failure, for example, even modest digoxin toxicity resulting from therapeutic doses is reported to cause hyperkalemia.[400] In fact, of drugs known to induce hyperkalemia, digoxin was the most frequently encountered among patients with hyperkalemic episodes,[380] and nearly one quarter of these had toxic digoxin levels.

Nonsteroidal anti-inflammatory drugs produce hyperkalemia best attributed to their antikaliuretic effect, which results in positive potassium balance.[401,402] No impairment of extrarenal potassium homeostasis has been directly demonstrated.[380,403,404]

Lithium intoxication in animals is associated with a progressive elevation in serum potassium and electrocardiogram abnormalities characteristic of hyperkalemia. However, only at concentrations of plasma lithium (>10 mEq/liter) many times the therapeutic lithium levels (1 mEq/liter) attained in manic-depressive patients[405] do these changes occur. Increments in serum potassium of under 1 mEq/liter have been reported during chronic lithium therapy,[406] but frank hyperkalemia is rarely observed.[407] Lithium may displace intracellular potassium from human red blood cells and from skeletal muscle.[406] Amphotericin B (including the liposomal formulation) can cause severe hyperkalemia due to potassium released from the intracellular compartment when the dose is excessive, the rate of infusion is rapid or renal function is impaired.[408]

Enhanced Extrarenal Disposal

Drug-induced lowering of serum potassium by exogenous insulin and beta-adrenergic-agonists was described in detail earlier. Increased circulating catecholamine levels, as well as enhancement of catechol stimulation of adenylate cyclase, also appear to mediate in part the effect of methylxanthine derivatives such as theophylline. Hypokalemia due to beta-adrenergic stimulation may occur with severe theophylline toxicity[409] in humans. Propranolol is reported to block hypokalemia due to theophylline toxicity in the dog.[409] Whether therapeutic levels of aminophylline are important in acutely lowering serum potassium in humans is unclear.[410] Other methylxanthines, such as caffeine, might also be expected to decrease potassium concentrations,[227] not only by stimulating release of catecholamines, but also by their blockade of high-affinity (A1) adenosine receptors, which normally act to inhibit adenylate cyclase.

Several clinical studies have reported minor decreases in serum potassium levels in patients treated with calcium-antagonists, sometimes associated with increased urinary potassium losses.[411] Severe hypokalemia with heart block may complicate overdosage of verapamil.[412] Enhanced extrarenal potassium disposal has been demonstrated with the calcium channel-blockers verapamil, nifedipine, and nitrendipine.[413–415] In one study,[415] pretreatment with either verapamil or nifedipine reduced by about 40% the increment in plasma potassium produced over 1 hour by the infusion of KCl in nephrectomized rats. The effect was not mediated by changes in pH, bicarbonate, insulin, aldosterone or the alpha- or beta-adrenergic systems. Diltiazem has been shown to reduce the interdialytic rate of increase in plasma potassium in patients with end-stage renal disease.[416] Diminished calcium-mediated potassium efflux from cells may be responsible, since increased intracellular calcium enhances potassium permeability *in vitro* (the Gardos effect)[417] in erythrocytes and other cells.[418] While this action would lower plasma potassium, the net effect of calcium channel-blockers in clinical practice is complicated by the fact that these agents also inhibit secretion of aldosterone,[419,420] which in turn would tend to produce potassium retention.

The increased use of thiopental infusions to achieve therapeutic barbiturate coma has been associated with extreme degrees of hypokalemia secondary to enhanced cellular uptake of potassium. Serious rebound hyperkalemia has ensued, moreover, following the administration of potassium to correct the hypokalemia and discontinuation of the thiopental.[421,422] The mechanism responsible for the hypokalemia is unknown, but could involve inhibition of voltage-dependent neuronal potassium currents. Overdosage of the antimalarial chloroquine has also been associated with hypokalemia, presumably from enhanced cellular uptake, but such cases are often confounded by concomitant administration of other medications.[423] High-dose intravenous methotrexate has been associated with the rapid development of tetraparesis and marked hypokalemia in one patient that appeared to be caused by enhanced extrarenal disposal of potassium.[424]

OTHER FACTORS

Two other factors that may clinically elevate serum potassium levels by affecting extrarenal potassium homeostasis are hyperosmolarity and cellular necrosis. Less well-described are the effects of barium, cesium, and body hypothermia to lower serum potassium levels by extrarenal shifts. A sudden increase in cell mass produced by rapid proliferation, moreover, may sequester potassium intracellularly and result in hypokalemia.

Hyperosmolarity

Hypertonic potassium-free solutions administered to normal human subjects fail to lower plasma potassium, despite expanding the extracellular fluid compartment.[425] This observation suggests that plasma potassium is maintained during the infusion by movement of potassium out of cells, impelled by an increase in its intracellular concentration, because of contraction of the intracellular volume. Potassium levels are maintained even when dilutional acidosis is prevented by incorporating bicarbonate into the hypertonic infusion.[426]

A modest rise in plasma potassium concentration (0.3–0.6 mEq/liter) can be produced in normal subjects by moderate increases in tonicity (10 mOsm/kg).[427] The effect is of clinical importance chiefly in diabetics, in whom plasma tonicity can be raised by 40–50 mOsm/kg during hyperglycemia, and who lack insulin-mediated potassium uptake. Glucose-induced hyperkalemia is more pronounced in diabetics deficient in aldosterone secretion[428] or during treatment with captopril,[429] but it may also be observed in diabetics with normal aldosterone responses. The standard 100 g oral glucose tolerance test produced an average increment of 1.3 mEq/liter in plasma potassium in four such patients.[430] The effect of hyperosmolarity on potassium homeostasis may also be present in patients with cerebral edema or with renal insufficiency when treated with large quantities of hypertonic mannitol.

Cellular Necrosis

When renal excretion and extrarenal disposal of potassium are exceeded, release of intracellular potassium into the extracellular compartment during cellular necrosis will result in hyperkalemia. The most common sources are muscle, tumor cells, and erythrocytes.

Traumatic muscle injury, due to motor vehicle accidents, alcoholism, cocaine abuse[431] or other etiologies, may produce life-threatening hyperkalemia, usually during rhabdomyolytic renal failure. Catabolic states, such as sepsis, compound fractures, burns, major surgery or overwhelming infections, result in protein breakdown to meet increased energy demands. Skeletal muscle, the source of protein loss, may release sufficient potassium to cause severe hyperkalemia, if renal excretory mechanisms are compromised.

Accelerated breakdown of a large leukemic tumor burden, especially during induction of chemotherapy, produces kaliuresis and may cause symptomatic hyperkalemia. Burkitt's lymphoma, a rapidly growing neoplasm, while not causing hyperkalemia even in azotemic patients prior to chemotherapy,[432] may result in hyperkalemia within hours of treatment, even in the absence of renal insufficiency. Fatal hyperkalemia has also been reported after initial tumor lysis therapy in acute lymphocytic leukemia, chronic lymphocytic leukemia, and lymphosarcoma. The tumor lysis syndrome is only rarely reported after treatment of non-lymphomatous solid tumors.[433] Intensive supportive therapy probably accounts for the absence of hyperkalemia reported in some series.[434]

Transient hyperkalemia, in the absence of renal failure, occasionally occurs during hemolytic states such as congenital or acquired hemolytic anemia, hemoglobinopathy or transfusion reactions. Conversely, plasma potassium may fall during the rapid proliferation of erythrocytes and their precursors when severe pernicious anemia is successfully treated.[435–437]

Barium

Barium is a well-known inhibitor of potassium exit channels in muscle at concentrations of 1–5 mM.[438] *In vitro*, Ba^{2+}-treated muscle develops flaccid paralysis and depolarization secondary to this change in potassium permeability.[439] Hypokalemia is therefore a feature of barium poisoning, as are cardiac arrhythmias and skeletal muscle paralysis,[440] associated with depolarization of muscle fibers.[438] Barium poisoning is thought to be responsible for "Pa Ping paralysis" reported in Chinese patients who had eaten salt or drunk wine with a high content of barium salts.[441,442]

Cesium

Cesium chloride has been marketed as part of an alternative therapy for malignancy. Cesium appears in the periodic table below rubidium and potassium with a positive valence of 1; its salts are extremely toxic, causing hypokalemia, cardiac arrhythmias, prolonged Q-T interval, and torsade de pointes, probably like barium, by blocking potassium exit channels.[443]

Fluoride

Exposure to toxic levels of inorganic fluoride can produce hyperkalemia that is refractory to standard measures to increase cellular uptake of potassium such as glucose, insulin, and bicarbonate. The mechanisms appear to be decreased potassium influx due to impairment of Na,K-ATPase, further aggravated by a subsequent increase in intracellular calcium that enhances potassium efflux via the Gardos effect.[444]

Hypothermia

Acute transient hypokalemia has been described in patients with hypothermia associated with accidental trauma or following surgery.[445,446] When body temperature returns to normal, the hypokalemia disappears.

Post-operative hypothermia ($<36.5°C$) was found in 40% of patients undergoing gastrointestinal and vascular surgery. Low serum potassium levels coincided with post-operative hypothermia in over half of these, whereas no patients with normothermia became hypokalemic. Urinary potassium losses did not account for the differences.[445] The hypokalemia of experimental hypothermia is not prevented by beta-adrenergic blockade.[447] It may be related to the alkalosis that regularly accompanies hypothermia because of the effect of lowered temperature to reduce the dissociation of carbonic acid.[448]

Race

The extrarenal disposal of an intravenous load of KCl is delayed in normal young African-Americans as compared with Caucasians, perhaps attributable to a racial tendency to lower Na,K-ATPase activity in the cells of African-Americans.[449]

References

[1] Rosa RM, Silva P, Young JB, Landsberg L, Brown RS, Rowe JW, et al. Adrenergic modulation of extrarenal potassium disposal. N Engl J Med 1980;302(8):431–4.

[2] Williams ME, Rosa RM, Silva P, Brown RS, Epstein FH. Impairment of extrarenal potassium disposal by alpha-adrenergic stimulation. N Engl J Med 1984;311(3):145–9.

[3] Keith NM, Osterberg AE, Burchell HB. Some effects of potassium salts in man. Ann Intern Med 1942;16:879–92.

[4] Keith NM, Osterberg AE, HE. King. The excretion of potassium by the normal and diseased kidney. Trans Assoc Am Physic 1940;55:219–22.

[5] Winkler AW, Hoff HE, Smith PK. The toxicity of orally administered potassium salts in renal insufficiency. J Clin Invest 1941;20:119–26.

[6] Bourdillon J. Distribution in body fluids and excretion of ingested ammonium chloride, potassium chloride, and sodium chloride. Am J Physiol 1937;120:411–9.

[7] Gonick HC, Kleeman CR, Rubini ME, Maxwell MH. Functional impairment in chronic renal disease. [3] Studies of potassium excretion. Am J Med Sci 1971;261(5):281–90.

[8] Keith NM, Osterberg AE. The tolerance for potassium in severe renal insufficiency. J Clin Invest 1947;26:773–83.

[9] Perez GO, Pelleya R, Oster JR, Kem DC, Vaamonde CA. Blunted kaliuresis after an acute potassium load in patients with chronic renal failure. Kidney Int 1983;24(5):656–62.

[10] Morita H, Fujiki N, Miyahara T, Lee K, Tanaka K. Hepatoportal bumetanide-sensitive $K^{(+)}$-sensor mechanism controls urinary $K^{(+)}$ excretion. Am J Physiol Regul Integr Comp Physiol 2000;278(5):R1134–9.

[11] Youn JH, McDonough AA. Recent advances in understanding integrative control of potassium homeostasis. Annu Rev Physiol 2009;71:381–401.

[12] Winkler AW, Smith PK. The apparent volume of distribution of potassium injected intravenously. J Biol Chem 1938;124:589–98.

[13] Perez GO, Oster JR, Pelleya R, Caralis PV, Kem DC. Hyperkalemia from single small oral doses of potassium chloride. Nephron 1984;36(4):270–1.

[14] Moore FD, Boling EA, Ditmore Jr. HB, Sicular A, Teterick JE, Ellison AE, et al. Body sodium and potassium. V. The relationship of alkalosis, potassium deficiency and surgical stress to acute hypokalemia in man; experiments and review of the literature. Metabolism 1955;4(5):379—402.

[15] Morgan DB, Cumberbatch M, Swaminathan R. The relation between plasma, erythrocyte and total body potassium in patients with hypokalemia. Miner Electrolyte Metab 1981;5: 233—9.

[16] Schwartz WB, Relman AS. Metabolic and renal studies in chronic potassium depletion resulting from overuse of laxatives. J Clin Invest 1953;32(3):258—71.

[17] Scribner BH, Burnell JM. Interpretation of the serum potassium concentration. Metabolism 1956;5(4):468—79.

[18] Knochel JP. Neuromuscular manifestations of electrolyte disorders. Am J Med 1982;72(3):521—35.

[19] Bilbrey GL, Herbin L, Carter NW, Knochel JP. Skeletal muscle resting membrane potential in potassium deficiency. J Clin Invest 1973;52(12):3011—8.

[20] Riecker G, Bolte HD, Rohl D. Hypokaliamie and membranpotential. Reanimation et Organes Artificiels 1954;1:41—50.

[21] Feig PU, Shook A, Sterns RH. Effect of potassium removal during hemodialysis on the plasma potassium concentration. Nephron 1981;27(1):25—30.

[22] Bergstrom J, Alvestrand A, Furst P, Hultman E, Sahlin K, Vinnars E, et al. Influence of severe potassium depletion and subsequent repletion with potassium on muscle electrolytes, metabolites and amino acids in man. Clin Sci Mol Med Suppl 1976;51(6):589—99.

[23] Patrick J, Bradford B. A comparison of leucocyte potassium content with other measurements in potassium-depleted rabbits. Clin Sci 1972;42(4):415—21.

[24] Giebisch G, Krapf R, Wagner C. Renal and extrarenal regulation of potassium. Kidney Int 2007;72(4):397—410.

[25] Miller H, Darrow D. Relation of muscle electrolyte to alteration in serum potassium and to the toxic effects of injected potassium chloride. Am J Physiol 1940;130:747—58.

[26] Spital A, Sterns RH. Paradoxical potassium depletion: a renal mechanism for extrarenal potassium adaptation. Kidney Int 1986;30(4):532—7.

[27] Sterns RH, Cox M, Feig PU, Singer I. Internal potassium balance and the control of the plasma potassium concentration. Medicine (Baltimore) 1981;60(5):339—54.

[28] Williams JA, Withrow CD, Woodbury DM. Effects of nephrectomy and KC1 on transmembrane potentials, intracellular electrolytes, and cell pH of rat muscle and liver in vivo. J Physiol 1971;212(1):117—28.

[29] Brown RS. Extrarenal potassium homeostasis. Kidney Int 1986;30(1):116—27.

[30] Cumberbatch M, Morgan DB. Erythrocyte sodium and potassium in patients with hypokalaemia. Clin Sci (Lond) 1983;64 (2):167—76.

[31] Levin ML, Rector Jr. FC, Seldin DW. Effects of potassium and ouabain on sodium transport in human red cells. Am J Physiol 1968;214(6):1328—32.

[32] Norgaard A, Kjeldsen K, Clausen T. Potassium depletion decreases the number of ^{3}H-ouabain binding sites and the active Na-K transport in skeletal muscle. Nature 1981;293(5835): 739—41.

[33] Akaike N. Sodium pump in skeletal muscle: central nervous system-induced suppression by alpha-adrenoreceptors. Science 1981;213(4513):1252—4.

[34] Harrop G, Benedict E. The role of phosphate and potassium in carbohydrate metabolism following insulin administration. Proc Soc Exp Biol Med 1923;20:430—1.

[35] Briggs A, Koechig I. Some changes in the composition of blood due to the injection of insulin. J Biol Chem 1924;58:721—30.

[36] Holler J. Potassium deficiency occurring during the treatment of diabetic acidosis. JAMA 1946;131:1186—9.

[37] Clausen T, Kohn PG. The effect of insulin on the transport of sodium and potassium in rat soleus muscle. J Physiol 1977;265 (1):19—42.

[38] Flatman JA, Clausen T. Combined effects of adrenaline and insulin on active electrogenic Na^+-K^+ transport in rat soleus muscle. Nature 1979;281(5732):580—1.

[39] Zierler KL. Effect of insulin on membrane potential and potassium content of rat muscle. Am J Physiol 1959;197:515—23.

[40] Berg T, Iversen JG. K^+ transport in isolated rat liver cells stimulated by glucagon and insulin in vitro. Acta Physiol Scand 1976;97(2):202—8.

[41] Burton SD, Mondon CE, Ishida T. Dissociation of potassium and glucose efflux in isolated perfused rat liver. Am J Physiol 1967;212(2):261—6.

[42] Lambotte L, Shoemaker W. Effect of insulin on hepatic K movements as influenced by hypothermia, barbiturate, and dibenzyline. Physiologist 1964;7: 184 A

[43] Gourley DR, Bethea MD. Insulin effect on adipose tissue sodium and potassium. Proc Soc Exp Biol Med 1964;115: 821—3.

[44] Groen J, Willebrands A, Kamminga E, Van Schothorst H, Godfried E. De invloed van toediening van glycose op het kaliumgehalte van het bloedserum bij normale personen en bij-niet-diabetische patienten. Ned Milit Geneeskd Tijdschr 1950;94:2187—201.

[45] Moore RD. Effects of insulin upon ion transport. Biochim Biophys Acta 1983;737(1):1—49.

[46] Fenn WO. The deposition of potassium and phosphate with glycogen in rat livers. J Biol Chem 1939;128:297—307.

[47] Zierler KL. Effect of insulin on potassium efflux from rat muscle in the presence and absence of glucose. Am J Physiol 1960;198:1066—70.

[48] Creese R. Sodium fluxes in diaphragm muscle and the effects of insulin and serum proteins. J Physiol 1968;197(2):255—78.

[49] Andres R, Baltzan MA, Cader G, Zierler KL. Effect of insulin on carbohydrate metabolism and on potassium in the forearm of man. J Clin Invest 1962;41:108—15.

[50] Kestens PJ, Haxhe JJ, Lambotte L, Lambotte C. The effect of insulin on the uptake of potassium and phosphate by the isolated perfused canine liver. Metabolism 1963;12:941—50.

[51] Zierler KL, Rabinowitz D. Effect of very small concentrations of insulin on forearm metabolism. Persistence of its action on potassium and free fatty acids without its effect on glucose. J Clin Invest 1964;43:950—62.

[52] Gourley DR. Separation of insulin effects on K content and O_2 consumption of frog muscle with cardiac glycosides. Am J Physiol 1961;200:1320—6.

[53] Manery JF, Dryden EE, Still JS, Madapallimattam G. Enhancement (by ATP, insulin, and lack of divalent cations) of ouabain inhibition of cation transport and ouabain binding in frog skeletal muscle; effect of insulin and ouabain on sarcolemmal (Na + K)MgATPase. Can J Physiol Pharmacol 1977;55(1): 21—33.

[54] Moore RD. Effect of insulin upon the sodium pump in frog skeletal muscle. J Physiol 1973;232(1):23—45.

[55] Resh MD, Nemenoff RA, Guidotti G. Insulin stimulation of (Na^+,K^+)-adenosine triphosphatase-dependent 86Rb + uptake in rat adipocytes. J Biol Chem 1980;255(22):10938—45.

[56] Fehlmann M, Freychet P. Insulin and glucagon stimulation of (Na^+-K^+)-ATPase transport activity in isolated rat hepatocytes. J Biol Chem 1981;256(14):7449—53.

[57] De Luise MA, Harker M. Insulin stimulation of Na^+-K^+ pump in clonal rat osteosarcoma cells. Diabetes 1988;37(1):33–7.

[58] Czech MP. Molecular basis of insulin action. Annu Rev Biochem 1977;46:359–84.

[59] Grinstein S, Erlij D. Insulin unmasks latent sodium pump sites in frog muscle. Nature 1974;251(5470):57–8.

[60] Gavryck WA, Moore RD, Thompson RC. Effect of insulin upon membrane-bound $(Na^{++}K^+)$-ATPase extracted from frog skeletal muscle. J Physiol 1975;252(1):43–58.

[61] Moore RD. Stimulation of Na:H exchange by insulin. Biophys J 1981;33(2):203–10.

[62] Clausen T, Flatman JA. Effects of insulin and epinephrine on Na^+-K^+ and glucose transport in soleus muscle. Am J Physiol 1987;252(4 Pt 1):E492–9.

[63] Sargeant RJ, Liu Z, Klip A. Action of insulin on $Na^{(+)}-K^{(+)}$-ATPase and the $Na^{(+)}-K^{(+)}-2Cl^-$ co-transporter in 3T3-L1 adipocytes. Am J Physiol 1995;269(1 Pt 1):C217–25.

[64] Gosmanov AR, Thomason DB. Insulin and isoproterenol differentially regulate mitogen-activated protein kinase-dependent $Na^{(+)}-K^{(+)}-2Cl^{(-)}$ co-transporter activity in skeletal muscle. Diabetes 2002;51(3):615–23.

[65] Boini KM, Graf D, Kuhl D, Haussinger D, Lang F. SGK1 dependence of insulin induced hypokalemia. Pflugers Arch 2009;457(4):955–61.

[66] Resh MD. Insulin activation of (Na^+,K^+)-adenosinetriphosphatase exhibits a temperature-dependent lag time. Comparison to activation of the glucose transporter. Biochemistry 1983;22(12):2781–4.

[67] Clausen T, Hansen O. Active Na-K transport and the rate of ouabain binding. The effect of insulin and other stimuli on skeletal muscle and adipocytes. J Physiol 1977;270(2):415–30.

[68] Erlij D, Grinstein S. The number of sodium ion pumping sites in skeletal muscle and its modification by insulin. J Physiol 1976;259(1):13–31.

[69] Al-Khalili L, Yu M, Chibalin AV. Na^+,K^+-ATPase trafficking in skeletal muscle: insulin stimulates translocation of both alpha 1- and alpha 2-subunit isoforms. FEBS Lett 2003;536(1–3):198–202.

[70] Weil-Maslansky E, Gutman Y, Sasson S. Insulin activates furosemide-sensitive K^+ and Cl^- uptake system in BC3H1 cells. Am J Physiol 1994;267(4 Pt 1):C932–9.

[71] Zierler K, Rogus EM. Rapid hyperpolarization of rat skeletal muscle induced by insulin. Biochim Biophys Acta 1981;640(3):687–92.

[72] Zierler KL. Increase in resting membrane potential of skeletal muscle produced by insulin. Science 1957;126(3282):1067–8.

[73] Beigelman PM, Hollander PB. Effects of hormones upon adipose tissue membrane electrical potentials. Proc Soc Exp Biol Med 1964;116:31–5.

[74] LaManna VR, Ferrier GR. Electrophysiological effects of insulin on normal and depressed cardiac tissues. Am J Physiol 1981;240(4):H636–44.

[75] Moore RD, Rabovsky JL. Mechanism of insulin action on resting membrane potential of frog skeletal muscle. Am J Physiol 1979;236(5):C249–54.

[76] Dorup I, Clausen T. Insulin-like growth factor I stimulates active $Na^{(+)}-K^+$ transport in rat soleus muscle. Am J Physiol 1995;268(5 Pt 1):E849–57.

[77] Wilde W. The distribution of potassium in the cat after intravascular injection. J Biol Chem 1939;128:309–17.

[78] DeFronzo RA, Felig P, Ferrannini E, Wahren J. Effect of graded doses of insulin on splanchnic and peripheral potassium metabolism in man. Am J Physiol 1980;238(5):E421–7.

[79] Bia MJ, DeFronzo RA. Extrarenal potassium homeostasis. Am J Physiol 1981;240(4):F257–68.

[80] Cox M, Sterns RH, Singer I. The defense against hyperkalemia: the roles of insulin and aldosterone. N Engl J Med 1978;299(10):525–32.

[81] Guerra SM, Kitabchi AE. Comparison of the effectiveness of various routes of insulin injection: insulin levels and glucose response in normal subjects. J Clin Endocrinol Metab 1976;42(5):869–74.

[82] Minaker KL, Rowe JW. Potassium homeostasis during hyperinsulinemia: effect of insulin level, beta-blockade, and age. Am J Physiol 1982;242(6):E373–7.

[83] Fineberg SE, Merimee TJ. Effects of comparative perfusions of equimolar, single component insulin and proinsulin in the human forearm. Diabetes 1973;22(9):676–86.

[84] McDonough AA, Thompson CB, Youn JH. Skeletal muscle regulates extracellular potassium. Am J Physiol Renal Physiol 2002;282(6):F967–74.

[85] Chen P, Guzman JP, Leong PK, Yang LE, Perianayagam A, Babilonia E, et al. Modest dietary K^+ restriction provokes insulin resistance of cellular K^+ uptake and phosphorylation of renal outer medulla K^+ channel without fall in plasma K^+ concentration. Am J Physiol Cell Physiol 2006;290(5):C1355–63.

[86] Yalow RS, Berson SA. Immunoassay of endogenous plasma insulin in man. J Clin Invest 1960;39:1157–75.

[87] Young DB. Analysis of long-term potassium regulation. Endocr Rev 1985;6(1):24–44 [Winter]

[88] DeFronzo RA, Sherwin RS, Dillingham M, Hendler R, Tamborlane WV, Felig P. Influence of basal insulin and glucagon secretion on potassium and sodium metabolism. Studies with somatostatin in normal dogs and in normal and diabetic human beings. J Clin Invest 1978;61(2):472–9.

[89] Allon M, Dansby L, Shanklin N. Glucose modulation of the disposal of an acute potassium load in patients with end-stage renal disease. Am J Med 1993;94(5):475–82.

[90] Hiatt N, Yamakawa T, Davidson MB. Necessity for insulin in transfer of excess infused K to intracellular fluid. Metabolism 1974;23(1):43–9.

[91] Pettit GW, Vick RL. Contribution of pancreatic insulin to extrarenal potassium homeostasis: a two-compartment model. Am J Physiol 1974;226(2):319–24.

[92] Santeusanio F, Faloona GR, Knochel JP, Unger RH. Evidence for a role of endogenous insulin and glucagon in the regulation of potassium homeostasis. J Lab Clin Med 1973;81(6):809–17.

[93] Silva P, Spokes K. Sympathetic system in potassium homeostasis. Am J Physiol 1981;241(2):F151–5.

[94] DeFronzo RA. Obesity is associated with impaired insulin-mediated potassium uptake. Metabolism 1988;37(2):105–8.

[95] de Weille JR, Fosset M, Mourre C, Schmid-Antomarchi H, Bernardi H, Lazdunski M. Pharmacology and regulation of ATP-sensitive K^+ channels. Pflugers Arch 1989;414(Suppl. 1):S80–7.

[96] Petersen OH, Dunne MJ. Regulation of K^+ channels plays a crucial role in the control of insulin secretion. Pflugers Arch 1989;414(Suppl. 1):S115–20.

[97] Dawson CM, Lebrun P, Herchuelz A, Malaisse WJ, Goncalves AA, Atwater I. Effect of temperature upon potassium-stimulated insulin release and calcium entry in mouse and rat islets. Horm Metab Res 1986;18(4):221–4.

[98] Dluhy RG, Axelrod L, Williams GH. Serum immunoreactive insulin and growth hormone response to potassium infusion in normal man. J Appl Physiol 1972;33(1):22–6.

[99] Davidson MB, Hiatt N. Effect of KCl administration on insulin secretion in dogs. Isr J Med Sci 1972;8(6):752–4.

[100] Hiatt N, Davidson MB, Bonorris G. The effect of potassium chloride infusion on insulin secretion *in vivo*. Horm Metab Res 1972;4(2):64–8.

[101] Pettit GW, Vick RL, Swander AM. Plasma K plus and insulin: changes during KCl infusion in normal and nephrectomized dogs. Am J Physiol 1975;228(1):107−9.

[102] Adrogue HJ, Chap Z, Ishida T, Field JB. Role of the endocrine pancreas in the kalemic response to acute metabolic acidosis in conscious dogs. J Clin Invest 1985;75(3):798−808.

[103] Blackard WG, Nelson NC. Portal and peripheral vein immuno-reactive insulin concentrations before and after glucose infusion. Diabetes 1970;19(5):302−6.

[104] Wolfson S, Ellis S. Effects of glucagon on plasma potassium. Proc Soc Exp Biol Med 1958;91:226−8.

[105] Massara F, Martelli S, Cagliero E, Camanni F, Molinatti GM. Influence of glucagon on plasma levels of potassium in man. Diabetologia 1980;19(5):414−7.

[106] Massara F, Cagliero E, Maccario M, Orzan F, Carini G. Pathophysiological doses of glucagon cause a transient increase of the hepatic vein potassium concentration in man. Miner Electrolyte Metab 1986;12(2):142−6.

[107] Finder AG, Boyme T, Shoemaker WC. Relationship of hepatic potassium efflux to phosphorylase activation induced by glucagon. Am J Physiol 1964;206:738−42.

[108] Lynch CJ, Bocckino SB, Blackmore PF, Exton JH. Calcium-mobilizing hormones and phorbol myristate acetate mediate heterologous desensitization of the hormone-sensitive hepatic Na^+/K^+ pump. Biochem J 1987;248(3):807−13.

[109] Cagliero E, Martina V, Massara F, Molinatti GM. Glucagon-induced increase in plasma potassium levels in type 1 (insulin-dependent) diabetic subjects. Diabetologia 1983;24(2):85−7.

[110] Muller WA, Faloona GR, Unger RH. Hyperglucagonemia in diabetic ketoacidosis. Its prevalence and significance. Am J Med 1973;54(1):52−7.

[111] Bilbrey GL, Faloona GR, White MG, Knochel JP. Hyperglucagonemia of renal failure. J Clin Invest 1974;53(3):841−7.

[112] Knochel JP. Role of glucoregulatory hormones in potassium homeostasis. Kidney Int 1977;11(6):443−52.

[113] D'Silva JL. The action of adrenaline on serum potassium. J Physiol 1934;82:393−8.

[114] Clausen T. Adrenergic control of $Na^+−K^+$-homoeostasis. Acta Med Scand Suppl 1983;672:111−5.

[115] Epstein FH, Rosa RM. Adrenergic control of serum potassium. N Engl J Med 1983;309(23):1450−1.

[116] Struthers AD, Reid JL. The role of adrenal medullary catecho-lamines in potassium homoeostasis. Clin Sci (Lond) 1984;66(4):377−82.

[117] Coats RA. Effects of apamin on alpha-adrenoceptor-mediated changes in plasma potassium in guinea-pigs. Br J Pharmacol 1983;80(3):573−80.

[118] D'Silva JL. Action of adrenaline on the perfused liver. J Physiol 1936;87:181−8.

[119] Todd EP, Vick RL. Kalemotropic effect of epinephrine: analysis with adrenergic agonists and antagonists. Am J Physiol 1971;220(6):1964−9.

[120] Todd EP, Vick RL, Bonner FM, Leudke DW. The influence of the rate of infusion on the kalemotropic effect of epinephrine. Arch Int Physiol Biochim 1969;77(1):33−45.

[121] Katz LD, D'Avella J, DeFronzo RA. Effect of epinephrine on renal potassium excretion in the isolated perfused rat kidney. Am J Physiol 1984;247(2 Pt 2):F331−8.

[122] Smythe CM, Nickel JF, Bradley SE. The effect of epinephrine (USP), l-epinephrine, and l-norepinephrine on glomerular fil-tration rate, renal plasma flow, and the urinary excretion of sodium, potassium, and water in normal man. J Clin Invest 1952;31(5):499−506.

[123] Powell Jr. WJ, Skinner Jr. NS. Effect of the catecholamines on ionic balance and vascular resistance in skeletal muscle. Am J Cardiol 1966;18(1):73−82.

[124] De La Lande IS, Manson J, Parks VJ, Sandison AG, Skinner SL, Whelan RF. The local metabolic action of adrenaline on skeletal muscle in man. J Physiol 1961;157:177−84.

[125] Grob D, Liljestrand A, Johns RJ. Potassium movement in normal subjects: effect on muscle function. Am J Med 1957;23(3): 340−55.

[126] Vick RL, Todd EP, Luedke DW. Epinephrine-induced hypoka-lemia: relation to liver and skeletal muscle. J Pharmacol Exp Ther 1972;181(1):139−46.

[127] Glitsch HG, Haas HG, Trautwein W. The effect of adrenaline on the K and Na fluxes in the frog's atrium. Naunyn Schmiedebergs Arch Exp Pathol Pharmakol 1965;250:59−71.

[128] Ballanyi K, Grafe P. Changes in intracellular ion activities induced by adrenaline in human and rat skeletal muscle. Pflugers Arch 1988;411(3):283−8.

[129] Clausen T, Flatman JA. The effect of catecholamines on Na-K transport and membrane potential in rat soleus muscle. J Physiol 1977;270(2):383−414.

[130] Evans RH, Smith JW. Mode of action of catecholamines on skeletal muscle. J Physiol 1973;232(2):81P−2P.

[131] Lockwood RH, Lum BK. Effects of adrenergic agonists and antagonists on potassium metabolism. J Pharmacol Exp Ther 1974;189(1):119−29.

[132] Hays ET, Dwyer TM, Horowicz P, Swift JG. Epinephrine action on sodium fluxes in frog striated muscle. Am J Physiol 1974;227(6):1340−7.

[133] Deibert DC, DeFronzo RA. Epinephrine-induced insulin resis-tance in man. J Clin Invest 1980;65(3):717−21.

[134] Pettit GW, Vick RL. An analysis of the contribution of the endocrine pancreas to the kalemotropic actions of catecho-lamines. J Pharmacol Exp Ther 1974;190(2):234−42.

[135] Bia MJ, Tyler KA, DeFronzo RA. Regulation of extrarenal potassium homeostasis by adrenal hormones in rats. Am J Physiol 1982;242(6):F641−4.

[136] Olsson A, Persson S, Schroder R. Effects of terbutaline and iso-proterenol on hyperkalemia in nephrectomized rabbits. Scand J Urol Nephrol 1977;12:35−8.

[137] Ahlquist RA. Study of the adrenotropic receptors. Am J Physiol 1948;153:586−600.

[138] Bia MJ, Lu D, Tyler K, De Fronzo RA. Beta adrenergic control of extrarenal potassium disposal. A beta-2 mediated phenome-non. Nephron 1986;43(2):117−22.

[139] Tannen RL. Potassium disorders. In: Kokko JP, Tannen RL, editors. Fluids and electrolytes. Philadelphia: Saunders; 1986. p. 150−228.

[140] DeFronzo RA, Bia M, Birkhead G. Epinephrine and potassium homeostasis. Kidney Int 1981;20(1):83−91.

[141] Ljunghall S, Joborn H, Rastad J, Akerstrom G. Plasma potas-sium and phosphate concentrations − influence by adrenaline infusion, beta-blockade and physical exercise. Acta Med Scand 1987;221(1):83−93.

[142] Vincent HH, Boomsma F, Man in't Veld AJ, Derkx FH, Wenting GJ, Schalekamp MA. Effects of selective and nonselec-tive beta-agonists on plasma potassium and norepinephrine. J Cardiovasc Pharmacol 1984;6(1):107−14.

[143] Vincent HH, Man in't Veld AJ, Boomsma F, Schalekamp MA. Prevention of epinephrine-induced hypokalemia by nonselec-tive beta blockers. Am J Cardiol 1985;56(6):10D−4D.

[144] Struthers AD, Reid JL, Whitesmith R, Rodger JC. The effects of cardioselective and non-selective beta-adrenoceptor block-ade on the hypokalaemic and cardiovascular responses to adrenomedullary hormones in man. Clin Sci (Lond) 1983;65(2):143−7.

[145] Weidmann P, De Chatel R, Ziegler WH, Flammer J, Reubi F. Alpha and beta adrenergic blockade with orally administered labetalol in hypertension. Studies on blood volume, plasma renin and aldosterone and catecholamine excretion. Am J Cardiol 1978;41(3):570−6.

[146] Clausen T, Flatman JA. Beta 2-adrenoceptors mediate the stimulating effect of adrenaline on active electrogenic Na-K-transport in rat soleus muscle. Br J Pharmacol 1980;68(4):749−55.

[147] Lockwood RH, Lum BK. Effects of adrenalectomy and adrenergic antagonists on potassium metabolism. J Pharmacol Exp Ther 1977;203(1):103−11.

[148] Sugarman A, Kaji DM, Stein RM, Kahn T. Extrarenal potassium transport and the beta 2-adrenergic system. J Lab Clin Med 1984;103(6):912−21.

[149] Brown MJ. Hypokalemia from beta 2-receptor stimulation by circulating epinephrine. Am J Cardiol 1985;56(6):3D−9D.

[150] Struthers AD, Reid JL. Adrenaline causes hypokalaemia in man by beta 2 adrenoceptor stimulation. Clin Endocrinol (Oxf) 1984;20(4):409−14.

[151] Hastwell G, Lambert BE. The effect of oral salbutamol on serum potassium and blood sugar. Br J Obstet Gynaecol 1978;85(10):767−9.

[152] Leitch AG, Clancy LJ, Costello JF, Flenley DC. Effect of intravenous infusion of salbutamol on ventilatory response to carbon dioxide and hypoxia and on heart rate and plasma potassium in normal men. Br Med J 1976;1(6006):365−7.

[153] Smith SR, Kendall MJ. Inhaled bronchodilators and hypokalaemia. Lancet 1983;2(8343):218.

[154] Smith SR, Ryder C, Kendall MJ, Holder R. Cardiovascular and biochemical responses to nebulised salbutamol in normal subjects. Br J Clin Pharmacol 1984;18(4):641−4.

[155] Thomas DJ, Dove AF, Alberti KG. Metabolic effects of salbutamol infusion during premature labour. Br J Obstet Gynaecol 1977;84(7):497−9.

[156] Braden GL, von Oeyen PT, Germain MJ, Watson DJ, Haag BL. Ritodrine- and terbutaline-induced hypokalemia in preterm labor: mechanisms and consequences. Kidney Int 1997;51(6):1867−75.

[157] Hurlbert BJ, Edelman JD, David K. Serum potassium levels during and after terbutaline. Anesth Analg 1981;60(10):723−5.

[158] Moravec MA, Hurlbert BJ. Hypokalemia associated with terbutaline administration in obstetrical patients. Anesth Analg 1980;59(12):917−20.

[159] Haalboom JR, Deenstra M, Struyvenberg A. Hypokalaemia induced by inhalation of fenoterol. Lancet 1985;1(8438):1125−7.

[160] Insel PA. Identification and regulation of adrenergic receptors in target cells. Am J Physiol 1984;247(1 Pt 1):E53−8.

[161] Clausen T, Everts ME. Regulation of the Na,K-pump in skeletal muscle. Kidney Int 1989;35(1):1−13.

[162] Cheng LC, Rogus EM, Zierler K. Catechol a structural requirement for (Na$^+$ + K$^+$)-ATPase stimulation in rat skeletal muscle membrane. Biochim Biophys Acta 1977;464(2):338−46.

[163] Buur T, Clausen T, Holmberg E, Johansson U, Waldeck B. Desensitization by terbutaline of beta-adrenoceptors in the guinea-pig soleus muscle: biochemical alterations associated with functional changes. Br J Pharmacol 1982;76(2):313−7.

[164] Bray JJ, Hawken MJ, Hubbard JI, Pockett S, Wilson L. The membrane potential of rat diaphragm muscle fibres and the effect of denervation. J Physiol 1976;255(3):651−67.

[165] Scheid CR, Honeyman TW, Fay FS. Mechanism of beta-adrenergic relaxation of smooth muscle. Nature 1979;277(5691): 32−6.

[166] Scheid CR, Fay FS. Beta-adrenergic stimulation of 42K influx in isolated smooth muscle cells. Am J Physiol 1984;246(5 Pt 1): C415−21.

[167] Kaibara K, Akasu T, Tokimasa T, Koketsu K. Beta-adrenergic modulation of the Na$^+$−K$^+$ pump in frog skeletal muscles. Pflugers Arch 1985;405(1):24−8.

[168] Desilets M, Baumgarten CM. Isoproterenol directly stimulates the Na$^+$−K$^+$ pump in isolated cardiac myocytes. Am J Physiol 1986;251(1 Pt 2):H218−25.

[169] Douglas WW. Stimulus-secretion coupling: the concept and clues from chromaffin and other cells. Br J Pharmacol 1968;34 (3):453−74.

[170] Baker PF, Rink TJ. Catecholamine release from bovine adrenal medulla in response to maintained depolarization. J Physiol 1975;253(2):593−620.

[171] Silberstein SD, Lemberger L, Klein DC, Axelrod J, Kopin IJ. Induction of adrenal tyrosine hydroxylase in organ culture. Neuropharmacology 1972;11(5):721−6.

[172] Vogt M. The secretion of the denervated adrenal medulla of the cat. Br J Pharmacol 1952;7(2):325−30.

[173] Opdyke DF, Carroll RG, Keller NE. Systemic arterial pressor responses induced by potassium in dogfish, *Squalus acanthias*. Am J Physiol 1981;241(3):R228−32.

[174] Hiatt N, Chapman LW, Davidson MB. Influence of epinephrine and propranolol on transmembrane K transfer in anuric dogs with hyperkalemia. J Pharmacol Exp Ther 1979;209(2): 282−6.

[175] Massara F, Tripodina A, Rotunno M. Propranolol block of epinephrine-induced hypokaliaemia in man. Eur J Pharmacol 1970;10(3):404−7.

[176] Brown MJ, Brown DC, Murphy MB. Hypokalemia from beta2-receptor stimulation by circulating epinephrine. N Engl J Med 1983;309(23):1414−9.

[177] Karlsberg RP, Cryer PE, Roberts R. Serial plasma catecholamine response early in the course of clinical acute myocardial infarction: relationship to infarct extent and mortality. Am Heart J 1981;102(1):24−9.

[178] Halter JB, Pflug AE, Porte Jr. D. Mechanism of plasma catecholamine increases during surgical stress in man. J Clin Endocrinol Metab 1977;45(5):936−44.

[179] Christensen NJ. Plasma norepinephrine and epinephrine in untreated diabetics, during fasting and after insulin administration. Diabetes 1974;23(1):1−8.

[180] Landsberg L, Young JB. Fasting, feeding and regulation of the sympathetic nervous system. N Engl J Med 1978;298(23): 1295−301.

[181] Carlsson E, Fellenius E, Lundborg P, Svensson L. beta-Adrenoceptor blockers, plasma-potassium, and exercise. Lancet 1978;2(8086):424−5.

[182] Williams ME, Gervino EV, Rosa RM, Landsberg L, Young JB, Silva P, et al. Catecholamine modulation of rapid potassium shifts during exercise. N Engl J Med 1985;312(13):823−7.

[183] Clausen T. Hormonal and pharmacological modification of plasma potassium homeostasis. Fundam Clin Pharmacol 2010;24(5):595−605.

[184] McKenna MJ, Schmidt TA, Hargreaves M, Cameron L, Skinner SL, Kjeldsen K. Sprint training increases human skeletal muscle Na$^{(+)}$−K$^{(+)}$-ATPase concentration and improves K$^+$ regulation. J Appl Physiol 1993;75(1):173−80.

[185] Zheng D, Perianayagam A, Lee DH, Brannan MD, Yang LE, Tellalian D, et al. AMPK activation with AICAR provokes an acute fall in plasma [K$^+$]. Am J Physiol Cell Physiol 2008;294(1):C126−35.

[186] Lands AM, Arnold A, McAuliff JP, Luduena FP, Brown Jr. TG. Differentiation of receptor systems activated by sympathomimetic amines. Nature 1967;214(88):597−8.

[187] Imura H, Kato Y, Ikeda M, Morimoto M, Yawata M. Effect of adrenergic-blocking or -stimulating agents on plasma growth hormone, immunoreactive insulin, and blood free fatty acid levels in man. J Clin Invest 1971;50(5):1069−79.

III. FLUID AND ELECTROLYTE REGULATION AND DYSREGULATION

[188] Westfall TC. Local regulation of adrenergic neurotransmission. Physiol Rev 1977;57(4):659–728.

[189] Jakobs KH, Saur W, Schultz G. Reduction of adenylate cyclase activity in lysates of human platelets by the alpha-adrenergic component of epinephrine. J Cyclic Nucleotide Res 1976;2(6):381–92.

[190] Jauchem JR, Vick RL. Phenylephrine-induced hyperkalemia: role of the liver. Proc Soc Exp Biol Med 1980;163(4):478–81.

[191] Wadstein J, Skude G. Does hypokalaemia precede delirium tremens? Lancet 1978;2(8089):549–50.

[192] McDonald Jr. RH, Goldberg LI, McNay JL, Tuttle Jr. EP. Effect of dopamine in man: augmentation of sodium excretion, glomerular filtration rate, and renal plasma flow. J Clin Invest 1964;43:1116–24.

[193] Meyer MB, McNay JL, Goldberg LI. Effects of dopamine on renal function and hemodynamics in the dog. J Pharmacol Exp Ther 1967;156(1):186–92.

[194] Finlay GD, Whitsett TL, Cucinell EA, Goldberg LI. Augmentation of sodium and potassium excretion, glomerular filtration rate and renal plasma flow by levodopa. N Engl J Med 1971;284(15):865–70.

[195] Granerus AK, Jagenburg R, Svanborg A. Kaliuretic effect of L-dopa treatment in parkinsonian patients. Acta Med Scand 1977;201(4):291–7.

[196] Williams M, Young JB, Rosa RM, Gunn S, Epstein FH, Landsberg L. Effect of protein ingestion on urinary dopamine excretion. Evidence for the functional importance of renal decarboxylation of circulating 3,4-dihydroxyphenylalanine in man. J Clin Invest 1986;78(6):1687–93.

[197] Carey RM, Thorner MO, Ortt EM. Effects of metoclopramide and bromocriptine on the renin–angiotensin–aldosterone system in man. Dopaminergic control of aldosterone. J Clin Invest 1979;63(4):727–35.

[198] Blevins RD, Whitty AJ, Rubenfire M, Maciejko JJ. Dopamine and dobutamine induce hypokalemia in anesthetized dogs. J Cardiovasc Pharmacol 1989;13(4):662–6.

[199] Bevilacqua M, Norbiato G, Raggi U, Micossi P, Baggio E, Prandelli M. Dopaminergic control of serum potassium. Metabolism 1980;29(4):306–10.

[200] Sager PT, DeFronzo RA. Dopaminergic regulation of extrarenal potassium metabolism. Miner Electrolyte Metab 1987;13(6):385–92.

[201] Zanella MT, Bravo EL. In vitro and in vivo evidence for an indirect mechanism mediating enhanced aldosterone secretion by metoclopramide. Endocrinology 1982;111(5):1620–5.

[202] Carey RM, Thorner MO, Ortt EM. Dopaminergic inhibition of metoclopramide-induced aldosterone secretion in man. Dissociation of responses to dopamine and bromocriptine. J Clin Invest 1980;66(1):10–8.

[203] Pratt JH, Ganguly A, Parkinson CA, Weinberger MH. Stimulation of aldosterone secretion by metoclopramide in humans: apparent independence of renal and pituitary mediation. Metabolism 1981;30(2):129–34.

[204] Sowers JR, Brickman AS, Sowers DK, Berg G. Dopaminergic modulation of aldosterone secretion in man is unaffected by glucocorticoids and angiotensin blockade. J Clin Endocrinol Metab 1981;52(6):1078–84.

[205] Whitfield L, Sowers JR, Tuck ML, Golub MS. Dopaminergic control of plasma catecholamine and aldosterone responses to acute stimuli in normal man. J Clin Endocrinol Metab 1980;51(4):724–9.

[206] Taylor P. Cholinergic agonists. In: Goodman AG, Goodman LS, Rall TW, Murad F, editors. The pharmacological basis of therapeutics. 7th ed. New York: MacMillan; 1985. p. 108.

[207] Adrenaline and potassium: everything in flux. Lancet 1983;2(8364):1401–1403.

[208] Donnelly T, Gray H, Simpson E, Rodger JC. Serum potassium in acute myocardial infarction. Scot Med J 1980;25:176.

[209] Madias JE, Shah B, Chintalapally G, Chalavarya G, Madias NE. Admission serum potassium in patients with acute myocardial infarction: its correlates and value as a determinant of in-hospital outcome. Chest 2000;118(4):904–13.

[210] Rolton H, Simpson E, Donnelly T, Rodger JC. Plasma potassium in acute myocardial infarction. Eur Heart J 1981;2(Suppl. A):21 A.

[211] Thomas R, Hicks S. Myocardial infarction: ventricular arrhythmias associated with hypokalemia. Clin Sci 1981;61:32p.

[212] Johansson BW, Dziamski R. Malignant arrhythmias in acute myocardial infarction. Relationship to serum potassium and effect of selective and non-selective beta-blockade. Drugs 1984;28(Suppl. 1):77–85.

[213] Nordrehaug JE, Johannessen KA, von der Lippe G. Serum potassium concentration as a risk factor of ventricular arrhythmias early in acute myocardial infarction. Circulation 1985;71(4):645–9.

[214] Struthers AD, Whitesmith R, Reid JL. Prior thiazide diuretic treatment increases adrenaline-induced hypokalaemia. Lancet 1983;1(8338):1358–61.

[215] Dyckner T, Helmers C, Lundman T, Wester PO. Initial serum potassium level in relation to early complications and prognosis in patients with acute myocardial infarction. Acta Med Scand 1975;197(3):207–10.

[216] Nordrehaug JE. Malignant arrhythmia in relation to serum potassium in acute myocardial infarction. Am J Cardiol 1985;56(6):20D–3D.

[217] Nordrehaug JE, Johannessen KA, von der Lippe G, Sederholm M, Grottum P, Kjekshus J. Effect of timolol on changes in serum potassium concentration during acute myocardial infarction. Br Heart J 1985;53(4):388–93.

[218] Amin DN, Henry JA. Propranolol administration in theophylline overdose. Lancet 1985;1(8427):520–1.

[219] Conci F, Procaccio F, Boselli L. Hypokalemia from beta2-receptor stimulation by epinephrine. N Engl J Med 1984;310:1329.

[220] Mikhailidis DP, Dandona P. Adrenaline and potassium. Lancet 1984;1(8369):170–1.

[221] Morgan DB, Young RM. Acute transient hypokalaemia: new interpretation of a common event. Lancet 1982;2(8301):751–2.

[222] Smith SK, Thompson D. The effect of intravenous salbutamol upon plasma and urinary potassium during premature labour. Br J Obstet Gynaecol 1977;84(5):344–7.

[223] Rohr AS, Spector SL, Rachelefsky GS, Katz RM, Siegel SC. Efficacy of parenteral albuterol in the treatment of asthma. Comparison of its metabolic side effects with subcutaneous epinephrine. Chest 1986;89(3):348–51.

[224] Rubinstein S, Hindi RD, Moss RB, Blessing-Moore J, Lewiston NJ. Sudden death in adolescent asthma. Ann Allergy 1984;53(4):311–8.

[225] Wilson JD, Sutherland DC, Thomas AC. Has the change to beta-agonists combined with oral theophylline increased cases of fatal asthma? Lancet 1981;1(8232):1235–7.

[226] Flack JM, Ryder KW, Strickland D, Whang R. Metabolic correlates of theophylline therapy: a concentration-related phenomenon. Ann Pharmacother 1994;28(2):175–9.

[227] Lindinger MI, Graham TE, Spriet LL. Caffeine attenuates the exercise-induced increase in plasma [K^+] in humans. J Appl Physiol 1993;74(3):1149–55.

[228] Beal AL, Deuser WE, Beilman GJ. A role for epinephrine in post-traumatic hypokalemia. Shock 2007;27(4):358–63.

[229] Bundgaard H, Kjeldsen K, Suarez Krabbe K, van Hall G, Simonsen L, Qvist J, et al. Endotoxemia stimulates skeletal muscle Na$^+$-K$^+$-ATPase and raises blood lactate under aerobic conditions in humans. Am J Physiol Heart Circ Physiol 2003;284(3):H1028−34.

[230] O'Brien WJ, Lingrel JB, Fischer JE, Hasselgren PO. Sepsis increases skeletal muscle sodium, potassium-adenosinetriphosphatase activity without affecting messenger RNA or protein levels. J Am Coll Surg 1996;183(5):471−9.

[231] Pedersen EB, Kornerup HJ. Relationship between plasma aldosterone concentration and plasma potassium in patients with essential hypertension during alprenolol treatment. Acta Med Scand 1976;200(4):263−7.

[232] Pedersen G, Pedersen A, Pedersen EB. Effect of propranolol on total exchangeable body potassium and total exchangeable body sodium in essential hypertension. Scand J Clin Lab Invest 1979;39(2):167−70.

[233] Waal-Manning HJ. Metabolic effects of beta-adrenoreceptor blockers. Drugs 1976;11(Suppl. 1):121−6.

[234] Bauer JH. Effects of propranolol therapy on renal function and body fluid composition. Arch Intern Med 1983;143(5):927−31.

[235] Steiness E. Negative potassium balance during beta-blocker treatment of hypertension. Clin Pharmacol Ther 1982;31(6):691−4.

[236] Petch MC, McKay R, Bethune DW. The effect of beta, adrenergic blockade on serum potassium and glucose levels during open heart surgery. Eur Heart J 1981;2(2):123−6.

[237] Pei Y, Richardson R, Greenwood C, Wong PY, Baines A. Extrarenal effect of cyclosporine a on potassium homeostasis in renal transplant recipients. Am J Kidney Dis 1993;22(2): 314−9.

[238] McCammon RL, Stoelting RK. Exaggerated increase in serum potassium following succinylcholine in dogs with beta blockade. Anesthesiology 1984;61(6):723−5.

[239] Arrizabalaga P, Montoliu J, Martinez Vea A, Andreu L, Lopez Pedret J, Revert L. Increase in serum potassium caused by beta-2 adrenergic blockade in terminal renal failure: absence of mediation by insulin or aldosterone. Proc Eur Dial Trans Assoc 1983;20:572−6.

[240] Arrizabalaga P, Montolio J, Martinez-Vea A, Andreu L, Lopez-Pedret J, Revert L. Increase in serum potassium caused by beta-2 adrenergic blockade in terminal renal failure: absence of mediation by insulin or aldosterone. Kidney Int 1983;24:427.

[241] Lundborg P. The effect of adrenergic blockade on potassium concentrations in different conditions. Acta Med Scand Suppl 1983;672:121−6.

[242] Ismail-Beigi F, Edelman IS. Effects of thyroid status on electrolyte distribution in rat tissues. Am J Physiol 1973;225(5): 1172−7.

[243] Kubota K, Ingbar SH. Influences of thyroid status and sympathoadrenal system on extrarenal potassium disposal. Am J Physiol 1990;258(3 Pt 1):E428−35.

[244] Lin SH, Lin YF. Propranolol rapidly reverses paralysis, hypokalemia, and hypophosphatemia in thyrotoxic periodic paralysis. Am J Kidney Dis 2001;37(3):620−3.

[245] Dias Da Silva MR, Cerutti JM, Arnaldi LA, Maciel RM. A mutation in the KCNE3 potassium channel gene is associated with susceptibility to thyrotoxic hypokalemic periodic paralysis. J Clin Endocrinol Metab 2002;87(11):4881−4.

[246] Schaafsma IA, van Ernst MG, Kouistra HS, Verkleij CB, Peeters ME, Boer P, et al. Exercise-induced hyperkalemia in hypothyroid dogs. Domest Anim Endocrinol 2002;22(2):113−25.

[247] Fenn WO, Cobb DM. The potassium equilibrium in muscle. J Gen Physiol 1934;17:629−56.

[248] Leibman J, Edelman IS. Interrelations of plasma potassium concentration, plasma sodium concentration, arterial pH and total exchangeable potassium. J Clin Invest 1959;38:2176−88.

[249] Swan RC, Pitts RF. Neutralization of infused acid by nephrectomized dogs. J Clin Invest 1955;34(2):205−12.

[250] Schwartz WB, Orning KJ, Porter R. The internal distribution of hydrogen ions with varying degrees of metabolic acidosis. J Clin Invest 1957;36(3):373−82.

[251] Burnell JM, Scribner BH, Uyeno BT, Villamil MF. The effect in humans of extracellular pH change on the relationship between serum potassium concentration and intracellular potassium. J Clin Invest 1956;35(9):935−9.

[252] Giebisch G, Berger L, Pitts RF. The extrarenal response to acute acid−base disturbances of respiratory origin. J Clin Invest 1955;34(2):231−45.

[253] Rogers TA. Tissue buffering in rat diaphragm. Am J Physiol 1957;191(2):363−6.

[254] Simmons DH, Avedon M. Acid−base alterations and plasma potassium concentration. Am J Physiol 1959;197:319−26.

[255] Brown Jr. EB, Goott B. Intracellular hydrogen ion changes and potassium movement. Am J Physiol 1963;204:765−70.

[256] Waddell WJ, Bates RG. Intracellular pH. Physiol Rev 1969;49(2):285−329.

[257] Adrogue HJ, Madias NE. Changes in plasma potassium concentration during acute acid−base disturbances. Am J Med 1981;71(3):456−67.

[258] Skou JC. Enzymatic basis for active transport of Na$^+$ and K$^+$ across cell membrane. Physiol Rev 1965;45:596−617.

[259] Breitwieser GE, Altamirano AA, Russell JM. Effects of pH changes on sodium pump fluxes in squid giant axon. Am J Physiol 1987;253(4 Pt 1):C547−54.

[260] Eaton DC, Hamilton KL, Johnson KE. Intracellular acidosis blocks the basolateral Na-K pump in rabbit urinary bladder. Am J Physiol 1984;247(6 Pt 2):F946−54.

[261] Altenberg GA, Aristimuno PC, Amorena CE, Taquini AC. Amiloride prevents the metabolic acidosis of a KCl load in nephrectomized rats. Clin Sci (Lond) 1989;76(6):649−52.

[262] Davies NW, Standen NB, Stanfield PR. The effect of intracellular pH on ATP-dependent potassium channels of frog skeletal muscle. J Physiol 1992;445:549−68.

[263] Magner PO, Robinson L, Halperin RM, Zettle R, Halperin ML. The plasma potassium concentration in metabolic acidosis: a re-evaluation. Am J Kidney Dis 1988;11(3):220−4.

[264] Oster JR, Perez GO, Vaamonde CA. Relationship between blood pH and potassium and phosphorus during acute metabolic acidosis. Am J Physiol 1978;235(4):F345−51.

[265] Vaamonde CA, Oster JR, Alpert HC, Rodriguez GR. Effect of potassium depletion on acidosis-induced changes in plasma potassium concentration. Miner Electrolyte Metab 1985;11(6):381−8.

[266] Schwarz KC, Cohen BD, Lubash GD, Rubin AL. Severe acidosis and hyperpotassemia treated with sodium bicarbonate infusion. Circulation 1959;19(2):215−20.

[267] Bettice JA, Gamble Jr. JL. Skeletal buffering of acute metabolic acidosis. Am J Physiol 1975;229(6):1618−24.

[268] Keating RE, Weichselbaum TE, Alanis M, Margraf HW, Elman R. The movement of potassium during experimental acidosis and alkalosis in the nephrectomized dog. Surg Gynecol Obstet 1953;96(3):323−30.

[269] Oster JR, Perez GO, Castro A, Vaamonde CA. Plasma potassium response to acute metabolic acidosis induced by mineral and nonmineral acids. Miner Electrolyte Metab 1980;4: 28−36.

[270] Tobin RB. Varying role of extracellular electrolytes in metabolic acidosis and alkalosis. Am J Physiol 1958;195(3):685−92.

[271] Rogers TA, Wachenfeld AE. Effect of physiologic acids on electrolytes in rat diaphragm. Am J Physiol 1958;193(3):623−6.

[272] Fulop M. Serum potassium in lactic acidosis and ketoacidosis. N Engl J Med 1979;300(19):1087−9.

III. FLUID AND ELECTROLYTE REGULATION AND DYSREGULATION

[273] Perez GO, Oster JR, Vaamonde CA. Serum potassium concentration in acidemic states. Nephron 1981;27(4–5):233–43.

[274] Kreisberg RA. Diabetic ketoacidosis: new concepts and trends in pathogenesis and treatment. Ann Intern Med 1978;88(5):681–95.

[275] Beigelman PM. Potassium in severe diabetic ketoacidosis. Am J Med 1973;54(4):419–20.

[276] Cohen AS, Vance VK, Runyan Jr. JW, Hurwitz D. Diabetic acidosis: an evaluation of the cause, course and therapy of 73 cases. Ann Intern Med 1960;52:55–86.

[277] Adrogue HJ, Lederer ED, Suki WN, Eknoyan G. Determinants of plasma potassium levels in diabetic ketoacidosis. Medicine (Baltimore) 1986;65(3):163–72.

[278] Arieff AI, Carroll HJ. Nonketotic hyperosmolar coma with hyperglycemia: clinical features, pathophysiology, renal function, acid–base balance, plasma-cerebrospinal fluid equilibria and the effects of therapy in 37 cases. Medicine (Baltimore) 1972;51(2):73–94.

[279] Madias NE. Lactic acidosis. Kidney Int 1986;29(3):752–74.

[280] Orringer CE, Eustace JC, Wunsch CD, Gardner LB. Natural history of lactic acidosis after grand-mal seizures. A model for the study of an anion-gap acidosis not associated with hyperkalemia. N Engl J Med 1977;297(15):796–9.

[281] Rodgrove HJ, Alabaster S. Lactic acidosis in seizures. N Engl J Med 1977;297(24):1352.

[282] Cooperman MT, Davidoff F, Spark R, Pallotta J. Clinical studies of alcoholic ketoacidosis. Diabetes 1974;23(5):433–9.

[283] Levy LJ, Duga J, Girgis M, Gordon EE. Ketoacidosis associated with alcoholism in nondiabetic subjects. Ann Intern Med 1973;78(2):213–9.

[284] Adler S, Fraley DS. Potassium and intracellular pH. Kidney Int 1977;11(6):433–42.

[285] Schwartz WB, Brackett Jr. NC, Cohen JJ. The response of extracellular hydrogen ion concentration to graded degrees of chronic hypercapnia: the physiologic limits of the defense of pH. J Clin Invest 1965;44:291–301.

[286] Nahas GG, Steinsland OS. Increased rate of catecholamine synthesis during respiratory acidosis. Respir Physiol 1968;5(1):108–17.

[287] Fenn WO, Asano T. Effects of carbon dioxide inhalation on potassium liberation from the liver. Am J Physiol 1956;185(3):567–76.

[288] Natalini G, Seramondi V, Fassini P, Foccoli P, Toninelli C, Caviliere S, et al. Acute respiratory acidosis does not increase plasma potassium in normokalaemic anaesthetized patients. A controlled randomized trial. Eur J Anaesthesiol 2001;18(6):394–400.

[289] Takahashi T, Kato A, Miura Y, Karube T, Sakai M, Amagasa S. [The effect of beta-adrenergic blockade on the plasma potassium elevation induced by acute respiratory acidosis during halothane or fentanyl anesthesia]. Masui 1994;43(4):479–86.

[290] Abrams WB, Lewis DW, Bellet S. The effect of acidosis and alkalosis on the plasma potassium concentration and the electrocardiogram of normal and potassium depleted dogs. Am J Med Sci 1951;222(5):506–15.

[291] Kim WG, Brown Jr. EB. Potassium transfer with constant extracellular pH. J Lab Clin Med 1968;71(4):678–85.

[292] Farley DS, Adler S. Isohydric regulation of plasma potassium by bicarbonate in the rat. Kidney Int 1976;9(4):333–43.

[293] Fraley DS, Adler S. Correction of hyperkalemia by bicarbonate despite constant blood pH. Kidney Int 1977;12(5):354–60.

[294] Bushinsky DA, Coe FL. Hyperkalemia during acute ammonium chloride acidosis in man. Nephron 1985;40(1):38–40.

[295] Williams ME, Rosa RM, Epstein FH. Hyperkalemia. Adv Intern Med 1986;31:265–91.

[296] Blumberg A, Weidmann P, Shaw S, Gnadinger M. Effect of various therapeutic approaches on plasma potassium and major regulating factors in terminal renal failure. Am J Med 1988;85(4):507–12.

[297] Mostellar ME, Tuttle Jr. EP. Effects of alkalosis on plasma concentration and urinary excretion of inorganic phosphate in man. J Clin Invest 1964;43:138–49.

[298] Singer RB, Clark JK, Barker ES, Crosley Jr. AP, Elkinton JR. The acute effects in man of rapid intravenous infusion of hypertonic sodium bicarbonate solution. I. Changes in acid–base balance and distribution of the excess buffer base. Medicine (Baltimore) 1955;34(1):51–95.

[299] Krapf R, Caduff P, Wagdi P, Staubli M, Hulter HN. Plasma potassium response to acute respiratory alkalosis. Kidney Int 1995;47(1):217–24.

[300] Edwards R, Winnie AP, Ramamurthy S. Acute hypocapneic hypokalemia: an iatrogenic anesthetic complication. Anesth Analg 1977;56(6):786–92.

[301] Sorensen MV, Matos JE, Sausbier M, Sausbier U, Ruth P, Praetorious HA, et al. Aldosterone increases KCa1.1 (BK) channel-mediated colonic K+ secretion. J Physiol 2008;586(Pt 17):4251–64.

[302] Sorensen MV, Matos JE, Praetorius HA, Leipziger J. Colonic potassium handling. Pflugers Arch 2010;459(5):645–56.

[303] Adler S. An extrarenal action of aldosterone on mammalian skeletal muscle. Am J Physiol 1970;218(3):616–21.

[304] Lim VS, Webster GD. The effect of aldosterone on water and electrolyte composition of incubated rat diaphragms. Clin Sci 1967;33(2):261–70.

[305] DeFronzo RA, Lee R, Jones A, Bia M. Effect of insulinopenia and adrenal hormone deficiency on acute potassium tolerance. Kidney Int 1980;17(5):586–94.

[306] Pan YJ, Young DB. Experimental aldosterone hypertension in the dog. Hypertension 1982;4(2):279–87.

[307] Young DB. Quantitative analysis of aldosterone's role in potassium regulation. Am J Physiol 1988;255(5 Pt 2):F811–22.

[308] Young DB, Jackson TE. Effects of aldosterone on potassium distribution. Am J Physiol 1982;243(5):R526–30.

[309] Sugarman A, Brown RS. The role of aldosterone in potassium tolerance: studies in anephric humans. Kidney Int 1988;34(3):397–403.

[310] Singhal PC, Desroches L, Mattana J, Abramovici M, Wagner JD, Maesaka JK. Mineralocorticoid therapy lowers serum potassium in patients with end-stage renal disease. Am J Nephrol 1993;13(2):138–41.

[311] Alexander EA, Levinsky NG. An extrarenal mechanism of potassium adaptation. J Clin Invest 1968;47(4):740–8.

[312] Spital A, Sterns RH. Extrarenal potassium adaptation: the role of aldosterone. Clin Sci (Lond) 1989;76(2):213–9.

[313] Schwartz WB. Potassium and the kidney. N Engl J Med 1955;253(14):601–8.

[314] Seldin DW, Carter NW, Rector Jr. FC. Consequences of renal failure and their management. In: Strauss MB, Welt LG, editors. Diseases of the kidney. Boston: Little, Brown; 1963. p. 173–217.

[315] Elkinton JR, Tarail R, Peters JP. Transfers of potassium in renal insufficiency. J Clin Invest 1949;27:378–88.

[316] Salem MM, Rosa RM, Batlle DC. Extrarenal potassium tolerance in chronic renal failure: implications for the treatment of acute hyperkalemia. Am J Kidney Dis 1991;18(4):421–40.

[317] Fernandez J, Oster JR, Perez GO. Impaired extrarenal disposal of an acute oral potassium load in patients with endstage renal disease on chronic hemodialysis. Miner Electrolyte Metab 1986;12(2):125–9.

[318] Sterns RH, Feig PU, Pring M, Guzzo J, Singer I. Disposition of intravenous potassium in anuric man: a kinetic analysis. Kidney Int 1979;15(6):651–60.

[319] Kahn T, Kaji DM, Nicolis G, Krakoff LR, Stein RM. Factors related to potassium transport in chronic stable renal disease in man. Clin Sci Mol Med 1978;54(6):661–6.

[320] Bia M, DeFronzo R. The medullary collecting duct (MCD) does not play a primary role in potassium (K) adaptation following decreased GFR. Clin Res 1978;26: [457 A]

[321] Tuck ML, Davidson MB, Asp N, Schultze RG. Augmented aldosterone and insulin responses to potassium infusion in dogs with renal failure. Kidney Int 1986;30(6):883–90.

[322] Goecke IA, Bonilla S, Marusic ET, Alvo M. Enhanced insulin sensitivity in extrarenal potassium handling in uremic rats. Kidney Int 1991;39(1):39–43.

[323] Adesman J, Goldberg M, Castleman L, Friedman IS. Simultaneous measurement of body sodium and potassium using Na22 and K42. Metabolism 1960;9:561–9.

[324] Bergstrom J, Alvestrand A, Furst P, Hultman E, Widstam-Attorps U. Muscle intracellular electrolytes in patients with chronic uremia. Kidney Int Suppl 1983;16:S153–60.

[325] Bilbrey GL, Carter NW, White MG, Schilling JF, Knochel JP. Potassium deficiency in chronic renal failure. Kidney Int 1973;4(6):423–30.

[326] Mitch WE, Wilcox CS. Disorders of body fluids, sodium and potassium in chronic renal failure. Am J Med 1982;72(3):536–50.

[327] Schultze G, Koeppe P, Molzahn M. Restoration of total body potassium in the course of long-term hemodialysis treatment. Miner Electrolyte Metab 1981;6:139–45.

[328] Spergel G, Bleicher SJ, Goldberg M, Adesman J, Goldner MG. The effect of potassium on the impaired glucose tolerance in chronic uremia. Metabolism 1967;16:581–5.

[329] Alvestrand A, Wahren J, Smith D, DeFronzo RA. Insulin-mediated potassium uptake is normal in uremic and healthy subjects. Am J Physiol 1984;246(2 Pt 1):E174–80.

[330] Westervelt Jr. FB. Uremia and insulin response. Arch Intern Med 1970;126(5):865–9.

[331] Cooke CR, Ruiz-Maza F, Kowarski A, Migeon CJ, Walker WG. Regulation of plasma aldosterone concentration in anephric man and renal transplant recipients. Kidney Int 1973;3(3):160–6.

[332] Schrier RW, Regal EM. Influence of aldosterone on sodium, water and potassium metabolism in chronic renal disease. Kidney Int 1972;1(3):156–68.

[333] Cooke CR, Horvath JS, Moore MA, Bledsoe T, Walker WG. Modulation of plasma aldosterone concentration by plasma potassium in anephric man in the absence of a change in potassium balance. J Clin Invest 1973;52(12):3028–32.

[334] Campese VM, Romoff MS, Levitan D, Lane K, Massry SG. Mechanisms of autonomic nervous system dysfunction in uremia. Kidney Int 1981;20(2):246–53.

[335] Henrich WL, Katz FH, Molinoff PB, Schrier RW. Competitive effects of hypokalemia and volume depletion on plasma renin activity, aldosterone and catecholamine concentrations in hemodialysis patients. Kidney Int 1977;12(4): 279–84.

[336] Botey A, Gaya J, Montoliu J, Torras A, Rivera F, Lopez-Pedret J, et al. Postsynaptic adrenergic unresponsiveness in hypotensive haemodialysis patients. Proc Eur Dial Trans Assoc 1981;18:586–91.

[337] Montoliu J, Lens XM, Revert L. Potassium-lowering effect of albuterol for hyperkalemia in renal failure. Arch Intern Med 1987;147(4):713–7.

[338] Allon M, Dunlay R, Copkney C. Nebulized albuterol for acute hyperkalemia in patients on hemodialysis. Ann Intern Med 1989;110(6):426–9.

[339] Stemmer CL, Perez GO, Oster JR. Impairment of beta 2-adrenoceptor-stimulated potassium uptake in end-stage renal disease. J Clin Pharmacol 1987;27(8):628–31.

[340] Martinez Vea A, Montoliu J, Andreu L, Torras A, Gaya J, Lopez-Pedret J, et al. Beta adrenergic modulation of extrarenal potassium disposal in terminal uraemia. Proc Eur Dial Trans Assoc 1983;19:756–60.

[341] Sugarman A, Kahn T. Parathyroid hormone impairs extrarenal potassium tolerance in the rat. Am J Physiol 1988;254(3 Pt 2): F385–90.

[342] Soliman AR, Akmal M, Massry SG. Parathyroid hormone interferes with extrarenal disposition of potassium in chronic renal failure. Nephron 1989;52(3):262–7.

[343] Izumo H, Izumo S, DeLuise M, Flier JS. Erythrocyte Na,K pump in uremia. Acute correction of a transport defect by hemodialysis. J Clin Invest 1984;74(2):581–8.

[344] Kramer HJ, Gospodinov D, Kruck F. Functional and metabolic studies on red blood cell sodium transport in chronic uremia. Nephron 1976;16(5):344–58.

[345] Krzesinski JM, Rorive G. Sodium–lithium countertransport in red cells. N Engl J Med 1983;309:987–8.

[346] Walter U, Becht E. Red blood cell sodium transport and phosphate release in uremia. Nephron 1983;34(1):35–41.

[347] Welt LG, Sachs JR, McManus TJ. An ion transport defect in erythrocytes from uremic patients. Trans Assoc Am Physic 1964;77:169–81.

[348] Zannad F, Kessler M, Royer RJ, Robert J. Effect of hemodialysis on red blood cell Na+–K+-ATPase activity in terminal renal failure. Nephron 1985;40(1):127–8.

[349] Zannad F, Royer RJ, Kessler M, Huriet B, Robert J. Cation transport in erythrocytes of patients with renal failure. Nephron 1982;32(4):347–50.

[350] Quarello F, Boero R, Guarena C, Rosati C, Giraudo G, Giacchino F, et al. Acute effects of hemodialysis on erythrocyte sodium fluxes in uremic patients. Nephron 1985;41 (1):22–5.

[351] Cole CH, Balfe JW, Welt LG. Induction of a ouabain-sensitive ATPase defect by uremic plasma. Trans Assoc Am Physic 1968;81:213–20.

[352] Cheng JT, Kahn T, Kaji DM. Mechanism of alteration of sodium potassium pump of erythrocytes from patients with chronic renal failure. J Clin Invest 1984;74(5):1811–20.

[353] Kaji D, Thomas K. Na+–K+ pump in chronic renal failure. Am J Physiol 1987;252(5 Pt 2):F785–93.

[354] Druml W, Kelly RA, May RC, Mitch WE. Abnormal cation transport in uremia. Mechanisms in adipocytes and skeletal muscle from uremic rats. J Clin Invest 1988;81(4):1197–203.

[355] Sangkabutra T, Crankshaw DP, Schneider C, Fraser SF, Sostaric S, Mason K, et al. Impaired K+ regulation contributes to exercise limitation in end-stage renal failure. Kidney Int 2003;63(1):283–90.

[356] Watson KR, O'Kell RT. Lack of relationship between Mg2+ and K+ concentrations in serum. Clin Chem 1980;26(3):520–1.

[357] Whang R. Magnesium and potassium interrelationships in cardiac arrhythmias. Magnesium 1986;5(3–4):127–33.

[358] Whang R, Oei TO, Hamiter T. Frequency of hypomagnesmia associated with hypokalemia in hospitalized patients. Am J Clin Pathol 1979;71:610.

[359] Solomon R. The relationship between disorders of K+ and Mg+ homeostasis. Semin Nephrol 1987;7(3):253–62.

[360] Ryan MP. Interrelationships of magnesium and potassium homeostasis. Miner Electrolyte Metab 1993;19(4–5):290–5.

[361] Alfrey AC. Disorders of magnesium metabolism. In: Seldin DWaG G, editor. The kidney: physiology and pathophysiology. New York: Raven Press; 1985. p. 1281–95.

III. FLUID AND ELECTROLYTE REGULATION AND DYSREGULATION

[362] Ladefoged K, Hagen K. Correlation between concentrations of magnesium, zinc, and potassium in plasma, erythrocytes and muscles. Clin Chim Acta 1988;177(2):157–66.

[363] Alfrey AC, Miller NL, Butkus D. Evaluation of body magnesium stores. J Lab Clin Med 1974;84(2):153–62.

[364] Manitius A, Epstein FH. Some observations on the influence of a magnesium-deficient diet on rats, with special reference to renal concentrating ability. J Clin Invest 1963;42(2):208–15.

[365] Shils ME. Experimental human magnesium depletion. Medicine (Baltimore) 1969;48(1):61–85.

[366] Whang R, Flink EB, Dyckner T, Wester PO, Aikawa JK, Ryan MP. Magnesium depletion as a cause of refractory potassium repletion. Arch Intern Med 1985;145(9):1686–9.

[367] Ryan MP, Whang R, Yamalis W, Aikawa JK. Effect of magnesium deficiency on cardiac and skeletal muscle potassium during dietary potassium restriction. Proc Soc Exp Biol Med 1973;143(4):1045–7.

[368] Whang R, Welt LG. Observations in experimental magnesium depletion. J Clin Invest 1963;42:305–13.

[369] Whang R, Oei TO, Aikawa JK, Ryan MP, Watanabe A, Chrysant SG, et al. Magnesium and potassium interrelationships, experimental and clinical. Acta Med Scand Suppl 1981;647:139–44.

[370] Kjeldsen K, Norgaard A. Effect of magnesium depletion on ^{3}H-ouabain binding site concentration in rat skeletal muscle. Magnesium 1987;6(1):55–60.

[371] Dorup I, Skajaa K, Clausen T, Kjeldsen K. Reduced concentrations of potassium, magnesium, and sodium-potassium pumps in human skeletal muscle during treatment with diuretics. Br Med J (Clin Res Ed) 1988;296(6620):455–8.

[372] Fischer PW, Giroux A. Effects of dietary magnesium on sodium-potassium pump action in the heart of rats. J Nutr 1987;117(12):2091–5.

[373] Findlay I. The effects of magnesium upon adenosine triphosphate-sensitive potassium channels in a rat insulin-secreting cell line. J Physiol 1987;391:611–29.

[374] Horie M, Irisawa H, Noma A. Voltage-dependent magnesium block of adenosine-triphosphate-sensitive potassium channel in guinea-pig ventricular cells. J Physiol 1987;387:251–72.

[375] Vandenberg CA. Inward rectification of a potassium channel in cardiac ventricular cells depends on internal magnesium ions. Proc Natl Acad Sci USA 1987;84(8):2560–4.

[376] Cannon-Babb ML, Schwartz AB. Drug-induced hyperkalemia. Hosp Pract (Off Ed) 1986;21(9A):99–107 111, 114-127

[377] Paice B, Gray JM, McBride D, Donnelly T, Lawson DH. Hyperkalaemia in patients in hospital. Br Med J (Clin Res Ed) 1983;286(6372):1189–92.

[378] Perazella MA. Drug-induced hyperkalemia: old culprits and new offenders. Am J Med 2000;109(4):307–14.

[379] Ponce SP, Jennings AE, Madias NE, Harrington JT. Drug-induced hyperkalemia. Medicine (Baltimore) 1985;64(6): 357–70.

[380] Rimmer JM, Horn JF, Gennari FJ. Hyperkalemia as a complication of drug therapy. Arch Intern Med 1987;147(5):867–9.

[381] Shemer J, Modan M, Ezra D, Cabili S. Incidence of hyperkalemia in hospitalized patients. Isr J Med Sci 1983;19(7):659–61.

[382] Brass EP, Thompson WL. Drug-induced electrolyte abnormalities. Drugs 1982;24(3):207–28.

[383] Gronert GA, Theye RA. Pathophysiology of hyperkalemia induced by succinylcholine. Anesthesiology 1975;43 (1):89–99.

[384] Iwatsuki N, Kuroda N, Amaha K, Iwatsuki K. Succinylcholine-induced hyperkalemia in patients with ruptured cerebral aneurysms. Anesthesiology 1980;53(1):64–7.

[385] Striker T, Morrow A. Effect of succinylcholine on the level of serum potassium in man. Anesthesiology 1968;29:214–5.

[386] Martyn JA, Richtsfeld M. Succinylcholine-induced hyperkalemia in acquired pathologic states: etiologic factors and molecular mechanisms. Anesthesiology 2006;104(1):158–69.

[387] Weintraub HD, Heisterkamp DV, Cooperman LH. Changes in plasma potassium concentration after depolarizing blockers in anaesthetized man. Br J Anaesth 1969;41(12):1048–52.

[388] George Jr. AL, Wood Jr. CA. Succinylcholine-induced hyperkalemia complicating the neuroleptic malignant syndrome. Ann Intern Med 1987;106(1):172.

[389] Krikken-Hogenberk LG, de Jong JR, Bovill JG. Succinylcholine-induced hyperkalemia in a patient with metastatic rhabdomyosarcoma. Anesthesiology 1989;70(3):553–5.

[390] Edelman S, Witztum JL. Hyperkalemia during treatment with HMG-CoA reductase inhibitor. N Engl J Med 1989;320(18): 1219–20.

[391] Grundy SM. HMG-CoA reductase inhibitors for treatment of hypercholesterolemia. N Engl J Med 1988;319(1):24–33.

[392] Alberti KG, Johnston H, Lauler D. The effect of arginine and its derivatives on potassium metabolism in the dog. Clin Res 1967;15:476.

[393] Hertz P, Richardson JA. Arginine-induced hyperkalemia in renal failure patients. Arch Intern Med 1972;130(5):778–80.

[394] Bushinsky DA, Gennari FJ. Life-threatening hyperkalemia induced by arginine. Ann Intern Med 1978;89(5 Pt 1): 632–4.

[395] Perazella MA, Biswas P. Acute hyperkalemia associated with intravenous epsilon-aminocaproic acid therapy. Am J Kidney Dis 1999;33(4):782–5.

[396] Edner M, Ponikowski P, Jogestrand T. The effect of digoxin on the serum potassium concentration. Scand J Clin Lab Invest 1993;53(2):187–9.

[397] Schmidt TA, Bundgaard H, Olesen HL, Secher NH, Kjeldsen K. Digoxin affects potassium homeostasis during exercise in patients with heart failure. Cardiovasc Res 1995;29(4):506–11.

[398] Bismuth C, Gaultier M, Conso F, Efthymiou ML. Hyperkalemia in acute digitalis poisoning: prognostic significance and therapeutic implications. Clin Toxicol 1973;6(2): 153–62.

[399] Smith TW, Willerson JT. Suicidal and accidental digoxin ingestion. Report of five cases with serum digoxin level correlations. Circulation 1971;44(1):29–36.

[400] Papadakis MA, Wexman MP, Fraser C, Sedlacek SM. Hyperkalemia complicating digoxin toxicity in a patient with renal failure. Am J Kidney Dis 1985;5(1):64–6.

[401] Clive DM, Stoff JS. Renal syndromes associated with nonsteroidal antiinflammatory drugs. N Engl J Med 1984;310 (9):563–72.

[402] Garella S, Matarese RA. Renal effects of prostaglandins and clinical adverse effects of nonsteroidal anti-inflammatory agents. Medicine (Baltimore) 1984;63(3):165–81.

[403] Clive D.M, Gurwitz J, Williams M, Rossetti R. Nonsteroidal antiinflammatory drugs (NSAID) do not impair potassium metabolism in normal humans. Paper presented at: 10th International Congress of Nephrology1990.

[404] Saris S, Lowenthal DT, Affrime MB, Rosenthal L, Swartz G. Lack of effect of nonsteroidsal anti-inflammatory drugs on exercise-induced hyperkalemia. N Engl J Med 1982;307(9): 559–60.

[405] Hariharasubramanian N, Devi D, Rao A. Serum potassium levels during lithium therapy of manic depressive psychosis. In: Johnson FN, Johnson S, editors. Lithium in medical practice. Baltimore: University Press; 1978. p. 205–8.

[406] McCusick V. The effect of lithium on the electrocardiogram of animals and relation of this effect to the ratio of the intracellular and extracellular concentrations of potassium. J Clin Invest 1954;33:598–610.

[407] Goggans FC. Acute hyperkalemia during lithium treatment of manic illness. Am J Psychiatry 1980;137(7):860–1.

[408] Groot OA, Trof RJ, Girbes AR, Swart NL, Beishuizen A. Acute refractory hyperkalaemia and fatal cardiac arrest related to administration of liposomal amphotericin B. Neth J Med 2008;66(10):433–7.

[409] Kearney TE, Manoguerra AS, Curtis GP, Ziegler MG. Theophylline toxicity and the beta-adrenergic system. Ann Intern Med 1985;102(6):766–9.

[410] Zantvoort FA, Derkx FH, Boomsma F, Roos PJ, Schalekamp MA. Theophylline and serum electrolytes. Ann Intern Med 1986;104(1):134–5.

[411] Trost BN, Weidmann P. Metabolic effects of calcium antagonists in humans, with emphasis on carbohydrate, lipid, potassium, and uric acid homeostases. J Cardiovasc Pharmacol 1988;12(Suppl. 6):S86–92.

[412] Minella RA, Schulman DS. Fatal verapamil toxicity and hypokalemia. Am Heart J 1991;121(6 Pt 1):1810–2.

[413] Davidovics Y, Peer G, Cabili S, Blum M, Serban I, Wollman Y, et al. Effect of verapamil on disposition of intravenous potassium in diabetic anephric uremic rats. Miner Electrolyte Metab 1993;19(2):99–102.

[414] Mimran A, Ribstein J, Sissmann J. Effects of calcium antagonists on adrenaline-induced hypokalaemia. Drugs 1993;46 (Suppl. 2):103–7.

[415] Sugarman A, Kahn T. Calcium channel blockers enhance extrarenal potassium disposal in the rat. Am J Physiol 1986;250 (4 Pt 2):F695–701.

[416] Solomon R, Dubey A. Diltiazem enhances potassium disposal in subjects with end-stage renal disease. Am J Kidney Dis 1992;19(5):420–6.

[417] Gardos G. The function of calcium in the potassium permeability of human erythrocytes. Biochim Biophys Acta 1958;30(3):653–4.

[418] Burgess GM, Claret M, Jenkinson DH. Effects of quinine and apamin on the calcium-dependent potassium permeability of mammalian hepatocytes and red cells. J Physiol 1981;317:67–90.

[419] Capponi AM, Lew PD, Jornot L, Vallotton MB. Correlation between cytosolic free Ca^{2+} and aldosterone production in bovine adrenal glomerulosa cells. Evidence for a difference in the mode of action of angiotensin II and potassium. J Biol Chem 1984;259(14):8863–9.

[420] Nadler JL, Hsueh W, Horton R. Therapeutic effect of calcium channel blockade in primary aldosteronism. J Clin Endocrinol Metab 1985;60(5):896–9.

[421] Bouchard PM, Frenette AJ, Williamson DR, Perreault MM. Thiopental-associated dyskalemia in severe head trauma. J Trauma 2008;64(3):838–42.

[422] Jung JY, Lee C, Ro H, Kim HS, Joo KW, Kim Y, et al. Sequential occurrence of life-threatening hypokalemia and rebound hyperkalemia associated with barbiturate coma therapy. Clin Nephrol 2009;71(3):333–7.

[423] Clemessy JL, Favier C, Borron SW, Hantson PE, Vicaut E, Baud FJ. Hypokalaemia related to acute chloroquine ingestion. Lancet 1995;346(8979):877–80.

[424] Thuss-Patience PC, Peters U, Jurkat-Rott K, Pink D, Kretzschmar A, Dorken B, et al. Acute hypokalemic tetraparesis induced by intravenous methotrexate. J Clin Oncol 2003;21(9):1896–7.

[425] Seldin DW, Tarail R. Effect of hypertonic solutions on metabolism and excretion of electrolytes. Am J Physiol 1949;159(1):160–74.

[426] Makoff DL, Da Silva JA, Rosenbaum BJ. On the mechanism of hyperkalaemia due to hyperosmotic expansion with saline or mannitol. Clin Sci 1971;41(5):383–93.

[427] Moreno M, Murphy C, Goldsmith C. Increase in serum potassium resulting from the administration of hypertonic mannitol and other solutions. J Lab Clin Med 1969;73 (2):291–8.

[428] Goldfarb S, Cox M, Singer I, Goldberg M. Acute hyperkalemia induced by hyperglycemia: hormonal mechanisms. Ann Intern Med 1976;84(4):426–32.

[429] Rado JP. Glucose-induced hyperkalemia during captopril treatment. Arch Intern Med 1983;143(2):389.

[430] Nicolis GL, Kahn T, Sanchez A, Gabrilove JL. Glucose-induced hyperkalemia in diabetic subjects. Arch Intern Med 1981;141(1):49–53.

[431] Singhal PC, Rubin RB, Peters A, Santiago A, Neugarten J. Rhabdomyolysis and acute renal failure associated with cocaine abuse. J Toxicol Clin Toxicol 1990;28(3):321–30.

[432] Cohen LF, Balow JE, Magrath IT, Poplack DG, Ziegler JL. Acute tumor lysis syndrome. A review of 37 patients with Burkitt's lymphoma. Am J Med 1980;68(4):486–91.

[433] Cech P, Block JB, Cone LA, Stone R. Tumor lysis syndrome after tamoxifen flare. N Engl J Med 1986;315(4):263–4.

[434] Tsokos GC, Balow JE, Spiegel RJ, Magrath IT. Renal and metabolic complications of undifferentiated and lymphoblastic lymphomas. Medicine (Baltimore) 1981;60(3):218–29.

[435] Hesp R, Chanarin I, Tait CE. Potassium changes in megaloblastic anaemia. Clin Sci Mol Med 1975;49(1):77–9.

[436] James GW, Abbott Jr. LD. Metabolic studies in pernicious anemia. I. Nitrogen and phosphorus metabolism during vitamin B12-induced remission. Metabolism 1952;1 (3):259–70.

[437] Lawson DH, Murray RM, Parker JL. Early mortality in the megaloblastic anaemias. Q J Med 1972;41(161):1–14.

[438] Sperelakis N, Schneider MF, Harris EJ. Decreased K^+ conductance produced by Ba^{++} in frog sartorius fibers. J Gen Physiol 1967;50(6):1565–83.

[439] Gallant EM. Barium-treated mammalian skeletal muscle: similarities to hypokalaemic periodic paralysis. J Physiol 1983;335:577–90.

[440] Roza O, Berman LB. The pathophysiology of barium: hypokalemic and cardiovascular effects. J Pharmacol Exp Ther 1971;177(2):433–9.

[441] Allen AS. Pa Ping, or Kiating paralysis. Chin Med J 1943;61:296–301.

[442] Huang K-W. Pa Ping (transient paralysis simulating family periodic paralysis). Chin Med J 1943;61:305–12.

[443] Dalal AK, Harding JD, Verdino RJ. Acquired long QT syndrome and monomorphic ventricular tachycardia after alternative treatment with cesium chloride for brain cancer. Mayo Clin Proc 2004;79(8):1065–9.

[444] McIvor ME. Acute fluoride toxicity. Pathophysiology and management. Drug Saf 1990;5(2):79–85.

[445] Bruining HA, Boelhouwer RU. Acute transient hypokalemia and body temperature. Lancet 1982;2(8310):1283–4.

[446] Koht A, Cane R, Cerullo LJ. Serum potassium levels during prolonged hypothermia. Intensive Care Med 1983;9(5):275–7.

[447] Sprung J, Cheng EY, Gamulin S, Kampine JP, Bosnjak ZJ. Effects of acute hypothermia and beta-adrenergic receptor blockade on serum potassium concentration in rats. Crit Care Med 1991;19(12):1545–51.

[448] Ellis RJ, Hoover E, Gay WA, Ebert PA. Metabolic alterations with profound hypothermia. Arch Surg 1974;109 (5):659–63.

[449] Suh A, DeJesus E, Rosner K, Lerma E, Yu W, Young JB, et al. Racial differences in potassium disposal. Kidney Int 2004;66(3):1076–81.

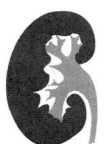

Regulation of K$^+$ Excretion

Gerhard Malnic[1], Gerhard Giebisch[2], Shigeaki Muto[3], Wenhui Wang[4], Matthew A. Bailey[5] and Lisa M. Satlin[6]

[1]Universidade de Sao Paulo, Instituto de Ciencias Biomedicas, Departamento de Fisiologie e Biofisica, Sao Paulo, Brazil

[2]Department of Cellular & Molecular Physiology, Yale University School of Medicine, New Haven, CT, USA

[3]Department of Nephrology, Jichi Medical School, Shimotsuke, Tochigi, Japan

[4]Department of Pharmacology, New York Medical College, Valhalla, NY, USA

[5]British Heart Foundation Centre for Cardiovascular Science, The University of Edinburgh, Edinburgh, UK

[6]Department of Pediatrics, Mt. Sinai School of Medicine, New York, NY, USA

OVERVIEW OF K$^+$ DISTRIBUTION AND EXCRETION–INTERNAL AND EXTERNAL BALANCE

As the most abundant cation in intracellular fluid, K$^+$ plays an important role in a variety of cell functions. High K$^+$ concentration in cells and low K$^+$ concentration in extracellular fluid is essential for many cellular processes, including determining the electrical properties of cell membranes in both excitable (nerve, muscle) and nonexcitable (transporting epithelia) tissues.[514,515] Cell K$^+$ also contributes importantly to the effective osmolality of intracellular fluid, and thus to the regulation of cell volume.[316,514,515,568] Changes in cell K$^+$ modify intracellular acidity, and thereby indirectly influence a variety of metabolic processes.[4,274] These important functions depend on the coordinated action of a variety of regulatory mechanisms that serve to maintain total K$^+$ content (50–55 mmol/kg body weight) and distribution.[4,154,274]

INTERNAL K$^+$ BALANCE

Figure 49.1 schematically shows several features of the distribution of K$^+$ in the body. More than 98% of body K$^+$ resides within cells, principally in skeletal muscle, whereas only 2% of total body K$^+$ is located in the extracellular fluid space. Maintenance of K$^+$ homeostasis is challenging, because the daily dietary intake of K$^+$ in the adult ($\sim$70 mEq) typically approaches the total K$^+$ content normally present within the extracellular fluid space ($\sim$70 mEq in 17 L of extracellular fluid, with a K$^+$ concentration averaging $\sim$4 mEq/l). To maintain zero balance in the adult, dietary intake of K$^+$ must be matched by its elimination, a task performed primarily by the kidney.

Ingested potassium enters the extracellular fluid by reabsorption from the small intestine, a process not subject to specific regulation.[264] K$^+$ that enters the extracellular fluid must temporarily and rapidly be translocated into cells to prevent dangerous increases in plasma K$^+$ levels. The buffering capacity of the combined cellular storage reservoirs, which includes muscle, liver, and red blood cells, is vast compared with the extracellular pool and is capable of sequestering large amounts of K$^+$. The biochemical and hormonal factors that influence the internal balance of K$^+$, typically by altering Na-K-ATPase activity, are listed in Figure 49.2.[7,259,479,480] Racial differences in K$^+$ distribution have also been reported.[495]

The steep K$^+$ concentration gradient across the cell membrane depends on the regulated interplay between active uptake by Na$^+$,K$^+$-ATPase and passive backleak through K$^+$ channels and carrier-mediated transport processes[514,515,568] (Figure 49.1b). When K$^+$ enters the extracellular fluid, active Na$^+$,K$^+$-ATPase-mediated K$^+$ uptake into cells occurs rapidly, and buffers against fluctuations of K$^+$ in the extracellular fluid. This process is efficient, and plasma K$^+$ concentration is kept

Seldin and Giebisch's The Kidney, Fifth Edition.
DOI: http://dx.doi.org/10.1016/B978-0-12-381462-3.00049-5

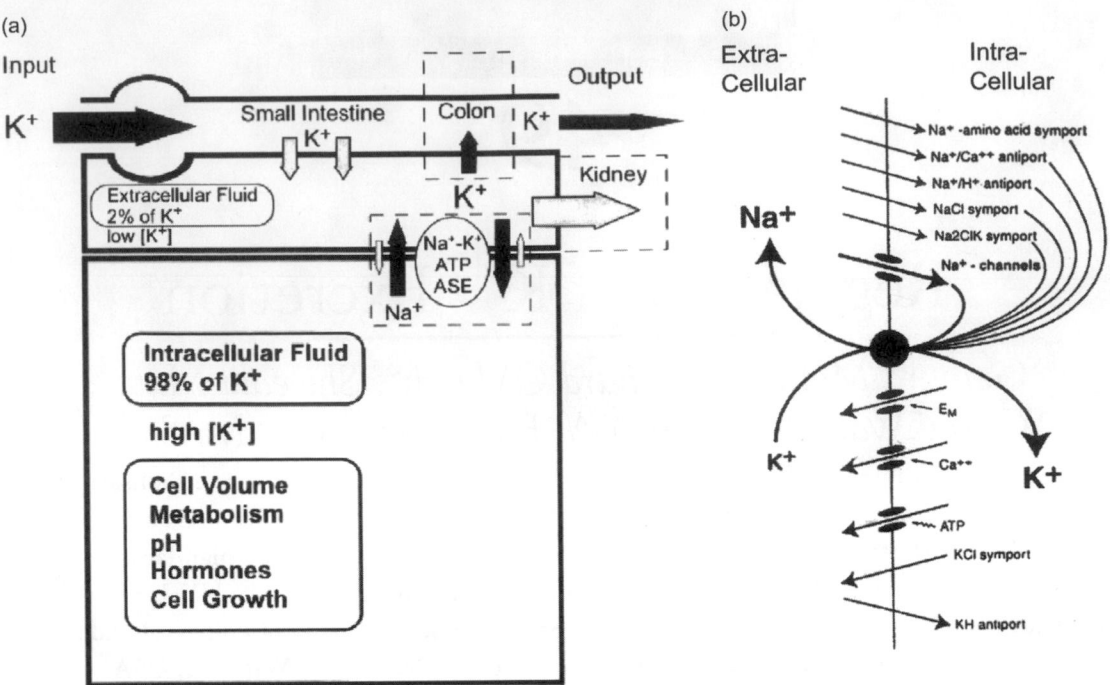

FIGURE 49.1 (a) Distribution of K⁺ in the body and pathways of K⁺ entry and exit. (b) Transporters involved in the distribution of K⁺ and Na⁺ across cell membranes. The activity of the Na⁺,K⁺-ATPase in cell membranes is opposed by several symporters, antiporters, and ion channels. *(From Giebisch, G. (2002). A trail of research on potassium. Kidney Int. **62**, 1498–1512, with permission.)*

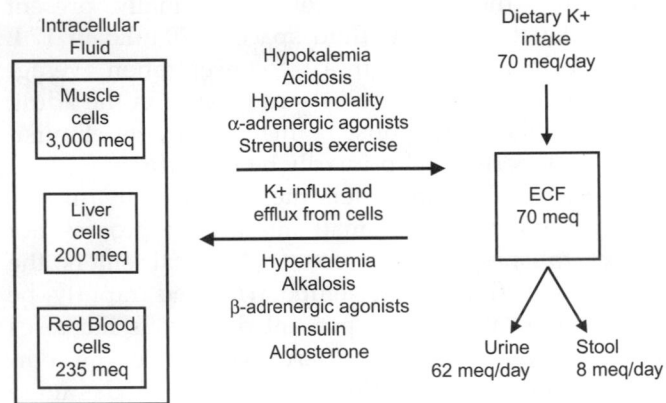

FIGURE 49.2 **Distribution of K⁺ between the intracellular and extracellular (ECF) fluid compartments.** Only ≈2% of the total body K⁺ is present in the ECF, with most of the remainder in intracellular fluid, here represented by three of the largest cellular compartments. The distribution of K⁺ represents a balance between active uptake into cells by the Na⁺,K⁺-ATPase and the passive leak of K⁺ out of cells. This balance is influenced by the K⁺ concentration of the ECF, as well as by the factors listed above and below the two arrows. A typical daily K⁺ intake of 70 meq/d is matched by the sum of a small excretion in the stool and the regulated excretion of K⁺ by the kidneys. *(From Giebisch, G. (2002). A trail of research on potassium. Kidney Int. **62**, 1498–1512, with permission.)*

remarkably constant in the range from 3.5 to 5.0 mM.[53–55,97,98,102,478,479] Variations in K⁺ intake are matched within hours by parallel adjustments in K⁺ excretion, most of which is mediated by the kidney.[49,177–185,473,579–583] However, during exercise and ischemia, extracellular K⁺ may quickly rise significantly. To minimize cell ATP decrease and loss of K⁺ production of AMP-activated protein kinase (AMPK), under these conditions, is stimulated by an increase in intracellular AMP-to-ATP ratio favoring translocation of K⁺ into cells in states of exercise and ischemia.[591,602] Although overshadowed by the kidney, the colon also excretes K⁺ and responds to stimuli calling for a change in excretion rate.[29,30,151,216]

EXTERNAL K⁺ BALANCE: THE ROLE OF THE KIDNEY

To accomplish excretion of the variable quantity of K⁺ ingested daily, the kidney must first extract K⁺ from blood in which K⁺ circulates at a rather low concentration. Indeed, dietary K⁺ may approximate that of sodium (80–120 mM/day), but the concentration of K⁺ in plasma, and therefore the rate at which it is filtered by glomeruli, is only one-thirtieth of that of sodium. Nevertheless, the glomerular filtration rate (GFR) is normally high enough so that K⁺ could be excreted by filtration alone. However, if the GFR is reduced to 10 to 15% of normal, as occurs with chronic renal failure, filtration alone would not be able to keep up with the normal dietary intake. Even if the GFR were reduced

TABLE 49.1 Main Features of Potassium Transport, Based on Clearance Experiments

1. K$^+$ secreted by renal tubules (excreted K$^+$ > filtered K$^+$)
2. K$^+$ excretion can be dissociated form the rate of glomerular filtration
3. Reabsorption of K$^+$ along the nephron precedes K$^+$ secretion
4. Secretion of K$^+$ occurs by exchange for Na$^+$
5. K$^+$ tolerance: Increased K excretion at relatively low K$^+$ in plasma
6. Reciprocal relation between urinary excretion of K$^+$ and H$^+$, carbonic anhydrase inhibitors induce kaliuresis
7. Adrenal steroids stimulate K$^+$ secretion

only by half, because not all filtered K$^+$ can escape reabsorption, it is likely that renal excretion would be inadequate and K$^+$ would be retained. Furthermore, even when GFR is normal, an excretion mechanism relying solely on filtration would have a limited capacity for adaptive increase, and could not achieve the 20-fold increase in K$^+$ excretion that has been observed in animals exposed to increased intake of K$^+$ by diets high in K$^+$ or parenteral infusions containing K$^+$. Indeed, net urinary K$^+$ excretion reflects not only glomerular filtration, but also tubular reabsorption and secretion. Clearance studies from as early as the 1940s revealed that the kidney is capable of secretion enabling the transfer of K$^+$ from plasma to tubule fluid.[48–52,177–186,187,292,330,345–347,379,473,474,583] Table 49.1 summarizes the main features of renal K$^+$ transport based on these studies.

A simplified but generally adequate view of renal K$^+$ handling is that proximal nephron segments between the glomerulus and the distal convoluted tubule (DCT) reabsorb a rather fixed fraction (80–90%) of the filtered K$^+$, whereas distal tubules and collecting ducts either secrete a variable quantity of K$^+$ into tubule fluid[49,177–187,221,320–324,379,485] or effectively reabsorb K$^+$.[119,179,325,371] By varying the rate and even the direction of K$^+$ transport, the distal nephron is able to respond homeostatically to changes in dietary K$^+$ intake or to changes in extracellular K$^+$ caused by other gains (parenteral administration, release from cellular pools) or losses (from the GI tract or skin). In people ingesting ≈70 mmol/day K$^+$, the usual rate of K$^+$ excretion in the postabsorptive period between meals is approximately 10–15% of the rate of K$^+$ filtration. In the hours following ingestion of K$^+$-rich meals, the rate of urinary excretion of K$^+$ can increase greatly to approach or even exceed the rate at which it is filtered. Such increments in K$^+$ excretion can be attributed to an increase in the quantity secreted by distal nephron segments. Increased secretion may not entirely account for increases in K$^+$ excretion in all cases, however, and variations in reabsorption by tubule segments, either proximal or distal to the main secretory sites, may become important in some circumstances.

If K$^+$ intake is reduced or eliminated (or if the body is depleted of K$^+$ by prior renal or nonrenal losses), urinary K$^+$ excretion declines rapidly as the deficit in total body K$^+$ increases. Within a few days K$^+$ excretion can be reduced to very low levels,[179,322–324] but K$^+$ conservation is less complete than that of sodium.[179]

General Aspects of K$^+$ Transport Along the Nephron

The generalization that filtered K$^+$ is largely reabsorbed by proximal nephron segments and that excreted K$^+$ is secreted by distal segments provides a useful framework for integrating information about renal handling of K$^+$, but a closer look at the cytologically distinct subdivisions of the nephron and the way each handles K$^+$ reveals a more complicated picture. K$^+$ is not continuously reabsorbed from all tubule segments proximal to the secretory sites in the distal tubules and collecting ducts. The rather constant fractional delivery of K$^+$ (10–20% of the filtered quantity) that has been found by collecting and analyzing samples of fluid from the earliest portion of the superficial DCT accessible to micropuncture is achieved by a sequence of reabsorption, secretion, and reabsorption as the glomerular filtrate travels through the proximal tubule and the loop of Henle.[179,322,323,324,325,466,470,471,473,579,583] Secretion of K$^+$ into loops of Henle has been documented only for the juxtamedullary nephron population[104,250,252,531]; however, it seems likely that the more superficial nephrons behave similarly.

Figures 49.3 and 49.4 represent schematic representations of the renal elements responsible for K$^+$ excretion. The location and naming of the subdivisions generally follow the scheme outlined by Kriz and Bankir.[281] Some features that distinguish superficial and deep nephrons are pictured. K$^+$ is filtered and reabsorbed from proximal convoluted tubules (PCT) of both superficial and deep nephrons. As the proximal straight tubule (PST) enters the outer medulla, the direction of K$^+$ transport reverses, and K$^+$ is secreted into the third proximal segment (S3) and the thin descending limb of the loop of Henle.[250–252] Higher K$^+$ concentrations are attained in loops of deeper nephrons that penetrate further into the inner medulla.

K$^+$ can be reabsorbed by thick ascending limbs (TALs), and net reabsorption probably occurs in both medullary and cortical TALs of both deep and superficial nephrons.[198,201,218] The portion of the distal tubule beyond the macula densa where each ascending limb contacts its parent glomerulus comprises several segments that are cytologically distinguishable. The DCT, extending beyond the

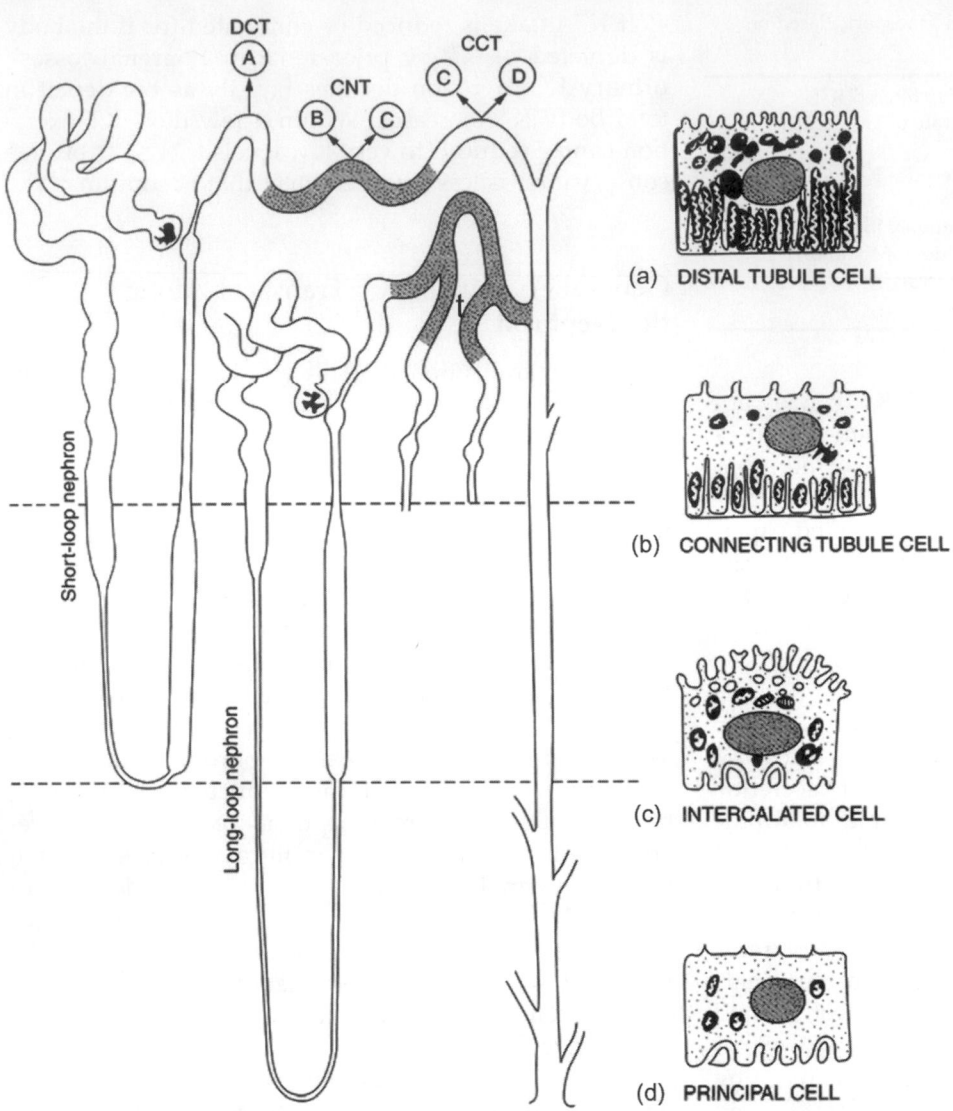

FIGURE 49.3 Schematic illustration of the distal nephron segments (CCT: cortical collecting tubule; CNT: connecting tubule; DCT: distal convoluted tubule). *(From ref. [244], with permission.)*

(a) DISTAL TUBULE CELL

(b) CONNECTING TUBULE CELL

(c) INTERCALATED CELL

(d) PRINCIPAL CELL

macula densa, is functionally distinct from the TAL segment, and probably contributes modestly to K$^+$ excretion.[451]

The next segment of the distal tubule – the connecting tubule (CNT), and the segment following it, the cortical collecting duct (CCD) – are major sites of K$^+$ secretion. In superficial nephrons, epithelium characteristic of the CCD appears some distance proximal to the first confluence of two distal tubules. This region has also been referred to as the late distal tubule or the initial collecting tubule (ICT).[28] In deeper nephrons, the CNTs frequently join to form arcades before flowing into the collecting duct. The separate segments of the distal tubule are discussed subsequently in more detail. K$^+$ is secreted into the collecting duct throughout the cortex, and probably in the outer stripe of the outer medulla as well.[485,486] However, in the inner stripe of the outer medulla, K$^+$ reabsorption appears once again and contributes to K$^+$ accumulation in the medullary interstitium. Both secretion and reabsorption of K$^+$ have been described along the terminal portions of the inner medullary collecting duct.[402,403,452,463,485–488]

K$^+$ Transport by Individual Nephron Segments

Glomerulus

K$^+$ ions that are free in plasma water pass across the glomerular capillary membrane with little hindrance. Nonfilterable proteins in plasma may bind a small fraction of K^{+294} and restrict filtration. The net negative charge on these plasma proteins tends to reduce K$^+$ concentration in glomerular filtrate relative to plasma water (Donnan equilibrium), but the concentration of

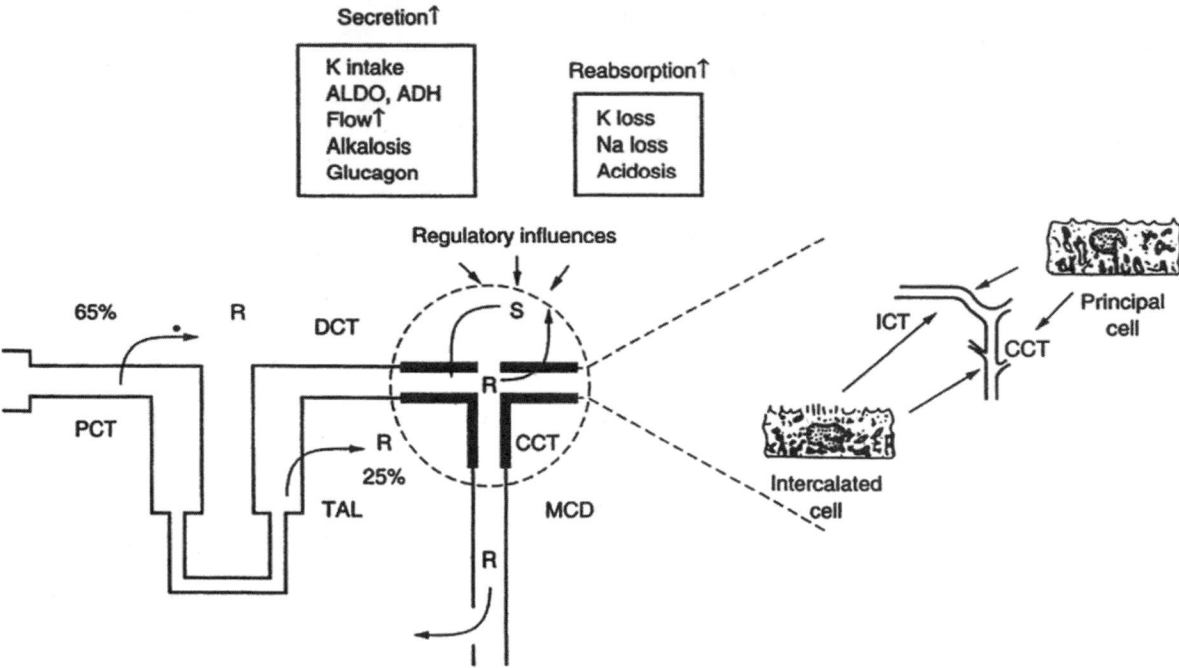

FIGURE 49.4   Overview of K$^+$ transport along the nephron. Secretion (S) largely determines the excretion of K$^+$ during normal and high K$^+$ intake; reabsorption (R) determines the excretion of K$^+$ in K$^+$ depletion. Note the cell heterogeneity in the distal nephron (see Figure 49.3) (ADH: antidiuretic hormone; ALDO: aldosterone; CCT: cortical collecting tubule; DCT: distal convoluted tubule; MCD: medullary collecting duct; PCT: proximal convoluted tubule; TAL: thick ascending limb of Henle). *(From Giebisch, G. (2002). A trail of research on potassium. Kidney Int.* **62***, 1498−1512, with permission.)*

K$^+$ in plasma is approximately 6% lower than in plasma water. These factors tend to cancel each other out, and the concentrations of K$^+$ in glomerular filtrate and in plasma or serum, are approximately equal.

Although variations in GFR do cause proportional variations in the rate of K$^+$ filtration, they do not usually result in large changes in K$^+$ excretion, because mechanisms promoting glomerulotubular balance tend to stabilize the rate of K$^+$ delivery out of the proximal tubule and the loop of Henle. In the 1950s, when renal clearance methods were first applied systematically to the study of K$^+$ regulation by the kidney, it was observed that rates of glomerular filtration and final K$^+$ excretion could be varied independently of one another.[49,100,346,347] However, if GFR is reduced enough to decrease sodium and water excretion, the rate of K$^+$ excretion will also decrease.[49,100]

Proximal Convoluted Tubule: Direction, Magnitude, and Mechanism of Transport

Transepithelial K$^+$ Transport

Information about the direction and magnitude of K$^+$ transport processes along the nephron was obtained in the 1960s by *in vivo* micropuncture techniques.[193] The main features of K$^+$ transport in various nephron segments are summarized in Figure 49.4. Collections of tubular fluid samples showed that about 50% of filtered K$^+$ reaches the last accessible surface segment of the PCT.[322] Collections from sites close to the glomerulus showed that reabsorption of K$^+$, which occurs over most of the accessible proximal tubule,[59,179,322,325,399,553] may be preceded by a small K$^+$ leak into the lumen.[516] The downstream reabsorption of K$^+$ along the proximal tubule, like that of sodium, generally proceeds without developing a large concentration difference across the proximal tubule as a roughly similar fraction of water is also absorbed. Although K$^+$ concentration has been reported to increase slightly[40] or to remain unchanged[109] along the proximal tubule, a few studies have provided evidence that proximal reabsorption of K$^+$ can proceed against an electrochemical gradient, and that tubular fluid K$^+$ concentration may decline (by about 10%) between early and late proximal segments in rat kidneys.[61,268]

Three mechanisms participate in K$^+$ reabsorption by the proximal tubule: solvent drag; diffusion; and apparent active transport. First, the consistently observed association between K$^+$ transport and fluid transport suggests that a fraction of proximal K$^+$ absorption depends on the simultaneous rate of fluid absorption.[61,62] This dependence of K⁺ transport on net fluid transport, and the finding of low reflection coefficients of K⁺,[550] support the notion of direct coupling of K⁺ and fluid through the same transport pathway: a solvent drag mechanism.

Second, diffusion of K⁺ from luminal to peritubular fluid may also occur because fluid absorption may raise the K⁺ concentration in the proximal tubule, thus creating a concentration difference favoring K⁺ absorption. *In vivo* microperfusion experiments show that proximal K⁺ transport is very sensitive to changes in luminal K⁺ concentration and transepithelial voltage.[61,62,550] The high K⁺ permeability in the proximal tubule,[270] and the dependence of K⁺ transport on the transepithelial electrochemical potential difference is consistent with diffusive movement through a paracellular pathway. However, barium, a potent K⁺ channel-blocker, has been shown to block a significant fraction of K⁺ reabsorption, implying possible participation of a transcellular route for reabsorption of K⁺.[270,528] However, little is known about this pathway.

Third, the direction of the electrochemical driving force for K⁺ in at least part of the proximal tubule, and the special microenvironment of the paracellular compartment between proximal tubule cells, provides theoretical support for apparent active K⁺ absorption. Such movement of K⁺ ions against an electrochemical potential gradient in the early proximal tubule is implied by experimental findings demonstrating both a concentration of K⁺ in the tubule lumen below that in arterial plasma, and a lumen-negative transepithelial potential.[162,268,518] Moreover, dissociation between sodium-driven fluid movement and K⁺ transport has also, albeit rarely, been observed. Micropuncture studies provide evidence that channel-dependent K⁺ fluxes mediate a secretory component of K⁺ movement into the early proximal tubule,[11,268,518] but K⁺ reabsorption further downstream exceeds such secretory K⁺ fluxes. Direct measurements of the electrochemical driving force for K⁺ across the apical cell membrane in amphibian proximal tubules also support active K⁺ reabsorption.[11,164] However, there is no evidence that K-H-ATPase activity identified in the apical membrane of mammalian proximal tubules[112,117] contributes to K⁺ reabsorption.[538a,592]

A cell model summarizing the complex mechanisms involved in proximal tubular K⁺ transport is pictured in Figure 49.5. It includes a sodium-K⁺ exchange pump (Na⁺,K⁺-ATPase) in the basolateral membrane, a K⁺ conductance in the apical membrane, and a pathway for K⁺ transport between cells. Two pathways for K⁺ exit across the basolateral membrane are shown: a conductive channel and a K-Cl co-transporter.[18,551] Note also that the transepithelial potential along the

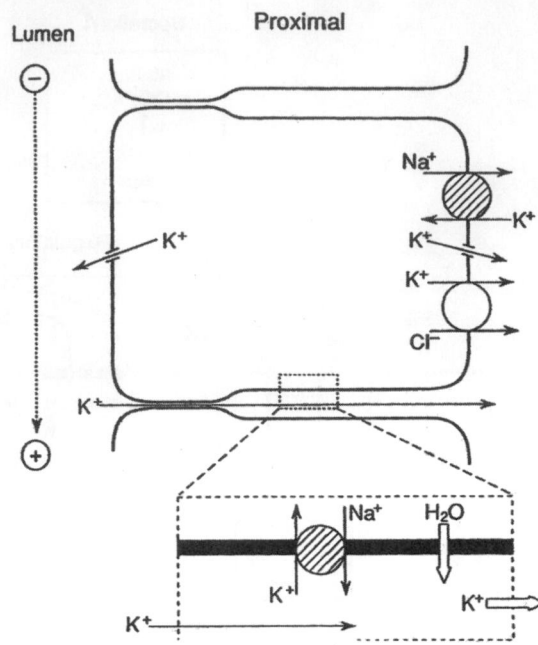

FIGURE 49.5 Model of proximal tubule cell. Transepithelial voltage is lumen-negative in S_1, and becomes lumen-positive in S_2. Enlargement of lateral membrane and the intercellular and extracellular spaces illustrates a postulated mechanism permitting absorption of potassium against a concentration gradient.

tubule changes from lumen-negative values in the early PCT to lumen-positive values in the late PCT.[162]

Weinstein has suggested that the apparent reabsorptive movement of K⁺ against an electrochemical driving force does not require an active, directly energy-driven reabsorptive maechanism for K⁺ in the apical cell membrane.[559] Given that Na⁺,K⁺-ATPase-driven uptake of K⁺ does occur in the cell membranes lining the paracellular compartment between cells, such transport could deplete this compartment of K⁺, particularly if the diffusion resistance to K⁺ across the basolateral exit was low. A situation could then develop in which the luminal fluid equilibrates with the low-K⁺ fluid in the interspace, effectively decreasing the K⁺ concentration in the lumen below peritubular plasma levels. Exit of K⁺ ions from the interspace into the peritubular fluid would be driven by bulk movement of fluid and K⁺ along the hydrostatic pressure gradient that normally develops along the interspace from its luminal to basolateral end.

In the later part of the PCT, the transepithelial potential difference becomes lumen-positive, providing an additional driving force for net K⁺ reabsorption.[162] It is likely that K⁺ movement driven by the transepithelial voltage occurs through the paracellular shunt pathway. *In vivo* microperfusion experiments using mannitol to vary tubular fluid osmolarity reveal that the direction of net K⁺ transport is dependent on that of net fluid transport.[61,62] Previous observations had already shown that inhibition of proximal sodium and water transport would also block K$^+$ reabsorption,[59,181,234,579,581] an effect consistent with entrainment of K$^+$ ions by sodium-dependent fluid reabsorption.

Transepithelial electrochemical gradients of K$^+$ demonstrate the effect of changes in the electrical potential difference on tubule K$^+$ concentration.[456] Marked differences were observed between K$^+$-replete and K$^+$-depleted animals: whereas a lumen-positive potential was recorded in replete animals, the transepithelial potential difference was reversed in K$^+$-depleted animals, and the K$^+$ concentration ratio across the late proximal tubule was significantly elevated. These data support the view that diffusion along an electrochemical gradient can play a critical role in transport of K$^+$ across the proximal tubule.

Cell K$^+$ Transport

In proximal tubule cells, steady-state levels of cell K$^+$ depend on the balance between active uptake from interstitial fluid and passive leakage from the cytosol, either to the interstitium or to the tubule lumen. K$^+$ ions are actively taken up by the ATP-driven Na$^+$-K$^+$ exchange pump located in the basolateral membranes. Microelectrode measurements of basolateral membrane voltage and of K$^+$ activities show that the electrical potential difference across cell membranes of both amphibian and mammalian tubule cells is too small to account for the measured intracellular K$^+$ activity by passive distribution. Also, inhibitor studies indicate that ATPase-driven accumulation of K$^+$ is responsible for high cell K$^+$ concentrations. Inhibition of Na$^+$,K$^+$-ATPase activity reduces intracellular K$^+$ concentrations and content.[48,49,83,124,233,284,420,421,514,515]

The basolateral sodium-K$^+$ pump operates in an electrogenic mode: the rate at which sodium ions are pumped out of the cell exceeds the rate at which K$^+$ ions are taken in. The contribution of such an electrogenic cation exchange to the steady-state voltage across the basolateral membrane is probably small; however, sudden activation of the pump, either by raising cell sodium, by increasing extracellular K$^+$ from low levels or by warming tubules previously cooled, leads to rapid hyperpolarization of the basolateral cell membrane to levels that can exceed the equilibrium potential that could be generated by passive diffusion of K$^+$ ions.[48,49,83,124,148,150,233,390,420,421]

Figure 49.6 illustrates additional transporters in the basolateral membranes of proximal tubule cells. K$^+$ channels are present in both cell membranes, and serve several functions. They generate the cell-negative electrical potential which constitutes an important driving force for the entry of positively-charged solutes and the basolateral exit of negatively-charged solutes. Sodium-coupled electrogenic glucose and amino acid transport across the apical membrane of proximal tubule cells is facilitated by the cell-negative potential. Chloride diffusion, electrogenic Na$^+$-HCO$_3$ cotransport and Ca^{2+}/Na$^+$ exchange are also modulated by the magnitude of the K$^+$-dependent basolateral membrane potential.[513–515]

K$^+$ channels are also involved in volume regulation of proximal tubule cells.[237,419] Both apical and basolateral K$^+$ channels are activated by cell swelling, either directly by stretching of the membrane or indirectly, by volume-dependent Ca^{2+} entry through non-selective cation channels.[150,381,419] Apical K$^+$ channels are also sensitive to changes in membrane voltage, with depolarization leading to increased activity. Apical K$^+$ channels in the proximal tubule are critical in stabilizing the cell-negative potential, especially during depolarizing Na$^+$-coupled transport (i.e., with glucose or amino acids). The K$^+$ channel KCNQ1 and the accessory protein KCNE1 have been localized to the brush border of the mid-to-late proximal tubule.[516] They have been proposed to play a role in net K$^+$ secretion in the early proximal tubule, and in polarizing the brush border membrane to maintain the electrical driving force for Na$^+$-coupled transport. In support of this view, mice lacking KCNE1 exhibit increased renal excretion of Na$^+$ and glucose, and signs of volume-depletion.[516]

Basolateral K$^+$ channels are inhibited by an increase in cell ATP, by a fall in pH, by cyclic AMP and taurine,[217] and they have been implicated in renal cell damage by hypoxia.[400]

Coupling Between Sodium Transport and Basolateral K$^+$ Channels

The constancy of intracellular K$^+$ in the presence of large changes in transepithelial net sodium transport depends on appropriate modulations of the basolateral K$^+$ conductance.[453,454] Because a major pathway for sodium reabsorption is transcellular and involves the basolateral sodium-K$^+$ exchange pump, large changes in the rate of basolateral sodium extrusion necessarily cause large changes in K$^+$ uptake. However, by varying the magnitude of the basolateral-leak conductance in proportion to changes in pump rate, cells in renal[35–39,56,57,79,241,290,561,564] and other transporting epithelia[194] are able to maintain cytosolic K$^+$ activity, and cell volume, within narrow limits.

Pump-Leak Coupling

Transport-related changes in the coupling between active sodium extrusion across the basolateral membrane and apical and basolateral K$^+$ conductances are depicted in Figure 49.7a and 49.7b. Changes in cell

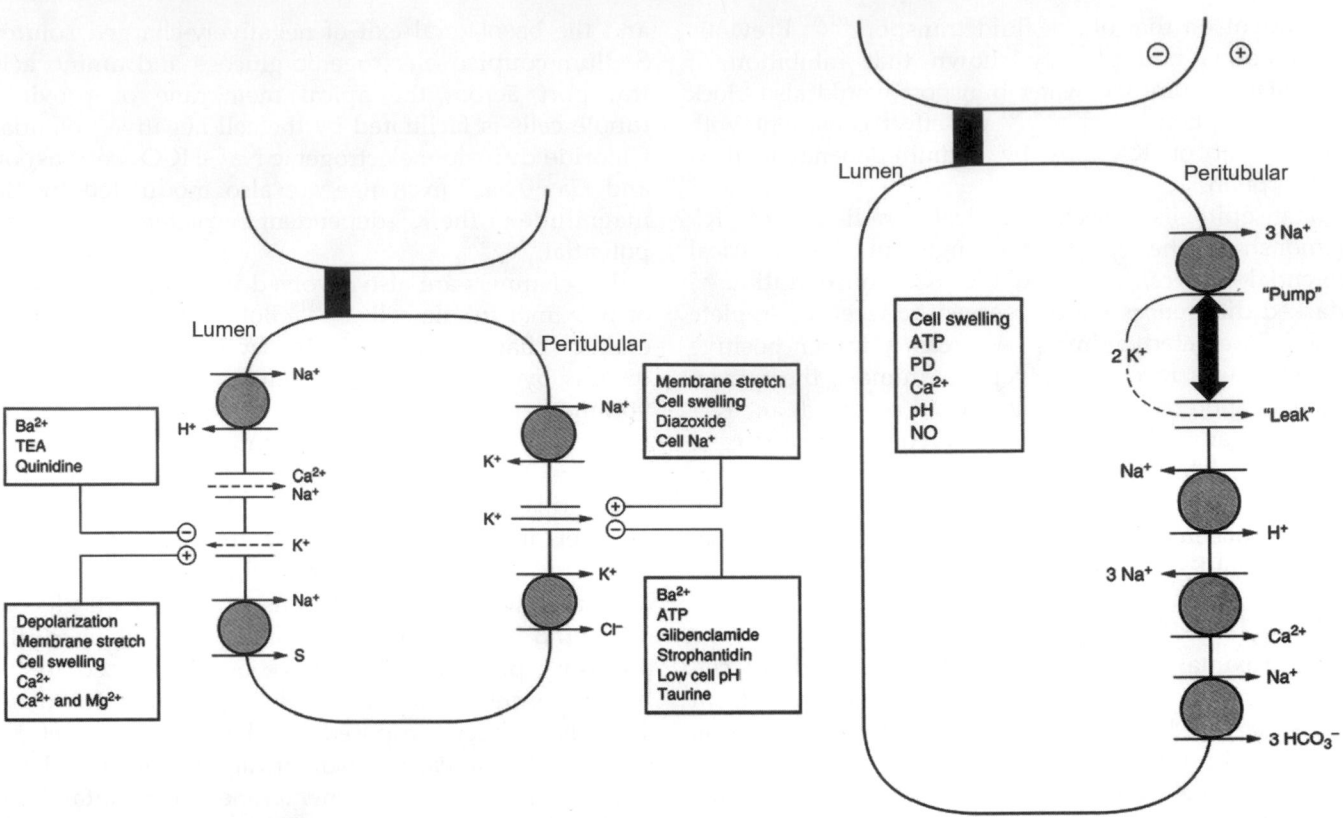

FIGURE 49.6   **Models of proximal tubule cells, including the main transport pathways and the apical and basolateral K⁺ channels** (ATP: adenosine triphosphate; TEA: tetraethylammonium; NO: nitric oxide). Left: Model of a proximal tubule cell. Right: Relationship between the activity of basolateral Na,K-ATPase and the leak through K channels. The two-headed arrow indicates linkage between the pump and K channels; as K uptake increases, permeability to K increases, and *vice versa*. Factors that regulate transport pathways (left) and mediate the pump-leak coupling (right) are indicated in individual boxes. Basolateral transporters that may alter these variables are also shown (ATP: adenosine triphosphate). (*From Malnic, G., Bailey, M. A. and Giebisch, G. (2004). Control of renal potassium excretion. In "The Kidney," 7th ed., Vol. 1, 453—496, Brenner, B. (ed.). WB Saunders, Philadelphia, with permission.*)

volume and pH have a significant effect on K⁺ channels, alkalosis increasing and acidosis decreasing the open probability.[35,210,282,286,362,446] During substrate-induced stimulation of proximal sodium transport, cell pH rises with a time-course that matches the observed increase in basolateral K⁺ conductance.[38]

Changes in the concentration of Ca²⁺ in tubule cells, especially those correlated with fluctuations in cell volume and nitric oxide, may also couple basolateral Na⁺, K⁺-ATPase activity to K⁺ permeability. Alterations in basolateral cell potential have also been implicated, since stimulation of electrogenic Na⁺,K⁺ pump activity hyperpolarizes tubule cells. Such membrane voltage changes are known to activate voltage-sensitive K⁺ channels.[543]

Renal K⁺ channel activity, including that of channels in the basolateral membrane of proximal tubule cells,[241,508] is also sensitive to alterations in cellular ATP.[35,36,508] Small amounts of ATP are required for the activity of some K⁺ channels in the renal tubule, but millimolar concentrations inhibit K⁺ channel activity. This effect is reversed by ADP,[217] and points to the involvement of the ATP/ADP ratio in the control of K⁺ channel activity. It appears that transport-related changes in cell ATP levels modify cell K⁺ conductance. Thus, stimulation of sodium transport in proximal tubules results in a significant fall in cell ATP, whereas inhibition of sodium transport increases cell ATP levels. This cross-talk mechanism, linking apical sodium transport to basolateral K⁺ channel activity, is shown in Figure 49.7.[241,508,561] Thus, transport-related changes in the basolateral membrane potential of tubule cells may be involved in coupling the K⁺ conductance to the pump activity. Measurements of the basolateral conductance of tubule cells,[233] as well as patch-clamp studies, in which the open probability of basolateral K⁺ channels was examined as a function of the membrane potential,[343] show an increase in K⁺ conductance with cell hyperpolarization. To the extent that stimulation of basolateral ATPase activity elevates the cell-negative potential, K⁺ conductance would also be expected to increase interaction between basolateral and apical membrane transport.

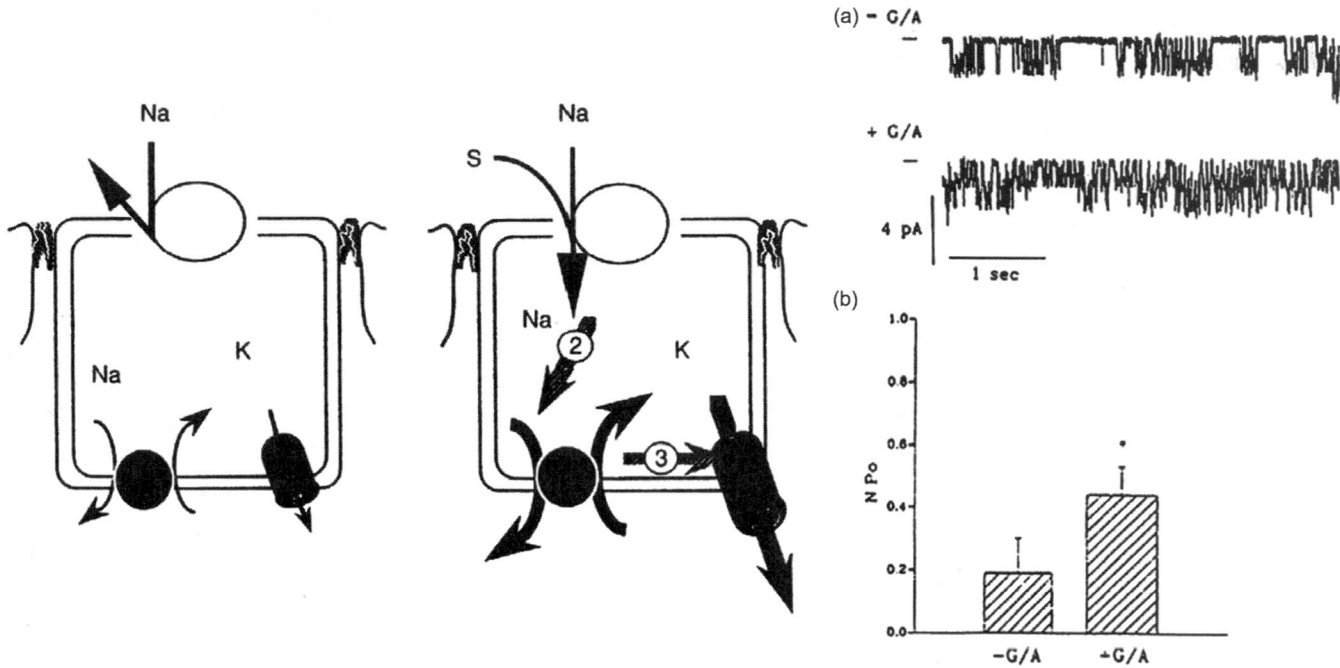

FIGURE 49.7 Left: Coupling between Na$^+$,K$^+$-ATPase activity and K$^+$ recycling in the basolateral membrane of proximal tubule cells.[36,37,198,512] Net rate of sodium transport was stimulated by addition of organic substrates (S; i.e., glucose or amino acid) to the lumen. Thus: (1) apical Na entry via Na-dependent substrate co-transporters is stimulated in the presence of substrates; (2) the Na$^+$, K$^+$-ATPase subsequently revs up so that active efflux of Na into the interstitium matches passive apical sodium entry; (3) ensuring that the increased active uptake of K$^+$ via the Na$^+$,K$^+$-ATPase will be efficiently recycled back across the basolateral membrane, K$^+$ channel activation ensues. *(Kidney Int. 1995; 48, 1017−1023.)* Right: (A) Patch-clamp analysis of basolateral K$^+$ channel activity in isolated perfused proximal tubule. Data for experiments before (−) and during (+) perfusion of glucose and alanine (G/A). Horizontal bars indicate zero current. (B) Effect of luminal addition of glucose and alanine on single-K channel open probability (NP$_o$). $p < 0.02$. *(Am. J. Physiol. Renal 1993; 264, F760−764.)*

Schultz has drawn attention to an additional relationship between transport events in the luminal and basolateral membrane of epithelial cells that involves changes in the pump-related K$^+$ conductance.[453,454] In leaky epithelia, such as the proximal tubule, stimulation of co-transport of sodium ions with organic solutes such as glucose or amino acids augments sodium entry across the apical membrane. Since the co-transporter carries positive current into the cell, the cell-negative electrical potential is reduced.[518] In tight epithelia, such as the CCD, mineralocorticoids increase apical sodium conductance, and thus bring about depolarization of the apical cell membrane.[64,65,275−277,356,358,361] The increase in K$^+$ conductance that occurs with stimulation of sodium pumping across the basolateral membrane also provides an important transport-sustaining feedback loop. The rise in potassium conductance hyperpolarizes the basolateral membrane and renders net transport more effective. An essential feature of these effects is that maneuvers that increase sodium transport tend to curtail further sodium entry, because the depolarization of the apical cell membrane reduces the electrochemical driving force for further sodium transport into the cell.

Loop of Henle: K$^+$ Recycling, Direction, Magnitude, and Mechanism of Transport

In vivo micropuncture and microperfusion studies show net reabsorption of K$^+$ between the last accessible segment of surface proximal tubules and the first accessible segment of surface distal tubules.[101,249,250,252,511−513] Thus, only a modest fraction, some 5−10% of the filtered K$^+$, reaches the early distal tubule (see Figure 49.4). As shown in Figure 49.3, this portion of the nephron comprises several morphologically and functionally distinct segments: the third segment of the proximal tubule (S3); the thin descending and thin ascending limbs; and the medullary and cortical thick ascending limbs of the loop of Henle.

The K$^+$ concentration in the loop of Henle fluid near the tip of the papilla can be as much as 10 times higher than the K$^+$ concentration in systemic plasma.[101,108,248−252] de Rouffignac and Morel[101] suggested that K$^+$ is added to tubule fluid along the descending limb of Henle's loop after being absorbed from the ascending limb and collecting duct. The phenomenon constitutes K$^+$ recycling (Figure 49.8). Jamison and coworkers further showed that K$^+$ delivery to the end of

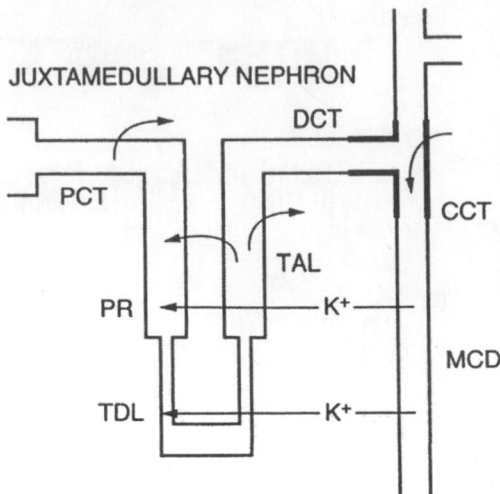

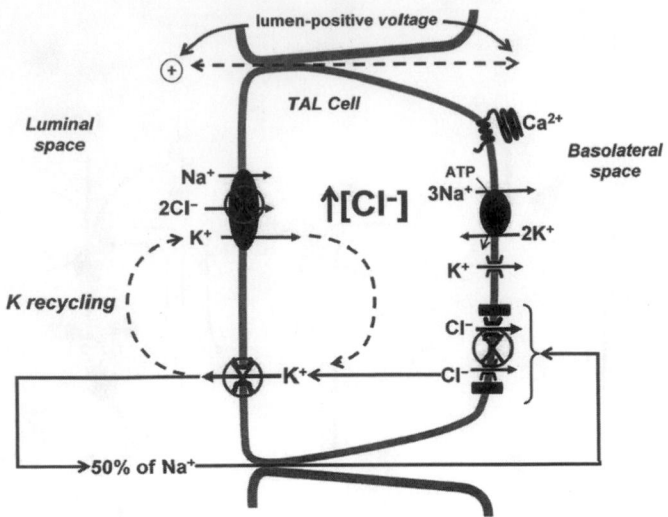

FIGURE 49.8   **Sites of K⁺ movement into and out of the nephron.** The diagram emphasizes the movement of K⁺ from the collecting ducts to the descending limbs of the loop of Henle via the medullary interstitium (CCT: cortical collecting tubule; DCT: distal convoluted tubule; MCD: medullary collecting duct; PCT: proximal convoluted tubule; PR: pars recta; TAL: thick ascending limb; TDL: thin descending limb). *(Field, M. J., and Giebisch, G. (1989). Mechanisms of segmental potassium reabsorption and secretion. In "The Regulation of Potassium Balance," 139–156, Seldin, D. W., and Giebisch, G. (eds.). Raven Press, New York, with permission.)*

FIGURE 49.9   **Model of a thick ascending limb cell, including the main transport pathways and the apical and basolateral ion channels.** Potassium may also leave the cell across the basolaterall membrane by KCl co-transport (not shown). Note that the lumen-positive transepithelial potential difference drives cation reabsorption through the paracellular pathway (AA: arachidonic acid; ATP: adenosine triphosphate; CaR: extracellular calcium-sensing receptor; cGMP: cyclic guanonine monophosphate; 20-HETE: 20-hydroxyeicosatetraenoic acid; NO: nitric oxide; PKA: protein kinase A; PKC: protein kinase C; TALH: thick ascending limb of Henle; V₂: receptor for arginine vasopressin). *(From Malnic, G., Bailey, M. A. and Giebisch, G. (2004). Control of renal potassium excretion. In "The Kidney," 7th ed., Vol. 1, 453–496, Brenner, B. (ed.). WB Saunders, Philadelphia, with permission.)*

the descending limb of deep nephrons could equal the rate of K⁺ filtration in normal rats,[252] and exceeded it in rats either fed a high-K⁺ diet[32] or infused acutely with K⁺.[15] The observation that isolated thin limbs of Henle lack a mechanism of active K⁺ secretion[245,246] supports the view that K⁺ enters the descending limb passively. If K⁺ is also secreted into the proximal straight tubule of superficial nephrons,[552,578] and the delivery of K⁺ to the DCT of deep nephrons is substantially less than the filtered quantity, then K⁺ must be reabsorbed by ascending limbs in both populations of nephrons. Thus, K⁺ is trapped in the medulla by countercurrent exchange between the ascending and descending limbs of the loop of Henle. Studies of isolated TAL perfused *in vitro* show that these segments are capable of absorbing K⁺.[74]

As originally postulated by Jamison et al.[249] and shown in Figure 49.8, the main pathway by which K⁺ can reach the renal medulla is absorption from the medullary collecting duct. Stokes[483–485] has shown that the outer medullary collecting duct is adequately permeable to both sodium and K⁺, and therefore could permit K⁺ reabsorption to occur passively. K⁺ secretion by cells of the distal tubule and the cortical collecting duct into the tubular fluid provide the source of K⁺ that accumulates in the renal medulla. Accordingly, more K⁺ recycles with stimulation of secretion, whereas suppression of secretion attenuates the

deposition of K⁺ in the renal medulla. Thus, K⁺ is secreted into tubule fluid in (at least) two sites along the nephron (see Figure 49.8), first into a proximal part of the nephron (the end-proximal tubule and descending limb), and second into a more distal region (the CT and CCD). When K⁺ intake is suddenly increased after a period of K⁺ deprivation, renal K⁺ excretion, distal K⁺ secretion, and K⁺ recycling[110,129,130,214,223,249,494] all increase. Stokes also proposed that rising medullary K⁺ concentrations inhibit NaCl and water absorption by the loop of Henle, and thus increase the flow rate and sodium concentration of fluid entering the distal tubule, providing optimum conditions for the distal segments to secrete K⁺.[484] Medullary recycling is thus responsible for maintaining high concentrations of K⁺ in the renal medulla. Such trapping of K⁺ is also expected to limit reabsorptive loss of K⁺ from the terminal collecting ducts.[579]

Thick Ascending Limb (TAL) Cell Transport Mechanisms

Studies of isolated mammalian TALs and amphibian (*Amphiuma*) early distal tubule have provided similar K⁺ transport models (Figure 49.9). The primary driving force for net K^+ reabsorption is again ATP-driven active Na^+-K^+ exchange across the basolateral membrane, which generates the steep sodium gradient for the entry of Na^+ across the apical cell membrane.

Apical Membrane

Entry of Na^+ is primarily mediated by an $Na^+ - 2Cl^- - K$ (or under certain conditions, Na,Cl) co-transport mechanism inhibited by the potent "loop" diuretics.[74-76,201-204,218,251,363,365-367,444] Also present in the apical membrane is a second pathway for sodium entry into cells, the Na-H exchanger (not shown in Figure 49.9). Conductive pathways for K^+ are found in both the apical and basolateral membranes.[201-204,218-220,363,365] The K^+ concentration gradient across the apical membrane favors K^+ secretion, which permits recycling of K^+ ions back to the tubule lumen. This back-diffusion provides a continuous luminal supply of K^+ for co-transport with sodium and chloride. The K^+ leak in the luminal membrane is also responsible for net K^+ secretion under those conditions in which the activity of the reabsorptive co-transport mechanism has been impaired.

Evidence supporting the operation of the $Na^+ - 2Cl^- - K^+$ co-transporter in the apical membrane includes the mutual dependence of these ions for transport. Net reabsorption of Na^+, K^+, and Cl^-, and the lumen-positive potential are abolished in the luminal absence of any of the three ions.[198,200-204] In addition, luminal application of furosemide also eliminates transport of all three ions, and collapses the transepithelial potential.[76,198,200,201,444] Interference with the co-transport system, either by appropriate luminal ion substitution or by administration of furosemide, lowers cell chloride and sodium activity, thereby supporting the view that the co-transport system is the main apical pathway for entry of these ions into the cell. Additional evidence for the requirement of a steady supply of luminal K^+ to safeguard $Na^+ - 2Cl^- - K^+$ co-transport in the cortical TAL is the observation that sodium reabsorption decreases sharply following the depletion of K^+ from the lumen or following the administration of K^+ channel-blockers.[537,538] These maneuvers also attenuate tubuloglomerular feedback.[519]

Morphological and electrophysiological criteria suggest the presence of at least two cell types in TALs, each with different permeability properties of the apical and basolateral cell membranes.[243,244,246] In the cortical TAL the K^+ permeability in the apical membrane exceeds that of the basolateral membrane, whereas the converse relationship was observed in the medullary TAL. These permeability differences may be associated with functional disparities, K^+ secretion being the prevalent transport mode in the cortical TAL, and reabsorption in the medullary TAL.[509]

Patch-clamp techniques have identified at least two K^+ channels in the apical membrane that mediate K^+ recycling.[58,217,540,544-547,548] The open probability of these apical K^+ channels is high, and they are inhibited by barium, low cell pH, millimolar concentration of ATP, and protein kinase C (PKC). Cell alkalinization and cyclic AMP, as well as NO and cyclic GMP, stimulate K^+ channels. Apical K^+ channels are also activated by furosemide, an effect mimicking the effects of aldosterone.[362,363,365,368] Aldosterone in amphibian early distal tubules, enhances apical Na-H exchange and alkalinizes cell pH. When furosemide is given, apical sodium entry is blocked and the intracellular sodium concentration decreases. As a consequence, the driving force for apical Na-H exchange increases and alkalinizes the cytoplasm. Because apical K^+ channels are stimulated by cell alkalinization, their activity increases.[362,363] This sequence of events explains why the full expression of the aldosterone effect on K^+ permeability depends on an intact Na-H exchange in the apical cell membrane.

A difference between the transport modes of cortical and medullary TAL segments has also been observed regarding the K^+ sensitivity of the apical co-transporter to K^+. Figure 49.10 shows two cell models in which vasopressin switches the apical sodium chloride transporter from a K^+-insensitive mode to one that depends critically on the presence of K^+ in the tubule lumen.[496a]

An interesting effect concerns the sequence of events following an increase in peritubular Ca^{2+}, which has been shown to inhibit both apical K^+ channels and $Na^+ - 2Cl^- - K^+$ co-transport.[217] Patch-clamp studies have demonstrated that the inhibitory effects of Ca^{2+} are mediated through activation of P450 and PKC.[539-542,546,547] It is likely that the extracellular Ca^{2+} ion-sensing receptor (CaSR) present on the basolateral membrane of the TAL[404,405] plays a role in this response. The CaSR is a G-protein-coupled surface receptor that is activated by increases in extracellular Ca^{2+} ion concentrations,[69] and has been shown to inhibit NaCl absorption and K^+ channels in the TAL by eicosanoids and P450 metabolites.[85,172]

Basolateral Membrane

As summarized in Figure 49.9, the basolateral membrane of TAL cells permits diffusion of both K^+ and chloride; however, the chloride conductance is dominant.[198,202,218,540] In addition to the K^+ conductance, $K^+ - Cl$ and the K^+-HCO_3^-[300] co-transport provide additional pathways for K^+ movement from cell to interstitium. Patch-clamp studies have defined a sodium-sensitive K^+ channel in the basolateral

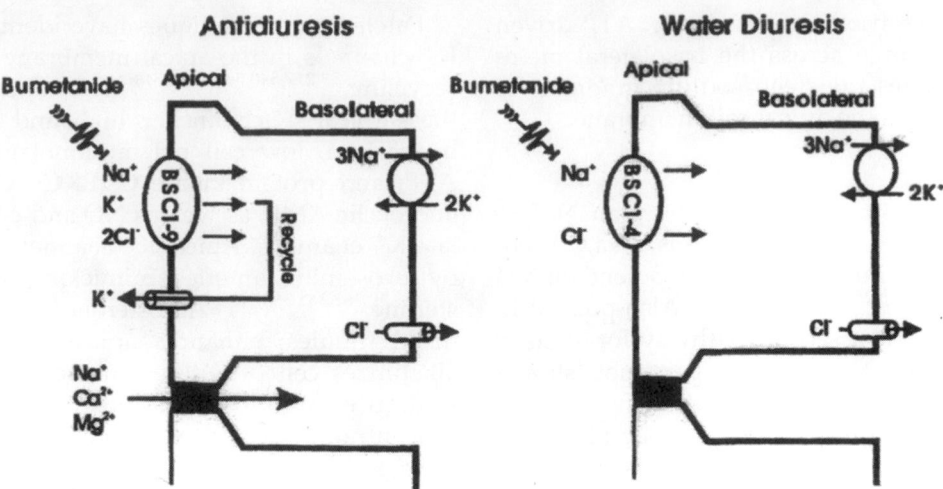

FIGURE 49.10   Proposed model for thick ascending limb (TAL) function. (a) Operation during water conservation. (b) Operation during maximal water diuresis. *(Am. J. Physiol. Renal 2001; **280**, F574—F582.)*

membrane.[383] These channels are stimulated by high cell sodium concentrations, providing coupling mechanisms between apical sodium uptake and basolateral ATP-dependent K$^+$ recycling. The Cl$^-$ concentration gradient across the basolateral membrane favors diffusion of chloride from interstitium into the cell. Thus, both the luminal K$^+$ conductance and the basolateral Cl$^-$ conductance tend to generate diffusion potentials oriented with the cell interior negative to the extracellular fluids. Because the K$^+$ concentration gradient across the apical membrane exceeds the Cl$^-$ concentration gradient across the basolateral membrane, the voltage across the apical membrane exceeds the voltage across the basolateral membrane. These unequal electrical potential differences arranged in series generate a lumen-positive transepithelial voltage, which provides a driving force for reabsorption of K$^+$ and other cations by passive diffusion through the paracellular shunt pathway. The magnitude of passive paracellular K$^+$ reabsorption is difficult to assess because the transepithelial electrochemical gradient for passive K$^+$ reabsorption along the cortico–medullary axis is poorly defined.

Overall K$^+$ reabsorption along the loop of Henle is the result of two opposing events: secretion into the descending limb of Henle's loop as a consequence of K$^+$ recycling (see Figure 49.8); and K$^+$ reabsorption along the TAL of Henle's loop. Stimulation of K$^+$ secretion into the descending limb and enhanced delivery to the tip of Henle's loop have been demonstrated during K$^+$-loading by puncture of juxtamedullary nephrons.[249,250]

Several factors modulate K$^+$ reabsorption along the loop of Henle.[511,512] K$^+$ reabsorption is enhanced by restricting dietary K$^+$ intake, provided a constant load

of fluid and K$^+$ is delivered into the loop of Henle; administration of a high-K$^+$ diet has the opposite effect.[511] Reabsorption of K$^+$ in perfused loops of Henle is stimulated by aldosterone R6TS.[107,465,468,473] However, no reduction in the rate of K$^+$ transport was observed in studies of perfused thick ascending limbs isolated from adrenalectomized animals.[577] Several factors modulate K$^+$ recycling and delivery into the distal tubule. Recycling of K$^+$ between the collecting duct and the descending limb of Henle's loop is enhanced following aldosterone administration in adrenalectomized animals.[223] Calcitonin reduced medullary recycling by inhibition of K$^+$ secretion into the distal tubule,[130] whereas vasopressin had the opposite effect.[129] Urea recycling increases delivery of fluid to principal cells and stimulates K$^+$ secretion.[214] Because ammonium ions may substitute for K$^+$ ions on the apical Na$^+$ − 2Cl$^-$ − K$^+$ co-transport site, hyperkalemia may inhibit ammonium accumulation in the renal medulla and impede its translocation into the collecting tubule.[121,122]

The amphibian diluting segment normally reabsorbs K$^+$, but it may secrete K$^+$ following K$^+$-loading,[364] administration of loop diuretics,[363,365] alkalinization of the peritubular fluid[436] or administration of aldosterone.[545,567] Aldosterone stimulates both cell K$^+$ uptake and release into the lumen, an effect that is reversed by exposure to amiloride.[516] Acidosis inhibits the Na-K pump, as well as the K$^+$ channel.[196,199,209] In contrast, alkalosis stimulates both pump-mediated uptake of K$^+$ into cells, and passive K$^+$ efflux from the cells of the diluting segment.[210] Apical K$^+$ channel activity also increases with cell volume.[210]

Reversal of the direction of K$^+$ transport, from reabsorption to secretion, frequently follows administration of loop diuretics. Free-flow micropuncture and loop perfusion studies[234,341] in the mammalian kidney, as well as perfusion of the amphibian diluting segment, show sharply reduced rates of K^+ reabsorption or reversal to net K^+ secretion following the inhibition of the apical $Na^+ - 2Cl^- - K^+$ co-transporter by furosemide,[74,76,511,512] torasemide,[512] ethacrinic acid,[75] and bumetanide.[512,523,524] The secretion of K^+ is the consequence of unopposed K^+ diffusion from the cell into the lumen.

Several experimental studies show that vasopressin enhances net sodium, chloride, and K^+ transport across the thick ascending limb of Henle.[218,220,319] Vasopressin action increases basolateral chloride permeability and accelerates chloride extrusion into the peritubular fluid. Vasopressin also enhances the affinity of the apical co-transporter for K^+ and augments the apical K^+ permeability. This increase in permeability speeds up apical membrane recycling of K^+ and stimulates $Na^+ - 2Cl^- - K^+$ co-transport. Loss-of-function mutations of the apical ROMK K^+ secretory channel can lead to Bartter's syndrome. Interference with recycling of K^+ ions in the apical membrane accounts for diminished sodium and K^+ reabsorption, and explains the urinary loss of sodium and K^+, hypokalemia, and high levels of aldosterone observed in this genetic disorder.[20,218]

Two mechanisms by which inhibition (or absence) of apical K^+ channels curtails sodium chloride and K^+ reabsorption in the TAL[20] are summarized in Figure 49.9. First, diminished K^+ recycling across the apical membrane lowers the turnover rate of $Na^+ - 2Cl^- - K^+$ co-transport. Second, the drastic reduction of the lumen-positive potential compromises the main driving force for passive movement of sodium through the paracellular pathway. Current flow across the basolateral membrane is largely carried by chloride ions which normally leave the cell along a favorable electrochemical gradient through chloride channels. Interference with such chloride exit from the cell is expected to increase its cell concentration and diminish apical activity of $Na^+ - 2Cl^- - K^+$ co-transport. This is illustrated in Bartter's Syndrome types 3, 4A, and 4B, in which either the basolateral chloride channels (CLCKA, CLCKB) or Barttin (BSDN) are mutated.[217]

DISTAL CONVOLUTED TUBULE CELL: DIRECTION, MAGNITUDE, AND MECHANISM OF TRANSPORT

The main pathways contributing to K^+ transport by DCT cells are shown in Figure 49.11. Two conductive pathways in the basolateral membrane allow for K^+

and Cl^- exit. K^+ is also able to exit the cell across the apical membrane, primarily through a K–Cl co-transporter, and, in some preparations, barium-sensitive K^+ channels.[590] The predominant path for sodium entry from the lumen is a Na–Cl co-transporter (slc12a3) that is blocked by thiazide diuretics, but not inhibited by bumetanide.[95,134,135,522–525] Amiloride-sensitive sodium channels may also be present in the apical membrane.[590] The junctional complexes between cells are cation-selective, and may permit diffusion of Na^+ and K^+ through the paracellular pathway from interstitium to lumen.

Evidence for the apical K-Cl co-transporter has come from microperfusion studies in rats.[134,135,522–525] K^+ secretion in this segment is increased when the luminal concentration of either K^+ or chloride is decreased. This increase in K^+ secretion occurs without a change in transepithelial voltage, and is not blocked by barium. Recirculation of chloride ions across the apical membrane is an important element of the mechanism of such K^+ secretion, particularly when luminal chloride concentrations are kept low by the administration of poorly-reabsorbable anions such as SO_4.[526] Under such conditions, thiazide diuretics, by blocking apical chloride entry via NaCl co-transport, inhibit K^+ secretion, consistent with K^+ ions entering the lumen by an electroneutral K-Cl co-transport mechanism.

Single channel analysis has demonstrated the presence of K^+ channels that modulate Na^+ and fluid reabsorption in this nephron segment (Figure 49.12). Of special interest is the function of KCNJ 10 Kir4.1 (KCNJ10), which provides an important pathway for basolateral K^+ recycling, especially by heteromerization with KCNJ 10 (Kir5.1).[287] This heteromeric complex is inhibited by low cell pH, and by activation of

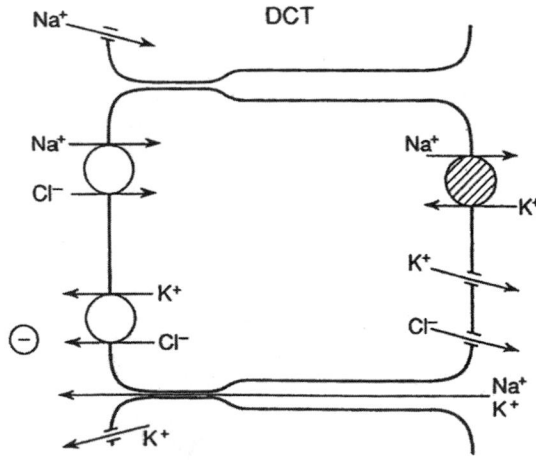

FIGURE 49.11 Model of distal convoluted tubule (DCT) cell. Some observations point to a lack of conductive pathways (channels) in the apical membrane; other studies have found evidence for Na and K conductances.

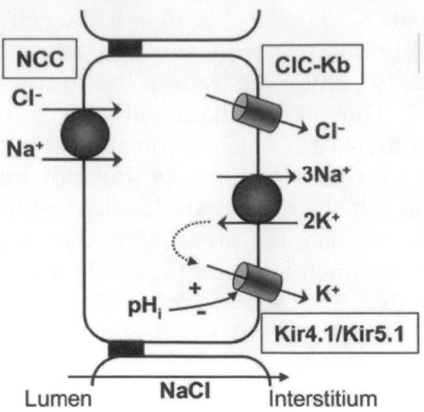

FIGURE 49.12 **Basolateral transport mechanisms in connecting tubule cells.** Note pH-sensitive K channels in the basolateral membrane. *(From ref. [24].)*

Ca^{2+} receptors.[24,287] Genetic dysfunction of this basolateral K$^+$ channel complex leads to salt-wasting due to diminished basolateral Na/K-ATPases activity, which results in high cell Na and a reduced driving force for passive Na entry across the apical membrane.[383a,401a]

Connecting Tubule and Cortical Collecting Duct Cells: Direction, Magnitude, and Mechanism of Transport

Two morphologically and functionally distinct cell types — principal cells and intercalated cells — determine K$^+$ transport in these segments, and play a major role in determining the magnitude of final urinary K$^+$ excretion (Figure 49.13). Principal cells, the most numerous cells in the initial collecting tubule (ICT), connecting tubule (CNT), and the cortical collecting duct (CCD) secrete K$^+$,[144–149,319–324,379–382,385,464,474] and are the cells subject to the most important regulatory influences. The less numerous intercalated cells also secrete K$^+$, but are capable of active K$^+$ reabsorption under certain conditions (dietary K$^+$ restriction) via an apical ATP-dependent electroneutral transport mechanism that mediates hydrogen ion secretion in exchange for K$^+$ reabsorption.[91,112,117,138,279,457–460,571,572]

K$^+$ Secretion

Figures 49.13–49.15 show the processes contributing to K$^+$ transport in the late DCT, CNT, and CCD. As pointed out above, the late distal convoluted tubule and collecting duct play a key role in K$^+$ homeostasis, but significant aldosterone-sensitive sodium reabsorption and K$^+$ secretion also occurs along the CNT. Collecting tubule K$^+$ secretion appears to become physiologically important whenever transport in the CNT is compromised or its transport capacity

overwhelmed during ingestion of a high-K$^+$ diet.[416,560] Theoretical analysis, based on known morphology and transport parameters, has also supported the importance of CNT-mediated K$^+$ transport in maintaining K$^+$ homeostasis.[560]

Figure 49.13 summarizes the main transport processes mediating K$^+$ secretion in principal (and intercalated) cells. K$^+$ uptake across the basolateral membrane is again coupled to active sodium extrusion by the Na$^+$, K$^+$-ATPase, and provides for coupling between transepithelial sodium reabsorption and K$^+$ secretion. From the rapid depolarization of the basolateral membrane voltage caused by addition of ouabain to the peritubular bathing solution, it has been concluded that the Na—K$^+$ exchange pump operates in an electrogenic fashion, particularly following stimulation by desoxycorticosterone (DOC) treatment.[275,276,424,425,436] The basolateral pump responds to several stimuli known to modulate net K$^+$ transport, such as acid—base disturbances, changes in plasma K$^+$, and mineralocorticoid hormones.[175,176,184,185,187,276,312,314,356,360,424–427,465–469] Figure 49.13 also indicates the presence of a K$^+$ conductance in the basolateral membrane which, along with

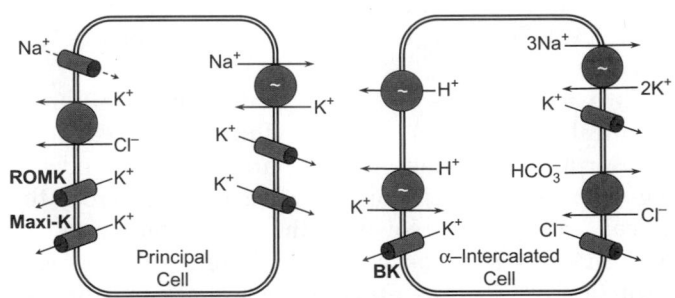

FIGURE 49.13 **Model of principal and intercalated cell, including apical and basolateral transport pathways.** Transcellular Na absorption proceeds through apical Na$^+$ channels and the basolateral Na$^+$-K$^+$ pump. K$^+$ secretion depends on K$^+$ uptake by Na$^+$-K$^+$ pump and movement through apical K$^+$ channels or K$^+$-Cl$^-$ cotransporter. In intercalated cells, K is actively reabsorbed in the apical membrane by K/H-ATPase activity, and leaves cells in the basolateral membrane by K channels.

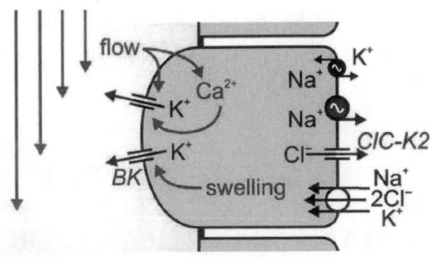

FIGURE 49.14 **Additional basolateral transport mechanisms (Na/2Cl/K transport) in principal and intercalated cells.** Note basolateral Na/2Cl/K transport. This model is consistent with passive paracellular Cl$^-$-secretion.[575]

the high electrochemical gradient for K$^+$ efflux, is largely responsible for the cell negativity. Stimulation of the electrogenic Na$^+$-K$^+$-ATPase by aldosterone may drive the cell negativity to values exceeding the K$^+$ equilibrium potential, and reverse the direction of K$^+$ movement through basolateral K$^+$ channels (see section on adrenal steroids). Microperfusion studies in isolated CCDs have also identified a significant contribution of bumetanide-sensitive K$^+$ entry across the basolateral membrane of both principal and intercalated tubule cells (Figure 49.14).[310] Such K$^+$ transport, mediated by Na-K-2Cl co-transport (Slc12a2), is stimulated by high flow rate, and contributes to the well-established increase in K$^+$ secretion through BK (or maxi-K) channels.[574,575]

The apical membrane has both sodium and K$^+$ conductances. The sodium concentration gradient between lumen and cell favors diffusion of sodium ions into the cells, reducing the cell-negative voltage across the

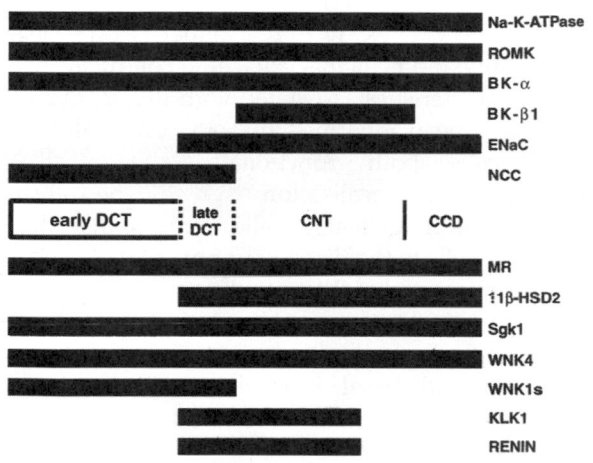

SODIUM AND POTASSIUM TRANSPORT IN THE DCT, CNT, AND CCD

Na-K-ATPase
ROMK
BK-α
BK-β1
ENaC
NCC

early DCT | late DCT | CNT | CCD

MR
11β-HSD2
Sgk1
WNK4
WNK1s
KLK1
RENIN

FIGURE 49.15 **Expression patterns of sodium and potassium transport systems and of their regulatory proteins along the distal convoluted tubule (DCT), connecting tubule (CNT), and cortical collecting duct (CCD).** In rat, mouse, and human, the sodium-chloride co-transporter (NCC) characterizes the DCT and co-localizes in the late DCT with the epithelial sodium channel (ENaC), which is also expressed in the CNT and CCD. The inwardly rectifying potassium channel (ROMK) and Na,K-ATPase are localized, respectively, in the apical and basolateral membrane along the aldosterone-sensitive distal nephron. Note that the expression of some regulatory proteins is restricted to the DCT and CNT, and does not extend to the CCD (MR: mineralocorticoid receptor; 11β-HSD2: 11β-hydroxysteroid dehydrogenase type 2; Sgk1: serum and glucocorticoid-inducible kinase; WNK4: with no lysine kinase 4; WNK1s: kidney-specific form with no lysine kinase 1; KLK1: tissue kallikrein). *(From Meneton, P., Loffing, J., and Warnock, D. G. (2004). Sodium and potassium handling by the aldosterone-sensitive distal nephron; the pivotal role of the distal and connecting tubule. Am. J. Physiol. Renal 287, F593—F601; and Pluznick, J. L., Wei, P., Grimm, P. R., and Sansom, S. C. (2005). BK-β1 subunit: Immunolocalization in the mammalian connecting tubule and its role in the kaliuretic response to volume expansion. Am. J. Physiol. Renal 288, F846—F854, with permission.)*

apical membrane relative to the voltage across the basolateral membrane. This asymmetrical electrical polarization of the apical and basolateral membranes favors diffusive movement of K$^+$ from cell to lumen, and is the source of the lumen-negative transepithelial potential difference which favors diffusive movement of K$^+$ from cell to lumen.

Sodium entry across the apical epithelial sodium channel (ENaC; see Chapter 7 by Palmer and Sackin) and its electrogenic basolateral extrusion by the Na-K pump play a critical role in regulating apical K$^+$ transport by their depolarizing effect on the apical membrane potential. In animals fed a normal K$^+$ diet, K$^+$ secretion in the CCD is generally dependent on sodium absorption.[155,156,160,161,342,382,489] However, in rats fed a high-K$^+$ diet for as little as 18 hours, a significant fraction of K$^+$ excretion becomes amiloride-insensitive, and thus ENaC-independent, an observation consistent with the activation of a non-principal cell-mediated pathway in α-intercalated cells.[161] Diminished K$^+$ reabsorption in the proximal tubule may further compensate for compromised distal tubule K$^+$ secretion, as it has been shown that hyperkalemia suppresses proximal fluid and K$^+$ reabsorption.[67]

The apical membrane voltage of principal cells is depolarized following administration of mineralocorticoids.[179,350,356,359,360] In contrast, amiloride blocks ENaC and hyperpolarizes the apical membrane. The reduction in the driving force for K$^+$ excretion explains the K$^+$-sparing effect of this diuretic.[275,357,358,361] The K$^+$ conductance of the apical membrane is variable and increased by high-K$^+$ intake,[350,352,356,358,375,376,424—427,437,438,441,443] and vasopressin.[437,438,443] The apical K$^+$ conductance is reduced by intracellular acidification,[350,472,498] consistent with the K$^+$-sparing effect of acute acidosis.[470,475] Coupling between basolateral Na$^+$,K$^+$-ATPase activity and apical K$^+$ and sodium channels has also been observed, as evidenced by the coordinated changes of basolateral Na$^+$-K$^+$-ATPase activity and apical membrane Na$^+$ and K$^+$ conductances.[351]

K$^+$ Channels in the Aldosterone-Sensitive Distal Nephron (ASDN)

The apical sodium as well as apical and basolateral K$^+$ channels have been extensively studied by applying the patch-clamp technique to cultured amphibian kidney cells and to cells of isolated mammalian collecting ducts[81,157—161,179,183,187,217,379—382,407,540—548,563] (see also Chapter 47 by Wang and Huang).

Figures 49.15 to 49.17 summarize our present state of knowledge about apical and basolateral K$^+$ channels in principal and intercalated cells. The apical low-conductance secretory K$^+$ channel (SK) are highly K$^+$ selective, and have a high open probability. They are

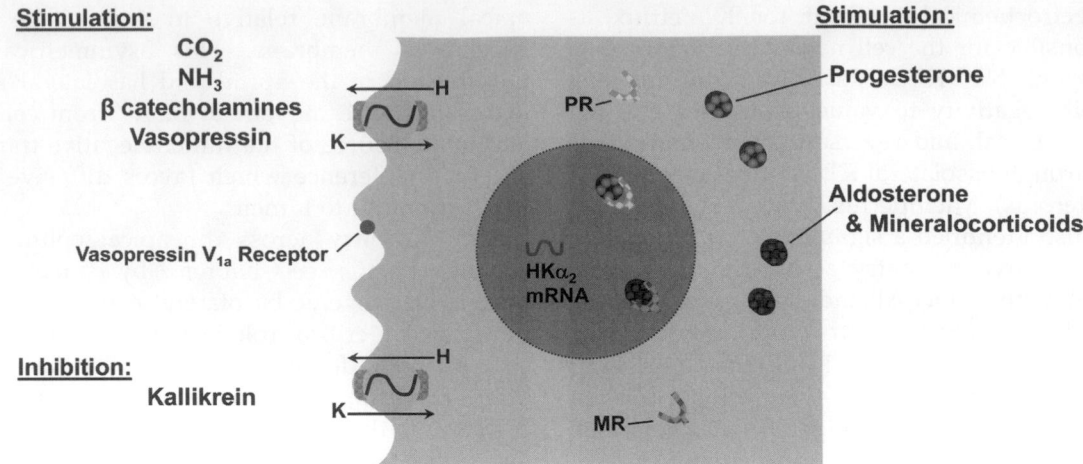

FIGURE 49.16   Model of acid secreting (A-type) intercalated cells in the ICT and CCD. These cells are the site of potassium absorption via an H,K-ATPase. Proton secretion is driven by an H-ATPase (not shown). *(Courtesy of Dr. Charles Wingo.)*

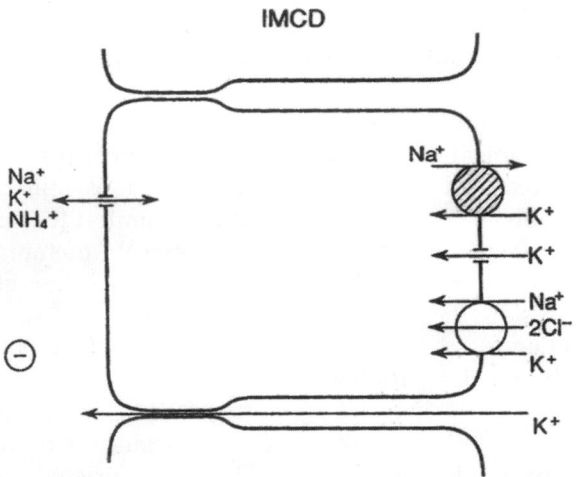

FIGURE 49.17   Model of inner medullary collecting duct (IMCD) cell. Apical cation channels are equally permeable to Na$^+$ and K$^+$.

stimulated by low concentrations of ATP and cyclic AMP-dependent protein kinase A, as well as by alkalinization of the cytoplasm. They are inhibited by barium, arachidonic acid, Ca^{2+}-calmodulin kinase II, millimolar concentrations of ATP, Ca^{2+}-dependent protein kinase C, and acidification of the intracellular fluid. The channel is sensitive to phosphorylation processes, so that protein phosphatase inhibitors are required to prevent channel "run-down," the decline in channel activity observed following excision of membrane patches. The open probability of the secretory K$^+$ channel is not markedly voltage-dependent, and Ca^{2+} ions do not directly affect channel activity in excised membrane patches. Increased channel activity is often reflected by recruitment of channels into the active apical membrane pool.[217] The K$^+$ channel is identical to ROMK (Kir1, KCNJ1), a

cloned, inwardly rectifying, low-conductance, ATP-regulated K$^+$ channel.[157,158,217,227,603]

Whereas the SK/ROMK channel is present solely in connecting and principal cells, high conductance channels with characteristics associated with BK or (maxi-K) channels have been identified in both principal and intercalated cells both functionally,[158,160,195,240,303,385–387,430] and by immunolocalization.[205–208,354] The density of BK channels in intercalated cells exceeds that detected in principal cells in the distal nephron.

The open-probability of BK channels, as defined in split-open, isolated connecting tubules and cortical collecting tubules, is quite low at the resting membrane potential and basal intracellular Ca^{2+} concentration, although their single-channel conductance is about five times that of ROMK.[158,303,377,430,432,440–443] Apical BK channels are activated by membrane depolarization, elevation of [Ca^{2+}], hypoosmotic stress, and/or membrane stretch,[120,160,224,239,377,490,491] and can be selectively blocked by iberiotoxin.[20,78,170] BK channels are generally comprised of pore-forming α-subunit, a member of the *slo* family of K$^+$ channels originally cloned from *Drosophila*, and a regulatory β-subunit.[17,131]

Cumulative evidence implicates the BK channel in mediating an important fraction of K$^+$ secretion in the CNT and CCD in response to high urinary flow rates[20,310,386,387,574,575] K$^+$-loading[20,354,385–387] and application of vasopressin to the lumen fluid,[10] and in the absence of ROMK in Bartter's syndrome.[20] BK channel-mediated K$^+$ secretion in the CCD is also dependent on a basolateral bumetanide sensitive chloride-dependent transport pathway, proposed to be NKCC1[310] (Figure 49.14). In support of this conclusion is the finding that mice with genetic disruption of NKCC1 exhibit higher serum potassium concentrations, with inappropriately low urinary potassium excretion, compared to wild-type mice.[334,533]

The density of BK channels in intercalcalated cells exceeds that detected in principal cells in the distal nephron. It remains unsolved as to how intercalated cells maintain a high steady state K concentration for sustained luminal K$^+$ secretion as there is little immunodetectable[418] and functional[34,44,116,380,434] Na$^+$-K$^+$ pump activity in intercalated cells. A K-independent Na-ATPase identified biochemically in kidney[468] and present in CA MDCK may serve as an exit pathway for Na brought in by the apical NBCDE or BL NKCC.

Flow activation of BK channels is associated with an increase in delivery to and reabsorption of Na$^+$ by the distal nephron.[269,342,574,575] This in turn increases the driving force for passive K$^+$ efflux by depolarizing the apical membrane potential. High tubular fluid flow rates also lead to an increase in [Ca^{2+}]$_i$, via luminal Ca^{2+} entry and IP3-mediated store release to concentrations sufficient to stimulate Ca^{2+}-sensitive BK channels.[574] It has been suggested that high flow rates along connecting and collecting tubules activates apical Ca^{2+} channels, which in turn stimulate Ca-sensitive maxi-K channels.[574,575]

An unresolved problem concerns the contribution of Ca^{2+}-sensitive BK$^+$ channels to K$^+$ secretion under physiological flow conditions. Single channel analysis by patch-clamp techniques is limited to "split-open" tubules in the absence of membrane stretch. This renders evaluation of BK$^+$ channel activity difficult in conditions mimicking physiological flow rates of tubule fluid.

The basolateral K$^+$ channels, shown in Figure 49.13, are also K$^+$ selective. Some are activated by membrane hyperpolarization; all are inhibited by barium. Basolateral K$^+$ channels are characterized by several factors that distinguish them from their apical homologs.[225,226,315] First, a subpopulation responds to hyperpolarization by increased activity,[543] which contributes to the increase in basolateral membrane K$^+$ conductance following stimulation of electrogenic Na$^+$-K$^+$-ATPase activity. Second, basolateral K$^+$ channels are stimulated by NO and cGMP.[225,226,315] The evidence for the involvement of NO is the decline in basolateral K$^+$ channel activity by inhibiting nitric oxide synthase, whereas donors of exogenous NO stimulate these channels. Application of cGMP analogs also activate basolateral K$^+$ channels, and hyperpolarize the basolateral membrane. This induces an increase in the apical membrane potential through current flow via the paracellular pathway, and stimulates sodium entry across the apical membrane of principal cells.[315] Features shared by these channels are their lack of inhibition by ATP and a biphasic effect of changes in cell Ca^{2+}: whereas low concentrations stimulate basolateral K$^+$ channels (via activation of cGMP), high levels of Ca^{2+} inhibit K$^+$ channels.[225,226,315,445]

Apical Co-Transport of KCl

Microperfusion studies of superficial distal tubules in the rat and isolated rabbit CCDs provide evidence for an electroneutral K$^+$ and chloride co-transport mechanism in the apical membrane,[8,132–135,521–525] also shown in Figure 49.13. The key evidence for this mechanism is that K$^+$ secretion into the distal tubule is stimulated when the lumen is perfused with solutions with a low chloride concentration. This effect occurs without changes in the transepithelial voltage across the distal tubule wall, and persists in the presence of barium, a K$^+$ channel inhibitor. K-Cl co-transport may contribute to K$^+$ secretion when the concentration of chloride in the lumen declines. This may occur with the delivery of poorly reabsorbable anions, such as sulfate, phosphate, and especially bicarbonate into the distal tubule.[8,264] The molecular identity of this KCl co-transporter is not known.

K$^+$ REABSORPTION

In the distal nephron, intercalated cells mediate K$^+$ reabsorption (Figure 49.14). They are scattered among the principal cells of the cortical and outer medullary collecting duct, and also among the cells of the distal tubule (infrequently in the distal convoluted tubule, and more commonly in the connecting tubule and initial collecting tubule).[99,255,318] Several types of intercalated cells have been recognized: A-type cells secrete hydrogen ions; and B-type cells secrete bicarbonate ions. A third, "mixed" type, containing both Cl$^-$–HCO$_3^-$ exchangers in the apical and basolateral membrane, has also been described.[558]

The A-type cells may also be responsible for K$^+$ reabsorption, as shown in Figures 49.14 and 49.16. Several important differences between intercalated cells and principal cells should be noted. Na$^+$, K$^+$-ATPase expression and activity in basolateral membranes of intercalated cells in tubules of the renal cortex is much lower than in principal cells.[258] However, it is possible but not yet proven that lack of this transport is compensated for by a K-independent, ouabain-insensitive Na$^+$-ATPase.[173,408] Moreover, intercalated cells also have low apical Na$^+$-conductances, but express large-conductance BK channels.[303,239,377,432]

Several isoforms of K$^+$-H$^+$-ATPase, distinguished by variable K$^+$/Na$^+$ sensitivities of the exchange processes, and by different sensitivities to inhibitors such as gastric K$^+$-H$^+$ blockers and ouabain, are responsible for active K$^+$ absorption in intercalated cells.[6,112,117,211,457–460,558,571,572] Two types of K$^+$-H$^+$-ATPase have been described in rat and mouse cortical and outer medullary collecting tubules, and they are structurally identical to isoforms of K$^+$-H$^+$-ATPases cloned from gastric and colonic mucosa. Their importance is suggested by numerous functional studies.[70,112,117,122] However, a recent study, based on experiments in gastric and colonic K$^+$-H$^+$-ATPase knockout mice has provided strong evidence for an as yet unidentified additional transport mechanism for linked K$^+$ reabsorption and hydrogen ion secretion that is distinct from known K$^+$-H$^+$-ATPases.[384a] The importance of this transporter is underscored by its ability to compensate effectively for the loss-of-function of both gastric and colonic K$^+$-H$^+$-ATPase. Similar results have also been reported using the mouse cortical collecting tubule. Thus, the contribution of individual K$^+$-H$^+$-ATPases and other not-yet-identified transporters to the maintenance of K$^+$ and hydrogen ion balance is not fully-understood.

Two inhibitors of the gastric K$^+$-H$^+$-ATPase, omeprazole and SCH28080, decrease both K$^+$ absorption and hydrogen secretion in the distal tubule and the outer medullary collecting duct. K$^+$-H$^+$ exchange is increased during metabolic acidosis,[404,460] experimental K$^+$ depletion,[70,112,117,122,457−460,571,572,592] and during administration of a low-sodium diet.[457,458] Increased sensitivity to K$^+$ depletion was reported in mice lacking the colonic isoform of K$^+$-H$^+$-ATPase, although the ability of renal K$^+$ conservation was quite well-preserved, and most of the loss of K$^+$ occurred by fecal excretion.[333]

Several factors modulate the activity of apical K-H exchange, and are summarized in Figure 49.16. They include acid−base-related factors such as stimulation by ammonium and CO$_2$, catecholamines, kallikrein, vasopressin, and adrenal steroids.[571] Moreover, progesterone is also important for effective retention during K$^+$ deprivation.[125,126] Interference with K-H exchange also compromises effective Na retention.[571]

Morphological studies of the apical cell membrane of intercalated cells in K$^+$-depleted rats have shown changes in fine structure, such as an increase in the number of rod-shaped particles and amplification of the microplicae.[254−257,481] These alterations in membrane structure are specific for the luminal membrane of intercalated cells. Intercalated cells also undergo marked morphological amplification of their apical membranes following acidification.[110a] These changes suggest that K$^+$ reabsorption and hydrogen ion secretion are functionally linked.

Medullary Collecting Duct Cells

Several sections of the medullary collecting ducts have been distinguished on the basis of morphological and functional differences. The outer medulla can be grossly separated into outer and inner stripes, and the inner medulla can be subdivided into outer and inner halves. The inner medullary collecting duct is separated into initial and terminal segments. Most of these collecting duct segments participate in the regulation of K$^+$ excretion.

The medullary collecting duct in the outer stripe resembles the cortical collecting duct. K$^+$ secretion and sodium reabsorption continue,[485−487] and the cells lining this segment have morphological and functional properties similar to principal and intercalated cells.[255]

The collecting duct in the inner stripe is characterized by a different transport pattern. K$^+$ secretion is absent when isolated tubule segments are perfused with symmetrical solutions, and the apical cell membrane lacks significant K$^+$ conductance.[464] However, when transepithelial K$^+$ gradients are applied, significant K$^+$ movement occurs, presumably via the paracellular transport route.[459,464,570] K$^+$ depletion increases the passive K$^+$ permeability.[464] The generation of electrical potentials also activates passive K$^+$ movement. For instance, a lumen-positive potential, generated by electrogenic hydrogen ion secretion, induces signficant K$^+$ reabsorption. This coupling between K$^+$ and hydrogen movement may explain why augmented proton secretion is frequently associated with enhanced K$^+$ reabsorption.

An active K$^+$-hydrogen exchange mechanism has also been detected in collecting ducts isolated from the inner stripe of the outer medulla in K$^+$-depleted rabbits. Activation of this transporter also contributes to the stimulation of K$^+$ reabsorption and hydrogen ion secretion that is observed in K$^+$ depletion.[569]

Both reabsorption and secretion of K$^+$ have been observed in the inner medullary collecting duct. Figure 49.17 summarizes some of the known transport properties of inner medullary collecting duct cells.[410] An important feature of inner medullary collecting duct cells is a nonspecific cation channel in the apical membrane.[305] Depending on the apical transmembrane electrochemical driving forces, this channel may mediate both sodium reabsorption and K$^+$ secretion. At very high lumen K$^+$ concentrations, passive reabsorption of K$^+$ may also take place. The presence of a furosemide-sensitive Na$^+$-2Cl-K$^+$ co-transporter in the basolateral membrane of inner medullary collecting duct cells has also been reported.[90a,209,410]

CONTROL OF RENAL K$^+$ TRANSPORT

General Aspects of Regulation of Renal K$^+$ Transport

Figure 49.18 illustrates the difference between two distinct K$^+$ mechanisms involved in renal K$^+$

homeostasis. First, feedback control of K$^+$ excretion depends on changes in plasma K$^+$ concentration which, either directly or by modulating aldosterone release, alters renal K$^+$ secretion. A second mechanism, feed-forward control of K$^+$ excretion, depends on the local increase of K$^+$ concentration in the gastrointestinal tract, the liver, and possibly the cerebral circulation.[591] Such feed-forward control of extracellular K$^+$ homeostasis minimizes changes of plasma K$^+$ concentrations, and may account for the rapid response of the kidney to changes in gastrointestinal K$^+$ uptake.[89,369,591] The nature of the intestinal and cerebral K$^+$ receptor and the signaling mechanisms effecting changes in renal K$^+$ excretion are not known. Attention should also be drawn to evidence that the central nervous system participates in controlling renal K$^+$ excetion. Examples include the rapid increase in K$^+$ excretion following unilateral nephrectomy, diurnal fluctuations of K$^+$ excretion, and aldosterone-independent changes in K$^+$ balance in hypo- and hyperkalemic conditions.[392−397] Figure 49.19 summarizes known agents modulating K$^+$ secretion.

Proximal Tubule

The proximal tubule is the main site of K$^+$ reabsorption, but does not play an important role in the physiological regulation of K$^+$ excretion.[179] K$^+$ transport is largely dependent on sodium and fluid movement, and changes with variations of proximal tubule sodium and fluid reabsorption. Increased delivery of K$^+$ into the loop of Henle occurs during osmotic diuresis and inhibition of proximal tubule sodium and fluid transport.

Secretory potassium entry into the proximal straight tubule has been reported[250,252] (Figure 49.8). Such secretory transport has been demonstrated in vitro,[260,261] but it is likely that modest K$^+$ secretion also occurs in vivo. Given the increase in medullary K$^+$ concentration along the corticomedullary axis, K$^+$ ions may enter the tubule lumen by diffusion as part of the process of medullary recycling.[248,249]

Thick Ascending Limb of Henle, Distal Convoluted Tubule, Connecting and Collecting Tubules

The TAL normally reabsorbs a significant fraction of filtered and recycled K$^+$. However, reabsorption may be significantly reduced or even replaced by net secretion, following inhibition of Na-2Cl-K co-transport or interference with apical K$^+$ recycling.[20,217,512] Diminished reabsorption of K$^+$ in the TAL may thus contribute to enhanced urinary excretion whenever TAL function is compromised.[20,234]

Modest rates of K$^+$ secretion have also been observed along the mammalian DCT, but changes in tubule flow rate and dietary K$^+$ intake do not affect K$^+$ secretion.[451] In vivo micropuncture and microperfusion experiments indicate that the DCT is the main site of action of thiazide diuretics.[94,95,522−525] An interesting relationship between sodium chloride and K$^+$ transport has been observed in microperfusion experiments. When apical sodium entry was stimulated by raising the Na concentration in the tubule lumen, K$^+$ secretion increased. It is likely that enhanced chloride entry increased cell chloride and stimulated K-Cl co-transport from cell to lumen.[521] Thus, recycling of chloride appears to play a significant role in K$^+$ secretion in DCT cells.

The CNT, ICT, and CCD are the main nephron sites that control K$^+$ excretion.[177−186,465,470,473,474,483−487,579−583,585] Information on the transport function of the ICT has been obtained by either free-flow or in vivo microperfusion studies. The CCD has also been investigated by in vitro microperfusion techniques. These tubule segments are distinguished by marked cell heterogeneity, and net transport of K$^+$ results from varying components of secretion and reabsorption of K$^+$. The most important systemic changes that affect these factors include K$^+$ intake, adrenal steroids, salt and water balance, and acid−base balance. Figure 49.19 summarized the main factors modulating K$_r$ transport in DCT, CNT, and CCD.

Changes in K$^+$ Intake

Both increases and decreases in K$^+$ intake, as well as acute loading with K$^+$-containing fluids, initiate appropriate adjustments in renal K$^+$ excretion. Increases in K$^+$ intake tend to raise plasma K$^+$ concentration, which both affects the kidney directly and stimulates the adrenal glands to secrete aldosterone.[31,66,118] Decreases in K$^+$ intake or losses of K$^+$ that exceed intake tend to reduce total body K$^+$ content, plasma K$^+$ concentration, and aldosterone secretion.

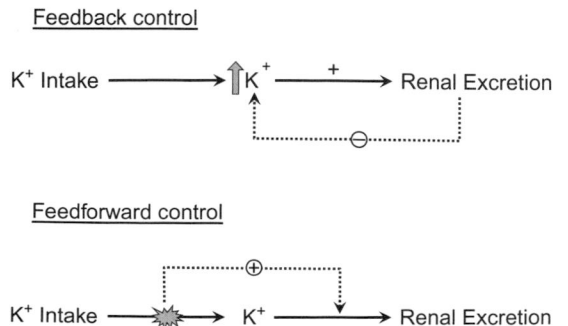

FIGURE 49.18 The main control mechanisms safeguarding K homeostasis.[591]

K⁺-Loading

Potassium secretion along the ICT rises sharply with parenteral administration of K⁺-containing solutions.[179,182,185,473,474,491,579,583,585] The stimulation of K⁺ secretion after acute K⁺-loading has been demonstrated in both free-flow and microperfusion studies. Factors contributing to increased rates of secretion include increases in plasma K⁺,[474,593] aldosterone levels,[66,118,145−147,166,482,487,585] and distal flow rate.[179,266,285,319,322] The independent and separate effects of these variables have been explored in microperfusion experiments in which flow rate, luminal ion concentrations, and the levels of both mineralocorticoids and glucocorticoids could be controlled.[121,123,154,155,416] Chronic K⁺-loading increases the secretory capacity of the distal nephron so that at a given plasma K⁺ level, renal K⁺ excretion is significantly accelerated.[2,48,49,50,52,345−348,466] Figure 49.20 illustrates relationships between plasma K⁺ concentration and either renal K⁺ excretion or distal K⁺ secretion in control animals, and in animals fed a high-K⁺ diet, and Figure 49.21 provides an overview of the cell messengers involved. Pretreatment with the high-K⁺ diet leads to powerful stimulation of K⁺ secretion and a more rapid onset of kaliuresis.[228,352,585] This stimulation of K⁺ secretion at normal or only slightly elevated plasma K⁺ levels following chronic elevation of K⁺ intake is a clear example of an adaptive change in renal function, and occurs even when plasma aldosterone is kept constant.[352] Full adaptation, though, does require an increase in mineralocorticoid levels.[140−147,381,382] Along with an enhanced rate of K⁺ uptake by nonrenal cells,[7,53] the increased secretory capacity of distal tubule cells promotes K⁺ tolerance — the ability of animals fed a high-K⁺ diet to survive an acute K⁺-load that would otherwise be fatal. As summarized in Figure 49.22, elevation of plasma K⁺ also inhibits proximal fluid absorption, thereby increasing the delivery of fluid and Na into the distal nephron.[67]

A further example of K⁺ adaptation is the ability of a reduced number of nephrons — such as in chronic renal failure — to sharply increase K⁺ secretion and to maintain K⁺ balance.[176] In addition to aldosterone, angiotensin II also increases ROMK activity, but only in animals fed a high-K diet.[556] A high-K diet increases not only the apical surface expression of ROMK, but also that of ENaC and of BK channels in both principal and intercalated cells in the CCD.[157] In contrast, NaCl co-transport expression in distal convoluted tubules was found to be decreased. Such redistribution of sodium reabsorption from NCC to nephron sites

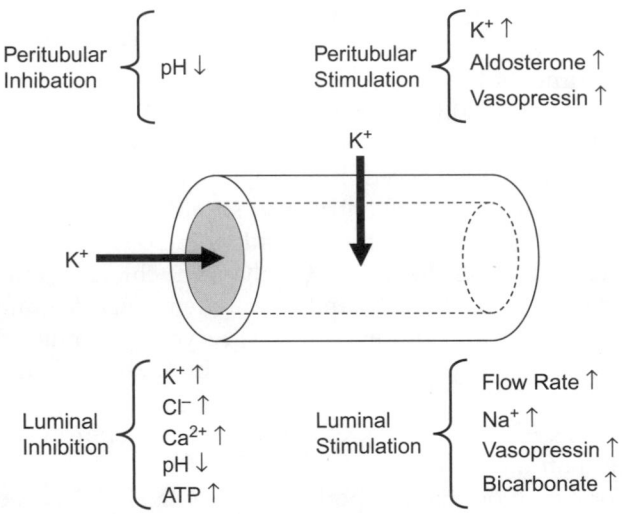

FIGURE 49.19 Summary of luminal and basolateral factors modulating K transport in connecting and collecting tubule cells.

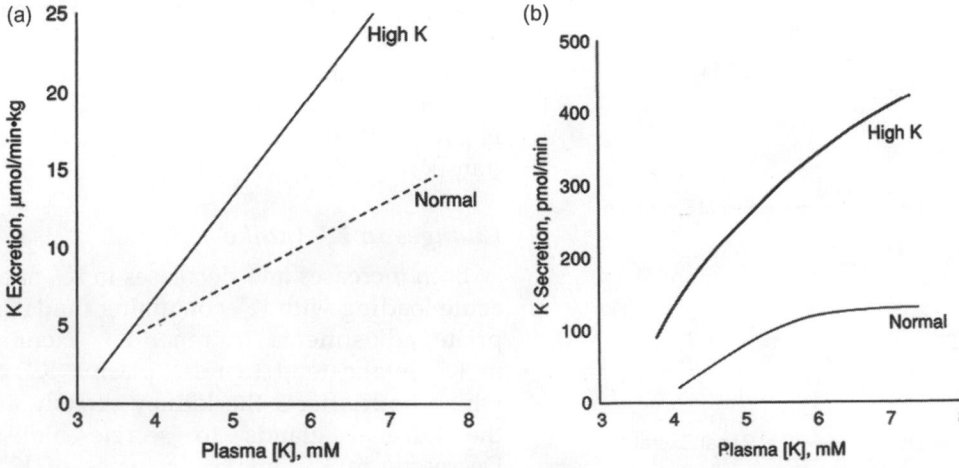

FIGURE 49.20 (a) Relation between plasma K⁺ concentration and renal K⁺ excretion in rats on a control and high-K diet; and (b) distal tubule K⁺ secretion.

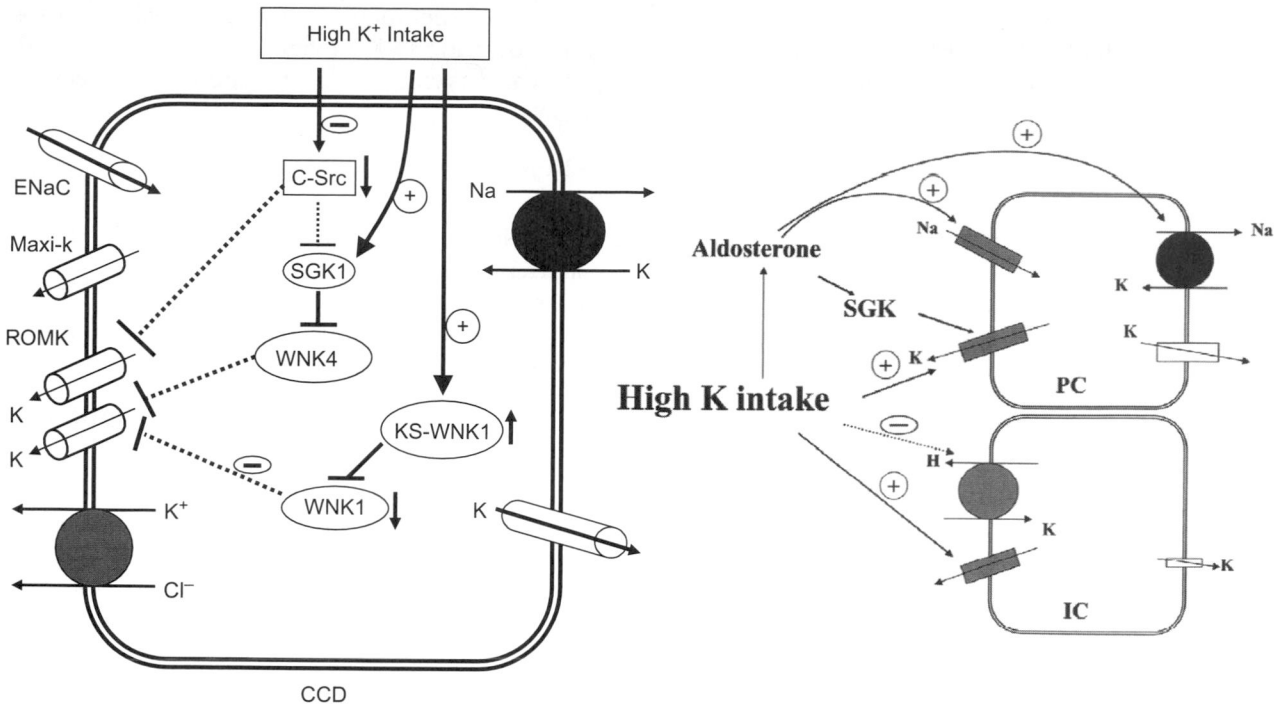

FIGURE 49.21 **Model of CCD cells illustrating the mechanisms by which high-K$^+$ diet increases K$^+$ secretion.** High-K$^+$ intake stimulates aldosterone secretion, which in turn activates ENaC and Na$^+$,K$^+$-ATPase in principle cells. Increased ENaC activity augments the driving force for K secretion, whereas stimulation of Na$^+$,K$^+$-ATPase can indirectly activate ROMK channel activity by a cross-talk mechanism. In addition, high K$^+$ intake can increase ROMK channel activity via modulation of the WNK pathway (see section on WNKs).

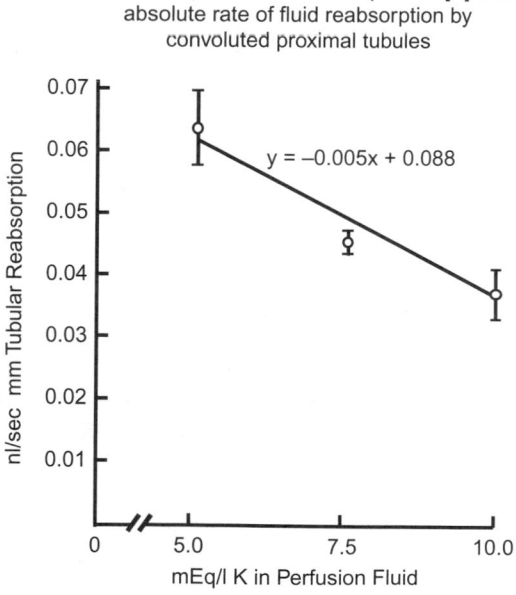

Relationship between arterial plasma [K] and absolute rate of fluid reabsorption by convoluted proximal tubules

$y = -0.005x + 0.088$

FIGURE 49.22 **Summary of the effects of changing peritubular K$^+$ concentration on proximal tubule fluid absorption.**[67]

with high ENaC expression provides an increase in the electrogenic driving force of K$^+$ secretion by the principal cell, and optimizes urinary K$^+$ excretion in hyperkalemic conditions.

Adaptive changes of K$^+$ transport have clear morphological and biochemical correlates in the distal tubule and CCD.[255−257,466,467,470] Proliferation of the basolateral cell membrane is highly significant in K$^+$-adapted animals, and is closely associated with a sharp increase in Na$^+$,K$^+$-ATPase.[113,114,156,163,254,296] Hyperkalemia and mineralocorticoids independently initiate the amplification of the basolateral membrane and the attendant increase in ATPase activity.[469] Thus, changes in basolateral membrane area, Na$^+$,K$^+$-ATPase content, and K$^+$ secretory rates are tightly coupled.[466,471,476] Morphological changes are apparent after 24 hours of increased K$^+$ intake and increase for about another week before a plateau is reached.[476] Increased K$^+$ excretion may continue beyond cessation of a high-K$^+$ intake.[348]

Principal cell basolateral membrane amplification also occurs with increased delivery of fluid and sodium ions to the ICT which occurs as a consequence of decreased proximal fluid absorption in hyperkalemic conditions[134,136,256,296,398] (Figure 49.22). The underlying mechanism appears to be stimulation of sodium reabsorption, which is linked to K$^+$ secretion. Another example is that chronic administration of furosemide to animals in which fluctuations of aldosterone and changes in electrolyte balance were prevented still leads to a sharp increase of K$^+$ secretion and sodium reabsorption.[469] Similar adaptation is observed in unilaterally nephrectomized animals: K$^+$ balance is maintained by redistribution of Na$^+$ reabsorption from proximal to distal nephron sites and increased delivery of fluid into the distal nephron of the remaining nephron population.[109,467] Again, amplification of the basolateral membrane occurs predominantly in the principal cell population.

High-K$^+$ feeding also increases the pool of active ROMK in principal cells by diminishing apical removal of channels by endocytosis[157,161,539,544,546,548] and redistributing BK channels from an intracellular pool to the plasma membrane.[354] Figure 49.21 summarizes the change in cell messenger activity in response to increased K$^+$ intake. An important element responsible for stimulation of K$^+$ secretion is an increase in aldosterone release.[354] However, the effect of dietary potassium on stimulation of ROMK and BK channel activity is not due a direct hormonal effect, but reflects the mineralocorticoid-induced increase in apical ENaC and basolateral Na-K-ATPase activity, leading to enhancement of the electrochemical gradient favoring potassium secretion. The contribution of the BK channel towards excretion of a dietary potassium-load has been underscored by the finding that mice with genetic ablation of the β1-subunit of the BK channel exhibit, at baseline, low urinary potassium and sodium clearances, conditions that are exacerbated when the animals are fed a high-K$^+$ diet.[205–208]

In animals fed a normal K$^+$ diet, K$^+$ secretion in the CCD is completely dependent on sodium absorption.[342,483,489] However, distal potassium secretion may occur via a sodium-independent pathway in animals loaded with potassium for as little as 18 hours.[156,382] Moreover, basolateral sodium uptake via the Na/H exchanger has been proposed to be able to sustain basolateral pump activity in principal cells and potassium secretion in the CCD in the absence of significant sodium absorption.[353]

Dietary-induced stimulation of K$^+$ secretion is mediated not only by the aldosterone-dependent mechanisms described above, albeit indirectly, but also by aldosterone-independent mechanisms, a notion suggested by microperfusion studies that reveal that a high-K$^+$ diet stimulates potassium secretion in CCDs isolated from adrenalectomized rabbits.[352] A high-K$^+$ diet stimulates the expression of renal CYP2C23, a major CYP-epoxygenase, and increases the concentration of 11,12-epoxyeicosatrienoic acid (EET), a product of CYP-epoxygenase-dependent arachidonic acid metabolism in the CCD, which in turn stimulates BK channel activity,[497] CYP-epoxygenase-dependent arachidonic acid metabolism has been proposed to mediate regulation of renal K$^+$ secretion in response to dietary K$^+$ intake.[547]

A high-K$^+$ diet may not only diminish K$^+$ reabsorption by lowering H-K exchange,[569] but also by enhancing apical recycling of K$^+$ in intercalated cells by BK channels.[380]

K$^+$-Deprivation

Renal K$^+$ excretion drops sharply after withdrawal of K$^+$ from the diet and aldosterone secretion is suppressed. Concurrently, distal tubule K$^+$ secretion is markedly depressed or disappears altogether[142,175,177,371] to be replaced by net reabsorption.[119,322,371] K$^+$ reabsorption involves both active and passive transport mechanisms. Active K-H exchange is significantly increased in cortical and medullary collecting tubule segments.[70,112,117,571] An increase in passive K$^+$ permeability in the OMCD has been reported in states of K$^+$-depletion, and could favor accelerated K$^+$ reabsorption if the electrochemical gradient were favorable.

Figure 49.23 provides an overview of some of the transport changes that take place following administration of a low-K$^+$ diet.[539,540,546] Tyrosine phosphorylation of ROMK by Src initiates the endocytotic removal of apical K$^+$ channels. Specific tyrosine phosphorylation on the C-terminus of ROMK is critical, and superoxide production is closely associated with the low-K$^+$ response.[546] Notably, the reduction of apical K$^+$ channel density in response to K$^+$-depletion is independent of aldosterone, and consistent with previous findings of a direct effect of K$^+$ intake on K$^+$ excretion.[352]

Interestingly, upregulation of Na$^+$,K$^+$-ATPase activity has also been observed in tubules following K$^+$-depletion.[72,113] The original hypothesis that Na,K-ATPase was relocated to the apical membrane to facilitate K$^+$ reabsorption was not supported by immunological studies.[258] Thus, increased Na$^+$,K$^+$-ATPase-mediated K$^+$ uptake across the basolateral membrane requires increased backleak through basolateral K$^+$ channels.[113] It is well-established that K$^+$-depletion stimulates renal growth, a condition in which Na$^+$, K$^+$-ATPase might be expected to increase, but this relationship requires further exploration.[254]

K$^+$-depletion also involves changes in the distribution of H-K ATPases in cortical and outer medullary collecting ducts.[12,231,259] As shown in Figure 49.24, the ouabain-insensitive isoform of H-K-ATPase (type I) is downregulated in K$^+$-depletion and replaced by the type III isoform that is sensitive to inhibition by ouabain, and less selective for K$^+$ compared to sodium.[70,106a,117] Furthermore, remodeling of H-K-ATPases in K$^+$-depletion involves their targeting to principal cells,[117] instead of intercalated cells.

Since ammonium can substitute for K$^+$ on both Na-K-ATPase and Na-2Cl-K transporters, changes in extracellular K$^+$ exert a significant effect on acid excretion.[175,176,534] The interactions between K$^+$ and

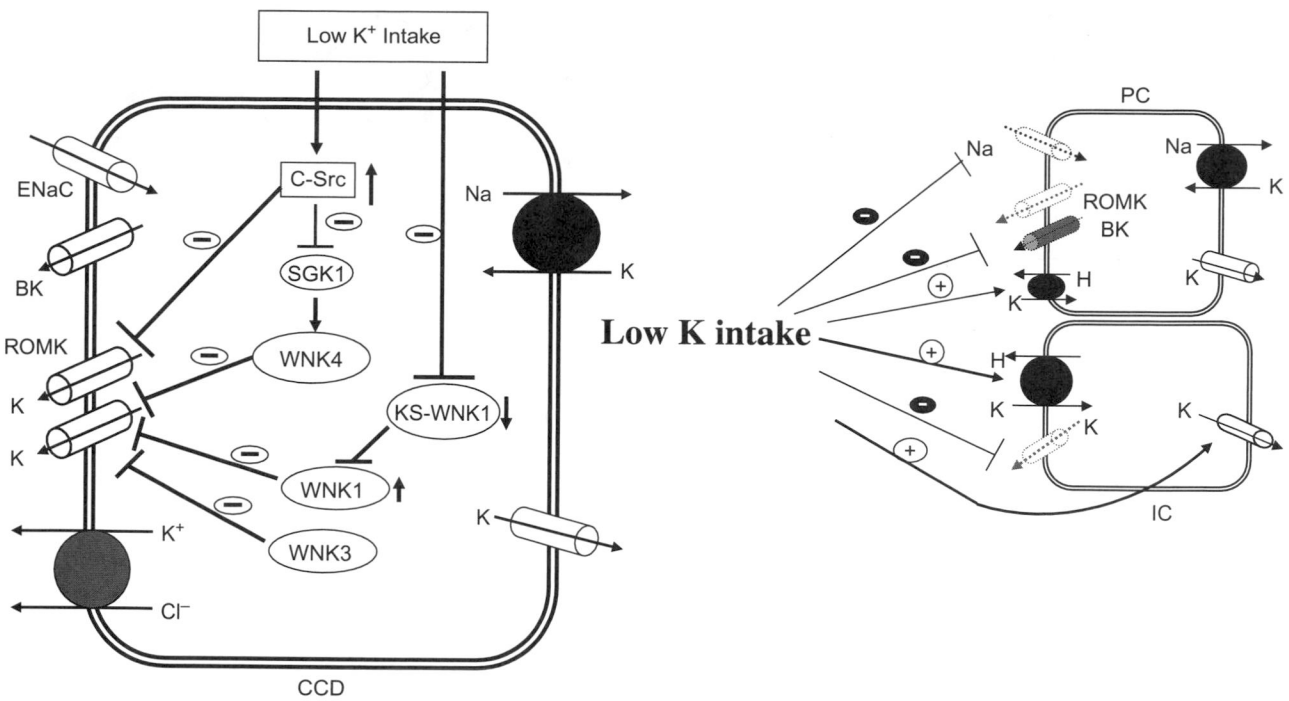

FIGURE 49.23 Model of CCD cells illustrating the mechanism by which low-K[+] diet decreases K[+] secretion. Low-K[+] intake reduces ROMK channel activity and thus K[+] secretion in principle cells via modulation of the WNK pathway and enhances apical H-K-ATPase activity in intercalated cells.

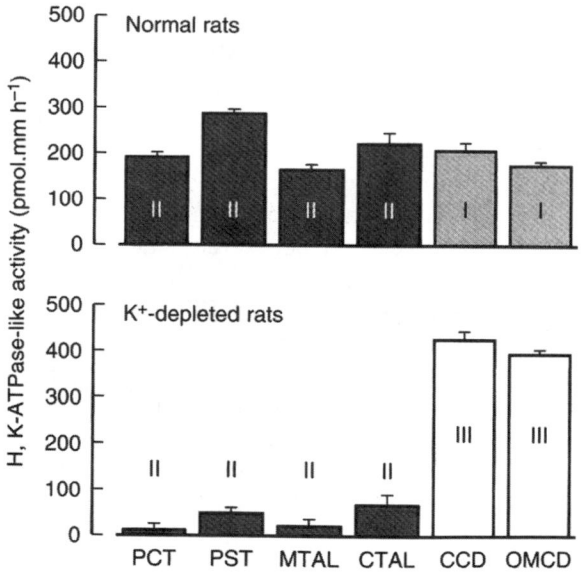

FIGURE 49.24 Distribution of three subtypes of H+,K+-ATPase-like activities, defined in the lower panel, along the nephron of normal rats and potassium-depleted rats.[117] All H-K-ATPase isoforms are sensitive to Sch28080. However, type I is insensitive to millimolar concentrations of ouabain whereas type III is sensitive to ouabain. Type II is inhibited by ouabain but is restricted in expression to the proximal tbule and thick ascending limb (TAL). Type III can be further distinguished from type II by its sensitivity to sodium and upregulation in response to K[+] depletion.[70,106a,117]

ammonium are summarized in Figure 49.25. Under conditions of K[+]-depletion, the interstitial concentration of K[+] declines, and Na[+]-K[+]-ATPase-mediated uptake of ammonium in inner and outer MCD increases. Enhanced supply of cell hydrogen ion increases apical secretion, in part through the H-K exchange mechanism, thus stimulating K[+] reabsorption. Net K[+] secretion decreases further, since tubule trapping of ammonium blocks ROMK.[215] Hyperkalemia has the opposite effect. K[+] ions replace ammonium on Na[+],K[+]-ATPase and the Na[+],K[+]-2Cl co-transporter, which leads to diminished cell acidification and hydrogen ion availability for apical secretion. As a consequence, hyperkalemia may induce metabolic acidosis.[176]

Changes in aldosterone modulate, but are not fully responsible for, the renal response to K[+]-deprivation. This mineralocorticoid modulates the urinary loss of K[+], but K[+] excretion continues to diminish when animals are put on a low-K[+] diet with clamped circulating aldosterone.[348–349]

In addition to aldosterone, progesterone has also been identified to be involved in the adaptive response to low-K intake.[126] Plasma concentrations of progesterone increase during K[+] restriction, and the efficiency of K[+] retention involves the stimulation of colonic H-K-ATPase in tubule cells.

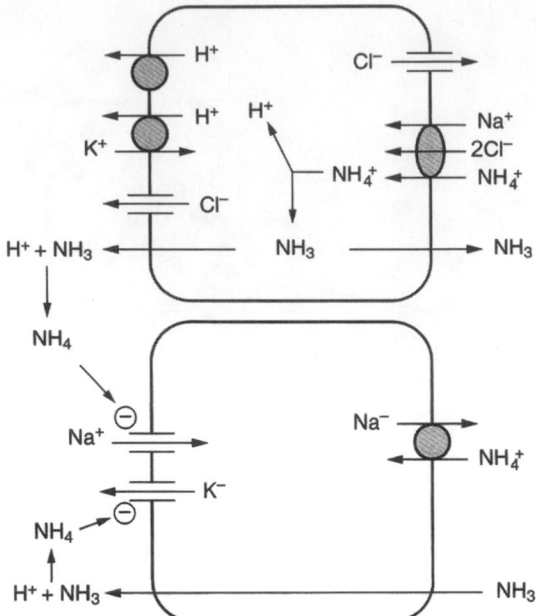

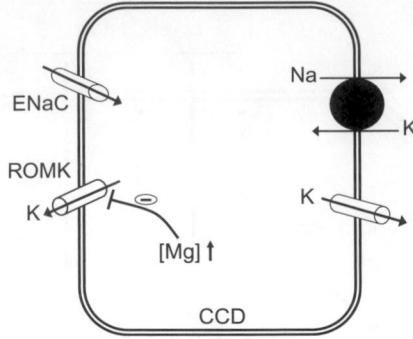

FIGURE 49.26 Effect of changes in intracellular magnesium on ROMK channels in principal cells.

FIGURE 49.25 Interaction between intercalated and principal cells. Active K⁺ reabsorption in the intercalated cell of the outer medullary collecting duct (OMCD) during K⁺ depletion. Note that NH₄ can bind to the extracellular K⁺ site of basolateral Na⁺K⁺-ATPase and the Na⁺-Cl⁻-K⁺ co-transporter and thereby stimulate H⁺ secretion and K⁺ reabsorption. Diffusion trapping of NH₄ in the tubule lumen directly inhibits K⁺ secretion. *(From Malnic, G., Bailey, M. A., and Giebisch, G. (2004). Control of renal potassium excretion. In "The Kidney," 7th ed., Vol. 1, 453–496, Brenner, B. (ed.). WB Saunders, Philadelphia; and Wall, S. M. (2000). Impact of K⁺ homeostasis on net acid secretion in rat terminal inner medullary collecting duct: Role of the Na-K-ATPase. Am. J. Kidney Dis. 36, 1079–1088, with permission.)*

Finally, angiotensin II also plays a role in the tubule response to changes in K⁺ intake. K-deprivation reduces apical ROMK activity, and patch-clamp experiments provide evidence for the involvement of AT1R receptor activation during inhibition of ROMK channels in rats given a low-K diet.[539,548]

Ultrastructural changes in medullary collecting ducts during K⁺-depletion are largely confined to the intercalated cell population, and include a marked increase in the length of the apical cell membrane, an increase in the number of rod-shaped particles in the apical membrane, and a fall in the number of subapical cytoplasmic vesicles.[471] These morphological observations suggest an increase in the number of apical K⁺ transporters, most likely the K,H-ATPase.

Interactions Between K⁺ Channels and Magnesium

Changes in magnesium metabolism affect the kidney's ability to maintain normal K⁺ balance. Magnesium deficiency tends to prevent restoration of K⁺ balance following K⁺ loss,[235] and recent evidence

has implicated involvement of apical ROMK channels in principal cells of the outer medulla[587]: a decrease in cell magnesium, during magnesium depletion, relieves K⁺ channel inhibition and promotes enhanced K⁺ secretion and kaliuresis whereas a rise in cell magnesium inhibits ROMK activity (Figure 49.26). Infusion of Mg decreases excretion of K⁺ in the human kidney.

Adrenal Steroids

Mineralocorticoids have long been known to stimulate sodium reabsorption and, under appropriate conditions, enhance K⁺ secretion. Figure 49.27 demonstrates the effects of aldosterone treatment on K⁺ excretion.[594] Results from experiments in which mineralocorticoids were administered for prolonged periods of time until a steady-state was reached are shown. Aldosterone significantly enhances the efficiency of K⁺ excretion, as evidenced by the fact that at each plasma K⁺ concentration, more K⁺ was excreted by animals with higher aldosterone levels. Expressed differently, as the aldosterone level rises, the same amount of K⁺ can be excreted at progressively lower plasma K⁺ levels. The direct stimulatory effect of mineralocorticoids on K⁺ secretion by the distal tubule and CCD has been amply demonstrated.[55,93,145–148,222,356] Enhanced uptake of K⁺ into extrarenal tissues has also been reported.[53,55,595]

The mechanism of aldosterone release from the adrenal glomerulosa involves two well-defined stimuli: cell depolarization by either an increase in extracellular K⁺ or angiotensin II.[90] Both maneuvers enhance Ca²⁺ entry and aldosterone-synthase activation.[90] Recent evidence reveals that K⁺ channel mutations characterized by diminished K⁺ selectivity (increased Na permeability) result in cell depolarization and enhanced aldosterone production.[90]

The effects of mineralocorticoids on cell K⁺ transport mechanisms of principal collecting duct cells are summarized in Figures 49.28a, 49.29 and 49.30. The effects of mineralocorticoids depend on the antecedent hormonal condition, the duration of hormone treatment, and the modifying effects of sodium ions on K⁺ transport.[96,146] Key aldosterone-sensitive transport mechanisms include the basolateral Na-K exchange pump, apical Na channels, and K⁺ channels in both apical and basolateral membranes. Mineralocorticoid hormone action occurs in several steps summarized in Figure 49.29b. They include binding of aldosterone to cytoplasmic receptors to form the aldosterone—receptor complex, activation of the gene to initiate transcription, synthesis of new aldosterone-induced proteins, and actions on apical and basolateral transport operations. This process can be divided into early and late phases.

In the early phase, mineralocorticoids activate the apical sodium conductance, and thus stimulate sodium entry. With this increase in sodium entry and cell sodium activity, the basolateral pump turnover increases and K⁺ secretion rises.[13,113,115,259,356,468,469] Enhanced sodium entry *per se* leads to rapid insertion of Na⁺-K⁺-ATPase units into the basolateral membrane from an enzyme pool whose magnitude depends on the antecedent aldosterone levels.[26,27,113,115,349] Thus, the acute effects of aldosterone include significant stimulation of Na⁺,K⁺-ATPase involving increased activity of individual pumps, and insertion of additional units.[115,259] Continued exposure to elevated mineralocorticoid levels results in late phase changes, including an additional increase in both K⁺ and sodium transport rates, insertion of additional basolateral Na-K pump units, and further enhancement of the apical sodium and K⁺ conductances.[153,276,356,424–427]

Also occurring in the late phase of mineralocorticoid administration are significant morphological changes in principal cells.[466–471,530,531] Mineralocorticoids have a direct effect on basolateral membrane amplification, independent of changes in K⁺ balance and plasma K⁺ levels.[469] However, sodium ions are required for full

Sites of Action of K and Aldosterone

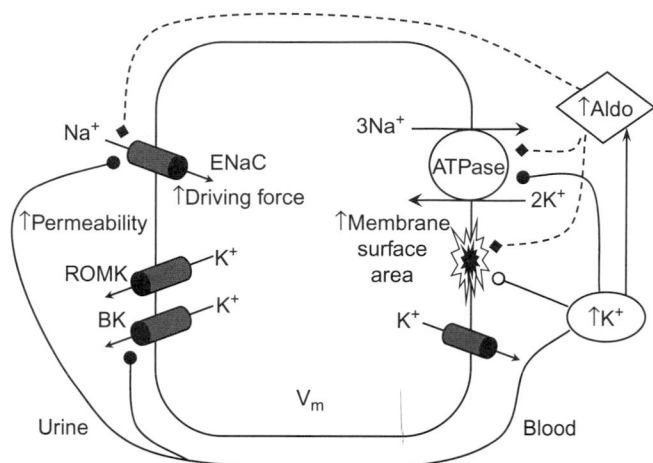

FIGURE 49.28 Factors involved in the regulation of K⁺ transport by aldosterone and peritubular K⁺. (1) Changes in peritubular K⁺ increase apical K⁺ and Na⁺ channel activity, stimulate Na⁺,K⁺-ATPase activity, and augment the basolateral membrane area. High K⁺ also activates the release of aldosterone. (2) Changes in aldosterone stimulate apical Na⁺ channels but enhance K⁺ channel activity only during chronic hyperkalemia. Similar to high K⁺, aldosterone stimulates Na⁺,K⁺-ATPase activity and increases the basolateral membrane area and Na⁺, K⁺-ATPase activity. (*From ref. [150], courtesy of S. Hebert.*)

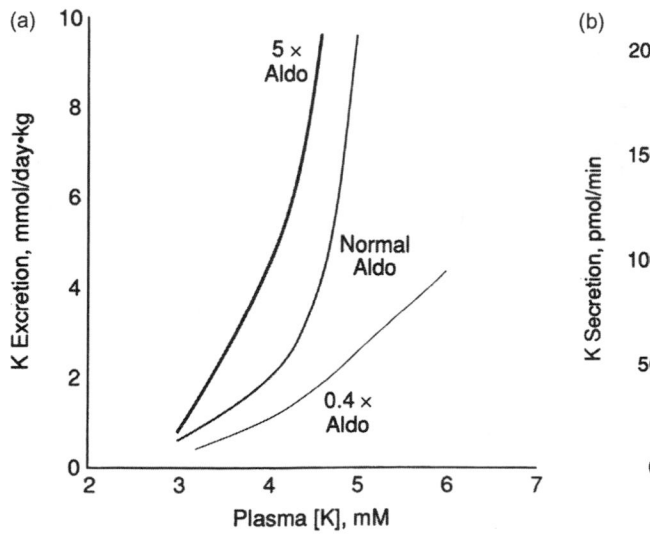

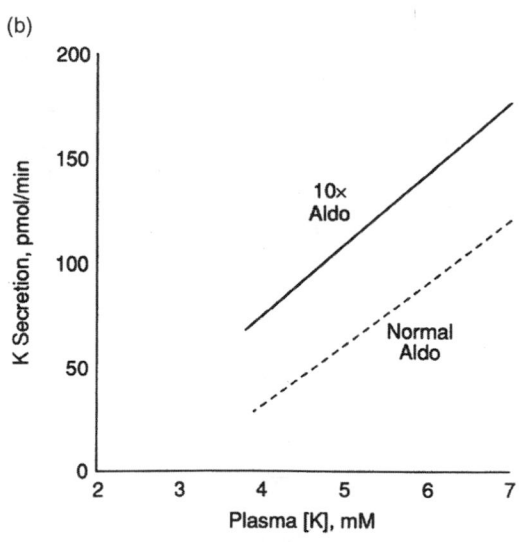

FIGURE 49.27 Relation between K excretion and plasma K at different levels of aldosterone. The relationship between plasma K⁺ concentration and renal K⁺ excretion (a) (*from ref. [415]*), and distal K⁺ secretion (b) (*from ref. [416]*) is affected by circulating aldosterone. Effects of increased and decreased aldosterone are shown with respect to normal levels.

mineralocorticoid effects: morphological changes fail to develop fully during administration of a low-sodium diet.[476] In contrast to the changes observed in principal and connecting tubule cells, significant changes in basolateral membrane area fail to occur in intercalated cells during either diet- or hormone-induced stimulation of tubular K+ secretion.[467,471]

The electrophysiological consequences of high-K+ and chronic mineralocorticoid administration are shown in Figure 49.30. The basolateral membrane voltage may hyperpolarize, and the direction of passive K+ transport may reverse.[276,324] The mineralocorticoid-induced increase in the basolateral electrogenic Na-K exchange and basolateral K+ conductance accounts for the rise in membrane potential above the K+ equilibrium potential. The increase in membrane voltage provides a driving force for K+ uptake into principal cells. This sequence of events suppresses the backflux of K+ from cell to peritubular fluid, and increases the efficiency of K+ secretion.

Measurements of proximal cell K+ levels in tubules harvested from chronically mineralocorticoid-treated animals do not show an increase in cell K+ content or activity.[375] This attests to the precise adjustments of basolateral pump activity to apical K+ conductance. Possible mechanisms of this interaction between basolateral and apical transport mechanisms are mineralocorticoid-induced changes in cell ATP, Ca^{2+}, and pH levels. Were the stimulation of basolateral Na-K exchange to reduce cell ATP concentrations, apical K+ channels would be released from inhibition. It is also possible that aldosterone activates basolateral Na-H exchange, alkalinizes the cytoplasm, and

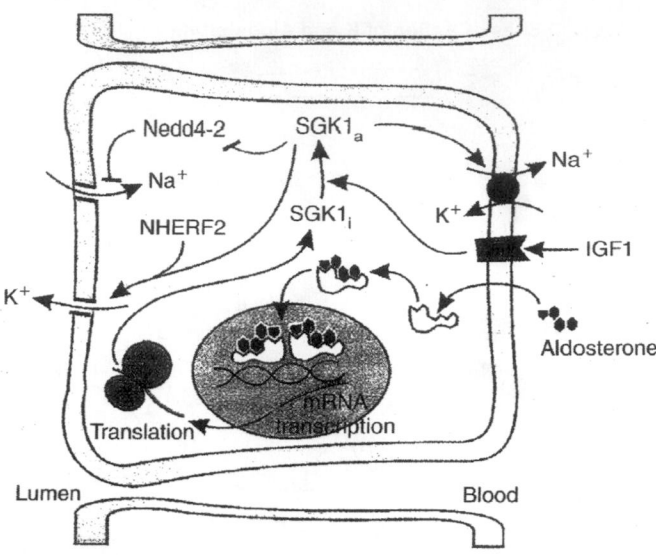

FIGURE 49.29 Effects of hormones on principle cell transport pathways. Aldo stimulate K+ secretion via pathways shown in this cell model.

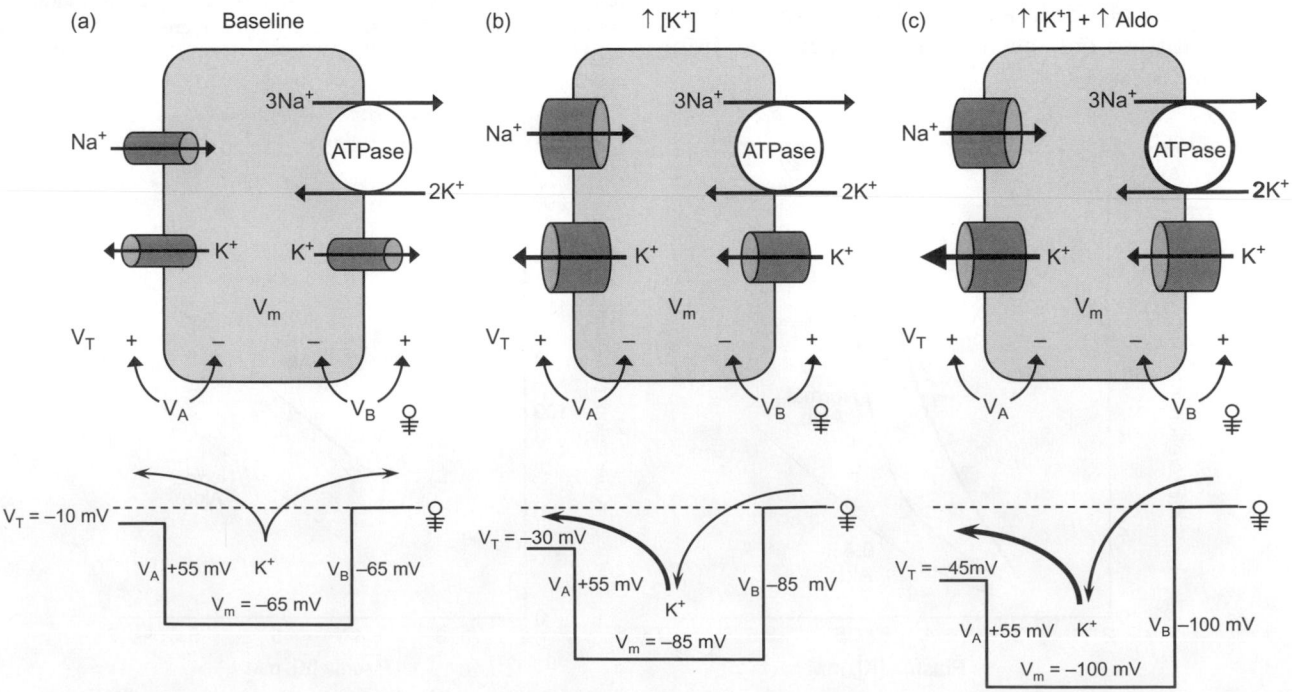

FIGURE 49.30 Schema of cortical collecting tubule cell with key site of potassium transport. Depending on the magnitude of the electrical potential difference across the basolateral cell membrane, potassium ions may either leave the cell (recycle) (a) or be taken up into the cell in parallel with pump-mediated potassium transport (b,c).

activates the apical secretory K$^+$ channels. Principal cells extrude hydrogen ions across the basolateral membrane by Na-H exchange,[86] and because aldosterone accelerates Na-H exchange in cells of the diluting segment,[362,368] this mechanism is an attractive possibility. Finally, cell Ca^{2+} changes could also be involved, owing to the effects of pump-induced alterations of cell sodium concentrations that affect Na$^+$/Ca^{2+} exchange.[445]

Sodium ions importantly modify the stimulating effect of mineralocorticoids on K$^+$ secretion. Thus, the kaliuretic effect of chronic desoxycorticosterone (DOC) treatment is effectively abolished by a low-sodium diet, and is amplified by a high-sodium intake.[455] Studies on single CCDs have confirmed the importance of an intact apical sodium entry mechanism, and an adequate lumen sodium supply, for the full stimulation of Na,K-ATPase activity that follows mineralocorticoid administration.[530,531] As pointed out above, switching from a low- to a high-cell-sodium environment induces a rapid increase of ATPase activity in proximal tubule cells.[113] Such prompt activation is consistent with a permissive role for Na in mineralocorticoid action mediated by the stimulating effect of sodium to insert pump units from a latent cytoplasmic pool into the basolateral membrane. Similarly, raising intracellular sodium concentrations enhances the cell surface expression of Na-K-ATPase α-subunit in mammalian cortical collecting duct principal cells. This process involves both c-AMP-dependent and cyclic-AMP-independent pathways.[113,188] Moreover, such activation of Na,K-ATPase is modulated by aldosterone, since cortical collecting ducts from aldosterone-depleted animals have a greatly diminished response to the change in ambient sodium, implying that the size of the cell sodium pool is strongly influenced by mineralocorticoids. In tubules from DOC-treated animals, amiloride significantly attenuates pump stimulation.[357] These results support the view that enhanced apical sodium entry into principal cells is necessary to allow full expression of mineralocorticoid stimulation of Na$^+$,K$^+$-ATPase activity. The efficacy of aldosterone-induced kaliuresis is also affected by urine flow rate.[145,147] Microperfusion experiments show that direct effects of aldosterone on K$^+$ transport are modified by simultaneous modulation of urine flow rate. Thus, although aldosterone enhances K$^+$ secretion in single distal tubules perfused at a constant rate, the antidiuretic effect of aldosterone may modulate the direct stimulation of aldosterone on K$^+$ excretion. On the other hand, dexamethasone does not stimulate potassium secretion in tubules perfused at a constant rate, but elicits K$^+$ transport stimulation through its enhancing effect on tubule flow rate.[147]

Aldosterone may act rapidly (<10 minutes) on renal distal nephron ion transport by a nongenomic mechanism. This is not affected by actinomycin D or spironolactone, and thus is independent of protein synthesis.[527] This nongenomic effect involves, primarily, stimulation of Na$^+$/H$^+$ exchange, and is thought to be mediated by specific membrane receptors for aldosterone. Membrane-binding sites of very low (0.1 nM) dissociation constant (Kd) for aldosterone which modulated Na$^+$/H$^+$ exchange were first described in human polymorphonuclear leucocytes. Such sites have no affinity for dexamethasone, corticosterone, ouabain, amiloride, and 18-hydroxyprogesterone.[140,505] Similar receptors for aldosterone were also found in pig kidney, but these had higher values of Kd for desoxycorticosterone acetate and corticosterone. These membrane receptors are different from the classical cytoplasmic mineralocorticoid receptors (MR), since MR knockout mice still display the nongenomic effect of aldosterone.[174] Activation of the nongenomic mechanism via membrane receptors includes a signaling path involving G-protein, inositol triphosphate, Ca^{2+}, and protein kinase C, as well as MAP-kinase.[527] ENaC-mediated current in isolated rabbit CCD is stimulated by nongenomic action of aldosterone.[527] Inasmuch as these nongenomic actions involve apical sodium channels, they could also have significant indirect effects on K$^+$ secretion.

Glucocorticoids

Abnormal function of the hypothalamic–pituitary–adrenal axis is often associated with deranged K$^+$ homeostasis.[63,123] In patients with low circulating levels of glucocorticoids, the excretory response to K$^+$-loading is blunted, even if aldosterone is normal. Glucocorticoid excess, in contrast, can be associated with kaliuresis and hypokalemia. The effect of glucocorticoids on urinary K$^+$ excretion largely reflects secondary stimulation of K$^+$ secretion in the distal nephron following glucocorticoid actions in proximal nephron segments. Glucocorticoids increase GFR, and also the delivery of sodium and fluid to the distal nephron[33]: these latter effects are strongly kaliuretic. Microperfusion experiments also support an indirect effect, since acute intravenous dexamethasone does not increase distal K$^+$ secretion when fluid and salt delivery are constant.

Nevertheless, studies suggest that chronically elevated glucocorticoids exert a direct mineralocorticoid-like effect on the distal nephron. Mineralocorticoid target genes are activated by glucocorticoid excess, even when aldosterone is normal, and patients with familial glucocorticoid receptor haploinsufficiency or apparent mineralocorticoid excess are hypokalaemic despite low circulating aldosterone. These conditions of corticosteroid cross-talk reflect the inherent affinity of the mineralocorticoid receptor for glucocorticoids.[16] As shown in Figure 49.31, the enzyme 11β-hydroxysteroid dehydrogenase type II (11βHSD2) converts active glucocorticoids to inactive metabolites. In the principal cell, 11βHSD2 brings mineralocorticoid receptor target proteins, such as ENaC, under the control of aldosterone.[16,22,280]

The 11βHSD2 barrier can be attenuated by mutations in the encoding gene or pharmacological inhibition of enzyme function: the hypokalemic hypertension of apparent mineralocorticoid excess or that following excess licorice consumption reflects glucocorticoid action in the distal nephron.[21,41] Micropuncture studies in rats confirm this,[23] and mice lacking 11βHSD2 maintain robust K$^+$ excretion despite severe hypokalemia.[22] Much of the K$^+$ excretion is amiloride-sensitive and is likely mediated by ROMK. However, kaliuresis is maintained after sodium handling is normalized and becomes resistant to amiloride. It is likely that such persistent K$^+$ excretion reflects BK-mediated K$^+$ secretion: 11βHSD2 null mice are severely polyuric and the increase in urine flow would activate BK channels.[20]

Some evidence suggests that glucocorticoids may also influence K$^+$ secretion by glucocorticoid receptor (GR) activation.[21,41] GR is expressed in the aldosterone-sensitive distal nephron of the rat, and it is this receptor, not MR, that translocates to the nucleus in response to physiological variations in aldosterone.[1,47] The physiological meaning of this is not resolved, but in mice with reduced levels of 11βHSD2 a high-salt diet causes hypokalemia and inappropriately high K$^+$ secretion in the distal nephron. The deranged K$^+$ homeostasis was prevented by GR blockade, and spironolactone was without effect.[41] In summary, there is strong evidence that chronic exposure to elevated glucocorticoids may directly influence K$^+$ secretion at this site, an effect above and beyond the kaliuresis triggered by rapid-onset events in more proximal segments.

WNKs (With No Lysine Kinase)

WNKs are serine/threonine protein kinases, and WNK1, 3, and 4 are expressed in the DCT and CCD.[127,229,253,331,562,598,604] A large body of evidence indicates that the WNK family plays an important role in the regulation of Na absorption and K$^+$ secretion. WNK4 suppresses the expression of the Na-Cl cotransporter (NCC) in the plasma membrane of the DCT, thereby inhibiting Na absorption.[253] In contrast, WNK1 stimulates NCC activity indirectly by antagonizing the inhibitory effect of WNK4. WNK1, 3, and 4 inhibit ROMK channel activity, and the effect of WNK on ROMK is mediated by stimulation of clathrin-dependent endocytosis. The inhibitory effect of WNK4 on ROMK1 does not require the kinase activity, because co-expression of the inactivated WNK4 inhibits expression of ROMK1 in *Xenopus* oocytes. The mutated gene products encoding inactivated WNK1 or WNK4 causes pseudohypoaldosteronism type II, a disease with characteristics of hypertension and low aldosterone levels. A kidney-specific splice form of WNK1 (KS-WNK1), in which an alternative 5′ exon replaces the first four exons of WNK1, is expressed in the DCT and CCD.[291] Unlike the long form of WNK1, KS-WNK1 lacks kinase activity and does not block ROMK channels. Moreover, KS-WNK1 can antagonize the inhibitory effect of WNK1. A high K$^+$ intake increases the expression of KS-WNK1, and accordingly attenuates the inhibitory effect of WNK1 on ROMK channels (Figure 49.32).[291,312] Thus, alteration of the ratio between the long and short forms of WNK1 may be an important mechanism by which a high-K intake stimulates ROMK channel activity. K$^+$ restriction has been reported to decrease the expression of KS-WNK1 and increase the long form WNK1. Consequently, the inhibitory effect of KS-WNK1 on WNK1 is diminished, and WNK1-mediated inhibition of ROMK channels is enhanced, in the CCD from animals fed a low-K diet.[236]

It should be noted that aldosterone is secreted both in the setting of intravascular volume depletion

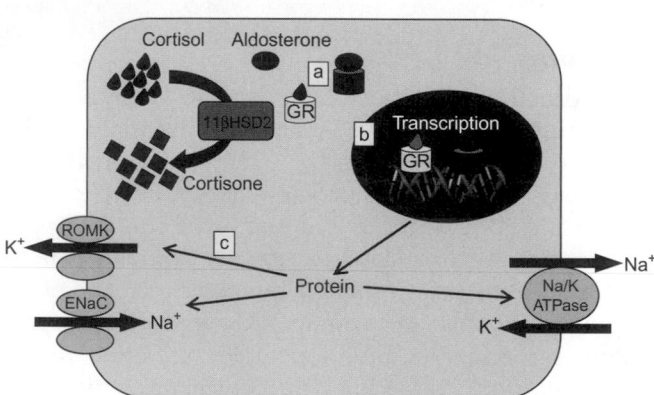

FIGURE 49.31 The enzyme 11β hydroxysteroid dehydrogenase type 2 (11βHSD2) is co-expressed with the mineralocorticoid receptor (MR) in aldosterone target tissues, such as the principal cell of the collecting duct. The enzyme converts cortisol, which is an agonist of the mineralocorticoid receptor (MR) to cortisone, which is not. This confers aldosterone-specificity on MR, placing transcription of aldosterone-induced proteins, such as ENaC, ROMK, and the basolateral Na/K-ATPase, under the control of the renin—angiotensin system. Recent data challenge the conventional view of corticosteroid action in the aldosterone-sensitive distal nephron, which expresses both the mineralocorticoid and glucocorticoid receptor (GR). As shown in (a), 11βHSD2 may also govern ligand access to GR, and GR translocation to the nucleus (b) is influenced by physiological changes in circulating aldosterone, and plays a permissive role in regulation of ENaC by aldosterone. Direct regulation of ROMK by GR is suggested (c) but the kaliuretic effects of glucocorticoids may also reflect activation of ENaC. *(Figure courtesy of Dr. Louise Evans.)*

(hypovolemia) and hyperkalemia. In the face of the hypovolemia, aldosterone promotes Na^+ retention and limits urinary K^+ loss. In hyperkalemia, aldosterone maximizes K^+ loss without Na^+ retention. This "aldosterone paradox" may be explained by changes in the relative expression and activities of WNK family members[127,229,236,253,331,493] (Figures 49.32 and 49.33).

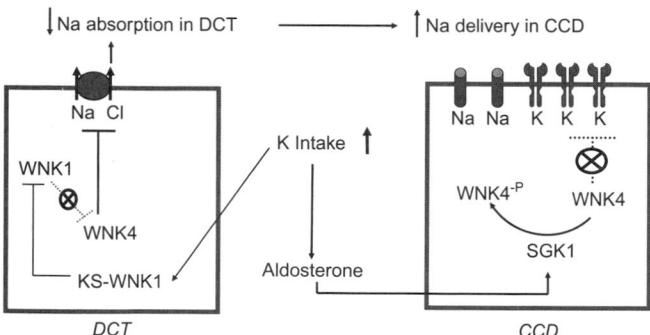

FIGURE 49.32 A cell scheme illustrates the mechanism by which increasing dietary potassium intake facilitates K secretion. A high-K intake increases KS-WNK4 expression which inhibits WNK1 function, thereby suppressing WNK1-mediated inhibition of WNK4. Thus, a high-K intake decreases NaCl co-transporter activity, and increases NaCl delivery to the connecting tubule and the CCD. A high-K intake also increases SGK1 activity which phosphorylates WNK4, thereby suppressing the WNK4-mediated inhibition of ROMK. Thus, a high-K intake stimulates K secretion in the connecting tubule and the CCD through increasing Na delivery and apical K^+ channel activity (CCD: cortical collecting duct; SGK1: serum-glucocorticoid-induced kinase 1; WNK: with-no-lysine kinase; KS-WNK1: kidney-specific WNK1).

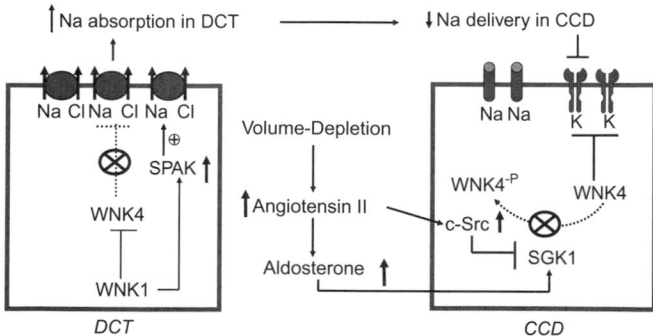

FIGURE 49.33 A cell scheme illustrating the role of angiotensin II in regulating ROMK channels during volume-depletion. Volume-depletion abolishes the inhibitory effect of WNK4 on the NaCl co-transporter through stimulation of SGK1-mediated WNK4, thereby increasing Na absorption in the distal nephron. Decreasing the Na delivery to the connecting tubule and the CCD diminishes the driving force for K secretion. In addition, the angiotensin II pathway inhibits SGK1-induced phosphorylation of WNK4 through activation of c-Src family protein tyrosine kinase, and leads to suppression of ROMK channel activity. A dotted line means a diminished effect (CCD: cortical collecting duct; DCT: distal convoluted tubule; SGK1: serum-glucocorticoid-induced kinase 1; WNK: with-no-lysine kinase).

Salt and Water Balance

K^+ excretion generally changes in association with modulation in sodium excretion. On the one hand, interventions that increase salt and water excretion — high-salt intake, extracellular volume expansion, saline infusion, administration of many diuretics acting upstream of the initial collecting tubule, and infusion of sodium salts of poorly-reabsorbable anions — all stimulate K^+ excretion.[59,180–186,234,267,326,399,470,582] On the other hand, maneuvers that diminish sodium excretion — rapid reduction of glomerular filtration rate, sodium-depletion, and volume-contraction — all decrease K^+ excretion. Thus, distal secretion of K^+ depends importantly on the delivery of sodium and tubule fluid to the sites of K^+ secretion.

Figure 49.34 illustrates the effect of different levels of sodium intake on the steady-state relationship between plasma K^+ and urinary K^+ excretion at clamped aldosterone levels.[596] K^+ excretion at a given plasma K^+ level is stimulated by augmenting sodium intake and a given rate of K^+ excretion occurs at lower plasma K^+ levels when sodium intake is elevated. This enhancement of K^+ excretion is thought to depend on increased delivery of fluid and sodium to the distal tubule and CCD.

Studies on single tubules, employing both micropuncture[260] and microperfusion[139,191,192,319] techniques, have fully confirmed that tubule fluid flow rate and luminal sodium concentration independently affect K^+ secretion. Figure 49.35 summarizes the effects of tubule flow rate and fluid sodium concentrations on K^+ secretion along the distal tubule. Increasing flow rate invariably stimulates K^+ secretion. For a given

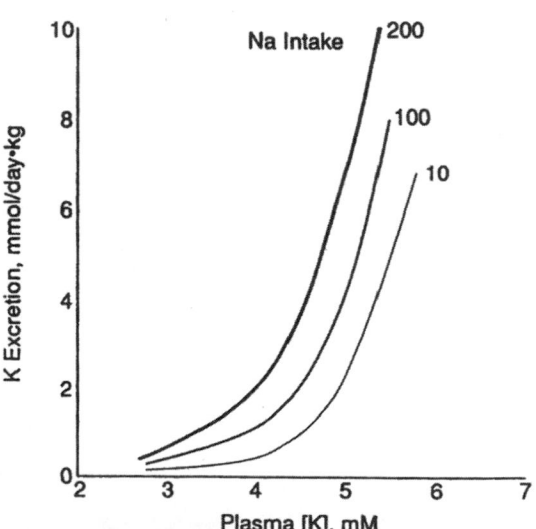

FIGURE 49.34 The relation between plasma K^+ concentration and renal K^+ excretion is affected by dietary Na intake. (*From ref [596], with permission.*)

flow rate, K$^+$ secretion is augmented in animals with a high-K intake[266] or after mineralocorticoid administration[123,183]; it is decreased in animals on a low-K$^+$ diet.[266]

Three separate mechanisms underlie the increase of distal K$^+$ secretion with enhanced flow rate. The first involves electrophysiological linkage between sodium absorption and K$^+$ secretion. Increasing fluid delivery into the distal tubule increases the sodium concentration in the lumen, which in turn stimulates sodium absorption[267] and depolarizes the apical cell membrane, thus creating a more favorable electrochemical gradient for K$^+$ secretion. This effect is of greatest importance when luminal Na concentration shifts from low to high levels.[48,139,192,319,485]

An increase in tubular fluid flow rate also stimulates sodium absorption due to an increase in the open probability of ENaC.[342,433]

Enhanced sodium entry from the lumen into principal cells during augmented delivery of fluid stimulates the basolateral Na,K-ATPase and accelerates K$^+$ translocation into cells from the peritubular fluid. Thus, as long as basolateral pump activity responds to increased lumen delivery of sodium with increased Na-K exchange, K$^+$ secretion continues at a high enough rate to either prevent (in the lower range of lumen flow rates) or to curtail (in the higher range of lumen flow rates) a decline in the concentration of K$^+$ in the tubule lumen. If K$^+$ concentrations decline less than flow rate increases, K$^+$ secretion rates increase. Experimental conditions in which lumen K$^+$ concentrations remain constant during diuretic conditions,[232] and in which the concentration difference between cell interior and lumen remain unaltered despite marked stimulation of K$^+$ secretion (see Table 24 in [415]), underscore the

importance of accelerated and coupled K$^+$ and sodium transport. By "clamping" the K$^+$ concentration in the lumen to fairly constant levels over the range of low physiological levels of tubule flow, the connecting and collecting tubule emerge as the major control site of K$^+$ excretion.[473]

A second mechanism that links increased delivery of fluid to the distal nephron to enhanced K$^+$ secretion may involve a flow-dependent fall of lumen K$^+$ concentration,[191,192] which increases the driving force for K$^+$ exit across the apical membrane. This mechanism permits K$^+$ secretion to increase under conditions in which increased sodium delivery into the distal tubule fails to stimulate basolateral Na-K-ATPase. Diminished apical sodium uptake and low lumen K$^+$ concentrations would hyperpolarize the apical membrane potential and tend to reduce the electrochemical driving force, favoring K$^+$ secretion. The functional state of the basolateral Na$^+$,K$^+$-ATPase transport system thus determines the extent to which increased fluid delivery stimulates K$^+$ secretion.

The third mechanism, illustrated in Figure 49.36, links changes in luminal flow to distal potassium secretion by activation of the BK channel. An increase in luminal flow rate transduces mechanical signals (circumferential stretch, shear stress, hydrodynamic bending moments on the cilium decorating the apical surface of virtually all renal epithelial cells) into increases in intracellular Ca^{2+} concentration, which in turn activate apical BK channels to secrete potassium, thereby enhancing urinary potassium excretion.[557,575]

Although apical sodium channels are a key pathway for entry of sodium into principal cells, K$^+$ excretion

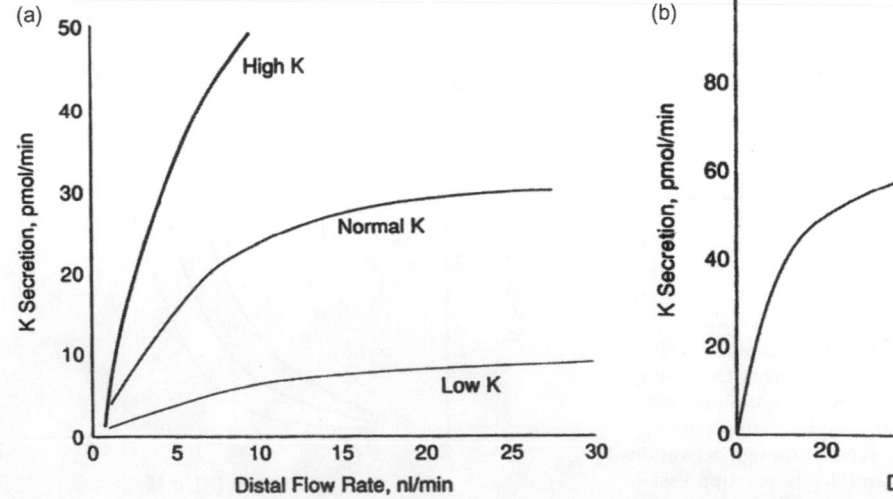

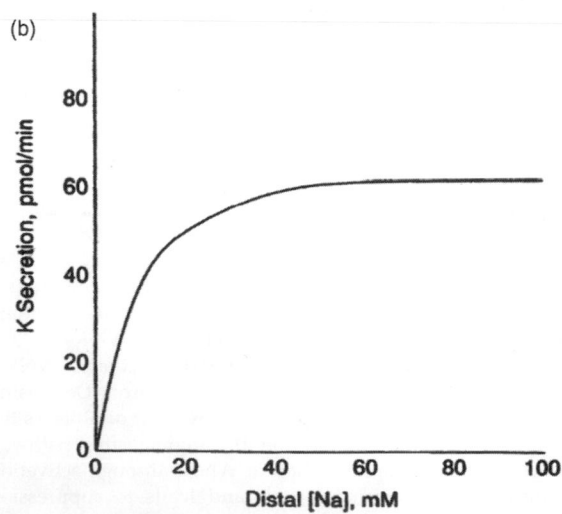

FIGURE 49.35 (a) Relationship between distal flow rate and distal K secretion as affected by K intake. (b) Distal K secretion requires a luminal Na$^+$ concentration exceeding 25–35 mM. The relation between flow rate of tubule fluid in distal tubule and distal K$^+$ secretion is affected by dietary intake: normal K$^+$ diet; low- K$^+$ diet; high- K$^+$ diet. (*From ref. [269], with permission.*)

appears not to be entirely dependent on apical sodium supply. Animals maintained on a low-sodium diet do respond with kaliuresis to acute K$^+$-loading,[384] as do animals given the ENaC inhibitior, amiloride.[589] Moreover, humans tolerate very well a diet high in K$^+$ and low in sodium.[374] An explanation for the apparent dissociation between apical sodium supply and maintained ability for K$^+$ secretion may be the presence of at least two additional sodium entry pathways in principal cells. These are located in the basolateral membrane, and include Na/H and Na/Ca^{2+} exchange.[86,295] Activity of these basolateral entry pathways may, at least in part, replace apical sodium supply and maintain K$^+$ secretion under conditions of low distal fluid and sodium delivery, especially under conditions of elevated levels of plasma K$^+$.[176] K$^+$ excretion independent of distal amiloride-sensitive Na transport has been confirmed in rats during high dietary K$^+$ intake.[156] Such Na-channel-independent K$^+$ excretion develops progressively during prolonged K-loading; it could be mediated, in part, by K$^+$ secretion in

intercalated cells[206,354] and/or by reduced K$^+$ reabsorption along the proximal tubule and thick ascending limb of Henle's loop as a consequence of high plasma K$^+$ levels. The latter have been shown to lower proximal tubule Na and fluid reabsorption.[67,302]

Recent evidence, based on distal tubule perfusion studies, suggests a significant component of electroneutral sodium reabsorption (Figure 49.37), resistant to amiloride inhibition but sensitive to hydrochlorthiazide. Mechanistically, the transport process involves the parallel action of sodium-dependent Cl/bicarbonate exchange and sodium-independent chloride-bicarbonate exchange (pendrin). The presence of this transport in ß-intercalated cells is significant, because it would uncouple K$^+$ secretion from electrogenic sodium transport via Na channels in principal cells.[127,128]

The ability of the distal tubule and CCD to maintain a fairly constant K$^+$ concentration in the lumen over the physiological range of flow rates has two important consequences. First, the marked flow

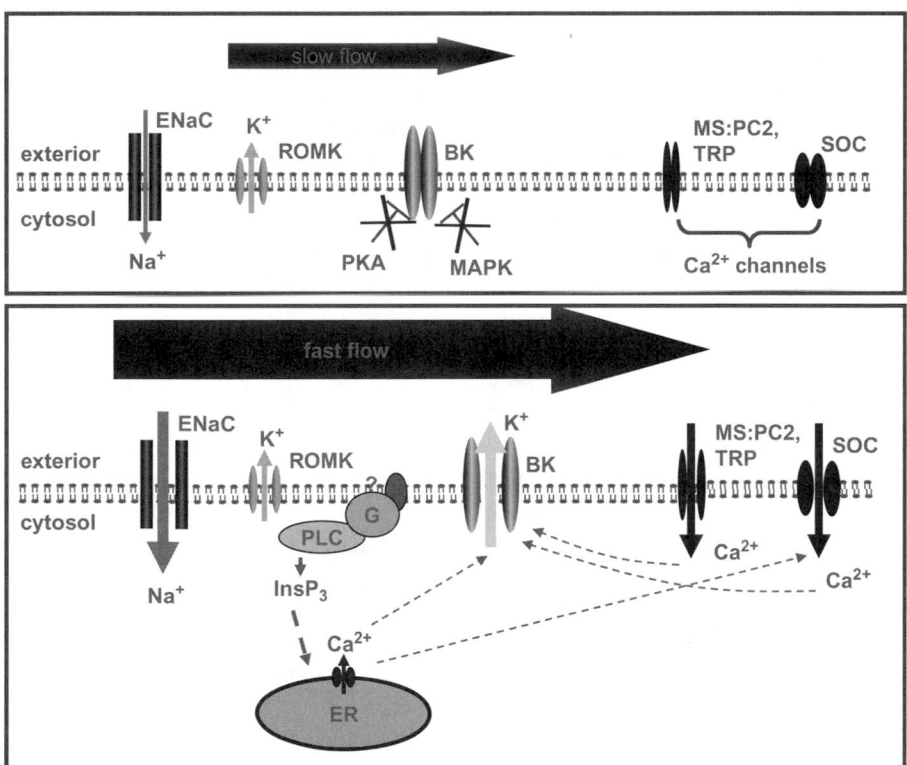

FIGURE 49.36 **Proposed model for the molecular physiology of flow-induced K$^+$ secretion (FIKS) in the distal nephron.** At slow "physiologic" flow rates, K$^+$ secretion requires electrogenic Na$^+$ absorption through ENaC, and is mediated by the SK/ROMK channel. The apical Ca^{2+}- and stretch-activated BK channel is tonically inhibited by PKA and MAPK. A rapid increase in tubular fluid flow rate associated with circumferential stretch of the CCD leads to shear or hydrodynamic impulses at the cilium or apical membrane and an increase in intracellular Ca^{2+} concentration ($[Ca^{2+}]_i$), due to luminal Ca^{2+} entry and internal store release. These hydrodynamic forces are associated with an increase in net Na$^+$ absorption and K$^+$ secretion, the latter mediated by Ca^{2+}-dependent activation of the BK channel. FIKS further requires microtubule integrity and possibly release of tonic channel inhibition. Mechanosensitive (MS) Ca^{2+} channels identified in the apical membrane of the distal nephron include polycystin 2, and the transient receptor vanilloid-4 (TRPV4) channels. Store-operated Ca^{2+} channels (SOC) also contribute to the flow-induced Ca^{2+} response.[574]

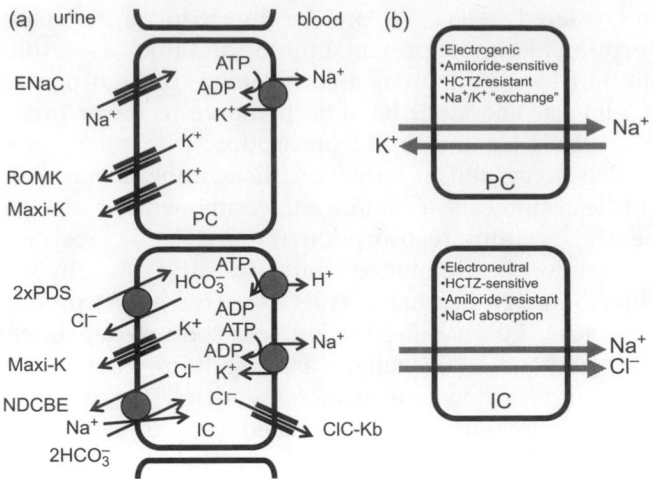

FIGURE 49.37   Overview of the two major Na⁺/* transport pathways in principal and intercalated cells, depicting electrogenic and electroneutral transport mechanisms. *(From ref. [128].)*

dependence of K⁺ secretion in the distal tubule and CCD endows the process of K⁺ secretion with great sensitivity to changes in the delivery of sodium and fluid. This tubule segment is thus responsible for the enhanced rate of K⁺ excretion that follows inhibition of sodium and fluid reabsorption upstream of the distal tubule and collecting duct ([234]; see "Diuretics" section below). Second, the ability of the distal nephron segments to "clamp" the K⁺ concentration has implications for the physiological importance of those components of K⁺ secretion that occur upstream during K⁺ recycling. K⁺ secreted upstream of the ICT determines the amount of K⁺ secreted along the DCT and ICT as the tubule fluid approaches the "late" distal tubule. Hence, with stimulation of medullary K⁺ recycling, the concentration of K⁺ in the early distal tubule rises and approaches the "clamped" concentration across the initial collecting tubule. Thus, a smaller fraction of excreted K⁺ is then contributed by distal secretion. Conversely, when medullary recycling of K⁺ is minimal, and the concentration of K⁺ in the fluid entering the distal tubule is low, a larger fraction of excreted K⁺ has to be secreted by the distal tubule and the CCD.

A non-invasive method for evaluation of the transtubule gradient of K⁺ (TTKG) in the CCD has been described.[565,566] Such estimates have been used to evaluate the effects of hormones, diuretics, and acid–base disturbances in patients. The method allows distinction between modulation of urine K⁺ excretion by changes in flow rate and/or direct effects on K⁺ secretion in principal cells. This approach has also shown that urea recycling, by enhancing flow rate in the cortical collecting tubule, provides a mechanism for aiding K⁺ excretion.[214]

Chronic enhancement of sodium delivery into the distal nephron, for instance during treatment with loop diuretics, leads to both functional and morphological adjustments in the downstream tubule segments; these changes increase the capacity for sodium absorption and K⁺ secretion in cells of the distal nephron.[136,257,296,344,466,467] Prolonged increased entry of sodium into cells of the distal tubule must be responsible for transport stimulation, because the functional and morphological changes persist when plasma aldosterone, vasopressin, and K⁺ are held constant.[466,470] Increased transport in collecting duct segments following chronic treatment with diuretics that act on the loop of Henle or the distal convoluted tubule may curtail sodium excretion as well as promote K⁺ secretion.[136] An increase in amiloride-sensitive K⁺ secretion has been observed following uninephrectomy, and is linked to an initial increase in plasma K⁺ concentration, and increased distal tubule fluid and sodium delivery.[25,46,109]

Renal sympathetic nerve activity affects renal K⁺ excretion, most likely mediated by changes in glomerular filtration rate (GFR) and sodium excretion.[422] Renal denervation was shown to increase GFR, accompanied by enhanced sodium excretion, significant kaliuresis, and lowering of plasma K⁺ concentration. Renal denervation lowers proximal sodium reabsorption, and the ensuing kaliuresis is best explained by enhanced sodium delivery to distal K-secreting nephron segments. An interesting observation concerns the relationship between distal tubule sodium reabsorption and K⁺ secretion in a rat model of nephrotic syndrome. Although displaying high rates of sodium reabsorption in collecting ducts, K⁺ secretion was not enhanced in tubules from such nephrotic rats. Inhibition of ROMK secretory K⁺ channels was traced to the presence of high albumin in the tubule lumen. Moreover, nephrotic rats were shown to be less able to excrete K⁺ when given a high-K⁺ diet, an observation consistent with compromised apical K⁺ channel activity.[149]

Non-chloride sodium salt also affects urinary K⁺ excretion. Thus, the kaliuretic effects of sulfate, phosphate, and bicarbonate are well-established. Prolonged fasting and the enhanced excretion of short-chain fatty acids and organic acid radicals also promote K⁺ loss.[306] Interestingly, infusion of sodium bicarbonate is more kaliuretic than similar amounts of sulfate.[80] It is generally assumed that the stimulating effect of poorly-reabsorbable anions on K⁺ secretion is mediated by their effects on the lumen-negative potential.[321] Although there is evidence that the transepithelial potential difference effectively alters K⁺ secretion,[179] it is unlikely that the effects of poorly-reabsorbable anions are solely mediated by changing the transepithelial potential, because sulfate-induced enhancement has been shown to continue in the presence of effective blockade of sodium and K$^+$ channels. This suggests that stimulation of K$^+$ secretion in the presence of sulfate is mediated by low tubule chloride, which stimulates electroneutral K$^+$ chloride co-transport.[526] Perfusion studies also provide support for the notion that lumen alkalinization and bicarbonate directly stimulate K$^+$ secretion through augmenting electroneutral secretory K$^+$ chloride co-transport.[8]

Acid−Base Balance

Acid−base derangements have long been known to affect the excretion of K$^+$, and losses of K$^+$, particularly in states of alkalosis, are well-documented.[14,48−52,68,176,179,182,320,470,472] Figure 49.38 shows the striking dependence of renal K$^+$ excretion and distal K$^+$ secretion on blood pH. It is apparent that alkalosis stimulates, and acidosis depresses, K$^+$ excretion.

Clearance, stop-flow, micropuncture, and microperfusion studies indicate that the DCT and CCD are the main nephron sites where acid−base changes affect K$^+$ secretion. The right panel of Figure 49.38 shows results of a microperfusion study in which tubule flow rate and solute composition of luminal fluid were kept constant. Metabolic acidosis caused distal K$^+$ secretion to decrease, whereas metabolic alkalosis had the opposite effect. Direct effects of acid−base disorders on K$^+$ transport in these nephron segments can be distinguished from indirect effects that include changes of: (1) distal flow rate; (2) composition of fluid reaching the distal tubule; and (3) aldosterone levels.[472] Changes

in plasma K$^+$ cannot be held responsible for acid−base related changes in K$^+$ excretion, because hyperkalemia is frequently associated with acidosis, whereas hypokalemia is commonly observed in alkalosis.[4,14,51,176,320]

The direct effects of acid−base disorders, summarized in Figure 49.39, involve modifications of both basolateral and apical transport functions in principal and intercalated cells. With regard to the basolateral membrane, alkalosis stimulates active K$^+$ uptake and increases the permeability to K$^+$ ions (Figure 49.40). The permeability increase in alkalosis shifts the membrane potential close towards the K$^+$ equilibrium potential, and minimizes K$^+$ loss from cells into the peritubular fluid. Acidosis has the opposite effect, including direct inhibition of basolateral Na$^+$,K$^+$-ATPase activity (Figure 49.41).[350] Acid−base related changes in the apical cell membrane are also observed and involve a striking sensitivity of both K$^+$ and sodium channel activity to cytosolic pH. Over a narrow and physiological pH range, acidosis (pH 7.0) suppresses and alkalosis (pH 7.4) stimulates sodium and K$^+$ channel activity.[158,159,217,544,546]

Additional stimuli modulating K$^+$ secretion in acid−base disturbances involve the delivery of tubule fluid with high Na$^+$ bicarbonate and low chloride concentrations to the distal nephron in metabolic alkalosis (Figure 49.42). Bicarbonate and other poorly-permeant anions act as osmotic diuretics and increase distal tubule flow rate and, as mentioned above, low lumen chloride concentration stimulates apical K-Cl secretion in distal convoluted and principal cells.[132,521,526] Bicarbonate also appears to activate K$^+$ excretion directly.[8,306] Figure 49.42 shows the results of *in vivo*

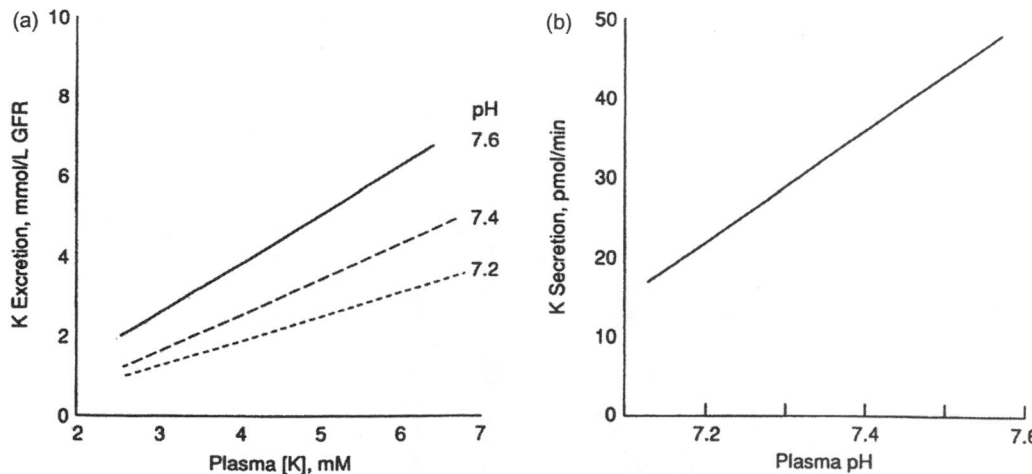

FIGURE 49.38 (a) The relationship between plasma K$^+$ concentration and renal K$^+$ excretion is affected by plasma pH. (*From Stanton, B. A., and Giebisch, G. (1991). Renal potassium transport. In "Handbook of Physiology: Renal Physiology," 813−874, Windhager, E. E. (ed.). Oxford University Press, New York, with permission.*) (b) Distal K$^+$ secretion is affected by plasma pH. (*From ref. [472], with permission.*)

microperfusion experiments in which luminal chloride was replaced with sulfate. Reducing luminal Cl concentration below 20 mM stimulates K$^+$ secretion into the distal tubule without changing the transepithelial voltage. Unidirectional flux measurements show that the increase in K$^+$ secretion occurs because the cell-to-lumen flux is enhanced. This enhanced secretory flux is not blocked by barium in the lumen.

Opposing effects of metabolic acidosis on K$^+$ excretion are summarized in Figure 49.41; metabolic acidosis may either inhibit or stimulate K$^+$ secretion. Direct actions of acidosis involve inhibition of K$^+$ secretion in distal nephron segments. In addition, indirect effects enhance K$^+$ secretion by elevating distal delivery of sodium-containing fluid following diminished proximal tubular bicarbonate transport. When flow rate along single distal tubules is kept constant, acidosis depresses K$^+$ secretion.[472] However, under free-flow conditions in intact tubules, K$^+$ secretion may rise as a consequence of increased fluid flow rate thought to result from inhibition of proximal transport during acidosis.[14] Such an increase in distal fluid and sodium delivery stimulates K$^+$ secretion during loading with ammonium chloride, in diabetic acidosis, and in proximal tubular acidosis. Taken together, it is clear that the effects of acid–base disturbances on K$^+$ excretion are mediated by two major components: direct effects related to pH, and secondary effects relating to the rate of delivery and composition of fluid entering the distal nephron. Increased aldosterone, possible related

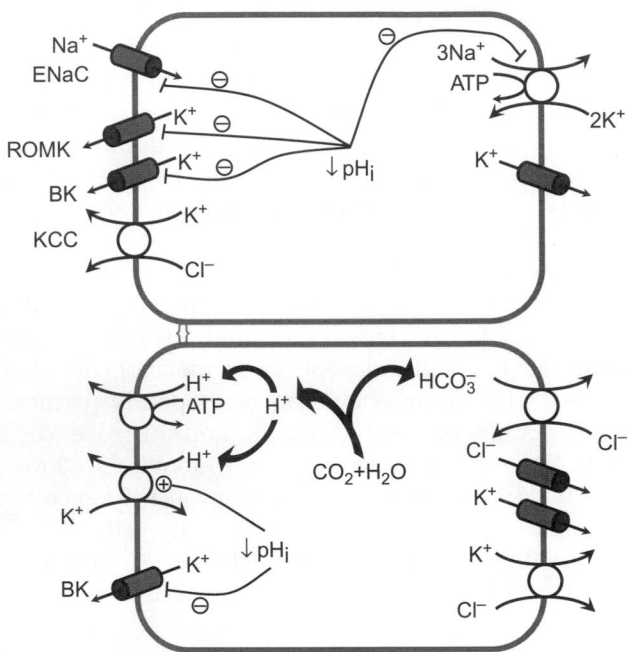

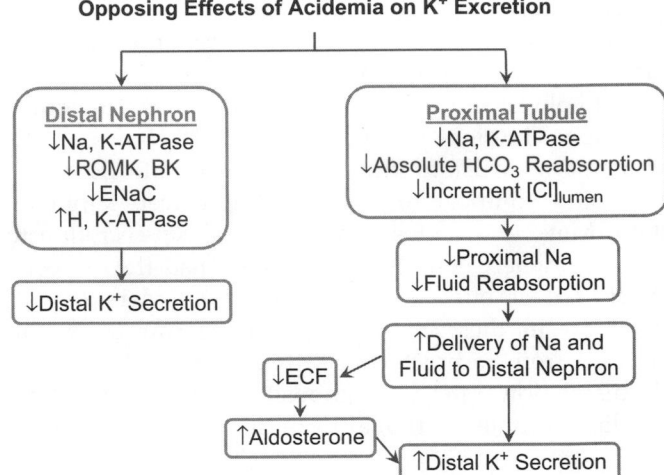

FIGURE 49.39   Effects of pH changes on K$^+$ transport in principal (top) and intercalated (bottom) cells. (From ref. [14].)

FIGURE 49.41   Complex effects of acidemia on proximal and distal tubule potassium transport.[14]

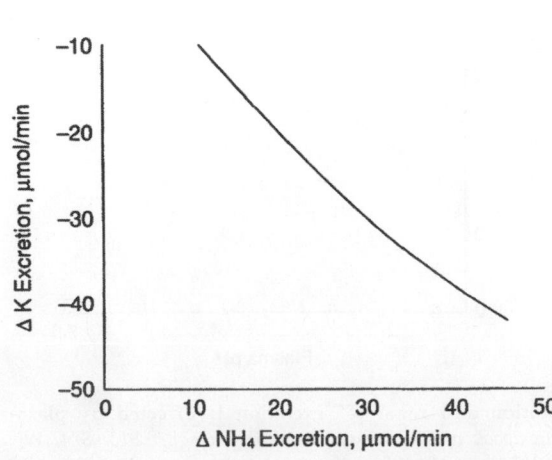

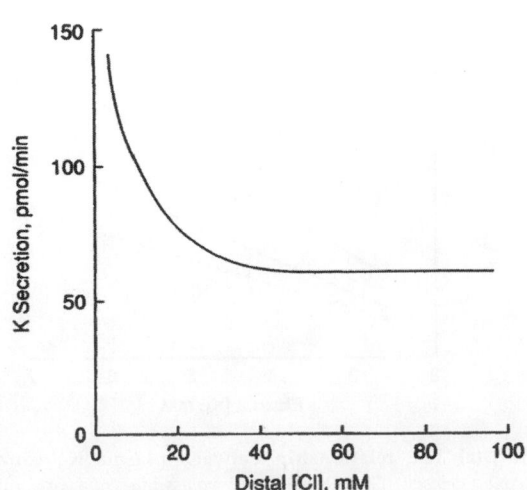

FIGURE 49.40   Effects of acute alkalemia on K$^+$ excertion.

to ECFV contraction, also contributes to kaliuresis during acidosis; K$^+$ excretion is reduced in acidosis when aldosterone levels are not allowed to increase.[473]

Metabolic alkalosis increases K$^+$ secretion by several mechanisms, both as a result of direct stimulation of K$^+$ secretion in principal cells and diminished K$^+$ reabsorption by K-H-ATPase in intercalated cells (Figure 49.40). Additionally, high delivery rates of bicarbonate-containing fluid into the distal tubule further promote K$^+$ secretion.[8,80,306]

It should be noted that the effects of respiratory acid—base disturbances on renal K$^+$ excretion are milder than those observed in metabolic acid—base disturbances.[14] In respiratory acidosis, the maintenance of significantly higher plasma bicarbonate concentrations sustains proximal tubule fluid reabsorption, and renal compensation of chronic respiratory acidosis restores plasma pH to normal more effectively than in metabolic acidosis.[14] Kaliuresis in respiratory alkalosis is also milder than that observed in metabolic alkalosis.

K$^+$ transport across the outer medullary collecting duct is also affected by changes in electrogenic hydrogen ion transport. Acidosis enhances electrogenic hydrogen secretion and tends to increase the lumen-positive potential, whereas alkalosis has the opposite effect. Passive K$^+$ reabsorption would thus be increased during acidosis and depressed in alkalosis. Independent of these indirect effects, metabolic acidosis has been shown to stimulate the activity of the apical K$^+$-H$^+$-ATPase in isolated rabbit CCDs.[458]

Renal production of ammonium is important not only to renal acid excretion, and therefore to maintenance of acid—base balance, but also to renal K$^+$ excretion. Tannen has drawn attention to the inverse relationship between urinary K$^+$ and ammonium excretion shown in Figure 49.42.[501,502] Studies in *in vivo* and isolated perfused kidneys have demonstrated that K$^+$ excretion is depressed when ammonium excretion is enhanced, an effect that has been localized in micropuncture studies to tubule sites beyond the ICT.[247] Studies of isolated perfused kidneys have systematically evaluated acid—base and endocrine factors modulating principal cell function.[445,446] The cell mechanism of the inhibitory effect of ammonium on K$^+$ excretion may involve competition between K$^+$ and ammonium at the K$^+$-binding site of the Na$^+$,K$^+$-ATPase in the basolateral membrane of principal tubule cells.[534]

Other Hormones

Vasopressin stimulates the secretion of K$^+$ ions across the distal tubule and CCD.[146,148,437,438,443,447] *In vivo* perfusion of the distal tubule and electrophysiological studies of K$^+$ transport in principal cells indicate that activation of K$^+$ secretion reflects an increase in apical sodium permeability.[443] Besides this effect on the driving force of K$^+$, patch-clamp studies have shown that vasopressin also increases the density of K$^+$ channels in the apical membrane of principal tubule cells.[82] The effects of vasopressin on K$^+$ secretion in cortical collecting ducts are sharply augmented by mineralocorticoid pretreatment.[438]

Luminal vasopressin also stimulates K$^+$ secretion via activation of V1 receptors.[10] This effect differs from the basolateral action, in that the V1 receptor is coupled to the phospholipase-IP3, Ca^{2+}-PKC signaling pathway, rather than cyclic AMP (Figure 49.43). A key role of Ca^{2+} was established by showing that chelators such as BAPTA abolished the luminal effects of vasopressin.

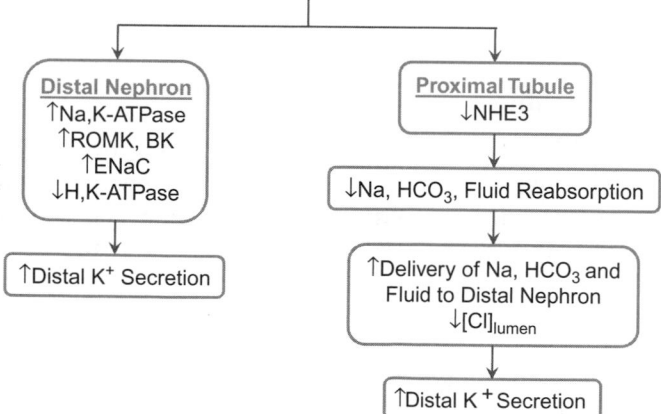

FIGURE 49.42 Relation between luminal NH$_4$ (left) and Cl$^-$ (right) concentration and K$^+$ secretion. Distal K$^+$ secretion is inhibited by the presence of Cl$^-$ in the tubule lumen and is stimulated when Cl$^-$ concentration falls below 20 mM. (*From Velazquez, H., Ellison, D. H., and Wright, F. S. (1987). Chloride-dependent potassium secretion in early and late distal tubules. Am. J. Physiol. Renal 253, F555—562, with permission.*) Changes in renal potassium excretion are negatively correlated with changes in ammonium excretion. (*From ref. [501,502], with permission.*)

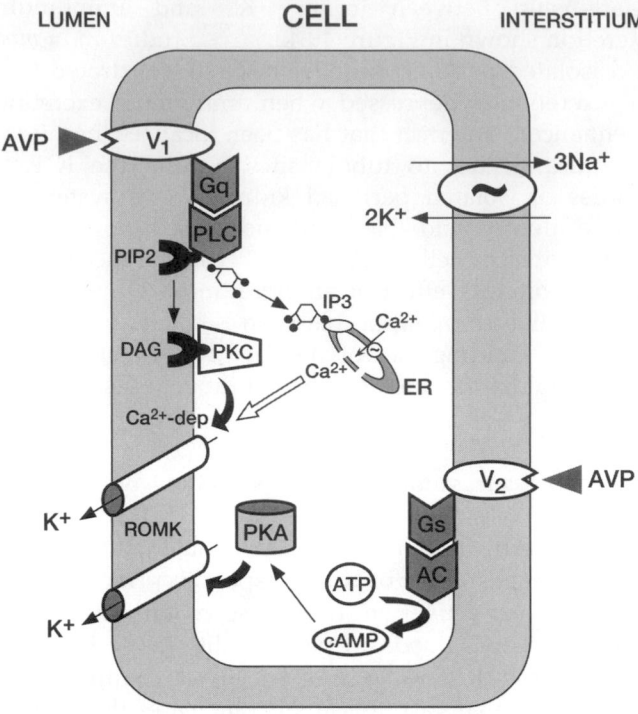

LUMEN **CELL** **INTERSTITIUM**

FIGURE 49.43   Signaling mechanisms of luminal (V1 receptors) and basolateral (V2 receptors) action of AVP (arginine vasopressin) (PLC: phospholipase C; ER: endoplasmic reticulum). *(From Amorim, J. B., Musa-Aziz, R., Mello-Aires, M., and Malnic, G. (2004). Signaling path of the action of AVP on distal K⁺ secretion. Kidney Int.* **66**, *696–704, with permission.)*

These observations strongly suggest that Ca^{2+}-sensitive B channels mediate the luminal effects of vasopressin. In contrast, the basolateral effects of vasopressin involve V2 receptors and the cAMP−PKA cascade which modulate ROMK channels.[82] The inhibitory effects on K^+ secretion of angiotensin and prostaglandins are similarly mediated by the phospholipase A-arachidonic acid pathway.[217]

Klotho, ATP, Catecholamines, Insulin, Glucagon, Kallikrein, and Guanilyn

Klotho, an age-suppressing agent, is expressed in distal tubule cells and regulates expression of ROMK channels in the kidney.[84] It not only increases ROMK abundance in HEK cells (human embryonic kidney cells), but also increases urinary K^+ excretion when given intravenously to rats. Diminished Klotho production associated with reduced renal mass and renal failure could contribute to impaired K^+ excretion. It is of interest that angiotensin II infusions curtail Klotho expression in the kidney. K^+ restriction activates the angiotensin II system, and its inhibitory effect on Klotho could account for diminished K^+ excretion during K-deprivation.[84]

Purinergic receptors and *ATP* affect K^+ transport in the kidney. Apical ATP reduces not only amiloride-sensitive Na transport,[128,297,298] but also decreases apical ROMK channel activity.[316] Consistent with inhibition of K^+ secretion by luminal ATP is the observation that mice lacking P2Y2 receptors display facilitated K^+ excretion accompanied by lower plasma K^+ concentrations.[406] A paracrine element of ATP-dependent regulation of tubule transport in collecting ducts has also been suggested: decreased Na reabsorption and diminished K^+ secretion as well as lowering of urinary ATP excretion result from ablation of renal purinergic receptors that are normally activated in intercalated tubule cells by enhanced tubule flow rate.[228a]

Both α- and β-adrenergic agonists affect K^+ transport by distal nephron segments. Care must be taken, however, to distinguish direct tubule effects from extrarenal effects, because epinephrine activates K^+ uptake in liver and muscle, and lowers plasma K^+ levels.[53,55] Nevertheless, when plasma K^+ levels are prevented from declining after epinephrine administration by infusion of K^+-containing fluids, renal K^+ excretion still falls. The epinephrine effect to suppress K^+ secretion or to enhance K^+ reabsorption has been localized to nephron sites beyond the initial collecting tubule.[104] Treatment with adrenergic agonists has been shown to reduce the lumen-negative voltage and chloride absorption in cortical collecting ducts.[242]

Insulin plays an important role in the regulation of extrarenal K^+ homeostasis,[53,103] but its renal effects are both modest and complex.[60,167,415] Insulin administration has been observed to reduce K^+ excretion,[104] but the role of changes of plasma K^+ and other hormones have proved difficult to resolve. In one clearance study, in which efforts were made to maintain constant K^+ levels in the blood, insulin modestly increased K^+ excretion.[415] In contrast, microperfusion of isolated CCDs with insulin *reduced* K^+ secretion.[167]

Glucagon has also been shown to have a significant effect on K^+ excretion. Its infusion induces a prompt increase in K^+ excretion, and it has been suggested that the effective excretion of K^+ following food intake may be related to glucagon release.[5]

Kallikrein is synthetized in distal connecting tubule cells,[87,128] and its release into the tubule fluid following a dietary K-load modulates downstream K^+ and Na transport.[137] Figure 49.44 illustrates its mode of action and that of other luminal agents. Following a dietary load of K, kallikrein is released into the tubule lumen and exerts its downstream action by inhibiting K^+ reabsorption by K/H exchange in intercalated cells. It also stimulates apical sodium channels in principal cells, depolarizing the apical membrane and enhancing the driving force for K^+ secretion. It is noteworthy that the prompt kaliuresis following food intake was not associated with increased urinary aldosterone excretion.[87]

Guanylin and *uroguanylin* are peptides found in the gut and urine, and renal function studies demonstrate their ability to promote an increase in sodium and fluid excretion.[9] Perfusion studies in single rat distal tubules show that these peptides also inhibit K⁺ secretion, most likely by modulating the activity of maxi-K channels. It is possible, but not certain, that guanilyn and uroguanylin are involved in the signaling between the gastrointestinal tract and the kidney with respect to changes in K⁺ balance.

Diuretics

Diuretic drugs, used primarily to promote excretion of salt and water, also affect renal K⁺ excretion.[73,134,135,171,181,186,201,234,345,524] Figure 49.45 illustrates the primary renal sites of action of compounds representative of three classes of diuretic drugs that act from the luminal side of tubule cells. Loop diuretics, such as furosemide, act mainly on the Na-K-2Cl co-transporter in the apical membrane of thick ascending limb cells.[74−76,198,201,234] Thiazide diuretics have their primary action on an Na-Cl co-transporter in cells of the distal convoluted tubule.[95,234,522−524] Loop and thiazide diuretics are both capable of increasing K⁺ excretion. K⁺-sparing diuretics, exemplified by amiloride and triamterene, block Na channels in principal cells of the ICT and

CCD.[19,73,119,232,357] Renal K⁺ excretion depends primarily on secretion by principal cells in the ICT and CCD. Amiloride targets these cells by a blocking ENaC, reducing the transepithelial potential difference and diminishing the driving focrce for K⁺ secretion. Luminal Ca²⁺ also blocks ENaC, and has similar inhibitory effects on K⁺ secretion.[372]

Loop diuretics increase renal K⁺ excretion, in part by direct effects on TAL cells, and also by secondary effects on principal cells in the ICT and CCD. Thus, furosemide inhibition of the Na-K-2Cl co-transporter leaves the cell-to-lumen K⁺ flux through apical membrane channels unopposed, resulting in either greatly reduced K⁺ absorption or even reversal to produce net K⁺ secretion, along the TAL.[201,511,512] The inhibition of Na and Cl absorption in the TAL also reduces medullary interstitial osmolality and results in decreased fluid absorption along the descending limb. Thus, loop diuretics not only decrease K⁺ reabsorption in the thick ascending limb but, in addition, increase the rate of fluid delivery out of the loop of Henle and provide a flow rate stimulus to K⁺ secretion along the distal tubule and collecting duct. Different degrees of kaliuresis have been observed in animal studies with furosemide and piretanide. The latter is less potent in promoting loss of K⁺, owing to stimulation of bradykinin production which curtails sodium entry into collecting duct principal cells.[71]

Thiazide diuretics also promote renal K⁺ excretion, largely via inhibition of the apical Na-Cl co-transporter in the DCT.[135,523−526] A likely explanation for the effect of thiazides to promote K⁺ excretion is the increase in distal sodium and fluid delivery through inhibition of sodium chloride co-transport. By decreasing carbonic anhydrase-dependent sodium and bicarbonate reabsorption in the proximal tubule, thiazides also tend to increase the flow rate of fluid into the distal nephron.[234,522]

Osmotic diuretics exert their kaliuretic action largely by increasing fluid and sodium delivery into the distal tubule following proximal tubule transport inhibition. As described above, poorly permeant anions such as sulfate, phosphate bicarbonate, ferrocyanide, and hippurate not only augment distal fluid and sodium delivery, but also facilitate K⁺ secretion by lowering lumen Cl⁻-concentration, thus stimulating K⁺-chloride co-transport.[8,132] It should be noted, though, that with increased fluid loads delivered to the distal nephron, larger fractions of K⁺ also enter the distal nephron. Additional mechanisms favoring K⁺ loss during administration of diuretic agents also involve hormonal effects. As extracellular volume shrinks owing to urinary loss of sodium chloride, aldosterone and vasopressin release stimulate K⁺ secretion.

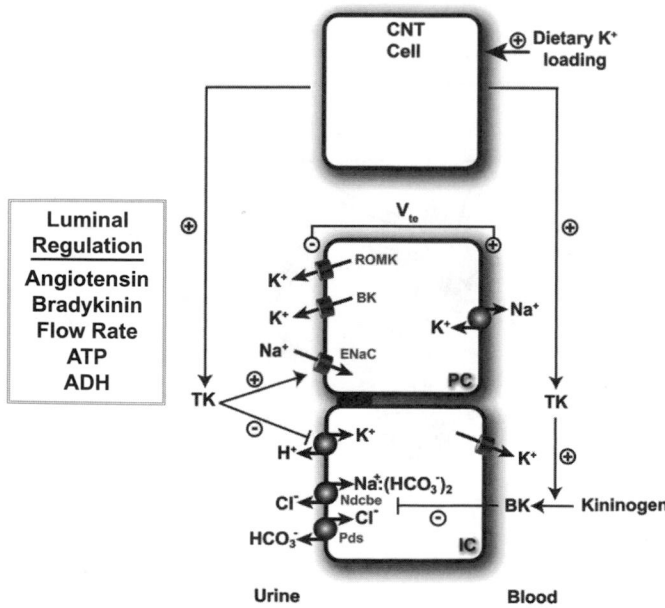

FIGURE 49.44 Regulation of distal tubule function by messengers. *(From ref. [128].)*

Maturation of K$^+$ Transport

Somatic growth after birth is associated with a predictable increase in total body potassium content[77,152] and maintenance of a state of positive potassium balance.[106,111,496] Renal potassium clearance is low in newborns, even when corrected for the low glomerular filtration rate prevailing early in life.[106,430,496] Although infants, like adults, can excrete urinary potassium at a rate that exceeds its glomerular filtration, reflecting the capacity for net tubular secretion, they are unable to excrete an exogenously administered potassium load as efficiently as the adult.[313,330,510] Micropuncture studies in young (2-week-old) rats[299] and clearance studies in saline-expanded dogs[271] provide additional evidence for a limited secretory and enhanced reabsorptive capacity of the distal nephron to potassium early in life.

The physiologic processes contributing to net urinary potassium excretion in the neonate are similar to those already described in the fully-differentiated kidney, and include glomerular filtration, reabsorption (predominant) along the proximal tubule and loop of Henle, and bidirectional transport in the distal nephron. The fraction of the filtered load of potassium reabsorbed along the proximal tubule of suckling (2-week-old) rats is similar to that reabsorbed along the same segment in the adult.[299,462] In contrast, the TALH appears to undergo a significant developmental increase in its capacity for potassium reabsorption and diluting capacity, as evidenced by the findings in rats of significant increases in the: (1) fractional reabsorption of potassium along this segment, expressed as a percentage of delivered load, between the second and sixth weeks of postnatal life;[299] and (2) osmolarity of early distal fluid between the second and fourth weeks of life.[605] Molecular studies identify postnatal increases in abundance of mRNA encoding NKCC2 and Na-K-ATPase in rodent kidney, and in particular, in the medulla,[450,588] and Na-K-ATPase activity in rabbit TALH.[448]

Potassium secretion in the distal nephron, and specifically in the mammalian cortical collecting duct

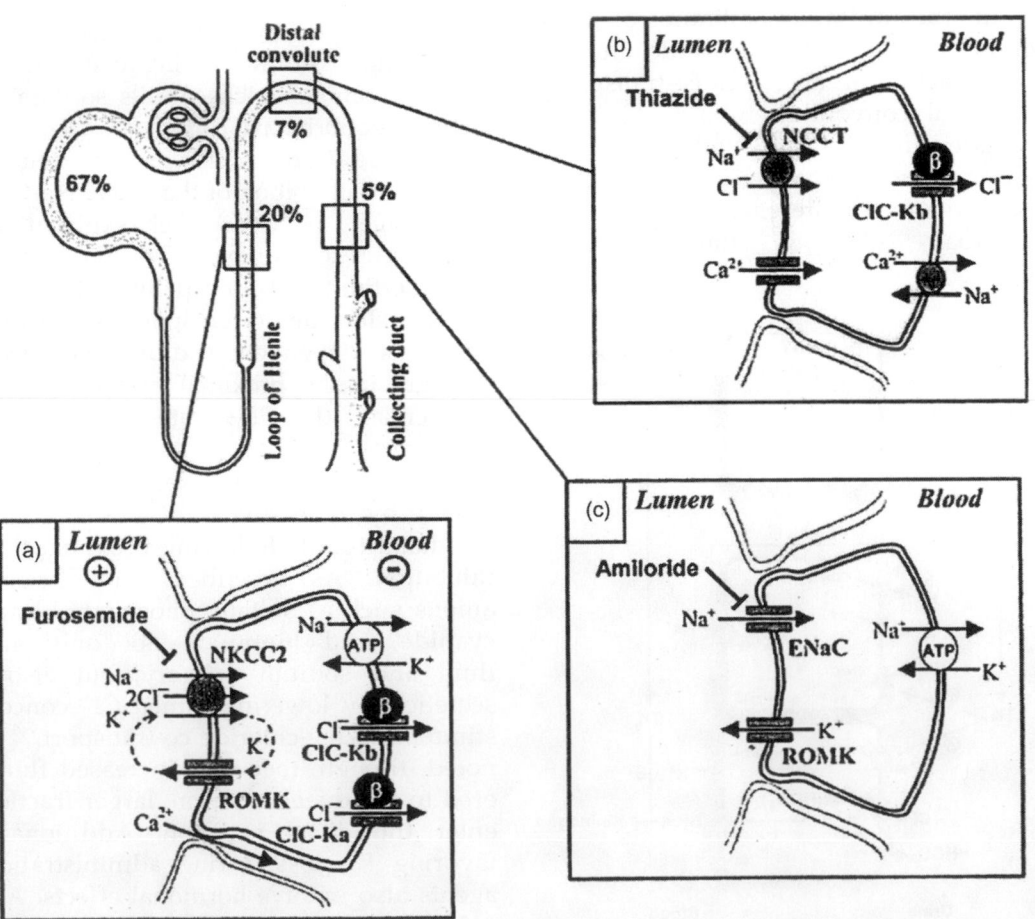

FIGURE 49.45 Distribution of NKCC2, ROMK, the ClC-ß-sub-unit Barttin, ClC-Kb, and NCCT along the nephron and site of action of the classic diuretic agents: (a) furosemide; (b) thiazide; and (c) amiloride. (*Acta Physiol. Scand.* 2004, 181, 513–521.)

(CCD) microperfused *in vitro*, is low early in life, and cannot be stimulated by high tubular (urinary) flow rates (Figure 49.46).[429,430] Indeed, basal potassium secretion cannot be detected in the rabbit CCD until after the third week of postnatal life, with potassium secretory rates increasing thereafter to reach adult levels by six weeks of age.[429] The limited capacity of the distal nephron for potassium secretion is due primarily to a paucity of apical conducting SK/ROMK channels in principal cells early in life.[431] The postnatal increase in apical channel activity reflects a developmental increase in number of channels, due to an increase in transcription and translation of channel proteins,[45,606] and not open probability which remained constant for all channels identified after the second week of life.[431] The electrochemical gradient favoring potassium secretion does not appear to be limiting early in life, as Na-K pump activity and the rate of net sodium absorption in the rabbit CCD at two weeks of age are 50–60% of that measured in the adult.[92,429,448] *In vivo* measurements of the sodium concentration in distal tubular fluid generally exceed 35 mEq/l both in healthy adult and suckling rats and thus should not restrict distal sodium secretion.[192,299,605]

Flow-induced potassium secretion, which is mediated by the Ca^{2+}- and stretch-activated BK channel, is a relatively late developmental event, first appearing in the rabbit CCD in the fifth week of postnatal life.[430,575] The detection of flow-induced potassium secretion coincides with the appearance of apical immunodetectable maxi-K channel α-subunit protein in this segment.[575] The absence of flow-induced potassium secretion early in life is not due to a limitation in the ability of the distal nephron to respond to an increase in luminal flow rate with an increase in net

sodium absorption and/or intracellular Ca^{2+} concentration, responses required for flow-stimulated net potassium secretion; these flow-induced responses in CCDs from young animals are equivalent to those detected in the adult by the second week of postnatal life.[575]

The paucity of apical potassium secretory channels and relatively robust basolateral Na-K-ATPase activity prevailing in the CCD early in life requires that potassium translocated into the cell by the Na-K pump be recycled back into the interstitium via basolateral potassium channels to maintain a constant intracellular potassium concentration. Thus, the postnatal increase in transepithelial potassium secretion likely requires not only activation of apical potassium channels, but also modification of the magnitude of basolateral potassium recycling. Little is known about the developmental expression and regulation of renal basolateral potassium channels. Immunodetectable Kir7.1, which co-localizes with Na-K-ATPase at the basolateral membrane of distal nephron and principal cells of the fully differentiated CCD,[374a] is first observed in the cortical and medullary TAL by the end of the first postnatal week in rat, appearing in the DCT and CCD at three weeks of age.[497a] As the postnatal appearance of Kir7.1 coincides with that of ROMK in the CCD, Kir7.1 is not a likely candidate for basolateral potassium recycling in the early postnatal period. Kir7.1 has been proposed to contribute to urinary potassium excretion in response to potassium-loading by generating a transepithelial potential difference for sodium reabsorption which, in turn, provides the driving force for potassium secretion.[497a]

While the distal nephron is limited in its capacity for potassium secretion early in life, clearance studies suggest that newborn dogs absorb 25% more of the distal potassium load than their adult counterparts.[313] Functional assays of apical H-K-ATPase in rabbit collecting duct reveal that pump activity in neonatal intercalated cells is equivalent to that measured in mature cells.[91] Although these data alone do not predict transepithelial potassium absorption under physiologic conditions, the high distal tubular fluid potassium concentrations measured *in vivo* in the young rat may[299] facilitate H-K-ATPase-mediated potassium absorption in this part of the nephron.

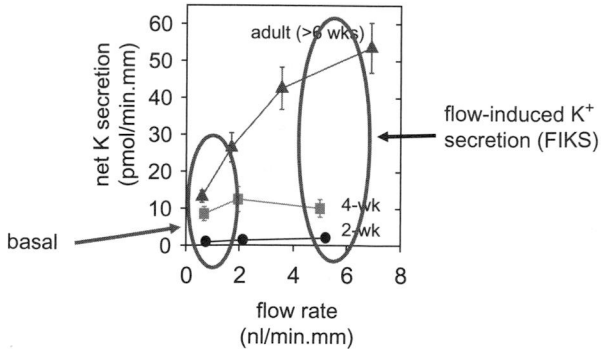

FIGURE 49.46 Developmental changes in basal and flow-induced (FIKS) K$^+$ secretion in microperfused rabbit CCDs. The maturing rabbit CCD is characterized by the relatively early appearance of basal K$^+$ secretion, mediated by SK/ROMK channels, at ~2 wks of age and, after the 4th week of postnatal life, BK channel-mediated FIKS. *Modified from ref. [429].*

Circadian Rhythm

Renal K$^+$ excretion varies during the 24-hour day.[337–339] Some of this variation occurs because of spacing between meals or other episodes of K$^+$ intake. However, even when K$^+$ ingestion is spread evenly throughout the day and night, a pattern of lower rates of K⁺ excretion at night and in the morning, and higher rates in the afternoon emerges.[337–339,397] Figure 49.47 shows the response of human subjects to an intravenous K⁺ load, given either starting at midnight or midday. The relationship between plasma concentration and rate of renal K⁺ excretion at different times of the day–night cycle is also summarized. It is apparent that the kaliuretic response was significantly diminished at night. Thus, higher concentrations of K⁺ were required at night to effect K⁺ excretion.

These daily fluctuations of K⁺ excretion have not been fully explained. As with other circadian rhythms, the periodicity is entrained by the light–dark cycle, and depends on both central and peripheral pacemakers.[337–339] Notably, the DCT and CCD express several regulatory "Clock" genes, indicating operation of a local, intrarenal, pacemaker.[607] ENaC-, aquaporin 2-, and vasopressin-receptors have marked circadian rhythms which could indirectly influence the excretion of K⁺. Also, it is likely that the changes in K⁺ excretion are produced by changes in distal secretion. It has been reported that changes in aldosterone are not required,[393–397] but that the higher K⁺ excretions during daytime may be related to enhanced bicarbonate loss in the urine.[477]

Integrated Regulation of K⁺ Homeostasis

Renal K⁺ excretion is regulated by multiple factors acting at several transport sites in response to influences originating outside the kidney. The final rate of excretion of K⁺ is determined by the net effect of mechanisms that may be cooperating or competing. In some situations the individual regulatory factors may act together, while in other cases they may change in directions that tend to cancel one another. Reasonable predictions of the rate of K⁺ excretion can be derived from knowledge of expected changes of individual factors.

Model calculations of tubule K⁺ transport have provided interesting insights between water and K⁺ transport. It was suggested that the increase in K⁺ concentration along both the water-permeable connecting and collecting tubule was not only mediated by net secretion in principal cells, but also by vasopressin-dependent fluid equilibration.[560] Indeed, it becomes apparent that the initial K⁺ concentration in both nephron segments may reach such high concentrations that they exceed the maximal transepithelial K⁺ gradient that can be achieved by K⁺ secretion in principal cells. As a consequence, both the CNT and CCD can become sites of modest, albeit significant, reabsorption of K⁺. Calculations based on these cell models also allowed an assessment of the interactions between axial flow rate along the CNT and CCD, the sodium-load,

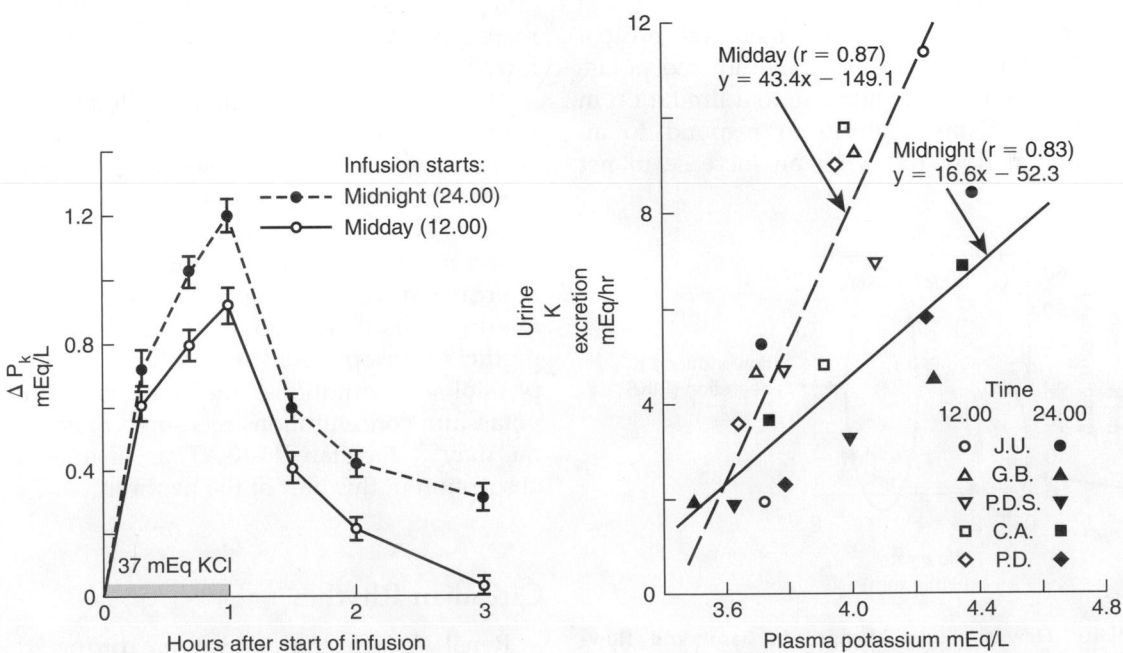

FIGURE 49.47 Left: Response of plasma potassium concentration (PK) in human subjects to intravenous infusion of 37 mEq of potassium chloride solution in 250 ml of water provided over 1 hour either starting at midnight (dashed line) or midday (solid line). Right: Relationship between plasma potassium concentration and rate of renal potassium excretion in human subject at midnight (dashed line) or midday (solid line). (*Am. J. Physiol.* 1986, **250**, R735–R752.)

transepithelial potential difference, and water permeability. It has also made possible an analysis of the factors leading to the typical kaliuresis produced by thiazides.[560]

An example of cooperative factors modulating K$^+$ transport is seen in the renal response to a high-K$^+$ intake. As noted previously, the increase in plasma K$^+$ concentration promotes K$^+$ uptake by K$^+$-secreting cells. It also stimulates the adrenal gland to secrete aldosterone, which in turn promotes K$^+$ secretion by cells of the distal nephron. Increased plasma K$^+$ concentration also inhibits sodium and fluid reabsorption by the proximal tubule, and thus increases flow rate into the distal nephron.

Evidence of the involvement of such factors in response to a change in K$^+$ intake was also obtained in a careful study employing human subjects.[391] Dietary K$^+$ was increased from 100 to 400 mmol/day. Renal K$^+$ excretion progressively increased so that external K$^+$ balance was restored within three days. During the first two hours after each meal, plasma K$^+$ rose by approximately 0.5 mM and then subsided, returning to the normal range before the next meal. Plasma aldosterone also increased after meals. The changes in plasma aldosterone (from 400 to 900 pM) were proportionately larger than the 10–20% increase in plasma K$^+$. Evidence that distal flow and sodium delivery increased after meals as well came from the observation that sodium excretion increased from 50 to 200 μmol/min. Thus, the concerted actions of multiple regulatory mechanisms improve the defense against the danger of hyperkalemia.

The effectiveness of aldosterone to stimulate K$^+$ secretion in principle cells is modulated by SGK1 (serum- and glucocorticoid-regulated kinase 1). This kinase affects several renal transport processes. Inspection of Figure 49.28 shows that the stimulation of apical sodium and K$^+$ channels, as well as of basolateral Na$^+$,K$^+$-ATPase through aldosterone, involves participation of SGK. Transcription and translation of SGK is upregulated by aldosterone,[89a,289,354a] and co-expression experiments in heterologous expression systems of SGK with Na$^+$ or K$^+$ channels, and with Na$^+$,K$^+$-ATPase, indicate increased activity of these transporters. It is significant that both the reabsorption of sodium, as well as the secretion of K$^+$, is impaired in SGK knockout mice. Compromised upregulation of urinary K$^+$ excretion during chronic K$^+$-loading was also demonstrated by maintenance of K$^+$ balance, but at elevated aldosterone levels.[520] SGK has been shown to enhance abundance of ROMK in the membrane of oocytes, a process that also involves the cooperative effect of NHERF (Na-H exchange regulating factor).[589a,589b] Increased activity of ROMK is also mediated by a significant shift in pH-sensitivity of the channel.[289]

Derangements in the regulation of aldosterone regulation can have important consequences for the maintenance of K$^+$ balance. The hypokalemia that appears in primary hyperaldosteronism has long been recognized.[175,176] Experimental administration of excess mineralocorticoid hormone (DOC) or aldosterone produces the effects seen in patients with adrenal overproduction of aldosterone. Sodium excretion falls initially, but within a few days it then increases until balance between intake and output is restored. Plasma sodium concentration does not change; however, arterial blood pressure is increased. The "escape" from the sodium-retaining effect of mineralocorticoid excess has been attributed to inhibition of Na reabsorption by factors related to extracellular fluid volume expansion,[213,273] and thiazide-sensitive Na-Cl co-transport has been defined as the key tubule transport that is downregulated during mineralocorticoid escape.[549] In contrast to sodium, K$^+$ excretion rises to levels exceeding K$^+$ intake, continues for a longer period, and results in hypokalemia. This continued stimulation of distal K$^+$ secretion appears to be related to the same volume-related inhibition of sodium reabsorption that limits the period of sodium retention. Inhibition of proximal sodium and fluid absorption leads to increased distal delivery of sodium and fluid, and therefore to a flow rate stimulus to K$^+$ secretion. Protective mechanisms, activated by the progressively increasing K$^+$ depletion, involve stimulation of K$^+$ reabsorption by H$^+$-K$^+$-ATPase which progressively restrains further K$^+$ loss.

It should be noted that some investigators are not satisfied that all stimuli acting to promote increased K$^+$ excretion have been identified. Rabinowitz and others have argued that increases in K$^+$ excretion after ingestion of K$^+$ are not fully-explained by changes in plasma K, circulating aldosterone or distal delivery of fluid and sodium.[105,168,393] These observations have recently been confirmed and extended, and it has been suggested that sensors in the gastrointestinal tract, the liver or the brain are involved in regulating K$^+$ homeostasis.[392–397] A gastrointestinal or hepatic K$^+$ sensor would explain the observation that a K$^+$-load given by infusion into the portal vein is more kaliuretic compared to the same amount of K$^+$ injected intravenously into the systemic circulation.[369] Moreover, by restricting the initial rise of K$^+$ to the hepatic circulation, kaliuresis could be induced without larger and potentially harmful fluctuations of K$^+$ in the general circulation.[89,343,369] Hepatic afferent nerve activity has been reported to increase with K$^+$ injection into the portal vein, but the mechanism modulating tubule transport of K$^+$ needs exploration.

When K$^+$ intake is restricted, reductions in plasma K$^+$ and circulating aldosterone withdraw the stimulus to K^+ secretion, and renal K^+ excretion tends to fall. However, in some circumstances the integrated actions of all factors, because of competing priorities, fail to maintain K^+ balance. For example, if K^+ intake is being restricted along with other food because an individual has just undergone an abdominal operation, stress-related stimulation of aldosterone secretion may put high aldosterone levels in competition with low plasma K^+ levels, and cause the rate of K^+ excretion to exceed the rate of intake. Furthermore, if saline infusions are maintaining extracellular fluid volume and urine flow, a high flow rate of tubule fluid may further compromise the ability of the kidney to retain K^+.

In other circumstances, competition among the regulatory factors may actually serve the cause of K^+ homeostasis. Changes in sodium intake are a relevant example. Although changes in sodium intake lead to changes in circulating aldosterone and extracellular fluid volume, they do not result in important deviations from K^+ balance. Lack of sodium enhances proximal fluid reabsorption, and may decrease distal flow rate and diminish K^+ excretion. However, the simultaneous stimulation of the renin—angiotensin—aldosterone system acts to promote K^+ excretion. Similarly, with deprivation of water alone, competition among regulatory factors may also act to stabilize K^+ excretion. The K^+-retaining influence of low luminal flow rate is opposed by the stimulatory influence on K^+ secretion of increased circulating vasopressin.

Finally, in some acid—base disturbances, the net result of several influences on K^+ secretion may cause the kidney to excrete K^+ at rates exceeding K^+ intake, and thus to deplete body K^+. In metabolic alkalosis, plasma K^+ concentration tends to be low because cell uptake of K^+ is enhanced. Aldosterone levels are often elevated and also tend to promote K^+ secretion. Increased distal delivery of bicarbonate, associated with increased distal flow, and high luminal bicarbonate concentration permits the distal Cl concentration to fall to low levels, and thus further favor K^+ secretion of KCl co-transport.

In acute metabolic acidosis, decreased uptake of K^+ by distal cells tends to reduce K^+ secretion. However, as acidosis proceeds, proximal fluid absorption is increasingly inhibited and distal flow rate begins to increase. An additional factor favoring K^+ secretion is the elevation of aldosterone that has been observed in chronic metabolic acidosis. Taken together, it is important to recognize that renal K^+ excretion has multiple determinants, and that they may not always be responding only to changes in K^+ balance.

Acknowledgments

We are grateful to Dr. Fred Wright, who was a major contributor and co-author of previous chapters in the earlier issues. Ms. Leah Sanders and Mr. Duncan Wong have also contributed by careful editing of the manuscript and preparation of the figures. We dedicate this chapter to Steve Hebert. He was an inspiration to all of us.

References

[1] Ackermann D, Gresko N, Carrel M, Loffing-Cueni D, Habermehl D, Gomez-Sanchez C, et al. *In vivo* nuclear translocation of mineralocorticoid and glucocorticoid receptors in rat kidney: differential effect of corticosteroids along the distal tubule. Am J Physiol 2010;299:F1473—1485.

[2] Adam WR, Dawborn JK. Potassium tolerance in rats. Aust J Exp Biol Med Sci 1972;50:757—86.

[3] Adams PR, Constanti A, Brown DA, Clark RB. Intracellular Ca^{2+} activates a fast voltage-sensitive K^+ current in vertebrate sympathetic neurones. Nature 1982;296:746—9.

[4] Adler S, Fraley DS. Potassium and intracellular pH. Kidney Int 1977;11:433—42.

[5] Ahloulay M, Dechaux M, Laborde K, Bankir L. Influence of glucagon on GFR and on urea and electrolyte excretion: direct and indirect effects. Am J Physiol 1995;269:F225—35.

[6] Ahn KY, Kone BE. Expression and cellular localization of mRNA encoding the "gastric"isoform of H^+-K^+-ATPase a-subunit in rat kidney. Am J Physiol 1995;268:F99—109.

[7] Alexander EA, Levinsky NG. An extrarenal mechanism for potassium adaptation. Clin Invest 1968;47:740—8.

[8] Amorin JB, Bailey MA, Musa-Aziz R, Giebisch G, Malnic G. Role of luminal anion and pH in distal tubule potassium secretion. Am J Physiol Renal 2003;284:F381—8.

[9] Amorim JBO, Musa-Aziz R, Lessa LMA, Malnic G, Fonteles MC. Effect of uroguanylin on potassium and bicarbonate transport in rat renal tubules. Can J Physiol Pharmacol 2006;84:1003—10.

[10] Amorim JBO, Malnic G. VI receptors in luminal action of vasopressin (AVP) on distal K^+ secretion. Am J Physiol 2000;278:F809—16.

[11] Anagnostopoulos T, Planelles G. Cell and luminal activities of chloride, potassium, sodium and protons in the late distal tubule of *Necturus* kidney. J Physiol 1987;393:73—89.

[12] Antes LM, Kujubu DA, Fernandez PE. Hypokalemia and the pathology of ion transport molecules. Semin Nephrol 1998;18:31—45.

[13] Aperia A, Holtback U, Syren ML, Svensson LB, Fryckstedt J, Greengard P. Activation/deactivation of renal Na^+,K^+-ATPase: a final common pathway for regulation of natriuresis. FASEB J 1994;8:436—9.

[14] Aronson PS, Giebisch G. Effects of pH on potassium: new explanations for old observations. J Am Soc Nephrol 2011;22:1981—9.

[15] Arrascue JF, Dobyan DC, Jamison RL. Potassium recycling in the renal medulla: effects of acute potassium chloride administration to rats fed a potassium-free diet. Kidney Int 1981;20:348—52.

[16] Arriza JL, Weinberger C, Cerelli G, Glaser TM, Handelin BL, Housman DE, et al. Cloning of human mineralocorticoid receptor complementary DNA: structural and functional kinship with the glucocorticoid receptor. Science 1987;237:268—75.

[17] Atkinson NS, Robertson GA, Ganetzky B. A component of calcium-activated potassium channels encoded by the *Drosophila* slo locus. Science 1991;253:551—5.

[18] Avison MJ, Gullans SR, Ogino T, Giebisch T. Na^+ and K^+ fluxes stimulated by Na^+-coupled glucose transport: evidence for a Ba^{2+}-insensitive K^+ efflux pathway in rabbit proximal tubules. J Membr Biol 1988;105:197—205.

[19] Baer JE, Jones CB, Spitzer SA, Russo HF. The potassium sparing and natriuretic activity of N-amindino-3.4-diamino-6-chloro-pytazine-carboxyamide hydrochloride dihydrate (amiloride hydrochloride). J Pharmacol Exp Ther 1967;157:472–85.

[20] Bailey MA, Cantone A, Yan Q, MacGregor GG, Leng Q, Amorim JBO, et al. Maxi-K channels contribute to urinary potassium excretion in the ROMK-deficient mouse model of Type II Bartter's syndrome and in adaptation to a high-K diet. Kidney Int 2006;70:51–9.

[21] Bailey MA, Mullins JJ, Kenyon CJ. Mineralocorticoid and glucocorticoid receptors stimulate epithelial sodium channel activity in a mouse model of Cushing syndrome. Hypertension 2009;54:890–6.

[22] Bailey MA, Paterson JM, Hodoke PW, Wrobel N, Bellamy CO, Brownstein DG, et al. A switch in the mechanism of hypertension in the syndrome of apparent mineralocorticoid excess. J Am Soc Nephrol 2008;19:47–58.

[23] Bailey MA, Unwin RJ, Shirley DG. In vivo inhibition of renal 11beta-hydroxysteroid dehydrogenase in the rat stimulates collecting duct sodium reabsorption. Clin Sci (Lond) 2001;101(2):195–8.

[24] Bandulik S, Schmidt K, Bockenhauer D, Zdebik AA, Humberg E, Kleta R, et al. The salt-wasting phenotype of EAST syndrome, a disease with multifaceted symptoms linked to the KCNJ10 K^+ channel. Pflugers Arch 2011;461:423–35.

[25] Bank N, Aynedjian HS. A micropuncture study of potassium excretion by the remnant kidney. J Clin Invest 1973;52:1480–90.

[26] Barlet-Bas C, Khadouri C, Marsy S, Doucet A. Enhanced intracellular sodium concentration in kidney cells recruits a latent pool of Na^+-K^+ATPase whose size is modulated by corticosteroids. J Biol Chem 1990;265:7799–803.

[27] Barlet-Bas C, Cheval L, Feraille E, et al. Regulation of tubular Na-KATPase. In: Hatano M, editor. Nephrology, Proceedings of the XIth International Congress of Nephrology. Berlin: Springer; 1991. p. 419–34.

[28] Barratt LJ, Rector Jr FC, Kokko JP, Tisher CC, Seldin DW. Transepithelial potential difference profile of the distal tubule of the rat kidney. Kidney Int 1975;8:368–75.

[29] Bastl C, Hayslett JP, Binder HJ. Increased large intestinal secretion of potassium in renal insufficiency. Kidney Int 1977;12:9–16.

[30] Bastl C, Kliger AS, Binder HJ, Hayslett JP. Characteristics of potassium secretion in the mammalian colon. Am J Physiol 1978;234:F48–53.

[31] Bassett MH, White PC, Rainey WE. The regulation of aldosterone synthase expression. Molec and Cellular Endocrinol 2004;217:67–74.

[32] Battilana CA, Dobyan DC, Lacy FB, Bhattacharya J, Johnston PA, Jamison RL. Effect of chronic potassium loading on potassium secretion by the pars recta or descending limb of the juxtamedullary nephron in the rat. J Clin Invest 1978;62:1093–103.

[33] Baylis C, Handa RK, Sorkin M. Glucocorticoids and control of GFR. Semin Nephrol 1990;10:320–9.

[34] Beck FX, Dorge A, Blumner E, Giebisch G, Thurau K. Cell rubidium uptake: a method for studying functional heterogeneity in the nephron. Kidney Int 1988;33:642–51.

[35] Beck JS, Breton S, Mairbaurl H, Laprade R, Giebisch G. Relationship between sodium transport and intracellular ATP in isolated perfused rabbit proximal convoluted tubule. Am J Physiol 1991;261:F634–9.

[36] Beck JS, Hurst AM, Lapointe JV, Laprade R. Regulation of basolateral K^+ channels in proximal tubule studied during continuous microperfusion. Am J Physiol 1994;264:F496–501.

[37] Beck JS, Laprade R, Lapointe J-Y. Coupling between transepithelial Na^+ transport and basolateral K^+ conductance in renal proximal tubule. Am J Physiol 1994;266:F517–27.

[38] Beck JS, Breton S, Giebisch G, Laprade R. Potassium conductance regulation by pH in rabbit proximal convoluted tubules. Am J Physiol 1992;263:F453–8.

[39] Beck JS, Potts DJ. Cell swelling, co-transport activation and potassium conductance in isolated perfused rabbit kidney proximal tubules. J Physiol 1990;425:369–78.

[40] Beck LH, Senesky D, Goldberg M. Sodium-independent active potassium reabsorption in proximal tubule of the dog. Clin Invest 1973;52:2641–5.

[41] Bailey MA, Craigie E, Livingstone DE, Kotelevtsev YV, Al-Dujaili EA, Kenyon CJ, et al. Hsd1 lb2 haploinsufficiency in mice causes salt sensitivity of blood pressure. Hypertension 2011;57:515–20.

[42] Bailey MA, Mullins JJ, Kenyon CJ. Mineralocorticoid and glucocorticoid receptors stimulate epithelial sodium channel activity in a mouse model of Cushing syndrome. Hypertens 2009;54:890–6.

[43] Bailey MA, Paterson JM, Hadoke PW, Wrobel N, Bellamy CO, Brownstein DG, et al. A switch in the mechanism of hypertension in the syndrome of apparent mineralocorticoid excess. J Am Soc Nephrol 2008;19:47–58.

[44] Beck FX, Dorge A, Blumner E, Giebisch G, Thurau K. Cell rubidium uptake: a method for studying functional heterogeneity in the nephron. Kidney Int 1988;33:642–51.

[45] Benchimol C, Zavilowitz B, Satlin LM. Developmental expression of ROMK mRNA in rabbit cortical collecting duct. Pediatr Res 2000;47:46–52.

[46] Bengele HR, Evan A, McNamara ER, Alexander EA. Tubular sites of potassium regulation in the normal and uninephrectomized rat. Am J Physiol 1978;234:F146–53.

[47] Bergann T, Fromm A, Borden SA, Fromm M, Schulzke JD. Glucocorticoid receptor is indispensable for physiological responses to aldosterone in epithelial Na^+ channel induction via the mineralocorticoid receptor in a human colonic cell line. Eur J Cell Biol 2011;90:432–9.

[48] Berliner RW. Renal secretion of potassium and hydrogen ions. Fed Proc 1952;11:695–700.

[49] Berliner RW. Renal mechanisms for potassium excretion. Harvey Lect 1961;55:141–71.

[50] Berliner RW, Kennedy TJ. Renal tubular secretion of potassium in the dog. Proc Soc Exp Biol Med 1948;67:542–5.

[51] Berliner RW, Kennedy TJ, Orloff J. Relationship between acidification of the urine and potassium metabolism. Am J Med 1951;11:274–82.

[52] Berliner RW, Kennedy Jr TJ, Hilton G. Renal mechanisms for excretion of potassium. Am J Physiol 1950;162:348–67.

[53] Bia MJ, DeFronzo RA. Extrarenal potassium homeostasis. Am J Physiol 1981;240:F257–68.

[54] Bia MJ, Tyler K, DeFronzo RA. The effect of dexamethasone on renal electrolyte excretion in the adrenalectomized rat. Endocrinology 1981;III:882–8.

[55] Bia MJ, Tyler KA, DeFronzo RA. Regulation of extrarenal potassium homeostasis by adrenal hormones in rats. Am J Physiol 1981;242:F461–8.

[56] Biagi B, Kubota T, Sohtell M, Giebisch G. Intracellular potentials in rabbit proximal tubules perfused in vitro. Am J Physiol 1981;240:F200–10.

[57] Biagi B, Sohtell M, Giebisch G. Intracellular potassium activity in the rabbit proximal straight tubule. Am J Physiol 1981;241:F677–86.

[58] Bleich M, Schlatter E, Greger R. K^+ channel of the thick ascending limb of Henle's loop. Pflugers Arch 1990;415:449–60.

[59] Bloomer HA, Rector Jr FC, Seldin DW. The mechanism of potassium reabsorption in the proximal tubule of the rat. J Clin Invest 1963;42:277–85.

[60] Boini KM, Graf D, Kuhl D, Haussinger K, Lang F. SGK1 dependence of insulin induced hypokalemia. Pflugers Arch 2009;457:955–61.

[61] Bomsztyk K, Wright FS. Effect of luminal potassium concentration and transepithelial voltage on potassium transport by the renal proximal tubule. Fed Proc 1983;42:304.

[62] Bomsztyk K, Wright FS. Dependence of ion fluxes on fluid transport by rat proximal tubule. Am J Physiol 1986;250: F680–9.

[63] Bouligand J, Delemer B, Hecart AC, Meduri G, Viengchareun S, Amazit L, et al. Familial glucocorticoid receptor haploinsufficiency by non-sense mediated mRNA decay, adrenal hyperplasia and apparent mineralocorticoid excess. PLoS One 2010;5: e13563.

[64] Boulpaep EL. Electrophysiology of the kidney [vol IVA] In: Giebisch G, Tosteson DC, Ussing HH, editors. Membrane transport in biology. Berlin: Springer-Verlag; 1979. p. 97–144.

[65] Boulpaep EL, Sackin H. Equivalent electrical circuit analysis and rheogenic pumps in epithelia. Fed Proc 1979;38:2030–6.

[66] Boyd JE, Mulrow PJ. Further studies of the influence of potassium upon aldosterone production in the rat. Endocrinology 1972;90:299–301.

[67] Brandis M, Keyes J, Windhager EE. Potassium-induced inhibition of proximal tubular fluid reabsorption in rats. Am J Physiol 1972;222:421–7.

[68] Brown EB, Goat B. Intracellular hydrogen ion changes and potassium movement. Am J Physiol 1963;204:765–70.

[69] Brown EM, Chattopadhyay N, Vassilev PM, Hebert SC. The calcium-sensing receptor (CaR) permits Ca^{2+} to function as a versatile extra-cellular first messenger. Recent Progr Horm Res 1998;53:257–80.

[70] Buffin-Meyer B, Younes-Ibrahim M, Barlet-Bas C, Cheval L, Marsy S, Doucet A. K depletion modifies the properties of Sch-28080-sensitive K-ATPase in rat collecting duct. Am J Physiol 1997;272:FI24.

[71] Buffin-Meyer B, Younes-Ibrahim M, El Mernissi G, Cheval L, Marsy S, Grima M, et al. Differential regulation of collecting duct Na$^+$K$^+$-ATPase and K$^+$ excretion by furosemide and piretanide: role of bradykinin. J Am Soc Nephrol 2004;15:876–84.

[72] Buffin-Meyer B, Verbatz JM, Cheval L, Marsy S, Younes-Ibrahim M, Le Moal C, et al. Regulation of Na$^+$, K$^+$ATPase in the rat outer medullary collecting duct during potassium depletion. J Am Soc Nephrol 1998;9:538–50.

[73] Bull MB, Laragh JH. Amiloride. A potassium-sparing natriuretic agent. Circulation 1968;37:45–53.

[74] Burg MB. Thick ascending limb of Henle's loop. Kidney Int 1982;22:454–64.

[75] Burg MB, Green N. Effect of ethacrynic acid on the thick ascending limb of Henle's loop. Kidney Int 1973;4:301–8.

[76] Burg MB, Stoner L, Cardinal J, Green N. Furosemide effect on isolated perfused tubules. Am J Physiol 1973;225:119–24.

[77] Butte NF, Hopkinson JM, Wong WW, Smith EO, Ellis KJ. Body composition during the first 2 years of life: an updated reference. Pediatr Res 2000;47:578–85.

[78] Candia S, Garcia ML, Latorre R. Mode of action of iberiotoxin, a potent blocker of the large conductance Ca$^{(2+)}$-activated K$^+$ channel. Biophys J 1992;63:583–90.

[79] Cardinal J, Lapointe J-Y, Laprade R. Luminal and peritubular ionic substitutions and intracellular potential of the rabbit proximal convoluted tubule. Am J Physiol 1984;247:F352–64.

[80] Carlisle EJF, Donnelly SM, Ethier JH, Quaggin SE, Kaiser UB, Vasuvattakul S, et al. Modulation of the secretion of potassium by accompanying anions in humans. Kidney Int 1991;39: 1206–12.

[81] Carrisoza-Gaytan R, Salvador C, Satlin LM, Liu W, Zavilowitz B, Bobadilla NA, et al. Potassium secretion by voltage-gated potassium channel Kv1.3 in the rat kidney. Am J Physiol Renal Physiol 2010;299:F255–64.

[82] Cassola AC, Giebisch G, Wang W. Vasopressin increases density of apical low-conductance K$^+$ channels in rat CCD. Am J Physiol 1993;264:F502.

[83] Cemerikic D, Wilcox CS, Giebisch G. Intracellular potential and K$^+$ activity in rat kidney proximal tubular cells in acidosis and K$^+$ depletion. J Membr Biol 1982;69:159–65.

[84] Cha S-K, Hu M-C, Kurosu H, Kuro-o M, Moe O, Huang C-L. Regulation of renal outer medullary potassium channel and renal K$^+$ excretion by Klotho. Molec Pharmacol 2009;76:38–46.

[85] Cha S-K, Huang C, Ding Y, Qi X, Huang C-L, Miller RT. Calcium-sensing receptor decreases cell surface expression of the inwardly-rectifying K$^+$ channel, Kir4.1. J Biol Chem 2011;286:1828–35.

[86] Chaillet JR, Lopes AG, Boron WE. Basolateral Na-H exchange in the rabbit cortical collecting tubule. J Gen Physiol 1985;86: 785–812.

[87] Chambrey R, Picard N. Role of tissue kallikrein in regulation of tubule function. Curr Opin Nephrol Hypertens 2011;20: 523–8.

[88] Cheema-Dhadli S, Lin S-H, Keong-Chong C, Kamel KS, Halperin ML. Requirements for a high rate of potassium excretion in rats consuming a low electrolyte diet. J Physiol 2006;572:493–501.

[89] Chen P, Guzman JP, Leong PKK, Yang LE, Perianayagam A, Babilonia E, et al. McDonough. Modest dietary K$^+$ restriction provokes insulin resistance of cellular K$^+$ uptake and phosphorylation of renal outer medulla K$^+$ channel without fall in plasma K$^+$ concentration. Am J Physiol Cell Physiol 2006;290:C1355–63.

[89a] Chen SY, Bhargava A, Mastroberardino L, Meijer OC, Wang J, Buse P, et al. Epithelial sodium channel regulated by aldosterone-induced protein sgk. Proc Natl Acad Sci USA 1999;96(5):2514–9.

[90] Choi M, Scholl UI, Yue P, et al. K$^+$ channel mutations in adrenal aldosterone-producing adenomas and hereditary hypertension. Science 2011;331:768–71.

[90a] Chou CL, Yu MJ, Kassai EM, Morris RG, Hoffert JD, Wall SM, et al. Roles of basolateral solute uptake via NKCC1 and of myosin II in vasopressin-induced cell swelling in inner medullary collecting duct. Am J Physicol Renal Physiol 2008;295:F192–201.

[91] Constantinescu A, Silver RB, Satlin LM. H-K-ATPase activity in PNA-binding intercalated cells of newborn rabbit cortical collecting duct. Am J Physiol 1997;272:F167–77.

[92] Constantinescu AR, Lane JC, Mak J, Zavilowitz B, Satlin R. Na$^+$-K$^+$-ATPase-mediated basolateral rubidium uptake in the maturing rabbit cortical collecting duct. Am J Physiol Renal Physiol 2000;279:F1161–1168.

[93] Cortney MA. Renal tubular transfer of water and electrolytes in adrenalectomized rats. Am J Physiol 1969;216:589.

[94] Costanzo LS. Comparison of calcium and sodium transport in early and late rat distal tubules: effect of amiloride. Am J Physiol 1984;246:F937–45.

[95] Costanzo LS. Localization of diuretic action in microperfused rat distal tubules: Ca and Na transport. Am Physiol 1985;248: F197–211.

[96] Coutry N, Blot-Chabaud M, Mateo P, Bonvalet JP, Farman N. Time course of sodium induced Na$^+$-K$^+$-ATPase recruitment in rabbit cortical collecting tubule. Am J Physiol 1992;263:C61–8.

[97] Cox JR, Platts MM, Horn ME, Adams R, Miller HE. The effect of aldosterone on sodium and potassium distribution in man. J Endocrinol 1966;36:103—14.

[98] Cox M, Sterns RH, Singer I. The defense against hyperkalemia: the roles of insulin and aldosterone. N Engl J Med 1978;299: 525—32.

[99] Crayen M, Thoenes W. Architektur und cytologische Charakterisierung des distalen Tubulus der Rattenniere. Fortschr Zool 1975;23:279—88.

[100] Davidson DG, Levinsky NG, Berliner RW. Maintenance of potassium excretion despite reduction of glomerular filtration during sodium diuresis. J Clin Invest 1958; 37:548—55.

[101] De Rouffignac C, Morel E. Micropuncture study of water, electrolytes and urea movements along the loops of Henle in *Psammomys*. J Clin Invest 1969;48:474—86.

[102] DeFronzo RA, Bia M, Birkhead G., Epinephrine and potassium homeostasis. Kidney Int 198; 20: 83-91.

[103] DeFronzo RA, Goldberg M, Agus Z. The effects of glucose and insulin on renal electrolyte transport. J Clin Invest 1976;58:83—90.

[104] DeFronzo RA, Stanton B, Klein-Robbenhaar G, Giebisch G. Inhibitory effect of epinephrine on renal potassium sectetion: a micropuncture study. Am J Physiol 1983;245:F303—11.

[105] Dekel B, Nakhoul F, Abassi Z, Aviv R, Winaver J, Szylman P. Complete adaptation to chronic potassium loading after adrenalectomy: possible humoral mechanisms. J Lab Clin Med 1997;129:453—61.

[106] Delgado MM, Rohatgi R, Khan S, Holzman IR, Satlin LM. Sodium and potassium clearances by the maturing kidney: clinical-molecular correlates. Pediatr Nephrol 2003; 18:759—67.

[106a] Dherbecourt O, Cheval L, Bloch-Faure M, Meneton P, Doucet A. Molecular identification of Sch28080-sensitive K-ATPase activities in the mouse kidney. Pflugers Arch 2006;451(6):769—75.

[107] Dietl P, Good D, Stanton B. Adrenal corticosteroid action on the thick ascending limb. Semin Nephrol 1990;10: 350—64.

[108] Diezi J, Michaud P, Aceves J, Giebisch G. Micropuncture study of electrolyte transport across papillary collecting duct of the rat. Am J Physiol 1973;224:623—34.

[109] Diezi J, Michaud P, Grandchamp A, Giebisch G. Effects of nephrectomy on renal salt and water transport in the remaining kidney. Kidney Int 1976;10:450—62.

[110] Dobyan DC, Lacy FB, Jamison RL. Suppression of potassium-recycling in the renal medulla by short-term potassium deprivation. Kidney Int 1979;16:704—9.

[110a] Dorup J. Structural adaptation of intercalated cells in rat renal cortex to acute metabolic acidosis and alkalosis. J Ultrastruct Res 1985;92:119—31.

[111] Dorup I, Clausen T. Effects of potassium deficiency on growth and protein synthesis in skeletal muscle and the heart of rats. Br J Nutr 1989;62:269—84.

[112] Doucet A. H+,K+-ATPase in the kidney: localization and function in the nephron. Exp Nephrol 1997;5:271—6.

[113] Doucet A. Functional control of Na-K-ATPase in single nephron segments of the mammalian kidney. Kidney Int 1998;34:749—60.

[114] Doucet A, Katz AI. Renal potassium adaptation: Na-K-ATPase activity along the nephron after chronic potassium loading. Am J Physiol 1980;238:F380—6.

[115] Doucet A, Katz AI. Short-term effect of aldosterone on Na-K-ATPase in single nephron segments. Am J Physiol 1981;241: F273—8.

[116] Doucet A, Katz AI, Morel F. Determination of Na-K-ATPase activity in single segments of the mammalian nephron. Am J Physiol 1979;237:FI05—13.

[117] Doucet A, Marsy S. Characterization of K-ATPase activity in distal nephron: stimulation by potassium depletion. Am J Physiol 1987;253:F418—23.

[118] Douglas JG. Effects of high potassium diet on angiotensin II receptors and angiotensin-induced aldosterone production in rat adrenal glomerulosa cells. Endocrinology 1980;106:983—90.

[119] Duarte CG, Chomety F, Giebisch G. Effect of amiloride, ouabain, and furosemide on distal tubular function in the rat. Am J Physiol 1971;221:632—9.

[120] Dube L, Parent L, Sauve R. Hypotonic shock activates a maxi K+ channel in primary cultured proximal tubule cells. Am J Physiol 1990;259:F348—56.

[121] DuBose Jr. TD. Hyperkalemic hyperchloremic metabolic acidosis: pathophysiologic insights. Kidney Int 1997;51:591—602.

[122] DuBose TD, Codina J, Burges A, Pressley TA. Regulation of H+-K+-ATPase expression in kidney. Am J Physiol 1995;269: F500—7.

[123] Dunbar DR, Khaled H, Evans LC, Al-Dujaili EA, Mullins LJ, Mullins JJ, et al. Transcriptional and physiological responses to chronic ACTH treatment by the mouse kidney. Physiological Genomics 2010;40:158—66.

[124] Edelman A, Curci S, Samarzija I, Frömter E. Determination of intracellular K+ activity in rat kidney proximal tubular cells. Pflugers Arch 1978;378:37—45.

[125] Elabida B, Edwards A, Salhi A, Azroyan A, Fodstad H, Meneton P, et al. A physiological role for progesterone in male: involvement in the renal adaptation to dietary K+ restriction. Kidney Int 2011; [in press]

[126] Elabida B, Edwards A, Salhi A, Azroyan A, Fodstad H, Meneton P, et al. Chronic potassium depletion increases adrenal progesterone production that is necessary for efficient renal retention of potassium. Kidney Int 2011;80:256—62.

[127] Eladari D, Chambrey R. WNKs: new concepts in the regulation of NaCl and K+ balance. J Nephrol 2007;20:260—4.

[128] Eladari D, Chambrey R, Peti-Peterdi J. A new look at electrolyte transport in the distal tubule. Annu Rev Physiol 2012;74:325—49.

[129] Elalouf J-M, Roinel N, de Rouffignac C. Effects of dDAVP on rat juxtamedullary nephrons: stimulation of medullary K+ recycling. Am J Physiol 1985;249:F291—8.

[130] Elalouf J-M, Roinel N, de Rouffignac C. Effects of human calcitonin on water and electrolyte movements in rat juxtamedullary nephrons: inhibition of medullary K+ recycling. Pflugers Arch 1986;406:502—8.

[131] Elkins T, Ganetzky B, Wu CFA. *Drosophila* mutation that eliminates a calcium-dependent potassium current. Proc Natl Acad Sci USA 1986;83:8415—9.

[132] Ellison DH, Velazquez H, Wright FS. Stimulation of distal potassium sectetion by low lumen chloride in the presence of barium. Am J Physiol 1985;248:F638—49.

[133] Ellison DH, Velazquez H, Wright FS. Unidirectional potassium fluxes in the renal distal tubule: effects of chloride and barium. Am J Physiol 1986;250:F885—94.

[134] Ellison DH, Velazquez H, Wright FS. Mechanisms of sodium, potassium and chloride transport by the renal distal tubule. Miner Electrolyte Metab 1987;13:422—32.

[135] Ellison DH, Velazquez H, Wright FS. Thiazide-sensitive sodium chloride cotransport in early distal tubule. Am J Physiol 1987;253:F546—54.

[136] Ellison DH, Velazquez H, Wright FS. Adaptation of the distal convoluted tubule of the rat: structural and functional effects

of dietary salt intake and chronic diuretic infusion. J Clin Invest 1989;83:113–26.

[137] El Moghrabi S, Houillier P, Picard N, Sohet F, Wootla B, Bloch-Faure M, et al. Tissue kallikrein permits early renal adaptation to potassium load. Proc Natl Acad Sci USA 2010;107:13526–31.

[138] Emmons C, Kurtz I. Functional characterization of three inter-calated cell subtypes in the rabbit outer cortical collecting duct. J Clin Invest 1994;93:417–23.

[139] Engbretson BG, Stoner LC. Flow-dependent potassium secretion by rabbit cortical collecting tubule in vitro. Am J Physiol 1987;253:F896–903.

[140] Engbretson BG, Beyenbach KW, Stoner LC. The everted renal tubule: a methodology for direct assessment of apical membrane function. Am J Physiol 1988;255:F1276–80.

[141] Estilo G, Liu W, Pastor-Soler N, Mitchell P, Carattino MD, Kleyman TR, et al. Effect of aldosterone on BK channel expression in mammalian cortical collecting duct. Am J Physiol Renal Physiol 2008;295:F780–8.

[142] Ethier JH, Kamel KS, Magner PO, Lemann Jr J, Halperin ML. The transtubular potassium concentration in patients with hypokalemia and hyperkalemia. Am J Kidney Dis 1990;15: 309–15.

[143] Evans LC, Mullins JJ, Kenyon C, et al. Progression of medullary atrophy and a urine concentrating defect in 11beta-hydroxysteroid dehydrogenase Type 2 knockout mice. Proc Physiol Soc 2010;19:PC248.

[144] Fang L, Garuti R, Kim B-Y, Wade JB, Welling PA. The ARH adaptor protein regulates endocytosis of the ROMK potassium secretory channel in mouse kidney. J Clin Invest 2009;119:3278–89.

[145] Field M, Giebisch G. Steroid effects on renal function. In: Laragh JH, Brenner BM, editors. Hypertension: pathophysiology, diagnosis and management. New York: Raven Press; 1990. p. 1273–85.

[146] Field MJ, Giebisch G. Hormonal control of renal potassium excretion. Kidney Int 1985;27:379–87.

[147] Field MJ, Stanton BA, Giebisch GH. Differential acute effects of aldosterone, dexamethasone and hyperkalemia on distal tubular potassium secretion in the rat kidney. J Clin Invest 1984;74:1792–802.

[148] Field MJ, Stanton BA, Giebisch GH. Influence of ADH on renal potassium handling: a micropuncture and microperfusion study in Brattleboro rats. Kidney Int 1984;25:502–11.

[149] Fila M, Brideau G, Morla L, Cheval L, Deschenes G, Doucet A. Inhibition of K$^+$ secretion in the distal nephron in nephrotic syndrome: possible role of albuminura. J Physiol 2011;14: 3611–21.

[150] Filipovic D, Sackin H. A calcium-permeable stretch-activated cation channel in renal proximal tubule. Am J Physiol 1991; 260:F119–29.

[151] Fisher KA, Binder HJ, Hayslett JP. Potassium secretion by colonic mucosal cells after potassium adaptation. Am J Physiol 1978;231:987–94.

[152] Flynn MA, Woodruff C, Clark J, Chase G. Total body potassium in normal children. Pediatr Res 1972;6:239–45.

[153] Fodstad H, Gonzalez-Rodriguez E, Bron S, Gaeggeler H, Guisan B, Rossier BC, et al. Effects of mineralocorticoid and K$^+$ concentration on K$^+$ secretion and ROMK channel expression in a mouse cortical collecting duct cell line. Am J Physiol Renal Physiol 2009;296:F966–75.

[154] Fraley DS, Adler S. Isohydric regulation of plasma potassium by bicarbonate in the rat. Kidney Int 1976;9:333–43.

[155] Frindt G, Houde V, Palmer LG. Conservation of Na$^+$ vs. K$^+$ by the rat cortical collecting duct. Am J Physiol Renal Physiol 2011;301:F14–20.

[156] Frindt G, Palmer LG. K$^+$ secretion in the rat kidney: Na$^+$ channel-dependent and -independent mechanisms. Am J Physiol Renal Physiol 2009;297:F389–96.

[157] Frindt G, Palmer LG. Effects of dietary K$^+$ on cell-surface expression of renal ion channels and transporters. Am J Physiol Renal Physiol 2010;299:F890–7.

[158] Frindt G, Palmer LG. Apical potassium channels in the rat collecting tubule. Am J Physiol Renal Physiol 2004;287:F1030–7.

[159] Frindt G, Palmer LG. Low-conductance K$^+$ channels in apical membrane of rat cortical collecting tubule. Am J Physiol 1989;256:F143–51.

[160] Frindt G, Palmer LG. Ca-activated K$^+$ channels in apical membrane of mammalian CCT, and their role in K$^+$ secretion. Am J Physiol 1987;252:F458–467.

[161] Frindt G, Shah A, Edvinsson J, Palmer LG. Dietary K$^+$ regulates ROMK channels in connecting tubule and cortical collecting duct of rat kidney. Am J Physiol Renal Physiol 2009;296: F347–54.

[162] Fromter E, Gessner K. Free flow potential profile along rat kidney proximal tubule. Pflugers Arch 1974;351:69–84.

[163] Fujii Y, Mujais SK, Katz AI. Renal potassium adaptation: role of the Na-K-ATP pump in rat cortical collecting tubules. Am J Physiol 1989;256:F79–284.

[164] Fujimoto M, Kubota I, Kotera K. Electrochemical profile of K$^+$ and CI ions across the proximal tubule of bullfrog kidneys. Contrib Nephrol 1977;6:114–23.

[165] Fujita T, Sato Y. Natriuretic and antihypertensive effects of potassium in DOCA-salt hypertensive rats. Kidney Int 1983;24:731–9.

[166] Funder JW, Blair-West JR, Coughlan JP, et al. Effect of plasma (K$^+$) on the secretion of aldosterone. Endocrinology 1969;85: 381–4.

[167] Furuya H, Tabei K, Muto S, Asano Y. Effect of insulin on potassium secretion in the rabbit cortical collecting tubule. Am J Physiol 1991;262:F30–5.

[168] Fuzman RI, Finkinshtein YA, Turner AY. Reflex mechanism of potassium homeostasis regulation. Nefrologia 1985;5:103–8.

[169] Gallazzini M, Attmane-Elakeb A, Mount DB, Hebert SC, Bichara M. Regulation by glucocorticoids and osmolality of expression of ROMK (Kir 1.1), the apical K$^+$ channel of thick ascending limb. Am J Physiol Renal Physiol 2003;284: F977–86.

[170] Galvez A, Gimenez-Gallego G, Reuben JP, Roy-Contancin L, Feigenbaum P, Kaczorowski GJ, et al. Purification and characterization of a unique, potent, peptidyl probe for the high conductance calcium-activated potassium channel from venom of the scorpion Buthus tamulus. J Biol Chem 1990;265:11083–90.

[171] Gamba G. The thiazide-sensitive Na$^+$-Cl$^-$ cotransporter: molecular biology, functional properties, and regulation by WNKs. Am J Physiol Renal Physiol 2009;297:F838–48.

[172] Gamba G, Friedman PA. Thick ascending limb: the Na$^{(+)}$:K $^{(+)}$:2CL$^{(-)}$ co-transporter, NKCC2 and the calcium-sensing receptor, CaSR. Pflugers Arch 2009;458(1):61–74.

[173] Garg LC, Narang N. Ouabain-insensitive K-adenosine triphosphatase in distal nephron segments of the rabbit. J Clin Invest 1988;81:1204–8.

[174] Garg LC, Knepper MA, Burg MB. Mineralocorticoid effects on Na,K-ATPase in individual nephron segments. Am J Physiol 1991;240:F536–44.

[175] Gennari FJ. Hypokalemia. N Engl J Med 1998;339:451–9.

[176] Gennari FJ, Cohen JJ. Role of the kidney in potassium homeostasis: lessons from acid–base disturbances. Kidney Int 1975;8: 1–5.

[177] Giebisch G, Wang W. Potassium transport: from clearance to channels and pumps. Kidney Int 1995;49:1624–31.

[178] Giebisch G. Cell models of potassium transport in the renal tubule [Potassium transport: Physiology and pathophysiology] In: Giebisch G, editor. Current topics in membranes and transport, vol. 28. Orlando, FL: Academic Press; 1987. p. 133

[179] Giebisch G. Renal potassium transport: mechanisms and regulation. Am J Physiol 1998;274:F817—33.

[180] Giebisch G. Some reflections on the mechanism of renal tubular potassium transport. Yale J Biol Med 1975;48:315—36.

[181] Giebisch G. Effects of diuretics on renal transport of potassium. Methods Pharmacol 1976;4A:121—64.

[182] Giebisch G. Renal potassium transport. In: Giebisch G, Tosteson DC, Ussing HH, editors. Membrane transport in biology, vol. IVA. Berlin: Springer-Verlag; 1978. p. 215—98.

[183] Giebisch G. Renal potassium channels: an overview. Kidney Int 1995;48:1004—9.

[184] Giebisch G. Recent advances in the field of renal potassium excretion: what can we learn from potassium channels? Yale J Biol Med 1998;70:311—22.

[185] Giebisch G, deMello-Aires M, Malnic G. Kinetics of potassium transport across single distal tubules of rat kidney. J Physiol 1973;232:47—70.

[186] Giebisch G, K1ein-Robbenhaar G, K1ein-Robbenhaar J, et al. Renal and extrarenal sites of actions of diuretics. Cardiovasc Drugs Ther 1993;7:11—21.

[187] Giebisch G, Wang W-H. Potassium transport — an update. J Nephrol 2010;23(S16):S97—104.

[188] Gonin S, Deschenes G, Roger F, Bens M, Martin PY, Carpentier JL, et al. Cyclic AMP increases cell surface expression of functional Na-K-ATPase units in mammalian cortical collecting duct principal cells. Mol Biol Cell 2001; 13:255—64.

[189] Good DW. Sodium-dependent bicarbonate absorption by cortical thick ascending limb of rat kidney. Am J Physiol 1985;248: F821—9.

[190] Good DW. Effects of potassium on ammonium transport by medullary thick ascending limb of the rat. Am J Physiol 1987;80:1358—65.

[191] Good DW, Velazquez H, Wright FS. Luminal influences on potassium secretion: low sodium concentration. Am J Physiol 1984;246:F609—19.

[192] Good DW, Wright FS. Luminal influences of potassium secretion: sodium concentration and fluid flow rate. Am J Physiol 1979;236:Fl92—205.

[193] Gottschalk CWO. Renal tubular function: lessons from micropuncture. Harvey Lect 1962-63;58:99—124.

[194] Grasset E, Gunter-Smith P, Schultz SG. Effects of Na-coupled alanine transport on intracellular K^+ activities and the K^+ conductance of the basolateral membranes of *Necturus* small intestine. J Membr Biol 1983;71:89—94.

[195] Gray DA, Frindt G, Zhang YY, Palmer LG. Basolateral K^+ conductance in principal cells of rat CCD. Am J Physiol Renal Physiol 2005;288:F493—504.

[196] Greenlee MM, Lynch IJ, Gumz ML, Cain BD, Wingo CS. Mineralocorticoids stimulate the activity and expression of renal H^+,K^+-ATPases. J Am Soc Nephrol 2011;22:49—58.

[197] Greenlee MM, Lynch IJ, Gumz ML, Cain BD, Wingo CS. The renal H,K-ATPases. Curr Opin Nephrol Hypertens 2010;19: 478—82.

[198] Greger R. Ion transport mechanisms in thick ascending limb of Henle's loop of mammalian nephrons. Physiol Rev 1985;65: 760—97.

[199] Greger R, Oberleithner H, Schlatter E, Cassola AC, Weidtke C. Chloride activity in cells of isolated perfused cortical thick ascending limbs of rabbit kidney. Pflugers Arch 1983;399:29—41.

[200] Greger R, Schlatter E. Presence of luminal K, a prerequisite for active NaCl transport in the cortical thick ascending limb of Henle's loop of rabbit kidney. Pflugers Arch 1981;392: 92—4.

[201] Greger R, Schlatter E. Cellular mechanism of the action of loop diuretics on the thick ascending limb of Henle's loop. Klin Woehensehr 1983;61:1019—27.

[202] Greger R, Schlatter E. Properties of the basolateral membrane of the cortical thick ascending limb of Henle's loop of rabbit kidney. A model for secondary active chloride transport. Pflugers Arch 1983;396:325—34.

[203] Greger R, Gogelein H. Role of K^+ conductive pathways in the nephron. Kidney Int 1987;31:1055—64.

[204] Greger R, Schlatter E. Properties of the lumen membrane of the cortical thick ascending limb of Henle's loop of rabbit kidney. Pflugers Arch 1983;396:315—24.

[205] Grimm PR, Foutz RM, Brenner R, Sansom SC. Identification and localization of BK-beta subunits in the distal nephron of the mouse kidney. Am J Physiol Renal Physiol 2007;293: F35—359.

[206] Grimm PR, Irsik DL, Liu L, Holtzclaw JD, Sansom SC. Role of BKbeta1 in Na^+ reabsorption by cortical collecting ducts of Na^+-deprived mice. Am J Physiol Renal Physiol 2009;297: F420—8.

[207] Grimm PR, Irsik DL, Settles DC, Holtzclaw JD, Sansom SC. Hypertension of Kcnmb1$^{-/-}$ is linked to deficient K^+ secretion and aldosteronism. Proc Natl Acad Sci USA 2009;106: 11800—5.

[208] Grimm PR, Sanson SC. BK channels and a new form of hypertension. Kidney Int 2010;78:956—62.

[209] Grupp C, Pavenstadt-Grupp R, Grunewald W, Bevan C, Stokes III JB, Kinne RK. A Na-K-CI cotransporter in isolated rat papillary collecting duct cells. Kidney Int 1989;36:201—9.

[210] Guggino WE, Oberleithner H, Giebisch G. The amphibian diluting segment. Am J Physiol 1988;254:F615—27.

[211] Gumz ML, Lynch IJ, Greenlee MM, Cain BD, Wingo CS. The renal H^+-K^+-ATPases: physiology, regulation, and structure. Am J Physiol Renal Physiol 2010;298:F12—21.

[212] Gunter-Smith PJ, Grasset E, Schultz SG. Sodium-coupled amino acid and sugar transport by *Necturus* small intestine. An equivalent circuit analysis of a rheogenic cotransport system. J Membr Biol 1982;66:25—39.

[213] Hall JE, Granger JP, Smith MJ, Premen AJ. Role of renal hemodynamics and 58: regulation of potassium excretion arterial pressure in aldosterone "escape.". Hypertension 1984;6(Suppl. 1):183—92.

[214] Halperin ML, Gowrishankar M, Mallie JP, Sonnenberg H, Oh M. Urea recycling: an aid to the excretion of potassium during antidiuresis. Nephron 1996;72:507—11.

[215] Hamm LL, Gillespie C, Klahr S. Ammonium chloride inhibits Na^+ and K^+ transport in the cortical collecting tubule. Contrib Nephrol 1985;47:125.

[216] Hayslett JP, Halevy J, Pace PE, Binder HJ. Demonstration of net potassium absorption in mammalian colon. Am J Physiol 1982;242:G209—14.

[217] Hebert SC, Desir G, Giebisch G, Wang WH. Molecular diversity and regulation of renal potassium channels. Physiol Rev 2005;85:319—71.

[218] Hebert SC, Andreoli TE. Control of NaCl transport in the thick ascending limb. Am J Physiol 1984;246:F745—56.

[219] Hebert SC, Friedman PA, Andreoli TE. Effects of antidiuretic hormone on cellular conductive pathways in mouse medullary thick ascending limbs of Henle: 1. ADH increases transcellular conductance pathways. Membr Biol 1984;80:201—9.

[220] Hebert SC, Andreoli TE. Effects of antidiuretic hormone on cellular conductive pathways in mouse medullary thick ascending limbs of Henle: II. Determinants of the ADH-mediated increases in transepithelial voltage and in net Cl$^-$ absorption. J Membr Biol 1984;80:221—33.

[220a] Heller BI, Hammarsten JF, Stutzman FL. Concerning the effects of magnesium sulfate on renal function, electrolyte excretion, and clearance of magnesium. J Clin Invest 1953;32:858—61.

[221] Hierholzer K. Secretion of potassium and acidification in collecting ducts of mammalian kidney. Am J Physiol 1961;201:318—24.

[222] Hierholzer K, Wiederholt M, Holzgreve H, et al. Micropuncture study of renal transtubular concentration gradients of sodium and potassium in adrenalectomized rats. Pflugers Arch 1965;285:193—210.

[223] Higashihara E, Kokko JP. Effects of aldosterone on potassium recycling in the kidney of adrenalectomized rats. Am J Physiol 1985;248:F219—27.

[224] Hirsch J, Leipziger J, Frobe U, Schlatter E. Regulation and possible physiological role of the Ca^{2+}-dependent K$^+$ channel of cortical collecting ducts of the rat. Pflugers Arch 1993;422: 492—8.

[225] Hirsch J, Schlatter E. K channels in the basolateral membrane of rat cortical collecting duct are regulated by a cGMP-dependent protein kinase. Pflugers Arch 1995;429:338—44.

[226] Hirsch J, Schlatter E. K channels in the basolateral membrane of rat cortical collecting duct. Kidney Int 1995;48:1036—46.

[227] Ho K, Nichols CG, Lederer WL, Lytton J, Vassilev PM, Kanazirska MV, et al. Cloning and expression of an inwardly rectifying ATP-regulated potassium channel. Nature 1993;362:31—8.

[228] Holtzclaw JD, Grimm PR, Sansom SC. Intercalated cell BK-alpha/beta4 channels modulate sodium and potassium handling during potassium adaptation. J Am Soc Nephrol 2010;21:634—45.

[228a] Holtzclaw JD, Cornelius RJ, Hatcher LI, Sansom SC. Coupled ATP and potassium efflux from intercalated cells. Am J Physiol Renal Physiol 2011;300:F1319—26.

[229] Hoorn EJ, Nelson JH, McCoprmick JA, Ellison DH. The WNK kinase network regulating sodium, potassium, and blood pressure. J Am Soc Nephrol 2011;22:605—14.

[230] Hoover RS, Angiotensin II. A candidate for an aldosterone-independent mediator of potassium preservation during volume depletion. Kidney Int 2011;79:377—9.

[231] Horisberger J-D, Doucet A. Renal ion translocating ATPases: the P type family 139. In: Seldin DW, Giebisch G, editors. The kidney: physiology and pathophysiology. 3rd ed. Philadelphia: Lippincott Williams & Wilkins; 2002. p. 139—70.

[232] Horisberger J-D, Giebisch G. Potassium-sparing diuretics. Renal Physiol 1987;10:198—200.

[233] Horisberger J-D, Giebisch G. Voltage dependence of the basolateral membrane conductance in the *Amphiuma* collecting tubule. J Membr Biol 1988;105:257—63.

[234] Hropot M, Fowler N, Karlmark B, Giebisch G. Tubular action of diuretics: distal effects on electrolyte transport and acidification. Kidney Int 1985;28:477—89.

[235] Huang C-L, Kuo E. Mechanism of hypokalemia in magnesium deficiency. J Am Soc Nephrol 2007;18:2649—52.

[236] Huang C-L, Yang S-S, Lin S-H. Mechanism of regulation of renal ion transport by WNK kinases. Curr Opin Nephrol Hypertens 2008;17:519—25.

[237] Hunter M. Stretch-activated channels in the basolateral membrane of single proximal cells of frog kidney. Pflugers Arch 1990;416:448—53.

[238] Hunter M, Cohen BJ, Forrest JA, et al. Patch-clamp recordings from cultured amphibian kidney cell (A6). Kidney Int 1984;25:303.

[239] Hunter M, Lopes A, Boulpaep E, Giebisch G. Regulation of single K-channels from apical membrane of rabbit collecting tubule. Am J Physiol 1986;251:F725—33.

[240] Hunter M, Lopes AG, Boulpaep EL, Giebisch GH. Single channel recordings of calcium-activated potassium channels in the apical membrane of rabbit cortical collecting tubules. Proc Natl Acad Sci USA 1984;81:4237—9.

[241] Hurst AM, Beck JS, Laprade R, Lapointe JY. Na$^+$ pump inhibition down regulates an ATP-sensitive K$^+$ channel in rabbit proximal convoluted tubule. Am J Physiol 1993;264:F760—4.

[242] Iino Y, Troy JL, Brenner BM. Effects of catecholamines on electrolyte transport in cortical collecting tubules. J Membr Biol 1981;61:67—73.

[243] Imai M. The connecting tubule: a functional subdivision of the rabbit distal nephron segments. Kidney Int 1979;15:346—56.

[244] Imai M, Nakamura R. Function of distal convoluted and connecting tubules studied by isolated nephron fragments. Kidney Int 1982;22:465—72.

[245] Imai M, Taniguchi J, Tabei K. Function of thin loops of Henle. Kidney Int 1987;31:565—79.

[246] Imai M, Taniguchi J, Yoshitomi K. Transition of permeability properties along the descending limb of long-loop nephron. Am J Physiol 1988;254:F323—8.

[247] Jaeger P, Karlmark B, Giebisch G. Ammonium transport in rat cortical tubule: relationship to potassium metabolism. Am J Physiol 1983;245:F593—600.

[248] Jamison R, Muller-Suur R. Potassium recycling. In: Giebisch G, editor. Current topics in membranes and transport, vol. 28. Orlando: Academic Press; 1987. p. 115—31.

[249] Jamison RL. Potassium recycling. Kidney Int 1987;31:695—703.

[250] Jamison RL, Lacy FB, Pennell JP, Sanjana VM. Potassium secretion by the descending limb of pars recta of the juxtamedullary nephron *in vivo*. Kidney Int 1976;9:323—32.

[251] Jamison RL, Sonnenberg H, Stein JH. Questions and replies: role of the collecting tubule in fluid, sodium, and potassium balance. Am J Physiol 1979;237:F247—61.

[252] Jamison RL, Work J, Schafer JA. New pathways for potassium transport in the kidney. Am J Physiol 1982;242:F297—312.

[253] Kahle KT, Ring AM, Lifton RP. Molecular physiology of the WNK kinases. Annu Rev Physiol 2008;70:329—55.

[254] Kaissling B. Structural aspects of adaptive changes in renal electrolyte excretion. Am J Physiol 1982;243:F211—26.

[255] Kaissling B, Kriz W. Structural analysis of rabbit kidney. Berlin: Springer; 1979.

[256] Kaissling B, LeHir M. Distal tubular segments of the rabbit kidney after adaptation to altered Na- and K-intake. 1. Structural changes. Cell Tissue Res 1982;224:469—92.

[257] Kaissling B, Stanton BA. Adaptation of distal tubule and collecting duct to increased sodium delivery. 1. Ultrastructure. Am J Physiol 1988;255:F1256—68.

[258] Kashgarian M, Biemesderfer D, Caplan M, Forbush III B. Monoclonal antibody to Na, K-ATPase: immunocytochemical localization along nephron segments. Kidney Int 1985;28:899—913.

[259] Katz AI. Renal Na-K-ATPase: its role in tubular sodium and potassium transport. Am J Physiol 1982;242:F207—19.

[260] Kaufman JS, Hamburger RJ. Potassium transport in the isolated proximal convoluted tubule. Am J Physiol 1982;244:F297—313.

III. FLUID AND ELECTROLYTE REGULATION AND DYSREGULATION

[261] Kaufman JS, Hamburger RJ. Passive potassium transport in the isolated proximal convoluted tubule. J Physiol 1985;248: F228—32.

[262] Kawahara K. A stretch-activated K^+ channel in the basolateral membrane of *Xenopus* kidney proximal tubule cells. Pflugers Arch 1990;415:624—9.

[263] Kawahara K, Hunter M, Giebisch G. Calcium-activated potassium channels in the luminal membrane of *Amphiuma* diluting segment: voltage-dependent block by intracellular Na^+ upon depolarisation. Pflügers Archiv 1990;416:422—7.

[264] Kaunitz JD, Barrett KE, McRoberts JA. Electrolyte secretion and absorption: small intestine and colon. In: 2nd ed. Yamada T, editor. Textbook of Gastroenterology, vol. 1. Philadelphia JB: Lippincott; 1995. p. 316—61.

[265] Keith NM, King HE, Osterberg AE. Serum concentration and renal clearance of potassium in severe renal insufficiency in man. Arch Intern Med 1943;71:675—701.

[266] Khuri RN, Strieder WN, Giebisch G. Effects of flow rate and potassium intake on distal tubular potassium transfer. Am J Physiol 1975;228:1249—61.

[267] Khuri R, Wiederholt M, Strieder N, Giebisch G. Effects of graded solute diuresis on renal tubular sodium transport in the rat. Am J Physiol 1975;228:1261—8.

[268] Khuri RN, Agulian SK, Bogharian K. Electrochemical potentials of potassium in proximal renal tubule of rat. Pflugers Arch 1974;346:319—26.

[269] Khuri RN, Strieder N, Giebisch G. Effects of flow rate and potassium intake on distal tubular potassium transfer. Am J Physiol 1975;228:1249—61.

[270] Kibble JD, Wareing M, Wilson RW, Green R. Effect of barium on potassium diffusion across the proximal convoluted tubule of the anesthetized rat. Am J Physiol 1995;268:F778—83.

[271] Kleinman LI, Banks RO. Segmental nephron sodium and potassium reabsorption in newborn and adult dogs during saline expansion. Proc Soc Exp Biol Med 1983;173:231—7.

[272] Knauf H, Mutschler E, Velazquez H, Giebisch G. Torasemide significantly reduces thiazide-induced potassium- and magnesium-loss despite supra-additive natriuresis. Eur J Clin Pharmacol 2009;65:465.

[273] Knox FG, Romero JE. Mechanism for escape from the sodium retaining effects of mineralocorticoids. In: Kaufman XI, Wambach G, Helber A, Meuer KA, editors. Mineralocorticoids and hypertension. Berlin: Springer-Verlag; 1983. p. 81—100.

[274] Koefoed-Johnsen V, Ussing HH. The nature of the frog skin potential. Acta Physiol Scand 1985;42:298—308.

[275] Koeppen BM, Biagi BA, Giebisch GH. Intracellular microelectrode characterization of the rabbit cortical collecting duct. Am J Physiol 1983;244:F35—47.

[276] Koeppen BM, Giebisch G. Mineralocorticoid regulation of sodium and potassium transport by the cortical collecting duct. In: Graves S, editor. Regulation and development of membrane transport processes. New York: Wiley; 1983. p. 89—104.

[277] Koeppen BM. Conductive properties of the rabbit outer medullary collecting duct: inner stripe. Am J Physiol 1985;248: F500—6.

[278] Kokko JP. Variations in the permeability and transport along the distal tubule. Proceedings of the VIIth international congress on nephrology. Basel: Karger; 1978 [225—233]

[279] Kone BE, Renal H-K-ATPase: structure, function, and regulation. Miner Electrolyte Metab 1996;22:349—65.

[280] Kotelevtsev Y, Brown RW, Fleming S, Kenyon C, Edwards CR, Seckl JR, et al. Hypertension in mice lacking 11beta-hydroxysteroid dehydrogenase type 2. J Clin Invest 1999;103: 683—9.

[281] Kriz XI, Bankir L. A standard nomenclature for structures of the kidney. Am J Physiol 1988;254:FI—8.

[282] Kubokawa M, Mori Y, Fujimoto K, Kubota T. Basolateral pH-sensitive K^+ channels mediate membrane potential of proximal tubule cells in bullfrog kidney. Jpn Physiol 1998; 48:1—8.

[283] Kubokawa M, Wang XI, McNicholas CM, Giebisch G. Role of Ca^{2+}/CaMK II in Ca^{2+}-induced K^+ channel inhibition in rat CCD principal cell. Am J Physiol 1995;268:F211—9.

[284] Kubota T, Biagi BA, Giebisch G. Intracellular potassium activity measurements in single proximal tubules of *Necturus* kidney. J Membr Biol 1983;73:51—60.

[285] Kunau RT, Webb ML, Botman SE. Characteristics of the relationship between the flow rate of tubular fluid and potassium transport in the distal tubule of the rat. J Clin Invest 1974;54:1488—95.

[286] Kuwahara M, Ishibashi K, Krapf R, Rector FC Jr, Berry CA. Effect of lumen pH on cell pH and cell potential in rabbit proximal tubules. Am J Physiol 1989;256:F1075—83.

[287] Lachheb S, Cluzeaud F, Bens M, Genete M, Hibino H, Lourdel S, et al. Kir4.1/Kir5.1 channel forms the major K^+ channel in the basolateral membrane of mouse renal collecting duct principal cells. Am J Physiol Renal Physiol 2008;294: F1398—407.

[288] Lalioti MD, Zhang J, Vollkman HM, Kahle KT, Hoffman KE, Toka HR, et al. Wnk4 controls blood pressure and potassium homeostasis via regulation of mass and activity of the distal convoluted tubule. Nature 2006;38:1124—32.

[289] Lang F, Shumilina E. Regulation of ion channels by the serum- and glucocorticoid-inducible kinase SGK1. FASEB J 2012; [Epub ahead of print].

[290] Lapointe JY, Garneau L, Bell PD, Cardinal J. Membrane cross-talk in the mammalian proximal tubule during alterations in transepithelial sodium transport. Am J Physiol 1990;258: F339—45.

[291] Lazrak A, Liu Z, Huang C-L. Antagonistic regulation of ROMK by long and kidney-specific WNK1 isoforms. Proc Natl Acad Sci 2006;103:1615—20.

[292] Leaf A, Camara AA. Renal tubular secretion of potassium in man. J Clin Invest 1949;28:1526—33.

[293] LeGrimellec E. Micropuncture study along the proximal convoluted tubule. Pflugers Arch 1975;354:133—50.

[294] LeGrimellec C, Poujeol P, de Rouffignac E. ^{3}H-inulin and electrolyte concentrations in Bowman's capsule in rat kidney. Pflugers Arch 1975;354:117—31.

[295] LeGrimellec C, Roinel N, Morel F. Simultaneous Mg, Ca, P K, Na and Cl analysis in rat tubular fluid. III. During acute Ca plasma loading. Pflugers Arch 1974;346:171—88.

[296] LeHir M, Kaissling B, Dubach UE. Distal tubular segments of the rabbit kidney after adaptation to altered Na- and K-intake. II. Changes in Na-K-ATPase activity. Cell Tissue Res 1982;224:493—504.

[297] Lehrmann H, Thomas J, Kim SJ, Jacobi C, Leipziger J. Luminal P2Y2 receptor-mediated inhibition of Na^+ absorption in isolated perfused mouse CCD. J Am Soc Nephrol 2002;13:10—8.

[298] Leipziger J. Control of epithelial transport via luminal P2 receptors. Am J Physiol Renal Physiol 2003;284:F419—32.

[299] Lelievre-Pegorier M, Merlet-Benicho C, Roinel N, de Rouffignac C. Developmental pattern of water and electrolyte transport in rat superficial nephrons. Am J Physiol 1983;245: F15—21.

[300] Leviel F, Borensztein B, Houillier P, Paillard M, Bichara M. Electroneutral K^+/HCO_3^- cotransport in cells of medullary thick ascending limb of rat kidney. J Clin Invest 1992;90: 869—78.

[301] Leviel F, Hubner CA, Houillier P, Morla L, El Moghrabi S, Brideau G, et al. The Na$^+$-dependent chloride-bicarbonate exchanger SLC4A8 mediates an electroneutral Na$^+$ reabsorption process in the renal cortical collecting ducts of mice. J Clin Invest 2010;120(5):1627—35.

[302] Levine DZ, Walker T, Nash LA, Raman S. Effects of KCl infusions on proximal tubular function in normal and potassium-depleted rats. Kidney Int 1973;4:318—25.

[303] Li D, Wang Z, Sun P, Jin Y, Lin DH, Hebert SC, et al. Inhibition of MAPK stimulates the Ca^{2+}-dependent big-conductance K$^+$ channels in cortical collecting duct. Proc Natl Acad Sci USA 2006;103:19569—74.

[304] Li Z, Cai T, Tian J, Xie JX, Zhao X, Liu L, et al. NaKtide, a Na/K-ATPase-derived peptide Src inhibitor, antagonizes ouabain-activated signal transduction in cultured cells. J Biol Chem 2009;284:21066—76.

[305] Light DB, McCann FV, Keller TM, Stanton BA. Amiloride-sensitive cation channel in apical membrane of inner medullary collecting duct. Am J Physiol 1988;255:F278—85.

[306] Lin S-H, Cheema-Dhadli S, Gowrishankar M, Marliss EB, Kamel KS, Halperin ML. Control of excretion of potassium: lessons from studies during prolonged total fasting in human subjects. Am J Physiol 1997;273:F796—800.

[307] Linas SL, Peterson LN, Anderson RJ, Aisenbrey GA, Simon FR, Berl T. Mechanism of renal potassium conservation in the rat. Kidney Int 1979;15:601—11.

[308] Lindinger MI, Franklin TW, Lands LC, Pedersen PK, Welsh DG, Heigenhauser GJ. NaHCO$_3$ and KHCO$_3$ ingestion rapidly increases renal electrolyte excretion in humans. J Appl Physiol 2000;88:540—50.

[309] Liu W, Pastor-Soler NM, Schreck C, Zavilowitz B, Kleyman TR, Satlin LM. Luminal flow modulates H$^+$-ATPase activity in the cortical collecting duct (CCD). Am J Physiol Renal Physiol 2011;302:F205—15.

[310] Liu W, Schreck C, Coleman RA, Wade JB, Hernandez Y, Zavilowitz B, et al. Role of NKCC in BK channel-mediated net K$^+$ secretion in the CCD. Am J Physiol Renal Physiol 2011;301: F1088—91.

[311] Liu W, Xu S, Woda C, Kim P, Weinbaum S, Satlin LM. Effect of flow and stretch on the [Ca^{2+}]$_i$ response of principal and intercalated cells in cortical collecting duct. Am J Physiol Renal Physiol 2003;285:F998—1012.

[312] Liu Z, Wang H-R, Huang C-L. Regulation of ROMK channel and K$^+$ homeostasis by kidney-specific WNK1 kinase. J Biol Chem 2009;284:12198—206.

[313] Lorenz JM, Kleinman LI, Disney TA. Renal response of newborn dog to potassium loading. Am J Physiol 1986;251: F513—9.

[314] Lourdel S, Paulais M, Cluzeaud F, Bens M, Tanemoto M, Kurachi Y, et al. An inward rectifier K$^+$ channel at the basolateral membrane of the mouse distal convoluted tubule: similarities with Kir4-Kir5.1 heteromereic channels. J Physiol 2002;538 (2):391—404.

[315] Lu M, Wang WH. Nitric oxide regulates the low-conductance K$^+$ channel in the basolateral membrane of the cortical collecting duct. Am J Physiol 1996;270:C1336—42.

[316] Lu M, Hebert SC, Giebisch G. Hydrolyzable ATP and PIP$_2$ modulate the small-conductance K$^+$ channel in apical membranes of rat cortical collecting duct. J Gen Physiol 2002;120: 603—15.

[317] Lynch IJ, Greenlee MM, Gumz ML, Rudin A, Xin S-L, Wingo CS. Heterogeneity of H-K-ATPase-mediated acid secretion along the mouse collecting duct. Am J Physiol Renal Physiol 2000;298:F408—15.

[318] Madsen KM, Tisher CE. Structural—functional relationships along the distal nephron. Am J Physiol 1986;250:F1—15.

[319] Malnic G. Berliner RW; Giebisch G. Flow dependence of K$^+$ secretion in cortical distal tubules of the rat. Am J Physiol 1989;256:F932—41.

[320] Malnic G, De Mello-Aires M, Giebisch G. Potassium transport across renal distal tubules during acid—base disturbances. Am J Physiol 1971;221:1192—208.

[321] Malnic G, Giebisch G. Some electrical properties of distal tubular epithelium in the rat. Am J Physiol 1972;223:797—808.

[322] Malnic G, Klose RM, Giebisch G. Micropuncture study of renal potassium excretion in the rat. Am J Physiol 1964;206: 674—86.

[323] Malnic G, Klose RM, Giebisch G. Microperfusion study of distal tubular potassium and sodium transfer in rat kidney. Am J Physiol 1966;211:548—99.

[324] Malnic G, Klose RM, Giebisch G. Micropuncture study of distal tubular potassium and sodium transport in rat nephron. Am J Physiol 1966;211:529—47.

[325] Marsh DJ, Ullrich KJ, Rumrich G. Micropuncture analysis of the behavior of potassium ions in rat renal cortical tubules. Pflugers Arch 1963;277:107—19.

[326] Matsumura Y, Cohen B, Guggino WE, Giebisch G. Regulation of the basolateral potassium conductance of the Necturus proximal tubule. J Membr Biol 1984;79:153—61.

[327] Mauerer UR, Boulpaep EL, Segal AS. Properties of an inwardly rectifying ATP-sensitive K$^+$ channel on the basolateral membrane of renal proximal tubule. J Gen Physiol 1998;111:139—60.

[328] Mauerer UR, Boulpaep EL, Segal AS. Regulation of an inwardly rectifying ATP-sensitive K$^+$ channel on the basolateral membrane of renal proximal tubule. J Gen Physiol 1998;111:161—80.

[329] McCance RA, Widdowson EM. Alkalosis with disordered kidney function. Lancet 1937;2:247—9.

[330] McCance R, Widdowson EM. The response of the new-born piglet to an excess of potassium. J Physiol 1958;141:88—96.

[331] McCormick JA, Yang C-L, Ellison DH. WNK kinases and renal sodium transport in health and disease. Hypertension 2008;51:588—96.

[332] Mello-Aires M, Malnic G. Renal handling of sodium and potassium during hypochloremic alkalosis in the rat. Pflugers Arch 1972;331:215—25.

[333] Meneton P, Schultheis PJ, Greeb J, Nieman ML, Liu LH, Clarke LL, et al. Increased sensitivity to K$^+$ deprivation in colonic H, K-ATPase-deficient mice. J Clin Invest 1998;101:536—42.

[334] Meyer JW, Flagella M, Sutliff RL, Lorenz JN, Nieman ML, Weber CS, et al. Decreased blood pressure and vascular smooth muscle tone in mice lacking basolateral Na$^+$-K$^+$-2Cl$^-$ cotransporter. Am J Physiol Heart Circ Physiol 2002;283: H1846—1855.

[335] Michell AR, Debnam ES, Unwin RJ. Regulation of renal function by the gastrointestinal tract: potential role of gut-derived peptides and hormones. Annu Rev Physiol 2008; 70:379—403.

[336] Molony DA, Reeves WB, Hebert SC, Andreoli TE. ADH increases apical NaK-2CI entry in mouse medullary thick ascending limbs of Henle. Am J Physiol 1987;252:F177—87.

[337] Moore-Ede MD, Meguid MM, Fitzpatrick GF, Boyden CM, Ball MR. Circadian variation in response to potassium infusion. Clin Pharmacol Ther 1978;23:218—27.

[338] Moore-Ede MD. Physiology of the circadian timing system: predictive versus reactive homeostasis. Am J Physiol 1986;250: R735—52.

[339] Moore-Ede MC, Herd JA. Renal electrolyte circadian rhythms: independence from feeding and activity patterns. Am J Physiol 1977;232:FI28—35.

[340] Morel F. Sites of hormone action in the mammalian nephron. Am J Physiol 1981;240:FI59—64.

[341] Morgan TO, Tadokoro M, Martin D, Berliner RW. Effect of furosemide on Na$^+$ and K$^+$ transport studied by microperfusion of the rat nephron. Am J Physiol 1970;218:292—7.

[342] Morimoto T, Liu W, Woda C, Carattino MS, Wei Y, Hughey RP, et al. Mechanism underlying flow-stimulation of Na absorption in the mammalian collecting duct. Am J Physiol 2006;291:F663—9.

[343] Morita H, Fujiki N, Miyahara T, Lee K, Tanaka K. Heptoportal bumetanide-sensitive K$^+$-sensor mechanism controls urinary K$^+$ excretion. Am J Physiol 2000;278:R1134—9.

[344] Morsing P, Velazquez H, Wright FS, Ellison DH. Adaptation of the distal convoluted tubule of the rat. II. Effects of chronic thiazide infusion. Am J Physiol 1991;261:FI37—43.

[345] Mudge GH, Ames 3rd A, Foulks J, Gilman A. Effects of drugs on renal secretion of potassium in the dog. Am J Physiol 1950;161:151—8.

[346] Mudge GH, Foulks J, Gilman A. The renal excretion of potassium. Proc Soc Exp Biol Med 1948;67:545—7.

[347] Mudge GH, Foulks J, Gilman A. Renal secretion of potassium in the dog during cellular dehydration. Am J Physiol 1950;161:159—66.

[348] Mujais WK. Renal memory after potassium adaptation: role of Na$^+$-K + -ATPase. Am J Physiol Renal 1988;254:F845.

[349] Mujais SK, Chekal MA, Jones WJ, Hayslett JP, Katz AI. Regulation of renal Na-K ATPase in the rat: role of the natural mineralo- and glucocorticoid hormones. J Clin Invest 1984;73:13—9.

[350] Muto S. Potassium transport in the mammalian collecting duct. Physiol Rev 2001;81:85—116.

[351] Muto S, Asano Y, Seldin D, Giebisch G. Basolateral Na$^+$ pump modulates apical Na$^+$ and K$^+$ conductances in rabbit cortical collecting ducts. Am J Physiol 1999;276:FI43—58.

[352] Muto S, Sansom SC, Giebisch G. Effects of high K$^+$ diet on the electrical properties of cortical collecting ducts from adrenalectomized rabbits. J Clin Invest 1988;81:376—80.

[353] Muto S, Tsuruoka S, Miyata Y, Fujimura A, Kusano E, Wang W, et al. Basolateral Na$^+$/H$^+$ exchange maintains potassium secretion during diminished sodium transport in the rabbit cortical collecting duct. Kidney Int 2009;75:25—30.

[354] Najjar F, Zhou H, Morimoto T, Bruns JB, Li HS, Liu W, et al. Dietary K$^+$ regulates apical membrane expression of maxi-K channels in rabbit cortical collecting duct. Am J Physiol Renal Physiol 2005;289:922—32.

[354a] Náray-Fejes-Tóth A, Canessa C, Cleaveland ES, Aldrich G, Fejes-Tóth G. sgk is an aldosterone-induced kinase in the renal collecting duct. Effects on epithelial Na$^+$ channels. J Biol Chem 1999;274(24):16973—8.

[355] Nichols CG, Ho K, Hebert SC. M$^+$-dependent inward rectification of ROMK1 potassium channels expressed in *Xenopus* oocytes. J Physiol 1994;476:399—409.

[356] O'Neil RG. Aldosterone regulation of sodium and potassium transport in the cortical collecting tubule. Semin Nephrol 1990; l0:365—74.

[357] O'Neil RG, Boulpaep EL. Effect of amiloride on the apical cell membrane cation channels of a sodium-absorbing, potassium-secreting renal epithelium. J Membr Biol 1979;50:365—87.

[358] O'Neil RG, Boulpaep EL. Ionic conductive properties and electrophysiology of the rabbit cortical collecting tubule. Am J Physiol 1982;243:F81—95.

[359] O'Neil RG, Hayhurst RA. Sodium-dependent modulation of the renal Na-K-ATPase: influence of mineralocorticoids on the cortical collecting duct. J Membr Biol 1985;85:169—79.

[360] O'Neil RG, Helman SI. Transport characteristics of renal collecting tubules: influences of DOCA and diet. Am J Physiol 1977;233:F544—58.

[361] O'Neil RG, Sansom SE. Characterization of apical cell membrane Na$^+$ and K$^+$ conductances of cortical collecting duct using microelectrode techniques. Am J Physiol 1984;247: FI4—24.

[362] Oberleithner H, Dietl P, Munich G, Weigt M, Schwab A. Relationship between luminal Na$^+$H$^+$ exchange and luminal K$^+$ conductance in diluting segment of frog kidney. Pflugers Arch 1985;405:5110—4.

[363] Oberleithner H, Giebisch G, Lang F, Wang W. Cellular mechanism of the furosemide sensitive transport system in the kidney. Klin Wochenschr 1982;60:1173—9.

[364] Oberleithner H, Guggino W, Giebisch G. Potassium transport in the distal tubule of *Amphiuma* kidney: effects of potassium adaptation. Pflugers Arch 1983;396:185—91.

[365] Oberleithner H, Guggino W, Giebisch G. The effect of furosemide on luminal sodium, chloride and potassium transport in the early distal tubule of *Amphiuma* kidney: effects of potassium adaptation. Pflugers Arch 1983;396:27—33.

[366] Oberleithner H, Lang F, Greger R, Wang W, Giebisch G. Effect of luminal potassium transport on cellular sodium activity in the early distal tubule of *Amphiuma* kidney. Pflugers Arch 1983;396:34—40.

[367] Oberleithner H, Lang F, Wang W, Giebisch G. Effects of inhibition of chloride transport on intracellular sodium activity in distal amphibian nephron. Pflugers Arch 1982;394:55—60.

[368] Oberleithner H, Weight M, Westphale HD, Wang W. Aldosterone activates Na/H exchange and raises cytoplasmic pH in target cells of the amphibian kidney. Proc Natl Acad Sci USA 1987;84:1464—88.

[369] Oh K-S, Oh YT, Kim S-W, Kita T, Kang I, Youn JH. Gut sensing of dietary K$^+$ intake increases renal K$^+$ secretion. Am J Physiol Integr Comp Physiol 2011;301:R421—9.

[370] Ohno-Shosaku T, Kubota T, Yamaguchi J, Fujimoto M. Regulation of inwardly rectifying K$^+$ channels by intracellular pH in opossum kidney cells. Pflugers Arch 1990; 416:138—43.

[371] Okusa MD, Unwin RJ, Velazquez H, Giebisch G, Wright FS. Active potassium absorption by the renal distal tubule. Am J Physiol 1992;31:F488.

[372] Okusa MD, Velazquez H, Ellison DH, Wright FS. Luminal calcium regulates potassium transport by the renal distal tubule. Am J Physiol 1990;258:F423—8.

[373] Okusa MD, Velazquez H, Wright FS. Effect of Na-channel blockers and lumen Ca on K$^+$ secretion by rat renal distal tubule. Am J Physiol 1991;260:F459—65.

[374] Oliver WJ, Cohen EL, Neel JV. Blood pressure, sodium intake, and sodium related hormones in the Yanomamo Indians, a "no-salt" culture. Circulation 1975;52:146.

[374a] Ookata K, Tojo A, Suzuki Y, Nakamura N, Kimura K, Wilcox CS, Hirose S. Localization of inward rectifier potassium channel Kir7.1 in the basolateral membrane of distal nephron and collecting duct. J Am Soc Nephrol 2000;11:1987—94.

[375] Ornt DB, Radke KJ, Scandling JD. Effect of aldosterone on renal potassium conservation in the rat. Am J Physiol 1996;270: EI003—1008.

[376] Ornt DB, Tannen RL. Demonstration of an intrinsic renal adaptation for K$^+$ conservation in short-term K$^+$ depletion. Am J Physiol 1983;245:F329—38.

[377] Pacha J, Frindt G, Sackin H, Palmer LG. Apical maxi K$^+$ channels in intercalated cells of cortical collecting tubule. Am J Physiol 1991;261:F696—705.

[378] Pallone TL, Cao C, Zhang Z. Inhibition of K$^+$ conductance in descending vasa recta pericytes by ANG II. Am J Physiol Renal Physiol 2004;287:F1213—22.

[379] Palmer LG, Choe H, Frindt G. Is the secretory K⁺ channel in the rat CCT ROMK?. Am J Physiol 1997;273:F404–10.

[380] Palmer LG, Frindt G. High-conductance K⁺ channels in intercalated cells of the rat distal nephron. Am J Physiol Renal Physiol 2007;292:F966–73.

[381] Palmer LG, Sackin H. Regulation of renal ion channels. FASEB J 1988;2:3061–5.

[382] Palmer L. Potassium secretion and the regulation of distal nephron K⁺ channels. Am J Physiol 1999;277:F821–5.

[383] Paulais M, Lachheb S, Teulon J. A Na⁺- and Cl⁻-activated K⁺ channel in the thick ascending limb of mouse kidney. J Gen Physiol 2006;127:205–15.

[383a] Paulais M, Bloch-Faure M, Picard N, Jacques T, Ramakrishnan SK, Keck M, et al. Renal phenotype in mice lacking the Kir5.1 (Kcnj16) K⁺ channel subunit contrasts with that observed in SeSAME/EAST syndrome. Proc Natl Acad Sci USA 2011;108(25):10361–6.

[384] Peterson LN, Wright FS. Effect of sodium intake on renal potassium excretion. Am J Physiol 1977;233:F225–34.

[384a] Petrovic S, Spicer Z, Greeley T, Shull GE, Soleimani M. Novel Schering and ouabain-insensitive potassium-dependent proton secretion in the mouse cortical collecting duct. Am J Physiol Renal Physiol 2002;282(1):F133–43.

[385] Pluznick JL, Sansom SC. BK channels in the kidney: role in K⁺ secretion and localization of molecular components. Am J Physiol Renal Physiol 2006;291:F517–29.

[386] Pluznick JL, Wei P, Carmines PK, Sansom SC. Renal fluid and electrolyte handling in BKCa-beta1⁻/⁻ mice. Am J Physiol Renal Physiol 2003;284:F1274–1279.

[387] Pluznick JL, Wei P, Grimm PR, Sansom SC. BK-β1 subunit: immunolocalization in the mammalian connecting tubule and its role in the kaliuretic response to volume expansion. Am J Physiol Renal Physiol 2005;288:F846–54.

[388] Praetorius HA, Leipziger J. ATP release from non-excitable cells. Purinergic Signalling 2009;5:433–46.

[389] Praetoriuis HA, Leipziger J. Intrarenal purineregic signaling in the control of renal tubular transport. Annu Rev Physiol 2010;72:377–93.

[390] Proverbio F, Whittembury G. Cell electrical potential during enhanced Na extrusion in guinea-pig cortex slices. J Physiol 1975;250:559–78.

[391] Rabelink TJ, Koomans HA, Hene J, Dorhout-Mees EJ. Early and late adjustment to potassium loading in humans. Kidney Int 1990;38:942–7.

[392] Rabinowitz L. Aldosterone and renal potassium excretion. Renal Physiol (Basel) 1979-80;2:229–43.

[393] Rabinowitz L. Homeostatic regulation of potassium excretion. J Hypertens 1989;7:433–42.

[394] Rabinowitz L, Aizman RI. The central nervous system in potassium homeostasis. Frontiers in Neuroendocrinol 1993; 14:1–26.

[395] Rabinowitz L, Berlin R, Yamauchi H. Plasma potassium and diurnal cyclic potassium excretion in the rat. Am J Physiol 1987;253:F1178–81.

[396] Rabinowitz L, Gunther RA. Renal potassium excretion in sheep during sodium sulfate, phosphate, and chloride infusion. Am J Physiol 1978;234:F371–5.

[397] Rabinowitz L, Wydner CJ, Smith KM, Yamauchi H. Diurnal potassium excretory cycles in the rat. Am J Physiol 1986;250:F930–41.

[398] Rastegar A, Biemesderfer D, Kashgarian M, Hayslett JP. Changes in membrane surfaces of collecting duct cells in potassium adaptation. Kidney Int 1980;18:293–301.

[399] Rector Jr FC, Bloomer HA, Seldin DW. Proximal tubular reabsorption of potassium during mannitol diuresis in rats. J Lab Clin Med 1964;63:100–5.

[400] Reeves WE, Shah SV. Activation of potassium channels contributes to hypoxic injury in proximal tubules. J Clin Invest 1994;94:2289–94.

[401] Reeves WE, Winters Q, Zimniak L, Andreoli TE. Medullary thick limbs: renal concentrating segments. Kidney Int 1996;50: S154–64.

[401a] Reichold M, Zdebik AA, Lieberer E, Rapedius M, Schmidt K, Bandulik S, et al. KCNJ10 gene mutations causing EAST syndrome (epilepsy, ataxia, sensorineural deafness, and tubulopathy) disrupt channel function. Proc Natl Acad Sci USA 2010;107(32):14490–5.

[402] Reineck HJ, Osgood RW, Ferris TF, Stein JH. Potassium transport in the distal tubule and collecting duct of the rat. Am J Physiol 1975;219:1403–9.

[403] Reineck HJ, Osgood RW, Stein JH. Net potassium addition beyond the superficial distal tubule of the rat. Am J Physiol 1978;235:F104–10.

[404] Riccardi D, Hall AE, Chattopadhyay N, Xu JZ, Brown EM, Hebert SC. Localization of the extracellular Ca²⁺-(polyvalent) cation-sensing receptor in kidney. Am J Physiol Renal Physiol 1998;274:F611–22.

[405] Riccardi D, Lee WS, Lee K, Segre GV, Brown EM, Hebert SC. Localization of the extracellular Ca²⁺-sensing receptor and PTH/PTHrP receptor in rat kidney. Am J Physiol 1996;271: F951–6.

[406] Rieg T, Bundey RA, Chen Y, Deschenes G, Junger W, Insel PA, et al. Mice lacking P2Y2 receptors have salt-resistant hypertension and facilitated renal Na⁺ and water reabsorption. FASEB J 2007;21:3717–26.

[407] Rieg T, Vallon V, Sausbier M, Sausbier U, Kaissling B, Ruth P, et al. The role of the BK channel in potassium homeostasis and flow-induced renal potassium excretion. Kidney Int 2007;72: 566–73.

[408] Rocafull MA, Romero FJ, Thomas LE, del Castillo JR. Isolation and cloning of the K⁺-independent, ouabain-insensitive Na⁺-ATPase. Biochim Biophys Acta 2011;1808:1684–700.

[409] Rocha AS, Kokko JP. Sodium chloride and water transport in the medullary thick ascending limb of Henle: evidence for active chloride transport. J Clin Invest 1973;52:612–23.

[410] Rocha AS, Kudo LH. Water, urea, sodium, chloride, and potassium transport in the in vitro isolated perfused papillary collecting duct. Kidney Int 1982;22:485–91.

[411] Rodan AR, Cheng C-J, Huang C-L. Recent advances in distal tubular potassium handling. Am J Physiol Renal Physiol 2011;300:F821–7.

[412] Rodan AR, Huang C-L. Distal potassium handling based on flow modulation of maxi-K channel activity. Curr Opin Nephrol Hypertens 2009;18:350–6.

[413] Rodriguez HJ, Hogan WE, Hellman RN, Klahr S. Mechanism of activation of renal Na⁺-K⁺-ATPase in the rat: effects of potassium loading. Am J Physiol 1980;238:F315–23.

[414] Rodriguez HJ, Sinha SK, Starling J, Klahr S. Regulation of renal Na⁺-K⁺ATPase in the rat by adrenal steroids. Am J Physiol 1981;241:F186–95.

[415] Rosetti L, Robbenhaar GK, Giebisch G, Smith D, DeFronzo R. Effect of insulin on renal potassium metabolism. Am J Physiol 1987;252:F60–4.

[416] Rubera I, Loffing J, Palmer LG, Frindt G, Fowler-Jaeger N, Sauter D, et al. Collecting duct-specific gene inactivation of αENaC in the mouse kidney does not impair sodium and potassium balance. J Clin Invest 2003;112:554–65.

[417] Rutledge JC, Rabinowitz L. Kaliuretic regulatory factors in the rat. Am J Physiol Renal Physiol 1987;253:F1182–96.

[418] Sabolic I, Herak-Kramberger CM, Breton S, Brown D. Na/K-ATPase in intercalated cells along the rat nephron

revealed by antigen retrieval. J Am Soc Nephrol 1999;10: 913—22.

[419] Sackin H. Stretch-activated potassium channels in renal proximal tubule. Am J Physiol 1987;241:F540—55.

[420] Sackin H, Boulpaep EL. Isolated perfused salamander proximal tubule. II. Monovalent ion replacement and rheogenic transport. Am J Physiol 1981;241:F540—55.

[421] Sackin H, Boulpaep EL. Rheogenic transport in rhe renal proximal tubule. J Gen Physiol 1983;82:819—51.

[422] Salman IM, Sattar MA, Abdullah NA, Ameer OZ, Basri F, Hussain NM, et al. Role of renal sympathetic nervous system in the control of renal potassium handling. J Nephrol 2010;23:291—6.

[423] Sampio MS, Bezerra IP, Pecanha FL, Fonseca PH, Capella MA, Lopes AG. Lack of Na^+,K^+-ATPase expression in intercalated cells may be compensated by Na^+-ATPase: a study on MDCK-C11 cells. Cell Mol Life Sci 2008;65:3093—9.

[424] Sansom SE, Agulian S, Muto S, Illig V, Giebisch G. K activity of CCD principal cells from normal and DOCA-treated rabbits. Am J Physiol 1989;256:F136—42.

[425] Sansom SE, Muto S, Giebisch G. Na-dependent effects of DOCA on cellular transport properties of CCDs from ADX rabbits. Am J Physiol 1987;253:F753—9.

[426] Sansom SC, O'Neil RG. Mineralocorticoid regulation of apical cell membrane Na^+ and K^+ transport of rhe cortical collecring duct. *Am J*. Am J Physiol 1985;248:F858—68.

[427] Sansom SE, O'Neil RG. Effects of mineralocorticoids on transport properties of cortical collecting duct basolateral membrane. Am J Physiol 1986;241:F743—57.

[428] Sastrasinh S, Tannen RL. Effect of potassium on renal NH3 production. Am J Physiol 1983;244:F383—91.

[429] Satlin LM. Postnatal maturation of potassium transport in rabbit cortical collecting duct. Am J Physiol 1994;266:F57—65.

[430] Satlin LM. Regulation of potassium transport in the maturing kidney. Semin Nephrol 1999;19(2):155—65.

[431] Satlin LM, Palmer LG. Apical K^+ conductance in maturing rabbit principal cell. Am J Physiol 1997;272:F397—404.

[432] Satlin LM, Palmer LP. The apical Na^+ conductance in the maturing rabbit principal cell. Am J Physiol 1996;279:F391—7.

[433] Satlin LM, Sheng S, Woda CB, Kleyman TR. Epithelial sodium channels are regulated by flow. Am J Physiol 2001;280:F1010—8.

[434] Sauer M, Flemmer A, Thurau K, Beck FX. Sodium entry routes in principal and intercalated cells of the isolated perfused cortical collecting duct. Pflugers Arch 1990;416:88—93.

[435] Scandling JD, Ornt DB. Mechanism of potassium depletion during chronic metabolic acidosis in the rat. Am J Physiol 1987;252:Fl22—130.

[436] Schafer C, Westphale HJ, Oberleithner H. Contrasting action of H^+ and Ca^{2+} on K^+-transport in diluting segment of frog kidney. Cell Physiol Biochem 1991;1:286—93.

[437] Schafer JA, Troutman SL. Effect of ADH on rubidium transport in isolated perfused rat cortical collecting tubule. Am J Physiol 1986;250:F1063—72.

[438] Schafer JA, Troutman SL, Schlatter E. Vasopressin and mineralocorticoid increase apical membrane driving force for K^+ secretion in rat CCD. Am J Physiol 1990;258:F199—210.

[439] Schafer JA, Work J. Transport properties of the pars recta. Nephrology 1985;1:186—95.

[440] Schlatter E, Bleich M, Hirsch J, Markstahler U, Fröbe U, Greger R. Cation specificity and pharmacological properties of the Ca^{2+}-dependent K^+ channel of rat cortical collecting ducts. Pflugers Arch 1993;422:481—91.

[441] Schlatter E, Lohrmann E, Greger R. Properties of the potassium conductances of principal cells of rat cortical collecting ducts. Pflugers Arch 1992;420:39—45.

[442] Schlatter E. Regulation of ion channels in the cortical collecting duct. Renal Physiol Biochem 1993;16:21—36.

[443] Schlatter E. Antidiuretic hormone regulation of electrolyte transport in the distal nephron. Renal Physiol Biochem 1989;12:65—84.

[444] Schlatter E, Greger R, Widtke C. Effect of "high ceiling" diuretics on active salt transport in the cortical thick ascending limb of Henle's loop of rabbit kidney. Correlation of chemical structure and inhibitory potency. Pflugers Arch 1983;396:210—7.

[445] Schlatter E, Haxelmans S, Ankorina I. Correlation between intracellular activities of Ca^{2+} and Na^+ in rat cortical collecting duct: a possible coupling mechanism between Na^+-K^+-ATPase and basolateral K^+ conductance. Kidney Blood Press Res 1996;19:24—31.

[446] Schlatter E, Haxelmans S, Hirsch J, Leipziger J. pH dependence of K^+ conductances of rat cortical collecting duct principal cells. Pflugers Arch 1994;428:631—40.

[447] Schlatter E, Schafer JA. Electrophysiological studies in principal cells of rat cortical collecting tubules. ADH increases the apical membrane Na^+-conductance. Pflugers Arch 1987;409: 81—92.

[448] Schmidt U, Horster M. Na-K-activated ATPase: activity maturation in rabbit nephron segments dissected *in vitro*. Am J Physiol 1977;233:F55—60.

[449] Schmidt U, Schmid J, Schmid H, Dubach UC. Sodium- and potassium-activated ATPase. A possible target of aldosterone. J Clin Invest 1975;55:655—60.

[450] Schmitt R, Ellison DH, Farman N, Rossier BC, Reilly RF, Reeves WB, et al. Developmental expression of sodium entry pathways in rat nephron. Am J Physiol 1999;276:F367—381.

[451] Schnermann J, Steipe B, Briggs JP. *In situ* studies of distal convoluted tubule in rat. II. K^+ secretion. Am J Physiol 1987;252: F970—6.

[452] Schon DA, Backman KA, Hayslett JP. Role of the medullary collecting duct in potassium excretion in potassium-adapted animals. Kidney Int 1981;20:655—62.

[453] Schultz SG. Homocellular regulatory mechanisms in sodium-transporting epithelia: avoidance of extinction by "flush-through". Am J Physiol 1981;21:F579—90.

[454] Schultz SG. Homocellular regulatory mechanisms in sodium-transporting epithelia: an extension of the Koefoed-Johnsen-Ussing model. Semin Nephrol 1982;2:343—7.

[455] Seldin DW, Welt LG, Cart JH. The role of sodium salts and adrenal steroids in the production of hypokalemic alkalosis. Yale J Biol Med 1956;29:229—47.

[456] Shirley DG, Walter SJ, Folkerd EJ, Unwin RJ, Bailey MA. Transepithelial electrochemical gradient in the proximal convoluted tubule during potassium depletion in the rat. J Physiol (Lond) 1998;513:551—7.

[457] Silver RB, Choe H, Frindt G. Low-NaCI diet increases H-K-ATPase in intercalated cells from rat cortical collecting duct. Am J Physiol 1998;275:F94—102.

[458] Silver RB, Frindt G, Mennitt P, Satlin LM. Characterization and regulation of H-K-ATPase in intercalated cells of rabbit cortical collecting duct. J Exp Zool 1997;279:443—55.

[459] Silver RB, Frindt G. Functional identification of H^+/K^+-ATPase in intercalated cells of cortical collecting tubule. Am J Physiol 1993;264:F259—66.

[460] Silver RB, Mennitt PA, Satlin LM. Stimulation of apical H-K-ATPase in intercalated cells of cortical collecting duct with chronic metabolic acidosis. Am J Physiol 1996;270: F539.

[461] Simon BB, Karel FE, Rodriguez-Soriano J, Hamdan JH, DiPietro A, Trachtman H, et al. Genetic heterogeneity of

Bartter's syndrome revealed by mutations in the K⁺ channel, ROMK. Nature Gen 1996;14:152—6.

[462] Solomon S. Absolute rates of sodium and potassium reabsorption by proximal tubule of immature rats. Biol Neonate 1974;25:340—51.

[463] Sonnenberg H. Medullary collecting duct function in antidiuretic and in salt- or water-diuretic rats. Am J Physiol 1974;226:501—6.

[464] Stanton BA. Characterization of apical and basolateral membrane conductances of rat inner medullary collecting duct. Am J Physiol 1989;256:F862—8.

[465] Stanton B. Regulation by adrenal corticosteroids of sodium and potassium transport in loop of Henle and distal tubule of rat kidney. J Clin Invest 1986;78:1612—20.

[466] Stanton B. Renal potassium adaptation: cellular mechanisms and morphology. In: Giebisch G, editor. Current topics in membranes and transport, vol. 28. Orlando: Academic Press; 1987. p. 225—67.

[467] Stanton B, Kaissling B. Adaptation of distal tubule and collecting duct to increased sodium delivery. II. Na⁺ and K⁺ transport. Am J Physiol 1988;255:FI269—1275.

[468] Stanton B, Giebisch G, Klein-Robbenhaar G, Wade J, DeFronzo RA. Effects of adrenalectomy and chronic adrenal corticosteroid replacement on potassium transport in rat kidney. J Clin Invest 1985;75:1317—26.

[469] Stanton B, Pan L, Deetjen P, Guckian V, Giebisch G. Independent effects of aldosterone and potassium on induction of potassium adaptation in rat kidney. Clin Invest 1987;79:198—206.

[470] Stanton BA. Renal potassium transport: morphological and functional adaptations. Am J Physiol 1989;257:R989—97.

[471] Stanton BA, Biemesderfer D, Wade JB, Giebisch G. Structural and functional study of the rat distal nephron: effects of potassium adaptation and potassium depletion. Kidney Int 1981;19:36—48.

[472] Stanton BA, Giebisch G. Effects of pH on potassium transport by renal distal tubule. Am J Physiol 1982;242:F544—51.

[473] Stanton BA, Giebisch G. Renal potassium transport Renal physiology In: Windhager EE, editor. Handbook of physiology. New York: Oxford University Press; 1991. p. 813—74.

[474] Stanton BA, Giebisch GH. Potassium transport by the renal distal tubule: effects of potassium loading. Am J Physiol 1982;243:F487—93.

[475] Stanton BA, Guggino WB, Giebisch G. Acidification of the basolateral solution reduces potassium conductance of the apical membrane. Ped Proc 1982;41:1006.

[476] Stanton BA, Janzen A, Klein-Robbenhaar G, DeFronzo RA, Wade J, Giebisch G. Ultrastructure of rat initial collecting tubule: effect of adrenal corticosteroid treatment. J Clin Invest 1985;75:1327—34.

[477] Sterns RH. Oscillations of plasma K⁺ and insulin during K⁺ infusion in awake anephric dogs. Am J Physiol 1982;243:F44—52.

[478] Sterns RH, Cox M, Feig PU, Singer I. Internal potassium balance and the control of the plasma potassium concentration. Medicine 1981;60:339—54.

[479] Sterns RH, Cox M, Feig PU, Singer I. Internal potassium balance and the control of the plasma potassium concentration. Medicine (Baltimore) 1981;60:339—54.

[480] Sterns RH, Feig PU, Pring M, Guzzo J, Singer I. Disposition of intravenous potassium in anuric man: a kinetic analysis. Kidney Int 1979;15:651—60.

[481] Stetson DL, Wade JB, Giebisch G. Morphologic alterations in the rat medullary collecting duct following potassium depletion. Kidney Int 1980;17:45—56.

[482] Stokes JB. Potassium intoxication: pathogenesis and treatment. In: Seldin DW, Giebisch G, editors. The regulation of potassium balance. New York: Raven Press; 1989. p. 269—302.

[483] Stokes JB. Potassium secretion by cortical collecting tubule: relation to sodium absorption, luminal sodium concentration, and transepithelial voltage. Am J Physiol 1981;241:F395—402.

[484] Stokes JB. Consequences of potassium recycling in the renal medulla. Effects on ion transport by the medullary thick ascending limb of Henle's loop. J Clin Invest 1982;70:219—29.

[485] Stokes JB. Ion transport by the cortical and outer medullary collecting tubule. Kidney Int 1982;22:473—84.

[486] Stokes JB. Na and K⁺ transport across the cortical and outer medullary collecting tubule of the rabbit: evidence for diffusion across the outer medullary portion. Am J Physiol 1982;242:F514—20.

[487] Stokes JB. Ion transport by the collecting duct. Semin Nephrol 1993;13:202—12.

[488] Stokes JB, Ingram MJ, Williams AD, Ingram D. Heterogeneity of the rabbit collecting tubule: localization of mineralocorticoid hormone action to the cortical portion. Kidney Int 1981;20:340—7.

[489] Stoner LC, Burg MB, Orloff J. Ion transport in cortical collecting tubule: effect of amiloride. Am J Physiol 1974;227(2):453—9.

[490] Stoner LC, Viggiano SC. Environmental KCl causes an upregulation of apical membrane maxi K⁺ and ENaC channels in everted Ambystoma collecting tubule. J Membr Biol 1998;162:107—16.

[491] Stoner LC, Viggiano SC. Elevation of basolateral K⁺ induces K⁺ secretion by apical maxi K⁺ channels in Abystoma collecting tubule. Am J Physiol 1999;276:R616—621.

[492] Stow LR, Gumz ML, Lynch IJ, Greenlee MM, Rudin A, Cain BD, et al. Aldosterone modulates steroid receptor binding to the endothelin-1 gene (edn1). J Biol Chem 2009;284:30087—96.

[493] Subramanya AR, Yang C-L, McCormick JA, Ellison DH. WNK kinases regulate sodium chloride and potassium transport by the aldosterone-sensitive distal nephron. Kidney Int 2006;70:630—4.

[494] Sufit CR, Jamison RL. Effect of acute potassium load on reabsorption in Henle's loop in the rat. Am J Physiol 1983;245:F569—76.

[495] Suh A, DeJesus E, Rosner K, Lerma E, Yu W, Young JB, et al. Racial differences in potassium disposal. Kidney Int 2004;66:1076—81.

[496] Sulyok E, Nemeth M, Tenyi I, Csaba IF, Varga F, Gyory E, et al. Relationship between maturity, electrolyte balance and the function of the renin—angiotensin—aldosterone system in newborn infants. Biol Neonate 1979;35:60—5.

[496a] Sun A, Grossman EB, Lombardi M, Hebert SC. Vasopressin alters the mechanism of apical Cl⁻ entry from Na⁺:Cl⁻ to Na⁺:K⁺:2Cl⁻ cotransport in mouse medulltary thick ascending limb. J Membr Biol 1991;120:83—94.

[497] Sun P, Liu W, Lin DH, Yue P, Kemp R, Satlin LM, et al. Epoxyeicosatrienoic acid activates BK channels in the cortical collecting duct. J Am Soc Nephrol 2009;20:513—23.

[497a] Suzuki Y, Yasuoka Y, Shimohama T, Nishikitani M, Nakamura N, Hirose S, Kawahara K. Expression of the K⁺ channel Kir7.1 in the developing rat kidney: role in K⁺ excretion. Kidney Int 2003;63:969—75.

[498] Tabei K, Muto S, Furuya H, Sakairi Y, Ando Y, Asano Y. Potassium secretion is inhibited by metabolic acidosis in rabbit cortical collecting ducts in vitro. Am J Physiol Renal 1995;268:F490—5.

[499] Taniguchi J, Imai M. Flow-dependent activation of maxi K^+ channels in apical membrane of rabbit connecting tubule. J Membr Biol 1998;164:35−45.

[500] Taniguchi J, Tsuruoka S, Mizuno A, Sato J, Fujimura A, Suzuki M. TRPV4 as a flow sensor in flow-dependent K^+ secretion from the cortical collecting duct. Am J Physiol Renal Physiol 2007;292:F667−73.

[501] Tannen RL. Effect of potassium on renal acidification and acid−base homeostasis. Semin Nephrol 1987; 7:263−72.

[502] Tannen RL. Potassium and acid−base balance. In: Giebisch G, editor. Current topics in membranes and transport, vol. 28. Orlando: Academic Press; 1987. p. 207−23.

[503] Teulon J, Anagnostopoulos T. Proximal cell K^+ activity: technical problems and dependence on plasma K^+ concentration. Am J Physiol 1982;243:FI2−8.

[504] Tian J, Xie Z-J. The Na-K-ATPase and calcium-signaling microdomains. Physiol 2008;23:205−11.

[505] Tomita K, Pisano J, Knepper MA. Control of sodium and potassium transport in the cortical collecting duct of the rat. Effects of bradykinin, vasopressin, and deoxycorticosterone. J Clin Invest 1985;76:132−6.

[506] Toussaint C, Vereerstraeten P. Effects of blood pH changes on potassium excretion in the dog. Am J Physiol 1962;202: 768−72.

[507] Tsai TD, Shuck ME, Thompson DP, Bienkowski MJ, Lee Ks. Intracellular H^+ inhibits a cloned rat outer medullary K^+ channel expressed in *Xenopus* oocytes. Am J Physiol 1995;268: C1173−8.

[508] Tsuchiya K, Wang W, Giebisch G, Welling PA. ATP is a coupling modulator of parallel Na^+/K^+ ATPase-K^+ channel activity in the renal proximal tubule. Proc Natl Acad Sci USA 1992;89:6418−22.

[509] Tsuruoka S, Koseki C, Muto S, Tabei K, Imai M. Axial heterogeneity of potassium transport across hamster thick ascending limb of Henle's loop. Am J Physiol Renal 1994;267:F121.

[510] Tudvad F, McNamara H, Barnett HL. Renal response of premature infants to administration of bicarbonate and potassium. Pediatrics 1954;13:4−16.

[511] Unwin R, Capasso G, Giebisch G. Potassium and sodium transport along the loop of Henle: effects of altered dietary potassium intake. Kidney Int 1994;46:1092−9.

[512] Unwin RJ, Capasso G, Giebisch G, et al. Loop of Henle (LOH) potassium transport and the urinary concentrating mechanism. In: DeSanto NG, Capasso G, editors. Acid−base and electrolyte balance. Naples: Institute Italy Pere Gli Studi Filosofici; 1995. p. 243−56.

[513] Unwin R, Capasso G, Giebisch G Water and electrolyte transport along the rat loop of Henle: effect of chronic dietary potassium adaptation and restriction. In: Proceedings of the 11th International Congress of Nephrology. Tokyo: 1990;493a.

[514] Ussing HH. The alkali metal ions in isolated systems and tissues. Handbuch der experimentellen Pharmakologie. Heidelberg: SpringerVerlag; 1960 [1−195]

[515] Ussing HH, Leaf A. Transport across multimembrane systems. In: Giebisch G, Tosteson DC, Ussing HH, editors. Membrane transport in biology, vol. 3. New York: Springer-Verlag; 1978. p. 1.

[516] Vallon V, Grahammer F, Richter K, Bleich M, Lang F, Barhanin J, et al. Role of KCNE1-dependent K^+ fluxes in mouse proximal tubule. J Am Soc Nephrol 2001;12:2003−11.

[517] Vallon V. P2 receptors in the regulation of renal transport mechanisms. Am J Physiol Renal Physiol 2008;294:F10−27.

[518] Vallon V, Grahammer F, Volkl H, Sandu CD, Richter K, Rexhepaj R, et al. KCNQ1-dependent transport in renal and

gastrointestinal epithelia. Proc Natl Acad Sci 2005;102(49): 17864−9.

[519] Vallon V, Osswald H, Blantz RC, Thomson S. Potential role of luminal potassium in tubuloglomerular feedback. J Am Soc Nephrol 1997;8:1831−7.

[520] Vallon V, Wulff P, Huang DY, Loffing J, Völkl H, Kuhl D, et al. Role of Sgk1 in salt and potassium homeostasis. Am J Physiol Regul Integr Comp Physiol 2005;288:R4−10.

[521] Velazquez H, Ellison DH, Wright FS. Chloride-dependent potassium secretion in early and late distal tubules. Am J Physiol 1987;253:F555−562.

[522] Velazquez H. Thiazide diuretics. Renal Physiol 1987;10: 184−97.

[523] Velazquez H, Giebisch G. Effects of diuretics on specific transport systems. Semin Nephrol 1988;8:295−304.

[524] Velazquez H, Wright FS. Control by drugs of renal potassium handling. Annu Rev Pharmacol Toxicol 1986;26:293−309.

[525] Velazquez H, Wright FS. Effects of diuretic drugs on Na, Cl, and K^+ transport by rat renal distal tubule. Am J Physiol 1986;250:FI013−l023.

[526] Velazquez H, Wright FS, Good DW. Luminal influences on potassium secretion: chloride replacement with sulfate. Am J Physiol 1982;242:F46−55.

[527] Verrey F. Early aldosterone effects. Exp Nephrol 1998;6:294−301.

[528] Vestri S, Malnic G. Mechanism of potassium transport across proximal tubule epithelium in the rat. Braz J Med Biol Res 1990;23:1195−9.

[529] Wade JB, Fang L, Coleman RA, Liu J, Grimm PR, Wang T, et al. Differential regulation of ROMK (Kir1.1) in distal nephron segments by dietary potassium. Am J Physiol Renal Physiol 2011;300:F1385−93.

[530] Wade JB, O'Neil RG, Pryor JL, Boulpaep EL. Modulation of cell membrane area in renal collecting tubules by corticosteroid hormones. J Cell Biol 1979;81:439−45.

[531] Wade JB, Stanton BA, Field MJ, Kashgarian M, Giebisch G. Morphological and physiological responses to aldosterone: time course and sodium dependence. Am J Physiol 1990;259: F88−94.

[532] Wagner CA. New roles for renal potassium channels. J Nephrol 2010;23(1):5−8.

[533] Wall SM, Knepper MA, Hassell KA, Fischer MP, Shodeinde A, Shin W, et al. Hypotension in NKCC1 null mice: role of the kidneys. Am J Physiol Renal Physiol 2006;290:F409−416.

[534] Wall SM, Koger LM. NH_4 transport mediated by Na^+K^+-ATPase in rat inner medullary collecting duct. Am J Physiol 1994;167:F660−70.

[535] Wang T. Renal outer medullary potassium channel knockout models reveal thick ascending limb function and dysfunction. Clin Exp Nephrol 2012;16:49−54.

[536] Wang T, Malnic G, Giebisch G, Chan YL. Renal bicarbonate absorption in the rat: 4. Bicarbonate transport mechanisms in the early and late distal tubule. J Clin Invest 1993;91:2776−84.

[537] Wang T, Wang W, Klein-Robbenhaar G, Giebisch G. Effects of a novel KATP channel blocker on renal tubule function and.K channel activity. J Pharmacol Exp Ther 1995;273:1382−9.

[538] Wang T, Wang W, Klein-Robbenhaar G, Giebisch G. Effects of glyburide on renal tubule transport and potassium-channel activity. Renal Physiol Biochem 1995;18:169−82.

[538a] Wang T, Yang CL, Abbiati T, Schultheis PJ, Shull GE, Giebisch G, et al. Mechanism of proximal tubule bicarbonate absorption in NHE3 null mice. Am J Physiol 1999;277(2 Pt 2): F298−302.

[539] Wang W, Giebisch G. Regulation of potassium (K) handling in the renal collecting duct. Pflugers Arch 2009;458:157−68.

[540] Wang W, Hebert SC, Giebisch G. Renal K$^+$ channels: structure and function. Annu Rev Physiol 1997;59:413−6.

[541] Wang W. Two types of potassium channels in thick ascending limb of rat kidney. Am J Physiol 1994;267:F599−605.

[542] Wang WH, Geibel J, Giebisch G. Mechanism of apical K$^+$ channel modulation in principal renal tubule cells. J Gen Physiol 1993;101:673−94.

[543] Wang WH. Regulation of the hyperpolarization-activated K$^+$ channel in the lateral membrane of the cortical collecting duct. J Gen Physiol 1995;106:25−43.

[544] Wang W, Geibel J, Giebisch G. Regulation of the small conductance K$^+$ channels in the apical membrane of rat cortical collecting tubule. Am J Physiol 1990;259:F494−502.

[545] Wang W, Henderson RM, Geibel J, White S, Giebisch G. Mechanism of aldosterone-induced increase of K$^+$ conductance in early distal renal tubule cells of the frog. J Membr Biol 1989;111:277−89.

[546] Wang WH. View of K$^+$ secretion through the apical K$^+$ channel of cortical collecting duct. Kidney Int 1995;48:1024−30.

[547] Wang WH, Lu M, Hebert SC. P450 metabolites mediate extracellular Ca^{2+}-induced inhibition of apical K$^+$ channels in the thick ascending limb of the rat kidney. Am J Physiol 1996;266:F813−22.

[548] Wang W-H, Yue P, Sun P, Lin D-H. Regulation and function of potassium channels in aldosterone-sensitive distal nephron. Curr Opin Nephrol Hypertens 2010;19:463−70.

[549] Wang XY, Masilamani S, Nielsen J, Kwon TH, Brooks HL, Nielsen S, Knepper MA. The renal thiazide-sensitive Na-Cl cotransporter as a mediator of the aldosterone-escape phenomenon. J Clin Invest 2001;108:215−22.

[550] Wareing M, Wilson RW. Kibble JD, Green R. Estimated potassium reflection coefficient in perfused proximal convoluted tubules of the anaesthetized rat in vivo. J Physiol 1995;488.1:153−61.

[551] Warnock DG, Eveloff J. K-Cl cotransport systems. Kidney Int 1989;36:412−7.

[552] Wasserman AG, Agus ZS. Potassium secretion in the rabbit proximal straight tubule. Am J Physiol 1983;245:FI67−74.

[553] Watson JF, Clapp IR, Berliner RW. Micropuncture study of potassium concentration in proximal tubule of dog, rat, and Necturus. J Clin Invest 1964;43:595−605.

[554] Wei Y, Babilonia E, Sterling H, Jin Y, Wang W-H. Mineralocorticoids decrease the activity of the apical small-conductance K$^+$ channel in the cortical collecting duct. Am J Physiol Renal Physiol 2005;289:F1065−71.

[555] Wei Y, Zavilowitz B, Satlin LM, Wang W-H. Angiotensin II inhibits the ROMK-like small conductance K$^+$ channel in renal cortical collecting duct during dietary potassium restriction. J Biol Chem 2007;282:6455−62.

[556] Wei Y, Zavilowitz B, Ren J, Liui W, Chan P, Estilio G, et al., Angiotensin type 2 (AT2) receptor regulates renal potassium secretory channel activity during high dietary potassium adaptation. (personal communication)

[557] Weinbaum S, Duan Y, Satlin LM, Wang T, Weinstein AM. Mechanotransduction in the renal tubule. Am J Physiol Renal Physiol 2010;299:F1220−1236.

[558] Weiner ID, Milton AE. H$^+$-K$^+$-ATPase in rabbit cortical collecting duct B-type intercalated cell. Am J Physiol 1996;270:F518−30.

[559] Weinstein AM. Modeling the proximal tubule: complications of the paracellular pathway. Am J Physiol 1988;254:F297−305.

[560] Weinstein AM. A mathematical model of rat distal convoluted tubule. II. Potassium secretion along the connecting segment. Am J Physiol Renal Physiol 2005;289:721−41.

[561] Welling PA. "Cross-talk" and the role of KATP channels in the proximal tubule. Kidney Int 1995;48:1017−23.

[562] Welling PA, Chang Y-PC, Delpire E, Wade JB. Multigene kinase network, kidney transport, and salt in essential hypertension. Kidney Int 2010;77:1063−9.

[563] Welling PA, Ho K. A comprehensive guide to the ROMK potassium channel: form and function in health and disease. Am J Physiol Renal Physiol 2009;297:F849−63.

[564] Welling PA, O'Neil RG. Cell swelling increases basolateral membrane Cl and K$^+$ conductances of the rabbit proximal straight tubule. Kidney Int 1987;31:452.

[565] West ML, Bendz O, Chen CB, Singer GG, Richardson RM, Sonnenberg H, et al. Development of a test to evaluate the transtubular potassium concentration gradient in the cortical collecting duct in vivo. Miner Electrolyte Metab 1986;12:226−33.

[566] West ML, Marsden PA, Richardson RM, Zettle RM, Halperin ML. New clinical approach to evaluate disorders of potassium excretion. Miner Electrolyte Metab 1986;12:234−8.

[567] Westphale HI, Schafer C, Oberleithner H. Aldosterone stimulates cellular K$^+$ uptake and K$^+$ release in the diluting segment of the frog kidney. Cell Physiol Biochem 1991;1:89−97.

[568] Whittembury G, Grantham RR. Cellular aspects of renal sodium transport and cell volume regulation. Kidney Int 1976;9:103−20.

[569] Wingo CS. Potassium transport by the medullary collecting tubule of the rabbit: effects of variation in K$^+$ intake. Am J Physiol 1987;253:Fl136−1141.

[570] Wingo CS. Potassium secretion by the cortical collecting tubule: effect of CI gradients and ouabain. Am J Physiol 1989;256:F306−13.

[571] Wingo CS, Cain BD. The renal H-K-ATPase: physiological significance and role in potassium homeostasis. Annu Rev Physiol 1993;55:323−47.

[572] Wingo CS, Straub SS. Active proton secretion and potassium absorption in the rabbit outer medullary collecting duct. Functional evidence for proton potassium-activated adenosine triphosphatase. J Clin Invest 1989;84:361−5.

[573] Wirz H. Untersuchungen ueber die Nierenfinktion in adrenalektomierten Katzen. Relv Physiol Pharmacol Acta 1945;3:589.

[574] Woda CB, Bragin A, Kleyman TR, Satlin LM. Flow-dependent K$^+$ secretion in the cortical collecting duct is mediated by a maxi-K channel. Am J Physiol 2001;280:F786−93.

[575] Woda CB, Miyawaki N, Ramalakshmi S, Ramkumar M, Rojas R, Zavilowitz B, et al. Ontogeny of flow-stimulated potassium secretion in rabbit cortical collecting duct: functional and molecular aspects. Am J Physiol Renal Physiol 2003;285:F629−639.

[576] Woodhall PB, Tisher CC. Response of the distal tubule and cortical collecting duct to vasopressin in the rat. J Clin Invest 1973;52:3095−108.

[577] Work I, Jamison RL. Effect of adrenalectomy on transport in the rat medullary thick ascending limb. J Clin Invest 1987;80:1160−4.

[578] Work I, Troutman SL, Schafer JA. Transport of potassium in the rabbit pars recta. Am J Physiol 1982;242:F226−37.

[579] Wright FS. Renal potassium handling. Semin Nephrol 1987;7:174−84.

[580] Wright FS. Increasing magnitude of electrical potential along the renal distal tubule. Am J Physiol 1971;220:624−38.

[581] Wright FS. Sites and mechanisms of potassium transport along the renal tubule. Kidney Int 1977;11:415−32.

[582] Wright FS. Flow dependent transport processes: filtration, absorption, secretion. Am J Physiol 1982;243:FI–ll.

[583] Wright FS, Giebisch G. Renal potassium transport: contributions of individual nephron segments and populations. Am J Physiol 1978;235:F515–27.

[584] Wright FS, Schnermann J. Interference with feedback control of glomerular filtration rate by furosemide, triflocin and cyanide. J Clin Invest 1974;53:1695–708.

[585] Wright FS, Strieder N, Fowler NB, Giebisch G. Potassium secretion by distal tubule after potassium adaptation. Am J Physiol 1971;221:437–48.

[586] Xu Z-C, Yang Y, Hebert SC. Phosphorylation of the ATP-sensitive, inwardly-rectifying K^+ channel, ROMK, by cyclic AMP-dependent protein kinase. J Biol Chem 1996;271:9313–9.

[587] Yang L, Frindt G, Palmer LG. Magnesium modulates ROMK channel-mediated potassium secretion. J Am Soc Nephrol 2010;21:2109–16.

[588] Yasui M, Marples D, Belusa R, Eklof AC, Celsi G, Nielsen S, et al. Development of urinary concentrating capacity: role of aquaporin-2. Am J Physiol 1996;271:F461–468.

[589] Yeyati NL, Etcheverry JC, Adrogue HJ. Kaliretic response to potassium loading in amiloride-treated dogs. Ren Physiol Biochem 1990;13:190–9.

[589a] Yoo D, Kim BY, Campo C, Nance L, King A, Maouyo D, Welling PA. Cell surface expression of the ROMK channel is regulated by the aldosterone-induced kinase, SGK-1, and protein kinase A. J Biol Chem 2003;278:23066–75.

[589b] Yoo D, Flagg TP, Olsen O, Raghuram V, Foskett JK, Welling PA. Assembly and trafficking of a multiprotein ROMK channel complex by PDZ interactions. J Biol Chem 2004;279:6863–73.

[590] Yoshitomi K, Shimizu T, Taniguchi I, Imai M. Electrophysiological characterization of rabbit distal convoluted tubule cell. Pflugers Arch 1989;414:457–63.

[591] Youn JH, McDonough AA. Recent advances in understanding integrative control of potassium homeostasis. Annu Rev Physiol 2009;71:381–401.

[592] Younes-Ibrahim M, Barlet-Bas C, Buffin-Meyer B, Cheval L, Rajerison R, Doucet A. Ouabain-sensitive and -insensitive K-ATPases in rat nephron: effect of K^+ depletion. Am J Physiol 1995;268:F1141–7.

[593] Young DB. Relationship between plasma potassium concentration and renal potassium excretion. Am J Physiol 1982;242:F599–603.

[594] Young DB. Quantitative analysis of aldosterone role in potassium regulation. Am J Physiol 1988;255:FI269–l275.

[595] Young DB, Jackson TE. Effects of aldosterone on potassium distribution. Am J Physiol 1982;243:R526–30.

[596] Young DB, Jackson TE, Tipayamontri U, Scott RC. Effects of sodium intake on steady-state potassium excretion. Am J Physiol 1984;246:F772–8.

[597] Young DB, Paulsen AW. Interrelated effects of aldosterone and plasma potassium on potassium excretion. Am J Physiol 1983;244:F28–34.

[598] Yue P, Lin D-H, Pan C-Y, Leng Q, Giebisch G, Lifton RP, et al. Src family protein tyrosine kinase (PTK) modulates the effect of SGK1 and WNK4 on ROMK channels. Proc Natl Acad Sci USA 2009;106:15061–6.

[599] Yue P, Sun P, Lin D-H, Pan C, Xing W, Wang W-H. Angiotensin II diminishes the effect of SGK1 on the WNK4-mediated inhibition of ROMK1 channels. Kidney Int 2010;79 (4):423–31.

[600] Zalups RK, Stanton BA, Wade JB, Giebisch G. Structural adaptation in initial collecting tubule following reduction in renal mass. Kidney Int 1985;27:636–42.

[601] Zeidel ML, Seifter JL, Lear S, Brenner BM, Silva P. Atrial peptides inhibit oxygen consumption in kidney medullary collecting duct cells. Am J Physiol 1986;251:F379–83.

[602] Zheng D, Perianayagam A, Lee DH, Brannan MD, Yang LE, Tellalian D, et al. AMPK activation with AICAR provokes an acute fall in plasma $[K^+]$. Am J Physiol Cell Physiol 2008;294: C126–35.

[603] Zhou HS, Tate S, Palmer LG. Primary structure and functional properties of an epithelia K^+ channel. Am J Physiol 1994;166: C809–24.

[604] Zhuang J, Zhang X, Wang D, Li J, Zhou B, Shi Z, et al. WNK4 kinase inhibits Maxi K^+ channel activity by a kinase-dependent mechanism. Am J Physiol Renal Physiol 2011;301:F410–9.

[605] Zink H, Horster M. Maturation of diluting capacity in loop of Henle of rat superficial nephrons. Am J Physiol 1977;33: F519–24.

[606] Zolonitskaya A, Satlin LM. Developmental expression of ROMK in rat kidney. Am J Physiol 1999;276:F825–36.

[607] Zuber AM, Centeno G, Pradervand S, Nikolaeva S, Maquelin L, Cardinaux L, et al. Molecular clock is involved in predictive circadian adjustment of renal function. Proc Natl Acad Sci USA 2009;106(38):16523–8.

III. FLUID AND ELECTROLYTE REGULATION AND DYSREGULATION

Physiopathology of Potassium Deficiency

Francesco Trepiccione, Miriam Zacchia and Giovambattista Capasso

Chair of Nephrology, Department of Internal Medicine, Faculty of Medicine, Second University of Naples, Italy

INTRODUCTION

Hypokalemia is a common clinical disorder that can be the end-result of: (1) potassium (K^+) redistribution between plasma and intracellular fluid (ICF); (2) insufficient K^+ intake; (3) disproportionate K^+ excretion. It is commonly defined as a plasma K^+ concentration less than 3.5 mmol/L, but this level infrequently causes trouble unless it has fallen rapidly: patients are usually symptomatic when plasma K^+ is lower than 2.5 mmol/L. Major muscle weakness have a tendency to occur at plasma K^+ less than 2 mmol/L.

The average K^+ intake in a typical western diet is roughly 70 mmol.[1] The intestine absorbs almost all of the ingested K^+; only negligible quantities of K^+ are excreted in the feces. The kidney plays an important role in K^+ balance, which is the result of glomerular filtration, extensive proximal tubule reabsorption, and highly regulated secretory/reabsorbtive processes located along the distal tubule and the collecting duct (CD).[2] Total body K^+ is roughly 55 mmol/kg of body weight, with 98% distributed to the intracellular fluid (primarily in muscle, liver, and erythrocytes) and 2% in the extracellular fluid. Na/K-ATPase actively pumps K^+ into the cell and preserves the electrochemical gradient between the intra- and extracellular pool.

NEW CONCEPTS ON THE INTEGRATIVE CONTROL OF K^+ HOMEOSTASIS

Feedback Control of K^+ Homeostasis

A large increase in plasma K^+ concentration triggers aldosterone release from the adrenal glands. Aldosterone, in turn, stimulates the activity and synthesis of both Na/K-ATPase and luminal K^+ channels in CD principal cells, thus promoting K^+ excretion.[3]

In addition, aldosterone enhances K^+ secretion in the distal colon, which can exert an essential role when renal function is reduced.[4]

On the other hand, if plasma K^+ concentration decreases as a consequence of reduced K^+ intake or increased K^+ excretion, then feedback regulation redistributes K^+ from ICF to plasma. At the same extent, skeletal muscle becomes insulin-resistant to K^+ (but not glucose) uptake, blocks the entry of K^+ from plasma into the cell. Hypokalemia also causes a decreased expression of skeletal muscle Na/K-ATPase 2 isoform, thus allowing a leak of K^+ from ICF to the plasma.[5] The low plasma K^+ concentration suppresses adrenal aldosterone release so that the kidney reduces urinary K^+ excretion.

Feedforward Control of K^+ Homeostasis

However, besides the classic feedback control, some findings suggest a feedforward control.[6] It is clear that plasma K^+ stimulates aldosterone secretion only at supra-physiological levels, with little effect within the physiological range.[7] Indeed, it has been shown that, in sheep, a meal intake produced a substantial kaliuresis in the absence of changes in plasma aldosterone concentration.[8] From these experiments it was concluded that the increased renal K^+ excretion following a meal cannot be explained by changes in aldosterone concentration, but it may be dependent on the existence of a kaliuretic reflex arising from *sensors* in the splanchnic bed (i.e., gut, portal circulation, and/or liver) (Figure 50.1).

One of the potential effectors of the feedforward control of serum K^+ is glucagon. Glucagon secretion is definitely stimulated after a protein-rich meal, and intraportal glucagon infusion produces significant increases in renal blood flow and glomerular filtration

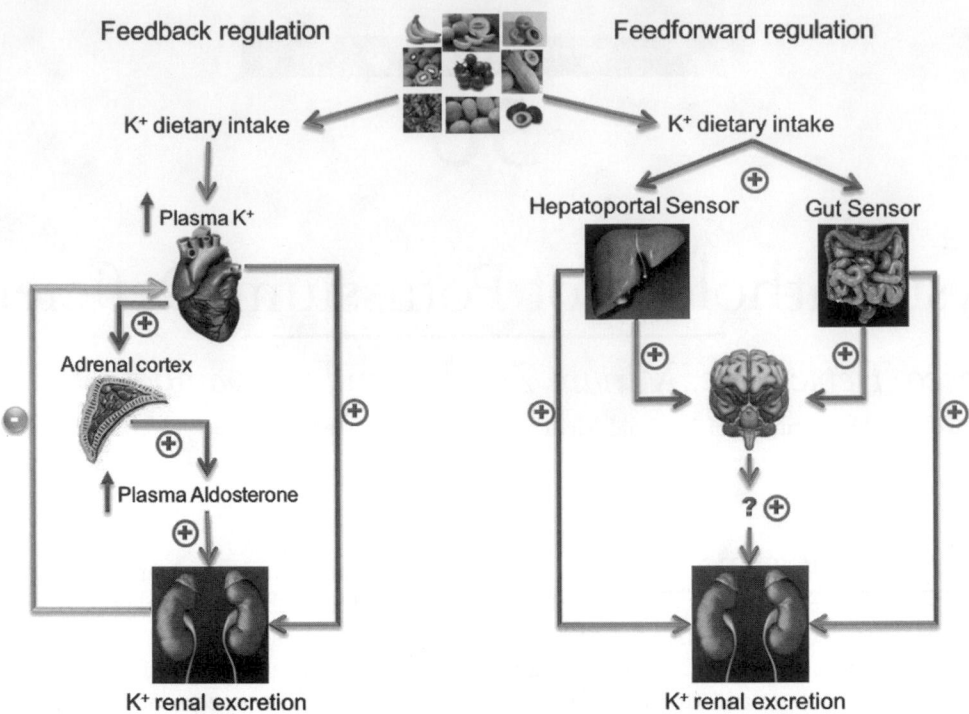

FIGURE 50.1 Schematic diagram illustrating feedback versus feedforward control of K⁺ homeostasis. Left: In feedback control, an increase in ECF [K⁺] is the signal that stimulates urinary K⁺ excretion. Right: In feedforward control, an increase in [K⁺] in the gut is sensed during K⁺ intake and stimulates urinary K⁺ excretion independently from a rise in ECF [K⁺].

rate (GFR), suggesting the existence of a hepatorenal axis.[9]

The feedforward regulation may act through three different mechanisms: (1) insulin release rapidly stimulates cellular K⁺ uptake into insulin-responsive tissues; (2) glucagon, through cAMP released from the liver, quickly increases renal K⁺ excretion after a protein-rich meal; (3) a yet-unidentified gut factor senses K⁺ ingestion and enhances renal K⁺ excretion. When plasma K⁺ level increases despite these layers of control, feedback regulation is activated. Aldosterone acts only after a certain time, it is not involved in rapid control of K⁺ homeostasis, but it can chronically increase K⁺ secretion until plasma K⁺ is normalized.[6]

Assessment of Urinary K⁺ Excretion

Several urine parameters are used to identify whether hypokalemia is dependent on renal loss. Renal K⁺ excretion can be assessed with a 24 hour urine collection or a spot urine test determining the K⁺: creatinine ratio. A 24-hour urinary K⁺ excretion lower than 15 mEq or a K⁺ (mmol)/creatinine (mmol) ratio <1 suggests an extrarenal cause of hypokalemia.

In the clinical practise, as an initial test to address the origin of K⁺ losses, a random urine K⁺ is used. However, this approach is hampered by the effect of renal water handling on urine K⁺ concentration. Determining the transtubular K⁺ gradient (TTKG) is still an accepted way to assess renal K⁺ handling:

$$TTKG = [uk/(uOsmolality/sOsmolality)]/sk$$

Tubular fluid K⁺ concentration in the last part of the CD is mainly dependent on aldosterone, because most K⁺ secretion takes place in the CD. Thereafter, urinary K⁺ concentration increases as a consequence of water reabsorption. The TTKG reflects the tubular fluid K⁺ concentration at the end of the cortical CD, by accounting for water reabsorption that takes place distal of where K⁺ secretion has ended.

However, there are few limitations to the clinical use of this formula.[10] First, the calculation assumes that there is no significant solute transport and only water reabsorption along the medullary CD. Any Na⁺ or urea reabsorption in this segment would tend to lower urine osmolality and cause the TTKG to overestimate the gradient for K⁺ secretion in the upstream CD. Second, there must be optimal conditions for K⁺ secretion at the time that the TTKG is measured. In this regard, urinary Na⁺ should be no less than 25 mEq/L, to guarantee that Na⁺ delivery to the CD is not rate-limiting in K⁺ secretion. In addition, urine osmolality should be equal to or higher than the plasma. A higher urine osmolality indicates increased vasopressin release, which is known to stimulate K$^+$ secretion in the CD.

Hypokalemia Associated With Intracellular Shift

The regulation of K$^+$ distribution between the intracellular and extracellular space is known as internal K$^+$ balance. Even though the kidney is in charge of the preservation of total body K$^+$, factors that adjust internal balance are central to the removal of acute K$^+$-loads. A large K$^+$ intake could potentially double extracellular K$^+$ concentration in the absence of a rapid shift into the cells. This process is mainly regulated by insulin and catecholamines, with a minor role of metabolic and respiratory alkalosis.

Hypokalemic periodic paralysis is a rare disorder characterized by muscle weakness or paralysis as a result of the sudden movement of K$^+$ into cells. Measurement of the TTKG at the time of the attacks typically shows values of $<$1. The attacks may be triggered by exercise, stress, intake of large quantities of carbohydrates, and increased release of catecholamines or insulin.[11]

This disorder is classified as primary, due to a genetic defect or acquired, due to drugs or glandular diseases. The genetic forms are associated with mutations in genes encoding for subunits of muscular sodium, calcium, and potassium channels. Mutations in the α-subunit of the calcium channel [dihydropyridine (DHP)-receptor] (CACNA1S) gene and the α-subunit of the sodium channel (SCN4A) have been described. Loss of function mutations of CACNA1S reduce current density. A mutation in the KCNJ2 gene encoding for the inward-rectifying potassium channel Kir2.1 causes Andersen-Tawil syndrome, characterized by the triad of periodic muscle weakness, cardiac arrhythmias, and multiple dysmorphic features (short stature, hypertelorism, micrognathia).[12] Whether hypokalemia determines the attack is not well-established. The onset of attacks occurs generally between 15 and 35 years of age; the severity of the clinical manifestations range from rare episodes in a lifetime to daily and severe attacks. The attacks can be triggered by all conditions which favor hypokalemia, such as physical exercise, a carbohydrate-rich meal, alcohol, and cold. Myalgia after the attack is a frequent complaint. The acquired form is mainly associated with thyrotoxicosis. Excess thyroid hormone may predispose to paralytic episodes by increasing Na/K-ATPase activity. The activity of this pump is further induced by catecholamines, which are typically increased in this setting. The underlying cause of thyrotoxicosis is most commonly Graves disease, but it can also be a solitary thyroid adenoma

(Plummer disease).[13] The acute attacks of hypokalemic periodic paralysis are best treated with intravenous KCl and propranolol.

It is important to administer KCl in non-dextrose-containing solutions, because glucose will stimulate insulin release, potentially exacerbating K$^+$ shift into the cells. Propranolol (a nonspecific adrenergic β-blocker) blocks the effects of catecholamines, and inhibits the peripheral conversion of T4 to T3.

Extrarenal K$^+$ Loss from the Body

Diarrhea is a common cause of hypokalemia due to gastrointestinal loss. Secretory diarrhea may be the consequence of two processes that can occur either alone or together. First, it may be related to inhibition of active intestinal NaCl and NaHCO$_3$ reabsorption and, second, it may be dependent on increased active secretion of Cl$^-$ coupled to passive secretion of an identical quantity of Na$^+$ in order to maintain the electrochemical balance. Under both circumstances, the stool electrolyte composition is analogous to plasma with a high concentration of NaCl and a much lower K$^+$ concentration. Despite the low K$^+$ concentration in the stool, large K$^+$ losses can take place in the setting of large fecal fluid volume.

Hypokalemia may also be associated with infectious diarrhea. In particular, malaria and leptospirosis may cause alterations in fluid and electrolyte balance. Hypokalemia is particularly frequent in children with severe malaria, and may arise within several hours of initiation of therapy. Hypokalemia develops in about one-third of patients with leptospirosis. Such patients are at risk of both gastrointestinal and renal losses. In the outer membrane of the organism there is a substance that has an inhibitory effect on the Na/K-ATPase within the nephron. It has been hypothesized that this inhibitory effect reduces Na$^+$ reabsorption along the proximal tubule, thus increasing distal Na$^+$ delivery, resulting in kaliuresis.[14] Hypokalemia may also be associated with watery diarrhea and achlorhydria, a condition secondary to hypersecretion of vasoactive intestinal polypeptide (VIP). In adults, this syndrome is most commonly a complication of pancreatic islet cell tumors, and sometimes of bronchogenic carcinoma, medullary thyroid carcinoma or retroperitoneal histiocytoma. There are now few reports describing chronic watery diarrhea and hypokalemia due to adrenal pheochromocytoma containing immunoreactive VIP.[15]

A recent report describes five consecutive patients with acute or subacute colonic pseudo-obstruction suffering a typical secretory diarrhea characterized by very high fecal K$^+$ concentrations (over 100 mEq/kg)

and low Na$^+$ concentration (Ogilvie syndrome). These elevated fecal concentrations of K$^+$ in large volume diarrhea induced important outputs of K$^+$ salts responsible for profound hypokalemia and decreased urinary excretion of K$^+$.[16]

RENAL K$^+$-LOSING SYNDROMES

Bartter Syndrome (BS)

BS results from a defect in any of the major components of NaCl reabsorbtive machinery along the TAL. So far, mutations of five genes have been described. The defect determines renal loss of water and electrolytes resulting in hypovolemia, with a compensatory increase in renin and aldosterone levels.

Genetic and Molecular Biology

BS type I is sustained by mutations of the SLC12A1 gene, encoding the kidney-specific furosemide-sensitive NKCC2.[17] A number of point mutations have been described in homozygosis or compound heterozygosis, mostly frameshift and non-conservative missense mutations. To date, over 30 mutations in the SLC12A1 gene have been reported[18]; phenotypic variability among patients with SLC12A1 mutations may be due to the effect of genetic mutations on protein function, and milder phenotypes may correlate with residual NKCC2 function.[19]

BS type II depends on inactivating mutations of the KCNJ1 gene, encoding the K$^+$ channel ROMK.[20] These channels are the main renal K$^+$ secretory channels. Along the TAL, ROMK mediates K$^+$ efflux to the lumen, which is critical for supporting Na/K-2Cl absorption via NKCC2. At this level of the nephron, ROMK channels contribute to the generation of the lumen-positive transepithelial voltage which allows paracellular calcium and magnesium absorption. An inactivating mutation of ROMK is thought to inhibit salt reabsorption along the TAL. Over 35 genetic mutations have been described, such as missense mutations, frameshift mutations, and stop codons which result in a truncated protein.[21] The majority of these mutations reduces or eliminates ROMK surface expression, as a consequence of misfolding and/or mistrafficking; others compromise K$^+$ permeation and channel regulation. Besides the TAL, ROMK channels are also expressed along the apical membrane of principal cells in the cortical CD, where they mediate K$^+$ secretion into the lumen. A defect in ROMK results in the classical BS phenotype, including the presence of hypokalemia. This finding brought attention to its role in K$^+$ secretion. Subsequent studies have demonstrated that, in the absence of functional ROMK channels, K$^+$ secretion is guaranteed by the upregulation of flux-sensitive Maxi-K channels along the CD in mice.[22]

BS type III depends on the mutation of the kidney-specific Cl$^-$ channel, CLC-K. Two genes belonging to the CLC family are involved in Cl$^-$ efflux across the basolateral membrane, CLCNKA and CLCNKB. Their products are nearly identical at protein level, and both channels are associated with the Barttin subunit, essential for their insertion on plasma membrane and their activity. These channels differ only in their distribution along the nephron, with CLC-Ka expressed predominantly along the TAL, while CLC-Kb is expressed along the DT.[23] CLCKNB defects are associated with a Bartter phenotype in humans; a high rate of deletions encompassing the entire gene has been described,[24] together with frameshift and splice-site mutations. These mutations are supposed to disrupt the protein, altering its function. The predominant location of CLCKb along the DT explains why this variant of BS is less commonly associated with a defect in concentrating mechanism, and with hypercalciuria. There is no evidence CLCKNA mutations may generate a Bartter like syndrome. ClCk1 (the ortholog of CLC-Ka)-deficient mice show a phenotype of nephrogenic diabetes insipidus.[25] However a combination of defects in both CLCNKA and CLCNKB genes result in a phenotype of antenatal BS.[23]

BS type IV refers to the mutations in the BSND gene product. In contrast to other BS variants, the gene does not encode for an ion channel or transporter, but for an accessory subunit of CLC-Ka and CLC-Kb, defined as Barttin. CLC-K/Barttin Cl$^-$ channels also localize in the cochlea, along the basolateral membrane of marginal cells of the stria.[26] Barttin has been found mutated in patients suffering from BS; different mutations generate phenotypes of varying severity. In heterologous expression, CLC-K channels do not yield currents in the absence of a functional Barttin subunit, suggesting that Barttin is essential for their function. As in the TAL, CLC-K channels participate in Cl$^-$ reabsorption in the inner ear. Recent studies have shown that the Barttin subunit is essential for the generation of endocochlear potential; in the absence of Barttin, the degeneration of cochlear outer cells and the collapse of endolymphatic space may contribute to the pathogenesis of deafness in this BS subtype.[27]

BS type V depends on the activating mutation of the calcium-sensing receptor (CaSR). The protein is expressed in the parathyroid and in the kidney, and it is mainly involved in calcium and magnesium homeostasis. Along the TAL the CaSR is expressed on the basolateral membrane and it can inhibit salt absorption. A case report showed that activating mutations of the CaSR gene associated with a BS phenotype inhibit ROMK, explaining the inhibition of salt absorption at this site.[28] A number of gain-of-function mutations of the CaSR gene have been identified as causing an inherited form of hypocalcemia/hypoparathyroidism (autosomal-dominant hypoparathyroidism). Whether those disarrangements lead to a different phenotype is still unknown.

Mutations in these five genes do not explain all cases of BS, and many patients do not get a genetic diagnosis. It is presumable that other genes are involved in the pathogenesis of this syndrome. Recently a role has been proposed for claudins, a family of transmembrane proteins expressed within the tight junction. Mutation in claudin-16 is associated with familiar hypomagnesemia with hypercalciuria and nephrocalcinosis. A single nucleotide substitution has been found in the extracellular domain of claudin-8 in four African-American BS patients.[29] The effect of the mutation on protein function has not yet been addressed.

Pathophysiology

The defective NaCl absorption along the TAL caused by mutations in any of these five genes leads to an increased salt delivery to the distal nephron. The subsequent volume-depletion leads to a compensatory hyper-reninemia. Mice models of BS type I and II show early onset of polyuria, metabolic alkalosis, increased calcium and magnesium urinary excretion, and hyper-prostaglandinemia, a phenotype which resembles the abuse of loop diuretics. The activation of RAAS leads to a compensatory increase in Na$^+$ absorption along the PT and the aldosterone-sensitive segments of the nephron. The latter favors K$^+$ secretion along the CD, enhancing the kaliuretic effect of the increased Na$^+$ delivery. Clinical differences among BS subtypes depend on the specific physiological role of the causative gene in the kidney and in other organs.

Type II BS is characterized by relatively mild hypokalemia compared with type I, and by the dual role of ROMK in the kidney in controlling NaCl absorption along the TAL (through K$^+$ recycling) and K$^+$ secretion along the CD. The presence of hypokalemia is ensured by the activation of the flux-sensitive Maxi-K channels which mediate urinary K$^+$ secretion along the distal nephron. However, newborn infants suffering from type II BS show transient hyperkalemia before developing normohypokalemia later in the infancy. This effect may be due to the delay in BK-dependent K$^+$ secretion, which later is responsible for urinary K$^+$ excretion.[30]

The widespread distribution of CLC-K channels along the distal nephron and the compensatory activation of Cl$^-$ absorption through other channels explains why CLCKNB mutations may result in a pure BS phenotype, GS phenotype or a combination of these.[23] Hypercalciuria and nephrocalcinosis are typical signs

of type I and II BS, but are rare in type III[24]; however, a broad spectrum of phenotypes has been associated with mutations of the CLCNKB gene, ranging from antenatal BS to classic BS and Gitelman-like syndrome, without any correlation with the type of genetic mutation. Additional studies are needed for a better understanding of the phenotypic variability.

The presence of deafness is a hallmark of type IV BS. Barttin, as pointed out above, is necessary for CLC-K channels trafficking to the membrane. ClCK-barttin complex is expressed in the kidney and in the inner ear. Mice lacking a functional CLC-Ka have a phenotype resembling nephrogenic diabetes insipidus, with high vasopressin plasma levels, and low osmolality of renal papilla even after water restriction, suggesting a role in the urinary concentrating mechanism. CLCKB-null mice show the classic form of BS, whereas only a defect of Barttin determines deafness. In the inner ear CLC-K/Barttin channels participate in Cl$^-$ transcellular extrusion across the basolateral membrane. It is possible that the absence of CLC-Kb could be compensated by the CLC-Ka-Barttin in the inner ear, while the absence of Barttin equals a double defect in CLC-k a and b, leading to deafness.[23] Hypercalciuria and nephrocalcinosis are the main features of type V BS. Activating mutation of the CaSR leads to autosomal dominant hypoparathyroidism, characterized by hypocalcaemia and hyperphosphoremia, with low-normal PTH levels.[31]

Clinical Presentation

Clinically, BS is divided into antenatal and classic BS with or without deafness.

Antenatal BS, or *hyper-prostaglandin E BS*, is the most severe form, characterized by polyhydramnios for excessive urinary output and premature birth. It is sustained by type I and II, and sometimes type III. After birth, patients have a life-threatening clinical course, with fever, vomiting, and lethargy. Biochemical analysis shows the presence of metabolic alkalosis, hypokalemia, isohypostenuria, and hypercalciuria. Nephrocalcinosis is frequent. High urinary prostaglandin excretion of E2 or its metabolites is typical of the antenatal form, and high levels of renin and aldosterone are secondary to volume-depletion. The reason for the high urinary and plasma prostaglandin levels is still unknown, but it seems to be secondary to the defect of NaCl absorption along the TAL.

Classic BS is sustained more often by type III BS. Clinical appearance occurs during infancy or childhood, in the absence of polyhydramnios and prematurity. The clinical course is milder than the antenatal subtype; patients manifest polyuria, polydipsia, vomiting, and dehydration. Nephrocalcinosis is an infrequent sign, and a less severe defect in urinary concentrating mechanism is present.

BS with sensorineural deafness. The presentation of patients with type IV BS shows remarkable variation, ranging from prenatal diagnosis with severe polyhydramnios and prematurity to late diagnosis.[32]

Gitelman Syndrome

Gitelman syndrome (GS) differs from BS because of the presence of hypocalciuria and hypomagnesaemia. It is often diagnosed in adulthood.

Genetics and Molecular Biology

The syndrome correlates with mutations of the SLC12A3 gene located on chromosome 16q, encoding the thiazide-sensitive sodium-chloride co-transporter (NCC). The transporter is expressed on the apical membrane of distal tubule, and represents the major NaCl transport pathway in this segment. More than 140 mutations have been described; the majority of mutations are missense substitutions, but frameshift and splice-site mutations have also been described.[33] Heterozygous subjects show a tendency for low blood pressure, while the complete GS phenotype occurs only in homozygosis. De Jong et al. have performed, in *xenopus laevis* oocytes, functional and immunohistochemical analysis of mutant human NCC of GS subjects.[34] This study has found class I mutants, characterized by the absence of significant metazolone-sensitive Na$^+$ uptake with undetectable protein distribution on the membrane, and class II mutants, which exhibited significant, albeit low, metazolone-sensitive Na$^+$ uptake, while NCC staining was equally present in plasma membrane and cytoplasm. These findings suggest that some mutations compromise NCC abundance in plasma membrane (class I), leading to a defect in protein activity; other mutations only partly impair NCC routing to the membrane, as suggested by the presence of mutant NCC both on plasma membrane and cytoplasm. However, different mechanisms are involved in the impaired trafficking for the two classes of mutations, and the precise mechanism has still to be established. Previous studies suggest the role of defective post-translational changes, such as protein glycosylation, which seems to be required for proper folding and trafficking to plasma membrane.[35] A minority of patients with GS phenotype show mutations in the CLCNKB gene, which is also responsible for BS type III.

Pathophysiology

Both NCC and CLC-Kb dysfunction result in decreased Na$^+$ and Cl$^-$ absorption along the DT. The volume-contraction resulting from defective NaCl absorption determines a compensatory activation of RAAS, which promotes electrogenic Na$^+$ absorption along the CD through ENaC. The latter enhances K$^+$ and H$^+$ secretion along the CD, favoring hypokalemia and metabolic alkalosis. The pathogenesis of hypocalciuria and hypomagnesemia refers to a not yet completely-elucidated mechanism. Micropuncture experiments have demonstrated an increased Ca^{2+} absorption along the proximal tubule (PT) after chronic administration of thiazides, whereas DT calcium absorption was unaffected.[36] This hypothesis is supported by the presence of thiazide-induced hypocalciuria in a mouse model lacking the calcium channel (TRPV5) along the DT. These findings demonstrate that increased calcium absorption parallels a compensatory increased Na$^+$ absorption along the PT secondary to volume-contraction. Other studies suggest that enhanced calcium absorption along the DT participates in the generation of hypocalciuria. In a mouse model of GS, the expression of TRPV5 and TRPV6 were increased, and TRPV5 is also overexpressed in renal tissue from patients with GS.[37]

Hypomagnesemia, another hallmark which distinguishes GS from BS, has a controversial origin. Magnesium is freely filtered by the glomerulus, and it is reabsorbed in a small fraction along the PT. The majority of Mg^{2+} is reabsorbed along the TAL, via paracellular pathway, and DT, via transcellular pathway. In the latter, Mg^{2+} reabsorption is mediated by the transient receptor potential cation channel, TRPM6. In NCC knockout mice a downregulation of TRPM6 in DT has been shown.[36] This effect could explain the defective Mg^{2+} absorption, and the subsequent hypomagnesemia.

The clinical phenotype in CLCNKB mutations is extremely variable; several reports have described subjects with phenotypic features of GS without any defect in SLC12A3 gene, carrying homozygous mutations of CLCNKB gene[38] or mixed BS-GS phenotype.[39]

Clinical Presentation

GS is characterized by an extreme inter- and intra-familial phenotype variability, varying from mild or undiagnosed forms to severe conditions complicated by growth retardation, ventricular arrhythmias, and neuromuscular symptoms. In most cases the diagnosis occurs in adulthood. The patients suffer from tetany, especially during conditions which determine further Mg^{2+} loss, like vomiting or diarrhea. Some patients experience fatigue which compromises daily activities, in relation to the degree of hypokalemia. In contrast with BS, those patients do not manifest polyuria and growth retardation. Chronic K$^+$ and Mg^{2+} deficiency may predispose to a higher risk for ventricular arrhythmias. However, lethal arrhythmias have been reported rarely in GS patients, and may be related to underlying triggering mechanisms besides hypokalemia. Riviera et al. have described a subgroup of GS patients with severe phenotype, characterized by early onset, and severe neuromuscular and cardiac symptoms.[40] Almost all patients of the subgroup were male, and showed a higher incidence of splicing mutation leading to a truncated transcript compared with mild and classic GS. This study suggests that male gender and splicing mutations, resulting in a severe protein dysfunction, may account for the clinical severity of GS. Biochemical analysis shows hypocalciuria, hypokalemia, and hypomagnesemia. Although hypocalciuria and hypomagnesemia have been considered necessary for the diagnosis of GS, recently a report of a GS patient with a proven mutation in the GS gene did not manifest those signs. Plasma renin and aldosterone levels are only slightly increased compared with BS.

Liddle Syndrome

Liddle syndrome (LS) is an autosomal dominant disease leading to hypertension. Besides the early onset of hypertension, it is characterized by hypokalemic metabolic alkalosis, with downregulation of RAAS. In the last 10 years the Lifton group has identified several mutations mapping in β- and γ-ENaC subunits, resulting in the expression of a higher number of channels in the plasma membrane.

Genetic and Molecular Biology

ENaC is comprised of three subunits, α, β, and γ, which are assembled at stoichiometry α2βγ. Several studies have suggested that also αβ and αγ are functional channels. The first description of Liddle syndrome (LS) in literature was correlated with the mutation in the gene encoding the β-ENaC subunit, resulting in a premature stop codon which leads to the loss of the last amino acids of the C-terminus.[41] Genetic screening of subjects suffering from LS has showed that the syndrome also segregates with mutations of the gene encoding for the γ-subunit. The expression of either truncated γ- or β-ENaC subunit increases amiloride-sensitive Na $^+$ uptake in oocytes.[42] These findings suggest that the C-terminus of β- and γ-subunits is a crucial region for the activity of the channel. Different investigations have found that most mutations resulting in LS phenotype are mapped on a highly-conserved PPPXY sequence (PPY motif) of the C-terminus in β and γ; disruption of the motif preserves the channel from inhibitory stimuli.

Pathophysiology

The amiloride-sensitive ENaC is an ion channel which mediates Na $^+$ absorption along the distal segment of CNT and CD. ENaC channels are positively regulated by aldosterone and vasopressin. In mice, aldosterone has been shown to activate ENaC via the ser/thr kinase Sgk1. This kinase induces ENaC activation partly through the inhibition of ENaC downregulation by the E3 ubiquitine ligase, Nedd4-2, which targets ENaC to degradation in cultured cells.[43] Sgk1 phosphorylates Nedd4-2 to an inhibitory site, thus preventing ENaC removal from the plasma membrane.[44] Mutations in β- and γ-subunits of ENaC in LS result in a constitutive activation of ENaC activity.[45] These mutations impair the PY motif in the C-terminus, which is required for Nedd4-2-mediated ENaC ubiquitination. In the absence of the binding site, Nedd4-2 fails to target the channel for degradation. However, these mutations increase the overall ENaC expression at the apical membrane, contributing to increased Na $^+$ absorption. The resulting volume-expansion explains the suppression of RAAS. Interestingly, mice bearing a LS deletion revealed normal aldosterone response.[46] Consistently, in cultured cell, aldosterone, vasopressin, and Sgk1 are still able to increase ENaC surface abundance in the presence of LS causative mutations,[47] suggesting that Nedd4-2 is not necessary for aldosterone-dependent increased ENaC activity. However, in LS patients, constitutive increased ENaC activity leads to volume-expansion, high blood pressure, and suppressed RAAS.[48] As a consequence of increased channel activity along the CD, patients do manifest hypokalemia and metabolic alkalosis. Mice bearing LS become hypertensive only when fed a high-salt diet.[49]

Clinical Presentation

LS was first described in 1963 as a condition resembling hyperaldosteronism, because of the coexistence of hypertension, hypokalemia, and metabolic alkalosis. However, due to the low/normal levels of plasma aldosterone this condition is described as pseudohyperaldosteronism of the second type. Hypertension usually develops at an early age in affected individuals, and worsens throughout the lifetime. Recently, Tapolyia et al. have proposed the presence of serum bicarbonate over 25 mmol/L, K $^+$ levels lower than 4 mEq/L, plasma renin activity lower than 0.35 μU/ml/h, and plasma aldosterone levels lower than 15 ng/dl as screening criteria for LS. Based on these criteria, this group found a prevalence of 6.7% patients that satisfied the criteria for likely LS in a cross-sectional investigation of 149 hypertensive patients with hypokalemia and metabolic alkalosis.[50] Hypertension is usually refractory to common antihypertensive drugs, while it is responsive to the use of the ENaC inhibitor, amiloride.

RENAL CHANGES IN K+ DEFICIENCY

Morphology

Experimental Studies

Hypokalemic states are associated with several renal morphological alterations. The severity and exposure time to hypokalemia are fundamental to the development of renal injuries. Mild hypokalemia ranging among 3.6 ± 0.2 is not associated with significant glomerular or tubular abnormalities in Sprague-Dawley rats.[51] Renal hypertrophy is a universal finding in studies of K+-depletion (KD) since the early report by Schraeder et al. in 1937. This renal growth has distinct morphologic characteristics. The increase in kidney mass is not uniform, being more prominent in the outer medulla, as reflected in the relative contribution of the different zones to total kidney weight in K+ deficient rats.[52]

The growth process consists of both hyperplasic and hypertrophic components. Despite the fact that hypokalemic mice present a different metabolic behavior (metabolic acidosis), they develop morphological abnormalities of CD similar to rats and humans. K+ deficient mice show morphological alterations in outer medulla CD (OMCD) after three days of a low-K+ diet. CD epithelial cells from K+ deficient mice have a higher proliferation rate than control mice. Intercalated cells show PCNA positive staining (proliferation marker) more than principal cells. No signs of cellular hypertrophy are detected at this time point in CD epithelial cells, despite IC already display an enlargement of the apical membrane domain. After 14 days of a low-K+ diet both principal and IC cells appear hypertrophic as evaluated at EM level. In hypokalemia-induced morphologic alteration of OMCD, hyperplasia precedes the development of cellular hypertrophy. Transcriptome analysis of OMCD suggests Gdf15 (growth differentiation factor 15) increases significantly from day 3 to day 14 of the low-K+ diet. It could be a potential candidate in driving the switch from hyperplasia to hypertrophy. Gdf15 belongs to the TGFβ superfamily, and it could be a growth-stop signal in OMCD.[53]

The growth-promoting effect of K+ deficiency is not limited by the state of the organ. It occurs in intact, as well as in previously damaged, kidneys. Peterson et al.[54] have shown that institution of K+ deficiency in a model of remnant kidney (5/6 nephrectomy) led to an increase in renal mass and RNA content beyond that expected of the surgical ablation alone.

CD is the main nephron site where morphologic alterations occur in K+ deficiency. Glomerular and vascular lesions have rarely been observed in pure K+ deficiency, and changes in proximal convoluted tubules have been limited to vacuolar degeneration.

While several studies demonstrate the occurrence of morphologic changes in individual CD cells, conflicting statements have been made regarding the proportion of cell types and number. Hansen et al.[55] observed extensive swelling of the epithelium of the CD involving both principal and intercalated cells along the OMCD (Figure 50.2). No changes were observed in either principal or intercalated cells of the initial CD.[56] Intercalated cells in the MCD segment develop extensive microplicae over the entire luminal surface with increased luminal surface boundary length,[55] whereas no change was observed in basolateral membrane length or in the luminal or basolateral aspects of principal cells[57] (Figure 50.3). This increased luminal surface could be due to the fusion of the cytoplasmic vesicles with the apical membrane domain. A large number of rod-shaped structures are opened in the lumen in this way. This event is thought to be useful for H+ secretion and K+ reabsorption through H+-ATPase or H+-K+-ATPase activity, respectively. There are conflicting findings about the proportion of intercalated and principal cells in any part of the CD in K+ deficiency. Evidences indicate the development of morphologic changes in individual cells as well as an increase in cell number.

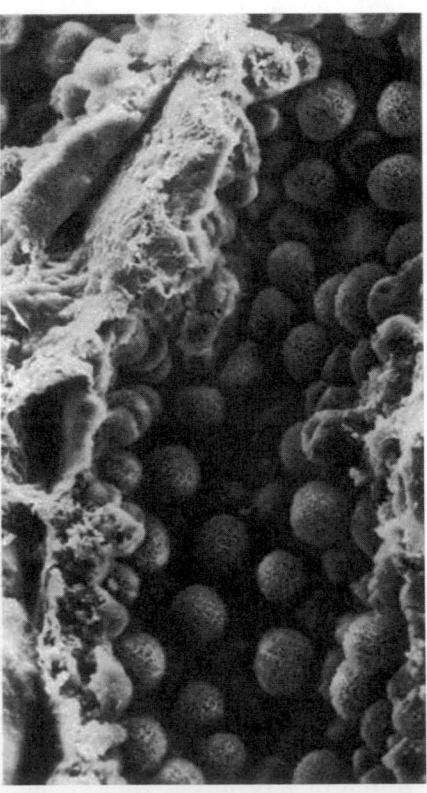

FIGURE 50.2 Electron microscopy of rat collecting duct in ISOM. This is a representative picture of hypertrophy of A-type-intercalated cells. *(With permission from Hansen, G. P. et al.[55])*

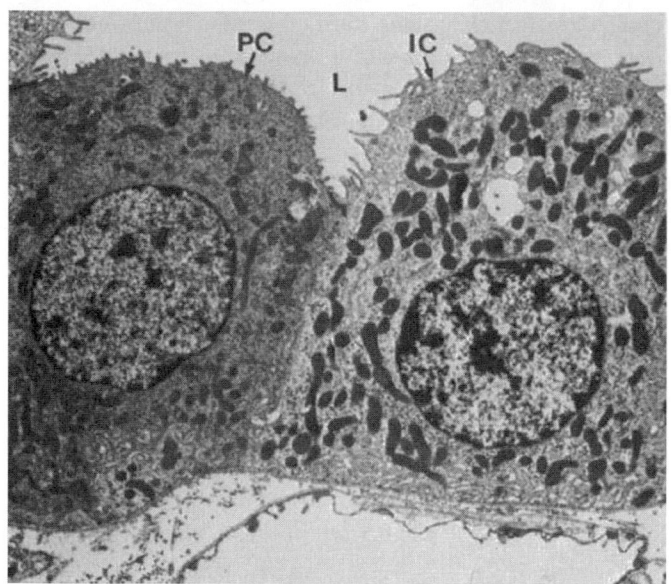

FIGURE 50.3 Electron microscopy of rat medullary collecting duct, showing a representative picture of hypokalemia-induced morphological changes in both principal and intercalated cells. *(With permission from Stetson, D. L. et al.* [57])

Recently, progressive capillary loss has been identified in hypokalemic nephropathy. This injury was first observed in the ISOM after 2 weeks of a K-restriction diet, expanded to the OSOM at 4 weeks, and then to the cortex by week 12. Capillary loss significantly correlated with local macrophage infiltration and low endothelial cell proliferation rate, an effect probably secondary to a decrease of VEGF and eNOS expression.[58]

The most remarkable ultrastructural change is the accumulation of cytoplasmic droplets in tubular cells of the medulla. The appearance of droplets starts from the CD at the tip of the papilla, and then extends upward into the outer medulla until the cortico-medullary junction. The extension depends on the duration of K$^+$ deficiency. Besides epithelial cells, interstitial and other cells in the medulla also show cytoplasmic droplets, with considerable enlargement of cell volume. With K$^+$ repletion, the droplets reversed progressively.[59] The droplets are believed to be the consequence of phospholipids dysregulation,[60] and their lysosomal origin is suggested by the presence of hydrolytic enzymes. It has been suggested that increased ammonia production secondary to hypokalemia may contribute to vacuolation of nucleated cells in KD.[61] In fact, ammonia has been shown to induce vacuolization of lysosomes, inhibition of endocytosis, and lysosomial protein degradation. Another hypothesis is that the cytoplasmic droplets could be related to a cellular autophagy phenomenon. Lipid droplets share common protein with the autophagosome in

hepatocytes and cardiac myocytes,[62] and those organelles may be an expression of autophagy. Ureteral ligation in K$^+$ deficient rats is followed by resolution of droplets, presumably because of increased renal medullary K$^+$ content.[63] The severity of droplet formation depends on the method of induction of K$^+$ deficiency, with minimal droplet formation developing with DOCA-induced compared with dietary deficiency.[64]

Tubular and interstitial apoptosis is observed during K$^+$ deficiency. Apoptotic cells are located mainly in the outer medulla. Bcl-2 protein distributed in the tubules of the outer medulla is significantly decreased in KD rats, while immunoreactivity for Bax protein tends to increase above control levels. These results suggest that apoptosis is associated with progression of cellular proliferation in hypokalemic nephropathy, and a decrease in bcl2 may be involved in promoting this apoptotic process.[65]

Human Studies

Unlike experimental studies where K$^+$ deficiency can be induced selectively, clinical observations are frequently based on complex conditions where K$^+$ deficiency is complicated by numerous other alterations, including Na$^+$ and acid—base homeostasis. The issue is even more complex if we consider additional factors like duration of disease, and therapeutic interventions that may substantially alter histopathologic manifestations in humans. Finally, clinical data are usually limited to cortical biopsies, and sampling of medullary and papillary structures may be lacking. An important observation comes from autopsy studies in healthy Thai adults who died of vehicular accidents. K$^+$ deficiency prevails among the healthy population of northeast Thailand. In this study, none of the patients had renal histopathological change compatible with a diagnosis of focal or diffuse interstitial nephritis, and there were minimal renal tubulo-interstitial changes.[66]

Glomerular changes consisted mostly of a reduction in capillary surface and Bowman capsule areas, and an increase in the mesangial space. The glomerular shrinkage was not associated with any alterations in cellular constitution of the tuft.[67] Of note is the increase in juxtaglomerular complex size in many of the patients to levels comparable to, or even exceeding, those observed in BS. Such findings underscore the non-specificity of this change, which is likely secondary to defective Cl$^-$ absorption in the thick ascending limb, rather than a characteristic feature of BS. Tubular vacuolization was not a frequent or pathognomic observation, although it was considered characteristic by Conn and Johnson, who coined the term kaliopenic nephropathy in 1956. More important for the prognosis of these patients is the occurrence of degenerative changes such as tubular atrophy, dilatation, epithelial flattening, and thickening of the basement membrane.[68] Again, these alterations are non-specific, and reflect evidence of chronic injury. Increased interstitial surface area and lymphocytic cellular infiltration were frequent. PAS-positive granules have been observed in some of these patients in all medullary cells when available in the specimen.

Taken together, these observations suggest that many of the renal changes seen in K^+ deficient animals have their counterparts in clinical cases. Some of these changes (glomerular shrinkage, tubular atrophy, interstitial fibrosis) indicate irreversible renal damage, and the occurrence of renal insufficiency in this group of patients has been convincingly demonstrated.[69] Indeed, in some young women the condition has led to end-stage renal disease.[70] Elements of the kaliopenic nephropathy mixed to morphological changes secondary to hypertension are also found in patients with primary aldosteronism. The apparently additive insults of hypertension and K^+ deficiency are illustrated in the study of 18 patients with primary aldosteronism by Danforth et al.[71] Moderate to severe hypertensive changes (fibrous thickening of small vessels and glomerular hyalinization) and kaliopenic lesions (vacuolization and degeneration of tubular epithelia) were observed in 14 (78%) and 16 (89%) patients, respectively. The hypertensive changes appeared to be more severe in this group than in subjects with primary hypertension of similar severity, suggesting a possible synergistic effect of K^+ deficiency.

Tubular Function

A heterogeneous pattern of structural and functional changes occurs along the nephron, with a progressive increase from proximal to distal segments.

Proximal Convoluted Tubule

SODIUM CHLORIDE

Transport along the proximal tubule has been extensively studied in both acute and chronic K^+ deficiency models with micropuncture and isolated tubule techniques. An acute change in K^+ concentration in the perfusion bath below 2.5 mM inhibits NaCl transport in isolated and perfused PT from rabbit.[72] Decrements in NaCl reabsorption, as evidenced by decreased net fluid absorption in this segment, have also been observed during capillary microperfusion with hypokalemic solutions in rats.[73] Studies in K^+ deficient animals show a different pattern of alterations in transport. Walter et al.[74] performed micropuncture studies on anesthetized rats which had been kept on a K deficient diet for 2 weeks. In these animals total glomerular filtration rate (GFR) and single-nephron filtration rate

were significantly lower than controls. Fractional reabsorption by the proximal convoluted tubule was enhanced, and end proximal fluid delivery was markedly reduced. These observations are in line with other studies showing reduced fractional excretion of lithium in K^+ deficiency,[75] presumably a surrogate measurement for enhanced proximal Na^+ reabsorption.

Chronic K^+ deficiency, but not an acute luminal exposure, leads to increased NaCl reabsorption. K^+ deficiency increased the expression of both the adrenergic receptor alfa$_{2B}$,[76] and AT1 (angiotensin II receptors)[77] in rat PT. These changes are coupled with an increase in renin and angiotensin II level, as demonstrated in many species. The higher Na^+ reabsorption could be in part transcellular, mainly driven by several Na^+ transporters upregulated in hypokalemia (vide infra).

Hypokalemic rats have an increased expression of Na-H exchanger 3 (NHE3) in membrane fractions of renal cortex and outer stripe of the outer medulla (OSOM). Immunohistochemistry confirms that NHE3 labeling is increased in the luminal membrane domain of the PT of hypokalemic rats.[78] However, Wang et al.[79] found no change in the expression of NHE3 mRNA and its cognate protein after 6 and 14 days in rats on a low-K^+ diet. The mRNA levels for NHE1, NHE2, and NHE4 also remained unchanged at 6 and 14 days of the low-K^+ diet. These apparent inconsistencies between protein expression and mRNA levels could be due to a posttranslational level of regulation of NHE3, as recently found in hypertensive models.[80] In parallel with Na^+ reabsorption, NHE3 promotes proton extrusion. This mechanism is functional for net bicarbonate reabsorption through the PT.

BICARBONATE

Chronic K^+ deficiency is associated with metabolic alkalosis and an increase in bicarbonate reabsorption, as demonstrated by free-flow micropuncture and microperfusion studies in rats.[81] In contrast, acute exposure of proximal tubules to ow (K^+ 2 mM) in capillary microperfusion experiments had no effect on bicarbonate reabsorption.[73] The mechanism of enhanced bicarbonate reabsorption is mediated by stimulation of NHE3 and the basolateral Na/3HCO$_3$-co-transporter.[75] In OKP cells, low-K medium causes a decrease in intracellular pH, which leads to increased NHE3 activity.[82] Accordingly, NHE3 total protein abundance and immunostaining along the apical membrane of PT and TAL were dramatically increased in hypokalemic rats.

The bicarbonate basolateral exit pathway from the PT cells is mediated by the sodium bicarbonate co-transporter (NBC1). During K$^+$ deficiency states both the activity and mRNA expression of NBC1 are increased.[83] It is not clear if the upregulation of NBC1 causes the lowering intracellular pH or whether it is a consequence of the higher bicarbonate reabsorption.

Angiotensin II could promote bicarbonate reabsorption in the PT. In fact, angiotensin II is found to increase NBC1 expression in rat PT, while it is debated whether it also regulates NHE3 function.[84]

AMMONIUM

Metabolic alkalosis developing during K$^+$ deficiency is also sustained by increased bicarbonate generation from the ammoniagenesis pathway in the PT. Chronic hypokalemia is associated with increased ammonium excretion in humans as well.[85] K$^+$ deficiency leads to a three-fold increase in ammonia production in the S1, and to a two-fold increase in S2 segments of PT.[86] No changes in ammonia production were observed in the S3 segment (pars recta) or in the thick ascending limb or distal convoluted tubule. The increased ammonia production in S1 occurred in both superficial and juxtamedullary nephrons, with a greater extent in the former. The primary mechanism by which K$^+$ deficiency stimulates renal ammonia production is not precisely known. Increased renal ammonia production and excretion, despite the simultaneous presence of metabolic alkalosis, suggest that intracellular factors, rather than extracellular pH, modulate renal ammonia metabolism. Intracellular acidosis that occurs in K$^+$ deficiency may initiate the adaptive response in ammoniagenesis. Both mitochondrial (glutamine transaminase activity) and cytosolic (phosphoenolypyruvate carboxykinase, PEPCK) enzymes involved in glutamine catabolism and gluconeogenesis are increased in the hypokalemic state.[87] This pathway induces a net gain of new bicarbonate production. K$^+$ repletion leads to prompt decreases in ammonia production.[88] Although mice present a species-different acid−base adaptation to hypokalemia, namely metabolic acidosis, they share a high urinary ammonium excretion with rats. Hypokalemic mice show an increase of glutamine transporter SNAT3. SNAT3, normally located in the S3 segment of the PT, spreads to S1 and S2 segments during K$^+$ deficiency, supporting the increase ammoniagenesis in the PT[89] (Figure 50.4).

PHOSPHATE

Chronic K$^+$ deficiency is associated with low serum phosphate (Pi) and an increase urinary Pi excretion in rats and mice. Key regulators of renal Pi excretion are the Na dependent co-transporter NaPi IIa and NaPi IIc, expressed almost exclusively in the

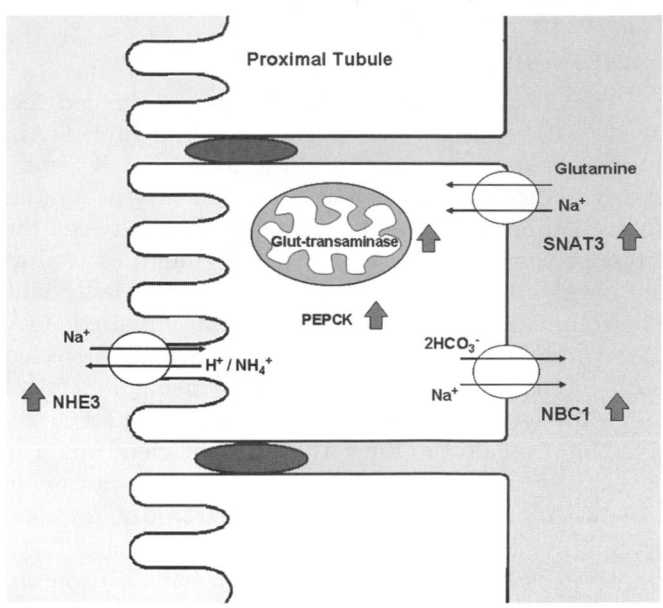

FIGURE 50.4 Hypokalemia increases ammoniagenesis in proximal tubule cells. Hypokalemia-induced ammoniagenesis is proved by an increased expression of PEPCK and glutamine transaminase.[87] Therefore, hypokalemic mice present an upregulation of SNAT-3, the sodium-coupled glutamine importer along the whole proximal tubule.[89] These effects are coupled to upregulation of NHE3[78] and NBC-1[145] transporters involved in proximal tubule bicarbonate reabsorption.

kidney. Another group of Pi transporters, Pit-1 and Pit-2, have been described.[90] In hypokalemia, a phosphaturic phenotype is associated with a differential regulation of the different NaPi transporters. NaPi IIa protein abundance in brush border membranes (BBM) and protein targeting to the apical membrane are increased, while NaPi IIc and PiT2 are decreased in animals fed with a low-K diet. In addition, NaPi IIc relocates from the apical membrane domain to cytoplasmic vesicles.[91] The downregulation of NaPi IIc seems to sustain the hypokalemia-induced urinary phosphate loss.

OTHER PROXIMAL TUBULE DYSFUNCTION

Chronic K$^+$ deficiency causes hypocitraturia. Urinary citrate excretion is mainly a function of citrate absorption along the proximal tubule, a process mediated by the Na-dicarboxilate co-transporter NaDC1, and citrate metabolism. Levi et al.[92] have shown an increased NaDC1 activity on renal cortical BBM from K$^+$ deficient rats. Hypokalemia may also participate in proximal tubular dysfunctions observed in children with primary distal renal tubular acidosis. Indeed, in these patients, correction of hypokalemia ameliorates low molecular weight proteinuria, phosphaturia, and generalized aminoaciduria.

Loop of Henle

SODIUM CHLORIDE

Eknoyan et al.[93] were the first to suggest that a defect in Na^+ transport by the thick ascending limb (TAL) could explain the concentrating defect of K^+ deficiency. Micropuncture and microperfusion studies showed diminished net Cl^- reabsorption between the latest proximal and earliest distal segment, as well as increased luminal Cl^- concentration at the latter site. These findings were consistent with impaired TAL absorption, and the defect was only partially corrected with indomethacin. Gutsche et al.,[94] using the micro stop-flow technique, have provided evidence for defective Na^+ transport in the TAL of K^+ deficient rats. The severity of the defect correlated with the decrease in plasma K^+ concentration, and was rapidly reversed with acute K^+ administration. In addition, net NaCl transport is inhibited by reduction in bath K^+ concentration in isolated perfused TAL.[95]

A more recent study has uncovered the molecular basis of the observed defects in electrolyte reabsorption in the TAL. In rats, NKCC2 mRNA expression in medulla is decreased about 56 and 51% after 6 and 14 days of K^+ restriction diet respectively. Functional studies in tubular suspensions of medullary TAL from K^+ deficient rats demonstrated a 45 and 37% decreased NKCC2 activity at 6 and 14 days, respectively. NKCC2 protein abundance of membrane fraction from renal ISOM is downregulated in rats fed for 4 days on a K^+ restricted diet. Immunohistochemical localization confirms a lower expression of NKCC2 in mTAL.[78] Na/K-ATPase plays a key role in the Na^+-dependent transport in this nephron segment. Despite the increase in the number of Na/K-ATPase units, the transport capacity of the Na/K pump, determined by ouabain-sensitive Rb uptake, was reduced in mTAL from K^+ deficient rats. Inhibition of the Na/K pump was the consequence of a reduced affinity for Na.[96]

BICARBONATE AND AMMONIUM

Basolateral and apical Na-H exchangers (NHEs) in TAL are involved in NH_4^+ and HCO_3^- absorption, respectively. The NH_4^+ absorption rate in Henle's loop is increased in K^+ deficiency, which may be secondary to the increased NH_4^+ concentration in luminal fluid and/or to an increased NH_4^+ absorptive capacity of TAL. HCO_3^- absorptive capacity in Henle's loop is unchanged in K^+ deficiency, despite the presence of metabolic alkalosis. The effects of K^+ deficiency on the expression of basolateral NHE-1 and the expression of apical NHE3 in TAL have been examined by Laghmani et al.[97] NHE1 protein abundance was similarly increased (approximately 90%) at 2 and 5 weeks of K^+ deficiency, while NHE1 mRNA amount in TAL cells was increased at 2 weeks, and returned to normal values by 5 weeks. NHE3 protein abundance and mRNA remained unchanged after 2 weeks of K^+ deficiency. NHE3 mRNA was reduced by approximately 50% at 5 weeks. In K^+ deficiency, the increased NHE1 expression may support an increased TAL NH_4^+ absorptive capacity. The lack of change in NHE3 expression, despite the presence of metabolic alkalosis, is in agreement with the unchanged HCO_3^- absorptive capacity of Henle's loop. Recently, an electro-neutral, Na-dependent HCO_3^--co-transporter (NBCn1) has been cloned and localized at the basolateral side of the mTAL. Several results show NBCn1 is fundamental for NH_4^+ reabsorption in the TAL. NH_4^+ entering the mTAL cell via the furosemide-sensitive NKCC2 transporter dissociates into H^+ and NH_3. The NH_3 leaves the cell via non-ionic diffusion preferentially through the basolateral membrane. The remaining proton may either be transported directly via a basolateral NHE1 and/or could be buffered by basolateral import of HCO_3^- through NBCn1. During hypokalemia, NBCn1 protein abundance is strongly upregulated in ISOM. In addition, in vitro perfusion of isolated mTAL shows hypokalaemia induced a three-fold upregulation of Na-coupled HCO_3^- influx[98] (Figure 50.5).

Distal Tubule

SODIUM CHLORIDE

Along the DT downregulation of the main Na^+ transporter has been reported. Rats fed a low-K^+ diet for 4 days present a downregulation of sodium chloride co-transporter (NCC) in the membrane fraction of cortex and OSOM. Immunoistochemistry confirms the reduced expression of NCC in the convolute distal tubule cells.[78]

BICARBONATE

In DT, the rate of bicarbonate absorption is not altered in K^+ deficiency, despite a lower delivery rate and the presence of a greater lumen-to-plasma bicarbonate concentration difference due to the higher plasma and lower luminal levels.[99] Micropuncture experiments have demonstrated that bicarbonate reabsorption along the distal tubule of K^+ deficient rats was increased when delivery rates of bicarbonate reached levels similar to those in controls. In the DT, bicarbonate reabsorption is relatively insensitive to peritubular alkalinization, and the systemic alkalosis does not affect acid secretion.[100] The mechanism, therefore, is not self-limiting, and no "braking" of the enhanced bicarbonate reabsorption occurs. This is due to enhanced electrogenic proton secretion (H^+-ATPase) as demonstrated by in vivo microperfusion of the superficial distal tubule in K^+ deficient animals.[101]

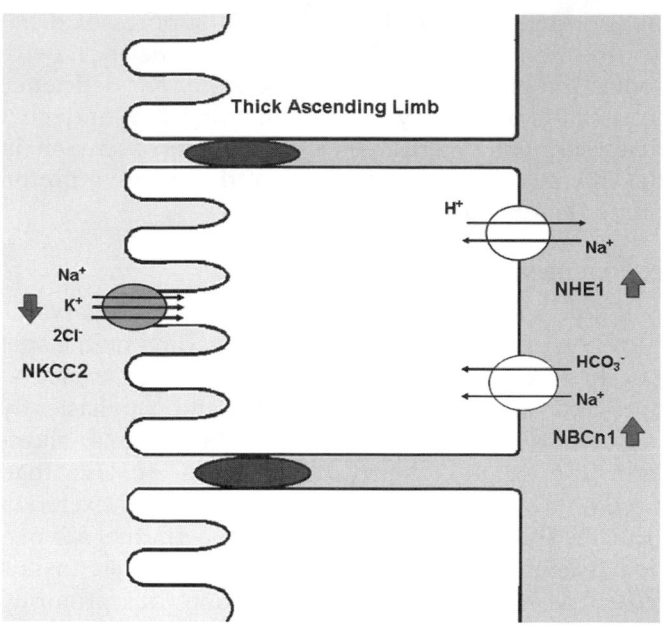

FIGURE 50.5 **Hypokalemia impairs sodium chloride absorption in the TAL, mainly inhibiting both the activity and expression of the NKCC2.**[78] The reduction of sodium chloride absorption in the TAL contributes to the urinary concentrating defect. Ammonium absorption is increased along the TAL, sustained by the upregulation of basolateral NHE1[97] and NBCn1.[98]

POTASSIUM

K$^+$ secretion in the segments of the distal nephron accessible to micropuncture (the early distal convoluted tubule, the connecting tubule, and the initial collecting tubule), is reduced to near zero in K$^+$ deficiency.[56]

Collecting Duct

This segment is the site of major structural changes in K$^+$ deficiency, and the alterations in its transport functions are primarily responsible for metabolic alkalosis and defective urinary concentrating ability.

SODIUM

Along the connecting tubule, as well as the cortical, outer, and inner medullary CD, Na$^+$ uptake occurs through the luminal amiloride-sensitive epithelial Na$^+$ channel (ENaC), and it is driven by the electrogenic potential induced by the basolateral Na/K-ATPase. During hypokalemic states, all ENaC subunits (α, β and γ) are downregulated in renal samples from cortex-OSOM, and in whole kidneys as well. This has been ascribed to the hypokalemia-induced inhibition of aldosterone secretion.[78] Despite this finding, K$^+$ deficiency produces a striking, time-dependent increase in Na/K-ATPase activity, mainly in the CD in ISOM. After 3 weeks of a K-free diet, Na/K-ATPase activity

was over four-fold higher than control animals.[102] The increased protein activity was larger than the extent of tubular volume or protein content, indicating that it is not merely a reflection of the concomitant hypertrophy observed in this region of the nephron. Na/K-ATPase activity returned to baseline after 7 days of K$^+$ repletion.[102] In association with the increased activity, it has been described that two weeks of K$^+$ deficiency induced a marked increase in the α1- and β1-subunits of Na/K-ATPase in medullary, but not in the cortical portion of the CD.[103] These observations are interesting, because enhanced activity of Na/K-ATPase would likely promote K$^+$ secretion and urinary loss, thus exacerbating the hypokalemia. Because the ISOM segment of the CD plays an important role in K$^+$ homeostasis, the upregulation of the Na/K-ATPase has been associated with a potential kaliferic function. To reconcile these observations, Hayashi and Katz[102] proposed that the induced Na$^+$ pumps were localized to the luminal domain, thus facilitating active K$^+$ reabsorption instead of secretion. Further evidence is needed to support this hypothesis. During a hypokalemic state, in the medullary interstitium a lower K$^+$ and an increased NH$_4^+$ concentration develop (see below). NH$_4^+$ and K$^+$ compete for the same transport site of the Na/K-ATPase. Upregulation of the Na/K-ATPase in the IMCD promotes ammonium uptake, primarily from the reduced interstitial K$^+$ concentration.[104] This phenomenon could be another explanation for the paradox of the Na/K-ATPase upregulation.

Proton Secretion

The development of metabolic alkalosis in sustained by the increased bicarbonate absorption and generation along the PT, as well as the enhanced proton secretion along the CD. Physiologically, the proteins responsible for proton secretion are mainly the H-ATPase and H/K-ATPase.

The effects of K$^+$ deficiency on the activity and distribution of the H-ATPase in the Sprague-Dawley rat were assessed by Bailey *et al.*[101] K$^+$ deficiency increased electrogenic H-ATPase activity in rat distal tubule, with an increased insertion of pumps into the apical membrane.[105] These findings were confirmed and expanded by Silver *et al.*[106] The rate of pH(i) recovery in intercalated cells (ICs) in response to an acute acid-load (a measure of plasma membrane H-ATPase activity) was three times larger after K$^+$ deficiency as compared to controls. This was associated with a change in the distribution of membrane-bound proton pumps in the IC population of cortical CD from K$^+$ deficient rats. Immunocytochemical analysis of rats CDs showed that K$^+$ deficiency increased the number of ICs with tight apical H-ATPase staining, and decreased the number of cells with diffuse basolateral H-ATPase staining. Taken together, these data indicate that chronic K⁺ deficiency induces a marked increase in plasma membrane H-ATPase activity in individual ICs.

The ability of A-ICs to secrete protons into the lumen is strictly coupled to bicarbonate extrusion on the basolateral side, and it is blocked when an impairment of bicarbonate extrusion occurs. The latter is mainly mediated by the anion exchanger-1 (AE-1) and other members of this family. During K⁺ deficiency, protein abundance of AE-1 increases in cortex and OSOM, and this is coupled with a strong upregulation of another anion exchanger, SLC26A7.[107] In MDCK cells, SLC26A7 was found to translocate from the endosomal compartment to the basolateral membrane in response to a low-K⁺ media.[108]

H/K-ATPase promotes luminal acidification and K⁺ reabsorption. Two isoforms, H/Kα1 (gastric) and H/Kα2 (colonic), are expressed along the entire length of the CD from the early connecting tubule to the inner medullary CD. This localization is consistent among species. In rat CD, H/K-ATPase is expressed mainly in intercalated cells.[109] Chronic K⁺ deficiency (3 weeks) led to a generalized increase in H/K-ATPases activity along the CD segments, with the greater increments occurring in CNT > CCD > MCD. This is in contrast to the morphologic changes that occur in the CD in K⁺ deficiency, which display a hypertrophic response with the hierarchy: MCD > CCD > CNT.[102] Studies from single H/Kα1 and H/Kα2 knockout mice show an impairment in acid secretion during normal diet, confirming the crucial role of this transporter in renal acid–base balance. Data from H/Kα2 null mice demonstrated increased fecal K⁺ loss, without significant differences in K⁺ urinary excretion. A compensatory activation of the H/Kα1 subunits might be responsible for K⁺ secretion in the absence of functional H/Kα2-subunits. Investigation of double H/Kα1 and H/Kα1,2-null mice on a K⁺ deficient diet will provide insight into the functional importance of H/K-ATPases in K⁺ deficient conditions.[109]

Pendrin belongs to a superfamily of Cl/anion exchangers, and has been localized in the apical side of non-type-A IC of the cortical CD. Reduced bicarbonate secretion was demonstrated in a pendrin knockout mouse model. In chronic K⁺ deficiency, known to elicit a metabolic alkalosis, pendrin protein levels are decreased and pendrin expression is shifted to an intracellular pool with the relative number of pendrin positive cells reduced. These results are in agreement with a potential role of pendrin in bicarbonate secretion and regulation of acid–base transport in the cortical CD.[110] These adaptations occurring during K⁺ deficiency are similar to those observed in chronic metabolic acidosis.

Considering that metabolic alkalosis suppresses distal acidification, the stimulation by K⁺ deficiency overcomes the effect of the alkalemic state. K⁺ deficiency thus exerts a primary, aldosterone and Na⁺-independent, stimulatory effect on hydrogen ion secretion in the CD, most likely at the level of the putative proton pump (Figure 50.6).

POTASSIUM

K⁺ deficiency results in a decrease in urinary K⁺ excretion of variable magnitude, depending on the species. In all species, however, the decline in K⁺ excretion does not match the reduced intake, and a persistently negative K⁺ balance is observed. In humans, short-term dietary K⁺ deprivation (intake of less than 1 mEq/day) induces a decline in urinary K⁺ excretion which is still higher than intake, with a gradual adaptation reaching a maximum within 5 to 7 days. In rats fed a low-K diet, urinary K⁺ excretion falls promptly and parallels intake by 72 to 96 hours after the institution of a K⁺ deficient diet.[111] The conservation of K⁺ can be conceived as being due to attenuation of kaliuretic mechanisms, in part by resistance to normally kaliuretic influences, and in part by activation of kaliferic ones. Both phenomena have to be examined in the context of renal and systemic adaptations to K⁺ deficiency, with differences in short-term and

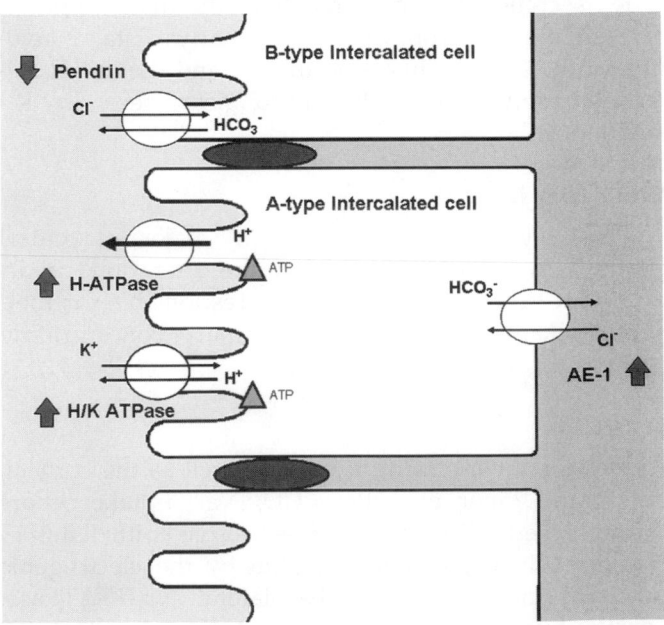

FIGURE 50.6 Hypokalemia led to a metabolic alkalosis in rats and humans. In addition to a proximal tubule effect, an increased acid secretion has been described in type-A-intercalated cells. Both H⁺-ATPase[106] and H⁺/K⁺-ATPase[146] showed increased expression, along with an upregulation of AE-1.[107] B-type-intercalated cells showed a reduced expression of the bicarbonate secreting transporter, pendrin.[110] This latter finding supports K⁺ depletion also impairing urinary bicarbonate secretion.

long-term K$^+$ deficiency. K$^+$ secretion in the CCD is markedly attenuated, but may not cease even with profound degrees of K$^+$ deficiency.[112] The reduced level of K$^+$ secretion is coupled with a decreased response to kaliuretic factors. Malnic *et al.*[112] have shown that K$^+$ deficient rats maintain their ability to increase K$^+$ secretion in response to increments in tubular flow, albeit at a much lower level. Finally, K$^+$ deficient humans are resistant to the kaliuretic influence of high urine flux, osmotic diuresis, and metabolic alkalosis. It has been suggested that an "escape" from kaliuretic influences may occur in K$^+$ deficient conditions, a concept which resembles the escape from the Na$^+$-retaining effects of chronic mineralocorticoid administration. Thus, no kaliuretic response is observed in rats when DOCA is administered 72 hours after initiation of K$^+$ deficiency.[111] In contrast, resistance to the kaliuretic effects of mineralocorticoids does not appear in short-term (7–10 days) K$^+$ deficient humans, in whom administration of DOCA is associated with a kaliuresis, despite the presence of hypokalemia and a large negative K$^+$ balance.

K restriction suppresses renal K$^+$ secretion and enhances its absorption.[113] This is achieved by both inhibiting apical K$^+$ channels in principal cells and stimulating K$^+$ absorption in intercalated cells. In CCD a molecular mechanism has been proposed to explain the inhibition of ROMK channels during severe and moderate hypokalemia. Low-K$^+$ intake increases renal superoxide anion generation, which stimulates PTK (protein tyrosine kinase) activity and MAPK (mitogen-activated protein kinase) phosphorylation. PTK inhibits ROMK activity through a tyrosine-mediated phosphorylation. MAPK can inhibit the activity of the ROMK-like SK and BK channels. Moreover, MAPK and PTK may have a positive feedback on each other. Since activation of PTK and MAPK inhibits the apical K-secretory channels, renal K$^+$ secretion is suppressed during K$^+$ restriction states[114] (Figure 50.7).

The decline in aldosterone levels and the increase of angiotensin II that accompany K$^+$ deficiency contribute to renal K$^+$ conservation. It has been proven that angiotensin II has an inhibitory effect on ROMK channels and, on the other hand, antagonists of the AT-1 receptor abolish the renal ability of K$^+$ conservation during K-restricted diet by preventing the tyrosine phosphorylation of the ROMK channels.[115] In K$^+$ deficiency states, the ratio of long versus kidney-specific Wnk1 isoforms represents a novel K-saving mechanism along the aldosterone-sensitive segments of the nephron (*vide infra*).

UREA

The concentrating defect of K$^+$ deficiency occurs in association with a reduced osmolality of the medullary

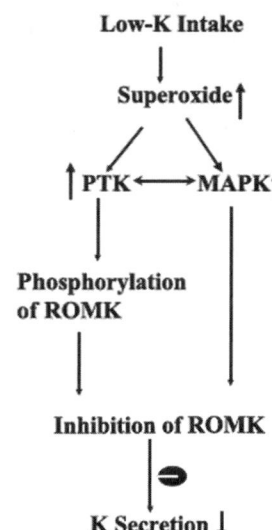

FIGURE 50.7 Cascade of events leading to the K$^+$-sparing effect in the CD during K$^+$ depletion states. Low extracellular K$^+$ stimulates an inactivating phosphorylation of ROMK channels through PTK and MAPK kinases.[114]

interstitium. Urea uptake in the kidney is mediated by a family of transporter proteins that include the renal urea transporter UT-A, and the erythrocyte urea transporter UT-B. UT-A1 and UT-A3 are localized in the distal part of the IMCD, and UT-A2 is localized in the descending thin limb of Henle's loop, while UT-B is localized in vasa recta. K$^+$ deficiency is associated with reduced expression of UT-A1, UT-A3, and UT-B, but with increased expression of UT-A2. These data suggest that the impairment of urea absorption in the terminal IMCD (UT-A1 and -A3), and the impairment of the vasa recta urea recycling, could play a key role in lowering the medullary osmolality of K$^+$ deficient mice.[116]

WATER

The concentrating defect of K$^+$ deficiency is manifest primarily as a limitation of maximal urinary concentrating ability, rather than persistent hyposthenuria. K$^+$ deficiency also results in polydypsia, thus accentuating polyuria independent of the urinary concentrating defect. In humans, thirst is a prominent symptom of experimental K$^+$ deficiency.[117] In rats, the increased water intake precedes the development of the urinary concentrating defect, and restriction of fluid intake in the initial phase attenuates the polyuria; however, it does not prevent the development of the urinary concentrating defect.[118]

In humans, the concentrating defect has been observed in pathologic and experimental K$^+$ deficiency. The degree of K$^+$ deficiency also relates to the severity of the urinary concentrating defect in the rat. The rat, however, is still capable of generating a maximally-concentrated urine for the first week,[118] while by 2 weeks the concentrating defect is fully established.[119]

Hypokalemic rats keep the basal water permeability at control level, whereas the response to vasopressin is significantly diminished.[120] These results are coupled with *in vitro* experiments where extracellular K^+ has been explored in rat renal papillary CD cells in culture.[121] Exposure of these cells to a K^+-free medium for more than 24 hours was associated with an attenuated cellular cAMP response to both vasopressin and forskolin. Hypokalemia results in decreased aquaporin-2 (AQP2) expression in principal cells of rat CD (cortical and medullary), in parallel with the development of polyuria. K^+ repletion is associated with normalization of AQP2 expression and urine output.[122]

Whether prostaglandin (PG) synthesis interferes with the action of vasopressin and the AQP2 system is not univocal among species. In rats, neither PGE_2 excretion nor papillary tissue content[118,123] is affected by K^+ deficiency. On the same line, indomethacin failed to reverse the concentrating defect, despite effective inhibition of medullary tissue prostaglandin synthesis.[118] The concentrating defect in K^+ deficiency is likely multifactorial; reduction in vasopressin response and in medullary interstitial osmolality are contributing mechanisms acting in a complementary fashion. Impaired NaCl reabsorption in the TAL and alteration in urea recycling limits the establishment of a hypertonic interstitium. The latter is a prerequisite for urine concentration, and it may be amplified by polydipsia and the consequent medullary washout. In addition, an impaired response of the CD to vasopressin contributes to the concentrating defect. Recently a tonicity-responsive enhancer-binding protein (TonEBP) has been identified as a transcriptional factor activated by hypertonicity. TonEBP, among other functions, plays a critical role in protecting renal medullary cells from the deleterious effects of hypertonicity. It is a key regulator of urinary concentration through the regulation of AQP2 and UT-A transcription, in a vasopressin-independent manner. K^+ deficiency conditions are associated with a downregulation of TonEBP in both inner and outer medullary CD and TAL. In the descending thin limb, TonEBP translocates from the nucleus to the cytoplasmic compartment where it is inactive. Lower interstitial osmolality occurring during K^+ deficiency could reduce TonEBP expression, and so contribute to the downregulation of AQP2 and UT-A[124] (Figure 50.8).

There is also evidence in K^+ deficiency for a decrease in inner medullary organic osmolytes which might precede the renal concentrating defect. Aldose-reductase (an osmoregulatory protein) mRNA abundance was reduced in K^+ deficiency.[125]

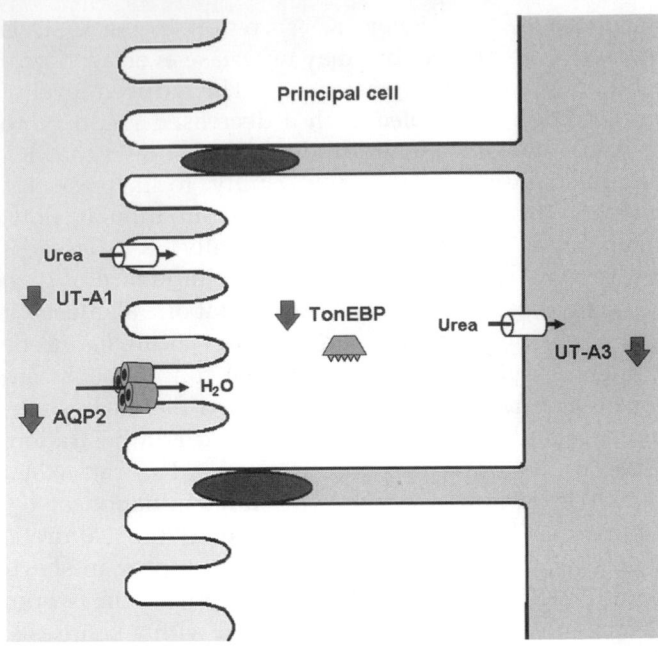

FIGURE 50.8 **A model of the urinary concentration impairment during K^+ deficiency.** In addition to a TAL-dependent low interstitial tonicity generation, principal cells along the CD play a key role. It has been described that K^+ deficiency downregulates AQP2 expression, mainly in cortical and OSOM CD.[122] In a mice model of K^+ deficiency, UT-A1 and UT-A3 are downregulated.[116] TonEBP could promote the downregulation of urea transporters and AQP2.[124]

System Biology Approach to Hypokalemia

Since the discoding of the human genome, a novel scientific approach has been widely diffuse in health science: so-called systems biology. Systems biology aims to observe any biological system in an holistic way. It examines multiple components of a biological system *simultaneously* through high-throughput techniques (transcriptomics, metabolomics, and proteomics), and integrates the data with mathematical models. Systems biology methods produce a vast amount of data to generate hypotheses on how the observed system works. It offers new opportunities to understand complex systems.

The OMCD transcriptome of hypokalemic mice has been compared with one from mice treated with an NH_4Cl-load. Data were determined by using the serial analysis for gene expression (SAGE) microassay; a cluster analysis of changed tags has been reported in this study. Hypokalemic mice showed overexpression of tags belonging to the cluster of proliferation and apoptosis, while tags of the transport cluster were predominant in NH_4Cl-induced acidotic mice. Several transcripts have been identified in these clusters, and they are listed in the study from Cheval *et al.*[126]

The proteome of kidneys from mild and severe hypokalemic mice has been examined by Thongboonkerd *et al.*[127] Chronic (8 weeks K$^+$ deficient diet) hypokalemic mice were compared with normokalemic mice. Two-dimensional gel-based MALDI-MS and/or Q-TOF MS/MS techniques were carried out on whole kidney samples. Thirty-three proteins induced by K$^+$ deficiency were identified. They are mainly metabolic enzymes and cytoskeletal proteins. Some of them are involved in the osmoregulatory process of the papillary interstitium, such as aldose reductase. A complete list of the altered proteins is also available.

SYSTEMIC EFFECTS OF K$^+$ DEPLETION

Healthy individuals may well tolerate short periods of mild K$^+$ deficiency; however, high K$^+$ deficiency may induce severe renal, cardiac, and neurologic injuries, and glucose intolerance. Indeed, reduced K$^+$ intake correlates directly with higher blood pressure in both normotensive and hypertensive individuals.

K$^+$ and Hypertension

Hypertension is a major health problem in developed countries. It has been extensively demonstrated that the occurrence of hypertension is associated with salt (NaCl) intake. There is evidence that dietary K$^+$ intake may participate in determining sensitivity to salt-induced hypertension.

Compared with our Paleolithic ancestors, the common Western diet contains a larger amount of Na$^+$ (150 versus 20 mmol per day), the majority (approximately 75%) is added to food products by manufacturers. While salt intake has been growing dramatically since the Paleolithic period, K$^+$ intake has been lessening (50 versus 320 mmol per day). This drop in K$^+$ intake is a consequence of reduced intake of fruits and vegetables in the diet. Epidemiologic studies have demonstrated that dietary K$^+$ is inversely related to the occurrence of hypertension, independently of salt intake.[128] An international study of electrolyte excretion and blood pressure performed on a large cohort of subjects, distributed in various countries, demonstrated that K$^+$ excretion is negatively and independently correlated with blood pressure.[129] Furthermore, K$^+$ supplementation (60 mmol KCl per day) decreased blood pressure in hypertensive patients with diuretic-induced hypokalemia.[130]

The role of dietary K$^+$ in controlling blood pressure has been assessed by the Dietary Approaches to Stop Hypertension (DASH) trial.[131] Slightly hypertensive individuals were arbitrarily assigned to either a control diet or to the DASH diet (a diet rich in vegetables, fruits, and low-fat dairy products); subgroups of participants on each diet were divided to ingest either low,

intermediate or high amounts of Na$^+$ (approximately 50, 100, and 150 mmol, respectively, per day). The DASH diet markedly reduced blood pressure, independent of Na$^+$ intake (Figure 50.9). According to a Scientific Statement issued by the American Heart Association, the beneficial blood pressure-lowering effect of the DASH diet is largely a function of its high K$^+$ content (about 120 mmol/day in the 2100 Kcal DASH diet versus approximately 60 mmol/day in the control diet).[132] The effect of K$^+$ supplementation on blood pressure was further confirmed in a meta-analysis of 33 clinical trials.[133]

The mechanisms by which low dietary K$^+$ intake increases blood pressure have been investigated.[134] It has been shown that the hypertensive effect of K$^+$ deficiency is prevented by lowering daily Na$^+$ intake. K$^+$ deficiency seems, at least partially, to enhance renal Na$^+$ reabsorption. This mechanism could be sustained by WNK1.[135]

New Physiologic Concepts in Aldosterone-Dependent Sodium and K$^+$ Handling

Aldosterone is an important regulator of the final composition of urine through its effects on the distal

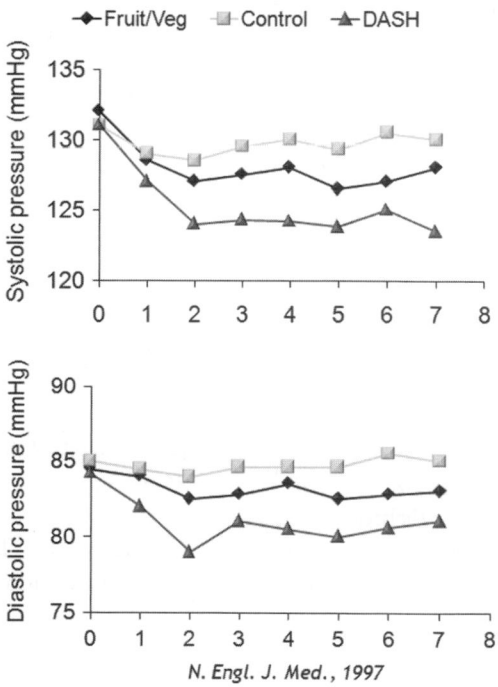

FIGURE 50.9 Progression of weekly blood pressure measurements during control diet, fruit- and vegetable-enriched diet and DASH diet. Control diet was typical of the diets of a substantial number of Americans with a K$^+$ content about 25th percentile of US consumption. The fruits- and vegetables-diet provided potassium and magnesium at levels close to the 75th percentile of consumption. The DASH diet had a K$^+$ content about 75th percentile of US consumption, and a reduced amount of saturated fat, total fat, and cholesterol. *(Adapted from Appel et al.[131])*

nephron. ENaC are activated by aldosterone, thus creating a lumen-negative potential. The luminal electronegativity supplies the driving force for Cl^- reabsorption through the paracellular pathway and K^+ and H^+ secretion. In such a way, Na^+ and K^+ homeostasis are finely tuned together. Aldosterone secretion is extremely sensitive to extracellular fluid volume depletion and hyperkalemia. In volume-depletion conditions, aldosterone increases salt reabsorption restoring extracellular fluid volume without generating hypokalemia. During hyperkalemia, aldosterone increases renal K^+ excretion, without concomitant renal salt retention.

The ability of the kidney to respond to increased aldosterone with two different physiologic adaptations (salt retention without K^+ secretion during volume-depletion states, and K^+ secretion without salt retention during hyperkalemia) is still a subject of debate. Recent data suggest a potential implication of the WNK kinase.[136] WNK (with no lysine) kinases are a novel family of large serine/threonine protein kinases that are conserved in multicellular organisms.[137] At present, there are four known mammalian WNK family members: WNK1, WNK2, WNK3, and WNK4. WNK4 is widely-expressed in epithelial tissues. Full-length WNK1 is ubiquitous, and is also known as long WNK1 (L-WNK1); an alternatively spliced WNK1 isoform is specifically expressed in the kidney and is, therefore, known as kidney-specific WNK1 (KS-WNK1). KS-WNK1 is an antagonist of L-WNK1.[138] L-WNK1 has been demonstrated to enhance the activity of both ENaC[139] and NCC; the latter occurs through the inhibition of WNK4, which in turn is capable of inhibiting NCC. Both L-WNK1 and WNK4 inhibit ROMK. Interestingly, KS-WNK1 antagonizes L-WNK1 with respect to its effects on ROMK, NCC, and ENaC. Therefore, a positive ratio of L-WNK1 to KS-WNK1 increases the rate of Na^+ reabsorption via ENaC and NCC, and decreases the rate of K^+ secretion by inhibiting ROMK. However, these effects uncouple Na^+ reabsorption from K^+ secretion. These mechanisms may be central to enlighten the hypotensive effect of K^+ supplementation in salt-sensitive hypertension. Indeed, high K^+ stimulates aldosterone secretion, which would be predicted to stimulate a hypertensive, rather than a hypotensive, effect. The abundance of ROMK in the apical membrane of distal nephron is regulated by dietary K^+ intake.[140] It has been reported that high- and low-K^+ intake increases and decreases KS-WNK1 expression, respectively. Low-K^+ intake also increases the expression of L-WNK1 in the kidney. The ratio of L-WNK1 to KS-WNK1 in the kidney is, therefore, increased when K^+ intake is low, and reduced when intake is high. So, by increasing the ratio of L-WNK1 to KS-WNK1, the kidney simultaneously conserves K^+ and Na^+ during K^+ deficiency (Figure 50.10). This effect could be implicated in the pathogenesis of salt-sensitive hypertension, and explain the positive action of high-K^+ intake on blood pressure.

K^+ Depletion and Glucose Intolerance

Insulin controls both K^+ and glucose homeostasis. It is possible that there is a common pathway between the two systems. Insulin-resistance is usually correlated with hyperinsulinemia, because pancreatic β-cells raise insulin secretion to balance insulin resistance.[141] The resulting hyperinsulinemia may induce hypokalemia from excessive cellular K^+ uptake, if the effect of insulin on K^+ uptake is not similarly reduced. In fact, a weakened insulin effect on K^+ fluxes in obesity and diabetes has been demonstrated,[142] which are both correlated with insulin resistance with respect to glucose metabolism.

There are data indicating that there are two distinct varieties of insulin resistance: resistance to cellular glucose uptake observed in type 2 diabetes; and resistance to cellular K^+ uptake observed during K^+ deficiency or fasting.

The molecular mechanisms involved in the differential regulation of glucose versus K^+ cellular uptake by insulin are not known. It is highly probable that these pathways are related to post-binding actions of insulin to its receptor, which is a common step in the regulation of K^+ and glucose uptake. The resistance of

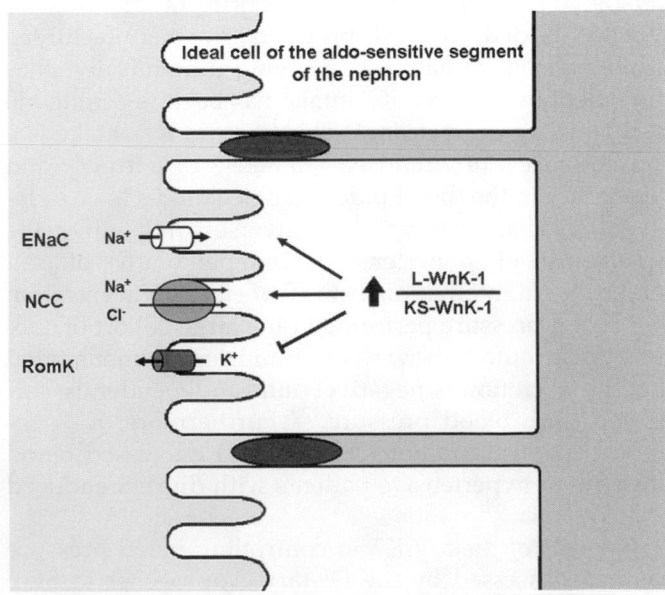

FIGURE 50.10　The role of WNK in Na^+ and K^+ handling along the aldosterone-sensitive segments. Hypokalemia induces an increase in the ratio of L-WNK1 to KS-WNK1 in the kidney, which decreases renal K^+ secretion in order to conserve K^+; however, this also causes reabsorption of Na^+ via ENaC and NCC.[140]

muscle cell glucose uptake during insulin resistance is attributed to an impairment of insulin signaling at the level of PI3-kinase, which involves GLUT4 trafficking.[143] Insulin has been suggested to trigger cellular K^+ uptake by activating the Na^+ pump.[144] It has also been anticipated that activation in the kidney, during K^+ deprivation, of NADPH oxidase, superoxide anion production, and PTK activities may affect insulin stimulation of K^+ cellular uptake.

Hypokalemia may play a role in the well-known association between the use of thiazide diuretics and the development of diabetes. It has been estimated that a decrease of 1 mEq/L K^+ may cause an approximately 10 mg/dl increase in glucose. These data are confirmed by the observation that glucose levels can be normalized after K^+ repletion in patients who have hypokalemia. The mechanism of thiazide-induced hyperglycemia is thought to be the consequence of decreased insulin released from the pancreatic beta cell. ATP-sensitive K^+ channels link cell metabolism to electrical activity, thereby playing an important role in the control of insulin secretion.

References

[1] Greenlee M, Wingo CS, McDonough AA, Youn JH, Kone BC. Narrative review: evolving concepts in potassium homeostasis and hypokalemia. Ann Intern Med 2009;150(9):619–25.

[2] Giebisch GH, Wang WH. Potassium transport – an update. J Nephrol 2010;23(Suppl 16):S97–104.

[3] Wang W. Regulation of renal K transport by dietary K intake. Annu Rev Physiol 2004;66:547–69.

[4] Giebisch G, Krapf R, Wagner C. Renal and extrarenal regulation of potassium. Kidney Int 2007;72(4):397–410.

[5] McDonough AA, Thompson CB, Youn JH. Skeletal muscle regulates extracellular potassium. Am J Physiol Renal Physiol 2002;282(6):F967–74.

[6] Youn JH, McDonough AA. Recent advances in understanding integrative control of potassium homeostasis. Annu Rev Physiol 2009;71:381–401.

[7] Rabinowitz L. Aldosterone and potassium homeostasis. Kidney Int 1996;49(6):1738–42.

[8] Rabinowitz L. Model of homeostatic regulation of potassium excretion in sheep. Am J Physiol 1988;254(2 Pt 2):R381–8.

[9] Bankir L, Martin H, Dechaux M, Ahloulay M. Plasma cAMP: a hepatorenal link influencing proximal reabsorption and renal hemodynamics? Kidney Int Suppl 1997;59:S50–6.

[10] Choi MJ, Ziyadeh FN. The utility of the transtubular potassium gradient in the evaluation of hyperkalemia. J Am Soc Nephrol 2008;19(3):424–6.

[11] El-Hennawy AS, Nesa M, Mahmood AK. Thyrotoxic hypokalemic periodic paralysis triggered by high carbohydrate diet. Am J Ther 2007;14(5):499–501.

[12] Finsterer J. Primary periodic paralyses. Acta Neurol Scand 2008;117(3):145–58.

[13] Tagami T, Usui T, Shimatsu A, Naruse M. Toxic thyroid adenoma presenting as hypokalemic periodic paralysis. Endocr J 2007;54(5):797–803.

[14] Sitprija V. Altered fluid, electrolyte and mineral status in tropical disease, with an emphasis on malaria and leptospirosis. Nat Clin Pract Nephrol 2008;4(2):91–101.

[15] Ikuta S, Yasui C, Kawanaka M, Aihara T, Yoshie H, Yanagi H, et al. Watery diarrhea, hypokalemia and achlorhydria syndrome due to an adrenal pheochromocytoma. World J Gastroenterol 2007;13(34):4649–52.

[16] Blondon H, Bechade D, Desrame J, Algayres JP. Secretory diarrhoea with high faecal potassium concentrations: a new mechanism of diarrhoea associated with colonic pseudo-obstruction? Report of five patients. Gastroenterol Clin Biol 2008;32(4):401–4.

[17] Simon DB, Karet FE, Rodriguez-Soriano J, Hamdan JH, DiPietro A, Trachtman H, et al. Genetic heterogeneity of Bartter's syndrome revealed by mutations in the K^+ channel, ROMK. Nat Genet 1996;14(2):152–6.

[18] Adachi M, Asakura Y, Sato Y, Tajima T, Nakajima T, Yamamoto T, et al. Novel SLC12A1 (NKCC2) mutations in two families with Bartter syndrome type 1. Endocr J 2007;54(6):1003–7.

[19] Pressler CA, Heinzinger J, Jeck N, Waldegger P, Pechmann U, Reinalter S, et al. Late-onset manifestation of antenatal Bartter syndrome as a result of residual function of the mutated renal Na^+-K^+-$2Cl^-$ co-transporter. J Am Soc Nephrol 2006;17 (8):2136–42.

[20] Simon DB, Karet FE, Rodriguez-Soriano J, Hamdan JH, DiPietro A, Trachtman H, et al. Genetic heterogeneity of Bartter's syndrome revealed by mutations in the K^+ channel, ROMK. Nat Genet 1996;14(2):152–6.

[21] International Collaborative Study Group for Bartter-like Syndromes. Mutations in the gene encoding the inwardly-rectifying renal potassium channel, ROMK, cause the antenatal variant of Bartter syndrome: evidence for genetic heterogeneity. Hum Mol Genet 1997;6(1):17–26.

[22] Bailey MA, Cantone A, Yan Q, MacGregor GG, Leng Q, Amorim JB, et al. Maxi-K channels contribute to urinary potassium excretion in the ROMK-deficient mouse model of Type II Bartter's syndrome and in adaptation to a high-K diet. Kidney Int 2006;70(1):51–9.

[23] Kramer BK, Bergler T, Stoelcker B, Waldegger S. Mechanisms of disease: the kidney-specific chloride channels ClCKA and ClCKB, the Barttin subunit, and their clinical relevance. Nat Clin Pract Nephrol 2008;4(1):38–46.

[24] Konrad M, Vollmer M, Lemmink HH, van den Heuvel LP, Jeck N, Vargas-Poussou R, et al. Mutations in the chloride channel gene CLCNKB as a cause of classic Bartter syndrome. J Am Soc Nephrol 2000;11(8):1449–59.

[25] Matsumura Y, Uchida S, Kondo Y, Miyazaki H, Ko SB, Hayama A, et al. Overt nephrogenic diabetes insipidus in mice lacking the CLC-K1 chloride channel. Nat Genet 1999;21(1):95–8.

[26] Estevez R, Boettger T, Stein V, Birkenhager R, Otto E, Hildebrandt F, et al. Barttin is a Cl^- channel beta-subunit crucial for renal Cl^- reabsorption and inner ear K^+ secretion. Nature 2001;414(6863):558–61.

[27] Rickheit G, Maier H, Strenzke N, Andreescu CE, De Zeeuw CL, Muenscher A, et al. Endocochlear potential depends on Cl^- channels: mechanism underlying deafness in Bartter syndrome IV. EMBO J 2008;27(21):2907–17.

[28] Watanabe S, Fukumoto S, Chang H, Takeuchi Y, Hasegawa Y, Okazaki R, et al. Association between activating mutations of calcium-sensing receptor and Bartter's syndrome. Lancet 2002;360(9334):692–4.

[29] Chen YH, Lin JJ, Jeansonne BG, Tatum R, Lu Q. Analysis of claudin genes in pediatric patients with Bartter's syndrome. Ann N Y Acad Sci 2009;1165:126–34.

[30] Welling PA, Ho K. A comprehensive guide to the ROMK potassium channel: form and function in health and disease. Am J Physiol Renal Physiol 2009;297(4):F849–63.

[31] Geibel JP. The calcium-sensing receptor. J Nephrol 2010;23 (Suppl 16):S130–5.

[32] Miyamura N, Matsumoto K, Taguchi T, Tokunaga H, Nishikawa T, Nishida K, et al. Atypical Bartter syndrome with sensorineural deafness with G47R mutation of the beta-subunit for ClC-Ka and ClC-Kb chloride channels, barttin. J Clin Endocrinol Metab 2003;88(2):781–6.

[33] Knoers NV, Levtchenko EN. Gitelman syndrome. Orphanet J Rare Dis 2008;3:22.

[34] de Jong JC, Van DV, van den Heuvel LP, Willems PH, Knoers NV, Bindels RJ. Functional expression of mutations in the human NaCl co-transporter: evidence for impaired routing mechanisms in Gitelman's syndrome. J Am Soc Nephrol 2002;13(6):1442–8.

[35] Kunchaparty S, Palcso M, Berkman J, Velasquez H, Desir GV, Bernstein P, et al. Defective processing and expression of thiazide-sensitive Na–Cl co-transporter as a cause of Gitelman's syndrome. Am J Physiol 1999;277(4 Pt 2):F643–9.

[36] Nijenhuis T, Vallon V, van der Kemp AW, Loffing J, Hoenderop JG, Bindels RJ. Enhanced passive Ca^{2+} reabsorption and reduced Mg^{2+} channel abundance explains thiazide-induced hypocalciuria and hypomagnesemia. J Clin Invest 2005;115 (6):1651–8.

[37] Yang SS, Lo YF, Yu IS, Lin SW, Chang TH, Hsu YJ, et al. Generation and analysis of the thiazide-sensitive $Na^+–Cl^-$ co-transporter (Ncc/Slc12a3) Ser707X knockin mouse as a model of Gitelman syndrome. Hum Mutat 2010;31(12):1304–15.

[38] Enriquez R, Adam V, Sirvent AE, Garcia-Garcia AB, Millan I, Amoros F. Gitelman syndrome due to p.A204T mutation in CLCNKB gene. Int Urol Nephrol 2010;42(4):1099–102.

[39] Jeck N, Konrad M, Peters M, Weber S, Bonzel KE, Seyberth HW. Mutations in the chloride channel gene, CLCNKB, leading to a mixed Bartter–Gitelman phenotype. Pediatr Res 2000;48 (6):754–8.

[40] Riveira-Munoz E, Chang Q, Godefroid N, Hoenderop JG, Bindels RJ, Dahan K, et al. Transcriptional and functional analyses of SLC12A3 mutations: new clues for the pathogenesis of Gitelman syndrome. J Am Soc Nephrol 2007;18 (4):1271–83.

[41] Shimkets RA, Warnock DG, Bositis CM, Nelson-Williams C, Hansson JH, Schambelan M, et al. Liddle's syndrome: heritable human hypertension caused by mutations in the beta subunit of the epithelial sodium channel. Cell 1994;79 (3):407–14.

[42] Schild L, Canessa CM, Shimkets RA, Gautschi I, Lifton RP, Rossier BC. A mutation in the epithelial sodium channel causing Liddle disease increases channel activity in the Xenopus laevis oocyte expression system. Proc Natl Acad Sci USA 1995;92 (12):5699–703.

[43] Abriel H, Loffing J, Rebhun JF, Pratt JH, Schild L, Horisberger JD, et al. Defective regulation of the epithelial Na^+ channel by Nedd4 in Liddle's syndrome. J Clin Invest 1999;103(5):667–73.

[44] Henry PC, Kanelis V, O'Brien MC, Kim B, Gautschi I, Forman-Kay J, et al. Affinity and specificity of interactions between Nedd4 isoforms and the epithelial Na^+ channel. J Biol Chem 2003;278(22):20019–28.

[45] Lifton RP. Molecular genetics of human blood pressure variation. Science 1996;272(5262):676–80.

[46] Dahlmann A, Pradervand S, Hummler E, Rossier BC, Frindt G, Palmer LG. Mineralocorticoid regulation of epithelial Na^+ channels is maintained in a mouse model of Liddle's syndrome. Am J Physiol Renal Physiol 2003;285(2):F310–8.

[47] Auberson M, Hoffmann-Pochon N, Vandewalle A, Kellenberger S, Schild L. Epithelial Na^+ channel mutants causing Liddle's syndrome retain ability to respond to aldosterone and vasopressin. Am J Physiol Renal Physiol 2003;285(3):F459–71.

[48] Warnock DG. Liddle syndrome: an autosomal dominant form of human hypertension. Kidney Int 1998;53(1):18–24.

[49] Pradervand S, Wang Q, Burnier M, Beermann F, Horisberger JD, Hummler E, et al. A mouse model for Liddle's syndrome. J Am Soc Nephrol 1999;10(12):2527–33.

[50] Tapolyai M, Uysal A, Dossabhoy NR, Zsom L, Szarvas T, Lengvarsky Z, et al. High prevalence of Liddle syndrome phenotype among hypertensive US Veterans in Northwest Louisiana. J Clin Hypertens (Greenwich) 2010;12(11):856–60.

[51] Reungjui S, Hu H, Mu W, Roncal CA, Croker BP, Patel JM, et al. Thiazide-induced subtle renal injury not observed in states of equivalent hypokalemia. Kidney Int 2007;72(12):1483–92.

[52] Ordonez NG, Toback FG, Aithal HN, Spargo BJ. Zonal changes in renal structure and phospholipid metabolism during reversal of potassium depletion nephropathy. Lab Invest 1977;36(1):33–47.

[53] Cheval L, Duong Van Huyen JP, Bruneval P, Verbavatz JM, Elalouf JM, Doucet A. Plasticity of mouse renal collecting duct in response to potassium depletion. Physiol Genomics 2004;19 (1):61–73.

[54] Peterson LN, Carpenter B, Guttierrez GA, Fajardo C, Levine DZ. Potassium depletion enhances renal compensatory hypertrophy in the nephrectomized rat. Miner Electrolyte Metab 1987;13(1):57–62.

[55] Hansen GP, Tisher CC, Robinson RR. Response of the collecting duct to disturbances of acid–base and potassium balance. Kidney Int 1980;17(3):326–37.

[56] Stanton BA, Biemesderfer D, Wade JB, Giebisch G. Structural and functional study of the rat distal nephron: effects of potassium adaptation and depletion. Kidney Int 1981;19(1):36–48.

[57] Stetson DL, Wade JB, Giebisch G. Morphologic alterations in the rat medullary collecting duct following potassium depletion. Kidney Int 1980;17(1):45–56.

[58] Reungjui S, Roncal CA, Sato W, Glushakova OY, Croker BP, Suga S, et al. Hypokalemic nephropathy is associated with impaired angiogenesis. J Am Soc Nephrol 2008;19(1):125–34.

[59] Sarkar K, Levine DZ. Ultrastructural changes in the renal papillary cells of rats during maintenance and repair of profound potassium depletion. Br J Exp Pathol 1979;60(2):120–9.

[60] Toback FG, Ordonez NG, Bortz SL, Spargo BH. Zonal changes in renal structure and phospholipid metabolism in potassium-deficient rats. Lab Invest 1976;34(2):115–24.

[61] O'Reilly DS. Increased ammoniagenesis and the renal tubular effects of potassium depletion. J Clin Pathol 1984;37 (12):1358–62.

[62] Shibata M, Yoshimura K, Furuya N, Koike M, Ueno T, Komatsu M, et al. The MAP1-LC3 conjugation system is involved in lipid droplet formation. Biochem Biophys Res Commun 2009;382 (2):419–23.

[63] Sarkar K, Nash LA, Levine DZ. Effects of ureteral ligation on renal medullary lesions of potassium depletion. Br J Exp Pathol 1983;64(6):677–83.

[64] Sarkar K, Levine DZ. Minimal medullary droplets in DOCA-induced potassium depletion of rats. Invest Urol 1978;15 (4):280–3.

[65] Kimura T, Nishino T, Maruyama N, Hamano K, Kubo A, Iwano M, et al. Expression of Bcl-2 and Bax in hypokalemic nephropathy in rats. Pathobiology 2001;69(5):237–48.

[66] Lelamali K, Khunkitti W, Yenrudi S, Panichaphongse V, Huiprasert L, Sitprija V, et al. Potassium depletion in a healthy north-eastern Thai population: no association with tubulointerstitial injury. Nephrology (Carlton) 2003;8(1):28–32.

[67] Riemenschneider T, Bohle A. Morphologic aspects of low-potassium and low-sodium nephropathy. Clin Nephrol 1983;19(6):271–9.

[68] Aithal HN, Toback FG, Dube S, Getz GS, Spargo BH. Formation of renal medullary lysosomes during potassium depletion nephropathy. Lab Invest 1977;36(2):107–13.

[69] Cremer W, Bock KD. Symptoms and course of chronic hypokalemic nephropathy in man. Clin Nephrol 1977;7(3):112–9.

[70] bdel-Rahman EM, Moorthy AV. End-stage renal disease (ESRD) in patients with eating disorders. Clin Nephrol 1997;47(2):106–11.

[71] Danforth Jr DN, Orlando MM, Bartter FC, Javadpour N. Renal changes in primary aldosteronism. J Urol 1977;117(2):140–4.

[72] Cardinal J, Duchesneau D. Effect of potassium on proximal tubular function. Am J Physiol 1978;234(5):F381–5.

[73] Chan YL, Biagi B, Giebisch G. Control mechanisms of bicarbonate transport across the rat proximal convoluted tubule. Am J Physiol 1982;242(5):F532–43.

[74] Walter SJ, Shore AC, Shirley DG. Effect of potassium depletion on renal tubular function in the rat. Clin Sci (Lond) 1988;75(6):621–8.

[75] Shirley DG, Walter SJ, Folkerd EJ, Unwin RJ, Bailey MA. Transepithelial electrochemical gradients in the proximal convoluted tubule during potassium depletion in the rat. J Physiol 1998;513(Pt 2):551–7.

[76] Huang L, Wei YY, Momose-Hotokezaka A, Dickey J, Okusa MD. Alpha 2B-adrenergic receptors: immunolocalization and regulation by potassium depletion in rat kidney. Am J Physiol 1996;270(6 Pt 2):F1015–26.

[77] Fryer JN, Burns KD, Ghorbani M, Levine DZ. Effect of potassium depletion on proximal tubule AT1 receptor localization in normal and remnant rat kidney. Kidney Int 2001;60(5):1792–9.

[78] Elkjaer ML, Kwon TH, Wang W, Nielsen J, Knepper MA, Frøkiaer J, et al. Altered expression of renal NHE3, TSC, BSC-1, and ENaC subunits in potassium-depleted rats. Am J Physiol Renal Physiol 2002;283(6):F1376–88.

[79] Wang Z, Baird N, Shumaker H, Soleimani M. Potassium depletion and acid–base transporters in rat kidney: differential effect of hypophysectomy. Am J Physiol 1997;272(6 Pt 2):F736–43.

[80] Riquier AD, Lee DH, McDonough AA. Renal NHE3 and NaPi2 partition into distinct membrane domains. Am J Physiol Cell Physiol 2009;296(4):C900–10.

[81] Capasso G, Kinne R, Malnic G, Giebisch G. Renal bicarbonate reabsorption in the rat. I. Effects of hypokalemia and carbonic anhydrase. J Clin Invest 1986;78(6):1558–67.

[82] Yang X, Amemiya M, Peng Y, Moe OW, Preisig PA, Alpern RJ. Acid incubation causes exocytic insertion of NHE3 in OKP cells. Am J Physiol Cell Physiol 2000;279(2):C410–9.

[83] Soleimani M, Burnham CE. Physiologic and molecular aspects of the Na$^+$:HCO$_3^-$ cotransporter in health and disease processes. Kidney Int 2000;57(2):371–84.

[84] Turban S, Beutler KT, Morris RG, Masilamani S, Fenton RA, Knepper MA, et al. Long-term regulation of proximal tubule acid–base transporter abundance by angiotensin II. Kidney Int 2006;70(4):660–8.

[85] Tizianello A, Garibotto G, Robaudo C, Saffioti S, Pontremoli R, Bruzzone M, et al. Renal ammoniagenesis in humans with chronic potassium depletion. Kidney Int 1991;40(4):772–8.

[86] Nonoguchi H, Takehara Y, Endou H. Intra- and inter-nephron heterogeneity of ammoniagenesis in rats: effects of chronic metabolic acidosis and potassium depletion. Pflugers Arch 1986;407(3):245–51.

[87] Fraley DS, Adler S, Rankin B, Curthoys N, Zett B. Relationship of phosphate-dependent glutaminase activity to ammonia excretion in potassium deficiency and acidosis. Miner Electrolyte Metab 1985;11(3):140–9.

[88] Sastrasinh S, Sastrasinh M. Renal mitochondrial glutamine metabolism during K$^+$ depletion. Am J Physiol 1986;250(4 Pt 2):F667–73.

[89] Busque SM, Wagner CA. Potassium restriction, high protein intake, and metabolic acidosis increase expression of the glutamine transporter SNAT3 (Slc38a3) in mouse kidney. Am J Physiol Renal Physiol 2009;297(2):F440–50.

[90] Murer H, Biber J. Phosphate transport in the kidney. J Nephrol 2010;23(Suppl 16):S145–51.

[91] Breusegem SY, Takahashi H, Giral-Arnal H, Wang X, Jiang T, Verlander JW, et al. Differential regulation of the renal sodium-phosphate co-transporters NaPi-IIa, NaPi-IIc, and PiT-2 in dietary potassium deficiency. Am J Physiol Renal Physiol 2009;297(2):F350–61.

[92] Levi M, McDonald LA, Preisig PA, Alpern RJ. Chronic K depletion stimulates rat renal brush-border membrane Na-citrate co-transporter. Am J Physiol 1991;261(5 Pt 2):F767–73.

[93] Eknoyan G, Martinez-Maldonado M, Suki WN, Richie Y. Renal diluting capacity in the hypokalemic rat. Am J Physiol 1970;219(4):933–7.

[94] Gutsche HU, Peterson LN, Levine DZ. In vivo evidence of impaired solute transport by the thick ascending limb in potassium-depleted rats. J Clin Invest 1984;73(4):908–16.

[95] Greger R. Cation selectivity of the isolated perfused cortical thick ascending limb of Henle's loop of rabbit kidney. Pflugers Arch 1981;390(1):30–7.

[96] Buffin-Meyer B, Marsy S, Barlet-Bas C, Cheval L, Younes-Ibrahim M, Rajerison R, et al. Regulation of renal Na$^+$,K$^{(+)}$-ATPase in rat thick ascending limb during K$^+$ depletion: evidence for modulation of Na$^+$ affinity. J Physiol 1996;490(Pt 3):623–32.

[97] Laghmani K, Richer C, Borensztein P, Paillard M, Froissart M. Expression of rat thick limb Na/H exchangers in potassium depletion and chronic metabolic acidosis. Kidney Int 2001;60(4):1386–96.

[98] Jakobsen JK, Odgaard E, Wang W, Elkjaer ML, Nielsen S, Aalkjaer C, et al. Functional up-regulation of basolateral Na$^+$-dependent HCO$_3^-$ transporter NBCn1 in medullary thick ascending limb of K$^+$-depleted rats. Pflugers Arch 2004;448(6):571–8.

[99] Capasso G, Kinne R, Malnic G, Giebisch G. Renal bicarbonate reabsorption in the rat. I. Effects of hypokalemia and carbonic anhydrase. J Clin Invest 1986;78(6):1558–67.

[100] Capasso G, Jaeger P, Giebisch G, Guckian V, Malnic G. Renal bicarbonate reabsorption in the rat. II. Distal tubule load dependence and effect of hypokalemia. J Clin Invest 1987;80(2):409–14.

[101] Bailey M, Capasso G, Agulian S, Giebisch G, Unwin R. The relationship between distal tubular proton secretion and dietary potassium depletion: evidence for up-regulation of H$^+$-ATPase. Nephrol Dial Transplant 1999;14(6):1435–40.

[102] Hayashi M, Katz AI. The kidney in potassium depletion. I. Na$^+$-K$^+$-ATPase activity and [^{3}H]ouabain binding in MCT. Am J Physiol 1987;252(3 Pt 2):F437–46.

[103] McDonough AA, Magyar CE, Komatsu Y. Expression of Na$^{(+)}$-K$^{(+)}$-ATPase alpha- and beta-subunits along rat nephron: isoform specificity and response to hypokalemia. Am J Physiol 1994;267(4 Pt 1):C901–8.

[104] Wall SM, Fischer MP, Kim GH, Nguyen BM, Hassell KA. In rat inner medullary collecting duct, NH uptake by the Na,K-

ATPase is increased during hypokalemia. Am J Physiol Renal Physiol 2002;282(1):F91—102.

[105] Bailey MA, Fletcher RM, Woodrow DF, Unwin RJ, Walter SJ. Upregulation of H$^+$-ATPase in the distal nephron during potassium depletion: structural and functional evidence. Am J Physiol 1998;275(6 Pt 2):F878—84.

[106] Silver RB, Breton S, Brown D. Potassium depletion increases proton pump (H($^+$)-ATPase) activity in intercalated cells of cortical collecting duct. Am J Physiol Renal Physiol 2000;279 (1):F195—202.

[107] Barone S, Amlal H, Kujala M, Xu J, Karet F, Blanchard A, et al. Regulation of the basolateral chloride/base exchangers AE1 and SLC26A7 in the kidney collecting duct in potassium depletion. Nephrol Dial Transplant 2007;22(12): 3462—70.

[108] Xu J, Worrell RT, Li HC, Barone SL, Petrovic S, Amlal H, et al. Chloride/bicarbonate exchanger SLC26A7 is localized in endosomes in medullary collecting duct cells, and is targeted to the basolateral membrane in hypertonicity and potassium depletion. J Am Soc Nephrol 2006;17(4):956—67.

[109] Gumz ML, Lynch IJ, Greenlee MM, Cain BD, Wingo CS. The renal H$^+$-K$^+$-ATPases: physiology, regulation, and structure. Am J Physiol Renal Physiol 2010;298(1):F12—21.

[110] Wagner CA, Finberg KE, Stehberger PA, Lifton RP, Geibisch GH, Aronson PS, et al. Regulation of the expression of the Cl$^-$/anion exchanger pendrin in mouse kidney by acid—base status. Kidney Int 2002;62(6):2109—17.

[111] Linas SL, Peterson LN, Anderson RJ, Aisenbrey GA, Simon FR, Berl T. Mechanism of renal potassium conservation in the rat. Kidney Int 1979;15(6):601—11.

[112] Malnic G, Berliner RW, Giebisch G. Flow dependence of K$^+$ secretion in cortical distal tubules of the rat. Am J Physiol 1989;256(5 Pt 2):F932—41.

[113] Wang W. Regulation of renal K transport by dietary K intake. Annu Rev Physiol 2004;66:547—69.

[114] Wang ZJ, Sun P, Xing W, Pan C, Lin DH, Wang WH. Decrease in dietary K intake stimulates the generation of superoxide anions in the kidney and inhibits K secretory channels in the CCD. Am J Physiol Renal Physiol 2010;298(6): F1515—22.

[115] Jin Y, Wang Y, Wang ZJ, Lin DH, Wang WH. Inhibition of angiotensin type 1 receptor impairs renal ability of K conservation in response to K restriction. Am J Physiol Renal Physiol 2009;296(5):F1179—84.

[116] Jung JY, Madsen KM, Han KH, Yang CW, Knepper MA, Sands JMJ, et al. Expression of urea transporters in potassium-depleted mouse kidney. Am J Physiol Renal Physiol 2003;285 (6):F1210—24.

[117] Garella S, Chang B, Kahn SI. Alterations of hydrogen ion homeostasis in pure potassium depletion: studies in rats and dogs during the recovery phase. J Lab Clin Med 1979;93 (2):321—31.

[118] Berl T, Aisenbrey GA, Linas SL. Renal concentrating defect in the hypokalemic rat is prostaglandin independent. Am J Physiol 1980;238(1):F37—41.

[119] Peterson LN. Time-dependent changes in inner medullary plasma flow rate during potassium-depletion. Kidney Int 1984;25(6):899—905.

[120] Carney S, Rayson B, Morgan T. A study in vitro of the concentrating defect associated with hypokalaemia and hypercalcaemia. Pflugers Arch 1976;366(1):11—7.

[121] Ishikawa S, Saito T, Kuzuya T. Role of potassium in vasopressin-induced production of cyclic AMP in rat renal papillary collecting tubule cells in culture. J Endocrinol 1987;113(2):199—204.

[122] Marples D, Frokiaer J, Dorup J, Knepper MA, Nielsen S. Hypokalemia-induced downregulation of aquaporin-2 water channel expression in rat kidney medulla and cortex. J Clin Invest 1996;97(8):1960—8.

[123] Beck N, Shaw JO. Thromboxane B2 and prostaglandin E2 in the K$^+$-depleted rat kidney. Am J Physiol 1981;240(2): F151—7.

[124] Jeon US, Han KH, Park SH, Lee SD, Sheen MR, Jung JY, et al. Downregulation of renal TonEBP in hypokalemic rats. Am J Physiol Renal Physiol 2007;293(1):F408—15.

[125] Nakanishi T, Yamauchi A, Yamamoto S, Sugita M, Takamitsu Y. Potassium depletion modulates aldose reductase mRNA in rat renal inner medulla. Kidney Int 1996;50(3):828—34.

[126] Cheval L, Morla L, Elalouf JM, Doucet A. Kidney collecting duct acid—base "regulon.". Physiol Genomics 2006;27 (3):271—81.

[127] Thongboonkerd V, Chutipongtanate S, Kanlaya R, Songtawee N, Sinchaikul S, Parichatikanond P, et al. Proteomic identification of alterations in metabolic enzymes and signaling proteins in hypokalemic nephropathy. Proteomics 2006;6(7): 2273—85.

[128] Langford HG. Dietary potassium and hypertension: epidemiologic data. Ann Intern Med 1983;98(5 Pt 2):770—2.

[129] Intersalt Cooperative Research Group 14. Intersalt: an international study of electrolyte excretion and blood pressure. Results for 24 hour urinary sodium and potassium excretion. BMJ 1988;297(6644):319—28.

[130] Kaplan NM, Carnegie A, Raskin P, Heller JA, Simmons M. Potassium supplementation in hypertensive patients with diuretic-induced hypokalemia. N Engl J Med 1985;312 (12):746—9.

[131] Appel LJ, Moore TJ, Obarzanek E, Vollmer WM, Svetkey LP, Sacks FM, et al. A clinical trial of the effects of dietary patterns on blood pressure. DASH Collaborative Research Group. N Engl J Med 1997;336(16):1117—24.

[132] Appel LJ, Brands MW, Daniels SR, Karanja N, Elmer PJ, Sacks FM. Dietary approaches to prevent and treat hypertension: a scientific statement from the American Heart Association. Hypertension 2006;47(2):296—308.

[133] Whelton PK, He J, Cutler JA, Brancati FL, Appel LJ, Follmann D, et al. Effects of oral potassium on blood pressure. Meta-analysis of randomized controlled clinical trials. JAMA 1997;277(20):1624—32.

[134] Grimm Jr RH, Neaton JD, Elmer PJ, Svendsen KH, Levin J, Segal M, et al. The influence of oral potassium chloride on blood pressure in hypertensive men on a low-sodium diet. N Engl J Med 1990;322(9):569—74.

[135] Huang CL, Kuo E. Mechanisms of disease: WNK-ing at the mechanism of salt-sensitive hypertension. Nat Clin Pract Nephrol 2007;3(11):623—30.

[136] Kahle KT, Wilson FH, Leng Q, Lalioti MD, O'Connell AD, Dong K, et al. WNK4 regulates the balance between renal NaCl reabsorption and K$^+$ secretion. Nat Genet 2003;35 (4):372—6.

[137] Xu B, English JM, Wilsbacher JL, Stippec S, Goldsmith EJ, Cobb MH. WNK1, a novel mammalian serine/threonine protein kinase lacking the catalytic lysine in subdomain II. J Biol Chem 2000;275(22):16795—801.

[138] Subramanya AR, Yang CL, Zhu X, Ellison DH. Dominant-negative regulation of WNK1 by its kidney-specific kinase-defective isoform. Am J Physiol Renal Physiol 2006;290(3): F619—24.

[139] Xu BE, Stippec S, Chu PY, Lazrak A, Li XJ, Lee BH, et al. WNK1 activates SGK1 to regulate the epithelial sodium channel. Proc Natl Acad Sci USA 2005;102(29):10315—20.

[140] Chu PY, Quigley R, Babich V, Huang CL. Dietary potassium restriction stimulates endocytosis of ROMK channel in rat cortical collecting duct. Am J Physiol Renal Physiol 2003;285(6):F1179−87.

[141] Bergman RN, Ader M, Huecking K, Van CG. Accurate assessment of beta-cell function: the hyperbolic correction. Diabetes 2002;51(Suppl 1):S212−20.

[142] Arslanian S, Austin A. Impaired insulin mediated potassium uptake in adolescents with IDDM. Biochem Med Metab Biol 1991;46(3):364−72.

[143] Graham TE, Kahn BB. Tissue-specific alterations of glucose transport and molecular mechanisms of intertissue communication in obesity and type 2 diabetes. Horm Metab Res 2007;39(10): 717−21.

[144] Benziane B, Chibalin AV. Frontiers: skeletal muscle sodium pump regulation: a translocation paradigm. Am J Physiol Endocrinol Metab 2008;295(3):E553−8.

[145] Soleimani M, Burnham CE. Physiologic and molecular aspects of the $Na^+:HCO_3^-$ co-transporter in health and disease processes. Kidney Int 2000;57(2):371−84.

[146] Mujais SK, Chen Y, Nora NA. Discordant aspects of aldosterone resistance in potassium depletion. Am J Physiol 1992;262 (6 Pt 2):F972−9.

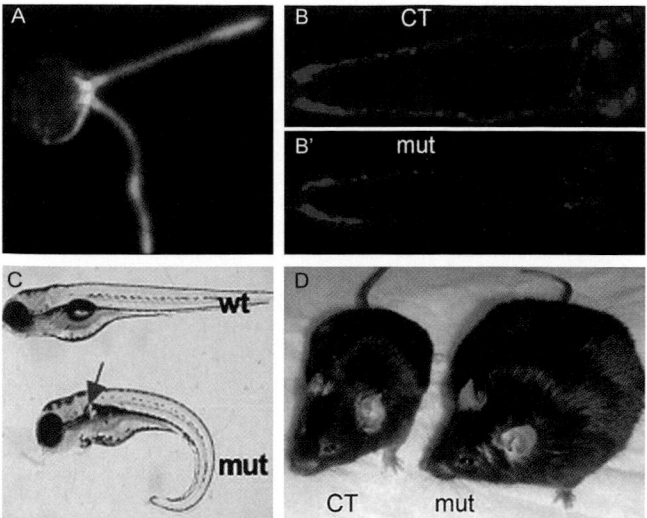

FIGURE 11.9   **Model systems to study cilia structure and function.** (A). *Chlamydomonas reinhardtii* expressing acetylated tubulin (green) in the flagella and IFT72/74 (red) in the cell body and basal bodies. *(Adapted from Pedersen et al. (2005). Curr Biol. Feb 8; 15(3), 262−266. With permission.)* (B) Dye filling of Control (CT) and (B′) cilia double mutant (mut) *Caenorhabditis elegans.* Note the dye-filling defective (dyf) phenotype of the mutant strain. *(Image: J. Pieczynski, unpublished.)* (C) Wild-type (top) and *seahorse* mutant *Dario reno* (zebrafish). The *seahorse* gene product, Lrrc6l, modulates Wnt and non-canonical Wnt signaling in zebrafish, and when mutated results in a cystic pronephros phenotype (red arrow). *(Image adapted with permission from Kishimoto et al. (2008). Dev. Cell Jun; 14(6), 954−961.)* (D) Control (CT, left) and BBS mutant (mut, right) mice (*Mus musculus*). Note the obesity phenotype found in BBS mutants. *(Image from Sharma et al. (2008). Curr. Top. Dev. Biol. 85, 371−427, with permission.)*

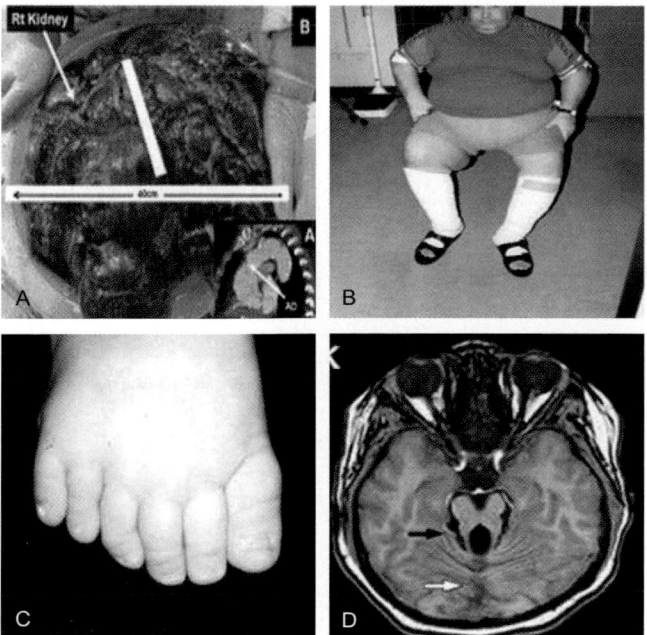

FIGURE 11.10   **Overlapping genes of ciliopathies.** A four-way Venn diagram showing the overlapping causative genes behind renal ciliopathies, creating a spectrum of disease phenotypes that include the kidney but may extend to other organs.

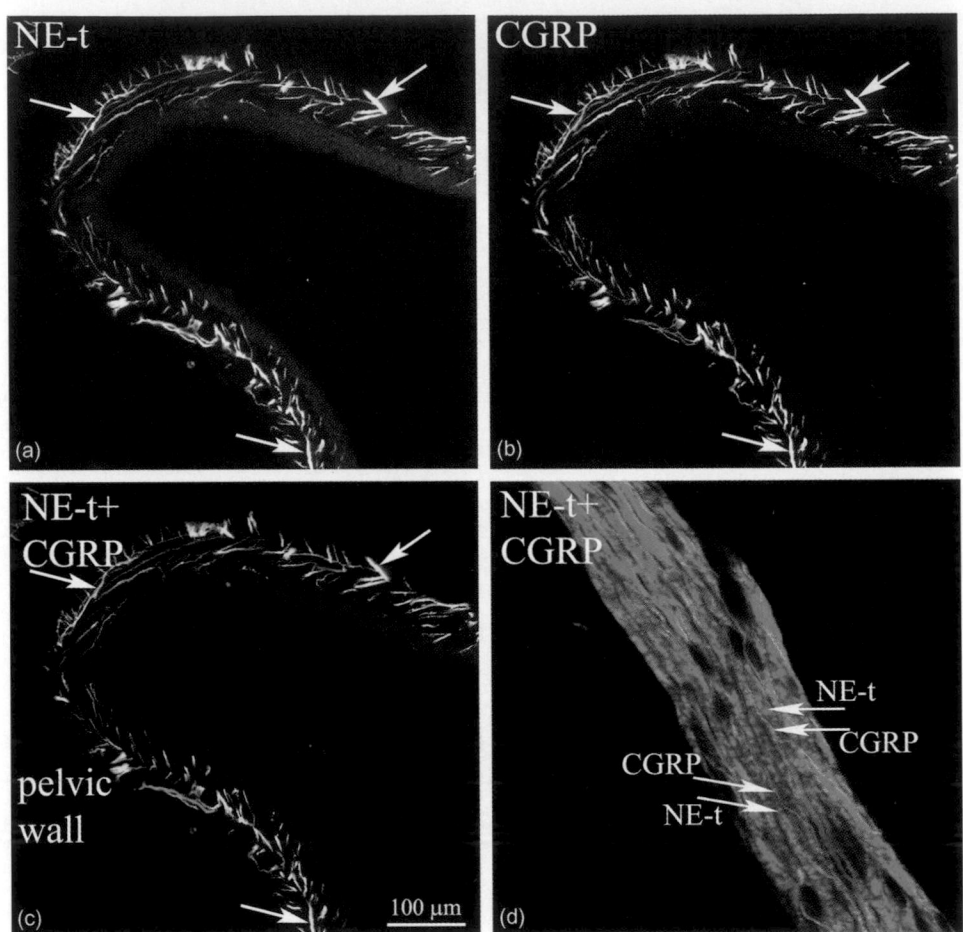

FIGURE 16.15 Applying antibodies against the norepinephrine transporter (NE-t) and the neuropeptide calcitonin gene-related peptide (CGRP) to kidney tissue to identify sympathetic and sensory nerve fibers, respectively (arrows) showed that the sympathetic nerves in the renal pelvic wall (a); are in close contact with the sensory nerves (b); as indicated by the color yellow (c). Higher magnification showed that the sympathetic and sensory nerves are separate fibers in close contact in the same nerve bundle (d). *(Modified from reference [159].)*

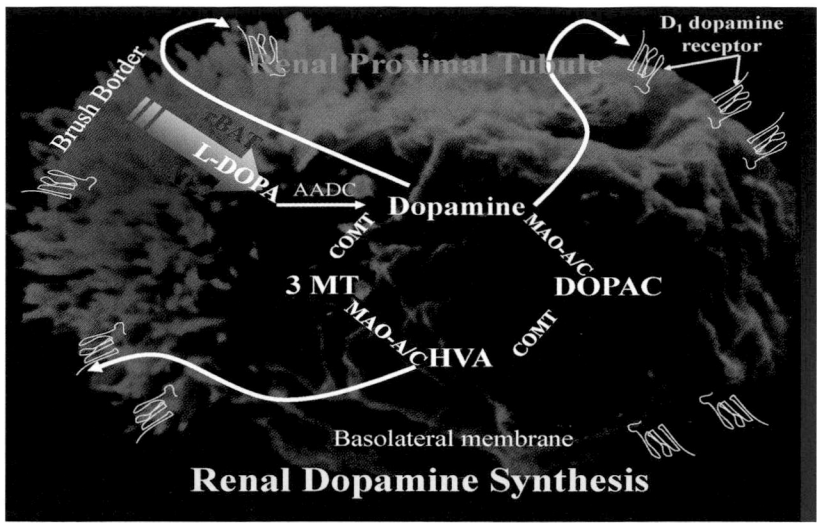

FIGURE 19.1 Dopamine synthesis inside a renal proximal tubule cell (scanning electron microscopy). The principal source of renal dopamine is from circulating L-dihydroxyphenylalanine (L-DOPA) which is found in the general circulation and is freely filtered by the glomerulus. Dopamine is produced in renal tubules following uptake by a sodium-independent and pH-sensitive L-type amino acid transporter (LAT2) and rBAT (related to Bo amino acid transporter), which is rate-limiting of the renal tubular dopamine synthesis. Renal proximal tubules convert L-DOPA to dopamine, via L-aromatic amino acid decarboxylase (AADC). In renal tubules, dopamine is not converted to norepinephrine, because unlike neural tissue renal tubules do not express tyrosine hydroxylase or dopamine b-hydroxylase (COMT: catechol-*O*-methyl transferase; MAO: monoamine oxidase; 3MT: 3 methoxytyramine; HVA: homovanillic acid; DOPAC: 3,4 dihydroxymandelic acid).

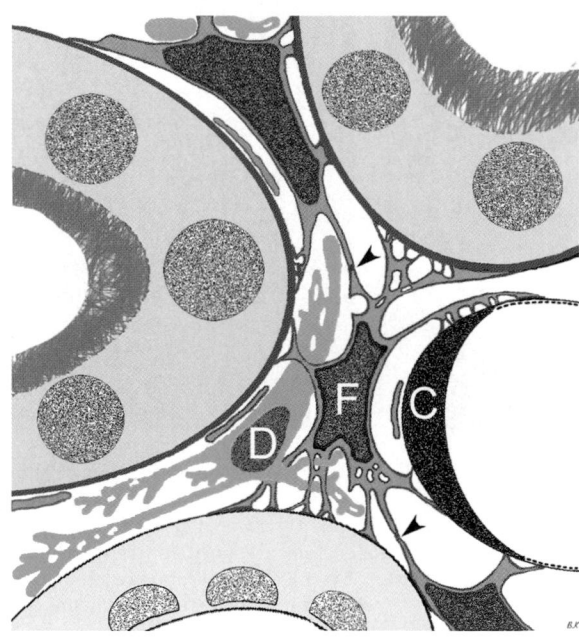

FIGURE 20.12 Schematic representation of cortical interstitial fibroblast (F) and dendritic cell (D) in the cortical interstitial space of a healthy kidney. The dark outline of fibroblasts indicates the f-actin layer under the plasma membrane (the nuclei cell organelles are not drawn); the fibroblasts are affixed to tubules and capillaries (C); the arrow heads indicate interconnection of fibroblasts by adhering junctions; the extensions of dendritic cells are narrowly intermingled with fibroblast cell processes.

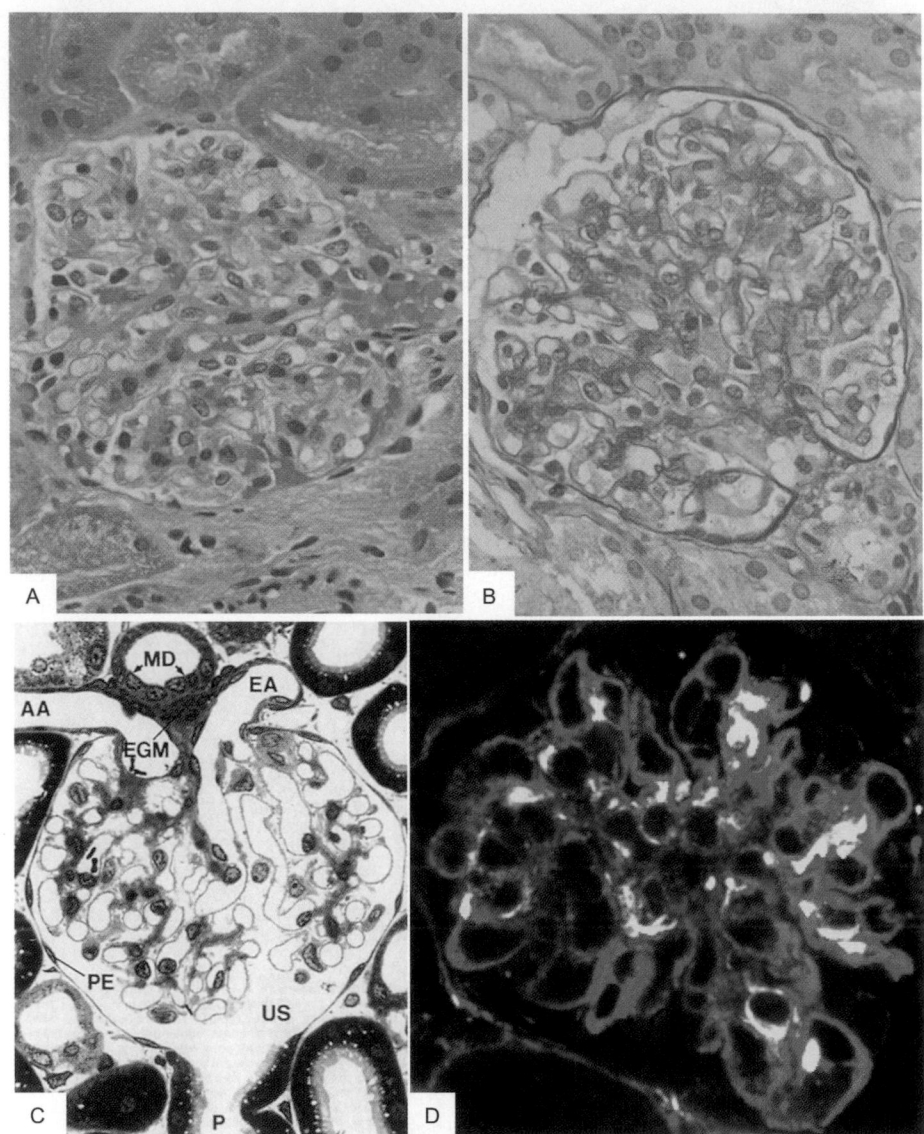

FIGURE 22.2 (A): Histology of normal human glomerulus. Hematoxylin-eosin (HE) staining showing patent capillary loops (CL) and vascular hilum (VH) (LM × 600). (B): Histology of normal human glomerulus. Periodic acid Schiff (PAS) staining (LM × 600). (C): Rat glomerulus sectioned through the vascular pole and the urinary pole. The afferent arteriole (AA), the efferent arteriole (EA), the extraglomerular mesangium (EGM), and the macula densa (MD) can be observed in this section. The orifice of proximal tubule (P) can be seen at the urinary pole (PE: parietal epithelial cells of Bowman's capsule; US: urinary space; LM × 490). (D): Immunostaining shows the three cell types found within the glomerular tuft (mouse glomerulus is shown) (Green: Zo-1 = podocytes; red: CD31 = endothelial cells; yellow: desmin = mesangial cells). The capillary loops are outlined by podocytes. Mesangial cells are located within the capillary tuft and connect capillary loops with each other (× 400). *(A and B: Courtesy of Dr. Paul S. Thorner, The Hospital for Sick Children, Toronto, ON.)*

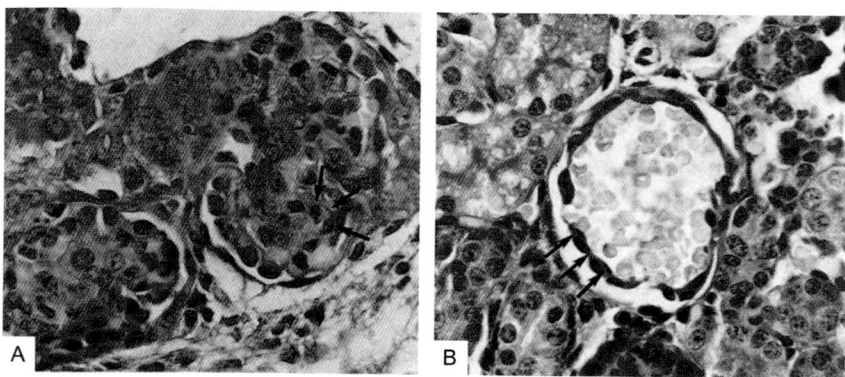

FIGURE 22.8 PAS stain of glomeruli from E17.5 mouse embryos. (A): Normal mouse glomerulus. Arrows show normal fold of the basement membrane. (B): Pdgfb$^{-/-}$ glomerulus shows a single open aneurysm-like capillary loop without any mesangium (failure of mesangial migration). There is no fold of basement membrane (arrows). *(From Betsholtz, C. (1995). Role of platelet-derived growth factor in mouse development. Int. J. Dev. Biol. **39**: 817–825 with permission.)*

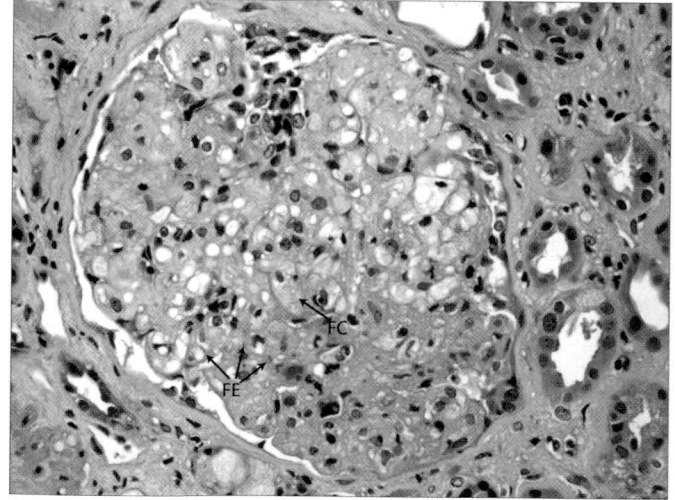

FIGURE 22.9 Glomerulus showing thrombotic microangiopathy from a patient who received anti-VEGF therapy, showing fragmentation of erythrocytes (FE: arrows) and foamy change (FC: arrow) of endothelium. *(Courtesy of Dr. Laura Barisoni, New York University School of Medicine, New York, NY.)*

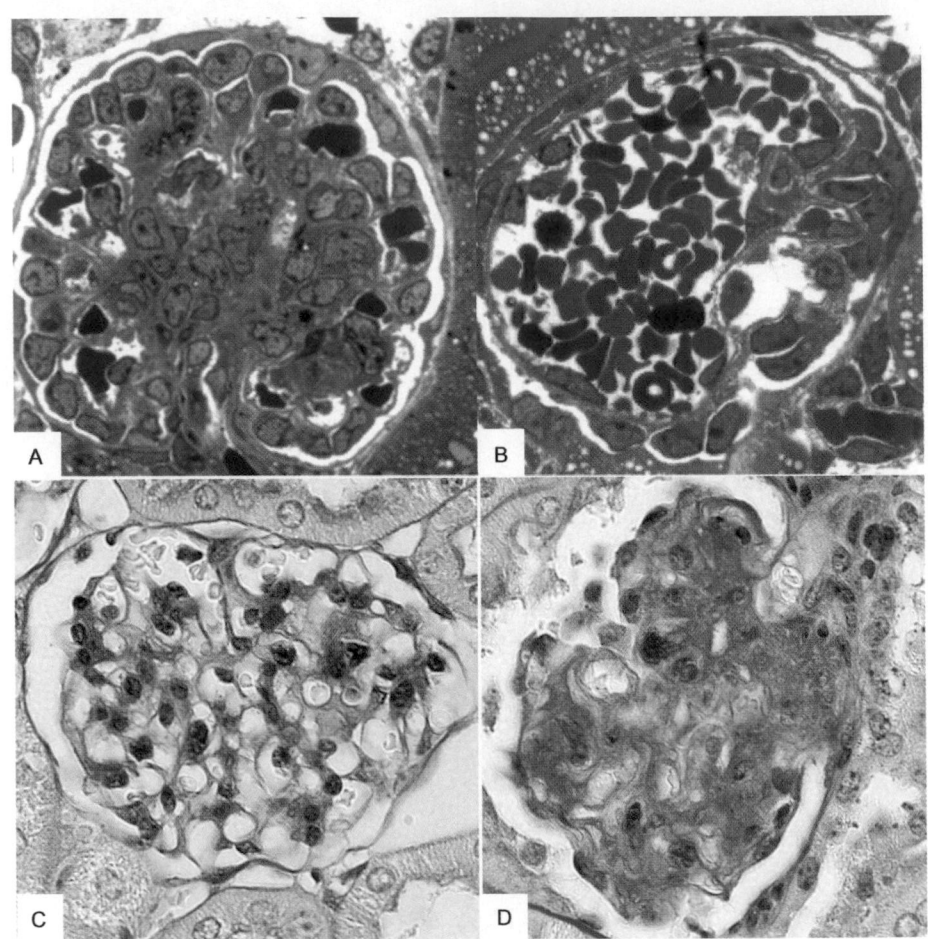

FIGURE 22.10 Conditional deletion of Angpt1 results in glomerular developmental defects and enhanced diabetic glomerular injury.
(A): A normal glomerulus at embryonic day 17.5 (E17.5). (B): Early conditional deletion of Angpt1 gene at embryonic day 10.5 (midgestation) results in some abnormal glomeruli with single open capillary loops similar to that of Pdgfb-null mouse at E17.5. (C) and (D): Late deletion of Angpt1 at E16.5 doesn't lead to any immediate phenotype. However, after 20 weeks of streptozotocin-induced diabetes, the diabetic mutant mice that carry Angpt1 deletion show an increase in mesangial matrix expansion and sclerosis (D) compared with that of diabetic controls (C) (LM × 1000). *(Courtesy of Dr. Marie Jeansson, Mount Sinai Hospital, Toronto, ON.)*

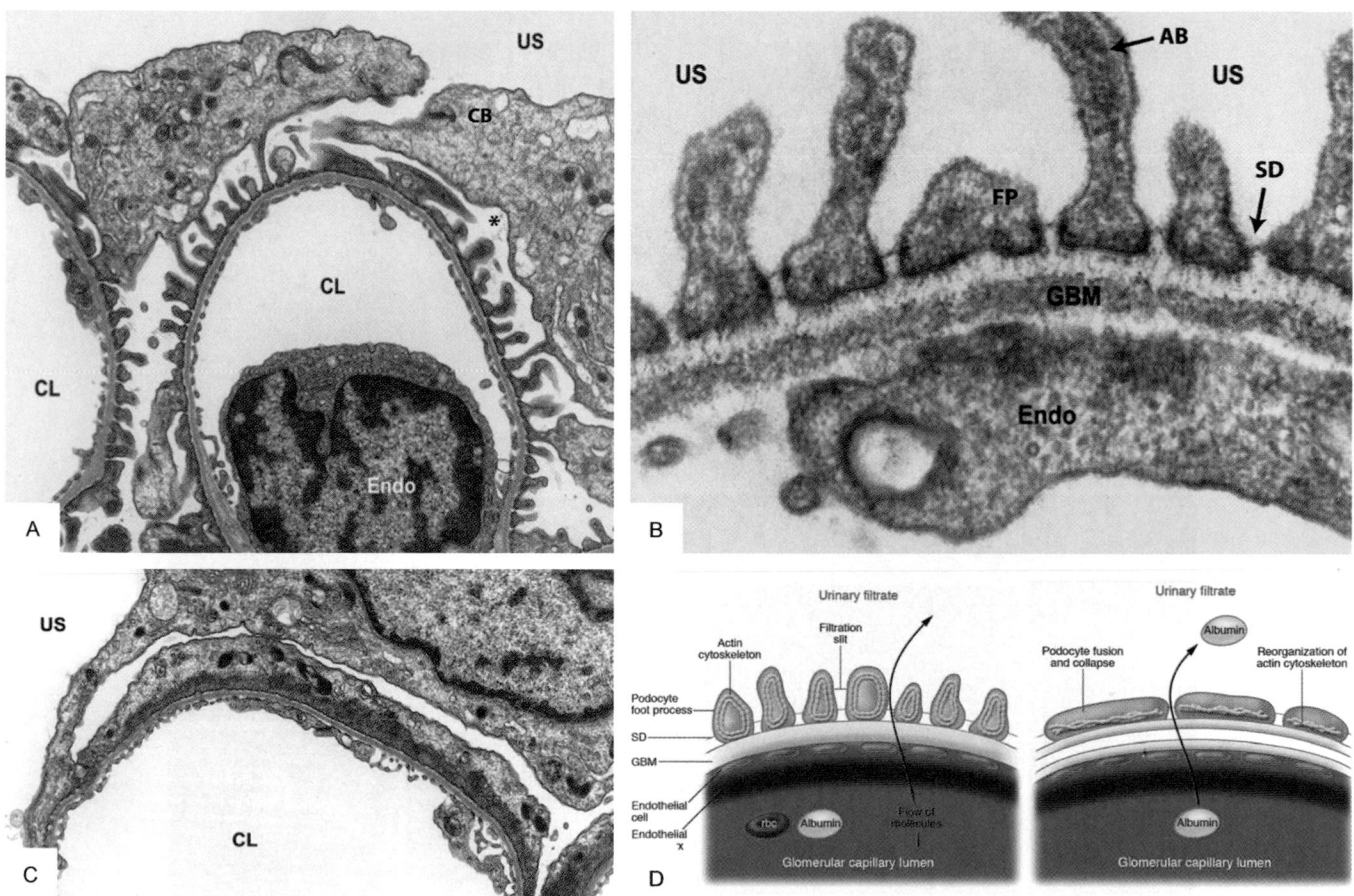

FIGURE 22.15 **Transmission electron micrograph of a normal and abnormal human podocytes.** (A): Coronal section of a podocyte intimately associated and lining a glomerular capillary loop (CL) cell body (CB) can be seen. Note the space (*) between the cell body and the basement membrane as the foot processes are the only point of contact between the podocyte and the GBM. (B): High power transmission EM shows podocyte foot processes (FP) attached to the glomerular basement membrane (GBM). Foot processes contain actin bundles (AB), and adjacent foot processes are attached by their slit diaphragms (SDs). (C): Transmission electron micrograph of podocyte foot process effacement in human focal segmental glomerulosclerosis (FSGS). (D): Scheme of podocyte foot process flattening. Left panel shows normal podocyte foot processes, actin cytoskeleton supports its elaborated shape. Once the actin cytoskeleton is disorganized, podocytes are no longer able to keep the foot process assembly, which results in fusion and flattening of foot processes (right panel). ((A)–(D): *Courtesy of Dr. Dontscho Kerjaschki, Medical University Vienna, Vienna, Austria; (E): From Ronco, P. (2007). Proteinuria: Is it all in the foot? J. Clin. Invest. 117: 2079–2082, with permission.)*

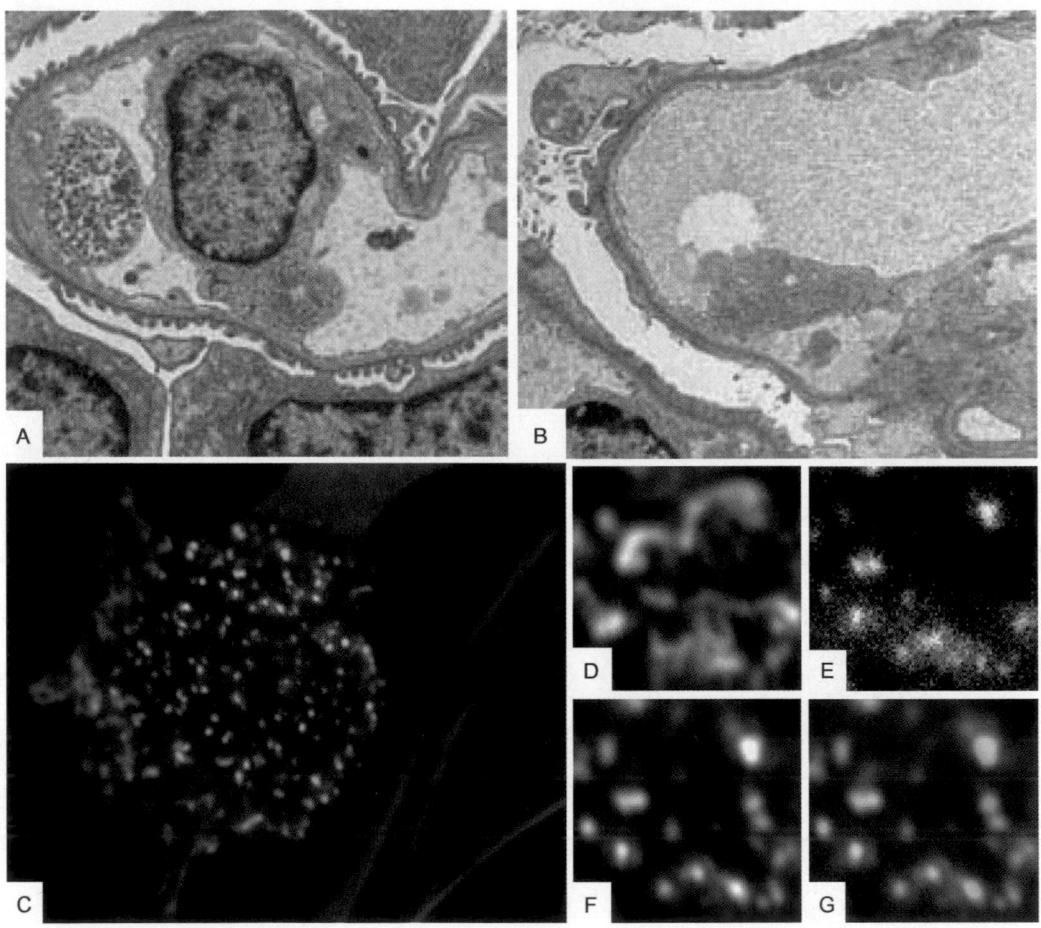

FIGURE 22.17 Transmission electron micrograph of distinct mouse podocyte foot-processes present at 4 days of birth (A), but absent in Nck knockout mice (B). (C)−(G): Cellular immunostaining showing co-localization of Nck2, nephrin at the actin tail. Nck-nephrin interaction is required for nephrin-dependent actin reorganization (Green: nephrin; purple: Nck2; red: palloidin = actin). (D), (E), and (F) show actin, nck2, and nephrin staining, respectively. ((A) and (B): *From Jones, N., et al. (2006). Nck adaptor proteins link nephrin to the actin cytoskeleton of kidney podocytes. Nature* **440**: *818−823, with permission; (C)−(G): Courtesy of Drs. Tony Pawson and Nina Jones.)*

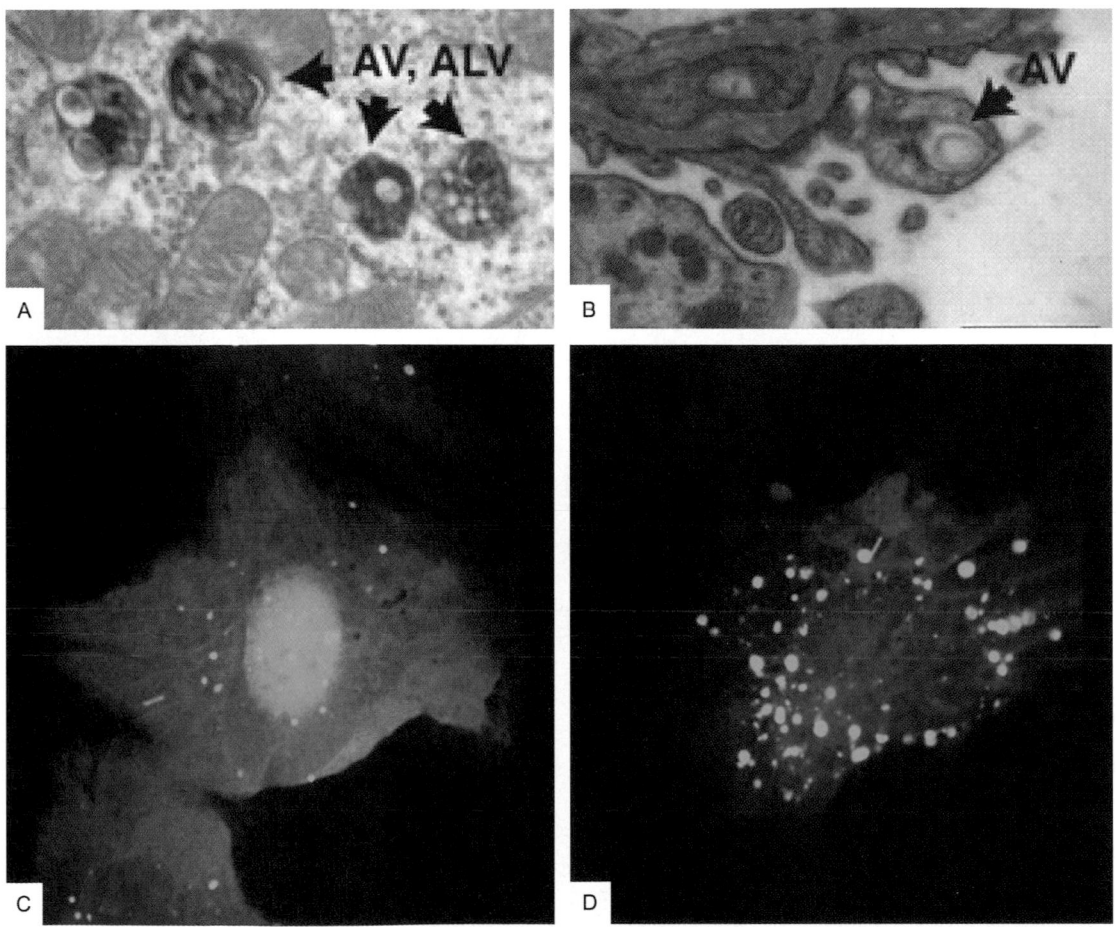

FIGURE 22.20 (A) and (B): Transmission electron micrographs of podocytes from 3 week old podocyte-specific mTor knockout mice showing an accumulation of autophagosomal vesicles (AV) and autophagolysosomal vesicles (ALV). *(From Cina, D. et al. (2012). Inhibition of MTOR disrupts autophagic flux in podocytes. J. Am. Soc. Nephrol. **23**: 412–420, with permission.)* (C): LC3 positive autophagosomes are visualized by green fluorescent protein in cultured human podocyte. (D): Treatment of the podocytes with rapamycin induces massive activation of autophagy.

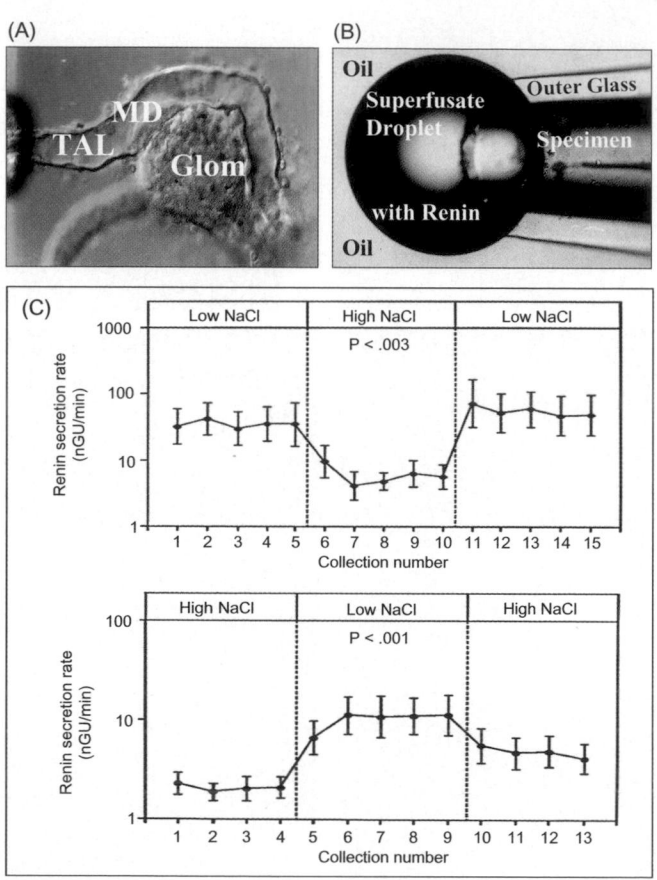

FIGURE 23.11 (A) Isolated perfused thick ascending limb (TAL) with attached glomerulus (glom); macula densa (MD) cells can be seen to protrude into the luminal space. (B) The perfused specimen is superfused through an outer glass pipette; emerging superfusate containing the secreted renin is collected under oil in defined time intervals [595]. (C) Macula densa-mediated changes in renin secretion showing the time course of changes in renin release to an increase (top) and decrease (bottom) in perfusate NaCl concentration[497,498].

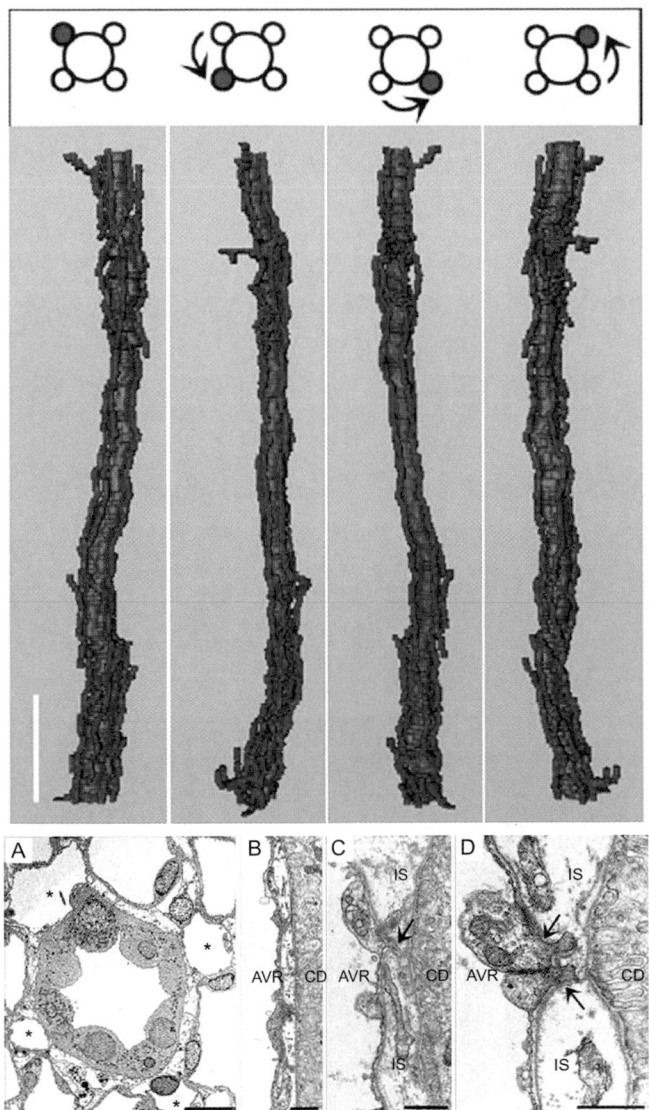

FIGURE 24.11 Relationship between vasa recta and collecting duct clusters. Upper panel: A single collecting duct (blue) with adjacent AVR (red) is shown in four 90° rotated views (Bar = 100 microns). Lower panel: (A)–(C) Electron micrographs of sections through a collecting duct (CD) and adjacent AVR, demonstrating the close apposition and interstitial space (IS). (D) Close approximation of AVR and CD where the two appear to be tethered with microvilli (arrows). *(Reproduced with permission from [25].)*

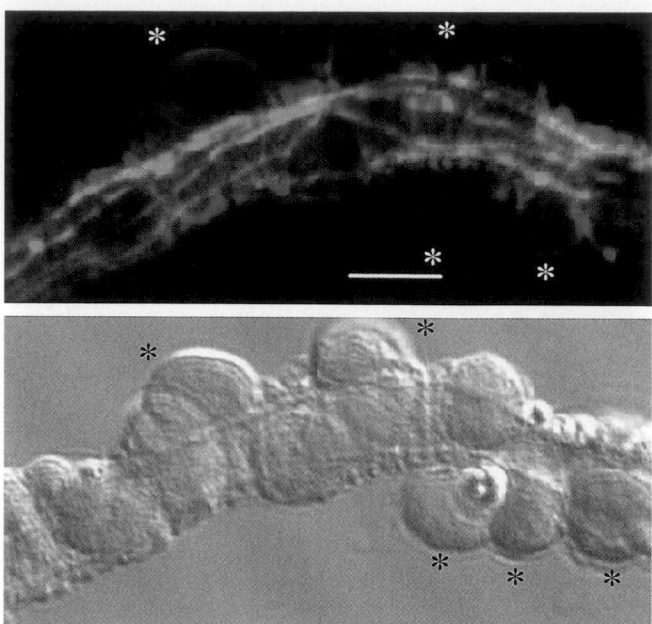

FIGURE 24.21 Connexin staining in DVR. Immunostaining with antibody directed against α-smooth muscle actin (SMA red, pericyte marker) or Cx40 (green) along with corresponding white light micrograph. Cx40 is linear and confined to the endothelium with very little SMA colocalization. Abluminal pericyte cell bodies (*) protrude from the outer rim of the vessel (Bar = 10 microns). *(Reproduced with permission from [364].)*

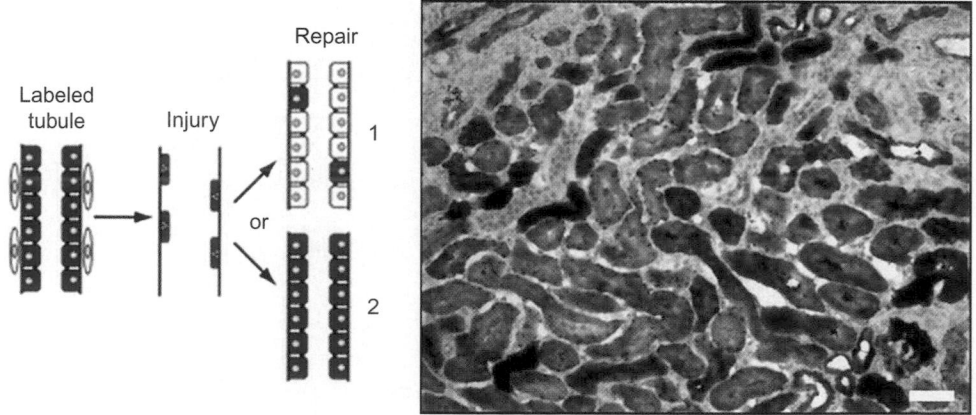

FIGURE 29.2 Surviving epithelial cells after injury generate new epithelial cells. (A) New cells after acute kidney injury in mice with genetically labeled epithelial tubules will not carry the label if they derive from cells outside the epithelial cell compartment (#1), but will carry the label if they derive from terminally differentiated epithelial cells (#2). (B) Fifteen days after transient ischemic injury and repair, there was no dilution on the number of labeled cells (dark) despite marked cellular proliferation, indicating that they derived from epithelial cells. *(From: Cell Stem Cell (2008). 2(3), 284–291.)*

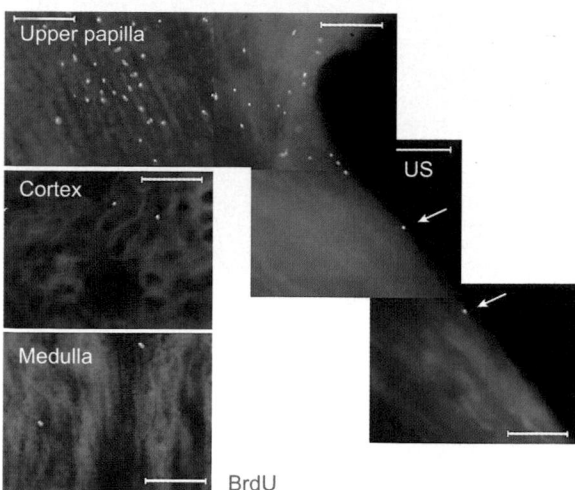

FIGURE 29.3 **Cellular proliferation was first detected in the upper papilla following kidney injury.** There was a selective increase of cells in S-phase in the upper papilla during the first hour after transient ischemic injury. Note abundant BrdU-labeled cells in the upper papilla, whereas the cortex and medulla revealed very rare BrdU-labeled cells (US: urinary space). Photomicrographs were done in 100 μm tissue sections obtained with a vibratome. *(From J. Am. Soc. Nephrol. (2009). 20(11), 2315−2327. Epub 2009 Sep 17.)*

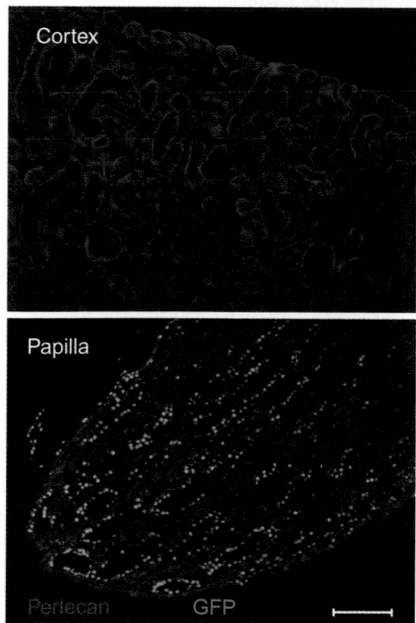

FIGURE 29.4 **Papillary LRCs in mice expressing histone 2B-GFP.** The kidney of an 11-week-old mouse pulsed with doxycycline during embryonic life showed low cycling cells (i.e., GFP- retaining) in the papilla but not the cortex or medulla. *(From J. Am. Soc. Nephrol. (2009) 20(11), 2315−2327. Epub 2009 Sep 17.)*

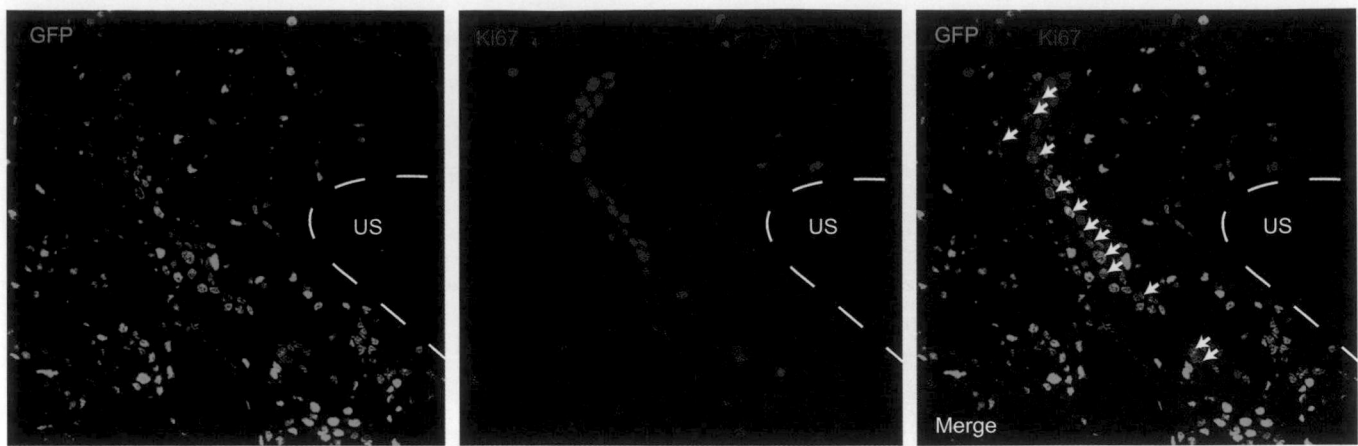

FIGURE 29.5   LRC in the upper papilla from chains of proliferating cells. LRCs (GFP$^+$: top) and proliferating cells (Ki67-positive: middle) in the upper papilla. The merged image shows that several cells are positive for both Ki67 and GFP (arrows). Broken white line depicts papillary edge (US: urinary space). *(From* J. Am. Soc. Nephrol. *(2009)* **20***(11), 2315−2327. Epub 2009 Sep 17.)*

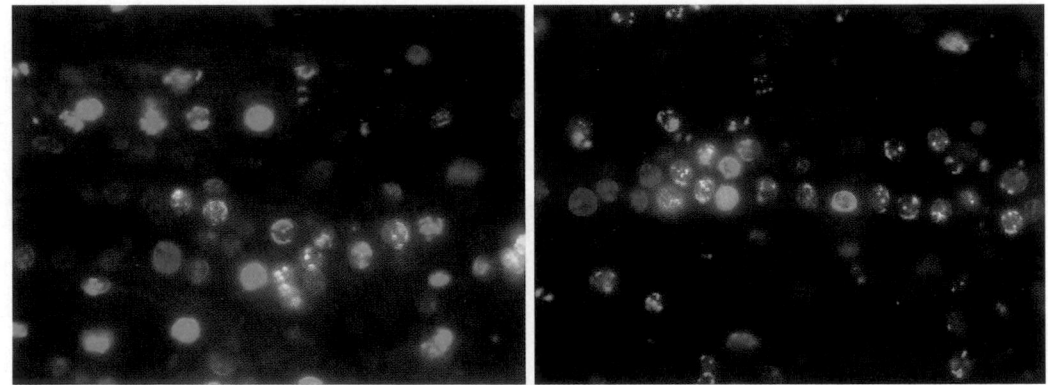

FIGURE 29.6   Proliferation of papillary LRC after transient ischemic injury. Cellular proliferation of papillary LRC after transient renal ischemia. Thirty-six hours after ischemic injury, many LRC of the papilla (FITC fluorescin) were cycling and labeled by a Ki67 antibody (rhodamine) (Scale bars: 50 μm). *(From* J. Clin. Invest. *(2004).* **114***(6), 795−804.)*

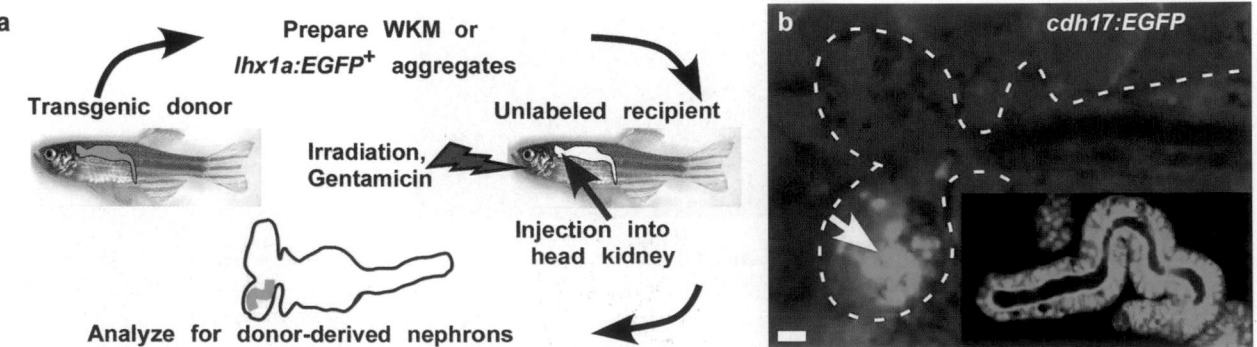

FIGURE 29.7   The kidney of the adult zebrafish contains progenitor cells that generate new nephrons. Left: Transplantation assay. Whole kidney marrow cells mostly comprising interstitial cells were isolated from genetically labeled donors. Right: Injection of the cells into recipients with damaged nephrons due to genatmicin injection resulted in donor-derived nephrons. *(From* Nature *(2011).* **470***(7332), 95−100. Epub 2011 Jan 26.)*